PATHOLOGIC BASIS *of* VETERINARY DISEASE

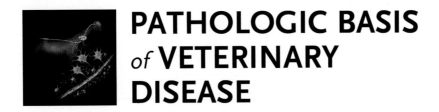

SIXTH EDITION

PATHOLOGIC BASIS *of* VETERINARY DISEASE

James F. Zachary, DVM, PhD, DACVP

Professor Emeritus of Veterinary Pathology
Department of Pathobiology
College of Veterinary Medicine
University of Illinois
Urbana, Illinois

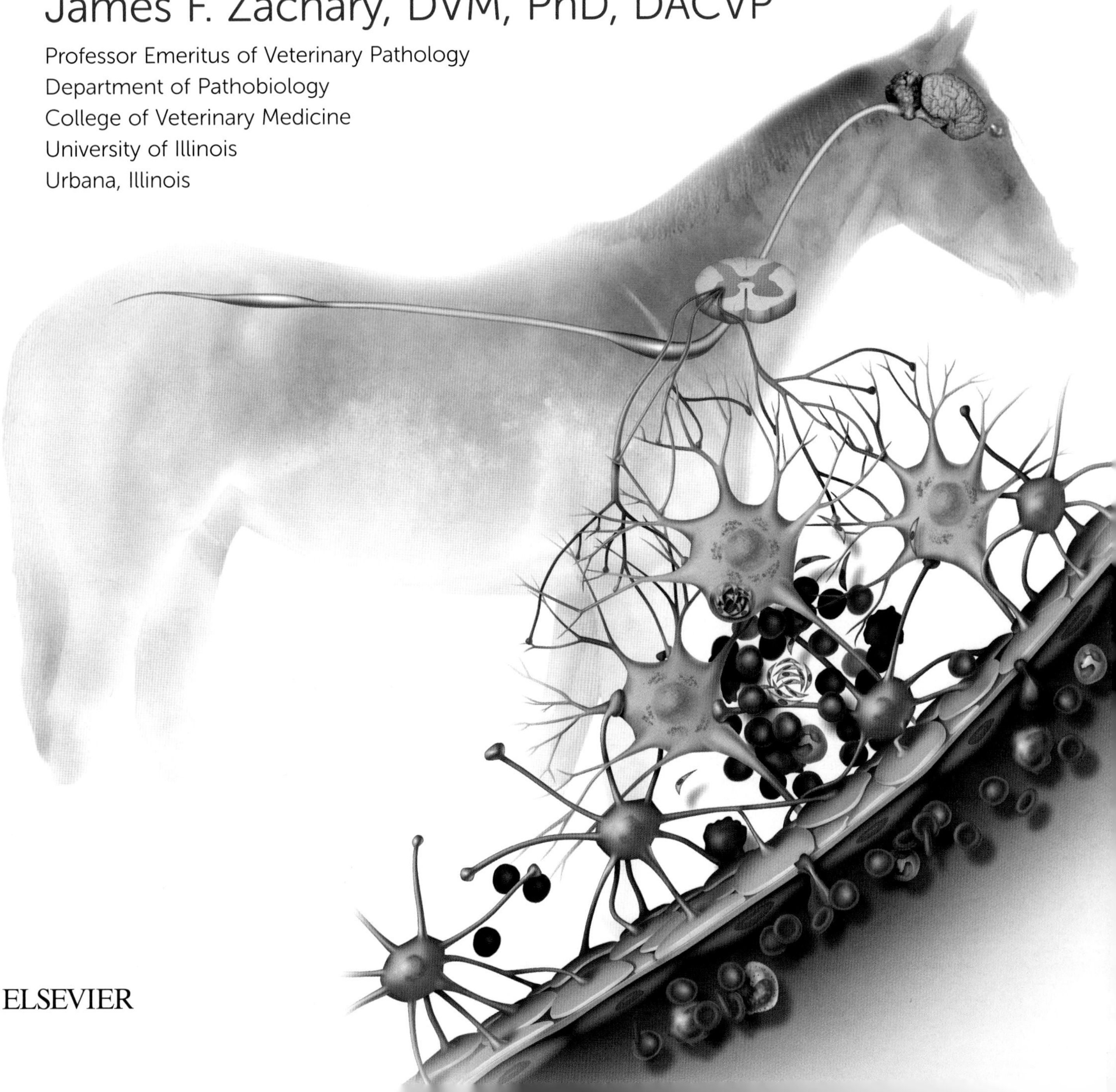

ELSEVIER

ELSEVIER

3251 Riverport Lane
St. Louis, Missouri 63043

PATHOLOGIC BASIS OF VETERINARY DISEASE, SIXTH EDITION ISBN: 978-0-323-35775-3

Library of Congress Cataloging-in-Publication Data

Names: Zachary, James F., editor.
Title: Pathologic basis of veterinary disease/ [edited by] James F. Zachary.
Description: Sixth edition. | St. Louis, Missouri : Elsevier, [2017] |
Includes index.
Identifiers: LCCN 2016021411 | ISBN 9780323357753 (hardcover: alk. paper)
Subjects: | MESH: Animal Diseases–pathology | Animals, Domestic
Classification: LCC SF769 | NLM SF 769 | DDC 636.089/607–dc23 LC record available at https://lccn.loc.gov/2016021411

Content Strategy Director: Penny Rudolph
Content Development Manager: Jolynn Gower
Associate Content Development Specialist: Laura Klein
Publishing Services Manager: Julie Eddy
Senior Project Manager: David Stein
Design Direction: Amy Buxton
Medical Illustrator: Theodore G. Huff
Medical Illustrator: Robert Britton
Cover Illustration: Giovanni Rimasti

Printed in China

Last digit is the print number: 9 8 7 6 5 4 3 2 1

Contributors

Mark R. Ackermann, DVM, PhD, DACVP
Professor, Department of Veterinary Pathology
Iowa State University
Ames, Iowa
Inflammation and Healing

Katie M. Boes, DVM, MS, DACVP
Clinical Assistant Professor
Department of Biomedical Sciences and Pathobiology
Virginia-Maryland Regional College of Veterinary Medicine
Virginia Polytechnic Institute and State University
Blacksburg, Virginia
Bone Marrow, Blood Cells, and the Lymphoid/Lymphatic System

Erin M. Brannick, DVM, MS, DACVP
Assistant Professor
Department of Animal and Food Sciences
University of Delaware
Newark, Delaware
Neoplasia and Tumor Biology

Melanie A. Breshears, DVM, PhD, DACVP
Associate Professor
Veterinary Pathobiology
Oklahoma State University
Stillwater, Oklahoma
The Urinary System

Danielle L. Brown, DVM, DACVP, DABT
Charles River Laboratories
Head, Specialty Pathology Services
Durham, North Carolina
Hepatobiliary System and Exocrine Pancreas

Cathy S. Carlson, DVM, PhD, DACVP
Professor
Veterinary Population Medicine
University of Minnesota
Saint Paul, Minnesota
Bones, Joints, Tendons, and Ligaments

Anthony W. Confer, DVM, MS, PhD, DACVP
Regents Professor
Endowed Chair of Food Animal Research
Veterinary Pathobiology
Oklahoma State University
Stillwater, Oklahoma
The Urinary System

John M. Cullen, VMD, PhD, DACVP, FIATP
Professor
Population Health and Pathobiology
North Carolina State University College of Veterinary Medicine
Raleigh, North Carolina
Hepatobiliary System and Exocrine Pancreas

Amy C. Durham, MS, VMD, DACVP
Assistant Professor
Department of Pathobiology
University of Pennsylvania
School of Veterinary Medicine
Philadelphia, Pennsylvania
Bone Marrow, Blood Cells, and the Lymphoid/Lymphatic System

Robert A. Foster, BVSc, PhD, MANZCVS, DACVP
Professor
Department of Pathobiology
Ontario Veterinary College
University of Guelph
Guelph, Ontario, Canada
Female Reproductive System and Mammae
Male Reproductive System

Arnon Gal, DVM, PhD, DACVIM, DACVP
Senior Lecturer in Small Animal Internal Medicine
Institute of Veterinary, Animal and Biomedical Services
Massey University
Palmerston North, New Zealand
Cardiovascular System and Lymphatic Vessels

Howard B. Gelberg, DVM, PhD, DACVP
Professor Emeritus of Pathology
Department of Biomedical Sciences
College of Veterinary Medicine
Oregon State University
Corvallis, Oregon;
Professor Emeritus of Pathology
Veterinary Diagnostic Laboratory
College of Veterinary Medicine
Oregon State University
Corvallis, Oregon
Alimentary System and the Peritoneum, Omentum, Mesentery, and Peritoneal Cavity

Ann M. Hargis, DVM, MS, DACVP
Affiliate Associate Professor
Department of Comparative Medicine
University of Washington
School of Medicine
Seattle, Washington;
Owner
Dermato Diagnostics
Edmonds, Washington
The Integument

Donna F. Kusewitt, DVM, PhD, DACVP
Research Professor
Department of Pathology
School of Medicine
University of New Mexico Health Sciences Center
Albuquerque, New Mexico
Neoplasia and Tumor Biology

Philippe Labelle, DVM, DACVP
Adjunct Professor
Department of Pathobiology
University of Illinois
Urbana, Illinois;
Anatomic Pathologist
Antech Diagnostics
Lake Success, New York
The Eye

Alfonso López, MVZ, MSc, PhD
Professor Emeritus
Department of Pathology and Microbiology
Atlantic Veterinary College
University of Prince Edward Island
Charlottetown, Prince Edward Island, Canada
Respiratory System, Mediastinum, and Pleurae

Shannon A. Martinson, DVM, MVSc, DACVP
Assistant Professor
Department of Pathology and Microbiology
Atlantic Veterinary College
University of Prince Edward Island
Charlottetown, Prince Edward Island, Canada
Respiratory System, Mediastinum, and Pleurae

M. Donald McGavin, MVSc, PhD, FACVSc, DACVP
Professor Emeritus of Veterinary Pathology
Department of Pathobiology
College of Veterinary Medicine
University of Tennessee
Knoxville, Tennessee
Photographic Techniques in Veterinary Pathology

Andrew D. Miller, DVM, DACVP
Assistant Professor
Department of Biomedical Sciences, Section of Anatomic Pathology
Cornell University College of Veterinary Medicine
Ithaca, New York
Nervous System

Lisa M. Miller, DVM, PhD, DACVP, MEd
Professor of Anatomic Pathology (retired, adjunct)
Department of Pathology and Microbiology
Atlantic Veterinary College
Charlottetown, Prince Edward Island, Canada
Cardiovascular System and Lymphatic Vessels

Margaret A. Miller, DVM, PhD, DACVP
Professor
Department of Comparative Pathobiology
Purdue University
West Lafayette, Indiana;
Pathologist
Indiana Animal Disease Diagnostic Laboratory
Purdue University
West Lafayette, Indiana
Mechanisms and Morphology of Cellular Injury, Adaptation, and Death
Endocrine System

Derek A. Mosier, DVM, PhD, DACVP
Professor
Diagnostic Medicine/Pathobiology
Kansas State University
Manhattan, Kansas
Vascular Disorders and Thrombosis

Sherry Myers, DVM, MVetSc, DACVP
Adjunct Professor
Veterinary Pathology
Western College of Veterinary Medicine
Saskatoon, Saskatchewan, Canada;
Diagnostic Pathologist
Prairie Diagnostic Services Inc.
Saskatoon, Saskatchewan, Canada
The Integument

Kimberly M. Newkirk, DVM, PhD, DACVP
Associate Professor
Department of Biomedical and Diagnostic Sciences
College of Veterinary Medicine
University of Tennessee
Knoxville, Tennessee
Neoplasia and Tumor Biology

Bradley L. Njaa, DVM, MVSc, DACVP
Associate Professor
Oklahoma Animal Disease Diagnostic Laboratory
Center for Veterinary Health Sciences
Oklahoma State University
Stillwater, Oklahoma
The Ear

Erik J. Olson, DVM, PhD, DACVP
Associate Professor
Department of Veterinary Population Medicine
College of Veterinary Medicine
University of Minnesota
St. Paul, Minnesota
Bones, Joints, Tendons, and Ligaments

Paul W. Snyder, DVM, PhD, DACVP, Fellow IATP
Senior Pathologist
Experimental Pathology Laboratories, Inc.
West Lafayette, Indiana
Diseases of Immunity

Beth A. Valentine, DVM, PhD, DACVP
Professor
Department of Biomedical Sciences
Oregon State University
Corvallis, Oregon
Skeletal Muscle

Arnaud J. Van Wettere, DVM, MS, PhD, DACVP
Assistant Professor
Department of Animal, Dairy & Veterinary Sciences
School of Veterinary Medicine
Utah State University
Logan, Utah
Hepatobiliary System and Exocrine Pancreas

James F. Zachary, DVM, PhD, DACVP
Professor Emeritus of Veterinary Pathology
Department of Pathobiology
College of Veterinary Medicine
University of Illinois
Urbana, Illinois
Mechanisms and Morphology of Cellular Injury, Adaptation, and Death
Mechanisms of Microbial Infections
Nervous System

Preface

The sixth edition of *Pathologic Basis of Veterinary Disease* continues the objectives of the fourth and fifth editions in keeping students up to date on the latest information concerning the pathogeneses of existing, new, and reemerging veterinary diseases. This edition has been revised and updated using the philosophy of earlier editions, "to explain pathology and its lesions in the context of understanding disease in a chronological sequence of events from both the morphologic and mechanistic perspectives with an emphasis on responses of cells, tissues, and organs to injury."

The textbook is divided into two sections: Section 1, *General Pathology*, and Section 2, *Pathology of Organ Systems*. *General Pathology* describes the underlying causes and mechanisms of cell and tissue injury and the resulting responses to injury (i.e., disease). Subject matter is divided into six chapters focusing on key concepts in the areas of cellular adaptations (degenerative, regenerative, or restorative) and cell death, vascular disorders, inflammation, mechanisms of infectious diseases, disorders of immunity, and neoplasia. *Pathology of Organ Systems* is the study of diseases that occur in specific tissues, organs, and organ systems. The material is divided among 15 chapters that cover disease and disease pathogeneses within each organ system.

New to This Edition

All 21 chapters in the sixth edition have been updated and revised; 10 of the chapters have been extensively rewritten and are a reflection of the efforts of contributors new to the sixth edition. Nearly all schematic materials have been replaced with new illustrations tailored to the practice of veterinary medicine. In addition, each chapter now has its own "Key Readings Index" to aid students in quickly identifying and locating information relevant to their coursework.

Each of the six *General Pathology* chapters includes new sections labeled "Essential Concepts" that concisely summarize "life-long learning" subject matter, for example, cell death, thrombosis, acute inflammation, portals of entry, inappropriate immune responses, and metastasis. Species-specific diseases in the chapters within *Pathology of Organ Systems* are described under headings of the major domestic animal affected—horses, ruminants (cattle, sheep, and goats), pigs, dogs, and cats. Those disorders and diseases not unique to a single species (i.e., those that occur in several species) are grouped under the heading "Disorders of Domestic Animals." In the sections of these chapters covering structure, function, dysfunction/responses to injury, portals of entry/pathways of spread, and defense mechanisms/barrier systems, new information on aging has been added and the full-color schematic diagrams and photographs of lesions have been updated and replaced as needed to emphasize pathogeneses of disease. Additionally, sections covering postmortem examination and evaluation procedures for each organ system are included in the ExpertConsult website. The sixth edition also includes the separation of Chapter 20, *The Ear and Eye* into two distinct chapters, Chapter 20, *The Ear*, and Chapter 21, *The Eye*.

Lastly, terminology in veterinary pathology continues to evolve with each new edition. In this edition, students will encounter in each chapter the use of different terms such as postmortem examination, necropsy, and autopsy (syn: necropsy) to describe methods used to examine tissues and organ systems. Although these terms are synonymous, this inconstancy reflects an ongoing discussion within the profession. There are strong opinions supporting each term and the proper terminology to use will likely take several editions to sort itself out.

Acknowledgments

The success of the fourth and fifth editions of *Pathologic Basis of Veterinary Disease* is a direct result of the substantive and sustained contributions made by a group of "educators" who, on a daily basis, succeed in transforming voluminous and challenging subject matter into understandable and meaningful concepts and then present them to students in a useful and "life-long learning format." These pathologists are dedicated to "student learning" and convey fundamental concepts about disease and disease processes and the dynamic and ever-changing discipline of veterinary pathology in an exciting, integrated, and well-organized manner. Additionally, they set the bar for excellence and establish the foundation for a student's clinical years and postprofessional school opportunities in veterinary medicine–related careers. These "teachers" are also internationally renowned veterinary pathologists who, by giving freely of their expertise, time, and resources to this book, inspire veterinary students to aim high and achieve excellence in career endeavors.

It is with great admiration that we recognize and honor the contributions of our colleagues in previous editions. Such contributions served in most instances as the foundation materials for the process of chapter revisions in subsequent editions.

5th Edition

Dr. Ronald K. Myers, *Chapter 1: Cellular Adaptations, Injury, and Death: Morphologic, Biochemical, and Genetic Bases*
Dr. M. Donald McGavin, *Chapter 1: Cellular Adaptations, Injury, and Death: Morphologic, Biochemical, and Genetic Bases*
Dr. John F. Van Vleet, *Chapter 10: Cardiovascular System and Lymphatic Vessels*
Dr. Shelley J. Newman, *Chapter 11: The Urinary System*
Dr. Krista M.D. La Perle, *Chapter 12: Endocrine System*
Dr. Michael M. Fry, *Chapter 13: Bone Marrow, Blood Cells, and the Lymphatic System*
Dr. M. Donald McGavin, *Chapter 13: Bone Marrow, Blood Cells, and the Lymphatic System*
Dr. M. Donald McGavin, *Chapter 15: Skeletal Muscle*
Dr. Steven E. Weisbrode, *Chapter 16: Bones, Joints, Tendons, and Ligaments*
Dr. Pamela Eve Ginn, *Chapter 17: The Integument*
Dr. Brian P. Wilcock, *Chapter 20: The Ear and Eye*

4th Edition

Dr. Laura J. Rush, *Chapter 6: Neoplasia and Tumor Biology*
Dr. Anthony W. Confer, *Chapter 11: The Urinary System*
Dr. Roger J. Panciera, *Chapter 11: The Urinary System*
Dr. Charles C. Capen, *Chapter 12: Endocrine System*

3rd Edition (as Thompson's Special Veterinary Pathology)

Dr. William W. Carlton, *Coeditor*
Dr. H. J. Van Kruiningen, *Chapter 1: Alimentary System*
Dr. Richard Dubielzeg, *Chapter 1: Section on Teeth: Alimentary System*
Dr. N. James MacLachlan, *Chapter 2: Liver, Biliary System, and Exocrine Pancreas*
Dr. Victor J. Ferrans, *Chapter 4: Cardiovascular System*
Dr. Gene P. Searcy, *Chapter 7: The Hemopoietic System*
Dr. Ralph W. Storts, *Chapter 8: The Nervous System*
Dr. Donald L. Montgomery, *Chapter 8: The Nervous System*
Dr. Cecil E. Doige, *Chapter 10: Bone and Joints*
Dr. Helen M. Acland, *Chapter 12: Reproductive System: Female*
Dr. Helen M. Acland, *Chapter 13: Reproductive System: Male*
Dr. James A. Render, *Chapter 14: The Eye and Ear*
Dr. William W. Carlton, *Chapter 14: The Eye and Ear*

In addition, we extend our deepest appreciation and thanks to colleagues throughout the world (truly an international effort), who have so generously provided their illustrative materials for use in the sixth edition. Although space limitations preclude listing them here, their names are cited in the figure legend credit for each illustration. We also extend our deepest appreciation to Drs. Barry G. Harmon, Elizabeth W. Howerth, and R. Keith Harris, who in their roles as Director of Noah's Arkive, College of Veterinary Medicine, The University of Georgia have supported our efforts over the last 2 decades. We have attempted to credit each illustration to its original source; however, inadvertent errors will be made in assembling a textbook of this size. Please address concerns about credits to <zacharyj@illinois.edu>. We will make every effort to confirm the origin of the photograph and correct the credit before the book goes into a subsequent printing.

Lastly, we thank the wide-ranging contributions of the Elsevier staff: Jolynn Gower, Content Development Manager; Brandi Graham, Content Development Specialist; Laura Klein, Associate Content Development Specialist; David Stein, Senior Project Manager; Lois Lasater and Dan Hays, Copy Editors; and Amy Buxton, Senior Book Designer. We also wish to thank our medical artists for their patience and dedication to the art for the sixth edition, Theodore G. Huff & Associates, Medical and Biological Illustration; Robert Britton, Medical Illustrator; and Giovanni Rimasti, GR Illustrations Inc. (cover illustration). We are also very grateful for the guidance of Penny Rudolph, Content Strategy Director, at Elsevier. Their hard work, patience, and collaboration have made the revision process manageable and successful.

ExpertConsult Website

An ExpertConsult website accompanies the sixth edition. This site includes all of the images from the book, plus additional materials that may be useful adjuncts for instructors in classroom and/or laboratory presentations.

To avoid adding length and weight to the book, information of historical value and basic clinical information have been removed from the printed book and can be found on the ExpertConsult website. Also included on the site are:

1. Suggested readings for each chapter.
2. Guidelines for performing systematic necropsies and appropriate sample acquisition for all organ systems.
3. A glossary of abbreviations and terms used for each chapter.
4. A listing of diseases with a real or suspected genetic basis for each organ system in Chapter 1.
5. Methods for gross specimen photography and photomicrography.

Additionally, all of the selected readings available on the ExpertConsult website are linked to original abstracts in PubMed.

The printed book will direct you to the ExpertConsult website when there is additional information available.

Finally, it is our hope that materials provided by ExpertConsult can serve as the basis for course development for instructors assigned the responsibility of teaching general, organ system, and diagnostic pathology in veterinary curricula and for instructors in related fields within university undergraduate and graduate curricula where the material is appropriate for course content.

About the Cover

Equine protozoal encephalomyelitis, an important and usually fatal disease of horses, is caused by the protozoan *Sarcocystis neurona*. The merozoite, the primary central nervous system (CNS) form of the protozoan, is small (3 to 5 μm in length), is crescent-shaped to round, has a well-defined nucleus, and is often arranged in aggregates or rosettes within the neuropil and/or within neurons and other neural cells. The disease can be characterized clinically by depression, behavioral changes, seizures, gait abnormalities, ataxia, facial nerve paralysis, head tilt, paralysis of the tongue, urinary incontinence, dysphagia, and atrophy of masseter, temporalis, quadriceps, and/or gluteal muscles, depending on the location(s) of the lesions.

Studies show that the opossum represents the definitive host; however, the natural intermediate host is unknown. Various mammals, including horses, represent aberrant intermediate hosts. Only the merozoite and schizont stages have been found in tissues within the aberrant intermediate hosts. It is unclear how the organism reaches the nervous system; however, it is speculated that following ingestion of sporocysts present in feed contaminated by opossum feces, the organism replicates in endothelial cells of the alimentary system. The developing schizonts eventually release merozoites, which are carried by leukocytes, likely macrophages, to the CNS.

Once in the CNS, merozoite-infected leukocytes appear to interact with endothelial cells, and the merozoites escape from and enter endothelial cells of the blood-brain barrier, where they develop into schizonts. Ligand-receptor interactions may determine tropism in the CNS and which areas of the vasculature are infected. Subsequently, schizogony results in lysis of these endothelial cells and release of merozoites into the neuropil, where they infect adjacent contiguous cells such as neurons, microglial cells, and endothelial cells. In the neuropil, merozoites occur extracellularly in cysts and intracellularly in neurons or macrophages. The mechanisms controlling the activation of cell lysis during schizogony are uncertain, but the outcomes, tissue destruction, and release of parasitic antigens are likely factors that initiate recruitment of inflammatory cells from the vascular system as part of a defense mechanism. These processes injure endothelium and neuropil, leading to inflammation, vasculitis, hemorrhage, and necrosis with the recruitment of macrophages and activation of resident microglial cells. Severe subacute inflammation characterized by accumulations of lymphocytes, macrophages, neutrophils, eosinophils, and a few multinucleated giant cells occurs in perivascular areas throughout the neuropil and leads to necrosis of both white and gray matter. Edema due to vascular injury accompanied by necrosis and hemorrhage can be quite prominent adjacent to blood vessels. Gross lesions are more common in the spinal cord, particularly the cervical and lumbar intumescences, than in the brain and appear grossly as regions of hemorrhage and malacia. In the brain, lesions are most commonly seen in the brainstem.

In Conclusion

No greater impact can be made on students in their veterinary education than by teachers, who are willing to share their expertise and knowledge with them. We hope the sixth edition of *Pathologic Basis of Veterinary Disease* and its mechanistic approach to disease will assist in this process, cultivate student interest in and understanding of disease pathogeneses, and perhaps transform the way pathology is taught in veterinary curricula.

James F. Zachary

In Appreciation: Dr. M. Donald McGavin

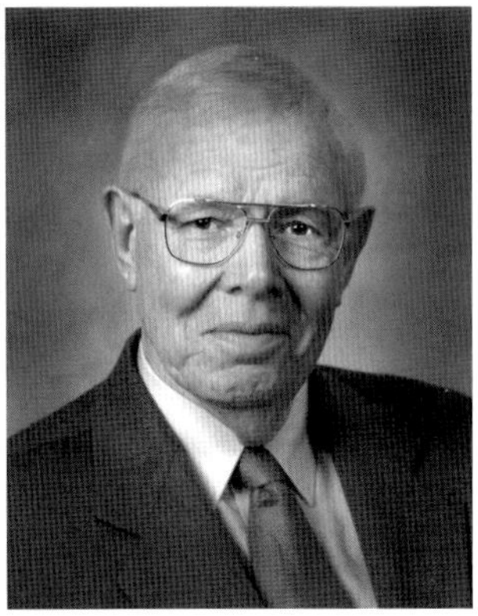

After working tirelessly and meticulously over the last three decades as an editor and a contributor, Dr. McGavin has chosen to step down from these roles and their demands to pursue other interests. It is an honor and a privilege to recognize him for his leadership role in the evolution of this book as well as for his sustained editorial and creative contributions to its philosophical style and informative and illustrative materials. His contributions include coauthoring Chapter 1, *Cellular Adaptations, Injury, and Death: Morphologic, Biochemical, and Genetic Bases;* Chapter 13, *Bone Marrow, Blood Cells, and the Lymphatic System;* and Chapter 15, *Skeletal Muscle* in the fifth edition. Moreover, he authored an appendix, *Photographic Techniques in Veterinary Pathology*, that provides detailed information on the proper methods to obtain the best photographic images from gross and histologic pathology specimens for the use in teaching, research, and publications. Additionally, in every edition, he served as a "hands-on" editor and assisted chapter contributors in organizing and revising the written elements of their chapters, as well as the figures and figure legends and ensuring that the complex field of veterinary nomenclature was used correctly within these components.

Dr. McGavin received his veterinary degree from the University of Queensland in 1952. He had been awarded a scholarship from the Queensland Department of Agriculture and, in return for the payment of tuition, he was required to serve in outback and rural areas for 6 years after graduation. In 1953, he was posted to Townsville, Queensland (a tropical area) as a field officer and worked with field investigations into tuberculosis, babesiosis, and mortalities from poisonous plants in beef cattle. In 1954, he was transferred to the Animal Health Station at Oonoonba, a small veterinary diagnostic laboratory outside of Townsville. As there was no histologic support in the laboratory, he learned to prepare his own histologic slides. This "on-the-job training" gave him an appreciation and empathy for histotechnicians preparing histologic sections, especially under tropical conditions without air conditioning and with the problems they encountered with routine fixation, processing, and staining of tissues. Additionally, Dr. McGavin was deeply appreciative of the mentoring he received early in his career from medical pathologists at the University of Queensland Medical School and Townsville General Hospital.

From 1956 to 1961, he was a diagnostic pathologist at the Animal Research Institute in Yeerongpilly, Brisbane, a superior veterinary diagnostic and research laboratory, fully staffed to provide bacteriologic, toxicologic, biochemical, parasitologic, and histologic support. Here, he completed neuropathologic studies of experimental Cycad poisoning, which produced ataxia in cattle from "dying back" in the spinal cord. To accomplish this goal, he developed a facility with special neurological stains such as the Marchi, silver stains such as the Sevier-Munger and Nauta and Gygax for nervous tissue, and Gordon and Sweets' reticulum stain. In parallel with this investigation, he also earned a Diploma in Photography from the Central Technical College, Brisbane to aid in black-and-white photomicrography and gross specimen photography.

He received a Fulbright Student Travel Grant in 1961 and was accepted into the graduate program in veterinary pathology at Michigan State University. For the next 3 years, he conducted experiments on the pathogenicity of what were then termed "atypical mycobacteria" (chiefly *Mycobacterium avium-intracellulare*) in cattle. He passed the examination to become a diplomate of the American College of Veterinary Pathologists in 1963 and was awarded a PhD in Veterinary Pathology in May 1964. He and his family returned to Brisbane, Australia; however, within a year he received invitations to return to the United States. After meeting stringent immigration requirements, he arrived in the United States in 1968 and began a faculty position at Kansas State University where he remained until 1976. During this period, he was involved in the pathology of several animal models including ovine progressive muscular dystrophy and sheep with congenital defects in the excretion of bilirubin (Gilbert's syndrome in mutant Southdown sheep and Dubin-Johnson syndrome in mutant Corriedale sheep).

In 1976, he accepted an invitation to be a foundation faculty member of the College of Veterinary Medicine, University of Tennessee as a full professor and remained there until retirement in 2002. During his tenure, he served as a foundation author for *Special Veterinary Pathology*, the first edition (1988) of this book, and as a coeditor on the second edition and senior editor on the third edition. He then served as senior editor for *Pathologic Basis of Veterinary Disease* (fourth edition) and as coeditor on the fifth edition. He also was a member of the Examination Committee of the American College of Veterinary Pathologists from 1975 to 1978 and Chairman of the Anatomic Pathology section in 1978; an Associate Editor (1983 to 1988) and Editor-in-Chief of the journal *Veterinary Pathology* from 1989 to 1993; a member of the Editorial Board of *Veterinary Dermatology* from 2002 to 2006; and a consultant on design of autopsy facilities in Australia, Canada, Ireland, Israel, and the United States. In 1988, in collaboration with Dr. S.W. Thompson, he published a book on gross specimen photography, *Specimen Dissection and Photography* (Springfield, IL, Charles C. Thomas publisher).

From 1990 to 2001, he was a member of the Faculty of Discussants of the Charles L. Davis DVM Foundation and lectured in the United States, Europe, the United Kingdom, Brazil, and Australia on the response of muscle to injury, photomicrography, and gross specimen photography. He received the Distinguished Lecturer Award from the Davis Foundation in 2008. In 1998, he was elected Fellow of the Australian College of Veterinary Scientists and in 2011 a Distinguished Member of the American College of Veterinary Pathologists.

Through these experiences, Dr. McGavin acquired his expertise in the practice of veterinary medicine, livestock disease outbreaks and losses, poisonous plants, histotechnology, diagnostic veterinary medicine, and veterinary pathology. He has personally observed, diagnosed, treated, and photographed diseases that for many have only been experienced by reading descriptions or viewing photographs in textbooks. Most importantly, Dr. McGavin was able to make the transition from practitioner to educator. He recognized and was challenged by the educational processes in veterinary curricula and veterinary pathology and sought to develop and implement new teaching methods to transmit information to students emphasizing the response of the tissue to injury and the sequence of these changes. As a consequence of the progression of his life experiences, Dr. McGavin has made *Pathologic Basis of Veterinary Disease* a leading textbook in veterinary pathology.

Lastly, Dr. McGavin is a kind, generous, and humorous man, willing to share his experiences and expertise selflessly to make this textbook a success. Therefore it is to Dr. McGavin we dedicate the sixth edition of *Pathologic Basis of Veterinary Disease*.

Contents

SECTION I

General Pathology

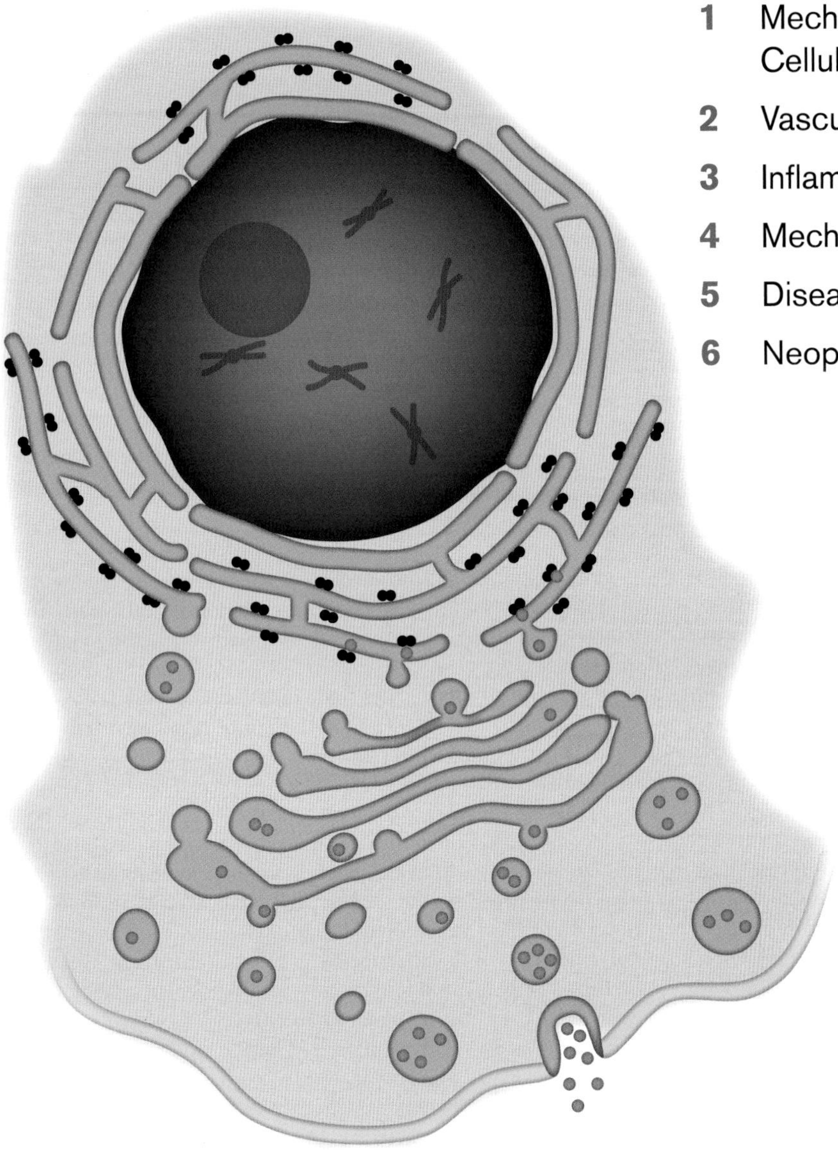

CHAPTER 1

Mechanisms and Morphology of Cellular Injury, Adaptation, and Death[1]

Margaret A. Miller and James F. Zachary

Key Readings Index

The goals of this chapter are to explain and illustrate the structure and function of cells and how they are interconnected with mechanisms of and responses to cell and tissue injury, such as adaptation, degeneration, and death. This information will serve as the underpinnings for materials presented in the remaining chapters covering general pathology and for comprehending materials presented on disease mechanisms and pathogeneses in subsequent chapters that cover pathology of organ systems.

Pathology is the study of disease from all perspectives. This pathology textbook begins with a 6-chapter general pathology section followed by 15 chapters of pathology of organ systems (systemic pathology). Although this layout parallels the instruction of pathology in many veterinary schools, the division into general pathology and systemic pathology is somewhat artificial. General pathology is the study of the reaction of cells or tissues to injury with a focus on the mechanisms of that response. In the first six chapters of this book, the response to injury is classified as cellular adaptations (degenerative, regenerative, or restorative), vascular disorders, inflammation, or neoplasia, with an additional chapter on the mechanisms of infectious diseases and one on disorders of immunity. These categorizations simplify the teaching and learning of general pathology. However, in the living body, cell injury provokes a variety of vascular, inflammatory, and immune-mediated responses in addition to disturbances of growth. These reactions not only extend beyond the injured cell to the organ or organismal level but also can occur simultaneously or in rapid succession. This first chapter is focused on the cellular responses to injury, not only on the degeneration that can progress to cell death but also on the adaptations of surviving cells. In subsequent general pathology chapters of Section I, more emphasis will be placed on the interaction among cells of different types, as well as the interaction of cells with their stroma, with other organ systems, and with circulating cells and molecules.

Systemic pathology is the study of systemic disease (i.e., disease that affects the system, meaning the entire organism). It is not a separate discipline from general pathology, but a different approach to the study of disease, in which the principles of general pathology are applied at the level of the tissue or organ or even the entire body. As for general pathology, the learning process is simplified by categorization, so Section II of this book is arranged in chapters based on a particular organ system. Again, this subdivision is arbitrary, and the student must bear in mind that disease seldom, if ever, affects only one organ or tissue. It also helps to remember that most organs or tissues respond in a similar way to a particular type of injury, hence the value in mastering the concepts of general pathology before the organ system approach. There is no optimum arrangement of the organ system chapters, so pathology of organ systems can be taught in different sequences in different curricula.

Pathologists are specialists in the discipline of pathology. Although general pathology and systemic pathology are educationally useful divisions of the discipline, pathologists are seldom categorized as general pathologists or systemic pathologists but, instead, are often classified as specialists in a particular organ system. For example, a dermatopathologist specializes in skin diseases; a neuropathologist, in diseases of the nervous system. In North America, pathologists are certified as anatomic pathologists, interested especially in the morphologic changes of gross (macroscopic) pathology and histopathology (microscopic pathology of tissues), or as clinical pathologists, who work more with microscopic and biochemical evaluations of blood, urine, and other bodily fluids or with cytologic samples, in which individual cells are studied rather than the intact tissue. Although there is overlap between anatomic and clinical

[1]For a glossary of abbreviations and terms used in this chapter see E-Glossary 1-1.

pathology, the focus of this book is anatomic pathology; clinical pathology is taught separately in most veterinary curricula. After certification, many anatomic pathologists specialize further in practice. Diagnostic pathologists are involved in autopsy (syn: necropsy; postmortem gross and histologic examination along with correlation of ancillary test results) and histologic examination of surgical biopsy specimens. Some diagnostic pathologists limit their practice to surgical (biopsy) pathology. Toxicologic and other experimental pathologists study the tissue, cellular, and molecular mechanisms of disease in a research setting.

In the practice of pathology the goal is to answer a question or solve a problem. The question depends on the nature of the investigation. In diagnostic pathology an autopsy (syn: necropsy) may be performed to determine the cause of death in an individual or in a group of animals or to explain decreased production in a herd, flock, kennel, or cattery. In forensic pathology the purpose of an autopsy is to determine the nature of death from a legal perspective. Surgical pathology (histologic examination of surgically excised tissue specimens) not only facilitates diagnosis and prognosis for a living animal but also can be the basis for therapy. Experimental pathologists contribute from the design to the end point of an investigation with the goal of correlating morphologic changes with clinical, functional, and biochemical parameters to elucidate the mechanisms of disease.

Most veterinary students will practice internal medicine or surgery, rather than pathology, yet pathology is an integral part of veterinary education and practice. Pathology is the link between basic sciences, such as anatomy and physiology, and clinical sciences and is the foundation for a lifetime of learning, diagnosing, and understanding disease in living and dead animals. The practicing veterinarian and the pathologist form a team at the forefront of animal and public health.

Basic Terminology

Information on this topic is available at www.expertconsult.com.

The Normal Cell

Knowledge of anatomy and of normal anatomic variations is prerequisite to lesion recognition and interpretation. Structure is covered briefly at the beginning of each of the organ system pathology chapters in Section II. The anatomic focus in this chapter is on the cell.

Components of Normal Cells and Their Vulnerabilities

A clear understanding of normal cell structure and function is essential to the study of cellular responses to injury. The cell can be visualized simplistically as a membrane-enclosed structure, subdivided into smaller functional units (organelles) by these membranes (Fig. 1-1). This interconnecting system of membrane-bound compartments is termed the *cytocavitary network*. The function of individual organelles depends in great part on the biochemistry of their membrane and intracellular matrix (i.e., gel component of the cytoplasm that supports the functions of the organelle). Cell membranes and organelles are targets for injury by microbes and various genetic, metabolic, and toxic diseases that are addressed in greater detail in the pathology of organ systems chapters.

Cell Membranes (Cytocavitary System)

Cell membranes are fluidic phospholipid bilayers that enclose cells and their organelles (Fig. 1-2). The two main functions of these membranes are (1) to serve as selective barriers (i.e., barrier systems [see Chapter 4]) and (2) to form a structural base for the membrane-associated proteins (enzymes and receptors) that determine cell function. The term fluidic indicates that proteins and lipids in the membrane are not immovable but can travel as part of the *cytocavitary system* (Fig. 1-3) throughout the physical extent of the cell. As an example of this process of "fluidic" movement, transmembrane proteins used as cell surface receptors are synthesized and assembled in the rough endoplasmic reticulum (rER), inserted into membranes in the Golgi complex, and moved (fluidic) to the cell's surface at the plasma membrane via the cytocavitary system (see Fig. 1-3).

The *plasma membrane* encloses the entire cell and thus is its first contact with harmful substances, agents, and infectious microbes. Microvilli and cilia (see Fig. 1-1) are specialized areas of the plasma membrane that are often altered in disease. Plasma membranes separate the interior of the cell from the external environment, neighboring cells, or the extracellular matrix (ECM). Surface proteins, such as fibronectin, play a role in cell-to-cell and cell-to-ECM interactions. *Transmembrane proteins* embedded in the phospholipid bilayer serve in a variety of essential structural, transport, and enzymatic functions (Fig. 1-4). Ligand-receptor interactions play key roles in these functions. Ligands are signaling molecules (also known as *first messengers*) (i.e., autocrine, paracrine, and endocrine signals [see Fig. 12-1]) that bind to receptors in the plasma membrane (cell surface receptors), cytoplasm (cytoplasmic receptors), or nucleus (nuclear receptors). Ligands may be cell associated, such as those on the surface of infectious microbes (see Fig. 4-31), or extracellular, such as hormones, growth factors, cytokines, cell recognition molecules, and neurotransmitters.

Cytoplasmic and nuclear receptors, through control of gene expression, regulate cellular development, homeostasis, metabolism, and aging. Ligands that bind these receptors include lipophilic substances, such as steroid hormones, vitamins, and xenobiotic endocrine disruptors that cross plasma and nuclear membranes by passive diffusion.

Cell surface receptors are central to the pathogenesis of many disorders discussed throughout this book. As an extension of a transmembrane protein, cell surface receptors receive and interpret extracellular signals (i.e., ligands) from the environment. When a ligand binds to an appropriate surface receptor, conformational changes in the transmembrane protein result in a process called signal transduction (signaling molecule → specific receptor protein on the plasma membrane → second messenger transmits the signal into the cell → physiologic response) and the activation (i.e., second messenger system [see later discussion]) or inhibition of the receptor's biochemical pathway. There are hundreds of different types of glycoprotein and lipoprotein transmembrane receptors; each type is linked to a specific intracellular biochemical pathway, and individual cells contain many of these receptors based on their function as determined by their genome. *Transmembrane receptors* are often used by infectious microbes to invade cells or use cell systems during their life cycles, thus initiating a process that can injure the host cell. These receptors and their roles in the mechanisms of infectious disease are discussed in detail in Chapter 4.

A unique transmembrane protein receptor is involved in the *notch-signaling pathway*. Ligand activation of notch signaling results in the formation of a cytoplasmic second messenger that enters the nucleus and modifies gene expression during embryonic development and homeostasis. During development, notch signaling allows specific types of cells and tissues to develop, organize, and grow. If a specific cell type expresses a trait essential for the development of a specific tissue type, ligands are released from the "essential" cell that bind notch receptors on adjacent cells. Signal transduction and

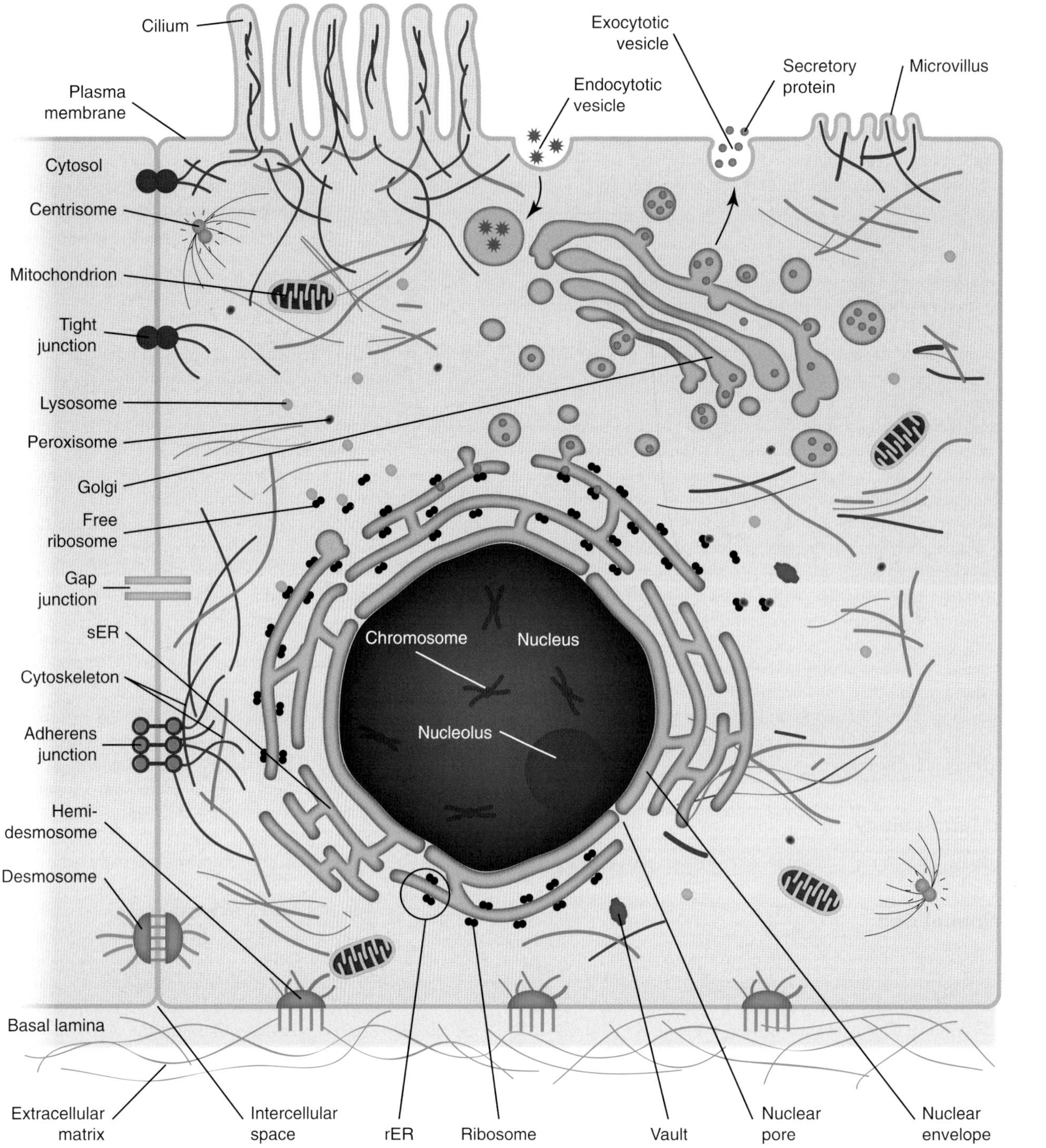

Figure 1-1 **Cell Structure and the Organization of Organelles, Cytoskeleton, and Membrane Enhancements.** *rER*, Rough endoplasmic reticulum; *sER*, smooth endoplasmic reticulum. (Courtesy Dr. M.A. Miller, College of Veterinary Medicine, Purdue University; and Dr. J.F. Zachary, College of Veterinary Medicine, University of Illinois.)

second messenger systems are activated, leading to the inhibition of division and development of affected "bystander" cells. This outcome allows specific types of cells to increase in number during development, while inhibiting other less essential cell types. Notch-signaling pathways are involved in the development of neural tissues, blood vessels, heart, pancreas, mammary gland, T lymphocytes, hematopoietic lineages, and other cell types. Notch-signaling pathways also play a role in mature animals. They appear to determine, for example, whether enteric stem cells differentiate into villous enterocytes with secretory or absorptive functions. Diseases that kill or injure enteric crypt stem cells (e.g., parvovirus) or villous enterocytes (e.g., coronaviruses) probably disrupt notch-signaling pathways, leading to a lack of secretory or absorptive enterocytes during healing with failure to return to "normal" function (see Chapter 7).

Second Messenger Systems. Cells are in continuous contact with a wide variety of extracellular molecules (see first messengers earlier). Examples of first messenger molecules include microbial ligands (see also Chapter 4), hormones, growth factors, neurotransmitters, and xenobiotics. First messenger interactions typically

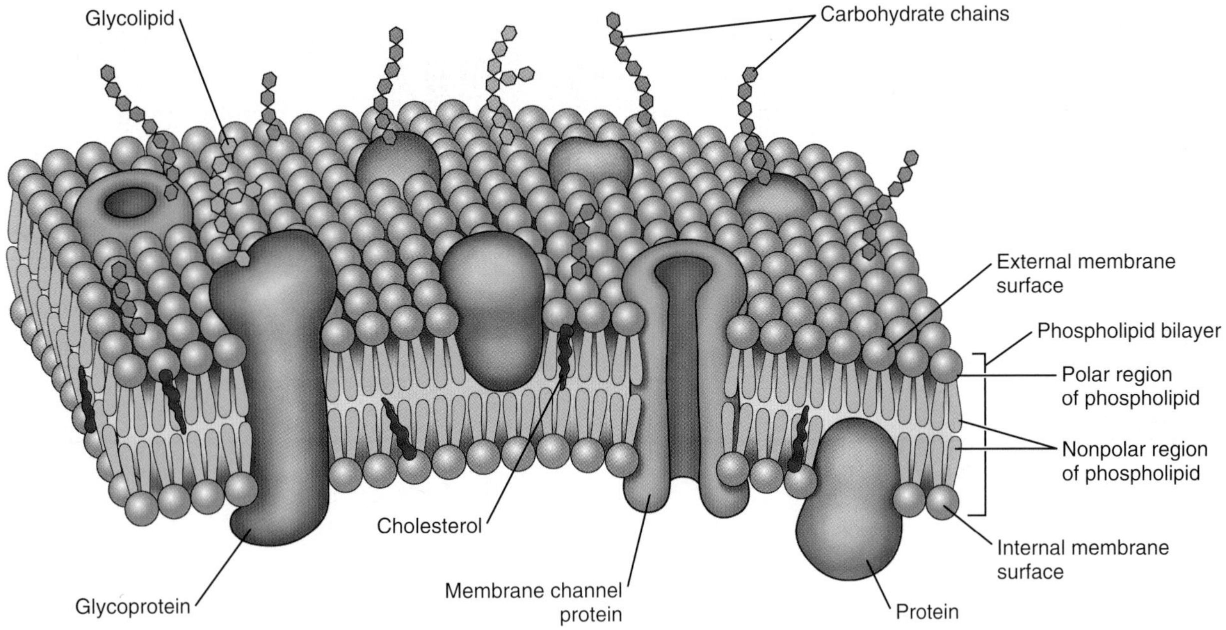

Figure 1-2 **Fluid Mosaic Model of Cell Membrane Structure.** The lipid bilayer provides the basic structure and serves as a relatively impermeable barrier to most water-soluble molecules.

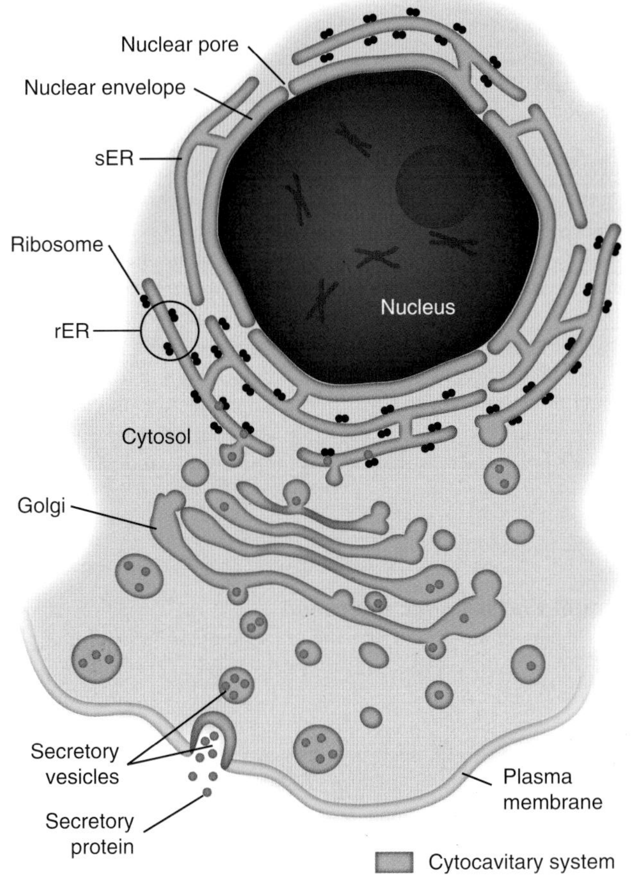

Figure 1-3 **Cytocavitary System.** The rough endoplasmic reticulum (rER) and Golgi complex function in synthesis of proteins and glycoproteins used in and secreted from cells. Transcription, translation, assembly, modification, and packaging of these molecules occur in an orderly sequence from the nucleus to the plasma membrane as shown. Smooth endoplasmic reticulum (sER) is involved in the synthesis of lipids, steroids, and carbohydrates and in the metabolism of exogenous substances. (Courtesy Dr. M.A. Miller, College of Veterinary Medicine, Purdue University; and Dr. J.F. Zachary, College of Veterinary Medicine, University of Illinois.)

involve the binding of a ligand to its transmembrane protein receptor, which activates a second messenger system (E-Fig. 1-1). Examples of second messenger molecules include Ca^{2+}, cyclic adenosine monophosphate (cAMP), cyclic guanosine monophosphate (cGMP), inositol triphosphate, diacylglycerol, arachidonic acid, and nitric oxide (NO). The second messenger initiates an intracellular signal transduction cascade that stimulates or alters a metabolic pathway. Thus second messenger systems translate "first messages" from the plasma membrane into specific actions within the cell and its organelles to maintain homeostasis or defend against infection or other injury.

Cytosol versus Cytoplasm

Whereas the term cytoplasm refers to the light microscopically visible portion of the cell that is inside the plasma membrane and outside the nuclear envelope (see the next section), the term cytosol specifies the cytoplasmic matrix (i.e., the gel portion of the cytoplasm that surrounds organelles). The cytosol contains water, dissolved ions, and macromolecules, such as proteins.

Nucleus

Animals are made of eukaryotic cells, meaning cells that have a nucleus, which, except in mammalian erythrocytes, is retained throughout the life of the cell. The nucleus (see Fig. 1-1) is readily visible by light microscopy because it contains chromatin (DNA complexed with histones), which is well stained by hematoxylin. Uncoiled chromatin is called *euchromatin* and is dispersed throughout the nucleus and actively involved in production of messenger RNA (mRNA). Tightly coiled chromatin is called *heterochromatin* and is clumped around the inner nuclear membrane and is inactive (see also E-Fig. 1-22). The nucleus is surrounded by an inner and an outer nuclear membrane that together form the nuclear envelope. The inner and outer nuclear membranes merge at the nuclear pore complexes, which allow bidirectional trafficking between the nucleus and the cytosol. The inner nuclear membrane is more "nuclear" in its biochemistry and serves to segregate and maintain the unique biochemistry of the nucleus, whereas the outer nuclear membrane has features more like those of the endoplasmic reticulum

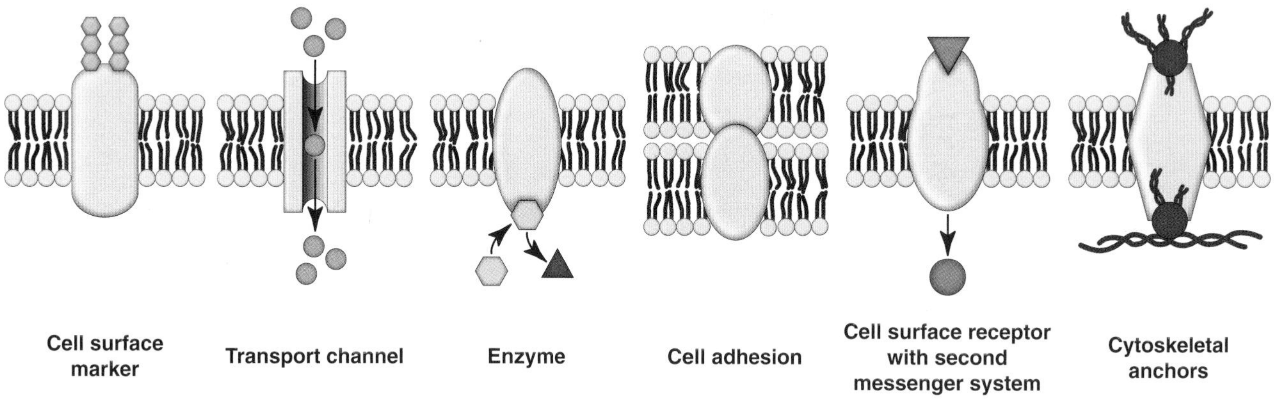

Figure 1-4 Functions of Transmembrane Proteins. Transmembrane proteins that span the phospholipid bilayer of cell membranes serve a variety of structural, transport, signaling, and enzymatic functions. (Courtesy Dr. M.A. Miller, College of Veterinary Medicine, Purdue University; and Dr. J.F. Zachary, College of Veterinary Medicine, University of Illinois.)

(ER), with which it is continuous. This differentiation and arrangement is essential for translation of genetic material (DNA and RNA) into gene products (proteins).

Nucleolus. The nucleolus (see Fig. 1-1) is a non–membrane-bound structure within the nucleus that forms around chromosomal loci of the ribosomal RNA (rRNA) genes known as nucleolar organizing regions (NORs). The nucleolus is the site of transcription and processing of rRNA and of assembly of preribosomal subunits. Thus it consists of ribosomal DNA, RNA, and ribosomal proteins, including RNA polymerases, imported from the cytosol. At the light microscopic level, the nucleolus can be inconspicuous in inactive cells or quite prominent in cells with high protein production.

Rough Endoplasmic Reticulum

The ER is a membrane-bound network of flattened saclike cisternae (see Figs. 1-1 and 1-3). The membrane of the rER is continuous with the outer nuclear membrane, so the luminal contents of the rER and of the nuclear envelope communicate. rER is so named because attached ribosomes impart a rough appearance (at the ultrastructural level) to its membrane as opposed to the appearance of the smooth ER (sER), which lacks surface ribosomes. The main function of rER is protein synthesis. Translation of mRNA with assembly of amino acids into peptides begins on ribosomes that are free in the cytosol. When the developing peptide is detected by a signal recognition particle, translation pauses until the ribosomal peptide–mRNA complex is attached to the outer surface of the rER. Protein formation continues in the membrane or lumen of the rER until a signal peptidase removes the signal peptide, at which time the newly formed protein can be transported to the cellular or extracellular site where it is needed or to the Golgi complex for further processing (see Fig. 1-3). Transmission electron microscopy is generally required to visualize the rER; however, cells that produce abundant protein and thus have abundant rER tend to have more basophilic cytoplasm because of the ample nucleic acid (RNA) in ribosomes.

Ribosomes. Ribosomes facilitate the synthesis of proteins in cells (i.e., translation) (see Figs. 1-1 and 1-3). Their function is to "translate" information encoded in mRNA into polypeptide chains of amino acids that make up proteins. There are two types of ribosomes, free and fixed (also known as membrane bound). They are identical in structure but differ in locations within the cell. Free ribosomes are located in the cytosol and are able to move throughout the cell, whereas fixed ribosomes are attached to the rER. Free ribosomes synthesize proteins that are released into the cytosol and used within the cell. Fixed ribosomes synthesize proteins that are (1) inserted into the cell membrane (transmembrane proteins) at the rER and subsequently moved (fluid mosaic membrane model) to their final destinations usually within the plasma membrane or (2) placed in membrane-bound vesicles and moved through the Golgi complex (see next paragraph) to the plasma membrane and released via exocytosis into the extracellular environment.

Golgi Complex

The Golgi complex, also commonly called the Golgi apparatus, is a series of flattened membrane-bound sacs with its inner face (*cis* or entry face) near the rER in a paranuclear position (see Fig. 1-3). Proteins made in the rER are delivered to the entry face of the Golgi complex by transport vesicles. As the proteins traverse the Golgi complex, they are processed (e.g., carbohydrate moieties added through glycosylation) and packaged into secretory vesicles to be released from the outer (*trans*) face of the Golgi complex into the cytosol, either for use by the cell that produced them, as in the case of lysosomal enzymes, or (more commonly) for delivery to the plasma membrane for export. Transmission electron microscopy is usually required to visualize the Golgi complex. However, an active Golgi complex, such as that needed for processing and packaging of immunoglobulin molecules, is large enough to impart a paranuclear eosinophilic pallor to plasma cells in a hematoxylin and eosin (H&E)–stained histologic section.

Smooth Endoplasmic Reticulum

sER is a membrane-bound network of tubules (see Figs. 1-1 and 1-3) without surface ribosomes. sER is not involved in protein synthesis. Its main function is the synthesis of lipids, steroids, and carbohydrates, as well as the metabolism of exogenous substances, such as drugs or toxins. Cells, such as hepatocytes, that are important for synthesis of lipids and metabolism of drugs or toxins have abundant sER, as do cells that produce steroid hormones, such as adrenocortical cells and certain testicular or ovarian cells. Cells with abundant sER have pale eosinophilic, finely vacuolated cytoplasm.

Mitochondria

Mitochondria are dynamic organelles that can change shape, undergo fission and fusion, and move about within the cell. They can be large enough (up to 1 μm) to resolve with the light microscope, especially in muscle from athletic animals such as racehorses. Because most cellular processes require "energy," a major mitochondrial function is the generation of energy as adenosine triphosphate (ATP) through oxidative phosphorylation. Mitochondria are also involved in programmed cell death (e.g., apoptosis), signaling, cell differentiation, and cell growth. Mitochondria contain their own genome (see later section on the Genetic Basis of Disease), which consists mainly of circular DNA that encodes transfer and rRNAs as well as some mitochondrial proteins. However, most of the genes that encode mitochondrial proteins are located in the nucleus of the cell. Mitochondria have a biochemically distinct inner and outer membrane. The inner membrane is folded into cristae that project into the central matrix of the mitochondrion (see Figs. 1-1 and 1-5). Some mitochondrial structural proteins and enzymes are made on free ribosomes and then imported from the cytosol to the appropriate mitochondrial compartment (outer membrane, intermembrane space, inner membrane, or matrix). Mitochondria also establish close contact, perhaps via tethering proteins, with the ER.

Oxidative Phosphorylation

Information on this topic is available at www.expertconsult.com.

Vaults

Vaults are rather recently discovered barrel-shaped organelles (see Fig. 1-1) that are thought to function in transporting large molecules (e.g., mRNA or proteins) between the nucleus and other intracellular locations. Their octagonal profile may facilitate docking at nuclear pores.

Lysosomes and Peroxisomes

Lysosomes are membrane-bound vesicles (see Fig. 1-1; also see E-Fig. 1-27, A) that contain enzymes (acid hydrolases) that can digest most chemical compounds (nucleic acids, carbohydrates, proteins, or lipids) endogenous to the cell or extracellular substances taken up by endocytosis or phagocytosis. Enzymes contained in lysosomes are synthesized by the rER (i.e., fixed ribosomes), processed and packaged in the Golgi complex, and released in vesicles from the outer surface of the Golgi complex into the cytosol.

Peroxisomes (see Fig. 1-1) are membrane-bound vesicles that are specialized for the β-oxidation of fatty acids and degradation by catalase of the hydrogen peroxide produced. They may be distinguished from lysosomes by an electron-dense core. Peroxisomes can import large protein complexes; their function depends on communication with the Golgi complex, mitochondria, and the cytosol. Peroxisomes are generated de novo by budding from the ER but are also capable of replication through fission. Enzymes contained in peroxisomes are synthesized on free ribosomes in the cytosol, then transported into peroxisomes.

The Cytoskeleton: Microfilaments, Intermediate Filaments, and Microtubules

The cytoskeleton (Fig. 1-5) is a structural network that regulates the shape and movement of the cell and its organelles, cell division, and biochemical pathways. It consists of three integrated components: actin microfilaments (6 to 7 nm in diameter), intermediate filaments (approximately 10 nm in diameter) of different types

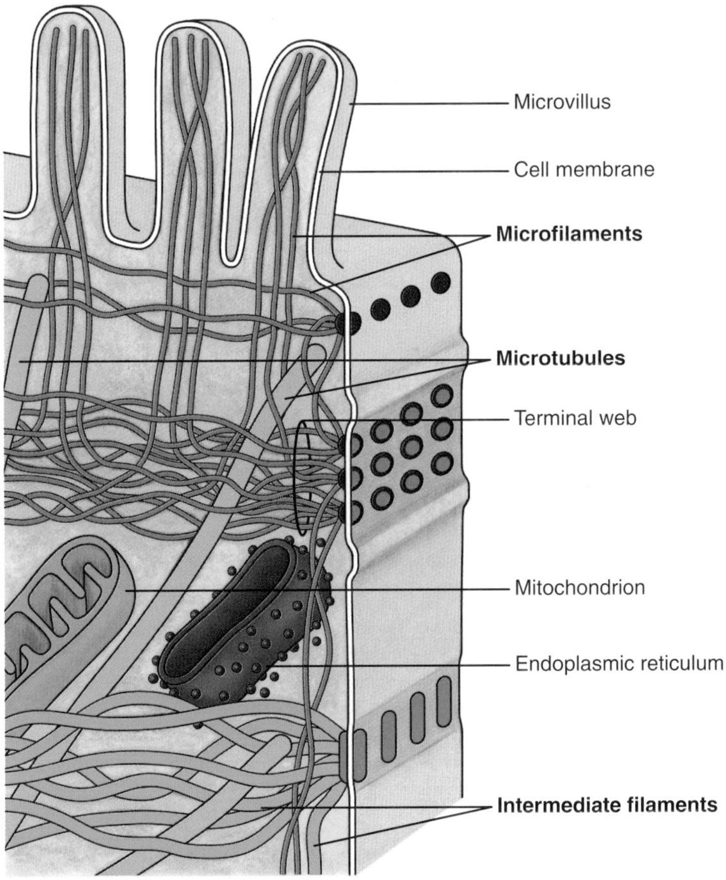

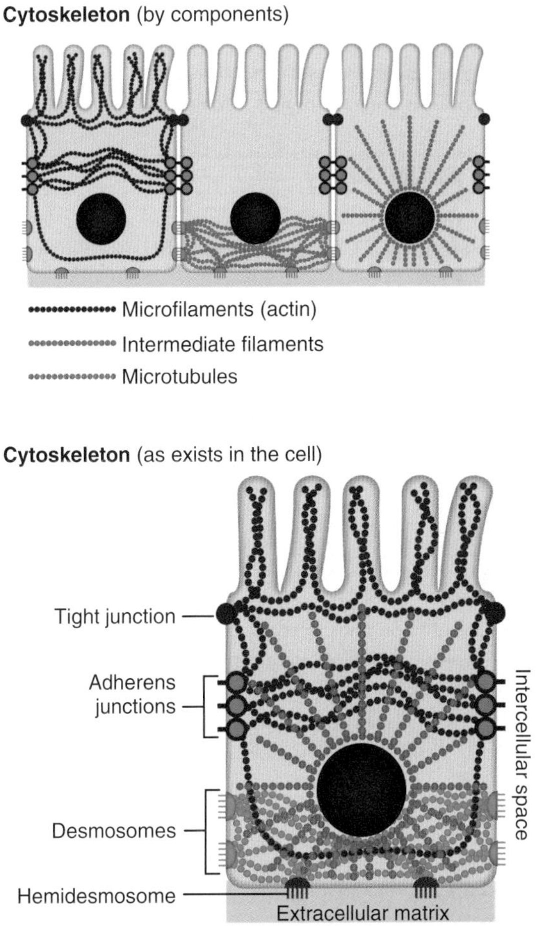

Figure 1-5 Cytoskeleton. The complexity and interrelations of microfilaments, intermediate filaments, and microtubules with the plasma membrane and other organelles are depicted.

depending on the cell type, and microtubules (approximately 25 nm in diameter). The function of most organelles requires their interaction with the cytoskeleton.

The following are general concepts: (1) microfilaments facilitate cell motility (e.g., ameboid movement [chemotaxis], cilia, pseudopodia); (2) intermediate filaments facilitate the physical strength and shape of cells and tissues, often via junctional complexes; and (3) microtubules move organelles and vesicles within the cytosol of a cell and chromosomes via mitotic spindles during cell division.

Cellular Inclusions

Cellular inclusions are composed of molecules, such as glycogen, proteins, nucleic acids, lipids, hemosiderin, and calcium, that accumulate as metabolic by-products, breakdown products of macromolecular complexes, or as a result of cell injury. Certain infectious microbes, especially viruses, can also produce intranuclear or cytoplasmic inclusions (see Figs. 1-11, 1-32, and 9-83). Cellular inclusions are "free" within the cytosol (i.e., not membrane bound).

Intercellular Junctions and the Extracellular Matrix

The cell connects and communicates with neighboring cells of the same type via intercellular junctions (Fig. 1-6). Certain cell types (e.g., basilar epithelial cells) also attach to a basal lamina and its contiguous connective tissue via hemidesmosomes, literally half a desmosome, in the ECM. These cell types interact with the ECM via integrin-mediated adhesions between ECM ligands, such as fibronectin or various collagens, and the cell's actin cytoskeleton. The ECM (see Chapter 3) is produced by fibroblasts and a variety of other supportive mesenchymal cells and includes such components as collagens and proteoglycans of basement membranes and the interstitium. Connections with neighboring cells and with the ECM are essential for normal cellular structure and function, including proliferation, migration, and signaling.

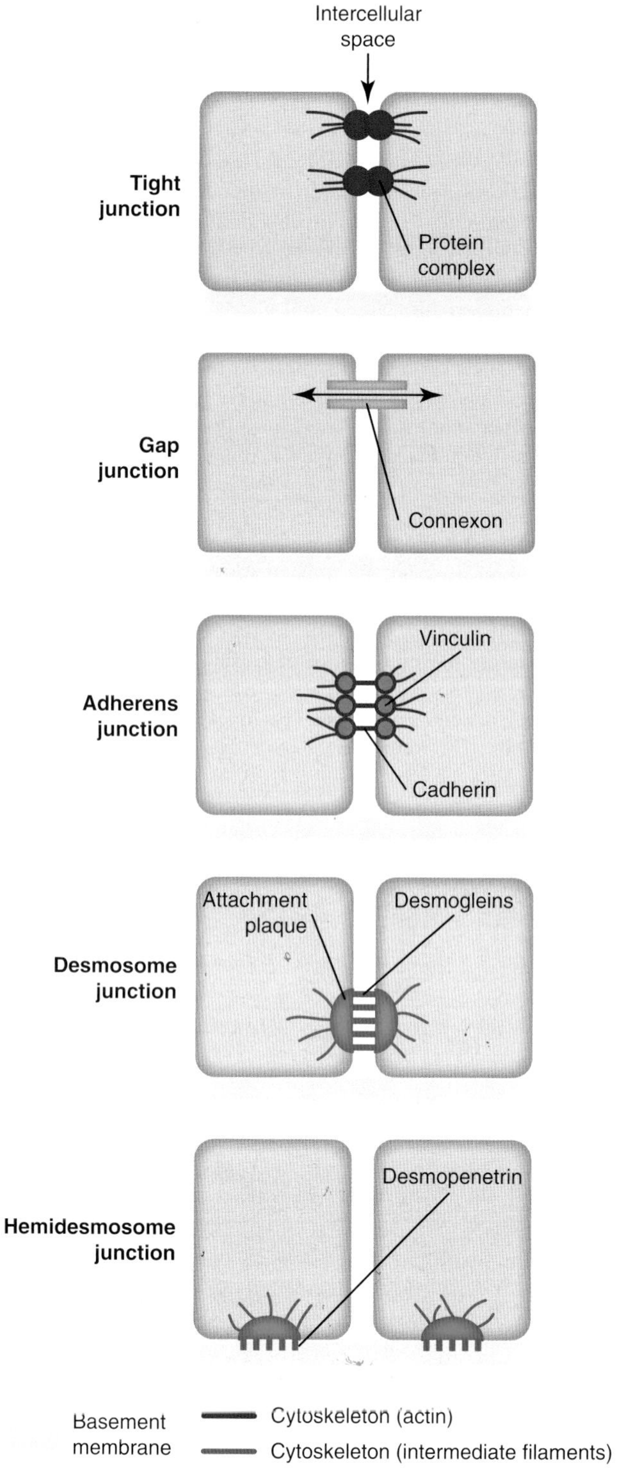

Figure 1-6 **Intercellular Junctions and Hemidesmosomes.** A variety of intercellular junctions connect certain cell types (e.g., epithelial cells) to each other and facilitate intercellular communication. Some types of cell (e.g., basilar epithelial cells) are connected to a basement membrane by hemidesmosomes. (Courtesy Dr. M.A. Miller, College of Veterinary Medicine, Purdue University; and Dr. J.F. Zachary, College of Veterinary Medicine, University of Illinois.)

Causes of Cell Injury

Injury to tissues and organs begins at the cellular level. Rudolf Virchow (1821-1902), known as the father of cellular pathology, based his study of diseased cells on the observation of structural alterations (morphologic lesions). However, Virchow also realized that biochemical changes in the cell, which preceded the appearance of lesions, more completely explained the functional disturbances in diseased cells and, in some cases, were the only detectable changes. Thus the pathologist must always correlate lesions with their biochemical bases and remember that a cell can be damaged functionally (biochemically) yet have no apparent morphologic alterations.

Simplistically, cell injury disrupts cellular homeostasis. Cells are injured by numerous and diverse causes (etiologic agents) from intrinsic and extrinsic sources; however, all of these causes, and they number in the thousands, activate one or more of four final common biochemical mechanisms leading to cell injury (Essential Concept 1-1). These fundamental underlying biochemical mechanisms of cell injury are (1) ATP depletion, (2) permeabilization of cell membranes, (3) disruption of biochemical pathways, and (4) damage to DNA. These four mechanisms will be discussed in greater detail in later sections of this chapter.

Cells have a limited repertoire of responses to injury, depending on the cell type and the nature of the injury. These responses can be categorized as (1) adaptation, (2) degeneration, or (3) death. A cell may adapt to a stimulus or sublethal injury positively, with increased efficiency or productivity, or undergo degeneration with diminished functional capacity. The response to injury can be reversible, with eventual restoration (i.e., healing) of normal or near-normal cellular structure and function, or irreversible with progression from degeneration to death of the cell (Fig. 1-7). Irreparable DNA damage can result in permanent growth arrest (senescence), cell death, or malignant transformation. Not surprisingly,

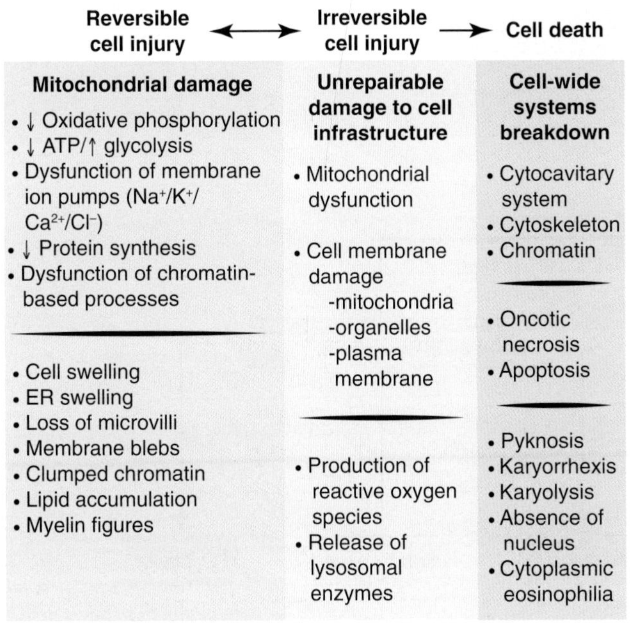

Figure 1-7 **Postulated Sequence of Events in Reversible and Irreversible Ischemic Cell Injury.** Although reduced oxidative phosphorylation and adenosine triphosphate (ATP) concentration have a central role, ischemia can damage membranes directly. *ER*, Endoplasmic reticulum. (Courtesy Dr. M.A. Miller, College of Veterinary Medicine, Purdue University; and Dr. J.F. Zachary, College of Veterinary Medicine, University of Illinois.)

ESSENTIAL CONCEPT 1-1 Mechanisms of Cell Injury

The fundamental pathogenesis of cell injury is a perturbation of homeostasis. Cell injury is initiated at the molecular level, and, although the specific causes are diverse and numerous, the basic mechanisms can be categorized as follows:

1. Adenosine triphosphate (ATP) depletion
2. Permeabilization of cell membranes
3. Disruption of biochemical pathways, especially those of protein synthesis
4. DNA damage

Although certain injurious agents can cause ATP depletion, membrane damage, pathway disruption, or DNA damage in isolation, more often there is interplay among these basic mechanisms. Anything that decreases the supply of oxygen and other nutrients to the cell or that damages mitochondria directly halts oxidative phosphorylation, leading to rapid depletion of ATP, even in those cells that can switch to anaerobic glycolysis. The ATP depletion results in additional cell damage by causing failure of energy-dependent enzymes, in particular the cell membrane adenosinetriphosphatase ion pumps that control cell volume and electrolyte balance. Mitochondria are the major site of ATP generation and are also one of the most vulnerable organelles of the cell. Importantly, mitochondrial injury results not only in ATP depletion but also in increased permeability of mitochondrial membranes with resultant loss of calcium homeostasis and activation of enzymes, such as phospholipases, proteases, and endonucleases, hence inflicting damage on mitochondrial and other cell membranes, structural and enzymatic proteins, and nucleic acids.

mitochondria, which are perhaps the organelles most susceptible to injury, are also thought to direct many of the processes of cellular adaptation, degeneration, and death through apoptosis or programmed necrosis (Fig. 1-8).

The more common causes (etiologic agents) of cellular injury are grouped, discussed, and illustrated in the following sections.

Oxygen Deficiency

Hypoxia, a reduction in oxygen supply, is one of the most common and most important causes of injury; indeed, it is often the ultimate cause of cell injury. Hypoxia can result from inadequate oxygenation of blood as a result of cardiac or respiratory failure, reduction of vascular perfusion (ischemia), reduced O_2 transport by erythrocytes (as in anemia or carbon monoxide [CO] toxicosis), or inhibition of respiratory enzymes of the cell (e.g., cyanide toxicosis).

Physical Agents

Physical agents of cell injury include mechanical trauma, temperature extremes, radiation, and electric shock. Trauma can damage cells directly (e.g., crushing or tearing), or indirectly by disruption of the blood supply to these cells and tissues. Low-intensity heat can damage blood vessels, accelerate certain cellular reactions, or halt those reactions with temperature-sensitive enzymes. Extreme heat denatures enzymes and other proteins. Cold causes vasoconstriction, limiting the blood supply to cells and tissues; extreme cold literally freezes cells with formation of ice crystals within the cytosol that disrupt cell membranes. Ionizing and ultraviolet radiation are the most important types of radiation causing cellular injury. Ionizing radiation, with its frequencies above the ultraviolet range, ionizes atoms or molecules, which then cause direct cell membrane or organelle damage or the production of free radicals that react with other cellular components, especially DNA. Ionizing radiation injury is a localized side effect of radiation therapy for cancer. Ultraviolet (frequencies just above that of visible light) radiation injury develops from exposure of sparsely haired and lightly pigmented skin (or other minimally pigmented tissues, such as the conjunctiva) to sunlight. Ultraviolet radiation can disrupt cellular bonds with the formation of reactive oxygen species (ROS). It also damages DNA, mainly through the formation of pyrimidine dimers. Electrical currents generate heat as they pass through tissues (e.g., skin, with high resistance), which can result in burns. Once the current enters the body, it is conducted through tissues of least resistance, especially the nervous system, where disruption of impulses in brainstem respiratory centers, the cardiac conduction system, or neuromuscular junctions results in indirect injury to cells and tissues.

Infectious Microbes

Infectious microbes (see also Chapter 4) differ from other injurious agents in that they can replicate once they gain access to cells or tissues. Infectious microbes range from protein molecules without nucleic acids (e.g., prions) through microbes (e.g., viruses and bacteria) to macroscopic parasites and injure cells in diverse ways. Viruses tend to subvert the host cell's DNA synthesis in the production of their own gene products; many bacteria produce toxins. Injury is exacerbated in many infectious diseases by the inflammatory (see Chapters 3 and 4) and immune (see Chapter 5) responses against the infectious microbe.

Nutritional Imbalances

Nutritional deficiencies, excesses, and imbalances all predispose the cell to injury. Animals can adapt to short-term dietary deficiencies in protein or calories through glycolysis, lipolysis, and catabolism of muscle protein; however, long-term starvation leads to atrophy of cells and tissues. In contrast, caloric excess can overload cells with glycogen and lipids and lead to obesity with metabolic disturbances that predispose the obese animal to a variety of diseases. Certain dietary deficiencies or imbalances of essential amino acids, fatty acids, vitamins, or minerals can lead to muscle wasting, decreased stature, increased susceptibility to infection, metabolic disturbances,

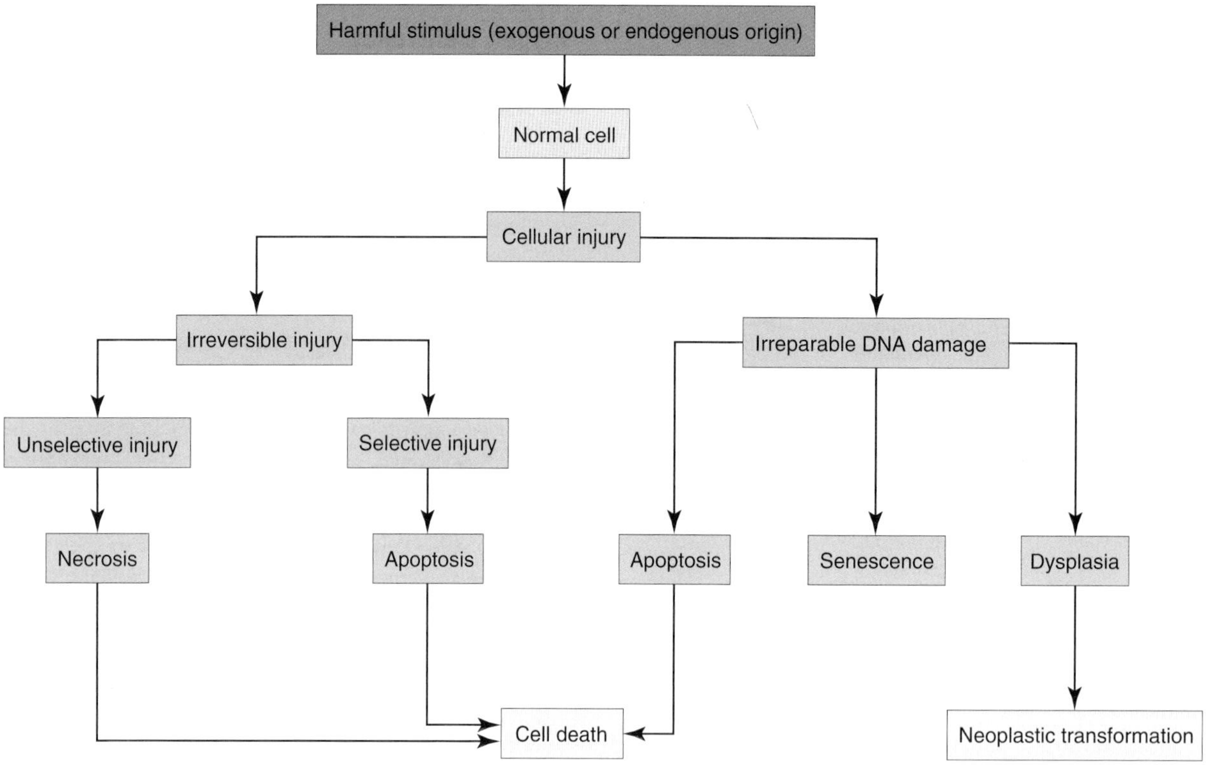

Figure 1-8 Stages in the Cellular Response to Irreversible Injury or Irreparable DNA Damage. (Courtesy Dr. M.A. Miller, College of Veterinary Medicine, Purdue University; and Dr. J.F. Zachary, College of Veterinary Medicine, University of Illinois.)

and a host of other diseases, depending on which elements are missing from or disproportionate in the diet.

Genetic Derangement

Selective breeding of domestic animals for a particular conformational or dispositional phenotype has resulted in decreased genetic diversity in purebred animals and increased prevalence of inherited diseases (see subsequent section on the Genetic Basis of Disease and pertinent chapters in Section II, Pathology of Organ Systems), as well as a familial predilection for disease conditions with more complex inheritance, such as metabolic abnormalities, neoplasia, autoimmune diseases, and increased susceptibility to infection. Since the sequencing of the genomes of domestic animals, the genetic basis has been discovered for more and more of these phenotypes and associated familial diseases. For example, a single insulin-like growth factor-1 (*IGF-1*) haplotype is common to toy and miniature dog breeds, but generally absent in giant breeds; a fibroblast growth factor 4 (*FGF4*) retrogene is associated with chondrodysplastic conformation. Some conformational phenotypes are strongly linked to pathologic conditions (e.g., a missense mutation in bone morphogenetic protein 3 [*BMP3*] is linked to the extreme brachycephalic phenotype of Cavalier King Charles spaniels and Brussels griffons). Interestingly, bone morphogenetic protein genes also determine patterning in the developing brain and spinal cord, so the brachycephalic conformation in these breeds is associated with Chiari-like malformation of the cerebellum and syringomyelia of the cervical spinal cord.

Workload Imbalance

Cells can compensate for increased workload with an increase in size (hypertrophy [e.g., muscle]) or, if capable, in number (hyperplasia [e.g., adrenal cortex]). Cells that cannot meet an increased demand may undergo degeneration or death. Conversely, cells that are no longer necessary or that no longer receive the stimulus of physical exercise, innervation, hormones, or growth factors tend to shrink as in the disuse atrophy or denervation atrophy in skeletal muscles or the physiologic atrophy of the mammary gland after weaning of the offspring. Excessive cells, for example, neurons in the developing brain, are also removed by programmed cell death (apoptosis).

Chemicals, Drugs, and Toxins

Chemicals, including drugs and toxins, can alter cellular homeostasis. The therapeutic effect of pharmaceutical agents (drugs) is achieved by perturbing the homeostasis of selected populations of cells, ideally within tolerable limits. Chemicals are considered toxins if they alter homeostasis in a harmful way (outside of tolerable limits) with no beneficial pharmaceutical effect. Of course, many chemicals are beneficial or therapeutic at certain doses and harmful at higher doses. Chemicals affect cells by binding receptors, inhibiting or inducing enzymes or otherwise altering metabolic pathways, producing free radicals, increasing membrane permeability, or damaging chromosomes or structural components of the cell. The susceptibility of a cell to chemical injury depends on such factors as its mitotic rate and its ability to bind, take up, concentrate, or metabolize the chemical.

Immunologic Dysfunction

Immunologic dysfunction can result in cell injury either through a failure to respond effectively (immunodeficiency) to infectious microbes (see Chapter 4) or other harmful foreign antigens or through an excessive response (allergic or hypersensitivity reaction) to a foreign antigen or an inappropriate reaction to self-antigens (autoimmune disease). See Chapter 5 for more complete information on immunodeficiencies, hypersensitivity reactions, and autoimmune diseases.

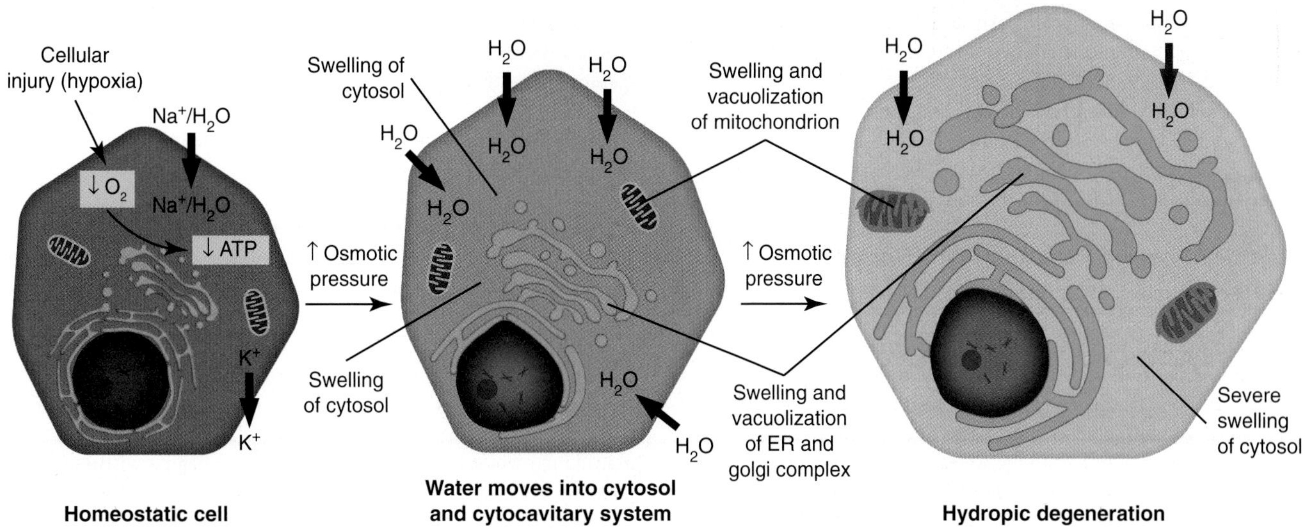

Figure 1-9 The Process of Acute Cell Swelling (Hydropic Degeneration). *ATP*, Adenosine triphosphate; *ER*, endoplasmic reticulum. (Courtesy Dr. M.A. Miller, College of Veterinary Medicine, Purdue University; and Dr. J.F. Zachary, College of Veterinary Medicine, University of Illinois.)

Aging

Cells and tissues age because of accumulated damage to their proteins, lipids, and nucleic acids. Much of the damage of aging is attributed to ROS, DNA mutations, and cellular senescence (see the subsequent section on Cellular Aging). Cumulative damage to DNA predisposes aged animals to the development of neoplasia. In cells that can replicate, the telomeres at the ends of chromosomes are shortened with each successive division, eventually causing the cell to stop dividing. Not surprisingly, many cancer cells have active telomerase to maintain the length of their telomeres. In cells with little regenerative capacity, such as neurons, accumulation of lipofuscin and other metabolic products contributes to their degeneration and loss, leading to cerebrocortical atrophy in the aging brain. However, many of the common "aging lesions" in geriatric animals (e.g., nodular hyperplasia in the liver [see Fig. 8-65], pancreas [see Fig. 8-91], or spleen [see Fig. 13-90; see E-Figs. 13-9, 13-14, and 13-15] of dogs; cholesterol granulomas in the choroid plexus of horses [see Fig. 14-87]; siderofibrotic plaques in the canine spleen [see Figs. 13-71 and 13-72; see E-Figs. 13-9 and 13-10]; even thyroid C-cell adenomas in horses [see Fig. 12-30]) are generally disregarded as incidental findings (i.e., not the cause of death) at autopsy.

Reversible Cell Injury

The initial response of the cell to perturbation of homeostasis is acute cell swelling. If the injury is not too severe or too prolonged, the cell can recover and return to normal structure and function. Therefore acute cell swelling is, up to a point, a reversible change (Essential Concept 1-2).

Acute Cell Swelling

Cell swelling, a fundamental and common expression of cell injury (Fig. 1-9), is also known as hydropic degeneration because it is the influx of water along with sodium ions when the sodium-potassium ion pumps fail that causes the swelling. If not stopped, acute cell swelling will cause lysis and death of the cell. The term *hydropic degeneration* is commonly used when the change occurs in certain types of cells, such as hepatocytes or renal tubular epithelial cells. In other tissues (e.g., keratinocytes in the epidermis), cell swelling from influx of water is called *ballooning degeneration*. In the central nervous system (CNS), cell swelling of glial cells, especially prominent in astrocytes, is termed cytotoxic edema. In any tissue, acute cell swelling is a degenerative change in which the cellular enlargement is the result of increased water volume. Acute cell swelling therefore is quite different from hypertrophy, in which the enlargement of cells is caused by an adaptive increase in number and/or size of organelles.

ESSENTIAL CONCEPT 1-2 Reversible Cell Injury

Cell injury is classified as reversible if the injured cell can regain homeostasis and return to a morphologically (and functionally) normal state. Acute cell swelling is the classic morphologic change in reversible injury; however, it is also the typical early change of irreversible cell injury. Irrespective of the nature of the initial injury, hypoxia is often the ultimate cause of acute cell swelling because it results in adenosine triphosphate depletion. The hypoxic cell then swells because of loss of volume control when membrane adenosine triphosphatase ionic pumps fail. Acute cell swelling is also a response to direct cell membrane damage from lipid peroxidation (by reactive oxygen species), binding of certain toxins, damage to ion channels, or insertion of transmembrane pore-forming complexes. Because acute cell swelling is a common early response to both reversible and irreversible injury, it is well to think of this morphologic change as a marker of *potentially reversible cell injury*. Cells, depending on their reparative or regenerative capacities, may recover from potentially irreversible cell injury; however, if the injury is severe or sustained, acute cell swelling becomes the initial step in the process of cell death. If the injury is not so severe as to be lethal, then the cell may not succumb but (again depending on the nature of the injury and of the cell) is unlikely to recover completely or to return to its "normal" structural and functional state.

Mechanisms of Acute Cell Swelling

In normal cells, sodium-potassium adenosine triphosphatases (Na^+/K^+-ATPases) function as ionic pumps, specifically, as active transporters of cations across cell membranes (see Fig. 1-9). For each ATP molecule hydrolyzed, the ionic pump exports (i.e., outside the cell) three Na^+ ions and imports (i.e., inside the cell) two K^+ ions. The resultant electrochemical gradient generates energy that is especially important in establishing and maintaining the membrane potential of neurons and of cardiac and skeletal muscle cells and pH homeostasis within the cytosol of the cell. Because water diffuses passively along the osmotic gradient, the ATPase pump also controls cell volume. The best-studied models of acute cell swelling are (1) hypoxia-induced failure of ATP synthesis (and hence the ATPase pumps) and (2) carbon tetrachloride (CCl_4)–induced membrane damage. Notably, the cardiac glycosides, digitalis and ouabain, specifically inhibit Na^+/K^+-ATPase pumps.

Acute Cell Swelling Resulting from Hypoxic Injury

Hypoxia is the end result of decreased oxygen concentration at any point in its passage from air into the respiratory tract through hemoglobin uptake and transport by the vasculature to cells, where it drives mitochondrial oxidative phosphorylation. Ischemia is a local decrease in blood supply to tissue with resultant decreased delivery of oxygen (hypoxia), glucose, and other nutrients to the cell, as well as decreased removal of metabolic wastes. Because any injury to the respiratory or cardiovascular system can lead to hypoxia, it is commonly the ultimate cause of acute cell swelling. When cellular oxygen is depleted, oxidative phosphorylation stops, and the cell must switch to anaerobic metabolism (i.e., glycolysis) or die. As production of ATP declines, the resultant drop stimulates hexokinases, phosphofructokinase 1 (PFK1), and other enzymes of glycolysis. PFK1 catalyzes the phosphorylation of fructose 6-phosphate to fructose 1,6-bisphosphate, another integral step in glycolysis. The end products of glycolysis are ATP and pyruvate and heat. This anaerobic generation of ATP (though less efficient than oxidative phosphorylation) contributes to short-term survival of the cell. In addition, pyruvate produced by glycolysis can enter the tricarboxylic acid (TCA) cycle. However, certain specialized cells (e.g., neurons) cannot generate ATP anaerobically and therefore need a continuous supply of oxygen and glucose. This dependency makes neurons one of the cells that are most susceptible to a deficiency or lack of oxygen.

The early events in acute cell swelling (see Figs. 1-7 and 1-9) caused by hypoxia or ischemia are potentially reversible if the injury is mild or of short duration. With the depletion of cellular oxygen, oxidative phosphorylation stops. The resultant deficiency of ATP causes failure of the Na^+/K^+-ATPase pumps with influx of Na^+, Ca^{2+}, and water into the cytosol, and loss of K^+ and Mg^{2+} from the cytosol. The electrolyte imbalance and influx of water expand the cytosol and swell mitochondria and the cytocavitary network. Ultrastructurally, chromatin is clumped, the cytosol is electron lucent, ribosomes detach from rER, and the ER becomes vesiculated. Damaged membranes coil into whorls (also known as "myelin figures"). Cytoskeletal damage causes the plasma membrane to lose microvilli or other specialized structures and to undergo blebbing (the formation of multiple irregular bulges). With light microscopy the acutely swollen cell has an expanded and rounded profile with pale eosinophilic or vacuolated cytoplasm. The cytoplasmic pallor and vacuolation is the result of dispersion of organelles and dilution of cytosolic proteins by the influx of water. The ATP deficiency also prompts a switch to anaerobic metabolism with production of ATP (and pyruvate) through glycolysis. Glycolysis depletes cellular glycogen, leads to an accumulation of lactate with decreased intracellular pH, and produces heat, which if excessive may also injure the cell.

Acute Cell Swelling Resulting from Specific Types of Cell Membrane Injury

Cell membranes can also be selectively injured by chemical modification of their phospholipids by free radicals (i.e., lipid peroxidation), by covalent binding of toxins to macromolecules, by interference with ion channels, and by insertion of transmembrane complexes. CCl_4 is an example of cell membrane injury caused by chemical modifications (see the following section). Cell membranes can also be injured directly by defensive molecules of the immune system and by bacterial cytotoxins (see later).

Carbon Tetrachloride and Cell Membrane Injury

Information on this topic is available at www.expertconsult.com.

Molecules of the Immune System and Cell Membrane Injury. Cell membranes can also be injured directly by the membrane attack complex (MAC) of the complement pathway, by bacterial cytolysins, and by molecules from natural killer (NK) cells (see Chapters 3, 4, and 5). The MAC, bacterial cytolysins, and NK cells exert their effect in part by forming a pore or channel that disrupts the lipid bilayers of the plasma membrane. The MAC is assembled from terminal components of the complement pathway, which are abundant in blood. Assembly of the MAC begins with enzymatic cleavage of complement fragment 5b (C5b) from complement component 5 (C5). Complement component 6 (C6) binds a labile site on C5b to produce a stable intermediate. Subsequent binding of complement component 7 (C7) renders the MAC precursor lipophilic. With binding of the α, β, and γ subunits of complement component 8 (C8), the MAC precursor penetrates a nearby cell membrane lipid bilayer. Binding and oligomerization of complement component 9 (C9) then completes formation of the MAC, which creates a lytic pore that is part of the innate immune response to bacteria. Cluster of differentiation 59 (CD59), a glycoprotein receptor on the surface of leukocytes, epithelial cells, and endothelial cells (and overexpressed on some cancer cells), blocks penetration of cell membranes by the C5b-8 precursor and blocks incorporation of C9 into the MAC, thereby protecting host cells against cell membrane injury.

Morphologic Changes: Their Detection and Evaluation

Information on this topic is available at www.expertconsult.com.

Morphology of Acute Cell Swelling

Gross Appearance. Acute cell swelling increases the volume and weight of parenchymal organs and imparts pallor to them. It is important to distinguish hydropic degeneration from more positive adaptations, such as hypertrophy or hyperplasia, which, if extensive, also increase the size of an organ. Liver and kidney (especially the renal cortex) are two organs in which the lesions of acute cell swelling can be striking (see Chapters 8 and 11). An affected liver weighs more than normal, appears pale and swollen with rounded edges, and has an accentuated lobular pattern (Fig. 1-10, *A*). In the CNS the cell swelling of cytotoxic edema has little effect on the color of neuroparenchyma but does increase the weight and volume of the affected tissue. Even a slight increase in volume of the brain has catastrophic consequences because there is little space in the cranium to accommodate swelling (see Chapter 14).

Microscopic Appearance. The influx of water in hydropic degeneration dilutes the cytosol, separates its organelles, and distends the cell, giving affected cells a swollen, pale, and finely vacuolated appearance. In renal proximal tubules, swollen epithelial cells impinge on the tubular lumen. In the liver, swollen hepatocytes and endothelial cells compress hepatic sinusoids.

Hydropic degeneration and cloudy swelling are terms for the microscopic appearance of acute cell swelling (see Fig. 1-10, *B*). In addition to endothelial cells, hepatocytes, and renal tubular epithelial cells, other epithelial cells, neurons, and glial cells are particularly prone to acute cell swelling. The clear cytoplasmic vacuoles in affected cells are mainly water-distended mitochondria or cisternae

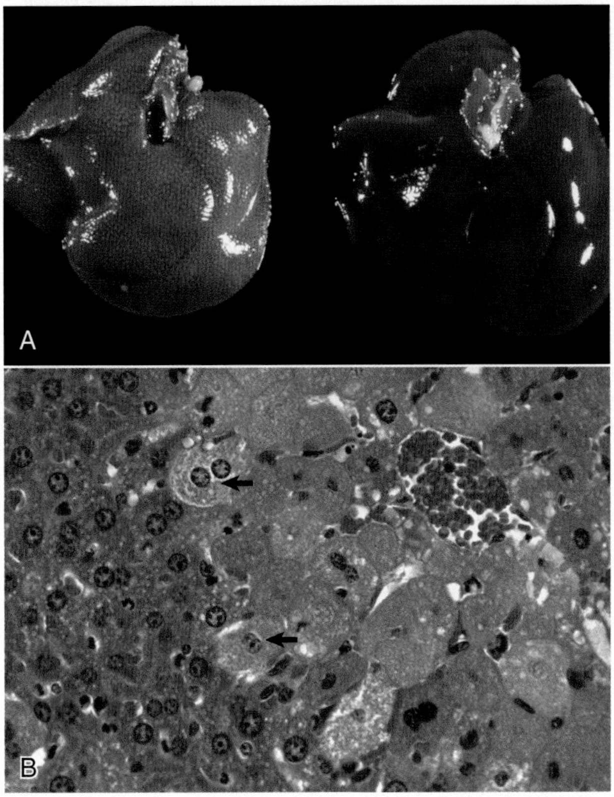

Figure 1-10 **Acute Cell Swelling, Liver, Mouse. A,** Hepatic swelling in a mouse exposed to chloroform 24 hours previously. The accentuated lobular pattern and slight pallor in the liver on the left are the result of acute cell swelling (hydropic degeneration) and necrosis of centrilobular hepatocytes. The right liver is normal. **B,** Liver from a mouse with chloroform toxicosis. Although many hepatocytes in the centrilobular areas *(at right)* are necrotic, several cells at the interface of normal and necrotic *(arrows)* are still undergoing acute cell swelling (hydropic degeneration). H&E stain. (Courtesy Dr. L.H. Arp.)

of the Golgi complex or ER; therefore these vacuoles are not labeled by histochemical techniques to detect fat or glycogen (two other causes of cytoplasmic vacuolation). Ballooning degeneration is an extreme variant of hydropic degeneration that is typically seen in keratinocytes of stratified squamous epithelium of the skin. Poxviruses are a classic cause of ballooning degeneration of keratinocytes of epidermal or mucosal (e.g., esophagus) stratified squamous epithelium (Fig. 1-11).

Ultrastructural Appearance. Ultrastructurally, the acutely swollen epithelial cell loses plasma membrane structures, such as cilia and microvilli, and develops cytoplasmic "blebs" at apical cell surfaces. The cytosol is electron lucent, mitochondria are swollen, and cisternae of the ER and Golgi complex are dilated. The cytocavitary network fragments into vesicles. Proteins and Ca^{2+} precipitate in the cytosol and in organelles, especially mitochondria. Acute cell swelling in the CNS has other distinctive features (see Chapter 14).

Significance and Fate of Acute Cell Swelling

If the injury is brief and mild, many cells can recover and regain normal or near-normal structure and function. Recovered cells can phagocytize their own damaged organelles (autophagy); these autophagosomes may ultimately appear as lipofuscin granules, indicative of previous injury. However, even with reversible injury, impaired regulation of water and electrolyte balance across cell membranes is generally accompanied by disruption of other cellular processes. The ultimate effect on the animal depends on the number of cells affected, reparative and regenerative abilities of the cell, and the importance of the disrupted biochemical processes, such as ATP synthesis. With severe, lengthy, or repetitive injury, acute cell swelling can progress beyond the "point of no return" and become an early stage in the process of cell death. In summary, the acute cell swelling of hydropic degeneration reflects potentially reversible, sublethal cell injury. However, unless the injury to essential cells in vital organs (e.g., brain, heart, lung, liver, or kidney) is stopped quickly, it can progress to cell and tissue death, loss of essential physiologic functions, and possibly death of the animal (Fig. 1-12).

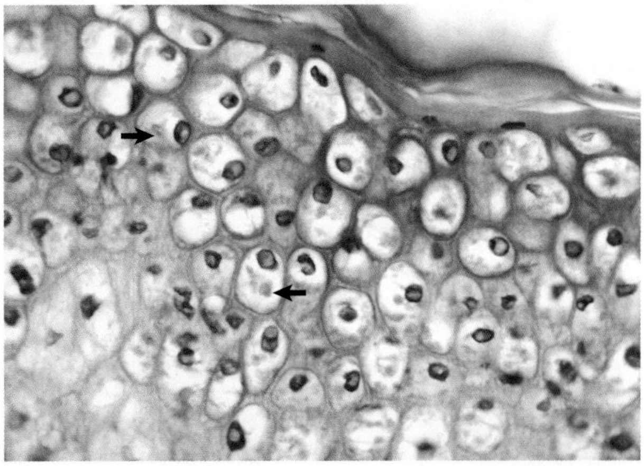

Figure 1-11 **Ballooning Degeneration, Papular Stomatitis, Oral Mucosa, Ox.** Cells infected by certain poxviruses (e.g., papular stomatitis virus) cannot regulate their volume and undergo hydropic degeneration at certain stages of the infection. These cells may become so distended (ballooning degeneration) that they eventually rupture. Note cytoplasmic viral inclusion bodies *(arrows)*. H&E stain. (Courtesy Dr. M.D. McGavin, College of Veterinary Medicine, University of Tennessee.)

Irreversible Cell Injury and Cell Death

Major mechanisms of acute cell swelling, as discussed and illustrated earlier, are (1) hypoxia, (including ischemia) and (2) membrane injury caused by lipid peroxidation or the formation of lytic pores through insertion of a MAC via the complement pathway or by bacterial cytolysins. The cellular response to injury depends on (1) the type of cell injured and its susceptibility and/or resistance to hypoxia and direct membrane injury and (2) the nature, severity, and duration of the injury. As examples, neurons, cardiac myocytes, endothelium, and epithelium of the proximal tubule of the kidney are cells that are extremely susceptible to hypoxia, whereas fibroblasts, adipocytes, and other mesenchymal structural cells are less susceptible.

The response to injury can be degenerative, adaptive, or completely reversible with restoration of normal structure and function for the affected cell; however, with more severe or persistent injury, acute cell swelling can progress to irreversible cell injury and cell death. The cellular alterations that differentiate reversible cell injury from irreversible cell injury have been and are being studied extensively.

Cell Death

The death of cells is an essential "value-added" part of embryonic development and maturation of the fetus and of homeostasis within populations of adult somatic cells. In these physiologic examples of

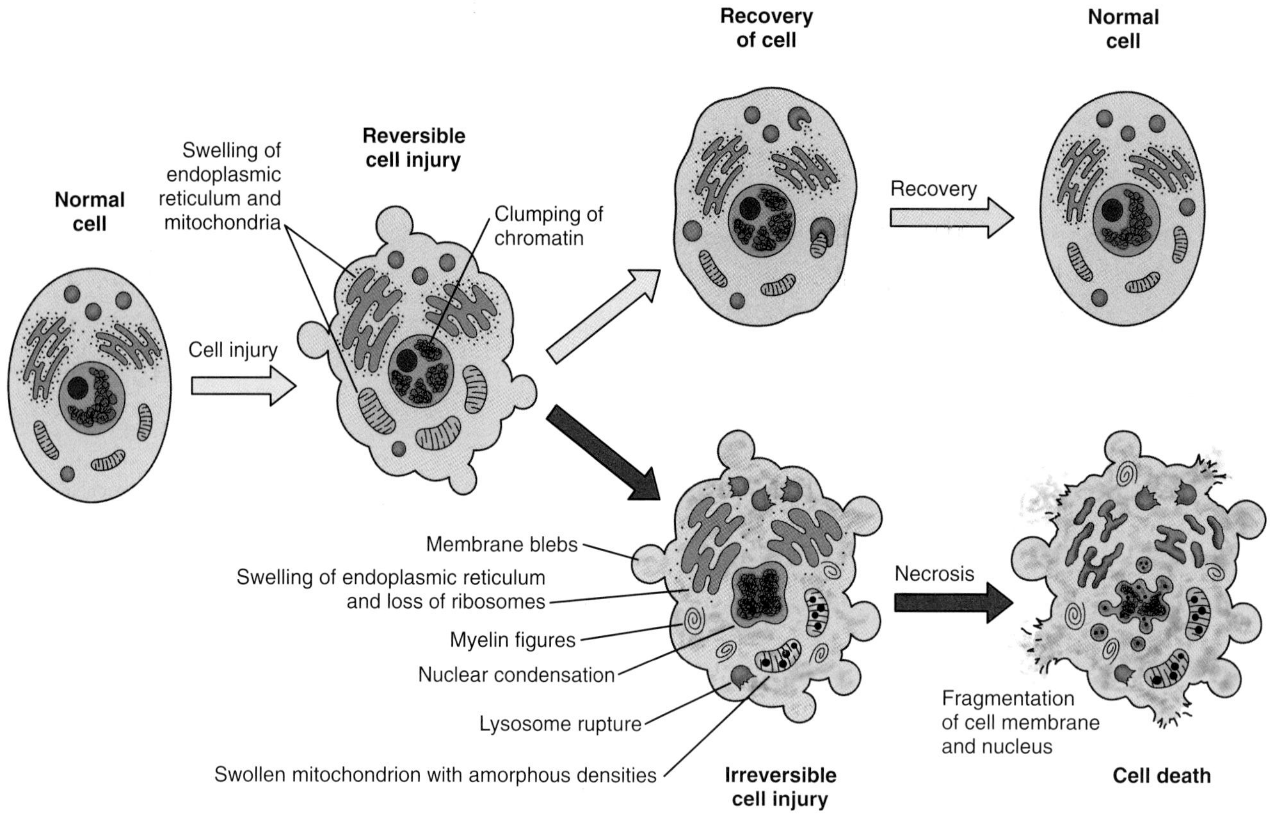

Figure 1-12 **Normal Cell and the Changes in Reversible and Irreversible Cell Injury.** Reversible injury is characterized by generalized swelling of the cell, its organelles (especially mitochondria), and the cytocavitary network. Other changes include blebbing of the plasma membrane, detachment of ribosomes from ER, and clumping of nuclear chromatin. Irreversible injury is characterized by increased cell swelling, disruption of lysosomes, formation of amorphous densities in mitochondria, membrane disruption in the cytocavitary network, and severe nuclear changes. Irreversible nuclear changes include pyknosis (severe condensation of chromatin), followed by karyorrhexis (nuclear fragmentation) and karyolysis (nuclear dissolution). Laminated structures (myelin figures) derived from injured cell membranes can appear during reversible injury, but become more pronounced in irreversibly injured cells.

cell death, cells that are no longer needed are removed during development or remodeling of tissues. However, cell death is also a point-of-no-return response to severe injury, and it is this pathologic form of cell death that is the topic of this section. Cell death typically assumes one of two morphologic forms (Fig. 1-13): necrosis or apoptosis. The term necrosis has evolved to mean death by swelling of the cell (oncosis) with eventual rupture of cell membranes. Necrotic cell death typically involves groups or zones of cells and elicits an inflammatory reaction because of the release of cell contents into the ECM. Apoptosis, in contrast, is directed by cellular signaling cascades and typically affects individual cells. Apoptosis is a process of condensation and shrinkage of the cell and its organelles with eventual fragmentation of the cell. Importantly, apoptotic cell fragments remain membrane bound; thus no cellular components that could induce inflammation are released. Autophagy is a third possible mechanism of cell death, but it is more commonly a means of cell survival. (See subsequent section on Autophagy under Chronic Cell Injury and Cell Adaptation.)

Whereas apoptosis has long been recognized as a regulated or programmed process, not only responsible for physiologic removal of surplus cells but also occurring as a reaction to certain injuries, necrosis was once considered an entirely accidental and random response to injury. However, with the discovery that inhibition of apoptosis could shift cells from apoptotic death to a regulated process of oncotic death, the idea arose that necrosis could, at least in certain situations, be regulated by cellular signaling pathways.

Cell Death by Oncosis (Oncotic Necrosis)

Oncotic cell death results from irreversible cell injury that, for example, is caused by hypoxia, ischemia, or direct damage to cell membranes (Essential Concept 1-3). Ischemia causes particularly extensive cell injury because the decreased perfusion results in not only an oxygen deficit (hypoxia) but also a deficiency of glucose and other nutrients, plus an accumulation of toxic metabolic by-products. Cell swelling, resulting from loss of volume control (see later), is the fundamental mechanism of oncotic necrosis and distinguishes it from apoptosis. Just as in reversible acute cell swelling, the initial O_2 deficit in irreversible acute cell swelling causes an uncoupling of oxidative phosphorylation and a switch to anaerobic glycolysis with accumulation of lactic acid and a resulting decrease in pH of the cytosol. The Na^+/H^+ exchanger exports the excess H^+ in exchange for Na^+. However, because glycolysis is less efficient in ATP production than oxidative phosphorylation, the decreased ATP concentration leads to failure of ionic ATPase pumps and a loss of volume control (i.e., failure of Na^+/K^+-ATPase pumps with influx of Na^+, Ca^{2+}, and water). In addition, the normal function of enzymes, contractile proteins, membrane pumps, and other protein-based mechanisms in the cell occurs in a very narrow pH range around 7.0. With glycolysis the cytosol becomes acidic, thus limiting or blocking these mechanisms and exacerbating cellular dysfunction.

Disruption of the intracellular calcium ion balance (Fig. 1-14) is integral to the transition from potentially reversible acute cell swelling to irreversible injury and cell death. The intracellular concentration of calcium is generally one-fourth that of extracellular calcium.

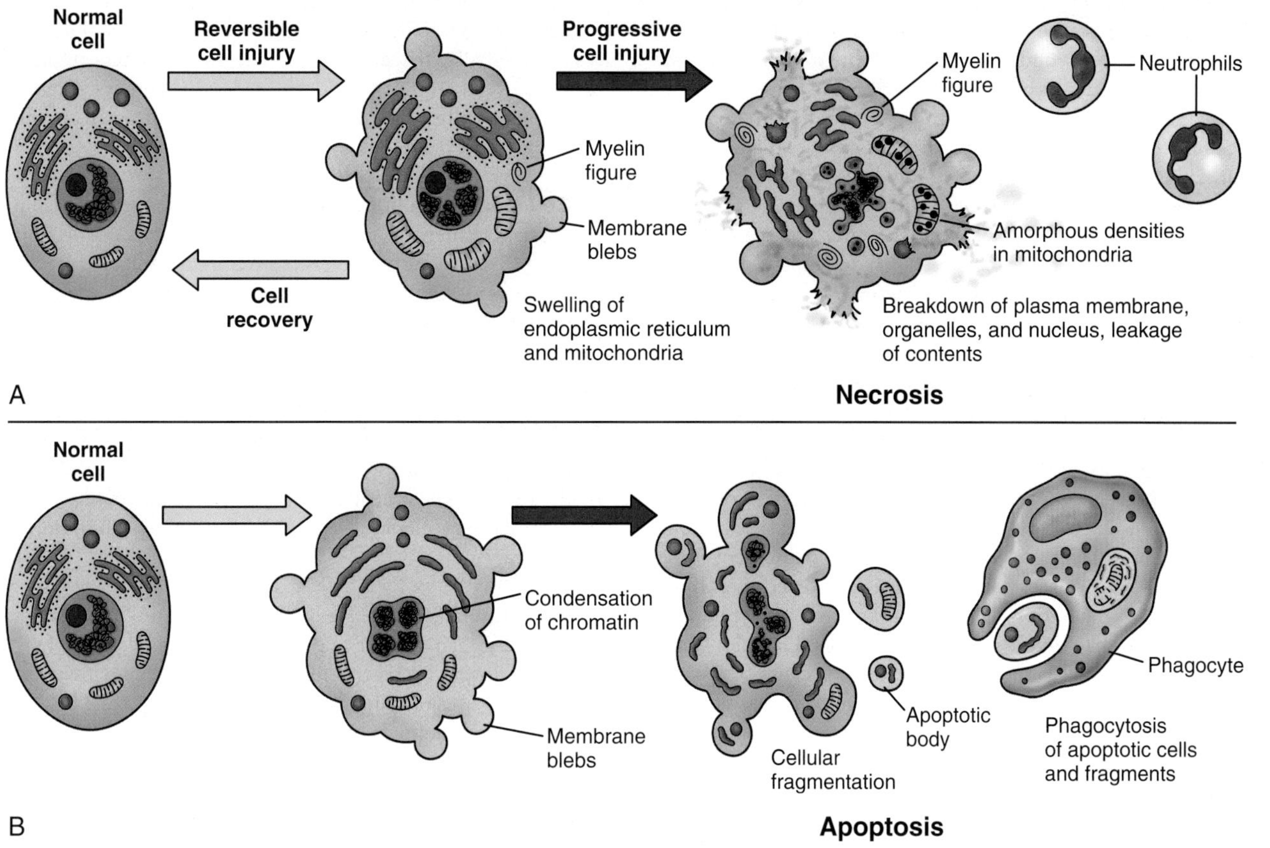

Figure 1-13 The Sequential Ultrastructural Changes of Necrosis and Apoptosis. **A,** In necrosis, leakage of cell contents through the ruptured plasma membrane into the extracellular matrix elicits inflammation. **B,** In apoptosis, cellular fragments are extruded as plasma membrane-bound apoptotic bodies that are recognized by phagocytes but do not cause inflammation.

ESSENTIAL CONCEPT 1-3 Cell Death

Severe or persistent injury can overwhelm the cell's capacity to restore homeostasis, in which case potentially reversible acute cell swelling can become irreversible and progress to cell death. The morphologic features of cell death change with the passage of time and depend on the manner of death (oncotic necrosis versus apoptosis) and the type of cell or tissue. *Oncotic necrosis* is a process of cell swelling and thereby distinct from cell death by apoptosis, which is a process of cellular shrinkage and fragmentation. If an acutely swollen cell fails to correct the electrolyte imbalance and loss of volume control, then potentially reversible cell injury can become the initial stage of oncotic necrosis. Once thought always to be unregulated, oncotic necrosis, like apoptosis, can be a programmed process (necroptosis). Programmed cell death, whether by necroptosis or apoptosis, has many extrinsic and intrinsic (acting mainly through mitochondria) triggers. Programmed cell death is a complex and varied process that includes stages of initiation, propagation, and execution. Cells that die by oncotic necrosis tend to do so in groups, whereas apoptosis commonly affects individual cells. Furthermore, oncotic necrosis results in rupture of cell membranes and release of cytoplasmic content into the extracellular matrix with ensuing inflammation. In contrast, the cell that dies by apoptosis shrinks and fragments, but the fragments remain membrane bound and therefore do not elicit an inflammatory response although they are marked for phagocytosis.

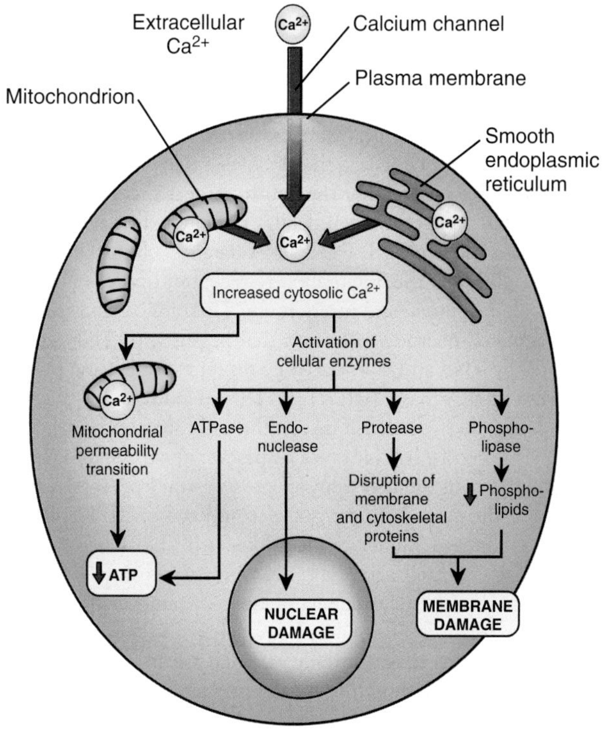

Figure 1-14 Sources and Consequences of Increased Cytosolic Calcium in Cell Injury. *ATP,* Adenosine triphosphate; *ATPase,* adenosinetriphosphatase.

In a normally functioning cell, calcium is sequestered into three major compartments: the cytosol (low concentration), ER (mid-range concentration), and mitochondria (high concentration). Each compartment has its own ATPase membrane pumps. Ischemia opens plasma membrane calcium channels, leading to increased intracellular calcium concentration in the cytosol, which activates protein kinase C, endonucleases, phospholipases, and various proteases, including calpains. Calpains abolish protein kinase C activity and cleave Na^+/Ca^{2+} exchangers in mitochondrial and plasma membranes, leading to decreased calcium efflux and reuptake by the ER with ensuing calcium overload in the cytosol and, even worse, in the mitochondria. Although the timing of the point of no return remains elusive, if the cell fails to restore mitochondrial function, acute cell swelling becomes irreversible, leading to cell death.

Paradoxically, restoration of blood flow and oxygen supply can exacerbate ischemic cell injury. This phenomenon is called *ischemia-reperfusion injury*, and it can continue for several days after reperfusion. It is attributed to "*oxidative stress*," which involves the formation of ROS, calcium imbalance, opening of the mitochondrial permeability transition (MPT) pore, endothelial damage, thrombogenesis, and arrival of leukocytes in the damaged tissue. Reperfusion injury correlates with the duration of ischemia, but the susceptibility of organs (brain > heart > kidney > intestine > skeletal muscle) varies. The brain is exquisitely sensitive to ischemia because of its high metabolic activity, absolute requirement for glucose, high concentration of polyunsaturated fatty acids, and release of excitatory neurotransmitters. A less susceptible tissue (e.g., adipose tissue, fibrous tissue) can, to an extent, undergo atrophy or enter a quiescent state in response to decreased perfusion, using autophagy and apoptosis as means to remove effete organelles or dead cells, respectively.

Once considered an unregulated process, necrosis can, at least in some circumstances, be regulated by signaling pathways. In fact, regulated necrosis may be the predominant form of oncotic cell death. A regulated process of necrotic cell death begins with a trigger (e.g., binding of TNF or Fas ligand [FasL] to a death receptor [DR; i.e., transmembrane protein of the plasma membrane]), followed sequentially by initiation, propagation, and execution. A cell can respond to binding of TNF to its receptor in at least three different ways: (1) survival through activation of nuclear factor κB (NFκB), (2) apoptosis, or (3) necrosis. Apoptosis is directed by caspases. Interestingly, it was the discovery that inhibition of caspases, rather than protecting the cell from death, could redirect it from apoptosis to necrotic cell death. The myriad triggers of regulated necrosis include TNF, FasL, DNA damage, cluster of differentiation 3 (CD3) via the T lymphocyte receptor, lipopolysaccharide via Toll-like receptors, and interferon γ. The term *necroptosis* refers to the regulated necrotic cell death that begins with TNF receptor activation by TNF and is initiated by receptor-interacting protein-serine/threonine kinase (RIPK) 1. The ubiquitination status of RIPK1 determines whether it directs the cell toward survival, apoptosis, or necroptosis. Inhibition of caspase-8, in particular, is important in redirecting the cell from apoptosis toward necroptosis with assembly of the so-called necrosome, composed of RIPK1, RIPK3, and mixed lineage kinase domain-like (MLKL). Though much remains to be learned about the necroptosis pathway, MLKL has been proposed as the main mediator downstream of RIPK3.

Another pathway of regulated necrosis is initiated by opening of the MPT pore, which entails an increase in permeability of inner and outer mitochondrial membranes and leads to mitochondrial swelling, production of ROS, and oxidized nicotinamide adenine dinucleotide (NAD^+) depletion. Mitochondrial production of ROS, mainly through reduced forms of nicotinamide adenine dinucleotide phosphate (NADPH) oxidases, is considered requisite to TNF-α–induced necrosis. ROS, along with Ca^{2+} dysregulation and depletion of NAD^+ and ATP, propagates the signal in regulated necrosis. Finally, the execution phase, with its catastrophic ATP depletion, cell swelling, lipid peroxidation, and lysosomal membrane permeability with release of cathepsins, leads to irreversible cell injury and death.

Cell Membrane Injury Leading to Cell Death. The failure to restore mitochondrial function and repair cell membrane damage is a critical component of irreversible cell injury. In particular, uncoupled oxidative phosphorylation and impaired mitochondrial calcium sequestration significantly increase the risk for cell death. Injured cell membranes have increased permeability, so when membrane ATPase ion pumps fail, extracellular calcium enters the cell. The calcium imbalance exacerbates the damage to mitochondria and to the cytoskeleton and activates endonucleases, proteases, and phospholipases. Phospholipase A catalytically hydrolyzes the phospholipids of the cell membranes, further exacerbating cell and mitochondrial membrane damage and the progression to irreversible cell injury.

Free Radical Injury. Free radicals contribute to mitochondrial injury and to cell death by oncotic necrosis, especially when ischemia is followed by reperfusion (see earlier section that discusses ischemia-reperfusion injury). Free radicals damage cell lipids (especially the phospholipids of cell membranes), proteins, and nucleic acids (Fig. 1-15). A free radical is any molecule with an unpaired electron. Free radicals include ROS (e.g., the superoxide radical [$O_2^{\cdot}$]) and reactive nitrogen species (e.g., NO). Such molecules are highly reactive, short-lived products of oxidative metabolism and occur in membranes of mitochondria and other organelles. NADPH oxidase, an enzyme complex found in membranes of a variety of cell types, especially phagocytes, such as neutrophils and macrophages, functions in the production of ROS.

Endogenous free radicals, such as reactive oxygen or nitrogen species, serve physiologic functions in cell signaling and in defense against microbes but also can harm cells, especially in the setting of ischemia/reperfusion injury. Free radicals, with their unpaired electron, are prone to extract a H^+ from the polyunsaturated fatty acids in cell membranes. The fatty acid that loses a H^+ becomes, itself, a free radical that can then be oxidized to an even more reactive radical that will extract a H^+ from the neighboring fatty acid, propagating a chain reaction that leads to membrane disintegration. Antioxidants, such as superoxide dismutase (SOD), catalase, glutathione peroxidase, and vitamins A, C, and E, are protective because they scavenge free radicals and can break the chain reaction of lipid peroxidation.

Morphologic Appearance of Necrotic Cells and Tissues (Oncotic Necrosis). The appearance of necrotic cells depends on the type of necrosis (see the next section), the tissue involved, the cause of cell death, and the time elapsed. In this chapter, necrosis (or necrotic) generally implies oncotic cell death.

Gross Appearance of Necrotic Tissue. Soon after death of the cell, necrotic tissue may have the same macroscopic features (gross appearance) as those of acute cell swelling, namely, swelling and pallor. With time, necrosis becomes more obvious with a loss of structural detail and demarcation from adjacent viable tissue. Zonal necrosis, such as centrilobular hepatic necrosis (see Fig. 8-15) or renal proximal tubular necrosis (see Figs. 11-11 and 11-12), particularly if diffuse rather than segmental or focal, can be indistinguishable in its early stages from reversible degeneration. In contrast, unifocal or multifocal (randomly distributed) necrosis or segmental

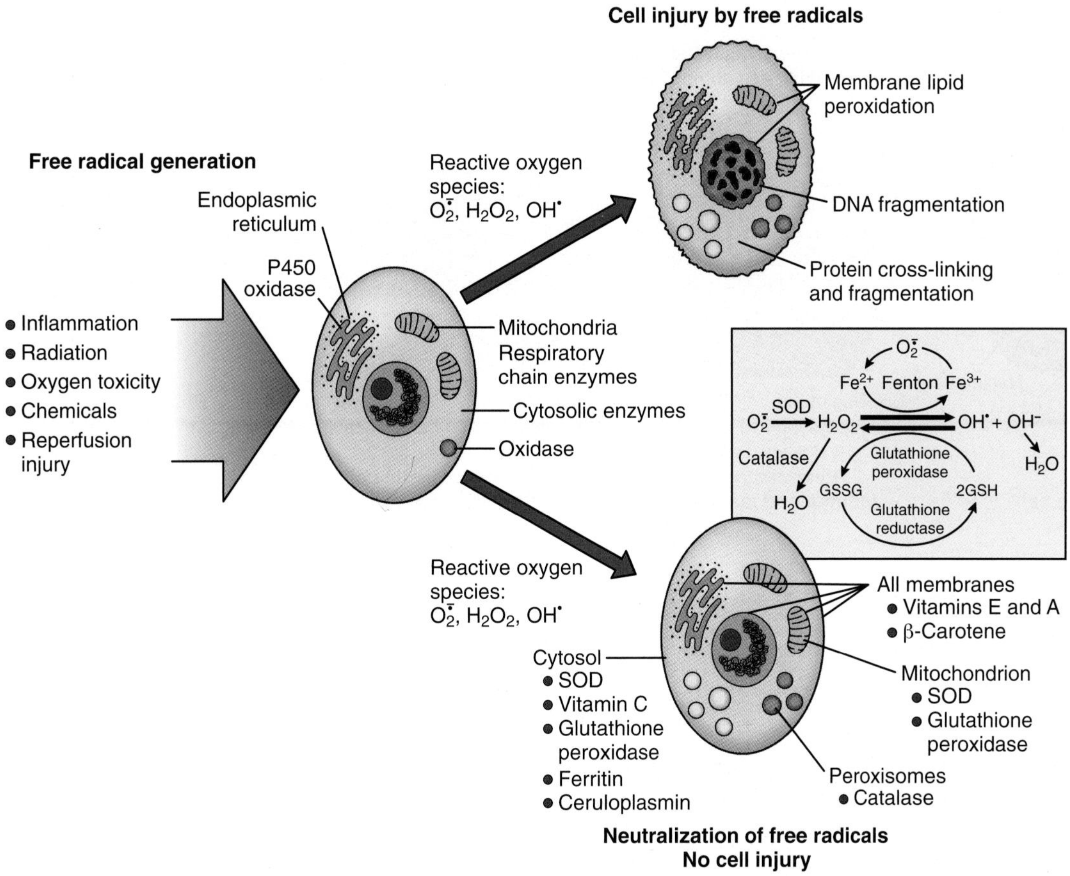

Figure 1-15 **The Role of Reactive Oxygen Species in Cell Injury.** *GSH,* Reduced glutathione; *GSSG,* oxidized glutathione; *SOD,* superoxide dismutase.

zonal necrosis is more easily recognized macroscopically precisely because it differs from adjacent viable tissue. Multifocal hepatic necrosis, for example, is recognizable in part because the necrotic foci differ from surrounding viable tissue and every hepatic lobule is not affected in the same manner. Likewise, segmental laminar cerebrocortical necrosis is recognized because only segments of the cerebral cortex are discolored or changed in texture or structure. An infarct, which is necrosis due to regional loss of blood supply, is recognized because it assumes the shape of the vascular field—rhomboidal in many tissues (e.g., lung or skin) or conical (wedge shaped in two dimensions) with its base at the edge of the spleen (see Fig. 13-64) or cortical surface of the kidney (see Figs. 2-37 and 2-38).

Histologic Changes in Necrosis (Oncotic Necrosis). The light microscopic changes of necrosis (Fig. 1-16) were described in the nineteenth century by Rudolf Virchow. The hallmarks are pyknosis (nuclear condensation with shrinkage and intense basophilia), karyorrhexis (nuclear fragmentation), or karyolysis (nuclear dissolution or loss). Dead cells also tend to have intense cytoplasmic eosinophilia because of the denatured protein and loss of ribosomes, hence loss of basophilia. Later the dead cell may have cytoplasmic pallor and become swollen, rounded, and detached from the basement membrane or from neighboring cells.

Ultrastructure of Necrotic Cells (Oncotic Necrosis). Initially the necrotic cell is swollen, rounded, and detached from adjacent cells and from the basal lamina, in the case of epithelium, or from the ECM, in the case of mesenchymal cells. Chromatin is clumped. The cytosol is electron lucent. Mitochondria are swollen and develop flocculent densities. The ER and the rest of the cytocavitary network swell and fragment into vesicles. Ultimately, cell swelling disrupts membranes, including the plasma membrane, at which point the cell literally explodes then collapses.

Types of Oncotic Necrosis. It can be diagnostically useful, though somewhat arbitrary, to classify necrosis by its morphologic features in tissue sections. This classification depends on the tissue involved, the nature of the injurious agent, and the time elapsed after cell death. Necrosis has been classified traditionally as coagulative, caseous, liquefactive or lytic, and gangrenous. The student should remember that the morphologic appearance of necrotic cells and tissues changes with time. For example, the morphologic features of coagulative necrosis can progress to those of lytic necrosis with liquefaction, particularly in certain tissues or when leukocytes arrive.

Coagulative Necrosis. The term coagulative necrosis refers to the denaturation of cytoplasmic proteins, which at the histologic level imparts an opaque and intense cytoplasmic eosinophilia to necrotic cells. Coagulative necrosis is a typical early response to hypoxia, ischemia, or toxic injury. It appears that the initial injury or the subsequent cellular acidosis denatures not only structural proteins, but also lysosomal enzymes in the affected cell. Normally, lysosomal enzymes would cause proteolytic disintegration of the entire cell, but as a result of this denaturation, proteolytic disintegration of the cell is delayed. However, the degradation of nucleic acids is not hindered. Thus a cell that has undergone coagulative necrosis has the expected nuclear features of cell death by oncosis (i.e., pyknosis, karyorrhexis, or karyolysis), but the cell outlines are still visible histologically (see Fig. 1-16). Coagulative necrosis is most easily recognized in the liver, kidney, myocardium, or skeletal

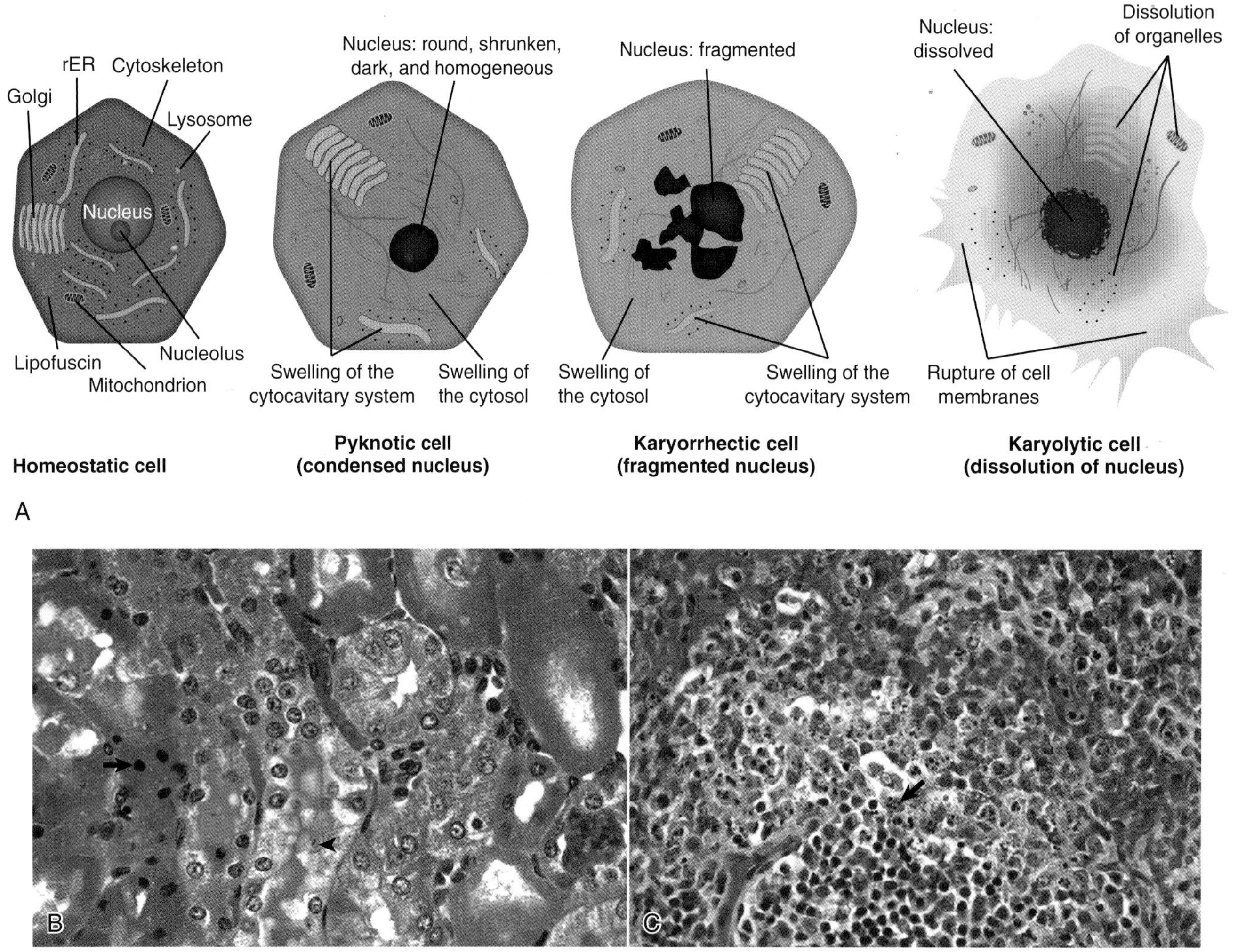

Figure 1-16 **Cytoarchitecture of Cellular Necrosis.** **A**, Schematic representation of nuclear and cytoplasmic changes in the stages of necrosis. *rER*, rough endoplasmic reticulum. **B**, Pyknosis and karyolysis, renal cortex, chloroform toxicosis, mouse. Some tubular epithelial cells have undergone hydropic degeneration; others are necrotic with pyknosis *(arrow)* or karyolysis *(arrowhead)*. H&E stain. **C**, Karyorrhexis, lymphocytes, spleen, dog. Necrotic lymphocytes have fragmented nuclei *(arrow)* because of parvovirus infection. H&E stain. (**A** courtesy Dr. M.A. Miller, College of Veterinary Medicine, Purdue University; and Dr. J.F. Zachary, College of Veterinary Medicine, University of Illinois; **B** and **C** courtesy Dr. L.H. Arp.)

muscle, in which the temporary preservation of cell outlines also preserves tissue architecture so that the outlines of hepatic plates, renal tubules, or muscle bundles are visible at the light microscopic level. Neurons also undergo coagulative necrosis before disappearing by lytic necrosis. Grossly, coagulative necrosis appears pale tan to pale gray, often sharply demarcated from the normal color of adjacent viable tissue, and solid (without apparent crumbling, sloughing, liquefaction, or other obvious loss of structure).

Infarction typically begins as coagulative necrosis, especially in tissues such as kidney (Fig. 1-17; E-Fig. 1-2), where scaffolding provided by tubular basement membranes and interstitial fibrous tissue maintains the tissue structure. Initially the tissue with loss of its blood supply is blanched, but within minutes blood enters the infarcted tissue because blood flow either was restored in the obstructed vessel or arrives from collateral circulation (therefore infarcts in organs with a dual blood supply, such as the lung, are typically hemorrhagic) or leaks from veins in unaffected tissue in and adjacent to the damaged tissue. In an end-artery organ, such as the kidney, macrophages remove the blood from acute hemorrhagic infarcts over the course of a few days, and the infarct becomes pale and sharply demarcated by a red rim, attributable to hyperemia, hemorrhage, and acute inflammation, from adjacent renal parenchyma.

Caseous Necrosis. Caseous, from the Latin word for cheese, refers to the curdled or cheeselike gross appearance of this form of necrosis. In comparison to coagulative necrosis, caseous necrosis is an older lesion with complete loss of cellular or tissue architecture (Fig. 1-18). Macroscopically, caseation may appear as crumbled, granular, or laminated yellow-white exudate in the center of a granuloma or a chronic abscess. Histologically, the lysis of leukocytes and parenchymal cells converts the necrotic tissue into a granular to amorphous—cell outlines are not visible—eosinophilic substance with basophilic nuclear debris. Calcification of the necrotic tissue can contribute to the basophilic granular appearance.

Caseous necrosis is prominent in the granulomas of bovine tuberculosis, caused by *Mycobacterium bovis*. *M. bovis* replicates within macrophages, protected by components of its cell wall from destruction by lysosomal enzymes until, with the development of cell-mediated (type IV) hypersensitivity, cytotoxic T lymphocytes destroy the infected macrophages, as well as parenchymal cells of the infected organ (see also Chapters 3, 4, and 5). *Corynebacterium pseudotuberculosis*, the cause of caseous lymphadenitis in sheep and

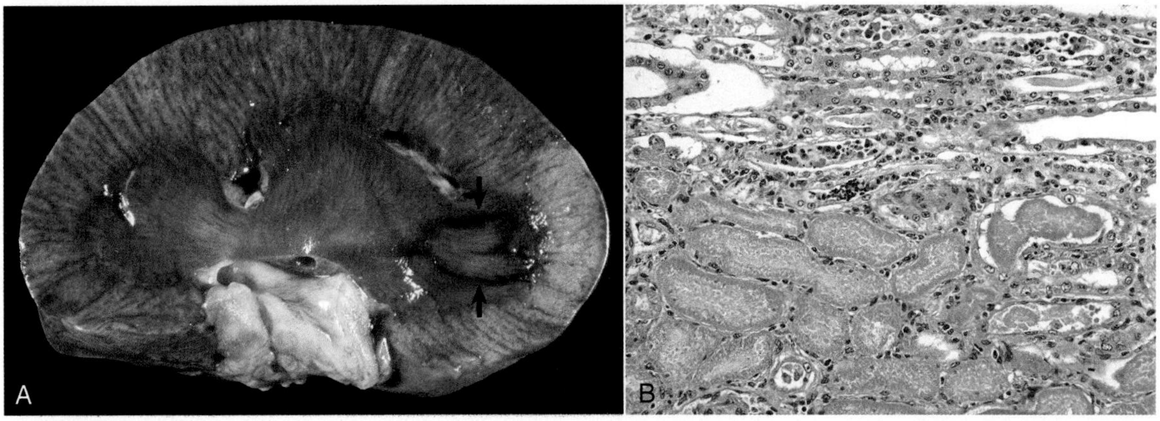

Figure 1-17 **Coagulative Necrosis, Infarct, Kidney, Ox. A,** A pale tan wedge of coagulative necrosis extends from the medulla to the capsular surface of the kidney. The apical (medullary) portion of this renal infarct has a dark red border of reactive hyperemia and inflammation *(arrows)*. **B,** Coagulative necrosis of renal tubular epithelial cells. Necrotic cells *(lower half of figure)* have homogeneous eosinophilic cytoplasm and pyknosis or karyolysis, but faint cell outlines and tubular architecture are retained. H&E stain. (**A** courtesy Dr. M.A. Miller, College of Veterinary Medicine, Purdue University. **B** courtesy Dr. J.F. Zachary, College of Veterinary Medicine, University of Illinois.)

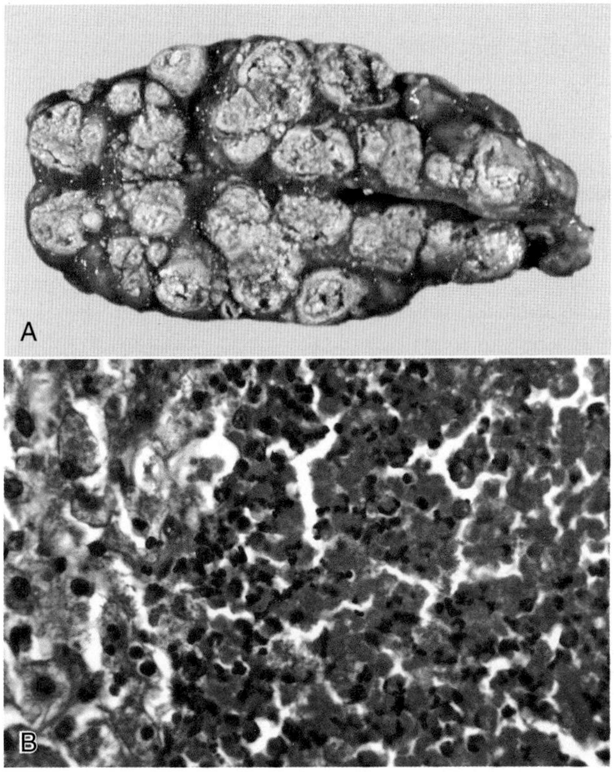

Figure 1-18 **Tuberculosis (Caseous Necrosis), Lymph Node, Transverse Section, Ox. A,** The lymph node contains coalescing caseated granulomas. Caseous necrosis is characterized by off-white, crumbly exudate. **B,** Granulomatous inflammation in caseous necrosis. Cell walls are disrupted, and tissue architecture is lost. Degenerated or lysed leukocytes, including many neutrophils, are at the center *(right)* of a granuloma; note epithelioid macrophages at left. H&E stain. (**A** courtesy Dr. M. Domingo, Autonomous University of Barcelona; and Noah's Arkive, College of Veterinary Medicine, The University of Georgia. **B** courtesy Dr. M.D. McGavin, College of Veterinary Medicine, University of Tennessee.)

goats, is another bacterium that can replicate in phagosomes of macrophages without being destroyed by lysosomal enzymes. The chronic stage of infection results in caseous abscesses in peripheral or internal lymph nodes (caseous lymphadenitis, see also Chapter 13 and Figs. 13-79 and 13-80) or other organs, such as the lungs.

Liquefactive Necrosis. In liquefactive necrosis, cells are lysed, and the necrotic tissue is converted to a fluid phase. This manifestation is typically the final stage of necrosis in parenchyma of the brain (Fig. 1-19; see also Chapter 14) or spinal cord because of the lack of a fibrous interstitium to uphold tissue structure and because cells of the CNS tend to be rich in lipids and lytic enzymes. The term for the macroscopic (gross) appearance of necrosis in the brain and spinal cord is malacia. Neurons are generally the cells most susceptible to necrosis, especially from hypoxia or ischemia, and develop (early in the process of cell death) the morphologic features of coagulative necrosis. With time, however, the glial cells also undergo necrosis and liquefaction of the neuropil begins. Initially malacia may merely result in a translucency of affected tissue, but within a few days necrotic tissue undergoes yellowing, softening, or swelling. Liquefaction progresses with arrival of macrophages (gitter cells) to phagocytize the myelin debris and other components of the necrotic tissue. Eventually the parenchymal cells are completely lysed or phagocytized, and all that remains is the vasculature with intervening spaces that are partially filled with lipid- and debris-laden gitter cells. In organs or tissues outside the CNS, liquefactive necrosis is most commonly encountered as part of pyogenic (pus-forming) bacterial infection with suppurative (neutrophil-rich) inflammation (see also Chapter 3) and is observed at the centers of abscesses or other collections of neutrophils.

Gangrenous Necrosis. Gangrene denotes a type of necrosis that tends to develop at the distal aspect of extremities, such as the limbs, tail, or pinnae, or in dependent portions of organs, such as the mammary glands or lung lobes. Gangrene can be designated as wet or dry; these forms are unrelated. If the dependent necrotic tissue is infected by certain bacteria, wet gangrene ensues. If those bacteria are gas forming (e.g., *Clostridium* spp.), then wet gangrene becomes gas gangrene. In the lung, wet gangrene is often a sequel to the lytic necrosis of aspiration pneumonia. The aspirated material could be foreign material (food or medicament) or gastric content (a mixture of ingesta and gastric secretions). Such materials can be caustic in their own right and are also likely to deliver bacteria from the environment or oropharynx into the lung. Staphylococcal infection of the ruminant mammary gland can result in gangrenous mastitis (Fig. 1-20, A; E-Fig. 1-3), a form of wet gangrene. Grossly, tissues with wet gangrene are red-black and wet. Histologically, the lesion of wet gangrene resembles that of liquefactive necrosis but is usually accompanied by more numerous leukocytes, especially neutrophils.

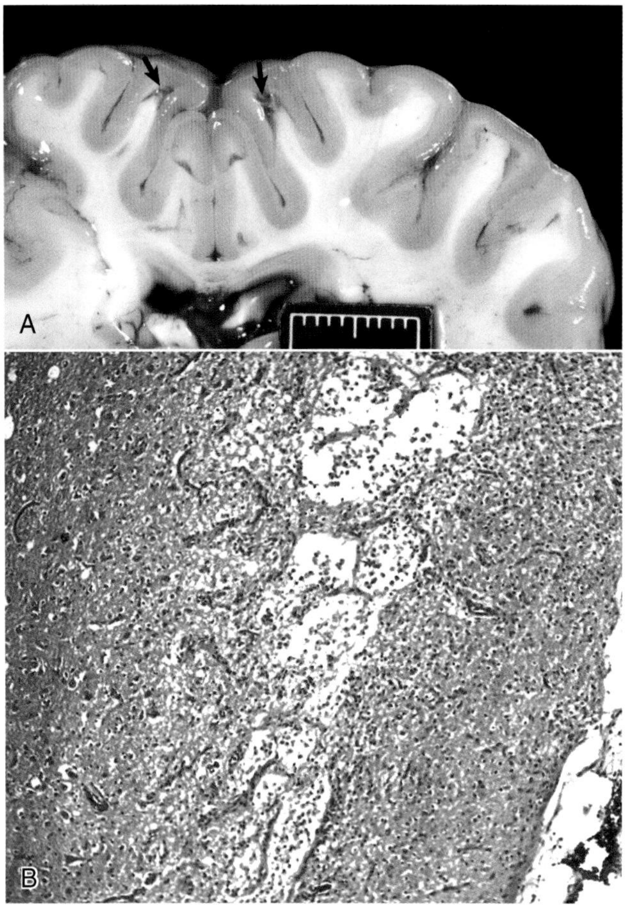

Figure 1-19 **Liquefactive Necrosis. A**, Acute polioencephalomalacia, brain, goat. A thiamine deficiency has resulted in cerebrocortical malacia, which microscopically is liquefactive necrosis with focal tissue separation *(arrows)*. Note yellow discoloration of affected cortex. Scale bar = 2 cm. **B**, Cortical necrosis, cerebrum, dog. The pale zone in deep laminae of the cerebral cortex is an area of *liquefactive necrosis* with loss of parenchyma. All that remains is the vasculature with gitter cells in intervening spaces. H&E stain. (**A** courtesy Dr. R. Storts, College of Veterinary Medicine, Texas A&M University. **B** courtesy Dr. L.H. Arp.)

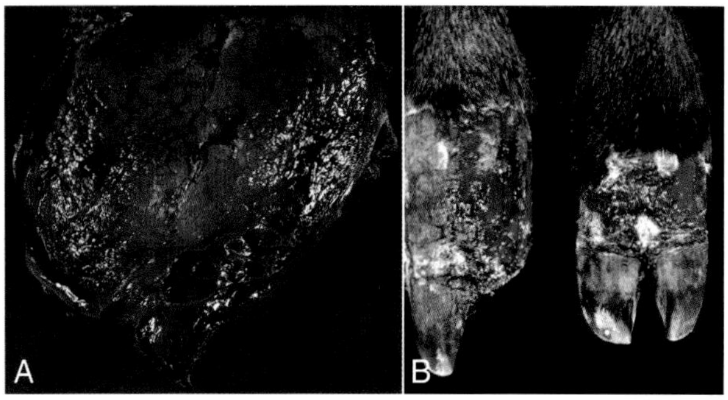

Figure 1-20 **Gangrenous Necrosis. A**, Wet gangrene, mammary gland (longitudinal section through the teat), sheep. Staphylococcal infection caused the gangrenous mastitis in this ewe. Note wet and hemorrhagic necrosis of mammary tissue and overlying skin, especially at the distal (ventral) aspect of the udder. **B**, Dry gangrene, digits, ox. Vasoconstriction from ergot alkaloids produced by endophyte-infected fescue grass caused this ischemic necrosis of the distal aspects of the hind limbs. Note that one of the claws *(left)* has been lost due to the process. (**A** courtesy Dr. M.A. Miller, College of Veterinary Medicine, Purdue University. **B** courtesy Dr. R.K. Myers, College of Veterinary Medicine, Iowa State University.)

Dry gangrene is the result of decreased vascular perfusion and/or loss of blood supply. It is a form of infarction resulting in coagulative necrosis that imparts a dry, leathery texture to the necrotic tissue, providing that it remains free of putrefactive bacteria. Arterial thrombosis (e.g., "saddle thrombus" formation at the iliac bifurcation of the aorta in cats) and frostbite are causes of dry gangrene of extremities. Dry gangrene is also the lesion of "fescue foot" in cattle (see Fig. 1-20, *B*), caused by the vasoconstrictive effect of the ergot alkaloids produced by endophyte-infected fescue grass.

Necrosis of Epithelium. Necrosis that develops in epithelial surfaces (e.g., epidermis or corneal epithelium) or epithelial linings (e.g., mucosal epithelium of the respiratory, digestive, or reproductive tracts) causes exfoliation or sloughing of dead cells, resulting in erosion of the epithelium, or, with full-thickness necrosis, in ulceration. Trauma, certain microbes (e.g., herpesviruses), and loss of blood supply are among the many causes of epithelial necrosis.

Necrosis of Adipose Tissue (Fat Necrosis). Fat necrosis can be classified etiologically as nutritional, enzymatic, traumatic, and idiopathic (see also Chapter 7). Nutritional fat necrosis, also known as steatitis or yellow fat disease, is usually the result of feeding a diet high in unsaturated fatty acids and low in vitamin E or other antioxidants, setting the stage for ROS production and lipid peroxidation. Yellow fat disease is often seen in carnivores, such as cats or mink, on a fish-based diet. Affected adipose tissue is firm, nodular, and yellow-brown.

Enzymatic necrosis of fat is seen mainly in peripancreatic adipose tissue, where it is attributed to release of lipases from necrotic pancreatic acinar cells (Fig. 1-21; see Figs. 8-88 and 8-89). Grossly, necrotic adipose tissue becomes firm and nodular with off-white chalky deposits, the result of saponification (soap formation). Microscopically, fat necrosis elicits inflammation that consists mainly of lipid-laden macrophages and variable number of neutrophils. Lipids are removed by solvents during histologic processing, so the cytoplasm of normal adipocytes is not stained, whereas necrotic adipocytes tend to have pale eosinophilic to amphophilic cytoplasm with scattered intensely basophilic soap deposits.

Traumatic fat necrosis is typically the result of blunt trauma or chronic pressure on adipose tissue against bony prominences, such as the subcutaneous adipose tissue compressed against the sternum in recumbent cattle. Ischemia is thought to contribute to the cell injury. Inflammation and saponification are inconspicuous in this form of fat necrosis.

Necrosis of abdominal fat in cattle is an example of idiopathic fat necrosis. This lesion tends to develop in the abundant adipose tissue of the mesentery and retroperitoneal tissue of overconditioned cows. Some have attributed retroperitoneal fat necrosis to ischemia associated with consumption of endophyte-infected tall fescue grass. Idiopathic fat necrosis is also encountered in the ventral parietal peritoneum of horses and ponies (see Fig. 7-15).

Sequelae to Oncotic Necrosis. Oncotic necrosis elicits an inflammatory reaction in most tissues. In the CNS the inflammatory reaction is slow to develop and consists mainly of an influx of macrophages that become gitter cells. In most other tissues a band of hyperemia (hemorrhage and acute inflammation) encircles the necrotic tissue and brings leukocytes to the site. The neutrophils and macrophages phagocytize and lyse the necrotic tissue, converting coagulative to liquefactive necrosis and hastening (in many cases) the removal of damaged tissue. In other cases, foreign material or bone fragments resist digestion and form a sequestrum. Smaller cavitations left by liquefactive necrosis may heal without scarring, depending on the regenerative capacity of the affected tissue. The liver is an organ with high regenerative capacity and, because of its dual blood supply, is not prone to infarction. In contrast, in renal

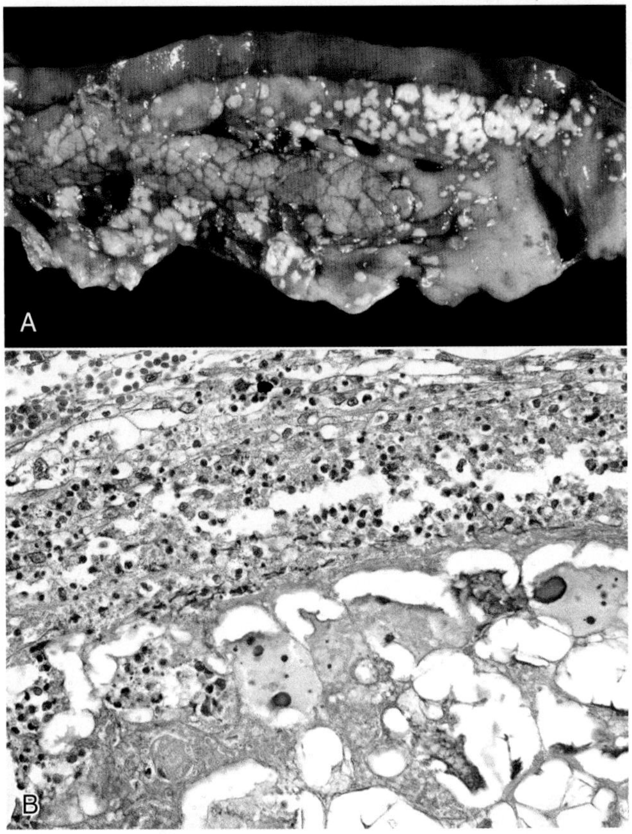

Figure 1-21 Fat Necrosis. **A**, Enzymatic necrosis of fat (fat necrosis); duodenum, pancreas, and peripancreatic adipose tissue, dog. Recurrent bouts of pancreatitis with leakage of lipases and other enzymes causes saponification of necrotic adipose tissue, giving it a chalky, off-white appearance. **B**, Peripancreatic adipose tissue, dog. Note the necrotic adipose tissue *(bottom)* with saponification (basophilic areas) and the border of neutrophils and macrophages *(top)*. H&E stain. (**A** courtesy Dr. J. Wright, College of Veterinary Medicine, North Carolina State University; and Noah's Arkive, College of Veterinary Medicine, The University of Georgia. **B** courtesy Dr. J.F. Zachary, College of Veterinary Medicine, University of Illinois.)

infarcts the lost nephrons are seldom successfully repaired and are usually replaced by a fibrous scar.

Focal epithelial necrosis that results in ulceration can be repaired by hyperplasia of adjacent normal epithelial cells without scarring if the defect is small or shallow and if basal or other progenitor cells remain nearby to fill the gap (i.e., healing in coronavirus or parvovirus infections of the small intestine [see Figs. 4-39 and 7-180]). Adipose tissue, in contrast, is ill equipped to replace necrotic fat lobules because of the low regenerative capacity of adipocytes.

Morphologic Appearance of Postmortem Changes

Information on this topic is available at www.expertconsult.com.

Cell Death by Apoptosis

In contrast to oncotic necrosis, in which the dying cell swells until it literally bursts, apoptotic cell death is a process of condensation and shrinkage. Apoptosis is a form of programmed cell death that is important in embryologic development, homeostasis, and involution of organs or tissues deprived of hormonal stimulation or growth factors. It is also a regulated form of cell death that is directed by signaling pathways in response to certain types of injury.

Triggers of Apoptosis. The triggers of apoptosis include binding of ligands such as TNF to cell surface DRs, various stresses or injury from toxins or ROS, nutrient deprivation or withdrawal of growth factors or hormones, DNA damage, or immune-mediated injury from cytotoxic T lymphocytes or NK cells. Apoptosis (Fig. 1-22) proceeds through an *extrinsic pathway* (initiated by the binding of a ligand to its DR) or an *intrinsic pathway* (initiated in mitochondria in response to various stresses or DNA damage) and almost always entails activation of *caspases*. Caspases are cysteine proteases that cleave peptides after aspartate residues. The initiator caspases that start the process of apoptosis include caspase-8 (activated by the death-inducing signaling complex (DISC) of the extrinsic pathway), caspase-9 (activated with the *apoptosome* in the intrinsic pathway), and caspase-2 (activated by p53 following DNA damage). The initiator caspases activate effector caspase-3, caspase-6, and caspase-7, which then execute apoptosis.

The Extrinsic (Death Receptor–Initiated) Pathway. Extrinsic apoptosis (see Fig. 1-22) begins with ligand-induced trimerization of a cell surface DR. The DRs include Fas, tumor necrosis factor receptor (TNFR) 1, and TNF-related apoptosis-inducing ligand receptor (TRAILR). The next step is internalization and recruitment of the intermediate membrane proteins TNF receptor–associated death domain (TRADD), Fas-associated death domain (FADD), and caspase-8 to form the cytoplasmic DISC. Remember that RIPK1, depending on its ubiquitination status, can associate with the trimerized DR and direct the cell toward regulated necrosis (if caspases are inhibited) or toward survival via activation of NFκB, and has an N-terminal death domain (DD) that links it to the apoptotic pathway through adaptor proteins such as TRADD or FADD. TRADD interacts with FADD, which in turn activates procaspase-8. Sufficient active caspase-8 then activates effector (executioner) caspase-3 and caspase-7 to execute apoptosis. Caspase-8 can also truncate Bid, a proapoptotic Bcl-2 protein, which translocates to mitochondria to trigger intrinsic apoptosis (see the next section). Importantly, the protein FLIP blocks the extrinsic pathway by binding procaspase-8 without activating it. If caspase-8 activity is insufficient, DR-mediated apoptosis can be augmented by mitochondria, almost always through Bcl-2 proteins, such as the proapoptotic Bak (Bcl-2 antagonist/killer) and Bax (Bcl-2–associated X protein). Even cells that cannot initiate or propagate apoptotic signaling can still die, but do so via caspase-independent pathways of cell death, such as regulated necrosis.

The Intrinsic (Mitochondrial) Pathway. The intrinsic or mitochondrial pathway of apoptosis (see Fig. 1-22) does not require ligation of a cell surface DR and can be triggered by a variety of cell stressors or by DNA damage that leads to activation of p53-upregulated modulator of apoptosis (PUMA). The key event of intrinsic apoptosis is mitochondrial outer membrane permeabilization (MOMP). MOMP can be triggered by activation, posttranslational modification, and upregulation of proapoptotic BH3-only proteins (e.g., PUMA protein). The BH3-only proteins usually induce MOMP via oligomerization of Bax and Bak to form channels in the outer mitochondrial membrane. This permeabilization of the outer mitochondrial membrane releases cytochrome *c* from the intermembrane space into the cytosol. Cytochrome *c* promotes the assembly of the *caspase-activating complex* or apoptosome, which consists of caspase-9 plus apoptotic protease activating factor 1 (Apaf-1). MOMP also releases the second mitochondrial activator of caspases (SMAC), as well as the catabolic hydrolases, apoptosis-inducing factor (AIF), and endonuclease G.

Recall from the section on regulated necrosis that opening of the MPT pore is a key event in cell death because it dissipates the proton gradient needed for oxidative phosphorylation. At low concentrations, opening of the MPT pore can induce protective autophagy to

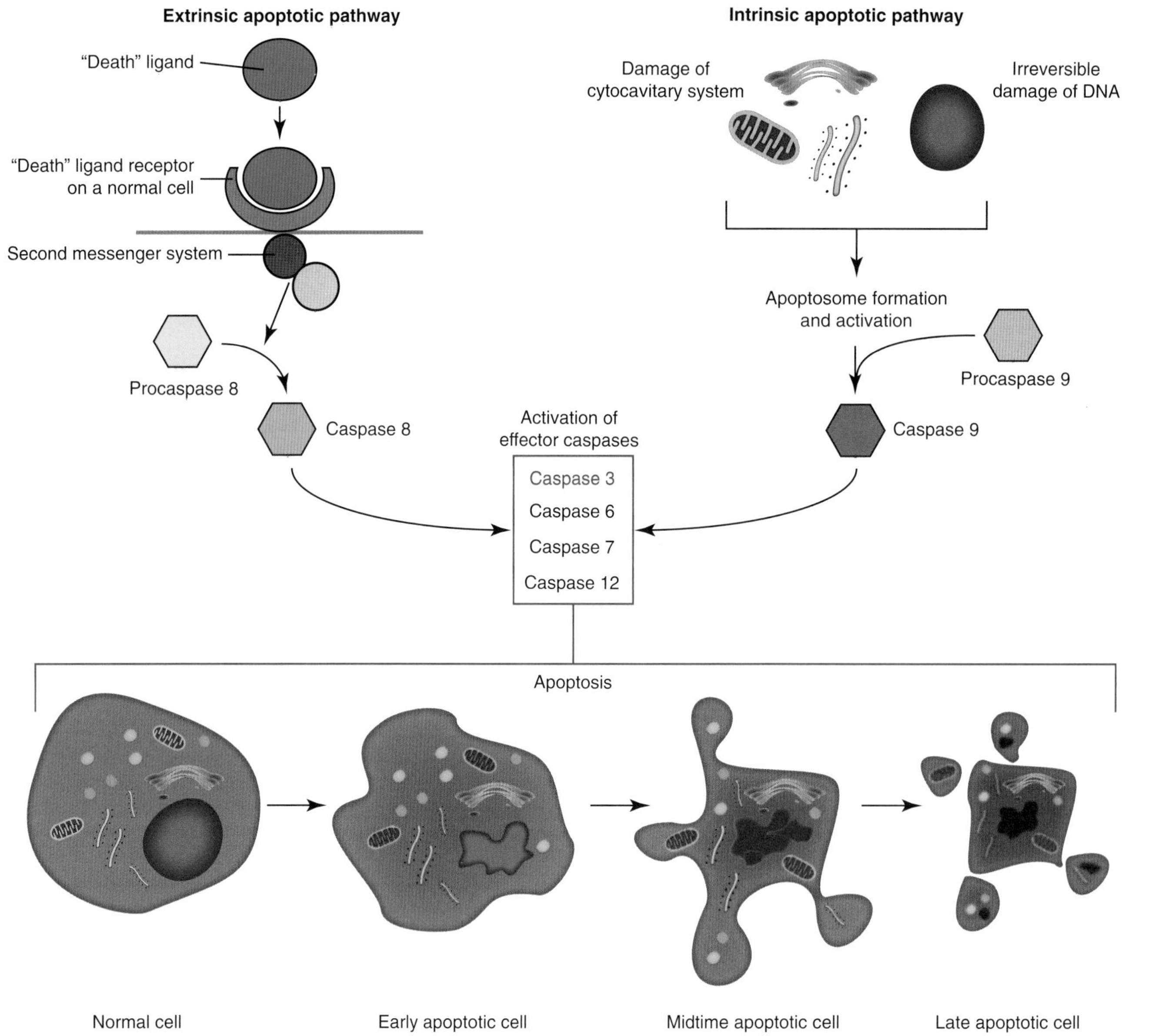

Figure 1-22 Apoptosis. In the extrinsic pathway *(left)*, apoptosis is triggered by binding of a ligand to a cell surface death receptor with subsequent formation of a cytoplasmic death-inducing signaling complex that activates an initiator caspase (e.g., caspase-8). The intrinsic pathway *(right)* of apoptosis is triggered by DNA damage or various cell stressors, especially those that result in permeabilization of the mitochondrial outer membrane, and leads to formation of the caspase-activating complex or apoptosome. The initiator caspase in the intrinsic pathway is usually caspase-9. In both the extrinsic and the intrinsic pathways, initiator caspases activate effector (executioner) caspases, resulting in cell death with the characteristic morphologic features of apoptosis (*shown at bottom*). (Courtesy Dr. M.A. Miller, College of Veterinary Medicine, Purdue University; and Dr. J.F. Zachary, College of Veterinary Medicine, University of Illinois.)

remove dysfunctional mitochondria. However, MOMP is a lethal permeabilization that initiates intrinsic apoptosis.

The Execution Phase of Apoptosis. Initiator caspases (2, 8, 9, or 10) cleave the downstream effector (executioner) caspases (mainly 3, 6, and 7), which then execute apoptosis by cleaving cell proteins after aspartate residues. Granzyme B from cytotoxic T lymphocytes and NK cells can also trigger apoptosis by activating caspase-3 and caspase-7. Effector caspases cleave nuclear and cytoplasmic proteins, leading to disintegration of the nucleus and disruption of the cytoskeleton.

Morphologic Appearance of Apoptosis. Morphologically, apoptotic cell death is a process of condensation and fragmentation of the nucleus (pyknosis and karyorrhexis) with blebbing of the plasma membrane to form membrane-bound apoptotic bodies that contain nuclear fragments, organelles, and condensed cytosol (Fig. 1-23; see Fig. 1-22). The plasma membrane that surrounds apoptotic bodies prevents the inflammation occurring with necrotic cell death but does express factors to attract phagocytes and stimulate heterophagy. Not surprisingly, apoptotic and necrotic cell death can coexist in the same tissue (E-Fig. 1-11).

Chronic Cell Injury and Cell Adaptations

In the previous section we considered reversible injury with acute cell swelling and irreversible injury with cell death. In this section

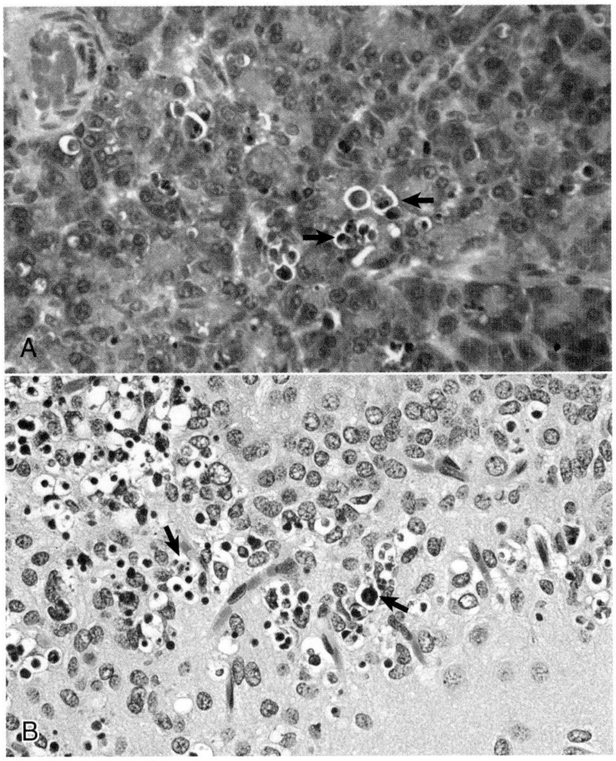

Figure 1-23 Apoptosis, Cytologic Features. A, Pancreas, rat. Individual acinar cells are shrunken, condensed, and fragmented *(arrows)*. Apoptotic bodies are in adjacent cells, but inflammation is absent. H&E stain. **B**, Hippocampus, brain, mouse. Individual neurons are shrunken, condensed, and fragmented *(arrows)*. H&E stain. (**A** courtesy Dr. M.A. Wallig, College of Veterinary Medicine, University of Illinois. **B** courtesy Drs. V.E. Valli and J.F. Zachary, College of Veterinary Medicine, University of Illinois.)

we examine chronic sublethal injury to which the cell may adapt by undergoing hypertrophy (increased cell size because of increase in the number and size of organelles), hyperplasia (increased number of cells due to proliferation of cells capable of mitosis), metaplasia (change in cell type), or dysplasia (development of cellular atypia). Alternatively, cells may undergo degenerative changes such as atrophy (diminished number and size of organelles with decreased cell size and tissue mass) or accumulation of normal or abnormal substances.

Cellular Survival during Sublethal Ischemia or Involution

Autophagy

Autophagy evolved as a cell survival mechanism during ischemia or involution in response to loss of growth factors or hormonal stimuli. In autophagy, cells consume their own damaged organelles, as a housekeeping function, and cytosolic proteins and carbohydrates, as a source of nutrients. Thus autophagy is distinct from heterophagy (Fig. 1-24), in which one cell phagocytizes another cell or parts thereof. Autophagy usually inhibits apoptosis; however, if uncontrolled, it can result in cell death. Autophagy can be categorized as macroautophagy, microautophagy (direct phagocytosis by the lysosome), and chaperone-assisted autophagy. In macroautophagy, portions of cytosol and organelles are enveloped in a double-membrane–bound *autophagosome*, which subsequently fuses with a lysosome to form a single-membrane–bound autophagolysosome.

The autophagy signaling pathway begins with formation of the ULK1 complex, composed of ULK1 (UNC-51–like kinase), FIP 200 (a kinase-interacting protein), and autophagy-related gene products (ATG) 13 and 101. The ULK1 complex drives the formation of the isolation membrane; mammalian target of rapamycin (mTOR), a protein-serine/threonine kinase, complex 1 inhibits the ULK1 complex. The Beclin 1-VPS34 (vacuolar protein sorting 34, a phosphatidylinositol-3 kinase) complex drives nucleation of the isolation membrane or phagophore, usually at the point of contact between mitochondria and ER, though other cell membranes may contribute. Transmembrane ATG9 and VMP1 (vacuolar membrane protein 1) recruit lipids to the isolation membrane. The double-layered isolation membrane wraps around a portion of cytosol with organelles. Two ubiquitin-like (UBL) protein conjugation systems—the ATG12-UBL system and the protein light chain (LC) 3-UBL system—cleave LC3 and catalyze the conjugation of ATG proteins. Finally, soluble NSF (*N*-ethylmaleimide–sensitive fusion protein) attachment protein receptor (SNARE)–like proteins are involved in docking and fusion of the lysosome to the autophagosome. The end result is a single membrane-bound autophagolysosome that contains a portion of the cytosol with dysfunctional organelles. See the later section on Intracellular Accumulations for the histologic appearance of autophagolysosomes.

In general, autophagy provides an escape from cell death by facilitating the removal of effete organelles and unnecessary cell proteins and by providing nutrients to the deprived cell. However, even when the autophagic cell dies (from apoptosis, oncotic necrosis, or uncontrolled autophagy), autophagy protects tissues from unnecessary inflammation by promoting the secretion of lysophosphatidylcholine, a chemotactic factor for phagocytes, and surface expression of phosphatidylserine, which marks the cell for heterophagy.

Adaptations That Change Cell Size, Number, or Appearance

Tissues adapt to chronic injury in positive or negative ways, depending on the nature of the injury and the type of cell (Essential Concept 1-4). Some changes, such as an increase in cell size (hypertrophy) or number (hyperplasia) can increase the function of the organ or tissue at least temporarily and are considered positive adaptations. In other cases, cells shrink (atrophy) and the organ or tissue has diminished function, but this seemingly negative adaptation can have the beneficial effect of avoiding cell death. A change in cell type (metaplasia) generally decreases normal cell function but can offer greater protection to underlying tissues. Dysplastic changes (dysplasia) in cell appearance, on the other hand, have little or no protective effect and can be a precursor to neoplasia. These changes are illustrated in Figure 1-25.

Atrophy

Atrophy is the decrease in the mass of a tissue or organ due to decreased size and/or number of cells after it has reached its normal size (see Fig. 1-25, *B*). Atrophy must be distinguished from hypoplasia, the term applied to tissues or organs that are smaller than normal because they never developed completely. The shrinkage of atrophied tissue is caused by decreased size or loss of its principal cells. The causes of cellular or tissue atrophy include nutrient deprivation or loss of hormonal stimulation, decreased workload (disuse atrophy), denervation (especially in skeletal muscles), and compression (e.g., adjacent to neoplasms, other masses, or distended body cavities). Autophagy and apoptotic cell death can contribute to the shrinkage or loss of cells, respectively, in an atrophied organ. Histologically, the principal cells of the tissue are small with little to no mitotic activity. Ultrastructurally, atrophied cells have few mitochondria or other organelles.

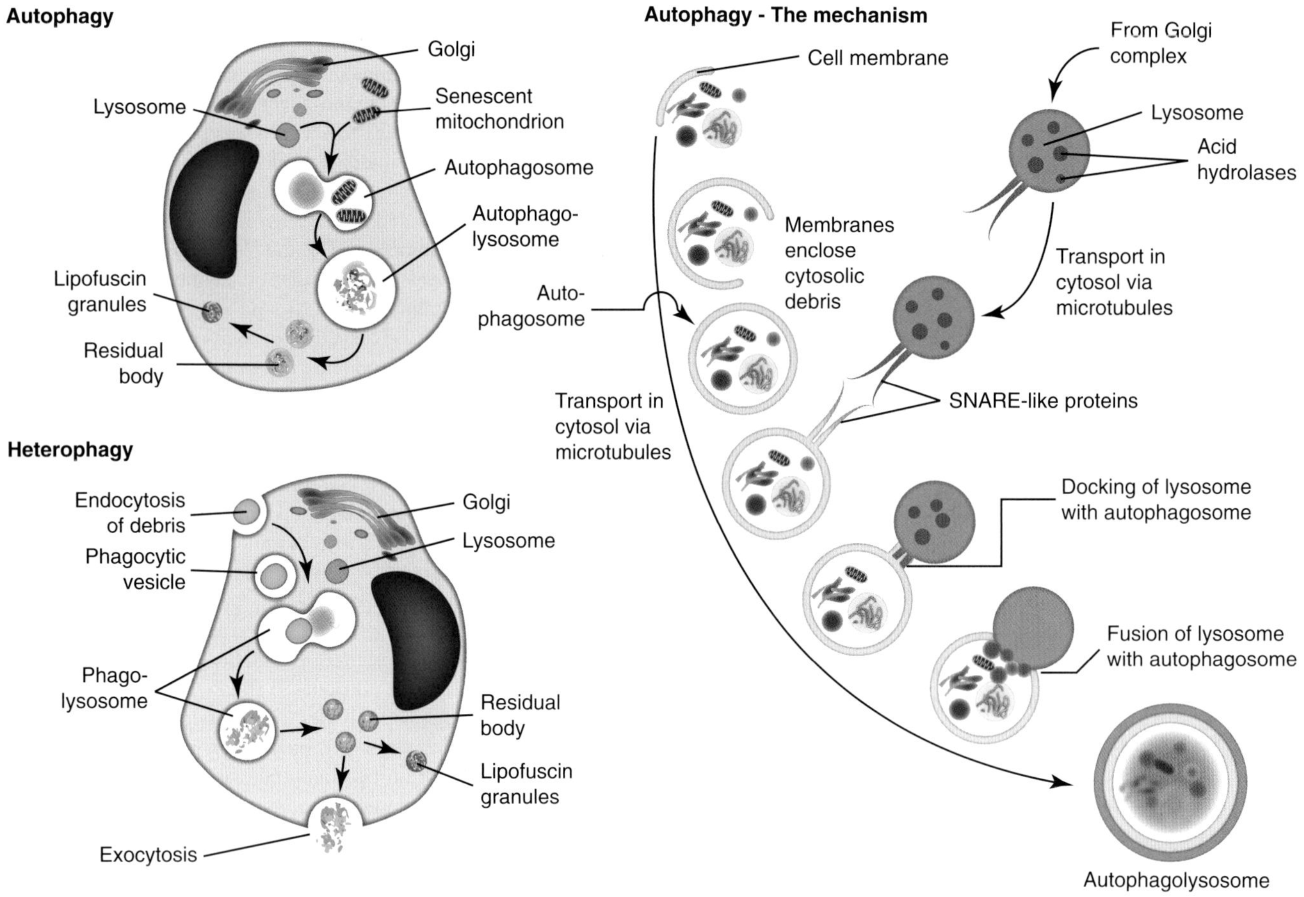

Figure 1-24 **Autophagy and Heterophagy.** Schematic comparison of autophagy *(top left)* and heterophagy *(lower left)*. The mechanism of autophagy is also illustrated. *SNARE*, Soluble NSF (*N*-ethylmaleimide–sensitive fusion protein) attachment protein receptor. (Courtesy Dr. M.A. Miller, College of Veterinary Medicine, Purdue University; and Dr. J.F. Zachary, College of Veterinary Medicine, University of Illinois.)

ESSENTIAL CONCEPT 1-4 Adaptations to Chronic Cell Injury

In the case of repetitive or continuous injury that is not inherently or immediately lethal, cells of many different types can survive, even without complete recovery, by adapting. Depending on the cell type—not all cells are capable of all possible responses—cellular adaptations to chronic injury include the following:

1. Hypertrophy, an increase in cell size by virtue of an increase in number and size of organelles
2. Hyperplasia, an increase in cell number that only those cells capable of mitosis can undergo
3. Metaplasia, a change from one differentiated cell type to another of the same germ layer (e.g., from ciliated epithelium to stratified squamous epithelium in the respiratory tract)
4. Dysplasia, abnormal differentiation with features of cellular atypia
5. Atrophy, a decrease in cell size by virtue of a decrease in number and size of organelles
6. Intracellular accumulations of endogenous or exogenous substances

Certain adaptations (e.g., myocardial hypertrophy) can increase the functional capacity of cells or tissues, at least temporarily, but more often cellular adaptations to chronic injury serve as means of protection (for example, keratinized stratified squamous epithelium offers more protection to underlying tissue than does pseudostratified ciliated epithelium) or survival (an alternative to cell death) and result in altered or diminished function of cells or tissues. Dysplasia is an adaptation without apparent advantages to the host. Indeed, dysplasia can be a precursor to malignant neoplasia (cancer).

Atrophy occurs in most organ systems of the animal body (see Pathology of Organ Systems chapters for details). Thyroid atrophy (Fig. 1-26) can be idiopathic or the result of autoimmune destruction of follicular cells (see Chapter 12). Because the portal vein provides most of the blood supply to the liver, a portosystemic shunt results in hepatic atrophy (E-Fig. 1-12; see also Chapter 8, Fig. 8-38). Atrophy can be particularly striking in the thymus, causing a rapid and drastic loss of tissue through apoptosis of lymphocytes. Thymic atrophy is so consistent and often severe in certain viral infections (e.g., canine distemper or canine and feline parvovirus infections) with a predilection for rapidly dividing cells that it serves as a diagnostically useful, but easily overlooked gross lesion (see also Chapter 13). The serous atrophy of fat in starving animals results in diminished volume and a translucent, semifluid to gelatinous appearance to adipose tissue throughout the body, but especially in the coronary groove of the heart (see Fig. 10-59) or in the marrow of long bones.

Hypertrophy

Hypertrophy, from the Greek word for increased growth, refers to an increase in size and volume of a tissue or organ due to increase in cell size (see Fig. 1-25, A). Importantly, the increased tissue mass is due to increased size of the parenchymal cells rather than stromal cells or leukocytes. Hypertrophy often accompanies an increase in cell number (hyperplasia) due to cellular proliferation but as a standalone phenomenon is observed mainly in organs or tissues such as the heart (E-Fig. 1-13; see Chapter 10) or skeletal muscle (see Chapter 15), in which the principal cells are postmitotic and incapable of replication. When the term hypertrophy is applied at the cellular level, it denotes an increase in cell size because of an increase in size or number of organelles as distinguished from increased cell size from hydropic cell swelling (loss of volume control) or from accumulation of endogenous or exogenous substances. Cellular hypertrophy is the process by which postmitotic cells, such as cardiomyocytes or skeletal myocytes, can grow as the juvenile animal grows. It is also the physiologic response of striated muscle to increased workload such as occurs in training of race horses. Smooth muscle cells (e.g., in the tunica media of arteries) also undergo hypertrophy in response to increased workload. Although muscular hypertrophy increases functional capacity in the short term, accompanying changes, such as increased fibrous stroma or decreased vascular perfusion, in myocardium, for example, can lead to decompensation of the affected organ.

Hyperplasia

Hyperplasia implies an increase in number of the principal cells of a tissue or organ (see Fig. 1-25, *A*). This response can occur only in a cell population that is capable of mitosis (see subsequent section on the Cell Cycle). Many epithelial cells (e.g., hepatocytes and epithelia of the epidermis and intestinal mucosae) are quick to undergo hyperplasia in response to hormonal stimulation, inflammation, or physical trauma. Hyperplasia of glandular epithelium (e.g., thyroid follicular epithelium) can be marked, resulting in striking gross enlargement of the thyroid gland (Fig. 1-27). Importantly, hyperplasia differs from neoplastic cellular proliferation in that it generally subsides if the stimulus is removed. Striated muscle and nervous system tissues have negligible capacity to proliferate and in general do not undergo hyperplasia. Other tissues, such as smooth muscle, bone, and cartilage, are intermediate in their ability to proliferate.

Hyperplasia is considered physiologic when it is a response to cyclic hormonal stimulation as in the endometrial or mammary development of pregnancy and lactation, respectively. The hyperplasia of wound healing is not a normal event, but it is an appropriate and compensatory response of fibroblasts and endothelial cells to traumatic injury. Likewise, hyperplastic goiter is not a normal change in the thyroid gland (see Fig. 1-27; see also Chapter 12) but is an appropriate response to generate thyroid hormones in the face of iodine deficiency. Idiopathic (of unknown cause) nodular hyperplasia is encountered rather commonly in certain organs (e.g., liver, pancreas, or spleen), especially in older dogs, and often is of no clinical significance. In contrast, inappropriate elevation of trophic hormones or growth factors can lead to persistent hyperplasia that can be a precursor to neoplastic transformation (see Chapter 6).

Metaplasia

Metaplasia (see Fig. 1-25, *B*) is a change from one differentiated (mature) cell type to another differentiated cell type of the same germline. Typically, squamous metaplasia is a reparative response to chronic inflammation (e.g., in mammary ducts in chronic mastitis), hormonal imbalance (e.g., estrogen-induced squamous metaplasia in the prostate gland; see Fig. 19-26, *C*), vitamin A deficiency (E-Fig. 1-14), or trauma. Although stratified squamous epithelium creates a protective barrier between the irritant and underlying tissue, there are negative consequences. For example, squamous metaplasia of respiratory epithelium in the trachea or bronchi entails a loss of ciliated cells and goblet cells, which are important for mucociliary clearance and resistance to pneumonic diseases.

Dysplasia

Dysplasia (see Fig. 1-25, *B*) implies an abnormality in formation of a tissue. For example, renal dysplasia (see Chapter 11) is the abnormal formation of the kidney; hip dysplasia (see Chapter 16) is the abnormal formation of the coxofemoral joint. When applied to epithelium, dysplasia implies an increase in the number of poorly differentiated or immature cells and can be a precursor to neoplasia (see Chapter 6). Microscopically, dysplastic epithelial cells have atypical features, such as abnormal variation in size (anisocytosis) and shape (poikilocytosis), hyperchromatic nuclei, increased nuclear size (karyomegaly), and increased number of mitotic figures.

Intracellular Accumulations

Injured cells can accumulate endogenous by-products and exogenous substances because of metabolic abnormalities, genetic mutations, or exposure to an indigestible exogenous substance. Some of these accumulations are relatively harmless; others promote cellular degeneration and can lead to death of the cell.

Lipids

Lipidosis (steatosis) is the accumulation of lipids within parenchymal cells. Intracellular lipid accumulation can develop in many organs and tissues, but because the liver is so important in lipid metabolism, hepatic lipidosis is particularly common (see Chapter 8). The causes of hepatic lipidosis (Fig. 1-28) include increased mobilization of free fatty acids, abnormal hepatocellular metabolism (of fatty acids, triglycerides, and apoproteins), and impaired release of lipoproteins. Grossly, hepatic lipidosis results in a swollen, yellowed liver, with a greasy texture (Fig. 1-29, *A*). Severe lipidosis can alter the specific gravity of hepatic parenchyma to the point that slices of liver float in formalin (or water). Histologically, lipid vacuoles (sharply defined and unstained because the lipid is leached by the solvents of histologic processing) distend the hepatocellular cytoplasm and displace the nucleus to the periphery of the cell (see Fig. 1-29, *B*).

Glycogen

In homeostasis, glycogen is stored mainly in hepatocytes and in skeletal muscle cells, though the stores are often depleted in starving or sick animals. In contrast, glycogen accumulation can be excessive in certain metabolic abnormalities in skeletal muscle (see Chapter 15), in various organs or tissues in the rare glycogen storage diseases, and in the liver in diabetes mellitus or canine hyperadrenocorticism (see Chapter 12). The hepatic response to hyperadrenocorticism, called glucocorticoid hepatopathy, imparts a swollen, pale brown, and mottled appearance (Fig. 1-30, *A*). Histologically, hepatocellular vacuoles of glycogen (see Fig. 1-30, *B*) are less sharply defined and more irregularly shaped than the vacuoles of hepatic lipidosis.

The amount of glycogen that can be demonstrated in hepatocytes microscopically is a function of its original concentration, the delay between death and fixation (during which time the glycogen is metabolized), and the fixation procedure. Although alcoholic fixatives have been recommended to preserve glycogen, fixation in 10% neutral buffered formalin at 4° C retains most of the glycogen without the excessive shrinkage and distortion of tissue seen with alcoholic fixatives, and it avoids polarization of the glycogen to one side of the cell. The periodic acid–Schiff (PAS) histochemistry technique can be used to demonstrate glycogen (Fig. 1-31; E-Fig. 1-15). The PAS reaction breaks 1,2-glycol linkages to form aldehydes, which are then revealed by Schiff's reagent. The glycol linkages occur in substances other than glycogen, so the PAS technique is often used with and without diastase pretreatment. Diastase digests glycogen and removes it from the histologic section. Thus, if glycogen is the PAS-positive material, pretreatment with diastase will remove it and render the PAS test negative.

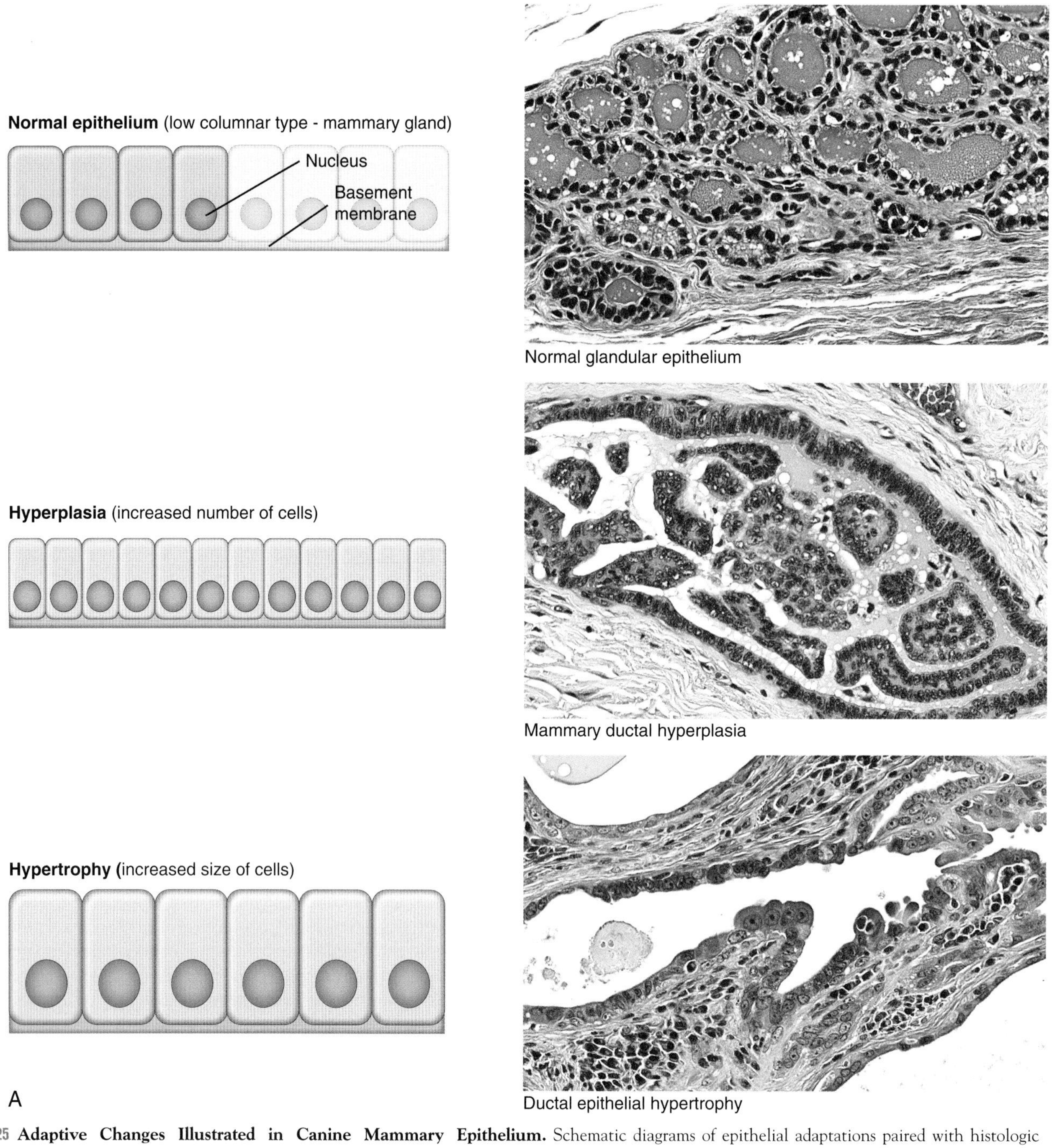

Figure 1-25 Adaptive Changes Illustrated in Canine Mammary Epithelium. Schematic diagrams of epithelial adaptations paired with histologic examples from canine mammary glands. **A**, Normal epithelium, hyperplasia, and hypertrophy.

Proteins

Histologically, proteins are eosinophilic; thus, depending on their biochemical nature (i.e., levels of structural organization [primary through quaternary]), proteins are pink to orange to red in an H&E-stained section.[2] In some diseases, proteins account for the *"hyaline"* appearance observed with H&E stain. The adjective hyaline is used to indicate a homogeneous, eosinophilic, and translucent appearance to a cellular or extracellular substance. Abnormal accumulations of intracellular hyaline proteins occur in various diseases. The protein resorption vesicles in the apical cytoplasm of proximal renal tubular epithelial cells in protein-losing nephropathy (see Chapter 11) appear as hyaline droplets (Fig. 1-32, *A*). Hyaline accumulations may also be a normal finding in specific types of cells (e.g., the globular Russell bodies [immunoglobulin-containing protein in distended rER] of plasma cells).

Defects in Protein Folding. After ribosomal synthesis, emerging proteins are moved into the ER lumen for folding and addition of disulfide bonds before translocation and packaging by the Golgi complex for secretion. Thus the ER is well developed in cells, such as hepatocytes, plasma cells, and pancreatic β cells that synthesize proteins for systemic export. Proteins can be folded into globular

[2]As a general rule in an H&E stain, hematoxylin dyes stain nucleic acids blue, and eosin dyes stain proteins red.

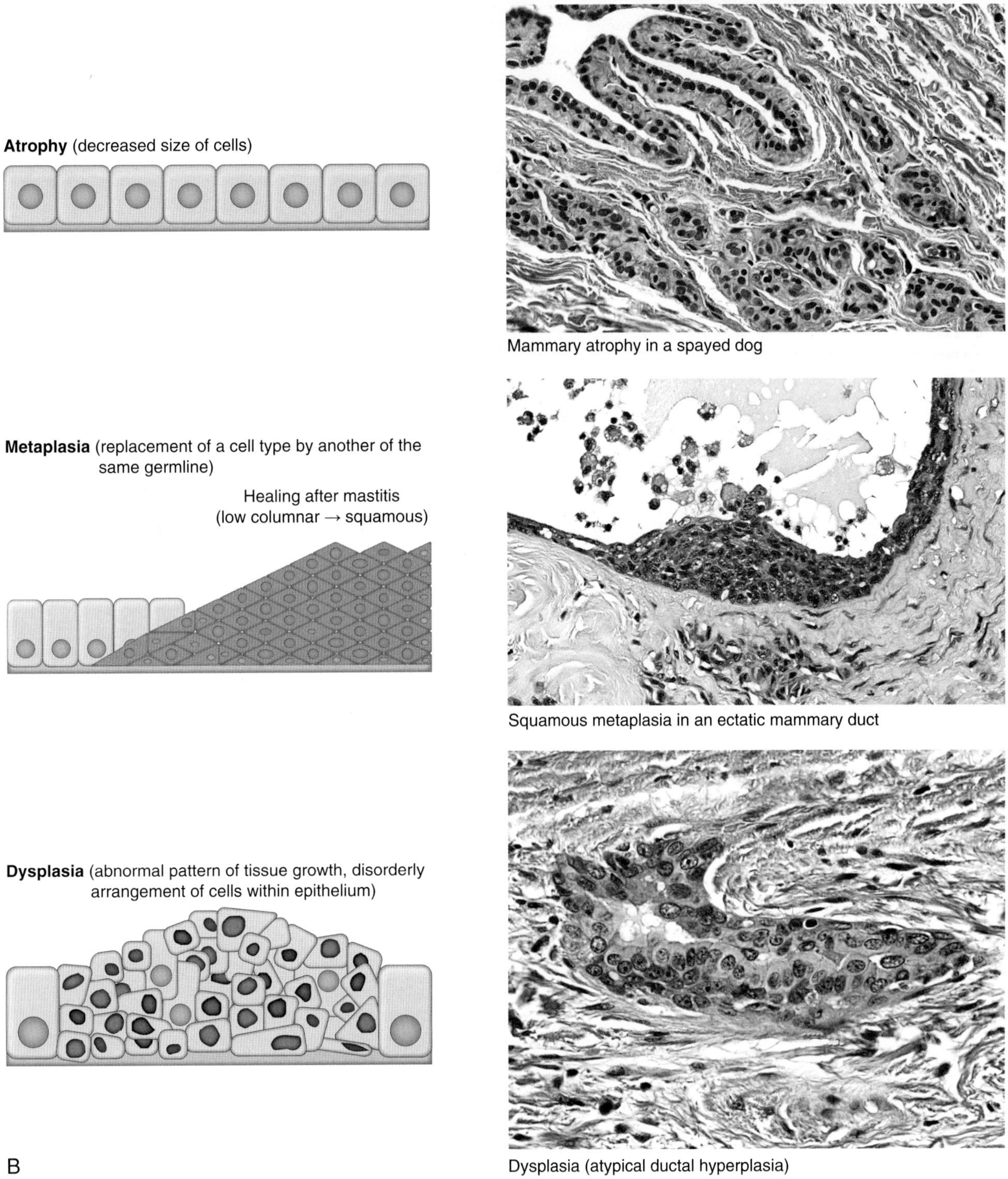

Figure 1-25, cont'd B, Atrophy, metaplasia, and dysplasia. H&E stain. (Courtesy Dr. M.A. Miller, College of Veterinary Medicine, Purdue University; and Dr. J.F. Zachary, College of Veterinary Medicine, University of Illinois.)

(e.g., myoglobin) conformation or exist in a relatively unfolded or disordered state (Fig. 1-33). Nevertheless, normal protein function requires correct three-dimensional conformation (i.e., correct folding in the ER and Golgi complex). Protein homeostasis is aided by molecular chaperones that foster the soluble and functional state of proteins, escort proteins to their site of action, assist in protein folding, target misfolded peptides for refolding or degradation, and generally protect against pathologic protein aggregation.

Hepatocytes, plasma cells, pancreatic islet cells, and other "professional" secretory cells have a sophisticated system that responds to the presence of unfolded proteins. Protein folding disorders develop when an ineffective response to unfolded proteins occurs in these cells. Unfolded proteins can result in "loss-of-function disorders"[3] and are usually managed and resolved by ubiquitination and degradation in a proteasome. In these "resolved"

[3]If a protein is not properly formed (folded), it is not able to complete its assigned function, and thus the outcome is called a "loss-of-function disorder."

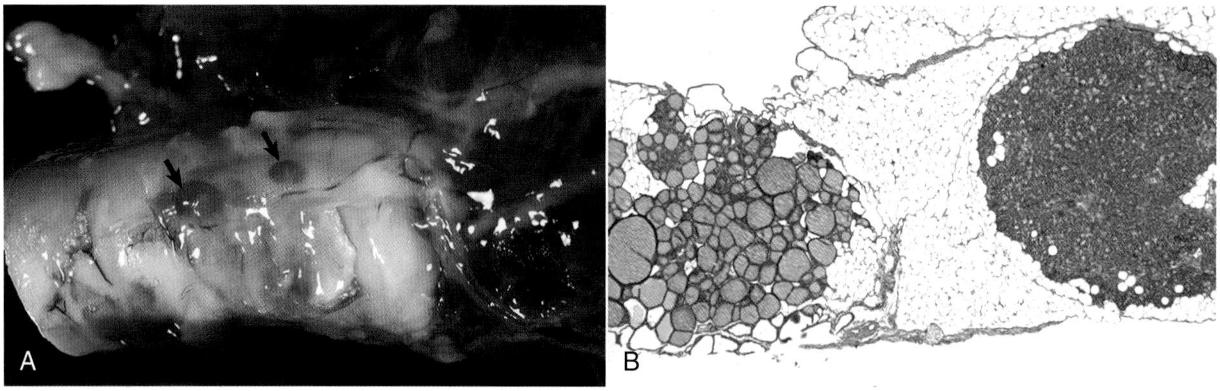

Figure 1-26 **Atrophy, Thyroid Gland, Trachea, Dog. A**, The thyroid gland is thin, translucent, and barely discernable. Note grossly normal parathyroid glands *(arrows)*. **B**, The atrophied thyroid follicles vary in size and colloid content but generally have a relative increase in luminal diameter and decrease in follicular epithelial height. Much of the supporting stroma has been replaced by adipose tissue. The parathyroid gland *(right)* is of normal size. H&E stain. (**A** courtesy Dr. W. Crowell, College of Veterinary Medicine, The University of Georgia; and Noah's Arkive, College of Veterinary Medicine, The University of Georgia. **B** courtesy College of Veterinary Medicine, University of Illinois.)

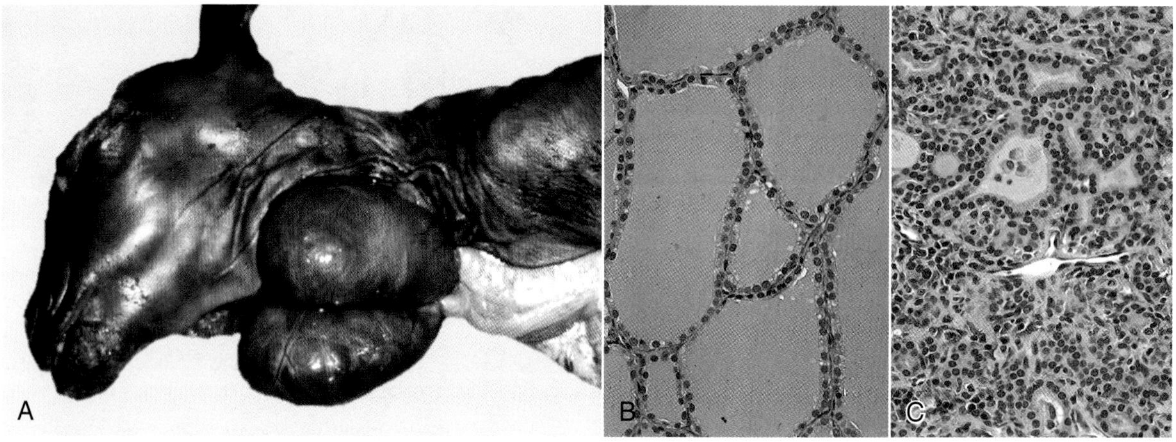

Figure 1-27 **Hyperplasia, Thyroid Gland, Goat. A**, Maternal iodine deficiency caused hyperplasia (and hypertrophy) of thyroid follicular epithelial cells in this neonatal goat, resulting in massive enlargement (goiter) of both lobes. **B**, Follicular epithelial cells from a normal thyroid gland. H&E stain. **C**, Thyroid follicular epithelial cells from a case of goiter. Note the increased number (and size) of the follicular epithelial cells. H&E stain. (**A** courtesy Dr. O. Hedstrom, College of Veterinary Medicine, Oregon State University; and Noah's Arkive, College of Veterinary Medicine, The University of Georgia. **B** and **C** courtesy Dr. B. Harmon, College of Veterinary Medicine, The University of Georgia; and Noah's Arkive, College of Veterinary Medicine, The University of Georgia.)

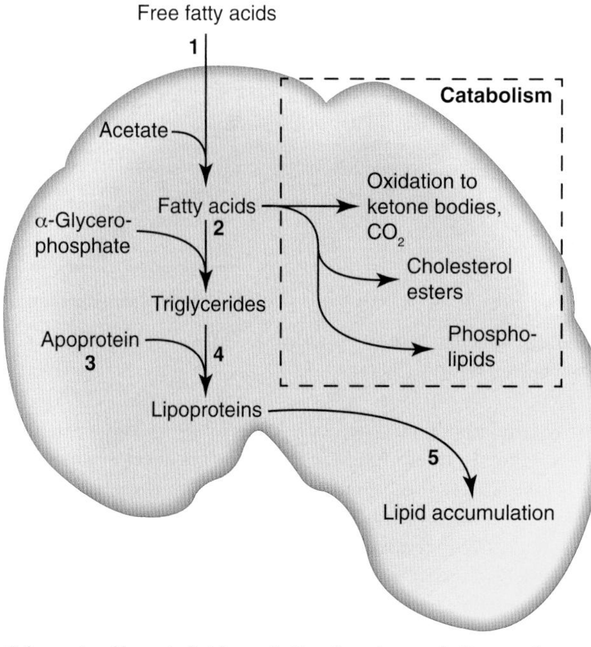

Figure 1-28 **Hepatic Steatosis (Lipidosis).** Schematic of hepatic lipid metabolism (uptake, catabolism, and secretion) and possible mechanisms resulting in lipid accumulation. *1*, Excessive delivery of free fatty acids (FFAs) from fat stores or diet. *2*, Decreased oxidation or use of FFAs. *3*, Impaired synthesis of apoprotein. *4*, Impaired combination of protein and triglycerides to form lipoproteins. *5*, Impaired release of lipoproteins from hepatocytes. (Courtesy Dr. M.A. Miller, College of Veterinary Medicine, Purdue University; and Dr. J.F. Zachary, College of Veterinary Medicine, University of Illinois.)

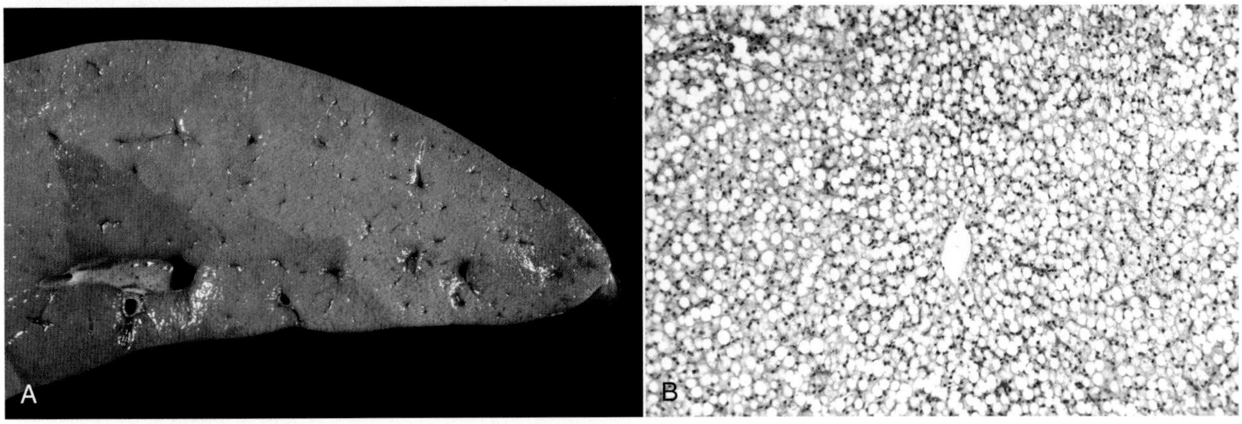

Figure 1-29 **Steatosis (Fatty Liver, Fatty Change, Hepatic Lipidosis), Liver, Ox. A**, Note the uniformly pale yellow-tan color. The liver is enlarged with rounded edges, bulges on incision, and may feel greasy. **B**, In this severely affected liver, all hepatocytes contain unstained, sharply defined cytoplasmic lipid vacuoles that displace the nucleus to the periphery of the cell. H&E stain. (Courtesy Dr. M.D. McGavin, College of Veterinary Medicine, University of Tennessee.)

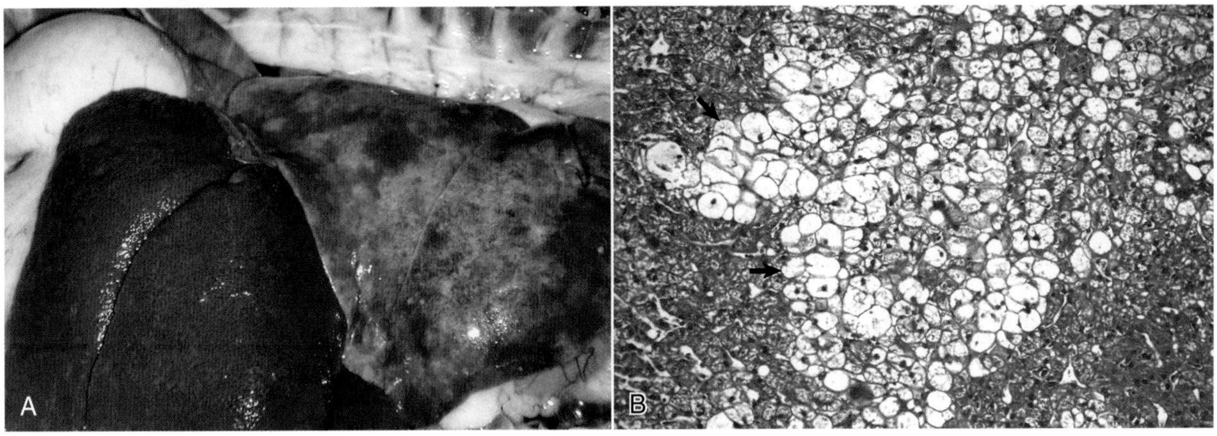

Figure 1-30 **Glucocorticoid Hepatopathy, Liver, Dog. A**, Extensive hepatocellular accumulation of glycogen leads to an enlarged and pale brown liver in dogs with glucocorticoid excess from endogenous or exogenous sources. **B**, Note the swollen hepatocytes *(arrows)* with extensive cytoplasmic vacuolation. H&E stain. (**A** courtesy Dr. K. Bailey, College of Veterinary Medicine, University of Illinois. **B** courtesy Dr. J.M. Cullen, College of Veterinary Medicine, North Carolina State University.)

situations, there is no accumulation of protein. However, certain protein-folding disorders result in intracellular accumulation or extracellular deposition (see the later section on Extracellular Accumulations) of relatively insoluble proteins, some of which, such as amyloid, are toxic to cells or tissues (see Fig. 1-33).

Other Intracellular Inclusions

Autophagic Vacuoles. Autophagy is a common response to sublethal cellular injury in which cell membranes are wrapped around portions of the cytoplasm to form an *autophagosome*. At the ultrastructural level, an autophagosome appears as a double-membrane–bound vesicle with a portion of cytosol and an organelle (e.g., mitochondrion) inside. At the light microscopic level, the autophagosome is an eosinophilic cytoplasmic inclusion. Subsequent fusion with a lysosome leads to at least partial digestion of the autophagolysosome. Residual material may be extruded from the cell or remain as lipofuscin (see later discussion of pigments).

Crystalline Protein Inclusions. Rhomboidal crystalline protein inclusions, also known as crystalloids (see Fig. 1-32, *B*), are common in hepatocytes and renal tubular epithelial cells of older dogs. Their significance, other than as a marker of aging, is unknown.

Viral Inclusion Bodies. Some types of viruses produce characteristic intranuclear or cytoplasmic inclusion bodies. Certain DNA viruses (e.g., herpesviruses, adenoviruses, and parvoviruses) exclusively produce intranuclear inclusions that are round to oval and vary from eosinophilic to basophilic or amphophilic. Other DNA viruses (e.g., poxviruses) produce large eosinophilic cytoplasmic inclusion bodies. The inclusion bodies of RNA viruses (e.g., rabies virus and canine distemper virus) are eosinophilic and cytoplasmic. The viral inclusions of rabies, called Negri bodies, are in the cytoplasm of neuronal soma. Canine distemper virus produces both cytoplasmic and intranuclear inclusions (see Fig. 1-32, C). The intranuclear location of inclusions in this RNA viral infection has been attributed to heat shock proteins.

Lead Inclusions. In some cases of lead poisoning, intranuclear inclusions develop in renal tubular epithelial cells. The inclusions are a mixture of lead and protein and are more easily

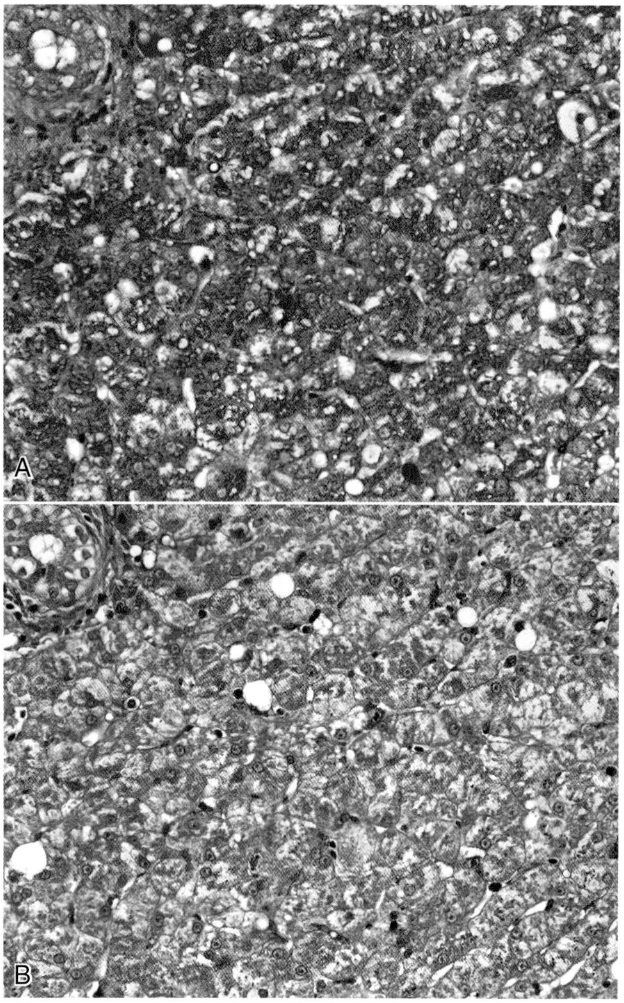

Figure 1-31 **Glycogen Accumulation, Liver, Dog. A**, Glycogen, accumulated in the cytoplasm of hepatocytes, appears as magenta granules with the periodic acid–Schiff technique. **B**, Hepatocellular glycogen was removed from the histologic section by pretreatment with diastase before application of the periodic acid–Schiff technique. (Courtesy Dr. M.A. Miller, College of Veterinary Medicine, Purdue University.)

observed with acid-fast stains than in H&E-stained sections (see Fig. 1-32, *D*).

Extracellular Accumulations

Hyaline Substances

Proteins account for the "*hyaline*" appearance in H&E-stained sections. Proteins are eosinophilic (i.e., have affinity for the eosin dye of the H&E stain). The word hyaline is used for intracellular (see previous section) or extracellular proteinaceous substances that take up eosin dye homogeneously. A variety of extracellular proteinaceous accumulations have a hyaline appearance in histologic sections. Examples include protein casts (albumin, hemoglobin, or myoglobin) in the lumen of renal tubules; serum or plasma in blood vessels; plasma proteins in vessel walls; collagen fibers in some scars or collagen fibers encrusted with proteins from degranulated eosinophils; thickened basement membranes; the "hyaline membranes" of diffuse alveolar damage in acute respiratory distress syndrome (see Chapter 9); fibrin thrombi in the microvasculature in disseminated intravascular coagulation (see Chapter 2); and amyloid (described next).

Amyloid. Increasingly diseases are recognized to be the result of misfolding of soluble and functional peptides or proteins, converting them into relatively insoluble and nonfunctional aggregates. Amyloidosis is one of the best-studied protein-misfolding disorders. Aggregated proteins can be rather amorphous ultrastructurally; however, in the case of amyloidosis, the misfolded and aggregated proteins have a characteristic highly organized fibrillar structure, even though their amino acid sequence varies. Thus amyloidosis is a biochemically diverse group of disorders that have a common pathogenesis (protein misfolding) and generic morphologic appearance. Not only is the biologic function of the misfolded protein generally lost, but the tissue in which amyloid is deposited may be damaged as well.

The mechanisms of amyloidosis (see Fig. 1-33) include (1) propagation of misfolded proteins that serve as a template for self-replication (e.g., prion diseases), (2) accumulation of misfolded precursor proteins due to failure to degrade them, (3) genetic mutations that promote misfolding of precursor proteins, (4) protein overproduction because of an abnormality or proliferation in the synthesizing cell (e.g., plasma cell dyscrasia or neoplasia), and (5) loss of chaperoning molecules or other essential components of the protein assembly process. Amyloid is typically formed from unfolded or partially unfolded proteins or peptide fragments and has a highly ordered, generic (independent of amino acid sequence) structure of fibrillar polypeptide chains that are rich in cross β-sheets (arranged perpendicular to the axis of the fibrils) and can self-replicate by virtue of this template formation. Amyloidosis was recognized as a disease by Virchow, who dubbed the offending material amyloid (starchlike) because the tissue deposits were stained with iodine. Iodine is still used on occasion as a gross technique to stain amyloid (see Fig. 11-40), even though amyloid deposits consist mainly of protein (typically associated with other molecules, such as carbohydrate moieties). If visible macroscopically, amyloid appears as yellow, waxy, coalescing nodular or amorphous deposits (Fig. 1-34). At the light microscopic level, amyloid is homogeneous to indistinctly fibrillar, and pale eosinophilic (Fig. 1-35, *A*). With the Congo red stain, amyloid takes a more orange-red hue (i.e., congophilia) (see Fig. 1-35, *B*). Because of its molecular periodicity, amyloid is anisotropic. Anisotropic substances are birefringent (i.e., they can refract polarized light into two rays that vibrate in perpendicular waves). Thus, when histologic sections are viewed through the microscope with polarized light (achieved by inserting a polarizing filter between the light source and the histologic section), amyloid deposits or other anisotropic substances (e.g., crystals, collagen) can rotate the plane of light so that it passes through the analyzer (a second polarizing filter between the histologic section and the oculars), whereas negligible light is passed through isotropic substances (most of the rest of the section). Amyloid has characteristic apple-green birefringence in polarized light, especially with the Congo red stain (see Fig. 1-35, C). Ultrastructurally amyloid appears as extracellular bundles of nonbranching filaments that are 7 to 10 nm in diameter.

Classification and Localization of Amyloidosis. Amyloid can be classified by the biochemical identity of its precursor peptide or protein. AL amyloid consists of immunoglobulin light chains derived from plasma cells. In light chain (AL) amyloidosis, abnormal plasma cells secrete the light chain fragments into the circulation, and the amyloid can be deposited almost anywhere in the body. Amyloidosis is considered primary when dyscrasias or neoplastic proliferations of plasma cells (see also Chapter 5) are the source of the amyloid. AL amyloidosis can be systemic, but in some extramedullary (e.g., cutaneous) plasmacytomas, amyloid deposition is limited to the stroma of the neoplasm. The localized deposits in nasal amyloidosis of

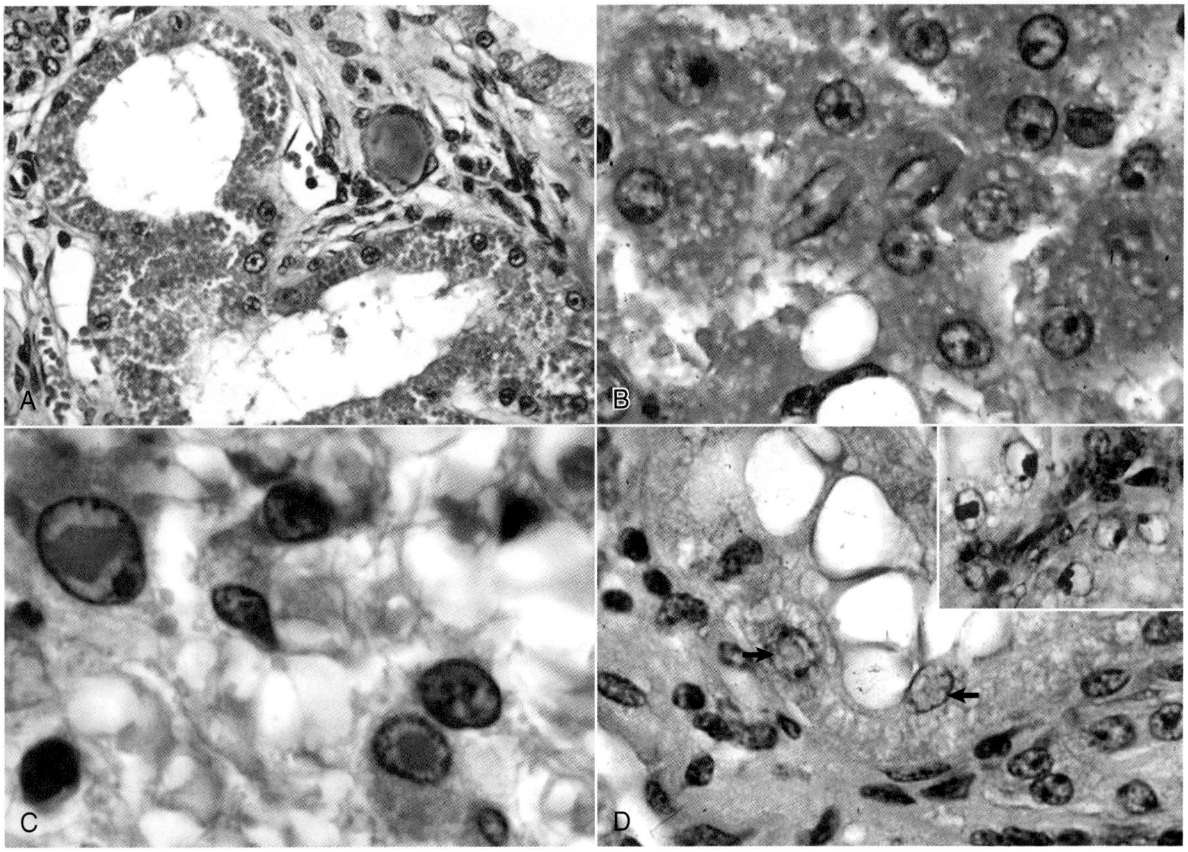

Figure 1-32 **Cell Droplets and Inclusion Bodies.** **A**, Protein resorption droplets, kidney, dog. The cytoplasm of proximal tubular epithelial cells is filled with eosinophilic droplets—protein that has been resorbed by the cells from the glomerular filtrate. H&E stain. **B**, Crystalloids, hepatocytes, dog. Note the elongated eosinophilic crystalline inclusions in the nucleus of two hepatocytes. **C**, Viral inclusion bodies, canine distemper, brain, dog. Note the intranuclear eosinophilic inclusion bodies in astrocytes. H&E stain. **D**, Lead inclusion bodies, kidney, dog. The intranuclear inclusions *(arrows)* in renal tubular epithelial cells are difficult to see with an H&E stain. *Inset,* The lead inclusion bodies are acid-fast *(red)* and easily observed with Ziehl-Neelsen stain. (**A** and **C** courtesy Dr. M.D. McGavin, College of Veterinary Medicine, University of Tennessee. **B** courtesy Dr. D.D. Harrington, College of Veterinary Medicine, Purdue University; and Noah's Arkive, College of Veterinary Medicine, The University of Georgia. **D** courtesy Dr. W. Crowell, College of Veterinary Medicine, The University of Georgia; and Noah's Arkive, College of Veterinary Medicine, The University of Georgia. Inset courtesy Dr. W. Crowell, College of Veterinary Medicine, The University of Georgia; and Noah's Arkive, College of Veterinary Medicine, The University of Georgia.)

horses (see Fig. 1-35) consist of AL amyloid. The conjunctiva (see Fig. 1-34) and skin are also affected in some horses with nasal AL amyloidosis. AL amyloid retains its congophilia and apple-green birefringence after pretreatment with potassium permanganate.

In systemic amyloidosis associated with chronic inflammation, and therefore classified as secondary, serum amyloid A (AA) protein (produced mainly by hepatocytes) is cleaved into fragments that are deposited as amyloid fibrils in various tissues, particularly the kidney (especially renal glomeruli; E-Fig. 1-16; see Chapter 11 and Figs. 11-32, 11-33, and 11-34), liver (especially the space of Disse; see Chapter 8 and Fig. 8-44), and splenic white pulp (see Fig. 13-61). Hereditary or familial forms of AA amyloidosis are also recognized. In Shar-Pei dogs and Abyssinian cats, AA amyloid deposits are typically most abundant in the renal medullary interstitium, rather than in renal glomeruli. Amyloid A is sensitive to potassium permanganate (i.e., congophilia and apple-green birefringence are lost or diminished after potassium permanganate pretreatment).

Amyloid deposits can be systemic (extracellular deposits in multiple organs or tissues, independent of the site of synthesis of the precursor protein) or localized (restricted to tissues in which the precursor protein or peptide is synthesized). Systemic amyloidosis is more likely to be life threatening, depending on the organs or tissues involved and on the volume of amyloid deposits. Thus diffuse and severe renal glomerular amyloidosis results in a protein-losing nephropathy (see Chapter 11).

In contrast to systemic amyloidosis, the severity of disease in localized amyloidosis may depend more on the biochemical nature of the amyloid fibrils. In fact, the precursor peptides or intermediate oligomers, rather than the mature amyloid fibrils, are thought to be the injurious agent at least in some forms of localized amyloidosis. The amyloid deposited in pancreatic islets of cats and human beings is derived from islet amyloid peptide and is secreted by the β cells. It can be associated with insulin-resistant (type 2) diabetes mellitus, but islet amyloidosis is also encountered in cats with normal glucose tolerance (see Chapter 12). Another example of localized amyloidosis is the accumulation of β-amyloid (Aβ) in the cerebral cortex of aged dogs with canine cognitive disorder and in human beings with Alzheimer's disease.

Other Extracellular Accumulations

Fibrinoid Change. Fibrinoid change is the result of leakage of plasma proteins, such as immunoglobulin, complement, or fibrin, into the wall of a blood vessel. This lesion is observed in septic or immune-mediated vasculitis. Injury, such as that caused by viruses or endotoxin, to endothelial cells, basement membrane, or smooth

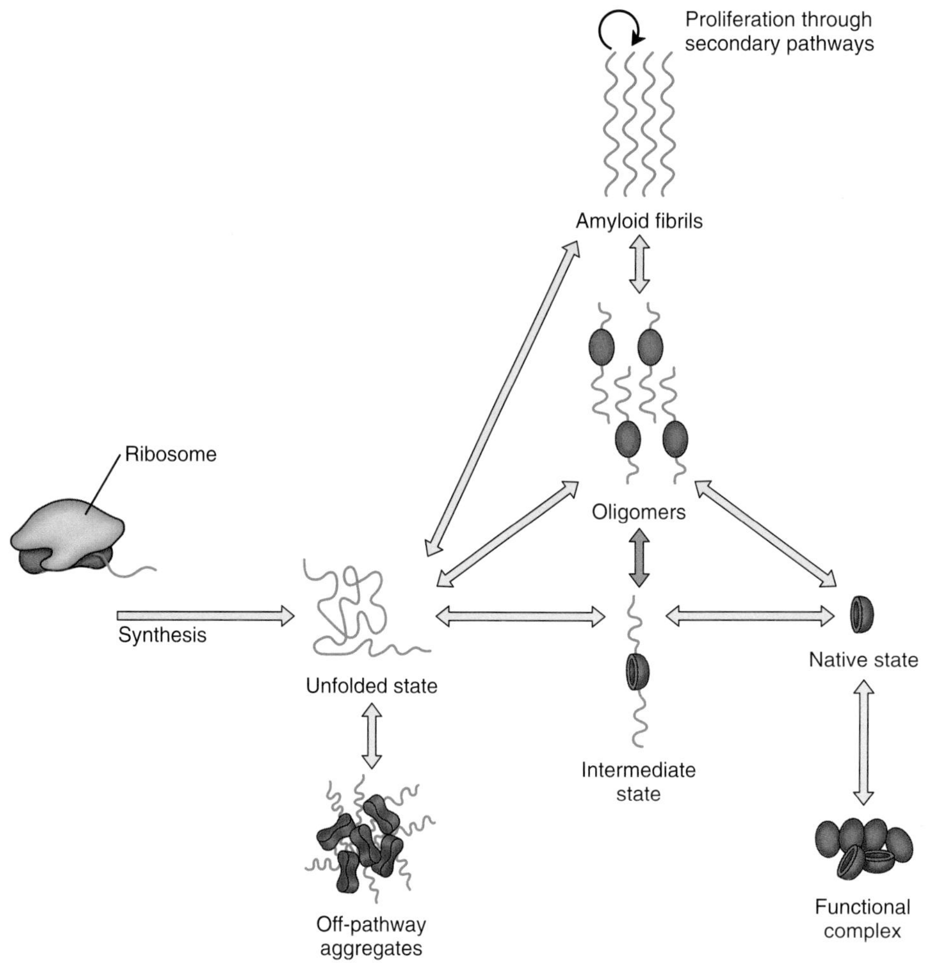

Figure 1-33 **Mechanisms of Protein Folding and the Unfolded Protein Response.** Proteins have different conformational states according to thermodynamic properties, rates of synthesis and degradation, interaction with chaperones, and posttranslational modifications. Amyloidosis is a protein folding disorder in which unfolded or partially unfolded peptides form fibrils that are rich in β-sheets and capable of self-replication.

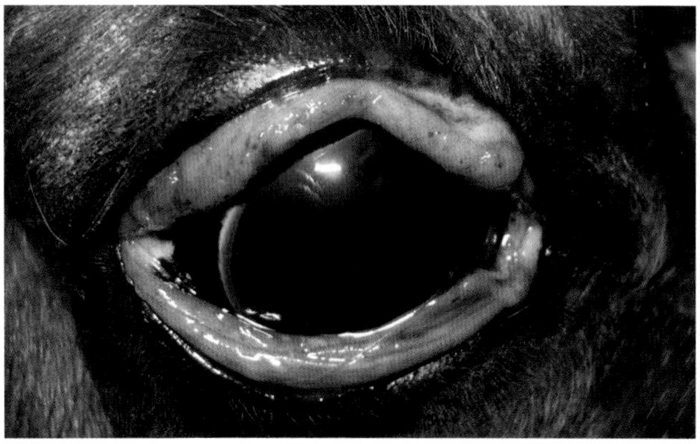

Figure 1-34 **Amyloidosis, Conjunctiva, Horse.** The palpebral conjunctiva (upper eyelid) in this horse with nasal and conjunctival amyloidosis is thickened by coalescing, waxy yellow nodules of amyloid in the subepithelial tissue. (Courtesy Dr. E.D. Conway, College of Veterinary Medicine, Purdue University.)

muscle cells of the tunica media can activate the acute phase inflammatory response leading to circumferential deposition of plasma proteins in blood vessel walls. These proteins, especially fibrin, are intensely eosinophilic and can be accompanied by leukocytic infiltration (Fig. 1-36; see also Chapter 3).

Collagen (Fibrosis). Fibrosis is an excess in fibrous collagen, predominantly type I collagen fibers, in the interstitium of organs or tissues. Necrosis, especially necrosis that destroys epithelial basement membranes, but also necrosis of mesenchymal tissues, tends to induce proliferation of fibroblasts. In many injured tissues, especially beneath ulcers or in wound healing, fibroblastic proliferation is accompanied by endothelial proliferation with formation of granulation tissue (fibrosis plus neovascularization [see Chapters 3 and 17]). As granulation tissue matures, the neovascularization subsides, fibroblasts become quiescent, collagen fibers remain, and scar tissue is the end result. In the liver (see Chapter 8), stellate cells are the source of the collagen in fibrosis. Macrophages (i.e., Kupffer cells in the liver, histiocytes, or other tissue macrophages) direct fibrosis by release of cytokines and growth factors such as TNF-α and TGF-β.

Fatty Infiltration. Fatty infiltration is an increase in the number and/or volume of adipocytes in the interstitium of an organ or tissue. Thus it is distinct from the intracellular accumulations known as lipidosis or steatosis. Normally adipocytes are present in small numbers in the myocardial interstitium, especially near the epicardium, and in skeletal muscle bundles. The adipocytes can increase in size and number in obesity and in certain cardiomyopathies (see Chapter 10) or skeletal myopathies (see Chapter 15 and Fig. 15-9). Adipocytes also accumulate in atrophied tissues, such as skeletal

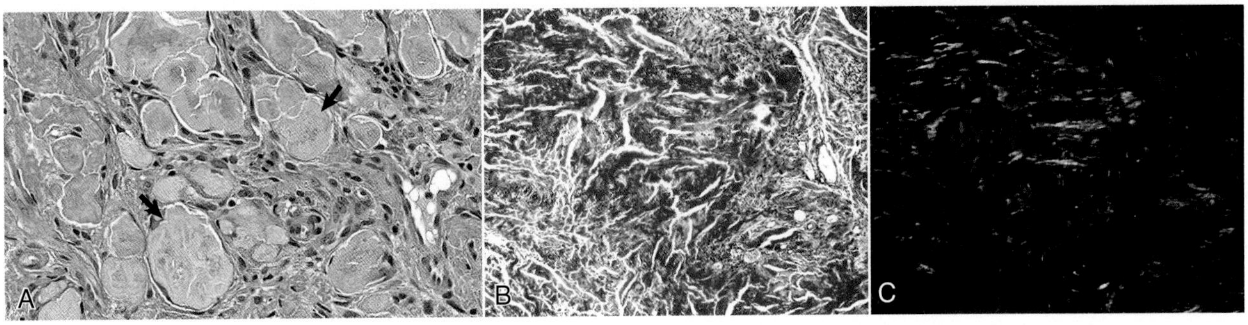

Figure 1-35 **Equine Nasal Amyloidosis. A**, The amyloid appears as homogeneous to faintly fibrillar, pale eosinophilic deposits *(arrows)* in the nasal mucosal interstitium. H&E stain. **B**, Congophilic substances, such as amyloid, are red-orange with Congo red stain. **C**, Viewed with polarized light, amyloid is birefringent and "apple-green." Congo red stain, same field and same magnification as in **B.** (Courtesy Dr. M.A. Miller, College of Veterinary Medicine, Purdue University.)

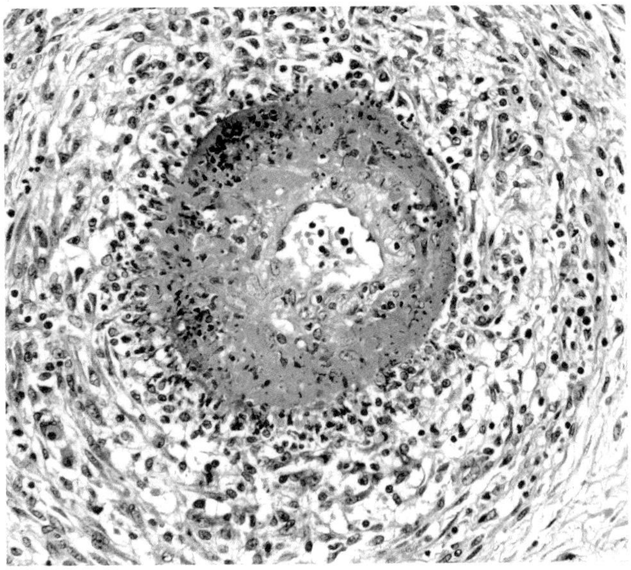

Figure 1-36 **Fibrinoid Change, Artery.** Note the deeply eosinophilic circumferential deposits in the arterial tunica media. The fibrinoid change is accompanied by leukocytic infiltration and medial necrosis. H&E stain. (Courtesy Dr. J.F. Zachary, College of Veterinary Medicine, University of Illinois.)

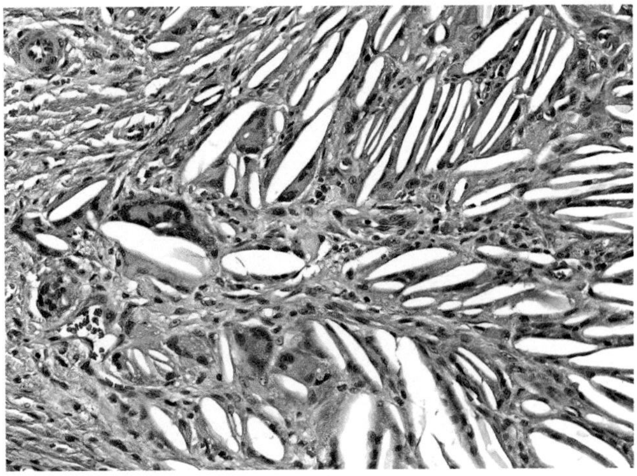

Figure 1-37 **Cholesterol Granuloma, Mammary Gland, Dog.** Note the acicular cholesterol clefts (cholesterol is removed from the histologic section in processing) with granulomatous inflammation. H&E stain. (Courtesy Dr. M.A. Miller, College of Veterinary Medicine, Purdue University.)

muscle (particularly when the result of denervation; see Chapter 15), thymus, and thyroid gland (see Fig. 1-26, *B*).

Gout

Gout has not been reported in domestic mammals but occurs in primates, birds, and reptiles. Information on this topic is available at www.expertconsult.com.

Pseudogout

Pseudogout has been reported in the dog but is rare. Information on this topic is available at www.expertconsult.com.

Cholesterol. Cholesterol crystals are dissolved out of the tissue specimen during histologic processing, leaving characteristic acicular (needle-shaped) clefts in histologic sections. In three dimensions the crystals are thin rhomboidal plates with a notched corner. Cholesterol crystals often form in tissue at sites of hemorrhage or necrosis. They are present in atheromas (degenerated arterial intima plaques in atherosclerosis); however, with the exception of hypothyroid dogs, atherosclerosis is not common in domestic mammals.

Cholesterol crystals typically elicit granulomatous inflammation (Fig. 1-37) and are common in the cholesterol granulomas ("cholesteatomas") in the choroid plexus of old horses; these can become large enough to obstruct the flow of cerebrospinal fluid but more often are an incidental finding. Grossly, the cholesterol granuloma appears as friable pale yellow nodules in the choroid plexus of the lateral or fourth ventricles (see Chapter 14 and Fig. 14-87).

Pathologic Calcification

Pathologic calcification refers to the deposition of calcium salts, typically as phosphates or carbonates, in soft tissues (i.e., tissues that would not be calcified in a healthy state). Soft tissue calcification as the result of elevated serum calcium concentration is termed metastatic calcification, whereas the calcification of dead tissue as part of the process of necrosis is called dystrophic calcification. If calcification is extensive, it appears grossly as chalky white deposits (Fig. 1-38) with a brittle or gritty texture. Calcium deposits that also contain hemosiderin or other blood pigments (see subsequent section on Pigments) may be discolored yellow-brown.

Dystrophic Calcification

A review of the biochemical events in cell death explains dystrophic calcification. Recall that loss of the ability to regulate cellular Ca^{2+} balance is a critical turning point that converts reversible to irreversible injury. Ischemia opens membrane calcium channels, leading to increased intracellular calcium concentration, which is normally sequestered in the cytosol, ER, and mitochondria, each with its own Ca^{2+}-ATPase membrane pumps. The increased intracellular calcium concentration activates calpains, which cleave Na^{+}/Ca^{2+} exchangers in mitochondrial and other cell membranes, leading to decreased efflux of Ca^{2+} and decreased reuptake of Ca^{2+} by the ER. Thus calcium overload is an expected sequel to cell death. Dystrophic calcification is most prominent in mitochondria and is first evident histologically as a basophilic stippling of the dead cell. With increasing deposition of calcium salts, the entire cell and even extracellular tissue can be calcified, resulting in more intense and widespread basophilia. Calcification is the gross lesion for which the myocardial and skeletal muscle necrosis of vitamin E or selenium deficiency in ruminants was named white muscle disease (see Fig. 1-38). Calcification is also prominent in other forms of necrosis (e.g., in the caseous necrosis of tuberculoid granulomas), in parasitic granulomas, and in necrotic fat or lipomas (benign neoplasms of adipocytes).

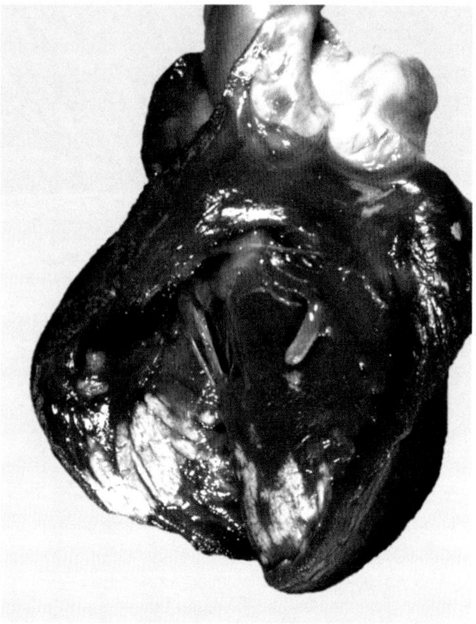

Figure 1-38 **Calcification, Vitamin E or Selenium Deficiency, Heart, Lamb.** The chalky white lesions are areas of myocardial necrosis that have been calcified. (Courtesy Dr. M.D. McGavin, College of Veterinary Medicine, University of Tennessee.)

Calcification of the skin (see Chapter 17) is categorized as (1) calcinosis cutis, a poorly understood form of epithelial and collagenous calcification seen mainly in canine hyperglucocorticoidism, and (2) calcinosis circumscripta. Calcinosis circumscripta is a localized deposit of calcium salts in the dermis or subcutis, and less often in other soft tissues or in the tongue. It is common over bony prominences of distal aspects of the limbs in young dogs of the large breeds but can occur in other species (e.g., horses). It is probably a form of dystrophic calcification and usually attributed to repetitive trauma.

Metastatic Calcification

Metastatic calcification targets the intima and tunica media of vessels, especially those in the lungs, pleura, endocardium, kidneys, and stomach. The primary defect is an imbalance in calcium and phosphate concentrations in the blood.

In chronic kidney disease, phosphate retention is the cause of the calcium-phosphate imbalance (see Chapter 11). In "uremic gastropathy" the damage to gastric arteries and arterioles results in ischemic injury and metastatic calcification in the gastric mucosa. The metastatic calcification of renal failure is also prominent in the lungs, pleura, and endocardium. In an H&E-stained section, metastatic calcification imparts a subtle basophilic stippling (Fig. 1-39, *A*). The von Kossa histochemical technique blackens the calcium phosphate or calcium carbonate salts (see Fig. 1-39, *B*).

Toxicosis with vitamin D or its analogues is also characterized by calcium-phosphate imbalance. *Cestrum diurnum*, a plant introduced from the West Indies to the Gulf Coast of the United States, is poisonous to herbivores because it contains glycosides of 1,25-dihydroxycholecalciferol (1,25-$(OH)_2D_3$) that cause elevated serum calcium concentration and often severe metastatic calcification of the lungs, kidney, and heart, especially the atrial endocardium and ascending aorta. Dogs and cats can be poisoned by consumption of rodenticides containing cholecalciferol.

Inappropriately elevated concentrations of parathyroid hormone (PTH) or secretion of PTH-related peptide cause hypercalcemia and metastatic calcification (see also Chapter 12). Primary hyperparathyroidism, usually the result of neoplasia of the parathyroid glands, is uncommon. Certain nonparathyroid neoplasms are associated with the so-called humoral hypercalcemia of malignancy

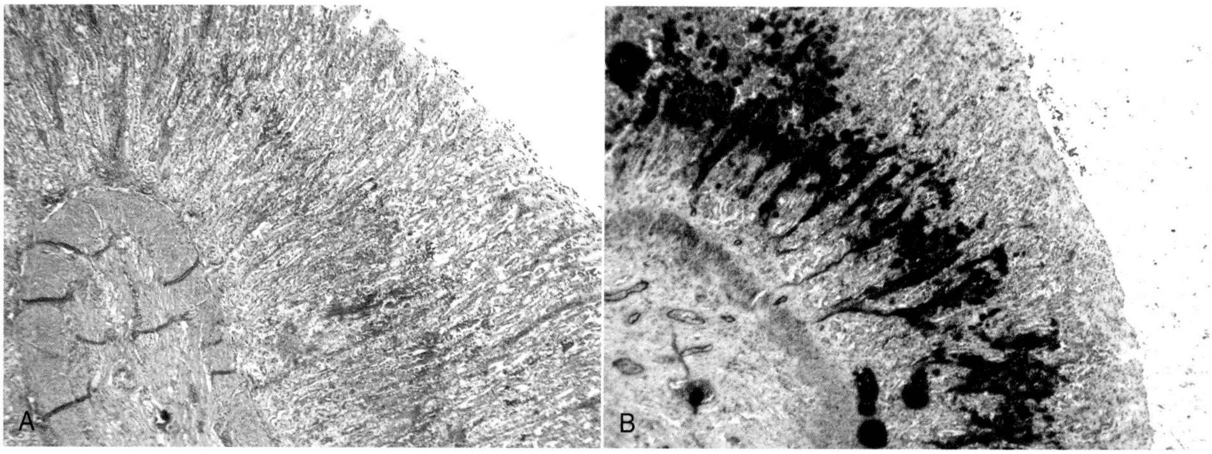

Figure 1-39 **Uremic Calcification, Stomach, Dog.** A band of calcification is in the middle of the gastric mucosa. **A**, The calcium salts are basophilic (stained blue with hematoxylin). H&E stain. **B**, The calcium salts are black with the von Kossa technique for mineralization. (**A** and **B** courtesy Dr. M.D. McGavin, College of Veterinary Medicine, University of Tennessee.)

(aka pseudohyperparathyroidism), either because the neoplastic cells secrete PTH-related peptide or because the neoplasm invades and lyses bone. Canine lymphoma and apocrine carcinoma of the anal sac glands are two tumors that can secrete PTH-related peptide.

Heterotopic Ossification

Heterotopic ossification is the formation of bony tissue at an extraskeletal site. It entails osteoid (bone matrix) deposition by osteoblasts with remodeling and mineralization to form bone. Although calcification is part of the process of ossification, whether skeletal or extraskeletal, and heterotopic ossification can develop in chronic lesions of soft tissue calcification, pathologic calcification of soft tissue does not necessarily entail ossification.

Heterotopic ossification appears grossly as hard spicules or nodules. Small bony spicules are commonly encountered as incidental findings in the pulmonary interstitium (Fig. 1-40) of old dogs. Nodular deposits of cartilage and bone may form the bulk of a canine mixed mammary tumor (see Chapter 18) in which the myoepithelial cells are thought to give rise to chondrocytes and osteoblasts.

Pigments

Various exogenous and endogenous substances can alter the color of tissues. These color changes may be evident clinically or at least macroscopically at autopsy and can be diagnostically useful. Though some pigmented substances disappear from histologic sections, others remain and must be interpreted by the pathologist.

Exogenous Pigmented Substances

Carbon and Other Dusts. Coal mine dust lung disease, also known as black lung, is the best-studied example of pneumoconiosis (lung disease due to inhalation of dusts; see Chapter 9). The major dust inhaled by coal mine workers is carbon, so this form of pneumoconiosis is called anthracosis. Carbon particles in the lung account for the black discoloration in anthracosis. Many cases, especially with the lower exposure in urban-dwelling people or animals that breathe polluted air, are not associated with clinical disease but impart a fine gray-black stippling to the lung (Fig. 1-41, A), visible through the visceral pleura, plus a dark gray discoloration of tracheobronchial lymph nodes. Carbon particles deposited in alveolar spaces are phagocytized by macrophages and then transported to bronchus-associated lymphoid tissue and on to tracheobronchial lymph nodes. Histologically, the indigestible carbon particles and other inhaled dusts appear as fine black granular material and crystalline material in macrophages in extracellular tissues adjacent to intrapulmonary airways and vasculature (see Fig. 1-41, *B*). This finding is usually incidental in older animals, but coal dust and other mineral dusts, especially silica,[4] can elicit an inflammatory response with release of TNF-α and interleukin 1 (IL-1) and interleukin 6 (IL-6). These cytokines can promote progressive fibrosis. Macrophages laden with carbon particles are also thought to have diminished capacity to phagocytize and destroy infectious agents.

Carotenoid Pigments. Carotenoid pigments, such as β-carotene, are abundant in leafy green plants and impart a yellow coloration to plasma, adipose tissue, and other lipid-laden cells. The deep yellow color of adipose tissue in herbivores on lush green pasture can be striking, especially in horses and dairy cattle of high milk-fat breeds, such as Jersey dairy cattle (Fig. 1-42). This discoloration is not a lesion but just a dietary indicator. Indeed, the carotenoids stored in fat are a source of antioxidants. Because carotenoids are fat soluble, they are removed from histologic sections by the solvents used in processing.

Tetracycline. The antibiotic tetracycline binds to calcium phosphate in teeth and bones. If administered to animals during the time of mineralization of the teeth, tetracycline results in permanent discoloration. Initially the staining is yellow, but after tooth eruption and exposure to light, oxidation changes the color to brown (Fig. 1-43). Yellowish discoloration (with bright yellow fluorescence under ultraviolet light) is also observed in bone.

[4]Silica crystals are colorless, so they are not an example of a pigmented substance.

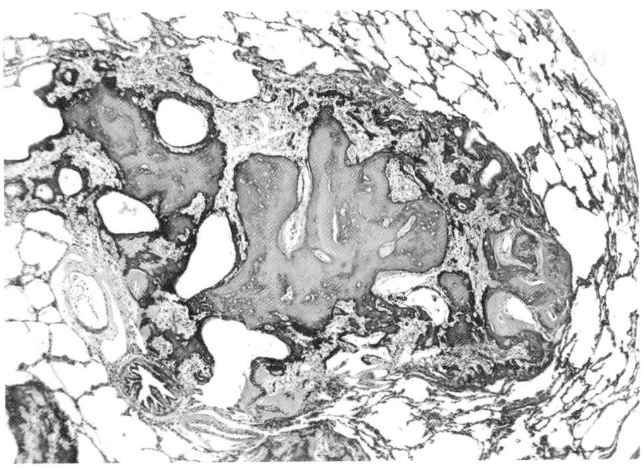

Figure 1-40 **Ectopic Bone, Lung, Dog.** A nodule of mature bone in the connective tissue of the lung. H&E stain. (Courtesy Dr. M.D. McGavin, College of Veterinary Medicine, University of Tennessee.)

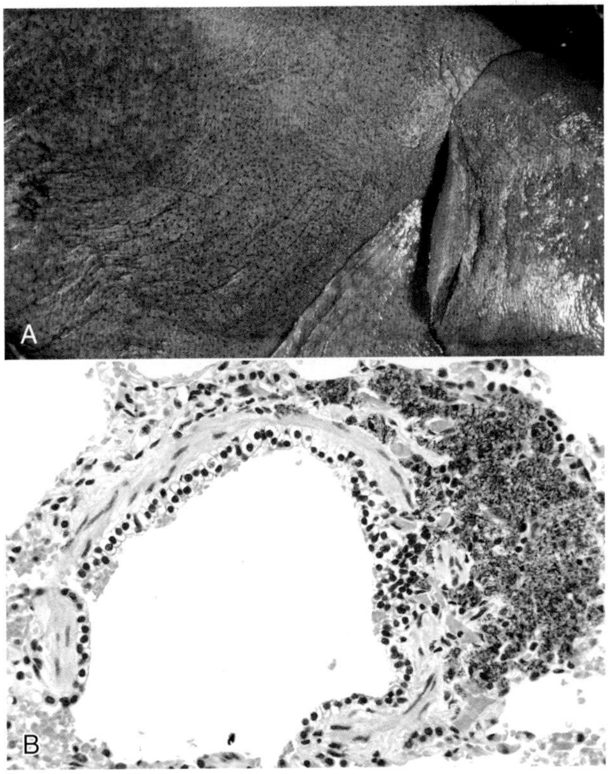

Figure 1-41 **Anthracosis, Lung, Aged Dog. A**, The fine black subpleural stippling represents peribronchiolar deposits of carbon. **B**, Inhaled carbon (*black*) has been phagocytized by macrophages and transported to the peribronchial/peribronchiolar tissue. H&E stain. (**A** and **B** courtesy Dr. M.D. McGavin, College of Veterinary Medicine, University of Tennessee.)

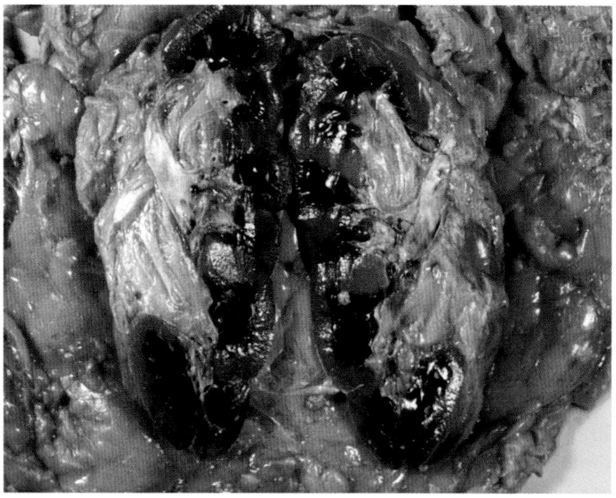

Figure 1-42 Carotenosis, Kidney and the Perirenal Fat, Jersey Ox. Accumulation of carotenoids in the adipocytes has colored the fat yellow to dark yellow. (Courtesy Dr. M.D. McGavin, College of Veterinary Medicine, University of Tennessee.)

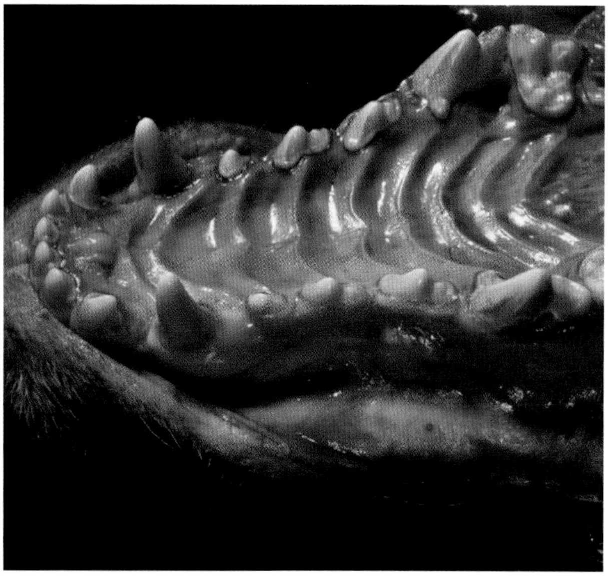

Figure 1-43 Tetracycline Staining, Teeth, Young Dog. The yellow-brown discoloration of the permanent teeth is the result of tetracycline therapy during their development. (Courtesy Dr. M.D. McGavin, College of Veterinary Medicine, University of Tennessee.)

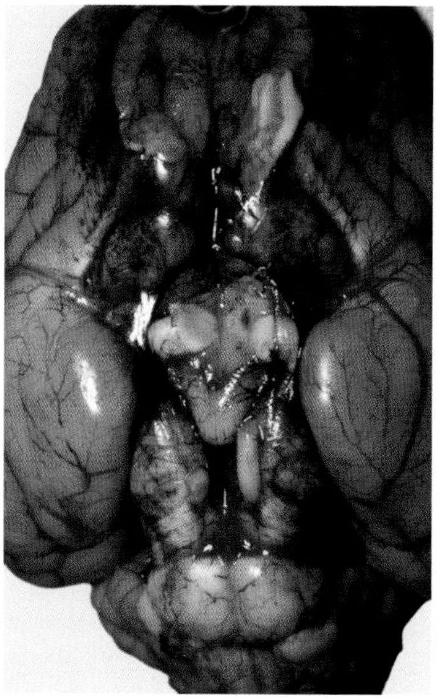

Figure 1-44 Congenital Melanosis, Leptomeninges, Suffolk Sheep. The leptomeninges have scattered black areas of melanin. This pigmentation is normal in black ruminants. (Courtesy Dr. M.D. McGavin, College of Veterinary Medicine, University of Tennessee.)

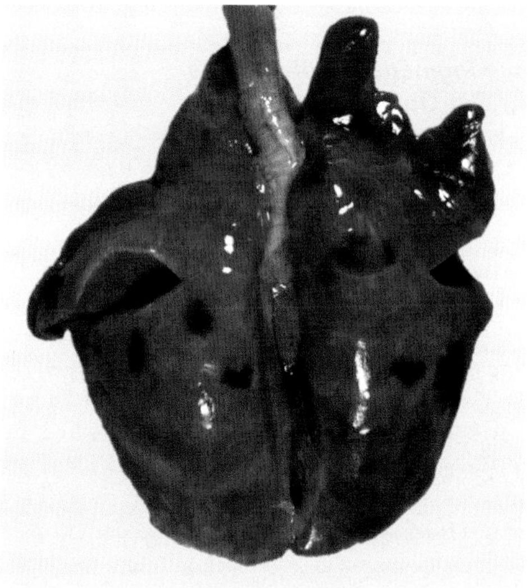

Figure 1-45 Congenital Melanosis, Lung, Pig. Melanin deposits are subpleural and extend into pulmonary parenchyma. This pigmentation, seen mainly in red or black pigs, has no detrimental consequences. (Courtesy Dr. M.D. McGavin, College of Veterinary Medicine, University of Tennessee.)

Nonhematogenous Endogenous Pigments

Melanin. Melanin is the pigment responsible for the color of the hair, skin, and iris. It also colors the leptomeninges in black-faced sheep (Fig. 1-44) and cattle and may be present multifocally in oral mucosa in various species. Localized deposits of melanin (melanosis) are common in the aortic intima in ruminants with pigmented coats and in the lungs (Fig. 1-45) of red or black pigs. The localized deposits in congenital melanosis are merely a color change and not a lesion because they are not a response to injury and have no ill effect on the animal.

The melanocytes that synthesize and secrete melanin are derived from the neural crest and migrate to the site of pigment production during embryonic development of the structure. In the skin, melanocytes reside in the stratum basale of the epidermis and follicular epithelium. Melanin is formed in organelles called melanosomes, then transferred through dendritic cell processes to adjacent keratinocytes. In the keratinocyte, melanin granules are mainly in the apical cytoplasm, where they may shield the nucleus from ultraviolet light. Histologically, melanin granules are small (usually less than 1 μm in diameter), brown, and nonrefractile.

Melanin pigment can be diminished or excessive in disease. The first step in melanin synthesis is the conversion of tyrosine to dihydroxyphenylalanine (DOPA), catalyzed by the copper-containing enzyme, tyrosinase. Thus a lack of tyrosinase results in albinism (lack of melanin pigmentation), and sheep and cattle with copper deficiency have defective tyrosinase and fading of coat color. Partial albinism in Chédiak-Higashi syndrome (CHS) (recognized in people, mink, Persian cats, mice, and other species) is caused by a mutation of the *LYST* gene that codes for a lysosomal trafficking regulator protein. The mutation causes abnormal lysosomal structure and function in leukocytes and in melanocytes. The melanocytes of animals with CHS have enlarged melanosomes, but the melanin pigment is not transferred effectively to keratinocytes, so coat color is a pastel shade of what it should have been. Normally pigmented skin and hair can also become depigmented because of an immune-mediated attack on melanocytes (vitiligo) or basilar keratinocytes (see Chapter 17). The dead keratinocytes spill their melanin into adjacent dermis in a process called pigmentary incontinence, where it is phagocytized by macrophages (melanophages).

The term hyperpigmentation implies excessive melanin. This finding can be a common epidermal response to chronic injury and appears as darkened skin. Endocrine skin disease, especially hyperadrenocorticism, is often associated with hyperpigmentation. Histologically, melanin granules are numerous, not only in the basilar keratinocytes, but in all layers of the epidermis, even the stratum corneum. Neoplasms of melanocytes can be darkly pigmented or not pigmented at all (amelanotic) (see Chapters 6 and 17).

Lipofuscin and Ceroid. Lipofuscin is a yellow-brown lipoprotein that accumulates as residual bodies in secondary lysosomes, especially in long-lived postmitotic cells, such as neurons and cardiac myocytes (Fig. 1-46), and especially in aged animals. It is known as a "wear and tear" pigment of aging—its accumulation in canine myocardium has a linear correlation with the age of the dog—and is generally thought to have little or no deleterious effect on the cell. Lipofuscin is autofluorescent with an excitation wavelength between 320 and 480 nm and emission wavelength between 460 and 630 nm. It is approximately two-thirds heterogeneous protein and one-third lipid (mainly triglycerides, free fatty acids, cholesterol, and phospholipids). Because of its lipid content, lipofuscin reacts with fat stains such as Sudan black B or Oil Red O; its carbohydrate moieties make it also PAS positive.

Ceroid is a lipofuscin-like (i.e., same morphologic appearance) pigment that accumulates in disease states, such as neuronal ceroid-lipofuscinosis (a group of hereditary lysosomal storage diseases), cachexia, vitamin E deficiency, or other oxidative stress. Ceroid can be grossly evident in the tunica muscularis of the small intestine of dogs with vitamin E deficiency (leiomyometaplasia [brown dog gut]; see Fig. 7-112) or dogs with ceroid-lipofuscinosis (Fig. 1-47).

Lipofuscin and ceroid have strikingly similar histologic and biochemical characteristics, yet are distinct. Both are autofluorescent lipoproteins with similar but not identical spectra. Ultrastructurally, lipofuscin has a granular appearance, whereas ceroid is more likely to form membranous stacks or whorls ("myelin figures"). Although both compounds are composed of proteins, lipids, dolichols, carbohydrates, and metals, their exact composition varies. Whereas the protein content of lipofuscin is heterogeneous, subunit c of mitochondrial ATP synthase is the predominant component of ceroid in neuronal ceroid-lipofuscinosis. Lectin histochemistry is useful to distinguish neuronal ceroid from lipofuscin by its sugar moieties.

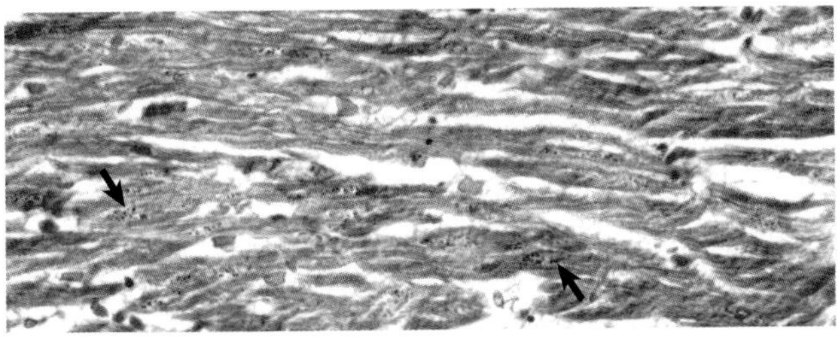

Figure 1-46 **Lipofuscinosis, Heart, Dog.** Note the brown lipofuscin granules *(arrows)* in the cytoplasm of cardiac myocytes. H&E stain. (Courtesy Dr. J.F. Zachary, College of Veterinary Medicine, University of Illinois.)

Hematogenous Pigments

Hematogenous pigments are derived from erythrocytes. They include hemoglobin, hematins, hemosiderin, hematoidin, bilirubin, biliverdin, and porphyrins.

Hemoglobin. The hemoglobin molecule consists of four globular protein subunits, each folded around and tightly associated with a central nonprotein, iron-containing heme group. Oxyhemoglobin, formed when oxygen binds to the heme group, gives oxygenated (arterial) blood its red color and imparts a pink tinge to well-perfused and well-oxygenated tissues. Deoxygenated hemoglobin explains the blue cast to venous blood and accounts for the blue to purple discoloration, known as cyanosis (Fig. 1-48), of hypoxic tissues. The word cyanosis comes from the Greek word for dark blue.

Toxic or Other Metabolic Disorders of Hemoglobin

Cyanide. Cyanide (CN^-) is a toxic compound that, when ingested, blocks oxidative phosphorylation in mitochondria by

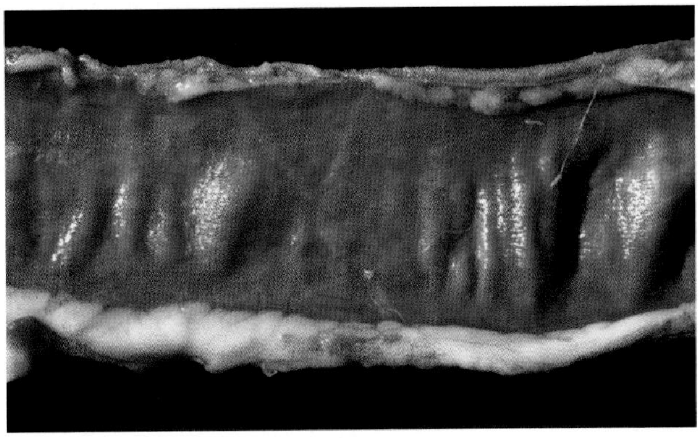

Figure 1-47 **Ceroid, Intestine, Serosal Surface, Dog.** Note the brown discoloration of the muscular layer. The condition has been called intestinal lipofuscinosis but is not age-related. (Courtesy Dr. M.D. McGavin, College of Veterinary Medicine, University of Tennessee.)

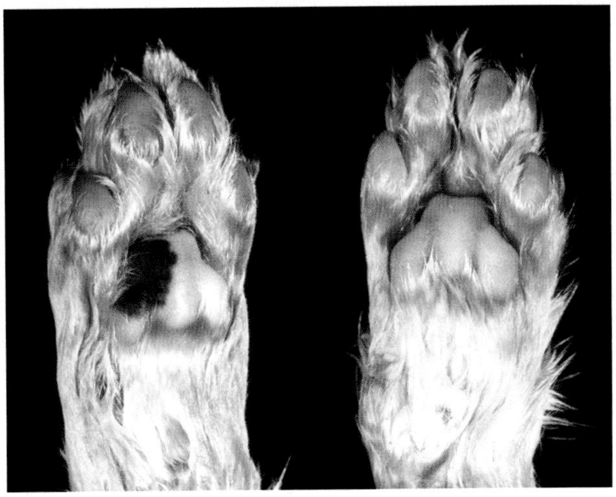

Figure 1-48 **Cyanosis, Paw, Cat.** The pads of the paw on the left are bluish due to deoxygenated hemoglobin, the result of obstruction of the iliac artery by a saddle thrombus at the aortic bifurcation. The pads of the normal paw (*on the right*) are pink. (Courtesy Dr. M.D. McGavin, College of Veterinary Medicine, University of Tennessee.)

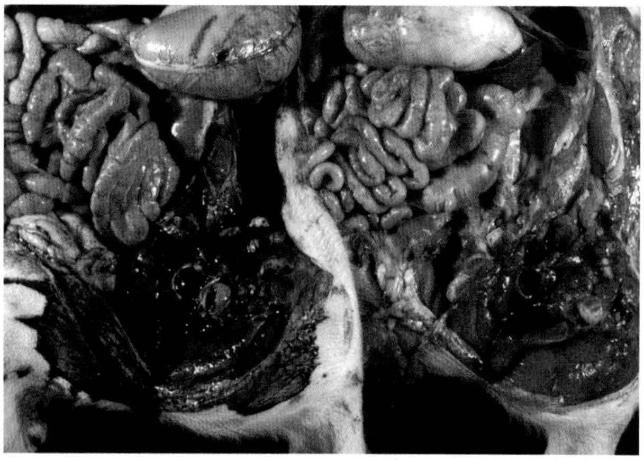

Figure 1-49 **Methemoglobinemia, Experimental Nitrite Poisoning, Hind Quarters, Pig.** *Left,* The methemoglobin has discolored the blood and musculature chocolate brown. *Right,* Normal control. (Courtesy Dr. L. Nelson, College of Veterinary Medicine, Michigan State University.)

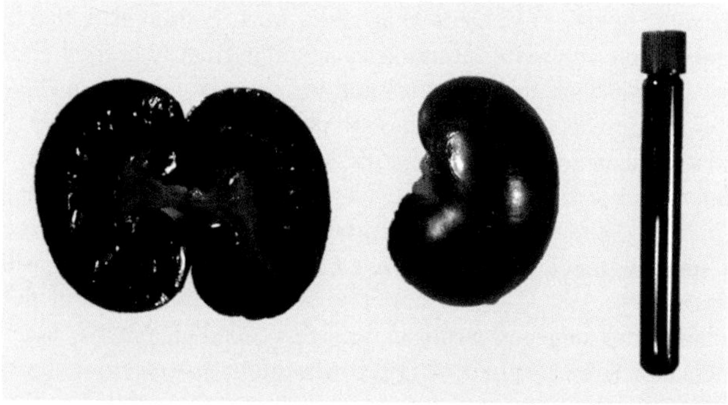

Figure 1-50 **Hemolytic Crisis in Chronic Copper Poisoning, Kidneys and Urine, Sheep.** The dark bluish color of the kidney and the dark red of the urine are caused by hemoglobinuria (hemoglobin excreted via the kidney). (Courtesy Dr. M.D. McGavin, College of Veterinary Medicine, University of Tennessee.)

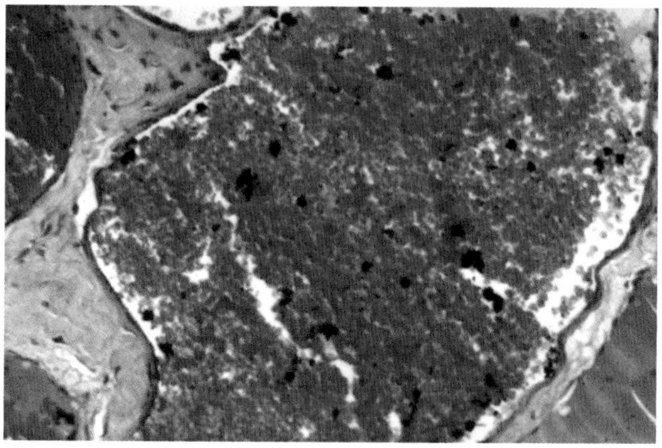

Figure 1-51 **Formalin Pigment, Blood.** Note the black specks of acid hematin on and around erythrocytes, the result of fixation in unbuffered (acidic) formalin. H&E stain. (Courtesy Dr. M.D. McGavin, College of Veterinary Medicine, University of Tennessee.)

binding cytochrome oxidase. As a result, cells cannot use the oxygen in hemoglobin, so venous blood in cases of cyanide poisoning tends to be as red as arterial blood. Cyanide poisoning in herbivores is usually the result of consumption of plants that contain cyanogenic glycosides.

Carbon Monoxide. Hemoglobin has a much higher affinity for CO than for oxygen, so even a small amount of CO reduces oxygen transport capacity. When hemoglobin binds CO, it forms carboxyhemoglobin, which colors the blood bright cherry red and imparts a bright pink color to the tissues even in fatal cases of CO poisoning (E-Fig. 1-17).

Nitrite Poisoning. Nitrite poisoning can be associated with consumption of nitrate-accumulating plants by livestock, usually ruminants, or from a water source contaminated with nitrate runoff from fertilized fields. Nitrate is converted in the rumen to nitrite, which can oxidize the iron in the heme group of the hemoglobin molecule to the Fe^{+3} (ferric) state, converting hemoglobin to *methemoglobin,* which has low affinity for oxygen. Methemoglobin turns the color of blood to a chocolate brown (Fig. 1-49).

Intravascular Hemolysis (Hemoglobinuria). If erythrocytes are lysed within vessels (intravascular hemolysis), the released hemoglobin imparts a transparent pink tinge to the plasma or serum. In the kidneys, intravascular hemoglobin passes through glomerular capillaries into the urinary filtrate with the formation of hemoglobin "casts" in renal tubules and reddish discoloration of the urine. Hemoglobinuria turns the color of renal parenchyma a dark red to gunmetal blue (Fig. 1-50; see Fig. 11-39, A and B). A similar or browner discoloration of kidney and urine occurs with myoglobinuria; the myoglobin is derived from injured skeletal muscle fibers.

Hematin. Hematin is a brown-black, Fe^{+3}-containing pigment formed by the oxidation of hemoglobin.

Acid Hematin (Formalin Pigment). The "acid" hematin that forms in tissues fixed in unbuffered, and therefore acidic ($pH < 6$), formalin appears as dark brown to nearly black, granular or crystalline material mainly in vessels or other areas of the tissue section where erythrocytes (and hemoglobin) are numerous (Fig. 1-51). The presence of acid hematin is a postmortem change and therefore not a lesion, but rather an indicator that the formalin solution was not properly buffered. Correctly prepared phosphate-buffered 10% formalin should have a pH of 6.8. Acid hematin can be so abundant in congested tissues that it hinders histologic evaluation. In these cases, hematin can be removed by soaking the dewaxed tissue section before H&E staining in a saturated alcoholic solution of picric acid.

Parasitic Hematin. Parasites that infect (e.g., *Plasmodium* spp.) or consume (e.g., *Haemonchus contortus*) erythrocytes liberate heme during the proteolysis of hemoglobin. Free heme is toxic, but the parasites have evolved to aggregate it into heme dimers called hemozoin or β-hematin. Hematin accounts for the blackening of the migration tracts of juvenile liver flukes (*Fascioloides magna*) in ruminants (Fig. 1-52; see also Figs. 8-60 and 8-61) and for the black speckling of the lungs in macaques infested with the lung mite, *Pneumonyssus simicola*.

Hemosiderin. Free iron is toxic to cells because it catalyzes the formation of ROS via the Fenton reaction. However, ferritin, a globular iron storage protein present in all tissues and particularly in the liver, spleen, and bone marrow, binds free iron and stores it in a nontoxic form available for use by the cell. Ferritin is mainly an intracellular protein, but serum concentrations correlate with iron stores. Accumulations of ferritin bound with iron, mainly in macrophages, are converted to golden brown granules of hemosiderin (Fig. 1-53, A). The Prussian blue reaction detects the iron in hemosiderin (see Fig. 1-53, B) in histologic tissue sections.

Hemosiderin is an intracellular iron storage complex, especially common in macrophages and less so in hepatocytes and renal

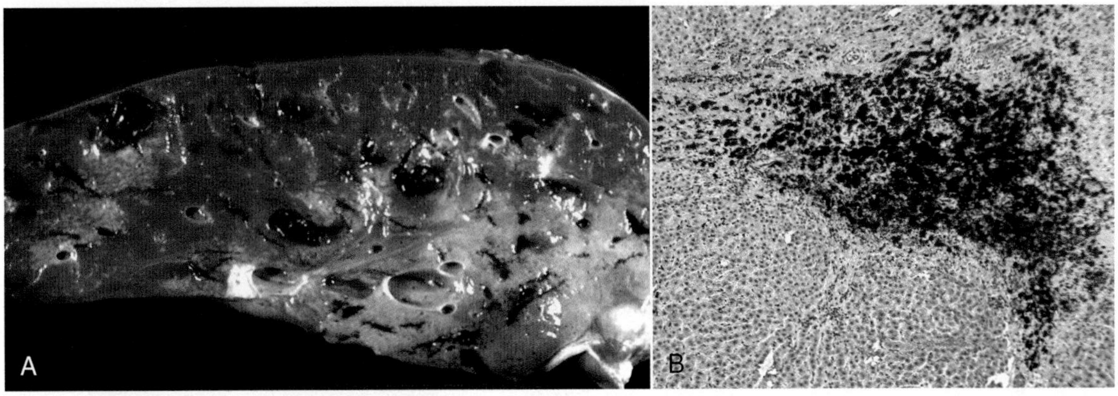

Figure 1-52 **Hematin pigment from *Fascioloides magna*, Liver, Ox.** **A**, Blackened areas in the liver are the result of hematin pigment excreted by migrating trematode larvae. **B**, Hematin *(black)* pigment in a fluke migration tract. H&E stain. (**A** courtesy Dr. J. Wright, College of Veterinary Medicine, North Carolina State University; and Noah's Arkive, College of Veterinary Medicine, The University of Georgia. **B** courtesy Dr. M.D. McGavin, College of Veterinary Medicine, University of Tennessee.)

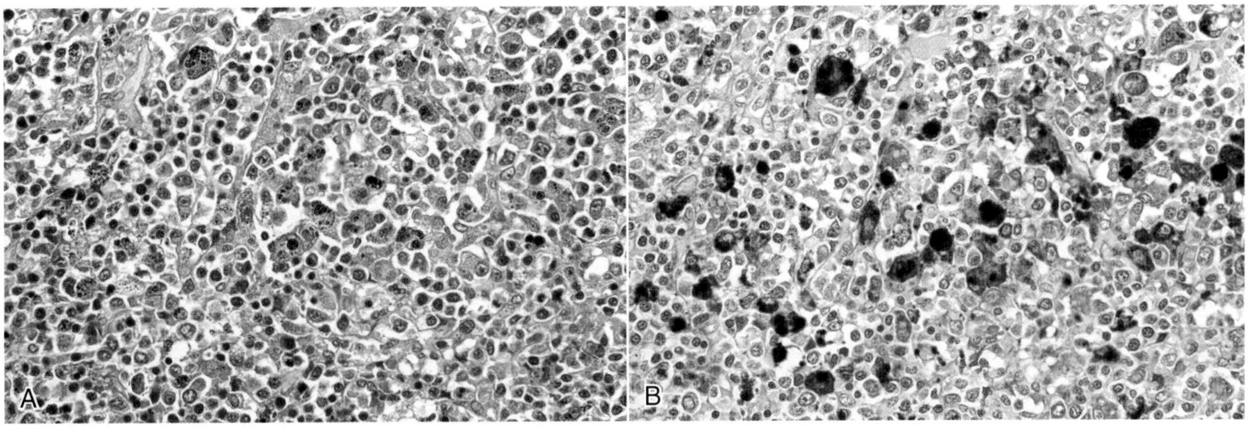

Figure 1-53 **Hemosiderosis, Spleen, Dog.** **A**, Hemosiderin appears as golden brown granules in macrophages. H&E stain. **B**, Granules of hemosiderin are stained blue by the Prussian blue reaction, which is specific for iron. Prussian blue reaction. (**A** and **B** courtesy Dr. J.F. Zachary, College of Veterinary Medicine, University of Illinois.)

tubular epithelial cells. Iron stores are most conspicuous in the spleen and are excessive (hemosiderosis) when there is an increased rate of destruction of erythrocytes. Rarely, excess iron can be derived from the diet (e.g., hemochromatosis, a more severe iron storage disease) or other external sources. The presence of hemosiderin-laden macrophages can also be an indicator of chronic passive congestion (Fig. 1-54, A). If abundant, hemosiderin imparts a brownish discoloration to tissues that should be pink (see Fig. 1-54, B). Hemosiderin is also one of the pigments that typifies a bruise (Fig. 1-55).

Hematoidin. Hematoidin is a bright-yellow crystalline pigment that is derived from hemosiderin, presumably within macrophages, but is free of iron. It is similar or identical to bilirubin, biochemically, and is deposited in tissues at sites of hemorrhage.

Bilirubin. Bilirubin is normally present in low amounts in the plasma as a breakdown product of erythrocytes (see Chapters 8 and 13). Effete erythrocytes are phagocytized and lysed by macrophages. The globular protein components of hemoglobin are broken down into amino acids. After removal of iron, the rest of the heme is converted by heme oxygenase to biliverdin, then by biliverdin reductase to bilirubin. The unconjugated bilirubin is released into the blood to be carried as an albumin-bilirubin complex to the liver for conjugation with glucuronic acid and secretion into the bile canaliculus, where it becomes a component of bile.

If the elevation in serum or plasma bilirubin level (hyperbilirubinemia) is sufficient, it will result in the yellow staining of tissues called icterus or jaundice. Icterus is often classified pathogenetically as prehepatic, hepatic, or posthepatic (see Chapter 8). Prehepatic icterus is caused by hemolysis or any process that increases the turnover of erythrocytes and delivers more unconjugated bilirubin to the liver than it can accommodate. Hepatic icterus is the result of hepatocellular injury that decreases the uptake, conjugation, or secretion of bilirubin. In posthepatic icterus, it is the outflow of bile from the liver into the intestine via the biliary system that is reduced by an obstruction.

Mutant Corriedale (Fig. 1-56) and Southdown sheep develop conjugated hyperbilirubinemia that is attributed to a defective ATP-dependent transport system for various organic anions, including bilirubin diglucuronide. Affected animals have a disease similar to the human Dubin-Johnson syndrome and can conjugate bilirubin but cannot secrete it into the bile efficiently.

Grossly, the yellow discoloration of icterus is easiest to see in pale or colorless tissues, such as plasma, the sclera, intima of the great vessels, adipose tissue (unless it is already yellowed by carotenoids), and even in a pale liver (Figs. 1-57 and 1-58, A). Icterus is not observed histologically but is often associated with cholestasis, the

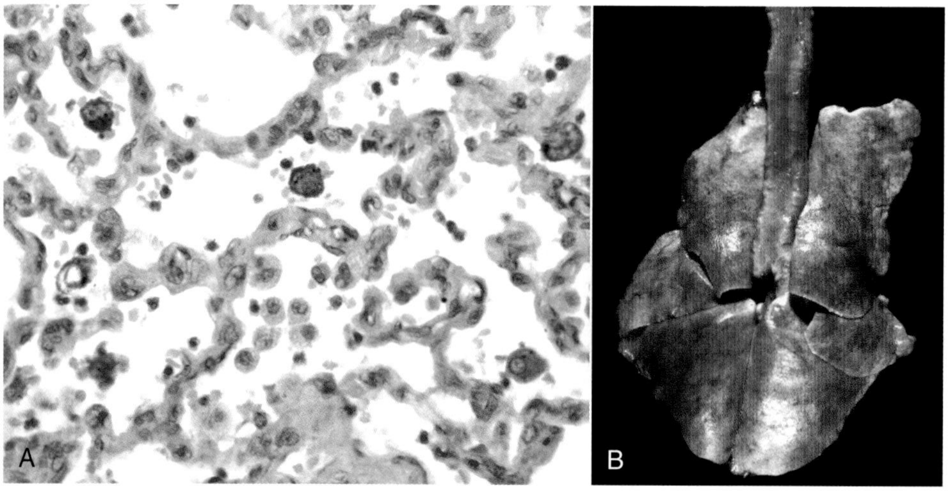

Figure 1-54 **Chronic Passive Congestion, Lung, Dog. A**, Macrophages containing hemosiderin *(blue)* are in the alveolar spaces. Prussian blue reaction. **B**, Chronic passive congestion of the lungs results in brownish discoloration because of the numerous hemosiderin-laden alveolar macrophages. Inflammatory mediators produced by these macrophages induce interstitial fibrosis, which caused the failure of the lungs to collapse upon opening of the thoracic cavity. Note the striped appearance of the lungs from rib imprints. (**A** courtesy Dr. M.D. McGavin, College of Veterinary Medicine, University of Tennessee. **B** courtesy College of Veterinary Medicine, University of Illinois.)

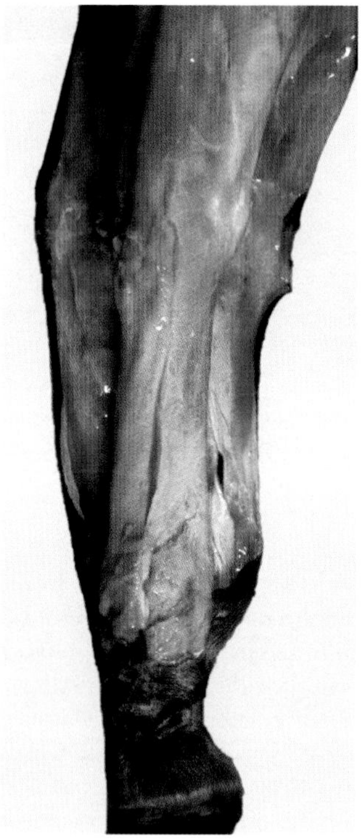

Figure 1-55 **Subcutis, Old Bruise, Leg, Horse.** The display of colors—red, yellow, and brown—is due to hemoglobin, bilirubin, and hemosiderin, respectively, from the breakdown of the erythrocytes. (Courtesy Dr. M.D. McGavin, College of Veterinary Medicine, University of Tennessee.)

distension of canaliculi by yellow-brown "casts" of bile (see Fig. 1-58, *B*).

Porphyria. Porphyrias are heme synthesis disorders that result in deposition of porphyrin pigments in tissues. The porphyrin ring in the hemoglobin molecule is composed of four pyrrole moieties linked together around the central iron ion. Congenital erythropoietic porphyrias of calves, cats, and pigs are the result of genetic defects caused by a deficiency of uroporphyrinogen III synthase. The disease name *pink tooth* comes from the discoloration of dentin and bone (Fig. 1-59; see also Chapter 7). Teeth, bone, and urine of

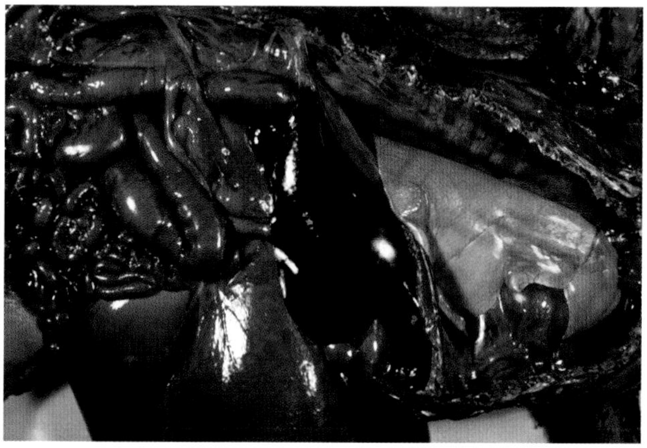

Figure 1-56 **Defective Bilirubin Excretion, Mutant Corriedale Sheep, Animal Model for Dubin-Johnson Syndrome.** Note the faint yellow discoloration of the lung from bilirubin. The other tissues are discolored dark green from phylloerythrin, which also has a similar defect in excretion in the liver. (Courtesy Dr. M.D. McGavin, College of Veterinary Medicine, University of Tennessee.)

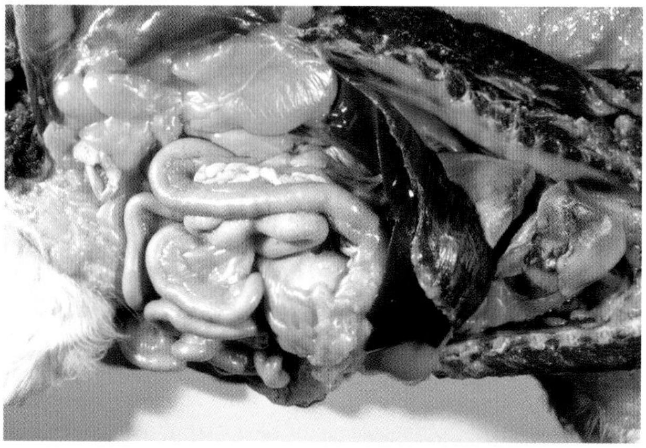

Figure 1-57 **Icterus, Hemolytic Anemia, Abdominal and Thoracic Viscera, Dog.** The yellow discoloration from the bilirubin is particularly evident in fat and mesentery. (Courtesy Dr. M.D. McGavin, College of Veterinary Medicine, University of Tennessee.)

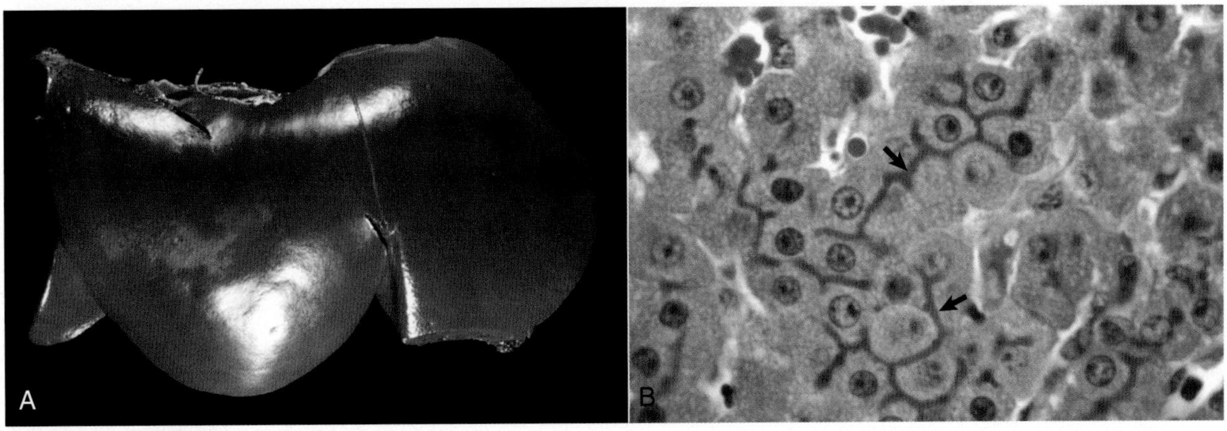

Figure 1-58 **Icterus.** **A**, Icterus, liver, cat. The liver is swollen with rounded edges and orange-brown discoloration caused by retained bilirubin. **B**, Acute hemolytic anemia, babesiosis, liver, cow. Bile casts distend canaliculi *(arrows)*. The cholestasis in this case was secondary to intravascular hemolysis with excessive delivery of unconjugated bilirubin to the liver. H&E stain. (**A** courtesy College of Veterinary Medicine, University of Illinois. **B** courtesy Dr. M.D. McGavin, College of Veterinary Medicine, University of Tennessee.)

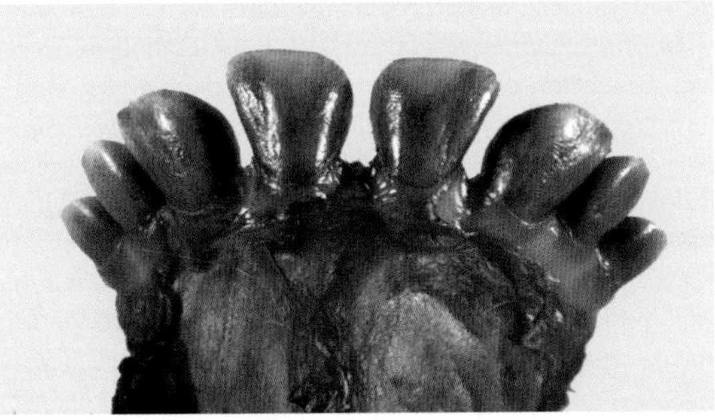

Figure 1-59 **Pink Tooth, Congenital Porphyria, Mandibular Incisor Teeth, Ox.** The teeth are discolored brown from the accumulation of porphyrins in the dentin. (Courtesy Dr. M.D. McGavin, College of Veterinary Medicine, University of Tennessee.)

affected animals are red-brown and fluoresce red under ultraviolet light. The feline disease has been mapped to two missense gene mutations in uroporphyrinogen III synthase.

Cell Cycle

Study of the cell cycle is fundamental to understanding development, homeostasis, and cellular proliferation in response to physiologic or pathologic stimuli, genetic disease, and the effects of cellular aging that include both the uncontrolled cellular proliferation of neoplasia and the permanent cessation of cellular replication known as senescence. The cell cycle (E-Fig. 1-18) consists of interphase (G_1, S, and G_2) and mitosis (M). Interphase, depending on the cell type, usually lasts at least 12 to 24 hours; in contrast, mitosis can be completed in as little as an hour or two. Cells enter the cell cycle in Gap 1 (G_1) in which they grow and produce protein, followed sequentially by the synthesis (S) phase in which DNA is replicated, a second (premitotic) gap (G_2) for continued growth and protein production, and finally the M phase for mitosis and cytokinesis, with partitioning of cellular contents between two daughter cells.

Because uncontrolled cellular replication perpetuates DNA damage and can lead to neoplasia, regulation of the cell cycle is essential. The cell cycle is controlled by a family of cyclin-dependent kinases (CDKs) that are activated by *cyclins*. Cells enter G_1 in response to growth factors that also cause the sequential accumulation of cyclins whose roles are to modulate the progress of G_1. Cyclin D activation of CDK4/6 results in phosphorylation of retinoblastoma (RB) protein, which in turn releases the transcription factor E2F and enables the cell to pass through the so-called restriction point in G_1, after which the cell is independent of extracellular growth signals. This restriction point is near the G_1 checkpoint, in which detection of damaged DNA results in growth arrest before S phase (i.e., before DNA replication). Other major checkpoints to interrupt the cell cycle occur in G_2 and M phases, if DNA is incorrectly replicated in the S phase or if the mitotic spindle is not properly formed in the M phase.

Growth arrest during the cell cycle is directed by many factors operating at checkpoints, but p53 plays a key role. Growth arrest can be a pause for the cell to repair damaged DNA and then resume cell division. Alternatively, if DNA is irreparably damaged, the cell dies, usually by apoptosis, or enters senescence, which is a permanent growth arrest (see subsequent section on Cellular Aging). Importantly, mutations in p53 are a common event in cancer (see also Chapter 6) and partly explain the uncontrolled proliferation that is the essence of neoplasia.

In health, most mature tissues are a mixture of continuously dividing (labile) cells, quiescent cells, terminally differentiated (postmitotic) cells, and stem cells. Homeostasis is a balance among cellular replication (of stem cells, labile cells, and quiescent cells), cellular differentiation, and cellular death. Labile tissues, such as epidermis, mucosal epithelium, and hematopoietic tissue, have germinal cells that cycle continuously throughout the life of the animal. These labile tissues are therefore quick to respond to physiologic or pathologic stimuli with an increased rate of cell division (hyperplasia).

Quiescent or stable tissues consist mainly of cells (e.g., the parenchymal cells of many organs, mesenchymal cells, or resting lymphocytes) that do not divide continuously and are said to reside in G_0 (i.e., outside the cell cycle). However, quiescent cells can reenter the cell cycle in response to hormonal stimuli or growth factors and are capable of striking proliferation in certain physiologic states (e.g., the pregnant uterus or the lactating mammary gland), as well as replacement of damaged tissue in disease (e.g., regeneration of hepatic tissue after lobectomy). The recruitment of quiescent cells into the cell cycle, a major mechanism to increase cellular replication, requires physiologic or pathologic signals to overcome barriers to proliferation.

Other adult tissues (e.g., the CNS, skeletal muscle, and myocardium) are composed mainly of terminally differentiated cells (e.g., neurons, skeletal myocytes, and cardiomyocytes) that no longer divide. Obviously, such cells must have a longer life span than the terminally differentiated cells of labile tissues, but if destroyed, they generally cannot be replaced by the same type of cell. That said, even relatively permanent tissues, such as those of the CNS, have stem cell niches.

The stem cells in adult tissues have an unlimited capacity to proliferate, although their rate of cell division is generally much lower than that of more differentiated cells. Importantly, stem cell division is asymmetric, producing one daughter cell that can differentiate into a variety of mature cell types and another daughter cell with stem cell properties.

The degree of cellular differentiation affects the size of a cell population and its proliferative potential. In labile tissues, such as bone marrow, epidermis, or mucosal epithelium, the mature cells are terminally differentiated, incapable of replication, and short-lived but are replaced by new cells arising from the germinal population, which cycles continuously. Most cells in stable tissues, such as hepatic or renal parenchyma, are in G_0 but retain the ability to proliferate on demand. In contrast, relatively permanent tissues, such as the brain, spinal cord, myocardium, or skeletal muscle, are composed mainly of terminally differentiated cells that are incapable of replicating.

Cellular Aging

With advanced age the function of cells and tissues diminishes from the molecular to the organismal level. DNA, especially telomeric DNA (see the following section), and metabolic pathway components affect the life span of cells in tissue culture and in laboratory mice. The stem cell theory of aging postulates that critical shortening of telomeres results in a DNA damage response (DDR) that activates p53 and leads to growth arrest, senescence, or apoptosis of the affected cell. A theory that combines genetic and metabolic pathways postulates that even indirect DNA damage through epigenetic changes, oxidative injury, or other cellular stresses can initiate the DDR, and that persistent DDR causes mitochondrial injury that generates a feed-forward loop.[5]

Genetic Basis of Aging

Telomeres

Since the discovery that functional telomeres were the limiting factor for replication of fibroblasts in cell culture, telomeres have been at the forefront of research on cellular aging. Most somatic cells have a finite number of cell divisions that, at least in part, is determined by the length of telomeres. Telomeres are repetitive nucleotide (TTA-GGG) sequences that cap the ends of linear chromosomes, providing a template for complete replication of the chromosomal DNA and preventing the chromosomal ends from being misinterpreted as double-stranded DNA breaks. Telomeric DNA is protected from inappropriate repair by associated proteins that form the *shelterin complex*. Telomeres are truncated (shortened) with each cell division because the DNA polymerases require a leading primer and so cannot replicate all the way to the end of the DNA molecule. In "immortal" cells, such as germ cells or certain stem cells, leukocytes (e.g., activated T lymphocytes), or cancer cells, active telomerase replenishes telomeres (E-Fig. 1-19). Telomerase consists of an RNA subunit template component (TERC) and a catalytic component (TERT), which is a reverse transcriptase. Mutations of either component have been associated with aging syndromes and other disorders. Dysfunctional telomeres signal the DDR with activation of p53 and arrest of the cell cycle. Arrest of the cell cycle can be a temporary pause for DNA repair or can progress to senescence (an irreversible growth arrest) or to cell death through apoptosis. DNA repair pathways that are triggered by dysfunctional telomeres tend to result in abnormal repair (e.g., chromosomal fusions) that exacerbates the DNA damage and elicits a persistent DDR.

A purely telomeric theory of aging does not explain the aging in tissues or organs composed mainly of quiescent postmitotic cells (e.g., neurons and muscle cells), in which telomeres would be less important. A broader theory combines DNA damage and metabolic abnormalities (E-Fig. 1-20) and proposes that endogenous and exogenous factors contribute to telomere dysfunction, impaired DDR, or increased ROS, each of which can independently activate p53, which in turn compromises mitochondrial function through repression of coactivators of peroxisome proliferator-activated receptor γ (PPARγ), a nuclear receptor that regulates many metabolic pathways. The interplay between the DDR and metabolism is complex; however, induction of a persistent DDR activates p53. Repression of PPARγ coactivators by p53 exacerbates oxidative injury and decreases energy production. Although p53 also represses the insulin/insulin-like growth factor-1 (IGF-1) and mTOR[6] pathways, this repression can protect cells by activating forkhead box protein O (FOXO) transcription factors and PPARγ coactivators that promote oxidative phosphorylation, antioxidant production, and p53 inactivation.

Cellular Senescence

The gradual decline in function in aging animals is associated with both degenerative and proliferative changes that are intricately linked to the stress response known as cellular senescence (E-Fig. 1-21). Genetically, senescence seems to be a situation of antagonistic pleiotropy, in which a group of genes are beneficial in early life, promoting survival during the reproductive years, yet the same genes contribute to debility and other diseases in aging animals.

The stresses that typically cause senescence include DNA damage (especially shortening of telomeres), epigenomic damage, oncogenes and other mitogenic stimuli, and activation of certain tumor suppressor genes. Notably, oxidative stress can indirectly cause double-stranded DNA breaks, especially in the guanine-rich telomeric DNA. Cellular senescence is an essentially irreversible arrest of the cell cycle, regulated by two tumor suppressor pathways: p53-p21 and p16^{INK4a}-RB. When the DDR becomes persistent, p53 causes growth arrest through the cell cycle inhibitor p21. A persistent DDR also, through p38 MAPK (a mitogen-activated protein kinase pathway component), protein kinase C, and ROS, activates p16^{INK4a}, which in turn activates RB protein, halting the cell cycle.

The benefits of cellular senescence are that it can prevent the formation of neoplasms and promote wound healing with less scarring. However, cellular senescence can also promote the degenerative diseases of old age and, ironically, can contribute to tumor progression in aging animals (see Chapter 6).

[5]A feed-forward loop is the positive or negative effect that a process or substance in a metabolic pathway may have on another substance or step in a process that occurs later in the pathway.

[6]Mammalian target of rapamycin (mTOR) is a growth regulator that can be inhibited by caloric restriction (or by rapamycin, hence the name) with a protective effect on mitochondria.

Structural and Biochemical Changes with Cellular Aging

In long-lived postmitotic cells, such as neurons and striated muscle cells, lipofuscin tends to accumulate with advancing age. Senescent cells (i.e., cells that were mitotic but have ceased to divide because of accumulated DNA damage or other factors) have cytologically detectable heterochromatin foci, increased volume, and a flattened profile if adherent to a basement membrane or other scaffolding.

Biochemically, senescent cells are recognized in part by their lack of expression of proliferation markers. Senescent cells take on what is known as a senescence-associated secretory phenotype (SASP). They overexpress the acidic lysosomal enzyme β-galactosidase. Another commonly used marker of senescence is $p16^{INK4a}$. The SASP is associated with secretion of numerous proinflammatory cytokines, as well as chemokines, growth factors, and proteases, including, as examples, growth-regulated oncogenes, vascular endothelial growth factor (VEGF), secreted frizzled related protein 1 that modulates Wnt, IL-6 and IL-8, and matrix metalloproteinases. Some SASP factors promote or inhibit proliferation depending on the setting. Other SASP factors can elicit inflammation or induce epithelial-to-mesenchymal transition, which can be part of the progression to invasive cancer. Importantly, not all senescent cells assume a SASP; it is mainly a response to DNA damage or epigenomic perturbations. NFκB has a positive effect on the SASP; p53, in contrast, restrains it.

Genetic Basis of Disease

Genetic diseases are caused by alterations in the number, structure, and/or function of chromosomes and their genes and gene products (proteins). Genes determine the differentiation, development, maturation, and aging of the 200 to 210 cell types in an animal's body and the tissues and organ systems they form. Additionally, they establish (1) the structural and functional roles each of these cell types plays in forming barrier systems and defense mechanisms against noninfectious and infectious diseases and (2) how each of these cell types and their organelles respond in homeostasis and to cellular adaptation, injury, aging, and neoplasia. Alterations in the structure and/or function of genes and gene products can have serious outcomes on cells, tissues, and organ systems that are reflected in patterns of lesions unique to affected cells and thus clinical signs reflective of the disease. Specific diseases with genetic bases are discussed in more detail in the Pathology of Organ Systems chapters; this section provides an "E-content" overview of (1) the structure and function of chromosomes and genes, (2) some basic mechanisms of genetic disorders, and (3) the outcomes of specific genetic diseases and includes:

- Chromosome Structure and Function
  - Nuclear Chromosomes
  - Mitochondrial Chromosomes
- Gene Structure and Function
- Mechanisms of Genetic Disorders
  - Single-Gene Disorders
    - Single-Gene Disorders of Somatic Cells
    - Single-Gene Disorders of Germ Cells
      - Autosomal Dominant Disorders
      - Autosomal Recessive Disorders
      - X-Linked Disorders
    - Single-Gene Disorders of Mitochondria
  - Chromosomal Disorders
    - Errors in Cell Division
      - Numeric Alterations
      - Structural Alterations
  - Complex Multigenic Disorders

The interaction of microbial genes with host genes in determining resistance to infectious diseases is discussed in Chapter 4. The role of genes in controlling immune responses and neoplastic transformation is discussed in Chapters 5 and 6, respectively. Examples of known or suspected genetic disorders in domestic animals are listed in E-Box 1-1 and are discussed in the chapters covering pathology of organ systems.

Information on this topic is available at www.expertconsult.com.

Types of Diagnoses

Anatomic and clinical pathologists endeavor to develop clear and concise morphologic diagnoses that describe lesions observed in "wet" tissues (postmortem examination-gross lesions) and in tissue sections and cytologic impressions (microscopic lesions). The nomenclature of a morphologic diagnosis attempts to describe and categorize lesions based on established patterns that most commonly characterize the following observations of the injury: degree, duration, distribution, exudate, modifiers, and tissue (DDDEMT). The nomenclature of each of these DDDEMT injury observations is described in more detail in Table 3-6 and Chapter 3.

Information on this topic is available at www.expertconsult.com.

Summary

This chapter is focused on the response to injury at the cellular level, but the student must remember that an injured cell is affected not only by its direct injury but also by neighboring and distant cells, stroma, and vasculature, and that the injured cell in turn affects cells and tissues around it (and at distant sites). In subsequent chapters we will see how blood flow, the inflammatory response, the immune response, and other factors come into play and realize that the whole body, not just one or a few cells, responds to injury.

Suggested Readings

Suggested Readings are available at www.expertconsult.com.

CHAPTER 2

Vascular Disorders and Thrombosis[1]

Derek A. Mosier

Key Readings Index

Free-living unicellular organisms obtain nutrients from and eliminate metabolic waste products directly into the external environment. Multicellular organisms require a circulatory system to deliver nutrients to and remove waste products from cells. The movement of fluid and cells through the circulatory system maintains homeostasis and integrates functions of cells and tissues in complex, multicellular organisms. In this chapter the basic abnormalities that affect fluid circulation and balance within an animal are described.

Circulatory System

The circulatory system consists of blood, a central pump (heart), blood distribution (arterial) and collection (venous) networks, and a system for exchange of nutrients and waste products between blood and extravascular tissue (microcirculation [also known as microvasculature]) (Fig. 2-1). A network of lymphatic vessels that parallel the veins also contributes to circulation by draining fluid from extravascular spaces into the blood vascular system.

The heart provides the driving force for blood distribution. Equal volumes of blood are normally distributed to the pulmonary circulation by the right side of the heart and the systemic circulation by the left side of the heart. The volume of blood pumped by each half of the heart per minute (cardiac output) is determined by the beats per minute (heart rate) and the volume of blood pumped per beat by the ventricle (stroke volume). Typically each half of the heart pumps the equivalent of the entire blood volume of the animal per minute.

Arteries have relatively large diameter lumens to facilitate rapid blood flow with minimal resistance. Artery walls are thick and consist predominantly of smooth muscle fibers for tensile strength and elastic fibers for elasticity (E-Fig. 2-1). Elastic fibers allow arteries to act as pressure reservoirs, expanding to hold blood ejected from the heart during contraction and passively recoiling to provide continuous flow and pressure to arterioles between heart contractions.

Arterioles are the major resistance vessels within the circulatory system; intravascular pressure can fall by nearly half after blood passes through an arteriole. Arterioles have relatively narrow lumens, the diameter of which is controlled by the smooth muscle cells that are the major component of their walls. Extrinsic sympathetic innervation and local intrinsic stimuli regulate the degree of arteriolar smooth muscle contraction, causing arterioles to dilate or constrict to selectively distribute blood to the areas of greatest need.

Capillaries are the site of nutrient and waste product exchange between the blood and tissue. Capillaries are the most numerous vessel in the circulatory system, with a total cross-sectional area nearly 1300 times that of the aorta. However, they normally contain only approximately 5% of the total blood volume. The velocity of blood flow through the capillaries is very slow, and red blood cells generally move through a capillary in single file to further facilitate the diffusion of nutrients and wastes. Capillaries have narrow lumens (approximately 3 to 10 μm) and thin walls (approximately 1 μm) consisting of a single epithelial cell layer (endothelium). At the junctions between capillary endothelia are interendothelial pores, which make the capillary semipermeable to facilitate diffusion of nutrients and waste products between the blood and tissues. There are three types of capillaries: continuous, fenestrated, and discontinuous. The basic functions and tissue locations of these types of capillaries are illustrated in Figure 2-2. They are discussed in greater detail in the chapters covering the diseases of organ systems.

The return trip of blood to the heart begins in the postcapillary venules. Venules have a composition similar to capillaries but may have thin layers of muscle as they become more distant from the capillary bed. Veins are composed mainly of collagen with smaller amounts of elastin and smooth muscle (see E-Fig. 2-1). Venules and veins provide a low-resistance pathway for the return of blood to the heart. Because of their distensibility, they can store large amounts of blood; nearly 65% of total blood volume is normally present within the systemic veins. Pressure and velocity of flow are low within venules and veins. Therefore other factors are necessary to help move venous blood toward the heart such as venous valves to prevent backflow of blood, skeletal muscle contraction, venous vasoconstriction, an increased pressure gradient due to decreased pressure in the heart during filling (cardiac-suction effect), and decreased

[1]For a glossary of abbreviations and terms used in this chapter see E-Glossary 2-1.

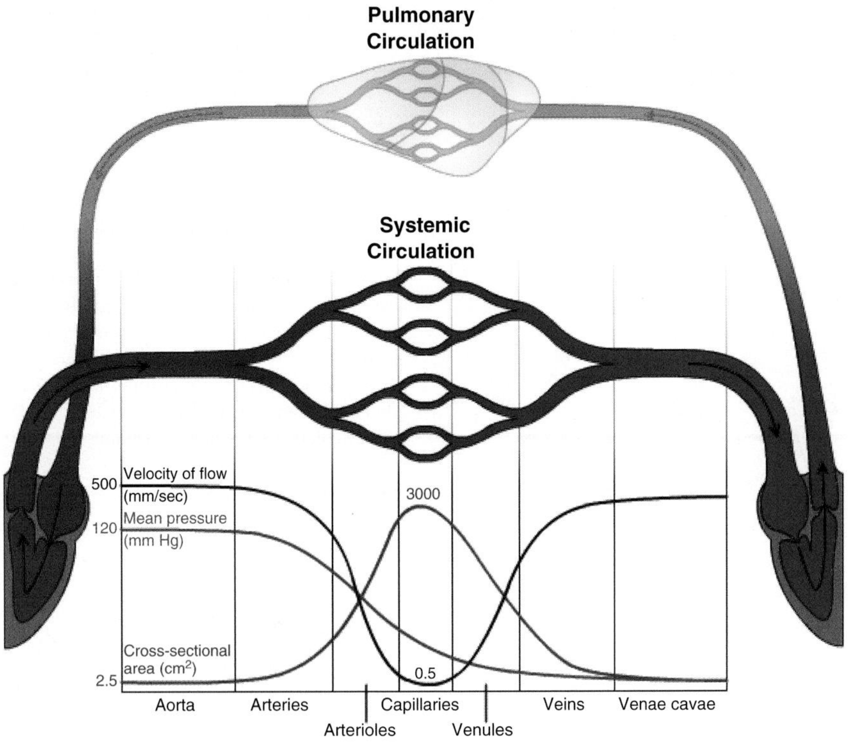

Figure 2-1 **The Vascular System.** Blood travels from the left to the right side of the heart via the systemic circulation, and from the right to the left side via the pulmonary circulation. Blood flow rate and pressure in the systemic arterial circulation decrease in conjunction with increased arterial cross-sectional area. In the venous systemic circulation, blood flow rate, but not pressure, increases in conjunction with decreased venous cross-sectional area. The flow, pressure, and cross-sectional area relationships are similar but reversed (i.e., veins deliver blood and arteries collect blood) in the pulmonary circulation. (Courtesy Dr. D.A. Mosier and L. Schooley, College of Veterinary Medicine, Kansas State University.)

pressure in the thoracic veins due to negative pressure within the thoracic cavity (respiratory pump).

The lymphatic system originates as blind-ended lymphatic capillaries, which permeate the tissue surrounding the microcirculation (arterioles, metarterioles, capillaries, and postcapillary venules [Fig. 2-3]). Lymphatic capillaries have overlapping endothelial cells and large interendothelial gaps so that external pressure allows movement of fluid and molecules into the vessel. However, intravascular lymphatic pressure forces these overlapping edges together to prevent the flow of lymph out of the vessel. Lymphatic capillary gaps are much larger than those between blood capillary endothelium, so they can accommodate movement of larger particles and substances. Lymphatic capillaries converge into progressively larger lymph vessels that drain into lymph nodes and then ultimately empty into the venous system. Similar to venous vessels, lymphatic vessels are distensible, low-pressure vessels that require lymphatic valves and contraction of surrounding muscles to facilitate return of fluid to the blood.

A single layer of endothelium lines all components of the circulatory system. Endothelium forms a dynamic interface between blood and tissue and is a critical participant in fluid distribution, inflammation, immunity, angiogenesis, and hemostasis (Fig. 2-4). Normal endothelium is antithrombotic and profibrinolytic and helps maintain blood in a fluid state, but when injured, endothelium becomes prothrombotic and antifibrinolytic. Endothelial activation by oxidative stress, hypoxia, inflammation, infectious agents, tissue injury, or similar events results in the production and release of numerous substances with wide-ranging roles in physiology and pathology (Box 2-1). Endothelial activation is typically localized to restrict a host response to a specific area, while not affecting the normal function of endothelium and flow of blood in other parts of the body.

Microcirculation, Interstitium, and Cells

The exchange of fluid, nutrients, and waste products between blood and cells takes place through the interstitium, the space between cells, and the microcirculation. The interstitium is composed of structural, adhesive, and absorptive components collectively referred to as the *extracellular matrix* (ECM). Type I collagen is the major structural component of the ECM and forms the framework in which cells reside. This is intimately associated with type IV collagen of cell basement membranes. Adhesive glycoproteins provide sites of attachment for structural components and also serve as receptors for cells, such as phagocytes and lymphocytes, which move through the interstitium. Absorptive disaccharide complexes (glycosaminoglycans) and protein-disaccharide polymer complexes (proteoglycans) are hydrophilic and can bind large amounts of water and other soluble molecules. In most cases, no more than 1.0 mm of interstitial space separates a cell from a capillary.

Fluid Distribution and Homeostasis

Water constitutes approximately 60% of body weight, of which approximately two-thirds is intracellular and one-third is extracellular (80% of which is in the interstitium and 20% is in the plasma). Physical barriers, as well as pressure and concentration gradients between each compartment, control the distribution of fluid-nutrients and waste products between the blood, interstitium, and cells. The cell's plasma membrane is a selective barrier that separates interstitial and intracellular compartments. Nonpolar (uncharged) lipid-soluble substances, such as O_2, CO_2, and fatty acids, move relatively freely across the plasma membrane based on their pressure or concentration gradients. Polar (charged) lipid-insoluble particles

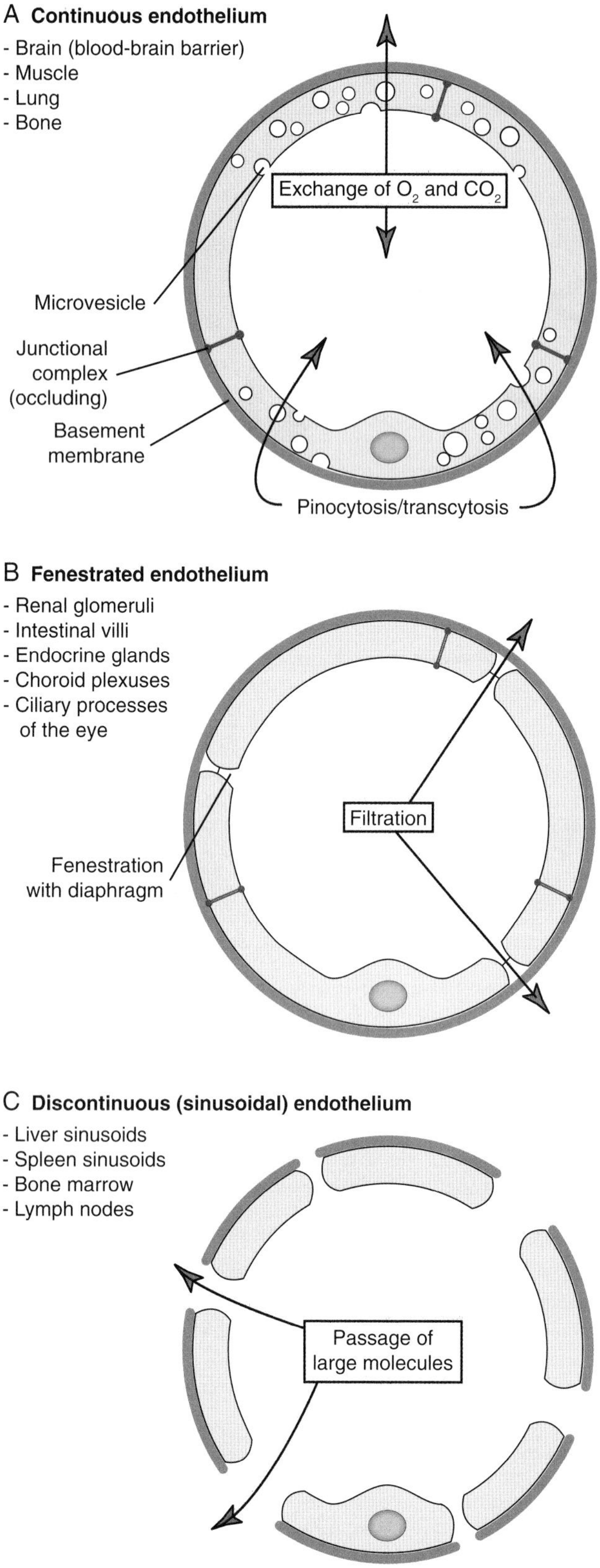

Figure 2-2 Types of Endothelium Lining Capillaries. **A**, Continuous endothelium. This type of endothelium forms a barrier system that strictly controls the transfer of molecules across the cell. It only allows transfer of H_2O, O_2, CO_2, and ions across the endothelium or through its junctional complexes. **B**, Fenestrated endothelium. This type of endothelium has fenestrae (pores) in endothelial cells that are bridged by a thin membrane. It allows controlled transfer of small molecules and limited amounts of protein across the fenestrae (filtration mechanism). **C**, Discontinuous (sinusoidal) endothelium. The junctional complexes in this type of endothelium have large "gap" openings (30 to 40 μm in diameter) between endothelial cells. These gaps allow "free" transfer of plasma proteins, red and white blood cells, water, and most molecules across endothelial cells in organs that need "mass" migration of materials such as the liver. Additionally, transfer of these molecules across the endothelium is facilitated by a discontinuous basal lamina (basement membrane). (Courtesy Dr. D.A. Mosier, College of Veterinary Medicine, Kansas State University; and Dr. J.F. Zachary, College of Veterinary Medicine, University of Illinois.)

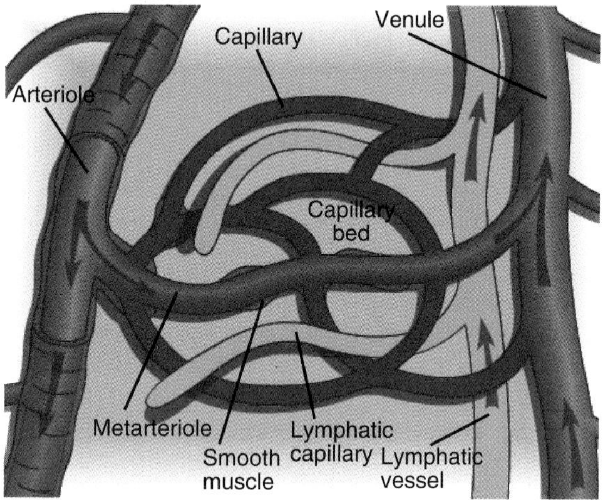

Figure 2-3 The Microcirculation. The microcirculation consists of arterioles (small arteries proximal to a capillary bed), metarterioles (arterial capillaries), capillaries (thin, semipermeable vessels that connect arterioles and venules), and postcapillary venules (small vessels that merge to form veins after collecting blood from a capillary network). Smooth muscle of the arterioles and metarterioles regulates flow of blood into the capillary bed. There is a dramatic drop in pressure and flow rate from the arterial to the venous side of the microcirculation, facilitating interactions between capillary blood and interstitial fluid. Blind-ended lymphatic vessels that originate near capillary beds interact intimately with the microcirculation. (Courtesy Dr. D.A. Mosier and L. Schooley, College of Veterinary Medicine, Kansas State University.)

and molecules, such as electrolytes, calcium, glucose, and amino acids, enter the cell by carrier-mediated transport. Water readily moves across the plasma membrane down its concentration gradient. Although approximately 100 times the volume of water in a cell crosses the plasma membrane in 1 second, cell fluid content remains relatively stable because of the activity of energy-dependent membrane pumps (e.g., Na^+/K^+-adenosine triphosphatase [ATPase] pump) and the balance between osmotic pressures exerted by interstitial and intracellular solutes.

The capillary wall is a semipermeable barrier that influences the movement of fluid, nutrients, and waste products between the blood and interstitium. Lipid-soluble substances can pass through capillary endothelium by dissolving in the membrane lipid bilayer, and large

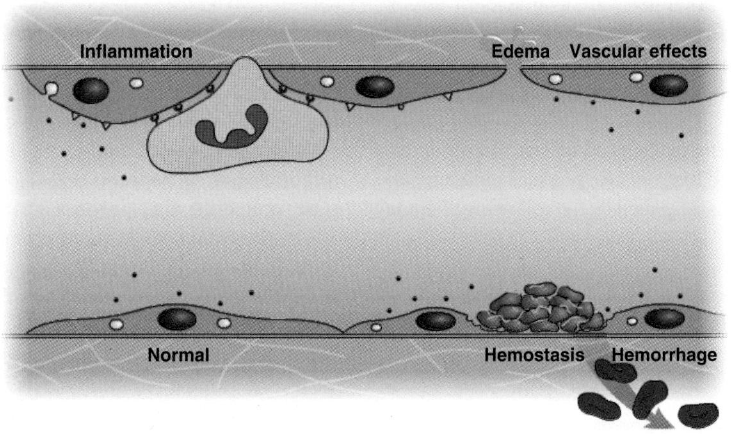

Figure 2-4 **Structure and Function of the Endothelium.** Endothelium is a physical barrier between intravascular and extravascular spaces, and it is an important mediator of fluid distribution, hemostasis, inflammation, and healing. (Courtesy Dr. D.A. Mosier and L. Schooley, College of Veterinary Medicine, Kansas State University.)

Box 2-1 Endothelial Cell Functions and Responses in Homeostasis and Disease

FLUID DISTRIBUTION AND BLOOD FLOW

Semipermeable membrane for fluid distribution
- Interendothelial junctions

Vasodilation
- Nitric oxide
- Prostacyclin (PGI_2)
- Endothelial-derived hyperpolarizing factor
- C-type natriuretic peptide

Vasoconstriction
- Endothelin
- Reactive oxygen species
- Angiotensin II
- Products of prostaglandin H_2 (e.g., thromboxane A_2)

HEMOSTASIS

Antihemostatic substances
- PGI_2
- Endothelial cell protein C receptor
- Tissue factor pathway inhibitor (TFPI)
- Tissue plasminogen activator (tPA)
- Heparan sulfate
- Adenosine diphosphatase (ADPase) and adenosine triphosphatase (ATPase)
- Protein S
- Thrombomodulin

Prohemostatic substances
- von Willebrand factor
- Tissue factor (TF) (factor III)
- Plasminogen activator inhibitor-1 (PAI-1)
- Protease-activated receptors (PARs)

INFLAMMATION

Cytokines
- Interleukin (IL) -1, IL-6, IL-8

Acute Phase Proteins
- C-reactive protein

Enhanced expression of TF

Expression of leukocyte adhesion molecules:
- Cell adhesion molecule family
  - Mucosal addressin cell adhesion molecule 1 (MAdCAM-1)
  - Intercellular adhesion molecule 1 (ICAM-1)
  - Vascular cell adhesion molecule 1 (VCAM-1)
  - Platelet endothelial cell adhesion molecule 1 (PECAM-1)
- Selectin family
  - P-selectin
  - E-selectin

GROWTH FACTORS

Platelet-derived growth factor (PDGF)
Colony-stimulating factor (CSF)
Fibroblast growth factor (FGF)
Transforming growth factor-β (TGF-β)
Heparin

FIBRINOLYSIS

Synthesis and secretion of fibrinolytic components under certain circumstances
Regulation of formation of plasmin
tPA
Urokinase plasminogen activator receptor
PAI-1
Annexin II

proteins can move through the cell by transport within vesicles. Most importantly, water and polar molecules move through interendothelial pores. Normally these pores are large enough to allow the passage of water, small nutrients (ions, glucose, amino acids), and waste products, yet small enough to prevent the movement of cells and large proteins (albumin and other plasma proteins such as complement, kinin, and coagulation proteins). Local stimuli, such as inflammation, can cause endothelial cells to contract to widen interendothelial pores and allow the passage of larger molecules. Under normal conditions the composition of plasma and interstitial fluid is very similar, with the exception of the large plasma proteins.

Movement of substances through interendothelial pores and cell membranes is generally passive in response to concentration and pressure gradients. Nutrient-rich arterial blood contains O_2, glucose, and amino acids that move down their pressure or concentration gradients into the interstitium, where they are available for use by cells. CO_2 and waste products generated by cells accumulate in the interstitium and move down their gradient into the venous blood. These gradients become larger in areas where cells are metabolically active.

Water distribution between the plasma and interstitium is determined mainly by osmotic and hydrostatic pressure differentials between the compartments and is described by the following formula (Fig. 2-5):

$$\text{Net filtration across the endothelium} = K[(P_{cap} - P_{int}) - \sigma(\pi_{cap} - \pi_{int})]$$

K = Capillary endothelial permeability constant
P = Hydrostatic pressure
σ = Reflection coefficient
π = Colloid osmotic pressure
cap = capillary
int = interstitium

Although sodium and chloride account for approximately 84% of the total osmolality of plasma, free movement of these electrolytes through interendothelial pores balances their concentrations in the plasma and interstitium, so their contribution to differences in osmotic pressure between these compartments is minimal. In contrast, nonpermeable, suspended plasma proteins make up less than 1% of the total osmolality of plasma. However, because these proteins (particularly albumin) do not readily move through interendothelial pores, they exert a colloidal osmotic pressure that is responsible for the majority of the difference in osmotic pressure between the plasma and interstitium.

In the microcirculation, intravascular and interstitial osmotic pressures and interstitial hydrostatic forces remain relatively constant and favor intravascular retention of fluid. However, high

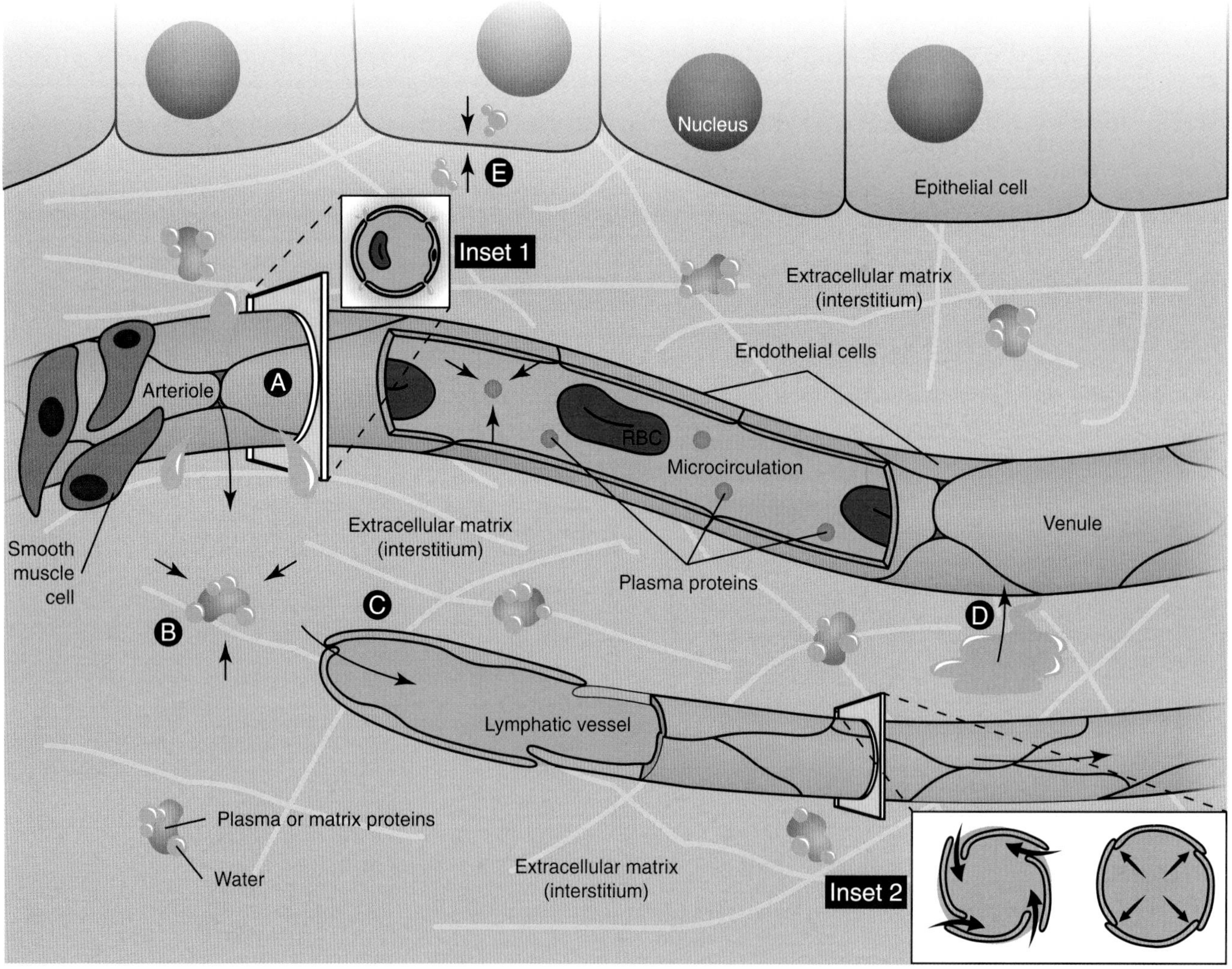

Figure 2-5 **Factors Affecting Fluid Balance in the Microcirculation.** Fluid distribution is determined by physical characteristics of the microcirculation and lymphatic vessels and osmotic and hydrostatic forces within the blood and interstitial fluid. Intercellular gaps between endothelium allow movement of fluid and small molecules between the blood and interstitial fluid *(insets 1 and 2)*. *A*, High arteriolar hydrostatic pressure forces fluid into the interstitium. *B*, Plasma proteins (e.g., albumin) and molecules within the extracellular matrix exert an osmotic effect to attract and retain water. *C*, Interstitial hydrostatic pressure forces interstitial fluid into lower-pressure venules. *D*, The slight excess of interstitial fluid not returned to the venules enters the lymphatic vessels to be drained from the area. *E*, Exchange of intracellular and interstitial fluid is balanced by osmotic forces and concentration gradients of electrolytes and other molecules across the cell plasma membrane. *Inset 1*, Cross section of a blood vessel capillary showing interendothelial junctions. Endothelium forms end-to-end junctions for movement of fluid and small molecules. *Inset 2*, Cross section of a lymphatic capillary showing the interendothelial junctions. Endothelium overlaps to allow movement of larger particles and closure when intravascular pressure forces overlapping endothelium together. (Courtesy Dr. D.A. Mosier and L. Schooley, College of Veterinary Medicine, Kansas State University.)

hydrostatic pressures within the arteriolar end of the capillary bed result in a net filtration of fluid into the interstitium. Lower hydrostatic pressures in the venular end of the capillary bed result in a net absorption pressure and reentry of fluid into the microvasculature. Alternatively, filtration and absorption may not occur because of a drop in hydrostatic pressure across individual capillary beds. Instead, filtration may occur across the entire length of capillary beds with high rates of blood flow, whereas absorption may occur across the entire length of capillary beds with low blood flow rates. The slight excess of fluid that is retained in the interstitium and any plasma proteins that have escaped the vasculature enter lymphatic capillaries to be drained from the area.

The constant flow of fluid between the microcirculation and interstitium allows exchange of nutrients and waste products between these two fluid compartments to support cell functions. Additionally, the interstitium provides a fluid buffer to either increase or decrease the plasma volume to ensure effective circulatory function. Excessive fluid intake will expand plasma volume and increase hydrostatic pressure, resulting in greater filtration into the interstitium to maintain a relatively constant plasma volume. Reduced fluid intake will decrease plasma volume, shifting the movement of water from the interstitium into the plasma to increase circulating fluid volume.

Abnormal Fluid Distribution

Alteration in any of the factors that regulate normal fluid distribution between the plasma, interstitium, and cells can lead to pathologic imbalances between these compartments.

Imbalance between Intracellular and Interstitial Compartments

Distribution of fluid between the interstitium and cells is generally dynamic but stable. This stability is necessary to maintain a relatively constant intracellular environment for cell function. Generalized conditions (e.g., alterations in plasma volume) and local stimuli (e.g., inflammation) can result in slight and usually transient shifts in fluid distribution between the interstitium and cells. Excess plasma volume (hypervolemia) results in movement of additional water into the interstitium and ultimately into the cell along both osmotic and hydrostatic gradients, causing cell swelling. In contrast, reduced plasma volume (hypovolemia) can result in a flow of water in the opposite direction, resulting in cell shrinkage and decreased interstitial volume. Increased interstitial volume will also cause a slight flow of fluid into cells in the affected region.

Disruption of any of the mechanisms that maintain proper fluid distribution between the cell and interstitium can have serious consequences for the cell. Failure to maintain proper osmotic balance as a result of cell membrane damage or failure of the energy-dependent plasma membrane pumps results in cell swelling, which if not quickly corrected can lead to cell death by osmotic lysis.

Imbalance between Intravascular and Interstitial Compartments (Edema)

Changes in the distribution of fluid between the plasma and interstitium are most commonly manifested as edema, which is an accumulation of excess interstitial fluid. Edema occurs by four major mechanisms: (1) increased microvascular permeability, (2) increased intravascular hydrostatic pressure, (3) decreased intravascular osmotic pressure, and (4) decreased lymphatic drainage (Box 2-2).

Box 2-2 Causes of Edema

INCREASED VASCULAR PERMEABILITY

Vascular leakage associated with inflammation
- Infectious agents
  - Viruses (e.g., influenza and other respiratory viruses, canine adenovirus 1, equine and porcine *Arterivirus*, *Morbillivirus*)
  - Bacteria (e.g., *Clostridium* sp., Shiga-like toxin–producing *Escherichia coli*, *Erysipelothrix rhusiopathiae*)
  - Rickettsia (e.g., *Ehrlichia ruminantium*, *Neorickettsia risticii*, *Anaplasma phagocytophilum*, *Rickettsia rickettsii*)
- Immune-mediated
  - Type III hypersensitivity (e.g., feline infectious peritonitis, purpura hemorrhagica)

Neovascularization

Anaphylaxis (e.g., type I hypersensitivity to vaccines, venoms, and other allergens)

Toxins (e.g., endotoxin, paraquat, noxious gases, zootoxins)

Clotting abnormalities (e.g., pulmonary embolism, disseminated intravascular coagulation)

Metabolic abnormalities (e.g., microangiopathy caused by diabetes mellitus, encephalomalacia caused by thiamine deficiency)

INCREASED INTRAVASCULAR HYDROSTATIC PRESSURE

Portal hypertension (e.g., right-sided heart failure, hepatic fibrosis)

Pulmonary hypertension (e.g., left-sided heart failure, high-altitude disease)

Localized venous obstruction (e.g., gastric dilation and volvulus, intestinal volvulus and torsion, uterine torsion or prolapse, venous thrombosis)

Fluid overload (e.g., iatrogenic, sodium retention with renal disease)

Hyperemia (e.g., inflammation, physiologic)

DECREASED INTRAVASCULAR OSMOTIC PRESSURE

Decreased albumin production (e.g., malnutrition or starvation, debilitating diseases, severe hepatic disease)

Excessive albumin loss (e.g., gastrointestinal disease [protein-losing enteropathies] or parasitism [haemonchosis or trichostrongylosis in sheep], renal disease [protein-losing nephropathies], severe burns)

Water intoxication (e.g., hemodilution caused by sodium retention, salt toxicity)

DECREASED LYMPHATIC DRAINAGE

Lymphatic obstruction or compression (e.g., inflammatory or neoplastic masses, fibrosis)

Congenital lymphatic aplasia or hypoplasia

Intestinal lymphangiectasia

Lymphangitis (e.g., paratuberculosis, sporotrichosis, epizootic lymphangitis of horses)

Mechanisms of Edema Formation

The formation of edema can be attributed to the four basic mechanisms, acting independently or in combination, described in the following sections (Essential Concept 2-1).

Increased Microvascular Permeability

Increased microvascular permeability is most commonly associated with the initial microvascular reaction to inflammatory or immunologic stimuli. These stimuli induce localized release of mediators that cause vasodilation and increased microvascular permeability.

ESSENTIAL CONCEPT 2-1 Edema (See Fig. 2-5)

Edema occurs when there is an imbalance in the distribution of water (fluid) between the interstitium, cells, and intravascular space resulting in the accumulation of excess fluid in these structures. It is manifested as interstitial edema (extracellular matrix, stroma), intracellular edema (cytosol/cytoplasm), or hypervolemia (blood plasma) and is diagnosed clinically and explained pathologically as disorders such as generalized edema, dependent edema, pulmonary edema, corneal edema, cerebral edema, lymphedema, and myxedema. The four most important factors involved in the occurrence of edema are hydrostatic pressure, oncotic (colloidal osmotic) pressure, vascular integrity (lymphatic and blood vessels), and cell membrane integrity (ion pumps). Hydrostatic pressure is the pressure exerted by intravascular fluid (i.e., blood plasma) or extravascular fluid on the wall (i.e., endothelium) of the blood vessel. Oncotic pressure is the pressure created by colloids (e.g., albumin) in a fluid that prevents the movement of water from one solution (i.e., plasma) across a semipermeable membrane (i.e., vascular endothelium) into another solution (i.e., interstitial fluid) or vice versa. Plasma proteins (e.g., albumin) and absorptive glycoproteins within the interstitium establish the oncotic pressure balance across the microvasculature. Vascular integrity refers to the normal structure and function of the barrier system formed by the microvasculature and their type of lining endothelium (i.e., continuous, fenestrated, and discontinuous) (see Fig. 2-2). Mechanistically, edema occurs from one or a combination of the following: (1) increased intravascular hydrostatic pressure, (2) decreased intravascular oncotic pressure, (3) increased microvascular permeability, and (4) decreased lymphatic drainage. Therefore (1) interstitial edema results from increased intravascular hydrostatic pressure, decreased intravascular oncotic pressure, increased interstitial oncotic pressure, or failure of lymphatic drainage; (2) intracellular edema (i.e., cell swelling) usually occurs as a result of cell injury (i.e., plasma membrane or membrane pumps) but could result from decreased interstitial oncotic pressure or increased intracellular oncotic pressure; and (3) hypervolemia may result from increased intravascular oncotic pressure, increased interstitial hydrostatic pressure, or decreased interstitial oncotic pressure. Damage to the microvasculature and their cell junctions, as well as cell membranes of any cell type (e.g., neurons), can result in substantial redistribution of fluid based on pressure or concentration gradients of fluids and colloids between intracellular, interstitial, and intravascular compartments.

Mediators such as histamine, bradykinin, leukotrienes, and substance P, which cause endothelial cell contraction and widening of interendothelial gaps, induce immediate increases in permeability. Subsequent release of cytokines such as interleukin 1 (IL-1), tumor necrosis factor (TNF), and interferon-γ induces cytoskeletal rearrangements within endothelial cells that result in endothelial cell retraction and more persistent widening of interendothelial gaps. Movement of intravascular fluid through these gaps into the interstitium results in localized edema that can dilute an inflammatory agent. The reaction terminates as localized edema and regresses when the stimulus is mild. However, most cases progress to the leakage of plasma proteins and emigration of leukocytes as early events in the formation of an acute inflammatory exudate.

Increased Intravascular Hydrostatic Pressure

Increased intravascular hydrostatic pressure is most often due to increased blood volume in the microvasculature. This can be the result of an active increased flow of blood into the microvasculature (hyperemia), such as occurs with acute inflammation. But more commonly it results from passive accumulation of blood (congestion), often caused by heart failure or localized venous compression or obstruction. Increased microvascular volume and pressure cause increased filtration and reduced or even reversed fluid absorption back into the vessel. When increased hydrostatic pressure affects a localized portion of microvasculature, the edema is localized. In the case of heart failure, congestion and increased hydrostatic pressure can occur in the portal venous system (right heart failure), causing ascites; in the pulmonary venous system (left heart failure), causing pulmonary edema; or in both venous systems (generalized heart failure), causing generalized edema. Generalized edema can result in a reduction of circulating plasma volume and renal hypoperfusion, which activate a variety of volume-regulating compensatory responses. Plasma volume is increased through sodium retention induced by activation of the renin-angiotensin-aldosterone pathways, and water retention mediated by antidiuretic hormone (ADH) release following activation of intravascular volume and pressure receptors. The resulting intravascular volume overload further complicates the dynamics of fluid distribution that accompany heart failure.

Decreased Intravascular Osmotic Pressure

Decreased intravascular osmotic pressure most commonly results from decreased concentrations of plasma proteins, particularly albumin. Hypoalbuminemia reduces the intravascular colloidal osmotic pressure, resulting in increased fluid filtration and decreased absorption and culminating in edema. Hypoalbuminemia is caused by either decreased production of albumin by the liver or excessive loss from the plasma. Decreased hepatic production most commonly occurs because of a lack of adequate protein for the synthetic pathway as a result of malnutrition or intestinal malabsorption of protein. Less often, severe liver disease with decreased hepatocyte mass or impaired hepatocyte function can result in inadequate albumin production. Loss of albumin from the plasma can occur in gastrointestinal diseases characterized by severe blood loss, such as that caused by parasitism. Renal disease, in which glomerular and/or tubular function is impaired, can result in loss of albumin into the urine and dilution of remaining albumin caused by sodium retention and expanded intravascular fluid volume (e.g., nephrotic syndrome). Plasma exudation accompanying severe burns is a less frequent cause of albumin loss. Because of the systemic nature of hypoalbuminemia, edema caused by decreased intravascular osmotic pressure tends to be generalized.

Decreased Lymphatic Drainage

Decreased lymphatic drainage reduces the ability of the lymphatic system to remove the slight excess of fluid that normally accumulates in the interstitium during fluid exchange between the plasma and interstitium. This can occur because of lymph vessel compression by a neoplastic or inflammatory swelling, lymph vessel constriction caused by fibrosis, or internal blockage of a lymph vessel by a thrombus. Edema occurs once the capacity of the damaged lymphatic vessels is exceeded and is localized to the area served by the affected lymphatic vessels.

Morphologic Characteristics of Edema

Edema is morphologically characterized by clear to slightly yellow watery fluid that may contain small amounts of protein and/or small numbers of inflammatory cells (transudate), which thickens and expands affected interstitium (Fig. 2-6). When edema occurs in tissues adjacent to body cavities or open spaces, such as alveolar lumens, the increased interstitial pressure often forces fluid into these cavities and spaces. The result can be fluid within alveolar

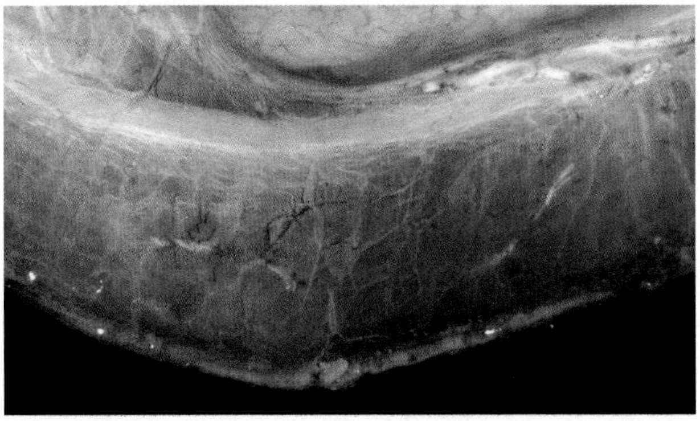

Figure 2-6 **Edema, Intestine, Submucosa, Horse.** Note the clear to slightly yellow fluid (which generally contains a small amount of protein [transudate]), which thickens and expands the affected submucosa. (Courtesy Department of Veterinary Biosciences, The Ohio State University; and Noah's Arkive, College of Veterinary Medicine, The University of Georgia.)

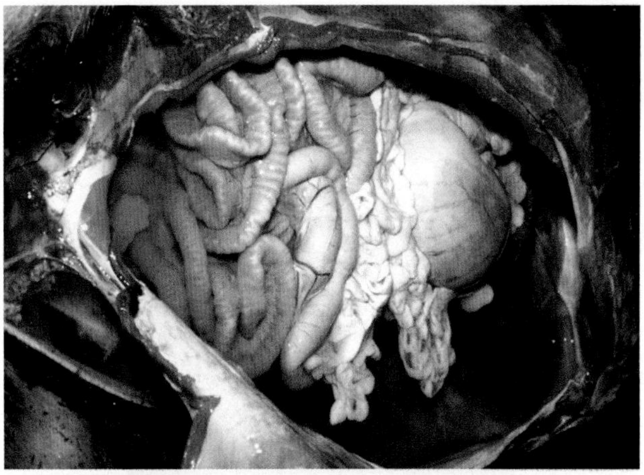

Figure 2-8 **Ascites (Hydroperitoneum), Peritoneal Cavity, Dog.** Slightly yellow fluid is present in the peritoneal cavity. When edema occurs in tissue adjacent to body cavities, the increased interstitial pressure forces the edema fluid, which is usually clear to slightly yellow (transudate), into these cavities. (Courtesy Dr. D.A. Mosier, College of Veterinary Medicine, Kansas State University.)

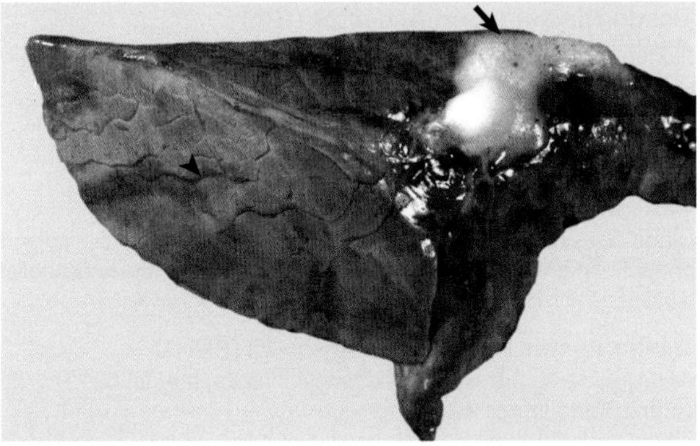

Figure 2-7 **Pulmonary Edema, Lung, Pig.** The lung failed to collapse and is heavy and firm due to edema fluid in alveoli and the interstitium. Note the prominent interlobular septa caused by edema *(arrowhead)* and the frothy edema fluid exuding from the bronchus *(arrow)*. (Courtesy Dr. M.D. McGavin, College of Veterinary Medicine, University of Tennessee.)

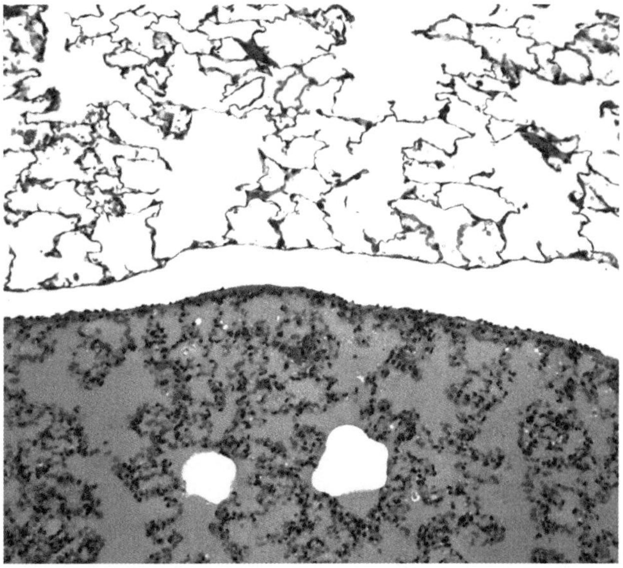

Figure 2-9 **Pulmonary Edema, Lung, Rat.** There is eosinophilic (pink staining) fluid distending the alveoli in the lower specimen. Histologically, edema is an amorphous, pale eosinophilic fluid, and the depth of the eosinophilia is proportional to its protein content. The fluid in this specimen has a high protein content. The upper specimen is normal rat lung. H&E stain. (Courtesy Dr. A. López, Atlantic Veterinary College; and Noah's Arkive, College of Veterinary Medicine, The University of Georgia.)

lumens (pulmonary edema; Fig. 2-7), the thoracic cavity (hydrothorax), the pericardial sac (hydropericardium), or the abdominal cavity (ascites or hydroperitoneum; Fig. 2-8). Histologically, edema is an amorphous, pale eosinophilic fluid (hematoxylin and eosin [H&E] stain) because of its low protein content (Fig. 2-9). The clinical significance of edema is variable, depending mainly on its location. Subcutaneous edema results in doughy to fluctuant skin and subcutis that is often cooler than adjacent unaffected tissue, but alone has minimal clinical significance (Fig. 2-10). Likewise, ascites does not generally have an impact on the function of abdominal organs. In contrast, edema of a tissue within a confined space, such as the brain in the cranial vault, can result in pressure within the organ that results in serious organ dysfunction. Similarly, filling a confined space with fluid, such as in hydrothorax or hydropericardium, can have a substantial impact on the function of the lungs and heart, respectively. In these situations, edema can have immediate and life-threatening implications.

Hemostasis

Hemostasis is the arrest of bleeding (Essential Concept 2-2). It is a physiologic response to vascular damage and provides a mechanism to seal an injured vessel to prevent blood loss. Hemostasis is a finely regulated process that predominantly involves interactions between endothelium, platelets, and coagulation factors. Physiologic hemostasis occurs only at the site of vascular injury, without affecting fluidity and flow of blood in normal undamaged vasculature. Disruption of the delicate balance of hemostasis can result in the pathologic states of blood loss (hemorrhage) or inappropriate hemostasis and thrombus formation (thrombosis).

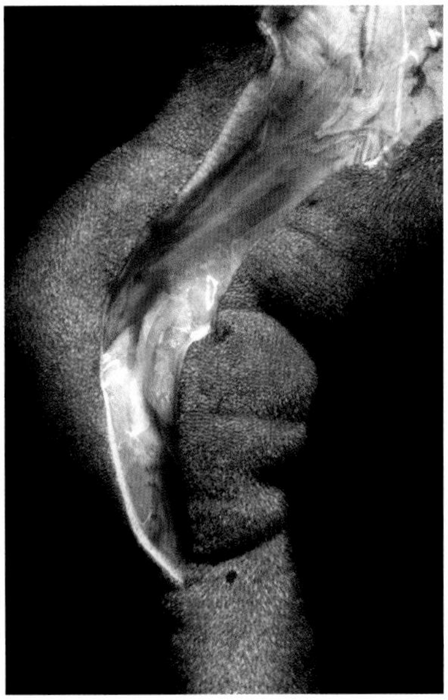

Figure 2-10 **Subcutaneous Edema, Congenital Lymphedema, Skin, Dog.** This form of edema results in doughy to fluctuant skin and subcutis. Edematous skin is often cooler than adjacent unaffected skin. In congenital lymphedema the lymph vessels are hypoplastic or aplastic. (Courtesy Dr. H. Liepold, College of Veterinary Medicine, Kansas State University.)

ESSENTIAL CONCEPT 2-2 Hemostasis (See Fig. 2-11)

Hemostasis is an immediate reparative response to injury of the vascular system designed to prevent blood loss. The response involves interdependent interactions between endothelium, platelets, and coagulation factors that are localized to the site of injury. Following vascular injury, hemostasis begins as a transient vasoconstriction and platelet aggregation to form a platelet plug at the site of injury (primary hemostasis). Narrowing of the vessel lumen reduces the volume of blood flowing through the damaged area and makes it easier for platelets to adhere to subendothelial tissues. Platelets mix with fibrinogen and form a loose aggregate covering the injury, and when injury is minimal, platelet aggregates contract into a dense "plug" that blocks the gap in the injured vessel and resolves the injury. If the injury is more severe, mediators released from the damaged area and aggregated platelets activate coagulation (see Fig. 2-11), leading to the formation of a fibrin-platelet aggregate (secondary hemostasis). Dissolution of the fibrin-platelet aggregate (thrombolysis/fibrinolysis) occurs concurrently with healing of the vessel wall and is initiated immediately following vessel injury, predominantly by the cleavage of the plasma protein plasminogen into plasmin, the major fibrinolytic protein (see Fig. 2-14).

Normal endothelium provides a surface that promotes the smooth, nonturbulent flow of blood. It produces and responds to mediators that enhance vasodilation and inhibit platelet activation and coagulation. In contrast, after injury or activation, endothelium produces or responds to mediators that induce vasoconstriction, enhance platelet adhesion and aggregation, and stimulate coagulation (Box 2-3).

Box 2-3 Endothelial Cell Mediators of Hemostasis

ANTICOAGULANT

Prostacyclin (PGI_2)
Maintains vascular relaxation and inhibits platelet adhesion and activation.

Nitric Oxide (NO)
Maintains vascular relaxation and inhibits platelet aggregation. Acts synergistically with the protein C pathway and antithrombin III (ATIII) to suppress thrombin production.

Thrombomodulin
Membrane protein that binds thrombin to initiate activation of protein C.

Protein S
Cofactor in protein C pathway; independently inhibits activation of factors VIII and X.

Heparin-Like Molecules
Heparan sulfate proteoglycans bind and concentrate ATIII on the endothelial surface.

Tissue Plasminogen Activator (tPA)
Activates fibrinolysis by stimulating plasminogen conversion to plasmin.

Adenosine Diphosphatase (ADP)
Degradation of ADP to inhibit its procoagulant effects.

Annexin V
Binds negatively charged phospholipids and calcium to displace phospholipid-dependent coagulation factors on the endothelial surface to inhibit formation of thrombin and factor Xa.

Tissue Factor Pathway Inhibitor-1 (TFPI-1)
A cell-surface protein that directly inhibits the factor TF:VIIa complex and factor Xa.

PROCOAGULANT

Tissue Factor
Produced after endothelial activation by substances such as cytokines, endotoxin, thrombin, immune complexes, and mitogens.

von Willebrand Factor
Released after endothelial exposure to substances such as thrombin, histamine, and fibrin.

Plasminogen Activator Inhibitor-1 (PAI-1)
Reduces fibrinolysis by inhibiting tPA and urokinase-like plasminogen activator (uPA).

Protease-Activated Receptors (PARs)
Serine protease (e.g., thrombin)–activated receptor resulting in endothelial cell activation.

VASCULAR REPAIR

Platelet-Derived Growth Factor (PDGF)
Stimulates mitogenesis of smooth muscle and fibroblasts.

Fibroblast Growth Factor (FGF)
Stimulates fibroblast proliferation.

Transforming Growth Factor-β (TGF-β)
Modulates vascular repair by inhibition of proliferation of various cell types, including endothelium.

Platelets are anucleate cell fragments derived from megakaryocytes that circulate as a component of blood. After vascular damage, platelets adhere to subendothelial collagen and other ECM components (e.g., laminin, fibronectin, and vitronectin). Adhered platelets express receptors that promote recruitment and aggregation of additional platelets and become activated to release the products of their cytoplasmic granules and produce other mediators of coagulation (Box 2-4). Platelet phospholipids that are exposed during platelet aggregation (particularly phosphatidylserine and phosphatidylethanolamine) play a critical role in establishing a biologic surface to localize and concentrate activated coagulation factors. In

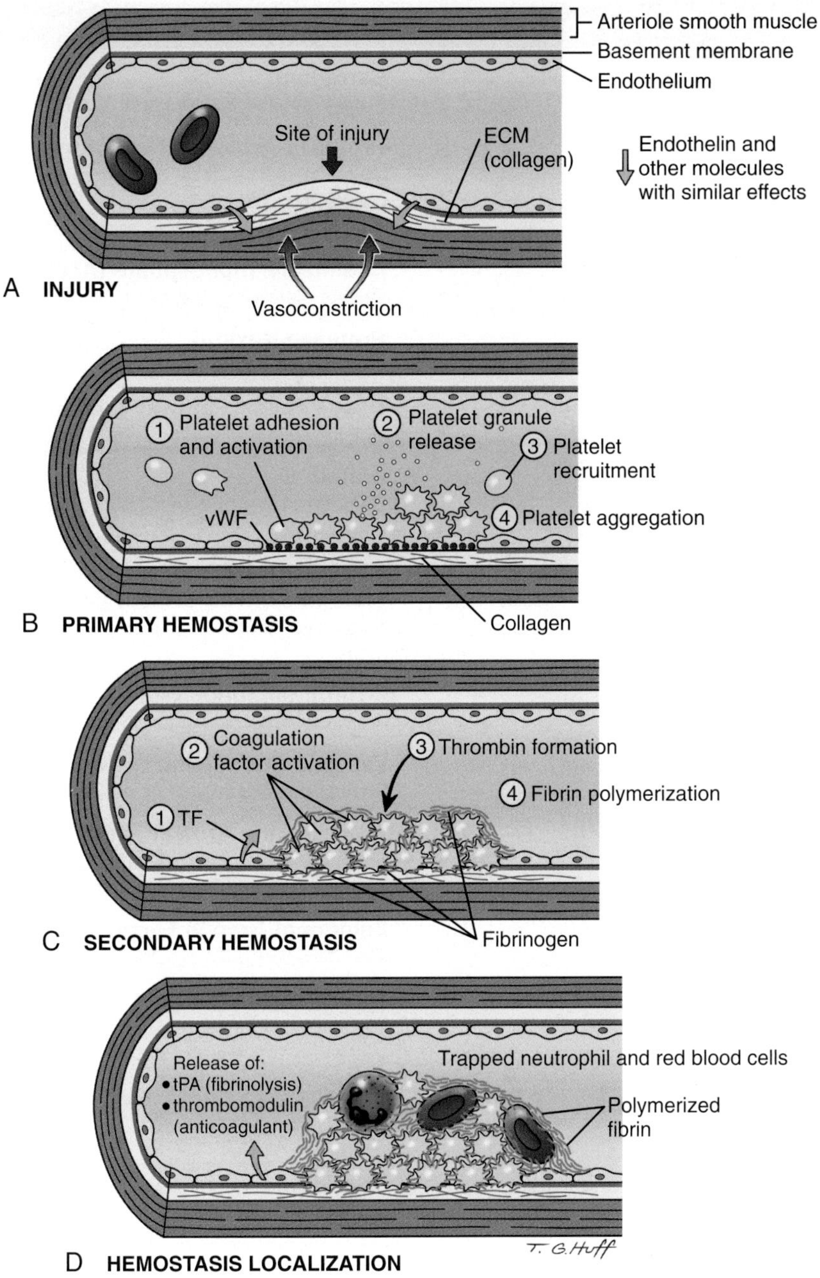

Figure 2-11 **Hemostatic Process. A**, Following vascular injury, local neural and humoral factors induce a transient vasoconstriction. **B**, Platelets adhere to the exposed subendothelial extracellular matrix (ECM) via von Willebrand factor (vWF) and become activated to release adenosine diphosphate, thromboxane A_2, and other procoagulant factors, resulting in aggregation of additional platelets and formation of a platelet plug (primary hemostasis). The numbers indicate the chronological order of events. **C**, Release of tissue factor (TF) and local activation of coagulation factors (resulting in conversion of prothrombin into thrombin) leads to fibrin polymerization that stabilizes the platelets into a platelet-fibrin meshwork (secondary hemostatic plug). The numbers indicate the chronological order of events. **D**, Regulatory mechanisms such as release of tissue plasminogen activator (tPA; fibrinolysis) and activation of thrombomodulin (anticoagulant) restrict the hemostatic process to the site of the vascular injury.

addition to their role in coagulation, platelets also participate in immunologic and inflammatory reactions.

Coagulation factors are plasma proteins produced mainly by the liver that are divided into (1) a structurally related and functionally interdependent contact group (prekallikrein, high-molecular-weight kininogen [HMWK], and factors XI and XII); (2) a vitamin K–dependent group (factors II, VII, IX, and X); and (3) a highly labile fibrinogen group (factors I, V, VIII, and XIII). Coagulation factors are activated by hydrolysis of arginine- or lysine-containing peptides to convert them to enzymatically active serine proteases (except for factor XIII, which has cysteine-rich active sites). The vitamin K–dependent coagulation factors play an important role in localizing coagulation by γ-carboxylating glutamic acid residues of N-terminal ends of precursor factors, so they can bind calcium to form calcium bridges with platelet phospholipids.

Hemostatic Process

The events that contribute to hemostasis are (1) transient vasoconstriction and platelet aggregation to form a platelet plug at the site of damage (primary hemostasis), (2) coagulation to form a meshwork of fibrin (secondary hemostasis), (3) fibrinolysis to remove the platelet/fibrin plug (thrombus retraction), and (4) tissue repair at

Box 2-4 Platelet Mediators in Hemostasis

PROCOAGULANT

Thromboxane A_2 (TXA_2)
Induces vasoconstriction and enhances platelet aggregation.

Phospholipids (i.e., phosphatidylserine and phosphatidylethanolamine)
Provide sites for coagulation reactions.

Adenosine Diphosphate (ADP)
Mediates platelet aggregation and activation.

Calcium
Cofactor in many coagulation reactions and promotes platelet aggregation.

Platelet Factor 4
Promotes platelet aggregation and inhibits heparin action.

Thrombospondin
Promotes platelet aggregation and inhibits heparin action.

Fibrinogen
Fibrin precursor, concentrated by binding to platelet receptor GpIIb-IIIa.

Factors V, XI, and XIII
Factors involved in coagulation reactions.

von Willebrand Factor
Promotes platelet adhesion to subendothelial collagen via platelet receptor GpIb.

α_2-Antiplasmin and α_2-Macroglobulin
Inhibition of plasmin.

Plasminogen Activator Inhibitor-1 (PAI-1)
Inhibits tissue plasminogen activator (tPA) and activated protein C to promote clot stabilization.

Thrombin-Activatable Fibrinolysis Inhibitor (TAFI; Procarboxypeptidase B)
Inhibits plasmin production by reducing binding of plasminogen/tPA to fibrin.

Serotonin
Promotes vasoconstriction.

Protease-Activated Receptors (PARs)
Serine protease (e.g., thrombin)–activated receptor resulting in platelet activation.

ANTICOAGULANT

Adenosine Triphosphate (ATP)
Inhibits platelet aggregation.

Protease Nexin II
Inhibits factor XIa.

Tissue Factor Pathway Inhibitor (TFPI)
Inhibits TF:factor VIIa of the extrinsic pathway.

Protein S
Cofactor in the protein C pathway for inhibition of factors Va and VIIIa.

VASCULAR REPAIR

Platelet-Derived Growth Factor (PDGF)
Stimulates mitogenesis of smooth muscle and fibroblasts for vessel repair.

β-Thromboglobulin
Promotes fibroblast chemotaxis for vessel repair.

Vascular Endothelial Growth Factor (VEGF)
Stimulates endothelial cell proliferation.

Transforming Growth Factor-β (TGF-β)
Modulates vascular repair by inhibition of proliferation of various cell types, including endothelium.

Epidermal Growth Factor (EGF)
Promotes fibroblast proliferation.

Thrombospondin
Inhibits angiogenesis.

the damaged site (Fig. 2-11). Although these events are traditionally described sequentially, there is considerable overlap and integration between these events.

Primary Hemostasis

Primary hemostasis includes the initial vascular and platelet response to injury. Neurogenic stimuli and mediators released locally by endothelium and platelets cause vasoconstriction immediately after damage (see Fig. 2-11, *A*). The nature and effectiveness of vasoconstriction is partially determined by the size of the affected vessel, the amount of smooth muscle it contains, and endothelial integrity. Narrowing of the vessel lumen allows opposing endothelial surfaces to come into contact with and sometimes adhere to each other to reduce the volume of blood flowing through the damaged area. Platelets can directly adhere to the exposed subendothelial matrix of collagen, fibronectin, and other glycoproteins and proteoglycans (see Fig. 2-11, *B*). However, more efficient adhesion occurs when von Willebrand factor (vWF; released by local activated endothelium or by cleavage from factor VIII) coats subendothelial collagen to form a specific bridge between collagen and the glycoprotein platelet receptor GPIb. At this stage and without further stimulation, adhered and aggregated platelets may disaggregate. Otherwise, mediators (e.g., thrombin) can cause additional platelet aggregation, stimulate release of the contents of platelet dense bodies and α-granules, and enhance production of procoagulant substances (e.g., thromboxane) that accelerate hemostasis. Adenosine diphosphate (ADP) released from platelet dense granules triggers the binding of fibrinogen to platelet receptor GPIIb-IIIa, resulting in the formation of fibrinogen bridges that link platelets into a loose aggregate. Platelet contraction along with small amounts of polymerized fibrin consolidates this loose aggregate into a dense plug, which covers the damaged area. When vascular injury is minimal, these plugs composed predominantly of platelets may be sufficient to fill the defect and prevent blood loss from the damaged area. If not, the presence of tissue factor (TF), aggregated platelet phospholipids, and small amounts of activated coagulation factors promote formation of fibrin (secondary hemostasis [see next section]) at the site.

Secondary Hemostasis

In many cases of vascular injury, fibrin is necessary along with the initial platelet plug for the prevention of blood loss. Fibrin is the end product of a series of enzymatic reactions involving coagulation factors, nonenzymatic cofactors, calcium, and phospholipids derived mainly from platelets (and possibly other cells like endothelium, monocytes, or smooth muscle) (see Fig. 2-11, *C*). Various models have been used to described fibrin formation, including the classic coagulation cascades (intrinsic, extrinsic, and common cascades [Fig. 2-12]), and a cell-based model (Fig. 2-13). Although each model provides a useful perspective for understanding fibrin formation, the complexity of the coagulation process and the multiple roles played by many of the reactants defies simple explanation by a single comprehensive model.

Initiation of coagulation is due to exposure of blood to TF (factor III). TF is present on perivascular cells (e.g., fibroblasts) and on microparticles derived from activated endothelium, platelets, monocytes, and/or apoptotic cells. Circulating factor VII or VIIa (approximately 1% of the circulating factor VII is in the activated [VIIa] state) of the extrinsic pathway forms a Ca^{2+}-dependent TF:VII complex on the surface of the injured area expressing TF and is activated to become TF:VIIa. The principal physiologic activator(s) of factor VII is unclear but may include factors XIIa, Xa, IXa, VIIa (autoactivation), thrombin, plasmin, and factor VII–activating protease. Subsequently, TF:VIIa (i.e., extrinsic tenase complex) directly activates factor X and factor IX, a key component of the intrinsic tenase complex (IXa/VIIIa). Activation of both the extrinsic and intrinsic tenase complexes results in the formation of small amounts of thrombin via the common coagulation pathway. Antithrombin III (ATIII) and tissue factor pathway inhibitor (TFPI) strictly regulate this initial phase of coagulation (based on the cell-based model) (see section on Coagulation Inhibitors). Although the amount of thrombin generated is insufficient to convert significant amounts of fibrinogen into fibrin, it does activate platelets that have bound to vWF or collagen at the site of injury (see section on primary hemostasis) and activates factors XI, VIII, V, and XIII on or near the platelet surface (amplification phase of the cell-based model). Factor XIa–induced formation of intrinsic tenase is 50 times more effective in activating factor X than TF:VIIa and plays the predominant role in the propagation phase of the cell-based model of coagulation and the formation of large amounts of thrombin. Thrombin concentrations are now high enough to begin to cleave substantial amounts of fibrinogen (factor I) that have accumulated between aggregated platelets into fibrinopeptides A and B to form fibrin monomers (E-Fig. 2-2). Removal of these fibrinopeptides reduces intermolecular repulsive forces so that fibrin monomers spontaneously form weak H^+ bonds and self-polymerize into soluble fibrin polymers. Factor XIIIa (activated by factor Xa and thrombin), catalyzes the formation of covalent bonds that cross-link adjacent fibrin molecules to make the polymer insoluble. Cross-linking of the fibrin network, along with concurrent platelet contraction and the presence of abundant calcium, thrombin, and adenosine triphosphate (ATP), causes retraction of the fibrin-platelet aggregate. Retraction reduces the size of the aggregate to allow blood flow to continue and to pull damaged vessel edges closer together for efficient healing.

Thrombolysis and Fibrinolysis

The purpose of a fibrin-platelet aggregate is to form a temporary patch that is dissolved (thrombolysis) after healing of the vessel. The rate of dissolution must be balanced so that it does not occur so quickly that bleeding returns but is not prolonged so that permanent healing of the vessel or vessel occlusion may occur. The most important aspect of thrombolysis is fibrin dissolution (fibrinolysis), which is initiated immediately after vessel injury by the cleavage of

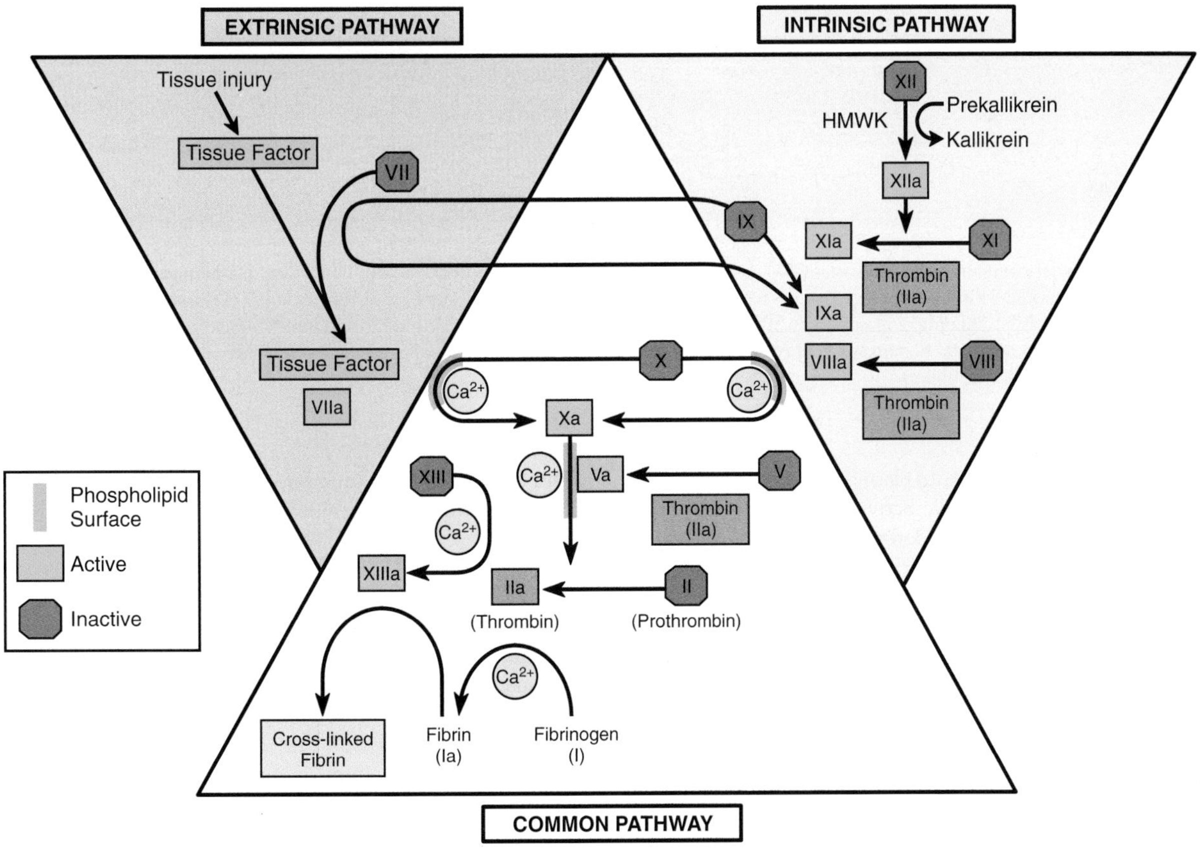

Figure 2-12 The Classic (Intrinsic, Extrinsic, and Common) Coagulation Cascades. The intrinsic and extrinsic pathways terminate with the formation of tenase complexes (factor IXa/factor VIIIa/Ca^{+2}/phospholipids and factor VIIa/TF on any TF-expressing surface/Ca^{+2} for the intrinsic and extrinsic pathways, respectively). Activation of factor X by these complexes initiates the common pathway. There is a common link between the intrinsic and extrinsic pathways at the concentration of factor IXa. *HMWK*, High-molecular-weight kininogen; *TF*, tissue factor.

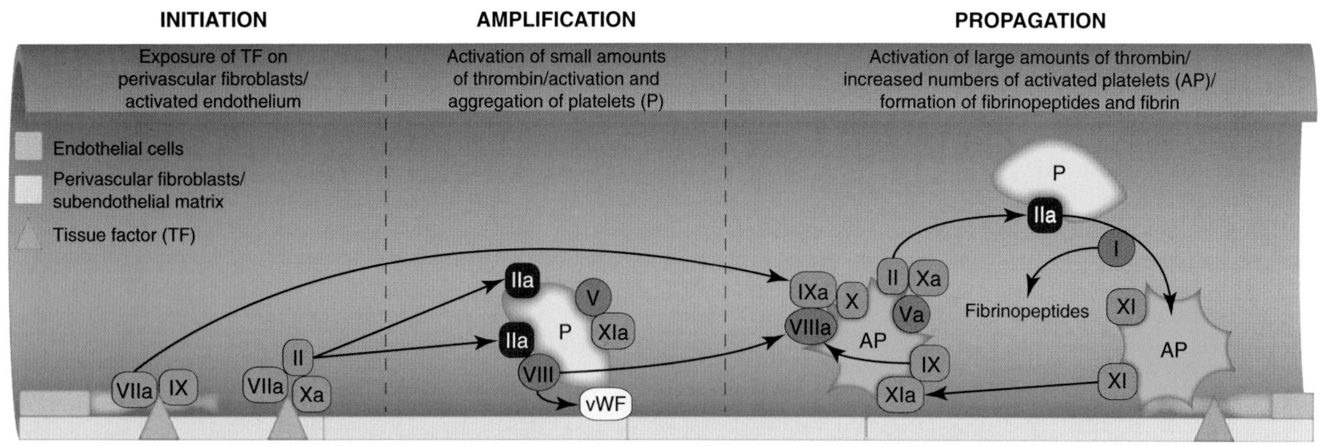

Figure 2-13 **Cell-Based Model of Coagulation.** Vascular damage results in tissue factor (TF) exposure and production of thrombin and factor IXa via the extrinsic pathway (initiation). The small amounts of thrombin formed during initiation cleave von Willebrand factor (vWF) from factor VIII, enhancing platelet adhesion to the damaged site. Thrombin activates platelets (P), which result in degranulation and the aggregation of additional platelets. Thrombin also results in the generation of factors Va, VIIIa and XIa (amplification). During propagation, activated platelet (AP) membranes support assembly of intrinsic tenase complex (IXa/VIIIa) that is rapidly induced from factor XIa. Factor Xa and its coreactants form prothrombinase to generate large amounts of thrombin, which is released directly onto platelets to cleave fibrinogen into fibrinopeptides, which cross-link to form fibrin. (Courtesy Dr. D.A. Mosier, College of Veterinary Medicine, Kansas State University; and Dr. J.F. Zachary, College of Veterinary Medicine, University of Illinois.)

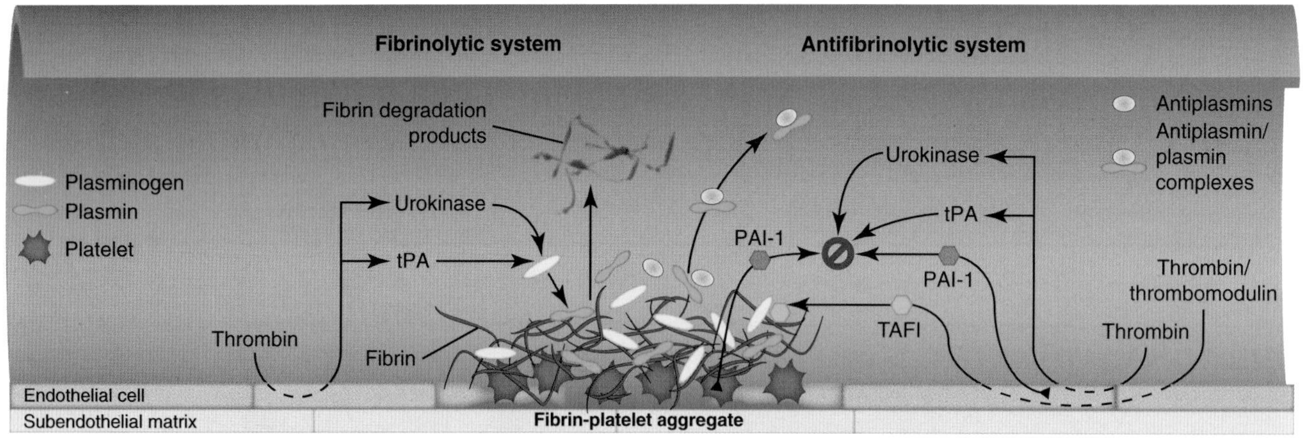

Figure 2-14 **Fibrinolysis.** Tissue plasminogen activator (tPa) and urokinase are major activators of fibrinolysis by cleaving plasminogen into plasmin. Plasminogen activator inhibitor-1 (PAI-1) inhibits these activators to decrease fibrinolysis. Other antifibrinolytic agents include (1) thrombin-activatable fibrinolysis inhibitor (TAFI), which inhibits binding of plasminogen/tPA to fibrin, and (2) antiplasmins, which bind to and inhibit activity of plasmin that has disassociated from the fibrin-platelet aggregate. (Courtesy Dr. D.A. Mosier, College of Veterinary Medicine, Kansas State University; and Dr. J.F. Zachary, College of Veterinary Medicine, University of Illinois.)

the plasma protein plasminogen into plasmin, an important fibrinolytic agent (Fig. 2-14). Physiologic activators of plasminogen are predominantly activators within endothelium (tPA) and activators present in the extracellular matrix and fluids (e.g., urokinase). A wide variety of other proteases, including activated contact group coagulation factors (e.g., factor XIIa), can also activate plasminogen. Plasminogen adsorbs to fibrin within a platelet-fibrin aggregate, so that upon activation the plasmin remains localized to the site. The presence of fibrin increases the efficiency of tPA-dependent plasmin generation by nearly twofold. Additionally, by binding to fibrin, plasmin is protected from its major inhibitor (α_2-antiplasmin). The bound plasmin restricts the size of the platelet-fibrin aggregate by degrading both cross-linked (insoluble) fibrin and fibrinogen, so that additional fibrin formation is inhibited. Dissolution of insoluble, but not soluble, fibrin by plasmin results in the formation of fibrin degradation products (FDPs). FDPs are various-sized fragments of fibrin and fibrinogen that can impair hemostasis. Collectively, FDPs inhibit thrombin, interfere with fibrin polymerization, and can coat platelet membranes to inhibit platelet aggregation.

Regulation of Hemostasis

The potent biologic effects of hemostatic products must be finely regulated to achieve appropriate hemostasis, without creating detrimental effects associated with too little or too much activity. Coagulation factors are continuously activated at low, basal concentrations to keep the system primed for a rapid response to an injurious stimulus. Proteins that inhibit or degrade activated hemostatic products are present in the plasma or are locally produced at the site of hemostasis. These products help confine hemostasis to a site of vascular damage and inhibit hemostatic reactions in normal vasculature. Regulation is also achieved by simple dilution of activated agents as blood removes them from the area, and the factors are removed from the circulation by the liver and spleen.

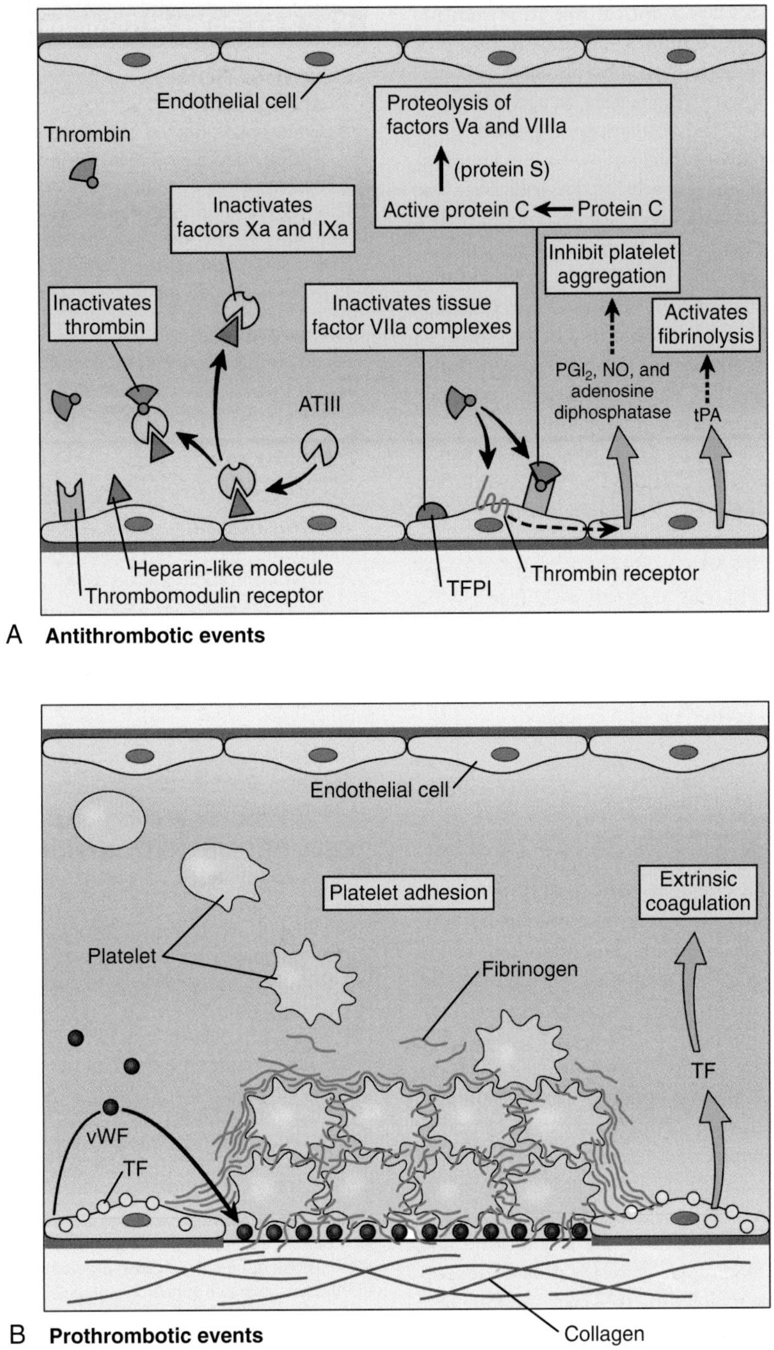

Figure 2-15 **Procoagulant and Anticoagulant Properties of Endothelium. A**, There are many properties of normal endothelium that create an anticoagulant state that inhibits thrombus formation. **B**, Injured endothelium releases von Willebrand factor (vWF) and tissue factor (TF), which stimulate platelet adhesion and coagulation, respectively, to promote thrombus formation. *ATIII*, Antithrombin III; *NO*, nitric oxide; *PGI*$_2$, prostacyclin; *TFPI*, tissue factor pathway inhibitor; *tPA*, tissue plasminogen activator.

Coagulation Inhibitors

The major anticoagulants on endothelial cells are molecules within the protein C–protein S–thrombomodulin system and endothelial heparan sulfate to which AT and TFPI are bound (Fig. 2-15). AT is the most potent and clinically significant of the coagulation inhibitors, accounting for nearly 80% of the thrombin-inhibitory activity of plasma. AT is a circulating serine protease produced by endothelium and hepatocytes that degrades to some extent virtually all activated coagulation factors (notably factors II, VII, IX, X, XI, XII), but it is most importantly recognized for inhibition of thrombin and factor Xa. AT can bind to heparan sulfate present on the surface of normal endothelium and platelets to localize it to the site where it is most needed to inactivate thrombin and factor Xa. Through this binding, heparin accelerates the rate of AT-induced inactivation of serine protease inhibitors by 2,000- to 10,000-fold. AT also inhibits fibrinolysis (by inactivating plasmin and kallikrein), kinin formation, and complement activation (by inactivating C1s). Although the major role of heparin is to bind and enhance the activity of AT, it also inhibits coagulation by enhancing the release of TFPI from endothelial cells and by interfering with binding of platelet receptors to vWF.

The protein C pathway also plays a critical role in preventing thrombosis. Proteins C and S are vitamin K–dependent glycoproteins that, when complexed together on phospholipid surfaces, potently inhibit coagulation by destroying factors Va and VIIIa. An important step in this process is the activation of protein C by thrombin, a reaction that normally occurs at a low basal concentration but that increases in efficiency nearly 20,000-fold after the binding of thrombin to the endothelial receptor thrombomodulin. This reaction is further enhanced by the presence of a protein C receptor on the surface of endothelial cells. Protein S, in addition to serving as a nonenzymatic cofactor with protein C, can independently inhibit factors VIIIa, Xa, and Va. Binding of thrombin to thrombomodulin also results in the loss of the procoagulant functions of thrombin. The protein C-S complex may also enhance fibrinolysis by neutralizing plasminogen activator inhibitors.

TFPI is a significant inhibitor of extrinsic coagulation, which functions synergistically with protein C and AT to suppress thrombin formation. TFPI is a plasma protein derived mainly from endothelium and smooth muscle cells that forms a complex with factor Xa on the endothelial-bound TF:VIIa molecule to inhibit subsequent factor X activation. TFPI can interact with factor VIIa without factor Xa but at a slow rate. Therefore, TFPI does not substantially inhibit extrinsic coagulation until factor Xa concentrations increase, after which TFPI provides negative feedback for further generation of factor Xa by the TF:VIIa complex.

Fibrinolytic Inhibitors

Major inhibitors of fibrinolytic agents include plasminogen activator inhibitor-1 (PAI-1) and antiplasmins, which include α_2-antiplasmin, α_2-macroglobulin, α_1-antitrypsin, AT, and C-1 inactivator (see Fig. 2-14). PAI-1 inhibits tPA and urokinase, thereby inhibiting fibrinolysis and promoting fibrin stabilization. PAI-1 also inactivates activated protein C, plasmin, and thrombin. Thrombin-activatable fibrinolysis inhibitor (TAFI; procarboxypeptidase B) circulates in the plasma or is released locally in small amounts by activated platelets. Thrombin/thrombomodulin complex–activated TAFI cleaves plasminogen/tPA binding sites (C-terminal lysine residues) from fibrin, resulting in reduced plasmin concentrations. TAFI also has antiinflammatory properties, such as the inactivation of bradykinin and complement fragments C3a/C5a (see Fig. 2-14). The antiplasmins function in a cooperative fashion to prevent excessive plasmin activity so that a fibrin-platelet aggregate can dissolve at a slow and appropriate rate. α_2-Antiplasmin is the first to bind and neutralize plasmin. When its binding capacity is saturated, excess plasmin is taken up by α_2-macroglobulin. α_2-Macroglobulin also binds to certain activated factors, such as thrombin, and physically entraps but does not degrade their active sites. When α_2-macroglobulin is saturated, plasmin binds to α_1-antitrypsin. α_1-Antitrypsin is a weak inhibitor of fibrinolysis, but a potent inhibitor of factor XIa. In addition to their fibrinolytic roles, α_1-antitrypsin and α_2-macroglobulin are the major plasma inhibitors of activated protein C.

Hemostasis and Other Host Responses

Hemostatic, anticoagulant, and fibrinolytic pathways are highly integrated, and many factors within the pathways have multiple roles, some of which result in opposite outcomes. Thrombin is the best example that demonstrates the complexity of these reactions (Box 2-5). Thrombin has a major procoagulant role to cleave fibrinogen to yield fibrin monomers. Thrombin also activates factors V, VIII, XI, and XIII and is a potent activator of platelets. However, high concentrations of thrombin destroy, rather than activate, factors V and VIII. Furthermore, when thrombin binds to thrombomodulin on endothelial surfaces, it activates protein C, a potent anticoagulant (see section on Coagulation Inhibitors and Fig. 2-15).

The role of coagulation proteins also extends beyond coagulation and hemostasis. Even though the contact factors of intrinsic coagulation are not considered to participate in physiologic hemostasis, they can still contribute to fibrin formation as well as kinin formation, complement activation, and fibrinolysis. In vivo activators of contact factors prekallikrein-HMWK-factor XII are not clearly known but may include collagen and long-chain inorganic polyphosphates derived from platelet dense granules or bacteria. Inorganic polyphosphates are of particular interest because they are also potent activators of prothrombin and factor XI and can contribute to thrombosis. During contact factor activation prekallikrein is converted to kallikrein, which is chemotactic for leukocytes, can

Box 2-5 Roles of Thrombin

COAGULATION

Procoagulant

Activates platelets via binding protease-activated receptors (PARs) (see Box 2-4 for properties of activated platelets)
Activate factors XI, VIII, and V on the platelet surface
Cleavage of fibrinogen into fibrinopeptides
Activates factor XIII to impact fibrin cross-linking
Stimulates microparticle formation (tissue factor [TF]–expressing cell membrane vesicles)

Anticoagulant

Binds endothelium thrombomodulin to activate protein C
Binds platelet GPIb to decrease platelet adhesion via von Willebrand factor (vWF)

Fibrinolytic

Stimulates release of tissue plasminogen activator

Antifibrinolytic

Stimulates release of plasminogen activator inhibitor-1 (PAI-1)
Activates thrombin-activatable fibrinolysis inhibitor (TAFI)

INFLAMMATION

Activates endothelium by binding endothelial cell PARs[2]
Activates monocytes and T lymphocytes
Stimulates mast cell degranulation
Enhances leukocyte chemotaxis/migration/adhesion
Increases vascular permeability
Activates complement
Chemotactic for macrophages and neutrophils

CELL PROLIFERATION/TISSUE REMODELING

Binds endothelial and smooth muscle PARs to stimulate mitogenesis
Stimulates angiogenesis (expression of matrix metalloproteinase-1 [MMP-1] and matrix metalloproteinase-2 [MMP-2], vascular endothelial growth factor [VEGF], angiopoietin 2)
Stimulates proliferation and migration of tumor cells
Activates collagen type IV degrading enzyme
Activates MMP-2
Activates fibroblasts
Enhances gene expression (proto-oncogenes, endothelin, vascular smooth muscle DNA)

[2]Properties of activated endothelium include, for example, increased expression of adhesions (see Box 2-3 for additional properties of activated endothelium). These adhesions include P-selectin and intercellular adhesion molecule (ICAM)/vascular cell adhesion molecule (VCAM) expression, platelet-activating factor (PAF) production, expression of cytokines (e.g., interleukin 1 [IL-1]).

directly cleave C5 to C5a and C5b, can cleave HMWK to form bradykinin, and can convert plasminogen into plasmin. Bradykinin contributes to vasodilation by stimulating production of tPA, nitric oxide, prostacyclin, and endothelial-derived hyperpolarizing factor. Plasmin results in fibrinolysis and can also cleave C3 to generate C3a and C3b, as well as activate additional XII. Additionally, both kallikrein and plasmin can directly activate factor XII to result in autoamplification of all factor XIIa pathways. Certain stimuli (e.g., misfolded proteins such as amyloid) activate inflammatory factor XII pathways (kallikrein-kinin) without concurrent activation of coagulation (via subsequent activation of factor XI).

A prothrombotic environment is also proinflammatory. Inflammatory stimuli, such as IL-1 and TNF, activate endothelium to produce TF and to increase their expression of leukocyte adhesion molecules. Thrombin and histamine released by degranulating mast cells also stimulate the expression of the adhesin P-selectin. In early stages of inflammation, leukocytes can loosely attach and roll along endothelium or adhered platelets by interacting with endothelial or platelet P-selectin. During this interaction the neutrophil $\alpha_M\beta_2$ integrin may localize neutrophils to fibrinogen on the surface of activated platelets to promote the conversion of fibrinogen into fibrin. An enhanced prothrombotic environment during inflammation also occurs because of decreased activity of thrombomodulin, protein C, and AT in response to inflammatory products such as endotoxin, IL-1, TNF, and TGF-β. Additionally, adhered or migrating neutrophils and platelets can release lysosomal proteases (e.g., elastase, collagenase, and acid hydrolases), which cleave many products on endothelial or platelet surfaces. Because coagulation and complement pathways are derived from the same ancestral system, they share many of the same activators and inhibitors. Complement components can be activated by the products of contact activation, but also by thrombin and factor Xa, whereas thrombomodulin–protein C will inhibit complement activation. Bacterial polyphosphates, through activation of contact factor pathways may result in generation of fibrin-rich microthrombi that are proposed to entrap bacteria, prevent their spread and tissue invasion, and enhance their removal by immunologic and inflammatory pathways (immunothrombosis). Mitogenic factors produced by activated endothelium and platelets (e.g., platelet-derived growth factor [PDGF], TGF-β, and vascular endothelial growth factor [VEGF]) can contribute to cell growth and angiogenesis associated with healing of damaged tissue. Other factors, such as HMWK, are antiproliferative, antiangiogenic, and proapoptotic. The diverse activities and numerous interactions between reactants in coagulation and inflammation demonstrate the fine balance and interrelatedness of these host responses.

Disorders of Hemostasis: Hemorrhage and Thrombosis

The purpose of hemostasis is to prevent blood loss after vascular damage, while at the same time maintaining blood in a fluid state so that it flows freely through a normal vasculature. Failure of hemostasis can result in the extravascular loss of blood (hemorrhage) or the inappropriate formation of intravascular clots (thrombosis).

Hemorrhage

Hemorrhage occurs because of abnormal function or integrity of one or more of the major factors that influence hemostasis—the endothelium and blood vessels, platelets, or coagulation factors.

Abnormalities in blood vessels can result from various inherited or acquired problems. Trauma can physically disrupt a vessel and cause hemorrhage by rhexis (*rhexis* = breaking forth, bursting).

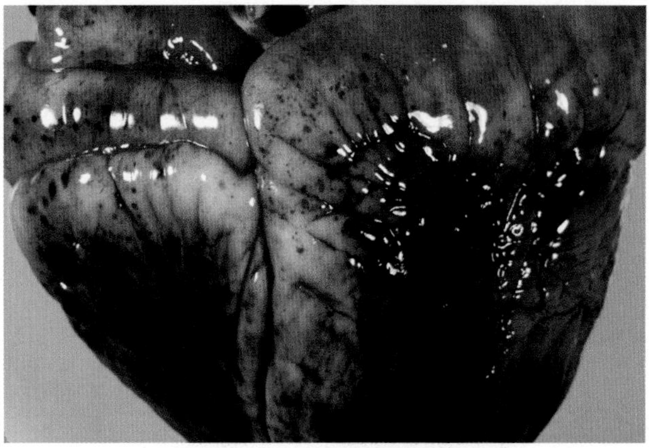

Figure 2-16 **Hemorrhage, Endotoxemia, Heart, Cow.** Note the epicardial and subepicardial hemorrhages in the fat of the coronary groove (a common site) from injury to the endothelium from endotoxin (component of the cell wall of Gram-negative bacteria). The smaller, pinpoint hemorrhages (1 to 2 mm) are petechiae. The larger, blotchy hemorrhages (3 to 5 mm) are ecchymoses. (Courtesy Dr. M.D. McGavin, College of Veterinary Medicine, University of Tennessee.)

Hemorrhage by rhexis can also occur following vascular erosion by inflammatory reactions or invasive neoplasms. Certain fungi commonly invade and damage blood vessels to cause extensive local hemorrhage (e.g., internal carotid artery erosion secondary to guttural pouch mycosis in horses). More commonly, minor defects in otherwise intact blood vessels allow small numbers of erythrocytes to escape by diapedesis (*dia* = through, *pedian* = leap). Endotoxemia is a common cause of endothelial injury that results in small widespread hemorrhages (Fig. 2-16). Infectious agents, such as canine adenovirus-1, or chemicals, such as uremic toxins, can also damage endothelium. Similarly, immune complexes can become entrapped between endothelial cells and activate complement and neutrophil influx to result in damage to the endothelium and vessel wall (type III hypersensitivity reaction). Developmental collagen disorders, such as the Ehlers-Danlos syndrome, are sometimes accompanied by hemorrhage. Affected blood vessels contain abnormal collagen in their basement membranes and surrounding supportive tissue, resulting in vascular fragility and predisposition to leakage or damage. Similar hemorrhages occur due to collagen defects in guinea pigs or primates with vitamin C deficiency.

Decreased platelet numbers (thrombocytopenia) or abnormal platelet function (thrombocytopathy) can cause hemorrhage. Thrombocytopenia can result from decreased production, increased destruction, or increased use of platelets. Decreased production generally occurs following megakaryocyte damage or destruction as a result of causes such as radiation injury, estrogen toxicity, cytotoxic drugs, and viral or other infectious diseases (e.g., feline and canine parvoviruses). Increased platelet destruction is often immune mediated. Autoimmune destruction due to antibody production against platelet membrane components, such as GPIIb and GPIIIa, can occur after immune dysregulation (e.g., systemic lupus erythematosus). Alteration of platelet membranes by drugs or infectious agents may also stimulate immune-mediated destruction or removal of platelets from the circulation. Isoimmune destruction of platelets in neonatal pigs has occurred after ingestion of colostrum containing antiplatelet antibodies. Viral diseases (e.g., equine infectious anemia and feline immunodeficiency syndrome) and arthropod-borne agents are often associated with platelet destruction and their removal by the spleen. An important cause of increased platelet use is diffuse endothelial damage or generalized platelet activation, which initiates disseminated intravascular coagulation (DIC). With disseminated intravascular coagulation there is widespread intravascular coagulation and platelet activation, which can result in consumption of platelets and coagulation factors (see section on Thrombosis). This outcome results in progressive thrombocytopenia and widespread hemorrhage as the syndrome escalates. Another platelet consumption disease that is not accompanied by coagulation is thrombotic thrombocytopenic purpura. In this condition, platelet aggregates form in the microvasculature, possibly the result of increased release of proagglutinating substances by normal or damaged endothelium.

Decreased platelet function is usually associated with an inability to adhere or aggregate at a site of vascular injury. Inherited problems of platelet function in human beings include deficiency of GPIb on the platelet surface (Bernard-Soulier syndrome), deficient or defective GPIIb and GPIIIa on the platelet surface (Glanzmann's thrombasthenia), and deficient release of platelet granule content ("storage pool disease"). Glanzmann's thrombasthenia is a rare disease that has been reported in otterhound and Great Pyrenees dogs and horses. Affected animals can have prolonged bleeding and hematoma formation from minor injury and spontaneous epistaxis because of a mutation affecting a Ca^{2+}-binding domain of the extracellular portion of GPIIb. Signal transduction disorders that result in abnormal platelet aggregation and synthesis or release of platelet granule content (calcium diacylglycerol guanine nucleotide exchange factor I platelet disorders) have been reported in Simmental cattle, dogs (spitz, basset hound, and American foxhounds), cats, and fawn-hooded rats. Defective platelet storage of ADP occurs in the Chédiak-Higashi syndrome (Aleutian mink, cattle, Persian cats, and killer whales). Acquired platelet inhibition and dysfunction is most often associated with administration of nonsteroidal antiinflammatory drugs such as aspirin. Aspirin inhibits the cyclooxygenase pathway of arachidonic acid metabolism, thus decreasing thromboxane production to result in reduced platelet aggregation. Platelet function is also inhibited by uremia because of renal failure. Secondary platelet dysfunction can also occur because of deficiencies of factors necessary for normal platelet function. In von Willebrand disease, or in autoimmune or myeloproliferative disorders in which autoantibodies against vWF are produced, the amount of functional vWF is decreased. This results in decreased platelet adhesion following vascular damage with either subclinical or severe hemorrhage.

Decreased concentrations or function of coagulation factors can also result in hemorrhage. Inherited deficiencies in coagulation factors have been recognized in many different breeds of dogs and less often in other species (E-Box 2-1). Most common are the X-linked hemophilias A and B. Less common (sometimes restricted to just a few families within a specific breed) are the autosomal factor deficiencies. Some coagulation factor deficiencies are not associated with increased bleeding tendencies (e.g., factor XII), some can result in severe hemorrhage (e.g., factor X), and others can range from subclinical to severe (e.g., factors VIII and IX). In many cases the coagulation factor deficiency is recognized because of prolonged bleeding after venipuncture or surgery but otherwise has minimal significance to the animal. In other cases, deficiencies can present as severe episodes of hemorrhage that begin soon after birth.

Acquired defects in coagulation can be caused by decreased production or increased use of coagulation factors. Severe liver disease results in decreased synthesis of most coagulation factors. Production of coagulation factors II, VII, IX, X and proteins C and S is reduced by vitamin K deficiency. Decreased vitamin K production, absorption, or function will reduce conversion of glutamic acid residues into γ-carboxyglutamic acid on these factors. Common substances that competitively inhibit this conversion include dicumarol in moldy sweet clover (*Melilotus alba*), warfarin-containing rodenticides, and sulfaquinoxaline (Fig. 2-17). An inherited deficiency of binding of γ-glutamyl carboxylase with vitamin K has been reported in British Devon rex cats. A common acquired cause of decreased coagulation factors is increased consumption associated with disseminated intravascular coagulation.

The appearance of hemorrhage depends on its cause, location, and severity. Hemorrhage within tissue is often characterized based on size. A petechia (pl. petechiae) is a pinpoint (1 to 2 mm) hemorrhage that occurs mainly because of diapedesis associated with minor vascular damage (see Fig. 2-16). An ecchymosis (pl. ecchymoses) is a larger (up to 2 to 3 cm in diameter) hemorrhage that occurs with more extensive vascular damage (Fig. 2-18), whereas suffusive hemorrhage affects larger contiguous areas of tissue than the other two types (Fig. 2-19). Hemorrhage that occurs in a focal, confined space

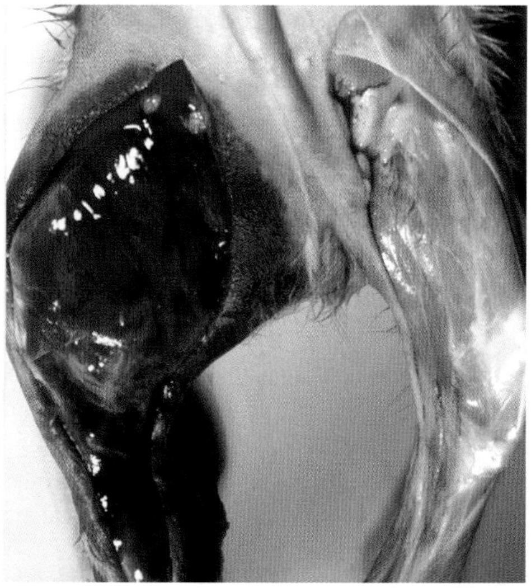

Figure 2-17 **Hemorrhage, Anticoagulant (Warfarin-Containing) Rodenticide Toxicosis, Skin and Subcutis, Medial Aspect of the Right Hind Leg, Dog.** There is a large area of extensive hemorrhage in the subcutis. This lesion was attributed to decreased production of coagulation factors II, VII, IX, and X and proteins C and S resulting from a deficiency of vitamin K induced by warfarin. (Courtesy Dr. D.A. Mosier, College of Veterinary Medicine, Kansas State University.)

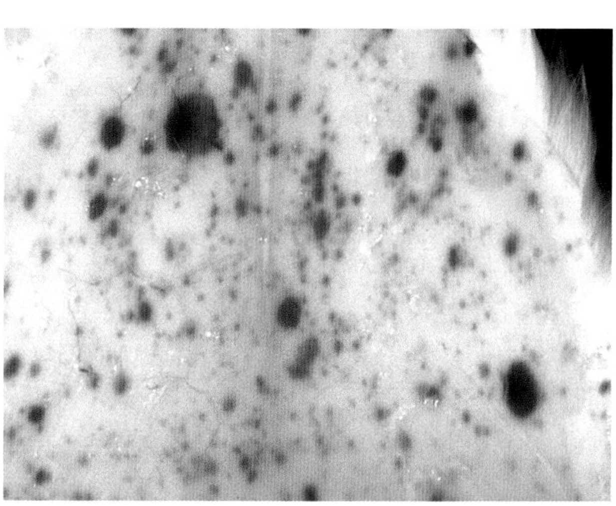

Figure 2-18 **Ecchymotic Hemorrhages (Ecchymoses), Subcutis, Rabbit.** Ecchymoses result from moderate injury to endothelial cells in the capillary beds. (Courtesy Dr. D.A. Mosier, College of Veterinary Medicine, Kansas State University.)

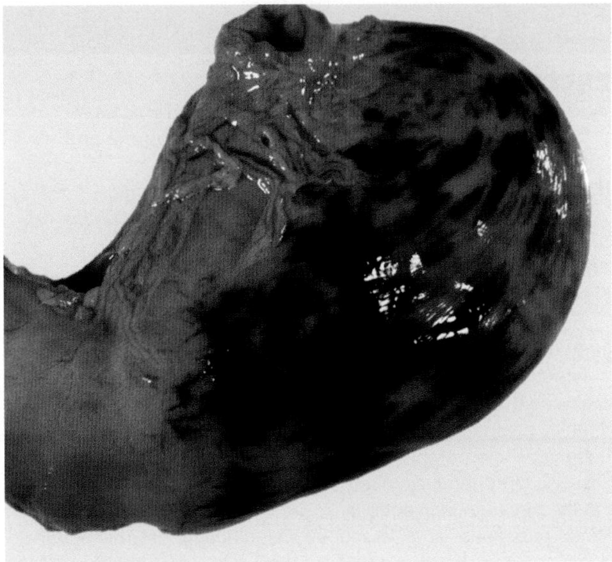

Figure 2-19 **Suffusive Hemorrhage, Serosa, Stomach, Dog.** Suffusive hemorrhage results from severe injury to endothelial cells in the capillary beds. (Courtesy Dr. D.A. Mosier, College of Veterinary Medicine, Kansas State University.)

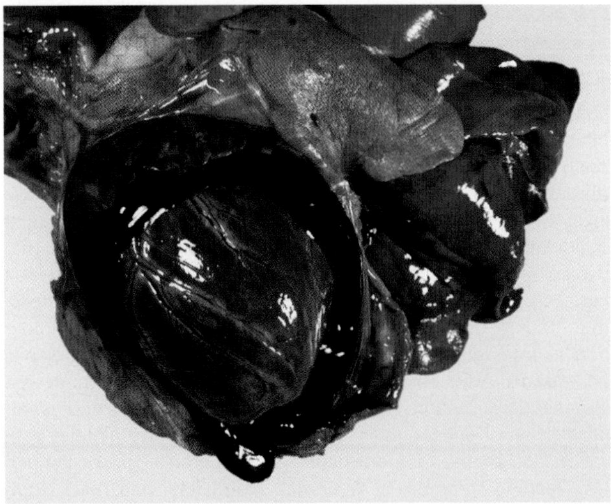

Figure 2-21 **Hemopericardium, Pericardial Sac, Dog.** Hemorrhage into the pericardial sac has caused its distention. Extensive hemopericardium can interfere with the dilation and contraction of the ventricles, causing cardiac tamponade. Both coagulated and noncoagulated blood are present in the pericardial sac. (Courtesy Dr. D.A. Mosier, College of Veterinary Medicine, Kansas State University.)

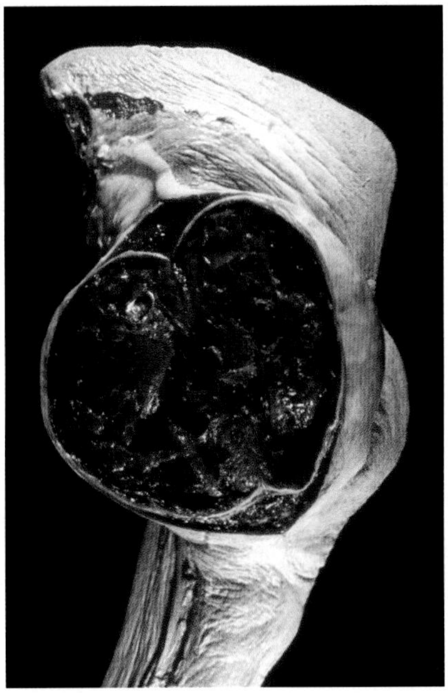

Figure 2-20 **Organizing Hematoma, Spleen, Horse.** Trauma to the spleen has caused damage to the splenic red pulp and its vessels, resulting in bleeding into the splenic parenchyma, forming a hematoma. Note that this hematoma is not acute but is several days old because the blood clot is being degraded. The hematoma is contained by the splenic capsule. (Courtesy Dr. H.B. Gelberg, College of Veterinary Medicine, Oregon State University.)

forms a hematoma. Hematomas are most common in the ears of long-eared dogs or pigs and in the spleen after trauma to the vasculature (Fig. 2-20). The hematoma grows in size until the pressure exerted by the extravascular blood matches that within the injured vessel or the vessel seals internally by hemostasis. Hemorrhage into body cavities results in pooling of coagulated or noncoagulated blood within the cavity and is classified by terms such as *hemoperitoneum* (blood in the peritoneal cavity), *hemothorax* (blood in the thoracic cavity), and *hemopericardium* (blood in the pericardial sac) (Fig. 2-21).

The significance of hemorrhage depends mainly on the amount, rate, and location of the blood loss. In most cases, blood loss occurs locally and is quickly stopped by hemostatic processes that seal the damaged vessel. In more severe cases, blood loss continues until local tissue pressure matches intravascular pressure and ends the hemorrhage (such as occurs with hematoma formation). When these mechanisms fail to stop blood loss, significant hemorrhage can occur externally or internally into body cavities. Rapid loss of substantial amounts of blood, such as occurs because of traumatic injury of a large vessel, can lead to hypovolemia, decreased tissue perfusion, and hypovolemic shock (see later discussion in this chapter). In contrast, slow rates of blood loss can be totally or partially compensated for by increased hematopoiesis. Many cases of gastric ulceration and hemorrhage are characterized by persistent but slow rates of blood loss. Some hemorrhages can create pressure that interferes with tissue function. This is most significant in vital organs or in tissue with little room to expand in response to the pressure, such as the brain and heart.

Thrombosis

Thrombosis is the term used to define the mechanisms involved in the formation of a thrombus in an injured blood vessel (Essential Concept 2-3). A thrombus (pl. thrombi) is an aggregate of platelets, fibrin, and other blood elements (e.g., erythrocytes and neutrophils) formed on a vascular wall. A "physiologic" thrombus is part of normal hemostasis and is usually rapidly resolved after vascular healing. A persistent or inappropriate thrombus forms on the wall of a blood or lymphatic vessel or heart (mural thrombus), or free in their lumens (thromboembolus). Major determinants of thrombosis are historically referred to as Virchow's triad and are the endothelium and blood vessels (vascular injury), coagulation factors and platelet activity (hypercoagulability), and the dynamics of blood flow (stasis or turbulence) (Fig. 2-22 and Box 2-6).

ESSENTIAL CONCEPT 2-3 Thrombosis

Thrombosis is the formation of an excessive or inappropriate fibrin-platelet aggregate on the endothelium of a blood or lymphatic vessel (mural thrombus), within the heart (cardiac thrombus), or free in the lumina of blood or lymphatic vessels (thromboembolus). Major factors involved in thrombosis include injury to the endothelium and blood vessels, excessive activity of coagulation factors and platelets (hypercoagulability), and the dynamics of blood flow (stasis or turbulence) (Virchow's triad; see Fig. 2-22). Of these, injury to the endothelium is the most important; causes of injury include trauma, vasculitis caused by infection or immunologic reactions, metabolic disorders, neoplasia, and toxins. Additionally, alterations in coagulation factors (i.e., increased production of procoagulant substances and decreased production of anticoagulant substances), excessive platelet activation, and altered proteoglycans in the endothelial glycocalyx can also lead to thrombosis. Abnormal blood flow can result from reduced flow (i.e., heart failure, vascular obstruction, or vascular dilation) and turbulence (disruption of laminar blood flow). Turbulence is usually greatest where vessels branch, there is narrowing of the vessel lumen, or at sites of venous or lymphatic valves. The color of a thrombus provides information about its genesis. Pale thrombi are composed predominantly of platelets and fibrin, whereas those containing many erythrocytes are red. Pale thrombi tend to form in areas of rapid blood flow where only firm platelet attachment and subsequent incorporation of fibrin occur. Rapid blood flow in the heart, arteries, and arterioles inhibits passive incorporation of erythrocytes into the thrombus (see Figs. 2-23 to 2-25). Red thrombi tend to form in areas of slow blood flow or blood stasis where erythrocytes are readily incorporated into the loose meshwork of fibrin and platelets (see Figs. 2-26 and 2-27). The significance of a thrombus is determined by its location, size, rate of development, and ability to produce ischemia due to decreased perfusion. In some cases a thrombus or portions of a thrombus can break loose and enter the circulation as an embolus (pl. emboli), a piece of free-floating foreign material within the blood. Thromboemboli (emboli derived from fragments of a thrombus) eventually obstruct a smaller downstream vessel as the vessel diameter reaches a size that prevents the passage of the embolus. Venous thromboemboli typically lodge in the pulmonary circulation, leading to pulmonary infarcts or right-sided heart failure, whereas arterial thromboemboli typically lodge within a smaller artery downstream from the site of the thrombus, resulting in infarction of the dependent tissue (see Figs. 2-37 to 39).

Box 2-6 Causes of Thrombosis

ENDOTHELIAL INJURY

Viruses (e.g., canine adenovirus 1, equine *Morbillivirus*, herpesvirus, and *Arterivirus*, ovine orbivirus, bovine and porcine pestivirus)
Bacteria (e.g., *Salmonella typhimurium, Mannheimia haemolytica, Erysipelothrix rhusiopathiae, Haemophilus somnus*)
Fungi (e.g., *Aspergillus, Mucor, Absidia, Rhizopus*)
Nematode parasites (e.g., *Strongylus vulgaris* larvae, *Dirofilaria, Spirocerca, Aelurostrongylus*, angiostrongylosis)
Immune-mediated vasculitis (e.g., purpura hemorrhagica, feline infectious peritonitis)
Toxins (e.g., endotoxin, *Claviceps*)
Vitamin E or selenium deficiency (microangiopathy)
Local extension of infection (e.g., hepatic abscesses, metritis)
Disseminated intravascular coagulation (DIC)
Faulty intravenous injections
Renal glomerular and cutaneous vasculopathy of greyhounds

ALTERATIONS IN BLOOD FLOW

Local stasis or reduced flow (e.g., gastric dilation and volvulus, intestinal torsion and volvulus, varicocele, external compression of vessel)
Cardiac disease (e.g., cardiomyopathy, cardiac hypertrophy)
Aneurysm (e.g., copper deficiency in pigs, *Strongylus vulgaris, Spirocerca lupi*)
Hypovolemia (e.g., shock, diarrhea, and burns)

HYPERCOAGULABILITY

Inflammation
Enhanced platelet activity (e.g., diabetes mellitus, nephrotic syndrome, malignant neoplasia, heartworm disease, uremia)
Increased clotting factor activation (e.g., nephrotic syndrome, disseminated intravascular coagulation, neoplasia)
Antithrombin III deficiency (e.g., disseminated intravascular coagulation, hepatic disease, glomerular amyloidosis)
Metabolic abnormalities (e.g., hyperadrenocorticism, hypothyroidism)
Glomerulopathies

Alterations in the endothelium are the most important factor in thrombosis and can result in increased production of procoagulant substances and decreased production of anticoagulant substances. Endothelial injury resulting in exposure of blood to TF and subendothelial components, such as collagen and laminin, is a potent stimulus for platelet aggregation and coagulation. Causes of injury vary widely and include trauma, vasculitis caused by infection or immunologic reactions (resulting in release of TNF and IL-1), metabolic disorders, neoplasia, and toxins (e.g., endotoxin). Endothelial activation typically results in the loss of anticoagulant properties of normal endothelium and enhanced expression of procoagulant substances to promote fibrin formation. Platelets may also adhere to intact activated endothelium by interacting with altered proteoglycans in the endothelial glycocalyx. Reduced prostacyclin synthesis may also increase platelet adhesion to endothelium.

Abnormal blood flow increases the risk for thrombosis. Reduced blood flow may occur systemically with heart failure or in a local region of congestion caused by vascular obstruction or vascular dilation. Reduced blood flow is most important in veins, in which the slow flow rate favors accumulation of activated coagulation factors and contact of platelets with the endothelium. Venous thrombosis is common in horses with occlusion of intestinal veins secondary to intestinal torsion. Inactivity can also lead to venous stasis and thrombosis in the limbs, a common problem in human beings but not in animals. Dilated heart chambers (e.g., dilated cardiomyopathy) or dilated vessels (e.g., aneurysms) are also areas in which reduced blood flow predisposes to thrombosis.

Turbulent blood flow also enhances the potential for thrombosis. Turbulence disrupts laminar blood flow, so the thin layer of plasma that normally separates the endothelium from cellular elements, particularly platelets, is disrupted, and platelets interact more readily with the endothelium. Similarly, turbulence results in mixing of the blood, which provides greater opportunity for interactions between coagulation factors. Turbulence can also physically damage endothelium, creating a strong stimulus for platelet adhesion and coagulation. Turbulence, along with increased risk for thrombosis, is usually greatest in areas in which vessels branch, there is narrowing of the vessel lumen, or at sites of venous or lymphatic valves.

Increased coagulability of blood (hypercoagulability) is another factor that predisposes to thrombosis. Hypercoagulability usually reflects an increase or decrease in the concentration of activated

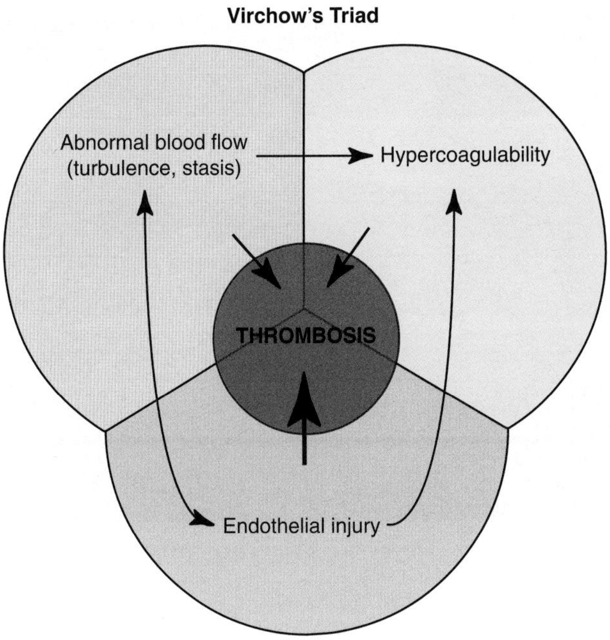

Figure 2-22 **Virchow's Triad in Thrombosis.** The components of Virchow's triad may act independently or may interact to cause thrombosis. However, injury of the endothelium is the single most important factor contributing to thrombosis. (Courtesy Dr. D.A. Mosier, College of Veterinary Medicine, Kansas State University; and Dr. J.F. Zachary, College of Veterinary Medicine, University of Illinois.)

hemostatic proteins (e.g., coagulation factors and coagulation or fibrinolytic inhibitors) caused by enhanced activation or decreased degradation of these proteins. Less often, an alteration in hemostatic protein function may influence coagulability. Activity of coagulation and fibrinolytic proteins can increase in certain conditions such as inflammation, stress, surgery, neoplasia, pregnancy, and renal disease (e.g., the nephrotic syndrome). Inflammation is the most common cause of hypercoagulability, resulting in a variety of changes such as increased TF, increased platelet activation, increased fibrinogen concentration, increased concentrations of membrane phospholipids (e.g., phosphatidylserine), increased concentration of PAI-1, and decreased thrombomodulin concentration. End products of complement activation can also increase coagulability of blood by inducing procoagulant and antifibrinolytic proteins (e.g., complement membrane attack complex induces TF expression). Transient increases in fibrinogen concentration can also occur with stress and tissue necrosis. Concentrations of factors I and VIII are elevated by trauma, acute illness, surgery, and increased metabolism that accompanies hyperthyroidism. Deficiency of AT, a major inhibitor of thrombin, occurs relatively often in dogs with the nephrotic syndrome. In this syndrome AT is depleted because of loss through damaged glomeruli. In affected dogs there is an increased incidence of venous thrombosis and pulmonary embolism. Increased platelet activation (e.g., heartworm disease, nephrotic syndrome, and neoplasia) can also contribute to hypercoagulability of blood.

The appearance of a thrombus depends on its underlying cause, location (artery, vein, or microcirculation), and composition (relative proportions of platelets, fibrin, and erythrocytes). Thrombi composed predominantly of platelets and fibrin tend to be pale, whereas those containing many erythrocytes are red. Cardiac and arterial thrombi are usually initiated by endothelial damage. This damage provides a site for firm platelet attachment and subsequent incorporation of fibrin. Rapid blood flow in these arteries and arterioles inhibits passive incorporation of erythrocytes into the thrombus (Fig. 2-23). Cardiac and arterial thrombi are dull, usually firmly attached to the vessel wall, and red-gray (pale thrombi) (Fig. 2-24). The thrombus may or may not occlude the vessel lumen, and large thrombi tend to have tails that extend downstream from the point of endothelial attachment. Cardiac and larger arterial thrombi often have a laminated appearance created by rapid blood flow and characterized by alternating layers of platelets, interspersed by fibrin intermixed with erythrocytes and leukocytes (lines of Zahn) (Fig. 2-25).

Venous thrombi often occur in areas of stasis, which results in increased activation of coagulation elements and reduced clearance rate of activated clotting factors. Increased erythrocytes in these areas can increase blood viscosity and enhance margination of platelets and leukocytes. Some erythrocytes express phosphatidylserine, which promotes thrombin generation; other erythrocytes decrease fibrinolysis by inhibiting plasminogen activation. Therefore specific interactions between erythrocytes, leukocytes, platelets, endothelium, and coagulation proteins may contribute to the loose meshwork of erythrocytes and fibrin that is characteristic of venous thrombi (Fig. 2-26). Venous thrombi are typically gelatinous, soft, glistening, and dark red (red thrombi) (Fig. 2-27). They are almost always occlusive and molded to the vessel lumen and often extend for a considerable distance upstream from their point of origin. They commonly have points of attachment to the vessel wall, but these are often very loose and difficult to discern. Venous thrombi are morphologically similar to postmortem clots (see E-Fig. 10-5). Compared with venous thrombi, postmortem clots are softer and do not have a point of vascular attachment. In larger vessels or in the heart, erythrocytes may settle to the bottom of the clot, leaving a yellow upper layer (chicken fat clot) indicative of postmortem formation. The presence or absence of associated lesions is often a major factor in distinguishing between an antemortem venous thrombus and a postmortem clot.

Microvascular thrombi (within the microcirculation; microthrombosis) are often due to systemic infection, neoplasia, response to emboli, or disseminated intravascular coagulation (discussed later in this section). Physiologic microthrombosis is proposed to occur as a defense against systemic infection (immunothrombosis). This process can be initiated by TF, factor XII, and neutrophil elastase to result in fibrin-rich microthrombi that may localize pathogens and host products (e.g., antimicrobial peptides and neutrophil products) to act as a mechanism of host defense against intravascular pathogens. However, excessive and widespread microthrombosis or immunothrombosis may rapidly progress to disseminated intravascular coagulation.

The significance of a thrombus is determined by its location and its ability to disrupt perfusion in a dependent tissue. Disruption of tissue perfusion is influenced mainly by the size of the thrombus, its rate of formation, its method of resolution or repair, and the number of vessels affected. In general, thrombi that rapidly develop are more detrimental than those that slowly develop. A slowly developing thrombus creates progressive narrowing of the vessel lumen, but the slow rate of development provides opportunity for collateral blood flow to increase into the affected area. Small thrombi are usually less damaging than large thrombi. Small thrombi are more easily removed by thrombolysis with little residual vessel damage or tissue compromise. In contrast, large thrombi substantially narrow the vessel lumen to restrict blood flow, are often occlusive, and are less readily dissolved by thrombolysis (Fig. 2-28). Occlusive thrombi block blood flow either into (occlusive arterial thrombus) or out of (occlusive venous thrombus) an area and often result in ischemia

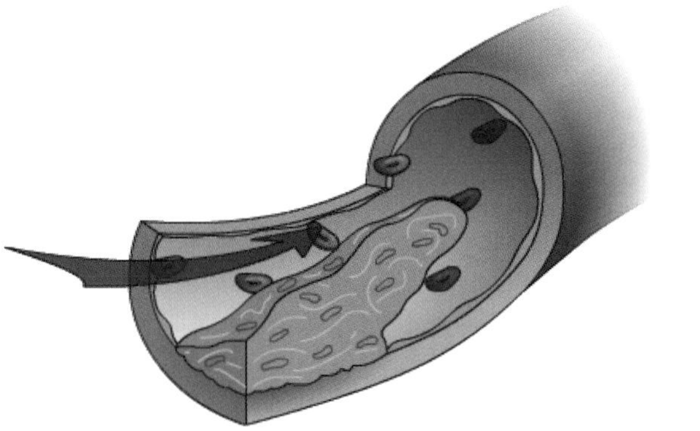

Figure 2-23 **Thrombus (Mural), Artery.** Thrombus formation is usually initiated by endothelial damage, forming a site of attachment for the thrombus. Growth of the thrombus is downstream, resulting in a tail that is not attached to the vessel wall. Portions of the tail can break off to form thromboemboli. (Courtesy Dr. D.A. Mosier and L. Schooley, College of Veterinary Medicine, Kansas State University.)

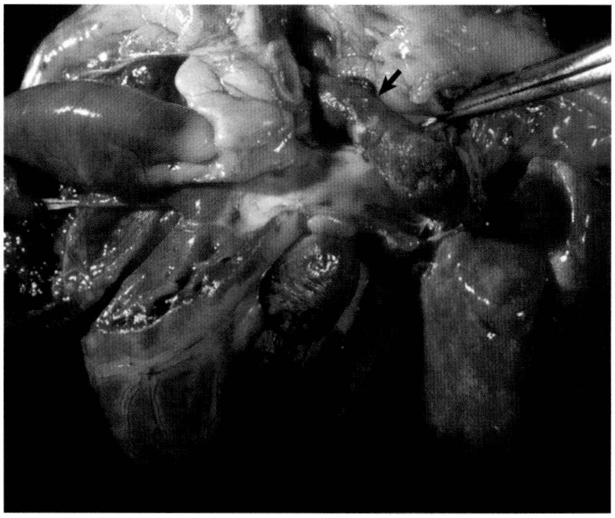

Figure 2-24 **Arterial Thrombus, Pulmonary Artery, Dog.** Arterial thrombi are composed primarily of platelets and fibrin because of the rapid flow of blood, which tends to exclude erythrocytes from the thrombus; thus they are usually tan to gray *(arrow)*. (Courtesy Dr. D.A. Mosier, College of Veterinary Medicine, Kansas State University.)

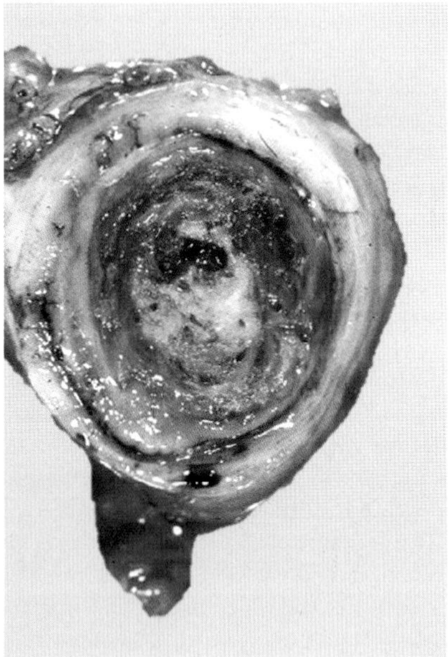

Figure 2-25 **Arterial Thrombus, Lines of Zahn, Cranial Mesenteric Artery, Horse.** Cardiac and larger arterial thrombi often have a laminated appearance characterized by alternating layers of platelets *(white-gray)* and fibrin *(white)* intermixed with erythrocytes and leukocytes (lines of Zahn). These lines are the result of rapid blood flow in the heart and arteries/arterioles that favors the deposition of fibrin and platelets and the exclusion of erythrocytes from the thrombus. This horse had verminous arteritis (*Strongylus vulgaris* fourth-stage larvae) in the affected artery. (Courtesy Dr. P.N. Nation, University of Alberta; and Noah's Arkive, College of Veterinary Medicine, The University of Georgia.)

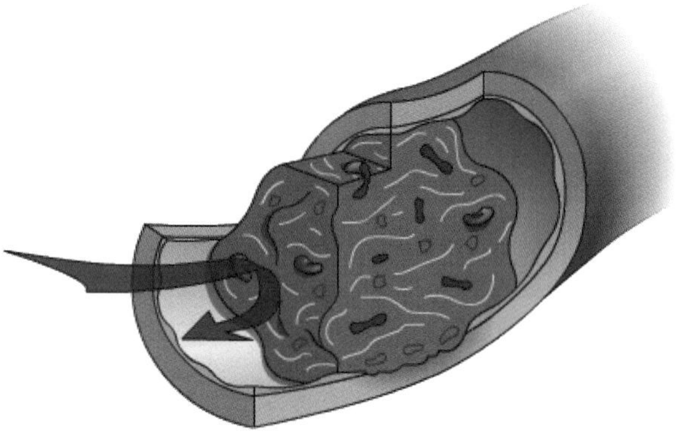

Figure 2-26 **Venous Thrombus.** Thrombus formation often occurs in areas of slow blood flow or stasis. Venous thrombi are dark red and gelatinous as a result of large numbers of erythrocytes that are loosely incorporated into the thrombus because of the slow blood flow. Most venous thrombi are occlusive. (Courtesy Dr. D.A. Mosier and L. Schooley, College of Veterinary Medicine, Kansas State University.)

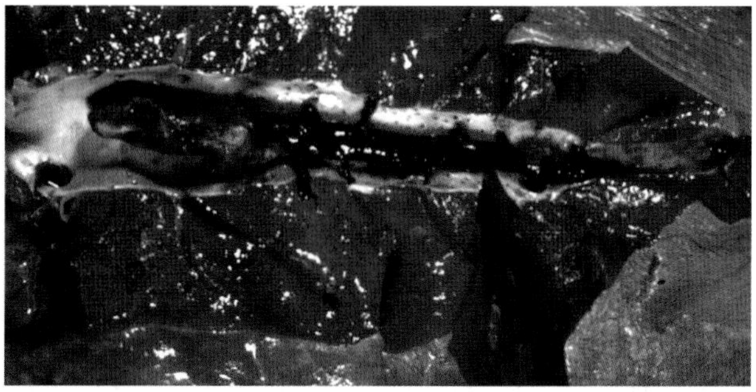

Figure 2-27 **Venous Thrombi, Pulmonary Vein, Lung, Horse.** Venous thrombi become molded to the shape of the lumen of the vein and grow upstream from the site of initiation. (Courtesy Dr. J. King, College of Veterinary Medicine, Cornell University; and Noah's Arkive, College of Veterinary Medicine, The University of Georgia.)

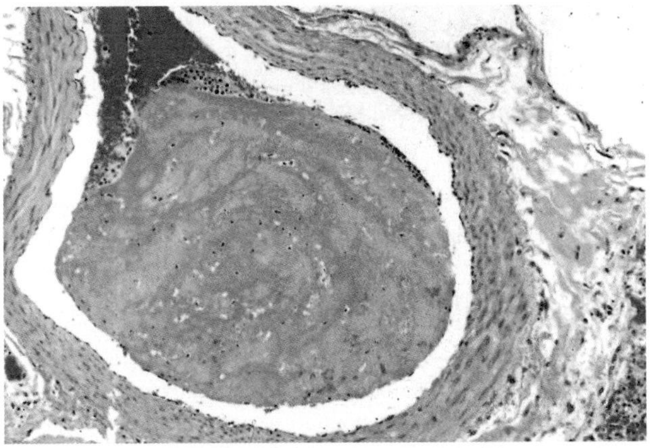

Figure 2-28 **Large Thrombus, Pulmonary Artery, Cow.** Large thrombi are less readily dissolved by thrombolysis and therefore heal by other methods. This thrombus consists of a large coagulum of fibrin that has undergone little to no resolution. H&E stain. (Courtesy Dr. M.A. Miller, College of Veterinary Medicine, University of Missouri; and Noah's Arkive, College of Veterinary Medicine, The University of Georgia.)

(decreased oxygenation of tissue) or infarction (necrosis of tissue caused by lack of oxygen).

Under most circumstances and after removal of the injurious stimulus, the well-regulated events of coagulation result in the return to normal structure and function of the affected vessel (Fig. 2-29, A). However, blood flow through a vessel containing a chronic large or occlusive thrombus can change over time. The thrombus provides an ongoing stimulus for platelet adhesion and coagulation, so thrombus propagation can result in progressive narrowing and possible occlusion of the vessel lumen. A thrombus can also be incorporated into the wall of the vessel by a process similar to that used to replace irreversibly damaged tissue. Products of the aggregated platelets stimulate permanent healing of the damaged area by recruiting fibroblasts to the damaged area. Thrombotic debris is removed by macrophages, and granulation tissue and subsequent fibrosis (organization) occur at the site of the thrombus. Concurrently, there is regrowth of endothelium over the surface of the scar. Although there is a permanent narrowing of the vessel lumen, the regrowth of endothelium over the healed thrombus decreases the stimulus for continued thrombosis (see Fig. 2-29, B). In occlusive and some large thrombi, this healing process may be accompanied by invasion and growth of endothelial-lined blood channels through the fibrotic area (recanalization) (see Fig. 2-29, C; Fig. 2-30). These channels provide alternate routes for blood flow to reestablish through or around the original thrombus. Although reestablishment of blood flow increases tissue perfusion, the permanent vascular narrowing and altered, more turbulent blood flow at the site of a healed thrombus result in an increased risk for subsequent thrombosis at the site.

In some cases a thrombus or portions of a thrombus can break loose and enter the circulation as an embolus (pl. emboli), a piece of free-floating foreign material within the blood. Thromboemboli (emboli derived from fragments of a thrombus) eventually become lodged in a smaller-sized vessel as the vessel diameter reaches a size that prevents the passage of the embolus, a process called *embolization*. Venous thromboemboli typically lodge in the pulmonary circulation, where they can cause pulmonary infarcts or right-sided heart failure. Arterial thromboemboli typically lodge within a smaller artery downstream from the site of the thrombus, often near sites of vascular bifurcation. Arterial emboli frequently result in infarction of dependent tissue, depending on the tissue and nature

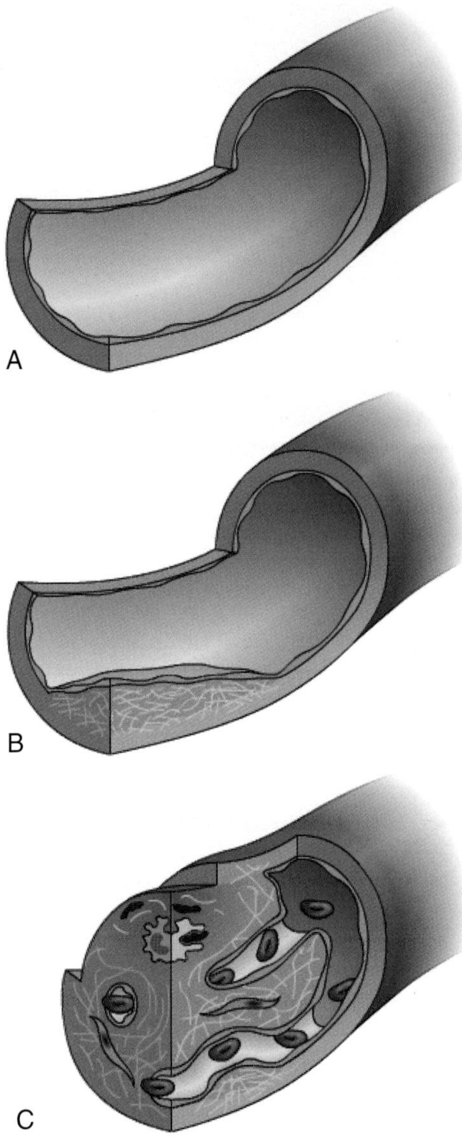

Figure 2-29 **Thrombus Resolution. A**, Small thrombi are removed by thrombolysis, and the blood vessel returns to normal structure and function. **B**, Larger, more persistent thrombi are resolved by removal of thrombotic debris by phagocytes with subsequent granulation tissue formation and fibrosis with regrowth of endothelium over the surface to incorporate the affected area into the vessel wall. **C**, In large mural or occlusive thrombi that are not removed by thrombolysis or phagocytosis of the thrombotic debris, the thrombus is organized by the invasion of fibroblasts and later by the formation of new vascular channels (recanalization), which provide alternate routes for blood flow through and around the site of the original thrombus. (**A**, **B**, and **C** courtesy Dr. D.A. Mosier and L. Schooley, College of Veterinary Medicine, Kansas State University.)

of its vascular supply. Cardiac thromboemboli usually lodge at the bifurcation of the external iliac arteries with a portion of the thromboembolus entering each iliac vessel to form a saddle thrombus (Fig. 2-31).

Emboli can also originate from substances other than thrombi. Fat from the bone marrow can be released into the circulation after the fracture of a long bone. Most fat emboli lodge in the pulmonary circulation. Fibrocartilaginous emboli consist of portions of an intervertebral disk, which are released after rupture of a degenerative disk. These can result in occlusion of local vessels and sometimes cause localized spinal cord infarction. Bacteria from inflammatory

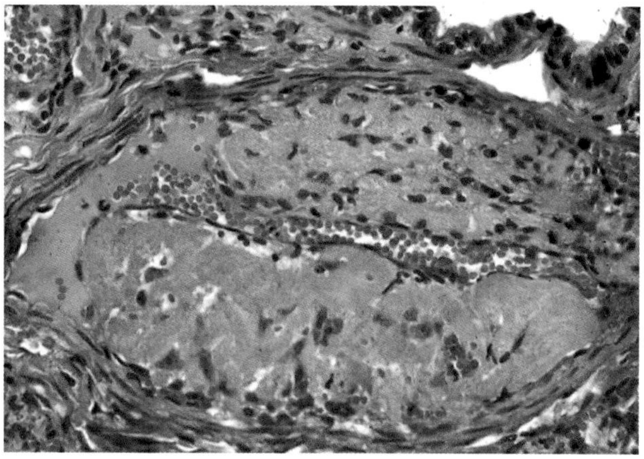

Figure 2-30 Occlusive Mural Thrombus, Recanalization, Cat. In occlusive and large thrombi the healing process may occur by fibrosis and the invasion and growth of endothelial-lined vascular channels through the fibrotic area (recanalization). Note the vascular channel, horizontally in the middle of the thrombus. This provides alternate routes for blood flow to reestablish through or around the original thrombus. The permanent vascular narrowing and altered, more turbulent blood flow at the site of a healed thrombus result in an increased risk for subsequent thrombosis at the site. H&E stain. (Courtesy Dr. B.C. Ward, College of Veterinary Medicine, University of Mississippi; and Noah's Arkive, College of Veterinary Medicine, The University of Georgia.)

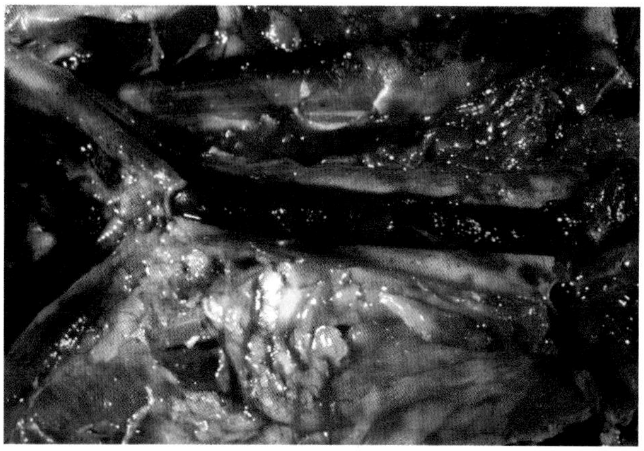

Figure 2-31 Saddle Thrombus, Iliac-Aortic Bifurcation, Cat. Cardiac thromboemboli usually lodge at the bifurcation of the aorta into the external iliac arteries with a portion of the thromboembolus entering each iliac vessel to form a saddle thrombus. A saddle thrombus is not attached to the wall of the aorta or iliac arteries and is easily removed at necropsy. The thromboembolus is composed of layers of platelets and fibrin in which there are enmeshed erythrocytes. (Courtesy Dr. M.D. McGavin, College of Veterinary Medicine, University of Tennessee.)

lesions, such as vegetative valvular endocarditis, or abscesses can enter the blood to form bacterial emboli. When these lodge within vessels, they may cause infarction and secondary sites of infection. Intravascular parasites, such as heartworms (e.g., *Dirofilaria*), or flukes (e.g., schistosomes) can form parasitic emboli. Malignant neoplasms that invade a vessel result in the formation of neoplastic emboli composed of neoplastic cells. Less common sources of emboli include hematopoietic cells from the bone marrow, amniotic fluid, agglutinated erythrocytes, clumps of other cells such as hepatocytes released after tissue trauma, or air bubbles (gas embolism) from intravenous injections. In any case the significance of these emboli is their potential to occlude a vessel and inhibit blood flow to dependent tissue.

A serious manifestation of abnormal coagulation is disseminated intravascular coagulation. This is a severe dyshomeostasis caused by the loss of localization of the coagulation process and generation of excess thrombin. Fundamental causes include widespread endothelial activation or injury and excessive concentrations of circulating TF, which are present in a wide variety of conditions, including extensive trauma or tissue damage, shock, systemic inflammation, vasculitis, sepsis, burns, neoplasia, heat stroke, surgery, or immunothrombosis that is unable to confine pathogens or damaged cells. Excess thrombin causes platelet aggregation and activation of coagulation factors (e.g., factors V and VIII) to form fibrin, resulting in widespread microvascular thrombi. Concurrently, the high concentrations of thrombin stimulate anticoagulant and fibrinolytic pathways by binding to thrombomodulin to activate protein C and by converting plasminogen into plasmin. The progression and outcome of disseminated intravascular coagulation is determined partially by the underlying cause and the nature of the imbalance between procoagulant and anticoagulant, and profibrinolytic and antifibrinolytic pathways. A fibrinolytic form of disseminated intravascular coagulation associated with excessive activation of tPA along with consumption of platelets and coagulation factors results in widespread hemorrhages. Conversely, a thrombotic form associated with excessive activity of PAI-1 results in widespread microthrombosis and multiple organ failure due to ischemia. Both forms share the fundamental imbalance between pro-coagulant and anticoagulant pathways that is characteristic of disseminated intravascular coagulation. The extreme imbalances associated with disseminated intravascular coagulation that result in widespread hemorrhages, microthrombosis, or both represents one of the most profound, rapidly progressive, and dramatic examples of dyshomeostasis in animals.

Normal Blood Flow, Distribution, and Perfusion

The heart provides the driving pressure for blood distribution. Baroreceptors in the carotid sinus and aortic arch signal the cardiovascular control center in the medulla to balance sympathetic and parasympathetic output to maintain appropriate blood pressure. Left atrial volume receptors and hypothalamic osmoreceptors also help regulate pressure by altering water volume and sodium balance. Sodium concentration is an important contributor to blood volume, osmolality, and pressure and is controlled by the renin-angiotensin-aldosterone system. Secretion of ADH by the hypothalamus in response to a water deficit increases renal tubular reabsorption of water to help maintain blood volume.

Distribution of blood within the circulatory system is highly variable. Organs that alter or recondition blood (e.g., lungs, gastrointestinal tract, kidney, and liver) receive substantially greater blood flow than is required for their metabolic needs. O_2 and CO_2 are exchanged in the lungs, nutrients are obtained from the gastrointestinal tract and processed by the liver, wastes are removed and electrolytes are balanced by the kidneys, heat is dissipated in the skin, and regulatory hormones enter from endocrine tissues. Systemic neural and hormonal influences can cause general changes in blood distribution. Blood vessel β_2-receptors, most abundant in cardiac and skeletal muscle, cause vasodilation and increased flow when stimulated by epinephrine. In contrast, vessel α-receptors, notably absent in the brain, induce vasoconstriction and reduced flow in most organs on stimulation with norepinephrine. Local intrinsic controls alter arteriolar diameter to adjust the blood flow to a tissue based on the metabolic needs of that tissue. These local controls generally override any central controls to maintain adequate blood flow to support normal cell function. At rest, more than 60% of the circulating blood volume is in the veins, providing a storage pool that can be quickly returned to the heart during periods of increased tissue need. In contrast, most capillary beds have minimal blood flow at any given time; blood flows through only approximately 10% of the total capillaries of resting skeletal muscle. The orchestration of central pressure, blood composition, and blood distribution is critical to meet the varying perfusion needs of all the cells in the body despite constantly changing conditions.

Alterations in Blood Flow and Perfusion

Increased Blood Flow

Hyperemia is an active engorgement of vascular beds with a normal or decreased outflow of blood. It occurs because of increased metabolic activity of tissue that results in localized increased concentrations of CO_2, acid, and other metabolites. These cause a local stimulus for vasodilation and increased flow (hyperemia). Hyperemia can occur as a physiologic mechanism within the skin to dissipate heat. It also occurs because of increased need such as increased blood flow to the gastrointestinal tract after a meal. Hyperemia is also one of the first vascular changes that occur in response to an inflammatory stimulus (Fig. 2-32). Neurogenic reflexes and release of vasoactive substances, such as histamine and prostaglandins, mediate the change to promote delivery of inflammatory mediators to the site. Tissues with hyperemic vessels are bright red and warm, and there is engorgement of the arterioles and capillaries.

Decreased Blood Flow

Congestion is the passive engorgement of a vascular bed generally caused by a decreased outflow with a normal or increased inflow of blood (see Fig. 2-32). Passive congestion can occur acutely (acute passive congestion) or chronically (chronic passive congestion). Acute passive congestion can occur in the liver and lungs in response to acute heart failure (Fig. 2-33), after euthanasia, or in organs in which relaxation of smooth muscle from barbiturate anesthesia or euthanasia results in dilation of the vasculature and vascular sinusoids such as in the spleen. Most passive congestion is recognized clinically as chronic passive congestion. It can occur locally because of the obstruction of venous outflow caused by a neoplastic or inflammatory mass, displacement of an organ, or fibrosis resulting from healed injury. Generalized passive congestion occurs because of decreased passage of blood through either the heart or the lungs. This is most often caused by heart failure or conditions (e.g., pulmonary fibrosis) that inhibit the flow of blood through the lungs. Right-sided heart failure causes portal vein and hepatic congestion (Fig. 2-34). Left-sided heart failure results in pulmonary congestion (Fig. 2-35). Chronically, there may be fibrosis caused by the hypoxia and cell injury that accompanies congestion (e.g., chronic hepatic congestion). Congested tissues are dark red, swollen (edema), and cooler than normal. The microvasculature is engorged with blood, and there is often surrounding edema and sometimes hemorrhage caused by diapedesis.

Decreased Tissue Perfusion

Reduced blood flow to an area is usually caused by a local obstruction of a vessel, local congestion, or decreased cardiac output. Local obstruction results in either reduced blood flow into an area or inadequate blood flow out of an area. Ischemia occurs when the perfusion of tissue in the affected area becomes inadequate to meet the metabolic needs of the tissue. Ischemia caused by arterial disease is most commonly the result of incomplete luminal blockage by a thrombus or embolus. The result is a decreased flow of oxygenated blood into the area. Arteriolar vasoconstriction, if prolonged, can

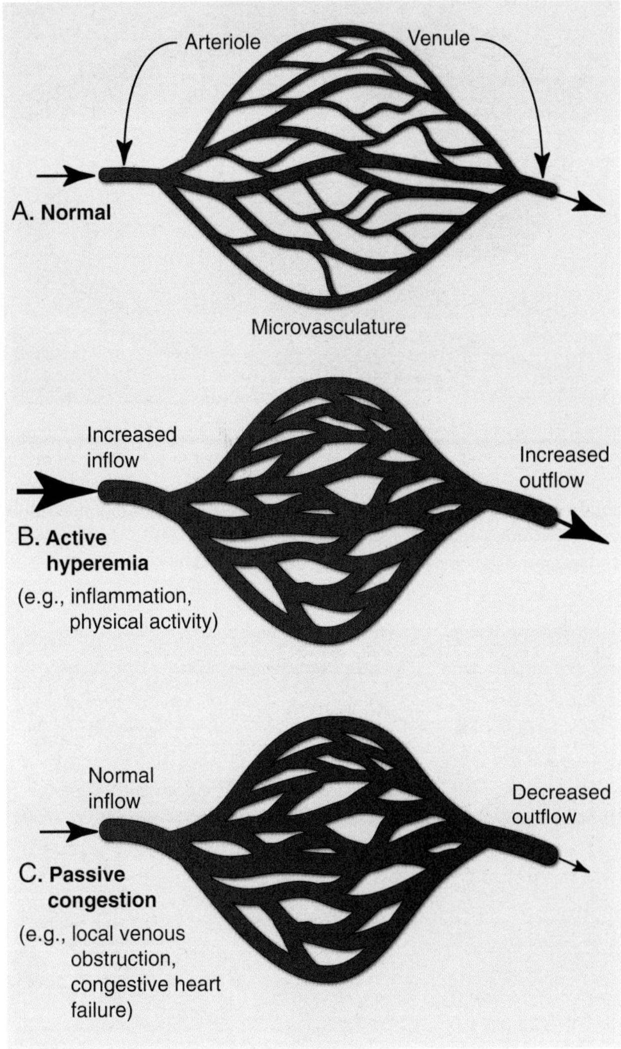

Figure 2-32 Active Hyperemia and Passive Congestion in Vascularized Tissue. Hyperemia and congestion are morphologically characterized by increased blood in the microvasculature of a tissue or organ. The terms active hyperemia and passive congestion are used to identify and characterize two distinct pathologic processes that can result in the same morphologic characteristics. **A**, Normal inflow, outflow, and distention of the microvasculature. **B**, Active hyperemia. There is increased inflow of well-oxygenated blood leading to distention of the microvasculature. Active hyperemia occurs in tissues with (1) acute inflammation or (2) increased metabolic activity such as ensues with muscle contraction. It occurs as a result of arteriolar distention when there is increased tissue demand for oxygenated blood, effector blood cells such as leukocytes, and other metabolites such as glucose and when there is need for removal of waste products such as carbon dioxide and lactic acid. **C**, Passive congestion. Passive congestion is a process in which microvasculature distention results from impaired (reduced) vascular outflow, (1) locally from an obstruction by a mass such as a tumor or (2) from heart failure leading to "backup" engorgement of the microvasculature systemically. Blood in passive congestion is deoxygenated, resulting in cyanosis. Passive congestion also occurs in two forms: acute and chronic. Acute passive congestion has a sudden onset and is observed in heart failure resulting from arrhythmias and after euthanasia (see Fig. 2-33). Chronic passive congestion occurs in animals when blood is retained in organs like the liver or lung for long durations leading to reparative healing responses such as fibrosis and loss of parenchymatous tissue (see Figs. 2-34 and 2-35). (Courtesy Dr. D.A. Mosier, College of Veterinary Medicine, Kansas State University; and Dr. J.F. Zachary, College of Veterinary Medicine, University of Illinois.)

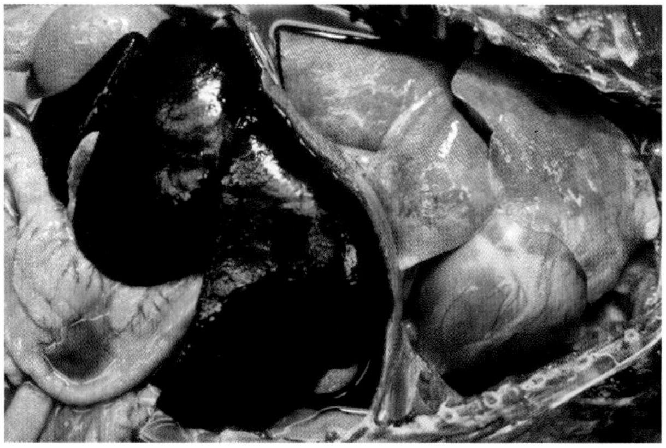

Figure 2-33 **Acute Passive Congestion, Liver, Dog.** The liver is enlarged and dark red. Acute passive congestion occurs in the vascular system and dependent organs (heart, lungs, portal system) when there is a sudden interruption of the return of blood to the heart, as occurs in heart failure resulting from arrhythmias and after euthanasia. (Courtesy Dr. D.A. Mosier, College of Veterinary Medicine, Kansas State University.)

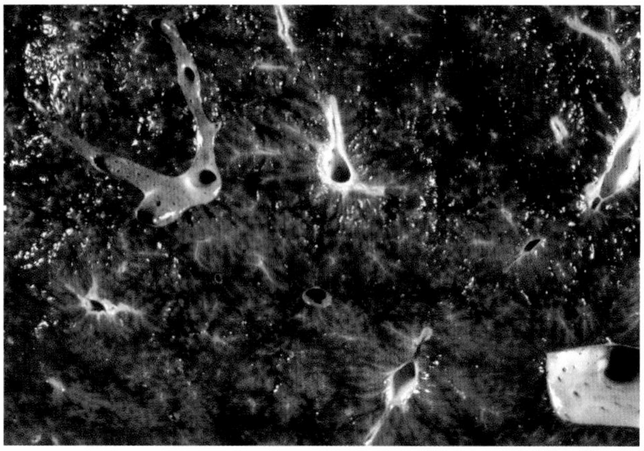

Figure 2-34 **Chronic Passive Congestion (Nutmeg Liver), Liver, Cut Surface, Dog.** The cut surface has a repeating pattern of red and tan mottling (an accentuated lobular pattern). Chronic passive congestion leads to persistent hypoxia in centrilobular areas and atrophy, degeneration, and/or eventually necrosis of centrilobular hepatocytes. The red areas are dilated central veins and adjacent areas of sinusoidal dilation and congestion caused by centrilobular hepatic necrosis. The tan areas are normal, uncongested parenchyma. (Courtesy Dr. D.A. Mosier, College of Veterinary Medicine, Kansas State University.)

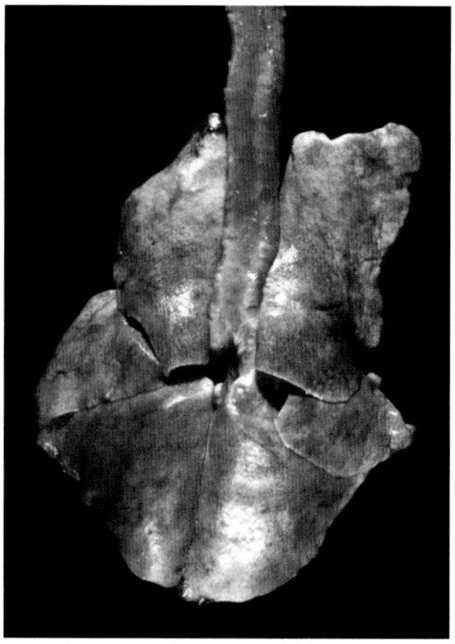

Figure 2-35 **Chronic Passive Congestion, Lung, Dog.** The lungs are moderately firm and yellow-brown because of alveolar macrophages containing hemosiderin. Inflammatory mediators produced by these macrophages also induce fibroplasia, thus there is extensive formation of interstitial collagen in the long term. This collagen is the reason the lungs fail to collapse after loss of negative pressure in the pleural cavity when the diaphragm is incised at necropsy. (Courtesy College of Veterinary Medicine, University of Illinois.)

also result in ischemia. Ischemia resulting from venous lesions can be caused by intraluminal obstruction such as a venous thrombus. However, external pressure that occludes the vein, such as inflammatory or neoplastic masses, is a common cause. Venous obstruction leads to congestion characterized by slowing and stagnation of blood flow, with loss of tissue oxygenation, local increased hydrostatic pressure, and leakage of fluid into the interstitium (edema). Increased interstitial pressure may partially inhibit arterial inflow into the area to compound the problem. Capillaries can also become occluded by thrombi or external pressure. The severity of ischemia is determined by the local vascular anatomy and degree of anastomoses and collateral circulation, the number of microcirculatory vessels and degree of resistance of the arteriole supplying the capillaries, the extent of the decreased perfusion, the rate at which the occlusion occurred, and the metabolic needs of the tissue. Ischemia can be tolerated to different concentrations by different tissues. The brain and heart are most susceptible because of a high need for O_2 and nutrients, combined with poor collateral circulation. In contrast, organs that recondition blood (e.g., lungs, gastrointestinal tract, kidneys, and skin) can tolerate substantial reductions in flow because they already receive more blood than necessary for their metabolic needs. Other tissues receive blood based on their immediate needs (e.g., skeletal muscle during physical activity). Rapid and complete occlusion that affects large areas of tissue is generally more severe because collateral circulation may not be able to reestablish flow to certain areas quickly enough to prevent tissue injury.

In tissue in which there has been a return of blood flow after brief ischemia, the tissue often returns to normal. The ATP of ischemic tissue is degraded to adenosine, a potent vasodilator, which relieves the ischemia and allows ATP production to resume. However, after prolonged ischemia the return of blood flow can result in a variety of detrimental effects. Reflow results in fluid loss to the interstitium, resulting in high tissue pressure, which compresses veins and inhibits local venous return. The congested capillaries hemorrhage, TF is released, and vessels are occluded by thrombi. In ischemic cells a breakdown product of ATP is hypoxanthine. In the absence of oxygen, this is nonreactive. However, on the return of oxygen, xanthine oxidase converts hypoxanthine into urates, hydrogen peroxide, and superoxide anions. Subsequent reaction of superoxide results in the formation of additional reactive oxygen species such as hydroxyl radicals. Collectively, these oxygen free radicals formed during reperfusion can induce damage, in addition to that caused by ischemia and energy depletion of the cell.

An infarct is a local area of peracute ischemia that undergoes coagulative necrosis. Infarction is caused by the same events that result in ischemia and is most common secondary to thrombosis or thromboembolism. The characteristics of an infarct are variable based on the type and size of vessel that was occluded (artery or vein), the duration of the occlusion, the tissue in which it occurs, and the prior perfusion and vitality of the tissue. Complete arterial blockage usually results in immediate infarction (Fig. 2-36). In

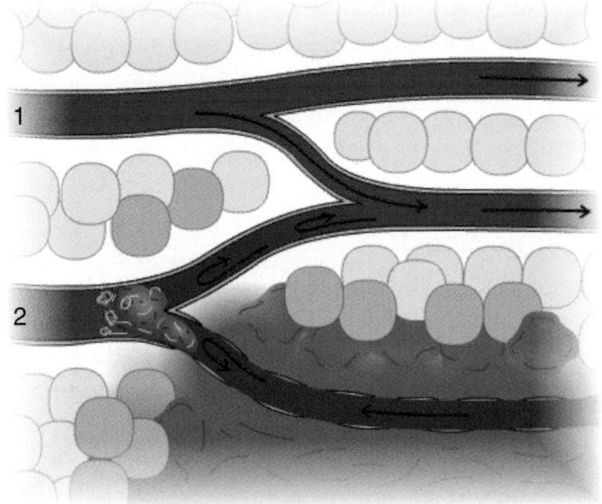

Figure 2-36 Infarction due to Arterial Obstruction. Arterial obstruction results in loss of blood flow to downstream tissue, resulting in abrupt coagulative necrosis. The amount of necrosis depends on factors such as the type and prior health of the tissue affected, its metabolic rate (neurons versus myocytes and fibroblasts), and amount of collateral circulation or alternative blood supply. *1*, Normal arterial flow; *2*, arterial flow obstructed by an arterial thrombus. (Courtesy Dr. D.A. Mosier and L. Schooley, College of Veterinary Medicine, Kansas State University.)

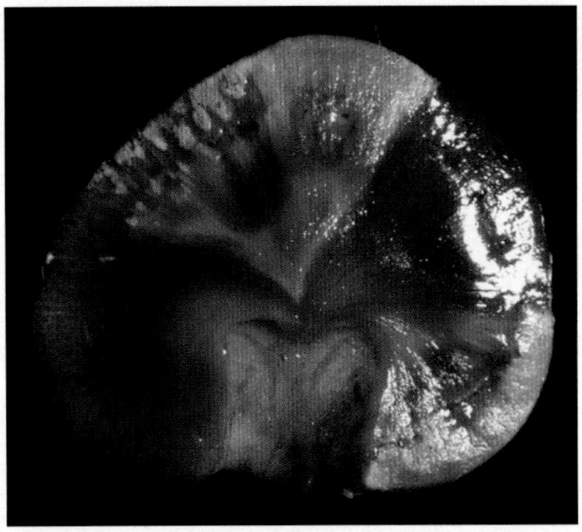

Figure 2-38 Acute Pale Infarcts, Kidney, Rabbit. Multiple, pale white to tan pyramidal-shaped infarcts extend from the renal cortex to the medulla. The infarcts bulge above the capsular surface *(center top)*, indicative of acute cell swelling. The glistening areas on the right are highlights from the photographic lamps. (Courtesy Dr. M.D. McGavin, College of Veterinary Medicine, University of Tennessee.)

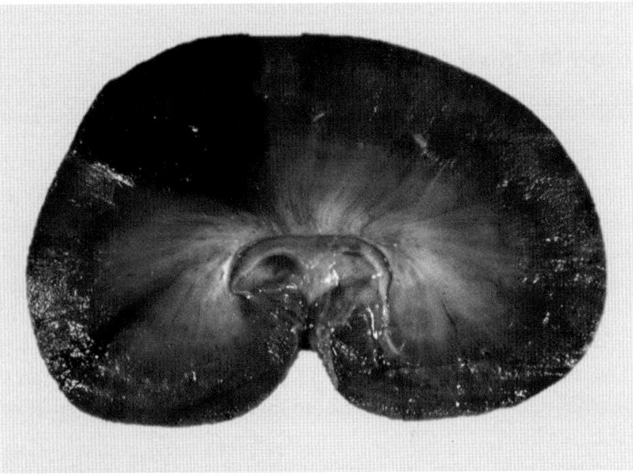

Figure 2-37 Acute Hemorrhagic Infarct, Kidney, Dog. There is a focal wedge-shaped hemorrhagic area of cortical necrosis. The capsular surface of the infarct bulges above that of the adjacent normal kidney, indicating acute cell swelling and hemorrhage. (Courtesy Dr. W. Crowell, College of Veterinary Medicine, The University of Georgia; and Noah's Arkive, College of Veterinary Medicine, The University of Georgia.)

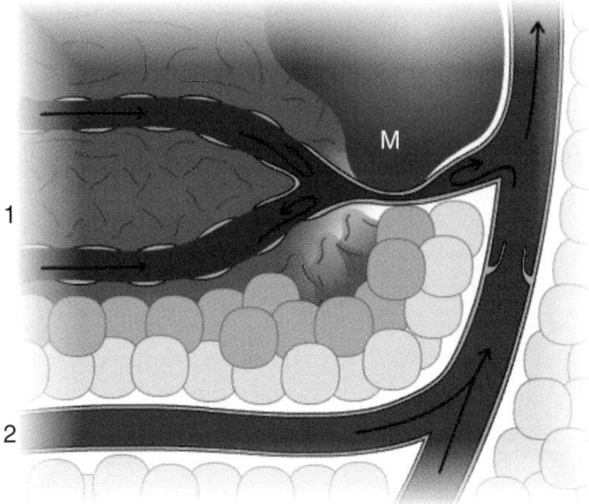

Figure 2-39 Infarction due to Venous Obstruction. Venous obstruction results in stagnation of blood flow and reduction or loss of venous return. There is progressive ischemia and ultimately coagulative necrosis of the tissue upstream of the site of vessel obstruction. The amount of necrosis depends on factors such as the type and prior health of the tissue affected, metabolic rate, and amount of collateral circulation or alternative blood supply. *1*, Venous return to a larger vein (note the valve) obstructed by a mass (M); *2*, normal venous return to a larger vein. (Courtesy Dr. D.A. Mosier and L. Schooley, College of Veterinary Medicine, Kansas State University.)

contrast, when venous obstruction occurs, such as from torsions or displacements of the bowel, there is extensive congestion and edema of the affected bowel that precedes and promotes infarction. Concurrent disease, decreased cardiovascular function, anemia, or decreased tissue vitality will increase the likelihood of localized areas of ischemia progressing to infarction. In tissue with a single blood supply and minimal anastomoses (e.g., brain, heart, kidney, and spleen), occlusion of nearly any sized vessel typically results in infarction of the dependent tissue (Fig. 2-37). In tissue with parallel blood supplies that have numerous anastomoses (e.g., skeletal muscle and gastrointestinal tract), occlusion is less serious unless it occurs in a large vessel. Tissues with dual blood supplies (e.g., liver and lung) are not commonly susceptible to infarction unless concurrent underlying disease compromises the overall blood supply.

Most infarcts are dark red soon after their occurrence because of hemorrhage from damaged vessels in the infarcted area and backflow of blood into the area from surrounding vessels (see Fig. 2-37). As cells undergo necrosis, there is swelling of the affected area, which can force blood out of the infarcted region, giving it a pale appearance (Fig. 2-38). Additionally, hemolysis of erythrocytes and degradation and diffusion of hemoglobin give the infarct a progressively paler appearance. This change in color can occur within 1 to 5 days depending on the tissue and extent of the infarction. Certain types of tissue that have a loose (spongy) consistency, such as the lungs and storage-type spleens (e.g., dogs and pigs), usually remain red because the interstitial areas are expandable and necrosis-induced pressure does not build up to force blood out of the infarcted region (Figs. 2-39 and 2-40). Parenchymal tissues with a less expansible interstitium (e.g., kidney) generally become pale over time because of the pressure that forces blood from the necrotic area.

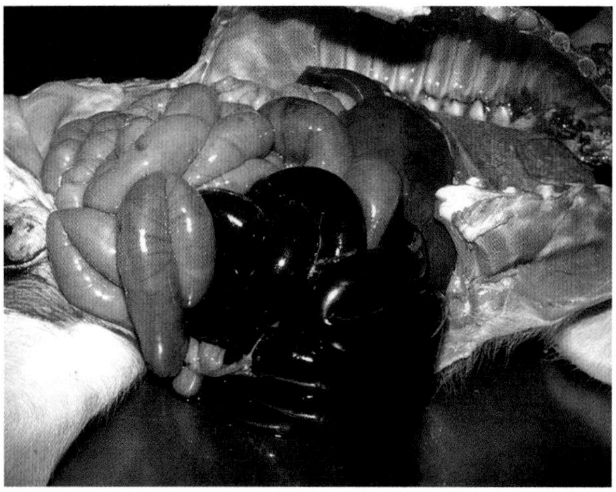

Figure 2-40 **Venous Infarction, Small Intestinal Volvulus, Pig.** Note the intensely congested loops of small intestine undergoing early venous infarction. The veins have been compressed by a volvulus that has compressed the veins but not the arteries, thus preventing the venous return. If the volvulus had rotated further, it would also have compressed the arteries. (Courtesy Dr. D.A. Mosier, College of Veterinary Medicine, Kansas State University.)

Inflammation occurs at the periphery of the dead tissue so that leukocytes, then macrophages, enter the area to clear the necrotic debris, and subsequently neovascularization and granulation occur to replace the necrotic region with fibrous tissue. This process can occur over a period of weeks or months depending on the extent of the damage. In contrast to the coagulative necrosis caused by infarction in most tissue, infarction in the brain and nervous tissue is characterized by liquefactive necrosis. Subsequently, there is glial cell removal of damaged tissue and astrocytic production of glial fibers (astrogliosis) to replace the affected area.

Shock

Shock (cardiovascular collapse) is a circulatory dyshomeostasis associated with loss of circulating blood volume, reduced cardiac output, and/or inappropriate peripheral vascular resistance. Although causes can be diverse (e.g., severe hemorrhage or diarrhea, burns, tissue trauma, endotoxemia), the underlying events of shock are similar. Hypotension results in impaired tissue perfusion, cellular hypoxia and a shift to anaerobic metabolism, cellular degeneration, and cell death (Fig. 2-41). Although the cellular effects of hypoperfusion are initially reversible, persistence of shock results in irreversible cell and tissue injury. Shock is rapidly progressive and life threatening when compensatory responses are inadequate. Shock can be classified into three different types based on the fundamental underlying problem: (1) cardiogenic, (2) hypovolemic, and (3) blood maldistribution. Shock attributed to blood maldistribution can be further divided into septic shock, anaphylactic shock, and neurogenic shock.

Cardiogenic Shock

Cardiogenic shock results from failure of the heart to adequately pump blood. Cardiac failure can occur due to myocardial infarction, ventricular tachycardia, fibrillation or other arrhythmias, dilated or hypertrophic cardiomyopathy, obstruction of blood flow from the heart (e.g., pulmonary embolism and pulmonary or aortic stenosis), or other cardiac dysfunctions. In all cases there is a decrease in both stroke volume and cardiac output. Major compensatory mechanisms (e.g., sympathetic stimulation of the heart), which increase heart contractility, stroke volume, total cardiac output, and heart rate, are only variably successful depending on the nature of the cardiac damage and the ability of the damaged heart to respond. Unsuccessful compensation leads to stagnation of blood and progressive tissue hypoperfusion.

Hypovolemic Shock

Hypovolemic shock arises from reduced circulating blood volume as the result of blood loss caused by hemorrhage or the result of fluid loss secondary to vomiting, diarrhea, or burns. Reduced circulating blood volume leads to decreased vascular pressure and tissue hypoperfusion. Immediate compensatory mechanisms (e.g., peripheral vasoconstriction and fluid movement into the plasma) act to increase vascular pressure and maintain blood flow to critical tissues such as the heart, brain, and kidney. Increased pressure provides an adequate driving force on which local mechanisms can draw to increase blood flow based on their needs. When the insult is mild, compensation is generally successful and the animal returns to homeostasis. Loss of approximately 10% of blood volume can occur without a decrease in blood pressure or cardiac output. However, if greater volumes are lost, adequate pressure and perfusion cannot be maintained and there is insufficient blood flow to meet the needs of the tissues. When blood loss approaches 35% to 45%, blood pressure and cardiac output can fall dramatically.

Blood Maldistribution

Blood maldistribution is characterized by decreased peripheral vascular resistance and pooling of blood in peripheral tissues. This is caused by neural or cytokine-induced vasodilation that can result from situations such as trauma, emotional stress, systemic hypersensitivity to allergens, or endotoxemia. Systemic vasodilation results in a dramatically increased microvascular area, and although the blood volume is normal, the effective circulating blood volume is decreased. Unless compensatory mechanisms can override the stimulus for vasodilation, there is pooling and stagnation of blood with subsequent tissue hypoperfusion. The three major types of shock caused by blood maldistribution are anaphylactic, neurogenic, and septic shock.

Anaphylactic shock is a generalized type I hypersensitivity. Common causes include exposure to insect or plant allergens, drugs, or vaccines. The interaction of the inciting substance with immunoglobulin E bound to mast cells results in widespread mast cell degranulation and the release of histamine and other vasoactive mediators. Subsequently, there is systemic vasodilation and increased vascular permeability, causing hypotension and tissue hypoperfusion.

Neurogenic shock may be induced by trauma, particularly trauma to the nervous system; electrocution, such as by lightning strike; fear; or emotional stress. In contrast to anaphylactic and endotoxic shock, cytokine release is not a major factor in the initial peripheral vasodilation. Instead, there are autonomic discharges that result in peripheral vasodilation, followed by venous pooling of blood and tissue hypoperfusion.

Septic shock is the most common type of shock associated with blood maldistribution. In septic shock, peripheral vasodilation is caused by components of bacteria or fungi that induce the release of excessive amounts of vascular and inflammatory mediators. The most common cause of septic shock is endotoxin, a lipopolysaccharide (LPS) complex within the cell wall of Gram-negative bacteria. Less often, peptidoglycans and lipoteichoic acids of Gram-positive organisms initiate shock. Local release of LPS from degenerating bacteria is a potent stimulus for many of the host responses

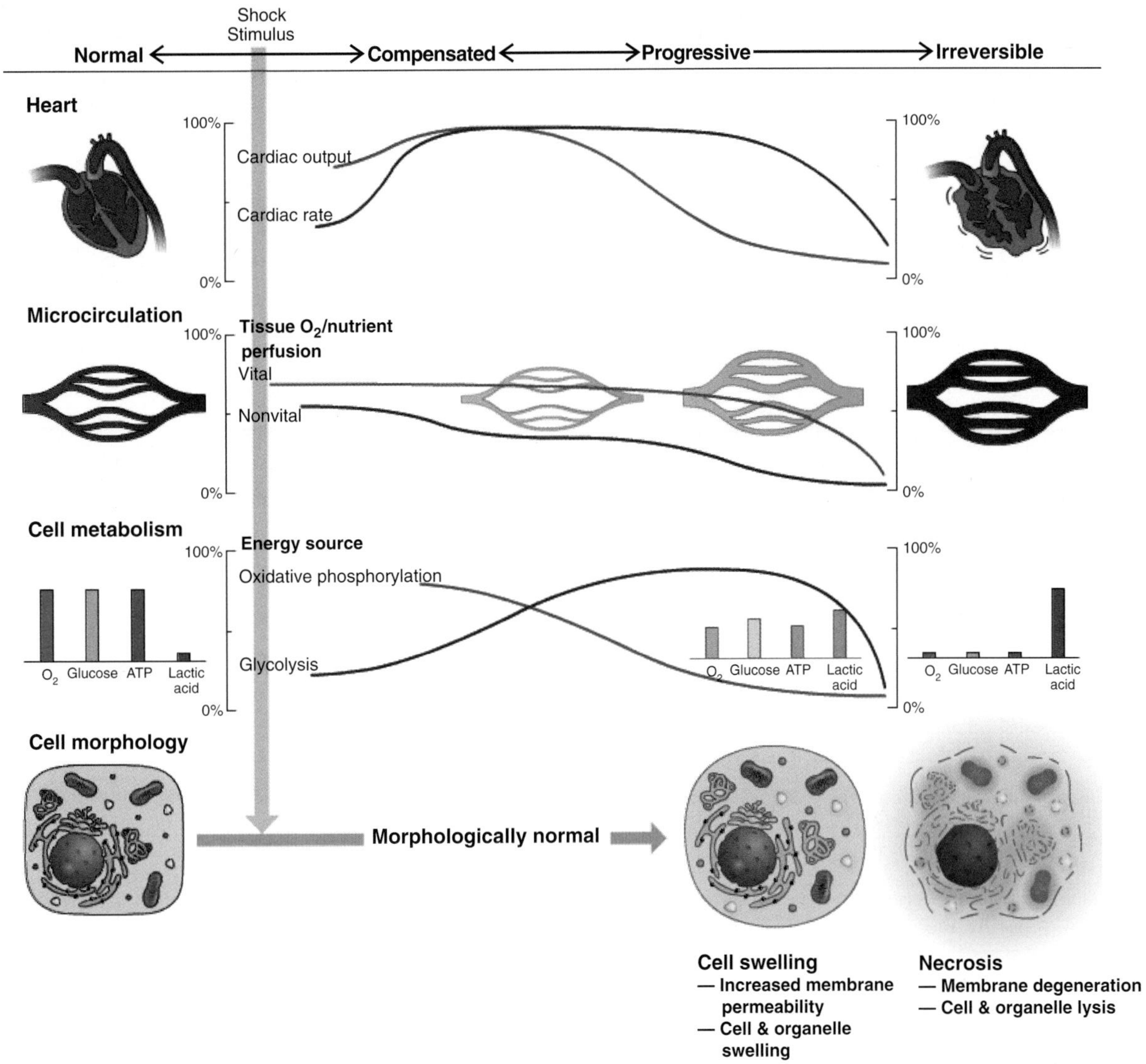

Figure 2-41 Shock. In hypovolemic shock, there is initially compensation characterized by increased cardiac rate and output, vasoconstriction of nonessential vascular beds, and predominantly oxidative metabolism by morphologically normal cells. With progression, cardiac output falls as peripheral vasodilation occurs, and cell metabolism shifts to glycolysis with progressive morphologic deterioration of cells. *ATP*, Adenosine triphosphate. (Courtesy Dr. D.A. Mosier and L. Schooley, College of Veterinary Medicine, Kansas State University.)

induced by the infectious agent. LPS often gains entry from microflora of the bowel, entering the circulation into the monocyte-macrophage system, then accumulating in the liver, spleen, alveoli, and leukocytes. LPS activates cells (mainly endothelium and leukocytes) through a series of reactions involving LPS-binding protein (an acute phase protein), CD14 (a cell membrane protein and soluble plasma protein), and Toll-like receptor 4 (TLR4, a signal-transducing protein). Endothelial activation by LPS inhibits production of anticoagulant substances (e.g., TFPI and thrombomodulin). Activation of monocytes and macrophages by LPS induces the direct or indirect release of TNF and IL-1 and other cytokines (e.g., IL-6, IL-8, chemokines). LPS directly activates factor XII to promote intrinsic coagulation and other factor XIIa–related pathways (kinins, fibrinolysis, complement). LPS can also directly activate the complement cascade to generate the anaphylatoxins C3a and C5a. Although these events are important for enhancing the inflammatory response to control localized infections associated with relatively low concentrations of LPS, they can be detrimental if the response becomes more pronounced and widespread. This may occur with overwhelming infections by bacteria (generating large concentrations of LPS), or when prolonged intestinal ischemia as the result of other types of shock results in breakdown of the mucosal integrity and leakage of bacteria and toxins into the blood. These higher concentrations of LPS induce even more production of TNF, IL-1, and other cytokines, and the secondary effects of these cytokines become more prominent. TNF and IL-1 induce TF expression and endothelial activation of extrinsic coagulation and enhance the expression of endothelial leukocyte adhesion molecules. IL-1 also stimulates the release of platelet-activating factor (PAF) and PAI to enhance platelet aggregation and coagulation. PAF released from leukocytes, platelets, and endothelium can cause platelet aggregation and thrombosis, increased vascular permeability, and similar to TNF and IL-1, stimulation of arachidonic acid metabolite production (particularly prostacyclin [PGI_2] and thromboxane). TNF and IL-1 induce nitric oxide production, which also contributes to vasodilation and hypotension. Neutrophils become activated by TNF and IL-1 to enhance their adhesion to endothelium, which further interferes with blood flow through the microvasculature. The end result of the activation of these myriad vascular, proinflammatory, and procoagulant alterations is the profound systemic vasodilation, hypotension, and tissue hypoperfusion characteristic of septic shock.

Stages and Progression of Shock

Regardless of the underlying cause, shock generally progresses through three different stages: (1) a nonprogressive stage, (2) a progressive stage, and (3) an irreversible stage.

Nonprogressive shock is characterized by compensatory mechanisms that counteract reduced functional circulating blood volume and decreased vascular pressure. Baroreceptors respond to decreased pressure by increasing medullary sympathetic nervous output and epinephrine/norepinephrine release, which increases cardiac output and causes arteriolar vasoconstriction (increased peripheral resistance) in most tissues in an attempt to raise vascular pressure. Notable exceptions are critical tissues, such as the heart, brain, and kidney, to which the blood flow is preserved. Left atrial volume receptors and hypothalamic osmoreceptors help regulate pressure by altering water and sodium balance. Reduced plasma volume stimulates ADH release and water retention and activates angiotensin II production by the renin-angiotensin system to result in aldosterone release and sodium retention. ADH and angiotensin II are also vasoconstrictors and help contribute to increased peripheral resistance. Vasoconstriction also results from endothelial release of endothelin, cold, increased O_2, or decreased CO_2. Decreased microvascular pressure results in a shift in fluid movement from the interstitium into the plasma to also help increase blood volume. The results of these and other responses are increased heart rate and cardiac output, as well as increased vascular pressure. This provides an adequate driving force on which local mechanisms can draw to increase blood flow based on their needs. When the insult is mild, compensation is generally successful and the animal returns to homeostasis.

In the case of severe or prolonged hypovolemia or cardiac damage that inhibits the ability of the heart to increase output, compensatory mechanisms are inadequate and shock enters the progressive stage. In this stage there is blood pooling, tissue hypoperfusion, and progressive cell injury. Cellular metabolism becomes less efficient and shifts from aerobic to anaerobic with pyruvate converted to lactate without entering the Krebs cycle. The deficient production of ATP and overproduction of lactic acid inhibits normal cell functions and results in cellular and systemic acidosis. Metabolic products (e.g., adenosine and potassium), increased local osmolarity, local hypoxia, and increased CO_2 eventually result in arteriolar relaxation and dilation. In the case of septic shock these events exacerbate preexisting cytokine- and mediator-induced vasodilation of the microvasculature. In hypovolemic and cardiogenic shock the decreased vascular resistance initiates pooling and stagnation of blood within previously closed vascular beds. Widespread arteriolar dilation caused by local influences overrides systemic controls and dramatically contributes to further decreases in vascular plasma volume and pressure. When oxygen and energy stores of the cell are depleted, membrane transport mechanisms are impaired, lysosomal enzymes are released, structural integrity is lost, and cell necrosis occurs. In addition to the detrimental metabolic effects of deficient oxygenation, cell and tissue injury occur in response to the dramatic accumulation of mediators that is characteristic of progressive shock, regardless of its underlying cause. These include histamine, kinins, PAF, complement fragments, and a wide variety of cytokines (e.g., TNF, IL-1, IL-8). These mediators are associated with inappropriate systemic inflammation and systemic activation of complement, coagulation, fibrinolysis, and kinin pathways.

The exact point at which shock enters the irreversible stage is not clear. At the cellular concentration, metabolic acidosis that results from anaerobic metabolism inhibits enzyme systems needed for energy production. Decreased metabolic efficiency allows vasodilatory substances to accumulate in the ischemic cells and tissues. Once these local products and reflexes override centrally mediated vasoconstriction to produce vasodilation, it is unlikely that shock will be reversed. The fall in peripheral resistance as the result of widespread peripheral vasodilation decreases vascular pressure even more. Irreversibility is generally ensured when shock progresses into the syndrome of multiple organ dysfunction. As each organ system fails, particularly the lung, liver, intestine, kidney, and heart, there is a reduction in the metabolic support each system provides to the others. Vicious cycles occur in which the failing function of one organ or tissue contributes to the failure of another (e.g., decreased cardiac output causes renal and pancreatic ischemia; electrolyte imbalances caused by renal ischemia then result in cardiac arrhythmias and myocardial depressant factor released by the ischemic pancreas, which contribute to even greater reductions in cardiac output). The end point of irreversible shock is often manifested as disseminated intravascular coagulation, which is the profound and paradoxic dysfunction of hemostasis.

Clinical and Morphologic Features of Shock

Clinical features of shock are rapidly progressive and include hypotension, weak pulse, tachycardia, hyperventilation with pulmonary rales, reduced urine output, and hypothermia. Organ and system failure occurs in later stages, each manifesting with signs specific to that organ or tissue.

The lesions of shock are variable and depend on the nature and severity of the initiating stimulus and the stage of progression of shock. Characteristically, there are vascular changes accompanied by cell degeneration and necrosis. Generalized congestion and pooling of blood are present in most cases, unless there has been substantial blood loss. Edema, hemorrhage (petechial and ecchymotic), and microthrombosis may be present as reflections of the vascular deterioration that accompanies shock. Microthrombosis and platelet plugging of capillaries is most common in septic shock. Vascular abnormalities are most obvious in those cases that progress to disseminated intravascular coagulation. Cell degeneration and necrosis are most prominent in those cells that are most susceptible to hypoxia, such as neurons and cardiac myocytes, and cells that do not obtain adequate preferential blood flow during shock. Hepatocytes, renal tubular epithelium, adrenal cortical epithelium, and gastrointestinal epithelium are often affected. With the exception of loss of neurons and myocytes, virtually all of these tissue changes can revert to normal if the animal survives. Specific changes may include severe pulmonary congestion, edema, and hemorrhage with alveolar epithelial necrosis, fibrin exudation, and hyaline membrane formation. Passive congestion and centrilobular hepatic necrosis, as well as renal tubular necrosis, are often present in these metabolically important organs. Intestinal congestion, edema, and hemorrhage with mucosal necrosis may occur. In the heart, myofibril coagulation is caused by hypercontraction of sarcomeres and is most likely a response to high sarcoplasmic calcium concentrations as the result of lack of energy and membrane damage. Cerebral edema and in some cases cerebrocortical laminar necrosis as a result of cerebral ischemia may be present.

Suggested Readings

Suggested Readings are available at www.expertconsult.com.

CHAPTER 3

Inflammation and Healing[1]

Mark R. Ackermann

Key Readings Index

Injury or death of cells caused by infectious microbes, mechanical trauma, heat, cold, radiation, or cancerous cells can initiate a well-organized cascade of fluidic and cellular changes within living vascularized tissue called *acute inflammation* (Fig. 3-1). These changes result in the accumulation of fluid, electrolytes, and plasma proteins, as well as leukocytes, in extravascular tissue and are recognized clinically by redness, heat, swelling, pain, and loss of function of the affected tissue. Inflammation is often a protective mechanism whose biologic purpose is to dilute, isolate, and eliminate the cause of injury and to repair tissue damage resulting from the injury. Without inflammation, animals would not survive their daily interactions with environmental microbes, foreign materials, and trauma and with degenerate, senescent, and neoplastic cells.

Acute inflammation is the progressive reaction of vascularized living tissue to injury over time. This process is usually a well-ordered cascade mediated by chemoattractants, vasoactive molecules, proinflammatory and antiinflammatory cytokines and their receptors, and antimicrobial or cytotoxic molecules. Acute inflammation has a short duration, ranging from a few hours to a few days, and its main characteristics are exudation of electrolytes, fluid, and plasma proteins and leukocytic emigration, principally neutrophils from the microvasculature, followed by rapid repair and healing. For convenience, acute inflammation is divided into three sequential phases: fluidic, cellular, and reparative.

Chronic inflammation is considered to be inflammation of prolonged duration, usually weeks to months and even years, in which the response is characterized predominantly by lymphocytes and macrophages, tissue necrosis, and accompanied by tissue repair, such as healing, fibrosis, and granulation tissue formation, all of which may occur simultaneously. Chronic inflammation can be a sequela to acute inflammation if there is failure to eliminate the agent or substance that incites the process. With such persistent substances the inflammatory reaction and exudates gradually transition from seroproteinaceous fluids and neutrophils to macrophages, lymphocytes, and fibroblasts with the potential for formation of granulomas. Alternatively, some inciting substances can invoke chronic inflammation directly and almost immediately. Examples include infections by *Mycobacterium* spp.; exposure to foreign materials, such as silicates and grass awns; and immune-mediated diseases, such as arthritis.

Evolution of the Current Understanding of Inflammation

Information on this topic, including E-Table 3-1, is available at www.expertconsult.com.

[1]For a glossary of abbreviations and terms used in this chapter see E-Glossary 3-1.

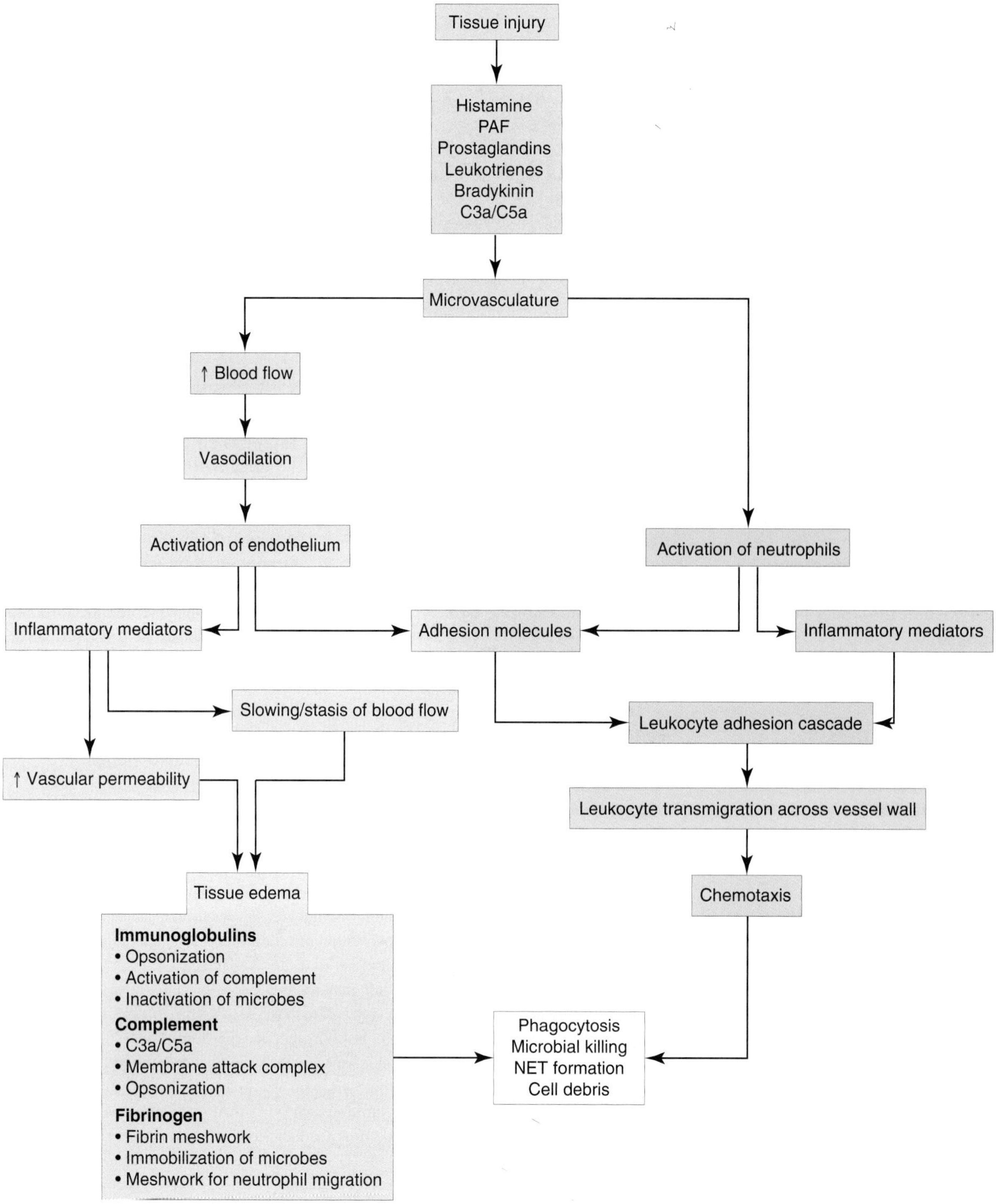

Figure 3-1 **Major Steps of Acute Inflammation.** *PAF*, Platelet-activating factor; *NET*, neutrophil extracellular trap. (Courtesy Dr. M.R. Ackermann, College of Veterinary Medicine, Iowa State University; and Dr. J.F. Zachary, College of Veterinary Medicine, University of Illinois.)

Beneficial and Harmful Aspects of Inflammation

In general, inflammatory responses are beneficial in the following ways:

- Diluting and/or inactivating biologic and chemical toxins
- Killing or sequestering microbes, foreign material, necrotic tissue (e.g., bone sequestrum), and neoplastic cells
- Degrading foreign materials
- Providing wound healing factors to ulcerated surfaces and traumatized tissue
- Restricting movement of appendages and joints to allow time for healing and repair
- Increasing temperature in the body or locally to induce vasodilation and inhibiting replication of some microbial agents

However, in some instances, an excessive and/or prolonged inflammatory response can be detrimental and even more harmful than that of the inciting agent/substance. In several disorders of human beings, such as myocardial infarction, cerebral thrombosis and infarction, and atherosclerosis, excessive and prolonged inflammatory responses can exacerbate the severity of the disease process.

Box 3-1 Selected Disorders That Are Induced or Exacerbated by Inflammatory Responses

DISORDERS IN WHICH THE MECHANISM OF INJURY IS INFLAMMATION

Human beings: Alzheimer's disease, atherosclerosis, atopic dermatitis, chronic obstructive pulmonary disease (COPD), Crohn's disease, gout, graft rejection, Hashimoto's thyroiditis, multiple sclerosis, pemphigus, psoriasis, rheumatoid arthritis, sarcoidosis, systemic lupus erythematosus (SLE), type I diabetes mellitus, ulcerative colitis, vasculitis (Wegener's granulomatosis, polyarteritis nodosa, Goodpasture's disease)
Cats: Eosinophilic stomatitis, lymphoplasmacytic syndrome, pemphigus
Dogs: Granulomatous meningoencephalitis, pemphigus, systemic and discoid lupus erythematosus
Common to many species: Anaphylaxis, spondylitis, asthma, reperfusion injury, osteoarthritis, glomerulonephritis

INFECTIOUS DISEASE EXACERBATED BY INFLAMMATION

Human beings: Dysentery, Chagas's disease, cystic fibrosis pneumonia, filariasis, *Helicobacter pylori* gastritis, hepatitis C, influenza virus pneumonia, leprosy, *Neisseria*/pneumococcal meningitis, poststreptococcal glomerulonephritis, schistosomiasis, sepsis, tuberculosis
Dogs: *H. pylori* gastritis
Cattle: *Mannheimia haemolytica* pneumonia, mastitis, *Mycobacterium bovis*, *Mycobacterium avium* subsp. *paratuberculosis*
Pigs: Circovirus
Ferrets/mink: Aleutian mink disease
Common to many species: Vegetative valvular endocarditis

CONDITIONS IN WHICH POSTINFLAMMATORY FIBROSIS OCCURS

Human beings: Bleomycin pulmonary fibrosis, allograft rejection, idiopathic pulmonary fibrosis, hepatic cirrhosis (postviral, alcohol, or toxin), radiation-induced pulmonary fibrosis
Dogs: Idiopathic pulmonary fibrosis (West Highland white dogs)
Cattle/sheep/horses: Plant toxins (hepatic fibrosis)

Modified from Nathan C: *Nature* 420:846-851, 2002.

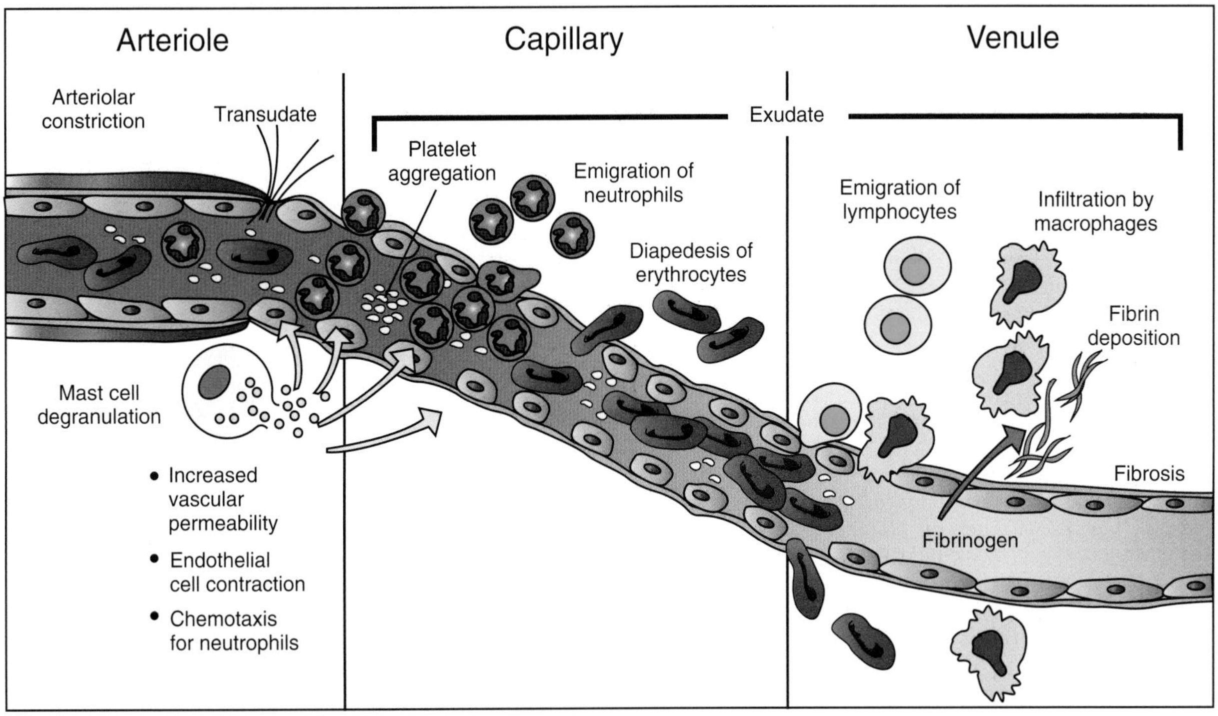

Figure 3-2 The Primary Vascular and Cellular Responses During Acute Inflammation. The majority of these responses occur in capillaries and postcapillary venules.

In veterinary medicine, exuberant or uncontrolled inflammatory responses occurring in the diseases listed in Box 3-1 can also result in increased severity of disease.

Acute Inflammation

The acute inflammatory response (Fig. 3-2; Essential Concept 3-1) can be initiated by a variety of exogenous and endogenous substances that injure vascularized tissue and affect the fluid clearance activities of sodium/potassium adenosinetriphosphatase (ATPase) pumps; sodium, cation, nucleotide-gated, and aquaporin channels; transcellular passage of chloride; and lymphatic drainage. The response to injury begins as active hyperemia, characterized by an increased flow of blood to injured tissue secondary to dilation of arterioles and capillaries (vasodilation), and it is this response that is responsible for redness and heat. It is facilitated by chemical mediators such as prostaglandins, endothelin, and nitric oxide (NO; Box 3-2). With vasodilation, vascular flow is slowed (vascular congestion), allowing time for fluid leakage that occurs as a result of changes in junctional complexes of endothelial cells induced by

ESSENTIAL CONCEPT 3-1 Acute Inflammation

Acute inflammation is a vascular response to cell and tissue injury triggered by numerous physical and biologic stimuli. In affected tissue its objectives are (1) to kill and/or eliminate the cause of injury (e.g., microbes, foreign material, thermal, radiation), (2) to phagocytose and remove debris, and (3) to repair the damage, thereby returning the tissue to normal structure and function. Acute inflammation progresses chronologically in sequence through three phases: fluidic, cellular, and reparative. The purpose of the fluidic phase is to dilute, surround (i.e., isolate), and contain (i.e., trap) the stimulus and the damage, thereby limiting the extent of involvement of adjacent normal cells and tissue. It is caused by direct or indirect injury of microvessels (capillaries) and results in increased vascular permeability and the "active" leakage of plasma proteins (e.g., fibrinogen, albumin) and edema fluid into affected tissue. Direct injury to microvessels (i.e., capillaries) is commonly caused by physical stimuli such as thermal injury (e.g., freeze/burn) or trauma, whereas indirect injury occurs in response to the release of biologic molecules from the inciting stimulus like microbes or from damaged cells. These molecules diffuse outwards from the site of injury in all directions and interact with capillaries in adjoining normal tissue to alter vascular permeability. Concurrently, these molecules also (1) initiate and facilitate the recruitment and movement of neutrophils through the walls of capillaries into affected tissue (i.e., cellular phase) and (2) form a "directional concentration gradient," greatest at the source and lowest at the periphery that guides (also known as chemoattractant molecules or chemoattractants) migrating neutrophils to the entrapped inciting stimulus. The purpose of the cellular phase is to kill and/or digest (inactivate) the stimulus, limit the extent and severity of the injury, and thus end the provoked microvascular response. The extent and intensity of this process causes varying degrees of injury to adjoining normal stroma and epithelium. Tissue injury evokes the reparative phase of acute inflammation and is characterized by the movement of macrophages into the areas of entrapped stimulus and injured tissue to further process and remove cellular debris. Once the debris is removed, macrophages release molecules that initiate tissue repair, leading to reepithelization of supporting stroma if tissue loss is minimal. If tissue loss is more extensive, reparative activities may include neovascularization, granulation tissue formation, reepithelialization, and scarring (reparative fibrosis). Because the triggering stimulus may spread from its initial focus to adjacent tissue, different areas of the tissue may be in different stages of acute inflammation, but each affected area progresses through all three phases in the same chronologic order.

vasoactive amines, complement components C3a and C5a, bradykinin, leukotrienes, prostaglandins, and platelet-activating factor (PAF), resulting in leakage of plasma and plasma proteins into the extracellular space (swelling and pain [stretching of pain receptors]) mainly from interendothelial cell gaps in the postcapillary venules.

The volume and protein concentration of leaked fluid is a function of the size of gaps between endothelial cells and the molecular weight, size, and charge of electrolytes and plasma proteins, such as albumin and fibrinogen. With more severe injury resulting in destruction of individual endothelial cells, hemorrhage, as well as plasma and plasma proteins, can leak directly through a breach in the wall of the capillary or venule. Once activated, endothelial and perivascular cells, such as mast cells, dendritic cells, fibroblasts, and pericytes, can produce cytokines and chemokines that regulate the expression of receptors for inflammatory mediators and adhesion molecules within the lesions.

Box 3-2 Key Responses of Acute Inflammation and the Principal Inflammatory Mediators That Mediate These Processes

VASODILATION
Nitric oxide
Bradykinin
Prostaglandins: PGD_2
Leukotrienes: LTB_4

INCREASED VASCULAR PERMEABILITY
Vasoactive amines: histamine, substance P, bradykinin
Complement factors: C5a, C3a
Fibrinopeptides and fibrin breakdown products
Prostaglandins: PGE_2
Leukotrienes: LTB_4, LTC_4, LTD_4, LTE_4
PAF, substance P
Cytokines: IL-1, TNF

SMOOTH MUSCLE CONTRACTION
Histamine
Serotonin
C3a
Bradykinin
PAF
Leukotriene D_4

CHEMOTAXIS, LEUKOCYTE ACTIVATION
Complement factors: C5a
Leukotrienes: LTB_4
Chemokines: IL-8
Defensins: α- and β-Defensins
Bacterial products: LPS, peptidoglycan, teichoic acid
Collagenous lectins: Ficolins, surfactant proteins A and D, mannan-binding lectin
Cytokines: IL-1, TNF
Surfactant proteins A and D

FEVER
Cytokines: IL-1, TNF, IL-6
Prostaglandins: PGE_2

NAUSEA
Cytokines: IL-1, TNF, high mobility group factors

PAIN
Bradykinin
Prostaglandins: PGE_2

TISSUE DAMAGE
Neutrophil and macrophage lysosomal/granule contents: Matrix metalloproteinases
Reactive oxygen species: Superoxide anion, hydroxyl radical, nitric oxide

C3a, Complement factor C3a; *C5a*, complement factor C5a; *IL-1*, interleukin 1; *IL-6*, interleukin 6; *IL-8*, interleukin 8; *LTB_4*, leukotriene B_4; *LPS*, lipopolysaccharide; *LTC_4*, leukotriene C_4; LTD_4, leukotriene D_4; LTE_4, leukotriene E_4; *PAF*, platelet-activating factor; *PGD_2*, prostaglandin D_2; *PGE_2*, prostaglandin E_2; *TNF*, tumor necrosis factor.

The plasma proteins and fluid that initially accumulate in the extracellular space in response to injury are classified as a transudate (Fig. 3-3). A transudate is a fluid with minimal protein (specific gravity < 1.012 [<3 g of protein/dL]) and cellular elements (<1500 leukocytes/mL) and is essentially an electrolyte solution similar to that of plasma. Most commonly, the formation of a transudate occurs with hypertension, hypoproteinemia, and/or early in the acute inflammatory response. With these conditions there is increased

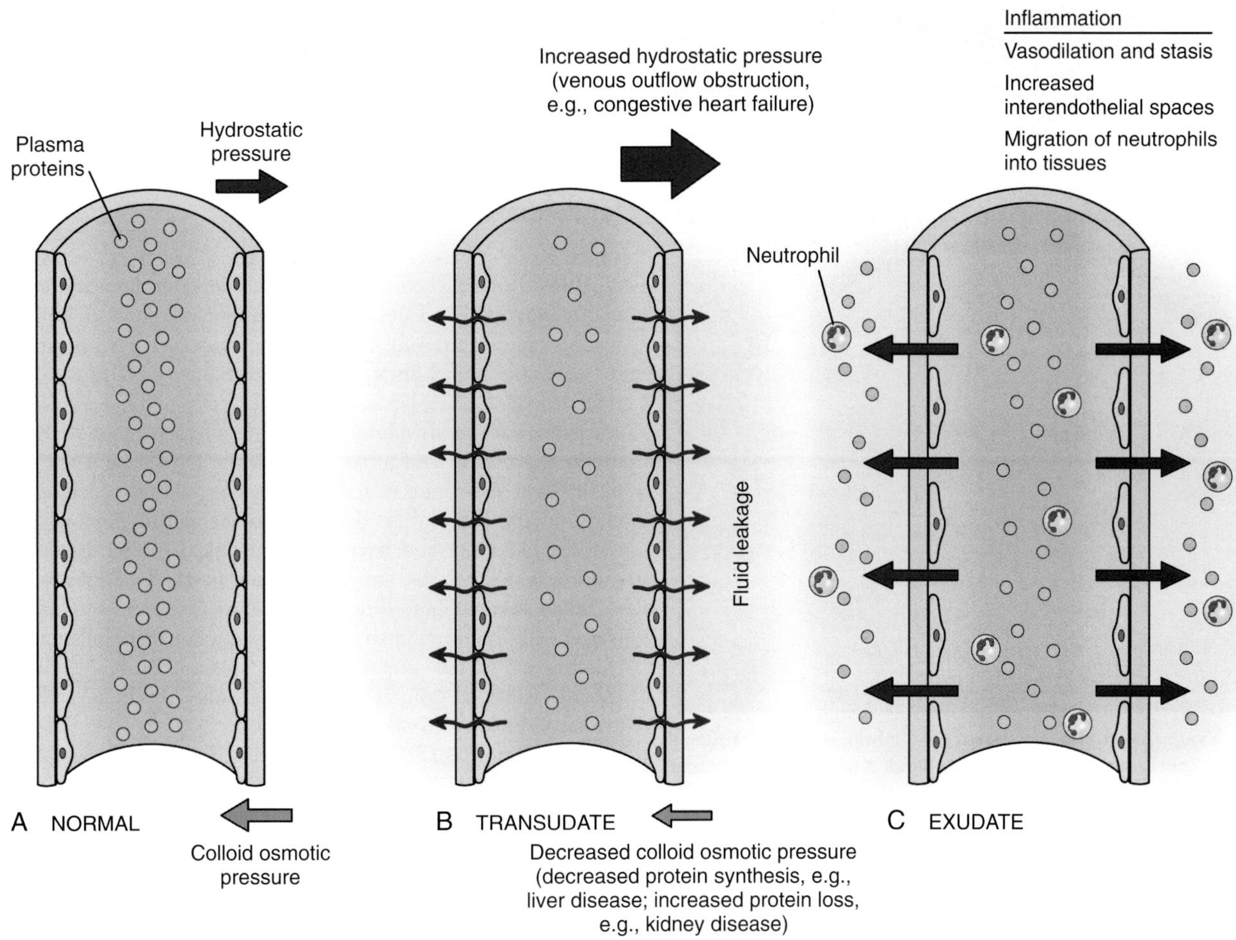

Figure 3-3 **Development of Transudates and Exudates. A,** Normal hydrostatic pressure *(blue arrow)* can lead to the outflow of fluid, but this is counterbalanced by the mean colloid osmotic pressure *(green arrow)*, which attracts fluid to the vascular lumen; therefore the net flow of fluid across the vascular bed is minimal. **B,** A transudate forms when fluid leaks out because of increased hydrostatic pressure or decreased osmotic pressure along with increased permeability across the endothelial cell layer. **C,** An exudate forms in inflammation because vascular permeability increases as a result of increased interendothelial spaces and damage to the endothelial layer.

permeability because of small physiologic gaps between endothelial cells. Hypertension in veins and capillaries can be secondary to arterial hypertension or venous/lymphatic obstruction. Hypoproteinemia is often due to loss of albumin, the major intravascular colloidal protein, and an inability of the liver to rapidly synthesize replacement albumin. The loss of albumin allows intravascular fluid to move toward the extravascular colloids (extravascular proteins). Loss of albumin and other intracellular proteins can occur secondary to renal disease (urinary loss), severe burns, and severe hepatic disease (decreased albumin production). During the early stages of the acute inflammatory response, intercellular gaps form between endothelial cells caused by endothelial cell contraction. The gaps are very small and allow only water and electrolytes to pass through them. With persistent and widening endothelial gap formation or with endothelial cell injury, neutrophils and additional protein can enter injured areas, resulting in the formation of an exudate (see Fig. 3-3). An exudate is an opaque and often viscous fluid (specific gravity > 1.020) that contains more than 3 g of protein per deciliter and more than 1500 leukocytes per milliliter. As discussed in a later section, the morphologic classification of inflammatory responses into categories, such as serous, fibrinous, and/or suppurative, is based on the character of the fluid that leaks from the vessel and of the leukocytes that migrate from the vascular lumen into the extracellular space.

Fibrinogen is an important plasma protein in exudates that polymerizes in extravascular tissues to form fibrin (Fig. 3-4). Plasma dilutes the effects of the inciting stimulus, whereas polymerized fibrin confines the stimulus to an isolated area, thus preventing its movement into adjacent tissue. This confinement provides leukocytes with a well-defined target for migration during the cellular phase of the acute inflammatory response. Neutrophils are the first leukocytes to enter the exudate, and their accumulation in the exudate after they liquefy is termed *pus*. Neutrophils have a variety of cytoplasmic granules, such as lysosomes, that contain antimicrobial peptides and proteins, as well as matrix metalloproteinases (MMPs), elastases, and myeloperoxidases. They kill pathogens and degrade foreign material by two mechanisms: (1) phagocytosis and fusion with primary and secondary lysosomes and (2) secretion of the contents of granules into the exudate. Because of the enzymes released, these cells can contribute to tissue injury. Fibrin and its products have additional activities, including chemotactic properties and blood clot formation. Fibrin also forms a framework/scaffold for fibroblast and endothelial cell migration during the initial stages of wound healing.

Neutrophils and other leukocytes leave capillaries and venules and migrate into tissue exudates in response to chemoattractant molecules released from host cells, microbes, foreign substances, and some neoplastic cells. As would be expected, the greatest

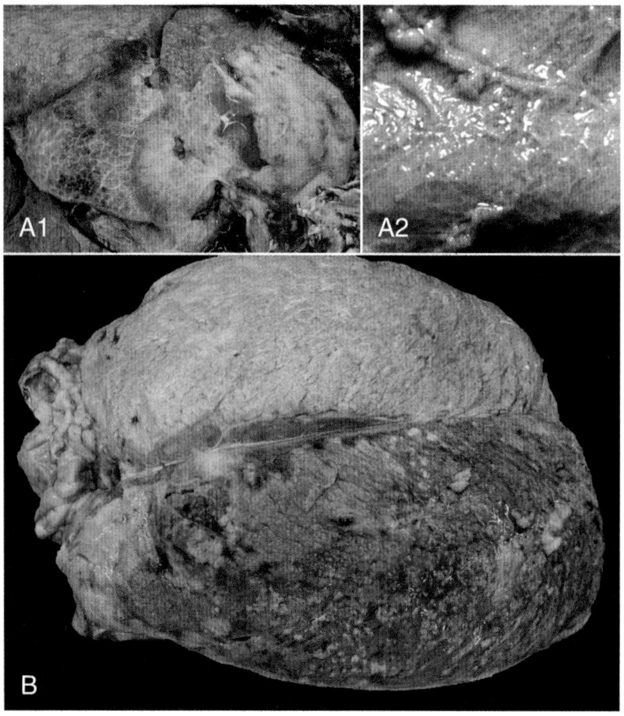

Figure 3-4 **Examples of the Appearance of Fibrin in Acute Inflammation in the Lung and Mammary Gland. A1,** Lungs (in situ) from an ox with acute pleuritis. The lungs have a thick mat of fibrin covering the cranioventral region. A small area of fibrin is torn away revealing the subjacent clear, yellow fluid subjacent. The fibrin coating the lung surface was released as fibrinogen from inflamed pleural vessels and polymerized on the serosal surface. The remaining lung surface is less affected. **A2,** Higher magnification of fibrin on the surface of the lung. **B,** Acute fibrinonecrotic mastitis, mammary gland, horizontal section, cow. The left quarters of the mammary gland *(lower half of the image)* are swollen as a result of edema and fibrin exudation and are reddened because of hyperemia, vascular congestion, and hemorrhage. The right quarters *(upper half of the image)* are unaffected. (**A1** and **B** courtesy Dr. J.S. Haynes, College of Veterinary Medicine, Iowa State University; **A2** courtesy Dr. M.D. McGavin, College of Veterinary Medicine, University of Tennessee.)

concentration of chemoattractant exists nearest the microbes or foreign substance, and the concentration decreases in a gradient-like manner with increasing distances from the source. This forms a "chemotactic gradient" that essentially creates a pathway for leukocytes to follow to reach the site of tissue injury. Chemoattractants activate receptors and molecules on neutrophils that result in (1) neutrophil movement and attachment to the luminal surface of capillaries and venules, (2) neutrophil migration through the intercellular junctions formed by gaps between endothelial cells, and (3) neutrophil migration within the exudate up the concentration gradient to the source of injury. This transmigration process, called the *leukocyte adhesion cascade*, has a well-characterized sequence of events occurring on the luminal surface of endothelial cells. These events, discussed in detail in a later section, lead to the transmigration of leukocytes into the exudate.

The reparative phase of the acute inflammatory response begins early and is completed only after the process or substance-causing injury is removed. In the reparative phase, necrotic cells and tissue are replaced by differentiation and regeneration of parenchymal and mesenchymal stem cells, coupled by filling the defect with connective tissue and covering denuded surfaces with a basement membrane and reepithelialization. When the acute inflammatory response has been completed in the proper sequence and the stimulus of injury removed, the inflammatory process is terminated. Failure to remove the stimulus can result in a persistent, unresolved lesion that becomes chronic and can form into granulation tissue or fibrosis.

Substances Inducing the Acute Inflammatory Response

There are two classes of substances, endogenous and exogenous, capable of injuring cells and tissue and inducing the acute inflammatory response. Endogenous substances include those that primarily cause autoreactive inflammatory responses, such as those induced by newly developed antigens and intracellular molecules released from degenerate, dysplastic, or neoplastic cells, and hypersensitivity reactions. Exogenous substances include microbes, such as viruses, bacteria, protozoa, and metazoan parasites; foreign bodies, such as plant fibers and suture material; mechanical actions, such as traumatic injury; physical actions, such as thermal or freezing injury, ionizing radiation, and microwaves; chemical substances, such as caustic agents, poisons, and venoms; and nutritive actions, such as ischemia and vitamin deficiencies. These substances or actions trigger cells to release mediators that lead to an acute inflammatory reaction and include preformed (in cytoplasmic granules) and synthesized (released from cell immediately after synthesis) chemical mediators from effector cells such as mast cells (histamine and tumor necrosis factor-α [TNF-α), leukocytes (cytokines, degradative enzymes), macrophages (cytokines), and endothelial and epithelial cells (chemokines, interferons). These cells also produce inflammatory mediators such as prostaglandins, leukotrienes, and PAF from products released from plasma membranes.

The acute inflammatory response to either endogenous or exogenous substances occurs simultaneously with activation of the innate immune system (see Chapter 5). Innate immunity is a nonspecific defense against potentially harmful environmental substances and consists of the following:

- Physical barriers and microenvironments provided by epithelia of the skin (low pH, lactic and fatty acids) and mucosae such as in the respiratory mucociliary escalator, reproductive tracts (secretions), and alimentary system (gastric and duodenal secretions, peristalsis, saliva).
- Molecular products released by mucosae, including lactoferrin, antimicrobial peptides (α- and β-defensins, cathelicidins), and collectins. These products have immune activity but also contribute to proinflammatory and antiinflammatory reactions, leukocyte activation, and wound healing.
- Effector molecules in the blood, such as plasma proteases (complement, kinin, and clotting systems) and inflammatory mediators released from nerve fibers (sensory fibers, C-reactive fibers), such as substance P.

The physical and biologic processes that activate the acute inflammatory and innate immune responses can exert their actions directly on the following:

- Effector cells in mucosae and vascularized connective tissue
- Effector molecules in the blood, on endothelial cells
- A combination of these components

The location, severity, and clinical signs of the acute inflammatory response depend on the route of exposure, such as dermal, alimentary, respiratory, urinary, or hematogenous, and the physical or biologic characteristics of the stimulus. More specifically, causes of the acute inflammatory response include but are not limited to the following:

- Visible and ultraviolet light spectra (sunburn and photosensitization)

- Radiation, blunt force trauma (abrasion, bruising, incision, and laceration)
- Thermal injury (hot and cold)
- Chemotherapeutics
- Environmental chemicals
- Microbial molecules (lipids and proteins)
- Venom (insect, snake, and reptile)
- Responses of the adaptive immune system (type I to IV hypersensitivities) to microbial and environmental antigens

These must either penetrate (light spectra, radiation, chemicals) or break/penetrate (microbes and foreign bodies) epithelial barriers of the skin and alimentary, urinary, and respiratory systems to irritate the tissue and incite an acute inflammatory response. Microbes have a few highly conserved ligands called *pathogen-associated molecular patterns* (PAMPs), and when in contact with mucosae, they immediately encounter cells that express membrane *pattern recognition receptors* (PRRs), which include Toll-like receptors (TLRs) nucleotide-binding oligomerization domain (NOD)-like receptors (NLRs) (and inflammasomes), C-type lectin receptors, and retinoic acid–inducible gene I (RIG-I)–like receptors, expressed on the cell surface or in its cytoplasm. These patterns include the lipopolysaccharide (LPS; Gram-negative bacterial cell wall), lipoteichoic acids (Gram-positive bacterial cell wall), mannose, peptidoglycan, bacterial DNA, *N*-formylmethionine (in bacterial proteins), double-stranded RNA (dsRNA; viruses), and glucans (fungal cell walls). When these molecular patterns are recognized by receptors on macrophages, leukocytes, and mucosal epithelia, they trigger the release of chemokines and cytokines and cellular activation, all of which initiate and/or participate in the acute inflammatory response and the innate immune response.

In contrast to the innate immune system, adaptive immunity results in an antigen-specific immune response characterized by the production of protective antibodies and effector leukocytes that attempt to eliminate the inciting cause of injury and the generation of memory cells that make subsequent adaptive immune responses against a specific microbial antigen more efficient and effective (see Chapter 5). Because acute inflammation is a vasocentric response, it would be reasonable to assume that just about any exogenous or endogenous cause could induce inflammation. This is true, but because the inflammatory response has numerous redundant checks and balances that regulate the occurrence and severity of expression of the response, harmful effects of inflammation are minimized.

The effects of inflammation are mediated through chemical mediators of inflammation, which include the following:

- Vasoactive amines such as histamine and serotonin
- Plasma proteases such as complement, kinin, and clotting system proteins
- Lipid mediators such as arachidonic acid metabolites and PAF
- Cytokines
- Chemokines
- Chemerin
- NO

Mast cells are rich in histamine and many of the chemical mediators listed previously and are widely distributed in connective tissue adjacent to blood vessels. Changes in the permeability of these vessels in the fluidic phase of the acute inflammatory response often occur as the result of mast cell activation. Histamine, preformed in mast cell granules, is released through a process called *degranulation*. Bradykinin, another vasoactive amine, is produced where there is vascular and/or endothelial cell injury. Both histamine and bradykinin cause changes in the caliber of arterioles, capillaries, and postcapillary venules and permeability in capillaries and postcapillary venules. These occur early in the fluidic phase of the acute inflammatory response and are quickly followed by the cellular phase.

Fluidic (Exudative) Phase of the Acute Inflammatory Response

The principal function of the fluidic phase of the acute inflammatory response is to dilute and localize the inciting agent/substance. In this phase there is an immediate vasocentric reaction (arterioles, capillaries, and postcapillary venules) to the inciting agent/substance. The sequence of vascular events in the acute inflammatory response includes the following:

- Increased blood flow (active hyperemia) to the site of injury
- Increased permeability of capillaries and postcapillary venules to plasma proteins and leukocytes through release of inflammatory mediators
- Emigration of leukocytes (via the leukocyte adhesion cascade) into the perivascular area

Initially, arterioles dilate and capillary beds in the affected area expand in volume to accommodate an increased blood flow (heat and redness) in response to the stimulus. Second, as a result of permeability changes induced by inflammatory mediators, blood flow through the capillary beds is slowed as a result of increased viscosity and hemoconcentration after leakage of water from capillary beds into extracellular space. Because of the reduced blood flow and pressure, microscopically, capillaries are often packed with erythrocytes, and the microenvironment facilitates leukocytic margination along the luminal surface of endothelial cells. This stage precedes leukocyte emigration through intercellular junctions of endothelial cells into the extravascular space. Inflammatory mediators induce endothelial cell contraction, resulting in the formation of interendothelial cell gaps, which further allow fluid leakage and leukocyte migration. In general, the endothelium of the normal vascular capillaries limits exchange of molecules to those less than 69,000 MW, the size of albumin. The exchange of small molecules and water between the vessel lumen and the interstitial space is extremely rapid. For example, the water of plasma is exchanged with the water of the interstitial space 80 times before the plasma can move the entire length of the capillary. Physiologically, increased amounts of fluid can pass across the vascular wall when there is (1) excessive hydrostatic pressure caused by hypertension and/or sodium retention, (2) decreased plasma proteins (colloid), or (3) lymphatic and/or venous obstruction. If fluid leakage is excessive, edema (transudate) develops (see Fig. 3-3). If the leakage is not excessive and postcapillary venules and lymphatic vessels are functioning normally, all of the fluid released from arterioles and small capillaries is returned to the circulation via paracellular gaps of postcapillary venular and lymphatic vessels. During acute inflammatory responses, there is a net outflow of fluid from arterioles, capillaries, and venules into extracellular tissue, which overwhelms the capacity for resorption by postcapillary venules and lymphatic vessels.

Endothelial Cell Dynamics during the Acute Inflammatory Response

Endothelial cells are the interface between plasma in the lumen and the perivascular connective tissue. They are polarized cells that have specific luminal versus abluminal surfaces, which serve the physiologic needs of the vascular bed of each organ. Transport across the endothelial cell layer occurs by (1) transcytosis (transcellular passage) via small vesicles and caveolae or (2) paracellular passage. Transcytosis, the process of transporting substances across the endothelium by uptake into and release from coated vesicles, facilitates the transport of albumin, low-density lipoproteins

(LDLs), metalloproteinases, and insulin. Paracellular passage allows transport of water and ions between cells (cell junctions). Paracellular passage is especially active in postcapillary venules. Roughly 30% of endothelial cell junctions in postcapillary venules can open to a width of 6 mm, roughly the width of a red blood cell. Leakage of fluid from the vasculature can occur within seconds after the acute inflammatory response is induced.

The mechanisms of leakage (Fig. 3-5) depend on the biologic and physical characteristics of the inciting agent or substance and include the following:

- Opening of junctional complexes (endothelial gaps) between endothelial cells responding to inflammatory mediators
- Direct injury that results in necrosis and detachment of endothelial cells, as occurs with certain viral, protozoal infections, toxins, and radiation
- Leukocyte-dependent injury that results in necrosis and detachment of endothelial cells and is induced by enzymes and mediators released from leukocytes during the transmigration phase of the acute inflammatory response
- Increased endothelial cell transcytosis mediated by vascular endothelial growth factor (VEGF)

Formation of Endothelial Cell Gaps

Endothelial gaps, resulting in vascular leakage, can occur (1) by contraction (actin/myosin) of adjacent endothelial cells and (2) through the reorganization of the cytoskeletal microtubule and microfilament proteins within the endothelial cells. With both of these changes, gaps result from the opening of junctional complexes between endothelial cells. Gaps by cell contraction occur in postcapillary venules where there is a high density of receptors for histamine, serotonin, bradykinin, and angiotensin II. Gaps formed by cytoskeletal reorganization occur most commonly in postcapillary venules and to a lesser extent in capillaries in response to cytokines, such as interleukin 1 (IL-1) and TNF, and hypoxia. Gap formation is transient and lasts 15 to 30 minutes after the stimulus occurs.

Vascular leakage resulting from direct injury to endothelial cells can cause detachment of the cell from the underlying basement membrane. Such damage establishes conditions favorable for the activation and attachment of platelets, clotting, and complement cascades. This type of extravasation usually occurs immediately after necrotizing injury induced by, for example, thermal injury, chemotherapeutic drugs, radiation, bacterial cytotoxins, and inhaled gases

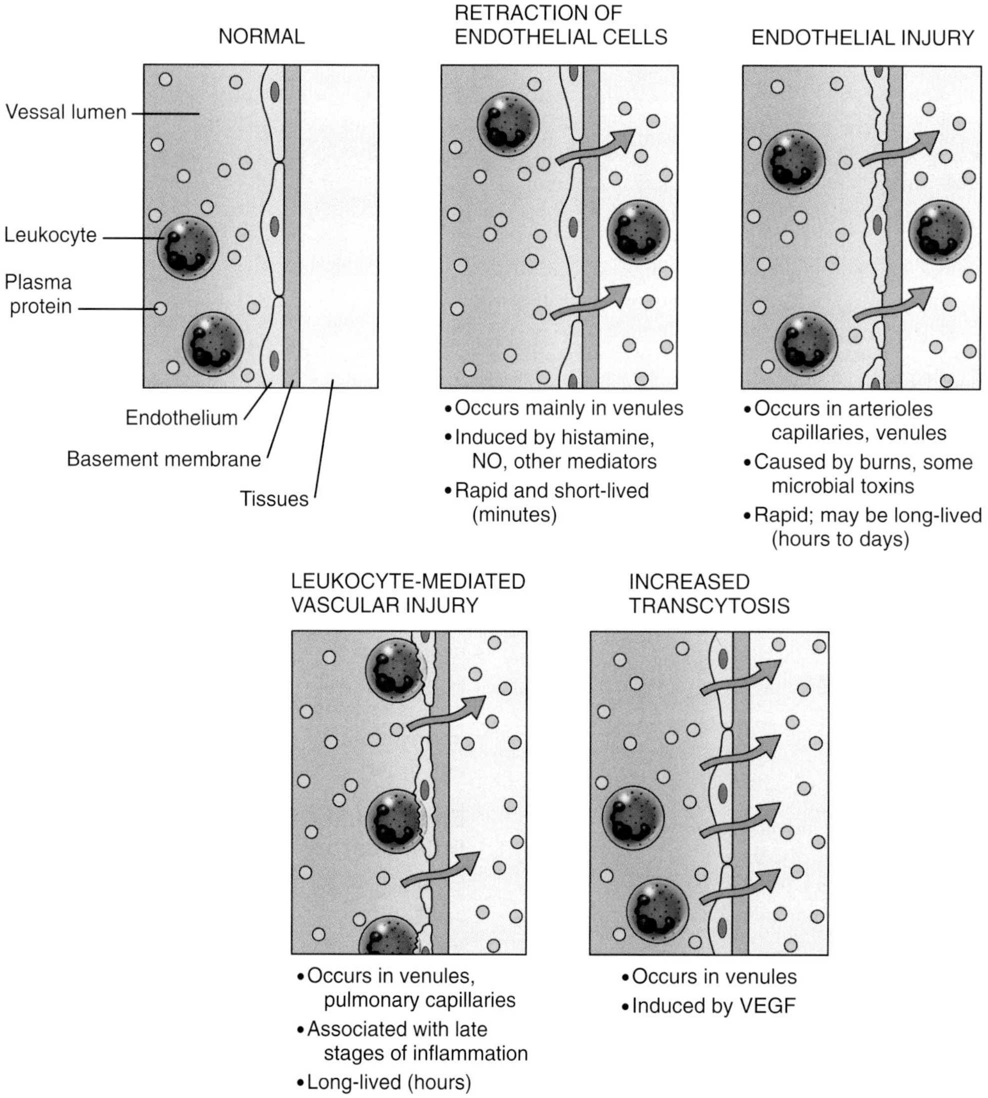

Figure 3-5 **Mechanisms of Increased Vascular Permeability with Inflammation.** *NO*, Nitric oxide; *VEGF*, vascular endothelial growth factor.

such as hydrogen sulfide. It affects arterioles, capillaries, and postcapillary venules. Vascular leakage resulting from leukocyte-induced damage occurs secondary to neutrophils and other leukocytes interacting with endothelial cells during the leukocyte adhesion cascade. Activated leukocytes release reactive oxygen species, such as singlet oxygen and oxygen free radicals, and proteolytic enzymes, such as matrix metalloproteinases (MMPs) and elastase from lysosomes during degranulation of the cells, which then result in endothelial cell necrosis and detachment and thus an increase in vascular permeability. This type of extravasation usually affects capillaries and postcapillary venules.

Cellular Phase of the Acute Inflammatory Response

The principal function of the cellular phase of the acute inflammatory response is to deliver leukocytes into the exudate at the site of injury so they can internalize agents/substances through phagocytosis and as required, for killing and/or degradation. Neutrophils, eosinophils, basophils, monocytes, mast cells, lymphocytes, natural killer T (NK-T) lymphocytes, and dendritic cells play an integral role in protecting mucosa, skin, and other surfaces of the body, as well as the pleura, pericardium, and peritoneum, from infection by microbes through phagocytosis or release of proteolytic degradative enzymes, chemical mediators, and reactive oxygen species. Neutrophils also have an important role in responding to foreign materials and toxins and in responding to neoplastic cells.

Leukocyte Adhesion Cascade

The movement of leukocytes from the lumina of capillaries and postcapillary venules into the interstitial connective tissue occurs through a process called the *leukocyte adhesion cascade* (Fig. 3-6). Chemokines, cytokines, and other inflammatory mediators influence this process by modulating the surface expression and/or avidity of adhesion molecules on both endothelial cells and leukocytes. It has a well-characterized sequence of events, including margination, rolling, activation and stable adherence (adhesion), and transmigration of leukocytes toward a chemotactic stimulus.

- *Margination*. As vessels vasodilate and have reduced hydrostatic pressure and blood flow, leukocytes exit the central region of the vascular lumen and move to the periphery of the vascular lumen near the endothelial cell surface (margination).
- *Rolling*. The initial contact between leukocytes and endothelial cells occurs by transient, weak binding interactions between the selectin family of adhesion molecules and their receptors. During rolling, leukocytes temporarily bind to endothelium and then release, which brings the leukocyte close to the endothelial cell surface and reduces the velocity of the traveling leukocyte. This process is mediated by selectins, including L-selectin expressed by neutrophils and P-selectin, a carbohydrate-binding molecule stored in Weibel-Palade bodies of endothelial cells and α-granules of platelets, as well as E-selectin expressed by endothelial cells. L-selectin is expressed on all leukocytes, but at low concentrations in normal human neutrophils and binds sialyl Lewis X receptor (and other receptors) on endothelial cells. P-selectin

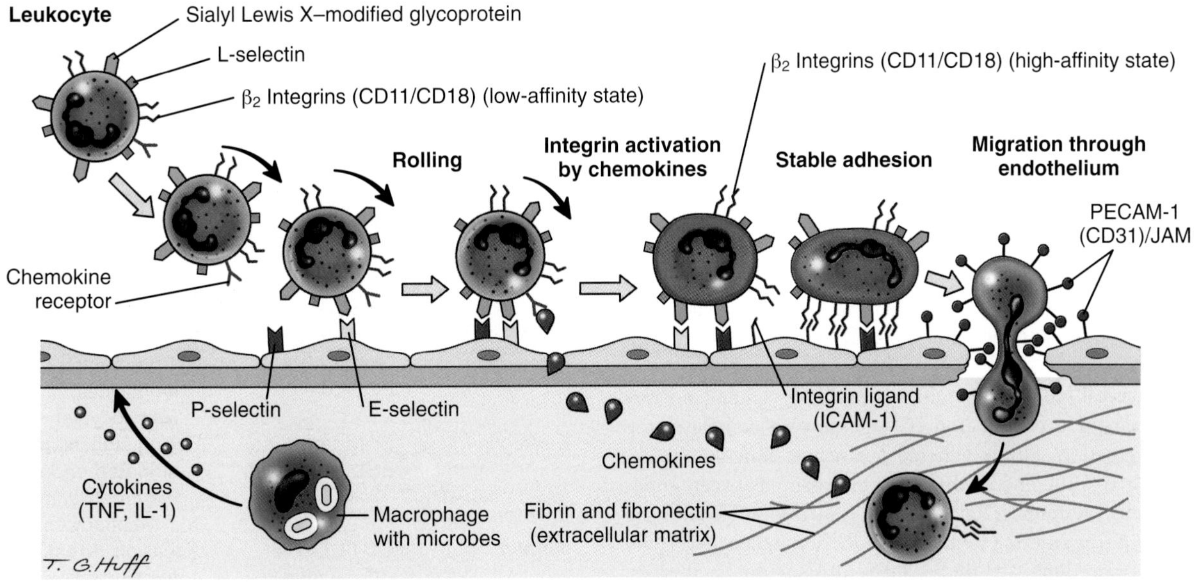

Figure 3-6 Leukocyte (Neutrophils) Adhesion Cascade. The leukocyte adhesion cascade illustrates the chronologic sequence of steps involved in the migration of neutrophils (leukocytes) through vascular endothelium. These steps include: (1) rolling, (2) activation by chemokines, (3) stable adhesion, and (4) migration through the endothelium. **Rolling**: Neutrophils have receptors, which bind to E- and P-selectin expressed on endothelial cells. L-selectin is also expressed by neutrophils to a varying degree in some species. Rolling slows neutrophil movement within capillaries and brings the neutrophil closer to the surface of vascular endothelial cells. **Activation**: Activation is induced by inflammatory mediators, including chemokines (e.g., interleukin 8 [IL-8]) and cytokines (e.g., interleukin 1β [IL-1β] and tumor necrosis factor-α [TNF-α]). Inflammatory mediators are released by neighboring leukocytes and endothelial cells. **Stable adhesion**: Inflammatory mediators by activating both neutrophils and endothelial cells induce conformational changes within integrins allowing enhanced binding avidity to integrin receptors and increased expression of additional adhesion molecules. Stable adherence of neutrophils to the endothelial cell surface occurs following binding of high-affinity β_2 integrins (Mac-1; CD11a/CD18) expressed by leukocytes to intercellular adhesion molecule 1 (ICAM-1) expressed by endothelial cells. **Migration**: Once neutrophils are attached to vascular endothelium, they adhere to platelet endothelial cell adhesion molecule 1 (PECAM-1) and other adhesion molecules present at the endothelial cell gap junction. They subsequently transmigrate through the junction into perivascular tissue, where they express β_1 integrins that adhere to extracellular matrix proteins such as laminin, fibronectin, vitronectin, and collagen. This process is mediated by chemokines (CXCL8; IL-8), complement fragments, vasoactive amines, cytokines, and membrane-derived mediators such as platelet-activating factor (PAF) and leukotrienes. *JAM*, Junctional adhesion molecule.

molecules expressed on endothelial cell surfaces bind to P-selectin glycoprotein ligand 1 (sialyl Lewis X–modified proteins) present on neutrophils, eosinophils, monocytes, and lymphocytes. E-selectin also mediates leukocyte–endothelial cell adherence and is expressed on endothelial cell surfaces for binding glycoprotein receptors expressed on leukocytes. Selectin-mediated attachments are formed at the leading edge of the rolling leukocyte and broken at the trailing edge. Even slight disturbances, such as surgical manipulation, heat, temporary ischemia, and mast cell products, induce rolling of neutrophils along the surface of endothelial cells. By slowing leukocyte transit time through capillaries and postcapillary venules, combined with the continual close proximity of slow rolling leukocytes to the endothelium, and the continued release of chemokines and proinflammatory cytokines, the proper microenvironment for progression to the "stable adhesion" stage occurs.

- *Stable adhesion*. For stable adhesion to occur, neutrophils and endothelial cells become activated by a variety of cytokines (such as IL-1, interleukin 6 [IL-6], TNF), complement factors (C5a), PAF, platelet-derived growth factor (PDGF), chemokines, and other inflammatory mediators. Once neutrophils are activated, L-selectin molecules are proteolytically cleaved from the neutrophil surface by ADAM17, and the neutrophils express a new set of membrane proteins (integrins) by rapid exocytosis of cytoplasmic vesicles. Firm adhesion of neutrophils to endothelial cells is mediated by binding of β_2 integrin molecules, such as macrophage-1 antigen (Mac-1) (CD11a/CD18), which are expressed on stimulated neutrophils in an active conformation, to intercellular adhesion molecule 1 (ICAM-1) and other ICAM molecules on endothelial cells. P- and E-selectin adherence also contributes to the process of firm adhesion. There are four β_2 integrins (lymphocyte function–associated antigen 1 [LFA-1], Mac-1, p150,95, and $\alpha d\beta_2$), which are heterodimers that differ only in their subunit CD11 a, b, c, and d for LFA-1, Mac-1, p150,95, and $\alpha d\beta_2$, respectively. CD18 (the β-subunit) is identical in all four β_2 integrins. Three β_2 integrins (LFA-1, Mac-1, and p150,95) are involved with leukocyte adherence; however, the β_2 integrin $\alpha d\beta_2$, which was first identified in dogs and subsequently in human beings, is apparently not meaningfully involved with the adherence of neutrophils or other leukocytes to endothelium. Once stable adherence is achieved, neutrophils move to endothelial cell junctions for transendothelial cell migration.
- *Transendothelial cell migration*. In postcapillary venules, neutrophil movement decreases from 10 μm/sec to a complete stop after margination. Firmly adhered leukocytes emigrate (transmigrate) across the endothelial layer by passing between endothelial cells. A number of leukocyte adhesion molecules are involved in this process (Table 3-1). Adhesion molecule activity and expression differ slightly for different tissues and cell types. In noninflamed skin, for example, there is a higher level of E- and P-selectin expression on endothelial cells, which facilitates rolling of leukocytes. In inflamed liver, CD44 of neutrophils binds serum-derived hyaluronan-associated protein (SHAP) that is bound to hyaluronic acid present on the luminal surface of endothelial cells. Nonactivated lymphocytes and monocytes use L-selectin to mediate adherence to high endothelial venules (HEVs) in lymph nodes. These cells also use $\alpha_4\beta_1$ (very late antigen-4 [VLA-4]) to mediate stable adherence to the endothelial ligand, vascular cell adhesion molecule 1 (VCAM-1). Neutrophils and other leukocytes transmigrate between endothelial cells at the intercellular junctions. Platelet endothelial cell adhesion molecule 1 (PECAM-1), a molecule that is present on endothelial cell membranes, and junctional adhesion molecules (JAMs) A, B, and C mediate adherence activities and the adherence process. Contributions to this process also include β_2 integrin binding of ICAM-1 and E-selectin binding. Pseudopodia of neutrophils and other leukocytes extend between endothelial cells and come into contact with and bind to the basement membrane (composed of laminin and collagens) and subjacent extracellular matrix (ECM) proteins (proteoglycans, fibronectin, and vitronectin). This binding interaction is mediated, at least in part, by the β_1 integrins. Neutrophils that pass across the vascular wall accumulate in the perivascular connective tissue stroma within the inflammatory exudate. Once within the perivascular stroma, neutrophils migrate along a pathway established by the chemotactic gradients and inflammatory mediators.

This process is actually initiated during the fluidic phase of the acute inflammatory response and is driven by chemokines, cytokines, and chemoattractant substances such as complement. Temporally, margination, rolling, activation and firm adhesion, and transmigration all occur concurrently, involving different leukocytes in the same capillaries and postcapillary venules. This process is largely mediated by the interaction of ligands expressed on the surface of neutrophils, lymphocytes, and macrophages and their receptors expressed on luminal surfaces of activated endothelial cells (see Table 3-1). Adhesion molecules are divided into (1) selectins (E-, L-, and P-selectin), (2) integrins (VLA family of β_1 integrins; β_2 integrins [Mac-1, LFA-1, p150,95, $\alpha d\beta_2$]), (3) cytoadhesin family (vitronectin, β_3 integrins, and β_7 integrins used predominantly by lymphocytes), (4) the immunoglobulin superfamily (ICAM-1 to ICAM-3, VCAM-1, PECAM-1) and mucosal addressin cell adhesion molecule 1 (MAdCAM-1), and (5) other molecules such as CD44 (E-Table 3-2).

Table 3-1 Endothelial Cell/Neutrophil Adhesion Molecules

Endothelial Molecule	Leukocyte Receptor	Major Role
P-selectin	Sialyl Lewis X PSGL-1	Rolling (neutrophils, monocytes, lymphocytes)
E-selectin	Sialyl Lewis X ESL-1, PSGL-1	Rolling, adhesion to activated endothelium (neutrophils, monocytes, T lymphocytes)
ICAM-1	CD11/CD18 (integrins) (LFA-1, Mac-1)	Adhesion, arrest, transmigration (all leukocytes)
PECAM-1	PECAM-1	Transendothelial cell migration
JAM A	JAM A, LFA-1	Transendothelial cell migration
JAM C	JAM B, Mac-1	Transendothelial cell migration

ESL-1, E-selectin ligand-1; *ICAM-1*, intercellular adhesion molecule 1; *JAM*, junctional adhesion molecule; *LFA-1*, lymphocyte function antigen-1; *Mac-1*, macrophage antigen-1; *PECAM-1*, platelet endothelial cell adhesion molecule-1; *PSGL-1*, P-selectin glycoprotein ligand-1; *VCAM-1*, vascular cell adhesion molecule 1; *VLA*, very late antigen.
From Cotran RS, Kumar V, Collins T, et al: *Robbins pathologic basis of disease*, ed 7, Philadelphia, 2005, Saunders.

Leukocyte Adhesion Deficiencies

Information on this topic, including E-Table 3-3 and E-Figs. 3-1 to 3-3, is available at www.expertconsult.com.

Therapeutic Strategies to Modulate Leukocyte Infiltration

Information on this topic is available at www.expertconsult.com.

Additional Regulation of Inflammation

Information on this topic is available at www.expertconsult.com.

Effector Cells of the Acute Inflammatory Response

Vascular Endothelial Cells

Central to the integrity of the vasculature and any type of acute inflammation is the endothelial cell. Once considered a cell that, in the most simplistic view, forms separation between the blood and the surrounding tissue, endothelial cells are now known to have an extremely sophisticated role in regulating (1) hemostasis/coagulation, (2) vascular pressure, (3) angiogenesis during wound healing, (4) carcinogenesis, (5) leukocyte homing, and (6) inflammation. Under physiologic conditions, transcytosis (transcellular passage) of albumin, LDLs, metalloproteinases, and insulin occur via small vesicles and caveolae in the cytoplasm of the endothelial cell. Paracellular passage (between cell junctions) of water and ions occurs with endothelial cell contraction secondary to physiologic stimuli and/or inflammatory mediators. Secondary to inflammatory mediators, endothelial cells are activated and contract, allowing fluid to leak into extravascular tissues. Vascular tone is held in check in part by endothelin, a vasoconstrictive molecule, and angiotensin II, both of which are produced by endothelial cells, along with vasodilatory substances such as NO and prostacyclin (PGI_2). Activated endothelial cells release these chemical mediators and express adhesion molecules and receptors, including E-selectin, P-selectin, L-selectin ligand, PECAM-1, JAM A, JAM B, and JAM C, and the immunoglobulin superfamily such as ICAM-1. These adhesion molecules serve as ligands for leukocyte adherence. With the onset of inflammation, endothelial cells tend to increase procoagulative properties through release of tissue factor and other procoagulative substances.

Mast Cells and Basophils

The origin and relationship between mast cells and basophils has been a traditional point of debate and confusion. Current research clearly indicates that mast cells and basophils represent distinct cell types even though they share several morphologic and functional characteristics. Mast cells and basophils, along with other granulocytes and monocytes, originate and differentiate in bone marrow from a common $CD34^+$ precursor cell. Differentiation of $CD34^+$ precursor cells into mast cells or basophils depends on stem cell factor, a glycoprotein that acts with other cytokines and is produced in the bone marrow by fibroblasts and vascular endothelial cells. There is no evidence to suggest that basophils differentiate into tissue mast cells.

Mammalian mast cells are normally distributed throughout connective tissue adjacent to small blood and lymphatic vessels of skin and mucous membranes. In this location they respond rapidly to foreign proteins, microbes, and other substances and contribute significantly to the initiation of acute inflammation. This location also allows mast cells to interact with resident dendritic cells and release inflammatory mediators that activate endothelial cells. Experimental studies suggest that cutaneous mast cells in tissue have a life span of 4 to 12 weeks, depending on their location. Mast cells represent an extremely heterogeneous population of cells. In the 1960s Enerback identified two separate types of mast cells: mucosal and connective tissue. The mucosal mast cells are typically located in the respiratory and intestinal mucosa and can increase in numbers during some types of T helper type 2 (T_H2) lymphocyte–dependent immune responses. In contrast, the connective tissue mast cells show little or no T lymphocyte dependence. Mast cells express high-affinity receptors (Fc ε-RI) for immunoglobulin E (IgE) on their surface, and the release of mast cell granules is stimulated by the cross-linking of IgE receptors and clustering of the Fc ε-RI receptors by antigens such as pollens, allergens, and parasites. Substance P released from sensory (C-reactive) nerve fibers and macrophages also causes degranulation of mast cells. Degranulation results in the release of preformed TNF-α histamine, neutral proteases, proteoglycans (chondroitin sulfates and heparin), serotonin (in rodent species but not human beings), tryptase, chymase, various cytokines and growth factors (TNF, IL-4, β fibroblast growth factor [βFGF], VEGF, transforming growth factor-β [TGF-β], nerve growth factor [NGF], IL-5, Il-6, IL-15), and stem cell factor into tissue. Histamine and substance P activity appears interrelated because histamine released by mast cells can downregulate the release of substance P by nerve fibers, thereby reducing excessive amounts of the two proinflammatory molecules. The mast cell–substance P fiber interrelationship is an often-cited example of the neuroinflammatory-neuroimmune pathway.

Mast cells also synthesize leukotriene (LT) C_4 (LTC_4), PAF, prostaglandin (PG) D_2 (PGD_2), numerous cytokines, serotonin (in some species), heparin, and CC chemokines (macrophage inflammatory protein [MIP]-1-α and macrophage chemotactic protein [MCP]-1). The release of these mediators contributes significantly to the initiation of the acute inflammatory response. In addition, at physiologic concentrations these products likely counteract the effects of dense populations of mast cells in tissue and thus assist in regulating vascular permeability. Mast cells also release proteolytic enzymes, such as tryptase and chymase, which are involved with remodeling of the ECM. Tryptase is mitogenic to epithelial cells and likely contributes to proliferation of epithelial cells during wound repair. Mast cell granules contain numerous lysosomal enzymes (hexosaminidase, glucuronidase, glucosaminidase, galactosides, arylsulfatase, cathepsins [B, C, L, D, E], histamine, serotonin, dopamine, polyamines, and carboxypeptidase A3 [CPA3]).

Basophils are similar to neutrophils and eosinophils in that they mature in the bone marrow, circulate in the peripheral blood, are recruited into the tissue, and have a life span of several days in tissue. Basophils express high-affinity IgE receptors, similar to mast cells, and release granules and inflammatory mediators. Basophils appear to lack heparin, have a more limited cytokine repertoire than mast cells, and release mainly IL-4 and IL-13. Basophils express CD40L and CCR3 (eotaxin receptor). The presence of these suggests that they have a role as a cell that can enter sites of inflammation, release regulatory cytokines where they upregulate VCAM-1 expression by endothelial cells, and switch B lymphocytes to produce IgE, further contributing to the IgE type of response. Basophils can be prominent in IgE-mediated leukocyte infiltration into the mucosa of the nose, sinuses, respiratory tract, and skin, and all of these sites are particularly predisposed to allergic conditions.

The role of mast cells and basophils in IgE-mediated hypersensitivity reactions has been known for decades. These cells are critical effector cells in disorders of IgE-dependent immediate type I hypersensitivities (see Chapter 5). The release of their granules and mediators at inflammatory concentrations in the lung, for example, results in mucus secretion, accumulation of seroproteinaceous fluid in airways, bronchoconstriction, and vasodilation. The excessive release of tryptase and chymase by mast cells may enhance degradation of the ECM, which contributes to fibrosis and tissue remodeling. Chemokines and cytokines from mast cells and basophils contribute to innate immune defenses through chemotaxis and release of antimicrobial peptides. The mediators also enhance adhesion molecule expression on endothelial cells of nearby blood vessels and leukocytes that enter the area.

Neutrophils

Neutrophils are often the first type of leukocyte recruited into the inflammatory exudate. Their purpose is (1) to kill microbes, such as bacteria, fungi, protozoa, and viruses; (2) to kill tumor cells; or (3) to eliminate foreign materials. The biologic activities of neutrophils are primarily designed to kill microbes through lysosomal degradation, but if killing does not occur, neutrophils can limit the growth of microbes, allowing time for adaptive immunologic responses to develop.

Neutrophils perform two important functions to accomplish their effects: (1) phagocytosis of microbes or foreign material and then fusion of the phagosome with primary lysosomes to form a phagolysosome in which the microbes or foreign material are killed or degraded, respectively (see Chapters 1 and 5; also see Fig. 4-13), and (2) secretion and/or release of the contents of their granules into the inflammatory exudate to enhance the acute inflammatory response. They also infiltrate areas of acute tissue necrosis, such as those that occur in infarcts and necrotic areas of tumors.

Neutrophils are produced in the bone marrow, circulate in the bloodstream, and if not recruited into tissue by an acute inflammatory response, can enter tissue, where they eventually are destroyed by macrophages via apoptosis and phagocytosis or are lost from the body by migration across mucosae such as the alimentary and respiratory tracts. The average transit time in the blood is 10 hours, and the half-life in the blood varies between species but ranges from 5 to 10 hours; neutrophils within tissue survive from 1 to 4 days. Cytokines, such as IL-1 and TNF, and growth factors, such as granulocyte-macrophage colony-stimulating factor (GM-CSF), granulocyte colony-stimulating factor (G-CSF), and IL-3 maintain neutrophil concentrations in a steady-state manner under normal physiologic conditions, but with acute inflammatory responses emergency granulopoiesis can increase the release of neutrophils from the bone marrow and induce granulopoiesis in 2 to 4 days through GM-CSF and G-CSF, which also prevent apoptosis of tissue neutrophils. Within areas of intense inflammation, neutrophils and other leukocytes must function under hypoxic conditions and do so through the stabilization of hypoxia-inducible factor-1α (HIF-1α). HIF-1α induces transcription of genes that promote phagocytosis, inhibition of apoptosis, release of antimicrobial peptides, granule proteases, VEGF, cytokine release, and inducible NO synthase (iNOS). Growth factor withdrawal, which occurs during resolution of acute inflammation, induces apoptosis, and this outcome can be accelerated by TNF. During apoptosis, neutrophils lose the capacity to degranulate and become activated, which prevents release of their lysosomal enzymes and thus excessive tissue damage and allows for their phagocytosis by macrophages.

Neutrophils entering activated venules can screen the area for activated platelets and inflammatory mediators, and then distribute receptors in a polarized manner that drives directed migration to the inflammatory site for phagocytosis, microbial killing, and release of inflammatory mediators. Inflammatory mediators bind receptors on neutrophils, such as receptors for PAF, C5a, IL-8, and substance P (the neurokinin-1 receptor), leukotrienes, kallikrein, GM-CSF, and cytokines such as TNF. Many of these mediators induce chemotaxis; when leukocyte adhesion molecules, such as the selectins and integrins, bind to their respective ligands, they induce mitogen-activated protein kinase (MAPK) and G proteins, resulting in migration of neutrophils, usually toward a chemotactic gradient and activation.

Neutrophils can internalize large particles up to 0.5 μm in diameter by phagocytosis, including microbes, foreign bodies, senescent cells, and debris. Although neutrophils can internalize nonopsonized particles, opsonization greatly facilitates phagocytosis. The principal opsonin receptors present on neutrophil membranes are complement (CR1 and CR3) and Fc receptors (Fc γ-receptor I, IIA, IIIB), which bind complement fragments (C3b and C3bi) and the Fc portion of immunoglobulins such as IgG1 and IgG3. Such binding initiates activity of the guanosine triphosphatase (GTPase) Rac1 and the β2 integrin Mac-1 (CD11b/CD18), which also binds complement fragment C3bi and initiates GTPase-ρ. Such binding-inducing proteins and lipid kinases (e.g., protein kinase C and phosphatidylinositol 3-kinase) mediate actin assembly for formation of filopodia or lamellipodia, which surround and then internalize particles via phagocytosis by activated neutrophils. The activation process also leads to the release of calcium stored in the endoplasmic reticulum, which induces a respiratory (oxidative) burst (Table 3-2). Oxidative burst is the process by which the reduced form of nicotinamide adenine dinucleotide phosphate (NADPH) oxidase composed of five phox protein subunits in the membrane of phagosomes is formed. It catalyzes the formation of superoxide free radical that is used to kill microbes or degrade internalized material. Superoxide can react to form hydrogen peroxide, and additional free radicals such as hydroxyl radical, and hypochlorous acid. Neutrophils also express iNOS, which generates NO, and myeloperoxidase, which also produces hypochlorous acid. Superoxide anion and NO can form peroxynitrite, which is highly reactive.

Once a particle is internalized, phagosomes can "mature" by fusing with lysosomes and endosomes or remove parts of internalized particles. The fusion process is likely mediated by calmodulin, a calcium-binding protein, and soluble *N*-ethylmaleimide-sensitive factor (NSF) attachment protein receptor (SNARE; a fusion protein) that bind ligands on another vesicle to bring the membranes together for fusion. The maturation process results in lowering of the pH within the phagosome and the activation of microbicidal enzymes, including NADPH oxidase and myeloperoxidase complexes. Smaller particles are internalized by receptor-mediator endocytosis.

The ability of neutrophils to kill microbes or to degrade foreign material depends largely on the contents of the neutrophil granules, which store degradative enzymes, peroxidative enzymes, adhesion molecules, and antimicrobial peptides and/or proteins (E-Box 3-1). Myeloperoxidase is an enzyme used to convert hydrogen peroxide to hypochlorous acid. Hypochlorous acid, hydrogen peroxide, and a halide cofactor (chloride) form the myeloperoxidase system, which is an effective microbicidal mechanism used by neutrophils to kill internalized microbes and degrade internalized substances. Defensins, cathelicidins, and antimicrobial proteins contribute to the degradation of microbes by forming pores in microbial membranes. They also affect chemotaxis and activation of the adaptive immune response. Lactoferrin inhibits the growth of phagocytosed bacteria by sequestering free iron, and elastase hydrolyzes bacterial cell wall proteins and tissue elastin. The enzymatic contents of granules, such as gelatinase (matrix metalloproteinase-9 [MMP-9]) and myeloperoxidase, and nonenzymatic substances, such as antimicrobial

Table 3-2 Antimicrobial Mechanisms in Phagocytic Vacuoles

Oxygen-independent antimicrobial mechanisms	
Cathepsin G and elastase	Damage to microbial membranes
Low-molecular-weight ***defensins***	
High-molecular-weight ***cationic proteins***	
Bactericidal ***permeability-increasing protein***	
Lactoferrin	Complex with iron
Lysozyme	Splits proteoglycan
Acid hydrolases	Degrade dead microbes
Oxygen-dependent antimicrobial mechanisms	
Reaction Sequence Generated by NADPH Oxidase:	
$\text{Glucose} + \text{NADP} + \xrightarrow{\text{Hexose monophosphate shunt}}$ Hexose monophosphate shunt $+$ HADPH $\text{NADPH} + O_2 \xrightarrow{\text{NADPH oxidase}} \text{NADP}^+ + O_2^-$	O_2 burst plus generation of superoxide anion
$2O_2^- + 2H^+ \xrightarrow{\text{Spontaneous dismutatione}} H_2O_2 + {}^1O_2$ $O_2^- + H_2O_2 \rightarrow \bullet OH + OH^- + {}^1O_2$	Spontaneous formation of further microbial agents
$H_2O_2 + Cl^- \xrightarrow{\text{Myeloperoxidase}} OCl^- + H_2O$ $OCl^- + H_2O_2 \rightarrow {}^1O_2 + Cl^- + H_2O$	Myeloperoxidase generation of microbicidal molecules
$2 \bullet O_2O_2^- + 2H^+ \xrightarrow{\text{Superoxide dismutase}} O_2 + H_2O_2$ $2H_2O_2 \xrightarrow{\text{Catalase}} O_2 + 2H_2O + O_2$	Protective mechanisms used by host and many microbes
Nitric Oxide Reaction Sequence	
$O_2 + \text{L-arginine} \xrightarrow{\text{NO Synthase}} NO^-$ $NO + O_2^- \rightarrow \bullet ONOO^-$	Reactive species
$NO + Fe/RSH \rightarrow Fe(RS)_2NO_2$	Complexes iron

Microbicidal species in bold letters. *Fe/RSH*, A complex of iron with a general sulfhydryl molecule; *$Fe(RS)_2$*, oxidized Fe/RSH; *O_2^-*, superoxide anion; *${}^1O_2$*, singlet (activated) oxygen; *•OH*, hydroxyl free radical; *NADPH*, reduced nicotinamide adenine dinucleotide phosphate; *$NADP^+$*, oxidized NADPH; *H_2O_2*, hydrogen peroxide; *OCl^-*, hypochlorite anion; *NO*, nitric oxide; *$\bullet ONOO^-$*, peroxynitrite radical.
From Goering R, Dockrell H: *Mims' medical microbiology*, ed 5, St. Louis, 2012, Saunders.

peptides and lactoferrin, are also commonly released by the cell into the extracellular space and contribute to killing of extracellular microbial pathogens and with degradation of the ECM. The effects of extracellular neutrophil proteases, if not inactivated, can cause serious injury to tissue; therefore protease inhibitors are present in plasma and are present in inflammatory lesions after vascular leakage.

Neutrophil granule formation begins during myeloid cell differentiation in the bone marrow (see E-Box 3-1). Granules are observed initially in myeloblasts and promyelocytes when immature transport vesicles bud from Golgi complex and fuse to form primary granules. Primary granules are also called *azurophilic granules* because of their affinity for the dye azure A. These granules contain myeloperoxidase, elastase, defensins, and small amounts of lysozyme. Myelocytes and metamyelocytes form secondary (specific) granules that contain defensins, lactoferrin, lysozyme, and lesser amounts of myeloperoxidase, CD11b/CD18, and elastase. Band cells, the penultimate stage of neutrophil development, form tertiary (gelatinase) granules that contain lysozyme, gelatinase (MMP-9), cysteine-rich secretory protein-3 (CRISP-3), and adhesion molecules CD11b/CD18 (Mac-1) but have smaller amounts of myeloperoxidase, lactoferrin, proteinase 3, elastase, and defensins. Band and mature neutrophils also have secretory vesicles that contain plasma proteins, alkaline phosphatase, and numerous CD antigens, including CD11b/CD18 adhesion molecules. The secretory vesicles are mobilized quickly after neutrophil activation, resulting in rapid expression of adhesion molecules, which mediate leukocyte infiltration.

Neutrophil granules have evolved phylogenetically and are specially adapted for each species. In most mammals, enzymes released into an exudate from neutrophil granules cause liquefaction of the exudate, and the process results in the formation of pus. Reptiles and birds either lack or have reduced concentrations of these enzymes, particularly myeloperoxidase, and cannot liquefy the exudate. Thus a caseous material forms to be degraded by the next available line of inflammatory cells, macrophages. Granules in chicken heterophils (the avian, rabbit, and guinea pig neutrophil equivalent is termed heterophils) have little myeloperoxidase, but concentrations are also reduced in neutrophils of cattle and pigs. Cattle and sheep neutrophils have limited lysozyme concentrations. α-Defensins are present in rabbits, guinea pigs, hamsters, rats, and cattle neutrophils but have not been identified in those of dogs, cats, mice, pigs, and horses. The effect of these granule differences in various animal species on host defense and neutrophil function is not fully understood.

On cell death, neutrophils can release neutrophil extracellular traps (NETs) composed of a DNA backbone embedded with antimicrobial peptides and proteins and peptides that include histones, primary granule contents, lactoferrin, gelatinase, cathelicidins, and α-defensins. NETs entrap bacteria and can be microbicidal. Some pathogens can evade NETs. *Staphylococcus aureus* can release enzymes to degrade NETs by releasing deoxyadenosine, which can induce apoptosis in nearby leukocytes through activation of caspase-3. Actin is also released from dead neutrophils, and in the lung it can increase the viscosity of respiratory mucus. This outcome may occlude airways in dehydrated animals.

Eosinophils

Eosinophils are recruited from the bloodstream into vascularized connective tissue of most organs in response to eosinophil chemoattractants present in allergic and parasitic diseases. Eosinophils frequently enter lesions during the transition from acute to chronic inflammation. Eosinophils have prominent granules that release basic proteins and when activated produce cytokines, chemokines, proteases, and oxidative radicals. This array of mediators is often released in response to helminthic infections, and eosinophilic infiltration has been more recently implicated in resistance to the development of some cancers. On the other hand, eosinophil products contribute to tissue damage in several organs, including the lungs (asthma), heart, skin, and gastrointestinal tract.

Eosinophils were first recognized as blood cells (leukocytes) having numerous cytoplasmic granules with affinity for acidic dyes such as eosin. Therefore the name *eosinophil* ("eosin-loving") was proposed by Ehrlich in the late 1800s for these unique cells. By 1939, eosinophils were postulated to have a role in the immune response to helminths, and by the 1970s, eosinophils were well known to increase in the blood (eosinophilia) in parasitic and allergic diseases. Eosinophils are slightly larger than neutrophils. The nucleus is lobulated (bilobed) and composed primarily of heterochromatin (condensed). Eosinophil granules are known for their large size, especially in horses, and are rich in arginine with reddish brown tinctorial properties.

Eosinophils have several types of granules listed in E-Table 3-4, including small granules, primary granules, and large specific granules (secondary granules). Large specific granules, the most important of the eosinophil granules, contain four distinct basic proteins: (1) major basic protein (MBP), (2) eosinophil cationic protein, (3) eosinophil-derived neurotoxin, and (4) eosinophil peroxidase. These proteins exert biologic effects on microbes and on the tissue in which the microbes replicate by damaging lipid membranes. In addition, histaminase and a variety of hydrolytic lysosomal enzymes, such as collagenase and gelatinase, are also present in the large specific granules. Small granules contain enzymes such as arylsulphatases, acid phosphatases, MMPs, and gelatinases. Eosinophils also elaborate cytokines such as IL-1 to IL-6, IL-8, IL-10, IL-12, IL-16, GM-CSF, TGF-α and TGF-β, and chemokines. The contents of eosinophil granules are released in response to inflammatory stimuli in a manner similar to those used to activate neutrophils. However, products of eosinophil granules can result in extensive tissue degradation, including the degradation of collagen, which is commonly seen in eosinophilic granulomas of cats, horses, and dogs. Nearly all mast cell tumors in dogs and some mast cell tumors in cats contain eosinophils.

Major chemoattractants for eosinophils include histamine and eosinophilic chemotactic factor A (from mast cells), C5a, cytokines (IL-4, IL-5, and IL-13), and chemokines (CCL5, known as *regulated on activation, normal T lymphocytes expressed and secreted* [RANTES], and CCL11 [known as *eotaxin*]) released from epithelial cells, eosinophils, mast cells, and helminths. 5-Oxo-6, 8, 11, 14-eicosatetraenoic acid (5-oxo-ETE) is a strong activator of human eosinophils with a chemotactic potency comparable with those of eotaxin and RANTES, both of which enhance 5-oxo-ETE–induced chemotaxis. 5-Oxo-ETE and these chemokines contribute to the accumulation of eosinophils in the respiratory system in diseases such as asthma.

Natural Killer Cells and Natural Killer T Lymphocytes

Natural killer (NK) cells are sentinels of the immune system named for lysis of tumor cells and virus-infected cells without previous encounter. These cells enter regions of acute inflammation hours and even days after initiation of the lesion. NK cells kill target cells through release of perforin from cytoplasmic granules. NK cells express CD161, a C-type lectin, but do not express CD3, the T lymphocyte antigen. Roughly 95% of NK cells express CD56 and produce interferon-γ (IFN-γ); these are type I NK cells. Type II NK cells lack CD56 expression and produce IL-4, IL-5, and IL-13, thus supporting a T_H2 response.

IL-21 regulates differentiation and apoptotic death induced by NK cells. Inactive NK cells can be stimulated by Flt-3 ligand, a hematopoietic cytokine that stimulates proliferation of dendritic cells and antitumor immune responses, and also by IL-4, IL-12, IL-15, and IL-21. Once activated, IL-21 induces NK cell differentiation and upregulation of CD16, the low-affinity IgG receptor necessary for antibody-dependent cellular cytotoxicity (ADCC), and also NK release of IFN-γ required for macrophage and dendritic cell activation. Finally, IL-21 initiates a delayed apoptotic program for death of the differentiated NK cell and prevents recruitment of uninvolved NK cells. NK-T lymphocytes are T lymphocytes (express CD3 antigen) that have T and NK cell properties. NK-T lymphocytes recognize CD1d molecule, which is an antigen-presenting molecule that binds self and foreign lipids and glycolipids, and on activation of the NK-T lymphocyte, induce release of IFN-γ, IL-4, and GM-CSF. Because of this close discretion of self and nonself, NK-T lymphocytes can have important roles in the development of autoimmune disease.

Monocytes and Macrophages

Macrophages arise from bone marrow–derived monocytes, which circulate hematogenously with some monocytes localizing in tissues physiologically. They enter acute inflammatory lesions roughly 12 to 48 hours after the initiation of a lesion, depending on the inciting agent/substance. Differentiation of monocyte stem cells into blood monocytes proceeds rapidly in the bone marrow (i.e., 1.5 to 3 days) and is regulated by growth and differentiating factors, cytokines, and adhesion molecules such as IL-3, colony-stimulating factors, and TNF. Under physiologic conditions, monocytes in the blood localize throughout the body and differentiate into tissue macrophages. Recently, nonclassical monocytes have been identified; they migrate slowly along the luminal side of endothelium and monitor healthy tissue. When these monocytes sense damage or infection, they migrate rapidly into the tissue.

There are two types of tissue macrophages: macrophages that reside within specific organs/tissue (free macrophages and fixed macrophages) and macrophages derived from monocytes in response to inflammatory stimuli. Macrophages residing in organs/connective tissue first enter these sites as blood monocytes under physiologic (rather than inflammatory) conditions. These macrophages form the monocyte-macrophage system and include macrophages in connective tissue (histiocytes [free macrophages]), liver (Kupffer cells [fixed macrophages]), lung (alveolar macrophages [free macrophages], and intravascular macrophages [fixed macrophages]), lymph nodes (free and fixed macrophages), spleen (free and fixed macrophages), bone marrow (fixed macrophages), serous fluids (pleural and peritoneal macrophages [free macrophages]), brain (microglial cells), and skin (histiocytes [fixed macrophages]). The number of macrophages in tissue is maintained by (1) influx of monocytes from the blood, (2) proliferation of recruited monocytes locally in tissue, and (3) biologic turnover of macrophages via apoptotic cell death (life span in tissue of less than 3 weeks). Recent work also shows that some adult tissue macrophage populations develop from embryonic progenitors (independent of bone marrow) and can self-renew throughout life.

During inflammatory responses, monocytes express receptors (IgG Fc-domains, C3b) for chemical mediators of inflammation that exert migratory, chemotactic, pinocytic, and phagocytic activities in response to inflammatory stimuli. Once within inflammatory lesions, monocyte receptors are bound by cytokines, antigens, and other stimuli, which rapidly activate the maturation of monocytes into macrophages. This process can occur virtually anywhere in the body and often sets the stage for the development of chronic inflammation. In chronic inflammatory lesions, macrophages are the cell of last resort and accumulate in sites of persistent antigen, persistent microbes, foreign material, or repeated injury. Functionally, macrophages are a component of the innate immune system in terms of their role in phagocytosis and cytokine release during the acute inflammatory response. However, macrophages are one of the main triggers of the adaptive immune response because of their ability to process and present antigen and regulate T lymphocyte activity. The Fc receptors of macrophages and dendritic cells are triggered by Ig binding. There are Fc receptors for IgM, IgA, IgG, and IgE. The IgG (γ) Fc receptor has various subtypes that are regulated by intracellular domains such as ITAM (immunoreceptor tyrosine-based activation motif) and ITIM (immunoreceptor tyrosine-based inhibition motif). The ITAM domain present in Fc γ-receptor I, mediates macrophage activation with Ig binding, whereas the ITIM domain, present on Fc γ-receptor IIB, inhibits activation.

Chemical Mediators of the Acute Inflammatory Response

Chemical mediators of the acute inflammatory response include molecules such as histamine, serotonin, bradykinin, and tachykinins (E-Appendix 3-1). Many are produced as preformed or synthesized molecules in the liver and in neutrophils, basophils, macrophages/monocytes, platelets, mast cells, endothelial cells, smooth muscle cells, fibroblasts, and most epithelial cells. Preformed molecules, such as histamine, are transcribed, translated, processed, and stored, often in granules or vacuoles within inflammatory cells. They can be released immediately on cellular activation and are therefore active in seconds. Other molecules, such as most cytokines, adhesion molecules, and prostaglandins, are largely synthesized after an inflammatory cell becomes activated or injured. Endothelial cells, for example, often express low, basal concentrations of the adhesion molecule ICAM-1, but after the cells become activated (by cytokines such as IL-1), they rapidly transcribe the ICAM-1 gene to generate ICAM-1 messenger RNA (mRNA), which is translated into ICAM-1 protein, that is, processed, transported, and expressed on the cell surface. This is a quick process, resulting in ICAM-1 expression within hours; however, it is not nearly as rapid as the release of histamine, which occurs in seconds. Inflammatory mediators originating from plasma proteins, such as kinin, and the coagulation and complement system proteins are constantly secreted by the liver in precursor forms that must be activated via proteolytic cleavage in the circulatory system to their active forms; however, once the proteolytic cleavage is initiated, kinin and complement activity is immediate, similar to histamine.

Inflammatory mediators, whether preformed, synthesized, or derived from plasma, generally bind to receptors on target cells and often activate target cells or cause the target cell to secrete additional inflammatory mediators. In the latter case, the mediators may amplify or suppress secretion by target cells of additional mediators. Once activated and released or secreted, most inflammatory mediators:

- Have short half-lives and decay rapidly
- Are destroyed enzymatically
- Are scavenged by protective mechanisms such as antioxidants
- Are blocked by endogenous inhibitors such as complement inhibitors and decoy receptors

This arrangement provides a check-and-balance system on the severity of the acute inflammatory response and also can be exploited in the development of drugs to inhibit excessive inflammatory responses. Inflammatory mediators, if excessively unregulated, have the potential to cause severe injury to tissue in and surrounding the acute inflammatory response.

In addition to histamine, other preformed inflammatory proteins include serotonin, bradykinin, and tachykinins (substance P and neurokinins). Mast cells and basophils are the principal sources of histamine and serotonin. Bradykinin is released by leukocytes and vascular endothelial cells, and substance P is released by mast cells, basophils, and C-reactive (sensory) nerve fibers. As indicated, the mediators are rapidly active (in seconds to minutes) and contribute to increased vascular permeability that lasts from minutes to hours.

Histamine rapidly enhances vascular permeability and is one of the earliest recognized mediators of inflammation. Experiments by Sir Thomas Lewis in 1927 and Dale and Laidlaw in 1911 indicated the potential role of histamine and other local mediators in acute inflammation. Histamine is derived from the amino acid histidine through the action of histidine decarboxylase. This enzyme catalyzes the decarboxylation of histidine to histamine and carbon dioxide. Histamine is stored in granules of mast cells, basophils, and platelets.

As a mediator of inflammation, major effects of histamine are (1) vasodilation (active hyperemia), (2) increased microvascular responses, (3) neural reflexes, vagal reflexes, bronchial constriction, (4) release of $PGF_{2\alpha}$, (5) pain and itching, (6) tachycardia, and (7) eosinophil chemotaxis (E-Table 3-5). The acute vascular effects of histamine are immediate (within minutes) and transient (last approximately 30 to 90 minutes). Whether histamine has a role in chronic inflammation is speculative, but it may act to modulate the inflammatory response and the reactivity of various leukocytes, including lymphocytes. There are four G protein–coupled receptors (GPCRs) for histamine. Two of these, H_1 and H_4, are present on leukocytes, whereas H_2 and H_3 are present on gastric mucosa and nerve terminals, respectively.

The release of histamine from mast cells is in response to a variety of stimuli, including IgE, C3a, C5a, heat, cold, substance P, adenosine triphosphate (ATP), and products from leukocytes, endothelial cells, and platelets. Free histamine reacts within minutes with H_1 receptors on venular endothelium to cause contraction and gap formation (cytoskeletal reorganization [actinomycin filaments]), resulting in increased vascular permeability. Histamine H_1-receptor activation may lead to the production of cytokines and antibodies by T lymphocytes and B lymphocytes, respectively. In addition, H_1 receptors are also found on a variety of blood leukocytes, such as T lymphocytes, B lymphocytes, and monocytes.

There is substantial overlap of activities by these receptors on many types of cells. Many of the actions of histamine can be mimicked by H_1- and H_2-receptor agonists (a molecule or drug that binds to a receptor and triggers a response by the cell), whereas these actions can be blocked by H_1 and H_2 antagonists, molecules or drugs that block a receptor and prevent a response by the cell. This latter effect is the basis for therapies used in veterinary medicine today. Histamine receptors, for example, are involved in the pathogenesis of allergies, and H_1-receptor antagonists (antihistamines) reduce symptoms associated with allergic rhinitis such as sneezing, pruritus, and rhinorrhea (runny nose). In allergic bronchiolitis of cats and horses, H_1-receptor activation results in increased vascular permeability leading to serous inflammation in the bronchi and bronchioles. If this response can be blocked, the effects of allergens can be minimized in affected patients. Eosinophils produce histaminases that degrade histamine.

Serotonin (5-hydroxytryptamine) is an important preformed vasoactive amine with actions similar to those described previously for histamine. Serotonin is also an important neurotransmitter. Serotonin is found in mast cell granules of rodents and platelets of mammals. Serotonin and histamine are released from platelets after they are activated by the following:

- Aggregation and after contact with collagen in an exposed basement membrane from areas of endothelial necrosis and detached cells
- Thrombin from activation of the coagulation cascade
- Adenosine diphosphate released from injured endothelial cells
- Immune complex activation of the complement cascade (C3a, C5a)

Kinins, such as the tachykinins and bradykinin, are chemical mediators of the acute inflammatory response and also act by modulating the responses of the clotting and complement cascades. Kinin system activation leads ultimately to the formation of bradykinin. Bradykinin, a prototype kinin and a vasoactive peptide, has proinflammatory (makes the disease worse) properties that result in the following:

- Increased vascular permeability
- Vasodilation (venules)
- Increased sensitivity to pain
- Smooth muscle contraction
- Increased arachidonic acid metabolism (stimulation of phospholipase A_2)
- Hypotension
- Bronchoconstriction

Kinins are formed by two distinct pathways: the plasma kinin pathway and the tissue kinin pathway. The plasma kinin pathway is activated by contact of a protein complex formed by high-molecular-weight kininogen (HMWK), factor XI, and prekallikrein with negatively charged surfaces, such as exposed basement membrane. When factor XII (Hageman factor [HF]) binds to this surface and interacts with the bound protein complex, there is reciprocal activation/generation of activated HF and kallikrein (contact activation system). Kallikrein then acts on HMWK to yield bradykinin, an oligopeptide containing nine amino acid residues.

The tissue kinin pathway is generated by the action of tissue kallikrein on a low-molecular-weight kininogen (LMWK) to produce lysyl bradykinin and finally bradykinin. Tissue kallikrein is chemically and antigenically distinct from plasma kallikrein, although it is capable of acting on either HMWK or LMWK to generate bradykinin. Bradykinin binds to two GPCRs, B1R in inflamed tissue and B2R in normal tissues. Control of the proinflammatory effects of kinins is through rapid inactivation of bradykinin and kallikrein. Bradykinin is broken down by aminopeptidase M, neutral endopeptidase, carboxypeptidase (kininase I), and angiotensin-converting enzyme (kininase II). Plasma kallikrein is inhibited by C1-INH esterase (serum α_2-macroglobulin), a member of the serpin family of proteases. This family of proteases forms approximately 20% of the proteins in blood plasma and includes α_1-antichymotrypsin, α_1-antitrypsin, and antithrombin III. They act to block proteolytic activity in the clotting and complement systems and thus serve as a regulatory check on these systems.

Tachykinins are a family of vasoactive neuropeptides that includes substance P, neurokinin A and B, neuropeptide Y, and hemokinin-1. Substance P and NK A and B are synthesized by sensory afferent nerve fibers of the lungs and alimentary system. These substances are involved in allergic reactions and asthma. Substance P can induce vasoconstriction, vasodilation, increased permeability changes leading to edema, leukocyte activation, and chemotaxis. Substance P also induces activation and degranulation of mast cells, basophils, and eosinophils and their release of histamine and other inflammatory mediators. The released histamine, in a feedback mechanism, binds the H_3 receptors of nerve fibers and partially inhibits the production of substance P, thus regulating the level of activity. One of the main receptors for substance P, neurokinin-1 receptor (NK-1R), is expressed on a variety of cells including mast cells, epithelial cells, endothelial cells, and macrophages. NK-1R is regulated by substance P expression. Frequently, increased concentrations of substance P result in decreased NK-1R expression. Neurokinin 2 and 3 receptors have a lower affinity for substance P than NK-1R.

The release of substance P from afferent sensory nerve fibers in skin and mucous membranes can also be induced by capsaicinoids such as capsaicin and dihydrocapsaicin. Capsaicinoids are natural compounds present in chile peppers of the genus *Capsicum*, which cause the burning sensation in commercial pepper sprays (less-than-lethal, self-defense weapons). Capsaicin binds the vanilloid receptor-1 of afferent sensory fibers, leading to release of substance P from these fibers. Thus the tachykinins induce inflammatory responses when released by activated and degranulated mast cells, basophils, and eosinophils and also from stimulated nerve fibers.

Complement Cascade

The complement cascade is a unique sequence of molecular events occurring within the vascular system in which inactive complement plasma proteins synthesized by the liver are activated after tissue injury (Fig. 3-7), inflammation, clotting, or immune responses. This cascade results in the generation of numerous biologically active molecules, which have effects that are proinflammatory, chemotactic, opsonizing, antigen solubilizing, antibody inducing, permeability enhancing, and microbicidal (cell lysis) and usually beneficial to the animal (Table 3-3). A large number of plasma proteins make up the complement system, and nearly 10% of serum proteins are complement factors. Divided by the "classical," "alternative," and lectin pathways, activation or "fixation" of complement proteins eventually results in formation of a membrane attack complex (MAC) that perforates the cell membranes of foreign invaders and naïve host cells alike. In the generation of MAC, a variety of complement components are elaborated that have important inflammatory and immune effects.

Complement proteins C1 through C9 are inactive components of plasma that are activated by substances, including microbial molecules such as endotoxins, aggregated immunoglobulin, complex polysaccharides, and venoms. The critical step in unleashing the biologic functions of the complement cascade in the classical pathway is activation of C3 through either the classical or alternative complement activation pathways. The classical pathway of the

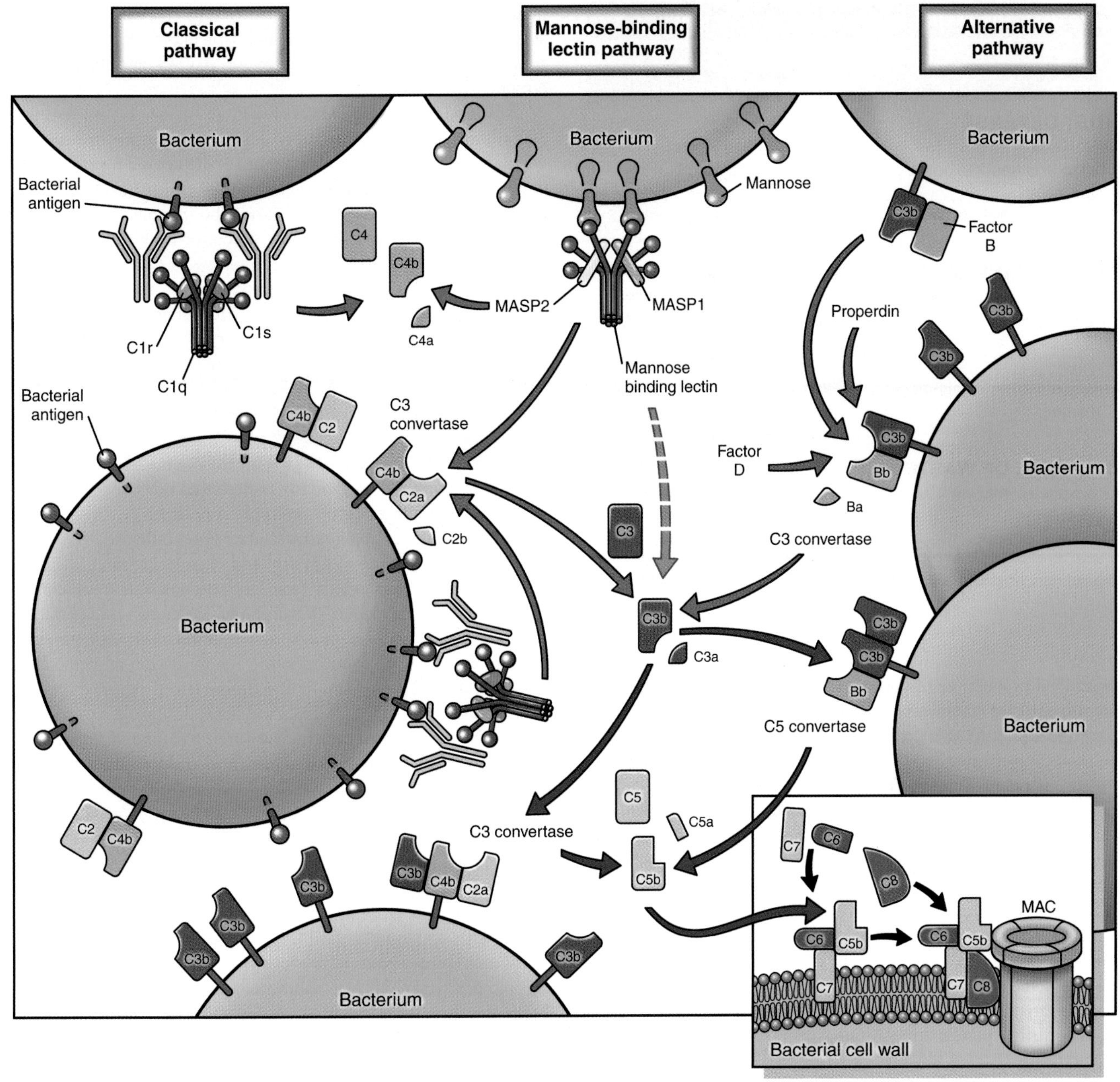

Figure 3-7 Activation of Complement Cascade. Complement is activated by classical, mannose-binding lectin, and alternative pathways. The classical pathway is triggered by antibody opsonization, the mannose-binding pathway is induced by binding of the mannose-binding lectin to mannose residue on the surface of microbes, whereas the alternative pathway is first initiated by binding of C3b to hydroxyl group residues of carbohydrates and proteins and subsequent factor D cleavage of C3b in plasma. After initiation by these three pathways, the complement cascade continues with formation of C5a and C3a, which induce inflammation through attraction of leukocytes; C3b, which opsonizes pathogens and induces phagocytosis; and formation of the membrane attack complex (MAC) that creates a pore in the microbial surface. (Redrawn from MJ Walport: Complement. *N Engl J Med* 344:1058-1066, 2001.)

complement cascade can be activated by antibody complexes. Activation occurs when IgG and/or IgM are cross-linked with C1. C1 has three components: C1q, r, and s. C1q binds the Fc regions of IgG and/or IgM and brings C1r, which is proteolytic, into proximity to C1s, which is cleaved, through interactions with C4 and C2. This leads to the formation of classical pathway C3 convertase (C4b2a) and the eventual formation of classical pathway C5 convertase (C4b2a3b). Classical pathway C3 convertase converts C3 to C3a, and classical pathway C5 convertase converts C5 to C5a.

The alternative pathway is initiated by products from microorganisms, including LPS from Gram-negative bacteria and polysaccharides from fungal cell walls (see Fig. 4-18). In addition, other activated plasma proteins, including kallikrein, plasmin, and activated factor XII, can cleave C3, resulting in its activation to C3b. C3b combines with factor B and coupled with factor D activity, forms the alternative pathway C3 convertase (C3bBb). Alternative pathway C3 convertase converts C3 to C3b. C3b combines with alternative pathway C3 convertase to form alternative pathway C5 convertase (C3bBb3b), which converts C5 to C5a. Because the alternative pathway can be activated by clotting and kinin factors, once the clotting or the kinin systems are activated, complement activity follows and vice versa. Therefore the clotting, kinin, and complement systems are closely interactive, and often activation of one system leads to activation of others (Fig. 3-8). When bound to

Table 3-3 The Main Functions of Complement

Activity	Associated Complement Protein
HOST DEFENSE	
Opsonization	C3 and C4 fragments
Chemotaxis and leukocyte activation	C5a, C3a, C4a, and leukocyte receptors
Lysis of microbial cell walls	Membrane attack complex (C5b-C9)
BRIDGING INNATE AND ADAPTIVE IMMUNITY	
Augmentation of antibody response	C3b, C4b immune complexes and antigen; C3 receptors on B lymphocytes and antigen-presenting cells
Enhancement of immunologic memory	C3b, C4b immune complexes and antigen; C3 receptors on follicular dendritic cells
DISPOSAL OF WASTE	
Clearance of immune complexes	C1q; C3 and C4 fragments
Clearance of apoptotic cells	C1q; C3 and C4 fragments

Adapted from Mackay IR, Rosen FS: *N Engl J Med* 344:1058, 2001.

a microbial product, mannose-binding lectins (MBLs) and ficolins can also activate complement through MBL-associated serine proteases (MASPs). MASP-2 cleaves C4 and C2 to activate steps of the classical pathway.

C3a increases vascular permeability by inducing histamine release from mast cells. C5a, once formed, is released into the inflammatory exudate and behaves as an anaphylatoxin (a molecule that causes the release of histamine and other chemical mediators from mast cells or basophils), a chemoattractant for leukocytes, and an inducer of adhesion molecule expression by endothelial cells. C3b and C3bi are important opsonins and enhance neutrophil phagocytosis through CR1 and CR3 receptors. C3 can covalently attach to some intracellular viral and bacterial pathogens and trigger mitochondrial antiviral signaling (MAVS) once the pathogens enter the cytosol. The plasma enzyme carboxypeptidase can degrade both C3a and C5b.

The MAC results from the cleavage of C5 by C5 convertase, leading to the formation of C5a and C5b. C5b serves as the anchor for the assembly of a single molecule composed of C6, C7, and C8. This MAC (C5b with C6, C7, C8) facilitates polymerization of C9 (up to 18 molecules of C9) into a tube that is inserted into the lipid bilayer of the plasma membrane of, for example, a bacterium. A channel is formed through the cell membrane allowing the passage of ions, small molecules, and water into the bacterium by osmosis. Bacterial lysis ensues. This process can also injure naïve host cells such as occurs in hemolytic anemia.

Arachidonic Acid Metabolites

When inflammation or inflammatory mediators injure cells, the cell membrane lipids are rapidly rearranged to create a variety of biologically active lipid mediators derived from arachidonic acid. Arachidonic acid metabolites are lipid-derived autocoid (acting as a local hormone [see Fig. 12-1]) mediators of inflammation that serve as intracellular and extracellular signals influencing the coagulation cascade and mediating nearly every step of the acute inflammatory response (Fig. 3-9). Effects are short-lived because these lipid metabolites decay rapidly or are destroyed by enzymes. Arachidonic acid metabolites include prostaglandins, leukotrienes, and lipoxins that are produced by cyclooxygenase (COX) and lipoxygenase enzyme pathways.

Arachidonic acid (eicosapentaenoic acid) is an essential 20-carbon, polyunsaturated fatty acid derived from linoleic acid, which is present in plasma membranes of dietary red meats. Arachidonic acid is an integral component of esterified membrane phospholipids that, when cleaved from the plasma membrane by phospholipase, serves as the major precursor for eicosanoids. Eicosanoids are synthesized by two main classes of enzymes: (1) COXs and (2) lipoxygenases and also (3) cytochrome P450 enzymes. Their respective products (eicosanoids) are (1) prostaglandins and thromboxanes and (2) leukotrienes and lipoxins. These molecules are synthesized in endothelial cells, leukocytes, and platelets and principally exert their biologic effects on vascular and airway smooth muscle cells, endothelial cells, and platelets during the acute inflammatory response.

Arachidonic acid is released from membrane phospholipids of many cell types, but particularly endothelial cells and leukocytes, through the action of cytoplasmic phospholipase A_2 ($cPLA_2$) and to a lesser degree, soluble (extracellular) phospholipase A_2 ($sPLA_2$). This occurs in response to physical and chemical stimuli, including C5a. $cPLA_2$ is translocated from the endoplasmic reticulum to plasma membrane when intracellular calcium concentrations increase. The activity of $sPLA_2$ also requires the participation of calcium; however, its contribution to the formation of intracellular arachidonic acid varies among the different cell types when compared with that of $cPLA_2$. Membrane phospholipids contain a glycerol backbone attached to which is often a saturated fatty acid at the sn-1 position, an unsaturated fatty acid at the sn-2 position, and a base at the sn-3 position. Arachidonic acid is often in the sn-2 position and released by $cPLA_2$ or $sPLA_2$ to become free arachidonic acid.

Free arachidonic acid is metabolized in one of three pathways: (1) the COX pathway for the formation of prostaglandins and thromboxanes, (2) the lipoxygenase pathway for the formation of leukotrienes and lipoxins, and (3) the cytochrome p450 pathway for the formation of epoxyeicosatrienoic acids (hydroperoxyeicosatetraenoic acid [HPETE] and hydroxyeicosatetraenoic acid [HETE]). There are three COX isoenzymes—COX-1, COX-2, and COX-3—that are actually components of prostaglandin H synthase and work in concert with a peroxidase heme group. The COX-1 isoenzyme is constitutively expressed, is present in almost all tissues, and is considered a housekeeping enzyme with physiologic roles in hemostasis and gastric mucosa protection. COX-2 isoenzyme expression is induced by exogenous and endogenous stimuli and occurs locally in sites of inflammation. It is present in leukocytes, endothelial cells of blood vessels, and synovial fibroblasts. COX-3 isoenzyme is a splice variant of COX-1 (and also termed *COX-1b* or *COX-1v*). It is present in greatest abundance in the cerebral cortex of dogs and human beings and is also detected in human aortas and rodent cerebral endothelia, heart, kidney, and neuronal tissues.

Prostaglandin Formation and Inhibition

Arachidonic acid metabolites from COX isoenzymes induce an intermediate prostaglandin, PGH_2, which is converted into at least five metabolites (PGD_2, PGF_2, PGE_2, PGI_2, and thromboxane A_2 [TXA_2]) by prostanoid synthase enzymes unique for each of these five metabolites. The relative concentration of each of these five types of prostaglandins synthesized after stimulation depends on the cell type stimulated. For example, PGI_2—a thromboresistant prostaglandin termed *prostacyclin*—is produced by endothelial cells via

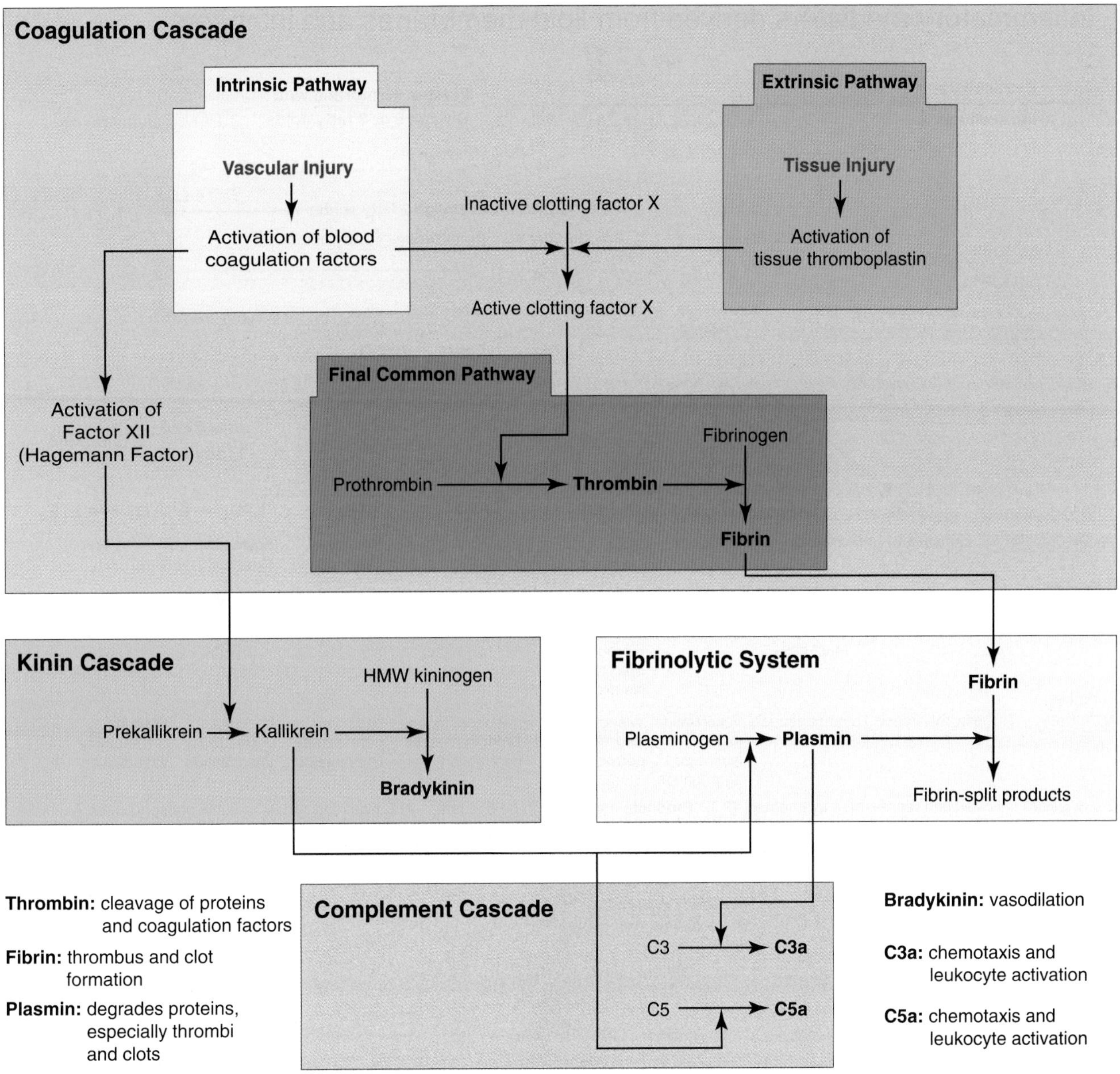

Figure 3-8 Interactions between the Four Plasma Mediator Systems. *HMW,* High-molecular-weight. (Courtesy Dr. M.R. Ackermann, College of Veterinary Medicine, Iowa State University; and Dr. J.F. Zachary, College of Veterinary Medicine, University of Illinois.)

PGI_2 synthase, whereas TXA_2—a thrombogenic prostaglandin termed *thromboxane*—is produced by platelets via TXA_2 synthase. PGD_2 is the major prostanoid produced by mast cells; PGE_2 is the major prostanoid produced by epithelial cells, fibroblasts, and smooth muscle cells. Specific prostaglandins inhibit (PGI_2) or induce (TXA_2) coagulation/thrombosis, whereas others affect vascular permeability (PGD_2 and PGE_2). Prostaglandins bind GPCRs that are specific for each prostaglandin. Activated prostaglandin receptors trigger cyclic adenosine monophosphate (cAMP) or increased cytoplasmic calcium. PGE_2 has been long known for immunomodulatory activity; mechanistically, recent work suggests that PGE_2 receptor EP4 promotes differentiation of both T helper type 1 (T_H1) and T helper type 17 (T_H17) $CD4^+$ T lymphocytes.

Prostaglandins contribute to the following:

- Fever (via PGE_2)
- Inflammatory tachycardia
- Adrenocorticotropic hormone (ACTH) response (neurons of the paraventricular nucleus of the brain release ACTH)
- Behavior stress syndrome (reduced movement and loss of social contact)
- Clotting/hemostasis (via prostacyclin and thromboxane)

Aspirin, indomethacin, ibuprofen, and naproxen are COX-1 inhibitors. Aspirin, naproxen, and ibuprofen also inhibit COX-2, as do the highly selective COX-2 inhibitor drugs celecoxib, rofecoxib, valdecoxib, lumiracoxib, and etoricoxib. Acetaminophen was thought to inhibit COX-3; however, acetaminophen's activity in human beings and rodents is not fully defined. Because COX-3 is present in greatest abundance in the cerebral cortex and acetaminophen crosses the blood-brain barrier (unlike other nonsteroidal anti-inflammatory drugs [NSAIDs]), these observations were initially thought to explain why acetaminophen was sometimes more effective for treating headaches and pain relief and less effective in

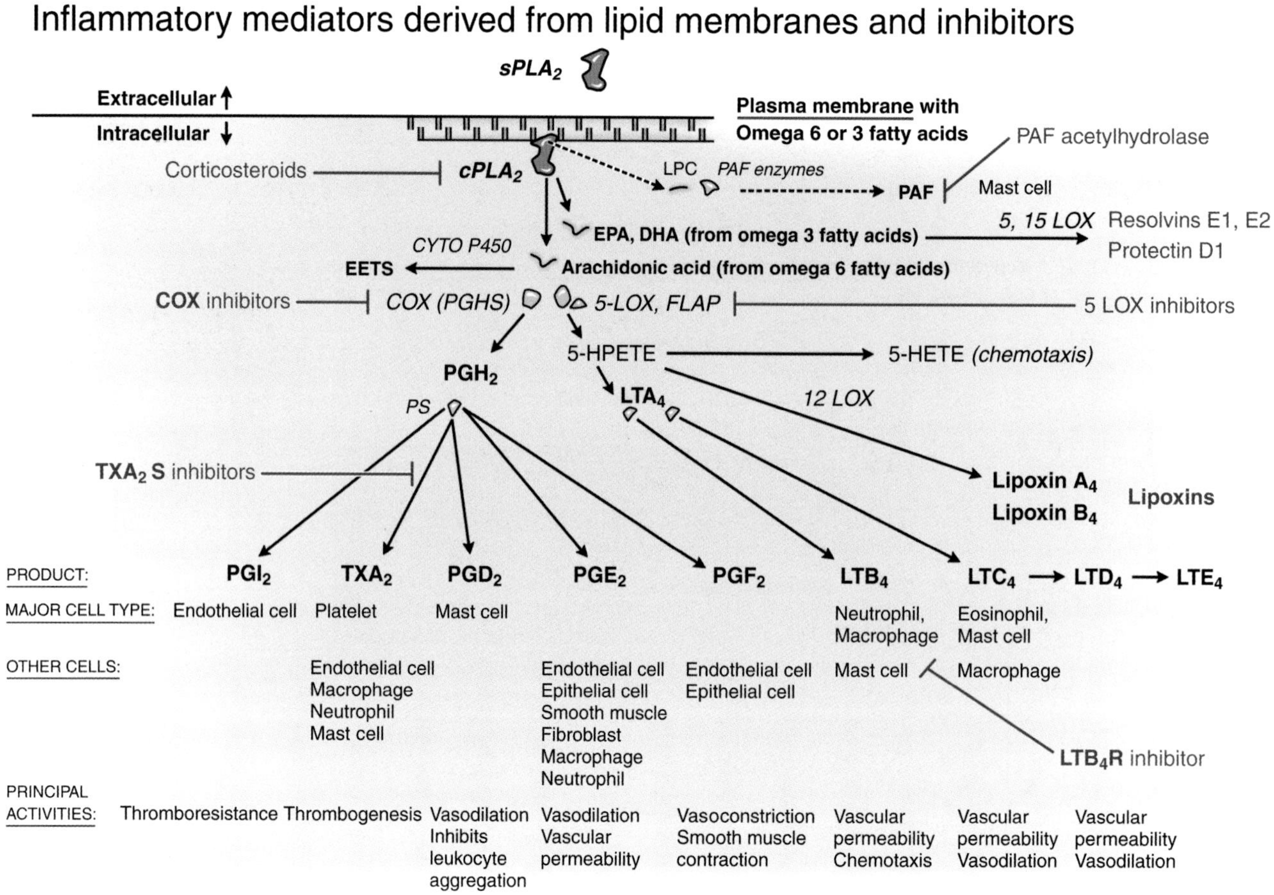

Enzymes are *italicized* and represented by shapes ( ). **Products** are written in bold letters. Abbreviations: $sPLA_2$, soluble phospholipase A2; $cPLA_2$ cytoplasmic phospholipase A2; LPC, lysophosphatidylcholine; PAF, platelet activating factor; AA, arachidonic acid; COX, cyclooxygenase; LOX, Lipoxygenase; FLAP, 5 LO activating protein; PG, prostaglandin; TX, thromboxane; LT, leukotriene; PS, prostanoid synthase; LTA4H, LTA4 hydrolase; LTC4S, LTC4 synthtase, EPA, eicosapentaenoic acid; DHA, docosapentaenoic acid. Inhibitors are listed in red and red lines with cross bars lead to sites of inhibition.

Figure 3-9 **Key Inflammatory Mediators Derived from the Plasma Membrane.** Cytoplasmic phospholipase A_2 ($cPLA_2$) activity on the plasma membrane leads to free arachidonic acid (AA) and lysophoshatidylcholine (LPC). Arachidonic acid metabolites include prostaglandins and leukotrienes, and LPC is a substrate for platelet-activating factor (PAF). The type of prostaglandin formed by a cell is dependent on the cell type. Platelets, for example, form thromboxane, whereas endothelial cells form prostacyclin. Leukotrienes are formed by leukocytes. Inhibitors specific to the various enzymes or products are indicated in red text and lines. COX, Cyclooxygenase; *CYTO P450*, cytochrome P450; *DHA*, docosapentaenoic acid; *EETS*, epoxyeicosatrienoics; *FLAP*, 5-lipoxygenase-activating protein; *HETE*, hydroxyeicosatetraenoic acid; *HPETE*, hydroperoxyeicosatetraenoic acid; *LOX*, lipoxygenase; *LTA_4*, leukotriene A_4; *LTA_4H*, leukotriene A_4 hydrolase; *LTB_4*, leukotriene B_4; *LTC_4*, leukotriene C4; *LTC_4S*, leukotriene C_4 synthase; *LTD_4*, leukotriene D_4; *LTE_4*, leukotriene E4; *PGD_2*, prostaglandin D_2; *PGE_2*, prostaglandin E_2; *PGF_2*, prostaglandin F_2; *PGH_2*, prostaglandin H_2; *PGI_2*, prostaglandin I_2 (also called prostacyclin); *PGHS*, prostaglandin H synthase; *PS*, prostanoid synthase; *$sPLA_2$*, soluble phospholipase A_2; *TXA_2*, thromboxane A_2. (Modified from Dr. M.R. Ackermann, College of Veterinary Medicine, Iowa State University.)

inhibiting inflammation in the body. Although this may be the case in dogs, the mechanistic basis of acetaminophen's activity in human beings is not fully understood at this time. Acetaminophen may inhibit COX-2 to a minor degree and also slightly inhibit COX-3 (COX-1b), and yet have other activity/activities. Much of the antiinflammatory effect of corticosteroids is due to their inhibition of phospholipase A_2, the enzyme that releases arachidonic acid from membrane phospholipids. Corticosteroids signal the cell to synthesize a polypeptide known as lipocortin (lipomodulin), which then acts to inhibit phospholipase A_2. Therefore the antiinflammatory effect of corticosteroids is delayed. A variety of other natural and synthetic compounds can inhibit phospholipase A_2.

Leukotriene Formation and Inhibition

Information on this topic is available at www.expertconsult.com.

Omega-3 Fatty Acids (Fish Oils) and Inhibition of Eicosanoid Activity

Information on this topic is available at www.expertconsult.com.

Platelet-Activating Factor

PAF is another potent molecule of phospholipid origin derived from cell membranes of platelets, basophils, mast cells, neutrophils, macrophages, and endothelial cells. PAF has potent pathophysiologic effects and contributes to inflammation, endotoxic shock, and allergic reactions (asthma) through vasoconstriction, bronchoconstriction, platelet aggregation, and leukocyte adhesion, chemotaxis, and degranulation. However, at low concentrations (experimentally induced), PAF can cause vasodilation and increased vascular permeability. PAF also contributes to the inflammatory response by increasing the oxidative burst in neutrophils following phagocytosis of bacteria and enhances the synthesis of eicosanoids by leukocytes. During IgE-mediated hypersensitivity reaction in the lung, PAF induces mast cell release of serotonin and histamine, as well as platelet aggregation. Thus platelet aggregation can increase vascular permeability in acquired immunologic responses and result in inflammation.

Two enzymes, lysoPAF acetyltransferase (lysoPAF-AT) and PAF-synthesizing phosphocholinetransferase (PAF-PCT), control the final synthesis of PAF from lipid membranes and thus promote PAF production. PAF mediates its effects on target cells through a single GPCR. These receptors have been identified on endothelium, neutrophils, eosinophils, macrophages, smooth muscle, and glial cells in the brain. PAF activity is reduced/regulated by PAF acetylhydrolase, which is expressed by cells expressing PAF receptor. PAF acetylhydrolase degrades PAF through hydrolysis of its acetate moiety in the sn-2 position of glycerol, which inhibits the proinflammatory activity of PAF. PAF acetylhydrolase is thus potentially an enzyme that could be used for the development of drugs to reduce inflammatory responses.

Cytokine Family

Overview in Inflammation and Induction of CD4 T_H Subsets

Cytokines are a group of proteins produced by many cell types, including lymphocytes, macrophages, endothelial cells, neutrophils, basophils, mast cells, eosinophils, epithelial cells, and connective tissue cells (see E-Appendix 3-1). The primary purpose of cytokines is to modulate, via enhancement or suppression, the functional expression of other cell types during the inflammatory response. Chemokines are produced from almost all cell types and are cytokines that promote leukocyte chemotaxis and migration across capillaries and postcapillary venules. Cytokines also play major roles in (1) hematopoiesis, including granulopoiesis by cytokines such as IL-3, G-CSF, and GM-CSF; and (2) adaptive immunity, such as the proliferation of lymphocytes by cytokines, including IL-2, and activation of T_H1 or T_H2 responses. The CD4 T_H cell response consists of subsets of T lymphocytes characterized by the secretion of different cytokines, including IFN-γ–producing T_H1 cells and IL-4–producing T_H2 cells, which are involved in cellular or humoral immunity, respectively. The cytokines have been organized into the following categories according to their principal functional activities:

- Hematopoietic growth factors, including IL-3, G-CSF, GM-CSF, possibly IL-9, IL-11, and stem cell factor
- Inflammatory mediators, which induce acute phase reactants and natural immunity (IL-1, IL-6, TNF-α, and TNF-β)
- Chemotactic cytokines (IL-8)
- T lymphocyte proliferation, activation, and differentiation cytokines (IL-2, IL-4, IL-5, IL-7, IL-9, IL-10, IL-12, and IL-17 on up to IL-29)

Stimuli that invoke expression of these families of cytokines are varied and secondary to activation of a wide variety of receptors, including soluble receptors, receptors on the cell surface, endosomal receptors, and cytoplasmic receptors, which activate nuclear factor κ B (NFκB), extracellular signal-related kinase (ERK), Jun, p38, and other signaling pathways.

Concerning T lymphocyte activity, there are cytokines and proteins that exert T lymphocyte regulatory activity (IFN-γ, TGF-β). Of particular importance is the presentation of antigen by dendritic cells to T lymphocyte cells that release cytokines, which mediate formation of lineages of T helper lymphocytes (T_H1, T_H2, T_H17, and T regulatory [T reg] lymphocytes). Dendritic cells are present in tissues that are in contact with the environment such as Langerhans cells of the skin and dendritic cells of the mucosal surfaces of the respiratory and alimentary systems. These dendritic cells are sentinels constantly monitoring for and phagocytosing microbes and foreign materials. In cooperation with lymphocytes and macrophages in lymphoid tissue, they act as antigen-presenting cells to activate T helper lymphocytes and cytotoxic T lymphocytes and B lymphocytes. The T_H1 lineage of CD4 T lymphocytes, normally driven by IL-12, expresses the transcription factor T-bet, releases IFN-γ, and induces cell-mediated immune responses within specific diseases such as the granulomatous inflammatory response to mycobacterial infections. Whereas T_H2 CD4 cells form in response to IL-4, IL-6, and thymic stromal lymphopoietin (TSLP); express transcription factor GATA-3; produce IL-4, IL-5, IL-10, and IL-13; and induce humoral responses and humoral-related diseases, such as asthma and atopy, T_H17 CD4 T lymphocytes form in response to TGF-β, IL-6, and IL-23, express transcription factor Rorγt, and release IL-17. These cells bridge innate and adaptive immune responses through the production of IL-17 cytokines, which promote inflammatory responses such as neutrophil recruitment and development of autoimmune responses. T reg lymphocytes develop in the thymus and also in response to antigenic stimulation in the presence of TGF-β, which induces transient or stabile expression of transcription factor forkhead box P3 (FOXP3). T reg lymphocytes modulate adaptive responses through the release of IL-10. Follicular CD4 T lymphocytes (T_{FH}) develop in the presence of IL-6 and IL-21, express transcription factor Bcl6 and cMaf (BLIMP-1 is inhibitory), and release IL-21. Through secretion of IL-21, T_{FH} cells support B lymphocyte development and antibody production. Follicular dendritic cells are present in the follicles of lymph nodes and present antigen to B lymphocytes.

Biochemically, cytokines can be divided into type I and type II cytokines. Type I cytokines have four α-helix units. Type II cytokines have six α-helix units and are likely derived from a single ancestral gene. Type I and II cytokines bind receptors specific for the I and II ligand structures. Despite the similarities within type I and type II cytokines and their receptors, there is still much diversity in structure and function of cytokines within each type.

Cytokine Receptors and Signaling

Information on this topic and E-Fig. 3-4 are available at www.expertconsult.com.

Inflammatory Proteins

Interferons. Interferons are glycoprotein cytokines produced by lymphocytes and many other cell types in response to viruses and virus-infected cells, parasites, and neoplastic cells. They inhibit viral replication within host cells, activate NK cells and macrophages, increase antigen presentation to T lymphocytes, and increase the resistance of host cells to viral infection. Type 1 interferons (IFN-α and IFN-β) bind IFN-α receptor (IFNAR), which has two subunits, IFNAR 1 and 2, to signal through JAK1 and TYK2 kinases. These kinases phosphorylate STAT1 and STAT2, which then dimerize and assemble with IFN regulatory factor 9 (IRF9) to form the complex IFN-stimulated gene factor 3 (ISGF3). ISGF3 binds IFN response elements in the DNA for transcription of IFN-stimulated genes (ISGs) to mediate antiviral responses; type II interferons (IFN-γ) bind IFN-γ receptors (IFNGR) 1 and 2 and signal through JAK1, JAK2, and STAT1 to induce T_H1 and T_H17 responses. Type III interferons bind IL-10 receptors and have been described, but their function is not fully clarified. Most cells produce IFN-β, but predominantly hematopoietic cells produce IFN-α, especially plasmacytoid dendritic cells. The antiviral activity of type I interferons involves expression activation of the ISGylation pathway, MxA protein, 2′,5′-oligoadenylate synthetase 1 (OAS1) activation of ribonuclease L (RNase L), and protein kinase R (PKR). ISGylation is a process in which interferon-stimulated gene 15 (ISG15) protein binds key interferon antiviral proteins (e.g., JAK1, STAT1, MxA, PKR, and RNase L) and prevents their degradation, thus enhancing the antiviral response. MxA protein binds and traps viruses. The OAS1/RNase L process cleaves viral RNA, and PKR protein dimerizes on itself and in the presence of viral RNA phosphorylates, thus inhibiting host cell translation initiation factor-2α (EIF-2α), which blocks viral replication.

Type III interferons include IFN-λ) 1, 2, and 3, also designated IL-29, IL-28A, and IL-28B, respectively. Respiratory and intestinal epithelial cells in response to viral infections produce these interferons. Release of triple phosphorylated viral RNA in infected cells can activate RIG-I, which can then mediate MAVS on mitochondria and peroxisomes, resulting in the activation of p38, NFκB, and IRF3 for the production of the type III IFNs. Type III IFNs bind unique receptors (IFNLR1 and IL10R2) for IFN response genes (ISGs) (e.g., IRF7, IRF3), leading to a response similar to type II IFNs (e.g., MxA, OAS, PKR).

IFN-ε is another family of IFNs that are produced in the female reproductive tract and mediate IFN responses.

High Mobility Group Box Protein 1. High mobility group box protein 1 (HMGB-1) is a proinflammatory cytokine released by monocytes and macrophages. It is a nonhistone nuclear protein that binds DNA to regulate gene expression and the chromosomal architecture. HMGB-1 is released by nearly all cells during necrosis, and once outside the cell, it is an alarmin, which is an endogenous molecule that triggers host inflammatory responses. HMGB-1 binds macrophage receptor for advanced glycosylation end products (RAGE) and TLRs 2 and 4, activating the innate immune system and pathologic responses that include release of IL-1, TNF-α, and IFN-γ. HMGB-1 and cytokines, such as IL-1, TNF, and IL-6, and prostaglandins, such as PGE_2, are involved with hypothalamic function in food aversion, hypophagia, anorexia, weight loss, and sickness behavior (see section on The Effect of Inflammation on the Febrile Response and Other Activities) and serve to amplify the inflammatory response.

Chemokines

Chemokines, released in response to inflammatory stimuli, are secreted proteins that induce leukocyte chemotaxis into inflammatory exudates (Fig. 3-10). They also activate inflammatory cells, induce antiviral activity, regulate immune responses, and induce hematopoiesis, angiogenesis, and cell growth. Chemokines are produced by all nucleated cells in the body, including epithelial cells, fibroblasts, macrophages, mast cells, keratinocytes, dendritic cells, and endothelial cells. Leukocytes secrete all types of chemokines, except for fractalkine (used for monocyte chemotaxis), which is produced by nonhematopoietic cells such as vascular endothelial cells.

Classification of Chemokines

Information on this topic and E-Tables 3-6 to 3-8 are available at www.expertconsult.com.

Chemokine Receptors and Signaling

Information on this topic is available at www.expertconsult.com.

Oxygen-Derived Free Radicals and Nitric Oxide

Free radicals, such as superoxide anion, hydroxy radical, and NO derivatives, can (1) injure vascular endothelial cells, leading to increased vascular permeability; (2) inactivate antiproteases, such as α_1-antitrypsin, resulting in damage to ECM proteins; (3) enhance cytokine and chemokine expression secondary to signaling changes and cell damage; (4) activate endothelial cells and increase adhesion molecule expression; and (5) increase the formation of chemotactic factors (LTB_4). They can also inactivate neurotransmitters (adrenaline and noradrenaline), leading to hypotension.

Oxygen-derived free radicals are released from neutrophils and macrophages after exposure to chemokines and immune complexes and after phagocytosis by the leukocyte (see Table 3-2). They damage cells through peroxidation of cell membrane lipids, cross-linking of proteins and oxidizing thiol groups on methionine and cysteine, cleaving glycoconjugates, directly damaging DNA phosphate backbone and bases, and inducing the formation of DNA adducts. Because of damage to proteins, the activity of key enzymes and transcription factors needed by the cell can be impaired. Fortunately, the body has antioxidants that are (1) enzymatic, such as superoxide dismutase (SOD) isoforms 1, 2, and 3, catalase, thioredoxin, peroxiredoxins, and glutathione reductase; (2) nonenzymatic endogenous substances, such as ceruloplasmin, transferrin, metallothionein, uric acid, and melatonin; and (3) nonenzymatic dietary substances, such as vitamins A, C, and E and lycopenes, flavonoids, resveratrol, genistein, anthocyanins, naringenin, and reserpines. All of these minimize the damage to tissue caused by free radicals.

NO is a chemical mediator of inflammation that causes vasodilation by relaxing vascular smooth muscle cells. In response to injury and inflammatory stimuli, NO derivatives are synthesized by endothelial cells, macrophages, and specific populations of neurons in the brain from L-arginine, molecular oxygen, NADPH, other cofactors, and the enzyme NO synthetase (NOS). There are three forms of NOS that mediate NO formation: neuronal (nNOS), iNOS, and endothelial (eNOS). In addition to its vasodilatory activities, NO inhibits platelet aggregation and adhesion, inhibits mast cell–induced inflammation, oxidizes lipids and other molecules, and regulates leukocyte chemotaxis.

Receptors for Exogenous and Endogenous Inflammatory Stimuli and Toll-Like Receptors

Inflammatory responses occur in response to endogenous and exogenous substances. The body's inflammatory reaction to exogenous pathogens has been understood and studied for many years. Increasingly it is clear that the body also produces inflammatory reactions to host endogenous molecules released under sterile conditions. Thus both endogenous and exogenous stimuli produce "danger" signals, termed *danger-associated molecular patterns* (DAMPs).

Exogenous microbial products, often with redundant molecular structure, are PAMPs and include substances such as LPS, peptidoglycan, and lipoteichoic acid. PAMPs can bind several types of PRRs (Fig. 3-11; Table 3-4; E-Fig. 3-5). These receptors include secreted receptors that circulate in the blood (LPS-binding protein), surface receptors (macrophage mannose receptors; and TLRs), NLRs, and endosomal receptors (TLR and endosomal viral receptors). These receptors have different mechanisms by which they activate the cell, and some work together. LPS, for example, is bound by LPS-binding protein (LBP), which in turn binds CD14 for endocytosis and TLR4 for cytokine and inflammasome responses. The formation of a PRR-PAMP complex initiates transmembrane signaling that often involves a MyD88 protein event leading to NFκB activation and MAPK (p38) signaling. The NFκB family of transcription factors initiates gene transcription and translation, resulting in the

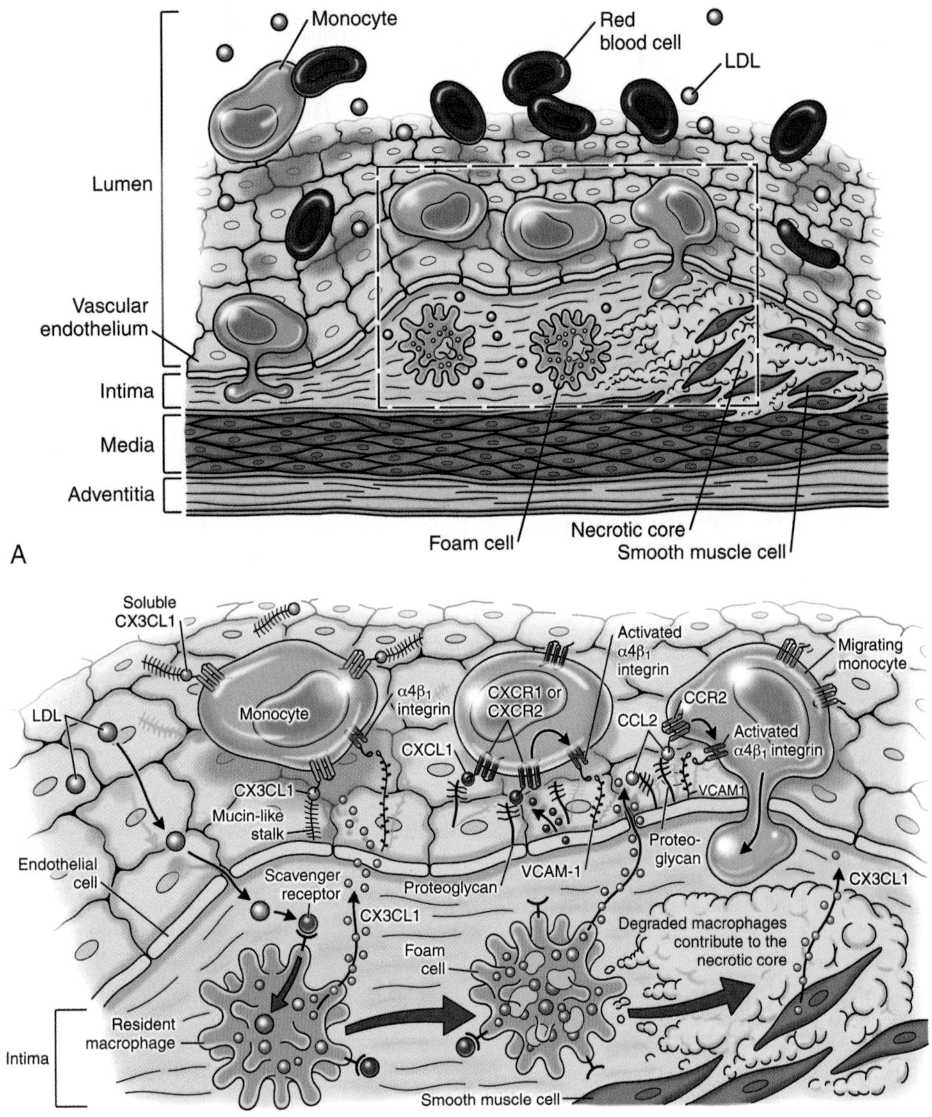

Figure 3-10 Chemokine Responses to Vascular Injury. **A,** The atherosclerotic plaque illustrates the interactions of chemokine ligands with their receptors during an inflammatory reaction. Whereas neutrophils respond to IL-8 (a CC chemokine), monocytes respond to CX3CL1, CXCL1, CCL2 and their respective receptors to attract cells along the vascular wall for adhesion molecule adherence and leukocyte infiltration. **B,** Higher magnification of the area defined by the box in **A**. *LDL*, Low-density lipoprotein; *VCAM-1*, vascular cell adhesion molecule 1. (Redrawn from Charo IF, Ransohoff RM: The many roles of chemokines and chemokine receptors in inflammation. *N Engl J Med* 354:610-621, 2006.)

expression of proteins involved in many cellular processes such as cell proliferation, differentiation, apoptosis, and cell responses to injury, stress, and external pathogens. NFκB and p38 then can induce phagocytosis by leukocytes, dendritic cell activation, release of inflammatory cytokines and chemokines, and the activation of the innate (defensin and antimicrobial peptide release) and adaptive (T_H1, T_H2, T_H17, T_{FH} activity) immune systems. Alternatively, TLR4 signaling does not engage MyD88 (MyD88-independent signaling) and results in the formation of IFN-β and IFN-inducible gene products.

In addition to LBP, other secreted PRRs that can trigger inflammatory reactions through complement activation or receptor binding include collagenous lectins such as mannan-binding lectins A and C, ficolins, surfactant proteins A (SP-A) and D (SP-D), and conglutinin (cattle), which bind glycans of chitin, bacterial capsules, viruses, C-reactive protein, and serum amyloid–binding protein. SP-A, for example, can bind, aggregate, and inhibit respiratory syncytial virus. SP-A can also activate macrophages.

Leukocytes, epithelia, mucosal-lining cells, and other cells can also express PRR on the plasma membrane, including TLR1, TLR2, TLR4, TLR5, TLR6, and TLR11. TLRs are a family of PRRs in mammals that can distinguish between chemically diverse classes of genetically conserved microbial products (see Table 3-4). For example, bacterial lipoprotein binds TLR1 and TLR2/6, flagellin binds TLR5, and LPS binds TLR4. These receptors have a central role in the release of inflammatory cytokines from the innate immune system in response to microbial structures, such as exogenous microbial substances and endogenous products (E-Fig. 3-6). Also, TLRs likely play a role in the adaptive immune response, which develops during the acute inflammatory response.

C-type lectin receptors are also present on the surface of monocytes, macrophages, neutrophils, and dendritic cells and include dectin-1, which binds β-1,3-glucan, as well as dectin-2, MBL, and dendritic cell–specific intercellular adhesion molecule-grabbing nonintegrins (DC-SIGNs) that bind high mannose and fructose; both glucans and mannose/fructose residues are produced and

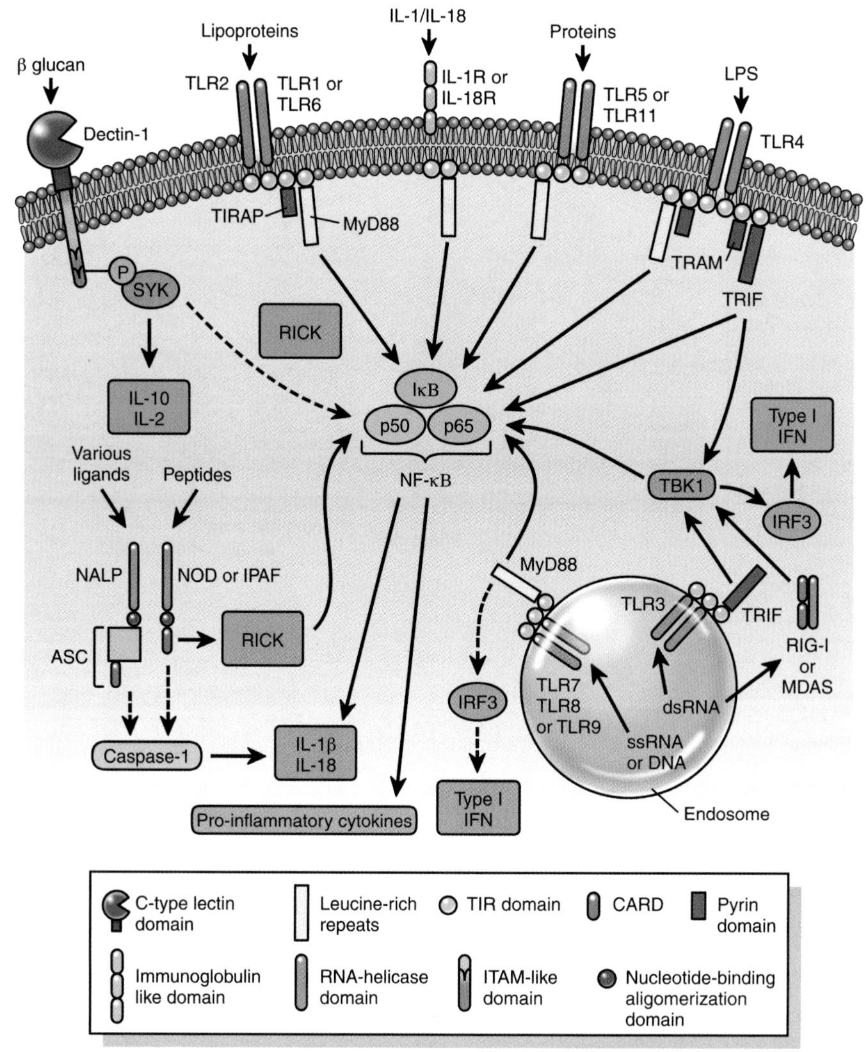

Figure 3-11 Pathogen-Associated Molecular Patterns (PAMPs), Pattern Recognition Receptors (PRRs), and Cellular Signaling. PAMPs such as lipopolysaccharide (LPS), teichoic acid, β-glucans, as well as microbial peptides, proteins, RNA, DNA, and CpG, bind specific receptors and trigger activation of the subjacent signaling cascade leading to transcription of proinflammatory genes (cytokines, interferons, chemokines). Receptors are present on the membrane surface (dectin-1, TLR1, 2, 4, 5, 6, 11; IL-1) in endosomes (TLR3, 7, 8, 9), and in the cytoplasm (nucleotide-binding oligomerization domain [NOD], NALP, retinoic acid–inducible gene 1 [RIG-1]). Toll-like receptors (TLRs) use MyD88 protein for signaling, except for TLR 3 and 4, which can be MyD88 independent. All pictured trigger NF κ B (NFκB), and some also induce interferon (IFN) responses. *CARD*, Caspase activation and recruitment domain; *dsRNA*, double-stranded RNA; *IL*, interleukin; *IRF*, interferon regulatory factor; *ITAM*, immuoreceptor tyrosine-based activation motif; *ssRNA*, single-stranded RNA; *TIR*, Toll/IL-1 receptor; *TRAM*, TRIF-related adaptor molecule; *TRIF*, TIR-containing adaptor inducing interferon-β. (Redrawn from Dale DC, Boxer L, Liles WC: The phagocytes: neutrophils and monocytes. *Blood* 112:935-945, 2008.)

released by mycobacterial and fungal organisms. Once bound, both TLR and C-type lectins regulate a wide range of innate and adaptive immune responses through NFκB, transcription factor activators protein-1 (TFAP-1), and interferon regulatory factors (IRFs).

Intracellular receptors, such as the NLRs, have a leucine-rich repeat domain that binds PAMPs and xenocompounds to induce and/or regulate inflammation. NOD1 is present in many cell types and binds to peptidoglycan-derived tripeptide structures (gamma-D-glutamyl-meso-diaminopimelic acid [iE-DAP]) of Gram-negative and some Gram-positive (*Listeria* and *Bacillus* spp.) bacteria. NOD2 is expressed predominantly by hematopoietic cells and intestinal epithelia and binds peptidoglycan-derived muramyl dipeptides. Bound NOD1 and NOD2 activate the receptor-interacting protein (RIP) family of serine/threonine protein kinase (RIPK2), which then induces NFκB activity and eventual secretion of antimicrobial peptides; inflammatory mediators such as TNF, IL-6, CCL2, IL-8, and CXCL2 invoking inflammation; and also activation of MAPK for gene transcription and regulation of autophagy in some cells.

Microbial products such as muramyl dipeptides and DAMPs can also bind NLRs, which, along with a variety of xenocompounds, can activate inflammasomes. Inflammasomes are multimeric protein units consisting of the NLR sensing molecule, adaptor protein ASC, and caspase-1. Through caspase-1 activation, inflammasomes mediate release of IL-1β, IL-18, and IL-33. NLRs of inflammasomes include NLRP1, NLRP3, NLRP6, NLRP7, and NLRP12 (or NNLRC4). LPS from Gram-negative bacteria binds TLR4, which activates NLR inflammasomes and produce IL-1β. LPS also binds CD14, which activates endocytosis. A recently identified LPS also binds caspase-11 in mice, activating a caspase-11 inflammasome.

PRRs for certain viral infections include RIG-I (e.g., Paramyxoviridae, influenza viruses) and melanoma differentiation-associated gene 5 (MDA5) (Picornaviridae). These molecules sense viral

Table 3-4 Types of Pathogen-Associated Molecular Pattern Exogenous Ligands, Their Pattern Recognition Receptors, and the Subsequent Action Related to Acute Inflammation

Exogenous PAMP Ligands	Secreted PRRs	Action
Mannose	MBL	Complement activation
Microbial membranes	CRP and SAP	Opsin, complement activation
LPS	LBP	LPS binding
	C1q	Complement activation
	Ficolins	Complement activation
Cell-Surface PRRs		
LPS, peptidoglycan	CD14	Nontranscriptional response; mediates endocytosis
Mannose	Macrophage mannose receptor	Phagocytosis
Bacterial cell walls	MARCO	Phagocytosis
β-glucan	Dectin-1	IL-10 and NFκB
Lipopeptides	TLR1	NFκB, MAPK
Lipoteichoic acid, lipoarabinomannan, zymosan	TLR2	NFκB, MAPK
LPS	TLR4	NFκB, MAPK
Flagellin	TLR5	NFκB, MAPK
Diacyl lipopeptides	TLR6	NFκB, MAPK
	TLR10	
	TLR11	
	TLR12	
	TLR13	
Intracellular PRRs		
DNA	TLR9	Type 1 IFN, NFκB
dsRNA	TLR3	Type 1 IFN, NFκB
ssRNA	TLR7/8, RIG-1, MDA5	Type 1 IFN, NFκB
Muramyl tripeptide peptidoglycan (Gram-negative bacteria)	NOD1	IL-1β
	NOD1	IL-1β
Peptidoglycan-muramyl dipeptide (Gram-positive and Gram-negative bacteria)	NALP3	IL-1β, IL-18, IL-33
Low K^+ concentration, uric acid, silica, amyloid β, microbial products, dsRNA		
Heparin sulfate, hyaluronic acid, heat shock protein 60 and 70, endoplasmic reticulum glycoprotein 96, fibronectin, fibrinogen, surfactant protein A, apoptotic cells, K^+ fluxes via P2X and pannexin 1, adenosine	Growth factor receptors, CD44, TLRs, TGF-βR, gp IIb/IIIa, surfactant protein receptor 210 (myosin XVIIIA), NALP3, adenosine receptor	Numerous cellular responses, including cellular activation, proliferation, and/or apoptosis, IL-1β, IL-18, IL-33 production, T_H2 responses

Endogenous inflammatory stimuli are those produced by host cells.
CRP, C-reactive protein; *dsRNA*, double-stranded RNA; *gp*, glycoprotein; *IFN*, interferon; *IL*, interleukin; *LBP*, LPS-binding protein; *LPS*, lipopolysaccharide; *MAPK*, mitogen-activated protein kinase; *MARCO*, class A scavenger receptor macrophage receptor with collagenous structure; *MDA5*, melanoma differentiation-associated gene 5; *MBL*, mannose-binding lectin; *NALP3*, NACHT, LRR and PYD domains-containing protein 3; *NFκB*, nuclear factor κ B; *NOD1*, nucleotide-binding and oligomerization domain; *PAMP*, pathogen-associated molecular pattern; *PRR*, pattern recognition receptor; *RIG-1*, retinoic acid–inducible gene-I; *SAP*, serum amyloid protein; *ssRNA*, single-stranded RNA; *TGF-βR*, transforming growth factor-β receptor; *TLR4*, Toll-like receptor 4.
Data from Medzhitov R: *Nat Rev Immunol* 1:135-142, 2001.

RNA, alter mitochondrial activity through MAVS, and invoke NFκB and IRF3 for IFN-α and IFN-β release and NFκB for inflammatory cytokine production, along with antimicrobial peptides.

Endosomes express PRRs that also have important roles in sensing viral infection and triggering a cellular response that often results in inflammatory and immune activity. TLR3, TLR7, TLR8, and TLR9 are present along the inner endosomal membrane and bind dsRNA (TLR3) or single-stranded RNA/DNA (ssRNA/DNA) (TLR7, TLR8, TLR9) and activate IRF7 and NFκB.

Endogenous molecules (not produced by microbes) are released in response to noninfectious injury (trauma, toxins, neoplasia, necrosis, or irritation). Because endogenous molecules can trigger an inflammatory reaction, they have been termed *alarmins*. Alarmins include sulfate, hyaluronan, heat shock protein (HSP) 60 (mitochondria), HSP70 (cytoplasm), Gp 96 (endoplasmic reticulum), fibronectin, fibrinogen, and SP-A, all of which can bind PRRs or other receptors and initiate cell signaling, inflammation, and activation of the innate immune system (see Table 3-4). These molecules are often overlooked when considering acute inflammation in the context of microbial infections because microbial products, such as teichoic acid and LPS, are very potent activators of acute inflammation. However, endogenous molecules likely have a significant role in inflammation generated against neoplastic cells, toxins, and mechanical injury. For example, a wide variety of xenocompounds, including apoptotic cells, toxins (maitotoxin, valinomycin, nigericin, aerolysin), stress molecules (ultraviolet radiation, monosodium urate, calcium pyrophosphate, beta amyloid fibrils), xenogeneic compounds (silicates, asbestos, aluminum hydroxide), as well as microbial products (lipoteichoic acid, LPS), can affect lysosomal function, which in turn induces NLRP3 (NALP3) activation

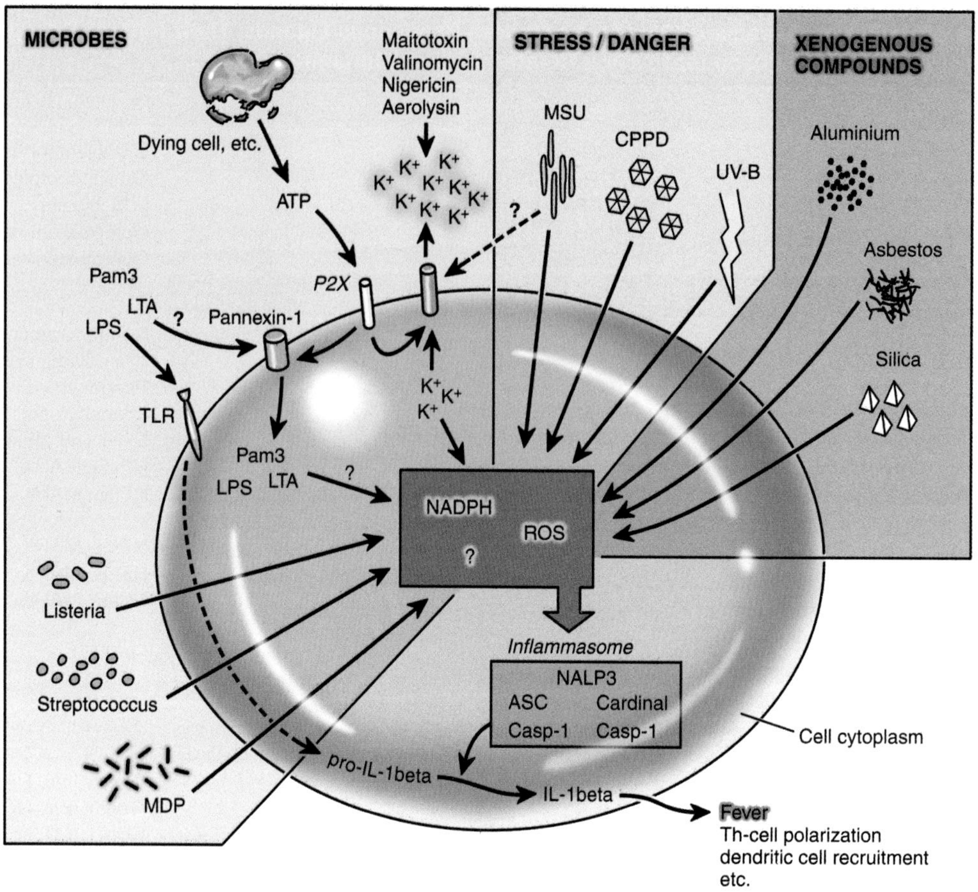

Figure 3-12 Inflammasome Activation by Exogenous and Endogenous Stimuli. Numerous stimuli can result in activation of the NALP3 inflammasome. Exogenous stimuli include lipopolysaccharide (LPS), lipoteichoic acid (LTA), toxins, monosodium urate (MSU) crystals, calcium pyrophosphate dihydrate (CPPD) crystals, ultraviolet (UV)-B waves, aluminum, asbestos, and silica. Endogenous stimuli include adenosine triphosphate (ATP), potassium, nicotinamide adenine dinucleotide phosphate (NADPH), and reactive oxygen species (ROS). Once engaged, NALP3 activates caspase-1, which cleaves pro-IL-1β into IL-1β and also activates IL-18 (not shown). *IL*, Interleukin; *MDP*, muramyl dipeptide; *TLR*, Toll-like receptor. (Redrawn from Benko S, Philpott DJ, Girardin SE: The microbial and danger signals that activate Nod-like receptors. *Cytokine* 43:368-373, 2008.)

(Fig. 3-12). Furthermore, adenosine, a by-product of cell injury CD39 hydroxylation of ATP, can bind adenosine receptors present on the surface membrane of leukocytes and modulate inflammatory and immune responses. Endogenous molecules mitigate the intensity of the inflammatory response by regulating signaling intensity.

Antimicrobial Peptides and Collectins

Antimicrobial peptides, such as the α- and β-defensins, cathelicidins, and others—such as anionic peptides, histantin, and dermacidins—are small peptides with microbicidal activity against Gram-negative and Gram-positive bacteria, fungi, mycobacteria, and some enveloped viruses such as human immunodeficiency virus (HIV) (E-Table 3-9). They are encoded by genes of the cells involved in the inflammatory response, especially neutrophils, and by epithelial cells forming the skin and the mucosal barriers of the respiratory and alimentary systems. The microbicidal activity likely occurs through the formation of pores within bacterial membranes and viral envelopes. In addition to the microbicidal activity, antimicrobial peptides are increasingly appreciated for their role in other nonmicrobial activities related to inflammation and wound repair. These activities include chemotaxis of leukocytes and dendritic cells, cell proliferation, wound repair, cytokine release, and the protease-antiprotease balance. There is also much evidence that antimicrobial peptides link the innate and adaptive immune responses.

There are a wide variety of antimicrobial peptides; however, the defensins have received the most attention for activities other than microbial killing. There are three types of defensins: the α-, β- and θ-defensins. α-Defensins are produced by neutrophils and Paneth cells. β-Defensins are produced by neutrophils and epithelial cells. θ-Defensins are produced in neutrophils of primates. The defensins are cationic proteins with three pairs of intramolecular disulfide bonds. α-Defensins and β-defensins can stimulate mast cell degranulation, induce IL-8 synthesis, induce T lymphocyte chemotaxis, and activate T lymphocytes, macrophages, and dendritic cells, thus interconnecting innate and adaptive immunity. The importance of defensins in immunity is underscored by the fact that HIV-1 infected individuals that are healthy and in "remission" have high concentrations of α-defensins, which are thought to enhance T lymphocyte activity and may also have direct anti–HIV-1 activity. Recent work has also shown that adipocytes in the dermis of skin express cathelicidins and other antimicrobial peptides to protect against infections caused by *Staphylococcus aureus*.

Acute Phase Proteins

Acute phase proteins are plasma proteins synthesized in the liver whose concentrations increase (or decrease) by 25% or more during inflammation. These proteins serve as inhibitors or mediators of the inflammatory processes and include C-reactive protein, α_1-acid glycoprotein, haptoglobin, mannose-binding protein, fibrinogen,

Table 3-5 Examples of Differing Types of Inflammatory and Clinical Responses to Substances

	TYPE OF INFLAMMATORY SUBSTANCES		
	Skin Allergen	Gram-Negative Bacterial Infection in Dermis	Gram-Negative Septicemia
Substance	Allergen	LPS, toxins	LPS, toxins
Site	Epidermis/dermis	Dermis	Blood
Molecular trigger	Immunoglobulin E–cross-linking, dendritic cell binding	TLR4, CD14, NOD1	Hageman factor, complement, TLR4
Major response	Histamine, leukotrienes	IL-1, IL-18, TNF, prostaglandins, PAF, neutrophil products	Kinins, bradykinin, PAF, prostaglandins, IL-1, TNF
Extent of response	Local	Local	Systemic
Clinical finding	Swelling, pruritus (bronchoconstriction)	Swelling, exudate (pus)	Fever, nausea, malaise
Desired resolution	Limited, resolves in hours/days	Limited, resolves in days	Transient, resolves
Possible sequelae	Severe wheal and flare, anaphylaxis	Cellulitis leading to ulceration, eventual fibrosis/granuloma	Septic shock

CD14 = receptor for LPS-binding protein.
Hageman factor = clotting factor.
IL-1, Interleukin-1; *IL-18*, interleukin 18; *LPS*, lipopolysaccharide (endotoxin); *NOD1*, nucleotide-binding and oligomerization domain; *PAF*, platelet-activating factor; *TLR4*, Toll-like receptor 4; *TNF*, tumor necrosis factor.

α_1-antitrypsin, and complement components C3 and C4. The concentration of these acute phase proteins usually increases during inflammation, whereas the concentration of prealbumin and albumin (also acute phase proteins) decreases in inflammation. Acute inflammatory conditions that are severe enough to raise blood plasma concentrations of cytokines, such as IL-1 and TNF, increase the blood concentrations of acute phase proteins, and elevation of fibrinogen concentration in the blood of cattle is used clinically as an indicator of systemic inflammation. C-reactive protein has recently received attention as a marker of inflammatory conditions, especially atherosclerosis in human beings. In addition to its diagnostic role, C-reactive protein binds to bacteria and fungi and also activates complement. Once concentrations of acute phase proteins and systemic concentrations of inflammatory cytokines are elevated, they affect the heart rate, blood pressure, and the hypothalamic regulation of temperature by directly or indirectly stimulating neurons within specific hypothalamic nuclei. The previously described changes also affect respiratory rates and gaseous exchange.

Antiinflammatory Mediators

Antiinflammatory mediators include adiponectin, lipoxins, resolvins, maresins, protectins, annexin A1, hydrogen sulfide, and regulatory cytokines. Regulation of these inflammatory mediators occurs by several mechanisms, which include (1) loss of the initiating inciting stimulus, (2) degradation of inflammatory mediators, (3) down-regulation of receptors, (4) dephosphorylation of signaling molecules, and (5) release of other mediators with antiinflammatory activity. Adiponectin is an adipokine, which in addition to its antiinflammatory activity also has potent insulin-sensitization, antilipotoxic, and antiapoptotic actions. Adiponectin binds two receptors, AdipoR1 and AdipoR2, which can decrease inflammation and oxidative stress in adipocytes. Lipoxins activate macrophages and alter neutrophil migration. Resolvins inhibit neutrophil transmigration across blood vessel walls. Maresins are lipids produced by macrophages that contribute to wound repair and reduce nerve sensitivity to painful stimuli. Protectins inhibit release of inflammatory mediators. Annexin A1 is released from neutrophils undergoing cell death and inhibits further neutrophil infiltration. Hydrogen sulfide is a gas that induces neutrophils to undergo apoptosis. IL-10 and many other cytokines regulate T lymphocytes and cells of the adaptive immune response.

Summary of the Chemical Mediators of Acute Inflammation

Various exogenous and endogenous stimuli can activate soluble, surface, or cytoplasmic and endosomal receptors or simply cause mechanical or other damage to invoke an acute inflammatory response. This response can occur very rapidly as the result of the release of preformed or rapidly activated inflammatory mediators such as histamine, kinins, complement factors like C3a and C5a, and tachykinins (substance P). These molecules generally affect vascular caliber and permeability and activate leukocytes and endothelial cells. Concurrently, lipid-based products, such as prostaglandins, leukotrienes, and PAF, contribute to chemotaxis, vascular tone, and leukocyte activity, all of which work in concert with chemokines and cytokines to activate endothelial cells and leukocytes and enhance neutrophil infiltration. NO released by macrophages and endothelia induce vasodilation and also can contribute to tissue damage caused by other reactive oxygen species. Inflammatory mediators bind receptors that subsequently induce cytoplasmic signaling and cellular activation, resulting in the production of additional cytokines, chemokines, adhesion molecules, antimicrobial peptides, and other inflammatory mediators that may either exacerbate or inhibit the inflammatory process. Activated neutrophils expressing leukocyte adhesion molecules, such as the integrins, enter inflamed tissue and can release hydrolytic enzymes and other granule contents that further damage tissue. Systemically, increases in acute phase proteins, cytokines, chemokines, complement, and inflammatory proteins can affect body temperature, cardiovascular function, locomotion, sleep, appetite, and other activities (Table 3-5).

Reparative Phase of the Acute Inflammatory Response

Outcomes of the Acute Inflammatory Response

The four main outcomes of acute inflammation are as follows:
- Resolution (the return to normal structure and function)
- Healing by fibrosis
- Abscess formation
- Progression to chronic inflammation

The severity of tissue damage, the ability of cells to regenerate, and the physical or biologic characteristics of the cause of the injury determine these outcomes. In the acute inflammatory response (Fig. 3-13), the desired outcome is resolution, that is, the complete return of normal structure and function. Resolution occurs if the following occur:

- The acute inflammatory response is completed in the correct sequence.
- Macrophages and lymphatic vessels remove the exudate.
- The inciting agent or substance is eliminated.
- The stroma (connective tissue) of the affected tissue is intact and can provide support for regeneration of epithelial cells.
- Ulcerated or necrotic epithelial cells are replaced by regeneration of adjacent epithelial cells on an intact basement membrane.

Mechanistically, the critical first stage of resolution involves the killing and/or removal of the inciting cause, removal of chemical mediators by neutralization or decay, return to normal vascular flow and capillary permeability, cessation of leukocyte emigration, apoptotic cell death of remaining neutrophils in the exudate, the removal of the exudate by monocyte-macrophage phagocytosis, and drainage to regional lymph nodes (Fig. 3-14). Inflammatory responses of neutrophils, monocytes, and macrophages are further inhibited by chemokine inactivation and release of products such as lipoxin A4, resolvins, annexin A, lactoferrin, and lysophosphatidylcholine.

Regeneration is the second stage of resolution and depends on the availability of progenitor epithelial cells and the presence of a supportive stroma and intact basement membrane for orderly

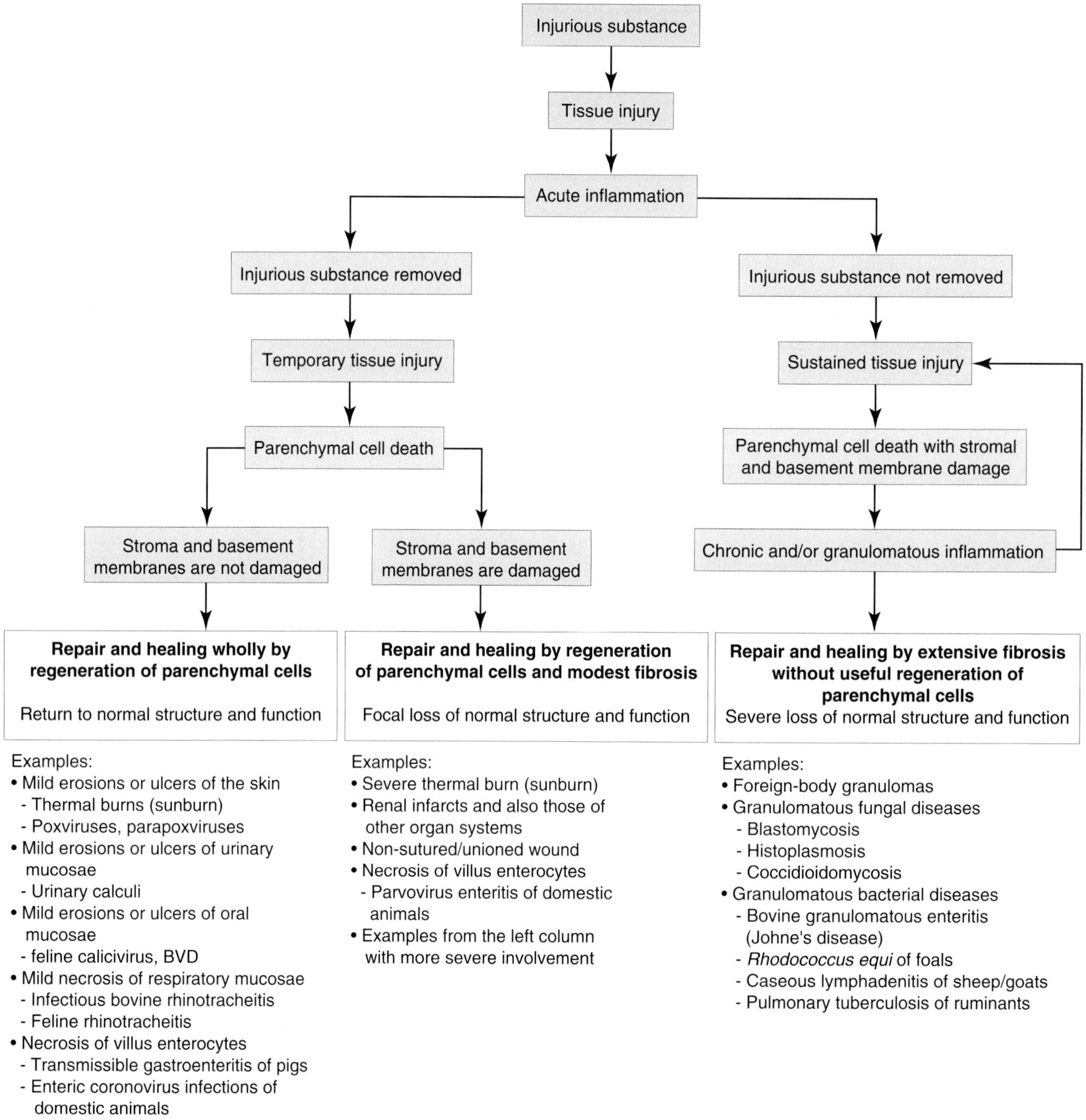

Figure 3-13 **Repair, Regeneration, and Fibrosis after Injury and Inflammation.** *BVD*, Bovine viral diarrhea. (Courtesy Dr. M.R. Ackermann, College of Veterinary Medicine, Iowa State University; and Dr. J.F. Zachary, College of Veterinary Medicine, University of Illinois.)

cellular migration. As an example, acute renal tubular necrosis can be caused by aminoglycoside antibiotics and results in detachment and necrosis of tubular epithelial cells from the tubular basement membrane. If the supporting stroma and basement membrane remain intact, progenitor epithelial cells can divide and migrate to replace lost cells and thus return the tubule to normal function. If the basement membrane is not intact to guide the proliferating cells, functional tubules will not form. Instead, regenerative tubular epithelial cells will atrophy or form into small aggregates with syncytial giant cells. Simultaneously, the microvascular supply to the region must be restored, which occurs mechanistically by the proliferation of endothelial cells in response to molecules such as VEGF.

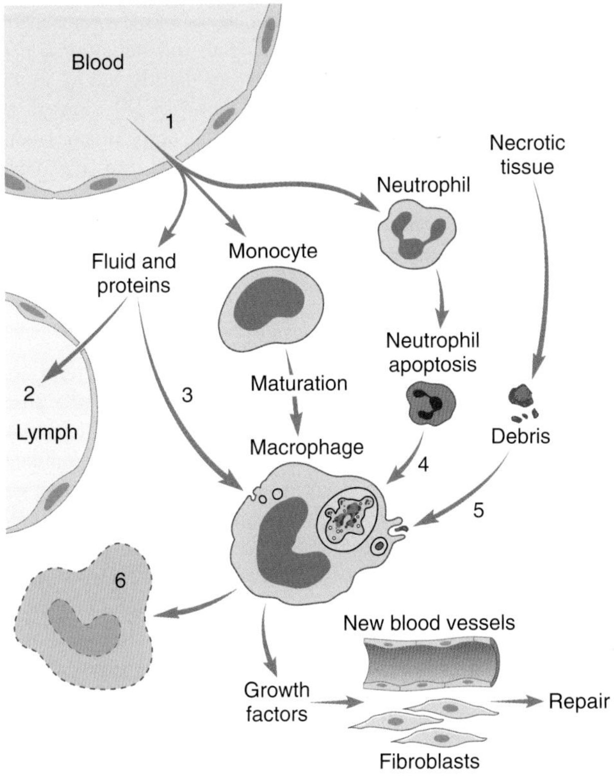

Figure 3-14 Events in the Resolution of Inflammation. *1*, Return to normal vascular permeability; *2*, drainage of edema fluid and proteins into lymphatic lymphatic vessels or *3*, by pinocytosis into macrophages; *4*, phagocytosis of apoptotic neutrophils and *5*, phagocytosis of necrotic debris; and *6*, disposal of macrophages. Macrophages also produce growth factors that initiate the subsequent process of repair. Note the central role of macrophages in resolution. (Redrawn from Haslett C, Henson PM: Resolution of inflammation. In Clark R, Henson PM, editors: *The molecular and cellular biology of wound repair*, New York, 1996, Plenum Press.)

Nomenclature of the Inflammatory Response (Morphologic Diagnoses)

Nomenclature, a system of names assigned to structures and processes in a scientific discipline, used in veterinary pathology provides clinicians with a morphologic diagnosis, a precise description of the process, type of inflammation, and disease. A morphologic diagnosis has six components listed in the following sequence: degree of severity, duration, distribution, exudate, modifier, and tissue (Table 3-6). Based on the results of a postmortem examination and/or histologic evaluation of tissue specimens, a pathologist will construct a morphologic diagnosis by including in sequential order the components of the nomenclature that best describe the specimens. For example, using the kidney as the injured tissue, the central component of a morphologic diagnosis is the name of the tissue derived from its Latin term, "nephro-." If the kidney is inflamed, the prefix "nephro-" is combined with the suffix "itis" (inflammation or disease of) to form the word "nephritis," meaning inflammation of the kidney. The other components of the morphologic diagnosis, such as degree, duration, distribution, exudate, and modifier, precede nephritis and are used to describe the characteristics of the inflammatory process. The pattern of distribution of the inflammatory lesion not only provides location but also in many instances implies a mechanism of injury. These patterns of distribution as shown in Fig. 3-15 include focal, multifocal, locally extensive, and diffuse. They are covered in greater detail in each organ system. The subtleties of this process

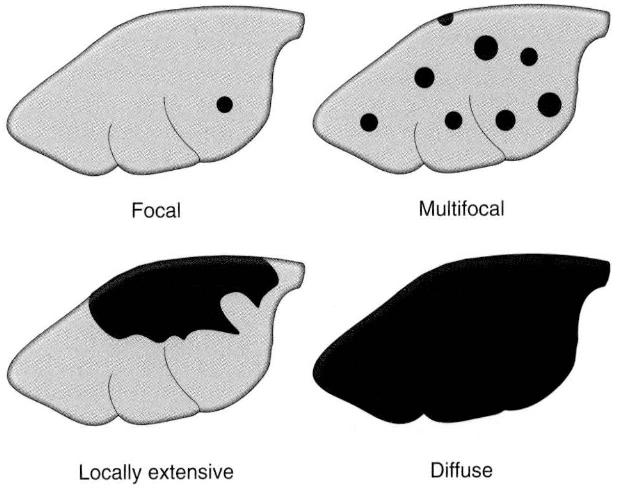

Figure 3-15 Patterns of Lesion Distribution Used to Construct Morphologic Diagnoses, as an Example, in the Lung. (Courtesy Dr. J.F. Zachary, College of Veterinary Medicine, University of Illinois.)

Table 3-6 The Nomenclature of a Morphologic Diagnosis

Degree	Duration	Distribution	Exudate	Modifier	Tissue
Minimal	Acute	Focal	Serous	Necrotizing	Nephritis
Mild	Subacute	Multifocal	Catarrhal	Bronchointerstitial	Cystitis
Moderate	Chronic	Locally extensive	Fibrinous	Hemorrhagic	Enteritis
Marked (severe)	Chronic-active	Diffuse (interstitial)	Suppurative	Embolic	Pneumonia*
		Cranioventral†	Granulomatous		Hepatitis

This table provides an example of how nomenclature can be used to construct a morphologic diagnosis. It is not intended to be all inclusive and may vary from schemes used in other veterinary colleges.
*In the lung, it is customary to use the term pneumonia to indicate inflammation of the lung.
†Used only for diseases of the lungs.

are learned through advanced training in the discipline of pathology, and terms describing the degree and duration evolve from years of professional experience and are not likely to be mastered by veterinary students during their professional training.

Morphologic diagnoses can also use the suffixes "osis" (diseased or abnormal condition) or "opathy" (disease). In this context, such diseases or conditions refer to those caused by degenerative or aging processes without inflammation. Therefore the same nomenclature can be used to diagnose a degenerative condition in the kidney by using the term *nephrosis* or the term *nephropathy*. The other components are then added to nephrosis or nephropathy to describe the characteristics of the degenerative process. Finally, some metabolic and neoplastic diseases do not fit into this nomenclature, but equally valid morphologic diagnoses can be constructed. An enlarged, soft and friable, yellow, and greasy liver can be morphologically diagnosed as "fatty liver" (hepatic lipidosis), whereas a solid, firm, white expansile mass in the liver could be morphologically diagnosed as "hepatic malignant lymphoma."

Morphologic Classification of Exudates in Acute Inflammatory Lesions

The gross and microscopic appearance of different types of acute inflammatory reactions in tissue can often be classified according to the vascular and cellular components of the response, thus providing a mechanistic basis for understanding the pathogenesis. Histopathologic lesions of acute inflammation are most commonly grouped into five categories: serous, catarrhal, fibrinous, suppurative or purulent, and hemorrhagic, or a combination of these lesions such as fibrinosuppurative. Similar histopathologic patterns of lesions also occur in chronic inflammation (lymphohistiocytic or granulomatous [macrophages, multinucleate giant cells (MGCs), lymphocytes, plasma cells, fibrosis]).

It should be recognized that the histopathologic lesions of acute inflammation often represent (1) a continuum of progressive changes of the same type of inflammation occurring over time or (2) different types of inflammatory responses occurring concurrently in the same or different areas of an affected tissue. Therefore rhinitis, for example, could progress in a sequence from serous to catarrhal to mucopurulent to purulent. If the inciting stimulus is severe, changes could progress rapidly from serous to fibrinous to hemorrhagic.

Serous Inflammation

Serous inflammation is the term used to describe a pattern of acute inflammation in which the tissue response consists of the leakage or accumulation of fluid with a low concentration of plasma protein and no to low numbers of leukocytes. This watery material is released from small gaps between endothelial cells and from hypersecretion of inflamed serous glands. This response is essentially a transudate (specific gravity < 1.012) and is seen with (1) thermal injury to skin, such as burns and photosensitization, in which the lesion can appear as a fluid-filled blisters, or (2) acute allergic responses characterized by watery eyes and a runny nose with a clear, colorless transudate.

Grossly, lesions, for example, with serous inflammation consist of tissue that (1) contains excessive clear to slightly yellow, watery fluid that leaks from the tissue on cut section or (2) forms raised fluid-filled vesicles protruding above the surface of the mucous membrane of the nasal cavity (serous rhinitis) or of the skin (Fig. 3-16). Microscopically, connective tissue fibers are separated, often widely, and capillaries and postcapillary venules are dilated with erythrocytes (active hyperemia). Endothelial cells lining these vessels can vary from flattened to hypertrophied.

Catarrhal Inflammation

Catarrhal inflammation, or mucoid inflammation, is the term used to describe a pattern of acute inflammation in which the tissue response consists of the secretion or accumulation of a thick gelatinous fluid containing abundant mucus and mucins from a mucous membrane. This response occurs most commonly in tissue with abundant goblet cells and mucous glands, such as in certain types of chronic allergic and autoimmune gastrointestinal diseases and with chronic inflammation of the airways of the respiratory system (chronic asthma). Grossly, the surface or cut surface of affected tissue may be covered with or contain a clear to slightly opaque, thick fluid (Fig. 3-17). Microscopically, the lesion can include hyperplastic epithelial cells of mucous glands and goblet cells, as well as connective tissue fibers separated by mucins.

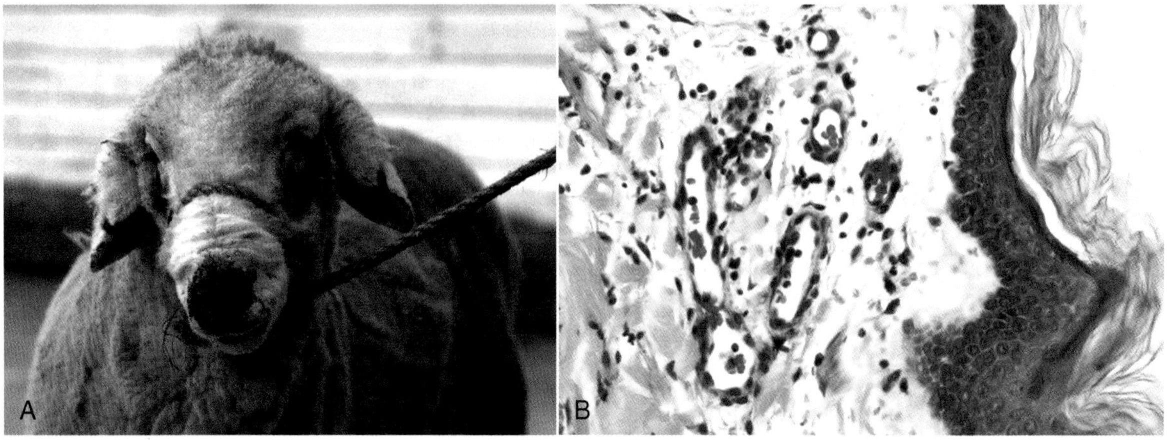

Figure 3-16 Serous Exudate/Subcutaneous Edema, Photosensitization, Skin of the Nose and Ears, Ewe. A, The nonhaired skin of the nose is covered by a crust resulting from dehydration of the serous exudate released from injured blood vessels following a short exposure to the sun. The ears are edematous and droopy. **B,** Microscopically, there is moderate expansion of the superficial dermis with edema secondary to vascular leakage (serous inflammation). The postcapillary venules are dilated (active hyperemia), and leukocytes have marginated on endothelial cells. H&E stain. (Courtesy Dr. M.D. McGavin, College of Veterinary Medicine, University of Tennessee.)

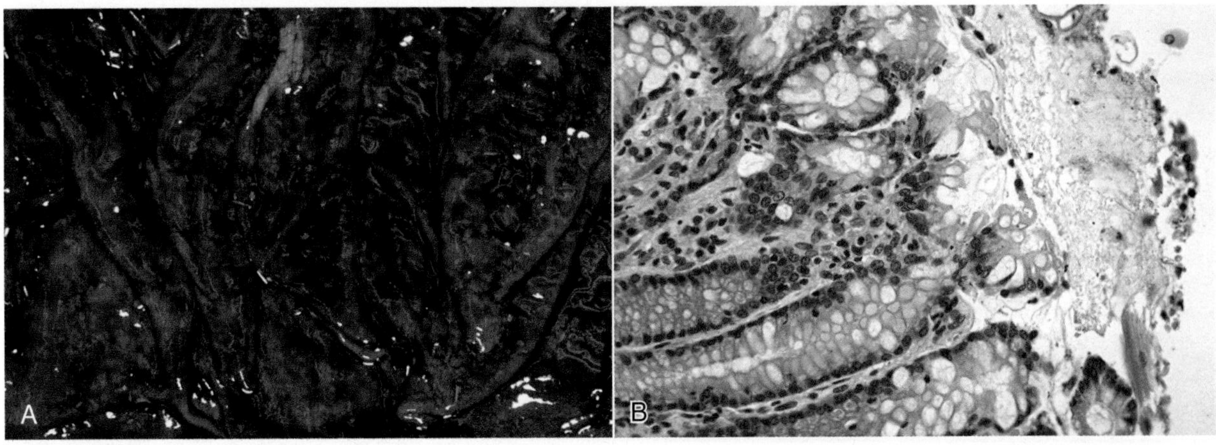

Figure 3-17 Catarrhal Inflammation. A, Abomasum, cow. The mucosal epithelium is moderately thickened, covered by a glistening layer of clear mucus, and has a subtle nodular appearance caused by accumulation of mucinous secretory products (catarrhal exudate) in the gastric pits. **B,** Colon, cow. Microscopically, there is a catarrhal colitis with hyperplasia of mucosal epithelial cells and increased accumulation of mucus on the mucosal surface. H&E stain. (Courtesy Dr. M.D. McGavin, College of Veterinary Medicine, University of Tennessee.)

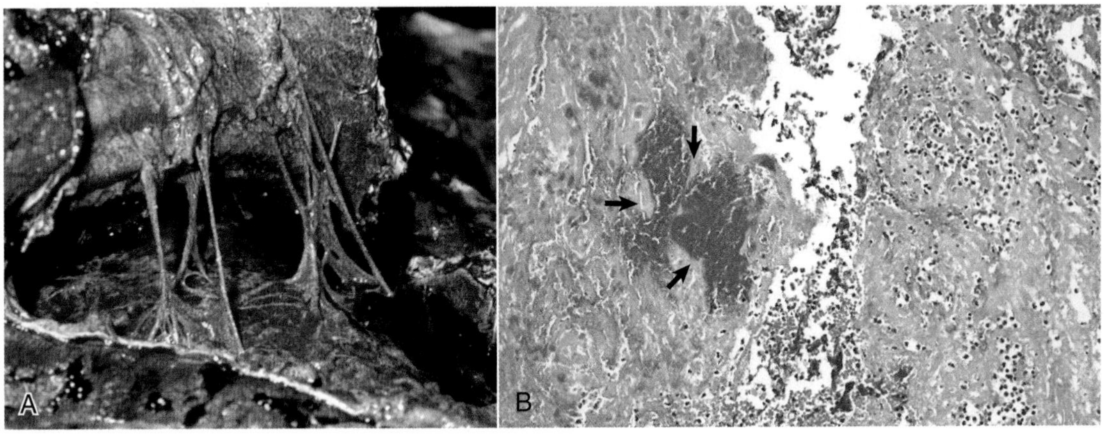

Figure 3-18 Fibrinous Inflammation, Pleural Cavity, Visceral and Parietal Pleurae, Horse. A, The pleural surfaces are covered by a yellow-gray, thick, friable exudate consisting of fibrin mixed with other plasma proteins. This exudate can be easily pulled apart and should not be confused with fibrous adhesions. The latter response occurs over time and consists of a similar appearing material that contains collagen fibers, which provide tensile strength to the material and form adhesions between opposing surfaces that can only be broken with some difficulty. **B,** Microscopically, there are layers of homogeneous red material (fibrin-fibrinous exudate) that contain occasional neutrophils and a focus of bacteria *(arrows)*. H&E stain. (Courtesy Dr. J.F. Zachary, College of Veterinary Medicine, University of Illinois.)

Fibrinous Inflammation

Fibrinous inflammation is the term used to describe a pattern of acute inflammation in which the tissue response consists of the accumulation of fluid with a high concentration of plasma protein (specific gravity > 1.02) and no to low numbers of leukocytes. This response is an exudate. Fibrinous inflammation occurs with more severe endothelial cell injury that allows leakage of large molecular weight proteins such as fibrinogen. Fibrinogen leaks from capillaries and postcapillary venules during the fluidic phase of the acute inflammatory response and polymerizes outside of the vessels to fibrin, a homogeneous and vividly pink (eosinophilic) protein when stained with hematoxylin and eosin (H&E). This lesion is most commonly caused by infectious microbes and is seen in the serous membranes of the body cavities, such as those lined by pleura (fibrinous pleuritis), pericardium (fibrinous pericarditis), peritoneum (fibrinous peritonitis), and in the synovial membranes of joints (fibrinous synovitis) and the meninges (fibrinous leptomeningitis). Common examples include the lesions in pulmonary alveoli in fibrinous pneumonia *(Mannheimia haemolytica)*, atypical interstitial pneumonia (3-methylindol), and respiratory viral infections (bovine herpesvirus 1 in cattle). When fibrin forms a distinct layer covering an ulcer, it is referred to as a *fibrinous pseudomembrane*, whereas when it lines the pneumonocyte surface of lung alveoli in a curvilinear fashion and is mixed with necrotic cell debris, such as occurs with bovine respiratory syncytial virus (BRSV) infection, it is called a *hyaline membrane*.

Grossly, the surfaces of affected tissue are red (active hyperemia) and covered with a thick, stringy, elastic, white-gray to yellow exudate that can be removed from the surface of the tissue (in contrast to a fibrous response) (Fig. 3-18; also see Fig. 3-4). A classic example of fibrinous inflammation occurs in fibrinous pneumonia caused by acute *M. haemolytica* infection, in which both alveoli and stromal connective tissue (interlobular septa and pleura) contain notable fibrinous exudate that rapidly becomes infiltrated by neutrophils, resulting in a fibrinosuppurative exudate. Another example of fibrinous inflammation occurs in bovine herpesvirus 1 infection. This virus injures epithelial cells of the respiratory tract, resulting

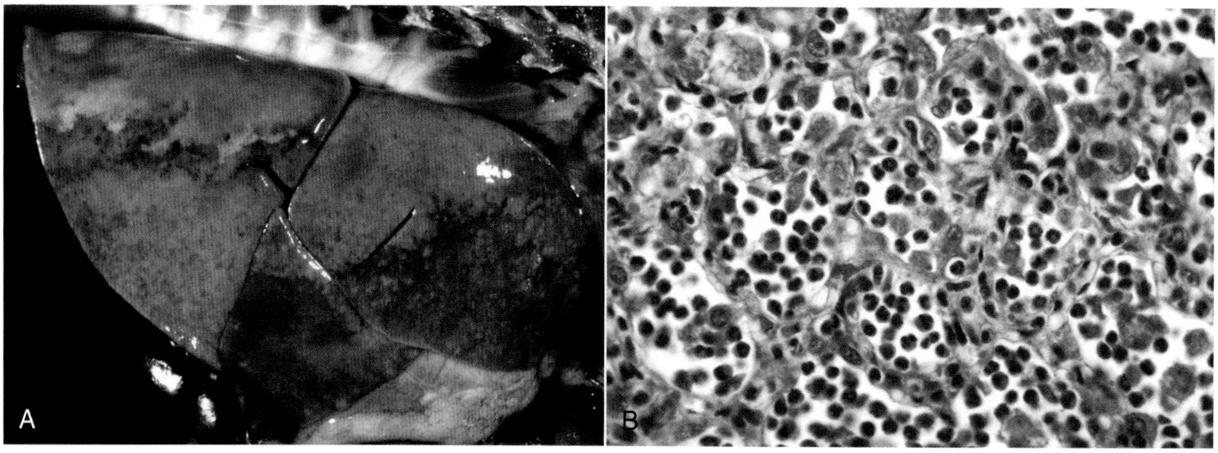

Figure 3-19 **Suppurative (Purulent) Inflammation, Secondary Bacterial Bronchopneumonia, Infectious Canine Distemper, Puppy. A,** The cranioventral areas of the lung are firm and beige to brown. This lesion is caused by neutrophils transmigrating into alveoli in an acute inflammatory response secondary to bacterial infection of the lung. **B,** Microscopically, alveoli contain numerous neutrophils (suppurative exudate) and sloughed pneumocytes. H&E stain. (Courtesy Dr. M.D. McGavin, College of Veterinary Medicine, University of Tennessee.)

in an acute fibrinous inflammatory response. Noninfectious causes, such as heat and smoke inhalation, can cause fibrinous exudate in the trachea. Microscopically, capillaries and postcapillary venules are dilated with erythrocytes (active hyperemia), and endothelial cells are reactive (hypertrophied). The stromal connective tissue or the mesothelial surfaces of the affected organ contains or is covered by red to vividly red layers of coagulated and/or polymerized fibrin, albumin, and other plasma proteins. The fibrinous exudate is often rapidly infiltrated by neutrophils, resulting in fibrinosuppurative inflammation.

Suppurative Inflammation

Suppurative inflammation is the term used to describe a pattern of acute inflammation in which the tissue response consists of the accumulation of fluid with a high concentration of plasma protein (specific gravity > 1.02) and high numbers of leukocytes, predominantly neutrophils. This material is an exudate commonly known as *pus*. Pus can be a creamy liquid, but if dehydrated, it can be more caseous and firm in consistency and occasionally laminated in diseases such as ovine caseous lymphadenitis. A collection of pus circumscribed by a fibrous capsule that is visible grossly is called an *abscess*, whereas if visible only microscopically, it is called a *microabscess*.

Dense neutrophil accumulation (pus) can also be distributed in tissue layers such as fascial planes and subcutaneous connective tissue and is referred to as *cellulitis* or *phlegmonous inflammation*. Instead of producing a focal abscess, the neutrophils evoke a watery suppurative exudate distributed along fascial planes and tissue spaces, as in some cases of blackleg or extensive Gram-positive (staphylococcal) infection. Suppurative inflammation, microabscesses, abscesses, and exudates are most commonly caused by bacteria, including *Staphylococcus* spp., *Streptococcus* spp., and *Escherichia coli*, and can occur in many organs. These genera can also cause suppurative bacterial meningitis in the central nervous system. Abscesses in the brains of horses caused by *Streptococcus equi* and microabscesses in the brains of cows caused by *Listeria monocytogenes* are good examples of suppurative inflammation. Bacteria-induced suppurative inflammation also occurs commonly in (1) the pelvis and tubules (pyelonephritis) of the kidney, (2) the bronchi of the lungs (bronchopneumonia), (3) the nasal and sinus cavities (rhinitis and sinusitis), (4) the glandular epithelium of the prostate (prostatitis), (5) the lumina of the gallbladder (cholecystis) and urinary bladder (urocystitis), and (6) the acini and ducts of the mammary gland (mastitis). Unresolved suppurative inflammation can progress to chronic inflammation.

Grossly, the surfaces and/or connective tissues of affected organs are hyperemic and covered by or contain, respectively, a thick white-gray to yellow pus (Fig. 3-19). In some cases pus will be mixed with fibrin, forming a fibrinosuppurative exudate. Microscopically, affected tissues have large numbers of neutrophils; many degenerate and often are mixed with necrotic cellular debris, bacteria, plasma proteins, and fibrin.

Chronic Inflammation

Chronic inflammation (Essential Concept 3-2) is inflammation of prolonged duration (weeks to months to years) that occurs (1) when the acute inflammatory response fails to eliminate the inciting stimulus, (2) after repeated episodes of acute inflammation, or (3) in response to unique biochemical characteristics and/or virulence factors in the inciting stimulus or microbe. Table 3-7 lists some of the most common causes of chronic inflammation in domestic animals. The underlying biologic mechanisms that result in chronic inflammation include persistence/resistance, isolation in tissue, unresponsiveness, autoimmunity, and unidentified mechanisms.

- Persistence/resistance: Persistent infections, such as those caused by *Mycobacterium* spp.; *Nocardia* spp.; deep-seated mycoses, such as *Blastomyces dermatitidis* (E-Fig. 3-7) and *Histoplasma capsulatum*; and parasites, such as *Toxocara canis* larvae, can avoid and/or resist phagocytosis by neutrophils and macrophages—or once internalized by these cells, can prevent fusion of primary and secondary lysosomes or killing by lysosomes. Such microbes also usually do not produce biologic molecules that cause severe tissue injury, but their presence continually incites chronic inflammatory and immune responses. Some microbial agents can induce macrophages to undergo apoptosis and subsequent internalization by adjacent macrophages. Tissue destruction, granulomatous inflammation, and fibrosis are common sequelae of persistent/resistant infectious agents.
- Isolation: Some microbes, such as *Streptococcus* and *Staphylococcus* spp., are not naturally resistant to phagocytosis and/or destruction but are able to isolate themselves from effective innate and adaptive immune responses and from antimicrobial drugs by "hiding" themselves in pus.

- Unresponsiveness: Certain foreign materials are virtually indestructible and therefore are unresponsive to phagocytosis and/or enzymic breakdown. These include plant material, grass awns, silica dust, asbestos fibers, some suture materials, and surgical prostheses.

ESSENTIAL CONCEPT 3-2 Chronic Inflammation

Chronic inflammation occurs (1) when the acute inflammatory response fails to eliminate the inciting stimulus, (2) after repeated episodes of acute inflammation in which there is extensive tissue injury and necrosis, or (3) in response to unique biochemical characteristics and/or virulence factors in the inciting stimulus or microbe. The underlying mechanisms that result in chronic inflammation include (1) persistence/resistance to phagocytosis by neutrophils and macrophages, (2) isolation ("hiding") from immune responses and antimicrobial drugs in exudates, (3) inability to destroy (or kill) via phagocytosis and/or enzymic breakdown, (4) "genetic" dysfunction of oxidative killing in leukocytes or in adaptive immune responses, and (5) unknown causes. Chronic inflammation is characterized microscopically by a shift of the cellular elements of the inflammatory response from neutrophils to lymphocytes, natural killer cells, macrophages, plasma cells, and multinucleated giant cells (e.g., granulomatous inflammation or granulomas) and by (1) proliferation of fibroblasts and deposition of collagen (desmoplasia and/or fibroplasia) and (2) angiogenesis and neovascularization (granulation tissue formation). Cytokines, chemokines, and other inflammatory mediators maintain the chronic inflammatory response. Chronic inflammation, characterized by two concurrently occurring processes: cellular infiltration and fibroplasia, attempts to overcome the inciting agent/substance via a variety of cells and the adaptive immune response and return the tissue to a state that is no longer harmful to the animal. If these responses fail, the inciting agent/substance is "isolated" by dense accumulations of chronic inflammatory cells and fibroblasts within a granulomatous exudate or within a granuloma. If this process fails, the inciting agent/substance is then "walled-off" with collagen produced by fibroblasts, encapsulating the agent/substance and functionally placing it "outside" of the body.

- Autoimmunity and leukocyte defects: Alterations in the regulation of adaptive immune responses to self-antigens result in autoimmune diseases, such as polyarteritis nodosa, with a chronic inflammatory response. Defects in leukocyte function can also result in chronic inflammation. For example, loss of NADPH oxidative function in human patients with chronic granulomatous disease impairs leukocyte free radical formation and oxidative killing, thus allowing persistence of microbial agents or internalized material.
- Unidentified mechanisms: In some diseases, such as canine granulomatous meningoencephalitis, the cause of chronic inflammation remains unknown.

The chronic inflammatory response is maintained by cytokines, chemokines, and other inflammatory mediators that are released and incite (1) ongoing inflammation mediated by infiltration and activation of lymphocytes, macrophages, plasma cells, and MGCs; (2) tissue destruction (necrosis); (3) proliferation of fibroblasts and deposition of collagen (desmoplasia and/or fibroplasia); (4) angiogenesis and neovascularization (granulation tissue formation); and (5) initiation of wound healing (reepithelialization and tissue repair).

Beneficial and Harmful Aspects of Chronic Inflammation

The body initially responds to injury through acute inflammation. Once the acute inflammatory response fails to overcome the inciting agent or persistent substance, chronic inflammation ensues as the body attempts to overcome the inciting agent/substance via a variety of cells such as NK cells, lymphocytes, macrophages and the adaptive immune response. If these responses fail, the inciting agent/substance is then "walled-off" with collagen produced by fibroblasts, encapsulating the agent/substance and functionally placing it "outside" of the body. Some types of responses, such as lepromatous (diffuse) granulomatous reactions, do not form defined fibrous capsules or walls and instead separate the agent/substance by dense accumulations of macrophages and fibroblasts that are arranged irregularly. Often, this response can be beneficial and in time can

Table 3-7 Selected Examples of Conditions That Can Cause or Lead to Chronic Inflammation in Domestic Animals

Microbial Agents	Toxins	Autoimmune Diseases	Foreign Bodies	Other
Bacteria: *Brucella* spp. *Mycobacteria* spp.: canine/feline leprosy *M. avium-intracellulare* *M. bovis tuberculosis* atypical (e.g., *M. marinum*) *Rhodococcus equi*	*Vicia villosa* (hairy vetch)	Lupus erythematosus Allergic contact dermatitis Irritant contact dermatitis Rheumatoid arthritis Polyarteritis nodosa	Retained suture Plant fibers Silica Asbestos Beryllium Inhaled smoke Inhaled dust	Canine granulomatous meningoencephalitis Lick granuloma Sterile nodular granuloma Sperm granuloma Chalazion Eosinophilic granulomas of dogs, cats, horses (see Table 3-8)
Virus: Porcine circovirus Fungi: *Trichophyton* spp. *Microsporum* spp. *Aspergillus* spp. Protozoa/parasites: *Leishmania* spp. *Trypanosoma* spp. *Draschia* spp. *Habronema* spp.				

lead to a return to normal activity. Small granulomas or abscesses in the lung, liver, or even in some areas of the skin, with time, eventually go unnoticed by the innate and adaptive immune systems and do not stimulate pain or mechanical interference to movement or function.

On the other hand, chronic inflammation can be detrimental. The mononuclear leukocyte infiltrates (macrophages, lymphocytes, and NK cells) within areas of chronic inflammation take up space and often displace, replace, and sometimes obliterate the original tissue. At the same time, new blood vessels form, fibroblasts proliferate and deposit collagen, and if the lesion expands, the inflammatory response can affect function of adjacent tissues and/or cells and ultimately the function of the entire organ. For example, chronic inflammatory lesions in the intestine of dogs and cats with inflammatory bowel disease (IBD) can induce progressive weight loss and debilitation. Also, chronic inflammation in the brains of dogs with granulomatous meningoencephalitis can destroy neurons and glia, impinge and obstruct flow of cerebrospinal fluid (CSF) in the ventricular system, and elevate the intracranial pressure, all of which can impair cognition and movement.

The extent of debilitation in animals with chronic inflammatory lesions depends on the location of the lesion and extent of tissue involvement. Even very small chronic lesions in the brain can rapidly incite clinical signs through either the destruction of neuroparenchyma or perhaps by impairing flow or resorption of CSF. In contrast, some widespread chronic inflammatory lesions, such as those in inflammatory bowel disease of dogs and cats and Johne's disease of cattle, can involve extensive areas of the intestine and often precede clinical signs (diarrhea) by months or even years. Yet other diseases, such as embolic hepatic or lung abscesses or disseminated tuberculoid granulomas, can be debilitating over time through the loss of parenchymal function and the continual release of inflammatory mediators, such as TNF and IL-1, both of which affect temperature and appetite.

In chronic inflammation, the first clinical intervention is to remove the inciting factor, if possible. Thus antibiotics and antifungal drugs are used against bacterial and mycotic infections. Some foreign bodies can be removed surgically, and it may be possible to identify, opsonize, chelate, or sequester immunologic allergens, antigens, and nondegradable substances. Unfortunately, few medical therapies completely resolve certain types of chronic inflammation, especially if granulomas and/or extensive scar tissue have developed. In the future, perhaps surgical debulking of large lesions may be followed by gene or stem cell therapy to effectively eliminate specific types of granulomas, such as those caused by mycobacterial infection or inducing apoptosis of fibroblasts, myofibroblasts, and macrophages.

Progression of the Acute Inflammatory Response to Chronic Inflammation, Fibrosis, and Abscess Formation

Acute inflammatory responses can either fully resolve with return of the tissue to normal structure and function or repair by healing (Fig. 3-20). If conditions do not allow for complete resolution of the acute inflammatory response, four outcomes can result: (1) progression to chronic/granulomatous inflammation, (2) healing by fibrosis, (3) healing with increased cellularity (cerebral gliosis, Kupffer cell hyperplasia, or glomerular mesangial cell hyperplasia), or (4) abscess formation. These outcomes are determined by the severity of tissue damage, the ability of cells to regenerate, and the biologic characteristics of the agent/substance (e.g., mycobacterial waxes, poorly degradable plant fibers) that caused the injury.

Progression to Chronic/Granulomatous Inflammation

Progression to chronic/granulomatous inflammation occurs when the acute inflammatory response fails. Failure is characterized by the following:

- Persistence of the inciting stimulus for a long period of time (weeks to months)
- Extensive tissue injury and necrosis (third-degree burn)

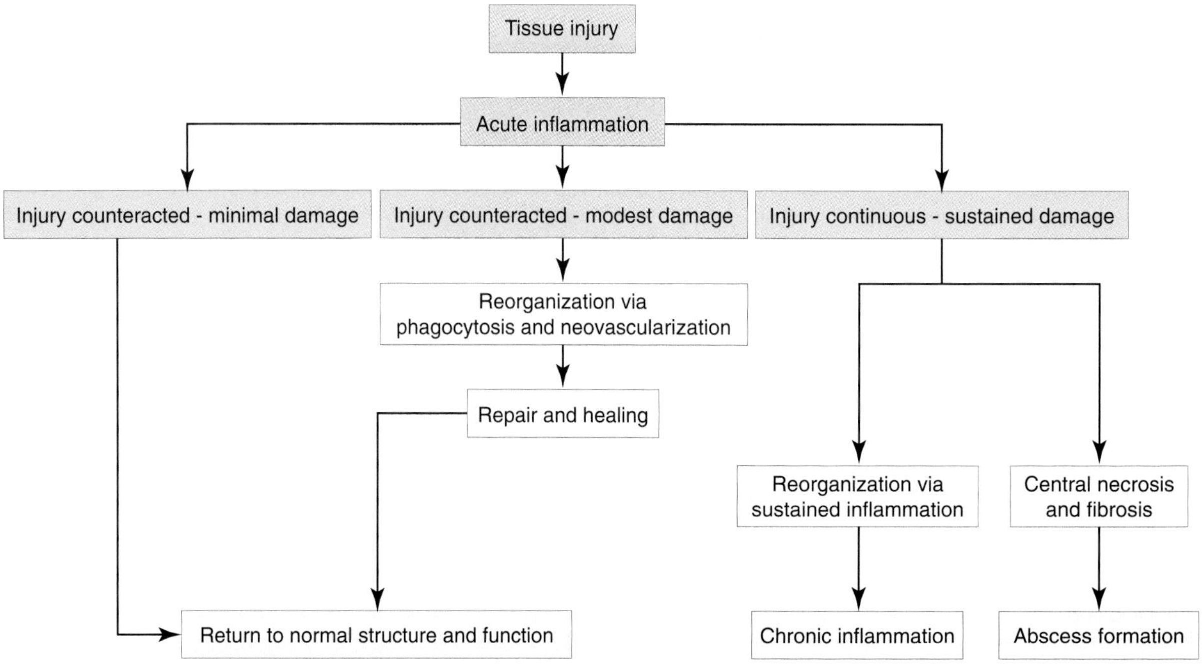

Figure 3-20 **The Outcomes of Tissue Injury and Unresolved Acute Inflammation.** (Courtesy Dr. M.R. Ackermann, College of Veterinary Medicine, Iowa State University; and Dr. J.F. Zachary, College of Veterinary Medicine, University of Illinois.)

- A shift of the cellular elements of the inflammatory response from neutrophils to lymphocytes, macrophages, and sometimes MGCs
- Extensive connective tissue reorganization followed by fibrosis (fibroplasia)

Examples of agents and substances that often result in chronic inflammatory responses include systemic mycoses, such as *B. dermatitidis* and *H. capsulatum*; intracellular bacterial pathogens, such as *Nocardia, Brucella, Mycobacterium*, or *Salmonella* spp.; protozoa, such as *Leishmania* or *Trypanosoma* spp.; parasites, such as *Toxocara* larvae or *Habronema*; autoantigens, such as those occurring in sperm granulomas or in autoimmune diseases like lupus erythematosus; and foreign bodies (plant awns, sticks, metals, asbestos, or suture material). Such agents continually induce the release of inflammatory mediators from indigenous parenchymal cells and leukocytes, leading to macrophage infiltration and activation; T lymphocyte, NK cell, and perhaps mast cell or eosinophil infiltration; and fibroblast and endothelial cell proliferation. Some of the inflammatory cytokines, such as TGF-β, may interfere with regeneration of epithelial and parenchymal cells (see section on Wound Healing and Angiogenesis).

Healing by Fibrosis

Healing by fibrosis occurs after tissue injury in which there is necrosis of the tissue framework provided by stromal elements (connective tissue) and of the epithelial cells required to regenerate and successfully reconstitute the parenchymatous elements of the tissue (Essential Concept 3-3). After necrosis, dead tissue and the acute inflammatory exudate are removed by macrophages (phagocytosis by cells of the monocyte-macrophage system), and the space is filled with fibrovascular tissue (granulation tissue) commonly seen in the healing process. Granulation tissue is eventually replaced by immature fibrous connective tissue that is poorly collagenized and then by mature connective tissue that is well collagenized, healing the wound and forming a scar (cicatrix). Structural integrity may be reestablished, but functional integrity depends on the extent of the loss of parenchymal cells. For example, with severe skin burns or extensive lacerations, dermal scarring eventually replaces lost dermal structures and to a limited extent restores structural integrity; however, the skin's functional integrity is extremely limited because of the loss of adnexal glands, hair follicles, and scar tissue that reduces the range of motion in joints of the limbs and digits. The degree and extent of fibroblast and myofibroblast proliferation in such wounds largely depends on mediators such as TGF-β and IL-13 (see the section on Wound Healing and Angiogenesis).

Abscess Formation

Abscess formation (Fig. 3-21) occurs when the acute inflammatory response fails to rapidly eliminate the inciting stimulus and the enzymes and inflammatory mediators from neutrophils in the exudate liquefy the affected tissue and neutrophils to form pus. Myeloperoxidase enzyme in neutrophils contributes to neutrophil necrosis and liquefaction. The presence of myeloperoxidase is an evolutionary phenomenon, and reptiles and birds lack this enzyme and are therefore unable to liquefy neutrophils into pus. Abscesses can have a septic or sterile origin. Septic abscesses most commonly originate from bacterial infection, whereas sterile abscesses arise from incompletely degraded foreign bodies or from the failure of injected medications to be completely absorbed. Pyogenic bacteria, such as *Staphylococcus* and *Streptococcus* spp., commonly cause septic abscesses. They enter tissue hematogenously or by direct extension from the skin following trauma. The pus within an abscess can range in consistency from serous to purulent to caseous and in color from white to yellow to green, depending on the inciting agent/substance. The color of the exudate often depends on the pigment produced by the inciting bacterium and the species; for example, yellow exudates are caused by abscesses formed by *Staphylococcus, Streptococcus* spp., and *Corynebacterium ovis;* green exudate is caused by abscesses formed by *Pseudomonas aeruginosa;* and red exudate is caused by abscesses formed by *Serratia marcescens*.

After an acute inflammatory response has been established, the development of an abscess in this site consists of a collection of

ESSENTIAL CONCEPT 3-3 Repair, Healing, and Sequestration of Tissue Injury

Tissue healing within the context of inflammation is a continuum of "reparative" responses that are triggered by the severity of tissue injury and by the metabolic conditions within the site of injury. The "healing" responses of affected tissues include (1) a return to normal structure and function, (2) healing by replacement fibrosis, and (3) healing by sequestration. The latter category includes healing by abscess or granuloma formation with or without encapsulating fibrosis, and healing by isolating and diluting the causative agent in a granulomatous exudate with or without fibrosis. Healing occurs in both acute and chronic inflammation, but the outcomes can be dramatically different and are based on the severity of tissue damage, the ability of cells to regenerate, and the biologic characteristics of the inciting agent/substance. Acute inflammation that is fully resolved often results in minimal damage to stroma and basement membranes (the tissue framework), and the affected tissue heals and returns to normal structure and function through regeneration, cell migration, and reepithelialization from stem cells in adjacent normal tissue (i.e., first and second intention wound healing). However, if there is necrosis and loss of tissue framework and the epithelial cells needed to reconstitute the basic structural elements of the tissue, then healing by fibrosis occurs. Exudate and debris are removed by macrophages, and the space is filled initially with immature fibrous connective and then by mature connective tissue (fibrosis) (i.e., scar) or granulation tissue. If the inciting agent/substance is not removed by acute inflammation, the inflammatory response transitions to chronic inflammation (see Essential Concept 3-2). If chronic inflammation is unable to remove the inciting agent/substance, then the affected tissue attempts to "heal" itself by using defensive mechanisms that act to isolate and sequester the lesion and limit the spread of additional tissue damage. Defensive sequestration healing includes (1) healing by abscess or granuloma formation with fibrosis and (2) healing by granulomatous inflammation with or without fibrosis. These outcomes are not healing that returns the tissue to normal structure and function but instead serve as compensatory defensive mechanisms to protect the animal against the cause. Healing by abscess formation occurs when enzymes and inflammatory mediators from neutrophils in the exudate liquefy the affected tissue and neutrophils to form pus but are unable to eliminate the inciting cause. Subsequently, fibroblasts produce collagen and extracellular matrix proteins that form a "thin" vascularized connective tissue wall and then if needed mature into a fibrous capsule surrounding (encapsulating) and isolating the cause. A similar process occurs in healing by granuloma formation, which again acts to isolate the cause. However, the granulomatous inflammatory response is characteristic of an inciting agent/substance that is difficult to kill and/or remove. In these latter cases, healing by fibrosis occurs, and the exudate is surrounded and encapsulated by connective tissue. The response is a last ditch attempt to isolate and dilute the cause; however, the healing outcome is usually unfavorable, and there is substantial tissue injury and loss with time.

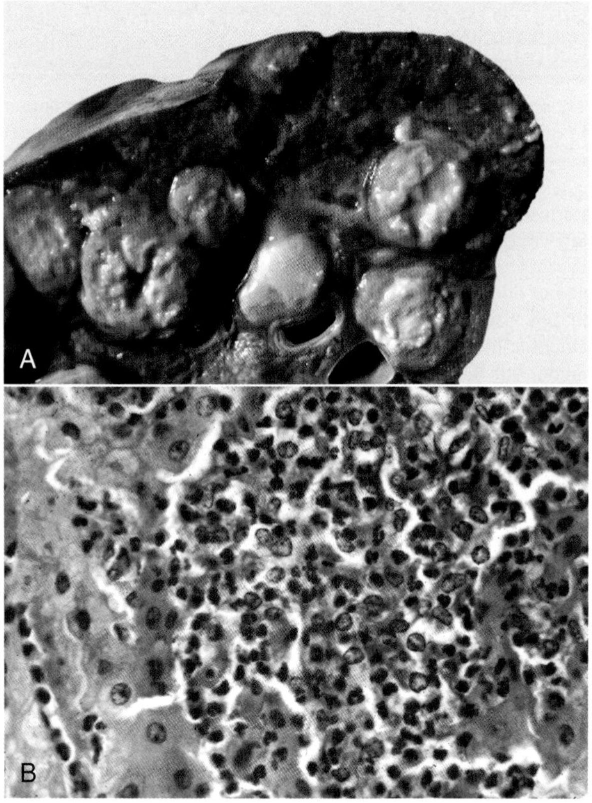

Figure 3-21 Abscess Formation. A, Abscess, lung, cow. A cut section of lung has numerous abscesses. Note the white to gray exudate and how it bulges from the cut surface. **B,** The exudate in **A** consists of cell debris and a large number of neutrophils admixed with lesser numbers of degenerating macrophages and lymphocytes, and bacteria (the latter not visible with H&E stain). H&E stain. (Courtesy Dr. M.D. McGavin, College of Veterinary Medicine, University of Tennessee.)

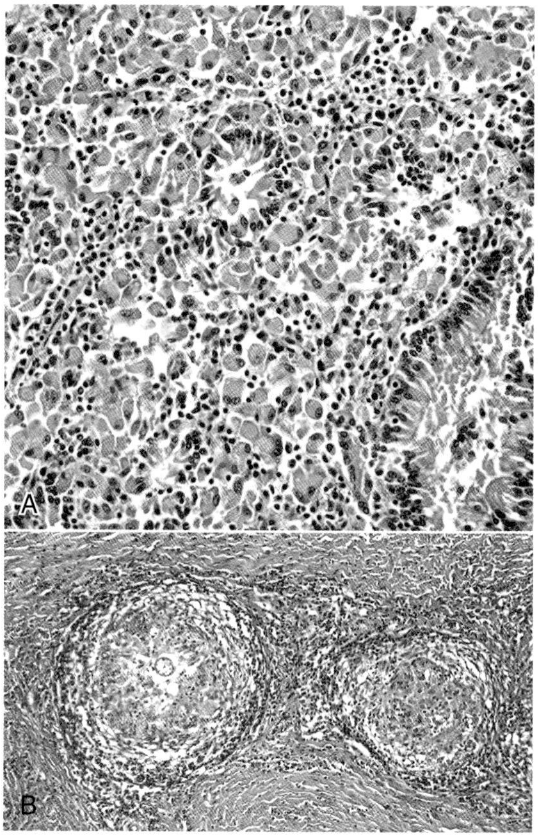

Figure 3-22 Granulomatous Inflammation and Granulomas. A, Granulomatous inflammation in Johne's disease, ileum. The lamina propria contains a solid sheet of granulomatous inflammatory cells, which is characteristic of lepromatous (diffuse) granulomatous inflammation. H&E stain. **B,** Nodular (tuberculoid) granuloma in coccidioidomycosis. Granulomas are round to oval with a central core of granulomatous inflammatory cells and a peripheral zone of fibroblasts, which may produce a fibrous capsule. The granuloma on the left contains a single central fungal element. H&E stain. (**A** courtesy Dr. J.F. Zachary, College of Veterinary Medicine, University of Illinois. **B** courtesy Dr. M.D. McGavin, College of Veterinary Medicine, University of Tennessee.)

neutrophils admixed with cell debris, macrophages, and fibroblasts with variable infiltrates of lymphocytes. Experimentally such a site can form in 2 to 3 days, depending on the agent/substance. Fibroblasts in this site begin to produce collagen and ECM proteins that can form into a "thin" vascularized connective tissue area. At this point antibiotics can penetrate this area and enter the exudate. If the septic abscess persists, the initial "thin" connective tissue area surrounding the exudates can mature into a fibrous capsule, which is thick and largely impermeable, in an attempt to "wall off" the exudates from normal tissue. A capsular wall takes weeks to form. Abscesses with this response can present serious problems in systemic (hematogenous) or local (topical diffusion) antibiotic treatments. In large abscesses with abundant pus, the pus itself may dilute the antibiotic and further prevent the drug from reaching the optimal concentration required to kill the bacteria. It is for these reasons that larger abscesses are often lanced to drain the pus. Sterile abscesses do not require antibiotics or other drugs to kill an inciting agent/substance, but they do require breakdown of the capsule by lancing or some other means.

Granulomatous Inflammation and Granuloma Formation

Granulomatous inflammation is a distinct type of chronic inflammation in which cells of the monocyte-macrophage system are predominant and take the form of macrophages, epithelioid macrophages (activated macrophages), and MGCs. In granulomatous inflammation the cells are dispersed as sheets of cells distributed at random (diffuse or lepromatous) within parenchymal and connective tissue planes (Fig. 3-22, *A*), whereas in a granuloma (tuberculoid granuloma) they are arranged in distinct masses or nodules (Fig. 3-22, *B*).

Granulomatous inflammation occurs secondarily in response to endogenous or exogenous antigens or idiopathically as in granulomatous meningoencephalitis of dogs. Development and regulation of granulomatous inflammation requires multiple factors: (1) the inciting agent, usually with indigestible, poorly degradable, and persistent antigens (e.g., *Mycobacteria* spp.); (2) the host immune response (e.g., T_H and macrophage response); and (3) the interplay of various cytokines, chemokines, and other proinflammatory and antiinflammatory mediators produced by cells within the chronic inflammatory lesion.

Classification of granulomatous inflammation by pathologists has evolved over the years because of the increased understanding of disease pathogenesis and advances in molecular biology. For simplicity, this chapter discusses two morphologic forms of granulomatous inflammation: diffuse (lepromatous) granulomas, which are currently thought to be consistent with a T_H2-biased immunologic response, and nodular (tuberculoid) granulomas, which are currently thought to be consistent with a T_H1-biased immunologic response. Both of these terms are derived from granulomatous lesions in human beings and are increasingly becoming defined and seen as distinct, both immunologically and molecularly.

Nodular (Tuberculoid) Granulomas (T_H1-Biased Granulomas)

Examples of nodular (tuberculoid) granulomas are those that have been classically caused by *Mycobacterium bovis* or *Mycobacterium tuberculosis* (Fig. 3-23) and by some deep fungal infections, such as coccidioidomycosis (E-Fig. 3-8). Grossly, nodular granulomas are often gray to white, round to oval, and firm to hard, whereas diffuse granulomatous inflammation is often gray to white, expansile but poorly demarcated from adjacent tissue, and firm. Tuberculoid (nodular) granulomas develop with a T_H1-type lymphocytic response and occur in many species but have been described extensively from lesions of infected human beings, cattle, and rhesus monkeys. Because the portal of entry is often the respiratory tract, these lesions involve the lung with secondary involvement of other parenchymal organs and induce the formation of granuloma. Microscopically, nodular (tuberculoid) granulomas may or may not have a central core of necrotic cell debris (caseating and noncaseating granulomas) (see Fig. 3-23). Granulomas of either type are often oval to round and can be irregular as well as multinodular, vary in size from microscopic to macroscopic, and very large.

Noncaseating granulomas are often round to oval and microscopically composed of numerous macrophages with variable numbers of epithelioid macrophages, perhaps MGCs, with a peripheral zone of fibroblasts, lymphocytes, and plasma cells. Caseating granulomas have the same morphologic features as noncaseating granulomas; however, the center is formed by a core of gray-white-yellow pasty (thick-dehydrated) necrotic debris resembling cheese (Latin caseus = cheese). Caseating granulomas most commonly occur in tuberculosis. Microscopically, caseating granulomas have a central core of cell debris, surrounded by a dense zone of macrophages that may contain epithelioid macrophages that are admixed increasingly in the outer layers of granuloma with lymphocytes, plasma cells, and fibroblasts.

The outermost zones of either a noncaseating or caseating granuloma are frequently similar and composed of fibroblasts that deposit collagen and ECM proteins that create a dense fibrous region that can form into a capsule. Thus a well-formed granuloma has three distinctive morphologic areas. The innermost area is often but not always a centrally located region of macrophages and MGCs in a

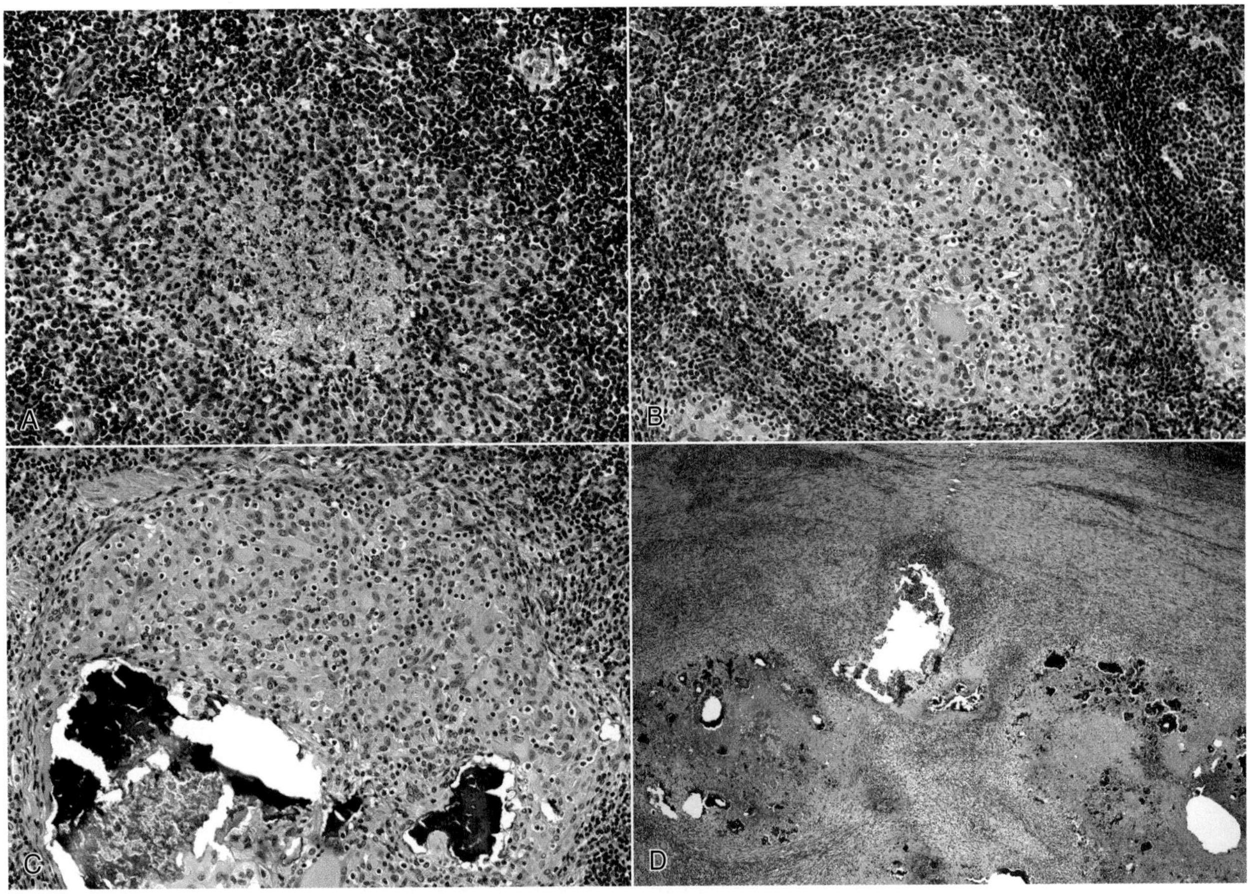

Figure 3-23 Nodular (Tuberculoid, T Helper Lymphocyte Type 1 [T_H1]) Type of Granulomatous Inflammation. A series of micrographs from lymph nodes of cattle experimentally infected with *Mycobacterium bovis* illustrate stages of T_H1 granuloma formation. **A,** Stage I granuloma. Initial lesions have a central region of cell debris with occasional neutrophils and macrophages that are surrounded by a zone of macrophages that are irregularly arranged and further surrounded by densely associated lymphocytes. **B,** Stage II granuloma. Days later, granulomas are composed of numerous macrophages aggregated in an oval region with occasional epithelioid macrophages and small multinucleate giant cells. This core is surrounded by dense infiltrates of lymphocytes. **C,** Stage III granuloma. The mature granuloma has a central area of mineralization along with numerous macrophages, multinucleate giant cells, and epithelioid macrophages. **D,** Stage IV granuloma. With long-term persistence of antigen, the granulomatous reactions with areas of mineralization coalesce and overtake additional surrounding tissue and are bordered by dense infiltrates of lymphocytes. H&E stain. (Courtesy Dr. M. Palmer, USDA/ARS-National Animal Disease Center, Ames, Iowa.)

noncaseating granuloma and cellular necrosis in a caseating granuloma, which is surrounded by a middle area containing macrophages, epithelioid macrophages, and MGCs. The outermost area surrounding the entire lesion consists of T and B lymphocytes, plasma cells, macrophages, and a fibrous capsule (Fig. 3-24).

Mycobacterial organisms and their antigens are very sparse in these granulomas and not commonly detected with acid-fast stains and immunohistochemical stains for mycobacterial antigens. Mineralization can occur in tuberculoid granulomas, but this outcome depends on the species of animal affected. It is common in cattle, present to a lesser degree in pigs, and uncommon in sheep. "Atypical" mycobacteria, such as *Mycobacterium marinum*, can also cause nodular (tuberculoid) granulomas in the subcutaneous tissues of dogs, cats, and other species, and very few organisms are detected with stains. Certain persistent, poorly degradable antigens, such as those in foreign bodies and in microbes, such as *Nocardia* spp., can have eosinophilic proteinaceous aggregates of immunoglobulin on their outer surfaces, which can be seen histologically and are termed *Splendore-Hoeppli proteins*.

Steps in formation of a tuberculoid (nodular) granuloma (see Fig. 3-23) are as follows:

1. Stage I granuloma. Days after infection, the lesion site is infiltrated by neutrophils, monocytes, macrophages, γ/δ T lymphocytes, and NK cells. Epithelioid macrophages also form.
2. Stage II granuloma. From roughly 48 hours to multiple days and weeks, lesions contain macrophages, epithelioid macrophages, thin rims of fibrous connective tissue, variable numbers of NK cells, and γ/δ T lymphocytes, as well as α/β T lymphocytes and B lymphocytes. MGCs can also form.
3. Stage III granuloma. From weeks to 1 month, the central area can caseate or become dense with macrophages and mineralize. Lymphocytes, plasma cells, a zone of fibroblasts, and a fibrous connective tissue capsule surround this core.
4. Stage IV granuloma. From several weeks to months, the lesion can be walled off by a dense capsule, and regions within the lesion can become mineralized and overtake the surrounding tissue. The capsule wall can sometimes become degraded when microorganisms are released from the inner regions of the lesion.

Diffuse (Lepromatous) Granulomas (T_H2-Biased Granulomas)

Mycobacterium leprae, the cause of human leprosy, produces noncaseating aggregates of macrophages and chronic inflammatory cells often around nerve fibers in the distal extremities and upper respiratory tract mucosa (sites in the body with temperatures lower than core body temperature) of infected human beings. This type of granulomatous inflammation appears to form with a predominantly T_H2 type of adaptive immune response that is seen in veterinary

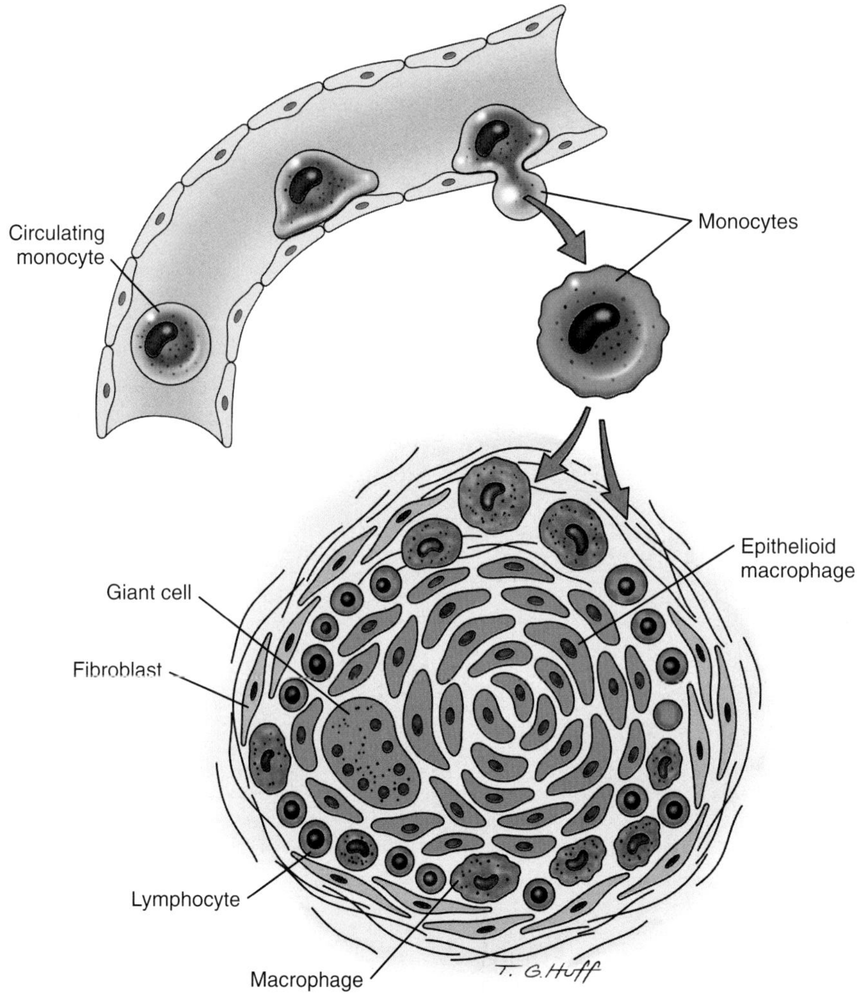

Figure 3-24 Formation of a Granuloma. Circulating monocytes that become attracted by chemokines and inflammatory mediators to the extravascular lesion adhere to the vascular wall and transmigrate between endothelial cells into the perivascular extracellular matrix stroma and migrate to form the granuloma.

medicine during the clinical stages of Johne's disease in cattle and sheep.

These lesions can be poorly delineated (e.g., poorly defined borders) and have a widespread distribution, a heavy intracellular bacterial burden, relatively few lymphocytes, numerous macrophages that extend into surrounding tissue often without a distinct capsule, variable degrees of fibrosis, and lack caseation. Similar granulomatous lesions are seen in animals. Feline leprosy and canine lepromatous-like granulomas are somewhat similar to human leprosy in lesion formation. *Mycobacterium avium* subsp. *paratuberculosis*—the cause of Johne's disease in cattle, sheep, and goats—also induces a diffuse (lepromatous) type of granulomatous inflammation consisting of diffuse sheets of macrophages with few lymphocytes and plasma cells. This lesion most commonly occurs in the lamina propria of the ileum and colon (Fig. 3-25) and in mesenteric lymph nodes. Special stains, such as acid-fast and immunohistochemical stains specific to bacterial antigens, can be used to identify these bacteria within the cytoplasm of macrophages and those that are extracellular (E-Fig. 3-9). Because bacteria are present in large numbers in these diseases, they are commonly identified by these techniques. Nodular (tuberculoid) granulomas, defined later, are not seen in Johne's disease lesions. Finally, *Mycobacterium avium* subsp. *paratuberculosis* infection also occurs in the lung and other organs of birds and often induces lesions with similar sheets of macrophages containing abundant bacteria detectable with special stains.

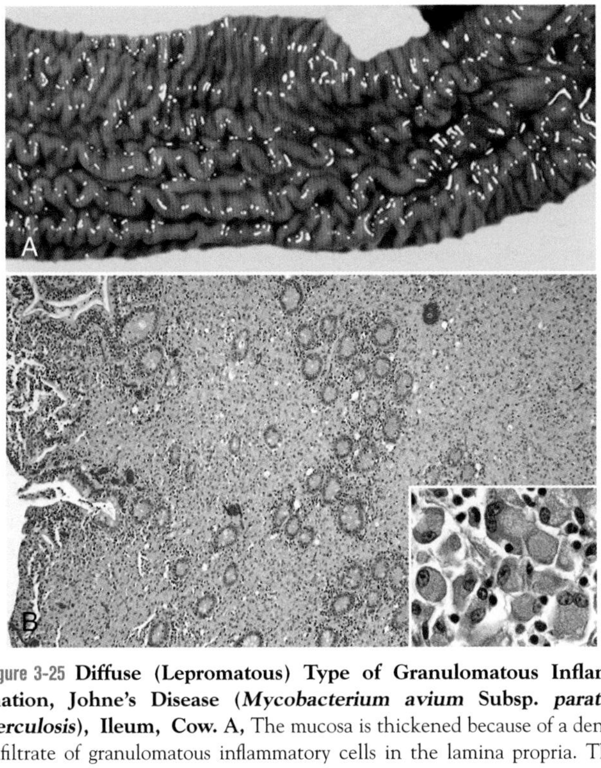

Figure 3-25 **Diffuse (Lepromatous) Type of Granulomatous Inflammation, Johne's Disease (*Mycobacterium avium* Subsp. *paratuberculosis*), Ileum, Cow. A,** The mucosa is thickened because of a dense infiltrate of granulomatous inflammatory cells in the lamina propria. The lumen of the intestine is to the left. **B,** The lamina propria contains numerous macrophages arranged in sheets. The ileal lumen is to the left; scattered crypts still remain in the central area of the specimen. H&E stain. **Inset,** Higher magnification of macrophages present in the granulomatous inflammatory exudate. H&E stain. (**A** courtesy Dr. M.D. McCracken, College of Veterinary Medicine, University of Tennessee; and Noah's Arkive, College of Veterinary Medicine, The University of Georgia. **B** courtesy Dr. J. Hostetter, College of Veterinary Medicine, Iowa State University. **Inset** courtesy Dr. M.D. McGavin, College of Veterinary Medicine, University of Tennessee.)

Sarcoids of Horses

Sarcoids of human patients are granulomatous-like lesions. In contrast, sarcoids of horses are not a correlate to sarcoids in human beings. Sarcoids that occur in the skin of horses are not granulomas as occur in human beings but are locally aggressive skin tumors, and the most common dermatologic neoplasm reported in horses. They are composed of proliferating fibroblasts and do not contain the numerous macrophages, lymphocytes, and plasma cells seen in human sarcoids. Bovine papillomavirus (BPV) types 1 and 2 and the major transforming protein, E5, are associated with equine sarcoids but appear not to produce infectious virions. E5 may contribute to the persistence of the virus and development of the lesion by down-regulating major histocompatibility complex (MHC) class I expression and thereby reducing immunosurveillance. The mode of transmission of BPV infection has not been determined.

Eosinophilic Granulomas

Certain types of chronic inflammation have dense infiltrates of eosinophils with macrophages, and varying numbers of lymphocytes and plasma cells (E-Fig. 3-10). Because of the presence of eosinophils, they are termed *eosinophilic granulomas* (Table 3-8). Some granulomas with numerous eosinophils develop in response to migrating parasites, such as *T. canis* (larva migrans). In eosinophilic granuloma of cats, eosinophilic stomatitis of dogs, and equine eosinophilic dermatitis of horses, it is suspected that these conditions form in response to antigen in a T_H2-directed manner; however, no specific antigen has been identified.

Grossly, eosinophilic granulomas in cats appear as papules, nodules, plaques (sometimes linear), and ulcers in the skin. They also occur as nodular or ulcerated lesions in the oral mucosae and footpads. Microscopically, the inflammatory response consists of eosinophils, macrophages, and areas of dense eosinophilia around collagen (Fig. 3-26). For many years, the densely eosinophilic, collagen-rich areas were considered regions of collagen degradation; however, the eosinophilic material is composed largely of MBP, a protein present in large amounts in the granules of eosinophils. Apparently eosinophils degranulate in these regions, releasing MBP, which accumulates over time. Some eosinophilic granulomas do not form distinct nodular granulomas, and the cellular content of the lesions (e.g., the numbers of macrophages and eosinophils) can vary widely. But the lesions are chronic in nature and contain enough macrophages and other chronic inflammatory cells to be classified as granulomas by most pathologists.

Other Chronic Inflammatory/ Granulomatous Conditions

Information on this topic, including visceral leishmaniasis and E- Figs. 3-11 and 3-12, is available at www.expertconsult.com.

Table 3-8 Eosinophilic Granulomas of Domestic Animals

Species	Type of Eosinophilic Granuloma
Feline	Eosinophilic plaque, granuloma, and dermatitis
Canine	Eosinophilic granuloma of the oral cavity of huskies and other dogs
Equine	Equine collagenolytic granuloma, axillary nodular necrosis, and unilateral papular dermatosis
All species	Eosinophilic (T_H2) granulomas secondary to parasitic infections

T_H2, T helper lymphocyte type 2.

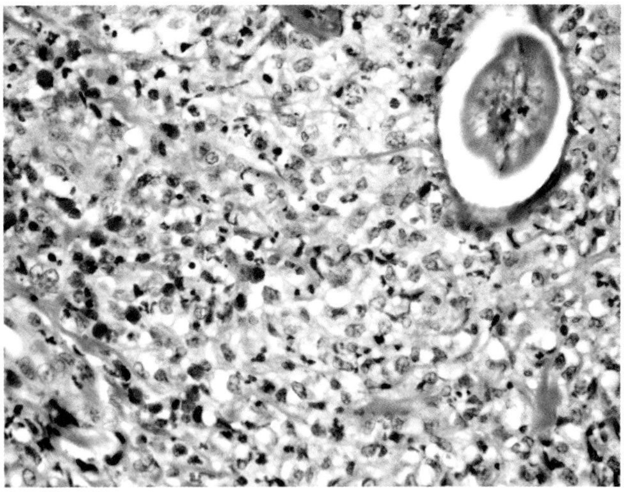

Figure 3-26 **Granuloma with Eosinophils.** A region of skin from a horse in which there is a parasitic organism (*Habronema* sp.) (upper right corner) that has invoked a marked granulomatous reaction of closely associated macrophages admixed with eosinophils (left third of photomicrograph). H&E stain. (Courtesy Dr. M.R. Ackermann, College of Veterinary Medicine, Iowa State University.)

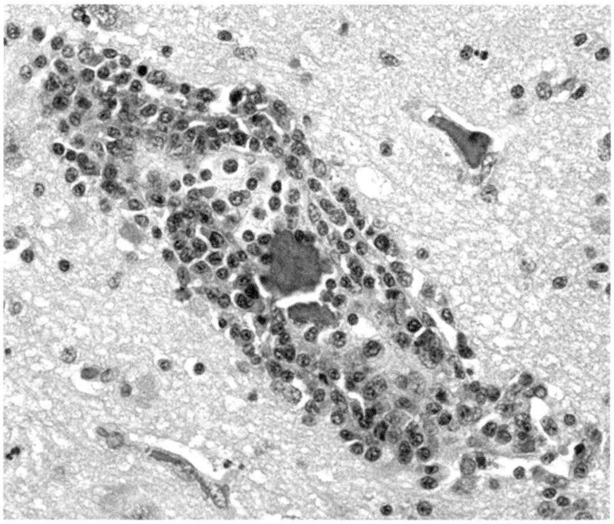

Figure 3-27 **Chronic Inflammation, Distemper, Brain, Raccoon.** In its simplest form, chronic inflammation, as seen with some viral infections, consists of an exudate of lymphocytes with occasional macrophages and plasma cells. In many tissues, especially in the central nervous system, these cells can have a perivascular pattern of distribution. In certain animal species (exotic wildlife species, horses) and specific disease categories (parasitic, protozoal, viral), perivascular chronic inflammatory exudates may also contain variable numbers of eosinophils. H&E stain. (Courtesy Dr. J.F. Zachary, College of Veterinary Medicine, University of Illinois.)

Gross and Microscopic Lesions and Nomenclature of the Chronic Inflammatory Response

The term *chronic inflammation* implies two underlying and often concurrently occurring processes: fibroplasia and cellular infiltration. Often one of these types of responses predominates. Fibroplasia, the formation of fibrous connective tissue, includes any stage of the process from the formation of fibrous connective tissue that includes newly formed "immature" connective tissue with newly formed blood vessels to "mature" connective tissue that contains well-collagenized and remodeled granulation tissue. Cellular infiltrates are composed of predominantly macrophages, lymphocytes, and plasma cells, depending on the inciting agent/substance and the duration of the inflammatory process. It is important to understand the mechanism of these processes to apply gross and histopathologic diagnoses. To clinicians these terms imply duration of illness, whereas to pathologists they imply the characteristics of the tissue's response to injury.

Grossly, chronic inflammatory lesions are often gray to white and firm and have either a nodular surface in the case of granulomas or an indented or pitted surface in the case of fibrosis. The gray to white color is largely a result of the infiltrates of macrophages and lymphocytes, proliferation of fibroblasts, and deposition of fibrous connective tissue. The firm texture is attributable to fibrous connective tissue (fibroblasts and endothelial cells) and the consolidation (i.e., solidification) of the leukocytes in the exudate. The irregular shape occurs because of the haphazard accumulation of leukocytes and the fibrosis/scarring and contraction of the lesion by myofibroblasts within the fibrous connective tissue (see section on Wound Healing and Angiogenesis).

The lungs of dogs with *B. dermatitidis* infection often have a nodular appearance because of the formation of numerous granulomas and/or pyogranulomas. The use of and distinction between terms such as *granuloma* and *pyogranuloma* depend on the number of neutrophils in the overall inflammatory exudate or in the center of the granuloma and often reflect the interpretation of the examining pathologist.

The pitted surface of kidneys of dogs, cats, or other species can be seen, for example, with chronic interstitial nephritis or chronic pyelonephritis. Frequently the pitted surfaces correspond to areas where fibrous tissue formed within renal parenchyma during the chronic inflammatory response that pulls the renal capsule into the parenchyma as part of the healing process. In chronic pyelonephritis the inflammatory bands often radiate from the renal medulla into the cortex and to the renal capsule and obliterate or surround and separate cortical tubules and glomeruli. Fibrous adhesions between the renal cortex and the capsule can occur. This fibrous connective tissue may also contain lymphocytes, plasma cells, and macrophages.

Grossly, abscesses, granulomas, and areas of fibrosis that occur with the persistence of chronic inflammation are often easily seen. Severe fibrosis results in an area that is generally gray to white with extensive contraction, whereas abscesses are often round with a fibrous capsule and a central area of pus. Grossly, the three main differential diagnoses for a white, firm, oval to irregular nodular mass are abscess, granuloma, and neoplasm. Most commonly, histopathology is required to differentiate the three because they can appear very similar grossly.

Microscopically, chronic inflammatory responses are classified into categories based on the types and distribution of the inflammatory cells in the exudate. These categories include (1) chronic lymphocytic/lymphohistiocytic inflammation, (2) fibrosing chronic inflammation, (3) chronic-active (purulent) inflammation, (4) granulomatous (noncaseating) inflammation, (5) pyogranulomatous inflammation, (6) granulomas, and (7) pyogranulomas.

- **Chronic inflammation** composed of lymphocytes and plasma cells admixed with macrophages occurs commonly in the body (Fig. 3-27). Sometimes lymphocytes and macrophages predominate over plasma cells, and such lesions can be called lymphohistiocytic. *Histiocytic* is a term used for macrophage infiltration;

however, some pathologists use the term *macrophagic*. This type of inflammatory response is characteristically seen in the early stages of the chronic inflammatory response and in response to specific microbes, such as viruses, and in mucosal surfaces in response to antigenic stimulation.

- **Fibrosing chronic inflammation** is a region of chronic inflammation that is predominantly composed of fibrous connective tissue. This can occur in chronic traumatic pericarditis (hardware disease) of cattle where there are areas of pericardial fibrosis covered by fibrin and in the chronic fibrosis that surrounds necrotic regions of lung and forms along the pleura of cattle with contagious bovine pleuropneumonia and chronic M. *haemolytica* pneumonia.
- **Chronic-active inflammation** has the same cellular components as chronic inflammation but also contains neutrophils, fibrin, and plasma proteins that are constituents of the acute inflammatory response. Chronic-active inflammation occurs when the inciting stimulus has not been removed from the exudate in the chronic inflammatory response, and it continues to elicit an acute inflammatory response. One should be careful not to confuse the morphologic diagnosis of chronic-active inflammation with the hepatic disease entity of dogs termed *chronic-active hepatitis*.
- **Granulomatous inflammation** has a basic cellular exudate consisting predominantly of activated macrophages and in some cases also epithelioid macrophages, MGCs, and lesser numbers of lymphocytes and plasma cells. Granulomatous inflammation can be arranged in a diffuse or haphazard manner as seen in the thickened intestinal mucosa (i.e., lamina propria) of cattle with Johne's disease (see Fig. 3-25). Although the presence of a few macrophages in a lesion is indicative of chronic inflammation, these are considered to be granulomatous inflammation when the macrophages aggregate and begin to replace portions of the normal stroma.
- **Pyogranulomatous inflammation** has the same cellular exudate as granulomatous inflammation but also contains multifocal/random infiltrates of neutrophils, fibrin, and plasma proteins, which are constituents of the acute inflammatory response. Pyogranulomatous inflammation occurs when the inciting stimulus has not been removed from the exudate in the granulomatous inflammatory response, and it continues to elicit an acute inflammatory response. A nodular-like granulomatous area with neutrophils is termed a *pyogranuloma* (see later). Pyogranulomatous inflammation is often seen with infections caused by *B. dermatitidis* and is frequently multinodular. Pyogranulomatous is sometimes used loosely, with little discretion. For example, it can be used in lesions that are in transition from acute inflammation to chronic inflammation or during the "clean-up" phase of healing.
- **Granulomas** are a distinct type of granulomatous inflammatory response that occurs when macrophage infiltration is present in a well-defined area and thus the aggregated macrophages form a distinct mass on gross observation. Granulomas can occur as noncaseating and caseating types, as described.
- A **pyogranuloma** is a nodular granuloma with a central area of neutrophils.

Cellular Mechanisms of Chronic Inflammatory Responses

Lymphocytes

Lymphocytes play a key role in most chronic inflammatory lesions, especially in autoimmune diseases and in diseases with persistent antigen. As with macrophages, lymphocytes enter unresolved areas of acute inflammation within 24 to 48 hours, being attracted by chemokines, cytokines, and other stimuli. Histologically, they are often aggregated around blood vessels and surround granulomas or are distributed haphazardly within injured tissue (see Fig. 3-27). In viral encephalitides, lymphocytes are commonly distributed in a perivascular pattern, primarily in the gray matter. In other types of conditions, such as lymphoplasmacytic stomatitis and pododermatitis of cats, lymphocytes and plasma cells are the predominant cell types in the lesions.

γ/δ T Lymphocytes

Information on this topic is available at www.expertconsult.com.

α/β T Lymphocytes (CD4/CD8)

Information on this topic is available at www.expertconsult.com.

T_H1, T_H2, T_H17, and T Reg Immunologic Responses

Information on this topic is available at www.expertconsult.com.

Monocytes/Macrophages

Monocytes/macrophages are the signature cell types of chronic inflammation (Fig. 3-28). They produce a wide variety of inflammatory mediators, including chemokines, cytokines, and NO, and are often situated at strategic locations within tissues of the body to (1) quickly sense the initial activity of acute inflammation, (2) migrate in response to chemotaxins, (3) remove and kill microbial agents by phagocytosis, (4) remove and degrade particulate matter by phagocytosis, (5) process antigens for presentation to effector cells of the adaptive immune response, and (6) facilitate angiogenesis and remodel the ECM (see Fig. 3-28).

Epithelium

Epithelial cells can contribute to chronic inflammatory responses in a variety of manners. For example, experimental models of granuloma formation have shown that mycobacteria release an early secretory antigen-6 (ESAT-6), which induces release of MMP-9 from epithelia that is vital for recruitment of macrophage infiltration. Epithelia can also release type I interferons, cytokines, antimicrobial peptides, and chemokines and express adhesion molecules.

Mononuclear Cell Maturation and Trafficking in the Chronic Inflammatory Response

The macrophage is key to the development and persistence of chronic inflammation. Monocytes, derived from the bone marrow, form the monocyte-macrophage system by entering tissues and differentiating into macrophages (e.g., Kupffer cells, alveolar macrophages, and microglial cells) and are central to innate and adaptive immune systems. Recent work also shows that the spleen is a significant reservoir of monocytes, which can exit en masse on tissue injury. Monocytes are then recruited from the bloodstream to enter tissue and differentiate into macrophages that can also respond to tissue injury. Under noninflammatory conditions, the replenishment of tissue macrophages occurs through local proliferation and not via monocyte influx. However, with inflammatory stimuli, monocytes are recruited from the blood into tissue in response to inciting agents/substances.

In noninflamed tissue, monocytes expressing CX3CR1 and CCR5 chemokine receptors are attracted to tissues expressing their respective ligands (i.e., fractalkine (CX3CL) and MIP-1-α [CCL3]). In areas of inflammation, monocytes expressing CCR2 chemokine

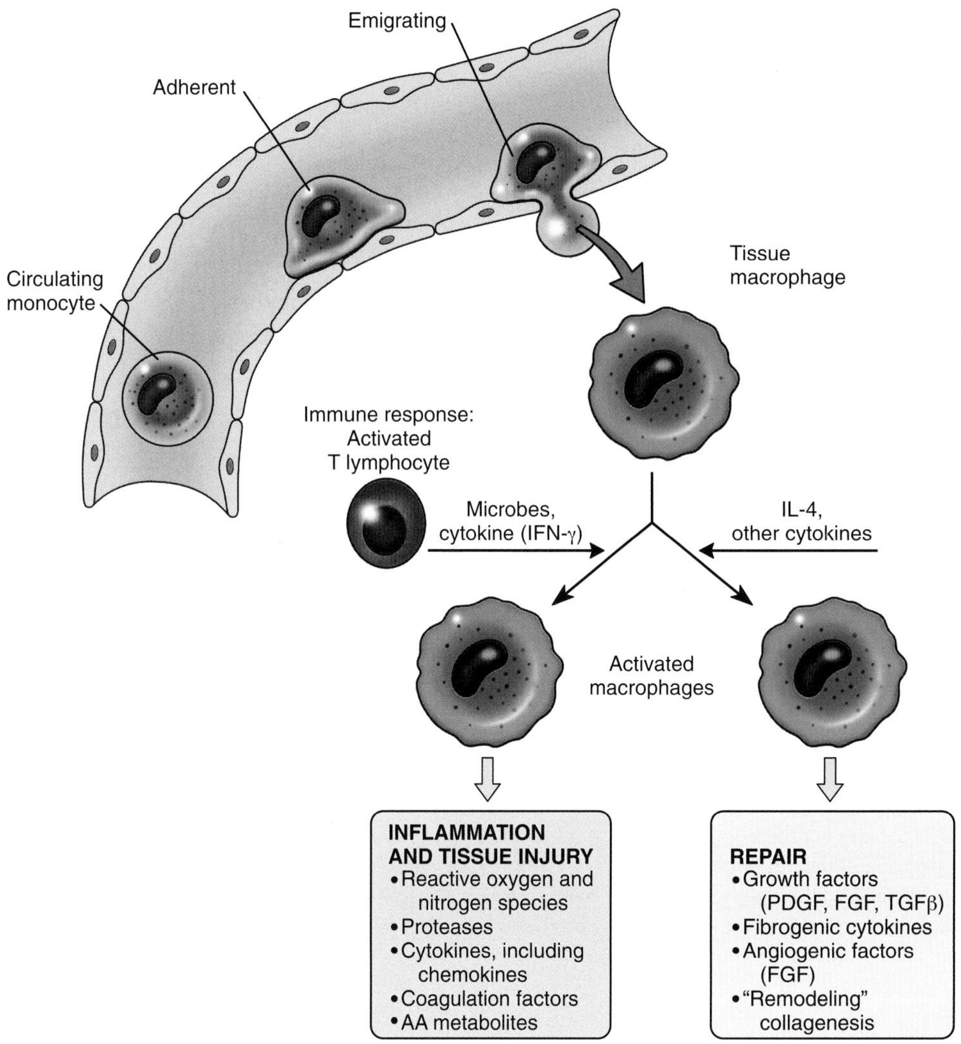

Figure 3-28 **The Roles of Activated Macrophages in Chronic Inflammation.** Macrophages are activated by microbial products or by cytokines from immune-activated T lymphocytes (particularly interferon-γ [IFN-γ]). These products further mediate inflammation and tissue injury, whereas macrophages activated by interleukin 4 (IL-4) released by T lymphocytes mediate fibrosis and repair. The products made by activated macrophages that cause tissue injury and fibrosis include arachidonic acid (AA), platelet-derived growth factor (PDGF), fibroblast growth factor (FGF), and transforming growth factor-β (TGF-β).

receptors are attracted by MCP-1 (CCL2). Attracted monocytes enter these areas in a manner similar to that described for the leukocyte adhesion cascade outlined for neutrophils. Slow rolling is mediated by E and P selectins, and firm adherence by monocytes to endothelial cells is largely mediated by LFA-1 (CD11a/CD18), VLA-4 ($\alpha_4\beta_1$-integrin), and also Mac-1 (CD11b/CD18) molecules that adhere to the respective endothelial cell ligands: ICAM-1/2, VCAM-1, and ICAM-1/2. Transmigration of monocytes between endothelial cells is mediated by leukocyte adhesion molecules expressed on the monocyte such as LFA-1, VLA-4, Mac-1, PECAM-1, and JAM A, JAM B, and JAM C. These molecules bind to adhesion molecules, such as PECAM-1, and the JAM molecules expressed by endothelial cells at the intracellular junction. As monocytes and other leukocytes pass between endothelial cells, they separate the tight junctions and vascular endothelial (VE)-cadherins to allow the passage of the leukocyte.

T_H1, T_H2, T_H17, and T reg lymphocytes, along with inflammatory mediators released by somatic cells and macrophages during injury and/or infection, affect the differentiation of monocytes and noncommitted macrophages to macrophages with specific function (see E-Fig. 3-13). In conditions favorable to T_H1 influence, macrophages respond to IFN-γ released by T_H1, NK lymphocytes, and TNF from antigen-presenting cells to form classically activated macrophages (Table 3-9). Under T_H2 conditions, macrophages respond to IL-4 released by T_H2 lymphocytes and granulocytes (e.g., mast cells, basophils) by forming wound-healing (tissue repair) type of macrophages. Under T reg secretion of IL-10 and other substances, such as immune complexes, prostaglandins, glucocorticoids, and apoptotic cells, macrophages differentiate into regulatory macrophages (antiinflammatory cells), which secrete IL-10 to suppress inflammation. Macrophages committed to the classical-activation, wound-healing/tissue repair, or regulatory pathways greatly influence the anatomic (histopathologic) structure and function of the chronic inflammatory response and granuloma formation (Fig. 3-29).

Macrophages activated within lesions enter lymphatic vessels that drain into nearby lymph nodes via the afferent lymphatic vessels. In addition, some macrophages from lesions within the caudal body can enter the thoracic duct, which drains into the cranial vena cava or one of its branches. Macrophages within the head and neck can enter right or left tracheal lymphatic ducts. The right tracheal lymphatic duct empties into the cranial vena cava, whereas the left tracheal duct empties into the thoracic duct. Once in the blood, the macrophages are disseminated throughout the body.

Table 3-9 Stimuli That Affect the Activation Status of Macrophages

Type of Activation	Activating Factor	Macrophage Response	Macrophage Activity
Innate activation to microbes	Toll-like receptor CD14 (LPS binding) β-Glucan receptor TREM	Costimulatory expression ROS, NO expression Cytokine release	Inflammation, antigen presentation to memory T lymphocytes
Humoral activation	Fc receptor Complement receptors	Ig/Fc internalization Cytolytic activity Cytokine release	Inflammation, antigen presentation to memory T lymphocytes
Classical activation T_H1	IFN-γ	MHC II expression Cytokine release (IL-1, IL-6, TNF) Respiratory burst NO release	Cell-mediated immunity Microbial killing DTH
Alternative activation T_H2	IL-4 IL-13	MHC II expression Mannose receptor expression	Humoral immunity Allergic response Response to parasites Arginase repair
Deactivation by innate/ adaptive stimuli	IL-10 TGF-β IFN-α, IFN-β GM-CSF CD47 CD200R CD36 (scavenger receptor) $\alpha_5\beta_3$-Integrin Glucocorticoid receptor Internalized ox LDL	MPH II downregulation PGE_2 release IL-10 release TGF-β release PPAR inhibition of NF κ B	Immunosuppress

DTH, Delayed-type hypersensitivity; *GM-CSF*, granulocyte-macrophage colony-stimulating factor; *IFN*, interferon; *Ig*, immunoglobulin; *IL*, interleukin; *MHC*, major histocompatibility complex; MPH, Macrophage; *NF*, nuclear factor, *NO*, nitric oxide; *ox LDL*, oxidized low-density lipoprotein; *LPS*, lipopolysaccharide; *PGE_2*, prostaglandin type E2; *PPAR*, peroxisome proliferator activated receptor; *ROS*, reactive oxygen species; *TGF*, transforming growth factor; *T_H1*, T helper type 1 lymphocyte response; *T_H2*, T helper type 2 lymphocyte response; *TNF*, tumor necrosis factor; *TREM*, triggering receptor expressed on myeloid cells.

The outcome of these different types of macrophage activation leads to the following specific responses (see Fig. 3-29):

- Innate activation can lead to release of reactive oxygen species, NO, and IFN-α and IFN-β.
- Classic activation with IFN-γ leads to expression of MHC II antigen, respiratory burst, release of IL-1 and TNF for microbial killing, cellular immunity, and delayed-type hypersensitivity.
- Alternative activation enhances MHC class II expression and mannose receptor expression for humoral immunity and allergic responses.
- Innate deactivation and reduced inflammatory responses can occur with the uptake of apoptotic cells or storage of oxidized LDLs in lysosomes and release of IL-10.

In addition to T reg lymphocytes and regulatory macrophages, recent work has shown that sialylated IgG molecules can regulate macrophage function. This stems from the observation that certain types of chronic inflammation, particularly autoimmune conditions of human beings, have responded favorably to polyclonal IgG given intravenously. The mechanism by which this therapy works is poorly understood. Recently evidence has suggested that the polyclonal IgG activity may be due to a subset of IgG molecules that are sialylated on the Fc chain of the IgG. The sialylated IgGs are thought to interact with sialic acid–specific receptors on regulatory macrophages and upregulate expression of Fc receptor IIB, which is inhibitory, on effector macrophages.

Formation of Epithelioid Macrophages and Multinucleate Giant Cells

Activated macrophages within tissues are relatively large cells histologically (20 to 25 mm in diameter) with abundant, often clear cytoplasm and a single, oval to polygonal, often slightly eccentric, reniform nucleus (Fig. 3-30). With time, activated macrophages can sometimes further differentiate into epithelioid macrophages and MGCs (Fig. 3-31).

Both epithelioid macrophages and MGCs often form in response to foreign bodies or persistent intracellular pathogens. The molecular mechanisms by which epithelioid macrophages and MGCs form are poorly understood. It is a fascinating biologic phenomenon that requires membrane fusion and integration of the cytoplasm and nuclei of multiple cells. Studies in human patients with sarcoidosis, a special type of granulomatous inflammation in human beings have elucidated some of the important factors and conditions that contribute to MGC formation. Epithelioid macrophages are larger than activated macrophages. They have abundant cytoplasm, and the cell membrane occasionally assumes a polygonal to elongated shape, forming sheets, and thus can resemble to a limited degree squamous epithelium. These cells have diminished phagocytic capacity, but they contain large amounts of rough endoplasmic reticulum (rER), Golgi complex, vesicles, and vacuoles. These latter structures suggest that the main function of epithelioid macrophages involves extracellular secretion; however, the physiologic activity of epithelioid macrophages is poorly understood and requires additional investigation.

MGCs are seen frequently in granulomatous inflammation. MGCs are syncytial cells formed by the fusion of two or more activated macrophages into one large cell with two or more nuclei (see Fig. 3-31). These nuclei can be distributed in the cell in a haphazard manner or aggregated in the center of the cytoplasm. This form is called a *foreign body type* of MGC. The nuclei can also be arranged in a horseshoe-like semicircle at the periphery of the cell. This form

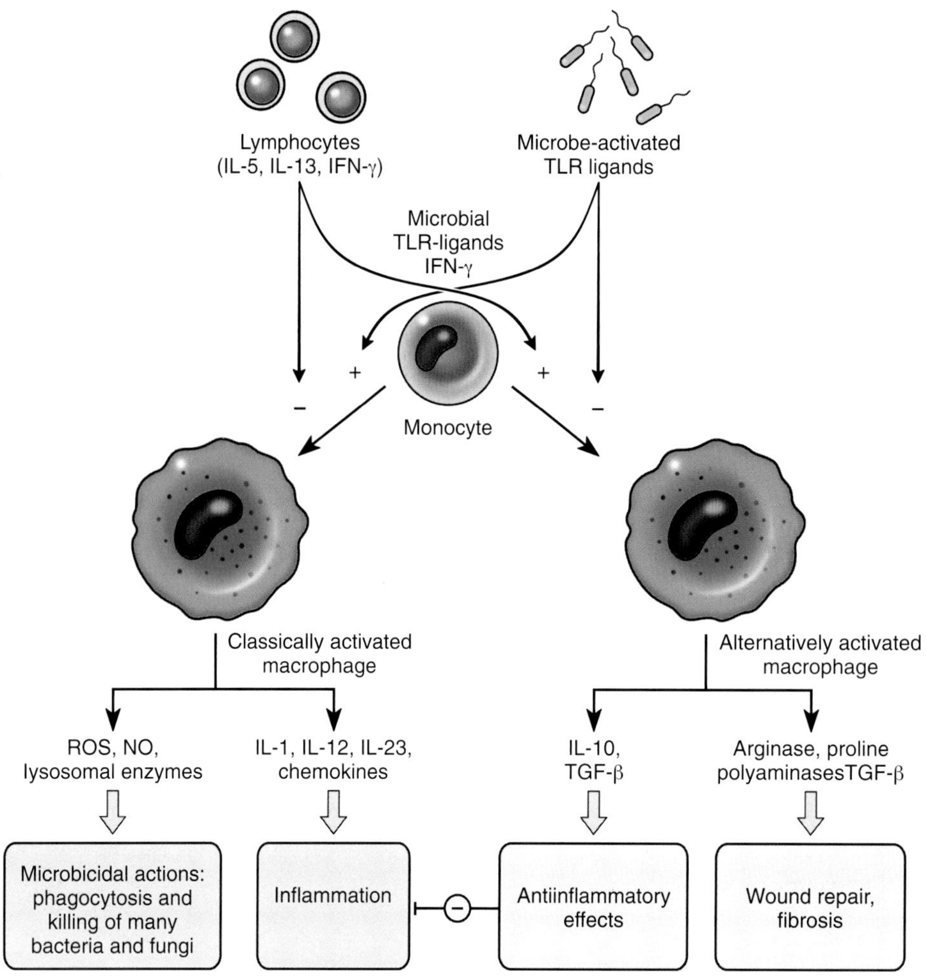

Figure 3-29 **Subsets of Activated Macrophages.** Functionally distinct populations of monocytes/macrophages arise in response to different stimuli such as microbial products and cytokines. Classically activated macrophages are induced by microbial products and cytokines, particularly interferon-γ [IFN-γ]. They act to phagocytose and kill microbes and are involved in inflammation. Alternatively activated macrophages are induced by cytokines (e.g., interleukin [IL]-5 and IL-13) and in response to helminths. These macrophages are important in tissue repair, the resolution of inflammation, and the defense against helminthic parasites. *NO*, Nitric oxide; *ROS*, reactive oxygen species; *TGF-β*, transforming growth factor-β; *TLR*, Toll-like receptor.

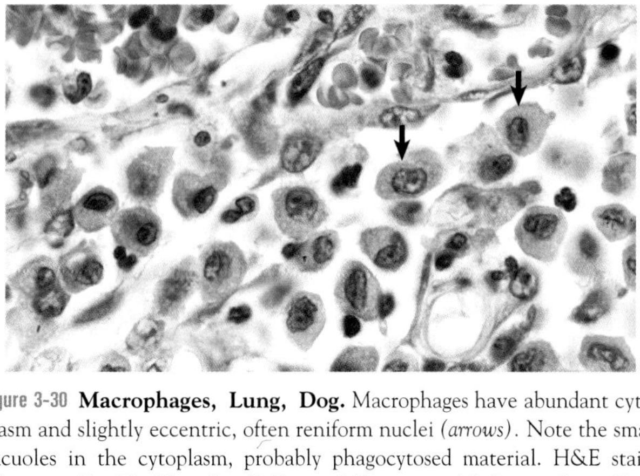

Figure 3-30 **Macrophages, Lung, Dog.** Macrophages have abundant cytoplasm and slightly eccentric, often reniform nuclei *(arrows)*. Note the small vacuoles in the cytoplasm, probably phagocytosed material. H&E stain. (Courtesy Dr. N. Cheville, College of Veterinary Medicine, Iowa State University.)

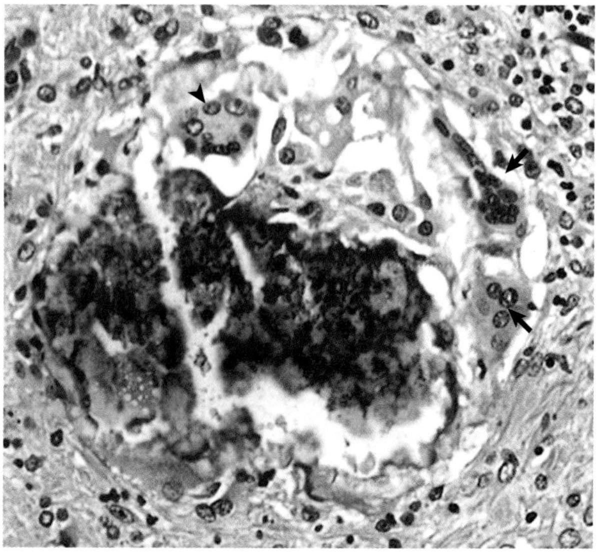

Figure 3-31 **Multinucleate Giant Cells, Chronic Granulomatous Inflammation, Central Nervous System, Rabbit.** This focus contains both foreign body-type *(arrows)* and Langhans-type *(arrowhead)* multinucleate giant cells. H&E stain. (Courtesy Dr. A. Loretti, Ontario Veterinary College, University of Guelph.)

is called a *Langhans-type cell*. The Langhans-type giant cell should not be confused with Langerhans cells, which are dendritic cells (see next discussion) of the skin. Although epithelioid macrophages, foreign body MGCs, and Langhans MGCs have distinct cellular morphology, their physiologic activity is poorly understood.

The process of MGC formation (macrophage fusion) is not fully understood. It requires that macrophages be present within a chronic inflammatory milieu and thus likely bathed in cytokines, such as IFN-γ, IL-3, IL-4, IL-13, and GM-CSF; pathogen factors, such as muramyl dipeptide, a peptidoglycan portion of bacterial cells walls; and other inflammatory mediators. In this close proximity the membranes of adjacent macrophages express fusionogenic molecules such as DC-STAMP (a seven transmembrane receptor), β_1 and β_2 integrins, CD44 (hyaluronic acid receptor), CD47 (integrin-associated protein), macrophage fusion receptor (MFR), fusion regulatory protein (FRP-1; CD98), and P2X7 (a ligand-gated ion channel activated by ATP that forms a pore). The fusion process has similarities to osteoclast formation.

Dendritic Cells

Dendritic cells are central to antigen processing, presentation, and the stimulation of adaptive immunity (Fig. 3-32). Functionally, they serve as sentinel cells of the adaptive immune response. Nearly all tissues and organs contain dendritic cells; however, they are most plentiful in tissues that cover the body, such as the skin and the mucous membranes that line the respiratory and alimentary tracts. Although dendritic cells have some resemblance to macrophages, they have numerous distinct filopodia, which extend from their surface (E-Fig. 3-14). Increasingly, several subtypes of dendritic cells are being identified (Table 3-10). In general, immature dendritic cells ($CD34^+$) migrate to sites of antigen exposure, take up antigen, and migrate to and mature in a lymphoid organ in which they present antigen to T and B lymphocytes. This migration process is mediated by chemokines and adhesion molecules, and most dendritic cells enter lymph nodes via the afferent lymphatic vessels in lymph fluid under the influence of chemokines, particularly CCL21. Once in the lymph node, dendritic cells often localize in the

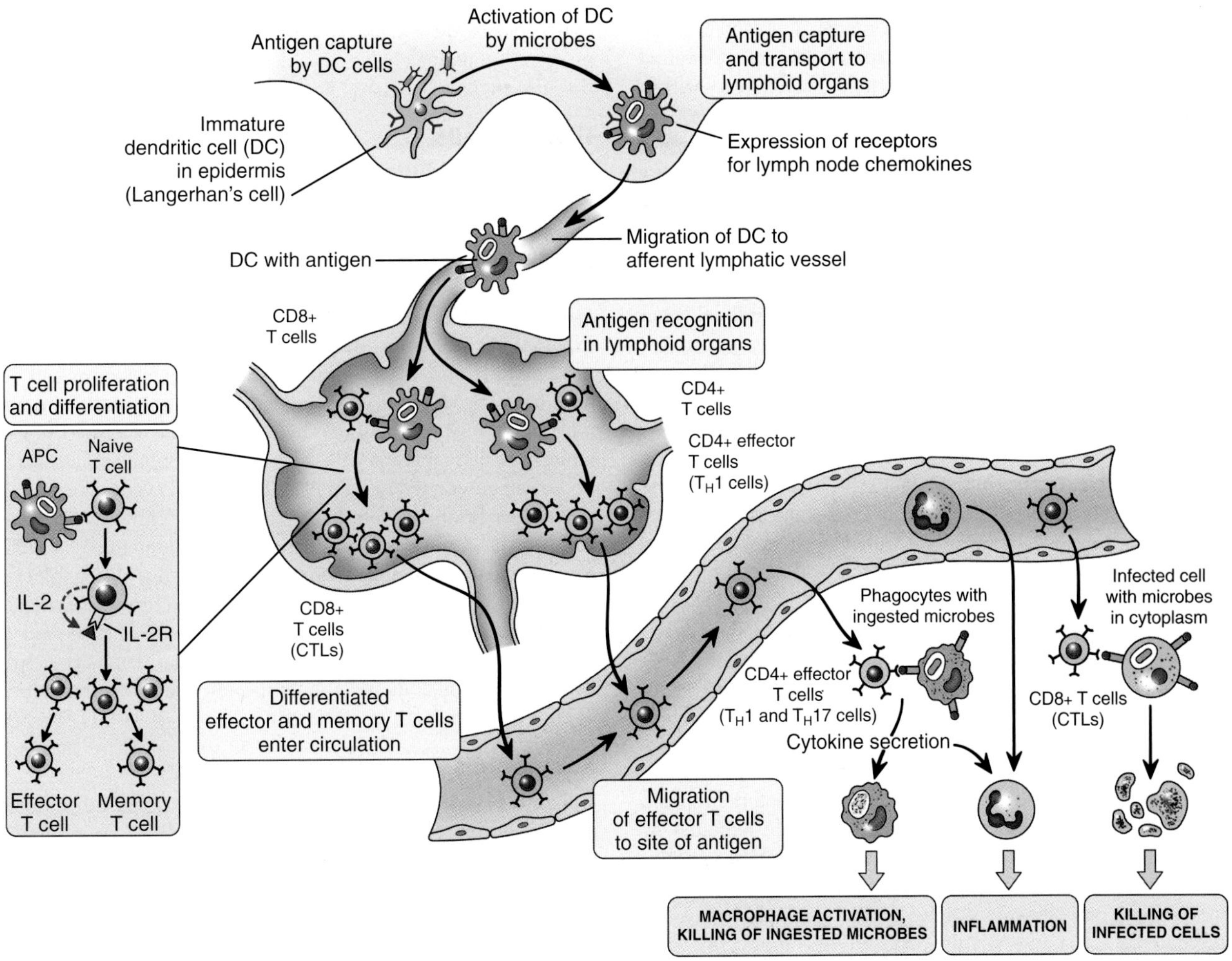

Figure 3-32 Dendritic Cells. Dendritic cells in mucosae, skin, and other tissues phagocytose or endocytose microbial antigens and transport them to regional and systemic lymph nodes. During this process, dendritic cells mature, and express high concentrations of major histocompatibility complex (MHC) molecules and costimulators. Naïve T lymphocytes recognize MHC-associated peptide ligands present on dendritic cells. T lymphocytes are activated to proliferate and differentiate into effector and memory cells, which migrate to sites of infection to facilitate cell-mediated immunity. $CD4^+$ effector T lymphocytes of the T helper lymphocyte type 1 [T_H1] subset recognize microbial antigens ingested by phagocytes and activate the phagocytes to kill the microbes and to induce inflammation. Additionally, $CD8^+$ cytotoxic T lymphocytes migrate from the vascular system into adjacent supporting tissues and kill cells infected with microbes. *APC*, Antigen-presenting cell; *IL*, interleukin. T cell or T cells are used as abridgements for the proper terms T lymphocyte or T lymphocytes.

Table 3-10 Subpopulations of Dendritic Cells and Activities

DC Subpopulation	Location	Activity	Other
$CD8^+$ DCs	T, S, LN, PP, L	$\downarrow T_H1$, $\uparrow T_H2$, $\downarrow$IL-12	Present antigen
$CD8^+$ DCs	T, S, LN, PP, L	$\uparrow T_H1$, $\downarrow T_H2$, $\uparrow$IL-12	Present antigen
$CD8^{int}$ DCs	LN	Enter LN via lymphatic vessels	
Langerhans cells	Skin epidermis	Antigen capture	Migrate to LN
Dermal DCs	Skin dermis	Antigen capture	Migrate to LN
Plasmacytoid DCs	T, S, LN, PP	Viruses induce type I IFN	Antiviral activity

DC, Dendritic cell; *IFN*, interferon; *IL-12*, interleukin 12; *L*, liver; *LN*, lymph node; *PP*, Peyer's patch; *S*, spleen; *T*, thymus; *T_H1*, T helper type 1 lymphocyte response; *T_H2*, T helper type 2 lymphocyte response.

parafollicular (T lymphocytes) area in the vicinity of HEVs, a site in which naïve T lymphocytes enter the node. In this location, dendritic cells activate naïve T lymphocytes. Follicular dendritic cells, localized in lymph node follicles, take up antigen from the lymphatic fluid for presentation to follicular B lymphocytes. In addition to their activity as antigen-presenting cells, dendritic cells also contribute to adaptive immune responses through release of chemokines and cytokines. Outside of lymph nodes, dendritic cells, cytokines, and chemokines also contribute to inflammatory and immune responses; however, their contribution to these responses are dwarfed by macrophages, because there are many more macrophages within inflammatory lesions than dendritic cells.

Although macrophages also present antigen to naïve T lymphocytes, macrophage antigen presentation is more efficient for memory T lymphocytes than for naïve T lymphocytes, the forte of dendritic cells. Through recruitment of naïve T lymphocytes within and outside of the lymph node and presentation of antigen, dendritic cells contribute to the ongoing persistence of a stimulus in chronic inflammatory lesions. In contrast, tolerogenic dendritic cells can suppress immune responses. They accomplish this activity through the sampling of small amounts of self-antigens, harmless environmental antigens, and inciting the deletion of self-reactive T lymphocytes.

Dendritic Cell Trafficking. Trafficking immature monocytic dendritic cells released from the bone marrow express chemokine receptors CCR1 and CCR5 and are recruited by chemokine ligands CCL3 and CCL4 released from lymphocytes and macrophages in tissue (see Fig. 3-32). There are several subtypes of dendritic cells, and those dendritic cells that express CD11c antigen express CCR2, which responds to CCL2, CCL7, CCL8, CCL12, and CCL13. After dendritic cells take up antigen and become exposed to an endogenous (e.g., TNF-α) or exogenous (a ligand for a TLR) mediator, the dendritic cell matures and expresses CCR7 (E-Fig. 3-15). Mature dendritic cells expressing CCR7 migrate from the site of the inflammatory lesion into the vasculature and then spread hematogenously throughout the body until they are recruited by HEVs in the paracortical areas of lymph nodes in which lymphocytes express CCL19 and CCL20. In this location, dendritic cells present antigen and thus contribute to the amplification of the adaptive immune response. Mature dendritic cells from lesion sites that enter the lymphatic vessels travel to the subtrabecular sinus of the lymph node, draining the lesion site and presenting antigen within paracortical regions. Some dendritic cells also drain via the lymphatic vessels to the thoracic duct and enter the blood. Follicular dendritic cells reside in the lymph node follicle and take up antigen present in the lymphatic fluid for presentation to B lymphocytes.

B Lymphocytes

B lymphocytes contribute to chronic inflammation in at least two major ways. B lymphocytes can (1) take up and present antigen and (2) differentiate into immunoglobulin-producing cells (plasma cells or immunocytes), which secrete immunoglobulins that bind to and opsonize antigens facilitating phagocytosis. B lymphocytes are present within chronic inflammatory lesions and granulomas. They also populate the medullary sinus of lymph nodes, in which they produce immunoglobulin locally or leave the medullary sinus through efferent lymphatic flow.

Plasma Cells

Under appropriate stimuli, such as intense antigenic stimulation and B lymphocyte presentation of antigens, B lymphocytes differentiate into plasma cells, which can secrete immunoglobulins that bind to and opsonize antigens and facilitate phagocytosis. Plasma cells form within lymph nodes, mucosal surfaces, and wound sites. The bone marrow also contains a resident population of plasma cells, which can increase in certain disease conditions. Clusters of these cells must be differentiated from neoplastic accumulations as can occur with multiple myelomas. Bone marrow plasma cells can easily migrate into venular walls in the bone marrow to enter the vasculature. Similarly, plasma cells within the medullary sinus of lymph nodes can enter efferent lymphatic vessels and eventually drain into the blood; however, peripheral blood often contains few plasma cells. In the chronic inflammatory exudate, plasma cells are usually found mixed with lymphocytes and macrophages, although in lesser numbers. Plasma cells predominate in certain chronic inflammatory conditions such as inflammatory bowel disease of dogs and cats, lymphoplasmacytic stomatitis and pododermatitis of cats, chronic dermatitis of any domestic animal species, and interstitial nephritis of dogs and cats.

Eosinophils

Different types of chronic inflammatory conditions and granulomas contain a low to high number of eosinophils. Eosinophils are recruited into and stimulated to proliferate within chronic inflammatory exudates by several mediators, most notably IL-5 and eotaxin. In some chronic inflammatory conditions that contain eosinophils, such as asthma in human beings, there is a T_H2 shift, resulting in increased concentrations of chemokines, such as eotaxin, in the tissue that contribute to the recruitment of additional eosinophils and exacerbates the T_H2 response. The same result is likely true for other as yet poorly characterized conditions such as the eosinophilic complex of cats, eosinophilic infiltrates in the base of the tongue of Siberian huskies and other dogs, eosinophilic enteritis in boxer dogs, and eosinophilic inflammatory lesions in the skin of horses. For these conditions it may be that some type of persistent yet unidentified T_H2-inducing antigen is present locally.

Mast Cells

Mast cells have a central role in triggering acute inflammatory reactions. In chronic inflammation, mast cells tend to look similar to macrophages in H&E-stained tissue sections and therefore are often not considered to be a part of the chronic inflammatory lesion. However, special stains, such as a Giemsa stain, of chronic or granulomatous inflammation frequently reveal a surprisingly large number of mast cells identified by their characteristic metachromatic granules. For example, chronic lung lesions (e.g., fibrosis and alveolar epithelial hyperplasia) that develop following severe M. *haemolytica* pneumonia often contain increased numbers of mast cells and reduced concentrations of substance P fibers, resulting in persistently altered immune responses.

The reason for the presence of mast cells in chronic inflammatory conditions likely relates to their production of proteolytic enzymes such as chymase and tryptase. Such enzymes likely help physiologically in remodeling and fine-tuning components of the ECM. With persistent inflammation and fibrosis, there can be increased proliferation of mast cells. Increased mast cell numbers in such lesions occur by increased infiltration and also by increased proliferation of mast cells in situ. With severe inflammation, there can be loss of substance P fibers, and mast cells can respond to this loss by increasing their expression of c-kit, an important regulator of mast cell proliferation.

Natural Killer Cells

NK cells are present in chronic inflammatory lesions, but their role varies based on the characteristics of the inflammatory stimulus. NK cells can kill cells recognized as foreign without prior exposure to antigen and thereby lacking antigen specificity as required by T lymphocytes. NK cells are activated by type I interferons and IL-12 and can activate macrophages and dendritic cells, thus contributing to chronic inflammation. NK-T lymphocyte activation can be triggered by lipid antigens in the presence of CD1d and can contribute to autoimmune responses.

Fibroblasts

Fibroblasts are multipurpose cells whose function is often overlooked in tissue responses to injury. Fibroblasts are elongated cells that contribute to the structural integrity of tissue and have abundant rER, which is used for the synthesis of collagen and ECM proteins. In addition, they also produce cytokines, MMPs, and chemokines that regulate the composition of the extracellular microenvironment in physiologic and pathologic conditions.

With tissue injury or certain hypoxic conditions, fibroblasts undergo proliferation in response to the release of fibroblast growth factors (FGFs), TGF-β, IL-13, PDGF, VEGF, and other mediators/molecules. Continued release of these substances in response to chronic inflammatory stimuli leads to the extensive fibrosis characteristic of chronic inflammation (Fig. 3-33; E-Fig. 3-16).

Endothelial Cells

Endothelial cells are essential for neovascularization of chronic inflammatory lesions. The process of angiogenesis (neovascularization) in chronic lesions is similar to that which occurs during wound healing (see section on Wound Healing and Angiogenesis) and is induced by hypoxia and release of endothelial cell growth factors, such as FGF, VEGF, and PDGF.

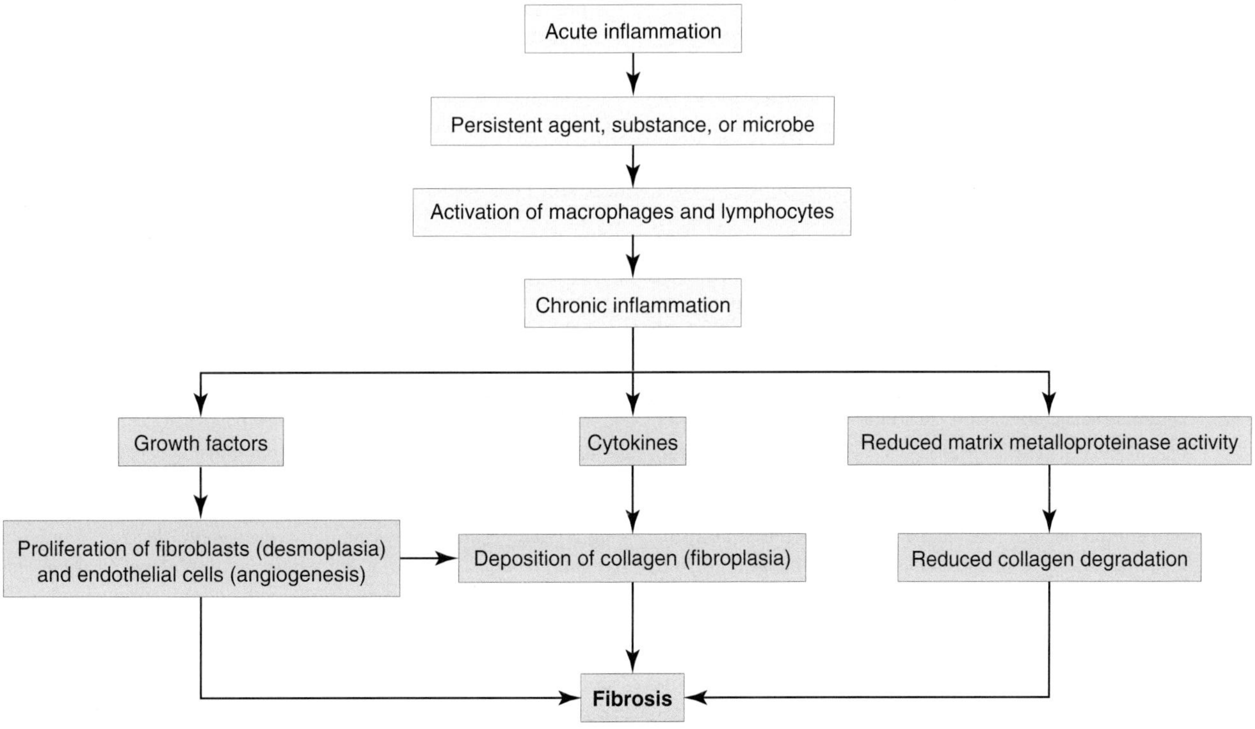

Figure 3-33 Development of Fibrosis in Chronic Inflammation. The persistent stimulus of chronic inflammation activates macrophages and lymphocytes, leading to the production of growth factors and cytokines, which increase the synthesis of collagen. Deposition of collagen is enhanced by decreased activity of metalloproteinases. (Courtesy Dr. M.R. Ackermann, College of Veterinary Medicine, Iowa State University; and Dr. J.F. Zachary, College of Veterinary Medicine, University of Illinois.)

Endothelial cells are interconnected by tight junctions composed of occludins, claudin, and JAMs, as well as adherens junctions composed of VE-cadherins. As leukocytes migrate between endothelial cells, leukocyte adhesion molecules bind some of these intercellular molecules. For example, LFA-1 molecule (CD11-α/CD18) binds JAM A, VLA-4 molecule (α-4/β-1) binds VCAM-1 and JAM B, and Mac-1 (CD11b/CD18) binds JAM C to mediate leukocyte passage between endothelial cells. These molecules are especially important for the transmigration of monocytes and lymphocytes through endothelial cell junctions into sites of chronic inflammation, by providing a stable yet temporary site of attachment of leukocyte filopodia and lamellipodia.

Trafficking of Naïve and Activated T and B Lymphocytes

Homing of Naïve Lymphocytes via High Endothelial Venules

Information on this topic is available at www.expertconsult.com.

Adherence and Transendothelial Migration of Activated T Lymphocytes

Information on this topic is available at www.expertconsult.com.

Inflammation and the Sensation of Pain

Information on this topic is available at www.expertconsult.com.

The Effect of Inflammation on the Febrile Response and Other Activities

Information on this topic is available at www.expertconsult.com.

Unique Types of Inflammation

Septicemia and Endotoxic Shock

Septicemia. Septicemia is a clinically significant form of bacteremia complicated by toxemia, fever, malaise, and often shock (see Table 3-5). Septicemia is characterized by the multiplication of microorganisms within the bloodstream and "seeding" into blood from fixed microcolonies present in one or more tissues. In septicemia, inflammation is not a localized reaction to injury, but instead mediators of inflammation are generated systemically, leading to diffuse "leakage" of plasma into the interstitium and sequestration of leukocytes in the microvasculature. Generation of cytokines, kinins, vasoactive amines, and lipid mediators of inflammation, combined with widespread endothelial damage, leads to profound circulatory disturbances. Because of the systemic nature of this host-microbial interaction, quantities of phagocytic cells, antibody, complement components, coagulation proteins, and platelets may become depleted unless septicemia is controlled in the early stages. Septic shock and disseminated intravascular coagulation (DIC) are the usual sequelae of advanced bacterial septicemia.

Septicemia should be differentiated from a bacterial embolism. For example, some strains of *Streptococcus* spp. may break free from vegetative lesions (valvular endocarditis), as large colonies are protected by cell debris and fibrin. The bacterial emboli may then mechanically lodge in the lung, liver, kidney, or brain to produce a secondary focus of infection (abscess), but the whole process remains subclinical. In such a case the blood sample taken for culture often lacks viable bacteria.

Septic (Endotoxic) Shock. The systemic interaction of microorganisms and their products (toxins) with a spectrum of host cells and chemical mediators results in a clinical syndrome recognized as sepsis or septic shock (see Table 3-5). The host mediators and amplification systems initiating the syndrome vary with the type of organism and the nature of the infectious process (local or systemic). Regardless of the specific cause, the major elements of septic shock form a continuum, including (1) hemodynamic derangements (reduced blood pressure and increased heart rate), (2) abnormal body temperature, (3) progressive hypoperfusion of the microvasculature, (4) hypoxic injury to susceptible cells, (5) quantitative adjustments in blood leukocytes and platelets, (6) disseminated intravascular coagulation, (7) multiple organ failure, and (8) death.

Bacterial endotoxin, the LPS from the outer membrane of Gram-negative bacteria, has been studied extensively as an initiator of septic shock. The peptidoglycan layer of Gram-positive bacteria and bacterial exotoxins can initiate many of the same host responses. Other important initiators are products of the interaction of neutrophils, macrophages, and platelets with microorganisms in the tissue. Endotoxin is bound in the serum by LBP that binds CD14. Endotoxin has numerous ways to induce systemic activation of inflammatory mediators. Three direct effects of endotoxin are the activation of Hageman factor (HF) (a clotting factor), the complement cascade, and induction of the TLR4 pathway. These pathways can ultimately activate bradykinin, PAF, arachidonic acid metabolites, and cytokines (IL-1 and TNF), all of which have a role in many of the coagulation, hemodynamic, thermoregulatory, and leukocyte derangements observed in septic shock. TNF is capable of producing most clinical and pathologic features of septic shock, including hypotension, metabolic acidosis, hemoconcentration, intestinal hemorrhage, fever, neutrophil and endothelial activation, and predisposition to thrombosis. IL-1 shares many of the biologic activities of TNF in the mediation of septic shock. Secretion of TNF by activated macrophages can be partially inhibited by pretreatment with glucocorticoids, such as dexamethasone, which have been used therapeutically, often with limited success. In addition, lethal shock is prevented with anti-TNF antibody or TNF-receptor inhibitors. Chelators of endotoxin and other bacterial products are also under development for use in therapeutic intervention.

In severe septicemia, a *systemic inflammatory response syndrome* (SIRS) can develop in which there is extensive accumulation of cytokines, activated neutrophils, and platelets in the circulatory system. This result leads to multiple organ failure (MOF) and shock. Most patients survive initial systemic inflammatory response syndrome insults, but these individuals are at increased risk for secondary or opportunistic infections termed *compensatory antiinflammatory response syndrome* (CARS). The initial activation of innate immunity can lead to decreased macrophage activity, T lymphocyte anergy, and apoptosis of lymphocytes contributing to compensatory antiinflammatory response syndrome.

Multiple organ dysfunction syndrome (MODS) represents a late stage in septic shock and accounts for much of the irreversibility of organ failure. Systemic tissue ischemia and hypoxia, associated with progressive cardiovascular derangements, increased vascular leakage, and disseminated intravascular coagulation, lead to generalized organ failure. Organs that are particularly sensitive to these effects include heart, brain, kidney, lung, liver, and intestinal mucosa. Cells injured by ischemia revert to anaerobic energy production (glycolysis), resulting in rapid depletion of substrates (glycogen, glucose), accumulation of lactate, and a deficiency of ATP. Without sufficient ATP, cell membrane ion pumps fail to maintain electrolyte balances, membrane integrity, and protein synthesis. The influx of sodium into cells with water causes cells to swell with further loss of function. Influx of calcium ions activates many intracellular enzymes, including phospholipase, which breaks down cellular membranes and generates arachidonic acid products. Loss of the proton gradient of the inner mitochondrial membrane makes oxidative phosphorylation impossible. Irreversible cell injury is believed to be closely related to generalized failure of mitochondria and loss of selective permeability of cell membranes. In dogs, sepsis of abdominal origin can induce multiple organ dysfunction syndrome, and dysfunction of any organ system is associated with increased risk for death, and mortality rates increase as the number of affected organs increase.

Animals dying of septic shock typically have evidence of fluid in the body cavities, pulmonary edema, petechial hemorrhages, congestion of the liver and intestines, and dehydration. Common microscopic lesions include acute necrosis of renal tubules, centrolobular hepatocytes, cardiac myocytes, adrenals, and tips of intestinal villi.

Wound Healing and Angiogenesis

Almost immediately after a wound develops, the process of healing begins (see Essential Concept 3-3). Injured tissue classically goes through four temporal phases to repair the wound: hemostasis, inflammation, proliferation, and remodeling (maturation and contraction). These phases occur in this sequence but may progress at different rates. Even in one lesion site, different areas may be in different phases of repair.

Hemostasis occurs immediately after injury unless there is a clotting disorder. Initially after injury, hemostasis is controlled via vasospasm, a process in which blood vessels constrict in response to injury. But this spasm subsides rapidly, and the injured (transected) blood vessels will subsequently relax, allowing additional bleeding if platelets do not become involved. During the initial period of vasoconstriction, platelets aggregate and adhere to exposed collagen, especially collagen in the basement membrane underlying injured endothelial cells. Once adhered, platelets secrete vasoconstrictive substances to (1) maintain constriction of the transected vessels, (2) initiate the process of thrombogenesis to "plug" the leak in the vessel and prevent additional bleeding, and (3) initiate blood vessel healing (angiogenesis) through, in part, the release of PDGF and TGF-β. This process also occurs with large blood vessels, but additional physiologic factors, such as blood shunting and decreased blood pressure, are involved.

By 24 hours after vascular injury, the inflammation phase (acute inflammation) of wound healing is fully established and can last up to 96 hours or longer if the healing process is disrupted by infection, trauma, or some other perturbation. It is in this phase that the "cardinal signs" of inflammation—redness, swelling, heart pain, and loss of function—are observed. Neutrophils and macrophages, through phagocytosis and their degradative enzymes, break down and remove ("clean-up") the cell debris resulting from tissue injury. Neutrophils release CXCL1, CXCL8, PDGF, and TGFβ, and macrophages secrete a variety of chemotactic and growth factors such as CS3CL1, CCL2, PDGF, VEGF, epidermal growth factor (EGF), IL-1, TNF-α, and TGF-α that establish the microenvironment for the proliferation (granulation) phase. The "clean-up" activity of neutrophils and macrophages within wounds is necessary, although excessive inflammatory cell infiltration reduces healing.

Some ECM molecules, such as some proteoglycans, have a negative charge, thus attracting and binding to more positive-charged growth factors, chemokines, cytokines, MMPs, and other molecules. In addition, fragments of collagen, fibrin, and other molecules in wounds can induce chemotaxis, cell proliferation, and angiogenesis. Thus, with degradation of the ECM in wounds, there is release of these molecules, which contribute to matrix degradation, chemotaxis, and cell proliferation.

During the proliferation phase, in tissues lined by epithelium, migration of basal cells from the overlying epithelium begins early in the healing process and does not require an underlying collagenous matrix. These cells arise from the transected edges of epithelium that border the wound, which rapidly undergo hyperplasia in response to EGF, FGFs, IL-1, hepatocyte growth factor (HGF), VEGF, IL-1β, and TGF-β, released by epithelial cells, endothelial cells, and fibroblasts. The migrating basal cells proliferate, spreading in attempt to bridge the wound, and some of these cells differentiate; however, once the cells differentiate, they cease to proliferate and migrate. The proliferation phase can last up to 3 to 4 weeks or longer depending on the size of the wound. This phase is characterized by the generation of new endothelium (angiogenesis), epithelium (epithelialization), and connective tissue stroma (fibroplasia/desmoplasia) to restore normal structure and function to the injured tissue. The healing of skin after third-degree burns or severe ulcerations is an excellent example of this process. The return to normal structure and function depends on (1) the retention of normal stromal elements of the ECM to provide the structural framework for repair and (2) normally functioning fibroblasts, myofibroblasts (contractile fibroblasts), endothelial cells, pericytes (nonendothelial components of blood vessels), and epithelial cells. Initial deposition of collagen and other key ECM molecules begins after fibroblasts have proliferated and fortified regions of the wound. Collagen fiber deposition alone is not sufficient for complete matrix repair without proliferative and functional fibroblasts.

The role of stem cells of epithelia and mesenchymal stroma in wound healing is increasingly understood. For epithelia, stem cells reside along the basal layer and are more clustered in specific regions. In the cornea of the eye, stem cells are located in the limbus. In skin, clusters are present in the bulge region of the hair follicle (roughly halfway down the follicular wall in the dermis). In lung, stem cells are present along the bronchiole-alveolar junction. In intestine, stem cells are present within the crypts. The stem cells are often in a quiescent (senescent) stage by the influence of bone morphogenic protein (BMP), which inhibits proliferation. β-Catenin (wnt) released from active stem cells in the dermal papilla of hair follicles, for example, induces proliferation of the quiescent cells that form new structures. Mesenchymal stromal cells subjacent to epithelia also undergo proliferation and communicate between epithelial cells and the subjacent inflammatory cells and stroma. The mesenchymal stromal cells function similarly to embryonic blastema cells.

The remodeling (maturation, contraction) phase begins approximately 3 to 4 weeks after injury, but only after the inflammation and proliferation phases have been successfully completed. This phase includes remodeling of granulation tissue by immature connective tissue and the conversion of immature connective tissue to mature connective tissue through extracellular collagen formation in response to TGF-β, PDGF, FGF-2, MMPs, and tissue inhibitors of MMP (TIMPs). Remodeling can last for 2 or more years. It essentially provides the time some tissues and organs, such as bone, need to return to the near-normal tensile strength required for normal axial and appendicular skeletal function.

A key component of wound repair is the ECM and stromal stem cells (fibroblasts, myofibroblasts). In mild or moderate injury, partially degraded collagen, proteoglycans, and elastin are completely degraded by MMPs and other enzymes removed by macrophages and then resynthesized by surviving fibroblasts. Simultaneously, fibroblasts and endothelial cells proliferate to fill tissue defects (granulation tissue), and epithelial cells, endothelial cells, and some parenchymal cells proliferate along basement membranes to restore the normal structure of the tissue. If basement membranes are degraded in the injury and the healing process disrupted, then complete healing is delayed because of a requirement for a new basement membrane to be deposited by endothelial cells that attach to and line the contiguous remaining basement membrane. Should healing be continually delayed (infection) or prevented (large tissue defect with loss of stroma and basement membrane), then dysregulated healing can occur in the form of extensive fibrosis (scars and hypertrophic scars) with haphazard arrangement and/or metaplasia of the overlying epithelial cells.

The four phases of wound healing described are applicable to all tissues and organ systems, but each system has its unique mesenchymal and parenchymal cell types that influence the process of healing. Bone healing with callus formation and skin healing with reepithelialization are good examples of healing and the specialization of cell types involved (see Chapters 16 and 17). Overall, the success of wound healing, especially in the skin, is often determined by whether the process occurs via first or second intention healing. Healing in other tissue is similar. In bone, for example, optimal healing occurs in bone fragments that are stabilized and in direct apposition.

First and Second Intention Healing

First intention healing (also called primary intention healing) in skin occurs when the edges of a wound site are directly apposed and reattach and heal to each other rapidly (Fig. 3-34). Wounds lacking such close, intimate apposition are termed *second intention healing* (also called secondary intention healing). In the simplest type of wound, such as a cut or incision in the skin by a surgeon, there is initial hemorrhage from the damaged vasculature and retraction and constriction of blood vessels. In the wound area there is deposition of fibrin, leakage of plasma proteins, clot formation, platelet aggregation, and neutrophil infiltration. The nature of repair depends on several factors, including the proximity of the cut edges to each other, the presence or absence of foreign bodies or infectious microbes, and the general health capacity of the animal to repair wounds. Under ideal conditions, such as in surgery, first intention healing is desired (see Fig. 3-34). First intention healing occurs in nonseptic wounds, whereas second intention healing occurs in septic wounds, with foreign bodies, or gaping wounds with nonopposed edges. If the wound healing process is disrupted or delayed, the process is shifted to second intention healing. First and second intention healing are also discussed in Chapter 17, The Integument.

First Intention Healing

First intention healing occurs in 2 to 3 days in the skin, if the cut edges of a nonseptic wound are positioned in close proximity to each other by sutures or bandages. During this time, the hemorrhage, plasma proteins, and cell debris within the wound are phagocytosed and removed by macrophages, new blood vessels sprout and grow into the lesion, and the ECM is synthesized to fill the gap between the apposed tissue edges. With time (weeks), this stable interconnection in the dermis is replaced by collagen fibers that undergo continual maturation, thus providing the skin with near-normal tensile strength after wound healing. Concurrently, basal cells of the squamous epithelium will undergo hyperplasia and cover the defect in 3 to 5 days. This type of repair leaves little trace of the wound, except for perhaps mild fibrosis in the superficial dermis and loss of adnexa (e.g., hair follicles, sebaceous glands, and sweat glands) at the site of the wound. The tensile strength is nearly the same as that of adjacent tissue. First intention healing is the goal of the surgeon for repair of incision sites made during surgery.

Second Intention Healing

Second intention healing occurs when the cut edges of the skin, for example, are not brought into appropriate apposition for healing (see Fig. 3-34). In such wounds, connective tissue is haphazardly synthesized and arranged, and there is little or no organization in the healing process; however, fibrous connective tissue fills the defect in the superficial and deep dermis. This disorganization can also delay or prevent the migration of epithelial cells that attempt to cover the surface of the wound and disrupt the orderly deposition of ECM in the wound. In addition, new fibrous connective tissue lacks adnexa (hair follicles, sebaceous and sweat glands). In some cases, fibrous connective tissue can form into granulation tissue (see later section) in which histologically, proliferating fibroblasts are arranged perpendicular to new capillaries, and the long axes of the new capillaries are arranged perpendicular to the surface of the skin (Fig. 3-35). Tensile strength of granulation tissue is diminished, and the lesions can tear or split. Thus with second intention healing the site can remain ulcerated and lack hair, and in some cases the fibrous connective tissue can undergo continuous proliferation and protrude from the skin surface as a hyperplastic scar.

Impaired Wound Healing

In addition to spontaneously occurring impairments of wound healing, such as foreign bodies, infection, and neoplasms, certain other conditions can prevent or impair wound healing, even first intention healing (see Essential Concept 3-3). Healing is affected by wound-specific variables (body site, infection, vascular supply/oxygenation, mechanical stress, and desiccation); systemic variables (nutrition, age, sex, and immobility); medications and environmental exposures (cancer drugs, NSAIDs, glucocorticoids, radiation, smoke/smoking, alcohol); and other diseases and body conditions. For examples, diabetes, autoimmune diseases, venous stasis, obesity, and neuropathies can affect healing. In addition, altered deposition of collagen and ECM proteins can occur with osteogenesis imperfecta because of impaired production of type I collagen. Similarly, impaired synthesis, cross-linking, hydroxylation, or posttranslational processing of collagen can delay wound healing in individuals with Ehlers-Danlos syndrome. Hyperglycosylation of proteins, which can occur with prolonged diabetes mellitus, can alter the vasculature, lead to diabetic ulcers, and inhibit wound healing.

As indicated, chemotherapeutic drugs can also prevent cellular proliferation and may reduce healing. Several new chemotherapeutic drugs specifically target endothelial cell proliferation, which may greatly influence the process of neovascularization so vital to efficient wound repair. In human beings, guinea pigs, and other species that require dietary vitamin C, deficiencies in intake can lead to scurvy, a disease in which there is decreased collagen hydroxyproline synthesis and poor wound healing. Extreme starvation, malnutrition, and cachexia from cancer or severe weight loss from chemotherapy can impair the synthesis and deposition of ECM proteins as a result of negative energy balance and a lack of amino acid substrates, normally synthesized in the liver. Additionally, such individuals and severe burn victims often lack adequate concentrations of serum proteins such as albumin, which results in lowered osmotic plasma pressure, impaired fluid resorption from the wound site, and enhanced edema fluid accumulation.

Expression of Genes Responsible for Wound Repair

Wound repair requires activation of genes of the viable cells such as macrophages, fibroblasts, and endothelial cells adjacent to the sites of tissue injury. As indicated, macrophages internalize through phagocytosis cell debris to "clean up" an area and degrade the ECM.

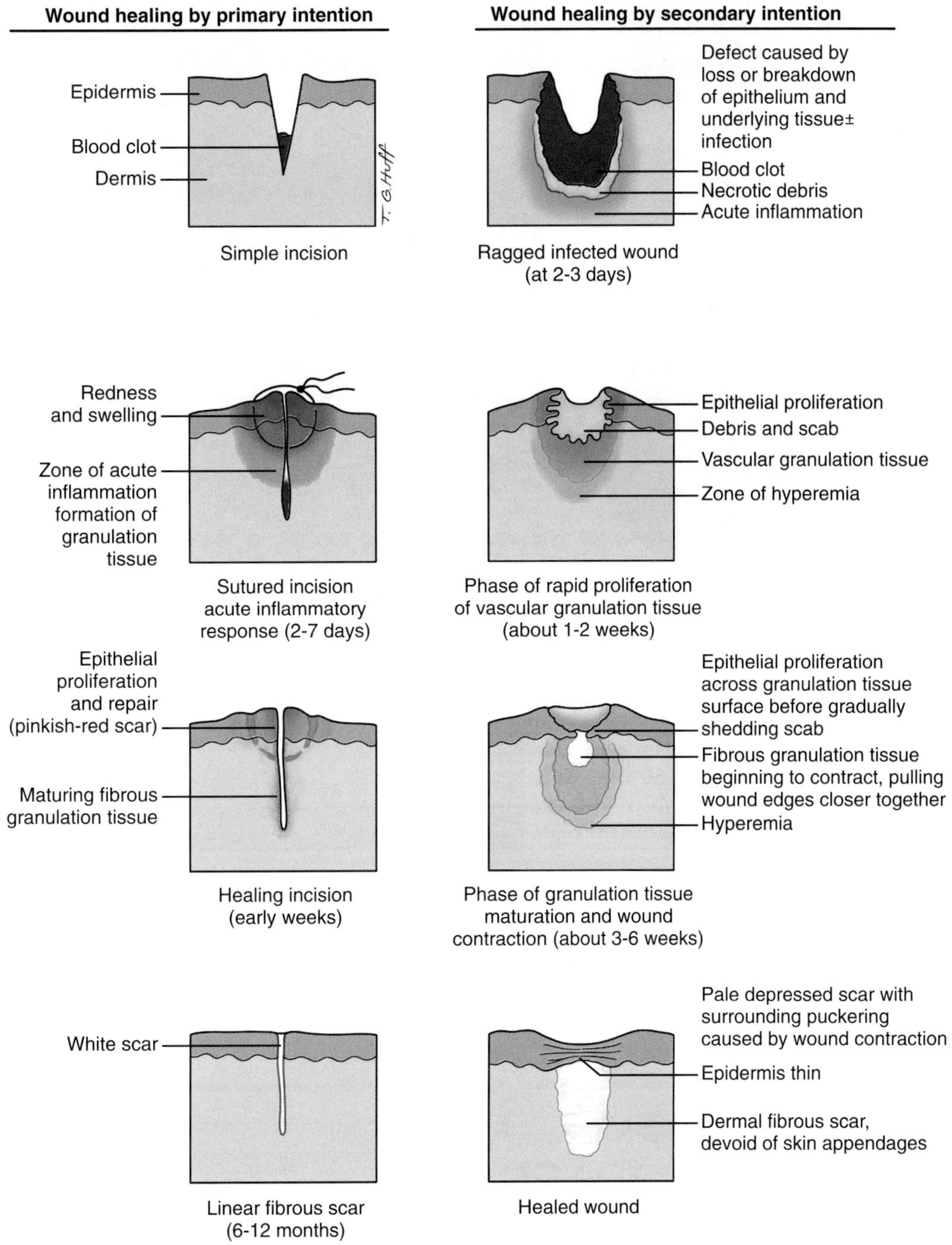

Figure 3-34 Phases of Wound Healing. Wounds can heal by primary intention *(left)* and/or secondary intention *(right)*. Primary intention healing occurs when the edges of affected tissues are brought together (sutured/glued) so they are adjacent to each other in a stable association. Secondary intention healing occurs when the edges of affected tissues are not closely associated and are unstable during the healing process. Healing occurs through the formation of abundant granulation tissue that bridges and fills gaps in the wound and stabilizes opposing surfaces so the other phases of healing may occur. Large amounts of granulation tissue and wound contraction can occur with healing by second intention. Wound healing is a dynamic process that passes through three phases: acute inflammation, epithelial proliferation, and maturation. It is not a "straight-line" process because wound healing often progresses backwards and forwards through the phases depending upon intrinsic (e.g., structural or functional deficiencies) and extrinsic (e.g., microbial infection) forces affecting healing. **Acute inflammation** is the normal response to injury. Blood vessels in the wound constrict and a blood clot is formed. Once hemostasis occurs, blood vessels dilate and acute inflammation ensues, leading to signs characteristic of acute inflammation: reddening (erythema), heat, edema, pain, and loss of function. Neutrophils and macrophages are active removing dead tissue. The **proliferation** phase follows in which granulation tissue composed of collagen, extracellular matrix, and blood vessels (angiogenesis) fills the defect and adheres opposing surfaces of the wound. Epithelial cells eventually resurface the wound (epithelialization). **Maturation** occurs when the wound has functionally and structurally closed and involves remodeling and strengthening of collagen, regression of angiogenesis and epithelialization, and resolution of inflammation.

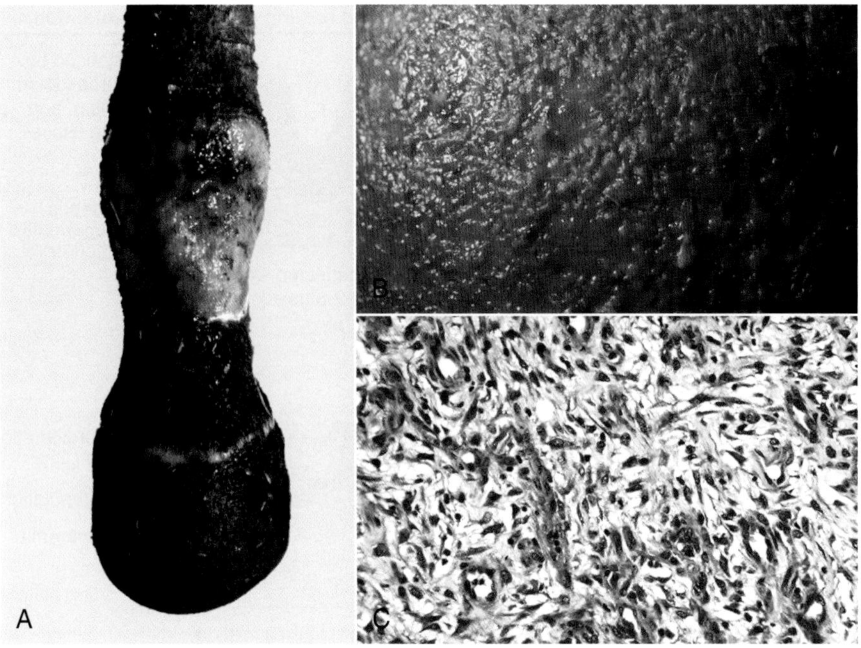

Figure 3-35 **Granulation Tissue, Nonhealing Ulcer, Skin, Distal Limb, Horse. A,** In the bed of the ulcer, there is extensive fibrosis and granulation tissue. **B,** Gross photograph of the surface of the granulation tissue. Note the fine nodules or "granulations" on the surface that gave rise to the term *granulation tissue*. These are a mixture of newly formed blood vessels, extracellular matrix (ECM), and fibroblasts, with minimal or no collagen deposition. It provides the support for wound repair and remodeling via fibroplasia and reepithelialization. **C,** Photomicrograph of granulation tissue. Note how the new fibroblasts are arranged perpendicularly to the newly formed blood vessels in a rich bed of ECM *(clear spaces)*. (Courtesy Dr. M.D. McGavin, College of Veterinary Medicine, University of Tennessee.)

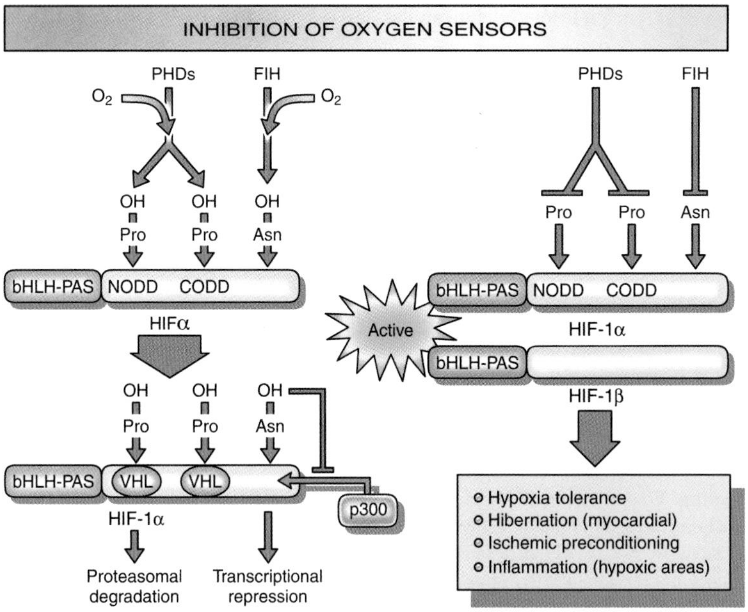

Figure 3-36 **Regulation of Hypoxia-Inducible Factor (HIF) Transcriptional Activity by Prolyl Hydroxylase Protein Domain-Containing Proteins (PHDs) and Factor-Inhibiting HIF (FIH).** With sufficient oxygen *(left)*, HIF-1α protein is hydroxylated by PHDs and FIH resulting in degradation. With insufficient oxygen *(right)* HIF-1α protein is not hydroxylated and forms an active complex with HIF-1β resulting in transcriptions of genes that contribute to wound healing and angiogenesis, including the transcription of vascular endothelial growth factor (VEGF). *bHLH-PAS*, Basic helix-loop-helix/PAS proteins; *CODD*, C-terminal oxygen degradation domain; *NODD*, N-terminal oxygen degradation domain; *VHL*, von Hippel-Linday tumor suppressor gene. (Redrawn from Fraisl P, Aragones J, Carmeliet P: *Nat Rev Drug Discovery* 8:139-151, 2009.)

In concert with fibroblasts, macrophages release growth factors that enhance the proliferation of (1) endothelial cells for neovascularization, (2) fibroblasts for deposition of a new ECM, (3) myofibroblasts for wound contraction, and (4) parenchymal cells for return to normal structure and function of the affected tissue.

Gene expression by cells in a wound is regulated to a large degree by oxygen concentrations (Fig. 3-36; E-Fig. 3-17). In the milieu of a wound there is generally a reduced oxygen tension caused by vascular damage. Normal tissues have oxygen concentrations above 90% oxygen saturation, and there is increased activity of nonheme iron–containing 2-oxoglutarate (2-OG)–dependent oxygenases that sense oxygen concentrations and use dioxygen as a cosubstrate. These include prolyl hydroxylase domain-containing protein-1 (PHD-1), PHD-2, PHD-3, and factor-inhibiting HIF (FIH). These enzymes place a hydroxyl group on proline and asparagine amino acids in HIF-1α protein. Hydroxylated HIF-1α is degraded by the ubiquitin pathway when oxygen concentrations are high. In hypoxic tissue, however, as occurs in wounds, within neoplastic masses, and areas of inflammation, there is reduced activity of PHDs and FIH and thereby less hydroxylation of HIF-1α. Nonhydroxylated HIF-1α aggregates with HIF-1β and induces transcription of hypoxia-responsive elements (HREs) in the genome.

The HREs include genes for growth factors, including VEGF, iron-binding proteins, regulators of apoptosis, erythropoiesis, angiogenesis, pH regulation, and glucose and energy metabolism. Early growth response gene-1 (EGR-1) is another transcription factor activated in wounds that leads to expression of growth factors and cytokines. Therefore both HIF-1α and EGR-1 activity in hypoxic conditions lead to increased cellular transcription that upregulates genes for energy (glucose transporters, hexokinase 1 and 2, lactate dehydrogenase, phosphofructokinase), endothelial and fibroblast proliferation (TGF-β, VEGF), and iron sequestration (ceruloplasmin, transferring receptor). These genes promote cell survival in hypoxic conditions, enhance cell proliferation, especially of cells vital to repair (endothelial cells, fibroblasts), and delay or alter differentiation of other cells (epithelia or parenchymal cells) until endothelial and fibroblast proliferation is well established.

Degradation of Cells and Tissue Components in Wounds

Wounds generally have a central core composed of (1) degenerate and/or necrotic cells, such as parenchymal cells, fibroblasts, and endothelial cells, as well as infiltrating leukocytes, such as neutrophils, platelets, lymphocytes, mast cells, and macrophages; (2) inflammatory products (cytokines, eicosanoids, chemokines, and their respective receptors); (3) serum proteins (albumin, acute phase proteins, complement); (4) clotting proteins (fibrin); and (5) ECM proteins and substances. Many of these cells and mediators need to be removed before optimal healing takes place. Phagocytic cells, such as neutrophils and macrophages, are very important in the clean-up process through phagocytosis of particulate matter and subsequent lysosomal degradation and the release of digestive enzymes into the tissue. In addition, macrophages have a major role in the uptake of apoptotic cells that form in response to TNF-α or other proapoptotic inflammatory stimuli. The ECM can be especially difficult to degrade. However, macrophages and fibroblasts are key to this process through the release of MMPs that degrade the ECM.

Degradation of the Extracellular Matrix in Wounds

The ECM is composed of (1) proteins and (2) the hydrated gel of proteoglycans in which they lie. It surrounds and interconnects cells in connective tissue such as fibroblasts, blood vessels, lymphatic vessels, resident mast cells, macrophages, dendritic cells, and nearby parenchymal cells and/or epithelia. The ECM influences cellular development, polarity (organization), and function of epithelial cells. Soluble proteoglycans and fragments of glycosaminoglycans (GAGs) can activate TLRs, and proteoglycans and hyaluronan can facilitate leukocyte adhesion. Also, ECM binds and sequesters cytokines, chemokines, and growth factors that are released during ECM degradation.

With tissue injury there is often destruction and degradation of the ECM. This process occurs through physical separation or tearing, dilution from plasma proteins, infiltration by inflammatory cells, and degradation by enzymes, largely the MMPs (E-Fig. 3-18). Macrophages, fibroblasts, mast cells, and most leukocytes produce MMPs (Table 3-11). Many MMPs were initially named after the type of ECM protein that they were found to degrade (e.g., collagenase), but because the MMPs are now known not to be uniquely specific for a particular ECM substrate, they have been reclassified in a numeric manner, MMP-1 to MMP-20.

Table 3-11 Matrix Metalloproteinase Activity, Regulation, and Cellular Production

Function: Degrade basement membrane and extracellular matrix proteins
Cofactors necessary: Zinc (Zn^{2+})
Regulation: Cellular synthesis, lysosomal degradation and release, and tissue inhibitors of metalloproteinases

Type of MMP	Cell Type
MMP 1, 2, 3, 11, 14	Fibroblasts
MMP 9, 12	Macrophages
MMP 9	Neutrophils
MMP 2, 3, 9	Endothelial cells
MMP 9	Pericytes
MMP 1, 3, 7, 9, 13	Some cancer cells

MMP, Matrix metalloproteinase.

For example, collagenase is MMP-1, gelatinase is MMP-2, stromelysin is MMP-3, and matrilysin is MMP-7. MMPs degrade collagen, gelatin, elastin, aggrecan, versican, proteoglycan, tenascin, laminin, fibronectin, and other ECM components. The MMP enzymatic domain contains three histidine residues that form a complex with zinc. A regulatory domain is responsible for latency and allows activation in the presence of zinc. MMP activity is also regulated by TIMP. ADAM (a disintegrin and metalloproteinase) is a family of zinc proteinases capable of degrading matrix molecules as can cathepsin G, tissue plasminogen activator (tPA), and urokinase plasminogen activator (uPA) (E-Box 3-2). Fragments of proteins degraded by MMP, tPA, uPA, and other degradative processes are removed from wounds by lymphatic drainage and phagocytosis by macrophages and neutrophils. Proteoglycans are largely degraded by lysosomal enzymes of macrophages and neutrophils that include hyaluronidases, heparinases, and galactosidases. As indicated, ECM degradative enzymes also (1) release latent growth factors and other latent molecules bound to ECM molecules, (2) inactivate some molecules present within the region, (3) break down basement membranes, and (4) cleave intercellular adhesion molecules between epithelial cells.

Resynthesis of the Extracellular Matrix with Wound Healing

Synthesis of Collagen and Matrix Proteins

As wounds repair, the body attempts to reestablish the ECM. The structural proteins of the ECM include several types of collagens, elastin, and adhesive type of proteins, including fibronectin, laminin, versican, tenascin, and vitronectin. The fibrillar collagens (types I, II, III, V, and XI) are triple-stranded helical structures aggregated into fibrils in the extracellular space and surrounded by collagens IX and XII, which interconnect the collagen fibrils with one another and the ECM. Most tissues have a predominance of one collagen type. For example, collagen type I is present in bone, skin, and tendon; collagen type II is present in cartilage and vitreous humor;

collagen type III is present in skin, around vessels, and in newly formed wounds; collagens type V and VI are present in interstitial tissues; collagen type VI is present near epithelia; collagen type VIII is present near endothelial cells; and collagens type X and XI are present in cartilage.

Collagen type IV is largely present in basal lamina along with laminin, entactin, a heparin sulfate proteoglycan, and perlecan. Throughout the ECM are molecules of elastin, which stretch, recoil, and allow flexibility in the tissue. Collagen fibers, laminin, fibronectin, tenascin, and other ECM proteins bind to cells in the connective tissue via extracellular domain of integrin molecules of cells by means of a specific amino acid sequence, the RGDS sequence. For example, laminin binds $\alpha_2\beta_1$-integrins of endothelial cells, some collagens bind $\alpha_6\beta_1$-integrins of epithelial cells, and fibronectin and vitronectin bind $\alpha_5\beta_3$-integrins. The intracellular portion of integrin molecules interact with the cellular cytoskeleton (i.e., actin assembly) and thereby link the extracellular milieu with cellular activities such as cell growth, differentiation, proliferation, and senescence.

Collagen Production by Fibroblasts

Collagen deposition within a site of wound repair provides a scaffold for reestablishment of the ECM and stroma. Fibroblasts are induced by TGF-β and other cytokines to synthesize collagen. Ribosomes in fibroblasts produce approximately 30 types of collagen α-chains that are composed of repetitive glycine-x-y segments. However, within the rER, praline and lysine residues in these chains are hydroxylated, and this hydroxylation process requires vitamin C. The chains are then glycosylated, arranged in a triple helix, and eventually released into the extracellular space as procollagen. The ends of procollagen are cleaved enzymatically, resulting in the formation of fibrils termed *tropocollagen*. Cross-linkages between collagen fibrils occur at lysine and hydroxylysine residues through the activities of the enzyme lysyl oxidase, and this cross-linking process provides the tensile strength of collagen.

Synthesis of Proteoglycans

Proteoglycans are produced by fibroblasts. They retain water and are vital to the hydration of the ECM. Proteoglycans have a protein backbone surrounded by a network of GAG chains (E-Fig. 3-19). The GAGs are negatively charged, often highly sulfated, polysaccharide chains covalently linked to the serine residues on a protein backbone. Most GAGs contain high concentrations of *N*-acetylglucosamine (E-Table 3-11). Hyaluronic acid lacks sulfation and is not connected to the protein backbone. GAGs are key to the water retention properties of proteoglycans and thus hydration of the extracellular milieu. Proteoglycan hydration of the ECM allows tissues to be pliable and have elasticity.

Heparin sulfate proteoglycans, such as syndecan, decorin, and perlecan, encircle and surround cells and basal laminae. Syndecan is an integral transmembrane protein that can bind chemokines. With inflammation, syndecan can release the chemokine, which then induces leukocyte infiltration.

Fibroblasts and the Mechanistic Basis of Fibrosis

Fibroblasts align along planes of tissue stress during development (Langer's lines or tension lines). In quadrupeds these lines are generally dorsoventral over the thorax and abdomen (axial body plane) and parallel to the long axis of the limbs (appendicular body plane). Surgical incisions along Langer's lines extend between, rather than transect, bands of fibrous connective tissue and tend to pull the margins of surgical skin incisions together. Such incisions reduce the degree of postsurgical scar formation.

Fibroblasts of cats appear to be especially responsive to injury and inflammation. In fact, injury of fibroblasts has been associated with their neoplastic transformation in cats. For example, traumatic lens rupture can lead to intraocular inflammation and fibroblast proliferation, and in some cases fibrosarcomas. In addition, fibroblast proliferation and fibrosarcomas are common in cats at vaccination sites.

Initially during the hemostasis and inflammation phases of wound repair, fibrin and serum proteins form a loose gel-like framework for the migration of fibroblasts and endothelial cells into the wound to form granulation tissue. Simultaneously, leukocytes and other cells, such as fibroblasts and endothelial cells, are stimulated by HIF-α and EGF to synthesize and release a variety of growth factors that result in fibroblast proliferation and migration. These factors include FGF-1 and FGF-2, PDGF, EGF, and TGF-β1, 2, and 3. FGF, PDGF, IL-13, and TGF-β induce fibroblasts to produce collagen, whereas FGF, VEGF, TGF-β, angiopoietin, and mast cell tryptase induce endothelial cells to proliferate and migrate and produce basement membrane for formation of new capillaries (E-Fig. 3-20).

With time the newly formed, provisional connective tissue is remodeled into a more mature matrix. In the entire process, TGF-β has a central role in fibroblast activity and collagen deposition because it is produced by platelets and macrophages and induces macrophage chemotaxis, fibroblast migration and proliferation, and synthesis of collagen and ECM proteins. TGF-β binds TGF-β receptor II (TGF-βRII), which dimerizes with TGF-βRI. The TGF receptor then phosphorylates R-SMAD and Co-SMAD to overcome inhibition of SMAD 7. This signaling process induces fibroblast activity, and regulation of the signaling may be useful in therapeutic strategies to control scarring and/or fibrosis (E-Fig. 3-21). Fibroblasts can undergo senescence through increased expression of cyclin-dependent kinase inhibitor p16 (INK 4a) and take on a senescence-associated secretory phenotype (SASP). These senescent fibroblasts can release PDGF-A, which enhances myofibroblast formation in wounds.

In addition to producing collagen, fibroblasts can migrate to a certain degree, and this process is mediated by adhesion molecules that bind to the ECM. This binding is a complicated event in which the adherence process is essential for migration of the cell and its anchoring to extracellular proteins. During wound repair, proliferating fibroblasts often align themselves parallel with lines of tension stress.

Morphology of Granulation Tissue and Fibrous Connective Tissue

Granulation Tissue

Some lesions develop a distinctive type of arrangement of connective tissue fibers, fibroblasts, and blood vessels termed *granulation tissue*. Granulation tissue is the exposed connective tissue that forms within a healing wound. It is often red and hemorrhagic and bleeds easily when bumped or traumatized because of the fragility of the newly formed capillaries (see Fig. 3-35). It is especially common in horses. When viewed with a magnifying glass, the surface of granulation tissue has a granular appearance, and thus the term granulation tissue arose. In granulation tissue, fibroblasts and connective tissue fibers grow parallel to the wound surface and are arranged perpendicularly to the proliferating capillaries. Often the penetrating blood vessels are evenly spaced. Excessive granulation can lead to a type of hypertrophic scar called *proud flesh*. In cats, fasciotomy and fascial excision induce formation of early granulation tissue in cutaneous wounds and may be effective in enhancing closure of secondary wounds.

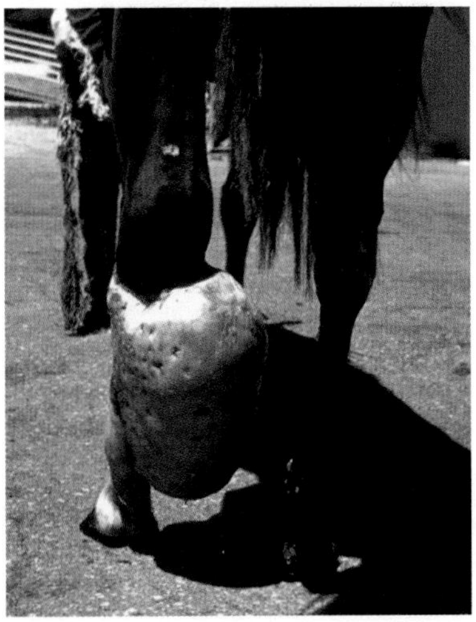

Figure 3-37 **Exuberant Granulation Tissue (Proud Flesh), Chronic Ulcer, Skin, Distal Hind Limb, Horse.** Note the large proliferating mass of fibrous tissue on the lower portion of the left hind limb. It often lacks superficial epithelium. (Courtesy Dr. M.D. McGavin, College of Veterinary Medicine, University of Tennessee.)

Hypertrophic Scars. Hypertrophic scars occur as a result of exuberant proliferation of fibroblasts and collagen in wounds that fail to heal properly. The best example of this condition occurs in skin wounds of the distal limbs of horses and is known as "proud flesh"; as indicated, proliferating connective tissue forms a large cauliflower-like mass that cannot be covered by epithelium (Fig. 3-37). Why this lesion most commonly occurs in horses is unclear; however, the epidermis of horses is often very "tight" with limited elasticity.

Keloid is a special type of excessive connective tissue deposit that occurs in human beings. It has an incidence of 5% to 16% after skin trauma in high-risk populations, such as blacks, Hispanics, and Asians. Clinical management of hypertrophic scars, proud flesh, and keloids can be difficult but includes intralesional corticosteroids, compression, occlusive dressings, pulsed-dye laser therapy, cryosurgery, surgical excision, radiation, fluorouracil chemotherapy, topical silicone, interferons, and drugs, such as imiquimod, that induce IFN-γ.

Fibrous Connective Tissue

Fibrous connective tissue is the dense accumulation of fibroblasts and collagen formed within a wound site. Histologic characteristics depend on wound severity and duration. Fibrous connective tissue contains variable numbers of fibroblasts and collagen along with inflammatory cells (Fig. 3-38). In recently formed wounds the collagen can be very immature and edematous with a variety of inflammatory cells, perhaps neutrophils. With time the fibrous connective tissue progresses into mature, densely packed collagen with few inflammatory cells. Once formed and matured, fibrous connective tissue often persists for years, perhaps life.

Wound Contraction

The Scirrhous Reaction

With severe thermal/chemical burns or extensive abrasions of a large surface area of the skin, the healing process and the formation of connective tissue becomes extensive. In time these areas of connective tissue contract and place tension on the surrounding normal skin, resulting in a scirrhous reaction that can cause immobility of

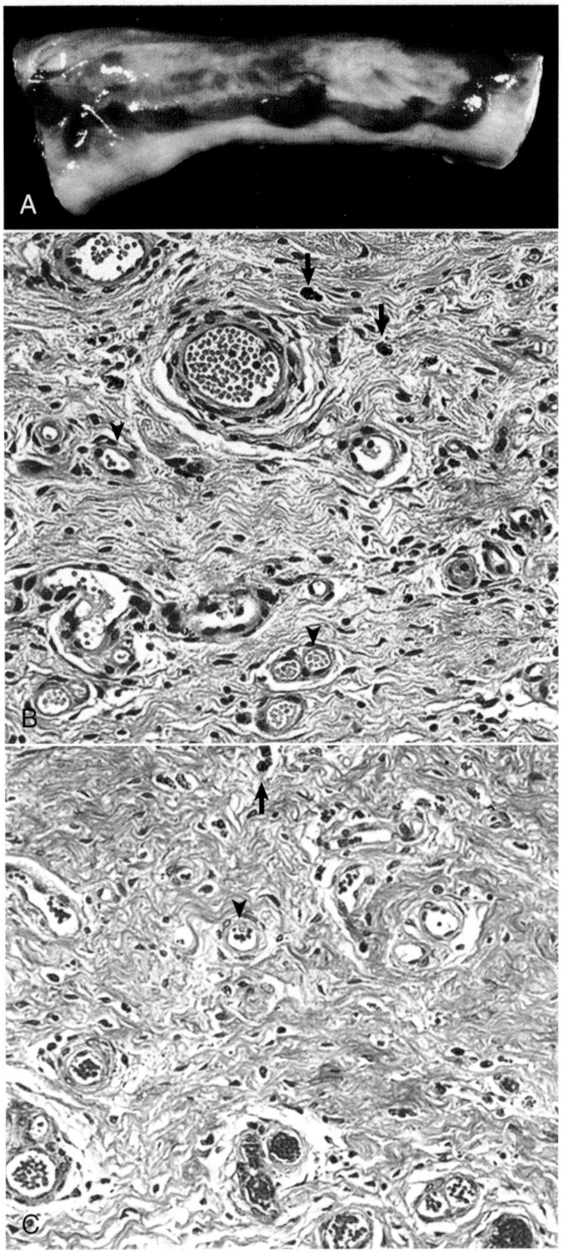

Figure 3-38 **Fibrous Connective Tissue. A,** Hemomelasma ilei, ileum, antimesenteric serosal surface, horse. This lesion is approximately 1 to 2 weeks old. *Strongylus edentatus*–induced injury to the serosal vasculature results in hemorrhage followed by wound healing. Note the raised areas of fibrosis *(raised gray-white areas)*, hemosiderosis *(yellow-brown areas)*, and hemorrhage *(red-brown areas)*. **B,** Healing response in hemomelasma ilei. Note the abundant newly formed capillaries *(arrowhead)* and intervening fibrous connective tissue *(bands of red fibers)*. This healing response is the next step following the granulation tissue phase demonstrated in Figure 3-35. Hemosiderin *(arrow)* is present in the connective tissue and is indicative of hemorrhage having occurred in the injury at an earlier time (weeks). H&E stain. **C,** Fibrous connective tissue in the healing response. Collagen is readily demonstrated in fibrous connective tissue by a Trichrome stain *(blue-stained fibers)*. Hemosiderin *(arrow)*; newly formed capillaries *(arrowhead)*. Masson trichrome stain. (Courtesy Dr. J.F. Zachary, College of Veterinary Medicine, University of Illinois.)

the surrounding skin and perhaps limbs along with pain and deformation. Contraction of such wounds is mediated largely by myofibroblasts.

Similarly, within areas of necrosis and/or inflammation in the liver, lung, spleen, and kidney, excessive fibrosis in parenchymal areas can result in the formation of connective tissue tracts between the healing area and capsular and interstitial connective tissue. When this new connective tissue contracts during the healing process, it grossly results in local indentation or pitting on the organ surface, such as occurs with chronic renal cortical infarcts. If there are multiple such areas, the organ surface develops an undulating and/or nodular appearance such as occurs in a cirrhotic liver. Contraction of such wounds is again mediated largely by myofibroblasts.

Myofibroblasts. Myofibroblasts are specialized fibroblasts with contractile activity. They form within wounds in response to tissue plane stress and the secretion of TGF-β by platelets and macrophages as wounds develop, and they increase in number with time and severity. Senescent fibroblasts and endothelial cells in wounds that have the senescence-assocated secretory phenocyte (SASP) can also induce myofibroblast formation and accelerate wound healing through the secretion of PDGF-AA. The myofibroblast function is to contract the wound and thus bring together injured tissue separated by edema and inflammation. Physiologically, myofibroblasts also occur in tissues with contractility such as uterine submucosa, intestinal villi, testicular stroma, the ovary, periodontal ligament, bone stroma, capillaries, and pericytes.

Myofibroblasts have stress fibers, actin and myosin fibers, gap junctions, and a fibronexus. The fibronexus is a mechanotransduction region of the plasma membrane, which is rich in integrin molecules. The fibronexus interconnects intracellular actin fibers with extracellular proteins such as fibronectin. This connection provides an anchor point during myofibroblast contraction. In contrast, fibroblasts lack contractile myofilaments and a fibronexus. Actin polymerization and contractility in myofibroblasts is stimulated by Rho GTPases. The Rho signaling that induces contractility in myofibroblasts results in continual contraction of filaments in myofibroblasts. Continual contraction by myofibroblasts differs from the periodic contractility that occurs in smooth muscle cells. Such contractions condense wound sites and are frequently beneficial to repair. But excess, as in severe burns, induces excessive contraction and sometimes loss of mobility of nearby joints requiring patients to undergo physical therapy to maintain the range of motion for limbs extending from affected joints.

Angiogenesis in Wound Repair

Angiogenesis is the formation of new blood vessels from preexisting vessels. It is a process essential for all living organisms with a cardiovascular system and involves a series of steps, as illustrated in Figure 3-39, for the formation of new capillaries, including the following:

- Proteolysis of the ECM and basement membrane of parental vessels at the margins of the wound so a new capillary "bud" can form and initiate cellular migration
- Migration of immature endothelial cells into the wound
- Proliferation of endothelial cells to form solid "endothelial tubes"
- Maturation of endothelial tubes into new capillaries with the formation of lumina
- Formation of stalk cells (proliferative endothelial cells lining developing vessels) and tip cells at the end of vascular buds
- Establishment of endothelial cell adhesion to adjacent cells and basal lamina and expression of the receptors/ligands responsible for the leukocyte adhesion cascade along the luminal surface of the endothelial cells
- Recruitment of pericytes and smooth muscle cells to support the final differentiation stage of the newly formed vessel

This process occurs because as wounds heal, new vessels are necessary to supply the injured site with oxygen, remove carbon dioxide and other waste products, drain excess fluid, and provide a vascular pathway for cells and stem cells into the wound. This same beneficial process has also been adapted by primary and metastatic neoplastic cells to grow and spread throughout tissues of the body.

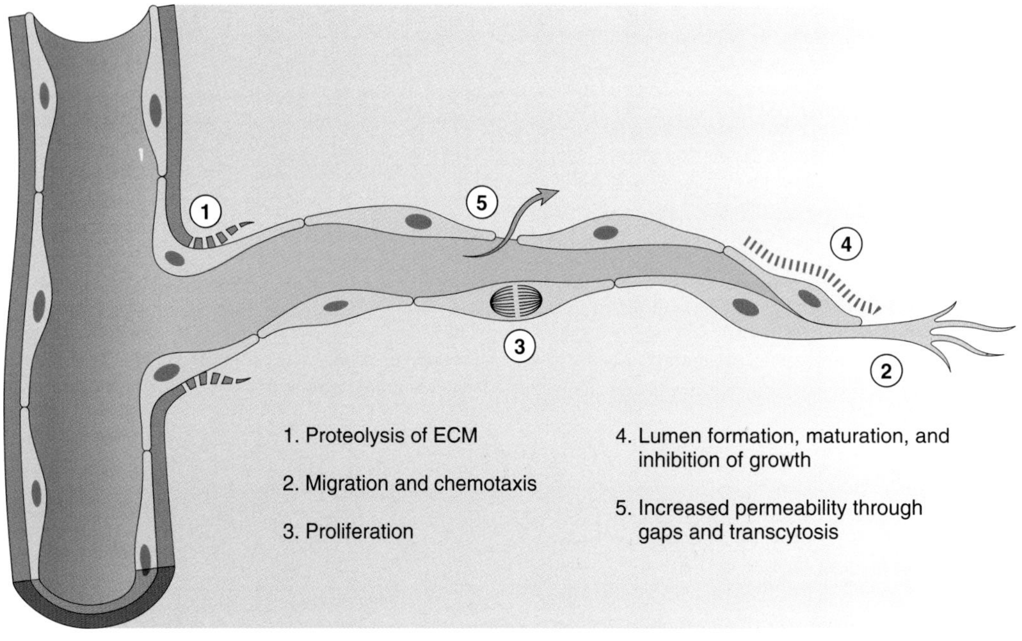

Figure 3-39 **Steps in the Process of Angiogenesis.** *ECM*, Extracellular matrix. (Redrawn from Motamed K, Sage EH: *Kidney Int* 51:1383, 1997.)

Initiation of Endothelial Cell Proliferation

Endothelial Cell Growth Factors. The formation of new blood vessels in wounds begins from the proliferation of endothelial cell buds from blood vessels in viable tissue adjacent to the wound or can be derived from bone marrow endothelial precursor cells (EPCs) (Fig. 3-40). These buds grow into the "healing" wound, form elongated vascular tubular structures within the wound, interconnect and revascularize the wound, and then eventually differentiate into mature vessels. Initially, endothelial cell buds form, and cells migrate into wounds under the autocrine influence of HIF-1α and EGF (see section on Expression of Genes Responsible for Wound Repair), which enhance expression of genes that improve cell survival in hypoxic conditions.

Concurrently, growth factors such as PDGF, FGF, VEGF-A, angiogenins, bone morphogenic protein (BMP), and ephrins released from macrophages, endothelial cells, and fibroblasts bind receptors on endothelial cells and induce vascular formation (Fig. 3-41). VEGF-A and its various isoforms stimulate the initial stages of endothelial cell proliferation through binding the VEGF-R2 receptor on endothelial cells. Proliferative effects of VEGF are regulated by Notch ligands and receptors. VEGF enhances expression of Dll4, a ligand in vascular tip cells produced by tip cells that bind to Notch receptors expressed by stalk cells. Dll4 binding of Notch receptor leads to expression of genes by the stalk cells that reduce VEGF-R expression and cellular proliferation. The secondary stages of endothelial cell proliferation involve angiopoietin 1 and its receptor, Tie2, both of which establish vascular stabilization through the recruitment of pericytes and smooth muscle cells and deposition of ECM proteins. Vascular stabilization is further advanced by PDGF and TGF-β. Recent work has shown that specific microRNA molecules, such as microRNA-92a (MiR-92a), control angiogenesis in mice. MiR-92a targets mRNAs with proangiogenic activity, binds these, and reduces their activity.

Endothelial Cell Migration Is Mediated by Integrins. Newly formed endothelial cells and fibroblasts migrate into wound sites and bind to fibrinogen and plasma proteins, as well as newly deposited ECM substances, such as heparin sulfate, chondroitin sulfate, type III collagen, laminin, vitronectin, and fibronectin. This adherence is mediated by adhesion molecules expressed by new endothelial cells and fibroblasts. These adhesion molecules include α_5- and β_3-integrins, which bind fibrin and fibronectin. It is interesting that for wound repair, enhancement of angiogenesis is beneficial and vital; however, in neoplasia, inhibition of angiogenesis and thus the growth of the tumor have potential therapeutic benefits.

Vascular Remodeling. Once blood vessels are initially formed, they are loosely arranged and require remodeling to become mature. With remodeling, endothelial cells produce a mature basement membrane. In addition, smooth muscle cells and pericytes can form within the wall, and fibroblasts can form adventitial fibers, depending on whether the vessel is a capillary, artery, vein, or lymphatic vessel. Other endothelial cell growth factors and receptors involved with vascular remodeling include angiopoietin 2, which also binds Tie2 and ephrin B2 (EphB2) and its receptor, EphB4. Proliferation of lymphatic endothelial cells is mediated largely by VEGF-C and its receptor, VEGF-R3, as well as by Prox-1 gene expression. During angiogenesis, BMP-1 inhibits Prox-1 and thus lymphangiogenesis.

Regulators/Inhibitors of Endothelial Cell Growth. Inhibitors of angiogenesis are produced by endothelial cells, macrophages, and fibroblasts. These inhibitors balance the proliferative healing

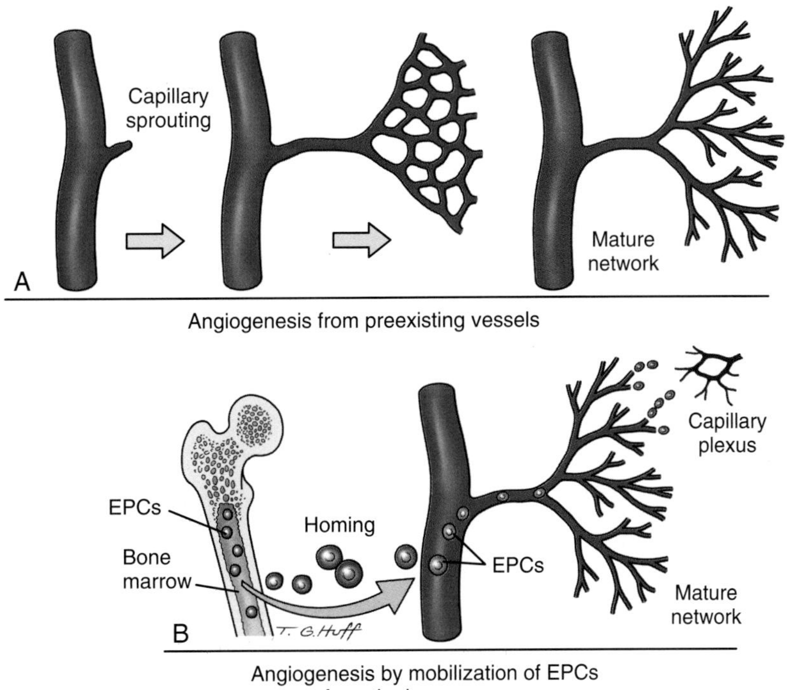

Figure 3-40 Angiogenesis by Mobilization of Endothelial Cell Precursors. **A,** Preexisting vessels (capillary sprouts). Capillary sprouts arise via angiogenesis from endothelial cell precursors in preexisting vessels that become motile and proliferate to form these sprouts. A new capillary network develops and matures with recruitment of pericytes and smooth muscle cells to form the periendothelial layer. **B,** Bone marrow. Progenitor cells for endothelial cell precursors (EPCs) migrate from bone marrow to a site of injury. The mechanisms are unclear. At sites of injury, EPCs differentiate and form endothelial cells and release proangiogenic factors to contribute to a mature capillary network by anastomosing with existing vessels.

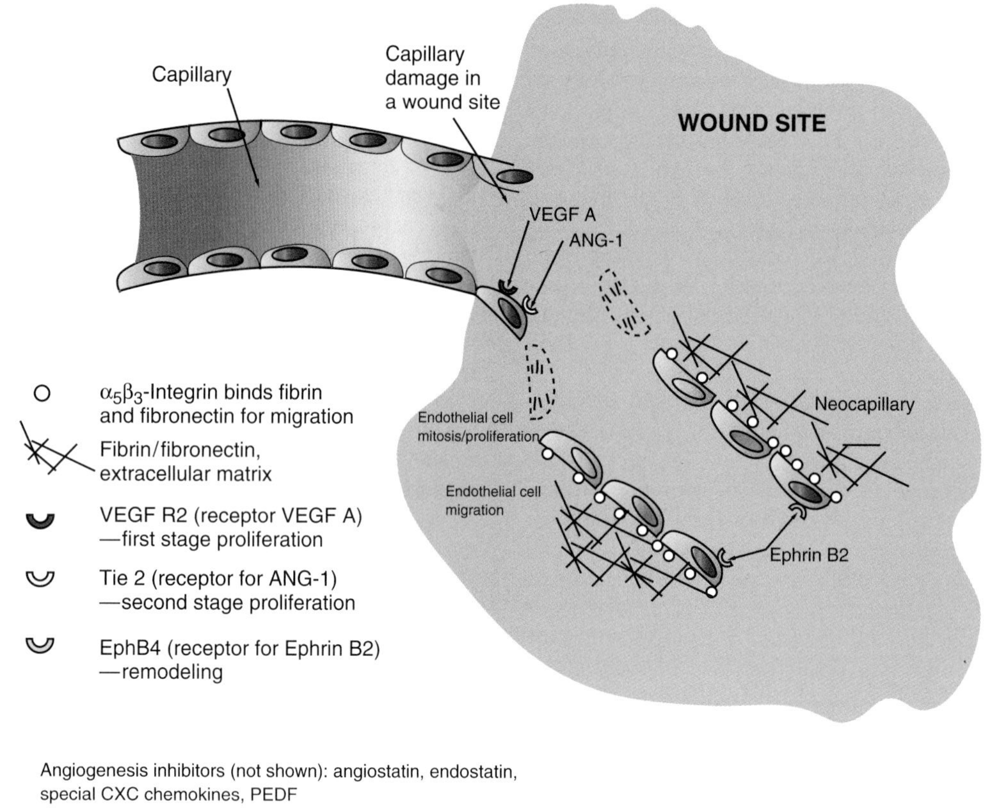

Figure 3-41 **Molecular Mechanisms of Angiogenesis.** Growth factors, such as vascular endothelial growth factor (VEGF-A) and angiopoietin (ANG-1), bind receptors on endothelial cells that induce proliferation and migration. The migration is mediated by $\alpha_5\beta_3$-integrins expressed by endothelial cells that bind molecules such as fibrin and fibronectin. Factors such as Ephrin B2 bind endothelial cell receptors Ephrin B4 and mediate vascular remodeling. *PEDF*, pigment epithelium-derived factor. (Redrawn from Dr. M.R. Ackermann, College of Veterinary Medicine, Iowa State University.)

responses of angiogenesis and prevent overexuberant proliferation of endothelial cells. These inhibitors include angiostatin, endostatin, thrombospondin, and specialized CXC chemokines (lacking ELR motif). In addition, certain isoforms of VEGF can bind VEGF receptors and reduce VEGF signaling and activity. Such inhibitors of angiogenesis are being studied intensely for their potential chemotherapeutic role against certain types of cancer and for exuberant vascularization that can occur in the retina, for example. Bevacizumab (Avastin, Genentech, Inc., South San Francisco) is an inhibitor of VEGF and can reduce vascularization in cancer and in the retina.

Epithelialization in Wound Repair

Epithelialization (reepithelialization) is the process by which the skin and mucous membranes replace superficial epithelial cells damaged or lost in a wound. Epithelial cells at the edge of a wound proliferate almost immediately after injury to cover the denuded area. Under normal conditions, this process is rapid, and first intention healing occurs in 3 to 5 days to repair the wound. During wound repair, keratinocytes and mucosal epithelial cells must move laterally across the wound surface to fill the void. Before this lateral movement can occur, epithelial cells must disassemble their connections to the underlying basement membrane and their junctional complexes with neighboring cells. They must also express surface receptors that permit movement over the ECM of the wound surface.

Intact Basement Membranes Enhance Reepithelialization

The presence or rapid deposition of basement membrane into the wound greatly facilitates proliferation of viable epithelial cells at the margins of the wound. For example, with initial loss of enterocytes that cover the surface of intestinal villi or renal tubular cells that line proximal convoluted tubules, the immediate response is for the adjacent normal epithelial cells to extend over the denuded basement membrane and to cover the area, if it is larger, by becoming thin, elongated cells. At the same time, there is proliferation (mitosis) of viable adjacent epithelial cells, and these cells migrate along the basement membrane to cover the denuded surface and replace lost cells. Without a basement membrane, proliferative cells lack a clear path of migration. The immature cells may loiter at the site of proliferation and fuse, thus forming syncytial cells, as can be seen with renal tubular injury and the failure of the tubular epithelium to migrate.

Similarly, regenerating skeletal muscle cells and transected axons will regenerate inside a tube surrounded by basal lamina and endoneurium. Components of the basement membrane, including laminin, type III collagen, and the associated proteoglycans, provide a substratum for epithelial and other cells to bind the basement membrane via integrins, proliferate, and migrate along the basement membrane surface.

Initiation of Cell Proliferation in Epithelia

Growth factors are vital for the proliferation of keratinocytes, mucosal epithelia, renal tubular cells, and other parenchymal epithelial cells. In skin and other surface epithelia, for example, keratinocyte growth factor (KGF) and EGF bind receptors on epithelial cells and induce signal transduction, which activates MAPK that induces cells in the nonproliferating G_0 phase of the cell cycle to enter the cycle and proliferate (see Chapters 1 and 6). Hepatocyte growth factor (HGF) induces proliferation of hepatocytes, and nerve growth factor (NGF) enhances growth of nerve fibers. Cell proliferation is regulated by (1) the amount of growth factor produced; (2) the level of expression of the growth factor receptor; (3) inhibitory signals from other growth factors; (4) the microenvironment, including the availability of oxygen and nutrients; and (5) integrin attachment to an established basement membrane. Although TGF-β induces fibroblast proliferation and collagen deposition, TGF-β inhibits proliferation of epithelial cells in many parenchymal organs.

Differentiation of Epithelia

Once epithelial cells have filled in a gap in the epithelium of a tissue or an organ, cellular differentiation is required for return of the tissue or organ to normal function. FGF-10 is a key initiator of wound repair in skin and lung epithelia. FGF-10 binds FGF-RIII, which through BMP-4 and sonic hedgehog (a signaling protein for developmental patterning) enhances expression of several transcription factors, including GATA-6, thyroid transcription factor-1 (TTF-1), hepatocyte nuclear factor-β (HNF-β), and hepatocyte factor homolog-4 (HFH-4). Each of these transcription factors enhances expression of genes, which regulate a specific function for a particular cell (E-Fig. 3-22). In the lung, for example, TTF-1 induces production of surfactant proteins A, B, and C, and HFH-4 stimulates cilia formation. Activity of these transcription factors is reduced in the presence of NFκB, an important mediator of inflammation. Therefore concurrent inflammation can impair differentiation of epithelial and parenchymal cells and thus inhibit or delay reepithelialization.

Metaplasia in Wound Repair

Some wounds do not heal properly and can turn into hypertrophic scars that impair epithelial and parenchymal cell growth. Such wounds may remain ulcerated or in parenchymal organs; the injured site may be replaced by fibroblasts and inflammatory cells rather than parenchymal cells. In either case, epithelial and parenchymal stem cells may continually attempt to cover or fill wound defects. With time, these cells may convert to another cell or tissue type. For example, regions of the lung constantly exposed to smoke can change from pseudostratified epithelium to stratified squamous epithelium, or regions of lower esophagus continually exposed to gastric acidity can undergo metaplasia into squamous cells. Osseous and chondroid metaplasia can occur in persistent wounds. In general, cells that undergo metaplasia have either (1) enhanced expression of an altered set of transcription factors and/or (2) decreased expression of transcription factors generally active for the affected tissue. The result is conversion of the cell's phenotype into a new phenotype. Often, if the initiating stimulus is removed, cells can revert to the original phenotype.

Suggested Readings

Suggested Readings are available at www.expertconsult.com.

CHAPTER 4

Mechanisms of Microbial Infections[1]

James F. Zachary

Key Readings Index

The goal of this chapter is to provide a mechanistic overview of the key steps involved in understanding the pathogeneses of infectious diseases caused by microbes (i.e., bacteria, viruses, fungi, protozoa, and prions). Coverage is not intended to be encyclopedic; specific diseases have been selected either because they illustrate a basic mechanism or because they are of primary importance to the practice of veterinary medicine. Because the knowledge base for some veterinary diseases is limited, certain sections of this chapter are conditional and are based on (1) extrapolations from known experimental systems, (2) established mechanisms of injury covered in the basic pathology chapters of this book, and (3) assumptions anchored in the characteristics of macroscopic and microscopic lesions that arise with each disease. This chapter will also discuss and illustrate selected "especially dangerous and contagious microbes" because diseases caused by these pathogens can have catastrophic impact on livestock health and production and on the economies of affected countries. The locations in this textbook of coverage of these diseases considered by the United States Department of Agriculture (USDA)/Animal and Plant Health Inspection Service (APHIS) and the World Organisation for Animal Health (OIE) as "Foreign Animal Diseases" or "OIE Reportable Diseases," respectively, are listed in E-Table 4-1.

Chronologic Sequence of Steps in Microbial Diseases

The following is a list in chronological order of the "typical" sequence of steps[2] leading to disease caused by microbes (Fig. 4-1):

1. Acquire access to a portal of entry
2. Encounter "targets" in mucosae, mucocutaneous junctions, or skin such as epithelial cells, tissue-associated leukocytes, or tissue-associated substances like mucus
3. Colonize targets to sustain and/or amplify the encounter[3] or cross the barrier system formed by mucosae, mucocutaneous junctions, or skin to gain access to targets located locally in the lamina propria, submucosa, or dermis/subcutis

[1]For a glossary of abbreviations and terms used in this chapter see E-Glossary 4-1.

[2]Depending on the microbe, only the first two or three steps may be required to cause a specific disease.

[3]Some microbes do not spread beyond cells encountered at portals of entry because these cells are their "final" target cells within mucosae, mucocutaneous junctions, or skin.

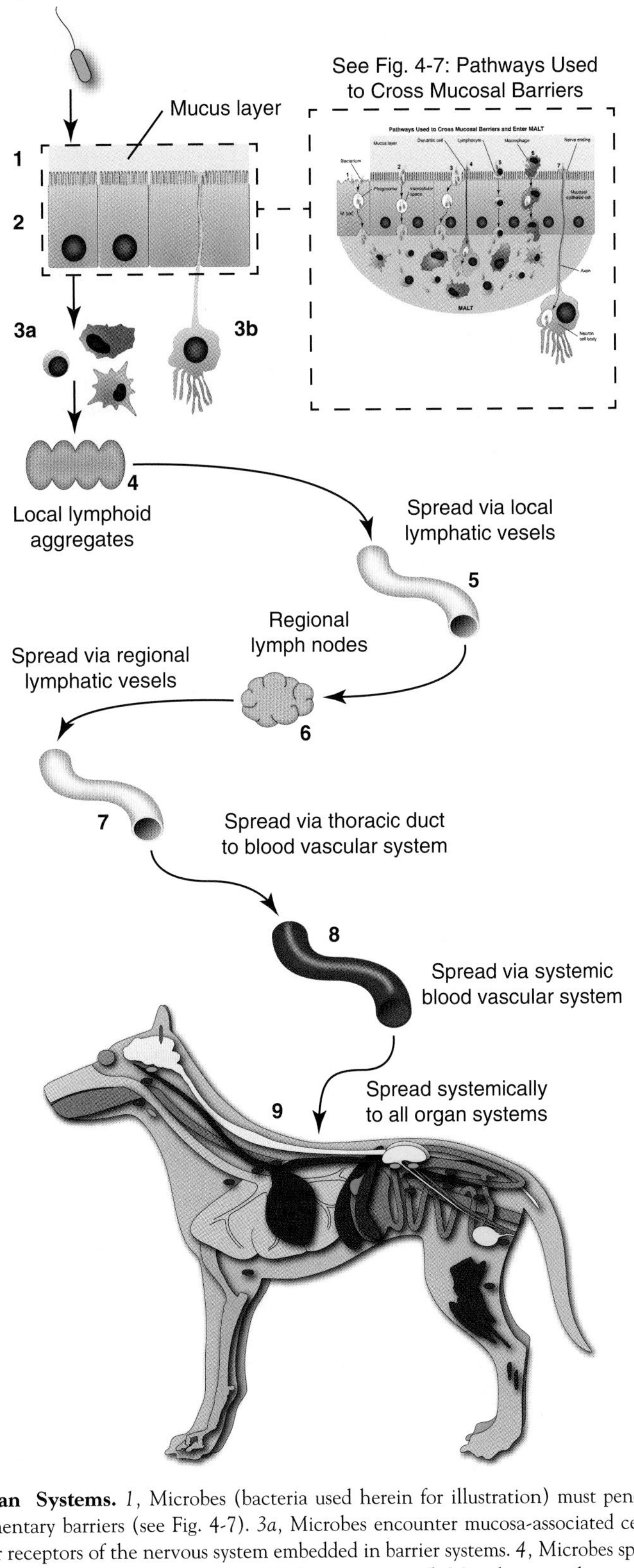

Figure 4-1 **Spread of Microbes to Organ Systems.** *1*, Microbes (bacteria used herein for illustration) must penetrate the mucus layer if present. *2*, Microbes cross mucosal, serosal, or integumentary barriers (see Fig. 4-7). *3a*, Microbes encounter mucosa-associated cells (e.g., lymphocytes, macrophages, and dendritic cells). *3b*, Microbes encounter receptors of the nervous system embedded in barrier systems. *4*, Microbes spread locally to lymphoid tissues (e.g., mucosa-associated lymphoid tissue [MALT] such as tonsils, Peyer's patches) in barrier system. *5*, Microbes spread regionally in afferent lymphatic vessels. *6*, Microbes encounter cells in regional lymph nodes. *7*, Microbes spread systemically in efferent lymphatic vessels to the thoracic duct and anterior vena cava. *8*, Microbes spread systemically in the blood vascular system. *9*, Microbes encounter target cells in systemic organ systems. (Courtesy Dr. J.F. Zachary, College of Veterinary Medicine, University of Illinois.)

4. Spread locally in the extracellular matrix (ECM) to encounter and colonize new populations of target cells, including lymphocytes, macrophages (monocytes), and dendritic cells, as well as blood and lymphatic vessels and their circulating cells
5. Enter blood and/or lymphatic vessels
   a. Travel inside lymphocytes, macrophages (monocytes), or dendritic cells within these vessels protected from the animal's defense mechanisms[4]
   b. Travel as "cell-free" microbes (i.e., not within or associated with a cell) within these vessels
6. Spread to regional lymph nodes and/or then systemically within the blood vascular system to encounter, colonize, and invade new populations of target cells that are unique to a specific organ system
7. Cause dysfunction and/or lysis of target cells and disease

These steps and thus the ability of microbes to cause disease (pathogenicity) are controlled by "virulence factors" expressed by their genes. The acquisition of new and/or more "virulent" genes through recombination and/or natural selection of mutated genes allows microbes to (1) complete one or more of the listed steps more rapidly and/or efficiently, (2) evade or reduce the effects of an animal's defense mechanisms, and/or (3) develop resistance to specific antibiotics. These outcomes may result in greater cell and tissue injury (and thus disease) within a targeted organ system of an individual animal or greater pathogenicity of a disease within a herd. Gene recombination also appears to account in part for "breakouts" of diseases thought to be contained by vaccination programs in farm and urban settings and, as an example, was also used as the scientific premise for the plot of the movie *Contagion*.

Portals of Entry

The portals of entry for microbes are the alimentary, respiratory, urogenital, and integumentary systems and the ear and eye (Fig. 4-2; Essential Concept 4-1). Microbes gain access to these portals via ingestion (alimentary system), inhalation (respiratory system), ascending entry (urogenital system), penetration (integumentary system, eye), and direct contact (integumentary system, ear, and eye). Following the initial entry, microbes may then gain access to (1) broader expanses of mucosa via normal physiologic processes such as ingestion (swallowing, peristalsis), inhalation (centrifugal forces, turbulence), ascension (reflux pressures, simple brownian movement [i.e., urogenital tract]), or direct contact (blink reflex, lacrimation) or to (2) deeper (and/or broader) expanses of skin and mucocutaneous junctions via traumatically induced abrasions or by penetration caused by insect bites or scratch and bite wound as examples.

[4]Some microbes enter nerve endings at portals of entry to gain access to the peripheral nervous system (PNS) and central nervous system (CNS).

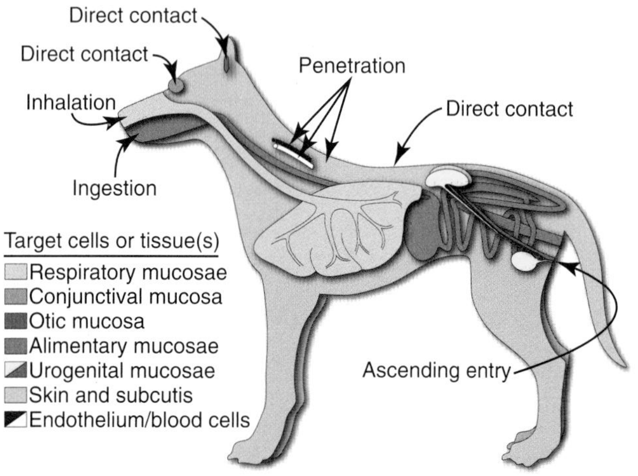

Figure 4-2 Portals of Entry. Microbes enter the body through ingestion, inhalation, direct contact, cutaneous penetration, and ascending infection and then encounter epithelial cells, macrophages, dendritic cells, and lymphocytes of barriers formed by mucosae, mucocutaneous junctions, or skin. (Courtesy Dr. J.F. Zachary, College of Veterinary Medicine, University of Illinois.)

A concept central to pathogeneses of infectious diseases is the ability of microbes to reach a site in the body that has "target cells or substances" suitable for their growth and replication. They will be discussed in a later section. Additionally, a second concept central to pathogeneses of infectious diseases is the phrase "virulence factor." Because this phrase will be used extensively in subsequent sections, its meaning needs to be summarized here but will be discussed in greater detail in sections that follow. Virulence factors are molecules (and thus genes) of microbes that enable them to replicate and cause disease. They include glycoprotein, glycolipid, or other types of molecules that are present in the structure of microbes, as well as molecules derived from transcription and/or translation of the microbial genome. Some of these virulence factors are integral to the biologic structure of microbes; other factors are synthesized by microbes using the metabolic processes of the target cell as needed to replicate. These factors serve to do the following:

- **Colonize** (e.g., adhesins) target substances, cells, and/or tissues at portals of entry
- **Invade** (e.g., invasins) target substances, cells, and/or tissues at portals of entry
- **Evade** (e.g., enzymes, toxic molecules) barrier systems and defense mechanisms
- **Suppress** (e.g., enzymes, toxic molecules) innate and adaptive immune responses
- **Acquire** (e.g., siderophores) nutrition from target substances, cells, and/or tissues.

The ability of microbes to replicate and cause disease is the result of their interactions with substances, cells, and/or tissues at portals

ESSENTIAL CONCEPT 4-1 Portals of Entry

Portals of entry are the gateways used by microbes to gain access to and enter an animal's body. They include the alimentary, respiratory, and urogenital systems; the skin; and the ear and eye. The locations of initial encounters within these portals consist of the following:

1. Mucosae and mucocutaneous junctions of the oral cavity (alimentary system), nasal cavity (respiratory system), and urethral orifice (urogenital system)
2. Epidermis (also dermis and/or subcutis via penetration) of the skin (integumentary system)
3. Epidermis of the external acoustic meatus of the ear (auditory system)
4. Corneal and conjunctival epithelia of the eye (ocular system)

The cells and substances (i.e., epithelia, immune cells, nerve endings, lamina propria, extracellular matrix proteins, and mucus) at these sites of initial encounters form "barrier systems" that function as defense mechanisms to protect the animal's cells against colonization and infection by microbes.

of entry. These interactions are facilitated by virulence factors under the control of the microbial genome.

Depending on the biologic behavior of the microbe (virulence factors expressed by their genes), a portal of entry and its target cell(s) or substance(s) may be located in the following areas:

- Locally (i.e., cells and tissues initially encountered by microbes at the portal of entry)
- Regionally (i.e., neighboring cells and tissues encountered by microbes as they spread in regional lymphatic vessels and lymph nodes that drain the portal of entry)
- Systemically (i.e., cells and tissues encountered by microbes as they spread distally in the circulatory and/or lymphatic systems to other organ systems)

Management practices and physical contact often place susceptible animals in close proximity to "contagious (carrier)" animals, where microbes can be spread in water droplets, aerosols, and body fluids such as snot, sputum, urine, and feces through direct contact, grooming, licking, scratch and bite wounds, sneezing, and other physiologic body processes. Except for contact with carrier animals, the chronologic sequence of events that leads to disease caused by microbes is not a random event. These events are well designed (virulence factors) and serve to colonize cells and tissues by inhibiting, altering, or evading defense mechanisms and barrier systems (see later section) that protect animals against infectious diseases.

Within each portal of entry, numerous sites (along the length of the entire system) contain potential target cells for "initial encounters" with microbes. Which target cells and what location in the portal of entry are colonized by what microbe depends upon the genes (virulence factors—see later section) of the microbe and the availability of target cells with appropriate substrates and/or receptors for the microbe and its microbial products. As an example, the alimentary system has diseases that occur in the oral cavity, tonsils, esophagus, stomach, small intestine, cecum, and large intestine. Therefore some microbes must travel within the alimentary system, often for a great distance, to reach their "initial encounter" target cells. Swine dysentery (*Brachyspira hyodysenteriae*) is a bacterial disease that colonizes the mucus layer and goblet cells of the colon and cecum. The microbe's portal of entry is the alimentary system, but its primary target cells are in distal segments of the system and therefore the microbe must travel a great length to reach them.

When microbes initially encounter cells and tissues at portals of entry, colonization (infection) depends on creating an initial "beachhead" to establish, sustain, amplify, and if needed spread the microbe. In these beachheads, some microbes attach to, enter, and replicate on or within mucosal, mucocutaneous, and cutaneous epithelial cells, whereas others pass through via endocytosis (phagocytosis) or between cells within intercellular junctions. In other cases, they encounter mucosa-associated leukocytes and dendritic cells, and via phagocytosis (or endocytosis) they are carried across the mucosa or skin. Through one of these mechanisms, microbes reach the basal side of epithelial cells and then encounter other mucosal, mucocutaneous, and cutaneous cells and tissues, including different tissue macrophages, lymphocytes, and dendritic cells, ECM, and nerve endings where they may again replicate to sustain, amplify, and/or spread the microbe. It is from these beachheads that microbes then spread locally (submucosa and dermis and associated lymphoid tissues), regionally (lymph nodes), and/or systemically (organ systems) to other target cells and cause disease.

Most commonly, the initial beachhead is established in mucosae or skin:

Mucosae (also mucocutaneous junctions)

- Alimentary system (oral cavity, oral pharynx, esophagus, stomach, small and large intestines [see Chapter 7])
- Respiratory system (nasal cavity, nasal pharynx, conductive component [see Chapter 9])
- Lower urinary system (urethra, bladder, ureters [see Chapter 11])
- Reproductive systems (reproductive tracts [see Chapters 18 and 19])
- Ear (external acoustic meatus [see Chapter 20])
- Eye (cornea, conjunctiva [see Chapter 21])

Skin (also mucocutaneous junctions)

- Epidermis/dermis, endothelial cells, blood and lymphatic vessels (see Chapters 10, 13, and 17)
- Mucocutaneous junctions, endothelial cells, blood and lymphatic vessels (see Chapters 7, 9, 10, 13, and 17)
- Subcutaneous ECM and immune system cells such as macrophages, lymphocytes, and dendritic cells (see Chapters 3, 5, 13 and 17)
- Subcutaneous muscle cells, endothelial cells, blood and lymphatic vessels (see Chapters 10, 13, 15, and 17)

Mucosae of the alimentary and respiratory systems are covered by a protective mucus gel secreted by goblet cells that forms a barrier system against colonization by microbes. This important barrier is discussed in more detail in a later section and in the following sections covering the alimentary and respiratory systems.

Alimentary System (Ingestion)

Microbes enter the alimentary system (see Chapter 7) through ingestion and gain access to mucosae, most commonly tonsillar epithelium, villus epithelium, crypt epithelium, and epithelium containing microfold cells (M cells) overlying Peyer's patches by chewing, swallowing, and peristalsis. They are trapped in the mucus layer of mucosae of the oral pharynx and intestines and must penetrate this layer to reach targets such as epithelial cells, macrophages, and dendritic cells. M cells of the small intestinal mucosa lack a mucus covering and therefore offer a unique portal to enter the alimentary system (see later section on Target Cells). Mucus in the alimentary system is produced by goblet cells distributed among mucosal epithelial cells in the villi and crypts where it covers and protects microvilli. The mucus layer is a (1) physical and (2) biologic barrier protecting the intestine against microbes via (1) its thickness and viscosity, (2) binding to bacterial adhesins, (3) serving as a reservoir for immunoglobulin A (IgA) and lysozyme, and (4) acting as a free radical scavenger. Additionally, the mucus layer is a favorable habitat for beneficial and competitive enteric microflora.

Generally there are more goblet cells in the large intestine than in the small intestine, more in crypts than in villi, and more in the ileum than in the jejunum or duodenum. It appears that mucus covers all intestinal epithelial surfaces to varying degrees of thickness and viscosity and is composed of an inner gel layer and an outer soluble layer. The mucus layer is thickest in the colon (≈830 μm) and thinnest in the jejunum (≈123 μm). It is less prominent over absorptive enterocytes with microvilli when compared to crypt enterocytes. A mucus layer does not cover M cells; therefore microbes can readily interact with their cell membranes. Once entrapped in the mucus layer, microbes must then penetrate it to gain access to target cells for infection. Additionally, microbes also encounter mucosal fluids, such as gastric acid, mucins, secretions such as lysozyme, and humoral mediators such as immunoglobulins, and must also compete with normal microflora for resources and for receptors expressed on target cells.

Mucosa-associated lymphoid tissue (MALT) is a general term used to categorize lymphoid nodules located in mucosae and submucosae of many organ systems. MALTs are important defense mechanisms of mucosae and are discussed in greater detail later. In the

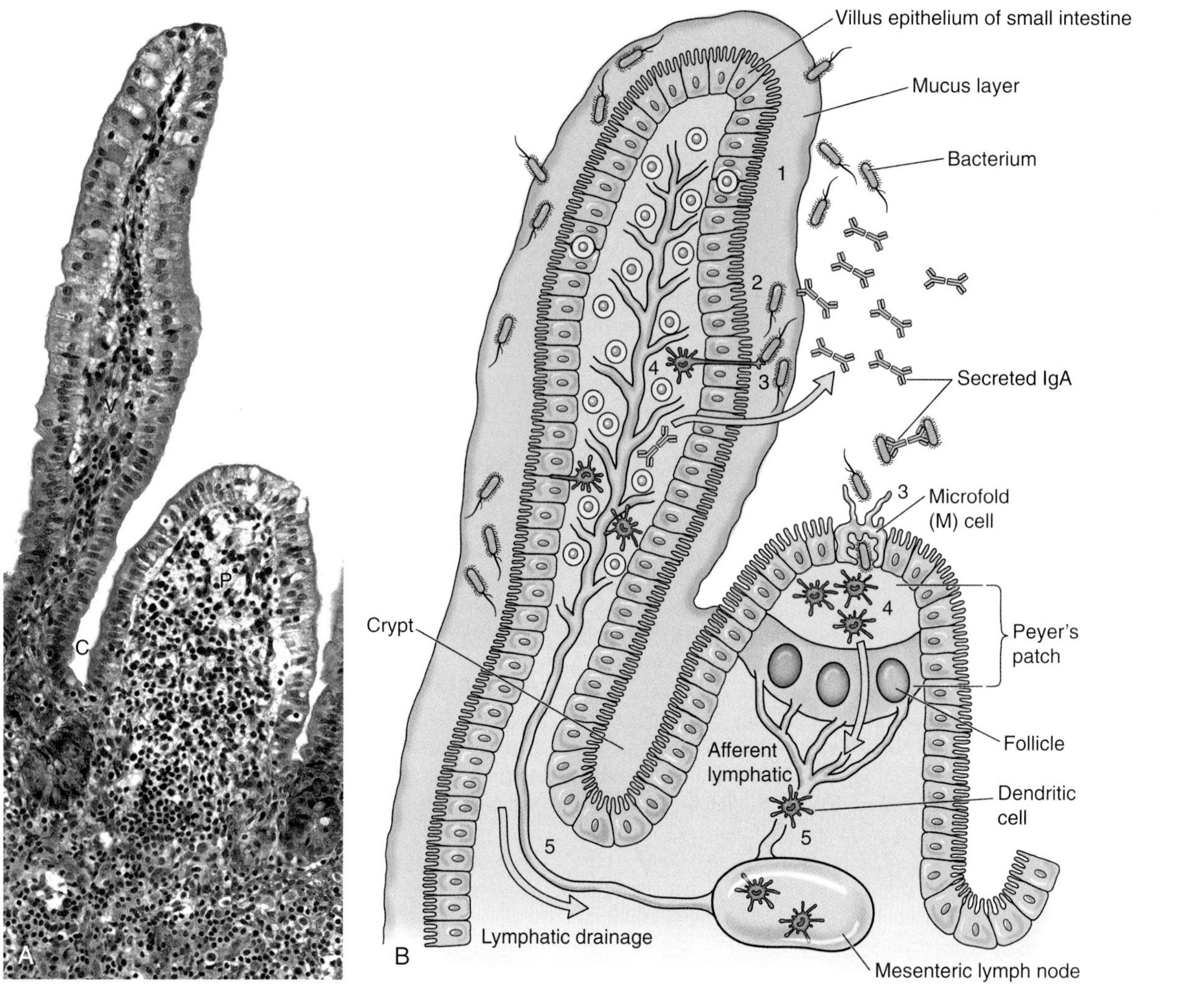

Figure 4-3 Microbial Interactions with a Barrier System: Intestinal Mucosa. A, Mucosa that cover intestinal villi *(V)* and Peyer's patches *(P)* and line crypts *(C)* form a barrier system that attempts to prevent the spread of microbes into the underlying lamina propria. H&E stain. **B,** Schematic diagram of the responses of bacteria (or viruses) trapped in the mucus layer *(1)*. Bacterial proteins (virulence factors) act to allow them to penetrate the mucus layer and come into contact with the mucosal epithelium *(2)*. Immunoglobulin (IgA) secreted by mature plasma cells in the lamina propria passes through mucosal epithelial cells into the lumen and can act as an "opsonizing" defense mechanism, thus preventing infection. Bacteria then interact with mucosal epithelial cells, dendritic cells, or microfold cells (M cells) *(3)*. They then encounter lymphoid cells in the lamina propria or Peyer's patches *(4)* and spread in lymphocytes or as free virus in lymph from this location via afferent lymphatic vessels to regional lymph nodes *(5)*. Note the absence of a mucus layer over M cells and follicle-associated epithelium. Also see Figure 4-7 for an example of barrier system: respiratory mucosae. (**A** courtesy Dr. J.F. Zachary, College of Veterinary Medicine, University of Illinois.)

alimentary system as an example, submucosal lymphoid nodules located in the distal jejunum and ileum that surround groups of intestinal crypts are assigned a specific name, gut-associated lymphoid tissue (GALT), but are also commonly known as Peyer's patches (Fig. 4-3). These nodules are composed of lymphocytes, macrophages, and dendritic cells. In GALT (Peyer's patches), nodules are covered by modified epithelial cells of intestinal crypts called follicle-associated epithelium (FAE) and its microfold cells (M cells). M cells are the interface between materials in the lumen of intestinal crypts and the lymphoid nodules and function to transfer antigens in the lumen of the intestine across the mucosa to dendritic cells and immune cells like macrophages and lymphocytes in the nodule. Peyer's patches (GALT) have afferent lymphatic vessels that drain to regional mesenteric lymph nodes. Cells similar to M cells likely cover lymphoid nodules in most mucosae and perform a similar function at the luminal interface.

Respiratory System (Inhalation)

In the respiratory system (see Chapter 9), microbes are inhaled through the nostrils (see Fig. 4-2) and are deposited on mucosae of the nasal turbinates, nasal pharynx, and/or the conductive system (trachea, bronchi) based on physical properties of the agent such as size, shape, weight, and electrostatic charge (Fig. 4-4). Groups of microbes ranked from smallest to largest include viruses (≈5 to 300 nm [1×10^{-9} m] in diameter), prions (≈16 nm in diameter), bacteria (≈0.5 to 5 μm [1×10^{-6} m] in diameter), fungi (≈5 to 60 μm in diameter), and protozoa (≈1 to 300 μm in diameter). Although it is convenient to compare microbes based on size, rarely are they inhaled as free organisms. Most commonly they are enclosed in fomites (i.e., inanimate objects or substances capable of carrying microbes) such as dust particles, soil, septum, or body fluids. Thus the physical properties of infectious fomites (i.e., fomites containing microbes) determine where they are deposited on mucosal surfaces of the respiratory system and cause disease. When inhaled, larger fomites, such as those containing bacteria and fungi, are deposited and trapped in the nasal turbinates, whereas in a gradient of descending size, smaller ones are able to reach the pharynx, larynx, trachea, and bronchi before they are deposited and trapped in mucosae. The nasal cavity and turbinates trap 70% to 80% of particulate matter approximately 3 to 5 μm or greater in diameter and 60% of particulate matter 2 μm or greater but cannot trap particles with sizes below 1 μm in diameter. In a normal functioning respiratory system, only fomites of approximately 1 μm or less in diameter, such as viruses and some bacteria, can be inhaled into bronchioles, alveolar ducts, and alveoli, which are the oxygen–carbon dioxide (O_2-CO_2) exchange portion of the respiratory system.

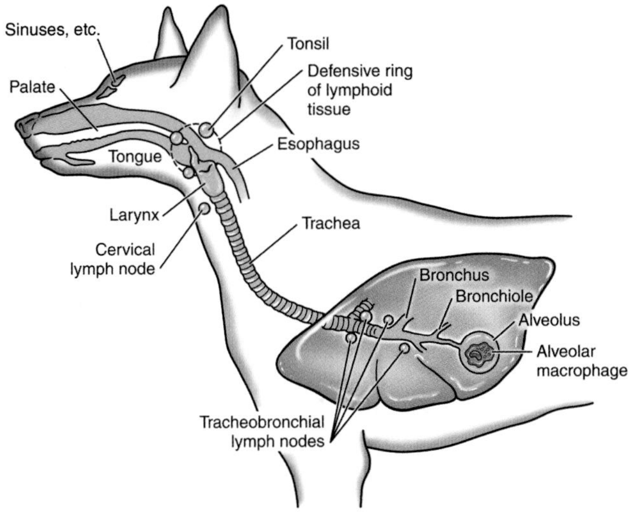

Figure 4-4 Deposition of Microbes. Microbes inhaled through the nostrils are deposited on mucosa of the nasal turbinates, nasal pharynx, and/or the conductive system of the respiratory tract. The site of deposition depends on the physical properties of the agent such as size, shape, weight, and electrostatic charge.

When infectious fomites are inhaled, they first encounter the nasal turbinates. The movement of air through the turbinates causes centrifugal turbulence that forces them against mucosae, where they are trapped in the overlying mucus layer for removal by the mucociliary apparatus. If the size of fomites allows them to pass through the turbinates and be carried to the pharynx, larynx, trachea, or bronchi, inertial turbulence forces fomites against airway mucosae, where they are trapped in the mucus layer for removal. Inertial turbulence occurs when a laminar stream of airflow is disrupted by a septum within the conductive portion of the respiratory system when airways branch. When the flow is split by a septum, the flow rotates centrifugally on either side of the septum and forces fomites against mucosae. Depending on the species, airways can branch 23 times en route from the trachea to the alveoli. The O_2-CO_2 exchange portion of the respiratory system (the bronchioles, alveolar ducts, and alveoli) is not ciliated and has no protective mucus layer because of its gas exchange function. The outcome of these turbulence mechanisms is to trap infectious fomites in the mucus layer overlying ciliated mucosal epithelial cells. When infectious fomites are trapped in the mucus layer, they are (1) acted on by other components of the innate immune system, such as phagocytes like alveolar macrophages and neutrophils, and microbicidal molecules, such as lysozyme and immunoglobulins, and (2) removed by the mucociliary apparatus (see Chapter 9).

The mucociliary apparatus is composed of the mucus layer and ciliated mucosal epithelial cells and is an important defensive mechanism in the respiratory system (Fig. 4-5). The mucus layer, produced by goblet cells and submucosal glands, is biphasic and consists of a luminal viscoelastic or gel layer used to trap infectious fomites and a serous inner layer in which the cilia of ciliated mucosal epithelial cells beat. The tips of the cilia just slightly enter the gel layer and their beating moves the gel and fomites. In the nasal cavity and sinuses, cilia move mucus and debris downward toward the pharynx for swallowing; in the conductive portion of the respiratory system, cilia move mucus and debris upward toward the pharynx for swallowing. The directionality of mucous flow is determined by the rhythmic unidirectional beating pattern of the cilia. If the mucus layer and/or the mucociliary apparatus are dysfunctional, gravity

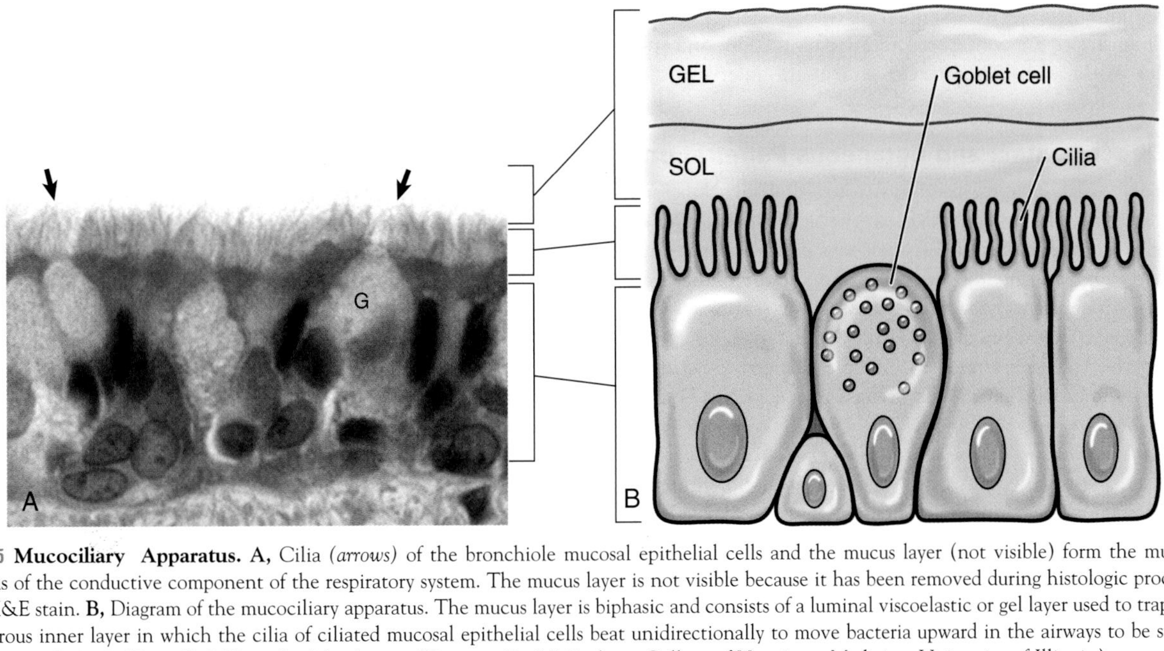

Figure 4-5 Mucociliary Apparatus. A, Cilia *(arrows)* of the bronchiole mucosal epithelial cells and the mucus layer (not visible) form the mucociliary apparatus of the conductive component of the respiratory system. The mucus layer is not visible because it has been removed during histologic processing of tissue. H&E stain. **B,** Diagram of the mucociliary apparatus. The mucus layer is biphasic and consists of a luminal viscoelastic or gel layer used to trap bacteria and a serous inner layer in which the cilia of ciliated mucosal epithelial cells beat unidirectionally to move bacteria upward in the airways to be swallowed or expectorated. G, Goblet cell; *SOL*, colloidal solution. (Courtesy Dr. J.F. Zachary, College of Veterinary Medicine, University of Illinois.)

influences the deposition of infectious fomites. The conductive portion of the respiratory system has an anterior and ventral flow pattern of distribution based on the effects of gravity. Therefore injury to mucosal epithelial cells by specific microbes, such as influenza and bovine rhinotracheitis viruses, can disrupt the function of the mucociliary apparatus, thereby exacerbating an existing disease or creating an opportunity for a secondary microbial infection of the dependent lung via settling attributable to gravity that is usually prevented by this clearance mechanism. The pathogenesis of many bronchopneumonias is based on this mechanism. Swallowing of infectious microbe-infected mucus may also be a mechanism to clear certain bacteria from the conductive portion of the respiratory system; however, it provides bacteria, such as *Rhodococcus equi*, the opportunity to gain access to the alimentary system and cause disease.

Mucosa of the conductive portion of the respiratory system contain dendritic cells and alveolar and tissue macrophages that commonly migrate through the mucosa and the mucus layer during their normal patterns of leukocyte trafficking (see Chapters 5, 9, and 13). Because these cells can phagocytose and kill microbes, they serve as a primary defense mechanism against infections. However, certain microbes have virulence factors that allow them to evade killing by phagocytes and use them like a "Trojan horse" to spread the agent and infect other cells and tissues. These cells are common targets for microbes and along with mucosal epithelia serve as the initial beachhead infection before microbes spread locally often to the tonsil, regionally to lymph nodes, and systemically to other organ systems. Bronchial-associated lymphoid tissues (BALTs) are submucosal lymphoid nodules located subjacent to ciliated mucosae, usually in areas in which inertial turbulence deposits foreign material on mucosae. Nodules are composed of lymphocytes, macrophages, and dendritic cells and function much like Peyer's patches. BALTs have afferent lymphatic vessels that drain to regional tracheobronchial lymph nodes.

Urogenital System (Ascending Infection)

Microbes can enter the lower urinary system and reproductive systems and encounter mucosae via ascending infection from coitus or the use of contaminated instruments, insemination straws, or semen. Traumatic injury of mucosae resulting in abrasions or penetrating wounds increases the likelihood of colonization by microbes. The mechanisms of encounter, colonization, infection, and spread are similar to those discussed earlier and in the later section on Pathways of Spread.

Skin (Direct Contact and Cutaneous Penetration)

For simplicity, this chapter uses the word "skin" in discussions. However, it should be remembered that the skin consists of epidermis, dermis, adnexa (hair follicles, sebaceous glands, sweat glands), and subcutis. Different microbes may use one or more of these components as portals of entry and will be discussed in sections covering specific diseases. The skin is a (1) thick and tenacious physical (especially the epidermis) and (2) biologic barrier protecting the body against microbes via (1) its dryness and acidity, (2) sebum (oils), and (3) normal bacterial flora, which compete against microbes for resources and for receptors expressed on target cells. Microbes encounter the skin (also mucocutaneous junctions) via direct contact and the dermis and subcutaneous tissues (see Chapter 17) via penetration through abrasions, scratches, and bite wounds or through bites (proboscis) of insect vectors like mosquitoes that spread the agent into subcutaneous tissues such as muscle, blood and lymphatic vessels, and ECM and connective tissue. In these tissues, microbes encounter a limited range of target cells such as epithelial cells in the skin, dendritic cells (Langerhans cells), tissue macrophages, nerve endings, endothelial cells of the vascular and lymphatic systems, and connective tissues and muscle of the dermis and subcutis. Microbes may also be deposited directly in the blood vascular system via penetration of a capillary, venule, or lymphatic vessel by an insect proboscis. Additionally in ECM of these tissues, microbes encounter body fluids, such as blood and plasma proteins, that serve as resources for survival, infection, and replication. The mechanisms of encounter, colonization, infection, and spread are similar to those discussed earlier and in the later section on Pathways of Spread.

Ear and Eye (Direct Contact and Cutaneous Penetration)

Microbes encounter the eye via direct contact with the cornea and conjunctiva (also lacrimal duct via its connection with the conjunctiva) and occasionally penetration, whereas they encounter the ear via direct contact with the external acoustic meatus. The mechanisms of encounter, colonization, infection, and spread are similar to those discussed earlier and in the later section on Pathways of Spread.

Target Cells and Substances

Microbes commonly colonize and injure specific populations of cells called "target cells" (and/or the biologic substances they synthesize and release into their surroundings) that are unique to a specific organ system (e.g., ciliated epithelial cells in the respiratory system) or to a cell lineage (e.g., M cells in the alimentary system) (Fig. 4-6; Essential Concept 4-2). The specific cells and substances used as targets by microbes are often based on ligand-receptor interactions in which proteins (ligands) expressed on the surface of microbes bind to receptors on membranes of target cells; mucus associated with these cells; vascularized ECM enclosing these cells; or macrophages, lymphocytes, and dendritic cells supporting these cells. Receptors expressed on target cells are usually those involved in normal function of cells and as examples may include receptors for complement, phospholipids, and carbohydrates. Once the proteins are bound to receptors, a sequence of steps facilitated by virulence factors is initiated that results in the colonization of the surface of these cells or invasion of the cells often through endocytosis/phagocytosis. The microbe then establishes control of the normal metabolic systems of these cells and uses them or their resources to replicate in and/or spread to other cells and/or organ systems. The outcome of this process is usually dysfunction and/or lysis of infected cells and thus clinical disease, and injury of specific targeted populations of cells in organ systems is often reflected in the results of serum biochemical analyses (e.g., elevated liver enzyme concentrations) and hematologic evaluations (e.g., leukopenia).

Target cells that are exploited by microbes can be placed into three functional groups:

- Target cells initially encountered at the portals of entry.
- Target cells used to spread microbes locally, regionally, or systemically.
- Target cells located systemically within other organ systems.

Microbes may use cells in one, some, or all of these groups to successfully complete their life cycles. As a general rule, target cells initially encountered at portals of entry (mucosae, mucocutaneous junctions, and skin) tend to be epithelial cells and mucosa-associated macrophages (monocytes), lymphocytes, dendritic cells, and nerve endings. Target cells used to spread microbes locally, regionally, or systemically tend to be macrophages (monocytes), lymphocytes, or dendritic cells that migrate through the body and encounter other

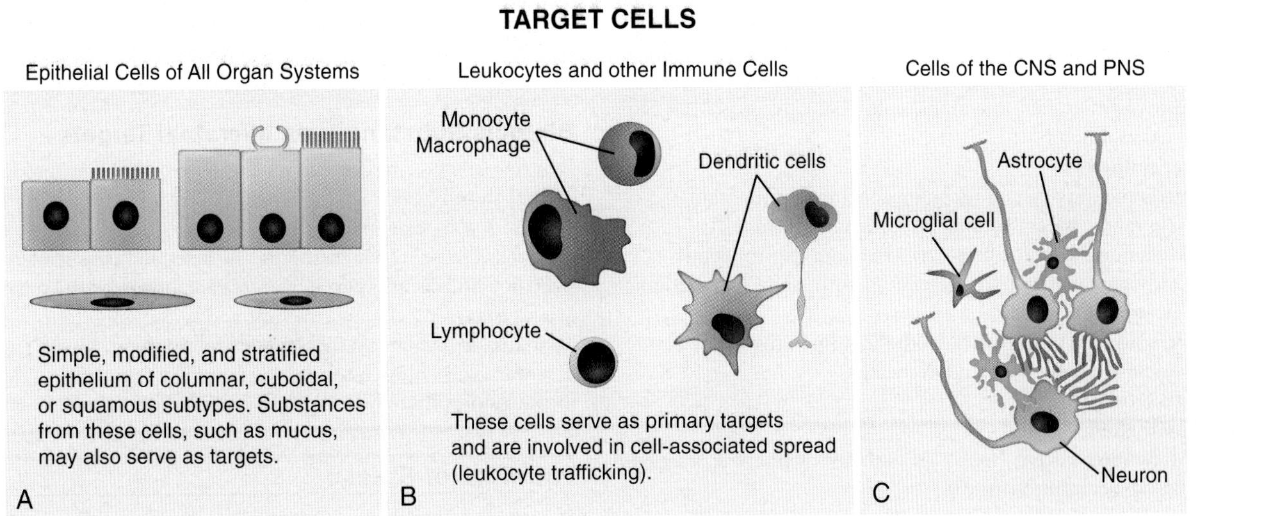
TARGET CELLS
Epithelial Cells of All Organ Systems
Simple, modified, and stratified epithelium of columnar, cuboidal, or squamous subtypes. Substances from these cells, such as mucus, may also serve as targets.
A
Leukocytes and other Immune Cells
Monocyte Macrophage
Dendritic cells
Lymphocyte
These cells serve as primary targets and are involved in cell-associated spread (leukocyte trafficking).
B
Cells of the CNS and PNS
Astrocyte
Microglial cell
Neuron
C

Figure 4-6 **Target Cells. A,** Target cells forming "barrier systems." Target cells encountered at portals of entry (i.e., barrier systems) and within organ systems of the body following systemic spread include simple or stratified epithelium (squamous, cuboidal, or columnar types). These cells cover and line surfaces (pleurae, pericardium, airways, ducts), form the parenchyma of organ systems such as hepatocytes in the liver, line organs (endothelium, synovium), and form glands (endocrine, exocrine [e.g., adrenal, pancreas]). Additionally, biologic substances, such as mucus, synthesized and released from these cells into their surroundings can be used by some microbes as target substances (not shown in figure). **B,** Target cells used to spread microbes. Target cells used by microbes to spread via leukocyte trafficking, regionally or systemically, to other organ systems include cells of the monocyte-macrophage system, lymphocytes, and dendritic cells. These cells may also be primary target cells for microbes in addition to being used as cells to travel in throughout the body. **C,** Target cells unique to the nervous system. Some microbes can enter nerve endings of the peripheral nervous system (PNS) (cranial and spinal nerves) in mucosa and dermis/subcutis at portals of entry and use retrograde and anterograde axonal transport to spread to and through neurons of the central nervous system (CNS). Other cells, including microglial cells (as part of the monocyte-macrophage system), and astrocytes can then become targets for infection. (Courtesy Dr. J.F. Zachary, College of Veterinary Medicine, University of Illinois.)

ESSENTIAL CONCEPT 4-2 Target Cells and Substances

Each kind of microbe requires a specific type of cell or substance in which to successfully replicate and complete its life cycle. Therefore the labels "target cells" and "target substances" are applied for the convenience of creating defined groups. Simple and stratified epithelial cells (squamous, cuboidal, or columnar types) are the cells most commonly used as targets by microbes at portals of entry. In organ systems these cells function as covering, lining, and glandular (including the liver) epithelia. Additionally, mucosa-associated leukocytes (lymphocytes, macrophages [monocytes], and dendritic cells) that form lymphoid aggregates and nodules (mucosa-associated lymphoid tissue [MALT]) in these organ systems can also serve as (1) "primary" target cells for diseases caused by some microbes or as (2) "secondary" targets used to spread microbes via leukocyte trafficking locally, regionally, or systemically to encounter epithelial cells (or substances) in other organ systems. Nerve endings embedded in epithelium may also be used as targets to enter the central nervous system (CNS) and peripheral nervous system (PNS). Substances, such as mucus produced by goblet cells, are often strong chemoattractants for specific types of microbes because they serve as physical matrices and chemical substrates for colonization. Colonization, invasion, and injury of target cells and/or substances are based on ligand-receptor interactions in which proteins (ligands) expressed on the surface of microbes bind to receptors on target cells or substances. Receptors on cells are usually transmembrane proteins involved in normal cell functions; receptors on substances are generally structural molecules. Once a microbe is bound, a sequence of steps is initiated that may result in colonization or invasion of cells (or substances). Thereafter the microbe may acquire control of some or all of the cell's metabolic systems, replicate, and complete its life cycle. The outcomes of successful microbial infections on target cells include cell death, directed cellular dysfunction, inflammation, structural injury, persistent infection, latent infection, cell proliferation, and malignant transformation.

organ systems. This mechanism of spread is called "leukocyte trafficking." From local sites, infected lymphocytes and macrophages spread via lymphatic vessels to regional lymph nodes, where additional cells are infected and then spread via lymphatic vessels to the thoracic duct and the circulatory system. From here, infected cells spread systemically to other organ systems in which specific target cells are infected, including lymphoid organs such as the spleen, lymph nodes, and bone marrow. Additionally, microbes can use nerve endings and fibers (that travel to and throughout all organ systems via the central nervous system [CNS] and peripheral nervous system [PNS]) to spread within the nervous system and/or systemically. Lastly, target cells located systemically within other organ systems tend to be epithelial cells, macrophages (monocytes), lymphocytes, dendritic cells, and/or neural cells. In some diseases, leukocyte trafficking ultimately returns the microbe back to mucosae, mucocutaneous junction, or skin initially encountered at the portal of entry. However, it is important to remember that the area of mucosa or skin involved in the initial beachhead encounter represents a very small percentage of the entire area of these organ systems; therefore there is always a large population of new target cells available for infection.

Epithelial Cells as Microbial Targets

Epithelial cells (and their ECM), the most common cell type used as targets by microbes, are categorized into two groups, simple epithelium (one layer of cells) or stratified epithelium (two or more layers of cells) (E-Fig. 4-1). Each group can be further subdivided into squamous, cuboidal, or columnar types based on morphologic structure (E-Table 4-2). However, for a better understanding of the mechanisms of microbial infections, epithelial cell targets can also be classified as follows:

Covering epithelium

- Integumentary system (skin, mucocutaneous junctions)
- Respiratory system (serosa: mesothelium [pleurae])[5]
- Alimentary system (serosa: mesothelium [peritoneum])[5]
- Cardiovascular system (serosa: mesothelium [pericardium/epicardium])
- Nervous system (serosa: mesothelium [meninges])
- Muscle (synovium of tendon sheaths)
- Eye (cornea)

Lining epithelium

- Alimentary system (mucosae: oral cavity, pharynx, esophagus, stomach, intestines)
- Respiratory system (mucosae: nasal cavity, pharynx, larynx, trachea, bronchi, lungs)
- Urinary system (mucosae: urethra, bladder, ureter, pelvis, tubules)
- Cardiovascular system (endothelium [blood vessels, endocardium, lymphatic vessels])[5]
- Reproductive system (mucosae: tracts)
- Skeletal system (synovium of joint capsules)[5]
- Eye (mucosa: conjunctiva)
- Ear (mucosa: external acoustic meatus)

Glandular epithelium

- Endocrine system (endocrine glands)
- Hepatobiliary system (liver [hepatic plates forming lobules], gallbladder)
- Alimentary system (exocrine [salivary] glands)
- Reproductive system (gonads, exocrine glands)

Mucosa-Associated Lymphoid Tissues as Microbial Targets

MALT is a general term used to categorize lymphoid nodules composed of lymphocytes, macrophages, and dendritic cells that are located in mucosae and submucosae of many organ systems. Each, some, or all of these cells types can serve as target cells for specific diseases. In some cases, these cells are the primary targets in which the microbe successfully completes its life cycle, whereas in other cases they serve as target cells used to spread microbes (leukocyte trafficking [see later section]) locally, regionally, or systemically and encounter cells and tissues in other organ systems. More specifically, MALT includes BALT, conjunctiva-associated lymphoid tissue (CALT), nose-associated lymphoid tissue (NALT), larynx-associated lymphoid tissue (LALT), and auditory tube–associated lymphatic tissue (ATALT), as well as lymphoid nodules (unnamed) in the genital tract, mammary gland, and urinary bladder mucosa. In GALT, nodules are covered by modified epithelial cells of intestinal crypts called microfold cells (M cells). M cells are the interface between materials in the lumen of intestinal crypts and the lymphoid nodules and function to transfer antigens in the lumen of the intestine across the mucosa to dendritic cells and immune cells like macrophages and lymphocytes in the nodule. Cells similar to M cells likely cover lymphoid nodules in most mucosae and perform a similar function at the luminal interface. MALT-like arrangements with similar functions to those in mucosae also exist in the skin.

[5]Endothelium and mesothelium (both derived from mesoderm) are considered epithelia by histologists, but in pathology such cell types are not considered true epithelium in the area of tumor diagnostics and thus are classified as sarcomas, not carcinomas.

Biologic Substances as Microbial Targets

In a few diseases, targets for infection are substances produced by epithelial cells, such as mucus by goblet cells of the alimentary system. As an example, swine dysentery (*B. hyodysenteriae*) is a bacterial disease in which the mucus layer and thus goblet cells of the colon and cecum (portal of entry) are targets for the spirochetes. Mucus is a strong chemoattractant and is also important as a physical matrix and chemical substrate for colonization. Mucus and swine dysentery will be discussed in several of the following sections and in the section that covers specific bacterial diseases.

Pathways of Spread

Microbes exploit a limited number of pathways to: (1) colonize cells, tissues, and/or substances at the site of initial encounter at the portal of entry and cause disease or (2) cross a "barrier system" such as mucosae of the alimentary or respiratory systems to reach and colonize cells, tissues, and/or substances located locally in mucosae and cause disease or to spread regionally or systemically to cells, tissues, and/or substances located in other organ systems and cause disease (Essential Concept 4-3; E-Figs. 4-2 and 4-3). Crossing a mucosal (or cutaneous) barrier system is an important step in the process, and microbes may use one or more of seven distinct mechanisms shown in Fig. 4-7 to accomplish this task:

1. Endosomes and transcytosis via M cells
2. Intercellular junctions
3. Endosomes and transcytosis via other types of epithelial cells (ciliated, microvillus border)
4. Mucosa-associated dendritic cells
5. Migrating mucosa-associated lymphocytes

ESSENTIAL CONCEPT 4-3 Pathways of Spread

Pathways of spread are the routes used by microbes to reach target cells or substances they require to replicate and complete their life cycles. For some microbes these pathways may begin and end at the portal of entry, whereas for others they may end in a distant organ system. In general, most pathways of spread follow this pattern: portal of initial encounter → cross a barrier system → encounter mucosa-associated leukocytes → spread to local lymphoid aggregates → afferent lymphatic vessels → regional lymph nodes → efferent lymphatic vessels → thoracic duct and anterior vena cava → blood vascular system → target cell in a systemic organ system.[9] Along these pathways, microbes encounter a variety of barrier systems, defense mechanisms, and cells and/or substances. As a result, they have acquired virulence factors that allow them to cross barrier systems (see later); evade defense mechanisms such as those involved in phagocytosis and microbial killing; and colonize and invade cells and/or substances via ligand-receptor interactions at the site of the initial encounter, at sites distant from portals of entry along pathways of spread, and in a targeted organ system. Mechanisms used to cross barrier systems include passage in M cells, microbial motility through intercellular junctions, passage through cells via endosomes (transcytosis), leukocyte trafficking, passage in blood and lymphatic vascular systems as cell-free microbes, and passage in nerve endings and processes.[10]

[9]See text for variations and exceptions.
[10]See text and Fig. 4-7 for greater detail.

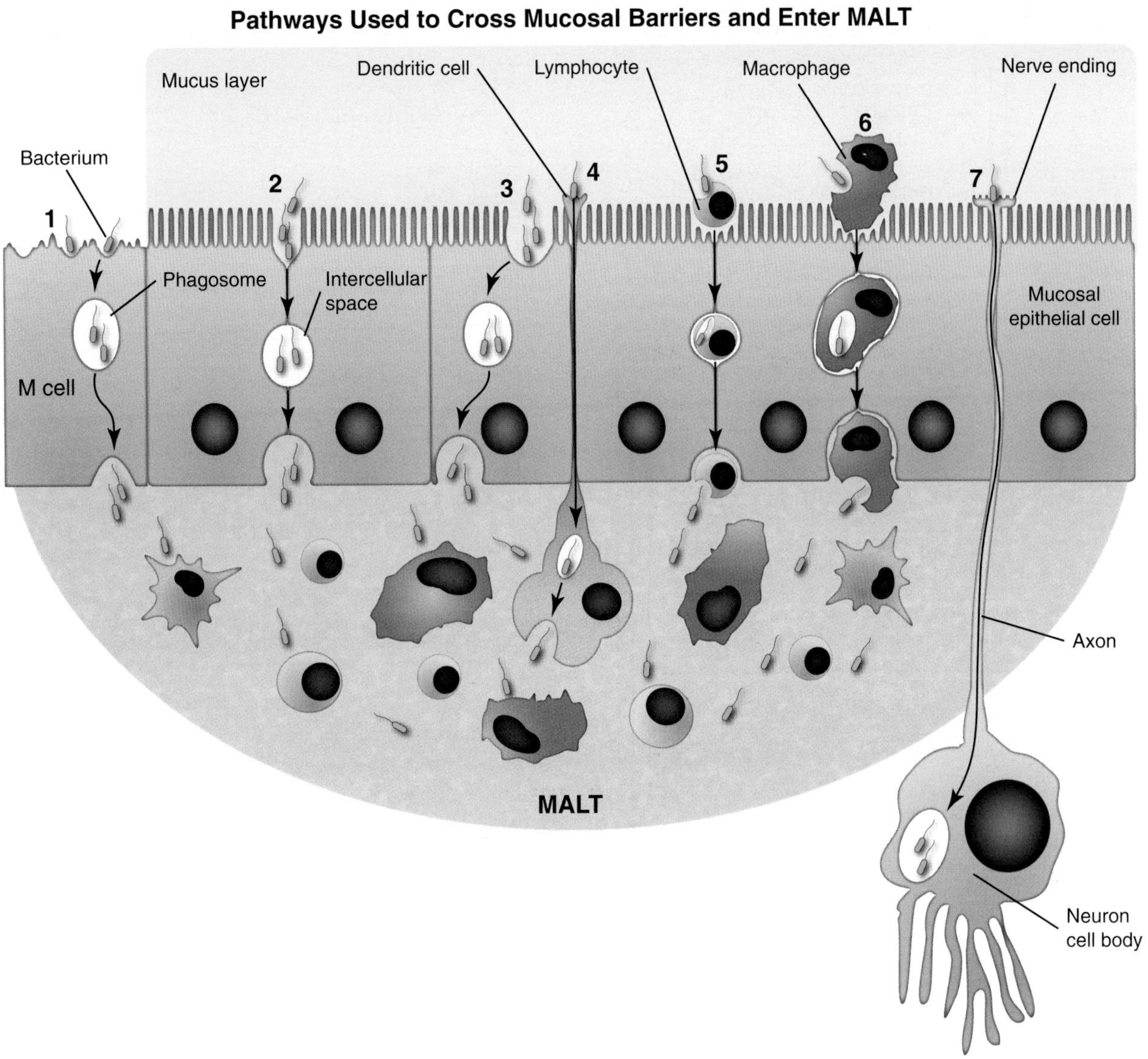

Figure 4-7 **Mechanisms Used to Cross Mucosal Barrier Systems.** *1,* Transcytosis (M cells, which lack a mucus layer). *2,* Microbial motility via intercellular junctions. *3,* Transcytosis. *4,* Processes of dendritic cells embedded in mucosae. *5,* Leukocyte trafficking (lymphocytes) via intercellular junctions. *6,* Leukocyte trafficking (monocytes or macrophages) via intercellular junctions. *7,* Nerve endings and nerve processes via axonal transport in cranial or spinal nerves. Once within MALT, microbes can interact with and/or be phagocytized by leukocytes to continue the processes of colonization and spread. Examples illustrated here are also, in general, applicable to skin and mucocutaneous junctions. Specific viruses, fungi, protozoa, or prions may use some of these mechanisms. *MALT,* Mucosa-associated lymphoid tissue; *M cell,* microfold cell. (Courtesy Dr. J.F. Zachary, College of Veterinary Medicine, University of Illinois.)

6. Migrating mucosa-associated macrophages
7. Mucosa-associated nerve endings

Transcytosis and endosomes (microvesicles) are covered in greater detail in the section on Transcytosis and Endocytosis/Exocytosis and in Chapter 1.

As examples, the pathways of spread for the alimentary and respiratory systems are shown in Fig. 4-8 and for the integumentary system (skin) in Fig. 4-9. For some microbes the mechanisms and pathways of colonization, replication, and spread occur at one location, usually restricted to mucosae or skin (also mucocutaneous junctions) at the site of the initial encounter; for others the processes involve multiple locations, including mucosae or skin at the site of the initial encounter, as well as tissues and cells located locally, regionally, and systemically. Although these latter processes occur at multiple locations, microbes have a limited number of "entry points" such as through M cells, within mucosa-associated leukocytes and dendritic cells (Trojan horse), via transcytosis (within endosomes [microvesicles]) within epithelial cells, or through nerve endings. Some motile microbes can also enter mucosae by moving directly through epithelial cells or between them through intracellular junctional complexes to spread to subjacent MALTs. Microbes use one or more pathways to reach their primary target cells or substances (i.e., cell or biologic substances in which they replicate) (see Figs. 4-1 and 4-7). These pathways and target cells and substances are discussed in greater detail later.

Mechanisms Used to Colonize Mucosae (or Biologic Substances) at Portals of Entry

Colonize Mucus (Goblet Cells)

Swine dysentery (*B. hyodysenteriae*) (see Figs. 7-171 and 7-172) is an example of a bacterial disease in which the mucus layer and thus goblet cells of the colon and cecum (portal of entry) are the primary targets for microbial colonization and replication. The encounter results in a mucohemorrhagic necrofibrinous colitis and typhlitis

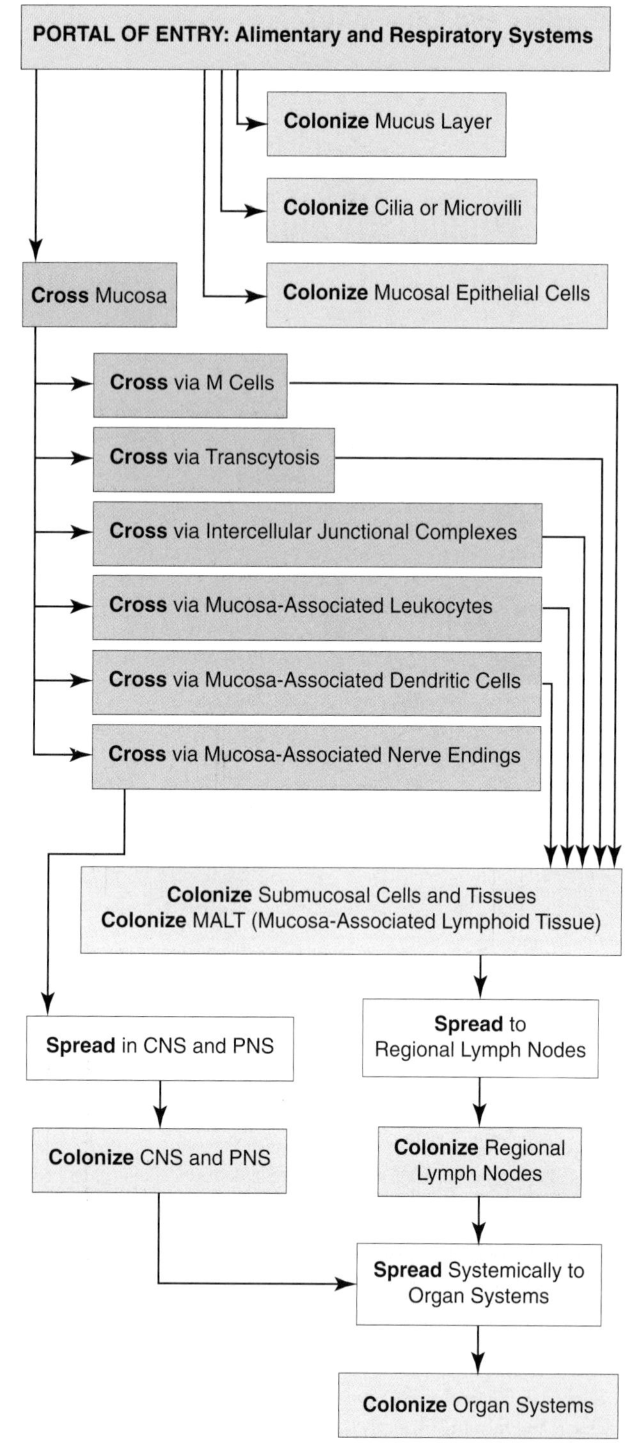

Figure 4-8 **Pathways of Spread Used by Microbes in the Alimentary and Respiratory Systems.** *CNS*, Central nervous system; *PNS*, peripheral nervous system. (Courtesy Dr. J.F. Zachary, College of Veterinary Medicine, University of Illinois.)

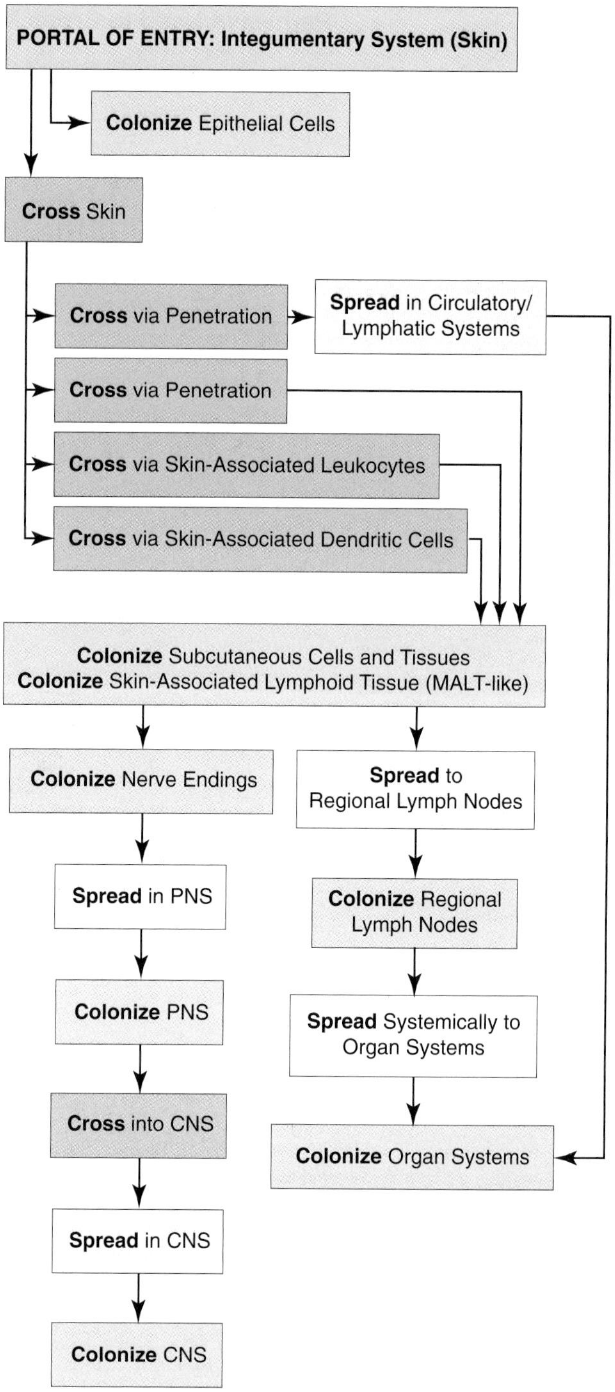

Figure 4-9 **Pathways of Spread Used by Microbes in the Integumentary System.** *CNS*, Central nervous system; *MALT*, mucosa-associated lymphoid tissue; *PNS*, peripheral nervous system. (Courtesy Dr. J.F. Zachary, College of Veterinary Medicine, University of Illinois.)

caused by bacterial hemolysins and proteases and from inflammation and its mediators and degradative enzymes. Mucus is a strong chemoattractant for spirochetes and is also important as a physical matrix and chemical substrate for colonization. This disease is discussed in greater detail in the section on Bacterial Diseases of Organ Systems; Alimentary System and the Peritoneum, Omentum, Mesentery, and Peritoneal Cavity; Disorders of Pigs; Swine Dysentery.

Colonize Cilia (or Microvilli) of Mucosal Epithelial Cells

Porcine enzootic pneumonia (*Mycoplasma hyopneumoniae*) (see Fig. 9-96 and E-Fig. 9-23) is an example of a bacterial disease in which cilia of ciliated mucosal epithelial cells in the respiratory system (or with a different bacterium the microvilli of the alimentary system) are the primary targets for microbial colonization and replication. The bacterium attaches to cilia of epithelial cells of the bronchi and bronchioles, and this interaction results in dysfunction of cilia (ciliostasis), lysis of the epithelial cells, reduced function of the mucociliary apparatus, and bronchopneumonia. Other bacteria such as *Mannheimia (Pasteurella) haemolytica* accomplish the same outcome after colonizing ciliated mucosal epithelial cells by producing toxins like neuraminidase (virulence factors) that injure and destroy the cilia and kill the ciliated epithelial cells. Porcine enzootic pneumonia is discussed in greater detail in the section on Bacterial Diseases of Organ Systems; Respiratory System, Mediastinum, and Pleurae; Disorders of Pigs; Porcine Enzootic Pneumonia (*Mycoplasma hyopneumoniae*).

Colonize the Cell (Endocytosis)

Proliferative enteritis/hemorrhagic bowel syndrome of pigs (*Lawsonia intracellularis*) (see Fig. 7-173) is an example of a bacterial disease in which the bacterium enters via endocytosis (phagocytosis) and colonizes epithelial cells of intestinal crypts located in the proliferative zone of the ileum. It resides in a phagosome within the cytoplasm but escapes from the phagosome before phagosome-lysosome fusion occurs and resides free in cell cytoplasm to then initiate the mechanism that causes cell proliferation. Proliferative enteritis/hemorrhagic bowel syndrome is discussed in greater detail in the section on Bacterial Diseases of Organ Systems; Alimentary System and the Peritoneum, Omentum, Mesentery, and Peritoneal Cavity; Disorders of Pigs; Porcine Proliferative Enteritis/Hemorrhagic Bowel Syndrome (*Lawsonia intracellularis*).

Mechanisms Used to Cross Mucosae at Portals of Entry

M Cell Entry

Postweaning multisystemic wasting syndrome (porcine circovirus type 2) (see Chapters 9 and 13) is an example of a viral disease in which the virus uses the alimentary system as its portal of entry to subsequently be physiologically transported through the system to reach the small intestine and encounter, enter, and cross the mucosa using M cells that overlie Peyer's patches (GALT). Via M cells the virus then gains access to and infects mucosa-associated lymphocytes and lymphocytes in GALT. Leukocyte trafficking spreads the virus systemically via lymphatic vessels to regional lymph nodes and then systemically through postcapillary venules or lymphatic vessels and the thoracic duct to the circulatory system to lymphocytes in the spleen, lymph nodes, and other lymphoid tissues. Postweaning multisystemic wasting syndrome (porcine circovirus type 2) is discussed in greater detail in the section on Viral Diseases of Organ Systems; Bone Marrow, Blood Cells, and Lymphatic System; Disorders of Pigs; Postweaning Multisystemic Wasting Syndrome (Porcine Circovirus Type 2, Nonenveloped DNA Virus).

Leukocyte Trojan Horse Entry

Rhodococcal pneumonia (*R. equi*) (see Fig. 9-82) is an example of a bacterial disease in which the bacterium crosses the mucosa and enters the respiratory system using leukocyte (Trojan horse) entry and subsequent trafficking. When inhaled, the bacterium is deposited in the mucus layer of mucosa of airways and then is phagocytosed by mucosa-associated macrophages (and likely mucosa-associated dendritic cells), carried via leukocyte trafficking to local lymphoid tissues, such as BALT (within lung tissue), and then to tracheobronchial lymph nodes (regional) via afferent lymphatic vessels. Rhodococcal pneumonia (*R. equi*) is discussed in greater detail in the section on Bacterial Diseases of Organ Systems; Respiratory System, Mediastinum, and Pleurae; Disorders of Horses; Rhodococcal Pneumonia (*Rhodococcus equi*).

Dendritic Cell Entry

Sheeppox and goatpox (poxviruses) (see Fig. 17-64) are examples of viral diseases in which each virus uses dendritic cells within mucosae of the respiratory and alimentary systems as portals of entry. Virus encounters oronasal mucosae via inhalation or ingestion, infects mucosa-associated dendritic cells, and then uses these cells to transfer across the mucosa into MALT and its leukocytes, including macrophages. Via leukocyte trafficking, virus spreads to regional lymph nodes, systemically to other lymph nodes, spleen, and bone marrow. Sheeppox and goatpox are discussed in greater detail in the section on Viral Diseases of Organ Systems, Integumentary System, Disorders of Ruminants (Cattle, Sheep, and Goats), Pox (Cowpox [Orthopoxvirus], Sheeppox and Goatpox [Capripoxvirus], Swinepox [Suipoxvirus], Enveloped DNA Virus).

Transcytosis Entry

Diamond skin disease of pigs (*Erysipelothrix rhusiopathiae*) (see Fig. 10-80) is an example of a bacterial disease that likely, but not fully proven, uses transcytosis entry. The bacterium likely interacts with the cell membrane at the luminal surface of the cell, enters a vesicle formed by an invagination of the membrane, crosses the interior of the cell in the vesicle, fuses with the basolateral membranes of the cell, and is then ejected from the vesicle into the tissues that surround the basolateral areas. The bacterium, a commensal organism that resides in a biofilm of the pharyngeal mucosae, replicates in sufficient numbers to colonize mucosae when pigs experience farm stress. It is spread via inhalation or ingestion to epithelia of the pharyngeal mucosae and the tonsil and to cells of MALT in susceptible pigs. The bacterium then spreads locally, regionally, and systemically via leukocyte trafficking to infect blood vascular endothelial cells of the skin and cause diamond skin disease. Diamond skin disease (*E. rhusiopathiae*) is discussed in greater detail in the section on Bacterial Diseases of Organ Systems, Integumentary System, Disorders of Pigs, Diamond Skin Disease (*Erysipelothrix rhusiopathiae*).

Direct Entry (Motility)

Leptospirosis (*Leptospira* spp.) (see Fig. 11-66) is an example of a bacterial disease that uses direct entry (motility) to cross mucosae. The bacterium is a highly motile spirochete and is able to move directly through mucosae or skin epithelial cells or between the cells via intracellular junctional complexes and reach well-vascularized ECM tissues. In ECM these spirochetes use invasive motility (a virulence factor) to penetrate endothelial cells and vascular walls of capillaries and postcapillary venules and gain access to the circulatory system and cause disease. Leptospirosis (*Leptospira* spp.) is discussed in greater detail in the section on Bacterial Diseases of Organ Systems, Urinary System, Disorders of Domestic Animals, Renal Leptospirosis (*Leptospira* spp.).

Nerve Ending Entry

Bovine herpesvirus meningoencephalitis (bovine herpesvirus 5) is an example of a viral disease that uses nerve endings located in mucosae to cross mucosae. Initially the virus is inhaled or ingested and deposited on mucosae of the oral, nasal, and pharyngeal cavities and the conductive component of the respiratory system. The virus enters nerve endings that extend onto the luminal surface of mucosae between epithelial cells. Through these nerve endings, virus enters neurons, such as the trigeminal and olfactory nerves, and spreads via retrograde axonal transport to other neurons and glial cells within the nervous system. Bovine herpesvirus meningoencephalitis is discussed in greater detail in the section on Viral Diseases of Organ Systems, Nervous System, Disorders of Ruminants

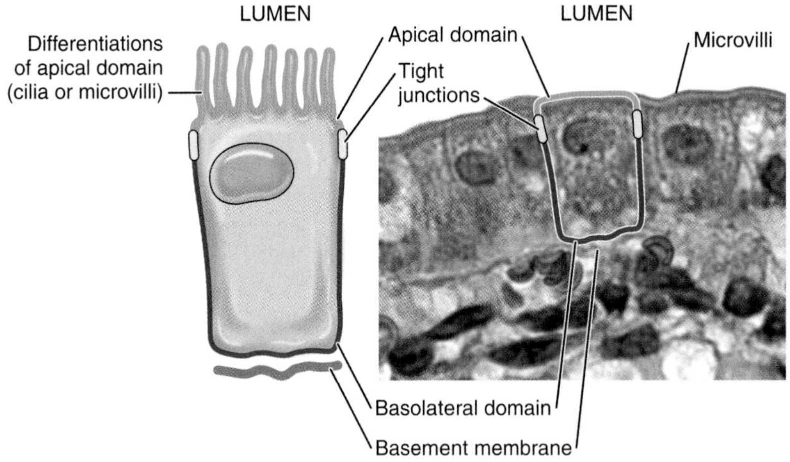

Figure 4-10 **Domains of Polarized Epithelial Cells in Mucosal Barriers.** Microbes use the apical or basolateral domains of mucosal epithelial cells to enter and exit from these cells. Apical or basolateral cell surface receptors may also facilitate entry into the cell. (Courtesy Dr. J.F. Zachary, College of Veterinary Medicine, University of Illinois.)

(Cattle, Sheep, and Goats), Bovine Herpesvirus Meningoencephalitis (Bovine Herpesvirus 5: Alphaherpesvirus, Enveloped DNA Virus).

Mechanisms of Adhesion, Colonization, Invasion, and Replication

Later in this chapter, diseases are grouped in sections under the headings Bacterial Diseases, Viral Diseases, Fungal Diseases (Mycoses), Protozoan Diseases, and Prion Diseases. At the beginning of each of these sections, the mechanisms used by microbes within each group to colonize cells and complete their life cycles are discussed and illustrated in greater detail.

Cell Polarity

In the alimentary and respiratory systems (and likely in other mucosae), the surface of an epithelial cell located above its junctional complexes and exposed to the lumen is called the *apical domain*, whereas the surface below junctional complexes on the sides and base make up the *basolateral domain* (Fig. 4-10). This relationship establishes a polarity to the cell, and it has been shown experimentally that such polarity is often reflected in the expression of different sets of cell membrane receptors that can potentially be used by microbes to attach to and enter the cells and also leave cells. As examples, parvoviruses use receptors expressed only on the basolateral surfaces to infect small intestinal crypt cells by spreading from cells located in Peyer's patches, whereas influenza viruses use receptors expressed only on apical surfaces to infect respiratory epithelial cells via the airway.

Transcytosis and Endocytosis/Exocytosis

Transcytosis is a normal function of epithelial cells, endothelial cells, and many other cell types of the body and is used to move macromolecules across cells in microvesicles (also known as endosomes) (see Chapter 1). By using specific virulence factors, microbes enter cells through a process called *receptor-mediated endocytosis*, most commonly at the apical surface, and exit the cell from the basolateral surface via a mechanism called *exocytosis* into the lamina propria and/or dermis and encounter mucosa- or dermis-associated lymphoid tissue (MALT) or other ECM tissues (see Fig. 4-7).

Systemic Spread

Systemic spread may occur (1) in a passive manner by dispersal of cell-free microbes in lymph via the lymphatic system or in plasma via the circulatory system to randomly encounter appropriate target cell(s) or (2) in an active manner through infection of mucosal or submucosal (also dermal/subcutaneous) macrophages, lymphocytes, and/or dendritic cells with dispersal of cell-associated microbes in the lymphatic or circulatory systems to randomly encounter appropriate target cell(s). This latter means of spread is called *leukocyte trafficking* (Fig. 4-11) and occurs as these cells migrate through all organ systems during their normal surveillance activities for the lymphoid (immune) system. When, during their migration, trafficking leukocytes encounter the appropriate target cell(s), a series of steps occur that allow cell-associated microbes to escape (often by lysing the trafficking cell) and then infect appropriate target cell(s) via ligand-receptor interactions (discussed later). For microbes that use leukocyte trafficking as a means of spread, the initial encounter with cells in mucosae, mucocutaneous junctions, or skin may be an initial and very limited beachhead step, where the sole purpose is to replicate microbes in sufficient numbers to infect appropriate leukocyte targets through phagocytosis or endocytosis for subsequent trafficking. An additional means of systemic spread for specific microbes is within the nervous system. Microbes can interact with nerve endings within mucosae, mucocutaneous junctions, or skin during the initial beachhead encounter, enter these nerve endings likely via endocytosis, acquire protection from the animal's defense mechanisms within the neuron, and then use retrograde and anterograde axonal transport mechanisms to be spread throughout the nervous system protected within neurons to reach their destination target cell (usually but not always located within the CNS or PNS).

Defense Mechanisms

At portals of entry, microbes run into a variety of structural, functional, physiologic, and innate defense mechanisms (Essential Concept 4-4).

Barrier Systems

Structural (Physical) Barriers

Structural barriers prevent microbes from gaining access to target cells and tissues. Although there are many important macroscopic structural barriers in the body, such as those formed by bone (calvarium, vertebral column) and meninges (dura mater) as examples, this section will focus on the microscopic structural barriers formed by mucosa, mucocutaneous junctions, and skin. Mechanisms such as trauma and penetrating wounds that allow microbes to cross

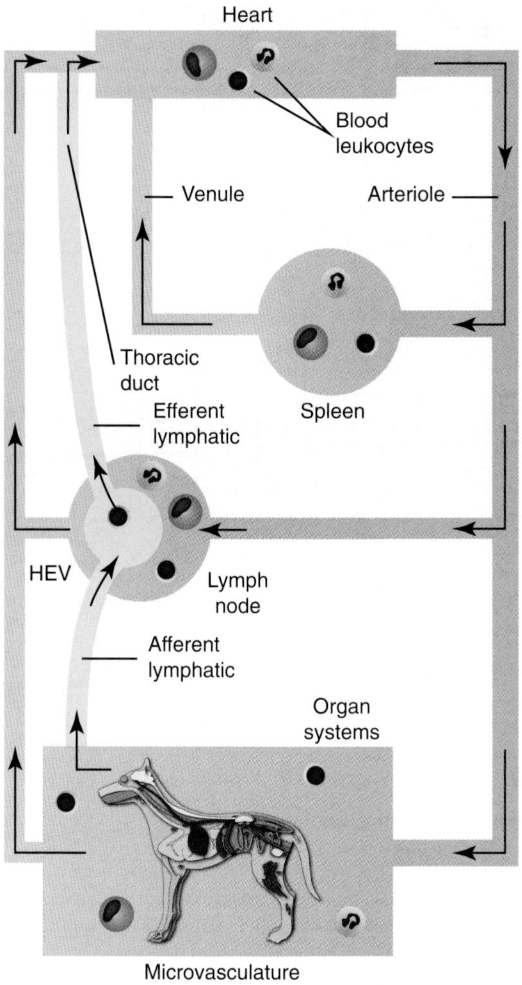

Figure 4-11 Leukocyte Trafficking. Microbes often use macrophages, lymphocytes, neutrophils, and/or dendritic cells to spread to other organ systems as these cells migrate through these systems as part of their normal immunologic surveillance activities. High endothelial venules (HEVs) are lined by specialized endothelial cells that allow lymphocytes circulating in the blood to enter the lymph node by crossing through the HEVs. (Courtesy Dr. J.F. Zachary, College of Veterinary Medicine, University of Illinois.)

structural barriers are relatively straightforward; other mechanisms used to cross mucosa, mucocutaneous junctions, and skin are much more stealthlike and are discussed herein.

Lining and covering epithelia (see earlier sections) of the alimentary, respiratory, integumentary, and urogenital systems, as well as the eye and ear, are the interface ("structural barriers") between the outside[6] and inside of the body and are held together (to each other) by occluding junctions such as tight junctions, desmosomes, and adherens junctions and to the basement membrane and ECM by anchoring junctions.

Skin is protected from microbes by (1) its physical thickness (five strata of stratified and pseudostratified epithelium) anchored by junctional complexes; (2) the keratinization, acidity, and oiliness (sebum) of the outer stratum corneum and stratum lucidum (antibacterial and antifungal properties); and (3) sloughing of keratinized cells into the environment from the stratum corneum. In contrast, the physical (thickness) defensive attributes of mucosae are not as substantial as those of the skin. Skin (in a dog as an example) ranges from 0.5 to 5.0 mm in thickness, whereas mucosae range from 10 to 100 μm in thickness. Thus skin is a substantial physical barrier to microbes when compared to mucosae.

[6]The alimentary, respiratory, and urogenital systems (also ear and eye) are functionally considered "outside" of the body because they have orifices that connect them with the outside.

ESSENTIAL CONCEPT 4-4 Defense Mechanisms and Barrier Systems

At portals of entry, along pathways of spread, and within organ systems, microbes encounter a variety of defense mechanisms and barrier systems. They are designed to prevent, limit, and/or delay microbial attachment to and/or colonization of cells and substances and then to isolate and contain their spread to allow acute inflammation and adaptive immunologic responses to control and eliminate them.

These defenses include the following:

1. Structural defenses such as those formed by the calvarium and vertebral column and the dura mater of the meninges
2. Structural and functional defenses such as those formed by mucosae, mucocutaneous junctions, and skin (epithelia) of barrier systems
3. Functional defenses such as mucus, bile, bacteriostatic/bactericidal molecules, lysozyme, defensins, surfactant, gastric acid, bile acids, and digestive enzymes
4. Physiologic defenses such as vomiting, exaggerated peristalsis (diarrhea), mucociliary clearance, lacrimation, and desquamation
5. Innate defenses such as those occurring in acute inflammation (e.g., phagocytosis, respiratory burst, antimicrobial granules, phagosome-lysosome fusion)

Acute inflammation dilutes, wall offs (isolates), and kills microbes via phagocytosis by neutrophils and macrophages (monocytes) recruited to the portals of entry or to sites along the pathways of spread. Additionally, these phagocytes present microbial antigens to lymphocytes, dendritic cells, and/or other cells involved in adaptive immune responses.

Functional (Biologic) Barriers

The functional (biologic) defense mechanisms of mucosae (alimentary, respiratory, and urogenital systems and the ear and eye) and of the skin are extensive. They include the physiologic functions of peristalsis (alimentary system, urinary system) and mucociliary clearance (respiratory system) and the biologic functions of substances such as mucus (alimentary, respiratory, and urogenital systems [discussed later]), bacteriostatic and bactericidal substances such as lysozyme, defensins, surfactant, gastric acid, bile acids, and digestive enzymes (alimentary and respiratory systems). Substances and processes such as tears (lacrimation [eye]), cerumen (ear), and desquamation of skin cells function to "flush" microbes off mucosae and skin and out of the organ system. Lastly, mucus provides nutrients for resident microflora that compete for resources needed by microbes and provides a suitable environment for mucosa-associated leukocytes that phagocytize and kill microbes.

Mucus Layer. Mucosae of the alimentary and respiratory systems are covered by a protective mucous gel composed predominantly of mucin glycoproteins synthesized and secreted by goblet cells (Fig. 4-12). The mucus layer forms a barrier system that attempts to do the following:

- Block microbes from reaching target cells
- Trap microbes so they can be phagocytosed by mucosal macrophages and neutrophils

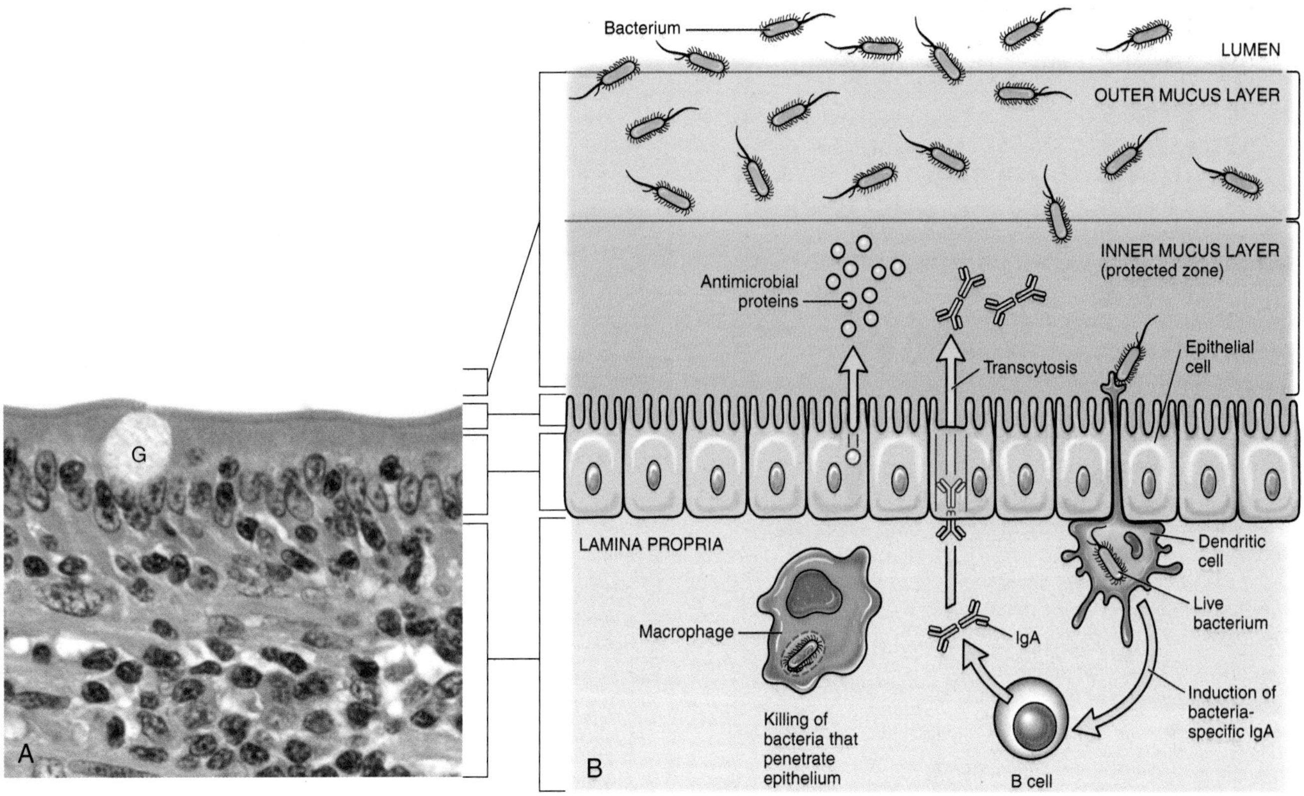

Figure 4-12 **Mucus Layer of Alimentary and Respiratory Mucosae. A,** Mucosae of the intestine (shown here) and of the conductive respiratory airways are covered by a mucus layer (not visible in H&E sections) secreted by goblet cells (*G*). The mucus covers the microvilli or cilia of these systems. H&E stain. **B,** The mucus layer has an outer layer that traps microbes (infectious and noninfectious) and other particles and an inner layer in which the cilia beat and which contains antimicrobial substances that diffuse into the outer layer. Dendritic cells and mucosa-associated macrophages and lymphocytes play central roles in preventing infection of mucosa. *IgA*, Immunoglobulin A. (**A** courtesy Dr. J.F. Zachary, College of Veterinary Medicine, University of Illinois.)

- Trap microbes so they can be exposed to bacteriostatic and bactericidal molecules sequestered in the mucin matrix
- Facilitate phagocytosis of microbes via mucosa-associated macrophages, mucosal dendritic cells, and microfold (M) cells
- Deliver microbial antigens to local lymphoid tissues like Peyer's patches or BALT and then to regional lymph nodes via afferent lymphatic drainage

Normal microflora such as bacteria are observed within the outer luminal zone of the mucus layer, indicating the importance of mucous gel in preventing direct adherence of bacteria to epithelial cells. Changes in the function of goblet cells and the chemical composition of mucus can occur through the release of bioactive factors from microbes or by activation of immune cells. Additionally, predisposing management stressors, such as dehydration, shipping, humidity, and ventilation, combined with weather changes can also change the function of goblet cells and the chemical composition of mucus, making mucosae more susceptible to infection.

Microbes use three mechanisms to penetrate the mucus layer and gain access to target cells. More information is known about the interactions of bacteria with the mucus layer, when compared to other microbes, especially viruses. These mechanisms include penetrating motility, digestion of mucus via enzymes and the consumption of mucus as an energy source, and evasion of the mucus layer in areas around Peyer's patches and M cells, areas devoid of mucus. Mucus also provides pathogenic advantages to bacteria as follows: (1) mucin oligosaccharides represent a direct source of carbohydrates, peptides, and exogenous nutrients, including vitamins and minerals; (2) bacteria that colonize mucus avoid rapid expulsion out of the alimentary system by peristalsis; and (3) adhesion to specific molecules within the mucin facilitates colonization of the mucus layer by microbes. Microbial mucolysis, the ability to enzymatically degrade mucus, appears to be a common trait among bacteria (virulence factor) and provides access to readily available sources of carbon and energy and enables bacteria to reach the surface of epithelial cells. Mucins are classified as neutral and acidic types, with the latter being further categorized as sulfated (sulfomucins) or nonsulfated (sialomucins). These biochemical differences likely explain some of the segmental target cell specificity (i.e., localization in one area of the organ over another) of some diseases of the alimentary and respiratory systems. Localization and colonization of specific zones of mucus by certain microbes likely occurs through the expression of adherence molecules unique to specific types of mucins.

As an example in cattle, a disease of the respiratory system, mannheimiosis, is caused by the bacterium *Mannheimia haemolytica*. One of its virulence factors is neuraminidase (a glycoside hydrolase enzyme), which reduces the viscosity of mucus, making it a less dense and more fluidic layer. This change allows the bacterium better access to cell membranes via gravity and random brownian movement. Concurrently, neuraminidase also cleaves sialic acid from the surface of cell membranes, thus decreasing the net negative surface charge and allowing closer contact of the bacterium with membranes in a functionally degraded mucus layer.

Innate and Adaptive Immune Responses

The innate (acute inflammation) and adaptive immune responses are covered in detail in Chapters 3 and 5. In summary, acute inflammation (see Chapter 3) is the first line of defense against the efforts of microbes to colonize and replicate in mucosa, mucocutaneous junctions, and skin (structural barriers). Acute inflammation is a response of vascularized tissue in these three structural barriers to cell injury and/or lysis and occurs when microbes attempt to colonize target cells. Molecules released from injured or dead cells (or cells in the area such as natural killer [NK] cells, basophils, mast cells, eosinophils, and platelets) initiate a cascade of humoral and cellular events designed to prevent or limit colonization by the microbe until phagocytes are recruited to the site and more effective defensive mechanisms are employed. Additionally, inflammasomes (see Chapters 3 and 5) are unique components of the innate immune system that detect microbes and are involved in the activation of inflammatory responses via pattern recognition receptors (PRRs), such as inflammasome sensor molecules. They activate a cascade of proinflammatory cytokines such as interleukin-1β (IL-1β) and IL-18.

With cell and tissue injury the fluidic phase (vascular phase) of acute inflammation dilutes, wall offs, and kills microbes via edema fluid, fibrin, and humoral factors of the complement and coagulation systems and other factors such as lactoferrin and transferrin, interferons, lysozyme, and IL-1. Some of these factors and microbial debris are chemotactic and recruit neutrophils and macrophages (monocytes) to the site. The fluidic phase hinders colonization and spread of microbes from the portal of entry and isolates them so they subsequently can be phagocytized and killed by neutrophils and macrophages (monocytes) during the cellular phase of the acute inflammatory response. Additionally, these phagocytes present microbial antigens to cells of the adaptive immune system such as macrophages (monocytes), lymphocytes, and dendritic cells.

Phagocytes interact with microbes using ligand-receptor interactions that are discussed in greater detail in sections covering specific classes of microbes such as bacteria, viruses, fungi, protozoa, and prions. Briefly, phagocytes bind (1) directly with microbes via ligands expressed specifically by the microbe or (2) indirectly with microbes by binding to biologic substances that coat the microbe during the fluidic phase of acute inflammation. In the first mechanism listed, microbial proteins called pathogen-associated molecular patterns (PAMPs) bind to PRRs (also known as Toll-like receptors [TLRs]) that are expressed on cell membranes of mucosa-associated phagocytes. PAMPs and PRRs play important roles in phagocytosis and killing ("activation") by phagocytes of specific types and classes of microbes. Additionally, these "activated" phagocytes release molecules such as inflammatory cytokines IL-1, IL-6, and tumor necrosis factor (TNF)-α that recruit additional phagocytic cells to the site. In the second mechanism listed , microbes become coated with a variety of biologic substances such as immunoglobulin G (IgG) antibody, C3b of complement, polyanions, and other molecules during the fluidic phase of acute inflammation. Phagocytes have cell membrane receptors for these ligands and attempt to phagocytose and kill these coated microbes.

The intended outcome of acute inflammation is to kill microbes and enable broad activation of an effective adaptive immune response. However, much of this chapter will discuss the processes used by microbes to block and evade innate and adaptive immune responses and to successfully complete their life cycles and cause disease in animals (Box 4-1).

Box 4-1 Mechanisms Used by Microbes to Block Defensive Activities of Phagocytes

Mechanism used by microbes	Effect on phagocytes
Avoidance	Gain access to tissues inaccessible to phagocytes
Stealth behavior	Avoid provoking an acute inflammatory (innate) response
Toxin	Inhibit chemotaxis by phagocytes
Polysaccharide capsule	Block encounter with phagocyte (prevents phagocytosis)
Opsonin	Block encounter with phagocyte (prevents phagocytosis)
Membrane trafficking molecules	Block fusion of phagosome with lysosome in phagocytic cell
Surface components or extracellular molecules	Block killing within the phagolysosome
Enzyme/toxin	Escape from phagosome or phagolysosome followed by replication in the cytoplasm
Toxin	Kill phagocyte before or after phagocytosis
Antioxidant	Resistance to killing by phagocytes

Monocyte-Macrophage System

The monocyte-macrophage system (also known as mononuclear phagocyte system [MPS]) is covered in detail in Chapter 5. Under normal conditions, tissue macrophages are derived from two sources: blood monocytes and tissue macrophage progenitor cells that are distributed throughout body tissues during organogenesis of the embryo. Precursor monocytes in bone marrow are capable of providing monocytes that migrate to and differentiate into macrophages in tissues. Tissue macrophages are also replenished locally and in large numbers by proliferation of tissue macrophage progenitor cells. These two populations of cells give rise to tissue macrophages that form the functional basis for innate and adaptive responses to microbes in tissues and organs (see Chapters 5 and 13).

In summary, cells of the monocyte-macrophage system are important in phagocytizing and killing microbes (Fig. 4-13) and then "presenting" microbial antigens to lymphocytes, dendritic cells, and/or other cells involved in the adaptive immune response. Cells of the monocyte-macrophage system originate in bone marrow and enter the circulatory system as blood monocytes. Monocytes (and macrophages) then (1) may be recruited into tissues along a chemotactic gradient during acute inflammation and differentiate into macrophages (see previous section) or multinucleated giant cells (fused macrophages) or (2) may migrate into the ECM and other types of supportive tissues in a wide variety of organ systems to establish and maintain a resident population of phagocytic cells. These latter cells include (1) lung (alveolar macrophages), (2) liver sinusoids (Kupffer cells), (3) lymph nodes (free and fixed macrophages), (4) spleen (free and fixed macrophages), (5) bone marrow (fixed macrophages), (6) connective tissue (histiocytes), (7) serous fluids (pleural and peritoneal macrophages), (8) skin (histiocytes), (9) mucosae (mucosa-associated macrophages), (10) brain (microglia cells), and (11) bone (osteoclasts) (Box 4-2). Monocytes and macrophages are also part of a systemic network of phagocytic and immune cells (lymphocytes, dendritic cells) that migrate through organs via the circulatory and lymphatic systems. This migratory process is called *leukocyte trafficking* (see Fig. 4-11), and these cells behave as "lookouts" for microbes and other matter such as cell debris (cells injured by microbes). When they encounter microbes, they facilitate responses like acute inflammation and "present" antigens for adaptive immunity to protect the animal against microbes. However, some microbes have acquired virulence factors that allow them to enter trafficking leukocytes and spread protected within them to target cells in other organ systems. This mechanism will be discussed in greater detail in later sections and in material covering individual diseases.

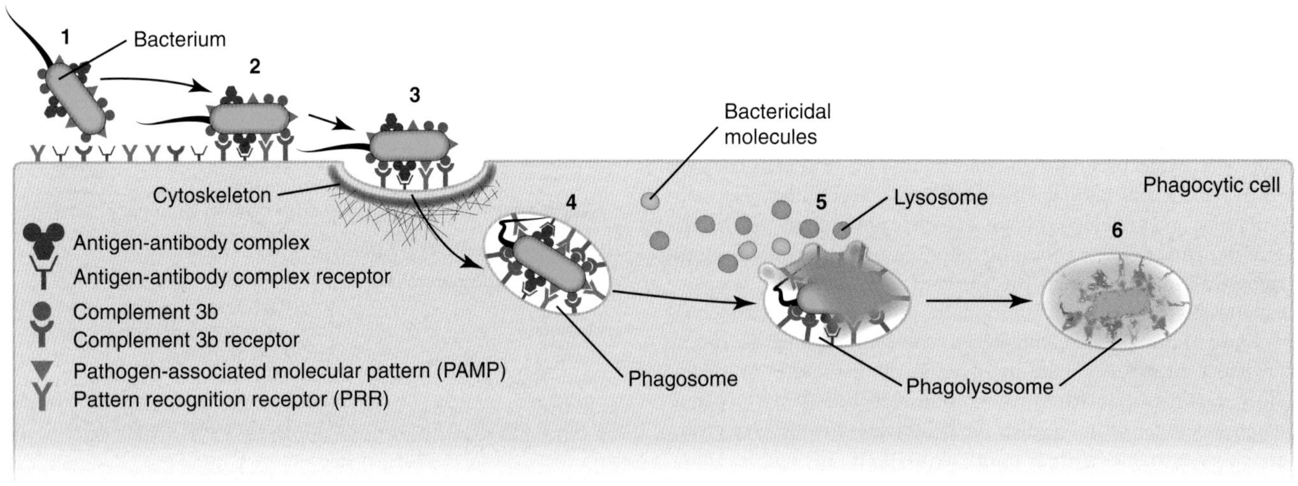

Figure 4-13 **Phagocytosis.** *1*, Microbes encounter phagocytic cells, such as macrophages and neutrophils, at portals of entry and extracellular matrix tissues. *2*, The surfaces of microbes contain a variety of ligands, such as opsonins, C3b, and pathogen-associated molecular patterns (PAMPs), that allow them to recognize and attach to phagocytes. Phagocytes have complementary receptors for these ligands. When ligand and receptors interact successfully, the microbe is firmly attached to the surface of the phagocyte. *3*, Ligand-receptor binding initiates a cascade of membrane second messengers and cytoskeletal elements (see Chapter 1) that begin the process of internalizing the microbe. *4*, The microbe is confined in the cytoplasm within a phagosome (phagocytic vacuole) and moved into the cell. *5*, The phagosome fuses with lysosomes and becomes a phagolysosome. Lysosomes contain a variety of enzymes and other microbiostatic and microbicidal molecules such as reactive oxygen species and nitric oxide. *6*, These molecules are released into the phagosome and act to kill the microbe. (Courtesy Dr. J.F. Zachary, College of Veterinary Medicine, University of Illinois.)

Box 4-2 Cells of the Monocyte-Macrophage System

Cell type	Location
Promonocyte	Bone marrow
Blood monocyte	Circulatory and lymphatic systems
Kupffer cell	Hepatic sinusoids
Mesangial cell	Renal glomerulus
Alveolar macrophage	Air-blood barrier of pulmonary alveolus
Tissue histiocyte	Extracellular matrix, surfaces covered by mesothelium
Microglial cell	CNS
Splenic macrophage	Red and white pulp of spleen
Tissue macrophage (histiocyte)	Medullary cords of lymph nodes
Mucosa-associated macrophages	Mucosae

CNS, Central nervous system.

Dendritic Cells

Dendritic cells are covered in detail in Chapters 3 and 5. In summary, dendritic cells are phagocytic antigen-processing and antigen-presenting cells that are commonly found intermixed with epithelial cells of mucosae and skin (e.g., Langerhans cells) as well as other tissues and organ systems. They play a central role in developing an adaptive immune response to microbes. However, because dendritic cells are phagocytic and migratory, microbes can also use them to complete their life cycles. Microbes use mechanisms similar to those used to infect macrophages to infect dendritic cells. Once infected, dendritic cells can migrate from mucosae and skin to local and regional lymphoid tissues via lymphatic vessels. Microbes through their surface proteins are able to bind to receptors expressed on the apical domains of these cells and infect them, then exit via the basolateral domain via exocytosis, gain access to lymphoid nodules (tissues commonly associated with dendritic cells), and establish a local infection in lymphocytes and macrophages. Infected lymphocytes and macrophages spread the agent via leukocyte trafficking from local sites to regional lymph nodes and then systemically to other organ systems.

Phagosome-Lysosome Fusion

Phagosome-lysosome fusion is an intracellular process used by phagocytes to kill microbes. Lysosomes are cellular organelles (see Chapter 1, Fig. 1-1, and Fig. 4-13) that contain an array of enzymes and toxic molecules. Microbes enter phagocytic cells via phagocytosis or endocytosis and are found in intracellular vesicles (phagosomes or endosomes). These vesicles fuse with lysosomes and these lysosomes release an array of degradative enzymes and toxic molecules into the fused vesicle, now called a phagolysosome that are designed to kill the microbe. Microbes have virulence factors that act to block phagosome-lysosome fusion or, if fusion occurs, to neutralize the effects of toxic molecules released from lysosomes and allow them to colonize cells and tissues, replicate, and complete their life cycles (Fig. 4-14). Examples of these mechanisms are discussed in the section covering Johne's disease (*Mycobacterium avium* subsp. *paratuberculosis*) and in other diseases in this chapter.

Genetic Resistance of Animals to Infectious Diseases

The resistance of animals to disease depends on the effective interplay of many structural and functional (physiologic) components of the body, including cutaneous and mucosal barrier systems and the immune system, respectively. Distinct networks of genes play central roles in structural and functional activities of the body. They control the development, maturation, and maintenance of epithelial cells, mucus, and supporting ECM tissues, such as collagen, that form the barrier systems. Additionally, they control similar structural activities for a variety of cell lineages of the innate and adaptive immune systems like T lymphocytes, macrophages, neutrophils, and dendritic cells and the expression of proteins that form PRRs in the membranes of these cells (see Chapter 5). These receptors recognize PAMPs expressed by microbes and are discussed

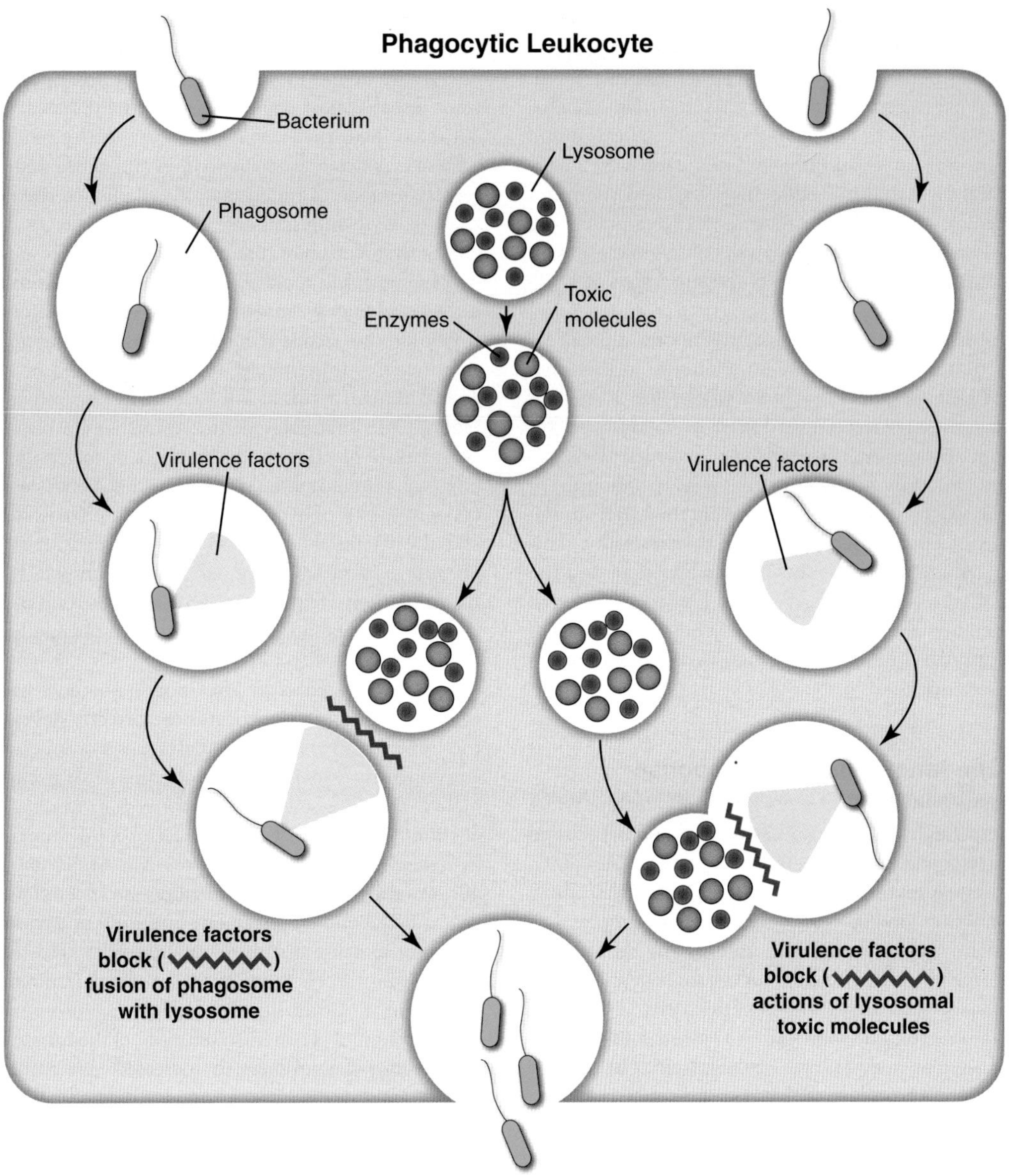

Figure 4-14 Virulence Factors Block Actions of Lysosomes in Phagocytes. Microbes enter leukocytes such as macrophages via phagocytosis and are protected within intracellular vesicles (phagosomes). As a defense mechanism, leukocytes have lysosomes that fuse with phagosomes and release an array of degradative enzymes and toxic molecules into the fused vesicle, now called a phagolysosome that are designed to kill the microbe. Microbes have virulence factors that act to block phagosome-lysosome fusion or if fusion occurs, to neutralize the effects of toxic molecules released from lysosomes and allow them to colonize cells and tissues, replicate, and complete their life cycles. (Courtesy Dr. J.F. Zachary, College of Veterinary Medicine, University of Illinois.)

in greater detail in Chapters 3 and 5. Genes also play a central role in functional processes of cells, including adhesion, chemotaxis, phagocytosis, phagosome-lysosome fusion, intracellular killing of microbes, and antigen processing (see Chapters 3 and 5) involved in innate and adaptive responses of the immune system. Thus genetic resistance to infectious diseases is a polygenic trait regulated mainly by the immune system and its interactions with barrier systems and environmental factors such as weather conditions and nutritional status.

In animals the genetics of disease resistance is most closely associated with the major histocompatibility complex (MHC), a tightly linked group of genes that encode proteins involved in immune responses. This genetic region in cattle has been given the abbreviated name *BoLA*, and similar regions have been identified in other animal species. Few specific genes or genetic markers related to disease resistance have been identified in domestic animals; however, genes involved in antigen processing appear to be important in resistance to infectious diseases.

Disorders of Barrier Systems

Barrier systems most commonly involved in infectious diseases of animals include the alimentary and respiratory mucosae and the skin and were discussed previously. Additionally, mucosae of the conjunctiva and urinary systems and skin of the ear also serve as barriers to microbes. These systems and their physical barriers develop embryologically under strict genetic control and when mature are functionally maintained, regulated, and repaired through processes dependent on transcription and translation of genes. Structural and/or functional alterations in these barriers can make animals more susceptible to microbes.

An example of a genetic disorder that predisposes animals to infectious disease that occurs because of an alteration in the development of the basic structure of a barrier is epitheliogenesis imperfecta. It is an autosomal recessive hereditary disease of young horses, cattle, and pigs characterized by loss of epithelium affecting the skin and mucosae of the oral cavity and tongue likely caused by alterations in the subbasal plate and its hemidesmosomes and laminin-5 (see Chapter 17). Loss of the skin or mucosae exposes underlying vascularized ECM tissues to environmental contamination with feces and other matter, allowing bacterial pathogens access to ECM and capillary beds.

An example of a genetic disorder that predisposes animals to infectious disease that occurs because of an alteration in the function of a barrier is primary ciliary dyskinesia of the dog. It appears to be an autosomal recessive hereditary disease of young dogs, but an autosomal dominant mutation has not been excluded. This disorder is caused by ciliary dysfunction attributable to immotile or dyskinetic cilia caused by defects of proteins in the outer and/or inner dynein arms of cilia, which give them their motility. This outcome leads to dysfunction of the mucociliary apparatus and the retention of microbes in the respiratory system leading to bacterial bronchitis and pneumonia. Other examples of genetic alterations of barrier systems that predispose animals to increased susceptibility to infectious disease are discussed in the organ system chapters of this book.

Disorders of the Innate Immune Response

The innate immune system (i.e., acute inflammation) provides animals with an immediate defense against microbes and is discussed in detail in Chapters 3 and 5 and in earlier sections of this chapter. In summary, this system involves the initial encounter of mucosae, mucocutaneous junction, and/or skin with microbes at a portal of entry. It is essentially acute inflammation and (1) the cellular and chemical mediators associated with the process, such as phagocytic cells like macrophages, neutrophils, and dendritic cells; (2) effector cells, such as T lymphocytes and mast cells; (3) chemical mediators of the complement system; and (4) the vascular system. The purpose of acute inflammation is to dilute and isolate microbes in edema fluid and fibrin, phagocytose and kill them, and process and present their antigens to effector cells of the adaptive immune response. When epithelial cells, endothelial cells, or mucosal or cutaneous macrophages of barrier systems are injured by or infected with microbes, they release large quantities of cytokines into the surrounding tissues. These cytokines recruit, via chemotaxis, inflammatory cells from capillaries in vascularized ECM tissues and cause vasodilation and increased permeability of these blood vessels (i.e., edema fluid and fibrin). Inflammatory cells also release cytokines and other chemical mediators that act to recruit additional inflammatory cells, activate the complement cascade to identify bacteria and kill microbes, promote phagocytosis of dead cells and microbes by phagocytic cells, and activate the adaptive immune system through antigen processing and presentation to immune cells such as T and B lymphocytes. Phagocytic and effector cells of the acute inflammatory response are recruited from capillaries and migrate along a chemoattractant gradient formed by chemical mediators and molecules released from microbes to the inflammatory focus. In inflammatory foci, these cells express TLRs, also known as *pattern recognition receptors* (PRRs), that recognize molecules on infectious agents called PAMPs (see Chapters 3 and 5). These cells also express IL-1 receptors that act in concert with PRRs to initiate and sustain the innate immune response through phagocytosis.

Genetic disorders can affect all of the steps involved in the innate immune response as summarized earlier from initial recognition of microbes to their phagocytosis and killing and are discussed in many chapters of this book. Examples of genetic disorders of the innate immune system that predispose animals to infectious disease, most commonly bacterial diseases, include leukocyte adhesion deficiencies and granulocytopathy syndromes. Leukocyte adhesion deficiency occurs in dogs and cattle and has an autosomal recessive mode of inheritance. It is characterized by alterations in the leukocyte adhesion cascade (see Chapter 3) involving deficiencies or dysfunction of integrins and selectins resulting in the inability of neutrophils to adhere to endothelial cells in the wall of blood vessels and migrate into sites of bacterial infection. Granulocytopathy syndrome occurs in dogs and cattle and has an autosomal recessive mode of inheritance. It is characterized by alterations in the ability of neutrophils to kill bacteria in phagosomes and is linked to reduced nicotinamide adenine dinucleotide phosphate (NADPH) concentrations that may arise from a metabolic anomaly in the hexose monophosphate shunt. This deficiency may lead to reduced concentrations of hydrogen peroxide in phagosome-lysosome fusion and the bactericidal capability of the neutrophil. The process of phagocytosis is usually normal. Affected animals have shortened life span, long-term febrile disease, dermatitis, oral ulcers, lymphadenitis, and poor healing, attributable to irresolvable and repeated bacterial infections.

Genetic disorders of the innate immune system can also be caused by failure of leukocytes to correctly develop and mature in the bone marrow. Cyclic hematopoiesis occurs in dogs and has an autosomal recessive mode of inheritance. It is caused by an abnormality of stem cells in the bone marrow resulting in periodic declines, every 10 to 12 days, in neutrophil concentrations followed by hyperplasia and a return to normal. Abnormal concentrations of purine and pyrimidine metabolites in affected stems cells suggest that a metabolic derangement in purine or pyrimidine metabolism may be the cause of this genetic disorder. This outcome increases susceptibility to bacterial infection, often leading to periodic fever, joint pain, or other signs of ocular, respiratory, or skin infections. Other examples of genetic alterations of the innate immune response that predisposes animals to increased susceptibility to infectious disease are discussed in the organ system chapters of this book.

Disorders of the Adaptive Immune Response

Genetic disorders of the adaptive immune response are disorders in which affected animals are incapable of generating antigen-specific immune responses (see Chapter 5). Such genetic diseases are closely associated with genes that regulate the expression of the MHC, especially those genes involved in antigen processing and presentation. Examples of this type of disorder include agammaglobulinemia (a B lymphocyte immunodeficiency) and severe combined immunodeficiency (a B and T lymphocyte immunodeficiency). T lymphocyte, macrophage, and complement immunodeficiencies also occur but are not discussed here. Agammaglobulinemia has an X-linked recessive mode of inheritance and thus is a disorder of young colts. It is likely caused by dysfunction of cytoplasmic tyrosine kinase resulting in blockage in the differentiation of B lymphocyte lineages and a nearly complete absence of B lymphocytes and plasma cells. Clinically, this type of immunodeficiency results in colts with chronic bacterial diseases leading to pneumonia, enteritis, dermatitis, arthritis, and laminitis. Severe combined immunodeficiency occurs in dogs and Arabian horses and has an autosomal recessive mode of inheritance. In dogs, an X chromosome–linked mode of inheritance has also been identified. Affected animals produce no antibodies after infection or immunization because of an absence of B lymphocytes and have no or nonfunctional T lymphocytes when present. This genetic disorder occurs when lymphocyte precursors fail to differentiate into mature T or B lymphocytes, which is likely because of the result of mutations within recombinase-activating genes or within genes encoding DNA-dependent protein kinase or when differentiated lymphocytes are incapable of completing signal transduction pathways because of defects in cell surface receptors for interleukins. Other examples of genetic alterations of the adaptive immune response that predisposes animals to increased susceptibility to infectious disease are discussed in the organ system chapters of this book.

Bacterial Diseases

Pathogenicity

The pathogenicity (i.e., ability to cause disease) of a bacterium is regulated by its virulence factors. In summary, virulence factors are used by microbes to kill phagocytic cells, block phagocytosis, evade fusion with lysosomes, block killing within phagocytes, and enhance replication within phagocytes. Virulence factors are molecules, often glycoproteins or glycolipids, derived from bacterial genes. Their expression establishes the processes used by bacteria to successfully colonize mucosae, infect cells, grow and replicate, and cause cell lysis.

Important actions of virulence factors and the biologic substances with which they interact include the following:

- Production of bacterial toxins that kill phagocytes
- Synthesis of bacterial proteins that prevent phagocytosis by blocking the interaction of opsonins with phagosomes
- Synthesis of a bacterial capsule that can block contact with the microbe and prevent phagocytosis
- Inhibition of fusion of the phagosome containing microbes with lysosomes
- Facilitate escape of the microbe into the cytoplasm before the microbe is killed in the phagolysosome
- Production of bacterial antioxidants (i.e., catalase) that block killing in phagolysosomes

The interaction between an animal and a bacterial pathogen is back and forth, each acting to influence the activities and functions of the other. The outcome depends on the virulence (i.e., virulence factors) of the pathogen and the resistance or susceptibility (i.e., genes) of the animal. Resistance or susceptibility to disease in healthy animals is derived from (1) innate defenses such as cellular and mucous barrier systems, acute inflammation (including neutrophil phagocytosis), the monocyte-macrophage system (phagocytosis), and normal bacterial flora and (2) adaptive defenses provided by the immune system such as passive immunity via colostrum and active immunity via T and B lymphocytes. In general, bacterial pathogenicity is determined by two characteristics: (1) the bacterium's ability to colonize cells and (2) its ability to produce toxins and damage cells and their ECM tissues such as collagen. To colonize cells, bacteria use mechanisms such as adhesion, multiplication, colonization, tissue invasion, and circumvention of animal defense mechanisms. To damage cells via toxins, microbes use mechanisms such as cytolysis and invasion of vascularized ECM tissues (locally or systemically) incited by bacteria-derived exotoxins (Gram-positive bacteria) and endotoxins (Gram-negative bacteria). Virulence factors determine the sum of the characteristics that allow bacteria to cause disease and thus provide a pathogenicity profile or fingerprint for each bacterium.

Virulence Factors

Bacterial virulence factors are molecules that influence interactions between bacteria and target cells and/or substances, including processes such as adherence to cell membranes; colonization and invasion of skin or mucosae; endocytosis and/or phagocytosis; growth, replication, and other metabolic processes; local, regional, and systemic spread; and cell injury and/or lysis (Fig. 4-15; Table 4-1). Furthermore, they inhibit innate and adaptive immune responses, allowing the bacterium to evade defense mechanisms and also to proliferate in harsh environments. Bacterial virulence factors act as proteases, lipases, deoxyribonucleases (DNases), toxins, physiologic mediators (inhibitors or enhancers), lytic agents, adhesion factors, biofilms, bacterial capsules made of carbohydrates, and antiphagocytic factors (see Table 4-1). Bacterial virulence is determined in part by the type and number of factors the bacterium expresses to successfully complete its life cycle in an animal. In general, virulence factors are coded for by more than one bacterial gene. Other things that can indirectly influence the success of these virulence factors include physical and environmental stressors, such as weather, access to food and water, and management (shipping) or housing conditions (ventilation, humidity, or overcrowding).

Initial Encounters at Portals of Entry

Before infecting epithelial cells in mucosae (except areas with M cells), bacteria must penetrate the mucus layer to gain access to these cells. Once in the mucus layer, bacteria may be phagocytized by macrophages, lymphocytes, and/or dendritic cells as they migrate in, on, and through the mucus. As these phagocytes containing bacteria migrate, they interact with epithelial cells, phagocytotic and immune cells in the lamina propria and submucosa, ECM, and endothelial cells. These interactions allow bacteria, if they "escape" from phagocytes, to interact with all of these cell types and infect those required for them to complete their life cycles. However, in many diseases, it is unclear how bacteria ultimately invade or penetrate the mucus layer to gain access to mucosal epithelial cells (target cells). Several mechanisms, some regulated by virulence factors, are likely used to reach mucosal epithelial cells, including (1) motility, (2) digestion and consumption of the mucus layer, and (3) random discovery of mucosae lacking a mucus layer. As examples in the alimentary system, some bacteria, such as the spirochetes, are motile and can penetrate the mucus layer and reach target cells. Other bacteria, such as *Clostridium septicum*, digest the mucus layer with bacterial enzymes and then consume oligosaccharides such as *N*-acetylglucosamine, galactose, and *N*-acetylgalactosamine in the mucus layer as a carbon source during intense periods of replication. Finally, some bacteria use M cells to gain access to target cells; these cells are not covered by mucus, and their surface membranes and receptors are available to passing microbes.

Adhesion, Colonization, Toxigenesis, and Invasiveness

Adhesion, colonization, toxigenesis, and invasiveness are processes that occur during initial encounters between bacteria and cells of mucosa/skin at portals of entry.

- **Bacterial adhesion**—the process of bacteria attaching to cells, tissue, and biologic substances.
- **Bacterial colonization**—the adherence, multiplication, and establishment of bacteria at a portal of entry.
- **Bacterial toxigenesis**—the ability of bacteria to produce toxins.
- **Bacterial invasiveness**—the ability of bacteria to invade tissues.

These processes, facilitated by bacterial virulence factors, are also affected by other factors that act indirectly to minimize the actions of the animal's defense mechanisms by enabling resistance to antibiotics, enhancing antiphagocytic properties, and weakening or inhibiting immune responses.

Virulence factors, derived from membrane proteins, polysaccharide capsules, secretory proteins, cell wall and outer membrane

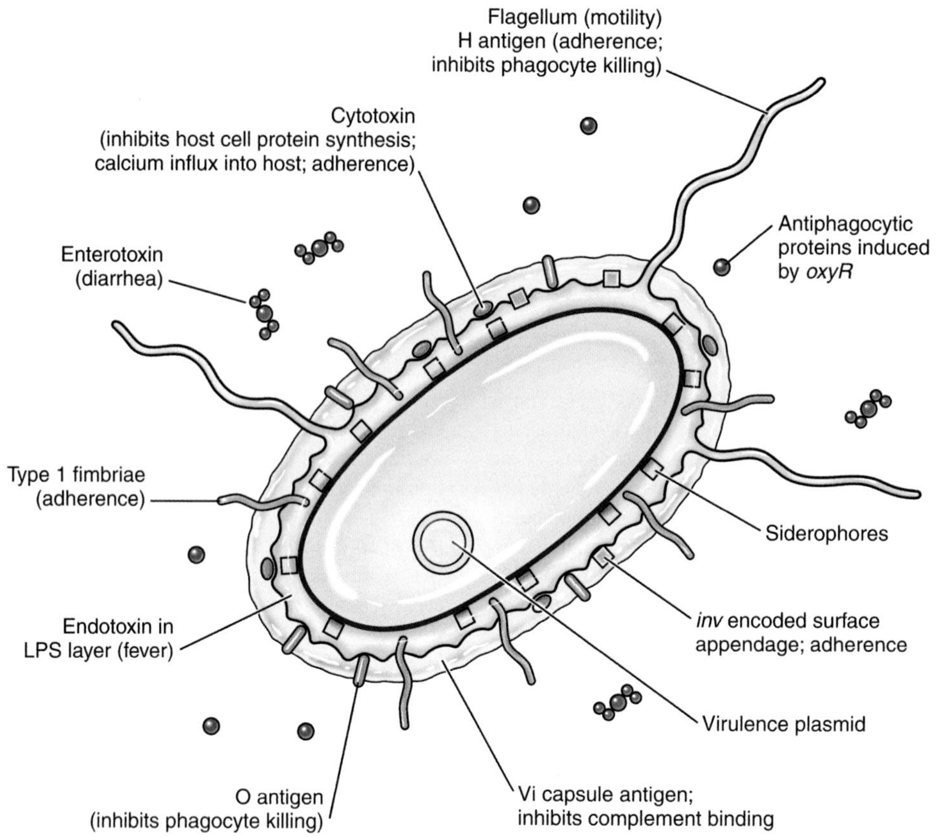

Figure 4-15 **Virulence Factors Used by Bacteria to Cause Disease.** *LPS*, Lipopolysaccharide.

Table 4-1 Examples of Virulence Factors and Their Biologic Actions

Virulence Factor(s)	Action
Adhesins	Attach to receptor(s) on cell membranes or on substances such as mucus, mucins, or ECM proteins; also facilitate entry into cell by endocytosis/phagocytosis
Invasins	Spread into and through cell membranes, cells, or tissue via ligand-receptor interactions, cell dysfunction and lysis, or breakdown of ECM
Endotoxins (lipopolysaccharides)	Stimulate macrophages and endothelial cells to secrete proinflammatory cytokines and nitric oxide; cause cell dysfunction and lysis
Exotoxins	Inhibit biochemical pathways within a cell
Excitotoxins	Dysfunction and lysis of neurons and other cell types
Mycotoxins	Dysfunction and lysis of cells
Immunoglobulin (Ig) proteases	Break down immunoglobins used in adaptive immune defense mechanisms
Hemolysins	Cell lysis
Lipases	Degrade cell lipids (cell membranes) and disrupt lipid metabolism
Hyaluronidases	Break down hyaluronan (hyaluronic acid) in ECM of mucosae, skin, connective tissue, and nervous tissue; some bacteria use hyaluronan as a carbon source for growth and replication; other bacteria may use hyaluronidase to spread though barrier systems and ECM
Collagenases	Break down collagen fibers of ECM, especially in muscle tissue
Neuraminidases	Degrade neuraminic acid (sialic acid) in cells and cell membranes; viral neuraminidase is used by influenza viruses to escape from target cells by budding from the cell membrane
Hemagglutinins	Attachment proteins located on the surface of influenza viruses that facilitate binding to cell membrane and entry into target cells
Kinases	Digest fibrin and prevent clotting of the blood needed to wall off bacteria
Lecithinases	Punch holes through or break down cell membranes
Phospholipases	Punch holes through or break down cell membranes

ECM, Extracellular matrix.

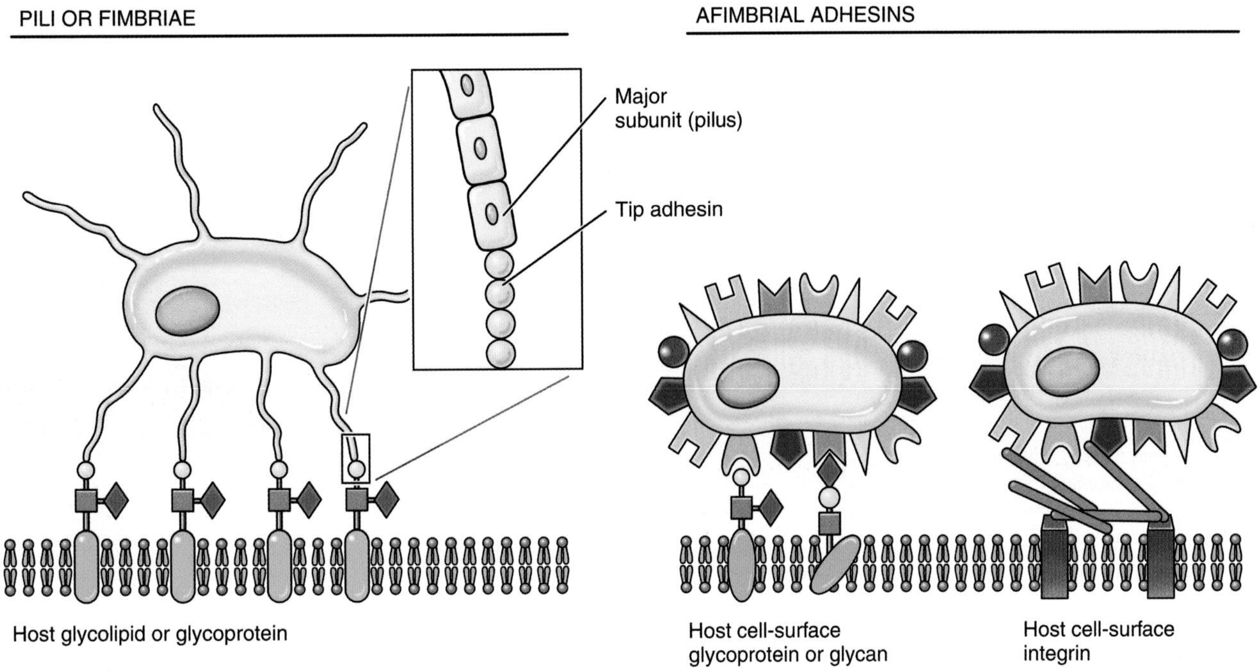

Figure 4-16 **Fimbrial (Pilus) and Afimbrial Adhesins.** These structures are used by microbes to attach and bind to protein receptors on membranes of target cells (especially mucosal epithelial cells) or to molecules of the mucus layer or vascularized extracellular matrix (connective) tissues.

components, and other miscellaneous proteins of bacteria, assist them in adhering to, colonizing, and invading epithelia at portals of entry (toxigenesis will be discussed in the next section). However, because epithelial cells of skin and mucosae are replaced continually (≈48-hour life span) and these systems have defensive mechanisms such as peristalsis, unidirectional mucociliary undulations, and micturition, bacteria must be able to adhere to, colonize (replicate), and/or invade into or between these epithelial cells in order to avoid being swept away. Attachment occurs when membrane proteins of bacteria called *adhesins* (a broad term) bind to receptors on cell membranes of mucosae and skin. Attachment is a typical ligand-receptor interaction; a protein on the bacterium binds to a receptor on a target cell. Some bacteria express adhesins, such as microbial surface cell recognition adhesion matrix molecules, that bind the bacterium to the surface of the cell. Other bacteria use extensions of their cell membranes called *fimbriae* or *pili* to bind to animal cells. Fimbriae and pili have adhesins, such as pilus-associated proteins, fimbrial antigens, or fimbrial adhesins that bind to receptors on microvilli of the glycocalyx or in the mucus layer (Fig. 4-16). Fimbriae and pili may also act to inhibit phagocytosis. For example, uropathogenic and enterotoxic *Escherichia coli*, causes of urinary tract infections and diarrhea in animals, express fimbrial (type 1, P, and S/F1C) and pilus (K99) adhesins, respectively. In the urinary tract, P fimbria is an important attachment adhesin and allows the bacterium to attach to the transitional epithelium (mucosa) of the bladder and cause the disease known as acute necrohemorrhagic urocystitis. Other virulence factors, such as α-hemolysin and cytotoxic necrotizing factor type 1, cause necrosis and hemorrhage later in the disease process. In the small intestine, K99 pilus adhesin allows *E. coli* to adhere to enterocytes and reduces their loss in number via intestinal peristalsis. When large numbers of *E. coli* are attached to the small intestine, they produce other virulence factors, such as enterotoxin, that act directly on enterocytes, leading to diarrhea.

Ligand-receptor interactions are likely common to most bacterial diseases; however, in many veterinary diseases, specific bacterial ligands and their target cell receptors have not been identified. The attachment of sufficient numbers of bacteria at the appropriate portal of entry initiates an early stage of bacterial infection termed *colonization*. After colonization, bacteria produce another group of virulence factors called invasins, or spreading factors. These factors include hyaluronidase, collagenase, kinases, lecithinase, and phospholipase and act to break down barrier systems formed by mucosae (mucus layer) and skin, cell junctional complexes, and ECM molecules like collagen. Additionally, other virulence factors that injure and/or kill cells include proteases and lipases; DNases, which break down DNA; and hemolysins that destroy cells, such as red blood cells. Invasiveness and invasins allow bacteria to spread rapidly into and through intercellular spaces and protect themselves in safe areas such lamina propria isolated from unfavorable host environments or host-derived defensive molecules. As examples, *Clostridium chauvoei*, the bacterium that causes blackleg in cattle, produces sufficient lecithinases and phospholipases to punch holes in cell membranes of skeletal muscle and cause lysis of myocytes and endothelial cells. *Listeria monocytogenes*, the cause of listeriosis in the nervous system of cattle, produces invasins that induce endocytosis of the bacterium for colonization by acting on target cell actin filaments. Other proteins of bacteria, such as surface components and polysaccharide capsules, are virulence factors that allow bacteria to avoid phagocytosis and evade recognition by cells of the innate and/or adaptive immune systems. They disrupt or block one or more steps used by neutrophils, monocytes, or macrophages in the phagocytic process such as initial contact, engulfment, phagosome formation, phagosome-lysosome fusion, and killing and digestion. As examples, *Streptococcus pyogenes*, a cause of bovine mastitis, uses M protein and a hyaluronic acid capsule to inhibit phagocytosis and the same hyaluronic acid capsule to evade recognition of the immune system. Finally, some bacteria

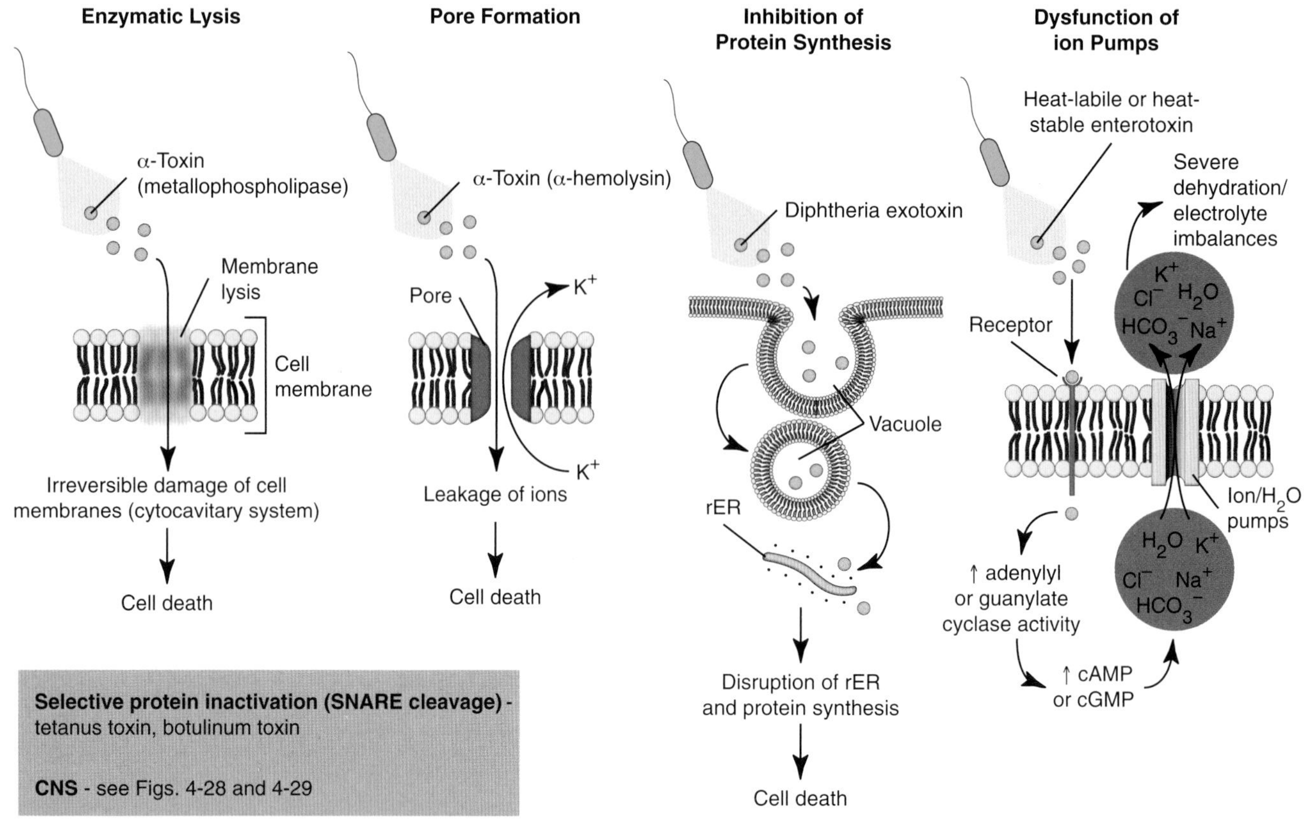

Figure 4-17 **Actions of Bacterial Toxins (Virulence Factors) on the Structure and Function of Target Cells** (see Fig. 4-6). Examples of such toxins in animals include the following (see text for greater detail): **enzymatic lysis:** clostridial myositis in horses (malignant edema; gas gangrene)—*Clostridium perfringens* α-toxin; **pore formation:** cutaneous superficial pyoderma in dogs—*Staphylococcus aureus* α-toxin; **inhibition of protein synthesis:** caseous lymphadenitis in ruminants—*Corynebacterium pseudotuberculosis* diphtheria-like toxin; **dysfunction of ion pumps:** enterotoxigenic enteritis in all domestic animal species—*Escherichia coli* heat-labile and heat-stable enterotoxins; **selective protein inactivation (SNARE cleavage):** tetanus in horses—*Clostridium tetani* tetanospasmin (neurotoxin); botulism in horses—*Clostridium botulinum* neurotoxin. *cAMP,* Cyclic adenosine monophosphate; *cGMP,* cyclic guanosine monophosphate; *rER,* rough endoplasmic reticulum; *SNARE,* soluble *N*-ethylmaleimide-sensitive factor attachment protein receptor. (Courtesy Dr. J.F. Zachary, College of Veterinary Medicine, University of Illinois.)

have virulence factors that are immunoglobulin proteases. They break down immunoglobins involved in adaptive immune responses and thus depress defensive mechanisms.

Toxigenesis (Toxins)

Certain virulence factors are toxins, including exotoxins, lipoteichoic acid, and endotoxins (lipopolysaccharide [LPS]). Exotoxins are secreted by living Gram-positive bacteria; lipoteichoic acid is released from dead Gram-positive bacteria (i.e., bacteriolysis from bactericidal molecules and antibiotics); and endotoxins are released from dead Gram-negative bacteria (i.e., normal bacterial turnover, bacteriolysis from bactericidal molecules and antibiotics). These toxins activate a large variety of biochemical cascades involving cell membrane systems and organelles that result in cell dysfunction and/or death (Fig. 4-17; Box 4-3). They are expressed by Gram-negative and Gram-positive bacteria (Fig. 4-18) and injure and/or kill cells and damage their ECM proteins, such as collagen. Structurally, these actions enable colonization and invasiveness. Functionally, these molecules also act to kill cells directly via cytolysis (e.g., pore formation) or apoptosis or indirectly through activation of acute inflammation, often initiated via the complement pathway. In certain diseases these toxins are named (and grouped) according to their biologic activity such as leukotoxins (bovine pneumonic pasteurellosis/mannheimiosis) and neurotoxins (botulism and botulinum toxin [*Clostridium botulinum*], tetanus and tetanospasmin [*Clostridium tetani*]) (see sections covering specific bacterial and viral diseases). Fungi also have virulence factors that produce toxins that cause tissue injury and lysis. Examples include mycotoxins/aflatoxins.

Exotoxins and Lipoteichoic Acid. Exotoxins (usually from Gram-positive bacteria) are secreted from viable bacteria and are potent toxins. Some act directly on cells to cause cytolysis; others act via the A-B toxin system and bind to cell membranes with a receptor (B subunit) and deliver a second toxic molecule (A subunit) into the cytoplasm. As examples, A-B toxin systems are used in botulism (*C. botulinum*), tetanus (*C. tetani*), and diseases caused by *Corynebacterium* spp. Vacuolating toxin of *Helicobacter pylori*, *E. coli* hemolysin, and superantigens belonging to *S. pyogenes* and *Staphylococcus aureus* are surface-acting exotoxins. Surface-acting exotoxins bind to cell membranes and form pores through which cell lysis occurs. *S. aureus* also has pore-forming cytotoxins called α-toxin. Another virulence factor, lipoteichoic acid, binds to endothelial cells, interacts with circulating antibodies, activates the complement cascade, and triggers the release of reactive oxygen and nitrogen species, acid hydrolases, highly cationic proteinases, bactericidal cationic peptides, growth factors, and cytotoxic cytokines from neutrophils and macrophages. Lipoteichoic acid is also located in the cell wall of Gram-positive bacteria like *S. aureus*. It behaves as a Gram-positive endotoxin because its actions mimic LPS.

Endotoxins. Gram-negative bacteria, such as *E. coli*, *Salmonella* spp., *Pseudomonas* spp., *Haemophilus* spp., and *Bordetella* spp. can

Box 4-3 Examples of the Effects of Toxins (Virulence Factors) Causing Diseases in Animals (see Fig. 4-17)

Biologic outcome	Disease	Pathogenesis
Enzymatic lysis	Clostridial myositis in horses (malignant edema; gas gangrene)	*Clostridium perfringens* α-toxin has phospholipase C activity and causes lysis of cell membranes (cell death).
Pore formation	Cutaneous superficial pyoderma in dogs	*Staphylococcus aureus* α-toxin has membrane-disrupting activities via a hemolysin that creates membrane pores and causes cell lysis (cell death).
Inhibition of protein synthesis	Caseous lymphadenitis in ruminants	*Corynebacterium pseudotuberculosis* diphtheria-like toxin inhibits protein synthesis by functioning as an RNA translational inhibitor and causes cell death.
Dysfunction of ion pumps	Enterotoxigenic enteritis in all domestic animal species	*Escherichia coli* heat-labile and heat-stable enterotoxins cause increased activity of membrane adenylyl and guanylate cyclase, resulting in increased intracellular cAMP and cGMP concentrations, respectively, leading to activation of ion and water pumps and loss of electrolytes and water from affected cells. These enterotoxins behave in a manner similar to cholera and pertussis toxins.
Selective protein inactivation (SNARE cleavage)	Tetanus and botulism in horses	*Clostridium tetani* tetanospasmin (neurotoxin) cleaves a SNARE protein, components of the synaptic fusion complex, preventing the release of inhibitory neurotransmitters glycine and γ-aminobutyric acid (GABA) into the synaptic cleft. This outcome results in exaggerated and frequent muscle twitches and "tetanic" contractions because the effects of the excitatory neurotransmitter (acetylcholine) are not effectively counterbalanced by those of inhibitory neurotransmitters. *Clostridium botulinum* neurotoxin cleaves a SNARE protein, components of the synaptic fusion complex, preventing the fusion of neurotransmitter vesicles (acetylcholine) with terminal membranes of the neuron and myoneural junctions. This outcome leads to muscle weakness, flaccid paralysis, and death attributable to respiratory failure.

cAMP, Cyclic adenosine monophosphate; *cGMP,* cyclic guanosine monophosphate; SNARE, soluble *N*-ethylmaleimide-sensitive factor attachment protein receptor

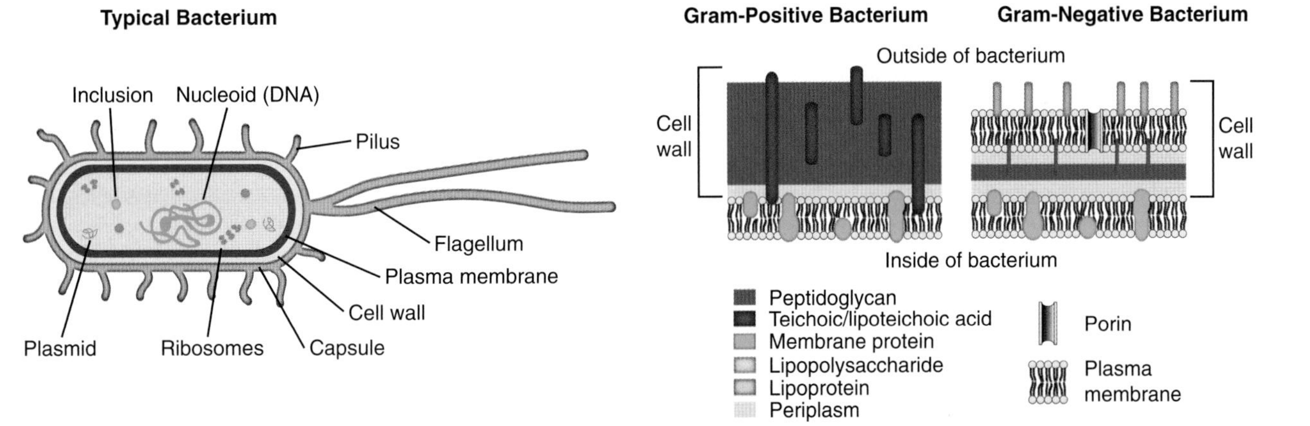

Figure 4-18 Morphologic Characteristics and Molecules of Gram-Positive and Gram-Negative Bacteria. The structure of a typical bacterium is shown on the left. The plasma membrane and cell wall of Gram-negative and Gram-positive bacteria contain molecules such as endotoxins (lipopolysaccharide [LPS]), exotoxins, and teichoic/lipoteichoic acid. They act as virulence factors (see Fig. 4-17) that damage target cells and their extracellular matrices such as collagen and thus are important in the pathogeneses of a wide variety of diseases. Gram-positive bacteria have a thick meshlike outer layer of peptidoglycan (also known as murein) that consists of sugars and amino acids. It provides structural strength in the formation of the cell wall. Gram-negative bacteria have a thin peptidoglycan layer and an outer membrane of LPS. Porins are cell membrane proteins that act as pores through which molecules can diffuse. (Courtesy Dr. J.F. Zachary, College of Veterinary Medicine, University of Illinois.)

release endotoxins into vascularized tissues when they die. Endotoxins is a general term used to characterize any outer membrane–associated toxin of the cell wall (see Figs. 4-15, 4-17, and 4-18). However, the term most commonly refers to LPS complex. Toxicity of LPS is attributable to the lipid A component of LPS, whereas immunogenicity (bacterin production [immunization]) is attributable to polysaccharide components of LPS. The outer membrane of the bacteria functions as a protective barrier against harmful large molecules and hydrophobic compounds in the environment such as bile salts, toxic molecules, lysozyme, and antimicrobial drugs. The membrane also functions to (1) impede phagocytosis by macrophages, (2) facilitate colonization of target cells, and (3) participate in the process of genomic variation (see section of viral diseases) in which the outer membrane acquires naïve polysaccharide components and evades host innate and acquired immune responses.

Endotoxins are released following destruction of the bacterial cell wall and are toxic to most animal cells (especially endothelial cells, platelets, and macrophages), tissues, and organs and can be lethal if large quantities are absorbed by or released into the circulatory system, causing the activation of proinflammatory cytokines and nitric oxide (NO) from macrophages and endothelial cells. This outcome leads to the activation of the complement and coagulation cascades and endotoxic shock (see Chapter 3) characterized by fever, hypoglycemia, thrombosis, (disseminated intravascular coagulation [DIC]), hypotensive shock, and death.

A-B Toxin. Some bacteria, such as *Bacillus anthracis* (anthrax) and *C. botulinum* (botulism), produce an exotoxin (virulence factor) called A-B toxin. A-B toxins are composed of two parts. Chronologically, the B part acts as a ligand and facilitates cell-surface recognition of target cells and entry of the A part into the cell via endocytosis. In the cell the A part carries out a toxic enzymatic reaction that interferes with one or more metabolic functions within the cell and allows the bacterium to colonize and replicate. For more detail see section on Bacterial Diseases of Organ Systems; Alimentary System and the Peritoneum, Omentum, Mesentery, and Peritoneal Cavity; Disorders of Domestic Animals; Alimentary Anthrax (*Bacillus anthracis*).

Other Virulence Factors

Secretion Systems. Secretion systems, of which six types (type I to VI) have been described, are bacterial organelles that secrete or inject bacterial-derived toxins into the cytoplasm of target cells. The type III secretion system is best known and occurs in some Gram-negative bacteria such as *Salmonella* spp. and *E. coli*. It injects, like a needle, specialized bacterial protein toxins like exotoxins into the cytoplasm of cells. These protein toxins often disrupt cell signal transduction and other cellular processes, leading to cell lysis.

Siderophores. Some bacteria require iron for colonization of mucosae. Iron is plentiful in cells but unavailable to bacteria because it is tightly bound in heme, ferritin, transferrin, or lactoferrin molecules. Siderophores are virulence factors that mediate the release of iron from intracellular iron stores (see Fig. 4-15). One example is enterobactin from *E. coli* and *Salmonella* spp.; this molecule scavenges bound iron from animal cells and makes it available for the bacteria. In another example, siderophores also play a role in the pathogenesis of the disease anthrax (*B. anthracis*). The bacterium releases two siderophores, bacillibactin and petrobactin, into the ECM, where they acquire iron for use by the bacterium.

Biofilms/Intracellular Bacterial Communities. Bacterial colonization can occur through virulence factors that form an exopolysaccharide matrix called a *biofilm* on mucosal surfaces lining the oral and nasal cavities and the mammary duct system as examples. Bacteria embedded in biofilms are not susceptible to phagocytosis by macrophages, and they can become resistant to antibiotics. A surface protein, biofilm-associated protein (Bap), has been implicated in the formation of a *S. aureus* biofilm in chronic bovine mastitis. Similarly, infections caused by certain strains of uropathogenic *E. coli* can result in the formation of intracellular bacterial communities affecting mucosal epithelial cells of the urinary bladder, which behave functionally much like a biofilm.

Capsules. Bacterial capsules are virulence factors that protect bacteria from phagocytosis by cells such as neutrophils and macrophages during acute inflammatory and adaptive immune responses. Capsules are secreted by the bacterium and are tightly adhered to the bacterial cell wall. They also aid with adhesion to mucosae and skin and are a reserve of nutrients, including water. Capsules are common in Gram-negative bacteria like *E. coli* and *Salmonella* spp., but also occur on fungi like *Cryptococcus neoformans*.

Role of Bacterial Genes in Susceptibility and/or Resistance to Disease

Microbes acquire through gene recombination (see later section) virulence genotypes and gene products (virulence factors) that allow them to escape defense mechanisms and spread locally, regionally, and/or systemically to encounter new target cell(s) and cause disease.

Virulence Factors

Virulence factors are encoded in and translated from genes in chromosomal DNA, bacteriophage DNA, or plasmids of bacteria. They can be readily transferred horizontally between bacteria (e.g., virulence factors for antibiotic resistance) via pathogenicity islands (PAIs) and/or virulence plasmids. PAIs are clusters of genes that code for virulence factors found in bacterial chromosomes. Virulence plasmids are clusters of self-replicating extrachromosomal genes for virulence factors located in plasmids within the cytoplasm of the bacteria. Most bacteria have only one chromosome but may contain hundreds of copies of a specific virulence plasmid. Plasmids replicate independently of cell division, and when a bacterium containing plasmids divides, the plasmids distribute randomly between the two resulting bacteria. Chromosomal or plasmid genes express virulence factors such as bacterial adhesins, colonization factors, protein toxins like hemolysins, other types of toxins, and molecules that affect the innate and adaptive immune responses. Strains of bacteria lacking PAIs and/or virulence plasmids usually do not cause disease. The number and type of virulence factors in a given bacterial strain are constantly changing, usually through genomic selection of those factors that favor the survival of the bacterium in the animal host. Each bacterial genera and strains within genera have their own unique virulence factor profile; therefore the total number of determinates that have been identified in all bacteria genera combined are in the hundreds. As an example, strains of *R. equi* that cause disease have chromosomal virulence factors for capsular polysaccharide, cholesterol oxidase, phospholipase C, lecithinase, and cell wall mycolic acids and plasmid virulence factors for virulence-associated protein (VAP).

Antibiotic Resistance

Antibiotic resistance, the ability of bacteria to withstand the static or lytic effects of antibiotics, evolves via natural selection of randomly mutated bacterial genes. These genes code for bacterial molecules (i.e., virulence factors) that cause resistance through the following four key mechanisms (Fig. 4-19):

1. Enzymatic deactivation (antibiotic inactivation or modification) as occurs with β-lactamases and extended-spectrum β-lactamases (resistant to cephalosporins and monobactams) produced by bacteria such as *Klebsiella pneumoniae*, *Pseudomonas aeruginosa*, *E. coli*, and *Salmonella typhimurium*
2. Alteration of antibiotic binding sites (penicillin-binding proteins [PBPs]) such as occurs in infections with methicillin-resistant *S. aureus* (MRSA) and other penicillin/methicillin/oxacillin-resistant bacteria such as *Streptococcus pneumoniae*, vancomycin-resistant enterococci (VRE), and penicillin-resistant *S. pneumoniae* (PRSP)
3. Alteration of a metabolic pathway, such as occurs with some sulfonamide-resistant bacteria that use preformed folic acid in place of *para*-aminobenzoic acid (PABA), a precursor for the synthesis of folic acid in bacteria inhibited by sulfonamides

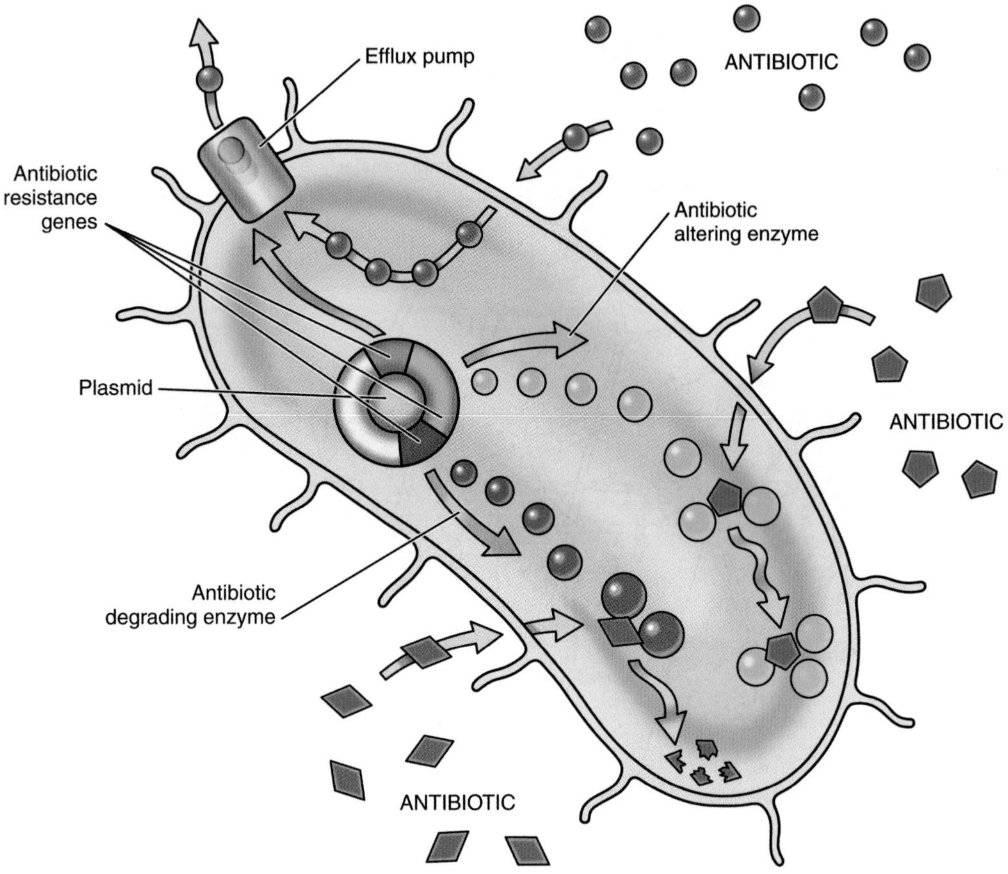

Figure 4-19 **Mechanisms Used by Bacteria to Establish Resistance to Antibiotics.**

4. Reduced antibiotic accumulation in bacteria through decreased membrane permeability to the antibiotic and/or enhanced efflux via membrane pumps

Bacterial Transfer of Antibiotic Resistance. The time required for bacteria to divide or a colony of bacteria to double in number is called the *generation time* and can be as short as 15 minutes. Although gene mutations for antibiotic resistance in bacteria are very rare steps, because of fast generation times and the ability to reach extremely high absolute numbers of bacteria via binary fission in short periods of time if unchecked, it does not take long before antibiotic resistance develops. The spontaneous mutation rate for antibiotic resistance is approximately 1×10^8 to 1×10^9. This means that one out of every 100 million to 1 trillion bacteria in an infection develops resistance through a mutation. The use of antibiotics is a form of environmental pressure on bacteria; those having a favorable genetic mutation (i.e., virulence factor for antibiotic resistance) survive therapy and continue to reproduce.

If a bacterium contains several antibiotic resistance genes, it is called a multiresistant microbe. Although a human disease, MRSA infections are beginning to appear in animals. Such pathogens have multiple resistance genes that protect them from most if not all broad-spectrum antibiotics commonly used to treat the disease. These resistance genes are transferred between and among bacteria of related and different genera by vertical and horizontal gene transfer.

Bacterial Gene Transfer

Vertical Gene Transfer. Vertical gene transfer is the process through which bacteria pass virulence factors such as antibiotic resistance to their offspring (asexual reproduction) during DNA replication. This transfer results in offspring fully resistant to an antibiotic. Because of this process, the overuse of broad-spectrum antibiotics in human beings and animals is a serious concern.

Horizontal Gene Transfer. Bacteria can also transfer antibiotic resistance genes between bacteria via horizontal gene transfer (Fig. 4-20) as follows:

1. Direct bacteria-bacteria contact (conjugation) via plasmids (the most common form)
2. Chromosomal DNA (transformation) in which pieces of DNA coded for antibiotic resistance and free in extracellular fluid as a result of lysis of its host bacterium are taken up by viable bacteria
3. Bacteria-specific viruses (bacteriophages) that transfer DNA (transduction) between two closely related bacteria

Mechanisms of Genomic Change

Mechanisms of genomic variation, antigenic drift (genetic drift), and antigenic shift are discussed in a later section on Viral Diseases, Mechanisms of Genomic Change. The concepts discussed are interchangeable with those that occur in bacterial diseases.

Bacterial Diseases of Organ Systems

Although the same bacterial disease often affects several different organ systems, diseases in this section are placed into a specific organ system based on which organ system demonstrates the primary gross lesion or lesions that are most commonly used to initially recognize and identify the disease. Bacterial diseases are identified by a primary mechanism of injury in E-Table 4-3.

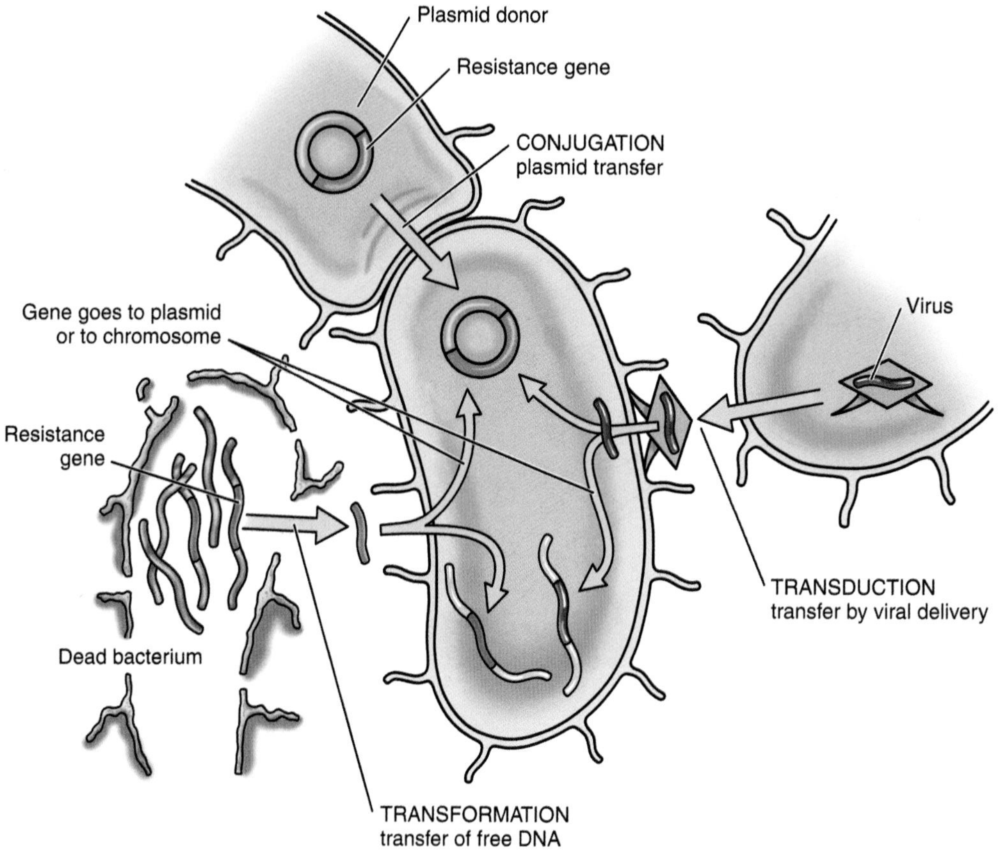

Figure 4-20 **Horizontal Gene Transfer.** Mechanisms used by bacteria to transfer resistance to an antibiotic to other bacteria.

Alimentary System and the Peritoneum, Omentum, Mesentery, and Peritoneal Cavity

Disorders of Domestic Animals

***Enteric Colibacillosis* (Escherichia coli).** *E. coli* strains that cause disease in animals have been named enterotoxigenic *E. coli* (ETEC), enteropathogenic *E. coli* (EPEC), and enterohemorrhagic *E. coli* (EHEC) based on the mechanisms and virulence factors that they use to cause diarrhea. In summary, the mechanisms of injury in enteric colibacillosis are (1) nonstructural alterations in the function of cell membrane ion and fluid transport systems (ETEC) and (2) structural alterations of cell membranes characterized by acute coagulative necrosis caused by bacterial toxins and by acute inflammation and its mediators and degradative enzymes (EPEC and EHEC). Enterotoxigenic and enteropathogenic strains do not invade mucosal enterocytes, whereas enterohemorrhagic strains do invade mucosal enterocytes. Enterotoxigenic strains secrete toxins that functionally, but not structurally, affect enterocytes, causing alterations in electrolyte and fluid secretion that result in a secretory diarrhea. Enteropathogenic strains structurally affect the microvillus border of enterocytes, causing alterations in electrolyte and fluid secretion that result in an osmotic diarrhea (malabsorption) and a less significant secretory diarrhea. Enterohemorrhagic strains structurally affect the enterocytes of the colon, causing cell lysis (necrosis), inflammation, and hemorrhage that lead to reduced absorption of colonic fluids and a malabsorption diarrhea. Endotoxins (LPS) likely directly or indirectly play a role in diseases caused by these three strains. There are no gross lesions in enterotoxigenic colibacillosis, whereas in enteropathogenic and enterohemorrhagic colibacillosis, mucosae are rough and granular (enterocyte necrosis, villus atrophy) with areas of hemorrhage, acute inflammation, and fibrin exudation.

Animals encounter *E. coli* through ingestion of bacteria in fomites contaminated with fecal material. The bacterium is swallowed and gains access via peristalsis to the mucus layer and mucosae of the intestines. It is likely that flagella expressed by some strains of *E. coli* facilitate their penetration of the mucus layer to gain access to microvilli of enterocytes.

Enterotoxigenic *Escherichia coli.* ETEC expresses K99 (F5) or F41 fimbrial adhesins that allow it to bind to receptor molecules in the mucus layer and to ganglioside and glycoprotein receptors on cell membranes of microvilli of enterocytes. When the mucosa is colonized, large numbers of bacteria are produced (Fig. 4-21), and they secrete heat labile (LT) and heat stable (ST) enterotoxins that diffuse in the mucus layer and microvilli, bind to specific receptors on the microvillus border of enterocytes, disrupt the function of cell membrane electrolyte and fluid transport systems, and cause secretory diarrhea. This process results in a functional lesion; no structural changes are observed grossly. LT and ST enterotoxins bind to glycolipid receptors on apical surfaces of enterocytes. After binding, these complexes are endocytosed and interact with a series of second messenger systems (epithelial cell signal transduction systems), which ultimately results in increased concentrations of intracellular cyclic adenosine monophosphate (cAMP, LT enterotoxin) and cyclic guanosine monophosphate (cGMP, ST enterotoxin). These molecules operate to open chloride channels (cystic fibrosis transmembrane regulator) in enterocyte cell membranes, thus acting irreversibly to move intracellular chloride ions extracellularly into the lumen of the intestine. Excessive chloride ion secretion also pulls water with it into the lumen of the intestine, thereby increasing the volume of fluid in the intestine. This volume ultimately exceeds the ability of the intestine to absorb the excessive fluid.

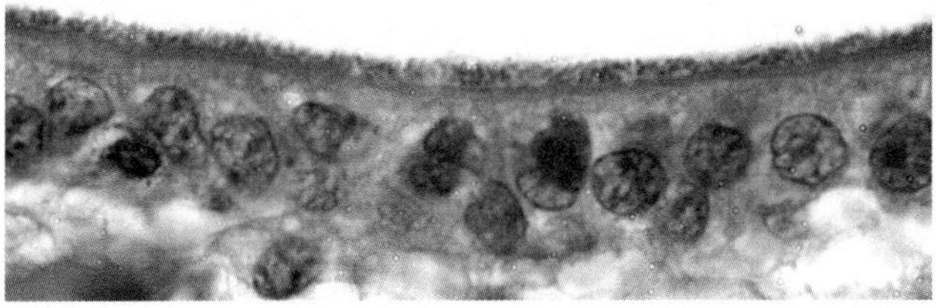

Figure 4-21 Colonization of Mucosa in Enteric Colibacillosis. *Escherichia coli* attach to microvilli, thus forming a uniform layer of blue-staining (hematoxylin) coccobacilli. Note the lack of epithelial cell injury. H&E stain. (Courtesy Dr. J.F. Zachary, College of Veterinary Medicine, University of Illinois.)

Enteropathogenic *Escherichia coli.* EPEC colonizes mucosae in a manner similar to that used by ETEC. EPEC does not produce LT or ST enterotoxins but does express adhesins such as P and S fimbriae, EPEC adherence factor, and intimin (nonfimbrial outer membrane protein). Integrins may serve as target cell membrane receptors for intimin, and this interaction appears to produce a tight bond between the bacterium and the enterocyte. After colonization and growth, bacterial virulence factors injure the brush border, leading to the loss of microvilli at the site of colonization. Such virulence factors appear to involve processes that disrupt cytoskeletal functions of the microvilli through interference with actin filaments, actin polymerization, and other cytoskeletal components and by causing alterations in intracellular calcium concentrations. This type of change has been called *attaching and effacing injury* and has resulted in naming the bacterium attaching and effacing *E. coli*. Injury to and loss of microvilli leads to decreased digestive enzyme activity in the glycocalyx (osmotic diarrhea) and disruption of ion transport systems (secretory diarrhea). EPEC also secretes bacterial proteins and likely injects them into the cytoplasm of enterocytes through a type III secretion system. These proteins, EspA, EspB, and EspD, activate a number of signal transduction pathways in the target cell, which appear to be involved in the pathogenesis of microvillus disruption. Additionally, acute inflammation occurs at the site of binding between the bacterium and the microvillus, likely contributing to the attaching and effacing lesion. Some attaching and effacing strains also secrete a virulence factor called *verotoxin*, which kills enterocytes and cells of the lamina propria (vascularized ECM tissues), leading to mucosal erosions and ulcers, intestinal edema and hemorrhage, and increased denuded mucosal surfaces for the absorption of endotoxins (LPS).

Enterohemorrhagic *Escherichia coli.* EHEC appears to colonize the mucus layer and mucosae in a manner similar to that used by the other two strains of the bacterium; however, enterocytes of the colon are the primary target cells. This specificity could be mediated through ligand-receptor interactions, and bacterial fimbriae have been shown to act as adhesins and attach to enterocyte cell membranes. Chemical gradients, such as the concentration of iron in target cells, could also provide the basis for colonic specificity. Once attached to colonic enterocytes, the bacterium replicates in large numbers and secretes a verotoxin that elicits an intense acute inflammatory response. It is also able to invade enterocytes, and verotoxin kills the cells. EHEC does not produce LT or ST enterotoxins, but Shiga toxins (Stxs) or Shiga-like toxins are virulence factors in some bacterial strains. Thus mucosal lesions (hemorrhagic colitis) characteristic of this strain of *E. coli* appear to result from a combination of inflammatory enzymes and mediators and toxins, all of which cause cell lysis and expose the underlying denuded lamina propria to a variety of harmful luminal molecules such as LPS that are readily available for absorption. Endotoxin, especially when in the blood, can lead to inflammation, capillary damage, vasculitis, thrombosis, intravascular coagulation, tissue degradation and infarction, endotoxic shock, and lysis. These mechanisms likely underlie the occurrence of acute adrenal cortical hemorrhage and necrosis (see E-Fig. 12-21) observed in endotoxemia with *E. coli* and other coliform infections.

Enterotoxemic and Septicemic Colibacillosis. Septicemic colibacillosis, likely resulting from an enteropathogenic strain of *E. coli*, may begin as an alimentary manifestation and then progress to enterotoxemic colibacillosis or septicemic colibacillosis. In these forms the enterotoxins (and the bacterium) most likely gain access to the circulatory system via invasion into and absorption through capillary beds in the lamina propria of injured intestinal mucosae. Enterotoxemic colibacillosis and its toxins cause edema disease of the nervous system (see section on Nervous System; also see Chapter 14) leading to fibrinoid arteriopathy/arteriolopathy of the brain and ischemia and malacia, whereas septicemic colibacillosis and its bacterium and toxins cause disease of the cardiovascular system (see Chapter 10) leading to lysis via toxic and endotoxic shock and cardiovascular collapse.

Salmonellosis (*Salmonella* spp.). The mechanism of injury in salmonellosis is acute coagulative necrosis of cells caused by bacterial toxins and by acute inflammation and its mediators and degradative enzymes. Three forms of salmonellosis occur: peracute, acute, and chronic. Gross lesions in the peracute form include petechiation and a blue discoloration (cyanosis) of the skin, fibrinous polyserositis, and disseminated intravascular coagulopathy (see Fig. 7-118). These lesions are rooted in injury of the vascular system with vasculitis and thrombosis caused by bacterial toxins. In the acute form, lesions affect mucosae of the small intestine, large intestine, and cecum (fibrinonecrotic ileotyphlocolitis) and are characterized by a rough and granular mucosal surface (necrosis) mixed with mucus, fibrin, and occasionally blood (see Fig. 7-118). The content is malodorous (septic tank odor). This pattern of injury is caused by bacterial toxins, acute inflammation, and their effects on enterocytes and blood vessels within the lamina propria. Many of these processes are enabled by virulence factors encoded on "Salmonella pathogenicity islands" on its chromosome. Bacteria can spread via the portal vein to the liver, leading to the formation of foci of bacteria- and toxin-induced necrosis and inflammation (paratyphoid nodules) (see Fig. 8-54). This spread likely occurs via leukocyte trafficking and infection of Kupffer cells, but bacteremia may also occur. Leukocyte trafficking also spreads the bacteria to mesenteric and systemic lymph nodes and the gallbladder (fibrinous cholecystitis). In the chronic form, injury is associated with discrete foci of necrosis and ulceration of mucosae (button ulcers). These lesions are rooted in injury of the vascular system with vasculitis and thrombosis caused by bacterial toxins diffusing within the submucosa of the intestine.

Animals encounter *Salmonella* spp. through ingestion of bacteria in fomites contaminated with fecal material. The bacterium is swallowed and gains access via peristalsis to the mucus layer and mucosae of the intestines. *Salmonella* spp. appear to use two mechanisms to colonize mucosae and gain access to the lamina propria and its capillary beds. The first mechanism uses M cells in intestinal crypts. Because a mucus layer is absent over M cells, the bacteria have direct contact with apically positioned cell membranes of M cells. The second mechanism uses apically positioned cell membranes of enterocytes to gain access to these cells; however, these cells are covered with a mucus layer. Because *Salmonella* spp. are motile bacteria (flagella—virulence factor), they likely can penetrate through the mucus layer and gain access to these membranes. The bacterium must adhere to the apical surfaces of M cells and enterocytes to begin the process of colonizing the intestine, which is a process mediated through ligand-receptor interactions. Although unproved, it is probable that one or some of the fimbriae possessed by *Salmonella* spp. are involved in the initial adherence between the bacterium and these cells. It is thought, though unconfirmed, that fimbriae may determine susceptibility of the various strains of *Salmonella* spp. for animal species and for specific target cells within each species. Which fimbriae (virulence factor) are used to bind to target cells may vary depending on whether the target cell is an M cell or an enterocyte. Additionally, PAMP and PRRs (also known as TLRs [Toll-like receptors]) are probably involved. Once bound to target cell membrane, a type III secretion system is used to inject bacterial proteins into the target cell that stimulate phagocytosis through the mobilization of actin filaments in the cytoplasm. Colonization of mucosae only occurs if LPS is present in the bacterial cell wall, and it likely plays a role in adherence to target cells through its participation in cell wall stability and resistance to bile salts, cell surface hydrophobicity, and the correct insertion and folding of membrane proteins such as those that occur in fimbriae.

Once the bacterium has reached the luminal (apical) surfaces of mucosal epithelial cells (villus epithelium or M cells), *Salmonella* spp. have several options in interacting with these cells. They can (1) colonize and replicate on apical surfaces, (2) enter via endocytosis and colonize and replicate within epithelial cells, or (3) migrate through cells via an endocytotic-exocytotic pathway to exit the basal side of the cell, enter the lamina propria, and colonize and replicate within cells such as those in GALT. Additionally, mucosa-associated macrophages and dendritic cells may interact with epithelial cells and bacteria and can phagocytize and carry bacteria via leukocyte trafficking to mucosa-associated lymphoid cells and in afferent lymphatic vessels to Peyer's patches.

Once the microbe is internalized via phagocytosis or endocytosis, *Salmonella* spp. survive and replicate within a "*Salmonella*-containing vacuole (SCV)". *Salmonella* spp. are able to inhibit phagosome-lysosome fusion, thereby blocking their killing within macrophages (see Fig. 4-14). If phagosome-lysosome fusion occurs, bacteria are able to block the effects of lysosomal enzymes, acidity, and free radicals. In fact, the bacterium resides and replicates in a phagosome and/or phagolysosome (SCV) until released from the macrophage after the lysis of the macrophage caused by toxins produced by the bacterium. Once in Peyer's patches, macrophages infected with bacteria die and release bacteria that will infect additional macrophages through ligand-receptor interactions. *Salmonella* spp. can kill macrophages via apoptosis using a type I secretory system that leads to activation of caspase-1 in macrophages. These macrophages are often recruited as monocytes from the systemic circulation as a component of the acute inflammatory response. Once infected with the bacterium, macrophages migrate in efferent lymphatic vessels via leukocyte trafficking to regional mesenteric lymph nodes using mechanisms similar to those described in Peyer's patches and then systemically via the thoracic duct and circulatory system. Macrophages also likely gain access to the systemic circulatory system through capillaries and postcapillary venules in lymph nodes. It also appears that dendritic cells in the intestinal mucosa are infected by the bacterium, and these cells likely spread the bacterium to Peyer's patches.

In all of these situations, acute inflammation occurs concurrently in response to bacterial toxins and antigens, resulting in vascular permeability changes and injury, and in the recruitment of neutrophils and their degradative enzymes, which can cause additional tissue injury. As part of this response, the interaction of M cells and enterocytes with bacteria appears to cause the release of chemokines and other chemoattractants for neutrophils into surrounding vascularized ECM. It appears that the form of disease (peracute, acute, or chronic) that occurs depends on which steps used in the chronology (as described previously) are emphasized through the expression of virulence factors by different strains of *Salmonella* spp. The peracute form likely favors spread to regional lymph nodes and then systemically with the release of toxins leading to vascular injury, failure of the circulatory system, and lysis. The acute form likely favors mucosal adherence and colonization leading to mucosal necrosis mediated by bacterial toxins. Through this process and the acute inflammation that ensues, capillary beds in the lamina propria are permeable and likely bacteria, bacterial toxins, and bacteria-infected macrophages enter the venous circulatory system and spread via the portal vein to the liver. The chronic form likely favors invasion of the lamina propria and submucosa (motile bacteria) with direct effects on the vasculature that supplies the intestine with blood. However, it is possible that button ulcers observed in this form are a manifestation of septicemia with attachment of bacteria to vascular endothelium resulting in vasculitis, thrombosis, ischemia, and infarction. The lesions and clinical signs that occur in diseases caused by *Salmonella* spp. are in part attributable to (1) an enterotoxin (exotoxin) that produces a secretory diarrhea, (2) a cytotoxin that inhibits protein synthesis, and (3) endotoxins and LPSs that cause membrane injury and cell lysis. Acute inflammation and cell and tissue injury that ensue are also important causes of the lesions.

Enterotoxemia (*Clostridium perfringens*). The mechanism of injury in enterotoxemia is acute coagulative necrosis of cells and tissues caused by bacterial toxins. Gross lesions include segments of the small intestine or the entire small intestine that are dark red to purple-black (hemorrhagic enteritis) and accompanied by mucosal, submucosal, and serosal edema and hemorrhage (see Figs. 7-121, 7-122, and 7-163). *Clostridium perfringens* attaches in a layered fashion to mucosal surfaces, and as toxins are released, it diffuses into the mucosa and lamina propria, causing in addition to necrosis, thrombosis of mucosal and submucosal vessels. Inflammation usually does not occur. *C. perfringens* causes disease syndromes that are categorized based on bacterial type (type A to E), toxin type (α-, β-, ε-, and ι-toxins), species affected, and/or age of the animal affected. These classification systems are always in a state of change as new toxins are identified in strains of the bacterium. At least 16 different toxins and enzymes (virulence factors) have been identified on chromosomes and plasmids of different clostridial strains; however, no single strain of the bacterium produces all of these factors. Further discussion of these classification systems is beyond the scope of this chapter.

Cattle, sheep, goats, pigs, and horses encounter *C. perfringens* through ingestion of bacterial spores in the soil or from contact with fomites contaminated with the vegetative form of the bacterium from carrier animals. The vegetative form of *C. perfringens* can be a normal inhabitant of the alimentary system of domestic animals. It appears that under the proper conditions in the intestine that are usually linked to changes in the diet or the ingestion of an energy source rich in carbohydrates, spores germinate into vegetative forms and proliferate or the ingested vegetative form proliferates. It has been shown experimentally that dietary trypsin can inactivate β-toxin, thus it is thought that diets deficient in trypsin may increase the likelihood of disease. Additionally, sudden dietary change can also alter the composition of normal intestinal microflora, providing opportunities for the vegetative form of the bacterium to proliferate and produce toxins. Vegetative forms are nonmotile and gain access to mucosae via random motion from peristalsis. They colonize the mucus layer by using bacterial proteases to expose receptors in mucus and then use bacterial adhesins to bind to these receptors. Within the mucus layer, bacteria are protected from acids and enzymes in intestinal content. The bacterium also consumes mucus as an energy source for bacterial growth and replication, and this process is thought to activate bacterial genes that regulate the production of toxins. Once the mucus layer is colonized, bacteria then interact with microvilli of enterocytes by attachment and retraction of type IV pili (gliding motility) and eventually attach to the apical surfaces of enterocytes. Attachment is likely mediated by ligand-receptor interactions.

Experimental studies suggest that bacterial toxins that diffuse across mucosae may first injure endothelial cells in capillaries of the lamina propria before the attachment of bacteria to the apical surfaces of enterocytes and that attachment may require changes in the membranes of apical enterocytes that are induced directly by the effect of toxins at the apical surfaces of enterocytes and indirectly by ischemia. At this phase of the disease, injury is primarily limited to enterocytes. Once mucosae are colonized, bacteria replicate in immense numbers, and the disease enters a second phase characterized by the production of abundant potent cytotoxins, which spread via diffusion as a wave into the mucosa, lamina propria, submucosa, and muscle layers. Some clinical forms of enterotoxemia remain in the first phase of the disease; others progress into the second phase. Discussion of these various clinical forms is outside the scope of this chapter. Potent cytotoxins produced by the bacteria include α-, β-, ε-, and ι-toxins (alpha [CPA], beta [CPB], epsilon [ETX], and iota [ITX]), which behave as enterocyte membrane toxins (α, β), such as phospholipases, lecithinases, and pore-forming toxins, as well as ECM toxins, such as collagenase, hyaluronidase, and sialidase. ε-Toxin has the unique ability to increase enterocyte and endothelial cell permeability by acting on the cytoskeleton and probably altering the function of junctional complexes, thus affecting the absorption of toxins by the vascular system, resulting in systemic effects. ι-Toxin disrupts the cytoskeleton, which leads to cell lysis. Because of the abundance of toxins produced in the second phase of enterotoxemia, toxins freely move in the intestinal lumen via peristalsis to interact with uncolonized normal enterocytes; thus the lesions are quickly spread to other areas within the intestine. Toxins cause lysis and sloughing of enterocytes of villi and crypts followed by further colonization by bacteria, additional proliferation and toxin production, and toxin-induced massive necrosis resulting in structural breakdown and hemorrhage of the entire intestinal wall. Because ε-toxin is a permease that alters cell permeability, the vascular beds in affected intestinal tissues readily absorb toxins from the lumen of the intestine into the circulatory system. Toxins are then carried to the brain, kidney, and other tissues in which the increase in vascular permeability leads to the release of blood plasma containing toxins into the interstitium and body cavities, resulting in edema and effusions. In the brain and kidney these toxins cause focal symmetric encephalomalacia (see Fig. 14-96) and pulpy kidney disease (see Fig. 11-49), respectively. However, it appears that the mechanisms leading to these two diseases occur in the first phase or early in the second phase of enterotoxemia before toxin-induced massive necrosis of the intestine occurs.

Alimentary Anthrax (*Bacillus anthracis*). The mechanism of injury in alimentary anthrax is acute coagulative necrosis of cells caused by bacterial toxins. Gross lesions include segments of the small intestine or the entire small intestine that are dark red to purple-black (hemorrhagic enteritis) and accompanied by mucosal, submucosal, and serosal edema and hemorrhage (see Fig. 7-124). Additionally, mesenteric lymph nodes can be enlarged, edematous, and hemorrhagic. The bacterium replicates in large numbers and is closely linked with mucosae of the small intestine; however, the mechanisms of adherence and colonization are uncertain. It produces an A-B toxin that diffuses into the mucosa and lamina propria, causing in addition to necrosis, thrombosis of mucosal and submucosal vessels. This latter lesion leads to ischemic necrosis (acute coagulative necrosis) of tissues supplied by these blood vessels. Inflammation usually does not occur.

Animals, most commonly cattle, encounter *B. anthracis* through the ingestion of fomites contaminated with endospores and/or vegetative forms of the bacterium. The bacterium exists most commonly in soil and water as an endospore, a dormant, nonreproductive form that is resistant to ultraviolet radiation, dehydration, extremely cold and hot temperatures, and chemical disinfectants. These conditions are harmful to the vegetative form, the form of the bacterium that produces toxin and causes disease. Animals can ingest endospores that subsequently germinate into vegetative forms in the alimentary tract. However, animals can also ingest vegetative forms as the result of environmental conditions that allow the vegetative form to persist for a limited period of time. Heavy rain after a drought can cause the germination of endospores in areas contaminated with endospores and the multiplication of vegetative forms. Endospores present in undercooked or poorly processed meat wastes and by-products can germinate into vegetative forms, persist for a limited period of time, and then be ingested when fed to animals.

Endospores and/or vegetative forms are swallowed, evade destruction by gastric acidity, and gain access to mucosae of the small intestine via peristalsis. The sequence of steps from ingestion of endospores or vegetative forms to the occurrence of lesions is largely unknown. It has been suggested that endospores can gain access to mucosae and lamina propria via ulcers, cuts, and puncture wounds of the alimentary system, geminate into vegetative forms, colonize the tissue, and secrete toxins causing disease. It is also likely that vegetative forms gain access to regional mesenteric lymph nodes via afferent lymphatic vessels as cell-free bacteria or within macrophages via phagocytosis that migrate via leukocyte trafficking in lymphatic vessels to these nodes. Vegetative forms probably use mechanisms discussed later to cause disease in the injured mucosae. Alternatively, the need for mucosal injury as an initiating step in the disease is conceivable. Hypothetically, three possible mechanisms could result in the production of vegetative forms, toxins, and lesions:

1. Endospores could be trapped in the mucus layer of the mucosa, endospores germinate to vegetative forms, vegetative forms use mucus to grow and replicate, and vegetative forms produce toxins that diffuse into the mucosa and submucosa, resulting in lesions.
2. Endospores could be trapped in the mucus layer of the mucosa, phagocytosed by macrophages or dendritic cells, and carried to Peyer's patches, where they germinate into vegetative forms, and vegetative forms produce toxins that diffuse into the mucosa and submucosa, resulting in lesions.
3. Endospores are phagocytosed by M cells and carried to Peyer's patches, where they germinate into vegetative forms, and vegetative forms produce toxins that diffuse into the mucosa and submucosa, resulting in lesions.[7]

Primary virulence factors produced by *B. anthracis* are in plasmid genes and include those that form the capsule and anthrax toxins. The capsule is important in establishing the infection, whereas anthrax toxins cause the lesions, disease, and lysis. The capsule consists of poly-D-glutamic acid that is nontoxic, protects the bacterium from destructive antibodies and bactericidal components of

---

[7]If vegetative forms are ingested, three similar mechanisms are proposed to occur in animals, but the time course of disease would likely be shortened.

plasma, and inhibits phagocytosis, killing, and digestion of vegetative forms of the bacterium by macrophages and neutrophils. Anthrax toxins behave as an A-B toxin system and consist of three exotoxins that act together to cause cell lysis. One exotoxin, called *protective antigen* (PA), the B part of the A-B toxin, facilitates the entry of itself into cells via endocytosis and then creates a pore in the cell membrane through which the remaining two toxins, *edema factor* (EF) and *lethal factor* (LF), the A component of the A-B toxin, can enter the cell. Exotoxins must first bind to receptors on target cells. PA binds to two different cell surface receptors, tumor endothelial marker 8 (TEM8) and capillary morphogenesis protein 2 (CMG2). These receptors appear to explain the vascular orientation of the disease and the circulatory system collapse that results. In addition to vascular tissues, these receptors are also commonly expressed on cells in many other organ systems, likely accounting for the various forms (inhalation, cutaneous, and gastrointestinal) of anthrax. Once inside cells, PA combines with edema factor to form edema toxin, which disrupts cell membrane water and electrolyte transport systems, resulting in edema, and also blocks phagocytosis of vegetative forms by neutrophils and macrophages. Additionally, PA combines with lethal factor to form lethal toxin. This toxin stimulates the production of a variety of cytokines that act to cause cell lysis, especially affecting phagocytic cells such as macrophages and endothelial cells of capillaries. Because of injury to mucosae and lamina propria, capillary beds in the ECM can absorb edema and lethal toxins, as well as a variety of intestinal endotoxins. Cytokines, anthrax toxins, and endotoxins have profound systemic effects on the cardiovascular system, all of which contribute to cardiogenic and circulatory shock and lysis. Chromosomal genes of the vegetative form of the bacterium also express a capsule virulence factor, which makes it resistant to phagocytosis by mucosa-associated tissue macrophages. Additionally, the bacterium has several chromosomal virulence factors for hemolysins, phospholipases, and iron acquisition proteins that can contribute to or cause cell lysis.

Disorders of Horses

Rhodococcal Enteritis (*Rhodococcus equi*). The pathogenesis of *R. equi* infection is also discussed in the section on Bacterial Diseases of Organ Systems; Respiratory System, Mediastinum, and Pleurae; Disorders of Horses. An overview is provided herein. Gross lesions include (1) ulcerative enteritis (see Fig. 7-138) characterized by discrete foci of ulceration and hemorrhage centered over Peyer's patches and (2) chronic active pyogranulomatous lymphadenitis (see Fig. 7-139) characterized by enlarged firm lymph nodes that on a cut surface have discrete and coalescing areas of yellow-white exudate infiltrating and compressing contiguous parenchyma.

In the alimentary system, foals encounter *R. equi* by swallowing mucus (sputum), exudate, and cellular debris contaminated with bacteria that move into the oral pharynx via the positive pressure of coughing and the upward rhythmic movement of cilia in the mucociliary apparatus. The bacterium then gains access to the alimentary system via intestinal peristalsis. Bacteria probably bind to receptors on luminal surfaces of M cells and are then transported in endocytotic vesicles to the basal membranes of the cell and released into the Peyer's patches, where they can be phagocytosed by tissue macrophages or dendritic cells. Unlike most other regions of the intestine, the luminal surface of M cells lacks a covering of mucus. Therefore bacteria have direct access to M cells. It is likely that ligand-receptor mechanisms (as discussed in the section on the Respiratory System, Mediastinum, and Pleurae) are applicable to M cells and tissue macrophages in Peyer's patches. Once tissue macrophages are infected, the pathogenesis of the disease appears to progress much like that which occurs in the lung resulting in pyogranulomatous enteritis and lymphadenitis. Mechanistically, *R. equi* has virulence factors in a PAI and in a plasmid that block (1) the fusion of phagosomes with lysosomes (virulence-associated proteins [Vaps]), (2) the actions of lysosomal enzymes and toxins, and (3) the respiratory burst used by macrophages to kill the bacterium. The bacterium can then replicate within the phagosome of macrophages. Pyogranulomatous enteritis is attributable to repeated cycles of phagocytosis, dysfunction of phagosomes, bacterial growth and replication, lysis of macrophages, release of large numbers of new bacteria, recruitment of additional naïve inflammatory cells, and reparative responses like fibrosis that likely perpetuate and expand the scope of the disease process. Ulcerative enteritis, characteristic of the alimentary form of the disease, occurs over affected Peyer's patches. Although unknown, it is probable that mediators and degradative enzymes from inflammation diffuse into contiguous tissues, causing direct injury to the mucosa or indirectly via vascular injury and occlusion leading to infarction and ulceration. Bacteria-infected tissue macrophages can also spread via leukocyte trafficking in afferent lymphatic vessels within the intestinal mesentery to mesenteric lymph nodes leading to a pyogranulomatous lymphadenitis and then systemically to lymph nodes and lymphoid tissues such as the spleen.

Tyzzer's Disease (*Clostridium piliforme* [*Bacillus piliformis*]). See Bacterial Diseases of Organ Systems, Hepatobiliary System and Exocrine Pancreas, Disorders of Horses, Tyzzer's Disease (*Clostridium piliforme* [*Bacillus piliformis*]).

Disorders of Ruminants (Cattle, Sheep, and Goats)

Johne's Disease (*Mycobacterium avium* ssp. *paratuberculosis* [MAP]). The mechanisms of injury in Johne's disease are (1) dysfunction and lysis of the epithelial cells and ECM proteins forming the junctional barrier systems of mucosae of the small intestine, (2) dysfunction of the drainage of afferent lymphatic vessels in the lamina propria of villi of the small intestine, and (3) lysis of cells of the monocyte-macrophage system and of all cell populations in the lamina propria of intestinal villi from chronic inflammation and its mediators and degradative enzymes. Gross lesions include granulomatous enteritis and mesenteric granulomatous lymphadenitis, lymphangitis, and lymphangiectasia (see Fig. 7-162). Granulomatous enteritis is characterized by a thickened intestinal wall, most commonly affecting the ileum and ileal-cecal junction with a yellow-white exudate exemplified by infiltrating granulomatous inflammatory cells. Mesenteric granulomatous lymphadenitis is characterized by enlarged mesenteric lymph nodes that on cut surfaces have discrete and coalescing areas of yellow-white caseous exudate, occasionally mineralized, infiltrating, and compressing contiguous parenchyma.

The young of cattle, sheep, and goats encounter *M. avium* ssp. *paratuberculosis* through ingestion of the bacterium in manure-contaminated fomites in the environment. It is unknown why young animals are more susceptible to this microbe. It has been suggested that the "open gut" that occurs during the first 24 hours after birth, where immunoglobulins in colostrum are absorbed by pinocytosis, is a mechanism that may also be used by the bacterium to cross the mucosal barrier and enter the submucosa. Young animals may also be more susceptible to infection because of immature innate and/or adaptive immune responses. Susceptibility is also probably strongly influenced by management and environmental factors and to a lesser extent by the genes of the animal.

The bacterium is swallowed and gains access via peristalsis to the alimentary system. Bacteria appear to bind to receptors on luminal (apical) surfaces of M cells and are likely translocated in endocytotic vesicles or phagosomes to the basal membranes of the cell and are released into Peyer's patches, where they can be phagocytosed by tissue macrophages. Unlike most other regions of the intestine, the luminal surface of M cells lacks a covering of mucus. Therefore bacteria have direct access to M cells. Lesions appear to have a segmental pattern of occurrence most commonly affecting the ileocecal intestine. Although attachment and phagocytosis of the bacterium by M cells likely involves ligand-receptor interactions, this mechanism does not explain why the lesions are most severe in ileocecal intestine. A second, but less likely, pathway of spread can also result from ingestion. Chewing of foodstuffs places *Mycobacterium*-infected fomites in contact with the palatine tonsils. Experimentally it has been shown that the bacterium can infect mucosal and submucosal cells of the tonsil, likely spread via leukocyte trafficking to regional lymph nodes, and then spread via leukocyte trafficking in efferent lymphatic vessels to mesenteric lymph nodes (ileocecal lymph nodes) and the mucosa and submucosa of the ileum and ileal-cecal junction areas.

M. *avium* ssp. *paratuberculosis* requires iron for growth inside phagosomes of tissue macrophages. For an unknown reason the concentration and availability of iron is greatest in tissue macrophages of the ileocecal intestine when compared to the concentration in other types of tissue macrophages. Therefore this gradient of iron appears to establish tissue specificity for lesions in Johne's disease. In macrophages, iron is stored as ferritin, but it is not accessible by the bacterium. Mycobacteria secrete iron-chelating proteins called exochelins, iron-reductases, and potentially siderophores (i.e., virulence factors) and use these enzymes to acquire iron from ferritin stored in macrophages. Additionally, as the severity of inflammation increases, there is a concurrent increase in the concentration of ferritin available for use by the bacterium in cells and tissues in the areas of inflammation. Mycobacterial siderophores or reductases may also serve to block iron-dependent bactericidal reactions of tissue macrophages such as Fe^{3+}-dependent conversion of H_2O_2 into highly toxic hydroxyl radicals.

In ileocecal tissues, phagocytosis of the bacterium by tissue macrophages likely involves ligand-receptor interactions. TLRs may also be involved in attachment and phagocytosis. The cell walls of mycobacteria contain a variety of complex lipoglycans, glycoproteins, and lipoproteins such as lipoarabinomannan (LAM), 19-kDa lipoprotein, and the mycolyl-arabinogalactan-peptidoglycan complex that can serve as ligands. The cell membranes of tissue macrophages express receptors for these specific molecules, and they are probably involved in the recognition, attachment, and adherence of the bacterium to the macrophage cell membrane. Additionally, complement receptors and other receptors, including mannose and CD14 receptors, expressed on tissue macrophages are the major receptors involved in phagocytosis of the bacterium, whereas integrin receptors, TLRs, mannose receptors, CD14 receptors, scavenger receptors, and immunoglobulin Fc receptors are involved in early recognition and cell signaling in response to interaction with the bacterium. Generally, these signaling pathways initiate production of a variety of cytokines, chemokines, and antimicrobial metabolites that control mycobacterial infections; however, the bacterium through these signaling pathways is able to attenuate macrophage activation responses induced by interferon-γ (IFN-γ) and the secretion of IFN-γ. Type 1 T helper lymphocytes, attempt to enhance the killing of intracellular mycobacterial organisms by releasing cytokines such as IFN-γ that activate macrophages to kill the bacterium.

These interactions do not involve opsonin-mediated phagocytosis; thus the induction of a respiratory burst to kill the internalized bacteria does not occur, and the bacterium persists in the phagosome. Receptors for opsonins expressed by tissue macrophages might also play a role in phagocytosis of the bacterium. Fibronectin may bind to the surface of macrophages and serve as a ligand to facilitate phagocytosis by macrophages. However, when employing opsonization as a means of entry into a phagosome, the bacterium must also use a mechanism to inhibit the respiratory burst to prevent its lysis.

The time from initial encounter with the bacterium to the expression of clinical disease is usually 12 months or longer. An explanation for this extended delay is unknown; it may simply be a slow-growing bacterium. However, bacterial growth likely involves the (1) interplay of bacterium-infected tissue macrophages and cells of the immune system mediated by proinflammatory and antiinflammatory cytokines, (2) migration of tissue macrophages locally from Peyer's patches into the lamina propria and submucosal tissues, (3) time it takes the bacterium to replicate in sufficient quantities to activate the adaptive immune response, and (4) progression of severity resulting from the lysis of bacterium-infected macrophages leading to the recruitment of additional macrophages.

After phagocytosis by tissue macrophages in Peyer's patches, the bacterium is confined within phagosomes and phagolysosomes (see Fig. 4-13). It appears to be able to disrupt phagosome-lysosome fusion and if fusion occurs, block the degradative actions of lysosomal enzymes and molecules via the structure and composition of its cell envelope and through the production of peroxidases. When a phagolysosome forms, the fused lysosome releases an acidic cytosol, proteases, and antibacterial substances, such as defensins and toxic oxygen and nitrogen intermediates, into the phagosome, all of which can injure and kill the bacterium. In general, mycobacterial species can (1) inhibit acidification of the phagosome, phagosome-lysosome fusion, and lysosomal enzyme activities; (2) block injury from toxic oxygen and nitrogen intermediates; and (3) suppress the ability of macrophages to be activated by cytokines such as INF-γ. Although highly probable, it is not known which or if any of these mechanisms are used by M. *avium* ssp. *paratuberculosis*. Tissue macrophages, once infected with the bacterium, are activated and begin to secrete proinflammatory cytokines that act to recruit and activate additional macrophages. Additionally, because the life span of fully differentiated tissue macrophages is approximately 10 to 30 days, lysis of these cells related to aging and bacterial-induced injury releases bacterium into adjacent tissue, where they are phagocytosed by newly recruited macrophages only to endlessly repeat this process. Granulomatous inflammation ensues, and multinucleated giant cells are noted histologically in the exudate (see Chapters 3 and 5).

The severity and extent of the inflammatory response, concurrently with tissue injury, grows through the recruitment of additional monocytes and tissue macrophages from the circulatory system and regional lymph nodes. This repetitive process accounts for the marked thickening of the mucosa and submucosa of the ileum and ileal-cecal junction characteristic of the gross lesion of Johne's disease. It also destroys the integrity of the mucosal barrier system, as well as lymphatic drainage, often resulting in a protein-losing enteropathy. This process is also probably an important factor contributing to severe malabsorption, diarrhea, weight loss, and emaciation that ensue. Bacteria-infected tissue macrophages can also spread via leukocyte trafficking in afferent lymphatic vessels within the intestinal mesentery to mesenteric lymph nodes (ileocecal lymph nodes), leading to a pyogranulomatous lymphadenitis and lymphangiectasia through the same progressive mechanism of inflammation.

Bovine Intestinal Tuberculosis (*Mycobacterium bovis*). The pathogenesis of *Mycobacterium bovis* infection is also discussed in the section on Bacterial Diseases of Organ Systems; Respiratory System, Mediastinum, and Pleurae; Disorders of Ruminants (Cattle, Sheep, and Goats). An overview is provided herein. The pathogenesis and lesions of bovine intestinal tuberculosis are identical to those observed in the pneumonic form. Also, see Johne's disease in the previous section because its pathogenesis is similar to that of intestinal tuberculosis. It appears that intestinal tuberculosis commonly begins as the pneumonic form and is spread to the intestine by (1) coughing up and swallowing sputum containing macrophages infected with bacteria and/or "free" bacteria and (2) hematogenous or lymphatic spread of infected macrophages via leukocyte trafficking to intestinal lymph nodes and Peyer's patches. Via the alimentary route, intestinal M cells and possibly dendritic cells are used to phagocytose bacteria and then release them via exocytosis from basolateral surfaces into Peyer's patches, where they are phagocytosed by macrophages and granulomatous inflammation and granuloma formation follow. Intestinal tuberculosis is associated with mucosal ulceration overlying Peyer's patches. Ulceration appears to result from vasculitis, thrombosis, ischemia, and infarction secondary to inflammation in Peyer's patches but could also be caused directly by inflammatory mediators released from granulomas diffusing to and acting on blood vessels or mucosae.

Wooden Tongue (*Actinobacillus lignieresii*). The mechanisms of injury in wooden tongue are persistent pyogranulomatous inflammation and fibrotic reparative responses. Gross lesions include a firm enlarged tongue that protrudes from the oral cavity. Cut surfaces have numerous randomly distributed yellow-white granulomas intermixed with broad bands of fibrous connective tissue (see Figs. 7-51 and 52). *Actinobacillus lignieresii* is a normal commensal bacterium of mucosae of the oral cavity of cattle and sheep, the species in which this disorder occurs most commonly. However, it has, although very rarely, been reported to occur in horses, pigs, and dogs. During chewing the bacterium is carried through the mucosa into submucosal connective tissues via penetrating wounds such as those caused by sharp foreign bodies like sticks or wires. The bacterium colonizes submucosal connective tissue, and LPS of the bacterial cell wall, in part, likely plays a role in the pyogranulomatous inflammatory and concurrent fibrotic responses that occur. Little is known about how virulence factors, ligand-receptor interactions, target cells, toxins, capsule antiphagocytic molecules, or other factors contribute to the pathogenicity of this bacterium. However, it appears likely that the bacterium is able to evade killing by neutrophils and macrophages, thus colonizing itself in abscesses in tissues of the tongue and oral cavity. Repeated cycles of phagocytosis, bacterial growth and replication, lysis of macrophages, release of large numbers of new bacteria, recruitment of additional naïve inflammatory cells, and reparative responses like fibrosis likely perpetuate and expand the scope of the disease process. Fibrosis and encapsulation occur concurrently and appear to represent a last-ditch attempt to isolate and wall off the bacterium from the vascularized tissue in the tongue and oral cavity. *A. lignieresii* can spread via lymphatic vessels to regional lymph nodes and cause a similar inflammatory response and lesion in these nodes.

Alimentary Anthrax (*Bacillus anthracis*). See Bacterial Diseases of Organ Systems; Alimentary System and the Peritoneum, Omentum, Mesentery, and Peritoneal Cavity; Disorders of Domestic Animals; Alimentary Anthrax (*Bacillus anthracis*).

Disorders of Pigs

Porcine Proliferative Enteritis/Hemorrhagic Bowel Syndrome (*Lawsonia intracellularis*). Although proliferative enteritis/hemorrhagic bowel syndrome is most commonly recognized as a disease of pigs, a syndrome resembling the proliferative form of this disease in pigs also occurs in horses (equine proliferative enteropathy [EPE]), and the pathogenesis is likely similar to that described in pigs. *L. intracellularis* appears to cause two distinct disease syndromes in a single disease continuum. The mechanism of injury of the first syndrome is characterized by pathologic processes that result in cell proliferation (i.e., proliferative enteritis), whereas the mechanism in the second syndrome is characterized by processes that result in cell lysis and hemorrhage (i.e., hemorrhagic bowel syndrome). It seems that the first syndrome can occur and resolve without transitioning into the second syndrome. The reverse scenario does not appear to occur. The proliferative form of this disease is also known as *porcine intestinal adenomatosis*, *proliferative ileitis*, *regional ileitis*, *garden hose disease*, and other similar names. The hemorrhagic form of this disease is also known as *necrotic enteritis* or *acute proliferative hemorrhagic enteropathy*. The mechanism of injury is initially cellular hypertrophy and hyperplasia (proliferation) that can be followed by cell lysis resulting from ischemia and necrosis. Gross lesions in proliferative enteritis include a circumferentially firm and thickened ileum with a mucosa that fills the lumen and bulges into the lumen on cut surface (see Fig. 7-173). Gross lesions in hemorrhagic bowel syndrome include segmental necrosis and hemorrhage with fibrinous diphtheritic membranes attached to the mucosa, luminal blood clots, and thinned intestinal walls (see Fig. 7-175).

Pigs encounter *L. intracellularis* through ingestion of the bacterium in manure-contaminated fomites from the environment. It is swallowed and gains access via peristalsis to mucosae of the small intestine. It is unclear how the bacterium initially colonizes the mucus layer and mucosae and why it targets epithelial cells in the ileum. Ligand-receptor interactions are likely involved in this ileal specificity and *Lawsonia* surface antigen (LsaA) may act as an adhesin or invasin early in colonization. Other specific bacterial adhesins or cell membrane receptors have not been identified. Alternatively, possibly in conjunction with ligand-receptor interactions, ileal specificity may be attributed to unidentified metabolic or growth factors required by the bacterium that are provided only by intestinal crypt cells (see later section for more detail). In addition, it is unclear how the bacterium is able to penetrate the mucus layer and gain direct access to the luminal membrane of epithelial cells. *L. intracellularis* is regarded as a nonmotile bacterium; however, there is scant experimental evidence suggesting that the bacterium develops a transient bacterial appendage that behaves as a flagellum and could provide motility into and through the mucus layer. Colonization also appears to be enhanced by the presence of other anaerobic bacterial species in the mucus layer. The significance of this finding is unclear but could be related to these species providing molecules required by *L. intracellularis* for colonization and replication.

L. intracellularis infects cells of the crypts located in the proliferative zone (Fig. 4-22). Following colonization, the bacterium interacts with the brush border and then is taken into the cell via endocytosis and resides in a phagosome within the cytoplasm. The bacterium rapidly escapes from the phagosome before phagosome-lysosome fusion occurs and resides free in cell cytoplasm. A phospholipase bacterial virulence factor, mediated through a type III secretion system, may be involved in the escape mechanism. Once free in the cytoplasm, bacteria remain in close proximity to the apical (luminal) cell membrane, where they grow and replicate within the cytoplasm (see Fig. 7-176). In this location, bacteria appear to aggregate near mitochondria; thus it has been suggested that they may need preformed triphosphates for growth.

A unique feature of the pathogenesis of proliferative enteritis is the finding that proliferation of bacteria intracellularly (growth and replication) occurs concurrently with proliferation of crypt enterocytes (hypertrophy and hyperplasia) (see Fig. 7-174). One process does not occur without the other. Under normal conditions, crypt cells within the proliferative zone are dividing cells that differentiate into nondividing cells of the differentiative zone as these cells migrate along basement membrane up the villus to its apex (see Fig.

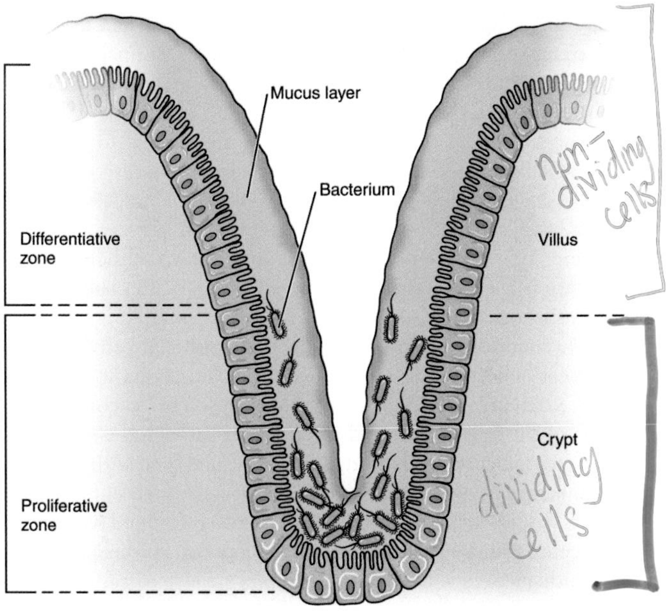

Figure 4-22 Pathogenesis of Proliferative Enteritis in Pigs. *Lawsonia intracellularis* infects cells of the crypts located in the proliferative zone.

4-22). It appears that once crypt cells of the proliferative zone are infected with bacteria, the bacterium is able to inhibit the normal maturation of crypt cells, probably through disruption of the cell cycle. Additionally, infection of crypt cells by bacteria dramatically increases the rate of crypt cell division.

Therefore, when crypt cells are infected, they do not mature but remain in an undifferentiated proliferative state and divide continuously, thus resulting in massive thickening of the mucosal surface by proliferating crypt cells. Proliferating cells continue to migrate to the apices of villi, where they die and their contents, including large numbers of bacteria, are extruded into the lumen of the intestine. This outcome provides a source of bacteria to infect additional uninfected crypt enterocytes and spread through feces into the environment. Normal villus structure is lost and replaced by a branching glandular pattern, where cells lining the hyperplastic glands are crowded into a mucosal layer of up to 10 to 15 epithelial cells in thickness. Mitotic activity is prominent. Inflammation does not occur.

The veterinary literature does not provide any discussion of the relationship between proliferative enteritis and hemorrhagic bowel syndrome and how the former transitions into the latter or if it does. Histologically, it has been shown that lesions occurring in necrotic enteritis (hemorrhagic bowel syndrome) include acute coagulative necrosis of the proliferating crypt epithelium. This lesion is consistent with ischemia or the direct effects of toxins (burnlike injury). Necrotic enteritis may simply be a manifestation of proliferating cells outgrowing an available blood supply, becoming ischemic, and then dying via acute coagulative necrosis. No cell in the body can survive if it is farther than 100 μm away from a source of oxygen, either from a capillary or highly oxygenated body fluid. Additionally, *L. intracellularis* is a Gram-negative bacterium, and endotoxin or other toxic molecules may directly cause injury and cell lysis consistent with acute coagulative necrosis. Acute inflammation with hemorrhage and fibrinogenesis commonly occur concurrently with acute coagulative necrosis.

Swine Dysentery *(Brachyspira hyodysenteriae)*. The mechanism of injury in swine dysentery is lysis of mucosal epithelial cells of the colon and cecum caused by bacterial hemolysins and proteases and from inflammation and its mediators and degradative enzymes. Gross lesions include a mucohemorrhagic necrofibrinous colitis and typhlitis with diphtheritic membranes covering intestinal mucosae formed by abundant mucus, hemorrhage, fibrin, plasma proteins, and cellular debris arising from necrotic mucosal epithelial cells and inflammatory cells (see Fig. 7-171).

Pigs encounter *B. hyodysenteriae* (previously named *Serpulina hyodysenteriae* and *Treponema hyodysenteriae*) through ingestion of the bacterium in manure-contaminated fomites in the environment. The bacterium is swallowed and gains access via peristalsis to the intestine, especially the cecum and colon. Virulence factors that block its destruction, by bile and digestive enzymes as examples, during transit in the small intestine to the cecum and colon are unknown. Goblet cell mucus is important as a physical matrix and as a chemical substrate for colonization by the bacterium; thus goblet cells play a central role in the pathogenesis of lesions affecting mucosal epithelial cells and their junctional complexes. *B. hyodysenteriae*, an anaerobic motile spirochete, is able to actively move through the mucus layer to gain access to mucosal epithelial and goblet cells. It is unclear why the bacterium infects the cecum and colon, but it appears that it prefers to initially replicate in mucigen droplets within goblet cells. Mucigen droplets fill the apical cytoplasm of goblet cells, and the nucleus is displaced to the basal region of the cell. Because the relative number of such cells is much greater in the cecum and colon when compared to other segments of the alimentary system, this quantitative difference may account for the location of the lesions. Additionally, mucins (e.g., the fucose and L-serine components) are strong chemoattractants for spirochetes, and because there are significant biochemical and pH differences in mucins, such as those that are synthesized and released from goblet cells, it is plausible that the chemical composition of the mucins may account for the locations of the lesions. Once the bacterium infects mucigen droplets within goblet cells, it appears to be able to activate the goblet cell to increase the production of mucus. Thus there is a large increase in the volume of mucus secreted by these cells so that mucosal surfaces are covered with a thick grayish gelatinous layer. It is unclear how the bacterium activates the goblet cell to produce and release large quantities of mucus. It is plausible that one or more bacterial virulence factors influence the cellular processes of transcription, translation, assembly, and packaging of mucigen droplets, thereby producing abundant quantities of mucus to enhance its opportunity to colonize the mucosa. Concurrently with infecting goblet cells, the bacterium begins the process of colonizing the thickened mucus layer covering the mucosal epithelium. It appears that mucus and its mucins are central to both the colonization and replication processes and result in the accumulation of large numbers of bacteria in close proximity to cell membranes and junctional complexes of mucosal epithelial cells.

Recently it has been demonstrated experimentally that more virulent strains of the bacterium express increased numbers of genes for carbohydrate and amino acid metabolism and transport that potentially could be linked to energy and carbon sources that are available in the mucus layer. Additionally, highly fermentable feeds favor colonization of the mucus layer by bacteria. Fermentation may provide the bacterium with an energy source or other molecules required for colonization and replication. Colonization is also enhanced by the presence of other anaerobic bacterial species in the mucus layer. The significance of this finding is unclear, but again could be related to these anaerobic species providing molecules required by *B. hyodysenteriae* for colonization and replication. Finally, because the bacterium is an anaerobe, it synthesizes high concentrations of nicotinamide adenine dinucleotide hydrogen (NADH) oxidase (a virulence factor) that is used to protect itself from oxidative stress and toxic oxygen molecules in the oxygen-rich environment of the mucus layer.

The bacterium does not attach to luminal (apical) membranes of colonic and cecal epithelial cells; however, experimental studies have reported that the bacterium invades the epithelium and the lamina propria because it has been identified in these areas. The largest quantity of bacteria appears to exist in the mucus layer just overlying the epithelium. Therefore it is unclear as to whether this invasion is a direct and targeted process or merely an innocent bystander phenomenon, in which the motility of the bacterium carries it into these locations to cause injury. Injury and lysis of colonic and cecal epithelial cells (enterocytes), as well as penetration through junctional complexes into the superficial lamina propria, are likely caused by one or more proteases and hemolysins and endotoxic effects of lipooligosaccharide (LOS) from the cell wall of the bacterium. Lysis and loss of the mucosal epithelium results in hemorrhage and the opportunity for other microbes, such as other anaerobic bacteria and the protozoan *Balantidium coli*, to invade the lamina propria. Denuded mucosa also provides a mechanism for the absorption of endotoxins, cytotoxins from inflammatory cells, and other toxic molecules that could cause endotoxic shock locally and systemically via the blood vascular system.

Porcine Polyserositis (*Haemophilus suis/parasuis, Actinobacillus suis, Streptococcus suis,* or *Escherichia coli*). See Bacterial Diseases of Organ Systems; Respiratory System, Mediastinum, and Pleurae; Disorders of Pigs; Porcine Polyserositis (*Haemophilus suis/parasuis, Actinobacillus suis, Streptococcus suis,* or *Escherichia coli*).

Hepatobiliary System and Exocrine Pancreas

Disorders of Domestic Animals

***Hepatic Leptospirosis* (*Leptospira* spp.).** The pathogenesis of hepatic leptospirosis begins as vascular leptospirosis caused by *Leptospira* spp. The pathogenesis is discussed in the section on Bacterial Diseases of Organ Systems, Cardiovascular System and Lymphatic Vessels, Disorders of Domestic Animals. The mechanisms used by *Leptospira* spp. to infect the liver are likely similar to those used in the kidney and are covered in the Urinary System section of this chapter. Gross lesions include discrete and coalescing white-to-gray foci of hepatic necrosis scattered at random throughout hepatic parenchyma that are intermixed with hemorrhage.

Disorders of Horses

Tyzzer's Disease (*Clostridium piliforme* [*Bacillus piliformis*]). The mechanism of injury in Tyzzer's disease is acute coagulative necrosis of hepatocytes, intestinal mucosal epithelial cells, and adjacent vascular and stromal tissues and from inflammation and its mediators and degradative enzymes. Gross lesions include hepatomegaly and numerous white-gray-yellow foci (<2-mm diameter) of hepatocyte necrosis distributed at random, usually throughout all lobes of the liver (see Fig. 8-53). In severe cases the center of these foci may be depressed and red (hemorrhage).

The young of all animal species can contract Tyzzer's disease; however, foals appear to be the most susceptible and encounter *Clostridium piliforme*, an obligate intracellular bacterium, through ingestion of spores present in soil or vegetative forms in fecal fomites from infected animals. The disease is less common in dogs, cats, and calves. Although the bacterium uses the intestinal mucosa as an initial beachhead, it ultimately infects, replicates in, and injures the liver. The mechanism of spread from ingestion to the liver is unclear. In other diseases caused by *Clostridium* spp., such as blackleg, cells of the monocyte-macrophage system and M cells are probably used to spread spores and/or vegetative forms and hide (sequester) from innate and adaptive immune responses. After ingestion, it is likely that spores or vegetative forms are carried by normal peristaltic activities through the oral pharynx, esophagus, and stomach to their final destination, the small intestine (ileum). It is unknown if and how the bacterium interacts with and gains access to intestinal mucosal epithelial cells and/or mucosal macrophages. Vegetative forms of the bacterium are motile and may be able to penetrate the mucus layer and encounter mucosal epithelial cells of the small intestine. How they enter these cells is unknown, although direct penetration or receptor-mediated endocytosis through ligand-receptor interactions could be involved. Spores could be taken up through endostosis by intestinal mucosal epithelial cells, but how the spores penetrate the mucus layer and gain access to epithelial cells is unknown. They could be phagocytosed by mucosal macrophages in the mucus layer and carried to or through the mucosa by leukocyte trafficking. Additionally, spores could bind with receptors on the surface of M cells, which lack a mucus layer, enter though endocytosis, germinate into vegetative forms, infect and replicate in these cells, and then spread to adjacent mucosal epithelial cells.

In either case, spores or vegetative form are able to infect mucosal epithelial cells of the intestine through their apical surfaces and then replicate in the cells. It is not known what type of ligand-receptor interactions are involved in this process of entry into the cell. The bacterium appears to adhere to the apical cell membrane, be phagocytosed, and then escape the phagosome to reside and replicate in the cytoplasm of the cell.

It has not been shown how the bacterium spreads from mucosal epithelial cells or from M cells systemically to the liver. Because *C. piliforme* is a motile bacterium, it has been suggested that it leaves epithelial cells of the intestine (possibly from their basal surfaces), enters subjacent lamina propria, encounters and penetrates capillaries, enters the circulatory system, and is carried in blood plasma via the portal vein to the liver. The bacterium could also potentially be transported to the liver within phagosomes in macrophages (leukocytic trafficking). If the bacterium is able to infect and replicate in M cells, the integration of M cells with Peyer's patches provides the opportunity for the bacterium to interact with macrophages or gain access to capillaries within submucosal ECM tissues. Macrophages could phagocytose the bacterium using ligand-receptor interactions and carry it via leukocyte trafficking in afferent lymphatic vessels to mesenteric lymph nodes and then systemically via the thoracic duct and venous system into the circulatory system and ultimately the liver via the hepatic artery. However, in a mouse model of Tyzzer's disease, depletion of macrophages did not change the course of infection. This outcome suggests that leukocyte trafficking may not be involved in the spread of the bacterium from the intestine to the liver.

Once in the liver, the bacterium encounters endothelial cells lining hepatic sinusoids. As a motile bacterium, it is free in the circulatory system and could (1) directly penetrate the endothelium and enter and infect hepatocytes, (2) infect and replicate in endothelial cells and then spread to adjacent hepatocytes, or (3) infect and replicate in Kupffer cells and then spread to adjacent hepatocytes. Hemorrhage occurs in Tyzzer's disease, and this lesion suggests that vascular injury occurs either from direct penetration of the blood vessels or by lysis of the endothelial cells after replication of the bacterium. Although direct penetration of endothelial cells and hepatocytes is a possible mechanism of entry into these cells, typical ligand-receptor interactions may also be involved. The bacterium enters hepatocytes probably via receptor-mediated endocytosis and then escapes the phagosome to reside and replicate in the cytoplasm. The replication of *C. piliforme* in hepatocytes eventually results in hepatocellular necrosis. The mechanisms causing necrosis are unknown. Bacterial cytotoxic proteins and several cellular cytokines like interleukin and TNF have been implicated as the cause of hepatocellular necrosis, but experimental results are inconclusive. It appears that the bacterium first causes acute hepatocyte necrosis, which then incites an acute inflammatory response with abundant neutrophils and occasional macrophages in affected tissues. In the same mouse model of Tyzzer's disease, the number of bacteria in hepatocytes and the severity of lesions were much worse in mice depleted of neutrophils and NK cells. This outcome suggests that the acute inflammation plays an important role as an innate defense mechanism in the disease.

Disorders of Ruminants (Cattle, Sheep, and Goats)

Bacillary Hemoglobinuria (*Clostridium haemolyticum*). The mechanism of injury in bacillary hemoglobinuria has a local component and a systemic component. Local injury is cell lysis (acute coagulative necrosis) of hepatocytes (necrotizing hepatitis), whereas systemic injury is lysis of erythrocytes in the blood vascular system. Injury in both components is caused by phospholipase C and other toxins released from *Clostridium haemolyticum*. Gross lesions include vasculitis, infarction, coagulative necrosis, and hemorrhage in the liver (see Fig. 8-73) and hemoglobinuria in the urinary system.

Cattle and sheep probably encounter *C. haemolyticum* through ingestion of spores present in the soil. Although the bacterium ultimately resides in and injures the liver, the mechanism of spread from ingestion to the liver is unknown. In other diseases caused by *Clostridium* spp., such as blackleg, cells of the monocyte-macrophage system, M cells, and dendritic systems are likely used to spread and to hide spores from immune responses and other defense mechanisms. It is plausible that after ingestion, spores are carried by normal peristaltic activities through the oral pharynx, esophagus, abomasum, and rumen to their final destination, the small intestine. It is unknown how spores interact with and gain access to epithelial cells and mucosal macrophages. The mucus layer of the small intestine probably presents a significant barrier to spores; therefore spores could bind with receptors on the surface of M cells or dendritic cells and through transcytosis gain access to macrophages and lymphocytes located in Peyer's patches contiguous with these cells. Mucosal-associated macrophages could also phagocytose spores using ligand-receptor interactions and carry the spores via leukocyte trafficking in afferent lymphatic vessels to mesenteric lymph nodes and then systemically via the thoracic duct into the circulatory system. Although unproved, spores are likely the form of the bacterium that spreads systemically to liver. Trafficking macrophages having spores in phagosomes could enter the sinusoids of the liver and transfer spores to Kupffer cells embedded in the endothelium. Spores then hide in Kupffer cells until they are activated to germinate and produce vegetative bacteria. Tropism for Kupffer cells is probably mediated by ligand-receptor interactions.

The occurrence of bacillary hemoglobinuria follows injury to the liver caused by migration of liver flukes (*Fasciola hepatica, Fascioloides magna*). Thus bacillary hemoglobinuria occurs only in geographic locations that have these flukes. The flukes migrate through the liver and injure intrahepatic veins, causing thrombosis, ischemia, and infarction of associated hepatocytes. Infarcted areas of liver are anaerobic and have a lowered oxidation-reduction (redox) potential required for germination of spores released from dead Kupffer cells. Spores germinate into vegetative bacteria, and they produce large quantities of phospholipase C (also known as *lecithinase* C, an α-toxin) and hemolysins that destroy cell membranes and cause hepatocyte lysis. These toxins are also absorbed into the venous system within viable liver, resulting in entry into the systemic circulation, leading to erythrocyte membrane injury, lysis of erythrocytes, release of hemoglobin, and hemoglobinuria.

Infectious Necrotic Hepatitis (*Clostridium novyi*). The pathogenesis and lesions of infectious necrotic hepatitis are similar to those of bacillary hemoglobinuria discussed in the previous section; however, the disease lacks hemoglobinuria, which is likely attributable to the absence of toxins that injure and lyse erythrocyte membranes.

Disorders of Pigs

Porcine Polyserositis (*Haemophilus suis/parasuis, Actinobacillus suis, Streptococcus suis,* or *Escherichia coli*). See Bacterial Diseases of Organ Systems; Respiratory System, Mediastinum, and Pleurae; Disorders of Pigs; Porcine Polyserositis (*Haemophilus suis/parasuis, Actinobacillus suis, Streptococcus suis,* or *Escherichia coli*).

Respiratory System, Mediastinum, and Pleurae

Disorders of Domestic Animals

Strep Zoo (*Streptococcus equi* subsp. *zooepidemicus*). The mechanism of injury in "strep zoo" is injury and lysis of mucosal and serosal epithelial cells and vascular endothelial cells from bacterial toxins and from inflammation and its mediators and degradative enzymes. Gross lesions include vasculitis leading to (1) a lung with a firm texture attributable to the leakage from injured blood vessels of variable quantities of fibrin into alveoli and alveolar septa (fibrinous pneumonia) and (2) the appearance of variable quantities of a gray-white friable material (fibrin) often mixed with hemorrhage on serosal surfaces (fibrinous polyserositis) of the lungs (fibrinous pleuritis), heart (fibrinous pericarditis), and abdominal cavity (fibrinous peritonitis) (see Fig. 10-60). The body cavities formed by these anatomic structures may also contain a fibrinous exudate and edema fluid mixed with hemorrhage. Facing serosal surfaces are often loosely attached to each other by fibrinous exudate, making normal physiologic processes such as respiration more difficult. The serosa and cavities of meninges, joints, and testis can also be affected. Information about the mechanisms used by this bacterium is limited. Some of this section is conditional and based on (1) what is known about virulence factors used by other members of the Streptococcaceae family, especially *Streptococcus equi* subsp. *equi*, to cause disease (see the section in this chapter on Bone Marrow, Blood Cells, and Lymphatic System, Disorders of Horses, Strangles [*Streptococcus equi* subsp. *equi*]) and (2) a reasonable probability that inflammation, responses to injury, and lesions that have been described in strep zoo are the result of underlying and known pathobiologic mechanisms.

S. equi subsp. *zooepidemicus* is a zoonosis. Horses and dogs likely encounter *S. equi* subsp. *zooepidemicus* through inhalation of the bacterium in fomites or fluid droplets from "carrier" or infected animals. The bacterium appears to be a commensal organism of mucous membranes of the nasal and oral pharynxes, probably existing in biofilms of healthy animals. Environmental stressors, such as overcrowding, poor ventilation and humidity, or abrupt changes in ambient air temperature, alter the mucus layer and the commensal relationship, allowing the bacteria to replicate in sufficient numbers to colonize the respiratory mucosae and spread the bacterium to other animals. Preceding or concurrent viral infections could also damage the mucociliary apparatus, allowing these bacteria to colonize the mucus layer or mucosae. In the respiratory system the bacteria are deposited on mucosae of the conductive component by centrifugal and inertial turbulence and trapped in the mucus layer. Although *S. equi* subsp. *zooepidemicus* can express many of the virulence factors expressed by *S. equi* subsp. *equi*, a causal link of these factors to disease is unclear. The bacterium is nonmotile, and it has not been clearly shown how it penetrates the mucus layer; gains access to mucosal epithelial cells or cilia; expresses virulence factors such as adhesins, capsular molecules, fimbriae, and outer membrane proteins (e.g., fibronectin-binding protein) required for ligand-receptor interactions; and colonizes the mucosa. Some strains of the bacterium have SzP, a surface M-like protein, which may through receptor-ligand phenomena determine which organ system is colonized and what types of cells in that organ system are colonized. Other strains of the bacterium may have putative virulence factors such as C5a peptidase, invasins, and fibronectin-binding protein that are thought to contribute to biofilm formation and cell adhesion. It has been shown that some of these virulence factors can be transferred between strains of the bacterium via PAIs through horizontal gene transfer. Once mucosae are colonized and epithelial cells are injured, acute inflammation ensues, leading to lysis of these cells and loss of the ciliated mucosal barrier. Injury to ciliated epithelial cells alters the function of the mucociliary apparatus, allowing the bacterium to gain access to terminal bronchioles and alveoli by dependent settling due to gravity. Herein, bacteria colonize mucosae of the terminal bronchioles and alveoli, spread into vascularized ECM tissues, interact with and injure blood vessels of the air-blood barrier, and leak fibrinogen into the alveoli (fibrinous pneumonia). This process accounts for a fibrinous pneumonia but may not satisfactorily account for the fibrinous polyserositis so characteristic of this disease.

By an undetermined mechanism, bacteria likely gain access to the lamina propria of the respiratory system and have direct access to the vascularized ECM. It has not been determined how bacteria actually cross this altered barrier, reach the capillary beds, penetrate the endothelium, and spread into the blood vascular system. Mechanisms, such as a cell-free bacteremia or leukocyte trafficking in alveolar or intravascular macrophages, lymphocytes, or dendritic cells, are hypothetical possibilities. The characteristic gross lesions of fibrinohemorrhagic polyserositis suggest these bacteria may have a tropism for vascular endothelial cells of serosae. It is unclear why this occurs, but it is probably linked to the expression of bacterial virulence factors and ligand-receptor interactions with host endothelial cells in specific locations of body systems. Additionally, it is possible that bacterial toxins may contribute to vascular injury and permeability changes leading to the leakage of fibrinogen and its polymerization to fibrin on serosal surfaces and in some cases to microthrombus formation and disseminated intravascular coagulation in other organ systems.

Disease caused by *S. equi* subsp. *zooepidemicus* in dogs appears to follow the same chronologic sequence of steps as in horses, but virulence factors involved in the disease appear to cause more severe lesions to the vascular system and a greater degree of hemorrhage.

Respiratory Anthrax (*Bacillus anthracis*). See Bacterial Diseases of Organ Systems; Alimentary System and the Peritoneum, Omentum, Mesentery, and Peritoneal Cavity; Disorders of Domestic Animals; Alimentary Anthrax (*Bacillus anthracis*) for detailed information on the pathogenesis and virulence factors.

The mechanism of injury in respiratory anthrax is cell lysis caused by bacterial toxins that act directly on cell membranes leading to acute coagulative necrosis. Gross lesions include pulmonary and lymph node edema, hemorrhage, and necrosis.

Animals encounter *B. anthracis* through inhalation of fomites contaminated with endospores from soil. Fomites containing endospores must be less than 5 μm in diameter to reach the O_2-CO_2 exchange portion of the respiratory system. Infected fomites are deposited on mucosae, where they are then phagocytosed either by alveolar macrophages migrating through and on the surface of mucosae or by dendritic cells. Infected macrophages and dendritic cells spread the bacterium to regional lymph nodes (bronchiolar and mediastinal) via afferent lymphatic vessels through leukocyte trafficking. During the migration process, endospores germinate into vegetative bacteria, so on arrival at the lymph nodes, bacteria are already producing anthrax toxins, which kill infected cells and release the bacteria into the ECM of the lymph nodes. In lymph nodes, bacteria continue to replicate and produce anthrax toxins killing additional lymphoid and endothelial cells, leading to edema and hemorrhage. The bacterium and its toxins enter lymphatic vessels and spread via the thoracic duct into the circulatory system as a septicemia, where endothelial cells and cells of other organ systems are injured, leading to edema, hemorrhage, and cell necrosis.

Disorders of Horses

Rhodococcal Pneumonia (*Rhodococcus equi*). See Bacterial Diseases of Organ Systems; Alimentary System and the Peritoneum, Omentum, Mesentery, and Peritoneal Cavity; Disorders of Horses; Rhodococcus Enteritis (*Rhodococcus equi*) for additional information on the pathogenesis and virulence factors.

The mechanism of injury in rhodococcal pneumonia is lysis of cells of the monocyte-macrophage system and of all cell populations in the respiratory system secondary to inflammation and its mediators and degradative enzymes. Gross lesions include (1) cranioventral chronic active pyogranulomatous pneumonia characterized by consolidated firm yellow-white lung parenchyma attributable to infiltrating inflammatory cells, abscesses, and granulomas in the affected lung tissue (see Fig. 9-82) and (2) necrotizing pyogranulomatous lymphadenitis of tracheobronchial lymph nodes of the lung typified by enlarged firm lymph nodes that on cut surface have discrete and coalescing areas of yellow-white exudate infiltrating and compressing contiguous parenchyma (see Fig. 7-139). The latter lesion occurs through leukocyte trafficking of bacteria-infected alveolar macrophages as described later.

Foals encounter *R. equi* through inhalation of the bacterium in manure-contaminated fomites or water droplets from the environment. It is a common bacterium of the soil, grows optimally at 30° C in the manure of most animal species, and has a very rapid generation time. When inhaled, the bacterium is deposited on mucosae of the conductive and exchange systems by centrifugal and inertial turbulence. Here, bacteria encounter cells of the monocyte-macrophage system, including alveolar macrophages and dendritic cells, which phagocytose bacteria in the mucus layer of the mucociliary apparatus. These cells carry bacteria via leukocyte trafficking to local lymphoid tissues, such as BALT, through peribronchiolar and alveolar septal connective tissue, and to regional lymph nodes via afferent lymphatic vessels. *R. equi* replicates intracellularly in alveolar and other tissue macrophages. Alveolar macrophages phagocytize *R. equi* through ligand-receptor interactions. The bacterium must initially adhere to macrophages and the bacterium must be opsonized with either antibody or complement fragments that occur through complement fixation and the activation of the alternative complement pathway. In nonimmune foals, complement is the primary opsonin. The bacterium also expresses uncharacterized surface molecules that bind to membrane receptors expressed on alveolar macrophages such as leukocyte complement receptor, Mac-1, other complement receptors, mannose receptors, and potentially TLRs before phagocytosis can occur.

Opsonized bacteria and the products of complement fixation facilitate the process of adhesion and invasion through phagocytosis into alveolar macrophages. Phagocytosis is mediated by bacterial virulence factors that appear to restrict tropism to specific types of phagocytic cells. After phagocytosis by alveolar macrophages, the bacterium is confined within phagosomes. Experimental results from studies on fusion of phagosomes with lysosomes to form phagolysosomes are contradictory. Some studies suggest that *R. equi* can block the fusion of lysosomes with phagosomes, which allows for the survival, persistence, and replication of bacteria intracellularly. Other studies suggest that *R. equi* is not able to block phagosome-lysosome fusion; however, the bacterium is able to produce molecules that suppress acidification of phagolysosomes, resulting in their survival and replication in alveolar macrophages. The mechanism used to block fusion is unknown but appears to involve bacterium-directed compartmentalization of the fusion process so that they are selectively isolated from lysosomal effector molecules, such as acid, reactive oxygen, NO compounds, and lysosomal hydrolases within phagosomes. Other proteins and molecules appear to contribute to persistence and replication in alveolar macrophages. For example, strains of *R. equi* that cause disease have chromosomal virulence factors for capsular polysaccharide, cholesterol oxidase, phospholipase C, lecithinase, and cell-wall mycolic acids and plasmid virulence factors (pathogenicity island) for VAP. It is also likely that mycolic acids from the bacterial cell wall are involved in the pathogenesis of the pyogranulomatous pneumonia characteristic of the disease.

Because *R. equi* is able to disrupt normal phagosome-lysosome killing (lysis) in alveolar macrophages and the generation of an oxidative burst that could kill the bacterium, it is able to persist and replicate. Studies suggest that rapid replication of bacterium within phagosomes and molecules such as cholesterol oxidase produced by the bacterium contribute to premature lysis of alveolar macrophages, leading to the release of large numbers of microbes into adjacent tissue. Additionally, because the life span of fully differentiated alveolar macrophages is approximately 10 to 30 days, lysis of these cells related to aging and bacteria-induced injury releases large numbers of bacteria into adjacent tissue, where they are phagocytosed by macrophages only to endlessly repeat the process. The severity and extent of the inflammatory response, concurrently with tissue injury, grows through the recruitment of additional monocytes and tissue macrophages from the circulatory system and regional lymph nodes.

Neutrophils are active in the acute inflammatory response against *R. equi*. They are able to phagocytose the bacterium, fuse the phagosome with the lysosome to form a phagolysosome, initiate an oxidative burst, and kill the bacterium. However, this process is an ineffective mechanism in controlling the disease and results in extensive tissue destruction through the release of lysosomal enzymes and reactive oxygen species, thus contributing to the cyclic and progressive destruction of pulmonary parenchyma. This damage allows large numbers of bacteria to gain access to the alveoli and bronchioles and encounter mucus of the mucous membranes and the mucociliary apparatus. In general, the mucociliary apparatus is not directly affected by *R. equi*; thus the bacterium is moved up the conductive system to the nasopharynx, where it is swallowed and gains access via peristalsis to the alimentary system (i.e., *Rhodococcus* enteritis).

Strep Zoo (*Streptococcus equi* subsp. *zooepidemicus*). See Bacterial Diseases of Organ Systems; Respiratory System, Mediastinum, and Pleurae; Disorders of Domestic Animals; Strep Zoo (Streptococcus equi subsp. *zooepidemicus*).

Strangles (*Streptococcus equi* subsp. *equi*). See Bacterial Diseases of Organ Systems; Bone Marrow, Blood Cells, and the Lymphatic System; Disorders of Horses; Strangles (*Streptococcus equi* subsp. *equi*).

Disorders of Ruminants (Cattle, Sheep, and Goats)

Bovine Respiratory Disease Complex. Bovine respiratory disease complex (BRDC) is the term applied to a group of respiratory diseases caused by four viruses and three bacterial strains acting jointly and concurrently in various combinations (i.e., polymicrobial respiratory diseases) to cause a variety of respiratory diseases in cattle (ruminants). It occurs in cattle of varying ages and management practices; the microbes involved also vary based on age, management practices, and geographic locations. It is typified by the interactions of a primary viral pathogen and a secondary bacterial pathogen. A primary viral pathogen may disrupt the function of the mucociliary apparatus and/or disrupt phagocytosis and killing by alveolar and intravascular macrophages. These outcomes allow a secondary bacterial pathogen to colonize and replicate within the respiratory system and disrupt mucociliary and macrophage function, resulting in disease. Acute inflammation may also contribute to injury of cells and tissues within the respiratory system. Viruses involved include infectious bovine rhinotracheitis (IBR) virus, bovine viral diarrhea (BVD) virus, parainfluenza virus (PI3), and bovine respiratory syncytial virus (BRSV). Bacteria involved include *Pasteurella multocida*, *M. haemolytica*, and *Histophilus somni*. The pathogeneses and mechanisms of injury for each of these microbes are discussed individually in other sections of this chapter.

Bovine Pneumonic Pasteurellosis/Mannheimiosis (*Mannheimia* [*Pasteurella*] *haemolytica*). Also see bovine respiratory disease complex discussed earlier. The mechanism of injury in bovine pneumonic pasteurellosis/mannheimiosis is injury and lysis (coagulative necrosis) of all cell populations in the respiratory system. In addition to injury caused by bacterial toxins (leukotoxin), acute inflammation and its mediators and degradative enzymes significantly contribute to the pathogenesis of the disease. *M. haemolytica* can cause severe pneumonic disease independent of other contributory factors; however, the susceptibility to and severity of disease can be enhanced by environmental stressors and earlier or concurrent viral infection. Gross lesions include severe fibrinonecrotic (often hemorrhagic) pneumonia and vasculitis attributable to necrosis and apoptosis, especially affecting type I pneumocytes and capillary endothelial cells forming the air-blood barrier of alveolar septa and the vascular system (severe necrotizing vasculitis) (see Figs. 9-72, 9-85, and 9-86).

Cattle (and probably sheep and goats) encounter *M. haemolytica* through inhalation of the bacterium in fomites or fluid droplets. The bacterium is a commensal organism that resides in the nasopharynx and tonsils of healthy animals, but environmental stressors, such as weaning, adverse weather conditions, changes in diet, and shipping, can alter the commensal relationship, allowing the bacteria to replicate in sufficient numbers to colonize the respiratory mucosae and spread the bacterium to other animals. Colonization appears to be a two-stage process, first affecting the conductive component (terminal bronchioles and alveoli), then affecting the O_2-CO_2 (terminal bronchioles and alveoli) exchange component. When inhaled, bacteria are deposited on and trapped in the mucus layer of mucosae of the conductive component by centrifugal and inertial turbulence. *M. haemolytica* is a nonmotile bacterium, and it has not been clearly shown how the bacterium penetrates the mucus layer to gain access to cilia of mucosal epithelial cells.

Several virulence factors have been identified in the pathogenesis of mannheimiosis including leukotoxin (LKT), LPS, adhesins, capsular polysaccharides, outer membrane proteins, and various proteases such as neuraminidase. Neuraminidase reduces the viscosity of the mucus, making it less dense and a more fluidic layer, thus allowing the bacterium better access to cell membranes via gravity and random brownian movement. Additionally, neuraminidase cleaves sialic acid from the surface of cell membranes, thus decreasing the net negative surface charge and allowing closer contact of the bacterium with membranes. Once in contact with cell membranes, bacteria adhere and bind to receptors using fimbria and pili adhesins via ligand-receptor interactions. This process results in bacterial colonization of mucosae. The types of adhesins (ligands) and receptors used in colonization have not been determined. Once colonization occurs, the bacteria replicate in large numbers in the conductive component of the respiratory system and produce enzymes (virulence factors), such as neuraminidase, and toxins (virulence factors), such as leukotoxin and LPS, that injure and disrupt the function of the mucociliary apparatus.

Additionally, polysaccharides of the bacterial capsule (virulence factor) inhibit phagocytosis of the bacterium by neutrophils and mucosal macrophages. Because of mucociliary dysfunction, bacteria spread via gravity to dependent portions of the lung, including terminal bronchioles and alveoli of the O_2-CO_2 exchange component. Once bacteria arrive in this location, the second stage of the process, which is more severe than the first stage, begins. The difference in severity is, in part, based on three factors: (1) extensive replication of bacteria in stage one that settle into the O_2-CO_2 exchange component and their subsequent amplification through replication, (2) the large surface area of lung tissue affected, and (3) the greater vulnerability of the air-blood barrier and septa in the O_2-CO_2 exchange component to injury. All of these factors contribute to the severity of the acute inflammatory responses and tissue injury.

The single most important virulence factor in bovine pneumonic mannheimiosis is leukotoxin. *Mannheimia* leukotoxin (LKT), a member of the RTX group of toxins, is a cytotoxin that causes lysis and apoptosis of alveolar macrophages and neutrophils. RTX toxins attach to cells through passive adsorption and cell surface β_2 integrin receptors, the latter being the transmembrane receptor CD18. At high concentrations, it causes necrosis by creating pores in cell membranes, leading to cell swelling and lysis (oncotic necrosis), whereas at lower concentrations, it causes apoptosis. Additionally, at lower concentrations, it activates neutrophils and induces the production of proinflammatory cytokines. When bacteria are phagocytosed by alveolar macrophages, leukotoxin is used to kill the macrophages and release the bacteria back into vascularized ECM tissue and alveolar spaces. Iron is also required for optimal growth of the bacterium and production of leukotoxin. LPS and leukotoxin also activate the complement system and the release of proinflammatory cytokines, resulting in vascular injury and severe acute inflammation. Vascular injury leads to permeability changes with edema and the release of fibrinogen that polymerizes to fibrin in alveolar spaces, interalveolar septa, interlobular and interlobar septa, and on pulmonary serosal surfaces (fibrinonecrotic pneumonia). Vascular injury can also lead to pulmonary hemorrhage.

Acute inflammation is characterized by the recruitment of large numbers of neutrophils from the circulation into affected lung tissue followed by activation of these cells via a respiratory burst and the release of degradative enzymes. The bacterium has several mechanisms (see later) to minimize the effects of neutrophils, but innocent bystander lung tissue, such as terminal bronchioles and cells that form the air-blood barrier, are severely injured by the molecules and enzymes released from activated neutrophils. Capsular polysaccharides, outer membrane proteins, and LPS of the bacterium are also important in the pathogenesis of the disease, especially as related to acute inflammation and vascular injury. Polysaccharides are virulence factors that facilitate adherence, colonization, and likely invasion of respiratory mucosae; inhibit phagocytosis by neutrophils; and disrupt complement-mediated lysis of bacteria. Outer membrane proteins are chemotactic for neutrophils, but when in contact with neutrophils, they disrupt phagocytosis and intracellular killing of bacteria. LPS binds with cell membrane CD14, β_2 integrins, and TLRs on alveolar macrophages, inducing the synthesis of proinflammatory cytokines, arachidonic acid metabolites, and NO that injure cells in inflammation. LPS may also injure endothelial cells directly and through molecules released from macrophages such as those listed in the previous sentence.

Pulmonary Histophilosis (*Histophilus somni*). Also see bovine respiratory disease complex discussed earlier.

The pathogenesis of pulmonary histophilosis is likely very similar to the mechanisms described earlier for bovine pneumonic pasteurellosis/mannheimiosis. Also see Bacterial Diseases of Organ Systems, Nervous System, Disorders of Ruminants (Cattle, Sheep, and Goats), Thrombotic Meningoencephalitis (*Histophilus somni*).

Bovine Enzootic Pneumonia (*Pasteurella multocida* subsp. *multocida* serogroup A). Also see bovine respiratory disease complex discussed earlier.

Mechanistically, the virulence factors and mechanisms used by *Pasteurella multocida* subsp. *multocida* to cause bovine enzootic pneumonia are very similar functionally to those used by *M. haemolytica* to cause bovine pneumonic mannheimiosis. However, in bovine enzootic pneumonia, bacterial pathogenicity is noticeably reduced and reflected by a slow onset and insidious inflammatory response and a nearly complete absence of cell necrosis, vasculitis, permeability changes, and fibrinogenesis. The mechanism of injury in bovine enzootic pneumonia is injury of all cell populations in the respiratory system attributable to inflammation and its mediators and degradative enzymes.

The susceptibility to and severity of bovine enzootic pneumonia caused by *P. multocida* subsp. *multocida* serogroup A can be enhanced by environmental stressors and a preceding or concurrent infection with a primary viral pathogen such as bovine respiratory syncytial virus, bovine viral diarrhea virus, infectious bovine rhinotracheitis virus, or parainfluenza III virus. Gross lesions include firm (consolidation) yellow-gray anterior-ventral lung lobes (see Fig. 9-69). Pleural surfaces are usually not involved, indicating that vascular injury and permeability changes and their association with the expression of bacterial virulence factors are not significant in the pathogenesis of the disease. In some cases, *Mycoplasma bovis* and *Mannheimia varigena* have been reported as secondary bacterial pathogens. The pathogenicity of the bacterial pathogen in bovine enzootic pneumonia/bovine respiratory disease complex is determined by its virulence factors, which may include protein adhesins, capsular polysaccharides, outer membrane proteins, iron-binding proteins, LPSs, LOSs, enzymes, and toxins.

Contagious Bovine Pleuropneumonia (*Mycoplasma mycoides* var. *mycoides* Small Colony). Little is known about the mechanisms used by *Mycoplasma mycoides* var. *mycoides* small colony (SC) to cause disease in the respiratory system of cattle; thus much of this section is conditional and based on a reasonable probability that lesions that occur are the result of underlying and known pathobiologic mechanisms. The mechanism of injury in contagious bovine pleuropneumonia is cell lysis likely caused by acute inflammation and its mediators and degradative enzymes and by vasculitis leading to thrombosis, ischemia, and infarction of lung tissue. Gross lesions include (1) fibrinous pleural effusion and fibrinous pleuritis with hemorrhage and (2) fibrinous pleuropneumonia with prominent interlobular septa filled with fibrinous effusion and fibrin thrombi (Fig. 4-23). Infarcts occur in affected lung tissues probably arising from vascular injury leading to permeability changes, vasculitis with activation of clotting cascades, thrombosis, and infarction. Infarcted lung often appears as sequestra likely arising from

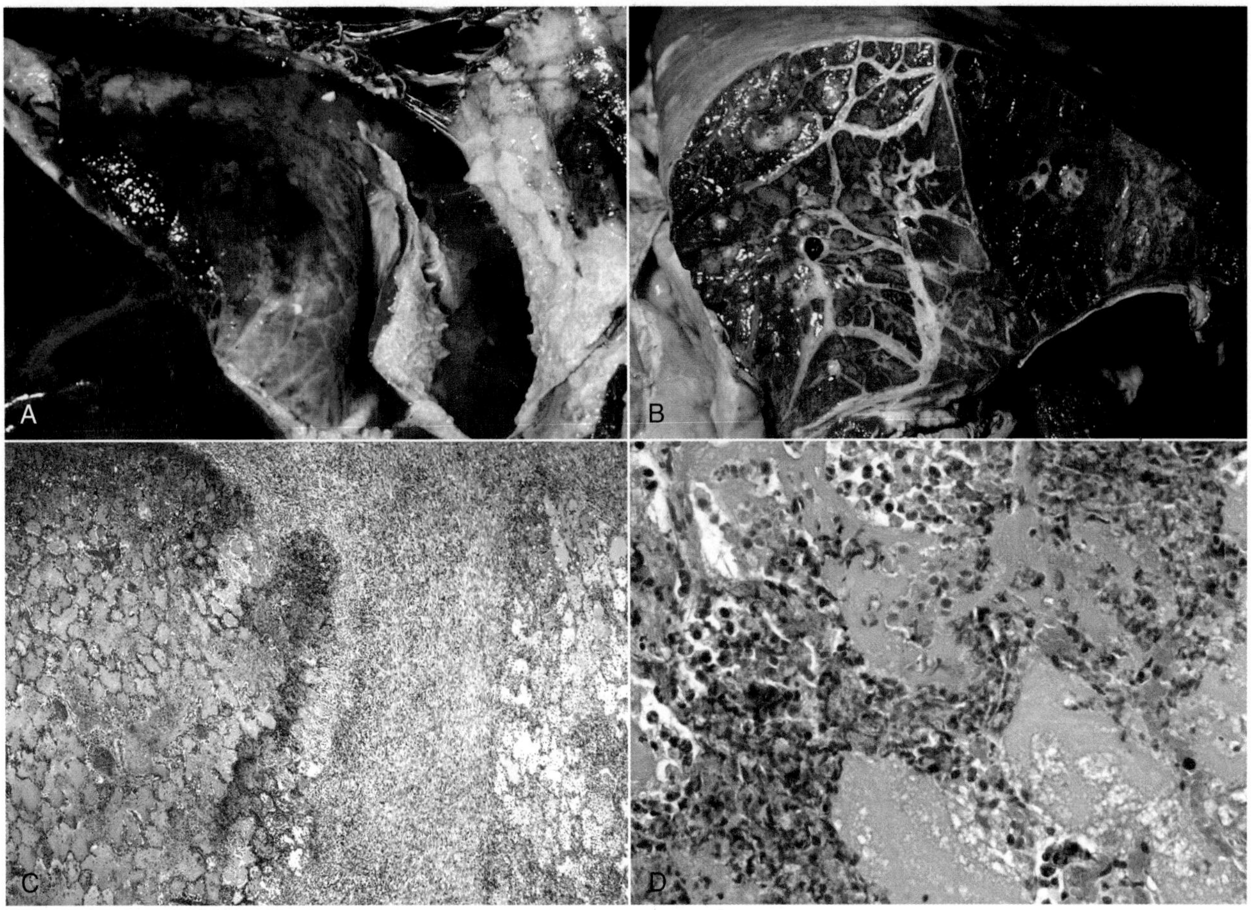

Figure 4-23 Contagious Bovine Pleuropneumonia. A, Thoracic cavity. The thoracic cavity is filled with a fibrinous pleural effusion, and the visceral and parietal pleurae are covered by fibrin (fibrinous pleuritis). Also note the areas of hemorrhage affecting the pleurae and the subjacent lung. **B,** Transverse section of lung. Note the prominent interlobular septa filled with fibrinous effusion and fibrin thrombi and additionally the area of hemorrhage *(right half of the section)*. Infarcts with pulmonary sequestra (not shown here) can occur in affected lung tissues, likely arising from vascular injury leading to infarction. **C,** The interlobular septum *(center)* is filled with acute inflammatory cells mixed with a fibrinous effusion. Alveoli are filled with highly proteinaceous edema fluid, fibrinous effusion, and acute inflammatory cells. There is extensive necrosis of all tissues at the interface between alveoli and the interlobar septum *(dark blue–staining band)*. H&E stain. **D,** Higher magnification of **C.** The dark blue color is attributable to necrosis of cells, including neutrophils, leading to escape and coagulation of nucleic acids from degenerate nuclei in the inflammatory exudate. Alveoli are filled with edema fluid and acute inflammatory cells. H&E stain. (**A** and **B** courtesy Dr. D. Gregg, Plum Island Animal Disease Center and Noah's Arkive, College of Veterinary Medicine, The University of Georgia. **C** and **D** courtesy Dr. J.F. Zachary, College of Veterinary Medicine, University of Illinois.)

reparative mechanisms that isolate the dead infarcted tissue via fibrosis. It is unclear how infarcts occur in lung tissue when it has a dual blood supply, unless infarcts occur in areas that lack a dual supply or vasculitis and thrombosis concurrently affect vessels of each arterial source.

Cattle (and probably sheep and goats) encounter *M. mycoides* var. *mycoides* SC through inhalation of infected fomites and fluid droplets. These droplets are deposited on mucosae of the conductive component of the respiratory system by centrifugal and inertial turbulence where they are trapped in the mucus layer and are subsequently phagocytosed by alveolar macrophages. Ligand-receptor interactions are probably involved in target cell specificity via adhesins. Alveolar macrophages in all probability spread the bacterium to local lymphoid tissue such as BALT, in which the bacterium replicates in large numbers and kills infected macrophages, releasing bacteria into bronchiolar and alveolar interstitium, causing severe acute inflammation and the characteristic fibrinous lesions and vasculitis. How the bacterium evades killing by phagosome-lysosome fusion, produces toxic molecules that injure and kill cells, spreads to blood vessels, and causes vasculitis and thrombosis are unknown. Bacterial membrane lipoprotein LppQ, a common antigen of *Mycoplasma mycoides* var. *mycoides* SC, could be involved in some of these processes. Highly virulent strains of the bacterium are known to produce and release large quantities of H_2O_2 that are cytotoxic for all cells. H_2O_2 release appears to be correlated with adhesion of the bacterium to target cell membranes. It also appears that macrophages may spread the bacterium via leukocyte trafficking systemically to lymph nodes and synovium and joint spaces such as the carpus where inflammation characteristic of the disease also occurs. As presumed virulence factors, outer surface proteins and/or plasma membrane proteins of *Mycoplasma* spp. contain lipoproteins, capsular polysaccharides (e.g., galactan), and carbohydrate biofilms that likely function to protect the microbe from defense mechanisms and to cause the acute fibrinoid inflammatory response so characteristic of the disease. Unique to *Mycoplasma mycoides* var. *mycoides* SC is the apparent lack of virulence factors that can be characterized as toxins or invasins. In fact, virulence factors appear to arise from metabolic or catabolic pathways within the bacterium or from intrinsic components of the bacterial outer surface and/or cell membrane such as capsular polysaccharides.

Bovine Tuberculosis (*Mycobacterium bovis*). The mechanism of injury in bovine tuberculosis is lysis of cells of the monocyte-macrophage system and of all cell populations in the lung and associated regional lymph nodes secondary to granulomatous inflammation and its mediators and degradative enzymes. Gross lesions include (1) enlarged lymph nodes that contain discrete and coalescing granulomas (tubercles) formed by dry and gritty (mineralized) yellow-white to green-white caseous exudate often encapsulated by fibrous connective tissue (see Fig. 1-18) and (2) lung parenchyma that contains similar granulomas distributed at random in some or all lung lobes (see Fig. 9-80 and E-Fig. 9-14).

Cattle (and probably sheep and goats) encounter *M. bovis* through inhalation of fomites and fluid droplets contaminated with the bacterium. These droplets are deposited on mucosae of the conductive component of the respiratory system by centrifugal and inertial turbulence where they are trapped in the mucus layer and are subsequently phagocytosed by alveolar and tissue macrophages. Ligand-receptor interactions are probably involved in target cell specificity via adhesins. Macrophages appear to use several routes to spread the bacterium across mucosal barriers and then to regional lymph nodes and the lung. In tonsillar mucosae, macrophages cross the mucosal barrier, migrate to the tonsil, and spread the bacterium to infect naïve macrophages in tonsillar tissues. In other mucosae of the pharynx, macrophages encounter and phagocytose bacteria and spread them to local lymphoid tissues and then via afferent lymphatic vessels to regional lymph nodes such as the retropharyngeal and parotid nodes to infect naïve macrophages in these nodes. Finally, in bronchi and bronchioles, bacteria that are deposited in the mucus layer of mucosae are phagocytosed by alveolar macrophages and spread to local lymphoid tissues (BALT) and then via afferent lymphatic vessels to regional lymph nodes, such as the tracheobronchial and mediastinal nodes, to infect naïve macrophages in these nodes.

The primary goal of *M. bovis* is to be phagocytized by macrophages. In the mucus layer, macrophages encounter trapped bacteria via random movement. Once bacteria are in contact with macrophages, bacteria adhere and bind to pathogen PRRs on macrophage cell membranes. The process used by macrophages to phagocytize *M. bovis* involves ligand-receptor interactions. In fact, the bacterium appears to use multiple membrane pathogen PRRs such as those for complement (CR1, 3, and 4), mannose, surfactant protein, and CD14 protein to enter macrophages. Some receptors are probably used in the early mucosal phases of infection when inflammation is minimal, whereas other receptors, such as those for complement, are used when vascular changes in lymph nodes and lung induced by acute inflammation result in permeability changes and the release of plasma proteins and complement into inflamed tissues.

M. bovis is able to activate the alternative pathway of complement and use C3b and C3bi fragments to opsonize its surface and then bind to complement receptors CR1, 3, and/or 4 on cell membranes of macrophages. This binding results in phagocytosis of the bacterium in phagosomes. Mannose receptors, surfactant proteins and receptors, and LAM and CD14 receptors are also involved in phagocytosis. It appears that the use of multiple ligands and pathogen PRRs ensures that the bacterium once inhaled or ingested can be phagocytosed by monocytes, macrophages, and/or even neutrophils that migrate to the site of local infection in response to chemokines secreted by infected macrophages. Subsequently, these cells can then be used to spread the infection to other regional or systemic sites, such as the liver, spleen, lymph nodes, and intestines, via leukocyte trafficking in the blood or lymphatic vascular systems.

Once present in a phagosome, *M. bovis* is able to disrupt phagosome-lysosome fusion and prevent activation of macrophage antimicrobial mechanisms such as production of reactive oxygen or nitrogen intermediates and phagosome acidification (see Figs. 4-13 and 4-14). The bacterium grows and replicates in phagosomes, but with cellular aging, infected macrophages die and release bacteria into the vascularized ECM tissues. This outcome results in repetitive cycles of inflammation and the recruitment of additional monocytes, macrophages, and neutrophils into the granuloma (tubercle). The formation of granulomas (tubercles) is covered in detail in Chapter 3, but components of the poorly digestible, waxy cell wall of the bacterium, such as sulpholipids and LAM, appear to contribute to the type of inflammatory response, chronic, that ensues and the formation of granulomas.

Ligand-receptor interactions are also important in initiating and prolonging the inflammatory response. PRRs on macrophages are activated by PAMPs on the bacterium. As a result, macrophages produce and release abundant proinflammatory cytokines and chemokines that act to recruit via chemotactic gradients additional macrophages/monocytes, neutrophils, and dendritic cells to the site. Because the life span of fully differentiated tissue macrophages is approximately 10 to 30 days, lysis of these cells related to aging and bacterial-induced injury releases bacterium into adjacent tissue, where they are phagocytosed by newly recruited macrophages only to endlessly repeat this process. Granulomatous inflammation ensues, and multinucleated giant cells are noted histologically in the exudate (see Chapters 3 and 5) as an attempt to degrade and eliminate the poorly digestible, waxy cell wall of the bacterium. Dendritic cells also phagocytose the bacterium, migrate to regional lymph nodes, and present mycobacterial antigens to lymphocytes for an adaptive immune response that ultimately is ineffective.

Disorders of Pigs

Porcine Respiratory Disease Complex. Porcine respiratory disease complex (PRDC) is the term applied to a group of respiratory diseases caused by three viruses and two bacterial strains acting jointly and concurrently in various combinations (i.e., polymicrobial respiratory diseases) to cause a variety of respiratory diseases in pigs. It occurs in pigs of varying ages and management practices; the microbes involved also vary based on age, management practices, and geographic locations. It is typified by the interactions of a primary viral pathogen and a secondary bacterial pathogen. A primary viral pathogen may disrupt the function of the mucociliary apparatus and/or disrupt phagocytosis and killing by alveolar and intravascular macrophages. These outcomes allow a secondary bacterial pathogen to colonize and replicate within the respiratory system and disrupt mucociliary and macrophage function, resulting in disease. Acute inflammation may also contribute to injury of cells and tissues within the respiratory system. Viruses involved include porcine reproductive and respiratory syndrome virus (PRRSV), swine influenza virus (SIV), and porcine circovirus type 2 (PCV2). Bacteria involved include *P. multocida* and *M. hyopneumoniae*. The pathogeneses and mechanisms of injury for each of these microbes are discussed individually in other sections of this chapter.

Porcine Pleuropneumonia (*Actinobacillus pleuropneumoniae*). The mechanism of injury in porcine pleuropneumonia is injury and lysis (coagulative necrosis) of all cell populations in the respiratory system, especially those of the vascular system (severe necrotizing vasculitis), secondary to the effects of bacterial toxins and to acute inflammation and its mediators and degradative enzymes. Gross lesions, attributable to vascular injury affecting lung and regional lymph nodes, include (1) edema and alterations in vascular permeability; (2) hemorrhage; and (3) fibrinous and hemorrhagic pneumonic, pleural, and pericardial effusions; and acute necrotizing inflammation and pneumonia (see Fig. 9-97). Although all lobes of the lung can be affected, a common site for lesions is the dorsal area of the caudal lung lobes. In fact, a large area of fibrinohemorrhagic pleuropneumonia involving the caudal lobe of a pig's lung is considered almost diagnostic for this disease.

Pigs encounter A. *pleuropneumoniae* through inhalation of the bacterium in contaminated fomites or fluid droplets. In the respiratory system the bacterium appears to initially colonize mucosal epithelial cells of the tonsils (likely in a biofilm) and then via inhalation is deposited on mucosae of the conductive system and probably of the exchange system by centrifugal and inertial turbulence. The characteristic distribution pattern (dorsal-diaphragmatic) of gross lesions may reflect the fact that droplet size and inertial turbulence results in the initial deposit being near branch points of conductive airways. The bacterium must first colonize mucosae by adhering and binding to the membranes of epithelial cells using ligand-receptor interactions mediated through type 4 fimbriae and likely adhesins (multiple-step binding process). The bacterium also binds to mucus, but the purpose of this act is unclear. Following colonization, A. *pleuropneumoniae* requires iron to grow and replicate and is capable of using porcine transferrin as a source of iron. However, it also appears that iron is obtained from lysis of red blood cells caused by bacterial hemolysins and proteases. After the lysis of red blood cells, LPS and outer membrane proteins of the bacterial cell wall can bind hemoglobin and assist in the transfer of the iron molecule required for growth and replication into the bacterium. In part, this requirement may explain the severe hemorrhage that occurs in this disease. Other virulence factors (LPSs, exotoxins) appear to be involved in the acquisition of essential nutrients required for colonization and replication.

It has been shown that the bacterium binds poorly to cilia and the epithelium of the trachea and bronchi, whereas it binds strongly to cilia and membranes of terminal bronchioles and membranes of alveolar epithelial cells (type I pneumocytes). This selective pattern of binding and inertial turbulence (see previous discussion) may account for the unique distribution of gross lesions involving the caudal lung lobes observed in porcine pleuropneumonia.

LPS and LOS are known to play important roles in the pathogenesis of Gram-negative infections; however, their role in porcine pleuropneumonia is unclear and may involve acting as ligands for adherence to target cell surfaces. Glycosphingolipids present in membranes of epithelial cells may serve as receptors for these ligands. It has not been determined if and how A. *pleuropneumoniae* penetrates the mucus layer to gain access to cilia and cell membranes of epithelial cells. The suppression of mucus production and ciliary activity increase the severity of porcine pleuropneumonia by decreasing clearance of the bacteria through the mucociliary apparatus mechanism. Phagocytosis and immunoglobulins appear to be important defense mechanisms in response to this bacterium in pigs. The bacterium is able to produce proteases that degrade IgA and IgG; however, the significance of this defense mechanism in the pathogenesis of the disease is uncertain. Therefore it appears that neutrophils, cells of the monocyte-macrophage system, phagocytosis, and phagosome-lysosome fusion are very important defense mechanisms against this bacterium.

Once A. *pleuropneumoniae* is bound to cilia and cell membranes of terminal bronchioles and alveolar epithelial cells, the bacterium is positioned to be phagocytized by alveolar, interstitial, and intravascular macrophages. Although all of these types of macrophages are phagocytic, intravascular macrophages also have strong cytolytic activities that may also account, in part, for the hemorrhage characteristic of pulmonary vascular lesions.

Neutrophils are not involved in the initial phagocytic response to the bacterium, but once the process has been started by macrophages and cytokines and chemokines (interleukins and TNF) are released from activated macrophages, neutrophils are recruited from the vasculature into the acute inflammatory response to phagocytize the bacteria. After phagocytosis, it has been shown that neutrophils can immediately kill A. *pleuropneumoniae*, whereas macrophages cannot. In fact, the bacterium can survive for more than 90 minutes in a phagosome of a macrophage, during which it grows, replicates, and synthesizes and releases Apx toxins, leading to the lysis of these macrophages and release of the bacterium. Additionally, during this time, infected macrophages can move into alveolar and lobular septa, alveolar lumina, and perivascular and peribronchiolar tissues. Thus, when an infected macrophage is killed, large numbers of bacteria are released into vascularized ECM, leading to more acute inflammation, recruitment of additional neutrophils and macrophages, and exacerbation of injury to surrounding tissues.

A. *pleuropneumoniae* has several virulence factors that allow it to survive in phagosomes and resist the effects of phagosome-lysosome fusion (see Fig. 4-14), including a polysaccharide capsule, cell-wall LPS, copper-zinc superoxide dismutase, stress proteins, and ammonia. The capsule, cell-wall molecules, and superoxide dismutase participate in removing oxygen free radicals. The bacterium produces ammonia within phagosomes through the release of a potent urease, which inhibits phagosome-lysosome fusion and disrupts acid hydrolase activity in lysosomes. Finally, Apx toxins, pore-forming exotoxins that lyse cells, are important virulence factors in the pathogenesis of the disease. At low concentrations and probably early in the disease process, Apx toxins (ApxI to ApxIII) produced by the bacterium also impair chemotaxis and phagocytosis by macrophages and neutrophils by likely acting to disrupt actin-myosin–directed movements of the cell or its organelles. At higher concentrations, such as those that occur after the bacteria has gone through several replication and kill cycles in macrophages, ApxI and ApxIII are highly toxic and ApxII is moderately toxic for macrophages and neutrophils. Additionally, ApxI to ApxIII are highly toxic to surrounding tissues, such as blood and lymphatic vessels, and ECM tissues, resulting in loss of barrier systems, increased vascular permeability with fibrin leakage and polymerization, hemorrhage, and vasculitis. In fact, it should be remembered that all of these infected cells and innocent bystander cells and tissues are within several hundred micrometers of one another and the vascular system. In particular, vascular injury appears to result from the activation and killing of intravascular macrophages and endothelial cells by Apx toxins and LPS. Activation results in the release of oxygen free radicals (superoxide anion, hydrogen peroxide, and hydroxyl radical) as well as proteolytic enzymes and various cytokines, all of which can injure endothelial cells of capillaries and postcapillary venules. Injury leads to activation of the coagulation, fibrinolysis, and kinin systems (see Chapters 2, 3, and 5) with concurrent hemorrhage, edema, effusions, platelet activation, and the formation of thrombi, ischemia, and subsequent coagulative necrosis of lung.

Atrophic Rhinitis (*Bordetella bronchiseptica* and *Pasteurella multocida*). Although *Bordetella bronchiseptica* and *P. multocida* can each separately cause clinical forms of atrophic rhinitis in pigs, the classic form of the disease from a pathologist's perspective appears to be caused by these two bacteria interacting synergistically. Information about the mechanisms used by *B. bronchiseptica* and *P. multocida* to cause atrophic rhinitis in pigs is limited. Thus portions of this section are conditional and based on (1) what is known mechanistically about other diseases of the respiratory system caused by *Pasteurella* spp. and (2) a reasonable probability that inflammation, responses to injury, and lesions that have been described in atrophic rhinitis are the result of underlying and known pathobiologic mechanisms. The mechanism of injury is (1) lysis of ciliated epithelial and stromal cells of turbinate mucosae and (2) concurrent activation and suppression of osteoclasts and osteoblasts, respectively, resulting in osteolysis of bone of the turbinates leading to turbinate atrophy. Gross lesions include varying degrees of loss (atrophy) and remodeling of turbinate scrolls and the nasal septum, with ventral scrolls usually being most severely affected (see Fig. 9-33).

Pigs encounter *B. bronchiseptica* and *P. multocida* through inhalation of the bacteria in fomites or fluid droplets. These bacteria are likely commensal microbes that reside in the nasopharynx of healthy pigs, but environmental stressors, such as overcrowding, poor ventilation and humidity, or abrupt changes in ambient air temperature, alter the commensal relationship, allowing the bacteria to replicate in sufficient numbers to colonize mucosae and spread the bacterium to other animals. Colonization appears to be a two-stage process, a *B. bronchiseptica* phase followed by a *P. multocida* phase. When inhaled, *B. bronchiseptica* is deposited on and trapped in the mucus layer of mucosae. The bacterium is nonmotile, and it has not been clearly shown how the bacterium penetrates the mucus layer, gains access to cilia of mucosal epithelial cells, and colonizes the nasal mucosae. *B. bronchiseptica* does produce a dermonecrotic toxin (DNT) (virulence factor) and possibly adenylate cyclase-hemolysin toxin that likely affect the mucus layer and ciliated epithelial cells, making them more susceptible to colonization. Eventually, the ciliated columnar epithelium of the nasal mucosa is replaced by stratified squamous epithelium. The types of adhesins (ligands) and receptors used in colonization have not been determined but may include adhesins such as filamentous hemagglutinin, pertactin, and fimbriae proteins. The bacterium has an outer membrane protein called pertactin that may act as an adhesin, allowing the bacterium to colonize turbinate mucosae that have been injured by DNT. Receptors for pertactin on mucosal epithelial cells have not been identified, but once in contact with cell membranes, bacteria likely adhere and bind to cell membrane receptors using fimbriae and pili. This process results in colonization of mucosae by *B. bronchiseptica*.

Under normal conditions, *P. multocida* has limited and weak virulence factors for attaching to and colonizing turbinate mucosae. Initial colonization by *B. bronchiseptica* leads to disruption of the mucus layer and the mucosal barrier system and results in mucosae that are more suitable for colonization by *P. multocida* in the second phase of infection. Mucosal lesions begin as focal erosions and ulcerations accompanied by acute inflammation (neutrophils), which subsequently spread into underlying lamina propria, ECM tissues, and bone of the turbinates. These lesions result in altered clearance mechanisms of ciliated epithelial cells and exposure of its lamina propria, where *P. multocida* can adhere to and colonize vascularized ECM tissues. Once mucosae and lamina propria are colonized, the primary virulence factor expressed by the bacterium is *P. multocida* toxin (PMT), a DNT. The toxin, a typical A-B toxin, causes turbinate atrophy and snout deformation through chronic inflammation leading to bone remodeling and fibrous osteodystrophy of periosteal fibroblast origin. Mechanistically, the toxin initially acts to stimulate osteoblasts, which in turn act to increase the numbers (hyperplasia) and activity of osteoclasts. As toxin concentrations increase, it acts by blocking the function of osteoblasts, and cell degeneration and lysis may ensue. Overall, PMT causes turbinate atrophy by increasing osteoclast numbers and activities through osteolysis of existing turbinate bone, as well as by inhibiting osteoblastic activities and the formation of new bone, both resulting in turbinate atrophy.

Porcine Enzootic Pneumonia (*Mycoplasma hyopneumoniae*). Also see porcine respiratory disease complex discussed earlier.

The mechanism of injury in porcine enzootic pneumonia is injury of ciliated epithelial cells of the bronchi and bronchioles, causing dysfunction and lysis of these cells. This outcome results initially in dysfunction of cilia, loss of cilia, and then cell lysis followed by a secondary bacterial infection leading to additional cell lysis of all cell types in the lung from chronic inflammation and its mediators and degradative enzymes. The susceptibility to and severity of porcine enzootic pneumonia can be enhanced by environmental stressors (abrupt or long-term changes in ventilation, temperature, and/or humidity) and earlier or concurrent viral (porcine reproductive and respiratory virus, swine influenza virus) or bacterial (*P. multocida*) infections. Gross lesions characteristic of this disease are firm (consolidation) yellow-tan-gray anterior-ventral lung lobes (see Fig. 9-96). Pleural surfaces are usually not involved, indicating that vascular injury and permeability changes and their association with the expression of bacterial virulence factors are not significant in the pathogenesis of the disease.

Pigs encounter *M. hyopneumoniae* through inhalation of the bacterium in fomites or fluid droplets. The bacterium is deposited on mucosae of the conductive component by centrifugal and inertial turbulence and trapped in the mucus layer. The bacterium is nonmotile, and it has not been clearly shown how it penetrates the mucus layer, gains access to cilia of mucosal epithelial cells, and colonizes mucosae. Colonization of the respiratory system appears to probably involve adherence and binding of the bacterium to cell membrane receptors, using fimbriae and pili by ligand-receptor interactions, because it has been shown that the bacteria attach to cilia and line up in parallel rows along the surface of the cells. A molecule called *cilium adhesin* expressed on the surface of the bacterium appears to be involved in the attachment and binding process, where it is thought to interact with glycosaminoglycan and heparin on cell membranes. Additionally, the bacterium probably expresses glycosaminoglycans, such as heparin, heparin sulfate, and chondroitin sulfate B, or coats itself with such molecules that bind to ECM molecules, such as fibronectin, vitronectin, laminin, and collagen, but little is actually known about this process. This interaction ultimately results in dysfunction of cilia (ciliostasis) and lysis of the epithelial cells and reduced function of the mucociliary apparatus. Secondly, there is an increase in mucus (from goblet cells) covering these ciliated epithelial cells. This outcome suggests the bacterium may use mucus in some as yet unknown manner to facilitate colonization of cilia, provide a source of nutrition, or protect itself against immune responses.

Virulence factors used by the bacterium to cause dysfunction and lysis of these cells have not been determined. *M. hyopneumoniae* does not produce toxins, but some mildly toxic molecules do occur. Because of dysfunction of the mucociliary apparatus, *M. hyopneumoniae* and other bacteria are able to reach distal aspects of terminal bronchioles and alveoli by dependent settling caused by forces of gravity. Bacteria replicate in these sites and cause chronic (active) anterior-ventral bronchopneumonia resulting from a continuum of concurrently occurring acute and chronic inflammation and their mediators and degradative enzymes.

Porcine Polyserositis (*Haemophilus suis/parasuis, Actinobacillus suis, Streptococcus suis*, or *Escherichia coli*). Several species of bacteria can cause porcine polyserositis, but it is most commonly associated with *Haemophilus suis/parasuis*, the bacterium that causes Glasser's disease. The mechanism of injury is vasculitis affecting serosal membranes and acute inflammation and its mediators and degradative enzymes. Gross lesions are characterized by variable quantities of a gray-white friable material (fibrin) on serosal surfaces (fibrinous polyserositis) of the lungs (fibrinous pleuritis), heart (fibrinous pericarditis), and abdominal cavity (fibrinous peritonitis) (see Fig. 7-17). Body cavities may also contain a fibrinous exudate and edema fluid. Facing serosal surfaces are often loosely attached to each other by the fibrinous exudate, making normal physiologic processes like respiration and cardiac contraction more difficult. With chronicity and healing, these opposing surfaces may adhere to each by fibrosis and consequently restrict normal "gliding" movements of serosal surfaces of the thoracic and pericardial cavities, thus impeding normal respiratory or cardiac function. The serosa and cavities of meninges, joints, and testis can also be affected. Information about the mechanisms used by these bacteria to cause porcine polyserositis is limited. Thus portions of this section are conditional and based on (1) what is known mechanistically about other diseases of the respiratory system caused by the Pasteurellaceae family of bacteria and (2) a reasonable probability that inflammation, responses to injury, and lesions that have been described in porcine polyserositis are the result of underlying and known pathobiologic mechanisms.

Pigs likely encounter these species of bacteria through inhalation in contaminated fomites or fluid droplets. They appear to behave as commensal microbes of respiratory mucosae existing in biofilms in the nasopharynx and tonsil of healthy pigs. Environmental stressors, such as overcrowding, poor ventilation and humidity, or abrupt changes in ambient air temperature, alter the mucus layer and the commensal relationship, allowing bacteria to replicate in sufficient numbers to begin colonization of respiratory mucosae and to spread to other animals. Preceding or concurrent viral infections (i.e., PRRSV or SIV) could also damage the mucociliary apparatus, allowing bacteria to more extensively colonize the mucus layer or mucosae. In the respiratory system the bacteria are deposited on mucosae of the conductive component by centrifugal and inertial turbulence and are trapped in the mucus layer. These bacteria are nonmotile, and it has not been clearly shown how they penetrate the mucus layer; gain access to cilia of mucosal epithelial cells; express virulence factors such as adhesins, capsular molecules, fimbriae, and outer membrane proteins required for ligand-receptor interactions; and colonize mucosae. It has been suggested that receptors necessary for colonization may be exposed by a molecule that behaves like neuraminidase. Once the mucus layer and/or mucosae are colonized, nonciliated and ciliated epithelial cells are injured by LPS and possibly by a purported neuraminidase and bacterial toxin. Acute inflammation quickly ensues and is followed to a limited extent by lysis of these cells.

It has also been suggested that bacteria gain access to the lamina propria by altering the function of junctional complexes, allowing them to move between adjacent mucosal epithelial cells. The outcome of these processes is the loss of normal mucosal barriers, which provide the bacteria with direct access to the vascularized ECM of the lamina propria. It has not been determined how the bacteria actually cross these altered mucosal barriers, reach capillary beds in ECM, encounter and penetrate the endothelium, and spread within the blood vascular system. Mechanisms, such as a cell-free bacteremia or leukocyte trafficking via alveolar or intravascular macrophages, lymphocytes, or dendritic cells, are hypothetical mechanisms of spread. A study of *Haemophilus suis* has shown that mucosal macrophages contain structures resembling phagolysosomes that are indicative of phagocytic activity. Lesions suggest these bacteria may have a tropism for vascular endothelial cells of serosae. It is unclear why this occurs, but it is probably linked to the expression of bacterial virulence factors and ligand-receptor interactions with host endothelial cells. Additionally, it is thought that bacterial endotoxins (LPS) may contribute to vascular injury and permeability changes leading to the leakage of fibrinogen and its polymerization to fibrin on serosal surfaces and in some cases to microthrombus formation and disseminated intravascular coagulation in other organ systems.

Disorders of Dogs

Acute Tracheobronchitis (*Bordetella bronchiseptica*). The mechanism of injury in acute tracheobronchitis is lysis of ciliated epithelial cells of mucosae of the trachea, bronchi, and bronchioles and acute inflammation and its mediators and degradative enzymes. Gross lesions are characterized by reddened, rough, and granular mucosae (necrosis) that may, depending on severity of injury, be covered with mucus, fibrin, and occasionally blood.

B. bronchiseptica is inhaled, deposited on, and trapped in the mucus layer of mucosae of the conductive component of the respiratory system through centrifugal and inertial turbulence. The bacterium colonizes ciliated epithelium via fimbrial and nonfimbrial adhesins such as filamentous hemagglutinin and pertactin. It has not been determined if and how it penetrates mucus layers to gain access to epithelial cells or if mucosal macrophages and/or dendritic cells are involved. Once ciliated cells are colonized, *B. bronchiseptica* releases exotoxins, such as adenylate cyclase-hemolysin and DNT and endotoxins, that further impair function of the mucociliary apparatus, allowing for additional colonization of mucosae by the bacterium at new sites. These outcomes, especially dysfunction of the mucociliary apparatus, contribute to "dependent settling" via gravity of bacteria into bronchi of dependent lung lobes, resulting in secondary bronchopneumonia. This damage results in an acute inflammatory response that further injures mucosae throughout the lung. *B. bronchiseptica* toxins may also disrupt phagocytosis and/or killing of bacteria by alveolar macrophages and neutrophils and suppress cellular and humoral immune responses. The bacterium can also invade epithelial cells, evade immunologic defense mechanisms, and establish a persistent infection.

Canine infectious tracheobronchitis is a disease in which there is primary injury caused by canine parainfluenza virus leading to increased susceptibility secondarily to infection with *B. bronchiseptica* (or other bacteria). The pathogeneses and mechanisms of injury in this and other respiratory diseases caused by *B. bronchiseptica* are also discussed in other sections of this chapter; see Viral Diseases of Organ Systems; Respiratory System, Mediastinum, and Pleurae; Disorders of Dogs; Canine Infectious Tracheobronchitis (Canine Cough, Kennel Cough; Canine Parainfluenza Virus, Enveloped RNA Virus); and also see Bacterial Diseases of Organ Systems; Respiratory System, Mediastinum, and Pleurae; Disorders of Pigs; Atrophic Rhinitis (*Bordetella bronchiseptica* and *Pasteurella multocida*).

Cardiovascular System and Lymphatic Vessels

Disorders of Domestic Animals

Embolic Vasculopathy/Vasculitis (*Actinobacillus equuli, Escherichia coli, Staphylococcus* spp., *Streptococcus* spp., *Fusobacterium necrophorum*). This section covers a variety of diseases in which the key component of the underlying pathogenesis is embolization through the blood vascular system, leading to vasculitis and potentially thrombosis and ischemia. Such embolic diseases most commonly begin in the skin/subcutis or mucosae but end in a wide variety of highly vascularized organ systems. Examples of embolic diseases include white spotted kidney disease (*E. coli*), embolic nephritis (foal shigellosis [*Actinobacillus equuli*]), milk spots in the liver (*E. coli*), bacterial endocarditis (*E. coli*), and bacterial hepatitis (*Fusobacterium necrophorum*). Embolization also occurs in diseases caused by angioinvasive fungi, and they are covered in the section on fungal diseases. The mechanism of injury in embolic vasculopathy/vasculitis is cell lysis, probably acute coagulative necrosis, caused by bacterial toxins and inflammation and its mediators and degradative enzymes. Gross lesions include gray-white foci of necrosis and inflammation (aggregates of acute inflammatory cells) distributed at random (vascular embolization pattern) in tissue such as those, which occur in renal actinobacillosis of foals (see Fig. 11-35).

Bacteria are able to enter and spread in the vascular system by three mechanisms: (1) direct entry into a blood vessel; (2) establishment of a local infection followed by invasion of the vascular system; and (3) leukocyte trafficking in macrophages, lymphocytes, and/or dendritic cells. The first category usually results from penetration of blood or lymphatic vessels from trauma, bite wounds, or lacerations; the second category from penetrating traumatic injury leading to local inflammation and abscess formation followed by vascular entry; whereas the last category results from endocytosis or phagocytosis of microbes by leukocytes. In the direct entry mechanism, access to the vascular system, embolization, and entrapment in capillary beds are likely physical interactions based on the anatomy of vascular distribution patterns (i.e., sharp angles [90-degree] of curvature), physiology of vascular flow and pressures, and probably the distribution and number of appropriate endothelial cell surface receptor molecules at final destinations. As an example in the cerebral cortices, lesions caused by bacterial emboli tend to be observed at the interface between gray and white matter. Anatomically, at this location, capillaries penetrate through the gray matter from the overlying meninges and as they run into the white matter, they make abrupt turns (90-degree), so capillaries can run parallel to fiber tracts in the white matter. This flow change causes vascular turbulence and endothelial cell surface perturbations, and under the proper conditions, activation of Virchow's triad can result in the formation of vascular endothelial surfaces that may be sticky or have receptors or attached fibrin that can bind or entrap bacteria, respectively. Many of the bacterial virulence factors discussed throughout this chapter, as well as ligand-receptor interactions, probably are involved to some extent in the origination and entrapment and growth of bacterial emboli in the direct entry mechanism.

In the establishment of a local infection mechanism, contamination of the umbilicus at birth and the skin/subcutis through management practices, such as tail docking, castration, and ear notching, are common means of establishing local infections. Injury of mucosae, such as occurs in the abomasum from lactic acidosis in grain overload, also provides opportunities for bacteria (and fungi) to enter the portal blood vascular system and then embolize to and colonize the liver. Finally, bacteria that induce biofilms or cause irresolvable inflammatory processes, such as in dermatitis, otitis, cellulitis, periodontal disease, arthritis, or abscesses, can serve as a site for intermittent bacteremia and embolization. Many of the bacterial virulence factors discussed throughout this chapter, as well as ligand-receptor interactions, probably are involved to some extent in the origination and entrapment and growth of bacterial emboli in the local infection mechanism. The third mechanism of entry and spread in the vascular system is leukocyte trafficking and has been discussed in earlier sections of this chapter.

Vascular Leptospirosis (*Leptospira* spp.). The mechanism of injury in vascular leptospirosis is cell lysis caused by (1) physical properties (penetrating movements from motility) of bacteria that disrupt functions of endothelial cells and (2) bacterial toxins that act directly on membranes of endothelial cells of small blood vessels, including capillaries of the systemic vasculature in all organ systems, leading to coagulative necrosis of affected cells. Gross lesions include acute vasculitis (endothelial cell necrosis) with systemic petechial and ecchymotic hemorrhages, edema, and disseminated intravascular coagulation affecting all organ systems and serosal surfaces (see Fig. 2-18).

Animals encounter *Leptospira* spp. through direct contact of oral or conjunctival mucosae or skin with leptospira-infected urine or with water from reservoirs or ponds into which infected urine drains. Ingestion may also serve as a portal of entry if water contaminated with leptospira is consumed and the bacteria encounter mucosae of the intestine. During chewing and swallowing, it is likely that mucosae of the oral pharynx trap the bacteria in its mucus layer. After swallowing and through intestinal peristalsis, the bacteria are moved into contact with villi and crypts, where they are probably trapped in the mucus layer and encounter enterocytes. In the conjunctiva, it is also likely that mucosae trap the bacteria in a mucus layer. For infection to occur, it has been suggested that the skin and mucosae must have small cuts or abrasions that allow the bacteria to penetrate into the vascularized lamina propria, dermis, submucosal, or subcutaneous connective tissues and gain access to capillaries and/or postcapillary venules. However, *Leptospira* spp. are motile bacteria and are probably able to penetrate mucus layers and move across mucosae by going directly through mucosal epithelial cells or between the cells through intracellular junctional complexes. In all of these portals of entry, the goal is for the bacteria to reach well-vascularized ECM tissues. As a group, these spirochetes are highly motile and invasive, and using their invasive motility (virulence factor), they are able to penetrate the vascular wall and endothelial cells of capillaries and postcapillary venules to gain access to the circulatory system. *Leptospira* spp. may also invade lymphatic vessels and through afferent and efferent branches and the thoracic duct eventually gain access to the circulatory system. *Leptospira* spp. are able to grow and replicate in the circulatory system, spread systemically, and attach to endothelial cell membranes in other organ systems via adhesins before invading these cells and underlying ECM. These encounters and the penetration of blood vessels result in systemic petechial and ecchymotic hemorrhages characteristic of vascular leptospirosis.

Surface-associated proteins (outer membrane leptospiral protein) appear to be involved in ligand-receptor interactions that facilitate adhesion to receptors like cell-adhesion molecules and ECM proteins (Len protein family) on endothelial cells. Adhesion also appears to cause an increased expression of adhesion receptors such as E-selectin on endothelial cells, resulting in additional adhesion of bacteria, platelets, and neutrophils (acute inflammatory response). This response may be attributable to bacteria wall LPS, peptidoglycans, and outer membrane proteins, thus promoting inflammation in capillaries leading to vasculitis and hemorrhage. Bacterial LPS likely activates cells by binding to TLRs on target cell membranes. *Leptospira* spp. also produce pore-forming hemolysins, proteases, sphingomyelinases, and collagenases that may assist in this process, but their role in causing endothelial cell injury remains to be determined.

Septicemic Anthrax (*Bacillus anthracis*). The sections in this chapter on alimentary and inhalation anthrax should be reviewed for background information pertinent to understanding septicemic anthrax (see Fig. 7-124). Once vegetative forms of the bacteria enter the circulatory system from the respiratory or alimentary systems, septicemia ensues and vascular collapse occurs, resulting from massive release of toxins into the blood plasma. Septicemic anthrax is characterized by animals found dead unexpectedly, often in a classic sawhorse stance and with hemorrhage (unclotted) from body orifices (Fig. 4-24). If inadvertently opened, the spleen will be enlarged and unclotted blood will exit from cut surfaces; lymph nodes will be enlarged, edematous, and hemorrhagic; and body tissues and serosal surfaces will be edematous and hemorrhagic (see

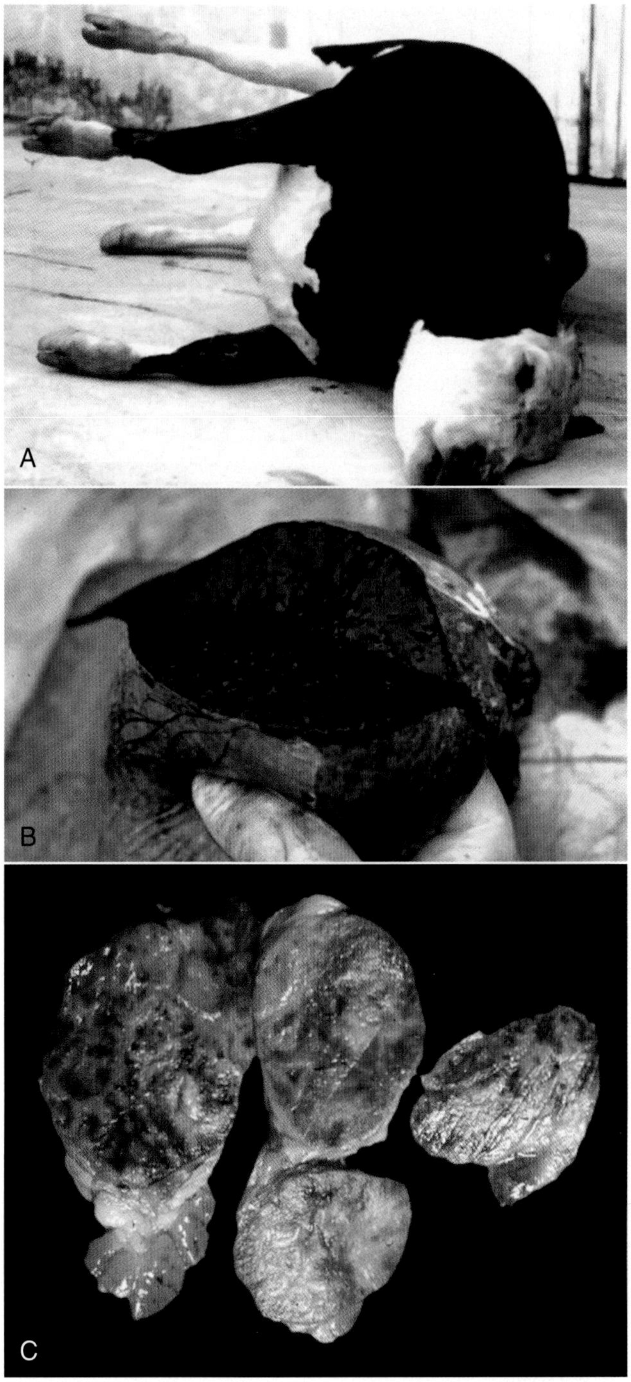

Figure 4-24 Anthrax, ox. A, Because of the high fever, cadavers of cattle dying of anthrax decompose rapidly with the usual result of excessive gas formation in the gastrointestinal tract, abdominal distention, and resultant "sawhorse" position of the legs. **B,** The spleen is enlarged and bloody (splenomegaly, bloody spleen). A postmortem examination should not be performed on an animal suspected of dying from anthrax. Air-dried impression smears of blood from external orifices or from an ear vein can be stained and the bacterium identified (see Fig. 7-124). **C,** Lymph nodes are also enlarged and bloody as a result of anthrax toxins that destroy vascular endothelial cells (see Fig. 13-57). Anthrax toxin can also cause severe injury to the intestines (see Fig. 7-124) and lungs. (**A** courtesy Dr. D. Driemeier, Federal University of Rio Grande do Sul, Brazil. **B** and **C** courtesy Dr. J. King, College of Veterinary Medicine, Cornell University.)

Fig. 4-24). Necropsies should not be performed on animals that are suspected of dying from anthrax because the vegetative form proliferates in large numbers in blood. When blood vessels are cut and blood drains onto the carcass or ground, the vegetative form quickly transforms into endospores, which contaminate the area long-term.

In the circulatory system, vegetative forms proliferate in large numbers and are arranged in long chains in the capillary beds of many organ systems, including the spleen (see Fig. 13-57). Large quantities of EF and LF toxins are released into the blood, causing dysfunction and lysis of endothelial cells and their barrier systems; thus the toxins increase the permeability of the capillary wall, leading to edema, vasodilation, and hemorrhage in affected organ systems. Anthrax toxins also disrupt the clotting cascade, likely through massive activation of disseminated intravascular coagulation and consumption of clotting factors. This outcome results in unclotted blood at body orifices (and within tissues and organs), a clinical (and gross) observation also characteristic of anthrax.

Disorders of Horses

Glanders (*Burkholderia mallei*; Farcy, Malleus, Droes). The mechanism of injury in glanders is cell lysis caused by pyogranulomatous inflammation and its mediators and degradative enzymes. It is a disease of lymphatic vessels (and local lymphoid tissues and skin) and of the respiratory system. Gross lesions include ulcers, pustules, and nodules that can affect skin of any part of the body but most frequently involves lymphatic vessels of the legs and flanks (cutaneous glanders), resulting in pyogranulomatous lymphangitis and lymphadenitis (Fig. 4-25). Nodules typically occur along the course of lymphatic vessels, resulting in a raised beaded appearance of the skin. They often rupture because of trauma to the skin or from pressure necrosis caused by an expanding volume of exudate within the nodules. This process results in craterlike ulcers of the skin that discharge a thick yellowish-white viscid and sticky purulent material containing abundant bacteria (see Fig. 4-25). In the respiratory system, pyogranulomas and ulcers occur in mucosae of the nasal cavity and in all lobes of the lungs (random pattern) (respiratory glanders).

Glanders is a zoonotic disease. Horses, mules, and donkeys probably encounter *Burkholderia mallei* most commonly via fomites arising from purulent exudate discharged from ulcerated lymphatic vessels of the skin. The skin and hair around draining ulcers becomes covered with exudate, which can be transferred to the skin of other animals via direct contact. Additionally, grooming behaviors may result in the bacterium being inhaled or ingested. Therefore the integumentary (skin), respiratory, and alimentary systems are portals of entry for the bacterium, whereas the integumentary and respiratory systems are final destinations for the bacterium. It is the intervening mechanisms involved in the potential pathways of spread that are unresolved.

At the skin, the epidermis and dermis impose structural and functional barriers blocking access to lymphatic vessels in the dermis and subcutis. It appears that the skin must be penetrated and the bacterium carried by direct extension into the dermis and subcutis for pyogranulomatous lymphangitis to develop. Thus the bacterium enters and acts locally. In the respiratory system, the potential pathway(s) of spread are more complicated. Following inhalation, the bacterium encounters mucus and mucosae of the nasal cavity and of the conductive component of the lung. The outcome of these interactions is likely controlled by virulence factors, which determine whether the nasal mucosa and lungs, lymphatic vessels of the skin, of both types of tissues are final targets for infection. In the nasal mucosa and lungs, the bacterium appears to enter and act

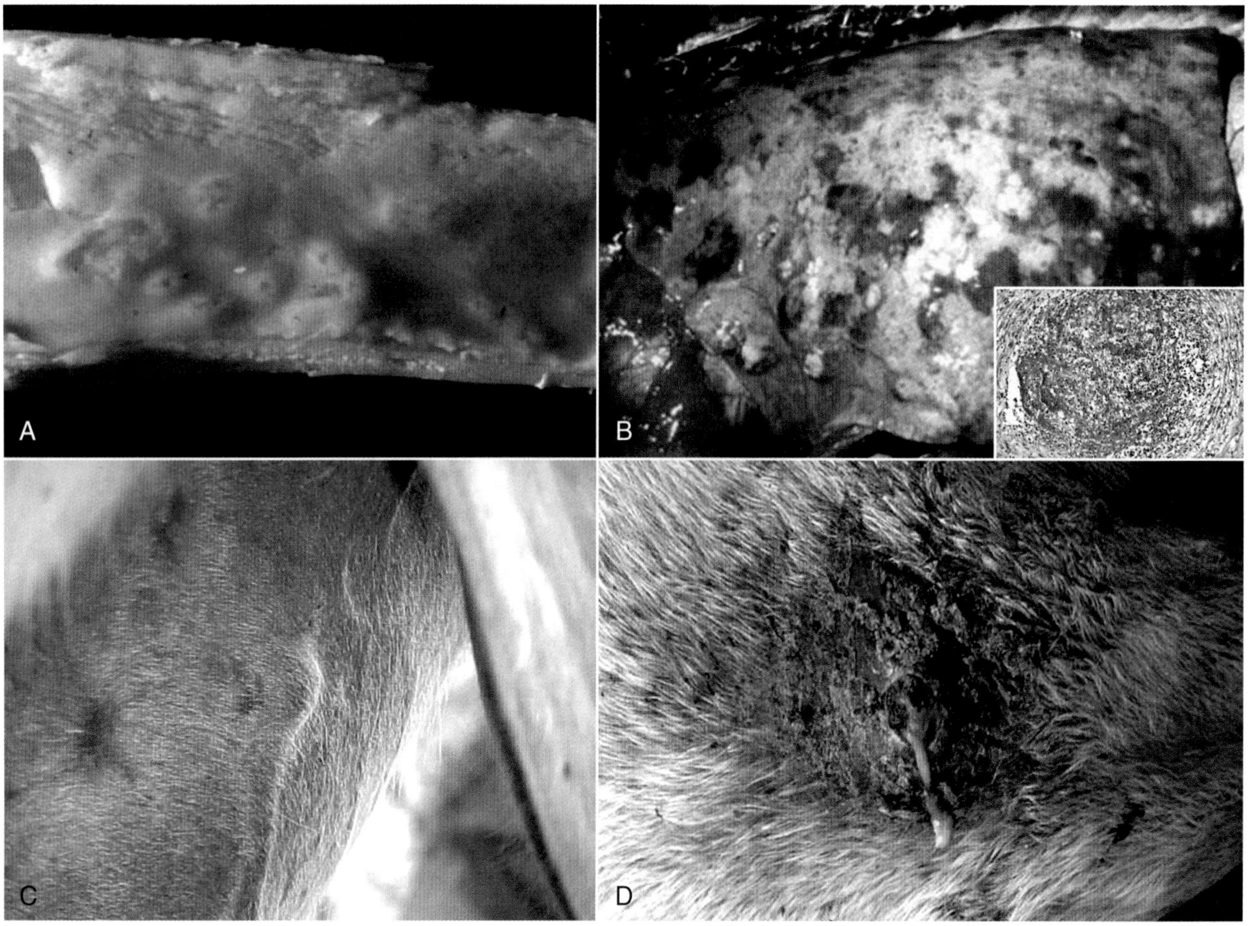

Figure 4-25 **Glanders Disease. A,** Mucosa, nasal turbinates, multiple nasal ulcers, and granulomas. *Burkholderia mallei* colonizes the nasal turbinates, resulting in pyogranulomatous inflammation, necrosis, and ulceration of the mucosa. **B,** When the bacterium colonizes the mucosa of the conductive system of the lung, it spreads into pulmonary parenchyma, resulting in the formation of pyogranulomas *(inset)* throughout the lung. *Inset,* H&E stain. **C,** When the bacterium spreads to the skin, it colonizes subcutaneous lymphatic vessels, resulting in the formation of pyogranulomatous nodules that typically occur along the course of lymphatic vessels (pyogranulomatous lymphangitis), resulting in a raised beaded appearance of the skin. **D,** These nodules frequently rupture because of trauma to the skin or from pressure necrosis due to the expanding volume of exudate within the nodules. This process results in crater-like ulcers of the skin that discharge a thick yellowish-white viscid and sticky purulent material containing abundant bacteria. (**A** courtesy Dr. D.D. Harrington, School of Veterinary Medicine, Purdue University; and Noah's Arkive, College of Veterinary Medicine, The University of Georgia. **B** courtesy United States Animal Health Association, St. Joseph, MO. Inset courtesy Dr. J. Tyler, College of Veterinary Medicine, University of Georgia and Noah's Arkive, College of Veterinary Medicine, University of Georgia. **C** courtesy Dr. D. Driemeier, Federal University of Rio Grande do Sul, Brazil. **D** courtesy Dr. R. Mota, Universidad Federal Rural de Pernambuco, Recife, Brazil, and Dr. M. Brito, Universidad Federal Rural do Rio de Janeiro, Brazil.)

locally. Whereas spread to the skin from the nasal mucosa requires a complicated series of steps, such as endocytosis, phagocytosis, and leukocyte trafficking (or cell-free bacteriemia) as examples, to cross the mucosa, spread, and reach and colonize target cells in cutaneous lymphatic vessels. Lastly, in the alimentary system, following ingestion and passage to the small intestine via swallowing and peristalsis, the potential pathway(s) of spread back to cutaneous lymphatic vessels (if they occur) are more complicated and largely unknown. Mechanisms potentially include virulence factors that facilitate crossing the mucus layer, crossing mucosal barriers at mucosal epithelial cells or M cells (endocytosis, phagocytosis, mucosa-associated macrophages), and leukocyte trafficking (or cell-free bacteriemia), as examples, to spread, reach, and colonize target cells in cutaneous lymphatic vessels.

Most of the mechanisms listed have been discussed and illustrated in earlier sections of this chapter and will not be detailed herein. However, a few important points will be discussed. It appears that the colonization process at mucosae may involve the development of a biofilm; adhesins, such as pili, have also been identified (virulence factors). An interaction of the bacterium with cell membranes is a prerequisite for infection to occur. A type IV pilin-like protein may be involved in the adherence of the bacterium to target cells. Secondly, the bacterium may have different sets of virulence factors that allow it to enter phagocytic cells (macrophages, dendritic cells) or nonphagocytic cells (mucosal and skin epithelial cells) via phagocytosis and endocytosis, respectively, and cross these barrier systems to gain access to BALT/GALT (MALT), and then spread systemically to the skin (lymphatic vessels) via leukocyte trafficking. In both macrophages and mucosal epithelial cells, type III and IV secretion systems (virulence factors) appear to be involved in cell invasion, actin-based motility, and transfer across cell membranes from cell to cell. Unique to nonphagocytic cells (mucosal and skin epithelial cells) are virulence factors that allow the bacterium to enter target cells through endocytosis, escape from endocytotic vesicles and replicate in target cell cytoplasm, move in cytoplasm to the cell membrane (actin-based motility), and enter new target cells via membrane protrusions (actin-based motility) that move bacteria from one cell to another. This later mechanism may be important when the bacterium interacts with endothelial cells of cutaneous lymphatic vessels in the skin, resulting in ulcerative pyogranulomatous lymphangitis.

Cells of the monocyte-macrophage system and possibly mucosal dendritic cells probably play a role in colonization, replication, and spread of the bacterium. Once in MALTs the bacterium could spread to regional lymph nodes in lymphatic vessels as (1) a cell-free bacteremia or (2) via leukocytic trafficking in macrophages, and after colonization of and replication in lymphoid tissues, the bacterium could then spread systemically via lymphatic vessels and the thoracic duct to the circulatory system. Via the circulatory system the bacterium ultimately arrives (cell-free or in macrophages) at capillary beds of the skin, passes through the endothelial cells (leukocytic trafficking, endocytosis, or transcytosis), enters the subcutaneous tissues, encounters endothelial cells of cutaneous lymphatic vessels, and elicits a pyogranulomatous inflammatory response in these tissues. Additionally, it is possible that pyogranulomas in the lung could arise from spread of the bacterium through the circulatory system as a cell-free bacteremia or in macrophages as described earlier.

In macrophages and multinucleated giant cells, how and if the bacterium evades killing by phagosome-lysosome fusion (see Figs. 4-13 and 4-14), replicates, and spreads to cutaneous lymphatic vessels via the circulatory system are unknown. Type III and IV secretion systems (virulence factors) may be possible mechanisms for the invasion, escape from lysosomes or phagolysosomes, and survival in target cells. The bacterium is surrounded by a type I O-antigenic polysaccharide (capsular) antigen, a virulence factor, that may also block phagocytosis or phagosome-lysosome fusion (see Figs. 4-13 and 4-14). LPS, which likely contains a lipid A component, may also play a role in tissue injury. Multinucleated giant cells occur in the inflammatory exudate, and it is thought that the bacteria has virulence factors that causes fusion of macrophages, allowing the bacterium to evade adaptive immune responses and replicate within these fused cells.

Disorders of Pigs

Edema Disease (*Escherichia coli*). The pathogenesis of edema disease begins as an alimentary enterotoxemia and ends as a fibrinoid arteriopathy/arteriolopathy of the vascular system, especially of the brain, leading to ischemia and malacia. The enterotoxemia phase is discussed in the section on bacterial diseases of the alimentary system; the nervous system phase is discussed in the section on bacterial diseases of the nervous system. The mechanism of injury is lysis (coagulative necrosis) of endothelial and smooth muscle cells of arteries and arterioles caused by Shiga toxin 2e (also known as *verotoxin 2e*) produced by hemolytic strains of *E. coli*. After colonization of the intestinal mucosae, the toxin is absorbed from the alimentary system and circulates in the blood vascular system. Cells susceptible to the effects of this toxin include endothelial and smooth muscle cells of arteries and arterioles that express receptors for the toxin such as globotetraosylceramide, galactosylgloboside, and globotriaosylceramide. Toxin acts to disrupt protein synthesis leading to vascular permeability changes and cell lysis and thus edema of affected organs, most notably the eyelids, ventral neck (jowls), the gastric and colonic mesenteries, and the nervous system (see Figs. 7-169 and 7-170). Additionally, endothelial injury caused by this toxin may lead to hemorrhage, intravascular coagulation, microthrombosis, and infarction.

Urinary System

Disorders of Domestic Animals

Necrohemorrhagic Urocystitis (*Escherichia coli, Corynebacterium renale, Pseudomonas* spp., *Proteus vulgaris*, or *Klebsiella pneumoniae*). Necrohemorrhagic urocystitis is a term used herein to group bacteria whose virulence factors can cause acute inflammation and hemorrhage of the mucosa of the urinary bladder, especially affecting transitional epithelial cells and the lamina propria and its capillary beds. Because of the complicated nature of structure and function involved in this disease, a brief overview is provided (also see Chapters 1 and 11). The uroepithelium (urothelium), a mucosa formed by transitional epithelium, is a unique barrier system between urine and its components in the urinary space and the underlying well-vascularized lamina propria. The mucosal epithelium forms a barrier to ions, solutes, and water flux, as well as microbes. Transitional epithelium is composed of three layers, umbrella, intermediate, and basal cell layers. The outermost umbrella layer is a single layer of highly differentiated and polarized cells with distinct apical and basolateral domains demarcated by tight junctions. The intermediate and basal cell layers are connected to each other and the overlying umbrella cell layer by desmosomes and, likely, by gap junctions. The basal layer is connected to a basement membrane and its underlying lamina propria via substrate adhesion molecules.

Because more is known about virulence factors for uropathogenic *E. coli* (UPEC), it is discussed in greater detail; however, the other bacteria listed in this group likely use similar or related mechanisms to cause disease in the urinary bladder. The mechanism of injury is probably cell lysis (coagulative necrosis) caused by bacterial toxins that act directly on mucosal epithelial cells and capillaries in the lamina propria of the bladder and acute and chronic inflammation and their effector molecules and degradative enzymes. Gross lesions of the bladder include mucosal edema and mucosae that are rough and granular, red to dark red, and covered with white-gray flecks of fibrin mixed with cellular debris from inflammation (see Fig. 11-57). Blood vessels in the wall and serosa of the bladder are prominent; this change is due to active hyperemia of the fluidic vascular phase of acute inflammation.

Animals encounter these bacteria through contact with them in fomites or fluid droplets of urinary or fecal origin. They commonly become commensal microbes that reside in the mucous membranes of the vagina and prepuce, likely in biofilms. Physical changes in pressure across the tubular components of the urinary and reproductive systems caused by parturition and breeding appear to force these commensal bacteria via reflux mechanisms into the urethra and urinary bladder. The length of the urethra, in part, appears to determine why females have cystitis more commonly than males. Environmental stressors, such as peak lactation, traumatic mucosal injury, and a high-protein diet that increases the pH of the urine, make mucosae more susceptible to colonization and alter the commensal relationship, allowing the bacteria to replicate in sufficient numbers to colonize mucosae of the urinary and reproductive systems and spread bacteria to other animals.

Once in the lumen of the urinary bladder, bacteria gain access to mucosal surfaces via random movement of the urine. The urinary mucosa lacks goblet cells; thus there is no mucus layer to penetrate. These bacteria encounter the apical surface of transitional epithelial cells, and using ligand-receptor interactions characteristic of other bacterial diseases, begin the process of adherence, binding, and colonization of the mucosa. UPEC expresses adhesins, such as type 1 fimbriae, P fimbriae, and S fimbriae that are involved in this process. These fimbriae (also known as *pili*) bind to hexagonal arrays of mannosyl-glycoprotein receptors called uroplakins. They are expressed on the apical (and luminal) surfaces of specialized transitional epithelial cells called *umbrella cells*. The tips of the type 1 fimbriae express a ligand called *FimH adhesin* that binds to uroplakin receptors. Uroplakins are integral membrane proteins of the umbrella layer, which can be used by microbes as adhesins (FimH adhesin protein) to colonize and invade the uroepithelium. Cells of the umbrella layer have one known receptor (UPIa) and other less well characterized receptors that are mannosylated proteins (integrins) for this adhesin (FimH). Similar processes of bacterial-induced internalization likely occur in the underlying intermediate and basal cell layers as a mechanism to cross the mucosal barrier. Once internalized, the bacterium apparently is able to replicate in endocytotic vesicles and can form intracellular bacterial communities where the bacteria are able to evade innate and adaptive immune defense mechanisms.

When uropathogenic *E. coli* adheres to and colonizes the apical surfaces of the umbrella cell layer, epithelial cells flatten and the bacterium is internalized via endocytosis. Endocytosis is a complicated process of entering and colonizing cells and mucosa, which occurs through a series of conformational changes in the apical surface of the umbrella cells and leads to cytoskeletal rearrangements and cell entry by a zipper mechanism. Bacterial flagella may also have a role in this mechanism. This process results in colonization of the mucosa and the development of a biofilm-like (or intracellular bacterial communities) arrangement affecting the mucosa. After formation of a biofilm, bacteria can kill infected umbrella cells via hemolysins that produce pores in membranes, thus releasing bacteria into the lumen of the bladder, where they colonize new umbrella cells and repeat the infective process or are released into the environment during urination.

The edema, hemorrhage, and necrosis characteristic of necrohemorrhagic urocystitis appear to be caused by acute inflammation and a variety of virulence factors in highly pathogenic strains of UPEC and likely the other bacteria listed earlier. Acute inflammation is probably induced via TLRs that recruit neutrophils from the vascular system into the lamina propria and mucosa and in response to cell necrosis, loss of the mucosal barrier, and interaction of the vascularized lamina propria with bacterial toxins. In umbrella cells infected by bacteria, bacterial toxins, such as LT and ST toxins, Shiga-like toxin, cytotoxins, and endotoxin, likely diffuse through the mucosa and cause membrane injury, leading to cell lysis (necrosis) and loss of the mucosal barrier system. These toxins may also stimulate apoptotic cell lysis, leading to release of bacteria into the urine. Once dead, these cells slough into the urine, and endotoxins and other toxic molecules can readily be absorbed into the highly vascularized lamina propria, resulting in injury to the capillaries and acute vasculitis with active hyperemia.

Other virulence factors that contribute to the pathogenesis of necrohemorrhagic urocystitis include bacterial surface molecules such as capsular K antigens and LPS that block phagocytosis and killing of the bacteria by neutrophils and macrophages. UPEC usually produces siderophores that play a role in iron acquisition for the bacteria during and after colonization. The lytic actions of hemolysins also increase the availability of iron and other nutrients for bacterial growth in colonized mucosa. Hemolysins also can kill lymphocytes and block phagocytosis and chemotaxis by phagocytic cells. Some strains of UPEC have a virulence factor for the production of urease, which hydrolyzes ammonia in urine into urea, resulting in alkaline urine that causes additional injury to mucosa. Finally, these bacteria can readily exchange genetic information with less virulent bacterial strains by transduction and conjugation using drug resistance, toxin, and other virulence plasmids. These factors are a few of the reasons why it is often difficult to treat and resolve certain types of acute and chronic bladder infections.

As a potential defensive mechanism, it has been shown that umbrella cells infected with bacteria undergo apoptosis, likely induced by LPS and TLRs, and affected cells are shed into the urine. This process may be a protective mechanism to remove infected cells; however, loss of apoptotic cells in the urine releases bacteria into the urine to encounter additional umbrella cells.

Renal Leptospirosis *(Leptospira* spp.*).* The pathogenesis of renal leptospirosis begins as vascular leptospirosis (see the section on Bacterial Diseases of Organ Systems, Cardiovascular System and Lymphatic Vessels, Vascular Leptospirosis [*Leptospira* spp.] for portals of entry) caused by *Leptospira* spp. The mechanism of injury in renal leptospirosis is cell lysis caused by (1) physical properties (penetrating movements) of bacteria that disrupt functions of endothelial cells, (2) bacterial toxins that act directly on membranes of renal tubular epithelial cells, and (3) acute and chronic inflammation and their effector molecules and degradative enzymes. Gross lesions include discrete and coalescing, often linear to radiating white to gray foci of acute tubular cortical necrosis and inflammation intermixed with hemorrhage (see Fig. 11-66). In chronic renal leptospirosis, lesions include discrete and coalescing, often linear to radiating white to gray foci of chronic inflammation and fibrosis (see Fig. 11-14).

In the kidney, primary target cells for infection appear to be epithelial cells of the proximal convoluted tubules (cortex) (Fig. 4-26, *A*) and then later, epithelial cells of the loops of Henle (medulla) (Fig. 4-26, *B*). Once *Leptospira* spp. gain access to the circulatory system, they disseminate in glomerular capillaries and then intertubular capillaries of proximal convoluted tubules. Bacteria could access proximal tubular cells via their apical or basolateral surfaces by two routes: (1) vascular by glomerular capillaries and migration into the lumen of the urinary space (apical) or (2) vascular via intertubular capillaries and migration into the interstitium (basolateral). Because glomerular changes are usually unremarkable and bacteria and inflammation are observed in the interstitium, it appears that epithelial cells of the proximal convoluted tubules are infected via the basolateral surfaces of the cells via migration through intertubular capillaries.

To infect tubular epithelial cells of the kidney, it appears that the bacterium must first attach to luminal (apical) surfaces of endothelial cell membranes, enter (endocytosis) and cross the cytoplasm (transcytosis), exit from basal surfaces (exocytosis), and gain access to underlying vascularized ECM adjacent to tubular epithelial cells. Bacteria likely attach to endothelial cell membranes of intertubular capillaries via adhesins then penetrate the vessel wall by moving directly through the cells or through their junctional complexes to gain access to the interstitium. In reality, the distance in the interstitium between capillaries and proximal tubular epithelial cells is probably no more than 100 μm, and it is likely that the flagella of these motile bacteria propel them to the tubular epithelial cells. It is unclear why the bacteria target proximal tubular epithelial cells for infection. *Leptospira* spp. initially spread through the vascular system to all tissues of the body and do not appear to specifically target the kidney via a tropism (attraction to a specific cell type or tissue) mechanism.

In the context of interacting with capillary endothelial cells and probably renal epithelium, surface-associated proteins (outer membrane leptospiral proteins) appear to be involved in ligand-receptor interactions that facilitate adhesion to target cell receptors like cell-adhesion molecules and ECM proteins (Len protein family). Adhesion to cells also appears to cause an increased expression of adhesion receptors such as E-selectin on endothelial cells, resulting in

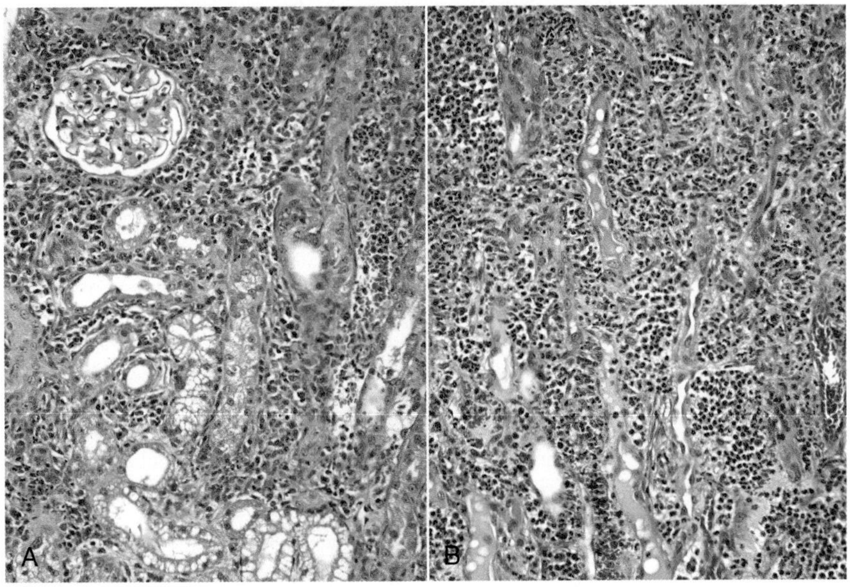

Figure 4-26 Renal Leptospirosis. A, Kidney, outer cortex. Note the infiltration of mononuclear cells, chiefly macrophages, lymphocytes, and plasma cells in the interstitium between the proximal convoluted tubules, the result of the leptospires infecting the proximal tubule cells after exiting the intertubular capillaries. H&E stain. **B,** Kidney (same as **A**), inner cortex. Numerous neutrophils distend the interstitium between the loops of Henle. This acute inflammatory response further down the nephron from the area in **A**, supports the concept that the cells of the loop of Henle are infected later than those in the proximal convoluted tubule. H&E stain. (**A** and **B** courtesy Dr. J.F. Zachary, College of Veterinary Medicine, University of Illinois.)

additional adhesion of bacteria as well as platelets and neutrophils (acute inflammatory response). This response may be attributable to bacteria wall LPS, peptidoglycans, and outer membrane proteins, thus promoting inflammation in capillaries leading to vasculitis and hemorrhage. Bacterial LPS likely activates cells by binding to TLRs on target cell membranes. *Leptospira* spp. also produce pore-forming hemolysins, proteases, sphingomyelinases, and collagenases that may assist in this process, but their role in causing endothelial cell injury remains to be determined. However, once epithelial cells are infected, the reason for dominance of lesions in these organs is unclear and may be related to some essential trophism (nourishment of tissues) provided by these cells to the bacteria for colonization and proliferation. Additionally, although undetermined, such specificity could be attributed to ligand-receptor interactions or to a chemical gradient, such as an iron concentration, that could be required for bacterial growth and replication.

The cause of lysis of proximal tubular cells is probably multifactorial, involving vasculitis and ischemia, trauma from physical injury caused by bacterial motility, inflammatory mediators and degradative enzymes, and bacterial toxins (LPS). The bacteria are present in the cytoplasm of these cells; endocytosis and phagosome-lysosome fusion are not involved in cell entry. It appears that the bacteria are able to directly enter these cells via their motility. Inflammatory cells in the lesion progress from neutrophils (suppurative) to lymphocytes, macrophages, and plasma cells (chronic) and provide an array of molecules that could injure ands lyse tubular epithelial cells. Biofilms (virulence factor) formed by *Leptospira* spp. may also play a role in tubular injury. Epithelial cells lining the loop of Henle could also be infected by an intertubular capillary–interstitial route. This mechanism has not been confirmed. Additionally and based on inflammatory cell responses, it is unclear why cells of the proximal tubules appear to be infected at an earlier point in the disease than those of the loop of Henle. However, when proximal tubular cells die, they may release bacteria into the urinary space where they are carried in urine and spread into the environment via urination. During this luminal transit, the bacteria also encounter the apical surfaces of epithelial cells lining the loop of Henle. It is plausible that *Leptospira* spp. infect epithelial cells of the loop of Henle via their apical surfaces projecting into the urinary lumen, using mechanisms similar to those previously described. Infection appears to result in the same cascade of cell alterations and inflammatory responses as those described for proximal tubular cells. These outcomes in both proximal tubular and loop of Henle cells serve as the basis for characterizing this disease as tubulointerstitial nephritis.

Disorders of Ruminants (Cattle, Sheep, and Goats)

Contagious Bovine Pyelonephritis (*Corynebacterium renale, Trueperella pyogenes* [formerly *Arcanobacterium pyogenes*], or *Escherichia coli*). Contagious bovine pyelonephritis is caused by the *Corynebacterium renale* group (*C. renale*, *Corynebacterium cystitidis*, and *Corynebacterium pilosum*) of bacteria, but *Trueperella pyogenes* (formerly called *Arcanobacterium pyogenes*) and *E. coli* may also cause this disease. Depending on the region, *T. pyogenes* may be most common. These bacteria are likely commensal microbes that reside, probably in a biofilm, in the mucous membranes of the vagina and prepuce. Mechanisms that contribute to the occurrence of cystitis that precede pyelonephritis are discussed in the section on necrohemorrhagic urocystitis and UPEC. Information about the mechanisms used by *C. renale* or *E. coli* to cause contagious bovine pyelonephritis in cattle is limited. Thus portions of this section are conditional and based on (1) what is known mechanistically about other diseases caused by *Corynebacterium* spp. or *E. coli* and (2) a reasonable probability that inflammation, responses to injury, and lesions that have been described in contagious bovine pyelonephritis are the result of underlying and known pathobiologic mechanisms.

The mechanism of injury in contagious bovine pyelonephritis is probably cell lysis (acute coagulative necrosis) caused by (1) bacterial toxins that act directly on transitional epithelium of bladder mucosa and on renal pelvic and tubular epithelium and by (2) acute and chronic inflammation and their effector molecules and degradative enzymes. Gross lesions include white-tan streaks often mixed with narrow red streaks (hemorrhage) that radiated from the pelvis, through the medulla, often extending to the cortical medullary junction or deeper into the cortex (see Fig. 11-46). In many ways, these lesions resemble inverted renal cortical infarcts with their bases against the pelvis and their apices extending into the medulla.

Cattle (and probably sheep and goats) encounter these bacteria through contact with contaminated fomites or fluid droplets of urinary or fecal origin. Environmental stressors such as parturition, peak lactation, traumatic mucosal injury, and a high-protein diet that increases the pH of the urine appear to alter the commensal (biofilm) relationship of bacteria in mucous membranes of the vagina and prepuce making them more suitable for colonization. It has been proposed that contagious bovine pyelonephritis occurs secondary to a chronic and often insidious cystitis (see section on Necrohemorrhagic Urocystitis [*Escherichia coli, Corynebacterium renale, Pseudomonas* spp., *Proteus vulgaris*, or *Klebsiella pneumoniae*]) likely resulting from reflux of bacteria into and up the urethra and then into the bladder via changes in urethral luminal pressures caused by parturition, breeding, or straining to defecate. Subsequently the bacterium must reach the renal pelvis via the ureters and then spread though the mucosal barrier formed by transitional epithelium of the renal pelvis to encounter the interstitium (vascularized ECM) of the renal medulla and renal tubules. How each of the steps occurs has not been specifically determined; however, ligand-receptor interactions characteristic of other bacterial diseases and their interaction with mucosae likely occur in contagious bovine pyelonephritis (see section on Necrohemorrhagic Urocystitis [*Escherichia coli, Corynebacterium renale, Pseudomonas* spp., *Proteus vulgaris*, or *Klebsiella pneumoniae*]).

Although *C. renale* is a nonmotile bacterium, some strains of *E. coli* are motile, and this virulence factor may help in ascension of the bacterium up the ureter to the kidney. It has been shown that pili are required for *C. renale* to adhere to transitional epithelium of the urinary system and to attach to and colonize mucosae of the reproductive system. Additionally, pili may serve to disrupt phagocytosis of the bacteria by neutrophils and macrophages. Putative adhesins such as FimH adhesin protein and other invasins are likely virulence factors (see section on Necrohemorrhagic Urocystitis [*Escherichia coli, Corynebacterium renale, Pseudomonas* spp., *Proteus vulgaris*, or *Klebsiella pneumoniae*]). Binding is strongest to mucosal epithelial cells of the vulva and vagina. This outcome allows for spread of the bacterium to other susceptible animals during breeding season or when other invasive management practices or examinations are performed. The receptors used by the bacterium to bind to mucosae have not been determined; however, once a bacterium is bound, colonization of mucosae begins. Once bacteria replicate in sufficient numbers, they spread by ascension to encounter and colonize mucosae of the urethra and bladder and then by vesicoureteral reflux to ascend to the ureters and renal pelvis. The development of a chronic insidious urocystitis is often an intervening stage in the disease that serves to produce large numbers of bacteria. After colonization of the renal pelvis, it is not known how bacteria cross mucosae to gain access to the medullary interstitium. Degradative enzymes and inflammatory mediators combined with bacterial virulence factors, such as Renalin, which is an extracellular cytolytic protein produced by *C. renale*, may facilitate spread across mucosal barriers and inflammation and cell lysis within the medulla. It has been suggested that lesions in the medulla (resembling inverted renal cortical infarcts) may actually begin as a vasculitis from inflammation resulting in thrombosis, ischemia, and necrosis. It has been shown that toxins (LPS) from *E. coli* may stimulate apoptotic cell lysis in renal tubular cells in pyelonephritis.

Pulpy Kidney (Overeating) Disease (*Clostridium perfringens*). The pathogenesis of pulpy kidney disease begins as an enterotoxemia of the alimentary system caused by *C. perfringens* and should be reviewed in the section on the alimentary system before reading this section. ε-Toxin appears to be an important virulence factor in the pathogenesis of pulpy kidney disease. Because ε-toxin is a permease that alters cell permeability (a pore-forming toxin), the vascular beds in affected intestinal tissues readily absorb toxins into the circulatory system. It appears that the sequence of steps leading to pulpy kidney disease occurs in the first phase or early in the second phase of alimentary enterotoxemia before toxin-induced massive necrosis of the intestine occurs. The mechanism of injury in pulpy kidney disease is cell lysis caused by ε-toxin that acts directly on renal endothelial cell membranes and tubular epithelial cell membranes, leading to vascular permeability changes and acute coagulative necrosis of tubular epithelial cells and likely endothelial cells. Microthrombosis and ischemia resulting from capillary endothelial injury are plausible but unproved mechanisms of tubular cell lysis. Gross lesions include soft pliable kidneys with hemorrhages; however, the lesions are often attributed to postmortem change. Experimental data suggest that vascular endothelial cells, such as those in the renal cortex supplying epithelial cells of renal tubules, express receptors (ligand-receptor interactions) for ε-toxin. Because ε-toxin is an angiotoxic permease, it increases the permeability of targeted endothelial cells, allowing plasma containing ε-toxin to leak into the ECM surrounding renal tubules. Renal tubular epithelial cells also express receptors for ε-toxin, and toxin binding may lead to membrane-mediated cytotoxicity and cell lysis.

Bone Marrow, Blood Cells, and Lymphatic System

Disorders of Domestic Animals

Brucellosis (*Brucella* spp.). The mechanism of injury in brucellosis is cell lysis caused by inflammation and its mediators and degradative enzymes. *Brucella* spp. do not have virulence factors for exotoxins or endotoxins that cause direct injury to cells. Gross lesions include chronic active pyogranulomatous lymphadenitis with enlarged firm lymph nodes that on a cut surface have discrete and coalescing areas of yellow-white exudate infiltrating and compressing contiguous parenchyma.

Animals (ruminants [cattle, sheep, and goats], pigs, and dogs) encounter *Brucella* spp. through inhalation or ingestion of bacteria in fomites contaminated with infected exudates from other organ systems such as the female reproductive tract. The bacterium encounters mucosae and their mucus layers through centrifugal turbulence and entrapment in the mucus layer of the nasal pharynx and through chewing, gravity, and entrapment in the mucus layer of the oral pharynx. Bacteria are phagocytosed by mucosa-associated macrophages or dendritic cells migrating through, on, or in mucosae and spread to local lymphoid tissues via leukocyte trafficking by lymphatic vessels, to regional lymph nodes via afferent lymphatic vessels, and then systemically to superficial and visceral lymph nodes and other organs such as spleen, liver, bone marrow, mammary glands, and reproductive organs. *Brucella* spp. can also enter and cross the mucosal barrier via endocytosis/transcytosis, exit the basal surface of mucosal epithelial cells through exocytosis, and spread cell-free in lymphatic vessels to local and regional lymph nodules and nodes, where they are phagocytosed by macrophages and then spread systemically as discussed earlier. Through ingestion, swallowing, and peristalsis, *Brucella* spp. can also reach the alimentary system where they encounter M cells. Bacteria infect M cells via endocytosis, undergo transcytosis, and exit the basal surfaces via exocytosis to gain access to macrophages within Peyer's patches. Macrophages within Peyer's patches are then infected with the bacteria and used to spread bacteria systemically. The goals of these three types of mucosal encounters are to provide *Brucella* spp. with ample opportunity to infect macrophages and subsequently gain access to local, regional, and systemic lymph nodules and nodes.

In lymph nodes, bacteria-infected macrophages are killed by the bacterium or die through aging, and the bacteria are released into vascularized ECM. These bacteria elicit an acute inflammatory response that is quickly replaced by a pyogranulomatous inflammation because of LPS in the bacterial cell wall. LPS is not readily degradable, and macrophages (as monocytes) are recruited from the systemic circulation to phagocytose and degrade such material and kill the bacteria. *Brucella* spp. are able to evade the killing mechanisms when phagocytosed by neutrophils and macrophages. Additionally, they are able to grow and replicate in macrophages and dendritic cells. Once *Brucella* spp. encounter cell membranes of macrophages, they use ligand-receptor interactions to attach to and enter cells; however, the details remain unclear. Outer membrane protein of the bacterial cell wall and class A scavenger receptors on target cells are likely involved but not necessarily with each other. TLRs are also likely involved in attachment and entry into macrophages. Entry occurs via endocytosis through a phagosome, but phagosome-lysosome fusion does not occur because bacteria are able to block fusion through rapid acidification of the phagosome (see Figs. 4-13 and 4-14). LPS (a PAMP), a type IV secretion system, and a long list of other putative virulence factors such as cyclic β-1,2-glucan and heat shock proteins may also be involved in blocking phagosome-lysosome fusion and promoting bacterial growth and replication. The virulence of Brucella spp. strains appears related to the LPS composition of its capsule, with the encapsulated smooth phenotypes generally being more virulent. Additionally, the presence of a smooth capsule enhances bacterial growth and replication in phagosomes.

When *Brucella* spp. spread via leukocyte trafficking systemically in macrophages, they are able to gain access to tissues in the male and female reproductive systems and the mammary gland (Fig. 4-27; also see Fig. 19-18). In summary, infected macrophages interact with and infect placental trophoblasts in placentomas and epithelial cells of other reproductive tissues. Once such cells are infected, the bacteria likely infect fetal macrophage-like cells that serve to spread the bacteria through the fetus and to other lymphoid tissues in reproductive organs (see Fig. 4-27, *C* and *D*). *Brucella* spp. also survive in macrophages of these tissues by inhibiting the phagosome-lysosome fusion. Bacterial growth and replication with concurrent lysis of bacteria-infected macrophages results in pyogranulomatous inflammation of these tissues and organ systems.

Disorders of Horses

Strangles (*Streptococcus equi* subsp. *equi*). The mechanism of injury in strangles is lysis (coagulative necrosis) of cells of lymphatic vessels, lymph nodes, and the monocyte-macrophage system attributable to acute suppurative inflammation and its mediators and degradative enzymes. Gross lesions include the formation of abscesses within regional lymph nodes resulting in enlarged firm lymph nodes that on cut surface have discrete and coalescing areas of yellow-white suppurative exudate infiltrating and compressing contiguous parenchyma (see Fig. 13-77). Affected retropharyngeal and mandibular lymph nodes may also have draining fistulous tracts between affected nodes and the surface of the skin, the guttural pouches, and the nasal cavities and sinuses, resulting in release of bacteria into the environment. This outcome occurs because degradative enzymes released from dead neutrophils in abscesses digest the capsule of the lymph node and the structures of all contiguous tissues until a fistulous tract is formed.

Foals encounter *S. equi* subsp. *equi* through inhalation or ingestion of fomites or body fluids contaminated with the bacterium. It is deposited on mucosae of the nasal (centrifugal turbulence) and oral pharynx and trapped in the mucus layer. The bacterium is nonmotile, and it has not been clearly shown how it penetrates the mucus layer and gains access to mucosal epithelial cells. Mucosal epithelial cells of the tonsils and tonsillar crypts appear to be important target cells for adherence and binding, and this specificity may be determined by unique ligand-receptor interactions. Once in contact with cell membranes, several bacterial cell wall surface proteins, such as M-like proteins (SeM, SzPSe), may act as adhesins and attach to receptors expressed on the membranes of these cells. The characteristics of these receptors are unknown. It has not been determined if the bacterium needs to first colonize the mucosal surface before spreading into subjacent local lymphoid tissues. Additionally, it has not been determined how the bacterium crosses the mucosal barrier of the tonsil. Mucosal macrophages could phagocytose the bacteria in the mucus layer and carry it via leukocyte trafficking through the mucosal barrier into the local lymphoid tissues, or once bound to target cell receptors, it could be transported through the cell via transcytosis and released via exocytosis from the basal membranes of the cells into local lymphoid tissues of the tonsil. Dendritic cells could also be involved in the spread of bacteria across the mucosal barrier and into local and regional lymphoid tissues and lymph nodes. In local lymphoid tissues of the tonsil, the bacterium is able to evade destruction by the innate immune system, replicate extracellularly, and then spread to regional lymph nodes such as the mandibular or retropharyngeal. Although unknown, the bacterium could spread by means of lymphatic vessels to these regional nodes in macrophages via leukocyte trafficking or through a bacteremia (cell-free migration). The bacterium multiplies extracellularly in the lymph tissues and nodes, and the exudate contains large numbers of viable bacteria.

Mechanistically, several bacterial virulence factors contribute to the character of this exudate (suppurative) and the large number of viable bacteria. Bacterial virulence factors that act as chemoattractants for neutrophils and that disrupt phagocytosis and killing by neutrophils appear to explain the abundance of exudate and viable bacteria, respectively. Early in the sequence of steps when bacteria encounter mucosal and tissue macrophages in local and regional lymphoid tissues and nodes, a bacterial cell wall protein, SeeH, interacts with these cells, resulting in the release of proinflammatory cytokines, increased vascular permeability, and edema. The occurrence of acute suppurative inflammation is also facilitated by several virulence factors. When peptidoglycan of the bacterial cell wall interacts with C3 of complement in edema fluid via the alternative complement pathway, it produces complement-derived chemotactic factors that attract large numbers of neutrophils from capillary beds into local vascularized connective tissues (ECM). Furthermore, bacterial streptokinase interacts with plasminogen in edema fluid to form active plasmin, which hydrolyzes fibrin. This process appears to increase the spread and dispersion of bacteria in tissue. Normally fibrin confines bacteria by isolating them within its polymerized fibrillar meshwork so they can be phagocytosed and killed by neutrophils and macrophages, but when fibrin is hydrolyzed, large numbers of bacteria can accumulate in the exudate of an abscess and be readily available for release into the environment (see later). The outcomes of these processes also contribute to the initiation of the cellular (leukocytic) phase of acute inflammation and the accumulation of suppurative exudate characteristic clinically of strangles.

The surface of *S. equi* subsp. *equi* is coated with numerous protein virulence factors, such as hyaluronic acid, SeM, and Se18.9 proteins

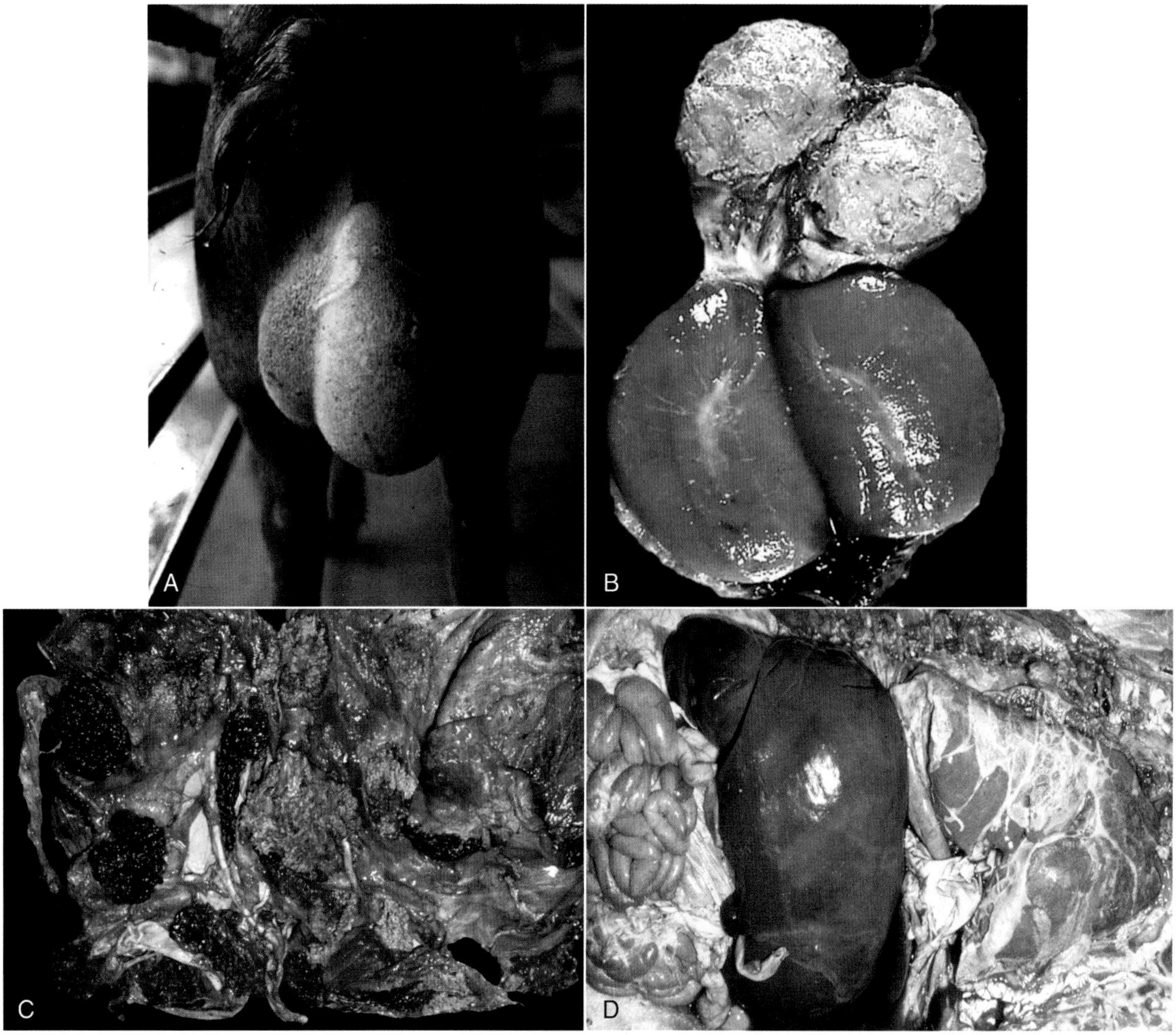

Figure 4-27 **Brucellosis.** Brucellosis is a disease in which the bacterium initially targets lymphocytes and macrophages in mucosa-associated lymphoid tissues, regional lymph nodes, systemic lymph nodes, and the spleen to replicate and grow in number. It uses macrophages to spread to and through these tissues and then systemically to infect cells and tissues in the placenta, sex organs of males and females, and fetuses. Therefore brucellosis is initially and long term characterized by a chronic active pyogranulomatous lymphadenitis with sequelae that affect the reproductive systems. **A,** Boar, swollen testis. The testis in enlarged due to chronic active pyogranulomatous inflammation. *Brucella* spp. spread in macrophages via leukocyte trafficking from lymphoid tissues systemically to the testis. **B,** The epididymis can be filled with pyogranulomatous exudate, which obstructs the flow of spermatozoa and causes infertility. Infected animals can also serve as carriers and spread the bacterium via sexual contact (also see Fig. 19-18). **C,** Fetal cotyledons. Note the roughened granular yellow-brown surface of cotyledons *(example: center of field)* infected with the bacterium. This lesion is caused by pyogranulomatous inflammation leading to severe necrosis of the affected cotyledons. Normal cotyledons are dark red and have a smooth shiny surface. **D,** Fetal brucellosis, hepatomegaly, and fibrinous polyserositis. The bacterium is thought to be spread from infected cotyledons to fetal organs via leukocytic trafficking in fetal macrophage-like cells. The bacterium causes extensive injury of the vascular system and organs through inflammatory responses induced in the fetus. (**A** courtesy Dr. C. Wallace, College of Veterinary Medicine, The University of Georgia; and Noah's Arkive, College of Veterinary Medicine, The University of Georgia. **B** courtesy Dr. K. McEntee, Reproductive Pathology Collection, University of Illinois; and Dr. J. King, College of Veterinary Medicine, Cornell University. **C** and **D** courtesy Dr. K. McEntee, Reproductive Pathology Collection, University of Illinois.)

that disrupt phagocytosis and killing. The bacterium also secretes leukocidal toxin and streptolysin S, a cell membrane pore-forming toxin, which kills leukocytes and disrupts phagocytosis. These processes lead to the accumulation of large numbers of viable bacteria in the exudate of lymphoid tissues and lymph nodes. Specific bacterial proteins are also chemoattractants and result in the recruitment of large numbers of neutrophils into the tissue and abscess formation. Additionally, hyaluronic acid in the capsule appears to block interactions between bacteria and neutrophils by increasing the negative charge and hydrophobicity of the bacterial surface and by producing a localized oxygen-reduced environment that protects the activity of oxygen-labile proteases and toxins such as streptolysin S. It is likely but undetermined that bastard strangles occurs because of spread of the bacterium to systemic lymph nodes and organ systems by leukocyte trafficking or bacteremia via efferent lymphatic vessels and/or capillaries or postcapillary venules in lymph nodes to gain access to the systemic circulatory system.

Rhodococcal Mesenteric Lymphadenitis (*Rhodococcus equi*). The pathogenesis of rhodococcal mesenteric lymphadenitis begins as an infection of the respiratory system (see section on

Bacterial Diseases of Organ Systems; Respiratory System, Mediastinum, and Pleurae; Disorders of Horses), followed by infection of the alimentary system (see section on Bacterial Diseases of Organ Systems; Alimentary System and the Peritoneum, Omentum, Mesentery, and Peritoneal Cavity; Disorders of Horses). The mechanism of injury in rhodococcal mesenteric lymphadenitis is lysis of cells of the monocyte-macrophage system and of all cell populations in the lymph node secondary to inflammation and its mediators and degradative enzymes. Gross lesions include chronic active pyogranulomatous lymphadenitis (see Fig. 7-139) with enlarged firm lymph nodes that on a cut surface have discrete and coalescing areas of yellow-white exudate infiltrating and compressing contiguous parenchyma. *R. equi* enters the alimentary system through M cells and is released into Peyer's patches, where it is phagocytosed by tissue macrophages. Bacteria-infected tissue macrophages spread via leukocyte trafficking in lymphatic vessels within the intestinal mesentery to mesenteric lymph nodes, leading to pyogranulomatous lymphadenitis, and then systemically via the thoracic duct and the blood vascular system to additional lymph nodes and lymphoid tissues such as the spleen. The pathogenesis of pyogranulomatous lymphadenitis appears to progress much like that which occurs in the lung (see section on the Respiratory System, Mediastinum, and Pleurae).

Caseous Lymphadenitis (*Corynebacterium pseudotuberculosis*). A disease similar to that which occurs in cattle, sheep, and goats also occurs in horses (see section on Bacterial Diseases of Organ Systems; Bone Marrow, Blood Cells, and Lymphatic System; Disorders of Ruminants [Cattle, Sheep, and Goats]; Caseous Lymphadenitis [*Corynebacterium pseudotuberculosis*]).

Disorders of Ruminants (Cattle, Sheep, and Goats)

Caseous Lymphadenitis (*Corynebacterium pseudotuberculosis*). The mechanism of injury in caseous lymphadenitis is cell lysis attributable to inflammation and its mediators and degradative enzymes affecting cells of the monocyte-macrophage system and cell populations in lymph nodes and other organ systems. Gross lesions include chronic active pyogranulomatous lymphadenitis (see Figs. 13-79 and 13-80) with enlarged firm lymph nodes that on a cut surface have discrete and coalescing areas of yellow-white caseous exudate infiltrating and compressing contiguous parenchyma and abundant connective tissue. In other organs, such as the lung, abscesses encapsulated by dense bands of fibrous connective tissue and containing yellow-white caseous exudate are common findings.

Sheep and goats encounter *Corynebacterium pseudotuberculosis* through penetrating wounds and potentially ingestion. The bacterium is a common contaminate of the environment usually from animals that have the cutaneous form of caseous lymphadenitis leading to fistulous tracts from draining cutaneous lymph nodes. Penetrating wounds most commonly involve the skin and mucous membranes of the oral cavity. Management practices, such as shearing, may cause skin abrasions, whereas objects like wire, sticks, and protruding barn or fence nails may puncture the skin. Similar types of injury may occur in the oral cavity by similar objects and mechanisms. Once the bacterium reaches the submucosa or dermis, it is phagocytosed by neutrophils and macrophages and spread via leukocyte trafficking to regional lymph nodes via afferent lymphatic vessels. The bacterium replicates in lymph nodes, and the inflammatory response results in multiple pyogranulomas (abscesses) that grow in size and with time, notably enlarge, and affect the entire lymph node. Macrophages infected with bacteria leave the lymph node via leukocyte trafficking and spread via efferent lymphatic vessels and probably the thoracic duct to the systemic circulation system or spread by entering the capillary or venous circulation within the node to gain access to the systemic circulatory system. Macrophages spread the bacterium to other visceral lymph nodes, especially the mediastinal and bronchial, and to tissues in a wide variety of organ systems, especially the lung. Because the bacterium is able to replicate in large numbers in macrophages and neutrophils, the lysis of these cells attributable to mycolic acid or cell aging results in the release of bacteria into vascularized ECM tissues. This process activates integrins and adhesins in vascular endothelium and causes massive recruitment of additional neutrophils and macrophages into the tissues as part of a chronic active inflammatory response, thus repeating the inflammatory process of forming pyogranulomas (abscesses).

The mechanisms used by *C. pseudotuberculosis* to gain access to lymph nodes via the alimentary system and ingestion (if it occurs) are unknown. Two potential pathways could be used, and both focus on macrophages and leukocyte trafficking. First, bacteria could interact with the mucus layer and mucosae of the oral pharynx, be phagocytized by mucosa-associated macrophages and carried to the tonsils, then to regional lymph nodes, and then systemically. Second, bacteria could be swallowed and via alimentary peristalsis encounter M cells of small intestinal crypts, spread via M cells to macrophages in contiguous Peyer's patches, then to regional lymph nodes, and then systemically. It is likely that the mechanisms and responses to injury described for the penetrating wounds portal of entry would also apply to these two scenarios.

C. pseudotuberculosis has two known bacterial virulence factors, phospholipase D and mycolic acid, that allow it to colonize tissues and produce pyogranulomas. Phospholipase D increases vascular permeability, which is thought to assist macrophages in migrating in and out of tissues infected with the bacterium, thus favoring the systemic spread of the bacterium. As a potent exotoxin, it also injures cell membranes, leading to macrophage and neutrophil dysfunction, disruption, and lysis, and interferes with neutrophil chemotaxis. *C. pseudotuberculosis* does not have a protective capsule but has a waxy mycolic acid coat on the cell wall surface. Mycolic acid induces acute inflammation, has a role in the formation of granulomas, is toxic for macrophages, and prevents killing of the bacterium with phagosome-lysosome fusion (see Fig. 4-14) likely by protecting against hydrolytic enzymes present within lysosomes.

Brucellosis (*Brucella* spp.). See the section on Bacterial Diseases of Organ Systems; Bone Marrow, Blood Cells, and Lymphatic System; Disorders of Domestic Animals; Brucellosis (*Brucella* spp.).

Disorders of Pigs

Rhodococcal Mesenteric Lymphadenitis (*Rhodococcus equi*). A disease similar to that which occurs in horses also occurs in pigs. See section on Bacterial Diseases of Organ Systems; Bone Marrow, Blood Cells, and Lymphatic System; Disorders of Horses; Rhodococcal Mesenteric Lymphadenitis (*Rhodococcus equi*).

Brucellosis (*Brucella* spp.). See section on Bacterial Diseases of Organ Systems; Bone Marrow, Blood Cells, and Lymphatic System; Disorders of Domestic Animals; Brucellosis (*Brucella* spp.).

Disorders of Dogs

Brucellosis (*Brucella* spp.). See section on Bacterial Diseases of Organ Systems; Bone Marrow, Blood Cells, and Lymphatic System; Disorders of Domestic Animals; Brucellosis (*Brucella* spp.).

Nervous System

Disorders of Domestic Animals

Botulism and Tetanus (*Clostridium botulinum, Clostridium tetani*). The mechanism of injury in botulism is disruption of neurotransmitter vesicle exocytosis at *myoneural junctions* by botulinum toxin resulting in flaccid paralysis. The mechanism of injury in tetanus is disruption of neurotransmitter vesicle exocytosis at *neural-neural junctions* by tetanospasmin toxin resulting in spastic paralysis. These toxins, categorized as neurotoxins, are produced in anaerobic microenvironments (a lowered oxidation-reduction [redox] potential) such as occur in necrotic tissue resulting from traumatic wounds (e.g., nail penetrating sole of the hoof, gastric ulcers, necrotic muscle). Gross or microscopic lesions are not observed in the nervous systems of animals with these diseases.

Animals encounter these bacteria through contact with bacterial endospores present in soil and resting on environmental objects. Spores are carried into wounds and with the appropriate anaerobic conditions they germinate to vegetative forms. Neurotoxins are produced by the vegetative form and are released into surrounding tissues. Examples of such wounds include penetration of the skin or sole of the hoof or gastric ulcers. In addition, botulinum neurotoxin can also be released from lysed vegetative forms in the anaerobic environment of decaying vegetable matter (e.g., spoiled silage, hay [equine grass sickness], grain) and decomposing carcasses and absorbed into the circulatory system from the alimentary system with their ingestion. From a wound (or the alimentary system), neurotoxins access myoneural (botulinum neurotoxin) and neural-neural (tetanus neurotoxin) junctions by two routes, either hematogenously (botulinum neurotoxin) or via retrograde axonal transport (tetanus neurotoxin).

Botulinum neurotoxin enters the blood from (1) wounds as it diffuses via a concentration gradient to the periphery of the wound to areas with adequate circulation in which it is absorbed into the blood via capillaries and (2) absorption through intestinal villi and transfer to capillary beds within the lamina propria of the villi. Botulinum neurotoxin gains access to myoneural junctions via capillary beds that supply muscular tissues. On its release from capillaries, the neurotoxin diffuses in interstitial fluids until contacting the cell membrane of peripheral nerves (e.g., lower motor neuron), where it enters the cytoplasm of the neuron through the formation of endocytotic vesicles.

In contrast, tetanus neurotoxin (tetanospasmin) enters the nervous system and gains access to neural-neural junctions by initially entering the cytoplasm of distal processes of neurons through the formation of endocytotic vesicles in viable nerve endings located in tissue surrounding the site of the wound. The endocytotic vesicles are transported into the CNS by retrograde axonal transport, and tetanus neurotoxin is released into the interstitial fluid of the neural-neural junctions by exocytosis. Free tetanus neurotoxin then binds to the cell membrane of inhibitory interneurons of the spinal cord, is internalized via endocytosis, and acts to disrupt the release of inhibitory neurotransmitters via the same mechanism used by botulinum toxin: disruption of the synaptic fusion complex. Presynaptic neurons (upper motor neurons) excite postsynaptic neurons (lower motor neurons) on a nearly continuous basis. Inhibitory interneurons acting on lower motor neurons serve to counterbalance and smooth the excitatory effects of acetylcholine released from presynaptic neurons (upper motor neurons) to excite the same lower motor neurons. Thus skeletal muscle groups (opposing flexor and extensor muscles) are given time to relax; as a result, skeletal muscle contractions initiated by lower motor neurons are well regulated and coordinated. Failure to have adequate inhibitory interneuron regulation of lower motor neurons leads to the spastic paralysis observed in tetanus.

Although botulinum and tetanus toxins gain access to targets in the nervous system by different mechanisms, from this point forward in the pathogenesis, both botulinum and tetanus neurotoxins share a common mechanism of injury, the disruption of neurotransmitter vesicle exocytosis by disrupting the synaptic fusion complex. The mechanisms are demonstrated in Figures 4-28 and 4-29 for botulinum toxin and tetanus toxin, respectively. Thus diseases (clinical signs) that occur are the direct result of disruption of the function of myoneural (flaccid paralysis) and neural-neural (spastic paralysis) junctions. Botulinum and tetanus toxins have heavy and light chains and behave as typical A-B toxins composed of two units: a binding B-domain (heavy chain) that mediates transport via endocytosis and exocytosis and an enzymatically active A-domain (light chain) that serves to cleave proteins within the target cell. The heavy chain binds to the neuronal membrane of myoneural junctions (botulinum toxin) and nerve endings (tetanus toxin), and the entire toxin molecule enters the neuron via receptor-mediated endocytosis. The A-domain is cleaved from the B-domain within the target cell endocytotic vesicle and then released into the cytoplasm where it is active. The A-domain (light chain), a zinc-containing endopeptidase, leaves the endocytotic vesicle and enters the cytoplasm of the neuron and acts to cleave proteins that form the synaptic fusion complex. This complex, formed by fusion of synaptic vesicle proteins with presynaptic plasma membrane proteins, serves to bring neurotransmitter vesicles into contact with the neuronal cell membrane at the myoneural (botulinum toxin) and neural-neural (tetanus toxin) junctions and facilitates membrane fusion and release of excitatory (acetylcholine) and inhibitory neurotransmitters (glycine and γ-aminobutyric acid [GABA]), respectively.

Different types of glycosylphosphatidylinositol-anchored protein(s) may be expressed on different types of neurons, which may explain why B-domain of tetanus toxin binds only to inhibitory interneurons and not other types of neurons. Disruption of the synaptic fusion complex prevents neurotransmitter vesicles from fusing with the membrane, which in turn prevents release of neurotransmitters into the synaptic cleft. Proteins that form the synaptic fusion complex (soluble *N*-ethylmaleimide-sensitive factor attachment protein receptor [SNARE] proteins) include neurotransmitter vesicle proteins (such as vesicle-associated membrane proteins [VAMPs]/synaptobrevin) and presynaptic plasma membrane proteins (syntaxin, synaptosomal-associated protein [SNAP-25]). Different types of *C. botulinum* produce different types of toxins (toxin type A to G), and these types target and cleave specific types of SNARE proteins, synaptobrevin (cleaved by toxin types B, D, F, and G), syntaxin (cleaved by toxin type C), and synaptosomal-associated protein (cleaved by toxin types A, C, and E). Botulinum toxin seemingly does not cross the blood-brain barrier; therefore neural-neural junction functions in the CNS remain intact. Notwithstanding the profound neurologic signs of spastic paralysis and flaccid paralysis that occur with tetanus (*C. tetani*) and botulism (*C. botulinum*), respectively, macroscopic or microscopic lesions are not observed in the nervous system.

Meningitis (*Escherichia coli* and Other Bacterial Species). The pathogenesis of meningitis shares many of the mechanisms discussed for porcine polyserositis (see section on Bacterial Diseases of Organ Systems; Respiratory System, Mediastinum, and Pleurae; Disorders of Pigs) and embolic vasculopathy/vasculitis (see section on Bacterial Diseases of Organ Systems, Cardiovascular System and Lymphatic Vessels, Disorders of Domestic Animals).

Disorders of Ruminants (Cattle, Sheep, and Goats)

Listeriosis (*Listeria monocytogenes*). The mechanism of injury in listeriosis is cell lysis caused by acute inflammation and its mediators and degradative enzymes. Gross lesions are often not observed, but when present consist of nodules and linear bands of gray-yellow

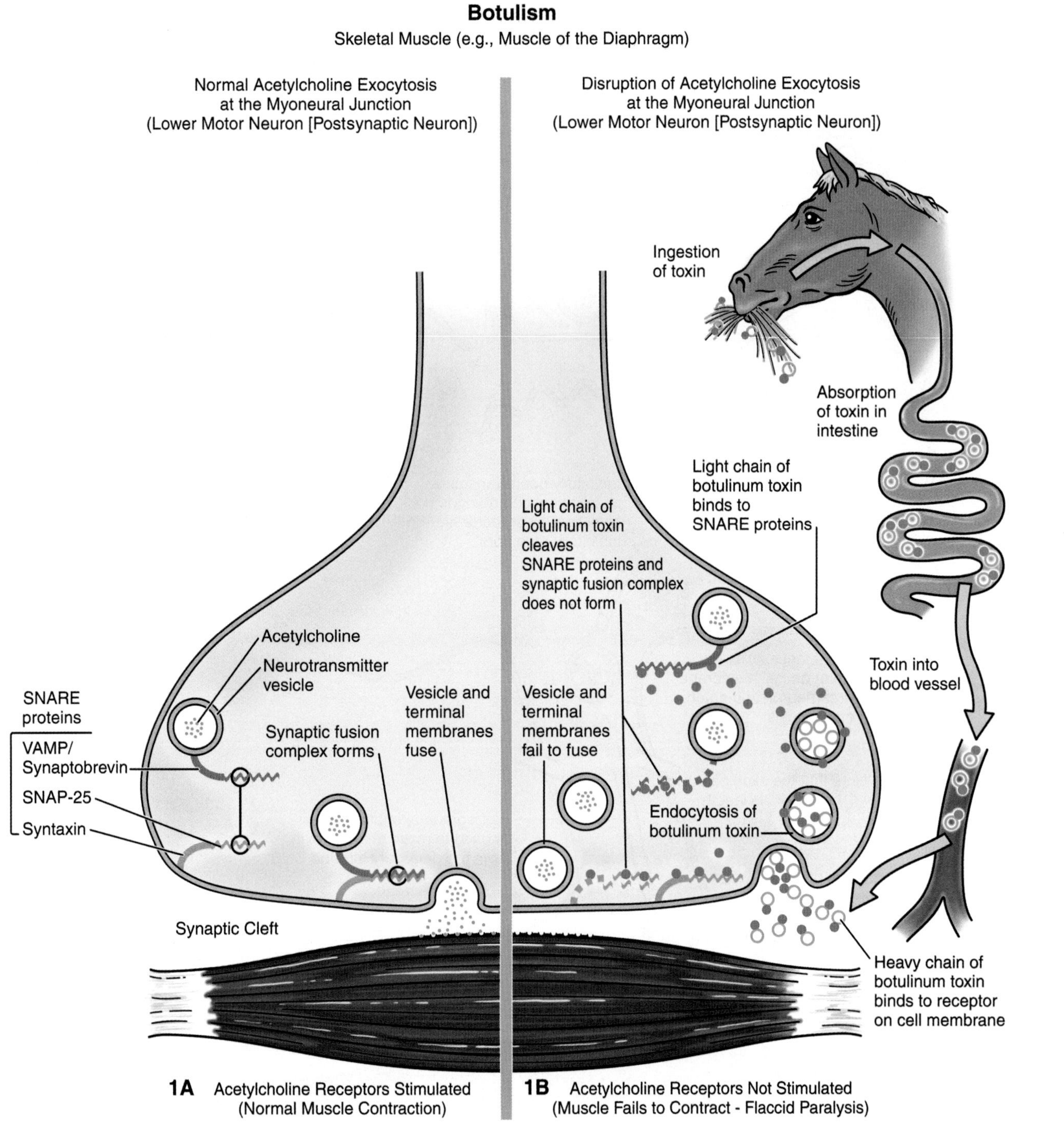

Figure 4-28 Mechanism of Myoneural Junction Dysfunction in Botulism. Note that botulinum toxin reaches the myoneural junction via the circulatory system. *SNAP,* Synaptosomal-associated protein; *SNARE,* soluble *N*-ethylmaleimide-sensitive factor attachment protein receptor; *VAMP,* vesicle-associated membrane protein. (Courtesy Dr. J.F. Zachary, College of Veterinary Medicine, University of Illinois.)

exudate (perivascular microabscesses formed by neutrophils) mixed with active hyperemia and/or hemorrhage commonly arranged in a perivascular pattern that are uniquely localized to the brainstem (see Fig. 14-88).

Cattle, sheep, and goats encounter *Listeria monocytogenes* in soil, animal feed, water, and feces; however, the greatest risk for contracting the disease occurs when ruminants are fed improperly stored silage in which the pH is not acidic enough to prevent overgrowth of the bacterium. Consumption of *L. monocytogenes*–contaminated silage is not sufficient to cause CNS disease, unless it occurs with a penetrating injury of the oral cavity caused by a stick or other sharp object (nail) that carries the bacterium in the silage into the submucosal connective tissue of the oral cavity or tongue. At this point the bacterium colonizes oral tissues, enters nerve endings in the oral cavity, and ascends into the CNS via retrograde axonal transport in cranial nerves. The oral cavity is primarily innervated by the trigeminal and other cranial nerves that terminate in the brainstem. Thus *L. monocytogenes* ultimately localizes to the brainstem (i.e., pons, medulla oblongata, and proximal cervical spinal cord). The mechanism of entry into nerve endings is unknown; however, it has

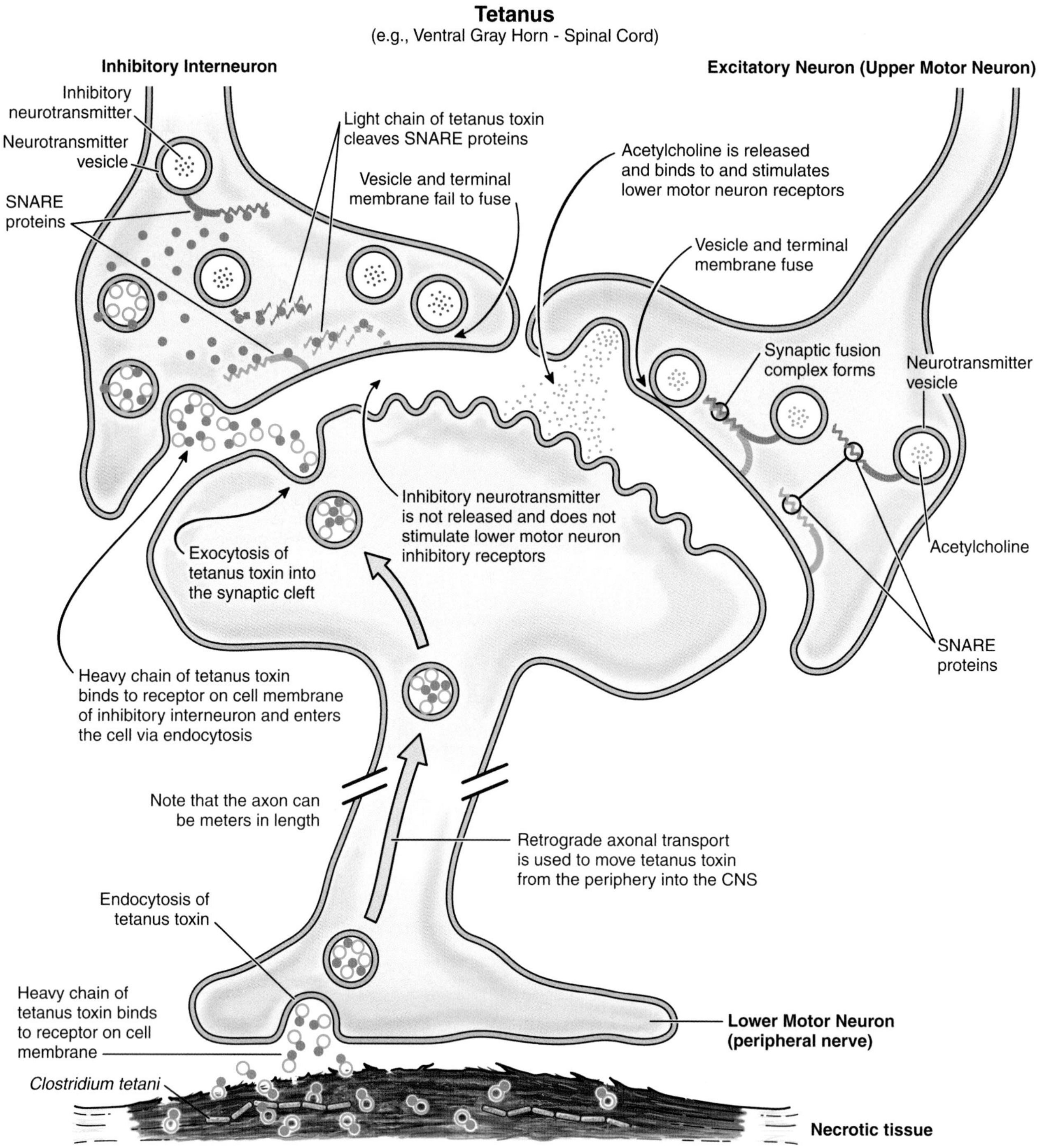
Tetanus
(e.g., Ventral Gray Horn - Spinal Cord)
Inhibitory Interneuron
Excitatory Neuron (Upper Motor Neuron)
Inhibitory neurotransmitter
Neurotransmitter vesicle
SNARE proteins
Light chain of tetanus toxin cleaves SNARE proteins
Vesicle and terminal membrane fail to fuse
Acetylcholine is released and binds to and stimulates lower motor neuron receptors
Vesicle and terminal membrane fuse
Synaptic fusion complex forms
Neurotransmitter vesicle
Acetylcholine
SNARE proteins
Inhibitory neurotransmitter is not released and does not stimulate lower motor neuron inhibitory receptors
Exocytosis of tetanus toxin into the synaptic cleft
Heavy chain of tetanus toxin binds to receptor on cell membrane of inhibitory interneuron and enters the cell via endocytosis
Note that the axon can be meters in length
Retrograde axonal transport is used to move tetanus toxin from the periphery into the CNS
Endocytosis of tetanus toxin
Heavy chain of tetanus toxin binds to receptor on cell membrane
Lower Motor Neuron (peripheral nerve)
Clostridium tetani
Necrotic tissue

Figure 4-29 **Mechanism of Neural-Neural Junction Dysfunction in Tetanus.** Note that tetanus toxin reaches the neural-neural junction via retrograde axonal transport. The selectivity of tetanus toxin for inhibitory interneurons is likely mediated by the expression of different glycosylphosphatidylinositol-anchored protein(s) on different types of neurons. The B-domain of tetanus toxin appears to bind only to the type of glycosylphosphatidylinositol-anchored protein expressed on inhibitory interneurons. *CNS*, Central nervous system; *SNARE*, soluble *N*-ethylmaleimide-sensitive factor attachment protein receptor; (Courtesy Dr. J.F. Zachary, College of Veterinary Medicine, University of Illinois.)

been shown experimentally in cell culture systems that *L. monocytogenes* gains entry into typically nonphagocytic cells through endocytosis and endocytic vesicles. Bacterial internalization, the entry process, is mediated by internalins (type A and B) that use target cell receptor E-cadherin, a transmembrane glycoprotein. Because *L. monocytogenes* resides in endosomes intracellularly within cell bodies of neurons when it arrives in the brainstem, it initially does not disrupt the blood-brain barrier and thus does not activate defense mechanisms provided by the innate (inflammation) and adaptive immune responses. The cytoplasm of infected neuron cell bodies appears to be permissive and allows free proliferation of the bacterium. This permissive environment also appears to be promoted by a bacterial virulence factor called *listeriolysin* O that inhibits immune responses and allows infected cells to hide from defense mechanisms.

Once free in the cytoplasm, the bacterium replicates to sufficient numbers and then begins the process of infecting other cells. In the cytoplasm the bacterium has a doubling time of approximately 1

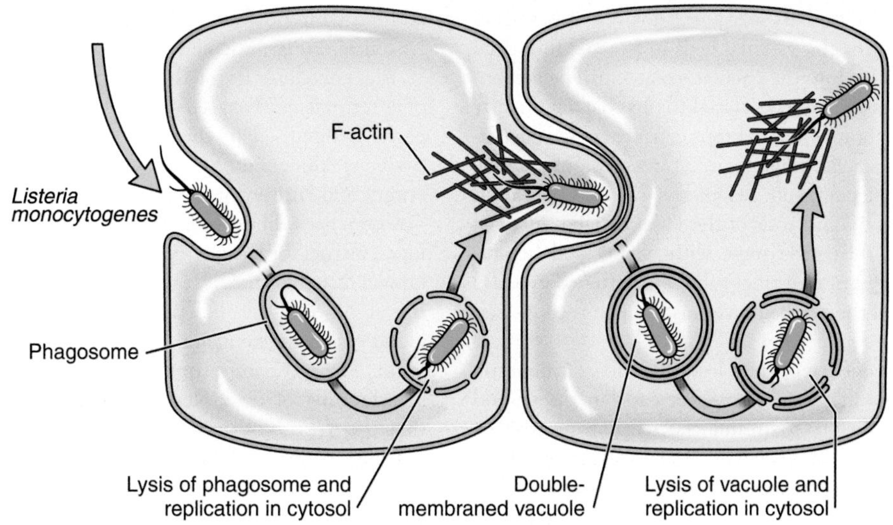

Figure 4-30 Mechanism of Infection in Listeriosis. *Listeria monocytogenes* propels itself via actin polymerization (*Listeria* actin-based motility) within a membrane pseudopod into cell membranes of adjacent neural cells forming invaginations of the membrane that ultimately result in double-membrane endocytotic phagocytic vesicles.

hour. When the number of bacterium in the cytoplasm reaches a level sufficient to facilitate infection of adjacent cells, bacteria move themselves, facilitated by a virulence factor in the cytoplasm, to the inner side of the cell membrane via polymerization and depolymerization of target cell actin filaments. Once near the cell membrane, aggregates of bacteria use a bacterial surface protein called *surface protein actA* to propel themselves via actin polymerization (listerial actin-based motility) and a pseudopod into cell membranes of adjacent cells, forming invaginations of the membrane that ultimately result in double-membrane endocytotic phagocytic vesicles (Fig. 4-30). This process is random, so it does not appear to target specific cells in the nervous system, only neighboring cells. These double-membrane endocytotic phagocytic vesicles are lysed by listeriolysin O, phospholipase C, and lecithinase, and the bacteria are released into the cytoplasm of newly infected cells. Experimentally, *L. monocytogenes* has been shown to infect neutrophils, macrophages, fibroblasts, endothelial cells, and various types of nerve cells, including neurons and microglial cells. It appears that infection of and injury to endothelial cells of capillaries initiates the inflammatory process. Once initiated, the blood-brain barrier is disrupted, and activation of the entire inflammatory cascade ensues. Neutrophils are the primary effector cells used by animal defense mechanisms to kill the bacterium. Experimentally, *L. monocytogenes*–infected endothelial cells express exuberant endothelial adhesion molecules (P- and E-selectin, intercellular adhesion molecule 1 [ICAM-1], and vascular cell-adhesion molecule 1 [VCAM-1]) resulting in activation of the neutrophil adhesion cascade and neutrophil binding, both components of the acute inflammatory response. The bacterium can also spread from macrophages to endothelial cells.

Thrombotic Meningoencephalitis (*Histophilus somni*). The pathogenesis of thrombotic meningoencephalitis (TME) begins as pulmonary histophilosis (see section on Bacterial Diseases of Organ Systems; Respiratory System, Mediastinum, and Pleurae; Disorders of Ruminants [Cattle, Sheep, and Goats]). The mechanism of injury in the nervous system is infarction (cell lysis) secondary to occlusive ischemia caused by bacterial-induced arteritis (vasculitis) and subsequent thrombosis caused by acute inflammation and its mediators and degradative enzymes. Gross lesions are red hemorrhagic infarcts of varied sizes distributed at random throughout nervous tissue, especially in the cerebral cortices (see Fig. 14-89).

Cattle encounter *Histophilus somni* (formerly *Haemophilus somnus*) via inhalation of fomites or water droplets contaminated with the bacterium. It likely exists in nasal or oral biofilms as a commensal bacterium of mucosae. Environmental stressors, such as overcrowding, combined with other factors, such as poor ventilation and humidity or abrupt changes in ambient air temperature, could alter the commensal relationship, allowing the bacteria to replicate in sufficient numbers to colonize mucosae and spread the bacterium to other animals. After colonization of the respiratory mucosae, the bacterium spreads to the lung (see section on Respiratory System, Mediastinum, and Pleurae; Disorders of Ruminants [Cattle, Sheep, and Goats]; Pulmonary Histophilosis) and then gains access to the vascular system in areas of pulmonary inflammation, embolizes to the CNS (septicemia), and colonizes and infects small arterioles likely via ligand-receptor interactions. The first encounter with endothelial cells of arterioles occurs at anatomic sites in the brain in which there are abrupt changes in the laminar flow of blood resulting in turbulence, such as occurs at the interface between gray and white matter in the cerebral cortex. Turbulence appears to make the luminal surface of endothelial cell membrane more adherent to the bacterium and platelets. Experimentally, *H. somni* and its membrane LOS (a truncated form of LPS) have been shown to activate bovine platelets and increase the expression of adhesion molecules, such as ICAM-1 and E-selectin and tissue factor (factor III) on endothelial cells (surface is procoagulant). Tissue factor is a protein necessary for activation of blood coagulation cascades. Thus, because strains of *H. somni* have virulence factors that enhance the adherence of the bacterium to endothelial cells, such areas are prone to endothelial injury, exposure of collagen, platelet aggregation and activation, activation of clotting cascades, arterial thrombosis and obstruction, and infarction (the lesion of thrombotic meningoencephalitis).

Focal Symmetric Encephalomalacia (*Clostridium perfringens*). The pathogenesis of focal symmetric encephalomalacia begins as an enterotoxemia caused by *C. perfringens* in the small intestine of the alimentary system (see section on Bacterial Diseases of Organ Systems; Alimentary System and the Peritoneum, Omentum, Mesentery, and Peritoneal Cavity; Disorders of Domestic Animals; Enterotoxemia (*Clostridium perfringens*). The mechanism of injury is acute coagulative necrosis of cells and tissues caused by bacterial toxins, especially ε-toxin. Because ε-toxin is a permease that alters cell permeability, the vascular beds in affected intestinal tissues readily absorb toxins into the circulatory system. The mechanism of injury is cell lysis caused by bacterial toxins that act directly on endothelial cell membranes and neurons causing acute coagulative necrosis of affected cells (angiotoxin). Gross lesions include bilaterally symmetric malacia (acute coagulative necrosis of neuron cell bodies) and liquefactive necrosis of the basal ganglia, internal capsule, thalamus, and substantia nigra with edema and hemorrhage. Cerebral edema causes indistinct sulci and flattened gyri and in severe cases, coning of the cerebellar vermis through the foramen magnum.

It appears that the sequence of steps leading to focal symmetric encephalomalacia occurs in the first phase or early in the second phase of enterotoxemia before toxin-induced massive necrosis of the intestine occurs (see section on Bacterial Diseases of Organ Systems; Alimentary System and the Peritoneum, Omentum, Mesentery, and Peritoneal Cavity; Disorders of Domestic Animals; Enterotoxemia [*Clostridium perfringens*]). Because microvascular beds of the alimentary system injured by enterotoxins are more permeable, they absorb large quantities of toxins that are carried to the brain via the blood vascular system. In the CNS they act to increase the permeability of capillary beds leading to release into the neuropil of blood plasma containing toxins, resulting in severe generalized vasogenic cerebral edema. Circulating ε-toxin likely accumulates preferentially in the brain via ligand-receptor interactions. Receptors expressed on different populations of endothelial cells in the body and within the brain may determine in part the specificity for certain neurons and nuclear groups within the nervous system. The cell membrane of cerebral endothelial cells is the probable site of toxin binding, and it appears that toxin-induced injury of endothelial cells leads to the expression of more receptors for circulating ε-toxin. Injury to the endothelium disrupts the integrity of the blood-brain barrier, leading to increased vascular permeability, vasogenic edema, and the diffusion of toxin into the neuropil, where it encounters neuron cell bodies. Acute coagulative necrosis of neuron cell bodies has been attributed to toxin-induced microthrombosis of capillaries, resulting in neuronal ischemia, and by direct cytotoxic action on neurons and other neural cells. The selective nature of neuronal lysis caused by ε-toxin may be explained by ligand-receptor interactions, selective metabolic vulnerability of specific populations of neurons, and/or the concentration of ε-toxin.

***Mannheimia* Meningoencephalitis (*Mannheimia haemolytica* A1).** The pathogenesis of *Mannheimia* meningoencephalitis shares many of the mechanisms discussed in the following sections: (1) Bacterial Diseases of Organ Systems; Respiratory System, Mediastinum, and Pleurae; Disorders of Ruminants (Cattle, Sheep, and Goats); Bovine Pneumonic Pasteurellosis/Mannheimiosis (*Mannheimia [Pasteurella] haemolytica*); (2) Bacterial Diseases of Organ Systems; Respiratory System, Mediastinum, and Pleurae; Disorders of Pigs; Porcine Polyserositis (*Haemophilus suis/parasuis*, *Actinobacillus suis*, *Streptococcus suis*, or *Escherichia coli*); and (3) Bacterial Diseases of Organ Systems, Cardiovascular System and Lymphatic Vessels, Disorders of Domestic Animals, Embolic Vasculopathy/Vasculitis (*Actinobacillus equuli*, *Escherichia coli*, *Staphylococcus* spp., *Streptococcus* spp., *Fusobacterium necrophorum*).

Disorders of Pigs

Edema Disease (*Escherichia coli*). See section on Bacterial Diseases of Organ Systems, Cardiovascular System and Lymphatic Vessels, Disorders of Pigs, Edema Disease (*Escherichia coli*); also see section on Bacterial Diseases of Organ Systems; Alimentary System and the Peritoneum, Omentum, Mesentery, and Peritoneal Cavity; Disorders of Pigs; Edema Disease (*Escherichia coli*).

Pigs encounter *E. coli* through ingestion followed by colonization of intestinal mucosae (enterotoxemia phase). The enterotoxemia phase is discussed in the section on Bacterial Diseases of Organ Systems; Alimentary System and the Peritoneum, Omentum, Mesentery, and Peritoneal Cavity; Disorders of Domestic Animals. This disease is caused by a specific strain of hemolytic *E. coli* having virulence factors for a bacterial enterotoxin called *Shiga toxin 2e* (also known as *verotoxin 2e*). It was initially called *edema disease principle*. It is absorbed in the alimentary system, circulates systemically in the blood vascular system, and is carried in the circulatory system to the brain. The mechanism of injury is lysis of endothelial and smooth muscle cells of arterioles (fibrinoid arteriopathy/arteriolopathy); thus the toxin biologically behaves as an angiotoxin. In the brain, vascular lesions are followed by secondary ischemia and necrosis of neural cells, particularly neurons in brainstem nuclei. Gross lesions include symmetric (bilateral) areas of yellow-gray malacia involving specific nuclei of the brainstem (see E-Fig. 10-27). It is unclear why lesions are symmetric; however, this observation suggests that ligand-receptor interactions or other targeting mechanisms are involved in cell specificity. Speculatively, receptors for Shiga toxin 2e could be expressed on specific populations of endothelial cells located within affected nuclei. Some endothelial and smooth muscle cells of arteritis and arterioles do express receptors for this toxin. This toxin causes vascular permeability changes and edema followed by endothelial injury and lysis leading to hemorrhage, intravascular coagulation, microthrombosis, and infarction (grossly malacia). Shiga toxin 2e acts to disrupt protein synthesis in affected cells leading to cell lysis.

Muscle

Disorders of Ruminants (Cattle, Sheep, and Goats)

Blackleg (*Clostridium chauvoei*). The mechanism of injury in blackleg is necrosis (acute gangrenous myositis) of muscle, connective tissues, and nervous tissues caused by α- and β-toxins released from vegetative forms of *C. chauvoei*. Gross lesions occur in large striated muscle groups and include dark red to black muscle that appears dry and contains gas bubbles (see Fig. 15-37). Affected muscle may have a rancid (spoiled butter) smell.

Cattle, sheep, and goats encounter spores through ingestion of plant matter and topsoil contaminated with spores often after disturbances (excavations) of the soil and pasture bed. Spores are carried by swallowing and peristalsis through the oral pharynx, esophagus, abomasum, and rumen to their final destination, the small intestine. It appears that spores can remain dormant in the small intestine or germinate into vegetative forms and become normal inhabitants of the alimentary system. How spores interact with mucosae and gain access to epithelial cells and mucosal macrophages is unknown. Other similar pathogens use M cells to enter Peyer's patches, so it is plausible that spores may gain access to M cells and use endocytosis/transcytosis to reach and infect macrophages in Peyer's patches. Although suggested but unproved, spores are likely the form of the bacterium that spread via M cells entry and then systemically by leukocyte trafficking to muscle and lie dormant in endosomes (or cytoplasm) of macrophages and dendritic cells. However, it is possible that vegetative forms of the bacterium spread to muscle as described earlier to ultimately "go dormant" and produce spores in macrophages and dendritic cells. If one or more of these mechanisms occurs, tropism for macrophages and dendritic cells of muscle is probably mediated by ligand-receptor interactions. Blackleg often follows some form of traumatic injury to muscle. It is thought that injury creates an anaerobic microenvironment with lowered oxidation-reduction (redox) potential suitable for germination of spores. It is likely that traumatic injury and anaerobic conditions cause lysis of infected macrophages and dendritic cells with release of spores into the microenvironment. Spores germinate into vegetative forms of the bacterium and produce large quantities of a variety of toxins such as *C. chauvoei* toxin A (pore-forming α-toxin), oxygen-stable hemolysin, DNase (β-toxin), hyaluronidase (δ-toxin), oxygen-labile hemolysin, and neuraminidase. These toxins diffuse out from the site of bacterial replication and coagulate muscle tissue and its vascular supply, resulting in acute gangrenous myositis.

Malignant Edema (*Clostridium septicum*). The pathogenesis of malignant edema is similar to that of blackleg discussed in the previous section regarding bacterial replication, the production of toxins, tissue injury, and gross lesions affecting striated muscle and blood vessels. However, the mechanism of spread to muscle is different. Cattle, sheep, and goats encounter spores through wounds caused by penetrating objects, such as a wire, which carries spores into the wound. Wounds caused by castration, tail docking, unsanitary vaccination, and other management practices can also be infected with spores. The injury must be sufficient to create an anaerobic microenvironment in the wound with lowering of the oxidation-reduction (redox) potential suitable for germination of spores. Once spores germinate, vegetative forms release toxins that injure and coagulate muscle and vascular tissues resulting in necrosis and edema much like in blackleg.

Big Head and Black Disease (*Clostridium novyi*). The pathogeneses of big head and black disease are very similar to malignant edema and blackleg, respectively. In big head of sheep, penetrating wounds of the skin of the head caused by horns during fighting establish the initial anaerobic microenvironment for spores to germinate. The resulting pathogenesis is similar to that which occurs in malignant edema. Black disease of cattle and sheep occurs because of fluke migration (*F. hepatica*) through the liver (see Figs. 8-60 and 8-61) that causes hepatocellular necrosis and establishes an anaerobic microenvironment suitable for germination of spores. Kupffer cells likely contain dormant spores. As in blackleg, spores are likely ingested, enter through mucosae (M cells) of the small intestine, become phagocytosed by cells of the monocyte-macrophage system, and spread via leukocyte trafficking to Kupffer cells of the liver.

Bone, Joints, Tendons, and Ligaments

Disorders of Ruminants (Cattle, Sheep, and Goats)

Lumpy Jaw (*Actinomyces bovis*). The mechanism of injury in lumpy jaw is cell lysis attributable to pyogranulomatous inflammation and its mediators. Gross lesions include misshapen bones of the mandible and/or maxilla resulting from abscesses, fibrosis, and fistulous tracts (i.e., pyogranulomatous osteomyelitis). Cut surface of affected bone has numerous randomly distributed discrete and coalescing yellow-white granulomas surrounded by remodeled bone intermixed with bands of fibrous connective tissue (see Fig. 16-55). *Actinomyces bovis* is a commensal bacterium of mucosae of the oral cavity of cattle and sheep, likely existing in a biofilm. The bacterium can infect bone by several routes: (1) genetic or developmental defects of the tooth root and/or socket that provide access to bone, (2) injury to a tooth and its socket opening a pathway into the bone, and (3) penetrating wounds that give the bacterium access to the bone and its periosteum. During chewing, the bacterium is carried by direct extension through the mucosa into submucosal connective tissues via penetrating wounds such as those caused by sharp foreign bodies like sticks or wires. The object may penetrate the periosteum and the bone, giving the bacterium direct access to these tissues. The bacterium colonizes submucosal connective tissue, and LPS of the cell wall, in part, likely plays a key role in the pathogenesis of the granulomatous inflammatory response. Little is known about virulence factors, ligand-receptor interactions, target cells, toxins, capsule antiphagocytic molecules, or other factors that may contribute to the pathogenicity of this bacterium. *A. bovis* can spread via lymphatic vessels to regional lymph nodes and cause a similar inflammatory response in these tissues.

Integumentary System

Disorders of Pigs

Greasy Pig Disease (*Staphylococcus hyicus*). The mechanism of injury in greasy pig disease is cell lysis and exfoliation of cells of the skin secondary to inflammation and its mediators and degradative enzymes. Gross lesions include areas of patchy red skin (active hyperemia of acute inflammation) followed by thickening of the reddened skin and the formation of reddish brown macules, vesicles, and pustules first around the eyes, nose, lips, and ears and then the flanks and abdomen (see Fig. 17-69). Affected skin, mostly through inflammation, exudes large quantities of a greasy exudate consisting of serum and sebum mixed with inflammatory cells, degradative enzymes, and cell debris. This exudate is the basis for naming the disease exudative epidermitis.

Pigs encounter *Staphylococcus hyicus* through fomites and body fluids contaminated with the bacterium. This bacterium is likely a commensal organism (biofilm) that resides in the skin and hair follicles of healthy pigs. Environmental stressors, such as skin trauma caused by overcrowding combined with other factors such as poor ventilation and humidity or abrupt changes in ambient air temperature, could alter the commensal relationship, allowing bacteria to replicate in sufficient numbers to colonize the skin, spread the bacterium to other animals, and cause disease. Infected droplets are deposited on the surface of the skin, but the bacterium under most conditions is not able to infect and colonize intact skin. It appears that skin trauma is usually a prerequisite for colonization because abrasions on the feet and legs or lacerations on the body often precede the onset of the disease.

The role of virulence factors, ligand-receptor interactions, and cells of the monocyte-macrophage system are poorly understood in the pathogenesis of the disease. Exfoliation-inducing as well as epidermitis-inducing exotoxins cause separation of epithelial cells of the stratum corneum and spinosum and aid in the invasion of the bacterium into the skin. It serves to expose vascularized ECM tissues in traumatized skin. Fibronectin-binding proteins expressed on the surface of the bacteria appear to act as adhesins, allowing the bacteria to bind to the fibronectin present in collagen, fibrin, and heparin sulfate proteoglycans of traumatized skin. Fibronectin is a glycoprotein of vascularized ECM tissues and is produced by cells such as fibroblasts. Once the skin is colonized, the infection appears to spread to the hair follicles, leading to suppurative inflammation and sebaceous gland hyperplasia and hypersecretion (i.e., greasy pig). It also appears that acute inflammation and its effector cells, such as neutrophils, play a central role in the onset and progression of the skin lesions. Capsule polysaccharides and protein A in the bacterial wall appear to block phagocytosis of the bacterium by neutrophils and increase the ability of bacteria to survive and replicate in vascularized ECM tissues of the skin.

Diamond Skin Disease (*Erysipelothrix rhusiopathiae*). The mechanism of injury in diamond skin disease is cell lysis and infarction of skin secondary to cutaneous vasculitis. Gross lesions include active hyperemia and red-purple skin affecting the ears, ventral abdomen, and legs followed by thrombosis, ischemia, and infarction resulting in rhomboidal (diamond) red-purple areas of skin (cutaneous infarcts) (see Figs. 17-70 and 10-80).

Pigs encounter *Erysipelothrix rhusiopathiae* through ingestion of fomites and body fluids contaminated with the bacterium. This bacterium is likely a commensal organism that resides in a biofilm of mucosae of the pharynx and tonsillar epithelia of healthy pigs. Environmental stressors, such as overcrowding combined with other factors such as poor ventilation and humidity or abrupt changes in ambient air temperature, can alter the commensal relationship, allowing the bacteria to replicate in sufficient numbers to colonize mucosae and spread the bacterium to other animals. Infected droplets are deposited on pharyngeal mucosae, where bacteria encounter the mucus layer and mucosal epithelial cells. It is unclear how this nonmotile bacterium is able to penetrate the mucus layer and gain direct access to the luminal membrane of epithelial cells. Additionally, it is unclear if and how the bacterium colonizes the mucus layer and mucosae. It appears that neuraminidase may be a virulence factor for *E. rhusiopathiae* potentially involved in initial interactions with and invasion of the mucus layer of pharyngeal mucosae. Neuraminidase acts to remove sialic acid from glycoproteins, glycolipids, and oligosaccharides expressed on target cells, potentially exposing new receptors for the bacterium. Also, it is probably important in the disease when the bacterium attaches to, colonizes, and invades cutaneous endothelial cells leading to vasculitis, thrombosis, infarction, and disseminated intravascular coagulation.

Other virulence factors involved in mucosal colonization and systemic spread of the bacterium include capsular polysaccharides (antiphagocytic properties), surface proteins (adhesins, antiphagocytic properties, biofilm formation), invasins such as hyaluronidase (invade ECM tissues), and enzymes such as superoxide dismutase and catalase (block the effects of the respiratory burst of phagocytosis and oxygen free radicals). Transcytosis could move bacteria through mucosal cells to the basal surface of mucosal epithelial cells to encounter local macrophages and lymphoid cells in the tonsils. Alternatively, mucosal macrophages could phagocytose bacteria in the mucus layer, migrate through the mucosal barrier, and spread them via leukocyte trafficking to the same cells.

Macrophages within the tonsil are likely used by the bacterium for replication and growth and then to spread bacteria via leukocyte trafficking in lymphatic vessels to regional lymph nodes to infect additional macrophages. Ligand-receptor interactions are likely involved, and bacterial surface proteins appear to serve as adhesins to macrophage and endothelial cell membrane receptors. Specific bacterial adhesins and target cell receptors on macrophages and endothelial cells have not been identified. Once bound to cell membrane, the bacterium is phagocytosed and retained in a phagosome within the cell cytoplasm. *E. rhusiopathiae* grows and replicates intracellularly in phagosomes and phagolysosomes. Capsular polysaccharides are able to inhibit phagocytosis of the bacterium by neutrophils and to a limited extent by macrophages. However, macrophages are used by the bacterium to isolate it from host innate and adaptive immune responses. Although it appears that phagosome-lysosome fusion occurs, capsular polysaccharides appear to block the oxidative burst and prevent killing of the bacterium by molecules present in the lysosome (see Figs. 4-13 and 4-14). Although undetermined, bacteria-infected macrophages in regional lymph nodes then probably spread the bacterium systemically via leukocyte trafficking using lymphatic vessels and the thoracic duct or postcapillary venules and the venous system to the systemic circulatory system and then to capillary beds within the skin. Cutaneous infarcts (also vascular-related lesions in other organs such as the kidney) suggest these bacteria may have tropisms for vascular endothelial cells. It is unclear why this occurs, but it is likely linked to the expression of bacterial virulence factors and ligand-receptor interactions with host endothelial cells. In addition to cell lysis attributable to direct infection of endothelial cells by the bacterium, bacterial neuraminidase may also activate the alternative complement pathway and induce thrombocytopenia, producing complement-derived chemotactic factors that could contribute to injury of capillary beds in local vascularized connective tissues. These mechanisms may contribute, in part, to the development of vegetative valvular endocarditis and arthritis that occurs in the chronic septicemic form of this disease.

Disorders of Dogs

Canine Pyoderma (*Staphylococcus intermedius*). The pathogenesis of canine pyoderma appears to be similar to that of greasy pig disease (see section on Bacterial Diseases of Organ Systems, Integumentary System, Disorders of Pigs, Greasy Pig Disease [*Staphylococcus hyicus*]). Skin trauma arising from pruritus and scratching or from existing skin disease leads to the exposure of vascularized ECM tissues and its colonization by bacteria. Although incompletely characterized, it is likely that a variety of virulence factors are involved in canine pyoderma, including surface proteins (colonization of host tissues); invasins such as leukocidin, kinases, hyaluronidase (promote bacterial spread in tissues); surface factors such as capsule polysaccharides and protein A (inhibit phagocytosis); and exotoxins and exfoliative toxins such as hemolysins, leukotoxin, and leukocidin (cause cell lysis).

Female Reproductive System and Mammary Gland

Disorders of Domestic Animals

Brucellosis (*Brucella* spp.). The pathogenesis of brucellosis begins as an infection of regional and systemic lymph nodes facilitated by entry through mucosae of the respiratory and alimentary systems (see section on Bacterial Diseases of Organ Systems; Bone Marrow, Blood Cells, and Lymphatic System; Disorders of Domestic Animals; Brucellosis [*Brucella* spp.] for more detail). The mechanism of injury is cell lysis caused by pyogranulomatous inflammation and its mediators and degradative enzymes. Gross lesions include aborted fetuses; necrosis, inflammation, and fibrinoid exudation of uterine caruncles and fetal cotyledons (see Fig. 4-27); and a yellow-white uterine exudate. Bacteria spread in macrophages via leukocyte trafficking from regional lymph nodes to the caruncular side of placentomas when they likely leave the vascular system to migrate into and through these tissues. Although it is unclear what additional cells in the placentoma are infected during transplacental spread to the fetus, trophoblasts are infected with bacteria. Other cell types may be involved. Bacteria then could spread in fetal macrophage-like cells within the fetal circulatory system to the fetus via the umbilical cord or within the allantoic and amniotic membranes and infect the fetus via contact with fetal mucosae of the respiratory or alimentary systems, but if this occurs or what cells facilitate this spread is unclear.

Disorders of Ruminants (Cattle, Sheep, and Goats)

Bovine Mastitis (*Staphylococcus aureus, Streptococcus agalactiae, Streptococcus dysgalactiae,* and *Escherichia coli*). The mechanism of injury in bovine mastitis is lysis of all cell populations in the mammary gland from (1) bacterial toxins, (2) inflammation and its mediators and degradative enzymes, and (3) induced reparative responses such as fibrosis. Gross lesions in acute mastitis include firm, swollen, edematous, and occasionally hemorrhagic glands and ectatic ducts and sinuses containing yellow-white exudate (see Figs. 18-49 to 18-51, 18-54, and 18-55). In chronic mastitis, tissues are firm and consist of large zones of fibrous connective tissue that have replaced and displaced remaining normal glands (see Fig. 18-52). Inflammatory exudate is difficult to observe unless abscesses have formed. Ducts and sinuses may be ectatic.

Animals encounter these bacteria through physical contact in fomites or fluid droplets from mammary gland, uterine, or fecal origin on milking equipment and human hands. They commonly become commensal microbes that reside in biofilms of the mucous membranes of the teat canal and mammary duct and sinuses. Trauma to mucosae in the gland induced by pressure changes acting on the duct system caused by milking likely makes mucosae more suitable for colonization and alters the commensal relationship, allowing the bacteria to replicate in sufficient numbers to spread the bacterium within the gland and to other animals mechanically during milking. Mastitis is an ascending infection, and milk in canals and sinuses is a suitable culture media for initial growth of bacteria. This environment is not suitable in the long term for survival of bacteria; thus they attempt to colonize mucosae to sustain the infection. Ligand-receptor interactions are likely involved in the adherence of these bacteria to receptors on mucosal epithelial cells; however, specific bacterial adhesins and target cell receptors have not been clearly identified. Once mucosae are colonized, bacteria employ mechanisms to sustain the infection. For example, *S. aureus* produces toxins, such as superantigens, leukocidins, hemolysins, coagulase, and likely α-, β-, and δ-toxins (virulence factors) that result in cell membrane injury and cell lysis and the activation of mucosal macrophages and inflammation. The severity of this lesion and its progression to gangrenous mastitis in the peracute and acute forms are dependent on the type and quantity of toxins secreted by the bacterium as determined by its virulence factors. Additionally, activated mucosal macrophages secrete proinflammatory cytokines resulting in the recruitment of neutrophils from the systemic circulation, through the mucosa, and ultimately into the milk, thus increasing the somatic cell count. With the focus of inflammation on the mucosa, epithelial cells and subjacent basement membrane are injured, killed, and sloughed, providing bacteria with access to vascularized ECM tissues of the gland. Using bacterial surface proteins, they are able to adhere to and colonize ECM tissues, likely using receptors expressed on molecules such as fibronectin, vitronectin, laminin, and collagen in the matrix. This process allows bacteria to evade many of the harmful actions of the innate and adaptive immune responses. Additionally, capsular polysaccharides block phagocytosis by neutrophils and macrophages. As a result, acute inflammation progresses with time to chronic inflammation with fibrosis (see Chapter 3), which is a common manifestation of mastitis caused by *S. aureus*.

Chronic mastitis is often linked to formation of mucosal biofilms. In mastitis caused by *Streptococcus agalactiae* and *Streptococcus dysgalactiae*, the bacteria use most of the mechanisms employed by *S. aureus* with one important exception. They lack virulence factors that injure the mucosa and allow the bacterium to invade vascularized ECM tissues and colonize this area. Thus the bacterium is limited to colonizing the mucosa and causing inflammation at the mucosal barrier. The outcome of this process is loss of mucosal epithelial cells lining glands, collapse of the glands, and replacement of the glands with fibrous connective tissue. In mastitis caused by *E. coli* and other coliforms, the bacterium uses most of the mechanisms discussed previously. However, in the initial phases of colonizing the mucosa, endotoxins (LPS) and other toxic molecules released from Gram-negative bacteria cause tissue injury and cell lysis, affecting the mucosa, lamina propria, submucosa, and capillary beds. The concurrent acute inflammatory response with neutrophils and their degradative enzymes exacerbate the severity of the injury. This outcome leads to tissue necrosis, edema, and hemorrhage. Endotoxin is also absorbed by the capillaries and can cause endotoxic shock of the circulatory system and death of affected animals (see Chapters 2 and 3).

Male Reproductive System

Disorders of Domestic Animals

Brucellosis (*Brucella* spp.). The pathogenesis of brucellosis begins as an infection of regional and systemic lymph nodes facilitated by entry through mucosae of the respiratory and alimentary systems (see Bacterial Diseases of Organ Systems; Bone Marrow, Blood Cells, and Lymphatic System; Disorders of Domestic Animals; Brucellosis [*Brucella* spp.] for more detail). The mechanism of injury is cell lysis caused by pyogranulomatous inflammation and its mediators and degradative enzymes. *Brucella* spp. spread in macrophages via leukocyte trafficking from regional lymph nodes to the testes, epididymides, and other male reproductive tissues. Gross lesions include enlarged and deformed testes and epididymides attributable to a yellow-white pyogranulomatous exudate resulting from the inflammatory response against the bacteria in the tissues (see Fig. 4-27).

Viral Diseases

Viruses are approximately a hundred times smaller than bacteria, and viruses, like bacteria, are genetically programmed to replicate endlessly, if all growth factors, metabolic needs, and microenvironments for replication are satisfactorily met. However, viruses are unable to produce energy and contain a limited number of enzymes; therefore they are completely dependent on target cells for such resources and thus are obligate intracellular parasites. They have evolved to specifically use target cells in animals that are susceptible to and suitable for completion of their viral replication cycles.

Target Cells

The term target cell assigns specificity to which cell(s) (see Fig. 4-6) of what organ system(s) are infected by viruses. This process is based on ligand-receptor interactions (see section on Target Cells and Substances at the beginning of this chapter), in which attachment and binding occur between envelope or capsid attachment proteins on the surface of viruses and receptors on target cell membranes (Fig. 4-31). Receptors are often expressed in unique patterns on target cells, and these patterns may determine the routes used by viruses to infect target cells. For example, parvoviruses and herpesviruses use specific receptors with specific distribution patterns to attach to and enter target cells. Parvovirus (canine parvovirus enteritis) infects intestinal crypt epithelial cells through receptors expressed on the basolateral surface of the cells, thus using a circuitous route via leukocyte trafficking to Peyer's patches and M cells to gain access to this surface. Although this route is not likely the most direct route to crypt epithelial cells, it may be advantageous for survival of the virus to avoid contact with gastric acids, bile, and other potentially toxic molecules in the intestinal lumen. Bovine herpesvirus 1 (infectious bovine rhinotracheitis [IBR]) infects epithelial cells of the respiratory system through receptors expressed on the apical and lateral surfaces of the cells. These receptors are distributed above junctional complexes formed with adjacent epithelial cells; therefore virus in the lumen of the respiratory tract can encounter appropriate receptors on mucosae.

In total, experimental studies suggest there are approximately 10^4 to 10^6 potential receptors for viruses expressed on a single target cell. This total is composed of many types or categories of receptors, so the total number of a specific kind of receptor is much less than this range. Receptors on target cells include those for complement, growth factors, neurotransmitters, integrins, adhesion molecules, complement regulatory proteins, phospholipids, and carbohydrates.

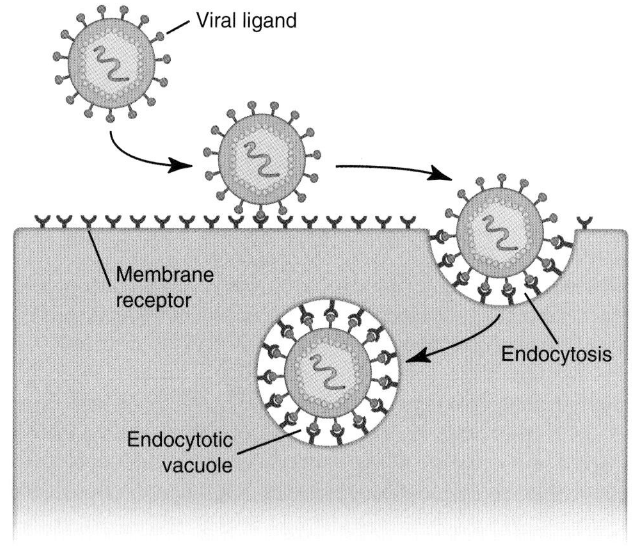

Figure 4-31 Ligand-Receptor Interactions. Ligand (viral envelope or capsid proteins)-receptor (target cell membrane proteins) interactions common to all cells are used by viruses to attach to and infect specific target cells. (Courtesy Dr. J.F. Zachary, College of Veterinary Medicine, University of Illinois.)

In general, specific viruses use one of these receptor types to infect a specific type of cell; however, some viruses use several receptors (coreceptors), which allows for invasion of a variety of cell types (i.e., pantropic viruses such as canine distemper virus).

In the context of diseases caused by viruses, target cells that allow replication of a virus are called *permissive cells*, whereas those that do not are called nonpermissive cells. Generally, virus-infected permissive cells are usually killed by the virus (cell lysis), whereas virus-infected nonpermissive cells are not killed. As an example, the pathogenesis of the lentiviral disease, maedi-visna, is determined, in part, by nonpermissive cells (immature progenitor monoblasts and promonocytes in bone marrow) and permissive cells (mature monocytes and macrophages in the blood vascular system and tissues). Infection of nonpermissive progenitor cells in bone marrow is used to provide a reservoir of immunologically protected virus-infected cells that become permissive when they mature into monocytes and macrophages in the vascular system and when they migrate into specific tissues and organs. These permissive macrophages are ultimately killed by virus replication, and the cell is lysed to release virus into areas with new target cells such as in the lung, brain, mammary gland, and synovia.

Viral Pathogenicity and Replication Cycle

Viral pathogenicity is a term used to express the relative severity of disease, clinical signs, and lesions caused by viruses. It is determined, in large part, by the expression of viral genes used to produce structural or functional proteins and other molecules needed to sustain or enhance replication of the virus. Similar to bacteria, viral genes and their proteins behave as virulence factors; however, the number of viral virulence factors is nowhere near the number, complexity, and diversity of those expressed by bacteria. In viruses the actions of virulence factors focus on (1) attachment to, replication in, and shedding from target cells and (2) the processes of modulating and/or evading host defense mechanisms. Thus the type, quantity, and arrangement of nucleic acid in viruses provide the bases for genomic diversity and the transfer of virulence factors among viruses (see later section on Mechanisms of Genomic Change).

During viral replication the pathogenicity of a disease and the survival of target cells are determined by (1) how the virus uses and/or alters the functions of cell organelles and the transcriptional and translational processes and (2) how it escapes from target cells such as by lysis. The phrase *virus replication cycle* is used herein to merge under a single key concept the chronologic sequence of steps that occurs when a virus encounters and enters cells, takes over the functions of cellular organelles and metabolic processes, produces new virus, and ultimately injures or lyses cells to cause disease. The outcome of encounters between viruses and target cells are often reflected in specific organ systems by clinical signs and alterations in biochemical analyses of blood samples.

The viral replication cycle has five key steps (Fig. 4-32):

- Attachment
  - Viruses have attachment proteins in their capsids or envelopes that bind to specific receptors on target cell membranes.
- Entry (Penetration)
  - Following binding, viruses enter cells via endocytosis/phagocytosis and release their contents into the cell.
- Spread (Uncoating)
  - Viral nucleic acid (RNA or DNA) and/or proteins are moved to specific locations within the cell.
- Replication
  - Viral nucleic acid (RNA or DNA) and/or proteins take over functions of normal cell processes to synthesize and aggregate additional copies of these components.
- Shedding (Release or Egress)
  - Viruses reassemble from resynthesized components and escape from cells by budding or cell lysis.

Specific groups of viruses (nonenveloped viruses) attach to target cells using a protein coat (viral coat, capsid, or capsomeres) (Fig. 4-33); others attach via a viral envelope (enveloped viruses) (see Fig. 4-33). Protein molecules, derived from viral genes and expressed in the protein capsid or envelope, are called *attachment proteins*. Attachment proteins are viral virulence factors that provided the basis for genomic diversity among viruses and play a central role in their replication and existence. However, the "infectious" advantages provided by attachment proteins for the virus are counterbalanced by specific disadvantages. Viral attachment proteins in the virus and present in infected target cells are recognized as foreign by the innate and adaptive immune systems via defense mechanisms provided by TLRs, NK cells, cytotoxic T lymphocytes, and acute inflammation, as examples. Once attachment occurs, viruses can enter target cells by one of two main mechanisms: (1) receptor-mediated endocytosis (phagocytosis) or (2) fusion. Once inside target cells, viruses initiate a variety of virus-specified processes to complete their replication cycles, such as replication of their genome, core proteins, and capsid and envelope proteins; assembly of new viruses; and release of new viruses from the cell.

When a DNA virus enters a target cell and its components are released into the cytoplasm, the DNA genome is transferred into the nucleus, where it uses target cell nuclear organelles to transcribe viral messenger RNA (mRNA) and later replicate new viral DNA (see Fig. 4-32). Viral mRNA leaves the nucleus and in the cytoplasm is translated into structural and nonstructural proteins of the virus by target cell organelles. After all viral proteins are translated in the target cell cytoplasm, new viral DNA is replicated (transcribed) and transferred into the cytoplasm, where it is assembled with structural and nonstructural proteins to form new virus.

When an RNA virus enters a cell and its components are released into the cytoplasm, the RNA genome, depending on the virus, can (1) replicate new viral RNA from the cytoplasmic viral RNA via

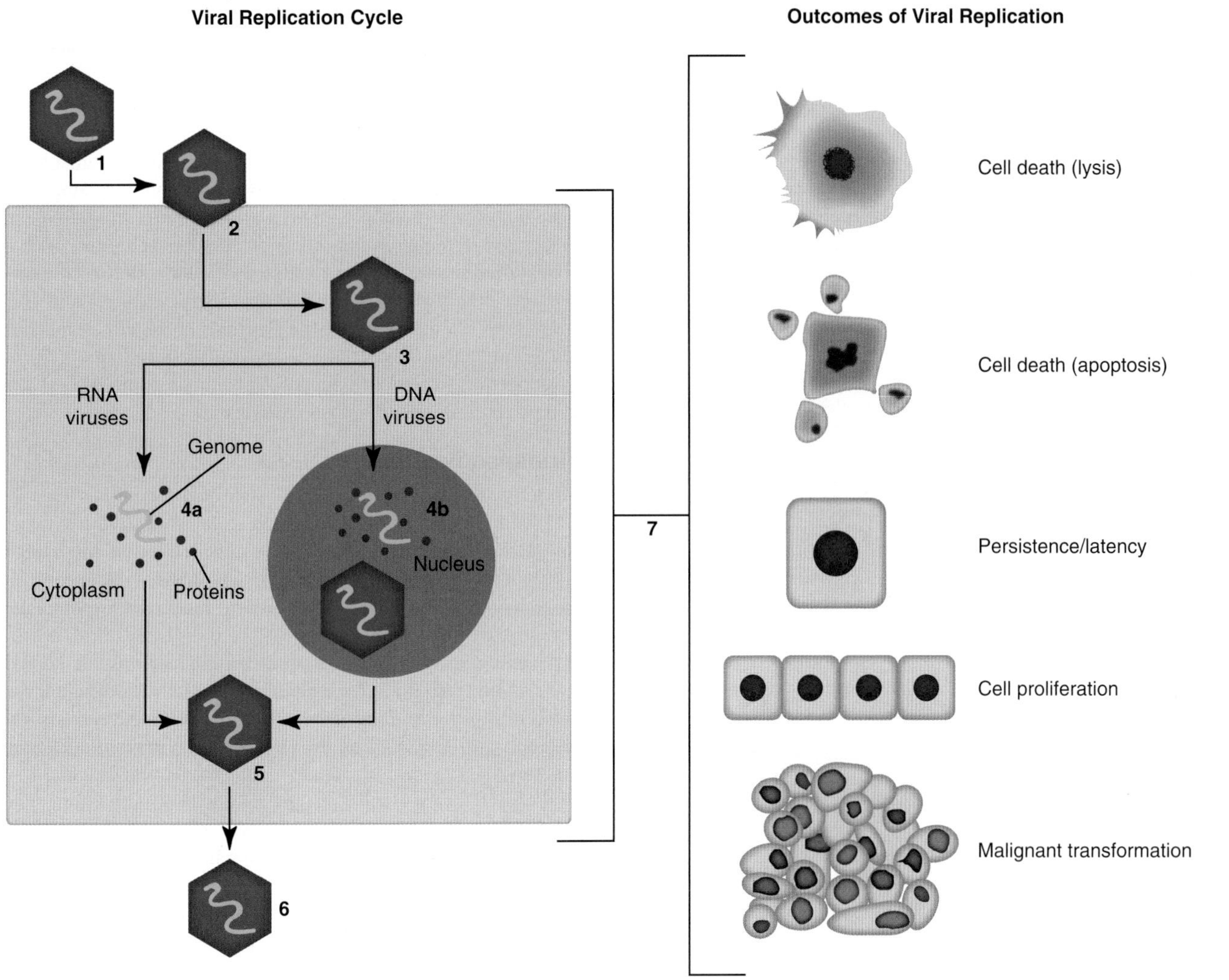

Figure 4-32 Viral Replication Cycles. Viruses do not replicate through division; in its place they use the organelles and biochemical processes of target cells to produce copies of their genome and proteins and assemble them into progeny. *1*, Interaction with and "recognition" of a target cell. *2*, Attach to the target cell membrane via ligand-receptor interactions (see Fig. 4-31). *3*, Enter the target cell via endocytosis/membrane fusion and spread genomic and protein components via "uncoating" to specific locations within the cell. *4a*, RNA viruses most commonly replicate in the cytoplasm. *4b*, DNA viruses most commonly replicate in the nucleus. *5*, RNA viruses reassemble in the cytoplasm; whereas DNA viruses are reassembled in the nucleus and transported through the cytocavitary system (see Fig. 1-3) for release at the cell membrane. *6*, Release of progeny from the target cell by budding or cell lysis. *7*, Outcomes of viral infection: cell death (lysis) (e.g., parvovirus—canine parvovirus enteritis); cell death (apoptosis) (e.g., morbillivirus—canine distemper); persistent infection (e.g., lentivirus—ovine progressive pneumonia); latent infection (e.g., herpesvirus—infectious bovine rhinotracheitis); cell proliferation (e.g., papillomavirus—sarcoids of horse skin); malignant transformation (e.g., retrovirus—feline leukemia). (Courtesy Dr. J.F. Zachary, College of Veterinary Medicine, University of Illinois.)

its own viral RNA-dependent RNA polymerase or (2) make viral DNA from viral RNA via RNA-dependent DNA polymerase (viral reverse transcriptase) and then use target cell nuclear and cytoplasmic organelles to transcribe and translate new proteins and viral RNA (see Fig. 4-32). Thus the genome of RNA viruses must express genes that code for enzymes such as RNA-dependent RNA polymerase and RNA-dependent DNA polymerase. Detailed coverage of these processes is outside the scope of this chapter and can be reviewed in virology textbooks; however, these replicative processes often lead to injury and cell lysis.

In general, nonenveloped viruses (viral protein coats or capsids) are released from target cells only when cell lysis occurs, whereas enveloped viruses are released from target cells by budding from cell membrane, and the cell usually does not lyse (a viable cell remains) except for infections with herpesviruses (see later). Enveloped viruses with envelope glycoproteins must acquire an envelope by budding through cellular membranes such as the plasma membrane, membranes of the Golgi complex or rough endoplasmic reticulum, or nuclear membrane. During transcription and translation of viral genes and proteins, new viral envelope glycoproteins are inserted into target cell membranes of the ER and Golgi apparatus as examples (i.e., cytocavitary system) and then moved to specific locations in cell membrane within the cell. These are the sites where virus buds from target cell membrane and acquires envelope glycoproteins. Most viruses that bud from the cell membrane do not cause cell lysis except for those that bud from the Golgi complex or rough endoplasmic reticulum (flavivirus, coronavirus, arterivirus, and bunyavirus) or the nuclear membrane (herpesvirus).

Virus capsid proteins and envelope glycoproteins are used immunologically as a means to clinically prevent (e.g., vaccination) or control (e.g., pharmaceutical products) diseases caused by viruses by developing strategies to block one of more of the steps in the viral attachment or replication cycle. Antibiotics have no effect on viruses; however, fortunately, viral infections (viral antigens) usually activate host innate and adaptive defense mechanisms and cause an immune response (cell-mediated), which can completely eliminate a virus or prevent an infection by a virus (vaccination). However, these defensive responses can also injure and lyse target cells, leading to disease. The list of structural and biochemical effects that viruses have on target cells is extensive. These effects are often called *cytopathic effects*, and as a general rule, many viral infections result in lysis of target cells. Depending on the virus and its replication cycle, injury to and lysis of target cells can occur at any point during the attachment, fusion, penetration, synthesis, assembly, or release phases. Generally viruses cause injury and lysis most commonly by two mechanisms: (1) as a result of taking over cell transcriptional and translational processes and (2) when they exit from infected cells. Additionally, causes of cell lysis include alterations in cell membrane structure and function, including direct damage to cell membranes (e.g., lytic phospholipids, endolysins, holins, and spanins), pore formation (viroporins), ion transport, and secondary messenger systems; alterations in metabolic processes, including activation cascades leading to altered cellular activities; alterations of target cell antigenic or immune properties, shape, and growth characteristics; inhibition of the synthesis of target cell macromolecules, including DNA, RNA, and protein; and direct (protein messenger molecules) and indirect (inflammatory mediators) activation of cell lysis and apoptosis cascades.

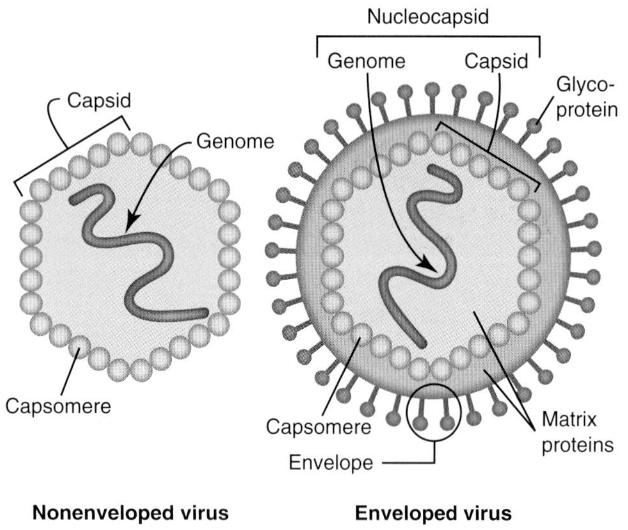

Figure 4-33 **Morphologic Characteristics of Viruses.** Nonenveloped viruses attach to target cells using capsomeres and capsids, whereas enveloped viruses attach using a viral envelope. (Courtesy Dr. J.F. Zachary, College of Veterinary Medicine, University of Illinois.)

Virulence Factors

Virulence factors also have been identified for viruses (see Table 4-1). The purpose of these factors is to improve a virus's ability to complete its replication cycle in the target cell, thus spreading and propagating the virus to naïve animals. Virulence factors control the processes involved in (1) replication, including attachment to, entering, replication in, and release of virus from target cells, and (2) evading, modulating, or suppressing the host's innate and adaptive immune responses. For example, feline immunodeficiency virus hides within the immune system and replicates and spreads within macrophages and T lymphocytes. Other viruses have evolved mechanisms to evade cytotoxic T lymphocyte and NK cell lysis of virus-infected target cells, disrupt complement activation, synthesize cytokine homologues that interfere with normal immunologic functions, and synthesize molecules that inhibit interferon responses or block the induction of apoptosis in virus-infected cells. Other viral virulence factors include viral proteins, as well as by-products of virus replication, such as caspases and caspase-like molecules, that accumulate in the cell and have toxin-like activities on target cells (Fig. 4-34; Box 4-4). As an example of a viral toxin,

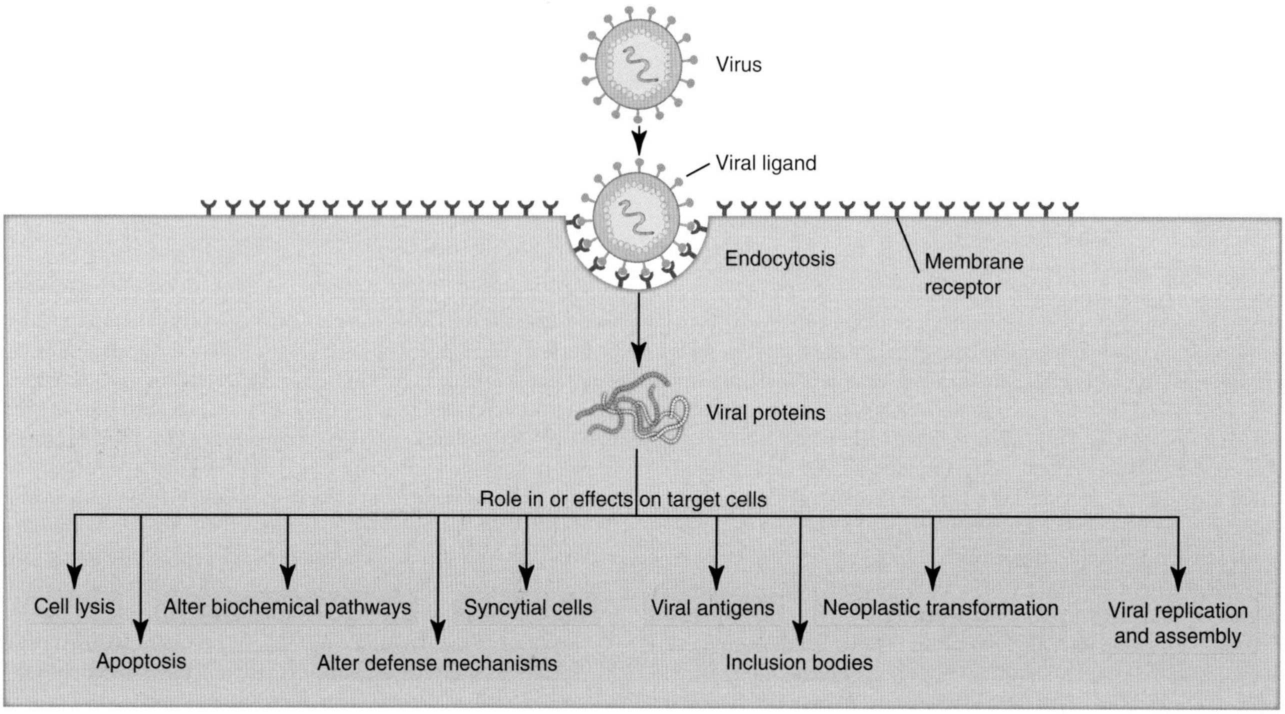

Figure 4-34 **Viral Proteins—Role in or Effects on Target Cells.** (Courtesy Dr. J.F. Zachary, College of Veterinary Medicine, University of Illinois.)

Box 4-4 Viral Proteins–Role in or Effects on Target Cells (see Fig. 4-34)

Role or effects	Proteins involved
Inclusion bodies	Aggregates of excessive production of viral proteins–cytoplasmic inclusions (RNA viruses) vs. intranuclear inclusions (DNA viruses))
Syncytial cells	Syncytia formation–viral fusion proteins (bovine respiratory syncytial virus)
Cell lysis	Viroporins, lytic phospholipids, endolysins, holins, and spanins
Apoptosis	Apoptotic proteins (inhibit or activate)–caspases
Viral replication and assembly	Replication cycle–target cell-adaptation proteins
	Structural proteins used in the construction of new progeny (membrane, capsid proteins)
	Structural proteins used to enter target cell (membrane and envelope proteins, membrane fusion proteins)
	Functional enzymes needed for viral genome transcription and replication (synthesized by the virus within the target cell) (e.g., RNA-dependent RNA polymerase, reverse transcriptase)
Viral antigens	Envelope and capsid proteins
Alter biochemical pathways	Inhibitory factors that stop host-cell DNA, RNA, and protein synthesis
Alter defense mechanisms	Inhibitory factors that block effects of interferon, phagocytosis, and acquired immune responses (immunoglobulin proteases)
Neoplastic transformation	Insert viral oncogenes directly into the target cell genome or insert viral genes that enhance the activity of existing oncogenic genes (proto-oncogenes) in the target cell genome

rotavirus-infected enterocytes secrete a viral-directed toxin called *NSP4* into the intestinal lumen. Adjacent enterocytes not infected with virus absorb this toxin, and it acts on a cytoplasmic messenger system to cause a secretory diarrhea. This diarrhea occurs before there is lysis of virus-infected enterocytes.

The number of virulence factors for viruses when compared to bacteria is extremely small and is directly related to the number of genes in the respective microbes. The number of genes in viruses ranges between 10^1 and 10^2, whereas the range in bacteria is 10^3 to 10^4 genes. Correspondingly, the number of virulence factors is low in viruses and much higher in bacteria. The introduction of a new viral virulence factor to a viral family results from genomic variation through genetic drift, reassortment, recombination, or defective interfering viruses (see section on Mechanisms of Genomic Change). Breaks in protection normally provided by commercial vaccines or the reemergence of a vaccinated/protected disease in certain regions of the country are often the result of genomic variation in the street virus and the introduction of a new viral strain such as have occurred with canine distemper and parvovirus infections.

Mechanisms of Genomic Change

Viruses are often classified as DNA or RNA viruses based on the nucleic acid used to form their genes. In general, the competitive advantages for infecting target cells favor RNA viruses because they have an extremely high mutation rate, which increases their chances of expressing virulence factors that improve their ability to complete their replication cycle. However, it is likely that this advantage is counterbalanced by their slower replication speed, allowing host defense mechanisms to intervene in the replication process and kill the virus and/or virus-infected cell. *Genomic variation* is a broad term used to categorize a group of biologic processes that allow viruses to acquire new virulence factors (genetic diversity) that favor their survival through infective and replicative mechanisms in target cells. The most common form of genomic variation is called *antigenic drift (genetic drift)*, a natural mutation in a viral genome over time. It is caused by a spontaneous point mutation of individual nucleic acid bases in viral DNA or RNA. These point mutations are usually silent and do not change the protein encoded by the affected gene; however, some mutations can result in a new protein (e.g., capsid or envelope proteins as examples), thus providing an opportunity for the virus to improve its chances of infectivity, replication, and spread during its replication cycle. As an example, a "new strain" of virus arising from antigenic drift may have a "new" attachment protein in its capsid or envelope. Because of the length of time it takes to develop an effective immune response to the new protein, the immune system is ineffective in defending the animal against viral attachment and entry into target cells. Similarly, mutations could occur in viral genes linked to biologic processes involved in spread, replication, or shedding, which could also make the virus more pathogenic.

Antigenic shift occurs when two or more different strains of the same virus or strains of two or more different viruses combine (also known as reassortment) to form a new virus that has a mixture of genes from two or more of the original virus strains. An example of antigenic shift occurs with influenza A viruses (RNA viruses) that cause influenza in horses, pigs, dogs, human beings, and other domesticated and wild animal species (see section on Viral Diseases of Organ Systems; Respiratory System, Mediastinum, and Pleurae; Disorders of Horses; Equine Influenza [Orthomyxovirus, Enveloped RNA Virus]). When target cells are infected concurrently with two different influenza viruses, each viral strain has genes that give it a competitive advantage to infect target cells and complete its life cycle. However, when the genes of both of these parental viruses intermix under genomic reassortment in a target cell, the newly emerging virus could acquire the most pathogenic genes from both parental strains. Thus, when the virus is reassembled, it may be significantly more pathogenic (virulence factors) than either parental strain (Fig. 4-35). This increased pathogenicity may provide, as an example, the new virus with attachment proteins (envelope glycoproteins) that are immunologically unique to the farm, region, or country. As a result, animals that are naïve to this new virus and whose innate and adaptive immune systems have not interacted with these proteins have no immune memory of them. Therefore defensive immune mechanisms provide a limited effective response against the pathogenicity of this new viral strain. Similarly, reassortment could also affect genes linked to processes involved in viral entry, uncoating, spread, replication, or shedding. Depending on the virulence and effect of the reassorted genes, the new virus could be significantly more pathogenic than either of the parental strains.

Reassortment occurs only in RNA viruses because they have discrete genomic segments, much like chromosomes, that behave independently of one another. These genomic segments can undergo reassortment during viral replication, resulting in new viruses with genomes different from the original infecting virus. Segmented genomes confer evolutionary advantages to RNA viruses. Antigenic shift also occurs from a process called *recombination*. Recombination occurs in DNA viruses and results in rearrangements within the viral genome and deletion or duplication of viral genes, as well as the acquisition of unrelated genetic material. Genetic recombination comes about when a strand of DNA is broken and then rejoined to

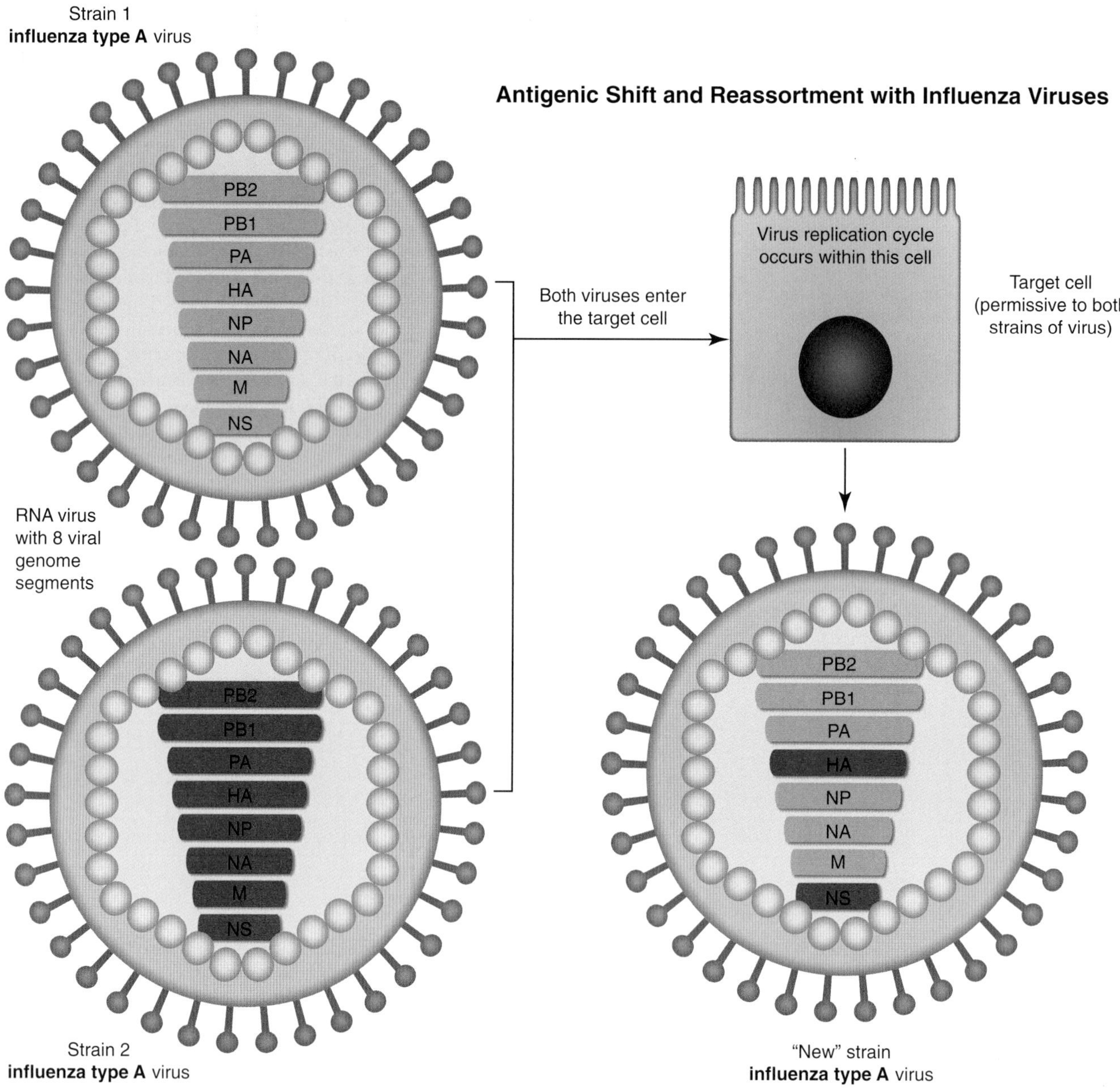

Figure 4-35 **Antigenic Shift in Influenza Virus.** Antigenic shift occurs when two different influenza viruses coinfect a target cell from an animal that is permissive for both viruses. When new virus is produced and released, it contains RNA strands resulting from the mixing of the strands of both infecting viruses, such that a hybrid virus is produced. In this example the hybrid virus contains new genetic information that allows it to more effectively attach and bind to target cells and to evade immunity that normally provides the animal with partial protection against infection. PB2 genome segment—viral polymerase involved in the replication cycle; PB1 genome segment—viral polymerase involved in the replication cycle; PA genome segment—viral polymerase involved in the replication cycle; HA genome segment—attachment and binding to the target cell; NP genome segment—structural protein for the virus; NA genome segment—attachment and binding to the target cell; M genome segment—regulates processes involved in the replication cycle; NS genome segment—evasion of immune defenses (blocks antiviral responses). (Courtesy Dr. J.F. Zachary, College of Veterinary Medicine, University of Illinois.)

the end of a different DNA molecule. A final mechanism for genomic change occurs in RNA and DNA viruses and involves *defective interfering viruses* that cannot replicate by themselves and therefore compete with nondefective viral genomes for a limited supply of replication enzymes. They can interfere with the replication of complete viruses in target cells and significantly decrease the numbers of newly replicated virus, thus favoring success of new mutants that may arise in the viral replication process.

Defense Mechanisms

Defense mechanisms include barrier systems, immunologic and biologic processes, effector cells (especially cytotoxic NK cells and cytotoxic T lymphocytes, which kill virus-infected target cells), and other effector molecules described in the opening sections of this chapter, in the sections covering bacteria, and in Chapters 3 and 5. The genome of the animal probably determines susceptibility to some viral infections via expression of or lack of expression of viral membrane receptors or through effects on the immune system. Stress (overcrowding), nutritional status, and environmental factors, such as temperature, humidity, and ventilation, also affect the susceptibility of animals to viral infections. Innate and adaptive immune mechanisms are actively involved in protection against viruses. However, it is important to remember that actions of the immune system, especially of T lymphocytes and NK cells, against viral infections have both beneficial and harmful outcomes. Beneficial outcomes include the return to normal structure and function of infected target cells and tissues and an animal that is free of and fully protected (vaccinated) against the virus. Harmful outcomes include the failure to return to normal structure and function of infected target cells because the cells and tissues, their stem cells, supporting stroma, basement membrane, and vascularized ECM tissues have been degraded by enzymes from neutrophils of acute inflammation or by macrophages of chronic inflammation and replaced by fibrous connective tissue. The innate immune system and TLRs, in response to viral antigens, induce inflammatory responses, cause secretion of cytokines and interferon, and activate the adaptive immune system.

Cell-mediated immunity (cytotoxic NK cells and cytotoxic T lymphocytes) and interferons are the most important adaptive defense mechanism against viral infections. The monocyte-macrophage system, through phagocytosis (endocytosis), is active in containing the spread of viruses, whereas phagocytosis by neutrophils does not play an important role. Antibody deficiencies usually do not affect the outcome of viral infections, whereas antibodies are important in preventing reinfection (autoimmunization or vaccination). Although viruses are obligate intracellular parasites, they have evolved sophisticated mechanisms to take over target cell transcriptional and translational processes. This approach to replication results in alteration of cell membranes that are now recognized as foreign by lymphocytes of the immune system. Virus replication and spread are abruptly stopped when virus-infected target cells are killed by cytotoxic NK cells and cytotoxic T lymphocytes. Interferons, a group of molecules that act on virus-infected cells to inhibit virus replication, function by inducing the synthesis of target cell proteins that inhibit translational activities of the virus (Fig. 4-36). The synthesis of interferon is induced by virus infection of target cells and by the action of proinflammatory molecules on these cells. Viral infection of target cells can also activate complement cascades independent of an antibody response. Complement components can act as opsonins (e.g., phagocytosis of viruses) and can cause lysis of viruses or virus-infected cells. Many of the viruses discussed in this chapter are able to infect cells of the lymphoid and monocyte-macrophage systems and dendritic cells. Under normal conditions such cells are migratory immunosurveillance cells, behaving as sentinel cells for the adaptive immune system and monitoring for the presence of foreign antigens expressed by microbes or microbe-infected target cells throughout the body. As part of their normal immunosurveillance functions, these cells migrate via lymphatic and blood vascular systems throughout all tissues and organs of the body, including the brain. It is through these normal migratory

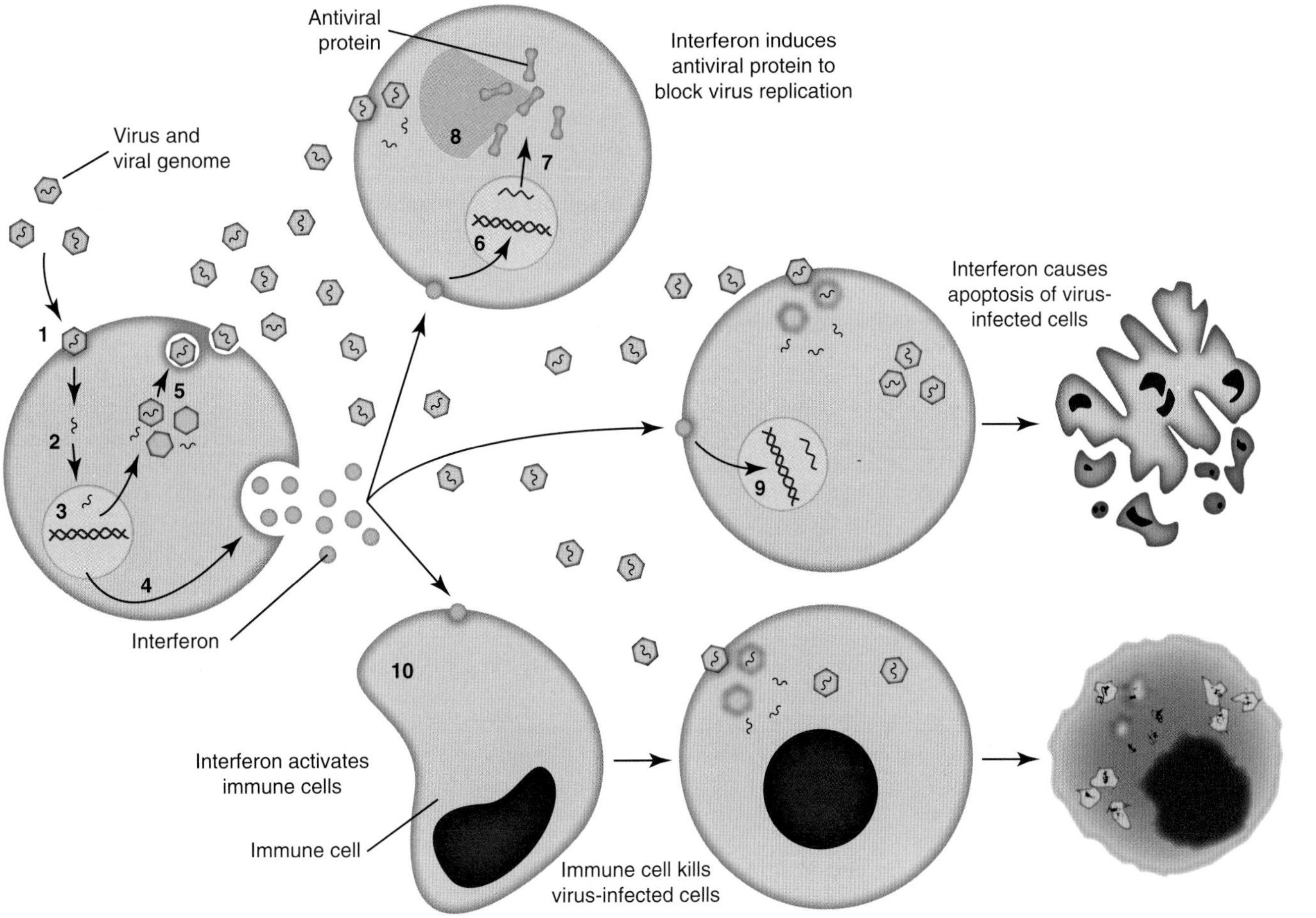

Figure 4-36 Actions of Interferon in Viral Infection of Target Cells. *1*, Virus attaches and enters the target cell. *2*, Viral genome enters nucleus for replication. *3*, Viral genome indirectly activates host genome to produce messenger RNA (mRNA) for interferon. *4*, Interferon is translated and secreted from the infected cell. *5*, Virus is reassembled and released from the cell to infect other target cells. *6*, Interferon stimulates the genome of the target cell to synthesize mRNA for an antiviral protein. *7*, Antiviral protein is translated and dispersed in the cytoplasm. *8*, Antiviral protein blocks the attachment, entry, and disassembly of the virus in the target cell. *9*, Interferon stimulates the genome of the target cell to undergo apoptosis. *10*, Interferon activates and modulates immune cells to kill virus-infected cells. (Courtesy Dr. J.F. Zachary, College of Veterinary Medicine, University of Illinois.)

pathways that viruses within these infected cells are able to spread to other tissues and organs. This process is termed *leukocyte trafficking* or *cell-associated* viremia. Viruses can also spread to other cells as a cell-free viremia in the blood vascular or lymphatic systems.

Viral Diseases of Organ Systems

Although viral diseases often affect several different organ systems, diseases in this section are placed into a specific organ system based on which organ system demonstrates the primary gross lesion (or lesions) that is most commonly used to initially recognize and identify the viral disease. The heading for each viral disease includes information on whether the virus is enveloped or nonenveloped (type of cell injury during viral shedding) and the type of nucleic acid (virulence factors, genomic diversity) it contains. This information is useful in understanding the mechanisms of injury in specific viral diseases. Viral diseases are identified by a primary mechanism of injury in E-Table 4-4.

Alimentary System and the Peritoneum, Omentum, Mesentery, and Peritoneal Cavity

Disorders of Domestic Animals

Rotavirus Enteritis (Rotavirus, Nonenveloped RNA Virus). The mechanism of injury and pathogenesis of rotavirus enteritis are similar to those of transmissible gastroenteritis in pigs (for more detail see section on Viral Diseases of Organ Systems; Alimentary System and the Peritoneum, Omentum, Mesentery, and Peritoneal Cavity; Disorders of Pigs; Transmissible Gastroenteritis [Coronavirus, Enveloped RNA Virus]). However, the clinical outcomes and pathogenicity (virulence factors) are much less severe (see Fig. 4-39). Viral capsid attachment proteins, VP4 and VP7, appear to be involved in the attachment and entry of virus into villus enterocytes through a multistage receptor-mediated process by binding to target cell membrane proteins such as sialic acids, integrins, heat shock proteins, and gangliosides located on apical surfaces. The replication of rotavirus in villus enterocytes results in the production of NSP4, an enterotoxin that (1) induces a secretory diarrhea, (2) stimulates the enteric nervous system and causes intestinal hypermotility, and (3) increases the concentration of intracellular calcium, disrupting the cytoskeletal system and tight junctions, and results in increased mucosal permeability. NSP4 also appears to cause dysfunction of cell membrane systems modulating electrolyte and water movement such as calcium ion–dependent chloride secretion, sodium-glucose transport proteins, brush-border membrane disaccharidases, and calcium ion–dependent secretion reflexes. Subsequently, rotavirus completes its replication cycle in infected enterocytes and is shed from these cells via cell lysis resulting in atrophy of intestinal villi and hyperplasia of crypt epithelial cells. Both the absorptive capacity of villi and their disaccharidase activity are impaired. Undigested and/or unabsorbed dietary disaccharides accumulate in the lumen of the intestine, thereby creating an osmotic gradient that draws fluids from the intestine into the lumen, leading to malabsorption and an osmotic diarrhea (see Chapter 7). Antigenic shift via reassortment of RNA segments of the viral genome from two or more strains of virus may be an important underlying mechanism in the emergence of new more pathogenic strains of rotavirus.

Vesicular Stomatitis (Vesiculovirus, Enveloped RNA Virus). Because the clinical signs of vesicular stomatitis are identical to those of foot-and-mouth disease (an especially dangerous microbe [see foot-and-mouth disease later]), affected animals must be carefully screened and the cause of the lesions identified. The mechanism of injury in vesicular stomatitis is cell dysfunction and lysis leading to intercellular edema with vesiculation, erosion, and ulceration of mucosae and skin. Gross lesions occur on the tongue, oral cavity, hoof coronary bands and interdigital skin, and teats. The pathogenesis has not been determined to an extent that results in an understanding of the chronologic sequence of steps leading to disease. The virus, an arbovirus, is spread to cattle, horses, and pigs primarily by sandflies and blackflies and rarely by instruments or equipment. Animals encounter the virus through the bite wounds of these insects, where the biting process injures blood vessels and capillaries, resulting in virus being deposited directly into plasma of blood vessels and/or into interstitial fluids (plasma leaked from vasopuncture) within vascularized submucosal and subcutaneous ECM (connective) tissues. It appears that vesicular lesions occur at or near the sites of insect bites, suggesting that the virus infects target cells locally and there is no systemic spread of virus to mucosae or skin through leukocyte trafficking or viremia. Squamous epithelial cells of mucosae and skin are the primary target cells for viral infection, but Langerhans cells (dendritic cells) and cells of the monocyte-macrophage system, although likely target cells for infection with virus, have not been clearly identified as target cells. In addition, it is likely but unproved that local migration of dendritic cells and cells of the monocyte-macrophage system spread virus to additional local target cells as described later. Lesions suggest that epithelial cells of the stratum basale and/or spinosum must be targets for virus infection, replication, and escape (through cell lysis). Lysis of these cells results in the formation of intercellular spaces that fill with fluid and form vesicles. Trauma likely ruptures the vesicles and leads to erosion/ulceration of the overlying mucosa or skin; however, acute inflammation may also contribute to the process. Virus appears to use envelope glycoprotein G as an attachment protein to bind with low-density lipoprotein (LDL) receptors on epithelial cells, enter the cells via endocytosis, replicate in the cytoplasm, and escape from the cell by cytolysis.

Disorders of Ruminants (Cattle, Sheep, and Goats)

Bovine Viral Diarrhea–Mucosal Disease (BVD Virus, Pestivirus, Enveloped RNA Virus). The variety of diseases caused by BVD virus is diverse and complex. Some of these diseases will be discussed in this chapter and other chapters of this book. Bovine viral diarrhea–mucosal disease as discussed herein refers to the disease that affects mucosae of the alimentary system from the oral cavity to the small intestine. The mechanism of injury in bovine viral diarrhea–mucosal disease is dysfunction and lysis of mucosal epithelial cells of the oral cavity and esophagus (stratified squamous epithelium) and of the small intestines (enterocytes [columnar epithelium]) preceded by dysfunction and lysis of submucosal lymphocytes in MALT, such as those in Peyer's patches. Gross lesions include erosion, ulceration, and hemorrhage of mucosae of oral/nasal cavities and pharynx, esophagus, and small intestine (see Figs. 7-34, 7-158, 7-159, and 7-160).

The typical pathogenesis of mucosal disease involves two forms of BVD virus, a *noncytopathic form* and a *cytopathic form*, acting synergistically to cause lesions. The noncytopathic form of the virus can be introduced into the herd in new stock, through commingling of cattle, semen, or other management practices that allow contact with carrier animals. When naïve pregnant cows (normal immune responses, unvaccinated, no prior exposure) have contact with carrier animals, they may become infected with the noncytopathic form of the virus. These cows are asymptomatic, but they functionally serve as a means for the virus to infect the fetus and establish "persistently infected (PI)" calves. These PI calves, present in small numbers, usually die before a year of age but serve as farm reservoirs for noncytopathic virus as they constantly shed virus in body secretions (saliva, tears) and feces into the environment. The cytopathic form of the virus commonly arises from a noncytopathic form that exists in the herd through mutations (antigenic drift or shift) of its viral genome, or it is introduced into the herd as a new virus via a carrier animal. The noncytopathic form makes cattle immunotolerant to cytopathic forms of BVD virus, and mucosal disease occurs when immunotolerant cattle are exposed to a cytopathic form. Cattle that have not been exposed to a noncytopathic form of the virus are not immunotolerant and develop a normal adaptive immune response to the cytopathic form. Thus they are usually able to prevent or limit the severity of mucosal disease that occurs unless the viral strain has several highly pathogenic virulence factors.

For convenience, let's begin the sequence of the steps that ultimately lead to mucosal disease with the exposure of pregnant cows to the noncytopathic form. Cows encounter the noncytopathic form in fomites from contaminated body fluids or wastes through direct contact with PI calves or carrier animals. The noncytopathic form is inhaled or ingested and deposited on mucosae of the oral, nasal, and pharyngeal cavities; especially favored are mucosae overlying the tonsil. It has not been determined if and how virus penetrates the mucus layer to gain access to mucosal epithelial cells or submucosal macrophages, lymphocytes, and/or dendritic cells, but this process could be facilitated via phagocytosis in the mucus layer by mucosa-associated macrophages, lymphocytes, and/or dendritic cells migrating through the mucosa. Noncytopathic virus probably infects and replicates in monocytes, macrophages, lymphocytes, and dendritic cells and is spread via leukocyte trafficking in lymphatic vessels from tonsil and submucosal lymphoid nodules to regional lymph nodes and then systemically to the caruncular side of placentomas. Noncytopathic virus can infect trophoblasts in the placentoma, and the virus likely completes a replication cycle in these cells. It is unclear how virus exits from trophoblasts and spreads to the fetus; however, fetal macrophage-like cells are likely involved. Virus probably infects these cells as they migrate into and through the caruncles and/or cotyledons and then enter the fetal vascular system and spread to the fetus. Additionally, noncytopathic virus can infect and spread within the allantoic and amniotic membranes and then infect the fetus, but it is unclear which cells facilitate this spread.

Bovine fetuses infected in utero become immunotolerant (see Chapter 5) to the noncytopathic form of the virus. They also do not recognize antigens from cytopathic forms of the virus as foreign, and as a result they fail to develop an effective adaptive immune response. Therefore, when exposed to cytopathic virus, mucosal disease ensues in these calves. Mechanistically, the sequence of steps that ultimately leads to mucosal disease begins when these immunotolerant calves inhale or ingest cytopathic virus and it is deposited on mucosa of the oral, nasal, and pharyngeal cavities and tonsil. The mechanism of infection and spread of the virus from the mucus layer systemically to MALT of the alimentary system, especially Peyer's patches (MALT), is similar to that described earlier for the noncytopathic virus. The cytopathic virus infects follicular dendritic cells and B lymphocytes in MALT and then spreads probably via leukocyte trafficking to infect and kill overlying stratified squamous epithelial cells and/or crypt enterocytes, resulting in mucosal erosions, ulcerations, and hemorrhage. In the small intestine, because of the lysis of crypt enterocytes, there is a failure of replacement of sloughed villus enterocytes after normal enterocyte turnover at the villus tip. This outcome may in part explain the mucosal lesions and initiate the formation of ulcers. Hemorrhage occurring with the ulcers could be the result of exposure of capillary beds to endotoxins or other toxic molecules absorbed through an open intestinal barrier system (cell junctions). Diarrhea could also occur secondary to the absorption of large quantities of endotoxins into the lamina propria and deeper supporting stroma that contains the enteric nervous system, resulting in an acquired dysautonomia (see Chapter 14). It has been recently reported that certain molecules released from lymphocytes and/or monocytes infected with cytopathic virus can initiate apoptosis in bystander lymphocytes and monocytes not infected with virus. The role of apoptosis in ulceration of mucosae has not been determined. Additionally, a vasculopathy involving arterioles and small arteries in submucosal tissue of Peyer's patches has been reported and is characterized by segmental necrosis of vascular walls and lymphohistiocytic perivasculitis. Potentially, such lesions could cause endothelial injury and occlusive thrombi, resulting in infarction of the mucosal enterocytes overlying Peyer's patches. Lymphoid cells in Peyer's patches initially proliferate when infected, but infection is followed by massive lysis of lymphocytes as part of the viral replication cycle, likely caused by a virus-induced apoptotic mechanism.

Ligand-receptor interactions are involved in encounters with both forms of the virus and with all types of its target cells. Studies suggest that glycoproteins (E1 and E2) present in the outer membrane of the virus may act as attachment proteins. Clathrin, lysosomal-associated membrane protein-2, and mannose receptors may be involved in entry into target cells via receptor-mediated endocytosis.

Rinderpest (Cattle Plague, Morbillivirus, Enveloped RNA Virus). Because of similarities in clinical presentations, lesions, causative viruses, and mechanisms of infection and spread between rinderpest and other viral diseases, the following materials should be reviewed: (1) morbilliviruses—local, regional, and systemic infection and spread and their target cells in the section on canine distemper; (2) bovine viral diarrhea–mucosal disease—clinical presentation and lesions; and (3) parvoviruses—mechanisms used to infect and spread between cells.

The mechanism of injury in rinderpest is dysfunction and lysis of mucosal epithelial cells, dendritic cells (Langerhans cells [oral cavity]), M cells, lymphocytes, and macrophages of the alimentary system from the oral cavity to the small intestine. Gross lesions include erosions, ulcerations, and hemorrhages of the oral cavity, including the gums, lips, hard and soft palate, cheeks, and base of the tongue, the esophagus, and the small intestine over Peyer's patches (Fig. 4-37). Lymph nodes, especially mesenteric nodes, are enlarged, hemorrhagic, and edematous.

Cattle (and likely sheep and goats) encounter the virus in fomites from body fluids and wastes, such as nasal-ocular fluids, salvia, urine, and feces, through direct contact with virus-infected cattle. Virus is inhaled, deposited on, and trapped in mucosae of the conductive and exchange components of the respiratory system through centrifugal and inertial turbulence. It has not been determined if and how virus penetrates the mucus layer to gain access to mucosal epithelial cells, mucosal macrophages, and/or dendritic cells. Virus probably infects and replicates in mucosal macrophages and dendritic cells as they migrate through the mucus layer and mucosae and then is spread by these cells locally through leukocyte trafficking to the submucosa, where they infect and replicate in tissue macrophages, lymphocytes, and dendritic cells. These cells then spread virus via leukocyte trafficking through afferent lymphatic vessels to regional lymph nodes. Similar cells are infected and used to spread the virus systemically via lymphatic vessels, the thoracic duct, and the blood vascular system systemically to lymph nodes and other organ systems, including the alimentary and respiratory systems. Systemically, primary target cells for infection include those cells in Peyer's patches of the small intestine and in lymphoid nodules, including Langerhans cells of the malpighian layer of stratified squamous epithelium of the oral cavity and esophagus.

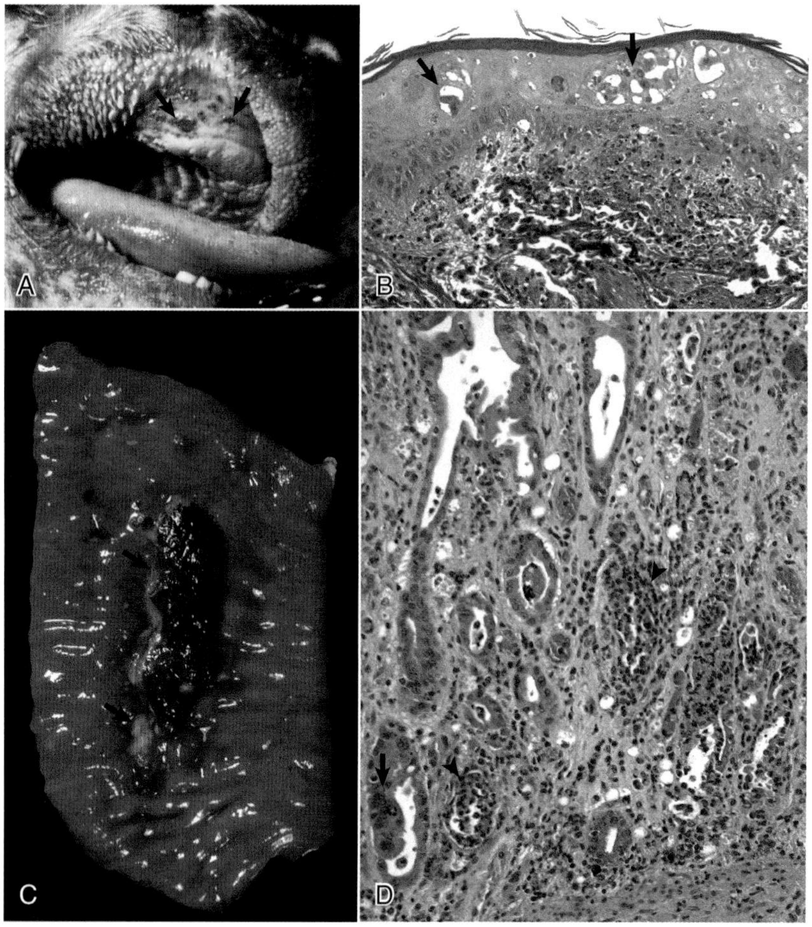

Figure 4-37 **Rinderpest. A,** Oral mucosa, dental pad. Note the erosions and ulcers *(arrows)* adjacent to the dental pad caused by rinderpest virus. **B,** Oral mucosa. Focal aggregates of epithelial cells in the mucosa are swollen, necrotic, and some are detached *(arrows)*. When abraded by ingesta or other trauma, the mechanical force applied to the lesion in **A** can separate the epithelium overlying the lesion, and it will grow and lead to ulcers or abrasions, depending on depth of the epithelial loss. Note the acute inflammatory response in the lamina propria. H&E stain. **C,** Ileum. The mucosa overlying Peyer's patches is ulcerated and covered with fibrin mixed with hemorrhage *(arrows)*. This lesion appears to result from spread of the virus from underlying lymphocytes in Peyer's patches to epithelial cells of the crypts. **D,** Epithelial cells of the crypts are hyperplastic and form syncytia *(arrow)*. In other areas, crypt enterocytes and cells in the adjacent lamina propria are necrotic *(arrowheads)* and accompanied by acute inflammation. This process leads to ulceration of the intestinal mucosa. H&E stain. (**A** and **C** courtesy Dr. C. Brown, College of Veterinary Medicine, The University of Georgia. **B** and **D** courtesy Dr. J.F. Zachary, College of Veterinary Medicine, University of Illinois.)

Erosive lesions in the oral-pharyngeal-lingual mucosae begin in the malpighian layer (stratum basale [germinativum], stratum spinosum, and stratum granulosum). Langerhans cells (dendritic cells) are located in the malpighian layer and are sentinel cells that migrate in and out monitoring for foreign antigens. Although unproved, Langerhans cells are likely infected with rinderpest virus via encounters with virus-infected macrophages migrating through these mucosae. Infected oral Langerhans cells also spread virus to contiguous squamous epithelial cells. Here the virus replication cycle results in lysis of infected squamous epithelial cells (oral-pharyngeal-lingual mucosal ulceration) and release of virus into the alimentary system. Erosive lesions in intestinal mucosae likely occur via a similar mechanism facilitated by the infection and migration of macrophages, monocytes, and dendritic cells systemically and into and through Peyer's patches and then to contiguous enterocytes. The entry of rinderpest virus into mucosal enterocytes has a polarized pattern restricted to their basolateral areas, the areas nearest Peyer's patches and M cells. The virus replication cycle results in lysis of infected enterocytes (small intestine mucosal ulceration) and release of virus into the alimentary system.

Similar to distemper virus, the rinderpest virus has envelope and hemagglutinin/fusion surface glycoproteins for attachment and fusion, respectively, to target cell membrane glycoprotein receptor CD150 (signaling lymphocyte activation molecule [SLAM]). SLAM has been demonstrated in membranes of lymphocytes, monocytes, and macrophages and of epithelial cells of the respiratory, alimentary, and integumentary systems.

Contagious Ecthyma (Orf, Sore Mouth, Pustular Dermatitis: Parapoxvirus; Enveloped DNA Virus). The mechanism of injury in contagious ecthyma is (1) dysfunction and lysis of squamous epithelial cells of the oral mucosa (squamous epithelium) and/or skin caused by viral replication and cytolysis and (2) exuberant hyperplasia (proliferation) of squamous epithelial cells of oral mucosa and/or skin through modulation of regulatory activities in the cell-division cycle by virulence factors expressed in the viral genome. Gross lesions include (1) macules, papules, vesicles, pustules, scabs, and scars and in cases having extensive injury resulting from vesicles and pustules (2) a reparative response with proliferation of mucosal squamous epithelial cells resulting in a thickened and granulation tissue–like appearance of affected mucosa (see Figs. 7-150 and

17-65). Lesions are most easily observed on wool-free or hair-free areas such as the muzzle (lips and mouth) and udder (teats) but also can occur in the skin of the perineum, groin, prepuce, scrotum, axilla, and vulva. This disease is zoonotic.

Sheep and goats encounter the virus in fomites of fluids from ruptured macules, vesicles, and pustules and from skin debris and scabs through direct contact with virus-infected animals. The virus can also be spread through mechanical contact with contaminated clothing, instruments, and clippers. Virus gains access to the malpighian layer of the squamous epithelium through traumatic abrasions, lacerations, or burns and infects Langerhans cells (dendritic cells) and capillary endothelial cells. Infection of additional Langerhans cells occurs when virus-infected dendritic cells migrate through the dermis and subcutis of the malpighian layer. Infection of endothelial cells may be facilitated by the migration of virus-infected dendritic cells through the capillary wall. Virus appears to use F1L envelope protein as an attachment protein to bind to glycosaminoglycan heparin sulfate receptor proteins on the surface of target cells. Endothelial cells are injured and lysed (killed) by virus, and injury is accompanied by vascular dilation, leakage (edema), and active hyperemia, likely contributing to formation of macules, vesicles, and papules in the skin. Reparative and regenerative responses contribute to proliferative lesions (hyperplasia) of mucosae and skin. Hyperplasia is apparently caused by (1) synthesis of vascular endothelial growth factor molecules from virus-infected capillary endothelial cells, (2) proliferation of new capillaries as occurs in angiogenesis, and (3) the concurrent proliferation of mucosal epithelial cells much like in the formation of granulation tissue. Virus also infects cells of the stratum basale (germinativum) that are regenerating (actively dividing [mitotic]) as a reparative response to the initial injury of mucosae; however, the relationship between infection of these epithelial cells and the proliferative response that ensues is unclear.

Bovine Papular Stomatitis (Parapoxvirus, Enveloped DNA Virus). The pathogenesis and mechanism of injury in bovine papular stomatitis are similar to those of contagious ecthyma discussed in the preceding section. The disease occurs primarily in cattle and also in sheep and goats (see Figs. 7-148 and 7-149).

Foot-and-Mouth Disease (Aphthovirus, Nonenveloped RNA Virus). The pathogenesis and mechanisms of injury in foot-and-mouth disease in cattle and pigs (less common in sheep and goats) are likely similar to that of swine vesicular disease and vesicular exanthema of pigs (see Viral Diseases of Organ Systems; Alimentary System and the Peritoneum, Omentum, Mesentery, and Peritoneal Cavity; Disorders of Pigs). In summary, virus encounters target cells through inhalation or ingestion and establishes a local infection in the oronasal-pharyngeal mucosae especially of the tonsil and subsequently in submucosal lymphoid cells, macrophages, and dendritic cells. It then spreads via leukocyte trafficking or cell-free viremia in afferent lymphatic vessels to regional lymph nodes to sustain and amplify the infection and then systemically via leukocyte trafficking or cell-free viremia to infect, replicate in, and lyse epithelial cells of the stratum spongiosum of stratified squamous mucosa and skin, resulting in vesicles (Fig. 4-38). Capsid proteins used by the virus to attach and bind to target cells appear to include VP1-4 attachment proteins, whereas α integrins (Vβ1, Vβ3, and Vβ6) expressed on target cells are used are receptors.

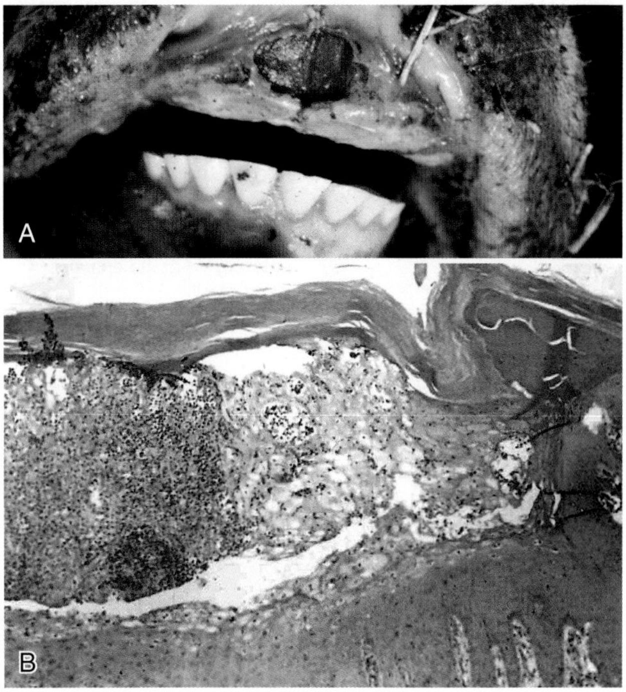

Figure 4-38 Foot-and-Mouth Disease. A, Ox. Note the ulcer on the mucosa of the upper dental pad. Such ulcers begin as fluid-filled vesicles that rupture, usually from the trauma of chewing or prehension. Vesicles and ulcers that result from their rupture may occur on all mucosae of the body, including the dental pad, tongue, gingiva, coronary bands, and teats, as examples. **B,** The mucosa has a large focus of a previous vesicle, which is now partially filled with edema fluid, fibrin, cellular debris, and acute inflammatory cells, forming a pustule. H&E stain. (**A** courtesy Dr. M. Adsit, College of Veterinary Medicine, The University of Georgia; and Noah's Arkive, College of Veterinary Medicine, The University of Georgia. **B** courtesy Dr. C. Brown, College of Veterinary Medicine, The University of Georgia.)

Disorders of Pigs

Transmissible Gastroenteritis (Coronavirus, Enveloped RNA Virus). The mechanism of injury in transmissible gastroenteritis (TGE) is dysfunction and lysis of epithelial cells (villus enterocytes) covering tips and sides of intestinal villi (Fig. 4-39, *A*). Gross lesions include congestion and thinning of the wall of the small intestine and shortening (atrophy) of villi (see Fig. 4-39, *B*; also see Figs. 7-166, 7-167, and 7-168).

Piglets encounter virus in fomites contaminated with feces through direct contact with virus-infected pigs. Virus is ingested, and swallowing and peristasis carry it through the oral pharynx, esophagus, and stomach to the small intestine, where it is trapped in the mucus layer. It is unclear how the virus is able to evade the actions of digestive enzymes, bile acids, and other microbial-lytic molecules. The mucus layer has mucins and mucin-like glycoproteins that contain sialic acid. The viral envelope contains S protein, an attachment protein, which binds to sialic acid in the mucus layer. It has not been determined how the virus penetrates the mucus layer to gain access to enterocytes. When in contact with cell membrane of enterocytes, S protein binds to a glycoprotein receptor, aminopeptidase N, which is expressed on apical surfaces of enterocytes located on the tips and sides of villi. E2 protein, also present in the envelope of the virus, is thought to facilitate entry of virus into the cytoplasm of the enterocyte. These interactions enable the attachment and entry of virus into the cytoplasm of villus enterocytes where the virus replicates. Virus then lyses enterocytes on the tips and sides of villi and escapes into the lumen of the small intestine to be passed in the feces. Injured and killed villus enterocytes are sloughed, resulting in collapse (atrophy) of the villus. Basement membranes are not injured, and crypt enterocytes divide and migrate up the denuded villus to cover exposed basement membrane (see

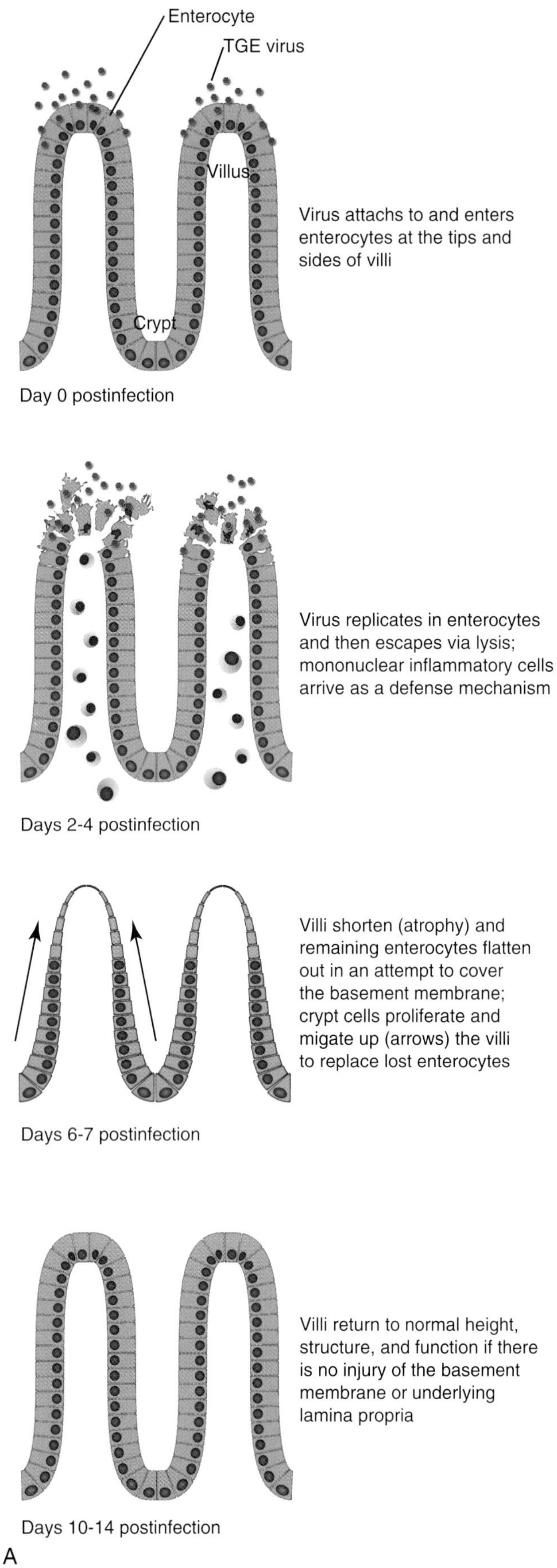
Enterocyte
TGE virus
Villus
Crypt
Virus attachs to and enters enterocytes at the tips and sides of villi
Day 0 postinfection
Virus replicates in enterocytes and then escapes via lysis; mononuclear inflammatory cells arrive as a defense mechanism
Days 2-4 postinfection
Villi shorten (atrophy) and remaining enterocytes flatten out in an attempt to cover the basement membrane; crypt cells proliferate and migate up (arrows) the villi to replace lost enterocytes
Days 6-7 postinfection
Villi return to normal height, structure, and function if there is no injury of the basement membrane or underlying lamina propria
Days 10-14 postinfection
A

Figure 4-39 **Mechanism of Viral Infections that Target Villus Absorptive Enterocytes. A,** Transmissible gastroenteritis (TGE) virus and rotavirus use similar mechanisms to infect villus enterocytes and cause disease. **B,** Small intestine, villus atrophy. Following the initial loss of tip enterocytes *(arrows)*, the villi contract, reducing the surface area to be reepithelialized. Note the crypt epithelium becomes hyperplastic with numerous mitoses, and the villi are covered by a less specialized, usually low cuboidal epithelium. Acute inflammatory cells infiltrate the villus lamina propria. H&E stain. (**A** and **B** courtesy Dr. J.F. Zachary, College of Veterinary Medicine, University of Illinois.)

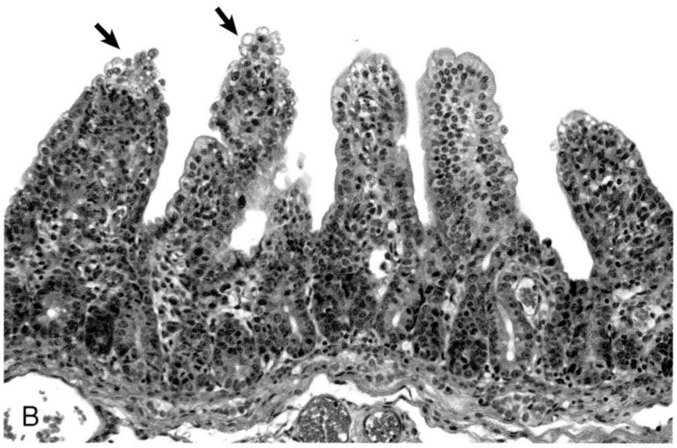
B

Fig. 4-39, A). Early in the reparative process, these migrating cells are flattened squamous-like cells stretched over the basement membrane. As the cells increase in density and maturity, they regain a more columnar structure. Additionally, the loss of enterocytes and exposure of basement membrane allows endotoxins and other potentially harmful molecules in digesta to cross into the lamina propria, enter capillary and lymphatic vessels, and through absorption cause systemic cardiovascular and hemodynamic effects. Finally, a malabsorption osmotic diarrhea also occurs because of the loss of enterocytes and the failure to digest carbohydrates (impaired hydrolysis) and other molecules in the digesta. The glycocalyx of the microvillus border (see Chapter 7) formed by affected enterocytes contains enzymes that are used to digest sugars. This activity is lost when enterocytes are lysed and sloughed into the intestinal lumen and leads to fermentation of substrates like glucose by resident bacterial flora (maldigestion). By-products of fermentation create on osmotic gradient that draws fluids across intestinal mucosa into the lumen to dilute the fermentation by-products. This process results in an osmotic diarrhea.

Porcine Epidemic Diarrhea (Coronavirus, Enveloped RNA Virus). Porcine epidemic diarrhea (PED) is an "especially dangerous and contagious disease" caused by porcine epidemic diarrhea virus (PEDV). Porcine epidemic diarrhea was diagnosed in the United States in May 2013, and in Canada in the winter of 2014. Additionally, a new viral strain, likely arising via antigenic drift and/or shift (see section on Viral Diseases, Mechanisms of Genomic Change), was detected in January 2014 in the state of Ohio. Economic losses to pork producers in the United States and Canada, as examples, at the time of this writing were undetermined but estimated to be substantial (≈ $900 million to $1.8 billion dollars). Virus affects "preweaning" piglets most severely; death losses of 75% to 100% are commonly reported in infected herds. The pathogenesis and mechanism of injury are very similar to those of transmissible gastroenteritis discussed in the previous section. Lesions in porcine epidemic diarrhea and transmissible gastroenteritis are similar (see Fig. 4-39); however, death losses are much more severe with porcine epidemic diarrhea infections because all animals exposed to the virus are "naïve" and have not acquired immune defense mechanisms via colostral antibodies (passive immunity) or through immunization (adaptive immunity) following natural exposure or vaccination (currently available only in South Korea, Japan, and China) as exist for transmissible gastroenteritis.

Swine Vesicular Disease (Enterovirus, Nonenveloped RNA Virus). The mechanism of injury in swine vesicular disease is cell dysfunction and lysis leading to intercellular edema (vesiculation), rupture of vesicles, and subsequent erosion and ulceration of mucosae and skin having vesicles. Gross lesions include vesicles, erosions, and ulcers on mucosae and skin of the snout, mouth, tongue, hoof coronary bands and interdigital skin, and teats. Pigs encounter virus through (1) contact with infected vesicular fluid, (2) contact with contaminated clothing or instruments, or (3) ingestion of contaminated pig offal, by-products, or meat products. It appears that the virus can enter the body through inhalation, ingestion, or contact with abraded skin.

Through inhalation or ingestion the virus encounters oronasalpharyngeal mucosae, especially of the tonsil. It has not been determined if and how the virus penetrates the mucus layer to gain access to mucosal epithelial cells, mucosal macrophages, and/or dendritic cells. The role of mucosal epithelial cells in infection is unclear. The virus probably infects and replicates in mucosal macrophages, lymphocytes, and/or dendritic cells as they migrate through the mucus layer and mucosae and then is spread by these cells locally through leukocyte trafficking to the lamina propria and submucosa, where they infect and replicate in macrophages, lymphocytes, and dendritic cells of lymphoid nodules and aggregates. From here the virus spreads via lymphatic vessels to regional lymph nodes and infects similar cells, spreads systemically in these cells to other organ systems, including mucosae and skin via lymphatic vessels, the thoracic duct, and the blood vascular system.

Through ingestion the virus encounters mucosa of the small intestine, most likely overlying Peyer's patches. Although unproved, the virus likely infects M cells, which spread virus to tissue macrophages, dendritic cells, and other cells in Peyer's patches. Here similar cells are infected, and they migrate via leukocyte trafficking to spread virus via lymphatic vessels to regional lymph nodes and then systemically to other organ systems, including mucosa and skin.

Finally, it has been suggested that virus can infect Langerhans (dendritic cells) or other cells of the malpighian layer if the skin of the coronary band of the hooves is traumatized and epithelial cells of the stratum basale and/or spinosum are exposed to the environment. Virus can replicate in these squamous epithelial cells and also likely in Langerhans cells. Thus they may serve as a site of local infection, followed by spread via leukocyte trafficking to regional lymph nodes via lymphatic vessels, and systemic spread to other organ systems, including mucosa and skin.

No matter which route is used to establish, sustain, and amplify the systemic infection, it appears that virus can infect, injure, and lyse squamous epithelial (mucosae) and dendritic cells of the skin, resulting in vesicle formation. The mechanisms involved in vesicle formation have not been identified but could be similar to those used in poxvirus infections or vesicular stomatitis. It is unclear whether spread is via a cell-free viremia or leukocyte trafficking; both mechanisms of virus spread have been demonstrated in enterovirus infections. Virus appears to use capsid proteins, VP1-4, as attachment proteins to bind to glycoprotein receptors, such as ICAM, expressed on the surface of target cells. When interacting with cell receptors, viral capsid proteins undergo conformational changes leading to fusion of virus to cell membrane and internalization of virus within the target cell. The diversity of ICAM receptors expressed on a variety of cell membranes probably determines target cell specificity. Additionally, coxsackievirus-adenovirus receptor and sulfated glycosaminoglycans, such as heparin sulfate, may also be used as receptors on target cells.

Vesicular Exanthema of Pigs (Calicivirus, Nonenveloped RNA Virus). The pathogenesis and mechanisms of injury in vesicular exanthema of pigs are likely similar to those of swine vesicular disease discussed in the previous section. Capsid proteins used by the virus to attach and bind to target cells and receptors for virus on target cells have not been clearly identified. Vesicles are shown in Figures 7-33.

Foot-and-Mouth Disease (Aphthovirus, Nonenveloped RNA Virus). See Viral Diseases of Organ Systems; Alimentary System and the Peritoneum, Omentum, Mesentery, and Peritoneal Cavity; Disorders of Ruminants (Cattle, Sheep, and Goats); Foot-and-Mouth Disease (Aphthovirus, Nonenveloped RNA Virus).

Disorders of Dogs

Parvovirus Enteritis (Parvovirus, Nonenveloped DNA Virus). Parvovirus enteritis is a general name used to group two closely related strains of parvovirus that cause canine parvovirus enteritis and feline panleukopenia (feline parvovirus enteritis). The mechanism of injury is lysis of crypt epithelial cells and lymphocytes, including lymphocytes in the bone marrow. Specificity for these mitotically active cells occurs because parvoviruses require a target cell–derived duplex transcription template, which is available only when cells divide during the S phase of the cell cycle. Parvoviruses are unable to turn on DNA synthesis in target cells, so they must wait for target cells to enter the S phase of the cell cycle (see E-Fig. 1-18) before infecting these cells. Gross lesions include segmental areas of the mucosa that are rough and granular (enterocyte necrosis, villus atrophy) with areas of hemorrhage, acute inflammation, and fibrin exudation (see Fig. 7-180).

Dogs and cats encounter parvoviruses in fomites from body fluids contaminated with fecal matter through direct contact with infected animals. The virus is inhaled or ingested; deposited on mucosae of the oral, nasal, and pharyngeal cavities; and trapped in the mucus layer. It has not been determined if and how virus penetrates the mucus layer to gain access to mucosal epithelial cells, mucosal macrophages, lymphocytes, and/or dendritic cells. Virus probably infects macrophages or dendritic cells migrating in the mucus layer and on the surface of mucosae. Virus replicates in these cells and is then spread via leukocyte trafficking to the lamina propria of the tonsils. Here additional macrophages and lymphocytes are infected and spread the virus via leukocyte trafficking in lymphatic and blood vascular systems to regional lymph nodes and systemically to the spleen, thymus, lymph nodes, bone marrow, and mucosa-associated lymphoid nodules such as Peyer's patches of the small intestine. Virus may also be spread as a cell-free viremia in lymph via lymphatic vessels to regional lymph nodes.

In these diseases the majority of virus-infected intestinal epithelial cells are found in crypts neighboring Peyer's patches in the small intestine. Experimental studies demonstrate that virus arrives at Peyer's patches before it reaches contiguous crypt enterocytes. Although not yet shown with canine or feline parvovirus, other similar viruses spread from Peyer's patches to M cells contiguous with Peyer's patches. Morphologically, M-cell processes extend into the mucosa and are contiguous with crypt enterocytes forming intestinal crypts. Additionally, virus entry into intestinal epithelial cells has a polarized pattern in which entry is restricted to the basolateral areas of crypt enterocytes, the areas nearest Peyer's patches and M cells. Collectively these findings suggest that virus initially spreads to the intestine and crypt cells via the blood vascular system and not in ingesta via peristalsis. It is unclear whether virus arrives as a cell-free viremia or within cells of the monocyte-macrophage and/or lymphoid systems; however, (1) virus infects such cells in the oral, nasal, pharyngeal mucosa, and tonsil and regional lymph nodes and (2) leukocyte trafficking is commonly used by other viruses to spread virus systemically to lymphoid and other organ systems, suggesting that parvovirus is spread to the intestine via leukocyte trafficking.

Infection is initiated through capsid-mediated attachment proteins to one or more glycosylated receptors on target cell membranes and is followed by entry via receptor-mediated endocytosis. It appears that canine transferrin receptor may need to present on target cells in canids. Parvoviruses also appear to use coreceptors for the attachment and entry processes. Attachment receptors may assist in aggregating virus near the cell membrane, and entry receptors may assist the virus in penetrating the cell membrane. In the dog this process requires capsid proteins to bind to transferrin receptors, whereas in the cat the process requires capsid proteins to bind to neuraminic acid and transferrin receptors. These receptors appear to determine which cells and which species of animal are infected by parvovirus strains. Parvoviruses are released from infected crypt enterocytes when the cell is lysed after the replication cycle is completed. Because of this outcome, parvovirus enteritis causes an osmotic malabsorption-maldigestion diarrhea. Diarrhea occurs because of the failure of replacement of absorptive enterocytes covering villi that are lost through normal turnover (≈48-hour life span). As a result, affected villi collapse, are atrophic, and all absorptive and digestive surfaces are lost; thus dietary carbohydrates are available for fermentation by intestinal bacteria. Under normal conditions, enterocytes covering villi are replaced by dividing crypt epithelial cells that move up and cover the villus. The loss of enterocytes covering villi also functionally opens a barrier system that normally prevents endotoxins from being absorbed by capillary beds in the lamina propria of the villi. Endotoxic shock and disseminated intravascular coagulation can result and kill the affected animal. Panleukopenia also occurs because of virus-induced cytolysis of rapidly dividing stem cells in the bone marrow. The effects of parvovirus on organs of the lymphatic system are discussed in the section on Viral Diseases of Organ Systems; Bone Marrow, Blood Cells, and Lymphatic System; Disorders of Dogs, and the effects of parvovirus on the heart are discussed in the section on Viral Diseases of Organ Systems, Cardiovascular System and Lymphatic Vessels, Disorders of Dogs.

Canine Enteric Coronavirus (Canine Coronavirus, Enveloped RNA Virus). The pathogenesis and mechanism of injury in canine enteric coronavirus are likely similar to but much less severe than those of canine parvovirus enteritis discussed in the previous section. Lysis of villus enterocytes may occur as the result of virus-induced apoptosis. Additionally, canine coronavirus may make villus enterocytes more susceptible to parvovirus infection. Thus coinfection may result in a disease more severe than that caused by either virus independently.

Canine Distemper (Morbillivirus, Enveloped RNA Virus). The pathogenesis and mechanisms of injury in canine distemper as related to the small intestine are discussed in the section on Viral Diseases of Organ Systems, Nervous System, Disorders of Dogs, Canine Distemper (Morbillivirus, Enveloped RNA Virus).

Disorders of Cats

Feline Infectious Peritonitis (Feline Infectious Peritonitis Virus, Nonenveloped RNA Virus). See the section on Viral Diseases of Organ Systems, Cardiovascular System and Lymphatic Vessels, Disorders of Cats, Feline Infectious Peritonitis (Feline Enteric Coronavirus/Feline Infectious Peritonitis Virus, Enveloped RNA Virus).

Parvovirus Enteritis (Parvovirus, Nonenveloped DNA Virus). The disease caused by parvovirus in cats is called feline panleukopenia or feline parvovirus enteritis. The pathogenesis and mechanisms of injury in feline parvovirus enteritis are likely very similar to those of canine parvovirus enteritis (see the section on Viral Diseases of Organ Systems; Alimentary System and the Peritoneum, Omentum, Mesentery, and Peritoneal Cavity; Disorders of Dogs; Parvovirus Enteritis [Parvovirus, Nonenveloped DNA Virus]).

Hepatobiliary System and Exocrine Pancreas

Disorders of Ruminants (Cattle, Sheep, and Goats)

Wesselsbron's Disease (Flavivirus, Enveloped RNA Virus). The mechanism of injury in Wesselsbron's disease is disruption and lysis of hepatocytes affecting young to very young sheep, cattle, and goats (ruminants). Gross lesions include an enlarged yellow to orange-brown liver (hepatomegaly) with randomly distributed white-gray foci (≈1 mm in diameter) of miliary necrosis of hepatocytes. Ruminants encounter this arbovirus through bite wounds from virus-infected mosquitoes; domestic herbivores likely serve as the animal reservoir. Seasonal variations in temperature and precipitation influence the population density of mosquitoes and thus the occurrence of disease. Virus can enter the circulatory system through direct penetration of a blood vessel during a bite wound, in which virus infects monocytes. It can also be deposited in vascularized ECM (connective) tissues, in which virus gains access to cutaneous blood and fluids, as well as Langerhans cells (dendritic cells) and trafficking tissue macrophages.

Through either route, virus-infected monocytes, macrophages, and/or dendritic cells spread virus via lymphatic vessels to regional lymph nodes, where similar cells are infected. These cells then spread virus systemically via lymphatic vessels and the thoracic duct or postcapillary venules to the blood vascular system and other lymphoid tissues, such as the spleen, and other organ systems, such as the liver. This virus uses hepatocytes and Kupffer cells (part of the monocyte-macrophage system) as target cells. Hypertrophy and hyperplasia of Kupffer cells has been reported experimentally; however, their role in the pathogenesis of Wesselsbron's disease has not been determined. The virus may also possibly spread via cell-free viremia. Although unidentified at this time, viral envelope glycoproteins probably serve as attachment proteins for receptors expressed on specific populations of target cells, thus probably determining cellular tropism for the virus.

Rift Valley Fever (Phlebovirus, Enveloped RNA Virus). The pathogenesis and mechanisms of injury in Rift Valley fever are similar to those of Wesselsbron's disease discussed in the previous section.

Disorders of Dogs

Infectious Canine Hepatitis (Canine Adenovirus Infection, Canine Adenovirus Type 1, Nonenveloped DNA Virus). The mechanism of injury in infectious canine hepatitis is cell lysis (cytolysis) affecting epithelial cells of the liver and kidney and endothelial cells of all organ systems. Gross lesions include randomly distributed white-gray foci (≈1 mm in diameter) of miliary necrosis, as well as mucosal and serosal hyperemia and hemorrhage, and edema of multiple organ systems, including the liver, kidney, lymph nodes, thymus, gastric serosa, pancreas, and subcutaneous tissues (see Fig. 8-79). Edema of the gallbladder wall is prominent and is likely the result of injury of vascular endothelial cells leading to changes in permeability. Tonsillar enlargement, characteristic of the disease, probably results from proliferation of lymphocytes as part of the innate and/or adaptive immune responses against virus-infected cells through hyperplasia of uninfected lymphocytes in response to inflammatory mediators or through recruitment of lymphocytes from other lymphoid tissues and organs.

Dogs encounter the virus in fomites from body fluids such as saliva, urine, or feces. Virus enters the body through ingestion and likely inhalation, and it is trapped in the mucus layer of oral and pharyngeal mucosae, especially of the tonsils. It has not been determined if and how virus penetrates the mucus layer to gain access to mucosal epithelial cells, mucosal macrophages, and/or dendritic cells. Virus probably infects and replicates in mucosal macrophages and dendritic cells as they migrate through the mucus layer and mucosae. It is then spread by these cells locally through leukocyte trafficking to the lamina propria and submucosa and tonsil, where they infect and replicate in additional tissue macrophages, lymphocytes, and dendritic cells and then spread via afferent lymphatic vessels to regional lymph nodes and infect similar cells. A cell-free viremia has also been proposed as a mechanism of spread.

Although undetermined, virus may also be swallowed and through peristalsis encounter and infect M cells and spread to and infect macrophages, dendritic cells, and lymphocytes in Peyer's patches and then be spread to regional mesenteric lymph nodes. It is unclear how the virus is able to evade the actions of digestive enzymes, bile acids, and other microbial-lytic molecules. A virus capsid protein called *fiber protein* has been identified and may serve as an attachment protein that binds to target cell receptors such as coxsackievirus-adenovirus or integrin receptors.

Using either the inhalation or ingestion route of infection and spread, virus spreads either within virus-infected macrophages or as a cell-free viremia from regional lymph nodes, systemically to infect endothelial cells and their contiguous epithelial cells in many organ systems, including liver, kidneys, spleen, and lungs. Infection of, replication in, and release of virus from endothelial and epithelial cells cause their lysis and subsequent necrosis. The attachment of virus or virus-infected macrophages to endothelial cells is likely facilitated by molecules of the leukocyte adhesion cascade (see Chapter 3). Virus infects and replicates in endothelial cells, leading to endothelial cell injury and lysis (necrosis-vasculitis). Depending on the severity of endothelial cell injury, vasculitis can be followed by hemorrhage and edema (increased vascular permeability) and disseminated intravascular coagulation. Infection of epithelial cells of the liver and kidney are likely facilitated by ligand-receptor interactions, although none have been identified. Infection and lysis of lymphocytes in lymphoid tissues and likely bone marrow may account for the leukopenia occurring early in the infection.

Respiratory System, Mediastinum, and Pleurae

Disorders of Horses

Equine Influenza (Orthomyxovirus, Enveloped RNA Virus). The mechanism of injury in equine influenza is lysis of epithelial cells of the oral, nasal, pharyngeal, and respiratory mucosae. Gross lesions include active hyperemia, hemorrhage, edema, and necrosis leading to mucosal erosions and ulcers often covered with a mucofibrinous membrane.

Horses encounter virus in fomites from body fluids contaminated with virus through direct contact with virus-infected animals. Virus is inhaled and deposited on and/or trapped in the mucus layer of mucosae of the nasal and pharyngeal cavities and of the conductive component of the respiratory system through centrifugal and inertial turbulence. Virus must penetrate the mucus layer to gain access to ciliated epithelial cells (mucociliary apparatus); however, mucus contains glycoprotein receptor molecules that bind to virus and prevent it from attaching to these cells. This defense mechanism allows virus to be removed via the mucociliary apparatus and phagocytosis and killing by mucosal macrophages. To counteract this defense mechanism, the virus has a neuraminidase (virulence factor) that destroys receptors that mimic viral glycoprotein receptors in the mucus. However, it has not been determined how virus penetrates the mucus layer to gain access to mucosal epithelial cells. When virus encounters these cells, hemagglutinin and neuraminidase glycoproteins in its viral envelope bind to target cell membrane receptors composed of sialyloligosaccharides. This ligand-receptor binding allows virus to attach to and enter ciliated epithelial cells. The overall structure of sialyloligosaccharide receptors, in part, determines the target specificity at the cellular and the species levels. Early in the encounter before lysis affects cell function, the mucociliary apparatus spreads virus to additional target cells. This mechanism of spread becomes less effective as virus lyses ciliated and nonciliated mucosal epithelial cells and the physiologic continuity of the mucociliary apparatus is disrupted. It also appears that virus can spread in lymphatic vessels to regional lymph nodes via cell-free viremia or leukocyte trafficking and infect lymphocytes and macrophages. It is likely that lysis of lymphoid cells (immunosuppression) and ciliated epithelial cells and disruption of the mucociliary apparatus makes horses more susceptible to secondary bacterial diseases of the respiratory system. Hemagglutinin (HA) and neuraminidase (NA) are surface glycoproteins of the RNA virus that are very important in its pathogenesis in all animal species. Reassortment (antigenic shift) of the segmented RNA genome usually involves genes for HA and NA, which are the two virulence factors most commonly associated with influenza epidemics and pandemics in human beings. Hemagglutinin is involved in ligand-receptor interactions that enable attachment to and entry of the virus into specific populations of target cells, whereas neuraminidase is involved in shedding of virus from infected cells.

A serious outbreak of equine influenza occurred in 2007 in Australia. A group of horses that entered the country for an exhibition carried a strain of influenza virus that was genetically different (antigenic drift and/or shift) than strains present in horses within the country; therefore resident horses had no or limited innate or adaptive immunity to this strain of virus. Additionally, antigenic drift and/or shift involving heterologous influenza viruses, including equine influenza virus, appear to be the underlying mechanism behind outbreaks of severe respiratory disease in racing greyhounds and English foxhounds. Experimentally it has been shown that canine and equine respiratory epithelium express similar sialyloligosaccharides. This finding suggests that receptors recognized by equine influenza virus are expressed on canine respiratory epithelial cells; nevertheless, subtle differences in receptor specificity may exist.

Equine Viral Rhinopneumonitis (Equine Herpesvirus, Alphaherpesvirus, Enveloped DNA Virus). The pathogenesis and mechanisms of injury in equine viral rhinopneumonitis are similar to those of infectious bovine rhinotracheitis; see Viral Diseases of Organ Systems; Respiratory System, Mediastinum, and Pleurae; Disorders of Ruminants (Cattle, Sheep, and Goats); Infectious Bovine Rhinotracheitis (Bovine Herpesvirus, Alphaherpesvirus, Enveloped DNA Virus).

Equine Viral Arteritis (Arterivirus, Enveloped RNA Virus). Because some clinical signs of disease caused by equine viral arteritis virus arise from alterations in the respiratory system, it has been commonly considered a respiratory disease. However, the primary target cells in the lung are endothelial cells and thus this disease is discussed in the section on Viral Diseases of Organ Systems, Cardiovascular System and Lymphatic Vessels, Disorders of Horses, Equine Viral Arteritis (Arterivirus, Enveloped RNA Virus).

Disorders of Ruminants (Cattle, Sheep, and Goats)

Infectious Bovine Rhinotracheitis (Bovine Herpesvirus, Alphaherpesvirus, Enveloped DNA Virus). Bovine herpesvirus targets cells of the respiratory system but can also infect cells of the nervous system (see Viral Diseases of Organ Systems, Nervous System, Disorders of Ruminants (Cattle, Sheep, and Goats), Bovine Herpesvirus Meningoencephalitis [Bovine Herpesvirus 5: Alphaherpesvirus, Enveloped DNA Virus]). The mechanism of injury in infectious bovine rhinotracheitis in the respiratory system is lysis of nonciliated and ciliated (mucociliary apparatus) epithelial cells of the oral, nasal, pharyngeal, and respiratory mucosae. Gross lesions include active hyperemia, hemorrhage, edema, and necrosis leading to large areas of mucosal erosions and ulcers often covered with a fibrinous membrane (see Fig. 9-22).

Cattle encounter bovine herpesvirus in fomites of body fluids contaminated with virus through direct contact with virus-infected animals. Virus can be (1) inhaled or ingested and deposited on and trapped in mucus layers of oral, nasal, and pharyngeal mucosae; (2) inhaled and deposited and trapped in the mucus layer of the mucosa of the conductive component of the respiratory system through centrifugal and inertial turbulence; or (3) deposited on conjunctival mucosa. It has not been determined if and how virus penetrates mucus layers of these mucosae to gain access to epithelial cells or if mucosal macrophages and/or dendritic cells are involved in trafficking virus to target cells. Viral envelope glycoproteins B, C, and D are used to attach to and enter a variety of target cells by binding to an array of glycosaminoglycan receptors, such as herpesvirus entry mediator A, nectin-1 and nectin-2 (herpesvirus entry proteins C and B), and 3-O-sulfated heparin sulfate, most commonly expressed on mucosal epithelial cells and also on sensory nerve endings that innervate the mucosa. These receptors have a polarized pattern of expression and are present only on apical and lateral surfaces of mucosal epithelial cells above junctional complexes; therefore inhalation of virus provides it with optimal opportunities for interactions with appropriate receptors. Virus infects nonciliated and ciliated mucosal epithelial cells, completes its replication cycle in these cells, buds from nuclear and cell membranes, and through cell lysis or budding from membranes is released from infected cells back onto mucosae to infect additional cells or to be spread in fomites into the environment. The mechanism of cell lysis is unclear; however, (1) budding from nuclear and cell membranes may be sufficient to eventually cause lysis of the cell and (2) the products of "lytic" viral genes transcribed and translated late in the viral replication cycle may also cause cell lysis.

Bovine herpesvirus can also attach to and enter sensory nerve endings of the trigeminal and olfactory nerves in the respiratory mucosae. It then spreads via retrograde axonal transport in these nerves to other neurons in the CNS. Neurons serve as reservoir cells in which virus establishes a latent infection. Additionally, because neurons express no MHC class II molecules and low concentrations of MHC class I molecules, they are less likely, even when infected with virus, to be recognized by and acted on by cytotoxic and helper T lymphocytes, macrophages trafficking through the nervous system, and by resident microglial cells. During latency, viral genomes are present in the nucleus of infected neurons, but no viral proteins (antigens) are synthesized. With activation, the virus reestablishes its replication cycle and through axonal transport mechanisms spreads back to nerve endings in mucous membranes to be released and infect adjacent mucosal epithelial cells and transmit the disease. Bovine herpesvirus produces proteins that (1) disrupt the synthesis of interferon, (2) block the recognition of virus-infected cells by cytotoxic T lymphocytes, and (3) block the homing of T lymphocytes to virus-infected cells. Virus can also infect and induce high levels of apoptosis in T helper lymphocytes, thus suppressing the adaptive immune response to the virus. It is likely that a combination of these immunosuppressive mechanisms and disruption of the mucociliary apparatus through lysis of virus-infected ciliated mucosal epithelial cells make affected animals more susceptible to many secondary bacterial diseases of the respiratory system, such as pasteurellosis or mannheimiosis, that follow an outbreak of infectious bovine rhinotracheitis.

Bovine Respiratory Syncytial Virus Pneumonia (Pneumovirus, Enveloped RNA Virus). The mechanism of injury in bovine respiratory syncytial virus pneumonia is dysfunction and lysis of cells of the respiratory mucosae, including ciliated cells of the conductive system and alveolar type II pneumocytes of the O_2-CO_2 exchange component from infection by virus and from acute inflammation and its mediators and degradative enzymes. Gross lesions include active hyperemia, interstitial edema and inflammation (proliferative and exudative bronchiolitis), and subpleural and interstitial emphysema. Syncytial cells with intracytoplasmic inclusion bodies are observed in microscopic lesions (see Fig. 9-83).

Cattle encounter bovine respiratory syncytial virus in fomites from body fluids contaminated with virus through direct contact with virus-infected animals. It is inhaled, deposited on, and trapped in the mucus layer of the mucosa of the conductive component of the respiratory system through centrifugal and inertial turbulence, but it has not been determined if and how virus penetrates mucus layers to gain access to epithelial cells or if mucosal macrophages and/or dendritic cells are involved. Virus infects and replicates in all epithelial cells; however, ciliated cells are the primary target cells. When virus encounters ciliated cells, it attaches and binds to membrane glycosaminoglycan receptors via heparin-binding domains on envelope glycoprotein G (attachment protein) and enters via envelope glycoprotein F (fusion protein). Fusion protein also appears to induce the formation of syncytial cells, a means by which cells infected with virus are able to interact with noninfected cells and spread the virus between cells. It has also been shown that virus can infect and replicate in lung dendritic cells and alveolar macrophages and cause the synthesis of interferons and interleukins. Infection of all target cell types appears to induce a cascade of proinflammatory chemokines and cytokines that recruit neutrophils, lymphocytes, and macrophages to the site, resulting in cell and tissue injury (inflammation). Additionally, TLR3 and TLR4 may initiate this cascade. In tissue culture experiments, virus appears to cause little or no injury to ciliated epithelial cells, suggesting that lesions may result in part from host defense mechanisms such as those modulated by the innate and adaptive immune responses. Bovine respiratory syncytial virus is part of bovine respiratory disease complex (shipping fever) (see section on Bacterial Diseases of Organ Systems; Respiratory System, Mediastinum, and Pleurae; Disorders of Ruminants (Cattle, Sheep, and Goats); Bovine Respiratory Disease Complex). This complex is characterized chronologically by (1) environmental or management stressors that suppress protective mechanisms in the respiratory system such as the production of protective mucus, (2) a primary viral infection that injures structural protective mechanisms such as the mucociliary apparatus, and (3) a secondary bacterial infection that causes severe inflammation often with fibrin exudation.

Bovine Influenza (Orthomyxovirus, Enveloped RNA Virus). The pathogenesis and mechanisms of injury in bovine influenza are similar to those of equine influenza (see section on Viral Diseases of Organ Systems; Respiratory System, Mediastinum, and Pleurae; Disorders of Horses; Equine Influenza [Orthomyxovirus, Enveloped RNA Virus]).

Ovine Progressive Pneumonia, (Maedi; Maedi-Visna Virus [Ovine Lentivirus], Enveloped RNA Virus). The mechanism of injury in ovine progressive pneumonia is dysfunction and lysis of cells of the respiratory system from infection with virus and from chronic-active granulomatous interstitial inflammation and its mediators and degradative enzymes. Ovine lentivirus persistently infects monocyte precursor cells, systemic monocytes, alveolar and tissue macrophages, and dendritic cells. Gross lesions include dense, rubbery, and enlarged lung lobes that are uniformly affected and grayish-yellow to grayish-blue (see Figs. 9-75 and 9-92). Cut surfaces bulge and are rubbery and are not edematous or exudative, but excessive mucus may be present in airways.

Sheep most likely encounter virus in fomites from respiratory fluids through direct contact with virus-infected animals. In the fluid, virus may be free or in alveolar macrophages. However, any condition that facilitates mechanical transfer of infected blood to the circulatory system or mucosae of uninfected animals can also serve to spread virus. It is inhaled, deposited on, and trapped in the mucus layer of the mucosa of the conductive component of the respiratory system through centrifugal and inertial turbulence. Inhaled free virus is probably phagocytized by alveolar macrophages in the mucus layer, whereas virus within inhaled macrophages is released by exocytosis or through lysis of the macrophage by the virus or the animal's immune cells. Following either of these processes, free virus is phagocytized by alveolar macrophages in the mucus layer. They then migrate to local lymphoid tissues (BALT) and release virus via exocytosis or cell lysis, and virus infects naïve macrophages. These macrophages then spread via leukocyte trafficking in afferent lymphatic vessels to regional lymph nodes, where additional macrophages are infected, and then systemically to all organ systems, including bone marrow.

In the bone marrow, virus infects immature monocyte precursor cells (monoblasts or promonocytes and likely similar cells in spleen and lymph nodes), where small numbers of infected precursor cells serve as biologic reservoirs for the distribution (via the circulatory and lymphatic systems) of virus-infected monocytes back into the blood. Infected monocytes migrate in the circulatory system to tissues where they enter ECM, mature into tissue macrophages, and release virus to infect resident tissue macrophages such as alveolar macrophages. Virus likely uses envelope glycoproteins to attach and bind to, and fuse with alveolar macrophages and other target cells that express small ruminant lentivirus receptors A or B or some other membrane receptor. All cells infected with virus are permanently infected (persistent infection) because virus inserts its genome into chromosomal DNA of target cells.

The ability of virus to replicate in a cell is directly related to the maturity of the permanently infected cell. Once in bone marrow, virus integrates into precursor monocytes (monoblasts or promonocytes) and persistently infects a very small number of these cells. However, it is not able to replicate in these precursor monocytes. As these cells differentiate into monocytes, they migrate to tissues and organ systems that use the services of the monocyte-macrophage system and in these tissues differentiate into macrophages. Virus-infected monocytes in the peripheral blood are not able to produce virus. However, when infected monocytes mature and differentiate into macrophages in tissues, virus is able to replicate in these cells and produce viral proteins and proinflammatory chemokines and cytokines that initiate and sustain inflammation as well as release virus into ECM. This virus can now infect and activate other susceptible types of tissue macrophages, such as alveolar macrophages, and this interaction initiates and sustains the chronic active granulomatous inflammatory process.

The chronic active granulomatous inflammatory response so characteristic of ovine progressive pneumonia is a recurring process linked to the life span of tissue macrophages, which normally ranges from 6 to 16 days but can be shortened because of the viral replication cycle. When tissue macrophages die from viral infection, virus and viral proteins are released into the ECM, initiate inflammation, and recruit additional macrophages into the site to phagocytize free virus. This cyclic process creates and sustains an extensive inflammatory response in affected tissues. As naïve tissue macrophages are recruited into the ECM, new monocytes infected with virus arrive from bone marrow, differentiate into tissue macrophages, replicate virus, and release virus into the ECM to infect these naïve tissue macrophages, consequently sustaining the virus and the inflammatory response against it that ensues. Additionally, virus within these newly arriving monocytes may have undergone genetic variation (antigenic drift/shift [reassortment]) in the bone marrow. Because affected animals have no or limited innate or adaptive immunity to this "new" strain of virus, the inflammatory process begins anew. Virus-infected monocytes travel throughout all tissues and organ systems of the body; however, chronic-active inflammation occurs only in specific tissues. It appears that selectivity and specificity of lung, brain, mammary gland, and synovia occur in tissues where tissue macrophages are permissive to genome integration. Kupffer cells in the liver are not permissive and do not allow transcription of viral RNA, and the liver does not develop lesions. Based on this mechanism, involvement of the lung (maedi) and brain (visna) should occur in the same sheep at the same time; however, this outcome is not common. The mechanism for this outcome is unknown.

Interstitial pneumonia results from virus-infected alveolar macrophages expressing high concentrations of proinflammatory chemokine, IL-8, that recruit inflammatory cells (not infected with virus) into the lung. These uninfected and recruited lymphocytes, plasma cells, macrophages, and neutrophils produce additional proinflammatory cytokines capable of sustaining inflammation and propagating the interstitial pneumonia. Thus a small number of virus-infected alveolar macrophages, responding to molecules through specific cell-membrane receptors, use a cascade of membrane, cytoplasmic, and nuclear messenger systems to control and sustain a large inflammatory response. Additionally, several studies suggest that lesions in ovine progressive pneumonia are, in part, immune mediated and that cytotoxic T lymphocytes may be important effector cells. Virus-infected macrophages present viral antigens to T lymphocytes, and activated T lymphocytes in turn release cytokines that lead to differentiation of monocytes to macrophages and recruitment of additional inflammatory cells. Host defense mechanisms are ineffective in ending virus infection because (1) the viral genome becomes part of the target cell genome, (2) viral infection of cells of the monocyte-macrophage system results in dysfunction of this system and an ineffective adaptive immune response (see Chapters 3 and 5), and (3) the parental virus can modify its progeny through repeated cycles of gene reassortment (genetic variation) so that these progeny are able to escape an effective adaptive immune response (cyclical [recurring] infection).

Caprine Pneumonia (Caprine Arthritis-Encephalitis Virus, Enveloped RNA Virus). The pathogenesis and mechanism of injury in caprine pneumonia are similar to those of ovine progressive pneumonia (see sections on Viral Diseases of Organ Systems; Respiratory System, Mediastinum, and Pleurae; Disorders of Ruminants [Cattle, Sheep, and Goats], Ovine Progressive Pneumonia [Maedi; Maedi-Visna Virus (Ovine Lentivirus), Enveloped RNA Virus]) and caprine encephalitis of goats (see Viral Diseases of Organ Systems, Nervous System, Disorders of Ruminants [Cattle, Sheep, and Goats], Caprine Encephalitis [Caprine Arthritis-Encephalitis Virus, Enveloped RNA Virus]).

Disorders of Pigs

Porcine Reproductive and Respiratory Syndrome (Mystery Swine Disease; PRRS Virus, Arterivirus, Enveloped RNA Virus). The mechanism of injury in porcine reproductive and respiratory syndrome (PRRS) is lysis of all cell populations in the lung and associated regional lymph nodes secondary to acute inflammation (interstitial pneumonia) and its mediators and degradative enzymes. Gross lesions include lung lobules distributed at random throughout all lung lobes that are firm (consolidation) and red-tan to beige with septal edema. Lymph nodes, especially those draining the lungs, are enlarged, firm, and edematous and have a beige-white cut surface that bulges. These lesions may, in part, be attributable to secondary infection with a bacterium like *P. multocida*.

Porcine reproductive and respiratory syndrome occurs in two sequential stages: an acute stage followed by a persistent stage (i.e., persistent infection). In the acute stage, pigs encounter virus in fomites from body fluids through direct contact with virus-infected pigs. It is inhaled, deposited on, and trapped in the mucus layer of the mucosa of the conductive and O_2-CO_2 exchange components of the respiratory system through centrifugal and inertial turbulence. Pulmonary alveolar macrophages probably phagocytize the virus in the mucus layer and then spread it via leukocyte trafficking to BALT, alveolar macrophages of pulmonary septa, pneumocytes of alveoli, and epithelial cells of bronchioles, where infection and replication occur and acute inflammation (acute interstitial pneumonia and alveolitis) ensues. In this context, virus appears to be able to escape being killed in these cells. Potential mechanisms are discussed later. Concurrently, virus-infected macrophages migrate via afferent lymphatic vessels to regional lymph nodes (tracheobronchial) and infect macrophages and lymphocytes. It has also been suggested, but unproved, that dendritic cells may be infected and spread the virus. Viral infection causes (1) hypertrophy and hyperplasia of macrophages and lymphocytes leading to enlarged lymph nodes; (2) production of proinflammatory cytokines resulting in lysis of infected cells, releasing virus into surrounding ECM to maintain the infection, acute inflammation, and edema; and (3) the initiation of an adaptive immune response. Spread to other systemic organ systems (potentially the reproductive system) occurs at this stage, but it is unclear if spread is cell-free or cell-associated in macrophages (the latter being the most likely). In these organ systems, virus also infects cells of the monocyte-macrophage system.

In the persistent stage, virus via leukocyte trafficking establishes reservoirs in tissues, such as the tonsil, spleen, lymph nodes, and lung and in cells of the monocyte-macrophage system, such as alveolar macrophages. In part, infection of cells of the monocyte-macrophage system is likely determined by ligand-receptor interactions and may be related to the presence of sialoadhesin, a glycoprotein macrophage-specific receptor, expressed on cells of monocyte-macrophage lineage as well as scavenger receptor CD163 and heparan sulfate receptors. As an enveloped virus, PRRSV escapes from cells without causing cell lysis, but infected alveolar macrophages release proinflammatory cytokines, leading to acute inflammation and the recruitment of additional inflammatory cells, followed by cell lysis attributable to mediators and degradative enzymes of the inflammatory response. As a result, alveoli become filled with neutrophils, necrotic cell debris arising from killing of cells by the degradative activities of inflammatory cell enzymes, and edema fluid. Acute inflammation may also cause limited injury of the mucociliary apparatus, leading to increased opportunities for secondary bacterial pneumonia caused by bacteria such as *Pasteurella* or *Mannheimia*.

It appears that PRRSV, possibly mediated via nucleocapsid proteins, has both suppressive and stimulatory activities on cells it infects in the immune system. On the one hand, it is able to alter functions of the innate and adaptive immune systems, specifically of cells of the monocyte-macrophage system, by suppressing the ability of these cells to (1) kill virus-infected cells, (2) phagocytose, kill, and present antigens to effector cells, (3) stimulate other effector cells, and (4) secrete cytokines such as IFN-α, and TNF-α that are necessary to implement an effective immune response. The virus also appears to be able to modulate and/or minimize the effects of interferon in activating immune cells to act against virus and virus-infected cells. On the other hand, during the acute phase of infection virus is able to stimulate cells to significantly increase the production of IL-10 from infected cells. This cytokine is immunosuppressive and interacts with a wide array of immune cells, including the cells of the monocyte-macrophage system and lymphocytes, resulting in inhibition of innate and adaptive immunity, particularly the cell-mediated immune responses.

Swine Influenza (Orthomyxovirus, Enveloped RNA Virus). The pathogenesis and mechanisms of injury in swine influenza are similar to those of equine influenza (see section on Viral Diseases of Organ Systems; Respiratory System, Mediastinum, and Pleurae; Disorders of Horses; Equine Influenza [Orthomyxovirus, Enveloped RNA Virus]).

Inclusion Body Rhinitis–Porcine Cytomegalovirus Infection (Herpesvirus-Cytomegalovirus, Enveloped DNA Virus). The pathogenesis of porcine cytomegalovirus infection has not been studied in sufficient detail to provide an evidence-based discussion of the chronologic sequence of steps characteristic of the disease. The mechanism of injury is probably dysfunction and lysis of epithelial cells of the nasal and respiratory mucosa via infection with virus, especially the epithelial cells that form the mucous glands of the nasal cavity and from acute inflammation and its mediators and degradative enzymes. Gross lesions can include active hyperemia and hemorrhage, congestion, and mucopurulent exudate covering mucosal surfaces of the nasal septum and turbinates.

Pigs encounter porcine cytomegalovirus in fomites from body fluids contaminated with virus through direct contact with virus-infected animals. It is inhaled, deposited on, and trapped in the mucus layer of the mucosa of the conductive component of the respiratory system, especially of the nasal cavity, through centrifugal and inertial turbulence, but it has not been determined if and how virus penetrates mucus layers of these mucosae to gain access to epithelial cells or if mucosal macrophages and/or dendritic cells are involved. Therefore it appears that virus encounters epithelial cells that form the mucous glands by direct contact of the virus with apical surfaces of these cells or via mucosa-associated macrophages (or dendritic cells) that carry the virus to these cells. The conjunctiva may also be a source of infectious virus that later infects the mucosa of the nasal turbinates and septum via the lacrimal duct. Envelope attachment and fusion glycoproteins of the virus and target cell membrane receptor proteins are likely involved in infection, virus replication, and spread of virus to other cells and tissues. It is unclear how virus spreads systemically from the nasal cavity to other organ systems; however, in other animal models and human beings, leukocyte trafficking and cells of the monocyte-macrophage system are involved in the spread of similar viruses. Also, virus appears to be able to persist in cells of the monocyte-macrophage system; target and infect endothelial cells, causing lysis and hemorrhage; and infect and injure erythroid precursor cells in bone marrow, resulting in neonatal anemia.

Disorders of Dogs

Canine Infectious Respiratory Disease Complex. Canine infectious respiratory disease complex is a disease in which there is primary injury of the conductive component of the respiratory system caused by a virus, leading to increased susceptibility to infection with other bacteria, such as *B. bronchiseptica*. See the next section, Canine Infectious Tracheobronchitis, for greater detail.

Canine Infectious Tracheobronchitis (Canine Cough, Kennel Cough; Canine Parainfluenza Virus, Enveloped RNA Virus). Canine infectious tracheobronchitis is a disease in which there is primary injury caused by canine parainfluenza virus, leading to increased susceptibility secondarily to infection with *B. bronchiseptica* (or other bacteria). Other viruses (canine adenovirus type 2, canine respiratory coronavirus, reovirus, canine herpesvirus, canine distemper virus) and other bacteria (*Mycoplasma* spp., *Streptococcus equi* subsp. *zooepidemicus*) have been implicated in canine infectious tracheobronchitis, thus the phrase *canine infectious respiratory disease complex* has been used to categorize this multifactorial pathogenesis. The mechanism of injury is dysfunction and lysis of ciliated epithelial cells of the mucociliary apparatus primarily from virus-induced cytolysis and secondarily from acute inflammation (bronchitis/bronchiolitis) and its mediators and degradative enzymes. Gross lesions include active hyperemia and granularity (necrosis) of the respiratory mucosae and concurrent inflammation of mucosae and submucosae (see Fig. 9-101).

Dogs encounter parainfluenza virus in fomites of oronasal-pharyngeal fluids through direct contact with virus-infected dogs. It is inhaled, deposited on, and trapped in the mucus layer of mucosae of the conductive component of the respiratory system through centrifugal and inertial turbulence, but it has not been determined if and how virus penetrates mucus layers of these mucosae to gain access to epithelial cells or if mucosal macrophages and/or dendritic cells are involved. Virus infects and replicates in all epithelial cells; however, ciliated mucosal cells are the primary target cells. It appears that virus attaches to and enters cells via viral attachment glycoproteins (HN and F glycoproteins) that bind to sialic acid receptors located on the apical and lateral surface of ciliated epithelia cells. Viral infection disrupts the normal function of the mucociliary apparatus. Therefore normal and injured ciliated and nonciliated epithelial cells have a greater opportunity to encounter and interact with secondary bacteria, especially *B. bronchiseptica*, because the bacterium is not successfully removed by mucociliary clearance from the conductive component of the respiratory system.

B. bronchiseptica is inhaled, deposited on, and trapped in the mucus layer of the mucosa of the conductive component of the respiratory system through centrifugal and inertial turbulence. The bacterium colonizes ciliated epithelium via fimbrial and nonfimbrial adhesins such as filamentous hemagglutinin and pertactin. It has not been determined if and how it penetrates mucus layers to gain access to epithelial cells or if mucosal macrophages and/or dendritic cells are involved. Once ciliated cells are colonized, *B. bronchiseptica* releases exotoxins, such as adenylate cyclase-hemolysin and DNT and endotoxins, that further impair function of the mucociliary apparatus, allowing for additional colonization of mucosae by the bacterium at new sites. These outcomes, especially dysfunction of the mucociliary apparatus, contribute to "dependent settling" via gravity of bacteria into bronchi of dependent lung lobes, resulting in secondary bronchopneumonia. This damage results in an acute inflammatory response that further injures mucosae throughout the lung. *B. bronchiseptica* toxins may also disrupt phagocytosis and/or killing of bacteria by alveolar macrophages and neutrophils and suppress cellular and humoral immune responses. The bacterium can also invade epithelial cells, evade immunologic defense mechanisms, and establish a persistent infection.

Canine Distemper (Morbillivirus, Enveloped RNA Virus). The pathogenesis and mechanisms of injury in canine distemper as related to the respiratory system are discussed in the section on Viral Diseases of Organ Systems, Nervous System, Disorders of Dogs, Canine Distemper (Morbillivirus, Enveloped RNA Virus).

Canine Influenza (Orthomyxovirus, Enveloped RNA virus). The pathogenesis and mechanisms of injury in canine influenza are similar to those of equine influenza (see section on Viral Diseases of Organ Systems; Respiratory System, Mediastinum, and Pleurae; Disorders of Horses; Equine Influenza [Orthomyxovirus, Enveloped RNA Virus]).

Canine influenza virus (H3N8) was originally diagnosed in racing greyhounds in January 2004 at a track in Florida, and the virus subsequently spread to 11 other states with dog racing tracks. Canine influenza virus (H3N8) appears to have resulted from mutation of the viral genome (antigenic drift/shift) of equine influenza virus (H3N8). Recently an outbreak of canine influenza occurred in the winter/spring 2015 in northern Illinois and midwestern states. The virus subsequently spread to New England and other areas. This outbreak was caused by canine influenza virus H3N2, which was originally limited within Korea, China, and Thailand.

When a new viral strain such as canine influenza virus H3N8 arises through recombination, natural selection, or antigenic drift/shift of viral genes such as those from equine influenza virus H3N8, infected dogs are exposed to a variety of new viral proteins. Many of these proteins behave as "new" virulence factors providing the virus with increased pathogenicity and thus the ability to cause disease. Other proteins serve only as immunogens unique to influenza viruses. When a new strain of virus occurs, dogs have limited innate and no acquired immune responses to use as defense mechanisms. However, if the dog was vaccinated with a vaccine based the H3N8 viral strain, the immune response may provide some cross-protection to newly introduced viral strains such as canine influenza virus H3N2.

Disorders of Cats

Feline Upper Respiratory Disease Complex. Feline upper respiratory disease complex is a syndrome caused by feline viral rhinotracheitis virus and feline calicivirus acting concurrently and synergistically to cause disease. The mechanism of injury is dysfunction and lysis of ciliated epithelial cells of the mucociliary apparatus primarily from virus-induced cytolysis and secondarily from acute inflammation (bronchitis/bronchiolitis) and its mediators and degradative enzymes. The pathogenesis and mechanisms of injury for each virus are discussed in the next two sections.

Feline Viral Rhinotracheitis (Feline Herpesvirus, Alphaherpesvirus, Enveloped DNA Virus). The pathogenesis and mechanisms of injury in feline viral rhinotracheitis are similar to those of infectious bovine rhinotracheitis and equine viral rhinopneumonitis discussed earlier. Additionally, virus also infects mucosal macrophages and spreads to and infects similar cells in regional lymphoid nodes and then systemically via leukocyte trafficking or cell-free viremia to infect bone, eye, and lung, resulting in lysis of osteoblasts and osteocytes in the turbinates, necrosis of conjunctival and corneal epithelial cells, and necrosis of alveolar macrophages, respectively. Viral envelope glycoprotein G has been shown to attach and bind to chemokine receptors on target cells.

Feline Calicivirus (Calicivirus, Nonenveloped RNA Virus). The pathogenesis and mechanisms of injury in feline calicivirus infection are similar to those of feline viral rhinotracheitis, infectious bovine rhinotracheitis, and equine viral rhinopneumonitis discussed earlier. Although the mechanism of injury is probably necrosis and cell lysis, experimental studies have suggested that synthesis of caspases can be induced in virus-infected cells, resulting in apoptosis of these cells. Virus infects and replicates in mucosal epithelial cells and likely mucosal macrophages and then spreads in lymphatic vessels to regional lymph nodes via leukocyte trafficking (or cell-free viremia) to infect additional lymphocytes and macrophages. These cells then spread virus systemically to infect synovial macrophages and pulmonary alveolar macrophages, leading to synovitis and probably interstitial pneumonia, respectively. Ligand-receptor interactions are likely involved in tropism for specific cell types. It is unclear whether interstitial pneumonia (1) results from inhalation and infection of apical membranes of mucosal epithelial cells and alveolar macrophages of mucosae of the conductive and O_2-CO_2 exchange components of the respiratory system, (2) is the result of leukocyte trafficking of virus-infected lymphocytes, macrophages, and monocytes back to the lung after infecting and being amplified in regional and systemic lymph nodes and lymphoid organs, or (3) is attributable to a combination of both mechanisms.

A syndrome termed *virulent systemic feline calicivirus infection* has been characterized clinically. In addition to epithelial cell tropism, this virulent strain has acquired tropism for endothelial cells. It causes systemic vascular injury, lysis of endothelial cells, microthrombosis, and disseminated intravascular coagulation, resulting in multiple–organ system failure. This change in viral pathogenicity likely occurred through reassortment of viral capsid genes (antigenic shift) leading to enhanced virulence factors that modulate attachment and entry and likely replication in endothelial cells. Furthermore, an additional virulence factor appears to contribute to an exuberant target cell cytokine response as a defense mechanism against virus-infected epithelial and endothelial cells. Thus vascular lesions may in part be immune mediated and worsened by the actions of cytokines.

Cardiovascular System and Lymphatic Vessels

Disorders of Horses

Equine Viral Arteritis (Arterivirus, Enveloped RNA Virus). The mechanism of injury in equine viral arteritis is lysis of endothelial cells, myocytes, and pericytes of small muscular arterioles and venules of multiple organ systems, especially of the lungs. Gross lesions include (1) congestion, edema, and hemorrhage in subcutaneous tissues of the limbs and abdomen; (2) hydroperitoneum, hydropericardium, and hydroabdomen; and (3) edema and hemorrhage in lymph nodes and intestines.

Horses inhale virus in fomites of body fluids, most commonly urine, through direct contact with virus-infected animals. It is deposited on mucosae of the conductive and O_2-CO_2 exchange systems through centrifugal and inertial turbulence and trapped in the mucus layer. Virus is likely phagocytosed by bronchiolar and alveolar macrophages as they migrate through the mucus layer and mucosae and spread locally through leukocyte trafficking to the submucosa (BALT), where they infect additional tissue macrophages. From here macrophages spread virus to regional lymph nodes via afferent lymphatic vessels, where additional macrophages are infected. Ligand-receptor interactions are probably involved in tropism for specific cell types. Virus expresses envelope glycoproteins and a nucleocapsid protein; however, their role in binding to target cells has not been clearly defined. Additionally, membrane receptors for the virus have not been identified. Macrophages leave regional lymph nodes and enter the circulatory system via postcapillary venules or lymphatic vessels and the thoracic duct. During vascular migration, infected macrophages encounter endothelial cells, myocytes, and pericytes of small arterioles (and venules), and their interactions are facilitated by molecules of the leukocyte adhesion cascade (see Chapter 3). Monocytes containing viral antigens have been observed adhering to endothelial cells, and virus appears to spread from monocytes to endothelial cells, myocytes, and pericytes of these vessels.

Migrating monocytes also encounter and infect hepatocytes, adrenal cortical cells, seminiferous tubular cells, and thyroid follicular cells. Virus-induced vascular injury leads to cell lysis characterized by endothelial swelling, degeneration, and necrosis, acute and chronic (lymphomonocytic) inflammation, necrosis of myocytes, and thrombus formation, leading to edema and hemorrhage in many tissues and organs. Virus replication occurs in endothelial cells, and the expression of envelope glycoproteins in endothelial cells likely activates acute inflammation, fibrinogenesis, the complement cascade, and the recruitment of neutrophils into vascular intima and tunica media and in severe cases results in fibrinoid necrosis and vasculitis. The role of proinflammatory chemokines and cytokines in vascular injury has not been defined. A lymphomonocytic inflammatory cell population is also commonly found in the tunica media and adventitia of blood vessels, suggesting that cytolytic T lymphocytes could induce cytolysis of virus-infected endothelial cells. Why lysis of endothelial cells and myocytes dominates over lysis of epithelial cells, such as those in renal tubules, is unknown. However, infection and lysis of renal tubular epithelial cells with release of virus into urine appear to be the mechanism by which virus is spread to naïve horses.

African Horse Sickness (Orbivirus, Nonenveloped RNA Virus). The pathogenesis and mechanism of injury in African horse sickness

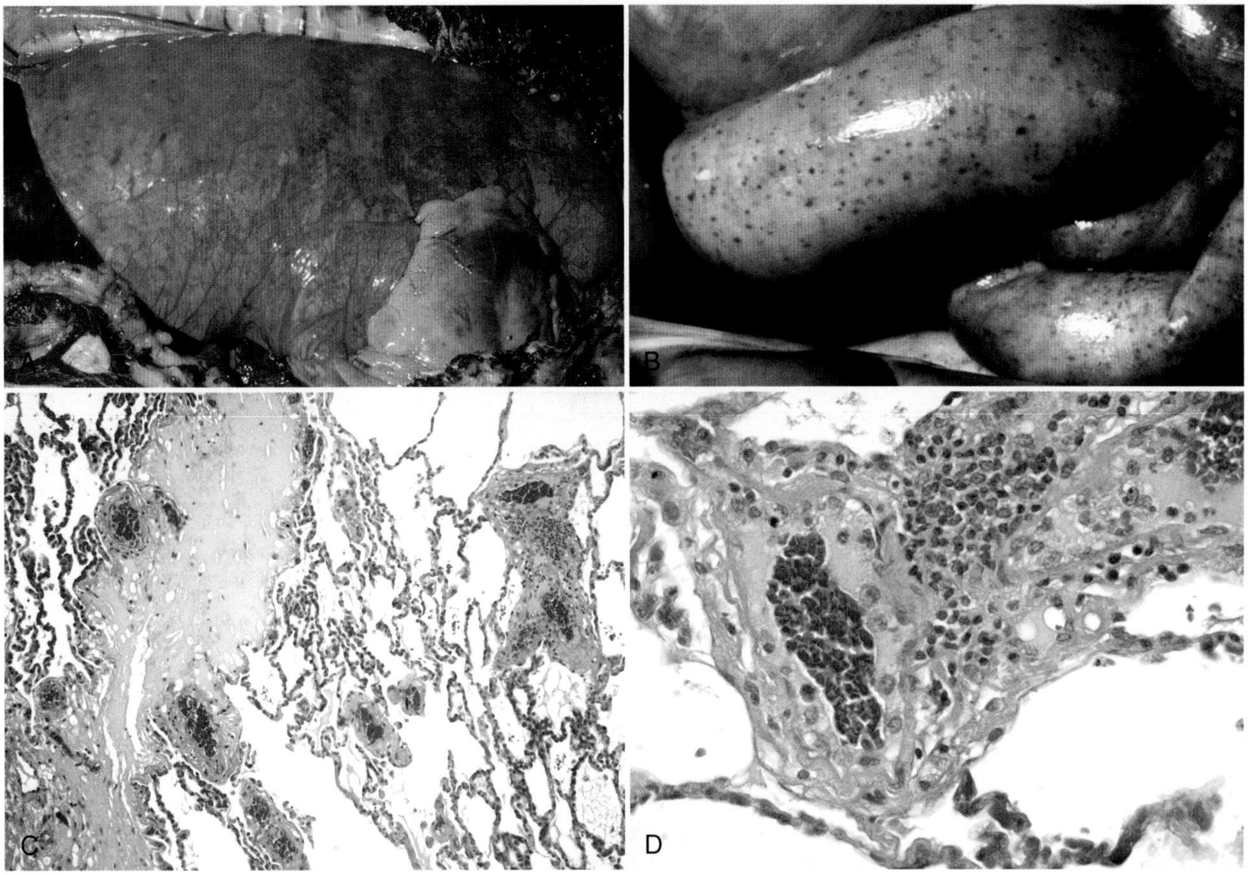

Figure 4-40 **African Horse Sickness. A,** Pulmonary edema. The interlobular septa are widely separated and distended with edema fluid. Edema fluid is also present in alveoli and alveolar septa. Also note the suffusive hemorrhage of the visceral pleura. These lesions are caused by infection of endothelial cells of the capillaries of the interlobular and alveolar septa by African horse sickness virus, resulting in endothelial cell barrier malfunction and lysis of endothelial cells. **B,** Colonic serosa, petechial and ecchymotic hemorrhages. These lesions are also caused by infection of and damage to endothelial cells. **C,** Lung, interlobular edema. The interlobular septum and alveoli contain edema fluid. Capillaries and venules are surrounded by bronchial-associated lymphoid tissue (BALT). H&E stain. **D,** Higher magnification of **C.** The endothelial cells of venules are swollen, have vacuolated and reticulated cytoplasm, and have large reactive nuclei consistent with responses to injury caused by infection of these cells by African horse sickness virus. Note the BALT. H&E stain. (**A** courtesy Dr. D. Gregg, Plum Island Animal Disease Center; and Noah's Arkive, College of Veterinary Medicine, The University of Georgia. **B** courtesy Dr. R. Breeze, Plum Island Animal Disease Center; and Noah's Arkive, College of Veterinary Medicine, The University of Georgia. **C** and **D** courtesy Dr. J.F. Zachary, College of Veterinary Medicine, University of Illinois.)

are similar to those of bluetongue disease discussed later. The mechanism of injury is endothelial cell barrier dysfunction and virus-induced dysfunction and lysis of endothelial cells. There are four clinical forms of African horse sickness; however, in each form the gross lesions are characteristic of vascular (endothelial cell) injury and include edema (pulmonary, systemic, subcutaneous, intramuscular, supraorbital fossae, eyelids, lips, cheeks, tongue, intermandibular space, and larynx), active hyperemia, petechial and ecchymotic hemorrhages (serosal [epicardial, endocardial], subcapsular [spleen], cortical [kidney], and mucosal [intestines]), hydrothorax, hydropericardium, ascites, and rhabdomyocytic necrosis (Fig. 4-40). The expression of these forms may be related to differences in viral tropism for different types of vascular endothelial cells within organ systems of the body or the permissiveness of different types of endothelial cells in allowing the virus to replicate efficiently or in large numbers. African horse sickness virus also infects cells of the dendritic, lymphoid, and monocyte-macrophage systems.

African horse sickness is a noncontagious disease of horses, donkeys, and mules. Animals encounter virus in bite wounds from midges. After skin penetration, virus can enter the circulatory system or be deposited in vascularized ECM (connective) tissues. If a blood vessel is penetrated, virus can enter the circulatory system and infect macrophages and lymphocytes or be carried cell-free to systemic lymphoid tissues. If deposited in connective tissue, virus gains access to cutaneous blood and fluids, as well as cutaneous dendritic cells (Langerhans cells) and tissue macrophages. Although unproved, it is likely that virus infects these cells, and virus-infected macrophages or dendritic cells spread the virus via leukocyte trafficking and lymphatic vessels to regional lymph nodes. Here virus infects lymphocytes and additional dendritic cells and macrophages. African horse sickness virus has two attachment proteins, capsid structural proteins (VP2 and VP5). These proteins bind to glycosaminoglycans on target cell membranes and facilitate attachment and entry of virus.

From regional lymph nodes, virus spreads systemically in macrophages via leukocyte trafficking to the circulatory system, through postcapillary venules and/or lymphatic vessels and the thoracic duct, to infect, injure, and kill vascular endothelial cells in the lungs, heart, spleen, lymph nodes, liver, and kidney. Infected macrophages likely interact with endothelial cells of these organs by adhering to and migrating through the endothelium, likely by activating the leukocyte adhesion cascade (see Chapter 3). Virus spreads from macrophages and infects and replicates in endothelial cells, resulting in direct injury and inducing an acute inflammatory response.

Vascular lesions are probably lytic and characterized by endothelial swelling, degeneration, and necrosis, and depending on the severity of injury, vasculitis can be followed by hemorrhage and edema (increased vascular permeability) affecting the lung and vascular thrombosis leading to tissue infarction. Necrosis of rhabdomyocytes in the heart has been attributed to the release of endogenous catecholamines, but experimental findings suggest that necrosis is caused by microthrombosis of myocardial capillaries, likely resulting in myocyte ischemia. Rarely, disseminated intravascular coagulation has been reported in African horse sickness. Additionally, NS3, a protein inserted in the target cell membrane by the virus, may be cytotoxic (acting as a viroporin that alters target cell membrane permeability) and involved in membrane damage and the release of virus from infected endothelial cells.

Disorders of Ruminants (Cattle, Sheep, and Goats)

Bluetongue (Orbivirus, Nonenveloped RNA Virus). The mechanism of injury in bluetongue is dysfunction and lysis of endothelial cells. Gross lesions include systemic hemorrhage, edema, and vasculitis. Such lesions are more severe in sheep when compared to cattle, apparently because there are species differences in the susceptibility of endothelial cells to infection and the severity of endothelial injury. Bluetongue is a noncontagious disease of sheep, cattle, and other ruminants (deer). The virus is encountered in fluids from hematophagous *Culicoides* (biting midges), which is the insect vector for the virus. After skin penetration, virus gains access to cutaneous blood and fluids, as well as cutaneous dendritic cells (Langerhans cells), monocytes, and tissue macrophages. Although unproved, virus probably infects these cells, and virus-infected monocytes and macrophages migrate to local lymph nodules and/or lymphoid aggregates, then to regional lymph nodes via afferent lymphatic vessels. Here virus infects lymphocytes and additional dendritic cells, monocytes, and macrophages. Macrophages then enter the blood vascular and lymphatic systems (blood vascular via the thoracic duct) and migrate in the vascular system to all organ systems. There they adhere to, migrate through, and reside in the walls of blood vessels and thus are in direct contact with endothelial cells. Virus lyses and escapes from these macrophages and binds to receptors on endothelial cells.

Bluetongue virus has two attachment proteins, capsid structural proteins (VP2 and VP5). These proteins bind to glycosaminoglycans in target cell membranes and facilitate attachment and penetration of virus into macrophages and likely into endothelial cells. Systemically the attachment of virus-infected macrophages to endothelial cells is likely facilitated by molecules of the leukocyte adhesion cascade (see Chapter 3). Virus in infected monocytes/macrophages that attach to endothelial cells escape (via cell lysis) from these monocytes/macrophages and adhere to, infect, and replicate in endothelial cells, leading to increased permeability of the endothelium as well as to endothelial cell injury and lysis (necrosis-vasculitis). Changes in permeability may also be attributable, in part, to the production of vasoactive cytokines such as TNF-α by virus-infected monocytes/macrophages, leading to increased permeability of the vascular endothelium. With excessive leakage of fluids, hypovolemic (circulatory) shock may occur. Finally, depending on the severity of endothelial cell injury, vasculitis can be followed by hemorrhage and edema affecting the lung and by vascular thrombosis leading to oral mucosal ulcerations, tissue infarction, and disseminated intravascular coagulation, which can kill the affected animal.

Bovine Malignant Catarrhal Fever (Ovine Herpesvirus 2 and Alcelaphine Herpesvirus 1 [γ-Herpesviruses], Enveloped DNA Virus). The mechanism of injury in bovine malignant catarrhal fever is dysfunction and lysis of vascular endothelial cells and hyperplasia, dysfunction, and lysis of lymphocytes in lymphoid tissues. Gross lesions include (1) erosive, ulcerative, and hemorrhagic lesions of mucosae of gingiva, tongue, oral papillae, hard and soft palate, oral pharynx, esophagus, turbinates, trachea, rumen, reticulum, and omasum (see Fig. 7-35); (2) enlargement of lymphoid organs and tissues followed by atrophy; and (3) increased size of visceral organs and tissues resulting from perivascular accumulations of lymphocytes (lymphoproliferative vasculitis).

Worldwide, sheep are the reservoir animal for sheep-associated ovine herpesvirus 2 (OvHV-2), which causes malignant catarrhal fever in cattle, bison, pigs, and deer. In Africa, blue wildebeest are the reservoir animal for wildebeest-associated alcelaphine herpesvirus 1 (AlHV-1), which causes malignant catarrhal fever in cattle. These viruses persist in carrier animals without ill effects.

The chronologic sequence of steps leading to malignant catarrhal fever has not been clearly determined. Animals probably encounter these viruses through inhalation and ingestion of fomites from oronasal-pharyngeal-ocular fluids (also seminal fluid) from reservoir animals that are actively shedding virus. In reservoir animals, OvHV-2 is shed predominantly through nasal secretions derived from turbinates, and shedding episodes are stress induced and occur more frequently in lambs than adult sheep. Virus is deposited on mucosae of the oral, nasal, and pharyngeal cavities; the conjunctiva; or the conductive component of the respiratory system through centrifugal and inertial turbulence. It is trapped in the mucus layer and apparently phagocytosed by mucosal macrophages and spread to submucosae and BALT via leukocyte trafficking. It has not been determined if dendritic cells are involved. In submucosae, virus infects lymphocytes (possibly B lymphocytes), macrophages, and monocytes and spreads in $CD8^+$ T lymphocytes via leukocyte trafficking to regional lymph nodes and then systemically to other organ systems and lymphoid tissues. Ligand-receptor interactions are probably involved in tropism for specific cell types, but viral envelope glycoproteins or cell receptors have not been identified.

Virus-infected $CD8^+$ T lymphocytes are distributed in intimal, medial, and adventitial tissues of blood vessels (vascular and perivascular pattern) in organ systems. This tropism may be determined by (1) ligand-receptor interactions or (2) permissiveness of specific vascular cells to viral infection and replication. As part of this tropism, virus-infected $CD8^+$ T lymphocytes produce proinflammatory cytokines and express viral glycoproteins in their cell membranes. Proinflammatory cytokines can act as cytotoxic molecules and may injure and kill bystander cells, such as those in the vasculature, and viral glycoproteins may recruit lymphocytes, macrophages, and monocytes and lesser numbers of neutrophils and plasma cells into perivascular and vascular tissues, leading to lymphoproliferative necrotizing vasculitis and vascular wall necrosis. It is not known if virus can infect, injure, and kill endothelial cells directly. The cause of the erosive, ulcerative, and hemorrhagic lesions has not been determined; however, infarction of mucosal blood vessels secondary to thrombosis induced by necrotizing vasculitis could potentially lead to these outcomes. Additionally, virus-infected large granular lymphocytes and other recruited cytotoxic lymphocytes and macrophages may play roles in vascular injury because they have been shown to be cytotoxic for vascular endothelial cells.

Atrophy of lymphoid tissues after viral infection is not likely caused by virus-induced cell lysis. Because lymphocytes are short-lived effector cells, atrophy is likely the result of normal cell aging and turnover that follows massive proliferation.

Apparently there is a lack of spread of virus between susceptible animals because they are dead-end hosts for these viruses. Virus spread appears to require cell-free virus in body fluids, and in

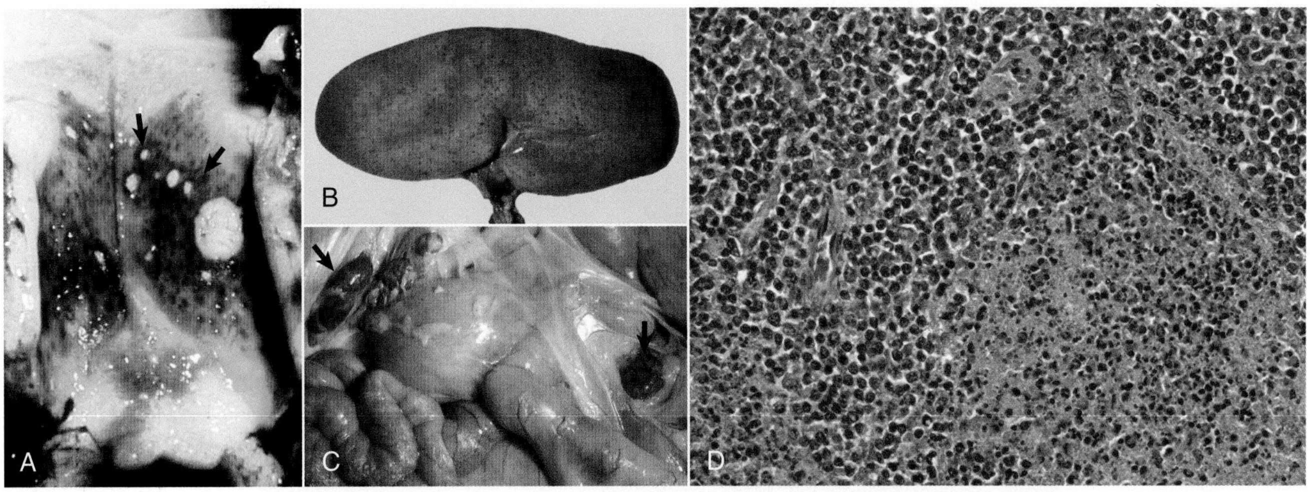

Figure 4-41 Classic Swine Fever (Hog Cholera). Lesions in classic swine fever are similar to those observed in African swine fever, but usually less severe. See Figure 4-42 for lesions of African swine fever. **A,** The tonsil (of the soft palate), a tissue of choice for isolation and identification of the virus, contains foci of hemorrhage and necrosis *(arrows)*, the result of necrosis of mucosal epithelial cells in tonsillar crypts and necrosis of the adjacent endothelial cells and lymphocytes in the lamina propria from infection with virus. **B,** Kidney. The cortical surface has numerous randomly distributed petechia caused by injury to and subsequent necrosis of endothelial cells following their infection with classic swine fever virus. **C,** Mesenteric lymph nodes *(arrows)* are enlarged and congested due to vascular injury caused by virus, resulting in blood in the subcapsular sinuses. **D,** Tonsillar crypt lymphoid nodules. Note the focal necrosis of lymphocytes *(right lower half of image)* in the nodules caused by infection with virus. H&E stain. (**A** courtesy Dr. R. Breeze, Plum Island Animal Disease Center; and Noah's Arkive, College of Veterinary Medicine, The University of Georgia. **B** courtesy Dr. D. Gregg, Plum Island Animal Disease Center and Noah's Arkive, College of Veterinary Medicine, The University of Georgia. **C** courtesy Dr. M.D. McGavin, College of Veterinary Medicine, University of Tennessee. **D** courtesy Dr. J.F. Zachary, College of Veterinary Medicine, University of Illinois.)

susceptible animals the virus replicates in a cell-associated manner (lymphocytes, macrophages, monocytes) and cell-free virus is not produced. Because virus-infected target cells do not produce infectious virus during the virus replication cycle, these species are unable to transmit virus to other animals (see carrier animals earlier).

Disorders of Pigs

Classic Swine Fever (Hog Cholera, Pestivirus, Enveloped RNA Virus). The mechanism of injury in classic swine fever is probably cytokine-induced dysfunction and lysis of endothelial cells of multiple organ systems, of macrophages and monocytes, and of hemopoietic cells in the bone marrow. Gross lesions include a red-blue discoloration of the skin; hydropericardium, hydrothorax, and hydroperitoneum; hemorrhage and necrosis of the palatine tonsil; and petechial and ecchymotic hemorrhages in most organs of the body, especially the kidney (Fig. 4-41).

Pigs encounter virus through (1) ingestion and likely inhalation of fomites from body fluids, body waste, or offal or other virus-contaminated pork products and (2) mechanical transfer from virus-contaminated vehicles, clothes/boots, instruments, and needles. Virus is deposited on mucosae of the oral and nasal pharynx, especially of the tonsil, where it infects and replicates in epithelial cells of tonsillar crypts. It has not been determined how virus penetrates the mucus layer to gain access to mucosal epithelial cells or if mucosal macrophages or dendritic cells phagocytose virus in the mucus layer and spread it through leukocyte trafficking to the lamina propria and submucosa. E^{rns} and E2 envelope glycoproteins and other viral envelope glycoproteins appear to be involved in binding to and entering mucosal epithelial cells and macrophages via cell surface glycosaminoglycan receptors such as heparin sulfate. Although unknown, virus likely buds from basal surfaces of tonsillar epithelial cells and infects subjacent mucosal macrophages in lymphoid aggregates (MALT). Infected macrophages migrate via leukocyte trafficking in afferent lymphatic vessels to regional lymph nodes such as the submandibular and pharyngeal. Here, through release of proinflammatory chemokines and cytokines, they likely recruit additional macrophages (i.e., monocytes) from the systemic circulation and also cause lymphoid hyperplasia in affected lymph nodes and lymphoid tissues. Virus-infected macrophages provide virus to infect these additional macrophages and lymphocytes. In addition to enlargement from hyperplasia, lymph nodes become edematous and hemorrhagic because of endothelial cell injury within capillaries caused by the actions of cytokines and mediators of acute inflammation (see later) initiated and modulated by virus-infected tissue macrophages.

Subsequently, virus-infected macrophages leave regional lymph nodes and enter the circulatory system via postcapillary venules or lymphatic vessels and the thoracic duct to migrate systemically to all organ systems. Infected macrophages probably interact with endothelial cells of all organs by adhering to and migrating into and through the endothelium, likely via cytokines (TNF-α and IL-1) and activation of the leukocyte adhesion cascade (see Chapter 3). Initially, lysis of endothelial cells was thought to be caused by viral replication in these cells; however, it is now thought that lysis is attributable to the effects of cytokines released from macrophages. Viral replication in macrophages (and lymphocytes) appears to result in the production and release of large amounts of proinflammatory cytokines into the ECM subjacent to endothelial cells from intact or lysed macrophages. This outcome results in injury to and lysis of endothelial cells by these cytokines and/or by mediators and degradative enzymes of the acute inflammatory response that ensues. Additionally, vascular lesions are characterized by endothelial swelling, degeneration, and necrosis (cytolysis); acute and chronic (lymphomonocytic) inflammation; necrosis of myocytes; and thrombus formation, leading to edema and hemorrhage in many tissues and organs. This pattern of injury serves as the basis for hemorrhage observed grossly and microscopically in lesions of the kidney.

Macrophages also spread virus to lymphoid tissues (spleen and lymph nodes) and bone marrow, where it either infects and lyses these cells or causes lysis via an apoptotic mechanism or a cytokine,

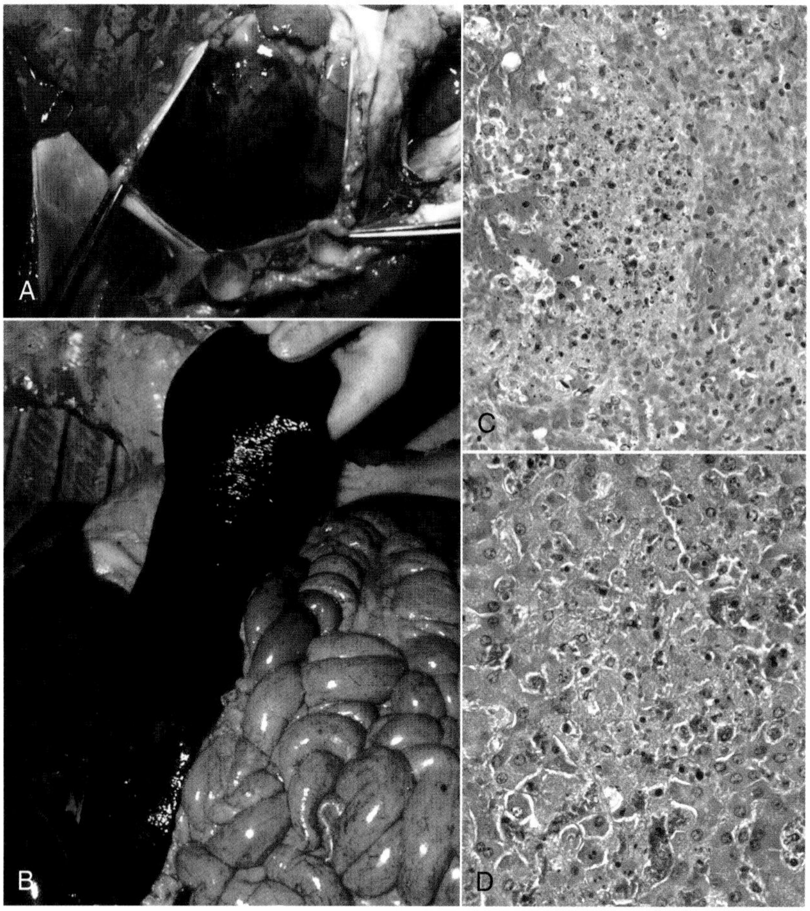

Figure 4-42 **African Swine Fever.** Lesions in African swine fever are similar to those observed in classic swine fever, but usually much more severe. See Figure 4-41 for lesions of classic swine fever. **A,** Epicardium and pericardial cavity. The epicardium and subjacent myocardium have numerous randomly distributed ecchymoses caused by injury to and subsequent necrosis of endothelial cells from infection with African swine fever virus. Note the accumulation of a fibrinous effusion in the pericardial cavity. **B,** Splenomegaly, bloody spleen. The spleen is congested with blood and friable as a result of vascular damage caused by the virus. Lymph nodes (not shown here) are also congested and edematous (see classic swine fever). **C,** Endothelial cells and lymphoid cells of white pulp of the spleen are necrotic (e.g., pyknosis, karyolysis). H&E stain. **D,** Endothelial cells lining sinusoids of the liver are necrotic (e.g., pyknosis, karyolysis). Also note the necrosis of some hepatocytes. H&E stain. (**A** courtesy Dr. C. Brown, College of Veterinary Medicine, The University of Georgia. **B** courtesy Dr. D. Gregg, Plum Island Animal Disease Center; and Noah's Arkive, College of Veterinary Medicine, The University of Georgia. **C** and **D** courtesy Dr. J.F. Zachary, College of Veterinary Medicine, University of Illinois.)

resulting in severely impaired adaptive immune responses with decreased neutralizing antibody production, decreased numbers of phagocytes, decreased cell-mediated immune responses, and decreased numbers of platelets. Virus also probably causes severe loss of monocytes, macrophages, and lymphocytes in all organ systems via cell lysis and apoptosis induced by proinflammatory cytokines. The impairment and loss of these defense mechanisms makes pigs more susceptible to other infectious diseases.

African Swine Fever (Asfivirus, Enveloped DNA Virus). The pathogenesis, mechanisms of injury, and clinical outcomes of African swine fever are very similar to those of classic swine fever discussed in the previous section. In summary, the pathogenicity (virulence factors) of lesions and disease caused by African swine fever virus are much more severe (Fig. 4-42). Additionally, African swine fever virus can also gain access to the blood vascular system and directly infect macrophages through bites of ticks. Virus envelope glycoproteins p12, p54, and p30 appear to be involved in attaching and binding to and entering target cells via cell receptors. Target cell receptors have not been clearly identified. Cytokines released from macrophages are probably the cause of lysis of endothelial cells in all organ systems, resulting in vasculitis, systemic petechial and ecchymotic hemorrhages, disseminated intravascular coagulation, collapse of the circulatory system, shock, and death of virus-infected pigs.

Disorders of Dogs

Parvovirus Myocarditis (Parvovirus, Nonenveloped DNA Virus). See the section on Viral Diseases of Organ Systems; Alimentary System and the Peritoneum, Omentum, Mesentery, and Peritoneal Cavity; Disorders of Dogs; Parvovirus Enteritis (Parvovirus, Nonenveloped DNA Virus) for information on the pathogenesis of viral spread and replication before spreading to the heart. The mechanism of injury in parvovirus myocarditis is cell lysis (necrosis of rhabdomyocytes) attributable to infection with virus. Gross lesions include gray-white areas of varied sizes distributed in the myocardium (see Fig. 10-81). It is likely that virus spreads via leukocyte trafficking or cell-free viremia in lymphatic or blood vessels from Peyer's patches to regional lymph nodes and then systemically in the circulatory system to capillary endothelial cells and rhabdomyocytes in the heart. Endothelial cells are dividing cells, and studies suggest that in the heart, virus initially infects and replicates in these cells and then spreads to infect contiguous cardiac rhabdomyocytes.

Rhabdomyocytes are also actively dividing cells in dogs under 15 days of age; therefore they can be infected with virus and are lysed with release of virus. This outcome results in necrosis of rhabdomyocytes and ectopic irritable foci, cardiac arrhythmias, and unexpected death of puppies. If puppies survive this stage, healing mechanisms cause cardiac fibrosis that can contribute clinically to dysfunction of the cardiac conduction system and contraction of the cardiac musculature later in life. Specificity for these mitotically active cells occurs because parvoviruses require a target cell–derived duplex transcription template, which is available only when cells divide during the S phase of the cell cycle (see the section on parvovirus enteritis for more detail). Ligand-receptor interactions are also probably involved, but unknown. It appears that canine transferrin receptor may need to present on target cells.

Canine Herpesvirus Infection (Canine Herpesvirus Type 1, Enveloped DNA Virus). The mechanism of injury in canine herpesvirus infection is lysis of endothelial cells of all organ systems and of epithelial cells of multiple organ systems (pantropic). Gross lesions include mucosal and serosal hemorrhage and randomly distributed white-gray foci (≈1 mm in diameter) of miliary necrosis within organ systems, especially the kidneys (see Fig. 11-67). Miliary necrosis can also be observed in spleen, lymph nodes, lung, and liver.

Puppies ingest and inhale virus in fomites from body fluids of the birth canal or nasal-oral cavity of bitches through grooming. It is deposited on mucosae of the nasal and oral pharynx, especially those of the tonsil, and is thought to infect mucosal epithelial cells. It has not been determined if and how virus penetrates the mucus layer to gain access to mucosal epithelial cells. Although it appears that virus infects lymphocytes in the tonsil, it has not been determined if and how virus spreads from mucosal epithelial cells to lymphocytes or if leukocyte trafficking via mucosa-associated macrophages or dendritic cells is involved. It is also unclear if or how virus migrates to regional or systemic lymphoid nodes, thymus, or spleen before it spreads systemically to infect endothelial and epithelial cells of other organ systems; however, virus appears to be spread systemically in lymphocytes via leukocyte trafficking. It has not been satisfactorily determined (1) how virus-infected lymphocytes interact with endothelial and epithelial cells or if this interaction is facilitated by molecules of the leukocyte adhesion cascade (see Chapter 3); (2) how virus infects and replicates in endothelial cells, leading to injury and cell lysis; and (3) if injury results in vasculitis and vascular thrombosis, leading to tissue infarction and disseminated intravascular coagulation. Additionally, the potential role of cytokines, derived from virus-infected lymphocytes or macrophages, in causing or contributing to endothelial cell injury and lysis has not been determined. Canine herpesvirus expresses envelope glycoproteins B, C, and D; however, their role in attaching and binding to target cells has not been clearly defined. Heparin sulfate may serve as a target cell receptor for canine herpesvirus. The disease is most severe in puppies less than 5 weeks of age; it is thought that low body temperatures of puppies increases the pathogenicity of the virus by improving its ability to enter cells, replicate, and spread.

Canine Circovirus Infection (Circovirus, Nonenveloped DNA Virus). This disorder of dogs was first recognized in the fall of 2013 in Ohio. Its mechanism of injury and pathogenesis are unknown; however, gross lesions characterized by a fibrinonecrotic vasculitis suggest that vascular endothelial cells are one of its target cells. Review of the earlier discussion of canine herpesvirus infection may be useful. It is unclear if this virus is the primary cause of this disorder or if it is the result of coinfection with other pathogens such as canine enteric coronavirus or one of six other pathogens.

Disorders of Cats

Feline Infectious Peritonitis (Feline Enteric Coronavirus/Feline Infectious Peritonitis Virus, Enveloped RNA Virus). A presumed mutation (antigenic drift/shift) of the 3c gene of feline enteric coronavirus genome appears to result in a "new" virulence form (biotype) virus, feline infectious peritonitis virus that causes feline infectious peritonitis (FIP). This mutation, which is thought to occur within mucosal macrophages and/or blood monocytes, seems to inhibit or block function(s) of the 3c gene, allowing the mutated virus to assume greater pathogenicity by enhancing cell tropism for and internalization and replication in macrophages. The mechanism of injury is chronic-active pyogranulomatous inflammation (vasculitis and perivasculitis) and its mediators and degradative enzymes. Gross lesions include gray-white nodules of varied sizes that have a perivascular pattern of distribution and in some cases a linear pattern following blood vessels in serosa and mesenteries (see Figs. 7-16, 11-68, and 14-105). Body cavities may contain a thick yellow exudate containing fibrin and pyogranulomatous inflammatory cells (see Fig. 7-16).

Cats encounter feline enteric coronavirus by ingestion of virus-contaminated fomites through two routes: (1) contact with virus-contaminated feces in litter boxes and (2) contact with carrier cats, usually queens. Fomites from saliva or respiratory droplets probably serve as a source of the virus to infect naïve cats via ingestion; therefore grooming behavior increases the likelihood that virus will enter the oral cavity. Feline enteric coronavirus is swallowed and moved via intestinal peristalsis to the alimentary system, where it gains access to mucosae. The replication of enteric coronavirus is primarily restricted to mature intestinal epithelial cells (terminally differentiated cells with a life span of 3 to 8 days); however, the virus can enter a carrier state and persist in unidentified cells of the intestinal mucosa. These cells are likely progenitor cells (i.e., crypt stem cells) with infinite life spans, so cell lysis through normal enterocyte turnover does not affect the carrier state of the virus. Feline enteric coronavirus spreads from enterocytes and carrier cells into the lamina propria and then to macrophages in Peyer's patches. It has not been determined if and how virus penetrates the mucus layer to gain access to mucosal epithelial cells or if mucosal macrophages, dendritic cells, or M cells are involved. Leukocyte trafficking to the submucosa by these cells would explain how virus spreads to macrophages in Peyer's patches.

Feline enteric coronavirus likely uses proteins, such as S1 protein, and potentially other glycoproteins such as S2, M, and E, to attach and bind to feline aminopeptidase-*N*, a cell membrane receptor on monocytes and macrophages. Other less well characterized attachment proteins and target cell receptors have been described in other strains of mutated virus. In mucosal macrophages of Peyer's patches and in blood monocytes, feline enteric coronavirus mutates into feline infectious peritonitis virus. Thus the genome of each new feline infectious peritonitis virus variant is unique to an individual cat. When feline enteric coronavirus mutates to feline infectious peritonitis virus, feline infectious peritonitis virus acquires virulence factors that allow it to infect and replicate in cells of the monocyte-macrophage system, resulting in rapid dissemination of the virus throughout the body.

Monocytes and macrophages infected with feline infectious peritonitis virus spread from Peyer's patches to regional lymph nodes via leukocyte trafficking in lymphatic vessels and infect additional macrophages. They then migrate in efferent lymphatic vessels through the thoracic duct into the circulatory system and to all tissues of the body and infect additional populations of free and fixed tissue macrophages. Virus-infected macrophages appear to target small and medium-sized veins of serosal membranes and tissues, cause damage to endothelial cells, and are recognized as foreign by the cat's innate (inflammation) and adaptive (cell-mediated and humoral) defense mechanisms (see Chapters 3 and 5). This process likely involves activation of the leukocyte adhesion cascade and binding of macrophages and monocytes to endothelial cells facilitated by ligand-receptor interactions and the activation of acute inflammation via proinflammatory cytokines released from activated macrophages and monocytes. All of these processes result in injury of vascular and perivascular tissues (vasculitis).

Cats with a strong cell-mediated response do not develop feline infectious peritonitis. Cats with a weak cell-mediated response have the dry (noneffusive) form; cats with no cell-mediated response have the wet form (effusive). An effective humoral response appears to increase the severity of disease. Tissue macrophages provide a source of viral antigens in and around venules, and if adequate antibody is present, antigen-antibody complexes form and a type III hypersensitivity response ensues. Where immune complexes are formed (i.e., basement membrane of endothelial cells) or whether they are free or cell associated is not clearly understood. These complexes activate complement, resulting in chemotaxis and accumulation of neutrophils via the leukocyte adhesion cascade. Additionally, they also activate tissue macrophages, leading to the secretion of a variety of proinflammatory cytokines that act on endothelial cells to increase neutrophil and mononuclear cell chemotaxis into the area and open tight junctions of endothelial cells (increased permeability), thereby allowing leakage of plasma and fibrin into body cavities. These mechanisms result in the vasocentric pyogranulomas and pyogranulomatous inflammation, fibrinous effusions, and fibrinous polyserositis (feline coronaviral polyserositis) so characteristic of feline infectious peritonitis. A type IV hypersensitivity reaction may be involved in the pathogenesis of some pyogranulomas. It appears that the commonly used categories of wet and dry forms and type III and type IV hypersensitivities are based more on clinical characteristics and immunologic tests, respectively, than on any morphologic criteria. Experimental studies have shown that there are no distinct histopathologic lesions that distinguish wet from dry cases, type III from type IV hypersensitivities, or acute/subacute cases from chronic cases.

Bone Marrow, Blood Cells, and Lymphatic System

Disorders of Horses

Equine Infectious Anemia (Equine Infectious Anemia Virus, Enveloped RNA Virus). The mechanism of injury in equine infectious anemia (EIA) is inflammation (and proliferation [hypertrophy and hyperplasia]) of the monocyte-macrophage and lymphoid systems, particularly in the spleen and lymph nodes, resulting in chronic-active splenitis and lymphadenitis. Virus does not cause cell lysis. Gross lesions include an enlarged spleen (splenomegaly) and lymph nodes (lymphadenomegaly) with abundant white-gray lymphoid tissue arranged in follicles and solid sheets of cells that often bulge from cut surfaces.

Equine infectious anemia is a bloodborne infection. Horses initially encounter virus through penetrating wounds of the blood vascular system in the skin, either from fly (horseflies, deerflies) or mosquito bites or from contaminated needles. Once in the bloodstream, free virus infects monocytes (nonpermissive cells), but because they are not fully differentiated macrophages, virus cannot fully replicate. Thus monocytes spread virus in the circulatory system via leukocyte trafficking to all organ systems. Infected monocytes then migrate through blood vessel walls and enter ECM of tissues, where they differentiate into tissue macrophages (permissive cells). In these cells, virus can replicate and serve to infect other macrophages and lymphocytes, especially in lymphoid tissues such as spleen and lymph nodes. It appears the virus has several envelope glycoproteins such as surface envelope protein (gp120) and gp90 (and likely others) that attach and bind to equine lentivirus receptor-1 present in cell membranes of monocytes and macrophages. Infected macrophages produce proinflammatory chemokines and cytokines that recruit additional monocytes and lymphocytes into organs; thus splenomegaly and lymphadenomegaly ensue. Virus does not cause cell lysis.

The two clinical phases of equine infectious anemia are acute and chronic. In the acute phase, horses have recurring fever, anemia, thrombocytopenia, and petechia with interspersed periods of quiescence. Fever is likely attributable to release of proinflammatory cytokines and endogenous pyrogens from activated macrophages during the leukocyte trafficking phases of the disease. Anemia occurs from phagocytosis and complement-mediated lysis of erythrocytes that have had their cell membranes altered by virus, antibody, complement, and/or fibrinogen. Pulmonary intravascular macrophages, Kupffer cells, and fixed macrophages lining vascular sinusoids in the spleen and lymph nodes are reservoirs for virus and release it continuously into the bloodstream. Cell-free virus adsorbs onto the surface of red blood cells (and likely platelets) in the circulatory system. Adsorbed viral proteins act as haptens that are recognized as foreign by cells of the monocyte-macrophage system and are phagocytosed. Additionally, the hapten is processed and presented to lymphocytes, leading to a humoral immune response and the generation of plasma cells that secrete antibody against the hapten and other antigens on the red blood cell membrane (type II hypersensitivity response). If the hapten-antibody complex fixes complement, red blood cells are lysed intravascularly. If complement is not fixed, red blood cells are phagocytosed by cells of the monocyte-macrophage system and lysed extravascularly. Both of these mechanisms result in severe anemia. The cause of thrombocytopenia is less clear and is thought to occur because of activation of platelets and concurrent binding of fibrinogen to the surface of platelets during acute viremic phases of the disease. It is likely that activated platelets are quickly phagocytosed by the monocyte-macrophage system, leading to thrombocytopenia. Petechial hemorrhages may be attributable to vascular injury caused by direct infection of endothelial cells by virus or more likely by secondary responses to injury induced by innate and adaptive immune defense mechanisms.

In chronic equine infectious anemia, recurrence of disease is caused by antigenic variation (antigenic drift/shift) of surface glycoproteins of the virus. This genetic variation results in "new" virus that expresses new surface glycoproteins, thus beginning anew the process of developing effective cell-mediated and humoral responses. Long-lasting "immunity" to equine infectious anemia appears to require that an adaptive immune response control the disease before antigenic variation occurs. Large quantities of virus are replicated in cells of the monocyte-macrophage system, and virus is not eliminated from these cells during the acute phase of the disease. As adaptive immune responses develop, cytotoxic T lymphocytes are thought to control, to a limited extent, viremia and virus replication in infected monocytes and macrophages. However, it appears that control of the disease (no or minimal anemia and thrombocytopenia) is linked to an effective antibody response against the virus that takes 6 to 8 months to develop.

Disorders of Ruminants (Cattle, Sheep, and Goats)

Enzootic Bovine Lymphoma (Lymphosarcoma, Bovine Leukosis Virus–Associated Malignant Lymphoma, Deltaretrovirus: Bovine Leukemia Virus, Enveloped RNA Virus). The mechanism of injury in enzootic bovine lymphoma is provirus-induced malignant transformation of B lymphocytes. Gross lesions include proliferation of neoplastic cells and their infiltration into perivascular spaces in organ systems resulting in (1) generalized enlargement of affected organs with increased pallor or (2) the formation of one or more solid white nodules distributed at random in the affected tissue (see Figs. 7-90, 10-46, 10-47, 13-60, 13-87, and 13-88). Additionally, cells can occupy and proliferate in confined spaces, causing compressive atrophy of tissue in these spaces such as axons in the spinal cord, hemopoietic cells in the bone marrow, and the retina in the eye. Organ systems commonly having lesions include superficial and visceral lymph nodes and thymus, skin, abomasum, heart, spleen, kidneys, uterus (caruncles), spinal meninges, retrobulbar lymphatic tissue, bone, and bone marrow. Malignant transformation is a sequence of steps in which normal cells acquire the biologic behaviors of neoplastic cells such as uncontrolled growth, tissue invasion, and metastasis. In cattle it takes several years for this transformation to occur and be manifested in overt lymphoma. This long prodromal period is likely caused by the complexity and interplay of injurious and reparative processes induced by the provirus that eventually result in dysfunction or mutation of regulatory cell cycle genes. Bovine leukemia virus infects B lymphocytes and thus is not free as a virus in blood or body fluids but is a provirus, cell associated, and integrated into the target cell's genome. When its replication cycle is completed, new virus is released from provirus-infected B lymphocytes. New virus serves to sustain and amplify the infection by infecting naïve B lymphocytes and cells of the monocyte-macrophage system.

Cattle and calves encounter provirus-infected B lymphocytes in blood, inflammatory exudates, and colostrum or milk. Provirus-infected B lymphocytes must gain access to the blood vascular and/or lymphatic systems and eventually to tissues and target cells suitable for infection. When they gain access to tissues, it is unclear whether B lymphocytes (1) behave as trafficking leukocytes and migrate into the vascular and/or lymphatic systems to spread new virus to other cells and tissues or (2) undergo cytolysis and release virus into tissues to infect local tissue macrophages, lymphocytes, or dendritic cells such as Langerhans cells. The use of needles or surgical instruments contaminated with blood (provirus-infected B lymphocytes) can transfer these cells directly into the vascular system or place them in vascularized subcutaneous tissues or muscle in close proximity to capillary and lymphatic vascular beds. Such exposure may require traumatic injury to skin or mucous membranes. Insect bites can apparently result in the same outcome. In either case, provirus-infected B lymphocytes, deposited in these locations, encounter cells of the monocyte-macrophage and lymphoid systems and dendritic cells. It has been shown that virus can infect these cells, but whether these cells spread virus or provirus to regional lymph nodes and then systemically via leukocyte trafficking in these cells or in B lymphocytes is unknown.

Transplacental spread of bovine leukemia virus from cows to calves also occurs through the blood. Provirus-infected B lymphocytes can also be present in inflammatory exudates, such as those occurring with postpartum metritis or vaginitis, and must gain access to capillary and lymphatic beds in host animals as previously described. Finally, provirus-infected B lymphocytes can be present in colostrum or milk, and it has been suggested that enzootic bovine lymphoma can result from virus entering the body via the alimentary system and gaining access to the blood vascular system. However, the role, as examples, of alimentary peristalsis, gastric acidity, mucosal mucous barrier systems, mucosal epithelial barrier systems, mucosal immunity, and M cells has not been adequately addressed in experimental studies. Although hypothetical, provirus-infected B lymphocytes in colostrum or milk could behave as typical trafficking leukocytes and thereby attach to and migrate through mucosae of the oral and nasal pharynx and gain access to local MALTs, lymphatic vessels, regional lymph nodes, and systemic lymphoid tissues.

It appears that whatever route is used by provirus-infected B lymphocytes to enter the body, they must gain access to the blood vascular system to establish, sustain, and amplify an infection regionally and systemically. Virus uses bovine leukemia virus envelope glycoproteins (gp51, gp30) to attach to and enter naïve host B lymphocytes that express a novel membrane protein called *bovine leukemia virus–binding receptor*. Other studies have shown that B lymphocytes expressing surface immunoglobulin M and cell surface markers CD5 and CD11b are more susceptible to infection with virus; however, the role of these molecules as receptors is unclear.

The mechanism of B lymphocyte transformation has not been established. Transformation may be linked to a mechanism called *gene transactivation*. When the genome of bovine leukemia virus (provirus) is integrated into the genome of a B lymphocyte, the provirus asserts control over the transcriptional and translational organelles and processes of the target cell. Genes of bovine leukemia provirus express a protein called bovine leukemia virus Tax protein (p34tax) that appears to stimulate the proliferation (increased mitoses) of B lymphocytes and increases viral replication in target cells. Tax protein also interacts with target cell genes and appears to transactivate genes that express proteins modulating target cell growth, such as cell division and differentiation, and are involved in regulatory steps of cell proliferation and longevity. Experimentally, Tax protein has been shown to be able to immortalize rat embryo fibroblasts in tissue culture and to cooperate with an oncogene to transform tissue culture cells that can then be grown as tumors in live animals. Collectively these findings suggest that transformation of B lymphocytes, leading to bovine lymphoma, is linked to the likely long-term actions of p34tax on target cell regulatory genes, but the chronologic stages of transformation are uncertain. Studies suggest that transformation may also result from Tax protein forming complexes with proteins expressed by tumor-suppressor genes such as p53, whereas other studies suggest that point mutations in the p53 gene may be one of the critical steps leading to lymphoma. The proteins translated from tumor-suppressor genes have an inhibitory effect on the regulation of the cell cycle and function to inhibit cell division, inhibit division of cells with damaged DNA, initiate apoptosis of cells with damaged DNA, and amplify cell adhesion (metastasis suppressors). When the activities of the p53 gene and its protein gene products are perturbed or inhibited, transformation of affected cells could occur.

Disorders of Pigs

Postweaning Multisystemic Wasting Syndrome (Porcine Circovirus Type 2, Nonenveloped DNA Virus). The mechanism of injury in postweaning multisystemic wasting syndrome (PMWS) is virus-induced dysfunction and lysis of lymphocytes leading to lymphocyte depletion and immunosuppression. Virus appears to require dividing cells, like lymphocytes, in the S phase of the cell cycle for infection and replication. Gross lesions include systemic enlargement of lymph nodes, normal-sized lymph nodes, and small atrophic lymph nodes, which are a continuum of changes in the response of lymphocytes to viral infection, replication, and release. Initial infection is likely correlated with viral replication and intense hyperplasia (lymphadenomegaly). Hyperplasia is followed by release of virus from infected lymphocytes, a process that kills lymphocytes and results in atrophy. Microscopic lesions are unique in the fact that inflammation is granulomatous with macrophage-derived syncytial giant cells.

Pigs encounter virus in fomites from oronasal-pharyngeal body fluids, feces, and urine from infected animals. Virus is inhaled or ingested and deposited on mucosae. In the respiratory system, virus is deposited on and trapped in the mucus layer by centrifugal and inertial turbulence and encounters mucosa of the tonsils. It has not been determined if and how virus penetrates the mucus layer to gain access to mucosal epithelial cells, mucosal macrophages, and/or dendritic cells. In the alimentary system, it is swallowed, gains access to the small intestine through peristalsis, and encounters M cells overlying Peyer's patches. M cells lack a mucus layer, and virus has direct access to cell membranes.

It appears that virus establishes an infection in lymphoid tissues of the tonsil and Peyer's patches by infecting mucosal dendritic cells, macrophages, and lymphocytes. Except for M cells, it is not clear how virus spreads through the mucosal epithelium to reach cells in lamina propria and submucosae (MALT), but leukocyte trafficking is likely involved. Spread through the mucosal epithelium could also occur through ligand-receptor interactions, followed by viral transcytosis to the basal surfaces with release on the abluminal side. Once macrophages, dendritic cells, and lymphocytes are infected locally, virus spreads by leukocyte trafficking in macrophages and dendritic cells via afferent lymphatic vessels to regional lymph nodes and then systemically through postcapillary venules or lymphatic vessels and the thoracic duct to the circulatory system to lymphocytes in the spleen, lymph nodes, and other lymphoid tissues.

Virus uses a viral capsid attachment protein to attach to heparin sulfate and chondroitin sulfate B (glycosaminoglycan [sialic acids] receptors) on macrophages, dendritic cells, and lymphocytes to enter and infect these cells. Macrophages are nonpermissive to virus and appear to serve primarily as trafficking cells to spread virus to other locations, whereas lymphocytes are permissive to virus and allow viral replication. Therefore lymphocytes are injured and killed during replication and release. Although virus-induced necrosis has been suggested as the mechanism for cell lysis, apoptosis may actually be the main cause through a viral protein that activates caspase pathways and apoptosis. Other studies suggest that lymphoid loss may result from reduced production of lymphoid cells in the bone marrow or reduced proliferation in secondary lymphoid tissues, resulting in depletion of all types of T and B lymphocytes, immunosuppression, and increased susceptibility to secondary opportunistic infections. Although there is no proof that it is the causal agent, porcine circovirus type 2 (PCV2) has also been linked to several other conditions, including PCV2 pneumonia, PCV2 enteritis, PCV2 reproductive failure, and PCV2 porcine dermatitis and nephropathy syndrome. Many of these conditions have concurrent infections caused by other microbes. These conditions have been grouped under the term PCV2-associated diseases and will not be covered in this chapter because of limited information.

Disorders of Dogs

Canine Distemper (Morbillivirus, Enveloped RNA Virus). See Viral Diseases of Organ Systems, Nervous System, Disorders of Dogs, Canine Distemper Canine Distemper (Morbillivirus, Enveloped RNA Virus) for discussion on pathogenesis and mechanisms of spread and injury. In summary, thymic atrophy and lymphoid depletion (lymphopenia) are manifestations of infection with canine distemper virus. Viral lymphotropism can lead to loss (lysis) of lymphoid cells (and macrophages), including specific types of T and B lymphocytes, resulting in severe immunosuppression. Additionally, loss of SLAM-positive lymphoid cells and specific cells that enable cell-mediated and humoral immunity likely contribute to this outcome. Loss of lymphocytes (and macrophages) appears to be caused by virus-induced cytolysis/apoptosis (not likely via the effects of cytokines) of infected lymphoid cells.

Disorders of Cats

Feline Leukemia (Feline Leukemia Virus, Retrovirus, Enveloped RNA Virus). The mechanism of injury in feline leukemia is virus-induced dysfunction, lysis, and/or neoplastic transformation of lymphoid cells leading to (1) lymphoma (lymphosarcoma) and leukemia, (2) malfunction of visceral organ systems, lymphoid tissues, or bone marrow, usually through compressive atrophy of parenchymal cells, in which the neoplastic cells proliferate, and (3) immunosuppression, resulting in increased susceptibility to other microbial diseases. Gross lesions include proliferation of neoplastic cells and their infiltration into perivascular spaces in organ systems resulting in (1) generalized enlargement of affected organs with increased pallor or (2) the formation of one or more solid white nodules distributed at random in the affected tissue (see Figs. 7-88, 13-83, and 13-94). Additionally, cells can occupy and proliferate in confined spaces, causing compressive atrophy of tissues such as axons in the spinal cord, hemopoietic cells in the bone marrow, and the retina in the eye. Discussion of the syndromes and lesions caused by feline leukemia virus (FeLV) is outside the scope of this chapter; however, they include (1) lymphoma (lymphosarcoma) and all of its forms (alimentary, thymic, anterior mediastinal, multicentric, atypical) based on anatomic distribution, (2) leukemia, (3) myeloproliferative disorders, (4) nonregenerative anemia, (5) panleukopenia-like syndrome, and (6) glomerulonephritis.

Cats encounter FeLV-A (see later) in fomites from body fluids, such as salivary and nasal secretions, through direct contact with virus-infected cats. Thus grooming behaviors are important in the transmission of the disease. Virus is ingested or inhaled and is deposited on mucous membranes of the oral and nasal pharynx, and it attaches to, infects, and replicates locally in mucosal epithelial cells and mucosa-associated macrophages and lymphocytes, especially in areas with tonsils. Virus spreads via leukocyte trafficking in lymphocytes and macrophages through afferent lymphatic vessels to pharyngeal lymph nodes (regional nodes), where it infects and replicates in additional lymphocytes and macrophages. It has not been determined how virus penetrates the mucus layer to gain access to and cross the mucosal epithelium or if dendritic cells are involved in infection or spread.

B lymphocytes appear to be the primary cells used to spread virus via leukocyte trafficking, whereas T lymphocytes appear to be the primary target cell for infection. Therefore T lymphocyte dysfunction is the principal cause of clinical signs of the disease. From regional lymph nodes, virus spreads systemically in B lymphocytes via leukocyte trafficking to the circulatory system, through postcapillary venules or lymphatic vessels and the thoracic duct to systemic lymph nodes and lymphoid organs, such as the spleen and Peyer's patches, and then to bone marrow and mucosa of the salivary glands. As stated earlier, salivary gland secretions and grooming behaviors spread the virus to naïve cats.

There are four known subgroups of FeLV, designated FeLV-A, FeLV-B, FeLV-C, and FeLV-T. For successful replication, virus requires rapidly dividing cells such as lymphocytes and the opportunity to establish a persistent infection in these cells. Clinical syndromes caused by FeLV arise from persistent infection of T lymphocytes in bone marrow. Persistent infections result from modulation of virus and cellular gene expression and modification of the cat's immune response by the virus. Persistence lasts for long periods, often the life of the cat, and occurs when the virus is not eliminated by the adaptive immune response because of dysfunction of cytotoxic T lymphocytes.

FeLV-A is the only subgroup that can be transmitted between cats. This occurs primarily through saliva. Once cats are infected with subgroup FeLV-A, the virus establishes a persistent infection of bone marrow cells, which are most likely T lymphocytes or their precursor cells. However, the virus is not integrated in the cat's genome. Because viral replication occurs continually in these cells, there is greater opportunity for genomic variation (antigenic drift/shift) to occur and new viral virulence factors to be introduced. Subgroup FeLV-B appears to have arisen through recombination (antigenic shift) of endogenous genes of subgroup FeLV-A, whereas subgroup FeLV-C appears to have arisen through point mutations (antigenic drift) of endogenous genes of subgroup FeLV-A. Cats may be infected with only subgroup FeLV-A or a combination of subgroup FeLV-A with FeLV-B and/or FeLV-C. In general, subgroup FeLV-A causes immunosuppression and is found in approximately 100% of virus-infected cats; subgroup FeLV-B causes neoplastic transformation and is found in approximately 50% of virus-infected cats; and subgroup FeLV-C causes anemia and is found in approximately 1% to 2% of virus-infected cats. FeLV-T arises through genomic variation of FeLV-A, infects T lymphocytes, and causes an immunodeficiency syndrome.

All subgroups of virus use envelope glycoproteins, probably surface glycoprotein (SU) and the transmembrane protein (TM), to attach to receptors on and enter T lymphocytes, other lymphocytes, and mucosal epithelial cells. Receptors for viral glycoproteins on target cells include (1) feline thiamine transport protein (FeTHTR1) as a receptor for FeLV-A; (2) feline phosphate transporter proteins 1 and/or 2 (FePit1 or FePit2) as receptors for FeLV-B; and (3) FeLV-C cellular receptor (FeLVCR), a heme transporter protein, as a receptor for FeLV-C. FeLV-T uses two proteins to attach to, enter, and infect cells. FePit1 is used as a receptor, whereas FeLIX, a protein secreted primarily by T lymphocytes, is used to restrict tropism to T lymphocytes. Retroviruses also have envelope glycoproteins that form membrane-spanning glycoprotein systems that attach to and bind with membrane-spanning receptors on lymphocytes. To infect T lymphocytes, FeLV-T expresses in its viral envelope a membrane-spanning glycoprotein that attaches to and binds with a target cell membrane-spanning receptor molecule (FePit1). It also appears that expression of a specific target cell receptor, the total number of receptors expressed on the cell, and the use of soluble cofactors play roles in determining which target cells are infected by FeLVs. Additionally, persistent infection of bone marrow cells by FeLV-A provides many opportunities for mutations in the envelope gene that result in the expression of new viral subgroups through mutations in viral envelope glycoproteins that recognize new target cell membrane receptors. It is likely that the clinical syndromes and lesions caused by these virus subgroups are related to genomic variation through the expression of envelope surface glycoproteins that determine and restrict attachment, entry, infection, and replication in target cells.

Immunosuppression and lymphopenia coincide with systemic involvement of lymphoid tissues, specifically T lymphocytes. Cats persistently infected with FeLV-A commonly die of secondary bacterial and viral opportunistic infections. Immunosuppression, targeted primarily to the cell-mediated immune system, appears to result from (1) a reduction in the number of lymphocytes, especially cytotoxic and helper cell T lymphocytes, through virus-induced cell lysis; (2) suppression of lymphokines (interferon-δ and interleukin) secreted by activated T lymphocytes that could eliminate virus and virus-infected cells; (3) production of FeLV protein p15, which suppresses lymphocyte function (controversial); (4) dysfunction of lymphokine-induced activation of macrophages; and (5) dysfunction of neutrophil phagocytosis. Estimates suggest that approximately 50% of cats with certain bacterial infections and hemobartonellosis (*Mycoplasma haemofelis*) and 75% of cats with toxoplasmosis (*Toxoplasma gondii*) are infected with and have their immune systems suppressed by FeLV. Additionally, virus-induced immunosuppression has also been associated with feline infectious peritonitis, chronic oral and gingival diseases, poor reparative responses in inflammation, recurrent abscesses and skin infections, respiratory diseases, acute enteritides, otitis, and virus-induced malignancies such as sarcomas.

Neoplastic transformation follows persistent infection of T lymphocytes, usually in bone marrow. Virus produces reverse transcriptase (a retrovirus) that transcribes viral RNA into proviral DNA and facilitates the insertion of proviral DNA into chromosomal DNA of T lymphocytes or other bone marrow cells. When virus has integrated its genome into the target cell DNA, the viral genome is passed to all new generations of cells when the cell is mitotic. Reverse transcriptase is carried by the virus and is released into target cell cytoplasm along with its viral RNA genome after attachment and entry. Neoplastic transformation of T lymphocytes or other bone marrow cells occurs when DNA provirus integrates into chromosomal DNA at critical regions that (1) contain oncogenes such as the cellular gene c-myc or (2) are near genes influencing the expression of c-myc genes. Activation of these genes and the expression of their gene products result in a series of alterations to the cell regulatory environment that leads to irreversible changes in cell behavior characteristic of neoplastic transformation (see Chapter 6). Feline oncornavirus-associated cell membrane antigen (FOCMA) is expressed on the cell membranes of transformed cells and is not found on normal (nontransformed) cells, even if they are infected with virus.

Feline Acquired Immunodeficiency Syndrome (Feline Immunodeficiency Virus, Lentivirus, Enveloped RNA Virus). The mechanism of injury in feline acquired immunodeficiency syndrome is provirus-induced dysfunction and lysis of $CD4^+$ T lymphocytes leading to immunosuppression. Gross lesions include transient lymph node enlargement (lymphadenomegaly) followed by the occurrence of secondary opportunistic microbial infections. Feline immunodeficiency virus causes persistent and gradual depletion of $CD4^+$ T lymphocytes (T helper [T_H] lymphocytes, effector T lymphocytes), resulting in an immunodeficiency syndrome characterized by chronic stomatitis and gingivitis, wasting syndrome (malnutrition), neurologic manifestations, and an increased incidence of lymphoma. The cause of $CD4^+$ T lymphocyte depletion is unknown. It may have a multifactorial basis, including lysis of cells caused directly by viral infection, lysis (turnover) after massive and rapid replication of virus-infected and noninfected cells stimulated by viral antigen and/or proinflammatory cytokines or other molecules, provirus-induced suppression of cell proliferation, lysis of provirus-infected $CD4^+$ T lymphocyte by adaptive immune responses, or apoptosis of provirus-infected cells.

Cats encounter the virus in blood, most commonly as a provirus in infected $CD4^+$ T lymphocytes, and much less commonly as free virus in fomites from saliva. During fights that result in bite wounds that bleed, blood contaminated with provirus-infected $CD4^+$ T lymphocytes encounters (1) oral mucosae (macrophages and dendritic cells), especially of the tonsils, through surface contamination and (2) macrophages and dendritic cells (Langerhans cells) of the skin through penetrating wounds. It appears that virus is able to establish a local infection in mucosal dendritic cells, macrophages, and lymphocytes; however, it is not clear how virus penetrates the mucus layer to gain access to mucosal epithelial cells, mucosal macrophages, and/or dendritic cells and migrates through the mucosal epithelium to reach cells in the lamina propria and submucosa (MALT). In mucosae, several proposed mechanisms of spread could be involved: (1) migration (leukocyte trafficking) of provirus-infected $CD4^+$ T lymphocytes through the epithelium into the submucosa, (2) infection of mucosal epithelial cells via a ligand-cell receptor endocytotic mechanism through virus released from provirus-infected $CD4^+$ T lymphocytes, (3) infection of mucosal epithelial cells via a ligand–target cell receptor mechanism by cell-free virus, or (4) transfer of cell-free virus via viral transcytosis, the process by which virus is transported across the interior of a cell in vesicles to be released from the basal surface on the abluminal side. In skin, free-virus or provirus-infected $CD4^+$ T lymphocytes could be carried via blood or saliva into penetrating wounds of the dermis and subcutis, where, through cell lysis, exocytosis, or direct extension, the virus or provirus could gain access to Langerhans cells and tissue macrophages.

It appears that by whatever route used by virus or provirus to enter the body, it must gain access to local mucosal (MALT) or skin-associated lymphoid tissues (MALT-like) and $CD4^+$ T lymphocytes, macrophages, and dendritic cells to establish an infection. Once these cells are infected, virus is then spread by leukocyte trafficking via afferent lymphatic vessels to regional lymph nodes and then systemically via leukocyte trafficking to the spleen and other lymphoid tissues through postcapillary venules or lymphatic vessels and the thoracic duct. Some studies suggest that virus may also spread to the oral cavity and tonsillar mucosa via saliva either by provirus-infected $CD4^+$ T lymphocytes or a cell-free viremia, especially if cats with chronic stomatitis and gingivitis are involved in grooming behavior or cat fights. Target cells for infection include $CD4^+$ T lymphocytes, $CD8^+$ T lymphocytes, B lymphocytes, cells of the monocyte-macrophage system, dendritic cells, megakaryocytes, and astrocytes. Virus envelope glycoproteins, probably surface glycoprotein (SU) and the transmembrane protein (TM), bind to target cell membrane receptors and serve to facilitate infection through virus attachment and entry into target cells. Different strains of virus appear to express different envelope glycoproteins (and other proteins); thus these molecules likely contribute to viral pathogenicity. Target cells express feline CD134 receptor and CXCR4 cofactor (chemokine receptor) in their membranes, both of which act as coreceptors and are needed for virus attachment, binding, and entry into target cells.

Nervous System

Disorders of Domestic Animals

Rabies (Lyssavirus, Enveloped RNA Virus). The mechanism of injury in rabies is neuronal dysfunction possibly caused by one of several mechanisms, including viral takeover of RNA transcription and translation in neurons, disruption of neurotransmitter functions, dysfunction of ion channels, and/or induction of the synthesis of NO. Rabies virus infects neurons of all mammalian species. Gross lesions are not present in nervous tissue; however, inclusion bodies (Negri bodies) and chronic lymphomonocytic perivascular inflammation characteristic of viral infections are observed (see Fig. 14-45). In addition to neurons, the virus infects glial cells in the nervous system and epithelial cells such as those in the salivary glands.

Animals encounter virus in fomites from saliva through a skin-penetrating bite wound from a rabid animal. Virus gains access to interstitial (extracellular) body fluids and plasma (bite wound hemorrhage); diffuses at random in this fluid; and encounters, attaches to, and enters striated muscles cells via binding of rabies virus envelope G protein to neurotransmitter receptors, such as acetylcholine receptors, located in muscle cell membranes. Envelope G protein is an important determinant of rabies neurovirulence and which neuron pathways are infected with virus in the nervous system. Virus then replicates in muscle, buds from cell membranes, enters interstitial fluids of myoneural (neuromuscular junction) junctions, and randomly encounters and binds to acetylcholine receptors, neuronal cell-adhesion molecule receptors, neurotrophin receptors, or other types of gangliosides in cell membranes of unmyelinated axon terminals (nerve endings) of lower motor neurons of peripheral nerves. Similar processes are also used to spread and replicate virus in cranial nerves after bite wounds to the face. Once bound, virus enters the cytoplasm of nerve endings through pinocytosis via clathrin-coated pits and the formation of vesicles. Virus in vesicles spreads centripetally from myoneural junctions to the cell body of the nerve via retrograde fast axonal transport, likely using the dynein light chain microtubule-based transport system (see Chapter 14; see E-Fig. 14-3). Virus replicates in the cell body of neurons and travels to dendrites via axonal transport where it buds from cell membrane of dendritic processes into synaptic clefts of neural-neural junctions. It randomly encounters receptors on motor nerve endings within the gray matter of the brain and ventral gray horns of the spinal cord. Mechanistically, viral replication and spread in motor neurons within the spinal cord and brain are identical to that in peripheral spinal nerves. The exact mechanism that facilitates transsynaptic spread of rabies virus is unknown. It may be linked in part to viral assembly where M protein encapsulates the virus and assists in moving the virus to cell membranes such as those in synapses that contain glycoproteins essential for formation of the viral envelope and viral budding. Envelope G protein is also required for attachment to cell membrane and transsynaptic spread of the virus to the next neuron in the neural pathway.

Virus uses axonal transport mechanisms to spread throughout the body via afferent and efferent neural pathways to infect epithelial cells of the salivary glands (see Fig. 14-44). Rabies virus, through these neural pathways, can also infect other cells such as those in taste buds, nasal cavity, skin and hair follicles, adrenal gland, pancreas, kidney, heart muscle, and the retina and cornea. In fact, the "furious" and "dumb" forms of rabies in domestic animals (see Chapter 14) are likely attributable to infection of specific neuronal populations and pathways such as those in the hippocampal formation or cerebellum, respectively. Virus spreads to salivary glands through axonal transport using parasympathetic nerves present in the facial (VII) and glossopharyngeal (IX) cranial nerves and sympathetic nerves in the thoracic segments of T1 to T3 spinal cord segments. In addition to spreading virus to the salivary glands, viral infection of parasympathetic and sympathetic nerves also results in increased salivary gland secretions: (1) directly through stimulating β-adrenergic receptors on the salivary acinar and ductal cells, leading to an increase in cAMP concentrations and the corresponding increase of saliva secretion, and (2) indirectly through stimulating nerves innervating blood vessels that supply the salivary glands. Virus buds from the cell membrane of these nerve terminals, infects salivary acinar epithelial cells through the envelope G protein–specific cell surface receptor mechanism, and replicates in and is amplified to large quantities in these cells. Virus then buds from apical (luminal) surfaces of salivary cell membranes, mixes with saliva, and can be transmitted in a bite wound. The apical specificity of viral budding is established during the assembly stage of viral replication. Viral genome and proteins form "envelope" complexes in the salivary epithelial cell cytoplasm that congregate at areas of the cell membrane that contain matching glycoprotein receptors and then bud from this membrane into the salivary gland lumen to eventually enter the duct system and saliva.

Disorders of Horses

Equine Polioencephalitis-Polioencephalomyelitis (Alphavirus, Enveloped RNA Virus). The mechanism of injury in equine polioencephalitis-polioencephalomyelitis is disruption and lysis of neurons in the CNS. Gross lesions include active hyperemia, vasculitis, hemorrhage, and yellow-white-gray areas of necrosis in gray matter of the nervous system, especially the spinal cord (see Fig. 14-79). Because neurons are the primary target cell, lesions are most commonly observed in gray matter (i.e., polio-), areas in which neuron cell bodies are located, and thus these diseases are classified as polioencephalitides or polioencephalomyelitides. Equine polioencephalitis-polioencephalomyelitis is used herein to group three closely related strains of alphaviruses that cause eastern equine encephalomyelitis, western equine encephalomyelitis, and Venezuelan equine encephalomyelitis. St. Louis encephalomyelitis is the human counterpart of these diseases in horses. Such diseases have also been called *arbovirus polioencephalitis-polioencephalomyelitis*. The term *arbovirus* is derived from the fact that these viruses are *ar*thropod-*bo*rne; this term was shortened to *arbo* and is used as a disease acronym.

Horses encounter viruses through skin-penetrating bite wounds from virus-infected mosquitoes. Mosquitoes are infected when they bite and consume infected blood from birds, the reservoir for the virus. Seasonal variations in temperature and precipitation greatly influence the population density of mosquitoes and thus the occurrence of disease. Following penetration of horse skin with their proboscis, virus-infected mosquitoes deposit virus directly into the circulatory system, where it infects blood monocytes, or into vascularized ECM (connective) tissue, where it infects dendritic cells (Langerhans cells) and tissue macrophages. In these cells, virus is spread via leukocyte trafficking to regional lymph nodes either by the circulatory system or afferent lymphatic vessels where it infects additional lymphocytes. It may also spread to regional lymph nodes via cell-free viremia in lymphatic vessels.

Viral envelope contains three membrane glycoproteins, E1, E2, and E3. Attachment protein E2 is used to attach to a target cell receptor, whereas viral envelope fusion protein E1 is used to enter target cells via endocytosis. Receptors for E1 and E2 proteins occur on a variety of cell types and probably determine which cells, such as lymphocytes, are used for leukocyte trafficking and ultimately which organ systems, such as the nervous system, are targeted for infection by virus. Virus then spreads systemically via leukocyte trafficking in lymphocytes and macrophages through postcapillary venules or lymphatic vessels and the thoracic duct to the circulatory system to systemic lymph nodes, spleen, thymus, bone marrow, Peyer's patches, pancreas, and skeletal muscle. Infection results in necrosis of myeloid cells in bone marrow and lymphocytes in lymph nodes and spleen. Proinflammatory cytokines, such as IFN-γ, and antiinflammatory cytokines, such IL-10 produced by infected lymphocytes, may cause cell lysis. Cytokines released into the blood vascular system may also act on the blood-brain barrier, making it more susceptible to viral infection via changes in its barrier functions and permeability. In eastern equine encephalomyelitis, osteoblasts appear to be the target cell used to amplify virus so it can spread to the nervous system. In this specific disease, dendritic cells, lymphoid cells, and cells of the monocyte-macrophage system are not as susceptible to infection, and thus systemic lymph nodes and spleen are infected to a limited degree with minimal injury and lysis. Although it is unclear how virus spreads to and enters the CNS, leukocyte trafficking by lymphocytes and macrophages (monocytes) appears to be the probable mechanism. Cell-free viremia may also occur.

West Nile Virus Polioencephalitis-Polioencephalomyelitis (Flavivirus, Enveloped RNA Virus). The pathogenesis and mechanism of injury in West Nile virus polioencephalitis-polioencephalomyelitis are similar to those of equine polioencephalitis-polioencephalomyelitis discussed earlier.

Equine Herpesvirus Myeloencephalopathy (Equine Herpesvirus 1: Alphaherpesvirus, Enveloped DNA Virus). The mechanism of injury in equine herpesvirus myeloencephalopathy is dysfunction and lysis of endothelial cells in small arterioles of the brain and spinal cord; however, the mechanism is uncertain but most likely caused by virus replication. Immune complexes (type III hypersensitivity reaction) and the fixation of complement (immune complex–induced vasculitis) have also been suggested. Gross lesions in the brain and spinal cord include randomly distributed foci of edema, hemorrhage, and vasocentric malacia (yellow-white-gray areas) consistent with vascular occlusion, resulting in infarction (see Fig. 14-80).

Horses encounter virus in fomites from body fluids through direct contact with virus-infected animals. It is inhaled or ingested and deposited on mucosae of the oral, nasal, and pharyngeal cavities or inhaled and deposited on mucosae of the conductive component of the respiratory system through centrifugal and inertial turbulence. Virus infects and replicates in mucosal epithelial and endothelial cells, next in contiguous mucosal and submucosal lymphocytes and likely macrophages, monocytes, and dendritic cells (MALT), and then spreads via leukocyte trafficking in afferent lymphatic vessels to regional lymph nodes. It has not been determined if and how virus penetrates the mucus layer to gain access to mucosal epithelial and endothelial cells or if or how mucosal macrophages and/or dendritic cells are involved, though their participation is very likely. Although specific ligands and receptors have not been identified, viral envelope glycoproteins likely attach to glycosaminoglycan receptors on target cell membranes and use this binding to enter the cells listed earlier. Infection appears to be sustained and amplified in lymphocytes and likely macrophages and monocytes of regional lymph nodes. Virus is then spread systemically through blood and lymphatic vessels in infected leukocytes via trafficking in the circulatory system. Infected lymphocytes and macrophages probably use envelope adhesion molecules to bind to receptors on vascular endothelium during migration via leukocyte trafficking through the wall of blood vessels and interact with their cell membranes. These interactions appear to lead to virus infecting and replicating in endothelial cells, myocytes, and pericytes of small arterioles in the brain and spinal cord, causing vasculitis and thrombosis. It is not known why these cells, especially endothelial cells, are targets for virus infection; however, ligand-receptor interactions or permissiveness of these cells is likely involved. Activation of endothelial and leukocyte adhesion molecules is an important step in spreading virus to endothelial cells and thus may contribute to endothelial cell tropism for viral infection.

Disorders of Ruminants (Cattle, Sheep, and Goats)

Bovine Cerebellar Hypoplasia (BVD Virus, Pestivirus, Enveloped RNA Virus). A syndrome, probably involving mechanisms similar to those that occur in animals infected in utero with parvovirus, occurs in calves infected in utero with bovine viral diarrhea–mucosal disease virus (see Fig. 14-36). For more detail, see the following sections:

- Viral Diseases of Organ Systems, Nervous System, Disorders of Cats, Parvovirus-Induced Cerebellar Hypoplasia
- Viral Diseases of Organ Systems; Alimentary System and the Peritoneum, Omentum, Mesentery, and Peritoneal Cavity; Disorders of Ruminants (Cattle, Sheep, and Goats); Bovine Viral Diarrhea–Mucosal Disease (BVD Virus, Pestivirus, Enveloped RNA Virus)
- Viral Diseases of Organ Systems; Alimentary System and the Peritoneum, Omentum, Mesentery, and Peritoneal Cavity;

Disorders of Dogs; Parvovirus Enteritis (Parvovirus, Nonenveloped DNA Virus).

Bovine Herpesvirus Meningoencephalitis (Bovine Herpesvirus 5: Alphaherpesvirus, Enveloped DNA Virus). Mechanistically, bovine herpesvirus 5 behaves much like bovine herpesvirus 1. It infects, spreads, and replicates in the same target cells but is more neurovirulent and induces severe and often fatal encephalitis. See the discussion of infectious bovine rhinotracheitis (bovine herpesvirus 1) in Viral Diseases of Organ Systems; Respiratory System, Mediastinum, and Pleurae; Disorders of Ruminants (Cattle, Sheep, and Goats). The mechanism of injury in bovine herpesvirus meningoencephalitis is dysfunction and lysis of neurons and astrocytes caused by viral replication and chemical mediators of inflammation. The latter consist of proinflammatory chemokines and cytokines arising from cytotoxic T lymphocytes as part of a lymphomonocytic inflammatory response (innate and adaptive immune responses). Gross lesions include randomly distributed areas of cerebral edema, active hyperemia, hemorrhage, and malacia.

Cattle encounter virus in fomites from body fluids through direct contact with virus-infected animals. It is inhaled or ingested and deposited on mucosae of the oral, nasal, and pharyngeal cavities and of the conjunctiva or inhaled and deposited on mucosae of the conductive component of the respiratory system through centrifugal and inertial turbulence. Viral envelope glycoproteins B, C, D, and E likely attach to receptors on sensory nerve endings that innervate these mucosae. They can also probably attach to receptors on a variety of other target cells. These receptors include glycosaminoglycan receptors such as herpesvirus entry mediator A, nectin-1 and nectin-2 (herpesvirus entry proteins C and B), and 3-O-sulfated heparin sulfate. It has not been determined how virus penetrates the mucus layer to gain access to mucosal sensory nerve endings. Through these nerve endings, virus enters neurons within the trigeminal and olfactory cranial nerves and spreads via retrograde axonal transport to other neurons and glial cells within the CNS. It appears that envelope glycoprotein E and 3-O-sulfated heparin sulfate receptors may amplify viral attachment, entry, and spread within the CNS. The mechanism of malacia remains unknown but does not appear to be caused by obvious vascular injury. Neuronal lesions are consistent with necrosis, likely caused by virus-induced injury and cell lysis or by chemical mediators of inflammation. In addition, overproduction of NO in virus-infected neurons and astrocytes could result in their dysfunction and lysis and that of contiguous noninfected cells. Bovine herpesvirus 5 can enter latency in the nervous system, through mechanisms likely identical for bovine herpesvirus 1.

Visna (Maedi-Visna Virus [Ovine Lentivirus], Enveloped RNA Virus). The chronologic sequence of steps that characterizes the pathogenesis of injury in visna is similar to that which occurs in ovine progressive pneumonia (maedi) of sheep. See the discussion of maedi in Viral Diseases of Organ Systems; Respiratory System, Mediastinum, and Pleurae; Disorders of Ruminants (Cattle, Sheep, and Goats). In the CNS the mechanism of injury is chronic-active (granulomatous) inflammation resulting in demyelinating encephalitis. Gross lesions include foci of yellow-white malacia distributed at random in the CNS. Virus is spread to the CNS by leukocyte trafficking of virus-infected monocytes and macrophages arising in the lung and bone marrow. Ovine lentivirus persistently infects cells of the monocyte-macrophage system, including microglial cells (local tissue macrophages in the CNS), and all of these cell types are central to the genesis of the inflammatory response in the CNS.

Caprine Encephalitis (Caprine Arthritis-Encephalitis Virus, Enveloped RNA Virus). The pathogenesis and mechanism of injury in caprine encephalitis are similar to those that occur in ovine progressive pneumonia (maedi) of sheep (see section on the Viral Diseases of Organ Systems; Respiratory System, Mediastinum, and Pleurae; Disorders of Ruminants [Cattle, Sheep, and Goats]); however, the initial route of exposure is by ingestion of virus-infected milk or colostrum. The mechanism of injury is chronic-active (granulomatous) inflammation of the CNS resulting in demyelinating myelitis. Gross lesions include foci of yellow-white malacia distributed at random in the CNS, especially the spinal cord (see Fig. 14-90). Caprine arthritis-encephalitis virus persistently infects cells of the monocyte-macrophage system; thus microglial cells (local tissue macrophages) and trafficking monocytes serve as the cell type central to the genesis of the inflammatory response. Kid goats are primarily exposed to virus through the ingestion of virus-infected milk or colostrum. Although not proven, virus likely infects M cells overlying Peyer's patches. Once the cells are infected, virus is transferred to and released from basilar surfaces of M cells to gain access to macrophages and lymphocytes within Peyer's patches. It is here that macrophages are infected with virus and then serve to spread virus to monocyte precursor cells in the bone marrow and ultimately to the CNS.

Disorders of Pigs

Pseudorabies (Aujeszky's Disease) (Alphaherpesviruses, Enveloped DNA Virus). The mechanism of injury in pseudorabies is disruption and lysis of neurons likely caused by the actions of immune cells, such as cytolytic T lymphocytes, interacting with virus-infected neurons. Because neurons (within neuron cell bodies) are the primary target of viral infection, lesions are most commonly observed in gray matter (polio-) and as a result, this disease is a polioencephalitis or polioencephalomyelitis. Gross lesions characteristic of injury are usually not observed but in severe cases could include randomly distributed areas of active hyperemia and hemorrhage.

Pigs encounter virus in fomites from oronasal-pharyngeal body fluids most commonly through inhalation and potentially through contamination of skin-penetrating bite wounds. When inhaled, virus is deposited on mucosae of the oral, nasal, and pharyngeal cavities, especially of the tonsil or on mucosae of the conductive component of the respiratory system through centrifugal and inertial turbulence. In the tonsil, virus may infect and replicate in mucosal epithelial cells, mucosal and submucosal macrophages, and dendritic cells (MALT). In the lung, virus also infects and replicates in similar cells (BALT), including alveolar macrophages, which it kills, resulting in a secondary bronchopneumonia. Virus attachment and entry is likely mediated by binding of viral envelope glycoproteins to target cell membrane receptors. In the nasal and pharyngeal mucosae and submucosae, especially of the tonsil, virus encounters and infects sensory nerve endings of the olfactory, glossopharyngeal, and trigeminal cranial nerves and uses retrograde axonal transport to enter the brain. Virus can spread transsynaptically throughout the CNS by using mechanisms similar to those described in rabies and infect and replicate in many types of neurons. Viral envelope glycoproteins C, B, D, H, and L are used to attach to, fuse with, and enter membranes of nerve endings. These glycoproteins are also involved in transsynaptic spread to other neurons in the CNS and to other neural cells, such as astrocytes, microglial cells, ependymal cells, and trafficking monocytes/macrophages, as well as in the formation of syncytial cells and the modulation of innate and adaptive immune responses.

Virus cannot replicate in neural cells; thus they are incapable of spreading infection to other cells in the CNS. This outcome may represent a local intrinsic and/or innate immune defense mechanism that isolates through phagocytosis the virus in astrocytes, monocytes-macrophages, and microglial cells and restricts spread of virus to other cells. Latent infections involve the trigeminal nerves and ganglia, but tonsillar lymph nodules may also be involved. Potentially, peripheral nerve endings in the skin, subcutis, and muscle may be exposed to infection via bite wounds and can be used by virus to gain access to and enter the CNS by mechanisms similar to those described in rabies.

Viral envelope glycoproteins in membranes of infected neurons are targets for neutralizing antibodies, cytotoxic T lymphocytes, and lymphokine-activated killer cells and are part of the chronic perivascular lymphomonocytic inflammatory response characteristic of viral infections. These cells appear to contribute in a large manner to neuronal injury and lysis in pseudorabies. Hypertrophy and hyperplasia of astrocytes, microglia, and monocytes-macrophages occur spatially and temporally with the severity of neuronal injury; however, the potential role of biologically active molecules, such as cytokines (e.g., TNF-α), from these cells is unclear.

Disorders of Dogs

Canine Distemper (Morbillivirus, Enveloped RNA Virus). The mechanism of injury in canine distemper, a pantropic virus,[8] is dysfunction and lysis of neuronal, epithelial, mesenchymal, neuroendocrine, and hematopoietic cells in many different tissues and organ systems. The nervous system is the primary organ system affected by distemper virus; however, the virus must infect and replicate in target cells of the respiratory and/or alimentary systems before spreading to the nervous system. As a result, canine distemper virus may also cause diseases of these organ systems. Gross lesions are not observed in the nervous system. Lymph nodes (and spleen) are initially enlarged, hemorrhagic, and edematous but then undergo cell lysis, resulting in loss of T and B lymphocytes in the spleen, lymph nodes, MALT, tonsil, and thymus (immunosuppression). Alterations in bone marrow are minimal; but thrombocytopenia may occur. Anterior-ventral regions of the lung may be firm (consolidation) and have yellow-tan-gray appearance (secondary bronchopneumonia); cut surfaces have discrete and coalescing areas of yellow-tan-gray exudate infiltrating and compressing contiguous lung parenchyma. Airways are hyperemic and often covered with mucopurulent exudate. Pleural surfaces may or may not be affected. The small intestine may be congested and have thin walls and shortened villi (atrophy).

Dogs encounter distemper virus in fomites from body fluids of the nasal and oral cavities, through direct contact with infected dogs. To reach the CNS the virus needs to infect mucosal lymphocytes, macrophages, and/or likely dendritic cells in one or more portals of entry and then spread via leukocyte trafficking to encounter target cells in the CNS (see later) and also in many other organ systems. The portals of entry, encounters with target cells, and pathways of spread include the oronasal pharynx, lung, and small intestine and are discussed at the end of this section. In summary, virus is inhaled and deposited in mucus and on mucosae of the pharynx and of the conductive (bronchi/bronchioles) and O_2-CO_2 exchange (alveoli) systems through centrifugal and inertial turbulence. It is also probably ingested and via swallowing and peristalsis encounters enterocytes (and mucus) and M cells (no mucus) of the small intestine.

Virus-infected lymphocytes and macrophages spread distemper virus via the blood vascular system to the CNS through leukocyte trafficking and cell-free viremia. At the blood-brain barrier, infected cells and virus likely interact with endothelial cells via the leukocyte adhesion cascade (see Chapter 3) and adhere to and migrate through the endothelium. Virus also infects and replicates in endothelial cells, resulting in a perivascular lymphomonocytic inflammatory response characteristic of viral infections in the CNS. Virus then infects and replicates in vascular pericytes, microglial cells, and perivascular astrocytic foot processes, as well as in choroid plexus epithelial cells. At this point, depending on how it is able to spread within the CNS, virus can cause disease in gray matter (neurons: polioencephalomyelitis), white matter (oligodendroglial cells: demyelinating leukoencephalomyelitis), or both. The location (i.e., gray matter versus white matter) of viral infection appears to be determined by the status of vaccination and adaptive immunity (degree of immunosuppression) in the infected dog and by the pathogenicity (virulence factors) of the strain of distemper virus. Additionally, the clinical signs accompanying infection of the CNS by distemper virus are most likely related, in part, to the degree of injury involving neurons and oligodendroglial cells, or a combination of both cell types.

- **Infection of neurons**—Neuronal infection likely arises after spread of virus to neurons from virus-infected pericytes and perivascular astrocytic foot processes. Virus-infected astrocytes may also serve as a reservoir for spreading virus within the CNS (see astrocytes in Chapter 14). Viral infection of neurons results in neuronal necrosis and subsequent neuronophagia via resident microglial cells and trafficking monocytes, macrophages, and lymphocytes.
- **Infection of oligodendroglial cells**—Spread of virus to oligodendroglial cells probably arises from infection of ependymal cells. Virus escapes from choroid plexus epithelium via cell lysis and is carried in cerebral spinal fluid (CSF) to infect ependymal cells via their apical surfaces and then spread via transcytosis to contiguous oligodendroglial cells in the subependymal white matter. However, infection through the blood vascular system, capillaries and postcapillary venules, and virus-infected pericytes and perivascular astrocytic foot processes has not been excluded as a potential infective mechanism. Involvement of oligodendroglial cells results in demyelinating leukoencephalomyelitis, which has an acute phase and a chronic phase. Two mechanisms have been proposed for the acute phase of demyelinating leukoencephalomyelitis: (1) lysis of oligodendroglial cells from infection or (2) a type II hypersensitivity reaction against proteins such as myelin basic protein and myelin-associated glycoprotein.
  - For a cell lysis mechanism, there is no evidence of virus-induced apoptosis or necrosis of oligodendroglial cells, and although virus can infect oligodendroglial cells, no viral proteins are present in these cells. Astrocytes and microglial cells can be infected and show activation such as hypertrophy and hyperplasia. It has been hypothesized that toxic molecules, such as proinflammatory cytokines produced by these glial cells, act to disrupt the function of oligodendroglial cells and kill the cells.
  - For a hypersensitivity reaction mechanism, microscopic lesions of vacuolization (intramyelinic edema) of myelin lamellae surrounding axons in white matter accompanied by reactive astrocytes, macrophages (monocytes), resident microglial cells, and occasional multinucleated giant cells are consistent with this type of immune-mediated injury. As this injury progresses, the inflammatory response becomes more intense and is characterized by perivascular mononuclear infiltrations. Myelin is phagocytosed by macrophages (monocytes) and microglial cells and the lesion is repaired by proliferation of astrocytic processes, thus forming dense plaques (astrocytic scars).

[8]The ability to infect many kinds of cells and tissues.

The chronic phase of demyelinating leukoencephalomyelitis appears to be a bystander mechanism involving inflammation and virus-induced immune responses, such as antibody-dependent cell-mediated reactions (cytotoxic T lymphocytes) against viral proteins expressed in oligodendroglial cell membranes, leading to macrophage-mediated separation, damage, and phagocytosis of myelin lamellae. Myelin damage is likely the result of proteolytic enzymes, oxygen free radicals, and cytokines from activated macrophages, monocytes, and resident microglia. Lipids from damaged lamellae stimulate an intense phagocytic response and likely initiate recruitment of additional monocytes and macrophages into the lesions. Disruption of the blood-brain barrier by proteolytic enzymes appears to play a role in the influx of inflammatory cells probably mediated by viral infection of astrocytes through their foot process involved in the structure and function of the blood-brain barrier.

Distemper virus can encounter and enter macrophages, lymphocytes, and/or dendritic cells through the respiratory and alimentary systems, especially at the oronasal pharynx; the bronchi, bronchioles, and lung; and the small intestine.

- **Oronasal pharynx**—Infection of the oronasal pharynx begins in the mucus layer, where virus is likely phagocytized by mucosa-associated lymphocytes and macrophages and likely dendritic cells and spread via leukocyte trafficking across the tonsillar mucosa to MALT of the tonsils. Here, naïve lymphocytes and macrophages are infected with virus and migrate in afferent lymphatic vessels to regional lymph nodes, where they infect new cells and then migrate systemically through postcapillary venules or efferent lymphatic vessels and the thoracic duct to the circulatory system. These infected cells leave the circulatory system and enter the spleen, thymus, lymph nodes, bone marrow, mucosa-associated lymphoid nodules and Peyer's patches, and liver (Kupffer cells) to infect additional naïve lymphocytes and macrophages. Infection of cells may also occur via a cell-free viremia and through virus-infected platelets. After infection of systemic lymphoid tissue, infected cells (leukocyte trafficking) or cell-free virus spreads to parenchymal organs, including the nervous, respiratory, alimentary, and urinary systems. Concurrently, massive lysis of lymphocytes may also occur, resulting in immunosuppression and dysfunction of immune responses to the virus. In these systems, virus infects a wide variety of epithelial and mesenchymal cells (pantropic virus) and lyses these cells as it replicates and escapes from them. Virus also gains access to ameloblasts during the embryonic development of adult teeth, infects and lyses these cells, and causes a condition known as *enamel hypoplasia* (see Fig. 7-45).
- **Lung**—Infection of the lung begins in the mucus layer of the conductive component of the respiratory system and in the O_2-CO_2 exchange component. Primary target cells are ciliated and nonciliated mucosal epithelial cells of bronchi and bronchioles. It has not been determined how virus penetrates the mucus layer to gain access to mucosal epithelial cells or whether this occurs via direct contact of virus with these cells or through contact with trafficking leukocytes. In bronchi and bronchioles, virus is able to infect mucosa-associated lymphocytes, alveolar macrophages, dendritic cells, and ciliated and nonciliated mucosal epithelial cells. Following replication, these cells are lysed, thereby disrupting the function of the mucociliary apparatus and the removal of particulate debris and secondary bacteria. This outcome contributes to a secondary suppurative bronchopneumonia. Furthermore, in the O_2-CO_2 exchange component, primary target cells are pneumocytes and alveolar macrophages and with replication and lysis of these cells, the function of the air-blood barrier and oxygenation of blood are also disrupted. Loss of the mucociliary apparatus, lysis of macrophages and lymphocytes leading to reduction in phagocytosis and antigen presentation by macrophages, and disruption of innate and adaptive immune responses contribute to secondary suppurative bronchopneumonia in dogs with distemper infections. Cell debris from lysis, viral antigens, and activation of T lymphocytes may also contribute to acute inflammation and the release of proinflammatory cytokines into ECM, perpetuating the inflammatory response. These mechanisms also cause substantial tissue injury and cell lysis.
- **Small intestine**—Infection of the small intestine and its spread of virus to the CNS is not well defined or characterized, if it occurs at all. However, the virus can cause disease of the alimentary system alone. Virus is thought to be ingested, and swallowing and peristasis carry it through the oral pharynx, esophagus, and stomach to the small intestine, where it is trapped in the mucus layer. It is unclear how the virus is able to evade the actions of digestive enzymes, bile acids, and other microbial-lytic molecules and then penetrate the mucus layer and encounter enterocytes. Virus is likely phagocytized by mucosa-associated lymphocytes and macrophages and likely dendritic cells and spread via leukocyte trafficking to and across enterocytes. Virus is probably able to replicate in enterocytes. However, they are lysed when virus replicates in them, leading to a malabsorption/osmotic diarrhea, which occurs because of the loss of enterocytes and the failure to digest carbohydrates (impaired hydrolysis) and other molecules in the digesta. Virus that crosses mucosa through leukocyte trafficking likely reaches MALT. Here similar cells are infected, and they migrate via leukocyte trafficking to spread virus via lymphatic vessels to regional lymph nodes and then systemically to other organ systems. Although unproved, the virus also likely infects M cells, which spread virus to tissue macrophages, dendritic cells, and other cells in Peyer's patches and then systemically to other organ systems by leukocyte trafficking as described earlier.

Virus uses two viral envelope proteins: an attachment protein called *viral H protein* and a fusion protein called *viral F protein* bind to cell membrane glycoprotein receptors. Viral fusion proteins are involved in the penetration of virus into uninfected lymphocytes, spread of virus from cell to cell, and formation of syncytial cells (e.g., CD9 transmembrane protein) characteristically seen in the lungs. It has been shown experimentally that when virus-infected lymphocytes encounter uninfected lymphocytes and other cell types, they are induced to express new and/or increased numbers of SLAM cellular receptors. Molecules secreted by virus-infected lymphocytes likely mediate this process and thus may serve as a means to amplify virus infection in dogs. Glycoprotein receptor CD150 (SLAM) occurs in membranes of lymphocytes, monocytes, macrophages, transitional epithelial cells, endothelial cells, and unspecified cells in the stomach, small intestine, and lung.

Disorders of Cats

Parvovirus-Induced Cerebellar Hypoplasia (Parvovirus, Nonenveloped DNA Virus). See parvovirus enteritis in the section on Viral Diseases of Organ Systems; Alimentary System and the Peritoneum, Omentum, Mesentery, and Peritoneal Cavity; Disorders of Dogs for information about mechanisms of viral spread and replication before involvement of the CNS.

In pregnant cats, parvovirus is able to cross the placenta and infect dividing cells in the developing cerebellum of kittens, resulting in cerebellar hypoplasia (see Fig. 14-35). Whether by leukocyte trafficking or cell-free viremia, parvoviruses are able to gain access to cells in the placenta. Virus infects and replicates in placental trophoblasts and spreads to, infects, and replicates in cytotrophoblasts and cells of the mesenchymal stroma of the fetal placenta. From these cells, virus then gains access to the fetal vascular system and spreads to, infects, and replicates in hematopoietic cells and other dividing cells. It has also been suggested that placental macrophages (or macrophage-like cells) and fetal endothelial cells are likely involved in the replication and spread of the virus to the developing CNS in the fetus. Although virus can infect a large number of different cells in the fetus, it is unclear why fetal infection is clinically dominated by injury to cells of the cerebellum, specifically cells of the external granular layer and Purkinje cells. Ligand-receptor interactions could contribute to this specificity; however, the ability of specific cells to divide and other unknown mechanisms are likely involved.

Parvoviruses infect and replicate in dividing cells. In the fetus, cells of the external granular layer of the cerebellum are dividing cells, whereas Purkinje cells are nondividing cells. However, cell lysis is observed in both of these cell types, although only one of them is a dividing cell population. Granule precursor cells of the cerebellar external granular layer are the major target cells for parvovirus replication during the perinatal period because they are able enter the S phase of the mitotic cycle. Purkinje cells are also infected, but they are nondividing postmitotic cells. It appears that virus infects Purkinje cells via a target cell membrane transferrin receptor that is commonly used by parvovirus for entering other types of target cells. Virus is unable to replicate in postmitotic Purkinje cells, but transcription of viral proteins does occur. It has been suggested that a nonstructural parvovirus protein NS1 is produced at low concentrations during the G_0 and G_1 phases of the cell cycle (see E-Fig. 1-18). Because NS1 is known to be highly cytotoxic and able to induce alterations of the cytoskeleton, this effect could result in injury and cytolysis of Purkinje cells during in utero infection with virus.

Embryologically, granule cells of the external granular layer are stem cells that contribute to formation of the cerebellum, especially the fully differentiated granule cell layer. This process is complicated and involves migration and differentiation of granule cells from the external layer into the cerebellar cortex, thus, in part, determining its "normal" size, shape, and structure. Infection and lysis of these cells by parvoviruses can severely alter the development of the cerebellum, resulting in cerebellar hypoplasia. The extent and severity of hypoplasia depends on how early in the process of migration and differentiation these cells are infected and lysed.

Although cerebellar hypoplasia is not commonly thought to occur from in utero infection of female dogs by canine parvovirus, a recent study has identified parvovirus DNA in brain tissue from puppies with the disease. However, the significance of this information remains unclear because parvovirus structural proteins were not identified in the same tissues. A similar syndrome, probably involving similar mechanisms, occurs in calves infected in utero with bovine viral diarrhea–mucosal disease virus (see Fig. 14-36).

Bone, Joints, Ligaments, and Tendons

Disorders of Ruminants (Cattle, Sheep, and Goats)

Caprine Arthritis (Caprine Arthritis-Encephalitis Syndrome, Enveloped RNA Virus). The mechanism of injury in caprine arthritis is chronic-active (granulomatous) inflammation of the synovium, resulting in proliferative synovitis. The chronologic sequence of steps that characterizes the pathogenesis of injury in caprine arthritis is similar to those that which occurs in ovine progressive pneumonia (maedi) of sheep (see section on Viral Diseases of Organ Systems; Respiratory System, Mediastinum, and Pleurae; Disorders of Ruminants [Cattle, Sheep, and Goats]; Ovine Progressive Pneumonia [Maedi; Maedi-Visna Virus (Ovine Lentivirus); Enveloped RNA Virus]).

Integumentary System

Disorders of Domestic Animals

Vesicular Stomatitis (Vesiculovirus, Enveloped RNA Virus). See section on vesicular stomatitis in the section on Viral Diseases of Organ Systems; Alimentary System and the Peritoneum, Omentum, Mesentery, and Peritoneal Cavity; Disorders of Domestic Animals; Vesicular Stomatitis (Vesiculovirus, Enveloped RNA Virus).

Foot-and-Mouth Disease (Aphthovirus, Nonenveloped RNA Virus). See foot-and-mouth disease in the section on Viral Diseases of Organ Systems; Alimentary System and the Peritoneum, Omentum, Mesentery, and Peritoneal Cavity; Disorders of Ruminants (Cattle, Sheep, and Goats); Foot-and-Mouth Disease (Aphthovirus, Nonenveloped RNA Virus).

Viral Papillomas (Warts, Sarcoids, Papillomaviruses, Nonenveloped DNA Virus). The mechanism of injury in viral papillomas is dysfunction of genes that regulate cell proliferation, differentiation, and adhesion, resulting in benign neoplastic transformation of virus-infected epithelial cells. Cells of stratum basale (germinativum) play a central role in the pathogenesis of viral papillomas. Gross lesions include the formation of exophytic and occasionally endophytic papillomatous fronds that arise from mucosae or skin (see Fig. 17-43). Papillomaviruses are species specific and cause (1) warts of the skin and papillomas of mucosae of the alimentary system, teats and udder, and penis in cattle; (2) sarcoids of the skin in horses, donkeys, and mules; and (3) papillomas of the mucosal epithelium of the oral cavity and reproductive system in dogs.

Animals encounter virus through direct contact with animals of the same species having warts, papillomas, or sarcoids. From these masses, virus is released into the environment via shedding and lysis of aged and virus-infected cells of the stratum lucidum and stratum corneum. Virus must then encounter cells of the stratum basale in naïve animals; therefore viral infection must be preceded by injury of the superficial layers of the stratified epithelium of mucosae or skin, resulting in the physical exposure of target cells in the stratum basale. Because of the short life span of cells in skin and mucosa, stem cells of the stratum basale are continuously dividing to replace cells in the suprabasilar layers. Maturation of these cells begins with the least differentiated layer, the stratum basale, and progresses outwardly through the suprabasilar layers: the strata spinosum, granulosum, lucidum, and corneum. Cells of the suprabasilar layers do not divide and therefore cannot be infected by virus. Virus likely uses capsid proteins, such as bovine L1 major capsid protein and L2 minor capsid protein, to attach and bind to and enter cells of the stratum basale. Viral receptors on cells of the stratum basale have not been clearly identified; however, an integrin (α_6 β_4) and potentially heparin sulfate proteoglycans mediate the attachment and entry of virions into target cells.

Dividing cells of the stratum basale are target cells for viral infection; however, they are nonpermissive cells. Because these cells have a life span for the duration of the animal's life, they serve as a reservoir for virus (i.e., persistent infection), and it replicates its genome to a limited extent within the nucleus of these stem cells. However, because these cells are nonpermissive, virus is unable to produce infective virions. Maturation of the virus occurs as cells of the stratum basale differentiate into cells of the strata spinosum, granulosum, lucidum, and corneum (suprabasilar layers). These differentiated cells are permissive and allow virus to complete its replication cycle and produce infective virions. Virus is released from cells of the stratum lucidum and stratum corneum into the environment to spread the disease, likely when these cells age and break down. A similar process probably occurs in infected mucosae of the alimentary system.

Neoplastic transformation of epithelial cells by papillomaviruses can result in the formation of benign tumors, such as papillomas, warts, and sarcoids, and malignant tumors, such as carcinomas. When virus infects stems cells of the stratum basale, the expression of viral genes is maintained at low numbers (approximately 20 to 100 extrachromosomal copies of viral DNA per cell) where it replicates in synchrony with the cell cycle as the cell divides. Normally, as epithelial cells leave the stratum basale and mature (differentiate), they turn off endogenous genes and the synthesis of proteins required for cell division. When virus-infected stem cells of the stratum basale divide, viral genomes are carried in cells that differentiate into cells of the suprabasilar layers. Viral proteins prevent these differentiated cells from stopping the cell cycle, thus cells of suprabasilar layers, especially the strata spinosum and granulosum, are now capable of division. Because cells of the suprabasilar layer are permissive and allow virus to complete its replication cycle and produce infective virions, large quantities of viral genes and regulatory proteins are present within these dividing target cells.

As a general rule, neoplastic transformation of virus-infected epithelial cells appears to be linked to the quantitative and qualitative expression of viral genes and gene products, such as oncoproteins, and how these molecules interact with target cell genes and gene products regulating cell proliferation, differentiation, and adhesion. It appears that strains of papillomavirus that are unable to integrate into target cell genes are most likely to cause benign transformation (papillomas, warts, and sarcoids) of virus-infected epithelial cells, whereas strains that are able to integrate into target cell genes are most likely to cause malignant transformation (carcinomas) of virus-infected epithelial cells. Therefore benign transformation involves nonpermissive cells of the stratum basale, whereas malignant transformation involves permissive cells of the suprabasilar layers. In nonpermissive cells, virus does not integrate into target cell genes and viral genes, and gene products like oncoproteins are expressed in low amounts. Thus the likelihood of papillomavirus (1) activating growth-promoting genes (oncogenes) in target cell DNA, (2) inactivating suppressor genes that would inhibit cell proliferation, and (3) altering the functional expression of genes that regulate apoptosis is very low. Malignant transformation is most likely to occur in suprabasilar cells where virus integrates into target cell genes and viral genes and gene products, such as oncoproteins, are expressed in high numbers. Thus the likelihood of virus (1) activating growth-promoting genes (oncogenes) in target cell DNA, (2) inactivating suppressor genes that would inhibit cell proliferation, and (3) altering the functional expression of genes that regulate apoptosis is very high. A similar process probably occurs in infected mucosae of the alimentary system.

Disorders of Ruminants (Cattle, Sheep, and Goats)

Pox (Cowpox [Orthopoxvirus], Sheeppox and Goatpox [Capripoxvirus], Swinepox [Suipoxvirus], Enveloped DNA Virus). The term pox is used herein to group diseases, such as bovine cowpox, sheeppox, goatpox, swinepox, and lumpy skin disease, that are caused by closely related strains of poxviruses. The mechanism of injury is dysfunction and lysis of dendritic and epithelial cells of the skin. Gross lesions include macules, papules, vesicles, pustules, scabs, and scars (see Figs. 17-64 and 17-68). Lesions are most easily observed on wool-free or hair-free areas (Fig. 4-43). In general, sheeppox and goatpox are more virulent and cause systemic disease, whereas bovine cowpox and swinepox usually do not cause systemic disease. In these latter species, spread of virus is the result of animal-to-animal contact or contact with clothing or tools/instruments

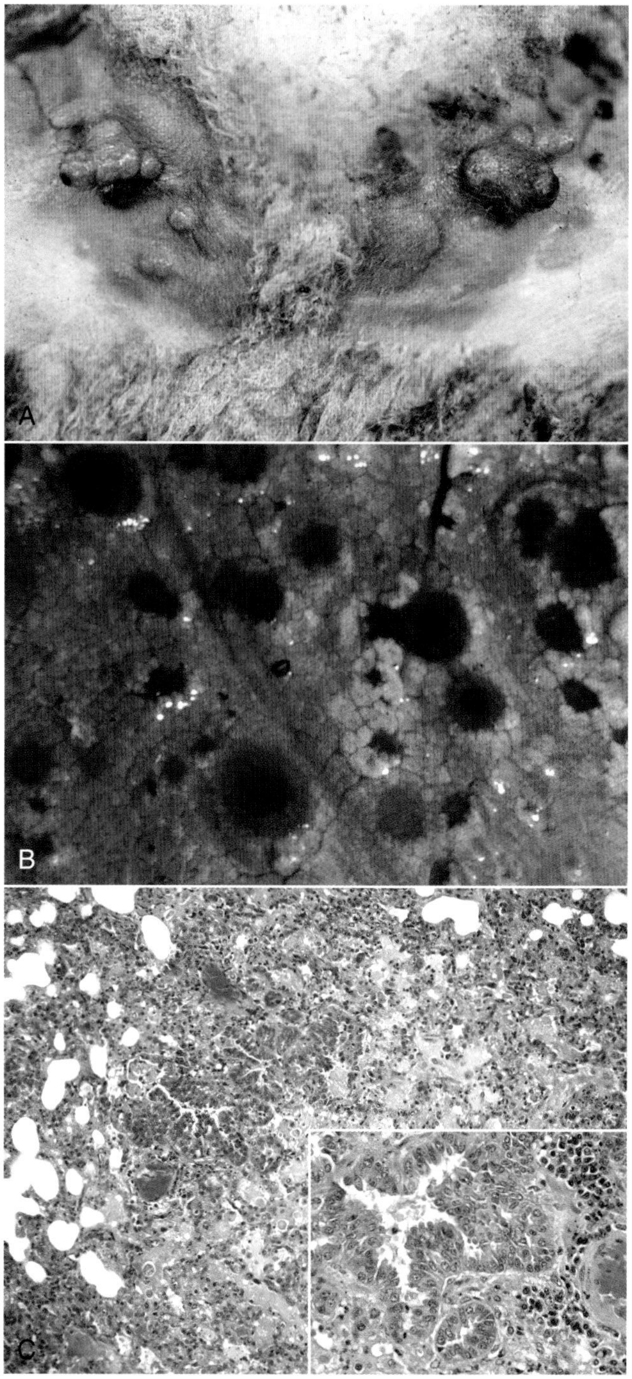

Figure 4-43 **Sheeppox and Goatpox. A,** Skin, teats, inguinal area. Macules, papules, vesicles, crusts (scabs), and papillomas (epidermal hyperplasia) are present on the skin of the inguinal area and teats. Additional information about the development and progression of poxvirus-induced lesions is schematically illustrated in Figure 17-32 and macroscopically and microscopically shown in Figures 17-64 (sheeppox) and 17-68 (swinepox). **B,** Lung, pox lesions. These circumferentially expanding dark red to plum-colored lesions of varied sizes are areas of proliferating bronchial and bronchiolar mucosal epithelial cells, necrotic epithelial cells, cell debris, and inflammation demonstrated in **C. C,** Lung, bronchiole. There is proliferation of mucosal epithelial cells of the lung's conductive system that are infected with poxvirus. Note the mononuclear inflammatory likely bronchial-associated lymphoid tissue (BALT) in adjacent supporting stroma. *Inset,* Higher magnification of **C.** H&E stain. (**A** courtesy Dr. D. Gregg, Plum Island Animal Disease Center; and Noah's Arkive, College of Veterinary Medicine, The University of Georgia. **B** courtesy Dr. R. Breeze, Plum Island Animal Disease Center; and Noah's Arkive, College of Veterinary Medicine, The University of Georgia. **C** courtesy Dr. J.F. Zachary, College of Veterinary Medicine, University of Illinois.)

contaminated with virus-infected skin, scabs, or other skin debris. It appears that skin must be injured (traumatic abrasions) so that capillary endothelial cells, trafficking leukocytes, or Langerhans cells (dendritic cells) are exposed, can encounter virus, and can be infected.

As examples, bovine cowpox most commonly occurs on the teats of dairy cows, the areas most commonly injured by milking trauma in a dairy herd. Insect bites result in penetrating skin wounds that can also carry virus into contact with susceptible target cells. However, in sheeppox and goatpox, animals encounter virus through inhalation or ingestion. It is deposited on mucosae of the oronasal pharynx, especially of the tonsil, and infects and replicates in epithelial cells, mucosal lymphocytes and macrophages, and dendritic cells (MALT). It has not been determined how virus penetrates the mucus layer to gain access to mucosal epithelial cells, macrophages, and/or dendritic cells, but it is likely virus is phagocytosed by leukocytes trafficking in the mucus layer when during migration these cells encounter virus. Macrophages of the lamina propria and submucosa are infected, and virus spreads in them via leukocyte trafficking and afferent lymphatic vessels to regional lymph nodes, such as the submandibular and pharyngeal. Here proinflammatory chemokines and cytokines are released from virus-infected macrophages, and they act to recruit naïve lymphocytes and macrophages, which are infected with virus. Virus then spreads systemically via leukocyte trafficking in these lymphocytes and macrophages through postcapillary venules or lymphatic vessels and the thoracic duct to the circulatory system and then to systemic lymph nodes, spleen, and bone marrow and infects and replicates in similar cells using mechanisms as described earlier. Virus then spreads from systemic lymphoid tissues via leukocyte trafficking to the skin, lung, liver, and other organ systems.

In the skin, virus spreads from migrating macrophages and lymphocytes and infects and replicates in endothelial cells, resulting in direct injury to the vasculature and an acute inflammatory response. Endothelial cell injury accompanied by vascular dilation, active hyperemia, and acute inflammation, in part, likely account for macules and papules observed in early skin lesions. Langerhans cells (dendritic cells) are in close contact with endothelial cells in the malpighian layer of the skin. It appears that virus from capillary endothelial cells and trafficking leukocytes is able to infect Langerhans cells and then spread virus to contiguous skin epithelial cells of the stratum basale and spinosum. All of these cells allow virus to replicate; thus when epithelial cells of the stratum basale and spinosum are killed, the space formerly occupied by these cells coalesces and is filled with cell debris and intercellular edema, forming vesicles. With injury, acute inflammation ensues, as does the pustular stage. Through adaptive immune responses, viral infection is resolved and pustular lesions heal as scabs over granulation tissue that becomes scars.

It is likely that both humoral and cell-mediated immunity are important in protecting against and resolving pox diseases; however, these responses can cause injury and lysis of virus-infected target cells. Similar lesions and lesion progression may affect oral mucous membranes. Pneumonia has been reported in systemic poxvirus-induced disease. Affected lungs have variable-sized and randomly distributed pock lesions in the form of large, irregularly shaped lobular areas of consolidation (see Fig. 4-43). This pattern is consistent with hematogenous spread of the virus via leukocyte trafficking in virus-infected macrophages to pulmonary endothelial cells and then to bronchiolar and alveolar epithelial cells followed by cell lysis and acute inflammation. Although reservoir hosts for poxvirus are wild rodents, cats are now the most commonly recognized reservoir. Cats are infected with virus through their skin by an indirect mechanism when hunting virus-infected rodents; however, infection, as previously described, via a direct mechanism (inhalation) and systemic spread in monocytes and macrophages has been reported.

Poxviruses use attachment proteins to bind to glycosaminoglycan receptor proteins on the surface of target cells. Because of the volume of information related to attachment proteins and receptors in poxvirus diseases, discussion of these protein molecules is outside the scope of this chapter.

Contagious Ecthyma (Orf Virus: Parapoxvirus, Enveloped DNA Virus). See contagious ecthyma in the section on Viral Diseases of Organ Systems; Alimentary System and the Peritoneum, Omentum, Mesentery, and Peritoneal Cavity; Disorders of Ruminants (Cattle, Sheep, and Goats).

Bovine Papular Stomatitis (Parapoxvirus, Enveloped DNA Virus). See bovine papular stomatitis in the section on Viral Diseases of Organ Systems; Alimentary System and the Peritoneum, Omentum, Mesentery, and Peritoneal Cavity; Disorders of Ruminants (Cattle, Sheep, and Goats).

Disorders of Pigs

Swine Vesicular Disease (Enterovirus, Nonenveloped RNA Virus). See swine vesicular disease in the section on Viral Diseases of Organ Systems; Alimentary System and the Peritoneum, Omentum, Mesentery, and Peritoneal Cavity; Disorders of Pigs.

Vesicular Exanthema of Pigs (Calicivirus, Nonenveloped RNA Virus). See vesicular exanthema of pigs in the section on Viral Diseases of Organ Systems; Alimentary System and the Peritoneum, Omentum, Mesentery, and Peritoneal Cavity; Disorders of Pigs.

Female Reproductive System

Disorders of Horses

Equine Herpesvirus Abortion (Equine Herpesvirus 1 and 4: Alphaherpesvirus, Enveloped DNA Virus). See equine viral rhinopneumonitis in the section on Viral Diseases of Organ Systems; Respiratory System, Mediastinum, and Pleurae; Disorders of Horses. In summary, gross lesions include abortions (born weak) and fetal lysis (mummification, stillbirths). Following inhalation, virus infects mucosal macrophages, lymphocytes, and/or dendritic cells, and these cells probably migrate in lymphatic vessels via leukocyte trafficking and spread virus to regional lymph nodes such as the tracheobronchial. Here it infects macrophages and lymphocytes and is spread systemically, via cell-free viremia or leukocyte trafficking through postcapillary venules or lymphatic vessels and the thoracic duct. Additionally, infection of vascular and lymphatic endothelial cells appears to occur. Within the circulatory system, virus ultimately reaches the uterus and placenta. It is not clear how virus spreads from the uterus, to the placenta, and then to the fetus, but some form of a fetal macrophage-like cell probably intervenes in the placentome. It is thought that abortions (also mummification and stillbirths) may result from (1) infection and lysis of cells within the fetus, (2) virus-induced vasculitis and thrombosis of the placental vasculature (infection of endometrial endothelium) resulting in placental separation, or (3) a combination of both mechanisms. Cell types involved and mechanism(s) of injury are undetermined, as are attachment proteins and target cell receptors in the fetus or endothelium of the uterus.

Coital Exanthema (Equine Herpesvirus 3: Alphaherpesvirus, Enveloped DNA Virus). The mechanism of injury in coital exanthema is dysfunction and lysis of skin and/or mucosal epithelial cells (mucocutaneous junctions) of the male and female reproductive systems. Gross lesions include active hyperemia; hemorrhage; and papules, vesicles, and pustules, resulting in erosions and ulceration of affected mucosae and an acute inflammatory response (see Fig. 18-31). Horses encounter virus through direct contact (venereal disease) with infected horses during breeding. Mucosae do not need to be injured for virus to infect cells. Virus can also spread mechanically via hands, gloves, instruments, palpation sleeves, and sponges, if contaminated with virus. Insect bites, especially fly bites, may also be a means of spreading the virus. Although unidentified, equine herpesvirus 3 probably expresses attachment proteins in its envelope that attach and bind to specific receptors on cells of reproductive mucosae.

Equine Viral Arteritis (Arterivirus, Enveloped RNA Virus). See equine viral arteritis in the section on Viral Diseases of Organ Systems, Cardiovascular System and Lymphatic Vessels, Disorders of Horses for information on portals of entry and initial encounters of virus with target cells. In summary, gross lesions include abortions (born weak) and fetal lysis (mummification, stillbirths). Virus-infected macrophages, arising at portals of entry, spread virus via leukocyte trafficking to the endometrium, where they encounter endothelial cells, lymphocytes, and macrophages. These cells are infected with virus. It is unclear how virus spreads from the uterus, to the placenta, and then to the fetus, but some form of a fetal macrophage-like cell probably intervenes in the placentome and spreads virus in the fetus. Furthermore, in the placentome, virus-infected endothelial cells and their supportive myocytes are lysed by virus, leading to a necrotizing vasculitis. Trophoblasts can also be infected with virus. It is thought that abortions (also mummification and stillbirths) may result from (1) infection and lysis of cells within the fetus, (2) virus-induced vasculitis and thrombosis of the placental vasculature (infection of endometrial endothelium), resulting in placental separation, or (3) a combination of both mechanisms. Cell types involved and mechanism(s) of injury are undetermined, as are attachment proteins and target cell receptors in the fetus or endothelium of the uterus.

Stallion semen is also a likely source of virus (accessory sex glands). It is deposited on mucosae, and virus likely infects and replicates in mucosal macrophages and as they migrate through the mucosa and then is spread by these cells locally through leukocyte trafficking to lamina propria and submucosae, where they infect and replicate in tissue macrophages and lymphocytes. These cells then migrate to blood vessels and injure endothelial cells of the endometrium/placentome as described earlier. Attachment proteins and target cell receptors in reproductive mucosae are unknown.

Disorders of Ruminants (Cattle, Sheep, and Goats)

Bovine Herpesvirus Abortion (Bovine Herpesvirus 1: Alphaherpesvirus, Enveloped DNA Virus). See infectious bovine rhinotracheitis in the section on Viral Diseases of Organ Systems; Respiratory System, Mediastinum, and Pleurae; Disorders of Ruminants (Cattle, Sheep, and Goats) for information on portals of entry and initial encounters of virus with target cells. In summary, gross lesions include abortions (born weak) and fetal lysis (mummification, stillbirths). From portals of entry, virus-infected mucosal macrophages, lymphocytes, or dendritic cells migrate in lymphatic vessels via leukocyte trafficking and spread virus to regional lymph nodes such as the tracheobronchial. Here it infects macrophages and lymphocytes, which spread it to the circulatory system and placenta via cell-free viremia or leukocyte trafficking through postcapillary venules or lymphatic vessels and the thoracic duct. It is not clear how virus spreads from the uterus, to the placenta, and then to the fetus, but some form of a fetal macrophage-like cell probably intervenes in the placentome. Experimental studies have shown that cells in the fetal liver are primary targets for viral infection. Additionally, but too a much lesser extent, endothelial cells of the heart, brain, and placenta are also infected. The role of virus-induced vasculitis and thrombosis of the placental vasculature (infection of endometrial endothelium) resulting in placental separation, if it occurs, has not been determined.

Infectious Pustular Vulvovaginitis/Balanoposthitis (Bovine Herpesvirus 1: Alphaherpesvirus, Enveloped DNA Virus). See infectious bovine rhinotracheitis in the section on Viral Diseases of Organ Systems; Respiratory System, Mediastinum, and Pleurae; Disorders of Ruminants (Cattle, Sheep, and Goats) for information on portals of entry and initial encounters of virus with target cells. In summary, gross lesions include erosion and ulcerations with hemorrhage of reproductive mucosae (see Fig. 18-29). From portals of entry, virus-infected mucosal macrophages, lymphocytes, or dendritic cells migrate in lymphatic vessels via leukocyte trafficking and spread virus to regional lymph nodes such as the tracheobronchial. Here, it infects macrophages and lymphocytes, which spread it to the circulatory system and placenta via cell-free viremia or leukocyte trafficking through postcapillary venules or lymphatic vessels and the thoracic duct. Virus then spreads to epithelial cells of the mucous membranes of the penis, prepuce, vulva, or vagina via cell-free viremia or leukocyte trafficking. Because virus causes lysis of infected cells and thus erosions and ulcerations of mucosae, it may also be spread via direct contact (venereal disease) of virus-infected mucosae from the penis or prepuce with mucosae of the vulva or vagina, or vice versa, during breeding.

Disorders of Pigs

Porcine Reproductive and Respiratory Syndrome (PRRS Virus, Enveloped RNA Virus). See porcine reproductive and respiratory syndrome in the section on Viral Diseases of Organ Systems; Respiratory System, Mediastinum, and Pleurae; Disorders of Pigs for information on portals of entry and initial encounters of virus with target cells. Although unknown, the mechanism and type of injury that occurs in the lung also probably affects a wide variety of cells in the placenta, fetal membranes, and fetus. Injury can be observed in fetal myocytes; however, it is unclear as to whether loss of myocytes is attributable to necrosis, apoptosis, or atrophy. Gross lesions include abortions (born weak) and fetal lysis (mummification, stillbirths). Virus probably spreads to the placenta in virus-infected macrophages within the circulatory system via leukocytic trafficking from an initial site of virus replication in another organ system such as the lung or uterus. It is likely that virus-infected macrophages transfer virus to fetal macrophage-like cells in the placentome, which then spread virus to all organ systems in the fetus. Although all fetuses in a litter may not be infected, it has been shown that pig fetuses in all stages of gestation can be infected with and support replication of virus resulting in normal, born weak, stillborn, and mummified fetuses.

Porcine Parvovirus Abortion (Parvovirus, Nonenveloped DNA Virus). See the following Viral Diseases sections for information on portals of entry and initial encounters of virus with target cells:

- Viral Diseases of Organ Systems; Alimentary System and the Peritoneum, Omentum, Mesentery, and Peritoneal Cavity; Disorders of Dogs; Parvovirus Enteritis (Parvovirus, Nonenveloped DNA Virus)
- Viral Diseases of Organ Systems, Cardiovascular System and Lymphatic Vessels, Disorders of Dogs, Parvovirus Myocarditis (Parvovirus, Nonenveloped DNA Virus)
- Viral Diseases of Organ Systems, Nervous System, Disorders of Cats, Parvovirus-Induced Cerebellar Hypoplasia (Parvovirus, Nonenveloped DNA Virus)

The mechanism of injury is dysfunction and potentially lysis of placental and fetal cells. Gross lesions include reproductive failure, embryonic lysis, fetal resorption, stillbirths, and mummified fetuses (see Fig. 18-56).

Pigs encounter virus through direct contact with fomites from fluids or tissues of the reproductive system, placenta, or aborted fetuses. Virus can also be transferred mechanically via hands, gloves, and instruments, if they are contaminated with virus-infected body fluids. It is ingested or inhaled and deposited on mucosae of the oral, nasal, and pharyngeal cavities, especially of the tonsil. It has not been determined if and how virus penetrates the mucus layer to gain access to tonsillar mucosal epithelial cells. Virus likely infects and replicates in mucosal macrophages and dendritic cells as they migrate through the mucus layer and mucosae and then is spread by these cells locally through leukocyte trafficking to mucosal epithelial cells and their lamina propria and submucosa, where they infect and replicate in tissue macrophages, lymphocytes, and dendritic cells of the tonsil (MALT). A cell-free viremia may also occur. These cells spread virus in afferent lymphatic vessels via leukocyte trafficking to regional lymph nodes, where they infect and replicate in similar cells. Then it spreads to the circulatory system and systemically to lymph nodes through postcapillary venules or lymphatic vessels and the thoracic duct.

From the circulatory system, it is unclear how virus interacts with and spreads from the uterus, to the placenta, and then to the fetus; however, studies suggest the spread of virus to the fetus occurs via leukocyte trafficking by fetal macrophage-like cells. Although unidentified, porcine parvovirus probably has capsid attachment proteins that bind to glycosylated cell membrane receptors (likely sialic acid–bearing cell surface receptors) of target cells in the uterus, placenta, and fetus. Virus has been identified in placental and fetal endothelial cells and in most tissues of virus-infected fetuses. Parvoviruses only infect and replicate in dividing cells because they require a target cell–derived duplex transcription template, which is available when cells divide during S phase of the cell cycle (see E-Fig. 1-18). Parvoviruses are unable to turn on DNA synthesis in target cells, so they must wait for target cells to enter the S phase of the cell cycle before they can infect cells. It is likely that the high mitotic rate of developing and growing fetal tissues is conducive to infection by virus. Virus-induced lysis of fetal cells during the first 35 days of gestation causes embryonic lysis (death) and fetal resorption, whereas infection between 35 and 70 days of gestation causes fetal death (stillbirths) and mummified fetuses.

Porcine Cytomegalovirus Abortion (Herpesvirus-Cytomegalovirus, Enveloped DNA Virus). See inclusion body rhinitis–porcine cytomegalovirus infection in the section on Viral Diseases of Organ Systems; Respiratory System, Mediastinum, and Pleurae; Disorders of Pigs for information on portals of entry and initial encounters of porcine cytomegalovirus with target cells. The pathways of spread and mechanisms and types of injury in the placenta, fetal membranes, and fetus are probably similar to those discussed earlier for porcine parvovirus abortion and porcine reproductive and respiratory syndrome.

Male Reproductive System

See the section on the Female Reproductive System.

Eye

Disorders of Cats

Feline Herpetic Keratitis (Feline Herpesvirus 1: Alphaherpesvirus, Enveloped DNA Virus). See the following Viral Diseases sections for information on portals of entry and initial encounters of herpes viruses with target cells:

- Viral Diseases of Organ Systems; Respiratory System, Mediastinum, and Pleurae; Disorders of Horses; Equine Viral Rhinopneumonitis (Equine Herpesvirus, Alphaherpesvirus, Enveloped DNA Virus)
- Viral Diseases of Organ Systems; Respiratory System, Mediastinum, and Pleurae; Disorders of Ruminants (Cattle, Sheep, and Goats); Infectious Bovine Rhinotracheitis (Bovine Herpesvirus, Alphaherpesvirus, Enveloped DNA Virus)
- Viral Diseases of Organ Systems; Respiratory System, Mediastinum, and Pleurae; Disorders of Cats; Feline Viral Rhinotracheitis (Feline Herpesvirus, Alphaherpesvirus, Enveloped DNA Virus)

The mechanism of injury in feline herpetic keratitis is lysis of epithelial cells of the cornea. Gross lesions include corneal ulcerations; however, with severe injury, involvement of the underlying corneal stroma can occur, leading to edema, neovascularization, collagenization, and inflammation. These secondary lesions are attributable to inflammation and its mediators, especially those derived from cytotoxic T lymphocytes. Cats encounter virus in fomites from body fluids, such as saliva and eye and nasal secretions, contaminated through direct contact (grooming behaviors) with virus-infected cats. Virus is deposited on mucosae of conjunctiva, where it infects and replicates in the epithelium. Viral envelope glycoproteins are used to attach to and enter these cells via glycosaminoglycan receptors on conjunctival epithelial cells. Virus replicates in these cells, and with cell lysis it is released to spread in conjunctival fluids. It is carried in these fluids and encounters additional conjunctival epithelial cells and corneal epithelial cells, where it replicates and escapes via cell lysis. In the latter cell type, if severely affected, the cornea can become inflamed, edematous, and ulcerated.

Fungal Diseases (Mycoses)

Portals of entry; target cells and substances; pathways of spread; virulence factors; mechanisms of adhesion, colonization, invasion, and replication; toxins; and defense mechanisms for fungal diseases are similar to those discussed in the opening sections of this chapter and in the sections on bacterial and viral diseases.

Fungi, microbes common in the environment and as microflora of mucosae, exist as yeasts or as branched filamentous pseudohyphal or hyphal forms (molds). Most fungi discussed in this section have both forms in their life cycles and are known as *dimorphic fungi* (Fig. 4-44). They have also be classified as superficial mycoses (candidiasis, aspergillosis) and systemic or deep mycoses (histoplasmosis, coccidioidomycosis, blastomycosis, angioinvasive fungi, and cryptococcosis) based on their relative "depth" of involvement in disease affecting one or more organ systems.

Fungi contain a variety of complex molecules that are arranged to form cell walls and capsules that aid in colonization of tissues and to protect the microbe against phagocytosis and other defense mechanisms. Because of this complexity, these molecules and cell walls cannot be completely degraded and removed by acute inflammation, and the response rapidly progresses to granulomatous inflammation. Specific molecules and their roles in disease mechanisms will be discussed in sections covering individual diseases. In summary, substances, such as glucans and glycoproteins, often act to block phagocytosis, and when they are phagocytized, they are often difficult to degrade to inert materials within macrophages and neutrophils because of their physical structure and biologic constituents. Because macrophages have short life spans (6 to 16 days), these nondegraded materials are released from dead macrophages into tissues and lead to the recruitment of additional macrophages into tissues to remove the debris. Furthermore, macrophages that phagocytize this debris are "activated," resulting in the synthesis and secretion of chemokines and cytokines that recruit additional macrophages from the

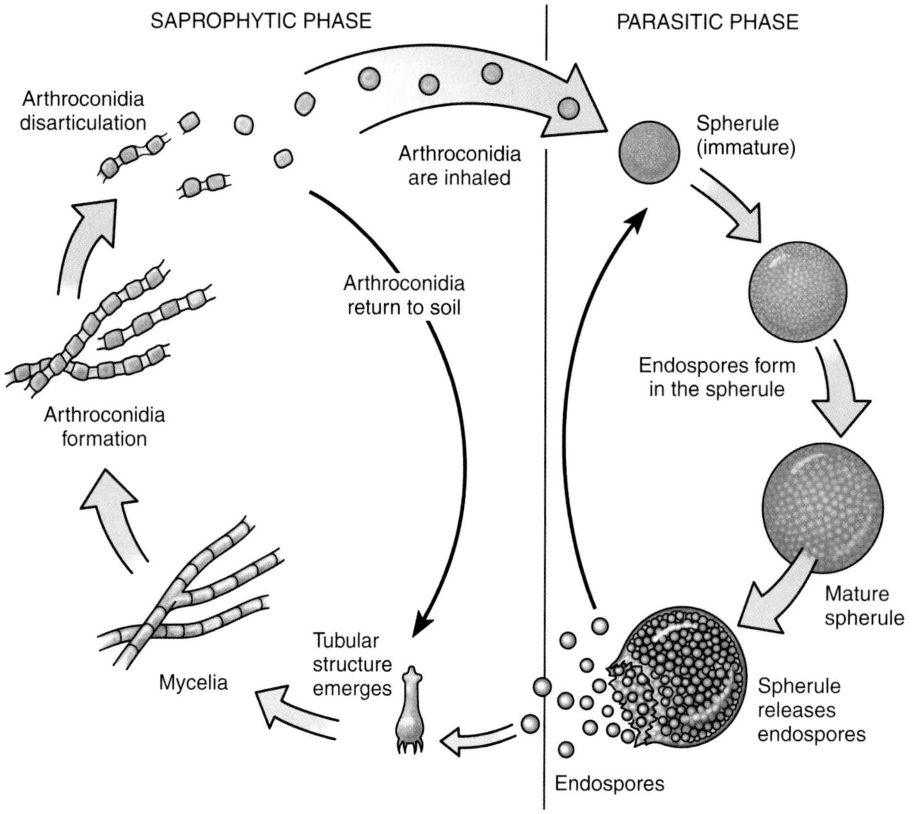

Figure 4-44 **Life Cycle of *Coccidioides immitis* and Other Dimorphic Fungi.**

vascular system into the site of inflammation. Because this process is repetitive with recurring cycles of replication in macrophages, death of macrophages and release of fungi and fungal debris and antigens, and phagocytosis of these materials by newly recruited and naïve macrophages, a granulomatous inflammatory response characteristic of fungal diseases occurs in affected tissues.

Fungal Diseases of Organ Systems

Alimentary System and the Peritoneum, Omentum, Mesentery, and Peritoneal Cavity

Disorders of Domestic Animals

Candida Glossitis–Oropharyngeal Candidiasis (Thrush) (*Candida albicans*). The mechanism of injury in candida glossitis is (1) proliferation and invasion of filamentous pseudohyphae and hyphae into lingual mucosa and (2) disruption and lysis of mucosa caused by inflammation and its chemical mediators and degradative enzymes. Gross lesions include acute pseudomembranous glossitis with an extensive white to yellow pseudomembrane consisting of desquamated epithelial cells, fibrin, and fungal hyphae covering the dorsal surface of the tongue (see Figs. 7-7 and 7-8).

Candida albicans can occur in two forms: (1) yeast that are commensal and nonpathogenic and (2) filamentous pseudohyphae and hyphae that are pathogenic. Animals encounter yeast through ingestion (and likely inhalation) where it persists as a commensal microbe that colonizes mucosa without causing injury or disease and becomes part of the normal microbial flora associated with mucosal surfaces (i.e., biofilm). The balance between commensalism and disease is tenuous, and perturbations of mucosae and/or changes in the physiologic status of the animal may shift this balance in favor of disease (i.e., the filamentous pseudohyphal and/or hyphal forms). Through a process called morphologic or phenotypic switching, the yeast form switches to the invasive and pathogenic filamentous pseudohyphal and/or hyphal form. Switching appears to occur through inducible chromosomal rearrangements in the genome of the yeast in response to changes in the mucosal environment. Switching appears to be reversible. Under normal conditions the temperature of mucosa in the oral cavity is near room temperature (25° C). This temperature favors the growth of yeast, whereas pseudohyphae and/or hyphae prefer to grow at 37° C. The yeast form is able to switch this temperature dependence for growth via chromosomal rearrangements, so that its pseudohyphae and/or hyphae forms can grow at 25° C. Switching is attributable to virulence factors selectively expressed under suitable predisposing conditions in the yeast (antigenic drift/shift) combined with the breakdown of mucosa, excessive use of broad-spectrum antibiotics and corticosteroids, hyperglycemia, tissue damage secondary to chemotherapy or radiation, or immunosuppression. Additionally, if innate (phagocytosis by neutrophils and macrophages) and adaptive (cell-mediated) immunity, important defense mechanisms in controlling candidiasis, are disrupted, switching is also favored.

A large group of virulence factors are involved in the processes of switching and infection and invasion, but no single factor accounts for virulence, and not all expressed virulence factors may be necessary for a particular stage of infection. The yeast form appears to have its own group of virulence factors; as does the pseudohyphal and hyphal form. Yeast persists in the oropharyngeal cavity by adhering to and colonizing mucosa via ligand-receptor and/or hydrophobic interactions. Yeast and pseudohyphal and hyphal forms have ligands in their cell walls such as those in the agglutinin-like (AL) family and hyphal wall protein (Hwp) family that allow these forms to adhere to epithelial cells and invade mucosa. Mannose and mannoproteins may also act as adhesins. Receptors expressed on mucosal epithelial cells can include E-cadherin, fibrinogen, fibronectin, thrombin, collagen, laminin, and vitronectin-binding proteins. The pseudohyphal and hyphal form adheres to and invades mucosa (epithelial cells) using virulence factors, such as fungal "invasin" proteins as examples. Pseudohyphae and hyphae also express new adhesin ligands and hydrolytic aspartyl proteinases that injure the mucosa and allow them to encounter new types of adhesin receptors and entry receptors in mucosa and submucosa and invade the layer. Although uncharacterized, epithelial damage, in addition to that produced by inflammation, may also be caused by apoptosis initiated by virulence factors in pseudohyphal and/or hyphal forms.

Disorders of Dogs

Histoplasmosis (*Histoplasma capsulatum*). The mechanism of injury in histoplasmosis is cell lysis via chronic granulomatous to pyogranulomatous inflammation and its effector molecules and degradative enzymes. *Histoplasma capsulatum* has a dimorphic life cycle; the mycelial (microconidia) phase occurs in extracellular environments (25° C), whereas the yeast phase occurs intracellularly within cells of the monocyte-macrophage system (37° C). Gross lesions include thickened walls of the small intestine and enlargement of the liver, lung, spleen, and mesenteric lymph nodes (see Figs. 7-182, 8-56, 13-91, and 14-48, C). Lesions are caused by the accumulation of granulomatous inflammatory cells in perivascular spaces, resulting in (1) generalized enlargement of affected organs with increased pallor or (2) the formation of one or more solid white-yellow nodules distributed at random in the affected tissue. Lesions are most prominent in the small intestine, where inflammatory cells accumulate in the lamina propria of villi and the submucosa, resulting in thickened walls and ulcerated mucosae. Systemic lymph nodes, bone marrow, and eyes may also become infected with fungus via leukocyte trafficking and acquire a granulomatous inflammatory response.

Dogs (and cats) encounter fungus through inhalation of microconidia (2- to 5-μm in diameter spores), which can reach the lower respiratory tract (i.e., bronchi and bronchioles). They are present in soil-derived aerosols from moist and humid environments. Microconidia are deposited on mucosae of the nasopharyngeal cavity and the conductive components of the respiratory system through centrifugal and inertial turbulence. Neutrophils and alveolar macrophages phagocytize microconidia trapped in the mucus layer of mucosae. Because microconidia can be killed by macrophages and neutrophils, there is a rapid transition to the yeast form because it provides protection against innate and adaptive immune responses. Recognition, attachment, and internalization of microconidia by phagocytes are likely mediated by ligand-receptor interactions, but specific molecules have not been identified. After phagocytosis and if not killed, microconidia germinate in phagosomes into the yeast form. Transitioning from microconidia to yeast is a requirement for fungal pathogenicity. Phagosomes attempt to kill the yeast by fusing with cellular lysosomes to form phagolysosomes. Lysosomes have an acidic pH and acid hydrolases that kill or restrict the growth of yeast. The yeast is able to prevent its lysis by synthesizing proteins that inhibit acidification of the phagolysosome and the activities of lysosomal proteases. The yeast form is protected against host defenses as long as it is hidden in phagosomes of viable macrophages. Yeast is spread in alveolar macrophages via leukocyte trafficking to local lymphoid tissues like BALT, where additional macrophages are infected. From here, infected macrophages spread via leukocyte trafficking in afferent lymphatic vessels to regional lymph nodes and then systemically via the lymphatic and vascular systems to mesenteric lymph nodes and Peyer's patches. It is likely that macrophages containing yeast spread from Peyer's patches into contiguous lamina propria and submucosa of the small intestine and via lymphatic vessels to mesenteric lymph nodes.

The ligand-receptor interactions that determine location specificity have not been identified. The innate immune system identifies fungi, in part, by recognition of PAMPs (see Chapters 3 and 5) formed by α- and β-glucan surface polysaccharides in yeast cell walls. Macrophages recognize these patterns through TLRs and other PRRs expressed on macrophages and use the information to develop an appropriate immune response. Fungi have developed mechanisms to evade and/or neutralize detection by PRRs on macrophages, neutrophils, and dendritic cells such as those leading to modifications in surface polysaccharides through genomic variation. Additionally, an array of suspected virulence factors have been identified, and they include adhesins and invasins, molecules involved in iron homeostasis, and molecules that may disrupt phagosome-lysosome fusion.

Because macrophages have short life spans (6 to 16 days), yeast and yeast-derived surface polysaccharide antigens are released from dead macrophages into the lamina propria of the small intestine. These polysaccharides and the chemokines and cytokines secreted by infected macrophages lead to recruitment of additional macrophages and pyogranulomatous inflammatory cells into the lamina propria. This process is repetitive; lesions characteristic of histoplasmosis ensue because of recurring cycles of replication in macrophages, death of macrophages and release of yeast, and phagocytosis of yeast by newly recruited and naïve macrophages. Thus the volume of inflammatory exudate grows with time, resulting in a thickened intestinal wall, disruption of lymphatic vascular drainage, and disturbances of junctional complexes of villus epithelial cells, all resulting in the protein-losing enteropathy characteristic of histoplasmosis clinically.

Disorders of Cats

Histoplasmosis (*Histoplasma capsulatum*). See earlier section on Histoplasmosis.

Respiratory System, Mediastinum, and Pleurae

Disorders of Domestic Animals

Aspergillosis (*Aspergillus fumigatus*). The pathogenesis of aspergillosis has similarities to those of other fungal diseases discussed in this section. The mechanism of injury is disruption and lysis of mucosae in the nasal cavity and respiratory system caused by inflammation, its mediators and degradative enzymes, and by the concurrent proliferation and invasion of fungal hyphae. Immunosuppression, impairment of phagocytosis, chemotherapy, or prolonged corticosteroid therapy may increase an animal's susceptibility to this fungus. Gross lesions include acute pseudomembranous rhinitis and sinusitis. An extensive gray-black pseudomembrane consisting of desquamated epithelial cells, fibrin, and fungal hyphae may cover the mucosal surfaces of turbinates, sinuses, and airways (see Fig. 9-34, A). The underlying bone and cartilage may also become necrotic as hyphae invade these tissues (see Fig. 9-34, B). In the lungs, yellow-white granulomas of varied sizes are distributed at random in lung parenchyma or may be oriented around airways.

Animals, especially dogs, encounter fungus through inhalation of conidia (≈2 to 3 μm in diameter) that are deposited on mucosae of the nasopharynx and the conductive component of the respiratory system through centrifugal and inertial turbulence. Fungus is a saprophyte of dead or decaying matter. With suitable growing conditions, the fungus produces conidia, which are inhaled and trapped in the mucus layer of mucosae. They interact with the mucociliary apparatus and defensive molecules (see Chapter 3) released from mucosal epithelial cells and are ultimately phagocytosed by neutrophils and alveolar and mucosal macrophages. Recognition, attachment, and internalization by phagocytes are likely mediated by ligand-receptor interactions such as sialic acid residues and molecular patterns (PAMPs) on conidia and by PRRs (TLRs) expressed on alveolar macrophages and neutrophils. In healthy animals this process results in the release of proinflammatory cytokines, which, in part, recruit additional neutrophils that phagocytize and kill conidia and hyphae that are trapped in the mucus. If an animal's phagocytes are unable to phagocytize and kill conidia (i.e., defective neutrophil functions), conidia germinate in the mucus layer and mucosae and begin the processes of colonizing mucosae of the nasal cavities and sinuses. Conidia and hyphae secrete proteases, gliotoxin, fumagillin, verruculogen, and helvolic acid that slow the beat of cilia in the mucociliary apparatus and injure ciliated mucosal epithelial cells. These outcomes lead to detachment and loss of ciliated epithelial cells and exposure and damage of underlying basement membrane (laminin). Thus when conidia germinate into hyphae, a denuded and disrupted mucosa and basement membrane provide a favorable environment for hyphae to invade mucosae. Fibrinogen, fibronectin, and complement C3 fragments from inflammation that cover exposed basement membrane as a reparative response, as well as exposed laminin and collagen, can serve as receptors for sialic acid and other conidial and hyphal glycoproteins, thus contributing to fungal pathogenicity by enhancing adhesion to and colonization and invasion of injured mucosae and basement membrane. Through these mechanisms, fungus is able to invade and spread in affected tissue and extensively damage normal tissues. Dendritic cells are also able to phagocytize conidia and hyphae and process antigens for effective innate and adaptive immune responses via proinflammatory cytokines. However, pathogenic strains of the fungus have virulence factors that appear to impair these immune responses by altering the functions of effector cells.

In dogs, aspergillosis occurs in the nasal cavities, paranasal sinuses, and/or the respiratory system. In other animal species, aspergillosis begins as an infection of the respiratory system, often asymptomatic, and then spreads to other sites likely via leukocyte trafficking of conidia-infected macrophages. These sites include the lung, mammary gland, and placenta in cattle; guttural pouches in horses; and lungs in cats. *Aspergillus* biofilms of mucosae of the respiratory tract may be involved in the pathogenesis of pulmonary disease. The ability to disseminate and spread systemically to other organs is modulated in part by the ability of conidia and hyphae to block immune responses and evade killing by phagocytes. Alveolar macrophages phagocytose conidia and hyphae through a process mediated by the recognition of PAMPs by PRRs (TLRs) expressed on alveolar macrophages and other phagocytic cells as described in the discussion of histoplasmosis. *Aspergillus fumigatus* uses β-glucans, melanin, and other molecules to block killing by reactive oxygen species, phagolysosomal acidification, and other mechanisms in macrophages and neutrophils.

Conidia and hyphae can spread systemically to other organ systems in macrophages via leukocyte trafficking. Hyphae can also disseminate via the circulatory system to other organ systems through a process called angioinvasion. They may invade endothelial cells lining capillaries, gain access to the circulatory system, break off into the bloodstream, circulate, and attach to and invade endothelium at other sites. Ligand-receptor interactions are probably involved in this process, determining which organ system and tissue types are targeted by the fungus.

Coccidioidomycosis (*Coccidioides immitis*). The pathogenesis of coccidioidomycosis is similar to that of histoplasmosis discussed earlier. The mechanism of injury is cell lysis via chronic granulomatous to pyogranulomatous inflammation and its effector molecules and degradative enzymes. It has a dimorphic life cycle (see Fig. 4-44). Gross lesions include pyogranulomatous interstitial pneumonia with yellow-white granulomas of varied sizes distributed at random in the lungs and similar appearing expansile granulomas in lymph nodes (see Fig. 3-22, *B* and E-Fig. 3-8). Bone marrow and eyes may also have granulomatous inflammation resulting from infection via leukocyte trafficking of infected macrophages (see E-Fig. 21-52). Fungus is present in the soil and with suitable growing conditions produces arthroconidia (≈3 to 6 μm in diameter) that are carried into the air by disruption of the soil, such as during construction or farming.

Animals encounter arthroconidia through inhalation, and they are deposited on and trapped in the mucus layer of mucosae of airways through centrifugal and inertial turbulence. In the mucus layer, arthroconidia can be phagocytosed and killed by neutrophils and alveolar macrophages. However, there is a rapid transition of arthroconidia to spherules because this latter form of the fungus provides protection against phagocytosis (virulence factor). Furthermore, transformation into spherules leads to the expression of additional virulence factors that cause acute inflammation resulting in mucosal injury and colonization. Spherules, trapped in the mucus layer, grow to approximately 20 to 60 μm in diameter (occasionally up to 100 μm) and form a small number of intraspherular endospores (≈1 to 5 μm in diameter) through a process called *endosporulation*. Spherules appear to escape phagocytosis because they are too large to be phagocytized by neutrophils, macrophages, and dendritic cells. When spherules are mature or are damaged by inflammatory cells, chemical mediators, and/or degradative enzymes, they release new endospores onto intact mucosa or into injured and denuded mucosa and its ECM. Endospores are approximately 1 to 5 μm in diameter and are capable of being phagocytosed by alveolar macrophages, mucosal macrophages, and dendritic cells. These endospores then grow into second-generation spherules protected within the cytoplasm of these cells. These spherules are now capable of producing an average of 200 to 300 endospores that are released onto and into mucosa when infected cells are lysed. This process rapidly amplifies the number of endospores and spherules in respiratory mucosae and the opportunity for successful colonization of the airways and lung.

Because endosporulation and cell lysis is a repetitive process, proinflammatory cytokines released from "activated" macrophages assist in recruiting additional macrophages and neutrophils into the lung (i.e., granulomatous inflammation). In addition, macrophages infected with endospores likely spread via leukocyte trafficking in lymphatic vessels and the circulatory system locally to lymphoid tissues, regionally to lymph nodes, and systemically to other tissues such as the skin, bone, muscle, lymph nodes, adrenal glands, and CNS. A primary skin infection can also occur by direct infection of damaged skin, but rarely. Each form of the fungus (arthroconidia, spherules, and endospores) has virulence factors that provide it with the opportunity to evade defense mechanisms and barrier systems, complete its portion of the fungal life cycle, and transition to the next form of the fungus. Virulence factors include the (1) production of a spherule outer wall glycoprotein that modulates the immune response and compromises cell-mediated immunity, (2) depletion of spherule outer wall glycoprotein on the surface of endospores, which prevents their phagocytosis, and (3) production of host tissue arginase I and coccidioidal urease, which contribute to tissue damage at sites of infection. Additionally, exposed laminin and collagen may serve as receptors for fungal ligands enhancing adhesion to and colonization and invasion of injured mucosae and basement membrane.

Blastomycosis (*Blastomyces dermatitidis*). The pathogenesis and mechanism of injury in blastomycosis are similar to those of histoplasmosis and coccidioidomycosis discussed earlier. Gross lesions include pyogranulomatous interstitial pneumonia with yellow-white granulomas of varied sizes distributed at random in the lungs (see Fig. 9-103) and similar-appearing expansile granulomas in lymph nodes. In the disseminated form, lymph nodes, skin, subcutaneous tissues, eyes, brain, and bone may also become infected by spread of yeast-infected macrophages via leukocyte trafficking and develop a pyogranulomatous inflammatory response. A primary skin infection can also occur by direct infection of damaged skin, but rarely.

Fungus is present in the soil and with suitable growing conditions, produces conidia (≈ 2 to 10 μm in diameter) that are carried into the air by disruption of the soil. Animals inhale conidia, which are deposited on and trapped in the mucus layer of mucosa of airways through centrifugal and inertial turbulence. In the mucus layer, conidia bind to alveolar macrophages via surface adhesins, such as BAD1 (*Blastomyces* adhesion factor 1). Several concurrent events may now occur, including (1) phagocytosis and killing of conidia by mucosal macrophages and neutrophils initiated by surface binding, (2) spread of conidia via leukocyte trafficking into and through mucosae, and (3) acute inflammation with tissue damage facilitated by proinflammatory cytokines released from macrophages. Inflammation with degradation of mucosa and ECM assist the fungus in encountering cells and tissues throughout lung parenchyma and spreading into lamina propria, submucosa, and deeper ECM tissues.

Because conidia are quickly killed by mucosal macrophages, they rapidly transition to the yeast form (≈12 to 15 μm in diameter) because it is more resistant to phagocytosis and killing by macrophages and neutrophils. Yeast accomplish this outcome by shedding their surface adhesins and/or produce masking capsules that allow them to avoid recognition by macrophages and neutrophils and evade phagocytosis and killing. However, because macrophages have short life spans (6 to 16 days), yeast and yeast-derived debris such as polysaccharides are released from dead macrophages into lung tissues. These materials act as chemokines and cytokines and help recruit additional macrophages and neutrophils into affected lung tissues. This process is repetitive, and lesions characteristic of blastomycosis ensue as the volume of pyogranulomatous inflammatory exudate grows within the lamina propria, submucosa, and deeper ECM tissues.

In the yeast phase the fungus has immune-modulating virulence factors (e.g., glucans) in its cell wall and other virulence factors (e.g., melanin) that provide resistance to phagocytosis and killing. Yeast evades the adaptive immune system by changing surface polysaccharides and by hiding in phagosomes. Additionally, yeast has the adhesion-promoting protein BAD1,which mediates adherence to CR3 and CD14 receptors on cell membranes of alveolar macrophages.

Disorders of Dogs

Histoplasmosis (*Histoplasma capsulatum*). See Fungal Diseases of Organ Systems; Alimentary System and the Peritoneum, Omentum, Mesentery, and Peritoneal Cavity; Disorders of Dogs; Histoplasmosis (*Histoplasma capsulatum*).

Blastomycosis (*Blastomyces dermatitidis*). See Fungal Diseases of Organ Systems; Respiratory System, Mediastinum, and Pleurae; Disorders of Domestic Animals; Blastomycosis (*Blastomyces dermatitidis*).

Cardiovascular System and Lymphatic Vessels

Disorders of Domestic Animals

Angioinvasive Fungi. Angioinvasive fungi include a group of microbes that have the ability to colonize and invade barrier systems such as mucosae and skin, invade the vascular system within these barrier systems, spread to other organ systems, and cause disease. Fungi in this group include *Aspergillus* spp., *Candida* spp., *Fusarium* spp., *Absidia* spp., *Rhizopus* spp., and *Mucor* spp. The spores or conidia of these fungi are common microflora of the skin, body fluids, mucosal surfaces, and intestinal content. To gain access to the vascular system, the barrier provided by skin or mucosa must be injured. Processes that result in abrasions, penetrating wounds, and cell lysis are commonly involved. Injury results in the loss of epithelial cells and the exposure of basement membrane and subjacent vascularized ECM connective tissue. Similar to what occurs with *Aspergillus fumigatus* (see Fungal Diseases of Organ Systems; Respiratory System, Mediastinum, and Pleurae; Disorders of Domestic Animals; Aspergillosis [*Aspergillus fumigatus*]), hyphae invade vascularized tissues and gain access to the circulatory system by growing in and invading through vessel walls and endothelial cells, gain access to the circulatory system, break off into the bloodstream, circulate, and attach to and invade endothelium and ECM of other organ systems. Leukocyte trafficking may also be used to spread the fungus systemically. Ligand-receptor interactions are likely involved in this process, and these interactions probably determine in certain diseases which organ systems and tissue types are targeted by fungi. In affected organ systems, the mechanism of injury is cell lysis via chronic granulomatous to pyogranulomatous inflammation and its effector molecules and degradative enzymes.

As an example, mycotic rumenitis (followed by mycotic hepatitis) of cattle is caused by several of the fungal species listed earlier. The disease is often initiated by farm management practices such as (1) diets high in grains such as corn or (2) the long-term use of antibiotics in feeds. In the first case, feedlot cattle are fed increasing quantities of corn that serve as a carbohydrate source for ruminal microflora, which convert it, in part, to lactic acid. Excessive grain in the diet (grain overload) increases the quantity of lactic acid (lactic acidosis) in the rumen, and if such animals are deprived of water, lactic acid can accumulate and result in a drop of the pH of fluids covering ruminal mucosa. This outcome results in acid burns followed by loss of the epithelium and exposure of the basement membrane and subjacent vascularized connective tissue of the lamina propria and ECM tissues. Additionally, the long-term use of antibiotics in feeds can disrupt the protective environment created by normal microbial flora and lead to colonization and invasion of the mucosa by these fungi. Angioinvasive fungi (i.e., fungal hyphae or other elements) are able to invade and colonize the injured mucosa (mycotic rumenitis and/or abomasitis) and invade the vasculature of the ECM, and then spread regionally to other organ systems such as the liver (granulomatous fungal hepatitis) (see Figs. 8-51 and 14-51). The biologic materials in cells walls of fungi characteristically elicit a granulomatous inflammatory response because they are difficult for phagocytes to degrade. Thus in this example, granulomatous fungal hepatitis ensues.

Nervous System

Disorders of Domestic Animals

Cryptococcosis (*Cryptococcus neoformans*). The pathogenesis of cryptococcosis has many similarities to those of histoplasmosis, coccidioidomycosis, and blastomycosis discussed earlier. The mechanism of injury is cell lysis likely caused by atrophy secondary to tissue distortion and compression from expanding cryptococcal cysts in brain neuropil. There is little or no inflammation in this disease. *C. neoformans* has a dimorphic life cycle. The mycelial (basidiospores) phase occurs in extracellular environments (25° C), whereas the yeast phase occurs intracellularly within cells of the monocyte-macrophage system (37° C). Gross lesions include the formation of expansile cystic spaces filled with a gelatinous matrix (the capsule) within the brain and spinal cord, leading to compression and distortion of the tissue (see Figs. 14-49 and 14-50).

Animals encounter *C. neoformans* (dimorphic fungus) through inhalation of blastoconidia, basidiospores, or poorly encapsulated yeast cells (≈1.8 to 3.0 μm in diameter), which can reach the lower respiratory tract and alveoli. They are present in soil-derived aerosols from moist and humid environments and from bird droppings and nests. Basidiospores are deposited on the surface of mucosae of the nasopharyngeal cavity and of the conductive component of the respiratory system through centrifugal and inertial turbulence. They are readily phagocytized and killed by neutrophils and alveolar macrophages. For survival, basidiospores quickly germinate to yeast in mucosae or within phagosomes of alveolar macrophages. Yeast-derived glucosylceramide synthase is essential for survival of the yeast in mucosae, but after phagocytosis by mucosa-associated alveolar macrophages, it is not needed because the yeast uses other means of evading killing (discussed later). Yeast cells also produce phospholipases that injure alveolar type II epithelial cells and hinder the production and function of surfactant, thereby enhancing their adhesion to pneumocytes and improving chances of being phagocytosed by alveolar macrophages.

Recognition, attachment, and internalization by macrophages are likely mediated by ligand-receptor interactions, but specific molecules have not been identified. The polysaccharide capsule of yeast has antiphagocytic properties and may be immunosuppressive. The degree of encapsulation provides resistance to phagocytosis and killing by macrophages. In mucosae, unencapsulated or poorly encapsulated yeast cells are readily phagocytosed and killed, whereas encapsulated yeast is more resistant to phagocytosis and killing. The capsule's negative charge inhibits phagocytosis and killing by neutrophils and macrophages and causes complement depletion, antibody unresponsiveness, and dysregulation of cytokine secretion by monocytes and macrophages. The capsule can also inhibit recognition of yeast by macrophages and neutrophils and inhibit chemotaxis of leukocytes from the bloodstream into areas of inflammation. This latter response may account for the lack of inflammation in cysts. After phagocytosis and phagosome-lysosome fusion, yeast synthesizes additional polysaccharide capsule within the phagolysosome of the macrophage. Capsule dilutes lysosomal hydrolases and other toxic contents and provides a physical separation between the yeast and the membrane of the phagosome in which microbicidal compounds are located. This process continues until macrophages are grossly distended with capsule (>30 μm in diameter) and is the underlying mechanism of the formation of expansile cysts filled with a gelatinous matrix observed grossly in the brain. The capsule is composed primarily of two polysaccharides, glucuronoxylomannan and galactoxylomannan, and a smaller quantity of mannoprotein. These molecules also suppress the immune response.

Yeast cells appear to spread from the nasopharyngeal cavity to the CNS by direct extension into the meninges and neuropil, following compressive remodeling and osteolysis of the cribriform plate from a local infection of the nasal sinuses. However, leukocyte trafficking from the respiratory system via yeast-infected macrophages in the circulatory system with spread into the neuropil may also occur. This mechanism is hypothetical but probable based on what is known about the biology of the fungus. It is likely that yeast-infected macrophages interact through ligand-receptor interactions with endothelial cells of capillaries in the CNS. Capsule polysaccharides are also likely used to adhere and bind to brain endothelial cells and mediate endocytosis across the blood-brain barrier into the neuropil.

Once in nervous tissue, macrophages migrate through the neuropil. Because macrophages have short life spans, yeast, yeast-derived antigens, and polysaccharide capsule are released from dead macrophages into the neuropil. This outcome and its associated chemokines and cytokines recruit additional macrophages into the nervous system. This process is repetitive; thus the volume of polysaccharide capsule increases, and expansile cystic spaces filled with a gelatinous matrix are observed grossly in the brain. Additionally, melanin is an important cryptococcal virulence factor, which facilitates yeast survival during infection of the CNS. It acts as an antioxidant and eliminates reactive oxygen species that could kill the yeast. In the nervous system, yeast may use neurotransmitters, such as dopamine, norepinephrine, and epinephrine, as substrates for melanin production.

Protozoan Diseases

Portals of entry; target cells and substances; pathways of spread; virulence factors; mechanisms of adhesion, colonization, invasion, and replication; toxins; and defense mechanisms for protozoan diseases are similar to those discussed in the opening sections of this chapter and in the sections on bacterial and viral diseases.

Protozoan Diseases of Organ Systems

Alimentary System and the Peritoneum, Omentum, Mesentery, and Peritoneal Cavity

Disorders of Domestic Animals

Cryptosporidiosis (*Cryptosporidium parvum*). The mechanism of injury in cryptosporidiosis is dysfunction and lysis of epithelial cells covering tips and sides of intestinal villi, resulting from (1) dysfunction of microvilli of the brush border, (2) cytolysis of villus enterocytes after the microbe is released from infected cells, and (3) degradative effects of inflammation and its chemical mediators. Gross lesions are not observed; however, microscopic lesions include necrosis of epithelial cells, atrophy of villi, and mucosal inflammation (see E-Fig. 7-20).

Animals encounter *Cryptosporidium parvum* through direct contact with oocysts in water and food contaminated with feces from infected animals. Oocysts are ingested and carried through the oral pharynx, esophagus, stomach, and small intestine by normal peristaltic activities where they interact with gastric acids, pancreatic enzymes, and bile salts. One or more of these substances may trigger a process called *excystation*, where sporozoites are released from oocysts and randomly encounter the apical brush borders (microvilli with glycocalyx) of villus enterocytes covering tips and sides of intestinal villi. Sporozoites have a tropism for villus enterocytes of the jejunum and ileum that is apparently mediated by ligand-receptor interactions involved in attachment, invasion, and intracellular development of the protozoan. Apical complex and surface proteins expressed by sporozoites act as ligands, whereas *C. parvum* sporozoite ligand (CSL [circumsporozoite-like glycoprotein]) and probably other cell membrane proteins expressed on the apical surfaces of villus enterocytes act as receptors. Furthermore, the apical ends of sporozoites also adhere to microvilli of brush borders of villus enterocytes via sporozoite-specific lectin adherence factors such as glycoprotein 900 (GP900). Sporozoites and merozoites also express other surface glycoproteins (e.g., sporozoite and merozoite cell surface protein gp15/40/60 complex, P23, TRAP-C1 [thrombospondin-related adhesive protein *Cryptosporidium* 1]), which are virulence factors that increase the pathogenicity of the organism.

Once bound to cell membrane, sporozoites infect villus enterocytes by a mechanism dependent on parasite motility ("gliding motility"), activities of its apical complex, and secretion of enzymes from its apical organelles. Sporozoites become surrounded by cell membranes of microvilli to form parasitophorous vacuoles. Such vacuoles are retained in the microvillus layer and do not enter, but directly communicate with, the cytoplasm of the villus enterocyte through a feeding organelle. Once in parasitophorous vacuoles, sporozoites differentiate into trophozoites and then undergo asexual multiplication to form schizonts that contain six to eight merozoites. Schizonts rupture their vacuoles to release merozoites, and thus infected villus enterocytes are lysed, resulting in cell death, disruption of cell junctions, and loss of barrier functions. Merozoites spread distally via alimentary peristalsis in the small intestine to infect additional villus enterocytes through ligand-receptor interactions. It is likely that such ligand-receptor interactions determine which "new" populations of epithelial cells and what segment of the small intestine are infected. Once infected, new schizonts are formed in villus enterocytes through (1) asexual multiplication to form schizonts and (2) sexual reproduction (gametogony) by differentiating into male microgamonts or female macrogamonts. Microgamonts release microgametes that fertilize macrogametes inside macrogamonts, resulting in the formation of oocysts with sporozoites that can reinfect additional "new" villus enterocytes or are passed in the feces to spread the infection to other animals. These multiplicative and reproductive processes cause additional cell lysis and villus atrophy and consequently amplify the severity of mucosal injury. It has also been suggested that lysis of cells and villus atrophy may be caused by cell dysfunction and damage induced by cytokines and inflammatory molecules released from T lymphocytes and macrophages in inflammation. This latter mechanism causes increased intercellular permeability and may alter secretory functions and impair absorption of villus enterocytes. Infection, injury, and loss of villus enterocytes result in diarrhea likely caused by a combination of mechanisms, including osmotic diarrhea (malabsorption), secretory diarrhea, and increased intercellular permeability from inflammation. Enterotoxins may be involved in the secretory diarrhea, but none have been identified.

Malabsorption likely occurs from dysfunction of digestive enzymes present in the brush border of villus enterocytes infected by sporozoites and the subsequent lysis of these cells, both leading to failure to digest carbohydrates (impaired hydrolysis) and other molecules in the ingesta. This outcome leads to bacterial fermentation of substrates and an osmotic diarrhea. Sporozoite-injured villus enterocytes are sloughed from the villi, resulting in collapse (atrophy) of the structure of the villus, whereas the basement membrane from under the sloughed villus enterocytes is usually unaffected and functionally normal. Because the basement membrane is not injured and remains structurally intact, villus enterocytes derived from regenerative crypt enterocytes can divide and replace sloughed cells. These regenerative cells migrate up the villus from the crypts to initially cover exposed basement membranes; thus they are recognized early in the reparative process as flattened squamous-like cells stretched over the basement membrane. As the cells increase in density and maturity, they regain a more normal columnar structure. Moreover, the loss of enterocytes allows endotoxins and other potentially harmful molecules to gain access to the capillary and lymphatic vessels in the lamina propria of the villi and through absorption cause systemic cardiovascular and hemodynamic effects.

Coccidiosis* (Eimeria *spp.,* Isospora *spp.). The pathogenesis of coccidiosis is similar in many ways to that of cryptosporidiosis discussed earlier. The mechanism of injury is adenomatous proliferation (hypertrophy and hyperplasia) of infected villus enterocytes covering tips and sides of small intestinal villi, followed by lysis resulting from release of protozoans from infected cells. Gross lesions include mucosae that are initially elevated from a focal adenomatous to cerebriform epithelial response subsequently followed by active hyperemia, hemorrhage, and necrosis often with fibrinous and/or fibrinohemorrhagic cylindrical casts formed within the lumen of the intestine (see Figs. 7-125 to 7-129).

Animals (cattle, sheep, goats, and pigs) encounter the protozoan in grass, soil, and/or floors or surfaces contaminated with unsporulated oocysts from feces of infected animals. Coccidian oocysts are not infective (unsporulated) and therefore survive in pastures and other holding areas. Under the proper conditions (oxygen concentrations, humidity, and temperature), oocysts sporulate and become infective. Sporulated oocysts are ingested and carried through the oral pharynx, esophagus, stomach, and small intestine by normal peristaltic activities where they excyst and sporozoites are released. In proximity to intestinal villi, sporozoites randomly encounter mucosal villus enterocytes covering tips and sides of intestinal villi. Sporozoites have tropisms for specific animal species and for specific populations of villus enterocytes in specific segments of the small and large intestine. This tropism is determined by surface microneme proteins (MICs) that appear to be unique to each species of the protozoan. Sialic acid, galactose, and many forms of these molecules act as receptors and are arrayed on enterocyte membranes. Patterns of these receptors likely determine the specificity for microneme proteins unique to individual species of coccidia. Other ligand-receptor interactions are probably involved in invasion and intracellular development of the protozoan. Sporozoites go through one or more asexual generations and a (single) sexual generation in different segments of the small intestine (see section on Cryptosporidiosis). The replication and release of generations of these protozoans in and from mucosal villus enterocytes, respectively, account for the lesions observed grossly.

Giardiasis* (Giardia *spp.). The pathogenesis of giardiasis is similar in many ways to those of cryptosporidiosis and coccidiosis discussed earlier. The mechanisms of injury in giardiasis are (1) dysfunction of microvilli and the glycocalyx of brush borders and (2) cell death via apoptosis of epithelial cells covering tips and sides of small intestinal villi. These outcomes result in increased permeability of the mucosal barrier system, chloride ion shifts probably via enterotoxin-mediated hypersecretion, dysfunction of digestive enzymes present in the brush border resulting in malabsorption diarrhea, and acute inflammation. Gross lesions are usually not observed; however, microscopic lesions may include loss of epithelial cells, atrophy of villi, and mucosal inflammation.

Animals (horses, cattle, sheep, goats, pigs, dogs, and cats) encounter *Giardia* spp. through direct contact with parasite cysts in water and food contaminated with feces from infected animals. Following ingestion, excystation occurs in the small intestine via the actions of gastric acid and pancreatic enzymes. An excyzoite is released into the intestinal lumen, where it matures into two trophozoites that subsequently attach to the brush border of villus epithelial cells by a cytoskeletal organelle called an *adhesive disk*. Trophozoites move via flagella but do not invade epithelial cells. The anatomic segment of intestine (duodenum, jejunum, or ileum) used for attachment is species specific, suggesting that colonization is facilitated by unique ligand-receptor interactions, especially by ligands in the outer membrane of the parasite. Trophozoites replicate attached to epithelial cells, encyst, and are then passed in feces.

Virulence factors for *Giardia* spp. have not been well characterized; however, colonization of specific segments of the small intestine involve genes for the adhesive disk, flagella, and variable small proteins (VSP) in the outer membrane of the parasite. Additionally, trophozoites appear to be able to cause apoptosis of colonized epithelial cells covering tips and sides of small intestinal villi through both the intrinsic and extrinsic apoptotic pathways and thus contribute to the outcomes discussed in the initial paragraph. Infection, injury, and loss of villus enterocytes result in (1) glucose malabsorption and bacterial fermentation with osmotic diarrhea; (2) Cl^- hypersecretion, and (3) systemic changes in other electrolyte (Na^+) and solute concentrations, leading to alterations in hydration and systemic vascular osmolarity. The cumulative effect of injury and giardia antigens also initiates an acute inflammatory response mediated by an array of chemical mediators, which contribute to dysfunction of cellular junctions and increased intercellular permeability and thus mucosal and intestinal edema.

Nervous System

Disorders of Horses

Protozoan Encephalomyelitis (*Sarcocystis neurona*). The mechanism of injury in protozoan encephalomyelitis is disruption and lysis of neurons and neural cells from replication and release of the protozoan and from inflammation and its chemical mediators and degradative enzymes. Gross lesions include yellow-white areas of malacia mixed with hemorrhage in gray and white matter of the brain and spinal cord (see Figs. 14-81 and 14-82).

The discussion that follows is provisional and is based, in part, on known mechanisms used by *T. gondii*, *C. parvum*, and other protozoans. Horses and other animals encounter sporocysts in feed, water, grass, or soil, and/or on floors or surfaces contaminated with feces from infected opossums. They are ingested and swallowed and through peristalsis gain access to mucosae of the intestines. Here sporozoites are released from sporocysts, which then must gain access to endothelial cells to mature to merozoites, the form that spreads to the CNS. Infection and involvement of endothelial cells appears to be a step central to the pathogenesis of the disease. However, little is known about the mechanism of interaction with mucosa or spread to the brain and spinal cord. Sporozoites could (1) be phagocytized by mucosa-associated macrophages (leukocyte trafficking) and subsequently spread locally to encounter endothelial cells within capillaries of the lamina propria supporting enterocytes or (2) interact with and penetrate the mucosa to gain direct access to endothelial cells in the lamina propria. It appears, but is unproven, that leukocyte trafficking via mucosa-associated macrophages is the mechanism most likely involved in spread to endothelial cells. Once in contact with endothelial cells, sporozoites enter them and mature to form schizonts containing merozoites, which eventually rupture and release merozoites into the blood and adjacent vascular ECM. They then infect adjacent endothelial cells and repeat the replicative process. Injury to endothelial cells likely causes focal vascular inflammation that recruits macrophages into the site of injury, where they may phagocytize merozoites.

At this local site there are three potential mechanisms for systemic spread to the CNS. First, cell-free merozoites may enter the venous system, navigate the heart, and be carried via the arterial system to the CNS to interact with endothelial cells. Second, cell-free merozoites may enter the lymphatic system, be carried to the thoracic duct and enter the venous system, navigate the heart, and be carried via the arterial system to the CNS to interact with endothelial cells. Third, merozoites could be phagocytized by macrophages and carried via leukocyte trafficking to encounter and enter capillaries in the lamina propria and spread systemically via the circulatory system to the CNS or be carried to Peyer's patches or by lymphatic vessels to regional lymph nodes, and then migrate via lymphatic vessels and the thoracic duct to the circulatory system and spread systemically to the CNS. Based on known mechanisms used by *T. gondii*, *C. parvum*, and other protozoans and the need to evade innate and adaptive immune responses, it seems more likely that sporozoites would attempt to gain access to intracellular locations in mucosal epithelial cells or mucosal-associated macrophages as early as possible in the disease. Thus the latter of the three mechanisms of spread appears most probable.

It is not known how merozoites enter the CNS; however, cell-free merozoites or merozoite-infected macrophages likely interact with endothelial cells in the CNS and are subsequently infected. Ligand-receptor interactions may determine tropism in the CNS and which areas of the vasculature are infected. Schizonts containing merozoites likely develop in endothelial cells of the CNS, and when these cells are lysed, merozoites are spread into the neuropil. This process undoubtedly injures the blood-brain barrier and causes inflammation. Additionally, macrophages via leukocyte trafficking may carry merozoites into the neuropil, where they could infect neurons, microglial cells, or other neuronal cells. In all of these infected cells, schizonts form containing merozoites that lyse the infected cell when merozoites are released. This process injures endothelium and neuropil, leading to inflammation, vasculitis and thrombosis, hemorrhage, and malacia and the recruitment of additional macrophages (from circulating monocytes) and activation of resident microglial cells, resulting in the lesions characteristic of protozoan encephalomyelitis.

Reproductive System

Disorders of Ruminants (Cattle, Sheep, and Goats)

Toxoplasmosis (*Toxoplasma gondii*). The mechanism of injury in toxoplasmosis is dysfunction and lysis of epithelial cells of the placenta and the fetus resulting in abortion, neonatal mortality, and fetal malformation predominantly in sheep and goats and less commonly in cattle. Toxoplasmosis in cats is usually inconsequential and will not be discussed here. Gross lesions include active hyperemia, rough and granular mucosae consistent with necrosis, and mineralization of caruncles of the uterus and cotyledons of fetal membranes (see Fig. 18-47). A component of this lesion includes acute inflammation. Intercaruncular and intercotyledonary tissues are unaffected.

Animals, other than cats, and human beings are intermediate hosts for *T. gondii* and encounter oocysts in contaminated soil. Cats are the definitive host; thus cat feces are the source of oocysts. Oocysts are resistant to degradation and may survive in the environment for years. Under the proper conditions (oxygen concentrations, humidity, and temperature), oocysts sporulate and become infective. Sporulated oocysts are ingested and carried by normal peristaltic activities through the oral pharynx, esophagus, and stomach to the small intestine, where they excyst and release sporozoites into the intestinal lumen in close proximity to intestinal mucosal villus enterocytes. Infections are characterized by the ability of the organism to cross barrier systems such as intestinal mucosae and the blood-brain barrier, blood-retina barrier, and placenta. This process appears to involve parasite motility (linear myosin, F-actin filaments, and gliding-associated proteins) and interactions between parasite adhesins and target cell receptors that facilitate transfer of the organism through mucosae. Mounting evidence also suggests that *T. gondii* uses migrating leukocytes to disseminate (leukocyte trafficking) throughout the animal while avoiding adaptive immune responses. Sporozoites infect villus enterocytes and complete an asexual replication in parasitophorous vacuoles forming tachyzoites. In parasitophorous vacuoles the protozoan initiates the production of the antiinflammatory cytokines IL-10 and transforming growth factor-β (TGF-β), which inhibit the production of proinflammatory cytokines IL-12 and TNF-α. Tachyzoites are released via cell lysis and infect and replicate in additional enterocytes and then invade subjacent lamina propria, infect cells of the monocyte-macrophage system, and enter lymphatic vessels. They spread locally to lymphoid tissues (likely Peyer's patches) and regionally to mesenteric lymph nodes via lymphatic vessels and then systemically via lymphatic vessels and the thoracic duct (or capillaries or postcapillary venules) to the circulatory system and then systemically to caruncular epithelial cells and cotyledonary trophoblasts.

T. gondii requires an intracellular site for growth and replication. Tachyzoite and likely sporozoite tropism for target cells appears to be mediated by ligand-receptor interactions. Infection of intestinal villus enterocytes by sporozoites and tachyzoites is a well-studied process that involves six steps that begin with the recognition of target cells and end with the formation of a parasitophorous vacuole within the same cell. Parasitophorous vacuoles are a mechanism used to modulate target cell functions in support of parasite replication and infection. Tachyzoites (and likely sporozoites) express glycosylphosphatidylinositol-linked surface proteins (SAGs) that serve as ligands, whereas intestinal villus enterocyte membrane receptors appear to include laminin, lectin, and SAG receptor proteins. Proteins, such as SAG1 and SAG3, are abundant on tachyzoites and function in target cell attachment and immune modulation and may also cause direct injury to intestinal epithelium.

When tachyzoites spread systemically from lymphoid tissues to other tissues such as the placenta, they encounter cells of the uterine caruncle and probably use ligand-receptor interactions and the six-step process described previously to infect cells of the caruncles and then spread to adjacent trophoblasts of the cotyledons. Tachyzoites replicate in these placental cells, eventually causing their lysis. Lysis leads to alterations in placental structure (necrosis and mineralization of caruncles and cotyledons), disturbances of vascular flow, and placental dysfunction that injures developing fetuses. Lesions caused by tachyzoites have also been described in the brain (inflammation and congenital malformations) and other tissues of the fetus. How and by what mechanism they spread from the placenta to the fetus is unknown (likely fetal macrophage-like cells); however, they appear to infect diverse populations of fetal cells, resulting in injury and lysis. If infection occurs early in gestation, fetal lysis and resorption occur. Infection in midgestation causes fetal lysis, leading to mummification mixed with live but weak fetuses. Infection in late gestation does not usually injure the fetus because of a good adaptive immune response.

Neosporosis (*Neospora caninum*). The pathogenesis and mechanisms of injury in neosporosis are similar to those of toxoplasmosis discussed earlier. The dog is the definitive host for *Neospora caninum*; all other animals are intermediate hosts. Much like in toxoplasmosis, abortion is the primary disease caused by *N. caninum* in cattle, sheep, goat, and pigs.

Prion Diseases

Portals of entry; target cells and substances; pathways of spread; virulence factors; mechanisms of adhesion, colonization, invasion, and replication; toxins; and defense mechanisms for prion diseases are similar to those discussed in the opening sections of this chapter and in the sections on bacterial and viral diseases.

Prion Diseases of Organ Systems

Nervous System

Disorders of Domestic Animals

Transmissible Spongiform Encephalopathies (Prion Diseases). The mechanism of injury in transmissible spongiform encephalopathies (TSEs) is metabolic dysfunction of neurons and neural cells caused by the conversion of normal cellular prion protein (PrP^C) to an abnormal form (PrP^{Sc}) and the accumulation of PrP^{Sc} in neurons, neural cells, and extracellularly within the neuropil (Fig. 4-45). Currently there is some research data that suggests a "potential" role for *Spiroplasma* spp., a group of small bacteria without cell walls,

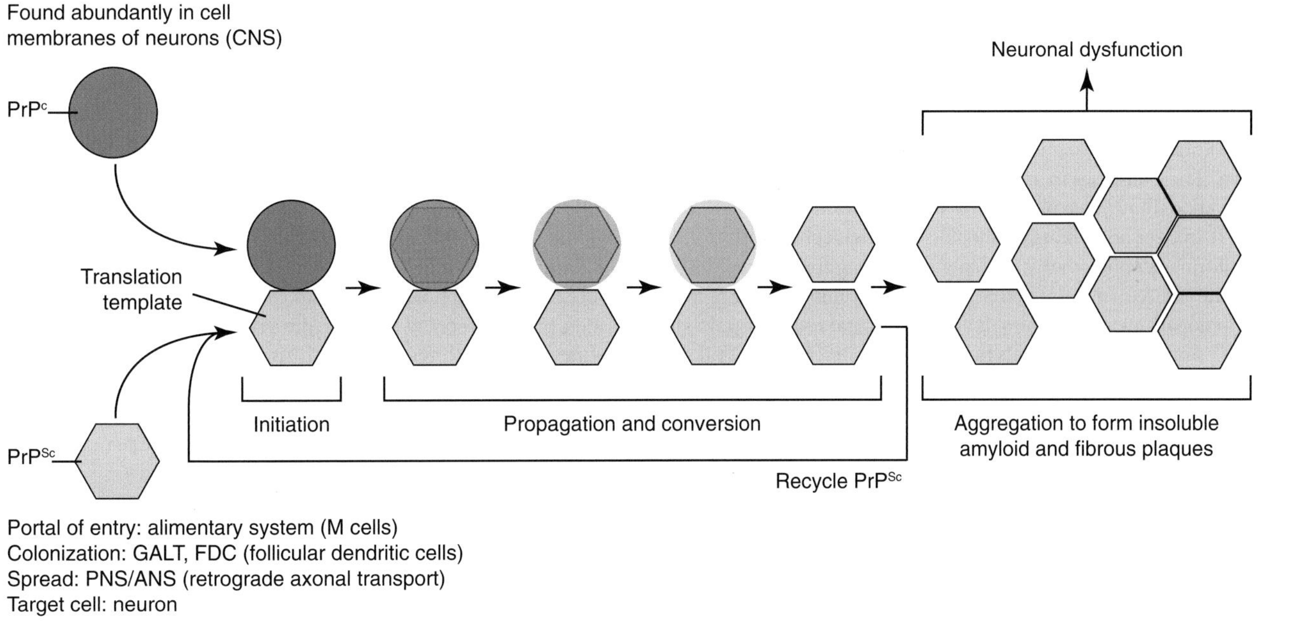

Figure 4-45 The Stepwise Process of Converting Prion Proteins to Amyloid and Fibrous Plaques. When the infectious form of prion protein (PrP^{Sc}) reaches the central nervous system (CNS) (see Fig. 4-46), it behaves as a translation template that converts normal PrP^C to PrP^{Sc}, a misfolded and aggregated β-sheet–rich isoform of PrP^C. Because neurons have large concentrations of PrP^C located in their cell membranes when compared to other cells of the body, PrP^{Sc} aggregation and accumulation affects the nervous system to a much greater extent. This outcome results in degeneration of neurons and the neuropil. Translation follows a stepwise process of initiation, propagation, conversion, and aggregation to end with the accumulation of large quantities of insoluble amyloid and fibrous plaques in neurons and the neuropil. Additionally, PrP^{Sc} that is not aggregated into the β-sheet–rich isoform is "recycled" to interact with PrP^C in a self-amplifying process resulting in the accumulation of high concentrations of PrP^{Sc}. The shapes of the prion proteins are used for illustrative purposes only and do not represent their molecular structure. *ANS*, Autonomic nervous system; *GALT*, gut-associated lymphoid tissue; *M cell*, microfold cell; *PNS*, peripheral nervous system. (Courtesy Dr. J.F. Zachary, College of Veterinary Medicine, University of Illinois.)

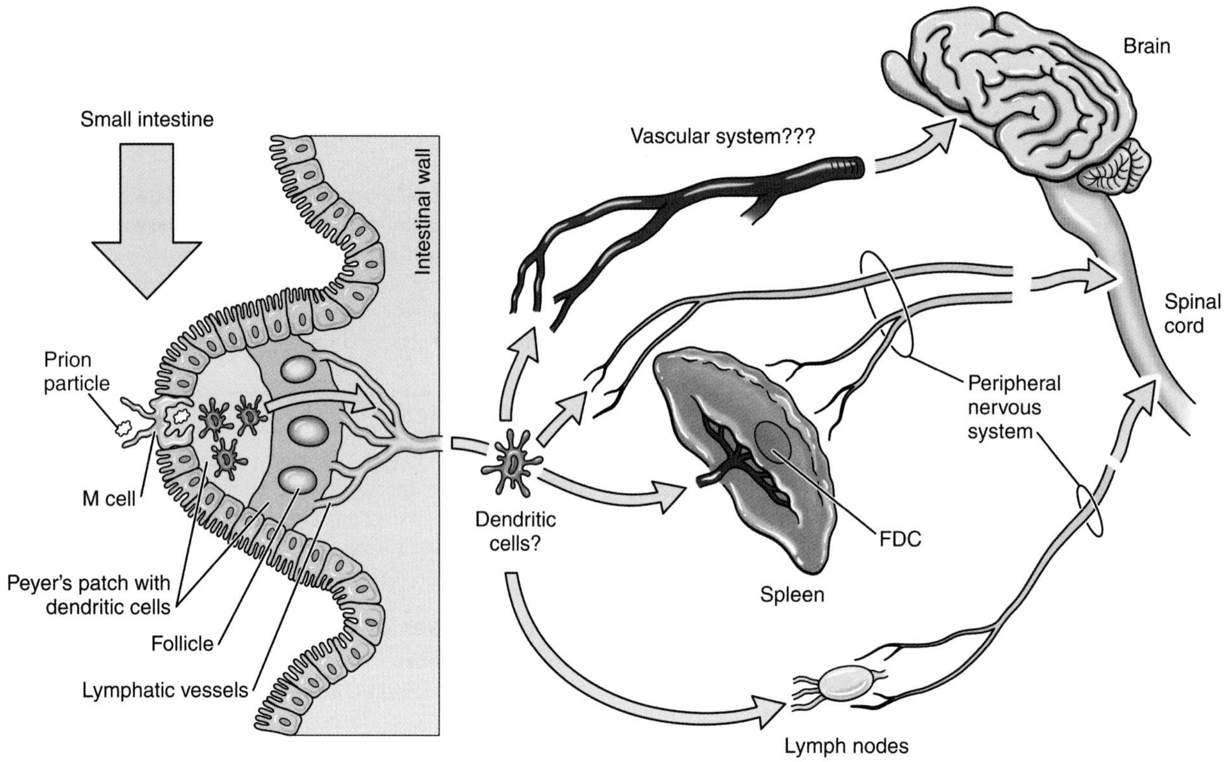

Figure 4-46 **Pathogenesis of Transmissible Spongiform Encephalopathies.** Prions appear to use microfold cell (M cells) (also macrophages) to enter Peyer's patches and infect dendritic cells as well as macrophages and lymphocytes. Dendritic cells (and likely macrophages) then spread prions through leukocyte trafficking in lymphatic vessels to local, regional, and systemic lymphoid nodules, lymph nodes, and/or spleen where infection is sustained and amplified, especially in follicular dendritic cells (FDCs) of the spleen and B lymphocytes. Prions released from dendritic cells are able to enter nerve endings in lymphoid tissues, and by retrograde and anterograde nerve transport they spread throughout the central nervous system (CNS). It has been hypothesized that prions may also spread to the CNS hematogenously, but the existence of this route is uncertain.

instead of prions in the pathogenesis of TSEs. These data are in dispute and will be sorted out over the next decade. Gross lesions are not observed except in chronic cases, in which atrophy of the brain may occur. Microscopic lesions characteristic of injury include intracytoplasmic vacuoles in neurons and neuropil (spongiform change), neuronal loss, gliosis, and an absence of leukocytic inflammation. These diseases in animals include scrapie (sheep and goats), bovine spongiform encephalopathy (BSE), chronic wasting disease (CWD) in deer and elk, transmissible mink encephalopathy, feline spongiform encephalopathy, and ungulate spongiform encephalopathy. The source of prions that spread transmissible spongiform encephalopathies among animals and the natural routes of transmission of prions between animals have not been determined. Soil may serve as a prion reservoir.

Animals probably encounter prions most commonly by ingestion. Alternatively, inhalation or direct contact (conjunctival mucous membranes) may also be important routes of spread in specific prion diseases such as scrapie and chronic wasting disease. Prions can be found in a tissue-free environment (urine, saliva, blood, and body waste) as a direct source of the microbe or in a tissue-associated environment (offal [i.e., entrails and internal organs of butchered animals], placentas, or decaying carcasses) as an indirect source of the microbe. This latter source appears to be the route that occurs primarily in cattle and mink. In the United Kingdom, cattle were infected with prions by ingesting offal derived from prion-infected sheep or cattle that had not been properly treated to kill the microbe. Mucosae of the oral pharynx, especially the tonsil, small intestine, nasal pharynx, and conjunctiva, are thought to be the probable locations of initial encounters with prions. It is unclear if and how prions are trapped in the mucus layer and, if so, how they gain access to mucosal epithelial cells, macrophages, and/or dendritic cells in the mucus layer. It appears that prions are able to attach to apical surfaces of mucosal epithelial cells, M cells, and possibly dendritic cells in tonsillar, alimentary, and respiratory mucosae, respectively. Transcytosis or dendritic cell migration (also potentially via macrophage migration) is probably used by prions to pass through mucosal epithelial cells and M cells to their basolateral surfaces and to gain access to and infect B and T lymphocytes, macrophages, and dendritic cells in Peyer's patches (GALT) or lymphoid nodules and aggregates like BALT. Prions are then probably spread systemically via leukocyte trafficking in lymphocytes, monocytes, and dendritic cells to other lymphoid organs such as the spleen and systemic lymph nodes. In lymphoid tissue, follicular dendritic cells and B lymphocytes are essential for prion replication, amplification, and accumulation in large numbers before spread to the nervous system.

Although in TSEs the final targets are neurons and the neuropil, the mechanisms used by specific TSEs to colonize and spread prions to reach these targets may vary based on animal species. In cattle, BSE prions encounter and colonize cells of MALT in the palatine tonsils and Peyer's patches of the distal ileum. They replicate in numbers sufficient to enter nerve endings in MALT. They then spread via retrograde axonal transport to the CNS and brain mainly following the parasympathetic and sympathetic nerve fibers of the autonomic nervous system. BSE prions amplify in large numbers almost exclusively in the CNS and PNS. In contrast in sheep, scrapie prions appear to amplify in large numbers in cells of the lymphoid and monocyte-macrophage systems before entering nerve endings and spreading to the brain via the autonomic nervous system.

Prions are able to infect nerve endings of the vagus nerve, sympathetic nerves, and sensory nerves that innervate lymphoid tissues and organs and then use retrograde axonal transport to gain access to the CNS and spread in the nervous system via synaptically linked neurons (Fig. 4-46). It is thought that prion-infected macrophages and dendritic cells deliver prions to these nerve endings; however, it is not known if endocytosis is involved in the entry of prions into nerve endings or in their spread between cell membranes in synapses. In macrophages and dendritic cells, prions are located in multivesicular endosomes (i.e., membrane-bound vesicles inside cells) and may be transferred between cells in exosomes (i.e., cell-derived extracellular vesicles). Such a mechanism may be involved in interneuronal spread within the nervous system. Attachment proteins of prions or membrane receptors on target cells have not been identified. However, Toll-like PRRs may serve as receptors for prion entry into cells. Prions have tropisms for different animal species that are likely determined by the tertiary and quaternary structure of prions, resulting in their binding to or interaction with different molecules (receptors) and thus different target cells. Cellular tropism may also be restricted to those cells that express a cofactor compatible with the respective prion strain.

Most cells in the body have PrP^{C}; however, the highest concentrations are present in the nervous system, especially in synaptic membranes as a neuronal membrane glycoprotein. PrP^{C} is also expressed in cells of the immune system (see Figs. 4-45 and 4-46). The function of PrP^{C} is unknown, but its physiologic function may include immunoregulation, signal transduction, copper binding, synaptic transmission, induction of apoptosis, or protection against apoptotic stimuli. In neurons, PrP^{Sc} serves as a translation template that converts (conformational change) normal PrP^{C} to PrP^{Sc}, a misfolded and aggregated β-sheet–rich isoform of PrP^{C}. This folding pattern makes PrP^{Sc} resistant to the action of proteases and causes it to aggregate and accumulate as an insoluble amyloid in neurons and neuropil in the form of large amyloid and fibrous plaques. It is not known how PrP^{Sc} causes neuronal degeneration; however, reduced antioxidant protection, increased oxidative stress, loss of function of normal PrP^{C}, or toxicity caused by PrP^{Sc}, all related to the accumulation of amyloid plaque, have been proposed. The activation (hypertrophy and hyperplasia) of microglial cells may also suggest that their biologic activities and effector molecules are involved in neuronal degeneration. There are no specific virulence factors for prions.

Suggested Readings

Suggested Readings are available at www.expertconsult.com.

CHAPTER 5

Diseases of Immunity[1]

Paul W. Snyder

Key Readings Index

General Features of the Immune System

The immune system is a defensive system whose primary functions are to protect against infectious organisms, such as bacteria, viruses, fungi, and parasites, and the development of cancer. The complexity by which these functions occur is evidenced not only by the cell types, recognition molecules, and soluble factors involved and interactions with other systems (e.g., endocrine, nervous) but also by the ability to recognize virtually any foreign antigen. Immunologic responses result in pathologic processes, primarily inflammatory responses, either as a result of normal immune responses to foreign antigens (e.g., microbial pathogens) or from aberrations of the immune system as in the case of hypersensitivity reactions and autoimmune diseases. Finally, the importance of a normal functional immune system cannot be more evident than in instances in which it is deficient as the result of a genetic defect or as the result of an acquired immunodeficiency disease.

Immunity is the result of nonspecific (innate) and specific (adaptive) responses that together provide effective protection. The immune system's recognition and response functional capabilities are key components of both innate and adaptive immune responses. The recognition capabilities are highly specific and allow immune responses to develop against a diverse group of foreign (nonself) antigens and prevent the development of immune responses to self-antigens. Innate and adaptive immune responses feature effector mechanisms for eliminating or neutralizing the antigen, whereas adaptive immunity has the additional feature of memory. A common paradigm shared by antigen nonspecific and specific mechanisms of immunity is the ability to polarize the responses in the direction of those most efficient in eliminating the pathogen. Unfortunately, this polarization can also be misdirected, resulting in inappropriate immune responses such as in allergy and autoimmunity. The emphasis of this chapter is on diseases that are the result of inadequate or inappropriate immune responses. Before one can understand the pathogenic mechanisms of these diseases, one must first have an understanding of the basic elements of the immune system. The chapter begins with an overview of our current understanding of innate and adaptive immunity, cells of the immune system, cytokines, and major histocompatibility complex (MHC) molecules. This overview facilitates the discussion of disorders of the immune system, which includes hypersensitivity reactions, autoimmunity, and immunodeficiency. This chapter concludes with a discussion of amyloidosis, a diverse group of conditions characterized by the deposition of a pathologic extracellular protein. One of the conditions is associated with the deposition of immunoglobulin components. Although the focus of this text is on the pathologic basis of veterinary diseases, with an emphasis on domestic species, in this chapter we use the vast knowledge base regarding human and rodent immunology (applicable to most mammalian species studied to date) as our basis and interject major known relevant species differences as appropriate.

Innate Immunity (Nonspecific Immunity)

As stated previously, the function of the immune system is to protect against infectious pathogens and the development of cancer. There are two categories of immune responses that are based in part on their specificity for the antigen: (1) innate immunity and (2) adaptive (specific) immunity (Fig. 5-1). Innate immune responses are considered the first-line defense mechanisms, are not specific to the antigen, and lack memory (Essential Concept 5-1). These defense mechanisms are the result of anatomic (e.g., skin, mucosal epithelia,

[1]For a glossary of abbreviations and terms used in this chapter see E-Glossary 5-1.

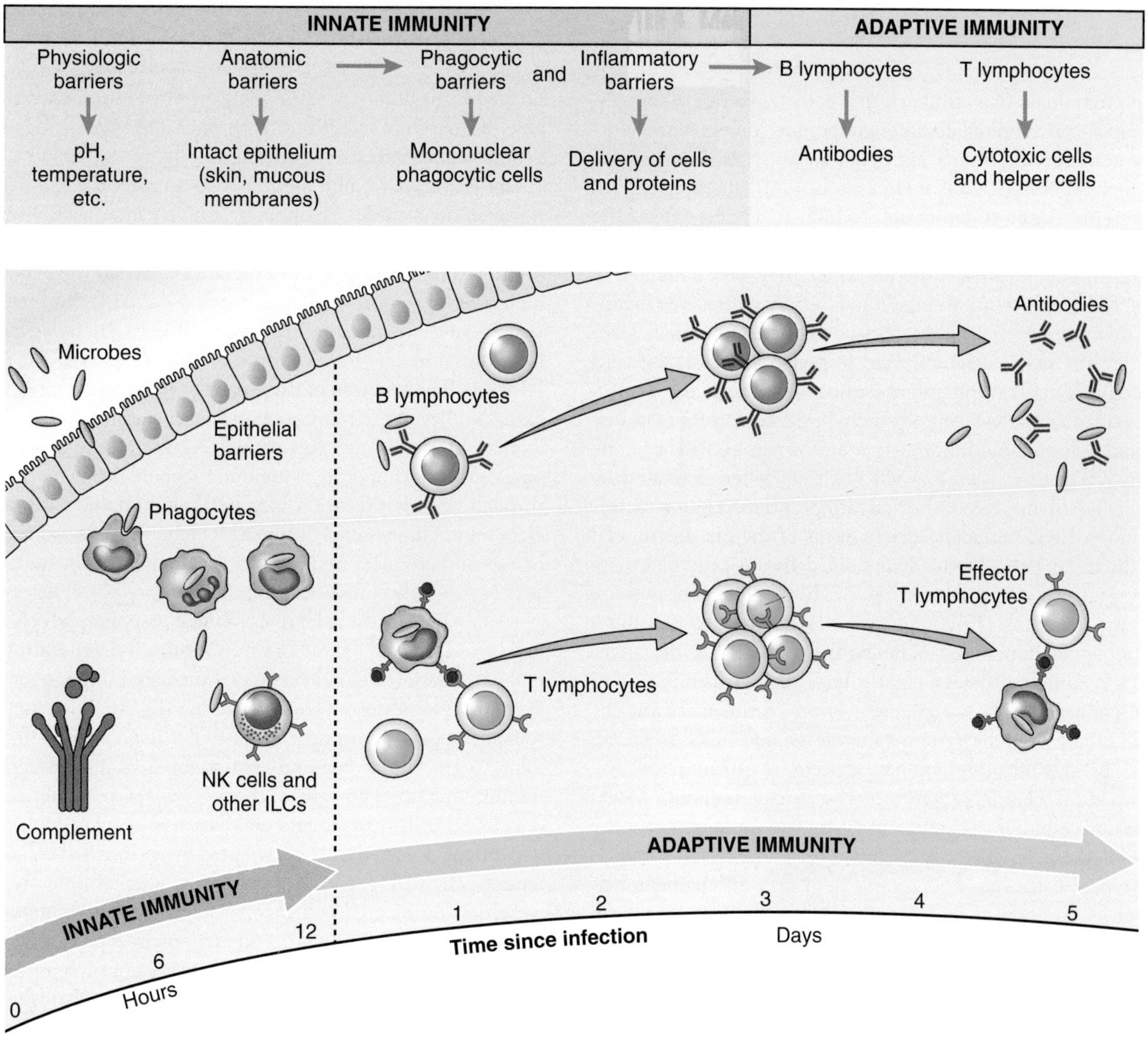

Figure 5-1 **Innate (Nonspecific) and Adaptive Immunity (Specific Immunity).** Innate immunity is the first-line defense against infectious organisms and comprises chemical and physical barriers, proteins like complement, and non–antigen-specific mononuclear cells like innate lymphoid cells (ILCs) and phagocytic cells. Adaptive immunity is the antigen-specific defense arm of immunity directed by T and B lymphocytes that have been "primed" by cells of innate immunity and result in effector mechanisms for eliminating infectious organisms. NK, Natural killer.

ESSENTIAL CONCEPT 5-1 Innate Immunity

Innate immunity is a group of nonspecific first-line defense mechanisms that occur immediately or within a very short time frame (i.e., minutes to hours) following exposure to antigens (from microbes [also tumor cells—see Chapter 6]). These defenses and mechanisms include (1) barrier systems (see Chapter 4) provided by skin or mucosae; (2) physiologic properties of these barriers such as pH, mucus layer, and body temperature; and (3) inflammatory and phagocytic responses within these barriers. Key structural components are epithelial cells of intact barriers; phagocytic cells such as neutrophils, monocytes, and tissue macrophages within these barriers; innate lymphoid cells (ILCs) and dendritic cells within these barriers; and plasma proteins, such as those of the complement system. When the epithelium of a barrier system is penetrated by a microbe, it subsequently encounters well-vascularized (endothelial cells) extracellular matrix in the lamina propria, submucosa, or dermis/subcutis.

Microbes express unique patterns of biologic molecules (ligands) on or in their membranes called *pathogen-associated molecular patterns* (PAMPs). PAMPs include molecules such as glycans, glycoconjugates, and lipopolysaccharide that are expressed across large groups of different types of microbes, thus making the innate immune response nonspecific to a particular individual genus of microbe as occurs in adaptive immunity. Endothelial cells, phagocytic cells, and ILCs have *pattern recognition receptors* (PRRs), including Toll-like receptors (TLRs), that recognize and respond to PAMPs and other cell surface molecules on microbes. These ligand-receptor interactions initiate acute inflammation and the recruitment of phagocytic cells from the vasculature and result in phagocytosis, phagosome-lysosome fusion, neutralization of toxins, and digestion of microbes. TLRs (1) regulate cell recruitment to sites of infection through adhesion molecules, chemokines, and chemokine receptors during an inflammatory response; (2) activate leukocytes (primarily neutrophils and natural killer cells of the innate immune system) and epithelial, endothelial, and hematopoietic cells; and (3) are essential for linking the innate immune response to the adaptive immune responses (see Essential Concept 5-2).

The innate immune system can also distinguish between intracellular (e.g., viruses) and extracellular (e.g., extracellular bacteria) microbes and initiate different types of responses to control them through cell-intrinsic and cell-extrinsic recognition mechanisms in infected cells or uninfected cells, respectively. ILCs are commonly located within skin or mucosae of barrier systems and act through PRR-PAMP interactions to initiate acute inflammation and other cytotoxic and noncytotoxic effects on microbes, as well as to initiate and sustain adaptive immune responses, primarily against microbes. Finally, the innate immune system can activate the complement system via the alternative or mannose/lectin pathways (see Chapter 3). This mechanism results in the formation of a membrane attack complex (see Chapter 3) that kills microbes by perforating their cell membranes.

cilia) and physiologic (e.g., stomach pH, body temperature) properties, and phagocytic and inflammatory responses. Major components of innate immunity are intact epithelial barriers, phagocytic cells, innate lymphoid cells (ILCs [see later discussion]), and a number of plasma proteins, the most important of which are the proteins of the complement system. Phagocytic cells are recruited to sites of infection during an inflammatory response, where they have a number of functions, two of which are to ingest and destroy pathogenic organisms and neutralize toxins. Neutrophils, monocytes, and tissue macrophages are the major cells involved in phagocytosis. These cells recognize components of microbial pathogens through the expression of several membrane receptors, including receptors for mannose residues and *N*-formyl-methionine–containing peptides and a family of pattern recognition receptors (PRRs) that, when activated by microbial components, signal the activation of transcription factors that facilitate the microbicidal mechanisms of the phagocytic cell and are discussed later. Innate lymphoid cells are cells of innate immunity and are also discussed later. The complement system, discussed in Chapter 3, is a complex cascade of proteins that has a number of biologic functions, including the formation of the membrane attack complex that efficiently lyses plasma membranes of microbial pathogens. The complement system can be activated by either the innate immune system (alternative and mannose/lectin pathways) or the adaptive immune system (classical pathway). Other important plasma proteins of the innate immune system include mannose-binding protein and C-reactive protein; two of the functions of these proteins are to facilitate phagocytosis through opsonization of pathogens and complement activation. Inflammatory responses comprise vascular, permeability, and cellular phases that act in response to damage to vascularized tissue. The features of the inflammatory response are also presented in Chapter 3.

Recognition Molecules of Innate Immunity

The recognition molecules of innate immunity provide an opportunity to recognize pathogens by cells other than lymphocytes. These germline-encoded molecules function to sense molecular structures shared by microbes and endogenous molecules associated with inflammation. The recognition molecules associated with microbes are generally referred to as *pathogen-associated molecular patterns* (PAMPs). The function of the innate immune system extends beyond microbial pathogen recognition to include endogenous molecules associated with cell damage and inflammation, which are generally referred to as danger- or damage-associated molecular patterns (DAMPs). The activation of the innate immune system through these invariant PRRs not only precedes lymphocyte activation but also is required to initiate the adaptive immune responses. The molecular patterns of PRRs are associated with microbial pathogens and classified as secreted, transmembrane, and cytosolic forms. Collectins and pentraxin are examples of secreted PRRs that largely function to bind to microbial surfaces and activate the complement system. Collectins, having properties of collagen and lectins, include mannose-binding lectins and pulmonary surfactants A and D. Pentraxin is composed of five identical subunits that form a pentamer and include C-reactive protein, an activator of the classical pathway of complement. Toll-like receptors (TLRs) and C-type lectins are examples of the transmembrane PRRs, and they have limited cellular distribution, including macrophages, natural killer (NK) cells, and dendritic cells. TLRs are expressed on the plasma membrane or in endosomal/lysosomal organelles. The cytosolic PRRs are more widely distributed, including all nucleated cells, and include retinoic acid–inducible gene (RIG)-I–like receptors (RLRs) and nucleotide-binding oligomerization domain (NOD) and NOD-like receptors (NLRs). These recognition molecules provide the host with the ability to sense "danger" either through PAMPs in the case of microbial infections or through DAMPs in the presence of cellular damage or stress. This allows the innate immune system to detect and initiate immune responses in response to infectious and noninfectious causes. NLR molecules as immune sensors are not unique to mammals because they have been found in plants and urchins. The molecules are designated based on the structure of the molecule NLR with a suffix of P (pyrin domain) or C (caspase activation and recruitment domains [CARD]), referring to the N-terminal moiety followed by a number (e.g., NLRP1, NLRP2, or NLRP3). The function of these pattern recognition molecules is also extended beyond the initiation of adaptive immunity to also include regulation of cell death (apoptosis). As is often the case in immunology, our understanding of immune responses is greatly enhanced through the identification of genetic immunologic disorders. Deficiencies in components of the NLRs have been described in human beings and are most frequently associated with inflammatory disorders (e.g., Crohn's disease and inflammatory bowel disease).

Analogous to the adaptive immune response, which has developed the ability to defend the host against a diverse array of microbial pathogens (humoral versus cell-mediated responses), the innate immune system is now seen as also having an ability to distinguish specific types of pathogens. Intracellular (e.g., viruses) and extracellular (extracellular bacteria) pathogens require different types of immune responses to control them. The innate immune system has developed cell-intrinsic and cell-extrinsic recognition mechanisms dependent on whether it is mediated by an infected cell or an uninfected cell. Cell-extrinsic recognition mechanisms are a way in which an uninfected cell can participate in the immune response and are mediated through transmembrane receptors (e.g., TLRs) on specialized cells of the innate immune system such as macrophages and dendritic cells. Cell-intrinsic recognition mechanisms are essential for recognizing intracellular pathogens and involve type I interferon (IFN) gene transcription signaling by members of the RLRs. Three members of the RLR family are RIG-I, melanoma differentiation-associated gene-5 (MDA-5), and laboratory of genetics and physiology gene 2 (LPG-2). In viral sensing the RLRs are highly discriminating with regard to the cytoplasmic localization and sensing of specific RNAs. They specifically detect RNA molecular patterns not normally present in the cytoplasm. Abnormal RNA patterns include chemical modifications, secondary or tertiary RNA conformations, specific RNA sequences, or double-stranded RNA. Although much of what is currently known about RLRs is centered around the sensing of RNA viruses, there is preliminary evidence that similar intracellular mechanisms may exist for sensing DNA viruses and some intracellular bacteria.

Members of the NLR are central regulators of immunity and inflammation largely through activation of transcription factors like nuclear factor (NF) κ B, interferon regulatory factor (IRF), or nuclear factor of activated T lymphocytes (NFAT). Some members of the NLR family form multiprotein complexes with the cysteine protease procaspase-1 and the adapter molecule ASC (apoptosis-associated speck-like protein [containing a CARD]) referred to as *inflammasomes* (also see Fig. 3-12). The inflammasome is a multiprotein complex that activates caspase-1. PAMPs and DAMPs are sensed through activation of the inflammasome complex, resulting in activation of caspase-1, which elicits effector functions through proteolytic cleavage of cytosolic proinflammatory cytokines (e.g., pro-interleukin [IL]-1β and pro-IL-18), which are then secreted in their active form. The inflammasome model is analogous to the model for the activation of the apoptotic caspases by CD95/Fas death–inducing signaling complex (DISC) and the Apaf-1 apoptosome. IL-1β functions in localized and systemic responses to infections and injury, to cause fever, activation of lymphocytes, and the extravasation of leukocytes at sites of injury or infection. IL-18 functions to induce IFN-γ by activated T lymphocytes and NK cells during a T helper lymphocyte type 1 (T_H1) response and to induce secondary inflammatory cytokines, chemokines, cell adhesion molecules, and nitric oxide (NO) synthesis. Other members of the NLR family are involved in inflammasome-independent (noninflammasome) innate immune responses and signal through different multicomponent signalosomes such as nodosomes, transcriptomes, and mito-signalosomes. Noninflammasome-mediated innate immune responses occur through NF κ B activation, mitogen-activated protein kinase (MAPK) activation, cytokine and chemokine production, antimicrobial reactive oxygen species production, IFN (IFN-α and IFN-β) production, and ribonuclease L activity.

Toll-Like Receptors

TLRs are the mammalian homologue of the Toll receptor originally identified in *Drosophila*. It has not only an embryologic function but also an immunologic function. In mammals, TLRs are membrane molecules that function in cellular activation by a wide range of microbial pathogens. TLRs are classified as PRRs because they recognize PAMPs and signal to the host the presence of an infection. Pathogen-associated molecules include lipopolysaccharide (LPS) from Gram-negative bacteria, peptidoglycan from Gram-positive bacteria, double-stranded RNA from viruses, or α-glucans from fungi (Table 5-1). In general, TLRs 1, 2, 4, and 6 recognize unique bacterial products that are found on the cell surface, and TLRs 3, 7, 8, and 9 are involved in viral detection and nucleic acid recognition within endosomes. The specificity of TLRs for microbial products depends on interactions between TLRs and non-TLR adapter molecules. All TLRs contain an extracellular domain characterized by a leucine-rich repeat motif flanked by a cysteine-rich motif (Fig. 5-2). They also contain a conserved intracellular signaling domain, Toll/IL-1 receptor (TIR), that is identical to the cytoplasmic domain of the IL-1 and IL-18 receptors. Figure 5-2 illustrates how TLRs function in the recognition of LPS. In the blood or extracellular fluid the binding of LPS to LPS-binding protein (LBP) facilitates the binding of LPS to CD14, a plasma protein and glycophosphatidylinositol-linked membrane protein present on most cells. The binding of LPS to CD14 results in the dissociation of LBP and the association of the LPS-CD14 complex with TLR4. An accessory protein, MD2, complexes with the LPS-CD14-TLR4 molecule and results in LPS-induced cell signaling.

Briefly, TLR signaling through the binding of PAMP to a TLR leads to the activation of TIR, which forms a complex with the cytoplasmic adapter protein MyD88, an IL-1 receptor–associated kinase (IRAK), and tumor necrosis factor (TNF) receptor–associated factor 6 (TRAF 6). Activated TRAF then activates the MAPK cascade, leading to the activation of NF κ B, a transcription factor. MyD88 is a universal signaling molecule for NF κ B activation, and MyD88-deficient mice are incapable of activation by TLR, IL-1, and IL-18. Recent information suggests that there are also signaling mechanisms unique to individual TLRs.

TLRs and their pathogen-associated ligands are important recognition molecules for the innate immune system and trigger a number of antimicrobial and inflammatory responses. Up to 15 different TLR genes have been identified. The importance of these receptors in immunity is further supported by the observation of polymorphisms in the genes encoding them.

Although the individual TLRs exhibit ligand specificity, they differ in their cellular expression patterns and the signal pathways

Table 5-1 Toll-Like Receptors (TLRs) and TLR Ligands and Their Microbial Source

TLR	Ligand	Microbial Source
TLR2	Lipoproteins	Bacteria
	Peptidoglycan	Gram-positive bacteria
	Zymosan	Fungi
	LPS	*Leptospira*
	GPI anchor	Trypanosomes
	Lipoarabinomannan	*Mycobacterium* spp.
	Phosphatidylinositol dimannoside	*Mycobacterium* spp.
TLR3	Double-stranded RNA	Viruses
TLR4	LPS	Gram-negative bacteria
	HSP60	Chlamydia
TLR5	Flagellin	Various bacteria
TLR6	CpG DNA	Bacteria, protozoans
TLR7	Single-stranded RNA	Viruses
TLR8	Single-stranded RNA	Viruses
TLR9	CpG DNA	Bacteria, viruses
TLR10	Unknown	Unknown
TLR11	Profilin	*Toxoplasma* spp., uropathogenic bacteria
TLR12	Profilin	*Toxoplasma* spp.
TLR13	rRNA	Various bacteria

CpG, Cytosine and guanine linked oligonucleotide; *GPI,* glycosylphosphatidylinositol; *HSP60,* heat shock protein 60; *LPS,* lipopolysaccharide.

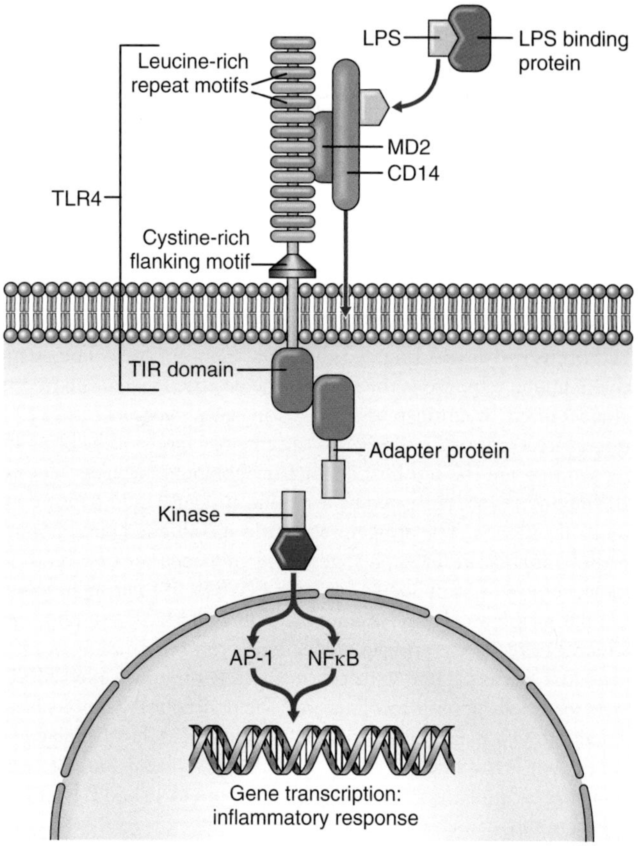

Figure 5-2 Toll-Like Receptor 4 (TLR4) Signaling in Response to Bacterial Lipopolysaccharide (LPS). LPS is transferred from the LPS-binding protein molecule to the TLR4, resulting in activation of cascade of signal transduction pathways leading to upregulation of genes that regulate inflammatory cellular and non-cellular responses. *NFκB,* Nuclear factor κB; *TIR,* Toll/interleukin 1 receptor.

they activate, similar to that described for cytokines, which exhibit pleiotropy, redundancy, synergy, and antagonism. There are constitutively and inducibly expressed TLRs in different tissues. TLRs regulate cell recruitment to sites of infection through the upregulation of the expression of adhesion molecules, chemokines, and chemokine receptors during an inflammatory response. TLRs activate leukocytes (primarily neutrophils and NK cells of the innate immune system) and epithelial, endothelial, and hematopoietic cells. TLRs are also hypothesized to be essential for linking the innate immune response to the adaptive immune responses. Central to this hypothesis is the TLR-dependent dendritic cell–mediated control of T lymphocyte activation. Dendritic cells are important antigen-presenting cells for T lymphocyte activation. Dendritic cells uptake microbial antigens in the peripheral tissues and migrate to regional lymph nodes, where they present peptide fragments, in the context of MHC molecules, to naïve T lymphocytes. In addition to the expression of the peptide-MHC signal, dendritic cells are also required to provide a second, costimulatory signal through the expression of B7, the ligand for the CD28 molecule on naïve T lymphocytes. The activation and maturation pathway related to the costimulatory signal occurs through TLR recognition of PAMPs.

There are species differences in the ligand specificity of TLRs and in the cellular responses elicited. Although sequences for canine, feline, and chicken TLR4 have been identified, no functional data have been published. With regard to domestic animals, a significant body of literature exists on TLRs of cattle.

Finally, TLRs have been implicated in "innate autoimmunity," with several reports of TLRs recognizing fibrinogen, heat shock proteins, or DNA. There are also reports of TLR binding of DNA as a factor in directing antibody production by autoreactive B lymphocytes, contributing to the pathogenesis of rheumatoid arthritis and systemic lupus erythematosus (SLE). Further studies are necessary to more fully understand these observations and the underlying immunopathogenesis.

Adaptive Immunity (Specific Immunity)

Adaptive immunity in general consists of cell-mediated immunity, mediated by T lymphocytes against intracellular pathogens, and humoral immunity, mediated by B lymphocytes against extracellular pathogens and toxins (Fig. 5-3; Essential Concept 5-2). The adaptive immune response is the second-line defense mechanism and is characterized by antigen specificity, diversity, memory, and self-/nonself-recognition. Antigen specificity and self-/nonself-recognition are the result of distinct membrane molecules. Mature B lymphocytes are activated by a specific antigen-binding molecule on its membrane. The antigen receptor is membrane-bound immunoglobulin. Mature T lymphocytes express a specific antigen-binding molecule, the T lymphocyte receptor (TCR), on their membrane. Unlike membrane-bound immunoglobulin on the B lymphocyte, which can recognize antigen alone, TCRs can recognize only antigens that are associated with cell membrane proteins called *MHC molecules*. Self-/nonself-recognition is the result of MHC molecules. There are two major classes of MHC molecules. Class I molecules are present on all nucleated cells, and class II molecules are present primarily on antigen-presenting cells. T lymphocytes and B lymphocytes are the major cells of adaptive immunity.

ESSENTIAL CONCEPT 5-2 Adaptive Immunity

Adaptive immunity is a group of specific second-line defense responses that occur days to weeks after exposure to microbial antigens during the innate immune response (see Essential Concept 5-1) at barrier systems provided by skin or mucosae (see Chapter 4). Unlike innate immune responses, adaptive responses are highly specific to antigens of the particular genera or species of microbe that induce them, and the response is "remembered" by the immune system. Adaptive immune responses are designed to destroy microbes and the toxins/enzymes they produce; therefore such responses must be against molecules that are foreign to the animal and not against structural and/or functional molecules of the animal itself. Through the MHC system, the adaptive immune system is able to distinguish foreign molecules from self-molecules. The defenses and mechanisms of adaptive immunity include (1) cell-mediated immunity, mediated by T lymphocytes against intracellular pathogens, and (2) humoral immunity, mediated by B lymphocytes against extracellular pathogens and toxins.

Innate immune responses and molecules expressed by innate lymphoid cells (ILCs) initiate and sustain responses of the adaptive immune system. Lymphocytes (ILCs and other types), dendritic cells, and other types of antigen-presenting cells at the site of injury in affected barrier systems deliver microbial antigens to local lymphoid tissues such as mucosa-associated lymphoid tissues and skin equivalents and then via lymphatic vessels to secondary lymphoid organs such as the spleen, lymph nodes, and lymph nodules. These tissues are responsible for immune responses to antigens, such as the production of antibody and cell-mediated immune reactions (see also Chapters 5 and 13). Lymphocytes are activated by microbial-specific antigens and undergo clonal selection, proliferation, and differentiation so they respond specifically to a unique species or genera of microbe. This process serves as the basis for immunizations in domestic animals.

Cells and Tissues of the Immune System

Innate Lymphoid Cells (ILCs)

Our understanding of how immune responses are initiated and sustained has been greatly enhanced through the identification of ILCs. ILCs are a heterogeneous population of non-B and non-T lymphocytes that are not antigen specific. ILCs develop in an Id2-dependent pathway and through additional transcriptional factors differentiate into subpopulations of cells that not only initiate and sustain immune responses, but also are important regulators in maintaining tissue integrity. The primary functions of ILCs involve defenses against infectious microbes, lymphoid tissue formation, and tissue remodeling following damage. Although first recognized as integral components of lymphoid tissue development, ILCs are now also recognized as important initiators of inflammation at mucosal and epithelial surfaces in response to microbial infection or tissue damage (Fig. 5-4). Similar to $CD4^+$ T helper cell subsets, ILCs can be polarized toward restricted cytokine profiles, allowing for tremendous plasticity (Fig. 5-5). This plasticity is driven by exogenous signals that are not fully understood but are in part directed by recognition molecules of innate immunity expressed on surfaces of ILCs. A common paradigm of both innate and adaptive immunity is the ability of exogenous signals (e.g., microbial antigen in the case of adaptive immunity) to polarize (i.e., focus) immune responses in most instances into a highly effective defensive response. It has now been recognized that these responses can also be polarized to undesirable responses (dysregulated) in some instances, contributing to the pathogenesis of certain allergic, inflammatory, and autoimmune diseases such as atopy, inflammatory bowel disease, and rheumatoid arthritis, respectively.

ILCs are one of three major cell populations that constitute innate immunity. The other two cell populations include phagocytic cells (macrophages and neutrophils) and dendritic cells. ILCs, like T and B lymphocytes, are derived from a common lymphoid precursor cell lineage. Unlike their adaptive lymphoid cell counterparts,

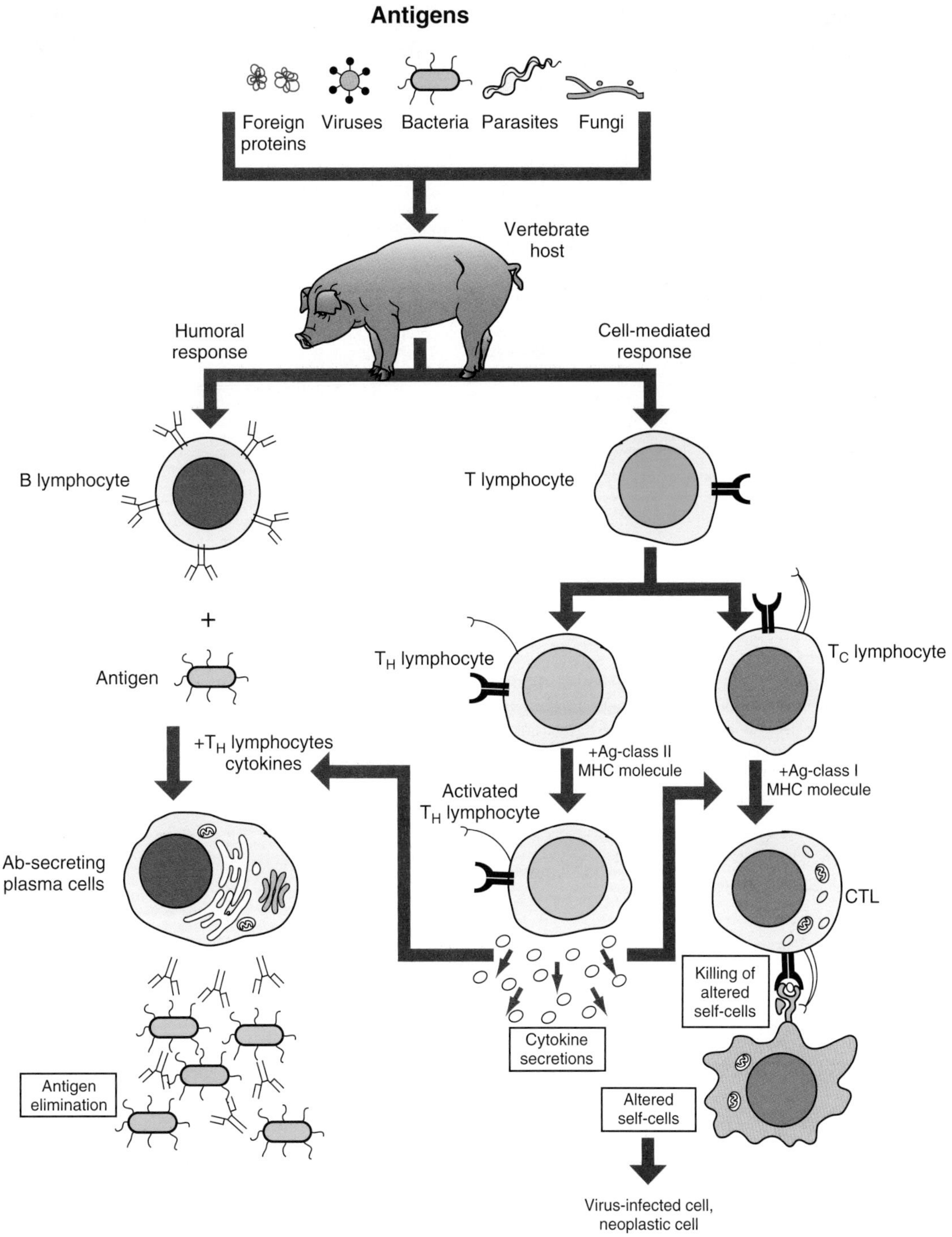

Figure 5-3 Overview of Humoral and Cell-Mediated Arms of Adaptive Immunity (Specific Immunity). *Ab,* Antibody; *Ag,* antigen; *CTL,* cytotoxic T lymphocyte; *MHC,* major histocompatibility complex; T_C, cytotoxic T lymphocyte; T_H, T helper lymphocyte. (Modified from Goldsby RA, Kindt TJ, Osborne BA: *Kuby immunology,* ed 4, New York, 2000, WH Freeman.)

ILCs lack recombination activating genes (RAGs) and RAG-mediated recombined antigen receptors and thus do not express antigen-specific receptors. Similar to their adaptive lymphoid cell counterparts, ILCs are often not defined by specific cellular markers but rather by cytokine profiles and in some instances transcriptional regulators that are involved in their development and function. ILCs are broadly classified as two distinct lineages: cytotoxic ILCs and noncytotoxic ILCs (Fig. 5-6). Cytotoxic ILCs are the conventional NK cells (cNK cells, also known as killer or cytotoxic ILCs), whereas the noncytotoxic ILCs are further subdivided into three distinct groups: group 1 ILCs, group 2 ILCs, and group 3 ILCs. Cytotoxic ILCs are discussed later. Group 1 ILCs are transcriptionally regulated by T-bet and produce IFN-γ and TNF. Group 1 ILCs are important defenses against intracellular bacteria and parasites. Group 2 ILCs are transcriptionally regulated by GATA-3 and produce IL-4, IL-5, IL-9, and IL-13. Group 2 ILCs are important defenses against helminths and contribute to the pathogenesis of certain types of asthma and allergic diseases. Group 3 ILCs are transcriptionally regulated by $ROR\gamma_t$ and are further subdivided by transcriptional regulator T-bet into lymphoid tissue inducer (LTi) cells that produce IL-17A, IL-22, and granulocyte-macrophage colony-stimulating factor (GM-CSF), and a second population that

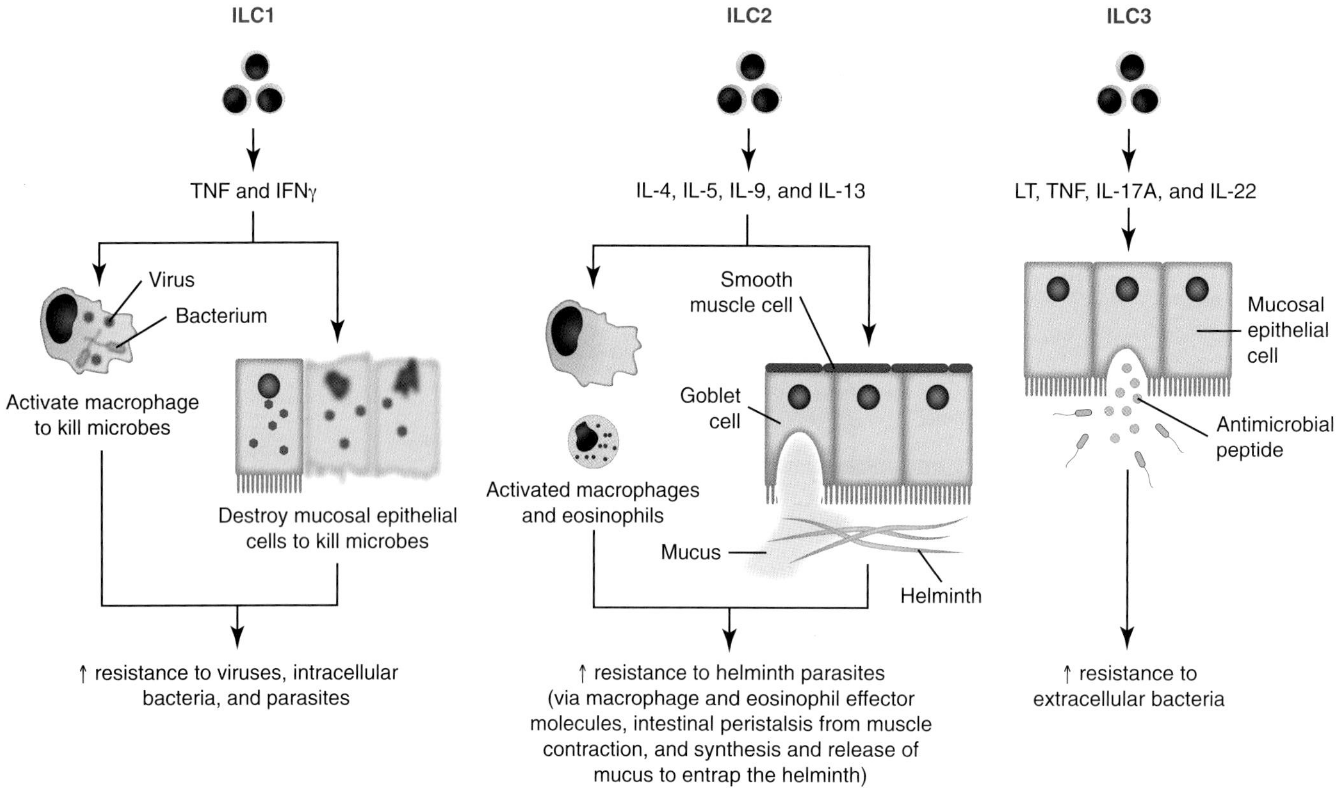

Figure 5-4 **Role of Innate Lymphoid Cells (ILCs) in Defenses Against Microbes.** ILCs have an important role in initiation of inflammatory responses at barrier surfaces in response to infectious organisms. Group 1 innate lymphoid cells (ILC1) provide increased resistance to viruses, intracellular bacteria, and parasites by producing tumor necrosis factor (TNF) and interferon-γ (IFN-γ). Group 2 innate lymphoid cells (ILC2) provide increased resistance to helminth parasites by producing interleukin (IL)-4, IL-5, IL-9 and IL-13. Group 3 innate lymphoid cells (ILC3) provide increased resistance to extracellular bacteria by producing lymphotoxin (LT), TNF, IL-17A, and IL-22. (Courtesy Dr. P.W. Snyder, School of Veterinary Medicine, Purdue University; and Dr. J.F. Zachary, College of Veterinary Medicine, University of Illinois.)

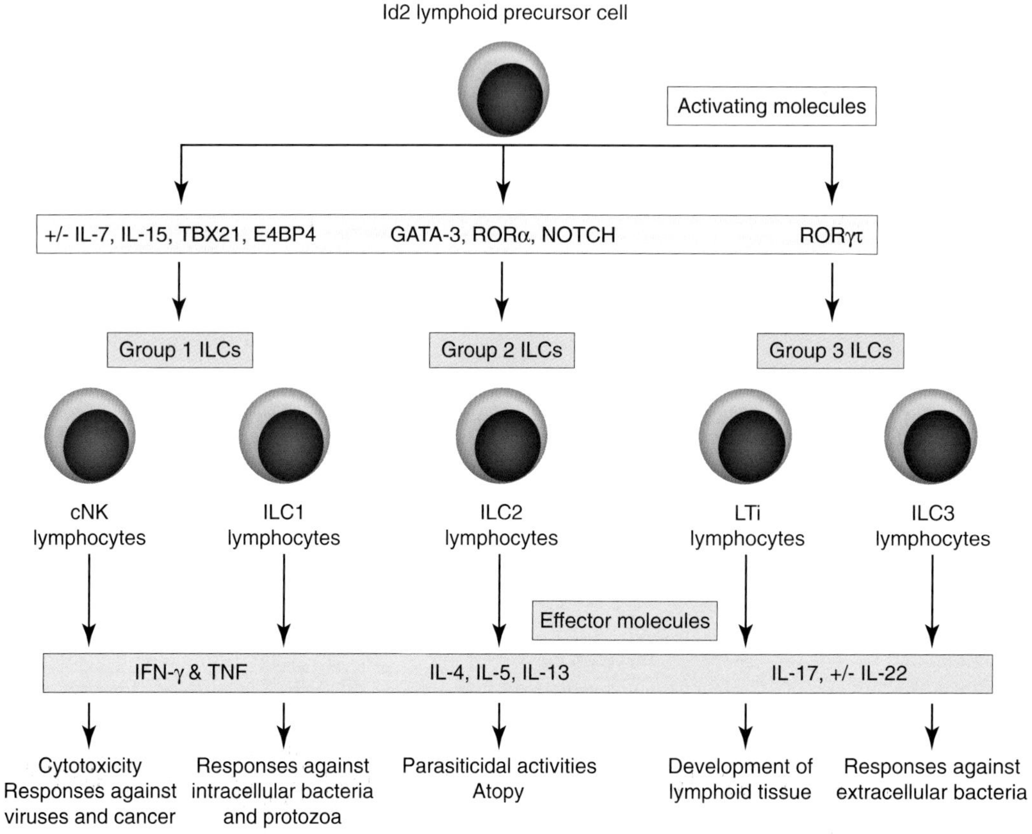

Figure 5-5 **Subclassification of Lymphocytes and Lymphoid Cells.** Innate lymphoid cells based on transcription factors and cytokine profiles, and their major effector molecules. (Courtesy Dr. P.W. Snyder, School of Veterinary Medicine, Purdue University; and Dr. J.F. Zachary, College of Veterinary Medicine, University of Illinois.)

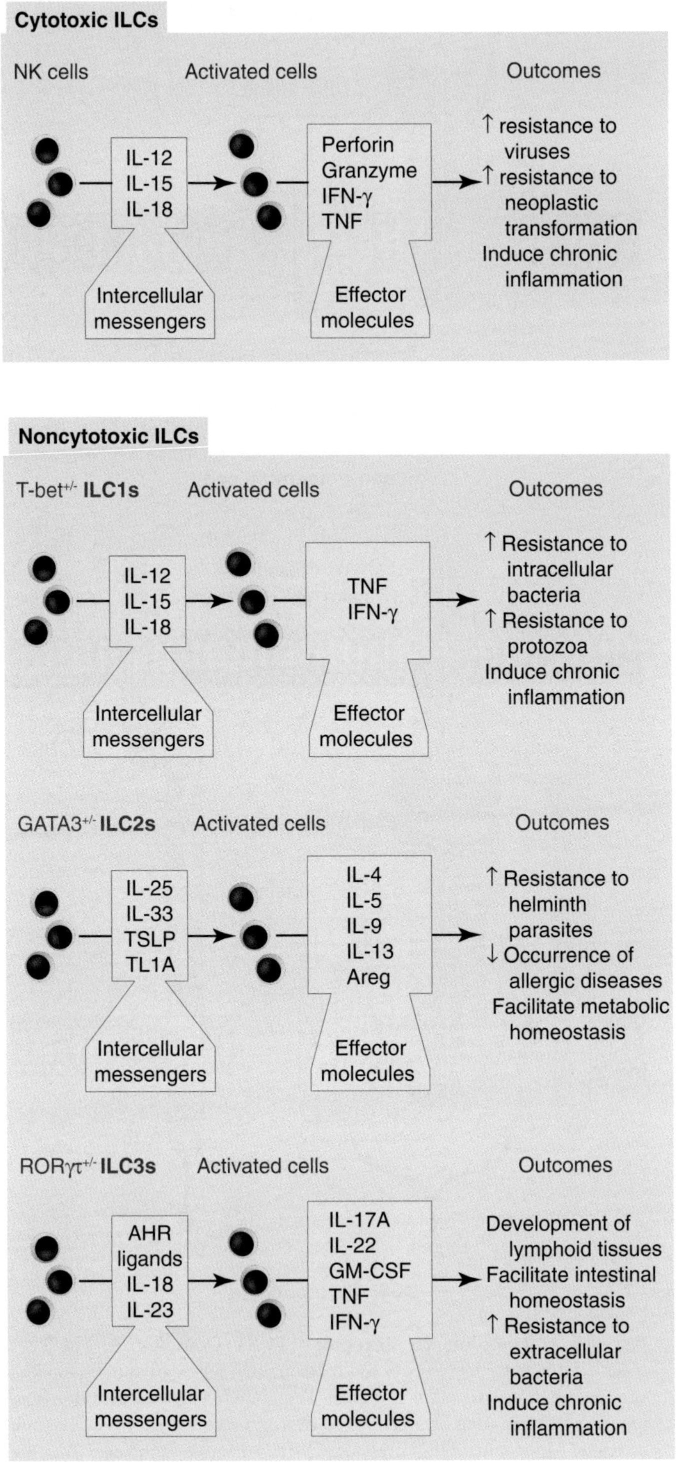

Figure 5-6 Cytotoxic and Noncytotoxic Innate Lymphoid Cells. Innate lymphoid cells (ILCs) are broadly classified as cytotoxic and noncytotoxic. Cytotoxic ILCs include natural killer (NK) cells that provide increased resistance to viruses and neoplastic transformation. Noncytotoxic ILCs are further classified Group 1 (ILC1), Group 2 (ILC2), or Group 3 (ILC3) based on cell surface markers, transcription factors (e.g., T-bet, GATA-3, and RORγt), and cytokine profiles. ILC1s provide increased resistance to intracellular bacteria and protozoa, and induce chronic inflammation. ILC2s provide increased resistance to helminth parasites and influence allergic diseases. ILC3s provide increased resistance to extracellular bacteria, function in lymphoid tissue development, and have a role in intestinal homeostasis. *AHR*, Aryl hydrocarbon receptor; *Areg*, amphiregulin; *GM-CSF*, granulocyte-macrophage colony-stimulating factor; *IFN-γ*, interferon-γ; *IL*, interleukin; *TL1A*, TNF-like ligand 1A; *TNF*, tumor necrosis factor; *TSLP*, thymic stromal lymphopoietin. (Courtesy Dr. P.W. Snyder, School of Veterinary Medicine, Purdue University; and Dr. J.F. Zachary, College of Veterinary Medicine, University of Illinois.)

produces TNF, IFN-γ, IL-22, and GM-CSF. Both populations of group 3 ILCs are involved in lymphoid tissue development and intestinal homeostasis and are important defense mechanisms against extracellular bacteria. In short, group 1 and 3 ILCs promote innate immune responses to viruses, intracellular bacteria and parasites, and fungi, whereas group 2 ILCs promote innate immune responses to extracellular helminths.

T Lymphocytes

T lymphocytes are small nongranular cells that constitute 50% to 70% of the peripheral blood mononuclear cells. They originate in the bone marrow and migrate to the thymus (thus the "T" designation), where they undergo differentiation, selection, and maturation processes before exiting to the periphery as effector lymphocytes. In secondary lymphoid tissues they are located primarily in the paracortical regions of lymph nodes and the periarteriolar lymphoid sheath (PALS) of the spleen. These specific anatomic sites elaborate chemoattractant cytokines (chemokines), for which the T lymphocytes express receptors. The definitive marker for T lymphocytes is the TCR, the polymorphic antigen-binding molecule. The antigen specificity of individual lymphocytes is attributed to their respective TCR, which is genetically determined. TCRs are classified as either αβ-TCR or γδ-TCR based on the composition of their disulfide-linked heterodimers. The individual polypeptide chains of the heterodimers contain variable (antigen-binding) and constant regions. In mammals, most peripheral blood T lymphocytes express αβ-TCR; however, in ruminants and pigs, these lymphocytes make up only 10% to 50%, and 10% of peripheral blood T lymphocytes, respectively. Both TCRs are associated with CD3, and together they form the TCR-CD3 complex. There are significant activation and functional differences between αβ-TCR– and γδ-TCR–expressing lymphocytes. Unlike membrane-bound immunoglobulin on B lymphocytes that can recognize soluble antigen, the αβ-TCR can only recognize antigen after it has been processed into peptide fragments and associated with MHC molecules (the MHC is discussed later). In most instances the antigen is associated with the MHC on the surface of an antigen-presenting cell, a virally infected cell, a neoplastic cell, or a cell of a foreign tissue graft. Individual αβ-TCRs are covalently linked to a cluster of five polypeptide chains, three constituting the CD3 molecule and two constituting the β-chain. The CD3 molecule and the β-chain are invariant, and although they do not bind antigen, they do function in the signal transduction after antigen binding by the TCR. Each T lymphocyte expresses a unique TCR with regard to structure and antigen specificity. The genes that encode α-, β-, γ-, and δ-chains of the TCR can undergo somatic rearrangements during their development in the thymus, resulting in tremendous diversity for antigen recognition. Not only are these rearrangements important for diversity, but also they can be used to molecularly phenotype proliferating populations of T lymphocytes as a diagnostic tool for the identification of clonal populations (neoplastic) and polyclonal populations (nonneoplastic) (see Chapter 6).

In most species a minority of T lymphocytes express γδ-TCR. The γδ-TCR lymphocytes develop in the thymus and migrate to the epithelium of the skin and intestine, mammary gland, and reproductive organs. Although these cells can be found within regional lymph nodes and the lamina propria, in these organs they primarily reside as intraepithelial lymphocytes. As stated, in some species, notably ruminants, γδ-TCR lymphocytes are the predominant circulating population of T lymphocytes. In contrast to the αβ-TCR lymphocytes, γδ-TCR lymphocytes can recognize native antigen in the absence of MHC binding, and they do not rely exclusively on the δ-chain as a signal transducer. Most γδ-TCR lymphocytes use the γ-chain for signal transduction after activation. The diversity of antigens recognized by γδ-TCR is limited in most species except ruminants and pigs, indicating their importance in these species. Some have suggested that they may provide early cell-mediated immune responses in neonates. The precise function of γδ-TCR lymphocytes remains unknown. Another small subset of T lymphocytes, called *NK-T lymphocytes*, expresses molecules found on NK cells in addition to a limited diversity of TCRs. NK-T lymphocytes primarily recognize glycolipids that are associated with an MHC-like molecule, CD1. The function of NK-T lymphocytes remains unknown.

Although all T lymphocytes express the TCR-CD3 complex, they are further classified according to accessory CD4 and CD8 molecules. These nonpolymorphic accessory molecules include CD4, CD8, CD2, integrins, and CD28. CD4 and CD8 functionally subdivide T lymphocytes into $CD8^+$ cytotoxic T lymphocytes (CTLs or T_C) and $CD4^+$ helper T lymphocytes (T_H). During antigen presentation, $CD4^+$ lymphocytes recognize only antigen bound to MHC class II molecules (Fig. 5-7), whereas $CD8^+$ lymphocytes recognize only antigen bound to MHC class I molecules. This coreceptor requirement is commonly referred to as *MHC class I and MHC class II restriction*, the basis for positive selection in the thymus.

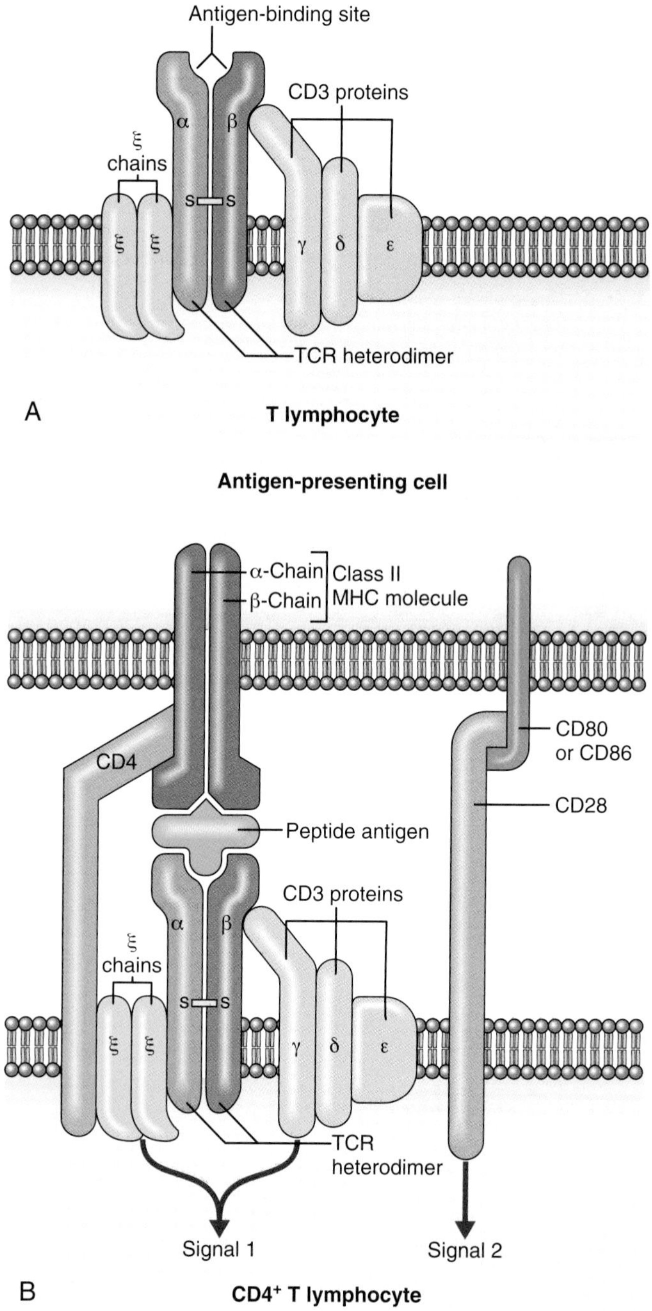

Figure 5-7 T Lymphocyte Receptor (TCR) Complex. A, The TCR complex in a heterodimer (αα and β chain) that forms an antigen-binding site and is linked to other proteins. The TCR recognizes peptides from processed antigens that are expressed on antigen-presenting cells in the form of major histocompatibility complex (MHC)–peptide complexes that are linked to other molecules essential to T lymphocyte activation. **B,** Additional molecules and their ligands are essential to fully activating the T lymphocyte (e.g., CD80 and CD80 ligand; CD4).

Although there have been reports in some species of CD4 lymphocytes that are functionally cytotoxic and CD8 lymphocytes that are functionally "helper"-like, these appear to be anomalies and for the purposes of this text are excluded. In most species, peripheral blood T lymphocytes express either CD4 or CD8. Except for ruminants and pigs, lymphocytes negative for both CD4 and CD8—"double-negative" lymphocytes—are rare in the peripheral blood. "Double-positive" lymphocytes, positive for both CD4 and CD8, are rare, except in pigs, where they can approach 25% of the T lymphocytes in the peripheral circulation. T lymphocytes require two signals for activation. Signal 1 is provided by the TCR and the MHC-antigen complex and the CD4 or CD8 MHC complex. Signal 2 is provided by another accessory molecule expressed by T lymphocytes, the CD28 molecule. The ligands for CD28 are B7-1 (CD80) and B7-2 (CD81) expressed on activated dendritic cells, B lymphocytes, and macrophages (see Fig. 5-6). An inability to deliver the second signal results in an unresponsive T lymphocyte that either undergoes apoptosis or remains anergic. These molecules provide an important costimulatory signal for T lymphocyte activation and are discussed in more detail later in the chapter regarding anergy and the development of tolerance with regard to autoimmunity. When T lymphocytes are activated by antigen and receive the appropriate costimulatory signals, they clonally expand as a result of their secretion of IL-2. This clonally expanded population of T lymphocytes, of the same antigen specificity, differentiates into populations of effector lymphocytes and memory lymphocytes.

T_H lymphocytes can be classified based on their functional capacity and ability to elicit primarily an antibody response or a cell-mediated immune response (Fig. 5-8). After activation of T_H lymphocytes, by recognition of antigen bound to MHC class II molecules on the surface of an antigen-presenting cell, there is clonal expansion of T_H lymphocytes of the same antigen specificity. These clonally expanded lymphocytes are important in directing the immune response as either primarily an antibody response or a cellular response. The type of response is dictated by a restricted cytokine profile that primarily activates B lymphocytes in the case of an antibody response or activates CTL and macrophages in a cellular response. The restricted cytokine profile for T_H lymphocytes allows for their classification as either T_H1 or T_H2 lymphocytes (E-Table 5-1). T_H1 lymphocytes synthesize and secrete IL-2 and IFN-γ, stimulating CTL and macrophages, and induce a cell-mediated immune response. T_H2 lymphocytes synthesize and secrete IL-4, IL-5, IL-6, and IL-13, which stimulate B lymphocytes to develop into antibody-secreting plasma cells and inhibit macrophage functions, and induce an antibody response. The type of immune response (antibody versus cell-mediated) can have a profound influence on the outcome of a disease. In the instance of an intracellular protozoal infection, a T_H2 type of response results in rapid proliferation of the organism and death of the host, whereas a T_H1 type of response results in elimination of the organism and survival of the host. Similarly, a T_H2 response to an allergen results in the elaboration of immunoglobulin (Ig) E, through IL-4 production, stimulation of eosinophils, through IL-5 production, and the development of an allergic reaction. The exact regulation of the T_H1 versus the T_H2 lymphocyte response is unknown, but studies suggest that IL-12 produced by activated macrophages stimulates the T_H1 response, whereas IL-4 inhibits the T_H1 response, allowing the T_H2 response to dominate. T_H lymphocytes predominantly drive the immune response to microbial pathogens by activating macrophages or B lymphocytes. Another functionally distinct subpopulation of $CD4^+$ T lymphocytes is the regulatory T (T reg) lymphocyte. T reg lymphocytes function to suppress the response of self-reactive CD4 lymphocytes that have escaped the negative selection process in the thymus. They are distinguished from other CD4 T lymphocytes by the expression of CD25 on the cell surface. Like T_H1 and T_H2 lymphocytes, T reg lymphocyte differentiation is driven by cytokine

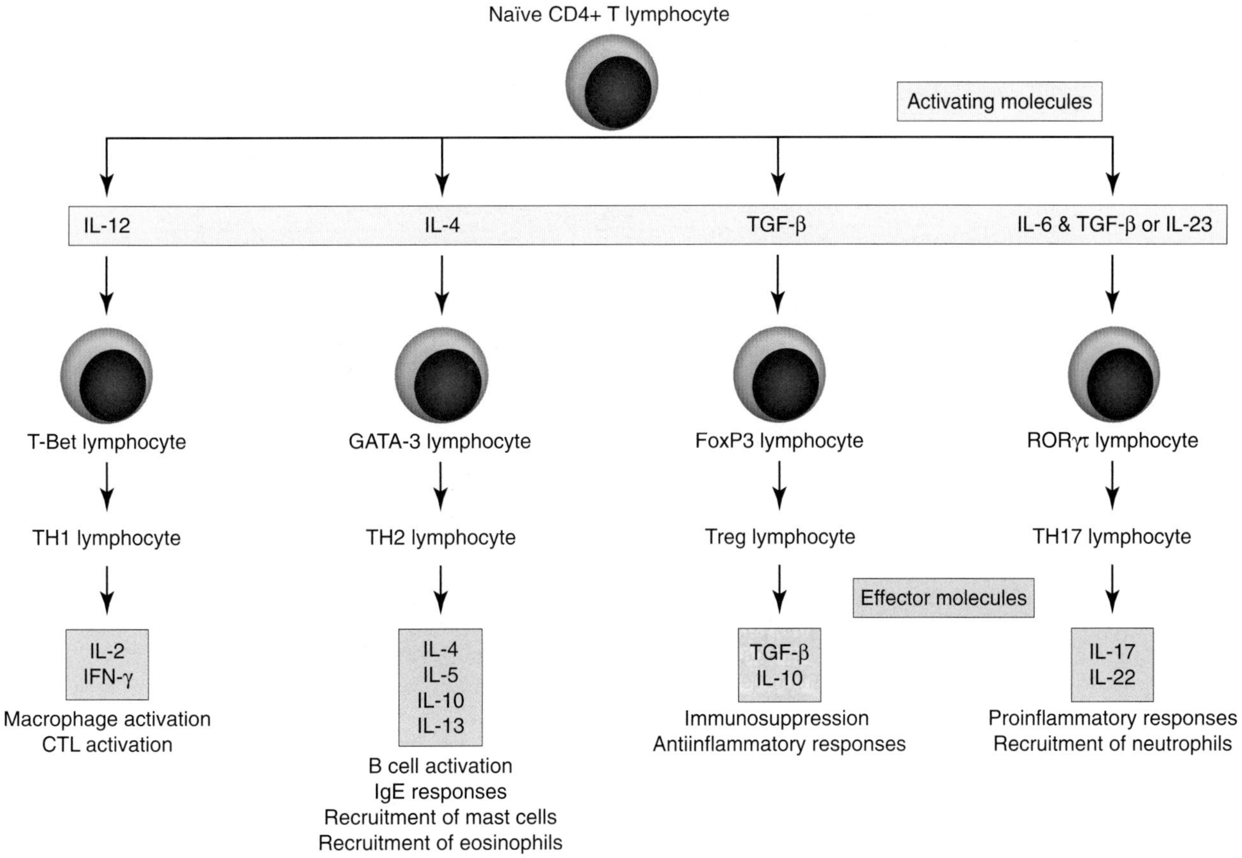

Figure 5-8 Subclassification of Lymphocytes and Lymphoid Cells. $CD4^+$ T lymphocyte based on transcription factors and cytokine profiles, and their major effector molecules and functions. (Courtesy Dr. P.W. Snyder, School of Veterinary Medicine, Purdue University; and Dr. J.F. Zachary, College of Veterinary Medicine, University of Illinois.)

environments; however, whereas T_H1 and T_H2 lymphocyte activation occurs through transcriptional activators T-bet and GATA-3, respectively, T reg lymphocytes are activated through the transcriptional repressor FoxP3 (see Fig. 5-8). This subpopulation of T reg lymphocytes is often referred to as FoxP3 lymphocytes and produces the immunosuppressive and antiinflammatory cytokines IL-4, IL-10, and transforming growth factor-β (TGF-β). FoxP3 lymphocytes are an intense area of investigation for their role as suppressor lymphocytes of immunity and inflammation. T reg lymphocytes have been shown to have a role in the prevention of organ-specific autoimmune diseases and in modulation of immune responses to microbial pathogens to prevent overwhelming inflammatory reactions. Finally, a subpopulation of CD4 lymphocytes characterized by the ability to produce IL-17 is designated as T_H17 lymphocytes. T_H17 lymphocyte differentiation is driven by TGF-β, IL-6, IL-1, and IL-23. T_H17 lymphocytes, through production of chemokines IL-17 and IL-22, induce the recruitment of monocytes and neutrophils to sites of inflammation. Again, one must recognize that this is an oversimplification of a complex regulatory mechanism and that as additional knowledge is gained about T_H1, T_H2, T reg, and T_H17 lymphocyte responses, we will be able to understand pathogenic mechanisms of diseases, which will lead to the development of more specific therapeutic targets.

B Lymphocytes

B lymphocytes constitute 5% to 20% of the peripheral blood mononuclear cells. B lymphocyte development occurs in two phases, an antigen-independent phase in the primary lymphoid tissues, followed by an antigen-dependent phase in secondary lymphoid tissues. B lymphocytes can be found in primary lymphoid tissues, such as the bone marrow and ileal Peyer's patches (a primary lymphoid tissue in some species because it is the site of B lymphocyte development, rather than the bone marrow), and in secondary lymphoid tissues, such as the spleen, lymph nodes, tonsils, and Peyer's patches. Within secondary lymphoid tissues, B lymphocytes are aggregated in the form of distinct lymphoid follicles, which on activation expand to form prominent pale regions called *germinal centers* (Fig. 5-9). This anatomic localization, similar to T lymphocytes in the PALS and paracortex, is the result of elaboration of chemokines for which the B lymphocyte has receptors. The antigen receptor of the B lymphocyte is the membrane-bound immunoglobulin. After the antigen-independent phase of development, B lymphocytes express IgM and IgD on their surface, which signifies a mature B lymphocyte. In the antigen-dependent phase, antigen-activated mature B lymphocytes differentiate into IgM-secreting plasma cells or switch to another antibody isotype. Immunoglobulins can be generated against an almost unlimited number of antigenic determinants through the rearrangement of genes encoding the light chain and heavy chain components. As in the case of the TCR, an evaluation of the rearranged genes of a B lymphocyte can be used to molecularly phenotype B lymphocyte neoplasms (see Chapter 6).

Like the T lymphocyte, the B lymphocyte also has accessory molecules that function to form the antigen receptor complex (Fig. 5-10). These nonpolymorphic molecules are nonpolymorphic

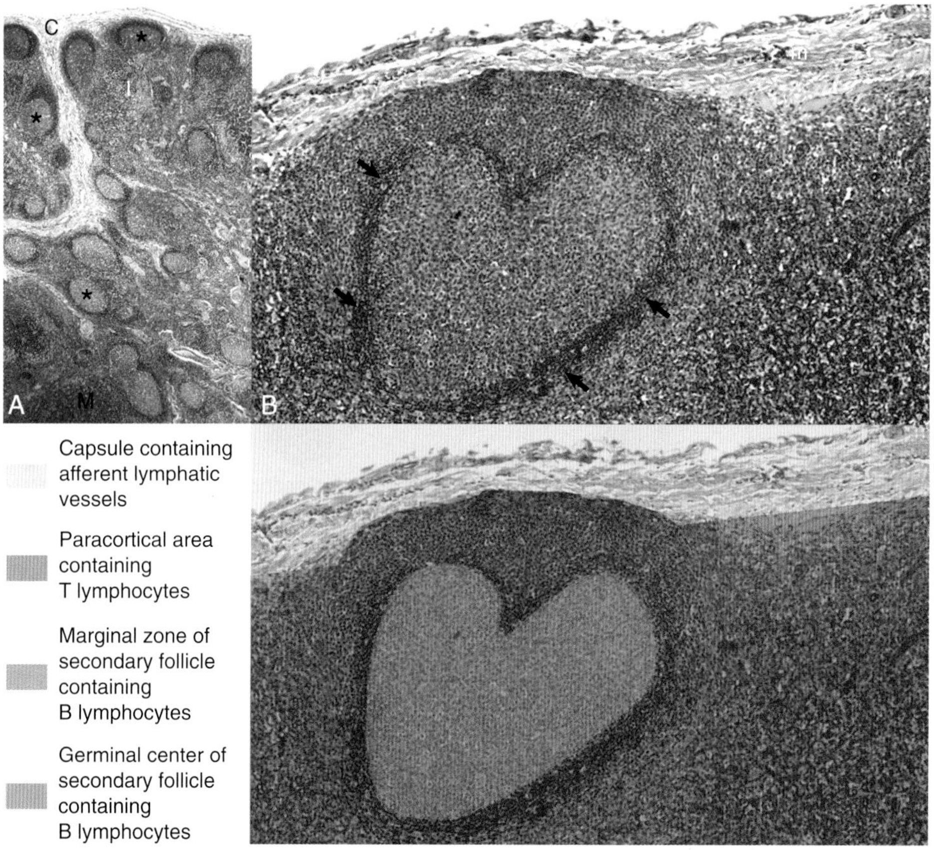

Figure 5-9 Hyperplastic Lymph Node. A, The outer cortex contains numerous secondary lymphoid follicles *(asterisks)*. Secondary follicles arise from primary follicles in the outer cortex that have been stimulated by antigens arriving via afferent lymphatic vessels in the capsule (*C*). H&E stain. **B,** Secondary follicle. It has a less cellular *(lighter staining)* central area called the germinal center, which is surrounded by a more cellular *(darker staining)* outer area called the marginal zone with its mantle *(arrows)*. H&E stain. *I,* Inner cortex; *M,* medullary cords. (Courtesy Dr. P.W. Snyder, School of Veterinary Medicine, Purdue University; and Dr. J.F. Zachary, College of Veterinary Medicine, University of Illinois.)

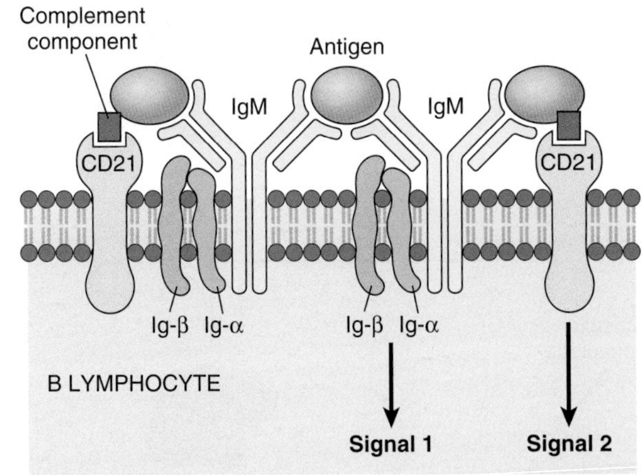

Figure 5-10 B Lymphocyte Antigen Receptor Complex. Membrane IgM (or IgD, not shown) and the signaling molecules Ig-α and Ig-β. CD21, also known as complement receptor-2, binds complement components and activates B lymphocytes. *Ig,* Immunoglobulin. (Courtesy Dr. Alex McPherson, University of California, Irvine.)

heterodimers composed of Ig-α (CD79a) and Ig-β (CD79b) that do not bind antigen but do interact with the transmembrane portion of surface immunoglobulin involved in cell activation. B lymphocytes, unlike T lymphocytes, can recognize soluble antigens. Additional nonpolymorphic molecules that are important to B lymphocyte functions are CD21 and CD40. The CD21 molecule is the complement receptor 2 molecule whose ligands are C3b and C3d. B lymphocyte responses to protein antigens are dependent on cytokines produced by activated T lymphocytes ($CD4^+$). The CD40 molecule interacts with CD40 ligand on the surface of T_H lymphocytes and functions to allow B lymphocyte development into antibody-secreting plasma cells. A failure to express CD40 ligand has been associated with an inability to isotype switch, resulting in a hyper-IgM syndrome. B lymphocytes activated by antigen develop into antibody-secreting plasma cells and memory lymphocytes of the same antigenic specificity.

Mononuclear Phagocytic System (Monocyte-Macrophage System)

The preferred term today for the functionally and phenotypically diverse population of mononuclear phagocytic cells is the *mononuclear phagocytic system* (MPS). It is also referred to as the monocyte-macrophage system. These cells have a broad range of functions contributing to immunity, inflammation, and tissue remodeling and repair. A brief history of the recognition of the defensive mechanism of phagocytosis not only facilitates our current understanding of how these cells play a crucial role in innate and adaptive immunity but also explains some of the terminology that often leads to confusion for students. Elie Metchnikoff (1845-1916), a comparative developmental zoologist, is credited with recognizing and establishing the process of phagocytosis, an important defensive mechanism for organisms. He recognized the association between the systemic clearance of microorganisms and the presence of the microorganisms in the spleen and liver. Subsequent studies evaluating the systemic clearance of dyes suggested that Kupffer cells and endothelial cells lining the sinusoids of the liver were responsible because both cell types internalized the dyes. Because the investigators considered macrophages (Kupffer cells) and endothelial cells to have a common biologic function, phagocytosis, they proposed that they be encompassed as a system, the reticuloendothelial system. We now understand that the mechanism of uptake by endothelial cells is not by phagocytosis, and as a result the term *reticuloendothelial system* is no longer used. The term *mononuclear phagocytic system* was developed to differentiate lymphoid cells (mononuclear T and B lymphocytes), granulocytes (polymorphonuclear leukocytes), and endothelial cells from the lineage-committed precursors in the bone marrow, blood monocytes and tissue macrophages, and dendritic cells that currently compose the MPS. It is very likely that as we learn more about the precursors and differentiated cells that constitute the MPS, there will be proposals for new, more specific classification schemes.

In general, a circulating MPS cell in the blood is designated as a monocyte, whereas the tissue-based cell is designated as a macrophage. The process of blood monocyte–to–tissue macrophage differentiation is well recognized, although the mechanisms that allow for differentiation of the circulating monocyte pool into the tissue-based pool are still largely unknown. The monocyte is a bone marrow–derived cell of the myeloid lineage that is the precursor cell to the terminally differentiated macrophage that has limited recirculation and replication capacity. The myeloid dendritic cell represents a specific type of mononuclear cell present in nonlymphoid tissues with unique migratory properties and is discussed separately. As opposed to granulocytic myeloid cells, macrophages are long lived (days to months) and can exist as quiescent "resident" cells widely distributed throughout the body. It is becoming increasingly clear that there is heterogeneity in the circulating monocyte pool that corresponds with the ultimate tissue localization of resident macrophages. The phenotypic characterization of the cells the MPS contains is often used in an attempt to identify specific populations of MPS (Fig. 5-11). Morphologically, monocytes are variably sized with an irregular shape, oval or kidney-shaped nucleus, prominent cytoplasmic vesicles, and a high cytoplasm to nucleus ratio. These features are not unique to monocytes, and as a result they are difficult to distinguish from circulating dendritic cells, activated lymphocytes, and NK cells based on morphologic features or by light scatter (flow cytometry). This section covers basic concepts attributable to monocytes, tissue macrophages, and myeloid dendritic cells and refers to specific organ systems. See additional chapters in the section on pathology of organ systems for details on organ-specific cells of the MPS. Certain organ systems have specific names for their resident macrophages, whereas other organ systems only refer to them as macrophages (Table 5-2).

Growth and differentiation of monocytes is regulated by specific growth factors, such as IL-3, colony-stimulating factor-1 (CSF-1), GM-CSF, IL-4, and IL-13, and inhibitors such as IFNs and TGF-β. CSF-1 is the most important because it controls the proliferation, differentiation, and survival of the monocyte. Monocytes represent approximately 4% to 10% of blood leukocytes and are identified in mammals, birds, amphibians, and fish. They are largely viewed as accessory cells that importantly link inflammation and innate immune responses to adaptive immunity.

Hematopoietic stem cells (HSCs) give rise to the common myeloid progenitor (CMP), the precursor cell to the granulocyte/macrophage progenitor (GMP) and macrophage/dendritic cell progenitor (MDP). The MDP is the common progenitor cell for monocytes, macrophages, and conventional dendritic cells. Monocytes express the CSF-1 receptor (CD115) and the chemokine receptor CX3CR1, are differentiated from polymorphonuclear cells (PMNs), NK cells, and lymphoid cells, and do not express CD3, CD19, or CD15. Monocyte heterogeneity based on surface marker expression and function has identified subsets that are an area of intense investigation and are best characterized in human beings and rodents. Subpopulations of blood monocytes can be phenotyped based on the expression of surface markers CD14 and CD16 (FcγR-III). Two additional subpopulations of blood monocytic cells are the myeloid

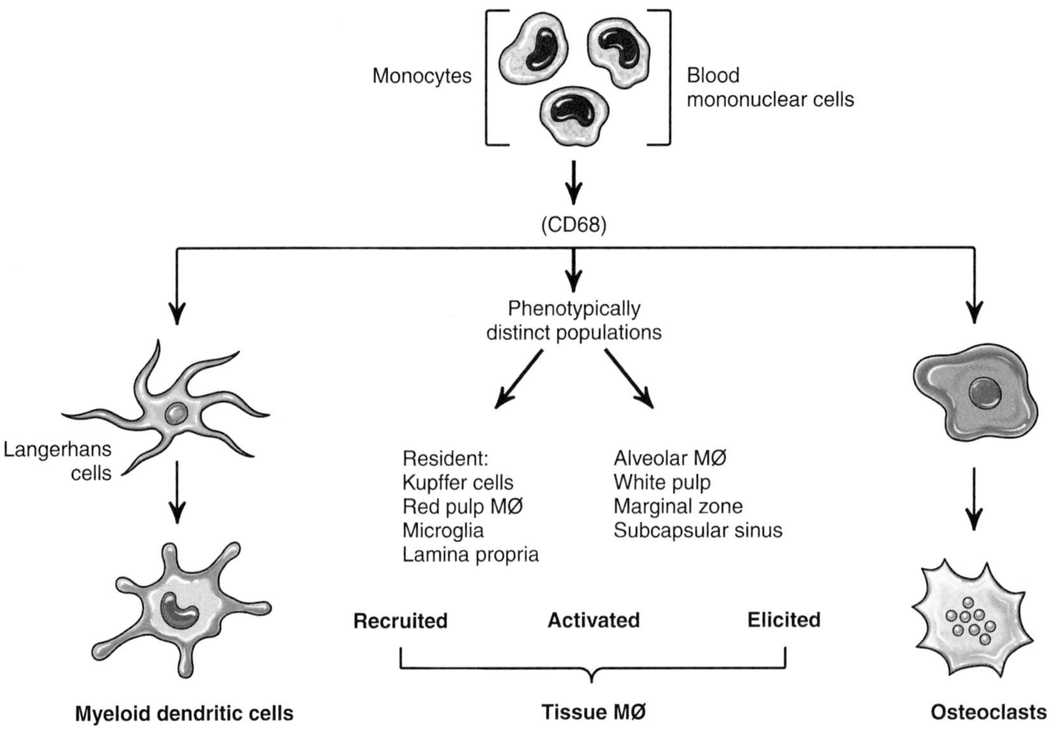

Figure 5-11 **Differentiation of Mononuclear Phagocytes Based on Antigen Markers.** *MØ,* Macrophage. (Modified from Paul WE: *Fundamental immunology*, ed 6, Philadelphia, 2008, Lippincott Williams & Wilkins.)

Table 5-2 Nomenclature and Location of Non-lymphoid Monocyte-Macrophage Cell Types

Organ/Tissue	Name	Location
Lung	Alveolar macrophages Pulmonary intravascular macrophages	Alveolar spaces Capillaries of the lung
Connective tissues	Histiocytes	Interstitium
Kidney	Mesangial cells	Glomerular tuft
Brain	Microglial cells	Neuroparenchyma and perivascular areas
Bone	Osteoclasts	Bone marrow
Blood	Monocytes	Circulation
Liver	Kupffer cells	Hepatic sinusoids

blood dendritic cells, which are negative for CD14 and CD16. In the mouse the main subset of $CD115^+$ monocytes are characterized as large cells expressing Ly6C, the chemokine receptor CCR2 and the adhesion molecule L-selectin (CD62L), and CX3CR1 (Fig. 5-12). These are referred to as inflammatory monocytes or inflammatory-monocyte–derived macrophages that are preferentially recruited to inflamed tissues and lymph nodes, where they produce high levels of TNF-α and IL-1. The emigration of $Ly6C^+$ monocytes from the bone marrow to the periphery depends on the chemokine receptor CCR2 and its ligands CCL7 and CCL2. Ly6C-negative monocytes have less of an influence on inflammatory reactions and appear to function more importantly as tissue resident cells and as cells involved in healing and regeneration associated with vascular injury. In those species characterized to date, there appear to be two major functional subpopulations of monocytes, one that is recruited and differentiated into macrophages at the site of inflammation and expresses higher levels of MHC class II and adhesion molecules and one that is responsible for repopulating resident tissue macrophages. Both populations can give rise to dendritic cells (see Fig. 5-12). Classification schemes are forever evolving, and there are definite species differences that may explain species differences in rates of infection and types of clinical disease associated with specific microbial agents. Similar phenotypic and functional heterogeneity exists with tissue-based macrophages.

The MPS of hematopoietic and lymphoid organs is diverse with functionally and phenotypically distinct parallel subpopulations in human beings, rodents, and pigs. In primary lymphoid organs, mature macrophages are involved in the production, differentiation, and destruction of all lineages of hematopoietic cells in the bone marrow, and in positive and negative selection processes in the thymus. In secondary lymphoid organs, macrophages are uniquely positioned to enhance their phagocytic properties to endogenous and exogenous material and to influence other cell types through their products. The resident macrophages in the spleen differ in microscopic localization, phenotype, and function. The reason for this complexity is largely attributable the spleen's role as a hematopoietic organ and as a secondary lymphoid organ. Distinct subpopulations of macrophages are present in the red pulp, white pulp, and marginal zone with some recognized species differences (see Chapter 13). The red pulp macrophage functions in the phagocytosis of hematogenous pathogens and senescent erythrocytes. Erythrophagocytosis primarily occurs in the spleen and liver and allows for the removal of senescent erythrocytes and recycling of iron, often evident as cytoplasmic accumulations of pigments. The white pulp macrophages are also actively phagocytic, and a morphologically distinct cell, the "tingible body macrophage," can often be easily identified histologically and represents macrophages involved in the uptake and removal of apoptotic T and B lymphocytes. The

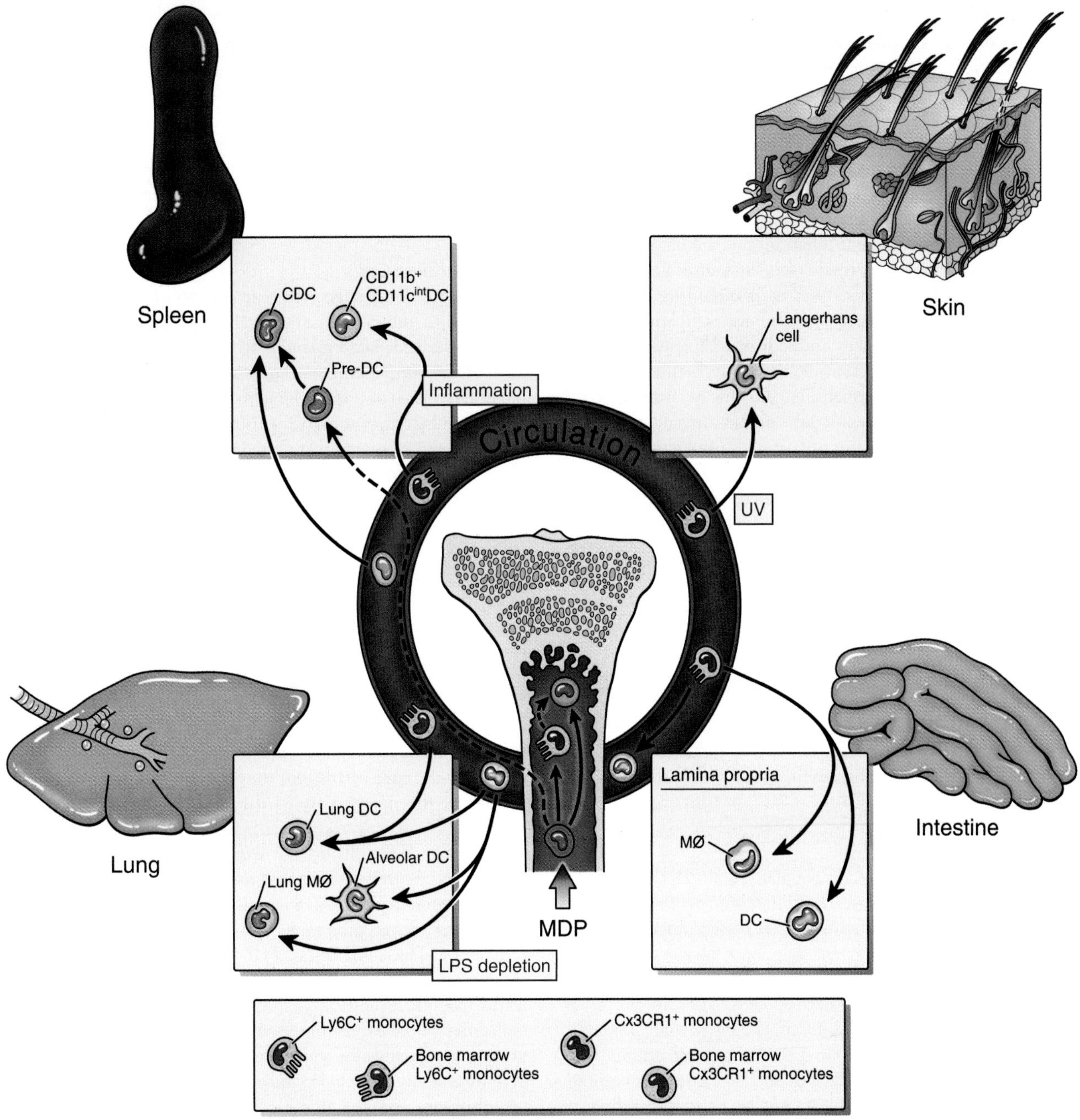

Figure 5-12 Monocyte Differentiation into Dendritic Cells (DCs) and Tissue Macrophages. *CDC,* Conventional dendritic cell; *LPS,* lipopolysaccharide; *MDP,* macrophage/dendritic cell progenitor; *MØ,* macrophage; *UV,* ultraviolet. (Redrawn and modified from Serbina NV, Jia T, Hohl HM, et al: *Ann Rev Immunol* 26:421-452, 2008.)

marginal zone of the spleen provides a complex environment for the interface for the red and white pulp, specifically an important transit area for cells leaving circulation and entering the white pulp, and for B lymphocyte differentiation. The development of granulomatous inflammatory reactions in the spleen as a response to hematogenous microorganisms often begins in the marginal zone. The two subpopulations of macrophages present in the marginal zone are the metallophilic macrophage and the marginal zone macrophage. Marginal zone macrophages express high levels of PRRs and scavenger receptors that facilitate the clearance of pathogens from the circulation. The function of metallophilic macrophages is unknown. Tissue macrophages are derived from a combination of precursors in the blood (monocytes) and from local proliferation of precursors that varies for individual organ systems.

Much has been written about the relationship between monocytes, macrophages, and dendritic cells. The inclusion of dendritic cells as a component of the MPS is in part attributable to the fact that they are derived from a common myeloid precursor, influenced by similar growth factors (e.g., CSF-1), express common surface markers, and have no unique properties as antigen-presenting cells that allow them to be differentiated from macrophages. Like macrophages, dendritic cells in specific organ systems may have a specific name or be designated only as dendritic cells preceded by the organ or in some instances a specific anatomic location within an organ. Dendritic cell subsets are also an intense area of investigation with regard to phenotypic and functional heterogeneity. The so-called conventional dendritic cells are present as immature cells in the interstitial tissues of all organs except the brain.

Macrophages

Mononuclear phagocytic cells include circulating monocytes and tissue-based macrophages. In the spleen, macrophages are located in the marginal zone, white pulp, and red pulp, where they function primarily as phagocytic cells. In the lymph node, macrophages are located in the subcapsular sinus, which is analogous to the marginal zone of the spleen, and the medulla. These physical locations, the subcapsular sinus of lymph nodes and marginal zone of the spleen, facilitate their exposure to potential antigens. Nonlymphoid tissue–based macrophages have different functions and are named according to the tissue in which they reside (see Table 5-2). One primary function of these cells is phagocytosis, as discussed in Chapter 3. Macrophages express Fc receptors (FcRs) for antibody and can phagocytose antigens opsonized by antibody or complement components. Another primary function is their involvement in the immune response as antigen-presenting cells. In this instance they phagocytose antigen and process it into peptide fragments, which are then presented to T lymphocytes, and the induction of cell-mediated immune responses. Although all nucleated cells express MHC class I molecules and could be considered antigen-presenting cells, only three cell types normally express MHC class II molecules and are regarded as the major antigen-presenting cells. They are the macrophage, dendritic cell, and B lymphocyte. Whereas B lymphocytes and dendritic cells constitutively express MHC class II molecules, macrophages only express MHC class II molecules on activation.

Macrophages also have an important role in the generation of a cell-mediated immune response and are essential to type IV hypersensitivity reactions. Activated T_H1 lymphocytes synthesize IFN-γ, a potent activator of macrophages. Under the influence of IFN-γ, macrophages have increased phagocytic activity and are more efficient at killing.

Dendritic Cells

Dendritic cells constitute a distinct population of cells that is characterized by elongate cell processes. Most dendritic cells are antigen-presenting cells, which process antigens and present fragments to T lymphocytes. They are more efficient than macrophages and B lymphocytes at antigen presentation. Antigen-presenting dendritic cells are nonphagocytic, bone marrow–derived cells. They are the most important antigen-presenting cell for initiating primary immune responses to protein antigens (Fig. 5-13). Antigen-presenting dendritic cells express a number of molecules, such as TLRs and mannose receptors, that make them efficient at capturing and responding to antigens. They also express high concentrations of MHC class II molecules and B7 costimulatory molecules. By expressing chemokine receptors similar to T lymphocytes, they have the ability to localize in T lymphocyte regions of lymphoid tissue. By colocalizing to these areas, they are uniquely positioned to present antigens to recirculating T lymphocytes. Antigen-presenting dendritic cells function to capture antigen and then migrate to T lymphocyte areas of secondary lymphoid organs, where they present fragments of the antigen on their surface and increase their expression of costimulatory molecules that activate T lymphocytes. Specifically, migrating dendritic cells, derived from Langerhans cells that have captured antigen, enter the lymph node through efferent lymphatic vessels and localize in lymphoid organs, where they present antigenic peptides to T lymphocytes that facilitate B lymphocyte activation and the production of antibody-secreting plasma cells. In addition to their function as antigen-presenting cells, they are also important in the process of negative selection in the thymus and in the maintenance of peripheral tolerance. The four types of antigen-presenting dendritic cells and their locations are listed in Table 5-3. Circulating dendritic cells, also known as *veiled cells*, make up less than 1% of peripheral blood mononuclear cells. The second type of dendritic cell, the follicular dendritic cell, is primarily located in lymphoid follicles. These cells are not derived from the bone marrow, do not express MHC class II molecules, and do not function as an antigen-presenting cell. Follicular dendritic cells have FcR and receptors for C3b. They store antigen-antibody and antigen-C3b complexes and are thought to be involved in the development and maintenance of memory B lymphocytes.

Natural Killer Cells

NK cells are nonspecific cytotoxic cells that are important in early responses to tumor cells and viral infections. NK cells are bone marrow–derived, large granular lymphocytes that make up 5% to 15% of the peripheral blood mononuclear cells. Their size, slightly larger than that of a small lymphocyte, and the presence of abundant granular cytoplasm distinguish them from T lymphocytes (Fig. 5-14). They are commonly referred to as large granular lymphocytes. The cytoplasm of NK cells and CTL is characterized by cytotoxic granules that contain perforin and granzymes, two potent pathways mediating lysis of the target cell. NK cells and T lymphocytes express numerous similar surface molecules and kill virus-infected cells and tumor cells by similar mechanisms. Two membrane molecules, CD16 and CD56, are commonly used to identify NK cells. NK cells express FcγR (CD16) and the β-subunit of the IL-2 receptor (CD2). They do not express antigen-specific TCR or CD3 molecules. In contrast to cytotoxic lymphocytes, NK cells are not MHC restricted, are constitutively cytolytic, and do not develop memory cells. Because NK cells are activated early in an immune response and do not require a previous sensitization phase to develop memory cells after activation, they are the cytotoxic cell of innate immunity, the counterpart to the CTL of the adaptive immune response.

Although NK cells do not express any antigen-specific molecules, they are very efficient at recognizing and killing altered or virally infected cells. NK cell activity is regulated through activating and inhibitory receptor molecules expressed on their cell surface (Fig. 5-15). These NK cell receptor molecules fall into two distinct categories: the immunoglobulin-like NK receptors and the C-type lectin-like NK receptors. Ligands for these receptors are cell surface molecules whose expression has been altered as a result of infection or damage. Ligands for activating receptors that stimulate NK cell activity commonly include viral and stress-induced proteins. Ligands for inhibitory receptors that block NK cell activity most commonly involve class I MHC molecules. A decreased expression of class I MHC molecules makes cells susceptible to NK cell–mediated lysis. A decrease in MHC class I expression often occurs in virus-infected cells and in neoplastic cells, making them susceptible to attack by NK cells. Normal cells are protected from NK cell killing because all nucleated cells express class I MHC molecules. This is an oversimplification of the "opposing-signals" model of NK cell regulation of how cytotoxic activity is limited to altered self-cells. Recent studies on the molecular mechanisms of NK cell regulation indicate that the absence of an inhibitory stimulus by itself is insufficient for triggering NK cell killing. NK cells also require triggering of activating receptors. Several activating receptors have been identified. One is the NKG2D receptor, a C-type lectin-like molecule that recognizes a number of stress-induced proteins. These stress-induced proteins are normally only constitutively expressed in the intestinal epithelium or as a result of cellular distress caused by infection or neoplastic transformation. There are a number of additional activating receptors, some of which recognize viral proteins, that are structurally similar to class I MHC molecules.

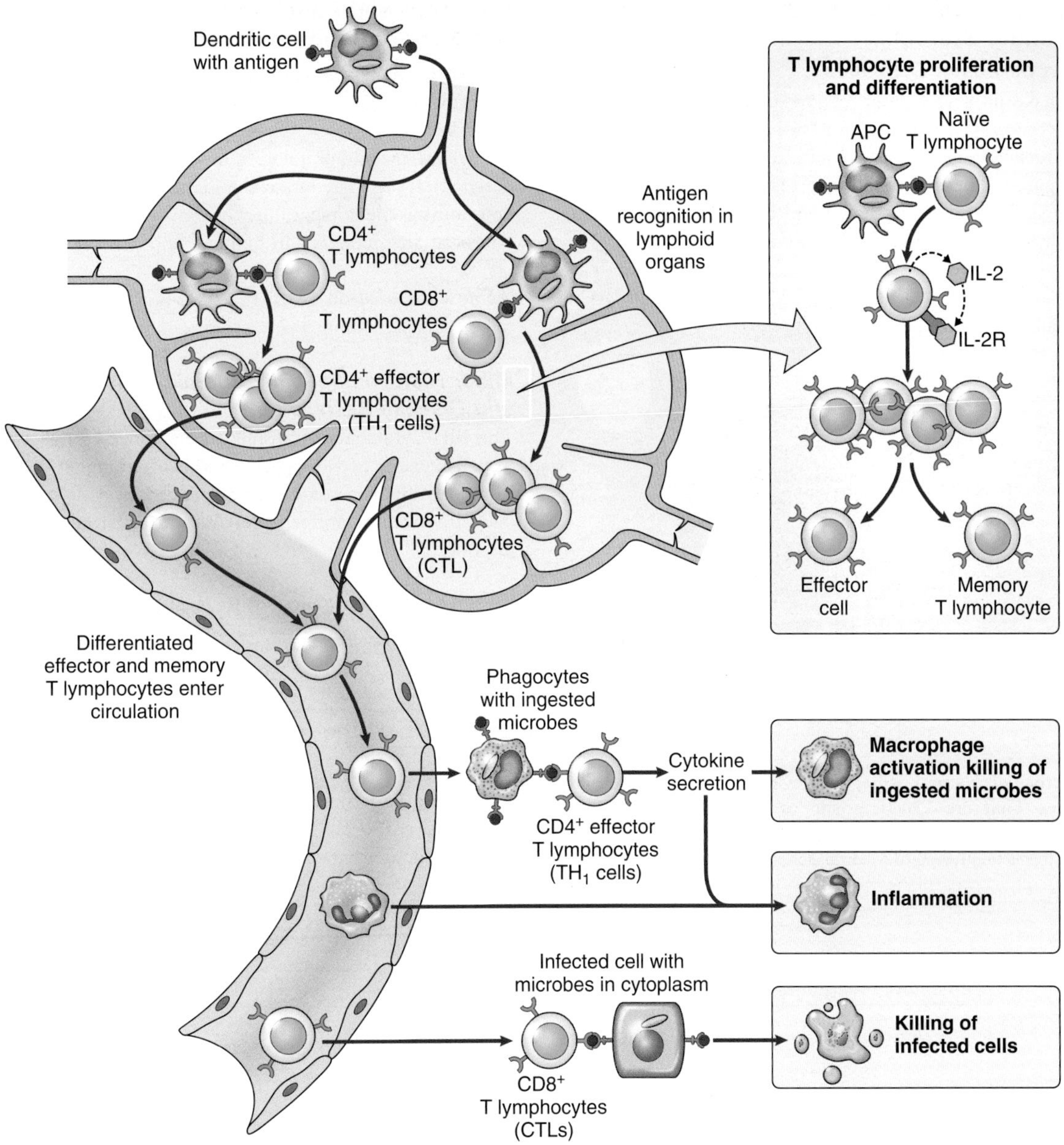

Figure 5-13 Dendritic Cell Functions. Dendritic cells are professional antigen-presenting cells that transport antigen from sites of infection to lymph nodes. Dendritic cells present peptide-MHC complexes to antigen-specific T lymphocytes present in specific areas of the lymph node and initiate the adaptive immune responses leading to cell-mediated immunity. *APC*, Antigen-presenting cell; *CTL*, cytotoxic T lymphocyte; *IL*, interleukin; *MHC*, major histocompatibility complex; T_H, T helper.

Table 5-3 Antigen-Presenting Dendritic Cells and Their Primary Location

Dendritic Cells	Location
Langerhans cells	Skin, mucous membranes, iris, ciliary body
Interstitial dendritic cells	Most major organs
Interdigitating dendritic cells	T lymphocyte area of secondary lymphoid tissue and thymic medulla
Circulating dendritic cells	Peripheral blood

Because NK cells express FcγR (CD16), they can also function in antibody-dependent cellular cytotoxicity (ADCC). In the case of NK cells, ADCC allows for antibody-bound targets to be identified and targeted for NK cell–induced lysis.

NK cells facilitate the early response to viral infections not only by responding to cytokines produced early in a viral infection, but also by producing cytokines that help direct the immune response. NK cells are activated by IFN-α and IFN-β, released by virus-infected cells, and by IL-12, released by macrophages. After activation, NK cells have the ability to produce IFN-γ, a major cytokine directing the development of T_H1-type immune response early in the infection. IL-2 and IL-15 stimulate NK cell proliferation, and IL-12 enhances NK cell killing.

Cytokines: Messenger Molecules of the Immune System

General Properties of Cytokines

Cytokines make up a vast group of low-molecular-weight soluble glycoprotein proteins that are produced by immune and nonimmune cells, are largely produced locally, and act locally to direct the immune response. The expression of cytokine receptors and their respective ligands is highly regulated and contributes to the complexity of the systemic organization of the immune response.

More Information on this topic is available at www.expertconsult.com.

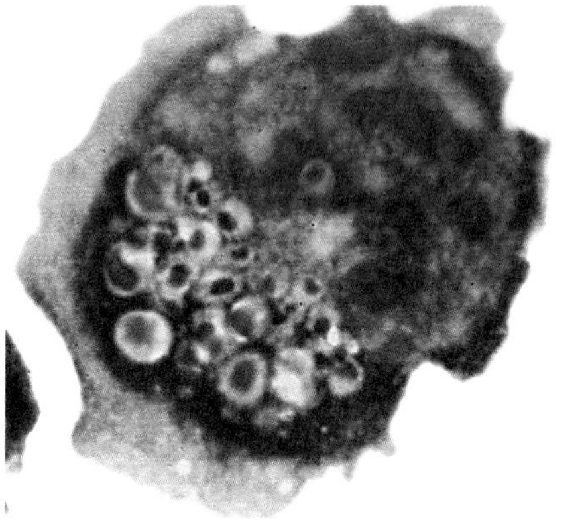

Figure 5-14 **Activated Natural Killer Cell with Numerous Cytoplasmic Granules That are Characteristic of These Large Granular Lymphocytes.** (Courtesy Dr. Noelle Williams, Department of Pathology, University of Texas Southwestern Medical School, Dallas.)

Structure and Function of Histocompatibility Antigens

The MHC represents a complex of genes that encode specialized molecules involved in intercellular recognition and the distinguishing of self from nonself. These cell surface molecules have immunologic and nonimmunologic functions. The histocompatibility designation originated from the identification of these molecules in determining the compatibility of transplanted tissues. The MHC is an essential component in humoral and cell-mediated immunity.

More information on this topic is available at www.expertconsult.com.

Major Histocompatibility Complex and Disease Association

The MHC influences transplant acceptance or rejection, immune responsiveness, and the pathogenesis of a number of diseases. The MHC represents a complex of genes that encode specialized molecules involved in antigen presentation and thus regulate immune responses.

More information on this topic is available at www.expertconsult.com.

Disorders of the Immune System

As has been discussed, immunity is a complex defensive system of recognition and effector mechanisms for protecting the host from infectious pathogens and cancer. During the normal immune response there are mechanisms for eliminating the inciting foreign

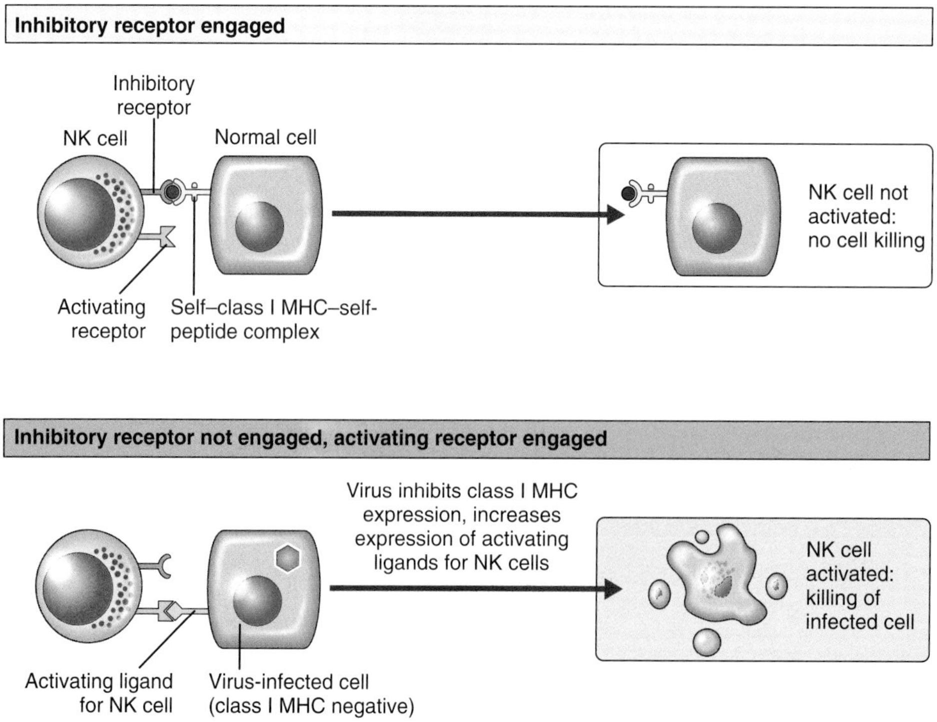

Figure 5-15 **Regulation of Natural Killer (NK) Cell Activity.** Activation of NK cells is mediated through activating and inhibitory receptors. Normal healthy cells express self-MHC molecules that function to inhibit the activation of NK cells. Abnormal or unhealthy cells fail to express self-MHC molecules and increase the expression of activating ligands that result in NK cell activation and killing of the abnormal or unhealthy cell. MHC, Major histocompatibility complex.

antigen, and associated with this is some degree of tissue damage that elicits an inflammatory response of appropriate duration and severity for the antigen. However, there are a number of instances in which the immune response elicits an inflammatory response that is not appropriate to the inciting antigen, and these fall into three general categories. The largest category is the hypersensitivity reactions, which are associated with a large number of diseases covered throughout this text. The second category is the autoimmune diseases, in which the immune response is inappropriately directed at a self-antigen, resulting in damage to normal organs or tissue. The third category is the immunodeficiency diseases, in which a genetic or acquired defect results in an inability to mount an immune response and thus control infections, resulting in severe systemic inflammation. The chapter now focuses on general features of immunologic tissue injury, with discussion of some specific immunologic diseases that are attributable to disorders of the immune system. Finally, we conclude with a discussion of amyloidosis, a condition that is the result of a number of mechanisms, some of which have an immunologic basis.

Mechanisms of Immunologic Tissue Injury: Hypersensitivity Reactions

A hypersensitivity reaction is defined as the altered reactivity to a specific antigen that results in pathologic reactions upon the exposure of a sensitized host to that specific antigen (Essential Concept 5-3). The designation of these immune responses as "hyper" is somewhat of a misnomer because the reactions elicited are better characterized as inappropriate or misdirected responses. An immune response can be either beneficial or harmful. By characterizing hypersensitivity responses as inappropriate or misdirected, we are not implying that these responses are any different from those that occur as a normal "beneficial" defense mechanism. To state it more clearly: If the immune response is beneficial, it is immunity, and if it is harmful, it is hypersensitivity. All hypersensitivity reactions are characterized by sensitization and effector phases. The sensitization phase requires that the host must have had either a previous exposure or a prolonged exposure to the antigen so that he or she can develop an immune response to the inciting antigen. The pathologic response associated with hypersensitivity reactions occurs in the effector phase and is most commonly manifested as an inflammatory reaction or as cell lysis.

Hypersensitivity reactions have historically been classified on the basis of the immunologic mechanism that mediates the disease as type I, type II, type III, or type IV. Types I, II, and III are mediated by antibody, and type IV is mediated by macrophages and T lymphocytes. Type I is also known as *immediate-type hypersensitivity* and most often is the result of an IgE response that is directed against an environmental or exogenous antigen (also known as an *allergen*). The result is the release of vasoactive mediators from IgE-sensitized mast cells, and these mediators produce an acute inflammatory response. Type II is also known as cytotoxic hypersensitivity and most often occurs when IgG or IgM is directed against either an altered self-protein or a foreign antigen bound to a tissue or cell. The result can lead to destruction of the tissue or cell by ADCC, complement-mediated lysis, or altered cellular function without evidence of tissue or cell damage. Type III is also known as *immune complex hypersensitivity* and is due to the formation of insoluble antibody-antigen complexes (also known as *immune complexes*). The result is activation of the complement system and the development of an inflammatory reaction at the sites of immune complex deposition. Type IV is also known as *delayed-type hypersensitivity* (DTH) and is the result of activation of sensitized T lymphocytes to a specific antigen. The resulting immune response is either mediated by direct cytotoxicity or by the release of cytokines that act primarily through macrophages. This original classification, as proposed by Gell and Coombs, was based largely on the primary initiating event involved in the individual reactions and not on the actual pathogenesis as it relates to what is seen clinically or pathologically.

Although the original classification of hypersensitivity reactions is still valid, "newer" versions that are based on the pathogenesis better illustrate the complexity of these reactions and the specific pathologic change (lesions) associated with them. For the purposes of our discussion, we will use the original version of the Gell and Coombs classification presented in Table 5-4, understanding that many of the diseases associated with hypersensitivity reactions are actually complex and may involve more than one type. In human beings, genetic mapping studies of most diseases characterized by a hypersensitivity reaction suggest that there are disease-associated susceptibility genes, further supporting the complex pathogenesis of these diseases. Finally, the pathogenesis of many diseases rarely involves a single hypersensitivity reaction, and in fact some diseases may begin as an immediate hypersensitivity but progress to be predominantly DTH. For clarity the hypersensitivity diseases are

ESSENTIAL CONCEPT 5-3 Hypersensitivity Reactions

Hypersensitivity reactions are inappropriate or misdirected responses to a specific antigen that result in harmful reactions upon exposure of a sensitized host to that specific antigen. Affected animals require a sensitization phase in which the animal must have had either a previous exposure or a prolonged exposure to the antigen so that it can develop an immune response to the inciting antigen. The harmful effects resulting from hypersensitivity reactions occur in the effector phase and are most commonly manifested through inflammation or cell lysis. Hypersensitivity reactions are classified on the basis of the immunologic mechanism that mediates the disease. Types I, II, and III are mediated by antibody, and type IV is mediated by macrophages and T lymphocytes.

Type I, also known as immediate-type hypersensitivity, is most often the result of an immunoglobulin (Ig) E response directed against environmental or exogenous antigens (allergens) causing the release of vasoactive mediators from IgE-sensitized mast cells and an acute inflammatory response. It can have systemic (e.g., anaphylaxis [bee sting]) and localized (e.g., allergic dermatitis) forms.

Type II, also known as cytotoxic hypersensitivity, most often occurs when IgG or IgM is directed against either an altered self-protein or a foreign antigen bound to a tissue or cell (a hapten) causing (1) destruction of the tissue or cell by antibody-dependent cellular cytotoxicity or complement-mediated lysis or (2) altered cellular function without evidence of tissue or cell damage.

Type III, also known as immune complex hypersensitivity, is caused by the formation of insoluble antibody-antigen complexes (immune complexes) resulting in activation of the complement system and the development of an inflammatory reaction at the sites of immune complex deposition. It can have generalized (e.g., rheumatoid arthritis and systemic lupus erythematosus) and localized (e.g., cutaneous Arthus reaction [blue eye anterior uveitis in dogs]) forms.

Type IV, also known as delayed-type hypersensitivity, is the result of activation of sensitized T lymphocytes to a specific antigen. The resulting immune response is either mediated by direct cytotoxicity by lymphocytes or by the release of cytokines that act primarily through macrophages to produce chronic inflammation. It is the underlying mechanism for tuberculin testing in cattle for bovine tuberculosis (*Mycobacterium bovis*) and for allergic contact hypersensitivity and granulomatous inflammatory responses.

Table 5-4 Mechanisms of Hypersensitivity Diseases

Type	Immunologic Component	Antigen	Prototype Disorder	Immune Mechanisms	Pathologic Lesions
Immediate (type I) hypersensitivity	IgE mediated	Allergens	Anaphylaxis; allergies (atopic forms)	Production of IgE antibody • Immediate release of vasoactive amines and other mediators from mast cells; recruitment of inflammatory cells (late-phase reaction)	Vascular dilation, edema, smooth muscle contraction, mucus production, inflammation
Antibody-mediated (type II) hypersensitivity	IgG and IgM mediated	Cell- or matrix-associated antigens Cell surface receptor	Autoimmune hemolytic anemia; neonatal isoerythrolysis; transfusion reactions; drug reactions; pemphigus	Production of IgG, IgM • Binds to antigen on target cell or tissue • Phagocytosis or lysis of target cell by activated complement or Fc receptors; recruitment of leukocytes	Cell lysis; inflammation
Immune complex-mediated (type III) hypersensitivity	IgG and IgM mediated	Soluble antigen (e.g., bacterial and viral antigens)	Systemic lupus erythematosus; some forms of glomerulonephritis; serum sickness; Arthus reaction	Deposition of antigen-antibody complexes • Complement activation • Recruitment of leukocytes by complement products and Fc receptors • Release of enzymes and other toxic molecules	Necrotizing vasculitis (fibrinoid necrosis); inflammation
Cell-mediated (type IV) hypersensitivity	T lymphocyte mediated	Soluble antigen (e.g., bacterial and viral antigens) Contact antigens Cell-associated antigen	Contact dermatitis; transplant rejection; tuberculosis; chronic allergic diseases	Activated T lymphocytes • Release of cytokines and macrophage activation • T lymphocyte–mediated cytotoxicity	Perivascular cellular infiltrates; edema; cell destruction; granuloma formation

IgE, Immunoglobulin E; *IgG,* immunoglobulin G; *IgM,* immunoglobulin M.

discussed in the context of their predominant mechanism except when it is appropriate to elaborate on the progression of a disease.

Type I Hypersensitivity (Immediate Hypersensitivity)

Type I hypersensitivity reactions are most commonly the result of an IgE-mediated immune response directed against environmental antigens (i.e., allergens) and parasite antigens. Harmful IgE-mediated responses to innocuous environmental antigens resulting in allergic reactions are termed *hypersensitivity,* whereas similar IgE-mediated protective responses to parasite antigens are considered immunity. This distinction emphasizes the fact that these are not unique immunologic reactions but rather misdirected or inappropriate "normal" immune responses.

Type I hypersensitivity occurs in a previously sensitized host and is initially manifested as acute inflammatory process that occurs within minutes ("immediate hypersensitivity") of exposure to the specific antigen. In many instances the reaction progresses from an early acute inflammatory response to a late-phase response and/or chronic inflammatory lesion that persists (Figs. 5-16 and 5-17). The basic pathogenesis involves a sensitization phase and an effector phase. The sensitization phase occurs during the initial exposure to an antigen when the host develops an antigen-specific IgE response, which results in sensitization of the host by the binding of the antigen-specific IgE to Fcε receptors on the surface of mast cells (Fig. 5-18). The host is now sensitized, and either through a second exposure or prolonged initial exposure to the IgE-specific antigen, there is cross-linking of two or more IgE molecules on the surface of the mast cell. This results in its activation and release of preformed and newly synthesized mediators, resulting in the effector phase. The effector phase can be limited to an acute inflammatory reaction (occurring within minutes), resulting primarily from the release of mast cell mediators, or can progress to a late-phase reaction (over a period of hours), or to a chronic reaction (persisting for days to years). The acute reaction is characterized by responses associated with release of preformed vasoactive amines from the mast cell and includes increased vascular permeability, smooth muscle contraction, and influx of inflammatory cells. The late-phase and chronic reactions, often associated with repeated or prolonged antigen exposures, are largely the result of a more intense inflammatory cell infiltration (primarily eosinophils, neutrophils, macrophages, and T lymphocytes) and tissue damage. Because the mast cell is central to the pathogenesis of a type I hypersensitivity reaction, its biologic features and primary functions are reviewed.

Mast cells are a heterogeneous population of bone marrow–derived cells that reside in vascularized tissue. Mast cells are easily identified by their abundant metachromatic cytoplasmic granules.

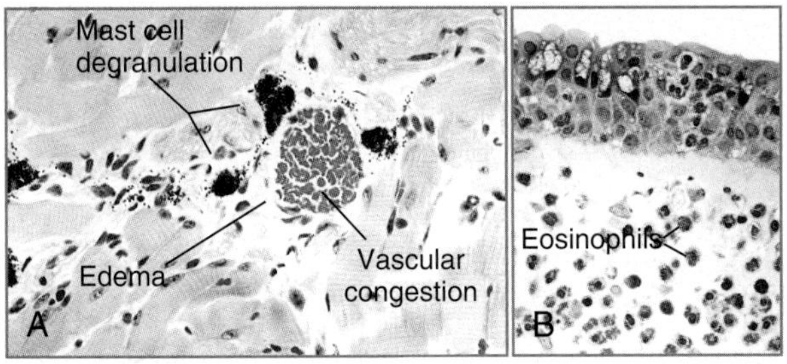

Figure 5-16 Immediate Hypersensitivity Reaction. A, Early reaction (minutes) is characterized by mast cell degranulation and release of preformed vasoactive substances that cause vasodilation and increased vascular permeability, resulting in edema of interstitial tissue. **B,** As the lesion progresses to the late phase (hours), the inflammatory infiltrate is primarily composed of eosinophils and fewer lymphocytes and neutrophils. (**A** and **B** courtesy Dr. Daniel Friend, Department of Pathology, Brigham and Women's Hospital, Boston.)

Metachromasia is defined as the staining of a tissue component so that the color (absorption spectrum) of the tissue-dye complex differs from the color of the original dye and of the other stained tissue. In other words, the metachromatic substance is a different color from those of the dye and the other stained tissue. For example, toluidine blue is a metachromatic dye, and it stains most tissues blue, but mast cell granules are purple. Other commonly used metachromatic dyes include methylene blue and thionine. Wright's and Giemsa's stains are dye mixtures that include a metachromatic dye. Mast cells can be divided into mucosal and connective tissue subpopulations, based not only on their location but also on their phenotypic, morphologic, histochemical, and functional characteristics. This suggests that individual subpopulations of mast cells may have specific functions in normal and pathologic responses that are a result of their activation. The tyrosine kinase receptor, c-kit, expressed on mast cells, their precursors, and its ligand—stem cell factor—is essential to mast cell development and function. Alterations in c-kit have been used to molecularly identify poorly differentiated mast cell tumors.

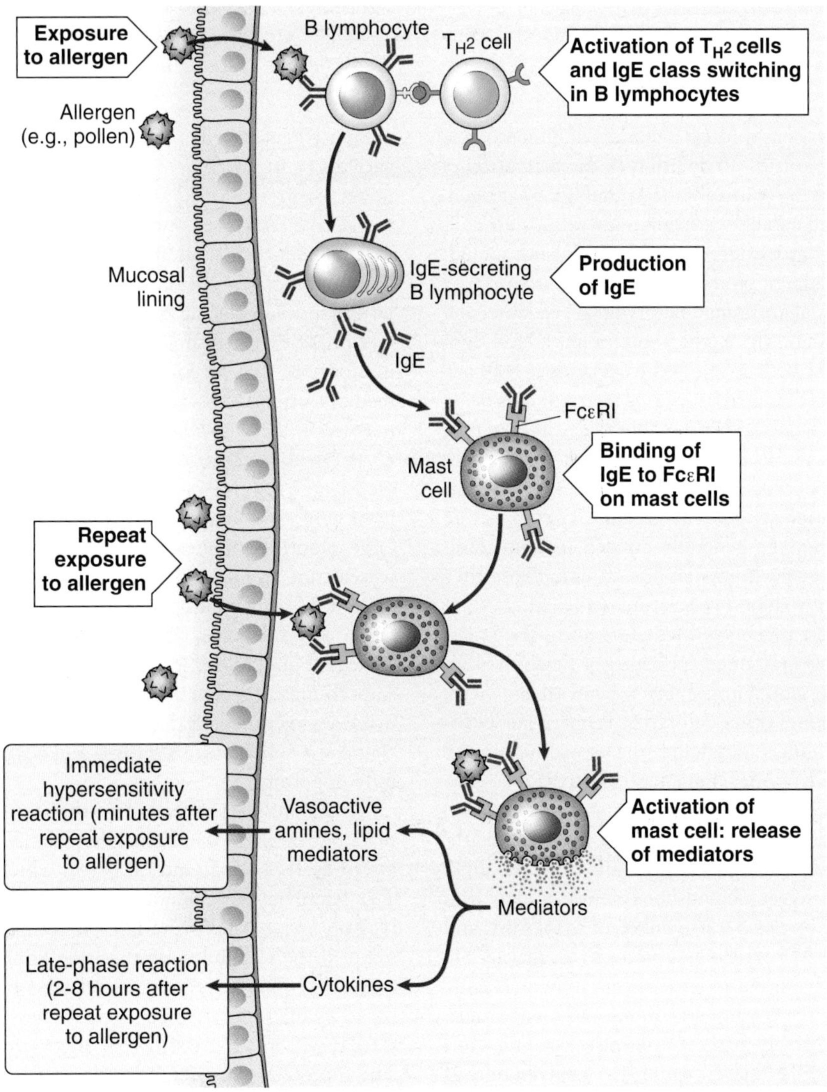

Figure 5-17 Type I Hypersensitivity Reaction. The pathogenesis of a type 1 hypersensitivity reaction begins with exposure to antigen (allergen) that results in activation of T helper lymphocyte type 2 (T_H2) lymphocytes and B lymphocytes, leading to the production of immunoglobulin E (IgE) and the sensitizing of mast cells. Continued or repeat exposure to antigen results in cross-linking of IgE bound to mast cells causing activation and release of inflammatory mediators.

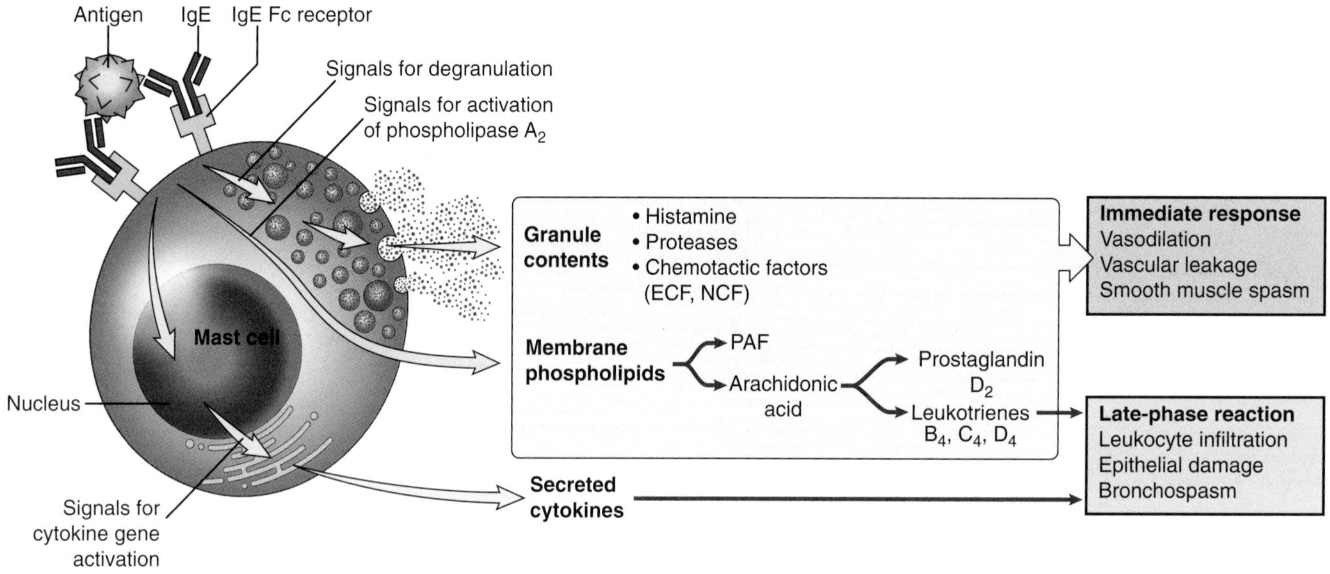

Figure 5-18 **Degranulation and Activation of Mast Cells.** When an animal is sensitized by antigen in a type 1 hypersensitivity reaction, it has immunoglobulin E (IgE) molecules bound to receptors on the surface of mast cells. When exposed to antigen, the bound IgE on the mast cell surface is cross-linked, resulting in activation of the mast cell. This leads to degranulation of preformed mediators and the synthesis of mediators largely though activation of phospholipase A_2, which lead to inflammatory responses. *ECF,* Eosinophil chemotactic factor; *NCF,* neutrophil chemotactic factor; *PAF,* platelet-activating factor.

Mast cell activation can occur through a number of immunologic and nonimmunologic mechanisms. In addition to the activation of mast cells through cross-linking of membrane-bound IgE by antigen, other substances and stimuli can also activate mast cells. Mast cells can be activated by Fcε receptor–independent mechanisms, including cytokines (IL-8), complement products (the anaphylatoxins C3a and C5a), drugs (nonsteroidal antiinflammatory drugs, codeine, and morphine), and physical stimuli (heat, cold, and trauma). Non–IgE-mediated activation of mast cells is referred to as an *anaphylactoid reaction,* whereas the IgE-mediated activation is referred to as *type I hypersensitivity*. There are species and tissue differences in how type I reactions are manifested, and these are attributable to the types and proportions of mediators produced by the mast cell. Mast cells are a heterogeneous population of cells with regard to their structure and function. Although they are generally divided into mucosal-based and connective tissue–based populations, in either case they are primarily found adjacent to blood vessels and nerves where their mediators have their greatest influence. Mediators released by mast cells are broadly classified as preformed (primary) or newly synthesized (secondary), and as presented in E-Table 5-3 and see Fig. 5-18, they influence local tissues and other cell types. Primary mediators are stored in cytoplasmic granules and include the vasoactive amines histamine, serotonin, and adenosine; chemotactic factors for eosinophils and neutrophils; enzymes, including neutral proteases and acid hydrolases; and proteoglycans, such as heparin and the chondroitin sulfates. Newly synthesized mediators consist largely of the lipid mediator products of cyclooxygenase and lipoxygenase metabolism of arachidonic acid (see Chapter 3), a number of cytokines, and platelet-activating factor (PAF). The major products of arachidonic metabolism are the prostaglandins and leukotrienes, of which prostaglandin D_2 and leukotrienes C_4, D_4, and E_4 are most important. The major cytokines released from mast cells during a type I reaction include IL-4, IL-5, IL-6, and TNF-α. IL-4 and IL-5 contribute to B lymphocyte activation and IgE synthesis. IL-5 is chemotactic for eosinophils. IL-6 and TNF-α are involved in the pathogenesis of shock during a systemic type I (anaphylactic) reaction. The biochemical events involved in IgE-mediated activation and mediator release by mast cells are similar to those described for leukocyte activation in Chapter 3. The primary actions of preformed and newly synthesized mediators are attributable to cellular infiltration, vasoactive responses, and smooth muscle contraction. PAF, which was first identified as an initiator of platelet aggregation and degranulation, functions not only in the acute phase by increasing vasodilation and vascular permeability but is also important early in the late phase by recruiting and activating inflammatory cells. Finally, it is of note that recent studies have identified TLR pathways that mediate interactions between dendritic cells, T lymphocytes, and mast cells, thus modulating type I responses.

A type I reaction begins as an acute inflammatory reaction mediated largely by the vasoactive amines released by degranulation of mast cells. It is during this early stage that mast cells also release large quantities of chemotactic factors and cytokines. These mediators recruit and activate the inflammatory cells that will not only sustain the inflammatory response in the absence of antigen but also cause tissue damage. The immediate response is characterized by increased blood flow, increased vascular permeability (edema), and smooth muscle spasm. As the reaction progresses, additional leukocytes are recruited, and they release biologically active substances that cause cell damage. Of these leukocytes, eosinophils are particularly important.

Eosinophils are recruited to the sites of type I hypersensitivity reactions by chemokines, such as eotaxin, and their survival is influenced by IL-3, IL-5, and GM-CSF, which are largely derived from T_H2 lymphocytes. Eosinophils recruited during the early response play an active role in the late-phase response by releasing components of their granules, synthesizing lipid mediators, and producing cytokines. The basic proteins released by eosinophils are toxic to parasites and host tissue. In particular, eosinophil major basic protein is toxic not only to parasites but also to tumor cells and normal cells. These proteins contribute to the epithelial cell damage associated with chronic type I reactions. Lipid mediators synthesized by activated eosinophils include PAF, leukotrienes, and lipoxins. Cytokines produced and released by eosinophils include growth factors, chemokines, cytokines involved in inflammation and repair, and regulatory cytokines. Macrophages and lymphocytes also participate in the late-phase response to varying degrees.

Epithelial cells further contribute to the inflammation by becoming activated and producing factors that recruit and activate additional inflammatory cells. It is this complex series of cell activation, recruitment, and mediator release that amplifies the immune response and sustains the inflammatory reaction long after the antigen has gone.

The factors that determine whether a host will develop a type I hypersensitivity reaction are complex. The genetic makeup of the host and the dose and route of antigen exposure are most important. These factors influence whether the individual will have a T_H1 or T_H2 response. The development of an IgE-secreting B lymphocyte from an immature (naïve) B lymphocyte depends on activated $CD4^+$ lymphocytes of the T_H2 type. The cytokines that define a T_H2-lymphocyte response have important roles in regulating the cells involved in a type I hypersensitivity reaction. IL-3, IL-4, and IL-10 influence mast cell production; IL-4 is involved in isotype switching to IgE; and IL-3 and IL-5 influence eosinophil maturation and activation. IL-13 promotes the production of IgE. The major cytokine that defines a T_H1 response, IFN-γ, inhibits the T_H2 response. Thus an animal that develops predominantly a T_H2 response to a particular antigen would be more likely to develop a type I hypersensitivity reaction as compared with one that develops predominantly a T_H1 response. The $CD4^+$ T lymphocyte plays a central role in the pathogenesis of a type I hypersensitivity. In human beings, additional genetic influences can be linked to the human leukocyte antigen (HLA)–linked immune response genes. These genes appear to control allergen-specific IgE responses. As mentioned previously, the association of specific class I MHC molecules with an increased susceptibility to atopy in the dog has been proposed. As with the mast cell and the eosinophil, a role for the $CD4^+$ T lymphocyte in the late-phase response has also been described. Studies suggest that the continued production of T_H2 cytokines contributes to the chronic inflammation associated with some chronic type I hypersensitivity reactions.

In summary, type I hypersensitivity is a complex disease process that occurs in sensitized hosts, which can result in three types of responses: (1) an acute inflammatory response, (2) a late-phase response, and (3) a chronic inflammatory response. In sensitized hosts the cross-linking of IgE on the surface of mast cells results in the immediate release of mediators that influence local tissue and recruit additional inflammatory cells. The acute response is dependent on resident mast cells, whereas the late-phase and chronic responses are dependent on recruited cells, especially the eosinophil. Central to the pathogenesis of a type I hypersensitivity reaction are the T_H2 lymphocytes and the cytokines they produce, which influence IgE production and the recruitment and activation of leukocytes.

Systemic and localized type I hypersensitivity reactions occur in animals. The pathogenesis of many infectious and noninfectious diseases involves the production of IgE and the development of a type I hypersensitivity reaction. Type I hypersensitivity is an allergic reaction that occurs within minutes of exposure to an antigen to which the host has been previously sensitized. Allergy has become synonymous with type I hypersensitivity. By definition, type I hypersensitivity reactions are mediated by IgE. Systemic type I hypersensitivity reactions are called *anaphylaxis*. Atopy is the genetic predisposition to develop localized type I hypersensitivity reactions to innocuous antigens. Atopy is often limited to an organ or tissue such as in allergic dermatitis and rhinitis, food allergies, and asthma. Non–IgE-mediated allergic-like reactions are referred to as anaphylactoid reactions.

Systemic Type I Hypersensitivity (Anaphylaxis). *Anaphylaxis* refers to an acute systemic hypersensitivity reaction to an antigen that is mediated by IgE and involves mast cell activation, resulting in a shocklike state often involving multiple organ systems. The clinical signs and pathologic changes attributable to a systemic anaphylactic reaction vary by species and often correlate to the primary shock organ in its most severe manifestation—death. This variation reflects differences in the distribution of the mast cells, the mediator content of their granules that are unique to individual species, and the primary target tissue. The primary target tissues are blood vessels and smooth muscle. Blood vessel beds and smooth muscles vary in their histamine receptor content, and therefore some are more susceptible than others to the influences of histamine. Because of this, the early signs of anaphylaxis can be varied. Cutaneous signs include pruritus, hyperemia, and angioedema. Cardiovascular signs include hypotension and an accompanying sinus tachycardia (characteristic of a vasovagal response). Respiratory signs include bronchospasms, laryngeal edema, and dyspnea. As the anaphylactic reaction progresses, hypotension or hypoxia may lead to unconsciousness. Fatal anaphylaxis may occur as the result of asphyxiation secondary to edema of the upper airway, circulatory failure as a result of dilation of the splanchnic vascular bed, or hypoxemia as a result of severe bronchospasms. In human beings a body of evidence also implicates human heart mast cells in myocardial anaphylaxis as a primary mechanism. Other than in cases with upper airway edema or pulmonary hyperinflation (emphysema), there are no pathognomonic lesions of anaphylaxis. The species most sensitive to the development of anaphylaxis is the guinea pig. The most common pathologic findings in most species are pulmonary edema and emphysema, except for dogs, for which the major shock organ is the liver, and severe hepatic congestion and visceral hemorrhage are the most common findings.

The types of antigens that can elicit a systemic anaphylactic reaction are diverse but most commonly include drugs (especially penicillin-based antibiotics), vaccines, venom of stinging insects, and heterologous sera. Although the greatest risk for the development of an anaphylactic reaction occurs during parenteral administration, it must be noted that in some cases even a small quantity of antigen in a highly sensitized host can elicit a systemic response.

Localized Type I Hypersensitivity. In a localized type I hypersensitivity reaction, the clinical signs and pathologic findings are restricted to a specific tissue or organ. Localized reactions most commonly occur at epithelial surfaces such as the surfaces of the skin and mucosa of the respiratory and gastrointestinal tract. As discussed previously, species differences on the location of mast cells, the mediators contained within them, and the histamine receptor distribution on target tissue may explain the different spectra of diseases seen among individual species.

Allergic dermatitis is a cutaneous manifestation of a type I hypersensitivity reaction that results in inflammation of the skin. The route of exposure to the antigen may be by inhalation, ingestion, or percutaneous absorption. If the allergic dermatitis is thought to have a genetic predisposition, then the disease is referred to as atopic dermatitis. Dietary type I hypersensitivity reactions in the dog and cat more commonly present as a cutaneous disease rather than a gastrointestinal disease. Other common cutaneous manifestations of type I hypersensitivity are flea and other arthropod bites and urticaria and angioedema (hives). All of these diseases are characterized by an acute inflammatory reaction, often perivascular, caused by mediators released from sensitized mast cells. In some instances, as in atopic dermatitis, the lesion may progress to a late-phase response or chronic inflammation characterized by more intense inflammatory infiltrates (e.g., atopic dermatitis) or to a type IV hypersensitivity reaction (arthropod bites). Other secondary changes, such as acanthosis, hyperpigmentation, sebaceous gland metaplasia, and pyoderma, occur in long-standing cases or in animals that have significant trauma related to pruritus.

Allergic rhinitis is a respiratory manifestation of a type I hypersensitivity reaction that most commonly develops in ruminants. The most common antigens are grass and weed pollens and mold spores (*Saccharopolyspora rectivirgula*). This disease also frequently progresses from an acute inflammatory disease to a late-phase response and chronic inflammation. In cattle, long-standing allergic rhinitis may progress to a type IV hypersensitivity reaction with the formation of nasal granulomas. Mold spores (*S. rectivirgula*) are more frequently associated with a type III hypersensitivity reaction, resulting in an allergic pneumonitis (extrinsic allergic alveolitis).

Although an inherited predisposition has been implicated in some species, the exact mode of inheritance remains to be determined. In human beings a link to genes encoding IL-4 and certain MHC antigens, important components of allergic diseases, has been made.

Type II Hypersensitivity (Cytotoxic Hypersensitivity)

In the original Gell and Coombs classification, the type II hypersensitivity reaction was designated as antibody-mediated cytotoxic hypersensitivity. This type of hypersensitivity most often occurs as the result of the development of antibodies directed against antigens on the surface of a cell or in a tissue, with the result that the cell or tissue is destroyed. Antigens may be either endogenous (normal cellular or tissue protein) or exogenous (e.g., a drug or microbial protein adsorbed to the cell). In some instances the antigen may be a cell surface receptor, and the antibody may activate or block the activation of the cell rather than cause cytotoxicity. The pathogenesis of many immune-mediated and autoimmune diseases is centered on the development of antireceptor or anti–surface antigen antibodies and a type II hypersensitivity reaction. The largest group of "cytotoxic" hypersensitivity reactions involves the hematologic diseases, with antibodies directed against antigens present on the surface of red blood cells and platelets. Type II hypersensitivity reactions are mediated by antibodies directed against antigens on the surface of tissue or cells so that the tissue or cell is destroyed or the function of the cell is altered. Type II hypersensitivity reactions most frequently involve IgM and IgG and occur within hours after exposure in a sensitized host.

There are three basic antibody-mediated mechanisms that result in type II hypersensitivity (Fig. 5-19). Complement-dependent reactions occur as a result of the complement-activating capability of IgG and IgM. Complement activation can mediate cytotoxicity by either the formation of the membrane attack complex, resulting in cell lysis, or the fixation of C3b fragments (opsonization) to the surface, facilitating phagocytosis (see Chapter 3). Antibody-dependent reactions can similarly opsonize cells, facilitating phagocytosis, or result in cell lysis by antibody-dependent cellular cytotoxicity. Opsonization of cells by antibody makes them susceptible to destruction by macrophages, neutrophils, NK cells, and eosinophils, all of which bear FcR. This is commonly referred to as *antibody-dependent cellular cytotoxicity* (ADCC). Finally, antibodies directed against surface receptors may result in altered cell or tissue function. The antireceptor antibodies can function as agonists, stimulating cell function, or as antagonists, blocking receptor function.

Diseases with a type II hypersensitivity pathogenesis are presented in Table 5-5. The physical and biochemical properties of red blood cells, platelets, and leukocytes make them susceptible to cytotoxic reactions. Two properties of red blood cells make them uniquely susceptible to being involved in type II reactions. First, their surface contains a complex array of blood group antigens that can become targets of antibody responses, as is commonly the case in transfusion reactions or immune-mediated hemolytic disease of the newborn. Second, the biochemical properties of red blood cells make them prone to adsorb substances such as drugs or antigenic components of infectious agents or tumors. In these instances the red blood cell may be either directly targeted because the substance alters a surface protein to an extent that it is now recognized as foreign, or indirectly targeted if there is an antibody response to the substance itself. Finally, in autoimmune forms of hemolytic anemia, agranulocytosis, and thrombocytopenia, there is a breakdown of tolerance and the subsequent development of antibodies to normal cells, and as a result they are destroyed.

The majority of cytotoxic type II diseases result in a decrease or loss of a population of cells (e.g., anemia, thrombocytopenia). Noncytotoxic type II diseases are initially characterized by activation or inhibition of cell or tissue function followed by inflammation, which may cause inflammatory damage to the targeted organ. In a type II reaction the pathogenesis commonly begins with cell surface antigens eliciting an antibody response, whereby the antibodies bind to the cell and either the cell is lysed or complement components attract phagocytic cells that damage tissues by releasing proteolytic enzymes.

Type III Hypersensitivity (Immune Complex Hypersensitivity)

Type III hypersensitivity is designated as immune complex hypersensitivity. This reaction occurs through the formation of antigen-antibody complexes that activate complement and result in tissue damage (Fig. 5-20). The cell or tissue injury is similar to a type II hypersensitivity reaction, although the underlying pathogenesis is different. With a type III reaction the cell or tissue is being destroyed not because the antibody is being directed against that cell or tissue, but rather because immune complexes either become "stuck" to that cell or are deposited in that tissue. Think of it as an "innocent bystander" reaction: The targeted tissue is not a direct target of the immune response. The pathogenesis begins with the formation of immune complexes that become lodged or are formed in or deposited in tissue and are capable of activating the complement system. Products of complement activation such as anaphylatoxins and chemotactic factors result in neutrophil infiltration and activation. On activation, neutrophils release their enzymes, and these result in tissue damage. Like type II hypersensitivity reactions, type III hypersensitivity reactions most frequently involve IgM and IgG and occur within hours after exposure in a sensitized host.

Antigen-antibody complexes form as a part of a normal immune response and usually facilitate the clearance of antigen by the phagocytic system without resulting in a type III hypersensitivity reaction. Although a number of factors determine whether a type III reaction will occur, the most important is the relationship of the antibody response to the quantity of antigen. When antibody is in great excess of antigen, the antigen-antibody complexes formed are large and insoluble and easily removed by the phagocytic system. When antigen is in great excess of the quantity of antibody, the antigen-antibody complexes formed are too small to be capable of becoming lodged in tissues or of activating the complement system. However, when antigen is in slight excess of antibody, these small soluble complexes can become lodged in tissue and activate the complement system. When this type of small soluble antigen-antibody complex is formed in the circulation, their accumulation in tissue is essentially the result of anatomic and physiologic processes and

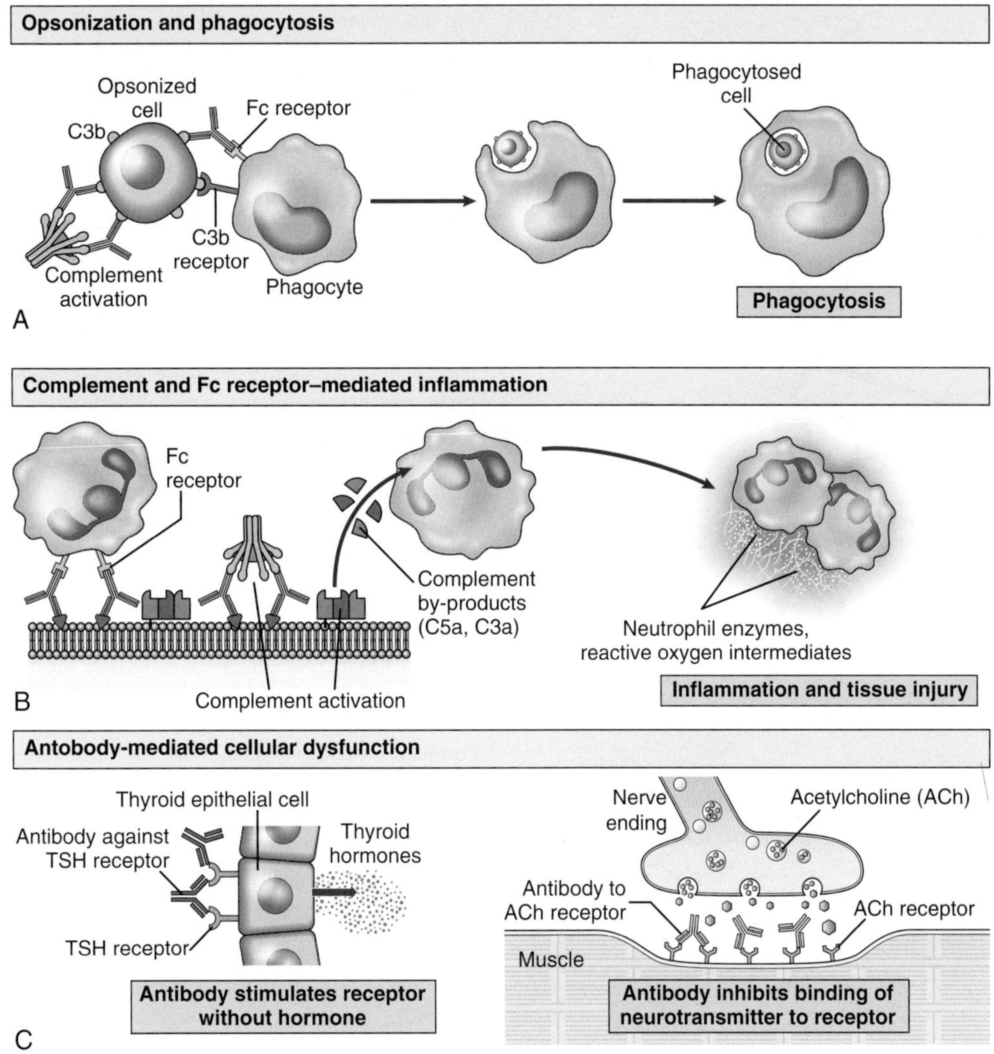

Figure 5-19 **The Three Major Mechanisms of an Antibody-Mediated (Type II Hypersensitivity) Injury.** The major mechanisms of tissue injury during a type II hypersensitivity reaction involve phagocytosis mediated by opsonization (A), complement and Fc receptor–mediated inflammation (B), and antibody-mediated cellular dysfunction through inhibition or activation of cellular receptors (C). *TSH*, Thyroid-stimulating hormone.

Table 5-5 Diseases with a Primary Cytotoxic Hypersensitivity (Type II Hypersensitivity) Pathogenesis

Disease	Target Antigen	Mechanisms of Disease	Clinicopathologic Manifestations
Autoimmune hemolytic anemia	Erythrocyte membrane proteins (blood group antigens)	Opsonization and phagocytosis of erythrocytes	Hemolysis, anemia
Neonatal isoerythrolysis	Erythrocyte membrane proteins (blood group antigens)	Opsonization and phagocytosis of erythrocytes	Hemolysis, anemia
Autoimmune thrombocytopenic purpura	Platelet membrane proteins (integrin GPIIb/IIIa)	Opsonization and phagocytosis of platelets	Bleeding
Pemphigus diseases	Proteins in intercellular junctions of epidermal cells (e.g., the epidermal cadherin desmoglein 1)	Antibody-mediated activation of proteases, disruption of intercellular adhesions	Vesiculobullous (diseases of the skin)
Vasculitis caused by ANCA	Neutrophil granule proteins, presumably released from activated neutrophils	Neutrophil degranulation and inflammation	Vasculitis
Myasthenia gravis	Acetylcholine receptor	Antibody inhibits acetylcholine binding, downmodulates receptors	Muscle weakness, paralysis
Pernicious anemia	Intrinsic factor of gastric parietal cells	Neutralization of intrinsic factor, decreased absorption of vitamin B_{12}	Abnormal erythropoiesis, anemia
Bullous pemphigoid	Collagen type XVII within hemidesmosomes	Antibodies against basal cells	Subepidermal vesicles characterized by basement membrane clefts

ANCA, Antineutrophil cytoplasmic antibody.

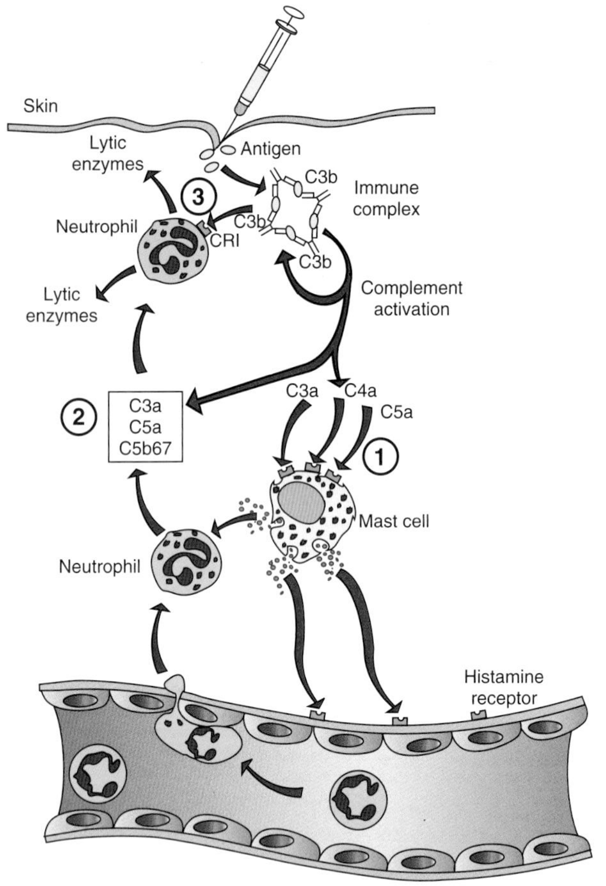

Figure 5-20 **A Localized Type III Hypersensitivity Reaction (Arthus Reaction) in the Dermis.** Antigen-antibody complexes, formed at the site of injection, activate the complement system to elaborate components that activate resident mast cells *(1)* and attract circulating neutrophils *(2)*. Inflammation is the result of tissue damage caused by mediators and enzymes released from both cell types *(3)*. *CRI*, Complement receptor 1. (Modified from Goldsby RA, Kindt TJ, Osborne BA: *Kuby immunology*, ed 6, New York, 2007, WH Freeman.)

has no immunologic basis. Finally, it has also been suggested that in some instances immune complex hypersensitivity may be the result of the normal phagocytic system being overwhelmed. Immune complex deposition can be localized to a tissue or generalized if the complexes are formed in circulation. Blood vessels, synovial membranes, glomeruli, and the choroid plexus are particularly vulnerable to deposition of immune complexes. The concentration and size of the complexes determine the sites of deposition.

Type III reactions can develop from antibody responses to endogenous or exogenous antigens, and immune complexes can be deposited in a number of tissues (Table 5-6). Although a number of diseases of domestic species involve a type III hypersensitivity pathogenesis, a majority of diseases are the result of persistent infections, autoimmune disease, or inhalation of foreign antigen. Organisms that result in persistent infections are often characterized by a weak antibody response and the development of immune complex formation. A number of autoimmune and immune-mediated diseases result in the development of antibody responses to self-antigens or antigens complexed to self-proteins, and these are capable of generating complement-activating immune complexes. Immune complexes formed against commonly inhaled environmental antigens can lead to the development of an allergic alveolitis. Type III hypersensitivity reactions are mediated by the formation of antigen-antibody complexes, which results in complement activation leading to an influx of neutrophils and subsequent cell or tissue destruction. Antigen-antibody complexes may be formed in the circulation and lodge in tissue or may be formed in the tissue directly. The cell or tissue injury is largely determined by physiologic or anatomic properties rather than an immunologic basis. The pathogenesis of a number of diseases of domestic animals have a type III hypersensitivity basis.

Localized Type III Hypersensitivity. Localized type III hypersensitivity reactions are best exemplified by the Arthus reaction (see Fig. 5-20). The parenteral administration of an antigen to an animal that has a circulating antibody specific for that antigen results in a localized acute inflammatory response. The complexes are formed either within the tissue at the site of antigen deposition or localized

Table 5-6 Diseases with a Primary Type III Hypersensitivity (Immune Complex Hypersensitivity) Pathogenesis

Disease	Antigen Involved	Clinicopathologic Manifestations
Systemic lupus erythematosus	DNA, nucleoproteins, others	Glomerulonephritis, arthritis, vasculitis
Blue eye	Canine adenovirus 1 antigen	Anterior uveitis
Equine infectious anemia	Viral antigens	Anemia, thrombocytopenia
Poststaphylococcal hypersensitivity	Staphylococcal cell wall antigens	Dermatitis
Cutaneous vasculitis	Bacterial antigens, viral antigens, drugs	Vasculitis
Poststreptococcal (*Streptococcus equi* subsp. *equi*) hypersensitivity	M protein	Purpura hemorrhagica, glomerulonephritis
Acute glomerulonephritis	Bacterial antigens; parasite antigens; viral antigens; tumor antigens	Nephritis
Reactive arthritis	Bacterial antigens	Acute arthritis
Arthus reaction	Various foreign proteins	Cutaneous vasculitis
Serum sickness	Various proteins (e.g., foreign serum)	Arthritis, vasculitis, nephritis
Hypersensitivity pneumonitis	Fungal spores, dust	Alveolitis, vasculitis
COPD	Fungal spores, dust	Bronchiolitis
Aleutian mink disease	Viral antigens	Glomerulonephritis, vasculitis
Rheumatoid arthritis	IgG	Erosive polyarthritis

COPD, Chronic obstructive pulmonary disease; *IgG*, immunoglobulin G.

within blood vessels, as the antigen and antibody diffuse into the vascular wall. Early, within hours, the reaction is characterized by margination and emigration of neutrophils to and from the blood vessels and progressively results in tissue and vascular damage. The quantity of antigen-antibody complexes formed in the wall of the vessel determines the extent of the tissue damage. Small quantities of complexes may result in only mild hyperemia and edema. Large quantities of complexes may result in tissue and vascular necrosis as a result of neutrophils releasing the contents of their granules. In some cases the damage to the wall may be so severe as to cause thrombosis and localized ischemic injury. The Arthus reaction is still used today as an experimental model of a localized type III reaction. Recent studies, using the cutaneous Arthus reaction in complement-deficient mice, document the requirement of FcR activation for eliciting an inflammatory response and a revision of the hypothesis of the mechanism of immune complex–mediated inflammation. Complement components, such as C5a, are generated as a result of FcR activation. Conversely, the use of FcR-deficient mice and the Arthus reaction establish the requirement of this receptor because immune complexes and C3 alone are not sufficient to trigger an inflammatory response and tissue damage.

Many diseases have a progressive clinical course, and immune complex reactions often play a role, even though they may not be involved in the initial immunologic response. There are limited clinical examples of diseases characterized primarily by a localized immune complex reaction. One dramatic example is blue eye in the dog, which is an anterior uveitis that develops in a small percentage of dogs naturally infected with or vaccinated against canine adenovirus type 1. Other organs commonly affected by localized immune complex disease include the lung and skin. In the lung, chronic exposure of the lower airways to inhaled antigens can lead to the development of antigen-specific antibodies that form complexes within alveolar walls. This form of allergic lung disease is commonly referred to as *allergic pneumonitis* (extrinsic allergic alveolitis). Common antigens include spore-forming organisms (e.g., some actinomycetes and fungi). Allergic diseases of the lower airways frequently lead to type II pneumocyte hyperplasia, emphysema, and fibrosis, which are all secondary to inflammation and tissue damage mediated by type III hypersensitivity. Chronic obstructive pulmonary disease (COPD) in horses may be caused in part by a localized type III reaction to spore-forming organisms or dust that results in bronchiolitis (see Chapter 9). In dogs, staphylococcal infections of the skin may develop a type I, III, or IV reaction. In the case of a type III reaction, a neutrophilic dermal vasculitis is often evident (see Chapter 17).

Generalized Type III Hypersensitivity. When antigen is present in the circulation at appropriate concentrations relative to circulating antibody concentrations (as discussed previously), the result is the formation of immune complexes capable of generating a type III hypersensitivity reaction. Serum sickness is the prototypical disease with a type III hypersensitivity pathogenesis. Early examples of this disease were the result of the administration of heterologous serum, which led to the formation of circulating immune complexes that became lodged primarily in blood vessels, glomeruli, and joints. The blood vessel, glomerulus, or joint was not a target of the immune response but rather an "innocent bystander" because the resulting inflammation occurred as a result of the complement-activating capacity of the immune complexes that lodged there.

The pathogenesis of a systemic immune complex disease is best illustrated in three phases as depicted in Fig. 5-21. The first phase, as discussed previously, occurs when the host develops an antibody response to an antigen so that the ratio of antigen to antibody is appropriate for the formation of small, soluble circulating complexes that are not adequately cleared by the monocyte-macrophage system. Because the formation of antigen-antibody complexes can be a normal component of an immune response, the presence of immune complexes in circulation by itself is not sufficient to diagnose an immune complex disease. In the second phase the complexes adhere to cells or lodge in tissues that are uniquely susceptible to circulating immune complexes. The biochemical properties of the antigen-antibody complexes (e.g., overall quantity and size, charge) and the physiologic and anatomic characteristics of some cells and tissues account for their unique susceptibility to immune complex deposition. Other factors may also contribute to the

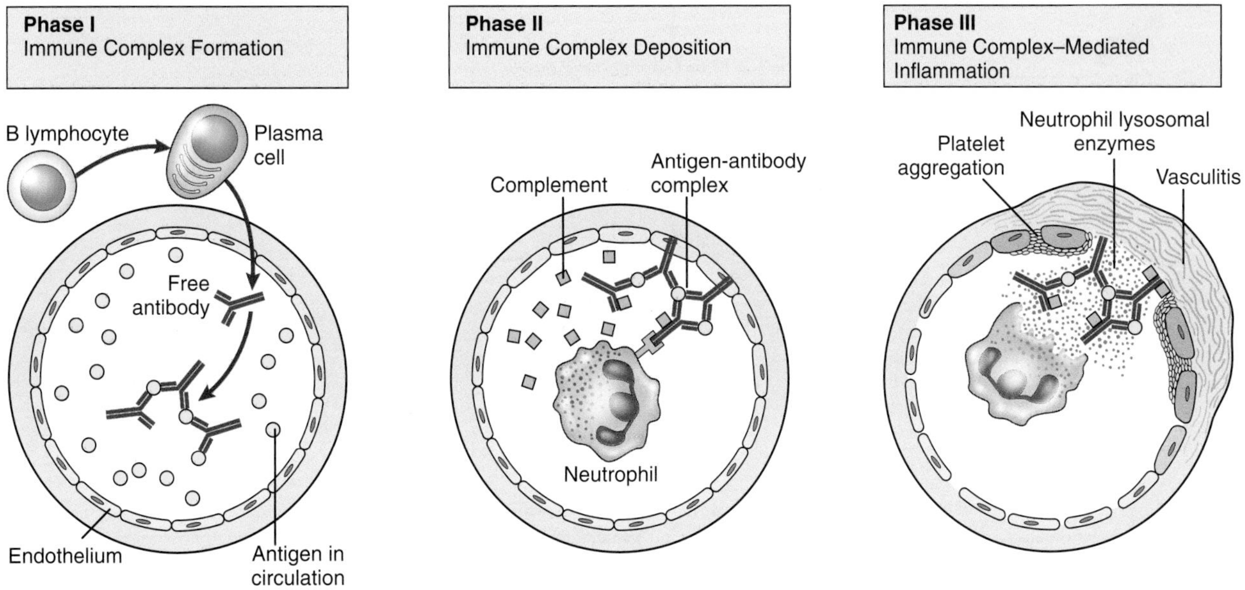

Figure 5-21 The Three Phases of A Systemic Type III Hypersensitivity Reaction. The three sequential phases of a type III hypersensitivity reaction are depicted from immune complex formation to immune complex deposition to immune complex–mediated inflammation.

formation or deposition of immune complexes in certain tissues. For example, in rheumatoid arthritis it has been proposed that lymphocytes within the joint may produce an altered IgG molecule that stimulates the production of rheumatoid factor (anti-IgG). Complexes become lodged within blood vessel walls and extravascular tissues as a result of the increased vascular permeability caused by the anaphylatoxins and vasoactive amines released from neutrophils, activated through the binding of antigen-antibody complexes to complement and FcR on their surface. The result is phase three: the activation of the complement system and the development of an acute inflammatory reaction centered on the vasculature. Neutrophils and macrophages are activated similarly through FcR and produce a number of inflammatory cytokines that attract and activate additional inflammatory cells. The inflammatory cells and mediators have been thoroughly discussed in Chapter 3. Immune complexes that lodge in blood vessels, glomeruli, or joints result in vasculitis, glomerulonephritis, and arthritis, respectively. The damage to the vessels also results in damage to the intima and exposure of collagen, which initiates the formation of microthrombi by the activation of the coagulation cascade and platelets.

The two primary cell types involved in a type III hypersensitivity reaction are FcR-bearing neutrophils and macrophages (Fig. 5-22). Complement activation leads to the elaboration of factors (primarily C5a) that are chemotactic and attract neutrophils and macrophages to the site. These cells are activated and produce a number of proinflammatory cytokines. Early in the response these cells release vasoactive amines that cause increased vascular permeability, allowing the immune complexes to lodge within the vessel wall. Many of these phagocytic cells are also stimulated to release their proteolytic enzymes and toxic free radicals, and these processes result in tissue and vascular damage. Platelets also contribute to the developing inflammatory reaction by releasing vasoactive amines and other proinflammatory constituents.

Diseases associated with type III hypersensitivity reactions are most commonly associated with a single exposure to a large quantity of antigen (e.g., administration of heterologous serum or from an immune response to systemic infections) or from continuous exposures to small quantities of antigen as in the case of autoimmune diseases (e.g., rheumatoid arthritis and systemic lupus erythematosus). In either of these instances the development of type III hypersensitivity depends on antigen in excess of antibody.

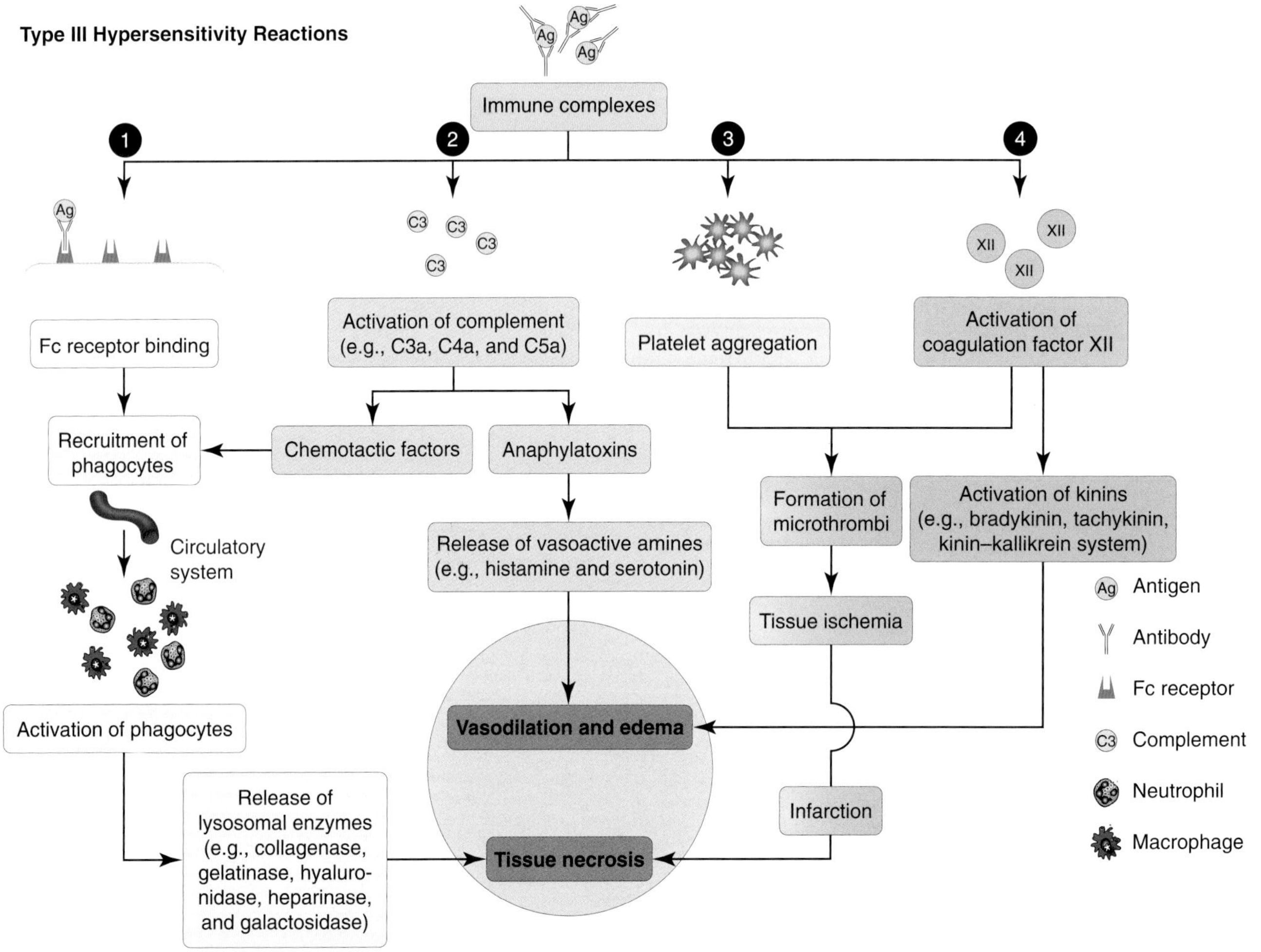

Figure 5-22 **Pathogenesis of Type III Hypersensitivity Reactions and the Morphologic Consequences.** Immune complexes can activate other inflammatory cascades and cellular processes, resulting in inflammation and tissue damage. *1*, Immune complex activation of phagocytic cells expressing Fc receptors, leading to tissue damage. *2*, Immune complex activation of the complement cascade, leading to the production of effector molecules of chemotaxis and anaphylaxis. *3*, Immune complexes activate platelet aggregation, leading to the formation of microthrombi that can result in tissue ischemia and infarction. *4*, Immune complexes activate the coagulation cascade, leading to the formation of inflammatory mediators, resulting in tissue damage. (Courtesy Dr. P.W. Snyder, School of Veterinary Medicine, Purdue University and Dr. J.F. Zachary, College of Veterinary Medicine, University of Illinois.)

Type IV Hypersensitivity (Delayed-Type Hypersensitivity)

Type IV hypersensitivity is also known as *cell-mediated hypersensitivity* because it is the result of the interaction of T lymphocytes and the specific antigen to which they have been sensitized. The resulting immune response is mediated either by direct cytotoxicity by CD8+ T lymphocytes or by the release of soluble cytokines from $CD4^+$ lymphocytes, which act through mediator cells (primarily macrophages) to produce chronic inflammatory reactions (Fig. 5-23). Because these responses are dependent on sensitized T lymphocytes and require 24 to 48 hours to develop, they are also referred to as *delayed-type hypersensitivity* (DTH). Unlike type I, II, and III hypersensitivity reactions, type IV hypersensitivity is not dependent on an antibody. We first discuss the response mediated primarily by activated $CD4^+$ lymphocytes. The prototypical DTH reaction is the localized tuberculin response. After an intradermal exposure of tuberculin, a purified protein derivative (PPD) of the tubercle bacillus, a previously sensitized host will develop a localized type IV reaction at the site of inoculation at 24 to 72 hours. The intradermal antigens are taken up and processed by dendritic Langerhans cells, which present antigenic peptides to antigen-specific $CD4^+$ lymphocytes that are activated to produce and secrete cytokines that attract and activate other inflammatory cells. Grossly the site appears as a swollen, firm nodule. Microscopically the nodule is composed of interstitial edema and a mononuclear infiltrate that is primarily centered around blood vessels. Early (<12 hours), the infiltrate is primarily neutrophilic, which is replaced largely by macrophages and lymphocytes (>12 hours). The DTH response is generally minimal and short lived because the concentration of PPD injected is small and rapidly degraded. A similar DTH reaction can be used to test for previous exposures to a number of intracellular organisms.

In addition to the tuberculin response, type IV hypersensitivity is the underlying pathogenesis for allergic contact hypersensitivity and granulomatous inflammatory responses. As mentioned with the other hypersensitivity reactions, the components of a type IV hypersensitivity reaction can be considered beneficial (protective immunity) when they occur as an appropriate response to intracellular organisms, or they can be considered harmful (hypersensitivity), for example, when they occur as an inappropriate response to exogenous chemicals or substances that are complexed with proteins, as in the case of allergic contact hypersensitivity.

In the tuberculin reaction the quantity of antigen limits the extent of the inflammatory response, and resolution of the inflammation generally occurs in 5 to 7 days. This is in contrast to chronic infections with persistent intracellular organisms or poorly degradable intracellular antigens (Table 5-7) that develop into a specific type of chronic inflammatory response called *granulomatous inflammation*. DTH reactions frequently occur in response to intracellular organisms and cause extensive tissue damage. These diseases are characterized by granulomatous inflammation. In this type of

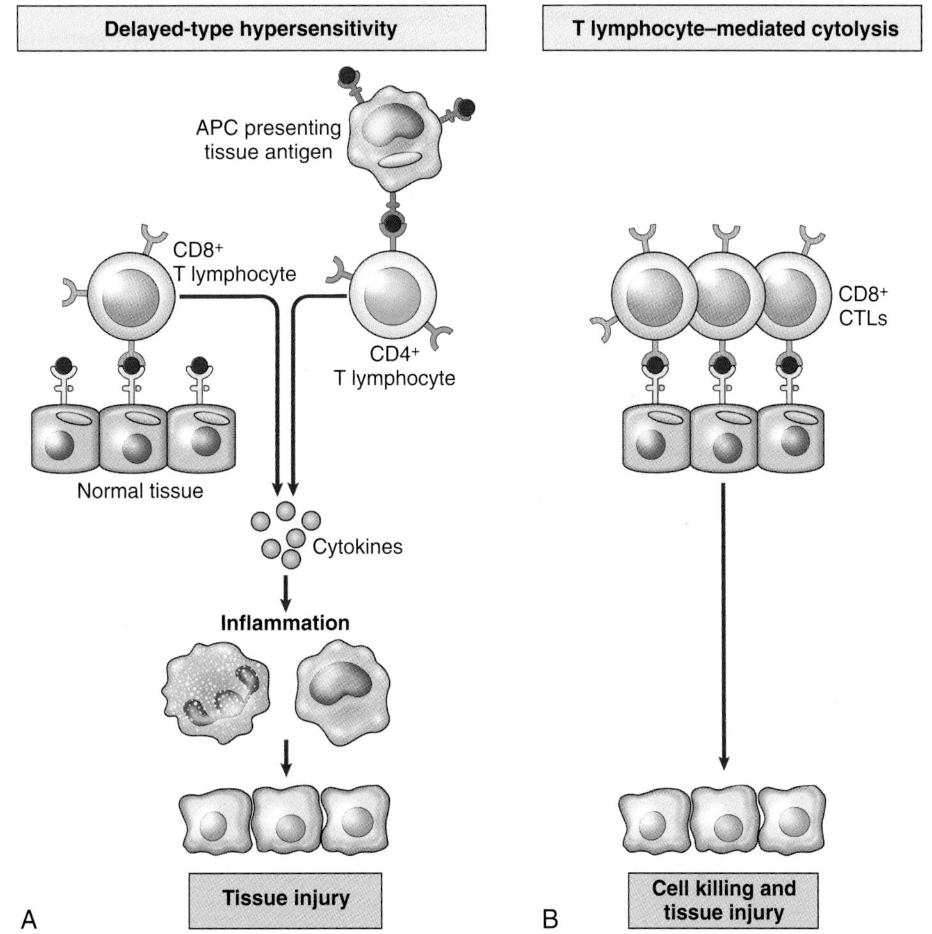

Figure 5-23 Type IV Hypersensitivity Reactions: the Mechanisms and Roles of T Lymphocytes. The pathogenesis of a type IV hypersensitivity is centered on activation of $CD4^+$ (T helper lymphocyte type 1) lymphocytes leading to activation of $CD8^+$ lymphocytes and the production of cytokines, resulting in tissue injury and cell killing. *A*, delayed-type hypersensitivity; *B*, T-lymphocyte-mediated cytolysis. *APC*, Antigen-presenting cell; *CTL*, cytotoxic T lymphocyte.

response the host is unable to destroy or eliminate the organism, resulting in antigen persistence. Compared with the tuberculin reaction, the type of inflammatory infiltrate is different. As discussed in Chapter 3, granulomatous inflammation designates that the inflammatory infiltrate has specific attributes, notably the presence of morphologically transformed macrophages into epithelial-like cells commonly called *epithelioid macrophages* (Figs. 5-24 and 5-25). Concurrently, there may be many multinucleated giant cells that represent fused macrophages. A number of fusion-related monocyte-macrophage surface proteins have been identified and include receptors for mannose and β_1 integrin, Src homology 2 domain-containing protein tyrosine phosphatase substrate 1 (SHPS-1), and the chemoattractant chemokine ligand 2. Lymphocytes can also represent a significant component of the inflammatory infiltrate. Generally, $CD4^+$ lymphocytes are interspersed with the macrophages, and $CD8^+$ lymphocytes are localized to the periphery. As these lesions progress, they may become organized into nodules commonly called *granulomas* (see Fig. 5-24, A). Depending on the inciting antigen, there may also be varying proportions of necrosis (often as a necrotic center), calcification of the necrotic tissue, and peripheral fibrous encapsulation. These features are largely the result of lytic enzymes released from activated macrophages. Nonimmunologic granulomas can occur in cases of foreign-body type granulomas, which typically have fewer lymphocytes. In either case, the body is trying to limit the spread or wall off the inciting antigen.

Table 5-7 Diseases with a Primary Type IV Hypersensitivity (Delayed-Type Hypersensitivity) Pathogenesis

Disease	Specificity of Pathogenic T Lymphocytes	Clinicopathologic Manifestations
Tuberculosis	*Mycobacteria* spp. antigens	Granuloma formation
Allergic contact dermatitis	Haptens	Perivascular dermatitis
Rheumatoid arthritis	Unknown antigen in joint synovium (type II collagen?); role of antibodies and type III hypersensitivity?	Chronic arthritis with inflammation, destruction of articular cartilage and bone
Johne's disease	*Mycobacterium paratuberculosis* antigens	Granulomatous enteritis
Allograft rejection	MHC molecules	Inflammation of graft tissue
Equine recurrent uveitis	Unknown	Uveitis

MHC, Major histocompatibility complex.

The type IV hypersensitivity reaction is immunologically specific and like all the hypersensitivity reactions involves a sensitization phase and an effector phase. The sensitization phase occurs with the initial exposure to the antigen and results in the development of antigen-specific memory T lymphocytes. These $CD4^+$ lymphocytes recognize peptides presented in the context of class II molecules on the surface of antigen-presenting cells. In this context the naïve $CD4^+$ T lymphocytes develop into functional T_H1 lymphocytes. These activated T_H1 lymphocytes are sometimes designated as T_{DTH} lymphocytes. Once the host is sensitized, a prolonged exposure or repeat exposure to the antigen results in the development of an effector phase. The effector phase can occur as a cytotoxic response mediated by $CD8^+$ lymphocytes or more commonly as a T_H1 response through the elaboration of cytokines by $CD4^+$ lymphocytes (see Fig. 5-25). T_H1 cytokines (most importantly, IL-2, IL-3, IFN-γ, and TNF-β) and chemokines (IL-8, macrophage chemotactic and activating factor, and macrophage-inhibition factor) enhance the function of cytokine-producing T lymphocytes (autocrine and paracrine fashion) and attract and activate macrophages. IL-2 induces the proliferation and long-term survival of T lymphocytes. IL-3 supports the growth and differentiation of T_H1 lymphocytes and NK cells. IFN-γ, the key mediator of type IV hypersensitivity, activates macrophages not only to enhance their phagocytic and killing mechanisms but also to enhance their ability to present antigen by inducing increased expression of class II MHC molecules. Activated

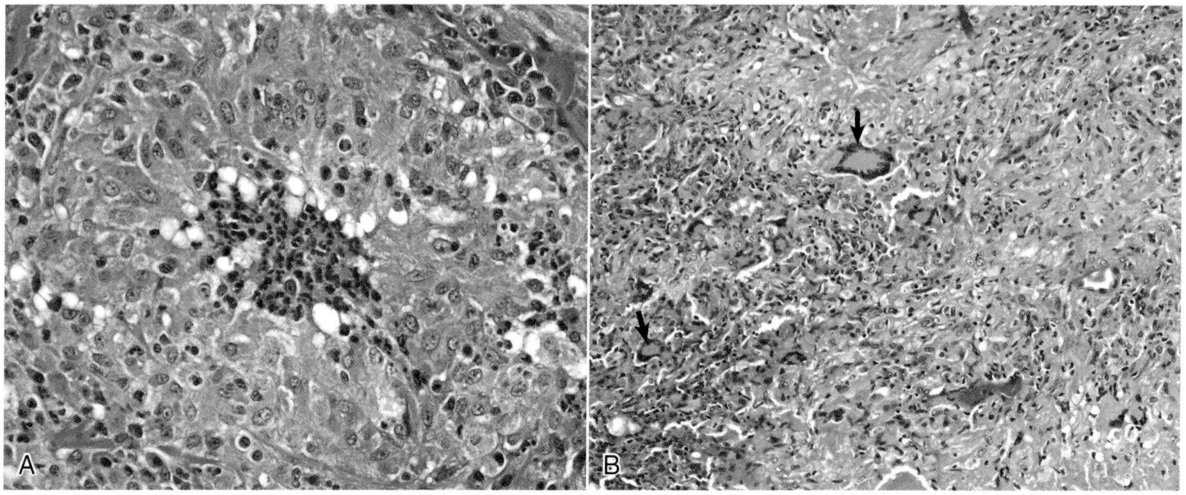

Figure 5-24 Granulomatous Inflammation Associated with Chronic Infections. A, Blastomycosis, skin, dog. Note the granuloma composed of sheets of epithelioid macrophages and the central focus of neutrophils. H&E stain. **B,** Mycobacteriosis, lung, gazelle. Numerous epithelioid macrophages and multinucleated Langhans-type giant cells *(arrows)* constitute the granulomatous tissue that has replaced normal lung parenchyma. H&E stain. (**A** and **B** courtesy Dr. P.W. Snyder, School of Veterinary Medicine, Purdue University.)

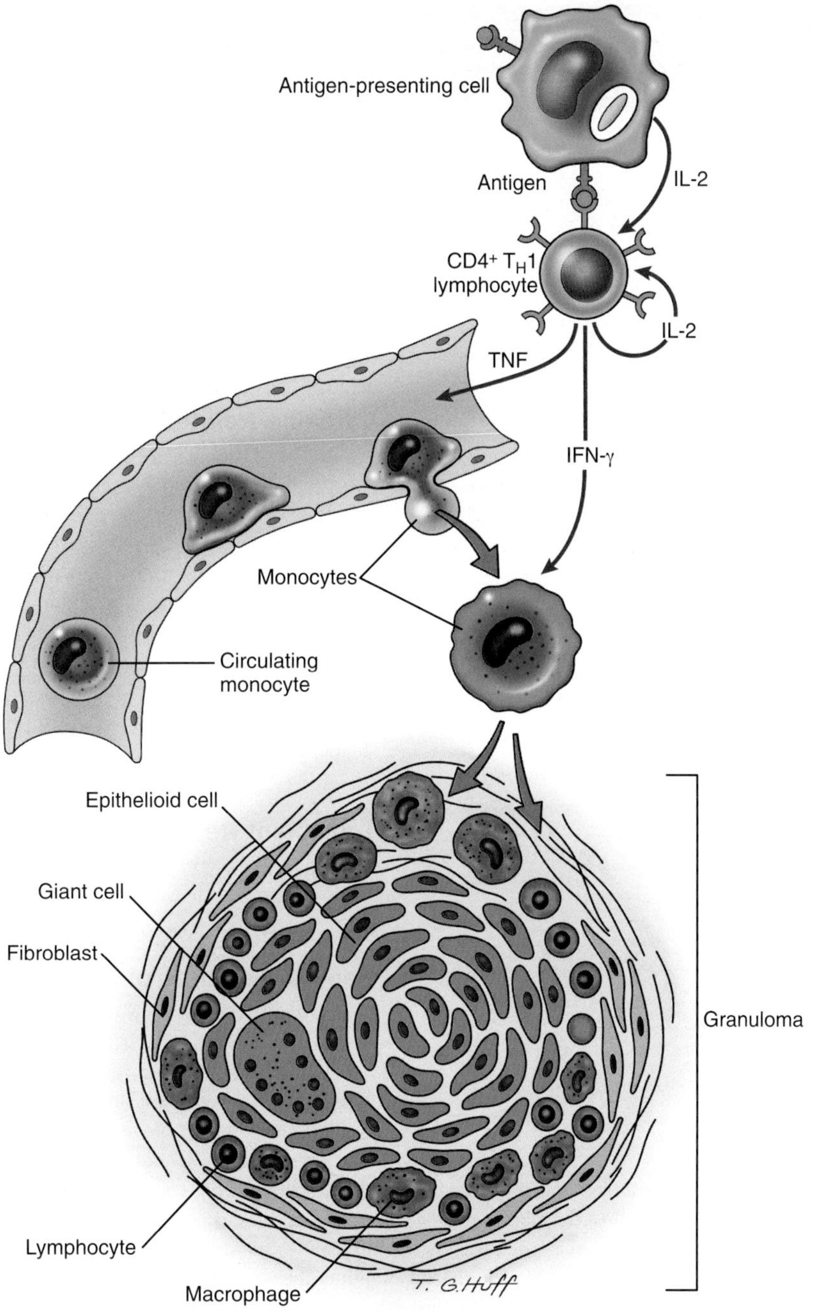

Figure 5-25 Granuloma Formation in a Type IV Hypersensitivity Reaction. The activated T helper lymphocyte type 1 (T_H1) is central to initiating the inflammatory response that characterizes the formation of a granuloma. *IFN-γ,* Interferon-γ; *IL,* interleukin; *TNF,* tumor necrosis factor.

macrophages and dendritic cells produce IL-12, which also facilitates the development of T_H1 lymphocytes. Activated macrophages also produce IL-1 and TNF-α, both of which act locally to increase the expression of adhesion molecules on endothelial cells, which further facilitates the extravasation of additional inflammatory cells. The production of cytokines and chemokines by the $CD4^+$ T_H1 lymphocytes influences macrophage function and mediates the production of cytokines that influence $CD4^+$ lymphocytes, resulting in a response that potentially goes from a beneficial protective response (immunity) to a harmful response that results in tissue damage (hypersensitivity).

The beneficial protective response of T lymphocyte–mediated hypersensitivity is not limited to intracellular organisms. It also can be a primary component of transplant rejection and immunity to cancer. There are other harmful T lymphocyte–mediated responses that result in disease. One example is allergic contact hypersensitivity. In allergic contact hypersensitivity the antigen is often too small to elicit an immune response by itself. These antigens must be complexed with other, larger proteins to become antigenic and are specifically referred to as *haptens* or generally called *contact antigens* (Box 5-1). Allergic contact hypersensitivity also depends on processing and presentation of the antigen by dendritic Langerhans cells to $CD4^+$ lymphocytes in regional lymph nodes. In the case of allergic contact dermatitis, the keratinocyte may also participate by producing a number of cytokines that activate Langerhans cells, mast cells, and other inflammatory cells. In the sensitization phase the protein-hapten complex is taken up and processed by Langerhans cells that migrate to regional lymph nodes. In the paracortex

Box 5-1 Pathogens and Contact Antigens Commonly Associated with Type IV Hypersensitivity Reactions in Domestic Animals

SOURCES OF ANTIGEN

Infectious Agents

Bacteria

- *Mycobacterium tuberculosis*
- *Mycobacterium bovis*
- *Mycobacterium avium* subsp. *paratuberculosis*
- *Mycobacterium avium* ssp.
- *Listeria monocytogenes*
- *Yersinia* spp.

Viruses

- Lymphocytic choriomeningitis virus

Fungi

- *Blastomyces dermatitidis*
- *Histoplasma capsulatum*
- *Cryptococcus neoformans*

Protozoa

- *Toxoplasma gondii*
- *Leishmania* spp.

Contact Antigens (Haptens)

Components of insecticides in:

- Flea collars
- Sprays
- Dips

Chemical components of plastics, leather, metals, and dyes
Components of shampoos
Topically applied drugs
Pollens
House plants

Allograft Tissues and Cells

MHC molecules

Neoplastic Cells

Tumor-associated antigens
Tumor-specific antigen

MHC, Major histocompatibility complex.

region of the lymph node (T lymphocyte area), they present antigenic components to $CD4^+$ lymphocytes. The host develops a population of memory lymphocytes and is now sensitized to the antigen. In a sensitized host, continuous exposure to the antigen, or more commonly, repeat exposure to the antigen, results in an effector phase response seen as epidermal vesicle formation with dermal and epidermal infiltrates of mononuclear inflammatory cells. The result is tissue damage that is disproportionate to any beneficial effects of the immune response.

Finally, as mentioned earlier, another form of DTH can occur that is mediated by direct cytotoxicity by $CD8^+$ T lymphocytes. This response is most commonly associated with viral infections. $CD8^+$ T lymphocytes, bearing viral antigen-specific TCRs, kill antigen-expressing target cells. These cells are commonly referred to as CTLs. The expression of viral proteins on the surface of an infected cell in association with class I MHC molecules serves as the recognition signal for the TCR-CD3 membrane complex. Following recognition of antigen by the CTL, there is upregulation of adhesion molecules on the CTL and the target cell, resulting in a CTL)–target cell conjugate. This stimulates an activating signal pathway that results in death of the target cell by apoptosis. The two principal mechanisms of CTL-mediated apoptosis are (1) the directional delivery of cytotoxic proteins and (2) the interaction of membrane-bound Fas ligand (FasL) on the CTL with the Fas receptor on the target cell. Both depend on the activation of caspases. Perforins and granzymes are preformed cytotoxic proteins contained in the cytoplasmic granules of CTL. Perforin, released between the conjugated CTL and the target cell, is polymerized in the presence of Ca^{2+} and forms pores in the plasma membrane of the target cell, not only causing lysis but also permitting the delivery of granzymes. Granzymes activate caspases, normally present in an inactive proenzyme form, that ultimately result in apoptotic death of the cell. The cross-linking of Fas by its ligand, membrane-bound FasL, results in the activation of the extrinsic (death-receptor–initiated) pathway of apoptosis, which is covered in greater detail in Chapter 1.

Cytokine-Related Diseases

A number of diseases are characterized by severe disruptions, either overproduction or underproduction, of cytokines or cytokine receptors. One of the most profound examples is the excessive elaboration of cytokines during bacterial septicemia and shock. The basic pathogenesis involves an infection with a Gram-negative, endotoxin-producing bacterium that stimulates macrophages to overproduce IL-1 and TNF-α, leading to systemic responses such as fever, disseminated intravascular coagulation (DIC), and shock.

More information on this topic is available at www.expertconsult.com.

Transplant Rejection

Information on this topic, including E-Fig. 5-5, is available at www.expertconsult.com.

General Features of Autoimmune Disease

Autoimmunity is by definition a specific immune response to self-antigens. Autoimmunity reflects a loss of immunologic tolerance to self-tissue or cellular antigens and is characterized by abnormal or excessive activity of self-reactive immune effector cells. Autoimmunity can be organ specific, localized, or systemic. Autoimmunity can be mediated by both autoantibodies and by self-reactive T lymphocytes. The cause of most autoimmune diseases remains elusive because they are often multifactorial and have a genetic and an environmental component. Criteria for diagnosing an autoimmune disease may include (1) direct proof, such as the fact that the disease can be transferred through cells or autoantibodies; (2) indirect proof, such as in identifying the antigen, then isolating the homologous antigen in an animal model, and reproducing the disease through administration of the antigen; (3) isolating self-reactive antibodies or T lymphocytes; and (4) circumstantial evidence, such as familial occurrence, lymphocyte infiltrate, MHC associations, and clinical improvement with immunosuppressive therapy. The complexity of autoimmune diseases is also supported by the fact that nonpathologic autoreactive T lymphocytes and antibodies can be found in normal individuals. Most autoimmune diseases have a tendency to be characterized by cyclic periods of alternating clinical disease and convalescence, an increased susceptibility of females, and a predisposition to multiple autoimmune phenomena as in the case of the mixed connective tissue disorders.

How does a loss of self-tolerance occur? To understand the mechanisms related to a loss of self-tolerance, one must first understand the basic concepts of maintaining immunologic tolerance to self-antigens.

Immunologic Tolerance

When exposed to an antigen, the immune system can be responsive and develop an immune response, or it can be nonresponsive and develop a state of tolerance. In either case, responsive or nonresponsive, the reaction is immunologically specific and has to be carefully regulated, because a response to a self-antigen or a nonresponse to a microbial pathogen could be equally detrimental. Immunologic tolerance is an active physiologic process and is not simply the lack of an immune response. Immunologic tolerance is defined as a failure of the immune system to respond to a specific antigen after previous exposure to that antigen. It is an absence of a functional response rather than a lack of any response at all. The development of autoimmunity (discussed later) can be simply described as an escape from the mechanism by which self-tolerance is maintained.

More information on this topic is available at www.expertconsult.com.

Central Tolerance. Central tolerance occurs during T lymphocyte development in the thymus, in which self-reactive T lymphocytes are clonally eliminated. Central tolerance has been most extensively studied in the thymus (see E-Fig. 5-6), where developing T lymphocytes undergo two selection processes that are essential for their development into mature effector cells and are based on the ability of developing lymphocytes to recognize self-peptides in association with MHC molecules. Positive selection is the clonal expansion of those cells capable of self-MHC restriction. Negative selection is the clonal deletion of those cells expressing TCRs capable of recognizing self-antigens in association with MHC molecules. Developing T and B lymphocytes expressing high avidity receptors for self-antigens are deleted from further development, resulting in a peripheral effector cell population lacking self-reactive cells. Self-reactive lymphocytes are eliminated by an apoptotic mechanism. For T lymphocytes it is the interaction of an immature lymphocyte and an antigen-presenting cell that triggers the process of clonal deletion of self-reactive T lymphocytes. This process of clonal deletion involves an apoptotic pathway mediated by the Fas-FasL. The exact molecular signals that trigger this apoptotic pathway remain elusive. The expression of peripheral antigens in the thymus is thought to be partially mediated by a protein called *autoimmune regulator* (AIRE), which is thought to be essential for the deletion of immature self-reactive T lymphocytes. Negative selection for developing B lymphocytes also occurs through a clonal deletion process involving an apoptotic pathway for those cells that have "excessive" stimulation of their antigen receptor molecules during development. Although the mechanisms regulating tolerance during lymphocyte development are very effective at identifying and eliminating self-reactive T and B lymphocytes, they are not perfect because self-reactive lymphocytes can be identified in normal individuals. Finally, the development of central tolerance requires exposure to the antigen during lymphocyte development, and many self-antigens are not present in the thymus or bone marrow. These self-antigens are commonly referred to as sequestered antigens because they are not seen by the developing lymphocytes. Some of the tissue antigens that fall into this class of antigens include myelin basic protein, lens proteins, and sperm protein, to mention a few. These antigens can be released as a result of infection or trauma and result in an immunologic response by self-reactive lymphocytes against myelin, lens, and sperm, respectively.

Because the development of self-reactive lymphocytes may escape the mechanisms of central tolerance, the immune system has developed peripheral tolerance mechanisms to prevent these cells from becoming activated and developing into effector cells capable of causing autoimmunity.

Peripheral Tolerance. In peripheral tolerance, self-reactive T lymphocytes that are not eliminated as a result of negative selection processes in the thymus have the potential to cause tissue injury when they exit the thymus and enter the peripheral tissues (see E-Fig. 5-6). Within the peripheral tissues there are mechanisms to prevent the activation of these self-reactive lymphocytes, and these occur as a consequence of the normal immune response to antigen and involve the same signals required for activation of lymphocytes during an immune response. Regulation of cellular activation occurs primarily by three mechanisms, which are briefly discussed next.

Anergy. Anergy is the functional inactivation of lymphocytes that encounter antigen. As previously discussed, two signals are required for the activation of naïve T lymphocytes by antigen-presenting cells. The first is generated by interaction of peptide antigen in association with MHC molecules on the surface of antigen-presenting cells within the TCR-CD3 complex, and the second is generated by the presence of costimulatory molecules. Costimulatory molecules are essential for the activation of naïve T lymphocytes and involve the interaction between T lymphocyte molecules (CD28) and their ligands (B7-1 and B7-2) on antigen-presenting cells. The interaction of CD28 with B7 results in T lymphocyte activation and its survival. However, if an antigen-presenting cell does not provide the costimulatory signal, the T lymphocyte receives a negative signal, and the cell becomes anergic (see E-Fig. 5-6). Another mechanism for inducing anergy involves the delivery of a specific inhibitory signal by CTLA-4 molecules on T lymphocytes that also bind to B7 molecules. The interaction of CTLA-4 with B7 results in inhibition of activation by blocking IL-2 production. The process of anergy is irreversible. The limited expression of costimulatory molecules by normal tissue facilitates the maintenance of peripheral tolerance to self-reactive lymphocytes. In general, CD28 is expressed on resting and activated T lymphocytes, whereas CTLA-4 is expressed only on activated T lymphocytes. What drives a T lymphocyte, expressing CD28 molecules, to recognize B7 molecules that lead to activation or to express CTLA-4 molecules that recognize the same B7 molecules that leads to anergy is unknown. Anergy of B lymphocytes occurs largely through the absence of specific T_H lymphocyte activation, although negative selection of mature self-reactive B lymphocytes is known to occur. An inability of B lymphocytes to receive appropriate signals from T_H lymphocytes, subsequent to antigen exposure, results in their deletion from lymphoid tissues.

Suppression by Regulatory T Lymphocytes. This mechanism of peripheral tolerance occurs through the activation of regulatory cells that prevent immune reactions to self-antigens. Suppression can occur as a result of cross-regulation of $CD4^+$ T_H1 lymphocytes by a specific population of $CD4^+$ T reg lymphocytes that were discussed previously. Specifically, $CD25^+$ and $CD4^+$ T reg lymphocytes producing IL-4, IL-10, and TGF-β downregulate T_H1 responses, effectively inhibiting lymphocyte activation and its effector function.

Clonal Deletion by Activation-Induced Cell Death. As discussed previously, one of the possible outcomes after lymphocyte activation as a result of antigen recognition during an immune response is lymphocyte proliferation. A second possible outcome after antigen exposure is cell death. For $CD4^+$ T lymphocytes, both outcomes—proliferation and death—are largely regulated by the expression of accessory costimulatory molecules. Activation-induced cell death (AICD) of T lymphocytes occurs by Fas-FasL signaling following persistent stimulation by antigen-presenting cells expressing antigen. During the normal immune response, AICD functions to downregulate immune responses and results in the return to immune homeostasis. Lymphocytes can be induced to express Fas (CD95), a member of the TNF-receptor family. The ligand for Fas, FasL, is expressed primarily on activated T lymphocytes. The binding of Fas to FasL results in apoptosis of activated T lymphocytes. Antigens that are expressed to a high level in normal tissue would result in persistent stimulation of self-reactive T lymphocytes, thus resulting in deletion through Fas-FasL–mediated apoptosis. In the case of an autoreactive B lymphocyte exposed to soluble antigen in the periphery, the cell becomes anergic. If the anergic autoreactive B lymphocyte is recognized by a T lymphocyte specific for the autoantigen, the interaction of the FasL on the T lymphocyte binding to the Fas molecule on the B lymphocyte results in activation-induced cell death of the B lymphocyte. Two strains of mice have been identified with a mutation in either the Fas molecule (lpr mice) or the FasL (gld mice). The lpr and gld strains have severe autoimmune disease develop with a phenotype similar to that of human beings with systemic lupus erythematosus.

Antigen Sequestration. Antigens that are not expressed in the thymus or are "cryptic" in nature have the potential to induce a self-reactive immune response. Certain physiologic characteristics of some tissue (e.g., testis, eye, and brain) are considered to render them as "immunologically privileged sites" because of the difficulty in eliciting an immune response to antigens in these tissues. Antigens in these sites cannot be seen by the immune system because they are sequestered. The sequestering of antigens may occur through the blood-brain barrier, an absence of lymphatic drainage, or the limited ability to express MHC molecules. A mechanism for the eye is referred to as the anterior chamber–associated immune deviation (ACAID), thought in part to be the result of inhibitory cytokines, such as TGF-β, produced by the cells of the iris and ciliary body. However, if the antigens in these tissues are released as the result of trauma or infection, they have the potential to cause a severe immune response as a consequence of activating self-reactive lymphocytes. Posttraumatic uveitis and orchitis are thought to be the result of the release of sequestered antigens.

Mechanisms of Autoimmunity

Although central tolerance is important in lymphocyte development, it is the mechanisms of peripheral tolerance that have a greater influence on the development of autoimmunity. We have described the complexities of central and peripheral tolerance, and thus it is understandable that the mechanisms responsible for allowing autoreactive lymphocytes to become activated and develop into self-reactive T lymphocytes or autoantibody-producing plasma cells are equally diverse and complex (Fig. 5-26). Although autoantigens have been described for a number of autoimmune diseases, it is the identification of the initiating antigen that remains elusive. The cause of most autoimmune diseases remains unknown, as they often are multifactorial and have genetic and environmental components (Fig. 5-27).

Failure of Peripheral Tolerance

The mechanisms of self-tolerance, as previously discussed, serve as a basis for presenting how a failure to maintain those mechanisms can contribute to the pathogenesis of autoimmunity.

Genetic Factors in Autoimmunity

The majority of autoimmune diseases in human beings have a strong genetic predisposition. The most well-studied genetic component centers around the MHC molecules. As previously discussed, MHC molecules are important in the development of lymphocytes and in the regulation of peripheral effector lymphocytes. Just as autoreactive lymphocytes have been identified in normal individuals without autoimmune disease, the presence of certain MHC molecules themselves is not sufficient to result in autoimmune disease. These observations would suggest that the expression of an autoimmune phenotype is not likely to be the result of a single-gene defect. Other genes that regulate proteins involved in other aspects of the immune response, or that are involved in the inflammatory or healing response, may also be involved. Additionally, experimental variations in the expression and activity of transcription factors can influence the expression of certain autoimmune diseases.

Several strains of mice with specific genetic mutations of factors involved in the maintenance of central and peripheral tolerance that result in autoimmune disease have been identified. Mice with defects of Fas or FasL have disruption of the activation-induced cell death signal in lymphocytes, resulting in autoimmune disease. Mice lacking the transcriptional factor AIRE, which is responsible for thymic expression of self-antigens, and mice defective in the expression of CTLA-4, the inhibitory receptor involved in T lymphocyte anergy, also develop autoimmunity. An important regulatory cytokine—IL-2, the major growth factor for lymphocytes—is also required for the development and function of T reg lymphocytes. Mice lacking either IL-2 or the IL-2 receptor develop autoimmune disease characterized by inflammatory bowel disease, anti-DNA antibodies, and autoimmune hemolytic anemia. The proposed mechanism of autoimmunity in these mice is thought to involve T lymphocytes and to be a result of a failure of suppression by T reg lymphocytes and a failure of activation-induced cell death, two mechanisms of peripheral tolerance. These mouse models of autoimmune disease have facilitated the identification of pathogenic mechanisms of autoimmunity. Although all of these mechanisms have now been identified in human autoimmune diseases, it is likely only a matter of time before they are identified in other species.

Of the domestic species, there have been a number of autoimmune diseases in dogs documented to have a familial tendency, and the mechanism is in part attributed to certain MHC alleles. These recognized associations of specific autoimmune diseases and MHC molecules have been limited to a few specific breeds. It should also be noted that other diseases of immunity, for example, immunodeficiency and atopy, also have a higher incidence in some breeds.

Microbial Agents in Autoimmunity

The recognition that certain infections may result in the development of an autoimmune disease is the result of two observations. First, experimentally, one can induce autoimmunity in specific strains of mice by infection with certain strains of virus. Second, many spontaneous autoimmune diseases occur after viral infections, although attempts to isolate and identify viral agents in patients with autoimmune diseases have been equivocal. Again, these observations would suggest that these diseases have a complex pathogenesis with a genetic and an environmental component.

The role of infections as environmental factors in the pathogenesis of autoimmune diseases may be explained by understanding how infectious agents may cause a breakdown of anergy to self-molecules (loss of self-tolerance). As discussed earlier, not all self-reacting B and T lymphocytes are eliminated during the differentiation and development process. These potentially self-reacting lymphocytes are regulated in the periphery by clonal anergy. Therefore a loss of this regulation could explain how autoimmune diseases develop. Plausible mechanisms of why infectious agents cause aberrations of peripheral clonal anergy are twofold (Fig. 5-28). One mechanism may be the result of nonspecific disruption of the regulatory cells, which results in the induction of costimulatory molecules on

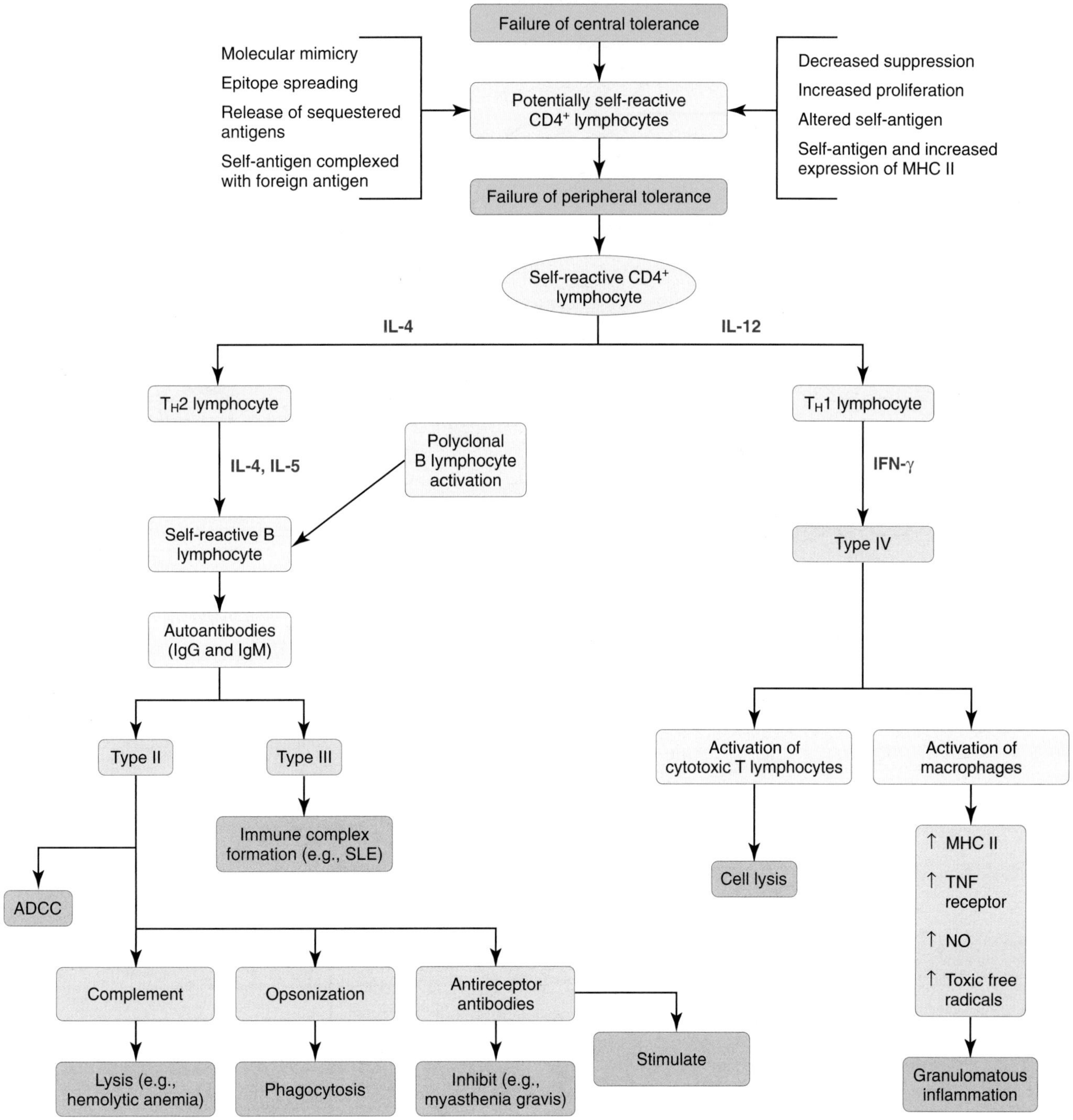

Figure 5-26 Autoimmunity. Pathogenetic mechanisms of autoimmunity mediated by activation of T lymphocytes ($CD4^+$). *ADCC*, Antibody-dependent cellular cytotoxicity; *IFN-γ*, interferon-γ; *Ig*, immunoglobulin; *IL*, interleukin; *MHC*, major histocompatibility complex; *NO*, nitric oxide; *SLE*, systemic lupus erythematosus; T_H, T helper lymphocyte; *TNF*, tumor necrosis factor.

antigen-presenting cells that are expressing self-molecules. This mechanism is not specific to the antigens of the infectious agent and is likely the result of the overall inflammatory response to the pathogen. Additionally, during an inflammatory response, some cells are induced by the inflammatory cytokine IFN-γ to increase their expression of MHC molecules. This can result in the expression of MHC molecules by cells that normally do not express them. Although the expression of MHC molecules in the absence of costimulatory molecules will not activate T lymphocytes, it does increase the potential to do so if costimulatory molecules are inappropriately expressed. The second mechanism is specific to the antigens of the infectious agent and is the result of cross-reactivity of T lymphocytes with an infectious agent's antigen and a self-antigen. Many infectious agents express antigens that have similar peptide sequences to those of normal peptides as a part of their immune evasion mechanism. Therefore the potential exists for any immune response to an infectious agent to cross-react with a normal peptide, resulting in an immune response directed against self-cells or self-tissues. This mechanism is called *molecular mimicry*. The result is the activation of T lymphocytes that recognize the infectious agent peptide–MHC complex. These T lymphocytes can potentially attack self-peptide–MHC complexes that are cross-reactive.

Once an autoimmune disease is initiated, the clinical course is generally progressive and characterized by cyclical periods of

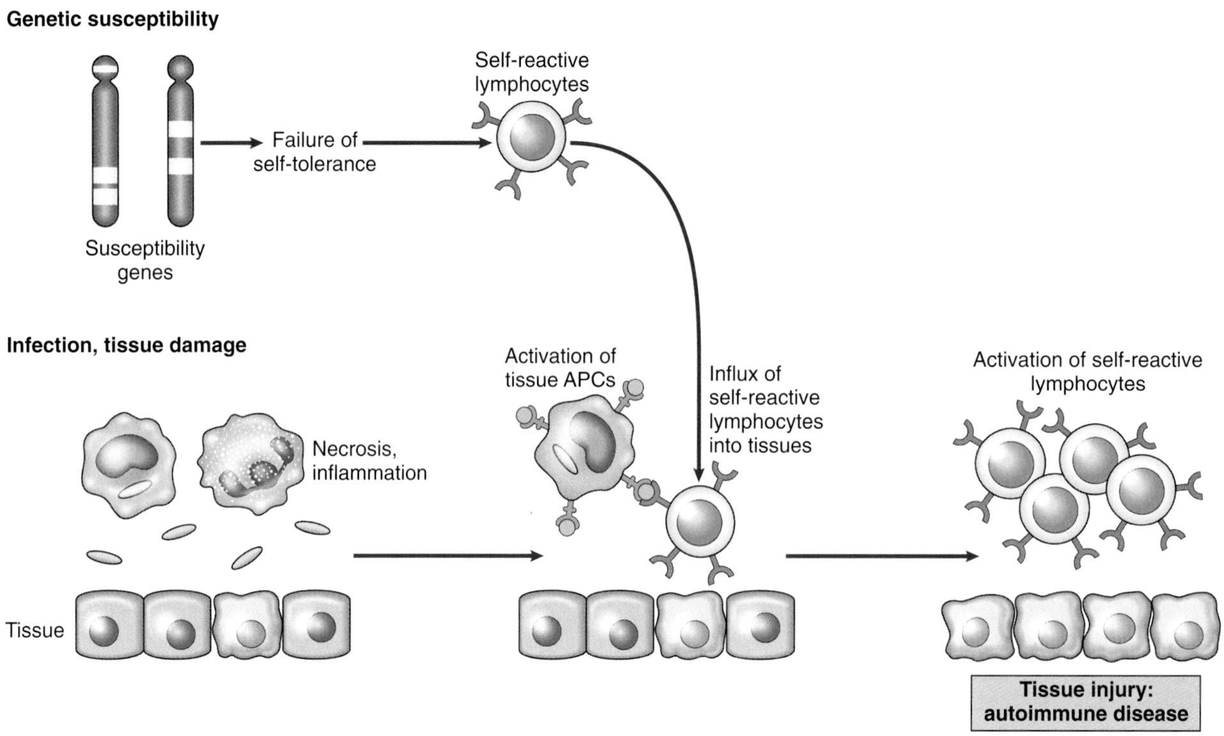

Figure 5-27 **Pathogenesis of Autoimmunity.** Autoimmunity is a multifactorial disease that involves genetic (tolerance) and environmental (e.g., infection) factors that results in the activation of self-reactive lymphocytes, leading to tissue damage. *APC*, Antigen-presenting cell.

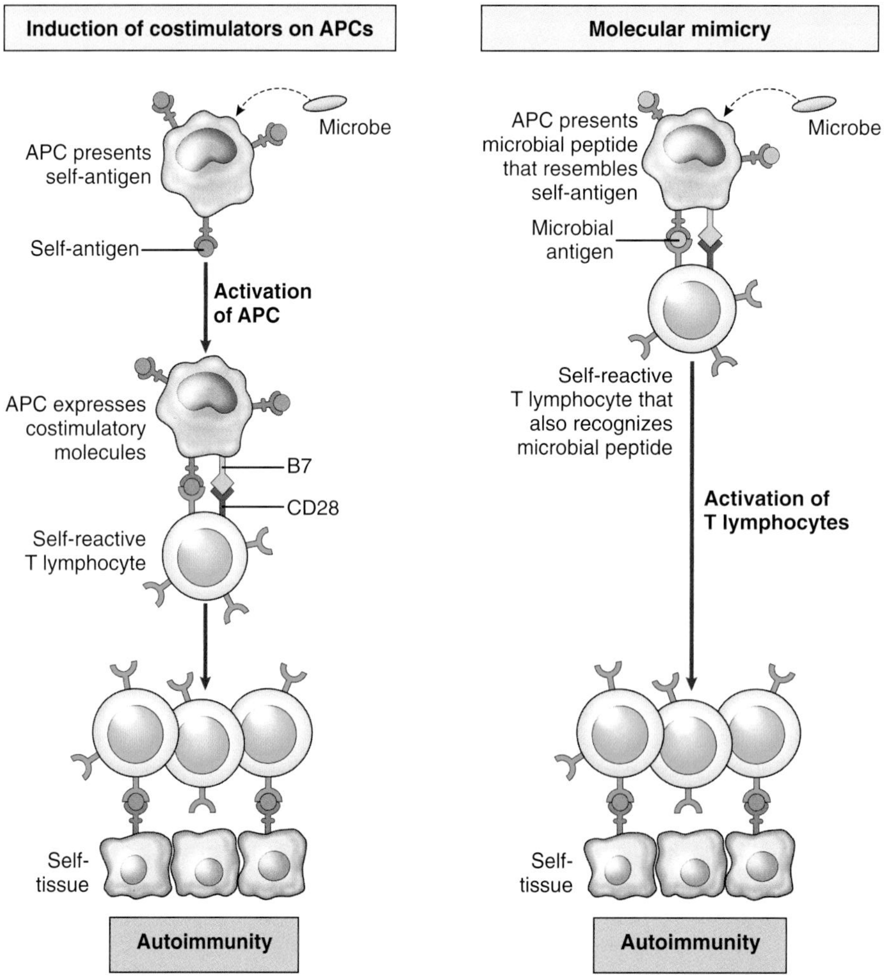

Figure 5-28 **The Potential Role of Microbial Infections in the Pathogenesis of Autoimmunity.** Microbes can lead to autoimmunity by inappropriately activating self-reactive lymphocytes or by activating lymphocytes that cannot distinguish between microbial peptides and self-peptides (molecular mimicry). *APC*, Antigen-presenting cell.

exacerbation and remission. As with any immune-mediated disease, antigen persistence is required to maintain the functional immune response. In autoimmune diseases, antigen persistence is thought in part to occur through epitope spreading. Epitope spreading is the process by which the immune response spreads from one epitope of an antigenic molecule to another, non–cross-reacting, epitope of the same antigenic molecule, or from one epitope of different peptides that are a part of a large complex. The epitopes involved are frequently ones that the immune response has not developed tolerance against because they are not normally presented by MHC molecules in sufficient concentrations. These so-called cryptic epitopes are normally not expressed at sufficient concentrations or are "hidden" during differentiation and development of lymphocytes. However, during an infection or inflammatory response, there may be tissue or cell damage that results in the release or expression of cryptic or hidden epitopes of self-antigens, and these become targets for the immune response. Because these epitopes were hidden, the immune system has not developed tolerance to them. Epitope spreading is thought to maintain the initiated immune response by means of the continued recruitment of autoreactive T lymphocytes specific for normal "cryptic" self-peptides.

With this basic understanding of self-tolerance and the possible molecular mechanisms involved in the pathogenesis of autoimmunity, we can present some of the more common autoimmune diseases of domestic species. Autoimmune diseases can be organ specific or systemic. With many of the organ-specific diseases, an immunologically mediated pathogenesis is suspected because of the finding of a lymphocytic inflammatory reaction within the affected tissue. Rarely, autoantibodies may be identified in the circulation. The organ-specific autoimmune diseases are discussed in the appropriate chapters covering individual organ systems. This chapter focuses on some of the systemic autoimmune diseases of domestic species, beginning with the multisystemic disease systemic lupus erythematosus.

Specific Autoimmune Diseases

Systemic Lupus Erythematosus

Systemic lupus erythematosus is one of the most well-studied systemic autoimmune diseases in human beings and is characterized by the production of autoantibodies directed against a wide array of normal tissue and cellular components. The predominant autoantibody, commonly known as *antinuclear antibody* (ANA), is directed against nuclear antigens. The disease has been described in human beings, nonhuman primates, mice, horses, dogs, cats, snakes, and iguanas. As with many autoimmune diseases, systemic lupus erythematosus has a highly variable and often progressive clinical course characterized by a variety of clinical and immunologic abnormalities. Unlike human beings, in whom the disease predominantly affects women, there is no clear sex predilection in domestic species. There are certain breeds of dogs that have a higher incidence. The average age of diagnosis is approximately 5 years. Epidemiologic data on other species are limited.

Etiology and Pathogenesis. The cause of systemic lupus erythematosus remains undetermined, although the presence of autoantibodies directed against a number of tissues and cellular components suggests that the underlying immunologic abnormality is a failure to maintain self-tolerance. Antibodies against nuclear and cytoplasmic components, which are neither organ specific nor species specific, and those directed against cell surface antigens, particularly red blood cell antigens, are central to the pathogenesis of the disease. Detection of autoantibodies also facilitates the diagnosis and monitoring of human patients with systemic lupus erythematosus. The autoantibodies and self-antigens form immune complexes, which can be deposited in glomeruli (glomerulonephritis), blood vessels (vasculitis), skin (dermatitis), and joints (arthritis), resulting in the major clinical signs associated with the disease.

ANAs are found in a high percentage of patients with systemic lupus erythematosus. In human beings, antinuclear antibodies are grouped into four categories: (1) antibodies against DNA, (2) antibodies against histones, (3) antibodies to nonhistone proteins bound to RNA, and (4) antibodies against nucleolar antigens. The most common method of measuring antinuclear antibodies is indirect immunofluorescence. The pattern of immunofluorescence is used to help identify the type of autoantibody present. Other methods can be used to more specifically identify the target of ANA. In human beings the majority of ANAs are directed against nucleic acids in native double-stranded DNA, in contrast to the dog, in which the majority of ANAs are directed against nuclear proteins such as histones and extractable nuclear antigens (ENAs). ANAs are also found in normal patients and in patients with other diseases; however, their frequency is much lower. In the dog the incidence of ANA in normal dogs and dogs with other canine diseases is 16% and 20%, respectively, compared with 97% to 100% in dogs with systemic lupus erythematosus. The indirect immunofluorescence test for ANA is sensitive but not specific because of the relatively high incidence in normal dogs and those with non–systemic lupus erythematosus diseases. Two anti-ENA antibodies appear to be specific for canine systemic lupus erythematosus. These are the anti-Sm and the anti-T1 antibodies.

Patients with systemic lupus erythematosus frequently have autoantibodies in an array of tissue and cells. Many patients have rheumatoid factors and thus have positive results for the Coombs test for anti-IgG antibodies. Antibodies directed against cellular antigens on red blood cells, platelets, and lymphocytes are frequently noted. In these instances they may lead to clinical signs of hemolytic anemia (anti–red blood cell antibodies), thrombocytopenia (antiplatelet antibodies), and immune system abnormalities (antilymphocyte antibodies). Other autoantibodies to components of muscle (myositis) and skin (dermatitis) are also frequently detected. Although there can be an extensive number of autoantibodies identified in patients with systemic lupus erythematosus, the major clinical signs are attributed to the deposition of immune complexes in the joint, skin, and kidney and the elaboration of a type III hypersensitivity reaction. The tissues most frequently involved are in the joint, skin, and kidney.

Canine lupus primarily affects middle-aged dogs, and in some studies has been reported to occur more frequently in males than females. Breeds overrepresented are the Shetland sheepdog, German shepherd, Old English sheepdog, Afghan hound, beagle, Irish setter, and poodle. Affected dogs usually present with a spectrum of clinical signs, and the disease has a progressive clinical course. Common clinical findings include fever, nonerosive polyarthritis, glomerulonephritis, mucocutaneous lesions, lymph node and splenic enlargement, and hematologic abnormalities (e.g., anemia, thrombocytopenia, and leukopenia). ANAs are the most common immunologic finding. In some reports, up to 100% of affected animals have been positive for ANAs. Dogs can also have antierythrocyte antibodies (Coombs' positive), anti-IgG antibodies (rheumatoid factor positive), and circulating immune complexes and deposits of these in the skin. Only the direct Coombs test is valid in the dog. In the dog, as in other species, the immunologic abnormalities involve both humoral and cellular immunity. The abnormalities in humoral immunity are largely attributed to the already discussed presence of autoantibodies and are centered on the activation of self-reactive B lymphocytes. The abnormalities in cellular immunity include a lymphopenia that is characterized by a decrease in the percentage and absolute number of $CD8^+$ lymphocytes and a concurrent increase in the percentage and a decrease in the absolute number of $CD4^+$ lymphocytes. This translates into a high $CD4^+$ to $CD8^+$ ratio (as high as 6:1 in dogs with systemic lupus erythematosus versus <2:1 in normal dogs).

Lesions of Systemic Lupus Erythematosus. A wide spectrum of morphologic lesions is associated with canine systemic lupus erythematosus. The most common finding, polyarthritis, is characterized as a nonerosive lesion that commonly affects the intervertebral, carpal, tarsal, and temporomandibular joints. The acute arthritis is characterized by exudation of neutrophils and fibrin into the synovial membrane and concurrent perivascular cuffing by mononuclear cells. The primary differential diagnosis for the arthritis is rheumatoid arthritis, which is an erosive lesion. The renal lesion, the result of immune complex deposition, involves the glomerulus, blood vessels, and the basement membranes of renal tubules (E-Fig. 5-7). The resulting glomerulonephritis is variable in appearance and ranges from slight mesangial alterations to diffuse proliferative lesions. The renal lesions have a common pathogenic mechanism that is a result of the deposition of immune complexes and the activation of complement (type III hypersensitivity). Glomerular lesions are often indicated by a persistent proteinuria (>0.5 g/dL).

Skin lesions are highly variable and nonspecific in canine systemic lupus erythematosus. The face, ears, and digital extremities are frequently involved and characterized by erythema, ulceration, and exfoliative dermatitis. The distribution of the lesions suggests that photosensitization may play a role. Histologically, the epidermis is characterized by basal cell vacuolation and necrosis, and the dermis is variably edematous with a superficial infiltration of mononuclear inflammatory cells at the dermal-epidermal junction (interface dermatitis). Additionally, there may be a panniculitis, composed primarily of lymphocytes and plasma cells, and vasculitis, with fibrinoid necrosis of the vessel wall. By indirect immunofluorescence there are deposits of immunoglobulin and complement components at the dermal-epidermal junction. Other dermatologic variants of lupus are covered in Chapter 17. The definitive diagnosis of systemic lupus erythematosus is based on accepted criteria rather than pathognomonic findings. Using 11 established criteria for the dog, modified from the American Rheumatism Association criteria for human beings, a definitive diagnosis requires the presence of four or more criteria. A "probable" diagnosis is based on the presence of three criteria or the presence of polyarthritis with the identification of ANAs. Other diagnostic schemes, using "major" and "minor" signs along with positive ANA or systemic lupus erythematosus prep test results, are also used to make definitive and probable diagnoses.

In the cat, systemic lupus erythematosus is less well recognized and manifests with fever, glomerulonephritis, dermatitis, and hemolytic anemia. The ANA test in cats is less reliable because many normal cats can have positive test results. Horses with systemic lupus erythematosus similarly present with generalized skin disease and may also have glomerulonephritis, arthritis, and hemolytic anemia.

Genetic Factors. Systemic lupus erythematosus in human beings is characterized as a disease with a complex genetic component with MHC and multiple non-MHC genes involved. Extensive genetic studies in domestic animals are lacking, yet it is reasonable to suggest that the disease in other species is also characterized by involvement of multiple genes. The association of systemic lupus erythematosus with certain MHC alleles in human beings indicates that the MHC genes that regulate the production of specific antibodies are involved—specifically, MHC alleles that are linked to the production of anti–double-stranded DNA, anti-Sm, and antiphospholipid antibodies. Other than the observation of breed predilections for the dog and cat and the report of an association with the canine MHC allele DLA-A7, there are no definitive genetic studies similar to those reported in human beings. Interestingly, a low percentage of human beings with systemic lupus erythematosus also have inherited deficiencies of complement components such as C2, C4, or C1q. Because complement components are important in the removal of circulating immune complexes by the monocyte-macrophage system, such a deficiency may contribute to the deposition of circulating complexes into tissue rather than to their removal. There is an increase in lupus-like autoimmunity in mice lacking certain complement components. Finally, a well-described animal model of systemic lupus erythematosus is the NZB ∞ NZW mouse strain, in which a number of genetic loci have been identified as being associated with the development of the disease.

Environmental Factors. In addition to the genetic factors, systemic lupus erythematosus in human beings has also been associated with a number of environmental factors. Specifically, drugs such as hydralazine, procainamide, and D-penicillamine can induce a systemic lupus erythematosus–like disease. In domestic animals, exposure to specific drugs and viral infections is suspected. Exposure to ultraviolet (UV) light is known to exacerbate the disease in the dog. These patients present with dermatologic manifestations localized to areas exposed to sunlight (e.g., face and dorsal regions) or areas lacking adequate hair coat (e.g., axillary region). A similar association has been noted in human beings with systemic lupus erythematosus. The influence of UV radiation may be attributed to tissue damage and inflammation that result in activation of keratinocytes and the elaboration of IL-1, or the modification of DNA through the induction of apoptosis that renders the DNA immunogenic. The influence of sex hormones on the occurrence and manifestations of systemic lupus erythematosus in human beings has not been documented in domestic species.

Immunologic Factors. As discussed previously, systemic lupus erythematosus is characterized by a number of immunologic abnormalities and is clinically noted to have manifestations attributable to specific immune components. It is therefore reasonable to suggest that the pathogenesis of systemic lupus erythematosus involves aberrations of humoral and/or cell-mediated immunity. Previously, as a result of the documentation of autoantibodies in patients with systemic lupus erythematosus, it was hypothesized that the pathogenesis centered on an intrinsic B lymphocyte defect. Additionally, polyclonal B lymphocyte activation is a common immunologic abnormality seen in patients with systemic lupus erythematosus and in animals that are models for the disease. Recent studies, however, indicate that the autoantibodies associated with the development of clinical systemic lupus erythematosus are not the result of polyclonal B lymphocyte activation but rather the result of antigen-specific T_H lymphocyte–dependent B lymphocyte responses. This observation is consistent with our overall understanding of autoimmunity, and the current hypothesis is that these diseases are more likely to be the result of an immunologic dysregulation centered on T_H lymphocytes. The currently proposed model for the pathogenesis of systemic lupus erythematosus is presented in Fig. 5-29. This model is an oversimplification of a complex disease with genetic and nongenetic factors that contribute to the development of a complex multisystemic disease with numerous clinical presentations, a progressive disease course, and an absence of specific cause.

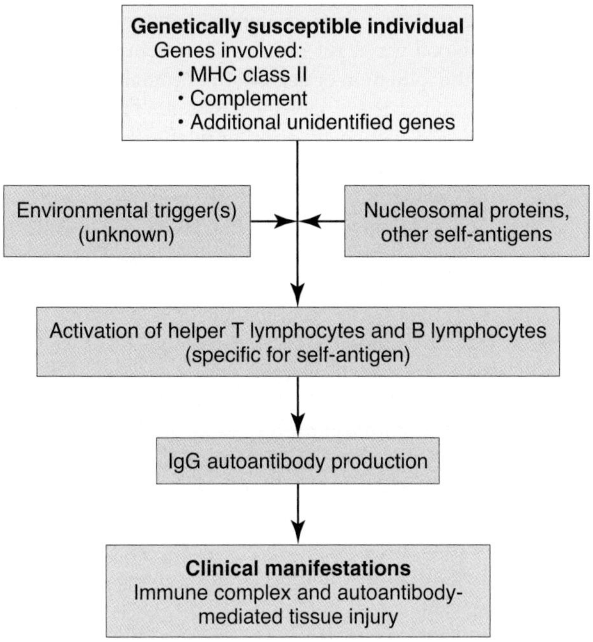

Figure 5-29 Systemic Lupus Erythematosus. Proposed model for the pathogenesis of systemic lupus erythematosus. *IgG*, Immunoglobulin G; *MHC*, major histocompatibility complex. (Modified from Kotzin BL: *Cell* 65:303-306, 1996.)

Although the underlying cause of autoantibody production in systemic lupus erythematosus remains unknown, the elaboration of antibody-peptide complexes is central to the mechanism of tissue damage. The majority of lesions in systemic lupus erythematosus are the result of immune complex disease (type III hypersensitivity). Antibodies directed against cell surface antigens also lead to the destruction of leukocytes, red blood cells, and platelets through direct cell lysis and enhanced removal by opsonization and phagocytosis. ANAs bind to cell-free nuclei to produce characteristic hematoxylin bodies or lupus erythematosus (LE) bodies. These bodies are frequently found in the skin, kidney, lung, lymph node, spleen, and heart of patients with systemic lupus erythematosus. These ANAs can also lead to the formation of LE cells, which are typically present in the bone marrow and are a phagocytic cell (macrophage or neutrophil) that has engulfed an opsonized nucleus. This phenomenon is also used as an in vitro diagnostic test to demonstrate the presence of ANA (LE test or LE prep).

In summary, systemic lupus erythematosus represents the prototypical multiorgan autoimmune disease with a highly variable clinical presentation, a complex cause, and pathogenesis involving multiple genetic and environmental factors and a multitude of immunologic abnormalities. The current pathogenesis suggests that these factors contribute to the activation of T and B lymphocytes, resulting in the production of autoantibodies directed against a number of self-constituents, namely molecules within the nucleus, in the cytoplasm, or on the cell surface.

Rheumatoid Arthritis

Rheumatoid arthritis is an autoimmune disease characterized by the presence of rheumatoid factors (anti-IgG antibodies) and is recognized in most species. The disease is discussed in Chapter 16.

Sjögren-Like Syndrome

Sjögren-like syndrome is a systemic autoimmune disease characterized by keratoconjunctivitis sicca, xerostomia, and lymphoplasmacytic adenitis. In human beings, Sjögren syndrome can manifest itself alone or in association with other autoimmune or immune-mediated diseases, such as rheumatoid arthritis, pemphigus, systemic lupus erythematosus, polymyositis, and immune-mediated thyroiditis. A Sjögren-like syndrome has been described in the dog and cat.

Etiology and Pathogenesis. The keratoconjunctivitis sicca (dry eyes) and xerostomia (dry mouth) result from the lymphocytic infiltration and fibrosis of lacrimal and salivary glands (lymphoplasmacytic sialoadenitis). In human beings the infiltrate is primarily composed of activated $CD4^+$ lymphocytes and fewer B lymphocytes and plasma cells. Affected dogs are frequently hypergammaglobulinemic and less frequently have identifiable ANAs and rheumatoid factors. Many human patients have ANAs, rheumatoid factors, and non–organ-specific autoantibodies. Two autoantibodies specific to Sjögren syndrome in human beings are directed against ribonucleoproteins, SS-A (Ro) and SS-B (La), which are considered serologic markers of the disease. Although autoantibodies can be identified, there is no direct evidence that they are the primary cause of tissue injury in any species evaluated to date. With the identification of autoantibodies and the presence of T lymphocytes within affected tissues, it is likely that the disease is the result of immunologic dysregulation centered on helper T lymphocytes. Sjögren syndrome in human beings also is weakly correlated with certain MHC alleles, suggesting that as in systemic lupus erythematosus, the presence of certain MHC alleles may predispose a patient to the development of the disease.

As with many autoimmune diseases, viruses are suspected as potential causal agents. In most species in which viruses have been implicated, the evidence is largely circumstantial and Koch's postulates have rarely been satisfied. The mechanisms by which infectious agents can induce autoimmunity were discussed earlier.

Clinical Signs and Lesions. Dogs with Sjögren-like syndrome have an adult onset of conjunctivitis and keratitis. Other findings include gingivitis and stomatitis. A case reported in the cat was characterized by dry eyes and enlarged salivary glands. The keratoconjunctivitis frequently leads to blepharospasm and conjunctival hyperemia. The xerostomia leads to dysphagia. Involvement of tissues other than salivary and lacrimal glands, as is reported in approximately one-third of human cases, has not been documented in the dog and cat. Human patients have lymph node involvement that is characterized as a pleomorphic infiltrate with increased mitoses and are at a fortyfold increased risk for developing lymphoid malignancies. Microscopically the salivary and lacrimal glands are infiltrated predominantly by lymphocytes (Fig. 5-30). In the cat, immunohistochemical analysis of lesions in these glands indicated that the predominant cell type was positive for CD79 (B lymphocyte marker) with fewer, scattered $CD3^+$ lymphocytes (T lymphocyte marker) and plasma cells. A mild interstitial fibrosis was also noted.

Inflammatory Myopathies

Inflammatory myopathies in domestic species constitute an uncommon, heterogeneous group of disorders that are characterized by skeletal muscle damage and inflammation. An immune-mediated pathogen is suspected. Four distinct disorders—masticatory muscle myositis, generalized inflammatory myositis, dermatomyositis, and extraocular myositis—are included in this category. They may occur alone or in association with other immune-mediated or autoimmune diseases. Of these diseases, only dermatomyositis is covered here; the remaining diseases are covered in Chapter 15.

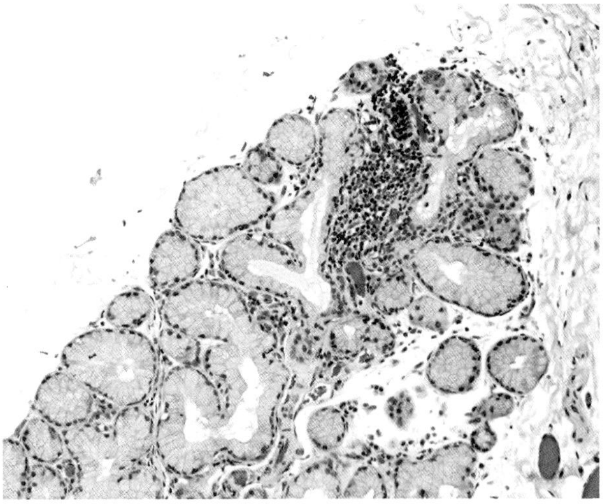

Figure 5-30 **Lymphoplasmacytic Sialoadenitis, Sjögren Syndrome, Salivary Gland, Cat.** Note the focus of lymphocytes and macrophages around a group of salivary acini. H&E stain. (Courtesy Dr. P.W. Snyder, School of Veterinary Medicine, Purdue University.)

Dermatomyositis. Dermatomyositis is an inflammatory disease of the skin, muscles, and vasculature affecting primarily young dogs. The cause and pathogenesis are unknown. The disease has a higher incidence in the collie and Shetland sheepdog breeds, and in these breeds it is often referred to as *canine familial dermatomyositis*, an inheritable inflammatory disease of the skin and muscle. The disease has also been diagnosed in a number of other breeds. A sex predilection has not been reported. The clinical and pathologic findings suggest that an immune-mediated or an autoimmune mechanism is involved in the pathogenesis.

Lesions. The dermatologic manifestations of the disease are variable but generally begin at an early age (between 2 and 6 months) and are characterized by alopecia and erythematous dermatitis that involve the face, ears, and bony prominences of the distal extremities. Erosions and ulcers are common early in the disease, and scarring and pigmentary changes are seen in chronic cases. Histopathologically, degeneration and necrosis of basal cells of the epidermis and follicular epithelium are characteristic. Frequently vacuolation of the basal epithelium leads to subepidermal cleft formation. Infiltration of the superficial dermis is often composed of lymphocytes, plasma cells, and macrophages with fewer mast cells and neutrophils. Follicular atrophy and secondary ulceration and fibrosis can also be noted. The skeletal muscle manifestations of the disease are a myositis composed of a variable infiltrate of primarily mononuclear inflammatory cells and occasional neutrophils. There are varying degrees of myofiber degeneration characterized by myofiber fragmentation, vacuolation, and hyalinization. In chronic cases there may be fibrosis and evidence of myofiber regeneration. The temporal and masseter muscles are commonly involved, although in severe cases there may be generalized muscle involvement. Involvement of the esophageal muscles can lead to the development of megaesophagus.

Vasculitis

Vasculitis is inflammation of the walls of blood vessels. It is most often seen as a component of an underlying systemic disease process (e.g., infectious or neoplastic) or as an adverse reaction to drug or vaccine administration. In these instances the pathogenesis involves a type III hypersensitivity reaction with the formation of immune complexes that are either formed in the vessel wall or formed in the circulation and lodge in the vessel wall. The inflammation of the blood vessel is not the result of an immunologic response to components of the blood vessel but rather an innocent bystander phenomenon with the formation or deposition of complexes in the wall and then activation of the complement system. The pathogenesis of a type III reaction was covered earlier in the chapter. An idiopathic febrile disease characterized by a systemic necrotizing vasculitis that occurs primarily in young (4 to 10 months of age) beagle dogs is suspected to be immune mediated, based on clinical signs, immunologic abnormalities, and pathologic findings. The syndrome has been designated as juvenile polyarteritis or beagle pain syndrome, and there appears to be a familial predisposition in some colonies. A similar syndrome has been reported in other breeds. Males and females are equally affected.

Clinical Signs and Immunologic Abnormalities. The classic presentation is a febrile (104° F to 107° F) young dog with anorexia, hunched stance, cervical pain, and an unwillingness to move the head and neck. The disease has a cyclic course, with two to seven periods of signs that resolve. They have a moderate to notable leukocytosis, with neutrophilia, nonregenerative anemia, and hypoalbuminemia. Cerebral spinal fluid analysis indicates a neutrophilic pleocytosis with mild to moderate increases in microprotein. On serum protein electrophoresis, they have a high α_2-globulin fraction. ANA tests, LE preparations, and rheumatoid factor tests are generally negative. Immunologic abnormalities include an increase in serum IgA concentration, an increase in the percentage of peripheral B lymphocytes, and a decrease in the percentage of total peripheral T lymphocytes, a marked suppression of the blastogenic response to mitogenic stimulation, an inability to generate immunoglobulin-secreting plasma cells after polyclonal activation, and evidence of monocyte-macrophage activation. There are increased concentrations of IL-6 in the serum of acutely affected dogs, and these return to baseline concentrations during periods of remission or after corticosteroid therapy.

Lesions. Severe necrotizing vasculitis and perivasculitis with thrombosis of small- to medium-sized blood vessels in the leptomeninges of the cervical spinal cord, cranial mediastinum, and heart are commonly seen (Fig. 5-31). In severe cases a more widespread distribution of vascular lesions occurs and commonly involves the thyroid gland, small intestine, testes, diaphragm, esophagus, and urinary bladder. Most patients experience multiple episodes, but some may have only one to two episodes before becoming normal,

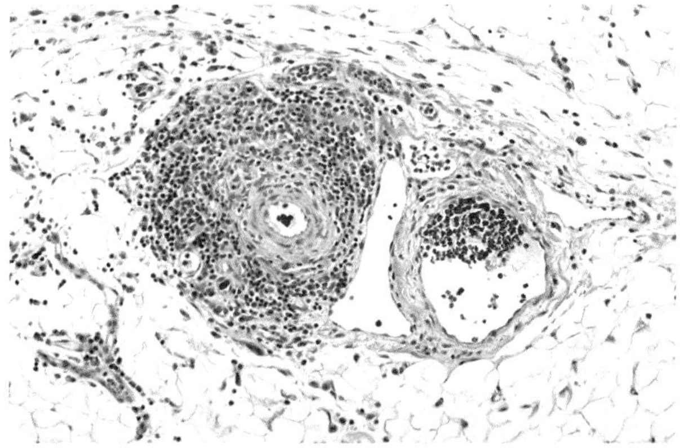

Figure 5-31 **Perivasculitis and Vasculitis, Polyarteritis, Beagle Dog.** Note the accumulation of lymphocytes and macrophages around the arteriole. H&E stain. (Courtesy Dr. P.W. Snyder, School of Veterinary Medicine, Purdue University.)

and clinical signs appear to resolve in all but the most severely affected patients by 12 to 18 months of age. Some dogs that experience repeated acute episodes develop splenic, hepatic, and renal amyloidosis. The pathogenesis of amyloidosis is attributed to serum amyloid A production and the development of reactive systemic amyloidosis secondary to the vascular inflammation.

Immunodeficiency Syndromes

Immunodeficiency diseases occur when there is a failure of the immune system to protect the host from infectious organisms or the development of cancer. An immunodeficiency syndrome that is the result of a congenital or genetic defect in a component of the immune system is called a primary immunodeficiency. Although the defect may be present at birth, the disease may not be manifested until later in life. An immunodeficiency syndrome that is an acquired loss of immune function as a complication of infections, malnutrition, or aging or a side effect of immunosuppression, irradiation, or chemotherapy for cancer or autoimmune disease is called a *secondary immunodeficiency*. It is important to differentiate between a primary and secondary state of immunodeficiency with respect to treatment and prognosis. In some instances it is useful to subclassify immunodeficiency diseases into those that affect adaptive (specific) or noninnate (nonspecific) immune responses. The study of immunodeficiency diseases has provided valuable insights and has enhanced our understanding of the complexities of the immune system. The ability to specifically identify the defective component provides great potential for the development of screening tests and of effective therapies. Naturally occurring and experimentally induced defects have made significant contributions to the field of immunology.

There are a greater number of well-characterized immunodeficiency diseases in human beings that likely have a domestic animal counterpart that have not yet been recognized. With the advent of new reagents and methodologies for characterizing cells and components of the immune system of domestic species, there should be a better chance of identifying immunodeficiency syndromes. Most primary immunodeficiency diseases are inherited, and the gene defect has been identified. There are additional forms of immunodeficiency that are the result of developmental defects that impair the function of an organ of the immune system. Finally, secondary immunodeficiency is a component of a large number of diseases of domestic species (ranging from malnutrition to viral infections that target lymphoid cells) and is beyond the scope of this chapter. This portion of the chapter covers some of the better characterized primary immunodeficiency diseases of domestic animals.

Primary Immunodeficiencies

Most primary immunodeficiency diseases are the result of a genetic defect (inherited or congenital) and affect specific (i.e., humoral and cell-mediated arms of the adaptive immune response) or nonspecific immunity (i.e., components of innate immune responses, such as complement, phagocytosis, NK cells, and so forth). Specific defects in adaptive immune responses can be divided into those affecting T lymphocytes or B lymphocytes or both (Fig. 5-32). As already discussed, interactions between B and T lymphocytes are necessary for the development of many immune responses. In some instances the clinical distinction between a primary B lymphocyte defect and a T lymphocyte defect may not be obvious with respect to humoral immunity. For example, T lymphocyte defects almost always result in impaired antibody synthesis and as such are indistinguishable from B lymphocyte defects or combined B lymphocyte and T lymphocyte defects. In general, most primary deficiencies manifest themselves early in life, and affected patients clinically have a failure to thrive and a susceptibility to recurrent infections. In many instances the type of infection suggests to some extent the likely component of the immune system that is defective (Table 5-8). It is beyond the scope of this chapter to present all of the forms of human and rodent immunodeficiency, and thus only a few are referenced for clarity to facilitate understanding diseases that have been characterized in domestic species.

Primary Immunodeficiencies of Specific Immunity

Severe Combined Immunodeficiency Disease. Severe combined immunodeficiency disease (SCID) is a family of genetic defects that have in common deficiencies in both humoral and cell-mediated immunity. In its extreme form, SCID results from a defect in the common lymphoid stem cell that results in defective cell-mediated and humoral immune responses. More commonly, SCID defects affect either T lymphocytes or B and T lymphocytes and are best characterized in human beings, mice, dogs, and horses. T lymphocyte defects often clinically have a combined immunodeficiency because there is a secondary impairment of humoral immunity that is the result of an inability of the T lymphocyte to provide the necessary signals for B lymphocyte activation. These defects result in an inability to generate a specific immune response and can have an autosomal recessive, X-linked, or sporadic inheritance pattern. The types of underlying defects are diverse and may involve enzyme systems or proteins necessary for lymphocyte development and differentiation, or signal transduction pathways involved in lymphocyte activation. Often the most common infectious manifestation of SCID is a viral or fungal infection. Immunity to viral and fungal infections is largely dependent on cell-mediated immunity. Immunity to most bacterial infections (especially extracellular bacteria) largely depends on humoral immunity, and neonates have adequate humoral immunity from the passive transfer of maternal antibodies that protect them.

SCID in horses is an autosomal recessive disorder described in the Arabian or Arabian-cross breed. The defect results in a severe lymphopenia (less than 1000/mm^3) attributed to an inability to produce functional T and B lymphocytes. At birth, before they acquire maternal antibodies via colostrum, affected animals are deficient in serum IgM, and after catabolism of passively transferred antibodies, they have agammaglobulinemia develop. Recurrent infections are typical, and death is commonly the result of infection with equine adenovirus, *Pneumocystis carinii*, *Cryptosporidium parvum*, or a variety of common equine bacterial pathogens. Grossly, the thymus is small and may be undetectable. Microscopically there is profound lymphoid hypoplasia of primary and secondary lymphoid tissue. Thymuses contain small lobules with no corticomedullary differentiation, few lymphocytes, Hassall's corpuscles, and occasional cysts. Spleens are characterized as having no lymphoid follicles, periarteriolar lymphoid sheaths, or plasma cells. Additionally, it has been noted that the lymphoid follicle sites in the spleen lack connective tissue stroma, and this characteristic can be used to differentiate hypoplasia from atrophy. Lymph nodes lack lymphoid follicles, plasma cells, and corticomedullary differentiation. The molecular basis for the defect has been identified as a spontaneous mutation in the gene encoding the catalytic subunit of a DNA-dependent protein kinase (DNA-PKcs) that is located on chromosome 9. Affected foals have a complete absence of functional DNA-PKcs. DNA-PK is required for the recombination of immunoglobulin heavy chain and TCR genes during development, which when defective results in an inability to form functional V regions. Interestingly, as a result of the DNA-PKcs mutation, affected horses also are defective in their DNA repair mechanisms. The importance of DNA repair mechanisms in preventing the development of

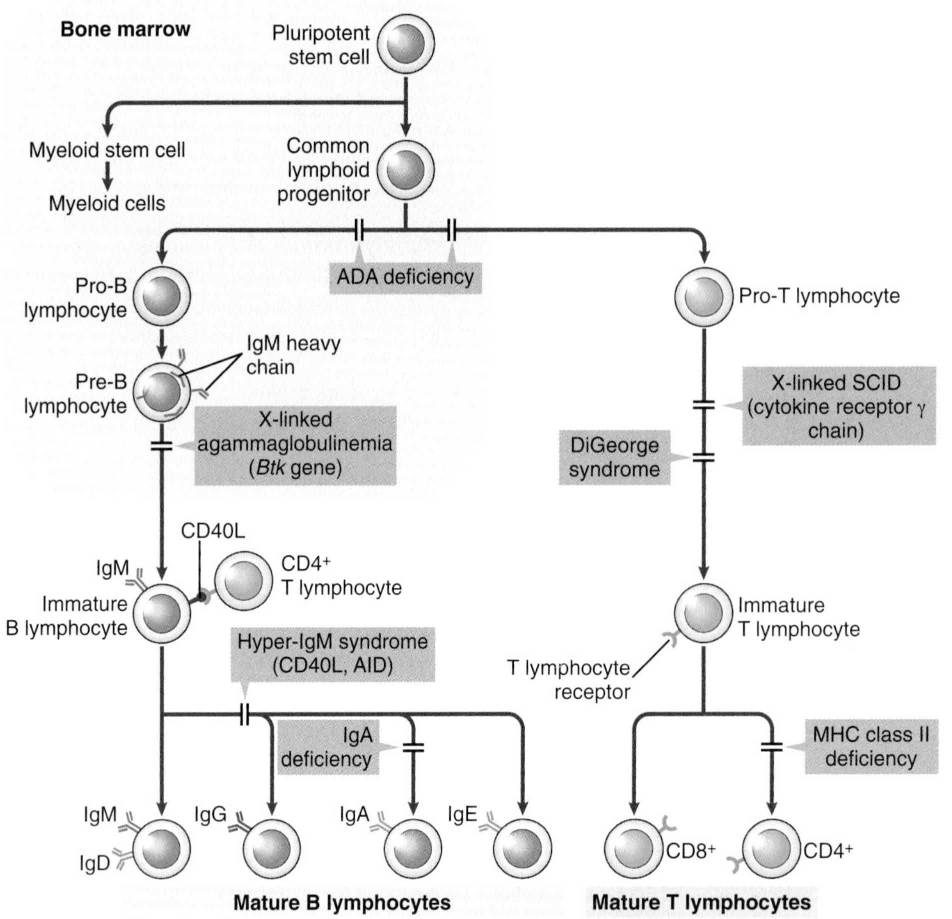

Figure 5-32 **Primary Immunodeficiency Diseases.** A simplified scheme of lymphocyte development and associated defects that result in primary immunodeficiency diseases. *ADA*, Adenosine deaminase; *AID*, activation-induced cytidine deaminase; *Ig*, immunoglobulin; *MHC*, major histocompatibility complex; *SCID*, severe combined immunodeficiency disease.

Table 5-8 Examples of Infections in Immunodeficiencies

Pathogen Type	T Lymphocyte Defect	B Lymphocyte Defect	Granulocyte Defect	Complement Defect
Bacteria	Bacterial sepsis	*Streptococcus* spp., *Staphylococcus* spp.	*Staphylococcus* spp., *Pseudomonas*	Pyogenic bacterial infections
Viruses	Cytomegalovirus, chronic infections with respiratory and intestinal viruses	Enteroviral encephalitis		
Fungi and parasites	*Candida*, *Pneumocystis carinii*	Intestinal giardiasis, aspergillosis	*Candida*, *Nocardia*, *Aspergillus*	
Special features	Aggressive disease with opportunistic pathogens, failure to clear infections, adverse reactions to attenuated vaccines	Chronic recurrent gastrointestinal infections, sepsis, meningitis	Neutrophilia	

cancer (see Chapters 1 and 6) would suggest that affected foals and heterozygous carriers would be at an increased risk for cancer. Although affected foals rarely live beyond 5 months of age, heterozygous carriers do, and they have been observed to be at a greater risk for developing sarcoids, a locally aggressive fibroblastic cutaneous neoplasm.

SCID in dogs was first described in basset hounds as an X-linked defect (XSCID) characterized by lymphopenia, with increased numbers of B lymphocytes and few to no T lymphocytes. The lymphopenia is not as profound as it is in foals with SCID. At approximately 6 to 8 weeks of age, as maternally derived antibody concentrations decline, they develop recurrent infections of the skin, respiratory, or gastrointestinal system. Phenotypically, there is a decrease in the number of circulating $CD8^+$ lymphocytes resulting in a $CD4^+$ to $CD8^+$ ratio of approximately 15 : 1 (compared with 2 : 1 in normal dogs) and normal percentages of B lymphocytes. Dogs with XSCID are hypogammaglobulinemic with normal serum IgM concentrations and decreased concentrations of IgG and IgA. Affected dogs rarely live past 4 months of age, and death is frequently attributed to septicemia or systemic viral infections. At

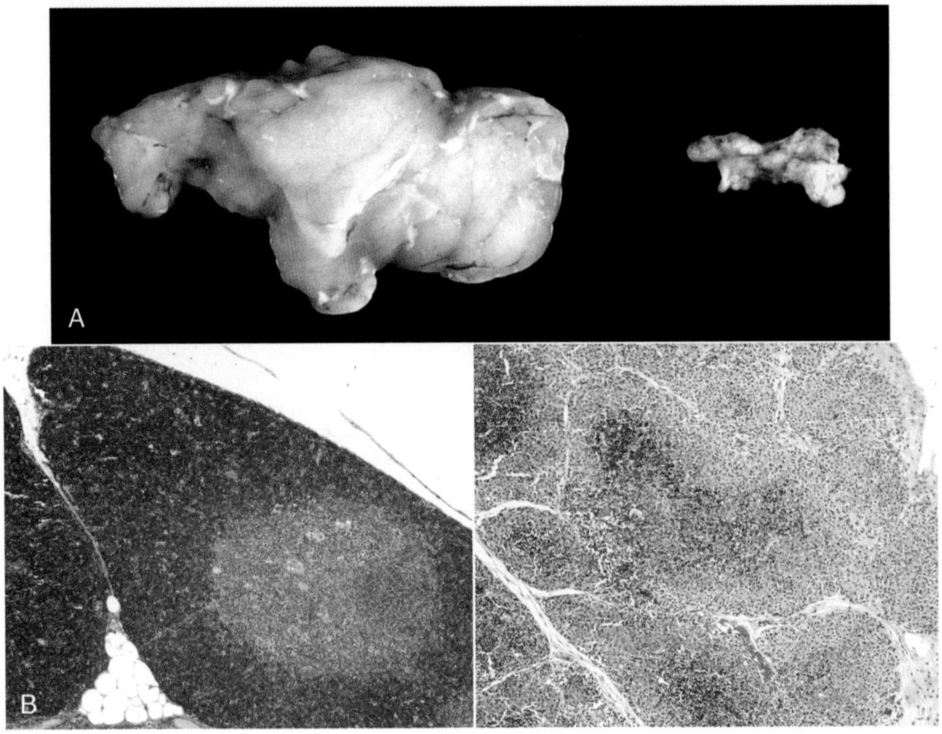

Figure 5-33 **X-linked Severe Combined Immunodeficiency Disease (XSCID) Thymuses, Normal Puppy and Littermate. A,** The gland from the normal puppy *(left)* weighed 7.4 g, and the gland from the XSCID puppy *(right)* weighed 0.2 g. **B,** Thymus from a normal neonatal dog *(left)* and from a neonatal dog with XSCID *(right)*. The normal thymic lobule has a pale medullary region and a dark cortical region that is densely packed with small lymphocytes. The XSCID thymus has small lobules with no corticomedullary distinction and a paucity of small lymphocytes. H&E stain. (**A** and **B** courtesy Dr. P.W. Snyder, School of Veterinary Medicine, Purdue University.)

necropsy, lymph nodes, tonsils, Peyer's patches, and the thymus are extremely small and may be undetectable.

Microscopically there is severe lymphoid hypoplasia with similar characteristic features as described previously for lymphoid tissues of the foal with SCID. Thymuses of affected puppies are small (approximately 10% the weight of age-matched controls) and are characterized by a lack of corticomedullary demarcation and small lobules with few to no lymphocytes (Fig. 5-33). Thymuses have markedly increased percentages of CD8/CD4 lymphocytes (46% versus 16% in age-matched controls), compatible with a block in T lymphocyte differentiation. Canine XSCID is due to a mutation in the common gamma (γ_c) subunit of the IL-2, IL-4, IL-7, IL-9, and IL-15 receptors. These receptors, for five immunologically different cytokines, belong to the type I cytokine receptor family. A four–base pair deletion results in a stop codon that prevents full translation of the γ_c messenger RNA (mRNA). T lymphocytes are nonfunctional because of an inability to express a functional IL-2 receptor. B lymphocytes are activated only by T lymphocyte–independent antigens, and although they are capable of synthesizing IgM, they are incapable of class-switching to IgG. A similar molecular form of XSCID has also been described in the Cardigan Welsh corgi breed. An insertional mutation, caused by the insertion of a cytosine in exon 4, also results in a stop codon preventing complete translation of γ_c mRNA. In human SCID, mutations of the γ_c are the most common molecular mechanism with numerous distinct point, insertion, and deletion mutations identified. An autosomal recessive form of SCID has been described in Jack Russell terriers that is the result of a mutation in DNA-PKcs similar to that described previously in the Arabian horse and the CB-17 mouse.

SCID in mice occurs in the CB-17 strain and is an autosomal recessive trait characterized by an absence of mature B and T lymphocytes. The molecular basis for the SCID phenotype is attributed to a defect resulting in decreased DNA-PK enzyme activity. Although mice are highly susceptible to opportunistic infections, they can be maintained in environments that minimize their exposure to pathogenic agents and kept alive for more than a year of age. An interesting, although poorly understood, immunologic finding in older (greater than 6 months of age) mice with SCID is the ability to produce small quantities of immunoglobulin and low numbers of mature T lymphocytes. This phenotype is referred to as *leaky SCID*. This leaky phenotype has not been described in other forms of SCID. As in other species with defective DNA repair mechanisms, there is an increased sensitivity to ionizing radiation damage.

Common Variable Immunodeficiency. Common variable immunodeficiency is a primary immunodeficiency disease characterized by an adult onset of hypogammaglobulinemia attributed to an intrinsic B lymphocyte defect, which results in an inability to produce much of the antibody. The disease has been described in a litter of miniature Dachshund dogs. The dogs were characterized as having an absence of B lymphocytes in lymphoid tissues and little to no serum immunoglobulins. At necropsy the affected animals had lesions characterized as atrophy of lymphoid tissue and pneumonia. Lymph nodes were further characterized as lacking lymphoid follicles. The pneumonia was caused by *P. carinii*, a common opportunistic pathogen in immunocompromised animals and human beings. In human beings there have been a number of identified defects intrinsic to B lymphocytes that prevent their terminal differentiation and affect their ability to produce immunoglobulin, thus the designation as variable immunodeficiency. A similar disease has also been described in a 12-year-old quarter horse, which was characterized by hypogammaglobulinemia and an absence of B lymphocytes in circulation, bone marrow, and spleen.

Agammaglobulinemia. Agammaglobulinemia is a primary immunodeficiency characterized by an inability to produce immunoglobulins and an absence of mature B lymphocytes and plasma cells. The disease has been described in thoroughbred, quarter horse, and standardbred breeds of horses. To date all cases have been males, suggesting that, as in the human disease, it is an X-linked trait. Microscopically there was an absence of plasma cells, primary follicles, and germinal centers in lymph nodes. Affected horses commonly have extracellular bacterial infections of the joints and respiratory system. In human beings there is a mutation of the *BTK* gene located on the X chromosome, which encodes a tyrosine kinase that results in an arrest of B lymphocyte development at the pre-B stage. The disease in human beings is referred to as X-linked agammaglobulinemia (XLA).

Selective Immunoglobulin Deficiencies. Selective deficiencies are represented by a number of diseases characterized by a deficiency of an individual class of immunoglobulin. Forms of these diseases have been identified and described in horses and dogs. The most common forms are selective IgM deficiency and selective IgA deficiency, characterized by a serum level of IgM or IgA, respectively, that is at least two standard deviations below normal. Serum concentrations of other classes of immunoglobulin are normal, and B lymphocyte numbers are normal. These deficiencies may not result in clinical signs until there is degradation of passively transferred maternal antibody. In horses there are distinct forms of selective IgM deficiency with most affected animals succumbing to septicemia or pneumonia by 10 months of age. A few affected foals live beyond 10 months and commonly die of recurrent respiratory infections before reaching adulthood. Some horses reach adulthood before they show clinical signs of selective IgM deficiency. Selective IgA deficiency has been described in a number of breeds of dogs, including the German shepherd, Shar-Pei, Irish setter, and beagle. Because of the importance of IgA in mucosal immunity, many affected animals have respiratory, gastrointestinal, and skin infections. Some affected dogs, like human patients with IgA deficiency, have a predisposition to developing atopic disease. In most instances there are normal numbers of IgA-producing plasma cells, suggesting an inability to synthesize or secrete IgA. Although the molecular basis for selective immunoglobulin deficiencies is unknown, they are thought to relate to the differentiation of naïve B lymphocytes into immunoglobulin-secreting plasma cells.

Thymic Hypoplasia. Thymic hypoplasia represents a number of immunodeficiency diseases characterized by a failure to develop a functional thymus, resulting in a T lymphocyte deficiency. Mice homozygous for the genetic trait nu (nu/nu) are hairless, and this athymic strain is commonly referred to as the nude mouse. Affected mice have a developmental arrest of the thymus, which occurs around day 12 of gestation and results in an absence of a functional thymus. Nude mice have defective cell-mediated immune responses and are unable to develop antibody responses. The immunologic abnormalities are attributed to a deficiency of T lymphocyte responses. Heterozygous (nu/+) animals are normal. The few circulating T lymphocytes in affected mice have TCRs of the γ/δ-type rather than the α/β-type. Under conventional housing conditions, mortality is high during the first 2 weeks of life; however, when maintained in germ-free environments, they can survive longer. This strain of mice is an important animal model, because they can tolerate allografts and xenografts. Similar, although less well-characterized, hairless and athymic conditions have been described in other species. A condition in human beings characterized by thymic hypoplasia is referred to as *DiGeorge syndrome*. DiGeorge syndrome is a T lymphocyte deficiency resulting from an embryologic defect affecting the development of the third and fourth pharyngeal pouches. Affected human beings have thymic (fourth pharyngeal pouch) and parathyroid (third pharyngeal pouch) defects. They have decreased circulating T lymphocytes, and T lymphocyte areas of lymphoid tissues (paracortical areas of lymph nodes and periarteriolar sheaths of the spleen) are depleted of lymphocytes. There is an absence of cell-mediated immune responses. DiGeorge syndrome is not familial but rather the result of the deletion of a specific gene that is a member of the T-box family of transcription factors. Specifically how or why this transcription factor influences the development of the thymus and parathyroid is unknown.

Primary Immunodeficiencies of Nonspecific Immunity

Deficiencies of the Complement System. The complement system contains more than 30 soluble and cell-bound proteins that influence immune and inflammatory responses. The pathways of complement activation, regulation of the complement system, and biologic consequences of complement activation have been previously covered in Chapter 3. In human beings, inherited deficiencies have been described for nearly all components and two of the inhibitors. Although a deficiency of C2 is the most common, human beings with deficiencies in components of the classical pathway have little to no increased risk for infections, suggesting that the alternative and lectin pathways of activation are sufficient for controlling infections. Deficiencies of the classical pathway components are associated with an increased incidence of systemic lupus erythematosus–like autoimmune disease, which has been attributed to impaired clearance of immune complexes by the monocyte-macrophage system. Although deficiencies of components of the alternative pathway (properdin and factors D and H) are rare, when they do occur they are associated with recurrent pyogenic infections. A deficiency of C3, which is required for all three pathways of complement, is the most serious deficiency and results in serious recurrent infections. An autosomal recessive trait resulting in a genetically determined deficiency of C3 has been described in the Brittany spaniel dog. Homozygous dogs have serum concentrations of C3 and also opsonic and chemotactic activities that are severely decreased compared with normal dogs. Affected dogs are predisposed to recurrent infections and type 1 membranoproliferative glomerulonephritis. Bacterial infections with *Clostridium* spp., *Escherichia coli*, and *Klebsiella* spp. resulting in pneumonia, septicemia, and pyometra, respectively, are the most common clinical manifestations.

The molecular basis for the deficiency has been identified as a deletion mutation that results in a premature stop codon, preventing adequate translation and resulting in decreased concentrations of mRNA. Heterozygous dogs have serum concentrations of C3 that are approximately 50% of normal, but these dogs are clinically normal. C3 deficiency has also been described in guinea pigs and rabbits.

An autosomal recessive trait resulting in a deficiency of factor H, a component of the alternative pathway of complement, has been described in the Norwegian Yorkshire breed of pig. Factor H is a regulator of complement activation that blocks the formation of C3 convertase and is a cofactor for cleavage of C3b by factor I. Deficiencies of factor H result in unregulated elaboration of C3b on activation of the alternative pathway. The most common clinical manifestation is renal disease. Affected pigs develop a type

II membranoproliferative glomerulonephritis characterized by glomerular changes consisting of thickened capillary walls, proliferation of mesangial cells, dense intramembranous deposits, and glomerular deposits of C3 components. The disease is commonly referred to as *porcine dense deposit disease*.

The molecular basis for the decreased serum concentrations of factor H has been reported to be the result of nucleotide sequence alterations in the factor H gene that cause a block in protein secretion. Hepatocytes of affected animals have increased intracellular concentrations of factor H. Hereditary factor H deficiency in human beings can be characterized by a variety of clinical manifestations ranging from recurrent bacterial infections to glomerular disease to hemolytic uremic syndrome. Deficiencies of the terminal components (C5, C6, C7, C8, and C9), which are required for the formation of the membrane attack complex and the lysis of cell membranes, do occur and generally result in increased bacterial infections.

Deficiencies of C1 inhibitor and other complement regulatory proteins, although described in human beings, have yet to be described in domestic animals. C1 inhibitor deficiency is an autosomal dominant trait that causes hereditary angioedema. C1 inhibitor is a protease inhibitor that targets C1r and C1s enzymes of the classical pathway of complement, Hageman factor (factor XII) of the coagulation pathway, and the kallikrein system. As indicated in Chapter 3, these three pathways are closely linked and result in the elaboration of vasoactive amines, notably bradykinin. Affected human patients develop episodes of edema involving the skin and mucosal membranes such as those of the larynx and gastrointestinal system. Deficiencies of membrane-bound regulator proteins, such as decay-accelerating factor and homologous restriction factor, result in paroxysmal nocturnal hemoglobinuria. In the absence of these regulatory factors, red blood cells can be more easily lysed by concentrations of complement that are much lower than normally required. The increased lysis of red blood cells causes chronic hemolytic anemia and hemoglobinuria.

Chédiak-Higashi Syndrome. Chédiak-Higashi syndrome is an inherited disease caused by defective lysosomes, melanosomes, platelet-dense granules, and cytolytic granules. The disease has been described in cats, cattle, killer whales, beige mice, rats, Aleutian mink, and human beings. Common clinical manifestations of the disease may include hypopigmentation, a bleeding tendency, ocular abnormalities, and recurrent infections. Some species are more susceptible to recurrent infections than others. The hallmark of the disease is the presence of enlarged granules within melanocytes, neutrophils, eosinophils, and monocytes. The enlarged granules are melanosomes (melanocytes), lysosomes (many cell types), or cytoplasmic granules (e.g., fused primary and secondary granules of neutrophils). Neutrophils containing giant granules have impaired functions such as defective chemotaxis and intracellular killing. NK cells are also defective and may also contribute to the increased susceptibility to infections reported in some species. Mink with Chédiak-Higashi syndrome have an increased susceptibility to Aleutian mink disease virus. The hypopigmentation is the result of an inability of melanocytes, containing abnormally large melanosomes, to migrate and release their contents, resulting in a deficiency of pigment most commonly evident in the skin, hair, and eye. The bleeding tendency is a coagulopathy resulting from defective platelets. Platelet counts are generally normal. In most species studied, most recently cattle, there is insufficient platelet aggregation because of a decreased response to collagen. Research suggests that the GPIa/IIa ($\alpha_2\beta_1$-integrin) glycoprotein or rhodocytin pathway of platelet activation may be defective. Ocular abnormalities identified in cattle, cats, mink, mice, and human beings are similar and are characterized by abnormal ocular pigmentation and an associated photophobia. Cats with Chédiak-Higashi syndrome frequently develop cataracts. The molecular basis for Chédiak-Higashi syndrome has been identified in some human forms and in beige mice and cattle to be a result of a mutation of the *Lyst* gene. The *Lyst* gene encodes a membrane-associated protein that is thought to regulate intracellular protein trafficking. Exactly how the protein regulates intracellular trafficking remains unknown.

Leukocyte Adhesion Deficiency. Leukocyte adhesion deficiency (LAD) is a primary immunodeficiency disease characterized by the inability of leukocytes to migrate from circulation into sites of inflammation, resulting in recurrent bacterial infections (see Chapter 3).

More information on this topic is available at www.expertconsult.com.

Amyloidosis

Although there is no evidence to suggest that amyloidosis is always the result of a primary immunologic abnormality, the pathogenesis of amyloidosis may involve components of the immune system. Primary amyloidosis is the most common systemic form of amyloidosis in human beings and is of the AL type (i.e., amyloid light chain [AL]), derived from immunoglobulin light chains of plasma cells. Many cases of AL amyloidosis are attributable to the presence of some type of immunocyte dyscrasia. The most common immunocyte dyscrasia associated with AL amyloidosis in domestic species is a neoplasm of plasma cells. Plasma cell–derived neoplasms include the extramedullary plasmacytoma and the myeloma or more common multiple myeloma that are most often limited to the bone marrow.

More information on this topic, including the classification, pathogenesis, and morphologic features of amyloidosis, is available at www.expertconsult.com.

Suggested Readings

Suggested Readings are available at www.expertconsult.com.

CHAPTER 6

Neoplasia and Tumor Biology[1]

Kimberly M. Newkirk, Erin M. Brannick, and Donna F. Kusewitt

Key Readings Index

Neoplasia is an important concern for veterinary practitioners, diagnosticians, and researchers. Tumor diagnosis and treatment for individual animals is becoming an increasingly prominent part of small animal practice. In farm animals, neoplasms caused by infectious or environmental agents can have a major impact on herd or flock health and result in economic losses due to carcass or organ condemnation. Furthermore, animal models of neoplasia provide important insights into the cause and treatment of cancer in human beings.

General Nomenclature

Neoplasia

Neoplasia is a process of "new growth" in which normal cells undergo irreversible genetic changes, which render them unresponsive to ordinary controls on growth exerted from within the "transformed" cell or by surrounding "normal" cells. With continued proliferation the cells expand beyond their normal anatomic boundaries, creating a macroscopically (grossly) or microscopically detectable *neoplasm*. Other common terms for neoplasms, such as *tumor* ("swelling") or *cancer* ("crab"), describe the clinical appearance or infiltrative behavior of these abnormal growths. In fact, *oncology*, the study of neoplasia, is derived from the Greek word *oncos* ("tumor"). Although the terms "neoplasm" and "tumor" may refer to either benign or malignant growths, the term "cancer" always denotes a malignant growth. It is important to note that a gross lesion described clinically as a "tumor" or "mass" may be a neoplasm or a nonneoplastic lesion like a granuloma.

Benign ("harmless") tumors do not invade surrounding tissue or spread to new anatomic locations within the body; thus these tumors are usually curable and are rarely responsible for death of the animal. *Malignant* ("harmful") tumors, if left untreated, invade locally, spread by *metastasis* ("change of place"), and ultimately kill the animal by interfering with critical body functions. Although nervous system tumors are often localized and very rarely metastasize, they may cause clinical signs and death by interrupting important neurologic pathways via compression of axons or critical clusters of neuron cell bodies (see Chapter 14).

Preneoplastic Changes

With the recognition that tumor development is a stepwise process, potentially preneoplastic changes, including hyperplasia, hypertrophy, metaplasia, and dysplasia, have assumed new diagnostic and clinical significance (Fig. 6-1). These preneoplastic changes often signal an increased risk or likelihood for progression to neoplasia in the affected tissue. *Hyperplasia* is an increase in the number of cells in a tissue through mitotic division of cells, in other words, through cellular proliferation. It must be distinguished from *hypertrophy*, which is an increase in individual cell size through the addition of cytoplasm (cytosol) and associated organelles. *Metaplasia*, the transformation of one differentiated cell type into another, is seen most commonly in epithelial tissues. For example, in several species of animals, vitamin A deficiency is characterized by transformation of columnar or cuboidal respiratory and digestive epithelium into squamous epithelium (squamous metaplasia). *Dysplasia* is an abnormal pattern of tissue growth and usually refers to disorderly arrangement of cells within the tissue.

In general, preneoplastic changes are reversible. They may arise in response to physiologic demands, injury, or irritation but often resolve with the removal of the inciting factor. For example, epidermal hyperplasia is a normal part of wound repair, and skeletal muscle

[1]For a glossary of abbreviations and terms used in this chapter see E-Glossary 6-1.

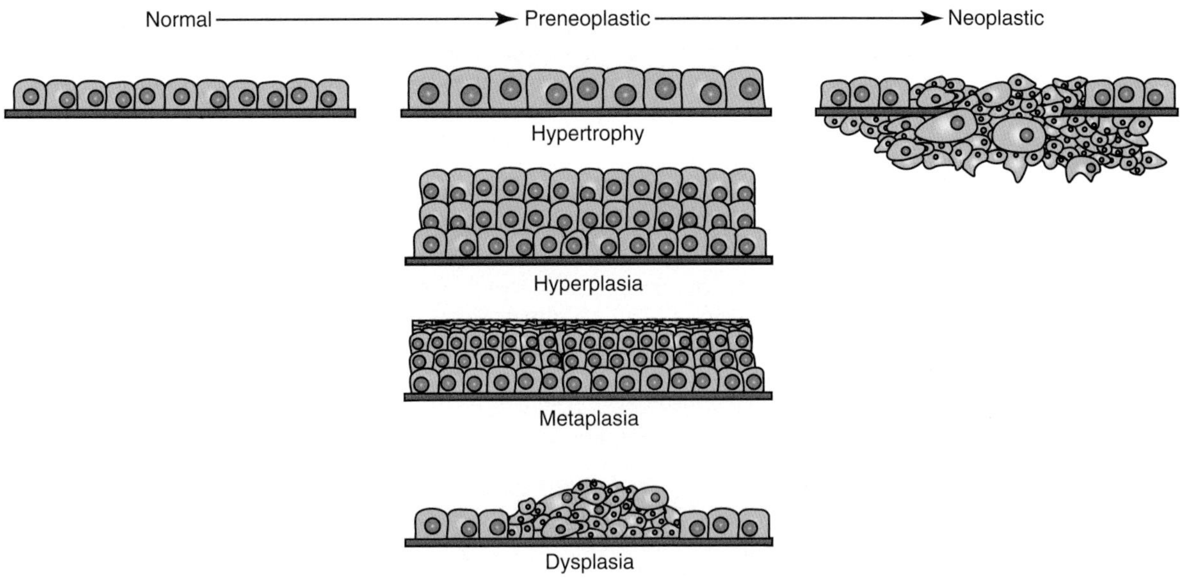

Figure 6-1 Preneoplastic Changes Preceding Tumor Emergence. Preneoplastic changes in tissues include alterations in cell size (hypertrophy), cell number (hyperplasia), and organization (metaplasia, dysplasia). In this example, preneoplastic changes are illustrated in simple cuboidal epithelium, although such changes may also be seen in other epithelial and mesenchymal tissue types. The metaplastic change shown is squamous metaplasia, that is, the conversion of simple cuboidal epithelium into stratified squamous epithelium. (Redrawn with permission from Dr. D.F. Kusewitt, Health Sciences Center, University of New Mexico.)

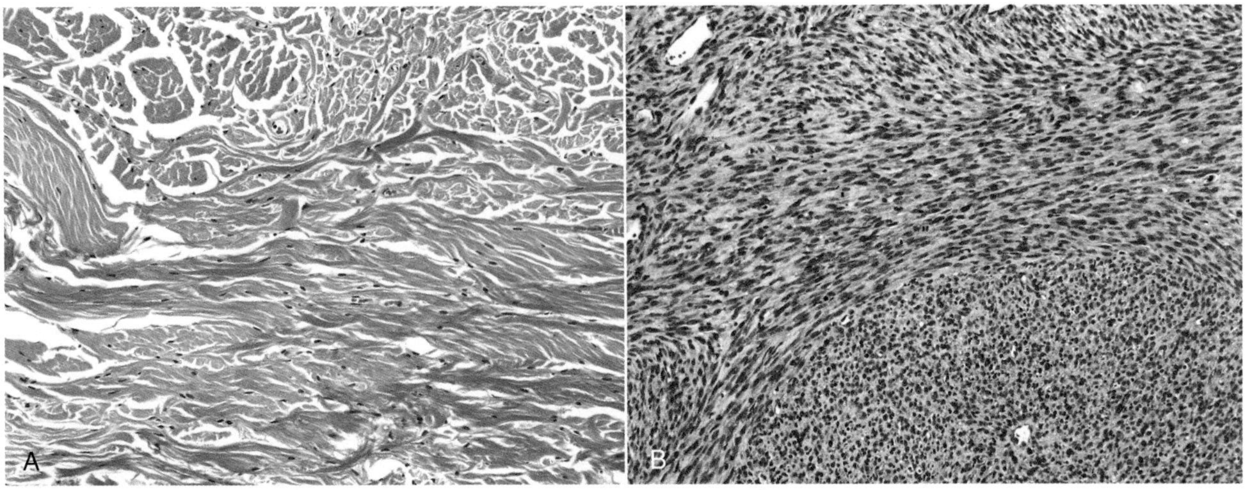

Figure 6-2 Comparison of Benign and Malignant Tumors of Fibroblast Origin. A, Fibroma, subcutis, dog. The benign fibroma is composed primarily of mature collagenous connective tissue with relatively few neoplastic fibroblasts that are indistinguishable from normal fibroblasts. H&E stain. **B,** Fibrosarcoma, subcutis, dog. The fibrosarcoma is composed of interlacing bundles of large fibroblasts with plump elongate nuclei and moderate amounts of eosinophilic cytoplasm; mature collagen is sparse to absent. H&E stain. (Courtesy College of Veterinary Medicine, University of Tennessee.)

hypertrophy is an adaptive response to increased workload. The terms "hyperplasia" and "hypertrophy" are not appropriate in descriptions of true neoplasms, but the terms "dysplasia" and "metaplasia" may describe changes that persist during the transition from preneoplasia to neoplasia. *Anaplasia* is the term used to describe loss of cellular differentiation and reversion to more primitive cellular morphologic features; anaplasia often indicates irreversible progression to neoplasia.

Tumor Types

Microscopically, most tumors consist of a single cell type, either mesenchymal or epithelial, and the name of the neoplasm reflects the cell type from which the tumor is thought to arise.

Mesenchymal Tumors

Mesenchymal tumors arise from cells of embryonic mesodermal origin. These tumors are generally composed of spindle cells arranged in streams and bundles. Benign tumors originating from mesenchymal cells are usually named by adding the suffix *-oma* to the name of the cell of origin. Thus a fibroma is a benign tumor of fibroblast origin (Fig. 6-2, *A*). A malignant tumor of mesenchymal origin is a *sarcoma* ("fleshy growth"). A prefix or modifier indicates the tissue of origin. For example, a fibrosarcoma is a tumor composed of malignant fibroblasts (see Fig. 6-2, *B*). The cells of the hematopoietic system are also mesenchymal; thus tumors arising from these cells are sarcomas. For instance, a malignant tumor of lymphocytes is called lymphosarcoma; by convention, lymphosarcoma is often shortened to lymphoma, but this term should not be mistaken for the name of a benign mesenchymal growth. These solid sarcomas of hematopoietic cell origin are composed of sheets of round cells (Fig. 6-3). Malignancies arising from circulating blood cells or their precursors are termed *leukemias* ("white blood") when characterized by large numbers of abnormal hematopoietic cells in the peripheral blood.

Epithelial Tumors

All three embryonic cell layers, endoderm, mesoderm, and ectoderm, can give rise to epithelial tissues and tumors derived from these tissues.

The terms *adenoma, papilloma,* and *polyp* refer to benign epithelial tumors. "Adenoma" denotes either a tumor arising from glandular epithelium like mammary epithelium or a tumor derived from nonglandular epithelial tissue that exhibits a tubular pattern microscopically, such as a renal tubular adenoma. The term "papilloma" refers to a benign, usually exophytic ("growing outward"), growth arising from a cutaneous or mucocutaneous surface, whereas a "polyp" is a grossly visible, benign epithelial tumor projecting from a mucosal surface (Fig. 6-4, *A*); however, the terms "polyp" and "papilloma" are sometimes used interchangeably.

All malignant tumors of epithelial origin are termed *carcinomas* ("cancers"). Tumors termed "carcinomas" may contain nests, cords, or islands of neoplastic epithelial cells, whereas the more specific term *adenocarcinoma* refers to carcinomas with a distinct glandular growth pattern, as indicated by the presence of tubules or acini (see Fig. 6-4, *B*). By definition, carcinomas are invasive and have the

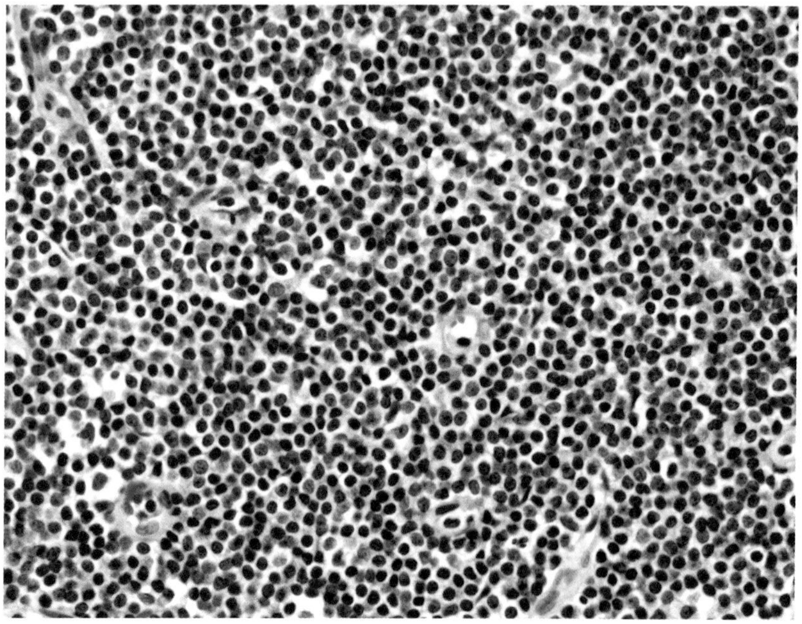

Figure 6-3 **Lymphoma (Lymphosarcoma), Lymph Node, Dog.** The tumor is composed of a solid sheet of neoplastic round cells (lymphocytes). The neoplastic cells are monomorphic, meaning that there is little variation in cell or nuclear size or shape. H&E stain. (Courtesy College of Veterinary Medicine, University of Tennessee.)

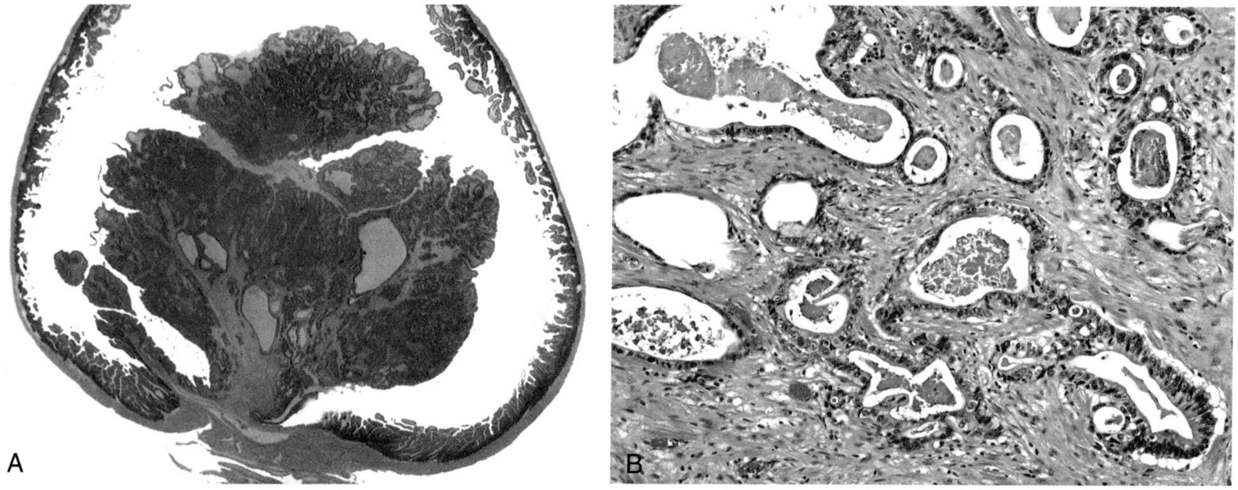

Figure 6-4 **Comparison of Benign and Malignant Epithelial Tumors. A,** Polyp, small intestine, mouse. The neoplastic growth arises from the mucosa and extends into the lumen of the intestine. There is no invasion of the intestinal wall. H&E stain. **B,** Adenocarcinoma (carcinomatosis), mesentery, cat. Irregular acini of neoplastic epithelial cells, presumably of biliary or pancreatic origin, have invaded mesenteric connective tissue. H&E stain. (**A** courtesy College of Veterinary Medicine, The Ohio State University. **B** courtesy College of Veterinary Medicine, University of Tennessee.)

potential to metastasize. The term *carcinoma* in situ, however, refers to a preinvasive form of carcinoma that remains within the epithelial structure from which it arises and that does not penetrate the basement membrane or invade underlying stroma.

As with mesenchymal tumors, the general terms "adenoma" and "carcinoma" may be further modified to indicate the organ of origin, as in "hepatocellular adenoma" or "hepatocellular carcinoma". In addition, these terms are frequently modified by prefixes or adjectives describing their microscopic appearance. For instance, the adjective "squamous" is applied to an epithelial neoplasm that demonstrates squamous differentiation similar to that seen in normal stratified squamous epithelia. The neoplastic epithelial cells of "mucinous" adenocarcinomas produce abundant mucin. Carcinomas that stimulate significant *desmoplasia*, the formation of abundant collagen in surrounding connective tissue, may be termed *scirrhous*.

Undifferentiated Tumors

The primitive or markedly heterogeneous microscopic appearance of some malignant tumors gives no clue to their cell of origin; thus they are termed *undifferentiated* or *anaplastic neoplasms*.

Mixed Tumors

A tumor containing multiple cell types is called a *mixed tumor*. Mixed tumors are believed to arise from a single pluripotent or totipotent stem cell capable of differentiating into a variety of more mature cell types. The benign mixed mammary gland tumor of dogs is a good example of a mixed tumor, because it typically contains a variable mixture of neoplastic epithelial or glandular elements, including luminal epithelium and myoepithelium, and mesenchymal elements, including fibrous connective tissue, fat, cartilage, and bone (Fig. 6-5). Teratomas and teratocarcinomas, which arise from totipotential germ cells, contain tissues normally derived from all three embryonic cell layers and thus may be composed of a bizarre mixture of adult and embryonic tissue types.

Tumor-Like Lesions

Several lesions may appear neoplastic grossly but are actually non-neoplastic growths when examined microscopically. *Hamartomas* are disorganized but mature mesenchymal or epithelial tissues found in their normal anatomic location (see Fig. 7-47). Many of the hamartomas identified in animals consist of abnormal proliferations of blood vessels. Hamartomas may be the result of aberrant differentiation in development rather than true neoplasia, and their behavior is completely benign. *Choristomas* are composed of normal mature tissue located at an ectopic site. An example is the dermoid, a mass consisting of mature skin and adnexa, which may be found in a variety of unusual sites, including the cornea (see Fig. 21-34 and E-Fig. 21-39).

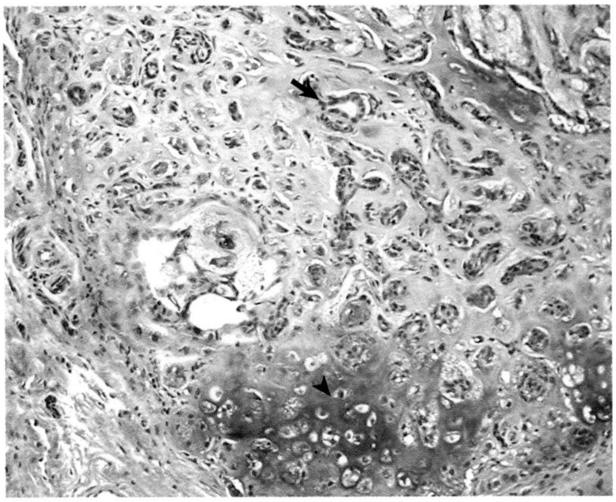

Figure 6-5 Mixed Mammary Tumor, Mammary Gland, Dog. Mixed mammary tumors of dogs contain both epithelial structures *(arrow)* and mesenchymal elements, such as cartilage and bone *(arrowhead)*. H&E stain. (Courtesy College of Veterinary Medicine, The Ohio State University.)

Veterinary Nomenclature

In Table 6-1 the names of common benign neoplasms in animals and their malignant counterparts are shown. The names given are those commonly employed in veterinary medicine. The terms used by veterinary pathologists to describe tumors in animals may differ from the terms used by medical pathologists to describe tumors in human beings. This inconsistency is partly because conventional usage plays an important role in tumor nomenclature; thus tumor nomenclature may be dictated by historic precedent rather than by logic. Moreover, attempts to standardize diagnostic terms for tumors in veterinary medicine have lagged far behind such efforts in human medicine. Thus more than one name for a given type of neoplasm may be reported in medical literature. For instance, a significant difference between veterinary and human nomenclature is that a benign tumor arising from melanocytes is termed a "benign melanoma" or "melanocytoma" by veterinary pathologists and a "nevus" by medical pathologists. Medical pathologists reserve the term "melanoma" for a malignant tumor of melanocyte origin, whereas veterinary pathologists term such tumors "malignant melanomas." Consideration of established precedents in tumor nomenclature and use of precise terminology are therefore critical for accurate communication among pathologists, practitioners, and researchers across medical disciplines.

Tumor Characteristics (Essential Concept 6-1)

Benign Versus Malignant Tumors

Benign tumors are generally expansile and may compress adjacent tissue, whereas malignant tumors are usually invasive. In malignant tumors, alterations in cell adhesion, motility, and protease production allow tumor cells to leave the tumor mass and penetrate surrounding tissue. Moreover, for malignant cells to invade and ultimately metastasize, they must become completely independent of local growth regulatory controls and acquire an independent blood supply. Acquisition of these features allows a tumor to spread well beyond its site of origin.

ESSENTIAL CONCEPT 6-1 Tumor Characteristics

Tumors may arise from virtually any normal tissue in the body. Benign tumors are expansile masses and may compress but do not invade surrounding tissue and do not spread to other sites in the body. In contrast, malignant tumors are locally invasive and have the potential to metastasize to distant sites. Tumor characteristics include the following:

1. Loss of differentiation as indicated by morphologic variability in tumor cells, abnormal tissue architecture, and loss of specialized cell function
2. Unlimited proliferative potential due to continuous cell division and resistance to cell death

Clinically, tumor grade (degree of differentiation) and stage (extent of spread) are used to establish prognosis and determine treatment options.

Table 6-1 Tumor Nomenclature

Origin	Tissue of Origin	Cell of Origin	Benign	Malignant
MESENCHYMAL				
Connective tissue and related tissue	Fibrous connective tissue	Fibroblast	Fibroma	Fibrosarcoma
	Fat	Adipocyte	Lipoma	Liposarcoma
	Cartilage	Chondrocyte	Chondroma	Chondrosarcoma
	Bone	Osteoblast	Osteoma	Osteosarcoma
Endothelium and related tissue	Blood vessel	Vascular endothelium	Hemangioma	Hemangiosarcoma
	Lymphatic vessel	Lymphatic endothelium	Lymphangioma	Lymphangiosarcoma
	Synovium	Synovial lining cell	Synovioma	Synovial sarcoma
	Mesothelium	Mesothelial cell	*	Mesothelioma
	Meninges	Meningeal connective tissue cell	Meningioma	Malignant meningioma
	Ovary	Modified mesothelium†	Adenoma	Adenocarcinoma
Hematopoietic and lymphoid tissue	Lymphoid tissue	Lymphocytes	*	Lymphoma
	Bone marrow	Leukocytes and erythrocytes	*	Leukemia
	Connective tissue	Mast cell	Mast cell tumor	Mast cell tumor
		Histiocytes	Histiocytoma	Histiocytic sarcoma (malignant histiocytosis)
Muscle	Smooth muscle	Smooth muscle cell	Leiomyoma	Leiomyosarcoma
	Skeletal muscle	Skeletal muscle cell	Rhabdomyoma	Rhabdomyosarcoma
EPITHELIAL				
Lining or covering epithelia	Skin	Squamous epithelial cell	Papilloma	Squamous cell carcinoma
		Adnexal cells	Adenoma	Adenocarcinoma Carcinoma
		Melanocyte	Benign melanoma (melanocytoma)	Malignant melanoma
	Upper alimentary tract (oral cavity, esophagus)	Squamous epithelial cell	Papilloma	Carcinoma
	Lower alimentary tract (intestine)	Columnar epithelium	Adenoma	Adenocarcinoma Carcinoma
	Upper respiratory tract (nasal cavity, trachea)	Columnar respiratory epithelium	Adenoma	Adenocarcinoma Carcinoma
	Lower respiratory tract (lung)	Columnar epithelium of bronchi and bronchioles	Adenoma	Adenocarcinoma Carcinoma
		Alveolar lining epithelium		
	Urinary tract	Transitional epithelium	Papilloma	Transitional cell carcinoma
	Uterus	Columnar epithelium	Uterine polyp	Endometrial carcinoma Endometrial adenocarcinoma
	Lining of glands or ducts	E.g., prostate, thyroid, bile ducts of liver	Adenoma	Adenocarcinoma Carcinoma
Solid epithelial organs	Glands	Pancreas, salivary gland, and others	Adenoma	Adenocarcinoma
	Liver	Hepatocyte	Hepatoma	Hepatocellular carcinoma
	Kidney	Renal tubular cell	Renal tubular adenoma	Renal cell carcinoma
	Testicle	Sertoli cell	Sertoli cell tumor	Malignant Sertoli cell tumor
		Interstitial cell	Interstitial/Leydig cell tumor	*
		Germ cell	Seminoma	Malignant Seminoma
			Teratoma	Teratocarcinoma
	Ovary	Stromal cell	Granulosa cell tumor	*
			Luteoma	*
			Thecoma	*
		Germ cell	Dysgerminoma	Dysgerminoma
			Teratoma	Teratocarcinoma
NERVOUS TISSUE				
Glial cells	Central nervous system	Astrocyte	*	Astrocytoma Glioblastoma
		Oligodendrocyte	*	Oligodendroglioma
		Microglial cell	*	Microgliomatosis
	Peripheral nervous system	Schwann cell	Benign peripheral nerve sheath tumor (schwannoma)	Malignant peripheral nerve sheath tumor (malignant schwannoma)

Table 6-1 Tumor Nomenclature–cont'd

Origin	Tissue of Origin	Cell of Origin	Benign	Malignant
Neural cells	Central nervous system	Neuron	*	Primitive neuroectodermal tumor
	Peripheral nervous system	Neuron	Ganglioneuroma	*
MIXED TUMORS				
Various	Mammary gland	Epithelium and myoepithelium	Adenoma Benign mixed mammary tumor (dog)	Adenocarcinoma Carcinoma Malignant mixed mammary tumor (dog)
	Testicle	Germ cell	Teratoma	Teratocarcinoma
	Ovary	Germ cell	Teratoma	Teratocarcinoma

*Not generally recognized.

†In contrast to the nomenclature for other mesenchymal tumors, tumors arising from modified ovarian mesothelium (i.e., surface epithelium, rete ovarii, or subsurface epithelial structures) are designated as adenomas/carcinomas based on the epithelioid cell morphology rather than spindle-shaped or round cell morphology of the tumor cells.

Table 6-2 Comparisons between Benign and Malignant Tumors

Characteristic	Benign	Malignant
Differentiation	Well-differentiated morphologic features and function	Poorly differentiated morphologic features and function
	Structure similar to tissue of origin	Tissue of origin sometimes unclear
	Little or no anaplasia	Variable degrees of anaplasia
Growth rate	Slow, progressive expansion	Rapid growth
	Rare mitotic figures	Frequent mitotic figures
	Normal mitotic figures	Abnormal mitotic figures
	Little necrosis	Necrosis if poor blood supply
Local invasion	No invasion	Local invasion
	Cohesive and expansile growth	Infiltrative growth
	Capsule often present	Capsule often absent or incomplete
Metastasis	No metastasis	Metastasis sometimes present

Although benign tumors are ultimately distinguished from their malignant counterparts based on invasiveness, a variety of morphologic and behavioral features are generally considered to predict the potential for malignant behavior (Table 6-2). Both benign and malignant tumors are composed of proliferating cells, but malignant tumors have essentially unlimited replicative potential. Malignant tumors are relatively independent of exogenous growth stimulatory molecules and are insensitive to growth inhibitory signals from their environment. Furthermore, malignant cells are better able than benign cells to evade apoptotic cell death (see Chapter 1). Compared with benign tumors, malignant tumors stimulate marked angiogenesis (the formation of new blood vessels), which ensures adequate tumor nutrition and promotes vascular invasion and metastasis. However, because of the rapid growth rate of many malignant tumors, areas of necrosis are often found within these tumors.

Because some benign tumors evolve into malignant neoplasms and some malignant tumors develop increasingly aggressive behavior over time in a process termed *malignant progression*, tumors may be graded to reflect where they lie on the continuum from benign to highly malignant or staged to indicate the extent of tumor spread. Together, the grade and stage of the tumor, discussed later in this chapter, indicate the risk the tumor poses to the animal and help determine a therapeutic strategy. It should be noted, however, that many benign tumors, such as sebaceous gland adenomas in dogs, have little or no malignant potential and rarely evolve into malignant tumors.

Differentiation

Morphology

Each normal, fully differentiated, mature tissue type has a characteristic gross and microscopic appearance that varies little from individual to individual of an animal species. To a variable extent, neoplastic tissues lose these mature differentiated features of cellular morphology and organization. In general, malignant tumors appear less differentiated than benign tumors. Many of the morphologic changes seen in neoplastic cells reflect frequent cell division, chromosomal abnormalities, and the active metabolic state that characterizes these cells.

Neoplastic cells often show considerable morphologic variability when compared with the normal tissue from which they are derived. Tumor cells, especially malignant tumor cells, may exhibit *anaplasia* or cellular *atypia*. Anaplastic cells are poorly differentiated cells with a wide variation in cell size (*anisocytosis*) and shape (*pleomorphism*). In some tumors, bizarre *tumor giant cells* with very large nuclei (*karyomegaly*) are observed (Fig. 6-6). There may also be extreme variability in nuclear size (*anisokaryosis*), shape, and pattern of chromatin distribution, and cells may contain multiple nuclei (Fig. 6-7). Anaplastic nuclei are often darkly staining (*hyperchromatic*) because of increased DNA content and are disproportionately large relative to cell size, resulting in an increased nuclear to cytoplasmic ratio. Prominent or multiple nucleoli may be present. The *mitotic figures* seen in dividing cells may be numerous, and atypical mitotic figures may be present.

Many tumor cells have noticeably basophilic cytoplasm as a result of the presence of large numbers of ribosomes required for rapid cell growth and frequent cell division. Neoplastic cells often exhibit loss of characteristic cytoplasmic features such as cilia or pigment. However, even in poorly differentiated tumors, special stains or immunohistochemical stains may be able to identify a characteristic morphologic feature retained in at least a subpopulation of tumor cells. For example, although poorly differentiated melanomas may lose their pigmentation, there is often positive

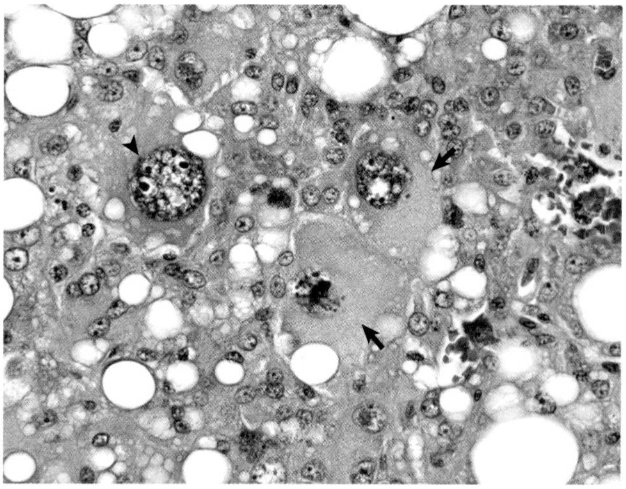

Figure 6-6 **Anaplastic Liposarcoma, Subcutis, Dog.** Anaplastic tumors of epithelial or mesenchymal cell origin often contain bizarre tumor giant cells such as the cells indicated by the arrows. Note also the large nuclei with abundant coarsely aggregated chromatin and multiple nucleoli *(arrowhead)*. The term "anaplastic" is used because the neoplastic cells bear very little resemblance to the adipocytes from which the tumor developed. H&E stain. (Courtesy College of Veterinary Medicine, University of Illinois.)

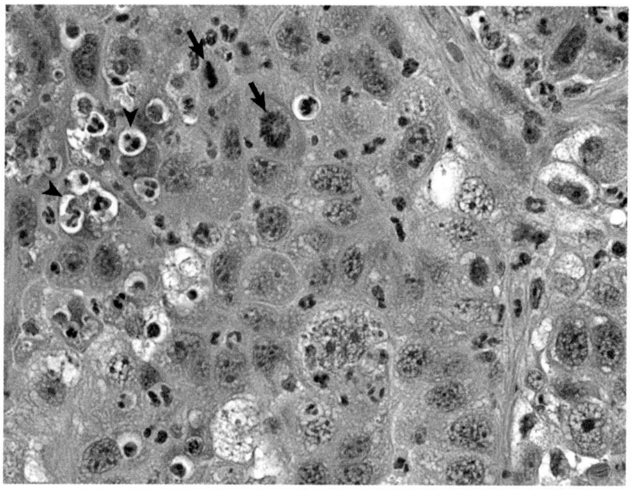

Figure 6-7 **Anaplastic Bronchoalveolar Carcinoma, Dog.** This tumor exhibits marked nuclear pleomorphism, as evidenced by the variation in nuclear and cellular size and shape. Note the prominent mitotic figures *(arrows)* and phagocytosis of neutrophils by the tumor cells *(arrowheads)*. H&E stain. (Courtesy Dr. J. F. Zachary, College of Veterinary Medicine, University of Illinois.)

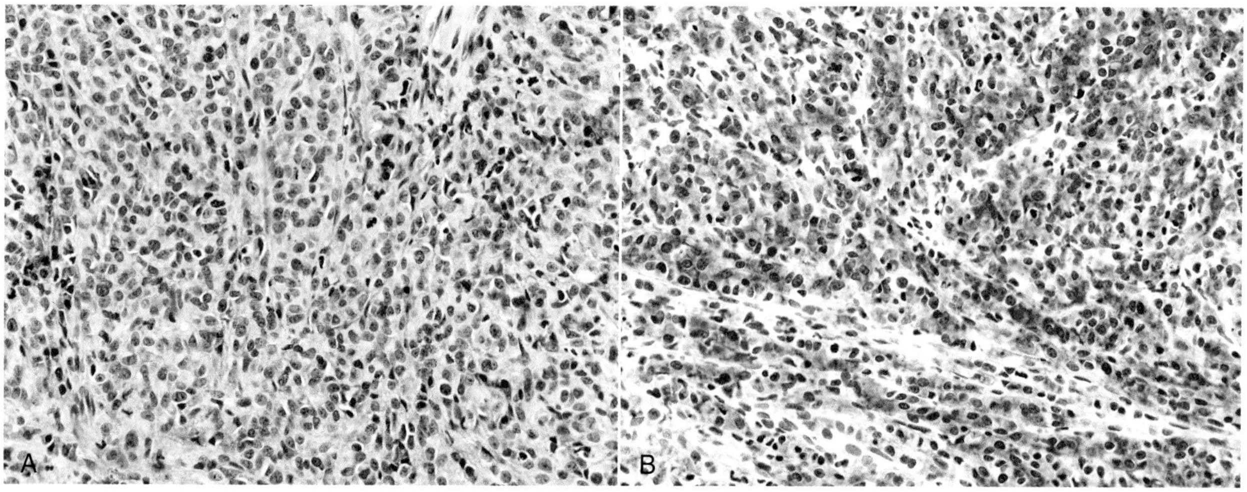

Figure 6-8 **Amelanotic Melanoma, Oral Cavity, Dog. A,** The tumor is composed of relatively uniform round to polygonal cells that lack obvious cytoplasmic pigmentation. H&E stain. **B,** Subsequent immunohistochemical staining for Melan A (red staining), a melanocyte marker, shows the tumor to be a melanoma. IHC for Melan A. (Courtesy College of Veterinary Medicine, University of Tennessee.)

immunohistochemical staining for the melanoma markers Melan-A (MART1) or dopachrome tautomerase (TYRP2) in amelanotic melanomas (Fig. 6-8).

In tumors, normal tissue organization is frequently lost. Increasing loss of normal architecture in tumors correlates with increasing independence of tumor cells from their surrounding tissues. As an example, lymphomas arising in lymph nodes often consist of solid sheets of neoplastic cells that partially or completely efface the normal follicular lymph node architecture (Fig. 6-9). In tissues that normally undergo continual renewal, such as the skin and oral mucosa, the normal maturation sequence may be altered. Thus in squamous cell carcinomas the orderly morphologic progression from basal cell layer to fully keratinized stratum corneum may not occur (Fig. 6-10).

Function

Loss of specialized function frequently accompanies loss of differentiated morphologic features in tumors. Neoplastic cells arising in the small intestinal epithelium may lack microvilli and thus lose their absorptive capabilities. However, in some tumors, aspects of normal function may be retained. For example, thyroid adenomas may continue to produce thyroid hormones, and plasma cell tumors may secrete immunoglobulins. However, in the majority of cases, these functions are no longer regulated appropriately because the neoplastic cells have lost responsiveness to and dependence on normal regulatory pathways. Thus thyroid adenomas may produce clinical hyperthyroidism, and plasma cell tumors may cause hypergammaglobulinemia.

Differentiation Therapy

Although tumor cells are generally less differentiated than normal cells, some tumor cells can be forced to differentiate into more mature, near-normal cells. Vitamin A derivatives are routinely employed to treat acute promyelocytic leukemia in human patients, vitamin D compounds are showing some promise in differentiation therapy of human epithelial tumors, and compounds that

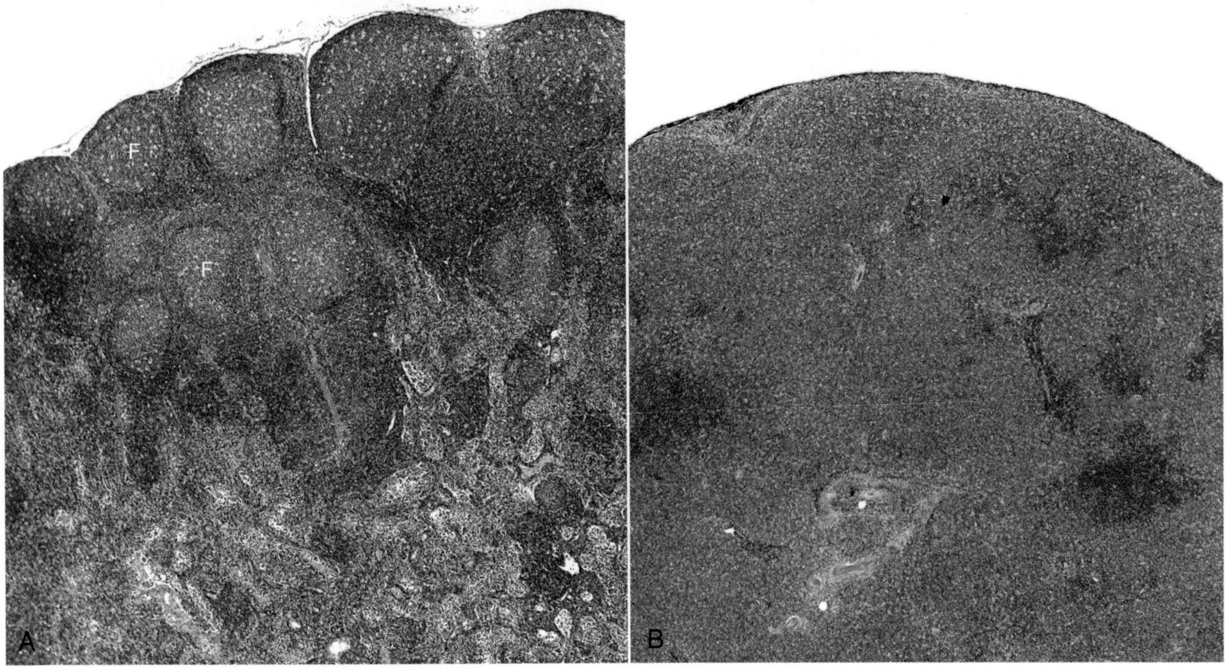

Figure 6-9 **Comparison of Lymphoid Hyperplasia and Lymphoma. A**, Lymphoid hyperplasia, lymph node, cat. Although there is an expansion of lymphoid elements in this lymph node, lymph node architecture is maintained, and several lymphoid follicles *(F)* are evident. Only two of several follicles are labeled. **B**, Lymphoma (lymphosarcoma), lymph node, dog. Solid sheets of neoplastic lymphocytes completely efface normal lymph node architecture. H&E stain. (Courtesy College of Veterinary Medicine, University of Tennessee.)

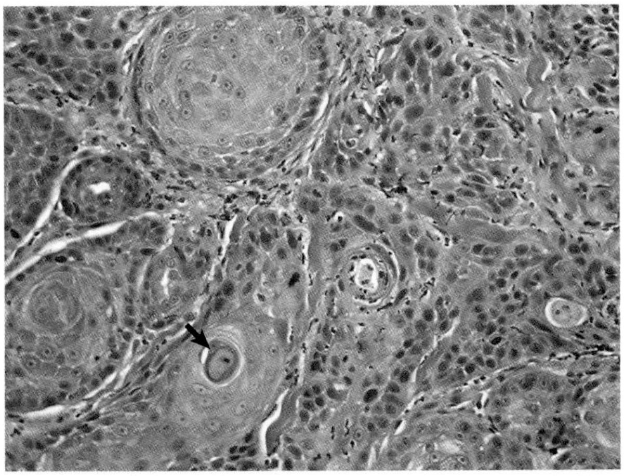

Figure 6-10 **Squamous Cell Carcinoma, Tongue, Cat.** The orderly pattern of epidermal maturation seen in normal oral mucosa is absent from this squamous cell carcinoma. An occasional "keratin pearl" *(arrow)* identifies the keratinized stratified squamous epithelial origin of this tumor. H&E stain. (Courtesy College of Veterinary Medicine, The Ohio State University.)

epigenetically alter tumor cells by modifying the histones in chromatin may also enhance differentiation of tumor cells. The assumption underlying differentiation therapies is that more differentiated tumor cells will have a less stem cell–like phenotype and will thus have reduced proliferative potential.

Proliferation

Tumor Growth

Essentially unlimited proliferative potential is a hallmark of neoplasia, especially of malignant neoplasms. Unlike normal cells, many tumor cells are immortal. In general, neoplastic cells escape normal limits on cell division, become independent of external growth stimulatory and inhibitory factors, and lose their susceptibility to apoptotic signals. These characteristics result in an imbalance between cell production and cell loss and a net increase in tumor size. However, it should be noted that the growth of a tumor is not completely exponential. A proportion of tumor cells is continually lost from the replicative pool because of irreversible cell cycle arrest, differentiation, and death.

Cell Division

Normal cell proliferation is largely controlled by soluble or contact-dependent signals from the microenvironment that either stimulate or inhibit cell division. An excess of stimulators or a deficiency of inhibitors leads to net growth. As discussed in Chapter 1, the cell cycle consists of G_1 (presynthetic), S (DNA synthetic), G_2 (premitotic), and M (mitotic) phases. Quiescent cells are in a physiologic state called G_0. In adult tissue, many cells reside in G_0 and are unable to enter the cell cycle at all or do so only when stimulated by extrinsic factors. In response to DNA damage, even actively dividing normal cells undergo cell cycle arrest, usually at one of several cell cycle checkpoints. Cell cycle arrest is initiated by the multifunctional tumor suppressor gene product p53 and gives the cell time to repair DNA damage, as discussed in more detail later in the chapter. Many neoplastic cells no longer respond to extrinsic or intrinsic signals directing them into G_0 and no longer express functional p53. Thus the cells move continuously through the cell cycle. Moreover, because the tumor cells do not undergo cell cycle arrest after DNA damage, they progressively accumulate potentially mutagenic DNA damage (Fig. 6-11).

The *mitotic index* is usually defined as the average number of tumor cells per 400× power microscopic field that contain condensed chromosomes and lack nuclear membranes (Fig. 6-12). Such cells are interpreted as being actively dividing, and the mitotic index of a tumor is considered to indicate its malignant potential. However, the mitotic index can be misleading. The fraction of tumor cells

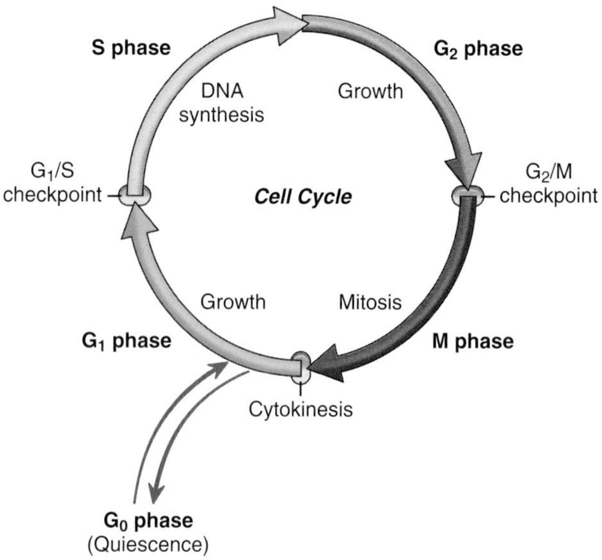

Figure 6-11 Cell Cycle Landmarks. This figure shows the cell cycle phases (G_1, S, G_2, and M). Prophase, metaphase, anaphase, and telophase constitute the M phase, whereas interphase encompasses G_1, S, and G_2. Actively dividing cells cycle continuously. Under the appropriate conditions, cells may exit the cell cycle to enter G_0, a quiescent state, or cells in G_0 may reenter the cell cycle. The G_1/S and G_2/M checkpoints are sites at which cell cycle arrest in response to DNA damage may occur.

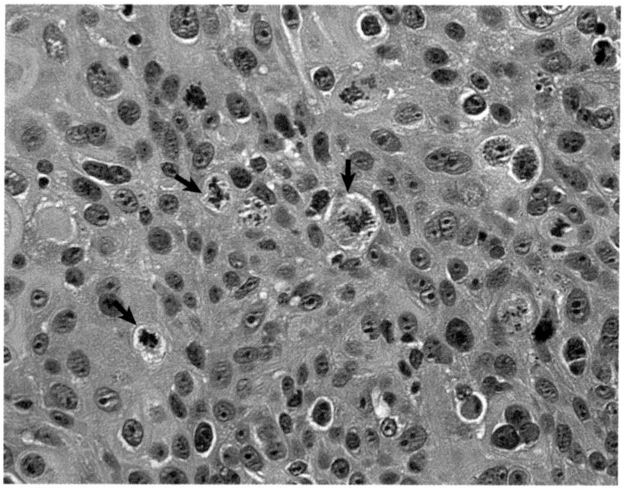

Figure 6-12 Anaplastic Neoplasm, Site Unknown, Dog. The arrows identify a few of the mitotic figures present. This tumor has a high mitotic index. H&E stain. (Courtesy College of Veterinary Medicine, University of Illinois.)

observed to be in mitosis depends not only on the number of cells undergoing mitosis but also on the length of time required to complete the process. In tumor cells the time required for completion of the cell cycle is generally as long as or even longer than for normal cells. Mitotic figures may persist in cancer cells that are unable to complete cell division; abnormal mitotic figures may also be observed.

For homeostasis to be maintained, normal cells must engage in a continual dialogue with their environment. There is a constant exchange of information among cells via soluble mediators, including growth stimulatory factors, growth inhibitory factors, and hormones (see Chapters 1 and 12). These soluble mediators tightly control the growth of nonneoplastic cells. Neoplastic cells, on the other hand, often lose both their dependence on extrinsic growth stimulatory substances and their susceptibility to growth inhibitory signals from their environment. The end result is that tumor cells are no longer responsive to the needs of the organism as a whole and develop the capacity to drive their own replication.

Cell Death

Senescence. In response to DNA damage, oxidative stress, and telomere shortening, proliferating cells may undergo a permanent arrest in the G_1 phase of the cell cycle termed *cellular senescence*. This growth arrest limits the life span of neoplastic cells and prevents unlimited tumor cell proliferation. Senescence is mediated by activation of the p53 or retinoblastoma pathways of cell cycle arrest. Senescent cells often express senescence-associated β-galactosidase.

Because DNA replication machinery is unable to duplicate the extreme ends of DNA templates, the telomeres that form the ends of chromosomes are shortened at each cell division. Embryonic cells express telomerase, a riboprotein enzyme that allows telomeres to be replicated and even expanded; however, most adult cells do not express this protein, and their telomeres shrink with each round of cell division. Very short telomeres are incompatible with continued cell division and trigger cellular senescence in normal cells. However, many neoplastic cells regain the ability to produce telomerase and thus to replicate their telomeres. Reexpression of telomerase appears to play an important role in the escape of tumor cells from senescence and their consequent immortality.

Apoptosis. *Apoptosis* is a form of "programmed cell death" that serves both as a normal physiologic process and as a response to injurious stimuli (see Chapter 1). In proliferative tissue, such as gut epithelium, terminally differentiated cells undergo apoptosis and are thus removed from the cell population. Apoptosis may occur in response to withdrawal of survival or growth factors from the cell environment or to binding of death factors, such as Fas ligand and tumor necrosis factor-α (TNF-α), to cell surface receptors. Cell hypoxia and lack of essential nutrients may end in apoptosis. DNA damage may also induce apoptosis; in this case, apoptosis is triggered by p53. Apoptosis may be stimulated by the activity of cytotoxic immune cells, including T lymphocytes and natural killer (NK) cells. Signals for apoptosis activate a variety of signaling pathways, many of which ultimately result in the release of cytochrome *c* from mitochondria. The final effectors of apoptosis are the caspases, intracellular proteases that selectively destroy cellular organelles and degrade genomic DNA into nucleosome-sized fragments (see E-Fig. 1-22). The morphologic hallmarks of apoptosis include margination of chromatin, condensation and fragmentation of the nucleus, and condensation of the cell with preservation of organelles. Ultimately, the cell breaks into membrane-bound apoptotic bodies that are engulfed by surrounding cells without stimulating an inflammatory response (Fig. 6-13).

Although virtually all normal cells in the body can undergo apoptosis in response to appropriate physiologic signals, many cancer cells acquire resistance to apoptosis. Because apoptosis is a major route of tumor cell loss, such resistance enhances the overall growth rate of the tumor. Many tumor cells circumvent apoptosis by functional inactivation of the *p53* gene, thus removing a key proapoptotic molecule. Additionally, tumor cells may constitutively activate survival signaling pathways, rendering the cells independent of exogenous survival factors. Finally, tumor cells may develop mechanisms for inactivating death factor signaling pathways, thus evading apoptosis in response to homeostatic signals from the cellular environment.

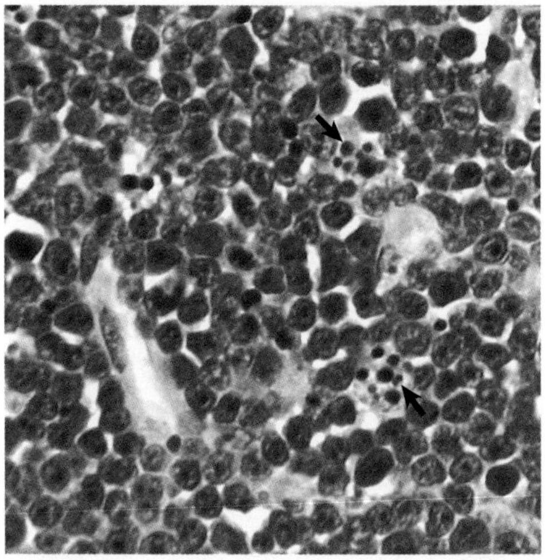

Figure 6-13 **Lymphoma (Lymphosarcoma), Lymph Node, Horse.** Histologically, apoptosis is characterized by condensation and fragmentation of nuclei *(arrows)*, cell shrinkage, and engulfment of apoptotic bodies by surrounding cells. Note the absence of associated inflammation. H&E stain. (Courtesy Dr. R. Tan, College of Veterinary Medicine, University of Illinois.)

Autophagy. *Autophagy* refers to degradation of a cell's own organelles within autophagosomes (see Fig. 1-24). Autophagy can be a mechanism for cell survival in the face of nutrient deprivation, because it salvages important cellular components for reuse; however, extensive autophagy can also lead to a form of programmed cell death. Autophagy plays a poorly understood and somewhat paradoxical role in tumor growth. In many tumors, autophagy is suppressed, thus presumably preventing autophagic tumor cell death. The mammalian target of rapamycin (mTOR) kinase is the major cellular inhibitor of autophagy, and mTOR inhibitors have shown limited promise as cancer therapeutics. However, in other tumors, increased autophagy may also enhance tumor cell survival under the conditions of reduced nutrient availability that arise during therapy.

Neoplastic Transformation (Essential Concept 6-2)

Latency

As illustrated in Figure 6-14, the *latent period* for a tumor is the time before a tumor becomes clinically detectable. The smallest clinically detectable mass is usually approximately 1 cm in diameter and contains approximately 10^9 cells. To form a tumor that size, a single transformed cell must undergo approximately 30 rounds of cell division, assuming all the progeny remain viable and capable of

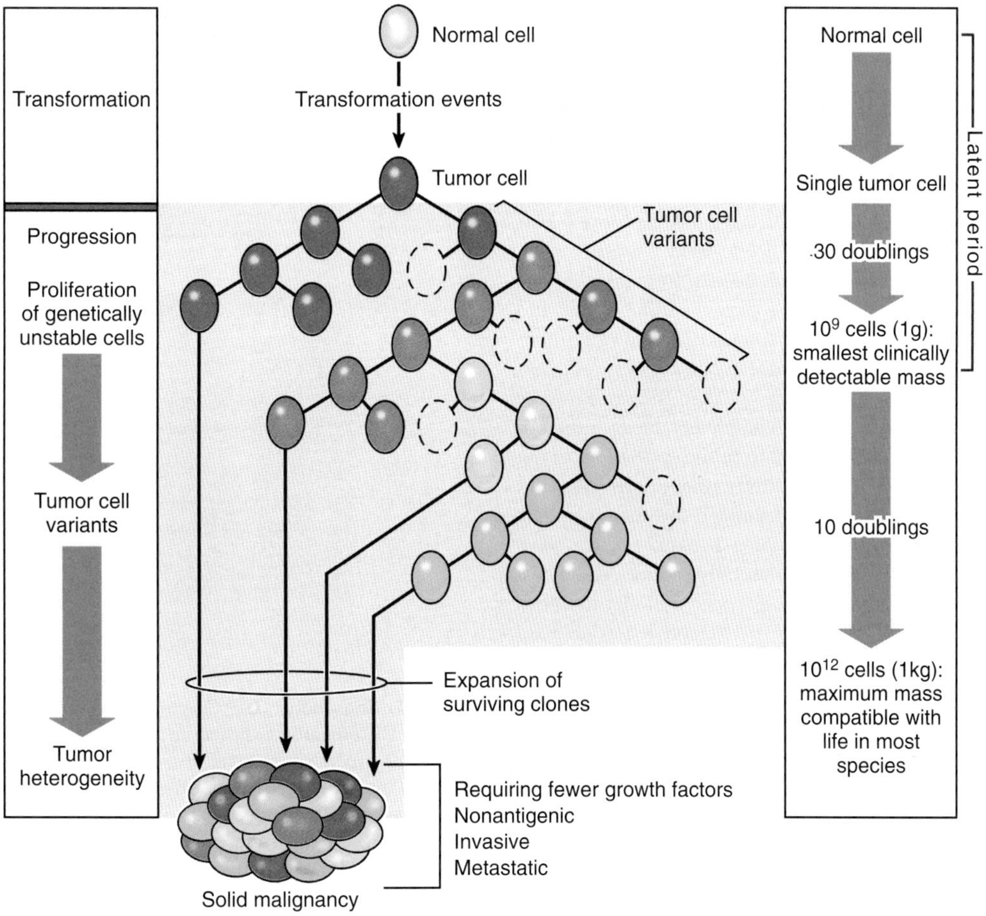

Figure 6-14 **Biology of Solid Tumor Growth.** The center panel illustrates clonal tumor evolution and generation of tumor cell heterogeneity. Subclones arise from descendents of the original transformed cell. As it grows, the tumor becomes enriched for those variant subclones that proliferate faster or are better able to evade host defenses; such subclones tend to be more aggressive, thus more invasive and likely to metastasize. The left panel shows the corresponding stages of tumor progression. The right panel shows, roughly, the tumor-cell doublings that precede the formation of a clinically detectable tumor. The maximum tumor size compatible with life depends to some extent on the species affected.

ESSENTIAL CONCEPT 6-2 Neoplastic Transformation

Neoplasia occurs by the step-wise transformation of normal cells into tumor cells able to escape ordinary mechanisms of growth control. Steps in neoplastic transformation include the following:

1. Initiation: An irreversible alteration of genetic material
2. Promotion: The selective outgrowth of initiated cells to form a benign tumor
3. Progression: The gradual development of features of malignancy due to a combination of genetic and epigenetic changes

replication. Thus, by the time most tumors become clinically evident, they have probably been developing in the host for many years. However, once tumors reach a clinically detectable size, their growth may appear to be very rapid, because only 10 subsequent doubling cycles are required to convert a 1-g tumor into a 1-kg tumor. Actually, volume doubling times for tumors vary considerably, depending on the rate at which tumor cells divide, the fraction of tumor cells that are replicatively competent, and the rate at which tumor cells die. In general, benign neoplasms grow more slowly than malignant tumors, although there is considerable variation among tumors. Moreover, tumors may grow erratically, depending on several additional factors, including blood supply, extrinsic growth-regulating factors such as hormones, the efficacy of the host immune response, and the emergence of subpopulations of particularly aggressive tumor cells.

Stepwise Tumor Development

Neoplasms develop as the result of multiple genetic and epigenetic changes that occur over a relatively long time course. It is the cumulative effect of these alterations that ultimately creates a tumor. Tumor development thus takes place in a gradual fashion and is described by the term *stepwise tumor development*. Another term applied to this process is *multistage carcinogenesis*. In many chapters in this book the less specific terms *neoplastic transformation* and *carcinogenesis* are used to describe the process of stepwise tumor development discussed here. The stepwise evolution of tumors has been studied most thoroughly in carcinomas. There are several types of carcinoma that develop in an orderly and predictable fashion. For instance, squamous cell carcinoma arises from the epithelium of the eyelid in many species of animals, including cattle, horses, cats, and dogs. In all species these tumors develop through the same sequence of steps: epidermal hyperplasia, carcinoma in situ, and invasive carcinoma. Extensive studies of experimentally induced squamous cell carcinomas in the skin of mice have revealed a similar morphologic pattern of tumor evolution (Fig. 6-15) and have led to a detailed model of stepwise carcinoma development (Fig. 6-16).

In a few well-studied tumor types, such as chemically induced skin tumors in mice and colonic carcinomas in human beings, the stepwise molecular changes that underlie morphologic changes in the tumors have also been determined, as discussed later in the chapter. Many of these genetic changes are associated with cell proliferation, DNA repair, angiogenesis, and invasiveness.

Initiation

The first step of carcinogenesis is *initiation*, the introduction of an irreversible genetic change into normal cells by the action of a mutagenic *initiating agent* or *initiator*. Initiators are chemical or physical carcinogens that damage DNA. Mutation induction requires not only the introduction of a DNA lesion, but also mispairing of the

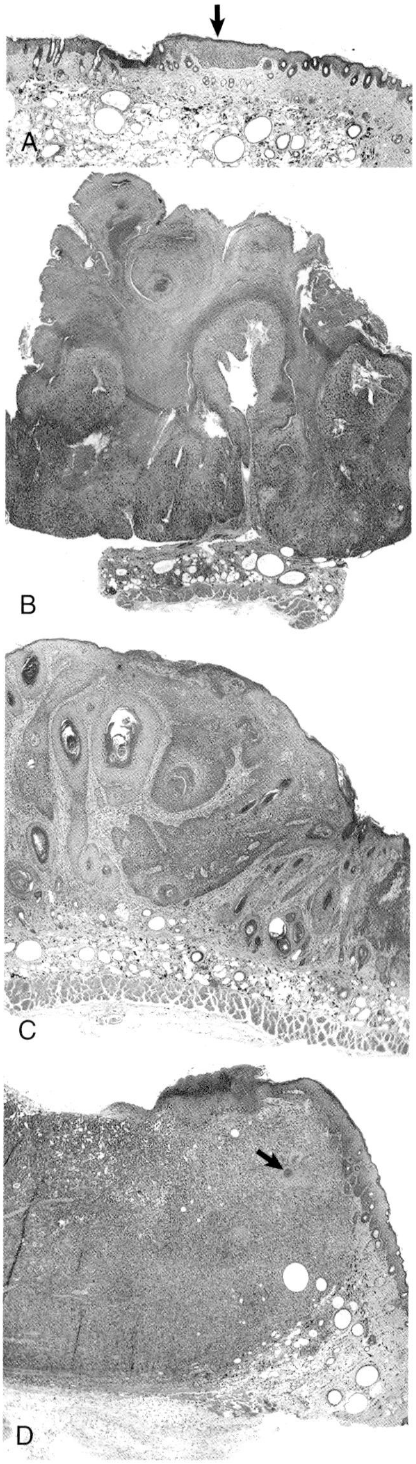

Figure 6-15 **Squamous Cell Carcinoma Development, Skin, Hairless Mouse Chronically Exposed to Ultraviolet Radiation. A,** A focus of epidermal hyperplasia *(arrow)* is the earliest lesion seen. **B,** This lesion develops into a papilloma, a benign exophytic papillary growth that is highly keratinized and does not penetrate the underlying dermis. **C,** As the papilloma undergoes conversion into a malignant squamous cell carcinoma, it begins to invade the dermis and to lose the regular pattern of epithelial differentiation. **D,** A fully developed squamous cell carcinoma has lost most differentiated characteristics and extends deep into the dermis and panniculus carnosus (muscle). Only a few keratin "pearls" *(arrow)* identify the origin of this tumor from the skin epidermis. All figures were taken at the same magnification. H&E stain. (Courtesy Dr. T.M. Oberyszyn, The Ohio State University.)

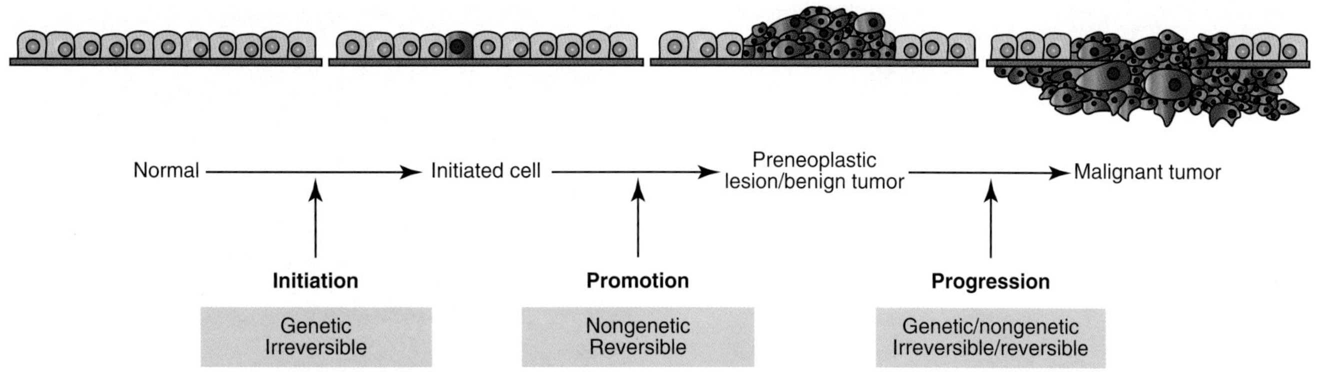

Figure 6-16 Stepwise Tumor Development. Initiated cells have irreversible genetic damage. In the presence of a promoter, these initiated cells expand to form a preneoplastic lesion or benign tumor. With further genetic and epigenetic alterations, a malignant tumor emerges from a subclone of cells within the benign precursor lesion. (Redrawn with permission from Dr. D.F. Kusewitt, Health Sciences Center, University of New Mexico.)

DNA lesion during subsequent DNA replication to produce an altered complementary DNA strand. Thus at least a single round of DNA replication is necessary for the genetic change to become permanent. Initiated cells may appear morphologically normal and may remain quiescent for years. However, these cells harbor mutations that could provide them with a growth advantage under special conditions. For example, the initiated cells may respond more vigorously to mitogenic signals or be more resistant to apoptosis-inducing stimuli than neighboring cells.

Promotion

The second stage of tumor development is *promotion*, the outgrowth of initiated cells in response to selective stimuli. Most of these selective stimuli, termed *promoting agents* or *promoters*, drive proliferation. In general, promoters are not mutagenic; instead, they create a proliferative environment in which initiated cells have a growth advantage. Because promoters are nonmutagenic, their effects are usually reversible. However, the proliferative response to promoters creates a large population of initiated cells at risk for further mutations. What emerges at the end of the promotion phase of tumor development is a benign tumor.

Progression

In *progression*, the final stage of tumor development, a benign tumor evolves into an increasingly malignant tumor in a process termed *malignant transformation*. Malignant tumors may ultimately become metastatic. Malignant transformation represents an irreversible change in the nature of the developing tumor. Progression is a complex and poorly understood process involving both genetic and epigenetic changes in tumor cells, as well as alterations in the tumor environment, that select for increasingly malignant clones of tumor cells. Genetic instability in tumor cells and increasing tumor cell heterogeneity are hallmarks of progression.

Tumor Heterogeneity and Clonal Selection

Most tumors are believed to be of *clonal* origin, that is, they are derived from a single transformed cell. Tumor cell heterogeneity is generated during the course of tumor growth by the progressive accumulation of heritable changes in tumor cells (see Fig. 6-14). With each new genetic alteration, the progeny of a single tumor cell with this new mutation will constitute a subclone of tumor cells. The generation of subclones is fostered by the marked genomic instability of tumor cells compared with normal cells. Successful subclones are those that have a high proliferative rate, are able to evade the animal's immune response, can stimulate the development of an independent blood supply, and become independent of exogenous growth factors. These characteristics give successful subclones a selective advantage over other subclones of cells within the tumor. A tumor subclone with a selective advantage will eventually predominate and, if acquiring certain additional traits, can metastasize from the tumor of origin. This overall process is referred to as *clonal selection* or *tumor evolution*.

Stem Cells and Cancer

Most tumors are composed of cells that lack fully differentiated morphologic, functional, and behavioral characteristics. Furthermore, many neoplastic cells acquire features similar to the embryonic cells that gave rise to the mature tissue in which the tumor originated. This similarity between embryonic cells and neoplastic cells may be accounted for in two different ways. First, normal mature cells may dedifferentiate as they evolve into tumor cells, leading to the reemergence of more primitive characteristics. Second, tumors may arise directly from the small population of *stem cells* found in all adult tissues; such stem cells are required for normal tissue renewal and often have unlimited replicative potential. The appearance and behavior of the tumor cells that develop from a neoplastic stem cell are determined by the stage of differentiation at which the malignant phenotype is manifested; the neoplastic stem cell is said to have undergone *maturation arrest* at that stage of its development. The diversity of cell types that can arise from a single progenitor stem cell is limited by the differentiation potential of that cell.

Totipotent stem cells, such as embryonic stem cells, can give rise to all tissues of the body, whereas multipotent or pluripotent stem cells can give rise to a smaller variety of tissue types. The plasticity of some adult stem cells is relatively restricted. Leukemias provide excellent examples of neoplasms arising from stem cells. Leukemia almost always arises from a single hematopoietic stem cell that has undergone neoplastic transformation. The progeny of this stem cell all exhibit the same genetic change, although the cell type and degree of differentiation of the progeny may vary. Thus in myelomonocytic leukemia a neoplastic multipotential stem cell may give rise to leukemic cells from both the granulocytic and monocytic series (Fig. 6-17). The concept of a stem cell origin for cancer explains not only the embryonic characteristics of neoplastic cells but also the success of certain treatment strategies that use differentiating agents such as retinoids, vitamin A derivatives that are used to induce maturation of some human leukemia cells.

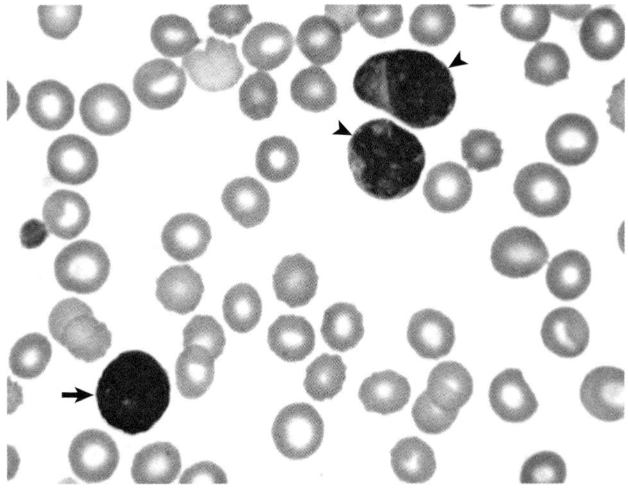

Figure 6-17 Myelomonocytic Leukemia, Peripheral Blood, Dog. In this unusual case, leukemic cells of both monocytic *(arrowheads)* and granulocytic (basophil) *(arrow)* origin were present in peripheral blood. The animal had a marked leukocytosis (103,000 white blood cells/μL) and thrombocytopenia. Wright's stain. (Courtesy Dr. M.J. Burkhard, College of Veterinary Medicine, The Ohio State University.)

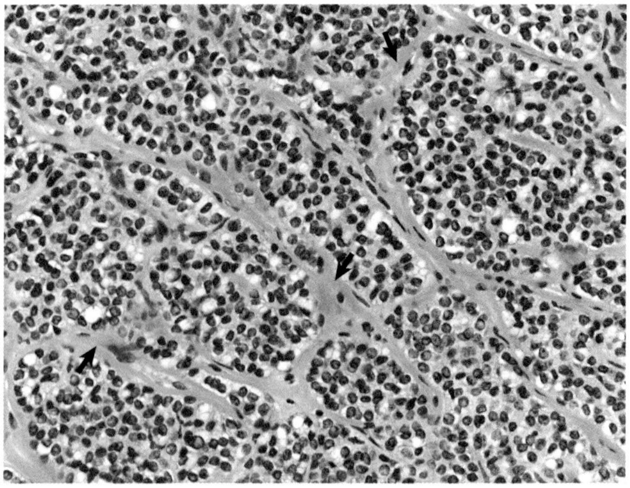

Figure 6-18 Trichoblastoma, Skin, Dog. Neoplastic basal epithelial cells are divided into incomplete lobules by the tumor stroma *(arrows)* composed of collagen and extracellular matrix components in which blood vessels, fibroblasts, and inflammatory and immune cells are embedded. H&E stain. (Courtesy College of Veterinary Medicine, University of Tennessee.)

Tumor Microenvironment (Essential Concept 6-3)

Tumor Stroma

Composition of the Stroma

A tumor consists of the tumor cells proper, termed the *parenchyma*, and a nonneoplastic supporting structure called the *stroma* (Fig. 6-18). The stroma is composed largely of extracellular connective tissue and consists of proteins and glycoproteins, such as collagen, embedded in a complex matrix of proteoglycans. This aggregate is called the *extracellular matrix* (ECM) throughout this book and is discussed in greater detail in Chapter 1. The stroma also contains the blood vessels that supply nutrients to the tumor, fibroblasts that synthesize collagen and other ECM components, and a variety of inflammatory and immune cells. The amount of stroma associated with tumors varies considerably. The extracellular material in the stroma of epithelial tumors is produced primarily by surrounding nonneoplastic mesenchymal cells, whereas many mesenchymal tumors produce their own stroma. For example, many osteosarcomas produce bone, a specialized form of connective tissue stroma. Stromal tissue may form a connective tissue *capsule* around tumors (Fig. 6-19), which may help to limit neoplastic spread. In general, encapsulated tumors have a better prognosis than unencapsulated tumors.

Rarely, the tumor stroma contains an amorphous eosinophilic substance termed *amyloid*. Amyloid consists of one of a variety of abnormal proteins arranged in β-pleated fibrils. The proteins that form amyloid are usually secreted by the tumor cells themselves. For example, λ-light chain protein secreted by neoplastic plasma cells forms the amyloid sometimes seen in the extramedullary plasmacytomas of various species. See Chapters 1 and 5 for more information on amyloid.

Tumor-Stromal Interactions

Tumor cells interact with their stroma in a complex fashion, exchanging a wide variety of signaling molecules, including growth factors, cytokines, hormones, and inflammatory mediators (Fig. 6-20). These exchanges modulate the growth rate, differentiation state, and behavior of both stromal cells and tumor cells. As an example, platelet-derived growth factor (PDGF) released by tumor cells stimulates tumor-associated fibroblasts to increase the production of collagen. In some cases this process leads to an extensive fibrous reaction, termed a "scirrhous" or "desmoplastic" response, in the stroma (Fig. 6-21). Some tumors produce transforming growth factor-α (TGF-α), which stimulates tumor-associated fibroblasts to differentiate into myofibroblasts, which have contractile capabilities. Tumor-associated fibroblasts may acquire special characteristics that distinguish them from normal fibroblasts. In some tumors, heritable genetic and epigenetic changes in tumor-associated fibroblasts

ESSENTIAL CONCEPT 6-3 Tumor Interactions with Other Tissues

Interactions between tumors and nonneoplastic tissues and organs of the body include the following:

1. Tumor-stromal interactions: A tumor consists of the tumor cells proper and a nonneoplastic supporting stroma composed of extracellular matrix, blood vessels, fibroblasts, inflammatory cells, and immune cells. Tumor cells and their stroma exert considerable mutual control. A particularly important effect of tumors on their stroma is the ability to stimulate angiogenesis, the formation of new blood vessels that support continued tumor growth.
2. Tumor immunity: The immune system may recognize tumor antigens as foreign and destroy tumor cells by a variety of mechanisms. Antitumor effector cells include those of the innate immune system (natural killer cells, macrophages) and the adaptive immune system (cytotoxic T lymphocytes, B lymphocytes). Tumor cells may employ a number of strategies to evade immunosurveillance.
3. Paraneoplastic effects: Once established, primary or metastatic tumors cause clinical disease through direct means, such as compression or effacement of normal tissues, or through paraneoplastic effects, such as the secretion of hormones by the tumor. Paraneoplastic effects important in veterinary medicine include cachexia, hypercalcemia, and anemia.

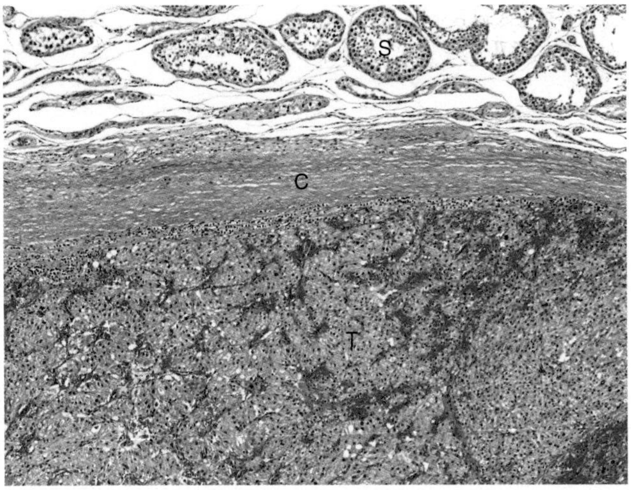

Figure 6-19 Interstitial Cell Tumor, Testis, Dog. This interstitial (Leydig) tumor (*T*) lies within the testis and is surrounded by a thick connective tissue capsule (*C*). Fibrous capsules are more common surrounding benign tumors than surrounding malignant tumors. *S*, Seminiferous tubule. H&E stain. (Courtesy College of Veterinary Medicine, The University of Tennessee.)

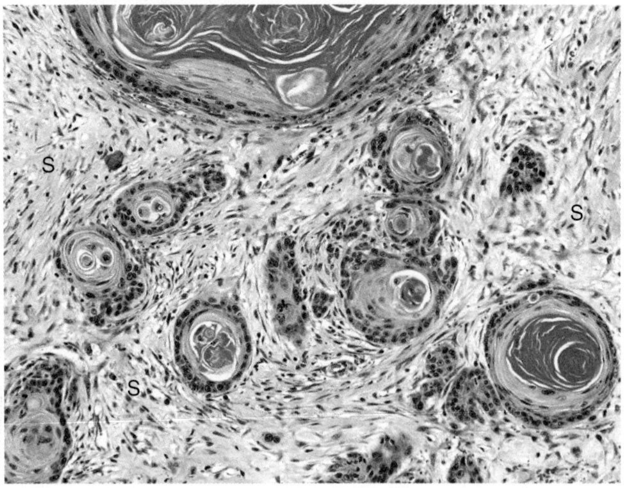

Figure 6-21 Squamous Cell Carcinoma. Carcinomas and adenocarcinomas that stimulate the formation of abundant collagen in surrounding connective tissue (desmoplasia) may be termed "scirrhous." Tumor-associated fibroblasts may secrete a fetal type of extracellular matrix and coevolve with adjacent tumor cells. In this photomicrograph, nests of squamous carcinoma cells with central keratin pearls are separated by abundant stroma containing large numbers of immature fibroblasts and collagen (*S*). H&E stain. (Courtesy College of Veterinary Medicine, The University of Tennessee.)

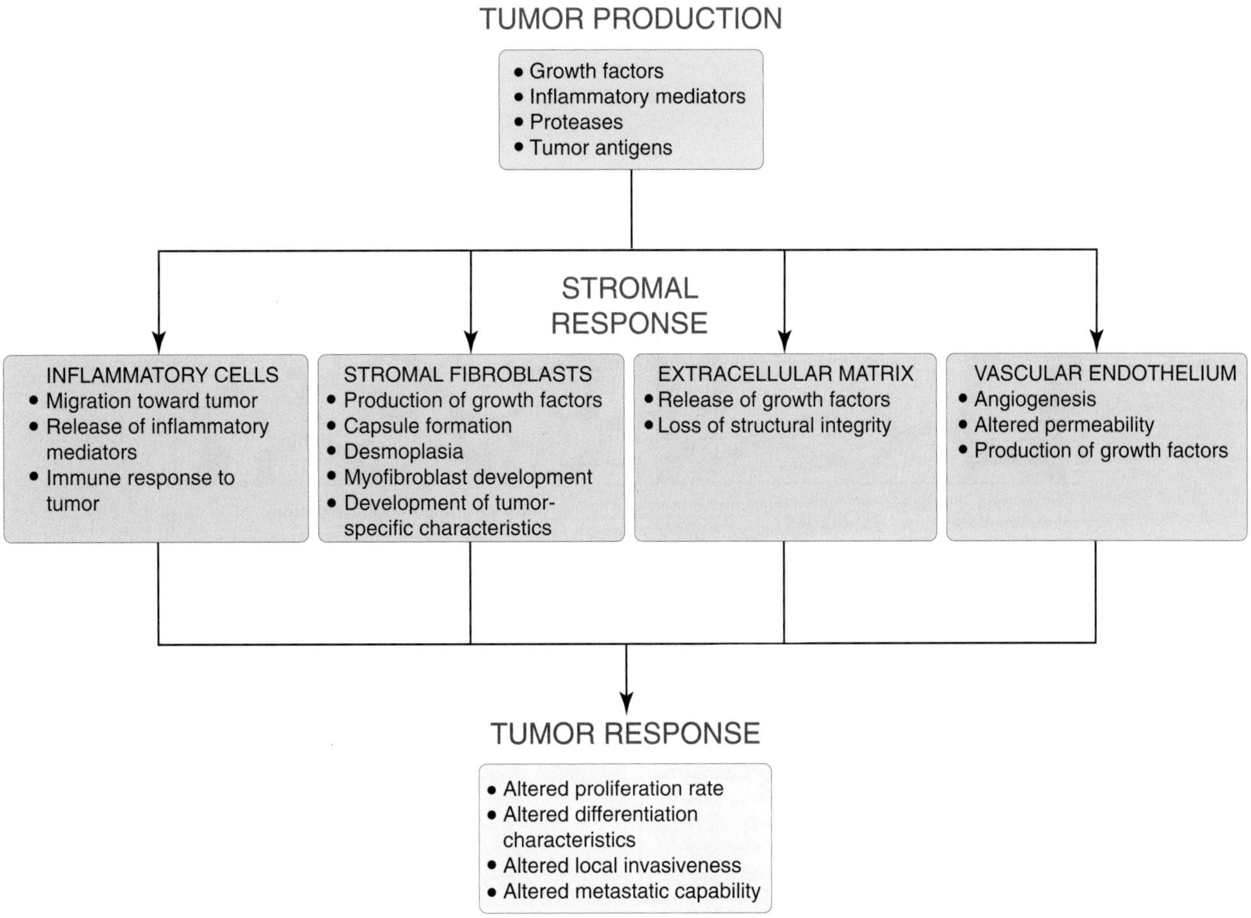

Figure 6-20 Tumor-Stromal Interactions. Tumor cells and the stroma in which they are embedded interact in a variety of ways that serve to modify the growth and behavior of both elements. Tumor stroma may both enhance and limit tumor development and spread. (Redrawn with permission from Dr. D.F. Kusewitt, Health Sciences Center, University of New Mexico.)

allow them to synchronize their growth with that of adjacent tumor cells. Tumor cells may induce surrounding stromal cells to produce cytokines that promote tumor cell proliferation and motility or attract inflammatory cells. Furthermore, growth factors are sequestered in the ECM of the stroma, where they bind to proteoglycans. Proteases secreted by tumor cells, stromal fibroblasts, or inflammatory cells can release these growth factors from the ECM, thus fostering tumor cell proliferation and migration.

Angiogenesis

Continued growth of solid tumors depends absolutely on an adequate blood supply to provide oxygen and nutrients to tumor cells. Without the development of new blood vessels, a process termed *angiogenesis* (see Chapter 2), tumors are limited to a maximum diameter of 1 to 2 mm. At some point during tumor development, an *angiogenic switch* occurs that allows tumor cells to induce and sustain new tumor vasculature. Angiogenesis is a complex process involving recruitment of endothelial cells from preexisting blood vessels, endothelial cell proliferation, directed migration of endothelial cells through the ECM, and maturation and differentiation of the capillary sprout. Angiogenesis is controlled by the balance between a plethora of angiogenesis-stimulating and angiogenesis-inhibiting factors. Tumors initiate angiogenesis by producing angiogenic factors, such as vascular endothelial growth factor (VEGF), or by downregulating production of antiangiogenic factors, such as thrombospondin. In addition, angiogenic and antiangiogenic factors bound to ECM components within the stroma can be released and activated by tumor protease activity. VEGF and fibroblast growth factors (FGFs) are among the most potent angiogenic factors produced by tumors. The tumor blood vessels that develop in response to angiogenic signals are usually more dilated, more tortuous, and more permeable (leaky) than normal blood vessels (Fig. 6-22).

In addition to supplying nutrients, tumor vasculature plays other roles in tumor development. Vessel leakiness allows perivascular deposition of a fibrin network that promotes formation of collagenous tumor stroma. The endothelial cells of tumor blood vessels produce growth factors, such as PDGF and interleukin-1 (IL-1), that stimulate tumor cell proliferation. Moreover, without access to the circulatory system, tumors cannot metastasize. Because solid tumor growth depends absolutely on an adequate blood supply, therapeutic strategies to inhibit angiogenesis have been developed; however, the clinical results using antiangiogenic agents have thus far been disappointing.

The development of lymphatic vasculature in tumors, termed *lymphangiogenesis*, shares many features with tumor angiogenesis. Tumor-associated lymphatic vessels sprout from preexisting lymphatic vessels in response to tumor-secreted factors such as VEGF. Tumor-associated lymphatic vessels are essential for metastasis of solid tumors to regional lymph nodes. In tumors of human beings, there is a strong correlation between the levels of VEGF expression and lymphatic metastasis; and in genetically engineered mice that do not express VEGF, lymphatic metastases do not occur.

Inflammation

Many tumors are heavily infiltrated with neutrophils, eosinophils, mast cells, lymphocytes, histiocytes, or a combination of these cells.

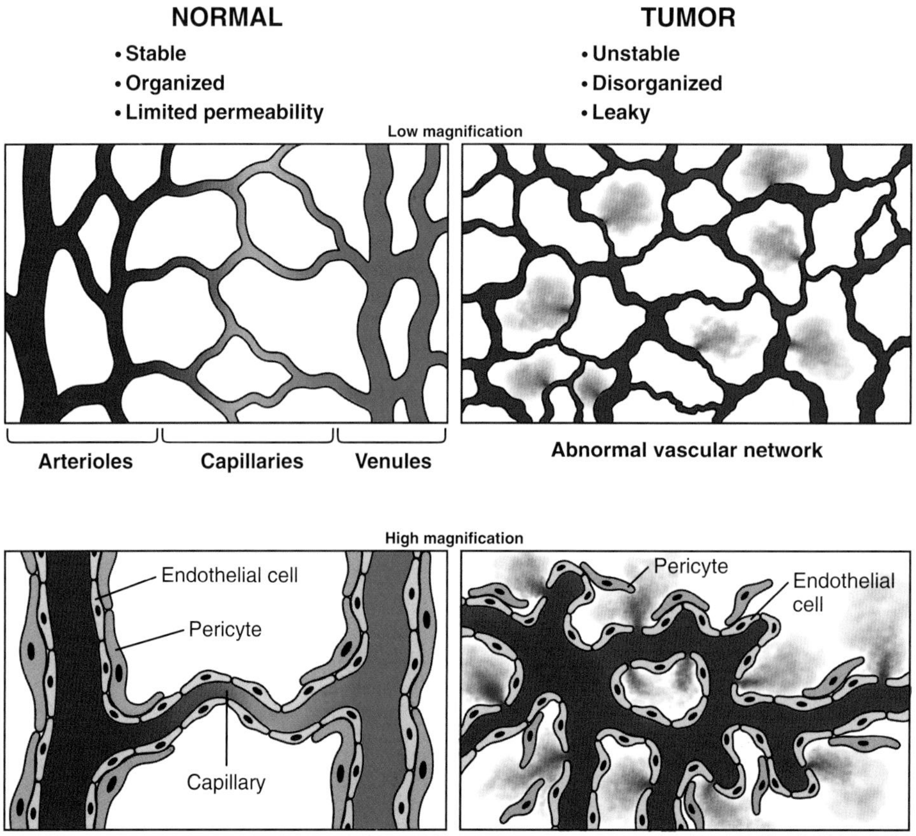

Figure 6-22 Tumor Angiogenesis. Compared with normal vessels *(left panels)*, tumor vessels are tortuous and irregularly shaped *(right panels)*. Arterioles, capillaries, and venules are clearly distinguishable in normal vasculature; in tumors, vessels are disorganized, and specific vessel types cannot be identified. In contrast to the stable vascular network of normal tissue, the networks formed by tumor vessels are unstable and leaky. Thus both the structure and function of tumor vasculature are abnormal.

Inflammatory cells are attracted to tumors by chemokines and cytokines released by tumor cells. Infiltrating inflammatory cells can then recruit additional leukocytes to the tumor. Inflammatory cells serve as a source of prostaglandins, leukotrienes, and reactive oxygen species. In general, inflammation does not appear to protect against tumors. In fact, many chronic inflammatory conditions increase the risk for cancer in affected organs. As an example, the development of vaccine-associated sarcomas in cats is clearly linked to the presence of inflammation at sites of inoculation. Moreover, in human beings, epidemiologic studies suggest that nonsteroidal antiinflammatory drugs (NSAIDs) reduce the incidence of some cancers.

Tumor Immunity (see Essential Concept 6-3)

Immunosurveillance

The vertebrate immune system evolved for the primary purpose of recognizing and destroying infectious organisms and the host cells they infect. However, the immune system also attacks tissue transplanted from genetically dissimilar animals of the same or different species. The same mechanisms used to identify and kill microbially infected cells or foreign cells can be directed against some self-antigens on tumor cells. This process is termed *immunosurveillance*. It is believed that effective immunosurveillance suppresses tumor development and that a failure of immunosurveillance allows tumors to emerge. The immunosurveillance hypothesis is supported by the dramatically increased tumor susceptibility of immunosuppressed human transplant recipients. The inability of these individuals to mount effective antitumor responses apparently allows the emergence of many tumors usually eliminated by immunosurveillance. The presence of lymphocyte and macrophage infiltrates within and around tumors of many types in many species also suggests that tumors can elicit an immune response. Finally, there is abundant experimental evidence that mice can mount an effective immune response against some chemically induced tumors.

Tumor Antigens

Tumor antigens are proteins, glycoproteins, glycolipids, or carbohydrates expressed on the surface of tumor cells (Fig. 6-23). They include both *tumor-specific antigens* restricted to tumor cells and *tumor-associated antigens* present on both tumor cells and normal cells. Tumor antigens can be exploited for both diagnostic and therapeutic purposes. Tumor antigens released into the bloodstream allow noninvasive detection of tumors and monitoring of tumor response to treatment. In combination with sophisticated imaging techniques, antibodies against tumor-restricted antigens can be used to identify the location of tumors and detect metastases. Some tumor antigens can serve as the targets of effective immunosurveillance. However, many tumor antigens are not appropriate therapeutic targets. The antigens may not be restricted solely to tumor cells or they may not elicit a strong cytotoxic response from immune cells.

Some tumor-specific antigens are newly expressed molecules, such as antigens derived from oncogenic viruses, or altered cellular products encoded by mutated genes. In these instances, productive viral infection or gene mutation is restricted to tumor cells and their progeny. Embryonic antigens or *oncofetal antigens*, normally not expressed in adult tissue but reexpressed in tumor tissue, may also behave as tumor antigens. For example, the developmental antigens, carcinoembryonic antigen (CEA) and α-fetoprotein, are

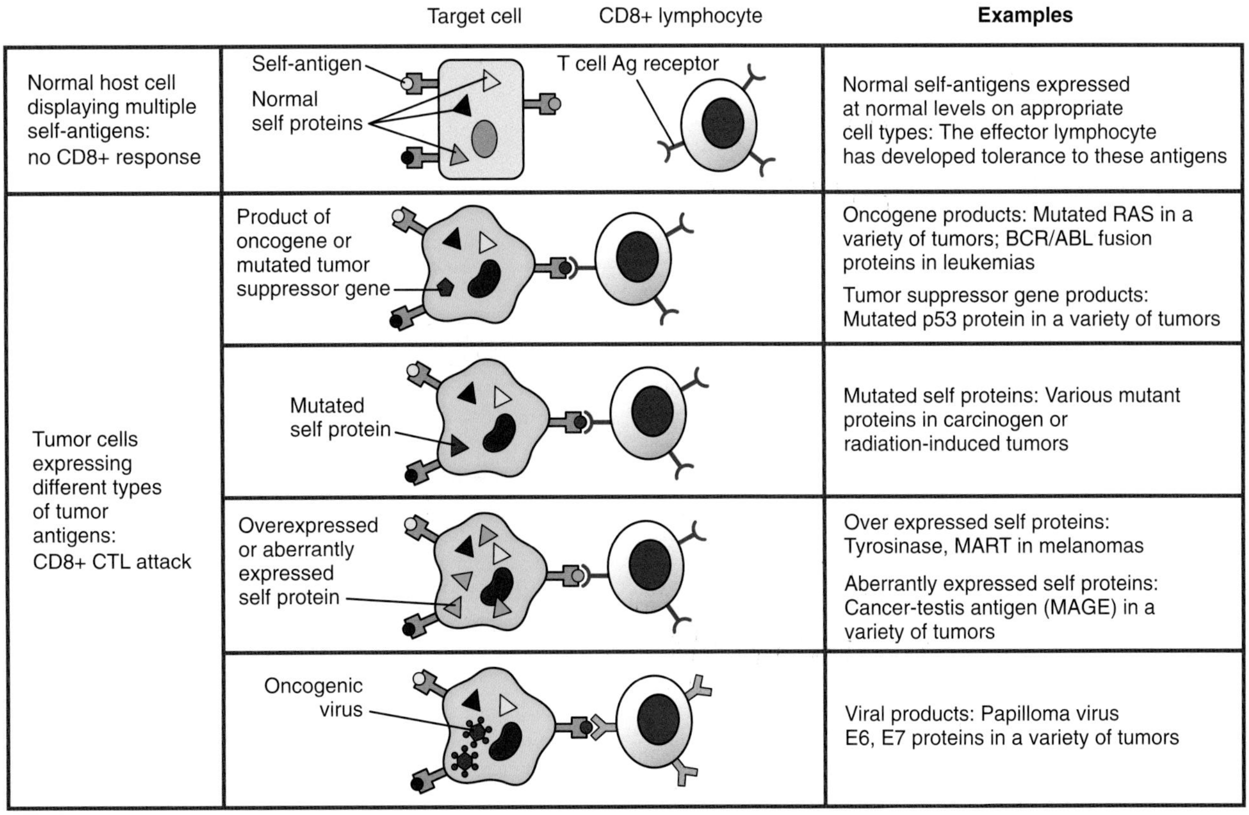

Figure 6-23 **Tumor Antigens Recognized by CD8⁺ T Lymphocytes.** All tumor cell target antigens are presented to cytotoxic CD8⁺ T lymphocytes by major histocompatibility complex class I molecules bound to the surface of the tumor cells. T lymphocyte receptors on the surface of the CD8⁺ lymphocytes recognize tumor antigens in this context but fail to recognize normal self-antigens to which the immune system has been tolerized.

reexpressed in some tumors in a variety of species and may be released into the circulation. Serologic testing for these antigens is widely used to test for recurrence of liver and intestinal tumors in human beings. *Tumor-specific shared antigens* are encoded by genes that have very limited expression in adult tissue but that are expressed by many types of tumor tissue. A striking example of useful tumor-specific shared antigens is the MAGE family of proteins, found in human beings and other animal species. These antigens are not present on the surface of normal adult cells; however, they are expressed by a wide variety of tumor types and are promising candidates for antitumor immunotherapy. *Tissue-specific antigens* are shared by tumors and the normal tissues from which they arise. In some cases these antigens are expressed only at specific stages of differentiation in the normal tissue and are thus termed *differentiation antigens*. When tissue-specific or differentiation antigens are expressed at considerably higher levels on tumor cells than normal cells, they may function much like tumor-specific antigens.

Antitumor Effector Mechanisms

The body may mount a variety of immune responses against tumor antigens, as illustrated in Fig. 6-24. For a more detailed discussion of immune responses, see Chapter 5. The type of immune response and its effectiveness against tumor cells are largely determined by the inherent immune responsiveness of the animal and the characteristics of the tumor antigen under attack. The least specific immune response to tumor cells is carried out by the *innate immune system*, which is responsible for immediate inflammatory responses. The innate immune response is believed to be the first line of defense against cancer cells. Antitumor effectors of the innate immune system, including NK cells and macrophages, do not require antigen-specific priming by dendritic cells. Innate immune responses do not create lasting antitumor immunity.

More specific immune responses are undertaken by the *adaptive immune system*, consisting of both cell-mediated and humoral components. The cell-mediated immune response is believed to mount the most effective antitumor defenses. Any adaptive antitumor immune response requires that tumor antigens be presented to appropriate immune effector cells in a recognizable context. Dendritic cells capture antigens that are secreted by viable tumor cells or released from dying tumor cells. The dendritic cells ingest these antigens, fragment them to a suitable size, link them to class I or class II major histocompatibility complex (MHC) antigens, and present them on the cell surface in association with appropriate costimulatory molecules. A dendritic cell can then interact with many different lymphocytes to prime their response to the specific tumor antigen presented by the dendritic cell. Antigen-activated $CD8^+$ and $CD4^+$ T lymphocytes develop into tumor-specific cytotoxic and T helper (T_H) lymphocytes, respectively, whereas B lymphocytes develop into immunoglobulin-secreting plasma cells. $CD8^+$ lymphocytes recognize tumor antigens in the context of MHC class I antigens, whereas $CD4^+$ cells recognize these antigens only in association with MHC class II molecules.

Natural Killer Cells

Natural killer (NK) cells are lymphocytes that lack many of the usual markers of T or B lymphocytes. NK cells display a variety of receptors, both inhibitory and activating, that recognize MHC molecules and stress-induced ligands on tumor cells. NK cells can kill a wide variety of neoplastic and virally infected cells. Cells that express MHC class I molecules are preferentially spared by NK cells, whereas cells lacking MHC molecules are specifically targeted. When an NK cell recognizes and attaches to its target cell, a well-organized structure, termed an *immunologic synapse*, is rapidly formed at the site of cell-to-cell contact and persists for more than an hour. At this interface the NK cell releases lytic granules containing perforin, a pore-forming protein, and granzymes, which are serine proteases. Perforin mediates the entry of granzymes into the target cell. Once inside the target cell, granzymes initiate both caspase-dependent and caspase-independent apoptosis. This mechanism of cell killing, termed *cytolysis*, is shared with T lymphocytes.

Macrophages

Macrophages are migratory phagocytic cells capable of killing tumor cells by releasing reactive oxygen intermediates, lysosomal enzymes, nitric oxide, and tumor necrosis factor. Their antitumor activity is stimulated by interferon-γ (IFN-γ), which is produced by both T lymphocytes and NK cells. Macrophage-mediated tumor cell killing is independent of MHC antigens, tumor-specific antigens, and the type of transformed cell being targeted, but direct contact between the macrophage and tumor cell is required.

Although macrophages have long been considered to be tumoricidal, recent evidence suggests that some macrophages actually promote tumorigenesis. It has been demonstrated experimentally that tumor-associated macrophages can promote angiogenesis and enhance tumor cell invasion and metastasis. In addition, macrophages may be immunosuppressive, blocking the antitumor activity of NK cells and lymphocytes. Early studies suggest that depleting tumor-associated macrophages may be useful as part of cancer therapy.

T Lymphocytes

Cytotoxic T lymphocytes (CTLs) are the primary effector cells of the adaptive antitumor immune response. Most CTLs are $CD8^+$ T lymphocytes that have been primed by dendritic cells to recognize and engage tumor antigens on the surface of tumor cells. Tumor cells are then killed by cytolysis. $CD4^+$ T_H lymphocytes enhance the function of $CD8^+$ CTLs and antigen-producing B lymphocytes by secreting cytokines, such as IL-2 and IFN-γ, which stimulate $CD8^+$ T lymphocyte proliferation and differentiation.

There is, however, one T cell population, composed of *regulatory T cells* (T reg), which actually protects tumors against attack by other immune cells. T reg cells accumulate in tumors, where they induce tolerance to tumor tissue. Tolerance is established via a complex set of interactions with other lymphocyte types, macrophages, and dendritic cells. These interactions are mediated by both soluble factors and cell-cell contact. In human beings, administration of antibodies that block the immunosuppressive effects of suppressor T cells allows a robust antitumor CTL response against melanoma.

B Lymphocytes

Many tumor antigens can incite both cell-mediated and humoral immune responses. Antibody-producing *B lymphocytes* mediate the humoral immune response to tumors. Antibodies that recognize tumor antigens kill tumor cells by binding to the cells and activating a local complement cascade (see Chapters 3 and 5). Activation of the complement cascade generates a *membrane attack complex* (MAC) that induces loss of tumor cell membrane integrity and rapid cell death with the morphologic hallmarks of necrosis. In addition, antitumor antibodies may be bound by their constant regions to NK cells or macrophages, leaving the variable regions of the immunoglobulins available for specific recognition of tumor antigens. This arrangement allows the effector immune cells to recognize, attach to, and kill tumor cells by the mechanism of *antibody-dependent cell-mediated cytotoxicity (ADCC)*.

<table>
<tr><th>Effector Cell</th><th></th><th>Activation/ Assistance</th><th>Target</th><th>Mode of Attack</th></tr>
<tr><td>NK cell</td><td>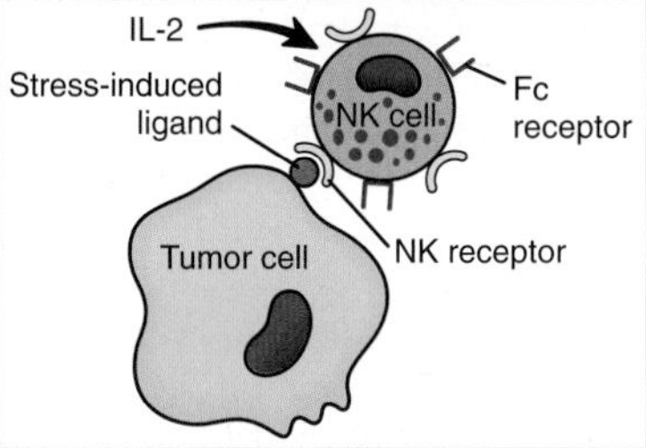
</td><td>IL-2</td><td>Stress-induced ligand</td><td>Immunologic synapse (perforin/granzymes)</td></tr>
<tr><td>NK cell (ADCC)</td><td>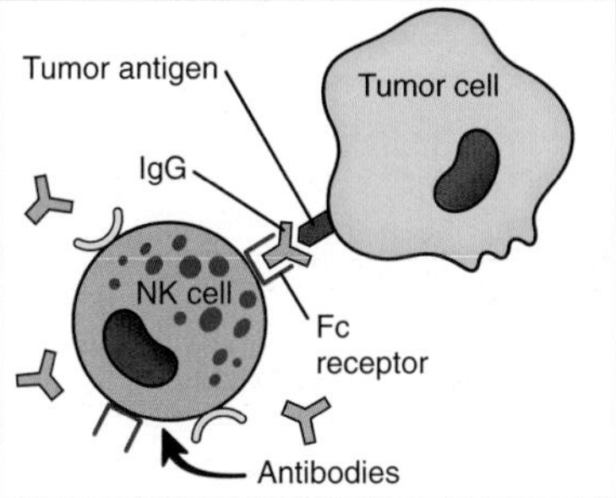
</td><td>Antibodies produced by B lymphocytes</td><td>Tumor antigen</td><td>Immunologic synapse (perforin/granzymes)</td></tr>
<tr><td>Macrophage</td><td>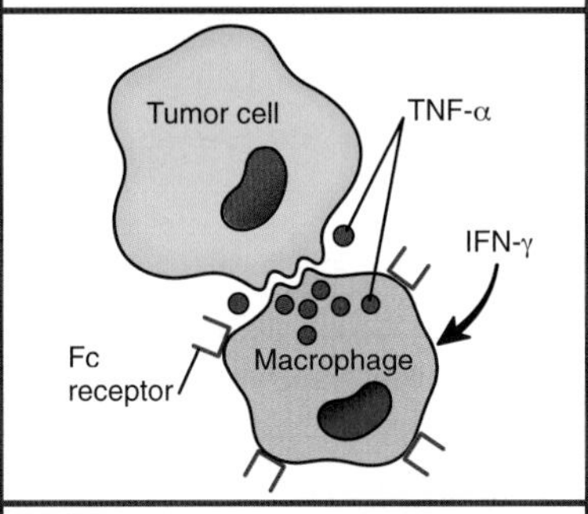
</td><td>IFN-γ activation</td><td>Tumor cell membrane</td><td>TNF-α, reactive oxygen species, nitric oxide, lysosomal enzymes</td></tr>
<tr><td>Macrophage (ADCC)</td><td>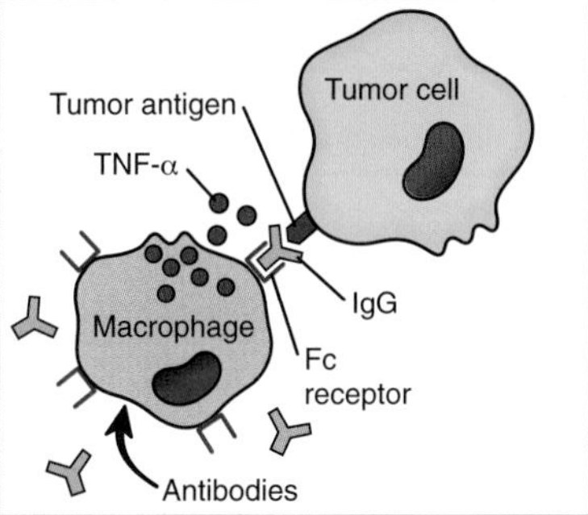
</td><td>Antibodies produced by B lymphocytes</td><td>Tumor antigen</td><td>TNF-α, reactive oxygen species, nitric oxide, lysosomal enzymes</td></tr>
<tr><td>T lymphocyte (CTL)</td><td>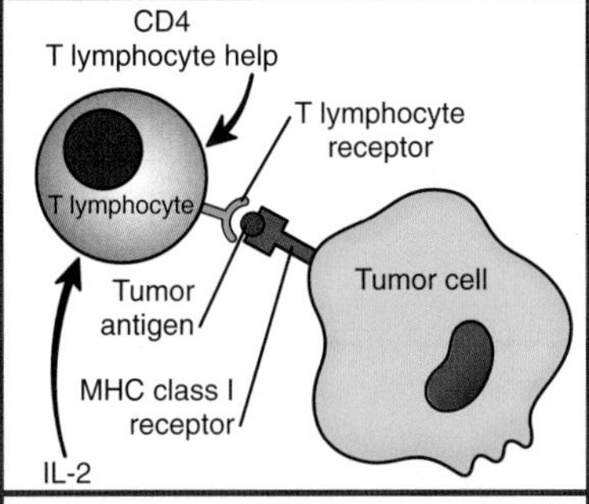
</td><td>Help by CD4 T lymphocyte, IL-2 activation</td><td>Tumor antigen presented in MHC class I context</td><td>Immunologic synapse (perforin/granzymes)</td></tr>
<tr><td>B lymphocyte</td><td>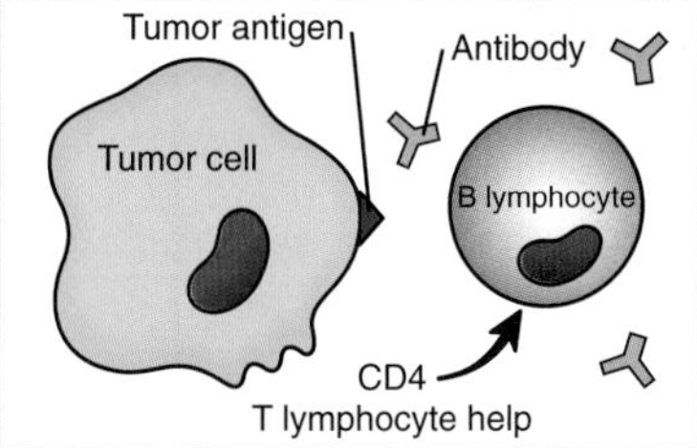
</td><td>Help by CD4 T lymphocyte</td><td>Tumor antigen</td><td>Membrane-attack complex (activated complement)</td></tr>
</table>

Figure 6-24 **Cells Involved in Immunosurveillance Against Tumors.** Antitumor responses involve a variety of immune cells, including natural killer (NK) cells, macrophages, and T and B lymphocytes. NK cells and macrophages can attack tumor cells directly or via the mechanism of antibody-dependent cell-mediated cytotoxicity (ADCC). In ADCC, macrophages and NK cells bind tumor-specific antibodies by their constant regions, allowing the variable regions of the antibodies to interact with specific tumor antigens. Most cytotoxic T lymphocytes (CTL) are $CD8^+$ lymphocytes.

Evasion of the Immune Response

Many tumors are able to evade immunosurveillance, using one or more of mechanisms illustrated in Fig. 6-25 and discussed in the following sections.

Altered Major Histocompatibility Complex Expression

CTLs recognize tumor antigens only on tumor cells that display the antigens in the context of MHC class I molecules. Thus tumor cells that lose or downregulate expression of class I MHC antigens may evade detection and have a distinct selective advantage. However, tumors that fail to express class I antigens are also more susceptible to NK cell killing. Tumors may also downregulate expression of class II MHC antigens. Class II antigens are required for activation of T_H lymphocytes that stimulate CTL differentiation, and loss of these antigens prevents the generation of an optimal antitumor CTL response.

Antigen Masking

Tumors may become invisible to the immune system by losing or masking their tumor antigens. The outgrowth of clonal tumor variants that do not express tumor antigens is favored during tumor evolution. Tumor antigens on the cell surface may be hidden from the immune system if they are complexed with glycocalyx molecules, fibrin, or even antibodies. Thus some humoral responses to tumor antigens may actually promote tumor survival by protecting tumor antigens from recognition by CTLs.

Tolerance

Although the immune system responds vigorously to nonself-antigens, it is tolerant to self-antigens. Thus tumor antigens shared with normal tissue usually are not able to evoke an immune response because the body has already been "tolerized" to the antigen. If nonself-antigens are presented in the absence of costimulatory molecules required for effective T lymphocyte activation, that is, in a "tolerogenic" context, tolerance may also result. Moreover, it has recently been shown that T reg cells in tumors can actively promote tolerance to tumor tissue.

Immunosuppression

Tumor cells or their secretory products may be immunosuppressive. Many tumors produce TGF-α, which inhibits the proliferation and function of lymphocytes and macrophages. Tumors may also produce Fas ligand. Fas ligand expressed by tumor cells binds to Fas receptors on nearby T lymphocytes and triggers their apoptosis. By this

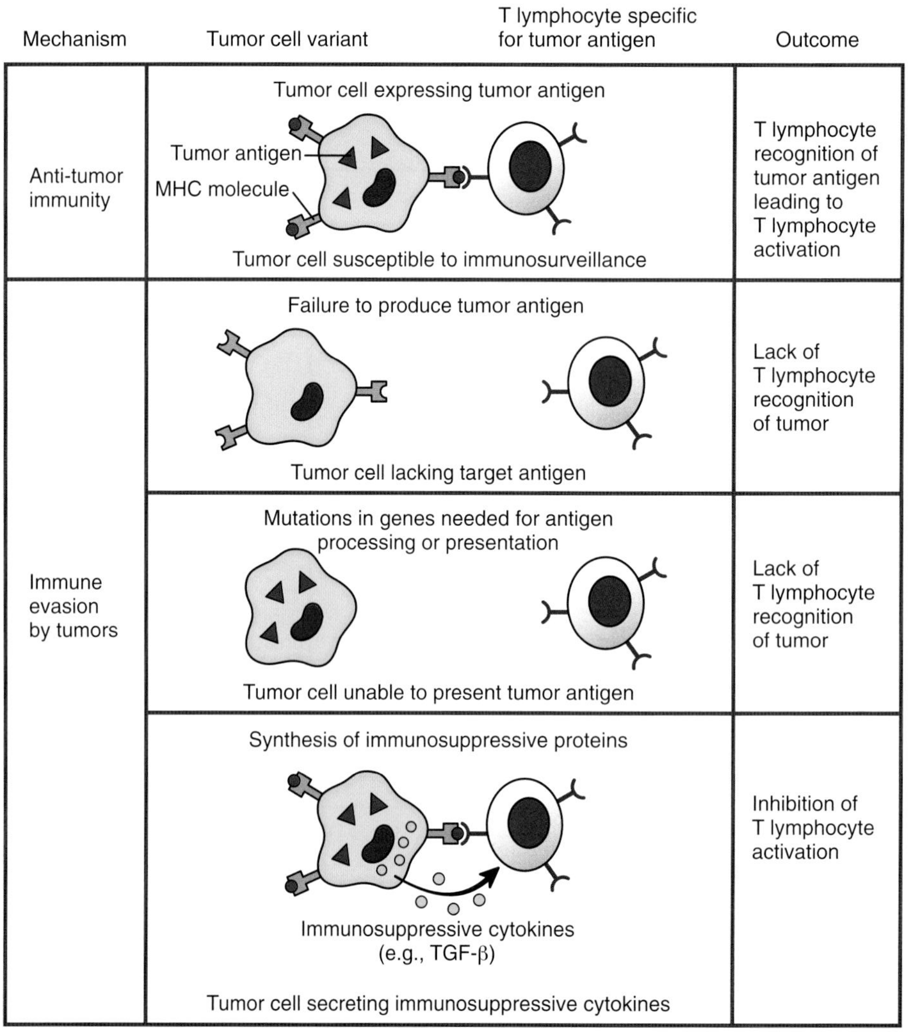

Figure 6-25 **Mechanisms by Which Tumors Evade the Immune System.** Tumors employ a variety of mechanisms to evade attack by cytolytic T lymphocytes. Tumor cells may cease expressing tumor antigens, fail to appropriately process these antigens, or lack expression of the major histocompatibility antigen necessary to present tumor cell antigens. Tumor cells may also secrete cytokines such as transforming growth factor-β (TGF-β) that inhibit cytolytic T lymphocyte activation.

mechanism, T lymphocyte clones that recognize a tumor may be specifically deleted, thus protecting the tumor from attack. Finally, tumor cells may release tumor antigens into the circulation that form immune complexes with antibodies, and these immune complexes may be immunosuppressive. In addition, tumor-associated macrophages and T reg cells have immunosuppressive functions that protect the tumor from immune attack.

Tumor Immunotherapy

The fact that an antitumor immune response attacks only the tumor cells and not normal tissue makes it an attractive candidate as a therapeutic modality. Moreover, effective immunotherapy would reduce or eliminate the need to use highly cytotoxic chemotherapeutic agents that indiscriminately target both normal and neoplastic dividing cells and thus cause significant morbidity and mortality in cancer patients. In general, immunotherapeutic strategies are aimed at (1) providing the patient with mature effector cells or antibodies that recognize and destroy tumors (passive immunotherapy) or (2) stimulating the immune response of the animal against the tumor (active immunotherapy).

Administration of monoclonal antibodies raised against tumor antigens generates rapid but short-lived passive tumor immunity. However, the coupling of toxins to monoclonal antibodies may allow targeted delivery of therapeutic agents to tumor cells. Monoclonal antibodies raised in other species have limited usefulness, because the tumor host may develop an immune response to these antibodies that abrogates their effectiveness. Antitumor lymphocytes are generated by removing lymphocytes from the human patient's blood or tumor and expanding them in vitro by incubation with IL-2; these autologous immune cells are then readministered to the patient.

Many approaches to stimulate the active immunity of human patients against their tumors have been attempted, including vaccination with tumor cells or tumor antigens to generate antitumor CTLs, administration of cytokines to increase effector cell number and function, and nonspecific stimulation of the immune system by treatment with proinflammatory substances, such as bacterial products. These approaches have proved particularly effective against malignant melanomas. A melanoma vaccine for dogs stimulates an immune response against human tyrosinase; antibodies against the human protein are formed that then attack canine melanocytes.

As mentioned earlier, blocking the activity of tumor-associated macrophages and T reg cells is a new and promising approach to tumor immunotherapy.

Tumor Dissemination (Essential Concept 6-4)

The Significance of Metastasis

Primary tumors are not usually the proximate cause of death for the animal or human cancer patient. Instead death is usually due to tumor metastasis to distant organs and interference with critical bodily functions. For example, widespread metastases to the lung from an osteosarcoma can result in death or euthanasia due to respiratory distress caused by interference with oxygen exchange. Indeed, it has been estimated that, in human beings, tumor metastasis is responsible for approximately 90% of cancer mortality from solid tumors. Fortunately, metastasis is a rather inefficient process. Very few cells within the primary tumor are capable of entering blood or lymphatic vessels, only a few of the circulating cells are able to exit vessels, and only a few of those that exit the vessels are able to survive at new sites within the body. In some cases, metastatic cancer cells enter a state of *dormancy* during which metastatic cells grow only slowly or not at all. However, dormant cancer cells can resume their growth at a later date, leading to cancer recurrence, sometimes after prolonged periods of remission. The mechanisms by which dormancy is established and the means by which dormant cancer cells are reactivated remain poorly understood.

ESSENTIAL CONCEPT 6-4 Tumor Dissemination

A tumor first grows locally, but acquisition of additional genetic and epigenetic changes allows the tumor to metastasize. Metastasis is responsible for most cancer mortality. Metastasis may occur through lymphatic vessels, via blood vessels, or by direct dissemination throughout a body cavity. To metastasize, tumor cells must escape the primary tumor mass through loss of intercellular attachments and acquisition of migratory and invasive capabilities. To avoid detection and elimination, tumor cells must also escape immunosurveillance. Once present at a distant site, tumor cells must be able to exit vessels and establish themselves in the new tissue.

Mechanisms of Tumor Invasion and Metastasis

A tumor's metastatic potential reflects the cumulative effect of a wide variety of genetic and epigenetic changes involving tumor cell adhesion, motility, and protease production.

Adhesion

As a first event in invasion and metastasis, tumor cells must detach from the main tumor mass, penetrate the basement membrane, and enter the ECM. For cells to separate from each other, intercellular adhesion structures, including desmosomes and adherens junctions, must be dismantled. In many tumor cells of epithelial origin, this process is due to loss of cadherins or catenins, molecules that are essential structural elements of intercellular junctions. At the same time that tumor cells detach from each other, they must also establish contacts with ECM elements within the tumor stroma. Integrins and other specific receptors on tumor cell membranes recognize and bind to a variety of ECM components such as fibronectin, laminin, collagen, and vitronectin. During invasion and metastasis, carcinoma cells often express increased numbers of these receptors. Tumor cells are also able to modulate the types and distribution of ECM receptors that they express, allowing them to adapt to the ECM of different microenvironments.

Migration

At many points during invasion and metastasis, tumor cells migrate actively. This migration is mediated by alterations in the cytoskeleton and the cellular adhesion structures to which the cytoskeletal components are anchored. Tumor cell migration is stimulated by autocrine growth factors, such as hepatocyte growth factor (HGF), also called "scatter factor," and by cleavage products of ECM components, including fragments of collagen.

Stromal Invasion

Epithelial cells normally rest on a specialized extracellular structure called the basement membrane, to which they are firmly attached by hemidesmosomes (see Figs. 1-5 and 1-6). In benign epithelial tumors, the basement membrane remains intact. In contrast, the neoplastic epithelial cells of malignant tumors actively degrade basement membrane and ECM components by increasing the net protease activity in their vicinity (Fig. 6-26). This allows them to penetrate the basement membrane and invade surrounding tissue. Net protease activity is determined by a variety of interacting factors, including the rate of protease synthesis and activation and

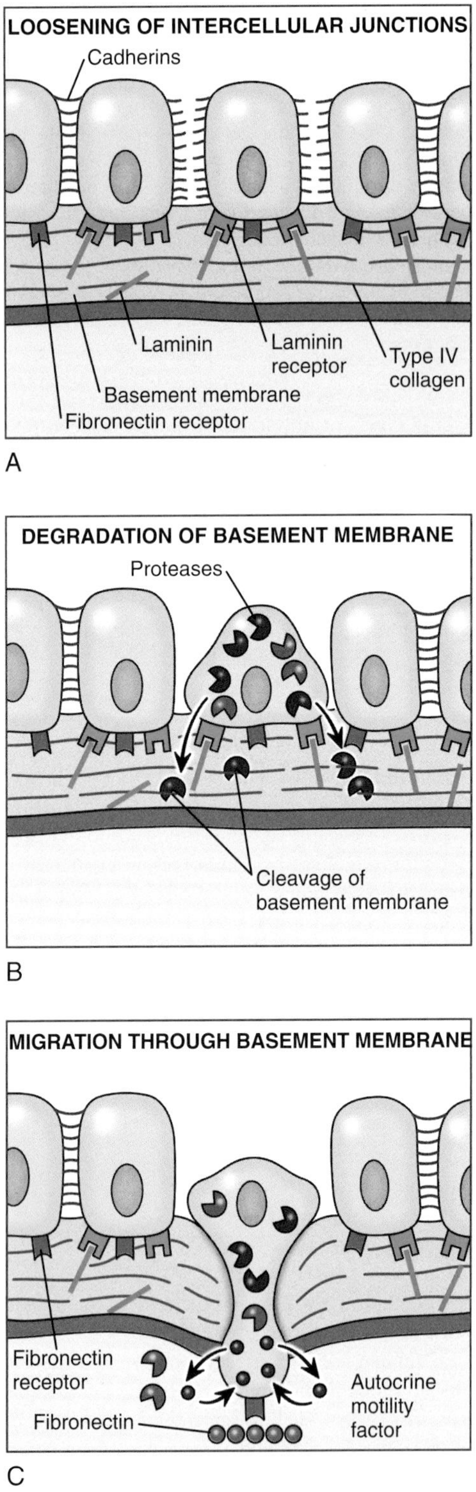

Figure 6-26 **Tumor Cell Invasion of Epithelial Basement Membrane.** **A,** Tumor cells detach from one another because of dissolution of intercellular junctions. **B,** Proteolytic enzymes, such as type IV collagenase and urokinase, secreted by tumor cells degrade the basement membrane. **C,** With degradation of the basement membrane, tumor cells are able to migrate into underlying tissue. Migration is enhanced by altered expression of receptors for extracellular matrix components on tumor cells and secretion of autocrine motility factors.

the rate at which protease inhibitors are produced. Proteases and antiproteases may be produced and activated by the tumor cells themselves, or tumor cells may induce nonneoplastic stromal cells to produce these enzymes. Proteases implicated in promoting tumor metastasis include matrix metalloproteinases, such as type IV collagenase, and urokinase, a serine protease.

Epithelial-Mesenchymal Transition

As they progress, some carcinomas undergo a change termed *epithelial-mesenchymal transition* (EMT). EMT is characterized by loss of intercellular adhesion structures, enhanced expression of proteases, acquisition of migratory capabilities, reduced expression of epithelial cytokeratins, and de novo expression of vimentin, a mesenchymal cell marker. During EMT, sessile neoplastic cells are transformed into motile fibroblast-like cells. Cells that have undergone EMT are typically spindle shaped and express little or no E-cadherin, a component of adherens junctions. EMT allows neoplastic epithelial cells to dissociate and migrate, thus fostering local invasion and distant metastasis. Most drivers of EMT are transcription factors, proteins that determine the timing and levels of DNA transcription into RNA. These transcription factors coordinate the expression of genes involved in cellular adhesion, migration, and protease production.

Intravasation

Cancer cells invade blood or lymphatic vessels by penetrating endothelial basement membranes and passing between or through endothelial cells into the vessel lumen (Fig. 6-27). This process is termed *intravasation*. Tumor cells are attracted to vessels by chemotactic factors produced by multiple cell types and migrate through the ECM with the aid of tumor-derived proteases. Tumor cell migration and vessel penetration are facilitated by tumor-associated macrophages that accompany the invading tumor cells.

Tumor Emboli

Once inside a lymphatic or blood vessel, tumor cells tend to clump together to form small emboli held together by shared adhesion molecules. While in the vessels, tumor cells may be recognized and attacked by host lymphocytes or may be surrounded by platelets. Interestingly, platelets may actually protect the tumor embolus from immune-mediated destruction, thereby increasing the potential for metastasis.

Extravasation

Intravascular tumor cells leave vessels by the process of *extravasation*. The site at which tumor cells exit the blood vascular or lymphatic system is largely determined by the ability of tumor cells to interact with adhesion molecules on endothelial cells. Once attached to vascular endothelium, tumor cells pass between or through endothelial cells and penetrate the basement membrane to enter the ECM, thus establishing a metastatic site. Metastatic sites must provide a suitable microenvironment for tumor cell growth, or metastatic tumor cells will not become established. Some tumors preferentially metastasize to specific sites; for example, prostate carcinomas in both human beings and dogs frequently spread to bone (Fig. 6-28).

Pathways of Tumor Metastasis

Lymphatic Spread

Most carcinomas and some sarcomas metastasize via the lymphatic system. The pattern of lymph node involvement is usually dictated by preexisting routes of normal lymphatic drainage. The lymph nodes closest to the tumor are usually affected first and develop the

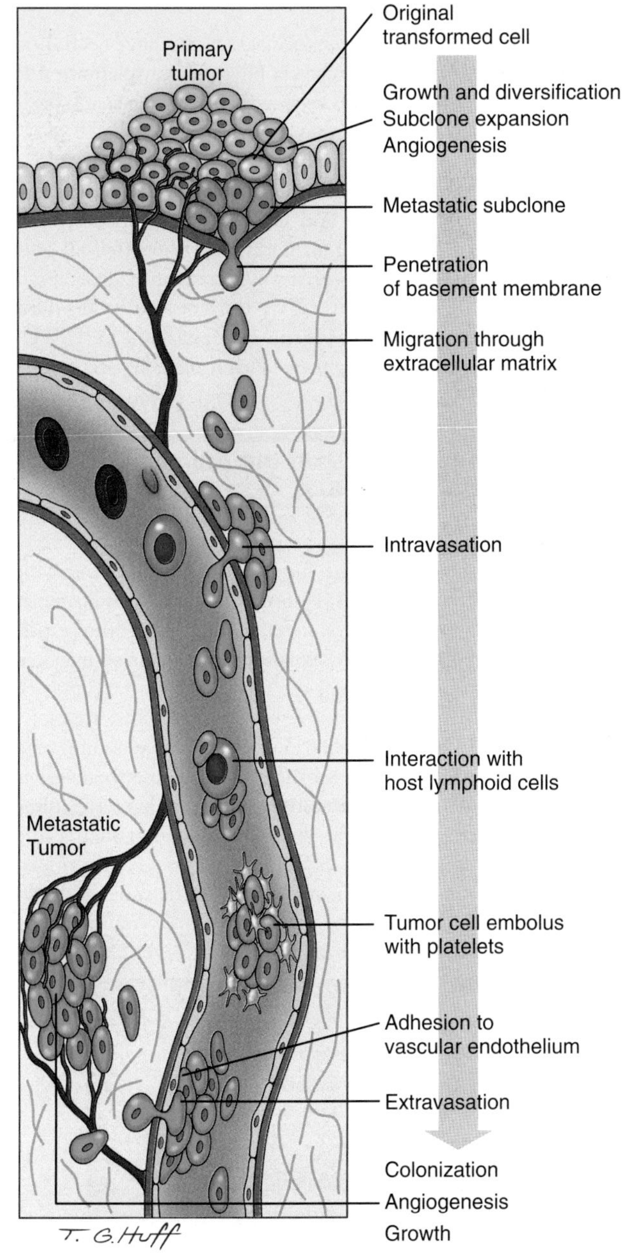

Figure 6-27 The Metastatic Cascade. Although this figure illustrates the sequential steps in the hematogenous spread of an epithelial tumor, similar steps occur during lymphatic spread. Metastasis is a complex process involving multiple steps and interactions of tumor cells with many different normal cell and tissue types. Failure at any point in the metastatic process prevents tumor spread; thus metastasis is usually an inefficient process.

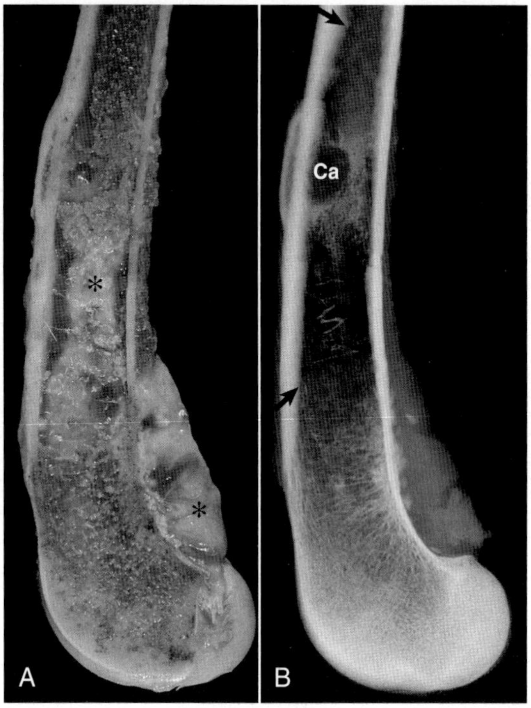

Figure 6-28 Prostate Carcinoma, Metastasis, Femur, Dog. A, The gross photograph of a sectioned femur reveals metastatic prostate carcinoma (*). B, The radiograph illustrates an osteolytic bone metastasis (*Ca*). In the region between the arrows, extensive proliferation of new bone has occurred in response to the tumor. (Modified from Rosol TJ, Tannehill-Gregg SH, LeRoy BE, et al: Animal models of bone metastasis. In Keller ET, Chung LWK, editors: *Cancer treatment and research*, Boston, 2004, Kluwer Academic Publishers.)

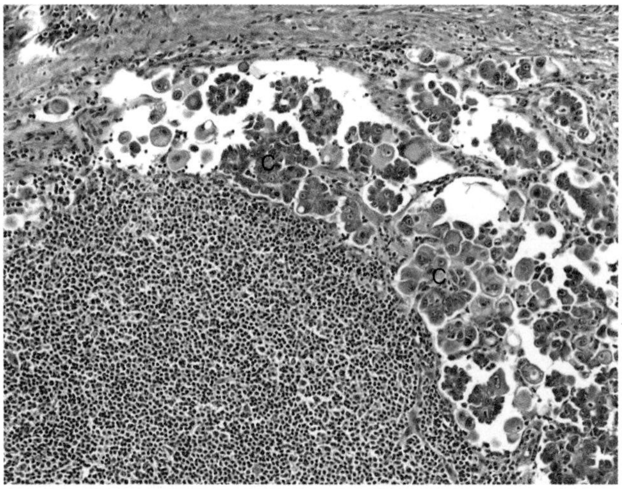

Figure 6-29 Mammary Carcinoma, Metastatic, Regional Lymph Node, Dog. Mammary carcinoma cells (*C*) are present in the subcapsular sinus of a lymph node that drains the affected mammary gland. Tumor cells spreading via lymphatic vessels typically lodge first at this location in lymph nodes draining the tumor site. H&E stain. (Courtesy College of Veterinary Medicine, The University of Tennessee.)

largest metastatic tumor masses (Fig. 6-29). For example, adenocarcinomas of the intestine usually metastasize first to the mesenteric lymph nodes and later to other lymph nodes within and outside the abdominal cavity. For many years it was assumed that cancers spread in a stepwise manner from the primary site to regional lymph nodes, then to distant sites such as the lung, and that regional lymph nodes acted as a mechanical barrier to the spread of cancer. Based on this assumption, it was believed that removal of all affected regional lymph nodes would prevent further spread of the tumor. However, regional lymph nodes may be bypassed as a result of natural, tumor-related, or treatment-induced anomalies in lymphatic drainage, resulting in distant metastases before the development of regional metastases. More recent studies suggest that lymphatic spread does not occur in an orderly fashion and that metastasis to regional lymph nodes indicates that systemic spread has likely already occurred.

Hematogenous Spread

Because lymphatic vessels connect with the vascular system, the distinction between lymphatic and hematogenous spread is somewhat artificial. However, sarcomas do tend to use the hematogenous route of spread more frequently than carcinomas. Tumors generally invade veins rather than arteries because venous walls are much thinner and easier to penetrate than arterial walls. Tumor cells that enter veins ultimately reach the vena cava, pass through the heart, and lodge in capillary beds, particularly in the lungs (Fig. 6-30). Tumors that invade portal vessels tend to lodge in the liver. Some tumors have a notable predilection for invading veins; for example, pheochromocytomas, particularly those arising from the right adrenal gland, frequently invade the adjacent caudal vena cava (see Figs. 12-40 and 12-41).

Transcoelomic Spread

When cancers arise on the surface of an abdominal or thoracic structure, they encounter few anatomic barriers to spread. Thus mesotheliomas may be confined to the peritoneal, pericardial, or pleural cavities, but the tumor cells within these cavities readily spread to cover visceral and parietal surfaces. In both human beings and dogs, ovarian and pancreatic adenocarcinomas preferentially spread transcoelomically, resulting in multiple tumor masses throughout the abdomen, a condition termed *carcinomatosis* (Fig. 6-31). Even in the absence of invasion into the underlying organs, tumors such as mesotheliomas and ovarian and pancreatic adenocarcinomas are extremely difficult to treat and are generally fatal.

Metastasis Suppression

Expression of some gene products in tumor cells appears to suppress metastasis. For example, sustained expression of E-cadherin, a transmembrane protein that forms part of adherens junctions, maintains adherence between tumor cells and prevents them from dissociating to invade surrounding tissues and lymphatic vessels. The E-cadherin gene is thus a candidate metastasis suppressor gene. Determining the expression levels of metastasis suppressor genes in tumors may provide valuable prognostic information. Moreover, drug-induced reactivation of metastasis suppressor genes is a potentially valuable therapeutic strategy.

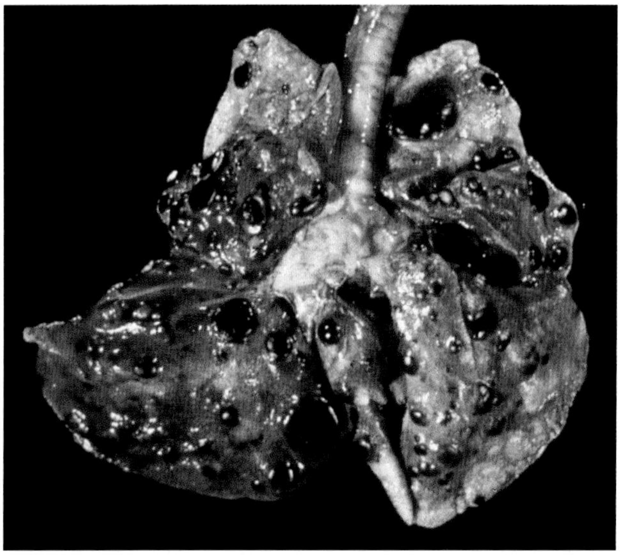

Figure 6-30 Melanoma, Metastatic, Lung, Dog. The multifocal (embolic) distribution of tumor nodules throughout the lung is characteristic of hematogenous metastasis. (Courtesy College of Veterinary Medicine, The University of Tennessee.)

Transmissible Tumors

A few tumors, termed *clonally transmissible cancers*, have been shown to spread beyond the original host via physical transplantation following direct physical contact between animals of the same species. Examples include the transmissible venereal tumor (TVT) of dogs and devil facial tumor disease (DFTD) of Tasmanian devils. In these syndromes, tumors isolated from multiple affected animals have essentially identical cytologic and genetic characteristics, which differ from those of the hosts. This finding indicates that all of the tumors arose from a single tumor that was subsequently disseminated to multiple animal hosts. Because TVT transmission occurs during mating, the tumors are found on the genitalia or face. DFTD is transmitted during territorial fighting; thus it tends to occur on the head and neck.

Systemic Clinical Effects on the Animal (see Essential Concept 6-3)

Direct Effects

Tumors directly compromise the function of the organs in which they arise by replacing (effacing) normal tissue and by disrupting normal anatomic relationships of affected organs. In both the tissue of origin and in metastatic sites, expanding tumor tissue may compress surrounding normal tissue or the blood vessels that supply this tissue, resulting in pressure atrophy or necrosis. This situation is particularly a problem in the calvarium, where an expanding tumor will quickly compress and damage the brain, because the overlying bone cannot expand to accommodate the growth of the tumor. Therefore even benign tumors arising in the brain that are not surgically accessible may prove fatal. Seizure activity is a common manifestation of brain tumors. Tumor invasion into the wall of a hollow

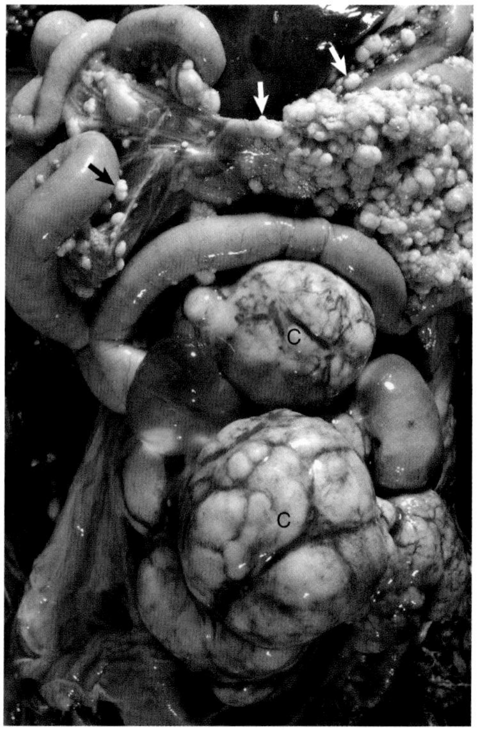

Figure 6-31 Ovarian Carcinoma, Coelomic Cavity, Chicken. This figure illustrates transcoelomic spread of an ovarian carcinoma. The primary tumor (*C*) has given rise to multiple tumor nodules (*arrows*) throughout the coelomic cavity. This condition is termed "carcinomatosis." (Courtesy College of Veterinary Medicine, The University of Tennessee.)

organ, such as the stomach, may create an obstruction or lead to organ rupture. Tumors may also erode blood vessel walls, causing acute hemorrhage, or extend into blood vessels, creating tumor emboli that may produce infarcts or metastases at distant sites.

Paraneoplastic Effects

In addition to the direct effects discussed earlier, tumors may cause a variety of systemic clinical signs termed *paraneoplastic syndromes*. Paraneoplastic disorders are indirect and usually remote effects caused by tumor cell products rather than by the "mass effect" of the primary tumor or its metastases. Approximately 75% of human cancer patients develop paraneoplastic syndromes, but the incidence in veterinary cancer patients is unknown. These syndromes are best described for the dog, although some affecting the cat and the horse have also been reported (E-Table 6-1). Recognition of paraneoplastic syndromes is important because (1) these syndromes may facilitate early tumor diagnosis if they arise in the initial stages of tumor development, (2) treatment of metabolic abnormalities associated with paraneoplastic syndromes may be required to ensure effective cancer management, and (3) the severity of paraneoplastic abnormalities may reflect the tumor burden; thus monitoring such abnormalities may be useful in determining tumor response to therapy and identifying tumor recurrence or spread.

Cachexia

Many animals with cancer show notable weight loss and debility, a condition referred to as *cachexia*. In cancer cachexia, both muscle and fat are lost, whereas in simple starvation fat is lost preferentially. The compensatory decrease in basal metabolic rate seen with starvation is not observed in cancer cachexia. Extra calories do not prevent or reverse the catabolic state of cancer cachexia. The etiology of cancer cachexia is complex. Cancer cachexia is due, in part, to cytokines and hormones, particularly TNF-α (also known as cachectin), IL-1, IL-6, and prostaglandins, which cause anorexia and debilitation. Other contributing factors include impaired digestion, nutritional demands of tumor tissue, nutrient loss in cancer-related effusions or exudates, and a variety of metabolic and endocrine derangements.

Endocrinopathies

Endocrine Tumors. A functioning endocrine tumor produces the hormonal products of the tissue of origin. For example, thyroid follicular tumors produce thyroid hormone. In endocrine glands with more than one cell type, such as the pancreatic islet, the anterior pituitary, the thyroid, and the adrenal, generally only a single cell type becomes neoplastic. Thus a pancreatic islet cell adenoma typically produces only a single hormone, such as insulin, glucagon, gastrin, or somatostatin, and not a combination of hormones. A functional tumor overproduces a hormone as the consequence of increased numbers of hormone-secreting tumor cells, increased production of hormone by individual neoplastic cells, or both.

Several clinically significant endocrinopathies occur commonly in veterinary medicine, and their effects and clinical presentations depend on the hormones being produced. Thyroid follicular adenomas in cats cause a syndrome of hyperthyroidism characterized by an increased metabolic rate. Functioning tumors of the pancreatic islet β-cells result in hyperinsulinemia with subsequent hypoglycemia. Because of the absolute dependence of the nervous system on glucose for energy, clinical signs of hypoglycemia are mostly neurologic and may include lethargy, incoordination, muscle weakness, and seizures. Profound hypoglycemia of unknown origin may also occur with other tumor types.

Nonendocrine Tumors. A variety of nonendocrine neoplasms may also produce hormonally active substances not normally found in the tissue of tumor origin. This relationship is termed *ectopic hormone production*. The hormone produced may be identical to the normal hormone, may be a modified form of the normal hormone, or may be the product of a gene that encodes a protein related to but not identical with the true hormone. In veterinary medicine the most common example of ectopic hormone production is secretion of parathyroid hormone–related peptide (PTHrP) by tumor cells, resulting in humoral hypercalcemia of malignancy. In dogs, *humoral hypercalcemia of malignancy* is seen most frequently with adenocarcinoma of the anal sac (≈90% of cases), lymphoma (≈20% of cases), and multiple myeloma (≈15% of cases). Hypercalcemia of malignancy in cats appears to be relatively rare. Like parathyroid hormone, PTHrP increases serum calcium level by increasing calcium release from bones, enhancing reabsorption of calcium in the kidneys, and stimulating absorption of calcium in the intestine. Clinical signs of hypercalcemia include muscle weakness, cardiac arrhythmia, anorexia, vomiting, and renal failure. Hypercalcemia and associated clinical signs may also occur as a result of excess production of parathyroid hormone by a parathyroid neoplasm. Hypercalcemia may also be due to tumor metastasis to bone and resultant bone resorption; however, this is not a true paraneoplastic disorder because it is a direct effect of the tumor.

Skeletal Syndromes

Hypertrophic osteopathy is a condition associated with extensive periosteal new bone growth, particularly on the extremities (Fig. 6-32). It is strongly associated with both neoplastic and nonneoplastic space-occupying thoracic lesions. This condition, which is seen in cats, dogs, and horses, presents as symmetric lameness. The cause of hypertrophic osteopathy is not known, although abnormalities of growth hormone production are suspected.

Another skeletal manifestation of neoplasia is *myelofibrosis*. Myelofibrosis results from overgrowth of nonneoplastic fibroblasts in

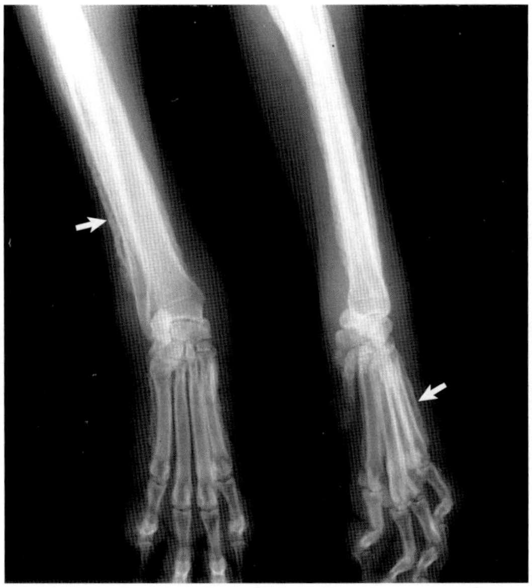

Figure 6-32 **Hypertrophic Osteopathy, Forelimbs, Dog with a Pulmonary Tumor.** On this radiograph the arrows indicate newly deposited bone that is less dense than normal cortical bone. Note that multiple bones on both limbs are affected and that new bone deposits are located primarily in the diaphyseal region of the long bones. (Courtesy Dr. J. Mattoon, College of Veterinary Medicine, The Ohio State University.)

the bone marrow, which impairs normal hematopoiesis and results in cytopenias. It may be associated with a local myeloproliferative disease like lymphoma or with distant tumors. The cause of myelofibrosis is also unknown.

Vascular and Hematologic Syndromes

Nonhematopoietic cancer in animals may result in a variety of vascular and hematologic syndromes, including eosinophilia and neutrophilia. The cause of these conditions is unclear, but they are likely due to alterations in circulating cytokine concentrations. Anemia is commonly seen in veterinary cancer patients. There are numerous potential causes for anemia in these animals, including anemia of chronic disease, bone marrow invasion, myelofibrosis, blood loss, and hemolysis. Polycythemia associated with ectopic production of erythropoietin has been reported. Thrombocytopenia is seen in approximately one-third of all dogs with cancer. Thrombocytopenia may be due to rapid consumption of platelets. For example, *disseminated intravascular coagulation* (DIC) leading to thrombocytopenia and concurrent anemia is frequently seen in dogs with hemangiosarcoma. In addition, platelets may display surface antigens similar to tumor antigens; antibodies directed against tumor antigens then cross-react with platelet antigens, resulting in an immune-mediated thrombocytopenia (see Chapter 5). Excessive immunoglobulin production by tumors, particularly monoclonal gammopathies caused by multiple myeloma, can result in massive hyperproteinemia and *hyperviscosity syndrome*, manifested as altered neurologic function, congestive heart failure, or bleeding disorders.

Miscellaneous Syndromes

Information on this topic, including E-Fig. 6-1, is available at www.expertconsult.com.

Heritable Alterations in Cancer (Essential Concept 6-5)

Cancer occurs as the result of the progressive accumulation of genetic and epigenetic abnormalities in cells. These abnormalities lead to changes in cell growth, cell death, apoptosis, alterations in cellular differentiation, defective DNA repair, and dysfunction of other critical pathways, endowing the cancer cell with its neoplastic characteristics. Alterations in DNA sequence, termed *mutations*, result from inaccurate DNA repair and are passed along to all progeny of the cancer cell (see Chapter 1). Some epigenetic alterations may also persist over multiple cell divisions. Thus, a cancer phenotype is *heritable*. Specific genes that play important roles in cancer development are discussed in a later section of this chapter.

ESSENTIAL CONCEPT 6-5 Heritable Alterations in Cancer

Cancer occurs as the result of the progressive accumulation of heritable genetic and epigenetic abnormalities in cells. The initial change in genetic material may be due to inherited germline mutations or to somatic mutations acquired as the result of DNA damage by a chemical carcinogen, radiation, or an oncogenic virus. Genetic changes that activate oncogenes like the *ras* genes or inactivate tumor suppressor genes like the *p53* gene are considered to be the mutations that drive cancer development. However, preexisting modifier genes, for example, genes that encode DNA repair enzymes, may affect cancer susceptibility and development, although less dramatically.

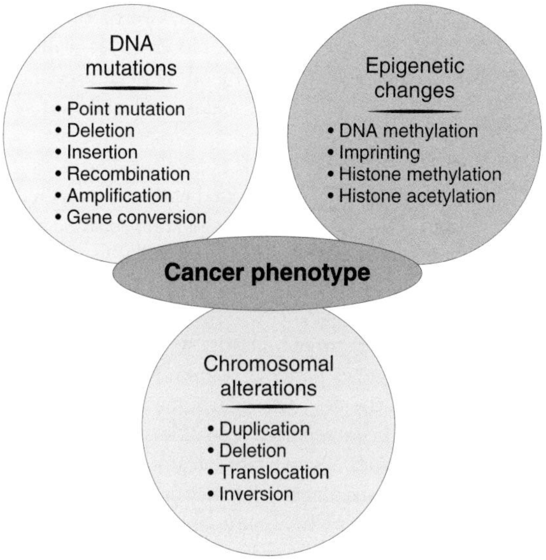

Figure 6-33 **Heritable Alterations Contributing to Carcinogenesis.** Many genetic changes caused by extrinsic and intrinsic DNA-damaging agents, normal physiologic processes, and aging alter the amino acid sequences of encoded proteins and the levels at which these proteins are expressed. It is these interacting alterations that are ultimately responsible for the neoplastic phenotype. (Redrawn with permission from Dr. D.F. Kusewitt, Health Sciences Center, University of New Mexico.)

Genetic Changes in Cancer

As illustrated in Fig. 6-33, DNA is susceptible to many types of chemical and physical alterations. Some of these alterations are caused by injurious endogenous and exogenous agents. In addition, DNA alterations also occur as part of normal processes of genome replication, repair, and rearrangement.

Point Mutations

DNA damage alone does not constitute mutation. However, when a DNA strand containing unrepaired or misrepaired damage is used as a template for the synthesis of a complementary DNA strand, DNA polymerases may insert an incorrect base in the newly synthesized DNA strand. The altered base sequence is reproduced in all subsequently synthesized DNA. This process is known as *mutation fixation*; at least one and sometimes two rounds of replication are required for mutations to become fully fixed in the genome.

If a point mutation occurs in an exon or at a splice site of a protein-coding gene, it may lead to an altered amino acid sequence in the gene product. A mutation located in a noncoding region of a gene may affect the level of gene transcription or the stability of the transcribed RNA, thus resulting in an altered level of expression of the encoded protein. Altered protein expression in turn may contribute to neoplastic transformation, tumor growth, invasion, and metastasis.

DNA Strand Breaks

Single- and double-strand breaks in DNA are caused by physical and chemical agents and viruses; they may also occur during normal physiologic processes such as recombination of immunoglobulin genes and T lymphocyte receptor genes. Although single-strand breaks are usually readily repaired, they sometimes trigger gene conversion, which is the replacement of a gene or part of a gene by DNA derived from a closely related gene. Gene conversion is one mechanism by which animals routinely generate diversity in large families of related genes, for example, genes encoding MHC antigens. Double-strand breaks produce unprotected, recombinogenic DNA ends and often lead to major chromosomal anomalies, including deletions and translocations. Clearly, such large-scale chromosomal changes have the potential to alter the gene expression repertoire of a cell in a dramatic fashion.

Insertions and Deletions

Insertions, or additions, of DNA bases into the genome may be as small as a single base or larger than a viral genome. *Deletions* involve loss of a DNA segment and range in size from one base pair to an entire chromosome arm. Heterozygous deletions occur on only one chromosome, whereas homozygous deletions occur on both chromosomes. Small deletions or insertions of one or two base pairs cause a shift in the reading frame during protein synthesis, a process termed *frameshift mutation*. Such mutations may alter the protein-coding sequences downstream from the site of deletion, eliminate or create splice sites, or generate premature stop codons, resulting in modified or truncated proteins (see Chapter 1).

Retroviral genomes replicate only after they insert into the animal genome, and these large insertions can interrupt the coding sequence of animal genes, abrogating their expression or leading to the production of abnormal gene products. On the other hand, juxtaposition of viral promoter elements adjacent to cellular coding sequences of the host can lead to dysregulated, often markedly increased, expression of cellular genes that drive tumorigenesis. Perhaps the best-studied example of insertional activation of host animal genes by a retrovirus is the mouse mammary tumor virus, which can integrate "upstream" of a variety of cellular genes to enhance their expression, leading ultimately to the formation of mammary adenocarcinomas.

Amplifications

Genomic *amplification* results in the presence of more than one copy of a DNA sequence. The amplified region can involve large segments of a chromosome and encompass millions of base pairs. Alternatively, the amplified region may be very small and contained within a portion of a single gene, such as the internal tandem duplication of the c-kit gene in canine mast cell tumors.

Unscheduled amplification of DNA segments is a poorly understood process by which multiple rounds of localized DNA replication produce hundreds or thousands of copies of DNA segments up to several megabases in length. Expansion or contraction of small regions of tandemly repeated DNA sequences can occur as the result of DNA polymerase slippage during replication.

Aneuploidy

Many cancer cells have abnormal numbers of chromosomes, a condition termed *aneuploidy*. Aneuploidy often results from deletion or duplication of one or multiple chromosomes or chromosome segments. Alterations in chromosome number are largely the result of mistakes in chromosome segregation caused by multipolar spindles, centrosome amplification, kinetochore malfunction, or abnormal cytokinesis. Cytogenetic analysis can determine the copy number of each chromosome. *Monosomy* is the term used when only one copy of a chromosome is present, instead of the usual two. *Trisomy* is the term used when three copies of a chromosome exist. For example, one-quarter of canine lymphomas show trisomy of chromosome 13. In mice, trisomy of chromosome 15 occurs in almost all T lymphocyte lymphomas and leukemias, suggesting that overexpression of a gene or genes on this chromosome plays an important role in tumor development.

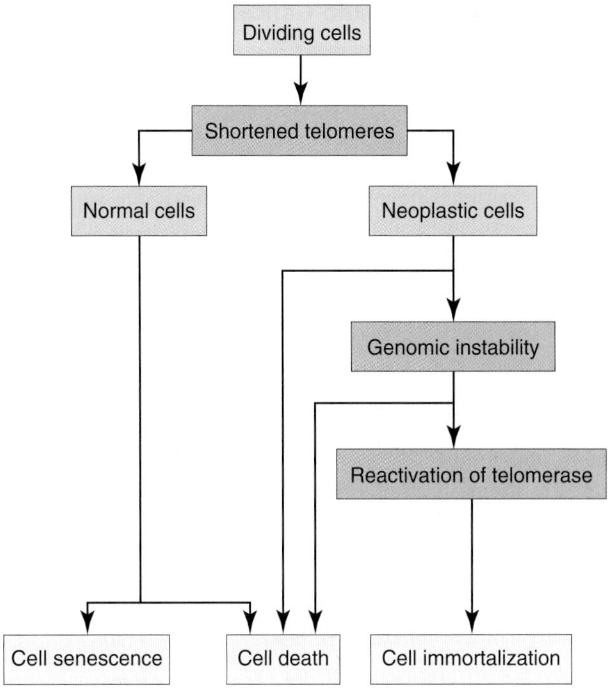

Figure 6-34 Cellular Responses to Telomere Shortening. This figure illustrates the difference between normal and neoplastic cells in their response to telomere shortening. In normal cells telomere shortening leads to cell death or senescence. In neoplastic cells, however, telomere shortening may lead to genomic instability, telomerase reactivation, and cell immortalization. (Redrawn with permission from Dr. D.F. Kusewitt, Health Sciences Center, University of New Mexico.)

Chromosomal Instability

The number and arrangement of chromosomes, termed the *karyotype*, of many tumor cells are extremely abnormal. These alterations are the result of chromosomal instability. In tumors with notable chromosomal instability, each cell may have a different karyotype and exhibit a remarkable array of duplications, deletions, and translocations. *Translocations* occur when pieces of two separate chromosomes break off and reattach inappropriately. As a result of the abnormal position of genes on the rearranged chromosomes, many cell processes are markedly disturbed.

Chromosomal instability often occurs when normal processes of DNA repair are disrupted. Dysfunctional telomeres also contribute to chromosomal instability (Fig. 6-34). Telomeres are DNA sequences that make up the ends of the chromosomes and help protect the DNA from damage. The precise mechanisms by which an intact DNA damage response and normal telomerase activity maintain chromosomal integrity are unclear.

In some cases, specific chromosomal abnormalities are associated with specific disease entities. The best-studied example of this is a reciprocal translocation between chromosomes 9 and 22 that yields an abnormal chromosome called the Philadelphia chromosome and results in chronic myeloid leukemia in human beings. This translocation fuses portions of the *BCR* and *ABL1* genes; the fusion gene thus produced encodes an abnormal protein that is responsible for the neoplastic transformation of myeloid cells.

Germline Mutations and Cancer Syndromes

Germline mutations affecting oncogenes or tumor suppressor genes are heritable. These mutations are transmitted to offspring and are present in all cells of affected progeny. Human families and genetically related animals with germline mutations that result in the development of a specific spectrum of tumor types are said to have a *cancer syndrome*. Inherited cancer syndromes due to germline mutations account for less than 10% of tumors in human beings. Characteristics of these heritable familial cancers include an early age of onset, formation of bilateral tumors in paired organs like the kidneys, occurrence of multiple primary tumors in unpaired organs like the colon, and a family history of cancer. Cancer syndromes generally show an autosomal dominant pattern of inheritance. However, some cancer syndromes have a recessive mode of inheritance. In such syndromes the affected individual must inherit the genetic defect from both parents. For instance, the mutant *ter* gene carried by strain 129/Sv-ter mice confers high susceptibility to testicular teratoma when present in the homozygous state but not when carried in the heterozygous condition.

Well-known inherited cancer syndromes in human beings include germline mutations of p53 in Li-Fraumeni syndrome associated with multiple tumor types, mutations of *NF1* and *NF2* that lead to neurofibromatosis, mutations of *BRCA1* and *BRCA2* associated with breast and ovarian cancers, and mutations in *MEN1* and *RET*, which are linked to multiple endocrine neoplasia. A well-documented veterinary cancer syndrome is the disease with the unwieldy name "hereditary multifocal renal cystadenocarcinoma and nodular dermatofibrosis" that occurs in the German shepherd dog. This disease is characterized by bilateral and multifocal renal tumors, uterine leiomyomas, and nodules in the skin (dermatofibrosis). The gene responsible has been mapped to a locus homologous to the human *BHD* locus; mutations in *BHD* cause a phenotypically similar human disease.

Acquired Somatic Mutations and Sporadic Cancers

In contrast to germline mutations, acquired *somatic mutations* are restricted to individual cells and the progeny of these cells. Such somatic mutations are responsible for sporadic tumors in the general population. Somatic mutations accumulate over time; thus the risk for cancer increases with age (Fig. 6-35). Somatic genetic alterations are caused by both intrinsic metabolic processes and extrinsic mutagens.

Epigenetic Changes in Cancer

In addition to the genetic changes that occur in cancer cells, there are also many epigenetic changes. The term *epigenetic* refers to a heritable change in gene expression in somatic cells resulting from something other than a change in the DNA sequence. Epigenetic alterations have recently come to light as being major players in tumor biology. The most frequently studied epigenetic changes are DNA cytosine methylation and histone modifications. These epigenetic modifications can enhance or suppress gene expression and can be transmitted to daughter cells during cell division. Although DNA methylation and histone modifications are carried out by normal cellular enzymes, the activity and specificity of these enzymes can be altered by exogenous agents such as carcinogens. Although epigenetic changes are usually stable and are readily transmitted from tumor cells to their progeny, they can be modulated or reversed by pharmacologic agents. This response makes them attractive targets for therapeutic intervention designed to restore gene expression to its normal state.

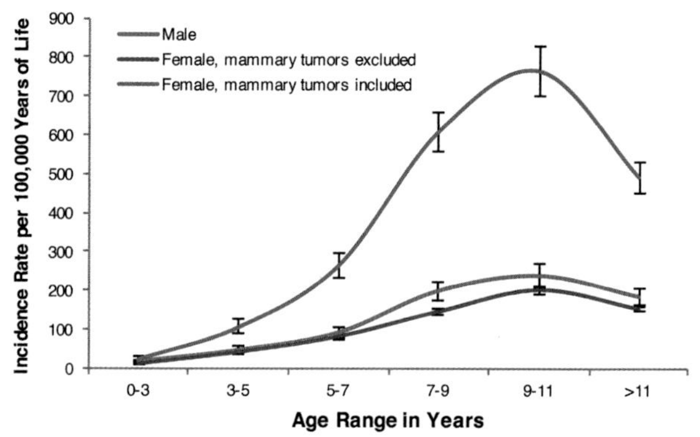

Figure 6-35 Cancer Incidence by Age in Dogs. This figure shows the incidence of tumors per 100,000 years of life for male *(green line)* and female *(red and blue lines)* dogs. The tumor incidence in female dogs is shown both for all tumors *(blue line)* and for all tumors with mammary tumors excluded *(red line)*. The difference between the incidence of all tumors in females dogs and the incidence of tumors exclusive of mammary gland tumors in females indicates the very large contribution of mammary gland tumors to overall tumor incidence in female dogs, especially if intact. For both sexes the tumor incidence increases with age until the age of 11 years. (Data courtesy Dr. D.F Merlo, National Cancer Research Institute, Genoa, Italy [Merlo DF, et al: *J Vet Intern Med* 22:976-984, 2008].)

DNA Methylation

DNA methylation involves the addition of a methyl group to carbon 5 of cytosine on cytosines located immediately 5′ to guanine (CpG dinucleotide). Methylation is essential for regulating gene expression in normal cells and is carried out by various methyltransferase enzymes. In general, hypomethylation of genes, particularly of promoter regions, leads to gene activation, whereas hypermethylation results in gene silencing. Cancer cells have lower levels of methylation in the genome, termed *global hypomethylation*, with a paradoxical increase in gene-specific methylation, termed *hypermethylation*, of clusters of CpG sites located in the promoter or first exon of genes (Fig. 6-36). Aberrant promoter methylation has been found in every type of human cancer studied.

Histone Modification

DNA is wound around histones to form chromatin (see E-Fig. 1-22). Loosely packed chromatin termed *euchromatin* is said to be in an open configuration; in this configuration, DNA is accessible to transcription factors. Chromatin in a closed, compact configuration is termed *heterochromatin*; in this state, DNA is inaccessible to transcription factors. Posttranslational histone modifications, such as acetylation, methylation, and phosphorylation, alter the transcription of associated DNA. These posttranslational histone modifications form the "histone code" that plays an important role in determining which genes are expressed and the level at which these genes are expressed. For example, the addition of a negatively charged acetyl group to certain lysine residues in a histone tail results in a weaker bond between the DNA and the histone. This histone acetylation results in a more relaxed chromatin configuration, making the DNA more accessible to transcription factors and thereby increasing transcription of the associated gene (Fig. 6-37).

Imprinting

Genomic imprinting refers to allele-specific expression of certain genes whereby only the maternal or paternal allele is expressed. This monoallelic expression is controlled in part by DNA methylation, but this regulation is sometimes lost in cancer. The loss of imprinting can allow a double dose of a growth-promoting gene product.

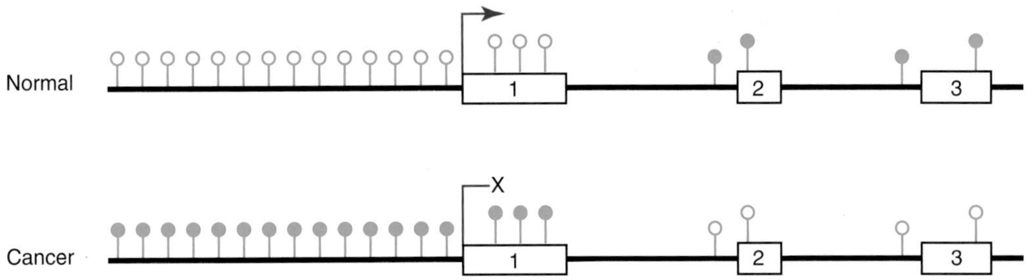

Figure 6-36 CpG Island Methylation. In most normal tissues the dense clusters of CpG sites in the 5′ regions of genes (CpG islands) are unmethylated *(open lollipops)*, whereas those in the body of the gene are methylated *(filled lollipops)*. The reverse is often seen in cancer where 5′ CpG islands become hypermethylated, and there is concurrent hypomethylation of CpG sites in the body of the gene. Unmethylated 5′ CpG islands are associated with active transcription *(arrow)*, whereas methylated 5′ CpG islands are associated with transcriptional repression *(x)*. The net effect is a heritable change in patterns of gene expression. (Redrawn with permission from Dr. L.J. Rush, College of Veterinary Medicine, The Ohio State University.)

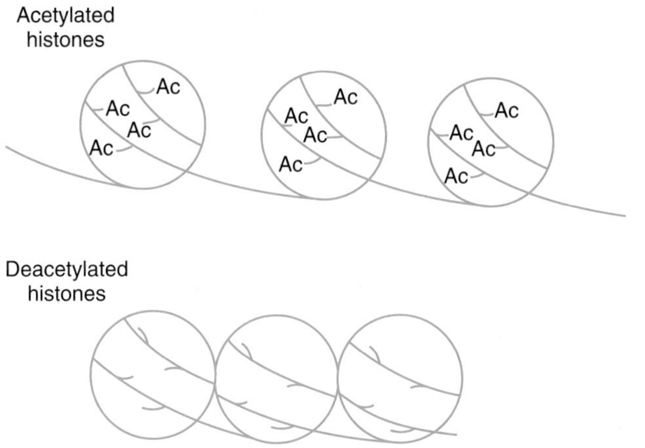

Figure 6-37 Histone Acetylation. DNA is wound around histones. The presence of acetyl groups *(Ac)* on histone tails is associated with relaxed chromatin, which allows gene transcription. Removal of acetyl groups by histone deacetylases results in a closed chromatin configuration that prevents gene transcription. (Redrawn with permission from Dr. L.J. Rush, College of Veterinary Medicine, The Ohio State University.)

For example, insulin-like growth factor-2 (IGF-2) is an imprinted gene that is expressed from only the paternal allele in most normal tissues. If a cancer cell undergoes relaxation of imprinting, the methylation-mediated silencing of the maternal allele is lost, enabling biallelic expression and higher than normal levels of this growth-promoting gene product.

Noncoding RNAs and Cancer

Although protein-coding genes constitute only approximately 2% of the mammalian genome, at least 90% of the genome is transcribed into RNA. Thus the vast majority of RNA transcripts do not encode proteins. Two classes of these *noncoding RNA* transcripts, short (less than 200 nucleotides long) and long (200 to several kilobases in length) noncoding RNAs, play important roles in regulating the transcription, stability, and translation of messenger RNA (mRNA) from protein-coding genes. Through these activities, noncoding RNAs modulate a variety of biologic processes, including normal growth and differentiation. Dysregulated expression of some noncoding RNAs contributes significantly to cancer development.

MicroRNAs (miRNAs) are the most thoroughly studied subclass of noncoding RNAs. These small noncoding RNA molecules post-transcriptionally regulate, usually by blocking, the expression of other genes. MiRNA genes are found throughout the genome, both within other known coding genes and within intergenic regions. MiRNA genes are transcribed into large precursor RNAs that undergo extensive enzymatic processing both within the nucleus and after export into the cytoplasm. Mature miRNAs are 18 to 25 nucleotides long and bind target mRNAs that have a complementary sequence. Once bound, miRNAs either trigger degradation of their target mRNAs or prevent translation of these mRNAs into proteins.

Approximately 1000 miRNA genes are present in the human genome, and each miRNA can regulate translation of approximately 200 target mRNA species. Overall, miRNAs control translation of perhaps one-third of all protein-coding genes in the human genome. The pattern of miRNA expression is extensively dysregulated in cancers by a wide variety of genetic and epigenetic mechanisms. Altered patterns of miRNA expression in turn create extensive changes in cellular processes related to neoplasia, including proliferation, apoptosis, invasiveness, and genomic stability. Intensive research effort is currently being focused on understanding how altered patterns of miRNA expression can be exploited for diagnostic and therapeutic purposes.

Molecular Determinants of Cancer

Although tumor cells may display a wide variety of genetic alterations, usually only a few of these alterations, termed *driver mutations*, are predominantly responsible for tumor development. Driver mutations frequently involve tumor suppressor genes or oncogenes. However, it is rare that a single driver mutation is responsible for cancer; instead multiple genetic and epigenetic changes collaborate to transform a normal cell into a tumor cell and to allow transmission of the neoplastic phenotype. The molecular changes that occur during cancer development are summarized in Fig. 6-38.

Oncogenes

Proto-oncogenes are normal cellular genes that regulate cell growth and differentiation. They often encode products such as growth factors and their receptors, cell cycle regulators, DNA-binding proteins, transcription factors, protein kinases involved in signal transduction, and others. When "activated" by overexpression or mutation, proto-oncogenes are termed *oncogenes*. Oncogenes drive proliferation and render the cell unresponsive to normal growth inhibitory signals, ultimately resulting in tumor formation.

There are a number of ways in which proto-oncogenes can be activated. The gene can be amplified, so that a signal to transcribe the gene results in the production of many more copies of mRNA than usual. Oncogenes can undergo mutations that cause constitutive activation of the encoded protein. In these cases the protein product is always "turned on" and is unresponsive to inhibitory

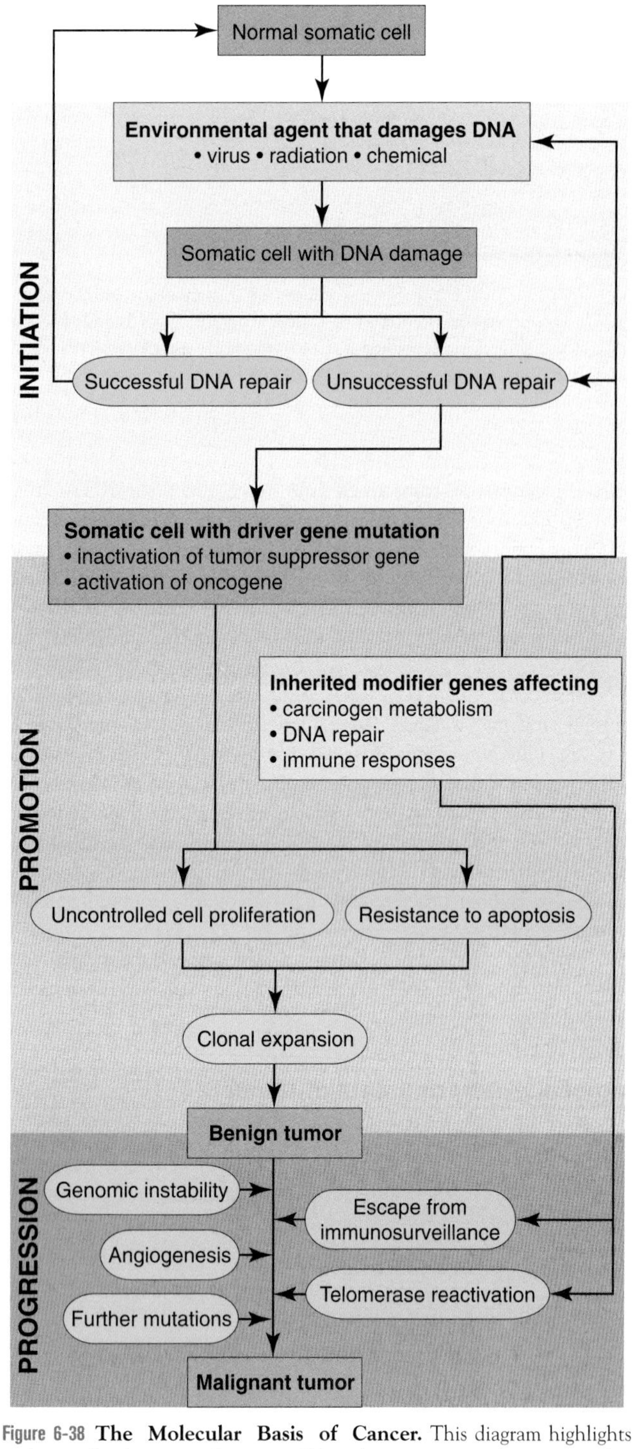

Figure 6-38 The Molecular Basis of Cancer. This diagram highlights multistep development of cancer. Although mutations in driver genes due to environmental DNA-damaging agents may initiate cancer, inherited modifier genes make significant contributions to tumor susceptibility and rate of growth. During the stage of tumor promotion, clones of initiated cells capable of continued cell proliferation and resistant to apoptosis emerge. A wide variety of additional genetic and epigenetic changes convert a benign tumor into an increasingly aggressive malignant tumor. (Courtesy Dr. D.F. Kusewitt, Health Sciences Center, University of New Mexico; and Dr. J.F. Zachary, College of Veterinary Medicine, University of Illinois.)

signals. This scenario is common for tyrosine kinase receptors, such as the epidermal growth factor receptor (EGFR). Activating mutations in genes encoding these receptors result in constitutive kinase activity even in the absence of appropriate triggers or ligands. Tumor cells may also synthesize large amounts of both tyrosine kinase receptors and their activating ligands, forming a growth-promoting autocrine loop.

The prototype of signal transduction oncogenes are the *ras* genes, which encode the RAS family of guanosine triphosphate (GTP)-binding proteins (G proteins) (Fig. 6-39). In normal cells, RAS proteins transmit growth stimulatory signals from growth factor receptors to the nucleus, ultimately activating transcription of genes that regulate cell proliferation. RAS is normally located on the cytoplasmic side of the cell membrane and is closely associated with farnesyl transferase. Inactive RAS binds guanosine diphosphate (GDP). Upon receiving a stimulatory signal from an activated growth factor receptor, RAS exchanges GDP for GTP. RAS bound to GTP is the active form, which triggers the RAS–RAF–mitogen-activated protein kinase (MAPK) signaling cascade and results in transcription of genes that promote cell division. The activation of RAS is normally short lived, because RAS has an intrinsic guanosine triphosphatase (GTPase) activity that hydrolyzes GTP to GDP and converts RAS to its inactive state. In many cancers, RAS mutation renders RAS activation independent of upstream growth factor receptor activation or abrogates RAS GTPase activity. RAS family members, the farnesyl transferase membrane anchor, and other components of the downstream MAPK signal transduction pathway are all attractive molecular targets for therapeutic intervention in cancer patients.

Tumor Suppressor Genes

The designation of *tumor suppressor gene* was originally given to genes that inhibited cell proliferation. Over time the class of tumor suppressor genes has expanded to include many different types of cancer-related genes that, when inactivated through genetic or epigenetic means, allow uncontrolled cell proliferation and tumor growth. Suppressor genes include genes that control cell cycle, apoptosis, DNA repair, and other fundamental pathways.

The pivotal concept of tumor suppressor genes was advanced by Alfred Knudson in 1971, based on his observations of children with familial and sporadic retinoblastoma, an uncommon tumor arising in the retina. According to Knudson's *"two-hit" hypothesis*, both alleles of a tumor suppressor gene must undergo mutation, a genetic "hit," for cancer to develop. When only one allele is inactivated, the remaining tumor suppressor allele prevents uncontrolled cell proliferation and tumor development. In inherited cancer syndromes a person is born with a germline mutation in one allele of the tumor suppressor gene in all cells of the body (E-Fig. 6-2). The second hit is acquired as a somatic mutation of the remaining tumor suppressor allele in a single cell. When both copies of the tumor suppressor gene are inactivated in the cell, a tumor arises from this cell. In contrast, development of a sporadic tumor in those born with two normal tumor suppressor alleles requires the much more unlikely event that a single cell sustains two hits, one on each allele of the tumor suppressor gene.

Loss of a tumor suppressor gene allele can occur by a variety of mechanisms, including point mutation in the allele, deletion of the allele or the chromosomal segment where it resides, deletion of the entire chromosome containing the allele, or mitotic recombination resulting in replacement of the normal allele by the mutant allele. In addition, DNA methylation is an alternative, epigenetic method of silencing tumor suppressor genes.

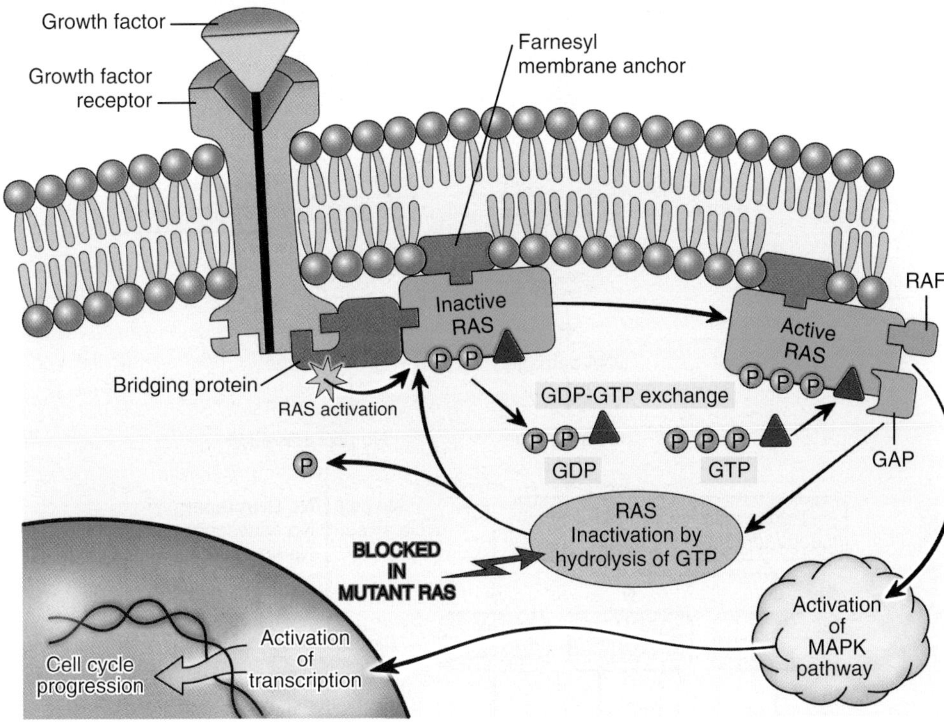

Figure 6-39 Model of RAS Action. When a normal cell is stimulated through a growth factor receptor, inactive RAS is activated to an active state by exchanging guanosine diphosphate (GDP) for guanosine triphosphate (GTP). Activated RAS in turn activates RAF-1 to stimulate signaling through the mitogen-activated protein kinase (MAPK) pathway, ultimately leading to transcription of genes that drive cell cycle progression. In normal cells, activated RAS is inactivated via guanosine triphosphatase (GTPase)–activating protein (GAP), which stimulates the GTPase activity of RAS, thus terminating signaling through the RAS-RAF-MAPK pathway. However, in cancer cells, mutant RAS proteins cannot be inactivated in this manner; thus they stimulate continual cell cycle progression. Anchoring of RAS to the cell membrane by the farnesyl moiety is essential for its action.

Although the classic definition of a tumor suppressor gene dictates that both alleles must be inactivated, recent evidence suggests that for certain genes inactivation of only one copy, a condition termed *haploinsufficiency*, is sufficient for tumor growth. Haploinsufficiency can contribute to tumor development by a number of mechanisms. One mechanism is a simple gene-dosage effect in which half the normal amount of a protein is insufficient to maintain the normal homeostatic balance in the cell. Alternatively, a mutation in one allele can give rise to a dominant-negative protein that blocks the function of the normal protein produced by the remaining normal allele.

Many tumor suppressor genes are key components of the cell cycle. One of the most widely studied tumor suppressor genes is *p53* (Fig. 6-40). It is inactivated, most commonly by mutation, in more than half of human cancers. It is a DNA-binding protein that regulates transcription of numerous genes and plays a critical role in cell cycle arrest and induction of apoptosis after DNA damage. Intracellular levels of p53 are rapidly elevated in response to DNA damage. Enhanced expression leads to increased transcription of p53 target genes, such as p21, which stop the cell cycle, allowing an opportunity for DNA repair. If DNA repair is unsuccessful, p53 directs cell death by activating BCL2-associated X protein (BAX), an important element of the apoptotic cascade. Therefore loss of functional p53 can have devastating consequences for maintaining integrity of the genome. Without p53, DNA damage goes unrepaired, the cell proceeds through division, and genetic changes become fixed in the genome. For these reasons, p53 has been called the "guardian of the genome."

Modifier Genes

In some cancer syndromes, such as the Li-Fraumeni syndrome and familial adenomatous polyposis in human beings, tumor risk is very markedly increased because of changes in a single driver gene; however, there are also a variety of tumor modifier genes that alter cancer susceptibility to a lesser extent. These so-called *modifier genes* or *quantitative trait loci* (QTL) alter the incidence and progression of tumors with driver mutations. In the absence of a driver mutation, modifier genes typically have no phenotype of their own. Indeed, many modifier genes represent polymorphic genes, such as those encoding drug-metabolizing enzymes or DNA repair enzymes, occurring naturally in the population. These cancer modifier genes only modestly alter the phenotype produced by cancer driver genes but may have a significant impact on cancer susceptibility. Their effects are substantially modified by interactions with each other and with the environment. For instance, sun exposure is the major etiologic factor in squamous cell carcinoma of the ears in white cats, but the lack of pigmentation in these cats contributes to their susceptibility to tumor development; thus genes that determine skin pigmentation are modifier genes for this cancer. Similarly, susceptibility to chemically induced skin cancer in mice is highly dependent upon the genetic background of the mouse strain. At least 13 skin cancer susceptibility genes have been identified that account for this strain-dependent variability. In the dog, a variety of cancer susceptibility patterns, presumably due to differences in modifier genes, have been identified (Table 6-3).

In many cases, tumor modifier genes are identified due to the association of their polymorphic variants with cancer susceptibility,

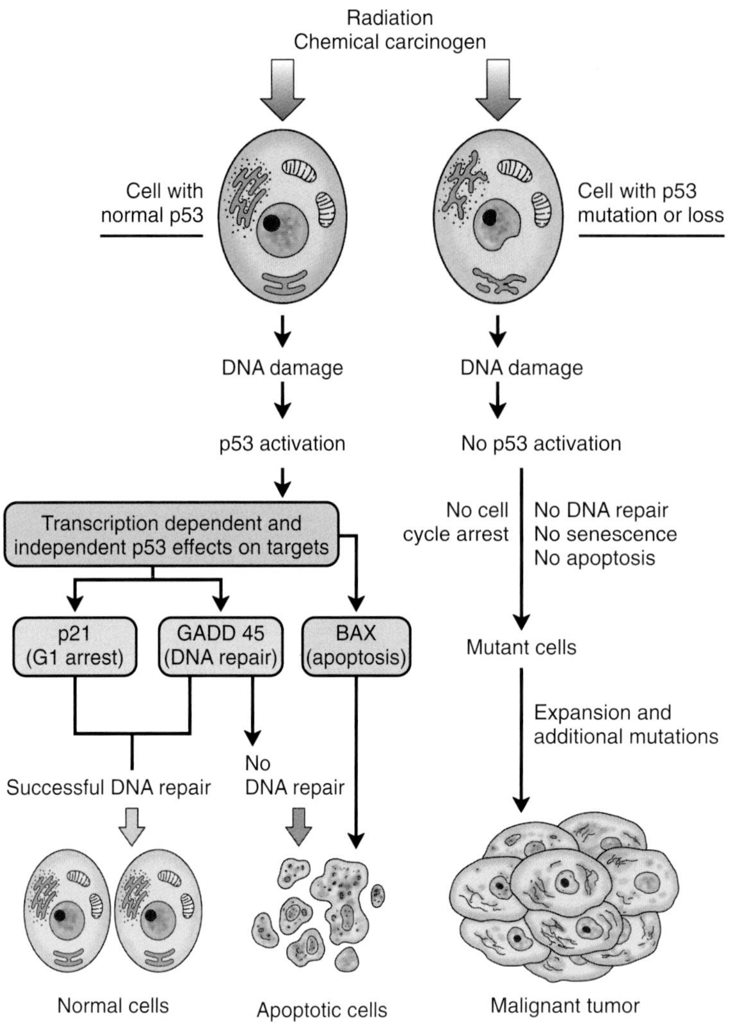

Figure 6-40 **p53 and Maintenance of Genome Integrity.** DNA damage activates normal p53. Activated p53 acts via both transcription-dependent and transcription-independent pathways to cause G_1 arrest via p21 and induction of DNA repair via growth arrest and DNA damage-inducible 45 (GADD45). Successful DNA repair allows cells to proceed through the cell cycle. However, if DNA repair fails, BCL2-associated X protein (BAX) promotes apoptosis. In contrast, DNA damage to cells with loss or mutation of p53 does not induce cell cycle arrest or DNA repair. The genetically damaged cells proliferate, accumulate mutations, and may eventually give rise to tumors.

and this association is determined by whole genome sequencing of large populations. Further studies are then required to determine the characteristics of the gene and the manner in which it influences tumor penetrance.

Defects in DNA Repair

Failure of DNA repair enzymes to function effectively results in DNA mutations and genomic instability. If these mutations inactivate tumor suppressor genes or activate oncogenes, the cell may develop an uncontrolled proliferative capacity. Specific types of DNA repair mechanisms have evolved to repair specific DNA lesions. *Mismatch repair* enzymes, such as MLH1 and MSH2 proofread DNA, much like the spell-check function on a computer, to locate and fix single nucleotide mismatches that occur on a regular basis during normal DNA synthesis. For example, if an adenine is mistakenly paired with a guanine during DNA replication, this error will be recognized and corrected. Some carcinogens create bulky DNA lesions. For example, ultraviolet (UV) light leads to cross-linking of pyrimidine residues and formation of pyrimidine dimers. Such lesions are repaired by *nucleotide excision repair*, which requires a large cohort of DNA repair proteins. This process is similar to the cut-and-paste function of a computer in that the DNA lesion is excised and the correct nucleotides are replaced. Additional DNA repair genes in human beings include such genes as *ATM*, *BRCA1*, and *BRCA2*.

As discussed earlier, intracellular p53 levels rise in response to DNA damage from any number of agents and stop the cell cycle to give the cell time to carry out repair processes. Failure of DNA repair can lead to mutation fixation with subsequent rounds of cell division. When function of the DNA repair gene itself is lost, through mutation, promoter methylation, or deletion, the result is an exponential increase in mutations throughout the genome, resulting in widespread genomic instability and, ultimately, increased cancer susceptibility.

Multistage Carcinogenesis

Some tumor types demonstrate an orderly morphologic progression through premalignant to malignant to invasive and metastatic disease. Molecular genetic investigations of these various stages have made important contributions to our understanding of cancer biology. The molecular events that occur in the development of familial adenomatous polyposis, a form of human colorectal cancer,

Table 6-3 Cancer Susceptibility in Dogs

Tumor Site	Tumor Type	Susceptible Breeds
Hematopoietic system	Lymphoma	Boxer
	Histiocytic sarcoma (malignant histiocytosis)	Bernese mountain dog, flat-coated retriever
Brain	Various gliomas	Boston terrier, boxer, bulldog
Chemoreceptor organs (aortic and carotid bodies)	Chemodectomas	Brachycephalic breeds (Boston terrier, boxer, bulldog, and others)
Skin	Mast cell tumor	Boxer, bulldog, retriever
Vasculature	Hemangiosarcoma	German shepherd, golden retriever, boxer
Mammary gland	Various	Boxer, Brittany spaniel, dachshund, English setter, Labrador retriever, pointer, springer spaniel
Nose and sinuses	Various	Airedale, collie, Scottish terrier
Oropharynx	Various	Boxer, cocker spaniel, golden retriever
Ovary	Carcinoma	Pointer
Pancreas	Carcinoma	Airedale terrier, poodle, boxer
	Insulinoma	Fox terrier, standard poodle, German shepherd, boxer
Thyroid	Carcinoma	Beagle, boxer, retrievers
Skeleton	Osteosarcoma	Giant breeds, boxer, Danish dog, German shepherd, Rottweiler
Testis		Boxer, collie, German shepherd
Urinary bladder	Carcinoma	Beagle, collie, Scottish terrier

Modified from McCullen JM, Page R, Misdorp W: An overview of cancer pathogenesis, diagnosis, and management. In Meuten DJ, editor: *Tumors in domestic animals,* ed. 5, Hoboken, NJ, 2010, John Wiley and Sons, with additional material from Meuten DJ, editor: *Tumors in domestic animals,* ed. 5, Hoboken, NJ, 2010, John Wiley and Sons, and Dobson JM: Breed-predispositions to cancer in pedigree dogs. *ISRN Vet Sci* 2013:941275, 2013.

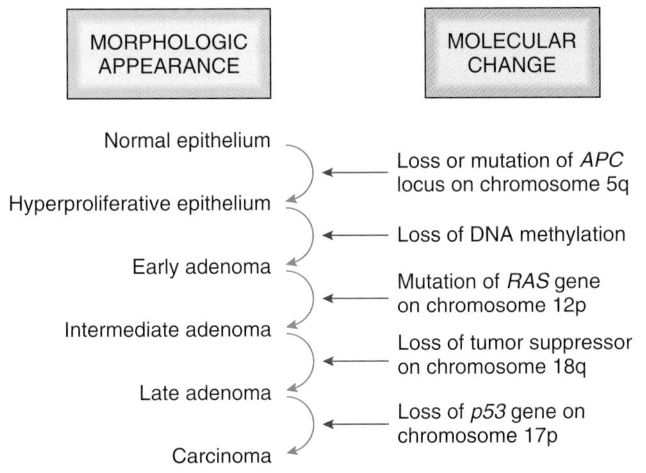

Figure 6-41 Evolution of Human Colorectal Cancers. Although adenomatous polyposis coli (*APC*) mutation is an early event and loss of *p53* occurs late in the process of tumorigenesis, the timing for the other changes may show variations. Note also that individual tumors may not have all of the changes listed. (Adapted from Vogelstein B, Kinzler KW: Colorectal tumors. In Vogelstein B, Kinzler KW, editors: *The genetic basis of human cancer*, New York, 2002, McGraw-Hill.)

provide an excellent example of the genetic evolution that underlies progressive morphologic changes in cancer (Fig. 6-41). The initiating event is loss or mutation of the adenomatous polyposis coli (APC) tumor suppressor gene, leading to the formation of an adenoma. This event is followed by an activating mutation of a RAS oncogene and loss of genetic material harboring additional tumor suppressor genes. Ultimately, a malignant carcinoma emerges.

Therapeutic Implications

Cancer is often treated using cytotoxic drugs or radiation therapy, neither of which discriminates between normal and tumor cells. Nonselective cell killing is responsible for many of the deleterious side effects of cancer treatment. Understanding the molecular basis of cancer is crucial for developing interventional strategies to kill neoplastic cells while leaving healthy cells unaffected. Examples of molecularly targeted therapies used in human beings include imatinib mesylate (Gleevec), which inactivates the BCR/ABL oncogene in chronic myeloid leukemia, and afatinib (Gilotrif), which targets the oncogenic EGFR in lung cancer. Specific molecular defects can also be exploited for early detection or early intervention at a stage when the tumor may be more responsive to treatment. Mutations in the *BRCA1* gene are associated with a high risk for development of breast and ovarian cancer in women. Identification of the carrier status gives women the option of prophylactic mastectomy or oophorectomy. Mutations and other molecular defects can also be used to stratify patients for treatment or prognostic purposes. Indeed, with the advent of whole genome sequencing, which allows identification of all mutations in a tumor, considerable emphasis in the human cancer field is now being placed on identifying and targeting specific driver mutations. The era of truly individualized cancer therapy has arrived.

Mechanisms of Carcinogenesis

Intrinsic Factors

As a by-product of ordinary cell metabolism, a variety of DNA-damaging metabolites, such as reactive oxygen species and organic acids, are produced. Additionally, in the course of many rounds of replication, DNA changes are introduced as a result of copying errors made by DNA polymerases. Illegitimate recombination and inappropriate nucleotide addition, activities carried out by normal cellular enzymes, can also lead to changes in DNA. Chromosomal abnormalities arise as a result of decreased telomere length, altered telomerase activity, and mistakes in chromosome segregation. The DNA lesions induced by these processes can result in mutations in critical cancer-related genes and ultimately in neoplasia.

Extrinsic Factors

Extrinsic factors that interact with DNA to cause cancer include chemical and physical environmental agents and oncogenic viruses. *Mutagens* are agents that create DNA damage that gives rise to mutations, whereas *carcinogens* are agents that cause cancer. Many mutagens are also carcinogens. However, there are carcinogens with unknown mechanisms of action; such carcinogens may or may not be mutagens.

Chemicals

A very wide variety of chemicals can cause cancer in animals. As an example, ptaquiloside, a toxin found in bracken fern, causes bladder cancer in cattle. Moreover, the susceptibility of mice and rats to chemically induced cancers is exploited for safety testing during drug development. *Direct-acting* chemical carcinogens are effective in the form in which they enter the body, but most carcinogens are procarcinogens that require metabolic activation by cellular enzymes, such as cytochrome P450 in hepatic microsomes, to form ultimate carcinogens. Such procarcinogens are thus termed *indirect-acting carcinogens*. Despite their varied composition, the effective form of most carcinogens binds covalently to DNA to form DNA adducts.

As discussed previously, experimental carcinogenesis studies have been critical in elucidating the stepwise development of cancer. Moreover, these studies have clearly defined the contribution of initiating versus promoting agents to cancer development (Fig. 6-42). In multistage tumorigenesis models, such as the skin carcinogenesis model in mice, the initiator must be administered before the promoting agent. Furthermore, the initiator is ineffective without subsequent application of a promoter. Often multiple, closely spaced promoter treatments are required to drive tumor emergence.

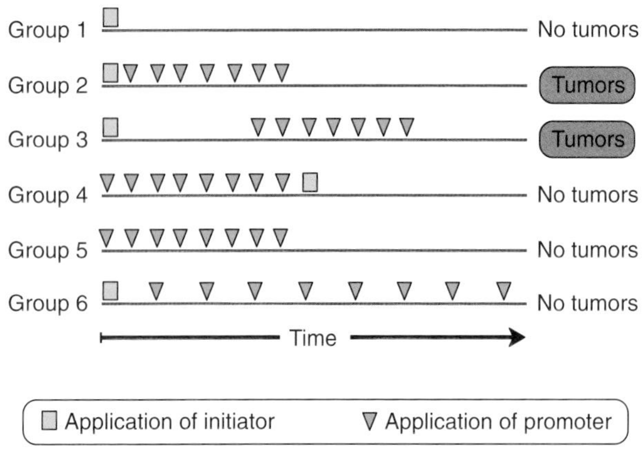

Figure 6-42 Experiments Demonstrating Initiation and Promotion Phases of Chemical Skin Carcinogenesis in Mice. Tumors arose only if application of an initiator was followed by multiple applications of a promoter. For group 2, application of the promoter was repeated twice weekly for several months. For group 3, application of the promoter was delayed for several months, and the promoter was then applied twice weekly. When the promoter was applied monthly rather than twice weekly (group 6), it did not effectively promote tumor emergence. In the absence of initiator (group 5) or promoter (group 1) application or if promoter treatment occurred before initiator application (group 4), no tumors developed. For these studies the initiator employed was a polycyclic hydrocarbon, and the promoter used was croton oil; however, similar results are seen with a variety of initiator and promoter combinations.

Radiation

Unlike chemicals, all forms of radiation are *complete carcinogens*, that is, they are able both to initiate and, with continued exposure, to promote tumorigenesis. For example, in both human beings and animals, secondary tumors may arise at sites previously treated for cancer by radiation. Direct DNA damage caused by ionizing radiation consists primarily of single- and double-strand breaks and base elimination. Absorption of UV radiation by DNA results in the formation of hallmark pyrimidine dimers, which are potentially mutagenic. Ionizing radiation and UV radiation, to a lesser extent, also generate reactive oxygen species from many cellular molecules. These highly reactive molecules cause many types of DNA damage, including altered bases, strand breaks, and DNA-protein cross-links. Because UV radiation is a component of sunlight, sun exposure can cause cancer in nonpigmented and relatively hairless areas in animals, such as the ears of white cats and the conjunctiva of Hereford cattle.

Viruses

Viruses that cause cancer are termed *oncogenic viruses*. Oncogenic viruses important in veterinary medicine are listed in E-Table 6-2). Oncogenic viruses employ a remarkable array of direct and indirect mechanisms to induce cancer.

Dominant Oncogene Mechanism. The genomes of many rapidly transforming oncogenic viruses include a dominant oncogene that drives tumor development. A virus may actually acquire an oncogene from the host animal cell, by incorporating a cellular proto-oncogene into the genome of the infecting virus and subsequently transmitting that oncogene to new animal cells. Once the oncogene becomes part of the viral genome, its expression is no longer subject to normal cellular controls. Uncontrolled production of oncoproteins from the viral oncogene drives cell proliferation and, ultimately, carcinogenesis. Examples of animal-derived oncogenes include the *fes*, *fgr*, *abl*, *fms*, and *kit* genes acquired by oncogenic sarcoma and leukemia retroviruses of cats. Viruses may also contain oncogenes not derived from the host target cell genome. For example, papillomavirus genomes include endogenous *E6* and *E7* genes that encode proteins that inhibit the tumor suppressor proteins p53 and pRb, respectively.

Insertional Mutagenesis Mechanism. Viruses that do not possess their own oncogenes can instead activate the expression of target cell oncogenes by a process called *insertional mutagenesis*. The insertion of viral DNA in these sites results in unregulated production of target cell–encoded oncoproteins responsible for carcinogenesis. For example, most tumors caused by the avian leukosis virus exhibit only a few sites of viral insertion near host proto-oncogenes, notably the *c-myc* gene, where viral promoters drive unregulated production of target cell–encoded oncoproteins.

Hit-and-Run Mechanism. In the two mechanisms discussed previously, the viral genome or portions of the genome persist in the host target cell. However, some viruses also cause tumors merely by transient residence in target cells. Bovine papillomavirus uses such a *hit-and-run* mechanism of cell transformation. In these instances the presence of the virus is necessary to initiate carcinogenesis, but the virus is typically no longer detectable in the tumor itself. The precise mechanism by which this might occur has not been elucidated.

Indirect Mechanisms. Viruses may also stimulate tumorigenesis by suppression of the animal's immune system or by stimulation of target cell proliferation. The herpesvirus that causes Marek's disease, a T cell lymphoma of poultry, is an example of a virus that suppresses the ability of the host to eliminate transformed cells; this suppression is believed to be due to cytolysis of B and T lymphocytes during the early lytic phase of viral infection. As a second example, the genome of the Shope fibroma virus, a poxvirus, encodes a homologue of the epidermal growth factor (*EGF*) gene, which drives host cell proliferation, thus promoting tumor development.

Cancer in Animals

Animal Models of Cancer

Animal models have been and remain critically important tools for understanding the cause of human cancer and for testing cancer therapeutic agents. Animal models of cancer include both experimentally induced and naturally occurring tumors. In experimentally induced cancer models, administration of carcinogenic substances or transplantation of human cancer cells results in *de novo* development of cancer in test animals. Naturally occurring models of cancer rely on the spontaneous development of tumors in the test animal.

Experimentally Induced Tumors

A major advantage of experimental model systems is the rapid and reproducible induction of cancer in a very large proportion of experimental animals. Rodents, mice in particular, are often used for such studies. Mice are small and relatively inexpensive to maintain, reproduce rapidly, and have genetics that are highly defined and readily manipulated. The mouse genome has been sequenced in its entirety and detailed comparative maps of the human and mouse genomes have been developed. Many inbred mouse strains, each consisting of genetically identical or syngeneic individuals, are available. Genetic homogeneity of mice standardizes responses and thus reduces the numbers of animals required for research studies. However, mice have several inherent shortcomings as models of human cancer. The genetic homogeneity of inbred mice does not reflect the high degree of genetic diversity within the general human population. Experimentally induced tumors in mice rarely metastasize, whereas metastasis is an important cause of morbidity and mortality in human beings. Finally, the short life span and small size of mice make them less than ideal for long-term testing of tumor therapies.

A number of inbred mouse strains have been developed that are particularly suited to specific needs in cancer research. Nude mice and other profoundly immunodeficient mouse strains accept tumor or normal tissue grafts from other species and provide an environment in which these xenografts can be maintained, manipulated, and studied. Sencar and hairless mice are highly susceptible to tumors of keratinocyte origin and have thus been employed for many skin carcinogenesis studies. Inbred mice have been used extensively to determine the carcinogenicity of chemical and physical agents and to test the safety and efficacy of anticancer therapeutics. Studies in mice, particularly studies of chemically induced skin cancer, have been critical in defining the stages of carcinoma progression. Differences in strain susceptibility to different experimentally induced cancers have been exploited to identify modifier genes that dramatically affect tumor incidence.

With the advent of effective means for creating genetically engineered mice, specific genes of interest can be introduced into or inactivated in the mouse genome. An exogenous gene introduced into the mouse genome is generally termed a *transgene*. A mouse lacking a functional normal gene is referred to as a *knockout* for that gene. Moreover, the timing, location, and level of gene expression in genetically engineered mice can now be precisely controlled, thus allowing gene expression to be turned on or off in particular tissues as required for specific studies. Gene expression modulated in this fashion is termed *conditional* gene expression. Genetically engineered mice have been essential for identifying the mechanisms by which specific genes act to retard or enhance tumor development, growth, and spread.

Naturally Occurring Tumors

Several naturally occurring cancers in animals, including avian leukosis, bovine lymphoma, and feline leukemia, have provided invaluable information about the cause, transmission, and prevention of virally induced cancers. However, virally induced cancers do not appear to account for a large proportion of human cancers.

Recently, the dog has become the focus of increasing attention as a useful animal model of human cancers. Sequencing of the canine genome and comparative alignment with human and murine genomes enhance the usefulness of dogs as a naturally occurring cancer model. The annual incidence rate for cancer in dogs is 381 per 100,000; this is comparable with the cancer incidence in human beings. With the large number of pet dogs in this country, many cancer cases are thus available for entry into clinical trials. Like human beings, dogs are outbred. Moreover, dogs share a common environment with human beings and are exposed to many of the same carcinogens. As in human beings, many canine tumors metastasize widely. Because tumors in dogs progress more rapidly than human tumors, studies can be completed within a reasonable time frame. On the other hand, the time course of tumor development is sufficiently long to allow meaningful comparison of response times in different treatment groups. Because dogs are relatively large, they provide abundant tumor tissue for diagnostic and experimental purposes. In addition, many therapeutic approaches that are difficult to test in small rodents can readily be examined using larger dogs. Clinical trials in dogs are much easier to initiate and much cheaper to carry out than comparable studies in human beings. Many dog owners are enthusiastic participants in clinical trials that may benefit their pets. Tumor types for which dogs are particularly good models of human cancer include osteosarcoma and lymphoma.

Tumor Diagnosis and Prognosis

Taken together, the tumor type, grade, stage, and completeness of excision are used by the veterinary clinician to develop the most appropriate treatment plan for the patient. As we learn more about the molecular pathogenesis of certain tumors, the need for specialized diagnostic tests will certainly increase, because targeted molecular therapies will only be effective if the target is present in the animal's tumor. A full description of molecular techniques used in cancer diagnosis is beyond the scope of this chapter. However, it is certain that their use will become more widespread and commonplace in veterinary medicine.

Histopathologic Diagnosis

A definitive diagnosis of cancer is frequently obtained by standard histopathologic evaluation of tumor biopsy specimens or cytologic studies of tumor aspirates. Biopsy specimens for histopathologic evaluation are analyzed by routine hematoxylin and eosin (H&E) staining, whereas cytologic samples are typically stained with Wright's or Diff-Quik stains. Cells are scrutinized for features of malignancy, including abnormal morphologic features, high mitotic index, presence of abnormal mitoses, high nuclear to cytoplasmic ratio, and evidence of invasion or metastasis. The degree of differentiation is also routinely evaluated. Malignant neoplasms are frequently poorly to moderately differentiated, and some may be so anaplastic that the cell of origin cannot be determined. The presence of cellular products, such as osteoid in osteosarcomas, may provide clues to the identity of the cell of origin for the tumor.

Immunohistochemistry for specific cell markers may be used to aid in the diagnosis of some tumors. For example, immunohistochemistry is commonly used to determine if a lymphoma originates from B or T lymphocytes (E-Fig. 6-3). This knowledge may be useful to the clinician in designing treatment or delivering a prognosis. The type of intermediate filaments present in an undifferentiated malignancy can indicate if the tumor is of epithelial (positive for cytokeratin staining) or mesenchymal (positive for vimentin staining) origin. Some neoplasms, such as mesotheliomas and synovial cell sarcomas, are often positive for both cytokeratin and vimentin. Carcinomas that have undergone EMT will have areas positive for cytokeratin or vimentin, and transition areas may be positive for both. An exhaustive list of antibodies is beyond the scope of this chapter, but immunohistochemical staining is becoming a widely used tool that assists pathologists in providing a more complete diagnosis in cases in which routine H&E evaluation does not provide a definitive diagnosis.

Histochemical stains can also aid in diagnosis. Poorly differentiated canine mast cells may have granules that are not clearly visible by H&E staining. Staining with toluidine blue often highlights the granules and confirms the diagnosis in otherwise challenging cases.

Other Diagnostic Techniques

Clonality Assays. Sometimes it is difficult to distinguish benign lymphoid hyperplasia from lymphoma by morphologic features alone. Most neoplasms are believed to be clonal, that is, they are ultimately derived from a single transformed cell. Thus, establishing that a lymphocyte population is clonal gives more weight to a diagnosis of a malignancy. Clonality can be assessed by analyzing the lymphocytes for T or B lymphocyte receptor rearrangement, using the polymerase chain reaction (PCR). If the entire lymphocyte population has a single rearrangement, the proliferation is clonal, and most likely neoplastic. Conversely, if each lymphocyte has a different receptor rearrangement, this indicates a polyclonal proliferation, which is more consistent with lymphoid hyperplasia. However, the presence of a clonal population of lymphocytes does not, by itself, guarantee lymphoma. Some nonneoplastic conditions, such as canine ehrlichiosis, can give rise to clonal lymphocyte populations. Therefore results must be interpreted in conjunction with clinical signs and other clinicopathologic data.

Cytogenetic Analysis. Cytogenetic analysis can be a useful tool for diagnosis, determining the presence of residual disease after treatment, and stratification of high- and low-risk patients. The discovery of recurrent chromosomal abnormalities and translocations, particularly in leukemias and lymphomas, will aid in diagnosis and understanding the pathogenesis of these diseases, as well as the design of targeted therapies.

Pedigree Analysis. Identification of genes involved in inherited cancers can be accomplished through the detailed analysis of well-described pedigrees, particularly in certain cancer-prone breeds. As is the case in human beings, the elucidation of these genes is important not only in the diagnosis and screening of high-risk animals but also in providing insight into the pathogenesis of sporadic tumors.

Molecular Diagnostic Techniques. Recently, new techniques have been developed that permit global gene expression analysis of tumors. Microarrays, which allow the measurement of thousands of mRNA transcripts simultaneously, are already available for a wide range of species. New techniques of high-throughput sequencing can determine the identity and abundance of all mRNAs in a tumor. High-throughput sequencing can also be used to sequence the entire genome of a tumor to identify potentially oncogenic mutations. Studies using these new techniques are likely to identify significant changes in gene sequence and gene expression, which can be used to facilitate diagnosis and therapy.

Grading

A tumor *grade* is assigned by a pathologist to provide some indication of how similar or dissimilar the neoplastic cells are to their normal counterparts. The underlying assumption is that this grade provides some indication about biologic behavior. This assumption is not universally true, however, and experience has demonstrated that tumor stage (see next section) is sometimes a more useful prognostic measure.

All grading schemes evaluate the degree of differentiation of tumor cells. The tumor grade classifications usually include well-differentiated (very similar to normal cells), moderately differentiated (somewhat similar to normal cells), and poorly differentiated (anaplastic) cells. These categories translate to low, medium, and high grade, or grades I, II, and III, respectively. Other criteria that may be included in grading schemes include the mitotic index, defined as the number of mitotic figures per 400× field (usually the average of 10 fields); the extent of tumor necrosis; tumor invasiveness; and overall tumor cellularity. Grading schemes vary depending on the tumor type. In an ideal scheme, grading criteria are easily identified on H&E-stained tumor sections, and the grade is strongly linked to prognosis or response to therapy. The criteria employed should be periodically reevaluated in light of new discoveries and diagnostic capabilities.

Staging

Tumor *stage* gives an indication of the extent of tumor growth and spread in the animal. In general, staging guides the clinician in developing a therapeutic plan and offering an estimate of prognosis to the client. One of the most widely used schemes is the TNM system, which is based on the size of the primary tumor (T), degree of lymph node involvement (N), and extent of metastasis (M). Within each category a number is assigned based on clinical, diagnostic, and histopathologic evaluations. A designation of T0 is given to carcinoma in situ, whereas T1 to T4 indicate increasing size of the primary tumor. N0 indicates the absence of detectable lymph node involvement, whereas N1 to N3 indicate progressive involvement. Similarly, M0 signifies no detectable metastasis, whereas M1 and M2 indicate metastasis to one and two organs, respectively.

Overall, TNM staging provides a standard measurement by which the natural course of disease and impact of treatment modalities can be compared. However, there is some variability in tumor staging at different institutions. This variability often reflects the availability of more sophisticated imaging modalities, such as computed tomography (CT) and magnetic resonance imaging (MRI), as well as more sensitive techniques of histologic detection, such as immunohistochemistry for cytokeratin to detect micrometastases in lymph nodes of carcinoma patients.

Surgical Margins

With *incisional biopsies* the intent is merely to get enough tissue to make a diagnosis, whereas *excisional biopsies* are performed with the intent of complete removal of the tumor mass to effect a cure. Microscopic evaluation of surgical margins to confirm that the tumor has been completely excised has long been a valuable service provided by the diagnostic pathologist (see Figs. 17-34, 17-35, and 17-36). Residual malignant cells at the surgical site may warrant a second surgical procedure. However, evaluation of margins is not always straightforward. It is often difficult for the pathologist to properly orient the gross specimen with respect to lateral, deep, and superficial margins. Using sutures or different colors of ink along with proper annotations is helpful in indicating which margin is which. It may also be difficult to distinguish true surgical margins from those produced at trimming. Inking of margins by the surgeon at the time of removal is often recommended to distinguish real margins from those created after sample removal. More importantly, having clean surgical margins on a histologic slide does not guarantee that the patient is free of tumor. Neoplasms are three-dimensional lesions and only a portion of the mass is examined in any one section. So although the margins examined may be free of neoplastic cells, in other areas the neoplastic cells may extend to the surgical margin. In addition, multifocal or *multicentric* lesions may not be submitted to the pathologist. Lastly, lymphatic or hematogenous spread may not be evident on the section or sections examined. Submission of regional lymph nodes is often helpful in determining if the tumor has spread.

Suggested Readings

Suggested Readings are available at www.expertconsult.com.

SECTION II

Pathology of Organ Systems

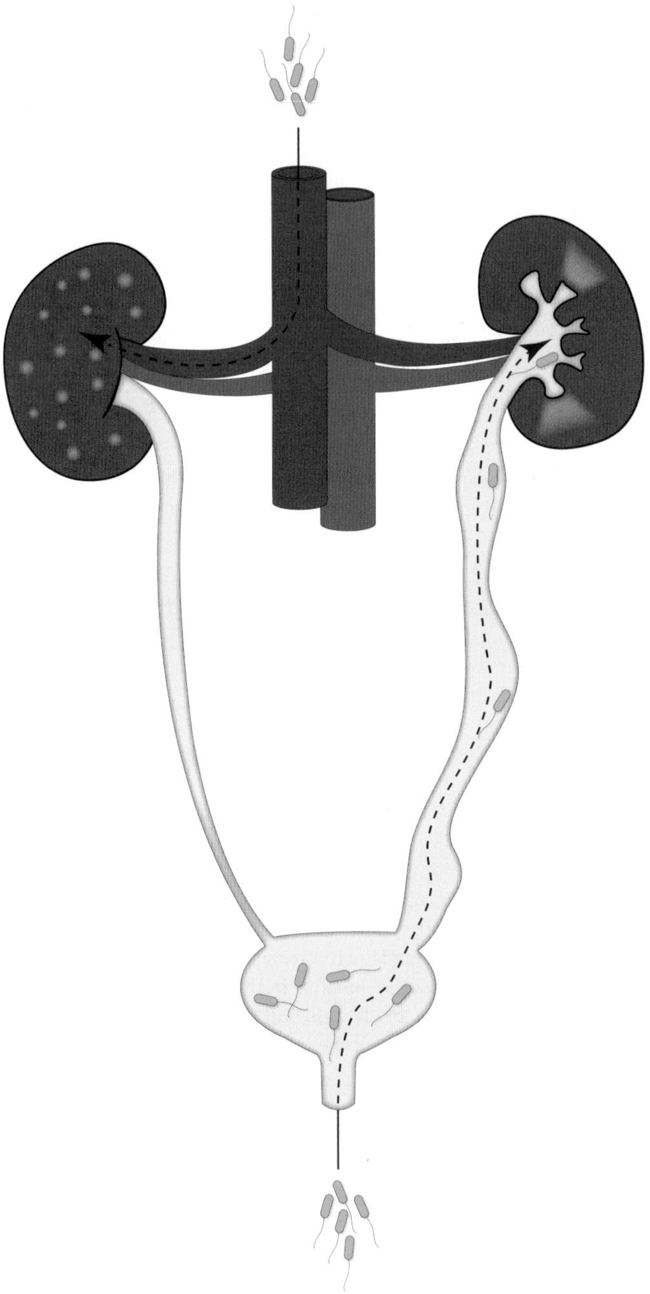

CHAPTER 7

Alimentary System and the Peritoneum, Omentum, Mesentery, and Peritoneal Cavity[1]

Howard B. Gelberg

Key Readings Index

The alimentary system is a long and complex tube that varies in its construction and function among animal species. For example, herbivores need a fermentation chamber (either a rumen or an expanded cecum) for the digestion of cellulose, a feature not present in carnivores. Although a large variety of gastrointestinal (GI) disturbances are clinically important in all species of animals, the predominant form of disease varies from species to species. Pet carnivores, partly because of their long life span, effective vaccines, and a lifestyle and diet similar to that of human beings, develop alimentary neoplasia far more often than herbivores. Meat-, milk-, and fiber-producing animals (ruminants and pigs) are host to a variety of infectious diseases that are largely resistant to vaccines. These pathogens may have evolved as a result of the herding instinct of these animals, giving the pathogens an opportunity to mutate within a large socially structured host population. Horses are most prone to displacements of alimentary viscera.

In general the alimentary system, including the salivary glands, pancreas, and liver, functions by adding water, electrolytes, and enzymes to ingested matter and then mixing and grinding it to facilitate its breakdown to water-soluble nutrients for absorption across mucous membranes into the blood circulation and subsequent distribution through the body. Although the alimentary tract is open ended, most ingested substances and secretions produced by the GI system are absorbed.

A large part of the practice of veterinary medicine is devoted to the diagnosis and treatment of alimentary disorders. Many of the newer molecular and imaging methods have been designed specifically to increase the clinician's ability to make accurate diagnoses of the various conditions of the alimentary system. Additionally, every physical examination includes the opportunity for a fecal analysis that allows the clinician a window into the functioning of the alimentary system as a whole.

The polymerase chain reaction (PCR) is a tool that allows the opportunity to rapidly diagnose an infectious cause of enteritis without having to culture the organism in the traditional manner. Diagnosis of the cause of an infectious disease of the alimentary system can also be made from examination of a biopsy sample by histologic and immunohistochemical staining or by *in situ* hybridization that allows demonstration of the pathogen within target cells.

Through the use of fiberoptic endoscopes inserted through the mouth or anus or through a small incision in the abdominal wall (laparoscopy), a thorough clinical examination of most of the alimentary system can be made. This knowledge is now a necessity in clinical practice because GI mucosa from the oral cavity, through the esophagus, stomach, duodenum, and the large colon and rectum and the entire serosal surface of the abdominal viscera can be viewed and sampled directly in the live animal.

For convenience of discussion and illustration, the alimentary system has been divided into the following anatomic subunits: oral cavity; teeth; tonsils; salivary glands; tongue; esophagus; rumen, reticulum, and omasum; stomach and abomasum; intestine; and the peritoneum, omentum, mesentery, and peritoneal cavity.

Structure and Function

The most important point to keep in mind when examining the alimentary system is that normal mucosal and serosal surfaces should be smooth and shiny (although there may be normal papilla, folds, and ridges). The exception to this rule is the rumen, whose papillae may normally have a roughened, dull surface appearance. When serosal and mucosal surfaces are not smooth and shiny, animals should be examined thoroughly to determine the reason.

[1]For a glossary of abbreviations and terms used in this chapter see E-Glossary 7-1.

The function of the alimentary system as a whole is to take ingested feedstuffs, grind them and mix them with a variety of secretions from the oral cavity, stomach, pancreas, liver, and intestines (digestion), and then to absorb the constituent nutrients into the bloodstream and lacteals. Undigested ingesta, effete neutrophils, fresh (hematochezia) or digested (melena) blood, and excess secretions are passed from the body into the alimentary lumen and thus become a component of the feces. The quality and quantity of the feces and clinical signs, such as regurgitation and vomiting, are often early indicators of alimentary dysfunction.

Oral Cavity

The physiologically normal oral mucosa is smooth, shiny, and pink. It is composed of variably keratinizing, stratified squamous epithelium (mucous membranes). In animals in which the oral mucosa is heavily pigmented (melanosis), assessment of circulatory function (capillary refill time) and color as an indicator of red blood cell concentration (packed cell volume) can be difficult. In these cases, examination of conjunctiva and rectal and urogenital mucosa can be substituted. The oral cavity is where ingested materials are masticated; mixed with digestive enzymes, such as those in saliva; and passed on through the oropharynx to the esophagus.

Teeth

Teeth provide mechanical advantage for prehension, tearing, and/or mastication of food. Among domestic animals there are differences in the growth pattern and numbers of teeth. Hypsodont teeth, such as in the horse, continue to grow throughout life, and appropriate leveling of the occlusive surfaces (floating) may be a necessary procedure to prevent malocclusion and sharp edges that can lacerate the adjacent buccal mucosa and interfere with appropriate mastication as the horse ages. Brachydont teeth, such as in carnivores, do not continue to grow after they are fully erupted. Most species of mammals have deciduous teeth that are replaced near maturity by permanent teeth. In many species the approximate age of the animal may be determined by eruption date and examination of wear patterns and shape of the teeth.

Molar teeth in general are designed for grinding feedstuffs, whereas incisors in ruminants (mandibular only) are for cropping forage. Canine teeth are designed for tearing flesh. Brachydont teeth consist of a crown, which is the portion above the gingiva; the neck, which is slightly constricted; and, just below the gingiva, the roots, which are embedded in the bony socket (alveolus) of the jaw. Enamel covers the crown, cementum covers the roots, and both cover the dentin. Besides carnivores, the incisor (lower) teeth of ruminants and porcine teeth, except the canines of the boar, are brachydont.

Hypsodont teeth have an elongated body, but the neck and roots may form later in life. Cementum covers the tooth, and enamel is beneath the cementum. Beneath the enamel is the dentin. The cementum and enamel invaginate into the dentin, forming the infundibula. Enamel crests result from normal wear, with enamel being the hardest of the layers. The cheek teeth of ruminants, tusks of boars, and the teeth of horses are hypsodont.

In simple-toothed animals, such as carnivores, the tooth root is not covered by enamel. Receding gingiva therefore expose the dentin, resulting in pain and invasion by bacteria. Domestic animal species seldom get caries, although buildup of plaque can result in gingival infections, osteolysis, and tooth loss.

Tonsils

The palatine tonsils are pharyngeal lymphoid structures covered by stratified squamous epithelium. Their function is uncertain, although it is likely they serve in lymphocyte production and antibody formation (see Chapters 5 and 13). In carnivores they are found in crypts or recesses at the dorsolateral aspect of the caudal oropharynx. In pigs they are flat and recognized by tiny pores in the surface epithelium of the caudal soft palate. Horses, ruminants, and pigs have lingual tonsils in addition to palatine tonsils.

Salivary Glands

Salivary glands are found in a variety of locations in the head and neck regions and vary in number and location from species to species. They arise from oral ectoderm. In all species the major salivary glands include the parotid, mandibular, and sublingual. Carnivores have a zygomatic gland as well. Minor salivary glands include buccal, labial, lingual, palatine, and others similarly named by location.

Most salivary glands are discrete aggregates of compound tubuloalveolar tissue. Saliva is a mixture of serous and mucoid secretions. Saliva lubricates the mouth and esophagus and moistens ingesta. Saliva also dissolves water-soluble components of food so the taste buds can function. The mucus in saliva binds to masticated food and creates a bolus that is more easily swallowed. Salivary mucus also coats the epithelium of the mouth, preventing mechanical damage to the tissue. Saliva, through its flushing action, reduces bacterial populations. Saliva contains a lysozyme that lyses bacteria. Carbohydrate digestion begins in the oral cavity as a result of the presence of α-amylase, which changes starch into maltose. There are very small quantities of this enzyme in carnivores and cattle. Saliva also is an effective buffer, especially in ruminants, whose forestomachs have no glands. In carnivores, evaporation of saliva is a major mechanism of thermoregulation.

Tongue

The tongue is a muscular organ covered by stratified epithelium and is functionally connected to the esophagus via the epiglottis. It is necessary for prehension, mastication, and swallowing of feedstuffs and water. The epithelial covering of the tongue is stratified squamous with various degrees of keratinization dorsally, but ventrally the epithelium is not keratinized and the tongue attaches to the floor of the oral cavity by a frenulum. Keratinized papillae are most prominent in ruminants and cats. There are various types of papillae, some with secondary lamellae. Vallate papillae, for example, are on the dorsal surface of the tongue near its origin and are flat structures completely surrounded by a cleft. Some surface macroscopic papillae contain taste buds. The tongue is a highly vascular (functioning in heat loss in many animals, especially carnivores that have no sweat glands) and sensitive organ containing a variety of serous and mucus glands and sensory cells (taste buds). The muscular part of the tongue is striated in randomly arranged bundles. A cordlike structure enclosed in dense collagen extending lengthwise near the ventral central surface of the tongue of carnivores is called the lyssa. Porcine and equine tongues have a similar structure. The lyssa appears to be a structure without a function. Historically the lyssa was removed as "prevention" for rabies. Lyssa bodies are synonymous with Negri bodies, and rabies used to be called lyssa. Adipose tissue becomes more abundant in the caudal part of the tongue in most species.

Esophagus

Under normal circumstances the esophageal lumen is a potential space. The wall collapses when the esophagus is not transporting ingesta. The esophagus extends from the aboral end of the oropharynx, passes through the mediastinum and the diaphragmatic hiatus, and ends at the stomach. The esophagus is lined by nonkeratinizing stratified squamous epithelium in carnivores and is keratinized in pigs, horses, and ruminants. Keratinization is greatest in ruminants, less in horses, and least in pigs. Longitudinal and oblique mucosal folds are present to varying degrees. Transverse, herringbone-like folds are present in the cat.

The tunica muscularis is completely striated in ruminants and dogs. In the horse the distal third of the esophagus contains smooth muscle. The pig is similar to the horse, except that the middle third of the esophagus contains a mixture of smooth and striated muscle. In cats, opossums, and primates, the distal two-thirds of the esophagus is composed of smooth muscle. The smooth muscle is arranged as an inner circular layer and an outer longitudinal layer. Horses are unable to vomit.

Mixed mucinous glands are present in the tunica submucosa of pigs and dogs. In pigs the glands are most abundant in the cranial half of the esophagus, and in dogs they are present throughout. Glands are present in cats, horses, and ruminants only at the junction of the esophagus and pharynx.

It is important to remember that unlike the rest of the tubular digestive tract, the esophagus is unique in that it lacks a serosa in all but the abdominal portion. This means that there is no serosa to leak serum and fibrin to seal a puncture wound from a perforation of a foreign body or a surgical incision. Likewise, sutures are not likely to seal an incision. Combine this with the strong muscular peristaltic contractions that characterize this organ and it is easy to understand why esophageal surgery is not often performed and is even less often successful. For the same anatomic reasons, perforating foreign bodies of the esophagus do not seal themselves off.

Esophageal innervation is from the vagus nerves. Esophageal smooth muscle contains myenteric ganglia. Striated muscle is innervated by motor end-plates via efferent fibers of the hypoglossal nerve along with contributory neurofibers from cranial nerves V, IX, and X, which control voluntary lingual function.

Rumen, Reticulum, and Omasum

The forestomachs of ruminants and camelids are dilations and modifications of the esophagus. They are designed to house the digestive flora responsible for breaking down cellulose into short-chain fatty acids. The rumen has small papillae that vary by diet up to 1.5 cm in length. Their length, shape, and degree of keratinization are affected by diet; they are longer with high-roughage diets and shorter with more concentrates in the ration. These changes are most obvious in the ventral compartment—the ventral ruminal sac. The reticulum has a honeycomb appearance, and the omasum consists of a series of approximately 100 longitudinal folds similar to the pages of a book. The non-glandular stratified squamous mucosa of the reticulum, rumen, and omasum can be acutely inflamed when their contents have an acid pH and the abnormal milieu permits bacterial and mycotic overgrowth.

The epithelial lining of the forestomach functions as a protective barrier for the forestomach and for the metabolism of ingesta and the absorption of volatile fatty acids, Na^+, and Cl^-. Because the reticulo-omasal orifice is more dorsal than the floor of the compartments, the reticulum can trap foreign bodies, especially dense metallic ones. These can irritate or penetrate the mucosa ("hardware disease"). Problems with motility and imbalances of rumen flora and fauna are the most frequent abnormalities of forestomach function. Often the changes in flora and fauna are precipitated by a change in ingested substrate, promoting the growth of particular organisms. These changes alter ruminal pH and thus affect the integrity of the mucosal lining of the compartments of the forestomach or cause the production of excessive gas, resulting in ruminal distention.

Parts of compartment one (C1) and C2 and C3 of the camelid forestomach are lined by mucinous glandular epithelium. Concretions of ingesta are sometimes found within the saccules that contain the glands. The saccules are also the sites of water and other solutes. The nonglandular portions of C1 and C2 are lined by non-keratinized stratified squamous epithelium without papillae. The forestomach of New World camelids contracts at two to three times the rate of ruminants (and in reverse order), and with each cycle, the saccules empty and refill. This results in high digestive efficiency across the saccules.

Stomach and Abomasum

The gastric mucosa of simple-stomached animals contains numerous folds or rugae that are flattened when the stomach is distended. Foveolae or gastric pits communicate with the lumen of the stomach and transport gastric cell secretions. The glandular stomach functions in the enzymatic and hydrolytic digestion of ingested food substances. The epithelial covering is one cell thick, and the cell types include columnar mucus and bicarbonate-secreting surface epithelial cells, mucous neck cells arranged in tubuloalveolar glands, acid-secreting parietal cells, pepsinogen-secreting chief cells, and neuroendocrine (enterochromaffin, argentaffin) cells that secrete gastrin, enteroglucagon, and somatostatin (Fig. 7-1). The neuroendocrine cells do not communicate with the gastric lumen. The mucous neck cells are the precursor cells for all the other epithelial types in the stomach and are responsible for the replacement of surface epithelial cells as they are lost, either at the end of their normal life span or from some type of insult.

Multiple submucosal lymphoid patches are present in monogastric animals. In ruminants a single lymphoid patch is present at the fold separating the omasum and abomasum.

In some species, such as the horse and rat, the cranial or orad part of the stomach (nonglandular part or pars nonglandularis) is lined by stratified squamous epithelium, whereas the distal portion (pars glandularis) is lined by glandular epithelium. In the horse the dividing line between the two is called the *margo plicatus*. The pars nonglandularis in the pig is a small square to rectangular area of stratified squamous epithelium surrounding the esophageal opening.

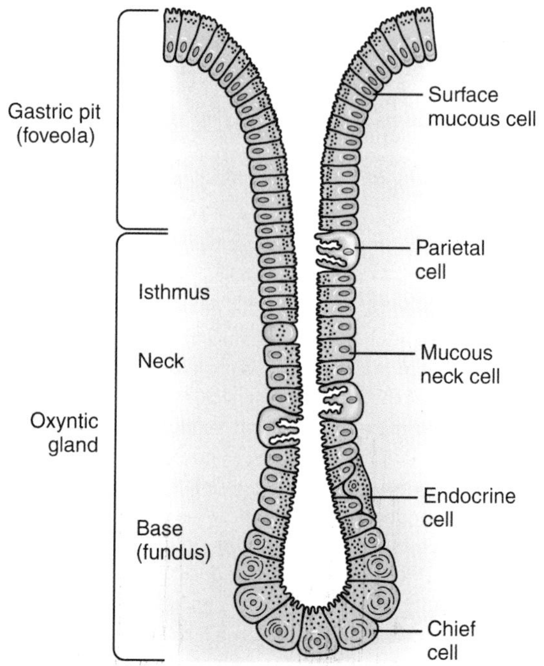

Figure 7-1 Microanatomy of the Stomach.

Although some differences exist, the stomachs of the simple-stomached animals and the abomasum of ruminants (third compartment of New World camelids) are very similar in structure and function. A fundus and body make up the cranial portion lined by numerous spiral folds and produce acid and pepsin. The aboral portion, the pyloric part, is lined by epithelium with mucous-secreting glands and G cells that produce gastrin. Stomachs have an indigenous flora. Most of these organisms cannot be cultured by traditional methods. C3 of New World camelids is more tubular than the abomasum, with more peristalsis-like rather than mixing motility. The first two-thirds of C3 is fermentative with a pH of approximately 6.5. At the caudal flexure the mucosa thickens to 7 to 10 mm and the pH is around 2.0. The final portion surrounding the torus pyloricus has an alkaline pH.

Intestine

The intestines might be thought of as a tube within the body cavity that carries material (ingesta/digesta) through the body. The overall anatomic and histologic organization of this digestive tube is illustrated in Figure 7-2. By the action of enzymes, resident flora, and added secretions from the liver and pancreas, ingesta are broken down, nutrients are absorbed into the body, and waste products are excreted. To perform these functions the intestine needs a very large surface area, which is accomplished by the following three means:

1. The intestine is coiled in the abdomen.
2. Numerous intestinal folds contain villi that notably increase the number of cells contacting the ingesta (Fig. 7-3, A and B).
3. Each enterocyte has a microvillous border, further increasing the surface area available for digestive and absorptive processes (see Fig. 7-3, C).

Herbivores have longer intestines than carnivores or omnivores and need a fermentation vat, either the rumen or cecum, to digest cellulose. Within the smooth muscle layers and villi are the neural network of the enteric nervous system.

The intestinal mucosa is composed of three layers—a single-cell-thick layer of epithelial cells lining the intestinal lumen,

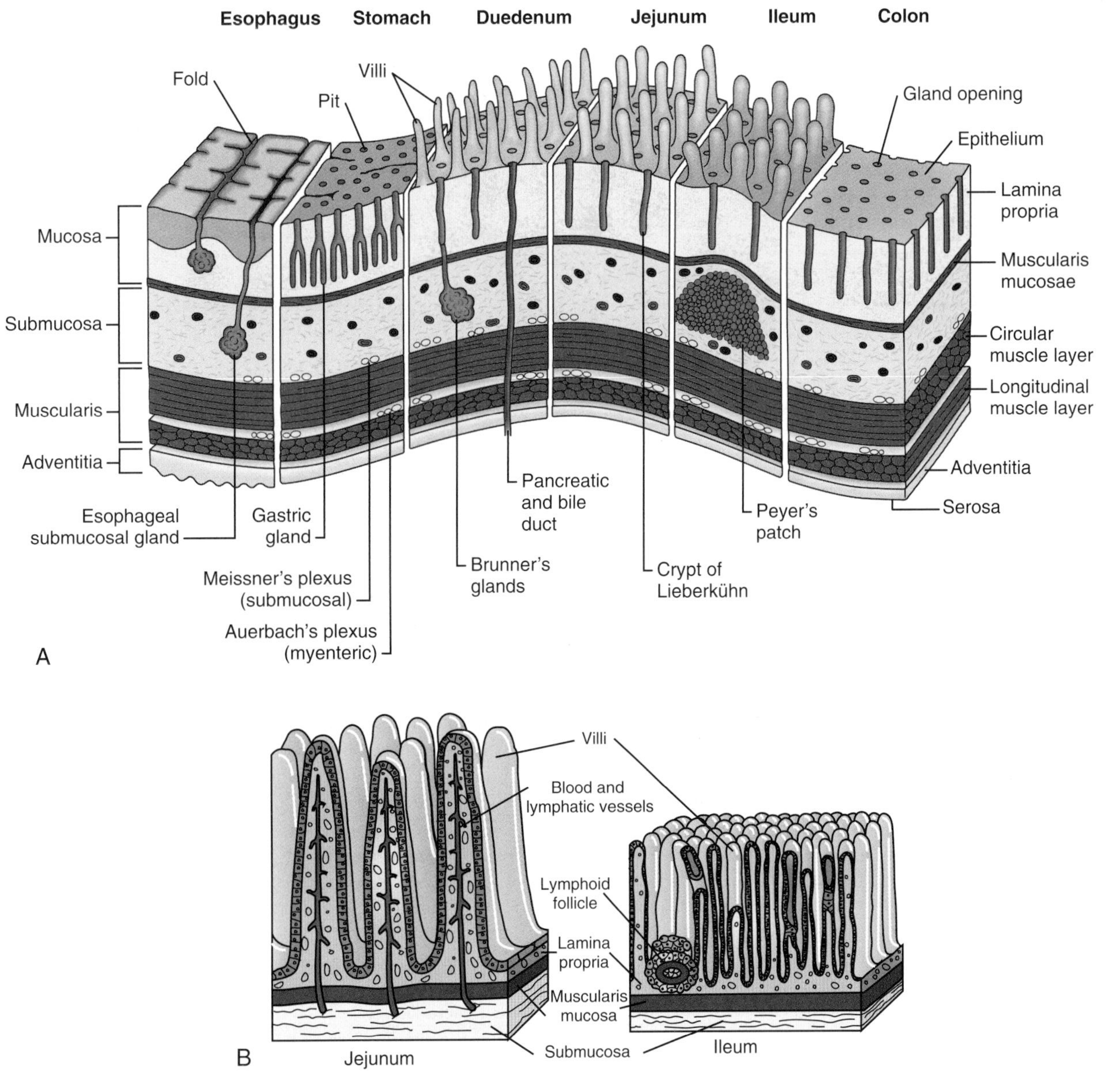

Figure 7-2 **Anatomic and Histologic Organization of the Digestive Tube. A,** Entire digestive tube. **B,** Higher magnification of the jejunum and ileum.

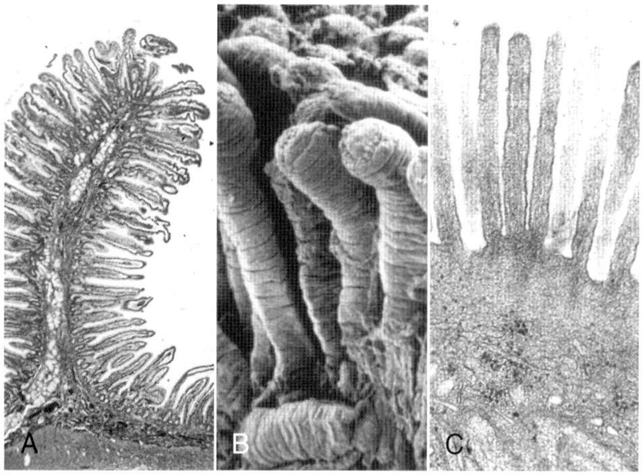

Figure 7-3 **Organization of the Intestine.** The digestive and absorptive surfaces of the intestine are markedly increased by the presence of villi and microvilli on the enterocytes. **A,** Intestinal villi. Villus epithelial cells are present on a basement membrane (not seen) on a core of lamina propria. Hematoxylin and eosin (H&E) stain. **B,** Small intestine, intestinal villi, scanning electron microscopy. Carbon sputter coat. **C,** Enterocyte microvilli. Transmission electron microscopy (TEM). Uranyl acetate and lead citrate stain. (From Damjanov I, Linder J: *Anderson's pathology*, ed 10, St. Louis, 1996, Mosby.)

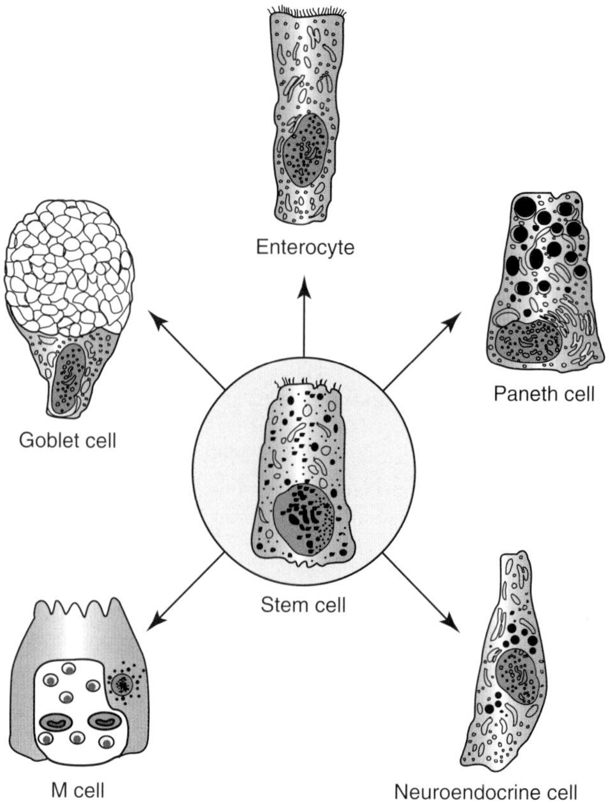

Figure 7-4 **Epithelial Cell types of the Small Intestine.** Progenitor cells, located in the intestinal crypts, give rise to all other epithelial cell types lining the crypt and covering the villi.

mesenchymal cells of the lamina propria, and the muscularis mucosa. Damage to any of these structures or to their innervation can result in digestive dysfunction and resultant diarrhea.

The epithelial cells function as a selectively permeable barrier allowing nutrient, electrolyte, and water absorption, while excluding pathogens, toxins, and other antigens. An understanding of these cell types and their functional roles in digestion and absorption is important in understanding the mechanisms of intestinal disease. Similarly, an understanding of the biology of these cell types is important in predicting clinical outcomes and designing therapeutic strategies for treating intestinal disease.

Epithelial Cells

There are six major types of polarized epithelial cells lining the intestine, all of which are produced by progenitor cells in the crypts via notch signaling. Notch and Wnt signals in combination are necessary for proliferation of enterocyte precursors, but differentiation of cell types is independent of Wnt. Wnt and notch synergy appears to induce intestinal adenomas. Notch pathways are used by cells (i.e., cell-cell communication) to regulate, via their genes, cell differentiation processes that occur during embryonic and adult life. In the gut, notch pathways influence whether intestinal epithelial stem cells differentiate into cells with secretory or absorptive functions. These pathways involve typical ligand-receptor interactions, in which the ligand is a transmembrane protein expressed in one cell type (see Chapter 1) that binds with a notch receptor (i.e., notch protein) present on or in the cell membrane of another cell type. This binding interaction results in modifications of gene expression in the cell expressing the receptor, such as facilitating its differentiation into an absorptive enterocyte. This ligand-receptor binding appears to result in cells organizing into groups of cell types as needed for their differentiation into specific tissues and organs.

The epithelial cells are enterocytes, undifferentiated or crypt epithelial cells, goblet cells, Paneth cells, enterochromaffin (neuroendocrine, argentaffin) cells, and microfold (M) cells (Fig. 7-4).

Enterocytes are tall and columnar with luminal microvilli. They contain a surface glycocalyx that houses the digestive and absorptive enzymes. The mature cells do not proliferate, but they provide feedback inhibition of mitosis to the crypt cells by chalones. The cells are attached to each other by tight junctions composed of more than 40 proteins anchored to actin filaments, the most predominant of which are occludin, junctional adhesion molecules, and claudins. Many nutrients are absorbed through the lateral intercellular spaces between cells. Enterocytes move up the crypt and intestinal villus to the extrusion zone at the villus tip, where effete enterocytes are discarded into the fecal mass by an apoptotic mechanism called *anoikis*. The turnover rate for enterocytes is the most rapid of any fixed-cell population in the body. In neonatal pigs, for example, the turnover rate is 7 to 10 days. In 3-week-old pigs that have achieved a mature or climax flora, that rate accelerates to 2 to 3 days. Enterocytes are pinocytotic in the neonate, which is important in colostrum uptake and transfer of passive immunity from the dam. Enterocytes contain class II major histocompatibility complex (MHC) molecules and a complement of biotransformation enzymes important in metabolizing xenobiotics. Inflammatory bowel disease in human beings is accompanied by downregulation of genes encoding some of these enzymes, such as colonic enterocyte cytochrome P450. Enterocytic microvilli shed receptor-laden alkaline phosphatase and catalase-containing vesicles, thus potentially interacting with pathogens that are subsequently shed in the feces. This is one means of intestinal protection from pathogens.

The microbiota/microbiome of the lower GI system consists of 100 trillion bacteria (10 times the number of cells in an animal) and 3.3 million genes (150 times the number of genes in an animal). These bacteria secrete bacteriocins (i.e., proteinaceous toxins that inhibit the growth of other bacteria) and compete for nutrients and for attachment sites, thus limiting potential pathogen growth. The microbiota promotes immune system maturation and contains biotransformation enzymes such as β-glucuronidases, β-glucosidases, demethylases, hydrolases, and reductases. It has been recently discovered that there are three enterotypes (i.e., types of bacteriologic ecosystems of the GI microbiome) in animals and that these biotypes may be in part responsible for susceptibility or resistance to certain diseases.

Undifferentiated crypt epithelial cells have little or no digestive capability. They are the progenitor cells that replace all of the other epithelial cell types. They have short, sparse microvilli. Crypt cells are the source of secretory component that acts as a receptor for immunoglobulin A (IgA) and immunoglobulin M (IgM) produced by plasmacytes in the intestinal lamina propria. The migration rate of crypt cells up the villus depends on several factors, one of which is an adaptation to gut microflora. In germ-free or gnotobiotic animals the enterocyte replacement rate is similar to that of the neonate. Crypt cells are a source of chloride ion secretion into the intestinal lumen.

Goblet cells secrete mucus. They occur in both villous and crypt regions. Their numbers tend to increase aborally throughout the length of the intestine. Mucus exerts a variety of protective effects, including trapping of bacteria with resultant passage in the fecal mass and lessening of shear forces of particulate matter on the enterocytes.

Paneth cells are located near the crypt base in some species, notably primates, horses, and rodents. It is not certain if Paneth cells are present in pigs. Unlike all the other cells of the intestinal surface, these cells migrate toward the crypts rather than the villus tips. Paneth cells are considered to have both secretory and phagocytic functions. Experimentally, Paneth cell function and microbial composition vary among strains of mice suggesting a genetic influence of the host.

Paneth cells produce cryptdins, lysins, peptidases and lysozymes. Some of these substances are toxic to bacteria and probably protect the proliferating crypt cells from infection. Paneth cells also act in a paracrine manner by opening anion channels in enterocytes, causing chloride secretion from crypt enterocytes. It has been suggested that Paneth cells play a role in elimination of heavy metals because they are selectively damaged by methylmercury. Collectively, Paneth cells constitute a cellular mass similar to that of the pancreas.

Enteroendocrine cells are also known as *enterochromaffin cells* and *argentaffin cells* because of their affinity for silver stains. The GI system is the largest endocrine organ in the body (Box 7-1). Enteroendocrine cells reside primarily in the crypts and produce serotonin, glucose-dependent insulotropic peptide, catecholamines, gastrin, somatostatin, serotonin, cholecystokinin, secretin, bombesin, enteroglucagon, and likely others in response to chemical and mechanical stimuli. They secrete these products into the tissue rather than the gut lumen and thus are truly endocrine. Serotonin, for example, activates both the intrinsic and extrinsic primary afferent neurons initiating peristalsis and secretory reflexes that are transmitted to the central nervous system (CNS). Occasionally enteroendocrine cells form neoplasms called *carcinoids*.

M cells (microfold [membranous] cells) occur in most species. These cells are located in the dome or follicle-associated epithelium of Peyer's patches or gut-associated lymphoid tissue (GALT). They are important in the uptake of antigens, including particulate toxins (e.g., asbestos) from the intestinal lumen, and transport to the lymphatic system. M cells have basal recesses that house lymphoid cells that allow more rapid interaction with phagocytosed antigens. They also allow bidirectional movement of lymphocytes between the lamina propria and intestinal lumen. M cells are exploited for the entry of a variety of pathogens such as *Salmonella*, *Yersinia*, *Rhodococcus*, and some viruses (bovine virus diarrhea). Figure 7-5 illustrates the anatomic and mechanistic relationships of M cells to the underlying lymphoid tissue.

Box 7-1 Enterochromaffin (Enteroendocrine, Argentaffin) Cells of the Gastrointestinal System

STOMACH	
Gastrin	Stimulates parietal cells to release HCl, ↑ motility
Ghrelin	Appetite regulator
Neuropeptide Y	↑ Food intake
Somatostatin	↓ Rate of gastric emptying and ↓ smooth muscle contractions and blood flow within the intestine ↓ Release of gastrin, cholecystokinin, motilin, secretin, vasoactive intestinal peptide, gastric inhibitory polypeptide
Enteroglucagon	↓ Release of pancreatic hormones ↓ Exocrine secretory action of the pancreas
Histamine	↑ Gastric acid secretion
Endothelin	Smooth muscle contraction
Glicentin	↑ Glycogenolysis in the liver
Glucagon	↑ Concentration of glucose in the blood
INTESTINE	
Serotonin (90% of body's total from GI tract)	Mood, appetite, sleep
Cholecystokinin	Gallbladder emptying, pancreatic secretion, satiety
Bombesin	Negative feedback for eating
Secretin	Regulates secretions of stomach, pancreas and water balance
Enteroglucagon	Delays gastric emptying
Enterogastrone–Brunner's gland	↓ HCl from stomach
Gastrin	Stimulates parietal cells to release HCl, ↑ motility
Fibroblast growth factor 19	Effects on liver (bile acid production, glucose, glycogen)
Substance P	Stimulates emetic center
Vasoactive intestinal polypeptide	Relaxes smooth muscle of stomach, esophageal and gastric sphincters, and gallbladder while also inducing contraction of enteric smooth muscle Increases water secretion, inhibits gastrin, and stimulates pancreatic secretion of bicarbonate
Gastric inhibitory peptide = glucose-dependent inhibitory peptide	↓ Gastrin, ↑ insulin
Motolin	Stimulates peristalsis
Peptide YY	↓ Motility
Neurotensin	↑ Pancreatic secretion, ↑ blood flow, ↓ motility
Glucagon-like peptide	↑ Insulin, ↓ gastric emptying, ↓ gastric secretion
Glicentin	↑ Glycogenolysis in the liver
Glucagon	↑ Concentration of glucose in the blood
Urogastrone	↓ HCl
Oxyntomodulin	↓ Gastric secretion, ↓ intestinal mucosal growth
Enkephalins	↑ Smooth muscle contraction, ↓ secretion of water and electrolytes

GI, Gastrointestinal; *HCl*, hydrogen chloride.

Mesenchymal Cells

The intestinal lymphoid tissue is 25% of the body's lymphoid mass (Fig. 7-6) and consists of lymphoid cells in the lamina propria and

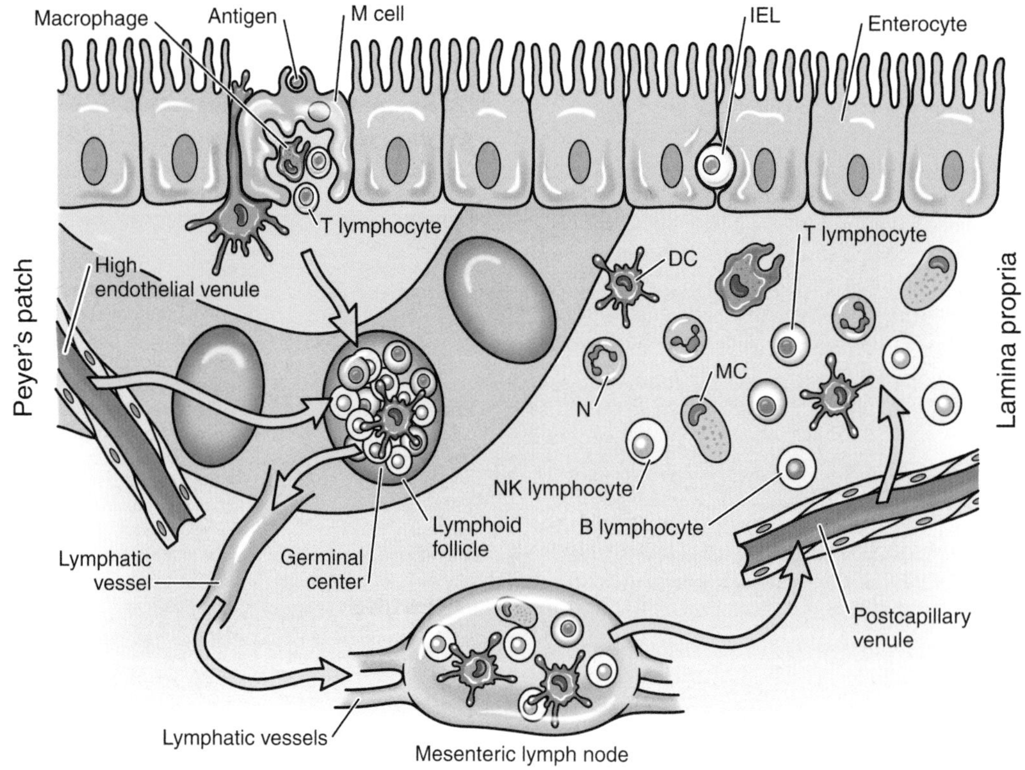

Figure 7-5 **Gut-Associated Lymphoid Tissue (GALT).** *DC*, Dendritic cell; *IEL*, intraepithelial lymphocyte; *M*, microfold; *MC*, mast cell; *N*, neutrophil; *NK*, natural killer.

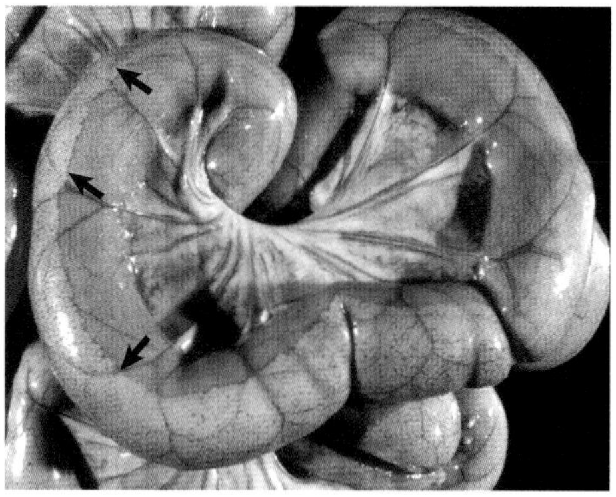

Figure 7-6 **Normal Gut-Associated Lymphoid Tissue (GALT), Intestine, Pig.** The lymphoid tissue on the antimesenteric surface of the intestine is outlined by arrows and makes up one-quarter of the animal's total lymphoid mass. (Courtesy Dr. H. Gelberg, College of Veterinary Medicine, Oregon State University.)

the GALT. This volume is larger than that of the spleen. In spite of the fact that the average person ingests 700 tons of antigens in a lifetime, the gut is adept at not responding to these food antigens. Laminal propria lymphocytes also play a role in intestinal crypt cell differentiation. Data are beginning to accumulate identifying the different effector and regulatory T lymphocyte types in the lamina propria and the functional organization of the GALT (see Fig. 7-5).

The classification and functions of innate immune cells are currently being elucidated. They arise from the same progenitor cell as natural killer (NK) T lymphocytes, do not contain T lymphocyte receptors, and produce a plethora of interleukins and other soluble mediators that parallel those of the antigen-specific immune effector cells. Current theory holds that the innate lymphoid cells hold infections in check until specific immune responses can be generated. Dendritic cells may be group 3 innate lymphoid cells and along with macrophages have toll-like receptors.

Mesenchymal cells reside in the lamina propria. They arise from primitive mesenchyme rather than from ectoderm or endoderm. Among these cells is a resident population of lymphocytes that increase with exposure to antigens, especially the microbiota. The immune system and microbiota have profound influences on each other in maintaining intestinal homeostasis.

Neutrophils are transient within the lamina propria of the intestine. Neutrophils are short-lived in the blood and tissues; their normal route of removal from the body is to migrate through the wall of the alimentary tract to the lumen and be digested or excreted from the body via feces. Human neutrophils spend approximately 5 days in the bloodstream and approximately 2 days in tissues. However, there is marked variation in neutrophil life span among species. In mice, for example, neutrophils live approximately 0.75 days.

Eosinophils, when present in the intestinal lamina propria and submucosa, indicate a hypersensitivity reaction, often to food antigens or parasites.

Mast cells comprise 2% to 3% of the cells of the lamina propria and under normal conditions help regulate the intestinal epithelial barrier. Intestinal mast cells differ in important ways from mast cells in other portions of the body. They lack membrane-bound immunoglobulin E (IgE) and release proinflammatory mediators through paracrine cytokines. Mast cells are very important in maintaining intestinal integrity and perform such functions as regulating the epithelial barrier, controlling blood flow, coagulation, smooth muscle contraction, stimulation of the enteric nervous system, peristalsis, and antibody-dependent recognition of parasites and microorganisms.

Globule leukocytes are large granular lymphocytes that are interepithelial or within the lamina propria. They are most common in parasitic infections. They are found in all species and occasionally form neoplasms, most notably in the cat. The normal function of these cells is unknown. Likewise, their origin is unknown. Theories include derivation from mast cells, plasma cells, large granular lymphocyte lineages, or from a distinct precursor.

Peritoneum, Omentum, Mesentery, and Peritoneal Cavity

The peritoneum is a membrane composed of a connective tissue stroma and a mesothelial cell component separated by a basement membrane. Mesothelial cells are permeable and function as a dialysis membrane. Their rapid regeneration after injury may be misinterpreted as neoplasia. It is speculated that mesothelial regeneration occurs from stem cells in the subserosal tissues rather than proliferation of adjacent uninjured mesothelial cells. Thus repair of a damaged peritoneum occurs across the whole of the damaged surface rather than from the edges such as occurs on epithelial-lined mucous membranes and skin. The peritoneum lines the abdominal cavity (parietal peritoneum) and reflects around and covers the visceral organs and scrotal cavity (visceral peritoneum). The omentum, mesenteries, and ligaments are doubled sheets of peritoneum that connect the visceral peritoneum to the parietal peritoneum. Nerves and vessels course through these structures into the various visceral structures. The visceral and parietal peritoneum receive afferent innervation from different sources. The visceral innervation is autonomic, responding with dull pain sensation to pressure and traction. In contrast, the parietal peritoneum receives afferent nerves from somatic and visceral sources, resulting in sharp pain when stimulation occurs. The peritoneal structures are an important site of fat storage and a site of serous atrophy when the animal is in negative energy balance. The kidneys are covered by peritoneum on only one surface and are thus termed *retroperitoneal*. Like other serous surfaces, peritoneal structures are smooth and shiny when not diseased.

Omenta (greater and lesser) connect the stomach to other organs or to the body wall. Ligaments course from the body wall to an organ or from organ to organ. A mesentery in its broad definition runs from the abdominal wall to the intestine or female reproductive system. The peritoneum and its connected structures produce a small amount of fluid, which is useful in lubrication of mesothelial surfaces. This fluid does not contain fibrinogen and therefore does not clot on exposure to air, except in pigs and camelids.

The omenta are capable of localizing infection and serve as an important source of revascularization of surgically altered tissues. Unfortunately, they also serve as a blood supply to metastatic tumors (i.e., carcinomatosis). Horses in general have a small omentum and thus are less able to wall off peritoneal infections than are ruminants. Omentectomy does not appear to have an adverse effect on general health.

Pacinian Corpuscles

Pacinian corpuscles are baroreceptors that are commonly present in the pancreatic interstitium (see Fig. 8-87) and in the mesentery of cats. They are often visible macroscopically and may whorl in a fingerprint pattern (E-Fig. 7-1) or appear as solid masses resembling parasites (see Fig. 8-87).

Dysfunction/Responses to Injury

Gastrointestinal Aging

Aging changes in the alimentary system are generally subtle and not of clinical significance and are most often recognized in dogs. In the oral cavity, significant changes occurring with aging are lacking with the exception of plaque buildup, which is generally more severe and more prone to advance to periodontitis in smaller breeds of pet carnivores. A variety of factors may account for this, including dental crowding, softer diets, and malocclusions. The end result may be alveolar bone resorption and dental loss.

In the intestinal tract, especially in dogs, increasing age results in decreased secretion of saliva and gastric acids. Hyperplasia of the mucus glands of the esophagus and leiomyometaplasia of the intestinal smooth muscle are most commonly seen in dogs. Villus size tends to decrease, gastric emptying and intestinal turnover slows, motility decreases, and there are changes in the microbiota. These changes, however, are not generally related to the digestive or absorptive functions of the gut. Experimentally, lifelong calorie restriction results in increased longevity in a variety of species, including dogs.

Oral Cavity

The oral cavity serves an important function in preventing many harmful xenobiotic substances (i.e., foreign chemical substances within an organism that are not produced by or expected to be present in the organism) from entering the body. It does this through "mouth feel" and taste. Caustic substances, heat, and electricity may result in chemical erosions or ulcerations of the oral mucosa, but mucous membranes in general heal rapidly.

Antibiotic use may kill normal flora within the oral cavity. This change and/or high blood glucose concentrations via intravenous fluid administration or metabolic disturbance such as diabetes mellitus may allow for colonization by organisms not generally present. This outcome may result in a condition, sometimes called thrush, caused by a surface growth of *Candida* spp. (Figs. 7-7 and 7-8).

Saliva contains electrolytes such as sodium, potassium, calcium, magnesium, chloride, bicarbonate, and phosphate; as well as iodine; mucus, which serves as a lubricant; antibacterial compounds such as thiocyanate and hydrogen peroxide; secretory IgA; epidermal growth factor (EGF); and the digestive enzymes α-amylase, lipase, and kallikrein. Antimicrobial enzymes secreted include lysozyme, lactoperoxidase, proline-rich proteins, class A and B acid phosphatases, *N*-acetylmuramoyl-L-alanine amidase, the reduced form of nicotinamide adenine dinucleotide phosphate (NAD[P]H) dehydrogenase (quinone), superoxide dismutase, glutathione transferase, class 3 aldehyde dehydrogenase, and glucose-6-phosphate isomerase. Saliva also contains a bacteria-rich flora and at least in human beings, opiorphin, an analgesic.

Teeth

Enamel is the only substance in the body incapable of turnover and repair. Advertisements by makers of toothpaste and other dental remedies notwithstanding, enamel is incapable of healing. Because enamel is deposited on teeth during amelogenesis (i.e., developmental formation of enamel on teeth) and is fully formed at the time of tooth eruption, pathogens and dietary supplementation such as those containing fluoride will not weaken or strengthen enamel once the tooth is erupted. Acid etching of enamel from vomition of gastric acid or eating and drinking of acidic substances such as carbonated beverages produces permanent loss of enamel.

In those species with hypsodont teeth, continual growth throughout life theoretically results in renewed occlusal surfaces to ensure grinding ability. In practice, however, continual growth has disadvantages such as uneven wear and the formation of ridges. For well-kept animals, this problem, especially in horses, is alleviated by mechanical evening of occlusal surfaces, a process known as "floating." The current popularity of motorized tools

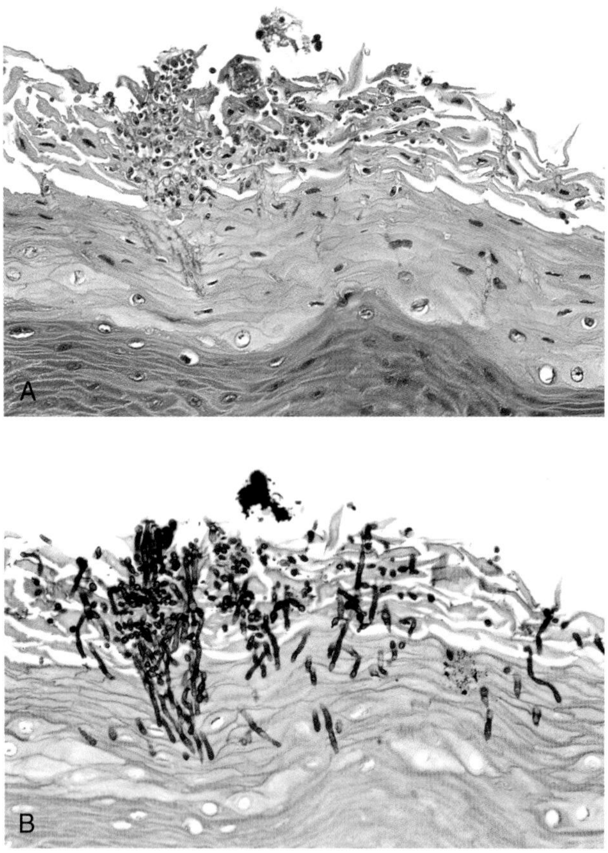

Figure 7-7 Thrush (Oral Candidiasis), Tongue, Foal. A, Hyphae of *Candida albicans* are growing in the superficial keratin of the tongue. H&E stain. **B,** Same specimen as **A.** Gomori's methenamine silver stain. (Courtesy Dr. J.F. Zachary, College of Veterinary Medicine, University of Illinois.)

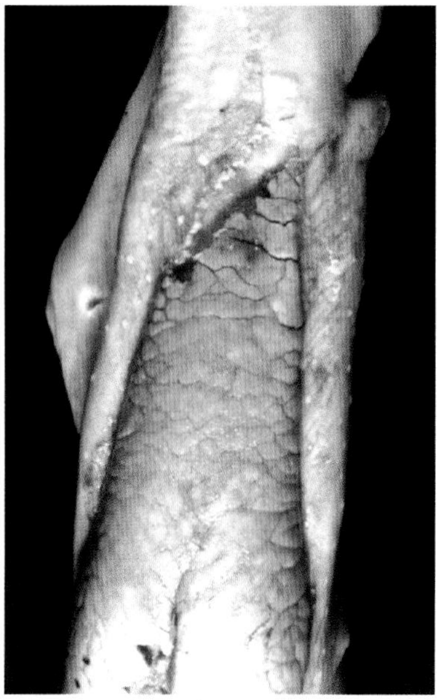

Figure 7-8 Thrush, Tongue, Foal. A pseudomembrane of hyphae of candida is present on the dorsal surface. It has been scraped off the rostral end of the tongue *(top)* to reveal normal mucosa beneath the fungal mat. (Courtesy Dr. H. Gelberg, College of Veterinary Medicine, Oregon State University.)

for this purpose has resulted in inexperienced and/or unlicensed operators causing considerable damage by overzealous application. In those species with brachydont dentition, loss of occlusal surfaces is irreversible.

Tonsils

Because the tonsils lack afferent lymphatic vessels, they do not act as a lymphoid filter for oral structures. Infections may be blood borne or by direct contact with substances dissolved in saliva. Therefore the tonsils may serve as antigen samplers and may be affected by pathogens in blood or oral secretions. The initial multiplication of some enteric viruses (e.g., feline parvovirus) occurs within the tonsillar tissues. Most neoplasms that develop in the tonsils are either from the epithelium (squamous cell carcinomas) or the lymphoid tissue (lymphoma).

Salivary Glands

Injury to the salivary gland is accompanied by incomplete regeneration, principally from ductular epithelium. There are often atrophy, fibrosis, and squamous metaplasia of secretory epithelium, sometimes resulting in blockage of ducts.

Tongue

The tongue is an important part of the oral cavity and provides for the mixing action of saliva with xenobiotics so that the taste buds can determine if the ingested material is worthy of swallowing. Likewise, nerve endings in the tongue provide data about the digestibility of ingesta.

Esophagus

Horses are unable to vomit, which is an important mechanism for eliminating toxic or otherwise undesirable ingesta from the alimentary system. Esophageal healing is relatively rapid; the normal epithelial turnover rate is 5 to 8 days.

Rumen, Reticulum, and Omasum

The three compartments of the ruminant forestomach are the reticulum, rumen, and omasum. Folds and compartments subdivide the forestomach. Normal forestomach motility, and thus innervation, is critical in maintaining digestive homeostasis. The ruminant forestomachs are aglandular. The resident flora and fauna are responsible for digestion and fermentation of cellulose. In general, the rumen is a large fermentation vat where microorganisms break down ingesta by mechanical and chemical action into short-chain fatty acids that are directly absorbed across the epithelial lining into the blood. These fatty acids supply more than half of the energy from nutrients absorbed by the alimentary tract. The reticulum and omasum act mechanically to further reduce the ingesta to fine particles.

Stomach and Abomasum

The gastric epithelial layer is one cell thick, and the turnover rate is 2 to 4 days. The parietal cells produce rennin that coagulates milk protein, intrinsic factor for vitamin B_{12} absorption, and hydrogen chloride (HCl). The low luminal pH destroys many ingested pathogens, but there is a resident bacterial flora that cannot be cultured by conventional methods. Chief cells produce zymogen and pepsin involved in digestion of feedstuffs, and enteroendocrine cells produce serotonin, gastrin, ghrelin, somatostatin, endothelin, histamine, enteroglucagon, and others involved in hormonal regulation (see Box 7-1). Mucus cells produce bicarbonate and an unstirred protective layer on the cell surface

Intestine

Inflammation

Chronic injury of the lamina propria that results in dense cellular infiltration can cause diarrhea in a variety of ways, none of which are completely understood. These mechanisms include simple physical impairment of mucosal diffusion by space-occupying cells, with resultant disruption of the overlying epithelium causing increased permeability. Examples of these diseases in domestic animals are canine histiocytic ulcerative colitis (boxer colitis), Johne's disease (paratuberculosis) of ruminants, amyloidosis, and lymphoma.

Necrotizing Processes

Primary necrotizing processes of the lamina propria generally involve necrosis of the GALT with extension to the overlying epithelium. Examples of diseases with these lesions include bovine viral diarrhea (BVD) of cattle and *Rhodococcus equi* infection of horses.

Lymphangiectasia

Dilation of lacteals is idiopathic or secondary to obstruction of flow. These lesions are seen most commonly as part of the syndrome resulting from space-occupying lesions of the lamina propria, such as occurs in Johne's disease and in lymphoma. In both cases there is obstruction to outflow of lymph—a granulomatous lymphangitis and lymphadenitis in Johne's disease and tumors in the lamina propria and lymph nodes in lymphoma. Endotoxemia that results in vascular damage and disseminated intravascular coagulopathy can cause thromboemboli in small vessels and hemorrhage, necrosis, and ulceration of the intestine.

Disorders of Innervation

Agangliosis and dysautonomia, malfunction of the cranial nerves, spinal nerves, ganglia, and/or autonomic nervous system, can have profound influences on intestinal motility. There are a great variety of agents that cause these changes, ranging from botulinum toxin to inflammatory diseases. Many cases are idiopathic or may be hereditary. In addition, there is a bidirectional neurohormonal interchange between intestinal microbiota and the brain. Thus alteration of the microbiota may result in changes in the gut-brain axis. Dysbiosis (also known as dysbacteriosis), a state of microbial imbalances in the alimentary system, has effects on early brain development in mice, irritable bowel syndrome, Crohn's disease, ulcerative colitis, demyelination in multiple sclerosis, hepatic encephalopathy, and psychiatric disorders such as early-onset autism. Finally, the interstitial cells of Cajal are of mesenchymal origin and are the pacemakers of the gut. Inflammation or loss of these cells affects coordinated movement of the alimentary system.

Diarrhea

Diarrhea is defined as secretion of abnormally fluid feces accompanied by an increased volume of feces and an increased frequency of defecation. Pathogens causing diarrhea fall into three major categories: those that induce intestinal secretion, such as enterotoxic, or enterotoxigenic, *Escherichia coli* (ETEC) (noninflammatory or secretory diarrhea); those that induce inflammation, such as *Lawsonia*; and those that are invasive, such as *Salmonella*. To simplify this further, there are two mechanistic "types" of diarrhea, noninflammatory and inflammatory. Noninflammatory diarrheas are produced by organisms that disrupt the absorptive or secretory mechanisms of the enterocytes without destroying the cells. Usually, but not always, noninflammatory diarrheas affect the more proximal portions of the bowel (enterotoxic *E. coli*, rotavirus, and *Cryptosporidium parvum*). Inflammatory diarrheas are produced by organisms that produce cytotoxins or are invasive and activate cytokines that initiate inflammatory cascades. The inflammatory diarrheas generally affect the ileum, cecum, or colon (*Salmonella*, *Brachyspira*, and *Lawsonia*). Combinations of these mechanisms are present in most enteric diseases and are as follows:

- **Malabsorption** with or without fermentation leads to osmotic diarrhea whether the cause is loss of digestive enzmes secondary to microvillus disruption, crypt or villus enterocyte death, or space-occupying lesions of the lamina propria. Generally this outcome is a problem of the small intestine, but secondary colonic malfunction can occur because of malabsorption of bile salts and fatty acids that stimulate fluid secretion in the large intestine. As examples, malabsorption occurs in rotavirus and coronavirus infections of neonates.
- **Chloride (Cl^-) hypersecretion** by the cystic fibrosis transmembrane regulator (CFTR) of a structurally intact mucosa. CFTR is regulated by kinases, which are dependent on cyclic adenosine monophosphate (cAMP), which acts as a second messenger. Prostanoids, bacterial toxins, and protein kinases all increase cAMP, thus increasing Cl^- secretion. Calcium ion (Ca^{2+}) also plays a role in opening Cl^- channels by increasing acetylcholine interaction with epithelial muscarinic receptors via cholenergic nerves in intestinal plexi. Through a different mechanism but also involving the CFTR, bicarbonate secretion is also increased. This osmotic activity results in a net efflux of fluid and electrolytes independent of permeability changes, absorptive capacity, or exogenously generated concentration gradients (i.e., osmotic diarrhea). As examples, chloride hypersecretion occurs in enterotoxic *E. coli* diarrhea.
- **Exudation** caused by an increased capillary permeability (protein-losing enteropathy) by leaky tight junctions between enterocytes. As examples, exudation occurs in some parasitic infections in which opening of the tight junctions allows macromolecules (antibodies) into the intestinal lumen.
- **Hypermotility** generally is involved in diarrhea but usually not as a primary mechanism in domestic animals. Hypermotility is defined as an increased rate, intensity, or frequency of peristalsis. Theoretically, with decreased mucosal contact time, digestion and absorption of nutrients and water should be less efficient. It is suspected that decreased motility in some diseases allows for increased bacterial proliferation (Fig. 7-9). Conversely, some enterotoxins can stimulate intestinal motitlity in some motility disorders of human beings such as achalasia, Hirschsprung's disease, and inflammatory bowel disease. Diarrhea occurs when there is an alteration in the network of interstitial cells of Cajal within the smooth muscle of the bowel wall. Whether this is a cause or effect of bowel motility disorders is not known.
- Toll-like receptors (TLRs) and related molecules produced by enterocytes and leukocytes are very important in the regulation of intestinal inflammation and in the host's response to intestinal pathogens. Intestinal inflammation can lead to neoplasia.
- M cells regulate the presentation of antigens to GALT.
- Other factors (prostaglandins, leukotrienes, and platelet-activating factor) act on enteric nerves to induce neurotransmitter-induced intestinal secretion by crypt cells.
- Cell damage is possibly a consequence of inflammation mediated by T lymphocytes or proteases and oxidants produced by mast cells. T lymphocytes also may affect epithelial cell maturation, causing villous atrophy and crypt hyperplasia.
- Cell death can result from pathogen invasion into enterocytes, multiplication of the pathogen, and extrusion of the affected enterocytes. These changes lead to notable distortion of villus

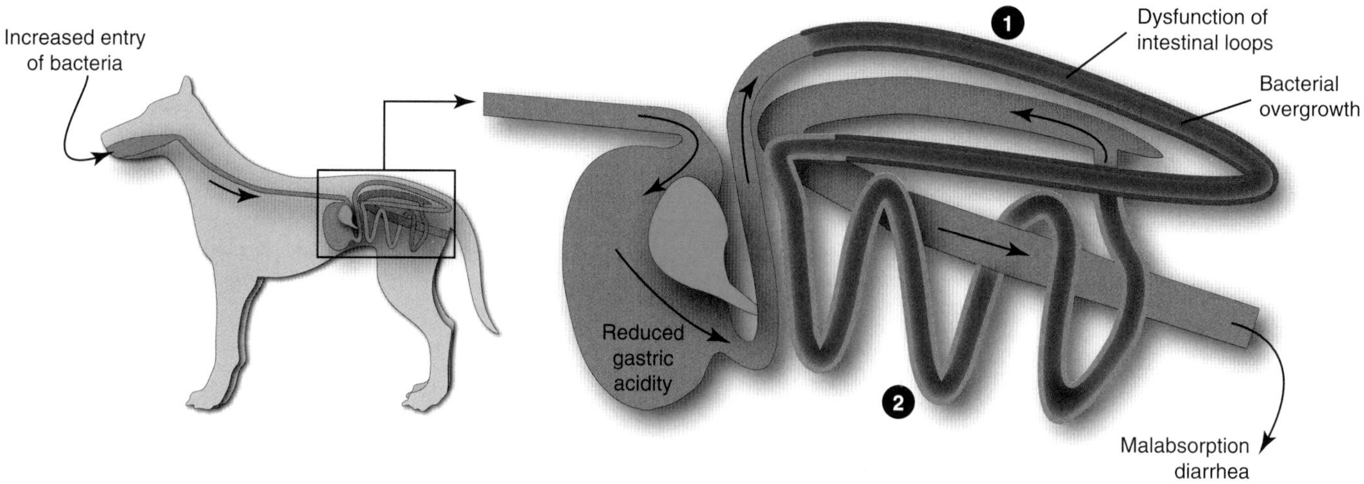

Figure 7-9 **Mechanism of How Intestinal Bacterial Overgrowth Causes Malabsorption and Diarrhea.** *1*, Bacterial overgrowth results from a combination of increased ingestion of bacteria, dysfunction of intestinal loops, and reduced clearance of bacteria. These processes result in excessive multiplication of bacteria and thus bacterial overgrowth in the intestines. *2*, Malabsorption and diarrhea occur as a result of bacterial overgrowth leading to bile salt deficiencies, excessive bacterial toxins, and overconsumption of resources by bacteria. (Courtesy Dr. H. Gelberg, College of Veterinary Medicine, Oregon State University; and Dr. J.F. Zachary, College of Veterinary Medicine, University of Illinois.)

architecture with a lack of mature absorptive enterocytes accompanied by nutrient malabsorption and osmotic diarrhea.
- Mast cells of the lamina propria are in close association with enteric neurons and the enteric vasculature. They release histamine, prostaglandins, 5-hydroxytryptamine (5-HT), and proteolytic enzymes that play a role in diarrhea production.

The nuts and bolts of the mechanisms listed are of course much more complicated. Pathogens enter or attach to enterocytes and may release enterotoxins. This action triggers the enterocytes to release cytokines (interleukin [IL]-8), which activate resident macrophages and recruit new blood-borne macrophages (e.g., monocytes) into the lamina propria. The activated macrophages release soluble factors (histamine, serotonin, adenosine) that increase intestinal secretion of chloride and water and inhibit absorption (Figs. 7-10 and 7-11). Recruitment of inflammatory cells to areas of injury results in release of a chemical milieu of cytokines (Fig. 7-12). Other factors (prostaglandins, leukotrienes, platelet-activating factor) act on enteric nerves to induce neurotransmitter-mediated intestinal secretion and hypermotility. The subsequent cell damage is possibly a consequence of inflammation mediated by T lymphocytes or proteases and oxidants secreted by mast cells (see Fig. 7-12). T lymphocytes also affect epithelial cell growth, producing villus atrophy and crypt hyperplasia. Cell death results from pathogen invasion, multiplication, and extrusion. The end result is marked distortion of villus architecture accompanied by nutrient malabsorption and osmotic diarrhea.

There are nonintestinal causes of diarrhea that must be considered in addition to diseases of the intestine. Among this group are hyperthyroidism, Addison's disease, pancreatic insufficiency, pancreatitis, chronic renal failure, and others. These diseases are discussed in their respective chapters of this book.

Consequences. Normal feces are 75% water. Diarrheal feces are greater than 85% water. The consequence of excess fluid loss in the feces through diarrhea is dehydration. Dehydration results in hypovolemia. Hypovolemia results in hemoconcentration that results in inadequate tissue perfusion. Energy therefore is generated in tissue by anaerobic glycolysis. The resultant hypoglycemia leads to ketoacidosis. Acidosis is, by definition, a reduction in blood and tissue pH. Acidosis causes a reduction in pH-dependent enzyme system functions. Acidosis is compounded by fecal bicarbonate loss in diarrhea and the results of inadequate renal excretion of hydrogen ions and inadequate absorption of bicarbonate, which is a late effect of inadequate renal perfusion. The resultant electrolyte imbalance results in an increase in intracellular hydrogen ion concentration and a decrease in intracellular potassium ion concentration. The imbalances decrease neuromuscular control of myocardial contraction, leading to a further decrease in tissue perfusion. A vicious cycle results, culminating in hypovolemic shock.

Peritoneum, Omentum, Mesentery, and Peritoneal Cavity

Ascites

Ascites or hydroperitoneum is defined as excess fluid in the peritoneal cavity. The quality of the fluid varies by cause from thick and syrupy in feline infectious peritonitis (FIP) to thin and watery in cases of hypoproteinemia (see Fig. 3-3). Ascites is nonspecific and can result from any cause of hypoproteinemia such as heart (see Fig. 10-6 and E-Fig. 10-10), liver, or kidney failure, protein-losing enteropathies such as Johne's disease, lymphangiectasia (Figs. 7-13 and 7-14, *A, B*), lymphatic blockage, ruptured lymph ducts, bladder rupture (uroperitoneum), and hypertension. Evaluation of fluid obtained by abdominocentesis is very helpful in the live animal in sorting out the various causes.

Fat Necrosis

There are four main categories of fat necrosis. They are nutritional, pancreatic, traumatic, and idiopathic, as follows:
- Nutritional fat necrosis, also called *steatitis* or *yellow fat disease*, results in peroxidation of lipids, including those in cell membranes. It is most common in cats but occurs in a variety of species. The free radicals produced evoke an inflammatory response. The inciting cause is generally a diet very high in lipids and low in vitamin E or other tocopherols. Although steatitis of cats has historically been a sequela of fish-based diets, anecdotal evidence suggests that it may also be caused by some unconventional diets being used today.
- Pancreatic or enzymatic fat necrosis is initiated by pancreatic enzyme release (lipase) from pancreatic necrosis (pancreatitis). Lipase converts triglycerides into fatty acids and glycerol. The

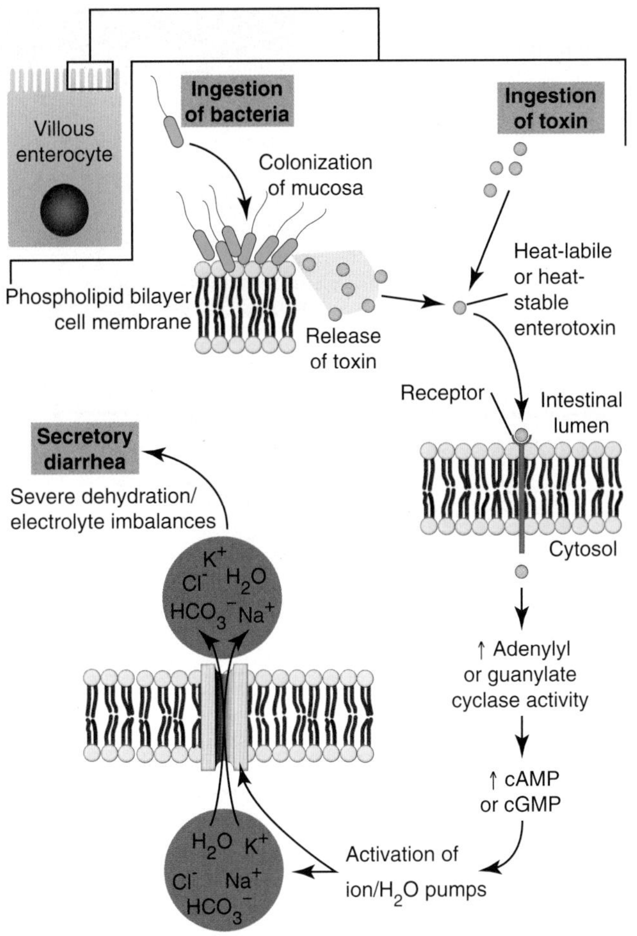

Figure 7-10 Mechanism of Action for Enterotoxin-Mediated Bacterial Diarrhea. *cAMP,* Cyclic adenosine monophosphate; *cGMP,* cyclic guanosine monophosphate. (Courtesy Dr. H. Gelberg, College of Veterinary Medicine, Oregon State University; and Dr. J.F. Zachary, College of Veterinary Medicine, University of Illinois.)

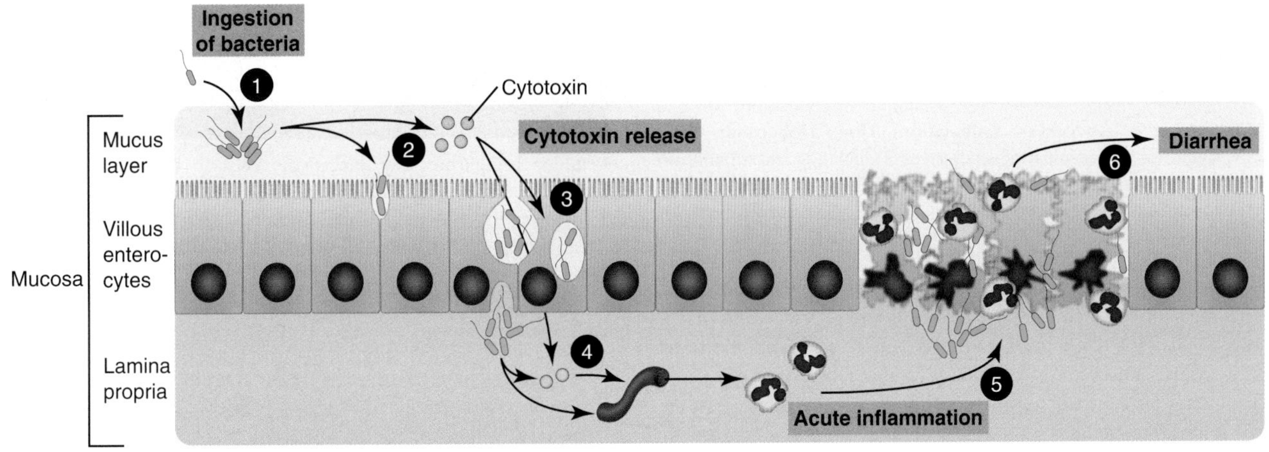

Figure 7-11 Mechanism of Invasive and Cytotoxin-Mediated Bacterial Inflammation. *1*, Colonization of the mucosa. *2*, Local production of cytotoxins and invasion of the mucosa by bacteria. *3*, Bacteria replicate in large numbers and spread to adjacent epithelial cells. *4*, Bacterial cytotoxins are released and injure adjacent mucosal endothelial cells and cause acute inflammation. *5*, Acute inflammation results in necrosis of the mucosa. *6*, Mucosal necrosis and bacterial toxins cause diarrhea. (Courtesy Dr. H. Gelberg, College of Veterinary Medicine, Oregon State University; and Dr. J.F. Zachary, College of Veterinary Medicine, University of Illinois.)

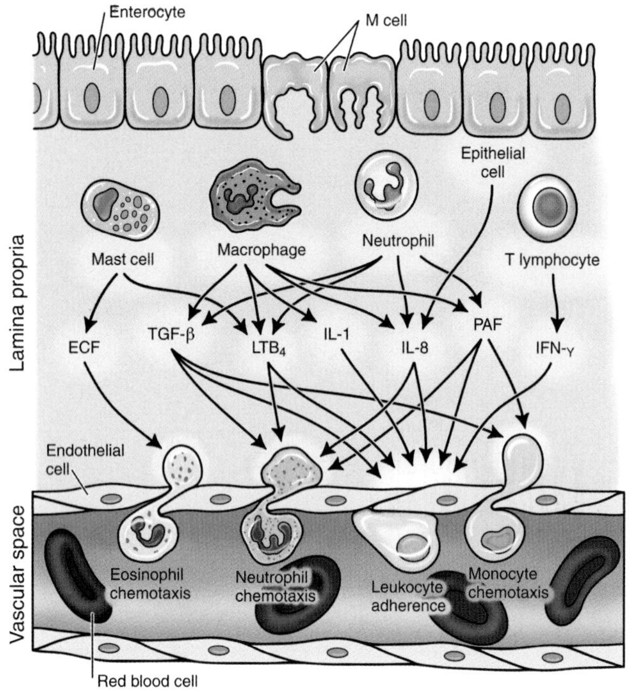

Figure 7-12 **Chemotactic Factors Active during Intestinal Inflammation.** *ECF,* Eosinophil chemotactic factor; *IFN-γ,* interferon-γ; *IL,* interleukin; *LTB_4,* leukotriene B_4; *PAF,* platelet-activating factor; *TGF-β,* transforming growth factor-β.

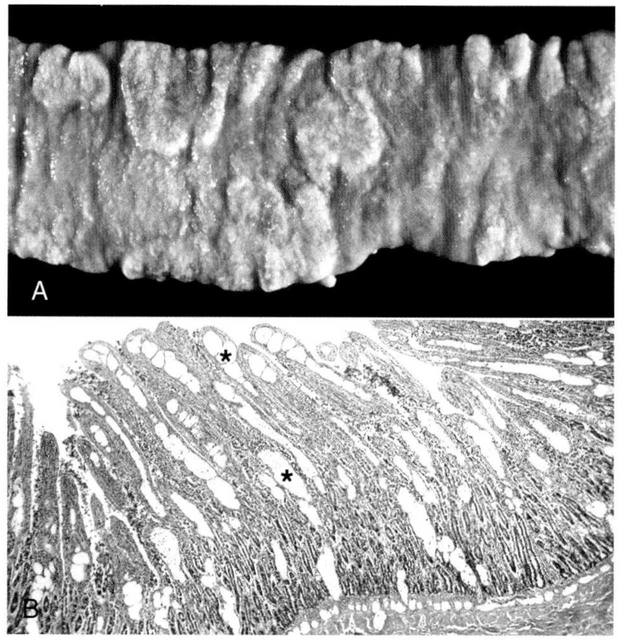

Figure 7-14 **Lymphangiectasia, Jejunum, Dog. A,** Intestinal villi are expanded by ectasia of the lymphatic vessels *(raised white areas).* Lymphangiectasia can be a congenital developmental disorder of the lymphatic vessels, or it can be acquired secondary to lymph vessel obstruction caused by granulomatous or neoplastic diseases. **B,** Lacteals are dilated *(asterisks),* thus resulting in diminished lymph absorption by lacteals in the lamina propria and subsequent loss of protein (hypoproteinemia) and other nutrients into the intestinal lumen. H&E stain. (**A** courtesy College of Veterinary Medicine, University of Illinois. **B** courtesy Dr. H. Gelberg, College of Veterinary Medicine, Oregon State University.)

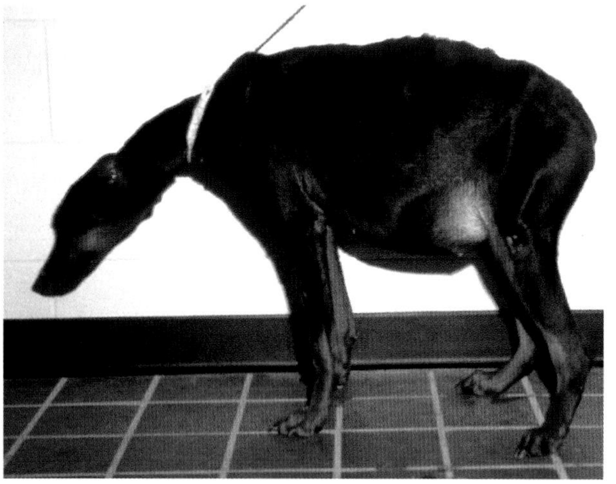

Figure 7-13 **Ascites, Abdomen, Emaciation, Dog, Doberman Pinscher.** Protein-losing enteropathy, secondary to idiopathic intestinal lymphangiectasia resulted in hypoproteinemia and then ascites. (Courtesy Dr. H. Gelberg, College of Veterinary Medicine, Oregon State University.)

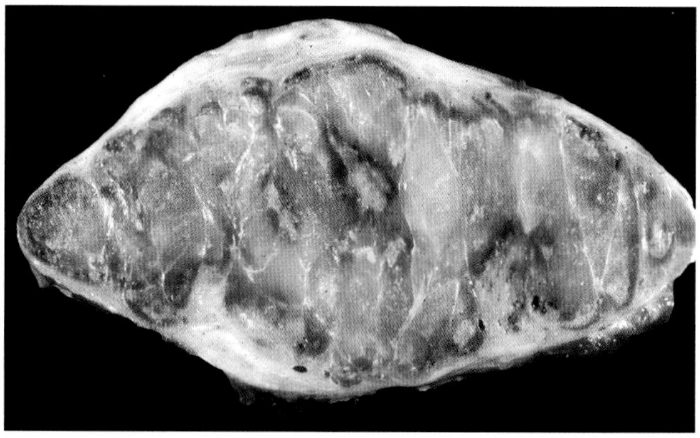

Figure 7-15 **Idiopathic Fat Necrosis, Ventral Parietal Peritoneum, Horse.** This cross section of necrotic fat is mottled by a mixture of areas of saponification and normal adipocytes. The cause of this sporadic condition is unknown. (Courtesy College of Veterinary Medicine, Cornell University.)

fatty acids combine with calcium, magnesium, and sodium ions, forming soaps resulting in chalky white deposits (see Figs. 1-38 and 8-90). This is a painful condition, and free lipid droplets are sometimes seen in fluids recovered from abdominocentesis.

- Traumatic fat necrosis results from direct, usually blunt, trauma to adipose tissue and is a relatively uncommon occurrence. Rupture of adipocytes releases triglycerides, which are hydrolyzed by tissue and/or serum lipases.
- Idiopathic fat necrosis can be focal or massive and occurs in all species of mammal but is seen primarily in large animal species, especially in sheep, horses (Fig. 7-15), and obese dairy cattle. With massive necrosis in cattle the hard lumps of dense necrotic fat can envelop intestinal loops, resulting in stricture and functional blockage of ingesta. The cause of this condition is unknown but may relate in some way to nutritional imbalances.

Damaged and necrotic adipose tissue frequently has a white, chalky or gritty appearance and texture caused by saponification and mineralization. Inflammatory cell presence and density vary based on the various causes of tissue damage and the area of fat sampled.

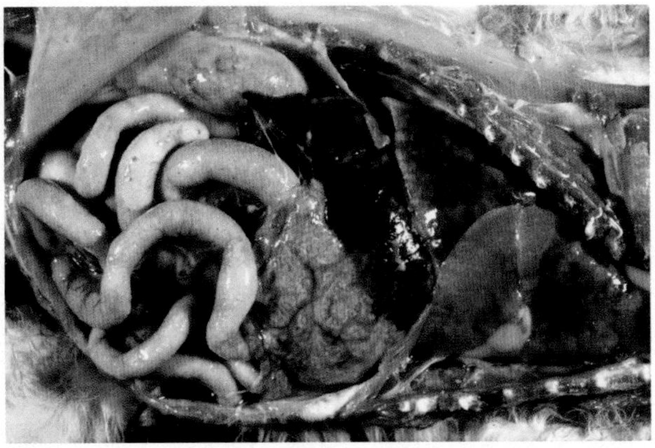

Figure 7-16 **Fibrinous Polyserositis, Abdomen, Cat.** Fibrin strands between viscera and mats of fibrin on organ surfaces are characteristic of the "wet form" of feline infectious peritonitis. The mesentery *(below and left of the liver)* has numerous white linear serpentine tracts, which are inflamed (type III hypersensitivity, immune complex) capillaries and venules. Note the small nodules (pyogranulomas) on the intestinal serosa and on the surface of the kidney. (Courtesy Dr. H. Gelberg, College of Veterinary Medicine, Oregon State University.)

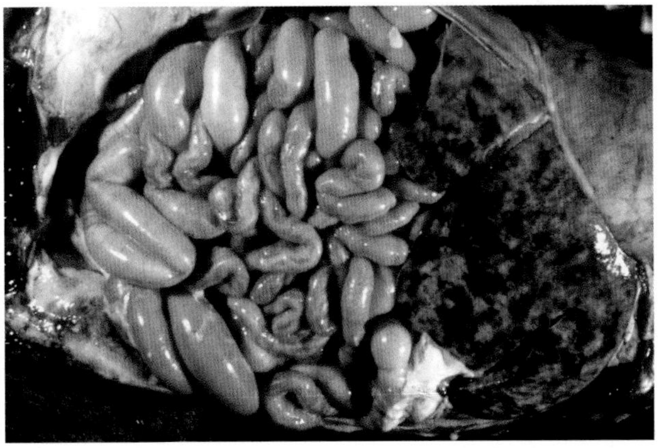

Figure 7-17 **Fibrinous Polyserositis, Abdomen, Pig.** Strands and clumps of fibrin are scattered throughout serosal surfaces. A milk-spotted liver is also present. Bacteria such as *Haemophilus suis/parasuis* (Glasser's disease), *Actinobacillus suis*, *Streptococcus suis*, or *Escherichia coli* can cause polyserositis. (Courtesy Dr. H. Gelberg, College of Veterinary Medicine, Oregon State University.)

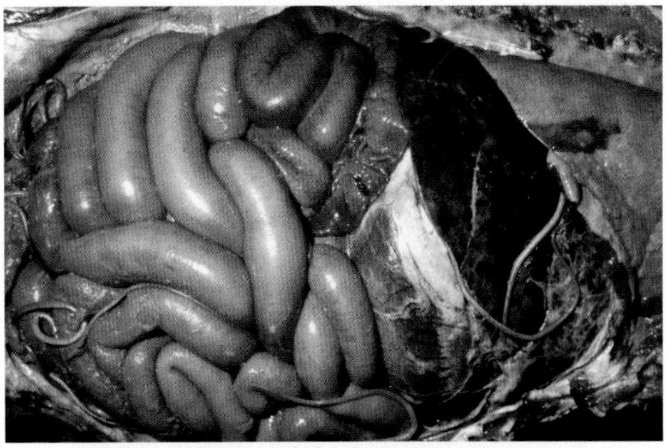

Figure 7-18 **Fibrinous Peritonitis, Abdomen, Pig.** The presence of fibrin in this pig's abdomen indicates that the intestinal rupture occurred antemortem. Ascarids are also present but do not help determine the time of rupture. (Courtesy Dr. M.D. McGavin, College of Veterinary Medicine, University of Tennessee.)

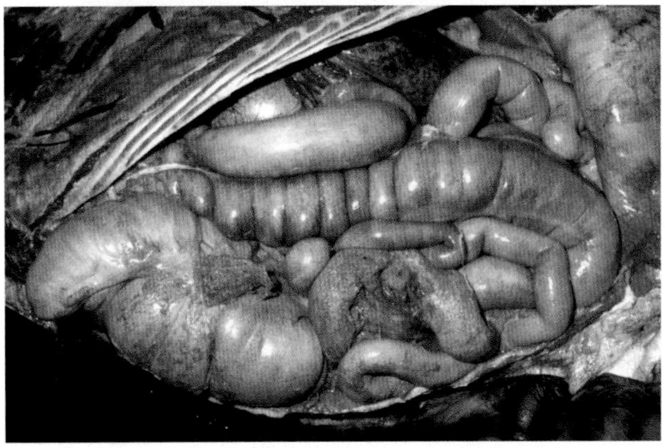

Figure 7-19 **Fibrinous Peritonitis, Abdomen, Horse.** The presence of fibrin and ingesta adherent to serosal surfaces indicates antemortem perforation or rupture of the intestine. (Courtesy Dr. M.D. McGavin, College of Veterinary Medicine, University of Tennessee.)

Inflammation: Peritonitis

Inflammation of the peritoneum, or peritonitis, is caused by a variety of agents varying from viral (feline infectious peritonitis) (Fig. 7-16) to bacterial (Fig. 7-17) to parasitic (ascarid migrations) (Fig. 7-18) to mechanical (hardware disease) to sterile (bile peritonitis) to organ rupture (Fig. 7-19). Peritonitis is also called *serositis*, and when multiple serous membranes like those of the meninges, joints, pleura, pericardium, peritoneum, and scrotum are affected, it is called a *polyserositis*. Glasser's disease of pigs is an example of a polyserositis (see Fig. 7-17). Different species vary in their stoicism and survival in the face of peritonitis, with horses showing the most pain and intolerance, whereas cattle and cats may live a long time with severe disease. The nature of the exudate includes those covered in Chapter 3 that result in suppurative peritonitis (Fig. 7-20) or fibrinous peritonitis (Fig. 7-21), as examples. Cytologic examination and bacterial culture are instrumental in determining a cause in the live animal. As in other diseases, the peritoneum responds to injury via acute inflammation (Fig. 7-22) and if needed, chronic inflammation (Fig. 7-23) and/or granulomatous inflammation (Fig. 7-24), if the source of the injury remains unresolved.

Parasitic Peritonitis. Aberrant migration of nematodes and trematodes in most species of animals can cause focal fibrosis in peritoneum and mesenteries when larvae travel through the abdominal cavity (see Fig. 8-52). Setaria, as an example, are nematodes that are sometimes found in the peritoneal cavity of ungulates and may cause mild focal peritonitis and rarely significant damage. Furthermore, a variety of cestodes may be found in the abdominal cavity of many animals. Some, such as *Echinococcus granulosus* (hydatid cysts) are zoonotic and may take 20 to 30 years to cause clinical signs in human beings. *Mesocestoides* and *Porocephalus* (pentastomiasis) are found in carnivores, where their migration may induce a pyogranulomatous reaction (Fig. 7-25).

Pneumoperitoneum

Spontaneous pneumoperitoneum is secondary to perforation of the GI or reproductive tracts. Causes include neoplasia, nonsteroidal

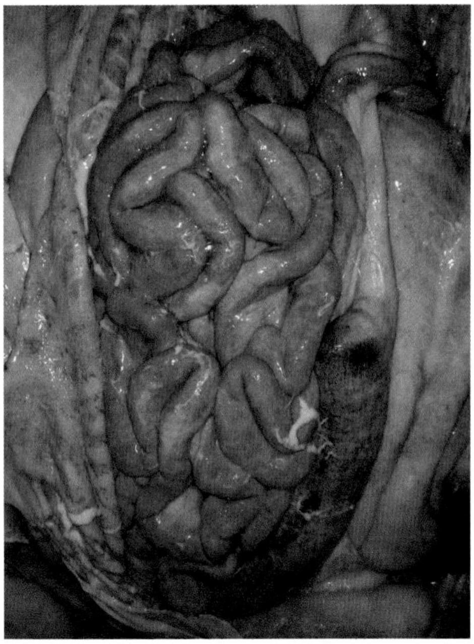

Figure 7-20 **Acute Suppurative Peritonitis, Bacterial Infection, Pig.** The surface of the peritoneum is rough and granular and covered with gray/white-yellow flecks of pus and fibrin. Red areas are indicative of active hyperemia and hemorrhage. (Courtesy College of Veterinary Medicine, University of Illinois.)

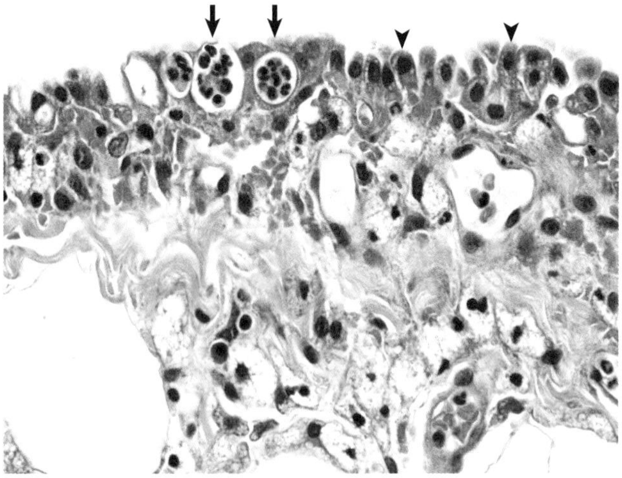

Figure 7-22 **Acute Peritonitis, Peritoneum, Dog.** The mesothelial cells are swollen, vacuolated, and misshapen *(arrowheads)*, indicating their response to injury. Capillaries under the mesothelial cells are dilated (active hyperemia and leukocyte adhesion cascade). Neutrophils are migrating through endothelial cell junctions and in the interstitium to reach the inflammatory stimulus in the abdominal cavity. Note the microabscesses in junctional spaces *(arrows)*. H&E stain. (Courtesy Dr. J.F. Zachary, College of Veterinary Medicine, University of Illinois.)

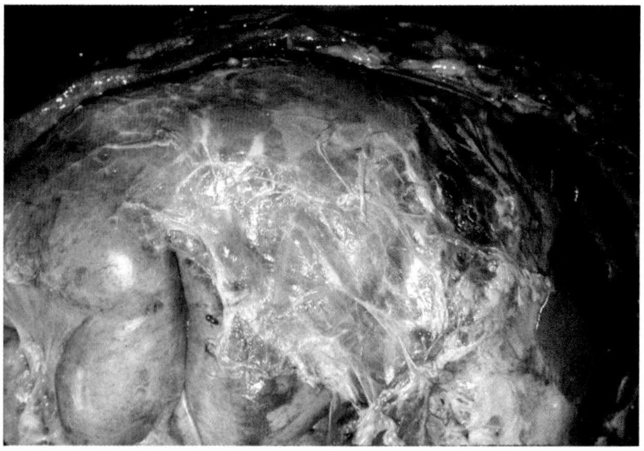

Figure 7-21 **Fibrinous Peritonitis, Acute Inflammation, Bacterial Infection, Cow.** This lesion was the result of extensive damage to capillaries in the peritoneum leading to leakage of fibrinogen and polymerization to fibrin on peritoneal surfaces. (Courtesy Dr. M.D. McGavin, College of Veterinary Medicine, University of Tennessee.)

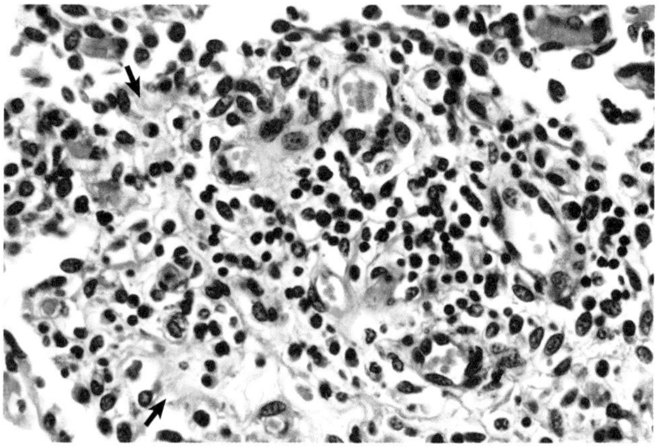

Figure 7-23 **Chronic Peritonitis, Peritoneum, Cow.** Because the inflammatory stimulus in the abdominal cavity has persisted, the inflammatory response has shifted to a chronic exudate in an attempt to resolve the damage. Note the abundance of immature collagen fibers *(arrows)* in the areolar tissue of the peritoneum. H&E stain. (Courtesy Dr. M.D. McGavin, College of Veterinary Medicine, University of Tennessee.)

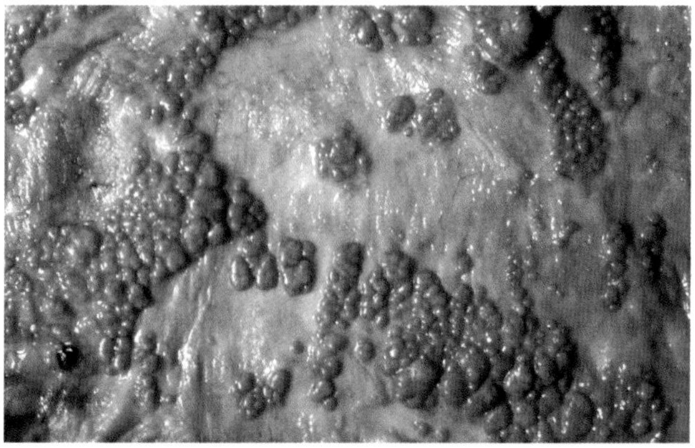

Figure 7-24 **Granulomatous Peritonitis, Peritoneum, Tuberculosis, Cow.** In long-standing cases of tuberculosis, granulomas can form on the peritoneum. (Courtesy Dr. M.D. McGavin, College of Veterinary Medicine, University of Tennessee.)

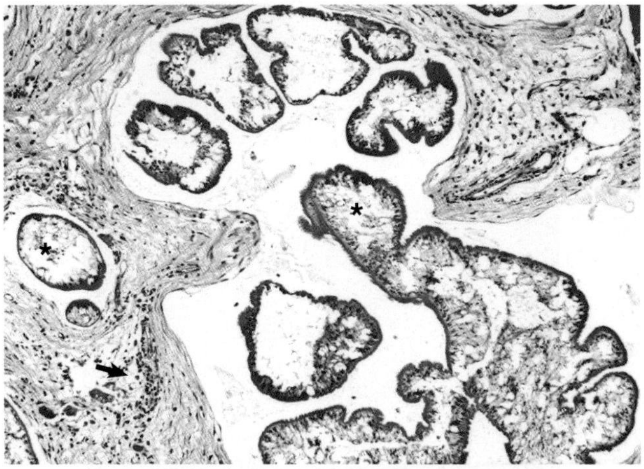

Figure 7-25 ***Mesocestoides* Infection, Peritoneum, Dog.** Encysted larval cestodes *(asterisks)* have elicited a granulomatous inflammatory reaction *(arrow)* in the peritoneum of this dog. H&E stain. (Courtesy Dr. C. Löhr, College of Veterinary Medicine, Oregon State University.)

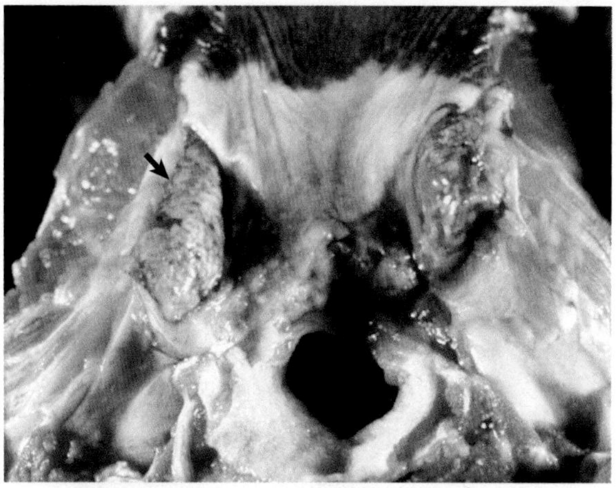

Figure 7-26 **Necrotizing Tonsillitis, Tonsils, Dog.** The palatine tonsils are enlarged and discolored. The right tonsil is covered by a diphtheritic membrane *(arrow)*, and the left tonsil is extensively ulcerated. Because there are no afferent lymphatic vessels to the tonsils, infection is either primary (by direct spread) or hematogenous. (Courtesy Dr. M.D. McGavin, College of Veterinary Medicine, University of Tennessee.)

Box 7-2 Portals of Entry in the Alimentary System

- Ingestion
- Coughed up from the lungs and swallowed
- Systemic blood-borne infections
- Parasite migration

antiinflammatory drugs (NSAIDs), and steroids. Traumatic pneumoperitoneum is caused by penetrating projectiles (e.g., bullets, knives, arrows), vehicular trauma, penetrating bite wounds, iatrogenic (surgery, peritoneal dialysis, positive pressure ventilation, urinary catheterization with penetration, penetrating gastrotomy, or percutaneous endoscopic gastrostomy [PEG] tubes), and idiopathic causes. Unless removed mechanically, it takes approximately 30 days for the air to be absorbed.

Portals of Entry/Pathways of Spread

There are limited numbers of ways that pathogenic agents gain entry into the alimentary system (Box 7-2). The most common, of course, is through ingestion. However, under certain circumstances, pathogens may be coughed up from the lungs into the pharynx and swallowed (*R. equi* in horses). Systemic blood-borne infections of viruses (viremia), bacteria (bacteremia), and systemic toxins (septicemia and toxemia) may make their way through the bloodstream and attach to specific receptors on the epithelial lining cells of the alimentary system. Parasites may migrate through various regions of the body to find a home within the mucosa or roam free in the lumen of the alimentary tract.

Oral Cavity

Any substance placed in the oral cavity has the opportunity to affect the mucosa. The fact that oral infections are relatively rare is evidence supporting the efficacy of oral secretions and the epithelial barrier. Mechanical penetration of oral mucosa allows pathogens the opportunity to spread through submucosal tissues and enter vascular channels or draining lymphatic vessels. Although most pathogens are halted and killed during their travels, some need epithelial surfaces (bovine viral diarrhea virus) or lymphoid tissues (parvoviruses of carnivores) to multiply.

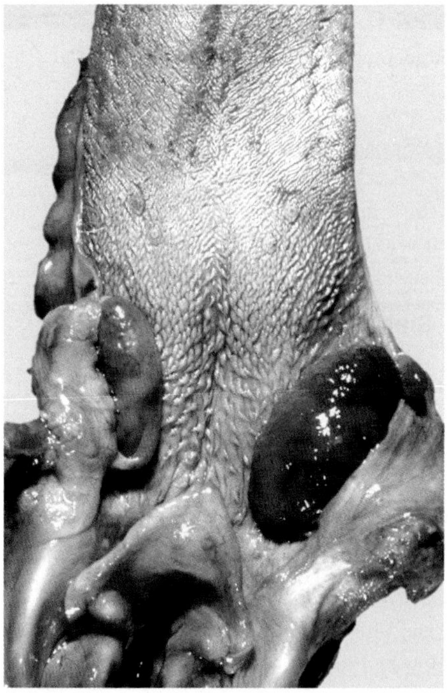

Figure 7-27 **Lymphoma (Lymphosarcoma), Tonsil, Dog.** Proliferation of malignant lymphocytes has expanded the tonsils so that they now protrude beyond their crypts and are pink-red because they are well vascularized. (Courtesy Dr. M.D. McGavin, College of Veterinary Medicine, University of Tennessee.)

Teeth

Enamel is inert and thus does not play a role in pathogen multiplication or spread, nor can it heal. Domestic animal species seldom develop caries, but plaque accumulation and periodontal disease can lead to gum loss, inflammation, bone resorption, and loss of teeth.

Tonsils

Tonsils do not possess afferent lymphatic vessels and do not serve as lymph filters. Therefore only primary (or direct) or hematogenous infections occur (tonsillitis) (Fig. 7-26), as well as primary neoplasms of either the lymphoid (lymphoma) (Fig. 7-27) or epithelial

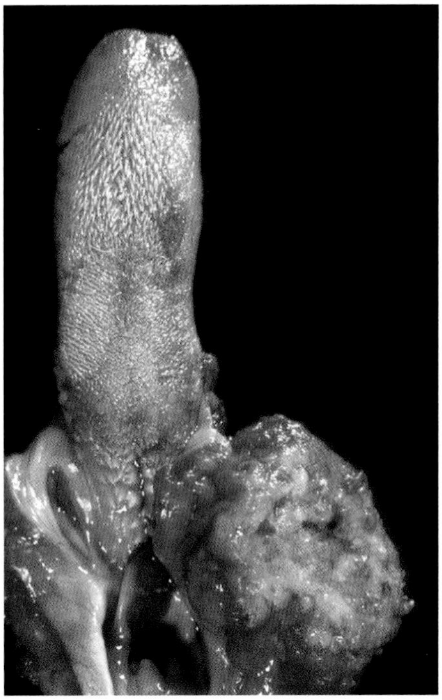

Figure 7-28 Squamous Cell Carcinoma, Tonsil, Cat. The right tonsil has been replaced by a large expansile neoplasm. The left tonsil is normal and remains in its crypt. (Courtesy Dr. R. Storts, College of Veterinary Medicine, Texas A&M University.)

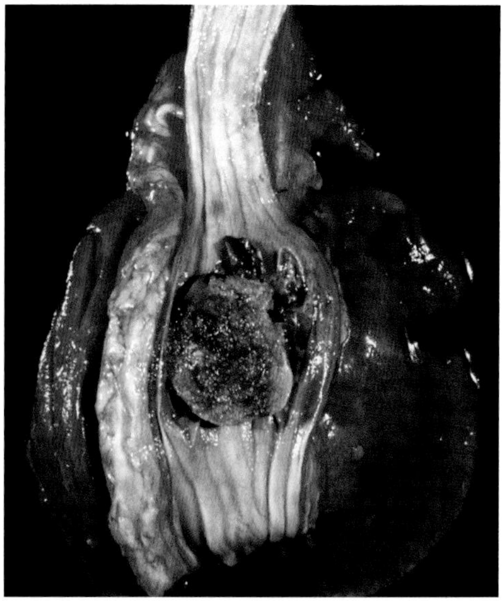

Figure 7-29 Foreign Body with Necrosis, Esophagus, Dog. A ham bone lodged in this dog's esophagus dorsal to the base of the heart has caused esophageal dilation and pressure necrosis of the esophageal mucosa. (Courtesy Dr. C.S. Patton, College of Veterinary Medicine, University of Tennessee.)

(squamous cell carcinoma) (Fig. 7-28) components. In many viremias of mammals, such as pseudorabies of pigs, virus may be isolated from the tonsils.

Salivary Glands

Salivary glands are generally affected by blood-borne pathogens, direct penetration by foreign objects, obstruction of the excretory ducts, or bite wounds. An important pathogen, rabies virus, is spread through saliva. In human beings, ascending infections from the salivary ducts occur, but there is no evidence that this occurs in domestic animals. The serous portions of the salivary glands are radiosensitive.

Tongue

Epitheliotropic viruses, many of which are foreign to the United States, such as foot-and-mouth disease, replicate in the epithelium of the oral cavity, including the tongue. Loss of lingual epithelium and exposure of nerves may result in pain, inappetence, ptyalism, and bruxism.

Esophagus

Materials, including caustic chemicals, from the oral cavity pass via the esophagus to the stomach or rumen. In the thoracic cavity, penetration or obstruction by foreign objects is the most common portal of entry into the mediastinum (Fig. 7-29). Some parasites spend part or all of their life cycles in the esophagus. Iatrogenic puncture of the esophagus is a not uncommon sequela to passage of stomach tubes. Gastric reflux is an additional portal of entry into the esophagus.

Rumen, Reticulum, and Omasum

The forestomachs in ruminants and camelids are dilations and modifications of the esophagus. They are designed to house a digestive flora necessary for producing short-chain fatty acids from forage that are subsequently directly absorbed into the bloodstream along with sodium and chloride. Most clinical disease of the forestomachs relates to disruptions in coordinated motility and changes in pH. Camelid forestomachs have glandular sacculations. Horses have stomachs that are divided into anterior stratified and aboral glandular portions. Pigs have only a small stratified portion that directly surrounds the esophageal os. The abomasum and C3 (a compartment comparable to the abomasum) of camelids function similarly to the stomachs of monogastric mammals.

Stomach and Abomasum

Gastric and abomasal ulcers occur in all species. Although the cause of ulcers, other than caustic agents and those caused by bacteria that can survive the extremely low pH of the stomach (*Helicobacter* spp.), is imprecisely understood, conditions necessary for ulcer development include local disturbances or trauma to the mucosal epithelial barrier, normal or high gastric acidity, and local disturbances to blood flow, including stress-induced and sympathetic nervous system–mediated arteriovenous shunts leading to ischemia. These physiologic changes allow pepsin and HCl into the submucosa. In addition, exogenous or endogenous steroids and NSAIDs depress prostaglandin E_1 (PGE_1) and prostaglandin E_2 (PGE_2), decreasing phospholipid secretions, which are gastroprotective, thus causing erosions and ulcers.

Intestine

Targets for Microbial Colonization or Destruction of Intestinal Mucosae

Mucosal targets include absorptive enterocytes, undifferentiated crypt cells, microvilli and glycocalyx, apical junctional complexes, unknown or nonspecific structures, and the lamina propria as illustrated in Figure 7-30.

Diseases of the Intestinal Epithelium

A number of diseases are characterized by colonization or destruction of the epithelial components of the intestinal mucosa. Although the disease-producing effects of pathogens are complex and multifactorial, a simplified understanding of the principal cell under

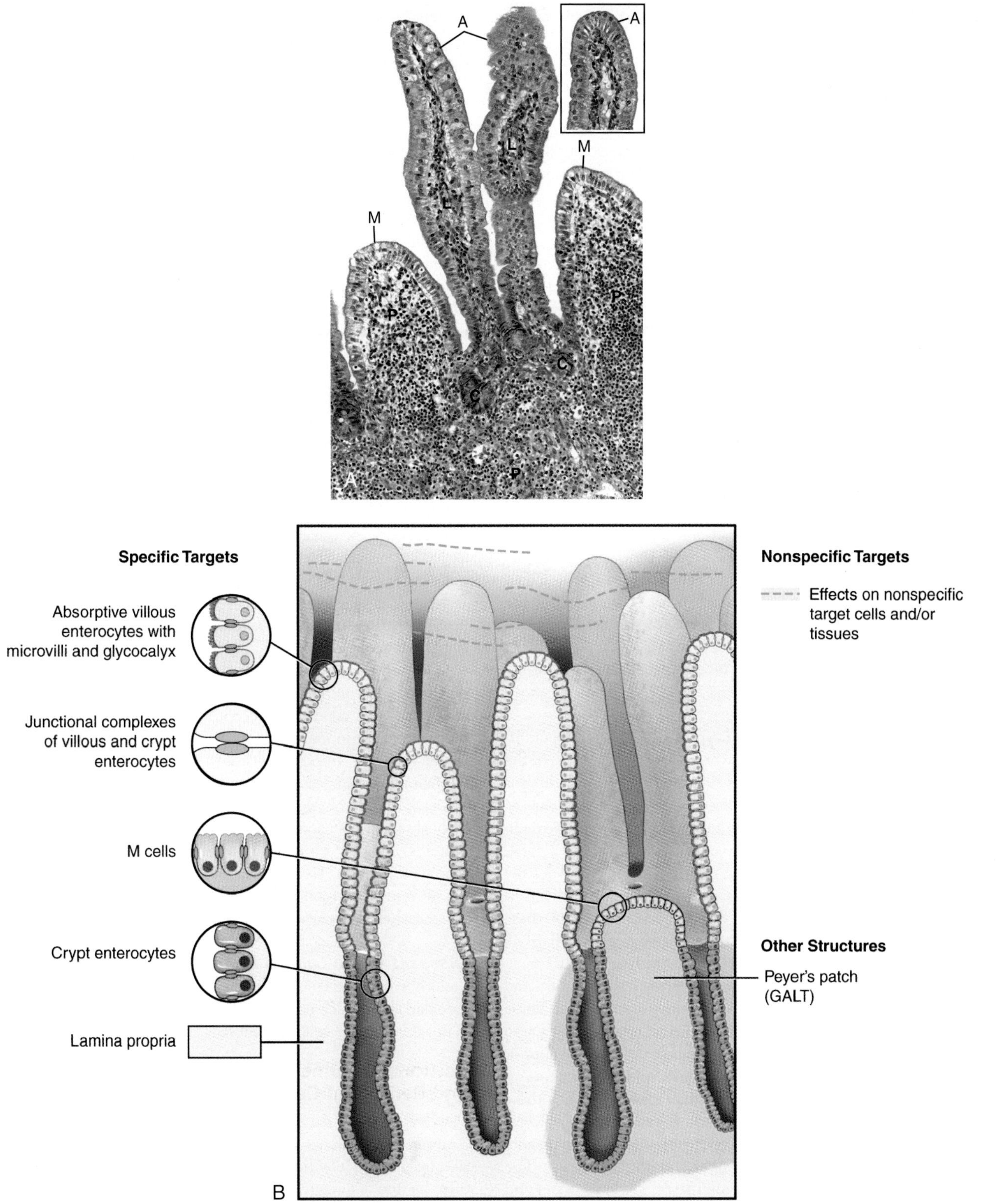

Figure 7-30 **Targets for Microbial Infection in the Intestine. A,** Photomicrograph of small intestinal mucosae identifying targets for infection. Compare with schematic diagram illustrated in **B.** *Inset,* Higher magnification of villus tip enterocytes with a microvillus border. **B,** Schematic diagram illustrating targets for infection. *A,* Absorptive enterocyte; *C,* undifferentiated crypt cells; *GALT,* gut-associated lymphoid tissue; *L,* lamina propria: *M,* M cells; *P,* Peyer's patch. (**A** and inset courtesy Dr. J.F. Zachary, College of Veterinary Medicine, University of Illinois.)

attack is helpful in predicting disease outcome and managing treatment.

Diseases of the Absorptive Enterocytes. A number of agents have a tropism for the absorptive cells lining the intestinal villi. These agents include viruses such as rotavirus, enteric coronavirus, and the coronavirus of transmissible gastroenteritis of pigs. Intracellular bacteria and parasites can likewise invade and multiply in absorptive epithelial cells. Examples include the agents of swine dysentery *(Brachyspira hyodysenteriae)*, coccidia, and cryptosporidium.

Some pathogens with a tropism for absorptive lining cells of the intestine cause destruction of these cells. This results in loss of enterocytes and at least temporary villous atrophy. The loss of the absorptive-digestive villous enterocytes causes maldigestion, and malabsorption results. Furthermore, because ingesta and normal alimentary secretions are unabsorbed, they are degraded further and fermented in the intestine by bacteria, increasing the osmolality of intestinal contents, with a subsequent increase in the fluid content of the bowel.

Because the regenerative crypt cells are not attacked by pathogens with tropism for villous enterocytes, diseases with villous enterocyte damage are not necessarily fatal. The denuded basement membrane contracts, causing villous atrophy. This contraction may be a function of the smooth muscle in the lamina propria. The functionally immature migrating crypt cells cover the villi. Often these immature cells become squamoid in an effort to cover the maximum area of basement membrane. However, if naked basement membranes contact each other, they will adhere, resulting not only in villous blunting but also in villous fusion, preventing the reformation of normal villi.

Diseases of Undifferentiated Crypt Cells. Loss of the undifferentiated epithelial cells in the base of the crypts means loss of the cells capable of mitosis, and thus regeneration of the epithelium is impaired. Therefore the clinical effect of crypt cell loss can be delayed for several days because the villi are initially still covered by enterocytes. This type of loss is more severe and often fatal, compared with villous enterocyte loss. Agents that target and destroy crypt cells are called *radiomimetic* because they mimic the effects of radiation on the rapidly dividing enterocytes. Examples of these agents include the parvoviruses of carnivores, bovine viral diarrhea virus, rinderpest virus, and some mycotoxins such as vomitoxin.

Enterotoxic *E. coli* infection of neonatal pigs, calves, lambs, and human beings causes what is known as a secretory diarrhea. These bacteria are able to colonize the small intestinal enterocytes by way of their surface or pilus antigens, which anchor them to the enterocytes. Different pilus antigens adhere to glycoconjugate receptors on enterocytes in different regions of the small intestine. Thus these bacteria are not washed out by peristalsis. Because the enterocytes are not damaged, no lesions are observed, although microscopically the bacteria can be seen attached to the epithelial surface. The bacteria produce a toxin that causes enterocytes to secrete water and electrolytes. Although cAMP and cyclic guanosine monophosphate (cGMP) mediate this process, the exact mechanism by which this secretion occurs is unknown. Some secretions, especially those of Cl^-, occur via the crypt cells. Intestinal secretion exceeds the ability of the colon to absorb the surplus fluid. The net result is diarrhea.

Abnormalities of the Microvilli and Glycocalyx. Because the microvilli and glycocalyx on villous enterocytes are largely responsible for the immense surface area and the enzymes responsible for nutrient digestion and absorption, it follows that damage to either of these structures can result in intestinal malfunction and resultant diarrhea. A prime example of this is human lactose intolerance. Such persons lack lactase in the glycocalyx. Because of this lack, they are unable to digest lactose from dairy products. The lack of lactase results in failure of uptake of milk sugar, and the lactose is fermented by bacteria in the colon. This results in an osmotic drain of fluid into the gut with resultant diarrhea. Thus the malabsorption in this case is limited to a single substrate. Histologically the intestine is normal.

Some bacteria, such as attaching and effacing *E. coli*, damage microvilli by their attachment. This attachment disrupts enzyme systems housed in microvilli and the glycocalyx and causes diarrhea. The antibiotic neomycin can similarly cause fragmentation of microvilli and destruction of the glycocalyx with resultant diarrhea. Cessation of neomycin therapy results in a return to normal structure and function.

Diseases in Which the Epithelial Targets Are Unknown or Nonspecific. In a number of enteric diseases the targeted epithelial cell is unknown or nonspecific. *Clostridium perfringens* type C is a pathogen of neonatal pigs, lambs, calves, and foals. Unlike enterotoxic *E. coli*, which produces a toxin affecting enterocytes, *C. perfringens* produces a nonspecific cytotoxin. This toxin causes necrosis of villous absorptive cells, which then extends to the lamina propria and blood vessels. The result is massive and acute necrohemorrhagic enteritis.

Separation of Apical Junctional Complexes. Apical junctional complexes, also called *tight junctions* or *zona occludens*, join enterocytes to each other. Transmembrane proteins, such as claudin, occludin, tricellulin, junction-associated molecules, and the coxsackievirus and adenovirus receptor (CAR), form tight junctions. Normally these junctions are a barrier to macromolecular transepithelial transport. In certain diseases, such as ostertagiasis, *Salmonella typhimurium in vitro*, *C. perfringens*, alimentary anthrax, and enterohemorrhagic *E. coli*, these tight junctions are pathologically opened through effects of bacterial toxins and products on transmembrane proteins, allowing transport of macromolecules into the intestinal (abomasal) lumen. This opening of tight junctions is also important in allowing macromolecules, such as immunoglobulin, into the lumen, where the pathogen can be attacked.

Diseases of the Lamina Propria

Lesions within the lamina propria can be infiltrative, necrotizing, or vascular, all of which can cause diarrhea even though the epithelium is not the primary cell type injured.

Peritoneum, Omentum, Mesentery, and Peritoneal Cavity

Most infections of the peritoneal cavity are traumatic in origin from a rupture in the alimentary, urinary, or reproductive systems. Extension from organ infection or neoplasia is another common source of introduction of foreign agents into the peritoneum. Traumatic injury to a body wall, such as by a projectile, can introduce foreign material or air (pneumoperitoneum). Traumatic injury to a vessel or to an organ or rupture from a tumor or ingestion or administration of anticoagulants may cause hemoperitoneum. The liver is particularly prone to rupture when infiltrated by fat or amyloid.

Defense Mechanisms/Barrier Systems

Considering the types of materials that are ingested by domestic animals, it is significant that they are not constantly ill. This

Box 7-3 Defense Mechanisms in the Alimentary System

- Taste buds
- Vomiting
- Saliva
  - Flushing action so potential pathogens are cleared from the oropharynx
  - Protective coating of the mucosa
  - Contains antimicrobial lysozyme, lactoferrin, lactoperoxidase, and immunoglobulins
- Gastric pH
- Microbiota/microbiome–lower GI tract (damaged by toxicants; carcinogen activation)
  - 100 trillion (anaerobic) bacteria (10 × host); 3.3 million genes (150 × host)
  - Bacteriocins
  - Compete for nutrients
  - Compete for attachment sites
  - Promote immune system maturation
  - Biotransformation
  - Enterotype
- Secreted immunoglobulins
- Extraintestinal secretions from the liver and pancreas
  - Lactoferrins
  - Peroxidase
- Intestinal proteolytic enzymes
- Intestinal biotransforming and metabolic enzymes
- Phagocytes and other effector cells within the submucosa
- High rate of epithelial turnover
- Shedding of receptor-laden ALP and catalase-containing vesicles from microvilli
- Large surface area
- Dilution with ingesta
- Increased peristalsis resulting in diarrhea
- Mucus–contains phages that destroy bacteria > 1×10^4
- Paneth cells (antimicrobial peptides, lysozymes, phospholipase A2, defensins-cryptdins)
- Innate lymphoid cells
- Adaptive immune system
- Kupffer cells (liver)
- Genetic polymorphisms (HLA) and host gene expression.

ALP, Alkaline phosphatase; *GI,* gastrointestinal; *HLA,* human leukocyte antigen.

resistance to disease occurs because the alimentary system is well suited to protect itself against most potentially pathogenic insults (Box 7-3). These protective mechanisms include oral secretions, such as saliva; "normal" resident flora and fauna; the gastric pH; opening of tight junctions between intestinal cells to allow macromolecules, such as immunoglobulins, into the lumen; vomiting; secretions from the liver and pancreas; intestinal proteolytic enzymes, macrophages, and other effector cells, such as neutrophils, within the submucosa, which are exuded into the alimentary lumen; the high rate of epithelial turnover; increased peristalsis resulting in diarrhea; Paneth cells; and the immune system. Paneth cells produce antimicrobial peptides and proteins, including lysozyme and secretory phospholipase A_2. They also produce α-defensins (cryptdins).

Oral Cavity

Defense mechanisms of the oral cavity include the stratified epithelial surface that is resistant to trauma and some irritants; taste buds, which reject potentially toxic materials based on taste and tongue feel; an indigenous bacterial flora that occupy attachment sites that would otherwise be available to pathogens; and saliva. Saliva provides a flushing action, so potential pathogens are cleared from the oropharynx and swallowed. Saliva also forms a protective coating of the mucosa and contains antimicrobial lysozyme in the zymogen granules of serous cells and immunoglobulins, especially IgA, in a manner analogous to cryptal enterocytes of the intestine, through the production of a secretory component. Migration through the alimentary tract, including the oral cavity, eliminates neutrophils at the end of their life span. In their absence, stomatitis results.

Teeth

In spite of the biophysical resistance of enamel and cementum to most pathogens, plaque accumulates on dental surfaces and may cause regression of gingiva (gingival recesses) as a result of bacterial colonization and inflammation (see Disorders of Domestic Animals, Teeth, Periodontal Disease).

Tonsils

The tonsils sample antigens dissolved in saliva and develop immune responses similar to other lymphoid tissues in the body. Barrier protection to the tonsils is provided by nonkeratinizing, stratified squamous epithelium.

Salivary Glands

Saliva contains electrolytes such as sodium, potassium, calcium, magnesium, chloride, bicarbonate and phosphate; iodine; mucus, which serves as a lubricant; antibacterial compounds such as thiocyanate and hydrogen peroxide; secretory immunoglobulin A; EGF; and the digestive enzymes α-amylase, lipase, and kallikrein. Antimicrobial enzymes secreted include lysozyme, lactoperoxidase, proline-rich proteins, class A and B acid phosphatases, *N*-acetylmuramoyl-L-alanine amidase, NAD(P)H dehydrogenase (quinone), superoxide dismutase, glutathione transferase, class 3 aldehyde dehydrogenase, and glucose-6-phosphate isomerase. Saliva also contains a bacteria-rich flora and at least in human beings, opiorphin, an analgesic.

Tongue

The thick, nonabsorptive, nonkeratinizing, stratified squamous epithelial barrier of the tongue is protective against most xenobiotics. Epitheliotropic viruses, direct penetrating wounds, and caustic agents can damage the epithelium. The tongue also manually removes substances from oral surfaces.

Esophagus

The lining stratified squamous epithelium of the esophagus is keratinized in pigs, horses, and ruminants and nonkeratinized in dogs and cats (carnivores). The epithelial cell turnover rate is 5 to 8 days; therefore healing is relatively rapid. The muscularis is striated in ruminants and dogs, smooth in horses (distal third), which are unable to vomit, and variably mixed in other species. Submucosal mucus glands are present throughout the esophagus in pigs and dogs and at the pharyngeal junction in cats, horses, and ruminants.

Rumen, Reticulum, and Omasum

A thick keratinizing stratified squamous epithelial lining provides protection against xenobiotics, including ingested roughage in the rumen, reticulum, and omasum. There is no secretory apparatus (i.e., goblet cells) in ruminant forestomachs such as in the abomasum, but absorption of volatile fatty acids occurs across the epithelium. The rich "normal" flora (i.e., microbiota) and alkaline pH provide a mechanism for preventing colonization by and multiplication of pathogens.

Stomach and Abomasum

The gastric mucosal barrier is significant in preventing autodigestion and bacterial overgrowth. There is, however, a resident flora that is difficult to grow on artificial media. Microorganismal overgrowth is prevented under normal physiologic conditions by abomasal or gastric motility, PGE_2, a protective layer of mucus and bicarbonate, secretory IgA, transforming growth factor-α (TGF-α), epidermal growth factor, an extremely acid luminal pH, and an effective pyloric sphincter that prevents regurgitation into the stomach or abomasum of duodenal, hepatic, and pancreatic secretions. An intact epithelial layer and adequate blood flow also prevent acid-induced damage.

Intestine

Defense mechanisms of the intestinal tract are diverse. They include indigenous (nonpathogenic) bacterial flora, intestinal and extraintestinal secretions, gastric acidity, intestinal motility, epithelial cell turnover, bile salts, immunologic mechanisms, and although a secondary mechanism, the Kupffer cells of the liver.

Secretions of the oral cavity, saliva, and intestine, called mucins, inhibit the adherence of organisms to the mucosa of the alimentary system. In addition to physically trapping pathogens, intestinal mucus serves to cover glycolipid and glycoprotein receptors on the surface of enterocytes (unstirred layer), thus preventing pathogen attachment and damage by toxins. Mucins are viscous and thus aid in protecting the epithelium from the shear forces of particulates driven against them by peristaltic waves. Because they are extensively glycosylated, mucins can cross-link and trap bacteria, making them more amenable to clearance by passage through the alimentary system. Mucus also contains bacteriophages (i.e., viruses that infect and replicate within bacteria) that destroy bacteria, reducing the population by more than 1×10^4.

Normal gastric acidity kills many organisms before they have the chance to reach the small intestine. Very young animals are achlorhydric; thus they may be more susceptible to some organisms such as pathogenic *E. coli*. Helical bacteria in the stomach are the single greatest cause of gastric ulcers in human beings. Although similar organisms occur in the stomachs of domestic animals, particularly carnivores, their role in gastritis of animals is less certain. Normal gastric acidity apparently does not kill all potentially pathogenic bacteria (helical bacteria) in the stomach and proximal small intestine of domestic animals.

Indigenous (nonpathogenic) bacterial flora (microbiota) competitively bind to putative attachment sites on the enterocytes, thus preempting pathogen attachment. These prokaryotic symbionts coevolved with their hosts and are an integral part of homeostatic mechanisms. Killing of these bacteria through the use of antibiotics sometimes allows pathogens to colonize the intestine and produce disease. Thus gnotobiotic animals are more susceptible to infection. The microbiome enhances the host's genome in contributing to normal physiologic functioning and disease resistance and susceptibility. Bacteria in the intestine outnumber the total somatic and germ cells of the body by approximately a factor of 10. Probiotics are "friendly bacteria" that are sometimes used therapeutically or prophylactically in a variety of products and nutraceuticals. These "friendly bacteria" also compete for substrate with pathogens, alter the microenvironmental pH, making the growth of competitive bacteria difficult, and produce short-chain fatty acids and inhibitory growth substances (bacteriocins) that are toxic to other bacteria. Colicins are bacteriocins produced by *E. coli*. Bacterial growth is also inhibited by lactoferrin and peroxidase from the pancreas and lysozyme and defensins from Paneth cells. Transferrin in serum and lactoferrin produced by enterocytes and neutrophils at sites of infection serve to sequester iron that is necessary for bacterial growth.

Intestinal peristalsis is protective in that loss of motility may lead to bacterial overgrowth in the intestine and increased susceptibility of enterocytes to toxins that are not moved out of the gut. Diarrhea can be in part a defense mechanism that rids the body of bacteria and toxins. Conversely, some bacteria secrete toxins that impair intestinal motility, thus allowing pathogens a greater opportunity to attach to enterocytes.

Epithelial cells of the intestine have the greatest turnover rate of any fixed-cell population in the body. In effect, this means that pathogens with a life cycle that exceeds that of the enterocytes will likely not be successful because their host cell will slough before the pathogen can reproduce. In addition, experimental evidence indicates that enterocyte microvilli form unilaminar vesicles containing digestive enzymes such as catalase and alkaline phosphatase on their surface. These vesicles are shed into the intestinal lumen, where they may interact with the pathogen(s), thus preventing contact of pathogens with enterocyte receptors because these vesicles are passed in the feces.

Bile salts inhibit the growth of many organisms. Kupffer cells of the liver act as a secondary line of defense. Because all the blood from the intestine enters the portal vein and percolates through the hepatic sinusoids, the Kupffer cells are perfectly positioned to phagocytose bacteria and endotoxins with which they come in contact. In pigs, goats, and cattle (artiodactyls), these functions are performed by intravascular pulmonary macrophages.

Secretory IgA and IgM constitute very important mechanisms of humoral immunity and function largely to prevent attachment of pathogens to intestinal epithelium. Crypt epithelial cells produce the secretory component of IgA. IgA functions through adhesion to M cells that regulates transepithelial movement of antigens while masking certain other antigens (Fig. 7-31).

Although in its infancy, research indicates that genetic polymorphisms of the host, including human leukocyte antigen (HLA), likely play a role in disease susceptibility and resistance.

Peritoneum, Omentum, Mesentery, and Peritoneal Cavity

Mesothelial cells produce a lubricant to allow serosal surfaces to slide easily against each other and prevent tumor cell adhesion. Mesothelial cells are also actively phagocytic, transport fluid and cells across serosal surfaces, and play a role in antigen presentation, inflammation, tissue repair, coagulation, and fibrinolysis.

Disorders of Domestic Animals[2]

Oral Cavity

The oral cavity is one of the places that can be examined directly by the clinician and pathologist and where they can use the same criteria for determining abnormality. The same can be said of the rectal mucosa.

Developmental Anomalies

There are a wide variety of developmental abnormalities in the oral cavity. Some are incompatible with life unless surgically corrected. Only a few of these congenital lesions have a proven hereditary component. Most are idiopathic. Thorough physical examination of

[2]See Necropsy Techniques in E-Appendix 7-1 for information on postmortem examination of the alimentary system.

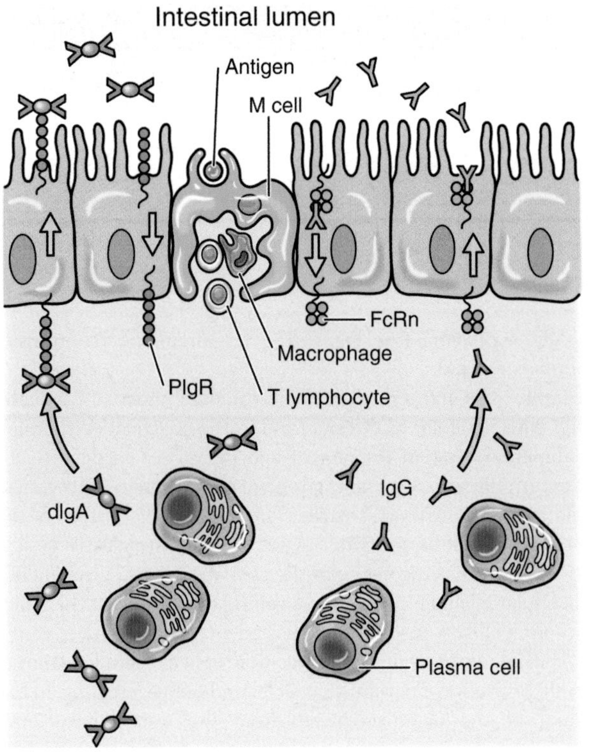

Figure 7-31 Immunoglobulin Secretion in the Intestine. Dimeric immunoglobulin A (dIgA), produced by plasma cells via interaction with polymeric IgR (PIgR) is transported across the intestinal epithelium in association with secretory component, which is a portion of PIgR secreted into the intestinal lumen. IgG transport is mediated by major histocompatibility complex class I (neonatal Fc receptor [FcRn]). IgG transport is bidirectional; IgA is not. M, Microfold.

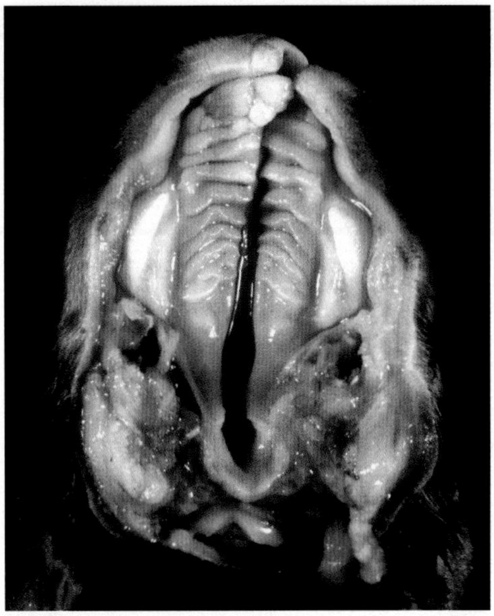

Figure 7-32 Palatoschisis and Cheiloschisis, Hard and Soft Palate, Puppy. The lateral palatine processes have failed to fuse during the first trimester of gestation (palatoschisis). In dogs, palatoschisis has been attributed to genetic abnormalities, excessive intake of vitamin A during gestation, and the administration of cortisone during gestation. The upper lip is also cleft (cheiloschisis). (Courtesy Dr. H. Gelberg, College of Veterinary Medicine, Oregon State University.)

neonates must include examination of the oral cavity for these defects.

Palatoschisis, or cleft palate, and cheiloschisis, or cleft lip, are among the most common developmental abnormalities of the oral cavity. Cheiloschisis is sometimes referred to as *hare lip* because this is a normal feature of the rabbit. It is a failure of fusion of the upper lip along the midline or philtrum. Palatoschisis can be genetic or toxic in origin. It results from a failure of fusion of the lateral palatine processes. It can be caused by steroid administration during pregnancy in primates, including human beings. Depending on the size of the defect, which may involve only the soft palate or both the soft and hard palates (Fig. 7-32), the lesion may be surgically correctable. It is a matter of some ethical concern whether to correct such defects without also sterilizing the patient because of the potential for cleft palate to have a genetic cause. Important sequelae to the host from cleft palate are starvation, as the result of the inability of the nursing animal to create a negative pressure in the mouth with a resultant failure to suckle, and aspiration pneumonia, because no effective separation is present between the oral and nasal cavities.

Stomatitis and Gingivitis

Stomatitis and gingivitis refer to inflammation of the mucous membranes of the oral cavity and gingiva, respectively. Because the oral cavity is constantly bombarded with ingested substances that are moved around by the tongue, the final result of a variety of insults to the lining of the oral cavity is a loss of mucosa—erosions, ulcerations, and necrosis. Thus, although inflammation is apparent, clues as to the initiating process may be absent. Lesions may be at different stages and are commonly classified as macules, papules, vesicles, erosions, abscesses, granulomas, and ulcers. These lesions can be caused by infectious agents, particularly viruses; chemical injury; trauma; intoxicants; or autoimmune or systemic disease. They often result in anorexia caused by painful mastication. Hypersalivation (ptyalism) is also apparent, whether from overproduction or a failure to swallow. In the cat, gingivitis is the first and most consistent sign of feline immunodeficiency virus (FIV) infection (immune system failure) associated with a reduction in CD4 lymphocytes, thymic atrophy, and lymph node atrophy.

Vesicular Stomatitides—Viral Diseases

Although vesicular stomatitis correctly refers to oral vesicles and blisters, the term is generally reserved for those lesions caused by epitheliotropic viruses. The vesicular stomatitides are listed in Table 7-1. Their genesis is from virus-induced epithelial cytolysis attended by fluid accumulation and subsequent rupture of the resultant vesicle. Blistering or vesiculation of the oral epithelium is present early in the course of these diseases. All of these diseases are virus induced, and all have identical appearances at gross and histopathologic examination. None of these conditions is fatal. They produce great economic loss because of poor weight gain in affected animals and sometimes abortions in gravid females. The exact cause of the abortions is unknown, but it is probably related to the stress induced by the painful oral, cutaneous, and pedal (hoof or foot) lesions. Secondary bacterial invaders, both Gram-negative and Gram-positive, of these lesions can result in endotoxemia. Several diseases, such as foot-and-mouth disease and vesicular exanthema, affect the coronary bands of the digits and interdigital clefts, resulting in lameness. Some of these diseases (foot-and-mouth disease, vesicular exanthema, and swine vesicular disease) are exotic to the United States and thus are reportable to state or federal authorities, or both, if the clinician or pathologist suspects the disease. This requirement

Table 7-1 Vesicular Stomatitides

Disease	Cause	Ruminant	Pigs	Horses
Foot-and-mouth disease	Picornavirus	+	+	–
Vesicular stomatitis	Rhabdovirus	++	+	+
Vesicular exanthema of swine	Calicivirus (vesivirus)	–	++	–
Swine vesicular disease	Enterovirus	–	++	–

+, Species in which disease occurs; –, species in which disease does not occur.

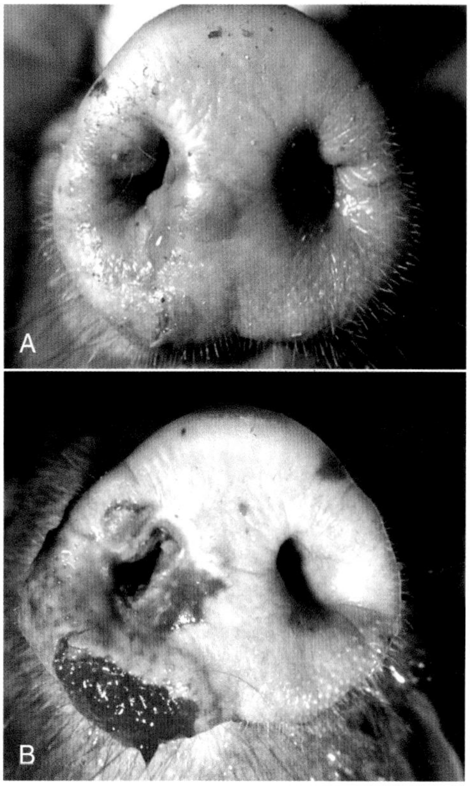

Figure 7-33 **Cutaneous Vesicles, Vesicular Exanthema, Snout, Pig. A,** Vesicles, both intact *(upper vesicle)* and ruptured *(lower vesicle)*, are present on the planum nasale and are caused by the infection of injured mucosal epithelial cells with vesicular exanthema of swine virus, a calicivirus (vesivirus). **B,** Ruptured vesicles with cutaneous ulceration, vesicular exanthema (later stage of the disease). Note the ruptured vesicles, which can cause pain, resulting in inappetence. (**A** from Gelberg H, Lewis RM: *Vet Pathol* 19:424-443, 1982. **B** courtesy Dr. H. Gelberg, College of Veterinary Medicine, Oregon State University.)

is due to the great expense involved in eradicating these diseases from the United States and their potential use as agents of agroterrorism. Nontariff export/import barriers designed to prevent the introduction of highly contagious agents, such as foot-and-mouth disease, into animal populations of countries with which we trade, are often put in place.

The gross lesions of the vesicular stomatitides are epithelial. Fluid-filled vesicles are present in the oral cavity, lips, rostral palate, tongue, and planum nasale (Fig. 7-33, A). Entry of virus in these cases is most likely oral into areas of temporary loss of mucosa as the result of normal mastication and trauma. The viruses are cytolytic, and the resultant release of virus from cells infects neighboring cells. The lesions enlarge centripetally, forming vesicles. Bullae result from coalescence, resulting in erosions and ulcers. These ulcers are typically hyperemic (see Fig. 7-33, *B*). Viremia, often transient, sometimes occurs.

Similar vesicular lesions occur in the nasal mucosa, particularly in pigs with vesicular exanthema and in the proximal epithelium of the alimentary system (esophagus and rumen) of cattle with foot-and-mouth disease. Some animals have conjunctivitis and vesicular dermatitis of the teats and vulva. The microscopic lesions of these four diseases (foot-and-mouth disease, vesicular stomatitis, vesicular exanthema, and swine vesicular disease) are similar. Virus-induced, intracellular edema progresses to swelling of the cells of the stratum spinosum, cell lysis and intercellular edema, and resultant vesicles. The epithelium overlying the virus-rich vesicular fluid is thin, and even slight friction can rupture vesicles and bullae, creating an ulcer. Healing of the ulcer progresses from the usual fibrin- and/or neutrophil-rich acute stages (scab) to the more chronic stages of granulation.

Lesions and signs of the vesicular stomatitides include vesicles, bullae, and detachment of patches of epithelium with resultant raw ulcers, ptyalism, lameness, fever, and anorexia. Besides the lesions that develop from the initially infected cells, the virus spreads centripetally to adjacent susceptible epithelium, causing repeated episodes of this infectious, lytic cycle. The vesicular stomatitides are tentatively diagnosed based on the clinical signs and lesions resulting from oral and nasal ulceration, conjunctivitis, and ulceration of the genitalia and mammary glands. Lameness is secondary to hoof involvement that is focused at the coronary band. Definitive diagnosis is important and performed at federal laboratories equipped to rapidly respond to suspected outbreaks. Federal quarantine of infected herds is an important control mechanism, followed by eradication, slaughter, and carcass disposal.

Foot-and-Mouth Disease. See Disorders of Ruminants (Cattle, Sheep, and Goats).

Vesicular Stomatitides

Vesicular Stomatitis. Vesicular stomatitis is common in calves, pigs, and some wildlife species but does not occur in sheep or goats. It is the only vesicular disease to which horses are susceptible. In northern latitudes, it is generally a warm weather disease, suggesting that insects act as vectors. As the name implies, vesicles in the oral cavity characterize the disease. Clinically the disease is often recognized by inappetence in the affected animal, accompanied by ptyalism.

Other Vesicular Stomatitides. Vesicular exanthema is a specific disease of pigs that is indistinguishable clinically and pathologically from foot-and-mouth disease. This disease is uniquely American and was believed eradicated from pigs in 1956 through enactment of federal laws requiring the cooking of garbage fed to pigs. The evidence indicates that vesicular exanthema of pig serovars are variants of San Miguel sea lion virus. This latter marine calicivirus (vesivirus) occurs in coastal sea lion and fur seal populations from California to Alaska (E-Fig. 7-2). Swine vesicular disease is indistinguishable from the other vesicular stomatitides and is exotic to the United States. Efforts are underway to develop DNA microarrays to facilitate rapid identification of specific vesicular diseases from a single sample.

Erosive and Ulcerative Stomatitides

Erosions are defined by a loss of part of the thickness of the surface epithelium, whereas ulcers are full-thickness epithelial losses exposing the basement membrane. Thus erosions may progress to ulcers, which in hollow organs may become perforating ulcers. Erosive and ulcerative stomatitis can have a variety of causes. Agents responsible include the viruses of bovine viral diarrhea (Fig. 7-34), rinderpest, malignant catarrhal fever (Fig. 7-35), feline calicivirus, and bluetongue, and in horses, NSAIDs. Other causes include uremia (Fig. 7-36); ingested foreign bodies, such as foxtail awns; the feline eosinophilic granuloma complex; and vitamin C deficiency in primates and guinea pigs (E-Fig. 7-3). Often the oral lesions must be evaluated in the context of the clinical signs, together with histopathologic findings and ancillary testing, to arrive at a definitive diagnosis. Additionally, the vesicular stomatitides can progress to ulceration secondary to abrasion to the point that they cannot be distinguished from the ulcerative stomatitides.

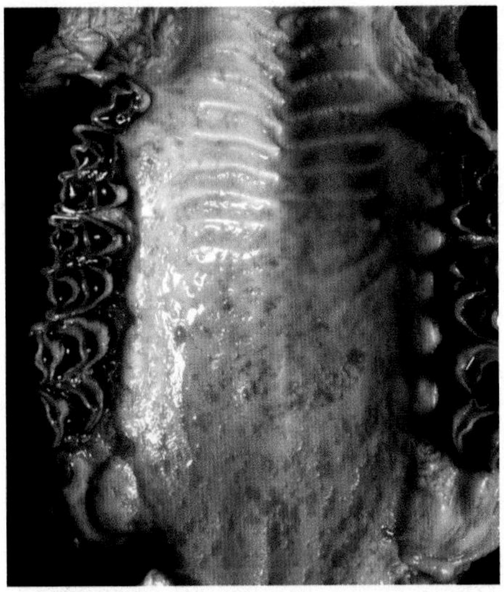

Figure 7-34 Erosions and Ulcers, Bovine Viral Diarrhea (BVD) Virus Infection, Hard Palate, Cow. Erosions and ulcers *(small red areas on mucosal surface)* caused by this pestivirus are particularly evident on the mucosal epithelial surface of the caudal hard palate. These lesions are characteristic of the ulcerative stomatitides, which, unlike the vesicular disease viruses, do not form vesicles. (Courtesy Dr. M.D. McGavin, College of Veterinary Medicine, University of Tennessee.)

Parapox Stomatitides

See Disorders of Ruminants (Cattle, Sheep, and Goats).

Necrotizing Stomatitides

Necrotizing stomatitis occurs in cattle, sheep, and pigs. In cattle it is sometimes referred to as *calf diphtheria* (Fig. 7-37). Necrotizing stomatitis is the end stage of all other forms of stomatitis when they are complicated by infection with *Fusobacterium necrophorum*, a filamentous-to-rodlike-to-coccoid, Gram-negative anaerobe. Bacterial toxins are responsible for the extensive lesions. Necrotizing stomatitis is characterized by yellow-gray, round foci surrounded by a rim of hyperemic tissue in the oral cavity, larynx, pharynx, or tongue. Well-demarcated foci of coagulation necrosis typify the histologic appearance of necrotizing stomatitis. As might be expected in foci of inflammation, there is a circumferential rim of leukocytes and hyperemia. Clinical signs include swollen cheeks, inappetence, pyrexia, and halitosis. Infection may become systemic if severe, resulting in lesions throughout the alimentary system and associated lymphoid tissue.

Noma is a severe form of oral ischemic necrosis with lesional spirochetes and fusiform bacteria. Although rare, it is seen most often in primates, including human beings, and dogs. It is characterized by severe necrotizing gingivitis that can extend into adjacent bone, causing osteolysis and sometimes death.

Ulcerative gingivitis (trench mouth), caused by anaerobic spirochetes, affects human beings, some nonhuman primates, and rarely,

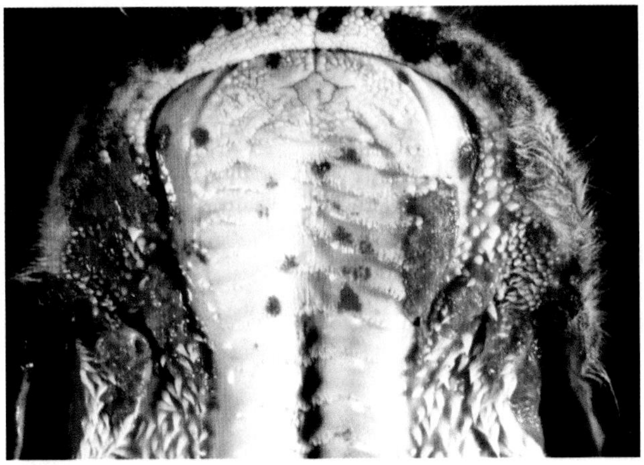

Figure 7-35 Erosions and Ulcers, Malignant Catarrhal Fever, Hard Palate, Dental Pad and Buccal Papillae, Cow. The erosions and ulcers *(red areas on mucosal surface)* are due to malignant catarrhal fever virus, a herpesvirus, but are characteristic of many ulcerative stomatitides. (Courtesy Dr. H. Gelberg, College of Veterinary Medicine, Oregon State University.)

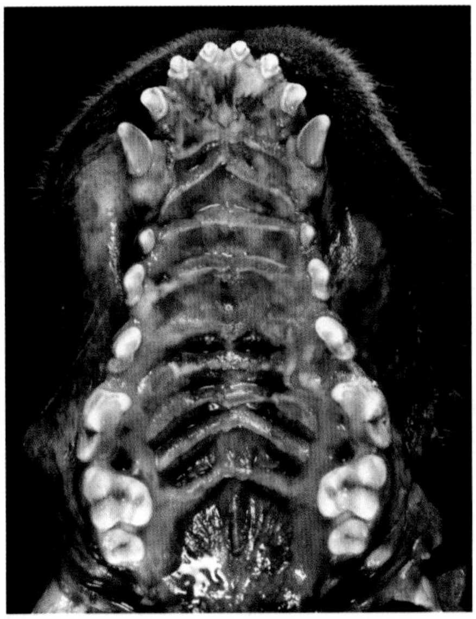

Figure 7-36 Uremic Ulcers, Hard Palate, Dog. Ulcers present on the transverse palatine ridges and periodontal gingiva are secondary to vascular damage associated with increased concentrations of plasma blood urea nitrogen and creatinine from kidney failure. Affected animals often have an ammoniacal or uremic odor to the breath. (Courtesy Dr. H. Gelberg, College of Veterinary Medicine, Oregon State University.)

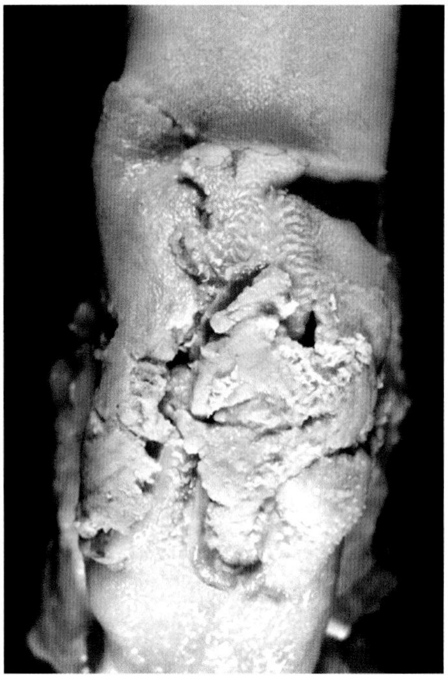

Figure 7-37 **Necrotizing Stomatitis, Calf Diphtheria, Tongue, Calf.** The dorsal surface of the tongue is ulcerated, and the ulcers are covered by a yellow-white diphtheric membrane. Calf diphtheria is caused by infection with the bacterium *Fusobacterium necrophorum* secondary to abrasion and/or trauma to the mucosal epithelium of the oral cavity or larynx. (Courtesy Dr. M.D. McGavin, College of Veterinary Medicine, University of Tennessee.)

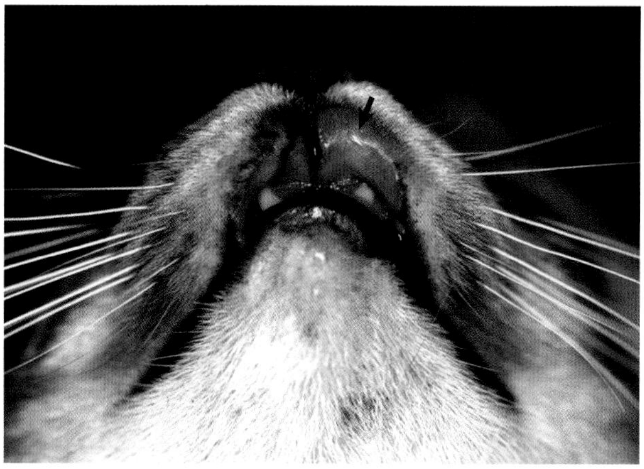

Figure 7-38 **Eosinophilic Granuloma, Skin, Upper Lip, Cat.** Bilateral ulceration of the upper lip is present. The upper left lip is more extensively affected *(arrow)*. (Courtesy Dr. Ann M. Hargis, DermatoDiagnostics.)

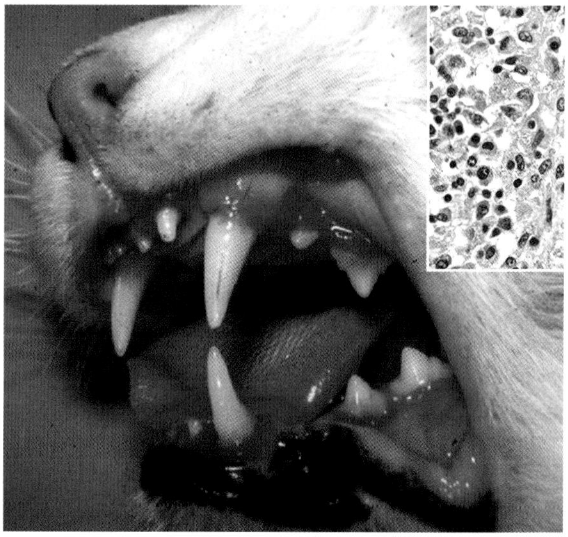

Figure 7-39 **Lymphoplasmacytic Stomatitis, Gingiva, Cat.** This chronic condition of cats is characterized by red, inflamed gums, fetid breath, and inappetence. The oral mucosa can also be hyperplastic and ulcerated. *Inset,* There is a florid infiltrate of mixed inflammatory cells, including many lymphocytes and plasma cells in the submucosa beneath the epithelium. H&E stain. (Figure courtesy Dr. C. Patrick Ryan, Veterinary Public Health, Los Angeles Department of Health Services; and Noah's Arkive, College of Veterinary Medicine, University of Georgia. Inset courtesy Dr. J.F. Zachary, College of Veterinary Medicine, University of Illinois.)

puppies. In addition to *Fusobacterium* spp., *Borrelia vincentii* may be causative. Debilitated animals and those with intercurrent infections are at increased risk for these secondary invaders, which may be part of normal oral flora. Similar clinically to necrotizing stomatitis, ulcerative gingivitis is characterized by acute inflammation and necrosis, oral ulceration and pain, halitosis, a fragile oral mucosa, and ptyalism. The morphologic diagnosis is an acute, necrotizing gingivitis. Unlike the case in necrotizing stomatitis, the causative agents are readily identified by tissue smears or by culture.

Eosinophilic Stomatitides

Oral granulomas or ulcers ("rodent ulcers") occur frequently in cats. Similar lesions occur sporadically in a variety of canine breeds. In cats they are termed *oral eosinophilic granulomas*. Although the cause of this condition is unknown, the histologic appearance of lesions suggests an immune-mediated mechanism, possibly a hypersensitivity reaction to an unknown antigen. Antibodies to intercellular material can often be demonstrated in affected cats. In the majority of cases of both dogs and cats, an increase in circulating eosinophils is present.

In cats, lip lesions are commonly visible near the philtrum and may extend through the adjacent haired skin (Fig. 7-38). Oral lesions may occur anywhere in the mouth, including the gingiva, hard and soft palates, oral and nasal pharynx, tongue, and occasionally draining lymphoid tissues, excluding the tonsils, which do not have afferent lymphatic vessels (see Fig. 17-22, C). In dogs, eosinophilic granulomas typically are raised, fungating masses on the ventral and lateral lingual epithelium and palate. Collagenolysis (because collagen is acellular, it cannot undergo necrosis) is characteristically central in the lesion. The surrounding inflammatory tissue contains mixed inflammatory cells with increased numbers of eosinophils, mast cells, and multinucleated giant cells (see E-Fig. 3-10). Lesions grouped as the eosinophilic granuloma complex of cats include eosinophilic ulcer, linear (collagenolytic) granulomas, and eosinophilic plaques. The latter two lesions are strictly cutaneous and do not affect the oral cavity. No proven etiologic link has been established among these cutaneous conditions (linear granulomas and eosinophilic plaques) and oral eosinophilic granulomas. The cause of the canine lesions is unknown.

Lymphoplasmacytic Stomatitis

Lymphoplasmacytic stomatitis is an idiopathic condition of the cat named on the basis of the histologic appearance of the lesions (Fig. 7-39). Associations have been hypothesized between this condition and the presence of bacteria or calicivirus associated with feline leukemia virus (FeLV) and/or FIV infection. It is a chronic condition characterized by red, inflamed gums, a fetid breath, and

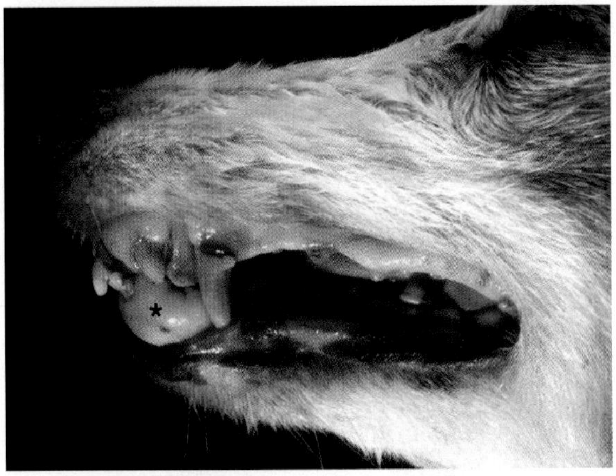

Figure 7-40 **Gingival Hyperplasia, Gingiva, Dog.** Hyperplastic gingiva *(asterisk)* has enveloped the lower incisor teeth. Dental calculus (tartar, *brown*) is also present on both upper and lower incisor, canine, and molar teeth. (Courtesy Dr. H. Gelberg, College of Veterinary Medicine, Oregon State University.)

inappetence. The oral mucosa may be hyperplastic and ulcerated. An inefficient immune response may be responsible for the persistence of oral bacteria and the accumulation of lymphocytes and plasma cells.

Chronic Ulcerative Paradental Stomatitis

Chronic ulcerative paradental stomatitis, a condition of dogs also known as *ulcerative stomatitis* and *lymphocytic-plasmacytic stomatitis*, is caused by apposition of "kissing ulcers" to dental plaque. The condition is painful with resultant inappetence and anorexia. Affected dogs drool and have halitosis. This condition occurs in older dogs of any breed, but Maltese dogs and Cavalier King Charles spaniels are particularly susceptible. The lymphocytic-plasmacytic lesions noted on histologic examination are suggestive of an inflammatory rather than infectious cause, possibly caused by mediators released from the plaque. If untreated, bone resorption may occur.

Oral Mucosal Hyperplasia and Neoplasia

Hyperplastic Diseases. Gingival hyperplasia is a simple overgrowth of gum tissue, principally the fibrous submucosa. The hyperplasia can become severe enough to bury incisor teeth (Fig. 7-40). Gingival hyperplasia is most common in brachycephalic dog breeds and is present in 30% of boxer dogs older than 5 years.

Grossly, gingival hyperplasia can be indistinguishable from an epulis (Fig. 7-41). Epulis is a nonspecific term that designates a growth of the gingiva. The several kinds of epulides can only be distinguished by histopathologic examination. These include fibromatous epulis of periodontal ligament origin—a benign tumor of dental mesenchyme. This distinction is not just an academic exercise because, although all epulides are considered benign, one form, acanthomatous epulis or acanthomatous ameloblastoma, invades bone and can be quite destructive. This growth arises from the epithelial rests of Malassez or epithelial tooth germ. Fortunately, this type of epulis can be managed therapeutically. Whether the epulides represent fibrous and epithelial hyperplasia or benign neoplasms of tooth germ is controversial.

Neoplasia. In the dog 70% of tumors of the alimentary system are in the oral cavity and oropharynx. These tumors run the gamut of biologic behavior from simple epithelial hyperplasia to malignant neoplasms with metastases to distant sites. Squamous cell

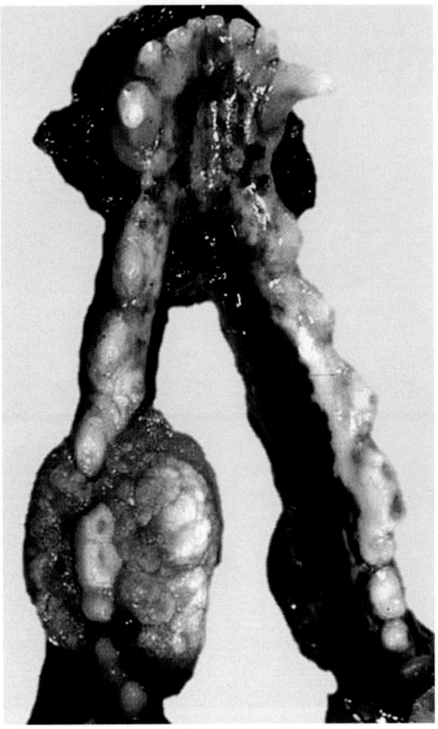

Figure 7-41 **Fibromatous Epulis, Left Mandible, Molar Teeth, Dog.** This growth is an epulis (fibromatous type); however, epulides are often grossly indistinguishable from gingival hyperplasia. Epulis is a term used to designate a growth of the gingiva that is firm, periodontal, and usually solitary, in contrast to gingival hyperplasia. This distinction is not just an academic exercise because, although all epulides are considered benign, one form, acanthomatous ameloblastoma, is locally invasive. It invades bone and can be quite destructive. (Courtesy Dr. J. King, College of Veterinary Medicine, Cornell University.)

carcinomas occur in the oral cavity, particularly in old cats, in which they account for 60% of oral neoplasms. They generally occur on the ventrolateral surface of the tongue and tonsils. Lingual squamous cell carcinomas occur more commonly in cats, and tonsillar squamous cell carcinomas are more common in dogs. Although often appearing histologically aggressive, only a small percentage of lingual neoplasms metastasize, most commonly to draining lymph nodes, the mandibular and medial retropharyngeal. Unfortunately, most tonsillar carcinomas metastasize, initially to regional lymph nodes and then to distant sites.

Squamous cell carcinomas vary both in size and in gross appearance—from flat to proliferative (Fig. 7-42). These tumors are often quite aggressive locally, invading subjacent tissues. Some tumors contain more differentiated cells, keratin, often in whorls (keratin pearls) and visible desmosomes (intercellular bridges), whereas others are less well differentiated but with significant mitotic activity. In these latter cases, intracellular immunohistochemical markers for cytokeratin are useful in determining a definitive diagnosis. The amount of fibrous tissue within an individual tumor is variable. Some carcinomas induce a scirrhous response, whereas others have areas of necrosis caused by rapid tumor growth, "collision necrosis," of the tightly packed proliferating cells and loss of contiguity with the blood supply.

Ninety percent of melanomas of the oral cavities of dogs are malignant. A breed predilection exists for Scottish terriers, Airedales, cocker spaniels, golden retrievers, Bedlington terriers, Duroc pigs, and others. Most melanomas contain copious intracellular pigment and are visibly black. Some melanomas without pigment,

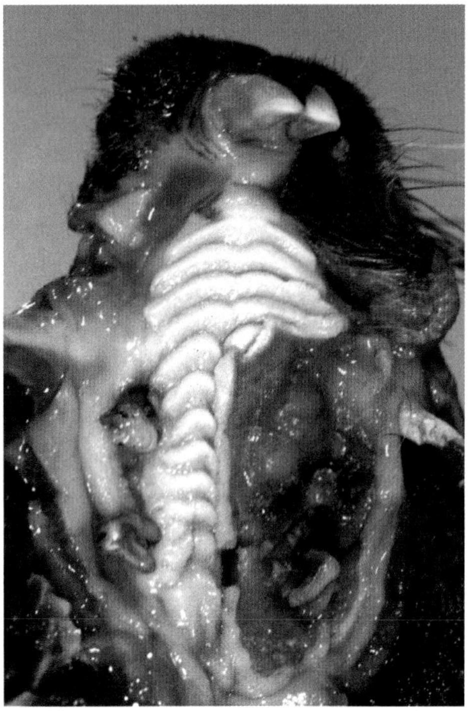

Figure 7-42 Squamous Cell Carcinoma, Palate, Woodchuck. A mass of proliferating neoplastic squamous epithelial cells has displaced and replaced the mucosa and underlying tissue of the left hard palate and gingiva. (Courtesy Dr. H. Gelberg, College of Veterinary Medicine, Oregon State University.)

termed *amelanotic melanomas*, present a greater diagnostic challenge to both the clinician and pathologist (Fig. 7-43). Immunohistochemical staining for tyrosinase-related proteins (TRP-1, TRP-2), Melan-A, and melanocytic antigen PNL2 are useful for immunohistochemically identifying amelanotic tumors. Melanomas are composed of melanocytes and are of neural crest origin. Cellular morphologic features within melanomas vary from spindloid to epithelioid. Thus some neoplasms are histologically difficult to differentiate from squamous cell carcinomas and others from fibrosarcomas.

Canine oral papillomatosis is a papovavirus-induced, transmissible condition that usually occurs in animals younger than 1 year. The lesions usually regress spontaneously. Immunity is long lasting. The lesions are papilliform or cauliflower-like and can become quite numerous. They are generally white and friable and occur on the mouth, tongue, palate, larynx, and epiglottis. These oral tumors are usually multiple, white to gray, raised, and pedunculated with a keratinized surface and a stromal core. The epithelial cells constituting the lesion can be acanthotic, hyperplastic, and rest on a hyperplastic, folded, connective tissue stroma. The stratum spinosum is also hyperplastic and ballooned. Cytoplasmic inclusion bodies are sometimes present.

Oral extramedullary plasmacytomas may occur anywhere in the mucous membranes of the oral cavity, and in the esophagus or intestine. In the oral cavity they are slow-growing neoplasms and in spite of often-recognized anisokaryosis, mitoses, and multinucleate cells, they rarely invade surrounding tissues and have not been reported to metastasize. Histologic examination is required for accurate diagnosis (see Fig. 13-84).

Fibrosarcomas arise from the collagen-producing cells (fibroblasts) of the oral cavity. Fibrosarcomas are most common in the cat, accounting for 20% of oral neoplasia in that species. They may occur anywhere in the oral cavity. In large-breed dogs, histologically

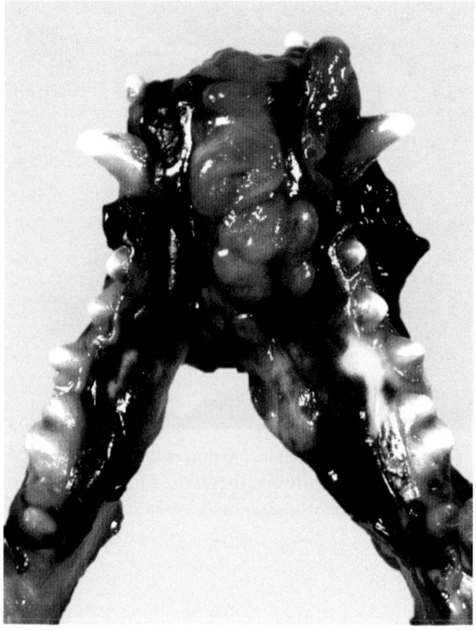

Figure 7-43 Amelanotic Melanoma, Mandibular Symphysis, Dog. A proliferative, ulcerated, nonpigmented mass is present on the oral mucosa at the mandibular symphysis and protrudes into the oral cavity, likely resulting in malocclusion. Incisor teeth have been lost. Note the absence of pigmentation (melanin) in this tumor. (Courtesy Dr. M.D. McGavin, College of Veterinary Medicine, University of Tennessee.)

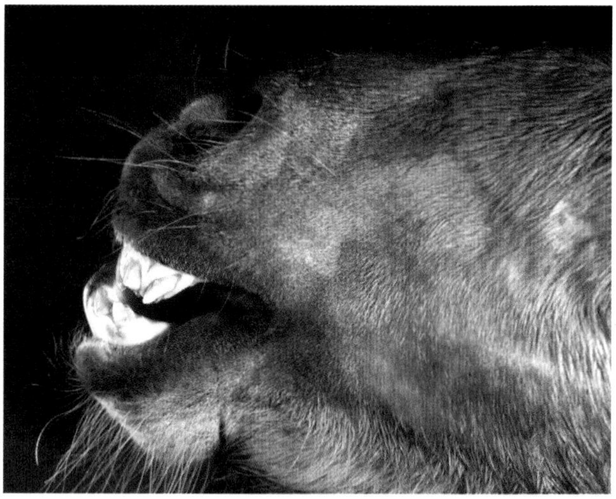

Figure 7-44 Prognathia, Head, Horse. The mandible is elongated when compared to the maxilla. (Courtesy Dr. H. Gelberg, College of Veterinary Medicine, Oregon State University.)

benign-appearing fibrosarcomas of the oral cavity invade bone and metastasize.

Teeth

Malocclusions

Abnormal development and positioning of the teeth may affect dental function. Malocclusion refers to a failure of the upper and lower incisors to oppose properly. This feature is "normal" for some dogs, particularly the brachycephalic breeds. In the extreme, malocclusions can lead to difficulty in the prehension and mastication of food. Malocclusions are named according to the position of the mandible. Protrusion of the lower jaw is termed *prognathia* (Fig. 7-44), whereas a short lower jaw with resultant protrusion of the upper jaw is termed *brachygnathia* and sometimes *hypognathia*. Sometimes these terms are incorrectly used, referring to brachygnathia as superior prognathia and prognathia as superior brachygnathia.

Malocclusions result from abnormal jaw conformation or rarely from abnormal tooth eruption patterns. In some animals, such as rodents and rabbits, the teeth continue to grow throughout the animal's lifetime. If these animals are not provided with sufficient roughage in their diets, the teeth (both incisors and cheek teeth) overgrow and either "lock" the jaw or because of a lack of occlusal grinding surfaces, prevent the animal from receiving proper nutrition (E-Fig. 7-4).

Anomalies of Tooth Development

In simple-toothed animals and rarely in other animals, agenesis of a tooth or teeth occurs and is generally of no clinical significance (see Fig. 17-37). Supernumerary tooth development is less common than tooth agenesis and is similarly of little clinical significance. Some animals, such as elasmobranches (sharks), continue to produce row on row of teeth as the outermost rows are lost. Dental dysgenesis may be primarily due to dysplasia of the enamel-forming organ or secondary to trauma, infection and hyperthermia, toxicosis, or other metabolic irregularities during odontogenesis.

Dentigerous cysts result from dental dysgenesis, and epithelial-lined, cystic structures in tissue, including the bone of the jaw, result. Dentigerous cysts develop from abnormal proliferation of the cell rests of Malassez. They appear as variably sized, sometimes fluctuant swellings of the mandible or maxilla. In the maxilla they sometimes invade the nasal sinuses. Although rare, dentigerous cysts are often painful, and although not usually neoplastic, they can destroy the jaw. Dentigerous cysts are epithelial lined and may become impacted with keratin. Rudimentary, malformed teeth may be found within these cysts, and painful fistulas may develop, especially in horses. These draining tracts are seen most often rostral and ventral to the ear ("ear tooth").

Segmental enamel hypoplasia occurs before eruption of the permanent teeth of dogs as a result of hyperthermia and viral infection, most often by canine distemper virus infection. Enamel is fully formed when the teeth erupt; therefore virus infection of ameloblasts must occur during enamel formation, which is before the dog is 6 months of age, if enamel hypoplasia is to occur. Canine distemper virus infection causes necrosis and disorganization of the enamel organ. After the virus is cleared, structure and function of the enamel organ return to normal. Thus segmental enamel hypoplasia results from the lack of enamel formation during the period of virus infection (Fig. 7-45). A similar condition in calves is caused by *in utero* bovine viral diarrhea virus infection.

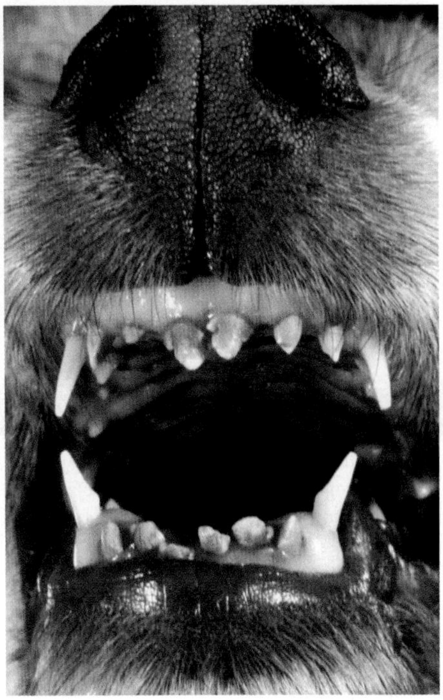

Figure 7-45 Enamel Hypoplasia, Permanent Incisor Teeth, Dog. There is a lack of enamel formation with resultant discrete deep pits and exposure of the dentin (light yellow to beige areas of the teeth), the result of infection with canine distemper virus and necrosis of the ameloblasts during enamel formation. Permanent adult teeth (shown in illustration) are infected with virus before their eruption and while they are still within their sockets (dental alveoli). (Courtesy Dr. H. Gelberg, College of Veterinary Medicine, Oregon State University.)

Chemicals, most notably tetracycline antibiotics ingested during the process of enamel mineralization, can cause yellowish, permanent discoloration (see Fig. 1-59). Congenital porphyria, a defect in red blood cell production, may result in incorporation of porphyrins into dentin, resulting in pink discoloration of the teeth ("pink tooth") (E-Fig. 7-5). Both tetracycline and porphyrins fluoresce under ultraviolet light, dramatically demonstrating these lesions.

Fluoride incorporation into the enamel and dentin occurs in fluoride toxicosis, particularly in cattle and sheep. A relationship exists in beef cattle between fluorosis and selenium supplementation, with selenium supplementation being protective in high fluoride areas such as those downwind from aluminum smelters or with high concentrations of fluoride in groundwater. Excessive dietary concentrations of fluorine during odontogenesis (from 6 to 36 months of age) may result in incorporation of the fluoride in the enamel and dentin of the permanent teeth. The result is soft, chalky, discolored enamel, usually yellow, dark brown, or black (E-Fig. 7-6). Occlusal grinding of affected soft teeth against more normal enamel results in rapid dental wear to the extent that severely affected sheep may have almost completely worn down their incisors. One wonders therefore about the cumulative effect of fluoride supplementation in municipal drinking water, vitamins with added fluoride, fluoride-supplemented toothpaste, fluoride treatment of teeth, reconstituted and bottled soft drinks made with fluoridated water, and so forth. It is difficult to calculate the total fluoride load ingested by individuals or what the effects may be of that fluoride supplementation.

Lesions Caused by Attrition and Abnormal Wear

Loss of normal dental structure and function often results from rapid and irregular and/or abnormal wear of occlusal surfaces in many species of domestic animals. In those species with hypsodont teeth, attention to the dentition as the animal ages is often a major factor in overall body conditioning and health (Fig. 7-46). Aggressive treatment of occlusal surface irregularity by filing of high points in the dental arcade (floating) can notably prolong an animal's life. Rock chewing or other compulsive oral behaviors in dogs may result in accelerated dental wear. Similarly, cribbing in horses and herbivorous animals grazing on sandy soils can cause premature dental wear. In all species, exposure of dentin or the pulp canal may lead to dental infection with serious consequences.

Miscellaneous Dental Disorders

Feline External Resorptive Neck Lesions. See Disorders of Cats.

Equine Odontoclastic Tooth Resorption and Hypercementosis. See Disorders of Horses.

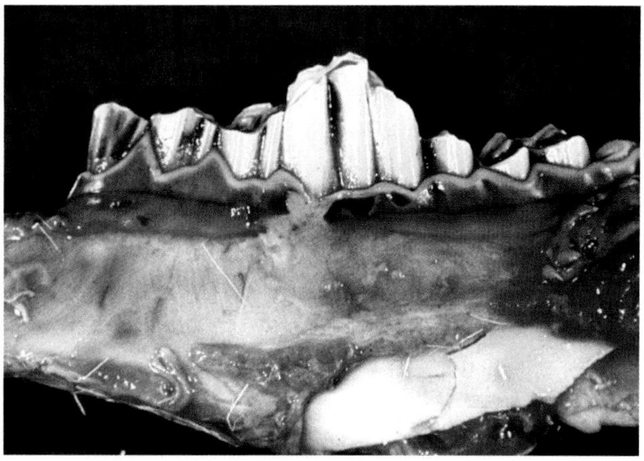

Figure 7-46 **Dental Attrition, Molar Teeth, Antelope.** Age-associated dental wear results in improper mastication of feedstuffs and malnutrition. This condition occurs most commonly in horses and is referred to as "step mouth" or "broken mouth." (Courtesy College of Veterinary Medicine, University of Tennessee.)

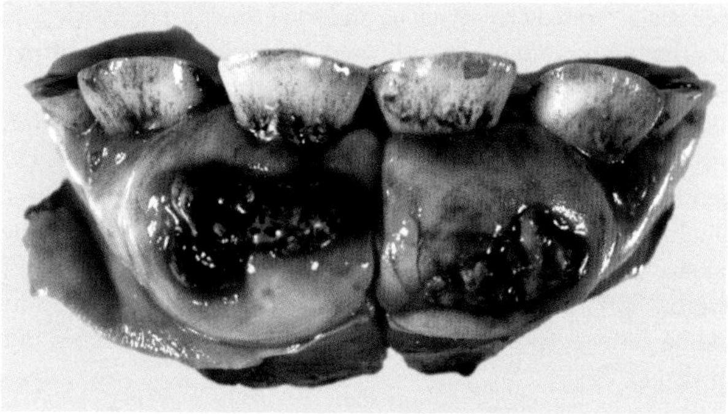

Figure 7-47 **Odontoma, Incisor Teeth, Cow.** This is a hamartoma (a benign tumor-like nodule) of the enamel organ that in this case has expanded bilaterally on the rostral mandibles. There is extensive hemorrhagic ulceration over the tumor. Diagnosis can be confirmed by radiographic and histopathologic examination. (Courtesy Dr. M.D. McGavin, College of Veterinary Medicine, University of Tennessee.)

Infundibular Impaction

Impaction of the infundibulum, also known as *infundibular necrosis* or *infundibular caries*, may cause serious dental disease in ruminants and more rarely in horses. Incomplete infundibular cementum formation before the tooth erupts likely predisposes to infundibular impaction. The pathogenic mechanism is comparable to dental caries in simple-toothed animals, which is uncommon in domestic animals. Feed material is ground into the infundibulum, where bacteria metabolize it to form acid, which causes demineralization. Bacterial enzymes digest the organic matrix of enamel and dentin. As a result of this destruction, the pulp cavity becomes exposed and infected, resulting in pulpitis and endodontitis. Dental abscesses and fistulous tracks may develop and rupture into the paranasal sinuses. The inflamed infundibular cavities often continue to become impacted with feed, creating a vicious cycle.

Periodontal Disease

More than 200 species of bacteria and fungi have been associated with dental plaque (a film of an organic matrix, food particles, and bacteria on the tooth surface). This plaque often becomes mineralized (tartar or dental calculus). The mineralized material contributes to atrophy and inflammation of the gingival mucosa and supporting stroma by acting as a nidus for additional plaque accumulation. Bacteria resident in films on the tooth surface produce acids and enzymes that may damage their enamel substrate (cavities) and also destroy the subjacent gingival tissue and periodontal ligament (periodontal disease).

The initial site for destructive inflammation is in the gingival crevice–forming pockets where bacteria lodge. With time, this inflammation spreads distally along the tooth, resulting in gingival-epithelial attachment only on the root of the tooth, deep in the alveolar socket. Progression of inflammation may destroy the connective tissue of the periodontal ligament, resulting in loosening of the tooth. The infection can spread, causing alveolar osteomyelitis and pulpitis and can result in apical abscesses and bacteremia. There is significant oral pain, reluctance to masticate, and halitosis. Periodontal disease is common in carnivores and human beings. Mildly abrasive diets and brushing of the teeth of pet carnivores, combined with regular dental examination, is preventive as it is in human beings.

Dental Neoplasia

Proliferative, cystic, or neoplastic diseases of the dental arcade can originate from cell rests that form from the dental lamina or the enamel organ (the cell rests of Malassez). Dental neoplasms usually arise close to the teeth, either deeply in the jaw or from the oral epithelium. There is a relatively precise method of naming dental neoplasms based on the tissue or cell of origin and the extent of differentiation and odontogenesis present within the neoplastic tissue. The histologic appearance of these neoplasms is complex; pathologists with considerable experience in differentiating these uncommon neoplasms should be consulted when a precise diagnosis is indicated.

Odontomas are hamartomas originating in the enamel organ and are usually seen in puppies and foals (Fig. 7-47). They usually contain well-recognizable dentin and enamel, as well as ameloblasts, odontoblasts, and dental pulp.

Ameloblastoma is a term applied to epithelial neoplasms of enamel organ origin. Several subtypes, distinguished histologically, are ameloblastic fibroma, ameloblastic odontoma, calcifying epithelial odontogenic tumor, peripheral odontogenic fibroma, and other rare tooth neoplasms. Ameloblastoma appears randomly in the dental arcade, usually in adult dogs. These neoplasms are often osteolytic and thus are locally invasive. Histologic examination by an expert is often necessary to distinguish ameloblastoma from acanthomatous epulis (acanthomatous ameloblastoma) and squamous cell carcinoma.

Tonsils

Tonsillitis is relatively rare in domestic species. Because they lack afferent lymphatic vessels, tonsils do not become secondarily affected by lymphatic drainage from infections elsewhere in the oral cavity. Tonsillitis may occur, however, as a result of saliva- and blood-borne agents such as infectious canine hepatitis and hog cholera. Epithelial tumors (squamous cell carcinomas) and lymphoid neoplasms occur in all species.

Salivary Glands

Inflammatory Diseases

Sialoadenitis, inflammation of a salivary gland, is relatively rare in veterinary medicine. Although diagnosis of systemic diseases is not made by examining the salivary gland, rabies and canine distemper are two very important diseases that cause inflammation of the salivary glands. Saliva is a particularly important medium of spread, by

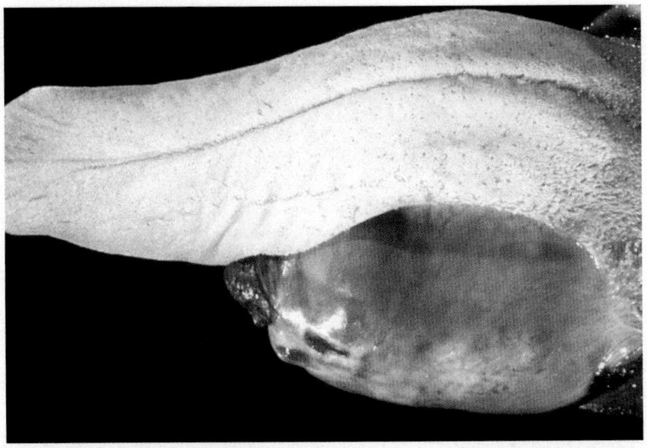

Figure 7-48 **Ranula, Mandibular Salivary Duct, Dog.** This is a cystic distention of the left mandibular salivary duct along the ventral-lateral aspect of the tongue. (Courtesy Dr. P. Stromberg, College of Veterinary Medicine, The Ohio State University.)

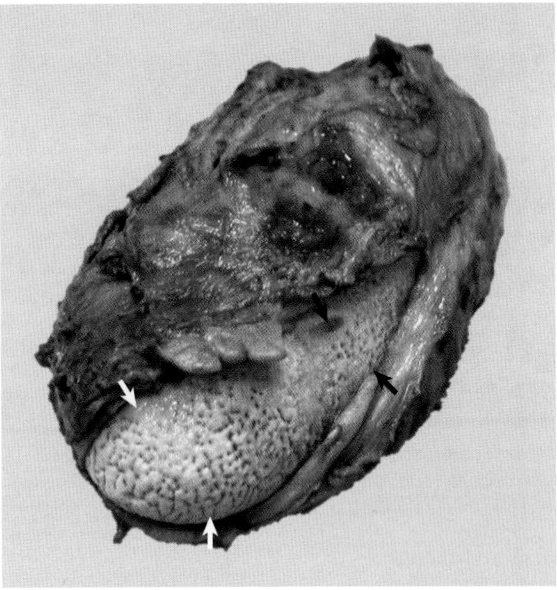

Figure 7-49 **Sialolith, Horse.** Pressure necrosis from this large stonelike mass *(arrows)* has destroyed the gland in which it formed. (Courtesy Dr. B. Cooper, College of Veterinary Medicine, Oregon State University.)

bite wounds, of the rhabdovirus that causes rabies. There are focal necrosis, mononuclear cell inflammation, and sometimes inclusions (Negri bodies) in the nuclei of ganglion cells. In the rat a coronavirus termed *sialodacryoadenitis virus* is responsible for inflammation of the salivary gland and some adnexal ocular glands. *Salmonella typhisuis* has caused suppurative parotid sialoadenitis in pigs.

Gross lesions of sialoadenitis are subtle and include swelling and edema. Sialoadenitis can be accompanied by pain on palpation. Abscesses occasionally occur, sometimes secondary to the migration of foreign bodies (grass awns), and are especially noticeable when they occur in the retrobulbar zygomatic gland where they may cause ocular protrusion (proptosis).

Miscellaneous Disorders

Changes in the salivary glands are uncommon in domestic animal species. A ranula is a cystic saliva-filled distention of the duct of the sublingual or submaxillary salivary gland that occurs on the floor of the mouth alongside the tongue (Fig. 7-48). It is thus epithelial lined. The cause is generally unknown, although some cases are due to sialoliths. A salivary mucocele, in contrast, is a pseudocyst not lined by epithelium but filled with saliva. The cause of this lesion is also unknown, but it may occur secondary to traumatic rupture of the duct of a sublingual salivary gland with resultant leakage and encapsulation of saliva by reactive connective tissue.

Sialoliths are rare in domestic animal species. When they do occur, they are considered to be caused by inflammation of the salivary gland with sloughed cells or inflammatory exudate forming a nidus for mineral accretion (Fig. 7-49). Thus they are one cause of ranula formation.

Neoplasia

Salivary gland neoplasms, both benign and malignant, are uncommon but occur in all species (Fig. 7-50). They are composed of glandular or ductular elements or a combination of epithelial and mesenchymal components similar to those in mixed mammary neoplasms. A grossly appearing similar condition, salivary gland infarction, occurs infrequently in cats and rarely in dogs. The cause of the infarction is unknown. The gross appearance of firmness and swelling of an infarcted gland must be distinguished microscopically from neoplasia (E-Fig. 7-7). In salivary gland infarction there are discrete foci of parenchymal necrosis with peripheral hemorrhage and inflammatory cells. Attempted incomplete regeneration of the gland

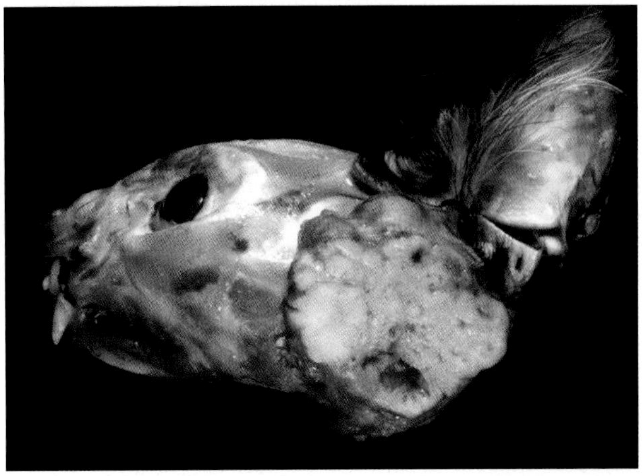

Figure 7-50 **Salivary Gland Carcinoma, Left Parotid Salivary Gland, Cat.** A large proliferative carcinoma of the salivary gland has replaced the normal gland. (Courtesy Dr. H. Gelberg, College of Veterinary Medicine, Oregon State University.)

from ductal epithelium can be mistaken for neoplasia unless one is familiar with the former condition.

Tongue

Developmental Anomalies

Congenital diseases of the tongue include epithelial defects such as fissures, epitheliogenesis imperfecta, macroglossia and microglossia, bifid tongue, and hair growing from the tongue (choristoma) (E-Fig. 7-8). Lethal glossopharyngeal defect, or bird tongue of dogs, is characterized by a pointed tongue that cannot wrap around a nipple and create the negative pressure required for nursing, and without intervention, starvation results. Ventral ankyloglossia, fusion of the tongue to the floor of the oral cavity, has been reported in related Anatolian shepherd dogs. The cause of these congenital lesions is not known, but they sometimes occur in association with other defects. As in the case of other congenital defects, ingestion of unknown teratogenic substances by the dam during gestation is an etiologic possibility, as is mutation of T-box genes.

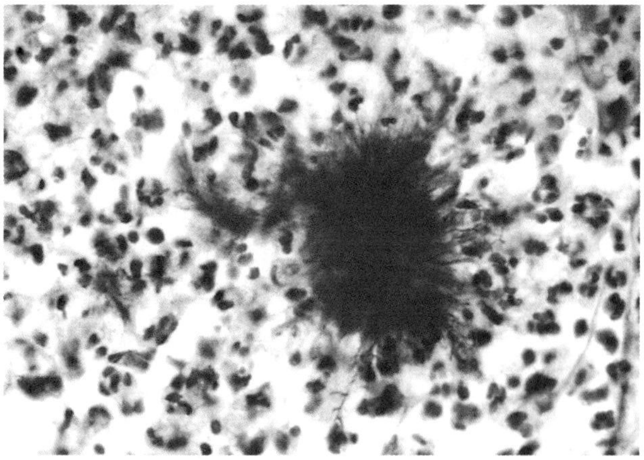

Figure 7-51 **Actinobacillosis (Wooden Tongue), Tongue, Cow.** Splendore-Hoeppli reaction (colony of bacteria with surrounding radiating "clubs" of immunoglobulin) is surrounded by suppurative inflammation. H&E stain. (Courtesy Dr. M.D. McGavin, College of Veterinary Medicine, University of Tennessee.)

Disease agents that principally target the tongue are relatively rare. The exception to this rule is *Actinobacillus lignieresii,* a Gram-negative bacillus that is a normal inhabitant of the oral cavity. It is an opportunistic invader of damaged lingual tissue, principally in cattle and occasionally in horses and small ruminants. The granulomas resulting from infection contain centrally located actinobacilli rimmed by radiating amorphic, eosinophilic, and clublike structures composed of immunoglobulin molecules from lesion plasmacytes (Fig. 7-51). Mixed mononuclear inflammatory cells, including multinucleated Langhans giant cells, often surround these foci (Splendore-Hoeppli phenomenon), and infection may drain and cause similar inflammation in submaxillary and retropharyngeal lymph nodes. The amount of fibrous tissue present depends on the duration of the inflammation and the swelling. Inflammation and fibrosis cause increased firmness and enlargement of the tongue called "wooden tongue" (Fig. 7-52). Horses are rarely affected by *A. lignieresii* infections, but when they are, lesions are cutaneous or lymph node abscesses, mastitis, and occasional glossitis.

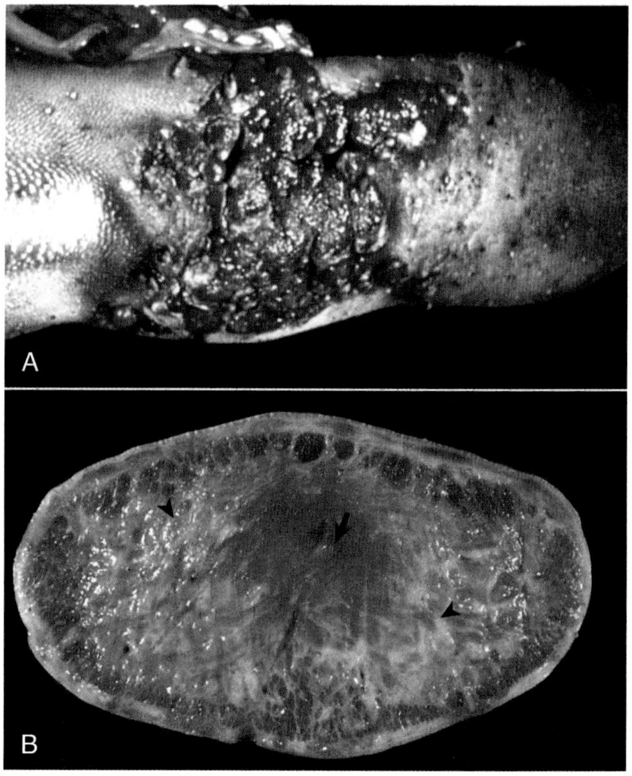

Figure 7-52 **Actinobacillosis, Tongue, Cow. A,** Dorsal surface. Proliferative and ulcerative chronic-active inflammatory lesions containing neutrophils mixed with mononuclear inflammatory cells (lymphocytes, macrophages, plasma cells) and fibrous tissue are present in the tongue. **B,** Chronic actinobacillosis (wooden tongue). Chronic inflammation results in loss of muscle of the tongue and its replacement by fibrous tissue during healing. Note the white interwoven bands of fibrous tissue *(arrowheads)* and the focus of granulomatous inflammation *(arrow)*. (**A** courtesy Dr. M.D. McGavin, College of Veterinary Medicine, University of Tennessee. **B** courtesy Dr. R.J. Panciera, School of Veterinary Medicine, Oklahoma State University; and Noah's Arkive, College of Veterinary Medicine, The University of Georgia.)

Systemic Disease: Secondary Involvement of the Tongue

Thrush is a *Candida albicans* (yeast) infection of intact mucous membranes of the tongue and esophagus (see Fig. 7-7). It occurs principally in ungulates but has also been seen in carnivores. Thrush is not a primary disease but often indicates an underlying debility, particularly in young animals. It occurs as a result of antibiotic treatment that kills normal flora, increased serum glucose concentrations as a result of diabetes mellitus, a high-sugar diet, or intravenous glucose therapy. The availability of iron is a limiting factor for the indigenous bacteria, which compete with yeast for mucosal colonization. Immunodeficiency states also contribute to the development of thrush. All of these scenarios provide tissue conditions suitable for the proliferation of yeast forms. Rarely, systemic infection may result. Factors predisposing to systemic infections include multiple antibiotic usage, indwelling catheters, and endotracheal tubes. This infection presents as a gray-green pseudomembrane that is easily scraped off the intact underlying mucosal surface (see Fig. 7-8).

Often, lingual lesions are manifestations of systemic diseases, such as bovine viral diarrhea, foot-and-mouth disease, multisystemic amyloidosis, and uremia (Fig. 7-53; also see Fig. 11-21). These diseases are discussed in more detail in this and other chapters of this book.

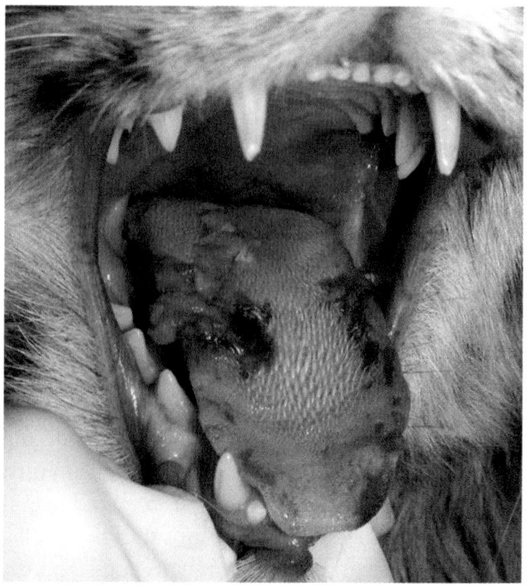

Figure 7-53 **Ulcerative Glossitis, Uremia (Uremic Glossitis), Tongue, Cat.** There is extensive ulceration of the mucosal epithelium of the tongue associated with increased concentrations of serum blood urea nitrogen and creatine from kidney failure. (Courtesy Drs. R.L. Fredrickson and R.A Doty, College of Veterinary Medicine, University of Illinois.)

Hyperplastic and Neoplastic Conditions

Lingual (glossal) neoplasms are rare but when they occur are generally of epithelial origin. Squamous cell carcinomas are most common (Fig. 7-54; also see Fig. 6-10), but papillomas (Fig. 7-55), rhabdomyomas, rhabdomyosarcomas, fibrosarcomas, melanomas, and granular cell tumors have all been reported in domestic animals.

Parasites

Parasites of the tongue are uncommon, with the exception of those that reside in muscles, such as *Sarcocystis* spp. in most species and *Trichinella spiralis* in pigs and occasionally in carnivorous wildlife such as polar bears. *Gongylonema* spp. can be present in the lingual mucosa of pigs and ruminants and are of no clinical significance.

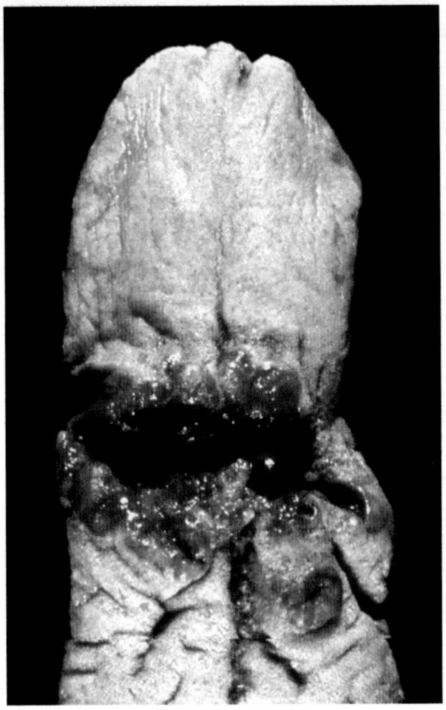

Figure 7-54 **Squamous Cell Carcinoma, Tongue (Dorsal Surface), Dog.** Note the proliferative, ulcerated, and hemorrhagic neoplasm growing transversely across the surface of the tongue. (Courtesy Dr. H. Gelberg, College of Veterinary Medicine, Oregon State University.)

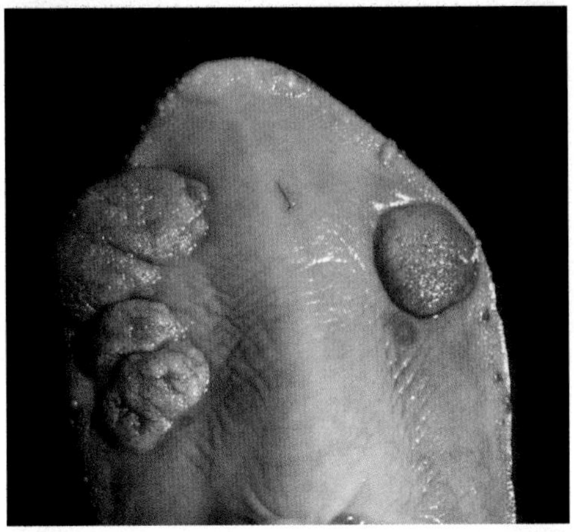

Figure 7-55 **Papillomas, Tongue (Ventral Surface), Cow.** Papillomas, often caused by bovine papillomavirus, are present on the ventral surface of the tongue. The virus infects traumatized mucosal epithelial cells and induces epithelial cell proliferation. (Courtesy Dr. M.D. McGavin, College of Veterinary Medicine, University of Tennessee.)

Esophagus

Developmental Anomalies

Achalasia. Esophageal motility disorders are termed *achalasia*. In this condition the sequential contractility of the esophagus is defective, and the lower cricopharyngeal sphincter fails to function properly. Achalasia results in difficulty in swallowing and may be responsible for regurgitation and weight loss.

Cricopharyngeal achalasia is a congenital, possibly neurogenic, disorder of the upper esophageal (cricopharyngeal) sphincter. It occurs in young, small-breed dogs, particularly terriers, cocker spaniels, and miniature poodles. Postweaning dysphagia and regurgitation after a meal of solid food is characteristic of this functional disorder. Liquids are generally swallowed without incidence. Gagging or choking behavior of the patient after swallowing is a good indicator in the appropriately aged dog of this condition.

Acquired canine achalasia is extremely uncommon. In this condition there is often a visible abnormality of the musculature of deglutition (cricopharyngeus). There does not appear to be a characteristic change in the affected musculature. Esophageal myotomy of the appropriate cricopharyngeal sphincter muscle is palliative for these idiopathic conditions.

Megaesophagus

Megaesophagus or esophageal ectasia is dilation of the esophagus because of insufficient, absent, or uncoordinated peristalsis in the mid and cervical esophagus. It has been described in dogs, cats, cows, ferrets, horses, and New World camelids. Causes include innervation or denervation disorders and partial physical obstructions and stenosis, secondary to inflammatory diseases of esophageal musculature or persistence of the right aortic arch. Many cases are idiopathic.

Congenital megaesophagus is usually due to partial blockage of the lumen of the esophagus by a persistent right fourth aortic arch. Because of the persistence of the arch, a vascular ring forms around the esophagus and trachea, preventing full dilation of the esophagus. The ring is formed by the aorta, pulmonary artery, and ductus arteriosus. This form of megaesophagus is unique in that the esophageal obstruction, and thus dilation, occurs cranial to the heart because of the location of the obstructing vascular ring (Fig. 7-56; also see Fig. 10-37. Persistent right aortic arch is likely hereditary in German shepherds, Irish setters, and greyhounds. All other forms of megaesophagus result in dilation cranial to the stomach.

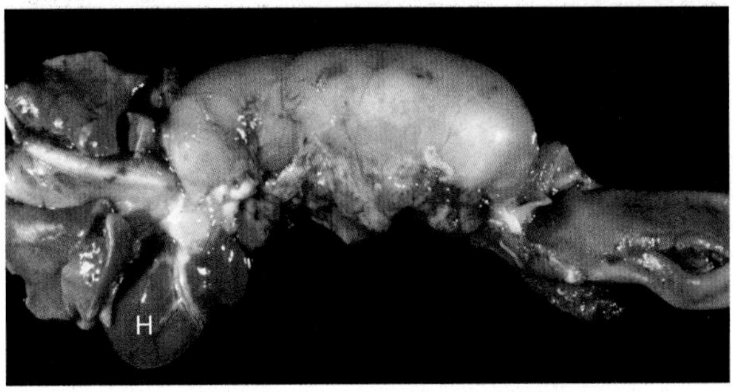

Figure 7-56 **Megaesophagus from a Persistent Right Aortic Arch, Esophagus, Dog.** Dilation of the esophagus cranial to the heart *(H)* is the result of failure of the right fourth aortic arch to regress during embryonic life (vascular ring abnormality). (Courtesy Dr. C.S. Patton, College of Veterinary Medicine, University of Tennessee.)

Congenital megaesophagus also occurs as an idiopathic denervation of the esophagus, most notably in great Danes, Irish setters, miniature schnauzers, Labrador retrievers, wire hair fox terriers, shar-peis, Newfoundlands, Siamese cats, and in some cases of vagal indigestion, in cattle. Some cases of myasthenia gravis (see later discussion) are congenital and may be of genetic origin.

Acquired megaesophagus (esophageal achalasia) is the result of failure of relaxation of the distal esophageal (cardiac) sphincter of the stomach. The obstruction and thus dilation occurs cranial to the stomach (Fig. 7-57). Although the gross appearance of acquired megaesophagus in animals is similar to that of human beings, the cause of the condition in animals does not involve the cardiac sphincter. Causes are idiopathic or secondary to polymyositis (inflammation of the esophageal muscle), myasthenia gravis (a congenital or autoimmune disease directed against acetylcholine receptors of the neuromuscular junction), hypothyroidism (which can result in muscle atrophy and denervation disease), congenital myopathy, lead and thallium poisoning (via effect on innervation), peripheral neuropathies, vagal indigestion, esophagitis, and recurrent gastric dilation. Increased risk in dogs is seen in German shepherds, golden retrievers, and Irish setters.

Megaesophagus is recognized clinically by regurgitation after ingestion of solid food. Thus congenital megaesophagus is often recognized at weaning. Often animals are thin and may have aspiration pneumonia. Radiographically, the esophagus is dilated anterior to the lesion and retains radiopaque dyes (E-Fig. 7-9). Dilation may vary from diffuse to locally extensive, depending on its cause. Putrid ingesta are sometimes found in the dilated, atonic portions of the esophagus. Although degenerate nerve fibers are occasionally found within vagus nerves, megaesophagus can occur without detectable histologic lesions.

Hiatal Hernia

Protrusion of the abdominal esophagus and cardia of the stomach through the diaphragm into the thoracic cavity is termed a *hiatal hernia*. This inversion is generally into the esophageal lumen and is self-reducing. Sometimes a gastroesophageal intussusception results.

Eosinophilic Esophagitis

Eosinophilic esophagitis is an emerging disease in human beings. In a single dog, clinical signs include regurgitation, dysphagia, and cough, accompanying a diffusely affected, friable, hyperemic, ulcerated, esophageal mucosa visible by endoscopy. Inflammation is dominated by granulocytes—half of which are eosinophils. Diagnosis is by elimination of other causes of inflammatory esophagitis. Seventy percent of human beings and the single dog described had concurrent allergic skin disease.

Esophageal Parasites

With notable exceptions, parasitic diseases of the esophagus are generally of no clinical importance. The more common parasites of the esophagus are *Gongylonema* spp., which affect ruminants, pigs, horses, primates, and occasionally rodents. These nematodes reside in the esophageal mucosa and are characteristically thin, red, and serpentine. They can be 10 to 15 cm in length and are easily visible (Fig. 7-58). The intermediate hosts are cockroaches and dung beetles.

Gasterophilus spp. occur in horses. These fly larvae have interesting life cycles because their eggs are laid on the skin in varying locations. The warmth and moisture from licking activates them. The larvae burrow into the oral mucosa, molt, and then migrate down the esophagus. They occur in both the distal esophagus and the stomach, where they attach to the mucosa via oral hooks. They eventually detach, leaving craters at the site of attachment, and pass in the feces.

Hypoderma lineatum is the larvae of the warble fly of ruminants. These parasites eventually migrate to the esophageal adventitia and then to the subcutaneous tissue of the back.

Spirocerca lupi of dogs is probably the most pathogenic of the esophageal parasites. These nematodes reach the esophageal submucosa after migrating from the stomach. They penetrate through the gastric mucosa to reach the adventitia of arteries and then migrate in the adventitia to the abdominal aorta and aborally to the caudal aorta, where they form a granuloma in the adventitia. From here they migrate to the adjacent esophageal submucosa. A passage forms between the esophageal lumen and the granuloma containing the parasite, allowing discharge of ova into the lumen of the alimentary system and eventually into the feces. Clinical sequelae of infestation

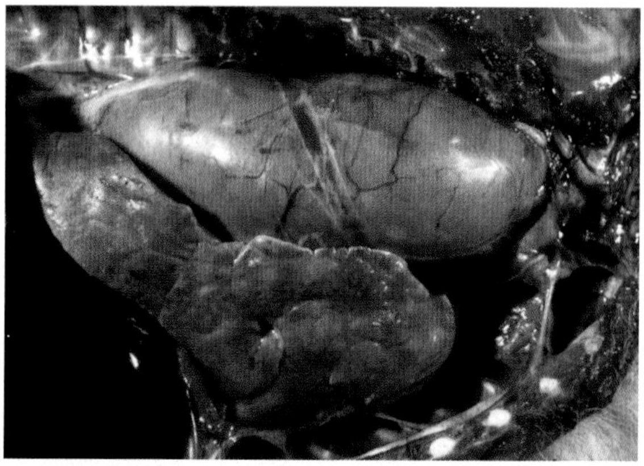

Figure 7-57 **Megaesophagus, Thoracic Esophagus, Dog.** A notably dilated thoracic esophagus cranial to the diaphragm has displaced the right lung caudally and ventrally. This form of megaesophagus is often attributable to an abnormality (mass, foreign body, innervation disorder) affecting the cardiac sphincter. (Courtesy Dr. H. Gelberg, College of Veterinary Medicine, Oregon State University.)

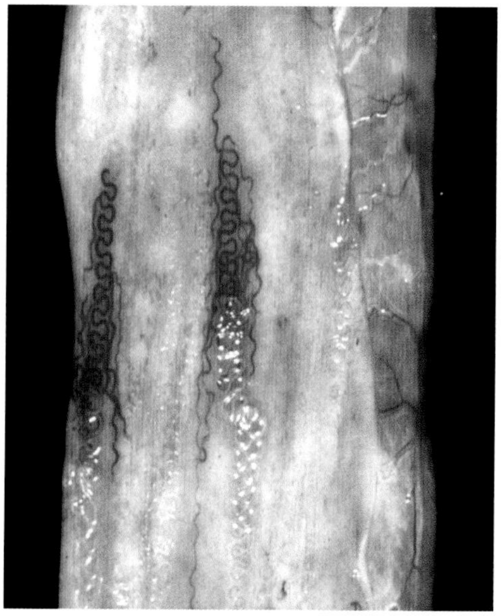

Figure 7-58 **Gongylonemiasis, Esophagus, Cow.** The red-white serpentine intramucosal nematodes are characteristic of *Gongylonema*, a nematode of the superfamily Spiruroidea. (Courtesy Dr. M.D. McGavin, College of Veterinary Medicine, University of Tennessee.)

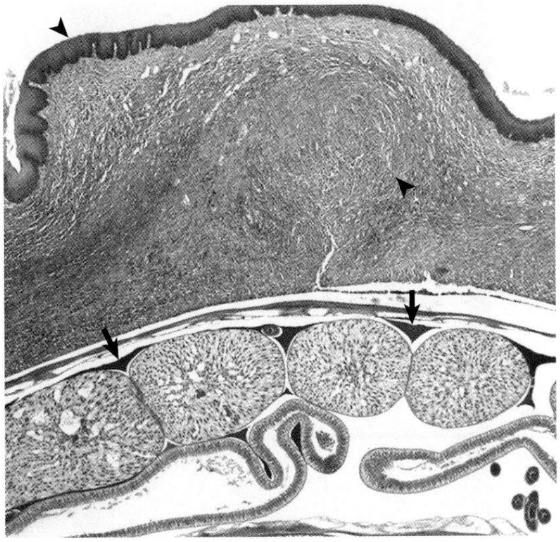

Figure 7-59 **Fibrosarcoma, Esophagus, Dog.** *Spirocerca lupi* (longitudinal section) *(arrows)* is present in the esophageal submucosa deep to the fibrosarcoma, which it has induced *(arrowheads)*. H&E stain. (Courtesy Dr. H. Gelberg, College of Veterinary Medicine, Oregon State University.)

include dysphagia, aortic aneurysms, hemothorax, and rarely esophageal fibrosarcomas or osteosarcomas (Fig. 7-59). Occasionally, chronic aortic granulomas will extend into the adjacent thoracic vertebral bodies of chronically affected dogs to cause spondylosis deformans adjacent to the aortic granulomas. *S. lupi* infestations occur in warmer climates. The intermediate hosts are dung beetles, and the paratenic hosts are chickens, reptiles, and rodents.

Miscellaneous Esophageal Disorders

Idiopathic muscular hypertrophy of the distal esophagus is a lesion peculiar to horses and pigs that can be quite spectacular at necropsy (Fig. 7-60) but usually is of no clinical significance. The esophageal musculature can be several centimeters thick, and the lesion can extend along the distal quarter of the esophagus. Rarely this condition plays a role in esophageal impaction. Similarly, dilation of the esophageal glands present throughout the esophagus of aged dogs can be a spectacular gross lesion of no clinical consequence. It is therefore important to carefully evaluate these lesions either at necropsy or by endoscopy in the live animal to determine whether what appear to be erosions and ulcers are instead mucosal elevations caused by glands filled with mucus. Because the lesions are subepithelial, the overlying mucosa is smooth and shiny. Dilated esophageal glands vary in number and location but are generally only a few millimeters in diameter (Fig. 7-61). They are most numerous in the distal esophagus.

Esophageal erosions and ulcers are relatively common and have a variety of causes. One of the more common causes of esophageal erosions and ulcers is reflux of stomach acid. This reflux of gastric acids causes chemical burning of the distal or aboral esophagus and is commonly called *acid reflux esophagitis* (Fig. 7-62) or clinically, heartburn in human beings. Other causes of esophageal ulcers include improper use of stomach tubes, which cause linear scraping on the crests of the longitudinal folds of the esophageal mucosa (Fig. 7-63), foreign bodies such as bones in dogs and infectious diseases, such as bovine viral diarrhea (Fig. 7-64), which cause mucosal injury in other locations as well.

Leukoplakia of the esophagus and stomach is characterized by discrete, flat, white mucosal elevations (epithelial plaques) of no clinical significance and of unknown cause. They are sometimes mistaken for thrush lesions or neoplasia. Unlike thrush lesions, they

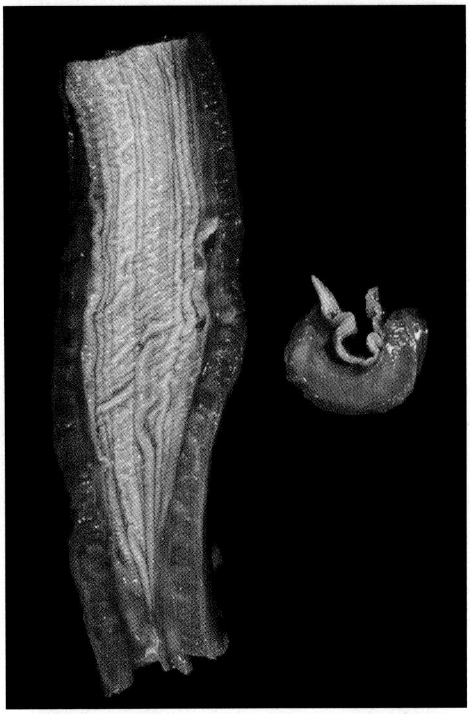

Figure 7-60 **Muscular Hypertrophy, Distal Esophagus, Horse.** Longitudinal *(left)* and transverse *(right)* sections of the esophagus demonstrate the marked increase in the thickness of the smooth muscle in the tunica muscularis of the distal esophagus. (Courtesy Dr. C.S. Patton, College of Veterinary Medicine, University of Tennessee.)

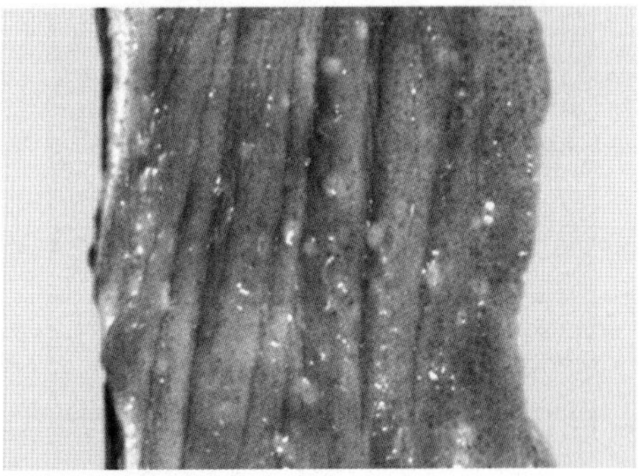

Figure 7-61 **Cystic Esophageal Glands, Distal Esophagus, Dog.** Multiple white mucosal cysts are present in the esophageal glands of the mucosa and submucosa. These cysts are common and insignificant findings in aged dogs. (Courtesy Dr. H. Gelberg, College of Veterinary Medicine, Oregon State University.)

do not scrape off easily, and their regularity, number, and location distinguish them from neoplasms. Histologically, the stratum basale and prickle cell layers are notably thickened, and the surface cells have pyknotic nuclei and some parakeratosis. In human beings approximately 5% of these lesions become cancerous. They are present in the oral cavity and esophagus of human beings and are believed related to chronic irritation most often associated with smoking or chewing tobacco. Alcohol consumption and restorative dental amalgams may also predispose to leukoplakia.

Choke

Choke is a clinical term referring to esophageal obstruction subsequent to stenoses or blockage. Choke most often occurs in anatomic locations in which the esophagus cannot fully expand.

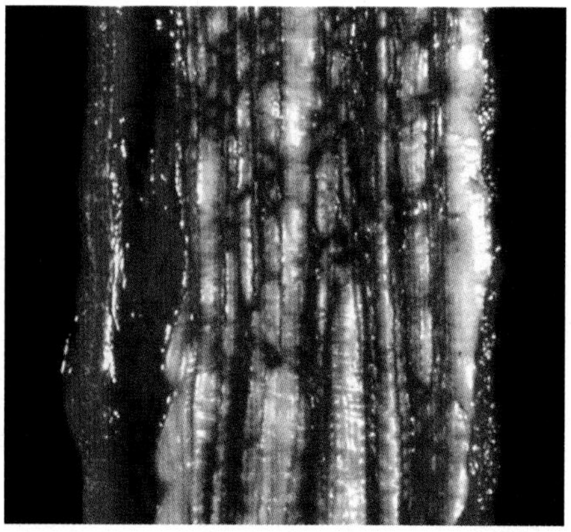

Figure 7-62 Acid Reflux Esophagitis, Esophagus, Horse. The dark red streaks on the surface of the esophagus are areas of epithelial loss secondary to gastric acid reflux. The white streaks and vertically linear areas on the surface of the esophagus are areas of unaffected and likely hyperplastic mucosal epithelium. As would be expected, erosions are most severe in the esophageal mucosa adjacent to the cardia and extend orad. This distribution is diagnostic of acid reflux esophagitis. (Courtesy Dr. H. Gelberg, College of Veterinary Medicine, Oregon State University.)

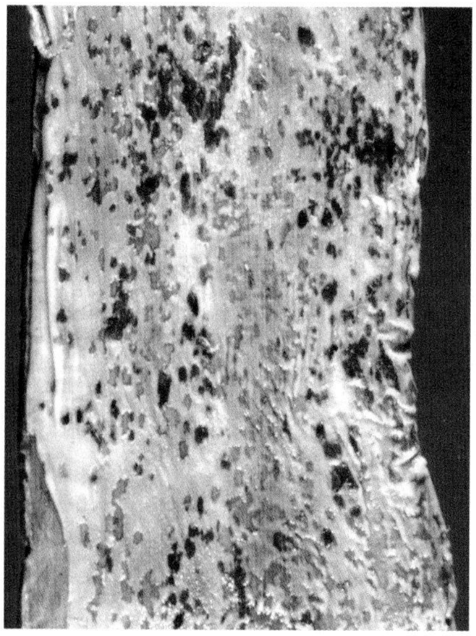

Figure 7-64 Ulcerative Esophagitis, Bovine Viral Diarrhea (BVD), Esophagus, Cow. Note the multiple variably sized (millimeter range) and variably shaped esophageal mucosal ulcers caused by the pestivirus of bovine viral diarrhea. (Courtesy Dr. H. Gelberg, College of Veterinary Medicine, Oregon State University.)

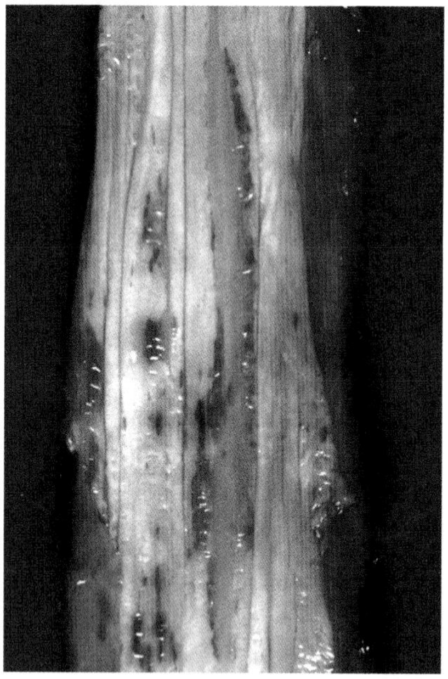

Figure 7-63 Trauma-Induced Esophageal Ulceration, Esophagus, Horse. These red linear ulcers are the result of abrasion from improper stomach tubing, either from an overly large diameter tube, from a too-vigorous insertion, or from a tube with a roughened edge. (Courtesy Dr. H. Gelberg, College of Veterinary Medicine, Oregon State University.)

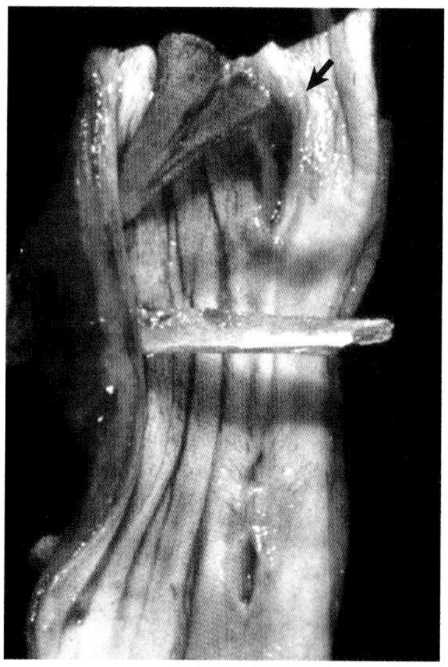

Figure 7-65 Ulcers and Perforation, Foreign Body, Esophagus, Dog. The esophagus has been perforated by an ingested chicken bone. Note that the end of the bone opposite the perforation site has caused a deep ulcer (*arrow*). There are also several chronic ulcers caudal to the perforation, presumably from abrasion by other bones as they moved down the esophagus. (Courtesy Dr. C.S. Patton, College of Veterinary Medicine, University of Tennessee.)

These locations are dorsal to the larynx, cranial to the first rib at the thoracic inlet, the base of the heart, and the diaphragmatic hiatus. Choke occurs most frequently as a result of ingestion of large foreign bodies, such as potatoes, apples, bones (Fig. 7-65), corn cobs (Fig. 7-66), or medicaments, such as large gelatin-filled capsules or tablets (dry boluses). If these bodies are lodged against the epithelium for longer than 2 days, the interaction often results in circumferential pressure necrosis of the esophageal mucosa (Fig. 7-67), which forms strictures during healing. These strictures then can cause reflex regurgitation after ingestion of food with possible starvation or aspiration pneumonia resulting.

In older horses, poor dentition causes feed to be incompletely masticated, resulting in impaction in the esophagus. Neoplastic or inflammatory lesions of the esophagus or periesophageal tissues also cause obstruction. Persistence of the right aortic arch has already been discussed as a cause of esophageal stenosis and megaesophagus.

Neoplasia

Neoplasms of the esophagus are rare. Bracken fern (*Pteridium aquilinum*) consumption, sometimes in association with papilloma

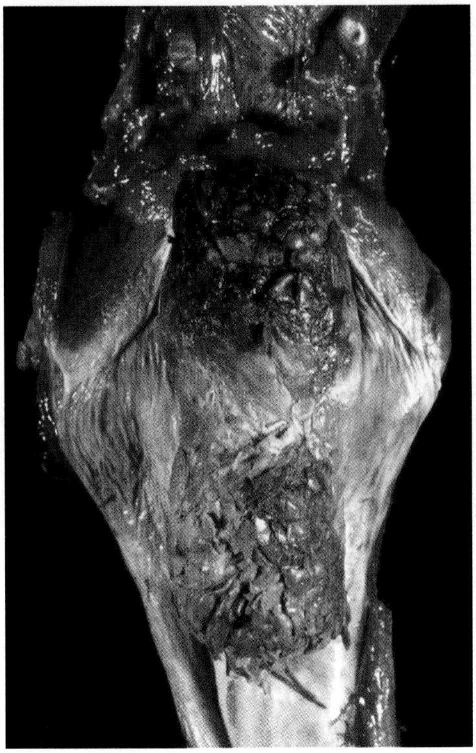

Figure 7-66 **Foreign Body (Choke), Esophagus, Cow.** A corn cob has lodged in the esophagus subjacent to the larynx. (Courtesy Dr. H. Gelberg, College of Veterinary Medicine, Oregon State University.)

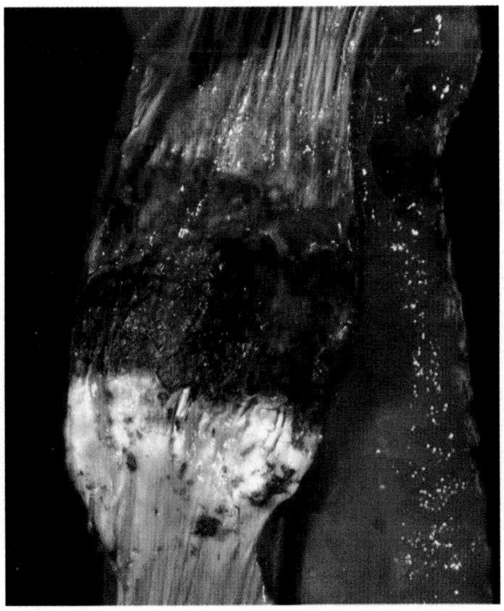

Figure 7-67 **Foreign Body (choke), Esophagus, Horse.** Pressure necrosis of the proximal esophageal mucosa adjacent to the larynx has occurred secondary to lodgment of a foreign body (compacted chaff). As a general rule, pressure necrosis usually occurs if the foreign body remains in place against the mucosal epithelium for longer than 2 days. (Courtesy Dr. M.D. McGavin, College of Veterinary Medicine, University of Tennessee.)

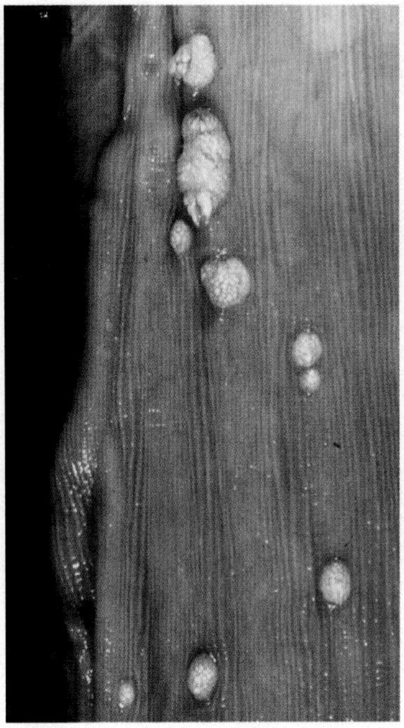

Figure 7-68 **Papillomatosis, Bovine Papillomavirus, Esophagus, Bull.** Multiple papillomas, characteristic of this viral-induced disease, occur following trauma to the esophageal mucosa and infection of mucosal epithelial cells. Oral papillomas may be present concurrently. (Courtesy Dr. M.D. McGavin, College of Veterinary Medicine, University of Tennessee.)

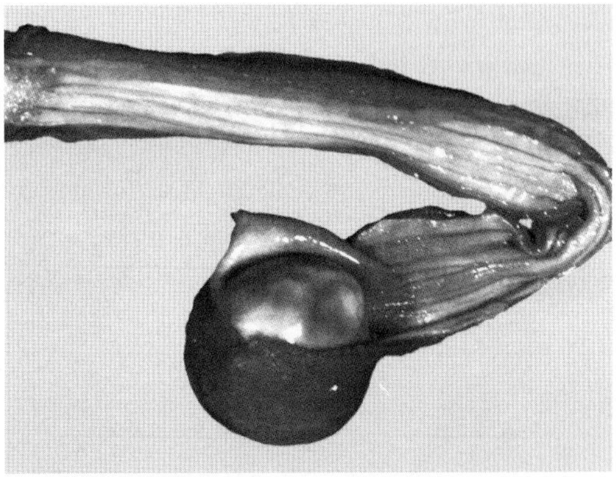

Figure 7-69 **Leiomyoma, Esophagus, Dog.** A mass consisting of submucosal proliferation of smooth muscle cells bulges into the distal esophageal lumen, causing obstruction. (Courtesy Dr. H. Gelberg, College of Veterinary Medicine, Oregon State University.)

viruses, has been associated with squamous cell carcinomas in cattle. The clinical signs are similar to those of other causes of esophageal blockage and include dysphagia, regurgitation, weight loss, and dilation of the esophagus proximal to the mass. Tumors of the esophagus are occasionally palpable but are most often intraluminal rather than mural. Epithelial tumors include papillomas (Fig. 7-68) and squamous cell carcinomas. The latter have wide metastatic potential. Smooth muscle tumors of the esophagus, whether benign or malignant, are also rare but may result in similar clinical signs (Fig. 7-69). Esophageal fibrosarcomas of dogs often develop in areas with *S. lupi* infestation. Esophageal lymphoma occurs sporadically in most species (Fig. 7-70).

Rumen, Reticulum, and Omasum

See Disorders of Ruminants (Cattle, Sheep, and Goats).

Stomach and Abomasum

Gastric Dilation and Volvulus

Simple gastric dilation occurs in a variety of animals (Fig. 7-71). In dogs, particularly in the large, deep-chested breeds, the acute gastric dilation and volvulus syndrome occurs. This lesion is life

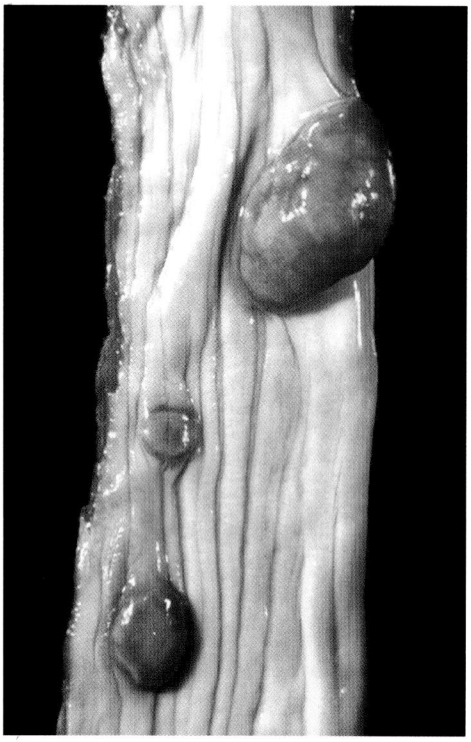

Figure 7-70 **Lymphoma (Lymphosarcoma), Esophagus, Dog.** Masses of submucosal proliferating malignant lymphocytes bulge into the esophageal lumen, causing partial obstruction. Note that the mucosal epithelium is intact (smooth and shiny). (Courtesy Dr. M.D. McGavin, College of Veterinary Medicine, University of Tennessee.)

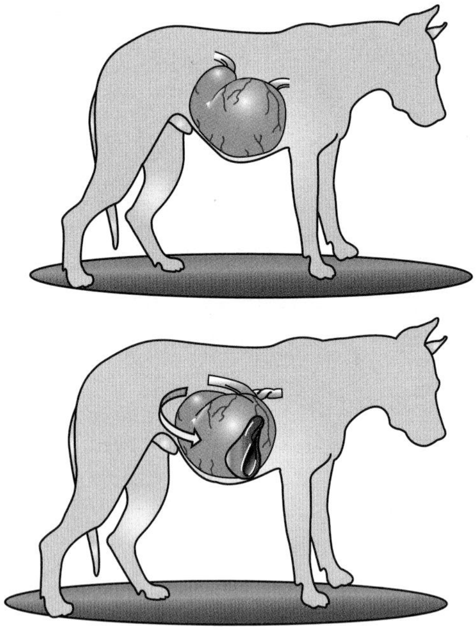

Figure 7-72 **Gastric Dilation and Volvulus, Stomach, Dog.** The stomach is distended with food and gas *(top example)*. It rotates *(arrow)* on the mesenteric axis *(bottom example)* clockwise (180, 270, or 360 degrees on a ventrodorsal axis when the abdomen is viewed from the ventral surface), resulting in a gastric volvulus with an obstructed esophagus that prevents eructation and thus further contributes to gastric dilation. The spleen, attached to the stomach by the gastrosplenic ligament, rotates with the stomach and is thus folded back upon itself and located in the right cranial abdomen against the diaphragm *(bottom example)*. The splenic vein is compressed, resulting in a congested spleen, because the arterial blood supply remains patent longer than venous drainage. (Modified from Van Kruiningen HJ, Gregoire K, Meuten DJ: *J Am Anim Hosp Assoc* 10:294-324, 1974.)

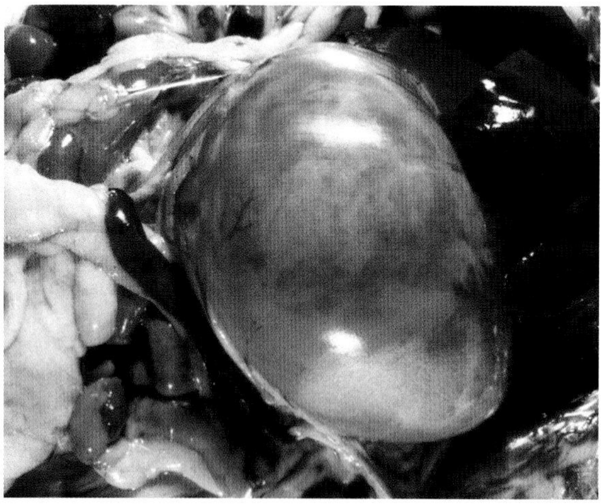

Figure 7-71 **Simple Gastric Dilation, Stomach, Rabbit.** The stomach is markedly dilated and filled with gas. Dilation occurs most commonly following aerophagia or overeating and is relieved by eructation or vomiting. (Courtesy Dr. H. Gelberg, College of Veterinary Medicine, Oregon State University.)

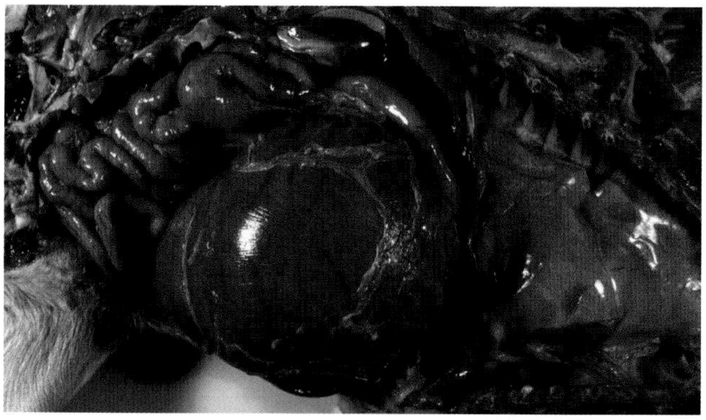

Figure 7-73 **Gastric Dilation and Volvulus, Abdomen, Dog.** The stomach is filled with gas and its serosa is congested *(dark red)*. The duodenum and engorged spleen have been displaced to the right. (Courtesy Dr. M.D. McGavin, College of Veterinary Medicine, University of Tennessee.)

threatening and should not be confused with simple gastric dilation, which is common in young puppies after overeating. Predisposing factors to acute gastric dilation include a source of distending gas, fluid, or feed; obstruction of the cardia that prevents eructation and emesis; and obstruction of the pylorus that prevents passage of gastric contents into the small intestine. The source of gas is not well understood. Theories include gas production by *C. perfringens*, spores of which are present in the feed, carbon dioxide from physiologic mechanisms of digestion, or simple aerophagia.

The result of repeated episodes of gastric dilation is stretching and relaxation of the gastrohepatic ligament. Recurrent dilation, combined with overfeeding, postprandial exercise, and perhaps a hereditary predisposition, results in gastric rotation. Gastric rotation is recognized by splenic displacement and a twisted esophagus and results in vascular compression and decreased venous drainage and hypoxemia (Figs. 7-72 and 7-73). The stomach generally is rotated clockwise on the ventrodorsal axis when the abdomen is viewed from the ventral surface. Rotation is 180 to 360 degrees. The combination of gastric hypoxemia, acid-base imbalance, obstruction of

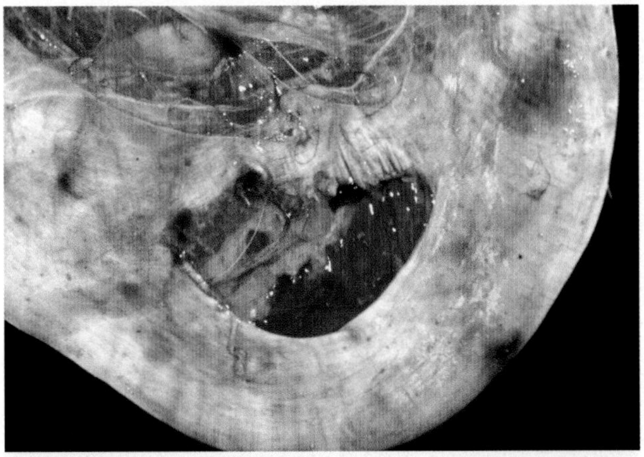

Figure 7-74 **Rupture, Abomasum, Calf.** Multifocal hemorrhages along the upper margin of the tear and subserosally adjacent to the greater curvature indicate that the rupture occurred antemortem. (Courtesy Dr. M.D. McGavin, College of Veterinary Medicine, University of Tennessee.)

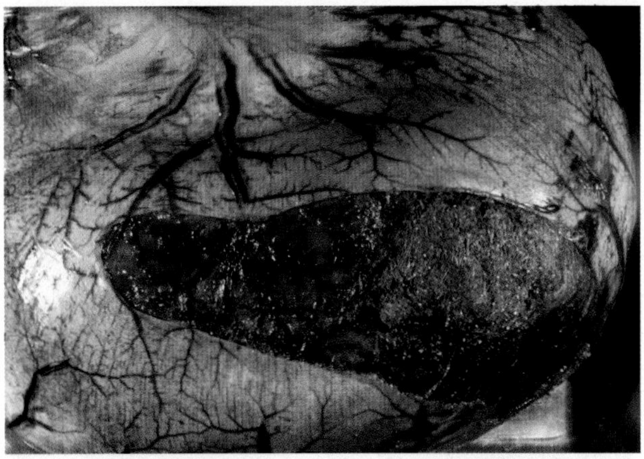

Figure 7-75 **Rupture, Stomach, Horse.** The hemorrhage visible on the right margin of the rupture indicates that the rupture occurred antemortem. Note also that the rent through the tunica muscularis is longer than that through the mucosa, which still covers the ingesta on the left and right sides. The mucosal and serosal surfaces are congested. (Courtesy Dr. H. Gelberg, College of Veterinary Medicine, Oregon State University.)

the pylorus and cardia, and increased intragastric pressure leads to antiperistaltic waves followed by atony, cardiovascular ischemia, arrhythmias, and shock. Decreased portal venous return leads to pancreatic ischemia and release of myocardial depressant factor, cardiac collapse, and death.

Epidemiologic evidence suggests that dry dog foods that list oils or fats among the first four ingredients increase the risk for the gastric dilation and volvulus syndrome. Gastric dilation and volvulus is sometimes associated with gastric eversion or intussusception into the distal esophagus. This latter condition can also occur independently of gastric dilation and volvulus.

Abomasal Displacement

See Disorders of Ruminants (Cattle, Sheep, and Goats).

Gastric Dilation and Rupture

Gastric dilation occurs in horses as a result of the ingestion of fermentable feeds or grain, a situation analogous to grain overload with lactic acidosis in cattle. Acute gastric dilation and rupture in horses occurs most frequently as a terminal event in intestinal obstruction and displacement. Because gastric dilation and rupture can occur after death, the diagnostic challenge is to determine if the rupture occurred ante mortem or post mortem. The only reliable indicator of the time of rupture, in relation to the death of the animal, is the presence of hemorrhage and evidence of inflammation, such as fibrin strands, along the margins of the rupture (usually the greater curvature) because such inflammatory responses occur only in live animals (Figs. 7-74 and 7-75).

In Northern Europe, acute gastric dilation occurs in horses on pasture as part of the syndrome called grass sickness or dysautonomia. The esophagus and stomach are often dilated and atonic. Although serologic evidence suggests an association of grass sickness with *C. perfringens* type A enterotoxin, noninflammatory degeneration of associated autonomic ganglia has also been described. This condition can be experimentally produced in the horse with whole blood from affected animals, suggesting that a soluble toxin may be the cause.

Chronic gastric dilation is also associated with ingestion of poorly digestible substances. Habitual cribbing and aerophagia may also be contributory.

Dysautonomia also occurs in pet carnivores secondary to ganglionic death in cranial nerves, spinal nerves, and autonomic nerves. Associated ganglionic peptide levels are reduced in an amount consistent with the functional aberrations. Ganglioneuritis creates a similar syndrome to dysautonomia in a variety of species and is infrequently diagnosed. GI signs of dysautonomia include xerostomia, decreased anal tone, vomiting, and regurgitation. See Chapter 14 for a description of the histologic lesions.

Chronic abomasal and/or ruminal dilation may occur in cows with overeating disease, dystocia, exhaustion, poor-quality or frozen feedstuffs, abomasal ulcers with or without abomasal lymphoma, and vagal indigestion. A sequela of abomasitis may be a mycotic infection similar to that which occurs in the rumen (Fig. 7-76).

In monkeys an increased frequency of acute gastric dilation often occurs during weekends, when there may be changes in feeding behavior secondary to unfamiliar keepers. Studies have implicated *C. perfringens* overgrowth secondary to an increase in fermentable feed consumption in the pathogenesis of gastric dilation in primates.

Chronic gastric dilation in dogs is usually secondary to gastric ulcer, mural gastric lymphomas, uremia affecting gastric structure and function, pyloric stenosis or obstruction, acute gastric dilation, intervertebral disk disease, or vagotomy. Chronic gastric dilation is characterized by reduced feed intake, diminished gastric motility, and increased gastric gas accumulation sometimes resulting in abdominal distention similar to that of bloat.

Abomasal Dilation and Tympany

See Disorders of Ruminants (Cattle, Sheep, and Goats).

Impaction

Impaction of the monogastric stomach and abomasum has a variety of causes. Intrathoracic lesions, such as pneumonia, pleuritis, lymphadenopathy, and lymphoma of mediastinal lymph nodes, can infiltrate and damage the vagal nerves, resulting in a problem with abomasal/gastric motility and emptying. Roughage, hairballs, and other foreign materials also cause impaction. Gastric trichobezoars and phytobezoars of monogastric animals are similar to those that occur in the rumen (E-Fig. 7-10).

Abomasal emptying defect can also cause impaction. It is principally a condition of Suffolk sheep 2 to 6 years of age. It is characterized by an impacted, dilated abomasum. Clinical signs include anorexia, weight loss, and increased ruminal chloride concentrations. The latter feature is believed to be secondary to

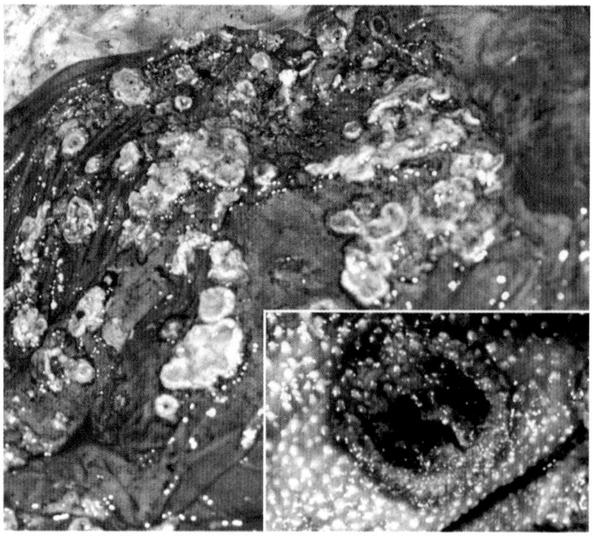

Figure 7-76 **Mycotic Abomasitis and Omasitis, Calf.** The mucosal surface of the abomasum has discrete and coalescing ulcers covered by yellow-white diphtheritic membranes and a red outer margin of active hyperemia and inflammation. These lesions are indicative of infarcts and are likely secondary to vasculitis and thrombosis by angioinvasive fungi such as *Aspergillus, Mucor, Rhizopus, Absidia,* and *Mortierella* spp. The diphtheritic membranes are a mixture of necrotic cellular debris from the infarct, inflammatory cells, and hyphae from the inciting fungus. *Inset,* Mycotic omasitis. The lesion is similar to the one in the abomasum. The diphtheritic membrane has been lost because of omasal peristalsis, but the necrotic center (infarct) and red outer margin of active hyperemia and inflammation are prominent. (Figure courtesy College of Veterinary Medicine, University of Illinois. Inset courtesy Dr. H. Gelberg, College of Veterinary Medicine, Oregon State University.)

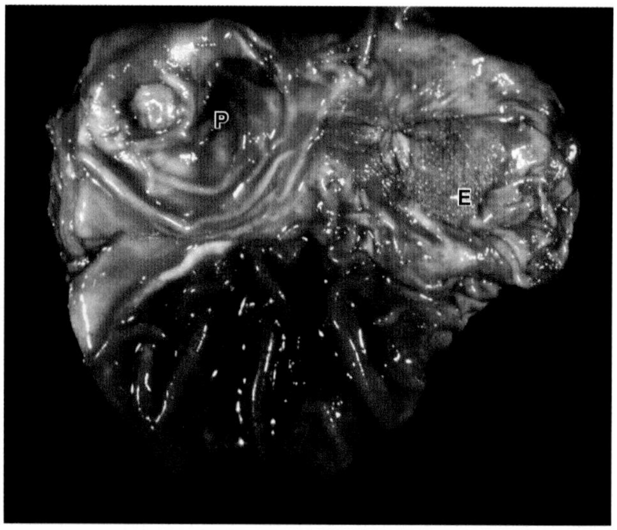

Figure 7-77 **Acute "Hemorrhagic Gastritis," Stomach, Pig.** The fundus of the stomach is hemorrhagic. This type of gastric change is often seen in the pig in acute septicemia, for example, from salmonella, and the severe congestion is attributed to venous infarction from endotoxemia. *E,* Esophageal os; *P,* pylorus. (Courtesy Dr. H. Gelberg, College of Veterinary Medicine, Oregon State University.)

abomasal reflux. Scattered chromatolysis and neuronal necrosis in the celiac and mesenteric ganglia are consistent changes from a neurotoxicosis. The process is likely mediated by excitotoxins, although viruses have not been ruled out. Clusters of affected animals in a single flock are suggestive of an environmental cause. Inflammation is minimal. Abomasal emptying defect may be a form of acquired dysautonomia.

Inflammatory Diseases

Inflammation of the simple stomach or abomasum is designated as gastritis and abomasitis, respectively, and must be differentiated from simple hyperemia and petechiae, which are often nonspecific agonal lesions. Gastritis is often associated clinically with vomiting, dehydration, and metabolic acidosis. Hemorrhage, edema, increased amounts of mucus, abscesses, granulomas, foreign body penetration, parasites, inflammatory cells of various types, erosions, ulcerations, and necrosis characterize the changes in the mucosal surface and subsequent inflammatory reaction.

Clostridium septicum is a cause of hemorrhagic abomasitis with submucosal emphysema of sheep and cattle, a disease known as *braxy*. Although this disease is most common in the United Kingdom and Europe, it occurs in North America as well. Generally, the disease follows ingestion of frozen feeds contaminated with the causative *Clostridium* spp. The lesions are produced by the exotoxin of the bacteria, and death therefore is due to an exotoxemia.

Sarcina-like organisms have been reported in association with abomasal bloat in several calves. Sarcinas are anaerobic, Gram-positive, nonmotile cocci found in rafts or packets. They are suspected gastric pathogens in a variety of animal species. The lesions are similar to braxy.

In many septicemias of pigs, bacterial emboli lodge in the vessels of the gastric submucosa and cause thrombosis, resulting in hyperemia, hemorrhage, infarction, and ulceration. This occurs in salmonellosis (Fig. 7-77), swine dysentery, Glasser's disease, and colibacillosis. Certain intoxicants such as vomitoxin produced by *Fusarium* spp. can cause similar lesions.

A deep mycosis that causes a granulomatous gastritis is due to *Histoplasma capsulatum* (see intestinal diseases of carnivores). Very rarely, *Mycobacterium tuberculosis* causes granulomatous gastritis in a variety of species. In granulomatous gastritis, epigastric discomfort after eating (postprandial), emesis, progressive cachexia, weakness, vomiting of blood (hematemesis), and pyloric obstruction caused by the space-occupying inflammatory reaction occur. In both histoplasmosis and tuberculosis, regional (gastric, splenic, and hepatic) lymph nodes may be affected. Nodular or diffusely thickened gastric and lymphoid lesions contain predominantly macrophages. Mononuclear inflammatory cells, fibroblasts, granulocytes (including eosinophils), and multinucleate giant cells are also present. Often the causative organisms can be demonstrated within the granulomatous inflammation, but special stains, such as acid-fast for mycobacteria and periodic acid–Schiff (PAS) reaction, or Gomori's methenamine silver stain may be necessary to demonstrate fungi.

Eosinophilic gastritis is uncommon in all species of domestic animals but has been reported in pet carnivores. In general, the etiologic basis for this condition is poorly understood. The three types of gastritis characterized by an influx of eosinophils are as follows:

- A characteristic focal eosinophilic infiltrate is sometimes associated with trapped, intramural nematode larvae, especially *Toxocara canis*. Larvae of *T. canis* pass to nursing puppies through the milk, through fecal soiling of bedding, or from dirt or other fomites harboring eggs or larvae. After ingestion the parasite's larval sheath, feces, and saliva are antigenic. In dogs and cats, tissue reaction to these larvae in the mucosal and submucosal intestine and gastric epithelial cell is hyperplasia, resulting in a polyp-like proliferation of the antral mucosa. Pyloric obstruction sometimes results.
- In other cases of eosinophilic gastritis the infiltration of eosinophils is more diffuse and is believed to be a hypersensitivity

reaction. The offending antigen is not known. In many of these cases there is a peripheral eosinophilia, especially when associated with eosinophilic infiltration of the small intestine (eosinophilic gastroenteritis). This form of eosinophilic gastritis may become transmural, with necrosis and scarring.

- The third type, scirrhous eosinophilic gastritis of dogs and cats, for the most part has unknown causes. The fibrosis associated with scirrhous changes in the stomach and lymph nodes results in persistent emesis, weight loss, and malnutrition.

The gross lesions of eosinophilic gastritis are rather nonspecific and consist of diffuse or nodular mural thickenings. Microscopic lesions are characterized by infiltrates of eosinophils in the mucosa and the submucosa and are seen extensively through the muscularis of the stomach. Similar lesions are sometimes present in segments of the small intestine and colon. In the dog there is sometimes necroproliferative eosinophilic perivasculitis and eosinophilic lymphadenopathy. In the scirrhous form the eosinophilic infiltrate is followed by transmural fibroplasia and scarring.

Hypertrophic or Hyperplastic Gastritis

Hypertrophic gastritis, characterized by thickened rugae, is the result of hyperplasia of the gastric glands. This effect is believed to be a response to chronic retention of gastric fluid and reflux of intestinal bile. Similar mucosal glandular changes are seen in immune-mediated lymphoplasmacytic gastritis of dogs. Hypertrophic gastritis has also been described in primates, horses, pigs, and rodents. The nematode *Nochtia nocti* causes this lesion in the stomachs of monkeys. Equine hypertrophic gastritis is a focal lesion or more diffuse lesion associated with the nematodes *Habronema* spp. and *Trichostrongylus axei*, respectively.

Chronic giant hypertrophic gastropathy of dogs affects the basenji, beagle, boxer, and bull terrier breeds, among others. The disease is similar to Ménétrier's disease in human beings. Clinical signs include weight loss, diarrhea, vomiting, and hypoproteinemia. The chronic gastritis results in increased mucosal permeability to serum proteins with subsequent protein-losing gastropathy. Unlike normal gastric mucosal folds, in giant hypertrophic gastropathy the mucosa does not flatten with distention of the organ (Fig. 7-78). Microscopically, the mucosa is hypertrophic and hyperplastic. The incorporation of folds of submucosa and muscularis mucosa is variable, as is the presence of inflammatory cells, principally lymphocytes and plasma cells. The cause of this condition is unknown.

Ulcers—Mucosal Defects

An ulcer is a mucosal defect in which the entire epithelial thickness, down to or through the basement membrane, has been lost. Penetration through the remaining tissue layers to the peritoneal cavity is termed a perforating ulcer. Partial-thickness epithelial loss is termed an *erosion*. Chronic ulcers differ from acute ulcers by the presence of an indurated rim caused by fibrosis and attempts at epithelial regeneration. The identification of gastric ulcers is not challenging, either at necropsy or by endoscopy. They are sharply bordered cavities, often coated with exudate. Thrombosis of blood vessels is sometimes adjacent to ulcers in ruminants with mycotic vasculitis secondary to ruminal lactic acidosis. Thus it is an infarct.

The pathogenesis of most gastric and duodenal ulcers in human beings has been demonstrated to be a result of infection with a helical bacterium, *Helicobacter pylori*. The same bacterium has been epidemiologically linked to gastric adenocarcinoma. *Helicobacter mustelae* acts similarly in ferrets. Although similar, gastric *Helicobacter*-like organisms are readily demonstrated in dogs and cats, their relationship with ulcer formation or neoplasia is not established. It appears that the stomachs of as many animals without gastritis or ulcers are as heavily colonized by these bacteria as are those of animals with ulcers (Fig. 7-79). More than 90% of cats are infected with two *Helicobacter* spp. *Helicobacter felis* can be cultured *in vitro*, but the noncultivatable *Helicobacter heilmannii* is the more frequent. Pathologic and clinical outcomes appear to depend on a number of bacterial virulence factors as well as on the host response to these agents. Investigations suggest there may be a link between the presence of *Helicobacter* and other diseases, including coronary and neurologic disease.

Theories abound as to the causes of most gastric ulcers in animals. None have been proved. There may be a heritable component to ulcer susceptibility. The conditions necessary for ulcer development boil down to an imbalance between acid secretion and mucosal protection. This imbalance occurs as a result of the following:

- Local disturbances or trauma to the mucosal epithelial barrier; this injury can be due to back flush of bile salts from the duodenum or ingestion of lipid solvents such as alcohol

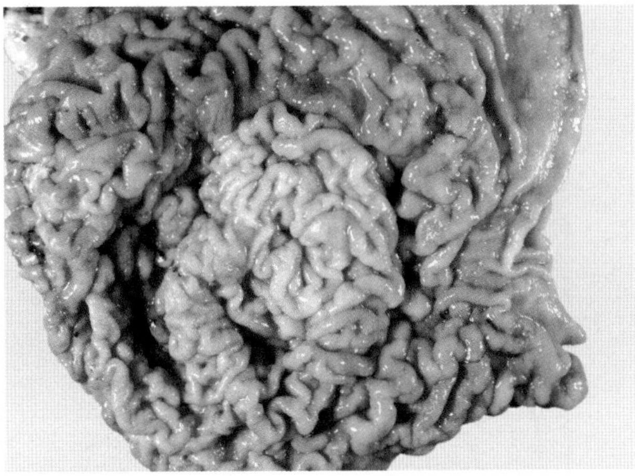

Figure 7-78 Chronic Giant Hypertrophic Gastropathy, Stomach, Dog. A cerebriform mass of redundant mucosa is present in the center of the gastric mucosa. Chronic inflammation in the mass results in increased mucosal permeability to serum proteins and a subsequent protein-losing gastropathy. (Courtesy College of Veterinary Medicine, Cornell University.)

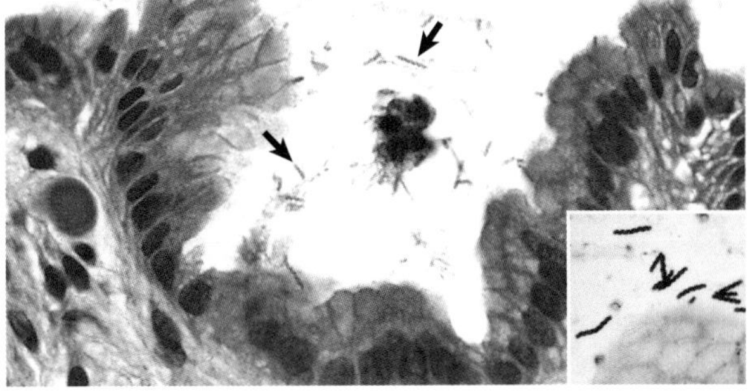

Figure 7-79 *Helicobacter* spp. Infection, Stomach, Cat. Numerous spiral bacteria *(arrows)* are present in the superficial mucous layer. There is no inflammation in the adjacent mucosa; however, in some areas the epithelium is hyperplastic. H&E stain. *Inset,* The helical shape of the helicobacter organisms is demonstrated with a Steiner's silver stain. (Figure courtesy Dr. H. Gelberg, College of Veterinary Medicine, Oregon State University. Inset courtesy Dr. C.S. Patton, College of Veterinary Medicine, University of Tennessee.)

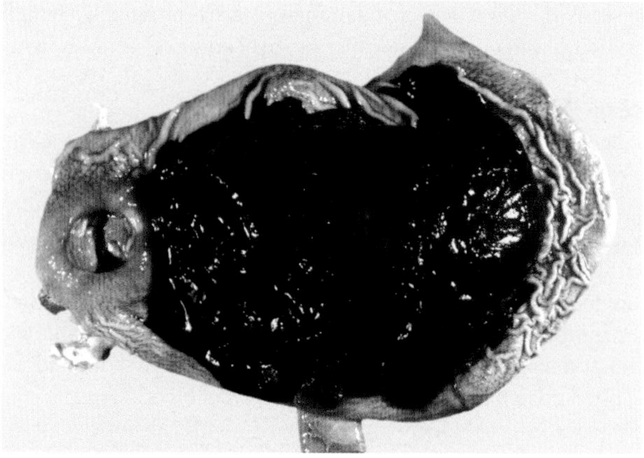

Figure 7-80 **Ulcer, Stomach, Dog.** The stomach contains a large volume of clotted and unclotted blood from a gastric ulcer (idiopathic) with rounded edges visible in the left side of the photograph. The hemorrhage was so severe that the dog died from exsanguination. (Courtesy Dr. H. Gelberg, College of Veterinary Medicine, Oregon State University.)

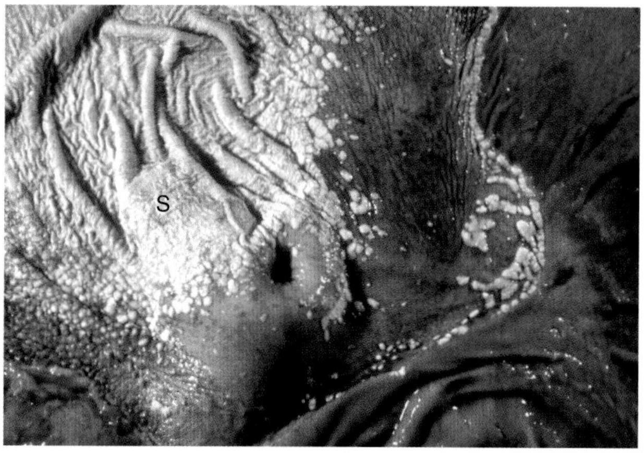

Figure 7-81 **Gastric Ulcers, Stomach, Horse.** Administration of nonsteroidal antiinflammatory drugs has caused extensive ulceration of the stratified squamous epithelium *(S)* of the nonglandular mucosa. The ulceration extends from the cardia *(center)* to the margo plicatus *(right)*. (Courtesy College of Veterinary Medicine, Cornell University.)

- Normal or high gastric acidity
- Local disturbances in blood flow (stress-induced and sympathetic nervous system–mediated arteriovenous shunts) resulting in ischemia
- Steroids and NSAIDs that depress prostaglandin formation (PGE_2, PGI_1) or concentration, thus decreasing phospholipid secretions, which are protective

All of these mechanisms allow pepsin and hydrochloric acid into the submucosa. Severe gastric hyperacidity and gastric ulcers are sometimes associated with the presence of islet cell tumors producing gastrin. Some of these gastrin-producing tumors arise in the duodenum, but the majority originate in the pancreas. These neoplasms release histamine into the bloodstream, which binds to receptors on parietal cells of the stomach, increasing HCl secretion. The gastric ulceration produced associated with these tumors is known as *Zollinger-Ellison syndrome*.

In dogs, gastric ulceration causes vomiting, inappetence, abdominal pain, and anemia secondary to gastric bleeding (Fig. 7-80). Melena (digested blood in feces) may also be present if the ulceration persists, and significant amounts of blood are lost to the GI system. Gastric ulcers in dogs and cats are generally idiopathic but can occur in those animals with mast cell tumors that stimulate gastric HCl secretion through histamine release and its effect on the surrounding blood vessels or other neoplasia that infiltrate and weaken the gastric wall.

Ulcers are idiopathic in foals. Foals with gastric ulcers may have abdominal pain, bruxism (grinding of the teeth), ptyalism, and gastric reflux and may lie in dorsal recumbency. Gastric ulcers associated with administration of NSAIDs are common in horses and to a lesser extent in other species (Fig. 7-81). Equine gastric ulcer syndrome occurs in 40% to 90% of competitive and performance horses, with the most severe ulcers occurring in those animals that are worked the hardest. More than one-third of horses used less strenuously develop mild ulcers.

Cattle with abomasal ulcers have partial or complete anorexia, decreased milk production, palpable discomfort on pressure applied to the right xiphoid area, and melena. In any species the vomiting of coffee grounds–like material (hematemesis) or passage of melena is highly suggestive of gastric ulcer disease. Abomasal ulcers of ruminants vary in significance from subclinical to fatal (Figs. 7-82 and 7-83). In calves, ulcers are associated with dietary changes or mechanical irritation of the abomasum by roughage. Dietary changes

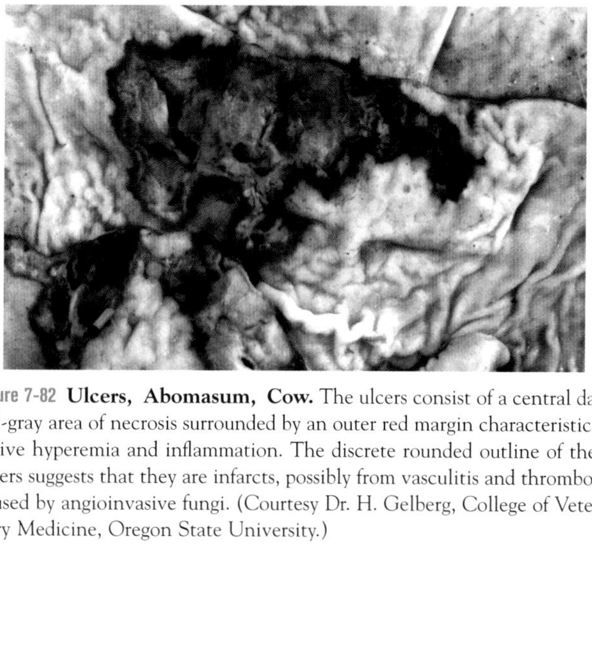

Figure 7-82 **Ulcers, Abomasum, Cow.** The ulcers consist of a central dark red-gray area of necrosis surrounded by an outer red margin characteristic of active hyperemia and inflammation. The discrete rounded outline of these ulcers suggests that they are infarcts, possibly from vasculitis and thrombosis caused by angioinvasive fungi. (Courtesy Dr. H. Gelberg, College of Veterinary Medicine, Oregon State University.)

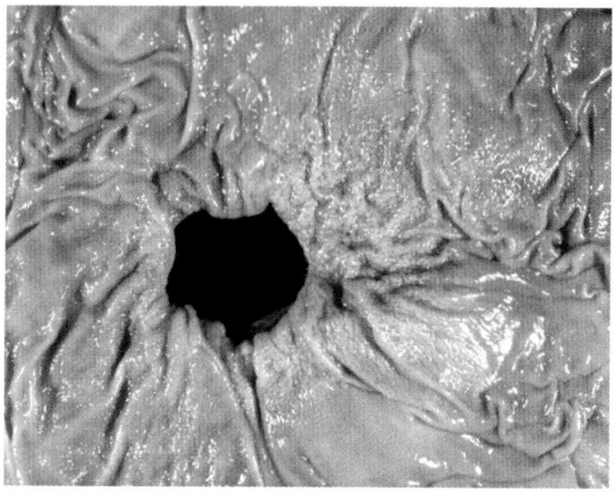

Figure 7-83 **Perforating Ulcer, Abomasum, Cow.** The rounded borders of the ulcer indicate an attempt at repair and therefore chronicity. Death was due to peritonitis. (Courtesy Dr. H. Gelberg, College of Veterinary Medicine, Oregon State University.)

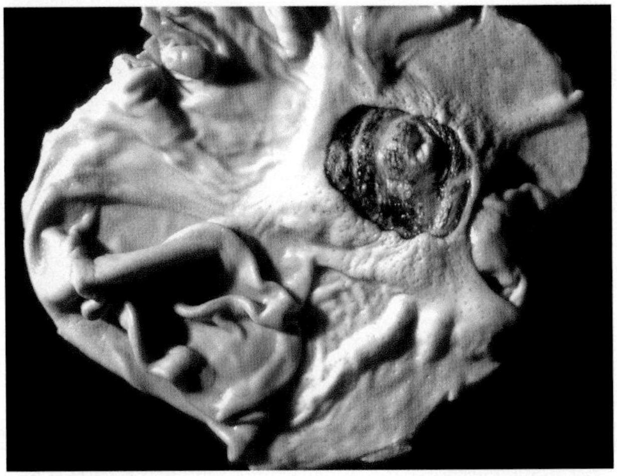

Figure 7-84 **Gastric Ulcer (Pars Esophagea), Stomach, Pig.** This type of gastric ulcer occurs exclusively in pigs and most commonly in confined growing pigs. The lesion is limited to the stratified squamous epithelium surrounding the cardia (pars esophagea). Ulcers in this location characteristically have a multifactorial cause, including the ingestion of finely ground grain or pelleted feed (possibly deficient in vitamin E), fermentation of sugars in the feed, and stress of confinement rearing. These ulcers frequently bleed and can cause exsanguination. (Courtesy Dr. M.D. McGavin, College of Veterinary Medicine, University of Tennessee.)

involve substitution of roughage for milk or milk replacer, together with the associated stress. In dairy cattle, ulcers are associated with heavy grain feeding (lactic acidosis) at the time of parturition, displacement of the abomasum, bovine viral diarrhea, impaction, torsion, and gastric lymphoma. Because cattle have an effective omentum that seals abomasal ulcers, they may live for a long time unless a large perforation occurs, resulting in septic peritonitis.

In pigs, gastric ulcers are common and occur in penned pigs fed finely ground grain. These ulcers always are limited to the stratified squamous epithelium of the esophageal portion of the gastric mucosa that surrounds the cardia (Fig. 7-84). Death can result from exsanguination into the gastric lumen. Evidence suggests that a high-carbohydrate diet alone is not sufficient to produce erosions and ulcers but rather that the appropriate diet in combination with fermentative commensal bacteria, such as *Lactobacillus* and *Bacillus* spp., produces lesions. Lesions progress from parakeratosis to hyperkeratosis through keratolysis to erosive gastritis or perforation of the stomach.

Miscellaneous Disorders

Uremic gastritis occurs most frequently in carnivores as a result of chronic renal disease (Fig. 7-85; also see Figs. 1-39, 11-22, and 11-23). In ungulates it is a rare event and is usually secondary to obstructive kidney disease (postrenal uremia). Uremic gastritis is characterized by mineralization of the glands, vessels, and lamina propria of the gastric mucosa and sometimes results in ulcer formation.

Amyloidosis occasionally is present in the stomach concomitant with systemic amyloid infiltrates. Generalized amyloid A (AA) amyloidosis with gastric deposits of amyloid has been reported in bats, Siamese and Abyssinian cats, goats, rhesus monkeys, sheep, and Siberian tigers.

Pyloric stenosis can be anatomic or physiologic because of an inability of the pyloric sphincter to function properly. This condition may be congenital or acquired. This lesion occurs most often in dogs (particularly brachycephalic breeds), Siamese cats, horses,

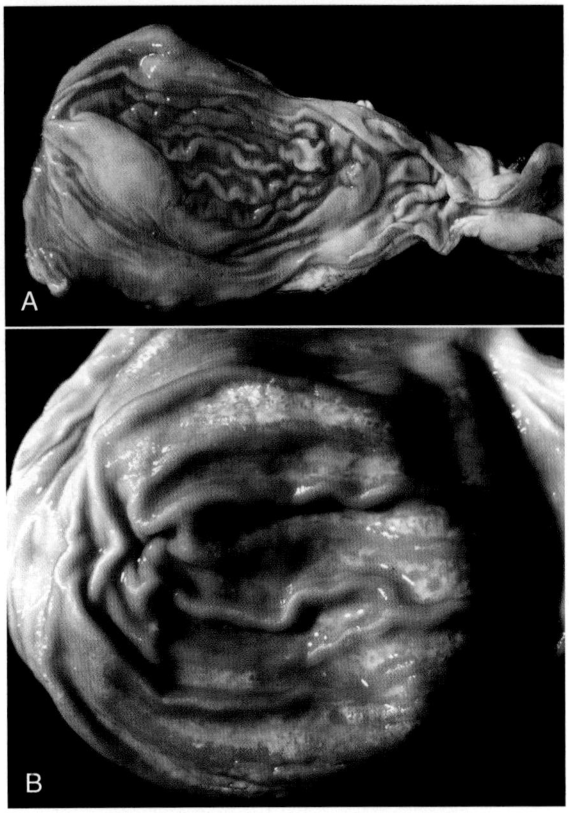

Figure 7-85 **Uremic Gastropathy (Also Called Uremic Gastritis), Stomach, Cat. A,** The major lesion is congestion and edema of the gastric mucosa caused by injury to capillaries within the lamina propria associated with elevated concentrations of nitrogen-derived metabolic waste products in the systemic circulation from kidney failure. **B,** With chronicity, there is mineralization of the gastric mucosa, visible as fine white stippling and lines in the mucosa. (**A** courtesy Dr. C.S. Patton, College of Veterinary Medicine, University of Tennessee. **B** courtesy Dr. M.D. McGavin, College of Veterinary Medicine, University of Tennessee.)

and human beings. Congenital pyloric stenoses may be hereditary, at least in human beings. Pyloric stenosis is often first recognized in recently weaned animals by projectile vomiting, retention of gastric contents, gastromegaly, and the presence of strong gastric peristaltic waves (E-Fig. 7-11). Pyloric muscular hypertrophy, variable submucosal edema, vascular ectasia, and degeneration of myenteric ganglion cells (dysautonomia) may be identified histologically in some cases. Functional pyloric stenosis can be a feature of vagus indigestion of ruminants. In general the many causes of pyloric stenosis are not well understood.

Giant hypertrophic pyloric gastropathy, not to be confused with giant hypertrophic gastropathy of basenjis and other dogs, is an idiopathic condition seen most often in older small-breed dogs. To the uninitiated the gross and microscopic features of this pyloric lesion strongly imitate those of carcinoma (Fig. 7-86). Microscopically, there is notable foveolar and glandular hyperplasia with variable hypertrophy of pyloric smooth muscle, small mucosal erosions, and ulcerations. There is usually a lymphoplasmacytic infiltrate of variable degree in the lamina propria.

Neoplasia

Gastric neoplasia, although uncommon, manifests in different ways in domestic animals. Leiomyoma and more rarely leiomyosarcoma arise from the tunica muscularis (Fig. 7-87). Lymphoma can be primary, metastatic, or multicentric in origin (Figs. 7-88 and 7-89);

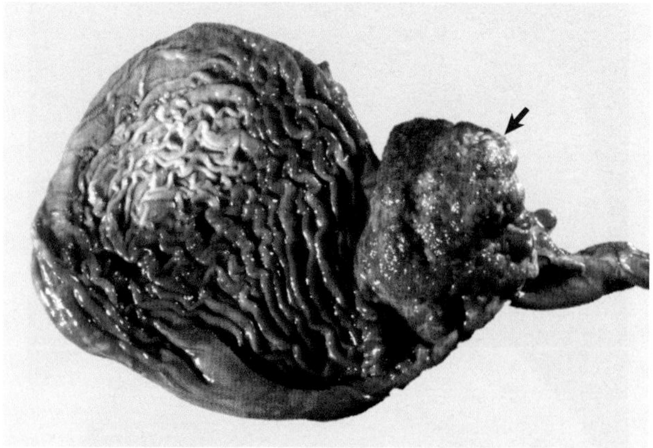

Figure 7-86 Giant Hypertrophic Pyloric Gastropathy, Stomach, Dog. The mass of hyperplastic glandular tissue *(arrow)* at the pylorus could be mistaken for a neoplasm. (Courtesy Dr. H. Gelberg, College of Veterinary Medicine, Oregon State University.)

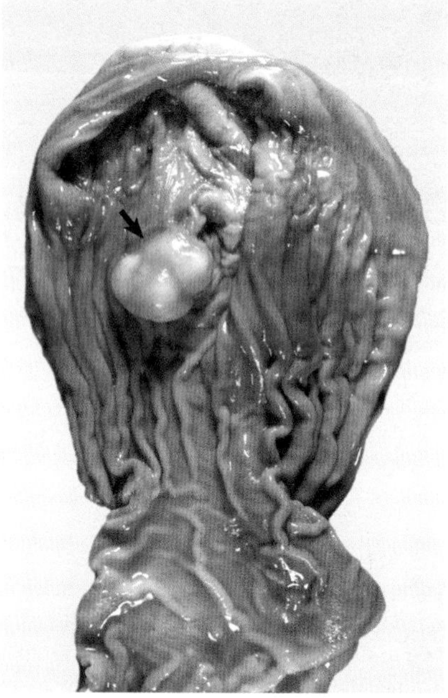

Figure 7-87 Leiomyoma, Stomach, Dog. This tumor *(arrow)* arose from smooth muscle in the tunica muscularis and is covered by intact mucosa. (Courtesy Dr. H. Gelberg, College of Veterinary Medicine, Oregon State University.)

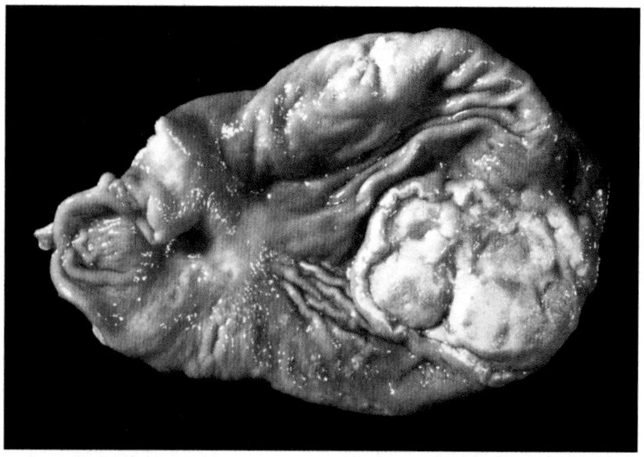

Figure 7-88 Lymphoma, Stomach, Cat. A large expansile white mass is present in the submucosa of the stomach *(top edge)* and is covered by an intact mucosal epithelium. Note the other lymphomatous white mass, which is ulcerated *(lower right)*. This latter lesion is somewhat atypical of this disease, because ulceration is uncommon and occurs in late-stage disease when the mass is quite large and protrudes into the gastric lumen. In most cases of gastric lymphoma the mucosal epithelium is intact and not ulcerated. (Courtesy Dr. C.S. Patton, College of Veterinary Medicine, University of Tennessee.)

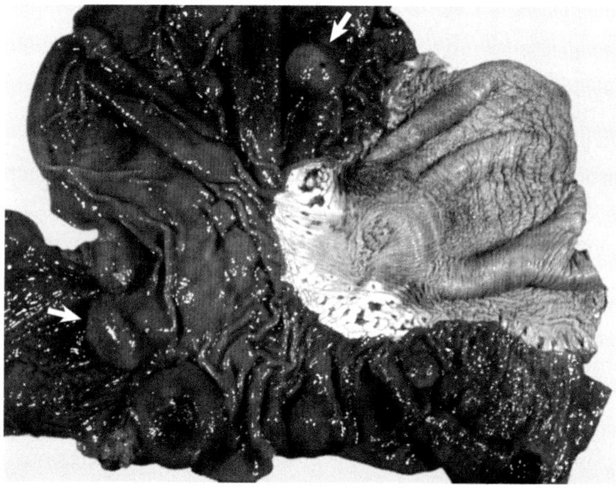

Figure 7-89 Lymphoma, Stomach, Horse. Large smooth-surfaced submucosal nodules *(arrows)*, two of which have a central hemorrhagic ulcer, are present in the glandular portion of the stomach. Ulcers in the stratified squamous portion *(white-gray areas)* of the stomach are sites of *Gasterophilus intestinalis* attachment. (Courtesy Dr. H. Gelberg, College of Veterinary Medicine, Oregon State University.)

also see Fig. 13-94). In cattle, lymphoma is often caused by the bovine leukemia virus and has a predilection for the abomasum, the right atrium, and uterus (Fig. 7-90). Squamous cell carcinoma of the stratified squamous (esophageal) portion of the stomach is relatively common in the horse (Fig. 7-91). Glandular neoplasms, adenomas, and adenocarcinomas occur in all species but are seen most often in dogs and cats. Dogs and rarely cats occasionally develop gastric mast cell tumors.

Intestine

Developmental Anomalies

Atresia. Occlusion of the intestinal lumen as the result of anomalous development of the intestinal wall is called *atresia* (Fig. 7-92). Atresia is generally named for the part of the bowel that is occluded, such as atresia ani or atresia coli. The causes of atresia in domestic animals are not completely understood, but they can be a result of mechanical lesions to fetal blood vessels in a portion of the gut, such as caused by malpositioning, that compromise circulation and results in vascular accidents and ischemia. Release of meconium into the abdominal cavity of the fetus may result in sterile peritonitis and may be responsible for some cases of atresia such as in cystic fibrosis of human beings. In still other cases the embryonic cells that normally occlude the lumen fail to break down, resulting in atresia. The end result is segmental atresia in which a segment of the bowel is either entirely missing or completely occluded because of a lack of epithelial development and confluence between two contiguous portions (Figs. 7-93 and 7-94).

Meckel's Diverticulum. Meckel's diverticulum is a remnant of the omphalomesenteric duct. Generally it disappears after the first

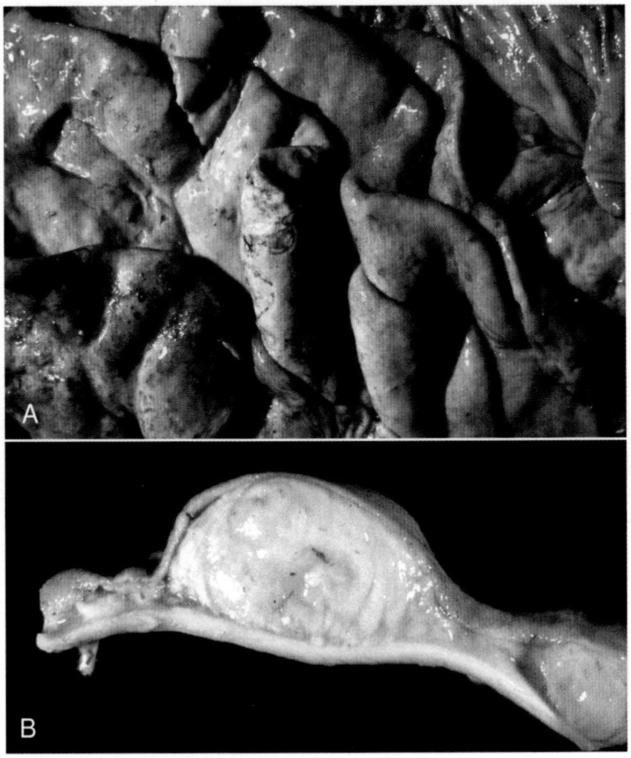

Figure 7-90 Lymphoma, Abomasum, Cow. A, Mucosal surface of abomasal folds. Note the folds are thickened and have a pale white-pink color resulting from the infiltration of neoplastic lymphocytes. Overlying mucosae are eroded and ulcerated. **B,** Transverse section. This cross section demonstrates a white, space-occupying submucosal mass. The intact mucosa is located at the top of the specimen. (**A** courtesy Dr. M.D. McGavin, College of Veterinary Medicine, University of Tennessee. **B** courtesy Dr. H. Gelberg, College of Veterinary Medicine, Oregon State University.)

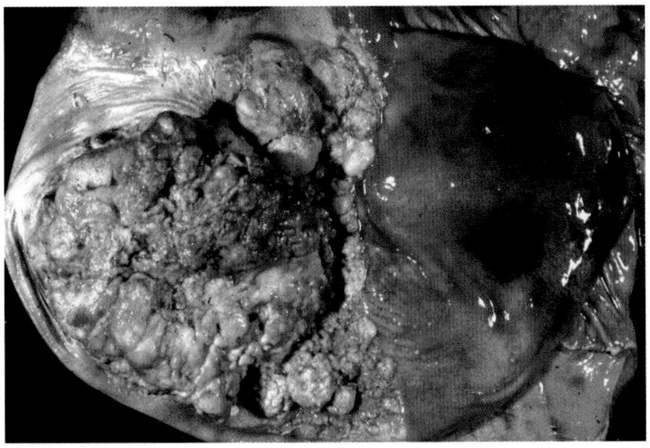

Figure 7-91 Squamous Cell Carcinoma, Stomach, Horse. A large proliferative, ulcerative mass has arisen from the epithelium of the nonglandular (squamous) mucosa of the stomach. (Courtesy Dr. A. Paulman, College of Veterinary Medicine, University of Illinois.)

trimester of gestation, but it can persist in all mammalian species. It is near the termination of the ileum, represents the stalk of the yolk sac, and because of its location and being blind ended, can be confused with the cecum.

Megacolon. Megacolon, as its name implies, is a large, usually fecal-filled colon (Figs. 7-95 and 7-96) that can be congenital or

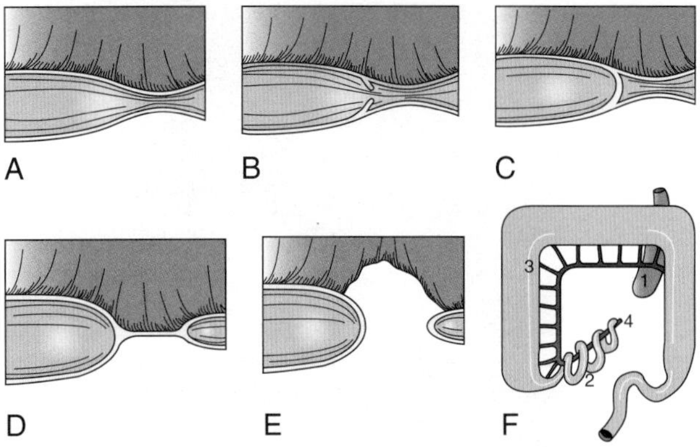

Figure 7-92 Types of Stenosis And Atresia. A, Stenosis. **B,** Stenosis with partial membrane. **C,** Membrane atresia. **D,** Cord atresia. **E,** Blind-end atresia. **F,** Christmas tree atresia (*1*, jejunum; *2*, ileum; *3*, colon; *4*, ileocolic artery). (Modified from van der Gaag I, Tibboel D: *Vet Pathol* 17(5):565-574, 1980.)

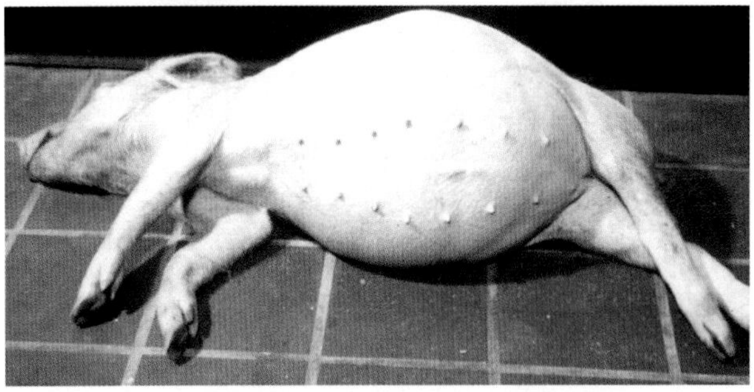

Figure 7-93 Abdominal Distention, Atresia Coli, Feeder Pig. This pig has been unable to defecate since birth because of an atretic developmental malformation of the distal colon. Note the greatly distended abdomen. (Courtesy Dr. J. King, College of Veterinary Medicine, Cornell University.)

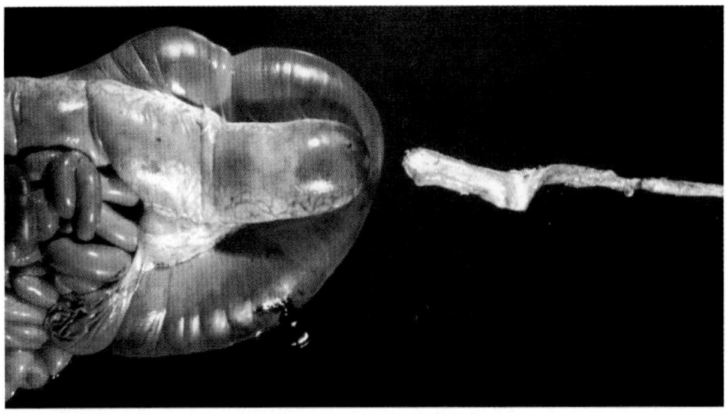

Figure 7-94 Atresia Coli, Colon, Cow. There is a blind-ended atretic segment of the spiral colon. The smaller segment at the right of the photograph is distal, the terminal part of the colon. (Courtesy Dr. H. Gelberg, College of Veterinary Medicine, Oregon State University.)

acquired. The congenital form occurs in pigs, dogs, cats, overo foals, and human beings from a developmental lack of myenteric plexuses (Hirschsprung's disease) secondary to the failure of migration of neuroblasts from the neural crest to the colorectal myenteric plexuses.

The equine overo pattern of spotting is defined by white patches of epidermis on the ventral or lateral abdomen and extends dorsally up to but not including the dorsal midline. The epidermis is also

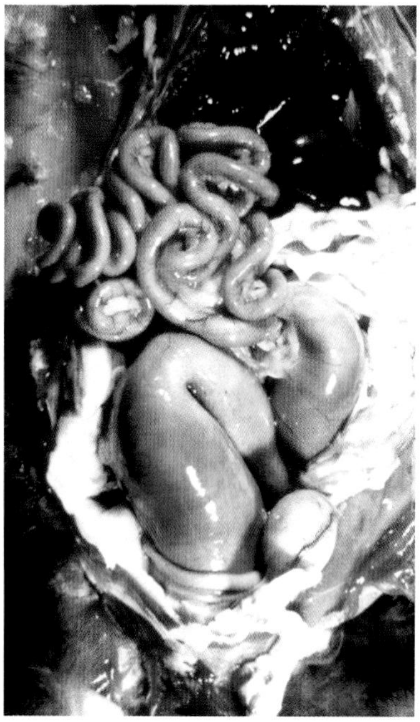

Figure 7-95 **Megacolon, Colon, Cat.** This disease may be congenital due to a lack of intestinal innervation or atresia of the distal colon or anus. It can also be acquired secondary to nerve injury. (Courtesy Dr. H. Gelberg, College of Veterinary Medicine, Oregon State University.)

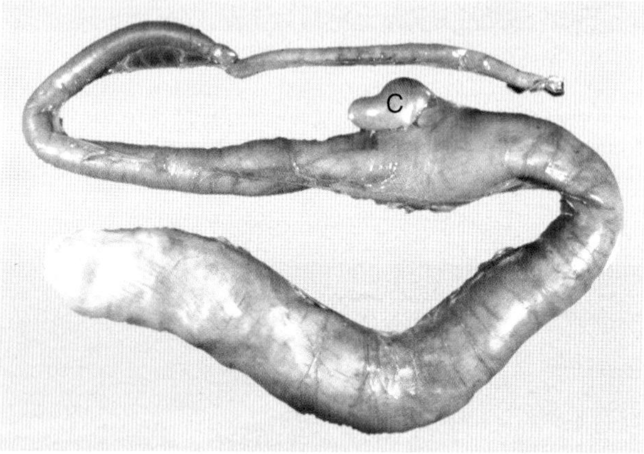

Figure 7-96 **Megacolon, Colon, Dog.** The large colon from the cecum (*C*) to the anus is dilated with feces. In dogs, this disease has pathogeneses similar to those described in cats (see Fig. 7-95). (Courtesy Dr. H. Gelberg, College of Veterinary Medicine, Oregon State University.)

nonpigmented on the lateral neck and flank. The overo pattern typically includes at least one pigmented leg. Affected foals are white and appear normal at birth. They do not pass meconium; subsequently they develop colic and die usually by 72 hours after birth. These white foals are nonperistaltic because of absence of the myenteric (Auerbach's) plexus or submucosal (Meissner's) plexus, particularly in the colon and rectum. Thus these anomalies can be termed aganglionosis. A congenital aganglionic megacolon is contracted and nonperistaltic. Dilation or megacolon occurs proximal to the aganglionic section of the gut. Acquired megacolon is secondary to damage to the colonic innervation. Such events are usually traumatic and most common in carnivores struck by automobiles. Atresia ani can also result in megacolon.

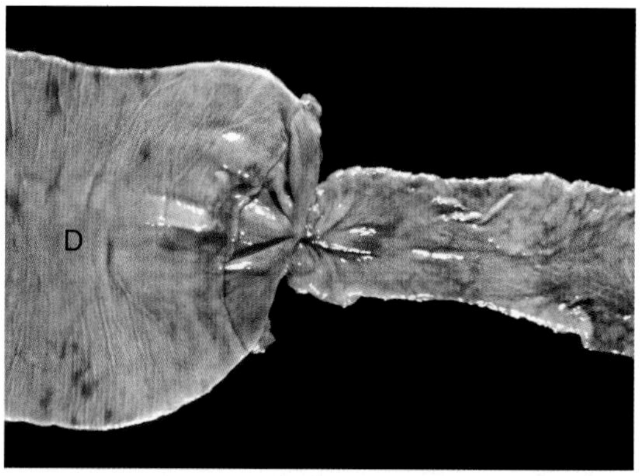

Figure 7-97 **Stricture, Intestine, Horse.** The dilated intestine (*D*) is proximal to the stricture. Such strictures can be caused by penetrating or nonpenetrating wounds of all kinds from the luminal surface or secondary to vascular injury. (Courtesy Dr. H. Gelberg, College of Veterinary Medicine, Oregon State University.)

Intestinal Obstruction

Mechanical obstruction of the intestinal tract occurs in all species of domestic and wild animals. Although foreign bodies of all types have been removed from animals at surgery, the long-term systemic effects of some foreign bodies are also important. These include copper and zinc toxicosis from ingestion of coins in dogs, seals, ruminants, and horses and lead poisoning in cattle from ingestion of old batteries. Primates caged in outdated facilities with lead paint or lead bars can also succumb to lead poisoning. *Pythium insidiosum* infection has caused intestinal obstruction in a puppy because of inflammation associated with the infection.

Enteroliths and Impaction. Enteroliths are rare in species other than the horse. The Arabian breed has an increased incidence. Generally, affected animals are more than 4 years old. The stones are usually formed by ammonium magnesium phosphate (struvite) and collect around a small central nidus, often a metallic foreign body (E-Fig. 7-12). Enteroliths vary greatly in size from several centimeters in diameter to greater than 20 cm, and they can weigh several kilograms. They generally lodge at the pelvic flexure or transverse colon. Diets high in magnesium and phosphorus predispose to enterolith formation. In the past, millers' horses (grain and feed mills) had access to large amounts of inexpensive bran, and thus their horses were more prone to enteroliths. In California the feeding of high-protein, magnesium-rich alfalfa hay may partially explain the higher incidence of enteroliths in California horses.

The presence of aggregated ingesta that cannot move along the intestinal tract (impaction) occurs in all species. It is especially common in horses after anthelmintic administration and is the result of the rapid die-off of large numbers of nematodes, particularly ascarids (E-Fig. 7-13). Cecal impaction occurs in old horses because of a high-roughage (indigestible) diet, debility, or poor dentition caused by a lack of mechanical leveling of the teeth (floating). Fibrous ingesta can also result in ileal impaction. Large amounts of ingested sand can accumulate anywhere in the equine colon, resulting in impaction (sand colic).

Strictures with Obstruction. Strictures are the result of narrowing of the lumen of a canal, which in the present case is the intestinal canal. They are generally the result of healing with scarring of penetrating and nonpenetrating wounds of all kinds or of a vascular injury causing infarction, followed by healing with fibrosis (Fig. 7-97). For example, rectal stricture is a sequela of salmonellosis

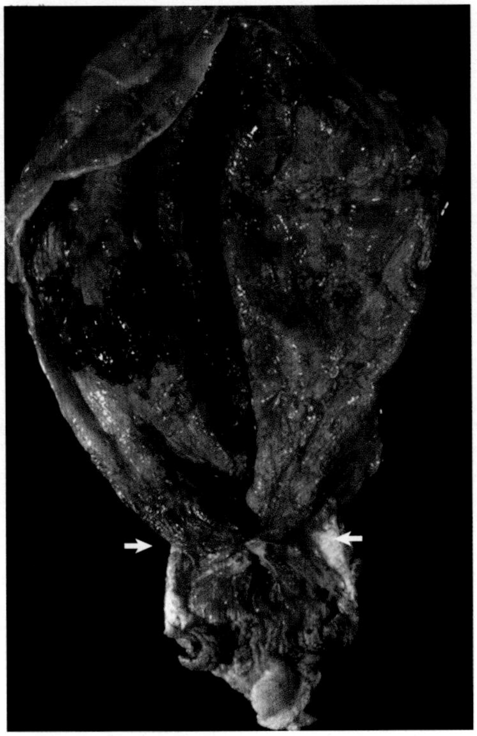

Figure 7-98 **Stricture, Colon, Pig.** This lesion *(between arrows)* in pigs has been attributed to thrombosis of the cranial hemorrhoidal artery from vasculitis and thrombosis caused by salmonella. (Courtesy Dr. C.S. Patton, College of Veterinary Medicine, University of Tennessee.)

in pigs and is the result in part of thrombosis of the cranial hemorrhoidal artery and lack of collateral circulation (Fig. 7-98) that could otherwise allow the intestinal segment to remain viable. Renal strictures obstruct the intestine.

Intussusception. When one segment of intestine becomes telescoped into the immediately distal segment of intestine, the lesion is called an *intussusception* (Figs. 7-99 and 7-100). The intussusceptum is the trapped segment, and the intussuscipiens is the enveloping portion of the intestine. The cause is generally unknown but is thought to be associated with intestinal irritability and hypermotility. Irritability and hypermotility can occur secondary to enteritis, irritation caused by parasites of all sorts, and general debility. Foreign bodies, neoplasms, and some parasites, such as the nodular worm of sheep (*Oesophagostomum* spp.), by means of the subserosal nodules it produces, can provide a toehold for the intestine to telescope into itself. In the dog, intussusception of the intestine has been related to, or caused by, handling of the small intestine during surgery, hypertrophied lymphoid nodules, granulomas secondary to inflammatory and parasitic diseases, linear foreign bodies (string) (Fig. 7-101, A), and ascarids.

In cattle and horses, tumors, abscesses, and granulomas may be causes of intussusceptions. In horses, verminous arteritis may uniquely cause intussusceptions. Ileoileal, ileocecal, cecocecal, and cecocolic intussusceptions are sometimes associated with *Anoplocephala perfoliata*. Rarely, duodenogastric and gastroesophageal intussusceptions occur.

Clinical features of intussusception are similar to those of intestinal obstruction. In small animals with thin abdominal walls, they can sometimes be palpated. Intussusceptions are enlarged, thickened segments of intestine that vary in length. Intussusceptions are grossly swollen, doughy-feeling segments of the intestine. They

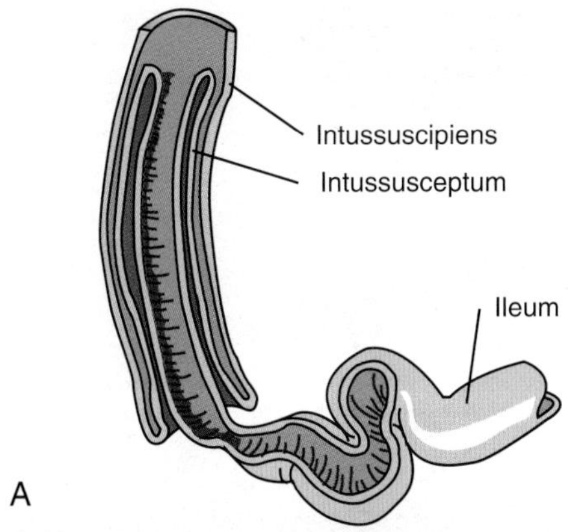

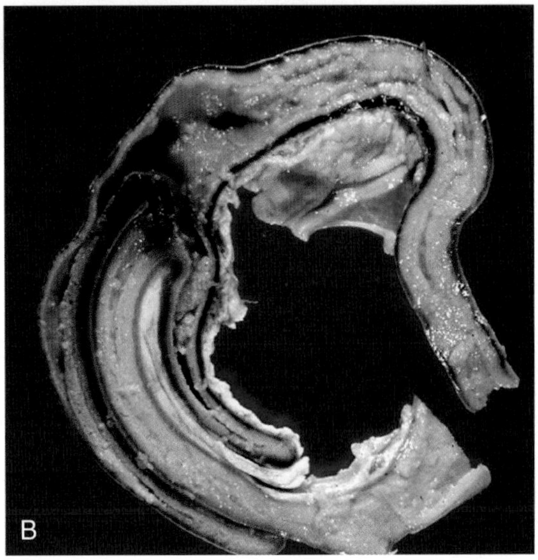

Figure 7-99 **Intussusception. A,** Schematic diagram showing the anatomic positioning of small intestinal segments in an intussusception. **B,** Longitudinal section of small intestinal intussusception demonstrating the position of the intussusceptum (trapped segment) and the intussuscipiens (the enveloping portion) of the small intestine. (**A** redrawn with permission from Dr. T. Boosinger. **B** courtesy Dr. T. Boosinger, College of Veterinary Medicine, Auburn University; and Noah's Arkive, College of Veterinary Medicine, The University of Georgia.)

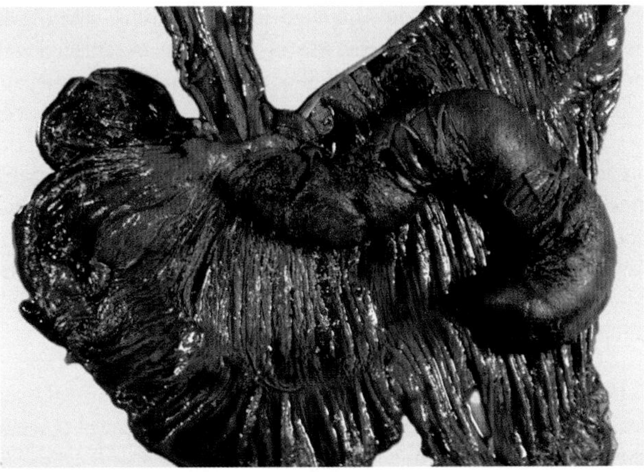

Figure 7-100 **Ileocecal Intussusception, Ileum, Horse.** The necrotic intussuscipiens is present in the lumen of the opened cecum. (Courtesy Dr. M.D. McGavin, College of Veterinary Medicine, University of Tennessee.)

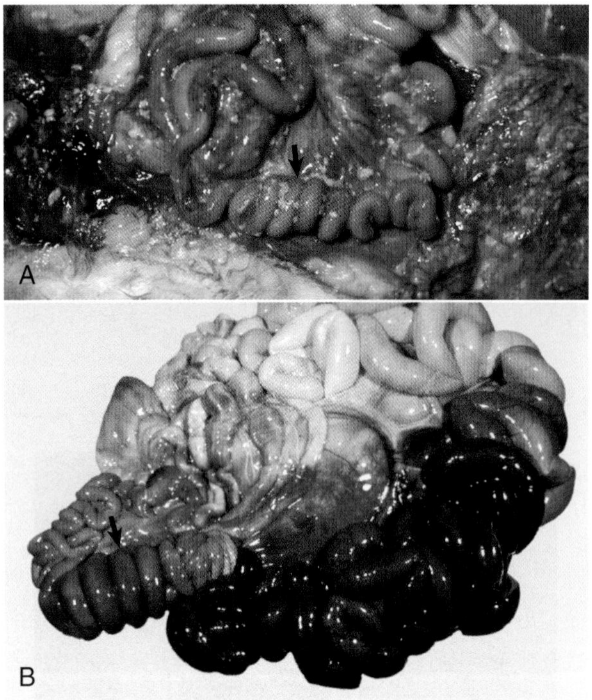

Figure 7-101 Accordion-Folded Intestines. A, Small intestine, cat. A linear foreign body (roast beef string) has caused the accordion-folded appearance of the small intestine *(arrow)*. Peristalsis of the intestine over the string, which is taut, in the intestinal lumen causes a sawing, abrasive effect and perforation of the intestine resulting in peritonitis. A white exudate is present on serosal surfaces. **B,** Intussusception, intestine, pig. The accordion-folded intussusception *(arrow)* is contiguous with infarcted red to dark red bowel, the result of vascular strangulation. (**A** courtesy College of Veterinary Medicine, University of Illinois. **B** courtesy Dr. H. Gelberg, College of Veterinary Medicine, Oregon State University.)

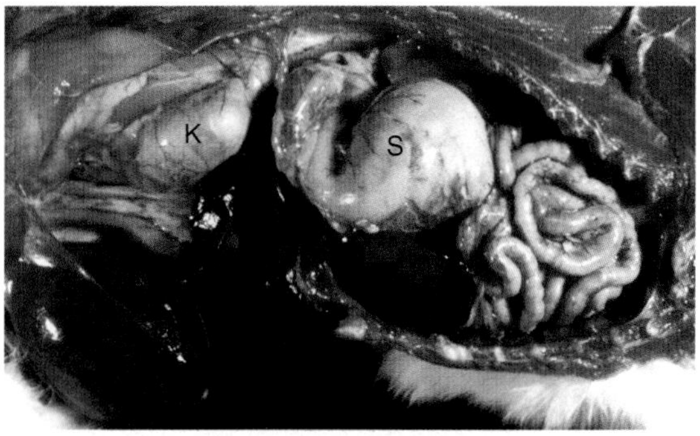

Figure 7-102 Diaphragmatic Hernia, Abdomen, Cat. Traumatic rupture of the diaphragm has allowed intestine, stomach *(S)*, and liver into the thoracic cavity, resulting in displacement and compression of the thoracic viscera and consequently compromise of cardiopulmonary function. *K,* Kidney. (Courtesy Dr. H. Gelberg, College of Veterinary Medicine, Oregon State University.)

resemble the folds of an accordion (see Fig. 7-101, *B*). Red to black discoloration depends on the degree of vascular compromise, ranging from congestion to hemorrhage and necrosis. The mesenteric attachment of the intussusceptum may be seen extending from the lesion. This occurs as the vascular mesentery gets pulled into the intussuscipiens compressing first the thinner-walled veins and then the arteries. Fibrin exudation, ischemic necrosis, congestion, and edema may occur in both the intussusceptum and intussuscipiens. On rare occasions, antemortem intussusceptions spontaneously reduce by sloughing of the infarcted intussusceptum, which then passes in the feces. Often the site of sloughing is replaced with fibrous tissue, and a circumferential scar or stricture forms. Because peristalsis continues after death, intestinal invaginations can occur post mortem. Before attributing death to intestinal obstruction caused by intussusception, there is a need to determine if the intussusception took place before or after death. Because inflammation occurs only in the living organism, postmortem invaginations are easily reduced because there are no adhesions and they are not accompanied by hyperemia or fibrin on the peritoneal surfaces, which remain smooth and glistening.

Ileus. Paralytic ileus (adynamic ileus) is a nonmechanical hypomotility resulting in a functional obstruction of the bowel (pseudo-obstruction). It can be due to paralysis of the bowel wall (generally the result of bowel manipulation at surgery), peritonitis from any cause, shock, severe pain, abnormal stimulation of splanchnic nerves, toxemia, electrolyte imbalances (especially hypokalemia), vitamin B–complex deficiency, uremia, tetanus, diabetes mellitus, or heavy-metal poisoning.

The gut is not paralyzed, but because of continuous nerve discharge, it becomes refractory, resulting in lack of tonic stimulation of the bowel musculature. In most cases of paralytic ileus, there are no gross lesions other than perhaps atonic dilation of the intestine. It occurs in most animal species.

Grass sickness of horses in Europe, southern South America, and rarely the United States is associated with dysphagia, GI hypomotility, and subsequent colic. Degenerative lesions of this idiopathic condition are present in the autonomic ganglia, suggesting it is an acquired dysautonomia. An occasional outbreak in horses is associated with the temporospatial occurrence of similar lesions in rabbits. Ingestion of *Clostridium botulinum* type C with subsequent toxin production is suspected to be the cause of this condition.

Intestinal Displacements

Intestinal displacements include herniations that lead to incarcerations (fixation) of the displaced bowel and finally strangulations (interference with blood flow) of the incarcerated segment of intestine and are categorized as internal or external. Internal herniations are displacements of intestine through a normal or pathologic foramen in the abdominal cavity. The most common of these displacements occur in horses and include herniation through the epiploic foramen and through mesenteric tears. The dorsal border of the epiploic foramen is formed by the caudate lobe of the liver and the caudal vena cava. The ventral boundary is the right lobe of the pancreas, the gastropancreatic ligament, and the portal vein. The cranial boundary is the hepatoduodenal ligament, and the caudal boundary is the junction of the pancreas and mesoduodenum. The epiploic cavity is only a potential space. It is proposed that in older horses the caudate lobe of the liver atrophies, enlarging the foramen and allowing loops of intestine to slip through and become incarcerated and strangulated (E-Fig. 7-14).

External hernias are formed when a hernial sac, formed by a pouch of parietal peritoneum, penetrates outside the abdominal cavity. Types of external herniation include umbilical, ventral, diaphragmatic (Fig. 7-102), hiatal, inguinal, scrotal (Fig. 7-103), and perineal, named for the location of the displaced viscera. Perineal hernias are seen in old male dogs with prostate gland enlargement and obstipation. Some of these herniations (diaphragmatic, perineal) are more correctly termed *eventrations* (protrusion of the intestine through the abdominal wall or diaphragm) because they are not accompanied by a peritoneal pouch. Postoperative wound

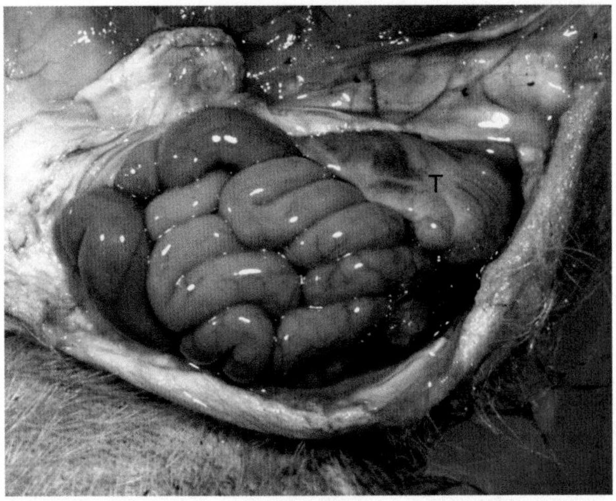

Figure 7-103 Scrotal Hernia, Scrotum, Pig. Loops of intestine within the scrotum entered through the inguinal canal to lie in the scrotal cavity and have displaced the testis *(T)* caudally. (Courtesy Dr. H. Gelberg, College of Veterinary Medicine, Oregon State University.)

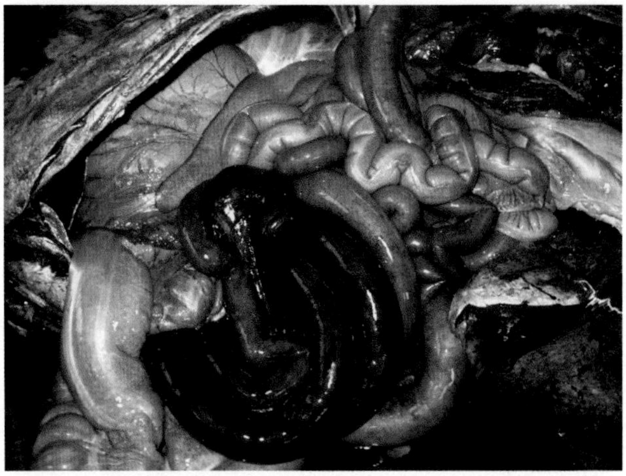

Figure 7-105 Infarction, Small Intestine, Horse. Volvulus of the intestine has resulted in vascular compromise and infarction *(dark red intestine)* of several loops of bowel. (Courtesy Dr. M.D. McGavin, College of Veterinary Medicine, University of Tennessee.)

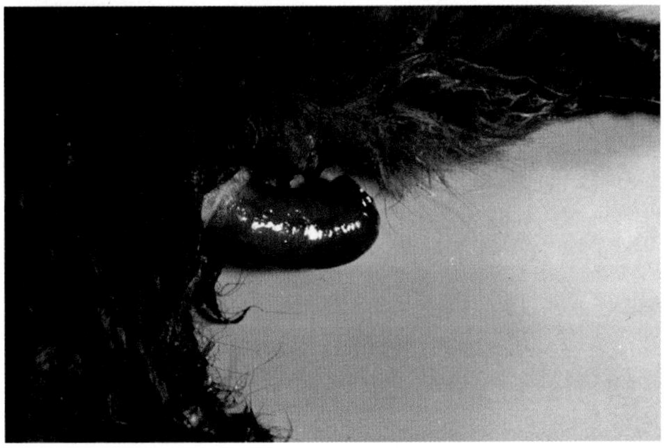

Figure 7-104 Prolapsed Rectum, Anus, Cat. Tenesmus caused the rectum to prolapse. (Courtesy Dr. M.D. McGavin, College of Veterinary Medicine, University of Tennessee.)

dehiscence of a ventral abdominal incision also causes eventration. It should be noted that umbilical hernias are generally caused by a defect in the abdominal wall and not by the chewing on the umbilical cord by the dam. Umbilical hernias may have a genetic basis, so it may be a matter of some ethical concern whether to surgically repair these hernias in show and breeding animals. In calves, umbilical infections are also associated with an increased risk for hernia development.

Rectal prolapse may occur secondary to tenesmus or excessive postpartum straining (Fig. 7-104).

Volvulus and Torsion. A volvulus is a twisting of the intestine on its mesenteric axis. A torsion is a rotation of a tubular organ along its long axis. The latter is most common in the cecum of cattle and horses and occasionally of the abomasum of calves (E-Fig. 7-15). Both volvulus and torsion result in compression of the mesenteric veins and arteries, resulting in ischemia initially followed by obstruction—veins first and later as the pressure on the mesenteric vessels increases, the arteries. Infarction is a result of occlusion of the thin-walled mesenteric veins. Because the mesenteric arterial supply is anatomically more resistant to occlusion, blood is pumped into the twisted segment but cannot drain. Edema, congestion, hemorrhage, and eventual necrosis result (Figs. 7-105 and 7-106). It is probable that the mechanism of intestinal twisting is secondary to movement of the walls of the abdominal cavity (i.e., the intestine stays still and the horse rolls or otherwise moves around the static intestine).

At surgery or necropsy the twisted segment of intestine is distended with gas and fluid and is discolored either dark red or black (see Fig. 2-40). There is usually a sharp line of demarcation between the affected and normal intestine. This line marks the site for surgical resection. A volvulus may result in a rotation of the intestine up to 720 degrees, either clockwise or counterclockwise on its mesenteric axis. Therefore surgical correction of a volvulus may be difficult and complex. It is very important to determine the viability of the bowel after reduction of a volvulus. The affected segment of intestine is often necrotic, congested, and hemorrhagic. Intestinal stasis and toxemia and/or bacteremia may result from bacterial overgrowth and anoxic bowel necrosis. Reperfusion injury may also occur. Toxemia and intestinal rupture may result in death.

Volvulus of the equine large intestine occurs most commonly in the left colon. In horses the left ventral colon is an extension of the right ventral colon beginning at the sternal flexure. The left ventral colon doubles back on itself in the pelvic inlet to form the left dorsal colon. This pelvic flexure can be palpated rectally. The left dorsal colon becomes the right dorsal colon at the diaphragmatic flexure. The diaphragmatic flexure lies cranial to the sternal flexure and usually contacts the ventral body wall. The left dorsal colon is sacculated with one taenia; the left ventral colon is sacculated with four taeniae. When twisting occurs, it is usually clockwise around the mesocolon and is thus a volvulus. Torsion of the large colon of mares accounts for half of their intestinal displacements in the peripartum period.

A peculiar type of intestinal strangulation occurs in horses in which lipomas, which are pedunculated, wrap around the intestinal mesentery or the bowel, causing ischemia, colic, and death (Fig. 7-107). Pedunculated lipomas may rotate about their pedicle, cutting off their own blood supply. When this occurs, they undergo mineralization and sometimes ossification. The stalk may become necrotic and break, leaving a free-floating lipoma within the abdominal cavity, where it apparently does no harm. However, most

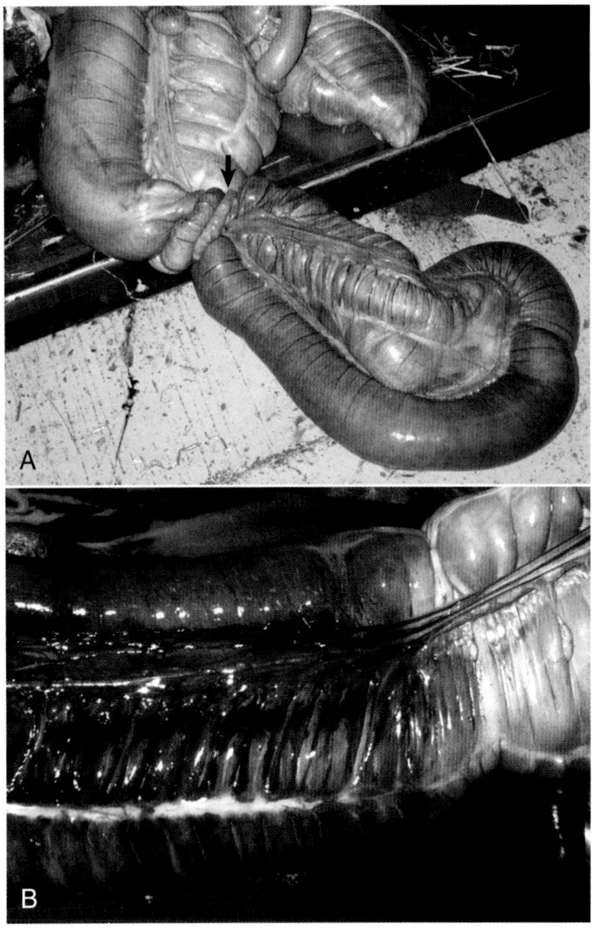

Figure 7-106 **Torsion, Large Colon, Horse. A,** Rotation of the colon on its long axis has resulted in severe colic with strangulation *(arrow)*. Note the red to blue discoloration of the colon distal to the torsion caused by obstruction of venous blood flow. **B,** Note the sharp line of demarcation (point where the torsion occurred) between viable colon *(to the right)* and nonviable colon *(to the left)* caused by obstruction of venous blood flow. In this case, the torsion was not found at the time of necropsy; however, a torsion will commonly untwist itself (reduce itself) during transport of the cadaver to the postmortem room. (**A** courtesy Dr. H. Gelberg, College of Veterinary Medicine, Oregon State University. **B** courtesy Dr. M.D. McCracken, College of Veterinary Medicine, University of Tennessee.)

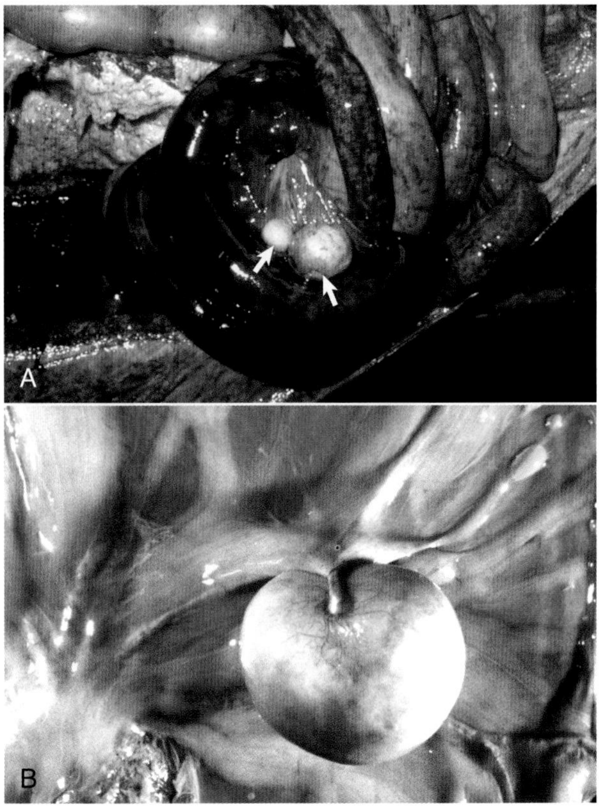

Figure 7-107 **Pedunculated Lipomas. A,** Intestinal strangulation by pedunculated lipomas, small intestine, horse. Two lipomas *(arrows)* have wrapped around the mesentery and strangled the bowel resulting in infarction *(dark red intestine)*. **B,** Mesentery, horse. Closer view of a pedunculated lipoma. (**A** courtesy College of Veterinary Medicine, Cornell University. **B** courtesy College of Veterinary Medicine, University of Illinois.)

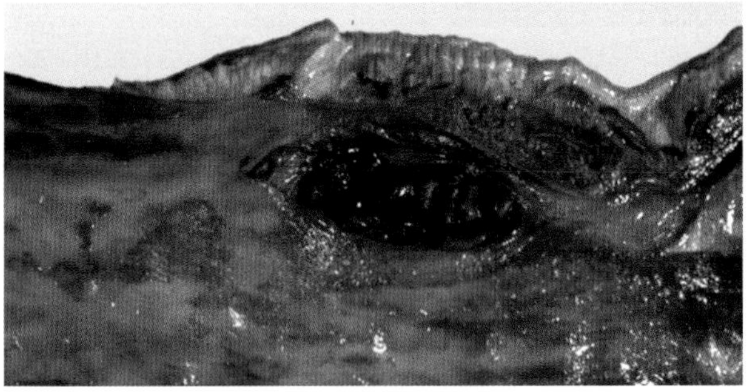

Figure 7-108 **Ulceration, Rectum, Horse.** Hemorrhage, ulcers, and tears in the rectum are often caused by inexperienced persons or overly vigorous rectal palpation. (Courtesy Dr. M.D. McGavin, College of Veterinary Medicine, University of Tennessee.)

mesenteric lipomas are of no clinical consequence. Rarely, intestinal strangulation by pedunculated lipomas has been reported in the dog.

Miscellaneous Disorders

Cecal or large intestinal rupture occurs most commonly in postparturient mares (see Fig. 7-19) but can also result from impaction and as a complication of anesthesia. The sites of rupture vary, and the mechanisms are unknown. Iatrogenic rectal tearing may occur secondary to rectal palpation (Fig. 7-108). The presence of blood on a rectal sleeve after palpation is cause for concern because peritonitis may be the result of penetration of the peritoneal cavity, especially if the tear occurs ventrally.

Diverticula (sing. diverticulum) are epithelium-lined cavities that are derived from mucosal epithelium that extend through the muscularis mucosa, submucosa, and muscularis and often reach the serosa, where they sometimes rupture, causing peritonitis (Figs. 7-109 and 7-110; E-Fig. 7-16). This can occur in any part of the tubular gut, including the esophagus and cecum.

Muscular hypertrophy of the distal ileum is an idiopathic condition of horses and pigs. Although generally an incidental finding, hypertrophy of the tunica muscularis can lead to impaction and rupture of the ileum. The lesion in horses is sometimes segmental, affecting the ileum and variably the jejunum. Often the lesion is a sequela of muscular hypertrophy caused by a damaged or stenotic ileocecal valve. Muscular hypertrophy of horses may also affect the duodenum and jejunum in association with diverticula in those gut segments. Horses with muscular hypertrophy of the distal ileum may have mild colic, occasional diarrhea, and weight loss. Often muscular hypertrophy is asymptomatic. Muscular hypertrophy of the ileum

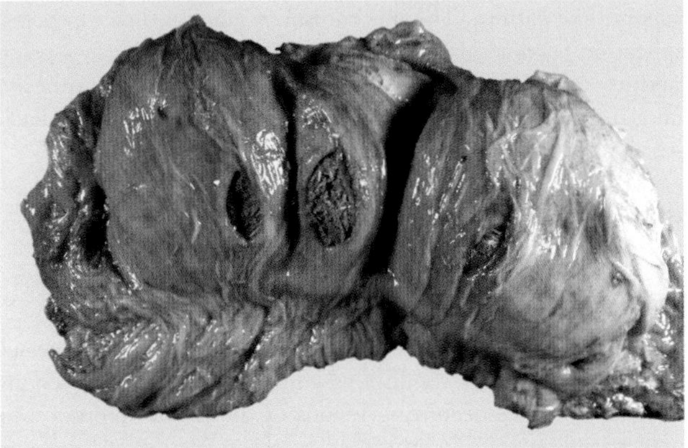

Figure 7-109 **Diverticula, Cecum, Horse.** Diverticula are mucosal outpouchings into the subjacent smooth muscle layers of the colon. They are filled with ingesta and lined by intact mucosa. (Courtesy Dr. H. Gelberg, College of Veterinary Medicine, Oregon State University.)

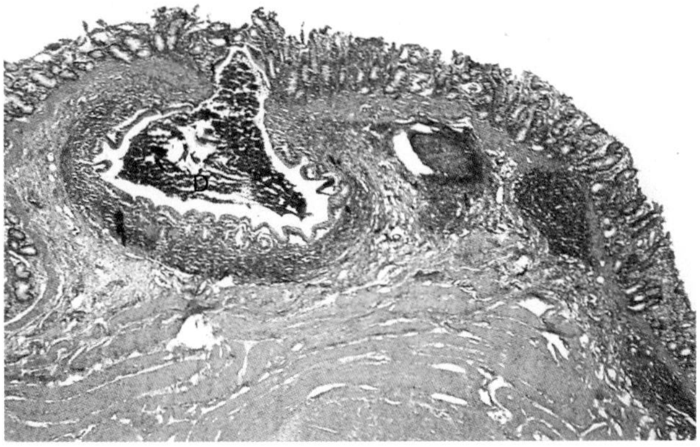

Figure 7-110 **Diverticulum, Colon, Cow.** A diverticulum *(D)* lined by superficial mucosa has penetrated through the submucosa to lie next to the muscularis. H&E stain. (Courtesy Dr. M.D. McGavin, College of Veterinary Medicine, University of Tennessee.)

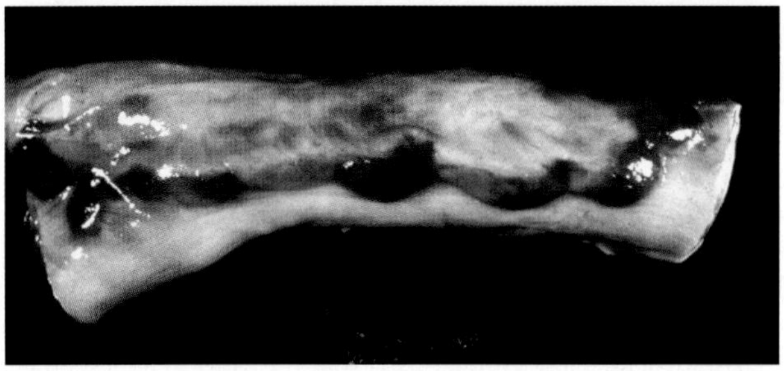

Figure 7-111 **Hemomelasma Ilei, Ileum, Horse.** Hemorrhagic and siderotic *(yellow-brown)* fibrovascular plaques on the antimesenteric serosa are attributed to strongyle larval migration *(Strongylus edentatus)*, but this association has never been demonstrated. (Courtesy Dr. H. Gelberg, College of Veterinary Medicine, Oregon State University.)

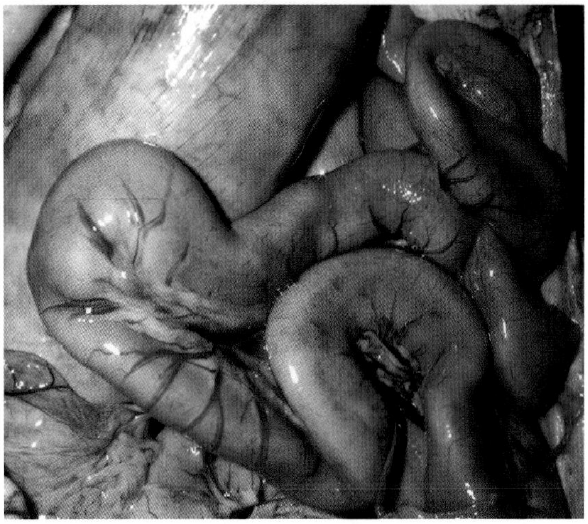

Figure 7-112 **Leiomyometaplasia, Intestine, Dog.** "Brown dog gut" is a rare condition caused by the accumulation of a brown pigment now known to be ceroid (formerly called *lipofuscin*) in the lysosomes of smooth muscle cells of the tunica muscularis. It is a dietary condition associated with vitamin E deficiency. (Courtesy Dr. L. Borst, College of Veterinary Medicine, University of Illinois.)

in pigs generally occurs as an idiopathic, asymptomatic lesion. Muscular hypertrophy of the tunica muscularis associated with diverticulosis of the ileum has been recorded in young Yorkshire pigs and in Romney Marsh and Hampshire sheep. The lesion is suspected to be secondary to a functional obstruction of the ileocecal valve. Diverticulosis and/or intestinal rupture may result.

Cats can have a severe hypertrophy of the inner, circular layer of the tunica muscularis of the ileum and sometimes the jejunum. In cats with hypereosinophilic syndrome, a disease characterized by intramural eosinophil infiltrates, hypertrophy of the gastric antrum and small intestinal musculature can occur. Muscular hypertrophy of the intestine and medial hyperplasia of the pulmonary arteries occur in cats given large oral doses of *Toxocara cati* larvae. These conditions are often accompanied by diarrhea and eosinophilic enteritis. Fibrosis of the lamina propria and hypertrophy of the inner layer of the tunica muscularis may result in a stiff, thickened intestine.

Another unique lesion in the horse is hemomelasma ilei. These lesions are pink to black plaques that vary in length from several millimeters to many centimeters and can occur anywhere in the intestinal subserosa but are generally limited to the ileum (Fig. 7-111; also see Fig. 3-38). They are attributed to larval migrations of strongyles (usually *Strongylus edentatus*) and are located on the antimesenteric serosal surface. However, parasites have never been reported in the lesions, and therefore the cause of hemomelasma ilei is unknown. The lesions are generally of no clinical consequence but can on occasion lead to intestinal strictures and intermittent colic.

Intestinal ceroidosis or leiomyometaplasia is also called *brown dog gut*. The discolored intestinal smooth muscle may occur in association with chronic enteritis and pancreatitis. Experimentally, leiomyometaplasia can be produced in dogs by vitamin E deficiency, in association with excess dietary lipids. The dietary requirement for vitamin E is proportional to the concentration of polyunsaturated fatty acids in the diet. Intestinal ceroidosis probably does not cause clinical signs but may be an indicator of a metabolic or nutritional disorder. In this condition the intestinal serosa varies from tan to dark brown (Fig. 7-112). The stomach and large bowel are variously affected, as is the small intestine. Accumulation of brown, granular, acid-fast–staining ceroid in the perinuclear lysosomes of the leiomyocytes is characteristic of this condition.

Amyloidosis occasionally is present in the intestinal and vascular walls of the lamina propria and muscularis in association with systemic amyloid A infiltrations in a variety of animal species of all ages.

Tiger striping is a nonspecific congestion of colonic ridges secondary to diarrhea and/or tenesmus (E-Fig. 7-17). The red and pale longitudinal stripes are formed by the congested tips of the folds alternating with the uncongested mucosa between them.

Small Intestinal Intoxicants

Because most toxins enter the body through ingestion, those that are irritants can cause contact lesions in the oral cavity, esophagus, stomach, and intestine. The lesions that result are generally those of hemorrhage and inflammation. In many cases of intoxication, induction of vomiting is contraindicated because what burns going down will also burn coming up. For some intoxicants, multidrug resistance (*MDR1*) gene products of enterocytes are part of the detoxification process. In addition, P450 enzymes are present on villus enterocytes, although in much lesser amounts than in the liver. They are in highest concentration in the jejunum and decrease aborally. In human beings, ingestion of grapefruit juice interferes with the function of these enzymes, sometimes resulting in enhanced oral drug availability.

The numbers and types of chemicals and intoxicants animals are exposed to make a listing of them a monumental undertaking. A few examples are phosphorus, arsenic, bracken fern (cattle), mercury, oak, copper, nitrate, thallium, and blister beetles. Blister beetles, a specific toxicity, are sometimes incorporated into crimped hay (Fig. 7-113). They contain a topical irritant called cantharidin. Lesions include sloughing of the epithelium of the stomach and enterocytes of the proximal small intestine (Fig. 7-114). In addition, cantharidin can cause hemorrhagic ulcers of the urinary bladder and myocardial necrosis.

Although not generally considered an intoxicant, corticosteroids cause colonic perforation in some treated dogs and can delay GI healing. They do this by decreasing cell turnover, decreasing mucus production, and stimulating gastrin secretion, leading to increased acid production. NSAIDs can cause *right dorsal colitis* in horses. This colitis is characterized by necrosis, resulting in erosions and ulcers. Epithelial loss may be severe, with only regenerating, rounded islands of normal mucosa remaining. The massive edema of the denuded intestine causes rupture of the submucosa in an elongated diamond-like pattern. The mechanism of injury is direct by topical application (oral administration) and through inhibition of prostaglandin synthesis. Neutrophils play a role by increasing synthesis of tumor necrosis factor-α, leukotriene B_4, and upregulation of leukocyte adhesion molecules.

Vascular Diseases of the Intestine

Strongylus Vulgaris. See Disorders of Horses.

Lymphangiectasia

Lymphangiectasia (i.e., pathologic *dilatation* of lymphatic vessels) may be congenital as a result of vascular malformations or acquired secondary to space-occupying lesions of the lamina propria. Most often it is idiopathic. It results in malabsorption, steatorrhea, and protein-losing enteropathy.

Innervation Disorders

See Dysfunction/Responses to Injury, Intestine, Disorders of Innervation.

Diseases Caused by Specific Pathogens

A number of pathogens affect different animal species in similar ways. The mechanism of damage is similar among these animal species and pathogens. Therefore it is useful to discuss the diseases caused by these organisms across species. Specific diseases that do not have analogues in other species are described later in this chapter. Depending on the mechanism of injury and repair, the morphologic types of infectious enteritis include necrotizing, hemorrhagic, fibrosing, lymphoplasmacytic, eosinophilic, granulomatous, proliferative, catarrhal, pseudomembranous, or combinations of these.

Viral Diseases

Group A Rotavirus Enteritis. Rotaviruses are ubiquitous pathogens present everywhere in the environment, including air and water. Each species of animal has its specific rotavirus, and although broad similarities exist in pathogenesis among viral infection of individual species, in general the viruses are not cross-infective among species. These viruses are important pathogens. Human group A rotavirus, for example, kills a million children a year in the

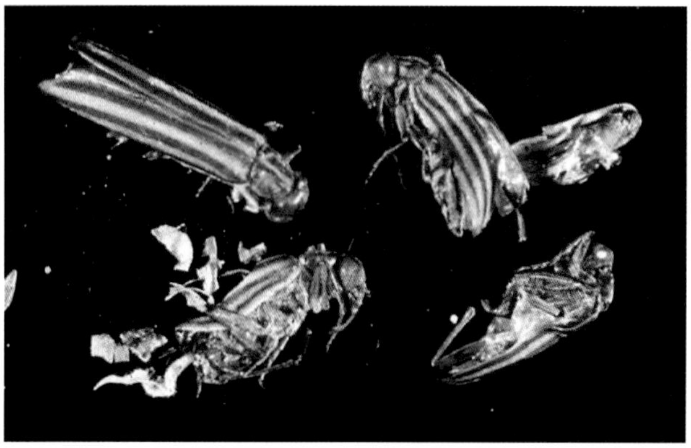

Figure 7-113 **Striped Blister Beetles.** Numerous species of blister beetles (*Epicauta* spp.), such as gray, black, and striped, can be found throughout the United States. They contain a vesicant (blister-causing substance) that causes inflammation and blistering of mucosal surfaces when they are ingested. Usually these beetles are trapped and crushed in crimped hay. (Courtesy Dr. W. Crowell, College of Veterinary Medicine, University of Georgia; and Noah's Arkive, College of Veterinary Medicine, University of Georgia.)

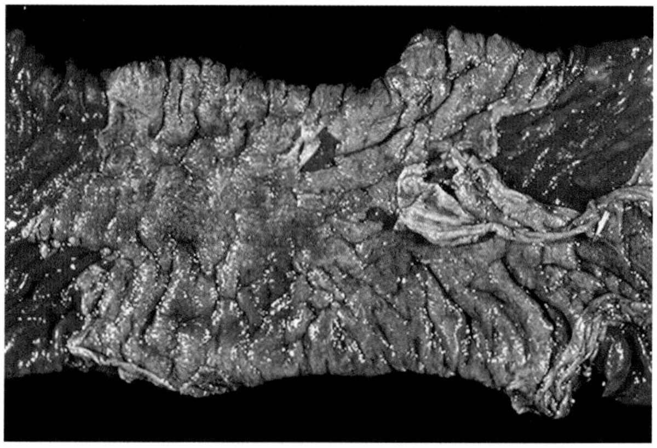

Figure 7-114 **Acute necrohemorrhagic Enteritis, Small Intestine, Horse.** The severe necrosis with sloughing of intestinal mucosa is the result of cantharidin, a toxin contained in ingested blister beetles. (Courtesy Dr. R. Panciera, School of Veterinary Medicine, Oklahoma State University; and Noah's Arkive, College of Veterinary Medicine, The University of Georgia.)

developing countries of the world. In all species these viruses cause disease in association with other enteropathogens of neonates.

In calves the disease is most important during the first week of life and in piglets in the first 7 weeks of life. These ages correspond to the reduction of colostral and milk-associated antirotavirus antibody titers that occur after weaning. Specific diagnosis of these diseases is difficult for a variety of reasons. The virus is ubiquitous and therefore can be isolated or detected in many animals, most of whom do not have clinical disease. Additionally, because the viruses are cytolytic, some animals with viral diarrhea can be negative for viruses because the cells harboring the virus have been shed previously in the feces.

Rotaviruses are approximately 70 nm in diameter and are trilayered. Only the complete triple-layered virion is infectious. Rotaviruses have double-stranded RNA at their core, and protein spikes project from the surface. The complete particle looks like a wheel, thus the appellation *rotavirus*. The route of infection is oral, and the target cells are villus enterocytes. Piglets and calves with rotavirus disease are dehydrated, have yellow, watery diarrhea, and are weak and depressed. Production of clinical disease depends on the amount of villous epithelium that is lost. This varies by host species.

Pathogenesis. The epithelial cells over the upper two-thirds of the affected villi of the proximal small intestine are infected first in those species that suffer with severe diarrhea from rotavirus infection (E-Fig. 7-18). Sloughing of villous cells results in shortening and sometimes fusion of villi, if basement membranes are exposed (Fig. 7-115). Interestingly, besides causing a malabsorptive diarrhea, rotaviruses produce a secretory enterotoxin nonstructural protein (NSP4) that increases chloride secretion through a calcium-dependent mechanism. This toxin also activates the enteric nervous system and blocks the intestinal sodium/glucose cotransporter. All of these increase fluid and the rate of peristalsis in the intestinal lumen. Depending on the degree of enterocyte loss, recovery may be delayed or incomplete, depending on the amount of absorptive surface that is permanently lost. When death occurs, it is generally associated with intercurrent infections with those organisms that also target villous epithelial cells such as coronavirus, *Cryptosporidium*, *E. coli*, coccidia, and others.

Coronavirus Enteritis. Coronaviruses responsible for calfhood enteritis (at 100 to 120 nm) are larger than rotaviruses. Their genetic core is single-stranded RNA. Peplomers project from the surface, resulting in the appearance of a corona, such as created by the sun; hence the appellation *coronavirus*. The clinical course of the disease, histologic lesions, mechanism of diarrhea production, and age of affected calves are very similar to those of rotavirus enteritis, although somewhat prolonged. Virus infection is more virulent than in rotavirus enteritis, and death is more common. Colitis occurs in addition to small intestinal involvement, but the principal disease signs and pathogenicity are related to the small intestinal lesions. In the colon, similar to the small intestine, enterocytes when lost are initially replaced by less mature and often squamoid cells.

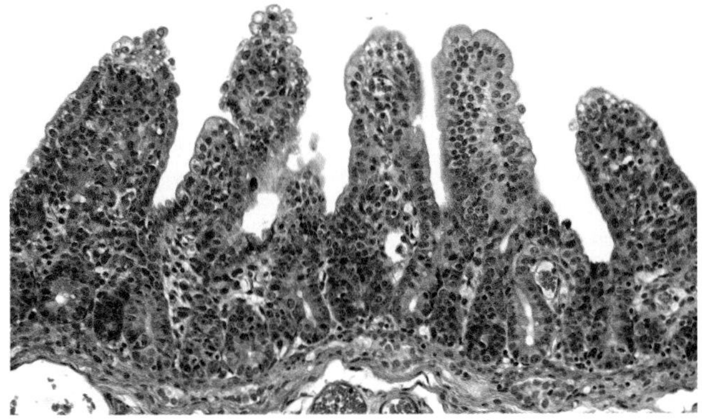

Figure 7-115 Rotavirus Enteritis, Jejunum, Piglet. There is notable blunting and fusion of intestinal villi secondary to virus-induced cytolysis of enterocytes covering the tips and sides of intestinal villi. H&E stain. (Courtesy Dr. J.F. Zachary, College of Veterinary Medicine, University of Illinois.)

Although generally a mild and self-limiting disease of neonates, feline enteric coronavirus has been associated with fatal enteritis in a series of cats. Lesions consist of degeneration and loss of enterocytes from jejunal villous tips. Cats 2 months to 7 years old are affected.

Pathogenesis. Unlike in rotavirus enteritis, crypt lumens contain cell debris and crypt cells may be focally hyperplastic, indicating attempts at enterocyte replacement and villus repair. The lamina propria and draining lymph nodes often contain increased numbers of inflammatory cells. A hemorrhagic form of the disease with extensive colitis has been reported.

Adenovirus Enteritis. Adenoviral infection occurs in cattle, sheep, pigs, goats, Spanish ibex, cervids, horses, and inland bearded dragons. Each species-specific virus causes inapparent respiratory disease and under some circumstances, clinical enteric disease. Other organs may also be affected, such as the liver and kidneys. Endothelial cells are often affected. In Arabian horses and Arabian crossbreeds, adenovirus enteritis occurs in association with combined immunodeficiency. Adenovirus is transmitted by aerosols, feces, and fomites. When enteritis is produced, characteristic basophilic to amphophilic intranuclear inclusion bodies are present in villous enterocytes, usually in young animals that are immunosuppressed. Endothelial cells also are affected and have similar inclusions. Loss of enterocytes results in villous blunting and fusion. In general, adenovirus infection is subclinical, although severe enteric disease may occur in calves.

Bacterial Diseases

Escherichia coli Diseases (Colibacillosis). Coliform bacteria arrive early among the normal flora that colonizes the intestinal tract of virtually all animals. Young animals are at highest risk for coliform diarrhea, especially pigs and calves. There is interplay of many intrinsic and extrinsic factors that act together to determine if disease will be produced by infection. Some of the factors are the genetic makeup of the host animals, the passive transfer of specific antibodies in the colostrums, the constant bathing of the intestine with milk-associated antibodies from nursing, environmental contamination, and the nutritional plane of the host. Environmental stressors predisposing to disease production include temperature extremes, crowding, and intercurrent infections with rotavirus, coronavirus, *Cryptosporidium*, coccidia, and others. The development of unique serotypes of *E. coli* may cause problems in individual environments. *E. coli* has a large number of mobile genetic elements. Gain or loss of these elements is responsible for the adaptability of *E. coli* as a commensal and pathogenic agent. In the past, autogenous vaccines, made to order for these environments, have been reasonably effective in controlling some disease outbreaks. Probiotics containing several *E. coli* types and/or *Lactobacillus* spp. have shown promise as a preventive in calves. Lytic phages have also been promising in eliminating infection.

There are a variety of classification schemes for the *E. coli* enteritides. They include enterotoxic (ETEC), septicemic (EIEC), edema disease (enterotoxemic), postweaning, enterohemorrhagic (EHEC),

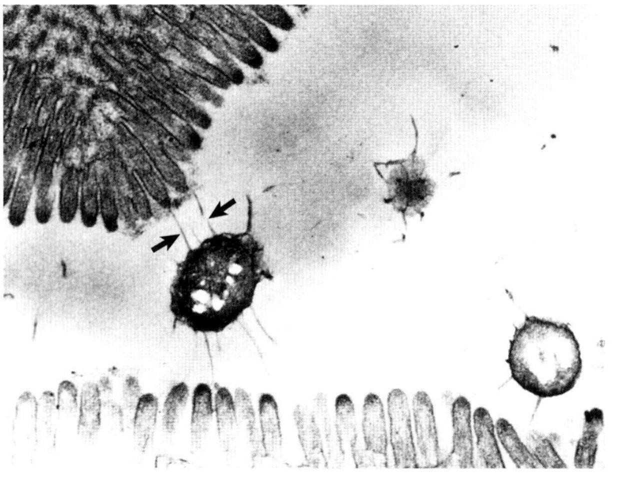

Figure 7-116 **Colibacillosis, Intestine, Piglet.** *Escherichia coli* pili *(arrows)* are attached to enterocytes. TEM. Uranyl acetate and lead citrate stain. (Courtesy Dr. R. Isaacson, College of Veterinary Medicine, University of Minnesota.)

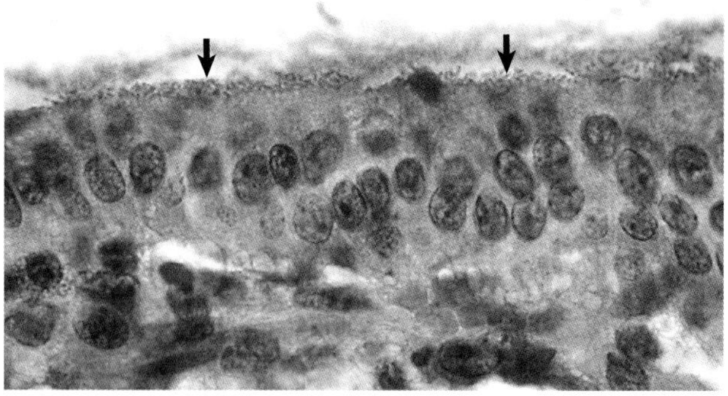

Figure 7-117 **Enterotoxic Colibacillosis, Jejunum, Piglet.** Mats *(arrows)* of *Escherichia coli* are attached to the microvillous surface of the enterocytes. H&E stain. (Courtesy Dr. H. Gelberg, College of Veterinary Medicine, Oregon State University.)

enteroinvasive, and enteropathogenic/attaching and effacing (EPEC/AAEC), among others (also see Chapter 4).

E. coli attaches to cells by a variety of pili or fimbriae (Fig. 7-116). Enterotoxic *E. coli* may have fimbrial antigens F4 (K88), F5 (K99), F6 (987P), 18, or 41 and may also produce up to three enterotoxins and Shiga toxins (STa, STb, LT). Fimbrial and nonfimbrial adhesins, such as adhesins involved in diffuse adherence (AIDA-1), may also be present. Many *E. coli* produce verotoxins (verotoxic *E. coli* [VTEC]) important in disease pathogenesis. More than 200 serotypes of verotoxic *E. coli* have been isolated from cattle alone. Diagnosis of toxin-producing *E. coli* is by selective culture properties of the bacteria, immunomagnetic separation, and other monoclonal-based immunoassays for the verotoxins and Shiga toxins. A more recent development is the use of real-time PCR to detect pathogenic gene sequences. Many of the virulence factors of *E. coli* can be exchanged among *E. coli* and other bacterial species by phages, as well as plasmids.

Enterotoxic Colibacillosis. Enterotoxic, or enterotoxigenic, colibacillosis (ETEC) (F18ac) occurs most often in animals 2 days to 3 weeks of age. Calves and piglets are most often affected. Why enterotoxic colibacillosis is a disease of neonates is not well understood. Some speculation is that enteric bacterial colonization is a function of gastric acidity and that the low pH of the stomach of postneonatal animals kills the bacteria.

The diarrhea that occurs is largely a function of bacterial endotoxin-induced cGMP-dependent and cyclic guanosine monophosphate-adenosine monophosphate (cGAMP)-dependent kinase-induced sodium and chloride secretion into the intestinal lumen. Water is drawn into the intestine to normalize the resultant sodium chloride. Thus the diarrhea is termed *secretory*. Diarrhea is voluminous, yellow to white, and watery to pasty. At necropsy the small intestine is dilated, flaccid, and filled with translucent, yellow fluid and sometimes gas. Chyle is present in the mesenteric lymphatic vessels similar to animals without enteric disease, indicating that unlike the malabsorptive diseases of the small intestine, absorption proceeds normally in cases of enterotoxic colibacillosis. Microscopically, the intestine is also normal. Diagnosis can be made by light microscopic examination in freshly dead animals by noting the presence of bacteria lining the luminal surface of the enterocytes (Fig. 7-117). Inflammation is absent. Affected animals are dehydrated, with a "tucked-up" abdomen. Subsequent to dehydration the eyes of affected animals may be recessed deeply into their sockets (sunken eyeballs). Animals that die from enterotoxic *E. coli* infection are often emaciated and have diarrheic feces pasted around their perineum.

Septicemic Colibacillosis. Septicemic or enteroinvasive colibacillosis (EIEC) is a disease of newborn calves, lambs, and occasionally foals that have not received sufficient colostrum to develop immunity. Although the lesions produced are generally those of septicemia, similar to those caused by other organisms, infection can localize in the intestine, causing enteritis. Diagnosis is generally made by finding fibrin in any location in the body such as the eye, joints, abdomen, heart sac, meninges, and/or thorax. The bacteria gain entry to the body through the respiratory system, oral cavity, or umbilicus. Fibrinous arthritis, ophthalmitis, serositis, meningitis (polyserositis), and white-spotted kidneys (cortical abscesses) characterize the septicemia (see Fig. 11-63). Mixed bacterial infections often occur with enterotoxic *E. coli*.

Edema Disease. See Disorders of Pigs.

Postweaning Colibacillosis. See Disorders of Pigs.

Enterohemorrhagic Colibacillosis. Enterohemorrhagic colibacillosis (EHEC) is described in human beings, laboratory animals, and occasionally cattle and pigs. It has not been reported as a field problem in livestock. The pathogenesis of the disease is similar to that of other invasive bacteria such as *Salmonella* spp. In human beings the colon is affected. A Shiga toxin gene, a locus for enterocyte effacement, and a plasmid encoding for hemolysin are produced by *E. coli*, which result in hemorrhagic colitis and sometimes the hemolytic uremic syndrome. These strains are also called *verotoxic E. coli*, which are strains based on the Vero (African green monkey kidney) cell line on which the bacteria are sometimes grown. Outbreaks of enteroinvasive colibacillosis in human beings are often food-borne illnesses. These organisms are pathogenic because of their acid resistance and ability to survive transport through the stomach. Shiga toxin–producing enterohemorrhagic *E. coli* O157:H7 rarely causes naturally occurring disease in domestic livestock but often contaminates ground beef. Surveys have indicated that the seroprevalence of *E. coli* O157:H7 in dairy herds is 38.5%, with an individual cow prevalence of 6.5%, and is most often isolated from the skin surface. This finding is an important reason not to eat undercooked ground beef. Steaks are a different matter because bacterial contamination is only a surface phenomenon, and bacteria are killed by surface searing of meat.

Experimentally, calves may develop necrohemorrhagic or mucohemorrhagic diarrhea. Human disease can be serious, resulting in hemorrhagic colitis, thrombocytopenic purpura, and the hemolytic uremic syndrome. Deer, sheep, cattle, horses, dogs, and rabbits, including laboratory rabbits, may be carriers. Stable flies and fecal contamination of a variety of substances may create fomites.

Attaching and Effacing *Escherichia coli.* Attaching and effacing *E. coli* (AAEC), also called enteropathogenic *E. coli* (EPEC), has been infrequently reported in rabbits, calves, pigs, lambs, dogs, and human beings. The actual incidence of this disease in domestic animals is unknown. Lesions are characterized by *E. coli* attachment to the microvillous border of enterocytes and gallbladder epithelium via cups and pedestals (E-Fig. 7-19). Intimin, a bacterial outer membrane protein, facilitates bacterial attachment to the host cell's membrane, resulting in attachment and effacement. These bacteria also alter a variety of tight junction proteins and therefore cause leakage of enterocyte tight junctions. Gross lesions are not present except that the intestine is dilated and fluid filled. Colonization of the epithelium by attaching and effacing *E. coli* is relatively common; disease occurs most often in association with other enteropathogens of calves of this age, namely rotavirus, *C. parvum*, enterotoxic *E. coli*, coronavirus, bovine viral diarrhea virus, and coccidia. In contrast to enterotoxic *E. coli* infection, in attaching and effacing *E. coli* infection the brush border of the enterocytes is disrupted and can be seen on select enterocytes in hematoxylin and eosin (H&E)-stained tissue sections. Microvillous disruption results in loss of the glycocalyx digestive enzymes, resulting in maldigestion, malabsorption, and diarrhea. Attaching and effacing *E. coli* also stimulates enterocyte apoptosis, Cl^- and mucus secretion, and toxin production. Attaching and effacing *E. coli* flagellin TLR5 stimulates interleukin (IL)-8 release by enterocytes, which initiates an inflammatory response resulting in cell death and fluid secretion.

Extraintestinal Pathogenic *Escherichia coli.* Extraintestinal pathogenic *E. coli* (ExPEC) are gut inhabitants with virulence genes that differ from strains of *E. coli* that are enteropathogens or commensal organisms of the intestine. They contain fimbrial adhesins for attachment, cytotoxins and hemolysins responsible for tissue necrosis and hemorrhage, and siderophore receptors to sequester iron. Extraintestinal pathogenic *E. coli* can be isolated from the feces of many healthy animals, particularly dogs and cats. When the animals are stressed, such as in group housing in shelters, aerosolized bacteria may be inhaled, resulting in fulminating necrohemorrhagic pleuropneumonia. Septicemia can result in urogenital infections. In addition, meningitis has been reported in human beings. There is concern about the zoonotic potential of these organisms.

Salmonellosis. *Salmonella* spp. are enteroinvasive bacteria. All known species of *Salmonella* are pathogenic, and salmonellosis is an important zoonosis and nosocomial infection. Salmonellosis is a significant cause of acute and chronic diarrhea and death in numerous animal species and in human beings. *S. typhimurium* is the second most common food-borne pathogen in human beings. In veterinary medicine, salmonellosis can occur epizootically, enzootically, or sporadically. The serovars most often isolated from diseased animals include *S. typhimurium*, *Salmonella enterica*, *Salmonella dublin*, *Salmonella choleraesuis*, and *Salmonella typhosa*.

The salmonellas are Gram-negative, aerobic to facultatively anaerobic, and motile. They survive and multiply within phagocytic cells, resulting in granulomatous inflammation. One way that they survive in the hostile environment of the phagosomes of professional phagocytes is by producing a nitrite transporter through their pathogenicity island (SPI-2) that neutralizes nitric oxide production by the phagocytosing cell. The form of salmonellosis that occurs—septicemic, acute enteric, or chronic enteric—depends on the challenge dosage of the bacterium, previous exposure to the bacterium, and stress factors such as overcrowding, transport, cold temperatures, feed changes, pregnancy, parturition, surgery, anesthesia, and antibiotic administration. Some recovered animals become carriers and shed the organism in their feces, particularly after stress. This may make diagnosis by culture difficult because carriers may not be ill. Conversely, antibiotic treatment of ill animals may create false-negative bacterial cultures. Although dogs and cats rarely get clinical salmonellosis, 10% are carriers and can infect their human companions. It has been documented that fatal salmonellosis may occur in cats in association with homemade, raw-meat diets.

The most common route of bacterial entry is fecal-oral. Effective hand washing is thus of paramount importance for food handlers ("typhoid Mary"). Besides being present in contaminated feed, water, and aerosols, salmonella can be transmitted by flies and fomites. Transplacental infection may also occur. After ingestion, salmonella may colonize regional lymphoid tissue in the oral cavity and gut through dendritic cells by means of pathogenicity islands, which are clusters of plasmid genes coding for virulence factors such as fimbriae, motility, lipopolysaccharide (LPS), and other secreted proteins. Some species of *Salmonella* are enteroinvasive.

S. choleraesuis and *typhimurium* in pigs have been shown to adhere to apical membranes of M cells, enterocytes, goblet cells, and sites of cellular extrusion. Salmonellas produce disease via enterotoxins, cytotoxins (verotoxins), and endotoxins, some of which block closure of Cl^- channels. In addition, inflammatory cells upregulate PGE_2, which results in hypersecretion of chloride. Secretory diarrhea results, as well as malabsorptive diarrhea from enterocyte death. Experimental infections of calves with *S. typhimurium* demonstrate upregulation of CXC chemokines (IL-8, growth-related oncogene-α [GRO-α], and granulocyte chemotactic protein-2 [GCP-2]), IL-1β, IL-1 receptor-α (IL-1Rα), and IL-4 associated with a neutrophilic influx. Once in contact with macrophages of the lamina propria or Peyer's patches, the organisms are phagocytosed and transported to regional lymph nodes or by way of the portal circulation to the liver. The organisms colonize the small intestine, colon, mesenteric lymph nodes, and gallbladder, which may serve as reservoirs in carrier animals. Salmonellosis infects the young more frequently; the young are more severely affected than are adults; and the young are more likely to succumb to septicemia.

Peracute *Salmonella* Septicemia. Peracute *Salmonella* septicemia is a disease of calves, foals, and pigs. Young animals are generally at greater risk than older animals, although the reasons for this difference are not understood. In foals the feces of affected animals are typically green. The serovar of *Salmonella* most often involved in septicemic salmonellosis is *S. choleraesuis*. Gross lesions of animals dying of peracute *Salmonella* septicemia are minimal and are caused by fibrinoid necrosis of blood vessels (Fig. 7-118). Necrosis of blood vessels causes widespread petechiation and a blue discoloration (cyanosis) of the extremities and ventrum of white pigs. Fibrinous polyserositis may be present. Peracute *Salmonella* septicemia is usually fatal in animals 1 to 6 months of age. Death is usually attributable to disseminated intravascular coagulopathy secondary to the generalized Shwartzman reaction.

Acute Enteric Salmonellosis. Acute enteric salmonellosis is caused most frequently by *S. typhimurium* and occurs in cattle, pigs, and horses. Carnivores are rarely affected. Characteristic of the disease is diffuse catarrhal enteritis with diffuse fibrinonecrotic ileotyphlocolitis. Intestinal contents are malodorous and contain mucus, fibrin, and occasionally blood. The feces have a septic tank odor. *Salmonella* are enteroinvasive through specific surface bacterial fimbrial (pilus adhesin) antigens. Receptor-mediated endocytosis then occurs. Membrane-bound vacuoles then translocate the bacteria to macrophages in the lamina propria. The intact *Salmonella* induce secretory diarrhea through interference with Cl^- channels. They also induce enterocyte apoptosis and recruit neutrophils.

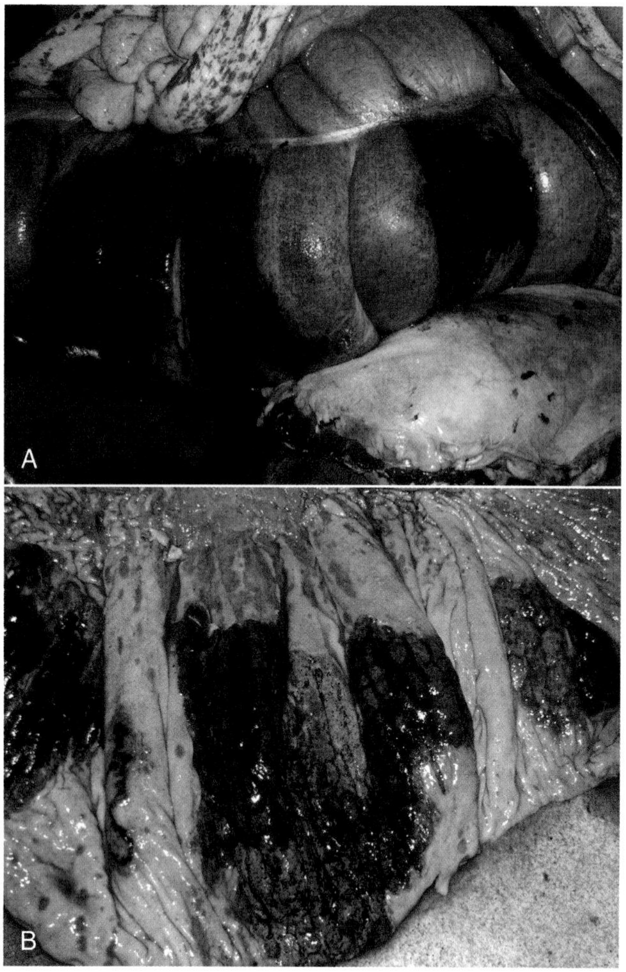

Figure 7-118 **Peracute to Acute Salmonellosis, Colon, Horse. A,** Serosal surfaces. Note the areas of hemorrhage and necrosis affecting multiple sacculations. This pattern is consistent with colonic infarcts secondary to ischemia caused by vascular thrombosis, which can occur with peracute and/or acute salmonellosis. **B,** Mucosal surfaces. Note the extensive mucosal edema and gray-white areas of mucosal necrosis. The green-stained tissue is postmortem imbibition. Mucosal erosions and ulcerations are also present. (Courtesy Dr. A. Gillen, College of Veterinary Medicine, University of Illinois.)

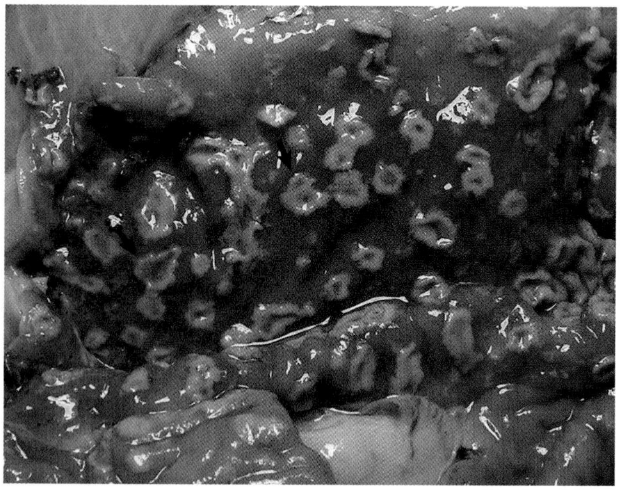

Figure 7-119 **Button Ulcers, Colon, Pig.** Multiple foci of necrosis (infarcts [*arrows*]) due to chronic enteric salmonellosis are termed *button ulcers* and are pathognomonic for this disease in North America and in other areas in which hog cholera has been eradicated. The morphologic features of this lesion are attributable to bacterial toxin-induced vasculitis and thrombosis of blood vessels in the lamina propria and submucosa resulting in focal intestinal infarcts. (Courtesy Dr. D. Driemeier, Federal University of Rio Grande do Sul, Brazil.)

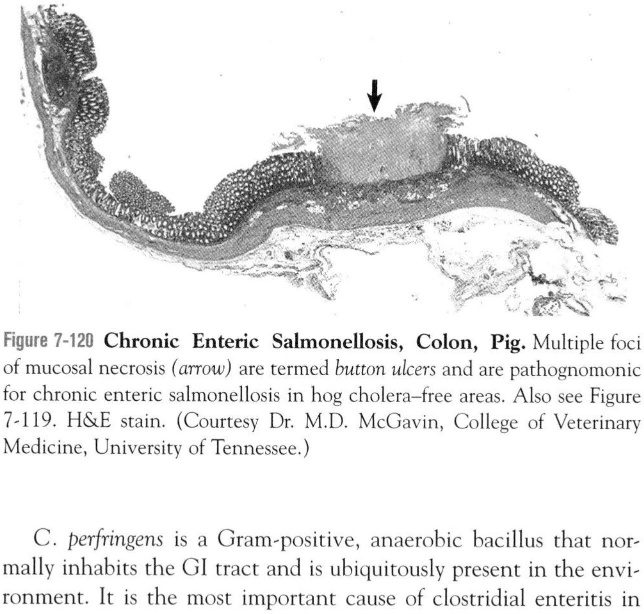

Figure 7-120 **Chronic Enteric Salmonellosis, Colon, Pig.** Multiple foci of mucosal necrosis (*arrow*) are termed *button ulcers* and are pathognomonic for chronic enteric salmonellosis in hog cholera–free areas. Also see Figure 7-119. H&E stain. (Courtesy Dr. M.D. McGavin, College of Veterinary Medicine, University of Tennessee.)

Endotoxins induce thrombosis. All these adherence and inflammatory changes are regulated by pathogenicity islands. Multiple foci of hepatocellular necrosis and hyperplasia of Kupffer cells (paratyphoid nodules), when present, are characteristic of acute enteric salmonellosis (see Fig. 8-54). Mesenteric lymphadenopathy is usually present. Fibrinous cholecystitis at necropsy is pathognomonic for acute enteric salmonellosis in calves (see Fig. 8-85).

Chronic Enteric Salmonellosis. Chronic enteric salmonellosis occurs in pigs, cattle, and horses. Lesions are seen principally in pigs that have discrete foci of necrosis and ulceration, principally in the cecum and colon. These are termed *button ulcers* (Figs. 7-119 and 7-120). Because salmonellosis causes vascular thrombosis and pigs have poor or no collateral blood supply to the rectum (cranial hemorrhoidal artery), in affected animals, rectal strictures develop, with resultant abdominal distention secondary to fecal retention.

Clostridial Enteritis. Clostridial organisms cause many diseases that affect animals and human beings. This discussion is limited to those clostridia that produce diarrheal disease. All clostridial enteritides produce enterotoxemias.

C. perfringens is a Gram-positive, anaerobic bacillus that normally inhabits the GI tract and is ubiquitously present in the environment. It is the most important cause of clostridial enteritis in domestic animals. At least 17 exotoxins have been described, but only 4 are believed to be involved in the pathogenesis of disease. Toxin genes are often present on plasmids. These spore-forming bacilli produce their toxins when circumstances provide them with an excess of nutrients that promote bacterial growth in an anaerobic environment. The four major toxins—α (CPA), β (CPB), ε (ETX), and ι (ITX)—are used to classify the toxigenic types of *C. perfringens* into five major groupings, A through E. The toxins are protein exotoxins, some of which are proenzymes, whereas others have enzymatic activity. *C. perfringens* type A produces the α-toxin responsible for necrotic enteritis of birds, enterotoxemia of calves and lambs, necrotizing enterocolitis of piglets, canine hemorrhagic enteritis, and possibly equine colitis. Type B produces α-, β-, and ε-toxins and the diseases lamb dysentery, hemorrhagic enteritis of neonatal calves and foals, and hemorrhagic enterotoxemia of sheep.

Type C produces α- and β-toxins and necrotic enteritis of birds, hemorrhagic enterotoxemia of neonatal farm animal species, and struck of sheep. Type D produces α- and ε-toxins and pulpy kidney disease of lambs and enterocolitis of goats of all ages. Type E produces α- and ι-toxins and enteritis of lagomorphs and possibly enterotoxemia in calves and lambs.

Enterotoxigenic strains of *C. perfringens*, particularly type A, are responsible for clostridial food poisoning. This generally occurs when cooked foods are improperly stored, and spores that survive the cooking environment germinate and produce enterotoxin.

Enterotoxemia. Enterotoxemia is produced by one of the five *C. perfringens* types described previously. Type D occurs most often. Clostridial enterotoxemia most often affects the better-fleshed animals within a group. Outbreaks often follow an abrupt change in the amount or quality of feed such as occurs in an animal being "finished" for sale or slaughter. In foals, enterotoxemia has been associated with feeding materials rich in carbohydrates and proteins. This diet leads to a change in the intestinal microbial balance. *C. perfringens* proliferates and produces abundant toxin. Clinical signs may be absent before death or may include diarrhea, sometimes with blood. Glycosuria occurs only in lambs with enterotoxemia and is a helpful feature in preliminary necropsy diagnosis. Enzyme-linked immunosorbent assay (ELISA) kits are available for toxin typing (CPA, CPB, ETX) and for the bacteria.

The small intestine, the target organ of clostridial enterotoxemia, typically has serosal and mucosal petechiae, ecchymoses, and paintbrush or diffuse hemorrhage similar in appearance to those of intestinal strangulation. The intestines are atonic and dilated. Emphysematous enteritis is variably present, as is coagulative necrosis of skeletal muscle. Congestive splenomegaly is present. On exposure to enterotoxin, villous tip enterocytes and midvillous enterocytes degenerate and are sloughed into the intestinal lumen, leaving denuded basement membranes. The exposed basement membranes allow fluid leakage and attract leukocytes into the lamina propria. Death is usually rapid.

***Clostridium perfringens* Type A.** *C. perfringens* type A is the most frequently occurring clostridium in mammals and birds. It is also the most common clostridium found in the environment. *C. perfringens* type A produces enteric disease in a great variety of animals. These diarrheal diseases are generally mild with minimal damage to the intestinal mucosa. In addition to enteritis, infection produces gas gangrene and other anaerobic wound infections. In the western United States, it causes hemorrhagic abomasitis in young ruminants, often accompanied by severe diarrhea. In the Pacific Northwest, principally in Washington and Oregon, a condition called yellow lamb disease is associated with *C. perfringens* type A. Death is rapid and accompanied by clinical and pathologic signs of hemolysis, hence the yellow discoloration of the carcass.

***Clostridium perfringens* Type B.** See Disorders of Ruminants (Cattle, Sheep, and Goats).

***Clostridium perfringens* Type C.** Enterotoxic hemorrhagic enteritis affects calves, lambs, and foals during the first few days of life and piglets during the first 8 hours of life. Adult horses may also be affected. Susceptibility of neonates is partially attributed to the antitrypsin activity of colostrum because β-toxin is susceptible to trypsin. Some foods also have antitrypsin effects, and trypsin is sometimes lacking in pancreatic disease. Clinical signs vary from none to bloody diarrhea. When piglets are affected, the whole litter dies. Lesions at necropsy include hemorrhagic or necrotizing enteritis of the small intestines, sometimes with gas in the lumen and within the walls of the intestine (Figs. 7-121 and 7-122). In piglets it has been demonstrated that β-toxin induces endothelial damage that is important in disease pathogenesis. Struck, which is also caused by *C. perfringens* type C, affects adult sheep, goats, and feedlot cattle in winter and early spring and is characterized by hemorrhagic enteritis with ulceration, ascites, and peritonitis.

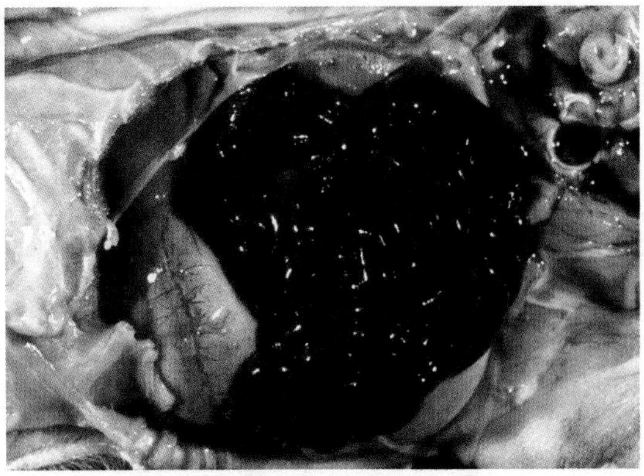

Figure 7-121 Enterotoxemia, Small Intestine, Piglet. The entire small intestinal mucosa is hemorrhagic. Necrosis can extend through the muscularis mucosa and is caused by toxins of the *Clostridium perfringens* type C group acting directly on the intestinal mucosa in the intestinal lumen. The entire litter of piglets was affected. (Courtesy Dr. H. Gelberg, College of Veterinary Medicine, Oregon State University.)

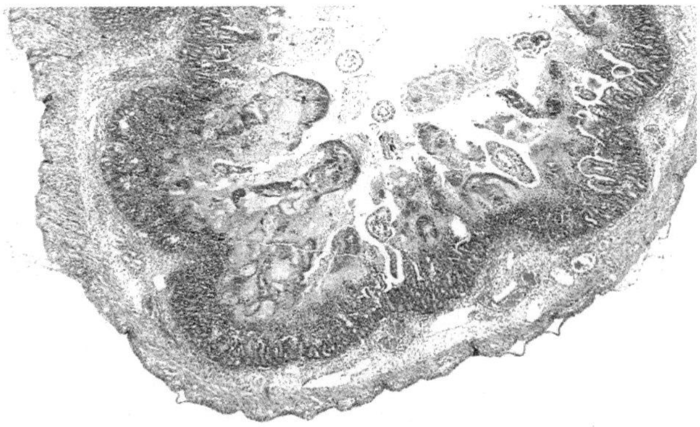

Figure 7-122 Clostridial Enteritis, Small Intestine, Pig. Nonspecific necrotizing enteritis results from the toxins produced by *Clostridium perfringens* type C. Note the disorganization, shortening, and pale staining (with H&E stain) of intestinal villi. H&E stain. (Courtesy Dr. H. Gelberg, College of Veterinary Medicine, Oregon State University.)

***Clostridium perfringens* type D.** See Disorders of Ruminants (Cattle, Sheep, and Goats).

***Clostridium perfringens* type E.** Case reports of necrohemorrhagic diarrhea associated with *C. perfringens* type E infection are poorly documented. It is safest to state that *C. perfringens* type E may rarely cause enterotoxemia of lambs, calves, and rabbits.

Peracute Hemorrhagic Gastroenteritis of Dogs. See Disorders of Dogs.

Lincomycin or Antibiotic Enteritis. Lincomycin or antibiotic enteritis is associated with antibiotic administration and is seen most commonly in rabbits and horses; both are cecal fermenters. It has been suggested but not proved that antibiotic administration causes death of normal enteric flora, which allows overgrowth of *C. perfringens* type A. Clinical signs and gross and microscopic lesions are similar to those observed in animals with *Clostridium* spp. enteritis, but bacterial organisms are often lacking.

Clostridium piliforme. *Clostridium piliforme* infects multiple mammalian species and is commonly called *Tyzzer's disease*. The target organs of *C. piliforme* vary among affected animals. Although

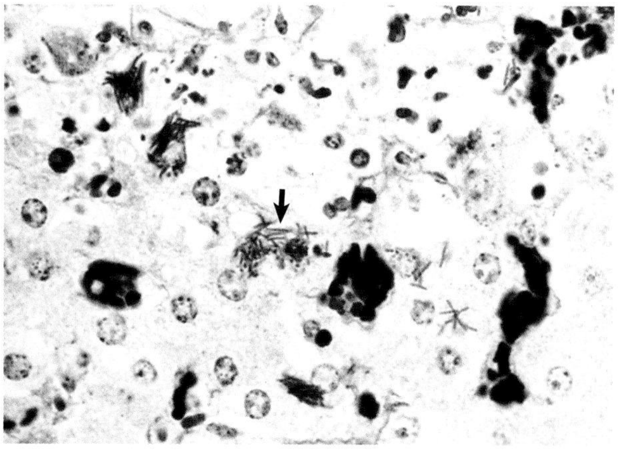

Figure 7-123 **Tyzzer's Disease, Liver, Foal.** Criss-crossed bacilli *(arrow)* resembling Chinese characters or pickup sticks are diagnostic of infection with *Clostridium piliforme*. Warthin-Starry stain. (Courtesy Dr. H. Gelberg, College of Veterinary Medicine, Oregon State University.)

pathogen entry is usually via the intestine, the principal target is the liver, but lesions also occur in the intestine and heart. Intestinal involvement is variable and most common in rodents and rabbits. The enteric manifestations of Tyzzer's disease are generally in the distal small intestine, particularly the ileum. Colitis occurs in some cats. Mucosal necrosis and edema extend into the muscularis. Definitive diagnosis is made by finding the causative bacillus (best done with silver stains such as Dieterle's or Steiner's) in the characteristic hepatic lesions (Fig. 7-123; also see Fig. 8-53).

Clostridium difficile. *Clostridium difficile* spores are common in the environment and in the intestinal tract of many mammals. They cause pseudomembranous colitis in primates, including human beings, hemorrhagic necrotizing enterocolitis in foals, necrotizing typhlocolitis in horses (colitis X) and possibly cats, and enteritis in a variety of laboratory animals. *C. difficile* also affects suckling pigs in outbreaks characterized by mesocolonic edema and typhlocolitis. Dogs, especially those hospitalized, may also shed the organism. The disease-producing ability of *C. difficile* in the dog is not understood, but its zoonotic potential may be important. The induction of disease by *C. difficile* is likely dose related, but the reasons for bacterial overgrowth, apart from those caused by oral antibiotic administration, are not known. The lesions are similar to those produced by *C. perfringens* infection.

Lawsoniasis. *Lawsonia intracellularis* is the cause of a proliferative segmental enteropathy in a variety of species, including human beings. *Lawsonia* are curved, Gram-negative, motile, and obligate intracellular bacteria that cannot be grown on artificial media. Lesions of proliferative enteropathy have been reported in pigs, dogs, horses, sheep, rabbits, guinea pigs, hamsters, rats, ferrets, foxes, cervids, monkeys, ostriches, and emus. In the dog the majority of cases occur in puppies younger than 3 months. The mechanism of enterocyte proliferation may relate to *Lawsonia*-induced altered transcription of host "alarm response" genes that affect regulation of the cell cycle and cell differentiation. Lesions consist of surface erosions and proliferation of cryptal enterocytes with the presence of bacteria in the apical cytoplasm of affected cells. Diagnosis depends on characteristic histologic findings of crypt cell proliferation and on the presence of comma-shaped bacteria in the intestinal crypt epithelial cytoplasm. Clinically, diarrhea is of 5 to 15 days' duration. The diarrhea is mucoid or watery, with or without blood, and is accompanied by partial anorexia, vomiting, and a slight fever.

Campylobacter. *Campylobacter* infections from asymptomatic poultry (*Campylobacter jejuni*) and pigs (*Campylobacter coli*) are an important issue in food safety and thus an important emerging zoonotic disease. Although *C. jejuni* is present in a high percentage of dogs without clinical signs, it has been associated with mild enterocolitis in kennels.

Yersiniosis. *Yersinia* are Gram-negative aerobic to facultative anaerobic coccobacilli. The species *enterocolitica* and *pseudotuberculosis* are normal gut inhabitants that may cause mild to severe diarrhea, septicemia, or lymphadenitis, primarily in ruminants. Pigs, cervids, horses, wild ungulates, poultry, and human beings (food borne) are also susceptible to infection and disease. Carrier states exist in many species, including dogs and cats, and cool climates support bacterial growth and environmental contamination. The bacteria invade the intestine through M cells overlying GALT via bacterial invasins and cell-associated β_1 integrins and then spread systemically. Microabscesses and granulomas, including giant cells, occur randomly in the intestinal lamina propria and crypts, and there is widespread lymphoid necrosis. The bacteria are extracellular and intracellular, and there is massive recruitment of host neutrophils. Histologic diagnosis with bacterial isolation is definitive.

Intestinal Mycobacteriosis. Intestinal tuberculosis, caused by *M. tuberculosis* and *Mycobacterium bovis*, is an uncommon disease in cattle, nursing calves, nonhuman primates, and human beings. Although historically associated with drinking unpasteurized milk, more recently, intestinal tuberculosis is an important acquired immunodeficiency syndrome (AIDS)-associated disease in human beings. The bacteria are ingested and then taken up by the M cells of the GALT, particularly in the distal ileum. Like Johne's disease of cattle, intestinal tuberculosis is a chronic wasting disease characterized by a roughened, rugae-like appearance to the intestine.

In small animals it is sometimes clinically possible to palpate the thickened intestine. A thickened colon is sometimes palpable rectally in large animals. Granulomatous lymphadenopathy is often present, sometimes with mineralization and necrosis. The intestinal lamina propria and submucosa, as in Johne's disease, are enlarged and the architecture distorted by epithelioid macrophages and giant cells. Fewer acid-fast organisms are present as compared with Johne's disease. In most cases of *Mycobacterium avium-intracellulare*–induced intestinal tuberculosis, lepromatous (noncaseating) granulomatous inflammation occurs similar to that of Johne's disease of small ruminants.

Pigs often contract intestinal tuberculosis as a result of the husbandry practice of feeding them avian litter as an inexpensive protein source. As might be expected, early lesions develop in the retropharyngeal lymph nodes.

Alimentary Anthrax. Anthrax occurs worldwide, principally in ruminants, but any mammal, including human beings, can be affected. In the United States it is a reportable disease and a potential agent of bioterrorism and agroterrorism. Most birds, along with amphibians, reptiles, and fish, are resistant to disease. Herbivores contact the disease by ingesting spore-contaminated vegetation, through a cutaneous wound, or by inhaling spores, whereas carnivores are usually infected by ingesting contaminated carcasses. Biting flies can also transmit the causative bacterium, *Bacillus anthracis*, or its spores. In peracute disease, generally in ruminants, bacteremia and septicemia result, and the blood may fail to clot because of toxin production from the bacteria. The spleen is often very large and bloody (blackberry jam spleen), and unclotted blood may ooze from any orifice. Blood or exudate smears often demonstrate the organisms as short chains of bacterial cells, thus avoiding the necessity of a necropsy. The spores are very resistant to environmental extremes and are infective. They have been known to survive the tanning process of hides. Pulmonary anthrax in human beings is also called *woolsorter's disease*. The type of infection that occurs is directly related to the route of infection: cutaneous, respiratory, or GI.

Alimentary anthrax is most common in horses, pigs, dogs, and cats and may be oropharyngeal or intestinal. The oropharyngeal type is characterized by oral or esophageal ulcers with infection of associated lymph nodes. The clinical signs are swelling, dyspnea, and dysphagia. The intestinal form is most severe in the terminal ileum or cecum and is characterized by abdominal pain, hematemesis, and fever. Mechanistically, alimentary infection requires that vegetative bacteria cross the intestinal epithelium. *In vitro*, anthrolysin O produced by *B. anthracis* disrupts the intestinal tight junction protein occludin. Cattle may develop ulcerative hemorrhagic abomasitis or small intestinal enteritis, as well as similar lesions in the large intestine (Fig. 7-124). The spleen and lymph nodes and mesentery are edematous and hemorrhagic. Pigs are relatively resistant to anthrax; they generally develop pharyngeal and neck swelling, but necrohemorrhagic enteritis may occur. Live attenuated livestock vaccines are safe and generally provide approximately 9 months of immunity.

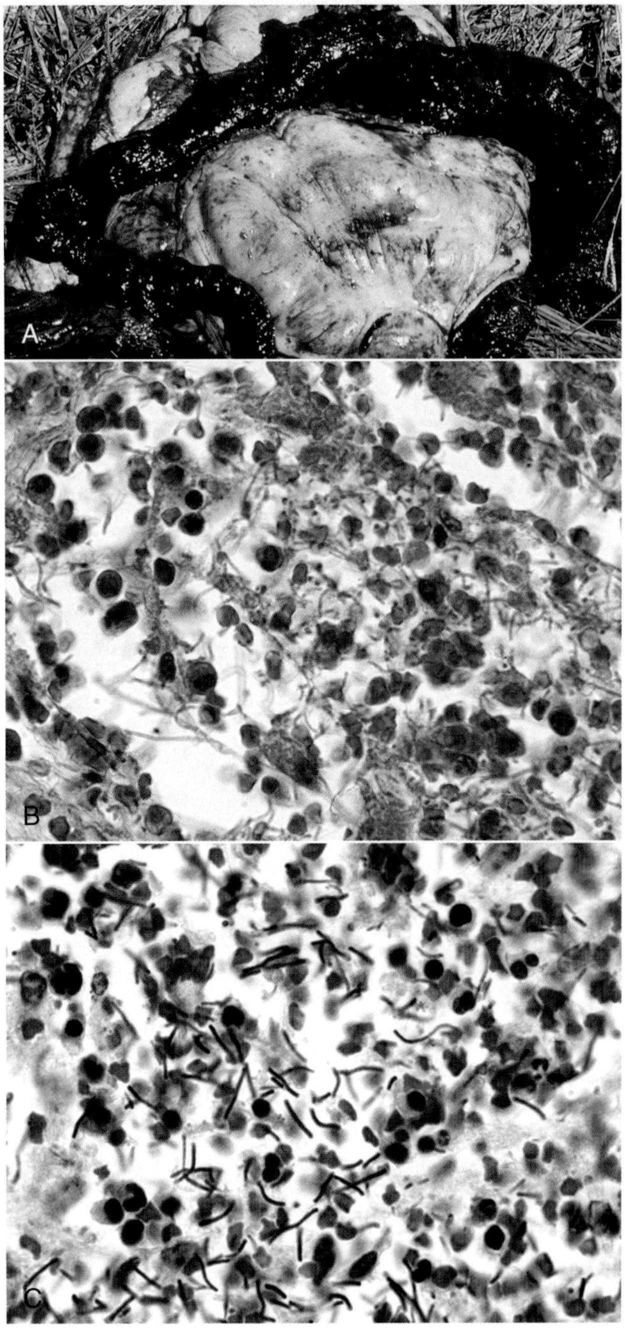

Figure 7-124 Necrohemorrhagic Enteritis, Intestine, Alimentary Anthrax, Cow. A, Note the massive transmural hemorrhage and necrosis caused by anthrax toxin. **B,** Tissue impression. The light blue bacilli in the debris are *Bacillus anthracis* bacteria. Some bacilli have blunted ends (presumably spores). H&E stain. **C,** Tissue impression. Note the dark blue bacilli (Gram-positive) in the debris. Gram stain. (**A** courtesy Dr. D. Driemeier, Federal University of Rio Grande do Sul, Brazil. **B** and **C** courtesy Drs. V. Valli and J.F. Zachary, College of Veterinary Medicine, University of Illinois.)

Parasitic Diseases. Parasites of the intestinal tract are legion in the various domestic animal species. Refer to a parasitology textbook for specific information regarding the life cycles and identification of the various species. Diagnosis of enteric parasitism is generally performed via fecal flotation or intestinal scrapings.

Amebiasis. *Entamoeba* spp. are obligate intracellular parasites with a direct life cycle. The portal of entry is oral. Trophozoites are produced that dwell in the intestinal lumen. They may also invade through the intestinal wall and go to many other organs, such as the liver, brain, and lung, especially in human beings, in whom microabscesses may form. Cysts are excreted with formed feces and continue their life cycle when ingested by another host. Trophozoites are more likely seen in diarrheic feces. Because cysts are the infective form, diarrheic feces of dogs are not usually considered to be especially dangerous to human beings or other animals. The trophozoites vary from 12 to 30 μm in diameter, and the cysts vary from 10 to 20 μm with four nuclei. Contact of ameba and host cells is likely mediated by adhesins. Soluble factors produced by the parasite mediate pathogenicity.

Entamoeba histolytica is zoonotic in human beings, other primates, dogs, cats, and other animals. Disease is serious in human beings. Lesions include colonic congestion, petechia, and ulceration (ulcerative colitis). This colitis may be acute or chronic, bloody or mucoid. In tissue, the amebas may be as large as 50 μm and often form typical flask-shaped ulcers spanning the mucosa and submucosa of the colon. After penetrating the surface mucus and adhering to the colonic enterocytes, *E. histolytica* releases amebapores (channel-forming peptides) that lyse the enterocytes without killing the ameba.

Balantidiasis (Balantidium coli). See Disorders of Pigs.

Trichomoniasis. *Tritrichomonas foetus* is a sexually transmitted pathogen of cattle. Cats, however, especially those less than a year of age housed in groups, have a tendency toward large bowel diarrhea when infected with this flagellate. Diagnosis is often made by visualization of motile flagellates on fecal wet mounts. Histologic diagnosis is most accurate when at least six biopsy sections of colon containing surface mucus are examined. PCR on paraffin-embedded tissue has also been successful, even in the absence of histologic evidence of the parasite. Infection occurs in the ileum, cecum, and colon. Lesions include mild to moderate colitis, with microabscesses and occasional extension of infection into the lamina propria. There may be colonic enterocyte attenuation and/or increased mitotic activity in the crypts. The 5- by 7-μm teardrop-shaped parasites can often be seen in surface mucus, within colonic glands, and occasionally within macrophages and lymphatic vessels. Thus the parasite is enteroinvasive under certain circumstances. Flagella are not visible on H&E staining. There is no effective treatment. The diarrheal disease in cats generally resolves within 2 years of onset.

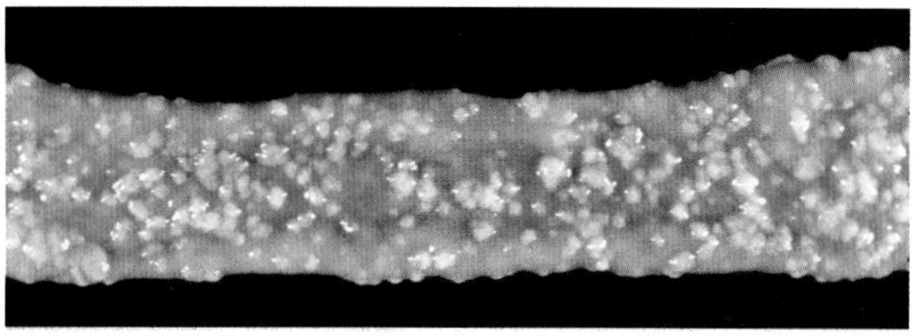

Figure 7-125 Multifocal Proliferative Enteritis, Small Intestine, Goat. Proliferative nodules (also see Fig. 7-129) in the small intestinal mucosa are characteristic of ovine and caprine coccidiosis. Sporozoites and merozoites infect enterocytes and replicate, stimulating hyperplasia of enterocytes. (Courtesy Dr. H. Gelberg, College of Veterinary Medicine, Oregon State University.)

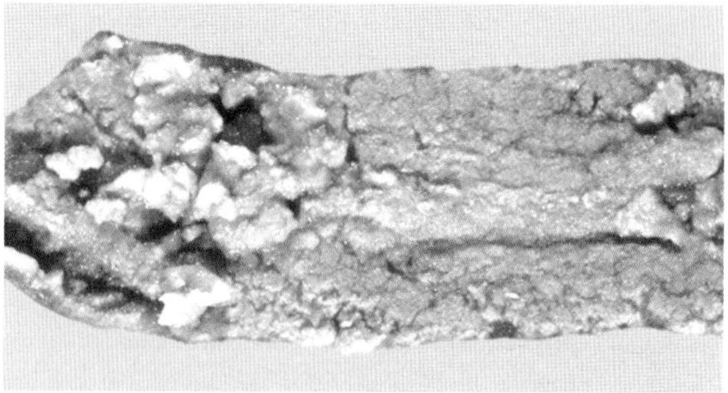

Figure 7-127 Fibrinonecrotic Enteritis, Small Intestine, Pig. Pseudomembranes are characteristic of porcine coccidiosis. (Courtesy Dr. H. Gelberg, College of Veterinary Medicine, Oregon State University.)

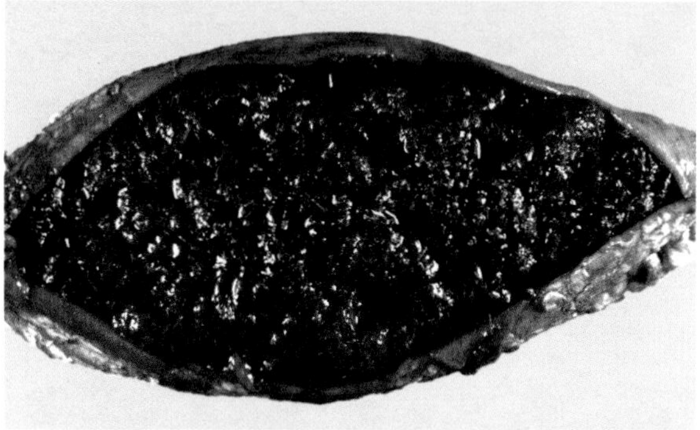

Figure 7-126 Necrohemorrhagic Enteritis, Small Intestine, Calf. Coccidiosis in cattle, dogs, and cats is characterized by intestinal hemorrhage. Hemorrhagic diarrheic feces may be visible on the perineum and hind legs. In severe cases there may be anemia, which will be evident as pale external mucous membranes. (Courtesy College of Veterinary Medicine, Cornell University.)

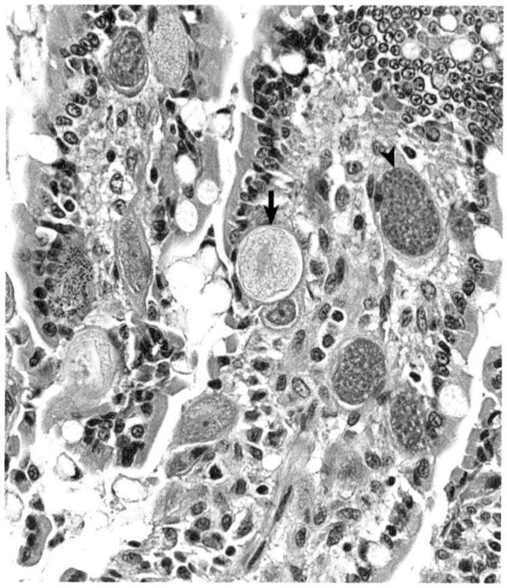

Figure 7-128 Sexual Stages of Intestinal Coccidiosis, Small Intestine, Cow. Note that the mucosal epithelial cells are distended with microgametes *(arrow)* and macrogametes *(arrowhead)*. H&E stain. (Courtesy Dr. J.F. Zachary, College of Veterinary Medicine, University of Illinois.)

Coccidiosis. Coccidia are exquisitely host- and tissue-specific protozoa. They are obligate intracellular pathogens. Lesions vary from proliferative in sheep and goats (Fig. 7-125) to hemorrhagic in dogs, cats, and cattle (Fig. 7-126). In pigs a fibrinonecrotic pseudomembrane, without blood, in 5- to 7-day-old animals is characteristic of enteric coccidiosis (Fig. 7-127). *Eimeria macusaniensis* is a relatively common cause of sickness and death in New World camelids of all ages. Gross lesions, even in heavily infested animals, are minimal to absent. In many cases, results of fecal examinations are negative.

Most species of *Eimeria* and *Isospora* infect villous or crypt epithelial cells, more rarely lacteals, the lamina propria, and regional lymph nodes. The coccidia undergo one or more asexual reproductive cycles within enterocytes. The resulting sporozoites produce schizonts containing merozoites, which infect additional enterocytes.

Merozoites produce gamonts that differentiate into microgametes and macrogametes (Fig. 7-128). Microgametes fertilize macrogametes, producing zygotes that develop into oocysts. When a small number of coccidia parasitize the intestine of otherwise healthy young growing animals, little disease results. However, when animals are in crowded conditions associated with poor sanitation, fecal-oral transmission of large numbers of organisms can occur. It is in these circumstances, compounded by malnutrition and intercurrent infections or parasitism, that clinical disease results. Enterocyte rupture occurs in all stages of the parasite's life cycle. Clinical disease depends on parasitic load and varies by animal species. Because of diminished epithelial turnover in young animals, they are most susceptible to disease.

Gross lesions of coccidiosis are variable by host species, parasite species, and intestinal location. Bleeding is variably present both within species and among species. Coccidiosis in sheep and goats is characterized by enterocyte proliferation that is visible grossly as mucosal nodules (Fig. 7-129). The large schizonts of some species are sometimes grossly visible as well. *Eimeria leuckarti* of horses is asymptomatic. In dogs and cats a slightly different organism, *Cystoisospora,* is responsible for disease. Intestinal toxoplasmosis of cats is an important zoonotic concern, especially for pregnant women.

"Poor doing" associated with diarrhea is characteristic of clinical coccidiosis. Depending on the host species and the region of intestine that is affected, infected fresh blood may be present in the feces. The presence of tenesmus is variable. Oocysts are usually demonstrable in the feces.

Cryptosporidiosis. C. *parvum* is a ubiquitous protozoan pathogen of mammals. Often waterborne, it is a significant cause of municipal water contamination. Although it causes a self-limiting infection in immunocompetent animals, the very young or

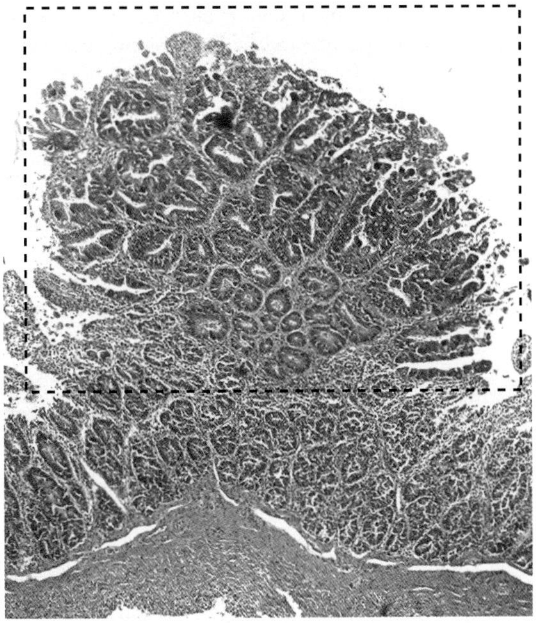

Figure 7-129 **Proliferative Enteritis, Small Intestine, Goat.** Coccidia-induced enterocyte hyperplasia results in nodule formation *(area identified by dashed lines)* as seen in Figure 7-125. Note the hyperplastic enterocytes lining crypts within the nodule. H&E stain. (Courtesy Dr. H. Gelberg, College of Veterinary Medicine, Oregon State University.)

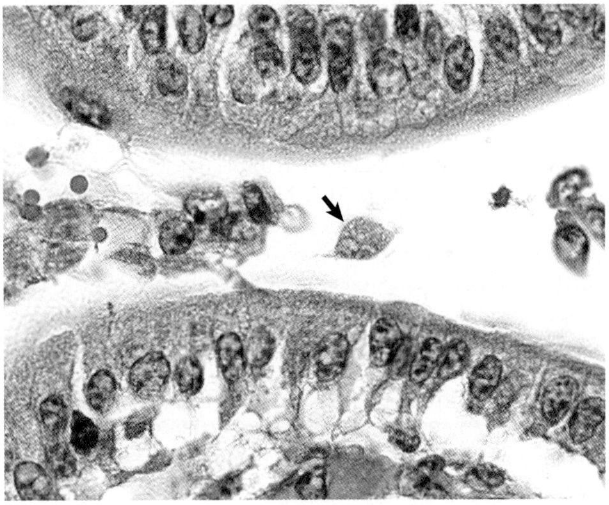

Figure 7-130 **Giardiasis, Small Intestine, Dog.** A single pear-shaped flagellated protozoa is readily visible in the intestinal lumen *(arrow)*. H&E stain. (Courtesy Dr. J.F. Zachary, College of Veterinary Medicine, University of Illinois.)

immunocompromised individuals, such as acquired immunodeficiency syndrome patients, suffer from intractable diarrhea. When treating calves, veterinarians and veterinary students are at particular risk for infection. Cryptosporidia attach to surface epithelial cells of the stomach, small intestine, or colon. The protozoa displace the microvilli and are enclosed by surface cell membranes. Thus the parasite lives in a unique environment described as intracellular but extracytoplasmic (E-Fig. 7-20). Microgametes, macrogametes, schizonts, trophozoites, meronts, merozoites, and oocysts can be demonstrated in the intestine adjacent to, or attached to, epithelial cells. Oocysts are 4 to 5 μm in diameter and are shed in the feces. Studies have indicated that there are species-specific tropisms or biotypes of cryptosporidia. Previously, fecal contamination of water supplies by ruminants was believed to be the cause of most human outbreaks. Molecular typing of the organism has shown in many disease outbreaks that contamination with human feces and human-specific cryptosporidia causes most human epidemics.

Oocysts can be identified in feces by Sheather's sucrose flotation and a modified acid-fast stain. Cryptosporidiosis causes subacute or chronic, sometimes bloody, watery diarrhea. The mechanism of diarrhea involves more than just cell loss. Prostaglandins, perhaps secreted by macrophages, increase anion (Cl^-) secretion through cAMP and inhibit sodium absorption and thus water absorption. In addition, *C. parvum* interferes with interferon-γ (IFN-γ) gene expression of host cells, thus contributing to immune evasion by the parasite. There is associated dehydration and electrolyte loss. Although the disease can be fatal, particularly in the presence of other pathogens, it is often self-limiting in immunocompetent individuals. In these cases the illness resolves spontaneously in approximately a week.

Affected portions of the GI tract are diffusely reddened and have fluid contents. The organisms appear as tiny blue (hematoxylinophilic) dots attached to the epithelial cells of affected segments. In addition to the dot forms, ring- and banana-shaped organisms are readily seen in Giemsa-stained sections. The lesions of enteritis or colitis consist of decreased mucosal (villous) height, irregular mucosal thickness, crypt necrosis, hyperemia, and an increase in lymphocytes and plasma cells in the lamina propria. Villous atrophy and fusion of the villi of the small intestine are the end result. Because of the intracellular, extracytoplasmic location of the parasite, chemotherapeutic intervention is ineffective. There are few chemicals that can decontaminate the environment. Clorox, for example, is used experimentally to purify the parasites.

Giardiasis. Giardiasis has been reported in many species, including human beings, dogs, cats, horses, cattle, rabbits, guinea pigs, hamsters, rats, mice, chinchillas, and parakeets. In clinical veterinary practice, giardiasis is frequently recognized in puppies and kittens and causes concern among owners because of its zoonotic potential. Prevalence of the parasite in human beings in the developed world is estimated at 2% to 5%. Giardiasis is caused by a pear-shaped protozoan with posterior flagella, a ventral sucker, and four nuclei, two of which resemble eyes (Fig. 7-130). *Giardia lamblia* (*Giardia intestinalis*, *Giardia duodenalis*) parasitizes the small intestine, particularly the duodenum. *Giardia* attach to the microvillous border of epithelial cells, producing membrane damage. Although generally asymptomatic, diarrhea may result in very young animals or in animals otherwise immunologically deficient.

Giardia spp. have been shown to induce apoptosis of enterocytes, thus increasing membrane permeability. In large numbers the parasites decrease the absorption of simple sugars and disaccharides secondary to microvillous destruction. Ingesta are then fermented by bacterial flora, creating gas and osmotically drawing water into the intestinal lumen. An enterotoxin stimulates intestinal Cl^- secretion. Clinical cases of giardiasis have brown, fluid diarrhea and abdominal discomfort without fever, weight loss, melena, and/or steatorrhea. The diagnosis is made by demonstrating *Giardia* in preparations of fresh feces or in histologic sections by identifying the organisms either with H&E or Giemsa stains.

Ascariasis. Ascarids are easily recognized as proximal-intestinal, luminal nematodes that are smooth and white. They are round on cross section, thus giving them the appellation of roundworms together with the other nematodes. They vary greatly in length; the larger the host species, the larger the ascarids. They are 3 to 4 cm long in small animals and attain lengths of 40 to 50 cm in pigs and horses. Ascarids of domestic animals belong to the genera *Ascaris* (pigs), *Parascaris* (horses), and *Toxocara* (dogs, cats, and human beings). The young of these species acquire larval ascarids by intrauterine transmission during the last 7 to 10 days of gestation, through the milk of the dam, and later in life through parasite ova contamination of the environment. After ingestion, infective larvae penetrate the intestine and migrate to the liver via the portal circulation. From there the larvae migrate via the caudal vena cava to the lungs. After leaving the circulation and entering the alveoli, the larvae undergo development and are coughed into the pharynx and swallowed. Development to adults occurs in the intestine. Ova passed in the feces complete the life cycle.

Alternatively, *Toxascaris leonina* of dogs and cats is ingested via an intermediate host. Hepatopulmonary migration does not occur. Lesions produced by ascarid larval migration include canine multifocal eosinophilic gastroenteritis and visceral larva migrans. Animals affected with heavy ascarid burdens lose weight, grow poorly as a result of competition for nutrients between luminal parasites and the host, and often have a pear-shaped abdomen when held vertically. Adult worms may be vomited or passed in the diarrheic feces. A hacking cough termed *thumping* is a sign of pulmonary larva migrans, especially in pigs. Anthelmintic administration can cause a rapid die-off of adult ascarids, resulting in intestinal occlusion (see E-Fig. 7-13). Ascarids continue to migrate after the death of the host and may be found in aberrant locations such as the bile duct, stomach, oral cavity, pancreatic duct, and abdomen (see Fig. 7-18).

Hookworm Disease. Parasitism by hookworms varies from asymptomatic to fatal based on the challenge dose of parasites, the host's age, nutritional status, and likely its immunologic state. When death occurs, it is by exsanguination because hookworms are blood eaters (Fig. 7-131). Challenge dosage is often exacerbated by poor nutritional and sanitary conditions, mild climatic conditions, and moisture. Hookworms are generally small nematodes, 1 to 1.5 cm long. Their habitat is usually the proximal small intestine. Genera include *Ancylostoma* and *Uncinaria* in dogs, *Bunostomum* in ruminants, *Globocephalus* in pigs, and *Ancylostoma* and *Necator* in human beings. *Ancylostoma caninum* in dogs has zoonotic potential. Environmental contamination occurs from the large number of eggs produced in the intestine. The first- through third-stage larvae feed on environmental bacteria. Third-stage larvae are infective and enter the host either by ingestion or direct dermal penetration. From either point of entry, they migrate through the pulmonary system, through somatic tissue to the uterus, or through mucosal tissue. Larvae may also be present in colostrum. The final destination is the intestine, where eggs are produced, completing the life cycle.

Because prenatal infections with hookworms do not become patent for 11 days, fecal examination results may be negative. Otherwise, fecal examination, especially in young animals with anemia, is diagnostic of this disease. Adult hookworms bury into the villous, ingesting tissue, mucus, and blood (Fig. 7-132). When the worm moves to another attachment site, blood may continue to flow from the wound for 30 minutes.

Trichuriasis. Trichurids, or whipworms, are long and slender at their anterior ends and may be numerous within the cecum and colon. Trichurids have a direct life cycle. The name *Trichuris* translates to "whip-tail," which is a misnomer because the parasite actually has a "whip-head" that invades and attaches to the mucosa of the cecum, colon, and rectum. Although the parasite ingests blood, anemia is rarely a clinical symptom. Bloody diarrhea may be present. Different species are parasites of carnivores, ruminants, pigs, and human beings. The disease in each species is similar. The horse does not have a whipworm.

Trichuris eggs are elongate, or football shaped, with an operculum at either end, and are very resistant to environmental conditions. Most infections are asymptomatic, and the complete life cycle may take up to 3 months. Therefore repeated dewormings are necessary to eliminate infection, even in the absence of fecal ova. Symptoms may be vague, with only paroxysmal diarrhea. Gross enteric lesions vary from mild to erosive and ulcerative.

Strongyloidosis. *Strongyloides* spp. are unique in having free-living and parasitic forms. Rhabditiform larvae may develop parthenogenetically. Free-living parasites are both male and female and undergo sexual reproduction. Enteritis can be severe; larvae or larvated eggs are in the feces of infected animals.

Strongyloides stercoralis of dogs is zoonotic. *Strongyloides* spp. also infect horses, pigs, and cats. Geographic differences in parasite populations account for differences in virulence within host species. Hyperinfection and autoinfection may occur, adding to the parasite

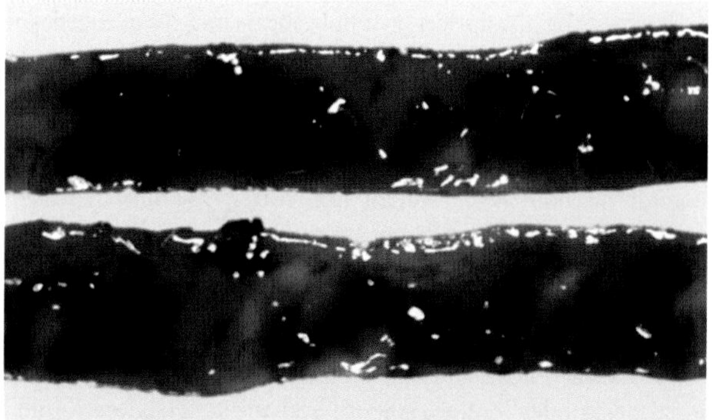

Figure 7-131 **Hookworms, Hemorrhagic Enteritis, Small Intestine, Dog.** Where hookworms have detached, hemorrhage is present. (Courtesy Dr. H. Gelberg, College of Veterinary Medicine, Oregon State University.)

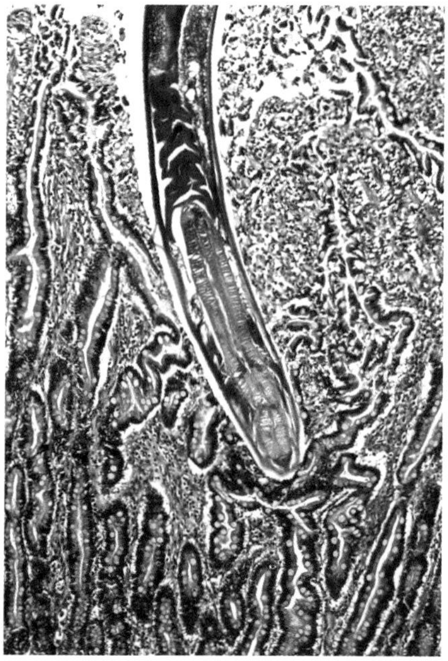

Figure 7-132 **Hookworm Enteritis, Intestine, Dog.** A hookworm has burrowed deep into and attached to the mucosa. H&E stain. (Courtesy College of Veterinary Medicine, Cornell University.)

burden. Larvae may enter the host by skin penetration, or less often by ingestion. *Strongyloides* spp. infection may be acquired *in utero* and through colostrum and milk. Larvae migrate to the bloodstream and lungs. When they gain access to alveoli, they subsequently migrate to airways, where they are carried, via the mucociliary elevator, to the pharyngeal cavity and are swallowed. Small intestinal parasitism is characterized by larvae residing within superficial mucosa (E-Fig. 7-21). Epithelial destruction by the parasites may result in villous atrophy and crypt hyperplasia. The nonspecific clinical signs include diarrhea, hypoproteinemia, weight loss, and dehydration. Rhabditiform dermatitis may also occur.

Pinworms. *Oxyuris equi* is the most common pinworm of domestic animals. The parasites occupy the lumen of the distal intestine of horses and occasionally cause rectal pruritus by laying their eggs on the perineal region. *Enterobius vermicularis* is the pinworm of primates and great apes. It is not zoonotic and is generally of little clinical consequence.

Cestodes. Tapeworms, although frequently found in the alimentary system, are generally of little clinical significance. They require two and sometimes three hosts, often including arthropods and other invertebrates, to complete their life cycles. Tapeworms attach to the gut wall by means of their anterior scolex, which may have hooks in addition to four suckers (Fig. 7-133). Although they can cause some damage at the site of attachment, generally they compete with the host for nutrients. Lacking an alimentary system, they absorb nutrients through their surface. Tapeworms are flat, segmented, and hermaphroditic, reproducing by addition of segments or proglottids. Examples of tapeworms are *Anoplocephala* spp. in horses, *Moniezia* spp. in ruminants, and *Diphyllobothrium* and *Dipylidium* spp. in dogs and cats. *Mesocestoides* spp. can infect dogs and cats. In some cases this parasite can perforate through the intestine and proliferate in the peritoneal cavity (see Fig. 7-25).

Taenia and *Echinococcus* spp. are the most destructive of the cestodes. Although carnivores are the definitive hosts, the larval forms reside in the viscera and body cavities of the intermediate hosts, usually ruminants, pigs, horses, or rodents (see Fig. 8-59). Human beings can also become infected, and sometimes it takes 20 or 30 years for clinical disease to appear. The damage in the intermediate hosts may be quite severe.

Trematodes. Trematodes are uncommon parasites of the alimentary tract. *Nanophyetus salmincola* uses a snail and a fish as intermediate hosts. It carries the rickettsia responsible for salmon poisoning in the Northwestern United States. Lesions of the intestine are hemorrhagic enteritis.

Alaria spp. can attach to the small intestine of dogs and cats but are generally innocuous. The mesocercariae can cause tissue damage during their migrations through body organs of the host. Paratenic hosts are frogs, snakes, and mice.

Schistosomiasis of ruminants, pigs, horses, and dogs can cause granulomatous intestinal lesions with protein loss secondary to the parasite's presence in mesenteric veins after migration through the liver. Parasites are acquired by direct penetration of the skin by cercariae.

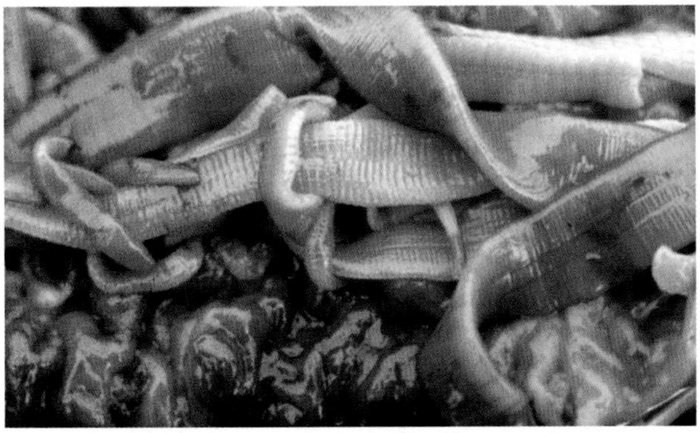

Figure 7-133 Cestodiasis, Small Intestine, Fur Seal. Segmented tapeworms are present in this otherwise normal intestine. (Courtesy Dr. H. Gelberg, College of Veterinary Medicine, Oregon State University.)

Acanthocephalans. The thorny-headed worm of pigs, *Macracanthorhynchus hirudinaceus*, is a small intestinal parasite with a soil-based arthropod intermediate host such as dung beetles. They are thus more common, as are many other parasites in a variety of mammalian species, in "free-range" animals. They are occasionally misidentified as tapeworms, which they superficially resemble. However, they are not truly segmented parasites. They occasionally penetrate the bowel wall at the site of parasite attachment, causing peritonitis. *Prosthenorchis* spp. are acanthocephalans of primates. Cockroaches are the intermediate hosts.

Intestinal Neoplasia

Neoplasms of various types occur in the GI system of domestic animals. Those of the oral cavity and stomach have already been discussed. Intestinal neoplasms are diagnosed most frequently in dogs and cats, in large part because of their longer life spans. Additionally, pets live in close harmony with their human companions, and thus it is possible that some of the same environmental factors that may contribute to human cancer may cause similar problems in animals.

In dogs, benign neoplasms of the intestinal tract are most commonly adenomas or polyps (see Fig. 6-4), and their malignant counterparts adenocarcinomas. Dogs and cats infrequently develop intestinal mast cell tumors and plasmacytomas. Smooth muscle neoplasms termed leiomyomas and leiomyosarcomas arise from existing intestinal muscular layers. An important caveat in diagnosing these spindle cell tumors is that some of them when examined immunohistochemically are composed of undifferentiated cells with an uncertain histogenesis. These neoplasms have been reported in dogs, horses, rats and primates. They are termed *GI stromal tumors* (GISTs). Supposition exists that these neoplasms arise from the interstitial cells of Cajal, which normally become the pacemaker cells of the gut. Most are KIT (CD117) positive (proto-oncogene c-kit).

Lymphoma can be solitary, metastatic, or multicentric. In cats the most common neoplasms include alimentary lymphoma (Fig. 7-134); mastocytomas (Fig. 7-135), which are associated with ulceration; adenomas; adenocarcinomas; and carcinoids. In dogs 5% to 7% of lymphomas are GI. Those of the GI tract are epitheliotropic and primarily T lymphocyte in origin. In human beings, most GI lymphomas are B lymphocyte in origin. In sheep, adenocarcinomas of the intestine are fairly common and are virus induced. In cows, alimentary lymphoma is most common. Horses rarely have intestinal neoplasms develop.

Algae

Chlorellosis and Protothecosis. Unicellular and sometimes achlorophyllic algae have been reported to opportunistically cause cutaneous or widely disseminated granulomatous disease in a variety of species, including human beings, dogs, cats, dromedaries, gazelle, a beaver, cattle, and sheep. These algae are found in a variety of

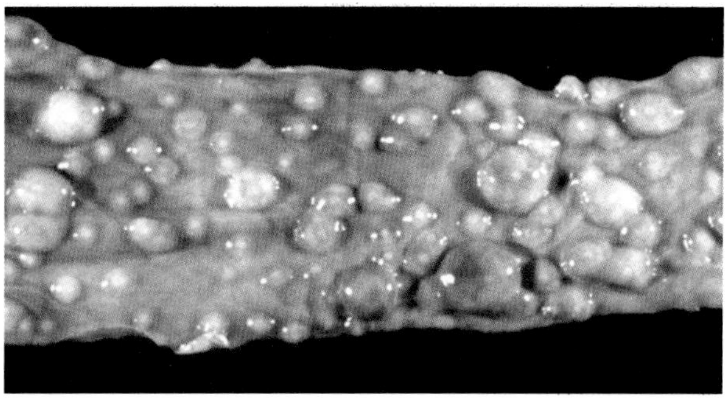

Figure 7-134 Lymphoma (Lymphosarcoma), Colon, Cat. Numerous submucosal nodules contain neoplastic lymphocytes. Note that the mucosal epithelium is intact (smooth and shiny) and not ulcerated. (Courtesy Dr. H. Gelberg, College of Veterinary Medicine, Oregon State University.)

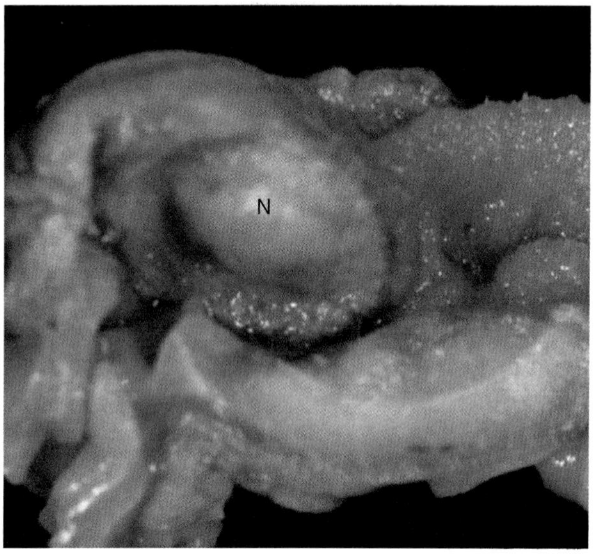

Figure 7-135 Mast Cell Tumor, Small Intestine, Cat. The submucosal nodule *(N)* contains neoplastic mast cells. (Courtesy Dr. H. Gelberg, College of Veterinary Medicine, Oregon State University.)

environmental locales, including both fresh and marine water. Primary infection is believed to be in the alimentary tract with chronic bloody diarrhea or through cutaneous wounds. Lesions are often tinted green if the algae contain chlorophyll. In the intestine the transmural lesions are those of granulomatous enteritis and lymphadenitis. Intracellular algae measuring 5 to 11 μm, including those in giant cells, are visualized by Gomori's methenamine silver or PAS staining of the thick capsule. *Chlorella*, unlike *Prototheca*, which is considered to be its achlorophyllous mutant, contains starch bodies and chloroplasts that are birefringent in H&E sections, PAS positive, and diastase negative. Internal septation of the organisms is present with 2 to 20 sporangiospores.

Peritoneum, Omentum, Mesentery, and Peritoneal Cavity

Parasitic Diseases

Aberrant migration of nematodes and trematodes in most species of mammals can cause focal fibrosis when they travel through the abdominal cavity (see Fig. 8-33). Setaria are nematodes that are sometimes found in the peritoneal cavity of ungulates and rarely cause significant damage in this location. Mild focal peritonitis is sometimes the result of their travels. A variety of cestodes may be found in the abdominal cavity of many species of mammal. Some, such as *E. granulosus* (hydatid cysts) are zoonotic. *Mesocestoides* and *Porocephalus* (pentastomiasis) are found in carnivores, in which their presence may induce a pyogranulomatous reaction (see Fig. 7-25).

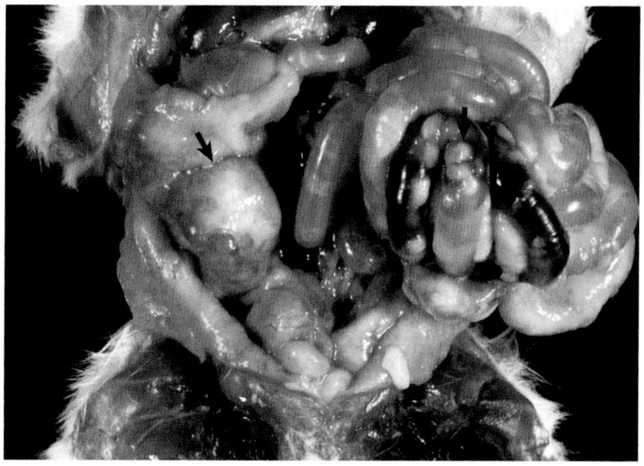

Figure 7-136 Mesothelioma, Abdominal Cavity, Rat. Raised nodules *(arrows)* of neoplastic mesothelial cells are present on serosal surfaces of the abdominal organs. (Courtesy College of Veterinary Medicine, University of Illinois.)

Neoplasia

Primary neoplasms of the peritoneum are uncommon with the exception of lipomas, which may become pedunculated and result in intestinal strangulation (see Fig. 7-107). Mesotheliomas occur sporadically in animals and more commonly in human beings (Fig. 7-136). In human beings, mesotheliomas are associated with asbestosis and other fibers with similar physicochemical properties and are considered an occupational hazard for some industries. Great efforts have been made to reduce occupational exposure to asbestos. Mesotheliomas have been reported in calves as a congenital disease. Tumors of mesothelial origin are all considered malignant because they may spread transcoelomically. They seldom metastasize to draining lymph nodes or distal sites. They are quite pleomorphic and vary from papillary and adenocarcinoma-appearing to spindloid and fibrosarcoma-like. It is extremely difficult to distinguish neoplastic mesothelium from hyperplastic, reactive mesothelium.

Disorders of Horses

For disorders occurring in two or more species of animals, see Disorders of Domestic Animals.

Oral Cavity

See Disorders of Domestic Animals, Oral Cavity.

Teeth

See Disorders of Domestic Animals, Teeth, Infundibular Impaction.

Equine Odontoclastic Tooth Resorption and Hypercementosis

Equine odontoclastic tooth resorption and hypercementosis (EOTRH) is an idiopathic disorder that affects incisor and canine teeth of aged horses. It is often painful with attendant periodontitis and resorption and/or proliferation of mineralized dental tissues. As the name implies, osteoclasts are mechanistically responsible for resorption, which is followed by hypercementosis (Fig. 7-137).

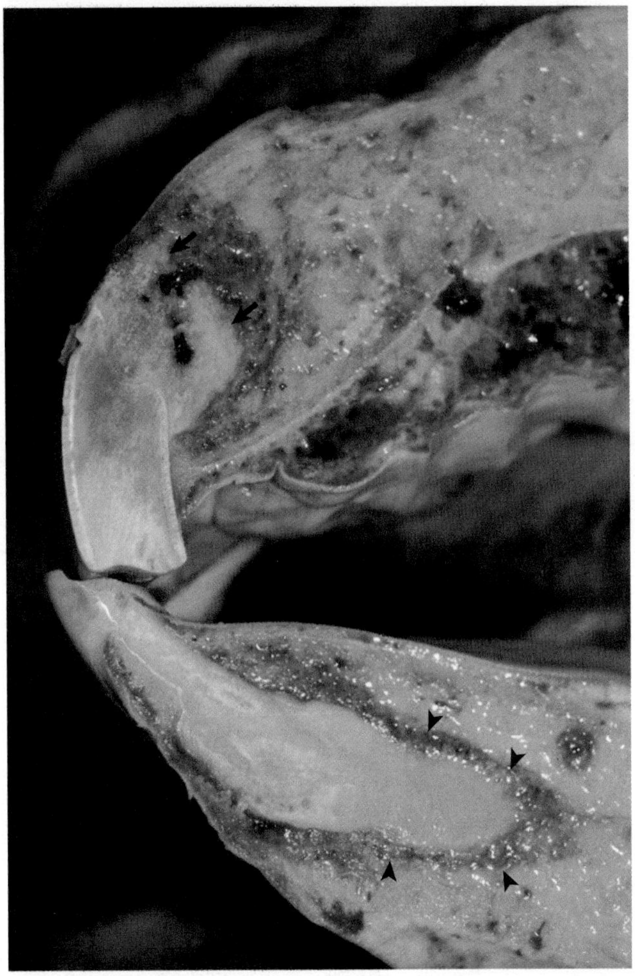

Figure 7-137 Equine Odontoclastic Tooth Resorption and Hypercementosis, Oral Cavity, Horse. This idiopathic disorder affects incisor and canine teeth of aged horses. It is often painful with attendant periodontitis *(arrowheads)* and resorption and/or proliferation of mineralized dental tissues *(arrows)*. (Courtesy Dr. H. Gelberg, College of Veterinary Medicine, Oregon State University.)

Tonsils

See Disorders of Domestic Animals, Tonsils.

Salivary Glands

Sialoadenitis is associated with strangles in horses.

See Disorders of Domestic Animals, Salivary Glands.

Tongue

See Disorders of Domestic Animals, Tongue.

Esophagus

Choke

See Disorders of Domestic Animals, Esophagus, Choke.

Stomach

See Disorders of Domestic Animals, Stomach and Abomasum.

Intestine

Intestinal Displacements

Renosplenic Entrapment. Renosplenic entrapment of the large colon in horses is due to left dorsal displacement of the left dorsal colon or left ventral colon between the spleen and left body wall. Entrapment occurs dorsally over the renosplenic ligament that runs between the left kidney and the spleen. The cause of the displacement is unknown but could occur secondary to rolling behavior in horses or gaseous distention of the large colon. If not corrected either by rolling the horse or by surgery, intestinal rupture and death may result.

Right Dorsal Displacement. In the equine condition right dorsal displacement, the left dorsal and ventral colons are displaced to the right of the cecum and may result in torsion with signs of colic. It is a surgically correctable disease.

Bacterial Diseases

***Rhodococcus equi* Enteritis.** *R. equi* is a soil saprophyte and a normal inhabitant of the equine intestine. The disease caused by this large, potentially zoonotic, Gram-positive, and facultatively anaerobic rod is often characterized by pulmonary pyogranulomas in foals under 6 months of age (see Fig. 9-82) and in immunocompromised adult horses and human beings, or those with intercurrent disease (acquired immunodeficiency syndrome patients). The bacterium is not resistant to neutrophil-mediated destruction but can resist the intracellular environment of macrophages. All pathogenic *R. equi* isolated from horses but not human beings have a large plasmid and the encoded surface-expressed lipoprotein VapA, which is associated with virulence. The frequent intercurrence of helminths and *R. equi* infection suggests that migrating larvae aid in distributing the bacterium through the body of the foal. Stringent control of helminth infections may therefore help to reduce or eliminate *R. equi* infections.

Equine abortion, pneumonia, and placentitis have been associated with infection, as have sporadic infections, sometimes fatal, of a wide variety of mammalian species. *R. equi* can be isolated from a large number of otherwise healthy mammals of different species.

When coughed up and swallowed in large numbers, the bacteria enter the intestinal M cells overlying the GALT, resulting in pyogranulomatous lymphadenitis of GALT and lymph nodes and pyogranulomatous ulcerative enterotyphlocolitis.

Intestinal infection commences in Peyer's patches, which are ultimately replaced by granulomatous inflammation, abscess formation, and necrotic tissue, and the patches are ulcerated. Infection then spreads to mesenteric lymph nodes with a similar result. Macrophages, often laden with intact bacteria, fill the intestinal lamina propria and submucosa, resulting in a markedly thickened, corrugated intestine. The grossly observable abscesses and foci of necrosis and ulceration often correspond to the distribution of GALT (Fig. 7-138).

Mesenteric, cecal, and colonic lymph nodes are enlarged, firm, and gray (Fig. 7-139). They, along with the spleen, may contain granulomas and abscesses (see Fig. 13-68). The large number of macrophages and multinucleated giant cells within the lamina propria and lymphoid tissue is characteristic of this infection. Bacteria may be seen within these cells with Giemsa and tissue Gram stains. The florid inflammatory infiltrate expands the intestinal villi and may distort the crypts of the entire intestinal tract.

Contamination of skin wounds by *R. equi* may result in cutaneous ulcerative lymphangitis in horses. Swine cervical lymphadenopathy may also be a result of infection.

Parasitic Diseases

Many parasites cause disease of the stomach, especially in ungulates.

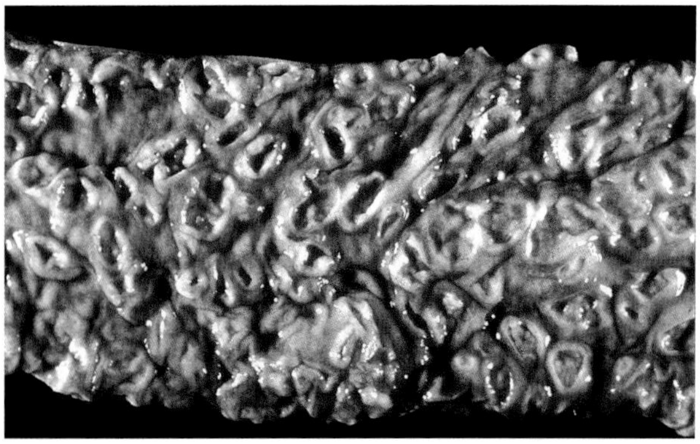

Figure 7-138 **Multifocal Ulcerative Colitis, Colon, Horse.** *Rhodococcus equi* infection causes multiple mucosal ulcers centered over gut-associated lymphoid tissue. (Courtesy Dr. H. Gelberg, College of Veterinary Medicine, Oregon State University.)

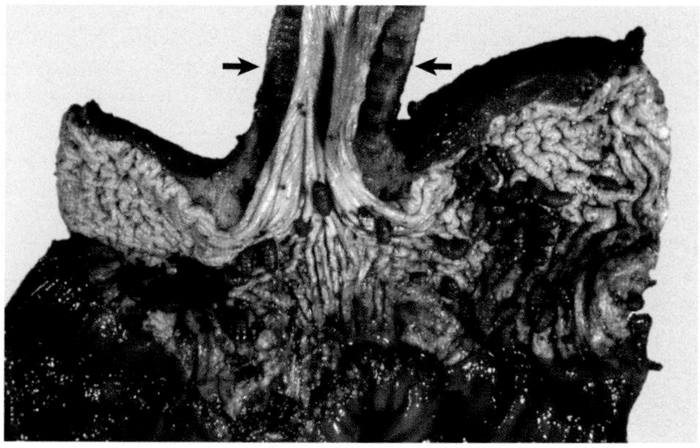

Figure 7-140 **Gasterophiliasis, Stomach, Horse.** Fly larvae (bots) of *Gasterophilus intestinalis* are attached to the epithelium of the nonglandular portion of the stomach. Note the muscular hypertrophy of the distal esophagus *(arrows)*. Although not shown in this illustration, *Gasterophilus nasalis*, another similar equine gastric parasite, attaches to the epithelium of the glandular portion of the stomach. (Courtesy Dr. H. Gelberg, College of Veterinary Medicine, Oregon State University.)

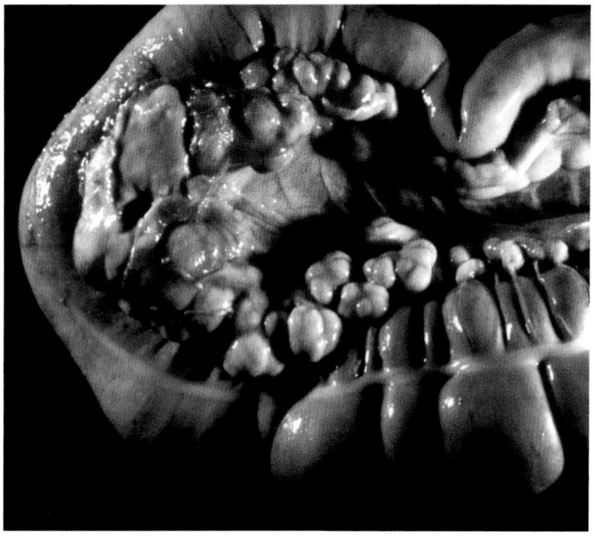

Figure 7-139 **Mesenteric Lymphadenitis, Colon, Horse.** Infection of colic lymph nodes with *Rhodococcus equi* causes pyogranulomatous lymphadenomegaly. (Courtesy Dr. H. Gelberg, College of Veterinary Medicine, Oregon State University.)

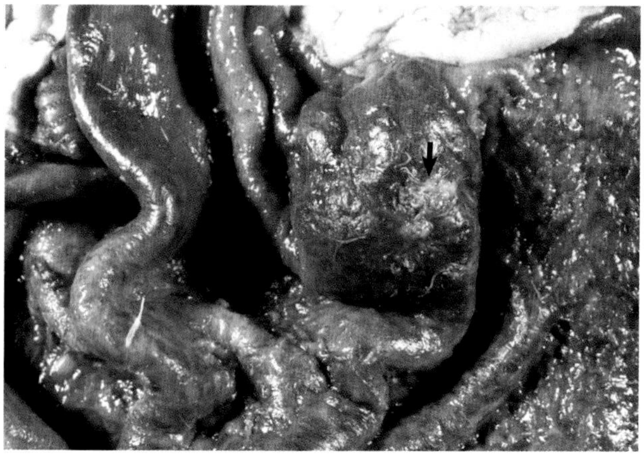

Figure 7-141 **Focal Granulomatous Gastritis, *Draschia* Brood Pouch, Stomach, Horse.** A large parasitic brood pouch is present in the glandular mucosa *(right center of illustration)* adjacent to the margo plicatus *(top right of illustration)*. Nematodes have been squeezed from the pouch and are visible on the surface *(arrow)*. Histologically, the mucosa is expanded by focal granulomatous inflammation containing clusters of adult *Draschia megastoma*. (Courtesy Dr. H. Gelberg, College of Veterinary Medicine, Oregon State University.)

Equine Bots. Equine bots, *Gasterophilus intestinalis* and *Gasterophilus nasalis*, are commonly seen in animals on inadequate deworming regimens (Fig. 7-140). Both species migrate in the tissues of the oral cavity and often reside in infected spaces adjacent to teeth. *G. intestinalis* colonizes the stratified portion of the stomach. The adult fly lays eggs on the hairs of the distal limbs of the horse. *G. nasalis* lays its eggs around the nose of the horse. The larvae hatch after being moistened and warmed by licking. They are swallowed and live in the glandular stomach and duodenum. Both species attach to the mucosa via their anterior pincers. The larvae pass in the feces, pupate, and develop into flies.

Draschia. *Draschia megastoma* is found in "brood pouches" in the glandular mucosa adjacent to the margo plicatus (Fig. 7-141). Infection is sometimes referred to as *habronemiasis*, based on antiquated taxonomic nomenclature in which these nematodes were classified as *Habronema* spp. Eggs produced in the cysts are extruded through a pore in the brood pouch to the gastric lumen. The eggs pass out with the feces and are consumed by fly larvae that are the intermediate hosts. Both *Draschia* and *Gasterophilus* spp. can cause gastric ulcers. Considering their location and means of survival in the stomach, it is remarkable that they do not cause serious damage more often.

Cyathostomiasis. In ponies and horses under 5 years of age in temperate climates, sudden emergence of massive numbers of fourth- and fifth-stage cyathostome larvae from the cecum and colon results in necroulcerative hemorrhagic typhlocolitis. Ova are generally not detected in feces, but larvae are often visible.

Rickettsial Diseases

Equine Monocytic Ehrlichiosis. Equine monocytic ehrlichiosis, also known as *Potomac horse fever,* was first reported in 1983. It appears that the disease was present for at least the previous 5 years. First described in the Potomac River valley of Maryland, Virginia, and Pennsylvania, it is now found throughout the United States and elsewhere. The common denominator is a proximity of horses to slow-moving bodies of water.

The causative agent, *Neorickettsia risticii*—an intracytoplasmic rickettsial pathogen of epithelial cells, macrophages, and monocytes—is found in trematodes in freshwater snails. A reduction in pollution levels of the Potomac River basin is believed to have resulted in an increase in the number of freshwater snails. Mayflies and caddis flies have been implicated in transmission. Horses are believed to become infected by eating the dead flies that may accumulate in water buckets and feed troughs, particularly those under artificial light. *Rickettsia* are often transmitted by arthropods, and this disease is seasonal in northern latitudes (May through September). Without treatment, one-third of cases with diarrhea die as a result of dehydration.

Experimental evidence indicates that *N. risticii* may be abortigenic. The gross lesions of Potomac horse fever are subtle, consisting of congestion, petechiae, and edema, primarily in the cecum and colon. There is a variable superficial necrotizing enterocolitis. Sometimes the small intestine is affected. Intestinal contents are tan, watery, and malodorous.

Because the experimental reproduction of clinical disease in germ-free animals has not been done, the microscopic appearance of lesions is not certain. Intercurrent bacteria may be responsible for some of the reported lesions. Interestingly, horses with Potomac horse fever have a mild necrotizing typhlocolitis similar in distribution to colitis X and enteric salmonellosis. The nature of the gross lesions is somewhat controversial because experimental infections produce variable results. Like hog cholera, Potomac horse fever is sometimes associated with concurrent *Salmonella* infection, perhaps accounting for the *Salmonella*-like lesions. Monocytes and macrophages in all layers of the intestine can be demonstrated with stains, such as Giemsa, to contain *Neorickettsia* organisms.

Clinical signs associated with Potomac horse fever include fever, watery diarrhea, depression, dehydration, variable colic, laminitis, and subcutaneous edema of the thorax, abdomen, and hind legs. Equine monocytic ehrlichiosis is apparently the same disease known as churrido equino (equine scours), which has been present for more than a century in Uruguay and Brazil.

Idiopathic Disorders

Equine Granulomatous Enteritis. Equine granulomatous enteritis is characterized by wasting and hypoalbuminemia and has been reported most often in thoroughbred and standardbred horses younger than 5 years of age. The pathogenesis of the disease is unknown. In a few cases *Mycobacterium avium* was isolated from lesions. The disease is characterized by diffuse or segmental transmural noncaseating granulomatous inflammation of the small and occasionally large intestines. Giant cells are present in approximately half the cases. The result is a notably thickened bowel (Figs. 7-142 and 7-143).

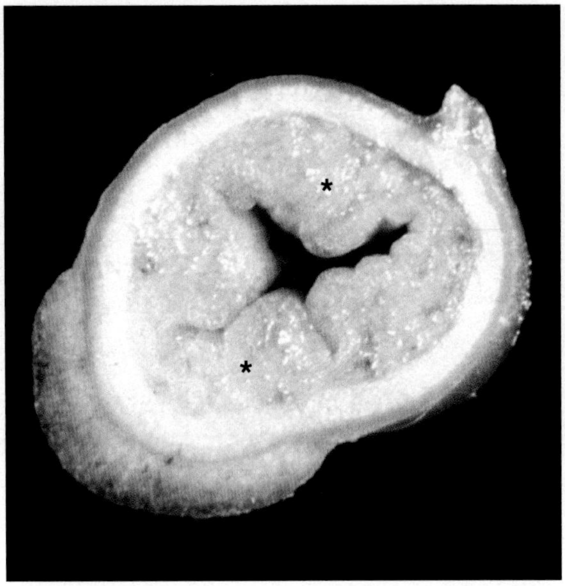

Figure 7-142 **Equine Granulomatous Enteritis, Small Intestine (Formalin Fixed), Horse.** The lamina propria *(asterisks)* is greatly thickened by granulomatous inflammatory cells. (Courtesy Dr. H. Gelberg, College of Veterinary Medicine, Oregon State University.)

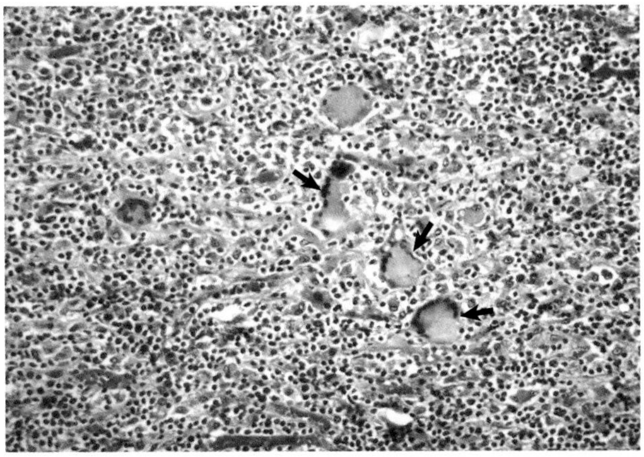

Figure 7-143 **Equine Granulomatous Enteritis, Small Intestine, Horse.** Mononuclear inflammatory cells (macrophages, lymphocytes, plasma cells) and multinucleate giant cells *(arrows)* are present in the lamina propria and submucosa. H&E stain. (Courtesy Dr. H. Gelberg, College of Veterinary Medicine, Oregon State University.)

Clostridial Enteritis (Colitis X). The severe diarrhea seen in cases of colitis X contains no blood and is rapidly fatal. The cause is unknown. However, the disease is associated with certain environmental and clinical variables. These include exhaustion; shock or other stressors; enterotoxemia, perhaps associated with overgrowth of *C. perfringens* type A (antibiotic enteritis); *Clostridium cadaveris*; *C. difficile*; anaphylaxis; or high protein–low cellulose diets. Lesions are limited to the mucosa of the cecum and colon and consist of edema, congestion, and hemorrhage (Fig. 7-144). The location and nature of these lesions overlap with those of acute enteric salmonellosis and equine monocytic ehrlichiosis. Therefore elimination of *Salmonella* spp. and *N. risticii* as causes is necessary before a diagnosis of colitis X can be made. Thus colitis X is a diagnosis made by exclusion of other causes. Appropriate lesions such as gelatinous edema of the intestinal wall, combined with variable intestinal congestion and hemorrhage, green, variably bloody diarrhea, and submucosal thromboses and detection of A-B toxins, are diagnostic. At necropsy, in addition to the intestinal lesions, evidence of endotoxic shock, such as disseminated intravascular coagulopathy, thrombosis, and hemorrhage of the adrenal cortices (Waterhouse-Friderichsen syndrome) can be present, as in salmonellosis and other septicemic diseases.

Hemorrhagic Fibrinonecrotic Duodenitis–Proximal Jejunitis. In hemorrhagic fibrinonecrotic duodenitis–proximal jejunitis, also known as *anterior enteritis* and *gastroduodenojejunitis*, the morphologic description of the lesions is the same as the name of this

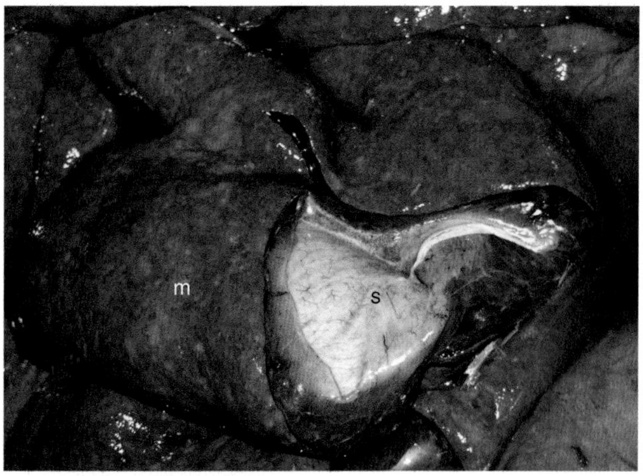

Figure 7-144 **Clostridial Enteritis, Colon, Horse.** Commonly called *colitis X*, this disease is characterized by mucosal edema, congestion, and hemorrhage. The lesions are attributed to endotoxemia caused by several species of clostridia, most likely *Clostridium difficile*. Note the punctate mucosal erosions and ulcerations. *s*, Serosa; *m*, mucosa. (Courtesy Drs. V. Hsiao and A. Gillen, College of Veterinary Medicine, University of Illinois.)

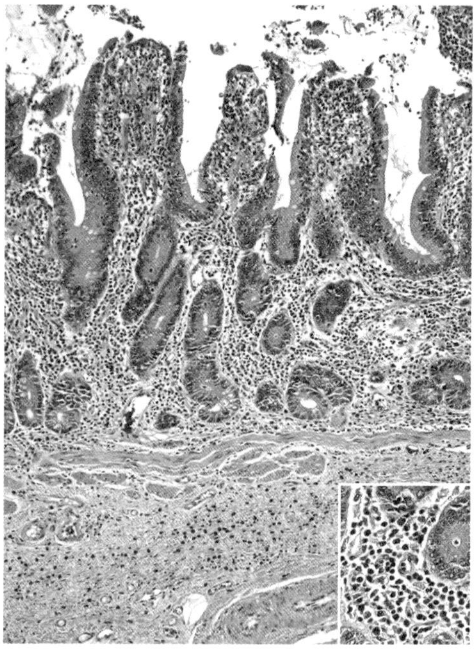

Figure 7-145 **Eosinophilic Enteritis, Small Intestine, Horse.** Eosinophils are numerous within the deep lamina propria, mucosal/submucosal interface, and superficial submucosa. Except in rare cases in which an etiologic agent is diagnosed and treated successfully, affected horses die. *Inset*, The lamina propria contains a mixture of eosinophils, lymphocytes, macrophages, and fibroblasts. H&E stain. (Courtesy Dr. H. Gelberg, College of Veterinary Medicine, Oregon State University.)

idiopathic disease. The disease is characterized microscopically by submucosal edema and a neutrophilic infiltrate of the submucosa and lamina propria. *Salmonella* and clostridial infections are suspected as the cause. This disease occurs in horses older than 9 years, and the definitive diagnosis is made at necropsy by the characteristic hemorrhagic necrotizing lesions in the small intestine. The duodenum is always involved; jejunal involvement is variable.

Chronic Eosinophilic Gastroenteritis and Multisystemic Eosinophilic Epitheliotropic Disease. Soft stools accompanied by weight loss characterize chronic eosinophilic gastroenteritis and multisystemic eosinophilic epitheliotropic disease, which are uncommon conditions. The inflammatory reaction consists of eosinophils among other inflammatory cells in both nodular and diffuse accumulations within all portions and layers of the GI system, salivary glands, and mesenteric lymph nodes (Fig. 7-145). A circulating eosinophilia may be present. The histologic findings of the condition, especially the presence of eosinophils, suggest a hypersensitivity reaction that in at least one instance was associated with *Pythium* spp. infection. With the exception of the rare cases with a specific etiologic agent, affected horses die. The disease is associated with an upregulated T helper lymphocyte type 2 response and increased IL-5 production.

Clinical signs relating to the GI system may include watery diarrhea and hypoproteinemia secondary to protein-losing enteropathy. In human beings and occasionally in horses the lymphoplasmacytic infiltrates in this condition are precursors to lymphoma.

Idiopathic Focal Eosinophilic Enteritis. Idiopathic focal eosinophilic enteritis is characterized by infiltration of eosinophils along with macrophages and fibroblasts in the mucosa and transmurally to the serosa (see Fig. 7-145). The cause of the condition is unknown and is associated with obstructive colic. Resection of the affected portion of the intestine is curative in most cases.

Cranial Cecal Impaction. In this uncommon condition, impaction of cecal cupula (cecal base) occurs without other cecal or intestinal involvement. Type I impactions are due to dry digesta; Type II are secondary to motility disorders such as ileus. Typical signs include mild colic without abnormalities being detected by rectal examination. Successful treatment is by typhlotomy and removal of the impacted material.

Anaphylactoid Purpura. Leukocytoclastic vasculitis associated with numerous discrete foci of necrosis and hemorrhage throughout the intestine and in the mucosa of the larynx and skeletal muscles is termed *anaphylactoid purpura* in the horse and *Henoch-Schönlein purpura* in human beings (see Fig. 15-32). Anecdotal evidence suggests that an Arthus-like hypersensitivity reaction to a streptococcal respiratory infection is the mechanism of lesion production.

Parasitic Enteritides

See Disorders of Domestic Animals, Intestine, Diseases Caused by Specific Pathogens, Parasitic Diseases.

Vascular Diseases of the Intestine

Strongylus vulgaris. In horses *Strongylus vulgaris* fourth-stage larvae are present in the wall of the cranial mesenteric artery, resulting in arteritis. So-called aneurysms (some with osseous metaplasia and bone marrow) and mural thromboses develop (Fig. 7-146; also see Fig. 10-73). In many cases even complete occlusion of the anterior mesenteric artery (see Fig. 2-25) does not result in bowel infarction because collateral circulation will develop if the vascular occlusion develops slowly (Fig. 7-147). Therefore it is important to ascertain if the colonic arteries are thrombosed before assigning the cause of bowel death to *S. vulgaris*. Severe colic and death often result from bowel infarction secondary to verminous arteritis and thrombosis.

Third-stage larvae are ingested and molt to fourth-stage larvae in the small intestine. They then invade small arterioles on their way to the anterior mesenteric artery. It takes 3 to 4 months in this

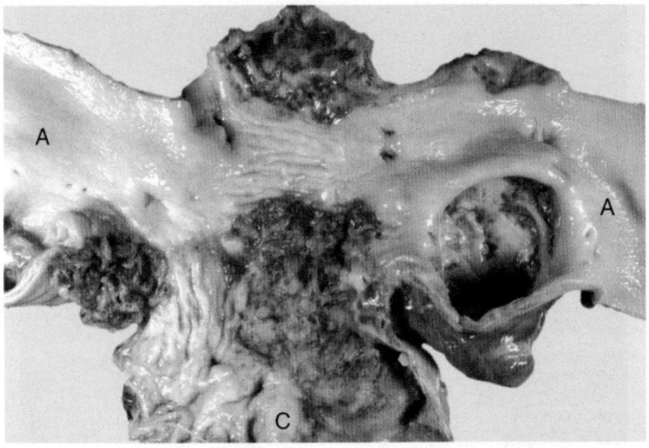

Figure 7-146 Verminous Arteritis, Cranial Mesenteric Artery *(C)*, Horse. Chronic proliferative arteritis and mural thrombosis have resulted from the migration of *Strongylus vulgaris* fourth-stage larvae through and within the vessel wall at or near its origin from the aorta *(A)*. The arteritis can lead to mural thrombosis, formation of aneurysms *(lower right)*, arterial mineralization, and infarction of the bowel. (Courtesy Dr. H. Gelberg, College of Veterinary Medicine, Oregon State University.)

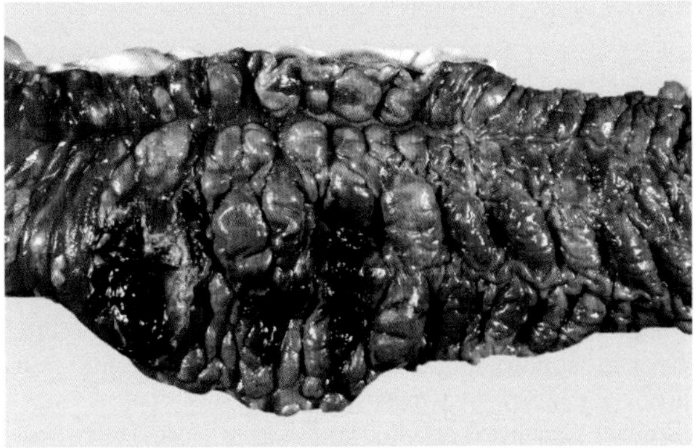

Figure 7-147 Infarcts, Small Intestine, Horse. Thromboemboli from sites of verminous arteritis in the cranial mesenteric artery will often lodge in end arteries of segments of the small intestine, resulting in sudden vascular occlusion and bowel infarction *(areas of red to dark red mucosa)*. (Courtesy Dr. H. Gelberg, College of Veterinary Medicine, Oregon State University.)

location until fifth-stage larvae are produced and migrate through the blood vessels to the cecocolonic subserosa. They may be walled off similarly to *Oesophagostomum* spp. in ruminants and pigs. In the lumen of the large intestine, adults develop. The entire cycle takes up to 6 months or more. Thus the prepatent period in foals is considerable, and by the time ova appear in the feces, significant vascular damage may have occurred. Modern deworming regimens have been quite effective and will hopefully succeed in making this disease of historic significance only.

Intestinal Neoplasia

See Disorders of Domestic Animals, Intestine, Intestinal Neoplasia.

Peritoneum, Omentum, Mesentery, and Peritoneal Cavity

See Disorders of Domestic Animals; Peritoneum, Omentum, Mesentery, and Peritoneal Cavity.

Disorders of Ruminants (Cattle, Sheep, and Goats)

For disorders occurring in two or more species of animals, see Disorders of Domestic Animals.

Oral Cavity

Viral Diseases

Foot-and-Mouth Disease. Foot-and-mouth disease is an extremely important disease and disease threat of artiodactyls worldwide but has not appeared in U.S. livestock since 1929, when it was eradicated after an outbreak in California. Virus spreads rapidly and principally by aerosol. The disease is characterized in its early stages by vesicles in the planum nasale, in the oral cavity, and tongue. The picornavirus of foot-and-mouth disease attaches to susceptible cells via integrins on the cell surface. Fluid from ruptured vesicles spreads to areas of abraded skin, for example, skin of a mammary gland. When coronary bands and hooves are affected, coronary band vesiculation may eventually lead to sloughing of the hoof. Although this disease is not fatal, the pain and accompanying inappetence lead to weight loss. If allowed to heal, the hoof will regrow into a ball-like structure. Young animals with foot-and-mouth disease frequently have a viral myocarditis without other signs. Vaccination is short-lived (6 months) and takes time to become effective in individual animals; thus immediate protection is not provided. Persistent infections occur in water buffalo and infected cattle that have been previously vaccinated.

Vesicular Stomatitides. See Disorders of Domestic Animals, Oral Cavity, Vesicular Stomatitides—Viral Diseases.

Erosive and Ulcerative Stomatitides. See Disorders of Domestic Animals, Oral Cavity, Erosive and Ulcerative Stomatitides.

Parapox Stomatitides. The two major diseases in this category, bovine papular stomatitis and contagious ecthyma, are zoonotic. Bovine papular stomatitis is recognized by papules on the nares, muzzle, gingiva, buccal cavity, palate, and tongue (Fig. 7-148). Lesions also occur in the esophagus, rumen, and omasum. Microscopically, acantholysis is responsible for the macule and ballooning degeneration of these cells, which may contain intracytoplasmic eosinophilic parapoxvirus inclusions at a later stage (Fig. 7-149; also see Fig. 1-11). Erosion of the infected cells accompanied by a neutrophilic infiltrate heals readily from the unaffected basal epithelium. The disease is more common in immunosuppressed animals such as those persistently infected with bovine viral diarrhea virus. In human beings the disease is called *milker's nodules* and is characterized by papules of the hands and arms.

Contagious ecthyma, sore mouth or infectious pustular dermatitis, is a condition of sheep and goats characterized by progression of the stages typical of poxviruses—macules, papules, vesicles, pustules, scabs, and scars in areas of skin abrasions, including the corners of the mouth (Fig. 7-150; also see Fig. 17-65), mouth, udder, teats, coronary bands, and anus. Occasionally the mucosa of the esophagus and rumen also can be affected. The virus is quite hardy and can survive for 50 to 60 days in the summer and longer in cold weather. At room temperature, scabs containing virus can be infective after 10 years. Eosinophilic cytoplasmic inclusion bodies are visible at microscopic examination of lesions early in the course of disease. The condition in human beings is called *orf*.

Teeth

See Disorders of Domestic Animals, Teeth.

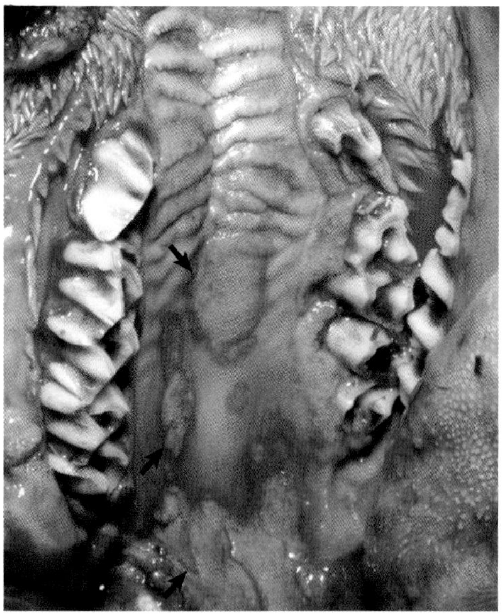

Figure 7-148 **Epithelial Plaques, Papular Stomatitis, Hard Palate Mucosa, Calf.** Virus-induced (parapoxvirus) epithelial plaques and papules are present on the mucosal epithelium of the hard palate and adjacent gingiva *(arrows)*. (Courtesy Dr. M.D. McGavin, College of Veterinary Medicine, University of Tennessee.)

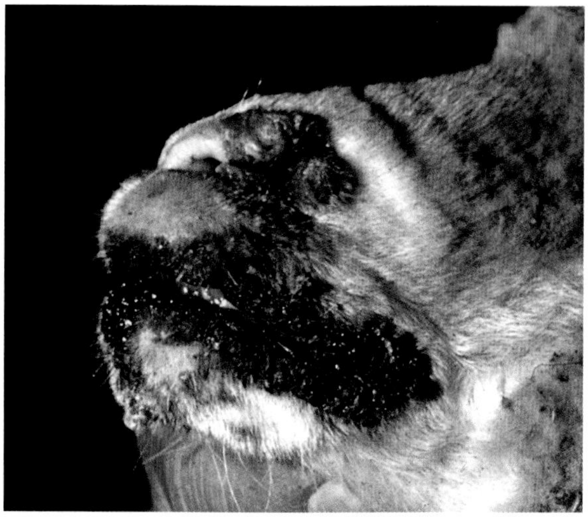

Figure 7-150 **Contagious Ecthyma, Oral Mucous Membranes, Lamb.** Note crusts around nose and lips. Multiple pustules and coalescing ruptured pustules covered by scabs are present on the skin. The parapoxvirus induces epithelial proliferation (acanthosis), followed by vesicle formation. These vesicles rupture and are quickly covered by scabs. Lesions develop at the sites of trauma, such as occur with a nursing lamb, where damage to the superficial oral epithelium allows entry of the virus into skin. (Courtesy Dr. M.D. McGavin, College of Veterinary Medicine, University of Tennessee.)

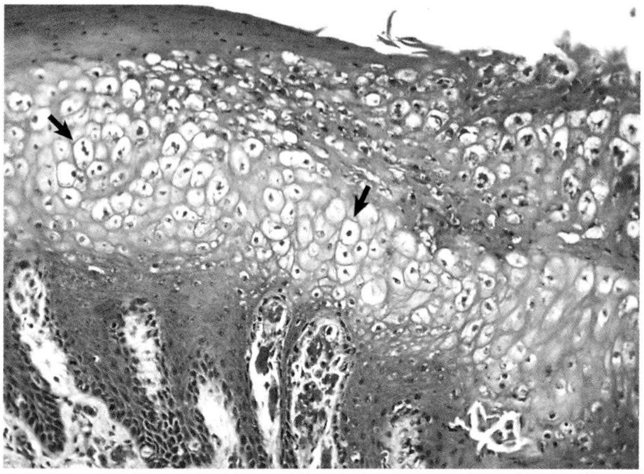

Figure 7-149 **Hydropic Change, Papular Stomatitis, Hard Palate Mucosa, Cow.** There is massive cytoplasmic swelling *(arrows)* of the epithelial cells of the stratum spinosum. At an earlier stage, these cells may contain intracytoplasmic eosinophilic parapoxvirus inclusions (not visible here). H&E stain. (Courtesy Dr. M.D. McGavin, College of Veterinary Medicine, University of Tennessee.)

Tonsils

See Disorders of Domestic Animals, Tonsils.

Bovine viral diarrhea and rinderpest viruses multiply in the tonsils.

Salivary Glands

See Disorders of Domestic Animals, Salivary Glands.

Tongue

See Disorders of Domestic Animals, Tongue.

Esophagus

See Disorders of Domestic Animals, Esophagus

Rumen, Reticulum, and Omasum

Bloat (Ruminal Tympany)

Ruminal tympany, or bloat, is by definition an overdistention of the rumen and reticulum by gases produced during fermentation. Mortality of affected animals is approximately 50%. A hereditary predisposition to bloat might exist in cattle because cases are on record of bloat in monozygotic twins. Bloat can be divided into primary tympany and secondary tympany.

Primary tympany is also known as *legume bloat, dietary bloat,* or *frothy bloat.* It generally occurs up to 3 days after animals begin a new diet. Certain legumes, such as alfalfa, ladino clover, and grain concentrates, promote the formation of stable foam. The nonvolatile acids of legume and ruminal fermentation lower the rumen pH to between 5 and 6, which is optimal for formation of bloat. Foam mixed with rumen contents physically blocks the cardia, preventing eructation and causing the rumen to distend with the gases of fermentation. Clinical signs include a distended left paralumbar fossa, a distended abdomen (see E-Fig. 1-8), increased respiratory and heart rates, and late in the disease, decreased ruminal movements. When death occurs, it is attributable to distention of the abdomen, which compresses the diaphragm, moving it cranially (orad), with resultant decreased pleural cavity size and respiratory embarrassment. There is also increased intraabdominal and intrathoracic pressure, resulting in decreased venous return to the heart and ultimately generalized congestion cranial to the thoracic inlet.

The lesions of primary tympany are often difficult to detect if there is an interval between death and postmortem examination because the foam can collapse. Conversely, fermentation can occur after death in a nonbloated animal, resulting in the production of abundant gas. The most reliable postmortem indicator of antemortem bloat is the sharp line of demarcation most evident in the mucosa between the pale, bloodless esophagus distal to the thoracic inlet and the congested proximal esophagus cranial (orad) to it. This line may sometimes form even after death before the blood clots. This division is known as a *bloat line* (Fig. 7-151).

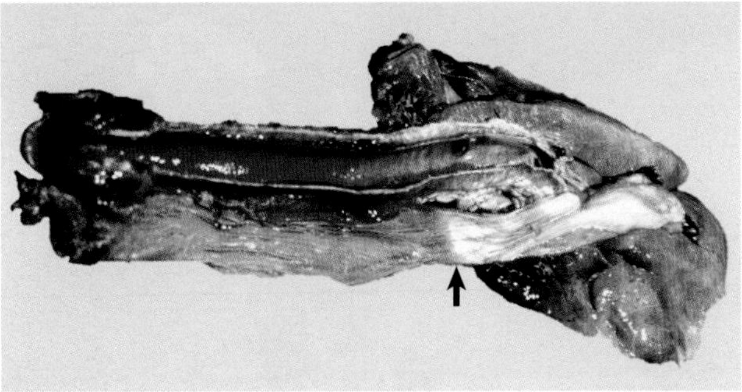

Figure 7-151 **Bloat Line, Esophagus and Trachea at the Thoracic Inlet, Cow.** There is a sharp demarcation between the caudal (blanched) and the cranial (congested) mucosa of the esophagus *(arrow)*. This demarcation is caused by compromised venous return, the result of a grossly distended rumen displacing the diaphragm cranially and causing increased intrathoracic pressure, thus preventing the flow of venous blood into the thorax. In this illustration, a similar demarcation can be seen on the mucosa of the trachea. The subcutaneous tissues of the neck and head are also congested. (Courtesy Department of Veterinary Pathology, Cornell University.)

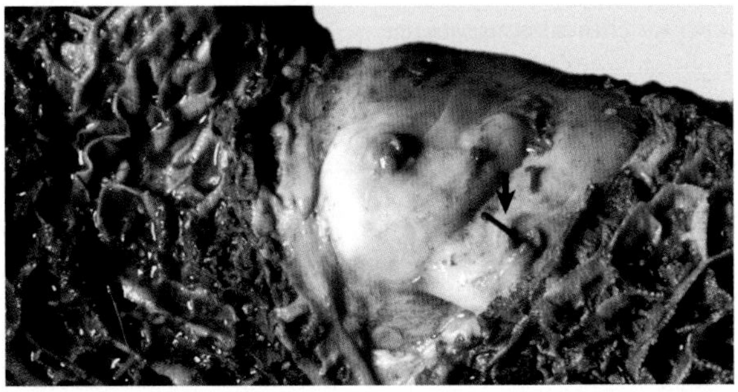

Figure 7-152 **Traumatic Reticulitis, Reticulum, Cow.** Several ingested wires have perforated the wall of the reticulum *(arrow)* and lodged in the tunica muscularis. Each wire is surrounded by a sinus tract draining to the surface of the reticulum. A chronic ulcer has formed around each area penetrated by the wires. (Courtesy Dr. M.D. McGavin, College of Veterinary Medicine, University of Tennessee.)

Secondary tympany is caused by a physical or functional obstruction or stenosis of the esophagus, resulting in failure to eructate. Examples of physical causes are esophageal papilloma, lymphoma, esophageal foreign bodies, and enlarged mesenteric or tracheobronchial lymph nodes, usually from lymphoma or tuberculosis. Vagus indigestion or other innervation disorders are examples of functional disorders.

It is questionable if New World camelids bloat.

Foreign Bodies

Foreign bodies can collect or lodge in the rumen. These include trichobezoars (hairballs) and phytobezoars (plant balls). Trichobezoars are sometimes a sequela to a habit of bucket-fed calves sucking on the skin of each other to satisfy their nursing instincts. Trichobezoars can form *in utero* because of hair circulating in the amniotic fluid and being swallowed by the fetus. Phytobezoars result from an excess of indigestible roughage. Ingestion of nails and wire, common where straw and hay bales are bound by wire, can result in perforation of the wall of the reticulum with resultant reticulitis, peritonitis, or eventually possible pericarditis (hardware disease) (Fig. 7-152). Often, in areas in the United States in which ruminants are at high risk for hardware disease because of farming practices, magnets are placed in rumens to prevent the ingested wires and nails from penetrating the reticular mucosa. Occasionally ruminants ingest plates from storage batteries and suffer lead poisoning.

Inflammatory Diseases

Inflammation of the rumen, rumenitis, is generally considered synonymous with lactic acidosis. Lactic acidosis is synonymous with grain overload, rumen overload, carbohydrate engorgement, and chemical rumenitis. All ruminants are susceptible. The pathophysiologic process of lactic acidosis usually involves a sudden dietary change to an easily fermentable feed or a change in the feed volume consumed. The latter scenario is most likely to occur during weather changes, especially among feedlot cattle, when a sudden cooling rainstorm will stimulate food intake of cattle that had previously lost appetite because of high environmental temperatures and humidity.

Ruminal microflora is generally rich in cellulolytic Gram-negative bacteria necessary for the digestion of hay. A sudden change to a highly fermentable, carbohydrate-rich feed promotes the growth of Gram-positive bacteria, *Streptococcus bovis*, and *Lactobacillus* spp. The lactic acid produced by the fermentation of ingested carbohydrates decreases the ruminal pH below 5 (normal, 5.5 to 7.5). This acidic pH eliminates normal ruminal flora and fauna and damages ruminal mucosa. Increased concentrations of dissociated fatty acids lead to ruminal atony. When death occurs, it is due to dehydration secondary to the increased osmotic effect of ruminal solutes (organic acids), causing movement of fluids across the damaged ruminal mucosa into the rumen, acidosis (from absorption of lactate from the rumen), and circulatory collapse. Mortality among animals with lactic acidosis ranges from 25% to 90% and usually occurs within 24 hours.

At necropsy the ruminal and intestinal contents are watery and acidic. Often, abundant grain is found in the rumen. The mucosa of the ruminal papillae is brown and friable and detaches easily, especially from the ventral ruminal sac. Caution must be exercised in interpreting this latter finding as a lesion because the ruminal mucosa often detaches easily in animals that have been dead for even a few hours at high environmental temperatures. Hydropic change and coagulative necrosis of the ruminal epithelium followed by an influx of neutrophils are common microscopic lesions. Animals surviving lactic acidosis develop stellate scars that are visible because of their color difference from the unaffected surrounding ruminal mucosa. Scars are pale; unaffected mucosa may be light to dark brown to black, depending on the original diet.

New World camelids appear to be more sensitive than ruminants to high-carbohydrate diets. Although their compartments do not have papillae, widespread ulceration of the squamous mucosa occurs in cases of lactic acidosis. New World camelids retain feed in their stomach longer than ruminants, possibly increasing fermentation and acid production. They rely on emptying of fluid to preserve milieu. High-energy feeds may quickly impede motility, promoting a drop in pH.

Bacterial rumenitis generally occurs secondary to lactic acidosis or mechanical injury to the ruminal mucosa. Bacteria that colonize the damaged ruminal wall can be transported into the portal circulation and to the liver, resulting in multiple abscesses. *Arcanobacterium (Corynebacterium) pyogenes* is a common cause of bacterial abscesses in the liver. *F. necrophorum*, also transported from the rumen to the liver, results in necrobacillosis, which has distinctive liver lesions.

Mycotic infections of the rumen also occur secondary to the damage to the ruminal mucosa caused by lactic acidosis and mechanical injury. Mycotic rumenitis also results from the administration of antibiotics, usually in calves but also in adult cattle, which reduce the numbers of normal flora and allow fungi to proliferate. In cases

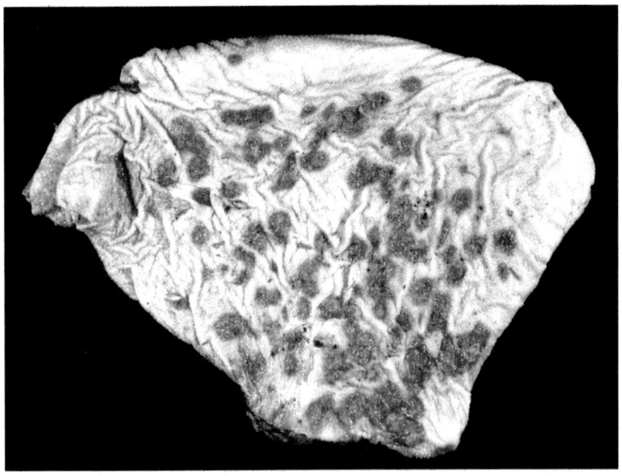

Figure 7-153 Mycotic Rumenitis, Rumen, Calf. Note the numerous well-demarcated red foci of necrosis and hemorrhage (infarcts) in the ruminal mucosa that can be caused by angioinvasive fungi such as *Aspergillus*, *Mucor*, *Rhizopus*, *Absidia*, and *Mortierella* spp. This type of mycotic infection is usually preceded by a chemical (lactic acid) rumenitis (overeating). (Courtesy Dr. H. Gelberg, College of Veterinary Medicine, Oregon State University.)

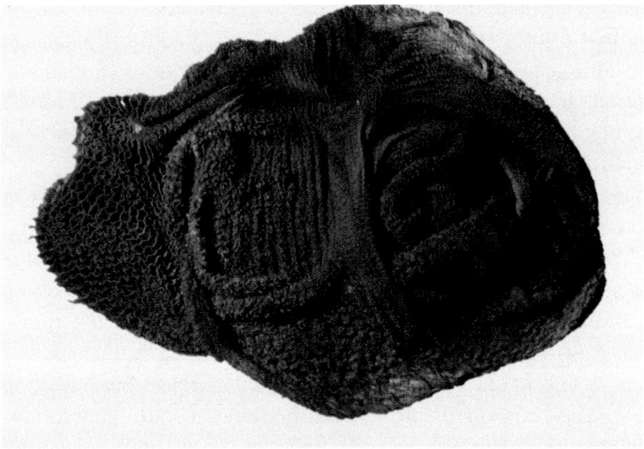

Figure 7-154 Parakeratosis, Reticulorumen, Calf. A diet that was almost devoid of roughage has resulted in atrophy and parakeratosis of ruminal papillae. Normal papillae are leaf shaped, but some of these papillae have become finger shaped, cauliflower shaped, or clumped. The parakeratotic epithelium has been stained brown to black by components of the feed because of the lack of abrasion by the ground feed. These lesions are most marked on the ventral floor of the ventral sac of the rumen. (Courtesy Dr. M.D. McGavin, College of Veterinary Medicine, University of Tennessee.)

of mycotic rumenitis, lesions are generally circular and well delineated and are caused principally by infarction from thrombosis secondary to fungal vasculitis (Fig. 7-153). Offending fungi include *Aspergillus*, *Mucor*, *Rhizopus*, *Absidia*, and *Mortierella* spp. These fungi can spread to the placenta hematogenously and cause mycotic placentitis, which leads to abortions.

Ruminal candidiasis occurs as an incidental finding at necropsy. There is usually an underlying debilitating condition, glucose therapy, milk-replacer overload (sour rumen), or an antibiotic-induced kill-off of resident flora and fauna. Ruminal candidiasis is seldom diagnosed in a live animal.

Miscellaneous Disorders

Ruminal papillae vary in length, becoming longer with high-roughage diets (Fig. 7-154). Such diets also can cause the papilla to

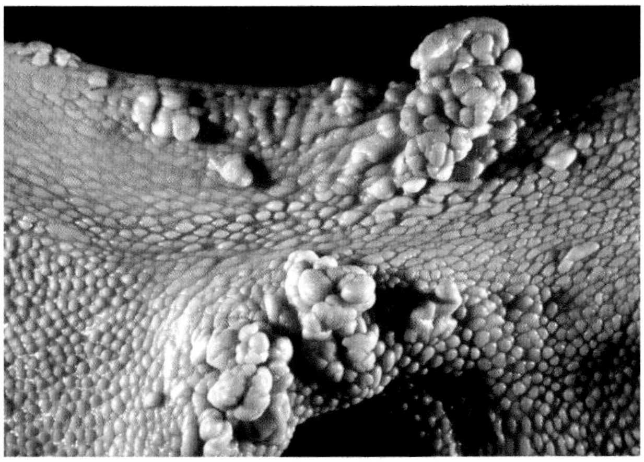

Figure 7-155 Papillomas, Rumen, Cow. Smooth-surfaced, squamous papillomas are present on the dorsal wall. (Courtesy Dr. H. Gelberg, College of Veterinary Medicine, Oregon State University.)

become tongue or leaf shaped. Animals consuming diets with less than 10% roughage can develop ruminal parakeratosis. These rumens have hard, brown, often clumped, papillae. This lesion has little to no clinical consequence.

Ruminal papillomas are papillomavirus induced in some cases, but in certain countries, bracken fern has been implicated as a cofactor in these forestomach neoplasms (Fig. 7-155).

Vagal Indigestion

Vagal indigestion results in a functional outflow problem from the forestomach. Damage to the vagus nerve can occur anywhere along its length and can result in functional pyloric stenosis and omasal dilation. Causes of vagal indigestion include damage to the vagus nerve due to traumatic reticuloperitonitis, liver abscesses with secondary peritonitis, volvulus of the abomasum, and bronchopneumonia. Mechanical obstruction of the forestomach or abomasal outflow can be due to abomasal lymphoma or papillomas or from blockage after ingestion of indigestible or foreign materials. Diet and dwarfism are sometimes associated with vagus indigestion. Many cases are idiopathic. Clinical signs include ruminoreticular distention. The presence of abomasal distention depends on the precise location of the damage to the vagus nerve. Vagal indigestion is divided into the following four types, based on the anatomic location of the functional obstruction.

- Type I is usually caused by inflammatory lesions around the vagal nerve at any location and is a failure of eructation, resulting in bloat.
- Type II is a functional or anatomic condition that results in failure of omasal transport into the abomasum. Usual causes are adhesions and abscesses on the medial wall of the reticulum associated with or secondary to traumatic reticuloperitonitis. Abomasal lymphoma and physical obstruction of the omasal canal (e.g., neoplasia or ingested placenta) may also be causative.
- Type III is caused by physical impaction of the abomasum by roughage and thus is dietary in origin. Abomasal displacements and volvulus are also potential causes.
- Type IV is pregnancy related, perhaps as a result of shifting of position of the abomasum secondary to the expanding uterus, causing compression of the abdominal branches of the vagus nerve.

Ruminal Parasitism

Paramphistomiasis is a fluke infestation of the ruminant forestomach in warmer latitudes around the world. These trematodes are in the

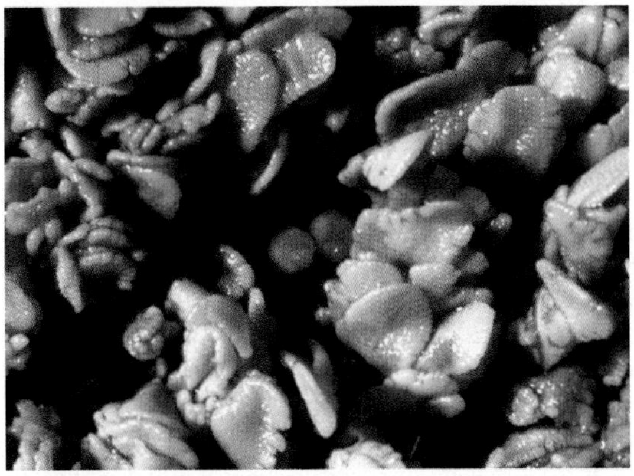

Figure 7-156 **Paramphistomiasis, Rumen, Cow.** The pink conical structures located in the center of the illustration are paramphistomes (ruminal flukes). They are considered to be innocuous, but massive numbers of immature flukes in the duodenum may cause a severe catarrhal duodenitis. Note the normal leaf-shaped ruminal papillae, indicative of a high-roughage diet. (Courtesy Dr. M.D. McGavin, College of Veterinary Medicine, University of Tennessee.)

genera *Paramphistomum*, *Calicophoron*, and *Cotylophoron*. They are similar in size and appearance to ruminal papillae (Fig. 7-156). Although the presence of adult organisms in the forestomach is usually of no clinical significance, heavy infestations of larvae in the proximal small intestine, before migration to the rumen and reticulum, can cause hypoproteinemia, anemia, and death. Larvae burrow deeply into and sometimes through the wall of the small intestine and can be found in the peritoneal cavity. The intermediate host is a snail. Cercariae encyst on aquatic vegetation and are eaten by the ruminant.

Abomasum

Abomasal Displacement

Normally the abomasum lies over the xiphoid process at the abdominal ventral midline. Abomasal displacement is usually to the left side, although right-sided displacements also occur (Fig. 7-157). Left-sided displacement of the abomasum is a generally nonfatal entity seen in high-producing dairy cattle during the 6 weeks after parturition. Strenuous activity can predispose nonpregnant cows to displacement. In the postcalving period, abomasal atony can occur as a result of heavy grain feeding (volatile fatty acids decrease motility) and hypocalcemia. Meanwhile, the gravid uterus may have displaced the rumen and abomasum cranially and to the left, rupturing the attachment of the greater omentum to the abomasum. The abomasum then occupies the cranial left quadrant of the abdomen and displaces the rumen medially. This change leads to partial obstruction of abomasal outflow. Metabolic alkalosis contributes to rumen atony and impaired movement of ingesta. The associated hypochloremia is a result of HCl secretion and is common along with hypokalemia. Abomasal ulcers and peritoneal adhesions can result in cases of chronic displacement.

Fifteen percent of abomasal displacements are right sided. The abomasum can be overdistended, displaced dorsally, and rotated on its mesenteric axis, and 20% of these cases develop abomasal volvulus. Right-sided displacements occur in postparturient dairy cows and in calves.

Clinical features of displaced abomasums, whether right sided or left sided, include anorexia, cachexia, dehydration, lack of feces, ketonuria, and a characteristic high-pitched ping subsequent to percussion over the abomasum. Idiopathic abomasal volvulus occurs occasionally in ruminants and calves (see E-Fig. 7-15).

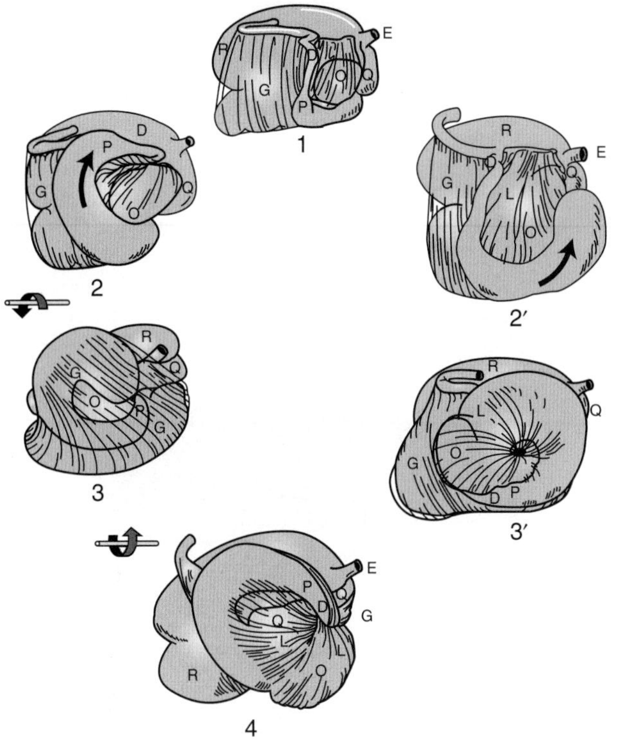

Figure 7-157 **Two Possible Modes of Rotation of the Omasum, Abomasum, and Cranial Part of the Duodenum in Volvulus.** *1*, Normal relations; *2*, simple dilation and displacement on the right; *3*, 180-degree volvulus around the longitudinal axis of the lesser omentum, counterclockwise as seen from the rear; *2′*, 90-degree rotation of the abomasum in a sagittal plane, counterclockwise as seen from the right; *3′*, 180-degree rotation of the abomasum and omasum around the transverse axis of the lesser omentum, drawing the duodenum cranially, medial to the omasum; *4*, 360-degree counterclockwise volvulus, final stage resulting from either mode of rotation. *D*, Duodenum; *E*, esophagus; *G*, greater omentum; *L*, lesser omentum; *O*, omasum; *P*, pylorus; *Q*, reticulum; *R*, rumen. (Modified from Habel RE, Smith DF: *J Am Vet Med Assoc* 179:447-455, 1981.)

Abomasal Dilation and Tympany

Abomasal dilation and tympany is a syndrome of young cattle that occurs most commonly in dairy breeds with a history of one or more of the following: only a single milk feeding per day, cold milk or milk replacer, lack of free choice water, inconsistency of feeding time, dosing with high-energy oral electrolyte solutions, and sometimes failure of passive transfer of immunity. The pathophysiologic process is presumed to be abomasal fermentation of high-energy ingesta by gas-producing bacteria. Hyperglycemia and a resultant glycosuria are present. Hemorrhage, edema, necrosis, and sometimes emphysema of the abomasum and other compartments of the forestomach are found at necropsy.

Abomasal Emptying Defect

See Disorders of Domestic Animals, Stomach and Abomasum, Impaction.

Braxy (Clostridium septicum)—Inflammatory Diseases

See Disorders of Domestic Animals, Stomach and Abomasum, Inflammatory Diseases.

Intestine

Viral Diseases

Bovine Viral Diarrhea. Bovine viral diarrhea, also known as *mucosal disease*, affects cattle of all ages but is most common in animals 8 months to 2 years of age. In this respect, clinical cases are typically younger than animals susceptible to Johne's disease. Animals, including New World camelids, infected *in utero* or early in life with noncytopathic bovine viral diarrhea pestivirus develop a persistent infection as a result of immunotolerance. They shed virus throughout their lives. Later in life, if exposed to cytopathic pestivirus, they may develop disease. Multifocal, sharply demarcated erosions and ulcers in the tongue, gingiva, palate (see Fig. 7-35), esophagus (Fig. 7-158), rumen, abomasum, and coronary bands of the hooves characterize bovine viral diarrhea. In the intestine the characteristic lesion is sharply demarcated foci of necrosis in the epithelium over the GALT (Figs. 7-159 and 7-160). Lesions in the stratified squamous epithelium begin in the stratum spinosum. Necrosis of the epithelium is soon followed by the formation of erosions and ulcerations. Villous and crypt enterocytes become necrotic. There is lympholysis in the GALT. Follicular medullary regions of intestinal lymphoid tissue may be filled with cell debris and dead enterocytes. There is commonly a fibrinonecrotic pseudomembrane over the damaged GALT.

Clinical signs may include anorexia, depression, profuse watery diarrhea with staining of the perineum and tail, agalactia, pyrexia, rumen atony, ptyalism, lacrimation, and a mucopurulent nasal discharge. Calves infected *in utero* may have cerebellar hypoplasia, cataracts, microphthalmia, or renal dysplasia and other congenital defects develop. Abortions, stillbirths, and mummified fetuses can also result from *in utero* infection in New World camelids, cervids, sheep, goats, and cattle. Aborted calves often have enlarged hemal lymph nodes. Morbidity in a herd varies from 2% to 50%. All affected animals die.

A more common outcome from bovine viral diarrhea infection occurs in immunocompetent animals that are seronegative at the time of exposure to either the cytopathic or noncytopathic virus. Variable signs develop, but they are mostly mild or subclinical. Most cattle in the United States have serologic evidence of exposure to nonvaccine bovine viral diarrhea virus. Exotic ruminants may also become infected. Under certain circumstances pigs may become subclinically infected. This is of interest because the viruses of bovine viral diarrhea and hog cholera are antigenically closely related. This may cause confusing serologic results when testing hogs for cholera. New World camelids may also succumb to bovine viral

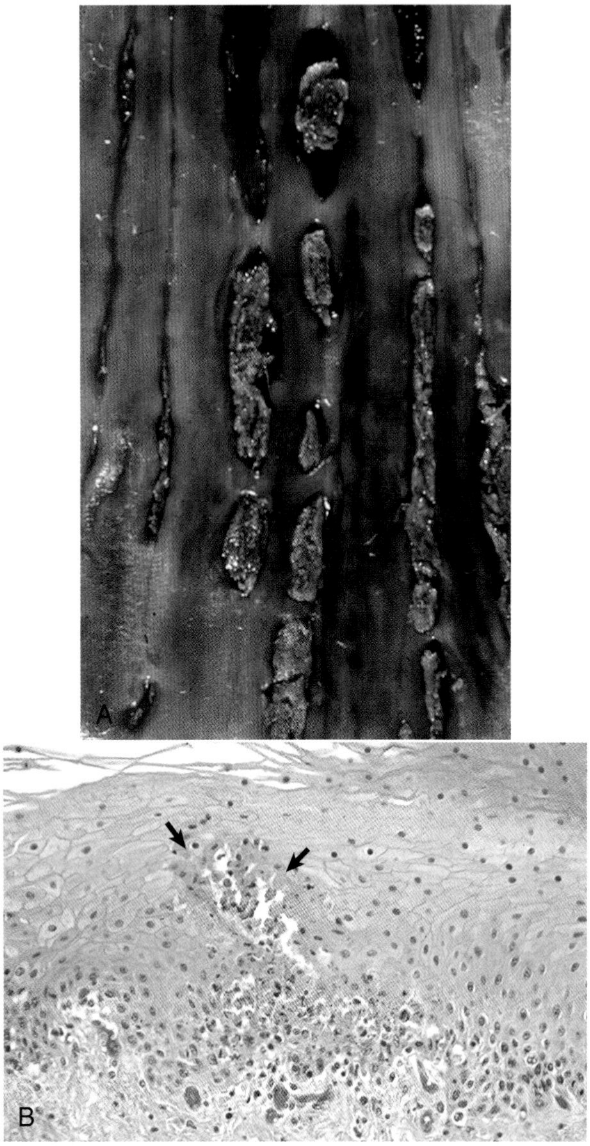

Figure 7-158 **Acute Multifocal Ulcers, Esophagus, Cow. A,** Grossly, there are multiple sharply demarcated ulcers *(vertically linear red streaks)* and similar areas covered by diphtheritic membranes *(vertically linear yellow-brown streaks)*. The cause is the pestivirus of bovine viral diarrhea. **B,** Microscopically, there is a focus of necrosis *(arrows)* of cells of the stratum basale and stratum spinosum caused by the pestivirus of bovine viral diarrhea. H&E stain. (**A** courtesy Department of Veterinary Biosciences, College of Veterinary Medicine, The Ohio State University; and Noah's Arkive, College of Veterinary Medicine, The University of Georgia. **B** courtesy Dr. J.S. Haynes, College of Veterinary Medicine, Iowa State University; and Noah's Arkive, College of Veterinary Medicine, The University of Georgia.)

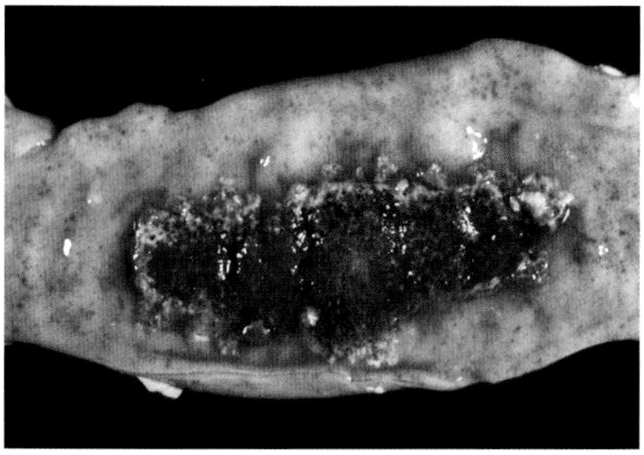

Figure 7-159 **Bovine Viral Diarrhea, Ileum, Mucosa, Cow.** Peyer's patches and the overlying epithelium are necrotic *(red to dark red elliptical area)* and covered with suppurative exudate *(yellow-white granular material)*. (Courtesy Dr. H. Gelberg, College of Veterinary Medicine, Oregon State University.)

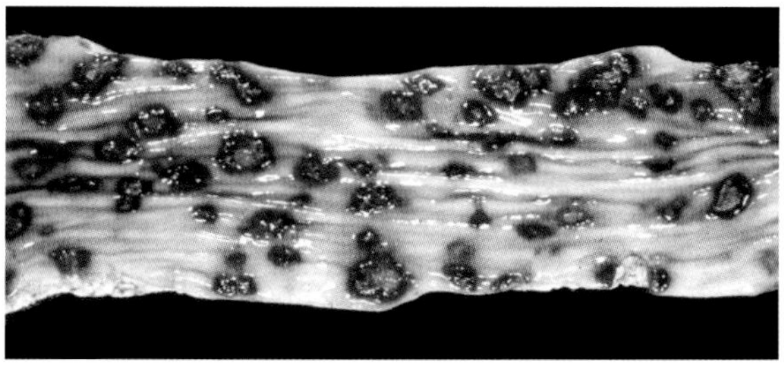

Figure 7-160 **Multifocal Ulcerative Colitis, Bison, Colon.** Multiple mucosal ulcers were caused by bovine viral diarrhea virus. (Courtesy Dr. H. Gelberg, College of Veterinary Medicine, Oregon State University.)

diarrhea infection, although infections are often subclinical. The diagnosis of persistent infection is by immunohistochemical examination of skin biopsies because calves shed large amounts of virus through the skin. Feedlot cattle that are persistently infected are believed to be more susceptible to mannheimiosis, chronic pneumonia and polyarthritis syndrome, salmonellosis, infectious bovine rhinotracheitis, bovine respiratory syncytial virus, and mycoses. Other diagnostic means are virus isolation, reverse transcription PCR (RT-PCR), and antigen-capture ELISA.

Rinderpest. Lesions similar to those of bovine viral diarrhea occur in cattle with rinderpest. The morbillivirus associated with rinderpest infects cattle, sheep, goats, pigs, water buffalo, giraffes, wildebeest, and other wild ruminants. Disease spread is via aerosolization and contact with other body secretions. Initial virus replication is in tonsils and pharyngeal and mandibular lymph nodes, resulting in viremia. Acute necrosis is typically severe in all lymph nodes and the epithelial lining of the alimentary, respiratory, and reproductive systems, including erosions and ulcers of the oral cavity and nasal planum. These lesions are particularly severe in regions of GALT, similar to bovine viral diarrhea. Pale eosinophilic, cytoplasmic, and perinuclear inclusion bodies surrounded by a halo are sometimes seen in epithelia and lymphoid tissue macrophages. Intranuclear inclusions are visible less often. The signature lesion is characteristic multinucleate enterocytes in epithelial tissues, including the intestinal lesions that do not occur in bovine viral diarrhea. Postinfection immunity is likely lifelong. Rinderpest does not occur in the United States or Europe but is a significant disease in Africa and Asia and is believed to be on the verge of eradication through effective vaccination. In immunologically naïve populations of animals, morbidity and mortality may be high.

Peste des Petits Ruminants. Peste des petits ruminants is a distinct morbillivirus disease of sheep and goats that causes ulcerative and pseudomembranous lesions of the oral cavity, similar to rinderpest, along with necrotizing tonsillitis, fibrinohemorrhagic enteritis, and bronchointerstitial pneumonia. Syncytial cells and nuclear and cytoplasmic inclusion bodies of epithelial and lymphoid tissues similar to those found in rinderpest are also present. Peste des petits ruminants is enzootic in the Middle East, the Indian subcontinent, and North Africa.

Border Disease. The pestivirus causing border disease in sheep and goats is antigenically related to the noncytopathic biotype of bovine viral diarrhea virus. Border disease is usually a congenital infection associated with reproductive failure or birth of abnormal lambs and kids. When subsequently infected with a cytopathic virus, they develop lesions similar to bovine viral diarrhea of cattle. Border disease has been reported in the British Isles, Australia, New Zealand, and the United States.

Malignant Catarrhal Fever. Malignant catarrhal fever, which is caused by closely related rhadinoviruses (γ-herpesviruses), occurs in a variety of species of ruminants, including cervids and bison. Persistent infection is common in host species, and disease occurs as a result of cross-species transmission. The African form of the disease, caused by alcelaphine herpesvirus 1 is common in wildebeests and other ruminants. In the United States and worldwide, ovine herpesvirus 2 (OvHV-2), caprine herpesvirus 2, and white-tailed deer herpesvirus are most often reported in ruminants. The respiratory form of the disease, associated with keratoconjunctivitis, is most commonly seen in cattle in the United States.

Lesions include widespread lymphadenomegaly, mucosal necrosis, lymphoplasmacytic necrotizing arteritis and phlebitis of the subcutis, and especially in the rete mirabile surrounding the base of the pituitary gland. Hoof walls may be shed. Coagulation necrosis is found in lymph nodes, and lymphoplasmacytic infiltrates are present in the retina, myocardium, brain, spinal cord, and meninges. The alimentary form of the disease is characterized as multifocal ulcerative stomatitis (see Fig. 7-35), glossitis, esophagitis, abomasitis, and enterotyphlocolitis associated with vasculitis. Hemorrhagic cystitis may also be present.

Winter Dysentery. Winter dysentery is a somewhat enigmatic, acute, generally nonfatal disease of adult cattle. Although its cause is unknown, a coronavirus has been implicated as causative and can sometimes be demonstrated immunohistochemically in colonic basal enterocytes of affected animals. As the disease progresses in a herd, virtually all members become ill. As the name implies, it is a seasonal disease and additionally occurs only in northern latitudes. Catarrhal ileitis and jejunitis characterize this highly contagious disease.

Mild lesions are noted in the rare animal that dies of winter dysentery. The intestinal mucosa is intact, but there is variable congestion and petechiae of the abomasum and small intestine. The intestine may be atonic. The colon may have congestion and hemorrhage of the colonic mucosal folds, a nonspecific lesion associated with tenesmus (tiger striping) (see E-Fig. 7-17).

Acute onset of profuse diarrhea, decreased milk production in dairy cattle, variable depression, and anorexia are characteristic. Malodorous green to black (melena) diarrhea lasts for up to 4 days and may contain fresh blood and mucus. Immunity in dairy herds is protective for years. Older animals are more severely affected than are younger ones. Calves appear to be refractory to disease development. Diagnosis is generally made by epizootic information, clinical signs, its seasonal occurrence, and lack of significant mortality.

Bovine Torovirus Diarrhea. The shedding of bovine torovirus (BoTV), or Breda virus, has been associated with diarrhea of neonatal veal calves. BoTV is a single-stranded, enveloped RNA virus, which currently cannot be grown in cell culture. BoTV is associated with the presence of other enteropathogens of neonates, including rotavirus, coronavirus, *Cryptosporidium*, *Salmonella*, and *Giardia*. Although it is not uncommon to have intercurrent infections producing diarrhea in calves, especially in the presence of immunosuppression, malnutrition, and other stressors, BoTV may cause disease independently. Necrosis and sloughing of enterocytes on the middle and lower villi, extending into the crypts, are noted on histologic examination. Diagnosis is confirmed by antigen-capture ELISA or RT-PCR in feces in the absence of evidence of other enteric pathogens. Death, when it occurs, is due to dehydration.

Coronavirus Colitis of Beef Calves. Recently a hemorrhagic and sometimes fatal colitis was reported from postweaning beef calves in Nebraska. A bovine coronavirus (clade 2) was associated with these lesions and was similar to clade 2 coronavirus isolated from the respiratory system of postweaned beef calves with pulmonary disease or without clinical symptoms.

Bacterial Diseases

***Clostridium perfringens* Type B.** *C. perfringens* type B is the cause of lamb dysentery. This is generally a disease of very young lambs, although older animals may be affected in prolonged disease outbreaks. Unexpected death is usual, but occasionally there is antecedent anorexia and abdominal pain with or without severe bloody diarrhea. Other young ruminants and foals may also be affected. This disease occurs sporadically in the United States but is more common in Europe, South Africa, and the Middle East.

Clostridium perfringens Type D. *C. perfringens* type D affects fattening sheep, goats, and calves. The disease is diet related and associated with grain overload or "overeating disease." The sudden change in diet promotes growth of organisms in the small intestine. The disease is often characterized by unexpected death, sometimes preceded by CNS signs or "blind staggers." Endothelial cell damage is produced by a bacterial toxin (angiotoxin). This lesion can result in bilateral symmetric encephalomalacia, which in sheep is similar in its regional distribution to edema disease of pigs (swine cerebral angiopathy) (see Fig. 14-96). Lesions of *C. perfringens* type D infection are multisystem hemorrhages, particularly of serosal surfaces. Fibrinonecrotic enterocolitis can also occur in association with the β-2 toxin, at least in goats. Pericardial effusion is present along with mild gastroenteritis. The angiotoxin produces "pulpy kidney disease" of sheep (see Fig. 11-42).

Paratuberculosis (Johne's Disease). Paratuberculosis, or Johne's disease, has been described in numerous ruminant species. Ruminants are infected from feces-contaminated soil. In cattle the disease is characterized by intractable diarrhea, emaciation, and hypoproteinemia in animals older than 19 months. In the average infected herd, 32% to 42% of animals are infected. In small ruminants (sheep and goats), the clinical disease is similar to that observed in cattle except that diarrhea does not occur. The pygmy goat is an exception to the course of disease in small ruminants in that some pygmy goats develop explosive diarrhea and die unexpectedly. In other ruminants the disease has a protracted course and is considered a wasting disease because of the loss of body mass (Fig. 7-161). The causative bacterium is *Mycobacterium avium* subsp. *paratuberculosis*.

The causative organisms are very resistant to environmental stressors, particularly in regions with acid soils. After ingestion the bacilli are transported through M cells and taken up by macrophages. Lesions in the lamina propria of the intestines, particularly in the ileum, include the accumulation of macrophages. There is little correlation between the severity of the gross lesions and the severity of clinical disease. An age-related immune resistance to

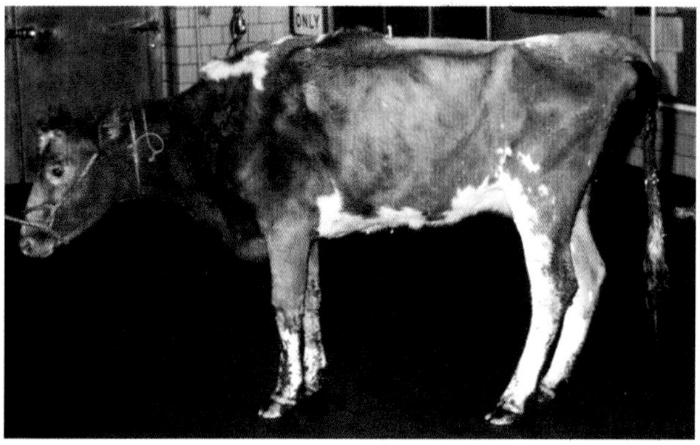

Figure 7-161 **Granulomatous Enteritis, Johne's Disease (*Mycobacterium avium* subsp. *paratuberculosis*), Cow.** There is chronic wasting and diarrhea in this 18-month-old heifer. The age at which this cow showed clinical signs is not typical of the disease. Signs usually occur 2 or more years after initial infection. (Courtesy College of Veterinary Medicine, Cornell University.)

infection and disease develops in animals older than 2 months. Fetuses can be infected, but disease is delayed until the animals are much older. Isolation of newborns from fecal contamination is a useful measure to reduce the incidence of infection in a particular herd.

Diagnosis is made by observing clinical signs together with the signalment. The gross lesion in Johne's disease is a chronic, segmental thickening of the ileum, cecum, and proximal colon (Fig. 7-162). The ileocecal valve region is usually affected. Affected segments have a variably thickened, rough, rugose mucosa, often with multiple foci of ulceration. There is mesenteric lymphadenopathy.

Noncaseating granulomas contain numerous foamy macrophages with large numbers of acid-fast organisms (see Fig. 7-162; also see Figs. 3-25 and 13-82). In contrast, sheep, goats, and deer may have tuberculoid (caseating) granulomas in the intestines, lymphatic vessels, and lymph nodes. These granulomas are sometimes mineralized and contain whorled accumulations of epithelioid macrophages with variable numbers of Langhans-type giant cells. It is more difficult to find acid-fast mycobacteria in these mature granulomas.

M. avium ssp. *paratuberculosis* can be isolated from feces of affected animals, from diseased intestines and regional lymph nodes, and sometimes from a variety of other tissues and fluids, including the liver, uterus, fetus, milk, urine, and semen. Acid-fast bacteria in rectal mucosal scrapings are found in 60% of the cases. Hepatic microgranulomas occur in approximately 25% of affected animals. Aortic and endocardial mineralization (arteriosclerosis), when it occurs in association with the clinical signs and lesions of paratuberculosis, is specific for Johne's disease in cattle (see Figs. 10-22 and 10-53). The pathogenesis of this vascular lesion is not well understood but is associated with the severe cachexia associated with the disease. The epizootiology of Johne's disease leads many to believe it is one of the most important diseases facing the dairy industry. Speculation has existed for many years that Johne's disease is zoonotic and somehow causative of Crohn's disease in human beings.

Hemorrhagic Bowel Syndrome of Dairy Cattle. Hemorrhagic bowel syndrome, also known as fatal jejunal hemorrhage syndrome, intraluminal-intramural hemorrhage of the small intestine, and jejunal hematoma, is characterized by intraluminal hemorrhage resulting in blood clots that lead to intestinal obstruction. It is characterized by dark, clotted blood in the feces; variable and multifocal distention of the small intestine; small intestinal ileus; and necrohemorrhagic jejunitis or enteritis (Fig. 7-163). This peracute fatal disease of dairy cattle during early lactation is tentatively associated with infections caused by *C. perfringens* type A and/or *Aspergillus fumigatus*. The clinical history usually includes a sudden loss of appetite, decreased milk production, abdominal distention, and melena. Usually the history includes a change in feed to a highly digestible, low-fiber ration.

Chlamydial Diseases

Chlamydiosis. Bovine chlamydia (*Chlamydophila pecorum*) has been recovered from spontaneous enteritis of young calves. After experimental inoculation, newborn calves develop fever and diarrhea within 24 hours and become moribund within 4 to 5 days. Grossly the ileum is most severely affected, but the jejunum and large intestine also have lesions. In diseased segments the mucosa is congested and marked with petechiae. The intestinal wall and mesentery are edematous. The lumen contains watery, yellow fluid mixed with a yellow, tenacious, fibrin-rich material attached to the surface. Colonic ridges are hyperemic and have small erosions. Bleeding from petechiae and ecchymoses of the colonic or rectal ridges occurs infrequently. Regional lymph nodes are enlarged.

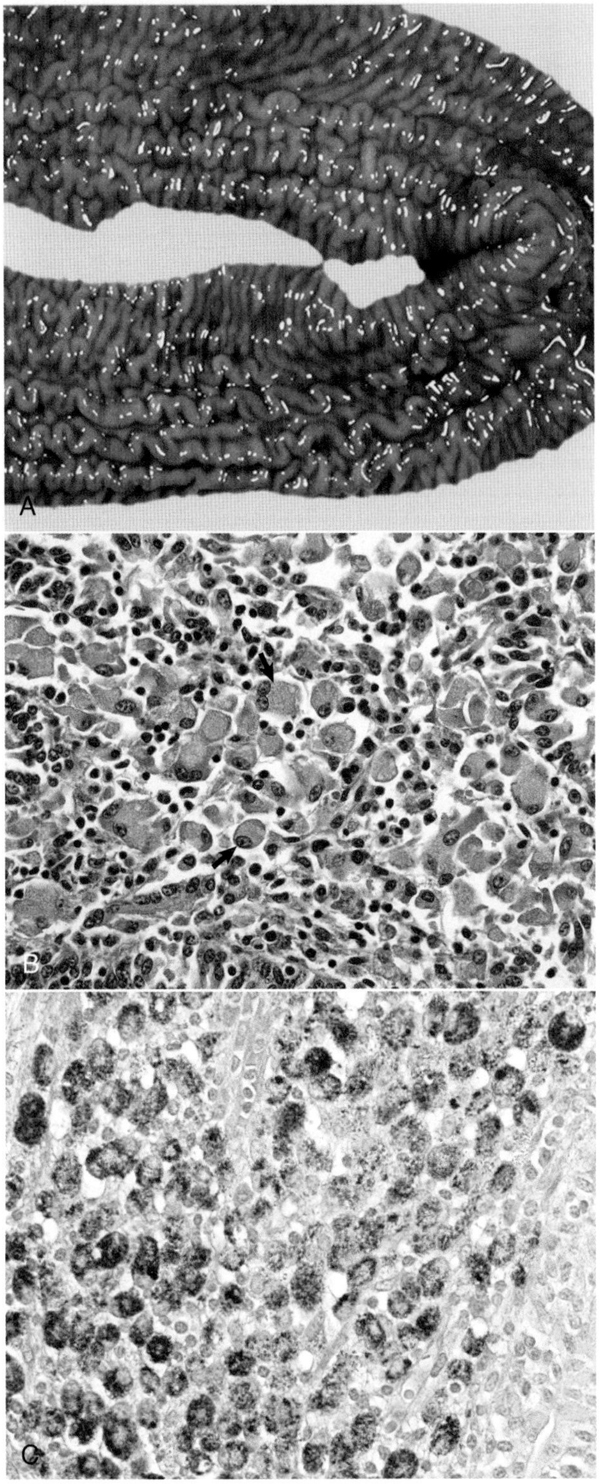

Figure 7-162 Granulomatous Enteritis, Johne's Disease (*Mycobacterium avium* subsp. *paratuberculosis*). A, Ileum, sheep. There is notable thickening of the mucosa, which is smooth and shiny (intact) and not ulcerated. **B,** Small intestine, cow. The lamina propria of the intestine is markedly expanded by granulomatous inflammatory cells (*arrows* = macrophages), which compress the crypts and eventually result in their loss (atrophy). H&E stain. **C,** Small intestine, cow. Mycobacterium-containing macrophages distend the lamina propria. Mycobacterium stain red with Ziehl-Neelsen stain. (**A** courtesy Dr. M.D. McCracken, College of Veterinary Medicine, University of Tennessee; and Noah's Arkive, College of Veterinary Medicine, The University of Georgia. **B** and **C** courtesy Dr. J.F. Zachary, College of Veterinary Medicine, University of Illinois.)

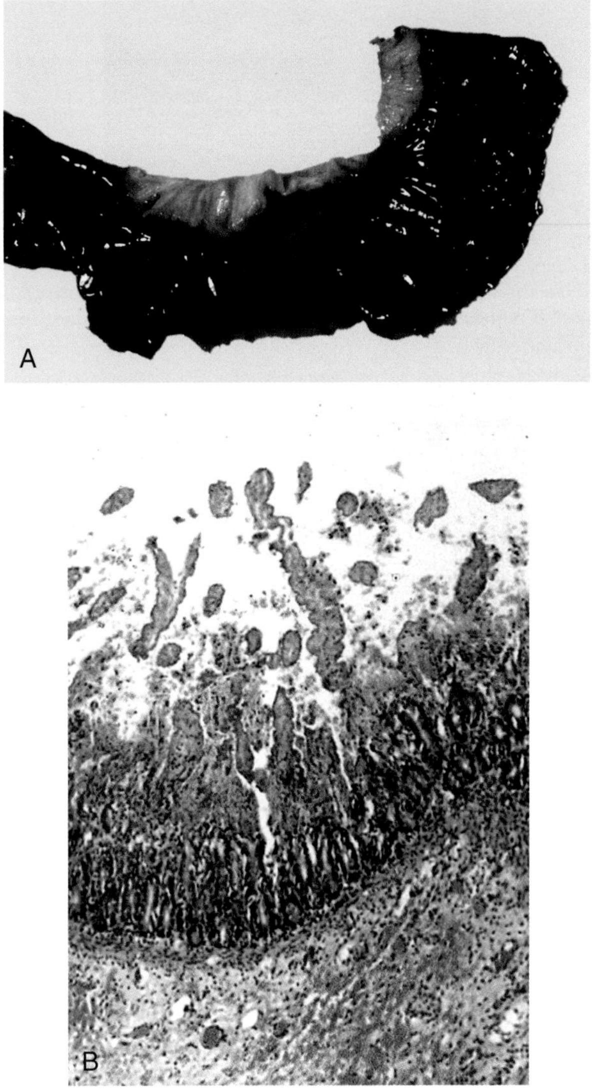

Figure 7-163 Necrohemorrhagic Enteritis, Hemorrhagic Bowel Syndrome, Small Intestine, Cow. A, The massive small intestinal hemorrhage and necrosis is characteristic of clostridial infections of the intestine. **B,** Note the horizontal linear "band" of acute coagulative necrosis affecting the superficial half of the mucosa *(light pink zone)* of the intestine caused by clostridial toxins. H&E stain. (**A** courtesy Dr. M.D. McGavin, College of Veterinary Medicine, University of Tennessee. **B** courtesy Dr. C.W. Qualls, College of Veterinary Medicine, Oklahoma State University, and Noah's Arkive, College of Veterinary Medicine, The University of Georgia.)

Microscopically, villous epithelial cells, enterochromaffin cells, goblet cells, macrophages, fibroblasts of the lamina propria, and endothelial cells of lacteals are parasitized by the chlamydia. The chlamydia are endocytosed and multiply in epithelial cell apices. They subsequently are liberated into the lamina propria. Villi are enlarged by dilated lacteals and infiltrates of mononuclear cells and neutrophils. Crypts of both small and large intestines are dilated and have sloughed epithelial cells and inflammatory exudate (colitis cystica superficialis). The centers of lymphoid follicles of Peyer's patches are necrotic. The mucosa and submucosa of the intestines are thickened by a diffuse granulomatous reaction. The abomasum also has lesions, and in some calves, foci of inflammation extend transmurally, thereby causing focal peritonitis. Affected calves have diarrhea, fever, anorexia, and depression.

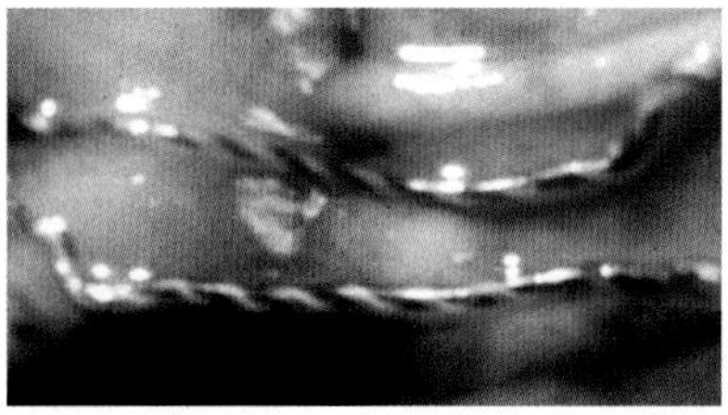

Figure 7-164 ***Haemonchus contortus*****, Abomasum, Sheep.** The white spiral reproductive tract wrapped around the blood-filled intestine is responsible for the striped appearance, hence the common name "barber's pole worm." (Courtesy Dr. H. Gelberg, College of Veterinary Medicine, Oregon State University.)

Parasitic Diseases

Haemonchus contortus. *Haemonchus contortus*, known as the *barber's pole worm*, is relatively common in ruminant abomasums. The common name of this parasite is related to the macroscopically visible entwining of the blood-filled intestine and white uterus in the female worm (Fig. 7-164). Hyperinfested pastures containing numerous third-stage larvae are the source of infection. Lambs are particularly at risk. Larvae on grasses are ingested by the host and enter the abomasum, where they may lie dormant within the gastric glands. After development to adults, they exit to the abomasal surface and attach via a buccal tooth. Eggs pass in the feces, completing the life cycle. *Haemonchus* are blood feeders and can cause severe anemia, hypoproteinemia, and resultant edema. This edema is characteristically present in the intermandibular space, resulting in a physical resemblance to a bottle ("bottle jaw"). As with any process resulting in anemia and hypoproteinemia, there are pale mucous membranes, stunting, and diarrhea. Diagnosis is by fecal egg counts and at necropsy by semiquantification of abomasal parasite load along with the attendant lesions of anemia and hypoproteinemia. At necropsy the carcass is pale and has generalized edema and fluid in all body cavities secondary to hypoproteinemia. Abomasal contents are fluid and discolored from free blood. Foci of mucosal hemorrhage are present at sites of worm attachment.

Ostertagiasis. In temperate climates, ostertagiasis is considered the most important parasitic disease in cattle (*Ostertagia ostertagi*) and small ruminants (*Ostertagia circumcincta*). Affected animals are unthrifty. *Ostertagia* spp. have a direct life cycle similar to that of *Haemonchus* spp. The nematodes are smaller than those of *Haemonchus* and are uniformly brown. Third-, fourth-, and fifth-stage larvae reside in the abomasal gastric glands. *Ostertagia* spp. are often present along with *Trichostrongylus* spp. in other GI locations. Intercurrent GI parasitism with other trichostrongyles has an additive effect on the clinical signs. Unthriftiness, lack of proper mentation, diarrhea, hypoproteinemia, and ventral edema may result. The multinodular appearance of the abomasum of heavily infested animals resembles morocco leather (Fig. 7-165). This cobblestone appearance is due to enlargement of the gastric glands because of mucous cell hyperplasia and hyperplasia of lymphoid nodules in the abomasal submucosa elevating the overlying mucosa. Abomasitis produced by *Ostertagia* spp. is characterized by an infiltration of mononuclear inflammatory cells and eosinophils in the lamina propria. There are also increased numbers of globule leukocytes, a decrease in the number of parietal and chief cells, and hyperplasia of abomasal mucous cells. Differential diagnoses include lymphoma.

Coccidiosis. Abomasal coccidiosis has been reported in a sheep. Mucosal lesions are nodular and hemorrhagic with hyperplasia of mucous neck cells, parietal cell atrophy, and lymphoplasmacytic fibrosis of the lamina propria associated with giant schizonts of uncertain taxonomy.

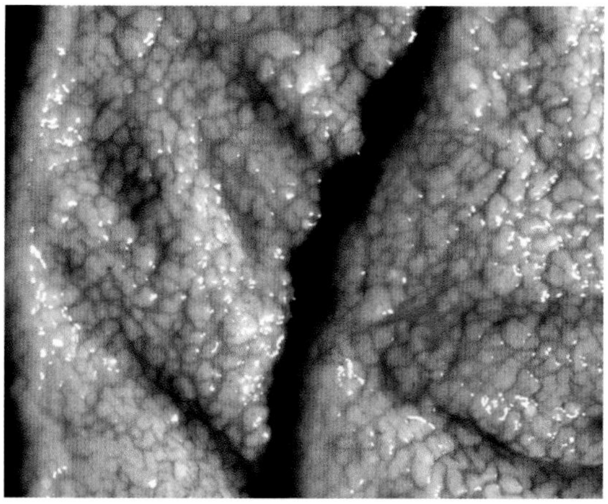

Figure 7-165 Ostertagiasis, Abomasum, Cow. The granular morocco leather appearance of the abomasal mucosa is characteristic of chronic ostertagiasis and is due to epithelial hyperplasia of the gastric glands, which may contain *Ostertagia* larvae and lymphoid hyperplasia. (Courtesy Dr. M.D. McGavin, College of Veterinary Medicine, University of Tennessee.)

Trichostrongylosis. Trichostrongyles are small nematodes that parasitize the small intestine of ruminants. Mild climates promote clinical disease. These parasites have a direct life cycle. Third-stage larvae are rendered infective in the acid environment of the abomasum. The larvae burrow in between crypt enterocytes but do not generally penetrate the basement membrane. Paradoxically, crypt hyperplasia is followed by villous atrophy. As with most other parasitisms, crowding, poor sanitation, and inadequate nutrition potentiate disease. Protein leakage into the intestinal lumen together with absorptive enterocyte loss leads to diarrhea, cachexia, and its metabolic consequences, which can be severe and widespread through many organ systems.

Nematodirosis. *Nematodirus* nematodes are parasites of the cranial small intestine of ruminants. The life cycle is direct. Unlike the case with other strongyles, *Nematodirus* larvae within ova are resistant to cold temperatures. In fact, the ova must overwinter to be infective. This is evolutionally interesting because it allows for a new crop of susceptible hosts, particularly lambs and calves each year. Fourth- and fifth-stage larvae reside in deeper layers of the mucosa than do the trichostrongyles. Villous atrophy of the cranial small intestine is the predominant histologic lesion. *Nematodirus* spp. do not generally cause disease except in association with other parasites. Signs include green diarrhea, weight loss, and hypoproteinemia secondary to weight loss and inappetence.

Cooperiasis. A small intestinal parasite of ruminants, *Cooperia* nematodes—unlike other trichostrongyles—do not burrow into the intestine. Rather, they reside between villi, causing pressure necrosis. Their life cycle and clinical signs are similar to those of the other strongyles already described.

Oesophagostomum. The nodular worms of ruminants (*Oesophagostomum columbianum, Oesophagostomum radiatum*) and pigs (*Oesophagostomum dentatum*) cause subserosal mineralized nodules that are characteristic of the disease. These nodules generally are of no clinical significance, but they make the intestines unsuitable for use as sausage casings. Occasionally they are associated with, and can be the cause of, intussusceptions.

Third-stage larvae of O. *columbianum* of sheep are ingested, penetrate deeply into the small intestinal wall, excyst, and molt to fourth-stage larvae, which mature in the colon. They may encyst in the colonic wall and become mineralized subserosal nodules or may mature to adults. Disease is more severe in nutritionally debilitated animals. Most infestations are asymptomatic. O. *radiatum* of cattle may produce inappetence, hypoproteinemia from damaged enterocyte tight junctions, and anemia and hemorrhage from consumptive coagulopathy induced by the parasites. Nodules may also form, as in sheep. Oesophagostomiasis in pigs is usually asymptomatic, although ill thrift and malaise secondary to typhlocolitis may occur.

Intestinal Neoplasia

Alimentary lymphoma is the most common alimentary neoplasm of ruminants. It has a propensity to develop in the abomasum. See Chapter 6 for more information.

Peritoneum, Omentum, Mesentery, and Peritoneal Cavity

See Disorders of Domestic Animals, Peritoneum, Omentum, Mesentery, and Peritoneal Cavity.

Disorders of Pigs

For disorders occurring in two or more species of animals, see Disorders of Domestic Animals.

Oral Cavity

See Disorders of Domestic Animals, Oral Cavity.

Viral Diseases

Vesicular Stomatitides. See Disorders of Domestic Animals, Oral Cavity, Vesicular Stomatitides—Viral Diseases.

Tonsils

Pseudorabies (Aujeszky's Disease)

The virus of Aujeszky's disease, or pseudorabies, initially replicates in the tonsils, which can be sampled to determine viral presence. See Chapter 4 for more information.

Salivary Glands

See Disorders of Domestic Animals, Salivary Glands.

Tongue

Epithelial hyperplasia of the lateral edges of the tongue is common in piglets before nursing, when the fringelike epithelium is rubbed off (E-Fig. 7-22).

Esophagus

See Disorders of Domestic Animals, Esophagus.

Stomach

See Disorders of Domestic Animals, Stomach and Abomasum.

In pigs, gastric ulcers are common and occur in penned pigs fed finely ground grain. These ulcers always are limited to the stratified squamous epithelium of the esophageal portion of the gastric mucosa that surrounds the cardia (see Fig. 7-84).

Intestine

Enteric diseases of pigs are a major cause of economic loss. Rapid and accurate on-farm diagnosis is critical in controlling disease outbreaks. If one takes into account the epizootiology of the outbreak, the age of the affected animals, and the location and nature of lesions, one can generally be fairly accurate in rendering an on-farm diagnosis, pending laboratory confirmation. This listing of specific infectious causes of enteritis in pigs is exclusive of those agents already discussed. When formulating a differential diagnosis, one must consider all causes of enteritis, including intestinal displacements, colibacillosis, rotavirus, *Salmonella*, clostridia, parasites, toxins, and so on.

Viral Diseases

Transmissible Gastroenteritis. Transmissible gastroenteritis (TGE) is an important disease in pigs younger than 10 days. Older animals apparently can compensate for the small intestinal damage through fluid and short-chain fatty acid absorption in the large intestine. The coronavirus that causes this disease cross-reacts with, but is distinct from, the coronavirus that causes feline infectious peritonitis. The virus is inactivated by sunlight; therefore transmissible gastroenteritis disease occurs mostly in winter. Target cells for the virus are villous enterocytes; therefore lesions consist of notable atrophy of villi of the small intestine (Fig. 7-166). In piglets, epithelial replacement time is much longer than in more mature animals, accounting for the high mortality. Diagnosis is by positive immunostaining of intestinal sections in piglets acutely ill with the disease.

Similar to rotavirus or non–transmissible gastroenteritis coronavirus infections, the virus is lytic, and sloughed enterocytes carry virus into the feces. The difference in pathogenicity between rotavirus and non–transmissible gastroenteritis coronavirus infections and transmissible gastroenteritis is the number of villous enterocytes destroyed by a virus. In transmissible gastroenteritis,

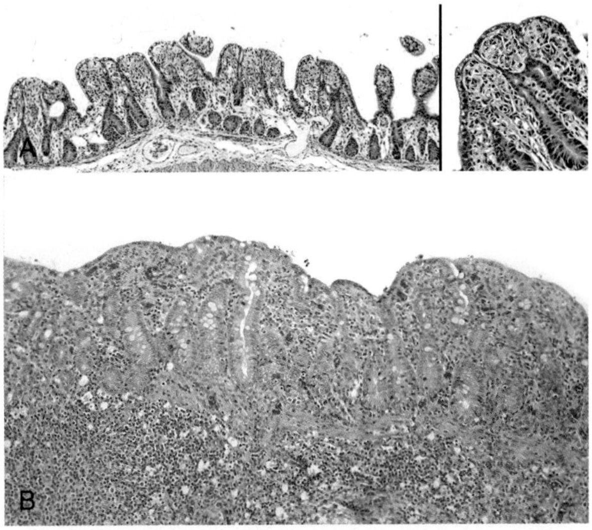

Figure 7-166 **Transmissible Gastroenteritis, Small Intestine, Piglet. A,** Early stage of the disease. Transmissible gastroenteritis virus targets epithelial cells of the tips and upper sides of intestinal villi, causing necrosis of the enterocytes and atrophy of the villi. These cells are sloughed and replaced by flattened epithelial cells migrating up the basement membrane from progenitor cells in the crypts. *Inset,* Note the flattened epithelial cells covering the tips and sides of the atrophic villi and the fusion of the adjacent villi. Inflammation is minimal. H&E stain. **B,** Later stage of the disease. There is severe blunting (marked villus atrophy) of intestinal villi with fusion of their basement membranes. Chronic inflammation is prominent in the lamina propria and submucosa. H&E stain. (**A** courtesy Dr. B.G. Harmon, College of Veterinary Medicine, The University of Georgia; and Noah's Arkive, College of Veterinary Medicine, The University of Georgia. **B** courtesy Dr. H. Gelberg, College of Veterinary Medicine, Oregon State University.)

most of the villous enterocytes are destroyed, and therefore the clinical disease is more severe.

The diarrhea contains odoriferous undigested milk. The loss of the majority of villous enterocytes results in continued significant intestinal malabsorption. Because of fusion of adjacent villi, the enterocyte mass may never fully be restored. Affected surviving animals remain chronic "poor doers."

Piglets dead from transmissible gastroenteritis are dehydrated, and their perineum is stained with liquid, yellow, fecal material. The small intestine is dilated and thin walled because of the loss of enterocytes and contains yellow fluid and gas (Fig. 7-167). Mesenteric lymph vessels are devoid of chyle as a result of malabsorption. The diagnosis is partially based on the presence of villous atrophy. The decrease in villous height to crypt depth ratio is marked and may be appreciated subgrossly (Fig. 7-168). Colibacillosis, coccidiosis, cryptosporidiosis, rotavirus infection, and non–transmissible gastroenteritis coronavirus infection are among the differential diagnoses.

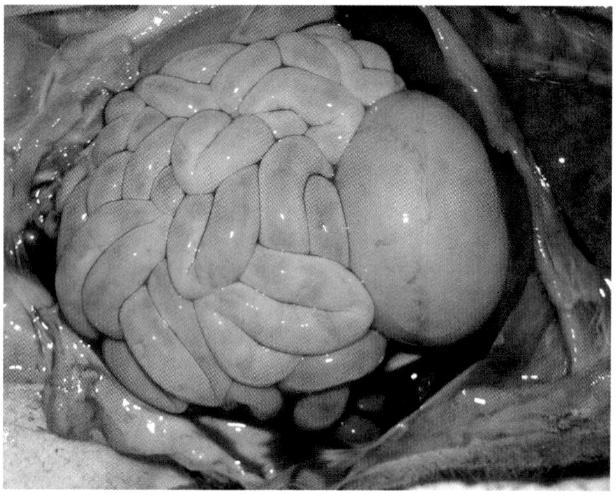

Figure 7-167 Transmissible Gastroenteritis, Small Intestine, Piglet. The small intestine is dilated by gas, is thin walled, and contains undigested milk. (Courtesy Dr. V. Hsiao, College of Veterinary Medicine, University of Illinois.)

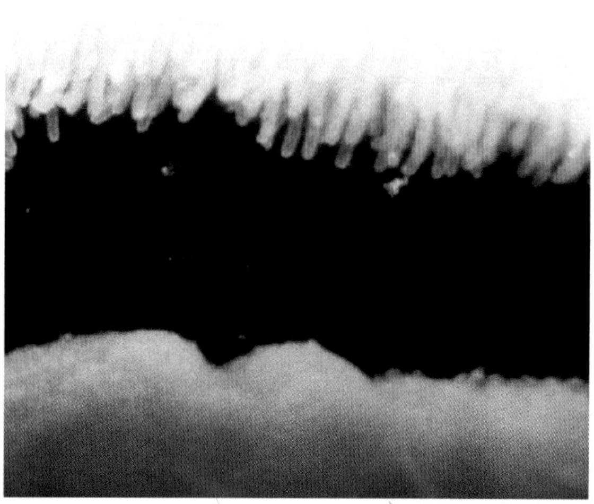

Figure 7-168 Wet Mount, Intestinal Villi, Transmissible Gastroenteritis, Small Intestine, Piglet. There is notable villous atrophy *(bottom)* compared with normal intestine *(top)*. (Courtesy Dr. H. Gelberg, College of Veterinary Medicine, Oregon State University.)

Piglets suffer from acute diarrhea, weight loss, vomiting, and dehydration. Morbidity and mortality, especially in neonates, approach 100% in susceptible herds. Death occurs within 48 hours to 5 days after the commencement of clinical signs. In feeder pigs, transmissible gastroenteritis virus infection causes transient clinical signs with eventual recovery. Sows are susceptible to the virus, and morbidity among the sows is 100%, but the clinical signs are mild and transient (fever, vomiting, inappetence, and agalactia), and none die. Immunity is solid.

Porcine Epidemic Diarrhea. Porcine epidemic diarrhea virus (PEDV) was first recognized in China in 2010 and rapidly spread worldwide, including at least 10 states in the Unites States in 2013. Porcine epidemic diarrhea virus is a coronavirus similar to the virus that causes transmissible gastroenteritis. Morbidity in naïve herds is 100%, and mortality among suckling and recently weaned piglets ranges from 50% to 100%. Transmission among pigs is rapid (36 hours) and by a variety of methods, including fecal-oral, fomites, and wind borne. Clinical signs are vomiting, inappetence, and watery, fetid diarrhea in all age pigs. Typical lesions are small intestinal atrophy with occasional epithelial syncytia. Severity of disease is variable and dependent on age with older animals having low mortality.

Porcine Circovirus Enteritis. Porcine circovirus (PCV) is ubiquitous in pigs worldwide. The small, single-stranded, nonenveloped, DNA genome of the virus is circular. Although PCV type 1 has been recognized as a nonpathogenic laboratory culture contaminant since 1982, in 1998 pathogenic variants emerged in commercial pigs and were designated PCV2 a and b. They were associated with a clinical syndrome termed postweaning multisystemic wasting syndrome. Porcine circovirus–associated disease (PCVAD) refers to the different disease manifestations associated with PCV2 infection, including enteritis. Seropositivity for PCV2 is ubiquitous and does not equate with clinical disease.

In confirmed clinical cases of porcine circovirus–associated disease, histologic lesions of lymphoid depletion and/or lymphohistiocytic to granulomatous inflammation must be present in affected organs and PCV2 must be identified within lesions by PCR or immunohistochemistry (IHC). The organs affected and the clinical signs vary greatly and are exacerbated by intercurrent infections by a variety of infectious agents.

Lesions in the intestine include depletion of germinal centers in GALT with replacement by histiocytes and multinucleated giant cells. Macrophages in Peyer's patches may contain botryoid, basophilic, intracytoplasmic inclusion bodies. Lymphohistiocytic to granulomatous inflammation may extend from GALT to the intestinal lumen of both the large and small intestines. In some cases the lesions are similar to those of *Lawsonia* infection. Virus is spread horizontally within a herd by all body secretions.

Bacterial Diseases

Edema Disease. Edema disease, also known as *enterotoxemic colibacillosis*, is an *E. coli* (F18ab) infection that is specific for pigs. Edema disease is caused by a bacterial enterotoxin (verotoxin) produced in the small intestine and spread hematogenously via induction of IL-8. This interleukin attracts neutrophils that carry the toxin throughout the body. It is generally a disease of pigs 6 to 14 weeks of age and is usually associated with dietary changes at weaning. It is often noted that the best pigs in a group are the ones affected. Edema disease is characterized by neurologic signs, including incoordination, poor balance, weakness, tremors, and convulsions.

Hemolytic *E. coli* proliferates in the small intestine subsequent to dietary changes and produces a heat-labile exotoxin called the *edema disease principle*. This systemic toxin (angiotoxin) causes generalized vascular endothelial injury of arterioles and arteries (see Fig. 10-69), resulting in fluid loss and edema. The edema can be found anywhere but is most characteristic in the gastric submucosa (see Fig. 10-79), eyelids (Fig. 7-169), forehead, gallbladder, and mesentery of the spiral colon (Fig. 7-170). In the brain, arterial damage causes focal malacia in the medulla, thalamus, and basal ganglia. These nervous tissue lesions are collectively known as focal symmetric encephalomalacia or swine cerebral angiopathy and are responsible for the variety of clinical signs. Death is due to an endotoxic shocklike syndrome. Some animals suffer from a Shwartzman-like bilateral renal cortical necrosis. Morbidity within a herd is approximately 35%, and all affected animals die.

Postweaning Colibacillosis. Postweaning colibacillosis is another specific disease of pigs caused by a hemolytic *E. coli*. The disease appears identical to enterotoxic colibacillosis of the neonate in that it produces a secretory diarrhea and therefore no lesions in the intestine, although gastric infarcts are common. It is a distinct strain of *E. coli*, however, and is associated with feed and management changes at weaning.

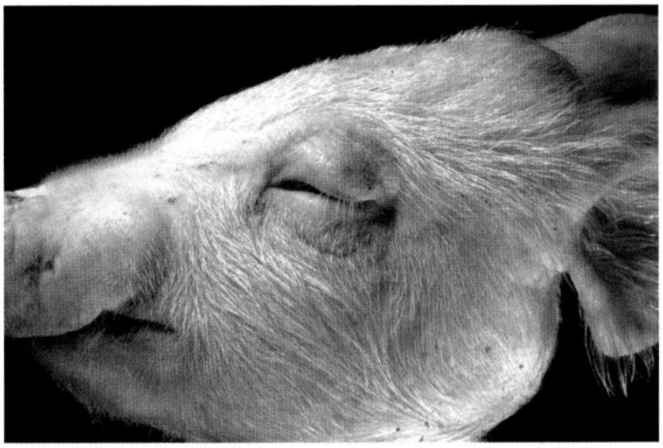

Figure 7-169 Edema Disease, Head, Pig. The skin of the eyelids, snout, and submandibular area are edematous as a result of production of angiotoxin by *Escherichia coli*, which increases the permeability of capillaries. (Courtesy Dr. H. Gelberg, College of Veterinary Medicine, Oregon State University.)

Swine Dysentery. Unlike most of the other diseases of the porcine gut, swine dysentery is generally confined to the large intestine. The causative bacterium, *Brachyspira hyodysenteriae*, previously known as *Treponema* and *Serpulina*, is a Gram-negative, flagellated, and anaerobic spirochete that acts synergistically with anaerobic colonic flora, such as *F. necrophorum* or *Bacteroides vulgatus*, to produce disease. This synergism is believed to be partially responsible for the age restriction (8 to 14 weeks old) of the disease because neonatal animals have not yet developed the appropriate anaerobic gut flora. *B. hyodysenteriae* produces a cytotoxic hemolysin, which is a virulence determinant.

The gross lesions of the disease closely approximate those of acute enteric salmonellosis except that bloody feces are more usual in dysentery. Weanling pigs 8 to 14 weeks old are usually affected, and the disease spreads rapidly through a herd. Morbidity approaches 90%, and mortality is around 30%. Lesions of mucohemorrhagic enteritis are present in the spiral colon, colon, cecum, and rectum. The intestine often has a fibrinonecrotic pseudomembrane that correlates with the severe diarrheic feces that contains blood, mucus, and fibrin (Fig. 7-171). The diarrhea and electrolyte loss that occur are caused by colonic absorptive failure.

B. hyodysenteriae is identified by impression smear (Fig. 7-172), dark-field microscopy, immunolabeling techniques, and PCR. It is assumed that a carrier state exists because the disease is enzootic in affected herds.

***Lawsonia* Enteritis.** *Lawsonia* enteritis manifests in a variety of ways, as indicated by the number of names applied to it: proliferative enteropathy, proliferative ileitis, intestinal adenomatosis, distal ileal hypertrophy, terminal ileitis, and proliferative hemorrhagic enteropathy. The genus of the causative agent has undergone several recent changes in nomenclature. For many years this disease was believed to be caused by *Campylobacter* spp. (*Campylobacter mucosalis*, *C. jejuni*, *Campylobacter hyointestinalis*). Newer methods of bacterial classification caused the name to be changed to *Ileobacter* and now *L. intracellularis*, the only species in the genus. Pigs older than

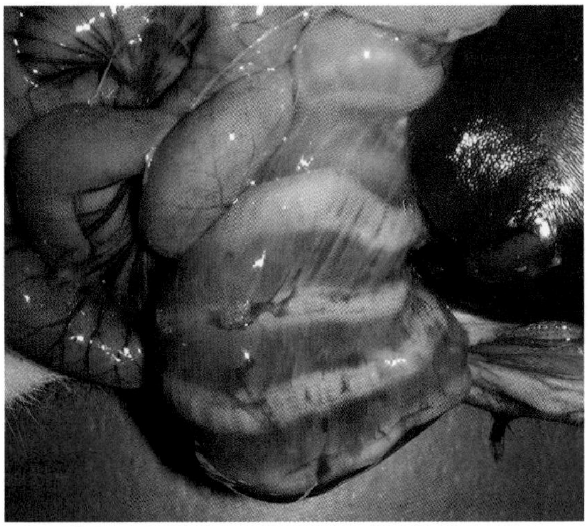

Figure 7-170 Edema Disease, Spiral Colon, Pig. Edema of the mesentery is a result of an angiotoxin produced by *Escherichia coli*. (Courtesy Drs. W. Haschek-Hock and L. Borst, College of Veterinary Medicine, University of Illinois.)

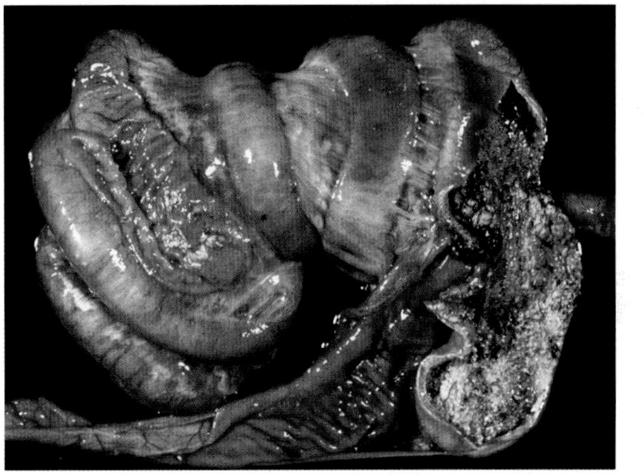

Figure 7-171 Necrohemorrhagic Enterocolitis, Swine Dysentery, Spiral Colon, Pig. There is marked necrosis and hemorrhage of the intestinal mucosa caused by the bacterium *Brachyspira hyodysenteriae*. (Courtesy Department of Veterinary Biosciences, College of Veterinary Medicine, The Ohio State University; and Noah's Arkive, College of Veterinary Medicine, The University of Georgia.)

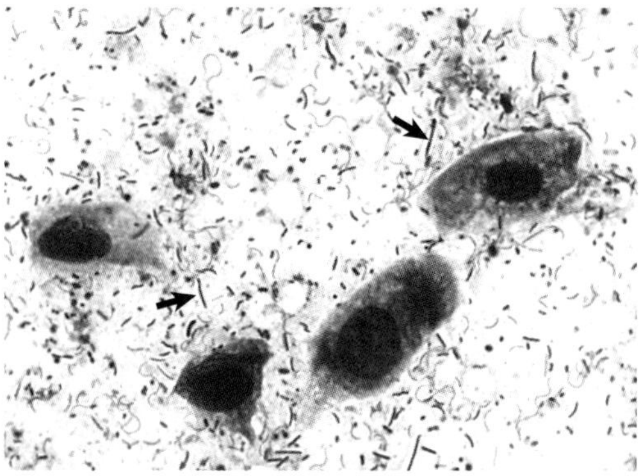

Figure 7-172 **Swine Dysentery, Colon, Pig.** This impression smear contains a few enterocytes and numerous bacteria. Note the spiral bacteria (*arrows*) consistent with *Brachyspira* spp. Diff-Quik stain. (Courtesy Dr. H. Gelberg, College of Veterinary Medicine, Oregon State University.)

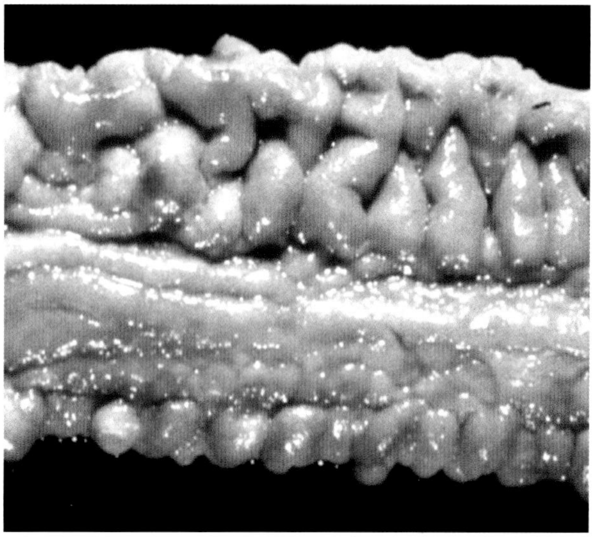

Figure 7-173 **Proliferative Enteritis, Ileum, Pig.** Note the marked mucosal expansion, the result of *Lawsonia*-induced epithelial hyperplasia. (Courtesy Dr. H. Gelberg, College of Veterinary Medicine, Oregon State University.)

4 weeks of age are susceptible; thus this condition is a postweaning disease. Disease is believed to be caused by an unknown interaction of *Lawsonia* with normal gut flora. The nature of the lesions is a function of the extent of intestinal mucosal necrosis. The disease begins as a bacteria-induced stimulation of small intestinal crypt epithelial cells, particularly in the ileum (Figs. 7-173 and 7-174), where lesions are generally most severe. With time the lesions progress to necrosis of the proliferating crypt cells with hemorrhage (Fig. 7-175). Thus the morphologic appearance of the lesions varies from case to case. The mechanism of lesion production is not well understood. Infection results in immunosuppression with a reduction in $CD8^+$ T and B lymphocytes. In the proliferative form of the disease, the causative bacteria may be seen in apical cytoplasm of enterocytes. The mechanism of enterocyte proliferation may relate to *Lawsonia*-induced altered transcription of host "alarm response" genes that affect regulation of the cell cycle and cell differentiation. The enterocyte hyperplasia that results may cause release of cytokines that attract macrophages. With severe disease, bacteria are present in macrophages in the lamina propria. This may cause release of tumor necrosis factor-α (TNF-α), resulting in vascular permeability and hemorrhage.

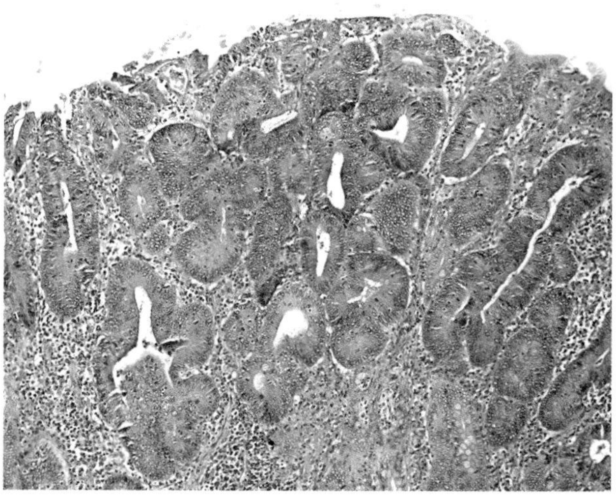

Figure 7-174 ***Lawsonia* Enteritis, Ileum, Pig.** There is notable hyperplasia of enterocytes, resulting in distortion of normal architecture and "collision necrosis" of tightly packed proliferating enterocytes. Also see Figure 7-173. H&E stain. (Courtesy Dr. J.F. Zachary, College of Veterinary Medicine, University of Illinois.)

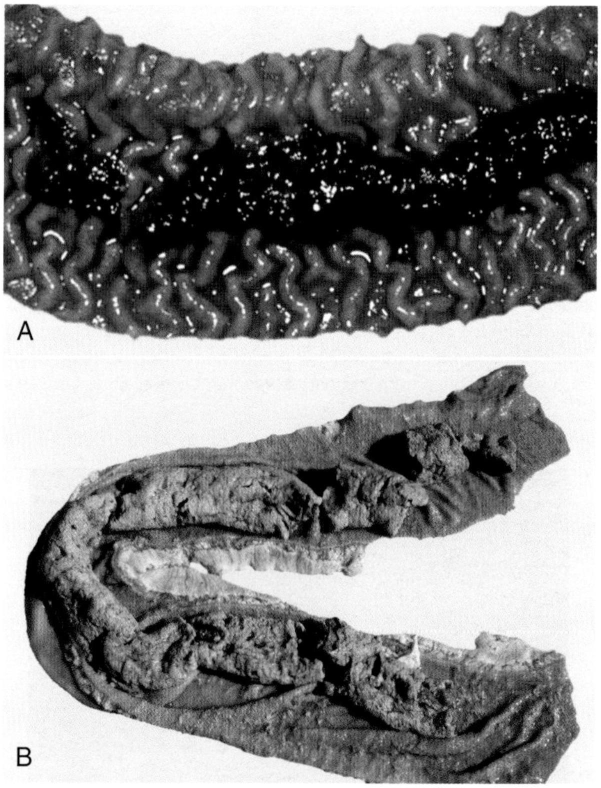

Figure 7-175 ***Lawsonia* Enteritis, Ileum, Pig. A,** Hemorrhagic bowel form. Note the prominent folds of hyperplastic mucosa and the concurrent hemorrhage forming a luminal cast. **B,** Necroproliferative form. Note the prominent necrosis of the ileal mucosa and its diphtheritic membrane (luminal cast) formed by cellular debris and inflammatory exudate. (**A** courtesy Dr. D.D. Harrington, School of Veterinary Medicine, Purdue University; and Noah's Arkive, College of Veterinary Medicine, The University of Georgia. **B** courtesy Dr. D. Driemeier, Federal University of Rio Grande do Sul, Brazil.)

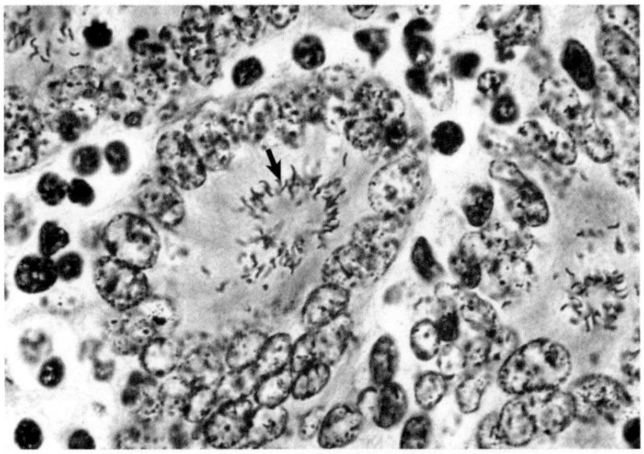

Figure 7-176 **Proliferative Enteritis, Ileum, Pig.** Curved *Lawsonia* spp. bacteria *(arrow)* are present in the apical cytoplasm of enterocytes. There is proliferation of crypt enterocytes. Warthin-Starry stain. (Courtesy Dr. H. Gelberg, College of Veterinary Medicine, Oregon State University.)

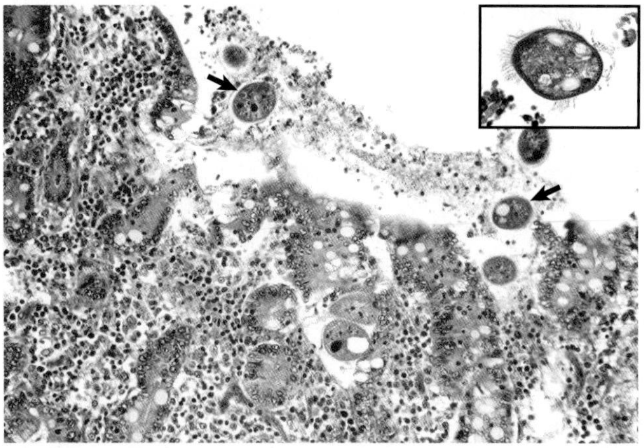

Figure 7-177 ***Balantidium coli*, Colon, Pig.** *B. coli* is an opportunistic flagellated protozoan that is normally present in the pig intestine (arrows). This pig had concurrent proliferative *(Lawsonia)* enteritis. H&E stain. *Inset,* Higher magnification of *B. coli*. H&E stain. (Courtesy Dr. C. Löhr, College of Veterinary Medicine, Oregon State University. Insert, Courtesy Dr. J.F. Zachary, College of Veterinary Medicine, University of Illinois.)

At clinical and necropsy examination, variable amounts of blood and intestinal casts are present in the feces. Microscopically, the comma-shaped bacteria are made visible with special stains, such as Steiner's, within the mitotically active cells of the small intestinal crypts (Fig. 7-176). The massive mitoses of crypt cells and resultant cryptal crowding and necrosis prevent maturation to absorbent villous enterocytes. There is resultant villous shortening. Mitosis can be so intense that the histologic features suggest neoplasia and a diagnosis of "intestinal adenomatosis."

Morbidity within a herd is 10% to 15%; mortality is around 50%. In fatal cases, affected pigs usually die within a day of the appearance of clinical signs. Pigs that recover are generally "poor-doers." A similar organism with associated intestinal proliferation is found in horses, hamsters, ostriches, cervids, sheep, ferrets, rats, and macaques.

Chlamydial Diseases

Chlamydiosis. *Chlamydia* has been found in enterocytes of normal pigs and pigs with diarrhea. In gnotobiotic pigs, *Chlamydia trachomatis* and *Chlamydia suis* infection result in villous atrophy and villous-tip necrosis. These lesions are most severe in the distal jejunum and ileum. Colonic infection has also been reported.

Parasitic Diseases

Balantidiasis (*Balantidium coli*). *Balantidium coli* is a normal inhabitant of the cecum and colon of primates, including human beings, and pigs. It is large (50 to 60 μm × 25 to 45 μm) and ciliated. Dogs with whipworm infestation may become infested after contact with infected pigs. In general, *Balantidium* is an opportunistic pathogen associated with enteric disease (Fig. 7-177).

Hyostrongylus rubidus. *Hyostrongylus rubidus* of pigs is a gastric parasite that causes a thickening of the mucosa, with mucus accumulation and mucous cell hyperplasia and inflammation of the lamina propria by lymphocytes, plasma cells, and eosinophils. The parasite is threadlike and red. Clinically, hyostrongylosis is associated with the "thin sow syndrome." Grossly, the gastric mucosa is thickened, catarrhal, and somewhat cobblestone, similar to ostertagiasis of ruminants. Microscopically, there is mucous metaplasia of parasitized and adjacent gastric glands. Submucosal lymphoid follicles develop in chronic infections.

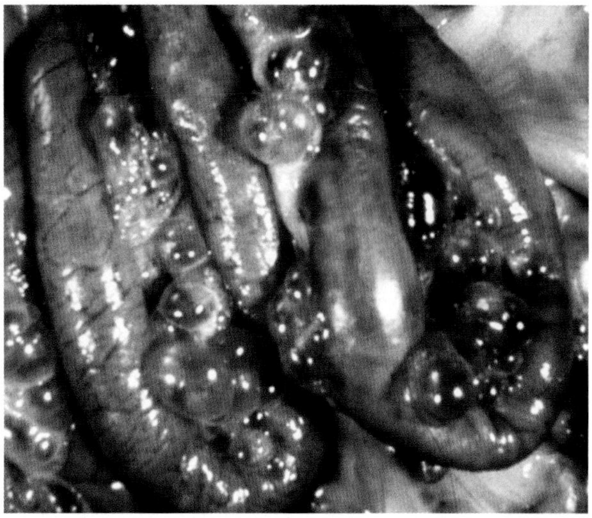

Figure 7-178 **Intestinal Emphysema, Intestines, Pig.** Gas bubbles dilate serosal and mesenteric lymphatic vessels. (Courtesy Dr. H. Gelberg, College of Veterinary Medicine, Oregon State University.)

Oesophagostomum. See Disorders of Ruminants (Cattle, Sheep, and Goats), Intestine, Parasitic Diseases, Oesophagostomum.

Miscellaneous Disorders

Intestinal Emphysema. Intestinal emphysema (pneumatosis cystoides intestinalis) of pigs and rabbits translates to gas-dilated lymphatic vessels of the intestinal serosa and mesentery. The cause of this condition is unknown, and it is not associated with clinical disease (Fig. 7-178).

Intestinal Neoplasia

See Disorders of Domestic Animals, Intestine, Intestinal Neoplasia.

Peritoneum, Omentum, Mesentery, and Peritoneal Cavity

Glasser's Disease

Glasser's disease is characterized by fibrinous polyserositis (pleuritis, pericarditis, peritonitis, arthritis, and leptomeningitis). Although not generally a diarrheal disease, it causes inflammation of the intestinal serosa (serositis). Lesions range from arthritis to peritonitis to leptomeningitis, depending on the serous surface infected. Glasser's disease generally occurs in 5- to 12-week-old pigs. Mortality of affected animals within a herd is high, but morbidity is low. Although classic Glasser's disease is caused by either *Haemophilus suis* or *Haemophilus parasuis*, porcine polyserositis can be caused by *Mycoplasma hyorhinis*, *Streptococcus suis* type II (zoonotic), septicemic salmonellosis, and septicemic *E. coli* (see Fig. 7-17).

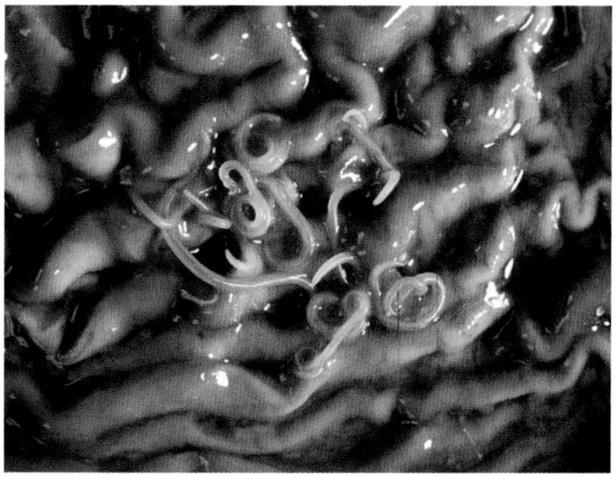

Figure 7-179 **Physalopteriasis, Stomach, Dog.** Stout coiled nematodes, *Physaloptera canis* are firmly attached to the gastric mucosa by dentate pseudolabia. (Courtesy Dr. M.D. McGavin, College of Veterinary Medicine, University of Tennessee.)

Disorders of Dogs

For disorders occurring in two or more species of animals, see Disorders of Domestic Animals.

Oral Cavity

See Disorders of Domestic Animals, Oral Cavity.

Eosinophilic Stomatitides

See Disorders of Domestic Animals, Oral Cavity, Eosinophilic Stomatitides.

Teeth

See Disorders of Domestic Animals, Teeth.

Tonsils

See Disorders of Domestic Animals, Tonsils.

Salivary Glands

See Disorders of Domestic Animals, Salivary Glands.

Tongue

See Disorders of Domestic Animals, Tongue.

Esophagus

Achalasia

See Disorders of Domestic Animals, Esophagus, Developmental Anomalies, Achalasia.

Stomach

Parasitic Diseases

Several genera of nematodes, principally *Ollulanus*, *Gnathostoma*, and *Cylicospirura*, cause gastritis in dogs and cats, but these infections are rare. *Physaloptera* spp. are often thought of as gastric parasites of carnivores because they are sometimes found in the stomach on endoscopic examination or at necropsy. They are occasionally responsible for vomiting. They appear similar to ascarids but generally attach by anterior hooks to the proximal duodenal mucosa at the gastric valve (Fig. 7-179). Intermediate hosts are coprophagous beetles.

Intestine

Lymphangiectasia

Lymphangiectasia, or lacteal dilation, is the most commonly reported cause of protein-losing enteropathy in dogs. Clinical signs include diarrhea, steatorrhea, hypoproteinemia, and ascites (see Fig. 7-13). Lymphangiectasia can be due to a congenital developmental disorder of the lymphatic vessels, or it can be acquired secondary to lymph vessel obstruction caused by granulomatous or neoplastic diseases. An inherited cause is suspected in some canine breeds. A special case is lipogranulomatous lymphangiectasia of the dog, the name of which is descriptive of the lesions present. Most cases of acquired lymphangiectasia are idiopathic. Gross and microscopic lesions are those of lymphangiectasia and include a thickened intestinal mucosa with dilated lymphatic vessels and lacteals (see Fig. 7-14). There are variable increases in lymphocyte and plasma cell numbers in affected tissue.

Viral Diseases

Parvovirus Enteritis. Also see Disorders of Cats, Intestine, Viral Diseases, Parvovirus Enteritis.

Parvovirus enteritis of dogs (and cats) is a severe, usually fatal disease. Because the target cells are those that are rapidly dividing, in the intestine the crypt cells are principally affected. This tropism is called *radiomimetic*. Initial virus replication occurs in lymphoid tissue. Although there is much overlap in the disease syndrome in dogs and cats, the dissimilarities warrant independent discussion of each species. To complicate matters further, there is a high mutation rate among canine and feline parvoviruses, and genetic recombination between the two viruses has been documented.

Canine parvovirus enteritis first appeared in Europe and the United States in 1978. The disease was initially recognized because the gross and microscopic lesions were identical to those of feline parvovirus enteritis. Panleukopenia vaccines were effective in preventing this disease in dogs and were used extensively until canine-specific parvovirus vaccines were developed. Rottweilers and Doberman pinschers, which are genetically related, are at increased risk for parvovirus disease even if properly vaccinated.

Canine parvovirus disease initially was described as occurring in three distinct syndromes. Puppies younger than 2 weeks of age had generalized disease with focal areas of virus-induced necrosis in those tissues with rapidly dividing cells. Thus multiple organs and tissues, such as the liver, kidney, heart, vessels, bone marrow, intestine, and lung, were affected. Puppies 3 to 8 weeks of age would sometimes have myocarditis develop for the same reason. Often, initial infection would go undetected, and these animals would die unexpectedly up to 5 months later because of myocardial scarring and conduction failure (see Fig. 10-81). In puppies 8 weeks or older, the disease is identical to that in the cat. Congenital cerebellar hypoplasia has not been induced in puppies.

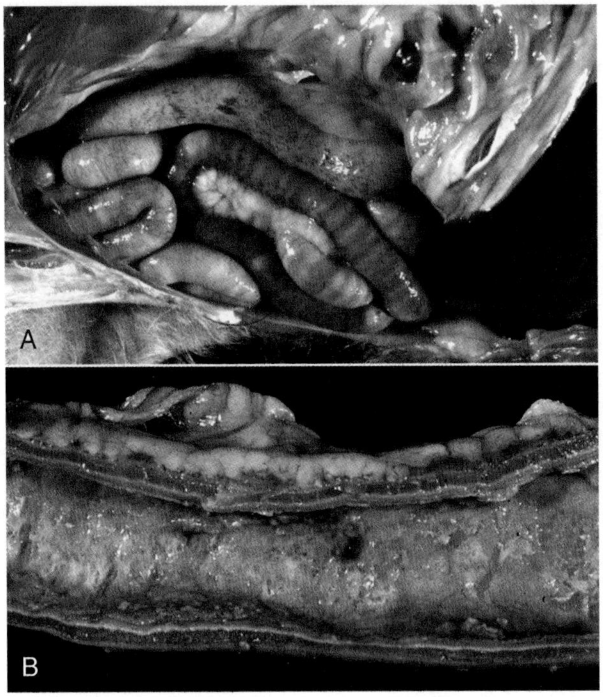

Figure 7-180 Parvovirus Enteritis, Small Intestine, Dog. A, Segments of the small intestine are diffusely reddened (active hyperemia of the mucosa), and the serosal surface is roughened, faintly granular, and petechiated. **B,** The mucosa of the small intestine is necrotic. Note the roughened, granular, focally petechiated, and focally sloughing mucosa. (**A** courtesy College of Veterinary Medicine, University of Illinois. **B** courtesy Department of Veterinary Biosciences, College of Veterinary Medicine, The Ohio State University; and Noah's Arkive, College of Veterinary Medicine, The University of Georgia.)

At necropsy the dilated, fluid-filled, flaccid, and hemorrhagic small intestine with serositis similar to that of panleukopenia is quite characteristic (Fig. 7-180). The contents of the small intestine are brown to red-brown and fluid with a fibrinous exudate, with or without hemorrhage (also see Fig. 7-185, *B*). Mesenteric lymphadenomegaly with variable hemorrhage is present. The bone marrow is depleted. Dogs but not cats may have coagulative lymphadenitis associated with severe lymphoid infection.

The intestinal lesion is necrosis of crypt epithelial cells. Surviving epithelial cells are not targets of the virus, but their morphologic configuration changes to squamoid to cover the surface of the denuded crypts and later to temporarily cover the denuded villous basement membrane, because replacement cells are not being produced, even though senile epithelial extrusion continues to occur from the villous tips. Severe lesions consist of partially denuded villi over debris-filled crypts, some of which lack an epithelial lining. Because the villous basement membrane is exposed during the continuing extrusion process, villous fusion occurs, resulting in lack of a scaffold for enterocyte replacement once the crypts recover. This results in permanent villous distortion and atrophy. Entrapped, hyperplastic crypt epithelium may therefore be present. Inclusion bodies are not present in lymphoid tissue. In bone marrow, erythropoiesis is normal, but granulopoiesis is reduced. Necrotizing colitis may occur but is much less important than the small intestinal lesions. Dogs with hemorrhagic parvovirus enteritis have bloody diarrhea and die from shock within 24 hours. Secondary bacterial infections with endotoxemia are believed to be associated with this syndrome.

Circovirus. Canine circovirus (dog CV) is associated with vomiting, hematochezia, hemorrhagic gastroenteritis, necrotizing vasculitis, and granulomatous lymphadenitis. Histologic lesions in pigs infected with porcine circovirus include viral inclusion bodies in macrophages and multinucleated giant cells, features not reported in dogs. Virus has been isolated from outbreaks of canine diarrhea, from heathy dogs, from dogs with a variety of other problems such as thrombocytopenia or neutropenia fever of unknown origin, and from some animals with tick bites. The virus is nonenveloped and round with a core of single-stranded, circular DNA. It is speculated that intercurrent pathogens potentiate disease in dog CV infections.

Minute Virus of Dogs. Canine parvovirus type 1 produces myocarditis and respiratory disease in young pups. The virus is widely distributed in the canine population, but disease is only diagnosed sporadically. The virus is spread via the oronasal route. Fetal death and embryo absorption occur between 25 and 35 days of gestation. Microscopically, intestinal lesions consist of enterocyte hyperplasia with eosinophilic or amphophilic intranuclear inclusion bodies in the enterocytes of the villous tips of the duodenum and jejunum. Crypt necrosis characteristic of canine parvovirus type 2 infection is not present.

Bacterial Diseases

Clostridial Enteritis

Peracute Hemorrhagic Gastroenteritis of Dogs. The cause of peracute hemorrhagic gastroenteritis of dogs, also known as canine hemorrhagic gastroenteritis, is undiscovered but is considered likely a result of infection with *C. perfringens* of unknown type. The disease most often occurs in dogs of toy and miniature breeds younger than 2 years. Blood is observed at the anus before death. As the name of the disease denotes, there is hemorrhagic necrosis of the GI mucosa anywhere from the stomach caudally. Numerous clostridial organisms are present in the intestinal debris but are not attached to intact mucosa. Unlike parvoviral enteritis, in which crypts are preferentially destroyed, the crypts are spared in peracute hemorrhagic gastroenteritis.

Histiocytic Ulcerative Colitis. Because of its occurrence in boxer dogs and the genetically related French bulldog, histiocytic ulcerative colitis has been called *boxer colitis*. *Granulomatous colitis* is another term for this disease, although true granulomas are not present. It generally occurs in dogs younger than 2 years. Dogs can have soft feces, but often no diarrhea or weight loss is observed. In some cases mucus and blood appear in the stool. The lesions, which are visible by proctoscopy, are raised ulcerative nodules (Fig. 7-181). Microscopically, the colon is ulcerated and has marked infiltration by macrophages containing PAS-positive material.

Large macrophages with abundant foamy eosinophilic cytoplasm are present in the colonic lamina propria and submucosa early in the disease process. There may be lesser numbers of smaller, mononuclear inflammatory cells, principally lymphocytes and plasmacytes. The PAS-positive material in macrophages has been visualized by tissue Gram stains, electron microscopy, and immunohistochemistry. They likely contain bacteria and the phagolysosomal remnants of digested cells. Evidence suggests that the bacteria are probably *E. coli*. The massive numbers of engorged macrophages within the lamina propria results in a space-occupying lesion that affects the overlying enterocytes. Enterocyte necrosis results in colonic erosion and ulceration. There is lymphadenopathy, both regional and generalized, characterized by an influx of foamy macrophages in the lymphatic sinuses.

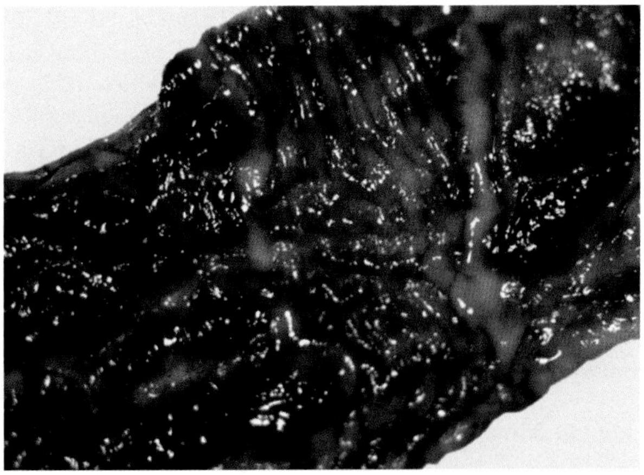

Figure 7-181 Histiocytic Ulcerative Colitis, Colon, Boxer Dog. There are numerous round and coalescing ulcers in the colon in this case of "boxer colitis." Research suggests *Escherichia coli* as the causative agent of boxer colitis. (Courtesy Dr. H. Gelberg, College of Veterinary Medicine, Oregon State University.)

***Citrobacter freundii* Enteritis.** Bacteremia and septicemia associated with *Citrobacter freundii* have been reported to cause mucohemorrhagic diarrhea in dogs with hemorrhagic lesions in the small intestine and colon. It is believed to be a condition of puppies and immunocompromised dogs. Being bacteremic and/or septicemic, many organs and tissues are affected besides the gut. The condition is more common in human beings as a nosocomial infection with a high mortality rate. In human beings the route of infection is through the urinary tract, gallbladder, GI tract, or cutaneous wounds. *Citrobacter* infections should be considered potentially zoonotic.

Fungal Diseases

Canine Histoplasmosis. Canine histoplasmosis occurs most often in the Ohio and Mississippi river valleys. This zoonotic systemic fungus can infect the intestine, but pneumonia is more common. Thus the route of infection is inhalation or ingestion. The reservoir is believed to be soil and bird feces. The yeast invades tissue, causes necrosis, and replicates in macrophages. Granulomatous lesions may be present in pulmonary, intestinal, lymphoid, hepatic, and other tissue. At necropsy or biopsy the intestine has a thickened and corrugated mucosa with ulceration. There is hepatomegaly and mesenteric lymphadenopathy and lymphadenomegaly. Scattered pulmonary granulomas may be present.

In the affected ileum and colon the lamina propria is widened by macrophages that contain *H. capsulatum* (Fig. 7-182). With time, infection may extend transmurally through the intestine and to the lymphoid system. There is hyperplasia of regional lymph nodes, and lymphoid sinuses contain numerous macrophages (see Figs. 13-59, 13-91, and 13-92). Multifocal granulomas with intracellular fungi are in the liver, presumably arriving via the portal vein (see Fig. 8-56).

Signs of intestinal histoplasmosis in the dog include intractable chronic diarrhea with anorexia and its attendant weight loss, lethargy, poor pelage, and anemia. Respiratory signs and peripheral lymphadenitis may be present.

Rickettsial Diseases

Salmon Poisoning. Salmon poisoning is an acute and fatal hemorrhagic granulomatous enterocolitis of the dog and fox that results from consuming salmon carrying the fluke *Nanophyetus salmincola*. When this trematode harbors *Neorickettsia helminthoeca*, a 0.3-μm coccoid rickettsia, disease may result. Lesions may extend from the pylorus to the anus. The enteric lesions consist of hemorrhage at sites of GALT necrosis, especially near the ileocecal valves. In the small intestine, trematodes may be embedded in the mucosa. Diagnosis is confirmed by visualizing macrophages in many tissues, including the lymph nodes, lamina propria, and brain, containing Giemsa- or Gram-stained elementary bodies (E-Fig. 7-23).

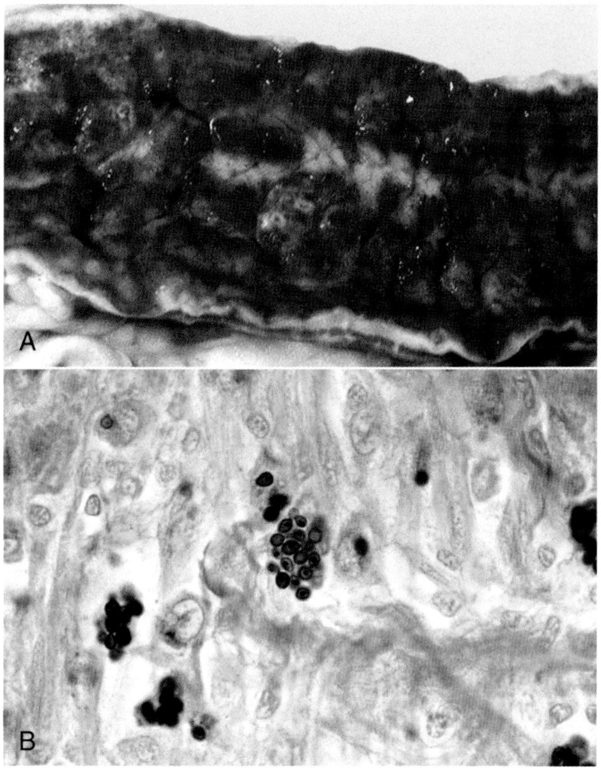

Figure 7-182 Histoplasmosis, Granulomatous Enteritis, Intestine, Dog. **A,** The mucosa is congested and greatly thickened from granulomatous inflammation that has expanded the lamina propria. **B,** Clusters of 3- to 5-μm *Histoplasma capsulatum* organisms (stained black) with a central nucleoid are in macrophages. Grocott-Gomori's methenamine silver stain. (**A** courtesy Dr. R. Panciera, School of Veterinary Medicine, Oklahoma State University; and Noah's Arkive, College of Veterinary Medicine, The University of Georgia. **B** courtesy Dr. H. Gelberg, College of Veterinary Medicine, Oregon State University.)

Six to eight days after eating parasitized fish, affected dogs become febrile and depressed. There is an oculonasal discharge, severe diarrhea, emesis, anorexia, and splenolymphadenopathy characterized by enlarged tonsils, spleen, and lymph nodes. The mesenteric lymph nodes are often more severely affected than peripheral nodes. Unless treated, affected animals die within 10 days.

Parasitic Diseases

Canine Multifocal Eosinophilic Gastroenteritis. Canine multifocal eosinophilic gastroenteritis is an uncommon disease of dogs generally younger than 4 years. It is caused by migrating larvae of *T. canis*. Therefore this disease occurs in association with poor parasite management.

Larvae of *T. canis* are ingested, invade the mucosa of the stomach and small intestine, and then become trapped and localized in their self-induced inflammation. Dormant larvae migrate into the uterus and fetuses during late pregnancy. Postpartum, larvae are secreted in the milk of the bitch or ingested from environmental feces. Ingested larvae penetrate the gastric and small intestinal mucosa, enter lymph vessels or the portal vein, and travel to the liver and lungs. They then develop into third-stage larvae and are coughed up and swallowed. In the GI tract they mature to adult ascarids. In the majority of puppies, ascarid larvae complete their life cycle in several weeks. Alternatively, the larvae are enveloped in granulomas that kill the parasite secondary to immune reactivity. These granulomas may occur anywhere along the parasite's migration tracts, including most abdominal organs, eyes, brain, and the lungs. Eosinophils are a prominent component of the inflammatory reaction and are attracted to the site of parasite entrapment by the waste products of the larvae. There may be subsequent mineralization of larvae, or they may remain viable for up to 4 years. This condition is especially common in aberrant host species and is called *visceral larval migrans*. It is an environmental danger where children play in sand or dirt contaminated by feces of infected animals. The ova are relatively resistant to environmental extremes.

Lesions are microscopic to macroscopic and may be quite numerous. As in other inflammatory diseases, there may be regional lymphadenopathy with or without nodules that vary from principally granulomatous to eosinophilic or a mix of the two. Larvae, when present, are surrounded by an eosinophilic, amorphous, fringed material that stains PAS positive (the Splendore-Hoeppli phenomenon).

In general, canine multifocal eosinophilic gastroenteritis is asymptomatic. However, chronic diarrhea, moderate weight loss, intermittent or persistent eosinophilia, and elevated serum γ-globulin concentrations may characterize this disorder. Serum albumin concentration and results of absorption tests and small bowel contrast radiographs usually are normal.

Immunologic Disorders

Inflammatory Bowel Disease. In dogs and cats inflammatory bowel disease is microscopically a lymphoplasmacytic enteritis. Diagnosis is made by biopsy. Breeds with a predilection for this disease include the basenji and the German shepherd. The cause is unknown, but the presence of numerous lymphocytes and plasma cells suggests an immunologic problem. Malabsorption and chronic protein-losing enteropathy can result from the marked infiltrate of lymphocytes and plasmacytes in the lamina propria. In dogs there are increased numbers of both B and T lymphocytes in the lamina propria of the small intestine (Fig. 7-183). In cats, but not dogs, dietary antigens cause some cases of inflammatory bowel disease; therefore control of the disease can be achieved by regulation of the diet. Anecdotal evidence suggests that lymphocytic plasmacytic enteritis in the cat can be a prelude to intestinal lymphoma.

Diffuse Eosinophilic Gastroenteritis. Although diffuse eosinophilic gastroenteritis has a predilection for the German shepherd breed, it occurs in other breeds of dogs and in cats. It is characterized by recurrent episodes of diarrhea associated with tissue and circulating eosinophilia. The increased concentration of eosinophils in the circulation and within lesions suggests a hypersensitivity reaction to some ingested substance or to parasites. The cause has not been identified. There are no gross lesions. Eosinophils, along with lymphocytes and plasma cells, heavily infiltrate all layers of the mucosa of the stomach and intestine (Fig. 7-184).

Wheat-Sensitive Enteropathy of Irish Setters. Wheat-sensitive enteropathy, a hereditable condition similar to gluten-sensitive enteropathy of human beings, is the first described dietary-induced enteropathy of dogs. It is characterized initially by increased numbers of intraepithelial lymphocytes and goblet cells and later by partial villous atrophy, particularly of the jejunum. Dietary therapy is palliative.

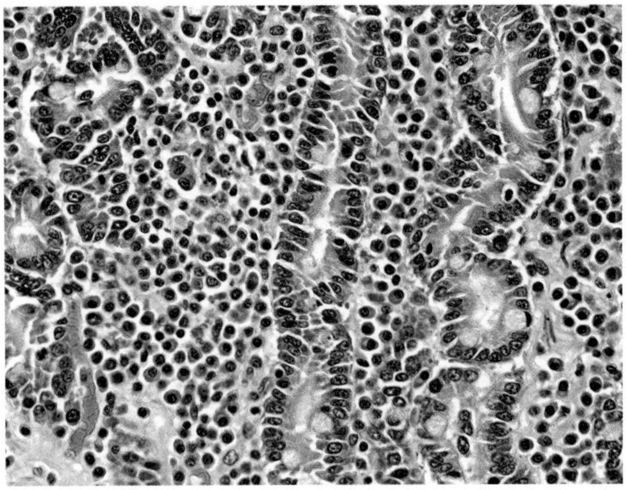

Figure 7-183 Lymphoplasmacytic Enteropathy, Intestine, Dog. The lamina propria is widened with lymphocytes and plasma cells. H&E stain. (Courtesy Dr. H. Gelberg, College of Veterinary Medicine, Oregon State University.)

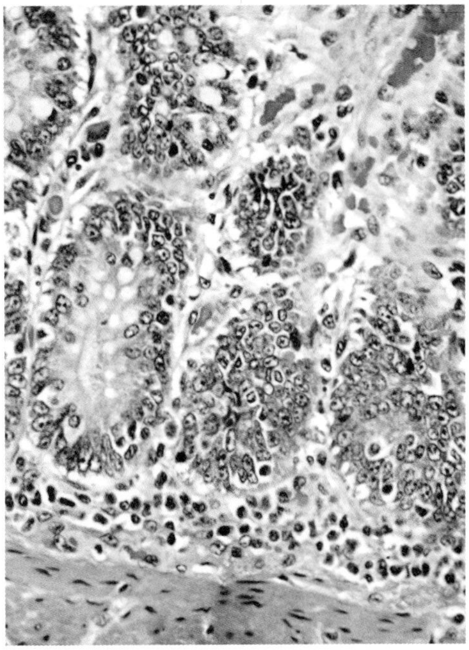

Figure 7-184 Diffuse Eosinophilic Enteritis, Small Intestine, Dog. Numerous eosinophils are present in the deep lamina propria and the mucosal-submucosal interface *(bottom quarter of image)*. The cause of this hypersensitivity reaction is not known. H&E stain. (Courtesy Dr. H. Gelberg, College of Veterinary Medicine, Oregon State University.)

Idiopathic Disorders

Canine Senile Gastrointestinal Amyloidosis. Amyloid located in and around vessels of the submucosal and muscular layers of the alimentary tract and within the mesentery has been reported in dogs. The mechanism and chemical nature of the amyloid deposition have not been determined. Dysfunction of the alimentary tract has not been reported to occur with canine senile GI amyloidosis.

Parasitic Enteritides

See Disorders of Domestic Animals, Intestine, Diseases Caused by Specific Pathogens, Parasitic Diseases.

Intestinal Neoplasia

See Disorders of Domestic Animals, Intestine, Intestinal Neoplasia.

Peritoneum, Omentum, Mesentery, and Peritoneal Cavity

See Disorders of Domestic Animals, Peritoneum, Omentum, Mesentery, and Peritoneal Cavity.

Sclerosing Encapsulating Peritonitis

Sclerosing encapsulating peritonitis is uncommon in dogs and rare in cats. Serous surfaces of the abdominal cavity are covered with granulation tissue and/or fibrous tissue, often encapsulating and sometimes distorting viscera. Multiple adhesions are present. In clinical patients it is sometimes possible to palpate the affected organs. Affected animals vomit, experience abdominal pain, and have ascites. The abdominal fluid contains variable numbers of erythrocytes, macrophages, mixed inflammatory cells, reactive mesothelial cells, and fibroblasts. The etiology in those cases that are not idiopathic includes steatitis, foreign bodies, and chronic bacterial infections.

Disorders of Cats

For disorders occurring in two or more species of animals, see Disorders of Domestic Animals.

Oral Cavity

Eosinophilic Stomatitides

See Disorders of Domestic Animals, Oral Cavity, Eosinophilic Stomatitides.

Feline rhinotracheitis and feline calicivirus may cause oral ulceration.

Teeth

Feline External Resorptive Neck Lesions

Cats suffering from feline external resorptive neck lesions often have pain upon chewing that may be reflected by inappetence and/or abnormal masticatory movements. External neck resorption of the cheek teeth of otherwise dentally normal cats is caused by odontoclastic resorption of cementum, particularly in the neck area or root of the tooth. Osteoclast ingrowths partially or completely line the resorption cavity. The resultant cavity may harbor bacterial plaque, resulting in intense inflammation and further osteoclastic resorption of dental tissue, including dentin and the root canal. The primary cause of this condition is not known.

Tonsils

See Disorders of Domestic Animals, Tonsils.

Salivary Glands

See Disorders of Domestic Animals, Salivary Glands.

Tongue

See Disorders of Domestic Animals, Tongue and Disorders of Cats.

Esophagus

See Disorders of Domestic Animals, Esophagus.

Stomach

See Disorders of Domestic Animals, Stomach and Abomasum.

Intestine

Viral Diseases

Parvovirus Enteritis. Also see Disorders of Dogs, Intestinal Disorders, Viral Diseases, Parvovirus Enteritis.

In the cat, mink, and raccoon, panleukopenia, cat distemper, feline enteritis, and mink enteritis are synonyms for this important disease. Early lesions in the course of the disease are lymphoid depletion and thymic involution. Later, lesions include flaccid, segmentally reddened intestine with serositis. Lesions are generally limited to the small intestine, but colitis occurs in some cats. Villous atrophy occurs secondary to crypt cell destruction (Fig. 7-185). Basophilic intranuclear inclusion bodies are present in enterocytes and lymphocytes early in infection. In germ-free cats with a low enterocyte turnover, the disease caused by feline parvovirus is much less severe. Intrauterine infection causes congenital cerebellar hypoplasia of kittens. The virus is cytolytic and infects dividing cells and thus alters the differentiation of layers in the cerebellum during organogenesis. The clinical disease is characterized by dehydration, depression, and diarrhea and vomiting. Because the bone marrow is a rapidly dividing tissue, panleukopenia dominates the clinical pathologic findings.

Immunologic Disorders

See Disorders of Dogs, Intestinal Disorders, Immunologic Disorders, Diffuse Eosinophilic Gastroenteritis.

Idiopathic Disorders

Inflammatory Bowel Disease. See Disorders of Dogs.

Feline Ulcerative Colitis. Feline ulcerative colitis is grossly and histologically analogous to its canine counterpart, histiocytic ulcerative colitis (Fig. 7-186). The cause is unknown.

Parasitic Enteritides

See Disorders of Domestic Animals, Intestine, Diseases Caused by Specific Pathogens, Parasitic Diseases.

Intestinal Neoplasia

See Disorders of Domestic Animals, Intestine, Intestinal Neoplasia.

Peritoneum, Omentum, Mesentery, and Peritoneal Cavity

Viral Diseases

Feline Infectious Peritonitis. Feline infectious peritonitis is a uniformly fatal disease of cats. A nearly identical coronaviral disease has been described in ferrets. Although it affects cats of all ages, the disease is principally found in the young and old. Twelve percent of feline deaths are associated with feline infectious peritonitis. The cause of the disease is a coronavirus related to the coronavirus of transmissible gastroenteritis of pigs. The coronavirus of feline infectious peritonitis in cats is believed to be a mutated enteric coronavirus. After entry into the body, the first round of viral replication takes place in the lymphoid system. Macrophages are infected and carry the virus systemically. Endothelial cells are activated secondary to upregulation of major histocompatibility complex class II. Observations suggest that activated monocytes are critical for development of vasculitis. Lesions are multifocal, and most organs, including the CNS, may be affected (see Figs. 14-105 and 14-106). The lesions in the vasculature of the eye are sometimes useful in making a

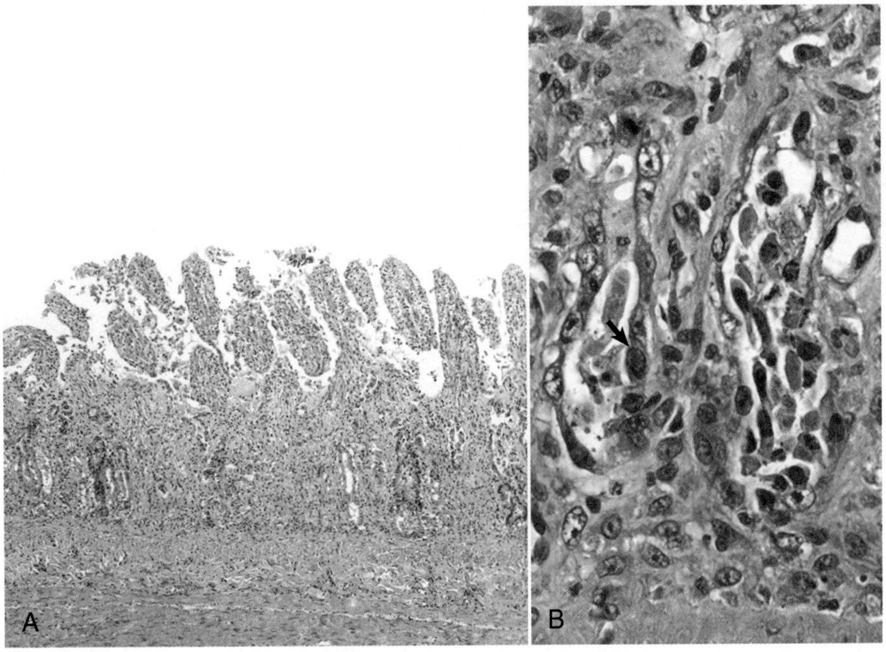

Figure 7-185 **Panleukopenia Virus Enteritis, Small Intestine, Cat. A,** Villi are denuded of epithelium and are atrophic. Note that because of the loss of epithelial cells in the crypts, they have collapsed, obliterating their lumens. Some crypts are dilated. H&E stain. **B,** Higher magnification of crypts. Note the sloughed necrotic epithelial cells in the crypt lumens and the lining of the crypts by squamoid epithelial cells and hyperplastic cells (some with intranuclear inclusion bodies) *(arrow)*, all indicative of attempts at epithelial repair and regeneration. Chronic inflammatory cells are present in the lamina propria. H&E stain. (**A** and **B** courtesy Dr. J.F. Zachary, College of Veterinary Medicine, University of Illinois.)

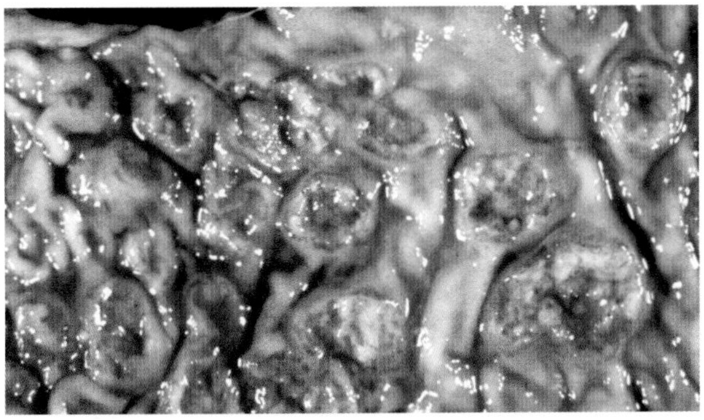

Figure 7-186 **Feline Ulcerative Colitis, Colon, Cat.** There are numerous round ulcers in the mucosa of this idiopathic disease. (Courtesy Dr. H. Gelberg, College of Veterinary Medicine, Oregon State University.)

tentative diagnosis of feline infectious peritonitis in the live cat, but other diseases, such as toxoplasmosis and systemic fungi, may cause similar lesions (see E-Figs. 21-11 and 21-75). The "wet form" of the disease is characterized by fibrinous polyserositis (see Fig. 7-16); the "dry form" is without the effusive process. Why one form develops rather than the other is not completely understood but may relate to the major type of immune effector cell. The disease often clusters in households, and virus spreads among cats by saliva on shared bowls and utensils or by mutation of an endogenous coronavirus.

Because of the presence of a nonneutralizing antibody, immune complexes develop and Arthus reactions localize in the vasculature. Complement is fixed, and inflammatory cell chemoattractants are produced. Vasculitis results in protein effusion. Thus lesions are vasocentric. The prodromal course of feline infectious peritonitis is shortened, and the development and extent of lesions are accelerated in seropositive cats. Feline infectious peritonitis is usually characterized by progressive wasting because of protein loss. It is unusual for a virus to result in pyogranulomatous lesions, but in feline infectious peritonitis the vasocentric deposition of immune complexes results in pyogranulomas. These lesions are single to multiple, white, and raised. On the surface of the kidney they often are linear, clearly following the renal surface vasculature (see Fig. 11-68). In its "wet form," feline infectious peritonitis is characterized by variable of amounts of thick, stringy, high-protein effusion in body cavities. When placed between gloved fingers, this transudate may be drawn out in strings as the fingers are separated. The transudate is sterile, eliminating most other causes of fibrinous peritonitis. The granulomas are translucent and less than 2 mm in diameter. The "dry form" of the disease is identical to the wet but contains only pyogranulomas and not the exudates.

Suggested Readings

Suggested Readings are available at www.expertconsult.com.

CHAPTER 8

Hepatobiliary System and Exocrine Pancreas[1]

Danielle L. Brown, Arnaud J. Van Wettere, and John M. Cullen

Key Readings Index

Liver and Intrahepatic Biliary System

Structure

Development

Early in embryogenesis, the origins of the liver are evident. The hepatic diverticulum, also termed the *liver bud*, arises from embryonic endoderm as a hollow outpouching of the primitive duodenum. Primitive hepatic epithelial cells of the hepatic diverticulum extend into the adjacent mesenchymal stroma and surround the vessels that form the vitelline venous plexus, a complex of vessels that drain the yolk sac. This close relationship between the epithelial cells of the liver and the small-caliber vitelline vessels is the earliest developmental form of the hepatic sinusoids. Subsequently, the caudal part of the hepatic diverticulum develops into the gallbladder and the cystic duct. Hepatic connective tissue is derived from the septum transversum, a sheet of cells that incompletely separates the pericardial and peritoneal cavity, and an ingrowth of mesenchymal cells from the coelomic cavity.

The biliary epithelium also arises from the hepatic diverticulum. Intrahepatic ducts develop from a structure, termed the *ductal plate*, which is composed initially of a single row of hepatoblasts that surround the portal vein branches and ensheathe the mesenchyme of the primitive portal tract. A second discontinuous outer layer of primitive hepatoblasts forms subsequently, and the two-cell-thick regions remodel into tubules and a few become the intrahepatic biliary ductular system. Superfluous cells of the ductal plate undergo apoptosis. Development of the ducts begins at the *porta hepatis* and extends to the margins of the liver until the later stages of gestation. Similarly, the hepatic artery also arises at the porta hepatis, and its extension into the portal tracts is typically concurrent with development of the mature bile ducts, suggesting an inductive process between the developing arteries and the bile ducts. The residual portions of the hepatic diverticulum persist to become the extrahepatic bile ducts.

It is known that hepatocytes and biliary epithelial cells share a common embryonic origin, but the factors that lead to the final characteristic morphology of the primitive hepatoblasts are not well understood. Epithelial-mesenchymal interactions are believed to play a role. Primitive hepatic epithelial cells in contact with vascular endothelium are destined to become hepatocytes, and those in contact with the developing mesenchyme of the portal tracts develop into bile ducts.

Macroscopic and Microscopic Structure

The liver is the largest internal organ in the body. In adult carnivores, the liver constitutes approximately 3% to 4% of the body weight. In adult omnivores and small ruminants, it is approximately 1.5% to 2% of the body weight, and in large herbivores, it is approximately 1% of the body weight. In the neonate of all species, the liver is a larger percentage of body weight than in the adult. In monogastric animals, the liver abuts the diaphragm and occupies the central area of the cranial abdomen. In ruminants, the liver is

[1]For a glossary of abbreviations and terms used in this chapter, see E-Glossary 8-1.

displaced to the right side of the cranial abdominal cavity. A series of ligaments maintains the liver in its position. The coronary ligament attaches the liver to the diaphragm near the esophagus. The falciform ligament attaches the midline of the liver to the ventral midline of the abdomen. The round ligament, a remnant of the umbilical vein, is embedded within the falciform ligament. The liver is supplied with blood from two sources. The portal vein drains the digestive tract and provides 70% to 80% of the total afferent hepatic blood flow. The hepatic artery provides the remainder of hepatic blood flow. Blood leaves the liver via the hepatic vein, which is very short, and enters the caudal vena cava. The liver has a smooth capsular surface, and the parenchyma consists of friable red-brown tissue that is divided into lobes. Gross subdivision of the liver into lobes differs among the domestic species. At the periphery, the lobes taper to a sharp edge.

The classic functional subunit of the liver is the hepatic lobule, a hexagonal structure, 1 to 2 mm wide (Figs. 8-1 and 8-2). At the center, the lobule has a central vein (also termed the terminal hepatic venule), which is a tributary of the hepatic vein, and at the angles of the hexagon, it has portal tracts (Figs. 8-3 and 8-4). The portal tracts contain bile ducts, branches of the portal vein, the hepatic artery, nerves, and lymph vessels, all supported by a collagenous stroma. The limiting plate, a discontinuous border of hepatocytes, forms the outer boundary of the portal tract. Divisions of the lobule are termed periportal, midzonal, and centrilobular (Fig. 8-5). Blood flows into the sinusoids from the terminal distributing branches of the hepatic artery and portal veins that leave the portal tracts and form an outer perimeter of the lobule (see Figs. 8-3 and 8-4). Portal blood and hepatic arterial blood mix in the sinusoids. Blood drains from the sinusoids into the central veins and to progressively larger sublobular veins and then into the hepatic veins.

Alternatively, when the liver is viewed as a bile-secreting gland, the acinus (vs. the hepatic lobule) is the anatomic subunit of the hepatic parenchyma (Fig. 8-6). Terminal afferent branches (penetrating vessels) of the portal vein and hepatic artery project into the parenchyma, like branches from the trunk of a tree, forming the long axis of the diamond-shaped acinus. Thus terminal afferent branches of the portal vein and hepatic artery are at the center of the acinus and the terminal hepatic venule is located at the periphery (see Figs. 8-3). Each terminal hepatic venule (central vein) receives blood from several acini. There are three zones within the acinus. Zone 1 is closest to the afferent blood coming from the hepatic artery and the portal vein. Zone 2 is peripheral to zone 1, and zone 3 borders the terminal hepatic venule (see Fig. 8-5). In this anatomic unit, bile flow begins in the canaliculi of the hepatocytes in zone 3 and flows through zones 2 and 1 and then into the interlobular bile ducts in the portal areas.

Additional perspectives of the subdivision of the liver architecture exist, such as portal lobules centered on a portal triad or the Matsumoto primary lobule.

The ultrastructural appearance of hepatocytes reflects the cell's active metabolism, bile secretion, and close contact with the plasma

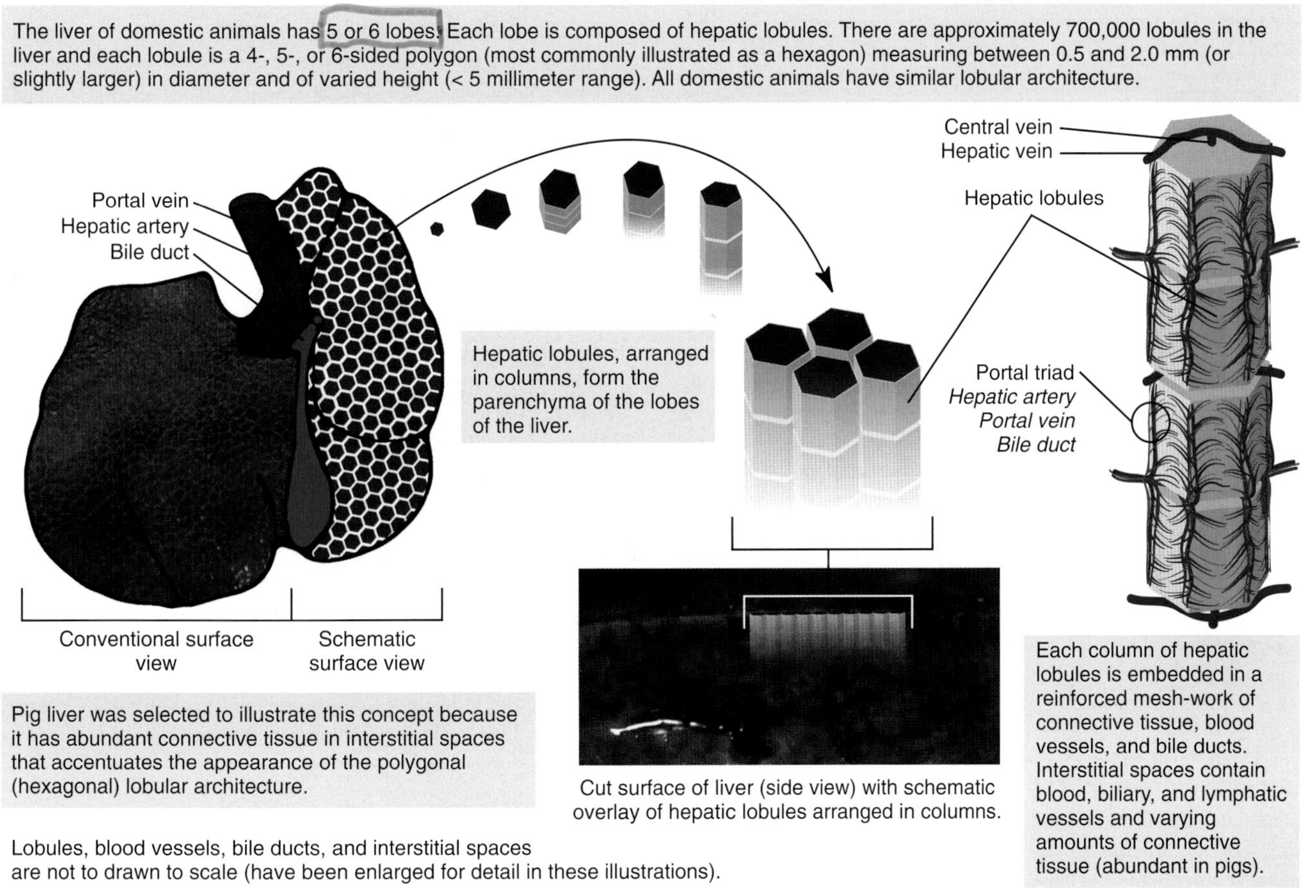

The liver of domestic animals has 5 or 6 lobes. Each lobe is composed of hepatic lobules. There are approximately 700,000 lobules in the liver and each lobule is a 4-, 5-, or 6-sided polygon (most commonly illustrated as a hexagon) measuring between 0.5 and 2.0 mm (or slightly larger) in diameter and of varied height (< 5 millimeter range). All domestic animals have similar lobular architecture.
Portal vein
Hepatic artery
Bile duct
Central vein
Hepatic vein
Hepatic lobules
Hepatic lobules, arranged in columns, form the parenchyma of the lobes of the liver.
Portal triad
Hepatic artery
Portal vein
Bile duct
Conventional surface view
Schematic surface view
Pig liver was selected to illustrate this concept because it has abundant connective tissue in interstitial spaces that accentuates the appearance of the polygonal (hexagonal) lobular architecture.
Cut surface of liver (side view) with schematic overlay of hepatic lobules arranged in columns.
Each column of hepatic lobules is embedded in a reinforced mesh-work of connective tissue, blood vessels, and bile ducts. Interstitial spaces contain blood, biliary, and lymphatic vessels and varying amounts of connective tissue (abundant in pigs).
Lobules, blood vessels, bile ducts, and interstitial spaces are not to drawn to scale (have been enlarged for detail in these illustrations).

Figure 8-1 Lobular Organization of the Liver in Domestic Animals. (Courtesy Dr. A.J. Van Wettere, School of Veterinary Medicine, Utah State University and Dr. J.F. Zachary, College of Veterinary Medicine, University of Illinois. Gross photomicrograph of the surface of the pig liver courtesy Dr. Edward (Ted) Clark, College of Veterinary Medicine, University of Calgary.)

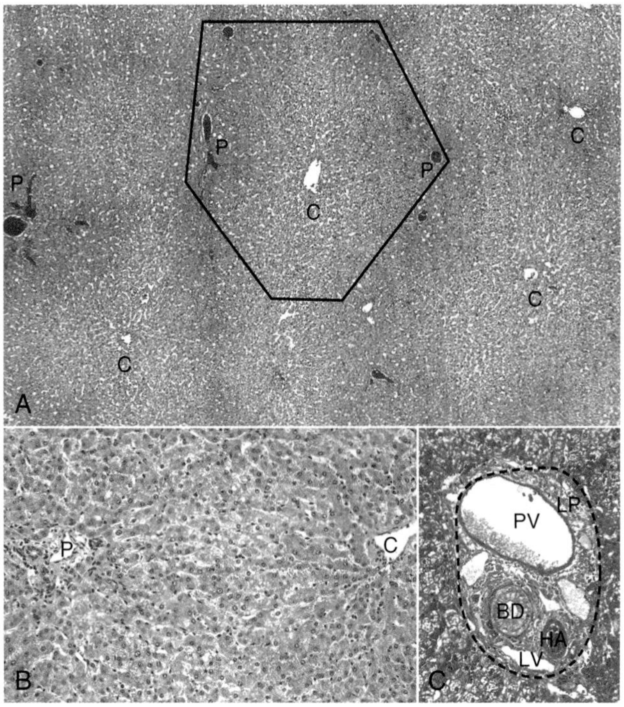

Figure 8-2 Liver, Hepatic Lobules, Normal Dog. **A,** Low magnification. A central vein *(C)* is located in the center of the lobule. Branches of the portal vein, hepatic artery, bile duct, and lymphatic vessels are located on the periphery of the lobule in portal tracts *(P)* (also Fig. 8-2, C). H&E stain. **B,** Higher magnification. Plates of hepatocytes arranged radially between portal tracts *(P)* to a central vein *(C)*. H&E stain. **C,** Higher magnification, portal tract. The normal portal tract contains the hepatic artery *(HA)*, bile duct *(BD)*, portal vein *(PV)*, and several lymphatic vessels *(LV)*. These structures are surrounded by a collagenous extracellular matrix that forms an abrupt border with a circumferential row of hepatocytes, termed the *limiting plate* (LP—*dotted line*). Note that the profile of the portal vein is typically larger than those of the hepatic artery and bile duct. H&E stain. (**A** and **C** courtesy Dr. J.M. Cullen, College of Veterinary Medicine, North Carolina State University. **B** courtesy Dr. J.F. Zachary, College of Veterinary Medicine, University of Illinois.)

(E-Fig. 8-1). The surface of the hepatocyte that faces the lumen of the sinusoid contains an abundance of microvilli. Basolateral aspects of hepatocytes are characterized by the presence of canaliculi, modified portions of the cell membrane of two adjacent hepatocytes, which form a lumen for bile secretion. The cytoplasm contains glycogen and a variety of organelles, including numerous mitochondria, lysosomes, and abundant smooth and rough endoplasmic reticulum.

Within the liver, hepatocytes are arranged in one-cell-thick branching plates, which extend radially from the terminal hepatic venule. Hepatic plates are separated by vascular sinusoids. Blood from the terminal afferent branches of the hepatic artery and portal vein mixes in the hepatic sinusoids and flows to the terminal hepatic venule. Hepatic sinusoids differ from capillaries in that they are lined by discontinuous (fenestrated) endothelial cells that lack a typical basement membrane (Fig. 8-7), whereas capillaries have a continuous endothelial lining and are ensheathed in the basement membrane. The sinusoids are critical for appropriate hepatic function. The architecture of the sinusoids enables efficient uptake of plasma constituents by hepatocytes and facilitates hepatocellular secretion. A fine scaffold of electron lucent basement membrane that contains collagen types III, IV, and XVIII and other extracellular matrix (ECM) components supports the sinusoidal endothelial cells (E-Fig. 8-2; also see Fig. 8-7). These elements collectively make up the "reticulin" of the liver (Fig. 8-8).

There is also a gap between the endothelial cells and hepatocytes. This critical anatomic feature of the liver is termed the space of Disse. Although blood cells are normally excluded from the space of Disse because they are too large to pass through endothelial gaps, the modified endothelial cells and basement membrane permit plasma to pass freely through this gap (see Fig. 8-7). Within this space, plasma constituents come into contact with the luminal surface of the hepatocytes. This surface of the hepatocytes is characterized by the presence of numerous microvilli, which increase the surface area of the hepatocytes and facilitate uptake of a variety of plasma-borne substances, as well as secretion of synthesized products. Any damage to this area has significant impact on hepatic function.

The lumen of the sinusoids contains hepatic macrophages, termed *Kupffer cells* (Fig. 8-9; also see Fig. 8-7). These cells are members of the monocyte-macrophage system, and they clear infectious agents and senescent cells, such as erythrocytes, particulate material, endotoxin, and other substances, from the sinusoidal blood. They are mobile and able to migrate along the sinusoids and into areas of tissue injury and regional lymph nodes. Kupffer cells are involved in cytokine-driven interactions with hepatocytes, endothelial cells, lymphocytes, and the stellate cells discussed later. They can express class II histocompatibility antigens and function as antigen-presenting cells, although they are not as efficient as the macrophages in other tissues. Phagocytosis and clearance of immune complexes are the primary roles of Kupffer cells. Kupffer cells are derived from in situ replication as well as recruitment of blood-borne monocytes.

Hepatic stellate cells (previously termed *Ito cells*) are found within the space of Disse and between hepatocytes at the edge of the space of Disse (E-Fig. 8-3; also see Fig. 8-7). Normally, hepatic stellate cells are primarily responsible for storing vitamin A in their characteristic cytoplasmic vacuoles. During hepatic injury, stellate cells alter their morphology and function. These activated hepatic stellate cells lose their vitamin A content, acquire a myofibroblast-like phenotype, and synthesize collagen and other ECM components that lead to hepatic fibrosis. Hepatic stellate cells also play significant roles in liver growth and regeneration by secretion of growth factors and in the hepatic immune response.

Bile flows within the lobule in the opposite direction to blood flow, which facilitates the concentration of bile. The biliary system commences as canaliculi within the centrilobular (periacinar) areas of the hepatic lobule. The walls of canaliculi are formed entirely by the cell membranes of adjacent hepatocytes. Just outside the limiting plate, canaliculi drain into the canals of Hering that are lined partially by hepatocytes and partially by biliary epithelium. These drain into cholangioles with low cuboidal biliary epithelium. The cholangioles converge into interlobular bile ducts that are lined with cuboidal epithelium and located in the portal areas. Bile then flows into the lobar ducts that unite to form the hepatic duct. The confluence of the common hepatic duct and the cystic duct from the gallbladder form the common bile duct by which bile is carried to the duodenum. The gallbladder is responsible for storage and concentration of bile in most species. It is absent in the horse, elephant, and rat.

Bipotential progenitor cells that have the ability to differentiate into hepatocytes or biliary epithelium are believed to reside in the area of the *cholangiole* (the canal of Hering). These cells may proliferate in circumstances in which mature hepatocytes or bile duct epithelium cannot replicate, such as severe injury or nutritional deficits. When these cells proliferate, they form islands or crude

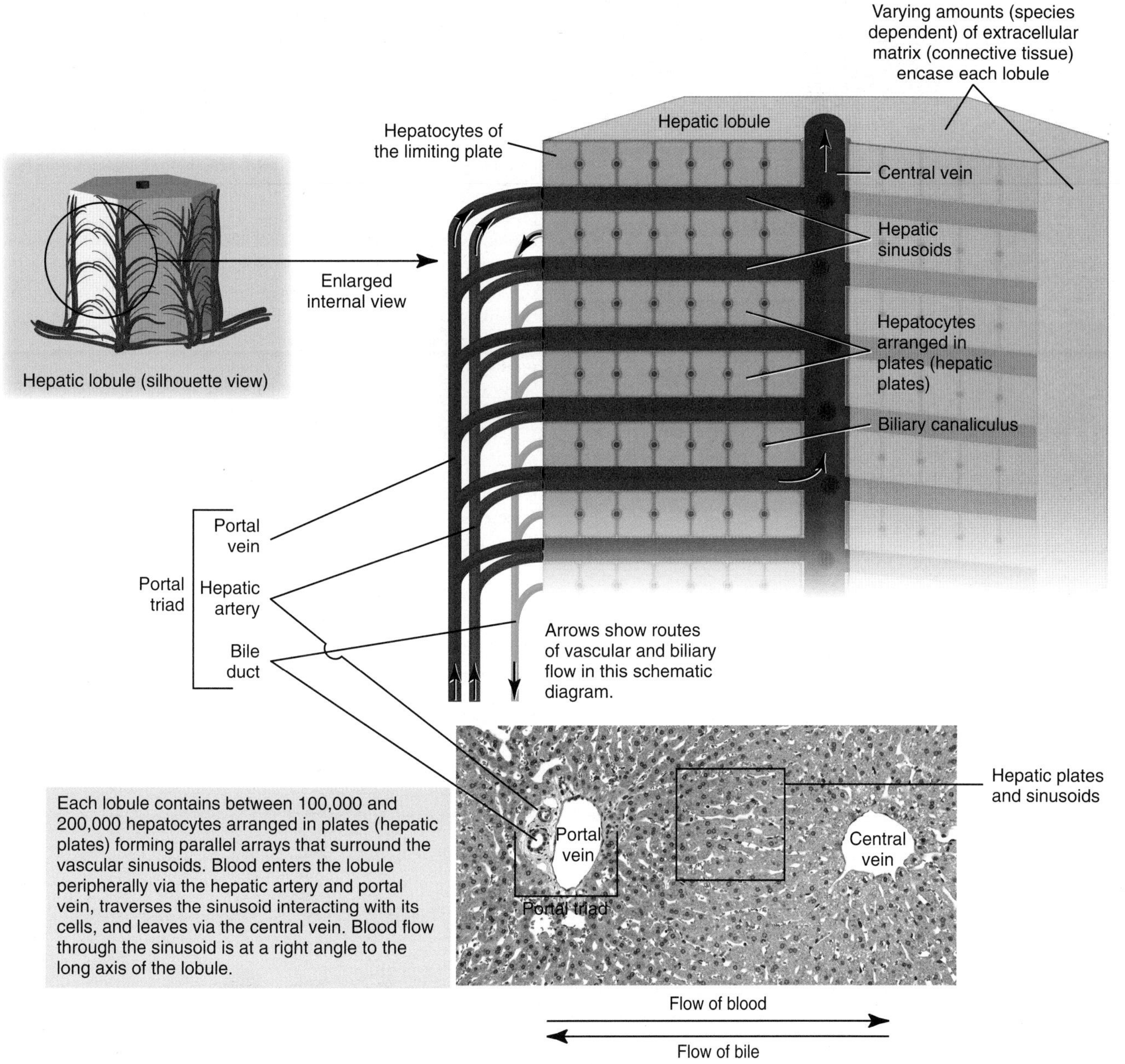

Figure 8-3 Blood and Bile Flow in Hepatic Lobules. Microscopic organization of the liver. A central vein is located in the center of the lobule with plates of hepatocytes arranged radially. Portal triads are located on the periphery of the lobule and contain branches of the portal vein, hepatic artery, and bile duct. Blood and bile flow in opposite directions within the hepatic lobule. Blood from the portal vein and hepatic artery perfuses and mixes within the sinusoids. Bile ducts drain bile from the biliary canaliculi that run between hepatocytes. (Courtesy Dr. A.J. Van Wettere, School of Veterinary Medicine, Utah State University and Dr. J.F. Zachary, College of Veterinary Medicine, University of Illinois.)

tubules of small basophilic cells found initially at the margin of the limiting plate. This proliferation is termed the *ductular reaction* and is a hallmark of severe injury.

Both sympathetic and parasympathetic nerves running along the portal vein and the hepatic artery innervate the liver. The nerve fibers enter the liver at the hilus and ramify to the level of the portal tracts and then extend along the sinusoids. Nerve supply is believed to affect sinusoidal blood flow, the balance of hepatic blood flow from the portal vein and the hepatic artery, and metabolic functions of the liver.

Postmortem Evaluation of the Liver

Information on this topic is available at www.expertconsult.com.

Function

Production and Excretion of Bile

Excretion of bile is the main exocrine function of the liver (Box 8-1). Bile is composed of water, cholesterol, bile acids, bilirubin, inorganic ions, and other constituents. Bile formation is continuous, but the rate of secretion can vary significantly. There are three major purposes for bile synthesis. The first purpose is excretory; many of the body's waste products, such as surplus cholesterol, bilirubin, and metabolized xenobiotics, are eliminated in bile. The second purpose is the facilitation of digestion; bile acids secreted into the intestine aid in the digestion of lipids within the intestine. The third purpose is to provide buffers to neutralize the acid pH of the ingesta as it is released from the stomach.

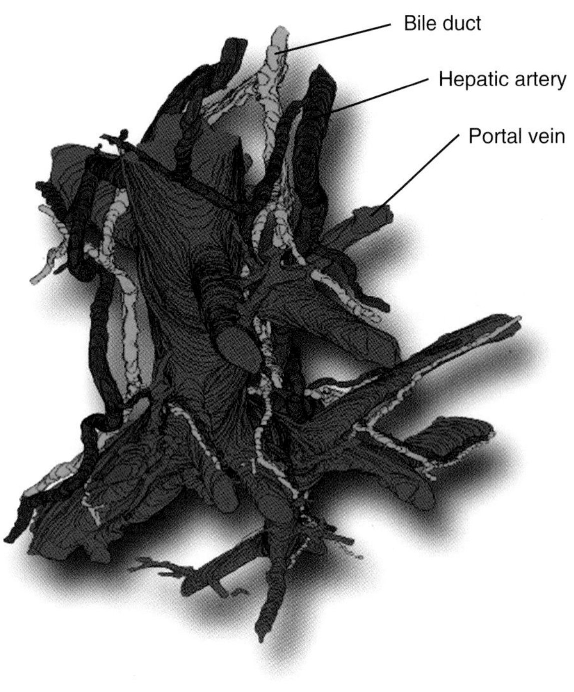

Figure 8-4 **Three-dimensional View of the Vascular and Biliary Structures within the Portal Triad.** Three-dimensional reconstruction of the structures of the normal portal tract of a dog demonstrating the relative size and position of the main components: portal vein *(blue)*, hepatic artery *(red)*, and bile duct *(green)*. (Courtesy of Drs. D.P. Livingston and J.M. Cullen, College of Veterinary Medicine, North Carolina State University.)

The three principal functions of bile acids, important constituents of bile, are maintenance of cholesterol homeostasis, stimulation of bile flow, and intestinal absorption of fats and fat-soluble vitamins. Bile acids are synthesized in the liver from cholesterol and are conjugated to glycine or taurine to facilitate their interaction with other components of bile and to prevent precipitation into calculi when they are secreted into the bile. The major bile acids are cholic acid and chenodeoxycholic acid, but there are various types and proportions of bile acids found in different species. Bile acids are actively secreted into the bile canaliculi from the hepatocyte cytoplasm by specific intramembranous molecular pumps against a concentration gradient, which creates an osmotic gradient, stimulating the inflow of water and solutes into the bile canaliculi. Conjugated bile acids are therefore the principal physiologic stimulus for bile production through a process termed *bile acid–dependent flow*. Bile acids are effective detergents that assist in the digestion of lipids within the intestine and increasing the solubility of lipids secreted into the bile. The quantities of bile acids required far exceed the liver's capacity to produce them. For this reason, bile acids are avidly reabsorbed from the ileum, extracted from the portal blood, and resecreted into bile via a process known as *enterohepatic circulation*. This process is a very efficient system. As much as 95% of secreted bile acids are recycled, and the proportion of reabsorbed bile acids in the liver greatly exceeds that of recently synthesized bile acids; bile acids may be recycled 15 times per day. Interruption of this process results in fat malabsorption and a deficiency of fat-soluble vitamins.

Bilirubin Metabolism

Bilirubin, a major component of bile, is produced from the metabolic degradation of hemoglobin and, to a lesser extent, other heme

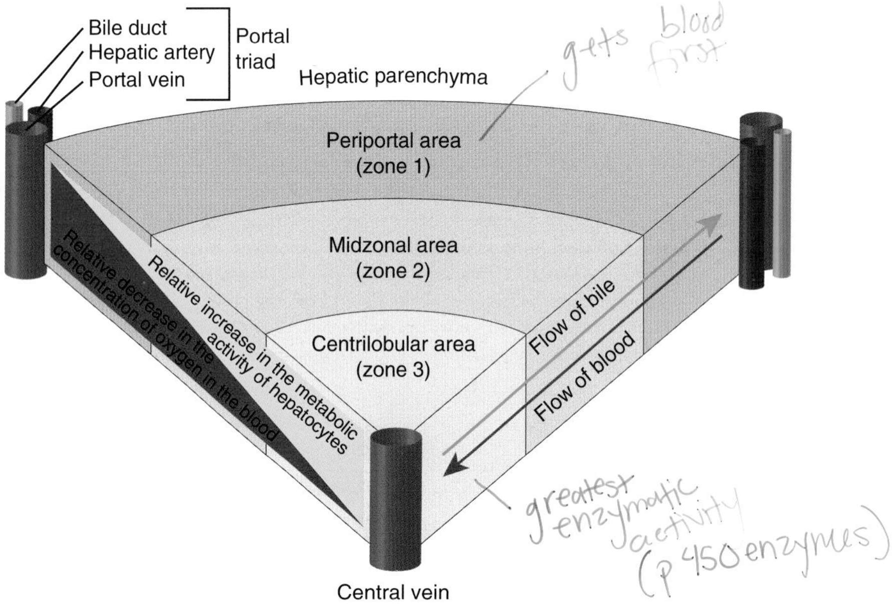

Figure 8-5 **Metabolic Zonation of Hepatic Lobules.** Functional organization of the liver. Both the lobule and the acinus are represented (see Fig. 8-6). The lobule is a hexagonal unit with portal areas at the margin and a terminal hepatic vein (central vein) at the center. The lobule is divided into the periportal, midzonal, and centrilobular areas. The acinus is a diamond-shaped structure with the distributing branches of the vessels from the portal areas as the center of the structure and central veins at the extremities. Zone 1 of the acinus is closest to the afferent blood supply, and zone 3 is at the tip of the diamond-shaped structure, closest to the terminal hepatic vein (central vein). Zone 2 is in between zones 1 and 3. Zone 3 receives the least oxygenated blood and is therefore more susceptible to hypoxia. In addition, zone 3 has the greatest enzymatic activity (mixed function oxidases) capable of activating many compounds into toxic forms. (Courtesy Dr. A.J. Van Wettere, School of Veterinary Medicine, Utah State University and Dr. J.F. Zachary, College of Veterinary Medicine, University of Illinois.)

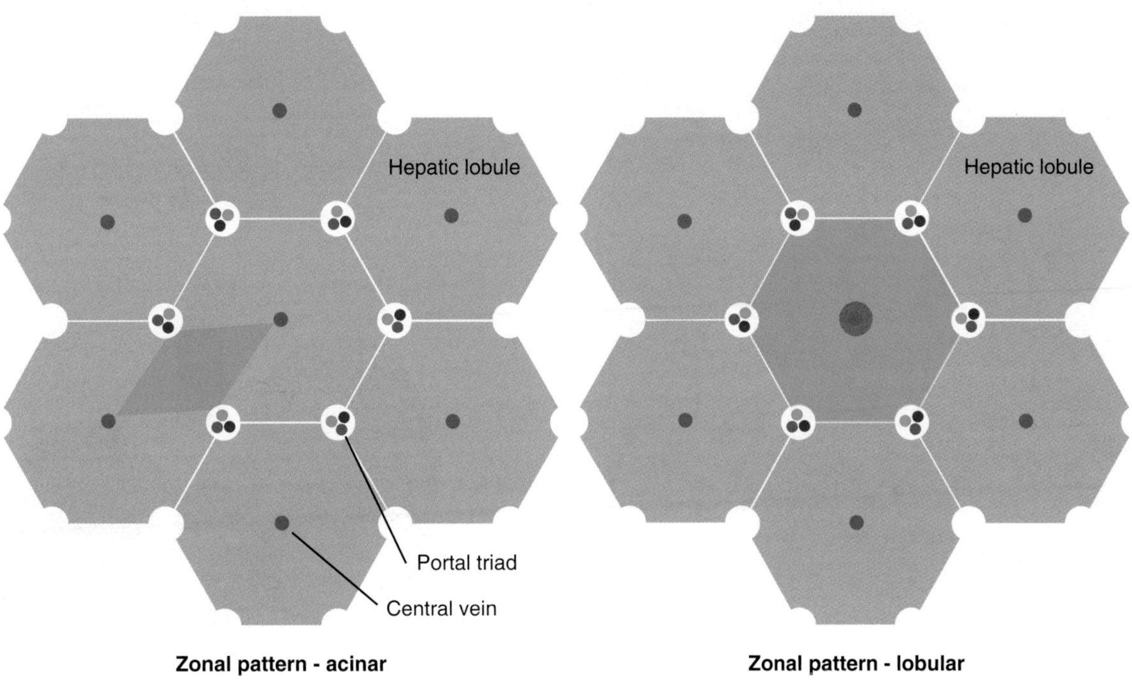
Hepatic lobule
Hepatic lobule
Portal triad
Central vein
Zonal pattern - acinar
Zonal pattern - lobular

Figure 8-6 **Concept of Hepatic Lobule and Acinus.** In the lobular model *(right)*, the terminal hepatic vein or central vein is at the center of a "lobule," while the portal tracts are at the periphery. In the acinar model, the acinus is centered on the terminal branches of the portal vein, hepatic artery, and bile ductule, while the central veins are at the points of the diamond. (Courtesy Dr. A.J. Van Wettere, School of Veterinary Medicine, Utah State University and Dr. J.F. Zachary, College of Veterinary Medicine, University of Illinois.)

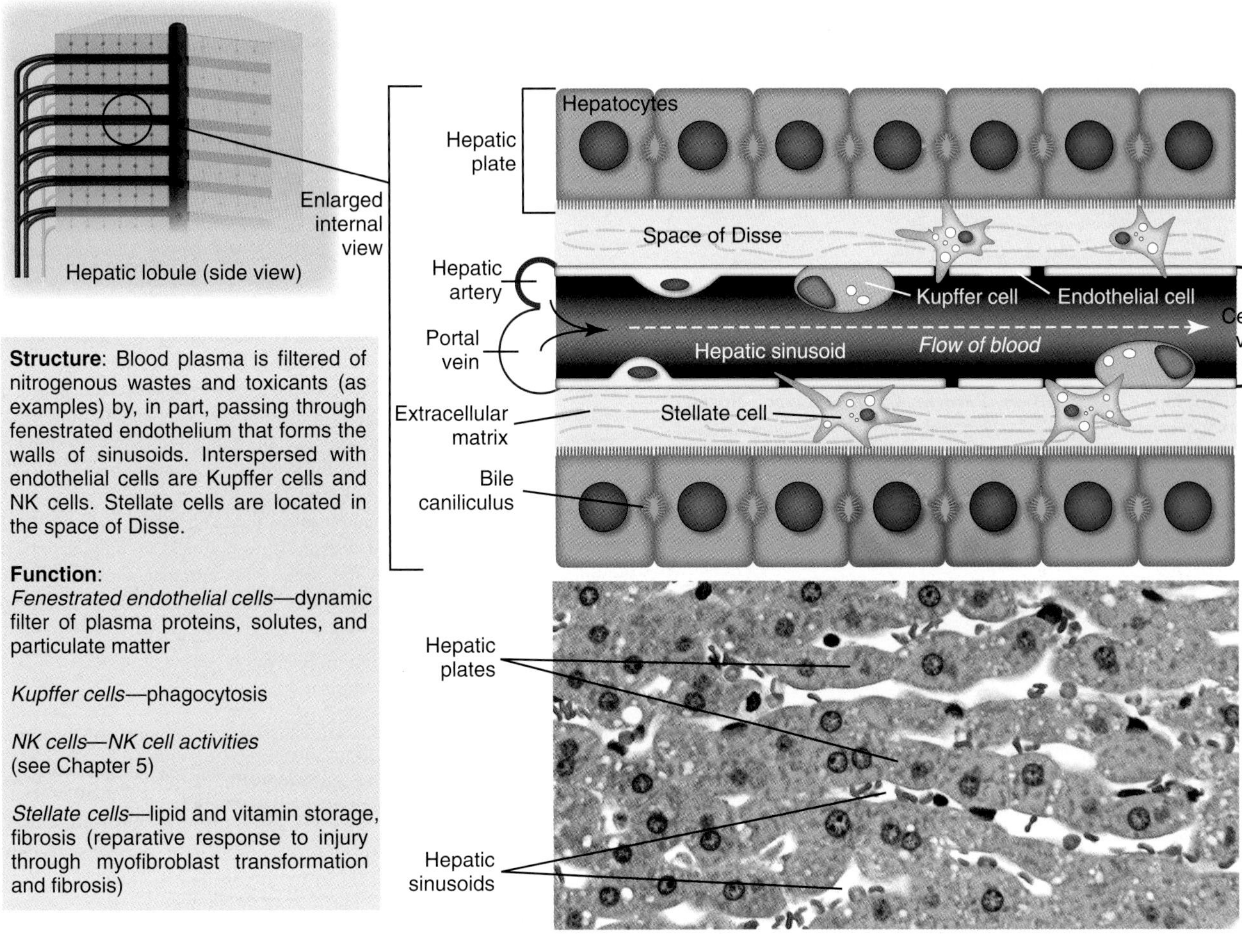
Hepatic lobule (side view)
Enlarged internal view
Hepatocytes
Hepatic plate
Space of Disse
Hepatic artery
Kupffer cell
Endothelial cell
Portal vein
Hepatic sinusoid
Flow of blood
Central vein
Extracellular matrix
Stellate cell
Bile caniliculus
Hepatic plates
Hepatic sinusoids
Structure: Blood plasma is filtered of nitrogenous wastes and toxicants (as examples) by, in part, passing through fenestrated endothelium that forms the walls of sinusoids. Interspersed with endothelial cells are Kupffer cells and NK cells. Stellate cells are located in the space of Disse.
Function:
Fenestrated endothelial cells—dynamic filter of plasma proteins, solutes, and particulate matter
Kupffer cells—phagocytosis
NK cells—NK cell activities
(see Chapter 5)
Stellate cells—lipid and vitamin storage, fibrosis (reparative response to injury through myofibroblast transformation and fibrosis)

Figure 8-7 **Hepatic Sinusoid.** Vascular spaces, termed sinusoids, run between the hepatic plates (cords). The vascular lumen is lined by discontinuous (fenestrated) capillaries. Blood within the sinusoids is supplied by both the hepatic artery and the portal vein, and the directional flow of blood is from the portal tract to the central vein. Kupffer cells rest on the sinusoidal endothelial cells and project into the sinusoid. Between the endothelial cells and the hepatocytes is a gap called the space of Disse. Microvilli extending from the luminal aspect of the hepatocytes are found in this space. Hepatic stellate cells are also situated within the space of Disse and extend between hepatocytes. Biliary canaliculi run between adjacent hepatocytes. (Courtesy Dr. A.J. Van Wettere, School of Veterinary Medicine, Utah State University and Dr. J.F. Zachary, College of Veterinary Medicine, University of Illinois.)

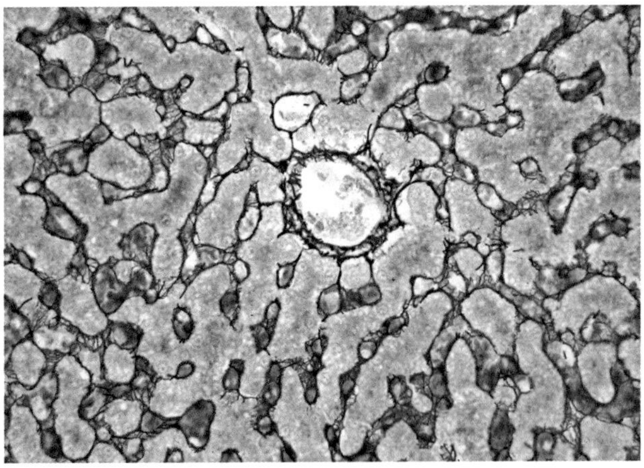

Figure 8-8 **Reticulin Fibers (Reticulin Stain), Hepatic Extracellular Matrix, Liver, Normal Dog.** This stain reveals "reticulin" *(black)*, composed of extracellular matrix found within the space of Disse that forms the scaffolding of the hepatic parenchyma. Note the radial arrangements of the hepatic plates and the single hepatocyte thickness of the plates. A central vein is evident in the center of the image. Gordon and Sweet's reticulin stain with a nuclear fast red counterstain. (Courtesy Dr. M.D. McGavin, College of Veterinary Medicine, University of Tennessee.)

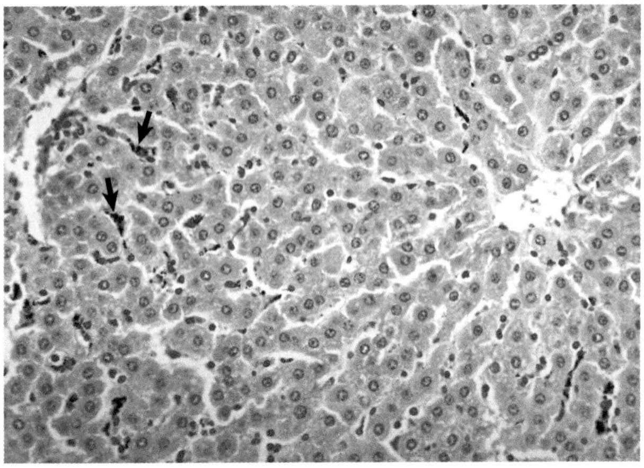

Figure 8-9 **Kupffer Cells, Carbon Particle Uptake, Liver, Normal Calf.** Carbon particles injected into the portal vein have been phagocytosed by Kupffer cells *(arrows)*, making them more easily detectable along the sinusoids of the liver. Nuclear fast red stain. (Courtesy Dr. M.D. McGavin, College of Veterinary Medicine, University of Tennessee.)

Box 8-1 Normal Functions of the Liver

- Production and excretion of bile
- Bilirubin metabolism
- Carbohydrate metabolism
- Lipid metabolism
- Xenobiotic metabolism
- Protein and urea synthesis
- Immune function

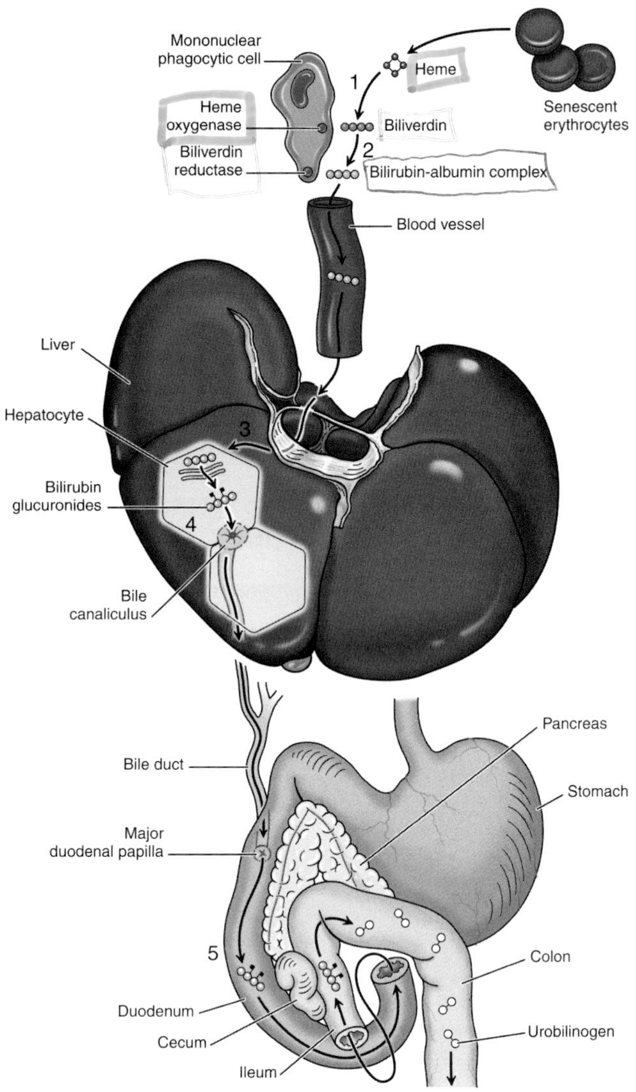

Figure 8-10 **Bilirubin Metabolism and Elimination (as Depicted in Human Beings).** *1*, Normal bilirubin production from heme (0.2 to 0.3 g per day) is derived primarily from the breakdown of senescent circulating erythrocytes, with a minor contribution from degradation of tissue heme-containing proteins. *2*, Circulating bilirubin is bound to serum albumin and delivered to the liver. *3*, Hepatocellular uptake. *4*, Glucuronidation in the endoplasmic reticulum generates bilirubin monoglucuronides and diglucuronides, which are water soluble and readily excreted into bile. *5*, Gut bacteria deconjugate the bilirubin and degrade it to colorless urobilinogens. The urobilinogens are excreted in the feces, with minimal reabsorption and excretion into urine. Residual urobilinogen is metabolized by bacteria into the brown pigment stercobilin, imparting the typical color to feces.

proteins including myoglobin and the hepatic hemoproteins, such as cytochromes (Fig. 8-10). The majority of bilirubin is derived from normal extrahepatic breakdown of senescent erythrocytes. Senescent erythrocytes normally are phagocytosed by macrophages of the spleen, bone marrow, and liver. Within the phagocyte, the globin portion is degraded and the constituents are returned to the amino acid pool. The heme iron is transferred to iron-binding proteins, such as transferrin, for recycling. The remaining portion of heme is first oxidized by heme oxygenase to biliverdin. In the next metabolic step, biliverdin reductase converts biliverdin to bilirubin. Subsequently, the bilirubin, which is poorly soluble in an aqueous medium, is then released into the blood in its unconjugated form and bound to albumin to increase its solubility in plasma.

The process of bilirubin elimination can be divided into three phases: uptake, conjugation, and secretion. Uptake refers to the process by which hepatocytes remove the bilirubin bound to albumin from the circulation. Unconjugated bilirubin is separated from albumin at the sinusoidal surface and bilirubin is taken up by hepatocytes by a carrier-mediated process. In the second phase of bilirubin metabolism, bilirubin is conjugated, principally with glucuronic acid, by bilirubin UDP-glucuronyltransferase in the endoplasmic reticulum. After conjugation, bilirubin becomes water soluble and less toxic. It is then excreted, in the third phase of bilirubin metabolism, into the bile by active transport through specialized portions of hepatocyte membranes that form the margins of the bile canaliculi. The excretion phase is the rate-limiting step in most species.

Within the gastrointestinal tract, conjugated bilirubin is converted to urobilinogen by bacteria and a minute fraction of urobilinogen is reabsorbed into the portal blood, a process called *enterohepatic circulation*, and returned to the liver. The majority of urobilinogen that is absorbed from the gastrointestinal tract is resecreted into bile. Urobilinogen has a small molecular weight and is freely filtered through the glomerulus, and small amounts are normally found in the urine. Urobilinogen that is not absorbed from the intestine becomes oxidized to stercobilin, which is responsible for the color of the feces.

Carbohydrate Metabolism

The liver has an important role in the regulation of plasma glucose concentrations. After eating, the liver removes carbohydrates (i.e., glucose and fructose) from the plasma and stores them as glycogen or fatty acids. In periods of need, energy balance is maintained by glycolysis of stored glycogen or by gluconeogenesis. Production of energy by oxidative phosphorylation and β-oxidation of fatty acids in hepatic mitochondria is used to sustain the activities of the hepatocyte.

Lipid Metabolism

The liver plays a central role in lipid metabolism. It is involved in the production and degradation of plasma lipids such as cholesterol, triglycerides, phospholipids, and lipoproteins. Cholesterol is synthesized, secreted, and degraded by hepatocytes. Hepatocytes can synthesize fatty acids when energy levels are high, and they can oxidize fatty acids as an energy source when necessary.

Xenobiotic Metabolism

Foreign substances (xenobiotics), such as many therapeutic drugs, insecticides, and endogenous substances—such as steroids that are lipophilic—require conversion to water-soluble forms for elimination from the body. The cytochrome P450 enzymes of the smooth endoplasmic reticulum (microsomes) of the hepatocytes serve as the major site of metabolism of these substances in preparation for excretion in bile or urine. This process is discussed in detail in the section on toxic liver injury.

Protein and Urea Synthesis

Synthesis of the majority of plasma proteins, mainly within the rough endoplasmic reticulum, is a principal function of the liver. Proteins produced in the liver include plasma proteins, such as albumin; a variety of transport proteins; lipoproteins; clotting factors II, V, and VII to XIII; fibrinolysis proteins; some acute phase proteins; and components of the complement system. The liver is responsible for synthesis of approximately 15% of body proteins.

The liver is also the principal site of ammonia metabolism. Highly toxic ammonia is generated through catabolism of amino acids. Metabolic conversion of ammonia into urea, a far less toxic compound, occurs through the urea cycle, which occurs almost exclusively in the liver. Urea then enters the systemic circulation (blood urea nitrogen) and is excreted in the urine.

Immune Function

The liver has a significant immune function. It is involved in systemic, local, and mucosal immunity. Hepatocytes participate in the response to systemic inflammation through the synthesis and release of acute phase proteins. Approximately 10% of the cells in the liver belong to the adaptive immune system (T and B lymphocytes) or the innate immune system (Kupffer cells, natural killer lymphocytes, and natural killer T lymphocytes). Compared with other organs, the liver is particularly enriched with cells of the innate immune system, likely a result of the fact it is the site where foreign antigens from the gastrointestinal tract first encounter the innate immune system defenses. The liver contains the largest pool of mononuclear phagocytes and natural killer cells in the body in most species. The Kupffer cells lining the sinusoids provide the first line of defense against infectious agents, endotoxin, and foreign material absorbed from the intestines before they gain access to the systemic circulation. Most blood-borne foreign material is cleared by Kupffer cells in all domestic species, except members of the Order Artiodactyla (pigs, goats, and cattle), in which this function is performed by intravascular macrophages in the pulmonary alveolar capillaries. Disposal of waste molecules (e.g., products of inflammation such as cytokines and immunoglobulins) and deletion of activated effector T lymphocytes are also important functions. The liver is also involved in transport of secretory immunoglobulin A (IgA), the primary immunoglobulin of the mucosal surfaces, from plasma cells into the biliary tree and intestine.

Dysfunction/Responses to Injury

The high metabolic rate of hepatocytes renders them highly susceptible to metabolic disturbances that lead to cellular degeneration and necrosis (Box 8-2). This section considers the patterns of hepatic degeneration, responses of the liver to injury, and inflammation of the liver.

Morphologic Classification of Hepatobiliary Disease

The nature and distribution of inflammatory lesions in the liver are usually dictated by the route of entry, the host inflammatory response, the nature of the infectious agent (e.g., virus, bacterium, or fungus), and any predilection they have for involvement with a particular cell type in the liver. The hematogenous route of infection tends to cause a random multifocal distribution of lesions. Infections, usually bacterial, that ascend the biliary tract from the intestine are typically centered in the bile ducts. Severe infections of the biliary tree may affect the entire portal tract and extend into the adjacent parenchyma. Penetrating wounds cause discrete areas of inflammation with or without necrosis that are evident on the capsule and extend into the hepatic parenchyma. Liver injury should be characterized by the pattern of involvement (multifocal random, zonal, or massive), type of inflammatory cells

Box 8-2 Mechanisms of Liver Injury

- Metabolic bioactivation of chemicals via cytochrome P450 to reactive species
- Stimulation of autoimmunity
- Stimulation of apoptosis
- Disruption of calcium homeostasis leading to cell surface blebbing and lysis
- Canalicular injury
- Mitochondrial injury

Data from Lee W: *N Engl J Med* 349:474-485, 2003.

involved (neutrophils, lymphocytes, plasma cells, eosinophils, and/or macrophages), evidence of necrosis or fibrosis, severity of these processes, evidence of regeneration, and the presence of an etiologic agent or agents. The type of inflammatory response and the duration of the injury can help identify the infectious agents.

Acute Hepatitis. Inflammation of the liver parenchyma is termed *hepatitis*. Acute hepatitis is characterized by inflammation, hepatocellular necrosis, and apoptosis. The proportion and type of inflammatory cells involved varies considerably, depending on the cause of inflammation, the host response, and the stage or age of the lesion. Characterization of the type of inflammation usually requires microscopic evaluation. In many forms of acute hepatitis, particularly bacterial and protozoal infections, neutrophils accumulate in response to the usual chemotactic stimuli. Random foci of neutrophilic hepatitis, as a consequence of embolic localization of bacteria, are relatively common in all species. In neonates—especially calves, lambs, and foals—bacteria, such as *Escherichia coli*, usually seed the liver via the umbilical veins or less often the portal venous or hepatic arterial systems. Acute hepatitis produced by viral infections, such as herpesvirus infection in many species, is more frequently characterized by a random distribution of necrosis and apoptosis with minimal inflammation or infiltrations of lymphocytes.

Chronic Hepatitis. Chronic hepatitis results when there is continued inflammation as a result of persistence of an antigenic stimulus. In the absence of such a stimulus, inflammation rapidly resolves. Chronic hepatitis is characterized by fibrosis; accumulation of mononuclear inflammatory cells, including lymphocytes, macrophages, and plasma cells; and, frequently, regeneration. Neutrophils often are present in chronic unresolved hepatic inflammation such as that which characterizes some forms of canine chronic hepatitis. The proportion and distribution of each of these elements varies with the inciting cause and host response. Local variation within the liver can also occur.

Different terms are used to distinguish separate types of chronic hepatitis. Granulomatous hepatitis may be obvious grossly if it produces discrete granulomas of sufficient size. These granulomas may be focal, multifocal, or diffuse. Chronic suppurative hepatitis is usually manifested as discrete or multiple abscesses. Focal lesions, such as abscesses or granulomas, often are sufficiently localized so that they do not alter hepatic function. In contrast, diffuse and severe chronic hepatitis, as seen in dogs, usually leads to loss of hepatic parenchyma and architectural distortion of the liver as a consequence of fibrosis and nodular parenchymal regeneration. This process can proceed to end-stage hepatic disease with hepatic failure and its associated constellation of clinical signs.

Nonspecific Reactive Hepatitis. Nonspecific reactive hepatitis is a diffuse process distributed throughout the liver in response to some systemic illness, most often within the gastrointestinal tract, or is the residuum of prior liver inflammation. Typically, there is a mild inflammatory infiltrate in the portal tract and possibly the parenchyma without evidence of necrosis. In acute cases, there is a minimal to mild infiltrate of neutrophils within the connective tissue of the portal tracts that may vary in intensity. Mononuclear cells, primarily lymphocytes and plasma cells, predominate in more chronic manifestations. Pigmented macrophages containing hemosiderin, lipofuscin, or both may be scattered throughout the parenchyma. Mononuclear inflammatory cells may also be evident within the hepatic parenchyma and at the periphery of central veins. Kupffer cells are usually reactive (i.e., they appear somewhat swollen because of abundant cytoplasm and display prominent nuclei as well).

Cholangitis. Inflammation of the biliary ducts (either intrahepatic or extrahepatic) is termed *cholangitis*. There are several patterns of cholangitis. The inflammatory cell population and the degree of fibrosis will vary with the type and duration of injury. Specific forms of cholangitis are discussed next.

Neutrophilic Cholangitis. Neutrophilic (suppurative) cholangitis is the most common type of cholangitis. It is characterized by the presence of neutrophils within the lumen or epithelium of the bile ducts (Fig. 8-11). Acute and chronic forms of this process can occur. Fibrosis and the addition of mononuclear inflammatory cells are characteristic of the chronic form. Rupture of affected bile ducts can lead to hepatic abscess formation. Most neutrophilic cholangitis is believed to be caused by ascending bacterial infections from the intestine. Bacterial culture from gallbladder bile is the most rewarding approach and most often reveals infection with enteric organisms such as *Escherichia coli*, *Enterococcus*, *Bacteroides*, *Streptococcus*, or *Clostridium*.

Lymphocytic Cholangitis. Lymphocytic cholangitis occurs most often in cats and is described in detail in the section on Disorders of Cats.

Destructive Cholangitis. Destructive cholangitis is an uncommon syndrome characterized by necrosis of the epithelium of bile ducts (Fig. 8-12). Inflammation is often present around the areas of biliary destruction and may extend along cholangioles outside of the portal tract. Pigmented macrophages are common within the portal tracts as well. Certain chemicals, such as trimethoprim-sulfa, have been implicated in this syndrome in dogs.

Cholangiohepatitis. Inflammation that affects both the biliary ducts and hepatic parenchyma is termed *cholangiohepatitis*. In most cases of intrahepatic disease, the primary focus of inflammation can be identified as affecting either the hepatocytes or the biliary tree, but occasionally both components of the liver are affected, usually as an extension of biliary disease, such as neutrophilic cholangitis, to involve the periportal hepatocytes; in that circumstance, the term *cholangiohepatitis* should be used.

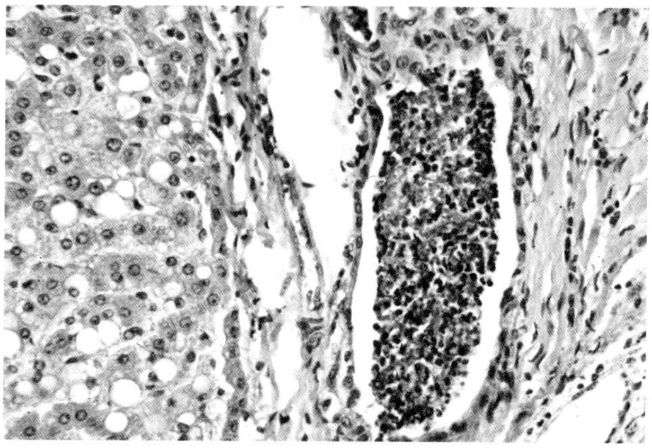

Figure 8-11 **Neutrophilic Cholangitis (Intrahepatic), Liver, Cat.** This condition is characterized by the presence of degenerate neutrophils within the lumen *(right center of image)* or the walls of bile ducts in the portal areas. The most common cause is ascending bacterial infection from the intestine via the common bile duct. H&E stain. (Courtesy Dr. M.D. McGavin, College of Veterinary Medicine, University of Tennessee.)

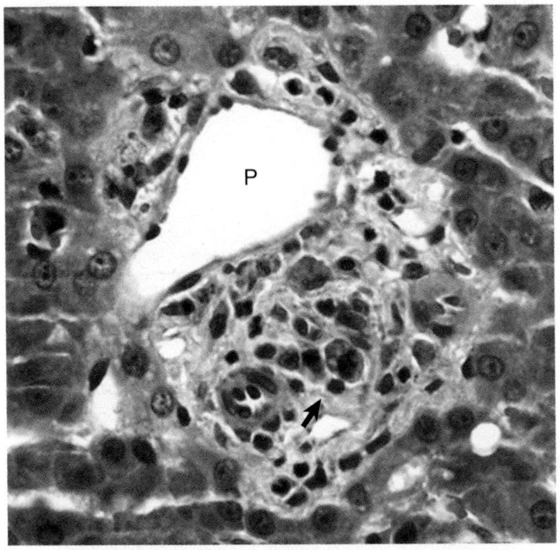

Figure 8-12 **Destructive Cholangitis, Liver, Dog.** This condition is an uncommon disorder affecting bile ducts *(arrow)* characterized by the destruction of bile duct epithelium, followed by regeneration in some instances. Necrotic or absent biliary epithelium, pigmented macrophages (hemosiderin), and small numbers of mononuclear inflammatory cells in portal tracts are the typical histologic findings. *P,* Portal vein. H&E stain. (Courtesy Dr. J.M. Cullen, College of Veterinary Medicine, North Carolina State University.)

Necrosis and Apoptosis

The epithelial cells of the liver, hepatocytes and biliary epithelium, are the principal targets of most liver diseases. Sublethal injury to hepatocytes is characterized by cell swelling (hydropic degeneration), steatosis, or atrophy. Cells that have sustained a sublethal injury often remove damaged organelles by forming autophagosomes. Material that cannot be digested further is retained as lipofuscin, which is why after sublethal injury, this pigment can often be found in affected cells and associated phagocytes.

By convention, cell death has been divided into two distinct processes. These processes are necrosis, which is characterized by cytoplasmic swelling, destruction of organelles, and disruption of the plasma membrane, and apoptosis, or programmed cell death, which is characterized by one of several active processes involving caspases that lead to cell shrinkage and an intact cell membrane. Necrosis is triggered by lethal injury. Necrotic cells typically swell and exhibit karyorrhexis followed by rupture and fragmentation of the cell body. Coagulative necrosis results from sudden denaturation of hepatocytes and produces swollen hepatocytes with a preserved eosinophilic cytoplasmic outline and karyorrhexis or karyolysis. Lytic necrosis is characterized by a loss of hepatocytes and an influx of erythrocytes and/or inflammatory cells into the vacant space or condensation of the reticular connective tissue (collagen and other ECM) scaffolding of the liver that once supported the hepatocytes.

Classic apoptosis is triggered by an interaction between tumor necrosis factor-α (TNF-α) or Fas ligand and specific receptors on the cell membrane leading to caspase activation, although other pathways, including those involving mitochondrial cytochrome *c,* have been identified. Apoptosis is recognized microscopically by the formation of apoptotic bodies, which are brightly eosinophilic, homogeneous, round structures that can be found between hepatocytes, within the lumen of sinusoids, or within macrophages or hepatocytes. A detailed review of cell death is beyond the scope of this section but is covered in Chapter 1. However, evidence has revealed that there may some overlap between necrosis and apoptosis, depending on the cell type and the type and dose of injurious agent. Thus both hepatic necrosis and apoptosis can be produced by the same agent and can occur in the same liver.

Box 8-3 Patterns of Hepatocellular Degeneration and/or Necrosis

- Random
- Zonal
  - Centrilobular
  - Paracentral/periacinar
  - Midzonal
  - Periportal
- Bridging
- Massive

Patterns of Hepatocellular Degeneration and Necrosis. Although the liver is subjected to a wide variety of different insults, the cellular degeneration and/or necrosis that results invariably occurs in one of three morphologic patterns (Box 8-3).

Random Hepatocellular Degeneration and/or Necrosis. Random hepatocellular degeneration and/or necrosis is characterized by the presence of either single cell necrosis throughout the liver or multifocal areas of necrotic hepatocytes. These areas are scattered randomly throughout the liver; there is no predictable location within a lobule. This pattern is typical of many infectious agents, including viruses, bacteria, and certain protozoa. Lesions may be obvious grossly as discrete, pale, or, less often, dark red foci that are sharply delineated from the adjacent parenchyma (Fig. 8-13, *A* and *B*). The size of such foci is variable, ranging from tiny (<1 mm) to several millimeters. Hepatocytes in affected areas are either damaged or necrotic because of the injurious effects of the infectious agents and the stage of the process (Fig. 8-13, *C*).

Zonal Hepatocellular Degeneration and/or Necrosis. Zonal hepatocellular degeneration and/or necrosis, or as it is more simply termed, *zonal change,* affects hepatocytes within defined areas of the hepatic lobule. The zones are centrilobular (periacinar), midzonal (between centrilobular and periportal areas), or periportal (centroacinar) areas. Extensive zonal change within the liver, regardless of location within the lobule, typically produces a liver that is pale and modestly enlarged with rounded margins, has increased friability, and characteristically has an enhanced lobular pattern on the capsular and cut surface of the organ (Fig. 8-14). Damaged hepatocytes swell, and when the majority of hepatocytes in a zone are affected, that portion of the lobule appears pale. In contrast, once the hepatocytes in a particular zone of the lobule have become necrotic, this results in dilation and congestion of sinusoids so that the affected zone appears red. Although zonal change typically produces an enhanced lobular pattern, microscopic examination is usually required to determine the type of zonal change. Specific forms of zonal change are described next.

Centrilobular Degeneration and/or Necrosis. Centrilobular degeneration and necrosis of hepatocytes is particularly common (Fig. 8-15), as this portion of the lobule receives the least oxygenated blood and is therefore susceptible to hypoxia, and it has the greatest enzymatic activity (mixed function oxidases) capable of activating compounds into toxic forms. Centrilobular necrosis can result from a precipitous and severe anemia or right side heart failure. Similarly, passive congestion of the liver results in hypoxia as a result of stasis of blood and produces atrophy of centrilobular hepatocytes.

Paracentral Cellular Degeneration and/or Necrosis. Paracentral cellular degeneration involves only a wedge of parenchyma around

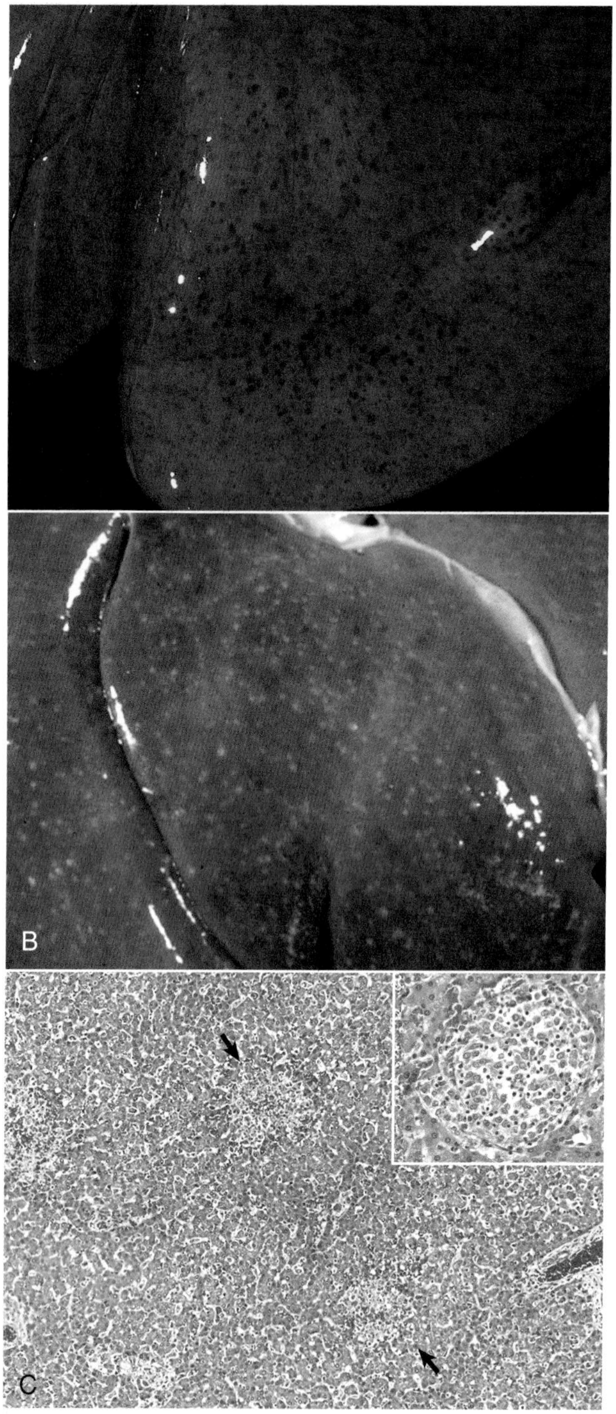

Figure 8-13 Random Hepatocellular Injury, Liver. A, Tyzzer's disease, horse. Random disseminated 1- to 2-mm red to dark red foci of necrosis due to *Clostridium piliforme* infection. **B,** Equine herpes virus infection, foal. Random white to gray foci of viral-induced lytic necrosis. **C,** Salmonellosis, focal necrosis and inflammation, pig. The random pattern of necrotic foci are infiltrated by macrophages and form discrete granulomas termed paratyphoid nodules *(arrows)* within the hepatic lobules. H&E stain. *Inset,* Higher magnification of a paratyphoid nodule. H&E stain. (**A** courtesy Dr. M. Stalker, College of Veterinary Medicine, University of Guelph; **B** courtesy Drs. J. King and L. Roth, College of Veterinary Medicine, Cornell University; **C** courtesy Dr. M.D. McGavin, College of Veterinary Medicine, University of Tennessee. Inset courtesy Dr. J. Simon, College of Veterinary Medicine, University of Illinois.)

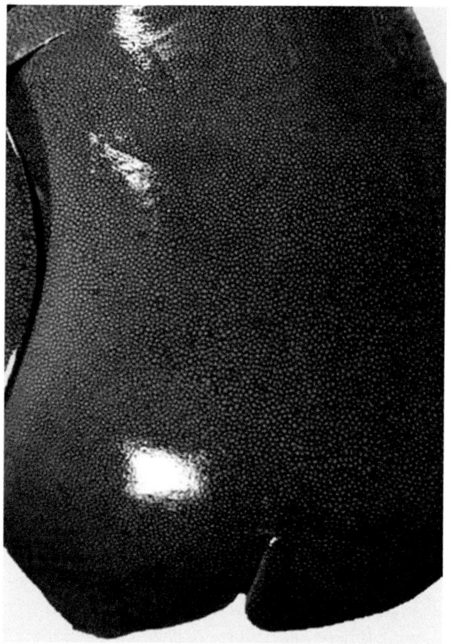

Figure 8-14 Zonal Hepatocellular Injury, Liver, Horse. Accentuation of the normal lobular pattern is evident on the capsular surface of the liver. It is not a specific change, as it may be associated with zonal hepatocellular degeneration and/or necrosis (regardless of lobular location), passive congestion, or diffuse cellular infiltration of the portal and periportal areas (often reflecting hepatic involvement of hematopoietic neoplasms, such as lymphoma and myeloproliferative disorders). (Courtesy Dr. J. King, College of Veterinary Medicine, Cornell University.)

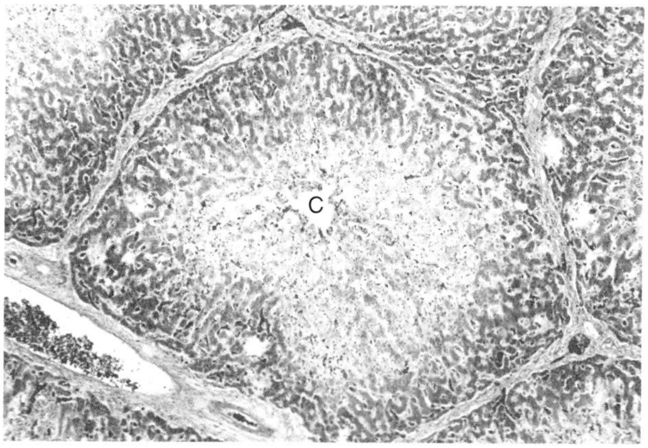

Figure 8-15 Centrilobular Necrosis, Zonal Hepatocellular Injury, Liver, Pig. Centrilobular necrosis is characterized by a circumferential zone of hepatocellular necrosis surrounding the terminal hepatic venule (central vein *[C]*). H&E stain. (Courtesy Dr. M.D. McGavin, College of Veterinary Medicine, University of Tennessee.)

the central vein because only the outer margin of one diamond-shaped acinus is affected, typically reflecting the action of a toxin that requires bioactivation (Fig. 8-16) or severe, acute anemia. Because several acini border on a single central vein (terminal hepatic venule), changes induced by hypoxia may not be present equally in all acini, and thus hepatocytes at the periphery of one acinus can have more severe change than those in adjacent acini.

Midzonal Degeneration and/or Necrosis. Midzonal degeneration and necrosis are unusual lesions in domestic animals but have been reported in pigs and horses with aflatoxicosis and cats exposed to hexachlorophene (Fig. 8-17).

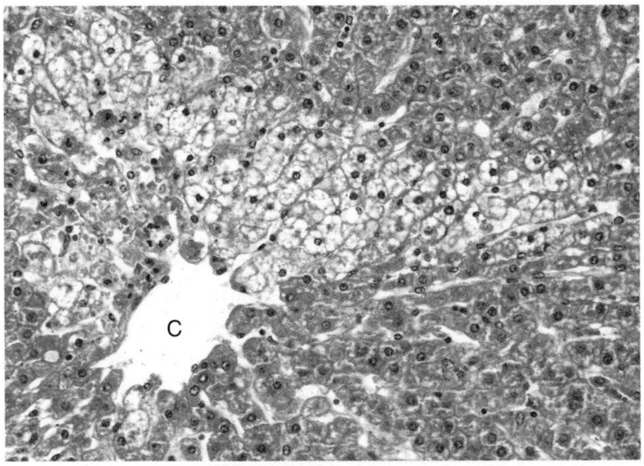

Figure 8-16 **Paracentral Degeneration and Necrosis, Zonal Hepatocellular Injury, Liver, Cow.** Rather than a pattern of complete circumferential necrosis, a wedge-shaped area of hepatocytes is damaged. In this case, the paracentral lesion consists of necrotic hepatocytes to the left and other hepatocytes with hydropic degeneration. This wedge is the apex of the diamond-shaped liver acinus (zone 3) and reflects the partitioning of the lobule based on the inflow of blood from each of the individual portal tracts that surround the lobule. This change can be seen as an early manifestation of hepatic hypoxia in animals with anemia or right-sided heart failure and precedes centrilobular necrosis. C, Central vein. H&E stain. (Courtesy Dr. M.D. McGavin, College of Veterinary Medicine, University of Tennessee.)

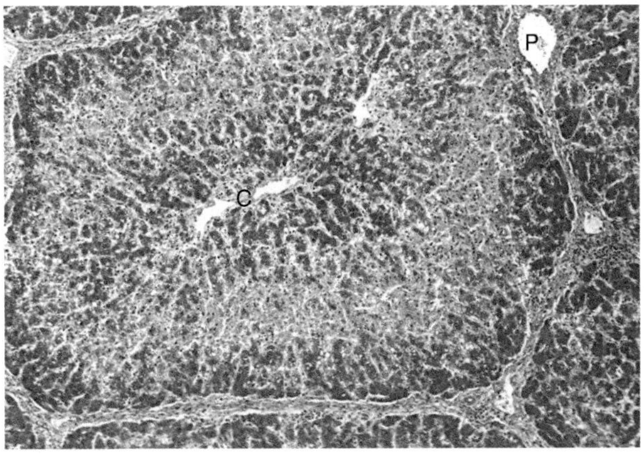

Figure 8-17 **Midzonal Necrosis, Zonal Hepatocellular Injury, Liver, Horse.** Midzonal necrosis is the least common pattern of hepatic injury. Hepatocytes in the middle portion of the lobule (zone 2) are affected, and hepatocytes in the other regions are spared. C, Central vein; *P*, portal vein. H&E stain. (Courtesy Dr. M.D. McGavin, College of Veterinary Medicine, University of Tennessee.)

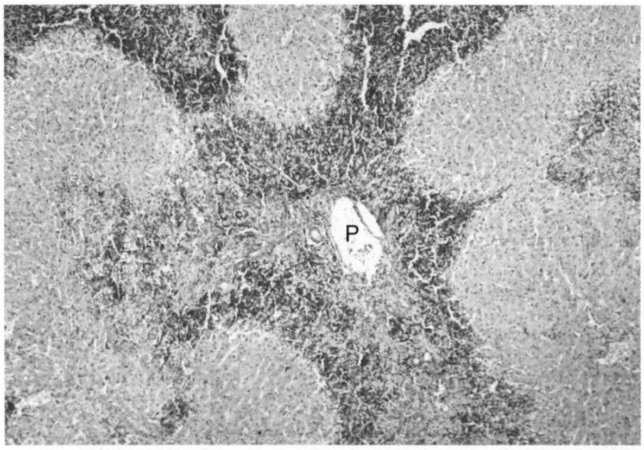

Figure 8-18 **Periportal Necrosis, Zonal Hepatocellular Injury, Liver, Horse.** Periportal (or zone 1) necrosis is an uncommon pattern of hepatocellular injury. Hepatocytes surrounding the portal tracts *(P)* are affected. H&E stain. (Courtesy Dr. M.D. McGavin, College of Veterinary Medicine, University of Tennessee.)

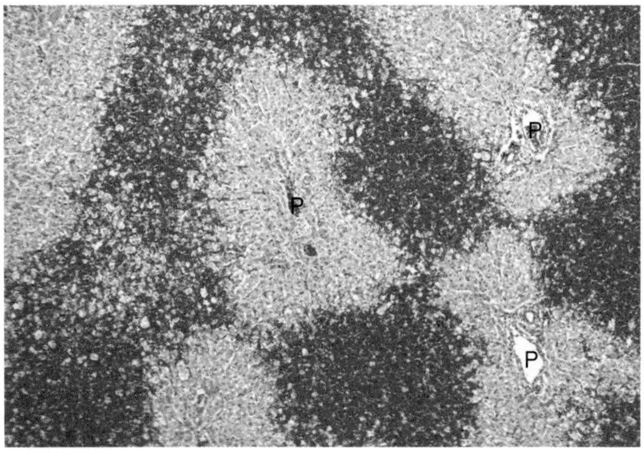

Figure 8-19 **Bridging Necrosis, Zonal Hepatocellular Injury, Liver.** Bridging necrosis refers to a pattern characterized by connection of areas of necrosis between different lobules. Three patterns of bridging necrosis are recognized: central to central, as seen here; portal to portal; and central to portal. *P*, Portal area. H&E stain. (Courtesy Dr. M.D. McGavin, College of Veterinary Medicine, University of Tennessee.)

Periportal Degeneration and/or Necrosis. Periportal degeneration and necrosis are also uncommon but may occur following exposure to toxins, such as phosphorus, that do not require metabolism by mixed function oxidases (most active in the centrilobular hepatocytes) to cause injury (Fig. 8-18). Some of these compounds may be metabolized to injurious intermediates by cytoplasmic enzymes found in periportal hepatocytes. Alternatively, some of these toxins may not require metabolism and produce hepatocyte injury in the first hepatocytes that they encounter as they flow from the portal areas.

Bridging Necrosis. Bridging necrosis is the result of confluence of areas of necrosis. Bridging may link centrilobular areas (central bridging) or centrilobular areas to periportal areas (Fig. 8-19).

Massive Necrosis. Massive necrosis is not necessarily, as the name might be taken to imply, necrosis of the entire liver but, rather, the term describes necrosis of an entire hepatic lobule or contiguous lobules (Fig. 8-20, *A*). All hepatocytes within affected lobules are necrotic. The gross appearance of the liver varies with the maturity of the lesion. If, in acute cases, the majority of the parenchyma is affected, the liver may initially be modestly increased in size with a smooth external surface and dark parenchyma because of extensive congestion. At first, necrotic hepatocytes lyse and the residual stroma becomes condensed. Regeneration does not occur as a rule because virtually all hepatocytes in the lobule are affected. Microscopically, affected areas consist of blood-filled spaces within a connective tissue stroma devoid of hepatocytes (see Fig. 8-20, *B*). Later in the course of the process, stellate cells or other ECM-producing cells from the portal and centrilobular areas that may survive or migrate to the site of injury contribute new collagen (collagen I, in particular). The final result is collapse of the lobule and replacement of the lost hepatic parenchyma with a scar consisting of condensed stroma, including variable amounts and types of collagen. Grossly the liver may be smaller than normal with a wrinkled capsule.

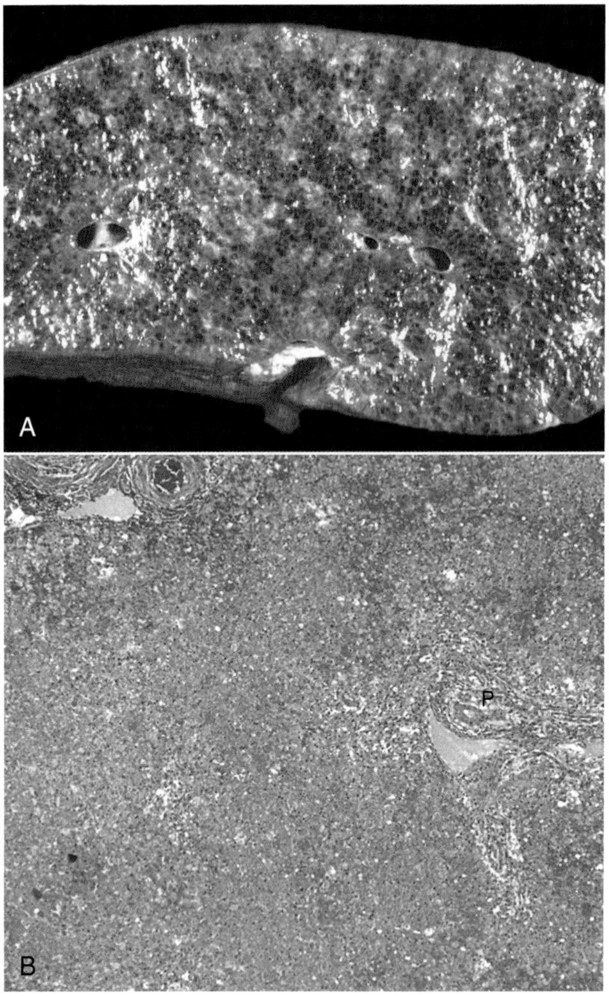

Figure 8-20 Massive Necrosis, Liver. A, Pig, cut surface. Massive necrosis refers to a pattern of necrosis that involves entire hepatic lobules, as shown here. **B,** Dog. The entire population of hepatocytes within many lobules have undergone necrosis. *P,* Portal area. H&E stain. (**A** courtesy Dr. D. Cho, College of Veterinary Medicine, Louisiana State University; and Noah's Arkive, College of Veterinary Medicine, The University of Georgia. **B** courtesy Dr. J.M. Cullen, College of Veterinary Medicine, North Carolina State University.)

Partial involvement of the liver is characterized by depressed areas of parenchymal necrosis and vascular congestion scattered throughout the organ.

Disturbances of Bile Flow and Icterus

Disturbance of flow of all of the constituents of bile is termed *cholestasis*, whereas *hyperbilirubinemia* refers specifically to an increased concentration of conjugated or unconjugated bilirubin in blood. For practical purposes, these processes can be considered together. Cholestasis can be divided into two types: intrahepatic and extrahepatic. Intrahepatic cholestasis can result from (1) a wide spectrum of liver injury affecting the ability of hepatocytes to metabolize and excrete bile; (2) hemolysis, which produces an abundance of bilirubin for excretion and diminishes the supply of oxygen for hepatocyte metabolism (also termed *prehepatic hyperbilirubinemia,* discussed later); or (3) inherited abnormalities of bile synthesis that inhibit the excretion of bile. Extrahepatic cholestasis is produced by obstruction of the extrahepatic bile ducts. It can occur by intraluminal obstruction (by calculi or possibly parasites) or extraluminal constriction by neoplasia or adjacent inflammation, often involving the pancreas. Cholestasis, if sufficiently severe, can produce a greenish brown discoloration to the liver (Fig. 8-21, *A*).

Histologically, acute intrahepatic cholestasis is characterized by formation of bile plugs within canaliculi (see Fig. 8-21, *B*). As intrahepatic cholestasis becomes more chronic, bile that has been released from hepatocytes is taken up by Kupffer cells and can be detected within their cytoplasm. Acute extrahepatic obstruction is characterized by edema of the portal areas, a mild neutrophilic inflammatory cell infiltrate, and a proliferative reaction by the biliary epithelium of the bile ducts. In chronic extrahepatic biliary obstruction, portal areas are enlarged by deposition of fibrosis, and there is a prominent laminar, circumferential fibrosis of bile ducts. Biliary hyperplasia characterized by proliferation of small-caliber bile ducts is often prominent (Fig. 8-22). Pigmented macrophages, containing bile, and mixed inflammatory infiltrates are also present. In severe cases, bridging fibrosis connecting portal tracts may develop.

Complete biliary obstruction leads to maldigestion of fats due to the reduction in bile acids and a characteristic clay-colored stool termed *acholic feces* because of the lack of normal dark pigment, stercobilin, the bilirubin-derived pigment produced by bacterial metabolism (Fig. 8-23).

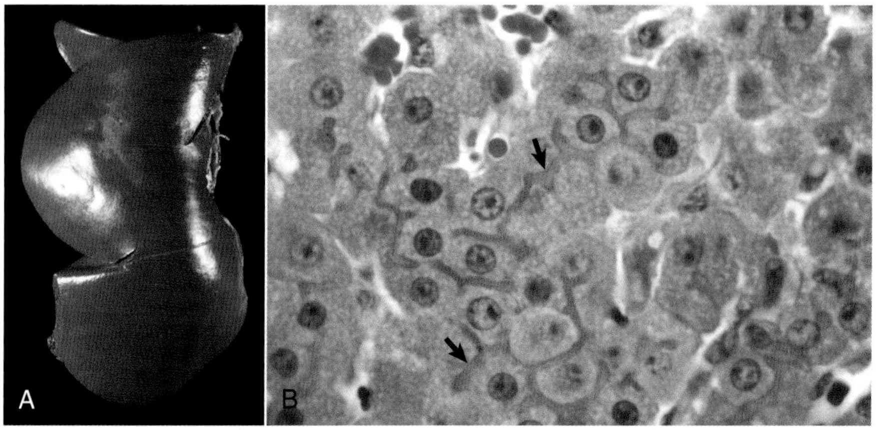

Figure 8-21 Hepatic Bilirubin Retention, Cholestasis, Liver. A, Cat. The liver is markedly yellowed by retained bilirubin. **B,** Canalicular bilirubin (*arrows*), acute hemolytic anemia, calf. Acute hemolysis caused by babesiosis has led to a dramatic increase in bilirubin production and distention of canaliculi, clearly demonstrating the location of canaliculi between hepatocytes. H&E stain. (**A** courtesy College of Veterinary Medicine, University of Illinois. **B** courtesy Dr. M.D. McGavin, College of Veterinary Medicine, University of Tennessee.)

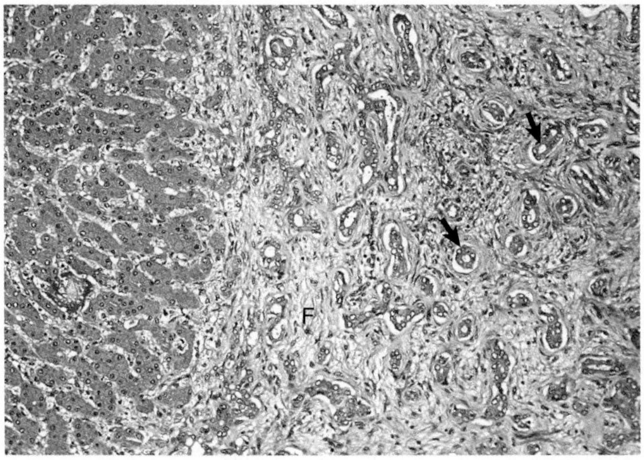

Figure 8-22 **Chronic Extrahepatic Cholestasis, Cholelithiasis, Liver, Horse.** There is reduplication of bile ducts *(arrows)* and extensive fibrosis *(F)* throughout the portal tract (biliary fibrosis) as a consequence of prolonged stasis and subsequent leakage of bile. H&E stain. (Courtesy Dr. J.M. Cullen, College of Veterinary Medicine, North Carolina State University.)

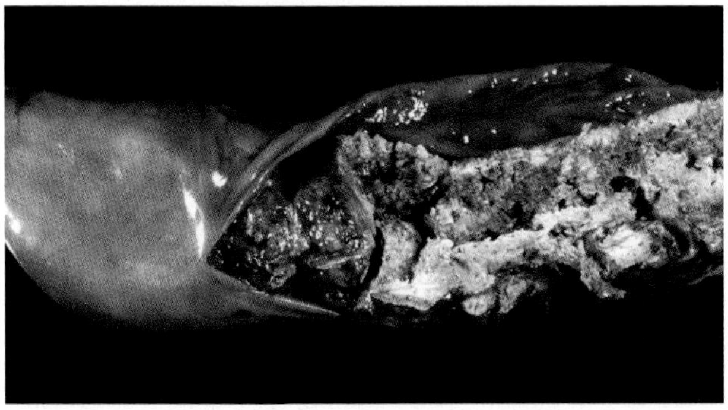

Figure 8-23 **Intrahepatic Biliary Obstruction, Intestine, Dog.** In cases of complete biliary obstruction, bile is unable to reach the intestine and as a result stool(s) lacks the characteristic dark color produced by bile pigments (white to pale gray feces). (Courtesy College of Veterinary Medicine, North Carolina State University.)

Icterus or *jaundice* is the yellowish discoloration of the tissues, particularly those with high elastic tissue content, including the sclera and aorta, due to an increase in bilirubin termed *hyperbilirubinemia* (Fig. 8-24). Before icterus develops, bilirubin concentrations usually must reach approximately 2 mg/dL. In most species, hyperbilirubinemia can occur once the concentration exceeds 0.5 mg/dL, and therefore the patient can be hyperbilirubinemic but not icteric. However, horses have a wider reference range for bilirubin and may not be hyperbilirubinemic at this concentration. Maximal accumulation of bilirubin in tissues takes approximately 2 days, and this explains why some animals with acute hepatic failure may have only slight icterus.

Hepatic dysfunction is not the only cause of hyperbilirubinemia and icterus. Prehepatic causes such as intravascular hemolysis can cause icterus. It is a common cause in ruminants and likely occurs more often than hepatic damage. Horses often manifest icterus with acute hepatic dysfunction or obstruction, but icterus may or may not occur in horses with chronic hepatic disease. Interestingly, "physiologic icterus" is also common in the horse, and horses deprived of feed for several days can become icteric because uptake of bilirubin from the plasma by hepatocytes is decreased. Icterus in carnivores occurs as a consequence of hemolysis, hepatic dysfunction, or biliary obstruction. Inherited metabolic abnormalities can also lead to abnormal concentrations of serum bilirubin, particularly in mutant

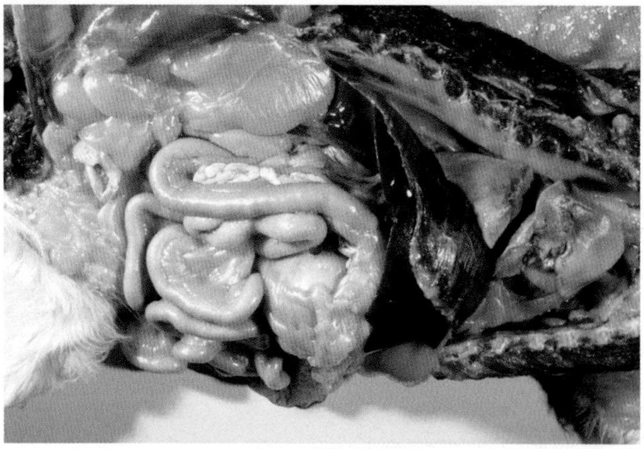

Figure 8-24 **Icterus, Dog.** Icterus and jaundice are terms that refer to the yellow discoloration of tissue by bilirubin, in this case evident in the fat and serosa. (Courtesy Dr. M.D. McGavin, College of Veterinary Medicine, University of Tennessee.)

sheep. In Southdown sheep with certain mutations (Gilbert syndrome), bile is ineffectively taken up from the circulation and a persistent unconjugated hyperbilirubinemia develops, although icterus is rarely apparent because there is sufficient excretion despite the mutation. Corriedale sheep may have a mutation that leads to deficient conjugated bilirubin excretion (Dubin-Johnson syndrome). Affected sheep have persistently elevated plasma bilirubin concentration, but jaundice is not apparent. Other compounds that are normally excreted through conjugation also accumulate in the liver of affected sheep. The livers are dark and discolored because of accumulated polymerized catecholamine metabolites that accumulate in lysosomes. These residues resemble lipofuscin histologically.

Biliary Hyperplasia and Ductular Reaction

Ductular reaction is the proliferation of bipotential progenitor cells found at the edges of the portal tract at the level of the cholangioles that can eventually mature into bile ducts and/or hepatocytes. These basophilic cells (also known as oval cells) initially form poorly defined tortuous small-caliber ducts and tubules that often lack a distinct lumen (Fig. 8-25). Ductular reaction can develop in injuries that inhibit proliferation of mature hepatocytes or bile duct epithelium, in cholestasis, and in regions of hypoxia. Consequently, ductular reaction can be a relatively nonspecific response to a variety of insults to the liver. Severe injury of hepatocytes or bile ducts often prompts the formation of prominent ductule formation in the hepatic parenchyma. In cholestasis, hyperplasia of bile ducts is a type of ductular reaction of portal and periportal ducts involving the proliferation of mature biliary epithelial cells (rather than progenitor cells). Histologically, ducts have variable calibers, often small, and may have piling up of the epithelium and a distorted shape (see Fig. 8-80). Biliary hyperplasia or ductular reaction can occur swiftly, particularly in young animals. These cells can mature as needed to replace hepatocytes or bile duct epithelium.

Regeneration

A characteristic feature of the liver is the ability to rapidly and efficiently regenerate lost hepatic mass. Experimentally, as much as two-thirds of the liver can be excised from a healthy animal without signs of hepatic dysfunction, and the liver mass is rapidly regenerated by compensatory hyperplasia. In addition to replication of hepatocytes, there is a wave of replication in bile duct epithelium, endothelium, and sinusoidal lining cells that is coordinated with hepatocyte replication.

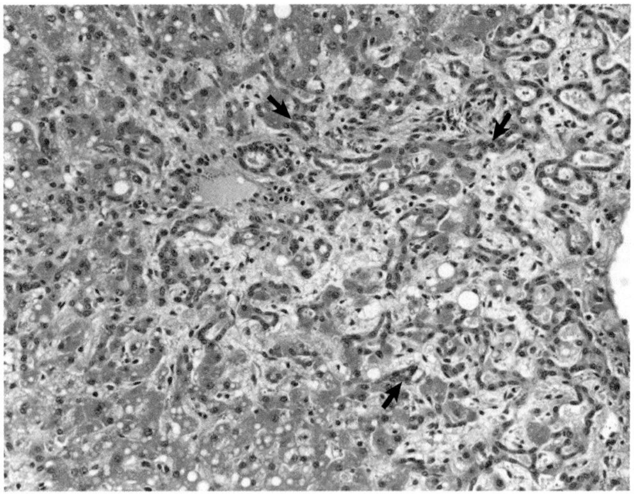

Figure 8-25 Ductular Reaction, Goat. Ductular reaction is characterized by the proliferation of basophilic progenitor cells *(arrows)* forming poorly defined small-caliber ducts that may lack a distinct lumen. H&E stain. (Courtesy Dr. J.M. Cullen, College of Veterinary Medicine, North Carolina State University.)

Regeneration usually takes place by replication of mature hepatocytes. In most circumstances, this leads to an increase in the size of existing lobules; however, recent data suggest that some new lobule formation can also occur through subdivision of existing lobules. After removal of liver lobes only, the remaining liver lobes persist, and no new lobe formation occurs.

Individual cell necrosis leads to local proliferation by regeneration of adjacent hepatocytes. Scattered foci of necrotic hepatocytes are quickly replaced through cell division of adjacent hepatocytes. Necrosis in the centrilobular area of the lobule leads to a wave of hepatocyte proliferation in the remaining areas of the lobule, particularly the periportal hepatocytes. In some circumstances, such as necrosis of nearly all hepatocytes or exposure to certain chemical toxicants that inhibit replication of mature hepatocytes, replacement of hepatocytes lost by necrosis occurs through the ductular reaction. This process is most prominent in experimental manipulations of laboratory rodents but also can be seen in naturally occurring cases of hepatotoxicity.

The body carefully orchestrates hepatic regeneration to replace lost hepatocyte mass along with bile ducts and vessels without producing excess liver. A variety of growth factors, including transforming growth factor-α (TGF-α) and hepatocyte growth factor (HGF), stimulate hepatocyte replication. Once normal hepatic mass has been established, macrophages release transforming growth factor-β (TGF-β), which, in concert with other less well characterized factors, stops hepatic parenchymal cell proliferation.

A single episode of extensive hepatic necrosis is usually followed by parenchymal regeneration without scarring, as long as the normal ECM (reticulin) scaffolding of the affected portion remains intact and has not collapsed. However, repetitive injury or massive necrosis can disrupt the normal lobular architecture, and there may be parenchymal collapse after removal of the dead hepatocytes and/or stromal collapse with repair by collagen synthesis (postnecrotic scarring) (Fig. 8-26). Even when necrosis of hepatocytes is continuous, the liver attempts to regenerate its functional mass. However, prolonged regenerative effort with damage to the normal ECM scaffolding of the liver often results in nodular proliferations of parenchyma, primarily in dogs, which architecturally distort the liver. Although regenerative nodules may reconstitute a proportionately large amount of hepatic mass, adequate function is rarely attained. Blood flow into the regenerative nodules and bile flow out of the nodules are abnormal, and as a result, sufficient hepatic function cannot be reestablished. As the nodules develop, the portal tract vessels and the central veins develop communications within the fibrous septa between nodules, which leads to vascular shunts between the portal vein and the central vein that bypass hepatocytes within the nodules.

Fibrosis

Fibrosis is one of the more common consequences of chronic liver injury. The pattern of fibrosis is frequently a useful indicator of the type of insult that produces the lesion. The significance of fibrosis depends on its effect on hepatic function and its reversibility. Despite the considerable regenerative capacity of the liver, hepatic fibrosis, when sufficiently severe, can be lethal.

In the normal liver, fibrillar collagens I and III are confined primarily to the connective tissue of the portal tracts and immediately around the terminal hepatic venule (central vein). Collagen IV is the most abundant collagen type in the reticulin framework of the sinusoids. A delicate scaffolding of collagen and other ECM components, which are produced by stellate cells, endothelial cells, and hepatocytes, make up the normal framework of the sinusoid. This stroma in the space of Disse supports the endothelial cells and maintains their spatial relationship to the hepatocytes.

Hepatic fibrosis is an overall increase in the ECM within the liver. In a fibrotic liver, there is an increase in the amount of ECM and a change in the types of collagen and their site of deposition. A severely fibrotic liver can contain up to six times as much collagen and proteoglycan as a normal liver. Hepatic fibrosis is characterized by an increase of fibrillar collagens, type I and type III, and nonfibrillar collagen type XVIII within the space of Disse, the portal areas, and the area surrounding the central veins. In addition to an increase in collagens, there is also a commensurate increase in the ECM components, proteoglycans, fibronectin, and hyaluronic acid.

The stellate cells (Ito cells) have a central role in hepatic fibrosis, although it should be noted that there are myofibroblastic cells with similar capabilities found within the connective tissue of the portal areas and connective tissue surrounding the central vein. In the normal liver, stellate cells occupy the space of Disse (a subendothelial position in the sinusoid) nestled between hepatocytes and around the circumference of the endothelium of the sinusoids. They have been likened to pericytes in other organs, such as the mesangial cells of the renal glomerulus. Hepatic stellate cells have been shown to have a role in the control of the diameter of the sinusoids and consequently the flow of blood through the sinusoids. Hepatic stellate cells are characterized by the presence of large lipid-containing vacuoles in their cytoplasm (see E-Fig. 8-3). The vacuoles are a primary storage site for retinyl esters, including vitamin A.

When the liver is injured, stellate cells go through a progressive phenotypic change from the typical lipid-storing cell to a cell with a myofibroblastic appearance (Fig. 8-27). When they are activated, they express α-smooth muscle actin, a marker usually found in muscle cells. Once these cells have switched to the myofibroblast phenotype, they begin synthesis of collagen types I, III, and IV. They also produce other ECM components, including fibronectin, laminin, and chondroitin sulfate proteoglycans. Hepatocytes synthesize few or no matrix proteins, and the large sum of matrix proteins is derived from the hepatic stellate cells. The type of hepatic injury does not seem to be important in the genesis of hepatic fibrosis. Chemical injury, biliary obstruction, and iron overload produce similar patterns of activation of hepatic stellate cells.

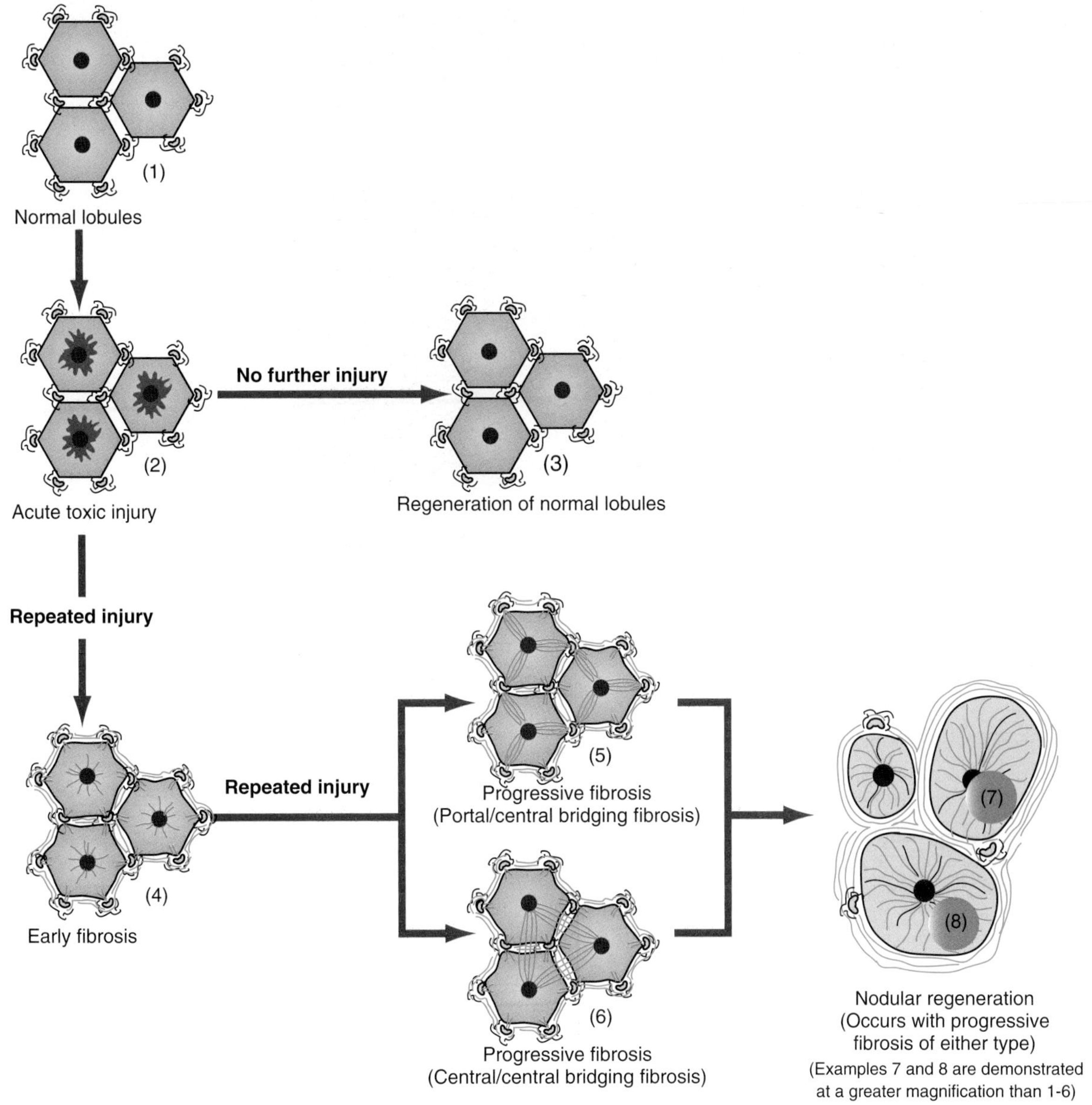

Figure 8-26 Effects of Hepatic Injury on the Development of Fibrosis. Acute hepatic centrilobular injury *(2)* that occurs only once usually resolves, and normal liver architecture returns *(1, 3)*. Repeated bouts of injury or severe injury can initiate hepatic fibrosis *(4)*. In the earliest stages, fibrosis may be reversible, but as fibrosis progresses, it reaches a point at which repair is not likely. Fibrosis often starts as fine branches of collagen deposition between portal areas or central areas or dissecting into the hepatic parenchyma *(5, 6)*. Over time, greater amounts of collagen and other extracellular matrix are deposited, and the lobular architecture becomes progressively distorted. In the end-stage liver, nodular regeneration and extensive, circumferential fibrosis are typical *(7, 8)*. The regenerative nodules shown here *(7, 8)* are at an early stage of regeneration. As shown in Fig. 8-27, they will regenerate to form nodules that will commonly exceed the size of normal hepatic lobules. These nodules will often compress *(7)* the central vein(s) of hepatic lobules within and adjacent to those from which they arose.

The site in which collagen is deposited in the liver has a significant impact on liver function. Perisinusoidal fibrosis can have a severe effect on hepatic function. In addition to collagen and ECM deposits, there is a loss of gaps in the endothelial cells and a loss of microvilli on the luminal surface of the hepatocytes. These changes have been termed *capillarization of the sinusoids* because the alterations in the sinusoids result in a vascular structure that more closely resembles a capillary than a sinusoid. The functional effect of this microanatomic change is profound. The ability of the liver to carry out its synthetic, catabolic, and excretory roles is severely compromised by the reduced exposure of hepatocytes to plasma.

Within the hepatic lobule, the site of fibrosis can be indicative of the type of insult. Most often, chronic toxic injury produces centrilobular (periacinar) fibrosis. This region is affected because the centrilobular hepatocytes are the site of metabolism for most drugs. Chronic passive hepatic congestion from long-standing right-sided heart failure can cause fibrosis in the centrilobular region as well. Periportal (centroacinar) fibrosis can result from chronic inflammatory conditions or a small group of toxicants that affect the periportal hepatocytes because they do not require metabolism by cytochrome P450 enzymes to produce an injurious metabolite. Fibrosis may be limited to individual lobules, but in more severe injuries, the areas of fibrosis can be more extensive. Bridging fibrosis, which is analogous to bridging necrosis, implies fibrosis that extends from one portal tract to another or from portal tracts to central veins. Bridging fibrosis is more likely to impair hepatic function than focal

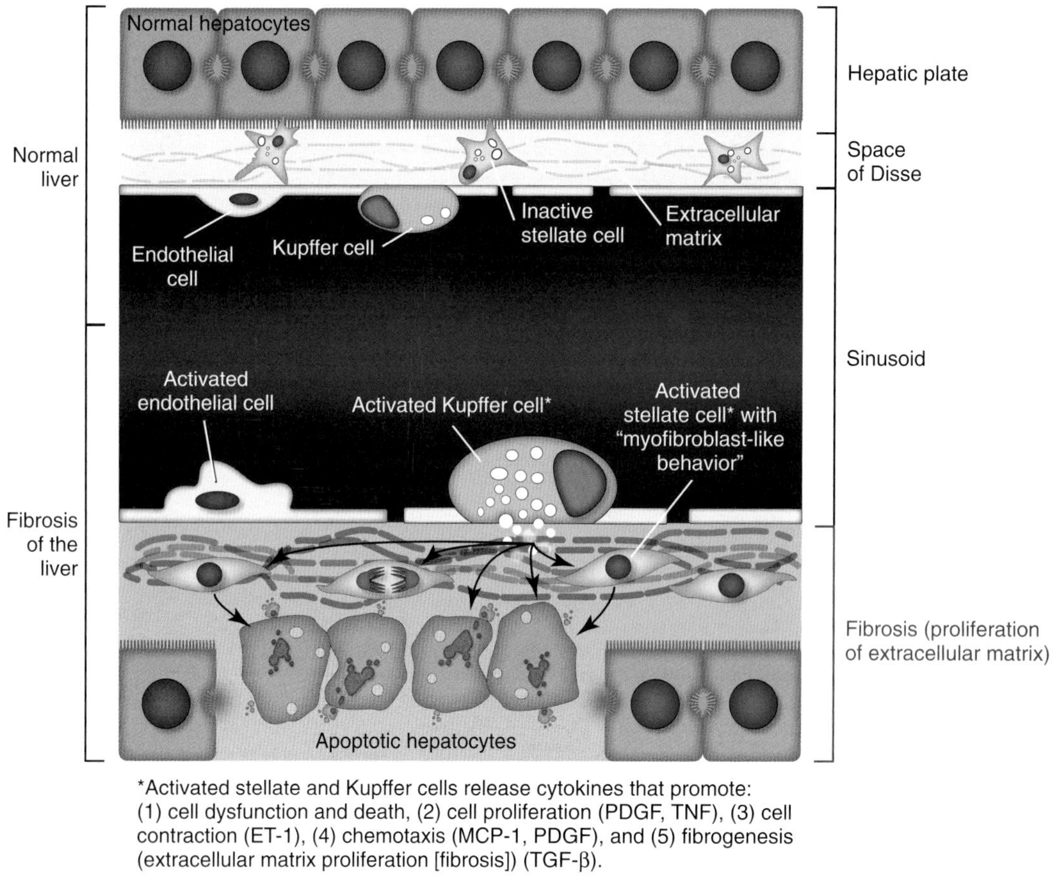

Figure 8-27 **Fibrotic Hepatic Sinusoid.** There are several events that occur during sinusoidal injury and fibrosis. The sinusoidal endothelial cells become activated and lose their fenestrations. Fibrosis of the liver *(bottom half of the diagram)* dramatically reduces contact between sinusoidal plasma and the hepatocytes. The space of Disse contains abundant collagen type I fibers that have been synthesized by activated hepatic stellate cells. The loss of endothelial fenestrations and the increased connective tissue beneath the endothelial cells leads to a condition termed *capillarization* of the sinusoids and is responsible for diminished hepatic function. Hepatic stellate cells have eliminated their lipid vacuoles and assumed a myofibroblastic morphology with cell extensions that often surround the endothelial cells (not shown here). Hepatocyte microvilli have been lost along the sinusoid, as shown on the apoptotic hepatocytes, and this loss begins with the onset of hepatocyte dysfunction and degeneration. Kupffer cells have also become activated and, together with activated stellate cells, release numerous proinflammatory cytokines. (Courtesy Dr. A.J. Van Wettere, School of Veterinary Medicine, Utah State University and Dr. J.F. Zachary, College of Veterinary Medicine, University of Illinois.)

forms of hepatic fibrosis, but all forms of hepatic fibrosis, if sufficiently severe, lead to impaired hepatic function. However, because of the enormous reserve capacity of the liver, fibrosis is usually quite extensive before there are clinical signs of hepatic dysfunction.

A single event of widespread hepatocellular necrosis is sometimes followed not by the usual regenerative response but, rather, by fibrosis and condensation of the preexisting connective tissue stroma that results in formation of bands of dense connective tissue. This process is referred to as *postnecrotic scarring*.

Other patterns of hepatic fibrosis can occur, including biliary fibrosis (centered on bile ducts in the portal triads), focal or multifocal hepatic fibrosis (randomly scattered throughout the hepatic parenchyma)—which is produced, for example, by migrating nematode larvae—and diffuse hepatic fibrosis (affects all regions of the lobule and is present throughout the liver). Different hepatic insults may produce different patterns of fibrosis, but when fibrosis is severe (end-stage liver disease), it frequently is impossible to determine either the cause or the initial pattern of fibrosis.

End-Stage Liver or Cirrhosis

The best accepted definition for cirrhosis was pronounced by the World Health Organization (WHO) in 1977 and is as follows: "a diffuse process characterized by fibrosis and the conversion of the normal liver architecture into structurally abnormal lobules" (Fig. 8-28). Because it is the final, irreversible result of any one of several different hepatic diseases, the term *end-stage liver* is appropriate, particularly because the term *cirrhosis* is neither descriptive nor precise in meaning and originally meant "tawny yellow." Another authority states that the hallmark is the total absence of any normal lobular architecture. The architecture of the liver is altered by loss of hepatic parenchyma, condensation of reticulin framework, and formation of tracts of fibrous connective tissue. Regeneration of hepatic tissue between fibrous bands leads to the formation of variably sized regenerative nodules (Fig. 8-29). The entire liver is thus distorted and consists of nodules of regenerating parenchyma separated by fibrous bands, which appear as depressions on the surface (see Fig. 8-28).

In addition to capillarization of the sinusoids, profound vascular abnormalities with serious consequences for the health of affected patients occur in this condition, including multiple abnormal vascular anastomoses between the portal vein and the systemic vasculature, known as acquired portosystemic shunts, as a consequence of the increased portal pressure. Also, venous shunts between the portal veins and the central veins and arteriovenous shunts between the hepatic arteries and the central veins can occur within the regenerative nodules or fibrous septa.

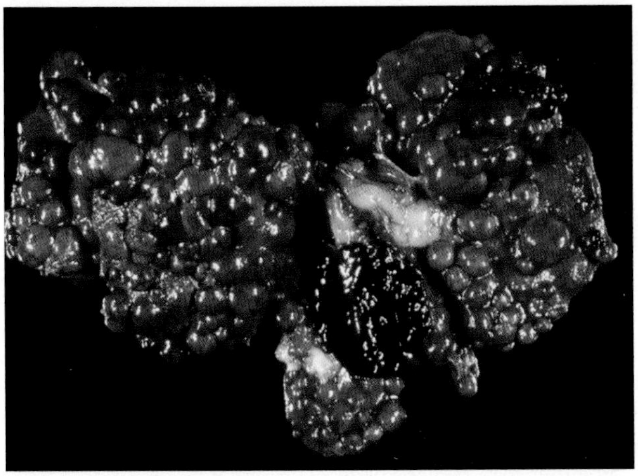

Figure 8-28 **End-Stage Liver (Cirrhosis), Dog.** End-stage liver from a dog that had received phenobarbital for many years. The liver is small, firm, and irregular with nodules of regenerative parenchyma separated by tracts of fibrous connective tissue. (Courtesy Dr. J.M. Cullen, College of Veterinary Medicine, North Carolina State University.)

The potential causes of an end-stage (cirrhotic) liver are numerous (Box 8-4). Chronic toxic insult results from the continued ingestion of any hepatotoxin (e.g., herbivores ingesting toxic plants, such as those that contain pyrrolizidine alkaloids, and the long-term administration of drugs with hepatotoxic potential, such as primidone for dogs). Chronic extrahepatic biliary obstruction and cholestasis leads to extensive fibrosis, which primarily affects the portal triads, but the fibrosis can eventually extend into the adjacent hepatic parenchyma. Chronic inflammation of the liver (hepatitis) or biliary tract (cholangitis) may lead to an end-stage liver. Although infection of the liver typically is focal or multifocal, diffuse hepatitis and subsequent fibrosis can occur in disease entities such as canine chronic hepatitis. Chronic passive hepatic congestion eventually leads to fibrosis near central veins, which is sometimes termed *cardiac sclerosis*, and can progress to cardiac cirrhosis, with fibrosis bridging between central veins. Abnormal storage or metabolism of metals, particularly copper, as occurs in Bedlington terriers and several other breeds, may produce chronic inflammation and an end-stage liver. Lobular dissecting hepatitis, a specific form of end-stage liver or cirrhosis, is usually seen in young dogs and is described further under specific diseases of dogs. A variety of more poorly defined disease entities can lead to progressive hepatocellular injury and hepatic fibrosis resulting in end-stage hepatic disease.

The end-stage liver obviously cannot perform its normal functions, so the clinical manifestations of hepatic failure invariably occur in affected animals. However, the cause of the hepatic damage that leads to the end-stage liver frequently cannot be determined at the time signs of hepatic failure are observed.

Hepatic Failure

The liver has considerable functional reserve and regenerative capacity. In healthy animals, more than two-thirds of the hepatic parenchyma can be removed without significant impairment of hepatic function, and normal hepatic mass can be regenerated in a matter of days. This process of tissue removal can be repeated several times, particularly in younger animals, and function is retained. In all species, clinical signs from hepatic derangement are similar, regardless of their cause. These clinical signs manifest, however, only when the liver's considerable reserve and regenerative capacity are depleted or when biliary outflow is obstructed. Only lesions that affect the majority of the hepatic parenchyma are likely to produce

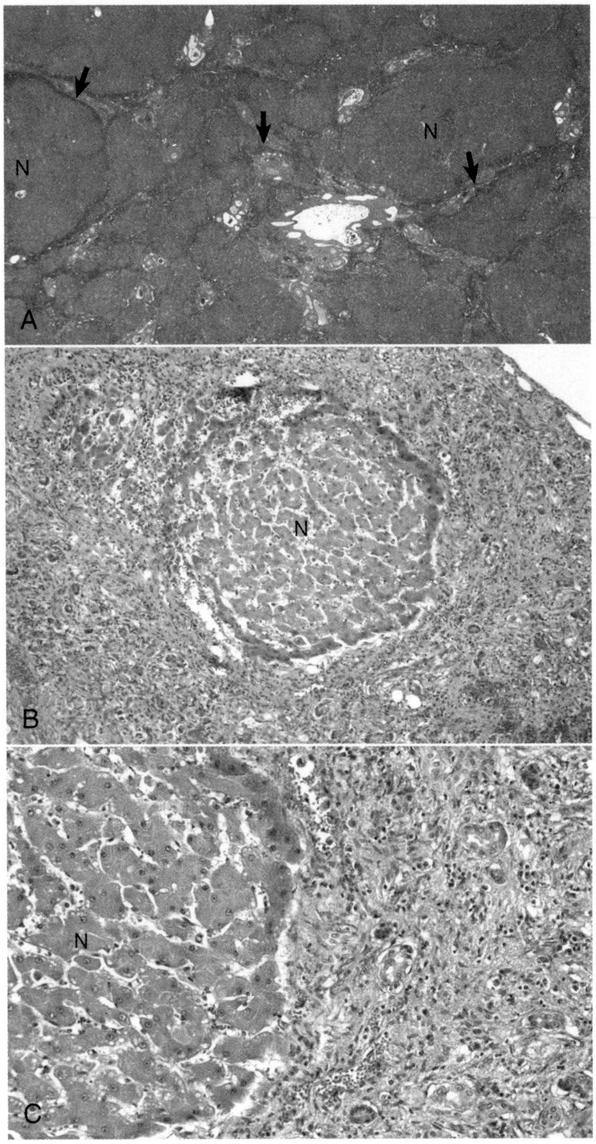

Figure 8-29 **End-Stage, Liver, Dog. A,** Histologic appearance of end-stage liver disease. Nodules of regenerative parenchyma *(N)* are separated by septa of collapsed reticulin and fibrous connective tissue *(arrows)*, which also contains numerous blood vessels and bile ducts. H&E stain. **B,** A single regenerative hepatic nodule *(N)* is surrounded by haphazardly arranged bands of fibrous connective tissue that contains numerous blood vessels and hypertrophied and hyperplastic bile ducts. H&E stain. **C,** Higher magnification of Fig. 8-29, *B*. Note the regenerative nodule *(N)*, bands of fibrous connective tissue, hyperplastic bile ducts, and mononuclear inflammatory cells. H&E stain. (**A** courtesy Dr. J.M. Cullen, College of Veterinary Medicine, North Carolina State University. **B** and **C** courtesy College of Veterinary Medicine, University of Illinois.)

Box 8-4 Causes of End-Stage Liver

- Chronic toxicity (therapeutic agents or naturally occurring toxins)
- Chronic cholangitis and/or obstruction
- Chronic congestion (right side heart failure)
- Inherited disorders of metal metabolism (copper or iron)
- Chronic hepatitis
- Idiopathic

the signs of hepatic failure because focal lesions rarely destroy sufficient parenchyma to deplete the liver's reserve. The term *hepatic failure* implies loss of adequate hepatic function as a consequence of either acute or chronic hepatic damage; however, all hepatic functions are not usually lost at the same time. The potential consequences of hepatic dysfunction are summarized in E-Box 8-1.

Hepatic Encephalopathy

Hepatic failure can result in a metabolic disorder of the central nervous system (CNS) termed *hepatic encephalopathy* (synonyms: hepatic coma or portosystemic encephalopathy). Elevated plasma ammonia concentration leading to abnormal neurotransmission in the CNS and the neuromuscular system is considered to be one of the main factors in the pathogenesis of hepatic encephalopathy.

Information on this topic is available at www.expertconsult.com.

Metabolic Disturbances of Hepatic Failure

Hepatic failure can be manifested by a variety of metabolic disturbances. The type and duration of the hepatic disorder may influence the nature of the metabolic perturbation.

Bleeding Tendencies

Information on this topic is available at www.expertconsult.com.

Hypoalbuminemia

Information on this topic is available at www.expertconsult.com.

Vascular and Hemodynamic Alterations of Hepatic Failure. Chronic hepatic injury typically is accompanied by extensive diffuse fibrosis of the liver, which increases resistance to portal blood flow through the liver. This resistance in turn elevates pressure within the portal vein (portal hypertension). With time, collateral vascular channels open to allow blood in the portal vein to bypass the abnormal liver (acquired portosystemic vascular anastomoses, which connect the portal vein and its tributaries to the systemic venous circulation). Shunting of portal vein blood directly to the central vein can also occur within the fibrous septa formed in the liver. In addition, the increased pressure within the hepatic vasculature causes transudation of fluid (modified transudate) into the peritoneal cavity to produce ascites in several species, except horses in most cases. Transudation of fluid into the peritoneal cavity can be enhanced by hypoalbuminemia because there is decreased colloid osmotic pressure in plasma. Hypoalbuminemia and reduced plasma colloid osmotic pressure can arise as a consequence of accelerated albumin loss into the lumen of the intestines as a result of portal hypertension or because of reduced hepatic synthesis of albumin and other plasma proteins by the diseased liver. Ascites associated with hepatic fibrosis in chronic liver disease (end-stage liver) or other causes of portal hypertension, such as right-sided heart failure, occur most commonly in the dog and cat, occasionally in sheep, and rarely in horses and cattle.

Cutaneous Manifestations of Hepatic Failure

Hepatocutaneous Syndrome (Necrolytic Migratory Erythema, Superficial Necrolytic Dermatitis)

Information on this topic, including E-Fig. 8-4, is available at www.expertconsult.com.

Cutaneous Manifestations of Hepatic Failure

Photosensitization

Information on this topic, including E-Fig. 8-5, is available at www.expertconsult.com.

Primary Photosensitization

Information on this topic is available at www.expertconsult.com.

Secondary Photosensitization

Information on this topic is available at www.expertconsult.com.

Congenital Porphyria

Information on this topic is available at www.expertconsult.com.

Immunologic Manifestations of Hepatic Failure. Chronic liver failure leads to an impairment of normal hepatic immune function. As a consequence, the affected patient frequently develops endotoxemia and an increased risk of systemic infection. For the most part, this impairment manifests as a reduction of blood filtration by Kupffer cells, which is primarily a result of shunting of portal blood rather than reduced phagocytic activity.

Aging

Studies have revealed that there are changes in liver structure and function with aging. The liver of aging animals has reduced weight, blood flow, regenerative ability, and ability to detoxify drugs or other toxicants. Microarray analysis of the liver of aged dogs has revealed increased genes related to inflammation and oxidative stress and reduced genes related to regeneration and xenobiotic metabolism. As a result of this, aged animals are more susceptible to a variety of hepatic insults, including inflammatory and toxic disorders.

Lipofuscin is an insoluble yellow-brown to dark brown pigment that is derived from the lipid component of membranous organelles. Amounts of lipofuscin present in the liver tend to increase with age, and it is particularly common in the centrilobular hepatocytes of aged cats. It is described in more detail under Metabolic Disturbances and Hepatic Accumulations.

Lipogranulomas are often observed in aged dogs and less commonly in other species. Microscopically, they present as discrete clusters of macrophages containing cytoplasmic lipid vacuoles and brown pigment (likely a mixture of lipofuscin, ceroid, and hemosiderin). Lipogranulomas tend to accumulate with age and hepatocellular turnover. They can also be seen in dogs with portosystemic shunts.

Hepatocellular nodular hyperplasia is common in the liver of aged dogs, often starting at approximately 6 years of age. Multiple hyperplastic nodules are frequently present. It is described in more detail in Proliferative Lesions of the Liver.

Portals of Entry/Pathways of Spread

The liver and biliary systems are exposed to infectious or otherwise injurious substances via three main routes: hematogenous, biliary, and direct penetration (Table 8-1). The liver receives the entire flow of the portal vein and as a consequence is bathed in potentially injurious microbes, which inhabit and penetrate the digestive system, and toxic substances that have been ingested or produced by the intestinal flora. The distribution of blood from the portal vein to the different lobes of the liver is most likely not uniform. So-called portal streaming refers to the concept that there is differential flow of portal blood from one segment of the digestive tract to particular lobes of the liver. This could explain why some lobes of the liver are more severely affected by toxins that are absorbed by the small intestine rather than the large intestine. Examples of this include the preponderance of injury to the left liver lobe of sheep that ingest the mycotoxin sporidesmin. Systemic infections or intoxications can also affect the liver through delivery of the blood from the hepatic artery. Neonates and fetal animals are also at risk from infections ascending the umbilical vein. Infectious agents, such as enteric

Table 8-1 Portals of Entry

	Liver	Biliary System	Exocrine Pancreas
DIRECT EXTENSION			
Penetrating trauma through the abdominal wall or rib cage	Yes	Yes	Yes
Penetrating trauma through the lumen of the gastrointestinal tract	Yes	Yes	Yes
HEMATOGENOUS			
Localization within the sinusoids via the portal vein, hepatic artery, or umbilical vein in neonates	Yes	No	No
Localization within Kupffer cells	Yes	No	No
Localization within capillary beds of the wall of the gallbladder or arteriolar rete of the biliary tree	No	Yes	No
Localization within capillary beds of the pancreatic parenchyma	No	No	Yes
RETROGRADE BILIARY TRANSPORT			
Ascending bacterial or parasitic infections gain access to the organ	Yes	Yes	No
RETROGRADE PANCREATIC DUCTULAR TRANSPORT			
Ascending bacterial or parasitic infections gain access to the organ	No	No	Yes

Table 8-2 Defense Mechanisms against Injury and Infectious Agents

	Liver	Biliary System	Exocrine Pancreas
STRUCTURAL AND FUNCTIONAL BARRIER			
Skin	Yes	Yes	Yes
Rib cage	Yes	Yes	Yes
Omentum (barrier that limits access of injurious material to the organ)	Yes	Yes	Yes
IMMUNOLOGIC RESPONSES			
Kupffer cells	Yes	No	No
Resident and migrating cells (recruited monocytes), which are part of the monocyte-macrophage system	Yes	Yes	Yes
Innate and adaptive immunologic responses (including secretory immunoglobulin A), which form the body's overall immune system	Yes	Yes	Yes
BIOCHEMICAL DEFENSES			
Enzyme inhibitors that reduce the risk of premature enzyme activation and tissue injury	No	No	Yes

bacteria and parasites, can also gain access to the liver through the biliary tree that is in direct connection with the duodenum. Finally, direct penetration of the body cavity or from the digestive tract (i.e., traumatic reticuloperitonitis or foreign bodies in the reticulum) can deliver infectious or traumatic insults.

Once an infectious or other injurious substance enters the liver, it can spread to additional hepatocytes or lobes of the liver via the sinusoids or biliary canaliculi, depending on the route of entry. Kupffer cells within the sinusoids are members of the monocyte-macrophage system and can work to clear the infectious agent or injurious substance. Agents or substances that are not cleared by the Kupffer cells can exit the liver through the hepatic veins and be carried to the heart and subsequently other tissues via the systemic circulation. Agents or substances can also spread through the biliary circulation and exit the liver via the common bile duct, entering the duodenum. The agent or substance can then be absorbed by the intestinal tract and enter the systemic circulation.

Defense Mechanisms/Barrier Systems

The liver is well defended from blood-borne injury by the Kupffer cells, resident macrophages that are distributed intermittently throughout the lumen of the sinusoids on the surface of endothelial cells (Table 8-2). They actively ingest and degrade bacteria and other organisms; senescent cells, such as erythrocytes; and particulate matter in the sinusoidal blood. They are very efficient and able to clear virtually all particulate matter in a single pass through the liver. Kupffer cells are particularly important in the removal of endotoxin from the portal blood.

The biliary tree, like the upper gastrointestinal tract, is defended from infection by secreted IgA as part of mucosal immunity. The majority of biliary IgA is synthesized by gastrointestinal plasma cells. The majority of released IgA is taken into lymph, and from there it enters the bloodstream. Hepatocytes in many species can transport IgA from blood across their cell membranes via a secretory component–mediated endocytosis. Subsequently, IgA molecules reach the bile by secretion into canaliculi. Concentrations of bile IgA are maintained by enterohepatic circulation. Within the biliary tree, IgA provides defense from infectious agents and clearance of harmful antigens as antibody-antigen complexes. In addition, the biliary tree is protected by the sphincter at the terminal end of the common bile duct, which provides a physical barrier to the ascent of enteric bacteria and the continuous flow of bile that assists in flushing bacteria out of the ducts.

The liver is protected from direct penetration by its anatomic location within the protection of the rib cage. The wall of the digestive tract also provides a certain degree of protection from penetration by ingested foreign bodies.

Gallbladder and Extrahepatic Bile Ducts

Structure

The structure of the gallbladder and major ducts of the biliary system is similar in all species (the gallbladder is absent in the horse, the rat, and the elephant). It consists of the adventitia, a muscular wall (tunica muscularis), and a mucosa lined by simple columnar epithelium. The epithelium and muscularis are separated only by the lamina propria because the gallbladder lacks a muscularis mucosa. Lobar ducts carry bile from different lobes of the liver; these ducts and the cystic duct from the gallbladder unite to form the common bile duct. The location of the opening of the common bile duct into the intestine differs somewhat among the domestic species; it is as little as 2 cm from the pylorus in the pig to as much as 70 cm from the pylorus in the cow.

Normal Function

The gallbladder stores and concentrates bile. When food containing fat enters the intestinal tract, it stimulates the secretion of cholecystokinin from the duodenum and jejunum. In response to cholecystokinin, the gallbladder contracts and releases its contents into the cystic duct, which then travels through the common bile duct and into the duodenum. The bile emulsifies fats and assists their absorption.

Considerable concentration (twentyfold to thirtyfold) of bile by active transport of sodium and anions across the gallbladder epithelial cells occurs in dogs and cats, whereas little concentration occurs in pigs and ruminants. The horse lacks a gallbladder and continuously releases bile into the duodenum.

Animals that have not eaten in 24 to 48 hours or that are starving or cachectic can have notably enlarged gallbladders (Fig. 8-30). The reason is that these animals lack the paracrine stimulus (i.e., cholecystokinin), and a number of other neural and hormonal stimuli, to contract the gallbladder and relax the sphincter at the termination of the common bile duct, which regulates flow of bile into the duodenum.

Dysfunction/Responses to Injury

When the entrance to the gallbladder or extrahepatic bile ducts become obstructed by a cholelith (gallstone), the gallbladder cannot release bile upon stimulation from cholecystokinin. Obstruction can lead to hyperbilirubinemia (discussed previously) and cholecystitis (inflammation of the gallbladder). If bile cannot be released from the gallbladder, maldigestion of fats will occur, leading to acholic feces (discussed previously). Larger choleliths can cause pressure necrosis and ulceration of the gallbladder mucosa or formation of saccular diverticula. In severe cases, the gallbladder can rupture. Rupture leads to leakage of bile into the peritoneal cavity, which is very irritating and can cause acute peritonitis.

Aging

There are no known age-related alterations of the gallbladder.

Portals of Entry/Pathways of Spread

Infectious agents or injurious substances can enter the gallbladder via reflux of intestinal bacteria into the cystic duct, particularly if there is dysfunction of or injury to the sphincter regulating bile flow into the intestine. Hematogenous entry from the hepatic circulation can also occur. Infectious agents or injurious substances can spread from the gallbladder through the venous circulation or through the bile into the intestine, where they can then be absorbed and distributed via the systemic circulation. As discussed previously, gallbladder rupture can lead to acute peritonitis due to leakage of irritating bile salts into the abdominal cavity.

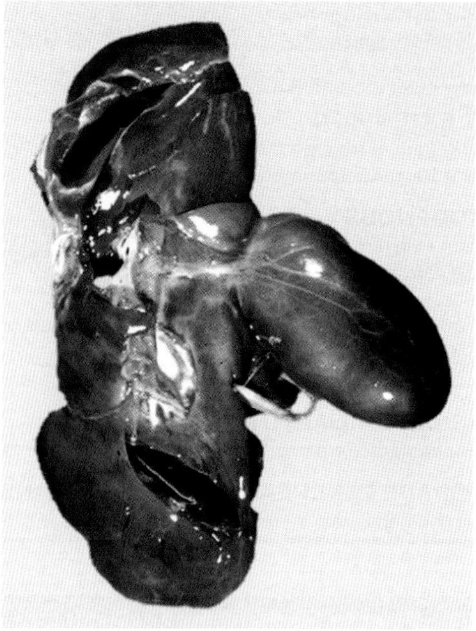

Figure 8-30 **Distended Gallbladder, Calf.** Note the distended gallbladder, which is common in all species after a prolonged period of fasting because there is no stimulus for emptying the gallbladder. Thus they are frequently seen at autopsy (syn: necropsy) of sick animals. (Courtesy Dr. J. King, College of Veterinary Medicine, Cornell University.)

Defense Mechanisms/Barrier Systems

The gallbladder, as the liver, is protected from direct penetration by its anatomic location within the protection of the rib cage. It is also somewhat physically protected by the surrounding liver lobes. In addition, the gallbladder is protected by the sphincter at the terminal end of the common bile duct, which provides a physical barrier to the ascent of intestinal bacteria and the continuous flow of bile that assists in flushing bacteria out of the ducts. Defense mechanisms for the gallbladder are similar to those listed for the hepatic biliary system (see Table 8-2).

Exocrine Pancreas

Structure

Development

The embryonic origin of the pancreas begins as a dorsal and a ventral bud of the duodenum. These buds fuse during embryogenesis to give rise to the entire pancreas. The major pancreatic duct arises from fusion of the ventral duct and the distal portion of the dorsal duct.

Macroscopic and Microscopic Structure

The pancreas is a lobulated, pink to gray, tubuloalveolar gland, a large portion of which is located in the mesentery immediately adjacent to the duodenum. The blood vessels, nerves, and lymph vessels that serve the pancreas are located within the delicate connective tissue septa that separate the lobules of pancreatic tissue. The pancreas contains both endocrine and exocrine elements, the endocrine portion being the islets of Langerhans. The exocrine portion constitutes the majority of the pancreas, up to 80% to 85% of the organ, and consists of acini composed of columnar to triangular secretory cells. The acinar cells have basally oriented nuclei and cytoplasm with a deeply basophilic basal margin and eosinophilic, granular zymogen granules occupying the apical portion. When the cells are appropriately signaled, the zymogen granules, containing the digestive enzymes of the pancreas, are released into the lumen of the acinus. The ductal system, in which secretions of the exocrine pancreas are conveyed to the intestinal tract, commences as fine radicals within acini and progresses to intralobular and interlobular ducts. These small ducts eventually drain into the main pancreatic duct or ducts. The arrangement of the major pancreatic ducts and how they empty into the duodenum varies among the domestic species. It is particularly variable in the dog, in which at least five different anatomic arrangements are recognized. In the cat, the major pancreatic duct enters the duodenum in close proximity to the common bile duct, and this relationship may predispose the cat to pancreatic injury.

Postmortem Examination

After opening the abdominal cavity, the pancreas and surrounding adipose tissue are evaluated and examined in situ for size, color changes, fat saponification, integrity, the presence of masses (e.g., granulomas and neoplasia), or other changes. Pancreatic ducts are also examined. Upon removal from the abdominal cavity, changes in color and consistency or presence of masses are evaluated and samples are collected for histology. If the presence of a small neoplasm such as an insulinoma is suspected but not detected at gross autopsy (syn: necropsy), the entire pancreas is formalin-fixed and later "bread sliced" to facilitate detection and sampling of small masses within the parenchyma. Pancreas samples for additional diagnostic investigation such as microbiology are collected as needed.

Autolysis of the pancreas is very rapid after death, particularly if the pancreas is traumatized. Postmortem release and activation of pancreatic proteolytic enzymes within the pancreas can hasten tissue breakdown. Thus autolysis may be advanced in the pancreas before it is evident in other organs. As autolysis progresses, the color of the gland may change from its normal pink to dark red or green. The metabolic activity of intestinal bacteria, which can easily gain access to the pancreas, can contribute to the discoloration of the pancreas through hemolysis and tissue decomposition.

Function

The exocrine pancreas produces secretions that contribute to digestion. The secretions contain a variety of enzymes that break down dietary lipids (lipase and phospholipase), proteins (trypsin and chymotrypsin), and carbohydrates (amylase). The secretions also contain electrolytes, which maintain the pH of the intestinal contents within a range that is optimal for enzymatic activity. Pancreatic enzymes act on the products of gastric digestion after they enter the duodenum. These enzymes often are released into secretions as inactive precursors (proenzymes), which helps prevent degradation of the pancreas by its own digestive enzymes. These are activated within the intestine. In addition, inhibitors of pancreatic enzymes are present in the pancreatic tissue. Secretion is controlled by neural stimulation regulated by the vagus nerve and by humoral factors. Secretin is one of the more important hormones involved in pancreatic secretion, and it stimulates water and bicarbonate secretion by duct cells. It is produced by neuroendocrine cells within the duodenal epithelium. The efflux of acid from the stomach and the presence of fatty acids in the duodenum stimulate its release. Cholecystokinin, another important hormone, stimulates the release of digestive enzymes from the acinar cells. It is produced by neuroendocrine cells of the duodenum in response to the presence of fatty acids, peptides, and amino acids.

Dysfunction/Responses to Injury

Dysfunction of the pancreas often manifests as pancreatitis. The pathogenesis of pancreatitis is discussed in detail later in this chapter (see Disorders of Domestic Animals—The Exocrine Pancreas). Pancreatic injury results in the release of pancreatic enzymes into the surrounding parenchyma, leading to further enzyme activation and autodigestion of the pancreatic tissue. One pancreatic enzyme in particular, trypsin, can activate the kinin system, complement, and clotting cascades, leading to overwhelming inflammation and necrosis. This outcome can eventually lead to disorders such as disseminated intravascular coagulopathy.

The pancreas possesses modest regenerative capacity after necrosis of exocrine pancreatic acinar cells, although more robust regeneration after partial pancreatectomy has been shown. Acinar cells can undergo replication in cases of limited injury, and precursor cells arise from cells within or adjacent to ductal epithelium in more severe injury. After acute pancreatic injury, there is usually little evidence of regeneration of the exocrine pancreas if there has been sufficient tissue destruction and fibrosis is the principal response. Proliferated ductules and atrophic exocrine pancreatic lobules are also found after significant pancreatic injury.

Aging

Reported age-related changes in the exocrine pancreas include decreased flow rates and decreased production of bicarbonate and pancreatic enzymes. However, studies have shown that these changes are not universally observed and do not progress continuously. They are also generally not associated with clinical signs.

Nodular hyperplasia of the exocrine pancreas is most common in older dogs and in cats, and it is occasionally seen in cattle. The lesion is of no clinical significance. It is described in more detail under Disorders of Domestic Animals—The Exocrine Pancreas.

Portals of Entry/Pathways of Spread

Portals of entry into the exocrine pancreas are listed in Table 8-1.

As discussed previously, damage to the pancreas results in activation of pancreatic enzymes and autodigestion of the pancreatic parenchyma. These activated enzymes, along with vasoactive peptides, inflammatory mediators, and embolic debris, can also be released into the systemic circulation, leading to inflammation and necrosis in other tissues such as the liver and lung and to systemic inflammatory response syndrome (SIRS). If pancreatitis is initiated by reflux of intestinal bacteria through the pancreatic duct(s), which is more common in human beings than in domestic animals, the infectious agent can also be released into systemic circulation, leading to septicemia.

Defense Mechanisms/Barrier Systems

Defense mechanisms for the exocrine pancreas are listed in Table 8-2. The pancreas is protected by the continuous flow of secretions into the duodenum, which prevents reflux of duodenal contents. The normal secretion of the pancreas contains trypsin, chymotrypsin, elastase, aminopeptidases, lipase, phospholipases, amylase, and nucleases. Trypsin is a critical enzyme because it has a role in the activation of several of the other pancreatic enzymes. Several mechanisms exist to protect the healthy pancreas from the effects of digestive enzymes it produces. Before secretion, enzymes are isolated from the acinar cell cytoplasm in membrane-bound zymogen granules. Most enzymes, except amylase and lipase, are secreted as proenzymes to prevent pancreatic injury. In particular, trypsin activation is tightly controlled because of its central role in activation of other enzymes. Consequently, the proenzyme trypsinogen is not normally activated until it enters the lumen of the duodenum through duodenal enteropeptidase. In addition, the chance of inappropriate trypsin activation in acinar cells or ducts of the pancreas is reduced by secretion of protective trypsin inhibitors. In circumstances in which trypsin or other enzymes are inappropriately activated, there are several other defenses in place. Acinar cells have an innate resistance to several of the digestive enzymes. Intrapancreatic release of active enzymes triggers the release of other enzymes that degrade the offending digestive enzymes, and lysosomal enzymes can degrade the zymogen granules when the pancreatic secretion is disturbed, reducing the burden of potentially injurious enzymes.

Disorders of Domestic Animals: The Liver and Intrahepatic Biliary System

Developmental Anomalies and Incidental Findings

Developmental anomalies of the liver occur in domestic animals, although most are of little consequence.

Congenital Biliary Cysts

Congenital biliary cysts are found most often within the livers of dogs, cats, and pigs, but presumably all domestic species can be affected. The cysts are usually an incidental finding and can be found in animals of any age. Grossly, the cysts can be single or multiple and are filled with clear fluid (Fig. 8-31). Histologically, cysts have a thin wall lined by a single layer of biliary epithelium. Congenital cysts must be distinguished from parasitic cysts, particularly cysticerci, because they also have a thin wall and are fluid-filled. The presence of the larval cestode within parasitic cysts assists in distinguishing the two structures.

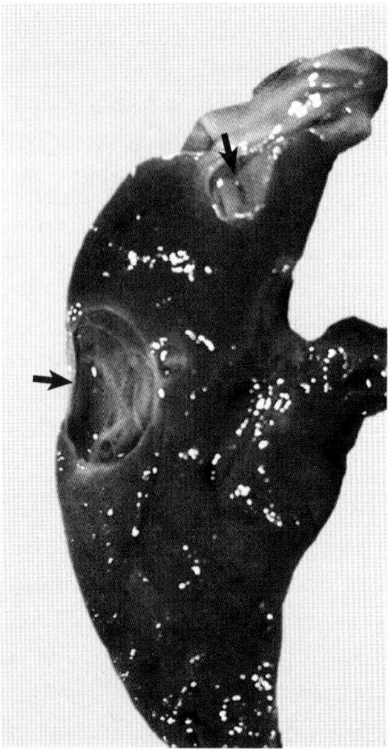

Figure 8-31 Biliary Cysts, Liver, Pig. Multiple biliary cysts *(arrows)* within the liver of a pig. Unilocular cysts replace a portion of the parenchyma in the affected portion of the liver. (Courtesy Dr. J. King, College of Veterinary Medicine, Cornell University.)

Multiple cysts that affect extensive areas of the liver occur in cats and occasionally dogs and are thought to represent developmental anomalies of the intrahepatic bile ducts. There are several types of these anomalies, which are collectively termed *ductal plate malformations*. Congenital polycystic disease, characterized by numerous epithelial-lined cysts in the liver, kidneys, and occasionally the pancreas, occurs in dogs, with Cairn terriers and West Highland white terriers predisposed; cats, with Persian cats believed to have a higher risk for the disorder; and goats and lambs. Affected animals can die of either liver or renal failure.

Different levels of the biliary tree can be affected, causing disorders of small-caliber ducts termed congenital hepatic fibrosis, intermediate-sized ducts causing polycystic liver disease, and large ducts causing Caroli syndrome.

Hepatic Displacement

Displacement of the liver into the thoracic cavity, called a *diaphragmatic hernia*, can occur when there is a defect in the diaphragm. A congenital malformation that leaves an opening in the diaphragm or a traumatic event that ruptures the diaphragm can cause this condition.

Tension Lipidosis (Steatosis)

Discrete, pale areas of parenchyma at the liver margins are common in cattle and horses (Fig. 8-32). These foci typically occur adjacent to the insertion of a ligament (serosal) attachment, and it is proposed that these attachments impede blood supply to the subjacent hepatic parenchyma by exerting tension on the capsule. Affected hepatocytes most probably accumulate fat within their cytoplasm (steatosis) as a consequence of hypoxia. The lesions are of no functional significance.

Capsular Fibrosis

Discrete fibrous tags or plaques are frequently present on the diaphragmatic surface of the liver and on the adjacent diaphragm of the horse (Fig. 8-33). Larval nematode migration tracts were originally believed to be the cause of this lesion, but this pathogenesis seems less likely in view of the widespread use of antiparasitic treatments and the continued prevalence of the lesion. Resolution of nonseptic peritonitis, possibly as a result of contact between the diaphragm and the adjacent liver capsule, has been proposed as the cause of these regions of capsular fibrosis.

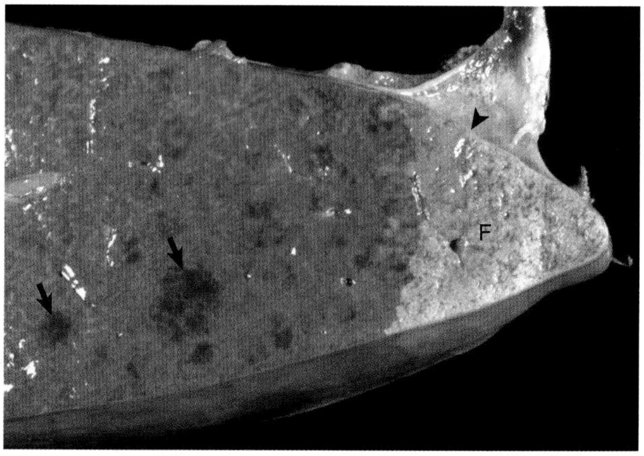

Figure 8-32 Tension Lipidosis (Steatosis), Liver, Cut Surface, Cow. Note the area of fatty infiltration *(F)*, the ligamentous attachment adjacent to the affected portion *(arrowhead)*, and the areas of telangiectasis *(arrows)*. (Courtesy College of Veterinary Medicine, North Carolina State University.)

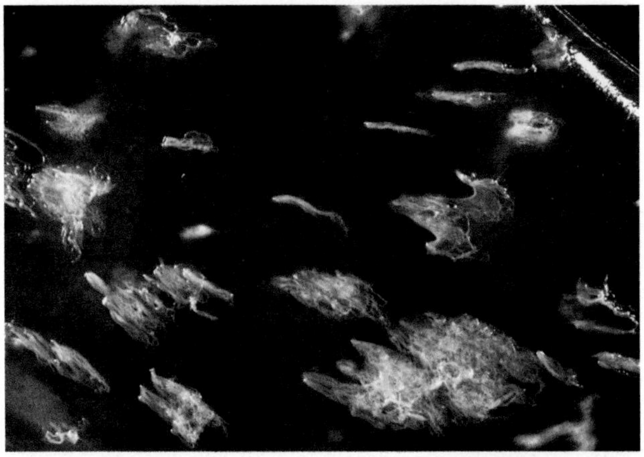

Figure 8-33 **Capsular Fibrosis, Liver, Horse.** Numerous white-gray fibrous tags are present on the diaphragmatic surface of the liver. The cause of these tags is not clear. (Courtesy College of Veterinary Medicine, North Carolina State University.)

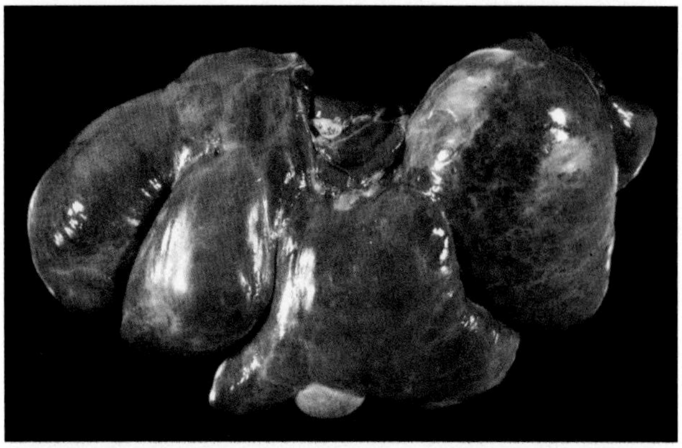

Figure 8-34 **Chronic Passive Congestion, Liver, Dog.** Chronic passive hepatic congestion in the liver of a dog with a heart base tumor that impeded venous return to the heart. Lobes of the liver are enlarged with rounded edges. (Courtesy College of Veterinary Medicine, North Carolina State University.)

Circulatory Disorders

Disturbances of Outflow

Passive Congestion (Acute and Chronic). Passive congestion of the liver can occur in any species and is almost always the consequence of cardiac dysfunction. Right-sided heart failure produces elevated pressure within the caudal vena cava that later involves the hepatic vein and its tributaries. Chronic passive congestion is particularly common in aged dogs and occurs secondary to right atrioventricular valve insufficiency resulting from valvular endocardiosis (myxomatous degeneration). Acute passive congestion, on the other hand, can occur as a consequence of acute right-sided heart failure, which has a wide variety of causes.

The appearance of the liver differs with the duration and severity of the congestion. Passive congestion initially causes distention of central veins and centrilobular sinusoids. Persistent centrilobular hypoxia leads to atrophy or loss of hepatocytes and eventually to centrilobular fibrosis. Fibrosis of the central vein (phlebosclerosis) may also occur.

Acute congestion of the liver produces slight enlargement of the organ, and blood flows freely from any cut surface. The intrinsic lobular pattern of the liver may be slightly more pronounced, particularly on the cut surface, because centrilobular areas are congested (dark red) in contrast to the more normal color of the remainder of the lobule.

Diffuse enlargement and rounded edges of liver lobes are the main features of chronic passive congestion (Fig. 8-34). Chronic passive congestion leads to persistent hypoxia in centrilobular areas, and because of oxygen and nutrient deprivation, the centrilobular hepatocytes atrophy, degenerate, or eventually may undergo necrosis. As a result, sinusoids in these areas are dilated and congested and grossly appear red, whereas periportal hepatocytes frequently undergo steatosis (fatty degeneration) because of relative hypoxia, thereby causing this area of the lobule to appear yellow. The result is accentuation of the lobular pattern of the liver, referred to as an *enhanced lobular* or *reticular pattern*. It is especially evident on the cut surface of the liver, and the enhanced lobular pattern that occurs with severe chronic passive congestion has been likened to the appearance of the cut surface of a nutmeg and is termed *nutmeg liver* (Fig. 8-35). This pattern is not unique to passive congestion, however, and is encountered with other processes such as zonal hepatic necrosis. In addition to an enhanced lobular pattern, chronic passive congestion is characterized by focal fibrous thickening of the capsule and, in severe cases, widespread hepatic fibrosis bridging between central veins (Fig. 8-36).

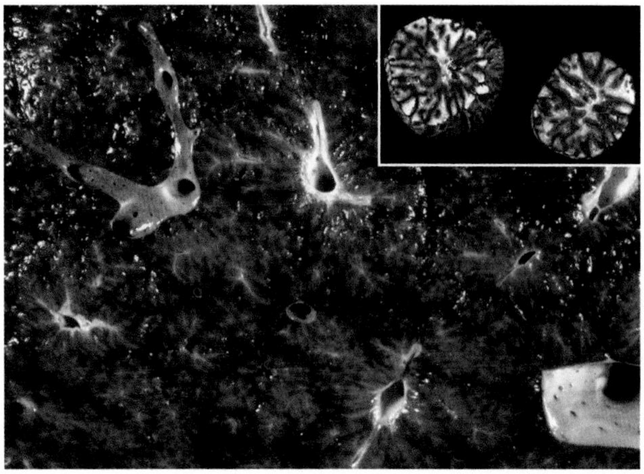

Figure 8-35 **Chronic Passive Congestion (Nutmeg Liver), Liver, Cut Surface, Cow.** The congestion in the centrilobular areas and the peripheral lipid accumulation give the liver a characteristic appearance that has been likened to that of the cut surface of a nutmeg, hence the term nutmeg liver. *Inset,* Cut surface of a nutmeg for comparison. (Figure courtesy Dr. D.A. Mosier, College of Veterinary Medicine, Kansas State University. Inset courtesy Dr. M.O. Howard, College of Veterinary Medicine, Iowa State University; and Noah's Arkive, College of Veterinary Medicine, The University of Georgia.)

Hepatic Veno-occlusive Disease. Intimal thickening and occlusion of the central vein by fibrous connective tissue characterize the distinctive lesions of this syndrome. The consequence is passive hepatic congestion and resultant hepatic injury, which may progress to hepatic failure and its associated constellation of signs. The lesion is not etiologically specific but can follow pyrrolizidine alkaloid or aflatoxin-induced hepatic injury. An extremely high incidence is recognized in captive exotic cats, such as cheetahs, possibly because of the ingestion of large amounts of vitamin A, although the mechanism for this lesion is not known.

Disturbances of Blood Flow into the Liver

Anemia. The centrilobular (periacinar) region of the lobule receives blood last; thus it is the least oxygenated, and the effects

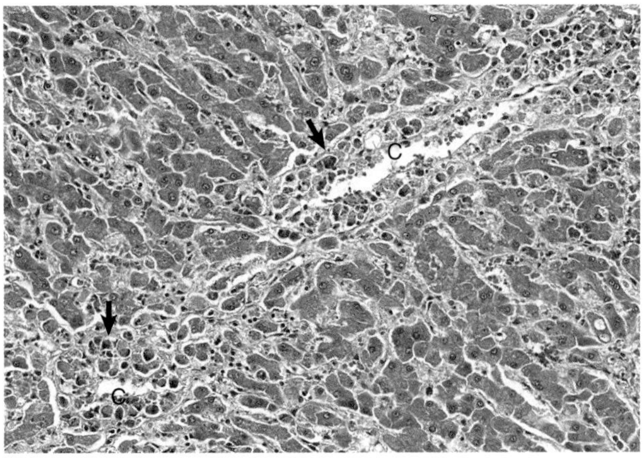

Figure 8-36 **Chronic Passive Congestion, Liver, Dog.** The liver is firm because of hepatic fibrosis that is most severe in centrilobular areas *(arrows)*. The central vein *(C)* is surrounded by a mild amount of connective tissue from which fine fibrous septa extend out into the lobule. Note the macrophages containing hemosiderin, the result of erythrocyte breakdown in this area as a result of chronic congestion. H&E stain. (Courtesy Dr. J.M. Cullen, College of Veterinary Medicine, North Carolina State University.)

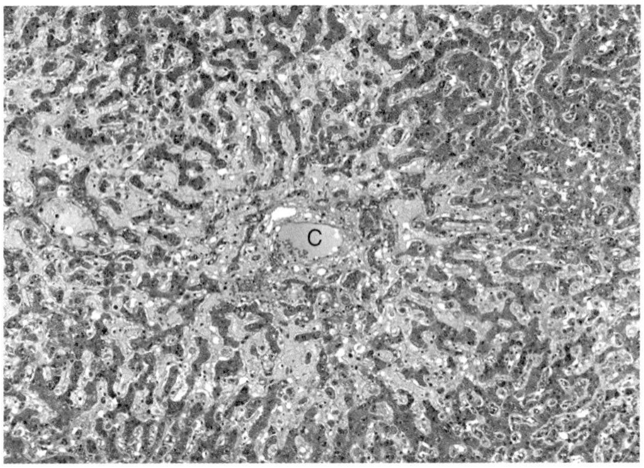

Figure 8-37 **Centrilobular Hepatocyte Atrophy, Liver, Dog.** In chronic anemia, centrilobular hepatocytes, which are the last hepatocytes in the lobule to receive oxygenated blood, become atrophic, and as a consequence, their sinusoids are more dilated. C, Central vein. H&E stain. (Courtesy Dr. J.M. Cullen, College of Veterinary Medicine, North Carolina State University.)

of hypoxia are usually manifested first in this area. Acute severe anemia, regardless of cause, can cause centrilobular or paracentral degeneration and even necrosis of hepatocytes. This typically occurs in severe anemias of precipitous onset. Chronic anemia can cause atrophy of centrilobular hepatocytes, which results in dilation and congestion of sinusoids (Fig. 8-37). Livers from animals with severe anemia, whether acute or chronic, typically have an enhanced lobular pattern that is evident on both the capsular and the cut surfaces of the organ.

Congenital Portosystemic Shunts. A congenital portosystemic shunt is an abnormal vascular channel that allows blood within the portal venous system to bypass the liver and to drain into the systemic circulation. A congenital shunt can be either intrahepatic or extrahepatic in location but is usually limited to a single relatively large-caliber vessel (Fig. 8-38, A). A variety of different shunts have been described. Typically, intrahepatic portosystemic

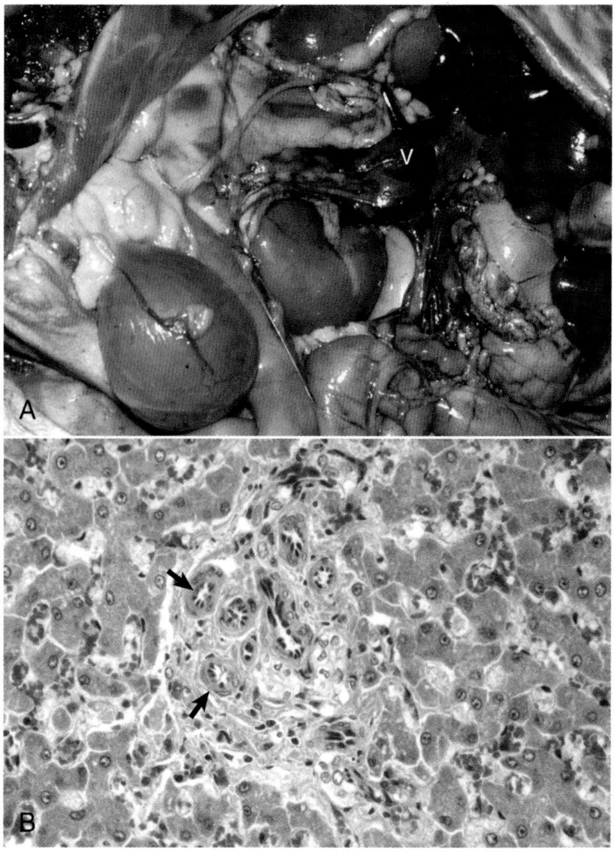

Figure 8-38 **Portosystemic Shunts, Liver, Dog. A,** A single anomalous vessel *(V)* that connects the portal circulation with the systemic circulation is the characteristic lesion of congenital portosystemic shunt. Note the small size but normal color of the liver (up under the rib cage). **B,** Congenital portosystemic shunt. Portal areas are abnormal because they lack a portal vein and contain numerous small-caliber arterioles *(arrows)*. H&E stain. (**A** courtesy Dr. J. Sagartz, College of Veterinary Medicine, The Ohio State University; and Noah's Arkive, College of Veterinary Medicine, The University of Georgia. **B** courtesy Dr. J.M. Cullen, College of Veterinary Medicine, North Carolina State University.)

shunts involve failure of closure of the ductus venosus at birth. The ductus venosus is a normal fetal vessel that conducts blood from the umbilical vein to the caudal vena cava. Intrahepatic shunts, such as the patent ductus venosus, are most often located in the left side of the liver and occur most commonly in large breed dogs. Extrahepatic congenital shunts, such as portal vein to caudal vena cava anastomoses and portal vein to azygous vein anastomoses, occur more often in small breeds of dogs and cats. Shunts have been described in several species but occur most commonly in the dog and cat. Affected animals are typically stunted and frequently develop signs of hepatic encephalopathy. The liver is small and may have a characteristic histologic appearance of small or absent portal veins within the portal tracts, reduplication of arterioles, and lobular atrophy (see Fig. 8-38, *B*). Microvesicular steatosis (lipidosis) and lipogranulomas can also be observed. Studies have shown that the histologic appearance of the liver is not a useful feature to assess prognosis in animals with congenital portosystemic shunts. The portal vein pressure is normal in congenital shunts, and ascites does not occur. Abnormal vascular anastomoses are often difficult to identify without benefit of antemortem imaging studies. Affected dogs frequently have abnormal plasma ammonia concentrations and, as a consequence, pass ammonium biurate crystals in their urine (Fig. 8-39). Note that the liver has a stereotypical response to

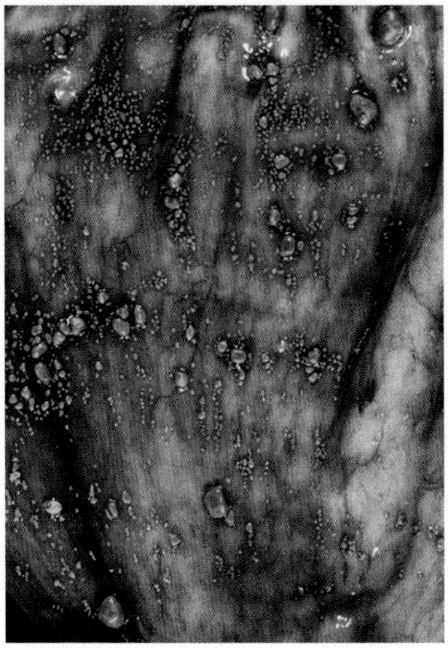

Figure 8-39 **Ammonium Biurate Crystals, Urinary Bladder, Dog.** The bladder contains ammonium biurate crystals. These green crystals can result from abnormal ammonia metabolism in dogs with portosystemic vascular anastomoses. (Courtesy College of Veterinary Medicine, North Carolina State University.)

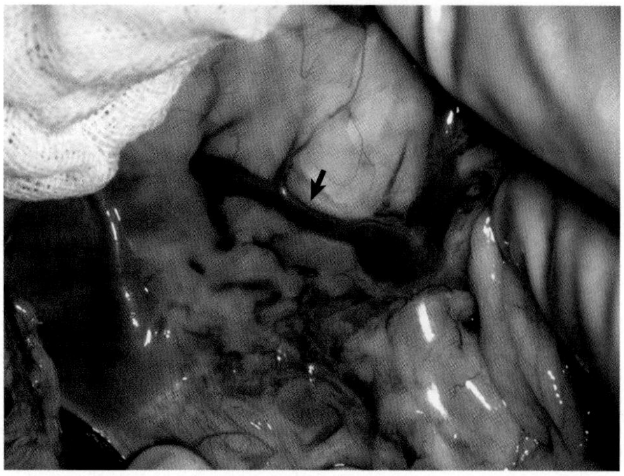

Figure 8-40 **Acquired Portosystemic Anastomoses, Abdomen, Dog.** Acquired portosystemic anastomoses secondary to portal hypertension (in this case as a consequence of chronic hepatitis in a dog). The numerous prominent veins *(arrow)* that are present over the surface of the kidney allow blood within the portal venous system to bypass the liver and directly enter the systemic circulation. (Courtesy Dr. L. Hardy, College of Veterinary Medicine, North Carolina State University.)

inadequate portal vein perfusion. Thus the histologic appearance of congenital portosystemic shunts and other vascular anomalies of the liver (discussed later) have considerable overlap. Clinical data, such as the presence or absence of shunt vessels and the determination of portal vein pressure, may be necessary to achieve a final diagnosis.

Portal Vein Thrombosis. Portal vein thrombosis refers to partial or total obstruction of blood flow into the liver caused by thrombosis within the extrahepatic portal venous system. It can lead to prehepatic portal hypertension (discussed next). Portal vein thrombosis is uncommon in all species, but it is reported most commonly in dogs. It can occur with diseases associated with hypercoagulability including liver disease, hyperadrenocorticism, protein-losing nephropathy, protein-losing enteropathy, neoplasia, and various immune-mediated and infectious diseases. It can also be induced by damage to the portal vein or by local inflammatory disorders, including pancreatitis.

Portal Hypertension. Increased pressure within the portal vein can arise from disturbances of venous blood flow in any of the following three sites:

- Prehepatic
- Intrahepatic
- Posthepatic

Prehepatic portal hypertension is relatively uncommon and occurs when blood flow through the portal vein is impaired before it enters the liver, such as occurs with portal vein thrombosis. Tumor emboli can also obstruct the portal vein. External compression by tumors or abscesses can restrict or obstruct portal vein flow as well. Portal vein hypoplasia (discussed later) affecting the extrahepatic segment of the portal vein is another cause.

Intrahepatic portal hypertension arises from increased resistance to blood flow to or within the sinusoids. Chronic liver disease that typically results in bridging collagenous septa, loss of normal lobular architecture, and regenerative nodule formation is the most common intrahepatic cause of portal hypertension. Sinusoidal fibrosis from diseases such as lobular dissecting hepatitis is another cause. Disorders such as veno-occlusive disease, amyloidosis, and schistosomiasis and other granulomatous disease processes can also produce intrahepatic portal hypertension. Arteriovenous fistulae (discussed later) within the hepatic parenchyma can also lead to intrahepatic portal hypertension.

Posthepatic causes of portal hypertension are uncommon and include any abnormalities that lead to increased resistance to venous outflow in the hepatic vein or adjacent vena cava. Partial or complete thrombosis of the hepatic veins (Budd-Chiari syndrome) or of the adjacent caudal vena cava are the most likely, although uncommon, causes of posthepatic portal hypertension. Congestive heart failure can also lead to portal hypertension.

Regardless of cause, persistent portal hypertension can lead to acquired portosystemic shunts with the exception of passive congestion, which rarely, if ever, results in the development of shunt vessels. These shunts are usually numerous and composed of distended thin-walled veins, which may connect the mesenteric veins and the caudal vena cava (Fig. 8-40). Ascites is common in conditions that develop acquired shunts because of the associated portal hypertension.

Vascular Anomalies that May Produce Portal Hypertension

Intrahepatic Arteriovenous Shunts (Anastomoses). Arteriovenous shunts, either acquired or congenital, occur in the dog and cat and are direct communications between the hepatic artery and branches of the portal vein. They may occur anywhere within the liver. Affected portions of the liver contain convoluted thick-walled arteries and distended portal vein branches. Shunting of blood from the arteries to the portal vein branches may lead to portal hypertension or reversal of the direction of portal blood flow, subsequent development of acquired portocaval shunts, and ascites. Clinical signs vary in intensity, most likely in relationship to the caliber of vessels that are affected, and are probably the result of the degree of portosystemic shunting of blood.

Portal Vein Hypoplasia (Microvascular Dysplasia, Noncirrhotic Portal Hypertension). Portal vein hypoplasia is a congenital vascular anomaly that occurs in dogs and occasionally in cats. Toy dog breeds, such as Yorkshire terriers and toy poodles, appear to be predisposed.

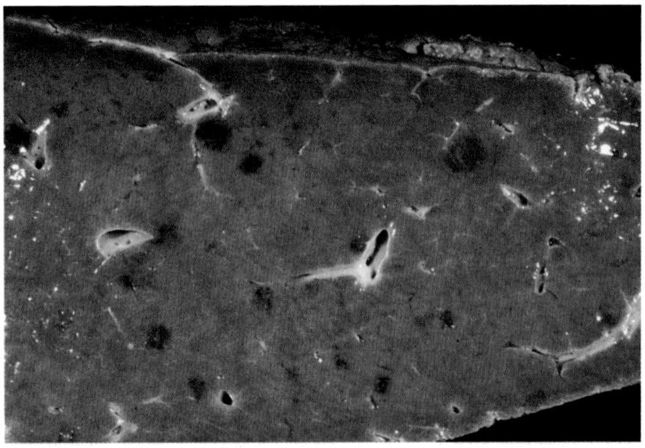

Figure 8-41 Telangiectasia, Liver, Cut Surface, Cow. Telangiectasia is a condition in which hepatic sinusoids become dilated and filled with blood. These lesions can be seen as red to dark red areas on the cut and capsular surface of the liver. (Courtesy Dr. M.D. McGavin, College of Veterinary Medicine, University of Tennessee.)

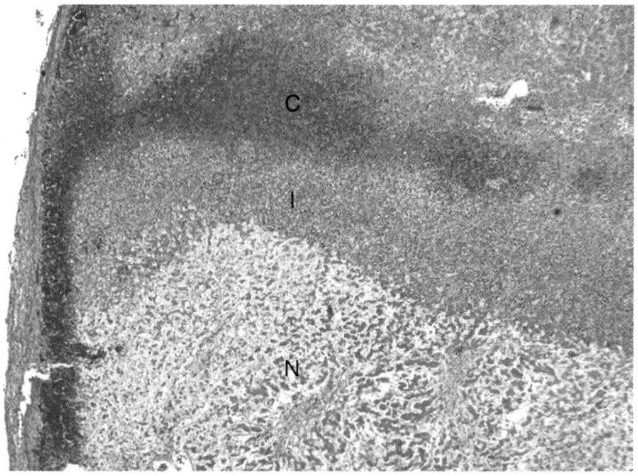

Figure 8-42 Hepatic Infarction, Liver, Dog. Hepatic infarction is uncommon and usually occurs at the margins of the liver where the terminal divisions of the blood supply are found. Infarction of the liver is characterized by a zone of coagulative necrosis *(N)* rimmed with inflammatory cells *(I)* and an outer zone of congestion *(C)* in the viable liver. H&E stain. (Courtesy Dr. J.M. Cullen, College of Veterinary Medicine, North Carolina State University.)

It is characterized by abnormally small extrahepatic or intrahepatic portal veins, which result in diminished hepatic perfusion by the portal vein blood flow and the potential for portal hypertension. Typically, affected animals have small livers and the typical histologic pattern of portal vein hypoperfusion: small or absent portal veins, proliferated hepatic arterioles (so-called reduplication), and hepatocyte atrophy. This disorder resembles portosystemic shunts histologically, but affected animals often have portal hypertension and resultant ascites. Portal fibrosis and biliary hyperplasia occur in approximately half of the cases. Because of the histologic similarities between portal vein hypoplasia and congenital portosystemic shunts, clinical data, such as imaging studies to determine the presence of a shunt vessel, are often required to make a final diagnosis from biopsy material.

Incidental Vascular Disorders

Telangiectasis. Telangiectasis is the notable dilation of sinusoids in areas where hepatocytes have been lost. Grossly, these areas appear as variably sized dark red-blue foci within the liver that vary from pinpoint to several centimeters in size (Fig. 8-41). Telangiectasis is particularly common in cattle and apparently is of no clinical significance. It also occurs in old cats, in which it can be mistaken for vascular tumors such as hemangioma or hemangiosarcoma. Histologically, there is ectasia of the sinusoidal space and a loss of hepatocytes. There is no evidence of inflammation or fibrosis associated with this lesion.

Infarction. Infarction of the liver occurs infrequently because of the organ's dual blood supply from the hepatic artery and portal vein. Infarcts are usually sharply delineated and may be either dark red when acute or pale as they age. They tend to occur at the margins of the liver, the terminal end of parenchymal perfusion, and can affect small wedges of only a few centimeters in length or larger portions of a lobe. The cut surface of infarcted liver tends to be dry and granular. Histologically, infarcted liver is characterized by a zone of coagulative necrosis bordered by a basophilic band of inflammatory cells and an outer band of hyperemia (Fig. 8-42). Torsion of individual lobes of the liver, which occurs infrequently, can result in vascular occlusion and infarction of the affected lobe.

Metabolic Disturbances and Hepatic Accumulations

Hepatocellular Steatosis (Lipidosis)

Lipids are normally transported to the liver from adipose tissue and the gastrointestinal tract in the form of either free fatty acids or chylomicrons, respectively. Within hepatocytes, free fatty acids can be esterified to triglycerides, converted to cholesterol or to phospholipids. Some oxidation of fatty acids to ketone bodies for energy production occurs within hepatocytes. Triglycerides can be complexed with apoproteins to form low-density lipoproteins, and these lipoproteins are released into the plasma as a readily available energy source for use by a variety of tissues. With the exception of ruminants, the liver also actively produces lipids from amino acids and glucose.

The presence of excessive lipid within the liver is termed *steatosis* or *lipidosis* (also known as fatty liver or fatty change) and occurs when the rate of triglyceride accumulation within hepatocytes exceeds either their rate of metabolic degradation or their release as lipoproteins. Hepatocellular steatosis is obviously not a specific disease entity but can occur as a sequel to a variety of perturbations of normal lipid metabolism. The potential mechanisms responsible for excessive accumulation of fat within the liver include the following (see also Hepatic Lipidosis in Chapter 1):

1. Excessive entry of fatty acids into the liver, which occurs as a consequence of excessive dietary intake of fat or increased mobilization of free fatty acids from adipose tissue because of increased demand (e.g., lactation, starvation, and endocrine abnormalities)
2. Excessive dietary intake of carbohydrates, resulting in the synthesis of increased amounts of fatty acids with formation of excessive triglycerides within hepatocytes
3. Abnormal hepatocyte function leading to accumulation of triglycerides within hepatocytes as a result of decreased energy for oxidation of fatty acids, as occurs with hypoxia or mitochondrial damage impairing oxidation of fatty acids
4. Increased esterification of fatty acids to triglycerides in response to increased concentrations of glucose and insulin, which stimulate the rate of triglyceride synthesis from glucose or from prolonged increases in dietary chylomicrons

5. Decreased apoprotein synthesis and subsequent decreased production and export of lipoprotein from hepatocytes
6. Impaired secretion of lipoprotein from the liver because of secretory defects produced by hepatotoxins or drugs

It must be stressed that the previous items are potential mechanisms (some being more significant than others, depending on the condition of the animal) and that more than one defect might occur in any given hepatic disorder. Regardless of cause, the gross appearance of the hepatocellular steatosis is highly characteristic. With progressive accumulation of lipid, the liver enlarges and becomes yellow (Fig. 8-43, *A*). In mild cases, lipids may only accumulate in specific portions of each lobule, such as centrilobular regions, thereby imparting an enhanced lobular pattern to the liver. In extreme cases, the entire liver is affected, and the organ may become considerably enlarged and have an extremely greasy texture. Histologically, hepatocellular lipid appears as a clear round vacuole. The vacuoles are clear because lipid is removed in routine processing of tissue for histologic review. Macrovesicular steatosis is most common and is characterized by large vacuoles that are larger than the nucleus and displace the nucleus of the hepatocyte (see Fig. 8-43, *B*). Microvesicular steatosis is characterized by multiple small, round, and clear vacuoles that do not displace the nucleus and can be associated with significant hepatocellular dysfunction. Frozen sections and special stains, such as Oil Red O, can be employed to identify lipid.

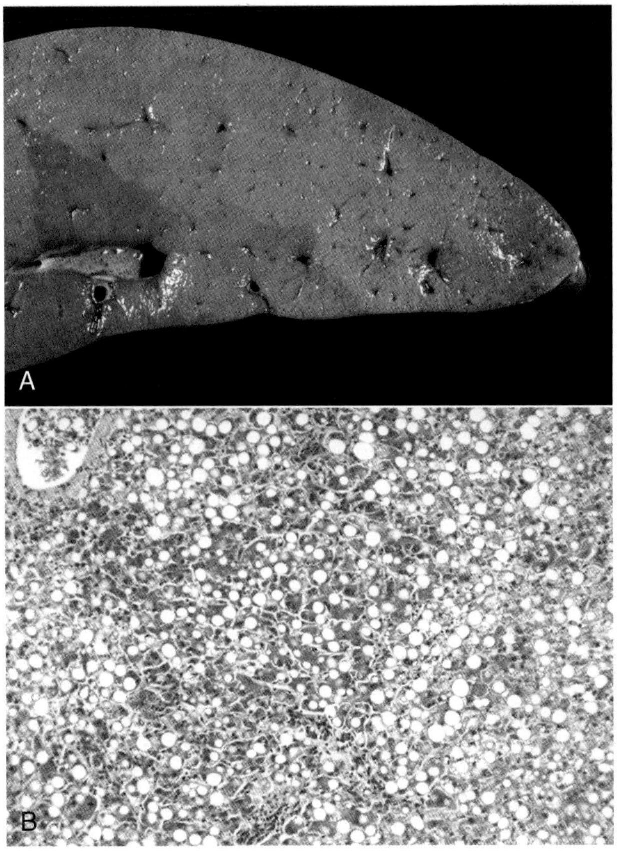

Figure 8-43 Fatty Liver Syndrome (Hepatic Steatosis). A, Cut surface, cow. The liver is swollen and yellow because of notable infiltration of lipid into hepatocytes. **B,** Steatosis or fatty degeneration, cat. Diffuse cytoplasmic accumulation of lipid is evident within the hepatocytes throughout the liver. H&E stain. (**A** courtesy Dr. M.D. McGavin, College of Veterinary Medicine, University of Tennessee. **B** courtesy Dr. J.M. Cullen, College of Veterinary Medicine, North Carolina State University.)

Specific causes and syndromes of hepatocellular steatosis in domestic animals include the following:

1. Dietary causes, including simple dietary excess in monogastric animals, such as a high-fat and/or high-cholesterol diet, or dietary deficiencies of cobalt and vitamin B_{12} in sheep and goats
2. Toxic and anoxic causes leading to sublethal (reversible) injury to hepatocytes
3. Ketosis, which is a metabolic disease that results from impaired metabolism of carbohydrate and volatile fatty acids. It is discussed in detail later in the chapter (see Disorders of Ruminants).
4. Bovine fatty liver syndrome, also known as *fatty liver disease*, which is mechanistically similar to ketosis and is especially common in ruminants with high energy demands. It is also discussed in detail later in the chapter (see Disorders of Ruminants).
5. Feline fatty liver syndrome, which is a distinct syndrome of idiopathic hepatocellular steatosis recognized in cats. It is discussed in detail later in the chapter (see Disorders of Cats).
6. Hepatocellular steatosis in ponies, miniatures horses, and donkeys, which is discussed in detail later in the chapter (see Disorders of Horses)
7. Endocrine disorders, such as diabetes mellitus and hypothyroidism, in a variety of species. In these cases, hepatocellular steatosis is obviously but one manifestation of abnormal metabolism. The accumulation of lipids in the liver in the diabetic animal is the result of increased fat mobilization and decreased use of lipids by injured hepatocytes.

Glycogen Accumulation

Glucose is normally stored within hepatocytes as glycogen and is often present in large amounts after feeding. Excessive hepatic accumulation of glycogen occurs with metabolic perturbations involving glucose regulation, including diabetes mellitus and the glycogen storage diseases. In these instances, hepatic involvement is just one manifestation of a systemic disease process. Excessive hepatic accumulation of glycogen is also observed in dogs secondary to excess glucocorticoids, which is explained further in the section Disorders of Dogs.

Grossly, glycogen accumulation in the liver can lead to variable degrees of pallor and swelling. Microscopically, hepatocytes are swollen with lacy vacuolated cytoplasm. Unlike lipid vacuoles, glycogen vacuoles are poorly defined and hepatocyte nuclei are not displaced to the periphery of the cell.

Lysosomal Storage Diseases

Vacuolation of hepatocytes and Kupffer cells can be observed in several types of lysosomal storage diseases. Lysosomal storage diseases often involve other tissues leading to vacuolation of neurons, other macrophages (particularly in the spleen), and/or other cells. Affected animals are usually young and have an abnormal pattern of growth and development.

Amyloidosis

Hepatic amyloidosis occurs in most species of domestic animals. Amyloidosis is not a single disease entity but, rather, a term used for various diseases that lead to the deposition of proteins that are composed of β-pleated sheets of nonbranching fibrils. Affected livers are enlarged, friable, and pale (Fig. 8-44, *A*). Histologically, hepatic amyloid appears as bright eosinophilic amorphous deposits that are usually found in the space of Disse along the sinusoids, but they can be found in the portal tracts and within blood vessel walls (see Fig. 8-44, *B*). Amyloid's physical properties are

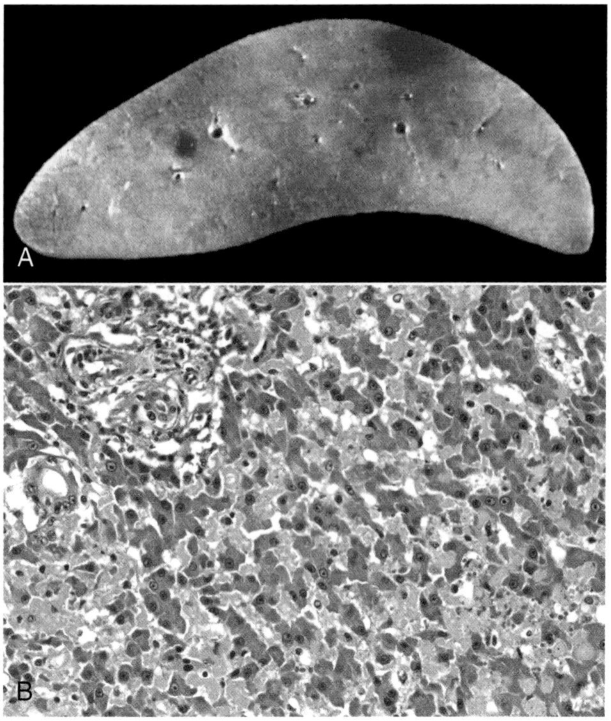

Figure 8-44 **Hepatic Amyloidosis, Liver. A,** Cut surface, duck. Hepatic amyloidosis has imparted a firm, waxy appearance and a pale brownish hue to the affected liver. **B,** Dog. The perisinusoidal spaces of Disse adjacent to the sinusoids are lined with a glassy eosinophilic (hyaline) material—amyloid. H&E stain. (**A** courtesy Drs. J. King and L. Roth, College of Veterinary Medicine, Cornell University. **B** courtesy Dr. J.M. Cullen, College of Veterinary Medicine, North Carolina State University.)

responsible for its characteristic apple green birefringence in Congo red–stained sections viewed under polarized light. As many as 15 distinct amyloid proteins have been identified, but the hepatic amyloid is usually derived from one of three types. In primary amyloidosis, the amyloid fibril is designated AL (amyloid light chain) and is composed of immunoglobulin light chains derived from the amino-terminal variable region of κ- and λ-light chains synthesized by plasma cell neoplasms. Secondary or reactive amyloidosis occurs as a consequence of prolonged inflammation such as chronic infection or tissue destruction. In secondary amyloidosis, by far the most common type to occur in veterinary medicine, the fibrils are composed of amyloid A (AA). The precursor protein is serum amyloid–associated (SAA) protein, an apolipoprotein that is an acute phase protein synthesized by the liver. Inherited or familial amyloidosis is uncommon in animals but occurs in Shar-Pei dogs and Abyssinian, Siamese, and other Oriental breeds of cats.

In severe cases of amyloidosis, affected animals may have clinical signs of either hepatic dysfunction or failure because the liver is more fragile; liver rupture and exsanguination may occur, especially in the horse. Frequently, amyloid is also deposited within the kidneys, particularly the glomeruli. Renal failure often occurs before signs of hepatic dysfunction are manifested.

Copper Accumulation

Copper toxicity is included as a metabolic disorder because hepatic injury in copper poisoning of domestic animals frequently is the result of progressive accumulation of copper within the liver. It occurs in domestic animals, especially sheep, in which storage of copper is poorly regulated. Also, disorders of copper metabolism have been described in various dog breeds and less commonly in cats.

Copper is an essential trace element of all cells, but even a modest excess of copper can be life-threatening because copper must be properly sequestered to prevent toxicosis. Normally, serum copper is bound to ceruloplasmin and the majority of hepatic copper is bound to metallothionein and stored in lysosomes. Excess copper, like excess iron, can lead to the production of reactive oxygen species that initiate destructive lipid peroxidation reactions that affect the mitochondria and other cellular membranes. In domestic animals, copper toxicosis usually occurs as a consequence of one of the following:

1. Simple dietary excess in ruminants, particularly sheep, and pigs occurring, for example, because of excessive dietary supplementation as an overcorrection for copper deficiency or from contamination of the pasture with copper from sprays or fertilizer. It also occurs in sheep that have access to copper-containing mineral blocks formulated for cattle.
2. Grazing animals on pastures with normal concentrations of copper but with inadequate concentrations of molybdenum, which antagonizes copper uptake.
3. Pasturing herbivores on fields with plants that contain hepatotoxic phytotoxins, usually pyrrolizidine alkaloids. *Heliotropium*, *Crotalaria*, and *Senecio* species are common examples of such plants (E-Table 8-1). Pyrrolizidine alkaloids prevent hepatocellular mitosis. This failure to replace necrotic hepatocytes leads to an ever-increasing copper load in surviving hepatocytes because these hepatocytes take up the copper released by the dying cells.
4. Metabolic disorders of copper metabolism, as occur in dogs. The disorder is best characterized in Bedlington terriers that have an autosomal recessive inheritance of a mutation in the COMMD1 gene that leads to impaired biliary excretion of copper, which results in progressive accumulation within the liver.

The consequences of excessive accumulation of copper within the liver of domestic animals are species-dependent. See specific species disease sections for more information.

Pigment Accumulation

Pigments are colored substances, some of which are normal cellular constituents, whereas others accumulate only in abnormal circumstances. They are covered in detail in Chapter 1.

Bile Pigments. Bile pigments may accumulate in excessive amounts as a consequence of either extrahepatic or intrahepatic cholestasis and typically produce icterus and green discoloration of the liver.

Hemosiderin. Hemosiderin is an iron-containing, golden-brown, granular pigment derived from ferritin, the initial iron-storage protein. As iron accumulates within the cell, aggregates of ferritin molecules form hemosiderin (E-Fig. 8-6). Most hemosiderin in Kupffer cells and other macrophages located in tissues throughout the body is derived from the breakdown of erythrocytes, whereas in health most hepatocellular hemosiderin is derived from iron present in transferrin and to a lesser extent hemoglobin. Hemosiderin forms in the liver when there is local or systemic excess of iron, such as when erythrocytic breakdown is excessive (e.g., hemolytic anemia), and within areas of hepatic necrosis. An excessive systemic load of iron that is characterized by abundant hemosiderin in a variety of tissues without impairment of organ function is called hemosiderosis. In contrast, hemochromatosis is an abnormally increased storage of iron within the body that can cause hepatic dysfunction. Notable accumulation of iron can produce a dark brown or even a black liver.

Lipofuscin. Lipofuscin is an insoluble pigment that is yellow-brown to dark brown and is derived from incomplete oxidation of lipids such as those in cell membranes (E-Fig. 8-7). Lipofuscin is progressively oxidized with time; thus it actually is a group of lipid pigments, all of which consist of polymers of lipid, phospholipids, and protein (and minimal carbohydrate in early forms). Amounts of lipofuscin present in the liver tend to increase with age.

Ceroid. Ceroid is a yellow-brown pigment similar to lipofuscin that is associated with peroxidation of fat deposits. It can be observed within fatty cysts that form in severe hepatocellular steatosis.

Melanin. Melanin is an endogenous pigment that is dark brown or black. Benign disorders of melanin pigmentation are usually designated as melanosis. Congenital melanosis of the liver occurs in pigs and ruminants and produces variably sized areas of discoloration of the liver. Acquired "melanosis" of sheep has been described in Australia and is associated with the ingestion of certain plants, but the pigment has not been proved to be melanin and may be derived from a component of the ingested plants.

Parasite Hematin. Liver flukes specifically produce very dark excreta that contain a mixture of iron and porphyrin. These excreta produce the characteristic discoloration that occurs in fascioliasis (*Fasciola hepatica*) and is especially pronounced in the migratory tracts produced by *Fascioloides magna* in bovine livers (see Fig. 8-61).

Infectious Diseases of the Liver

Viral Diseases

Herpesvirus Infections. Herpesvirus infections of the liver typically occur in neonates or fetuses. A variety of abortigenic herpesviruses are described, each animal species being affected by a specific virus. Examples of these viruses include the abortigenic equine herpesvirus (*equine herpesvirus 1*), infectious bovine rhinotracheitis virus (*bovine herpesvirus 1*), caprine herpesvirus, canine herpesvirus (*canine herpesvirus 1*), feline viral rhinotracheitis virus (*feline herpesvirus 1*), and pseudorabies virus (*suid herpesvirus 1*).

Infection can occur via several routes, including transplacental exposure, passage through the birth canal, contact with infected littermates, and contact with oronasal secretions from the dam. In neonates, initial infection often occurs in the oronasal epithelium where virus replication first takes place. After local replication, the virus enters the bloodstream via infected mononuclear phagocytic cells. Viremia leads to dissemination of the virus to a variety of organs, and viral infection is cytolytic.

The abortigenic herpesviruses characteristically induce multifocal, randomly distributed, small (<1 mm) areas of necrosis in several fetal organs, including the liver (Fig. 8-45, *A*). Similar lesions occasionally are present in neonates infected with herpesviruses.

Histologically, herpesvirus can produce multifocal hepatic necrosis with scant inflammation in fetuses and neonates (see Fig. 8-45, *B*). The liver is often affected, but foci of necrosis are more consistently present in the kidneys, lungs, and spleen. The virus most often affects neonates in the first 2 weeks of life and is most severe before they develop competent thermoregulation. Animals that are able to maintain a normal body temperature are less likely to be affected.

Other Viral Infections. Infectious canine hepatitis, Rift Valley fever, and Wesselsbron disease are discussed under species-specific disease sections later in the chapter.

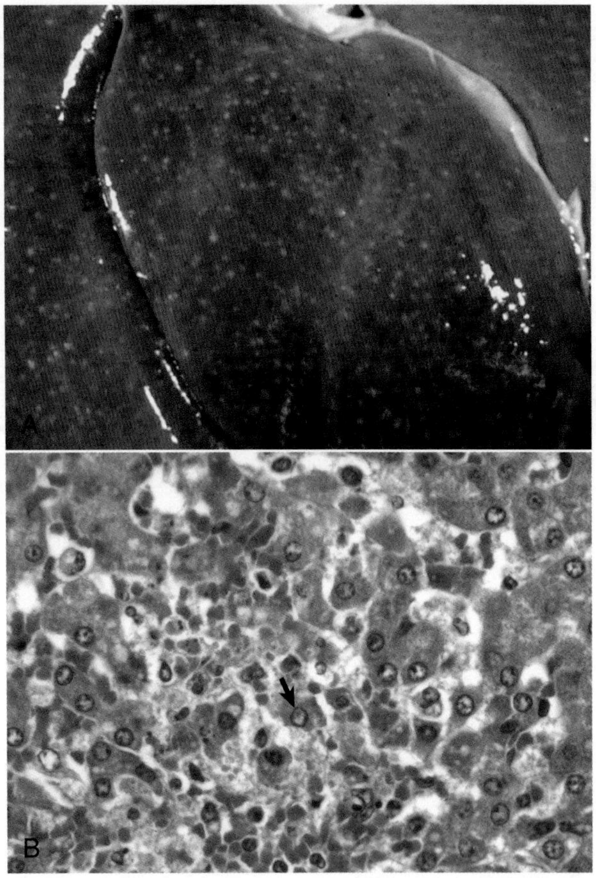

Figure 8-45 **Equine Herpesvirus Hepatitis, Hepatic Necrosis, Liver, Foal. A,** Note the randomly distributed gray-to-white foci of random hepatocellular necrosis caused by equine herpesvirus. **B,** Infection of hepatocytes with equine herpesvirus produces characteristic acidophilic intranuclear inclusions surrounded by a clear zone that separates them from the marginated chromatin (*arrow*). Note the individual cell necrosis. H&E stain. (**A** courtesy Drs. J. King and L. Roth, College of Veterinary Medicine, Cornell University. **B** courtesy Dr. J.M. Cullen, College of Veterinary Medicine, North Carolina State University.)

Certain viral diseases may involve the liver, but the hepatic involvement either does not occur invariably or it may be but one manifestation of a systemic process. Such diseases include feline infectious peritonitis (FIP) that is characterized by foci of pyogranulomatous vasculitis or perivascular accumulations of lymphocytes and plasma cells within multiple organs, sometimes including the liver. Subacute and chronic forms of equine infectious anemia are characterized by cellular accumulations, particularly lymphocytes, in sinusoids and the space of Disse. Systemic adenoviral infection of lambs, calves, and goat kids may produce multifocal areas of hepatocellular necrosis, cholangitis, and necrosis of biliary epithelium. *Porcine circovirus* type 2 injures hepatocytes and Kupffer cells and can cause mild to severe necrosis.

Bacterial Diseases

Liver Abscesses and Granulomas. Bacteria can reach the liver via a number of different routes and form abscesses (Figs. 8-46 to 8-48). Routes include the following:

- The portal vein
- The umbilical veins from umbilical infections in newborn animals
- The hepatic artery, as part of a generalized bacteremia
- Ascending infection of the biliary system
- Parasitic migration

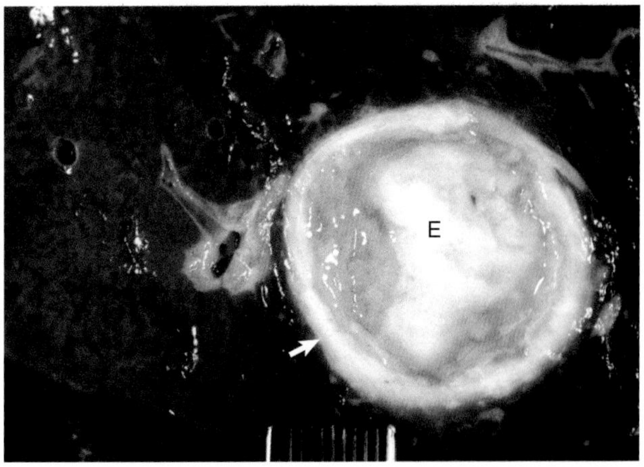

Figure 8-46 Chronic Hepatic Abscesses, *Corynebacterium Pseudotuberculosis*, Liver, Sheep. Note the thick fibrous capsule *(arrow)* and the characteristic pale caseous exudate *(E)* produced by *Corynebacterium pseudotuberculosis* in sheep. (Courtesy College of Veterinary Medicine, North Carolina State University.)

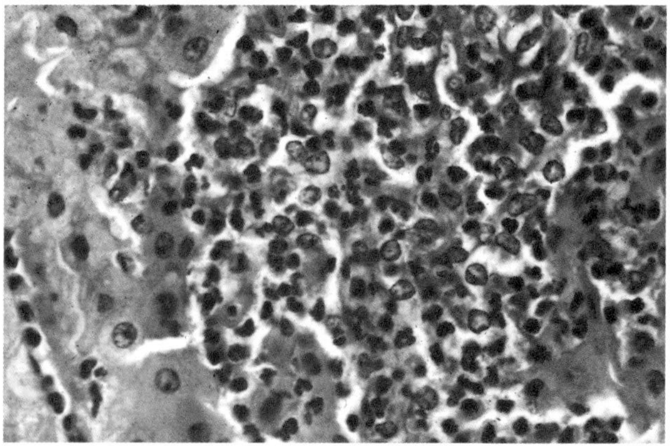

Figure 8-48 Hepatic Abscess, Liver, Cow. An abscess in the liver is similar to those in other tissues and consists of an infiltrate of neutrophils, degenerating neutrophils, and necrotic tissue debris. H&E stain. (Courtesy Dr. M.D. McGavin, College of Veterinary Medicine, University of Tennessee.)

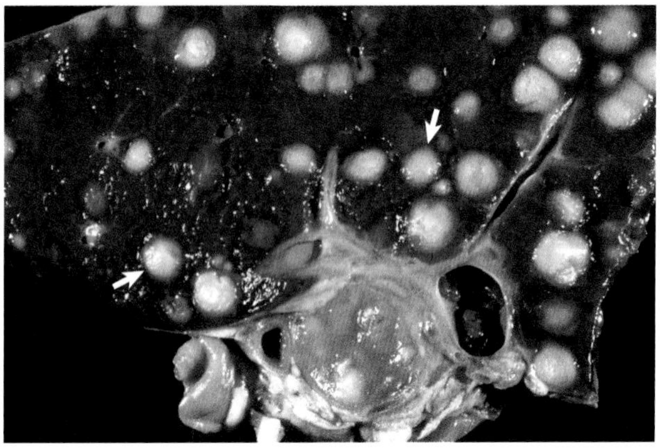

Figure 8-47 Hepatic Abscesses, *Rhodococcus Equi*, Liver, Goat. Disseminated hepatic abscesses *(arrows)* in a goat caused by *Rhodococcus equi*. This lesion is more commonly found in foals. (Courtesy Dr. P. Stromberg, College of Veterinary Medicine, The Ohio State University.)

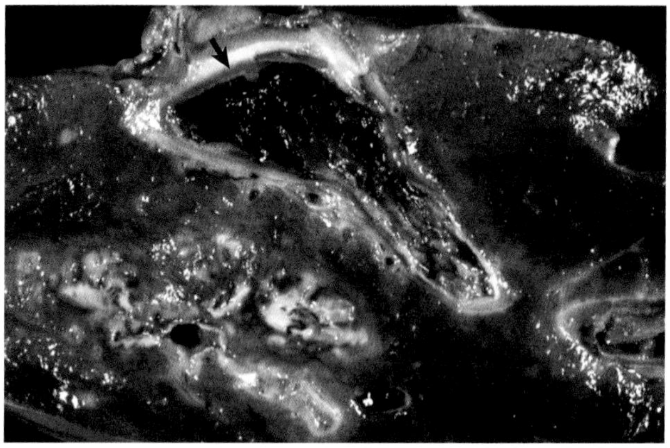

Figure 8-49 Hepatic Abscess, *Fusobacterium Necrophorum*, Liver, Cow. Foci of necrosis and abscess formation *(arrow)*. Abscesses, such as this one, can erode the wall of a hepatic vein or the caudal vena cava, rupture, and release their contents into the bloodstream. (Courtesy Dr. P. Stromberg, College of Veterinary Medicine, The Ohio State University.)

- Direct extension of an inflammatory process from tissues immediately adjacent to the liver, such as the reticulum

Both Gram-positive and Gram-negative organisms can cause hepatic abscesses. In adult small animals, hepatic abscesses are often caused by any of a variety of enteric species, as well as *Francisella* spp., *Nocardia asteroides*, and *Actinomyces* spp. Bacterial infections of the liver and subsequent formation of hepatic abscesses or foci of necrosis are especially common in neonatal foals and ruminants, in addition to feedlot cattle. In feedlot cattle, hepatic abscesses usually occur as a sequel to toxic rumenitis because damage to the ruminal mucosa allows ruminal microflora, particularly *Fusobacterium necrophorum*, to enter the portal circulation. After initially localizing within the liver, bacteria proliferate and produce focal areas of hepatocellular necrosis and hepatitis that can in time develop into hepatic abscesses (Fig. 8-49). Liver abscesses of cattle frequently are incidental lesions, but they can cause weight loss and decreased milk production. Less commonly, a hepatic abscess encroaches on the lumen of either a hepatic vein or the caudal vena cava. It can cause phlebitis that results in mural thrombosis, and because of the obstruction of the outflow to the venous drainage of the liver, passive congestion of the liver and portal hypertension can occur (Fig. 8-50). Detachment of portions of these mural thrombi can produce septic thromboemboli that lodge in the lungs. Rupture of hepatic abscesses directly into the hepatic vein or into the caudal vena cava occurs sporadically in cattle and may result in fatal septic embolization of the lungs. Sometimes death can be sudden from the blockage of large areas of pulmonary capillaries by the exudate. Hepatic abscesses derived from bacteria arriving via the portal vein may not be evenly distributed throughout the liver, possibly because of selective distribution of portal blood into different liver lobes, termed *portal streaming*. Occasionally, fungi, such as *Mucor* sp., that proliferate in areas of ruminal ulceration invade the portal circulation and are carried to the liver, where they cause extensive areas of necrosis and inflammation (Fig. 8-51).

Tuberculosis (*Mycobacterium bovis*) has been eradicated from almost all of the United States, but its occurrence in other countries varies with the effectiveness of control efforts. The primary site of the disease is pulmonary with subsequent dissemination to other organs, including the liver. Other domestic animal species can be infected with *Mycobacterium bovis*, and it is also a zoonotic microbe. *Mycobacterium avium-intracellulare* complex can occur in domestic animals, especially dogs, in the southern areas of the United States.

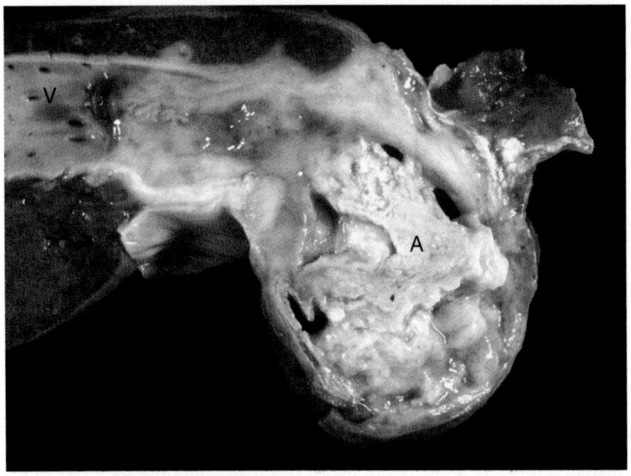

Figure 8-50 Hepatic Abscess, Caudal Vena Cava, Cow. A hepatic abscess *(A)* has eroded the wall of the vena cava, ruptured, and released its contents into the caudal vena cava *(V)*. (Courtesy College of Veterinary Medicine, North Carolina State University.)

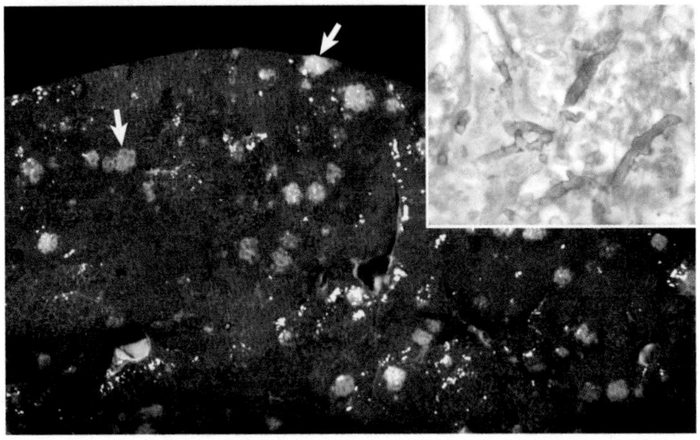

Figure 8-51 Multiple Necrotic Foci, Disseminated Fungal Infection (*Mucor* Spp.), Liver, Cow. *Mucor* spp. enter the portal blood after ulcerative rumenitis and cause focal necrosis and inflammation in the liver (granulomas *[arrows]*). *Inset,* The hyphae of the causative organism *(pink)* are usually evident within the granuloma. Periodic acid–Schiff *(PAS)* reaction. (Figure courtesy College of Veterinary Medicine, University of Illinois. Inset courtesy Dr. M.D. McGavin, College of Veterinary Medicine, University of Tennessee.)

Granulomas are randomly distributed (i.e., hematogenous spread) in the liver. They have a central core of cell debris, caseation, and granulomatous inflammation surrounded by a fibrous capsule (Fig. 8-52).

Tyzzer's Disease. This disease is caused by *Clostridium piliforme* (formerly *Bacillus piliformis*), a Gram-negative obligate intracellular parasite. It is well recognized in laboratory animals but occurs only sporadically in domestic animals. Infection is most common in foals but has been described in calves, cats, and dogs and many other species. Typically, only very young or immunocompromised animals are affected. The bacteria are found in the intestinal tract of rodents. Infection is most likely through the oral route. The mechanisms of attachment and entry into host cells are unknown. After colonization of the gastrointestinal tract, organisms penetrate into the portal venous drainage and enter the liver. The disease is characterized by enlarged, edematous, and hemorrhagic abdominal lymph nodes; hepatic enlargement; and the presence of randomly distributed, pale foci of hepatocellular necrosis surrounded by a variably intense

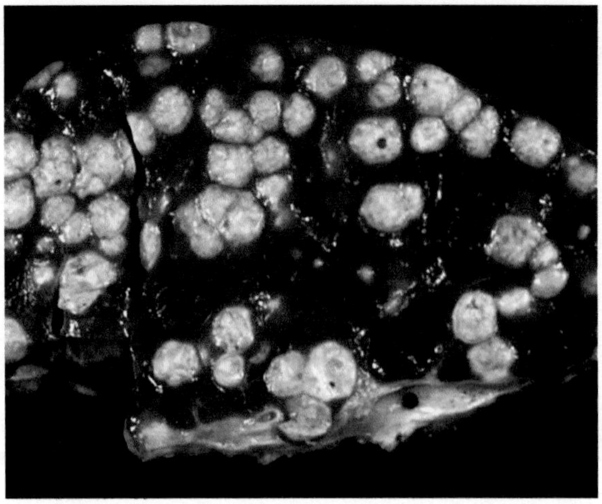

Figure 8-52 Multiple Caseous Granulomas, Tuberculosis, *Mycobacterium Bovis*, Liver, cow. Hepatic tuberculosis is characterized by random multifocal pale white-to-yellow caseous granulomas on the capsular and cut surfaces. (Courtesy Dr. M. Domingo, Autonomous University of Barcelona; and Noah's Arkive, College of Veterinary Medicine, The University of Georgia.)

inflammatory infiltrate of neutrophils and mononuclear cells (Fig. 8-53, *A*). Diagnosis requires the demonstration of the characteristic, elongated large bacilli within viable hepatocytes at the margins of necrotic foci (see Fig. 8-53, *B*). Silver stains, such as Warthin-Starry or Gomori's silver stain, are frequently used for this purpose (see Fig. 8-53, *C*).

Leptospirosis. Leptospirosis is caused by infection with the Gram-negative, thin, spiral, and motile bacterium of the genus *Leptospira.* There are two species, of which *Leptospira interrogans* is capable of causing disease in animals. The taxonomy of these organisms is complicated because there are more than 23 antigenically distinct pathogenic serogroups and more than 200 serovars. Each serovar can differ with respect to the species affected, organs affected, and severity of disease. Leptospires enter the body through the mucous membranes or through the skin if its barrier functions have been disrupted. Contaminated water, bedding, and soil are common sources of infection because the organism is shed in urine. Fetuses can develop transplacental infection and are often aborted. Infection can involve red blood cells, kidney, liver, and a number of other tissues, depending on the infecting serovar. The liver is often involved in acute, severe leptospirosis of all domestic species because a number of serovars cause intravascular hemolytic anemia leading to ischemic injury to centrilobular areas. Furthermore, organisms can be seen in large numbers in the liver after silver staining methods, although the direct effects of leptospira toxins on hepatocytes are less well established.

Gross lesions include icterus when animals are infected with serovars that produce hemolysis. Hepatic hemorrhage and ascites can occur, depending on the course of infection and the serovar involved. In some cases, acute infection can cause focal necrosis in addition to or instead of centrilobular necrosis. A common but nonspecific change in the liver of infected dogs is dissociation of hepatocytes. Affected cells become rounded and have eosinophilic granular cytoplasm and dark, shrunken hyperbasophilic nuclei. Bile casts in canaliculi are often apparent. Kupffer cells may contain abundant hemosiderin. Infection of dogs with *Leptospira grippotyphosa* has been reported to produce chronic (chronic-active) hepatitis, but it is unlikely that leptospira are involved in the pathogenesis of many cases of spontaneous chronic hepatitis.

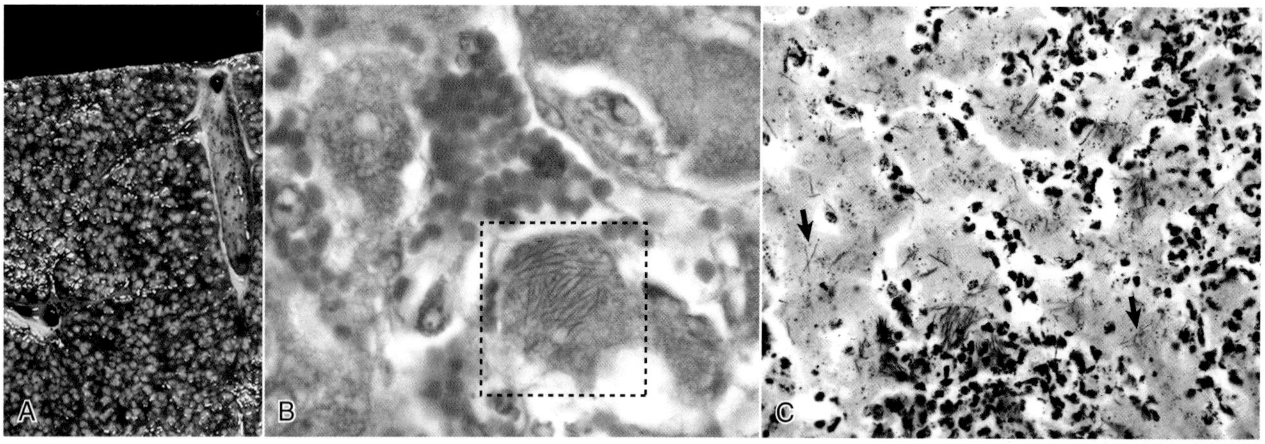

Figure 8-53 **Tyzzer's Disease (*Clostridium Piliforme*). A,** Liver, horse. Disseminated gray-white 1- to 2-mm foci of necrosis surrounded by suppurative inflammation. **B,** Foal. *Clostridium piliforme* can be identified by the haphazard distribution of filamentous bacteria *(dashed box)* in the cytoplasm of hepatocytes. Giemsa stain. **C,** Foal. *Clostridium piliforme (arrows)* can be readily seen with special stains such as Giemsa and Warthin-Starry. Warthin-Starry stain. (**A** courtesy Dr. R.C. Giles, University of Kentucky; and Noah's Arkive, College of Veterinary Medicine, The University of Georgia. **B** and **C** courtesy Dr. M.D. McGavin, College of Veterinary Medicine, University of Tennessee.)

Other Bacterial Infections. These diseases are grouped together because they all arise from a bacteremia that occurs during a systemic infection. A comprehensive list of systemic infections that may produce hepatocellular necrosis and hepatitis is beyond the scope of this chapter, but examples include *Yersinia pseudotuberculosis*, *Salmonella* spp. (lesions present within the liver are discrete accumulations of mixed mononuclear inflammatory cells, which often are referred to as paratyphoid nodules), and *Brucella* spp. infection in many species (Fig. 8-54). *Haemophilus agni*, *Mannheimia haemolytica*, and *Bibersteinia trehalosi* can present as infections in sheep. Other infections include *Trueperella pyogenes* (*Arcanobacter pyogenes*) of the bovine fetus and neonate, *Campylobacter fetus* subsp. *fetus* in fetal and neonatal lambs (Fig. 8-55), *Actinobacillus equuli* infection of neonatal foals, and *Nocardia asteroides* infection of dogs. *Francisella tularensis*, the cause of tularemia, can occur in cats, dogs, sheep, and many other species. These bacterial infections may produce lesions within the liver that range from small foci of hepatic necrosis to multiple, large abscesses. Determination of the specific causative agent often depends on bacterial isolation and characterization.

Bacillary hemoglobinuria and infectious necrotic hepatitis, both due to species of *Clostridia*, are described in detail in the section on Disorders of Ruminants.

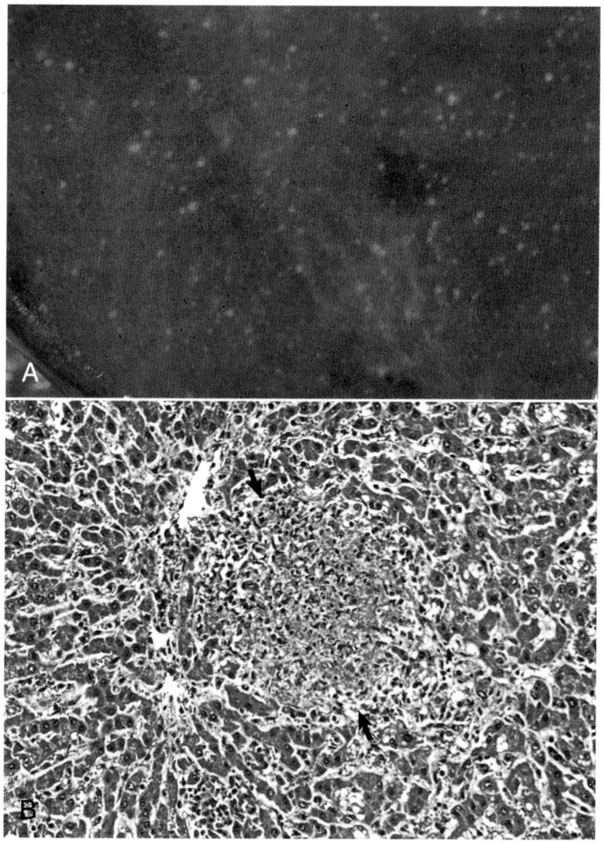

Figure 8-54 **Hepatic Salmonellosis, Liver, Cow. A,** Diaphragmatic surface of liver. Random gray-white 1- to 2-mm foci of focal necrosis in a cow with *Salmonella septicemia*. Multiple pale subcapsular foci of necrosis are evident. **B,** Necrotic focus infiltrated by macrophages *(arrows)*, forming a discrete granuloma. These lesions are termed paratyphoid nodules. H&E stain. (**A** courtesy Dr. M.D. McGavin, College of Veterinary Medicine, University of Tennessee. **B** courtesy Dr. A.J. Van Wettere, School of Veterinary Medicine, Utah State University).

Protozoal Diseases

The liver can be involved in systemic infections with *Toxoplasma gondii*, *Neospora* sp., and other less common protozoa (E-Fig. 8-8). Liver lesions are usually characterized by multifocal necrosis and inflammation. Inflammatory cells include neutrophils, macrophages, and smaller numbers of other cells. Free tachyzoites or cysts containing bradyzoites can be found within necrotic areas or adjacent to them. Although there are subtle physical differences between the organisms, molecular or immunohistochemical tests are more reliable means to separate the two organisms.

Fungal Diseases

Systemic involvement with fungi often includes the liver. Several genera of fungi may involve the liver, including *Blastomyces*, *Coccidioides*, *Aspergillus*, and *Histoplasma*. Histoplasmosis is a fungal disease that is endemic in the United States and Canada and can occur occasionally in other areas. It is caused by *Histoplasma capsulatum*, a soil-dwelling organism. Dogs are affected most often. The route of infection is primarily through inhalation, although ingestion is also a possible route. In some circumstances, pulmonary infections become disseminated and affect a variety of visceral organs, including the liver. Lesions in the liver consist of a multifocal distribution of granulomas with intralesional yeast forms of the

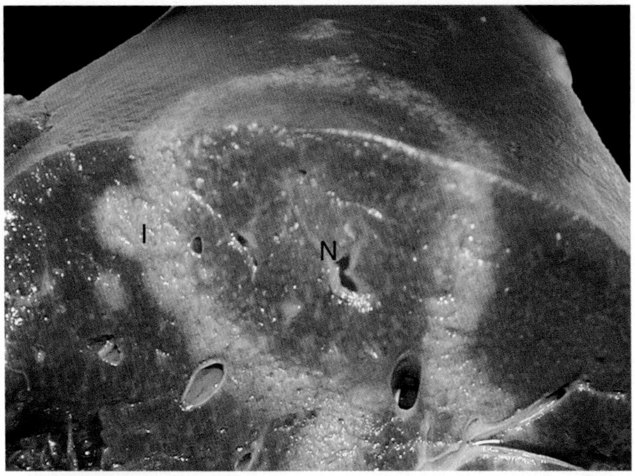

Figure 8-55 Hepatic Campylobacteriosis, Multifocal Necrotizing Hepatitis, Liver, Capsular and Cut Surfaces, Lamb Fetus. The lesion consists of a necrotic center (coagulation necrosis) *(N)*, which in older lesions is distinctly tan and depressed. This center is surrounded by a white to gray rim of inflammatory cells *(I)*. The cut surface illustrates the same changes and the extent of the necrosis into the hepatic parenchyma. (Courtesy Drs. C. Lichtensteiger and R. Doty, College of Veterinary Medicine, University of Illinois.)

organism. Numerous yeast forms can be found in the cytoplasm of macrophages and can be readily stained with the periodic acid–Schiff (PAS) reaction (Fig. 8-56, *A* and *B*).

Parasitic Diseases

Nematodes. Migration of larvae through the liver is a common component of a nematode's life cycle in domestic animals. As larvae travel through the liver, they produce local tracts of hepatocellular necrosis that are accompanied by inflammation. These tracts are eventually replaced with connective tissue that matures into fibrous scars, which are especially prominent on the capsular surface (Fig. 8-57). These capsular scars appear as pale areas, and the term *milk-spotted liver* has been used to describe livers in pigs scarred by migrating larvae of *Ascaris suum*. Larvae occasionally become entrapped within the liver or its capsule and are walled off within abscesses or granulomas. Examples of chronic hepatitis or hepatic scarring as a consequence of larval migration include migration of ascarids in several species of domestic animals, such as *Stephanurus dentatus* in pigs and *Strongylus* spp. in the horse. Infection of the liver with adult nematodes is considerably less common than larval migration. *Calodium hepaticum* (*Capillaria hepatica*) occasionally may be found in the hepatic parenchyma of dogs and cats where the ova provoke granulomatous inflammation.

Dogs with heartworm infection (*Dirofilaria immitis*) occasionally develop vena caval syndrome, also known as postcaval syndrome, which is characterized by DIC, intravascular hemolysis, and acute hepatic failure. The syndrome typically occurs in dogs, with large numbers of adult worms in the vena cava and their more usual location within the right side of the heart and pulmonary artery (Fig. 8-58). The liver is engorged with blood as a consequence of severe passive congestion from partial blockage of the caudal vena cava. It is proposed that mechanical factors produced by the presence of large numbers of worms in the right atrium or caudal vena cava are the cause of intravascular hemolysis, which characterizes vena caval syndrome, although other theories suggest that there may be a hypersensitivity reaction to antigens released by the worms.

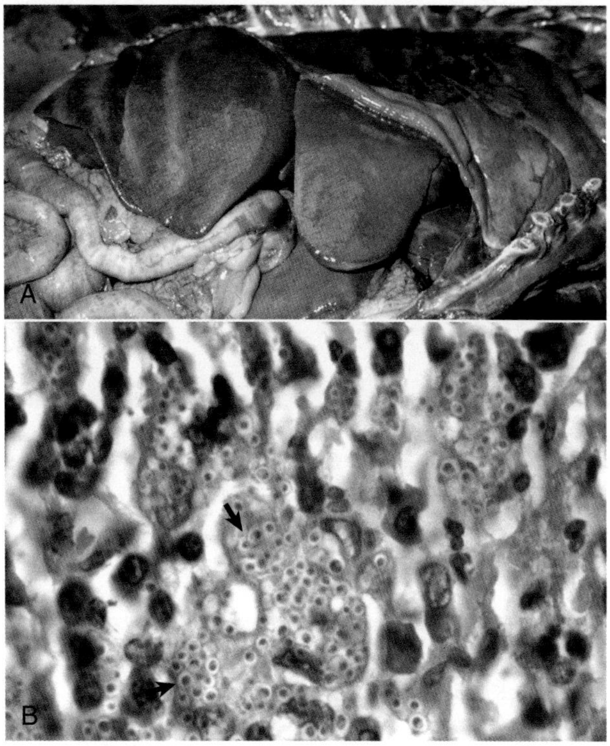

Figure 8-56 Hepatic Histoplasmosis, Liver, Dog. A, In disseminated cases, *Histoplasma capsulatum* can involve the liver. Affected livers tend to be enlarged and pale mahogany from the diffuse hypertrophy and proliferation of Kupffer cells and other macrophages. **B,** Note the yeast form of *Histoplasma (arrows)* in the cytoplasm of Kupffer cells and other macrophages. H&E stain. (**A** courtesy College of Veterinary Medicine, University of Illinois. **B** courtesy Dr. J. Simon, College of Veterinary Medicine, University of Illinois.)

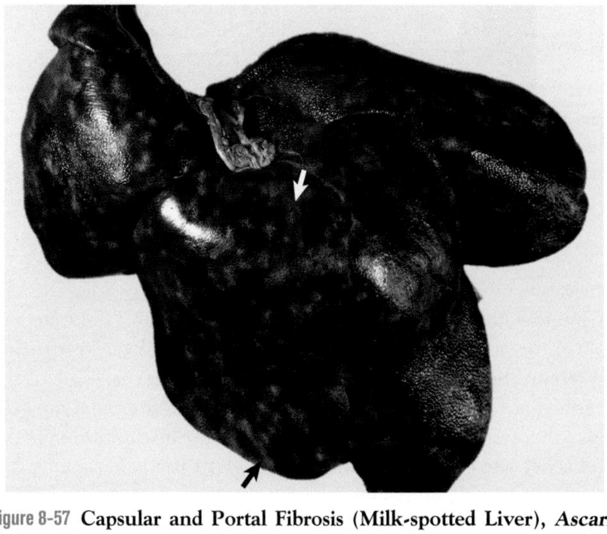

Figure 8-57 Capsular and Portal Fibrosis (Milk-spotted Liver), *Ascaris Suum* Larval Migration, Liver, Diaphragmatic Surface, Pig. Fibrous tissue (scars) has been deposited in the migration tracks of the ascarid larvae and in adjacent portal areas *(arrows)*. (Courtesy Dr. M.D. McGavin, College of Veterinary Medicine, University of Tennessee.)

Cestodes. A number of cestodes occur within the hepatobiliary system of domestic animals. Those cestode parasites of greatest clinical significance develop encysted forms within the liver of the intermediate hosts. The most important are larval cestodes of the genus *Taenia*; adults inhabit the gastrointestinal tract of carnivores and

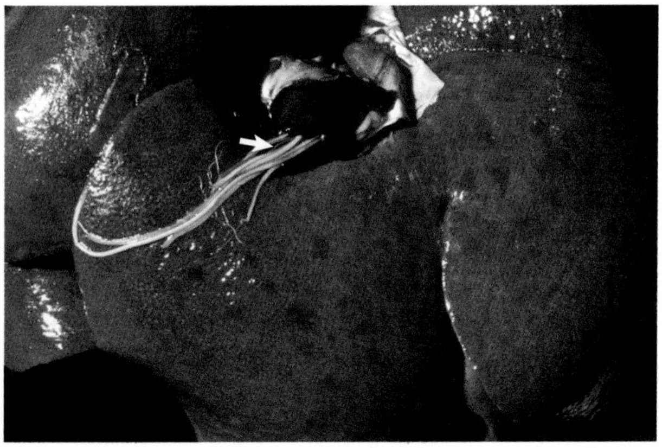

Figure 8-58 **Dirofilariasis, Vena Caval Syndrome, Caudal Vena Cava at the Level of the Liver, Dog.** Large collections of adult *Dirofilaria immitis (arrow)* are present in the caudal vena cava. The condition is rapidly fatal unless the nematodes are removed. (Courtesy Dr. C.S. Patton, College of Veterinary Medicine, University of Tennessee.)

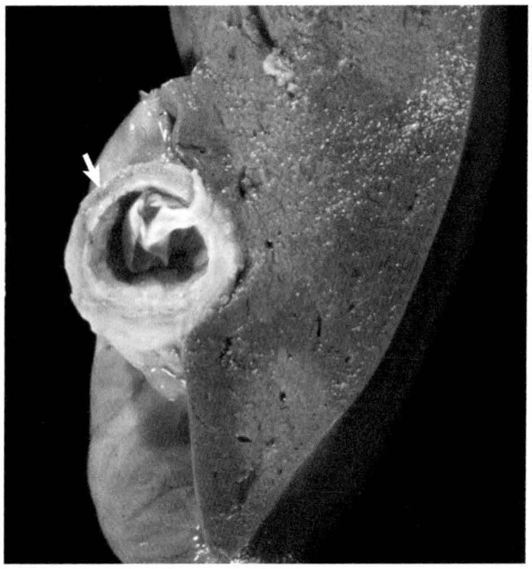

Figure 8-59 **Cysticercosis, Liver, Cut Surface, Sheep.** The thick fibrous capsule *(arrow)* usually indicates the death of the larva. (Courtesy Dr. K. Read, College of Veterinary Medicine, Texas A&M University; and Noah's Arkive, College of Veterinary Medicine, The University of Georgia.)

usually are innocuous to their definitive host. The ova ingested by an intermediate host develop into embryos, which penetrate the wall of the gut and then are distributed via the blood to virtually any site in the body. Parasitic cysts develop within the tissue of the intermediate host, and the life cycle of the parasite is completed when the cysts are ingested by the definitive host. Although the liver is but one organ in the intermediate host that may be affected, hepatic involvement is common because portal blood, in which embryos migrate, drains into the liver before flowing to the systemic circulation.

The adult cestode *Taenia hydatigena* shows up in the small intestine of dogs, whereas its intermediate stage, *Cysticercus tenuicollis*, appears in the peritoneal cavity of a variety of species, including horses, ruminants, and pigs (Fig. 8-59). Immature cysticerci migrate in the liver and can induce extensive damage if infection is heavy; lesions present are comparable to those induced by migration of immature *Fasciola hepatica*.

Hydatid liver disease is common in some countries. *Echinococcus granulosus* is a cestode that parasitizes canids as the definitive host, and hydatid cysts can develop in many different intermediate host animal species, including human beings. The dog-sheep cycle is most important in many geographic areas. Pastured cattle are also commonly affected in other geographic locations. Adult worms in the intestines of dogs pass proglottids into the dog's stool and thereby contaminate pastures. Ova are then ingested by sheep, cattle, or other species. Embryos may develop into hydatid cysts in virtually any organ in the intermediate host, but the liver and lungs are commonly affected. These cysts are usually less than 10 cm in diameter but can attain quite a spectacular size, particularly in human beings. Hydatid cysts, even when present in large numbers, rarely cause overt clinical signs of disease in domestic animals.

Cestode adults occurring within the hepatobiliary system include *Stilesia hepatica*, *Stilesia globipunctata*, and *Thysanosoma actinoides*, all of which can inhabit the bile duct of ruminants. Infections with these parasites may result in chronic inflammation of the biliary tract, but they usually do not produce clinical signs of hepatic dysfunction.

Trematodes. The majority of parasitic hepatic injury caused by trematodes is produced by members of three major families: Fasciolidae, Dicrocoelidae, and Opisthorchidae.

The principal liver fluke disease of sheep and cattle and occasionally other species is caused by *Fasciola hepatica*. Hepatic fascioliasis occurs throughout the world in areas where climatic conditions, typically in low swampy areas, are suitable for the survival of aquatic snails, which serve as intermediate hosts for the parasites. Adult *Fasciola hepatica* are leaf-shaped parasites that inhabit the biliary system; their eggs pass via the bile to the intestinal tract and eventually are passed in the feces. Larvae (miracidium) then must develop in the snail intermediate host (genus *Lymnaea*). Cercariae that leave the snail encyst on herbage, where they develop into infectious metacercariae. Metacercariae are ingested by the ruminant host and penetrate the wall of the duodenum to enter the peritoneal cavity and subsequently enter the liver. They migrate within the liver before taking up residence within the bile ducts. Migration of immature flukes through the liver produces hemorrhagic tracts of necrotic liver parenchyma. These tracts are grossly visible and in acute infection are dark red, but with time they become paler than the surrounding parenchyma. Repair is often by fibrosis. A variety of untoward sequelae can follow these migrations, including acute peritonitis; hepatic abscesses; death of the host as a consequence of acute, widespread hepatic necrosis produced by a massive infiltration of immature flukes; and the proliferation of spores of *Clostridium haemolyticum* or *Clostridium novyi* in necrotic tissue, which causes the subsequent development of bacillary hemoglobinuria or infectious necrotic hepatitis, respectively.

Mature flukes reside in the larger extrahepatic and intrahepatic bile ducts and cause cholangitis. Chronic cholangitis and bile duct obstruction lead to ectasia and stenosis of the ducts and periductular fibrosis that thickens the walls so that the ducts become increasingly prominent. Mineralization may occur, producing the classic "pipe-stem" appearance of diseased bile ducts. The contents of the bile ducts are often dark brown and viscous caused by a combination of abnormal bile, cellular debris, and the iron-porphyrin pigment excreted by the flukes. Obstruction of the ducts leads to cholestasis. Animals with chronic liver fluke disease are often in poor body condition.

Fasciola gigantica and *Fascioloides magna* are important causes of liver fluke disease of ruminants in some areas of the world. *Fasciola gigantica* is most common in areas of Africa and surrounding countries, and *Fascioloides magna* is found in North America. The adults of *Fasciola gigantica* and *Fasciola hepatica* reside in the bile ducts

(Fig. 8-60). In contrast, adult *Fascioloides magna*, whose normal hosts are elk and white-tailed deer, reside in the hepatic parenchyma in aberrant hosts, such as cattle and sheep. In cattle, the immature *Fascioloides magna* flukes cause extensive tissue damage as they migrate through the liver (Fig. 8-61), but the adults are enclosed by fibrous connective tissue in cysts containing a black fluid. In sheep and goats, the flukes continuously migrate through the liver, causing extensive damage and eventual death.

Other trematodes that may inhabit the bile ducts include *Dicrocoelium dendriticum* in horses, ruminants, pigs, dogs, and cats; *Eurytrema pancreaticum* and *Eurytrema coelomaticum* in ruminants; *Opisthorchis tenuicollis* in pigs, dogs, and cats and *Opisthorchis felineus* in dogs and cats; and *Pseudamphistomum truncatum*, *Metorchis conjunctus*, *Metorchis albidus*, *Parametorchis complexus*, *Concinnum* (*Eurytrema*) *procyonis*, and *Platynosomum fastosum* in dogs and cats. All are capable of inducing changes similar to but usually considerably milder than those caused by *Fasciola hepatica*. In addition, they occasionally cause obstruction of the biliary ducts.

Cats, and less often dogs, can develop pronounced chronic cholangitis from infections with flukes, most often Opisthorchiidae and *Platynosomum fastosum*. Microscopically, larger intrahepatic bile ducts are dramatically thickened by concentric fibrosis and the duct lumen is usually dilated, often with papillary projections of biliary epithelium into the lumen (Fig. 8-62). A mild to moderate inflammatory infiltrate of neutrophils and macrophages is often found in and around the ducts, and the portal tracts are infiltrated by neutrophils, lymphocytes, and plasma cells. Eosinophils are generally uncommon. It is often difficult to detect adult flukes or ova in affected animals.

Dogs can be infected with the schistosome *Heterobilharzia americana*, which is normally a parasite in raccoons. Ova shed into water from feces passed by infected raccoons release miracidia, which penetrate host snails. Dogs become infected when their skin is penetrated by cercariae, which are released from the intermediate snail hosts. Granulomatous lesions of the liver, pancreas, intestines, and mesentery result when ova released by adult schistosomes lodge in affected tissue and incite an inflammatory reaction. Recently, horses have been shown to be susceptible to hepatic granulomas induced by *Heterobilharzia americana* as well, although the infection was subclinical in all cases.

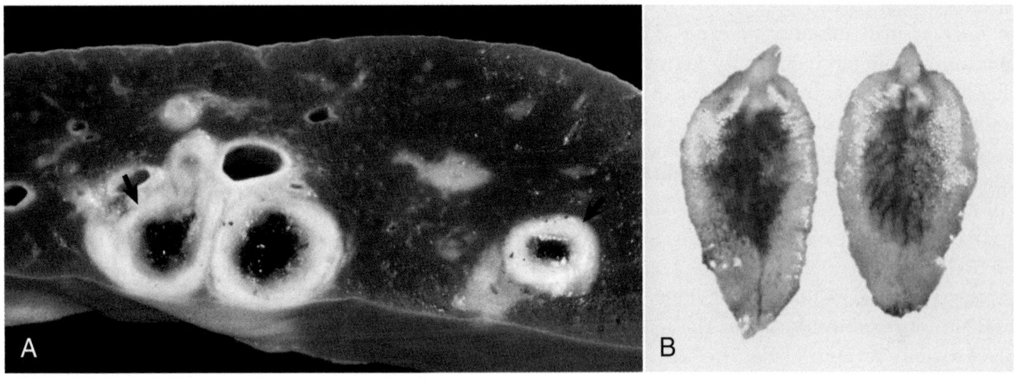

Figure 8-60 ***Fasciola Hepatica* Infection. A,** Chronic intrahepatic cholangitis (*Fasciola hepatica*), liver, cow. When *Fasciola hepatica* metacercariae are ingested, they migrate to the liver and then take up residence within the bile ducts. Mature flukes reside in the larger extrahepatic and intrahepatic bile ducts and cause chronic cholangitis and bile duct obstruction that lead to ectasia and stenosis of the ducts and periductular fibrosis that thickens the walls so that the ducts become increasingly prominent, as shown here *(arrows)*. **B,** Adult *Fasciola hepatica* are leaf-shaped flukes that inhabit the biliary system; their eggs pass via the bile into the intestinal tract and eventually are passed in the feces. (**A** courtesy Dr. K. Read, College of Veterinary Medicine, Texas A&M University; and Noah's Arkive, College of Veterinary Medicine, The University of Georgia. **B** courtesy Dr. T. Boosinger, College of Veterinary Medicine, Auburn University; and Noah's Arkive, College of Veterinary Medicine, The University of Georgia.)

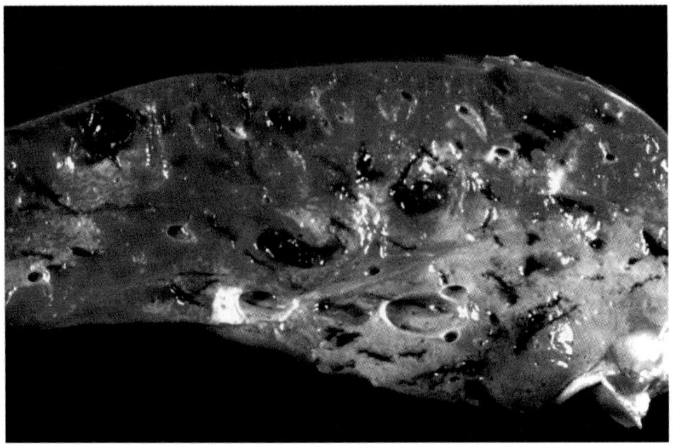

Figure 8-61 Fluke Migration Tracts, Fascioloidiasis, Liver, Cow. Migration of *Fascioloides magna* through the bovine liver produces extensive parenchymal damage. A black excretory pigment deposited by the fluke discolors the migration tracks black. (Courtesy Dr. J. Wright, College of Veterinary Medicine, North Carolina State University; and Noah's Arkive, College of Veterinary Medicine, The University of Georgia.)

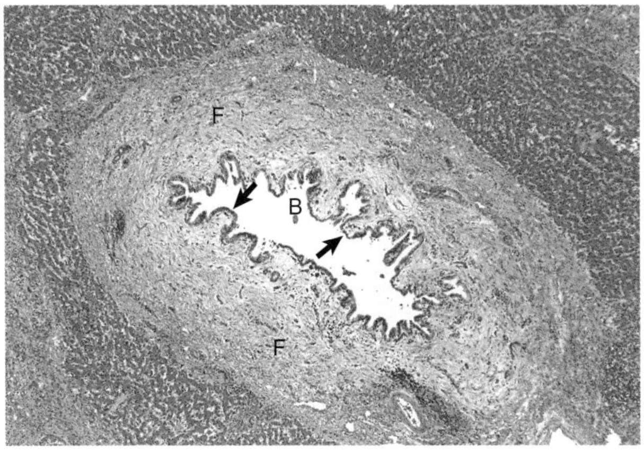

Figure 8-62 Chronic Intrahepatic Cholangitis, Liver, Cat. Fluke infections of the biliary tree of cats produce a characteristically pronounced periductular fibrosis *(F)*, dilated bile duct *(B)*, and papillary projections *(arrows)* of biliary epithelium, although flukes may be difficult to find. H&E stain. (Courtesy Dr. J.M. Cullen, College of Veterinary Medicine, North Carolina State University.)

Toxicant-Induced Liver Disease

The liver is subjected to toxic injury more often than any other organ. This susceptibility is not surprising because the portal vein blood that drains from the absorptive surface of the intestinal tract flows directly to the liver. Thus the liver is exposed to virtually all ingested substances, including plant, fungal, and bacterial products, and metals, minerals, drugs, and other chemicals that are absorbed into the portal blood. Hepatotoxic injury can range along a spectrum from pure hepatocellular injury to pure biliary injury and a mixed pattern of injury that involves both components of the liver.

Hepatotoxic drugs can be divided into two basic categories. Predictable hepatotoxicants are those that affect the large majority of animals that are exposed, and the effect is evident within a similar dose range. The majority of recognized hepatotoxicants in veterinary medicine fall into this category; acetaminophen and pyrrolizidine alkaloids are examples of predictable hepatotoxicants. Toxic injury, even with predictable toxicants, is not always uniform, however. A variety of factors influence the severity of injury induced by a toxicant, including age, sex, diet, endocrine function, genetic constitution, and diurnal factors. It is therefore not surprising that responses of individual animals exposed to the same toxicant can vary considerably. Idiosyncratic drug reactions are characterized as responses seen in only a small minority of exposed individuals. There are a number of possible mechanisms for idiosyncratic drug reactions, including atypical metabolism as a result of inheritance of rare genes encoding enzymes involved in drug metabolism, deletions of genes encoding certain enzymes, or immunologic responses to drugs or modified hepatocyte proteins (haptens). Interactions with other drugs or effects of diet and health status can also play a role in idiosyncratic toxicity. Diazepam toxicity in cats is an example of an idiosyncratic toxicity.

The response of the liver to acute hepatotoxic injury depends on the mechanism and site of toxic insult. By far the most common pattern of acute liver toxicity is centrilobular necrosis. The mechanisms for this pattern of injury involve metabolism by the cytochrome P450 system and are discussed later. Certain chemicals that are uncommonly encountered produce periportal necrosis. These chemicals are able to produce a toxic effect without requiring metabolism by the cytochrome P450 system and include white phosphorus (once used as a rodenticide) and allyl alcohol.

It should be kept in mind that a single episode of nonlethal hepatotoxic injury in an otherwise healthy animal is difficult to detect histologically within the first day after the episode. Within 48 to 72 hours, macrophages clear cell debris, and hepatocytes begin to undergo mitosis to replace the lost cells. Within a week or less, the liver regains a normal histologic appearance, unless there is massive necrosis, which can lead to collapse of the hepatic connective tissue scaffolding and subsequent fibrosis surrounding the central vein. Chronic toxic liver injury, manifested as either repeated bouts of toxicant exposure or more consistent daily exposure (e.g., through dietary contamination), can lead to activation of hepatic stellate cells within the space of Disse or related myofibroblasts in the portal areas and the connective tissue of the central vein area, which may then initiate synthesis of extracellular matrix leading to hepatic fibrosis. In addition, chronic liver injury can lead to disruption of the normal framework that supports the hepatic architecture and leads to hepatic fibrosis. Sufficient injury also can produce nodules of regenerative hepatocytes that are surrounded by bands of fibrosis that connect central vein areas to each other, connect portal tracts to each other, or bridge portal tracts to centrilobular areas. This pattern is recognized as cirrhosis.

Hepatocytes are not the only cell type in the liver that can be affected by toxic drugs. The biliary epithelium is susceptible to injury from trimethoprim-sulfa and the mycotoxin, sporidesmin, Kupffer cells to endotoxin, sinusoidal endothelial cells to arsenicals and some pyrrolizidine alkaloids, and the hepatic stellate cells to vitamin A excess. Bile duct necrosis can disrupt bile flow. Activated Kupffer cells can release cytokines that affect the type and degree of inflammation within the liver. Hepatic stellate cells play a central role in hepatic fibrosis, as is discussed later. Damage to endothelial cells can affect blood flow through the liver.

Hepatotoxic liver injury can be classified into the following six categories based on the cellular target involved:

1. The most frequent mechanism of hepatocellular injury involves production of injurious metabolites by the cytochrome P450 system. This family of enzymes is located in the smooth endoplasmic reticulum (microsomes) of hepatocytes primarily, although they are also found in many other cells of the body. A major role of cytochrome P450 enzymes is to metabolize lipid-soluble chemicals into water-soluble compounds for excretion from the body in bile or urine. In the first step of this three-step process, termed *biotransformation*, chemicals are bioactivated to a high-energy reactive intermediate molecule, termed *phase I*, in preparation for the second step, *phase II*, which involves formation of covalent bonds with polar molecules, such as glucuronic acid. This conjugation forms a water-soluble metabolite that can be excreted. *Phase III* involves the transport of these molecules across the cell membrane into the lumen of the canaliculus by molecular pumps. In some circumstances, such as an overdose, the high-energy reactive metabolites can form covalent bonds with other cellular constituents, such as proteins, and nucleic acids termed adducts. In acute toxicity, adducts with essential cellular enzymes may lead to cell injury or death. Toxic hepatocellular injury of this category occurs most often in the centrilobular area of the liver because this area is the region of the liver with the highest concentration of cytochrome P450 enzymes. For example, acetaminophen is metabolized by cytochrome P450 enzymes to *N*-acetyl-*p*-benzo-quinone imine (NAPQI), a free radical that is responsible for the toxicity of the parent compound. Lesions induced by acetaminophen are most severe in the centrilobular (periacinar) areas, where the active form of the chemical is present in greatest concentration. Many plant toxicities cause hepatic injury by this mechanism.
2. Adduct formation between drugs and cellular enzymes, other proteins, or nucleic acids can alter the cellular constituents sufficiently that they become neoantigens, as may be the case with toxicity following exposure to halothane, an inhalant anaesthetic agent used previously. These neoantigens, like other foreign antigens, can be processed in the cytoplasm, transported to the cell surface, presented as antigens, and recognized by the immune system. Consequently, the immune system may develop an inflammatory response toward hepatocytes or biliary epithelium that contain the adducts. Both cellular and humoral immunity can be involved. Injury can occur through direct cellular cytotoxicity and antibody-dependent cellular cytotoxicity. Although this mechanism is not well characterized in clinical veterinary medicine, it is likely to occur on occasion.
3. Certain toxicants, including retained or excess hydrophobic bile acids, can trigger apoptosis (individual cell necrosis) by direct stimulation of proapoptotic pathways in the hepatocytes. Alternatively, apoptosis can be stimulated by immune-mediated events, such as those discussed previously, which lead to the release of TNF-α or activate Fas pathways.
4. Injury that damages cell membranes and disables enzymes responsible for calcium homeostasis, as seen in carbon tetrachloride toxicity, can lead to an influx of calcium. One consequence of

the increased intracellular calcium is activation of proteases that damage actin filaments. Blebbing and lysis of the cell membranes can result.

5. Chemicals that bind to and disrupt the molecular pumps that secrete bile constituents into the canaliculi, such as estrogen and erythromycin, can produce cholestasis. More extensive hepatocellular injury that affects canalicular pumps and hepatocytes may produce cholestasis by disrupting the actin filaments situated around the bile canaliculi and preventing the normal pulsatile contractions that move bile through the canalicular system to the bile ducts.
6. Hepatocyte injury or death can follow mitochondrial damage, as seen with some toxic antiviral nucleosides or intravenous tetracycline administration. Chemical or reactive oxygen species–induced injury to mitochondrial membranes, enzymes, or DNA can inhibit or disrupt mitochondrial function. Disruption of the electron transport chain can release reactive oxygen species, such as superoxide, which can produce widespread cellular damage. Damaged mitochondria do not produce sufficient adenosine triphosphate (ATP) to power the essential functions of the hepatocytes. Also, β-oxidation of lipids is reduced once the mitochondria are damaged, which leads to intrahepatic lipid accumulation (microvesicular steatosis) and diminished energy production. Damaged mitochondria may release cytochrome c, triggering apoptosis, or if disruption of mitochondrial function is sufficient, hepatocyte necrosis ensues.

Hepatotoxic Agents

Hepatotoxic Cyanobacteria (Blue-Green Algae). Cyanobacteria are classified in the kingdom Monera, phylum Cyanobacteria; are considered to be more closely related to bacteria; and are no longer considered members of the plant family. Several genera of cyanobacteria, including *Anabaena, Aphanizomenon, Microcystis,* and *Nodularia*, can cause lethal poisoning of livestock and less commonly small animals such as dogs and cats. Cyanobacterial (algal) blooms usually occur in late summer or early fall because of the warm temperatures, long hours of sunlight, and abundance of essential nutrients. Dead and dying cyanobacteria, which contain preformed toxins such as microcystin LR, a cyclic heptapeptide, accumulate on the surface of bodies of water and are ingested by livestock. Secondary bacterial growth in dying algae may contribute to toxin formation. Microcystin binds to protein phosphatases 1 and 2A causing hyperphosphorylation of cytoskeletal proteins, redistribution of actin filament, and ultimately cytoskeletal collapse and cell death. Signs develop rapidly and include diarrhea, prostration, and death. Gross lesions include hemorrhagic gastroenteritis and a red, swollen, hemorrhagic liver. Histologically, centrilobular, or even massive, hepatic necrosis and hemorrhage are evident. Animals that survive the acute manifestations may develop clinical signs of chronic liver disease. Other preformed toxins that affect different organ systems, including the nervous system, have also been identified in cyanobacteria.

Hepatotoxic Plants. Toxic plants of great variety cause hepatic injury in domestic animals. A comprehensive discussion of each is beyond the scope of this chapter.

Pyrrolizidine Alkaloid-Containing Plants. Pyrrolizidine alkaloids are found in many plant families, including Compositae, Leguminosae, and Boraginaceae, that occur throughout much of the world. The most important genera are *Senecio, Cynoglossum, Amsinckia, Crotalaria, Echium, Trichodesma,* and *Heliotropium.* Approximately 100 different alkaloids are recognized; toxic effects depend on which alkaloids are present within ingested plants. Ingested alkaloids are converted to pyrrolic esters by hepatic cytochrome P450 enzymes. These esters are alkylating agents, which react with cytosolic and nuclear proteins and nucleic acids. Pigs are particularly susceptible to pyrrolizidine alkaloid intoxication, sheep and goats considerably less so, and cattle and horses are intermediate in susceptibility. Most cases of intoxication arise from chronic intoxication, and the gross lesion is typically hepatic fibrosis (Fig. 8-63, A). The characteristic histologic lesions of pyrrolizidine alkaloid intoxication are megalocytosis, hepatic fibrosis, biliary proliferation, and, in some circumstances, nodular regeneration of parenchyma. Megalocytes are hepatocytes with enlarged nuclei and increased cytoplasmic volume and may be many times the size of normal hepatocytes (see Fig. 8-63, B). Megalocytes are the result of the antimitotic effects of pyrrolizidine alkaloids, which prevent cell division but not DNA synthesis because the hepatocytes attempt to divide to replace those that have undergone necrosis. This change, although indicative of pyrrolizidine alkaloid intoxication, is not

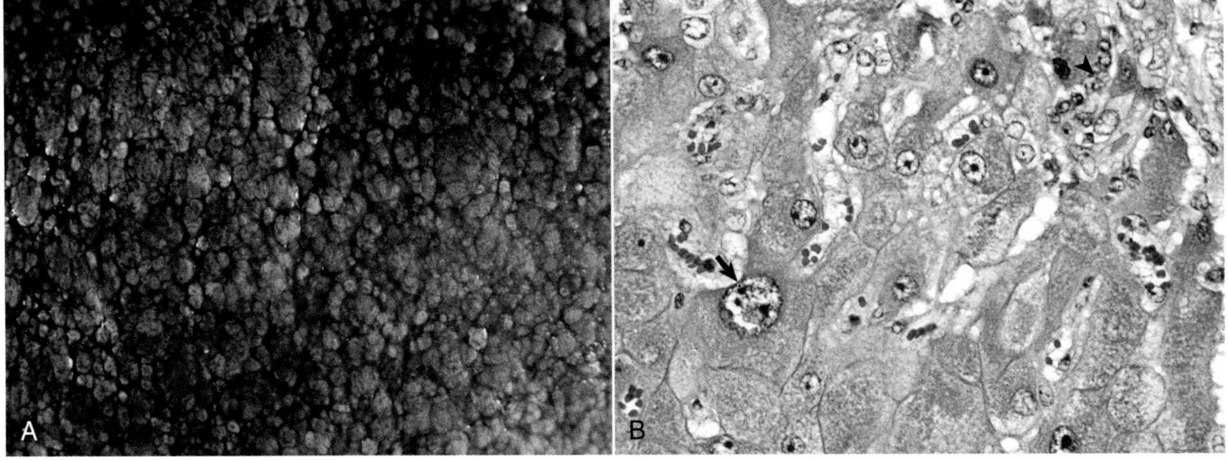

Figure 8-63 **Chronic Pyrrolizidine Hepatotoxicity, Cow. A,** Chronic pyrrolizidine intoxication produces a fibrotic and sometimes distorted liver with an irregular capsular surface. **B,** Greatly enlarged hepatocytes (megalocytes) *(arrow)* and hyperplasia of biliary epithelium *(arrowhead)* in the persisting parenchyma are typical of pyrrolizidine toxicity. H&E stain. (**A** courtesy Dr. P. Carbonell, School of Veterinary Science, Melbourne. **B** courtesy Dr. M.D. McGavin, College of Veterinary Medicine, University of Tennessee.)

pathognomonic because it can also be observed with other toxins such as aflatoxins and nitrosamines. Nodular regeneration does not always occur because hepatocyte proliferation can be inhibited by pyrrolizidines; however, exposure is not likely to be constant, and there may be periods during which hepatocyte replication can occur, such as the end of the dry season when more desirable plant species reappear. Species differences may also have an effect on the hepatic response to pyrrolizidines because cattle have regenerative nodules more often than horses. Chronic hepatic damage can lead to hepatic failure and its associated constellation of signs (described in detail previously).

Cycads. Cycads are primitive palmlike plants that inhabit tropical and subtropical regions. They contain cycasin and macrozamin, nontoxic glycosides, which after ingestion are deconjugated by intestinal bacteria to release a toxic metabolite, methylazoxymethanol. After absorption into the portal vein, hepatic metabolism of this compound yields alkylating agents, leading to acute or chronic liver injury. Acute injury is manifested as acute centrilobular necrosis. Chronic hepatic lesions in cattle include hepatocellular megalocytosis caused by the mitoinhibitory effects of alkylating agents, nuclear hyperchromasia, and varying degrees of hepatic fibrosis. In addition to hepatic disease, clinical signs indicative of gastrointestinal disease are frequent. Cycads also contain the neurotoxin β-methylamino-L-alanine (BMAA) and an unidentified neurotoxin. This unidentified neurotoxin is thought to be the cause of neurologic disease in cattle with chronic cycad poisoning, where progressive proprioceptive deficits in the hind legs are attributed to "dying back" (axonal degeneration) in the dorsal funiculus and the spinocerebellar and corticospinal tracts. Acute intoxication is more common in sheep than in other species and produces acute gastrointestinal dysfunction and centrilobular hepatic necrosis. Dogs can also be intoxicated by cycads.

Cholestatic Plant Intoxications. The ornamental shrub *Lantana camara* produces toxic pentacyclic triterpenes—lantadene A, B, and C—that primarily produce a syndrome of chronic cholestasis in grazing animals. Bile accumulation is evident within the canaliculi, hepatocytes, and Kupffer cells.

In Australia and New Zealand, cattle and sheep grazing *Brassica* species plants (e.g., turnips, rape, and kale) during the late summer and fall have developed cholestasis and secondary (hepatogenous) photosensitization. Microscopically, cholangiectasis (dilation) and peribiliary fibrosis of small to medium-sized bile ducts is present in the liver. The clinical signs often mimic those of sporidesmin toxicity. The hepatotoxic phytochemical in brassica is unknown.

Primarily in South Africa, *Tribulus terrestris* (puncture vine) ingestion by sheep can produce a fatal disorder (geeldikkop) characterized by icterus, biliary injury, and secondary photosensitization. Histologically, there is abundant crystalline material within and obstructing the bile ducts. Crystals may also be found in Kupffer cells. In various areas of the world, a similar pattern of crystal deposition can be seen in sheep and goats that graze a number of grass species, including *Panicum* sp., that contain steroidal sapogenins. Ruminal metabolism gives rise to metabolites that complex with calcium leading to crystal formation.

Secondary photosensitization and icterus can occur in all of these conditions as the result of impaired bile secretion.

Mycotoxins. Mycotoxins are secondary metabolites of fungi—that is, their production is not necessary for the survival of the fungus. The amount of toxin synthesized by a given strain of fungus reflects the genetic constitution of the particular strain and the presence of appropriate substrate, temperature, humidity, and available nutrients. There are several hepatotoxic mycotoxins of veterinary significance.

Aflatoxin. The fungus *Aspergillus flavus* is the most important source of aflatoxins. Aflatoxin B1 is the most common form and is also the most potent aflatoxin and carcinogen. Aflatoxins are usually elaborated during storage of fungus-contaminated feed, particularly in humid conditions, and may be present in many crops, including corn, peanuts, and cottonseed. They can be incorporated into commercial food, leading to significant outbreaks of acute toxicity in dogs. Aflatoxins are converted to toxic intermediates by hepatic cytochrome P450 enzymes. Carcinogenic, toxic, and teratogenic effects of aflatoxins reflect binding of the toxic intermediates to cellular DNA, RNA, or proteins. Pigs, dogs, horses, calves, and avian species (e.g., ducks and turkeys), especially younger animals, are sensitive to the toxic effects of aflatoxins, whereas sheep and adult cattle are more resistant. Acute aflatoxin intoxication is rare in horses and cattle because an inordinately large amount of contaminated feed would have to be ingested to achieve a sufficient dose. Acute aflatoxicosis in dogs is characterized by hemorrhagic central to massive necrosis. Steatosis and biliary proliferation also may occur. Chronic intoxication is more common than acute intoxication and results in ill-thrift, increased susceptibility to infection, and occasionally signs of hepatic failure. Affected livers are firm and pale and microscopically are characterized by steatosis and necrosis of hepatocytes, biliary hyperplasia, centrilobular to bridging fibrosis, and cellular atypia of hepatocytes, characterized by variable cell size and variable nuclear size (Fig. 8-64, *A* and *B*).

Phomopsins. Phomopsins are toxic metabolites of the fungus *Diaporthe toxica* (formerly *Phomopsis leptostromiformis*). The fungus grows on lupines (*Lupinus* sp.), and cattle, sheep, and occasionally horses that graze contaminated lupine stubble develop hepatic injury. Hepatic dysfunction is usually chronic, and the liver is atrophic and fibrotic. The microscopic appearance of affected livers is characterized by diffuse scattered hepatocyte necrosis with a background of mitotic figures, often appearing to be arrested in metaphase. Later in the course of the disease, diffuse fibrosis and biliary hyperplasia predominate. Signs of hepatic failure, including photosensitization, may occur in affected animals. This mycotoxicosis should not be confused with the condition known as *lupinosis*, which is caused by naturally occurring alkaloids (e.g., anagyrine) in lupines that are capable of inducing skeletal deformities but not obvious hepatic injury in calves and lambs following in utero exposure.

Sporidesmin. The mycotoxin sporidesmin is produced by *Pithomyces chartarum*, a fungus that grows particularly well in dead ryegrass (*Lolium perenne*), a common pasture plant in New Zealand and Australia. The majority of the toxin is concentrated into the fungal spores, and when a sufficient amount of the spores is ingested by sheep and, to a lesser extent, cattle, the toxin is secreted into the biliary tree in an unconjugated form that produces necrosis of the epithelium of large intrahepatic and extrahepatic biliary ducts with minimal inflammation. Cholestasis with a concurrent failure to excrete phylloerythrin frequently leads to photosensitization with skin lesions predominantly on the head, thus the common name facial eczema. Acute cases are characterized by a bile-stained liver with prominent small-caliber bile ducts. Ducts are dilated by bile in the lumens and surrounded by periductal edema. In chronic cases of facial eczema, the bile ducts become thickened by fibrosis secondary to biliary epithelial necrosis and subsequent inflammation (chronic cholangitis). Perhaps because of streaming of blood in the portal vein, the left lobe of the liver (although this lobe occupies the ventral portion of the ruminant liver), which may have an increased proportion of blood draining from the small intestine, is usually most

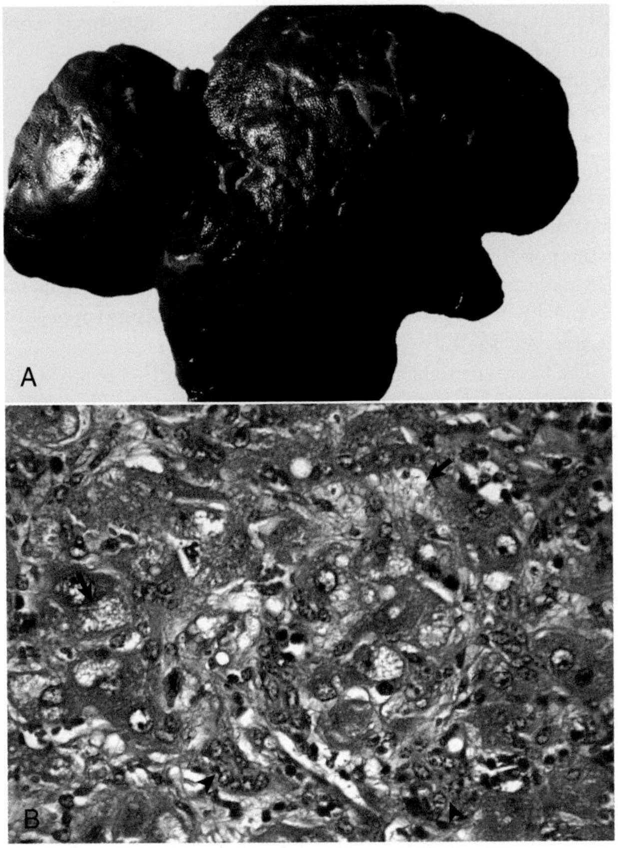

Figure 8-64 **Chronic Hepatic Aflatoxicosis. A,** Postnecrotic scarring, pig. Chronic aflatoxicosis produces a shrunken and fibrotic liver from collapse of areas of massive necrosis and condensation of the fibrous stroma. **B,** Histologic appearance. Chronic aflatoxicosis is characterized by variable amounts of steatosis (fatty change *[arrows]*), biliary hyperplasia *(arrowheads)*, and cellular atypia in hepatocytes. H&E stain. (**A** courtesy Dr. M.D. McGavin, College of Veterinary Medicine, University of Tennessee. **B** courtesy Dr. J. Simon, College of Veterinary Medicine, University of Illinois.)

severely affected and in severe cases undergoes atrophy and fibrosis.

Mushrooms. Poisonous mushrooms, such as *Amanita* sp. and others, can cause acute fatal liver necrosis. Intoxication by *Amanita phalloides*, known as the death cap, is caused by a group of toxins termed toxic cyclopeptides. This species is particularly toxic; a single gram of this mushroom is sufficient to kill a human being, and even smaller amounts are likely to prove fatal to dogs. The octopeptide amatoxin is in particular responsible for hepatocellular injury. The mechanism of injury is attributed to inhibition of RNA polymerase II function disrupting DNA and RNA transcription. Gross lesions usually consist of hepatic hemorrhage and a shrunken liver because of the loss of hepatocytes. Hepatocellular steatosis, hemorrhage, and centrilobular to massive necrosis are the typical lesions. Death from liver failure may occur 3 or 4 days after the onset of clinical signs. Phalloidin, a toxic heptapeptide found in *Amanita* sp., causes disruption of intracellular actin filaments, leading to cell injury or death. It is a less significant toxin in natural exposure because of the limited absorption from the digestive tract. Other mushroom species contain different toxic agents.

Hepatotoxic Chemicals

Xylitol. The artificial sweetener xylitol is used in various food items and snacks prepared for diabetics or dieters. Xylitol also prevents oral bacteria from producing acids that damage the surfaces of teeth and is therefore included in sugar-free gums, toothpastes, and other oral care products. Although innocuous to human beings (e.g., people consuming more than 130 g per day may develop diarrhea but no other abnormalities), xylitol can be acutely toxic to dogs. After ingesting as little as 0.5 g/kg, affected dogs can develop hyperinsulinemia, hypoglycemia, icterus, and liver failure. Clinical signs include vomiting, lethargy, and weakness. Dogs with severe hypoglycemia may present with seizures. The liver changes are characterized by severe centrilobular or midzonal to massive necrosis and periportal vacuolar degeneration. Over time, there is moderate to marked centrilobular hepatocyte loss and atrophy, lobular collapse, and disorganization. The mechanism for liver damage is not fully understood but is thought to be related to either ATP depletion during xylitol metabolism or the production of reactive oxygen species.

Phosphorus. Phosphorus occurs in two forms: red phosphorus and white phosphorus. Red phosphorus is unimportant as a toxicant, but white phosphorus was previously used as a rodenticide. The mechanism of phosphorus toxicity is unclear, although it apparently is directly toxic. Poisoning is first indicated by signs of gastroenteritis and subsequently by microscopic lesions of steatosis of hepatocytes and periportal necrosis. The pattern of periportal necrosis is unusual because most toxic liver injury occurs in the centrilobular region of the liver. This difference is explained by the fact that white phosphorus does not require metabolic transformation to a reactive intermediate by cytochrome P450 enzymes, which are most concentrated in the centrilobular region of the liver lobule.

Carbon Tetrachloride. Carbon tetrachloride is the classic example of a hepatotoxicant that must be bioactivated by the mixed function oxidase system to produce a toxic intermediate form. Historically, it was used for a variety of purposes, including as an anthelmintic. Carbon tetrachloride produces centrilobular hepatic necrosis and steatosis of surviving hepatocytes (see Chapter 1).

Metals. Several metals can cause toxic hepatic injury. Excessive iron supplementation in animals may result in excessive storage of iron and subsequently hepatic disease caused by iron overload, termed *hemochromatosis*. Two specific syndromes of iron poisoning are iron-dextran intoxication of piglets and ferrous fumarate intoxication of newborn foals. Severe cases of these two toxicities are characterized by massive hepatic necrosis. Intoxication of foals with ferrous fumarate occurred after its use as a component of a specific dietary supplement, and it was characterized by massive necrosis and also a remarkable amount of hyperplasia of bile ducts and cholangioles, possibly with hepatic progenitor cell (oval cell) proliferation, despite the short clinical course of the disease. Iron-dextran is frequently administered intramuscularly to suckling pigs to prevent anemia, but administration of iron-dextran has occasionally resulted in significant mortality, and affected pigs die soon after injection.

Copper toxicity is discussed in separate sections on Disorders of Ruminants and Canine Chronic Hepatitis.

Hepatotoxic Therapeutic Drugs. There are a variety of drugs that have a proven therapeutic application but can cause significant acute or chronic hepatic injury in some animals. A partial list of hepatotoxic therapeutic drugs in dogs and cats is presented in E-Table 8-2. Clearly, these drugs would not be used if the proportion of injured animals was high, but it is important to keep in mind that many drugs have the potential to cause hepatic injury in some patients. The mechanisms by which these drugs cause injury vary by species and by individual. Some therapeutic drugs are predictable toxicants, and all members of a particular species are susceptible to liver injury if a sufficient dose is given. However, because the therapeutic effect occurs at a lower dose than the toxic dose, liver injury occurs only when overdoses are ingested. Hepatic metabolism (bioactivation) of these compounds is likely to be involved because the site of liver injury is typically centrilobular. Cats are more susceptible than dogs to intoxication by many chemicals because they are relatively deficient in hepatic glucuronyltransferase activity. This phase II enzyme forms conjugates between bioactivated (phase I) xenobiotics and glutathione. When phase II metabolism is overwhelmed, injurious bioactivated products cause liver injury. Cats are more sensitive to acetaminophen intoxication than dogs because of this relative enzyme deficiency. Other therapeutic drugs are idiosyncratic toxicants, and they affect only a small minority of patients. The mechanism of injury is not known but may be a consequence of inherited differences in hepatic enzyme content and activity, atypical immune reactions to drug metabolites, or novel antigens created when drug metabolites bind to cellular proteins. For example, the antiinflammatory drug carprofen can occasionally cause acute hepatic necrosis in a variety of dogs, but certain breeds of dogs, such as Labrador retrievers, may be affected more often than others. The tranquilizer diazepam can cause acute fatal hepatic injury in some cats, but the majority of treated cats are unaffected, and dogs do not seem to be adversely affected.

Chronic liver toxicity has been described in dogs receiving any of the anticonvulsants—primidone, phenytoin, and phenobarbital—for prolonged periods. The mechanism of hepatotoxicity is unknown. Only a small proportion of dogs receiving these drugs are affected, and these dogs frequently have signs of hepatic failure. The liver is small and has widespread hepatic fibrosis and nodular regeneration (end-stage liver).

Hepatic Injury as a Consequence of Systemic Disease

A variety of extrahepatic disorders, usually affecting the gastrointestinal tract, can result in hepatocellular injury and hepatic dysfunction. Acute hemorrhagic pancreatitis of dogs, for example, sometimes is accompanied by icterus and increased activities of hepatic enzymes in serum. Release of various toxins and inflammatory mediators from the injured pancreas into the portal vein showers the liver with a variety of injurious substances. Similarly, movement of hepatotoxic substances, such as endotoxins, into the portal vein can occur as a consequence of diseases that disrupt the mucosal barrier of the intestine. Some cases of chronic inflammation of the colon can result in chronic hepatic inflammation as well. Accumulation of inflammatory cells within the portal triads may accompany blood-borne infection or abdominal sepsis (nonspecific reactive hepatitis).

The liver is particularly susceptible to the effects of hypoxia; thus any disease that causes anemia can produce centrilobular or paracentral degeneration and necrosis. Also, the hepatocytes in hemolytic anemias must remove and conjugate the increased amounts of circulating bilirubin and hemoglobin, and Kupffer cells must remove either erythrocytes during extravascular hemolysis or erythrocytic fragments during intravascular hemolysis.

Proliferative Lesions of the Liver

A summary of the identification and differentiation of nodular lesions of the liver can be found in Table 8-3.

Hepatocellular Nodular Hyperplasia

Hepatocellular nodular hyperplasia is common only in the dog. The incidence increases with age, starting at approximately 6 years of age, without predilection for either sex or breed. Nodular hyperplasia is not the result or the cause of significant hepatic dysfunction, but nodular hyperplasia should be distinguished from regenerative nodules and hepatic neoplasms, with which they are often confused. Multiple hyperplastic nodules are frequently present. Nodules that can be seen on the capsular surface are typically raised and

Table 8-3 Differentiation of Nodular Lesions in the Liver

Lesion	Species Affected	Gross Appearance	Histologic Appearance
Nodular hyperplasia	Mainly older dogs, occasionally cats	Often multiple Friable Well-demarcated Compressive	Contains all elements of normal lobule Fewer portal tracts and central veins than normal liver Hepatocytes often vacuolated
Regenerative nodules	Mainly dogs, not age-related	Rest of liver is abnormal (fibrotic)	Usually only contain a single portal tract
Hepatocellular adenoma	All species	Usually single Unencapsulated Compressive Red-brown	Well-differentiated hepatocytes Plates 2 or 3 cells thick No portal tracts or central veins
Hepatocellular carcinoma	All species	Usually single Can be large (can involve entire lobe) Intrahepatic metastases may be present Friable White-gray to yellow-brown Subdivided by fibrous bands	Irregular plates >3 cells thick Can have a pseudoglandular pattern Cells can be bizarre Look for invasion at margins
Cholangiocellular adenoma	Most common in cats	Discrete Firm Gray-white Can be cystic Compressive	Well-differentiated biliary epithelium forming tubules Can be cystic Well-developed fibrous stroma
Cholangiocellular carcinoma	All species	Large single mass or multiple nodules Often central depression (umbilicated) Gray-tan Unencapsulated Often see metastasis in other tissues	Well-differentiated have tubular or acinar arrangement Poorly differentiated have solid masses of cells Abundant fibrous stroma Multiple sites of invasion at margins

hemispherical, yellow to tan (although they can be dark red when congested), 0.5 to 3 cm in diameter, and are more friable than normal liver. On incision, the hyperplastic nodules are well demarcated from normal parenchyma and usually compress adjacent parenchyma (Fig. 8-65, *A* and *B*). Hyperplastic nodules contain all the elements of normal liver, but the lobular pattern is distorted. The lobules in areas of nodular hyperplasia contain an increased proportion of hepatocytes and decreased numbers of portal tracts and central veins compared with a normal liver. Hepatocytes are variably sized and frequently contain cytoplasmic lipid or glycogen-containing vacuoles (Fig. 8-65, *C*).

Regenerative Nodules

Regenerative nodules are another type of nodular hepatocellular lesion. Regenerative nodules are unlikely to be related to nodular hyperplasia because regenerative nodules arise from the proliferation of hepatocytes in response to loss of hepatocytes, and the incidence is not related to age. Often the insult is unknown, but the response of some dogs to anticonvulsant drugs, such as phenobarbital or phenytoin, is a well-recognized cause. Regenerative nodules are readily distinguished from nodular hyperplasia because the process occurs in the presence of significant fibrosis and disruption of normal hepatic parenchymal architecture. Because these lesions result from the outgrowth of surviving hepatocytes, there is usually only a single portal tract apparent in sections of the regenerative nodules.

Hepatic Neoplasia

Primary neoplasms of the hepatobiliary system can arise from epithelial elements, including hepatocytes, biliary epithelium of bile ducts or the gallbladder, mesenchymal elements such as connective tissue and blood vessels, and neuroendocrine cells. The liver is a common site of metastasis for many malignant tumors; in fact, the majority of neoplasms within the liver are metastases from other organs.

Hepatocellular Adenoma. Hepatocellular adenomas are benign neoplasms of hepatocytes. Hepatocellular adenomas have been described most commonly in young ruminants, although hepatic adenomas are likely underdiagnosed in older dogs, in which they may be diagnosed as well-differentiated hepatocellular carcinomas. The neoplasms usually are single, unencapsulated, variably sized, and red or brown masses that compress adjacent parenchyma. They are typically spherical but may be pedunculated (Fig. 8-66). They are composed of well-differentiated hepatocytes, which form

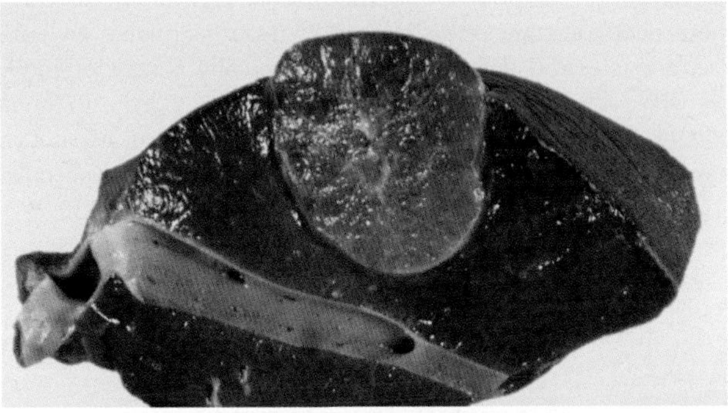

Figure 8-66 **Hepatocellular Adenoma, Liver, Dog.** Hepatocellular adenomas form discrete masses of hepatocytes that compress adjacent normal parenchyma. (Courtesy Dr. J.M. Cullen, College of Veterinary Medicine, North Carolina State University.)

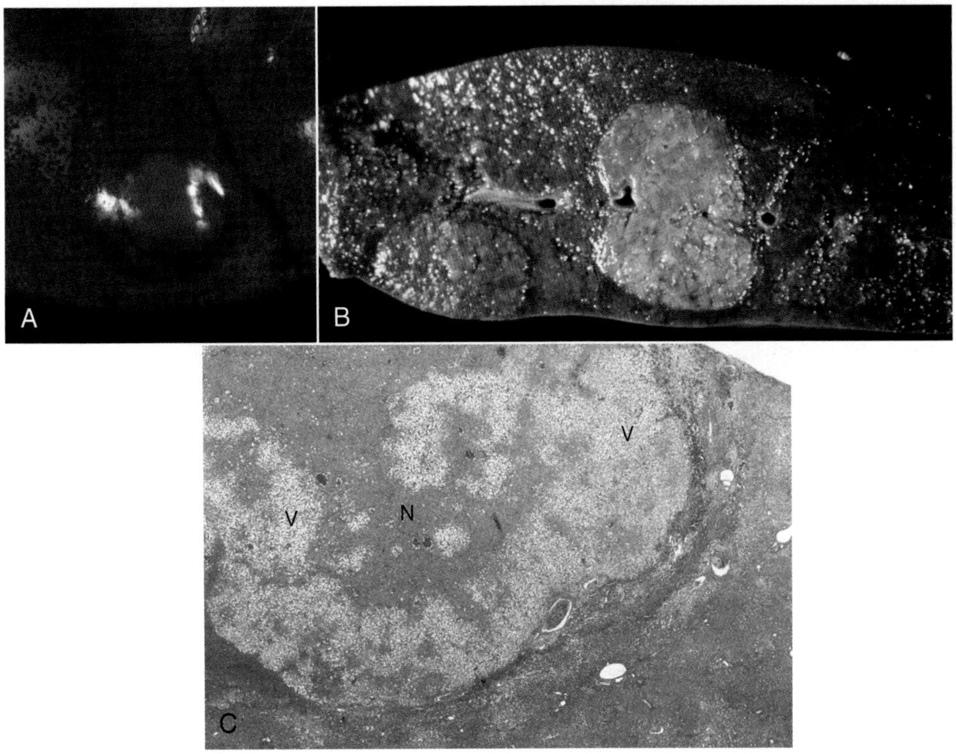

Figure 8-65 **Hepatic Nodular Hyperplasia, Liver, Dog. A,** A nodule protrudes above the surface of the adjacent, normal parenchyma. **B,** Nodular hyperplasia, cut surface of liver. Two pinkish-red hyperplastic nodules are shown. **C,** A single expanding hyperplastic nodule (*N*) compresses adjacent normal hepatocytes, and the hepatocytes of the nodule can be prominently vacuolated (*V*) as in this case. H&E stain. (**A** courtesy Dr. M.D. McGavin, College of Veterinary Medicine, University of Tennessee. **B** courtesy Dr. R. Fairley, Lincoln University. **C** courtesy Dr. J.M. Cullen, College of Veterinary Medicine, North Carolina State University.)

uniform plates that may be two or three cells thick. Hepatic plates in adenomas tend to abut normal adjacent hepatocytes at right angles. Portal tracts and central veins are scarce within the neoplasm, if they can be found at all. Diagnostic criteria to distinguish hepatocellular adenomas from hepatocellular nodular hyperplasia can be somewhat subjective because both arise in livers with no background abnormality, unlike regenerative nodules that arise in damaged livers. Histologically, adenomas are characterized by only one or very few portal tracts, whereas hyperplastic nodules retain normal lobular architecture elements, although the portal tracts are more separated than normal.

Hepatocellular Carcinoma. Hepatocellular carcinomas are malignant neoplasms of hepatocytes. They are uncommon in all domestic species but may occur more frequently in ruminants, particularly sheep, and dogs. Occurrence in cats, pigs, and horses is rare. These neoplasms are often solitary, frequently involve an entire lobe, and are well demarcated. They typically consist of friable, gray-white or yellow-brown tissue, which is subdivided into lobules by multiple fibrous bands (Fig. 8-67, *A*). Malignant hepatocytes characteristically form irregular and variable plates (trabeculae) three or more cells thick, and vascular spaces are present between the trabeculae (see Fig. 8-67, *B*). Crude acini forming a pseudoglandular pattern of neoplastic cells are sometimes present. Within an individual tumor, trabecular, pseudoglandular, and solid patterns may be found. Cells present in the neoplasm range from well-differentiated hepatocytes to atypical or bizarre forms. In the absence of metastasis, which is obviously indicative of malignancy, distinction of well-differentiated carcinoma from adenoma can be difficult, although invasion by malignant hepatocytes at the margin of the adjacent compressed normal hepatocytes, mitotic figures, and hepatocellular atypia are useful indicators of malignancy. Distant metastasis is uncommon but may occur to a variety of sites, particularly to lymph nodes within the cranial abdomen, lungs, and seeding into the tissue of the peritoneal cavity. Some hepatocellular carcinomas extensively spread within the liver (intrahepatic metastasis).

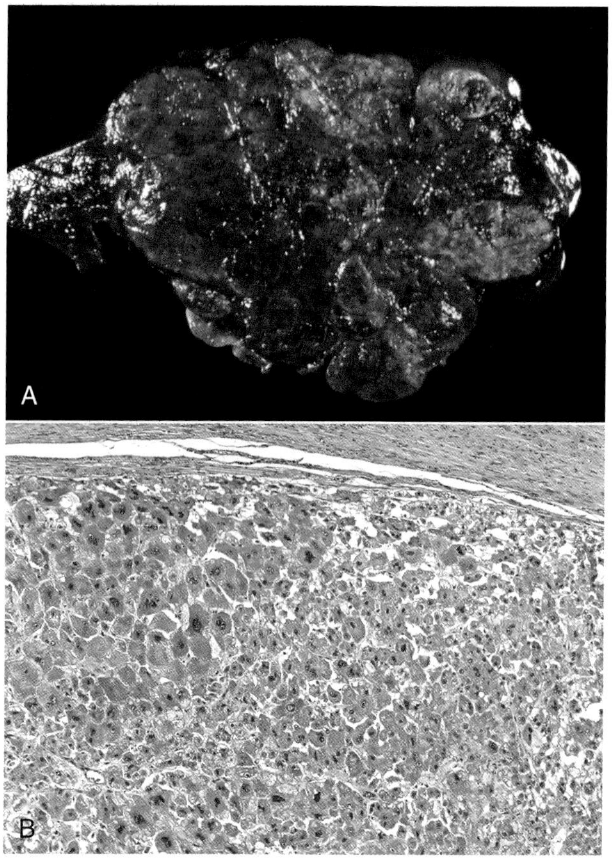

Figure 8-67 Hepatocellular Carcinoma, Liver, Dog. A, A multilobular carcinoma has replaced much of the normal liver. **B,** Hepatocellular carcinomas contain pleomorphic hepatocytes that can form trabeculae, a glandular-like pattern or solid sheets of cells, as in this case. H&E stain. (**A** courtesy College of Veterinary Medicine, North Carolina State University. **B** courtesy Dr. J.M. Cullen, College of Veterinary Medicine, North Carolina State University.)

Intrahepatic Biliary Neoplasia

Cholangiocellular (Bile Duct) Adenoma. Adenomas of the biliary ducts are uncommon in most species. They are usually discrete, firm, and gray or white masses consisting of well-differentiated biliary epithelium. Cholangiomas are glandlike structures formed by tubules lined with cuboidal epithelium and moderate amounts of stroma. The tubules may have narrow lumens or may be distended by fluid-forming cystic structures of variable sizes. Hepatocytes are usually compressed at the margins and not entrapped by expanding cysts. Cystic variants, termed *biliary cystadenomas* by some, are more likely developmental anomalies of the biliary tree.

Congenital biliary cysts are multiloculated and can involve extensive areas of the liver. Typically, they have flattened epithelium and varying amounts of fibrous tissue, and islands of hepatocytes are often scattered between the cysts.

Cholangiocellular (Bile Duct) Carcinoma. Cholangiocellular carcinomas are malignant neoplasms of biliary epithelium, which usually arise from the intrahepatic ducts, but extrahepatic bile ducts can be affected. These neoplasms occur in all species. A large single mass or multiple nodules may be present within the liver; these typically are firm, raised, often with a central depression (umbilicated), pale gray to tan, and unencapsulated (Fig. 8-68, *A*). The tumors are composed of cells that retain a resemblance to biliary epithelium. Characteristically, well-differentiated carcinomas are organized into a tubular or acinar arrangement. In less differentiated neoplasms, some acinar arrangements can be detected among solid masses of neoplastic cells. Poorly differentiated carcinomas are composed of packets, islands, or cords, and areas of squamous differentiation can occur. The epithelial components of the neoplasms are usually separated by fibrous connective tissue (see Fig. 8-68, *B*). The amount of connective tissue varies among tumors, but an abundant deposition of collagen, termed a *scirrhous response*, is relatively common and is responsible for the firm texture of these neoplasms. The margins of cholangiocarcinomas are characterized by multiple sites of local invasion by tumor cells of surrounding hepatic parenchyma. Multiple sites of hepatic necrosis are also common in the adjacent parenchyma.

Metastasis to extrahepatic sites is common, particularly to the adjacent lymph nodes of the cranial abdomen, lungs, or by seeding into the abdominal cavity. Metastasis into the peritoneal cavity can produce variably sized nodules within the mesentery and on the serosal surface of the abdominal viscera. A unique cutaneous paraneoplastic syndrome can be observed in cats with pancreatic adenocarcinoma or cholangiocarcinoma. This syndrome manifests grossly as symmetric alopecia of the ventral trunk and limbs with a glistening appearance. Histologically, affected areas have marked follicular

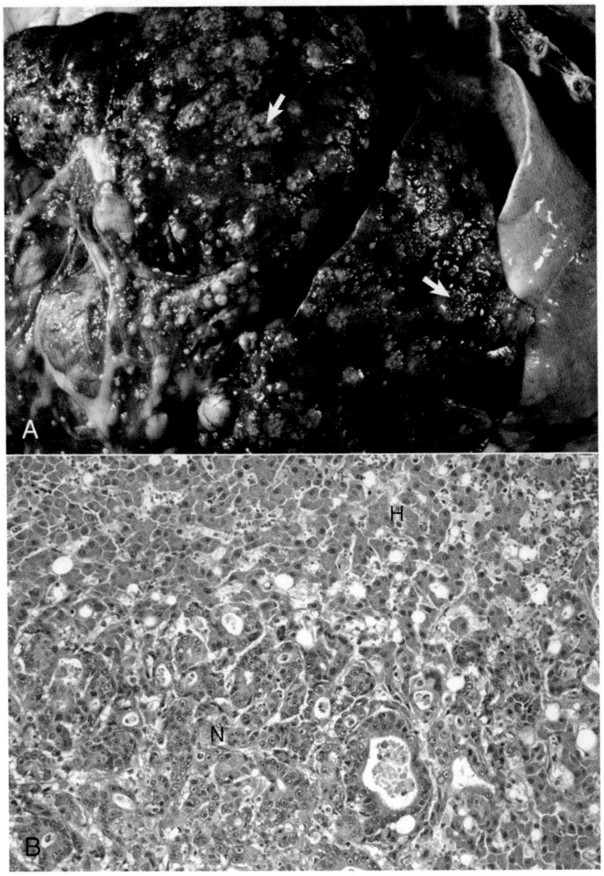

Figure 8-68 **Cholangiocellular (Bile Duct) Carcinoma, Liver. A,** Dog. Multiple nodules of tumor, some of which are umbilicated *(arrows)*. **B,** Cat. Cords and acini of neoplastic bile duct epithelial cells *(N)* invade the adjacent normal hepatic parenchyma *(H)*. H&E stain. (**A** courtesy Dr. M.D. McGavin, College of Veterinary Medicine, University of Tennessee. **B** courtesy Dr. J. Simon, College of Veterinary Medicine, University of Illinois.)

and adnexal atrophy and loss of the stratum corneum of the epidermis.

Carcinoids

Carcinoids are uncommon tumors that are believed to arise from neuroendocrine cells that lie within the biliary epithelium. They can form within the intrahepatic or extrahepatic biliary system. Often, they form a single mass, but multiple nodules can occur, probably secondary to intrahepatic metastasis. Cells tend to be small, elongated, or spindle-shaped and form ribbons or rosettes (Fig. 8-69). Immunohistochemical detection of neuroendocrine markers, such as chromogranin A, can be used to confirm the diagnosis.

Miscellaneous Primary Mesenchymal Neoplasms of the Liver

Primary neoplasms can arise from any of the cellular constituents of the liver, including mesenchymal neoplasms derived from the liver's connective tissue (fibrosarcoma, leiomyosarcoma, and osteosarcoma) and endothelium (hemangioma and hemangiosarcoma). Primary hepatic hemangiosarcoma is well recognized in dogs, although it is a relatively uncommon site of origin for this neoplasm compared with the skin, spleen, and heart. Primary mesenchymal neoplasms of the liver must be distinguished from metastases; the presence of disseminated masses throughout the liver is more typical of metastatic sarcomas than of primary hepatic sarcomas.

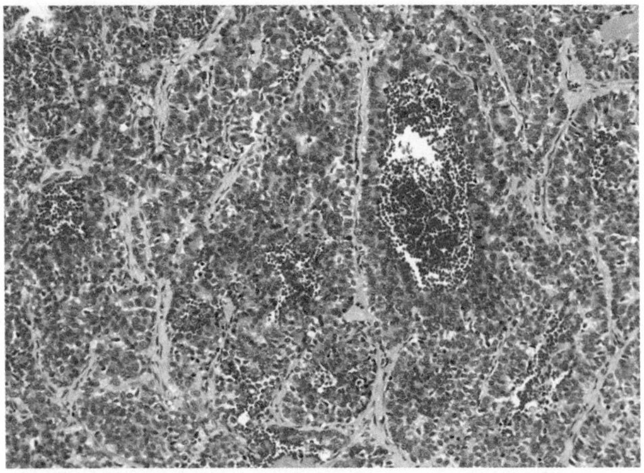

Figure 8-69 **Neuroendocrine Tumors, Carcinoid, Liver, Dog.** Carcinoids are malignant neoplasms of neuroendocrine cells, including those of the liver or bile ducts. Histologically, the tumor is composed of small elongated or spindle-shaped basophilic cells that form ribbons or rosettes and contain numerous vascular spaces. H&E stain. See Chapter 12 and Figs. 12-45 and 12-46 for more information on carcinoids (β-cell adenoma). (Courtesy Dr. J.M. Cullen, College of Veterinary Medicine, North Carolina State University.)

Metastatic Neoplasms

The liver and the lung are the two most common sites for metastatic spread of malignant neoplasms. Metastatic neoplasms must be distinguished from primary hyperplasia or neoplasia of the hepatobiliary tissue. Therefore, when evaluating a neoplasm within the liver, it is important to determine if a neoplasm is present at some extrahepatic site that might be the primary neoplasm. The animal's medical history should also be reviewed to determine if masses have been removed previously. Malignant lymphoma is the most common metastatic neoplasm found in the liver of most, if not all, species.

Some metastatic neoplasms have a typical appearance within the liver; for example, melanomas frequently are black because of the presence of melanin, and hemangiosarcomas are usually dark red to brown because of blood. Hematopoietic neoplasms, such as lymphoma and the myeloproliferative disorders, can diffusely expand the liver and can be diffusely infiltrative (Fig. 8-70, A), producing hepatomegaly and an enhanced lobular pattern on the cut surface, or may have a nodular appearance (see Fig. 8-70, B). This characteristic appearance of diffuse involvement is attributable to centrilobular hepatocellular degeneration because of anemia in both lymphoma and myeloproliferative disorders and because of the specific location of accumulations of neoplastic cells; locations include portal and periportal for lymphomas (see Fig. 8-70, C) and sinusoidal for myeloproliferative disorders. Metastatic carcinomas often have an umbilicated appearance similar to that seen with cholangiocellular carcinomas, but umbilication is rarely a feature of sarcomas.

Hepatosplenic and Hepatocytotropic T Cell Lymphoma

Two distinct types of T cell lymphoma, described mainly in dogs, involve the liver in the absence of peripheral lymphadenopathy: hepatosplenic lymphoma and hepatocytotropic lymphoma. In hepatosplenic lymphoma, neoplastic lymphocytes are centered on the hepatic and splenic sinusoids, and affected animals present with hepato- and/or splenomegaly, regenerative anemia, thrombocytopenia, and hypoproteinemia. In hepatocytotropic lymphoma, the neoplastic cells are present within hepatic cords in addition to sinusoids. Bone marrow and lungs are consistently but variably involved in hepatosplenic lymphoma.

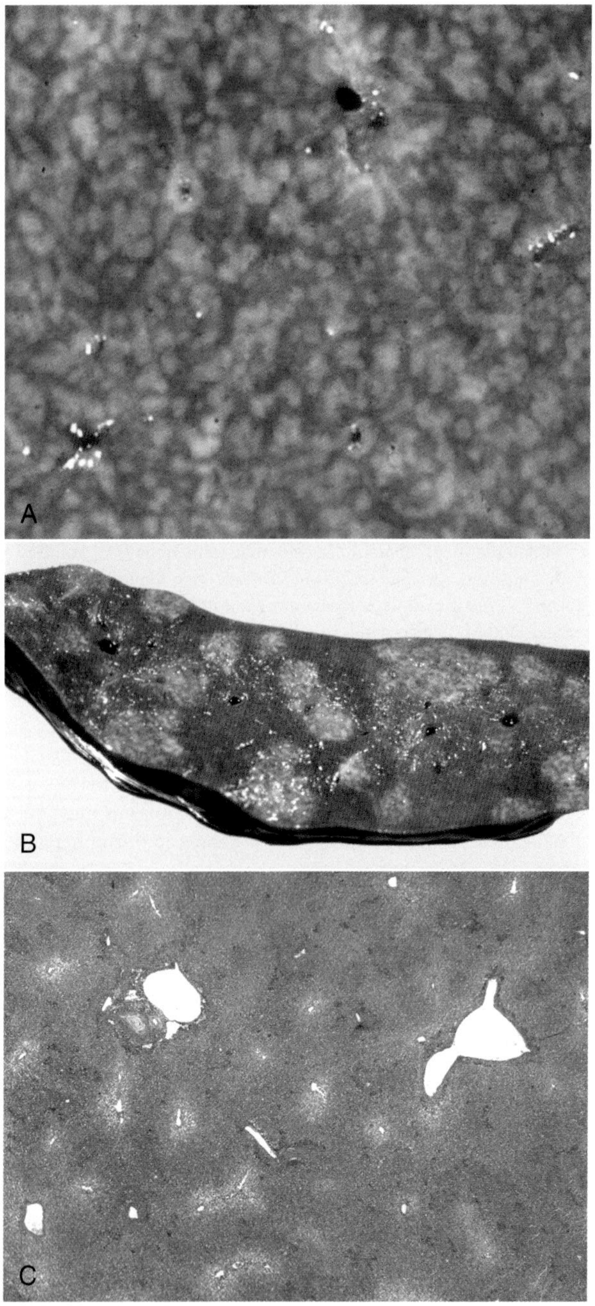

Figure 8-70 Hepatic Lymphoma, Liver. A, Cut surface, high magnification, dog. The entire liver is enlarged (not shown here), and there are multiple pale gray-white foci caused by infiltrating neoplastic lymphocytes. The regular distribution of neoplastic foci apparent on the cut surface is due to the preferential infiltration of the portal tracts by neoplastic cells. **B,** Cow. As shown here, hepatic lymphoma can have a nodular rather than a diffuse pattern, as seen in Fig. 8-70, *A*. **C,** Dog. Neoplastic lymphocytes *(blue areas)* are typically distributed within and around the portal tracts and central veins. H&E stain. See Chapter 6 and Figs. 6-3, 6-9, and 6-13 and E-Figure 6-3 for more information on lymphomas. (**A** and **C** courtesy Dr. J.M. Cullen, College of Veterinary Medicine, North Carolina State University. **B** courtesy College of Veterinary Medicine, University of Illinois.)

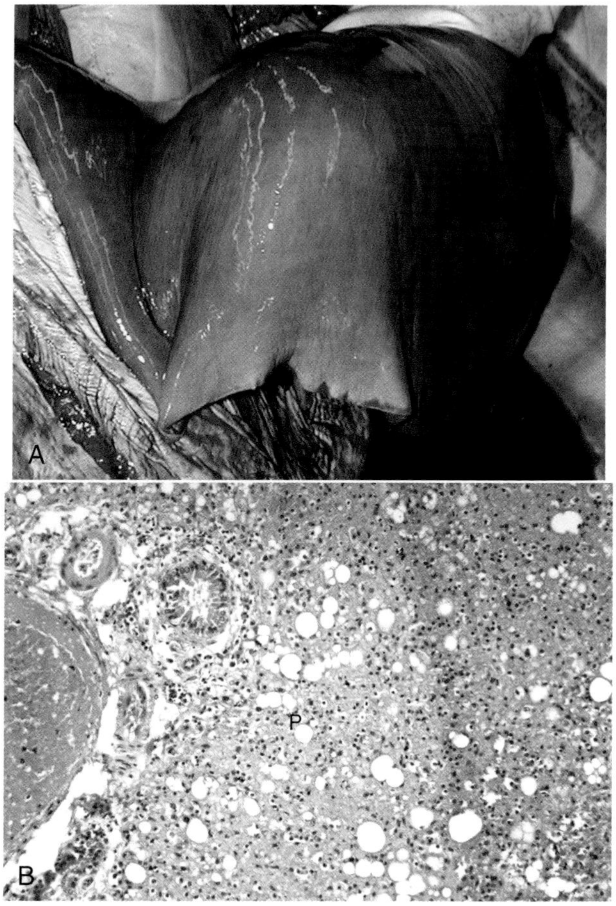

Figure 8-71 Equine Serum Hepatitis, Liver, Horse. A, Livers from horses affected with equine serum hepatitis can be small, flabby, and pale or discolored by bile pigment. **B,** In horses with equine serum hepatitis, most hepatocytes are necrotic, although there may be a few remaining hepatocytes with lipid-containing vacuoles in the periportal regions *(P)*. Inflammation consists of mononuclear cells predominantly. H&E stain. (**A** courtesy Dr. K. Bailey, College of Veterinary Medicine, University of Illinois. **B** courtesy Dr. J.M. Cullen, College of Veterinary Medicine, North Carolina State University.)

Disorders of Horses

Equine Serum Hepatitis

Equine serum hepatitis was first described by Theiler in South Africa at the beginning of the twentieth century but is now recognized in many countries. It occurs frequently but not invariably in horses that have received an injection of a biologic that contains equine serum—for example, equine antisera such as tetanus antitoxin or pregnant mare serum gonadotropin. Recent studies have investigated the possibility of an infectious etiology; however, a causative infectious agent has not been definitively identified. The incubation period is prolonged, but the clinical course of the disease is very rapid and is invariably fatal. Affected horses typically have hepatic failure, which manifests as hepatic encephalopathy and icterus. Intravascular hemolysis occurs in the terminal stages of the disease. The livers of affected animals may be normal size or even enlarged but are typically small, flabby, and discolored greenish brown to dark brown (Fig. 8-71, *A*). The liver of affected animals has an enhanced lobular pattern because of diffuse centrilobular degeneration and necrosis of hepatocytes and subsequent congestion of these necrotic areas (see Fig. 8-71, *B*). Frequently, only narrow rims of periportal hepatocytes survive, and these cells may be prominently vacuolated with lipid. The centrilobular areas usually contain only remnants of necrotic hepatocytes, apoptotic bodies, pigmented Kupffer cells, and dilated sinusoids. Sometimes the portal areas contain proliferating tubules or columns of small basophilic cells, which are probably a regenerative response of bipotential hepatic progenitor cells, termed a *ductular reaction*.

Equine Hepatocellular Steatosis

A form of hepatocellular steatosis occurs in ponies, miniatures horses, and donkeys. Shetland ponies and donkeys are predisposed. The condition usually occurs in overweight pregnant or lactating mares, characteristically after an event that causes stress or anorexia. In addition to notable hepatocellular steatosis, affected ponies are usually hyperlipemic and may also manifest signs of renal failure and hepatic rupture. In severe cases, hepatic encephalopathy and/or terminal DIC can occur. Mechanisms of hepatocellular steatosis have been discussed previously.

Disorders of Ruminants (Cattle, Sheep, and Goats)

Ketosis

Ketosis is a metabolic disease that results from impaired metabolism of carbohydrates and volatile fatty acids. In times of energy demand, free fatty acids are released from body fat stores, and the free fatty acids are esterified into fatty acyl CoA in the liver. Ketone bodies (acetoacetic acid and β-hydroxybutyric acid) are derived from fatty acyl CoA by oxidation in the mitochondria. In pregnant and lactating animals, there is a continuous demand for glucose and amino acids, and ketosis results when fat metabolism, which occurs in response to the increased energy demands, becomes excessive. Ketosis is characterized by increased concentrations of ketone bodies in blood (hyperketonemia), hypoglycemia, and low concentrations of hepatic glycogen. Ketosis is common in ruminants and usually occurs during peak lactation, whereas ketosis of sheep usually occurs in late gestation, particularly in ewes carrying twins; this latter disease is known as pregnancy toxemia.

Bovine Fatty Liver Syndrome

Bovine fatty liver syndrome, also known as *fatty liver disease*, is mechanistically similar to ketosis and is especially common in ruminants with high energy demands. In dairy cattle, the disease is usually encountered in obese animals in late gestation, within a few days after parturition or peak lactation, and is often precipitated by an event that causes anorexia, such as retained placenta, metritis, mastitis, abomasal displacement, or parturient paresis. In beef cattle, affected animals are typically overweight and the disease occurs within a few days before parturition. Accumulation of lipid within the liver is the result of both increased mobilization of lipids from adipose tissue, which results in increased influx of fatty acids to the liver, and, in severe cases, defective hepatocytic function, which results in decreased export of lipoprotein from the liver.

Copper Toxicosis

In ruminants, particularly sheep, copper can accumulate within the liver over a period of time due to dietary excess or insufficient molybdenum to antagonize bioavailability of copper. When such sheep ingest hepatotoxins, such as pyrrolizidine-containing plants or mycotoxins, the resultant hepatocellular injury can, when sufficiently serious, trigger a sudden release of copper, which is followed by acute, severe intravascular hemolysis and additional hepatocellular necrosis, mostly because of acute anemia. Necrosis of the liver is extensive and affects centrilobular and midzonal regions most consistently because of hypoxia, but massive necrosis can occur in severe cases. Affected animals are icteric with swollen pale to orange livers, and hemoglobinuria is prominent. Despite the acute and fulminant nature of the terminal event, this process is referred to as *chronic copper poisoning* to distinguish it from disease caused by simple copper intoxication that causes gastroenteritis.

Rift Valley Fever

Rift Valley fever is an acute, arthropod (mosquito)-transmitted zoonotic viral disease that principally affects ruminants, causing extensive mortality among calves and lambs and abortion in ewes and cows, although adults can also be affected. The causative virus is a member of the family Bunyaviridae in the genus *Phlebovirus*. The disease is enzootic in southern and eastern Africa, but significant outbreaks can spread throughout much of Africa and extend into the Middle East. It is especially prevalent after periods of unusually high rainfall. Disease manifestations are typically more severe in the epidemic outbreaks than in enzootic cases. In severe cases, affected animals are febrile, may abort, and have respiratory and gastrointestinal signs, including prominent diarrhea. Mortality is highest in sheep, with lambs most severely affected, but even in cattle up to one-third of calves may die.

Hepatic involvement is consistently present in fulminant cases, typically in neonates, and is characterized by hepatomegaly with a yellow-orange discoloration. Areas of congestion may be present. In older animals, pale, 1- to 2-mm randomly scattered foci of hepatocellular necrosis impart a mottled appearance and sometimes an enhanced lobular pattern. Microscopic lesions are characterized by the presence of both randomly distributed foci of hepatocellular necrosis and apoptosis. Secondarily, more widespread zonal necrosis, which ranges from centrilobular to midzonal, can develop (Fig. 8-72). These lesions, particularly random hepatic necrosis, are more severe and widespread in young animals and aborted fetuses. Fibrin deposition within sinusoids is common, but cholestasis is not a consistent feature. Eosinophilic intranuclear inclusion bodies may be present in degenerate hepatocytes in areas of necrosis.

Diffuse petechiae and ecchymoses are also characteristic of the disease, as are edema and hemorrhages of the intestinal tract and the wall of the gallbladder. DIC probably contributes to the hemorrhagic diathesis and perhaps to the development of zonal hepatic necrosis.

Wesselsbron Disease

Wesselsbron disease of sheep is caused by Wesselsbron virus, a flavivirus, and like Rift Valley fever, is a zoonotic arthropod (mosquito)-transmitted viral disease that occurs in Africa. The virus can cause

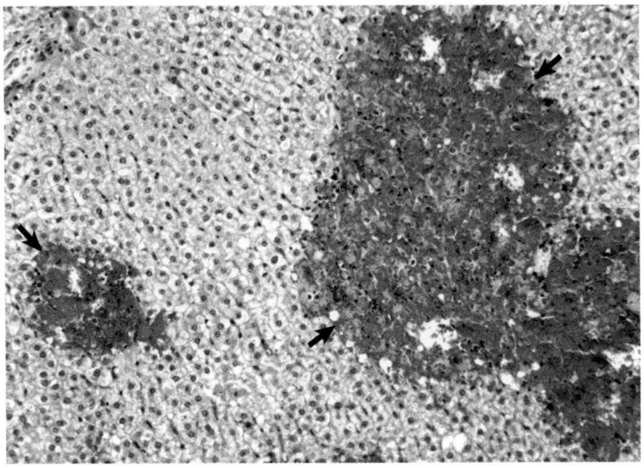

Figure 8-72 Focal Hepatic Necrosis, Rift Valley Fever, Liver, Sheep. This disease produces randomly distributed focal areas of necrosis *(arrows)* in the liver of lambs and fetuses, often with a central area of older necrosis surrounded by a rim of hepatocytes, which have been killed at a later stage in the infection. H&E stain. (Courtesy Armed Forces Institute of Pathology.)

disease in newborn lambs and abortion in ewes, but adults rarely have apparent clinical signs. Affected lambs have multifocal areas of generalized petechiae, intestinal hemorrhage, and an enlarged pale to orange liver. Icterus may develop. Canalicular cholestasis is often apparent and is occasionally prominent. Scattered individual hepatocyte and sinusoidal lining cell necrosis accompanied with pigmented macrophages and mononuclear inflammatory cells within the parenchyma are typical. Eosinophilic inclusions can be found in hepatocytes. In Wesselsbron disease, foci of hepatic necrosis are typically less extensive than in Rift Valley fever, although cholestasis is usually more prominent.

Bacillary Hemoglobinuria

Bacillary hemoglobinuria is an acute and highly fatal disease of cattle and sheep that occurs in various areas of the world and can be endemic in those regions in which liver fluke, particularly *Fasciola hepatica*, infection also occurs. Spores of *Clostridium haemolyticum*, the causative agent of bacillary hemoglobinuria, are ingested and come to reside within Kupffer cells, but they proliferate only in areas of low oxygen tension. Migration of immature liver flukes, or less commonly other parasites, or an event such as liver biopsy produces a nidus of necrotic hepatic parenchyma in which bacterial spores can germinate. Bacteria proliferate and release exotoxins, including the beta toxin phospholipase C, which induces the hepatocellular necrosis, intravascular hemolysis, anemia, and hemoglobinuria that characterize the disease. Grossly, these foci (or often a large single lesion), which have been misnamed infarcts, are sharply delineated from the adjacent parenchyma and usually are pale and surrounded by an intensely hyperemic zone (Fig. 8-73). The causative organisms, Gram-positive spore-containing rods, may be visible in histologic sections. Migration tracts of the immature flukes that typically precipitate the disease may be present. Serous cavities (pleura, peritoneum, and pericardium) can be flecked with fibrin.

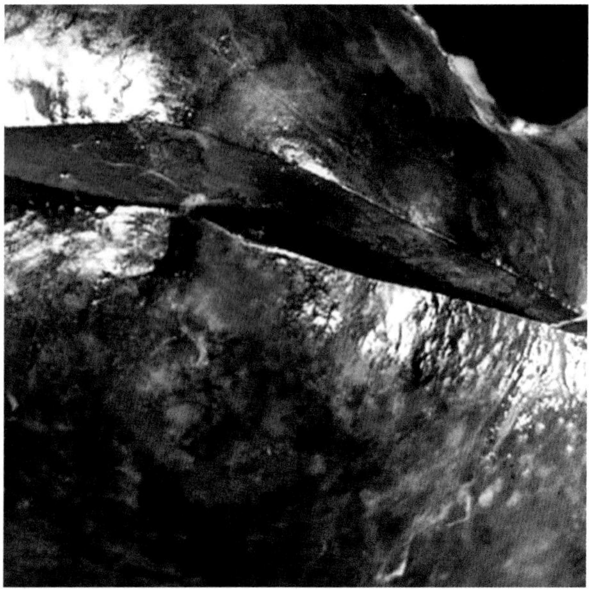

Figure 8-73 Focal Hepatic Necrosis, *Clostridium Haemolyticum* (Bacillary Hemoglobinuria), Liver, Cut Surface, Cow. These large areas of necrosis are sharply delineated from the adjacent parenchyma, usually pale, and surrounded by an intensely hyperemic zone of acute inflammation. (Courtesy Dr. J. King, College of Veterinary Medicine, Cornell University.)

Infectious Necrotic Hepatitis

Infectious necrotic hepatitis, also known as black disease, is most common in sheep and cattle but also occurs in pigs and horses. This disease is somewhat analogous to bacillary hemoglobinuria in that dormant spores of *Clostridium*—in this circumstance, *Clostridium novyi* (type B)—germinate in areas of lowered oxygen tension and release exotoxins that produce discrete foci of coagulation necrosis and hemorrhage within the liver, hemolysis, and eventually death of the host. In endemic areas, germination of spores is usually initiated by hepatic necrosis caused by the migration of immature liver flukes; however, a variety of other initiating factors that produce low oxygen tension within the liver parenchyma have been described. Parasitic migration tracts are usually present within the affected liver. Other lesions that may be present include diffuse venous congestion and accumulation of fluid within the pericardial sac and pleural and peritoneal cavities. Affected animals typically have one or more areas of hepatocellular necrosis, which usually manifests as discrete, pale areas of variable size. A zone of intense hyperemia often surrounds these foci. Histologically, well-demarcated areas of necrosis with peripheral neutrophils and subjacent, abundant Gram-positive rods within the necrotic areas are found. The carcass of affected animals typically putrefies rapidly because of high fever before death.

White Liver Disease

White liver disease derives its name from the pale, fatty livers in sheep that develop from a nutritional deficiency caused by insufficient cobalt intake. Animals grazing on soil that is depleted in cobalt either by natural deficiency or by previous use of the area for plants, such as potatoes, that deplete soil of cobalt are affected. Cobalt is a necessary cofactor in the synthesis of vitamin B_{12} and other enzymes. Deficiency of vitamin B_{12} can lead to anemia, and the liver lesions may be attributed to the effects of anemia.

Disorders of Pigs

Hepatosis Dietetica

Hepatosis dietetica (nutritional hepatic necrosis) is a syndrome of acute hepatic necrosis that occurs in young, rapidly growing pigs. It is but one manifestation of a variety of disorders that are likely to be at least in part caused by deficiency of vitamin E and/or selenium. The pathogenesis of hepatosis dietetica is incompletely defined. Although it is apparent that affected animals respond to the provision of vitamin E or selenium, it has been difficult, on an experimental basis, to produce the syndrome consistently by feeding diets deficient in vitamin E and selenium. Because vitamin E and selenium-containing enzymes are antagonists of free radical formation and are therefore important for the maintenance of stability and integrity of cellular membranes, it is believed that oxidative injury leads to hepatocyte necrosis.

Regions of massive necrosis in the affected liver are initially distended, deep red, and friable. Hepatosis dietetica is characterized by hemorrhagic centrilobular to massive hepatic necrosis (Fig. 8-74, A and B). The appearance of the liver reflects the extent of hepatic necrosis, the severity of the hemorrhage, and the duration of the deficiency. Later, in animals that survive the acute disease, parenchymal collapse and dense tracts of connective tissue (postnecrotic scarring) are usually evident.

Cresols

Cresols once were incorporated in clay pigeons and asphalt shingles. If pigs ingest cresols, centrilobular to massive hepatic hemorrhage

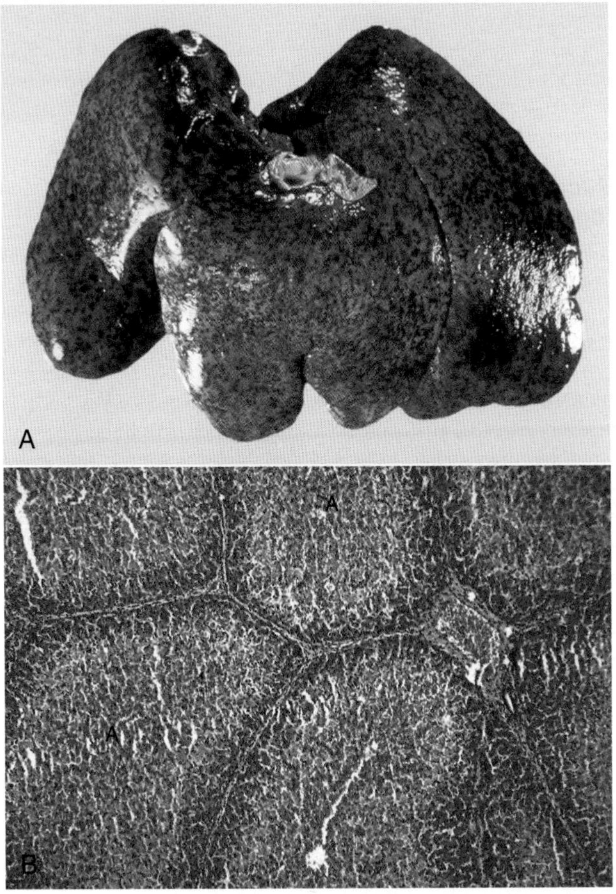

Figure 8-74 **Massive Necrosis, Hepatosis Dietetica, Liver, Pig. A,** Areas of hemorrhagic centrilobular necrosis and massive necrosis appear as dark regions of different size scattered throughout the liver. **B,** Acute centrilobular necrosis *(A)* is the principal lesion of this disorder. (**A** courtesy Dr. R. Michel, College of Veterinary Medicine, University of Tennessee. **B** courtesy College of Veterinary Medicine, North Carolina State University; Dr. A.R. Doster, University of Nebraska; and Noah's Arkive, College of Veterinary Medicine, The University of Georgia.)

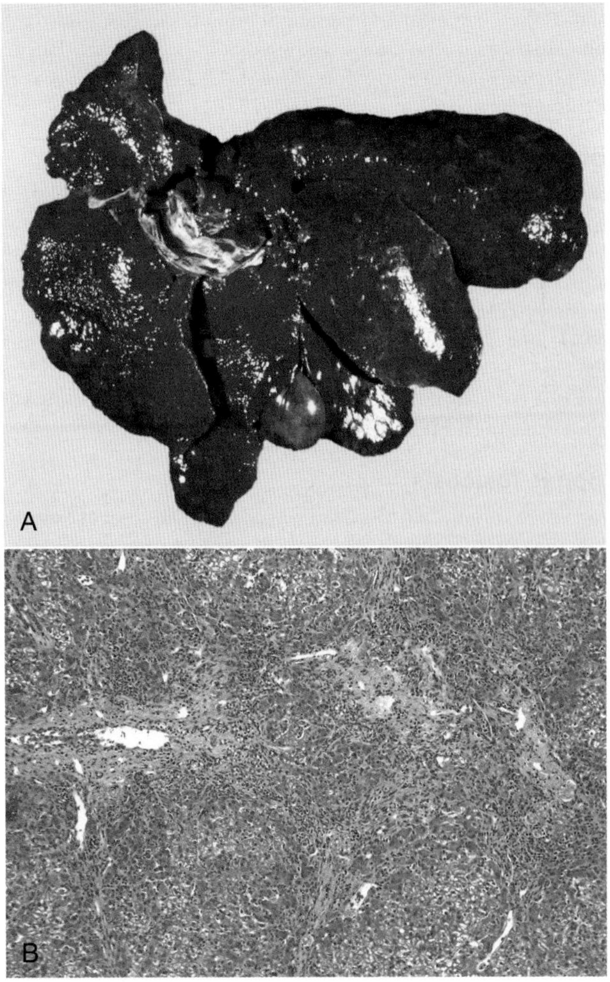

Figure 8-75 **Chronic Hepatitis. A,** Liver, diaphragmatic surface, dog. The liver is characterized by scattered regenerative nodules of different sizes and extensive fibrosis that gives the liver an irregular surface. **B,** End-stage liver with chronic hepatitis (also see Fig. 8-29). The liver lobular architecture is replaced by irregular nodules of regenerative parenchyma separated by tracts of connective tissue with an inflammatory infiltrate and pigment accumulation. H&E stain. (**A** courtesy College of Veterinary Medicine, University of Illinois. **B** courtesy Dr. J.M. Cullen, College of Veterinary Medicine, North Carolina State University.)

and necrosis result, a pattern that can also be seen in pigs with hepatosis dietetica or in those that ingest cottonseed meal.

Disorders of Dogs

Canine Chronic Hepatitis (Chronic-Active Hepatitis)

Chronic hepatitis in dogs is poorly understood. The terminology of this entity, in keeping with the inflammatory process, has been a persistent topic of dispute. *Chronic-active hepatitis* is a descriptive term that has been used to identify a particular pattern of inflammation in the human liver. Originally, the purpose of this classification was to identify hepatic lesions, regardless of cause, that were predictive of a progressive course of inflammation and fibrosis. This term was adopted by veterinary pathologists and used to indicate hepatic disorders of the dog that have microscopic changes similar to those seen in human livers. Based on usage, the term *chronic-active hepatitis* has incorrectly evolved from a morphologic description into a disease entity. The appropriateness and usefulness of this designation is conjectural in human beings and dogs. Recent publications in the medical literature have argued that this terminology should be abandoned because it is no longer regarded as useful in predicting the course of liver disease, and it ignores the cause of the liver inflammation. Accordingly, the term *chronic hepatitis* is preferred to describe this entity in dogs.

Chronic hepatitis, with modifiers indicating the type and degree of inflammation and fibrosis, is used to fully characterize the activity and stage of the lesion. If the cause of the inflammation is known, it should be included in the diagnosis. The cause of most of the spontaneous cases of canine chronic hepatitis is uncertain. Some cases have been hypothesized to be caused by leptospira infection or experimental canine adenovirus I infection. Immune-mediated, toxin, or drug-related mechanisms and metabolic abnormalities with breed predispositions have also been described.

Excessive copper retention is the best characterized and the most common recognizable cause of chronic hepatitis in dogs and is discussed in detail later.

The liver in cases of chronic hepatitis is usually small, often with an accentuated lobular pattern; severely affected livers are characterized by architectural distortion, which ranges from a coarsely nodular texture to an end-stage liver (Fig. 8-75, A). Chronic hepatitis, depending on the duration of inflammation and injury, is characterized by portal and periportal mononuclear cell inflammation, intrahepatic cholestasis, and fibrosis of portal areas that may extend into adjacent periportal areas of the lobule, leading to the prominent lobular pattern (see Fig. 8-75, *B*).

Lobular Dissecting Hepatitis

Lobular dissecting hepatitis is a form of cirrhosis usually seen in young dogs. The condition is frequently fatal and has no known cause. Affected livers tend to be smooth and small, rather than the multinodular livers seen in typical cirrhosis. Histologically, the livers are characterized by fine septa with increased fibrosis that dissect the hepatic plates, distort the lobular architecture, and isolate small aggregates or individual hepatocytes (Fig. 8-76). Inflammation in the tissue is usually mild to moderate, and the inflamed area contains mononuclear cell infiltrates.

Copper Toxicosis

Progressive chronic hepatitis has been described in cases of excessive copper retention leading to toxicosis in a variety of breeds. Bedlington terriers are the only breed with a recognized mutation linked to the disorder. Copper accumulates continuously in the livers of Bedlington terriers shown to have a mutation (deletion of exon 2) or other mutations in the COMMD1 gene, which encodes a chaperone protein involved in copper excretion by hepatocytes. Several breeds appear to have a familiar involvement with copper retention, including Dobermans, Labrador retrievers, Skye terriers, West Highland white terriers, and Dalmatians. The cause of the abnormal concentrations of hepatic copper is not well understood, but it is likely related to dietary copper intake. Although copper is excreted in bile, extrahepatic cholestasis does not seem to significantly increase hepatic copper levels. Copper can be detected within hepatocytes and in macrophage or Kupffer cell aggregates using special stains such as rhodanine. Copper accumulates in the centrilobular regions of the liver and leads to ongoing necrosis of hepatocytes, chronic inflammation, replacement fibrosis, and eventually to an end-stage liver and signs of hepatic failure (Fig. 8-77).

The significance of copper in the development of chronic hepatic disease is not always clear, and the level of copper and intensity of hepatic injury do not always correlate. Some dogs may have an idiopathic chronic hepatitis rather than injury driven by copper retention. As a general rule, hepatic copper concentrations of more than 2000 ppm dry weight are expected before liver disease can clearly be attributed to copper retention.

Glucocorticoid-Induced Hepatocellular Degeneration (Steroid Hepatopathy)

Glucocorticoid-induced hepatocellular degeneration is a specific disorder characterized by excessive hepatic accumulation of glycogen (Fig. 8-78, *A*). Glucocorticoids induce glycogen synthetase and so enhance hepatic storage of glycogen. Glycogen accumulation leads to pronounced swelling of hepatocytes (up to 10 times normal volume), particularly those in the midzonal areas (see Fig. 8-78, *B*). In severe cases of glucocorticoid-induced hepatocellular degeneration (often referred to as *steroid-induced hepatopathy*), the liver is enlarged and pale but otherwise unremarkable. The disorder occurs in dogs and frequently is iatrogenic but can also be a consequence of hyperadrenocorticism. The diagnosis can be confirmed on the basis of the characteristic microscopic appearance of the liver and identification of the source of the excess glucocorticoids.

Infectious Canine Hepatitis

Infectious canine hepatitis is, as the name implies, a viral infection of the liver of dogs and other canids, including foxes and coyotes. The disease is caused by *canine adenovirus 1*. The majority of infections are asymptomatic, and infections that result in disease may not be fatal. Young dogs, in the first 2 years of life, are more likely to die of the infection than older dogs. The virus has a predilection for hepatocytes, vascular endothelium, and mesothelium; fulminant disease is characterized by hepatic necrosis and widespread serosal hemorrhage that can affect a variety of organs.

Exposure of susceptible dogs is most often via the oral route by contact with urine from infected dogs. Viremia lasts for 4 to 8 days, but virus is shed in the urine of infected dogs for prolonged periods. Virus multiplication initially occurs in the tonsils and produces tonsillitis, which can be severe, with spread to local lymph nodes and then to the systemic circulation. Viremia is associated with leukopenia and fever. Spread of virus to the liver, endothelial cells, and mesothelial cells follows. Infection of Kupffer cells may precede

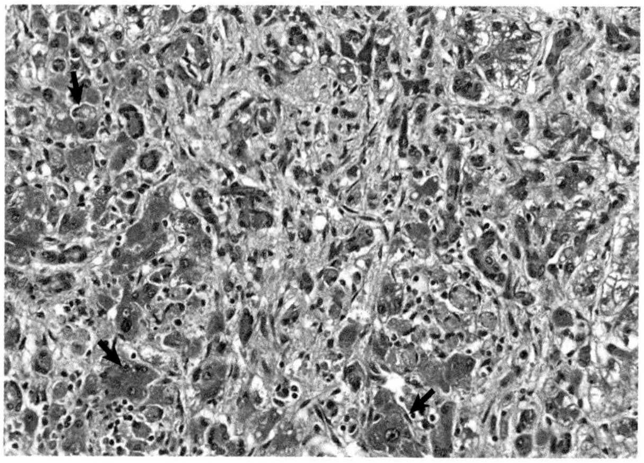

Figure 8-76 **Lobular Dissecting Hepatitis, Liver, Dog.** Lobular dissecting hepatitis is a form of end-stage liver characterized microscopically by fine septa of extracellular matrix (chiefly collagen) that divide hepatocyte plates into small clusters or individual hepatocytes *(arrows)*. Because of the disruption of blood flow through the liver and the failure of hepatocytes to come in contact with blood, there is profound hepatic dysfunction. H&E stain. (Courtesy Dr. J.M. Cullen, College of Veterinary Medicine, North Carolina State University.)

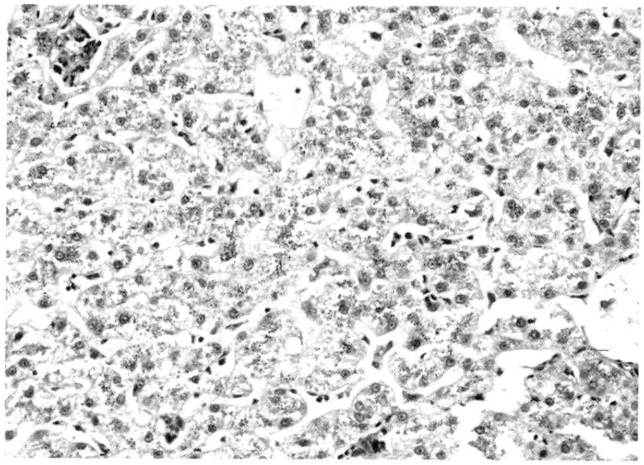

Figure 8-77 **Hepatic Copper, Liver, Dog.** The red-brown copper-containing granules are indicative of excess copper in the lysosomes of hepatocytes. Copper is not readily visible with H&E staining but can be confirmed by special stains. Rhodanine stain. (Courtesy Dr. J.M. Cullen, College of Veterinary Medicine, North Carolina State University.)

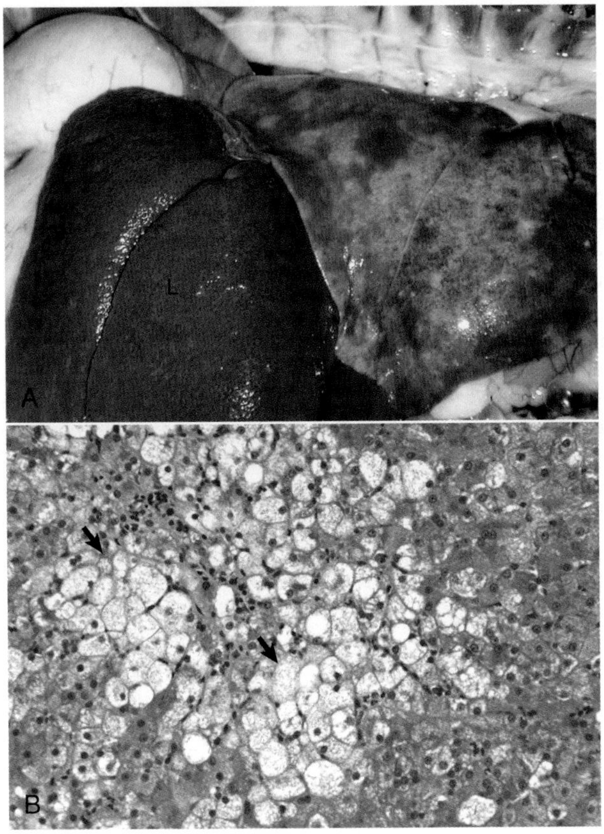

Figure 8-78 **Glucocorticoid-induced Hepatopathy, Liver, Dog. A,** In dogs with glucocorticoid excess (Cushing's disease) from endogenous or exogenous sources, an extensive accumulation of glycogen in hepatocytes results in an enlarged, pale-brown to beige liver *(L)*. **B,** Note the swollen hepatocytes *(arrows)* with extensive cytoplasmic vacuolation from glycogen accumulation. H&E stain. (**A** courtesy Dr. K. Bailey, College of Veterinary Medicine, University of Illinois. **B** courtesy Dr. J.M. Cullen, College of Veterinary Medicine, North Carolina State University.)

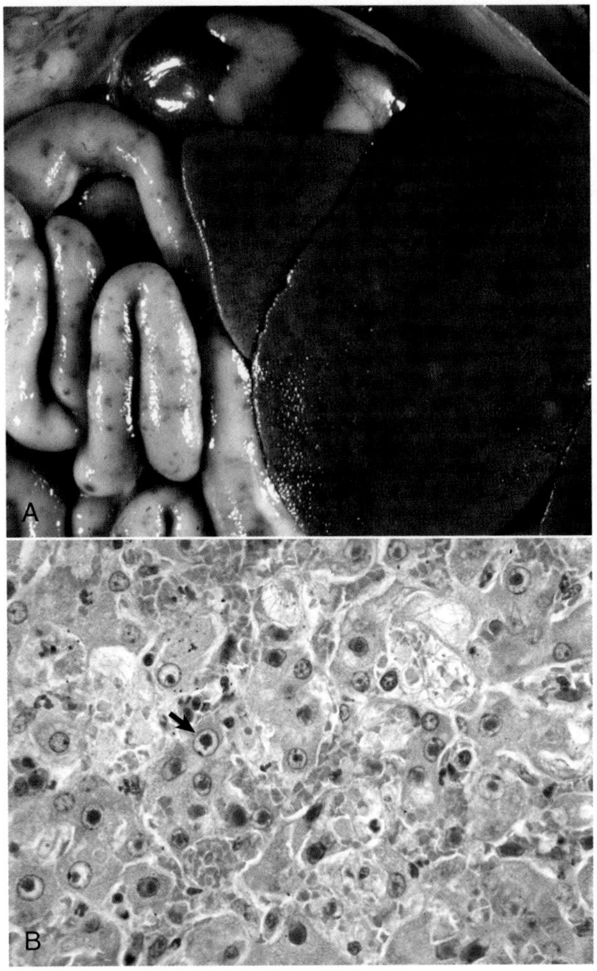

Figure 8-79 **Infectious Canine Hepatitis, Hepatic Necrosis, Liver, Dog. A,** The liver from a dog infected with infectious canine hepatitis (*ICH*) can be slightly enlarged and friable with a blotchy yellow discoloration. Sometimes, fibrin is evident on the capsular surface. Note the petechiae on the serosal surface of the intestines caused by vascular damage from canine adenovirus type I infection. **B,** Infection of hepatocytes and endothelial cells with canine adenovirus type I produces characteristic deeply eosinophilic to amphophilic intranuclear inclusions surrounded by a clear zone that separates them from the marginated chromatin *(arrow)*. H&E stain. (**A** courtesy Dr. W. Crowell, College of Veterinary Medicine, The University of Georgia; and Noah's Arkive, College of Veterinary Medicine, The University of Georgia. **B** courtesy Dr. M.D. McGavin, College of Veterinary Medicine, University of Tennessee.)

hepatocellular injury. Adenoviruses are cytolytic and cause necrosis of infected cells.

Lesions of infectious canine hepatitis include widespread petechiae and ecchymoses, accumulation of clear fluid in the peritoneal and other serous cavities, the presence of fibrin strands on the surface of the liver, and enlargement and reddening of the tonsils and lymph nodes (Fig. 8-79, *A*). The liver is moderately enlarged and friable and may contain small foci of hepatocellular necrosis centered on centrilobular areas. An enhanced lobular pattern is sometimes evident because of the centrilobular hepatic necrosis. Characteristically, the wall of the gallbladder is thickened by edema. Foci of hemorrhage in the lung, brain, kidneys, and the metaphysis of the long bones may also be evident.

The severity of microscopic lesions present in individual dogs may reflect the duration of the disease. Susceptible puppies rapidly succumb to infection and have only scattered foci of hepatocellular necrosis, whereas fulminant disease in more mature dogs often produces both randomly scattered foci of hepatocellular necrosis and widespread centrilobular necrosis. The predilection for centrilobular necrosis may be related to the virus's penchant for infection and necrosis of endothelial cells that may lead to vascular stasis and local hypoxia rather than to any increased propensity for the virus to damage centrilobular hepatocytes, although this issue is not resolved. Large deeply eosinophilic to amphophilic intranuclear inclusions are found in hepatocytes, vascular endothelium, and Kupffer cells (see Fig. 8-79, *B*). Inflammation tends to be mild, and neutrophils are the most abundant cell type. Virus-induced endothelial damage may lead to DIC and hemorrhagic diathesis, which contribute to the hemorrhage observed in affected dogs. Some dogs recovering from infectious canine hepatitis develop an immune-complex uveitis (type III hypersensitivity), which produces degeneration and necrosis of the corneal endothelium and resultant corneal edema clinically known as "blue eye."

Hepatocerebellar Degeneration

Hepatocerebellar degeneration is an autosomal recessive genetic variant of cerebellar abiotrophy in the Bernese mountain dog characterized by a combination of cerebellar and hepatocellular degeneration. Clinical signs usually become evident by 6 to 8 weeks of age and are mainly related to the cerebellar lesion (ataxia, intention tremors, etc.), although ascites is also possible. Histologically, there is hepatocellular vacuolation, degeneration, and regenerative nodule formation. There is no treatment, and affected dogs usually die by 6 months of age.

Disorders of Cats

Feline Fatty Liver Syndrome

Feline fatty liver syndrome is a distinct syndrome of idiopathic hepatocellular steatosis recognized in cats. Typically, affected cats are obese and have been exposed to a stressful event (e.g., moving to a new house, introduction of a new pet, and sudden dietary change) or suffer from a disease (e.g., pancreatitis) that resulted in anorexia. Cats with this type of hepatocellular steatosis frequently develop hepatic failure, icterus, and subsequently hepatic encephalopathy, unless they are treated medically. (See also hepatocellular steatosis under Metabolic Disturbances and Hepatic Accumulations.)

Lymphocytic Cholangitis

Lymphocytic cholangitis, a relatively common disorder of cats, is slowly progressive and chronic. There are several synonyms of this disorder in the literature, including lymphocytic cholangiohepatitis, lymphocytic portal hepatitis, nonsuppurative cholangitis, and feline cholangiohepatitis syndrome; however, the favored terminology to date is lymphocytic cholangitis. Affected cats are usually older than 4 years of age and may have icterus as a consequence of intrahepatic cholestasis. Small lymphocytes infiltrate the portal tracts and usually center on bile ducts directly. The intensity of the infiltration can make it difficult to identify the original bile duct within an affected portal tract. Often, by the time a biopsy is obtained, the liver is characterized by extensive aggregations of inflammatory cells, typically lymphocytes and plasma cells in portal tracts, and surrounding numerous small bile ducts (Fig. 8-80).

Inflammation usually is accompanied by bile duct proliferation, damage to the larger bile ducts, hepatic or biliary fibrosis, and intrahepatic cholestasis. The cause or causes of this syndrome are unknown. The disease might have an immunologic basis. The main differential diagnosis is lymphoma. Lymphocytic cholangitis should be distinguished from chronic suppurative cholangitis, which is caused most often by ascending bacterial infection of the biliary tree and typically includes at least small numbers of neutrophils within the bile ducts.

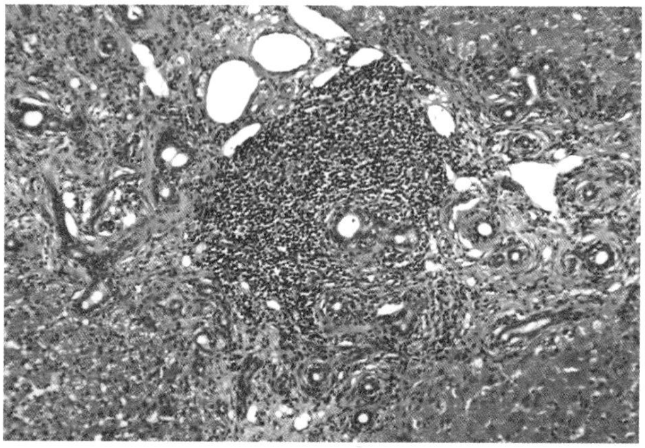

Figure 8-80 **Feline Lymphocytic Cholangitis, Liver, Cat.** Large numbers of lymphocytes surrounding bile ducts and biliary hyperplasia in portal areas are the hallmarks of this disease (central area of image). The inflammation most often affects the periphery of the bile ducts and could be termed a pericholangitis, but the syndrome is referred to as cholangitis. H&E stain. (Courtesy Dr. J.M. Cullen, College of Veterinary Medicine, North Carolina State University.)

Neutrophilic (Suppurative) Cholangitis

Neutrophilic cholangeitis is a disorder in mature cats (and occasionally dogs) most frequently associated with bacteria ascending from the gastrointestinal tract. It is characterized by accumulation of neutrophils within and surrounding bile ducts. When there is clear tissue injury and degeneration of neutrophils, the term suppurative cholangitis can be used. If inflammation extends into the adjacent hepatic parenchyma, the term cholangiohepatitis is appropriate. There is often accompanying degeneration of bile duct epithelium and/or periportal hepatocellular necrosis. Over time, the inflammatory infiltrate can become more mixed, with lymphocytes and plasma cells accompanying the neutrophils. It can eventually lead to peribiliary fibrosis. This disorder is most common in cats 11 to 15 years of age and often occurs in conjunction with pancreatitis and inflammatory bile disease (clinically referred to as "triaditis").

Disorders of Domestic Animals–The Gallbladder and Extrahepatic Bile Ducts

Developmental Abnormalities

Developmental anomalies of the gallbladder may be most common in the cat; bilobed and occasionally trilobed gallbladders can occur (Fig. 8-81). These anomalies usually are of no clinical significance but rarely can be associated with cholecystitis or cholelithiasis.

Biliary atresia, a congenital anomaly in which the extrahepatic bile ducts are nonpatent or absent, has been reported rarely in all domestic animal species. It leads to hyperbilirubinemia and jaundice.

In animals with polycystic kidney disease, cysts can also occur in the liver, affecting extrahepatic bile ducts. Biliary cysts may also occur in the liver without accompanying renal involvement. Congenital biliary cysts have been discussed in more detail previously.

Cholelithiasis

Choleliths, or *gallstones* as they are commonly called, occur infrequently in all the domestic species, but they are especially well described in ruminants. Choleliths are concretions of normally soluble components of bile (Fig. 8-82). They form when these components become supersaturated and precipitate. Choleliths in the gallbladder usually do not become clinically significant unless they migrate and obstruct the extrahepatic bile ducts. However,

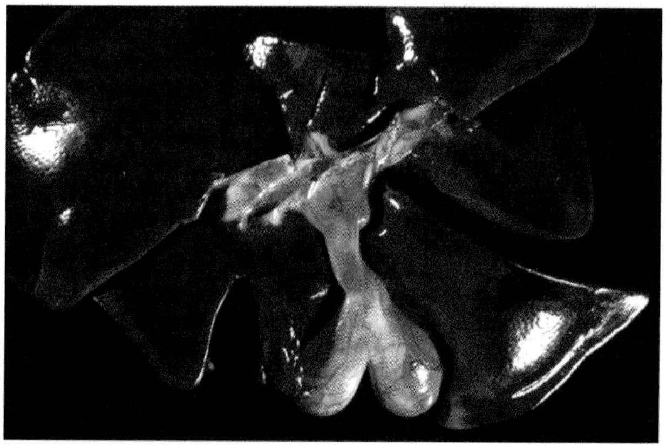

Figure 8-81 **Bilobed Gallbladder, Liver, Cat.** Bilobed gallbladders are developmental anomalies that have little or no clinical significance and are found most often in cats. (Courtesy College of Veterinary Medicine, University of Illinois.)

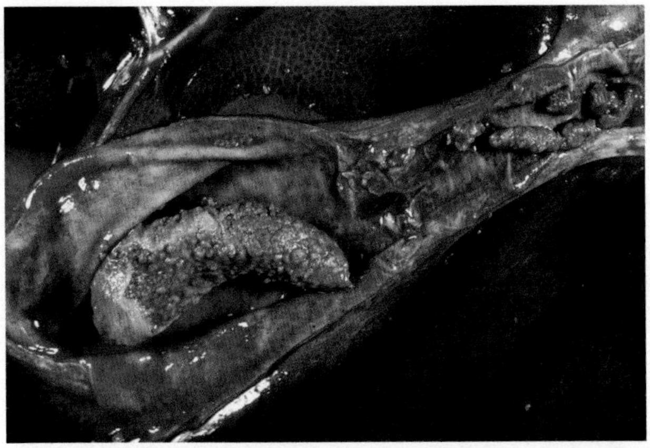

Figure 8-82 Choleliths, Gallbladder, Pig. Choleliths are concretions formed from the constituents of bile. (Courtesy Dr. M.D. McGavin, College of Veterinary Medicine, University of Tennessee.)

larger choleliths can lead to pressure necrosis and inflammation (cholecystitis).

Cholecystitis

Cholecystitis is inflammation of the gallbladder and can be acute or chronic. Acute inflammation of the gallbladder may be produced by viral infections, such as Rift Valley fever in ruminants and infectious canine hepatitis, and produces characteristic edema and hemorrhage in the gallbladder. Several types of bacteria, either derived from the blood or ascended from the intestine, can cause acute or chronic cholecystitis. Chronic cholecystitis typically accompanies prolonged bacterial infection of the biliary tree or ongoing irritation from choleliths or parasites of the gallbladder. Rupture of the gallbladder is rare but can occur as a result of acute or chronic infection. The resultant release of bile, with or without accompanying bacteria, can cause life-threatening peritonitis because of the irritating effect of bile on the serosal surfaces of the abdomen.

Hyperplastic and Neoplastic Lesions

Cystic Mucinous Hyperplasia of the Gallbladder

Cystic mucinous hyperplasia of the gallbladder mucosa has only been reported in dogs and sheep. There are no apparent abnormalities evident from the exterior of the gallbladder, and the features of cystic hyperplasia can only be appreciated by opening the gallbladder and draining residual bile that may obscure the mucosa. When the bile is rinsed away, affected mucosa is gray-white and has a diffusely thickened, spongelike consistency. Sessile or polypoid masses or large cysts are occasionally found, and they are evident as papillary projections into the lumen of the gallbladder (Fig. 8-83). Numerous 1- to 3-mm cysts within the hyperplastic mucosa impart the characteristic appearance. Histologically, the hallmark of cystic hyperplasia of the gallbladder is the abundance of variably sized cystic spaces that distort and thicken the entire mucosa of the gallbladder. Most of the cysts contain a copious amount of mucus. The majority of the lining cells are typical of the normal gallbladder epithelium (i.e., tall columnar with abundant apical cytoplasmic mucus). The entire mucosa may be affected. These lesions are usually of no significance to the host. In all likelihood, cystic hyperplasia of the gallbladder frequently goes undetected visually. The cause is not known.

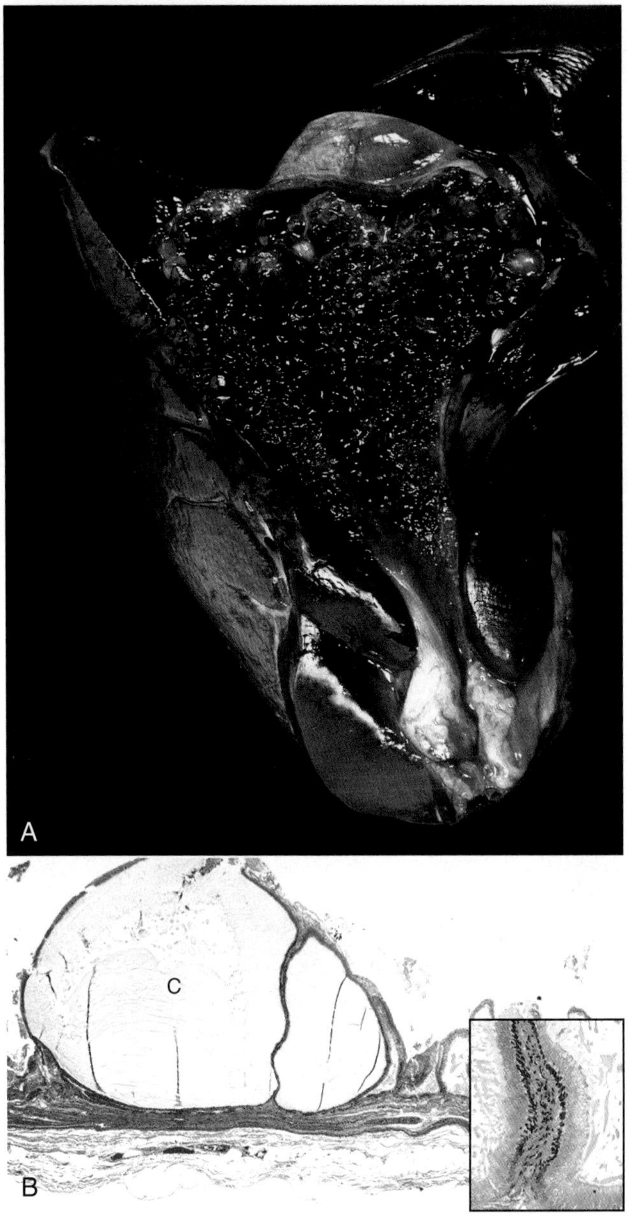

Figure 8-83 Cystic Mucinous Hyperplasia, Gallbladder, Dog. A, The gallbladder mucosa is thickened and contains multiple mucous cysts. **B,** The mucosa contains a mucous cyst (C). H&E stain. *Inset,* The mucosa is hyperplastic with prominent goblet cells that produce the mucus that fills the cysts. H&E stain. (**A** courtesy Dr. T. Cecere, Virginia-Maryland Regional College of Veterinary Medicine. **B** and inset courtesy Dr. M.D. McGavin, College of Veterinary Medicine, University of Tennessee.)

Adenoma

Adenomas of the gallbladder are rare neoplasms but are most common in young cattle and have also been described in dogs, cats, and sheep. They are multinodular or papillary masses that protrude from the mucosal surface and consist of a loose connective tissue stalk that is lined with well-differentiated biliary epithelium (Fig. 8-84).

Carcinoma

Malignant neoplasms of the gallbladder epithelium are rare in domestic animals but have been described in dogs, cats, and cattle. They typically are composed of mucin-secreting epithelial cells and often have a papillary arrangement. Carcinoma of the gallbladder may invade the liver by direct extension and may metastasize to the hepatic lymph nodes and to more distant sites.

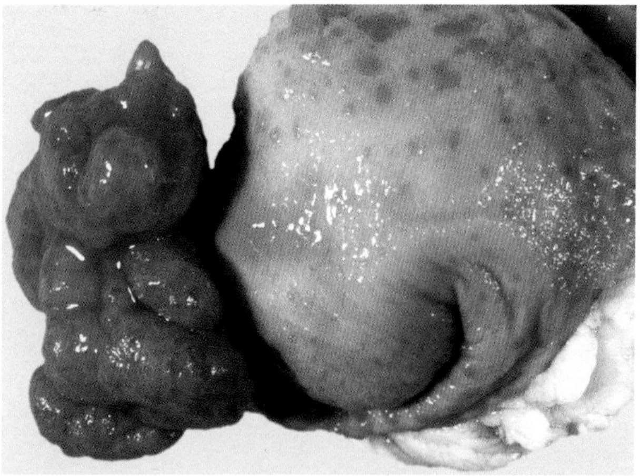

Figure 8-84 **Adenoma, Gallbladder, Dog.** Papillary projections of proliferating mucosa *(left third of the image)* bulge into the lumen of the gallbladder. (Courtesy Dr. M.D. McGavin, College of Veterinary Medicine, University of Tennessee.)

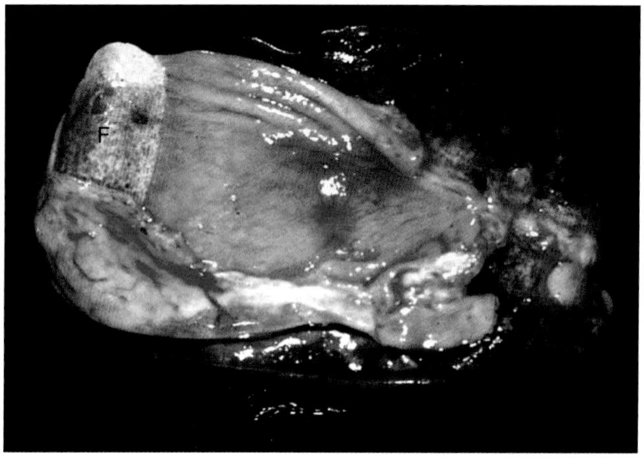

Figure 8-85 **Fibrinous Cholecystitis, Gallbladder, Cow.** Fibrinous cholecystitis caused by *Salmonella enteritidis* serotype *Dublin* has produced a fibrinous cast *(F)*, which is evident in the lumen of the gallbladder. (Courtesy Dr. D.A. Mosier, College of Veterinary Medicine, Kansas State University.)

Disorders of Ruminants (Cattle, Sheep, and Goats)–The Gallbladder and Extrahepatic Bile Ducts

Salmonella Infection

Fibrinous cholecystitis may occur in calves with acute salmonellosis, particularly that caused by *Salmonella enteritidis* serotype *Dublin* (Fig. 8-85). It occurs in conjunction with lesions in other tissues, such as the intestinal tract.

Disorders of Pigs–The Gallbladder and Extrahepatic Bile Ducts

Mulberry Heart Disease

Mulberry heart disease occurs in weaning piglets; the pathogenesis is unclear but likely involves disruption of metabolism with free radical formation and lack of sufficient free radical scavenging antioxidants such as vitamin E, resulting in oxidative cell injury. As the disease name implies, the characteristic lesion is extensive hemorrhages on the surface of the heart. Edema of the wall of the gallbladder and marked congestion of the liver can also be seen in pigs with this disorder.

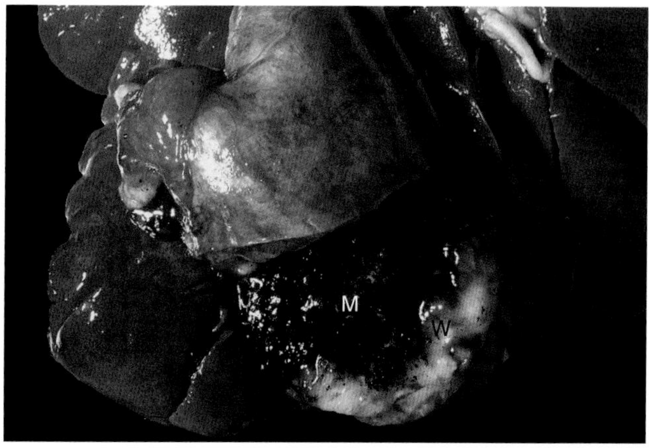

Figure 8-86 **Gallbladder Mucocele, Dog.** The gallbladder lumen is distended with thick mucoid *(M)* contents and the wall *(W)* is thickened. (Courtesy of Dr. A. Talley)

African Swine Fever

African swine fever (ASF) is a viral disease of swine characterized by edema and hemorrhage in multiple internal organs. As a part of the disease, edema is often observed within the walls of the gallbladder, and the vessels of the wall are often engorged.

Disorders of Dogs–The Gallbladder and Extrahepatic Bile Ducts

Thrombosis and Infarction of the Gallbladder

Occasionally, infarction without significant inflammation of the gallbladder can be seen in dogs. Thrombi can be found in the arteries of the muscular wall of the affected gallbladders. Rupture of the gallbladder can occur secondarily to the infarction of the wall. The cause is not known.

Gallbladder Mucocele

Gallbladder mucocele refers to a syndrome in dogs characterized by a distended gallbladder filled with tenacious mucus (Fig. 8-86) that can be associated with signs of biliary obstruction and that can occasionally be associated with thrombosis and gallbladder rupture. Smaller dog breeds appear to be predisposed, particularly Shetland sheepdogs. The mucosa of the gallbladder is usually hyperplastic. Occasionally, the common bile duct is similarly affected and cholestasis can develop. The pathogenesis of gallbladder mucocele is uncertain, although dogs with hyperadrenocorticism are reported to have a higher incidence of the disorder than other dogs.

Infectious Canine Hepatitis

Infectious canine hepatitis, a disorder caused by *canine adenovirus 1*, causes characteristic lesions in the liver that have been described in detail previously. In addition to the liver lesions, the wall of the gallbladder of infected dogs becomes thickened by edema. It may also contain intramural hemorrhages.

Disorders of Domestic Animals–The Exocrine Pancreas

Developmental Anomalies and Incidental Findings

Anomalies of the Duct System

The arrangement of the major pancreatic duct or ducts varies between and within species, so a variety of normal arrangements occur. Sheep, for example, have only one pancreatic duct that drains into the common bile duct, whereas cattle and horses typically have two ducts, and several distinct arrangements of the pancreatic ducts have been described in dogs. The pancreatic duct of cats enters the duodenum immediately adjacent to or confluent with the common bile duct. Specific anomalies include congenital stenosis of the pancreatic ducts and cystic dilation of the ducts.

Ectopic Pancreatic Tissue

Nodules of ectopic pancreatic tissue sometimes are present in the duodenum or other sections of the small bowel, stomach, spleen, gallbladder, and mesentery of the dog and cat. This type of anomaly, normal tissue in an abnormal location, is termed a *choristoma.*

Ectopic Splenic Tissue

Nodules of ectopic splenic tissue have been reported in the pancreas of dogs and cats. The lesions are usually firm, well-demarcated, dark red, spherical masses. Microscopically, they are composed of normal splenic tissue. It is an uncommon, incidental finding that should not be mistaken for pancreatic neoplasia.

Pacinian Corpuscles

Pacinian corpuscles are normally present within the interlobular connective tissue of the pancreas and mesentery of the cat, and they appear as discrete 1- to 3-mm nodules (Fig. 8-87 and E-Fig. 7-23). The corpuscles should not be mistaken for abnormal structures.

Pancreatic Calculi

The formation of concretions or "stones" within the pancreatic duct system is termed pancreatolithiasis and occurs uncommonly in cattle. It is usually an incidental finding at slaughter, and apparently it is slightly more common in cattle older than 4 years of age than in younger animals. Pancreatitis secondary to pancreatolithiasis occurs rarely.

Stromal Fat Cell Infiltration

Fat cell infiltration of the interstitial connective tissue of the pancreas occurs occasionally, especially in obese cats. The pancreas itself is usually unaffected, so exocrine pancreatic function is normal, but the dispersion of the parenchyma creates the impression that the pancreas has been replaced by adipose tissue.

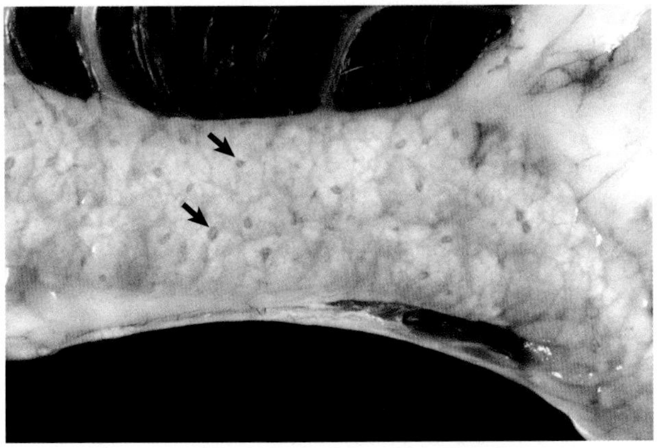

Figure 8-87 Pacinian Corpuscles, Pancreas, Cat. The feline pancreas contains numerous pacinian corpuscles *(arrows)*, which may be visible grossly as approximately 1-mm clear foci. (Courtesy College of Veterinary Medicine, North Carolina State University.)

Pancreatic Pseudocysts

Pancreatic pseudocysts are fluid-filled nonepithelialized fibrous sacs containing cellular debris and pancreatic enzymes that form within the pancreas or adjacent to the organ following pancreatic inflammation. They are described in dogs and cats. They should be distinguished from abscesses, cystic neoplasms, and congenital cysts seen with polycystic disease.

Cysts

Cysts can occasionally be observed in the pancreas as a component of congenital polycystic disease, which occurs in dogs, with Cairn terriers and West Highland white terriers predisposed; cats, with Persian cats believed to have a higher risk for the disorder; and goats and lambs. Cysts in the pancreas are usually incidental and of no functional significance.

Pancreatic Degeneration and Atrophy

Degeneration of the acinar cells of the exocrine pancreas is a nonspecific process that can occur as a consequence of a variety of local and systemic diseases. For example, starvation results in loss of zymogen granules within the cytoplasm of acinar cells of the exocrine pancreas because the rate of synthesis of the granules is diminished, and available protein is used to maintain serum protein concentrations when dietary protein is limited. Obstruction of the pancreatic ducts, whatever the cause, can also cause degeneration and atrophy of the exocrine pancreas. Obstruction of the pancreatic duct(s) can be caused by neoplasms or chronic inflammation and associated fibrosis that compress the duct or by foreign bodies, such as parasites or pancreatoliths, that occlude the ductal lumen. Exocrine pancreatic atrophy also may occur secondary to widespread interstitial fibrosis of the pancreas, as occurs, for example, in dogs with chronic pancreatitis.

Lysosomal Storage Diseases

Vacuolation of exocrine pancreatic acinar cells can be observed in several types of lysosomal storage diseases, including congenital disorders and toxic causes (i.e., α-mannosidosis due to swainsonine-containing plants). This lesion is most often seen in addition to vacuolation of neurons, macrophages, hepatocytes, and/or other cells.

Pancreatitis/Pancreatic Necrosis

Pancreatitis is a condition characterized primarily by necrosis and varying degrees of inflammation of the pancreas, and it can be either acute or chronic. The predominance of necrosis over inflammation in acute cases supports using the term *acute pancreatic necrosis* over acute pancreatitis for dogs and cats in most instances. Obese, sedentary bitches are especially predisposed.

Pathogenesis

The three major proposed mechanisms of pancreatitis are as follows (Fig. 8-88):

- Obstruction of the duct(s)
- Direct injury to acinar cells
- Disturbances of enzyme trafficking within the cytoplasm of acinar cells

Obstruction of ductal flow by calculi or parasites can lead to interstitial edema that compresses small-caliber vessels and compromises local blood flow, leading to ischemic damage to acinar cells. Direct damage to acinar cells can be caused by a few specific agents in animals, including compounds found in *Cassia occidentalis* and T-2 toxin, a trichothecene mycotoxin produced by *Fusarium* species that affects pigs and sheep, and zinc toxicosis of dogs, veal

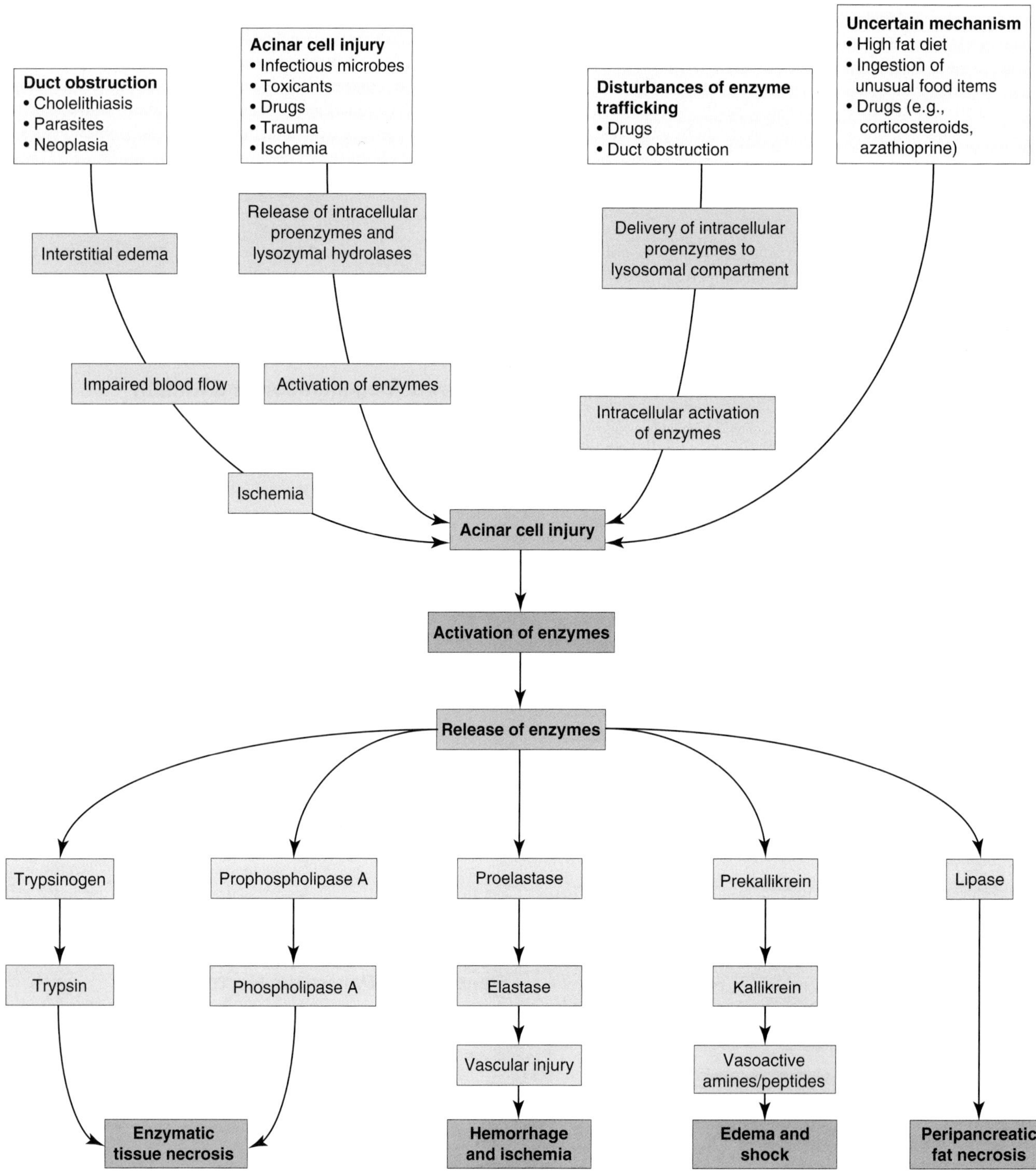

Figure 8-88 **Proposed Mechanisms of Acute Pancreatitis.** There are several proposed mechanisms of acute pancreatitis, with the main mechanisms being duct obstruction, acinar cell injury, and disturbances of enzyme trafficking. There are also several unknown mechanisms. Regardless of the mechanism, all converge on acinar cell injury leading to activation and release of pancreatic enzymes. These enzymes lead to tissue necrosis, hemorrhage and ischemia, edema, shock, and peripancreatic fat necrosis. (Courtesy Dr. A.J. Van Wettere, School of Veterinary Medicine, Utah State University and Dr. J.F. Zachary, College of Veterinary Medicine, University of Illinois.)

calves, and sheep. Certain therapeutic drugs, such as sulfonamides and potassium bromide–phenobarbital combinations, can damage the pancreas in dogs, and other species are probably similarly affected. Ischemia to the pancreas from a variety of causes may also produce direct injury to the acinar cells. A third mechanism involves aberrant transport of proenzymes within the acinar cells, leading to inappropriate activation of the enzymes within the cells. The association between corticosteroid administration in dogs and an increased risk of acute pancreatitis could possibly be explained by this mechanism. However, many cases of acute pancreatitis commonly occur after dogs have consumed a meal high in fat or some other dietary indiscretion, and the specific mechanism triggering the disease remains unclear. Pancreatitis is occasionally initiated by trauma, usually in dogs and cats as a consequence of some accidental crushing or impact trauma to the abdomen or surgical trauma. Acute pancreatitis in dogs occurs as a consequence of release of activated pancreatic enzymes into the pancreatic parenchyma and adjacent tissue producing autodigestion. Trypsin is believed to be a key player in pancreatitis. Once activated, trypsin in turn can activate proelastase and prophospholipase into elastase and phospholipase A. These enzymes digest pancreatic tissue and adjacent fat and damage blood vessels. Trypsin also activates prekallikrein, leading to involvement of the kinin system, complement, and clotting cascades in affected tissue. These systems in turn amplify the process, promote thrombosis and hemorrhage, attract inflammatory cells, and lead to the production of reactive oxygen species. Major factors that then play a role in progression of disease include altered pancreatic microcirculation, ischemia-reperfusion injury, a shift from acinar cell apoptosis to necrosis, and the complex interaction of the multiple inflammatory pathways outlined previously.

Acute Pancreatitis

Acute pancreatitis occurs less often in cats than dogs but more often in cats than most other species. Pancreatitis has been described in a variety of species, although the cause is usually different in each. In dogs, an increased incidence of acute pancreatitis has been observed in cocker spaniels.

The gross lesions of acute pancreatitis are referable to proteolytic degradation of pancreatic parenchyma, vascular damage and hemorrhage, and necrosis of peripancreatic fat by lipolytic enzymes of the pancreas. Mild cases of pancreatitis are characterized by edema of the interstitial tissue of the pancreas. Acute hemorrhagic pancreatitis is more severe, and characteristically, the pancreas is edematous and contains areas that are gray-white, the result of coagulation necrosis, and other areas that are dark red or blue-black, which are hemorrhagic (Fig. 8-89, A). Areas of fat necrosis are manifest as chalky-white foci as a result of saponification of necrotic adipose tissue in the mesentery adjacent to the pancreas. Portions of normal pancreatic parenchyma may be interspersed between affected portions. The peritoneal cavity frequently contains blood-stained fluid, which may contain droplets of fat in the early stage. Peritonitis is manifest by fibrinous adhesions between the affected portions of the pancreas and adjacent tissues.

The microscopic appearance of acute hemorrhagic pancreatitis reflects the gross lesions just described. Characteristic lesions include focally extensive areas of hemorrhage, influx of leukocytes, and coagulation necrosis of the pancreatic parenchyma; accumulation of fibrinous exudate in the interlobular septa; and necrosis and inflammation of fat in the mesentery adjacent to the affected portions of pancreas (see Fig. 8-89, B).

Species differences in acute pancreatitis are recognized. For example, in cats, there appear to be two distinct syndromes of acute pancreatitis, one characterized by an acute pancreatic necrosis and a distinct suppurative pancreatitis that is most likely the consequence of ascending bacterial infection. Pancreatitis in cats also often coexists with inflammatory bowel disease, neutrophilic (suppurative) cholangitis, or both (often clinically termed "triaditis").

Acute pancreatitis is usually characterized by vomiting, diarrhea, anorexia, and abdominal tenderness. Acute, severe pancreatitis also produces systemic effects secondary to the release of inflammatory mediators and activated enzymes from the damaged pancreas; these effects include widespread vascular injury and subsequent hemorrhage, shock, and DIC. The liver also is affected in many cases of pancreatitis, as indicated by increased concentrations of serum hepatic enzymes (e.g., alanine aminotransferase) and, sometimes, focal hepatic necrosis.

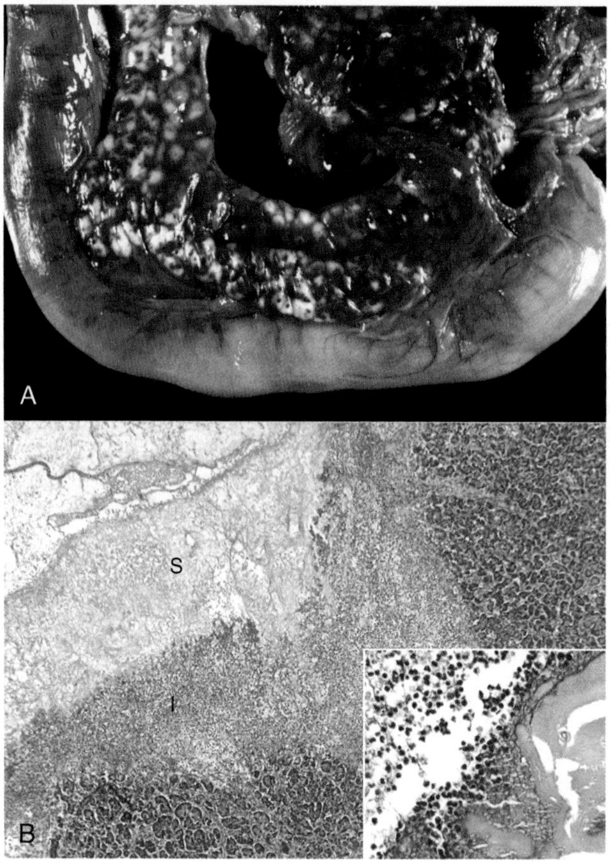

Figure 8-89 **Acute Pancreatic Necrosis, Acute Pancreatitis, Pancreas, Dog. A,** Note the expansion of the pancreas by areas of hemorrhage and edema. **B,** Acute pancreatitis (histologic appearance of the pancreas depicted in **A**). Note the accumulation of fibrinous exudate and edema within the interlobular septa *(S)* and inflammatory cell infiltrate *(I)*. H&E stain. *Inset,* Higher magnification of acute pancreatitis. Note the abundant neutrophils and the area of "saponification" of fat *(lower right)*. H&E stain. (**A** courtesy Dr. R. Fairley. **B** courtesy Dr. J.M. Cullen, College of Veterinary Medicine, North Carolina State University. Inset courtesy Dr. M.D. McGavin, College of Veterinary Medicine, University of Tennessee.)

Acute pancreatitis sufficient to cause clinical disease apparently is considerably less common in species other than the dog and cat. Acute pancreatic necrosis and pancreatitis have been described in the horse, but the pathogenesis of pancreatitis in this species differs from that in the dog and cat. Necrosis and inflammation are the result of migration of strongyle larvae through the pancreas, which results in the release of pancreatic enzymes and enzymatic digestion of the pancreas and surrounding tissue.

Chronic Pancreatitis

Chronic pancreatitis is typically accompanied by fibrosis and parenchymal atrophy. It can occur in all species as a consequence of obstruction of the pancreatic ducts and presumably all of the other mechanisms associated with acute pancreatitis. In the dog, pancreatic fibrosis and chronic pancreatitis are the result of progressive destruction of the pancreas by repeated mild episodes of acute pancreatic necrosis and pancreatitis. An increased incidence of chronic pancreatitis has been reported in cocker spaniels, cavalier King Charles spaniels, collies, and boxer dogs. The pancreas has modest regenerative capacity and responds to injury with replacement fibrosis and atrophy of persisting parenchyma. Thus ongoing destruction of pancreatic tissue causes progressive loss of glandular tissue without replacement (Fig. 8-90). Grossly, the pancreas in affected animals is a distorted, shrunken, nodular mass with fibrous adhesions to adjacent tissue. If a significant portion of the pancreas is affected, dogs may develop signs of exocrine pancreatic insufficiency, with or without signs of endocrine pancreatic insufficiency (diabetes mellitus). However, destruction of pancreatic tissue frequently is not of sufficient magnitude to cause exocrine pancreatic insufficiency, and pancreatic fibrosis is sometimes found as incidental lesions at autopsy (syn: necropsy) of dogs with apparently normal digestive function. The microscopic appearance of chronic pancreatitis in dogs may also differ by breed. A recent study illustrated that in English cocker spaniels, chronic pancreatitis is characterized by interlobular and periductular fibrosis and inflammation and a marked absence of interlobular ducts, whereas in other breeds such as cavalier King Charles spaniels, the disease is intralobular and there is ductular hyperplasia. In cats, chronic pancreatitis almost always manifests as extensive fibrosis, with little inflammation, and is the most common cause of exocrine pancreatic insufficiency in this species. Fibrosis of the exocrine pancreas also occurs after the necrosis of exocrine pancreatic cells from zinc toxicosis in sheep. Ectasia of the pancreatic ducts with cyst formation also is relatively common in cats with interstitial pancreatic fibrosis.

Chronic pancreatitis and replacement fibrosis occurs sporadically in the horse, usually as a consequence of either parasitic migration or from ascending bacterial infection of the pancreatic ducts. In addition, pancreatitis may occur in horses with chronic eosinophilic gastroenteritis. However, chronic pancreatitis usually is not clinically apparent in the horse because signs of exocrine pancreatic insufficiency rarely, if ever, occur in this species. Chronic inflammation of the pancreas, characterized by lymphoplasmacytic infiltrates, is most common and important in the dog, but it does occur in the cat, horse, and cattle, in which it is rarely of clinical significance.

Parasitic Infections

A variety of parasites may inhabit the pancreatic ducts of domestic animals. Parasitic infections of the pancreatic ducts are important if they occlude the ducts, either by direct physical obstruction or by inducing inflammation within and around ducts. Examples include flukes of the families Opisthorchiidae (*Opisthorchis tenuicollis*, *Opisthorchis viverrini*, *Clonorchis sinensis*, *Metorchis albidus*, and *Metorchis conjunctus*) and Dicrocoeliidae (*Eurytrema pancreaticum*, *Concinnum procyonis*, and *Dicrocoelium dendriticum*), which may inhabit the pancreatic ducts of a variety of animal species and occasionally cause fibrosis and/or pancreatitis. Nematodes, particularly ascarids, and cestodes are common gastrointestinal parasites of the domestic species; occasionally, they may lodge within the pancreatic ducts.

Hyperplasia and Neoplasia

Pancreatic Nodular Hyperplasia

Nodular hyperplasia of the exocrine pancreas occurs in dogs, cats, and cattle. It is especially common in older dogs and cats. The lesion is of no clinical significance, but it must be distinguished from neoplasms of the endocrine and exocrine pancreas.

These hyperplastic nodules typically are multiple, raised, smooth, and a uniform gray or white on cut surface (Fig. 8-91, *A*). The

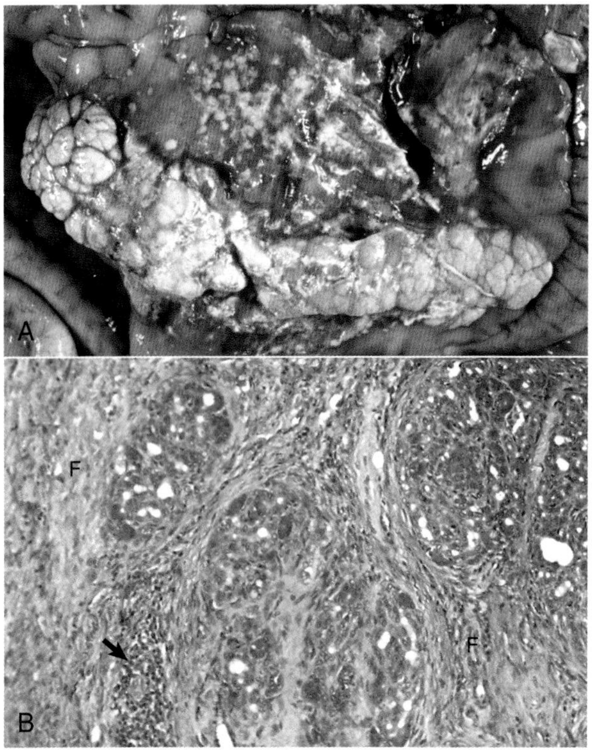

Figure 8-90 **Chronic Pancreatitis, Pancreas, Dog. A,** Lobules are more prominent as the result of fibrosis, and the pancreas is paler (gray-white) than normal. The white, raised, granular areas in the pancreas and mesentery are foci of fat necrosis that result from enzymatic digestion of lipids that then become mineralized. **B,** Remaining exocrine pancreatic cells are separated into small lobules by abundant fibrous connective tissue (*F*), which contains chronic inflammatory cells (*arrow*). H&E stain. (**A** courtesy College of Veterinary Medicine, North Carolina State University. **B** courtesy Dr. J.M. Cullen, College of Veterinary Medicine, North Carolina State University.)

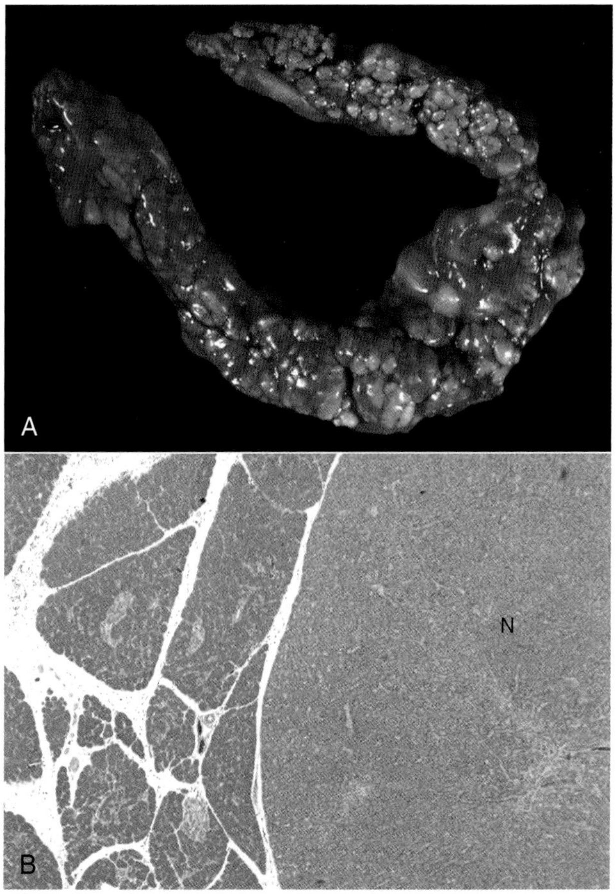

Figure 8-91 **Pancreatic Nodular Hyperplasia, Exocrine Pancreas, Dog. A,** Hyperplastic nodules are pale beige to white and project above the surface. **B,** Microscopically hyperplastic nodules (*N*) are composed of numerous small acini, most of which, in this case, lack typical zymogen granules. H&E stain. (**A** courtesy Dr. M.D. McGavin, College of Veterinary Medicine, University of Tennessee. **B** courtesy Dr. J.M. Cullen, College of Veterinary Medicine, North Carolina State University.)

nodules may be firmer than the adjacent normal pancreas. Microscopically, these nodules consist of unencapsulated aggregates of acinar cells that may lack zymogen granules or contain an abundance of them (see Fig. 8-91, *B*). Some nodules contain a mixture of the two types of acinar cells. The distinction between hyperplasia and adenoma of the exocrine pancreas is poorly defined in domestic animals.

Pancreatic Adenoma

Adenomas of the exocrine pancreas are extremely rare but have been described in the cat. Those of acinar cell origin share all the features of hyperplastic nodules but are single and larger than normal pancreatic lobules, whereas hyperplastic nodules are not larger than normal lobules; this distinction clearly is somewhat arbitrary. Rarely, these neoplasms can be cystic and are diagnosed as pancreatic cystadenoma, although this lesion may actually represent congenital cystic disease.

Pancreatic Carcinoma

Carcinoma of the ductular epithelium or acinar cells of the exocrine pancreas is uncommon in all species. It is most often reported in the dog and cat. The neoplasms may consist of single or multiple nodules of variable size within the pancreas, each of which consists of gray or yellow tissue. Lesions may consist of a single nodule or affect the organ diffusely. Tumors are typically grayish-white to pale yellow with a firm to hard consistency (Fig. 8-92, *A*). Tumors are often gritty when cut. Areas of hemorrhage, mineralization, or necrosis may be present within the neoplasm. The neoplasm is usually firmer than the adjacent pancreas because of proliferation of fibrous connective tissue. Adhesion of the affected pancreas to adjacent tissue may occur. This neoplasm often invades adjacent tissue and seeds the peritoneal cavity. Peritoneal implants form nodules over the mesentery, omentum, and serosa of the abdominal viscera. Metastasis to the regional lymph nodes (pancreatoduodenal, which is inconstantly present and the right hepatic lymph node) is also common, and some carcinomas metastasize widely.

Microscopic features of carcinomas of the exocrine pancreas range from well-differentiated adenocarcinomas with tubular patterns to undifferentiated carcinomas with solid patterns. The amount of fibrous stroma varies considerably and usually is greatest in poorly differentiated neoplasms (see Fig. 8-92, *B*). Zymogen granules similar to those present in normal acinar cells of the pancreas are often absent within the cytoplasm of the neoplastic cells. Mitotic figures are common.

A unique cutaneous paraneoplastic syndrome can be observed in cats with pancreatic adenocarcinoma or cholangiocarcinoma. It manifests grossly as symmetric alopecia of the ventral trunk and limbs with a glistening appearance. Histologically, affected areas have marked follicular and adnexal atrophy and loss of the stratum corneum of the epidermis.

Disorders of Ruminants (Cattle, Sheep, and Goats)–The Exocrine Pancreas

Pancreatic Hypoplasia

Hypoplasia of the exocrine pancreas occurs sporadically in calves. The endocrine pancreatic tissue is normal. Grossly, the organ is small, pale, and may appear only as small wisps of white-cream tissue within the mesentery. Microscopically, acinar tissue is present but scarce, organized in small clusters of cells. Many of the cells are poorly differentiated and lack zymogen granules. Affected calves have clinical signs of exocrine pancreatic insufficiency.

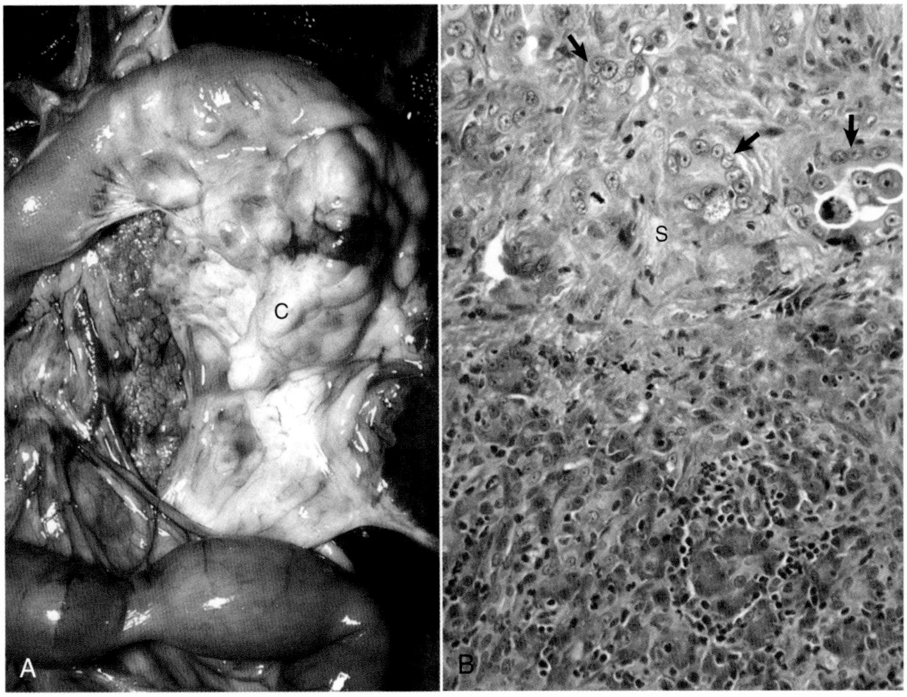

Figure 8-92 **Pancreatic Carcinoma. A,** Stomach and pancreas *(center)*, ventral-dorsal view, dog. Pancreatic carcinoma *(C)* has invaded the mesentery, wall of the stomach, and gastrosplenic ligament. Note the lobulated appearance of the mass, which is formed by neoplastic exocrine pancreatic epithelial cells and scirrhous connective tissue. Proximal duodenum *(bottom)*, liver *(top)*, and spleen *(right [left anatomically])*. **B,** Pancreas, cat. Pancreatic carcinoma tends to form crude acini or tubules *(arrows)* that aggressively invade adjacent normal tissue. Prominent fibrosis, termed scirrhous response *(S)*, is commonly caused by this type of tumor. H&E stain. (**A** courtesy College of Veterinary Medicine, University of Illinois. **B** courtesy Dr. M.D. McGavin, College of Veterinary Medicine, University of Tennessee.)

The distinction between atrophy and hypoplasia can be difficult to determine because both processes lead to an abnormally small organ with diminished function. Cells of the hypoplastic exocrine pancreas do not usually contain lipofuscin, which can be seen in atrophic cells.

Disorders of Dogs–The Exocrine Pancreas

Exocrine Pancreatic Atrophy (Juvenile Pancreatic Atrophy)

A distinct syndrome characterized by a dramatically diminished exocrine pancreas has been recognized in several breeds of dog. It is particularly common in the German shepherd dog and rough-coated collies, in which it appears to be inherited. Inheritance was originally believed to be autosomal recessive but has recently been shown to be more complex, likely involving multiple genes (including alleles of the major histocompatibility complex) and environmental factors. This lesion is most likely one of atrophy rather than hypoplasia, given recent evidence that suggests that an autoimmune pancreatitis (lymphocytic infiltration) precedes the loss of normal pancreatic parenchyma. The pancreas in affected dogs is small (Fig. 8-93), but islands of normal exocrine pancreatic tissue usually remain. Histologically, there is marked depletion of exocrine pancreatic acinar cells with relative non-involvement of endocrine islet cells. Young animals are affected, usually between 6 and 12 months of age. Affected dogs have signs typical of maldigestion secondary to exocrine pancreatic insufficiency and rapidly lose weight despite a voracious appetite.

A recent entity of juvenile pancreatic atrophy has been reported in greyhounds, in which atrophy of both the exocrine and the endocrine pancreas is observed.

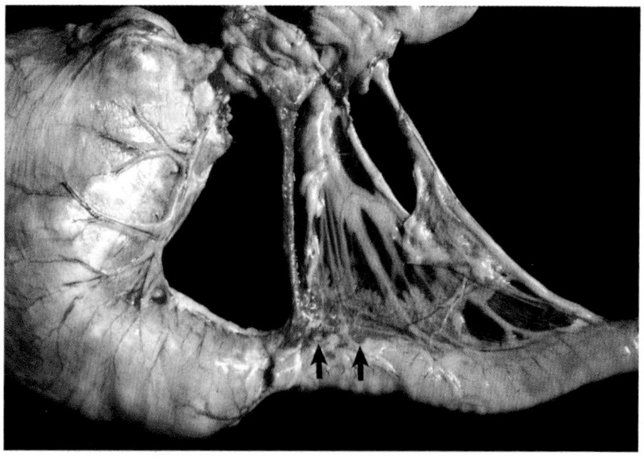

Figure 8-93 **Pancreatic Atrophy/Hypoplasia, Pancreas, Dog.** Virtually no pancreatic tissue is present in this case. Pancreatic remnants are indicated by *arrows*. (Courtesy Dr. M.D. McGavin, College of Veterinary Medicine, University of Tennessee.)

Disorders of Cats–The Exocrine Pancreas

The most common disorder of the exocrine pancreas in cats is chronic pancreatitis, which has been described previously.

Suggested Readings

Suggested Readings are available at www.expertconsult.com.

CHAPTER 9

Respiratory System, Mediastinum, and Pleurae[1]

Alfonso López and Shannon A. Martinson

Key Readings Index

Diseases of the respiratory system (respiratory apparatus) are some of the leading causes of morbidity and mortality in animals and a major source of economic losses. Thus veterinarians are routinely called to diagnose, treat, and implement health management practices to reduce the impact of these diseases. In companion animals, diseases of the respiratory tract are also common and, although of little economic significance, are important to the health of the animals and thus to clinicians and pet owners. In the past few years, animal shelters have been recognized as a major risk factor for respiratory diseases in dogs and cats, a comparable situation to what is reported in human beings with nosocomial infections.

Structure and Function

General Structure

To facilitate the understanding of the structure and function, it is convenient to arbitrarily divide the respiratory system into conducting, transitional, and gas exchange systems (Fig. 9-1).

Conductive System

The conducting system includes nostrils, nasal cavity, paranasal sinuses, nasopharynx, larynx, trachea, and extrapulmonary and intrapulmonary bronchi, all of which are largely lined by pseudostratified, ciliated columnar cells, plus a variable proportion of secretory goblet (mucous) and serous cells (Figs. 9-2 and 9-3 and E-Fig. 9-1).

Transitional System

The transitional system of the respiratory tract is composed of bronchioles, which are microscopic structures that serve as a transition zone between the conducting system (ciliated) and the gas exchange (alveolar) system (see Fig. 9-1). The disappearance of cilia in the transitional system is not abrupt; the ciliated cells in the proximal bronchiolar region become scarce and progressively attenuated, until the point where distal bronchioles no longer have ciliated cells. Normal bronchioles also lack goblet cells but instead have other types of secretory cells, notably Club cells (formerly Clara cells) and neuroendocrine cells. Club cells, also referred to as secretory bronchiolar cells, contain numerous biosynthetic organelles that play an active role in detoxification of xenobiotics (foreign substances), similar to the role of hepatocytes (Fig. 9-4). Club cells are also critical stem cells in the repair and remodeling of not only the bronchioles but also of most of the respiratory tract. In addition, Club cells contribute to the innate immunity of the lung by secreting protective proteins (collectins) and pulmonary surfactant (see Fig. 9-4, *B*). In carnivores and monkeys, and to a much lesser extent in horses and human beings, the terminal portions of bronchioles are lined not only by cuboidal epithelium but also by segments of alveolar capillaries. These unique bronchioloalveolar structures are known as respiratory bronchioles (Fig. 9-5; also see Fig. 9-1).

Exchange System

The gas exchange system of the respiratory tract in all mammals is formed by alveolar ducts and millions of alveoli (Fig. 9-6; also see Fig. 9-1). The surface of the alveoli is lined by two distinct types of epithelial cells known as type I (membranous) pneumonocytes and type II (granular) pneumonocytes (Fig. 9-7).

All three—the conducting, transitional, and exchange systems of the respiratory system—are vulnerable to injury because of constant exposure to a myriad of microbes, particles and fibers, and toxic gases and vapors present in the air. Vulnerability of the respiratory system to aerogenous (airborne) injury is primarily because of (1) the extensive area of the alveoli, which are the interface between the blood in alveolar capillaries and inspired air; (2) the large volume of air passing continuously into the lungs; and (3) the high concentration of noxious elements that can be present in the air (Table 9-1). For human beings, it has been estimated that the surface of the pulmonary alveoli is approximately 200 m^2, roughly the area

[1]For a glossary of abbreviations and terms used in this chapter, see E-Glossary 9-1.

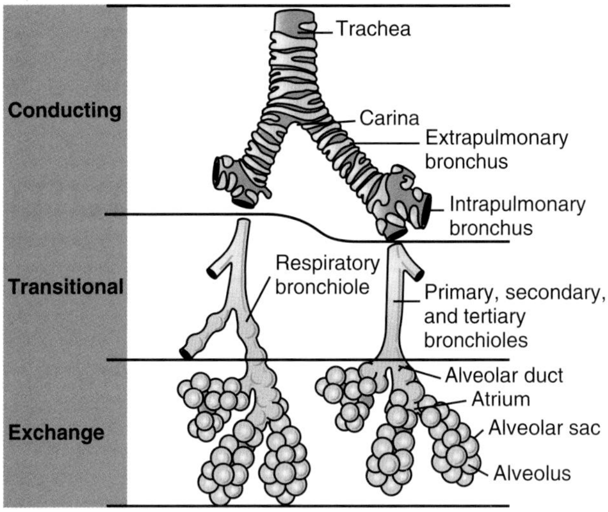

Figure 9-1 Airways From the Trachea to the Alveoli. Conducting, transitional, and exchange components of the respiratory system. The transitional zone (bronchioles) is not as equally well developed in all species. (Adapted from Banks WJ: *Applied veterinary histology*, ed 3, St. Louis, 1993, Mosby.)

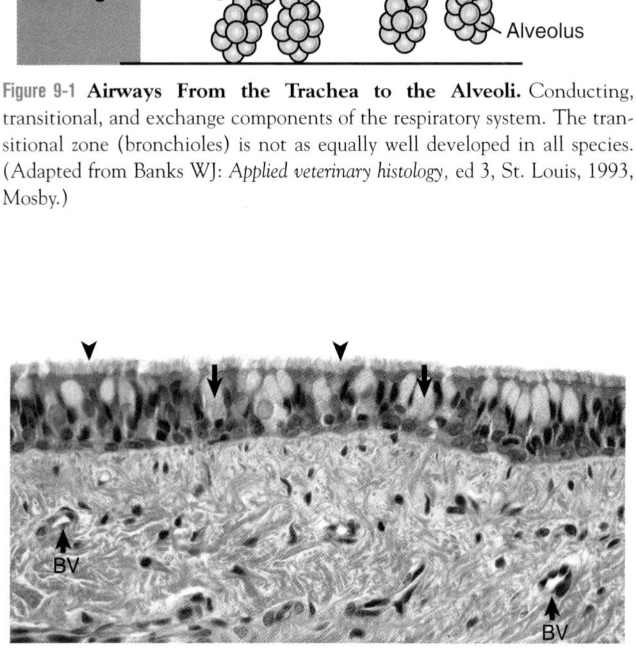

Figure 9-2 Normal Mucosa, Trachea, Dog. Mucosa consists of ciliated and nonciliated secretory cells. Goblet cells have a pale staining cytoplasm *(arrows)*. The proportion of ciliated to nonciliated cells varies depending on the level of airways. Ciliated cells *(arrowheads)* are more abundant in proximal airways, whereas secretory cells are proportionally more numerous in distal portions of the conducting and transitional systems. The submucosa of the conducting system (nasal to bronchi) has abundant blood vessels *(BV)*. H&E stain. (Courtesy Dr. J.F. Zachary, College of Veterinary Medicine, University of Illinois.)

of a tennis court. The alveolar surface of the equine lung is estimated to be approximately 2000 m^2. It has also been estimated that the volume of air reaching the human lung every day is approximately 9000 L. Lungs are also susceptible to blood-borne (hematogenous) microbes, toxins, and emboli. This fact is not surprising because the entire cardiac output of the right ventricle goes into the lungs, and approximately 9% of the total blood volume is within the pulmonary vasculature. The pulmonary capillary bed is the largest in the body, with a surface area of 70 m^2 in the adult human; this area is equivalent to a length of 2400 km of capillaries, with 1 mL of blood occupying up to 16 km of capillary bed.

Normal Flora of the Respiratory System

The respiratory system has its own normal flora (microbiota), as does any other body system in contact with the external environment. If a sterile swab is passed deep into the nasal cavity of any healthy

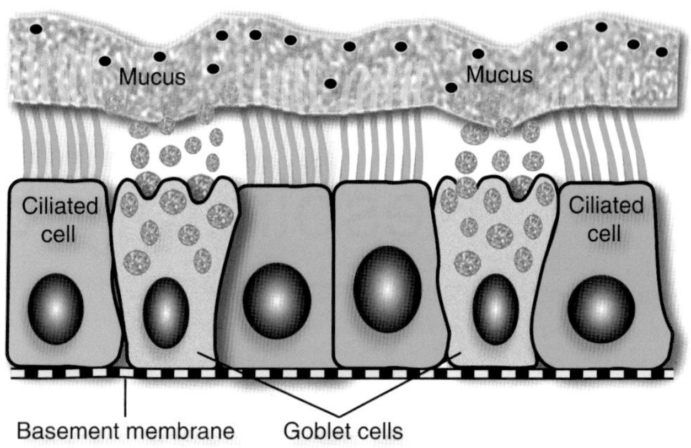

Figure 9-3 Mucociliary Apparatus of the Conducting System. Both ciliated and goblet cells rest on the basement membrane. Mucus produced and released by goblet cells forms a carpet on which inhaled particles *(black dots)* are trapped and subsequently expelled into the pharynx by the mucociliary apparatus. (Courtesy Dr. A. López, Atlantic Veterinary College.)

animal and cultured for microbes, yeasts, and fungi, many species of bacteria are recovered, such as *Mannheimia (Pasteurella) haemolytica* in cattle; *Pasteurella multocida* in cats, cattle, and pigs; and *Bordetella bronchiseptica* in dogs and pigs. The organisms that constitute the normal flora of the respiratory tract are restricted to the most proximal (rostral) region of the conducting system (nasal cavity, pharynx, and larynx). The thoracic portions of the trachea, bronchi, and lungs are considered to be essentially sterile. The types of bacteria present in the nasal flora vary considerably among animal species and in different geographic regions of the world. Some present in the nasal flora are pathogens that can cause important respiratory infections under some circumstances. For instance, *Mannheimia (Pasteurella) haemolytica* is part of the bovine nasal flora, yet this bacterium causes a devastating disease in cattle—pneumonic mannheimiosis (shipping fever). Experimental studies have established that microorganisms from the nasal flora are continuously carried into the lungs via tracheal air. Despite this constant bacterial bombardment from the nasal flora and from contaminated air, normal lungs remain sterile because of their remarkably effective defense mechanisms.

Dysfunction/Responses to Injury and Patterns of Injury

Conductive System (Nose, Paranasal Sinuses, Larynx, Trachea, and Bronchi)

The conducting portion of the respiratory system is lined by pseudostratified columnar ciliated epithelium (most of the nasal cavity, paranasal sinuses, part of the larynx, and all of the trachea and bronchi), olfactory epithelium (part of the nasal cavity, particularly ethmoidal conchae), and squamous epithelium (nasal vestibulum and parts of the larynx). The pattern of injury, inflammation, and host response (wound healing) are characteristic for each of these three types of epithelium independent of its anatomic location.

Pseudostratified ciliated epithelium, which lines most of the nasal cavity and nasopharynx, part of the larynx, and all of the trachea and bronchi, is exquisitely sensitive to injury. When these cells are irreversibly injured, whether caused by viral infection, trauma, or inhalation of toxic gases, the ciliated cells swell, typically lose their attachment to underlying basement membrane, and rapidly exfoliate (Fig. 9-8). A transient and mild exudate of fluid, plasma proteins, and neutrophils covers the ulcer. In the absence of

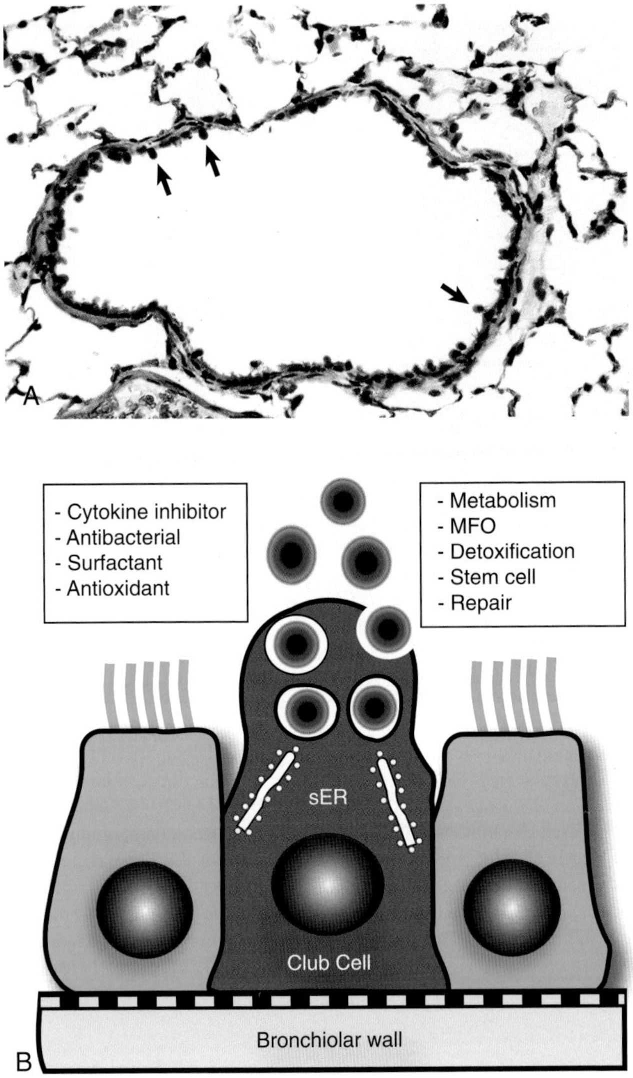

Figure 9-4 **Normal Bronchiole, Rat. A,** Bronchiole showing a thin wall composed of a basement membrane, smooth muscle, and connective tissue. On the luminal surface of the bronchiole, note dome-shaped Club (Clara) cells *(arrows)* protruding into the lumen. H&E stain. **B,** Schematic representation of a Club cell showing abundant smooth endoplasmic reticulum *(sER)* and cytoplasmic granules, which are extruded into the bronchiolar lumen. MFO, Mixed function oxidases. (Courtesy Dr. A. López, Atlantic Veterinary College.)

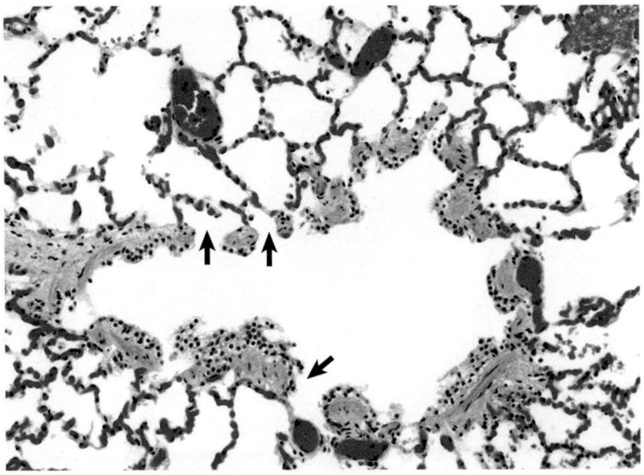

Figure 9-5 **Normal Respiratory Bronchiole, Dog.** The wall of the bronchiole is covered by ciliated epithelium, which is supported by smooth muscle and connective tissue. Terminally, the wall becomes interrupted, forming lateral communications between the bronchiolar lumen and alveoli *(arrows)*. H&E stain. (Courtesy Dr. A. López, Atlantic Veterinary College.)

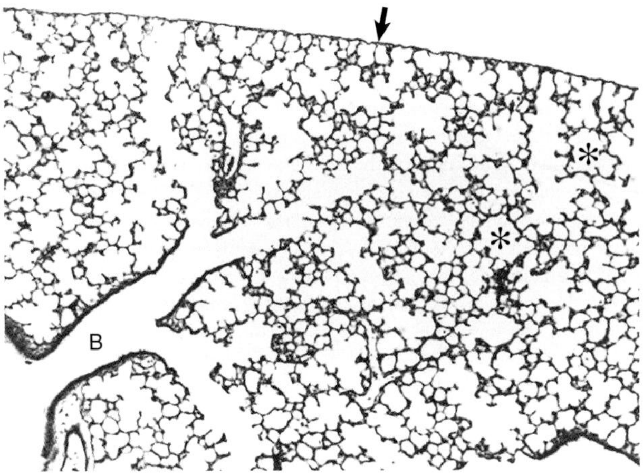

Figure 9-6 **Lung, Rat.** Lungs were fixed by intratracheal perfusion of fixative to retain normal distention of airways. Note the dichotomous branching of the bronchioles *(B)* that terminate as alveoli *(asterisks)* and the thin visceral pleura *(arrow)* covering the surface of the lungs. H&E stain. (Courtesy Dr. J. Martinez-Burnes, Atlantic Veterinary College.)

complications or secondary bacterial infections, a specific type of progenitor cells known as basal cells or *nonciliated secretory cells* (preciliated cells), which are normally present in the mucosa, migrate to cover the denuded basement membrane and undergoes mitosis, eventually differentiating into new ciliated epithelial cells (see Fig. 9-8). Cellular migration, proliferation, and attachment are regulated by locally released interleukins (IL-1β, IL-2, IL-4, and IL-13), growth factors, integrins and extracellular matrix (ECM) proteins such as collagen, and fibronectin. The capacity of ciliated epithelium to repair itself is remarkably effective. For example, epithelial healing in an uncomplicated ulcer of the tracheal mucosa can be completed in only 10 days. This sequence of cell degeneration, exfoliation, ulceration, mitosis, and repair is typically present in many viral infections in which viruses replicate in nasal, tracheal, and bronchial epithelium, causing extensive mucosal ulceration. Examples of transient infections of this type include human colds (rhinoviruses), infectious bovine rhinotracheitis (bovine herpesvirus 1), feline rhinotracheitis (felid herpesvirus 1), and viruses of the canine infectious respiratory disease (CIRD) group such as canine adenovirus 2 (CAV-2) and canine parainfluenza virus (CPIV).

If damage to the mucociliary blanket becomes chronic, goblet cell hyperplasia takes place, leading to excessive mucus production (hypersecretion) and reduced mucociliary clearance, and when there is loss of basement membrane, repair is by fibrosis and granulation tissue (scarring). In the most severe cases, prolonged injury causes squamous metaplasia, which together with scarring causes airway obstruction and an impediment to mucociliary clearance. In laboratory rodents, hyperplastic and metaplastic changes, such as those seen in nasal polyps and squamous metaplasia, are considered a prelude to neoplasia.

The second type of epithelium lining the conducting system is the sensory olfactory epithelium, present in parts of the nasal mucosa, notably in the ethmoidal conchae. The patterns of degeneration, exfoliation, and inflammation in the olfactory epithelium are similar to those of the ciliated epithelium, except that olfactory

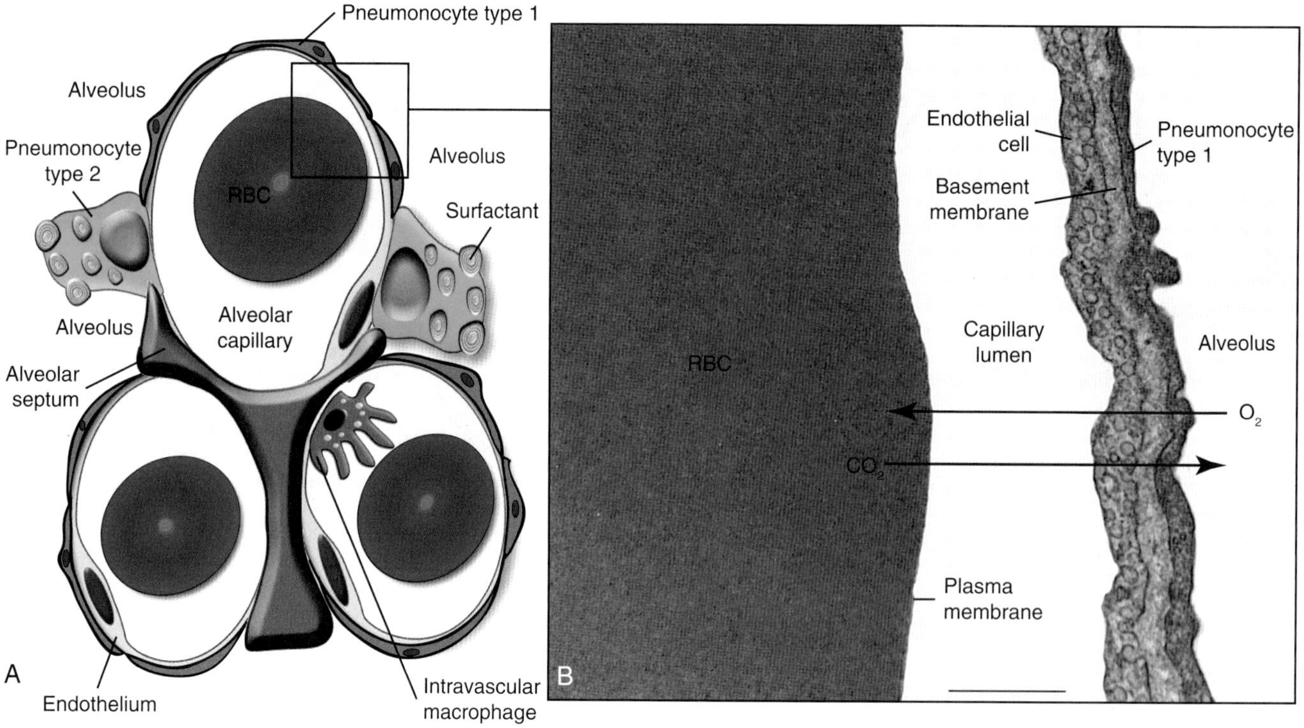

Figure 9-7 **The Blood-Air Barrier. A,** In this schematic diagram, note the thin membrane (blood-air barrier) separating the blood compartment from the alveoli. Type I (membranous) pneumonocytes are remarkably thin and cover most of the alveolar wall. Note the endothelial cells lining the alveolar capillary. Alveolar interstitium supports the alveolar epithelium on one side and the endothelium on the other side of the blood-air barrier. Type II (granular) pneumonocytes appear as large cuboidal cells with lamellar bodies (surfactant) in the cytoplasm. A pulmonary intravascular macrophage, a component of the monocyte-macrophage system, is depicted on the wall of an alveolar capillary. A red blood cell *(RBC)* is present inside the lumen of the alveolar capillary. **B,** Alveolar wall. The blood-air barrier consists of cytoplasmic extensions of (1) type I (membranous) pneumonocytes, (2) a dual basal lamina synthesized by type I pneumonocytes, and (3) cytoplasmic extensions of endothelial cells. TEM. Uranyl acetate and lead citrate stain. Bar = 500 nm (0.5 μm). (**A** courtesy Dr. A. López, Atlantic Veterinary College. **B** courtesy Dr. A.G. Armien, Diagnostic Ultrastructural Pathology Service, College of Veterinary Medicine, University of Minnesota.)

Table 9-1 Common Pathogens, Allergens, and Toxic Substances Present in Inhaled Air

Category	Agents
Microbes	Viruses, bacteria, fungi, protozoa
Plant dust	Grain, flour, cotton, wood
Animal products	Dander, feathers, mites, insect chitin
Toxic gases	Ammonia (NH_3), hydrogen sulfide (H_2S), nitrogen dioxide (NO_2), sulfur dioxide (SO_2), chlorine (Cl)
Chemicals	Organic and inorganic solvents, herbicides, asbestos, nickel, lead

epithelium has only limited capacity for regeneration. When olfactory epithelium has been irreversibly injured, olfactory cells swell, separate from adjacent sustentacular cells, and finally exfoliate into the nasal cavity. Once the underlying basement membrane of the olfactory epithelium is exposed, cytokines are released by leukocytes and endothelial cells, and inflammatory cells move into the affected area. When damage is extensive, ulcerated areas of olfactory mucosa are replaced by ciliated and goblet cells or squamous epithelium, or by fibrous tissue, all of which eventually cause reduction (hyposmia) or loss of olfactory function (anosmia). Repair of the olfactory epithelium is slower and less efficient than repair of the respiratory epithelium. Neurons in the olfactory mucosa have the unique ability to regenerate, a fact that is being explored as a potential source of new neurons in the treatment of spinal cord injury.

Squamous epithelium, located in the vestibular region of the nose (mucocutaneous junction), is the third type of epithelium present in the nasal passages. Compared with ciliated and olfactory epithelia, nasal squamous epithelium is quite resistant to all forms of injury. The pharyngeal mucosa, composed of squamous epithelium, has similar patterns of necrosis and inflammation as the oral mucosa (see Chapter 7).

Bronchi

The patterns of necrosis, inflammation, and repair in intrapulmonary bronchi are similar to those previously described for the nasal and tracheal epithelium. In brief, injury to ciliated bronchial epithelium may result in degeneration, detachment, and exfoliation of necrotic cells. Under normal circumstances, cellular exfoliation is promptly followed by inflammation, mitosis, cell proliferation, cell differentiation, and finally by repair (Fig. 9-9 and see Fig. 9-8). Depending on the type of exudate, bronchitis can be fibrinous, catarrhal, purulent, fibrinonecrotic (diphtheritic), and sometimes granulomatous. When epithelial injury becomes chronic, production of mucus is increased via goblet cell hyperplasia (chronic catarrhal inflammation). This form of chronic bronchitis is well illustrated in habitual smokers who continually need to cough out excessive mucus secretions (sputum). Unfortunately, in some cases, excessive mucus cannot be effectively cleared from airways, which

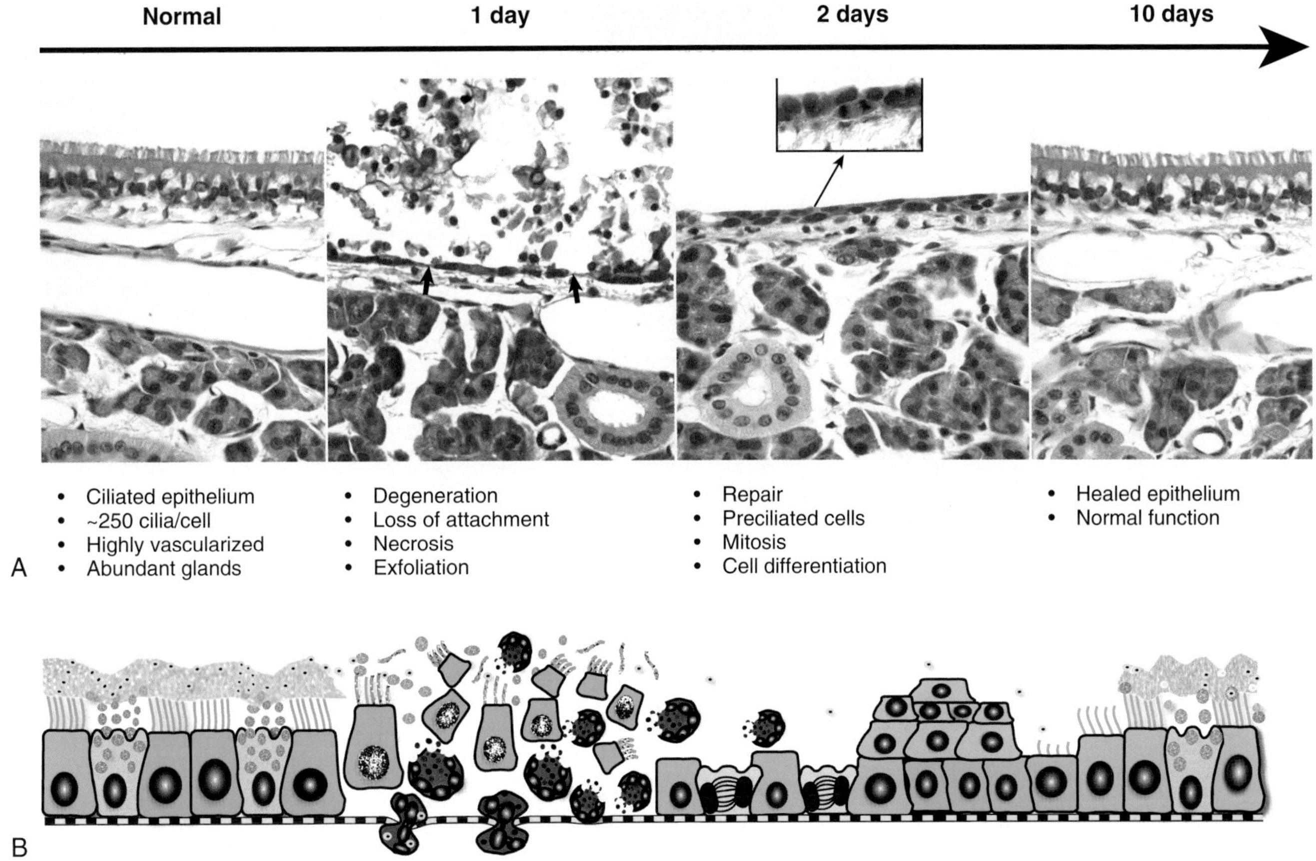

Figure 9-8 Normal and Injured Nasal Epithelium Following Exposure to Air Containing an Irritant Gas (Hydrogen Sulfide), Nasal Concha, Rats. A, Normal ciliated epithelium composed of tall columnar cells with numerous cilia. Day 1: Note detachment and exfoliation of ciliated cells, leaving a denuded basement membrane *(arrows)*. This same type of lesion is seen in viral or mechanical injury to the mucosa of the conducting system. Two days after exposure, the basement membrane is lined by rapidly dividing preciliated cells, some of which exhibit mitotic activity *(inset)*. Ten days after injury, the nasal epithelium is completely repaired. H&E stain. **B,** Schematic representation of the events of injury and repair in the respiratory mucosa of the conducting system. Blue cell, ciliated mucosal epithelial cell; pink cell, goblet cell; red cell, neutrophil. (**A** from López A, Prior M, Yong S, et al: *Am J Vet Res* 49:1107-1111, 1988. **B** courtesy Dr. A. López, Atlantic Veterinary College.)

leads to chronic obstructive bronchitis and emphysema (see Fig. 9-9). Chronic bronchial irritation causes squamous metaplasia of highly functional but vulnerable ciliated epithelium to nonfunctional, but more resistant, squamous epithelium. Squamous metaplasia has a calamitous effect on pulmonary clearance because it causes a structural loss and functional breakdown of portions of the mucociliary escalator. Hyperplasia of bronchial glands occurs frequently in chronic bronchitis, which translates to an increase of the Reid index (bronchial-gland to bronchial-wall ratio) (E-Fig. 9-2). This index is less than 30% in the healthy human lung and in the lungs of most domestic species, except for cats, which generally have an index higher than 40%. The term *airway remodeling* encompasses all the structural changes that accompany chronic bronchitis such as hypertrophy and hyperplasia of smooth muscle, submucosal glands, and goblet cells; fibrosis; and increased bronchial vascularity.

Bronchiectasis is one of the most devastating sequelae to chronic remodeling of the bronchi. It consists of a pathologic and permanent dilation of a bronchus with rupture of the bronchial wall as a result of obstruction or chronic inflammation. Destruction of walls occurs in part when proteolytic enzymes and oxygen radicals released from phagocytic cells during chronic inflammation degrade and weaken the smooth muscle and cartilage (chondromalacia) that help to maintain normal bronchial diameter (Fig. 9-10). Bronchiectasis may be saccular when destruction affects only a small localized portion of the bronchial wall or cylindrical when destruction involves a large segment of a bronchus. Grossly, bronchiectasis is manifested by prominent lumps in the lungs (bosselated appearance or having rounded eminences) resulting from distention of bronchi with exudate, which results in a concurrent obstructive atelectasis of surrounding parenchyma (Fig. 9-11). The cut surfaces of dilated bronchi are filled with purulent exudates; for this reason, bronchiectasis is often mistaken for pulmonary abscesses. Careful inspection, usually requiring microscopic examination, confirms that exudate is contained and surrounded by remnants of a bronchial wall lined by squamous epithelium and not by a pyogenic membrane (connective tissue) as it is in the case of a pulmonary abscess. The squamous metaplasia further interferes with the normal function of the mucociliary escalator.

Transitional System (Bronchioles)

The epithelial lining of the bronchiolar region (transitional zone) is exquisitely susceptible to injury, particularly to that caused by some respiratory viruses (bovine parainfluenza virus 3, bovine respiratory syncytial virus, adenovirus, or canine distemper virus), oxidant gases (nitrogen dioxide [NO_2], sulfur dioxide [SO_2], or ozone [O_3]), and toxic substances (3-methylindole or paraquat). The precise explanation as to why bronchiolar epithelium is so prone to injury is still not clear, but it is presumably due in part to (1) its high vulnerability to oxidants and free radicals; (2) the presence of

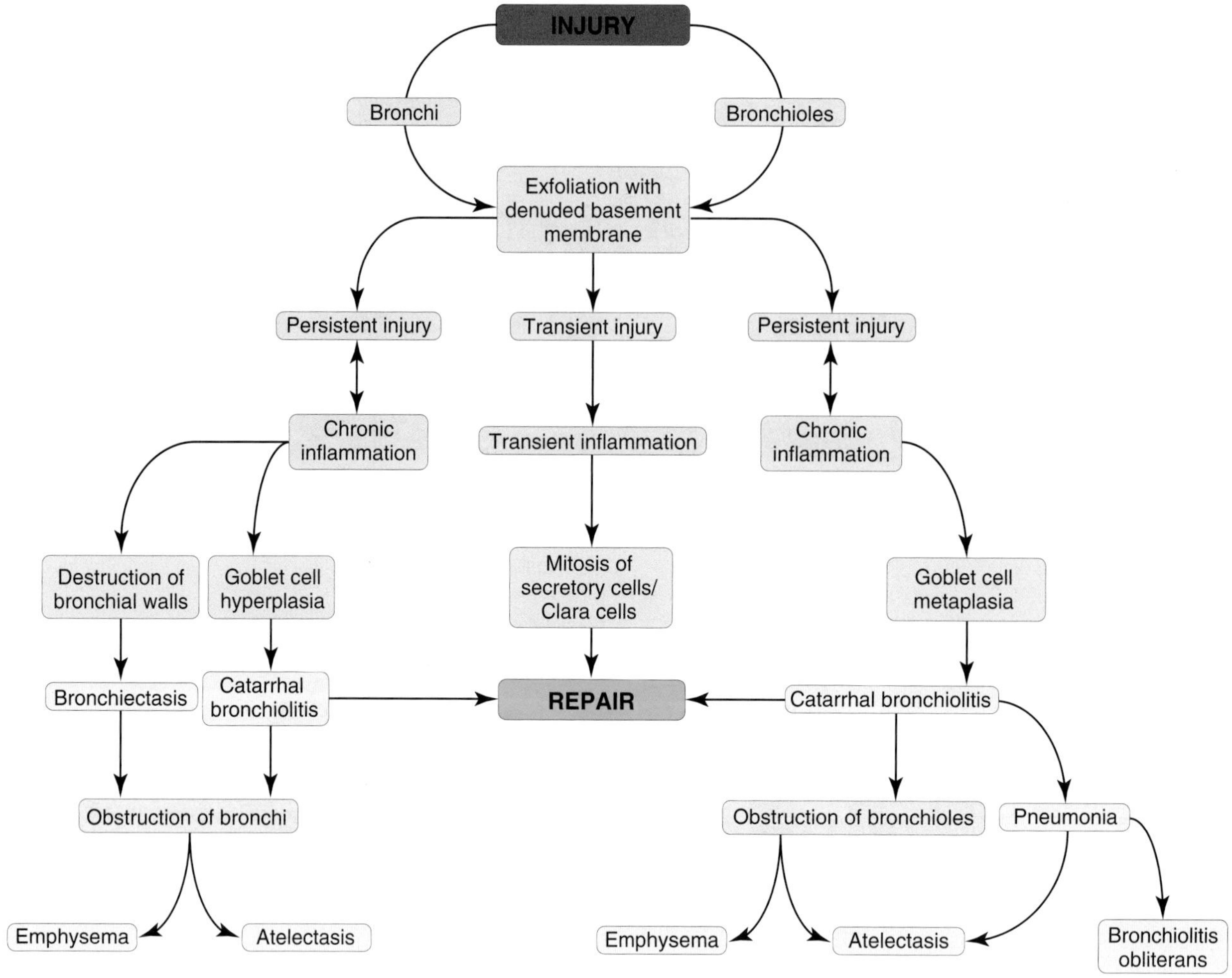

Figure 9-9 **Patterns of Host Response and Possible Sequelae to Bronchial and Bronchiolar Injury.** (Courtesy Dr. A. López, Atlantic Veterinary College.)

Club (Clara) cells rich in mixed function oxidases, which locally generate toxic metabolites (see Fig. 9-4); and (3) the tendency for pulmonary alveolar macrophages and leukocytes to accumulate in this region of the lungs. Depending on the types of injury and inflammatory response, bronchiolitis is classified as necrotizing, suppurative, catarrhal (mucous metaplasia), or granulomatous.

Repair in Acute and Mild Bronchiolar Injury

Once injury to bronchiolar ciliated cells becomes irreversible, the cells degenerate and exfoliate into the bronchiolar lumen, leaving a denuded basement membrane. Repair in the bronchiolar region is similar to, but less effective than, that in the tracheal or nasal mucosa. Under normal circumstances, recruited phagocytic cells remove exudate and cell debris from the lumina of affected bronchioles, thus preparing the basement membrane to be repopulated with new, undifferentiated cells originating from a rapidly dividing pool of Club (Clara) cells. After several days, these proliferating cells fully differentiate into normal bronchiolar cells.

Repair in Acute and Severe Bronchiolar Injury

In severe acute injury, such as that caused by aspiration pneumonia or by highly pathogenic microorganisms, exudate attaches and cannot be removed from the basement membrane of bronchioles. The exudate becomes infiltrated by fibroblasts, which form small nodular masses of fibrovascular tissue that develop into well-organized, microscopic polyps inside the bronchiolar lumen. The external surface of the exudate eventually becomes covered by ciliated cells. This lesion is referred to as *bronchiolitis obliterans*, and the polyps may become so large as to cause airflow impairment (Fig. 9-12 and see Fig. 9-9).

Repair in Chronic Bronchiolar Injury

In mild but persistent bronchiolar injury, goblet cells normally absent from bronchioles proliferate from basal cells, resulting in goblet cell metaplasia and causing a profound alteration in the physicochemical properties of bronchiolar secretions (Fig. 9-13). The normally serous bronchiolar fluid released by Club (Clara) cells becomes a tenacious material when mucus produced by goblet cells is added. As a result of increased viscoelasticity of the mucus, bronchiolar secretions cannot be removed effectively by ciliary action, leading to plugging and obstruction of distal airways. Under such conditions, often grouped as chronic obstructive pulmonary disease, coughing is required to clear mucus from obstructed bronchioles. Pulmonary emphysema and atelectasis are further sequelae to bronchiolar metaplasia and mucous hypersecretion blocking or partially blocking the lumens of these bronchioles. These two inflation abnormalities are characteristically present in chronic obstructive pulmonary disease (COPD), which is called “recurrent airway obstruction (RAO or “heaves”) in horses (see Recurrent Airway Obstruction, under Disorders of Horses). Peribronchiolar

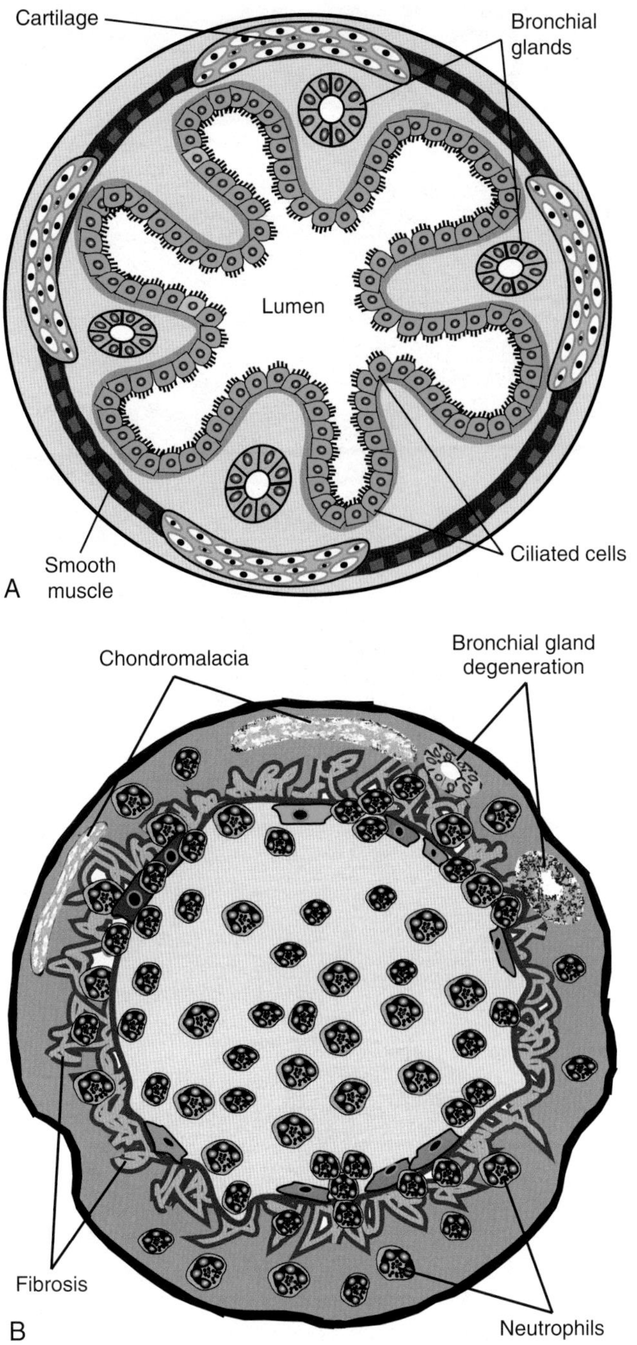

Figure 9-10 **Schematic Illustrations of Bronchiectasis. A,** Normal bronchus showing mucosa, submucosa, bronchial glands, and cartilage. **B,** Bronchiectasis. The affected bronchus is dilated and has lost its normal projections of the mucosa into the lumen. Note the inflammation, loss of mucosa, destruction of bronchial wall, and fibrosis with atrophy of cartilage and bronchial glands. (Courtesy Dr. A. López, Atlantic Veterinary College.)

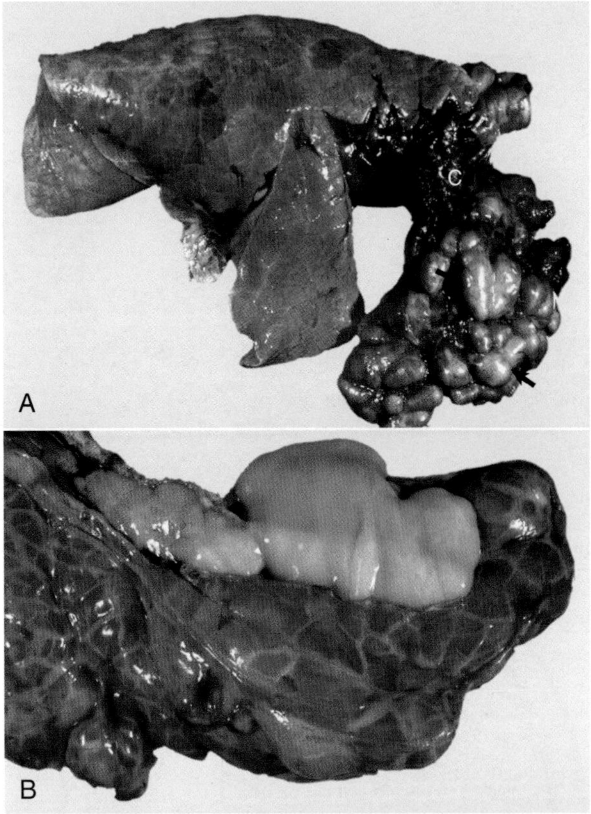

Figure 9-11 **Severe Bronchiectasis with Chronic Bronchopneumonia, Right Lung, Calf. A,** Note the segmentally distended (bosselated) bronchi (*arrows*) supplying the ventral portion of the cranial lung lobe. The lumens of affected bronchi are filled with purulent exudate. The surrounding lung parenchyma supplied by these bronchi is atelectatic (*C*). Bronchiectatic bronchi resemble pulmonary abscesses, but unlike abscesses, which are composed of pyogenic exudate within a fibrous capsule, the exudate in bronchiectasis is largely mucopurulent and contained within the remnants of the dilated bronchial wall. **B,** These distended bronchi are filled with mucopurulent exudate (gray-white material) that exudes from airways when they are cut. (**A** courtesy Ontario Veterinary College. **B** courtesy Dr. M.D. McGavin, College of Veterinary Medicine, University of Tennessee.)

proliferation of lymphocytes (BALT hyperplasia) is also a common microscopic lesion seen in chronic bronchiolitis.

Airway Hyperresponsiveness

Airway hyperresponsiveness, or hyperreactive airway disease, is another sequela of bronchiolar injury arising from gene-environment interactions. It develops in human beings and animals (experimentally) after a transient and often innocuous viral infection of the lower respiratory tract or from exposure to certain allergens. Experimental work has shown that airway hyperreactivity in postviral bronchiolitis is associated with increased expression of TLRs and unusual susceptibility to inhaled endotoxin. Hyperreactive animals typically have an increased number of mast cells, eosinophils, and T lymphocytes in the airway mucosa. Clinically, airway hyperresponsiveness is characterized by an exaggerated bronchoconstriction after natural exposure to mild stimuli, such as cold air, or after animals are experimentally exposed to aerosols of histamine or methacholine.

Exchange System (Alveoli)

Because of their extremely delicate structure, alveoli are quite vulnerable to injury once the local defense mechanisms have been overwhelmed. The alveolar wall is a thin membrane formed by a core of interstitium supporting an extensive network of alveolar capillaries. Fibroblasts (septal cells), myofibroblasts, collagen, elastic fibers, and few interstitial macrophages and mast cells constitute the alveolar interstitium. The wall of the alveolar capillaries facing the airspace is remarkably thin and has three layers composed of vascular endothelium, basal lamina, and alveolar epithelium. These three layers of the alveolar capillaries constitute what is customarily referred to as the *blood-air barrier* (see Fig. 9-7). The epithelial side of the alveolus is primarily lined by rather thin type I

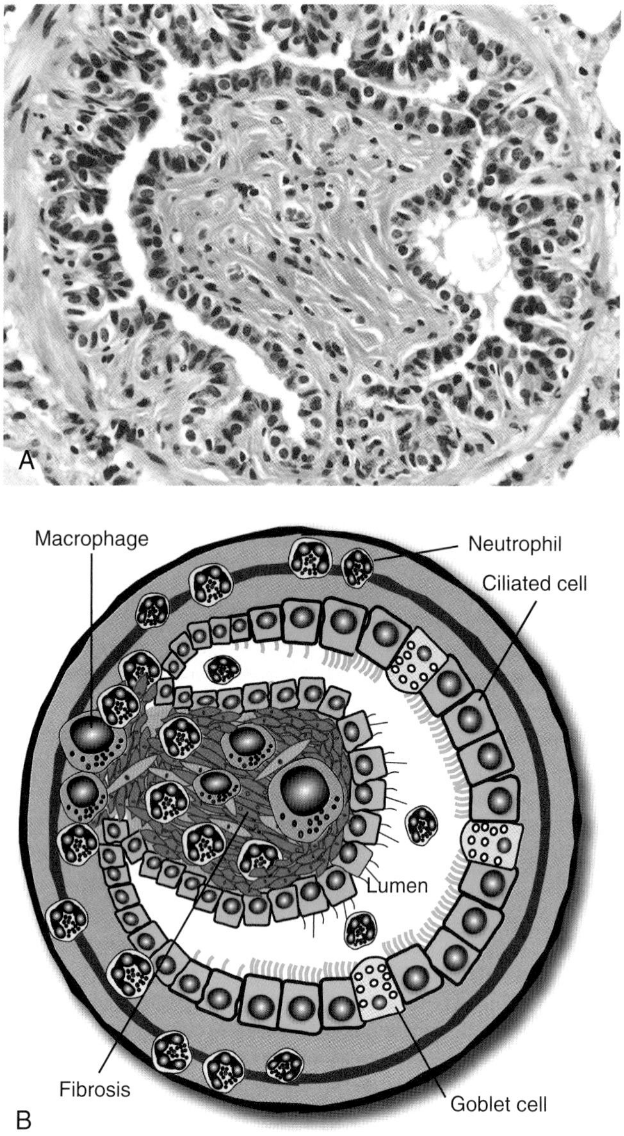

Figure 9-12 Bronchiolitis Obliterans. A, Chronic inflammation in the bronchiolar wall resulting in the formation of a nodular mass *(center)* of granulation tissue firmly attached to the airway wall, protruding into the bronchiolar lumen and lined by bronchial epithelium. H&E stain. **B,** Diagram illustrating organized exudate, formed by connective tissue, macrophages, lymphocytes, and neutrophils, that is attached to the bronchiolar wall and covered by respiratory ciliated cells. (Courtesy Dr. A. López, Atlantic Veterinary College.)

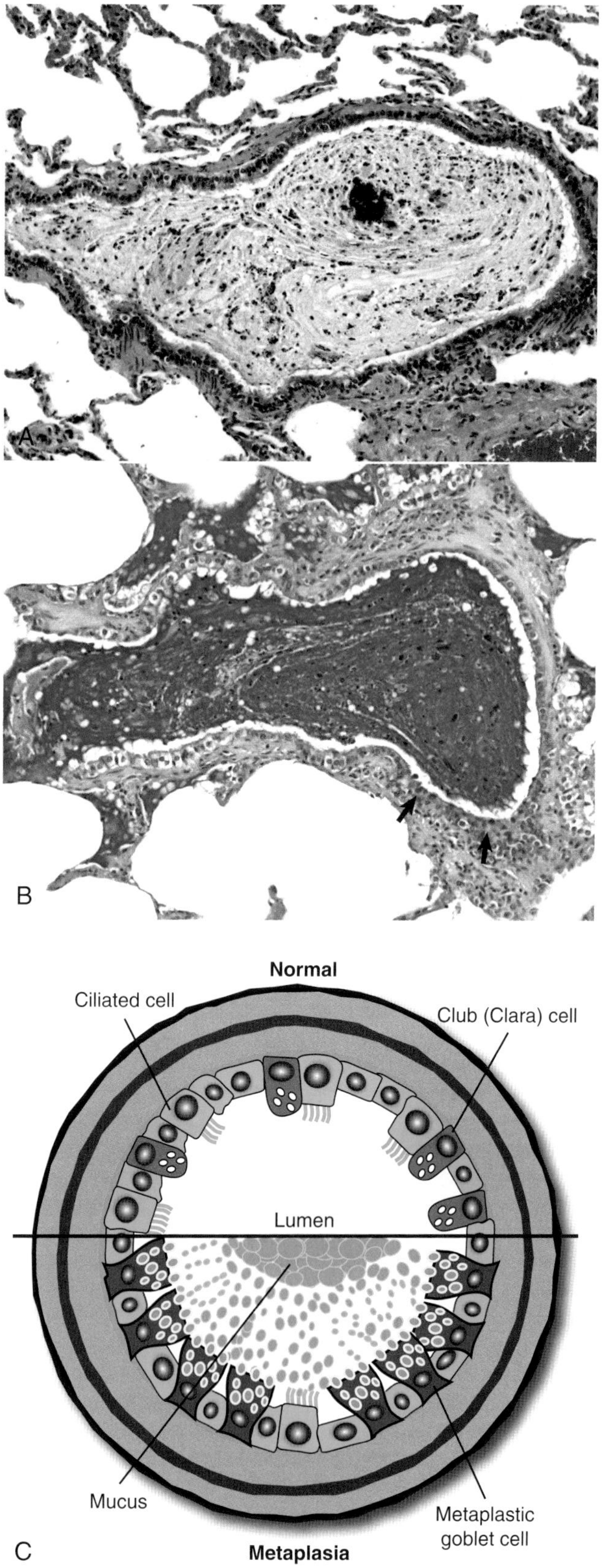

Figure 9-13 Chronic Obstructive Pulmonary Disease (Heaves), Recurrent Airway Obstruction (RAO), Bronchiole, Lung, Horse. A, This 15-year-old horse had a history of recurrent and progressive dyspnea unresponsive to treatment. Note how the bronchiole is plugged with mucus admixed with cell debris and a few neutrophils. H&E stain. **B,** The bronchiole is filled with mucus, and several goblet cells *(arrows)* are present in the mucosa. Healthy bronchioles do not have goblet cells or mucus. Alcian blue stain. **C,** Schematic diagram of a normal bronchiole *(top half of the diagram)* lined with Club cells and some ciliated cells. Bronchiole with severe goblet cell metaplasia *(bottom half of the diagram)* showing abundant metaplastic goblet cells *(purple cells)* and mucus accumulation in the lumen causing chronic obstructive pulmonary disease. (**A** and **B** courtesy Dr. A. López and Dr. C. Legge, Atlantic Veterinary College. **C** courtesy Dr. A. López, Atlantic Veterinary College.)

pneumonocytes, which are arranged as a very delicate continuous membrane extending along the alveolar surface (see Fig. 9-7). Type I pneumonocytes are particularly susceptible to noxious agents that reach the alveolar region either aerogenously or hematogenously. Injury to type I pneumonocytes rapidly causes swelling and vacuolation of these cells (Fig. 9-14). When cellular damage has become irreversible, type I cells detach, resulting in denudation of the basement membrane, increased alveolar permeability, and alveolar edema. Alveolar repair is possible as long as the basement membrane remains intact and lesions are not complicated by further injury or infection. Within 3 days, cuboidal type II (granular) pneumonocytes, which are the precursor cells and more resistant to injury, undergo mitosis and provide a large pool of new undifferentiated cells (Fig. 9-15 and see Fig. 9-14). These new cells repave the denuded alveolar basement membrane and finally differentiate into type I pneumonocytes. When alveolar injury is diffuse, proliferation

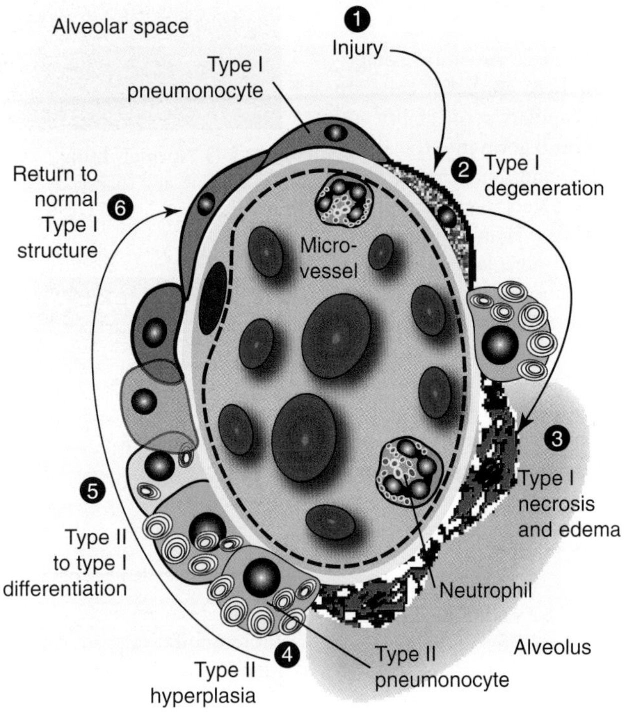

Figure 9-14 Cellular Events during Injury and Necrosis of Type I Pneumonocytes. Severe injury *(1)* can cause degeneration and necrosis of type I pneumonocytes *(2)*. Necrosis of these cells leads to transient alveolar edema *(area that is pink)* *(3)*, which is followed by hyperplasia of type II pneumonocytes *(4)*, stem cells that differentiate *(5)* into type I pneumonocytes as part of alveolar repair and healing *(6)*. (Courtesy Dr. A. López, Atlantic Veterinary College.)

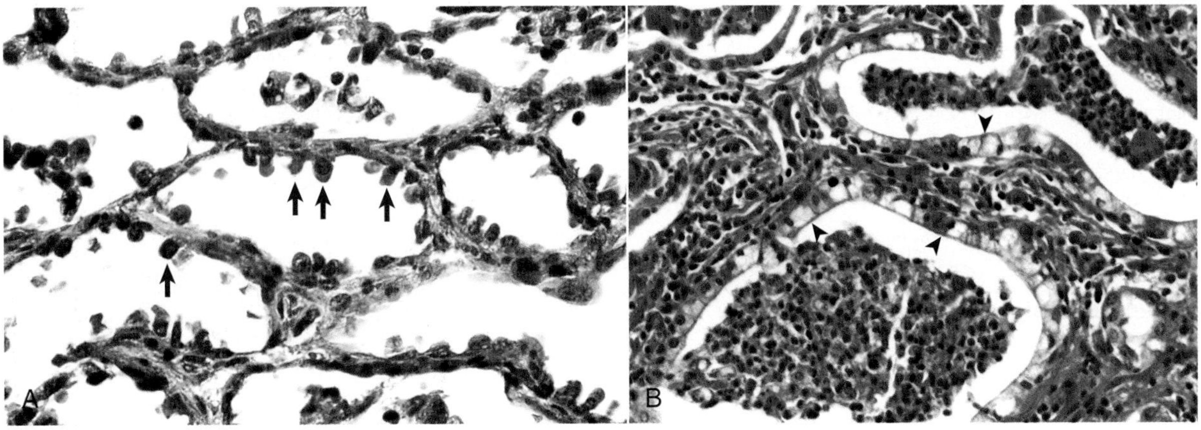

Figure 9-15 Hyperplasia of Type II Pneumonocytes. A, Acute alveolar injury, crude oil aspiration, cow. Note proliferation of cuboidal epithelial cells (type II pneumonocytes) *(arrows)* along the luminal surface of the alveolar wall. During alveolar repair, type II pneumonocytes are the precursor cell for necrotic and lost type I pneumonocytes. H&E stain. **B,** Chronic alveolar injury, interstitial pneumonia, horse. Note entire alveolar membrane lined with cuboidal type II pneumonocytes *(arrowheads)*. The alveolar interstitium is expanded with inflammatory cells, and the alveolar lumens contain cell debris mixed with leukocytes. H&E stain. (**A** courtesy Dr. A. López, Atlantic Veterinary College. **B** courtesy Dr. G. Hines, Provincial Veterinary Laboratory, New Brunswick, and Dr. A. López, Atlantic Veterinary College.)

of type II pneumonocytes becomes so spectacular that the microscopic appearance of the alveolus resembles that of a gland or fetal lung; this lesion has been termed *epithelialization* or *fetalization*. Although it is part of the normal alveolar repair, hyperplasia of type II pneumonocytes can interfere in gas exchange and cause hypoxemia. In uncomplicated cases, type II pneumonocytes eventually differentiate into type I pneumonocytes, thus completing the last stage of alveolar repair (see Fig. 9-14). In some forms of chronic interstitial lung injury, the surface of the alveolar basement membrane could become populated with migrating bronchiolar cells, a process known as alveolar *bronchiolization* or *lambertosis*. In severe cases, lambertosis, a metaplastic change, can be mistaken microscopically with alveolar adenomas.

Type I pneumonocytes are one of the three structural components of the blood-air barrier, so when these epithelial cells are damaged, there is an increase in alveolar capillary permeability and transient leakage of plasma fluid, proteins, and fibrin into the alveolar lumen (see Fig. 9-14). Under normal circumstances, these fluids are rapidly cleared from the alveolus by alveolar and lymphatic absorption, and necrotic pneumonocytes (type I) and fibrin strands are phagocytosed and removed by pulmonary alveolar macrophages. When there is persistent and severe injury, fibroblasts and myofibroblasts may proliferate in the alveolar walls (alveolar interstitium), causing alveolar septal fibrosis, whereas in other forms of severe injury, fibroblasts and myofibroblasts actively migrate from the interstitium into the alveolar spaces, causing intraalveolar fibrosis. These two types of alveolar fibrosis are most commonly seen in toxic and allergic pulmonary diseases and have a devastating effect on lung function.

Endothelial cells are also major players in the normal and abnormal physiology of the alveolus (see Figs. 9-7 and 9-14). These cells trap and share circulating antigens with intravascular and interstitial macrophages. The junction between alveolar endothelial cells is not as tight as that of the type I pneumonocytes, allowing some movement of fluid and small-size molecular weight proteins into the alveolar interstitium. Endothelial cells maintain an intimate cell contact with erythrocytes and leukocytes passing through the lung, since the lumen of alveolar capillaries is slightly smaller (5.0 μm) than the diameter of red and white blood cells. Erythrocytes are easily deformable, so their transit time through the alveolar capillaries is shorter than that of leukocytes, which are less deformable cells. This longer transit time of leukocytes and their close cellular contact with alveolar endothelial cells have major impacts in lung inflammation and acute respiratory distress syndrome (ARDS).

On a minute-to-minute basis, the pulmonary defense mechanisms deal effectively with noxious stimuli and mild tissue injury without the need for an inflammatory response. However, if normal defense mechanisms are ineffective or insufficient (overwhelmed), the inflammatory process is rapidly turned on as a second line of defense.

Postmortem Examination of the Respiratory Tract

Postmortem examination of the respiratory tract should always be conducted in a thorough and systematic manner and include the conducting system (trachea, bronchi, and bronchioles), the lungs, and the thoracic cavity and pleura. Detailed record keeping and photographic documentation are essential elements of a thorough examination. Normal lungs typically have a homogeneous pink color (Fig. 9-16) and are slightly deflated from loss of negative intrathoracic pressure. The E-sections that follow describe a systematic approach to this process.

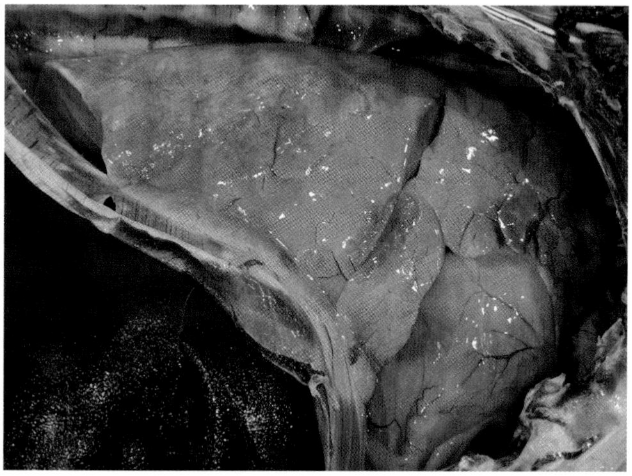

Figure 9-16 **Normal Lung, Dog.** The lung parenchyma appears homogeneously pink and slightly deflated from loss of negative intrathoracic pressure. (Courtesy Dr. A. López, Atlantic Veterinary College.)

Table 9-2 Portals of Entry into the Respiratory System

Route	Agents
Aerogenous (inhalation)	Virus, bacteria, fungi, toxic gases, and pneumotoxicants
Hematogenous (blood)	Virus, bacteria, fungi, parasites, toxins, and pneumotoxicants
Direct extension	Penetrating wounds, migrating awns, bites, and ruptured esophagus or perforated diaphragm (hardware)

More information on postmortem examination of the lung can be found at www.expertconsult.com.

Histopathology and Biopsies

Information on this topic is available at www.expertconsult.com.

Bronchoalveolar Lavage and Transtracheal Wash

Information on this topic is available at www.expertconsult.com.

Portals of Entry/Pathways of Spread

Microbes, toxins, and pneumotoxicants can gain access into the respiratory system by the following routes (Table 9-2; also see Table 9-1): aerogenous, hematogenous, direct extension, and by local production of free radicals and toxic metabolites.

Aerogenous

Pathogens, such as bacteria, mycoplasmas, and viruses, along with toxic gases and foreign particles, including food, can gain access to the respiratory system via inspired air. This is the most common route in the transmission of most respiratory infections in domestic animals.

Hematogenous

Some viruses, bacteria, parasites, and toxins can enter the respiratory system via the circulating blood. This portal of entry is commonly seen in septicemias, bacteremias, and with protozoa and viruses that target endothelial cells. Also, circulating leukocytes may release infectious organisms such as retroviruses and *Listeria monocytogenes* while traveling through the lungs.

Direct Extension

In some instances, pathogenic organisms can also reach the pleura and lungs through penetrating injuries, such as gunshot wounds, migrating awns, or bites, or by direct extension from a ruptured esophagus or perforated diaphragm.

Local Production of Free Radicals and Toxic Metabolites

The lungs, particularly the bronchioles and alveoli, are vulnerable to endogenous injury caused by the local generation of free radicals during inflammation or by toxic metabolites generated by Club (Clara) cells (see Fig. 9-4, *B*).

Pathways of Spread from the Respiratory System (Locally, Regionally, and Systemically)

Inflammatory processes in the respiratory system, particularly those caused by infectious organisms, can spread to contiguous or distant tissues. For instance, rhinitis may spread into the sinuses causing rhinosinusitis. Similarly, laryngeal inflammation may spread into the lungs when exudate in the larynx is aspirated. Lung disease can have profound systemic effects when cytokines, produced locally during necrosis or inflammation, are released into circulation. As a result of the enormous vascular bed present in the lung, sepsis and septic shock often develop when proinflammatory molecules overwhelm the antiinflammatory response during the so-called "cytokine storm."

Defense Mechanisms/Barrier Systems

Defense Mechanisms Against Aerogenous Injury

It is axiomatic that a particle, microbe, or toxic gas must first gain entry to a vulnerable region of the respiratory system before it can induce an adaptive immune response or have a pathologic effect. The characteristics of size, shape, dispersal, and deposition of particles present in inspired air are studied in aerobiology. It is important to recognize the difference between deposition, clearance, and retention of inhaled particles. Deposition is the process by which particles of various sizes and shapes are trapped within specific regions of the respiratory tract. Clearance is the process by which deposited particles are destroyed, neutralized, or removed from the mucosal surfaces. The difference between what is deposited and what is cleared from the respiratory tract is referred to as *retention*. The main mechanisms involved in clearance are sneezing, coughing, mucociliary transport, and phagocytosis (Table 9-3). Abnormal retention of particles resulting from increased deposition, decreased clearance, or a combination of both is the underlying pathogenetic mechanism in many pulmonary diseases (Fig. 9-17).

The anatomic configuration of the nasal cavity and bronchi plays a unique role in preventing or reducing the penetration of noxious material into the lungs, especially into the alveoli, which is the most vulnerable portion of the respiratory system. The narrow nasal meatuses and the coiled arrangement of the nasal conchae generate enormous turbulence of airflow, and as a result, physical forces are created that forcefully impact particles larger than 10 μm onto the surface of the nasal mucosa (Fig. 9-18). Although particles smaller than 10 μm could escape trapping in the nasal cavity, these medium-sized particles meet a second barrier at the tracheal and bronchial

Table 9-3 Main Defense Mechanisms of the Respiratory System

Regions of the Respiratory System	Defense Mechanisms
Conducting system (nose, trachea, and bronchi)	Mucociliary clearance, antibodies, lysozyme, mucus
Transitional system (bronchioles)	Club cells, antioxidants, lysozyme, antibodies
Exchange system (alveoli)	Alveolar macrophages (inhaled pathogens), intravascular macrophages (circulating pathogens), opsonizing antibodies, surfactant, antioxidants

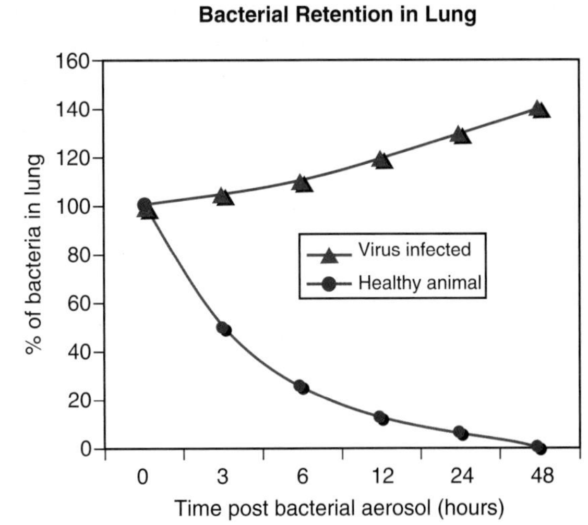

Figure 9-17 **Pulmonary Clearance and Retention of Bacteria Following Inhalation of an Experimental Aerosol of Bacteria.** When large numbers of bacteria are inhaled, the normal defense mechanisms promptly eliminate these microorganisms from the lungs (*blue line*). However, when the defense mechanisms are impaired by a viral infection, lung edema, stress, and so forth, the inhaled bacteria are not eliminated but colonize and multiply in the lung (*red line*). (Courtesy Dr. A. López, Atlantic Veterinary College.)

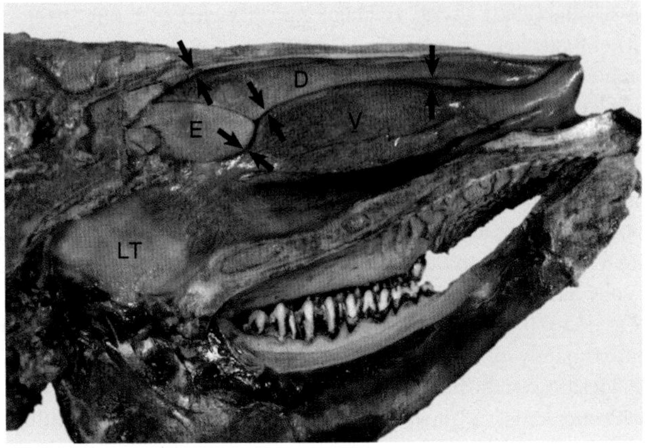

Figure 9-18 **Dorsal *(D)*, Ventral *(V)*, and Ethmoidal *(E)* Conchae, Midsagittal Section of Head, Cow.** These meatuses (*spaces between arrows*) are narrow, and the air turbulence produced in them by the coiled arrangement of the conchae causes suspended particles to impact on the mucus covering the surface of the nasal mucosa. These particles are then moved caudally by the mucociliary apparatus to the pharynx and finally swallowed. Note the abundant lymphoid tissue (*LT*) in the nasopharynx. (Courtesy Dr. R.G. Thomson, Ontario Veterinary College.)

bifurcations. Abrupt changes in the direction of air (inertia), which occurs at the branching of major airways, cause particles in the 2- to 10-μm size range to collide with the surface of bronchial mucosa (see Fig. 9-1). Because the velocity of inspired air at the level of the small bronchi and bronchioles has become rather slow, inertial and centrifugal forces no longer play a significant role in the trapping of inhaled particles. Here, in the transitional (bronchiolar) and exchange (alveolar) regions, particles 2 μm or smaller may come into contact with the mucosa by means of sedimentation because of gravitation or by diffusion as a result of Brownian movement. Infective aerosols containing bacteria and viruses are within the size range (0.01 to 2 μm) that can gain access to the bronchiolar and alveolar regions.

In addition to size, other factors, such as shape, length, electrical charge, and humidity, play an important role in mucosal deposition, retention, and pathogenicity of inhaled particles. For example, particles longer than 200 μm may also reach the lower respiratory tract provided their mean aerodynamic diameter is less than 1 μm. Asbestos is a good example of a large but slender fiber that can bypass the filtrating mechanisms by traveling parallel to the airstream. Once in the terminal bronchioles and alveoli, asbestos fibers cause asbestosis, a serious pulmonary disease in human beings. In summary, the anatomic features of the nasal cavity and airways provide an effective barrier, preventing the penetration of most large particles into the lungs.

Once larger particles are trapped in the mucosa of conducting airways and small particles are deposited on the surface of the nasal, tracheal, or bronchoalveolar mucosa, it is crucial that these exogenous materials be promptly removed to prevent or minimize injury to the respiratory system. For these purposes, the respiratory system is equipped with several defense mechanisms, all of which are provided by specialized cells operating in a remarkably well-coordinated manner.

Conducting System (Nose, Trachea, and Bronchi) and the Transitional System (Bronchioles)

Mucociliary clearance is the physical unidirectional movement and removal of deposited particles and gases dissolved in the mucus from the respiratory tract. Mucociliary clearance, also referred to as the *waste disposal system*, is provided by the mucociliary blanket (mucociliary escalator) and is the main defense mechanism of the conducting system (nasal cavity, trachea, and bronchi) (see Figs. 9-2 and 9-3). Mucus acts primarily as a barrier and a vehicle, and it is a complex mixture of water, glycoproteins, immunoglobulins, lipids, and electrolytes. These substances are produced by goblet (mucous) cells, serous cells, submucosal glands, and fluid from transepithelial ion and water transport. Once serous fluid and mucus are secreted onto the surface of the respiratory mucosa, a thin, double-layer film of mucus is formed on top of the cells. The outer layer of this film is in a viscous gel phase, whereas the inner layer, which is in a fluid or sol phase, is directly in contact with cilia (see Fig. 9-3 and see E-Fig. 9-1). The respiratory system of a healthy human produces approximately 100 mL of mucus per day. Each ciliated cell in the conducting system has approximately 100 to 200 motile and chemosensory cilia (6 μm long), beating metachronously (forming a wave) at a ciliary beat frequency of approximately 1000 strokes per minute, and in a horse, for example, mucus moves longitudinally at a rate of up to 20 mm per minute. Rapid and powerful movement of cilia creates a series of waves that, in a continuous and synchronized manner, propel the mucus, exfoliated cells, and entrapped particles out of the respiratory tract to the pharynx. The mucus is finally swallowed or, when present in large amounts, is coughed up out of the conducting system. If mucus flow were to move at the same rate in all levels of a conducting system, a "bottleneck" effect would be created in major airways as the minor but more numerous airways enter the bronchi. For this reason, the mucociliary transport in proximal (rostral) airways is physiologically faster than that of the distal (caudal) ones. Ciliary activity and mucus transport increase notably in response to stimuli such as in respiratory infections.

The mucociliary blanket of the nasal cavity, trachea, and bronchi also plays an important role in preventing injury from toxic gases. If a soluble gas contacts the mucociliary blanket, it mixes with the mucus, thus reducing the concentration of gas reaching deep into the alveoli. In other words, mucus acts as a "scavenger system," whereby gases are solubilized and subsequently cleared from the respiratory tract via mucociliary transport. If ciliary transport is reduced (loss of cilia) or mucus production is excessive, coughing becomes an important mechanism for clearing the airways.

In addition to the mechanical barrier and physical transport provided by the mucociliary escalator, other cells closely associated with ciliated epithelium contribute to the defense mechanism of the conducting and transitional systems. Among the most notable are the microfold (M) cells, which are modified epithelial cells covering the bronchial-associated lymphoid tissue (BALT), both of which are strategically situated at the corner of the bifurcation of bronchi and bronchioles, where inhaled particles often collide with the mucosa because of inertial forces. From here, inhaled particles and soluble antigens are phagocytosed and transported by macrophages, dendritic cells, and other professional antigen-presenting cells (APCs) into the BALT, thus providing a unique opportunity for B and T lymphocytes to enter into close contact with inhaled pathogenic substances. Pulmonary lymphocytes are not quiescent in the BALT but are in continual traffic to other organs and contribute to both cellular (cytotoxic, helper, and suppressor T lymphocytes) and humoral immune responses. Immunoglobulin A (IgA), produced by mucosal plasma cells, and, to a lesser extent, immunoglobulin G (IgG) and M (IgM) play important roles in the local immunity of the conducting and transitional systems, especially with regard to preventing attachment of pathogens to the cilia. Chronic airway diseases, especially those caused by infectious agents such as mycoplasmas or retroviruses, are often accompanied by severe hyperplasia of the BALT.

The mucociliary clearance terminates at the pharynx, where mucus, propelled caudally from the nasal cavity and cranially from the tracheobronchial tree, is eventually swallowed and thus eliminated from the conducting system of the respiratory tract. Some respiratory pathogens, such as *Rhodococcus equi*, can infect the intestines after having been removed and swallowed from the respiratory tract into the alimentary system.

Exchange System (Alveoli)

Alveoli lack ciliated and mucus-producing cells; thus the defense mechanism against inhaled particles in the alveolar region cannot be provided by mucociliary clearance. Instead, the main defense mechanisms of alveoli (exchange system) are phagocytosis provided by the pulmonary alveolar macrophages and antimicrobial molecules of the alveolar lining fluid (Fig. 9-19). Pulmonary alveolar macrophages are highly phagocytic cells, which are not to be confused with pulmonary intravascular macrophages, and are derived largely from blood monocytes and, to a much lesser extent, from a slowly dividing population of interstitial macrophages. After a temporary adaptive stage within alveolar interstitium, blood monocytes reduce their glycolytic metabolism and increase their oxidative metabolism to function in an aerobic rather than an anaerobic environment. Pulmonary alveolar macrophages contribute to the

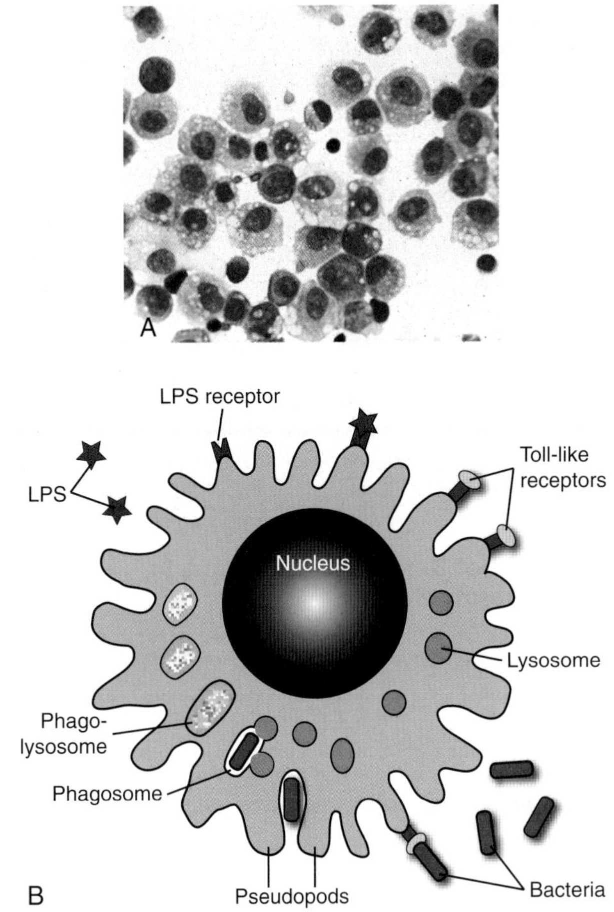

Figure 9-19 **Pulmonary Alveolar Macrophages. A,** Bronchoalveolar lavage, healthy pig. Alveolar macrophages characterized by abundant and vacuolated cytoplasm are the predominant cell in lavages from healthy lungs. Mayer's hematoxylin counter stain. **B,** Schematic representation of a pulmonary alveolar macrophage. Note receptors in cell membrane, attachment of bacteria to cell receptor, bacteria being engulfed by cytoplasmic projections (pseudopods), formation of cytoplasmic phagosomes, and fusion of lysosomes with phagosome (phagolysosomes), which finally kill the ingested bacteria. (**A** courtesy Dr. L.A. Rijana-Ludbit, Tübingen. **B** courtesy of Dr. A. López, Atlantic Veterinary College.)

pulmonary innate and adaptive immune response by rapidly attaching and phagocytosing bacteria and any other particles reaching the alveolar lumens. The number of free macrophages in the alveolar space is closely related to the number of inhaled particles reaching the lungs. This ability to increase, within hours, the number of available phagocytic cells is vital in protecting the distal lungs against foreign material, particularly when the inhaled particle load is high. Unlike that of tissue macrophages, the life span of alveolar macrophages in the alveoli is notably short, only a few days, and thus they are continuously being replaced by newly migrated blood monocytes.

Alveolar phagocytosis plays a prominent role in the innate defense mechanism against inhaled bacteria without the need of an inflammatory reaction. Bacteria reaching the alveoli are rapidly phagocytosed, and bactericidal enzymes present in lysosomes are discharged into the phagosome containing the bacteria (see Fig. 9-19, *B*). Except for some facultative pathogens that are resistant to intracellular killing (e.g., *Mycobacterium tuberculosis*, *Listeria monocytogenes*, *Brucella abortus*, *Rhodococcus equi*, and some *Salmonella* spp.), most bacteria reaching the lungs are rapidly destroyed by activated alveolar macrophages. Similarly, inhaled particles, such as dust, pollen, spores, carbon, or erythrocytes from intraalveolar hemorrhage, are all phagocytosed and eventually removed from alveoli by pulmonary alveolar macrophages. Most alveolar macrophages leave the alveoli by migrating toward the bronchiolar (transitional) region until the mucociliary blanket is reached. Once there, pulmonary macrophages are removed in the same way as any other particle: along the mucociliary flow to the pharynx and swallowed. In the cat, as many as 1 million macrophages per hour move out from the alveoli into the conducting system and pharynx.

Destruction and removal of inhaled microbes and particles by alveolar macrophages is a well-orchestrated mechanism that engages many cells, receptors (i.e., Toll-like receptors [TLRs]), and pulmonary secretions in the lung. The cell-to-cell interactions are complex and involve pulmonary alveolar macrophages, pneumonocytes, endothelial cells, lymphocytes, plasma cells, natural killer (NK) cells, and dendritic cells. Antibodies are also important in the protection (acquired immune response) of the respiratory tract against inhaled pathogens. IgA is the most abundant antibody in the nasal and tracheal secretions and prevents the attachment and absorption of antigens (immune exclusion). IgG and, to a lesser extent, IgE and IgM promote the uptake and destruction of inhaled pathogens by phagocytic cells (immune elimination). IgG is the most abundant antibody in the alveolar surface and acts primarily as an opsonizing antibody for alveolar macrophages and neutrophils. In addition to antibodies, there are several secretory molecules locally released into the alveoli that constitute the alveolar lining material and contribute to the pulmonary defense mechanisms. The most important of these antimicrobial products are transferrin, anionic peptides, and pulmonary surfactant (Table 9-4).

To facilitate phagocytosis and discriminate between "self" and "foreign" antigens, pulmonary alveolar macrophages are furnished with a wide variety of specific receptors on their cell surfaces. Among the most important ones are Fc receptors for antibodies; complement receptors (for C3b, C3a, and C5a); tumor necrosis factor (TNF) receptor; and CD40 receptors, which facilitate phagocytosis and destruction of opsonized particles. Toll-like receptors (TLRs) recognize microbial components, and apoptosis stimulating fragment (FAS) receptors are involved in apoptosis and in the phagocytosis of apoptotic cells in the lung. "Scavenger receptors," which are responsible for the recognition and uptake of foreign particulates, such as dust and fibers, are also present on pulmonary alveolar macrophages.

Defense Mechanisms Against Hematogenous (Blood-Borne) Injury

Lungs are also susceptible to hematogenously borne microbes, toxins, or emboli. The hepatic (Kupffer cells) and splenic macrophages are the primary phagocytic cells responsible for removing circulating bacteria and other particles from the blood of dogs, some rodents, and human beings. In contrast, the cell responsible for the removal of circulating particles, bacteria, and endotoxin from the blood of ruminants, cats, pigs, and horses is mainly the pulmonary intravascular macrophage, a distinct population of phagocytes normally residing within the pulmonary capillaries (see Fig. 9-7). In pigs, 16% of the pulmonary capillary surface is lined by pulmonary intravascular macrophages. In ruminants, 95% of intravenously injected tracer particles or bacteria are rapidly phagocytosed by these intravascular macrophages. Studies have shown that an abnormally reduced number of Kupffer cells in diseased liver results in a compensatory increase in pulmonary intravascular macrophages, even in animal species in which these phagocytic cells are normally absent from the lung. In some abnormal conditions, such as sepsis,

Table 9-4 Defense Mechanisms Provided by Some Cells and Secretory Products Present in the Respiratory System

Cells/Secretory Products	Action
Alveolar macrophage	Phagocytosis, main line of defense against inhaled particles and microbial pathogens in the alveoli
Intravascular macrophage	Phagocytosis, removal of particles, endotoxin, and microbial pathogens in the circulation
Ciliated cells	Expel mucus and inhaled particles and microbial pathogens by ciliary action
Club (Clara) cells	Detoxification of xenobiotics (mixed function oxidases) and protective secretions against oxidative stress and inflammation; production of surfactant
Mucus	Physical barrier; traps inhaled particles and microbial pathogens and neutralizes soluble gases
Surfactant	Protects alveolar walls and enhances phagocytosis
Lysozyme	Antimicrobial enzyme
Transferrin and lactoferrin	Inhibition and suppression of bacterial growth
α_1-Antitrypsin	Protects against the noxious effects of proteolytic enzymes released by phagocytic cells; also inhibits inflammation
Interferon	Antiviral agent and modulator of the immune and inflammatory responses
Interleukins	Chemotaxis, upregulation of adhesion molecules
Antibodies	Prevent microbe attachment to cell membranes, opsonization
Complement	Chemotaxis; enhances phagocytosis
Antioxidants*	Prevent injury caused by superoxide anion, hydrogen peroxide, and free radicals (ROS) generated during phagocytosis, inflammation, or by inhalation of oxidant gases (ozone, nitrogen dioxide [NO_2], sulfur dioxide [SO_2])

*Superoxide dismutase, catalase, glutathione peroxidase, and oxidant free radical scavengers (tocopherol and ascorbic acid).

excessive release of cytokines by pulmonary intravascular macrophages may result in acute lung injury.

Defense Mechanisms Against Oxidants and Free Radicals

Existing in an oxygen-rich environment and being the site of numerous metabolic reactions, the lungs also require an efficient defense mechanism against oxidant-induced cellular damage (oxidative stress). This form of damage is caused by inhaled oxidant gases (e.g., nitrogen dioxide, ozone, sulfur dioxide, or tobacco smoke), by xenobiotic toxic metabolites produced locally, by toxins reaching the lungs via the bloodstream (e.g., 3-methylindole and paraquat), or by free radicals (reactive oxygen species) released by phagocytic cells during inflammation. Free radicals and reactive oxygen species (ROS) not only induce extensive pulmonary injury but also impair the defense and repair mechanisms in the lung. Oxygen and free radical scavengers, such as catalase, superoxide dismutase, ubiquinone, and vitamins E and C, are largely responsible for protecting pulmonary cells against peroxidation. These scavengers are present in alveolar and bronchiolar epithelial cells and in the extracellular spaces of the pulmonary interstitium.

In summary, the defense mechanisms are so effective in trapping, destroying, and removing bacteria that, under normal conditions, animals can be exposed to aerosols containing massive numbers of bacteria without any ill effects. If defense mechanisms are impaired, inhaled bacteria colonize and multiply in bronchi, bronchioles, and alveoli, and they produce infection, which can result in fatal pneumonia. Similarly, when blood-borne pathogens, inhaled toxicants, or free radicals overwhelm the protective defense mechanisms, cells of the respiratory system are likely to be injured, often causing serious respiratory diseases.

Impairment of Defense Mechanisms in the Respiratory System

For many years, factors such as viral infections, toxic gases, stress, and pulmonary edema have been implicated in predisposing human beings and animals to secondary bacterial pneumonia. There are many pathways by which the defense mechanisms can be impaired; only those relevant to veterinary species are discussed.

Viral Infections

Viral agents are notorious in predisposing human beings and animals to secondary bacterial pneumonias by what is known as viral-bacterial synergism. A good example of the synergistic effect of combined virus-bacterial infections is documented from epidemics of human beings with influenza virus in which the mortality rate has been significantly increased from secondary bacterial pneumonia. The most common viruses incriminated in predisposing animals to secondary bacterial pneumonia include influenza virus in pigs and horses; bovine herpesvirus 1 (BoHV-1), bovine parainfluenza virus 3 (BPIV-3), and bovine respiratory syncytial virus (BRSV) in cattle; canine distemper virus (CDV) in dogs; and felid herpesvirus 1 (FeHV-1) and feline calicivirus (FCV) in cats. The mechanism of the synergistic effect of viral-bacterial infections was previously believed to be the destruction of the mucociliary blanket and a concurrent reduction of mucociliary clearance, but in experimental studies, viral infections did not significantly reduce the physical removal of particles or bacteria out of the lungs. Now, it is known that 5 to 7 days after a viral infection, the phagocytic function of pulmonary alveolar macrophages and, to a lesser extent, the mucociliary clearance are notably impaired (see Fig. 9-8). Other mechanisms by which viruses impair defense mechanisms are multiple and remain poorly understood (Box 9-1). Immunization against viral infections in many cases prevents or reduces the synergistic effect of viruses and thus the incidence of secondary bacterial pneumonia.

Toxic Gases

Certain gases also impair respiratory defense mechanisms, rendering animals more susceptible to secondary bacterial infections. For instance, hydrogen sulfide and ammonia, frequently encountered on farms, especially in buildings with poor ventilation, can impair pulmonary defense mechanisms and increase susceptibility to bacterial pneumonia. The effects of environmental pollutants on the defense mechanisms of human beings and animals living in crowded and polluted cities remain to be determined.

Box 9-1 Postulated Mechanisms by Which Viruses and Mycoplasma May Impair the Defense Mechanisms of the Respiratory Tract

- Reduced mucociliary clearance
- Injured epithelium enhances attachment for bacteria
- Enhanced bacterial attachment predisposes to colonization
- Decreased mucociliary clearance prolongs resident time of bacteria favoring colonization
- Injured epithelium prevents mucociliary clearance and physical removal of bacteria
- Lack of secretory products facilitates further cell injury
- Break down the antimicrobial barrier in mucus and cells (β-defensins and anionic peptides)
- Ciliostasis caused by inflammation or by some pathogenic organisms (mycoplasmas)
- Dysfunction of pulmonary alveolar macrophages and lymphocytes
- Consolidation of lung causes hypoxia resulting in decreased phagocytosis
- Infected macrophages fail to release chemotactic factors for other cells
- Infected macrophages fail to attach and ingest bacteria
- Lysosomes become disoriented and fail to fuse with phagosome-containing bacteria
- Intracellular killing or degradation is decreased because of biochemical dysfunction
- Altered cytokines and secretory products impair bacterial phagocytosis
- Viral-induced apoptosis of alveolar macrophages
- Altered CD4 and CD8 lymphocytes
- Toll-like receptors (TLRs) in virus-infected macrophages increase proinflammatory response to bacteria

Immunodeficiencies

Immunodeficiency disorders, whether acquired or congenital, are often associated with increased susceptibility to viral, bacterial, and protozoal pneumonias. For example, human beings with acquired immunodeficiency syndrome (AIDS) are notably susceptible to pneumonia caused by proliferation of *Pneumocystis (carinii) jirovecii*. A similar ubiquitous organism, which under normal circumstances is not pathogenic, is also found in the pneumonic lungs of immunosuppressed pigs, foals, dogs, and rodents. Pigs infected with the porcine reproductive and respiratory syndrome (PRRS) virus frequently develop *Pneumocystis carinii* infection (Fig. 9-20). Arabian foals born with combined immunodeficiency disease easily succumb to infectious diseases, particularly adenoviral pneumonia. Combined infections with two respiratory viruses, such as canine distemper virus (CDV) and canine adenovirus 2 (CAV-2), are sporadically reported in immunosuppressed puppies. Also, large doses of chemotherapeutic agents, such as steroids and alkylating agents, cause immunosuppression in dogs, cats, and other animals, increasing susceptibility to secondary viral and bacterial infections.

Other Conditions that Impair Defense Mechanisms

Stress, uremia, endotoxemia, dehydration, starvation, hypoxia, acidosis, pulmonary edema, anesthesia, and ciliary dyskinesia are only some of the many conditions that have been implicated in impairing respiratory defense mechanisms and consequently predisposing animals to develop secondary bacterial pneumonia. The mechanisms by which each of these factors suppresses pulmonary defenses are diverse and sometimes not well understood. For example, hypoxia and pulmonary edema decrease phagocytic function of pulmonary alveolar macrophages and alter the production of surfactant

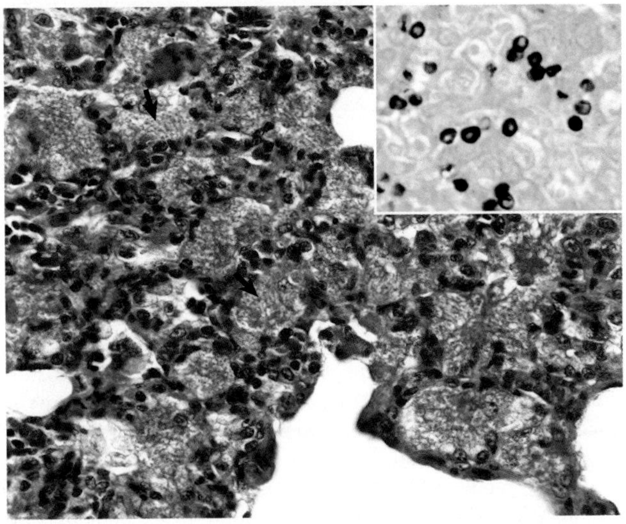

Figure 9-20 Pneumocystosis *(Pneumocystis carinii)*, Lung, Pig. Alveoli are filled with a foamy eosinophilic proteinaceous material in which numerous punctiform organisms *(arrows)* are present. H&E stain. *Inset,* Silver-stained oval bodies typical of *Pneumocystis carinii*. Pneumocystosis is generally a microscopic diagnosis because this condition does not cause remarkable gross lesions. Gomori's methenamine silver stain. (Courtesy Dr. A. López, Atlantic Veterinary College.)

by type II pneumonocytes. Dehydration is thought to increase the viscosity of mucus, reducing or stopping mucociliary movement. Anesthesia induces ciliostasis with concurrent loss of mucociliary function. Ciliary dyskinesia, an inherited defect in cilia, causes abnormal mucus transport. Starvation, hypothermia, and stress can reduce humoral and cellular immune responses.

Disorders of the Conducting System

Disorders of the Nasal Cavity and Paranasal Sinuses in Domestic Animals

Anomalies[2]

Localized congenital anomalies of the nasal cavity are rare in domestic animals and are often merely part of a more extensive craniofacial deformity (e.g., cyclops) or a component of generalized malformation (e.g., chondrodysplasia). Congenital anomalies involving the nasal cavity and sinuses, such as choanal atresia (lack of communication between the nasal cavity and pharynx), some types of chondrodysplasia, and osteopetrosis, are incompatible with life. Examples of nonfatal congenital anomalies include cystic nasal conchae, deviation of the nasal septum, cleft upper lip (harelip and cheiloschisis), hypoplastic turbinates, and cleft palate (palatoschisis) (see Fig. 7-32). Bronchoaspiration and aspiration pneumonia are common sequelae to cleft palate. Nasal and paranasal sinus cysts are slowly growing and expansive lesions that mimic neoplasia and cause severe cranial deformation in horses. As in other organs or systems, it is extremely difficult to determine the actual cause (genetic vs. congenital) of anomalies based on pathologic evaluation.

Metabolic Disturbances

Metabolic disturbances affecting the nasal cavity and sinuses are rare in domestic animals.

[2]See E-Box 1-1 for potential, suspected, or known genetic disorders.

Nasal Amyloidosis. Amyloidosis, the deposition of amyloid protein (fibrils with a β-pleated configuration) in various tissues, has been sporadically reported as a localized lesion in the nasal cavity of horses and human beings (see Nasal Amyloidosis, in Disorders of Horses).

Circulatory Disturbances

Congestion and Hyperemia. The nasal mucosa is well vascularized and is capable of rather dramatic variation in blood flow, whether passively as a result of interference with venous return (congestion) or actively because of vasodilation (hyperemia). Congestion of the mucosal vessels is a nonspecific lesion commonly found at necropsy and presumably associated with the circulatory failure preceding death (e.g., heart failure, bloat in ruminants in which the increased intraabdominal pressure causes increased intrathoracic pressure impeding the venous return from the head and neck). Hyperemia of the nasal mucosa is seen in early stages of inflammation, whether caused by irritation (e.g., ammonia and regurgitated feed), viral infections, secondary bacterial infections, toxemia, allergy, or trauma.

Hemorrhage. *Epistaxis* is the clinical term used to denote blood flow from the nose (nosebleed) regardless of whether the blood originates from the nasal mucosa or from deep in the lungs, such as in horses with "exercise-induced pulmonary hemorrhage." Unlike blood in the digestive tract, where the approximate anatomic location of the bleeding can be estimated by the color the blood imparts to fecal material, blood in the respiratory tract is always red. This fact is due to the rapid transport of blood out of the respiratory tract by the mucociliary blanket and during breathing. Hemorrhages into the nasal cavity can be the result of local trauma, can originate from erosions of submucosal vessels by inflammation (e.g., guttural pouch mycosis), or can be caused by neoplasms. Hemoptysis refers to the presence of blood in sputum or saliva (coughing or spitting blood) and is most commonly the result of pneumonia, lung abscesses, ulcerative bronchitis, pulmonary thromboembolisms or hemorrhage, and pulmonary neoplasia.

Inflammation (Rhinitis and Sinusitis)

Inflammation of the nasal mucosa is called *rhinitis*, and inflammation of the sinuses is called *sinusitis*. These conditions usually occur together, although mild sinusitis can be undetected. Clinically, rhinosinusitis is characterized by nasal discharge.

Rhinitis. The occurrence of infectious rhinitis presupposes an upset in the balance of the normal microbial flora of the nasal cavity. Innocuous bacteria present normally protect the host through a process called *competitive exclusion*, whereby potential pathogens are kept at a harmless level. Disruption of this protective mechanism can be caused by respiratory viruses, pathogenic bacteria, fungi, irritant gases, environmental changes, immunosuppression, local trauma, stress, or prolonged antibacterial therapy.

Inflammatory processes in the nasal cavity are not life-threatening and usually resolve completely. However, some adverse sequelae in cases of infectious rhinitis include bronchoaspiration of exudate leading to bronchopneumonia. Chronic rhinitis often leads to destruction of the nasal conchae (turbinates), deviation of the septum, and, eventually, craniofacial deformation. Also, nasal inflammation may extend into the sinuses causing sinusitis; into facial bones causing osteomyelitis; through the cribriform plate causing meningitis; into the Eustachian tubes causing otitis media or guttural pouch empyema (eustachitis) in horses; and even into the inner ear causing otitis interna and vestibular syndrome (abnormal head tilt and abnormal gait), which in severe cases may lead to emaciation.

Based on the nature of exudate, rhinitis can be classified as serous, fibrinous, catarrhal, purulent, or granulomatous. These types of inflammatory reactions can progress from one to another in the course of the disease (i.e., serous to catarrhal to purulent), or in some instances exudates can be mixed, such as those seen in mucopurulent, fibrinohemorrhagic, or pyogranulomatous rhinitis. Microscopic examination of impression smears or nasal biopsy, and bacterial or fungal cultures are generally required in establishing the cause of inflammation. Common sequelae of rhinitis are hemorrhage, ulcers, and, in some cases, nasopharyngeal polyps (hyperplasia) arising from inflamed mucosa. Rhinitis also can be classified according to the age of the lesions as acute, subacute, or chronic; to the severity of the insult as mild, moderate, or severe; and to the etiologic agent as viral, allergic, bacterial, mycotic, parasitic, traumatic, or toxic.

Serous Rhinitis. Serous rhinitis is the mildest form of inflammation and is characterized by hyperemia and increased production of a clear fluid locally manufactured by serous glands present in the nasal submucosa. Serous rhinitis is of clinical interest only. It is caused by mild irritants or cold air, and it occurs during the early stages of viral infections, such as the common cold in human beings, upper respiratory tract infections in animals, or in mild allergic reactions.

Catarrhal Rhinitis. Catarrhal rhinitis is a slightly more severe process and has, in addition to serous secretions, a substantial increase in mucus production by hypersecretion of goblet cells and mucous glands. A mucous exudate is a thick, translucent, or slightly turbid viscous fluid, sometimes containing a few exfoliated cells, leukocytes, and cellular debris. In chronic cases, catarrhal rhinitis is characterized microscopically by notable hyperplasia of goblet cells. As the inflammation becomes more severe, the mucus is infiltrated with neutrophils, giving the exudate a cloudy appearance. This exudate is referred to as *mucopurulent*.

Purulent (Suppurative) Rhinitis. Purulent (suppurative) rhinitis is characterized by a neutrophilic exudate, which occurs when the nasal mucosa suffers a more severe injury that generally is accompanied by mucosal necrosis and secondary bacterial infection. Cytokines, leukotrienes, complement activation, and bacterial products cause exudation of leukocytes, especially neutrophils, which mix with nasal secretions, including mucus. Grossly, the exudate in suppurative rhinitis is thick and opaque, but it can vary from white to green to brown, depending on the types of bacteria and type of leukocytes (neutrophils or eosinophils) present in the exudate (Fig. 9-21). In severe cases, the nasal passages are completely blocked by the exudate. Microscopically, neutrophils can be seen in the submucosa and mucosa and form plaques of exudate on the mucosal surface. Neutrophils are commonly found marginated in vessels, in the lamina propria, and in between epithelial cells in their migration to the surface of the mucosa.

Fibrinous Rhinitis. Fibrinous rhinitis is a reaction that occurs when nasal injury causes a severe increase in vascular permeability, resulting in abundant exudation of plasma fibrinogen, which coagulates into fibrin. Grossly, fibrin appears as a yellow, tan, or gray rubbery mat on nasal mucosa. Fibrin accumulates on the surface and forms a distinct film of exudate sometimes referred to as *pseudomembrane* (Fig. 9-22). If this fibrinous exudate can be removed, leaving an intact underlying mucosa, it is termed a *croupous* or *pseudodiphtheritic rhinitis*. Conversely, if the pseudomembrane is difficult to remove and leaves an ulcerated mucosa, it is referred to as *diphtheritic* or *fibrinonecrotic rhinitis*. The term *diphtheritic* was derived from human diphtheria, which causes a severe and destructive inflammatory process of the nasal, tonsillar, pharyngeal, and laryngeal mucosa.

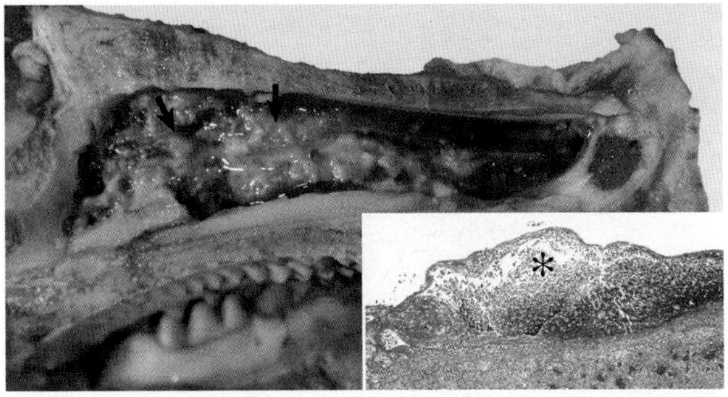

Figure 9-21 Suppurative Rhinitis, Midsagittal Section of Head, Pig. The nasal septum has been removed to expose nasal conchae. The nasal mucosa is hyperemic and covered by yellow-white purulent exudate *(arrows)*. *Inset,* Histological section showing submucosal congestion and edema and also large aggregates of neutrophils on the superficial mucosa *(asterisk)*. H&E stain. (Courtesy Dr. A. López, Atlantic Veterinary College.)

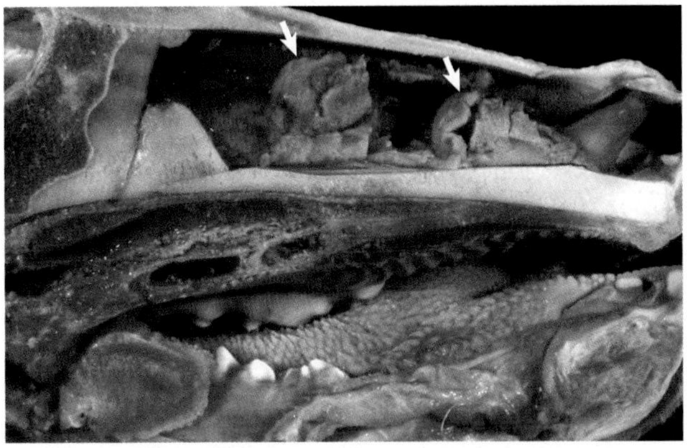

Figure 9-22 Fibrinous Rhinitis, Midsagittal Section of Head, Calf. Infectious bovine rhinotracheitis (IBR; bovine herpesvirus 1). The nasal septum has been removed to expose nasal conchae. The nasal mucosa is covered by diphtheritic yellow membranes consisting of fibrinonecrotic exudate *(arrows)*. Removal of these fibrinous membranes reveals focal ulcers in the underlying mucosa. (Courtesy Dr. Scott McBurney, Atlantic Veterinary College.)

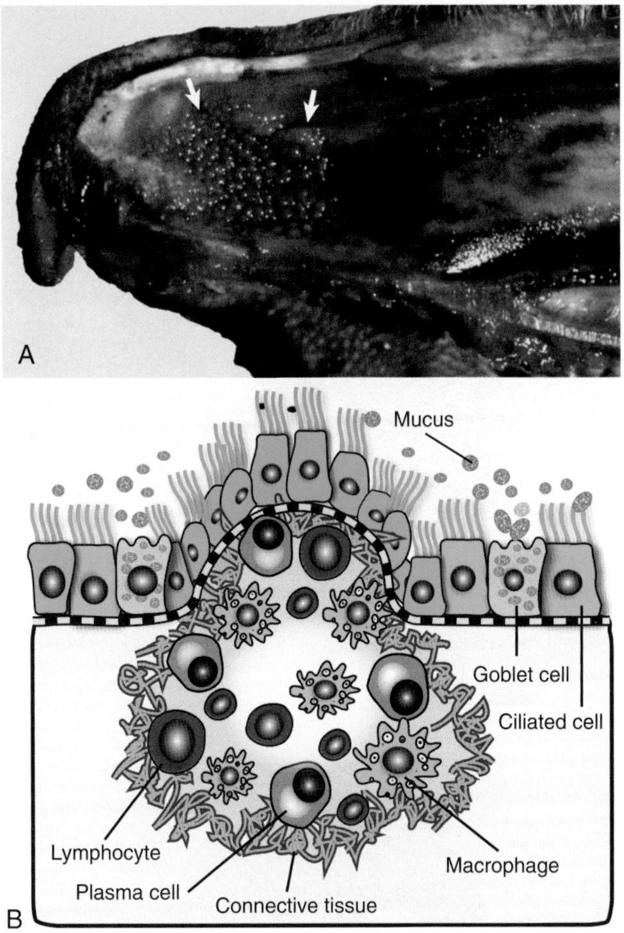

Figure 9-23 Granulomatous Rhinitis, Midsagittal Section of Head, Cow. A, Note multiple and often confluent granulomas *(arrows)* arising from the nasal mucosa. **B,** Schematic representation of a nasal granuloma showing the outer wall of the granuloma composed of connective tissue enclosing the center, which has been infiltrated with lymphocytes, plasma cells, and macrophages. (**A** courtesy Ontario Veterinary College. **B** courtesy of Dr. A. López, Atlantic Veterinary College.)

Microscopically, the lesions include a perivascular edema with fibrin, a few neutrophils infiltrating the mucosa, and superficial plaques of exudate consisting of fibrin strands mixed with leukocytes and cellular debris covering a necrotic and ulcerated epithelium. Fungal infections, such as aspergillosis, can cause a severe fibrinonecrotizing rhinitis.

Granulomatous Rhinitis. Granulomatous rhinitis is a reaction in the nasal mucosa and submucosa that is characterized by infiltration of numerous activated macrophages mixed with a few lymphocytes and plasma cells (Figs. 9-23 and 9-24). In some cases, chronic inflammation leads to the formation of polypoid nodules that in severe cases are large enough to cause obstruction of the nasal passages (Fig. 9-25). Granulomatous rhinitis is generally associated with chronic allergic inflammation or infection with specific organisms, such as fungi (see Fig. 9-24), tuberculosis, systemic mycosis (see section on Granulomatous Pneumonia), and rhinosporidiosis (Fig. 9-26; also see Fig. 9-25). In some cases, the cause of granulomatous rhinitis cannot be determined.

Sinusitis. Sinusitis occurs sporadically in domestic animals and is frequently combined with rhinitis (rhinosinusitis), or it occurs as

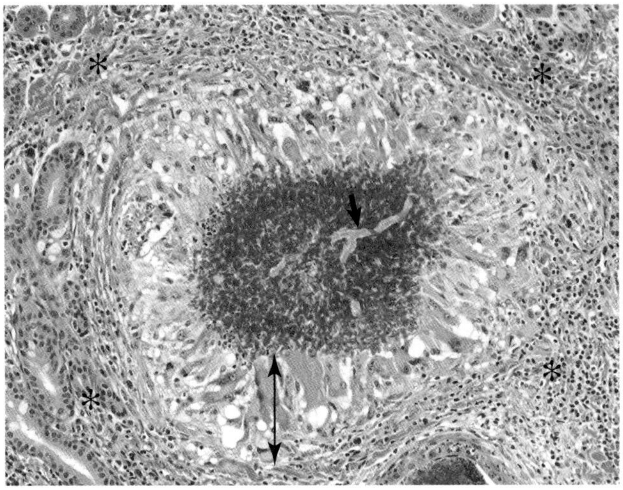

Figure 9-24 Nasal Mucosa, Granulomatous Rhinitis, Mycotic Infection, Ewe. The granuloma is composed of three distinct layers: an outer layer of fibroblasts, lymphocytes, and plasma cells *(asterisks)*; a middle thick layer of epithelioid macrophages *(double-headed arrow)*; and a necrotic center of cellular debris containing a fungal hypha *(arrow)*. H&E stain. (Courtesy Dr. A. López, Atlantic Veterinary College.)

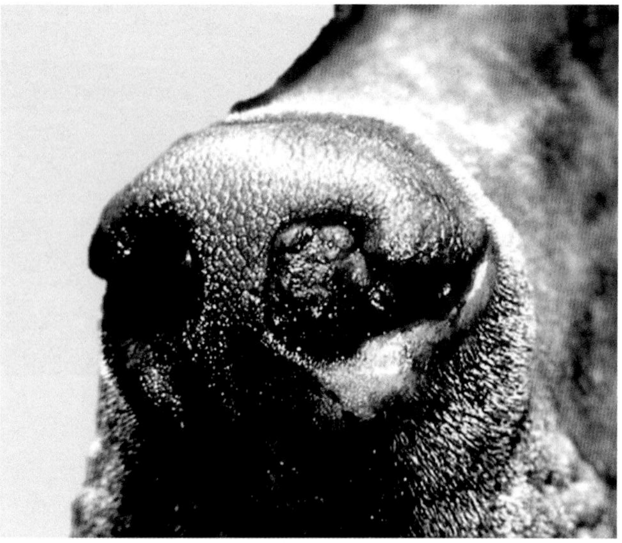

Figure 9-25 **Granulomatous Rhinitis (*Rhinosporidium seeberi*), Nasal Cavity and Nostril, Dog.** A polypoid granulomatous mass fills the rostral part of the left nasal cavity. (Courtesy Dr. C. Bridges, College of Veterinary Medicine, Texas A&M University, and Dr. J.M. King, College of Veterinary Medicine, Cornell University.)

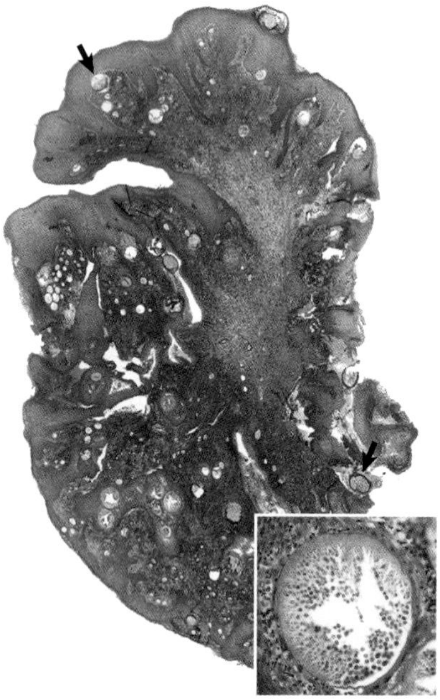

Figure 9-26 **Exophytic Granulomatous Mass Surgically Removed From the Nasal Mucosa (*Rhinosporidium seeberi*), Mule.** Large pedunculated mass of granulomatous tissue containing numerous sporangia *(arrows)*. *Inset,* Sporangium. Note a large encapsulated cyst filled with a myriad of *Rhinosporidium seeberi* endospores. H&E stain. (From Berrocal A, López A: *Can Vet J* 48:305-306, 2007.)

a sequela to penetrating or septic wounds of the nasal, frontal, maxillary, or palatine bones; improper dehorning in young cattle, which exposes the frontal sinus; or maxillary tooth infection in horses and dogs (maxillary sinus). Based on the type of exudate, sinusitis is classified as serous, catarrhal, fibrinous (rare), purulent, or granulomatous. Paranasal sinuses have poor drainage; therefore exudate tends to accumulate, causing mucocele (accumulation of mucus) or empyema (accumulation of pus) (Fig. 9-27). Chronic sinusitis may

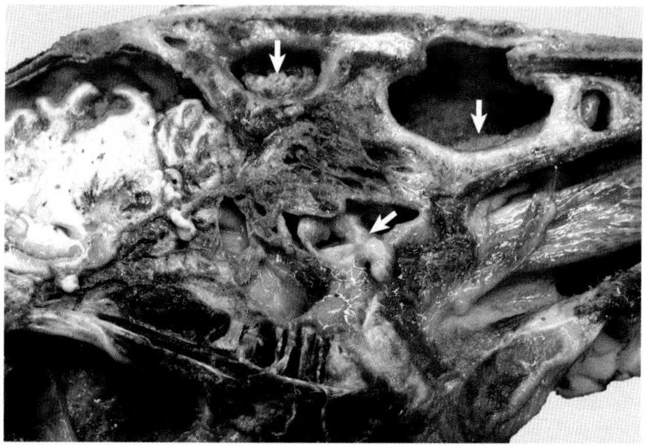

Figure 9-27 **Fibrinosuppurative Sinusitis, Midsagittal Section of Head, Donkey.** Note that the paranasal sinuses are filled with fibrinopurulent exudate *(arrows)*. (Courtesy Facultad de Medicina Veterinaria y Zootecnia, Universidad Nacional Autónoma de México.)

extend into the adjacent bone (osteomyelitis) or through the ethmoidal conchae into the meninges and brain (meningitis and encephalitis).

Species-Specific Diseases of the Nasal Cavity and Paranasal Sinuses

Disorders of Horses

Metabolic Disturbances

Nasal Amyloidosis. Amyloidosis, the deposition of amyloid protein (fibrils with a β-pleated configuration) in various tissues, has been sporadically reported as a localized lesion in the nasal cavity of horses. Unlike amyloidoses in other organs of domestic animals where amyloid is generally of the reactive type (amyloid AA), equine nasal amyloidosis appears to be of the immunocytic type (amyloid AL). Affected horses with large amyloid masses have difficulty breathing because of nasal obstruction and may exhibit epistaxis and reduced athletic performance; on clinical examination, large, firm nodules resembling neoplasms (amyloidoma) can be observed in the alar folds, rostral nasal septum, and floor of nasal cavity. Microscopic lesions are similar to those seen in other organs and consist of a deposition of hyaline amyloid material in nasal mucosa that is confirmed by a histochemical stain, such as Congo red.

Circulatory Disturbances

Progressive Ethmoidal Hematoma. Progressive ethmoidal hematoma (PEH) is important in older horses and is characterized clinically by chronic, progressive, often unilateral nasal bleeding. Grossly or endoscopically, an ethmoidal hematoma appears as a single, soft, tumor-like, pedunculated, expansive, dark red mass arising from the mucosa of the ethmoidal conchae (Fig. 9-28). Microscopic examination reveals a capsule lined by epithelium and hemorrhagic stromal tissue infiltrated with abundant macrophages, most of which are siderophages.

Viral Infections. Viruses, such as equine viral rhinopneumonitis virus, influenza virus, adenovirus, and equine picornavirus, cause mild and generally transient respiratory infections in horses. The route of infection for these respiratory viruses is typically aerogenous. All of these infections are indistinguishable clinically; signs consist mainly of malaise, fever, coughing, conjunctivitis, and nasal

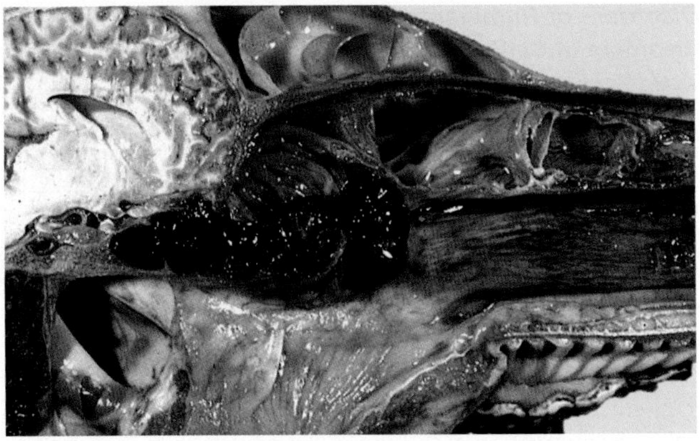

Figure 9-28 **Ethmoidal Hematoma, Midsagittal Section of Head, Horse.** A large amount of dark-red hemorrhage *(left center of image)* overlying the ethmoid conchae conceals an underlying hematoma in these conchae. (Courtesy Dr. J.M. King, College of Veterinary Medicine, Cornell University.)

discharge varying from serous to purulent. Viral respiratory infections are common medical problems in adult horses.

Equine Viral Rhinopneumonitis. Equine viral rhinopneumonitis (EVR) is caused by two ubiquitous equine herpesviruses (EHV-1 and EHV-4) and may be manifested as a mild respiratory disease in weanling foals and young racehorses, as a neurologic disease (myeloencephalopathy), or as abortion in mares. The portal of entry for the respiratory form is typically aerogenous, and the disease is generally transient; thus the primary viral-induced lesions in the nasal mucosa and lungs are rarely seen at necropsy unless complicated by secondary bacterial rhinitis, pharyngitis, or bronchopneumonia. Studies with polymerase chain reaction (PCR) techniques have demonstrated that, like other herpesviruses, EHV-1 and EHV-4 persist in the trigeminal ganglia for long periods of time (latency). Reactivation because of stress or immunosuppression and subsequent shedding of the virus are the typical source of infection for susceptible animals on the farm.

Equine Influenza. Equine influenza is a common, highly contagious, and self-limiting upper respiratory infection of horses caused by aerogenous exposure to type A strains of influenza virus (H7N7 [A/equi-1] and H3N8 [A/equi-2]). Equine influenza has high morbidity (outbreaks) but low mortality, and it is clinically characterized by fever, conjunctivitis, and serous nasal discharge. It occurs mainly in 2- to 3-year-old horses at the racetrack. As with human influenza, equine influenza is usually a mild disease, but occasionally it can cause severe bronchointerstitial pneumonia with pulmonary edema. In some horses, impaired defense mechanisms caused by the viral infection are complicated by a secondary bacterial bronchopneumonia caused by opportunistic organisms (*Streptococcus zooepidemicus*, *Staphylococcus aureus*, or *Bacteroides* sp.) found in the normal flora of the upper respiratory tract. Uncomplicated cases of equine influenza are rarely seen in the postmortem room. Equine influenza virus (H3N8) recently did an equine to canine "host-jump" causing extensive outbreaks of respiratory disease in dogs (see Pneumonias of Dogs).

Other Equine Respiratory Viruses. Equine picornavirus, adenovirus, and parainfluenza virus produce mild and transient upper respiratory infections (nasopharynx and trachea) in horses, unless complicated by secondary pathogens. In addition to reduced athletic performance, infected horses may have a temporary suppression of cell-mediated immunity leading to opportunistic infections such as *Pneumocystis carinii* pneumonia. Fatal adenoviral infections with severe pneumonia or enteritis occur commonly in immunocompromised horses, particularly in Arabian foals with inherited combined immunodeficiency disease.

Bacterial Infections. Strangles, glanders, and melioidosis of horses are all systemic bacterial diseases that cause purulent rhinitis and suppuration in various organs. These diseases are grouped as upper respiratory diseases because nasal discharge is often the most notable clinical sign.

Strangles. Strangles is an infectious and highly contagious disease of Equidae that is caused by *Streptococcus equi* ssp. *equi* (*Streptococcus equi*). It is characterized by suppurative rhinitis and lymphadenitis (mandibular and retropharyngeal lymph nodes) with occasional hematogenous dissemination to internal organs. Unlike *Streptococcus equi* ssp. *zooepidemicus* (*Streptococcus zooepidemicus*) and *Streptococcus dysgalactiae* ssp. *equisimilis* (*Streptococcus equisimilis*), *Streptococcus equi* is not part of the normal nasal flora. Infection occurs when susceptible horses come into contact with feed, exudate, or air droplets containing the bacterium. After penetrating through the nasopharyngeal mucosa, *Streptococcus equi* drains to the regional lymph nodes—mandibular and retropharyngeal lymph nodes—via lymphatic vessels. The gross lesions in horses with strangles (mucopurulent rhinitis) correlate with clinical findings and consist of copious amounts of mucopurulent exudate in the nasal passages with notable hyperemia of the nasal mucosa. Affected lymph nodes are enlarged and may contain abscesses filled with thick purulent exudate (purulent lymphadenitis). The term *bastard strangles* is used in cases in which hematogenous dissemination of *Streptococcus equi* results in metastatic abscesses in such organs as the lungs, liver, spleen, kidneys, or brain or in the joints. This form of strangles is often fatal.

Common sequelae to strangles include bronchopneumonia caused by aspiration of nasopharyngeal exudate; laryngeal hemiplegia ("roaring"), resulting from compression of the recurrent laryngeal nerves by enlarged retropharyngeal lymph nodes; facial paralysis and Horner syndrome caused by compression of sympathetic nerves that run dorsal to the medial retropharyngeal lymph node; and purpura hemorrhagica as a result of vasculitis caused by deposition of *Streptococcus equi* antigen-antibody complexes in arterioles, venules, and capillaries of the skin and mucosal membranes. In severe cases, nasal infection extends directly into the paranasal sinuses or to the guttural pouches via the Eustachian tubes, causing inflammation and accumulation of pus (guttural pouch empyema). Rupture of abscesses in the mandibular and retropharyngeal lymph nodes leads to suppurative inflammation of adjacent subcutaneous tissue (cellulitis), and in severe cases the exudate escapes through cutaneous fistulas.

Strangles can affect horses of all ages, but it is most commonly seen in foals and young horses. It is clinically characterized by cough, nasal discharge, conjunctivitis, and painful swelling of regional lymph nodes. Some horses become carriers and a source of infection to other horses.

Glanders. Glanders is an infectious World Organization for Animal Health (OIE)-notifiable disease of Equidae caused by *Burkholderia mallei* (*Pseudomonas mallei*) that can be transmitted to carnivores by consumption of infected horsemeat. Human beings are also susceptible, and untreated infection is often fatal. This Gram-negative bacterium has been listed as a potential agent for biologic warfare and bioterrorism. In the past, *Burkholderia mallei* was found throughout the world, but today, glanders has been eradicated from most countries, except for some areas in North Africa, Asia, and eastern Europe. There also have been sporadic outbreaks reported in Brazil. The pathogenesis of glanders is not fully understood. Results from experimental infections suggest that infection occurs via the ingestion of contaminated feed and water and, very rarely, via inhalation of infectious droplets. The portals of entry are presumed to be the oropharynx or intestine, in which bacteria penetrate the mucosa and spread via lymph vessels to regional lymph nodes, then to the bloodstream, and thus hematogenously to the internal organs, particularly the lungs.

Lesions in the nasal cavity start as pyogranulomatous nodules in the submucosa; these lesions subsequently ulcerate, releasing copious amounts of *Burkholderia mallei*–containing exudate into the nasal cavity (see Fig. 4-25, A). Finally, ulcerative lesions in conchal mucosa heal and are replaced by typical stellate (star-shaped), fibrous scars. In some cases, the lungs also contain numerous gray, hard, small (2 to 10 mm), miliary nodules (resembling millet seeds) randomly distributed in one or more pulmonary lobes because of the hematogenous route. Microscopically, these nodules are typical chronic granulomas composed of a necrotic center, with or without calcification, surrounded by a layer of macrophages enclosed by a thick band of connective tissue infiltrated with macrophages, fewer giant cells, lymphocytes, and plasma cells. Cutaneous lesions, often referred to as equine farcy, are the result of severe suppurative lymphangitis characterized by nodular thickening of extended segments of lymph vessels in the subcutaneous tissue of the legs and ventral abdomen (see Fig. 4-25, C). Eventually, affected lymph vessels rupture and release large amounts of purulent exudate through sinuses to the surface of the skin.

Melioidosis (Pseudoglanders). Melioidosis (pseudoglanders) is an important, life-threatening disease of human beings, horses, cattle, sheep, goats, pigs, dogs, cats, and rodents caused by *Burkholderia pseudomallei* (*Pseudomonas pseudomallei*). This disease in horses is clinically and pathologically similar to glanders, hence the name *pseudoglanders*. In human beings, this infection can cause severe sepsis and septic shock and has also been considered to have potential for biologic welfare. Melioidosis is currently present in Southeast Asia and, to a much lesser extent, in northern Australia and some European countries where the causative organism is frequently found in rodents, feces, soil, and water. Ingestion of contaminated feed and water appears to be the main route of infection; direct transmission between infected animals and insect bites has also been postulated as a possible mechanism of infection. After gaining entrance to the animal, *Burkholderia pseudomallei* is disseminated by the bloodstream and causes suppuration and abscesses in most internal organs, such as nasal mucosa, joints, brain and spinal cord, lungs, liver, kidneys, spleen, and lymph nodes. The exudate is creamy or caseous and yellow to green. The pulmonary lesions in melioidosis are those of an embolic bacterial infection with the formation of pulmonary abscesses, which can become confluent. Focal adhesive pleuritis develops where abscesses rupture through the pleura and heal.

Parasitic Infections

Rhinosporidiosis. The protistan parasite, *Rhinosporidium seeberi*, causes nasal infection in human beings, horses, mules, cattle, dogs, and cats. Gross lesions vary from barely visible granulomas to large expansive polypoid nodules that may be mistaken as tumors. These granulomatous nodules are detected by direct observation when present in the nasal mucosa close to the nares or by rhinoscopy when located in the deep nasal cavity. The offending organism, *Rhinosporidium seeberi*, is readily visible in histologic preparations and in impression smears, appearing as a large (400 μm), oval sporangium containing thousands of endospores (see Fig. 9-26). *Rhinosporidium seeberi* was once considered a mycotic agent, but recent phylogenetic investigations suggest that it is an aquatic protistan parasite of the class Mesomycetozoea.

Disorders of Ruminants (Cattle, Sheep, and Goats)

Disorders of Cattle

Viral Infections

Infectious Bovine Rhinotracheitis. Infectious bovine rhinotracheitis (IBR), or "rednose," occurs worldwide and is a disease of great importance to the cattle industry because of the synergism of the IBR virus with *Mannheimia haemolytica* in producing pneumonia. The causative agent, bovine herpesvirus 1 (BoHV-1), has probably existed as a mild venereal disease in cattle in Europe since at least the mid-1800s, but the respiratory form was not reported until intensive management feedlot systems were first introduced in North America around the 1950s. Typically, the disease is manifested as a transient, acute, febrile illness, which results in inspiratory dyspnea caused by obstruction of the airways by exudate only in very severe cases. Other forms of BoHV-1 infection include ulcerative rumenitis; enteritis; multifocal hepatitis in neonatal calves; nonsuppurative meningoencephalitis; infertility; and in experimental infections, mastitis, mammillitis, and ovarian necrosis. Except for the encephalitic form, the type of disease caused by BoHV-1 depends more on the site of entry than the viral strain. Like other herpesviruses, BoHV-1 also can remain latent in nerve ganglia, with recrudescence after stress or immunosuppression. This virus also causes bovine abortion, systemic infections of calves, and genital infections such as infectious pustular vulvovaginitis (IPV) and infectious balanoposthitis (IBP).

The respiratory form of IBR is characterized by severe hyperemia and multifocal necrosis of nasal, pharyngeal, laryngeal, tracheal, and sometimes bronchial mucosa (Fig. 9-29 and see Fig. 9-22). As in other respiratory viral infections, IBR lesions are microscopically characterized by necrosis and exfoliation of ciliated cells followed by repair. Secondary bacterial infections of these areas of necrosis result in the formation of a thick layer of fibrinonecrotic material (diphtheritic) in the nasal, tracheal, and bronchial mucosa (see Fig. 9-22). Intranuclear inclusion bodies, commonly seen in herpesvirus infections, are rarely seen in field cases because inclusion bodies occur only during the early stages of the disease.

The most important sequela to IBR is bronchopneumonia, which is caused either by direct aspiration of exudate from airways or as a result of an impairment in pulmonary defense mechanisms, thus predisposing the animal to secondary bacterial infection, most frequently *Mannheimia haemolytica* (see pneumonic mannheimiosis discussion). Postmortem diagnosis of IBR is confirmed by isolation of the virus or its identification by immunohistochemistry or PCR in affected tissues.

Other Causes of Rhinitis. Nasal granulomas occur in cattle presumably as a result of repeated exposure to an unidentified inhaled antigen. Nasal granulomas (atopic rhinitis) are reported mainly in cattle in Australia, South Africa, and the United Kingdom, where affected cattle develop multiple, small, pink or red, polypoid nodules, starting in the nasal vestibule that in time extend into the caudal aspect of the nasal septum (see Fig. 9-23). These nodules are composed of fibrovascular tissue mixed with lymphocytes (granulation tissue) superficially lined by hyperplastic epithelium with abundant mast cells and eosinophils in the lamina propria (nasal eosinophilia). The microscopic features suggest that hypersensitivity type I (immediate), type III (immune complex), and type IV (delayed) may be involved in nasal granulomas of cattle. Bovine (idiopathic) nasal granuloma must be differentiated from nasal mycetomas, nasal rhinosporidiosis, and nasal schistosomiasis, which also cause the formation of nodules in the nasal mucosa of cattle. An eosinophilic material consistent with the Splendore-Hoeppli phenomenon is occasionally observed in bovine mycotic granulomas. This phenomenon seen in some mycotic or bacterial infections is microscopically

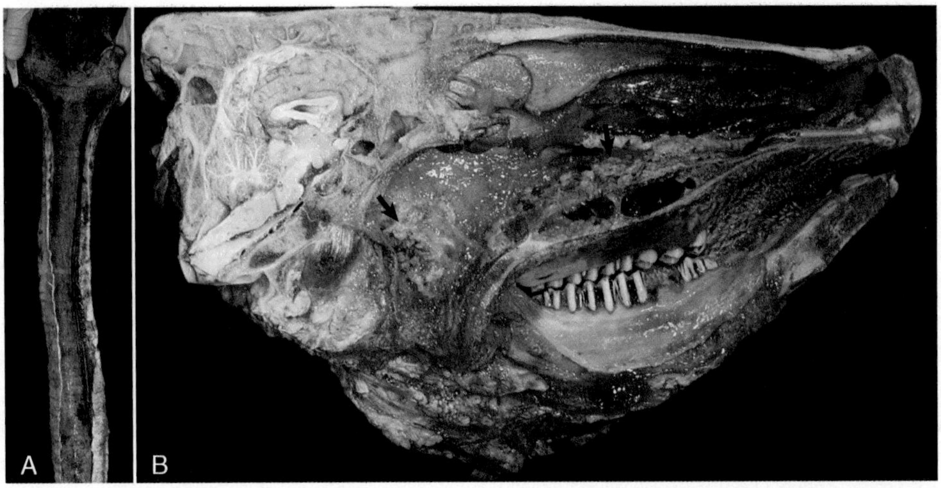

Figure 9-29 **Fibrinonecrotic Rhinitis, Pharyngitis, Laryngitis, and Tracheitis, Infectious Bovine Rhinotracheitis (IBR; Bovine Herpesvirus 1), Longitudinal (Dorsal) Section of Larynx and Trachea (A) and Midsagittal Section of Head (B), Calf.** Thick plaques of fibrinonecrotic exudate cover the nasal *(right arrow)*, pharyngeal *(left arrow)*, laryngeal, and tracheal mucosae. (Courtesy Dr. A. López, Atlantic Veterinary College.)

characterized by a deeply eosinophilic homogeneous material surrounded by bacteria or mycelia. It is thought to result from a localized antigen-antibody response in tissue.

Disorders of Sheep and Goats

Parasitic Infections

Oestrus ovis. *Oestrus ovis* (Diptera: Oestridae; nasal bot) is a brownish fly about the size of a honeybee that deposits its first-stage larvae in the nostrils of sheep in most areas of the world. Microscopic larvae mature into large bots (maggots), which spend most of their larval stages in nasal passages and sinuses, causing irritation, inflammation, and obstruction of airways. Mature larvae drop to the ground and pupate into flies. This type of parasitism in which living tissues are invaded by larvae of flies is known as *myiasis* (Fig. 9-30). Although *Oestrus ovis* is a nasal myiasis primarily of sheep, it sporadically affects goats, dogs, and sometimes human beings (shepherds). The presence of the larvae in nasal passages and sinuses causes chronic irritation and erosive mucopurulent rhinitis and sinusitis; bots of *Oestrus ovis* can be found easily if the head is cut to expose the nasal passages and paranasal sinuses. Rarely, larvae of *Oestrus ovis* penetrate the cranial vault through the ethmoidal plate, causing direct or secondary bacterial meningitis.

Other Causes of Rhinitis. Infectious rhinitis is only sporadically reported in goats, and most of these cases are caused by *Pasteurella multocida* or *Mannheimia haemolytica*. The lesions range from a mild serous to catarrhal or mucopurulent inflammation. Foreign body rhinitis caused by plant material is sporadically seen cattle, sheep, and goats (Fig. 9-31).

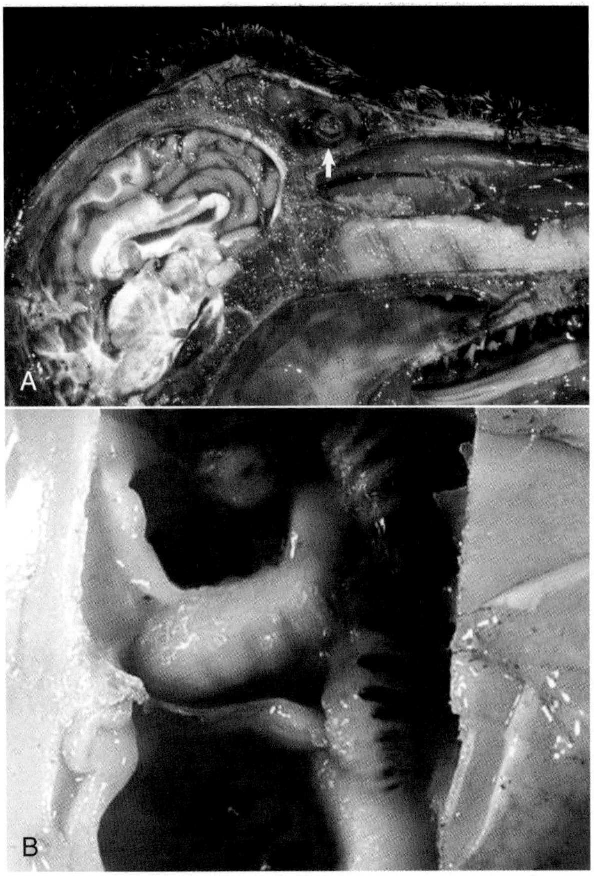

Figure 9-30 ***Oestrus ovis*, Sheep. A,** Frontal sinus. Note the parasitic (fly) larvae in the frontal sinus *(arrow)*. **B,** Nasal cavity. Higher magnification view of larvae of *Oestrus ovis* in a nasal cavity. (**A** courtesy Dr. M.D. McGavin, College of Veterinary Medicine, University of Tennessee. **B** courtesy Dr. M. Sierra and Dr. J. King, College of Veterinary Medicine, Cornell University.)

Disorders of Pigs

Viral Infections

Inclusion Body Rhinitis. Inclusion body rhinitis is a disease of young pigs with high morbidity and low mortality caused by a porcine cytomegalovirus (suid herpesvirus-2) and characterized by a mild rhinitis. This virus commonly infects the nasal epithelium of piglets younger than 5 weeks and causes a transient viremia. Because this disease is seldom fatal, lesions are seen only incidentally or in euthanized animals. In uncomplicated cases, the gross lesion is hyperemia of the nasal mucosa, but with secondary bacterial infections, mucopurulent exudate can be abundant. Microscopic lesions are typical and consist of a necrotizing, nonsuppurative rhinitis with giant, basophilic, intranuclear inclusion bodies in the nasal epithelium, particularly in the nasal glands (Fig. 9-32). Immunosuppressed piglets can develop a systemic cytomegalovirus infection characterized by necrosis of the liver, lungs, adrenal glands, and brain with intralesional inclusion bodies. Inclusion body rhinitis is clinically

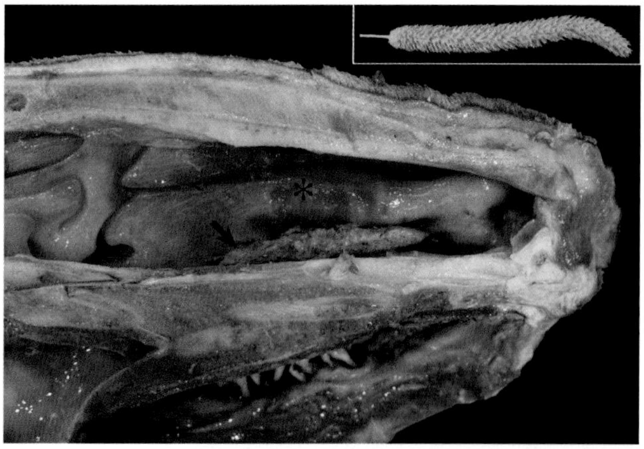

Figure 9-31 **Foreign Body Rhinitis, Midsagittal Section of Head, Nasal Cavity, Timothy Grass, Sheep.** Locally extensive ulceration and inflammation of maxillary concha *(asterisk)*. Note a spikelet of Timothy grass (*Phleum pratense*) covered by mucopurulent exudate in the ventral meatus *(arrow)*. A fresh spikelet of Timothy grass is shown at the *top right*. (Courtesy Dr. A. López, Atlantic Veterinary College.)

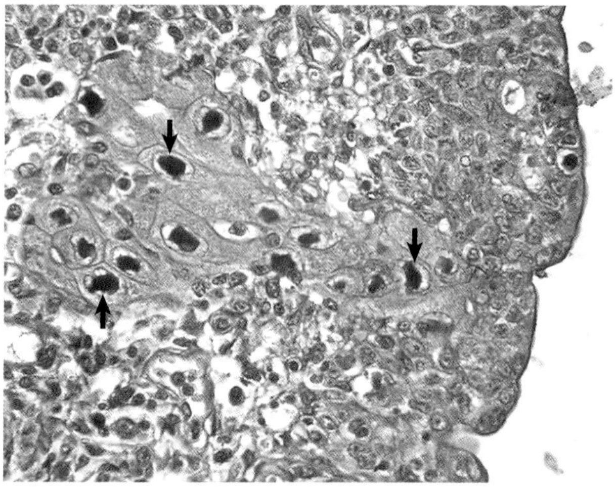

Figure 9-32 **Inclusion Body Rhinitis Caused by Cytomegalovirus Infection, Nasal Conchae, 3-Week-Old Pig.** Epithelial cells of mucosal glands contain large basophilic intranuclear inclusion bodies *(arrows)*. H&E stain. (Courtesy Dr. A. López, Atlantic Veterinary College.)

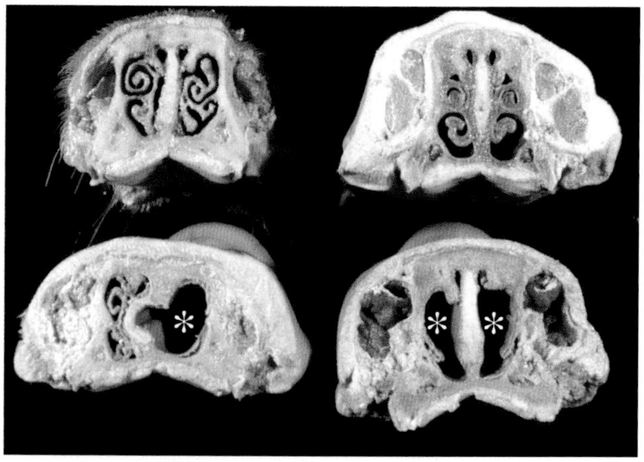

Figure 9-33 **Atrophic Rhinitis, Transverse Sections of Nasal Passages and Sinuses, Caudal Surfaces, Level of the First or Second Premolar Teeth, Pigs.** *Top left,* Normal nasal cavity showing complete conchae (turbinates) that fill most of the nasal cavity and form narrow air passages (meatuses). *Top right,* Mild, symmetric atrophy of nasal conchae. *Bottom left,* Severe, unilateral atrophy of the right ventral nasal concha *(asterisk)* with deviation of the nasal septum to the left and widening of the ventral meatus. *Bottom right,* Severe, bilateral atrophy with complete loss of nasal conchae and extensive widening of the meatuses *(asterisks)*. (Courtesy Dr. A. López, Atlantic Veterinary College.)

characterized by a mild and transient rhinitis, causing sneezing, nasal discharge, and excessive lacrimation.

Bacterial Infections

Atrophic Rhinitis. A common worldwide disease of pigs, atrophic rhinitis (progressive atrophic rhinitis) is characterized by inflammation and atrophy of nasal conchae (turbinates). In severe cases, atrophy of the conchae may cause a striking facial deformity in growing pigs because of deviation of the nasal septum and nasal bones. The etiopathogenesis of atrophic rhinitis is complex and has been a matter of controversy for many years. Pathogens historically associated with atrophic rhinitis include *Bordetella bronchiseptica*, *Pasteurella multocida*, *Haemophilus parasuis*, and viral infections such as porcine cytomegalovirus (inclusion body rhinitis). In addition, predisposing factors have included genetic makeup, environment, and nutritional deficiencies. The cause of atrophic rhinitis is currently believed to be a combined infection by specific strains of *Bordetella bronchiseptica* producing dermonecrotic toxin and toxigenic strains of *Pasteurella multocida*. The only lesion associated with infection with *Bordetella bronchiseptica* alone is a mild to moderate turbinate atrophy (nonprogressive atrophic rhinitis), but this bacterium actively promotes the colonization of the nasal cavity by *Pasteurella multocida*. The toxigenic strains of *Pasteurella multocida* produce potent cytotoxins that inhibit osteoblastic activity and promote osteoclastic reabsorption in nasal bones, particularly in the ventral nasal conchae, where abnormal bone remodeling results in progressive atrophy of conchae.

The degree of conchal atrophy in pigs with atrophic rhinitis varies considerably, and in most pigs, the severity of the lesions does not correspond to the severity of the clinical signs. The best diagnostic method of evaluating this disease at necropsy is to make a transverse section of the snout between the first and second premolar teeth. In normal pigs, conchae are symmetric and fill most of the cavity, leaving only narrow airspaces (meatuses) between coiled conchae. The normal nasal septum is straight and divides the cavity into two mirror-image cavities. In contrast, the septum in pigs with atrophic rhinitis is generally deviated and the conchae appear smaller and asymmetric (Fig. 9-33). Conchal atrophy causes dorsal and ventral meatuses to appear rather enlarged, and in the most advanced cases, the entire nasal conchae may be missing, leaving a large, empty space.

It may seem logical to assume that after loss of conchae in an obligate nasal breather, such as the pig, the filtration defense mechanism of the nasal cavity would be impaired, thus enhancing the chances of aerogenous infections in the lung. However, the relationship between atrophic rhinitis, pneumonia, and growth rates in pigs is still controversial.

Osteoclastic hyperplasia and osteopenia of the conchae are the key microscopic lesions in atrophic rhinitis. Depending on the stage of the disease, mucopurulent exudate may be found on the surface of the conchae. Hyperplastic or metaplastic changes can occur in the nasal epithelium and glands, and infiltrates of lymphoplasmacytic cells can be present in the lamina propria. In summary, atrophic rhinitis is an important disease in pigs worldwide; morphologic diagnosis is simple, but additional understanding of the pathogenesis will be necessary before effective preventive measures can be established.

Atrophic rhinitis is clinically characterized by sneezing, coughing, and nasal discharge. Obstruction of the nasolacrimal duct is common and results in accumulation of dust and dried lacrimal secretions on the skin inferior to the medial canthus of the eye.

Disorders of Dogs

Viral Infections. Dogs have no specific viral infections affecting exclusively the nasal cavity or sinuses. Acute rhinitis and sinusitis occurs as part of the canine infectious respiratory disease (CIRD) group caused by several distinct viruses, such as canine distemper virus, CAV-1 and -2, canine parainfluenza virus, reovirus, and canine herpesvirus. The viral lesions in the respiratory tract are generally transient, but the effect of the virus on other tissues and cells can be fatal, as in distemper encephalitis in dogs.

Bacterial Infections. As in other species, secondary bacterial rhinitis, sinusitis, and pneumonia are possible sequelae of respiratory viral infections; *Bordetella bronchiseptica*, *Escherichia coli*, and *Pasteurella multocida* are the most common isolates in dogs with bacterial rhinitis.

Mycotic Infections. *Aspergillus* spp. and *Penicillium* spp. cause mycotic rhinitis and sinusitis in dogs (canine nasal aspergillosis) (Fig. 9-34). Nasal biopsies reveal extensive necrosis of the nasal epithelium and thick plaques of fibrinopurulent exudate mixed with many fungal hyphae. *Cryptococcus neoformans* and *Blastomyces dermatitides* infections of the nasal cavity occur sporadically in dogs (Fig. 9-35). Lesions are characterized by mucosal granulomas containing periodic acid–Schiff (PAS)-positive fungal organisms, and the infection is clinically characterized by mucopurulent nasal discharge.

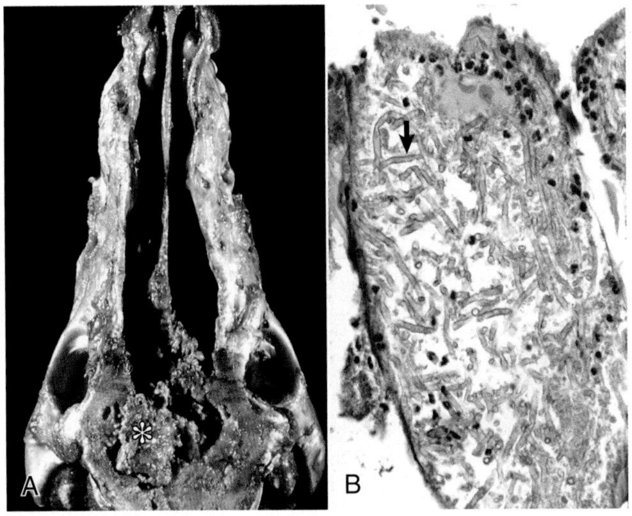

Figure 9-34 Granulomatous Rhinitis, Aspergillosis, Dorsal View of Nasal Cavities, Nasal and Frontal Bones Removed, Dog. A, The nasal conchae have been destroyed by chronic granulomatous inflammation. Mycotic exudate *(asterisk)* remaining in the caudal aspect of the nasal cavity is yellow-green and granular. **B,** Hyphae *(arrow)* of *Aspergillus* spp. were isolated from the granulomatous inflammatory exudate. Note the neutrophils at the periphery of the fungal mat. PAS stain. (**A** courtesy College of Veterinary Medicine, University of Illinois. **B** courtesy Dr. M.A. Wallig, College of Veterinary Medicine, University of Illinois.)

Parasitic Infections

Linguatula serrata. *Linguatula serrata* is a rare but highly specialized pentastomid parasite that shares some morphologic features with arthropods and annelids and causes infection when dogs consume uncooked ruminant meat containing infective larvae. It occurs primarily in carnivores, although sheep and goats may become aberrant hosts. Human beings can also acquire the infection by ingesting raw ovine or caprine meat. The adult parasite is found throughout the nasal passages and sometimes can reach the sinuses and middle ear by moving through the exudate in the Eustachian tubes. In common with other nasal parasites, *Linguatula serrata* acts as an irritant, causing sneezing, catarrhal inflammation, and epistaxis. The eggs of this parasite leave the host in the exudate, which is coughed up or swallowed and eliminated in the feces.

The nasal cavity and paranasal sinuses of dogs can occasionally be infested with other parasites, including mites (*Pneumonyssus caninum*) and *Rhinosporidium seeberi* (see Figs. 9-25 and 9-26).

Allergic Rhinitis. Allergic rhinitis (hay fever; nasolacrimal urticaria), which is so common in human beings sensitized and reexposed to inhaled pollens or allergens, has been reported only sporadically in dogs and cats. Hay fever in human beings and animals is a type I hypersensitivity reaction in which an IgE-mediated degranulation of mast cells results in an acute rhinitis and conjunctivitis. Microscopically, the nasal mucosa is edematous and infiltrated with numerous eosinophils, neutrophils, and some macrophages. Clinically, allergic rhinitis is characterized by profuse serous nasal discharge and lacrimation.

Other Causes of Rhinitis. A nonspecific (idiopathic) chronic lymphoplasmacytic rhinitis is occasionally seen in dogs. Immotile cilia syndrome (ciliary dyskinesia), a congenital disease, reduces mucociliary clearance and is an important factor in recurrent canine rhinosinusitis, bronchitis, bronchiectasis, and pneumonia.

Disorders of Cats

Viral Infections

Feline Viral Rhinotracheitis. Feline viral rhinotracheitis (FVR) is a common, worldwide respiratory disease of cats caused by felid herpesvirus 1 (FeHV-1). The disease causes an impairment of pulmonary defense mechanisms predisposing cats to secondary bacterial pneumonia or to a coinfection with feline calicivirus. The virus also can remain latent in ganglia. The vast majority of cats that recover from FVR become carriers and shed FeHV-1, either spontaneously or following stress. Susceptible animals, particularly kittens with low maternal immunity, become infected after exposure to a diseased or carrier cat. Replication of FeHV-1 in the nasal, conjunctival, pharyngeal, and, to a lesser extent, tracheal epithelium causes degeneration and exfoliation of cells.

Lesions caused by FeHV-1 are fully reversible, but secondary infections with bacteria, such as *Pasteurella multocida*, *Bordetella bronchiseptica*, *Streptococcus* spp., and *Mycoplasma felis*, can cause a chronic, severe suppurative rhinitis and also conjunctivitis. Intranuclear inclusion bodies are rarely seen in cats with FVR because inclusions are only present during the early stages of infection and have already disappeared by the time the cat is presented for diagnosis.

Respiratory sequelae to FVR can include chronic bacterial rhinitis and sinusitis with persistent purulent discharge; lysis of nasal bones, which can lead to conchal atrophy; permanent damage to the olfactory epithelium; and secondary bacterial pneumonia. In addition to rhinitis and interstitial pneumonia, FVR also causes ulcerative keratitis, hepatic necrosis, emaciation, abortion, and

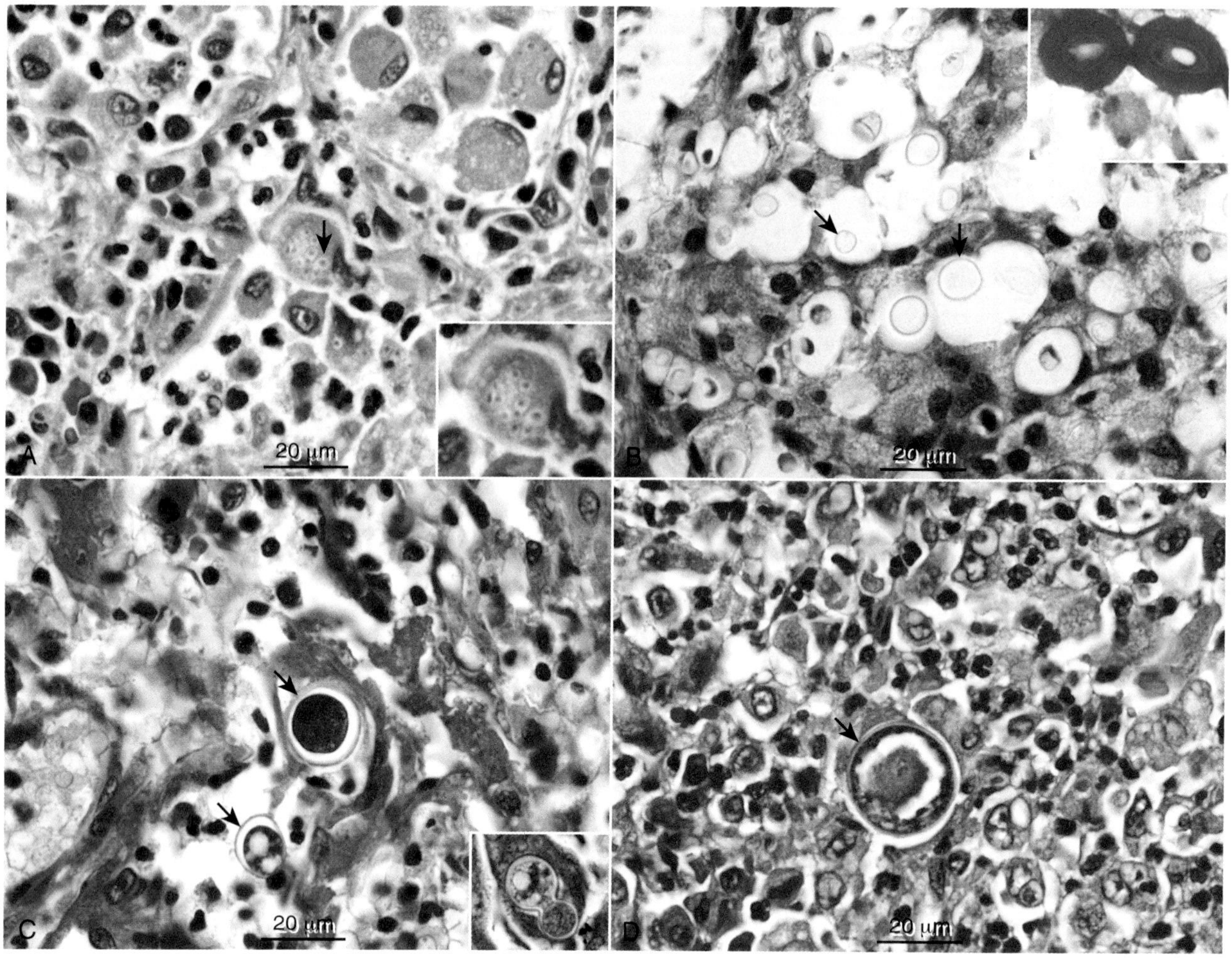

Figure 9-35 **Systemic (Deep) Mycoses. *Histoplasma capsulatum, Cryptococcus neoformans, Blastomyces dermatitidis,* and *Coccidioides immitis* Photographed All at the Same Magnification for Comparative Purposes. A,** *Histoplasma capsulatum,* located intracellularly, is spherical to slightly elongated, 5 to 6 µm in diameter *(arrow).* H&E stain. **B,** *Cryptococcus neoformans,* spherical, 2 to 10 µm in diameter *(arrows),* usually surrounded by a thick mucus capsule, which can increase the overall diameter up to 30 µm, intracellular or extracellular location. H&E stain. *Inset,* The mucus capsule does not stain with H&E but becomes visible with mucicarmine stain. **C,** *Blastomyces dermatitidis,* 8 to 25 µm in diameter, broad-based budding spherical yeast-like organisms *(arrows),* intracellular or extracellular location. *Inset,* Budding yeast typical of this fungus. H&E stain. **D,** *Coccidioides immitis,* spherules, 20 to 30 µm in diameter, containing endospores (<5 µm in diameter) *(arrow),* intracellular or extracellular location. H&E stain. (**A, B, C,** and **D** courtesy Dr. A. López and Dr. M. Forzán, Atlantic Veterinary College. Inset **B** courtesy of Dr. M.D. McGavin, College of Veterinary Medicine, University of Tennessee.)

stillbirths. Clinical signs of FVR infection are characterized by lethargy, oculonasal discharge, severe rhinitis, and conjunctivitis.

Feline Calicivirus. Feline rhinitis can be caused by different strains of feline calicivirus (FCV). It is an important infection of the respiratory tract of cats, and depending on the virulence of the strain, lesions vary from a mild oculonasal discharge to severe rhinitis, mucopurulent conjunctivitis, and ulcerative gingivitis and stomatitis. The lesions, in addition to rhinitis and conjunctivitis, include acute, diffuse interstitial pneumonia with necrotizing bronchiolitis (see Pneumonias of Cats) and in some cases prominent ulcers of the tongue and hard palate. Primary viral lesions are generally transient, but secondary bacterial infections (*Bordetella bronchiseptica, Pasteurella multocida,* or *Escherichia coli*) are a common complication. Some kittens develop lameness after infection or vaccination with calicivirus because of an acute and self-limiting arthritis ("limping kitten syndrome"). Carrier state and virus shedding from oronasal secretions and feces are natural sequelae after recovery from the acute phase of the disease. Clinical and pathologic features of FCV disease are strikingly similar but not identical to those of FVR; these two viral infections account for 80% of all cases of feline respiratory diseases. A febrile systemic hemorrhagic syndrome with high mortality (up to 50%) has been reported in cats infected with virulent strains of FCV.

Bacterial Infections

Feline Chlamydiosis. Feline chlamydiosis is a persistent respiratory infection of cats caused by *Chlamydophila felis.* Infection results in a conjunctivitis (similar to the conjunctivitis seen in human trachoma caused by *Chlamydia trachomatis*) and serous or mucopurulent rhinitis. In the past, *Chlamydophila felis* was incriminated as the agent responsible for "feline pneumonitis," but its role in causing bronchointerstitial pneumonia in cats has been seriously challenged in recent years (see Pneumonias of Cats).

Mycotic Infections. The most common mycotic infection in the feline nasal cavity is caused by *Cryptococcus neoformans* and *Cryptococcus gatti,* but not all animals exposed to these fungi necessarily develop cryptococcosis unless they are immunosuppressed.

The lesions vary from discrete nasal granulomas to large confluent masses of mucopurulent exudate filling the entire nasal cavity and paranasal sinuses. Microscopic examination of the exudate reveals the typical thick-walled PAS-positive organisms (see Fig. 9-35).

Other Causes of Rhinitis and Sinusitis. *Mycoplasma felis* can also cause mucopurulent conjunctivitis and a mild upper respiratory infection, with clinical signs and lesions overlapping those seen with chlamydiosis, FVR, and FCR infections. Respiratory infections and bronchopneumonia in cats may also be associated with the immunosuppressive effects of feline retroviruses such as feline leukemia virus (FeLV) and feline immunodeficiency virus (FIV). Nasal aspergillosis and allergic rhinosinusitis are sporadically reported in cats (see Disorders of the Conducting System: Species-Specific Diseases of the Nasal Cavity and Paranasal Sinuses: Disorders of Dogs: Mycotic Infections).

Neoplasia of the Nasal Cavity and Paranasal Sinuses

Neoplasms of the nasal cavity and paranasal sinuses may arise from any of the tissues forming these structures, including bone (osteoma or osteosarcoma), cartilage (chondroma or chondrosarcoma), connective tissue (fibroma or fibrosarcoma, myxoma or myxosarcoma), and blood vessels (hemangioma or hemangiosarcoma), and from all the different types of cells of glands and lining epithelium (adenoma, carcinoma, or adenocarcinoma). Nasal tumors originating from stromal tissues, such as bone, cartilage, and connective tissue, are morphologically indistinguishable from those seen in other sites. In general, nasal neoplasms are rare in domestic animals, except for enzootic ethmoidal tumor (retroviral) in sheep and goats, which can occur in several animals in a herd (see the next section).

In companion animals, nasal neoplasms are most common in dogs, particularly in medium to large breed dogs such as the collie, Airedale terrier, basset hound, and German shepherd. The cat and the horse are less frequently affected. The main sites in order of frequency are the nasal passages and sinuses for dogs, the tip of the nose and nasal passages for cats, and the maxillary sinus and nasal passages for horses.

The majority of neoplasms in the nasal cavity are malignant. Benign nasal neoplasms (papilloma and adenoma) are rare and generally are either solitary or multiple, well-delineated nodules. In contrast, nasal carcinomas and nasal sarcomas are generally larger but vary in size and are often pale and multilobulated masses composed of fleshy to friable tissue (Figs. 9-36 and 9-37). Malignant neoplasms are locally invasive and tend to infiltrate sinuses, meninges, frontal brain, olfactory nerves, and vessels resulting in epistaxis. Carcinomas vary from anaplastic (poorly differentiated) to well differentiated, in which cell and tissue morphology retains some glandular (adenocarcinoma) or squamous cell patterns. Because nasal tumors in dogs and cats are usually large and invasive at the time of diagnosis, prognosis is usually poor and survival times are short. Sarcomas originating in the nasal cavity and paranasal sinuses are less common than carcinomas. Mesenchymal tumors can arise from bone (osteoma or osteosarcoma), cartilage (chondroma or chondrosarcoma), blood vessels (hemangioma or hemangiosarcoma), and connective tissue (fibroma or fibrosarcoma). Overall, benign epithelial and mesenchymal tumors are less common than their malignant counterparts. Secondary tumors in the nasal cavity are rare, with lymphoma being the most common secondary tumor in the nasal cavity of domestic animals (Fig. 9-38).

Nasal neoplasms become secondarily infected by bacteria, and clinical signs often overlap with those of infectious rhinitis and include catarrhal or mucopurulent nasal discharge, periodic hemorrhage, increased lacrimation as a result of obstruction of nasolacrimal ducts, and sneezing. In some instances, it is not possible to clinically or grossly differentiate neoplasms from hyperplastic nodules or granulomatous rhinitis. Some neoplasms may infiltrate adjacent bone structures and produce notable facial deformities, loss of teeth, exophthalmus, and nervous signs. Large neoplasms also project into the meatuses, narrow the lumen, and interfere with airflow, causing stertorous breathing (see Figs. 9-36, 9-37, and 9-38). Biopsies, as well as brush and imprint cytology, have proven effective in the antemortem diagnosis of nasal neoplasms, particularly in those of epithelial lineage.

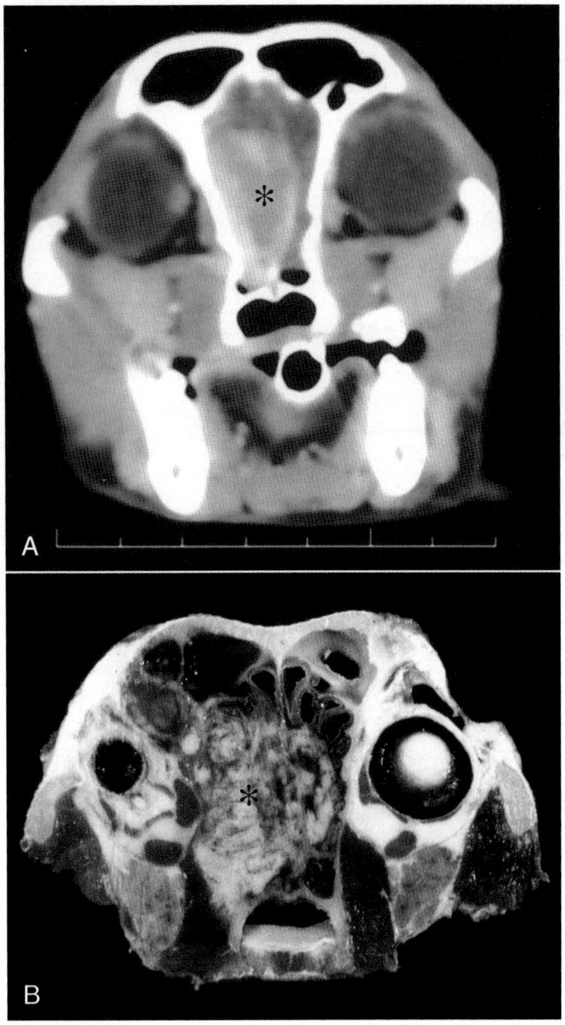

Figure 9-36 **Nasal Carcinoma, Transverse Section of Nasal Passages and Sinuses, 10-Year-Old Dog. A,** Computerized tomography shows a large neoplastic mass *(asterisk)* infiltrating the nasal cavity and displacing the nasal septum laterally. Scale bar units in centimeters. **B,** Transverse section of head showing tumor diffusely infiltrating the nasal conchae and obliterating the meatuses *(asterisk)*. (**A,** courtesy Atlantic Veterinary College. **B** courtesy Dr. A. López, Atlantic Veterinary College.)

Enzootic Nasal (Ethmoidal) Tumors

A unique group of nasal carcinomas (enzootic nasal tumors, enzootic intranasal tumors, and enzootic nasal carcinoma) of sheep and goats arise from the surface epithelium and glands of the ethmoidal conchae. These types of carcinomas are caused by betaretroviruses in sheep (ENTV-1) and goats (ENTV-2). The enzootic nasal tumor has been successfully transmitted to susceptible animals by

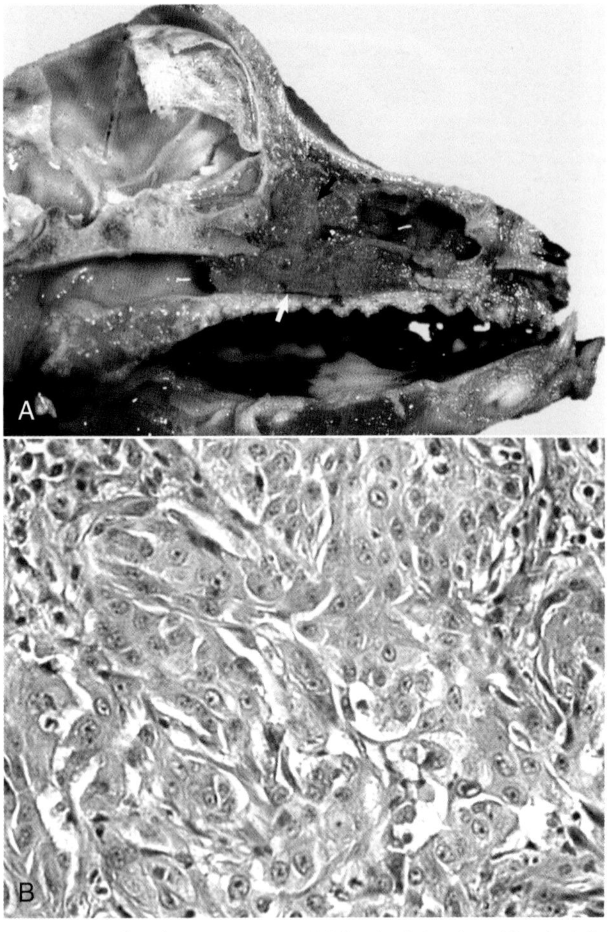

Figure 9-37 **Nasal Adenocarcinoma, Midsagittal Section, Head, Adult Dog. A,** A large neoplastic mass *(arrows)* has arisen from the ethmoidal concha and has infiltrated along the nasal passages. **B,** Multiple clusters of neoplastic epithelial cells with abundant eosinophilic cytoplasm and prominent nucleoli. H&E stain. (**A** courtesy Dr. J.M. King, College of Veterinary Medicine, Cornell University. **B** courtesy Dr. A. López, Atlantic Veterinary College.)

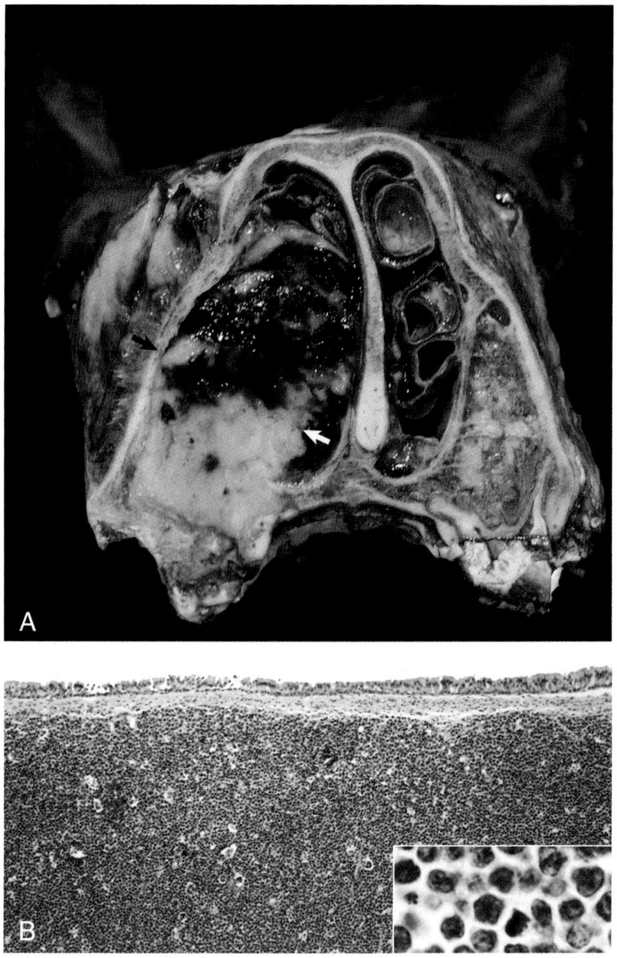

Figure 9-38 **Lymphoma *(Arrows)*, Right Nasal Cavity, Horse. A,** Tumoral mass occludes the right nasal cavity and invades the conchae and maxillary bone. **B,** Note diffuse infiltration of the nasal submucosa with neoplastic lymphocytes. H&E stain. *Inset,* Close-up of neoplastic lymphocytes. H&E stain. (Courtesy Dr. S. Martinson and Dr. C. Lopez-Mendez, Atlantic Veterinary College.)

inoculation of cell-free tumor filtrates. Enzootic nasal tumors are typically invasive but do not metastasize (Fig. 9-39). In some regions of the world, ethmoid tumors have been reported in horses and pigs, particularly in those farms where the endemic nasal tumors of ruminants are known to occur.

Nasal Polyps and Nasal Cysts Resembling Neoplasms

Nonneoplastic exophytic masses that resemble neoplasms are commonly found in horses, cats, and, to a lesser extent, other species. In horses, polyps tend to form in the ethmoidal region, whereas in cats, polyps are most frequently found in the nasopharynx and Eustachian tubes. The pathogenesis of these benign growths is uncertain, although in many cases they follow chronic rhinitis or sinusitis. Most recently, lymphatic obstruction secondary to inflammation has been postulated as the main culprit. Grossly, polyps appear as firm, pedunculated nodules of various sizes protruding from the nasal mucosa into the nasal passages or nasopharynx (Fig. 9-40); the surface may be smooth, ulcerated, secondarily infected, and hemorrhagic. Microscopically, polyps are characterized by a core of well-vascularized stromal tissue that contains inflammatory cells and are covered by pseudostratified or squamous epithelium (see Fig. 9-40).

Nasal and paranasal sinus cysts are common idiopathic lesions in horses and are medically important because they clinically mimic neoplasms or infections. Although not considered a neoplastic growth, cysts are expansive and cause deformation or destruction of the surrounding bone. These cysts are typically composed of an epithelial cell capsule filled with yellow or hemorrhagic fluid and do not recur after surgical removal. Ethmoidal hematomas also resemble nasal tumors in horses.

Disorders of the Pharynx, Guttural Pouches, Larynx, and Trachea in Domestic Animals

Anomalies[3]

Congenital anomalies of the pharynx, guttural pouches, larynx, and trachea are rare in all species. Depending on their location and severity, they may be inconsistent with postnatal life, pose little or no problem, interfere with quality of life, or manifest themselves in later life. If clinical signs of respiratory distress, such as stridor, coughing, dyspnea, or gagging, do occur, they are usually exacerbated by excitement, heat, stress, or exercise.

Brachycephalic Airway Syndrome. See Disorders of the Conducting System: Species-Specific Diseases of the Pharynx, Guttural

[3]See E-Table 1-1 for potential, suspected, or known genetic disorders.

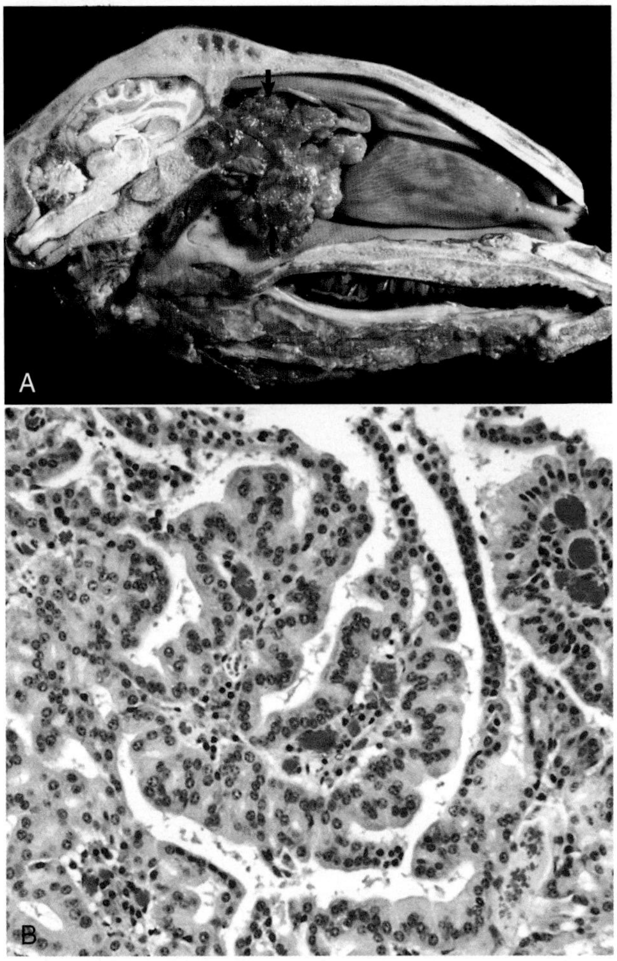

Figure 9-39 Nasal Adenocarcinoma *(Arrows)*, Midsagittal Section of the Head, Sheep. A, The tumor has occluded the right nasal passage and choanae. The location (ethmoturbinates) and type of tumor (carcinoma) are typical of retrovirus-induced "enzootic nasal carcinoma." **B,** Neoplastic cells forming conspicuous papillary growths *(center of image)*. (**A** courtesy Dr. L.E. Craig, College of Veterinary Medicine, University of Tennessee. **B** courtesy Dr. A. López, Atlantic Veterinary College.)

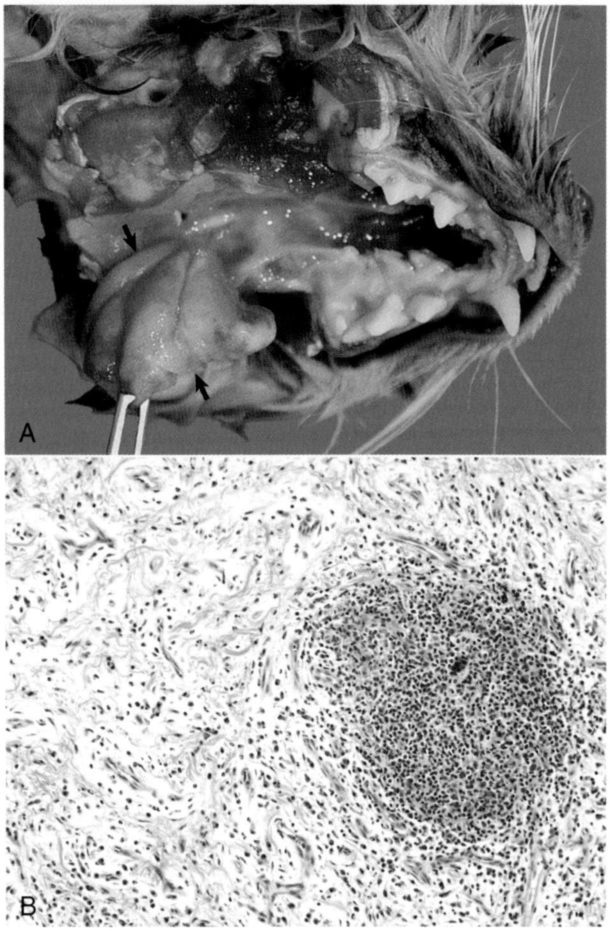

Figure 9-40 Nasopharyngeal Polyp, Oral Cavity, Cat. A, Large polypoid mass arising from the nasopharyngeal mucosa *(arrows)*. **B,** Loose connective tissue infiltrated with lymphocytes and plasma cells forms the core of the mass *(right side of figure)*. H&E stain. (Courtesy Dr. F. Marrón and Dr. A. López, Atlantic Veterinary College.)

Pouches, Larynx, and Trachea in Domestic Animals: Disorders of Dogs: Anomalies: Brachycephalic Airway Syndrome.

Hypoplastic Epiglottis, Epiglottic Entrapment, and Dorsal Displacement of the Soft Palate. See Disorders of the Conducting System: Species-Specific Diseases of the Pharynx, Guttural Pouches, Larynx, and Trachea: Disorders of Horses: Anomalies: Hypoplastic Epiglottis, Epiglottic Entrapment, and Dorsal Displacement of the Soft Palate.

Tracheal Collapse and Tracheal Stenosis. Tracheal collapse with reduction in tracheal patency occurs in toy, miniature, and brachycephalic breeds of dogs, in which the condition is also called *tracheobronchial collapse* or *central airway collapse*. The defect also occurs in horses, cattle, and goats. By radiographic, endoscopic, or gross examination, there is dorsoventral flattening of the trachea with concomitant widening of the dorsal tracheal membrane, which may then prolapse ventrally into the lumen (Fig. 9-41). Most commonly, the defect extends the entire length of the trachea and only rarely affects the cervical portion alone. Affected segments with a reduced lumen contain froth and even are covered by a diphtheritic membrane. In horses, the so-called scabbard trachea is characterized

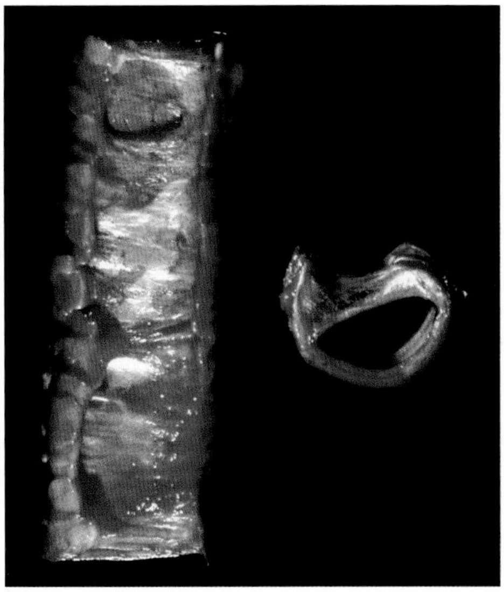

Figure 9-41 Tracheal Collapse, Trachea, Pony. *Left specimen*, The dorsal surface of the trachea is flattened dorsoventrally, the dorsal ends of the C-shaped tracheal rings are widely separated, and the dorsal ligament between the two ends is lengthened and thinned. *Right specimen* (transverse section), The ends of the tracheal rings are widely separated, and the dorsal wall of the trachea is formed by the lengthened and thinned dorsal ligament. (Courtesy Dr. C.S. Patton, College of Veterinary Medicine, University of Tennessee.)

by lateral flattening so that the tracheal lumen is reduced to a narrow vertical slit.

Segmental tracheal collapse causing stenosis has been associated with congenital and acquired abnormalities. In severe cases, abnormal cartilaginous glycoproteins and loss of elasticity of tracheal rings causes the trachea to collapse. In some other cases, it is an acquired tracheal lesion that follows trauma, compression caused by extraluminal masses, peritracheal inflammation, and flawed tracheotomy or transtracheal aspirate techniques.

Other tracheal anomalies include tracheoesophageal fistula, which is most commonly found in human beings and sporadically in dogs and cattle. Congenital fistulas can occur at any site of the cervical or thoracic segments of the trachea. Acquired tracheoesophageal fistula can be a complication of improper intubation, tracheotomy, or esophageal foreign body.

Degenerative Diseases

Laryngeal Hemiplegia. Laryngeal hemiplegia (paralysis), sometimes called *roaring* in horses, is a common but obscure disease characterized by atrophy of the dorsal and lateral cricoarytenoid muscles (abductor and adductor of the arytenoid cartilage), particularly on the left side. Muscular atrophy is most commonly caused by a primary denervation (recurrent laryngeal neuropathy) of unknown cause (idiopathic axonopathy) and, to a much lesser extent, secondary nerve damage (see the section on Denervation Atrophy in Chapters 14 and 15). Idiopathic laryngeal hemiplegia is an incurable axonal disease (axonopathy) of the cranial laryngeal nerve that affects mostly larger horses. Secondary laryngeal hemiplegia is rare and occurs after nerve damage caused by other pathologic processes such as compression or inflammation of the left recurrent laryngeal nerve. The medial retropharyngeal lymph nodes are located immediately ventral to the floor of the guttural pouches. As a result of this close anatomic relationship, swelling or inflammation of the guttural pouches or retropharyngeal lymph nodes often results in secondary damage to the laryngeal nerve. Common causes of secondary nerve damage (Wallerian degeneration) include guttural pouch mycosis, retropharyngeal abscesses, inflammation because of iatrogenic injection into the nerves, neck injury, and metastatic neoplasms involving the retropharyngeal lymph nodes (e.g., lymphosarcoma).

Grossly, the affected laryngeal muscle in a horse with laryngeal hemiplegia is pale and smaller than normal (muscle atrophy) (Fig. 9-42). Microscopically, muscle fibers have lesions of denervation atrophy (see Chapters 14 and 15). Atrophy of laryngeal muscles also occurs in dogs as an inherited condition (Siberian husky and Bouvier des Flanders), as a degenerative neuropathy in older dogs, secondary to laryngeal trauma in all species (e.g., choke chain damage), or secondary to hepatic encephalopathy in horses.

The abnormal inspiratory sounds (roaring) during exercise in horses with laryngeal hemiplegia are caused by paralysis of the left dorsal and lateral cricoarytenoid muscles, which cause incomplete dilation of the larynx, obstruction of airflow, and vibration of vocal cords.

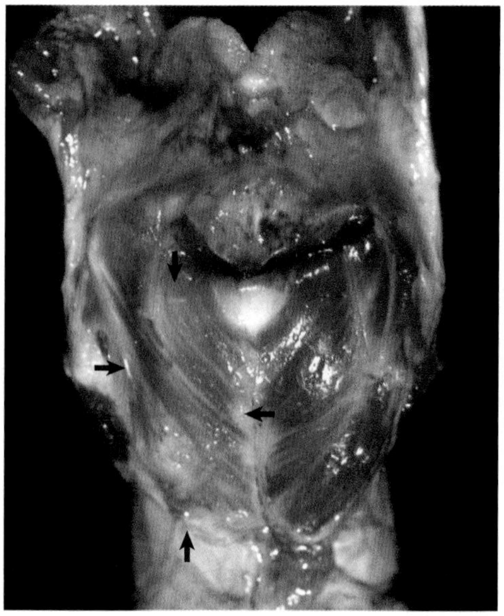

Figure 9-42 Laryngeal Hemiplegia, Larynx, Dorsal Surface, 2-Year-Old Horse. The left cricoarytenoideus dorsalis muscle is pale and atrophic *(arrows)*, whereas the right cricoarytenoideus dorsalis muscle is normal. (Courtesy Dr. A. López, Atlantic Veterinary College.)

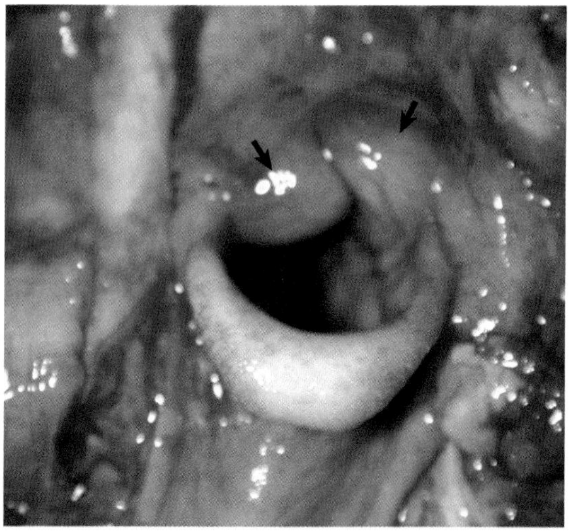

Figure 9-43 Laryngeal Edema, Larynx, Mature Cow. Note the edematous thickening of the laryngeal mucosa of the vocal cords *(arrows)*, which can cause respiratory distress due to the narrowing of the laryngeal lumen (rima glottidis). (Courtesy Dr. J. Andrews, College of Veterinary Medicine, University of Illinois.)

Circulatory Disturbances

Laryngeal Edema. Laryngeal edema is a common feature of acute inflammation, but it is particularly important because swelling of the epiglottis and vocal cords can obstruct the laryngeal orifice, resulting in asphyxiation. Laryngeal edema occurs in pigs with edema disease; in horses with purpura hemorrhagica; in cattle with acute interstitial pneumonia; in cats with systemic anaphylaxis; and in all species as a result of trauma, improper endotracheal tubing, inhalation of irritant gases (e.g., smoke), local inflammation, and allergic reactions. Grossly, the mucosa of the epiglottis and vocal cords is thickened and swollen, often protrudes dorsally onto the epiglottic orifice, and has a gelatinous appearance (Fig. 9-43).

Laryngeal and Tracheal Hemorrhage. Hemorrhages in these sites occur as mucosal petechiae and are most commonly seen in coagulopathies; inflammation; septicemia and sepsis, particularly in pigs with classical swine fever (hog cholera); African swine fever or salmonellosis; and horses with equine infectious anemia. Severe dyspnea and asphyxia before death can cause congestion, ecchymosis, and petechiae in the laryngeal and tracheal mucosa; this lesion must be differentiated from postmortem imbibition of hemoglobin in autolyzed carcasses (see Chapter 1).

Tracheal Edema and Hemorrhage Syndrome of Feeder Cattle. See Disorders of Cattle.

Inflammation (Pharyngitis, Laryngitis, and Tracheitis)

Inflammation of the pharynx, larynx, and trachea are important because of their potential to obstruct airflow and to lead to aspiration pneumonia. The pharynx is commonly affected by infectious diseases of the upper respiratory and upper digestive tracts, and the trachea can be involved by extension from both the lungs and larynx.

Inflammation and Trauma of the Pharynx (Pharyngitis)

Pharyngeal Obstruction and Perforation. Intraluminal foreign bodies in the pharynx, such as medicament boluses, apples, or potatoes, can move down and obstruct the larynx and trachea. Also, pharyngeal obstruction can be caused by masses in the surrounding tissue, such as neoplasms of the thyroid gland, thymus, and parathyroid glands.

A number of nonspecific insults can cause lesions and clinical signs. Trauma may take the form of penetrating wounds in any species: perforation of the caudodorsal wall of the pharynx from the improper use of drenching or balling guns in sheep, cattle, and pigs; choking injury because of the use of collars in dogs and cats; and the shearing forces of bite wounds. The results of the trauma may be minimal (local edema and inflammation) or as serious as complete luminal obstruction by exudate. Foreign bodies may be lodged anywhere in the pharyngeal region; the location and size determine the occurrence of dysphagia, regurgitation, dyspnea, or asphyxiation. Pigs have a unique structure known as the *pharyngeal diverticulum* (4 cm long in adult pigs), which is located in the pharyngeal wall rostral and dorsal to the esophageal entrance. It is important because barley awns may lodge in the diverticulum, causing an inflammatory swelling that affects swallowing. The diverticular wall may be perforated by awns or drenching syringes, which results in an exudate that can extend down the tissue planes between muscles of the neck and even into the mediastinum. The pharynx of the dog may also be damaged by trauma from chicken bones, sticks, and needles, resulting in the formation of a pharyngeal abscess.

Equine Pharyngeal Lymphoid Hyperplasia. See Disorders of the Conducting System: Species-Specific Diseases of the Pharynx, Guttural Pouches, Larynx, and Trachea: Disorders of Horses: Inflammation: Equine Pharyngeal Lymphoid Hyperplasia.

Inflammation of Guttural Pouches. See Disorders of the Conducting System: Species-Specific Diseases of the Pharynx, Guttural Pouches, Larynx, and Trachea: Disorders of Horses: Inflammation: Inflammation of Guttural Pouches.

Inflammation of the Larynx (Laryngitis)

Necrotic Laryngitis. See Disorders of the Conducting System: Species-Specific Diseases of the Pharynx, Guttural Pouches, Larynx, and Trachea: Disorders of Ruminants (Cattle, Sheep, and Goats): Inflammation: Necrotic Laryngitis.

Laryngeal Contact Ulcers. See Disorders of the Conducting System: Species-Specific Diseases of the Pharynx, Guttural Pouches, Larynx, and Trachea: Disorders of Ruminants (Cattle, Sheep, and Goats): Inflammation: Laryngeal Contact Ulcers.

Inflammation of the Trachea (Tracheitis). The types of injury and host inflammatory responses in the trachea are essentially the same as those described for the nasal mucosa. Although tracheal mucosa is prone to aerogenous injury and necrosis, it has a remarkable capacity for repair. According to the exudate, tracheitis in all animal species is classified as fibrinous, catarrhal, purulent, or granulomatous (Figs. 9-44 and 9-45). Chronic polypoid tracheitis occurs in dogs and cats, probably secondary to chronic infection.

The most common causes of tracheitis are viral infections, such as those causing infectious bovine rhinotracheitis (see Fig. 9-29), equine viral rhinopneumonitis, canine distemper, and feline rhinotracheitis. Viral lesions are generally mild and transient but often become complicated with secondary bacterial infections. At the early stages, the mucosa is notably hyperemic and can show white foci of necrosis. In the most severe cases, the affected mucosa detaches from the underlying basement membrane, causing extensive tracheal ulceration.

Chemical tracheitis is also commonly seen after aspiration (see Fig. 9-45). Also, inhalation of fumes during barn fires can cause extensive injury and necrosis of the tracheal mucosa. In forensic cases, the presence of carbon pigment in the mucosal surface of trachea, bronchi, and bronchioles indicates that the burned animal was alive during the fire.

Parasitic Diseases of the Larynx and Trachea. Parasitic infections of the larynx and trachea can cause obstruction with dramatic consequences, but burdens sufficient to cause such effects are not commonly seen in veterinary practice.

Besnoitiosis (Besnoitia Spp.). Besnoitiosis (*Besnoitia* spp.) is caused by several species of this apicomplexan coccidian parasite, whose life cycle is still unknown. This parasite can cause pedunculated lesions on the skin, sclera, mucosa of the nasal cavity, and larynx of horses and donkeys, cattle, goats, and wild animals. Besnoitiosis has been reported from Africa, Central and South America, North America, and Europe. Grossly, pale, round, exophytic nodules up to 2 cm in diameter can be observed protruding from mucosal surfaces. Microscopically, these nodules consist of finger-like projections covered by hyperplastic and sometimes ulcerated epithelium containing numerous thick-walled parasitic cysts with little inflammatory response.

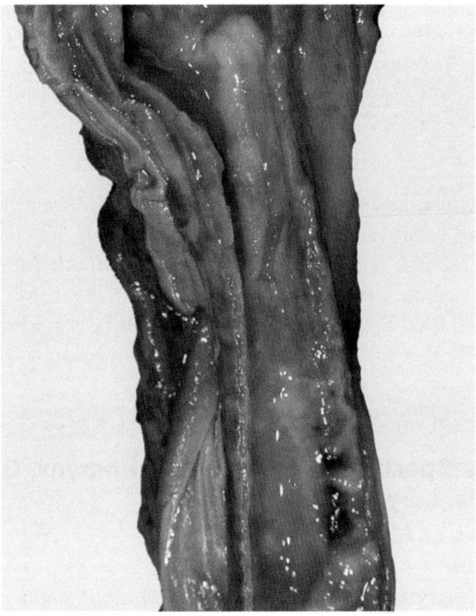

Figure 9-44 **Fibrinopurulent Tracheitis, Cat.** Note uniform plaque of yellow-gray fibrinopurulent exudate covering the entire tracheal mucosa. This cat also had suppurative bronchopneumonia, and *Pasteurella multocida* was isolated from the trachea and lung. (Courtesy Dr. L. Miller and Dr. A. López, Atlantic Veterinary College.)

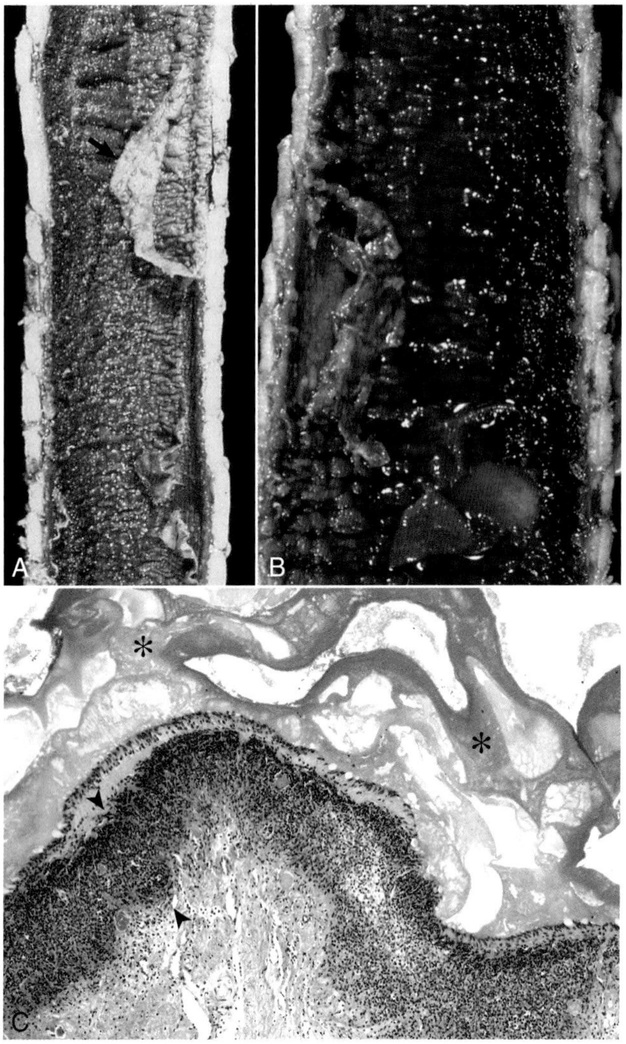

Figure 9-45 **Chemical Tracheitis, Accidental Drenching with Disinfectant, Cow. A,** Tracheal mucosa is diffusely covered with fibrinonecrotic exudate. Note a diphtheritic membrane peeling from the mucosa *(arrow)*. **B,** Close-up of the fibrinonecrotic exudate in a location of the trachea different from that shown in A. **C,** Section of mucosa showing a dark rim of neutrophils *(arrowheads)* and a thick layer of fibrin *(asterisks)*. H&E stain. (Courtesy Dr. A. López, Atlantic Veterinary College.)

Mammomonogamus (Syngamus) Spp. *Mammomonogamus (Syngamus) laryngeus* is a nematode that is seen attached to the laryngeal mucosa of cattle in tropical Asia and South America, and cats (gapeworm: *Mammomonogamus ierei*) in the Caribbean and southern United States. Occasionally, human beings with a persistent cough or asthma-like symptoms have the parasite in the larynx or bronchi.

Oslerus (Filaroides) osleri. See Disorders of Dogs.

Species-Specific Diseases of the Pharynx, Guttural Pouches, Larynx, and Trachea

Disorders of Horses

Anomalies[4]

Hypoplastic Epiglottis, Epiglottic Entrapment, and Dorsal Displacement of the Soft Palate. Anomalies, such as hypoplastic epiglottis, epiglottic entrapment, and dorsal displacement of the soft palate, are important causes of respiratory problems and reduced athletic performance in horses. An undersized epiglottis is prone to being entrapped below the arytenoepiglottic fold, causing an equine syndrome known as *epiglottic entrapment*. This syndrome also occurs in horses with lateral deviation and deformity of epiglottis, epiglottic cysts, or necrosis of the tip of the epiglottis. Hypoplastic epiglottis also occurs in pigs. Dorsal displacement of the soft palate, particularly during exercise, narrows the lumen of the nasopharynx and creates abnormal air turbulence in the conducting system of horses. Epiglottic entrapment is clinically characterized by airway obstruction, exercise intolerance, respiratory noise, and cough.

Subepiglottic and Pharyngeal Cysts. Anomalous lesions, such as subepiglottic and pharyngeal cysts, are occasionally seen in horses, particularly in Standardbred and Thoroughbred racehorses. These cysts vary in size (1 to 9 cm) and occur most commonly in the subepiglottic area and to a lesser extent in the dorsal pharynx, larynx, and soft palate. Cysts are lined by squamous or pseudostratified epithelium and contain thick mucus. Large cysts cause airway obstruction, reduced exercise tolerance, or dysphagia and predispose to bronchoaspiration of food.

Inflammation

Equine Pharyngeal Lymphoid Hyperplasia. Equine pharyngeal lymphoid hyperplasia, or pharyngitis with lymphoid follicular hyperplasia, is a common cause of partial upper airway obstruction in horses, particularly in 2- and 3-year-old racehorses. Lymphoid hyperplasia is also seen in healthy horses as part of a response to mild chronic pharyngitis, which in many instances tends to regress with age in older animals. The cause is undetermined, but chronic bacterial infection combined with environmental factors may cause excessive antigenic stimulation and lymphoid hyperplasia. The gross lesions, visible endoscopically or at necropsy, consist of variably sized (1 to 5 mm) white foci located on the dorsolateral walls of the pharynx and extending into the openings of the guttural pouches and onto the soft palate. In severe cases, lesions may appear as pharyngeal polyps. Microscopically, the lesions consist of large aggregates of lymphocytes and plasma cells in the pharyngeal mucosa. Clinical signs consist of stertorous inspiration, expiration, or both.

Inflammation of Guttural Pouches. The guttural pouches of horses are large diverticula (300 to 500 mL) of the ventral portion of the auditory (Eustachian) tubes. These diverticula are therefore exposed to the same pathogens as the pharynx and have drainage problems similar to the sinuses. Although it is probable that various pathogens, including viruses, can infect them, the most common pathogens are fungi, which cause guttural pouch mycosis and guttural pouch empyema in the horse. Eustachitis is the term used for inflammatory processes involving the Eustachian (pharyngotympanic) tube. Because of the close anatomic proximity of guttural pouches to the internal carotid arteries, cranial nerves (VII, IX, X, XI, and XII), and atlantooccipital joint, disease of these diverticula may involve these structures and cause a variety of clinical signs in horses.

Guttural pouch mycosis occurs primarily in stabled horses and is caused by *Aspergillus fumigatus* and other *Aspergillus* spp. Infection is usually unilateral and presumably starts with the inhalation of spores from moldy hay. Grossly, the mucosal surfaces of the dorsal and lateral walls of the guttural pouch mucosa are first covered by focal, rounded, raised plaques of diphtheritic (fibrinonecrotic) exudate, which with time can become confluent and grow into a large fibrinonecrotic mass (Fig. 9-46). Microscopically, the lesions are severe necrotic inflammation of the mucosa and submucosa with widespread vasculitis and intralesional fungal hyphae. Necrosis of the

[4]See E-Box 1-1 for potential, suspected, or known genetic disorders.

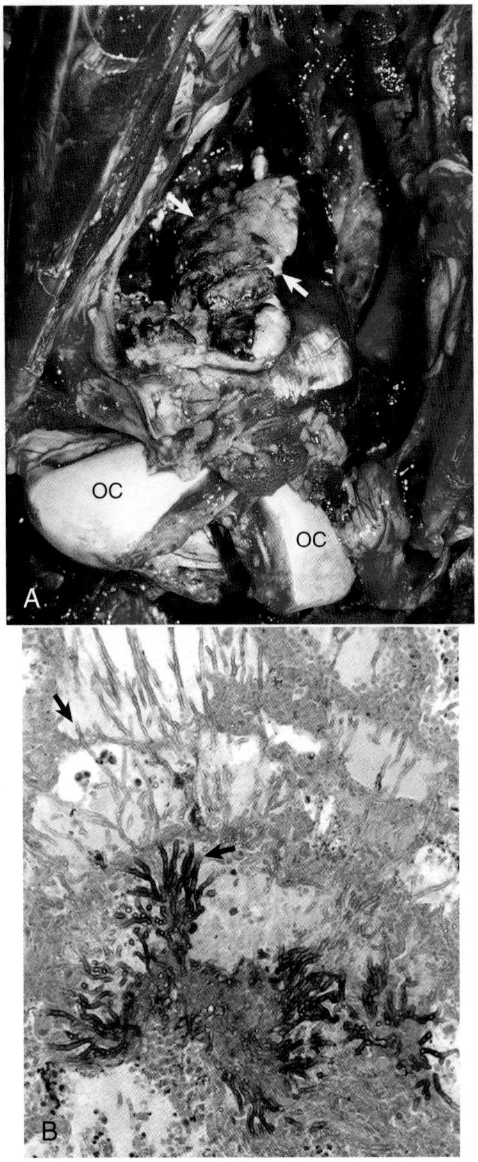

Figure 9-46 **Guttural Pouch Mycosis, Ventral View of the Head, Horse. A,** Note the large mass filling the right guttural pouch *(arrows)*. It is firmly attached to the wall and composed of fibrinonecrotic exudate and surrounded by clotted blood. OC, Occipital condyles. **B,** Fungal hyphae *(arrows)* are admixed with necrotic exudate. H&E stain. (Courtesy Dr. A. López, Atlantic Veterinary College.)

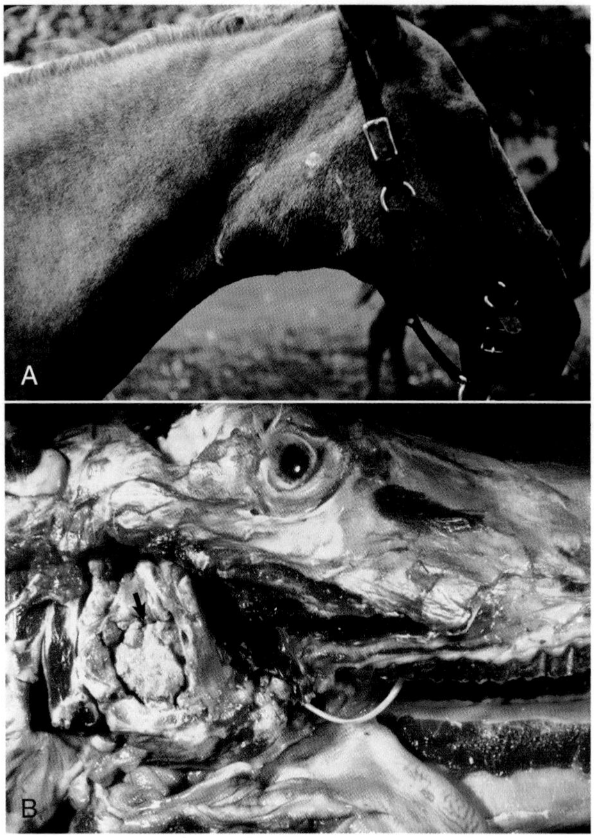

Figure 9-47 **Guttural Pouch Empyema, Guttural Pouch, Horse. A,** Note the swollen right neck *(outlined in yellow)* in this horse with guttural pouch empyema. **B,** The guttural pouch is filled with masses of inspissated purulent exudate *(arrow)*. (**A** courtesy College of Veterinary Medicine, University of Illinois. **B** courtesy Dr. M.D. McGavin, College of Veterinary Medicine, University of Tennessee.)

wall of the guttural pouches can extend into the wall of the adjacent internal carotid artery causing hemorrhage into the lumen of the guttural pouch and recurrent epistaxis. Invasion of the internal carotid artery causes arteritis, which can also lead to formation of an aneurysm and fatal bleeding into the guttural pouches. In other cases, the fungi may be angioinvasive, leading to the release of mycotic emboli into the internal carotid artery, generally resulting in multiple cerebral infarcts. Dysphagia, another clinical sign seen in guttural pouch mycosis, is associated with damage to the pharyngeal branches of the vagus and glossopharyngeal nerves, which lie on the ventral aspect of the pouches. Horner's syndrome results from damage to the cranial cervical ganglion and sympathetic fibers located in the caudodorsal aspect of the pouches. Finally, equine laryngeal paralysis (hemiplegia) can result from damage to the laryngeal nerves as previously described in the section on Laryngeal Hemiplegia.

Empyema of guttural pouches is a sequela to suppurative inflammation of the nasal cavities, most commonly from *Streptococcus equi* infection (strangles). In severe cases, the entire guttural pouch can be filled with purulent exudate (Fig. 9-47). The sequelae are similar to those of guttural pouch mycosis except that there is no erosion of the internal carotid artery. It is clinically characterized by nasal discharge, enlarged retropharyngeal lymph nodes, painful swelling of the parotid region, dysphagia, and respiratory distress.

Guttural pouch tympany develops sporadically in young horses when excessive air accumulates in the pouch from the one-way valve effect caused by inflammation or malformation of the Eustachian tube. Arabian and German warm-blooded horses are particularly susceptible to develop guttural pouch tympany. It is generally unilateral and characterized by nonpainful swelling of the parotid region.

Disorders of Ruminants (Cattle, Sheep, and Goats)

Circulatory Disturbances

Tracheal Edema and Hemorrhage Syndrome of Feeder Cattle. Tracheal edema and hemorrhage syndrome of feeder cattle, also known as the *honker syndrome* or *tracheal stenosis of feedlot cattle*, is a poorly documented acute disease of unknown cause, most often seen during the summer months. Severe edema and a few hemorrhages are present in the mucosa and submucosa of the dorsal surface of the trachea, extending caudally from the midcervical area as far as the tracheal bifurcation. On section, the tracheal mucosa is diffusely thickened and gelatinous. Clinical signs include inspiratory dyspnea that can progress to oral breathing, recumbency, and death by asphyxiation in less than 24 hours.

Inflammation

Necrotic Laryngitis. Necrotic laryngitis (calf diphtheria, laryngeal necrobacillosis) is a common disease of feedlot cattle and cattle affected with other diseases, with nutritional deficiencies, or housed under unsanitary conditions. It also occurs sporadically in sheep and pigs. Necrotic laryngitis, caused by *Fusobacterium necrophorum*, is part of the syndrome termed *necrotic stomatitis* or *laryngeal necrobacillosis*, which can include lesions of the tongue, cheeks, palate, and pharynx. An opportunistic pathogen, *Fusobacterium necrophorum* produces potent exotoxins and endotoxins after gaining entry either through lesions of viral infections, such as IBR and vesicular stomatitis in cattle, or after traumatic injury produced by feed or careless use of specula or balling guns.

The gross lesions, regardless of location in the mouth or larynx (most common in the mucosa overlying the laryngeal cartilages), consist of well-demarcated, dry, yellow-gray, thick-crusted, and fibrinonecrotic exudate (Fig. 9-48) that in the early stages is bounded by a zone of active hyperemia. Deep ulceration develops, and if the lesion does not result in death, healing is by granulation tissue formation. Microscopically, the necrotic foci are first surrounded by congested borders, then by a band of leukocytes, and finally the ulcers heal by granulation tissue and collagen (fibrosis). The lesions can extend deep into the submucosal tissue. Numerous bacteria are evident at the advancing edge.

There are numerous and important sequelae to calf diphtheria; the most serious is death from severe toxemia or overwhelming fusobacteremia. Sometimes, the exudate may be copious enough to cause laryngeal obstruction and asphyxiation or be aspirated and cause bronchopneumonia. The clinical signs of necrotic laryngitis are fever, anorexia, depression, halitosis, moist painful cough, dysphagia, and inspiratory dyspnea and ventilatory failure because of fatigue of the respiratory muscles (diaphragmatic and intercostal).

Laryngeal Contact Ulcers. Ulcerative lesions in the larynx are commonly found in feedlot cattle. Grossly, the laryngeal mucosa reveals circular ulcers (up to 1 cm in diameter), which may be unilateral or bilateral and sometimes deep enough to expose the underlying arytenoid cartilages. The cause has not been established, but causal agents, such as viral, bacterial, and traumatic, have been proposed, along with increased frequency and rate of closure of the larynx (excessive swallowing and vocalization) when cattle are exposed to market and feedlot stresses such as dust, pathogens, and interruption of feeding. Contact ulcers predispose a calf to diphtheria (*Fusobacterium necrophorum*) and laryngeal papillomas. Ulceration of the mucosa and necrosis of the laryngeal cartilages have also been described in calves, sheep, and horses under the term *laryngeal chondritis*. Laryngeal abscesses involving the mucosa and underlying cartilage occur as a herd or flock problem in calves and sheep, presumably caused by a secondary infection with *Trueperella* (*Arcanobacterium*) *pyogenes*.

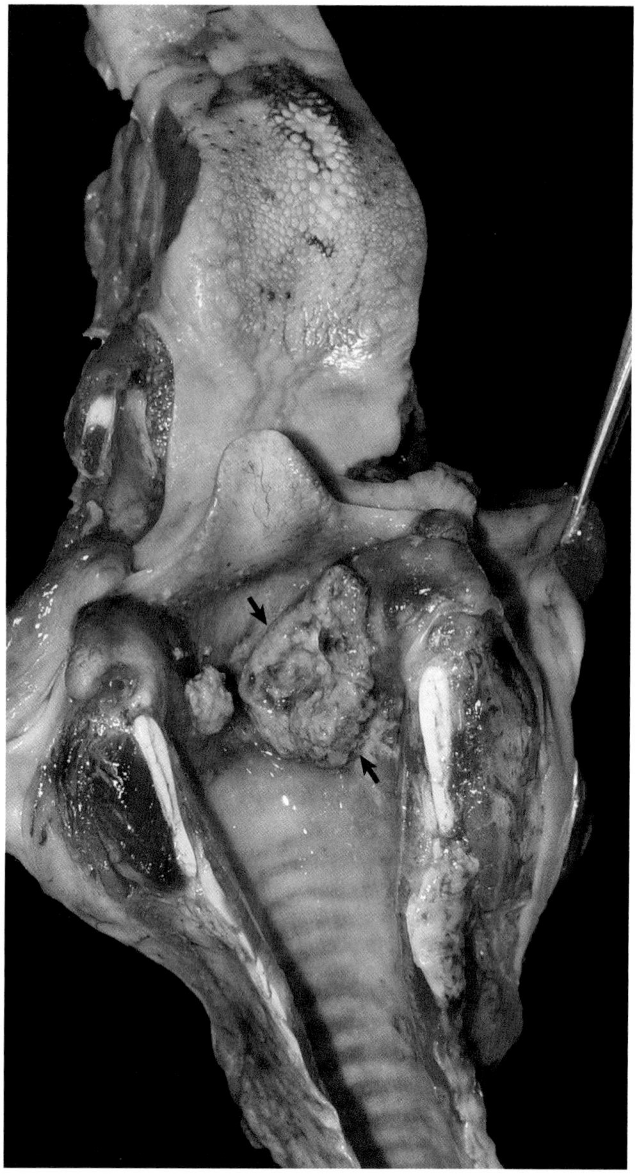

Figure 9-48 **Necrotic Laryngitis, Calf Diphtheria *(Fusobacterium necrophorum)*, Larynx, Calf.** Plaques of fibrinopurulent exudate are present on the mucosa of the arytenoid cartilages *(arrows)*. Pieces of the exudate can be aspirated into the lungs and cause bronchopneumonia. (Courtesy Dr. A. López, Atlantic Veterinary College.)

Disorders of Dogs

Anomalies[5]

Brachycephalic Airway Syndrome. Brachycephalic airway syndrome is a clinical term that refers to increased airflow resistance caused by stenotic nostrils and nasal meatuses and an excessively long soft palate. These abnormalities are present in brachycephalic canine breeds such as bulldogs, boxers, Boston terriers, pugs, Pekingese, and others. The defects are a result of a mismatch of the ratio of soft tissue to cranial bone and the obstruction of airflow by excessive length of the palatine soft tissue. Secondary changes, such as nasal and laryngeal edema caused by forceful inspiration, eventually lead to severe upper airway obstruction, respiratory distress, and exercise intolerance.

Tracheal Hypoplasia. Tracheal hypoplasia occurs most often in English bulldogs and Boston terriers; the tracheal lumen is decreased in diameter throughout its length.

Inflammation

Canine Infectious Respiratory Disease. Canine infectious respiratory disease (CIRD), formerly called canine tracheobronchitis or kennel cough, is a highly contagious group of infectious diseases characterized clinically by an acute onset of coughing notably exacerbated by exercise. The term is nonspecific, much like the

[5]See E-Box 1-1 for potential, suspected, or known genetic disorders.

"common cold" in human beings or bovine respiratory disease complex (BRDC) in cattle. The infection occurs commonly as a result of mixing dogs from different origins such as occurs at commercial kennels, animal shelters, and veterinary clinics. Between bouts of coughing, most animals appear normal, although some have rhinitis, pharyngitis, tonsillitis, or conjunctivitis; some with secondary pneumonia become quite ill.

The pathogenesis of CIRD is complex, and many pathogens and environmental factors have been incriminated. *Bordetella bronchiseptica*, canine adenovirus-2 (CAV-2), and canine parainfluenza virus-2 (CPIV-2) are most commonly implicated. The severity of the disease is increased when more than one agent is involved or if there are extreme environmental conditions (e.g., poor ventilation). For example, dogs asymptomatically infected with *Bordetella bronchiseptica* are more severely affected by superinfection with CAV-2 than those not carrying the bacterium. Other agents are sometimes isolated but of lesser significance and include canine adenovirus-1 (CAV-1: infectious canine hepatitis virus), reovirus type 1, canid herpesvirus-1 (CaHV-1), canine respiratory coronavirus (CRCoV), and *Mycoplasma* species.

Depending on the agents involved, gross and microscopic lesions are completely absent or they vary from catarrhal to mucopurulent tracheobronchitis, with enlargement of the tonsils and retropharyngeal and tracheobronchial lymph nodes. In dogs with *Bordetella bronchiseptica* infection, the lesions are suppurative or mucopurulent rhinitis and tracheobronchitis, and suppurative bronchiolitis. In contrast, when lesions are purely viral, microscopic changes are focal necrosis of the tracheobronchial epithelium. Sequelae can include spread either proximally or distally in the respiratory tract, the latter sometimes inducing chronic bronchitis and bronchopneumonia.

Oslerus (Filaroides) osleri. *Oslerus* (*Filaroides*) *osleri* is a nematode parasite of dogs and other Canidae that causes characteristic protruding nodules into the lumen at the tracheal bifurcation. They are readily seen on endoscopic examination or at necropsy. In severe cases, these nodules can extend 5 cm cranially or caudally from the tracheal bifurcation and even into primary and secondary bronchi. The disease occurs worldwide, and *Oslerus osleri* is considered the most common respiratory nematode of dogs.

The gross lesions are variably sized, up to 1 cm, submucosal nodules that extend up to 1 cm into the tracheal lumen (Fig. 9-49, *A*). Microscopically, nodules contain adult parasites with a mild mononuclear cell reaction; with the death of the parasite, an intense foreign body reaction develops with neutrophils and giant cells (Fig. 9-49, *B*). Clinically, it can be asymptomatic, although it most often causes a chronic cough that can be exacerbated by exercise or excitement. Severe infestations can result in dyspnea, exercise intolerance, cyanosis, emaciation, and even death in young dogs.

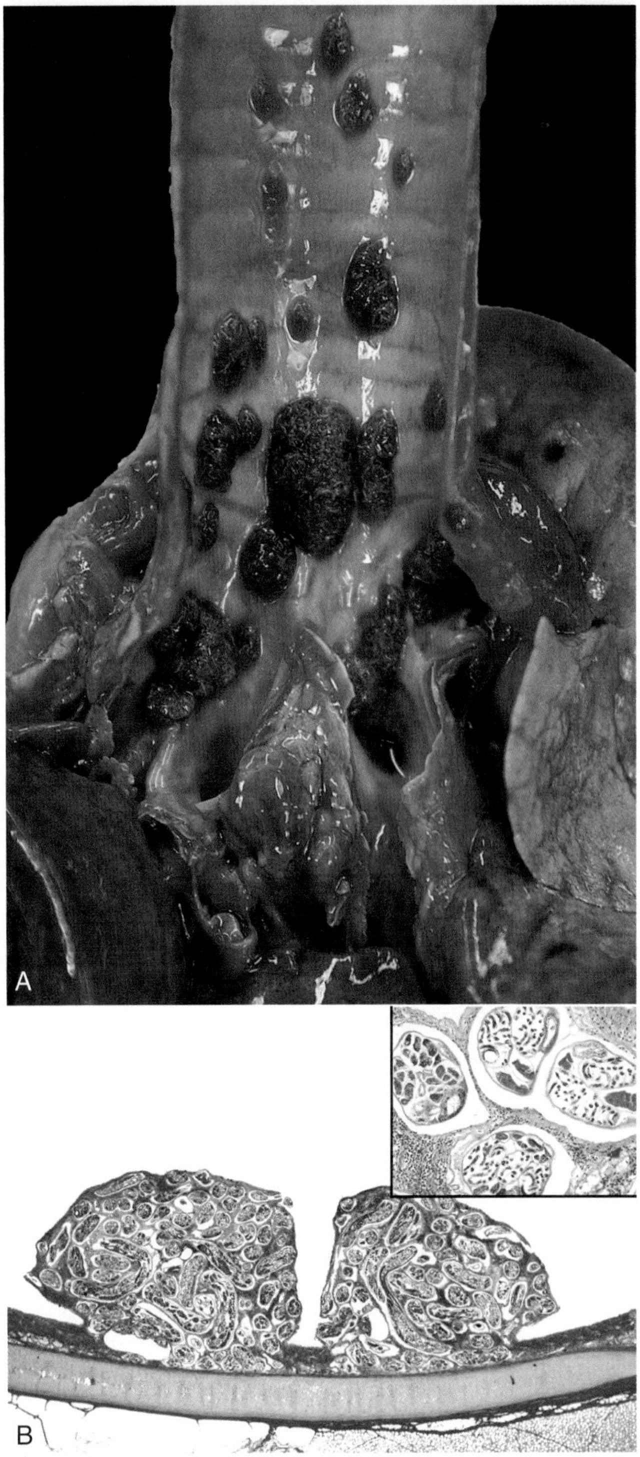

Figure 9-49 Parasitic Tracheobronchitis (*Oslerus osleri*), Trachea and Main Bronchi, Dog. A, Note the numerous large red-brown parasitic nodules on the mucosal surface of the distal trachea and main bronchi. These nodules cause clinical signs only in severe infections. **B,** Two parasitic nodules in the tracheal mucosa. *Inset,* Filarial forms of *Oslerus osleri* can be seen in the lamina propria of the tracheal mucosa. Numerous chronic inflammatory cells are also present. H&E stain. (**A** courtesy Facultad de Medicina Veterinaria y Zootecnia, Universidad Nacional Autónoma de México. **B** courtesy Dr. P.-Y. Daoust and Dr. A. López, Atlantic Veterinary College.)

Neoplasms of the Guttural Pouches, Larynx, and Trachea

Neoplasms of the Guttural Pouches

Neoplasms of the guttural pouches occur rarely in horses and are usually squamous cell carcinomas.

Neoplasms of the Larynx and Trachea

Laryngeal neoplasms are rare in dogs and extremely so in other species, although they have been reported in cats and horses.

The most common laryngeal neoplasms in dogs are papillomas and squamous cell carcinomas. Other less common tumors are laryngeal rhabdomyoma, previously referred to as *laryngeal oncocytoma*, and chondromas and osteochondromas. Lymphoma involving the laryngeal tissue is sporadically seen in cats.

When large enough to be obstructive, neoplasms may cause a change or loss of voice, cough, or respiratory distress with cyanosis, collapse, and syncope. Other signs include dysphagia, anorexia, and exercise intolerance. The neoplasm is sometimes visible from the oral cavity and causes swelling of the neck. The prognosis is poor because most lesions recur after excision.

Tracheal neoplasms are even more uncommon than those of the larynx. The tracheal cartilage or mucosa can be the site of an osteochondroma, leiomyoma, osteosarcoma, mast cell tumor, and carcinoma. Lymphoma in cats can extend from the mediastinum to involve the trachea.

Disorders of the Lungs

Species Differences

Each lung is subdivided into various numbers of pulmonary lobes (see Fig. 9-16). In the past, these were defined by anatomic fissures. However, in current anatomy, lobes are defined by the ramification of the bronchial tree. Following this criterion, the left lung of all domestic species is composed of cranial and caudal lobes, whereas the right lung, depending on species, is composed of cranial, middle (absent in horse), caudal, and accessory lobes. Each pulmonary lobe is further subdivided by connective tissue into pulmonary lobules, which in some species (cattle and pigs) are rather prominent and in others are much less conspicuous. From a practical standpoint, identification of the lungs among different species could be achieved by carefully observing the degree of lobation (external fissures) and the degree of lobulation (connective tissue between lobules). Cattle and pigs have well-lobated and well-lobulated lungs; sheep and goats have well-lobated but poorly lobulated lungs; horses have both poorly lobated and poorly lobulated lungs and resemble human lungs; finally, dogs and cats have well-lobated but not well-lobulated lungs. The degree of lobulation determines the degree of air movement between the lobules. In pigs and cattle, movement of air between lobules is practically absent because of the thick connective tissue of the interlobular septa separating individual lobules. This movement of air between lobules and between adjacent alveoli (via the pores of Kohn) constitutes what is referred to as collateral ventilation. This collateral ventilation is poor in cattle and pigs and good in dogs. The functional implications of collateral ventilation are discussed in the section on Pulmonary Emphysema.

The lungs have an interconnecting network of interstitial stromal tissue supporting the blood and lymphatic vessels, nerves, bronchi, bronchioles, and alveoli. For purposes of simplicity, the pulmonary interstitium can be anatomically divided into three contiguous compartments: (1) bronchovascular interstitium, where main bronchi and pulmonary vessels are situated; (2) interlobular interstitium separating pulmonary lobules and supporting small blood and lymph vessels; and (3) alveolar interstitium supporting the alveolar walls that contain pulmonary capillaries and alveolar epithelial cells (no lymphatic vessels here) (see discussion on the blood-air barrier in the section on Alveoli). Pulmonary changes, such as edema, emphysema, and inflammation, may affect one or more of these interstitial compartments.

Disorders of the Lung (Bronchioles, Bronchi, and Alveoli) in Domestic Animals

Anomalies[6]

Congenital anomalies of the lungs are rare in all species but are most commonly reported in cattle and sheep. Compatibility with life largely depends on the type of structures involved and the proportion of functional tissue present at birth. Accessory lungs are one of the most common anomalies and consist of distinctively lobulated masses of incompletely differentiated pulmonary tissue present in the thorax, abdominal cavity, or subcutaneous tissue virtually anywhere in the trunk. Large accessory lungs can cause dystocia. Ciliary dyskinesia (immotile cilia syndrome, Kartagener's syndrome) is characterized by defective ciliary movement, which results in reduced mucociliary clearance because of a defect in the microtubules of all ciliated cells and, most important, in the ciliated respiratory epithelium and spermatozoa. Primary ciliary dyskinesia often associated with situs inversus has been reported in dogs, which as a result usually have chronic recurrent rhinosinusitis, pneumonia, and infertility. Pulmonary agenesis, pulmonary hypoplasia, abnormal lobulation, congenital emphysema, lung hamartoma, and congenital bronchiectasis are occasionally seen in domestic animals. Congenital melanosis is a common incidental finding in pigs and ruminants and is usually seen at slaughter (Fig. 9-50). It is characterized by black spots, often a few centimeters in diameter, in various organs, mainly the lungs, meninges, intima of the aorta, and caruncles of the uterus. Melanosis has no clinical significance, and the texture of pigmented lungs remains unchanged. Congenital emphysema is sporadically seen in dogs (E-Fig. 9-4).

Metabolic Disturbances

Pulmonary Calcification ("Calcinosis"). Calcification of the lungs occurs in some hypercalcemic states, generally secondary to hypervitaminosis D or from ingestion of toxic (hypercalcemic) plants, such as *Solanum malacoxylon* (Manchester wasting disease), that contain vitamin D analogs. It is also a common sequela to uremia and hyperadrenocorticism in dogs and to pulmonary necrosis (dystrophic calcification) in most species. Calcified lungs may fail to collapse when the thoracic cavity is opened and have a characteristic "gritty" texture (Fig. 9-51). Microscopically, lesions vary from calcification of the alveolar basement membranes (see

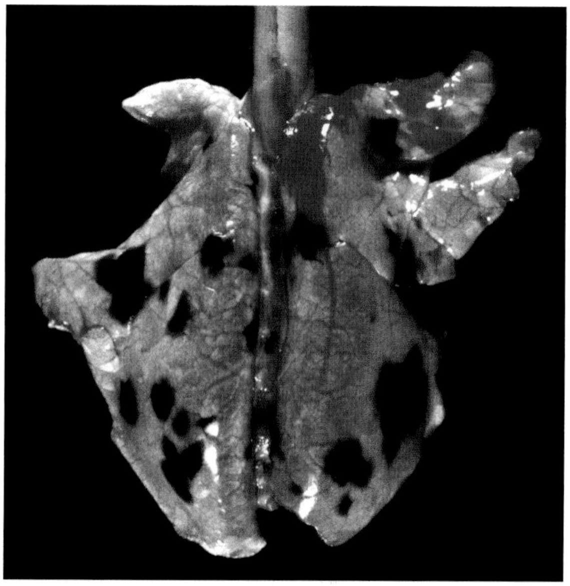

Figure 9-50 **Pulmonary Melanosis, Lungs, Pig.** Note the areas of black (melanin pigment) discoloration of the pleural surface. This pigmentation extends into the lungs and is an incidental finding that has no clinical or pathologic significance. It is most common in "black-face" breeds of animals, especially sheep. (Courtesy College of Veterinary Medicine, University of Illinois.)

[6]See E-Box 1-1 for potential, suspected, or known genetic disorders.

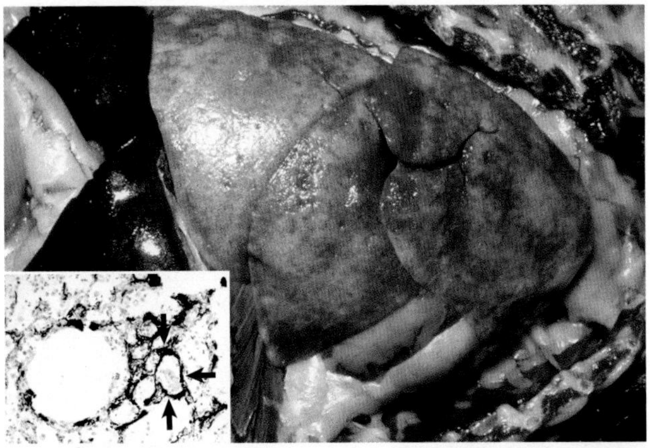

Figure 9-51 **Uremic Pneumopathy From Chronic Renal Failure, Lung, 4-Year-Old Dog.** The lungs have failed to collapse when the thorax was opened because of extensive mineralization of alveolar walls. *Inset,* Calcification *(black)* of alveolar septa. Note the linear deposits of mineral in the alveolar septa *(arrows)*. von Kossa stain with nuclear fast red counterstain. (Courtesy Dr. A. López, Atlantic Veterinary College.)

Fig. 9-51) to heterotopic ossification of the lungs (E-Fig. 9-5). In most cases, pulmonary calcification in itself has little clinical significance, although its cause (e.g., uremia or vitamin D toxicosis) may be very important.

Alveolar Filling Disorders

Alveolar filling disorders are a heterogeneous group of lung diseases characterized by accumulation of various chemical compounds in the alveolar lumens. The most common are *alveolar proteinosis*, in which the alveoli are filled with finely granular eosinophilic material; *pulmonary lipidosis*, in which alveoli are filled with macrophages containing endogenous or exogenous lipid; and *alveolar microlithiasis*, in which the alveoli contain numerous concentric calcified "microliths" or "calcospherites." A similar but distinct concretion is known as *corpora amylacea*, which is an accumulation of laminated bodies composed of cellular debris, lipids, proteins, and possibly amyloid. For most alveolar filling disorders, there is little host response, and in many cases, it is an incidental finding. Most of the alveolar filling disorders originate from inherited metabolic defects in which alveolar cells (epithelial or macrophages) cannot properly metabolize or remove lipids or proteins, whereas others result from an excessive synthesis of these substances in the lung.

Endogenous Lipid (Lipoid) Pneumonia. Endogenous lipid pneumonia is an obscure, subclinical pulmonary disease of cats and occasionally of dogs, which is unrelated to aspiration of foreign material. Although the pathogenesis is not understood, it is presumed that lipids from pulmonary surfactant and from degenerated cells accumulate within alveolar macrophages. Accumulation of surfactant lipids can occur in metabolic abnormalities of alveolar macrophages or in bronchial obstruction where surfactant-laden macrophages cannot exit the lungs via the mucociliary escalator. The gross lesions are multifocal, white, firm nodules scattered throughout the lungs (E-Fig. 9-6). Microscopically, the alveoli are filled with foamy lipid-laden macrophages accompanied by interstitial infiltration of lymphocytes and plasma cells, fibrosis, alveolar epithelialization, and, in some cases, cholesterol clefts and lipid granulomas.

Lipid (lipoid) pneumonia occurs frequently in the vicinity of cancerous lung lesions in human beings, cats, and dogs. The reason for this association remains unknown and frequently unrecognized by pathologists. Recent investigations suggest that excessive lipid originates from the breakdown products of neoplastic cells. Bronchial and bronchiolar obstructions such as those caused by lungworms can also cause alveolar lipidosis. The pathogenesis relates to the inability of alveolar macrophages that normally remove part of the surfactant lipids to exit the lung via the mucociliary escalator.

Exogenous Lipid Pneumonia. Another form of lipid pneumonia occurs accidentally in cats or horses given mineral oil by their owners in an attempt to remove hairballs or treat colic (aspiration pneumonia).

Inflation Disturbances of the Lung

To achieve gaseous exchange, a balanced ratio of the volumes of air to capillary blood must be present in the lungs (ventilation/perfusion ratio), and the air and capillary blood must be in close proximity across the alveolar wall. A ventilation-perfusion mismatch occurs if pulmonary tissue is either collapsed (atelectasis) or overinflated (hyperinflation and emphysema).

Atelectasis (Congenital and Acquired). The term *atelectasis* means incomplete distention of alveoli and is used to describe lungs that have failed to expand with air at the time of birth (congenital or neonatal atelectasis) or lungs that have collapsed after inflation has taken place (acquired atelectasis or alveolar collapse) (Figs. 9-52 and 9-53).

During fetal life, lungs are not fully distended, contain no air, and are partially filled with a locally produced fluid known as fetal lung fluid. Not surprisingly, lungs of aborted and stillborn fetuses sink when placed in water, whereas those from animals that have breathed float. At the time of birth, fetal lung fluid is rapidly reabsorbed and replaced by inspired air, leading to the normal distention of alveoli. Congenital atelectasis occurs in newborns that fail to inflate their lungs after taking their first few breaths of air; it is caused by obstruction of airways, often as a result of aspiration of amniotic fluid and meconium (described in the section on Meconium Aspiration Syndrome) (see Fig. 9-52). Congenital atelectasis also develops when alveoli cannot remain distended after initial aeration because of an alteration in quality and quantity of pulmonary surfactant produced by type II pneumonocytes and Club (Clara) cells. This infant form of congenital atelectasis is referred to in human neonatology as infant respiratory distress syndrome (IRDS) or as hyaline membrane disease because of the clinical and microscopic features of the disease. It commonly occurs in babies who are premature or born to diabetic or alcoholic mothers and is occasionally found in animals, particularly foals and piglets. The pathetic, gasping attempts of affected foals and pigs to breathe have prompted the use of the name "barkers"; foals that survive may have brain damage from cerebral hypoxia (see Chapter 14) and are referred to as "wanderers" due to their aimless behavior and lack of a normal sense of fear.

Acquired atelectasis is much more common and occurs in two main forms: compressive and obstructive (see Fig. 9-53). Compressive atelectasis has two main causes: space-occupying masses in the pleural cavity, such as abscesses and tumors, or transferred pressures, such as that caused by bloat, hydrothorax, hemothorax, chylothorax, and empyema (Fig. 9-54). Another form of compressive atelectasis occurs when the negative pressure in the thoracic cavity is lost because of pneumothorax. This form generally has massive atelectasis and thus is also referred to as lung collapse.

Obstructive (absorption) atelectasis occurs when there is a reduction in the diameter of the airways caused by mucosal edema and inflammation, or when the lumen of the airway is blocked by

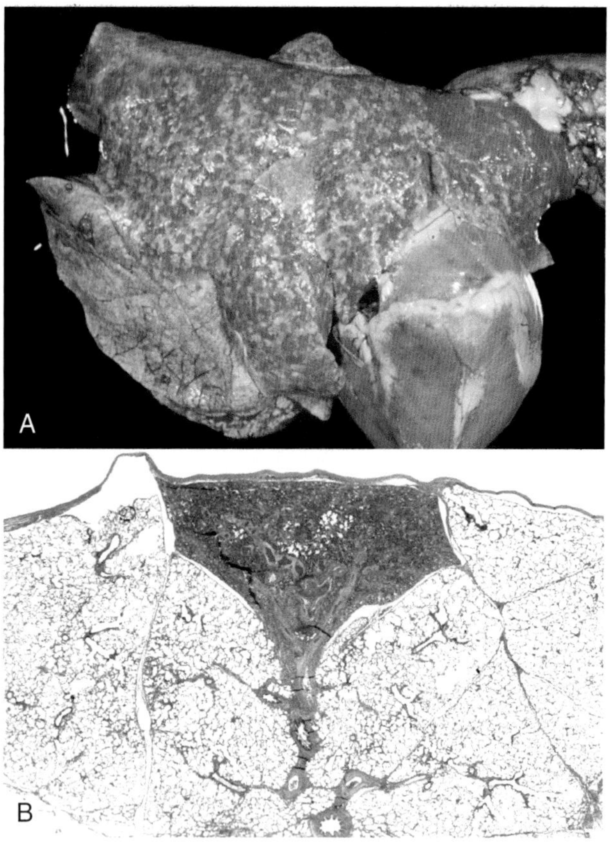

Figure 9-52 **Pulmonary Atelectasis. A,** Multifocal neonatal atelectasis of the lung from 1-day-old calf. Note the prominent mosaic pattern of normally inflated *(lighter)* and atelectatic, uninflated *(darker)* lobules. Neonatal atelectasis is caused by aspiration of amniotic fluid, meconium, and squamous epithelial cells, causing obstruction of small bronchi and bronchioles at the time of birth. All pulmonary lobes are involved. Although focal lobular atelectasis is commonly seen in neonates, this lesion suggests that the fetus was acidotic and aspirated amniotic fluid. **B,** Atelectasis of a superficial pulmonary lobule *(upper center of image)* in a cow. Note the absence of air in alveoli of this lobule that has resulted in its collapse and thus its darker color as shown in **A.** H&E stain. (**A** from López A, Bildfell R: *Vet Pathol* 29:104-111, 1992. **B** courtesy Dr. M.D. McGavin, College of Veterinary Medicine, University of Tennessee.)

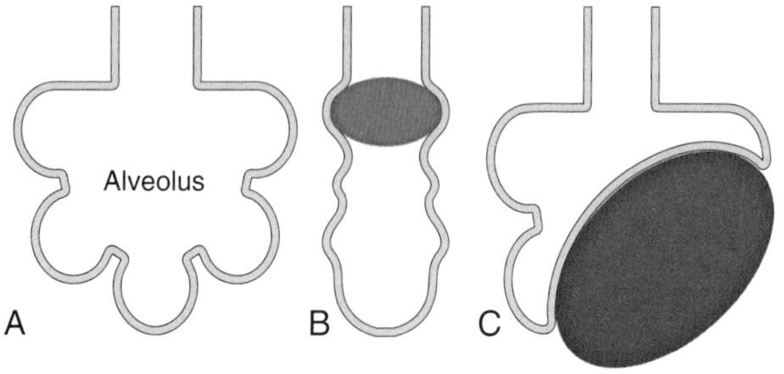

Figure 9-53 **Types of Atelectasis. A,** Normal alveolar distention. **B,** Obstructive atelectasis; obstruction of airways (i.e., exudate or parasite) affecting airflow and causing alveolar collapse. **C,** Compressive atelectasis; mass (i.e., abscess or tumor) compressing the lung parenchyma and causing alveolar collapse. (Redrawn from Dr. A. López, Atlantic Veterinary College.)

mucus plugs, exudate, aspirated foreign material, or lungworms (see Fig. 9-53). When the obstruction is complete, trapped air in the lung eventually becomes reabsorbed. Unlike the compression type, obstructive atelectasis often has a lobular pattern as a result of blockage of the airway supplying that lobule. This lobular

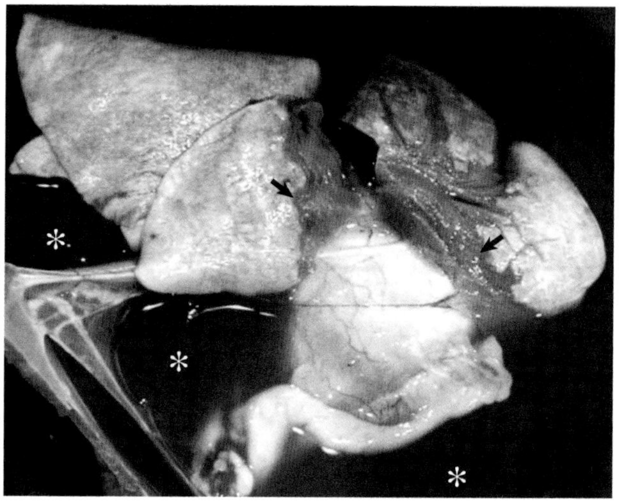

Figure 9-54 **Compressive Atelectasis and Hydrothorax, Lungs, Dog.** Atelectatic lung appears as dark depressed pulmonary tissues *(arrows)*. Also note a large volume of transudate in the ventral pleural cavity *(asterisks)*. (Courtesy Atlantic Veterinary College.)

appearance of atelectasis is more common in species with poor collateral ventilation, such as cattle and pigs. The extent and location of obstructive atelectasis depends largely on the size of the affected airway (large vs. small) and on the degree of obstruction (partial vs. complete).

Atelectasis also occurs when large animals are kept recumbent for prolonged periods, such as during anesthesia (hypostatic atelectasis). The factors contributing to hypostatic atelectasis are a combination of blood-air imbalance, shallow breathing, airway obstruction because of mucus and fluid that has not been drained from bronchioles and alveoli, and from inadequate local production of surfactant. Atelectasis can also be a sequel to paralysis of respiratory muscles and prolonged use of mechanical ventilation or general anesthesia in intensive care.

In general, the lungs with atelectasis appear depressed below the surface of the normally inflated lung. The color is generally dark blue, and the texture is flabby or firm; they are firm if there is concurrent edema or other processes, such as can occur in ARDS or "shock" lungs (see the section on Pulmonary Edema). Distribution and extent vary with the process, being patchy (multifocal) in congenital atelectasis, lobular in the obstructive type, and of various degrees in between in the compressive type. Microscopically, the alveoli are collapsed or slitlike and the alveolar walls appear parallel and close together, giving prominence to the interstitial tissue even without any superimposed inflammation.

Pulmonary Emphysema. Pulmonary emphysema, often simply referred to as *emphysema*, is an extremely important primary disease in human beings, whereas in animals, it is always a secondary condition resulting from a variety of pulmonary lesions. In human medicine, emphysema is strictly defined as an abnormal permanent enlargement of airspaces distal to the terminal bronchiole, accompanied by destruction of alveolar walls (alveolar emphysema). This definition separates it from simple airspace enlargement or hyperinflation, in which there is no destruction of alveolar walls and which can occur congenitally (Down syndrome) or be acquired with age (aging lung, sometimes misnamed "senile emphysema"). The pathogenesis of emphysema in human beings is still controversial, but current thinking overwhelmingly suggests that destruction of alveolar walls is largely the result of an imbalance between proteases released by phagocytes and antiproteases produced in the lung as a defense mechanism (the protease-antiprotease theory). The destructive process in human beings is markedly accelerated by defects in the synthesis of antiproteases or any factor, such as cigarette smoking or pollution, that increases the recruitment of macrophages and leukocytes in the lungs. This theory originated when it was found that human beings with homozygous α_1-antitrypsin deficiency were remarkably susceptible to emphysema and that proteases (elastase) inoculated intratracheally into the lungs of laboratory animals produced lesions similar to those found in the disease. More than 90% of the problem relates to cigarette smoking, and airway obstruction is no longer considered to play a major role in the pathogenesis of emphysema in human beings.

Primary emphysema does not occur in animals, and thus no animal disease should be called simply emphysema. In animals, this lesion is always secondary to obstruction of outflow of air or is agonal at slaughter. Secondary pulmonary emphysema occurs frequently in animals with bronchopneumonia, in which exudate plugging bronchi and bronchioles causes an airflow imbalance where the volume of air entering exceeds the volume leaving the lung. This airflow imbalance is often promoted by the so-called one-way valve effect caused by the exudate, which allows air into the lung during inspiration but prevents movement of air out of the lung during expiration.

Depending on the localization in the lung, emphysema can be classified as alveolar or interstitial. Alveolar emphysema characterized by distention and rupture of the alveolar walls, forming variably sized air bubbles in pulmonary parenchyma, occurs in all species. Interstitial emphysema occurs mainly in cattle, presumably because of their wide interlobular septa, and lack of collateral ventilation in these species does not permit air to move freely into adjacent pulmonary lobules. As a result, accumulated air penetrates the alveolar and bronchiolar walls and forces its way into the interlobular connective tissue, causing notable distention of the interlobular septa. It is also suspected that forced respiratory movements predispose to interstitial emphysema when air at high pressure breaks into the loose connective tissue of the interlobular septa (Fig. 9-55). Sometimes these bubbles of trapped air in alveolar or interstitial emphysema become confluent, forming large (several centimeters in diameter) pockets of air that are referred to as *bullae* (singular: bulla) (see E-Fig. 9-4); the lesion is then called *bullous emphysema*. This lesion is not a specific type of emphysema and does not indicate a different disease process but, rather, is a larger accumulation of air at one focus. In the most severe cases, air moves from the interlobular septa into the connective tissue surrounding the main stem bronchi and major vessels (bronchovascular bundles), and from here it leaks into the mediastinum, causing pneumomediastinum first, and eventually exits via the thoracic inlet into the cervical and thoracic subcutaneous tissue causing subcutaneous emphysema.

Note that mild and even moderate alveolar emphysema is difficult to judge at necropsy and by light microscopy unless special techniques are used to prevent collapse of the lung when the thorax is opened. These techniques include plugging of the trachea or intratracheal perfusion of fixative (10% neutral-buffered formalin) before the thorax is opened to prevent collapse of the lungs. Important diseases that cause secondary pulmonary emphysema in animals include small airway obstruction (e.g., heaves) in horses and pulmonary edema and emphysema (fog fever) in cattle (see Fig. 9-55) and exudates in bronchopneumonia. Congenital emphysema occurring secondary to bronchial cartilage hypoplasia with subsequent bronchial collapse is occasionally reported in dogs.

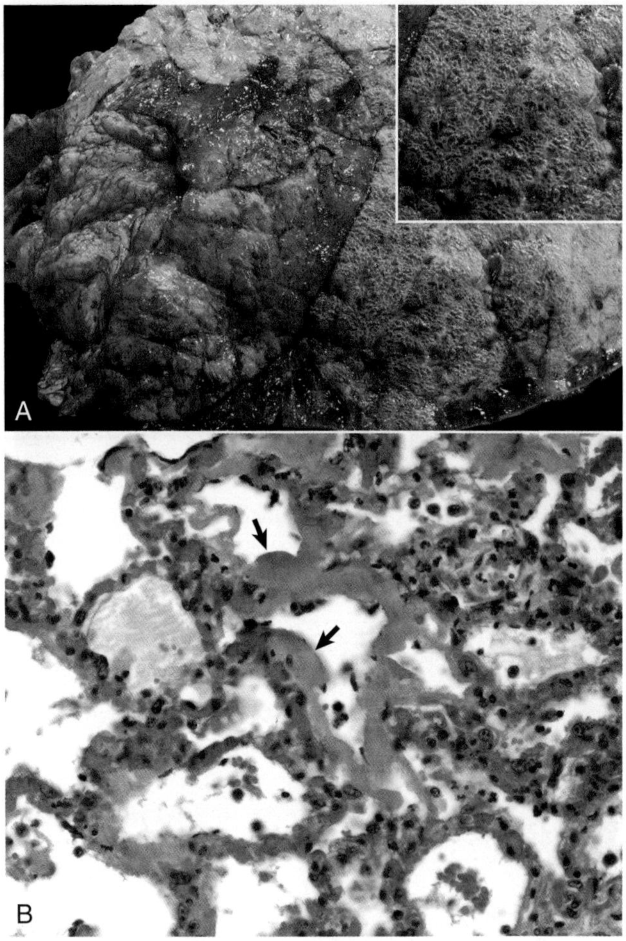

Figure 9-55 Bovine Pulmonary Edema and Emphysema (Fog Fever), Lung, Cow. A, Emphysema, edema, and interstitial pneumonia involving all pulmonary lobes. Note the variably sized air bubbles in the interlobular septa and pulmonary parenchyma. The texture of these lungs would be notably crepitus as a result of the accumulation of air in pulmonary parenchyma. *Inset,* Closer view of air bubbles in the parenchyma. **B,** Note the thick eosinophilic hyaline membranes *(arrows)* lining the alveoli. The alveoli are dilated and also contain some edema fluid, occasional pulmonary macrophages, and necrotic alveolar cells. H&E stain. (Courtesy Dr. A. López, Atlantic Veterinary College.)

Circulatory Disturbances of the Lungs

Lungs are extremely well-vascularized organs with a dual circulation provided by pulmonary and bronchial arteries. Disturbances in pulmonary circulation have a notable effect on gaseous exchange, which may result in life-threatening hypoxemia and acidosis. In addition, circulatory disturbances in the lungs can have an impact on other organs, such as the heart and liver. For example, impeded blood flow in the lungs because of chronic pulmonary disease results in cor pulmonale, which is caused by unremitting pulmonary hypertension followed by cardiac dilation, right heart failure, chronic passive congestion of the liver (nutmeg liver), and generalized edema (anasarca).

Hyperemia and Congestion. Hyperemia is an active process that is part of acute inflammation, whereas congestion is the passive process resulting from decreased outflow of venous blood, as occurs in congestive heart failure (Fig. 9-56). In the early acute stages of pneumonia, the lungs appear notably red, and microscopically, blood vessels and alveolar capillaries are engorged with blood from

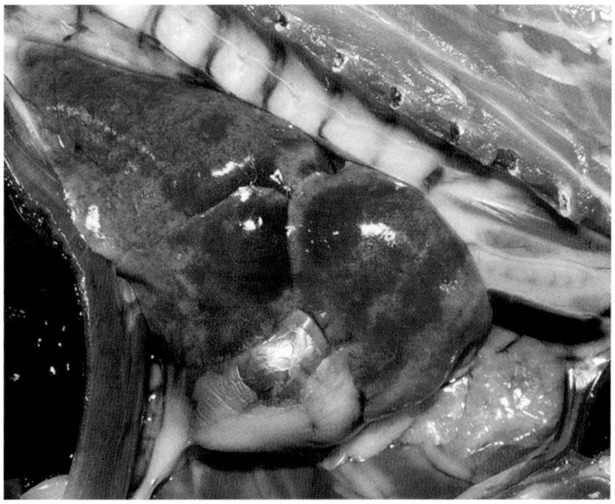

Figure 9-56 **Acute Pulmonary Congestion, Lungs, Dog.** The lung parenchyma is red because of congestion of pulmonary vasculature and alveolar capillaries. (Courtesy Dr. A. López, Atlantic Veterinary College.)

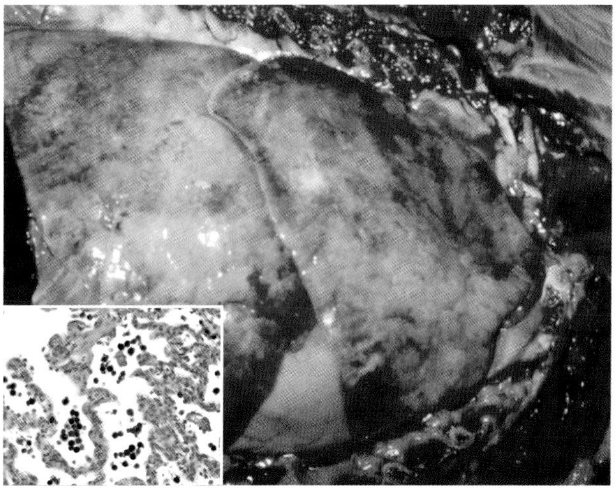

Figure 9-57 **Chronic Pulmonary Congestion and Edema Because of Chronic Heart Failure (Dilative Cardiomyopathy), Lungs, 5-Year-Old Dog.** The lungs have failed to collapse (fibrosis) and have a mottled and yellow-brown appearance (hemosiderosis). *Inset,* Microscopic view of alveoli. Large numbers of macrophages containing hemosiderin (heart failure cells *[blue color]*) are present in alveoli. During heart failure, red blood cells gain access to alveoli where they are rapidly phagocytosed by pulmonary macrophages and the iron of the hemoglobin molecule is converted to hemosiderin. Hemosiderin gives a positive reaction for iron with the Prussian blue reaction. Prussian blue (iron) reaction with nuclear fast red counterstain. (Courtesy Dr. A. López, Atlantic Veterinary College.)

hyperemia. Pulmonary congestion is most frequently caused by heart failure, which results in stagnation of blood in pulmonary vessels, leading to edema and egression of erythrocytes into the alveolar spaces. As with any other foreign particle, erythrocytes in alveolar spaces are rapidly phagocytosed (erythrophagocytosis) by pulmonary alveolar macrophages. When extravasation of erythrocytes is severe, large numbers of macrophages with brown cytoplasm may accumulate in the bronchoalveolar spaces. The brown cytoplasm is the result of accumulation of considerable amounts of hemosiderin; these macrophages filled with iron pigment (siderophages) are generally referred to as *heart failure cells* (Fig. 9-57). The lungs of animals with chronic heart failure usually have a patchy red appearance with foci of brown discoloration because of accumulated hemosiderin. In severe and persistent cases of heart failure, the lungs fail to collapse because of edema and pulmonary fibrosis. Terminal pulmonary congestion (acute) is frequently seen in animals euthanized with barbiturates and should not be mistaken for an antemortem lesion.

Hypostatic congestion is another form of pulmonary congestion that results from the effects of gravity and poor circulation on a highly vascularized tissue, such as the lung. This type of gravitational congestion is characterized by the increase of blood in the lower side of the lung, particularly the lower lung of animals in lateral recumbency, and is most notable in horses and cattle. The affected portions of the lung appear dark red and can have a firmer texture. In animals and human beings who have been prostrated for extended periods of time, hypostatic congestion may be followed by hypostatic edema, and hypostatic pneumonia as edema interferes locally with the bacterial defense mechanisms.

Pulmonary Hemorrhage. Pulmonary hemorrhages can occur as a result of trauma, coagulopathies, and disseminated intravascular coagulation (DIC), vasculitis, sepsis, and pulmonary thromboembolism from jugular thrombosis or from embolism of exudate from a hepatic abscess that has eroded the wall and ruptured into the caudal vena cava (cattle). A gross finding often confused with intravital pulmonary hemorrhage is the result of severing both the trachea and the carotid arteries simultaneously at slaughter. Blood is aspirated from the transected trachea into the lungs, forming a random pattern of irregular red foci (1 to 10 mm) in one or more lobes. These red foci are readily visible on both the pleural and the cut surfaces of the lung, and free blood is visible in the lumens of bronchi and bronchioles.

Rupture of a major pulmonary vessel with resulting massive hemorrhage occurs occasionally in cattle when a growing abscess in a lung invades and disrupts the wall of a major pulmonary artery or vein (Fig. 9-58). In most cases, animals die rapidly, often with spectacular hemoptysis, and on postmortem examination, bronchi are filled with blood (see Fig. 9-58).

Pulmonary Edema. In normal lungs, fluid from the vascular space slowly but continuously passes into the interstitial tissue, where it is rapidly drained by the pulmonary and pleural lymphatic vessels. Clearance of alveolar fluid across the alveolar epithelium is also a major mechanism of fluid removal from the lung. Edema develops when the rate of fluid transudation from pulmonary vessels into the interstitium or alveoli exceeds that of lymphatic and alveolar removal (Fig. 9-59). Pulmonary edema can be physiologically classified as cardiogenic (hydrostatic; hemodynamic) and noncardiogenic (permeability) types.

Hydrostatic (cardiogenic) pulmonary edema develops when there is an elevated rate of fluid transudation because of increased hydrostatic pressure in the vascular compartment or decreased osmotic pressure in the blood. Once the lymph drainage has been overwhelmed, fluid accumulates in the perivascular spaces, causing distention of the bronchovascular bundles and alveolar interstitium, and eventually leaks into the alveolar spaces. Causes of hemodynamic pulmonary edema include congestive heart failure (increased hydrostatic pressure); iatrogenic fluid overload; and disorders in which blood osmotic pressure is reduced, such as with hypoalbuminemia seen in some hepatic diseases, nephrotic syndrome, and protein-losing enteropathy. Hemodynamic pulmonary edema also occurs when lymph drainage is impaired, generally secondary to neoplastic invasion of lymphatic vessels.

Permeability edema (inflammatory) occurs when there is excessive opening of endothelial gaps or damage to the cells that constitute the blood-air barrier (endothelial cells or type I pneumonocytes).

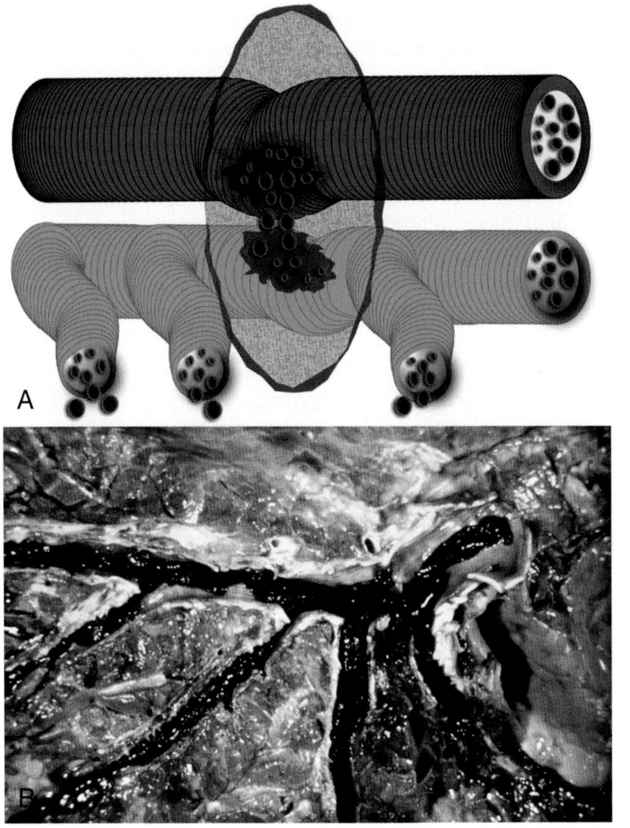

Figure 9-58 Fatal Pulmonary Hemorrhage. A, Schematic of an abscess *(green)* eroding the wall of a major pulmonary artery *(red)* and causing bleeding into the airways *(blue)*. **B,** Cut surface of lung, cow. Major bronchi and the trachea are filled with clotted dark red blood. This cow died unexpectedly, with severe respiratory distress and blood coming from the nose and mouth. A large abscess in the lung had eroded through the wall of a major pulmonary vessel. (**A** courtesy Dr. A. López, Atlantic Veterinary College. **B** courtesy Dr. R. Curtis, Atlantic Veterinary College.)

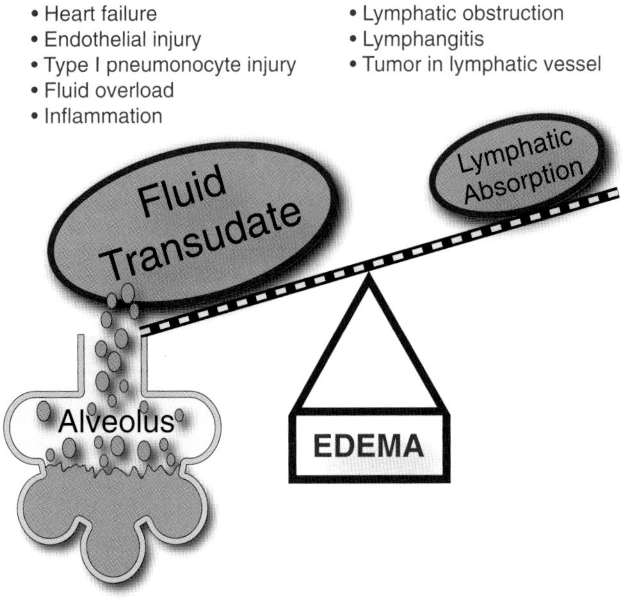

Figure 9-59 Pathogenesis of Pulmonary Edema. (Courtesy Dr. A. López, Atlantic Veterinary College.)

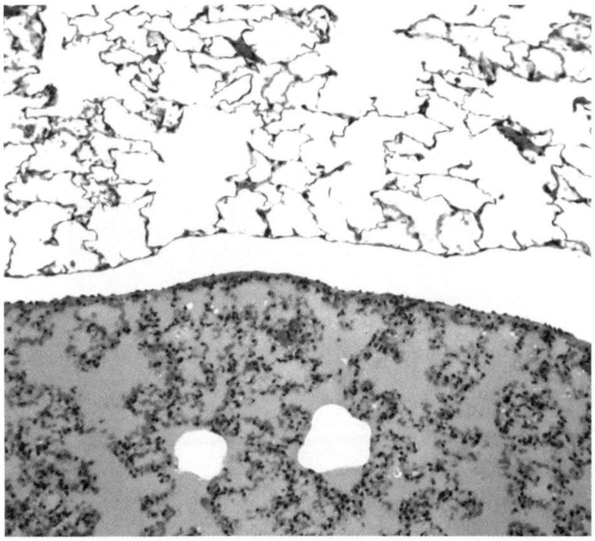

Figure 9-60 Pulmonary Edema, Lung, Rat. Normal lung with alveoli filled with air *(top)* and lung with severe pulmonary edema characterized by transudation of protein-rich fluid (deeply eosinophilic *[pink-red]*) filling the alveoli and congested alveolar septa *(bottom)*. H&E stain. (Courtesy Dr. A. López, Atlantic Veterinary College.)

This type of edema is an integral and early part of the inflammatory response, primarily because of the effect of inflammatory mediators, such as leukotrienes, platelet-activating factor (PAF), cytokines, and vasoactive amines released by neutrophils, macrophages, mast cells, lymphocytes, endothelial cells, and type II pneumonocytes. These inflammatory mediators increase the permeability of the blood-air barrier. In other cases, permeability edema results from direct damage to the endothelium or type I pneumonocytes, allowing plasma fluids to move freely from the vascular space into the alveolar lumen (Fig. 9-60 and see Fig. 9-14). Because type I pneumonocytes are highly vulnerable to some pneumotropic viruses (influenza and BRSV), toxicants (nitrogen dioxide [NO_2], sulfur dioxide [SO_2], hydrogen sulfide [H_2S], and 3-methylindole), and particularly to free radicals, it is not surprising that permeability edema commonly accompanies many viral or toxic pulmonary diseases. A permeability edema also occurs when endothelial cells in the lung are injured by bacterial toxins, sepsis, ARDS, DIC, anaphylactic shock, milk allergy, paraquat toxicity, adverse drug reactions, and smoke inhalation (E-Fig. 9-7).

The concentration of protein in edematous fluid is greater in permeability edema (exudate) than in hemodynamic edema (transudate); this difference has been used clinically in human medicine to differentiate one type of pulmonary edema from another. Microscopically, because of the higher concentration of protein, edema fluid in lungs with inflammation or damage to the blood-air barrier tends to stain more intensely eosinophilic than that of the hydrostatic edema from heart failure.

Grossly, the edematous lungs—independent of the cause—are wet and heavy. The color varies, depending on the degree of congestion or hemorrhage, and fluid may be present in the pleural cavity. If edema is severe, the bronchi and trachea contain considerable amounts of foamy fluid, which originates from the mixing of edema fluid and air (Fig. 9-61). On cut surfaces, the lung parenchyma oozes fluid like a wet sponge. In cattle and pigs that have distinct lobules, the lobular pattern becomes rather accentuated because of edematous distention of lymphatic vessels in the interlobular septa and the edematous interlobular septum itself (Fig. 9-62). Severe pulmonary edema may be impossible to differentiate from peracute pneumonia;

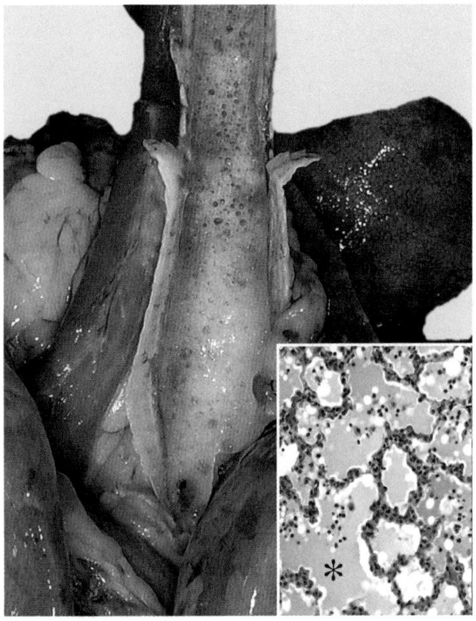

Figure 9-61 **Pulmonary Edema, Lungs and Trachea, Sepsis, Sheep.** Note large amounts of foamy fluid in the trachea and uncollapsed lungs with wet appearance. *Inset,* Alveoli filled with protein-rich edematous fluid *(light pink color [asterisk])* admixed with few inflammatory cells. H&E stain. (Courtesy Dr. C. Legge and Dr. A. López, Atlantic Veterinary College.)

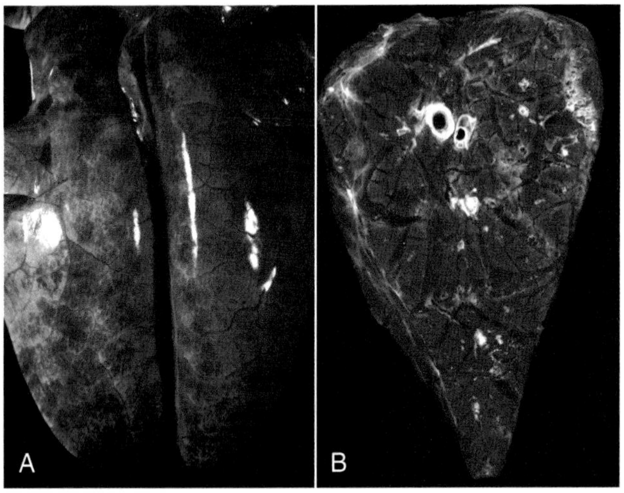

Figure 9-62 **Pulmonary Edema, Lungs, Pig. A,** The lungs are distended by edema fluid, which has resulted in rounded edges and edematous distention of the interlobular septa. **B,** The cut surface is wet and the interlobular septa are markedly distended with edema fluid. Lung lobules are also congested. (**A** and **B** courtesy College of Veterinary Medicine, University of Illinois.)

this fact is not surprising because pulmonary edema occurs in the very early stages of inflammation (see E-Fig. 9-7). Careful observation of the lungs at the time of necropsy is critical because diagnosis of pulmonary edema cannot be reliably performed microscopically. This is due in part to the loss of the edema fluid from the lungs during fixation with 10% neutral-buffered formalin and in part to the fact that the fluid itself stains very poorly or not at all with eosin because of its low protein content (hemodynamic edema). A protein-rich (permeability) edema is easier to visualize microscopically because it is deeply eosinophilic in hematoxylin and eosin (H&E)-stained sections (see Fig. 9-60), particularly if a fixative such as Zenker's solution, which precipitates protein, is used.

Acute Respiratory Distress Syndrome. Acute (adult) respiratory distress syndrome (ARDS; shock lung) is an important condition in human beings and animals characterized by pulmonary hypertension, intravascular aggregation of neutrophils in the lungs, acute lung injury, diffuse alveolar damage, permeability edema, and formation of hyaline membranes (Fig. 9-63). These membranes are a mixture of plasma proteins, fibrin, surfactant, and cellular debris from necrotic pneumonocytes (see Fig. 9-55, *B*). The pathogenesis of ARDS is complex and multifactorial but in general terms can be defined as diffuse alveolar damage that results from lesions in distant organs, from generalized systemic diseases, or from direct injury to the lung. Sepsis, major trauma, aspiration of gastric contents, extensive burns, and pancreatitis are some of the disease entities known to trigger ARDS. All these conditions provoke "hyperreactive macrophages" to directly or indirectly generate overwhelming amounts of cytokines causing what is known as a "cytokine storm." The main cytokines that trigger ARDS are TNF-α, interleukin (IL)-1, IL-6, and IL-8, which prime neutrophils previously recruited in the lung capillaries and alveoli to release cytotoxic enzymes and free radicals. These substances cause severe and diffuse endothelial and alveolar damage that culminates in a fulminating pulmonary edema (see Fig. 9-63). ARDS occurs in domestic animals and explains why pulmonary edema is one of the most common lesions found in many animals dying of sepsis, toxemia, aspiration of gastric contents, and pancreatitis, for example. A familial form of ARDS has been reported in Dalmatians. The pulmonary lesions in this syndrome are further discussed in the sections on Interstitial Pneumonia and Aspiration Pneumonia in Dogs.

Neurogenic pulmonary edema is another distinctive but poorly understood form of life-threatening lung edema in human beings that follows CNS injury and increased intracranial pressure (i.e., head injury, brain edema, brain tumors, or cerebral hemorrhage). This type of pulmonary edema can be experimentally reproduced in laboratory animals by injecting fibrin into the fourth ventricle. It involves both hemodynamic and permeability pathways presumably from massive sympathetic stimulation and overwhelming release of catecholamines. Neurogenic pulmonary edema has sporadically been reported in animals with brain injury or severe seizures or after severe stress and excitement.

Pulmonary Embolism. With its vast vascular bed and position in the circulation, the lung acts as a safety net to catch emboli before they reach the brain and other tissues. However, this positioning is often to its own detriment. The most common pulmonary emboli in domestic animals are thromboemboli, septic (bacterial) emboli, fat emboli, and tumor cell emboli.

Pulmonary thromboembolism (PTE) refers to both local thrombus formation and translocation of a thrombus present elsewhere in the venous circulation (Fig. 9-64). Fragments released inevitably reach the lungs and become trapped in the pulmonary vasculature (Fig. 9-65 and see Fig. 9-64). Small sterile thromboemboli are generally of little clinical or pathologic significance because they can be rapidly degraded and disposed of by the fibrinolytic system. Larger thromboemboli may cause small airway constriction, reduced surfactant production, pulmonary edema, and atelectasis resulting in hypoxemia, hyperventilation, and dyspnea. Parasites (e.g., *Dirofilaria immitis* and *Angiostrongylus vasorum*), endocrinopathies (e.g., hyperadrenocorticism and hypothyroidism), glomerulopathies, and hypercoagulable states can be responsible for pulmonary arterial thrombosis and pulmonary thromboembolism in dogs (E-Fig. 9-8). Pieces of

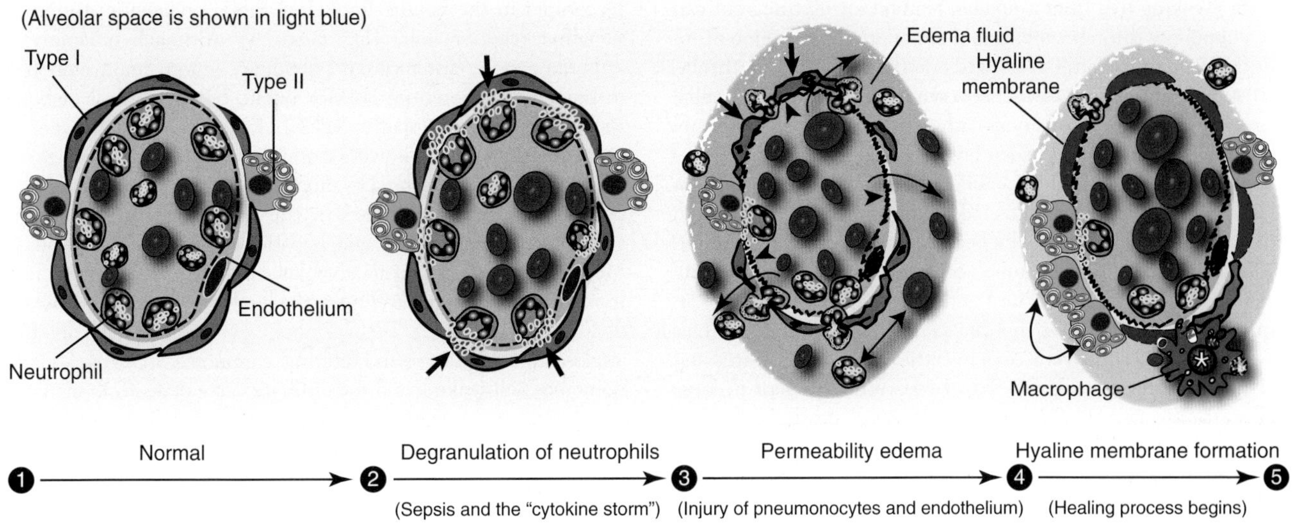

Figure 9-63 Cellular Events Leading to Acute Respiratory Distress Syndrome (ARDS) (Also See Fig. 9-104**).** *1,* Normal alveolar capillary externally covered by type I and type II pneumonocytes and internally by vascular endothelium (see Fig. 9-14 for more detail). *2,* At the early stages of sepsis, proinflammatory cytokines (interleukin 1 [IL-1] and tumor necrosis factor [TNF]) cause circulating neutrophils to adhere to the endothelial surface. Following a "cytokine storm," the marginated neutrophils further activated by inflammatory mediators suddenly release their cytoplasmic granules (proteolytic enzymes and elastases myeloperoxidase) into the surrounding milieu *(arrows)*. *3,* Enzymes released by these neutrophils cause injury to type I pneumonocytes *(arrows)* and endothelial cells *(arrowheads)*, disrupting the blood-air barrier and causing permeability edema *(curved arrows)*, alveolar hemorrhage *(double-headed arrow)*, and exocytosis of neutrophils into the alveolar space *(double-headed arrow)*. *4,* Extravasated plasma proteins admixed with surfactant and cell debris form thick hyaline membranes along the alveolar wall. *5,* In the unlikely event that the animal survives, the healing process starts with alveolar macrophages removing cellular debris, reabsorption of edema, and hyperplasia of type II pneumonocytes *(double-headed curved arrow)* that subsequently differentiate into type I pneumonocytes (see Fig. 9-14). (Courtesy Dr. A. López, Atlantic Veterinary College.)

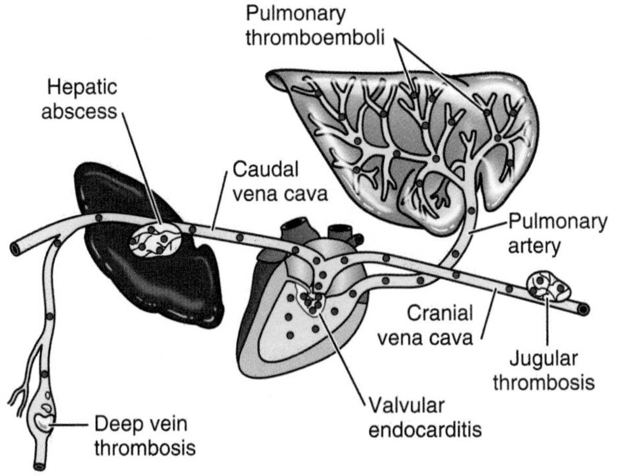

Figure 9-64 Sources of Pulmonary Emboli. Schematic diagram of pulmonary emboli *(red dots)* arising from (1) rupture of a hepatic abscess into the caudal vena cava, (2) vegetative valvular endocarditis (tricuspid valve), (3) jugular thrombosis, and (4) deep vein thrombosis. Pulmonary infarcts are rare and often of little clinical significance because of the lung's dual arterial circulation (i.e., pulmonary and bronchial arteries). (Redrawn with permission from Dr. A. López, Atlantic Veterinary College.)

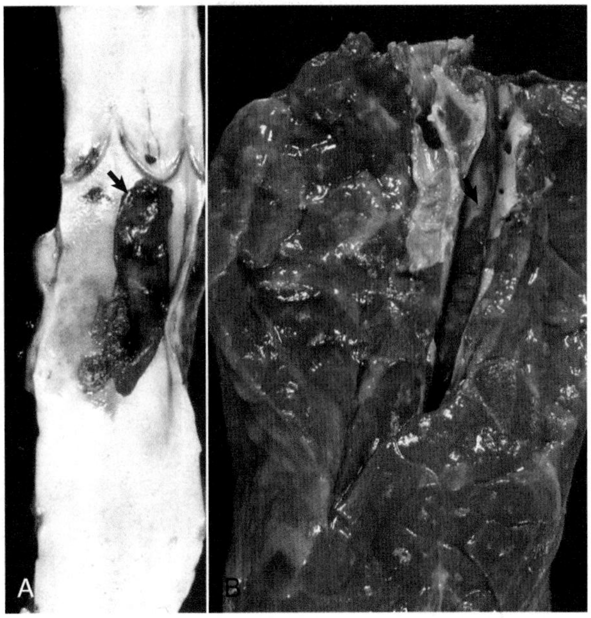

Figure 9-65 Jugular Thrombophlebitis and Pulmonary Thromboembolism, Jugular Vein and Lung, Cut Surface, Cow. A, The jugular vein has a large thrombus *(arrow)* attached to the wall at the site of prolonged catheterization. **B,** The pulmonary artery contains a large thrombus *(arrow)*, presumably a thromboembolus that has broken off the jugular mural thrombus. Note that the pulmonary thromboembolus is not attached to the wall of the pulmonary artery. (Courtesy Dr. A. López, Atlantic Veterinary College.)

thrombi breaking free from a jugular, femoral, or uterine vein can cause pulmonary thromboembolism. Pulmonary thromboembolisms occur in heavy horses after prolonged anesthesia (deep vein thrombosis), recumbent cows ("downer cow syndrome"), or in any animal undergoing long-term intravenous catheterization in which thrombi build up in the catheter and then break off (see Fig. 9-65).

Septic emboli, pieces of thrombi contaminated with bacteria or fungi and broken free from infected mural or valvular thrombi in the heart and vessels, eventually become entrapped in the pulmonary circulation. Pulmonary emboli originate most commonly from bacterial endocarditis (right side) and jugular thrombophlebitis in all species, hepatic abscesses that have eroded and discharged their contents into the caudal vena cava in cattle, and septic arthritis and omphalitis in farm animals (see Fig. 9-64). When present in large numbers, septic emboli may cause unexpected death because of massive pulmonary edema; survivors generally develop pulmonary arteritis and thrombosis and embolic (suppurative) pneumonia, which may lead to pulmonary abscesses.

Bone marrow and bone emboli can form after bone fractures or surgical interventions of bone. These are not as significant a problem in domestic animals as they are in human beings. Brain emboli (i.e., pieces of brain tissue) in the pulmonary vasculature reported in severe cases of head injury in human beings have recently been recognized in the bovine lung after strong pneumatic stunning at slaughter (captive bolt) (Fig. 9-66, *A*). Although obviously not important as an antemortem pulmonary lesion, brain emboli are intriguing as a potential risk for public health control of bovine spongiform encephalopathy (BSE). Fragments of hair can also embolize to the lung following intravenous injections (see Fig. 9-66, *B*). Hepatic emboli formed by circulating pieces of fragmented liver occasionally become trapped in the pulmonary vasculature after severe abdominal trauma and hepatic rupture (see Fig. 9-66, *C*). Megakaryocytes trapped in alveolar capillaries are a common but incidental microscopic finding in the lungs of all species, particularly dogs (see Fig. 9-66, *D*). Tumor emboli (e.g., osteosarcoma and hemangiosarcoma in dogs and uterine carcinoma in cattle) can be numerous and striking and the ultimate cause of death in malignant neoplasia. In experimental studies, cytokines released during pulmonary inflammation are chemotactic for tumor cells and promote pulmonary metastasis.

Pulmonary Infarcts. Because of a dual arterial supply to the lung, pulmonary infarction is rare and generally asymptomatic. However, pulmonary infarcts can be readily caused when pulmonary thrombosis and embolism are superimposed on an already compromised pulmonary circulation such as occurs in congestive heart

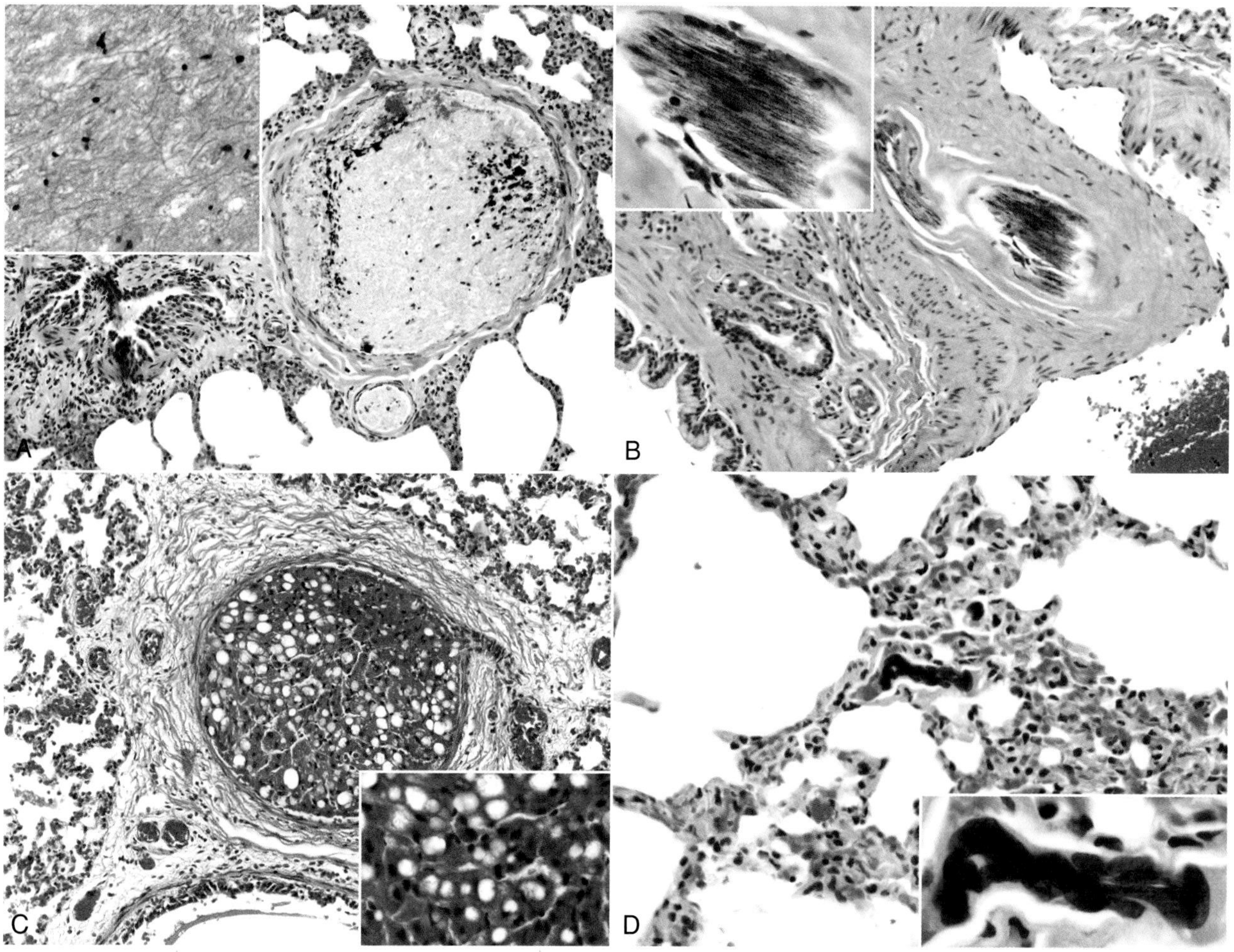

Figure 9-66 **Types of Pulmonary Emboli, Microscopic Appearance, Lung. A,** Brain embolism to the lung that resulted from severe head trauma. *Inset*, Note brain neuropil. H&E stain. **B,** Hair embolism to the lung (incidental finding) that resulted from an intravenous injection. *Inset*, Note pigmented hair shaft lodged in pulmonary vessel. H&E stain. **C,** Liver embolism to the lung that resulted from severe abdominal trauma caused by forced obstetric extraction of a foal. *Inset*, Vacuolated hepatocytes. H&E stain. **D,** Megakaryocyte lodged in alveolar capillary. *Inset*, Higher magnification of the megakaryocyte. This is a common incidental finding in the lungs of animals, particularly dogs. H&E stain. (Courtesy of Dr. A. López, Atlantic Veterinary College.)

failure. It also occurs in dogs with torsion of a lung lobe (Fig. 9-67). The gross features of infarcts vary considerably, depending on the stage, and they can be red to black, swollen, firm, and cone or wedge shaped, particularly at the lung margins. In the early acute stage, microscopic lesions are severely hemorrhagic, and this is followed by necrosis. In 1 or 2 days, a border of inflammatory cells develops, and a few days later, a large number of siderophages are present in the necrotic lung. If sterile, pulmonary infarcts heal as fibrotic scars; if septic, an abscess may form surrounded by a thick fibrous capsule.

General Aspects of Lung Inflammation

In the past three decades, an information explosion has increased the overall understanding of pulmonary inflammation, with so many proinflammatory and antiinflammatory mediators described to date that it would be impossible to review them all here (see Chapters 3 and 5).

Pulmonary inflammation is a highly regulated process that involves a complex interaction between cells imported from the blood (platelets, neutrophils, eosinophils, mast cells, and lymphocytes) and pulmonary cells (type I and II pneumonocytes; endothelial and Club [Clara] cells; alveolar and intravascular macrophages; and stromal interstitial cells, such as mast cells, interstitial macrophages, fibroblasts, and myofibroblasts). Blood-borne leukocytes, platelets, and plasma proteins are brought into the areas of inflammation by an elaborate network of chemical signals emitted by pulmonary cells and resident leukocytes. Long-distance communication between pulmonary cells and blood cells is largely done by soluble cytokines; once in the lung, imported leukocytes communicate with pulmonary and vascular cells through adhesion and other inflammatory molecules. The best known inflammatory mediators are the complement system (C3a, C3b, and C5a), coagulation factors (factors V and VII), arachidonic acid metabolites (leukotrienes and prostaglandins), cytokines (interleukins, monokines, and chemokines), adhesion molecules (ICAM and VCAM), neuropeptides (substance P, tachykinins, and neurokinins), enzymes and enzyme inhibitors (elastase and antitrypsin), oxygen metabolites (O_2•, OH•, and H_2O_2), antioxidants (glutathione), and nitric oxide (E-Table 9-1). Acting in concert, these and many other molecules send positive or negative signals to initiate, maintain, and, it is hoped, resolve the inflammatory process without causing injury to the lung.

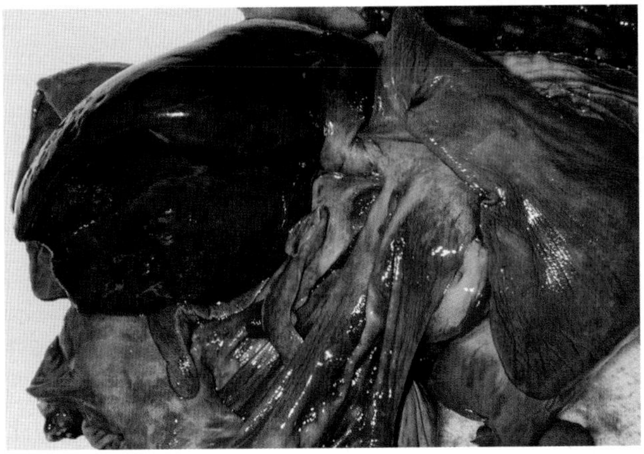

Figure 9-67 Lobe Torsion, Middle Lobe, Lung, Dog. The right middle lung lobe *(dark red)* is markedly congested and hemorrhagic from complete torsion. Although the right middle lobe is most frequently affected, other lobes can also rotate and undergo torsion. (Courtesy Dr. R. Fredrickson, College of Veterinary Medicine, University of Illinois.)

Pulmonary macrophages (alveolar, intravascular, and interstitial), which have an immense biologic armamentarium, are the single most important effector cell and source of cytokines for all stages of pulmonary inflammation. These all-purpose phagocytic cells modulate the recruitment and trafficking of blood-borne leukocytes in the lung through the secretion of chemokines (see E-Table 9-1).

Before reviewing how inflammatory cells are recruited in the lungs, three significant features in pulmonary injury must be remembered: (1) Leukocytes can exit the vascular system through the alveolar capillaries, unlike in other tissues, where postcapillary venules are the sites of leukocytic diapedesis (extravasation); (2) the intact lung contains within alveolar capillaries a large pool of resident leukocytes (marginated pool); and (3) additional neutrophils are sequestered within alveolar capillaries within minutes of a local or systemic inflammatory response. These three pulmonary idiosyncrasies, along with the enormous length of the capillary network in the lung, explain why recruitment and migration of leukocytes into alveolar spaces develops so rapidly. Experimental studies with aerosols of endotoxin or Gram-negative bacteria have shown that within minutes of exposure, there is a significant increase in capillary leukocytes, and by 4 hours the alveolar lumen is filled with neutrophils. Not surprisingly, the BAL fluid collected from patients with acute pneumonia contains large amounts of inflammatory mediators such as TNF-α, IL-1, and IL-8. Also, the capillary endothelium of patients with acute pneumonia has increased "expression" of adhesion molecules, which facilitate the migration of leukocytes from capillaries into the alveolar interstitium and from there into the alveolar lumen. In allergic pulmonary diseases, eotaxin and IL-5 are primarily responsible for recruitment and trafficking of eosinophils in the lung.

Movement of plasma proteins into the pulmonary interstitium and alveolar lumen is a common but poorly understood phenomenon in pulmonary inflammation. Leakage of fibrinogen and plasma proteins into the alveolar space occurs when there is structural damage to the blood-air barrier. This leakage is also promoted by some types of cytokines that enhance procoagulant activity, whereas others reduce fibrinolytic activity. Excessive exudation of fibrin into the alveoli is particularly common in ruminants and pigs. The fibrinolytic system plays a major role in the resolution of pulmonary inflammatory diseases. In some cases, excessive plasma proteins leaked into alveoli mix with necrotic type I pneumonocytes and pulmonary surfactant, forming microscopic eosinophilic bands (membranes) along the lining of alveolar septa. These membranes, known as *hyaline membranes*, are found in specific types of pulmonary diseases, particularly in ARDS, and in cattle with acute interstitial pneumonias such as bovine pulmonary edema and emphysema and extrinsic allergic alveolitis (see Pneumonias of Cattle).

In the past few years, nitric oxide has been identified as a major regulatory molecule of inflammation in a variety of tissues, including the lung. Produced locally by macrophages, pulmonary endothelium, and pneumonocytes, nitric oxide regulates the vascular and bronchial tone, modulates the production of cytokines, controls the recruitment and trafficking of neutrophils in the lung, and switches on/off genes involved in inflammation and immunity. Experimental work has also shown that pulmonary surfactant upregulates the production of nitric oxide in the lung, supporting the current view that pneumonocytes are also pivotal in amplifying and downregulating the inflammatory and immune responses in the lung (see E-Table 9-1).

As the inflammatory process becomes chronic, the types of cells making up cellular infiltrates in the lung change from mainly neutrophils to largely mononuclear cells. This shift in cellular composition is accompanied by an increase in specific cytokines, such as

IL-4, interferon-γ (IFN-γ), and interferon-inducible protein (IP-10), which are chemotactic for lymphocytes and macrophages. Under appropriate conditions, these cytokines activate T lymphocytes, regulate granulomatous inflammation, and induce the formation of multinucleated giant cells such as in mycobacterial infections.

Inflammatory mediators locally released from inflamed lungs also have a biologic effect in other tissue. For example, pulmonary hypertension and right-sided heart failure (cor pulmonale) often follows chronic alveolar inflammation, not only as a result of increased pulmonary blood pressure but also from the effect of inflammatory mediators on the contractibility of smooth muscle of the pulmonary and systemic vasculature. Cytokines, particularly TNF-α, that are released during inflammation are associated, both as cause and as effect, with the systemic inflammatory response syndrome (SIRS), sepsis, severe sepsis with multiple organ dysfunction, and septic shock (cardiopulmonary collapse).

As it occurs in any other sentinel system where many biologic promoters and inhibitors are involved (coagulation, the complement and immune systems), the inflammatory cascade could go into an "out-of-control" state, causing severe damage to the lungs. Acute lung injury (ALI), extrinsic allergic alveolitis, ARDS, pulmonary fibrosis, and asthma are archetypical diseases that ensue from an uncontrolled production and release of cytokines (cytokine storm).

As long as acute alveolar injury is transient and there is no interference with the normal host response, the entire process of injury, degeneration, necrosis, inflammation, and repair can occur in less than 10 days. On the other hand, when acute alveolar injury becomes persistent or when the capacity of the host for repair is impaired, lesions can progress to an irreversible stage in which restoration of alveolar structure is no longer possible. In diseases, such as extrinsic allergic alveolitis, the constant release of proteolytic enzymes and free radicals by phagocytic cells perpetuates alveolar damage in a vicious circle. In other cases, such as in paraquat toxicity, the magnitude of alveolar injury can be so severe that type II pneumonocytes, basement membranes, and alveolar interstitium are so disrupted that the capacity for alveolar repair is lost. Fibronectins and transforming growth factors (TGFs) released from macrophages and other mononuclear cells at the site of chronic inflammation regulate the recruitment, attachment, and proliferation of fibroblasts. In turn, these cells synthesize and release considerable amounts of ECM (collagen, elastic fibers, or proteoglycans), eventually leading to fibrosis and total obliteration of normal alveolar architecture. In summary, in diseases in which there is chronic and irreversible alveolar damage, lesions invariably progress to a stage of terminal alveolar and interstitial fibrosis.

Species-Specific Disorders of the Lung (Bronchi, Bronchioles, and Alveoli) in Domestic Animals

For pneumonia, see section Species-Specific Pneumonia of Domestic Animals.

Disorders of Horses

Circulatory Disturbances

Exercise-Induced Pulmonary Hemorrhage. *Exercise-induced pulmonary hemorrhage* (*EIPH*) is a specific form of pulmonary hemorrhage in racehorses that occurs after exercise and clinically is characterized by epistaxis. Because only a small percentage of horses with bronchoscopic evidence of hemorrhage have clinical epistaxis, it is likely that EIPH goes undetected in many cases. The pathogenesis is still controversial, but current literature suggests laryngeal paralysis, bronchiolitis, and extremely high pulmonary vascular and alveolar pressures during exercise, alveolar hypoxia, and preexisting pulmonary injury as possible causes. EIPH is seldom fatal; postmortem lesions in the lungs of horses that have been affected with several episodes of hemorrhage are characterized by large areas of dark brown discoloration, largely in the caudal lung lobes. Microscopically, lesions are alveolar hemorrhages, abundant alveolar macrophages containing hemosiderin (siderophages), mild alveolar fibrosis, and occlusive remodeling of pulmonary veins.

Inflammation with Mucosal Injury in the Lung

Recurrent Airway Obstruction. Recurrent airway obstruction (RAO) of horses, also referred to as COPD, heaves, chronic bronchiolitis-emphysema complex, chronic small airway disease, alveolar emphysema, and "broken wind," is a common clinically asthma-like syndrome of horses and ponies. RAO is characterized by recurrent respiratory distress, chronic cough, poor athletic performance, airway neutrophilia, bronchoconstriction, mucus hypersecretion, and airway obstruction. The pathogenesis is still obscure, but genetic predisposition, T_H2 (allergic) immune response, and the exceptional sensitivity of airways to environmental allergens (hyperreactive airway disease) have been postulated as the basic underlying mechanisms. What makes small airways hyperreactive to allergens is still a matter of controversy. Epidemiologic and experimental studies suggest that it could be the result of preceding bronchiolar damage caused by viral infections; ingestion of pneumotoxicants (3-methylindole); or prolonged exposure to organic dust, endotoxin, and environmental allergens (molds). It has been postulated that sustained inhalation of dust particles, whether antigenic or not, upregulates the production of cytokines (TNF-α, IL-8, and monokine-inducible protein [MIP-2]) and neuropeptides (neurokinin A [NKA], neurokinin B [NKB], and substance P), attracting neutrophils into the bronchioloalveolar region and promoting leukocyte-induced bronchiolar injury. Summer pasture-associated obstructive pulmonary disease (SPAOPD) is a seasonal airway disease also reported in horses with similar clinical and pathologic findings. More recently, the term *inflammatory airway disease (IAD)* has been introduced in equine medicine to describe RAO-like syndrome in young horses 2 to 4 years old.

The lungs of horses with heaves are grossly unremarkable, except for extreme cases in which alveolar emphysema may be present. Microscopically, the lesions are often remarkable and include goblet cell metaplasia in bronchioles; plugging of bronchioles with mucus mixed with few eosinophils and neutrophils (see Fig. 9-13); peribronchiolar infiltration with lymphocytes, plasma cells, and variable numbers of eosinophils; and hypertrophy of smooth muscle in bronchi and bronchioles. In severe cases, accumulation of mucus leads to the complete obstruction of bronchioles and alveoli and resultant alveolar emphysema characterized by enlarged "alveoli" from the destruction of alveolar walls.

Disorders of Cats

Inflammation with Mucosal Injury in the Lung

Feline Asthma Syndrome. Feline asthma syndrome, also known as *feline allergic bronchitis*, is a clinical syndrome in cats of any age characterized by recurrent episodes of bronchoconstriction, cough, or dyspnea. The pathogenesis is not well understood but is presumed to originate, as in human asthma, as a type I hypersensitivity (IgE–mast cell reaction) to inhaled allergens. Dust, cigarette smoke, plant and household materials, and parasitic proteins have been incriminated as possible allergens. This self-limited allergic disease responds well to steroid therapy; thus it is rarely implicated as a primary cause of death except when suppressed defense mechanisms allow a secondary bacterial pneumonia. Bronchial biopsies from affected cats at the early stages reveal mild to moderate inflammation characterized by mucosal edema and infiltration of leukocytes, particularly eosinophils. Increased numbers of circulating eosinophils (blood eosinophilia) are present in some but not all cats with feline asthma.

In the most advanced cases, chronic bronchoconstriction and excess mucus production may result in smooth muscle hyperplasia and obstruction of the bronchi and bronchioles and infiltration of the airway mucosa by eosinophils. A syndrome known as *canine asthma* has been reported in dogs but is not as well characterized as the feline counterpart.

Classification of Pneumonias in Domestic Animals

Few subjects in veterinary pathology have caused so much debate as the classification of pneumonias. Historically, pneumonias in animals have been classified or named based on the following:

1. Presumed cause, with names such as viral pneumonia, Pasteurella pneumonia, distemper pneumonia, verminous pneumonia, chemical pneumonia, and hypersensitivity pneumonitis
2. Type of exudation, with names such as suppurative pneumonia, fibrinous pneumonia, and pyogranulomatous pneumonia
3. Morphologic features, with names such as gangrenous pneumonia, proliferative pneumonia, and embolic pneumonia
4. Distribution of lesions, with names such as focal pneumonia, cranioventral pneumonia, diffuse pneumonia, and lobar pneumonia
5. Epidemiologic attributes, with names such as enzootic pneumonia, contagious bovine pleuropneumonia, and "shipping fever"
6. Geographic regions, with names such as Montana progressive pneumonia
7. Miscellaneous attributes, with names such as atypical pneumonia, cuffing pneumonia, progressive pneumonia, aspiration pneumonia, pneumonitis, farmer's lung, and extrinsic allergic alveolitis

Until a universal and systematic nomenclature for animal pneumonias is established, veterinarians should be acquainted with this heterogeneous list of names and should be well aware that one disease may be known by different names. In pigs, for instance, enzootic pneumonia and *Mycoplasma* pneumonia refer to the same disease caused by *Mycoplasma hyopneumoniae*.

The word *pneumonitis* has been used by some as a synonym for pneumonia; however, others have restricted this term to chronic proliferative inflammation generally involving the alveolar interstitium and with little or no evidence of exudate. In this chapter, the word *pneumonia* is used for any inflammatory lesion in the lungs, regardless of whether it is exudative or proliferative, alveolar, or interstitial.

On the basis of texture, distribution, appearance, and exudation, pneumonias can be grossly diagnosed into four morphologically distinct types: bronchopneumonia, interstitial pneumonia, embolic pneumonia, and granulomatous pneumonia. By using this classification, it is possible at the time of a necropsy to predict with some degree of certainty the likely cause (virus, bacteria, fungi, or parasites), routes of entry (aerogenous vs. hematogenous), and possible sequelae. These four morphologic types allow the clinician or pathologists to predict the most likely etiology and therefore facilitate the decision as to what samples need to be taken and which tests should be requested to the diagnostic laboratory (i.e., histopathology, bacteriology, virology, or toxicology). However, overlapping of these four types of pneumonias is possible, and sometimes two morphologic types may be present in the same lung.

The criteria used to classify pneumonias grossly into bronchopneumonia, interstitial pneumonia, embolic pneumonia, and granulomatous pneumonia are based on morphologic changes, including distribution, texture, color, and general appearance of the affected lungs (Table 9-5). Distribution of the inflammatory lesions in the lungs can be (1) cranioventral, as in most bronchopneumonias; (2) multifocal, as in embolic pneumonias; (3) diffuse, as in interstitial pneumonias; or (4) locally extensive, as in granulomatous

Table 9-5 Morphologic Types of Pneumonias in Domestic Animals

Type of Pneumonia	Portal of Entry (e.g., Pathogens)	Distribution of Lesions	Texture of Lung	Grossly Visible Exudate	Disease Example	Common Pulmonary Sequelae
Bronchopneumonia: Suppurative (lobular)	Aerogenous (bacteria)	Cranioventral consolidation	Firm	Purulent exudate in bronchi	Enzootic pneumonia	Cranioventral abscesses, adhesions, bronchiectasis
Bronchopneumonia: Fibrinous (lobar)	Aerogenous (bacteria)	Cranioventral consolidation*	Hard	Fibrin in lung and pleura	Pneumonic mannheimiosis	BALT hyperplasia, "sequestra," pleural adhesions, abscesses
Interstitial pneumonia	Aerogenous or hematogenous (virus, toxin, allergen, sepsis)	Diffuse	Elastic with rib imprints	Not visible, trapped in alveolar septa	Influenza, extrinsic allergic alveolitis, PRRS, ARDS	Edema, emphysema, type II pneumonocyte hyperplasia, alveolar fibrosis
Granulomatous pneumonia	Aerogenous or hematogenous (mycobacteria, systemic mycoses)	Multifocal	Nodular	Pyogranulomatous, caseous necrosis, calcified nodules	Tuberculosis, blastomycosis, cryptococcosis	Dissemination of infection to lymph nodes and distant organs
Embolic pneumonia	Hematogenous (septic emboli)	Multifocal	Nodular	Purulent foci surrounded by hyperemia	Vegetative endocarditis, ruptured liver abscess	Abscesses randomly distributed in all pulmonary lobes

ARDS, Acute respiratory distress syndrome; *BALT*, bronchial-associated lymphoid tissue; *PRRS*, porcine reproductive and respiratory syndrome.
*Porcine pleuropneumonia is an exception because it often involves the caudal lobes.

pneumonias (Fig. 9-68). Texture of pneumonic lungs can be firmer or harder (bronchopneumonias), more elastic (rubbery) than normal lungs (interstitial pneumonias), or have a nodular feeling (granulomatous pneumonias). Describing in words the palpable difference between the texture of a normal lung compared with the firm or hard texture of a consolidated lung can be a difficult undertaking. An analogy illustrating this difference based on touching the parts of the face with the tip of your finger has been advocated by some pathologists. The texture of a normal lung is comparable to the texture of the center of the cheek. Firm consolidation is comparable to the texture of the tip of the nose, and hard consolidation is comparable to the texture of the forehead. The term *consolidation* is frequently used to describe a firm or hard lung filled with exudate.

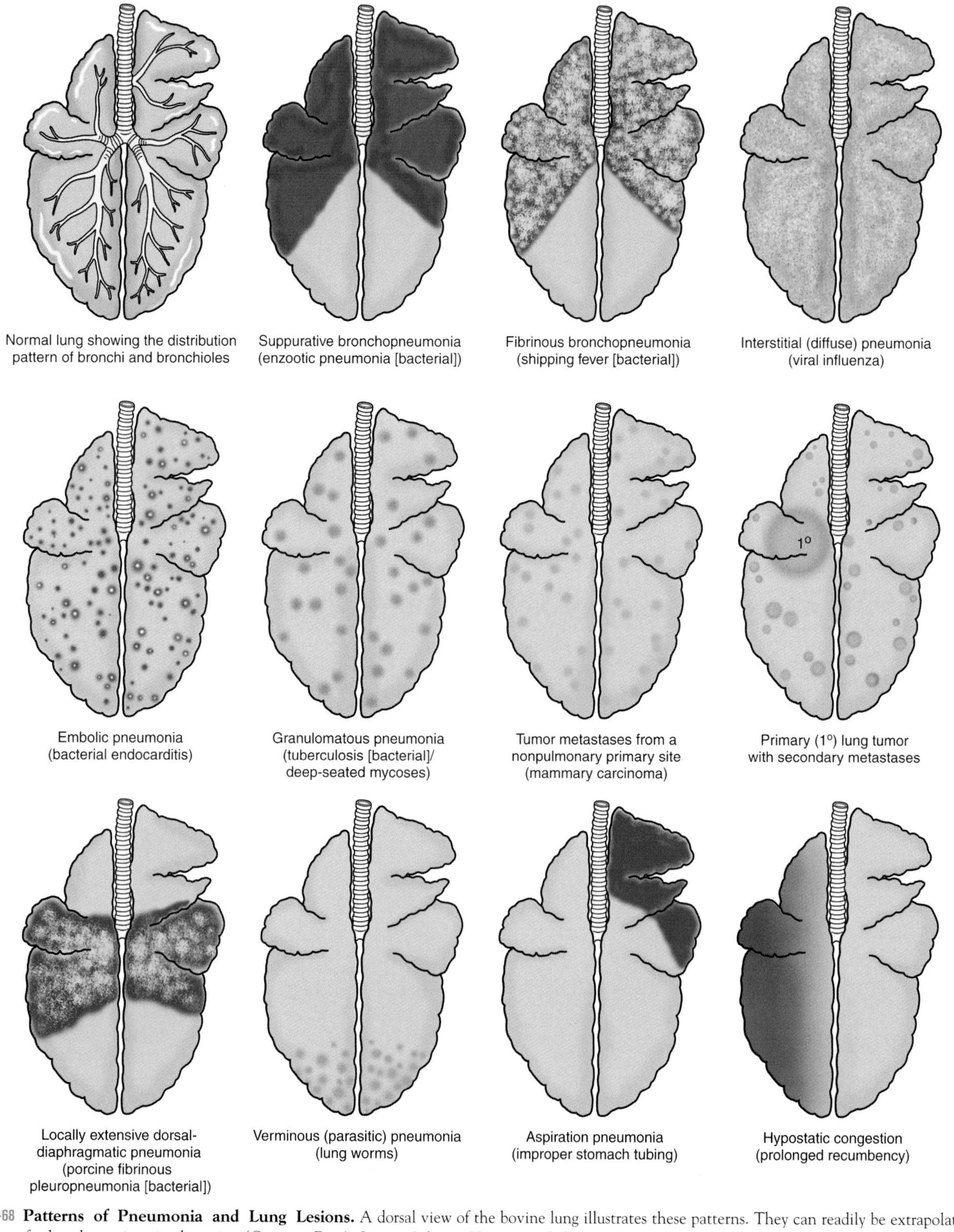

Figure 9-68 **Patterns of Pneumonia and Lung Lesions.** A dorsal view of the bovine lung illustrates these patterns. They can readily be extrapolated to the lungs of other domestic animal species. (Courtesy Dr. A. López, Atlantic Veterinary College and Dr. J.F. Zachary, College of Veterinary Medicine, University of Illinois.)

Changes in the gross appearance of pneumonic lungs include abnormal color, the presence of nodules or exudate, fibrinous or fibrous adhesions, and the presence of rib imprints on serosal surfaces (see Fig. 9-68). On cut surfaces, pneumonic lungs may have exudate, hemorrhage, edema, necrosis, abscesses, bronchiectasis, granulomas or pyogranulomas, and fibrosis, depending on the stage.

Palpation and careful observation of the lungs are essential in the diagnosis of pneumonia. (For details, see the section on Examination of the Respiratory Tract.)

Bronchopneumonia

Bronchopneumonia refers to a particular morphologic type of pneumonia in which injury and the inflammatory process take place primarily in the bronchial, bronchiolar, and alveolar lumens. Bronchopneumonia is undoubtedly the most common type of pneumonia seen in domestic animals and is with few exceptions characterized grossly by cranioventral consolidation of the lungs (Fig. 9-69 and see Fig. 9-68). The reason why bronchopneumonias in animals are almost always restricted to the cranioventral portions of the lungs is not well understood. Possible factors contributing to this topographic selectivity within the lungs include (1) gravitational sedimentation of the exudate, (2) greater deposition of infectious organisms, (3) inadequate defense mechanisms, (4) reduced vascular perfusion, (5) shortness and abrupt branching of airways, and (6) regional differences in ventilation.

The term *cranioventral* in veterinary anatomy is the equivalent of "anterosuperior" in human anatomy. The latter is defined as "in front (ventral) and above (cranial)." Thus, applied to the lung of animals, "cranioventral" means the ventral portion of the cranial lobe. However, by common usage in veterinary pathology, the term *cranioventral* used to describe the location of lesions in pneumonias has come to mean "cranial and ventral." Thus it includes pneumonias affecting not only the ventral portion of the cranial lobe (true cranioventral) but also those cases in which the pneumonia has involved the ventral portions of adjacent lung lobes—initially the middle and then caudal on the right and the caudal lobe on the left side.

Bronchopneumonias are generally caused by bacteria and mycoplasmas, by bronchoaspiration of feed or gastric contents, or by improper tubing. As a rule, the pathogens causing bronchopneumonias arrive in the lungs via inspired air (aerogenous), either from infected aerosols or from the nasal flora. Before establishing infection, pathogens must overwhelm or evade the pulmonary defense mechanisms. The initial injury in bronchopneumonias is centered on the mucosa of bronchioles; from there, the inflammatory process can spread downward to distal portions of the alveoli and upward to the bronchi. Typically, for bronchopneumonias, the inflammatory exudates collect in the bronchial, bronchiolar, and alveolar lumina leaving the alveolar interstitium relatively unchanged, except for hyperemia and possibly edema. Through the pores of Kohn, the exudate can spread to adjacent alveoli until most or all of the alveoli in an individual lobule are involved. If the inflammatory process cannot control the inciting cause of injury, the lesions spread rapidly from lobule to lobule through alveolar pores and destroyed alveolar walls until an entire lobe or large portion of a lung is involved. The lesion tends to spread centrifugally, with the older lesions in the center, and exudate can be coughed up and then aspirated into other lobules, where the inflammatory process starts again.

At the early stages of bronchopneumonia, the pulmonary vessels are engorged with blood (active hyperemia), and the bronchi, bronchioles, and alveoli contain some fluid (permeability edema). In cases in which pulmonary injury is mild to moderate, cytokines locally released in the lung cause rapid recruitment of neutrophils and alveolar macrophages into bronchioles and alveoli (Fig. 9-70 and see Fig. 9-69). When pulmonary injury is much more severe, proinflammatory cytokines induce more pronounced vascular changes by further opening endothelial gaps, thus increasing vascular permeability resulting in leakage of plasma fibrinogen (fibrinous exudates) and sometimes hemorrhage in the alveoli. Alterations in permeability can be further exacerbated by structural damage to pulmonary capillaries and vessels directly caused by microbial toxins. Filling of alveoli, bronchioles, and small bronchi with inflammatory exudate progressively obliterates airspaces, and as a consequence of this process, portions of severely affected (consolidated) lungs sink to the bottom of the container when placed in fixative. The replacement of air by exudate also changes the texture of the lungs, and depending on the severity of bronchopneumonia, the texture varies from firmer to harder than normal.

The term *consolidation* is used at gross examination when the texture of pneumonic lung becomes firmer or harder than normal as a result of loss of airspaces because of exudation and atelectasis. (For details, see the discussion of lung texture in the section on Classification of Pneumonias in Domestic Animals). Inflammatory consolidation of the lungs has been referred to in the past as *hepatization* because the affected lung had the appearance and texture of liver. The process was referred to as *red hepatization* in acute cases in which

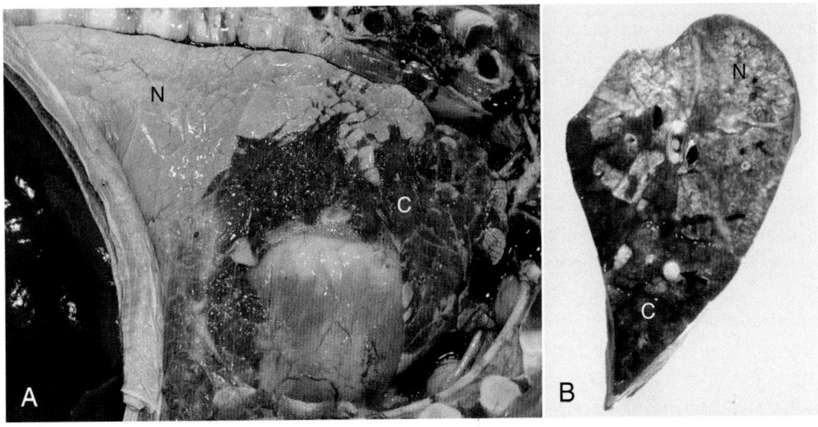

Figure 9-69 Suppurative Bronchopneumonia, Enzootic Pneumonia, Lung, Calf. A, Cranioventral consolidation *(C)* of the lung involves approximately 40% of the pulmonary parenchyma. Most of the caudal lung is normal *(N)*. **B,** Cut surface. Consolidated lung is dark red to mahogany *(C)*, and a major bronchus contains purulent exudate *(arrow)*. *N*, Normal. (**A** courtesy Dr. A. López, Atlantic Veterinary College. **B** courtesy Ontario Veterinary College.)

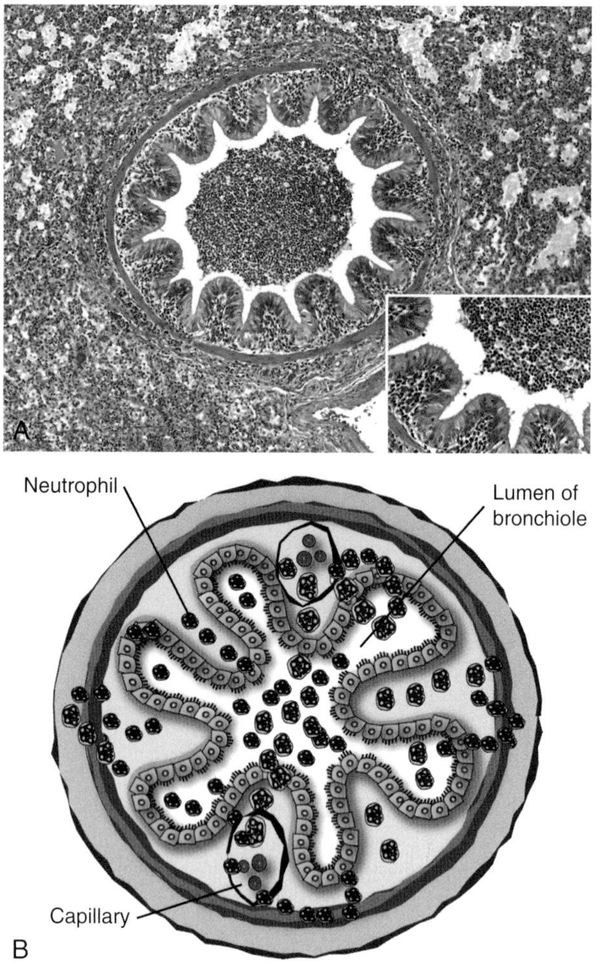

Figure 9-70 **Suppurative Bronchopneumonia, Lung, Pig. A,** Note the bronchiole in the center of the figure plugged with purulent exudate. The adjacent alveoli are filled with leukocytes and edema fluid. *Inset,* Higher magnification of wall of bronchiole. H&E stain. **B,** Schematic diagram of acute bronchiolitis. Note the neutrophils exiting the submucosal capillaries (leukocyte adhesion cascade; see Chapter 3) and moving into the walls of the bronchioles (blue cells = ciliated mucosal epithelium) and then into the bronchiolar lumen. (Courtesy Dr. A. López, Atlantic Veterinary College.)

there was notable active hyperemia with little exudation of neutrophils; conversely, the process was referred to as *gray hepatization* in those chronic cases in which hyperemia was no longer present, but there was abundant exudation of neutrophils and macrophages. This terminology, although used for and applicable to human pneumonias, is rarely used in veterinary medicine primarily because the evolution of pneumonic processes in animals does not necessarily follow the red-to-gray hepatization pattern.

Bronchopneumonia can be subdivided into *suppurative bronchopneumonia* if the exudates are predominantly composed of neutrophils and *fibrinous bronchopneumonia* if fibrin is the predominant component of the exudates (see Table 9-5). It is important to note that some veterinarians use the term *fibrinous pneumonia* or *lobar pneumonia* as a synonym for fibrinous bronchopneumonia, and *bronchopneumonia* or *lobular pneumonia* as a synonym for suppurative bronchopneumonia. Human pneumonias for many years have been classified based on their etiology and morphology, which explains why pneumococcal pneumonia (*Streptococcus pneumoniae*) has been synonymous with lobar pneumonia. In the old literature, four distinct stages of pneumococcal pneumonia were described as (1) congestion, (2) red hepatization (liver texture), (3) gray hepatization, and (4) resolution. Because of the use of effective antibiotics and prevention, pneumococcal pneumonia and its four classic stages are rarely seen; thus this terminology has been largely abandoned. Currently, the term *bronchopneumonia* is widely used for both suppurative and fibrinous consolidation of the lungs because both forms of inflammation have essentially the same pathogenesis in which the pathogens reach the lung by the aerogenous route, injury occurs initially in the bronchial and bronchiolar regions, and the inflammatory process extends centrifugally deep into the alveoli. It must be emphasized that it is the severity of pulmonary injury that largely determines whether bronchopneumonia becomes suppurative or fibrinous. In some instances, however, it is difficult to discriminate between suppurative and fibrinous bronchopneumonia because both types can coexist (fibrinosuppurative bronchopneumonia), and one type can progress to the other.

Suppurative Bronchopneumonia. Suppurative bronchopneumonia is characterized by cranioventral consolidation of lungs (see Figs. 9-68 and 9-69), with typically purulent or mucopurulent exudate present in the airways. This exudate can be best demonstrated by expressing intrapulmonary bronchi, thus forcing exudate out of the bronchi (see Fig. 9-69). The inflammatory process in suppurative bronchopneumonia is generally confined to individual lobules, and as a result of this distribution, the lobular pattern of the lung becomes notably emphasized. This pattern is particularly obvious in cattle and pigs because these species have prominent lobulation of the lungs. The gross appearance often resembles an irregular checkerboard because of an admixture of normal and abnormal (consolidated) lobules (see Fig. 9-69). Because of this typical lobular distribution, suppurative bronchopneumonias are also referred to as lobular pneumonias.

Different inflammatory phases occur in suppurative bronchopneumonia where the color and appearance of consolidated lungs varies considerably, depending on the virulence of offending organisms and chronicity of the lesion. The typical phases of suppurative bronchopneumonia can be summarized as follows:

1. During the first 12 hours when bacteria are rapidly multiplying, the lungs become hyperemic and edematous.
2. Soon after, neutrophils start filling the airways, and by 48 hours the parenchyma starts to consolidate and becomes firm in texture.
3. Three to 5 days later, hyperemic changes are less obvious, but the bronchial, bronchiolar, and alveolar spaces continue to fill with neutrophils and macrophages, and the affected lung sinks when placed in formalin. At this stage, the affected lung has a gray-pink color, and on cut surface, purulent exudate can be expressed from bronchi.
4. In favorable conditions where the infection is under control of the host defense mechanisms, the inflammatory processes begin to regress, a phase known as *resolution*. Complete resolution in favorable conditions could take 1 to 2 weeks.
5. In animals in which the lung infection cannot be rapidly contained, inflammatory lesions can progress into a chronic phase. Approximately 7 to 10 days after infection, the lungs become pale gray and take a "fish flesh" appearance. This appearance is the result of purulent and catarrhal inflammation, obstructive atelectasis, mononuclear cell infiltration, peribronchial and peribronchiolar lymphoid hyperplasia, and early alveolar fibrosis.

Complete resolution is unusual in chronic bronchopneumonia, and lung scars, such as pleural and pulmonary fibrosis; bronchiectasis as a consequence of chronic destructive bronchitis (see bronchiectasis [Dysfunction/Responses to Injury and Patterns of Injury]); atelectasis; pleural adhesions; and lung abscesses may remain unresolved for a long time. "Enzootic pneumonias" of ruminants and pigs are typical examples of chronic suppurative bronchopneumonias.

Microscopically, acute suppurative bronchopneumonias are characterized by hyperemia, abundant neutrophils, macrophages, and cellular debris within the lumen of bronchi, bronchioles, and alveoli (see Fig. 9-70). Recruitment of leukocytes is promoted by cytokines, complement, and other chemotactic factors that are released in response to alveolar injury or by the chemotactic effect of bacterial toxins, particularly endotoxin. In most severe cases, purulent or mucopurulent exudates completely obliterate the entire lumen of bronchi, bronchioles, and alveoli.

If suppurative bronchopneumonia is merely the response to a transient pulmonary injury or a mild infection, lesions resolve uneventfully. Within 7 to 10 days, cellular exudate can be removed from the lungs via the mucociliary escalator, and complete resolution may take place within 4 weeks. In other cases, if injury or infection is persistent, suppurative bronchopneumonia can become chronic with goblet cell hyperplasia, an important component of the inflammatory process. Depending on the proportion of pus and mucus, the exudate in chronic suppurative bronchopneumonia varies from mucopurulent to mucoid. A mucoid exudate is found in the more chronic stages when the consolidated lung has a "fish flesh" appearance.

Hyperplasia of BALT is another change commonly seen in chronic suppurative bronchopneumonias; it appears grossly as conspicuous white nodules (cuffs) around bronchial walls (cuffing pneumonia). This hyperplastic change merely indicates a normal reaction of lymphoid tissue to infection. Further sequelae of chronic suppurative bronchopneumonia include bronchiectasis (see Figs. 9-10 and 9-11), pulmonary abscesses, pleural adhesions (from pleuritis) (Fig. 9-71), and atelectasis and emphysema from completely or partially obstructed bronchi or bronchioles (e.g., bronchiectasis).

Clinically, suppurative bronchopneumonias can be acute and fulminating but are often chronic, depending on the etiologic agent, stressors affecting the host, and immune status. The most common pathogens causing suppurative bronchopneumonia in domestic animals include *Pasteurella multocida*, *Bordetella bronchiseptica*, *Trueperella* (*Arcanobacterium*) *pyogenes*, *Streptococcus* spp., *Escherichia coli*, and several species of mycoplasmas. Most of these organisms are secondary pathogens requiring a preceding impairment of the pulmonary defense mechanisms to allow them to colonize the lungs and establish an infection. Suppurative bronchopneumonia can also result from aspiration of bland material (e.g., milk). Pulmonary gangrene may ensue when the bronchopneumonic lung is invaded by saprophytic bacteria (aspiration pneumonia).

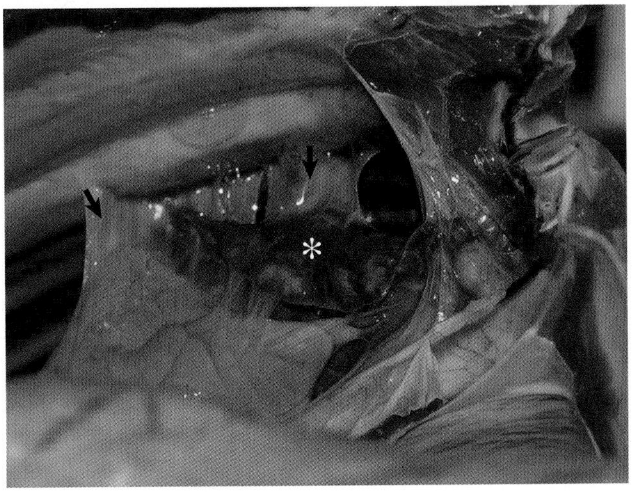

Figure 9-71 Pleural Adhesions, Chronic Bronchopneumonia, Steer. Note thick bands *(arrows)* of connective tissue between the visceral and parietal pleura. The cranial lobe *(asterisk)* appears consolidated and dark red. (Courtesy Dr. A. López, Atlantic Veterinary College.)

Fibrinous Bronchopneumonia. Fibrinous bronchopneumonia is similar to suppurative bronchopneumonia except that the predominant exudate is fibrinous rather than neutrophilic. With only a few exceptions, fibrinous bronchopneumonias also have a cranioventral distribution (Fig. 9-72 and see Fig. 9-68). However, exudation is not restricted to the boundaries of individual pulmonary lobules, as is the case in suppurative bronchopneumonias. Instead, the inflammatory process in fibrinous pneumonias involves numerous contiguous lobules and the exudate moves quickly through pulmonary tissue until the entire pulmonary lobe is rapidly affected. Because of the involvement of the entire lobe and pleural surface, fibrinous bronchopneumonias are also referred to as lobar pneumonias or pleuropneumonias. In general terms, fibrinous bronchopneumonias are the result of more severe pulmonary injury and thus cause death earlier in the sequence of the inflammatory process than suppurative bronchopneumonias. Even in cases in which fibrinous bronchopneumonia involves 30% or less of the total area, clinical signs and death can occur as a result of severe toxemia and sepsis.

The gross appearance of fibrinous bronchopneumonia depends on the age and severity of the lesion and on whether the pleural surface or the cut surface of the lung is viewed. Externally, early stages of fibrinous bronchopneumonias are characterized by severe congestion and hemorrhage, giving the affected lungs a characteristically intense red discoloration. A few hours later, fibrin starts to permeate and accumulate on the pleural surface, giving the pleura a ground glass appearance and eventually forming plaques of fibrinous exudate over a red, dark lung (see Fig. 9-72). At this stage, a yellow fluid starts to accumulate in the thoracic cavity. The color of fibrin deposited over the pleural surface is also variable. It can be bright yellow when the exudate is formed primarily by fibrin, tan when fibrin is mixed with blood, and gray when a large number of leukocytes and fibroblasts are part of the fibrinous plaque in more chronic cases. Because of the tendency of fibrin to deposit on the pleural surface, some pathologists use the term *pleuropneumonia* as a synonym for fibrinous bronchopneumonia.

On the cut surface, early stages of fibrinous bronchopneumonia appear as simple red consolidation. In more advanced cases (24 hours), fibrinous bronchopneumonia is generally accompanied by notable dilation and thrombosis of lymph vessels and edema of interlobular septa (see Fig. 9-72, *B*). This distention of the interlobular septa gives affected lungs a typical marbled appearance. Distinct focal areas of coagulative necrosis in the pulmonary parenchyma are also common in fibrinous bronchopneumonia such as in shipping fever pneumonia and contagious bovine pleuropneumonia. In animals that survive the early stage of fibrinous bronchopneumonia, pulmonary necrosis often develops into pulmonary "sequestra," which are isolated pieces of necrotic lung encapsulated by connective tissue. Pulmonary sequestra result from extensive necrosis of lung tissue either from severe ischemia (infarct) caused by thrombosis of a major pulmonary vessel such as in contagious bovine pleuropneumonia or from the effect of necrotizing toxins released by pathogenic bacteria such as *Mannheimia haemolytica*. Sequestra in veterinary pathology should not be confused with "bronchopulmonary sequestration," a term used in human pathology to describe a congenital malformation in which whole lobes or parts of the lung develop without normal connections to the airway or vascular systems.

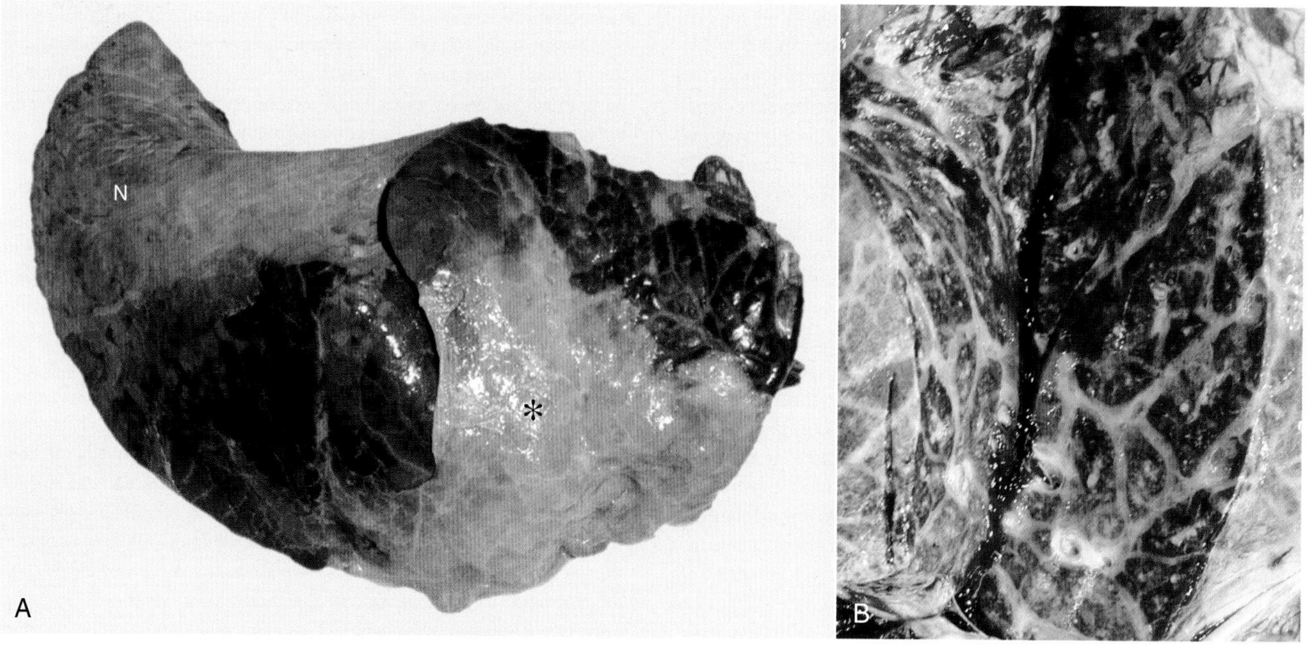

Figure 9-72 **Fibrinous Bronchopneumonia (Pleuropneumonia), Right Lung, Steer. A,** The pneumonia has a cranioventral distribution that extends into the middle and caudal lobes and affects approximately 80% of the lung parenchyma. The lung is firm, swollen, and covered with yellow fibrin *(asterisk)*. The dorsal portion of the caudal lung is normal *(N)*. **B,** Cut surface. Affected parenchyma appears dark and hyperemic compared with more normal lung *(top quarter of figure)*. Interlobular septa are prominent as yellow bands due to the accumulation of fibrin and edema fluid. This type of lesion is typical of *Mannheimia haemolytica* infection in cattle (shipping fever). (**A** courtesy Ontario Veterinary College. **B** courtesy Dr. A. López, Atlantic Veterinary College.)

Microscopically, in the initial stage of fibrinous bronchopneumonia, there is massive exudation of plasma proteins into the bronchioles and alveoli, and as a result, most of the airspaces become obliterated by fluid and fibrin. Leakage of fibrin and fluid into alveolar lumina is due to extensive disruption of the integrity and increased permeability of the blood-air barrier. Fibrinous exudates can move from alveolus to alveolus through the pores of Kohn. Because fibrin is chemotactic for neutrophils, these types of leukocytes are always present a few hours after the onset of fibrinous inflammation. As inflammation progresses (3 to 5 days), fluid exudate is gradually replaced by fibrinocellular exudates composed of fibrin, neutrophils, macrophages, and necrotic debris (Fig. 9-73). In chronic cases (after 7 days), there is notable fibrosis of the interlobular septa and pleura.

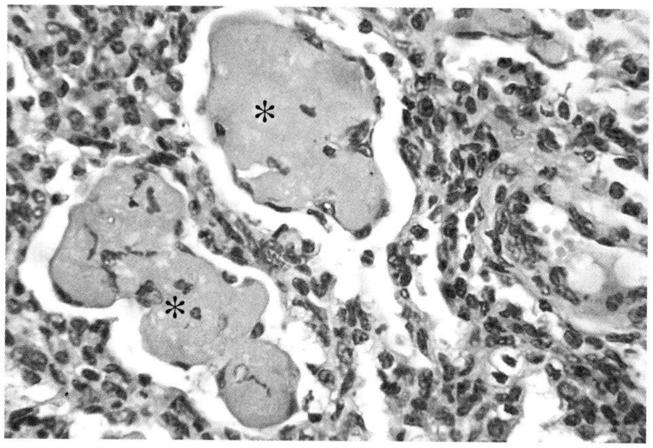

Figure 9-73 **Fibrinous Bronchopneumonia, Chronic, Lung, Calf.** Note large aggregates of condensed fibrin *(asterisks)* surrounded and infiltrated by phagocytic cells. H&E stain. (Courtesy Dr. A. López, Atlantic Veterinary College.)

In contrast to suppurative bronchopneumonia, fibrinous bronchopneumonia rarely resolves completely, thus leaving noticeable scars in the form of pulmonary fibrosis and pleural adhesions. The most common sequelae found in animals surviving an acute episode of fibrinous bronchopneumonia include alveolar fibrosis and bronchiolitis obliterans, in which organized exudate becomes attached to the bronchiolar lumen (see Fig. 9-12). These changes are collectively referred to as *bronchiolitis obliterans organizing pneumonia* (BOOP), a common microscopic finding in animals with unresolved bronchopneumonia. Other important sequelae include pulmonary gangrene, when saprophytic bacteria colonize necrotic lung; pulmonary sequestra; pulmonary fibrosis; abscesses; and chronic pleuritis with pleural adhesions. In some cases, pleuritis can be so extensive that fibrous adhesions extend onto the pericardial sac. Pathogens causing fibrinous bronchopneumonias in domestic animals include *Mannheimia* (*Pasteurella*) *haemolytica* (pneumonic mannheimiosis), *Histophilus somni* (formerly *Haemophilus somnus*), *Actinobacillus pleuropneumoniae* (porcine pleuropneumonia), *Mycoplasma bovis*, and *Mycoplasma mycoides* ssp. *mycoides* small colony type (contagious bovine pleuropneumonia). Fibrinous bronchopneumonia and pulmonary gangrene can also be the result of bronchoaspiration of irritant materials such as gastric contents.

Fulminating hemorrhagic bronchopneumonia can be caused by highly pathogenic bacteria such as *Bacillus anthracis*. Although the lesions in anthrax are primarily related to a severe septicemia and sepsis, anthrax should always be suspected in animals with sudden death and exhibiting severe acute fibrinohemorrhagic pneumonia, splenomegaly, and multisystemic hemorrhages. Animals are considered good sentinels for anthrax in cases of bioterrorism.

Interstitial Pneumonia

Interstitial pneumonia refers to that type of pneumonia in which injury and the inflammatory process take place primarily in any of the three layers of the alveolar walls (endothelium, basement membrane, and alveolar epithelium) and the contiguous bronchiolar interstitium (see Fig. 9-7). This morphologic type of pneumonia is the most difficult to diagnose at necropsy and requires microscopic confirmation because it is easily mistaken in the lung showing congestion, edema, hyperinflation, or emphysema.

In contrast to bronchopneumonias, in which distribution of lesions is generally cranioventral, in interstitial pneumonias, lesions are more diffusely distributed and generally involve all pulmonary lobes, or in some cases, they appear to be more pronounced in the dorsocaudal aspects of the lungs (see Fig. 9-68). Three important gross features of interstitial pneumonia are (1) the failure of lungs to collapse when the thoracic cavity is opened, (2) the occasional presence of rib impressions on the pleural surface of the lung indicating poor deflation, and (3) the lack of visible exudates in airways unless complicated with secondary bacterial pneumonia. The color of affected lungs varies from diffusely red in acute cases to diffusely pale gray to a mottled red, pale appearance in chronic ones. Pale lungs are caused by severe obliteration of alveolar capillaries (reduced blood-tissue ratio), especially evident when there is fibrosis of the alveolar walls. The texture of lungs with uncomplicated interstitial pneumonia is typically elastic or rubbery, but definitive diagnosis based on texture alone is difficult and requires histopathologic examination. On a cut surface, the lungs may appear and feel more "meaty" (having the texture of raw meat) and have no evidence of exudate in the bronchi or pleura (Fig. 9-74). In acute interstitial pneumonias, particularly in cattle, there is frequently pulmonary edema (exudative phase) and interstitial emphysema secondary to partial obstruction of bronchioles by edema fluid and strenuous air gasping before death. Because edema tends to gravitate into the cranioventral portions of the lungs, and emphysema is often more obvious in the dorsocaudal aspects, acute interstitial pneumonias in cattle occasionally have a gross cranioventral-like pattern that may resemble bronchopneumonia, although the texture is different. Lungs are notably heavy because of the edema and the infiltrative and proliferative changes.

The pathogenesis of interstitial pneumonia is complex and can result from aerogenous injury to the alveolar epithelium (type I and II pneumonocytes) or from hematogenous injury to the alveolar capillary endothelium or alveolar basement membrane. Aerogenous inhalation of toxic gases (i.e., ozone and NO_2) or toxic fumes (smoke inhalation) and infection with pneumotropic viruses (influenza, herpesviruses, or canine distemper virus) can damage the alveolar epithelium. Inhaled antigens, such as fungal spores, combine with circulating antibodies and form deposits of antigen-antibody complexes (type III hypersensitivity) in the alveolar wall, which initiate a cascade of inflammatory responses and injury (allergic alveolitis). Hematogenous injury to the vascular endothelium occurs in septicemias, sepsis, DIC, larva migrans (*Ascaris suum*), toxins absorbed in the alimentary tract (endotoxin) or toxic metabolites locally generated in the lungs (3-methylindole and paraquat), release of free radicals in alveolar capillaries (ARDS), and infections with endotheliotropic viruses (canine adenovirus and classical swine fever [hog cholera]).

Interstitial pneumonias in domestic animals and human beings are subdivided based on morphologic features into acute and chronic. It should be kept in mind, however, that not all acute interstitial pneumonias are fatal and that they do not necessarily progress to the chronic form.

Acute Interstitial Pneumonias. Acute interstitial pneumonias begin with injury to either type I pneumonocytes or alveolar capillary endothelium, which provokes a disruption of the blood-air barrier and a subsequent exudation of plasma proteins into the alveolar space (see Fig. 9-14). This leakage of proteinaceous fluid into the alveolar lumen constitutes the exudative phase of acute interstitial pneumonia. In some cases of diffuse alveolar damage, exuded plasma proteins mix with lipids and other components of pulmonary surfactant and form elongated membranes that become partially attached to the alveolar basement membrane and bronchiolar walls. These membranes are referred to as hyaline membranes because of their hyaline appearance (eosinophilic, homogeneous, and amorphous) microscopically (see Figs. 9-55 and 9-63). In addition to intraalveolar exudation of fluid, inflammatory edema and neutrophils accumulate in the alveolar interstitium and cause thickening of the alveolar walls. This acute exudative phase is generally followed a few days later by the proliferative phase of acute interstitial pneumonia, which is characterized by hyperplasia of type II pneumonocytes to replace the lost type I pneumonocytes (see Fig. 9-15). Type II pneumonocytes are in fact progenitor cells that differentiate and replace necrotic type I pneumonocytes (see Fig. 9-14). As a consequence, the alveolar walls become increasingly thickened. This process is in part the reason why lungs become rubbery on palpation, what prevents their normal collapse after the thorax is opened, and why the cut surface of the lung has a "meaty" appearance (see Fig. 9-74).

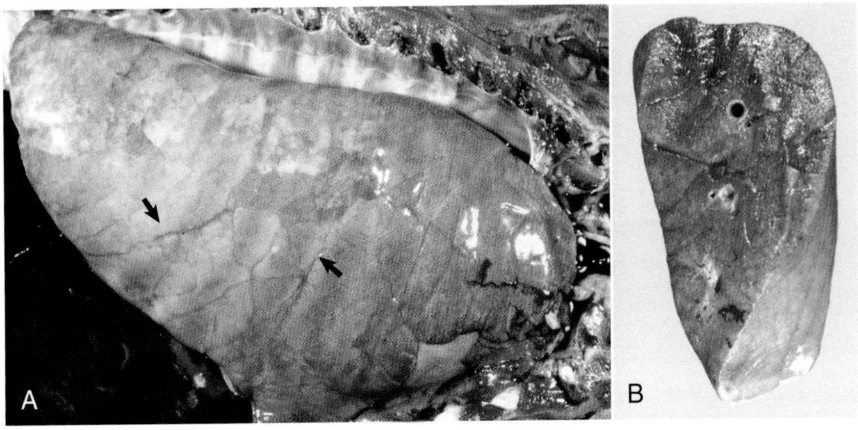

Figure 9-74 **Interstitial Pneumonia, Lung, Feeder Pig. A,** The lung is heavy, pale, and rubbery in texture. It also has prominent costal (rib) imprints (*arrows*), a result of hypercellularity of the interstitium and the failure of the lungs to collapse when the thorax was opened. **B,** Transverse section. The pulmonary parenchyma has a "meaty" appearance and some edema, but no exudate is present in airways or on the pleural surface. This type of lung change in pigs is highly suggestive of a viral pneumonia. (Courtesy Dr. A. López, Atlantic Veterinary College.)

Acute interstitial pneumonias are often mild and transient, especially those caused by some respiratory viruses, such as those responsible for equine and porcine influenza. These mild forms of pneumonia are rarely seen in the postmortem room because they are not fatal and do not leave significant sequelae (see the section on Defense Mechanisms/Barrier Systems). In severe cases of acute interstitial pneumonias, animals may die of respiratory failure, usually as a result of diffuse alveolar damage, a profuse exudative phase (leakage of proteinaceous fluid) leading to a fatal pulmonary edema. Examples of this type of fatal acute interstitial pneumonia are bovine pulmonary edema and emphysema, and ARDS in all species.

Chronic Interstitial Pneumonia. When the source of alveolar injury persists, the exudative and proliferative lesions of acute interstitial pneumonia can progress into a morphologic stage referred to as *chronic interstitial pneumonia*. The hallmark of chronic interstitial pneumonia is fibrosis of the alveolar walls (with or without intraalveolar fibrosis) and the presence of lymphocytes, macrophages, fibroblasts, and myofibroblasts in the alveolar interstitium (Figs. 9-75 and 9-76). In other cases, these chronic changes are accompanied by hyperplasia and persistence of type II pneumonocytes, squamous metaplasia of the alveolar epithelium, microscopic granulomas, and hyperplasia of smooth muscle in bronchioles and pulmonary arterioles. It should be emphasized that although the lesions in interstitial pneumonia are centered in the alveolar wall and its interstitium, a mixture of desquamated epithelial cells, macrophages, and mononuclear cells are usually present in the lumens of bronchioles and alveoli. Ovine progressive pneumonia, hypersensitivity pneumonitis in cattle and dogs, and silicosis in horses are good veterinary examples of chronic interstitial pneumonia. Pneumoconioses (silicosis and asbestosis), paraquat toxicity, pneumotoxic antineoplastic drugs (bleomycin), and extrinsic allergic alveolitis (farmer's lung) are well-known examples of diseases that lead to chronic interstitial pneumonias in human beings. Massive pulmonary migration of ascaris larvae in pigs also causes interstitial pneumonia (Fig. 9-77).

There is an insidious and poorly understood group of chronic idiopathic interstitial diseases, both in human beings and in animals, that eventually progress to terminal interstitial fibrosis. These were originally thought to be the result of repeated cycles of alveolar injury, inflammation, and fibroblastic/myoblastic response to an unknown agent. However, aggressive antiinflammatory therapy generally fails to prevent or reduce the severity of fibrosis. Now, it is

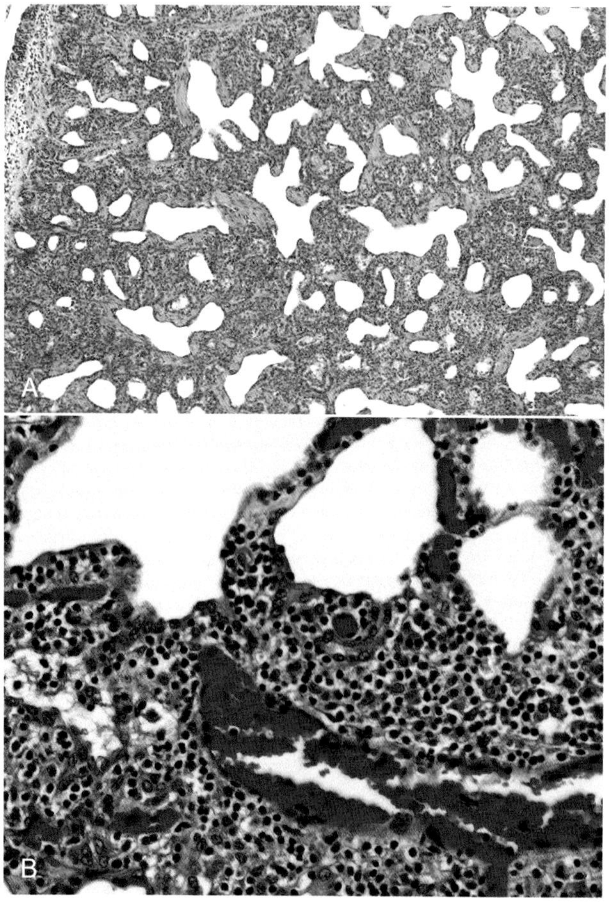

Figure 9-75 Interstitial Pneumonia, Lung, Aged Ewe. A, The alveolar septa are notably thickened by severe interstitial infiltration of inflammatory cells. H&E stain. **B,** Higher magnification of **A** showing large numbers of lymphocytes and other mononuclear cells infiltrating the alveolar septal interstitium. H&E stain. (**A** courtesy Western College of Veterinary Medicine. **B** courtesy Dr. A. López, Atlantic Veterinary College.)

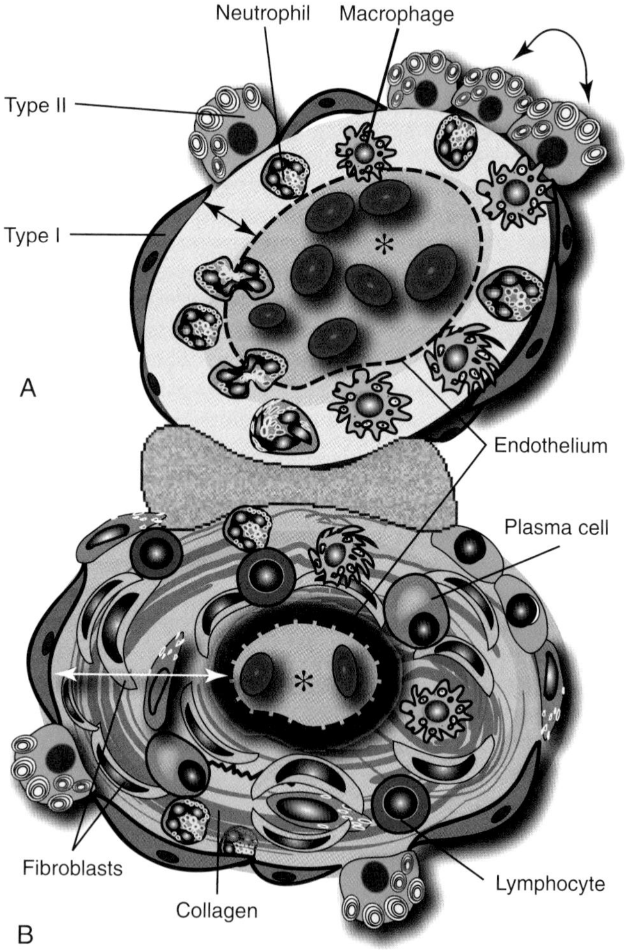

Figure 9-76 Acute and Chronic Interstitial Pneumonia. A, Acute interstitial pneumonia. Thickening of the alveolar septum caused by edema *(double-headed arrow)*, infiltration of neutrophils and macrophages, and hyperplasia of type II pneumonocytes *(double-headed curved arrow)*. Note the relative diameter of the capillary lumen *(asterisk)*. **B,** Chronic interstitial pneumonia. Thickening of the alveolar septum with notably reduced diameter of the capillary lumen *(asterisk)* caused by proliferation of connective tissue (fibroblasts, ECM, and collagen fibers) and infiltration of lymphocytes and plasma cells *(double-headed white arrow)*. In severe cases, the alveolar capillary may be totally obliterated. (Courtesy Dr. A. López, Atlantic Veterinary College.)

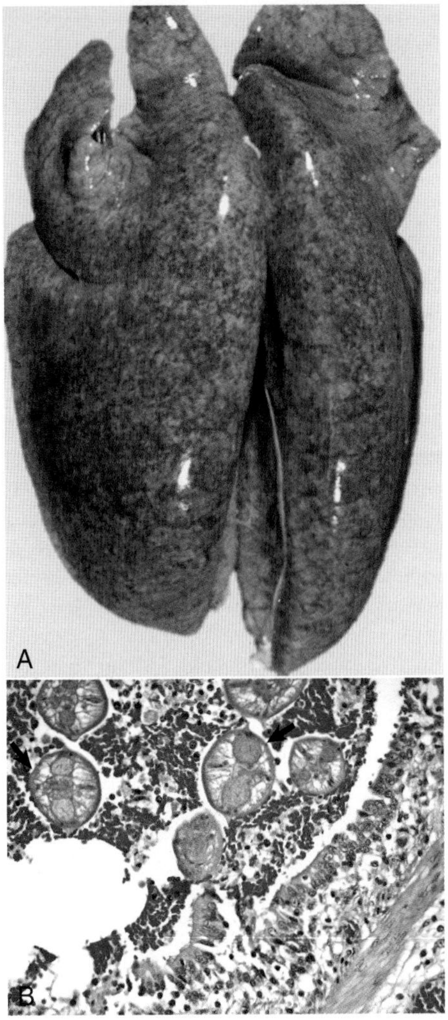

Figure 9-77 **Interstitial Pneumonia, Edema, and Hemorrhages, Lungs, *Ascaris suum* Larvae, Pig. A**, This pig had migrating *Ascaris suum* larvae. The lungs are heavy and wet and failed to collapse when the thorax was opened, as a result of pulmonary edema. The mottled appearance of the lungs is due to the presence of numerous petechiae scattered in the pulmonary parenchyma. Petechiae are likely alveolar hemorrhages caused by migrating larvae. Larvae leave the bloodstream to enter the alveoli by penetrating and rupturing alveolar capillaries and thus damage the air-blood barrier of alveolar septa. **B**, Multiple ascarid larvae *(arrows)*, erythrocytes, and small numbers of inflammatory cells are present within the lumen of a bronchus. H&E stain. (**A** courtesy Dr. J.M. King, College of Veterinary Medicine, Cornell University. **B** courtesy Dr. S. Martinson, Atlantic Veterinary College.)

proposed that a genetic mutation alters the cell-cell communication between epithelial and mesenchymal cells in the lung. This aberrant cellular communication leads to an overexpression of inflammatory and repair molecules (i.e., IL-4, IL-13, TGF-β1, and caveolin), leading to increased apoptosis and interstitial deposition of extracellular matrix (ECM). The chronic interstitial (restrictive) diseases in human medicine include "idiopathic pulmonary fibrosis," "nonspecific interstitial pneumonia," "unusual interstitial pneumonia," and "cryptogenic organizing pneumonia," also referred to as idiopathic *bronchiolitis obliterans organizing pneumonia* (idiopathic BOOP). Feline idiopathic pulmonary fibrosis is an example of this type of progressive interstitial disease in veterinary medicine. It has been reported that in rare cases, chronic alveolar remodeling and interstitial fibrosis can progress to lung cancer.

The term *bronchointerstitial pneumonia* is used in veterinary pathology to describe cases in which microscopic lesions share some histologic features of both bronchopneumonia and interstitial pneumonia (E-Fig. 9-9). This combined type of pneumonia is in fact frequently seen in many viral infections in which viruses replicate and cause necrosis in bronchial, bronchiolar, and alveolar cells. Damage to the bronchial and bronchiolar epithelium causes an influx of neutrophils similar to that in bronchopneumonias, and damage to alveolar walls causes proliferation of type II pneumonocytes, similar to that which takes place in the proliferative phase of acute interstitial pneumonias. It is important to emphasize that bronchointerstitial pneumonia is a microscopic not a gross diagnosis. Examples include uncomplicated cases of respiratory syncytial virus infections in cattle and lambs, canine distemper, and influenza in pigs and horses.

Embolic Pneumonia

Embolic pneumonia refers to a particular type of pneumonia in which gross and microscopic lesions are multifocally distributed in all pulmonary lobes. By definition, lung injury is hematogenous, and the inflammatory response is typically centered in pulmonary arterioles and alveolar capillaries. Lungs act as a biologic filter for circulating particulate matter. Sterile thromboemboli, unless extremely large, are rapidly dissolved and removed from the pulmonary vasculature by fibrinolysis, causing little, if any, ill effects. Experimental studies have confirmed that most types of bacteria when injected intravenously (bacteremia) are phagocytosed by pulmonary intravascular macrophages, or they bypass the lungs and are finally trapped by macrophages in the liver, spleen, joints, or other organs. To cause pulmonary infection, circulating bacteria must first attach to the pulmonary endothelium with specific binding proteins or simply attach to intravascular fibrin and then evade phagocytosis by intravascular macrophages or leukocytes. Septic thrombi facilitate entrapment of bacteria in the pulmonary vessels and provide a favorable environment to escape phagocytosis. Once trapped in the pulmonary vasculature, usually in small arterioles or alveolar capillaries, offending bacteria disrupt endothelium and basement membranes, spread from the vessels to the interstitium and then to the surrounding lung, finally forming a new nidus of infection.

Embolic pneumonia is characterized by multifocal lesions randomly distributed in all pulmonary lobes (see Fig. 9-68 and E-Figs. 9-10 and 9-11). Early lesions in embolic pneumonia are characterized grossly by the presence of very small (1 to 10 mm), white foci surrounded by discrete, red, hemorrhagic halos (Fig. 9-78). Unless emboli arrive in massive numbers, causing fatal pulmonary edema, embolic pneumonia is seldom fatal; therefore these acute lesions are rarely seen at postmortem examination. In most instances, if unresolved, acute lesions rapidly progress to pulmonary abscesses. These are randomly distributed in all pulmonary lobes and are not restricted to the cranioventral aspects of the lungs, as is the case of abscesses developing from suppurative bronchopneumonia. The early microscopic lesions in embolic pneumonias are always focal or multifocal (Fig. 9-79); thus they differ from those of endotoxemia or septicemia, in which endothelial damage and interstitial reactions (interstitial pneumonia) are diffusely distributed in the lungs.

When embolic pneumonia or its sequela (abscesses) is diagnosed at necropsy, an attempt should be made to locate the source of septic emboli. The most common sources are hepatic abscesses that have ruptured into the caudal vena cava in cattle, omphalophlebitis in farm animals, chronic bacterial skin or hoof infections, and a contaminated catheter in all species (see Fig. 9-64). Valvular or mural endocarditis in the right heart is a common source of septic emboli and embolic pneumonia in all species. Most frequently, bacterial isolates from septic pulmonary emboli in domestic animals are *Trueperella (Arcanobacterium) pyogenes* (cattle), *Fusobacterium necrophorum* (cattle, pigs, and human beings), *Erysipelothrix rhusiopathiae* (pigs, cattle, dogs, and human beings), *Streptococcus suis* (pigs), *Staphylococcus aureus* (dogs and human beings), and *Streptococcus equi* (horses).

Granulomatous Pneumonia

Granulomatous pneumonia refers to a particular type of pneumonia in which aerogenous or hematogenous injury is caused by organisms or particles that cannot normally be eliminated by phagocytosis and that evoke a local inflammatory reaction with numerous alveolar and interstitial macrophages, lymphocytes, a few neutrophils, and sometimes giant cells. The term *granulomatous* is used here to describe an anatomic pattern of pneumonia typically characterized by the presence of granulomas.

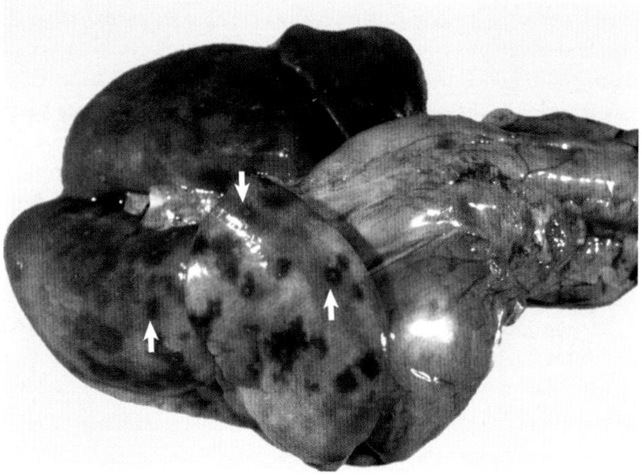

Figure 9-78 **Embolic Pneumonia, Lungs, 6-Week-Old Puppy.** Large hemorrhagic foci are scattered relatively uniformly throughout all pulmonary lobes *(arrows)*. These hemorrhagic foci are the sites of lodgment of *Pseudomonas aeruginosa* emboli (septic) that originated from necrotizing enteritis. Note the multifocal distribution of the inflammatory foci, which is typical of embolic pneumonia. Septic emboli were also present in the liver. (Courtesy Atlantic Veterinary College.)

The pathogenesis of granulomatous pneumonia shares some similarities with that of interstitial and embolic pneumonias. Not surprisingly, some pathologists group granulomatous pneumonias within one of these types of pneumonias (e.g., granulomatous interstitial pneumonia). What makes granulomatous pneumonia a distinctive type is not so much the portal of entry or site of initial injury in the lungs but, rather, the unique type of inflammatory response that results in the formation of granulomas, which can be easily recognized at gross and microscopic examination. As a rule, agents causing granulomatous pneumonias are resistant to intracellular killing by phagocytic cells and to the acute inflammatory response, allowing prolonged persistence of these agents in tissues.

The most common causes of granulomatous pneumonia in animals include systemic fungal diseases, such as cryptococcosis (*Cryptococcus neoformans* and *Cryptococcus gatti*), coccidioidomycosis (*Coccidioides immitis*), histoplasmosis (*Histoplasma capsulatum*), and blastomycosis (*Blastomyces dermatitidis*) (see Fig. 9-35). In most of these fungal diseases, the port of entry is aerogenous, and from the lungs the fungi disseminate systemically to other organs, particularly the lymph nodes, liver, and spleen. Filamentous fungi such as *Aspergillus* spp. or *Mucor* spp. can also reach the lung by the hematogenous route.

Granulomatous pneumonia is also seen in some bacterial diseases, such as tuberculosis (*Mycobacterium bovis*) in all species and *Rhodococcus equi* in horses. Sporadically, aberrant parasites such as *Fasciola hepatica* in cattle and aspiration of foreign bodies can also cause granulomatous pneumonia (E-Fig. 9-12). Feline infectious peritonitis (FIP) is one of a few viral infections of domestic animals that result in granulomatous pneumonia (see Pneumonias of Cats).

Granulomatous pneumonia is characterized by the presence of variable numbers of caseous or noncaseous granulomas randomly distributed in the lungs (see Fig. 9-68). On palpation, lungs have a typical nodular character given by well-circumscribed, variably sized nodules that generally have a firm texture, especially if calcification has occurred (Fig. 9-80). During postmortem examination, granulomas in the lungs occasionally can be mistaken for neoplasms. Microscopically, pulmonary granulomas are composed of a center of necrotic tissue, surrounded by a rim of macrophages (epithelioid cells) and giant cells and an outer delineated layer of connective tissue commonly infiltrated by lymphocytes and plasma cells (Fig. 9-81). Unlike other types of pneumonias, the causative agent in granulomatous pneumonia can, in many cases, be identified

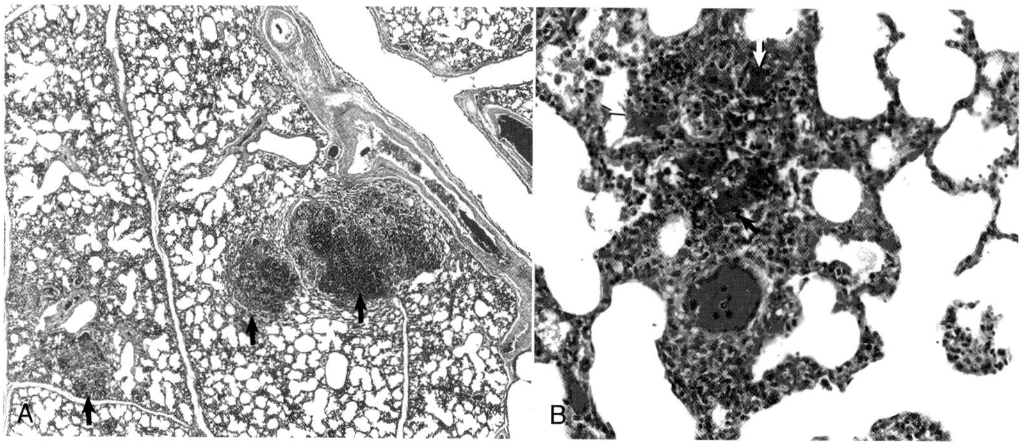

Figure 9-79 **Embolic Pneumonia, Lung, Cow. A,** Foci of necrosis and infiltration of neutrophils *(arrows)* resulting from septic emboli. Note the multifocal distribution of the lesion, which is typical of embolic pneumonia. Vegetative endocarditis involving the tricuspid valve was the source of septic emboli in this cow. H&E stain. **B,** Embolic focus in the lung. Note bacterial colonies *(arrows)* mixed with neutrophils and cellular debris. H&E stain. (Courtesy Dr. A. López, Atlantic Veterinary College.)

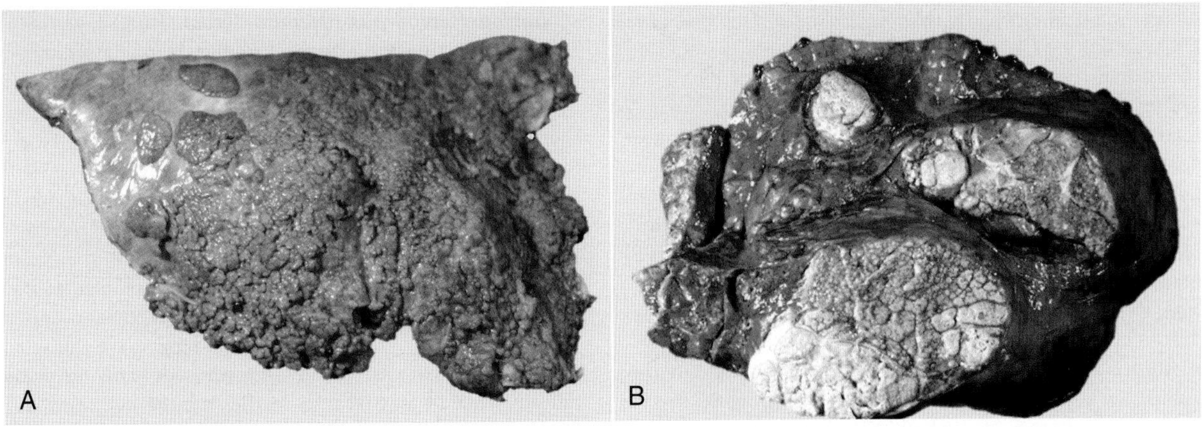

Figure 9-80 Pulmonary Tuberculosis, Lung, Aged Cow. A, Multifocal, coalescing granulomatous pneumonia involves most of the lung, except for the dorsal portion of the caudal lung lobe. **B,** Transverse section. Large multifocal to confluent caseating granulomas are present in the pulmonary parenchyma. Note the caseous ("cheesy," pale yellow-white) appearance of the granulomas, which is typical of bovine tuberculosis. (**A** courtesy Facultad de Medicina Veterinaria y Zootecnia, UNAM, México. **B** courtesy Dr. J.M. King, College of Veterinary Medicine, Cornell University.)

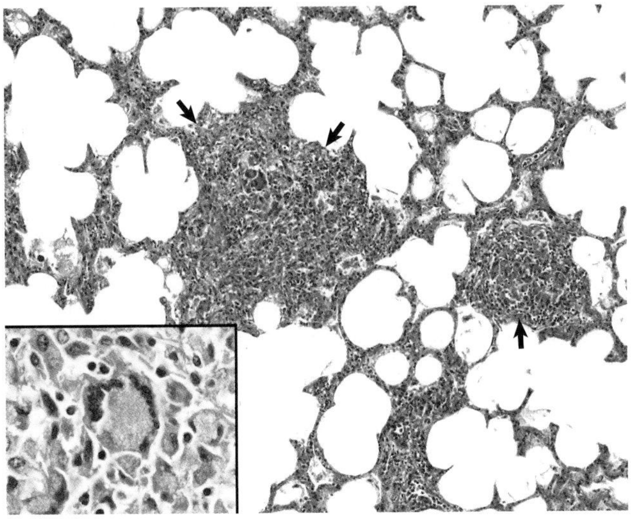

Figure 9-81 Granulomatous Pneumonia, Lung, Cow. Confluent noncaseous granulomas *(arrows)* with a small necrotic center filled with neutrophils, surrounded by histiocytes and mononuclear cells, and with an outer rim of connective tissue. H&E stain. *Inset,* Epithelioid macrophages and a large multinucleated giant cell *(in center of figure)*. H&E stain. (Courtesy Dr. A. López, Atlantic Veterinary College.)

microscopically in sections by PAS reaction or Grocott-Gomori's methenamine silver (GMS) stain for fungi or by an acid-fast stain for mycobacteria.

Species-Specific Pneumonias of Domestic Animals

Pneumonias of Horses

Viral infections of the respiratory tract, particularly equine viral rhinopneumonitis and equine influenza, are important diseases of horses throughout the world. The effects of these and other respiratory viruses on the horse can be manifested in three distinct ways. First, as pure viral infections, their severity may range from mild to severe, making them a frequent interfering factor in training and athletic performance. Second, superimposed infections by opportunistic bacteria, such as *Streptococcus* spp., *Escherichia coli*, *Klebsiella pneumoniae*, *Rhodococcus equi*, and various anaerobes, can cause fibrinous or suppurative bronchopneumonias. Third, it is possible but yet unproven that viral infections may also predispose horses to airway hyperresponsiveness and recurrent airway obstruction (RAO).

Viral Pneumonias

Equine Influenza. Equine influenza is an important and highly contagious flulike respiratory disease of horses characterized by high morbidity and low mortality and explosive outbreaks in susceptible populations. It is an OIE-notifiable disease. Two antigenically unrelated subtypes of equine influenza virus have been identified (H7N7 [A/equi-1] and H3N8 [A/equi-2]). The course of the disease is generally mild and transient, and its importance is primarily because of its economic impact on horse racing. The types of injury and host response in the conducting system are described in the section on disorders of the nasal cavity and paranasal sinuses of horses. Uncomplicated lesions in the lungs are mild and self-limiting bronchointerstitial pneumonia. In fatal cases, the lungs are hyperinflated with coalescing areas of dark red discoloration. Microscopically, there is a bronchointerstitial pneumonia characterized by necrotizing bronchiolitis that is followed by hyperplastic bronchiolitis, hyperplasia of type II pneumonocytes, hyaline membranes in alveoli, and sporadic multinucleated giant cells. The microscopic changes are ARDS in severe and fatal cases. The influenza virus antigen can be readily demonstrated in ciliated cells and alveolar macrophages. Clinical signs are characterized by fever, cough, abnormal lung sounds (crackles and wheezes), anorexia, and depression. Secondary bacterial infections (*Streptococcus equi*, *Streptococcus zooepidemicus*, *Staphylococcus aureus*, and *Escherichia coli*) commonly complicate equine influenza.

Equine Viral Rhinopneumonitis. Equine viral rhinopneumonitis (EVR), or equine herpesvirus infection, is a respiratory disease of young horses that is particularly important in weanlings between 4 and 8 months of age and to a much lesser extent in young foals and adult horses. The causative agents are ubiquitous equine herpesviruses (EHV-1 and EHV-4) that in addition to respiratory disease can cause abortion in pregnant mares and neurologic disease (equine herpes myeloencephalopathy) (see the section on disorders of the nasal cavity and paranasal sinuses of horses).

The respiratory form of EVR is a mild and a transient bronchointerstitial pneumonia seen only by pathologists when complications with secondary bacterial infections cause a fatal bronchopneumonia

(*Streptococcus equi*, *Streptococcus zooepidemicus*, or *Staphylococcus aureus*). Uncomplicated lesions in EVR are seen only in aborted fetuses or in foals that die within the first few days of life. They consist of focal areas of necrosis (0.5 to 2 mm) in various organs, including liver, adrenal glands, and lungs. In some cases, intranuclear inclusion bodies are microscopically observed in these organs. Outbreaks of interstitial pneumonia in donkeys have been attributed to multiple strains of asinine herpesviruses (AHV-4 and -5). Clinically, horses and donkeys affected with the respiratory form of EVR exhibit fever, anorexia, conjunctivitis, cough, and nasal discharge.

Equine Viral Arteritis. Equine viral arteritis (EVA), a pansystemic disease of horses, donkeys, and mules caused by an arterivirus (equine arteritis virus [EAV]), occurs sporadically throughout the world, sometimes as an outbreak. This virus infects and causes severe injury to macrophages and endothelial cells. Gross lesions are hemorrhage and edema in many sites, including lungs, intestine, scrotum, and periorbital tissues and voluminous hydrothorax and hydroperitoneum. The basic lesion is fibrinoid necrosis and inflammation of the vessel walls (vasculitis), particularly the small muscular arteries (lymphocytic arteritis), which is responsible for the edema and hemorrhage that explain most of the clinical features. Pulmonary lesions are those of interstitial pneumonia with hyperplasia of type II pneumonocytes and vasculitis with abundant edema in the bronchoalveolar spaces and distended pulmonary lymphatic vessels. Viral antigen can be detected by immunoperoxidase techniques in the walls and endothelial cells of affected pulmonary vessels and in alveolar macrophages.

Clinical signs are respiratory distress, fever, abortion, diarrhea, colic, and edema of the limbs and ventral abdomen. Respiratory signs are frequent and consist of serous or mucopurulent rhinitis and conjunctivitis with palpebral edema. Like most viral respiratory infections, EVA can predispose horses to opportunistic bacterial pneumonias.

African Horse Sickness. African horse sickness (AHS) is an arthropod-borne, OIE-notifiable disease of horses, mules, donkeys, and zebras that is caused by an orbivirus (family Reoviridae) and characterized by respiratory distress or cardiovascular failure. AHS has a high mortality rate—up to 95% in the native population of horses in Africa, the Middle East, India, Pakistan, and, most recently, Spain and Portugal. Although the AHS virus is transmitted primarily by insects (*Culicoides*) to horses, other animals, such as dogs, can be infected by eating infected equine flesh. The pathogenesis of African horse sickness remains unclear, but this equine orbivirus has an obvious tropism for pulmonary and cardiac endothelial cells and, to a lesser extent, mononuclear cells. Based on clinical signs (not pathogenesis), African horse sickness is arbitrarily divided into four different forms: pulmonary, cardiac, mixed, and mild.

The pulmonary form is characterized by severe respiratory distress and rapid death because of massive pulmonary edema, presumably from viral injury to the pulmonary endothelial cells. Grossly, large amounts of froth are present in the airways, lungs fail to collapse, subpleural lymph vessels are distended, and the ventral parts of the lungs are notably edematous (see Fig. 4-40). In the cardiac form, recurrent fever is detected, and heart failure results in subcutaneous and interfascial edema, most notably in the neck and supraorbital region. The mixed form is a combination of the respiratory and cardiac forms. Finally, the mild form, rarely seen in postmortem rooms, is characterized by fever and clinical signs resembling those of equine influenza; it is in most cases transient and followed by a complete recovery. This mild form is most frequently seen in donkeys, mules, and zebras and in horses with some degree of immunity. Detection of viral antigen for diagnostic purposes can be done by immunohistochemistry in paraffin-embedded tissues.

Equine Henipavirus (Hendra Virus). Fatal cases of a novel respiratory disease in horses and human beings suddenly appeared in approximately 1994 in Hendra, a suburb of Brisbane, Australia. This outbreak was attributed to a newly recognized zoonotic virus that was tentatively named equine *Morbillivirus*. Now called Hendra virus (HeV), this emerging viral pathogen is currently classified as a member of the genus *Henipavirus* (includes Hendra virus and Nipah virus), in the family Paramyxoviridae. Fruit bats (flying foxes) act as natural reservoirs and are involved in the transmission by poorly understood mechanisms. The lungs of affected horses are severely edematous with gelatinous distention of pleura and subpleural lymph vessels. Microscopically, the lungs have diffuse alveolar edema associated with vasculitis, thrombosis, and the presence of multinucleated syncytial cells in the endothelium of small pulmonary blood vessels and alveolar capillaries. The lymphatic vessels are notably distended with fluid. The characteristic inclusion bodies seen in other paramyxovirus infections are not seen in horses; however, the virus can be easily detected by immunohistochemistry in pulmonary endothelial cells and alveolar epithelial cells (pneumonocytes). Clinical signs are nonspecific and include fever, anorexia, respiratory distress, and nasal discharge.

Equine Multinodular Pulmonary Fibrosis. Equine multinodular pulmonary fibrosis is a lung disease characterized by well-demarcated fibrotic nodular lesions in the lung (E-Fig. 9-13). Until recently, the pathogenesis was unclear, but recent studies proposed equine herpesvirus 5 (EHV-5) as the putative etiology. Grossly, the lungs show multifocal to coalescing, firm tan nodules scattered in all pulmonary lobes, which resemble pulmonary neoplasia. Microscopically, alveolar walls are thickened due to collagen deposition, infiltration of lymphocytes and macrophages, and cuboidal cells lining the alveolar walls. The alveolar lumens contain neutrophils and macrophages, some of which may contain a large eosinophilic intranuclear inclusion body. Typical clinical signs include weight loss, low-grade fever, and progressive exercise intolerance. This condition has a poor prognosis.

Bacterial Pneumonias

Rhodococcus equi. *Rhodococcus equi* is an important cause of morbidity and mortality in foals throughout the world. This facultative intracellular Gram-positive bacterium causes two major forms of disease: The first involves the intestine, causing ulcerative enterocolitis, and the second severe and often fatal bronchopneumonia. Although half of foals with pneumonia have ulcerative enterocolitis, it is rare to find animals with intestinal lesions alone. Occasionally, infection disseminates to lymph nodes, joints, bones, the genital tract, and other organs. Because *Rhodococcus equi* is present in soil and feces of herbivores (particularly foals), it is common for the disease to become enzootic on farms ("hot spots") where the organism has been shed earlier by infected foals. Serologic evidence of infection in horses is widespread, yet clinical disease is sporadic and largely restricted to young foals or to adult horses with severe immunosuppression. Virulence factors encoded by plasmids (virulence-associated protein A [*vapA* gene]) are responsible for the survival and replication of *Rhodococcus equi* in macrophages, thus determining the evolution of the disease. This bacterium has also been sporadically incriminated with infections in cattle, goats, pigs, dogs, and cats, and quite often in immunocompromised human beings, for example, those infected with the AIDS virus, after organ transplantation, or undergoing chemotherapy.

It is still debatable whether natural infection starts as a bronchopneumonia (aerogenous route) from which *Rhodococcus equi* reaches the intestine via swallowed sputum or whether infection starts as an enteritis (oral route) with a subsequent bacteremia into the lungs.

The results of experimental studies suggest that natural infection likely starts from inhalation of infected dust or aerosols. Once in the lung, *Rhodococcus equi* is rapidly phagocytosed by alveolar macrophages, but because of defective phagosome-lysosome fusion and premature lysosomal degranulation, bacteria survive and multiply intracellularly, eventually leading to the destruction of the macrophage. Interestingly, *Rhodococcus equi* appears to be easily killed by neutrophils but not macrophages. Released cytokines and lysosomal enzymes and bacterial toxins are responsible for extensive caseous necrosis of the lungs and the recruitment of large numbers of neutrophils, macrophages, and giant cells containing intracellular Gram-positive organisms in their cytoplasm.

Depending on the stage of infection and the immune status and age of affected horses, pulmonary lesions induced by *Rhodococcus equi* can vary from pyogranulomatous to granulomatous pneumonia. In young foals, the infection starts as a suppurative cranioventral bronchopneumonia, which progresses within a few days into small variable-size pulmonary abscesses. These abscesses rapidly transform into pyogranulomatous nodules, some of which become confluent and form large masses of caseous exudate (Fig. 9-82). Microscopically, the early lesion starts with neutrophilic infiltration, followed by an intense influx of alveolar macrophages into the bronchoalveolar spaces. This type of histiocytic inflammation persists for a long period of time because *Rhodococcus equi* is a facultative intracellular organism that survives the bactericidal effects of equine alveolar macrophages. In the most chronic cases, the pulmonary lesions culminate with the formation of large caseonecrotic masses with extensive fibrosis of the surrounding pulmonary parenchyma. PCR analysis of tracheobronchial aspirates has successfully been used as an alternative to bacteriologic culture in the diagnosis of *Rhodococcus equi* infection in live foals.

Clinically, *Rhodococcus equi* infection can be acute, with rapid death caused by severe bronchopneumonia, or chronic, with depression, cough, weight loss, and respiratory distress. In either form, there may be diarrhea, arthritis, osteomyelitis, or subcutaneous abscess formation.

Parasitic Pneumonias

Parascaris equorum. *Parascaris equorum* is a large nematode (roundworm) of the small intestine of horses; the larval stages migrate through the lungs as ascarid larvae do in pigs. It is still unclear whether migration of *Parascaris equorum* larvae can cause significant pulmonary lesions under natural conditions. Experimentally, migration of larvae results in coughing, anorexia, weight loss, and small necrotic foci and petechial hemorrhages in the liver, hepatic and tracheobronchial lymph nodes, and lungs. Microscopically, eosinophils are prominent in the interstitium and airway mucosa during the parasitic migration and in focal granulomas caused by dead larvae in the lung.

Dictyocaulus arnfieldi. *Dictyocaulus arnfieldi* is not a very pathogenic nematode, but it should be considered if there are signs of coughing in horses that are pastured together with donkeys. Donkeys are considered the natural hosts and can tolerate large numbers of parasites without ill effects. *Dictyocaulus arnfieldi* does not usually become patent in horses, so examination of fecal samples is not useful; BAL is only occasionally diagnostic because eosinophils (but not parasites) are typically found in the lavage fluid. Mature parasites (up to 8 cm in length) cause obstructive bronchitis, edema, and atelectasis, particularly along the dorsocaudal lung. The microscopic lesion is an eosinophilic bronchitis similar to the less acute infestations seen in cattle and sheep with their *Dictyocaulus* species.

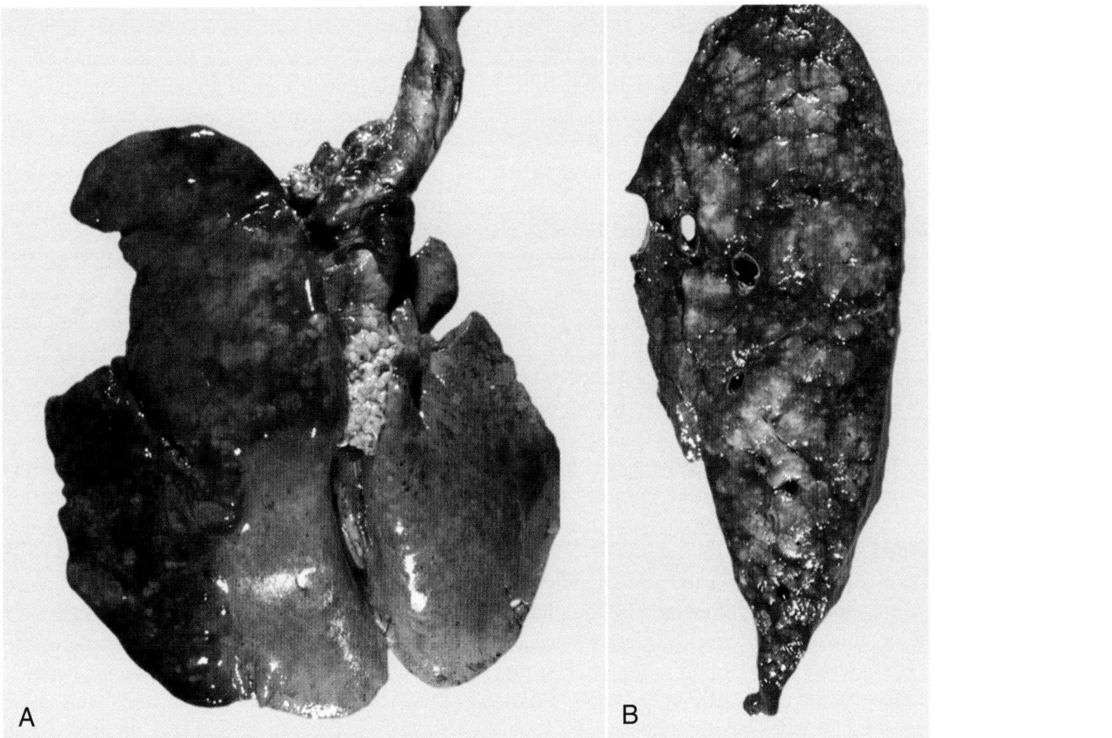

Figure 9-82 Granulomatous Pneumonia *(Rhodococcus equi),* Lungs, Foal. A, Cranioventral consolidation of the lungs with subpleural granulomas. Note that the pneumonic lesions in this foal are unilateral. This was an experimental case in which a foal was intratracheally inoculated with a suspension of *Rhodococcus equi*. **B,** Cut surface. Note the numerous, large, confluent, caseated white-brown granulomas. (Courtesy Dr. J. Yager and Dr. J. Prescott, Ontario Veterinary College.)

Aspiration Pneumonia. Aspiration pneumonia is often a devastating sequela to improper gastric tubing of horses, particularly exogenous lipid pneumonia from mineral oil delivered into the trachea in treatment of colic. Gross and microscopic lesions are described in detail in the section on aspiration pneumonias of cattle.

Other Causes of Pneumonia

Opportunistic Infections. *Chlamydophila* (*Chlamydia*) spp., obligatory intracellular zoonotic pathogens, can cause systemic infection in many mammalian and avian species; in horses, they can also cause keratoconjunctivitis, rhinitis, pneumonia, abortion, polyarthritis, enteritis, hepatitis, and encephalitis. Serologic studies suggest that infection without apparent disease is common in horses. Horses experimentally infected with *Chlamydophila psittaci* develop mild and transient bronchointerstitial pneumonia. There are unconfirmed reports suggesting a possible association between these organisms and recurrent airway obstruction in horses. Detection of chlamydial organisms in affected tissue is not easy and requires special laboratory techniques such as PCR, immunohistochemistry, and fluorescent antibody tests.

Horses are only sporadically affected with mycobacteriosis (*Mycobacterium avium* complex, *Mycobacterium tuberculosis*, and *Mycobacterium bovis*). The intestinal tract and associated lymph nodes are generally affected, suggesting an oral route of infection with subsequent hematogenous dissemination to the lungs. The tubercles (granulomas) differ from those in ruminants and pigs, being smooth, gray, solid, sarcoma-like nodules without grossly visible caseous necrosis or calcification (E-Fig. 9-14). Microscopically, the tubercles are composed of macrophages, epithelioid cells, and multinucleated giant cells. Fibrosis increases with time, accounting in part for the sarcomatous appearance.

Adenovirus infections occur commonly in Arabian foals with combined immunodeficiency (CID), a hereditary lack of B and T lymphocytes. In cases of adenoviral infection, large basophilic or amphophilic inclusions are present in the nuclei of tracheal, bronchial, bronchiolar, alveolar, renal, and intestinal epithelial cells. As it occurs in other species, infection with a unique fungal pathogen known as *Pneumocystis carinii* typically occurs in immunosuppressed or immunoincompetent individuals such as Arabian foals with CID (see Fig. 9-20). Diagnosis of *Pneumocystis carinii* requires microscopic examination of lungs and special stains.

Idiopathic Interstitial Pneumonia. Interstitial and bronchointerstitial pneumonias of undetermined cause that can progress to severe pulmonary fibrosis have been reported in foals and young horses. The gross and microscopic lesions are reminiscent of those of bovine pulmonary edema and emphysema or ARDS. The lungs are notably congested and edematous and microscopically are characterized by necrosis of the bronchiolar epithelium, alveolar edema, hyperplasia of type II pneumonocytes, and hyaline membranes. The cause of this form of equine interstitial pneumonia is not known, but toxic and particularly viral causes have been proposed.

Pneumonias of Cattle

Bovine respiratory disease complex (BRDC) and acute undifferentiated respiratory disease are general terms often used by clinicians to describe acute and severe bovine respiratory illness of clinically undetermined cause. These terms do not imply any particular type of pneumonia and therefore should not be used in pathology reports. Clinically, the BRD complex includes bovine enzootic pneumonia (multifactorial etiology); pneumonic mannheimiosis (*Mannheimia haemolytica*); respiratory histophilosis (*Histophilus somni*), previously known as respiratory hemophilosis (*Haemophilus somnus*); *Mycoplasma bovis*; respiratory viral infections, such as infectious bovine rhinotracheitis (IBR)/bovine herpes virus 1 (BoHV-1), bovine parainfluenza virus 3 (BPIV-3), and bovine respiratory syncytial virus (BRSV); and noninfectious interstitial pneumonias, such as bovine pulmonary edema and emphysema, reinfection syndrome, and many others.

Bovine Enzootic Pneumonia. Enzootic pneumonia, sometimes simply referred to as *calf pneumonia*, is a multifactorial disease caused by a variety of etiologic agents that produces an assortment of lung lesions in young, intensively housed calves. The host-microbial-environmental triad is central in the pathogenesis of this disease. Morbidity is often high (up to 90%), but fatalities are uncommon (>5%) unless management is poor or unless new, virulent pathogens are introduced by additions to the herd. Enzootic pneumonia is also called *viral pneumonia* because it often begins with an acute respiratory infection with BPIV-3, BRSV, or possibly with one or more of several other viruses (adenovirus, BoHV-1, reovirus, bovine coronavirus [BCoV], and bovine rhinitis virus). Mycoplasmas, notably *Mycoplasma dispar*, *Mycoplasma bovis*, *Ureaplasma*, and possibly *Chlamydophila*, may also be primary agents. Following infection with any of these agents, opportunistic bacteria, such as *Pasteurella multocida*, *Trueperella* (*Arcanobacterium*) *pyogenes*, *Histophilus somni*, *Mannheimia haemolytica*, and *Escherichia coli*, can cause a secondary suppurative bronchopneumonia, the most serious stage of enzootic pneumonia. The pathogenesis of the primary invasion and how it predisposes the host to invasion by the opportunists are poorly understood, but it is likely that there is impairment of pulmonary defense mechanisms. Environmental factors, including air quality (poor ventilation), high relative humidity, and animal crowding, have been strongly incriminated. The immune status of the calf also plays an important role in the development and severity of enzootic pneumonia. Calves with bovine leukocyte adhesion deficiency (BLAD), which prevents the migration of neutrophils from the capillaries, are highly susceptible to bronchopneumonia.

Lesions are variable and depend largely on the agents involved and on the duration of the inflammatory process. In the acute phases, lesions caused by viruses are those of bronchointerstitial pneumonia, which are generally mild and transient, and therefore are seen only sporadically at necropsy. Microscopically, the lesions are necrotizing bronchiolitis, necrosis of type I pneumonocytes with hyperplasia of type II pneumonocytes, and mild interstitial and alveolar edema.

In the case of BPIV-3 and BRSV infection, intracytoplasmic inclusion bodies and the formation of large multinucleated syncytia, resulting from the fusion of infected bronchiolar and alveolar epithelial cells, can also be observed in the lungs (Fig. 9-83). Airway hyperreactivity has been described in calves after BRSV infection; however, the significance of this syndrome in relation to enzootic pneumonia of calves is still under investigation.

The mycoplasmas also can cause bronchiolitis, bronchiolar and alveolar necrosis, and an interstitial reaction, but in contrast to viral-induced pneumonias, mycoplasmal lesions tend to progress to a chronic stage characterized by striking peribronchiolar lymphoid hyperplasia (cuffing pneumonia). When complicated by secondary bacterial infections (e.g., *Pasteurella multocida* and *Trueperella pyogenes*), viral or mycoplasmal lesions change from a pure bronchointerstitial to a suppurative bronchopneumonia (Fig. 9-84). In late stages of bronchopneumonia, the lungs contain a creamy-mucoid exudate in the airways and later often have pulmonary abscesses and bronchiectasis (see Fig. 9-11).

Note that the same viruses and mycoplasmas involved in the enzootic pneumonia complex can also predispose cattle to other diseases, such as pneumonic mannheimiosis (*Mannheimia*

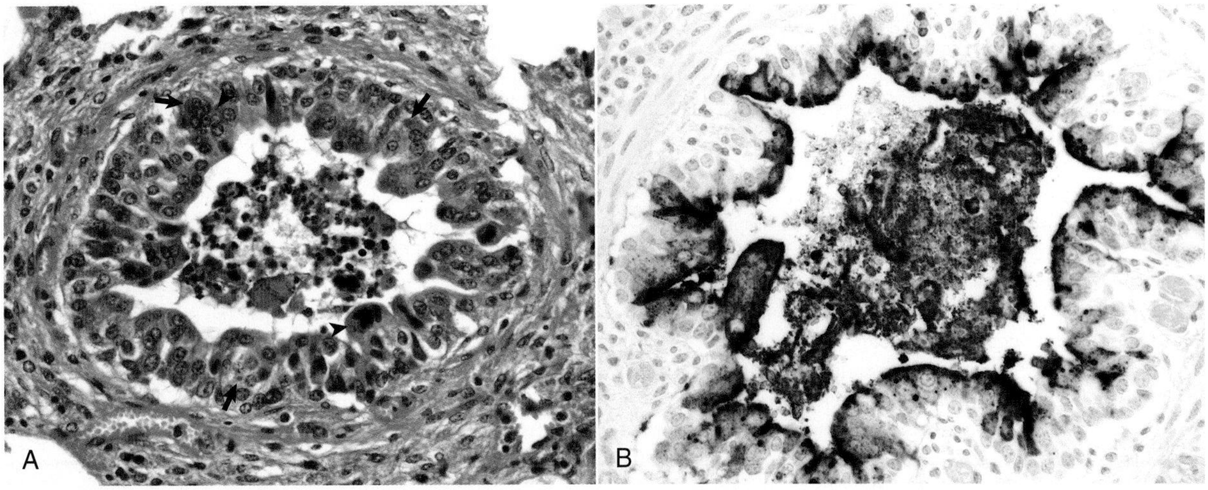

Figure 9-83 **Necrotizing Bronchiolitis, Bovine Respiratory Syncytial Virus, Lung, 5-Week-Old Calf.** This is the reparative stage of necrotizing bronchiolitis and is characterized by epithelial hyperplasia and exfoliation of necrotic cells into the bronchiolar lumen. **A,** Epithelial cells are swollen, some are multinucleated *(arrowheads)*, and the cytoplasm of some cells contains eosinophilic inclusion bodies surrounded by a clear halo *(arrows)*. Many of these hyperplastic bronchiolar cells eventually undergo apoptosis during the last stage of bronchiolar repair. H&E stain. **B,** Necrotizing viral bronchiolitis, immunohistochemistry. Note positive staining for bovine respiratory syncytial virus antigen in bronchiolar cells and in exfoliated necrotic material in the bronchiolar lumen. Immunoperoxidase stain. (**A** and **B** courtesy Dr. A. López, Atlantic Veterinary College.)

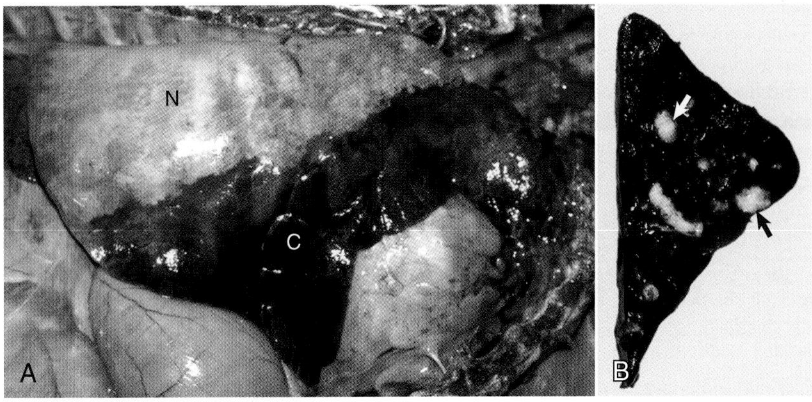

Figure 9-84 **Suppurative Bronchopneumonia, Right Lung, Calf. A,** Approximately 40% of the lung parenchyma is consolidated and includes most of the cranial lung lobe and the ventral portions of the middle and caudal lung lobes, a distribution often designated as cranioventral. Note the dark color of the consolidated lung (C) and the normal appearance of the dorsal portion of the caudal lung lobe *(N)*. **B,** Transverse section of the cranial lung lobe showing bronchi filled with purulent exudate *(arrows)*. (Courtesy Ontario Veterinary College.)

haemolytica). Clinically, enzootic pneumonia is usually mild, but fatal cases are occasionally seen even in farms with optimal health management.

Bacterial Pneumonias

Pneumonic Mannheimiosis (Shipping Fever). Shipping fever (transit fever) is a vague clinical term used to denote acute respiratory diseases that occur in cattle several days or weeks after shipment. The disease is characterized by a severe fibrinous bronchopneumonia, reflecting the fact that death generally occurs early or at an acute stage. Because *Mannheimia haemolytica* (formerly *Pasteurella haemolytica*) is most frequently isolated from affected lungs, the names pneumonic mannheimiosis and pneumonic pasteurellosis have been used synonymously. It is known that pneumonic mannheimiosis can occur in animals that have not been shipped and that organisms other than *Mannheimia haemolytica* can cause similar lesions. Therefore the term *shipping fever* should be relinquished in favor of more specific names, such as pneumonic mannheimiosis or respiratory histophilosis.

Pneumonic mannheimiosis (shipping fever) is the most important respiratory disease of cattle in North America, particularly in feedlot animals that have been through the stressful marketing and assembly processes. *Mannheimia haemolytica* biotype A, serotype 1 is the etiologic agent most commonly responsible for the severe pulmonary lesions. A few investigators still consider that *Pasteurella multocida* and other serotypes of *Mannheimia haemolytica* are also causes of this disease.

Even after many years of intense investigation, from the gross lesions to the molecular aspects of the disease, the pathogenesis of pneumonic mannheimiosis remains incompletely understood. Experiments have established that *Mannheimia haemolytica* A1 alone is usually incapable of causing disease because it is rapidly cleared by pulmonary defense mechanisms. These findings may explain why *Mannheimia haemolytica*, despite being present in the nasal cavity of healthy animals, only sporadically causes disease. For *Mannheimia haemolytica* to be established as a pulmonary infection, it is first required that stressors impair the defense mechanisms and allow the bacteria to colonize the lung (see section on Impairment of Defense

Mechanisms). These stressors include weaning, transport, fatigue, crowding, mixing of cattle from various sources, inclement weather, temporary starvation, and viral infections. Horizontal transmission of viruses and *Mannheimia haemolytica* occurs during crowding and transportation of cattle.

Viruses that most commonly predispose cattle to pneumonic mannheimiosis include BoHV-1, BPIV-3, and BRSV. Once established in the lungs, *Mannheimia haemolytica* causes lesions by means of different virulence factors, which include endotoxin, lipopolysaccharide, adhesins, and outer membrane proteins; however, the most important is probably the production of a leukotoxin (exotoxin), which binds and kills bovine macrophages and neutrophils. The fact that this toxin exclusively affects ruminant leukocytes probably explains why *Mannheimia haemolytica* is a respiratory pathogen in cattle and sheep but not in other species. During *Mannheimia haemolytica* infection, alveolar macrophages, neutrophils, and mast cells release maximum amounts of proinflammatory cytokines, particularly TNF-α, IL-1, IL-8, adhesion molecules, histamine, and leukotrienes. By locally releasing enzymes and free radicals, leukocytes further contribute to the injury and necrosis of bronchiolar and alveolar cells.

The gross lesions of acute and subacute pneumonic mannheimiosis are the prototypic fibrinous bronchopneumonia, with prominent fibrinous pleuritis (Fig. 9-85 and see Fig. 9-72) and pleural effusion. Lesions are always cranioventral and usually ventral to a horizontal line through the tracheal bifurcation. The interlobular septa are distended by yellow, gelatinous edema and fibrin. The "marbling" of lobules is the result of intermixing areas of coagulation necrosis, interlobular interstitial edema, and congestion (Fig. 9-86).

Microscopically, lung lesions are evident 4 hours after experimental infection in which neutrophils fill the bronchial, bronchiolar, and alveolar spaces. Within 24 to 48 hours, the cytotoxic effect of *Mannheimia haemolytica* is manifested by necrosis of individual alveolar cells and fibrin begins to exude into the alveoli from increased permeability of the air-blood barrier. These changes are exacerbated by endothelial swelling, altered platelet function, increased procoagulant activity, and diminished profibrinolytic activity in the lungs. By 72 hours, alveolar macrophages start to appear in the bronchoalveolar space. At this time, large and irregular areas of coagulative necrosis are typically bordered by a rim of elongated cells often referred to as *oat-shaped cells* or *oat cells* that are degenerating neutrophils mixed with a few alveolar macrophages (see Fig. 9-86). In the early stages of necrosis, there is no evidence of vascular thrombosis, suggesting that necrosis is primarily caused by the cytotoxin of *Mannheimia haemolytica* and is not the result of an ischemic change. The interlobular septa become distended with protein-rich edematous fluid, and the lymphatic vessels contain fibrin thrombi. The trachea and bronchi can have considerable amounts of blood and exudate, which are transported by the mucociliary escalator or coughed up from deep within the lungs, but the walls of the trachea and major bronchi may or may not be involved. Because of the necrotizing process, sequelae to pneumonic mannheimiosis can be serious and can include abscesses, encapsulated sequestra (isolated pieces of necrotic lung), chronic pleuritis, fibrous pleural adhesions, and bronchiectasis.

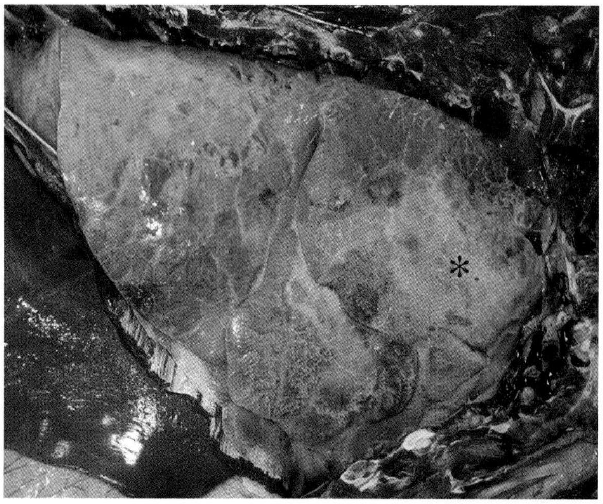

Figure 9-85 Fibrinous Bronchopneumonia (Pleuropneumonia), Pneumonic Mannheimiosis *(Mannheimia haemolytica)*, Right Lung, Steer. Note the cranioventral pneumonia involving approximately 85% of the lung parenchyma. The affected lung is firm and swollen, and the pleura is covered with a thick layer of fibrin *(asterisk)*. (Courtesy Dr. A. López, Atlantic Veterinary College.)

Clinically, pneumonic mannheimiosis is characterized by a severe toxemia that can kill animals even when considerable parts of the lungs remain functionally and structurally normal. Cattle usually become depressed, febrile (104° to 106° F [40° to 41° C]), and anorexic and have a productive cough, encrusted nose, mucopurulent nasal exudate, shallow respiration, or an expiratory grunt.

Hemorrhagic Septicemia. Pneumonic mannheimiosis should not be confused with *hemorrhagic septicemia* (septicemic pasteurellosis) of cattle and water buffalo (*Bubalus bubalis*) caused by inhalation or ingestion of serotypes 6:B and 6:E of *Pasteurella multocida*. This OIE-notifiable disease does not occur in North America and currently is reported only from some countries in Asia, Africa, and recently in Germany. In contrast to pneumonic mannheimiosis, in which lesions are always confined to the lower respiratory tract, the bacteria of hemorrhagic septicemia always disseminates hematogenously to other organs. At necropsy, typically, generalized petechiae are present on the serosal surfaces of the intestine, heart, and lungs and in skeletal muscles. Superficial and visceral lymph nodes are swollen and hemorrhagic. Variable lesions include edematous and hemorrhagic lungs with or without consolidation; hemorrhagic enteritis; blood-tinged fluid in the thorax and abdomen; and subcutaneous edema of the head, neck, and ventral abdomen. Bacteria can be cultured from blood, and animals have high fever and die rapidly (100% case fatality).

Respiratory Histophilosis (Haemophilosis). Respiratory histophilosis is part of the *Histophilus somni* (*Haemophilus somnus*) disease complex, which has at least eight different clinicopathologic forms, each one involving different organs. This complex includes septicemia, encephalitis (known as *thrombotic meningoencephalitis* [TME]), pneumonia (respiratory histophilosis), pleuritis, myocarditis, arthritis, ophthalmitis, conjunctivitis, otitis, and abortion. The portals of entry for the different forms of histophilosis have not been properly established.

The respiratory form of bovine histophilosis is the result of the capacity of the bacterium to induce both suppurative and fibrinous bronchopneumonia (E-Fig. 9-15). The latter is in some cases indistinguishable from that of pneumonic mannheimiosis. The pathogenesis of respiratory histophilosis is still poorly understood, and the disease cannot be reproduced consistently by administration of *Histophilus somni* alone. Like *Mannheimia haemolytica*, it requires predisposing factors such as stress or a preceding viral infection. *Histophilus somni* is often isolated from the lungs of calves with enzootic pneumonia. The capacity of *Histophilus somni* to cause septicemia and localized infections in the lungs, brain, eyes, ear, heart, mammary gland, male and female genital organs, or placenta is perhaps attributable to specific virulence factors, such as immunoglobulin-binding proteins (IgBPs) and lipooligosaccharide (LOS). Also, *Histophilus*

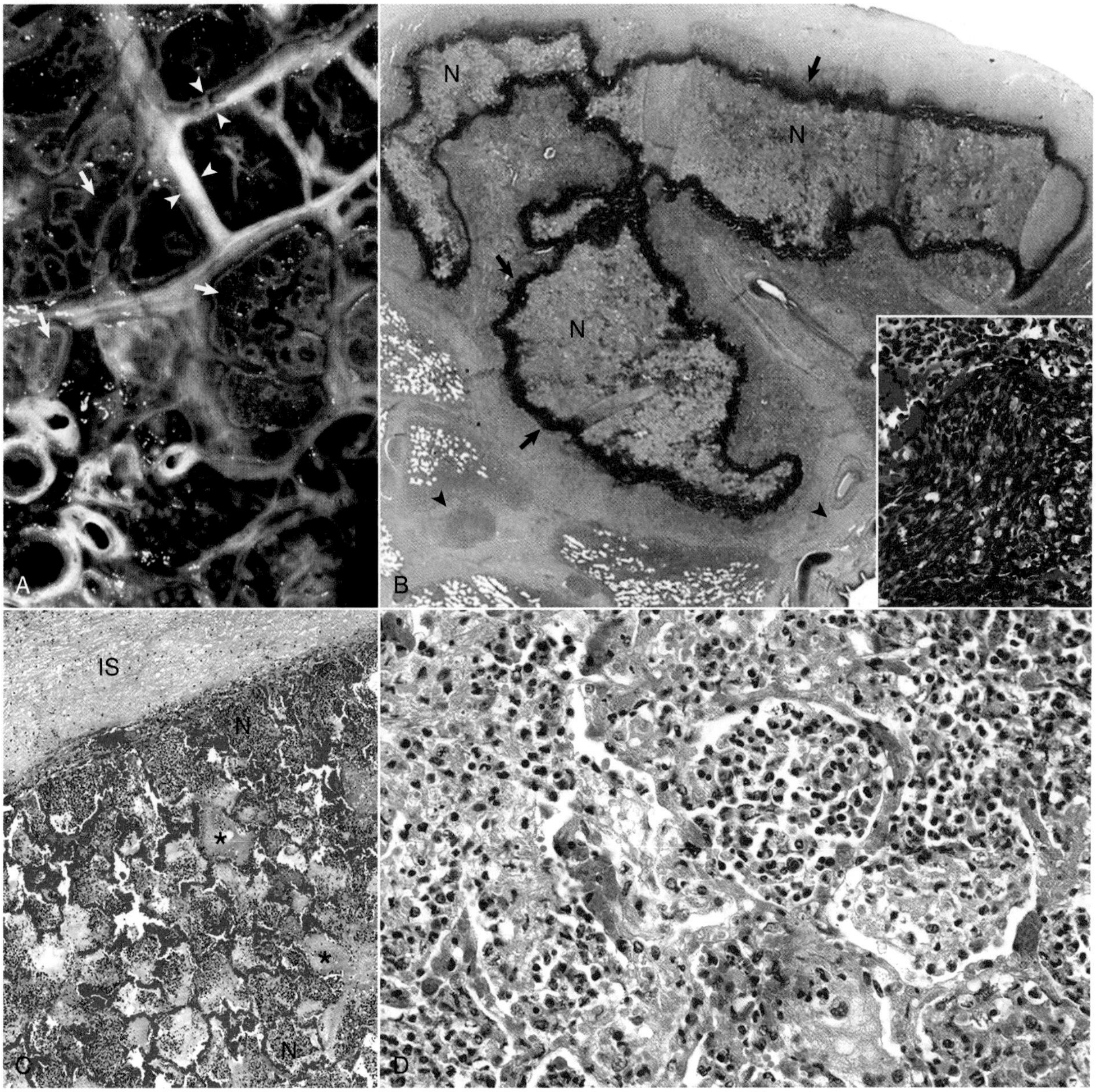

Figure 9-86 **Pneumonic Mannheimiosis (*Mannheimia haemolytica*), Lung, Steer. A,** Cut surface. Interlobular septa *(arrowheads)* are notably distended by edema and fibrin. In the lung parenchyma are irregular areas of coagulative necrosis *(arrows)* surrounded by a rim of inflammatory cells. **B,** Note a large irregular area of necrosis *(N)* of the pulmonary parenchyma. Typically, these necrotic areas are surrounded by an outer dense layer of inflammatory cells *(arrows)*. The interlobular septa are distended *(arrowheads)*. Inset *(bottom right corner)* shows the typical elongated and basophilic appearance of degenerated neutrophils known as oat cells. H&E stain. **C,** Note alveoli filled with fibrin *(asterisks)* and with neutrophils *(N)*. The interlobular septum *(IS)* is distended with proteinaceous fluid. H&E stain. **D,** *Mannheimia haemolytica* produces leukotoxin (cytotoxic for ruminant leukocytes) and lipopolysaccharide. Note the accumulation of cells, chiefly neutrophils, in the alveoli. Also note the active hyperemia of acute inflammation of the alveolar capillaries. H&E stain. (**A, B,** and **C** courtesy Dr. A. López, Atlantic Veterinary College. **D** courtesy Dr. J.F. Zachary, College of Veterinary Medicine, University of Illinois.)

somni has the ability to undergo structural and antigenic variation, evade phagocytosis by promoting leukocytic apoptosis, inhibit intracellular killing, reduce transferrin concentrations, and induce endothelial apoptosis in the lungs of affected calves. Mixed pulmonary infections of *Histophilus somni*, *Mannheimia haemolytica*, *Pasteurella multocida*, *Trueperella pyogenes*, and mycoplasmas are fairly common in calves.

***Mycoplasma bovis* Pneumonia.** *Mycoplasma bovis* is the most common *Mycoplasma* sp. isolated from pneumonic lungs of cattle in Europe and North America. Pulmonary infection is exacerbated by stress or any other adverse factor (e.g., viral infection) that depresses the pulmonary defense mechanisms. Lung lesions are typically those of a chronic bronchopneumonia with numerous well-delineated caseonecrotic nodules (Fig. 9-87 and E-Fig. 9-16). Microscopically, lesions are quite characteristic and consist of distinct areas of pulmonary necrosis centered on bronchi or bronchioles. The lesion is formed by a core of fine eosinophilic granular debris surrounded by a rim of neutrophils, macrophages, and fibroblasts (see Fig. 9-87). Although the origin of the caseonecrotic lesions is under investigation, recent studies incriminate reactive oxygen species (ROS) and reactive nitrogen species (RNS) as the major contributors for cell injury in the lung. The diagnosis is confirmed by isolation or

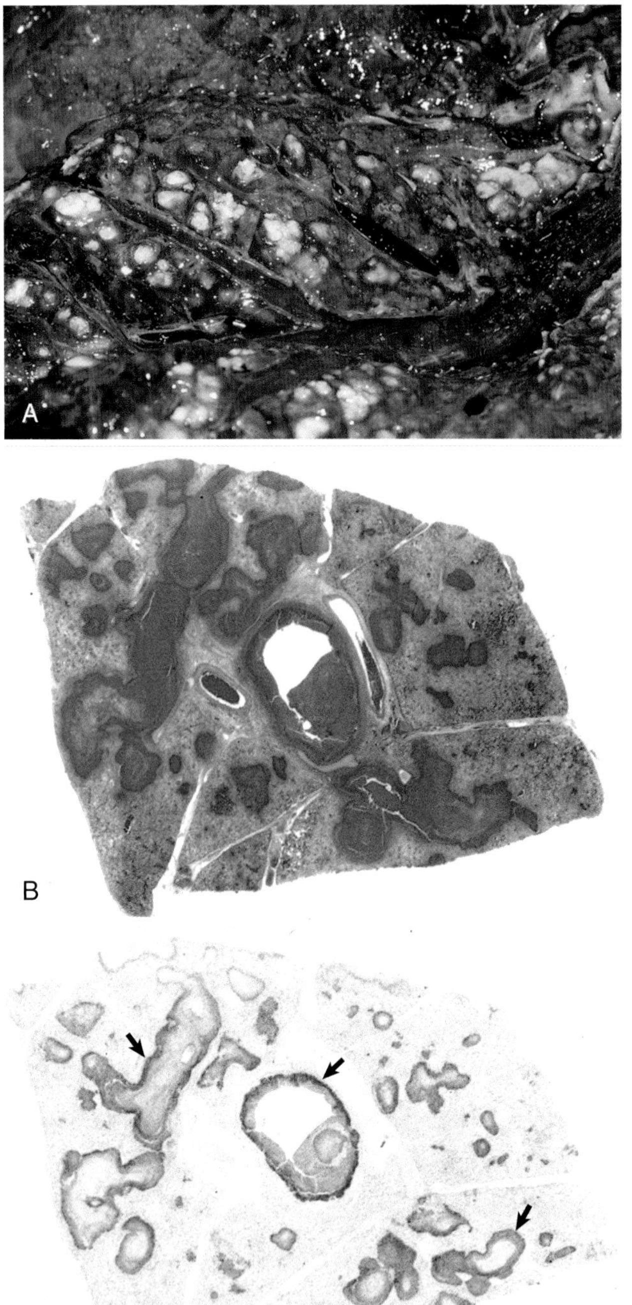

Figure 9-87 Chronic Bronchopneumonia (*Mycoplasma bovis*), Steer. **A,** Cut surface of lung showing multifocal to coalescing yellow-white caseonecrotic nodules. **B,** Section of lung showing large rounded areas of necrosis filled with hypereosinophilic *(pink-red)* granular debris. H&E stain. **C,** Necrotizing bronchopneumonia, immunohistochemistry. Note positive staining *(brown)* for *Mycoplasma bovis* antigen in the margin of the necrotic lung *(arrows)*. Immunoperoxidase stain. (**A** courtesy Dr. A. López, Atlantic Veterinary College. **B** and **C** courtesy Dr. A. López and Dr. C. Legge, Atlantic Veterinary College.)

immunohistochemical labeling of tissue sections for *Mycoplasma* antigens. *Mycoplasma bovis* is also incriminated in arthritis, otitis, mastitis, abortion, and keratoconjunctivitis.

Contagious Bovine Pleuropneumonia. Contagious bovine pleuropneumonia is an OIE-notifiable disease of historic interest in veterinary medicine because it was the object of early national control programs for infectious disease. It was eradicated from North America in 1892 and from Australia in the 1970s, but it is still enzootic in large areas of Africa, Asia, and eastern Europe. The etiologic agent, *Mycoplasma mycoides* ssp. *mycoides* small colony type, was the first *Mycoplasma* isolated and is one of the most pathogenic of those that infect domestic animals. Natural infection occurs in cattle and Asian buffalo. The portal of entry is aerogenous, and infections occur when a susceptible animal inhales infected droplets. The pathogenic mechanisms are still inadequately understood but are suspected to involve toxin and galactan production, unregulated production of TNF-α, ciliary dysfunction, immunosuppression, and immune-mediated vasculitis. Vasculitis and thrombosis of pulmonary arteries, arterioles, veins, and lymphatic vessels lead to lobular infarction.

The name of the disease is a good indication of the gross lesions. It is a severe, fibrinous bronchopneumonia (pleuropneumonia) similar to that of pneumonic mannheimiosis (see Figs. 9-72 and 9-85) but having a more pronounced "marbling" of the lobules because of extensive interlobular edema and lymphatic thrombosis. Typically, 60% to 79% of lesions are in the caudal lobes (not cranioventrally), and pulmonary sequestra (necrotic lung encapsulated by connective tissue) are more frequent and larger than pneumonic mannheimiosis. Unilateral lesions are common in this disease. Microscopically, the appearance again is like that of pneumonic mannheimiosis, except that vasculitis and thrombosis of pulmonary arteries, arterioles, and capillaries are much more obvious and are clearly the major cause of the infarction and thrombosis of lymphatic vessels in interlobular septa. *Mycoplasma mycoides* ssp. *mycoides* small colony type remains viable in the sequestra for many years, and under stress (e.g., starvation), the fibrous capsule may break down releasing mycoplasma into the airways, thus becoming a source of infection for other animals. Clinical signs are those of severe sepsis, including fever, depression, and anorexia followed by severe respiratory signs such as opened-mouth breathing, dyspnea and coughing, and crepitation and pleural friction on thoracic auscultation. Vaccination is highly effective in preventing the disease.

Bovine Tuberculosis. Tuberculosis is an ancient, communicable, worldwide, chronic disease of human beings and domestic animals. It continues to be a major problem in human beings in underdeveloped countries, and it is on the rise in some industrialized nations, largely because of the immunosuppressive effects of AIDS, immigration, and movement of infected animals across borders. The World Health Organization (WHO) estimates that more than 1 million people die of tuberculosis and 8 million new cases appear each year, mostly in developing countries. *Mycobacterium tuberculosis* is transmitted between human beings, but where unpasteurized milk is consumed, *Mycobacterium bovis* from the milk of cattle with mammary tuberculosis is also an important cause of human tuberculosis. *Mycobacterium bovis* infections have also been reported in a number of domestic and wild mammalian species; in some countries, wildlife reservoirs exist and may act as a source of infection for cattle.

Bovine tuberculosis is primarily caused by *Mycobacterium bovis*, but infection with *Mycobacterium tuberculosis*, the pathogen of human tuberculosis, and *Mycobacterium caprae* (formerly *Mycobacterium bovis* ssp. *caprae*/*Mycobacterium tuberculosis* ssp. *caprae*) can occur sporadically. Tuberculosis can be acquired by several routes, but infection of the lungs by inhalation of *Mycobacterium bovis* is the most common in adult cattle, whereas ingestion of infected milk is more predominant in young animals. Organisms belonging to the *Mycobacterium avium* complex can also infect cattle, but for infection caused by these organisms, the term *atypical mycobacteriosis* (not tuberculosis) is currently preferred.

Respiratory infection usually starts when inhaled bacilli reach the alveoli and are phagocytosed by pulmonary alveolar macrophages. If these cells are successful in destroying the bacteria, infection is averted. However, *Mycobacterium bovis*, being a facultative pathogen of the monocytic-macrophage system, may multiply intracellularly, kill the macrophage, and initiate infection. From this first nidus of infection, bacilli spread aerogenously via airways within the lungs and eventually via the lymph vessels to tracheobronchial and mediastinal lymph nodes.

The initial focus of infection at the portal of entry (lungs) plus the involvement of regional lymph nodes is termed the *primary (Ghon) complex* of tuberculosis. If the infection is not contained within this primary complex, bacilli disseminate via the lymph vessels to distant organs and other lymph nodes by the migration of infected macrophages. Hematogenous dissemination occurs sporadically when a granuloma containing mycobacteria erodes the wall of a blood vessel, causes vasculitis, and allows the granuloma to discharge mycobacteria into the alveolar circulation. If dissemination is sudden and massive, mycobacteria are widely disseminated and numerous small foci of infection develop in many tissues and organs and the process is referred to as miliary tuberculosis (like millet seeds). The host becomes hypersensitive to the mycobacterium, which enhances the cell-mediated immune defenses in early or mild infections but can result in host-tissue destruction in the form of caseous necrosis. The evolution and dissemination of the pulmonary infection are closely regulated by cytokines and TNF-α production by alveolar macrophages.

Unlike abscesses that tend to grow rather fast, granulomas evolve slowly at the site of infection. The lesion starts with few macrophages and neutrophils ingesting the offending organism, but because mycobacterium organisms are resistant to phagocytosis, infected macrophages eventually die, releasing viable bacteria, lipids, and cell debris. Cell debris accumulates in the center of the lesion, whereas viable bacteria and bacterial lipids attract additional macrophages and a few lymphocytes at the periphery of the lesion. Some of these newly recruited macrophages are activated by local lymphocytes and become large phagocytic cells with abundant cytoplasm resembling epithelial cells, thus the term *epithelioid macrophages*. Multinucleated giant cells (also macrophages) appear at the edges of the lesion, and finally the entire focus of inflammatory process becomes surrounded by fibroblasts and connective tissue (see Fig. 9-81). It may take weeks or months for a granuloma to be grossly visible.

Bovine tuberculosis, the prototype for granulomatous pneumonia, is characterized by the presence of a few or many caseated granulomas (see Fig. 9-80). The early gross changes are small foci (tubercles) most frequently seen in the dorsocaudal, subpleural areas. With progression, the lesions enlarge and become confluent with the formation of large areas of caseous necrosis. Calcification of the granulomas is a typical finding in bovine tuberculosis. Single nodules or clusters occur on the pleura and peritoneum, and this presentation has been termed *pearl disease*. Microscopically, the tubercle is composed of mononuclear cells of various types. In young tubercles, which are noncaseous, epithelioid and Langhans' giant cells are at the center, surrounded by lymphocytes, plasma cells, and macrophages. Later, caseous necrosis develops at the center, secondary to the effects of cell-mediated hypersensitivity and enclosed by fibrosis at the periphery. Acid-fast organisms may be numerous but more often are difficult to find in histologic section or smears.

Clinically, the signs of tuberculosis relate to the dysfunction of a particular organ system or to general debilitation, reduced milk production, and emaciation. In the pulmonary form, which is more than 90% of bovine cases, a chronic, moist cough can progress to dyspnea. Enlarged tracheobronchial lymph nodes can contribute to the dyspnea by impinging on airways, and the enlargement of caudal mediastinal nodes can compress the caudal thoracic esophagus and cause bloating.

Interstitial Pneumonias. Atypical interstitial pneumonia (AIP) is a vague clinical term well entrenched in veterinary literature but one that has led to enormous confusion among veterinarians. It was first used to describe acute or chronic forms of bovine pneumonia that did not fit in any of the "classic" forms because of the lack of exudate and lack of productive cough. Microscopically, the criteria for diagnosis of AIP in cattle were based on the absence of obvious exudate and the presence of edema, interstitial emphysema (see the section on Pulmonary Emphysema), hyaline membranes, hyperplasia of type II pneumonocytes, and alveolar fibrosis with interstitial cellular infiltrates. At that time, any pulmonary disease or pulmonary syndrome that had a few of the previously mentioned lesions was traditionally diagnosed as AIP, and grouping all these different syndromes together was inconsequential because their etiopathogenesis were then unknown.

Field and laboratory investigations have demonstrated that most of the bovine syndromes previously grouped under AIP have rather different causes and pathogeneses (Fig. 9-88). Furthermore, what was "atypical" in the past has become so common that it is fairly routine nowadays to find "typical cases" of AIP. For all these reasons, investigators, largely from Britain, proposed that all these syndromes previously clustered into AIP should be named according to their specific cause or pathogenesis. The most common bovine syndromes characterized by edema, emphysema, hyaline membranes, and hyperplasia of type II pneumonocytes include bovine pulmonary edema and emphysema (fog fever), "extrinsic allergic alveolitis" (hypersensitivity pneumonitis), "reinfection syndromes" (hypersensitivity to *Dictyocaulus* sp. or BRSV), milk allergy, ingestion of moldy potatoes, paraquat toxicity, toxic silo gases, mycotoxins, and others.

Acute Bovine Pulmonary Edema and Emphysema (Fog Fever). Acute bovine pulmonary edema and emphysema (ABPEE), known in Britain as fog fever (no association with atmospheric conditions), occurs in cattle usually grazing "fog" pastures (i.e., aftermath or foggage, regrowth after a hay or silage has been cut). Epidemiologically, ABPEE usually occurs in adult beef cattle in the fall when there is a change in pasture from a short, dry grass to a lush, green grass. It is generally accepted that L-tryptophan present in the pasture is metabolized in the rumen to 3-methylindole, which in turn is absorbed into the bloodstream and carried to the lungs. Mixed function oxidases present in the nonciliated bronchiolar epithelial (Club) cells metabolize 3-methylindole into a highly pneumotoxic compound that causes extensive and selective necrosis of bronchiolar cells and type I pneumonocytes (Fig. 9-89 and see Fig. 9-88) and increases alveolar permeability, leading to edema, thickening of the alveolar interstitium, and alveolar and interstitial emphysema. 3-Methylindole also interferes with the lipid metabolism of type II pneumonocytes.

The gross lesions are those of a diffuse interstitial pneumonia with severe alveolar and interstitial edema and interlobular emphysema (see Fig. 9-55, *A*). The lungs are expanded, pale, and rubbery in texture, and the lesions are most notable in the caudal lobes. Microscopically, the lesions are alveolar and interstitial edema and emphysema, formation of characteristic hyaline membranes within alveoli (see Fig. 9-55, *B*), and in those animals that survive for several days, hyperplasia of type II pneumonocytes and alveolar interstitial fibrosis.

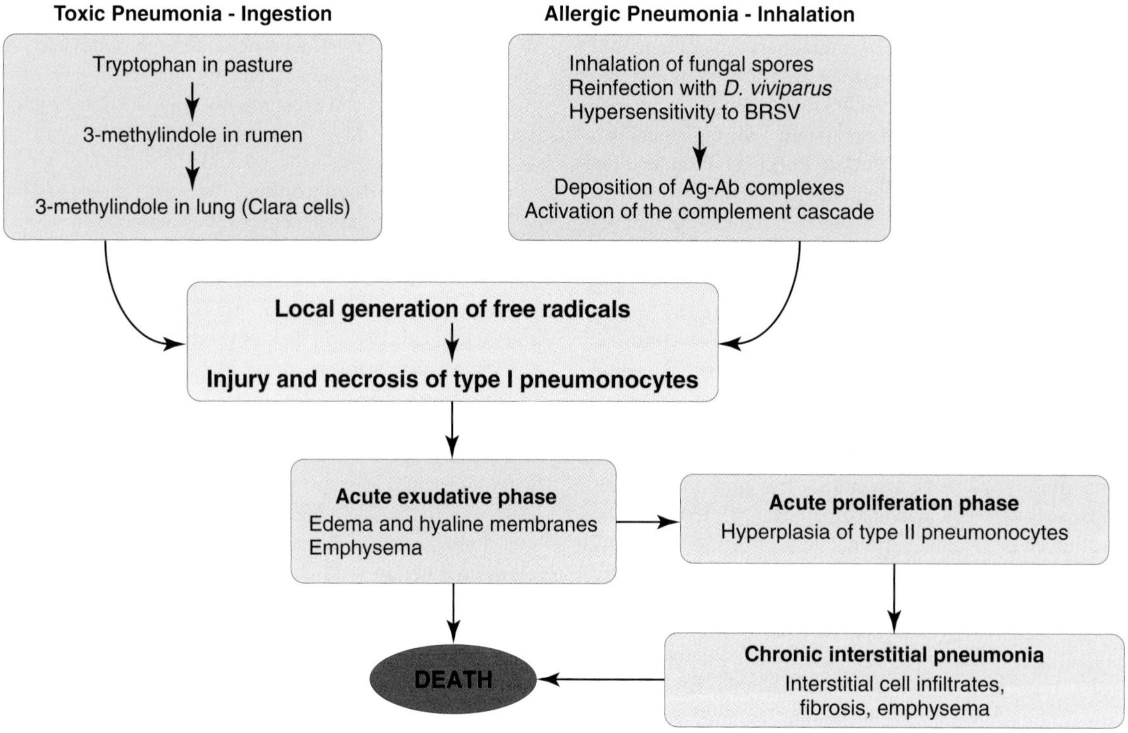

Figure 9-88 **Pathogenesis of Toxic and Allergic Pneumonias ("Atypical Interstitial Pneumonias") in Cattle.** (Courtesy Dr. A. López, Atlantic Veterinary College.)

Clinically, severe respiratory distress develops within 10 days of the abrupt pasture change, and cattle develop expiratory dyspnea, oral breathing, and evidence of emphysema within the lungs and even subcutaneously along the back. Experimentally, reducing ruminal conversion of L-tryptophan to 3-methylindole prevents the development of ABPEE.

A number of other agents cause virtually the same clinical and pathologic syndrome as is seen in ABPEE. The pathogenesis is assumed to be similar, although presumably other toxic factors are specific for each syndrome. One of these pneumotoxic factors is 4-ipomeanol, which is found in moldy sweet potatoes contaminated with the fungus *Fusarium solani*. Mixed function oxidases in the lungs activate 4-ipomeanol into a potent pneumotoxicant capable of producing irreversible oxidative injury to type I pneumonocytes and bronchiolar epithelial cells, presumably through lipoperoxidation of cell membranes. Similarly, purple mint (*Perilla frutescens*), stinkwood (*Zieria arborescens*), and rapeseed and kale (*Brassica* species) also cause pulmonary edema, emphysema, and interstitial pneumonia.

Extrinsic Allergic Alveolitis. Extrinsic allergic alveolitis (hypersensitivity pneumonitis), one of the most common allergic diseases in cattle, is seen mainly in housed adult dairy cows in the winter. This disease shares many similarities with its human counterpart known as *farmer's lung*, which results from a type III hypersensitivity reaction to inhaled organic antigens, most commonly microbial spores, mainly of the thermophilic actinomycete, *Saccharopolyspora rectivirgula* (*Micropolyspora faeni*), commonly found in moldy hay. This is followed by an antibody response to inhaled spores and local deposition of antigen-antibody complexes (Arthus reaction) in the lungs (see Fig. 9-88). Because it affects only a few animals of the herd or the sporadic person working in a farm, it is presumed that intrinsic host factors, such as dysregulation of dendritic cells, T lymphocytes, IgG, interleukins, IFN-γ, and surfactant, are involved in the pathogenesis of the disease.

Grossly, the postmortem lesions vary from subtle, gray, subpleural foci (granulomatous inflammation) to severe lesions, in which the lungs are firm and heavy and have a "meaty appearance" because of interstitial pneumonia (E-Fig. 9-17) with type II pneumonocyte hyperplasia, lymphocytic infiltration, and interstitial fibrosis. Characteristically, discrete noncaseous granulomas formed in response to the deposition of antigen-antibody complexes are scattered throughout the lungs. Chronic cases of extrinsic allergic alveolitis can eventually progress to diffuse fibrosing alveolitis. Clinically, it can be acute or chronic; the latter has a cyclical pattern of exacerbation during winter months. Weight loss, coughing, and poor exercise tolerance are clinical features. Full recovery can occur if the disease is recognized and treated early.

Reinfection Syndrome. Hypersensitivity to reinfection with larvae of *Dictyocaulus viviparus* is another allergic syndrome manifested in the lungs that causes signs and lesions indistinguishable from ABPEE, with the exception of eosinophils and possibly larvae in the alveolar exudate. The hypersensitivity reaction in the lung causes diffuse alveolar damage and edema, necrosis of type I pneumonocytes, and hyperplasia of type II pneumonocytes. In the later stages of the disease, there is formation of small granulomas with interstitial infiltrates of mononuclear cells.

It has been suggested but not confirmed that emphysema with diffuse proliferative alveolitis and formation of hyaline membranes can also occur sporadically in the late stages of BRSV infection in cattle. Presumably, this disease shares many similarities with "atypical" infections occasionally seen in children with respiratory syncytial virus (RSV human strain), in which a hypersensitivity to the virus or virus-induced augmentation of the immune response results in hypersensitivity pneumonitis (see Fig. 9-88). BRSV infection is also known to enhance hypersensitivity to environmental allergens in cattle.

Other Forms of Bovine Interstitial Pneumonia. Inhalation of manure ("pit") gases, such as nitrogen dioxide (NO_2), hydrogen

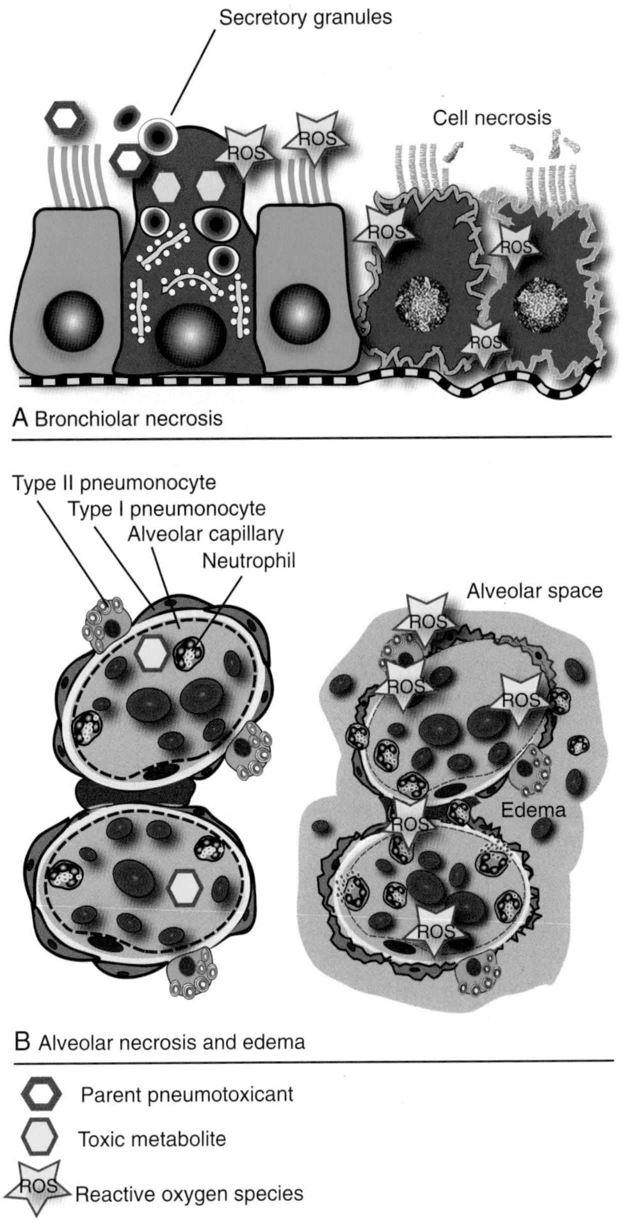

Figure 9-89 Bronchiolar and Alveolar Injury Caused by Pneumotoxicants. A, Inhaled pneumotoxicants, such as paraquat or 3-methylindole, are metabolized into toxic metabolites and reactive oxygen species *(ROS)* by bronchiolar Club cells. ROS reach adjacent bronchiolar cells *(blue)* by diffusion and cause injury and necrosis *(right two cells)*. Secretory granules released by Club cells contain several proteins, such as surfactant-like protein, antiinflammatory protein (CC10), and bronchiolar lining proteins. **B,** ROS produced by Club cells are also absorbed into capillaries within the lamina propria and are transferred by the circulatory system to pulmonary capillaries where they disrupt the air-blood barrier, causing degeneration and necrosis of type I pneumonocytes. This process leads to leakage of plasma fluid (alveolar edema *[pink color]*) and extravasation of erythrocytes (alveolar hemorrhage) and neutrophils (inflammation). Ingested pneumotoxicants can be metabolized by the liver, leading to release of ROS into the circulatory system that then disrupts the air-blood barrier in a similar manner. (Courtesy Dr. A. López, Atlantic Veterinary College.)

sulfide (H_2S), and ammonia (NH_3), from silos or sewage can be a serious hazard to animals and human beings. At toxic concentrations, these gases cause necrosis of bronchiolar cells and type I pneumonocytes and fulminating pulmonary edema that causes asphyxiation and rapid death (see Fig. 9-60). Like other oxidant gases, inhalation of NO_2 (silo gas) also causes bronchiolitis, edema, and interstitial pneumonia and, in survivors, bronchiolitis obliterans ("silo filler's disease").

Smoke inhalation resulting from barn or house fires is sporadically seen by veterinarians and pathologists. In addition to skin burns, animals involved in fire accidents suffer extensive thermal injury produced by the heat on the nasal and laryngeal mucosa, and severe chemical irritation caused by inhalation of combustion gases and particles in the lung. Animals that survive or are rescued from fires frequently develop nasal, laryngeal, and tracheal edema, and pulmonary hemorrhage and alveolar edema, which are caused by chemical injury to the blood-air barrier or by ARDS caused by the excessive production of free radicals during the pulmonary inflammatory response (see E-Fig. 9-7). Microscopic examination of the lungs often reveals carbon particles (soot) on mucosal surfaces of the conducting system.

Parasitic Pneumonias

Verminous Pneumonia (Dictyocaulus viviparus). Pulmonary lesions in parasitic pneumonias vary from interstitial pneumonia caused by migrating larvae to chronic bronchitis from intrabronchial adult parasites, to granulomatous pneumonia, which is caused by dead larvae, aberrant parasites, or eggs of parasites. In many cases, an "eosinophilic syndrome" in the lungs is characterized by infiltrates of eosinophils in the pulmonary interstitium and bronchoalveolar spaces and by blood eosinophilia. Atelectasis and emphysema secondary to the obstruction of airways by parasites and mucous secretions are also common findings in parasitic pneumonias. The severity of these lesions relates to the numbers and size of the parasites and the nature of the host reaction, which sometimes includes hypersensitivity reactions (see section on Reinfection Syndrome). A common general term for all of these diseases is *verminous pneumonia,* and the adult nematodes are often visible grossly in the airways (Fig. 9-90).

Dictyocaulus viviparus is an important pulmonary nematode (lungworm) responsible for a disease in cattle referred to as *verminous pneumonia* or *verminous bronchitis*. Adult parasites live in the bronchi of cattle, mainly in the caudal lobes, and cause severe bronchial irritation, bronchitis, and pulmonary edema, which in turn are responsible for lobular atelectasis and interstitial emphysema. Atelectasis is confined to the lobules of the lungs ventilated by the obstructed bronchi (dorsocaudal). Interstitial emphysema (interlobular) is caused by forced expiratory movements against a partially obstructed single bronchus. In addition to the inflammation of bronchial mucosa, bronchoaspiration of larvae and eggs also causes an influx of leukocytes into the bronchoalveolar space (alveolitis). Verminous pneumonia is most commonly seen in calves during their first summer grazing pastures that are repeatedly used from year to year, particularly in regions of Europe that have a moist cool climate. The parasite can overwinter in pastures, even in climates as cold as Canada's, and older animals may be carriers for a considerable length of time.

At necropsy, lesions appear as dark or gray, depressed, wedge-shaped areas of atelectasis involving few or many lobules usually along the dorsocaudal aspect of the lungs. On cut surface, edematous foam and mucus mixed with white, slender (up to 80-mm long) nematodes are visible in the bronchi (see Fig. 9-90). In the most severe cases, massive numbers of nematodes fill the bronchial tree. Microscopically, the bronchial lumens are filled with parasites admixed with mucus because of goblet cell hyperplasia, and there is squamous metaplasia of the bronchial and bronchiolar epithelium because of chronic irritation. There are also inflammatory infiltrates in the bronchial mucosa; alveolar edema; hyperplasia of BALT

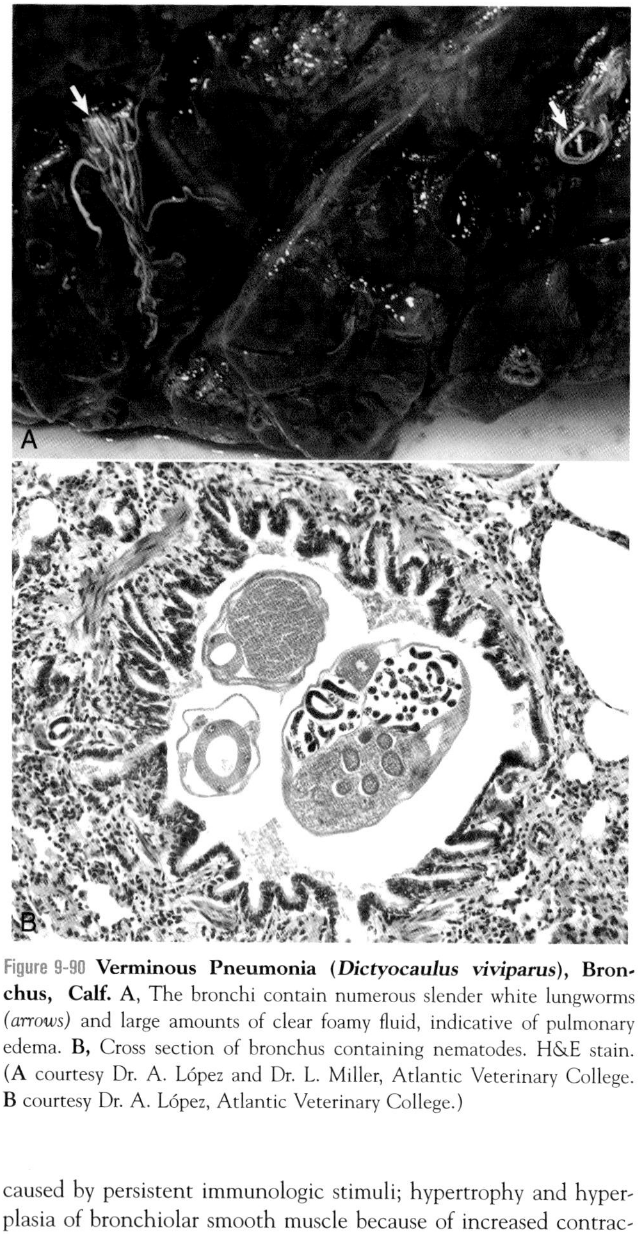

Figure 9-90 **Verminous Pneumonia (*Dictyocaulus viviparus*), Bronchus, Calf.** **A,** The bronchi contain numerous slender white lungworms *(arrows)* and large amounts of clear foamy fluid, indicative of pulmonary edema. **B,** Cross section of bronchus containing nematodes. H&E stain. (**A** courtesy Dr. A. López and Dr. L. Miller, Atlantic Veterinary College. **B** courtesy Dr. A. López, Atlantic Veterinary College.)

caused by persistent immunologic stimuli; hypertrophy and hyperplasia of bronchiolar smooth muscle because of increased contraction and decreased muscle relaxation; and a few eosinophilic granulomas around the eggs and dead larvae. These granulomas, grossly, are gray, noncaseated nodules (2 to 4 mm in diameter) and may be confused with those seen at the early stages of tuberculosis.

The clinical signs (coughing) vary with the severity of infection, and severe cases can be confused clinically with interstitial pneumonias. Expiratory dyspnea and death can occur with heavy parasitic infestations when there is massive obstruction of airways.

A different form of bovine pneumonia, an acute allergic reaction known as *reinfection syndrome*, occurs when previously sensitized adult cattle are exposed to large numbers of larvae (*Dictyocaulus viviparus*). Lesions in this syndrome are those of a hypersensitivity pneumonia as previously described.

Other Lung Parasites. *Ascaris suum* is the common intestinal roundworm of pigs; larvae cannot complete their life cycle in calves, but the larvae can migrate through the lungs and cause severe pneumonia and death of calves within 2 weeks of infection. Infection is usually acquired from the soil on which infested pigs were previously kept. The gross lesions are a diffuse interstitial pneumonia with hemorrhagic foci, atelectasis, and interlobular edema and

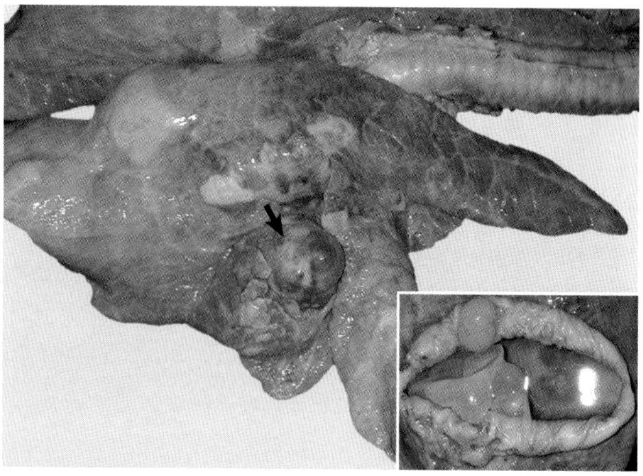

Figure 9-91 **Hydatidosis (Echinococcosis), Lung, Sheep.** A large hydatid cyst *(arrow)* is present in the pulmonary parenchyma. *Inset,* Hydatid cyst, cut-open section. The cyst contains fluid and larvae and is enclosed by a fibrous capsule. (Courtesy Dr. Manuel Quezada, Universidad de Concepción, Chile.)

emphysema, similar to what is seen in the lungs of pigs (see Fig. 9-77). Microscopically, there are focal intraalveolar hemorrhages caused by larvae migrating through the alveolar walls. Some larvae admixed with edematous fluid and cellular exudate (including eosinophils) may be visible in bronchioles and alveoli. The alveolar walls are thickened because of edema and a few inflammatory cells. Clinical signs include cough and expiratory dyspnea to the point of oral breathing.

Hydatid cysts, the intermediate stage of *Echinococcus granulosus*, can be found in the lungs and liver and other viscera of sheep and to a lesser extent in cattle, pigs, goats, horses, and human beings. The adult stage is a tapeworm that parasitizes the intestine of Canidae. Hydatidosis is still an important zoonosis in some countries, and perpetuation of the parasite life cycle results from animals being fed uncooked offal from infected sheep and consumption of uninspected meat. Hydatid cysts are generally 5 to 15 cm in diameter, and numerous cysts can be found in the viscera of affected animals (Fig. 9-91). Each parasitic cyst is filled with clear fluid; numerous daughter cysts attach to the wall, each containing several "brood capsules" with protoscolices inside. Hydatid cysts have little clinical significance in animals but are economically important because of carcass condemnation.

Aspiration Pneumonias. The inhalation of regurgitated ruminal contents or iatrogenic deposition of medicines or milk into the trachea can cause severe and often fatal aspiration pneumonia. Bland substances, such as mineral oil, may incite only a mild suppurative or histiocytic bronchopneumonia, whereas some "home remedies" or ruminal contents are highly irritating and cause a fibrinous, necrotizing bronchopneumonia. The right cranial lung lobe tends to be more severely affected because the right cranial bronchus is the most cranial branch and enters the ventrolateral aspect of the trachea. However, the distribution may vary when animals aspirate while in lateral recumbency. In some severe cases, pulmonary necrosis can be complicated by infection with saprophytic organisms present in ruminal contents, causing fatal gangrenous pneumonia. Aspiration pneumonia should always be considered in animals whose swallowing has been compromised—for example, those with cleft palate or hypocalcemia (milk fever). On the other hand, neurological diseases such as encephalitis (e.g., rabies) or encephalopathy (e.g., lead poisoning) should be investigated in animals in which the cause of aspiration pneumonia could not be explained otherwise. Depending on the nature of the aspirated material, histopathologic evaluation generally reveals foreign particles such as vegetable cells, milk droplets, and large numbers of bacteria in bronchi, bronchioles, and alveoli (E-Fig. 9-18). Vegetable cells and milk typically induce an early neutrophilic response followed by a histiocytic reaction with "foreign body" multinucleated giant cells (see E-Fig. 9-12). Special stains are used for the microscopic confirmation of aspirated particles in the lung (e.g., PAS for vegetable cells and Oil Red-O for oil or milk droplets).

Pneumonias of Sheep and Goats

Viral Pneumonias

Maedi (Visna/Maedi). Maedi is an important, lifelong, and persistent viral disease of sheep and occurs in most countries, except Australia and New Zealand. Maedi means "shortness of breath" in the Icelandic language, and it is known as *Graaff-Reinet disease* in South Africa, *Zwoegerziekte* in The Netherlands, *La bouhite* in France, and *ovine progressive pneumonia* (OPP) in the United States. More recently, the disease has also been referred to as *ovine lentivirus-induced lymphoid interstitial pneumonia* or simply *lymphoid interstitial pneumonia* (LIP).

Maedi is caused by visna/maedi virus (VMV), a nononcogenic small ruminant lentivirus (SRLV) of the family Retroviridae that is antigenically related to the lentivirus causing caprine arthritis-encephalitis (CAE). Seroepidemiologic studies indicate that infection is widespread in the sheep population, yet the clinical disease seems to be rare.

The pathogenesis is incompletely understood, but it is known that transmission occurs largely vertically, through ingestion of infected colostrum, and horizontally, via inhalation of infected respiratory secretions. Once in the body, the ovine lentivirus causes lifelong infections within monocytes and macrophages, including alveolar and pulmonary intravascular macrophages; clinical signs do not develop until after a long incubation period of 2 years or more.

Pulmonary lesions at the time of death are severe interstitial pneumonia and failure of the lungs to collapse when the thorax is opened. Notable rib imprints, indicators of uncollapsed lungs, are often present on the pleural surface (Fig. 9-92). The lungs are pale, mottled, and typically heavy (two or three times normal weight), and the tracheobronchial lymph nodes are enlarged. Microscopically, the interstitial pneumonia is characterized by BALT hyperplasia and thickening of alveolar walls and peribronchial interstitial tissue by heavy infiltration of lymphocytes, largely T lymphocytes (see Fig. 9-75). Recruitment of mononuclear cells into the pulmonary interstitium is presumably the result of sustainable production of cytokines by retrovirus-infected pulmonary macrophages and lymphocytes. Hyperplasia of type II pneumonocytes is not a prominent feature of maedi, likely because in this disease there is no injury to type I pneumonocytes, but there is some alveolar fibrosis and smooth muscle hypertrophy in bronchioles. Secondary bacterial infections often cause concomitant bronchopneumonia. Enlargement of regional lymph nodes (tracheobronchial) is due to severe lymphoid hyperplasia, primarily of B lymphocytes. The virus can also infect many other tissues, causing nonsuppurative encephalitis (visna), lymphocytic arthritis, lymphofollicular mastitis, and vasculitis.

Maedi is clinically characterized by dyspnea and an insidious, slowly progressive emaciation despite good appetite. Death is inevitable once clinical signs are present, but it may take many months.

Caprine Arthritis-Encephalitis. Caprine arthritis-encephalitis (CAE) is a retroviral disease of goats (small ruminant lentivirus) that has a pathogenesis remarkably similar to that of visna/maedi in sheep. It was first described in the United States in the 1970s, but it also occurs in Canada, Europe, Australia, and probably elsewhere. This disease has two major clinicopathologic forms: One involves the central nervous system of goat kids and young goats and is characterized by a nonsuppurative leukoencephalomyelitis; the other form involves the joints of adult goats and is characterized by a chronic, nonsuppurative arthritis-synovitis. In addition, infection with CAE virus can cause chronic lymphocytic interstitial pneumonia.

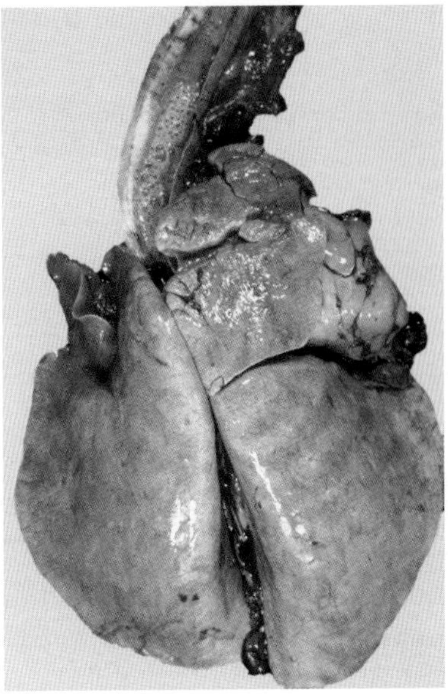

Figure 9-92 **Interstitial Pneumonia (Unknown Etiology), Lung, Sheep.** The lungs are heavy, rubbery, and show costal (rib) imprints on the visceral pleural surface. The diffuse distribution is typical of interstitial pneumonia. The trachea contains froth (edema fluid). (Courtesy Western College of Veterinary Medicine.)

The lentivirus of CAE, caprine arthritis and encephalitis virus (CAEV), is closely related to visna/maedi virus and, in fact, cross infection with CAE virus in sheep has been achieved experimentally. Similar to maedi, CAE infection presumably occurs during the first weeks of life when the doe transmits the virus to her offspring through infected colostrum or milk. Horizontal transmission between infected and susceptible goats via the respiratory route has also been described. After coming into contact with mucosal cells at the portal of entry, the virus is phagocytized by macrophages, which migrate to the regional lymph nodes. Infected macrophages are disseminated hematogenously to the central nervous system, joints, lungs, and mammary glands. Like maedi, there is some evidence that the recruitment of lymphocytic cells results from dysregulation of cytokine production by infected macrophages and lymphocytes in affected tissues. It can take several months before serum antibodies can be detected in infected goats.

Grossly, the interstitial pneumonia is diffuse and tends to be most severe in the caudal lobes. The lungs are gray-pink and firm in texture with numerous, 1- to 2-mm, gray-white foci on the cut surface. The tracheobronchial lymph nodes are consistently enlarged. Microscopically, the alveolar walls are thickened by lymphocytes and conspicuous hyperplasia of type II pneumonocytes (Fig. 9-93). One important difference between the pneumonias of CAE and maedi is that in CAE the alveoli are filled with proteinaceous eosinophilic material (alveolar proteinosis), which in electron micrographs has structural features of pulmonary surfactant. The pulmonary form of CAE can be mistaken for parasitic pneumonia (*Muellerius capillaris*) because these two diseases have lymphocytic interstitial pneumonia and can coexist in the same goat.

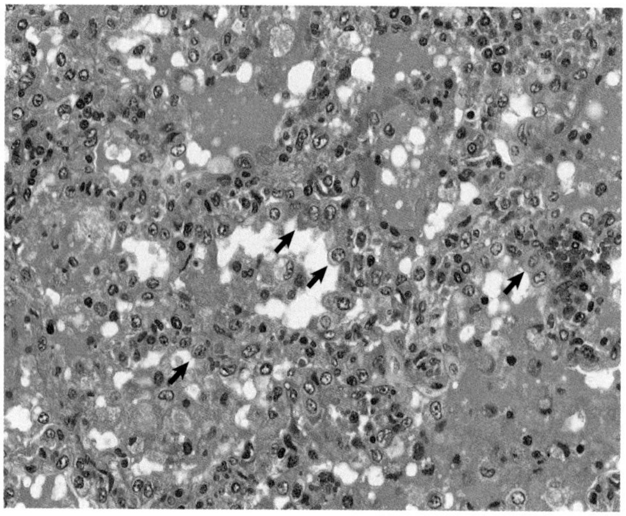

Figure 9-93 **Interstitial Pneumonia, Caprine Arthritis-Encephalitis, Lung, Goat.** Thickening of alveolar septa with hyperplasia of type II pneumonocytes *(arrows)*. The alveolar lumens are filled with protein-rich fluid admixed with occasional macrophages or exfoliated cells. H&E stain. (Courtesy Joint Pathology Center, Conference 201, Case 02 20222026.)

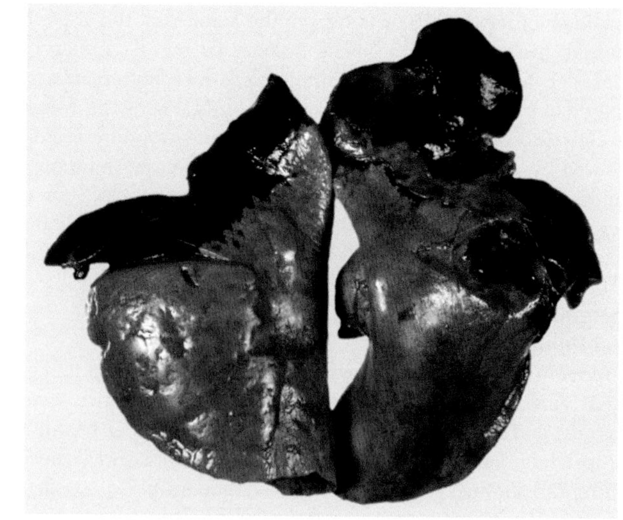

Figure 9-94 **Acute Fibrinous Bronchopneumonia (Pleuropneumonia), Pneumonic Mannheimiosis *(Mannheimia haemolytica)*, Lungs, Lamb.** The cranioventral aspects of the lung are red, swollen, and very firm (consolidated), with some fibrin on the pleural surface. Note that the consolidated lung resembles liver, a change that was previously referred to as "hepatization." (Courtesy Ontario Veterinary College.)

Clinically, goats are active and afebrile but progressively lose weight despite normal appetite. The encephalitic or arthritic signs tend to obscure the respiratory signs, which are only evident on exertion. Secondary bacterial bronchopneumonia is common in affected animals.

Bacterial Pneumonias. In the past, *Pasteurella haemolytica* was incriminated in four major ovine diseases known as (1) *acute ovine pneumonic pasteurellosis* (shipping fever), (2) *enzootic pneumonia* (nonprogressive chronic pneumonia), (3) *fulminating septicemia*, and (4) *mastitis*. Under the new nomenclature, *Mannheimia haemolytica* is responsible for ovine pneumonia resembling shipping fever in cattle (ovine pneumonic mannheimiosis), septicemia in young lambs (younger than 3 months of age), and ovine enzootic pneumonia and sporadic severe gangrenous mastitis in ewes. *Bibersteinia (Pasteurella) trehalosi* (formerly *Pasteurella haemolytica* biotype T) is the agent incriminated in septicemia in lambs 5 to 12 months old.

Chronic Enzootic Pneumonia. In sheep, this entity is a multifactorial disease complex that, in contrast to ovine pneumonic mannheimiosis, causes only a mild to moderate pneumonia and it is rarely fatal. It generally affects animals younger than 1 year of age. Significant costs associated with chronic enzootic pneumonia include reduction of weight gain, labor costs, veterinary fees, and slaughterhouse waste. The modifier "chronic" is used here to avoid any confusion with pneumonic mannheimiosis ("acute enzootic pneumonia"). It is also sometimes called atypical pneumonia, chronic nonprogressive pneumonia, proliferative pneumonia, or other names.

Chronic enzootic pneumonia is a clinical epidemiologic term and does not imply a single causal agent but is the result of a combination of infectious, environmental, and managerial factors. The list of infectious agents involved in ovine enzootic pneumonia includes *Mannheimia haemolytica*, *Pasteurella multocida*, parainfluenza virus 3 (PI-3), adenovirus, reovirus, respiratory syncytial virus (RSV), chlamydiae, and mycoplasmas (*Mycoplasma ovipneumoniae*).

In the early stages of enzootic pneumonia, a cranioventral bronchointerstitial pneumonia is characterized by moderate thickening of alveolar walls because of hyperplasia of type II pneumonocytes. In some cases, when lungs are infected with secondary pathogens, such as *Pasteurella multocida*, pneumonia may progress to fibrinous or suppurative bronchopneumonia. One might expect some specific evidence pointing to the infectious agents (e.g., large intranuclear inclusion bodies in epithelial cells with adenoviral infection), but this is often not the case, either because examination is seldom done at the acute stage when the lesions are still present or because secondary bacterial infections mask the primary lesions. In the late stages, chronic enzootic pneumonia is characterized by hyperplastic bronchitis, atelectasis, alveolar and peribronchiolar fibrosis, and marked peribronchial lymphoid hyperplasia (cuffing pneumonia).

Ovine Pneumonic Mannheimiosis. Ovine pneumonic mannheimiosis is one of the most common and economically significant diseases in most areas where sheep are raised. It is caused by *Mannheimia haemolytica* and has a pathogenesis and lesions similar to those of pneumonic mannheimiosis of cattle. Colonization and infection of lungs are facilitated by stressors such as changes in weather; handling; deworming; dipping; viral infections such as parainfluenza virus 3 (PIV3), respiratory syncytial virus (RSV), and adenovirus; and probably chlamydiae and *Bordetella parapertussis* infections. Lesions are characterized by a severe fibrinous bronchopneumonia (cranioventral) with pleuritis (Fig. 9-94 and E-Fig. 9-19). Subacute to chronic cases progress to purulent bronchopneumonia, and sequelae include abscesses and fibrous pleural adhesions. A similar form of pneumonic mannheimiosis has been reported with increased frequency in bighorn sheep.

Septicemic Pasteurellosis. Septicemic pasteurellosis, a common ovine disease, is caused by *Bibersteinia trehalosi* (formerly *Pasteurella trehalosi or Mannheimia haemolytica* biotype T) in lambs 5 months of age or older or by *Mannheimia haemolytica* (biotype A) in lambs younger than 2 months of age. Both organisms are carried in the tonsils and oropharynx of clinically healthy sheep, and under abnormal circumstances (particularly under stress from dietary or environmental changes) bacteria can invade adjacent tissues, enter the bloodstream, and cause septicemia. Gross lesions include a distinctive necrotizing pharyngitis and tonsillitis; ulcerative esophagitis (E-Fig. 9-20); severe congestion and edema of the lungs; focal hepatic necrosis; and petechiae in the mucosa of the tongue, esophagus, and intestine and particularly in the lungs and pleura.

Microscopically, the hallmark lesion is a disseminated intravascular thrombosis often with bacterial colonies in the capillaries of affected tissues. The alveolar capillaries contain bacteria and microthrombi, and the alveolar lumens have fibrin and red blood cells. *Mannheimia haemolytica* and *Bibersteinia trehalosi* are readily isolated from many organs. Affected animals usually die within a few hours of infection, and these animals only rarely have clinical signs such as dullness, recumbency, and dyspnea.

Contagious Caprine Pleuropneumonia. A number of *Mycoplasma* spp., often referred to as the "mycoides cluster," can produce respiratory tract infections in goats; however, only *Mycoplasma capricolum* ssp. *capripneumoniae* is considered to cause contagious caprine pleuropneumonia. This disease is the goat counterpart of contagious bovine pleuropneumonia in cattle; sheep do not have a corresponding disease. This OIE-notifiable disease is important in Africa, the Middle East, and areas of Asia, but it is also seen elsewhere.

The gross lesions caused by *Mycoplasma capricolum* ssp. *capripneumoniae* are similar to those of the bovine disease and consist of a severe, often unilateral fibrinous bronchopneumonia and pleuritis; however, distention of the interlobular septa (which are normally not as well developed in goats as in cattle) and formation of pulmonary sequestra are less obvious than in the bovine disease. Clinically, contagious caprine pleuropneumonia is similar to contagious bovine pleuropneumonia, with high morbidity and mortality, fever, cough, dyspnea, and increasing distress and weakness.

Other Small Ruminant Mycoplasmas. Pneumonia, fibrinous polyarthritis, septicemia, meningitis, mastitis, peritonitis, and abortion are possible manifestations of disease caused by *Mycoplasma mycoides* ssp. *mycoides* large colony type and *Mycoplasma mycoides* ssp. *capri*. The pathogenicity of other mycoplasmas, such as *Mycoplasma ovipneumoniae*, *Mycoplasma arginini*, and *Mycoplasma capricolum* ssp. *capricolum*, in sheep and goats is still being defined and specific description of the lesions would be premature. These organisms probably cause disease only in circumstances similar to those for enzootic pneumonia, where host, infectious, and environmental factors create a complex interaction in the pathogenesis of the disease. It has been suggested that IgG antibodies directed against ovine mycoplasmal antigens cross-react with ciliary proteins, causing inflammation and ciliary dysfunction, a condition in lambs referred to as *coughing syndrome*.

Tuberculosis. Although tuberculosis has generally been considered uncommon in sheep and goats, caprine tuberculosis has become a significant disease in areas of Spain and Europe. *Mycobacterium caprae* (formerly *Mycobacterium bovis* ssp. *caprae*/*Mycobacterium tuberculosis* ssp. *caprae*) is the most common cause, but infection with *Mycobacterium bovis* or with the *Mycobacterium avium* complex does occur when the disease is prevalent in other species in the locality. The pulmonary form, similar to that seen in cattle, is characterized by a granulomatous pneumonia with multiple, large, caseous, calcified, and well-encapsulated granulomas scattered throughout the lungs. Intralesional acid-fast organisms within macrophages are not as abundant as in bovine tuberculosis.

Staphylococcus aureus. Young sheep (2 to 12 weeks old) are susceptible to *Staphylococcus aureus* septicemia (tick pyemia). This bacterium causes disseminated inflammation and abscesses in the joints, heart, liver, kidneys, and CNS, and in the lung it can also produce bronchopneumonia and pulmonary abscesses (E-Fig. 9-21).

Parasitic Pneumonias

Dictyocaulus filaria. *Dictyocaulus filaria*, also called the *large lungworm*, is a serious, worldwide, parasitic disease of the lungs, most commonly of lambs and goat kids but occurring in adults as well. The life cycle and lesions are similar to those of *Dictyocaulus viviparus* of cattle. As seen in cattle with *Dictyocaulus viviparus*, areas of atelectasis secondary to bronchiolar obstruction are present, particularly along the dorsal caudal aspects of the caudal lung lobes. Microscopically, affected lungs are characterized by a catarrhal, eosinophilic bronchitis, with peribronchial lymphoid hyperplasia and smooth muscle hyperplasia of bronchi and bronchioles. Bronchioles and alveoli can contain edematous fluid, eosinophils, and parasitic larvae and eggs. Microscopic granulomas caused by aspirated eggs can be observed in the distal lung. The clinical signs (cough, moderate dyspnea, and loss of condition) and lesions relate mainly to obstruction of the small bronchi by adult worms and filaria. Anemia of undetermined pathogenesis and secondary bacterial pneumonia are common in small ruminants with this parasitic disease.

Muellerius capillaris. *Muellerius capillaris*, also called the *nodular lungworm*, occurs in sheep and goats in most areas of the world and is the most common lung parasite of sheep in Europe and Northern Africa. It requires slugs or snails as intermediate hosts. The lesions in sheep are typically multifocal, subpleural nodules that tend to be most numerous in the dorsal areas of the caudal lung lobes (Fig. 9-95, A). These nodules are soft and hemorrhagic in the early stages but later become gray-green and hard or even calcified. Microscopically, a focal, eosinophilic, and granulomatous reaction occurs in the

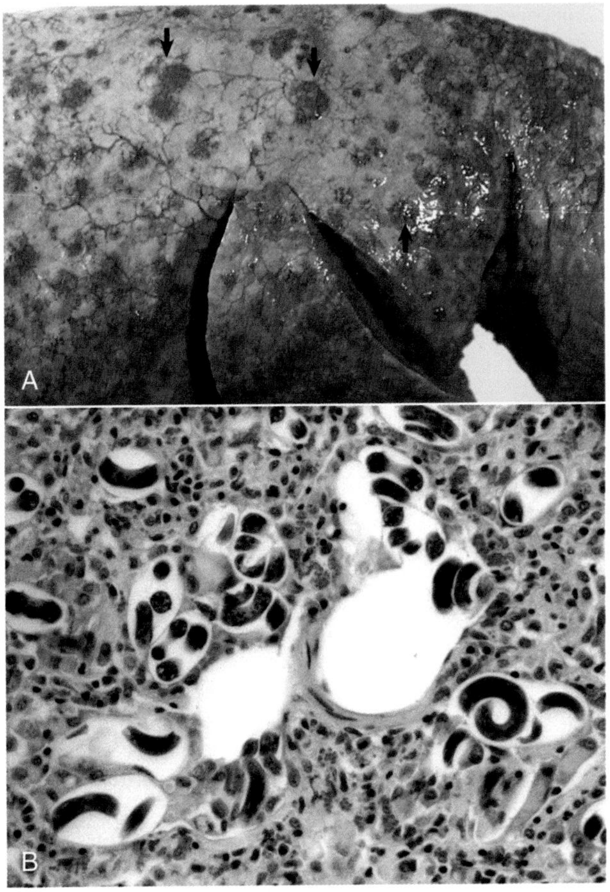

Figure 9-95 Multifocal Granulomatous Pneumonia, Lungworm (*Muellerius* spp.), Lungs, Sheep. A, Multiple gray-red nodules (granulomas) (*arrows*) are scattered throughout the pulmonary parenchyma. On palpation, the lungs have a nodular texture. **B,** Coiled larvae of *Muellerius* spp. in the lung. Note also mononuclear cells extending into the surrounding pulmonary interstitium. H&E stain. (**A** courtesy Dr. J. Edwards, Texas A&M University, Olafson Short Course, Cornell Veterinary Medicine. **B** courtesy Dr. A. López, Atlantic Veterinary College.)

subpleural alveoli where the adults, eggs, and coiled larvae reside (Fig. 9-95, *B*). Clinical signs are usually not apparent.

Goats differ from sheep by having diffuse interstitial rather than focal lesions, and the reaction to the parasites seen microscopically varies from almost no lesions to a severe interstitial pneumonia with heavy infiltrates of mononuclear cells in alveolar walls resembling CAE or mycoplasmal infections. Secondary effects of *Muellerius capillaris* infection in sheep and goats include decreased weight gain and possibly secondary bacterial infections.

Protostrongylus rufescens. *Protostrongylus rufescens* is a worldwide parasite of sheep, goats, and wild ruminants. It requires an intermediate snail as a host. Infection is usually subclinical, but *Protostrongylus rufescens* can be pathogenic for lambs and goat kids and can cause anorexia, diarrhea, weight loss, and mucopurulent nasal discharge. The adult parasite lives in bronchioles as *Dictyocaulus* spp., but it causes pulmonary nodules similar to those of *Muellerius capillaris*.

Pneumonias of Pigs

Porcine pneumonias are unequivocally a major obstacle for the contemporary swine industry. The incidence, prevalence, and mortality rates of pneumonias in pigs depend on a series of complex, multifactorial interactions. Among the most commonly recognized elements linked to porcine pneumonias are the following:

- Host (age, genetic makeup, immune status)
- Infectious agents (viruses, bacteria)
- Environmental determinants (humidity, temperature, ammonia concentrations)
- Management practices (crowding, mixing of animals, air quality, nutrition, stress)

Because of the nature of these multifactorial interactions, it will become obvious in the following paragraphs that more often than not a specific type of pneumonia frequently progresses to or coexists with another. The term *porcine respiratory disease complex* (PRDC) has been introduced in clinical practice to describe pigs with signs of respiratory infection involving combined bacterial and viral infections. Commonly implicated microbes include porcine reproductive and respiratory syndrome virus (PRRSV), swine influenza virus (SIV), porcine circovirus 2 (PCV2), porcine respiratory coronavirus (PRCoV), *Mycoplasma hyopneumoniae*, and *Pasteurella multocida*.

Viral Pneumonias

Swine Influenza (Swine Flu). Swine influenza is a highly contagious acute respiratory viral disease of swine that is caused by swine influenza virus (SIV), a type A influenza virus of the family Orthomyxoviridae. It is generally accepted that swine influenza resulted from adaptation of the type A influenza virus that caused the human influenza pandemic during World War I. The most common subtypes of SIV currently circulating in pigs are H1N1, H1N2, and H3N2. Swine influenza is enzootic worldwide and is known to infect human beings who are in close contact with sick pigs. In 2009, an outbreak of swine-human influenza (H1N1), presumably transmitted from pigs to human beings, emerged in Mexico and rapidly spread to many countries throughout the world. This new "pandemic" was attributed to a triple-reassortant of influenza A virus containing gene segments of swine, Eurasian avian, and human strains. Human infection with this novel strain affected mainly children and young adults, as well as individuals of any age with an underlying debilitating condition.

Transmission between influenza-infected and susceptible pigs occurs mainly by aerosol or oral route. SIV attaches to and replicates within epithelial cells of the upper respiratory tract; the infection of epithelial cells spreads rapidly throughout the nasal, tracheal, and bronchial mucosa, with the more severe outbreaks reflecting more involvement of intrapulmonary airways and secondary infection with *Pasteurella multocida*, *Trueperella* (*Arcanobacterium*) *pyogenes*, or *Haemophilus* spp. Although uncommon, human beings infected with swine influenza (H1N1) can transmit the virus to pigs; therefore it is important that veterinarians or workers with influenza-like illness stay away from pig farms. Natural transmission of H1N1 and H5N1 from human beings to ferrets (*Mustela putorius furo*) and from human beings to cats and dogs has also been reported.

Pulmonary lesions caused by influenza virus alone are rarely seen in the postmortem room because this disease has a very low mortality rate unless complicated with secondary bacterial infections. Grossly, a copious catarrhal to mucopurulent inflammation extends from the nasal passages to the bronchioles, with the volume of mucus being sufficient to plug small airways and cause a lobular or multilobular atelectasis in the cranioventral regions of the lungs. The appearance can be similar grossly, although not microscopically, to that of *Mycoplasma hyopneumoniae*. Fatal cases have severe alveolar and interstitial pulmonary edema. Microscopically, the lesions in uncomplicated cases are typical of a virus-induced, necrotizing bronchitis-bronchiolitis, which in severe cases extends into the alveoli as bronchointerstitial pneumonia. It is characterized by necrosis of the bronchial/bronchiolar epithelium, thickening and infiltration of the alveolar wall with mononuclear cells and aggregates of macrophages, neutrophils, mucus, and some necrotic cells within the alveolar lumen. If these changes are extensive enough, the lumen of bronchioles can be occluded by exudate, causing lobular atelectasis. Viral antigen can be demonstrated in infected epithelial cells by immunoperoxidase techniques. In the later stages of alveolar inflammation, neutrophils are progressively replaced by intraalveolar macrophages, unless the pneumonia is complicated by secondary bacterial infections. Recent serologic surveys indicate that infection is also prevalent in wild pigs.

Clinically, a sudden onset of fever, nasal discharge, stiffness, labored breathing, weakness or even prostration, followed by painful and often paroxysmal coughing, is seen in animals of all age groups and may affect most of the herd. The outbreak subsides virtually without mortality within 1 or 2 weeks; the clinical appearance is much more alarming than the pathologic changes, unless the pigs have secondary infection with bacteria. Infection can be confirmed using PCR in secretions collected with nasal swabs. The most important effect of most outbreaks of influenza is severe weight loss, but pregnant sows may abort or give birth to weak piglets.

Porcine Reproductive and Respiratory Syndrome. A disease originally named *mystery swine disease* was first recognized in the United States in 1987. In 1990, it was seen in Europe, and the disease now occurs worldwide in most major pig-raising countries. In 1991, Dutch investigators isolated a virus as the etiologic agent; porcine reproductive and respiratory syndrome virus (PRRSV) is currently classified in the genus *Arterivirus* of the family Arteriviridae.

As its name implies, PRRS is characterized by late-term abortions and stillbirths and respiratory problems. The respiratory form is generally seen in nursery and grow/finish pigs. The pathogenesis has not been completely elucidated, but it is presumed that there is a mucosal portal of entry with virus replication in macrophages of the lymphoid tissue, followed by viremia and finally dissemination of infected macrophages to the lungs and other organs, such as the thymus, liver (Kupffer cells), spleen, lymph nodes, and intestine. The pulmonary alveolar and intravascular macrophages are the major targets for PRRS virus, which induces apoptosis of these cells. The virus also downregulates the innate immune response by inhibiting interferons and deregulates the adaptive immune response, thus interfering with the normal defense mechanisms predisposing pigs to septicemia and bacterial pneumonia. The most common opportunistic organisms are *Streptococcus suis*, *Salmonella* Cholerae-suis, *Mycoplasma hyopneumoniae*, *Haemophilus parasuis*, *Bordetella bronchiseptica*, *Pasteurella multocida*, and *Pneumocystis carinii*. Dual viral infections with PRRSV and porcine circovirus 2 (PCV2), SIV, and porcine respiratory coronavirus (PRCoV) are commonly found in pigs, and such coinfections increase the severity of disease.

On postmortem examination, pulmonary lesions vary from very mild changes characterized by failure of the lung to collapse when the thorax is opened and the presence of rib imprints (see Fig. 9-74) to severe changes manifested by consolidation of the lung in cases that have been complicated with bacterial pneumonia. Tracheobronchial and mediastinal lymph nodes are typically enlarged. Microscopically, pulmonary changes are those of interstitial pneumonia characterized by thickening of alveolar walls by infiltrating macrophages and lymphocytes and mild hyperplasia of type II pneumonocytes. Necrotic cells are scattered in the alveolar lumens. Unlike some other viral infections, bronchiolar epithelium does not appear to be affected. Diagnosis of PRRS in tissue collected at necropsy can be confirmed by immunohistochemistry and PCR techniques. Infected pigs may become carriers and transmit the infection through body fluids and semen. Clinically, PRRS in nursery and young growing animals is characterized by sneezing, fever, anorexia, dyspnea, cough, and occasional death. Some piglets develop severe cyanosis of the abdomen and ears, which explains why this syndrome was named *blue ear disease* when first described in Europe.

Porcine Circovirus-Associated Disease. Another emerging porcine syndrome, characterized clinically by progressive emaciation in weaned pigs, was originally described in the 1990s in Canada, the United States, and Europe. Since then, it has disseminated to many countries, causing economic devastation in pig farms worldwide. Because of the clinical signs and lesions in many organs, this syndrome was named *postweaning multisystemic wasting syndrome* (PMWS). Porcine circovirus 2 (PCV2) has been incriminated as the etiologic agent and is a member of the Circoviridae family. PCV2 has been associated with a number of syndromes in pigs, including systemic PCV2 infection (the preferred term for PMWS because it may also affect mature pigs), PCV2-associated pneumonia, PCV2-associated enteritis, porcine dermatitis and nephropathy syndrome (PDNS), PCV2-associated reproductive failure, and, most recently, PCV2-associated cerebellar vasculitis. The diseases caused by PCV2 are now collectively known as porcine circovirus-associated disease (PCVAD); the most common manifestations are systemic PCV2 infection (PMWS) and PCV2-associated pneumonia as part of the porcine respiratory disease complex. All of these manifestations affect more than one organ, and there is substantial overlap between the syndromes.

At necropsy, pigs with systemic PCV2 infection (PMWS) and PCV2-associated pneumonia are often in poor body condition, and the most remarkable changes, not considering other possible secondary infections, are enlargement of the superficial and visceral lymph nodes and a mild interstitial pneumonia characterized by failure of the lungs to collapse when the thorax is opened. Jaundice is occasionally observed. Microscopically, the lymphoid tissues show lymphoid depletion, histiocytic replacement of follicles, and notable proliferation of parafollicular histiocytes, some of which fuse and form syncytial cells (granulomatous lymphadenitis); necrosis of the lymphoid follicles is seen less often. In some cases, large basophilic inclusion bodies are present singly or as grapelike clusters (botryoid inclusions) within the cytoplasm of macrophages, particularly in Peyer's patches, spleen, and lymph nodes (E-Fig. 9-22). Similar inclusions are occasionally seen in bronchial glandular and renal epithelial cells. The lungs show thickening of the alveolar walls because of hyperplasia of type II pneumonocytes and interstitial infiltrates of mononuclear cells, peribronchiolar fibrous hyperplasia, and necrotizing bronchitis/bronchiolitis. Circovirus can be confirmed in affected tissue by immunohistochemical or PCR techniques.

Dual infections with PCV2 and PRRSV frequently occur in pigs, and secondary infections with *Pneumocystis carinii* are commonly seen in pigs with this coinfection. Characteristically, alveoli are filled with a distinctive foamy exudate that contains the organism, which is not visible in H&E-stained sections but is easily demonstrated with Gomori's methenamine silver stain (see Fig. 9-20). In human beings, *Pneumocystis* (*carinii*) *jirovecii* pneumonia (pneumocystosis) is one of the most common and often fatal complications in AIDS patients. As in AIDS patients, abnormal populations of $CD4^+$ and $CD8^+$ T lymphocytes have been incriminated as the underlying mechanism leading to pneumocystosis in foals and pigs.

Nipah Virus. Nipah virus belongs to the Paramyxoviridae family and shares a genus (*Henipavirus*) with the closely related Hendra virus (see section on Pneumonias of Horses). Another emerging zoonotic disease, Nipah virus caused a major epidemic with significant human mortality in Southeast Asia in 1998 and 1999. People handling pigs were primarily affected. Similar to Hendra virus, fruit bats (flying foxes) act as natural reservoir and are involved in the transmission to pigs by poorly understood mechanisms. In pigs, this virus infects the respiratory system resulting in pneumonia with syncytial cells occurring in the vascular endothelium and in the respiratory epithelium at all levels of the lung. Disease is spread to human beings via the respiratory route. Human-to-human transmission of this virus has been reported in more recent outbreaks.

Other Viral Pneumonias of Pigs. Porcine respiratory coronavirus (PRCoV) is sporadically incriminated in pneumonia in pigs. This viral pneumonia is generally mild, and most pigs fully recover if the pneumonia is not complicated with other infections. Lesions in the lung are those of bronchointerstitial pneumonia with necrotizing bronchiolitis. Interestingly, infections with porcine and other respiratory coronaviruses have been used to investigate the pathogenesis of severe acute respiratory syndrome (SARS), an emerging and highly contagious condition in human beings that is attributed to a novel human coronavirus (SARS-CoV). The relationship between SARS-CoV and animal coronavirus is still under investigation.

Other viruses rarely incriminated in porcine respiratory disease complex (PRDC) include paramyxovirus, encephalomyocarditis virus, hemagglutinating encephalomyocarditis virus, and adenovirus. Petechial hemorrhages in the lung and pulmonary edema may be seen with African swine fever, classical swine fever, and pseudorabies virus infections.

Bacterial Pneumonias

Porcine Enzootic Pneumonia. Porcine enzootic pneumonia, a highly contagious disease of pigs caused by *Mycoplasma hyopneumoniae*, is grossly characterized by suppurative or catarrhal bronchopneumonia (Fig. 9-96 and E-Fig. 9-23). When its worldwide prevalence and deleterious effect on feed conversion are taken into account, this disease is probably the most economically significant respiratory disease of pigs. Although an infectious disease, it is very much influenced by immune status and management factors, such as crowding (airspace and floor space), ventilation (air exchange rate), concentrations of noxious gases in the air (ammonia and hydrogen sulfide), relative humidity, temperature fluctuations, and mixing of stock from various sources. It has been demonstrated with

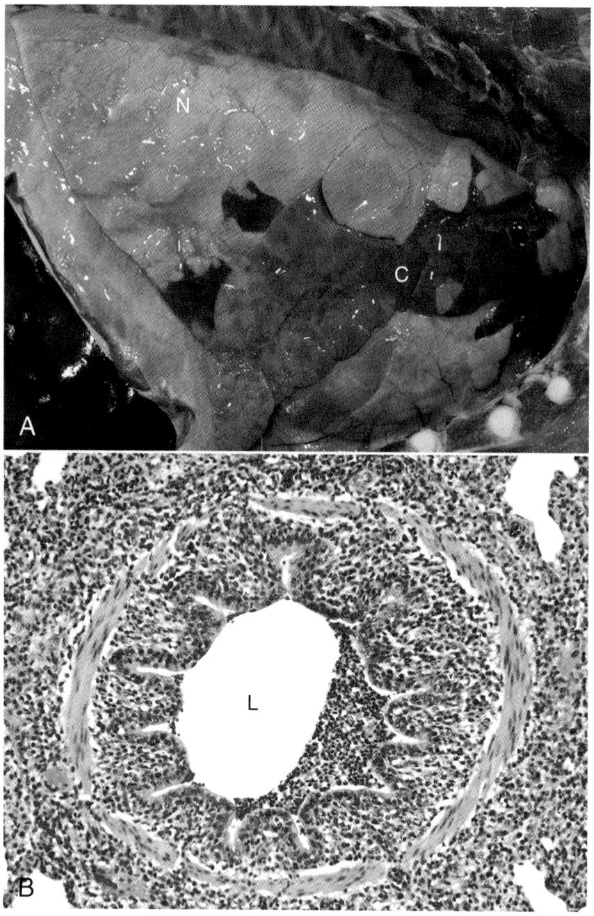

Figure 9-96 Chronic-Active (Suppurative) Bronchopneumonia (Enzootic Pneumonia), *Mycoplasma hyopneumoniae*, Lung, Pig. A, Cranioventral consolidation of 40% to 50% of the pulmonary parenchyma. Consolidated lung *(C)* is firm, and the outlines of the lobules are accentuated by edema of the interlobular septa. *N*, Normal lung. **B,** Lymphocytes and histiocytes infiltrate the bronchiolar lamina propria and peribronchiolar and alveolar interstitium. The bronchiolar lumen also contains neutrophils and erythrocytes. *L*, lumen of the affected bronchiole. H&E stain. (Courtesy Dr. A. López, Atlantic Veterinary College.)

PCR that *Mycoplasma hyopneumoniae* is present in the air of infected farms.

The causative agent, *Mycoplasma hyopneumoniae*, is a fastidious organism and very difficult to grow; thus the final diagnosis is frequently based on interpretation of lesions alone or supported by ancillary tests to detect this mycoplasma in affected lungs by immunohistochemistry, immunofluorescence, or PCR. The bronchopneumonic lesions of porcine enzootic pneumonia are in most cases mild to moderate, and thus mortality is low unless complicated with secondary pathogens, such as *Pasteurella multocida, Trueperella (Arcanobacterium) pyogenes, Bordetella bronchiseptica, Haemophilus* spp., *Mycoplasma hyorhinis*, and other mycoplasmas and ureaplasmas. Although the pathogenesis of porcine enzootic pneumonia is not completely elucidated, it is known that *Mycoplasma hyopneumoniae* first adheres to the cilia of the bronchi by means of a unique adhesive protein, produces ciliostasis, and finally colonizes the respiratory system by firmly attaching to the ciliated epithelial cells of the trachea and the bronchi of the cranioventral regions of the lungs. Once attached to the respiratory epithelium, it provokes an influx of neutrophils into the tracheobronchial mucosa; causes extensive loss of cilia (deciliation); stimulates an intense hyperplasia of lymphocytes in the BALT; and attracts mononuclear cells into the peribronchial, bronchiolar, and alveolar interstitium. Additional virulence factors include the ability of *Mycoplasma hyopneumoniae* to cause immunosuppression, reduce the phagocytic activity of neutrophils in the lung, and change the chemical composition of mucus. All of these functional alterations can predispose the lung to secondary bacterial infections.

The lesions caused by *Mycoplasma hyopneumoniae* start as a bronchointerstitial pneumonia and progress to a suppurative or mucopurulent bronchopneumonia once secondary pathogens are involved (commonly seen at necropsy). In most pigs, gross lesions affect only portions of the cranial lobes, but in more severely affected pigs, lesions involve 50% or more of the cranioventral portions of the lungs (see Fig. 9-96). The affected lungs are dark red in the early stages but have a homogeneous pale-gray ("fish flesh") appearance in the more chronic stages of the disease. On cut surface, exudate can easily be expressed from airways, and depending on the stage of the lesions and secondary infections, the exudate varies from purulent to mucopurulent to mucoid. Microscopic lesions are characterized by an influx of macrophages and neutrophils into the bronchi, bronchioles, and alveoli, and with time there is also notable BALT hyperplasia (see Fig. 9-96, *B*). In some cases, accumulation of exudate can be severe enough to cause occlusion of bronchioles and atelectasis of the corresponding lobules. The suppurative bronchopneumonia may be accompanied by a mild fibrinous pleuritis, which is often more severe if other organisms, such as *Mycoplasma hyorhinis, Pasteurella multocida*, or *Actinobacillus pleuropneumoniae*, are also involved. Abscesses and fibrous pleural adhesions are sequelae of chronic complicated infections.

Clinically, enzootic pneumonia occurs as a herd problem in two disease forms. A newly acquired infection of a previously clean herd causes disease in all age groups, resulting in acute respiratory distress and low mortality. In a chronically infected herd, the mature animals are immune and clinical signs are usually apparent only in growing pigs at times of particular stress such as at weaning. In such herds, coughing and reduced rate of weight gain are the most notable signs.

Porcine Pasteurellosis. Porcine pasteurellosis is an infectious disease complex with unclear pathogenesis that includes primary infections by *Pasteurella multocida* alone (primary pasteurellosis) or, more frequently, after the defense mechanisms are impaired and a secondary bacterium colonizes the lung (porcine pneumonic pasteurellosis). In rare cases, *Pasteurella multocida* causes acutely fatal septicemias in pigs (primary septicemic pasteurellosis). It is important to remember that *Pasteurella multocida* serotypes A and D are both part of the normal nasal flora and are also causative agents of bronchopneumonia, pleuritis, and atrophic rhinitis in pigs.

Pasteurella multocida is one of the most common secondary pathogens isolated from the lungs of pigs with swine influenza virus (SIV), porcine reproductive and respiratory syndrome virus (PRRSV), porcine circovirus 2 (PCV2), pseudorabies (SuHV-1), classical swine fever (hog cholera), enzootic pneumonia, and porcine pleuropneumonia. Secondary infections with *Pasteurella multocida* notably change the early and mild bronchointerstitial reaction of enzootic and viral pneumonias into a severe suppurative bronchopneumonia with multiple abscesses and sometimes pleuritis. The other important role of *Pasteurella multocida* in porcine pneumonias is as a cause of a fulminating, cranioventral, fibrinous bronchopneumonia (pleuropneumonia) after influenza virus infection or stress from inadequate ventilation resulting in high levels of ammonia in the air. The nature of the lesion and the predisposing factors of poor management or coexisting viral infections suggest that fulminating porcine pasteurellosis has a pathogenesis similar to that of pneumonic mannheimiosis of cattle. Pharyngitis with subcutaneous cervical edema, fibrinohemorrhagic polyarthritis, and focal lymphocytic interstitial nephritis are also present in porcine pneumonic pasteurellosis. Sequelae of porcine pneumonic pasteurellosis include fibrous pleuritis and pericarditis, pulmonary abscesses, so-called sequestra, and usually death. In contrast to ruminants, *Mannheimia haemolytica* is not a respiratory pathogen for pigs, but in some instances, it can cause abortion in sows.

Porcine Pleuropneumonia. Porcine pleuropneumonia is a highly contagious, worldwide disease of pigs caused by *Actinobacillus (Haemophilus) pleuropneumoniae* (APP), which is characterized by a severe, often fatal, fibrinous bronchopneumonia with extensive pleuritis (pleuropneumonia). Survivors generally develop notable residual lesions and become carriers of the organisms. Porcine pleuropneumonia is an increasingly important cause of acute and chronic pneumonias, particularly in intensively raised pigs (2 to 5 months old). Transmission of *Actinobacillus pleuropneumoniae* occurs by the respiratory route, and the disease can be reproduced experimentally by intranasal inoculation of the bacterium. Considered a primary pathogen, *Actinobacillus pleuropneumoniae* can sporadically produce septicemia in young pigs and otitis media and otitis interna with vestibular syndrome in weaned pigs. Two biovars and 15 serotypes of the organism have been identified; all serotypes can cause the disease, but differences in virulence exist. The pathogenesis is not yet well understood, but specific virulence factors, such as RTX toxins (hemolytic/cytolytic toxins Apx I to Apx IV), capsular factors, fimbriae and adhesins, lipopolysaccharide, and permeability factors have been identified. These factors allow *Actinobacillus pleuropneumoniae* to attach to cells; produce pores in cell membranes; damage capillaries and alveolar walls, resulting in vascular leakage and thrombosis; impair phagocytic function; and elicit failure of clearance mechanisms.

The gross lesions in the acute form consist of a fibrinous bronchopneumonia characterized by severe consolidation and a fibrinous exudate on the pleural surface. Although all lobes can be affected, a common site is the dorsal area of the caudal lobes. In fact, a large area of fibrinous pleuropneumonia involving the caudal lobe of a pig's lung is considered almost diagnostic for this disease (Fig. 9-97). On cut surface, consolidated lungs have notably dilated interlobular septa and irregular but well-circumscribed areas of necrosis caused by potent cytotoxins produced by *Actinobacillus pleuropneumoniae*. Except for the distribution, pulmonary lesions of porcine pleuropneumonia are identical to those of pneumonic mannheimiosis of cattle. The microscopic lesions are also very similar and include areas of coagulative necrosis surrounded by a thick cluster of "streaming (oat-shaped/oat cell) leukocytes" and notable distention of the interlobular septa because of severe edema and lymphatic thrombosis. Bronchioles and alveoli are filled with edematous fluid, fibrin, neutrophils, and few macrophages (see Fig. 9-97). Pigs with the chronic form have multiple pulmonary abscesses and large (2 to 10 cm) pieces of necrotic lung encapsulated by connective tissue (sequestra)—changes frequently seen in slaughterhouses.

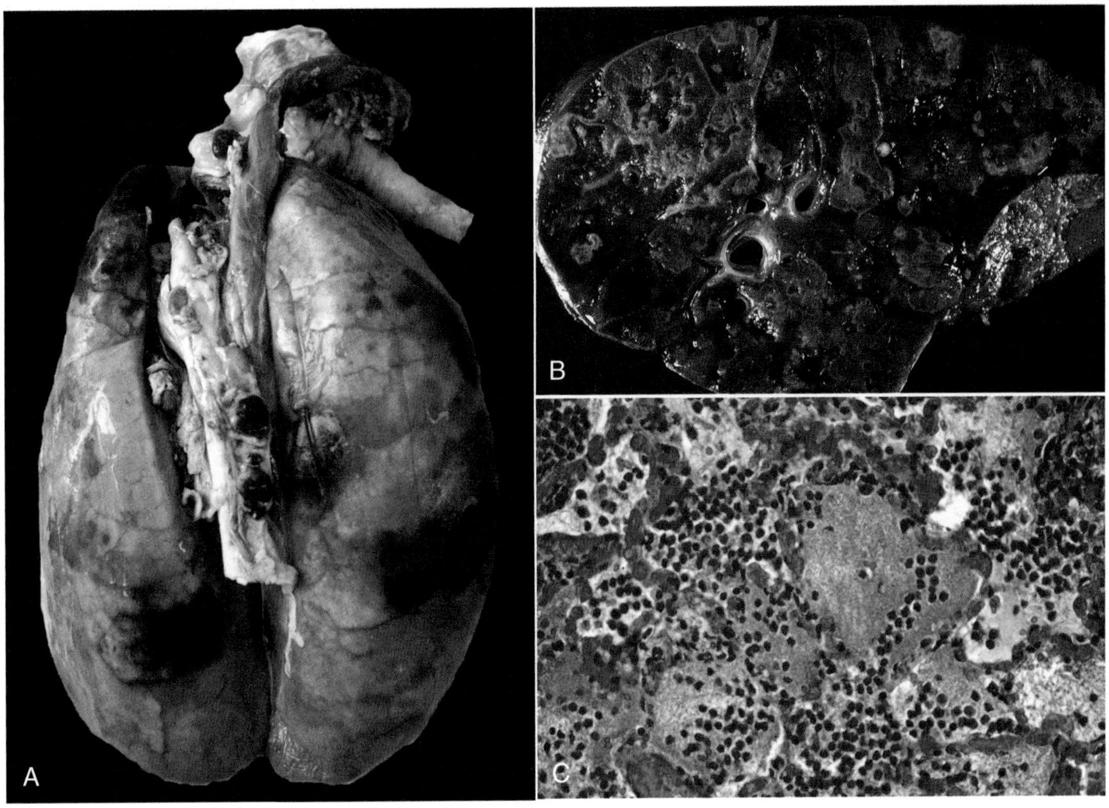

Figure 9-97 **Porcine Pleuropneumonia (*Actinobacillus pleuropneumoniae*), Lung, Pig. A,** In peracute porcine pleuropneumonia, the red to dark red pneumonic lesions are locally extensive in the dorsal aspects of the caudal lung lobes. There is lobular congestion, consolidation, and interlobular edema. As the disease progresses and becomes acute to subacute, the lesions expand in size and severity. **B,** The cut surface has numerous discrete and coalescing zones of lobular inflammation and necrosis (*upper left*), which are pale pink to white and often surrounded by a white margin (inflammation). There is extensive congestion (active hyperemia) and hemorrhage throughout the section. **C,** Alveoli are filled with fibrin, edema fluid, and neutrophils. Capillaries in alveolar septa are congested (active hyperemia), and in many cases, there is necrosis of alveolar septa (not visible at this magnification). (**A** courtesy Facultad de Medicina Veterinaria y Zootecnia, Universidad Nacional Autónoma de México. **B** and **C** courtesy Dr. A.R. Doster, University of Nebraska; and Noah's Arkive, College of Veterinary Medicine, The University of Georgia.)

Clinically, porcine pleuropneumonia can vary from an acute form with unexpected death and blood-stained froth at the nostrils and mouth to a subacute form characterized by coughing and dyspnea accompanied by clinical signs of sepsis such as high fever, hypoxemia, anorexia, and lethargy (E-Fig. 9-24). A chronic form is characterized by decreased growth rate and persistent cough. Animals that survive often carry the organism in the tonsils, shed the organism, and infect susceptible pigs.

Haemophilus Pneumonia. In addition to Glasser's disease characterized by polyserositis (pericarditis, pleuritis, peritonitis, polyarthritis, and meningitis) (E-Fig. 9-25), some serotypes of *Haemophilus parasuis* (originally *Haemophilus influenzae suis*) can also cause suppurative bronchopneumonia that in severe cases can be fatal. The causal organism, *Haemophilus parasuis*, is usually carried in the nasopharynx of normal pigs and requires abnormal circumstances such as those following stress (weaning and cold weather) or viral infections (swine influenza or PCV2). Specific pathogen-free (SPF) pigs seem to be particularly susceptible to Glasser's disease (arthritis and serositis) but not to pulmonary infection (bronchopneumonia).

Streptococcal Pneumonia. *Streptococcus suis* is a common cause of porcine disease worldwide and a serious zoonosis capable of causing death by septic shock or meningitis and residual deafness in butchers, veterinarians, and pig farmers. Typically, *Streptococcus suis* gains entrance to the susceptible young pig through the oropharyngeal mucosa and is carried in the tonsils, nasal mucosa, and mandibular lymph nodes of healthy animals, particularly in survivors of an outbreak. Infected sows can abort or vertically transmit the infection to their offspring. Some serotypes of *Streptococcus suis* cause neonatal septicemia, and this can result in suppurative meningitis, otitis, arthritis, polyserositis, myocarditis, valvular endocarditis, and embolic pneumonia (Fig. 9-98). Other serotypes of *Streptococcus suis* can reach the lung by the aerogenous route and cause a suppurative bronchopneumonia, in combination with *Pasteurella multocida*, *Escherichia coli*, or *Mycoplasma hyopneumoniae*, or in combination with *Actinobacillus pleuropneumoniae*, which causes a fibrinous bronchopneumonia. Coinfections of *Streptococcus suis* with PCV2 and PRRSV are also frequently seen in some farms.

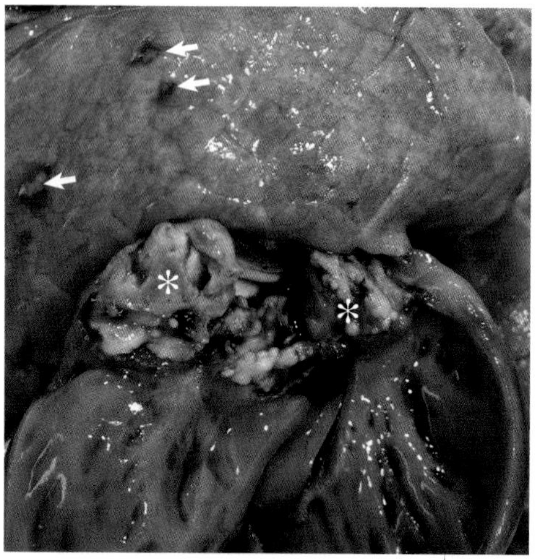

Figure 9-98 **Vegetative Endocarditis, Heart and Multiple Embolic Lesions, Lung, Pig.** Note the large vegetative (cauliflower-like) mass attached to the tricuspid valve *(asterisks)*. The lung *(top half of figure)* shows multifocal well-circumscribed nodules *(arrows)*, the result of emboli being released from the tricuspid valve. (Courtesy Dr. A. López, Atlantic Veterinary College.)

Tuberculosis. Tuberculosis is an important disease in domestic and wild pigs that has a much greater prevalence in pigs than in cattle or other domestic mammals in many countries. Porcine tuberculosis is attributed to infection with *Mycobacterium bovis* and porcine mycobacteriosis to infection with *Mycobacterium avium* complex. A common scenario in small mixed-farming operations is the diagnosis of avian tuberculosis at the time that pigs are slaughtered, and the source is ingestion of tuberculous chickens or contaminated litter. As would be expected, granulomas are found in the mesenteric, mandibular, and retropharyngeal lymph nodes; to a lesser extent in the intestine, liver, and spleen; and only in rare cases in the lung. The route of infection in pulmonary tuberculosis and mycobacteriosis of pigs is most often hematogenous after oral exposure and intestinal infection. Lung lesions are those of a granulomatous pneumonia. The microscopic lesions are basically those of tubercles (granulomas), but the degree of encapsulation, caseation, and calcification varies with the type of mycobacterium, age of the lesion, and host immune response.

Other Bacterial Pneumonias of Pigs. Septicemias in pigs often cause petechial hemorrhages in the lung and pulmonary edema. Salmonellae, *Escherichia coli*, and *Listeria monocytogenes* can cause severe interstitial pneumonia in very young animals. *Salmonella* Choleraesuis causes a necrotizing fibrinous pneumonia similar to porcine pleuropneumonia, and *Salmonella* Typhisuis causes a chronic suppurative bronchopneumonia. In high health herds, *Actinobacillus suis* may cause fibrinohemorrhagic pleuropneumonia and is easily confused with porcine pleuropneumonia.

Parasitic Pneumonias of Pigs

Metastrongylosis. *Metastrongylus apri* (*elongatus*), *Metastrongylus salmi*, and *Metastrongylus pudendotectus* (lungworms) of domestic and feral pigs occur throughout most of the world and require earthworms as intermediate hosts for transmission. The incidence of disease has therefore decreased with development of confinement housing. The importance of pig lungworms is mainly because infection results in growth retardation of the host. Clinical signs include coughing because of parasitic bronchitis.

The gross lesions, when noticeable, consist of small gray nodules, particularly along the ventral borders of the caudal lobes. The adult worms are grossly visible in bronchi, and microscopically, the parasites cause a catarrhal bronchitis with infiltration of eosinophils and lobular atelectasis (Fig. 9-99).

Ascaris suum. The larvae of *Ascaris suum* can cause edema, focal subpleural hemorrhages, and interstitial inflammation (see Fig. 9-77). Along their larval migration tracts, hemorrhages also occur in the liver and, after fibrosis, become the large white "milk spots" seen so frequently as incidental findings at necropsy. It has been reported that *Ascaris suum* may cause immunosuppression in severely affected pigs. Pigs can be killed if exposed to an overwhelming larval migration.

Other Causes of Pneumonia. Foreign body granulomatous pneumonia occurs frequently in pigs after inhalation of vegetable material (starch pneumonia), presumably from dusty (nonpelleted) feed. Lesions are clinically silent but are often mistaken for other pneumonic processes during inspection at slaughterhouses. Microscopically, pulmonary changes are typical of foreign body granulomatous inflammation in which variably sized feed particles are surrounded by macrophages and neutrophils, and often have been phagocytosed by multinucleated giant cells. Feed (vegetable) particles appear as thick-walled polygonal cells that stain positive with PAS because of their rich carbohydrate (starch) content (see E-Fig. 9-12).

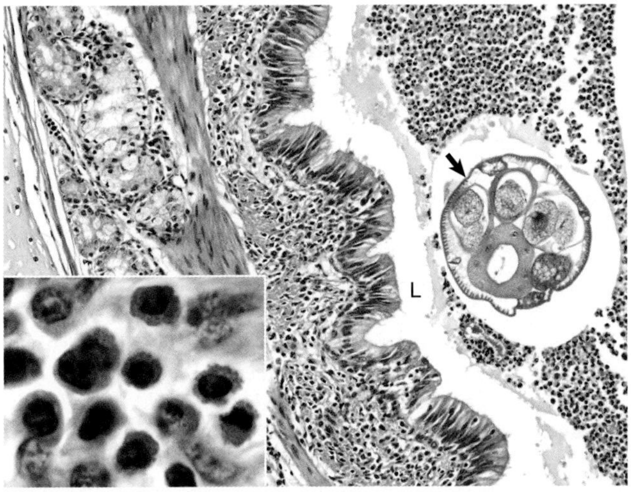

Figure 9-99 **Acute Verminous Bronchitis (*Metastrongylus apri*), Bronchus, Cross Section, Pig.** Cross section of a nematode (*Metastrongylus apri*) *(arrow)* admixed with mucus, neutrophils, and eosinophils (not visible at this magnification) within the lumen *(L)* of the bronchus. H&E stain. *Inset,* Eosinophils with distinct red granules infiltrate the lamina propria. H&E stain. (Courtesy Dr. S. Martinson and Dr. A. Lopez, Atlantic Veterinary College.)

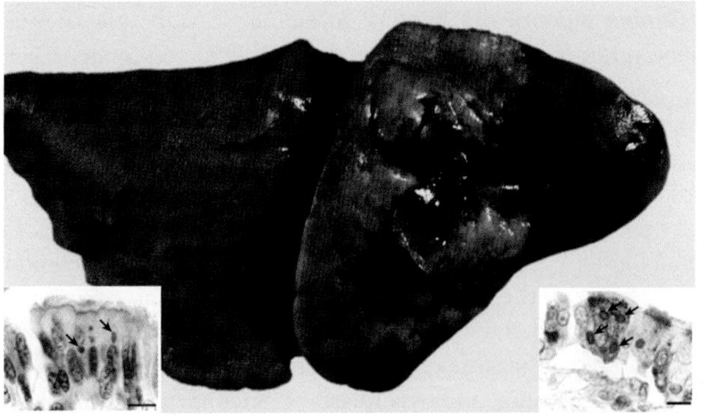

Figure 9-100 **Interstitial Pneumonia, Canine Distemper, Lungs, Dog.** The lungs are heavy, edematous, and rubbery, with costal (rib) imprints on the pleural surface. *Inset, left,* Bronchial epithelial cells contain intracytoplasmic eosinophilic inclusion bodies *(arrows)*. H&E stain. *Inset, right,* Immunohistochemistry revealing canine Morbillivirus antigen *(arrows)* in the cytoplasm and apical borders of bronchial epithelial cells. Immunoperoxidase stain. Bars = 20 μm. (From Berrocal A, López A: *J Vet Diagn Invest* 15:292-294, 2003.)

Pneumonias of Dogs

In general, inflammatory diseases of the lungs are less of a problem in dogs than in food-producing species and can be subdivided in two major groups, infectious and noninfectious pneumonias. "*Canine infectious respiratory disease*" (CIRD) is the term currently used by clinicians to describe a heterogeneous group of respiratory infections in dogs; these diseases were previously clustered under the name of infectious tracheobronchitis or "kennel cough." CIRD is the canine counterpart of BRD and PRD complexes in cattle and pigs, respectively. The most common viruses in CIRD include canine parainfluenza virus (CPIV), canid herpesvirus 1 (CaHV-1), canine adenovirus-2 (CAV-2), canine respiratory coronavirus (CRCoV), canine distemper virus (CDV), and canine influenza virus (CIV). *Bordetella bronchiseptica, Streptococcus equi* ssp. *zooepidemicus*, and *Mycoplasma* spp. are the most frequent bacterial isolates in CIRD. It has been recently recognized that animal shelters are an important source of viral and bacterial infections for dogs and cats. Uremia and paraquat toxicity are perhaps the two most notable noninfectious causes of canine respiratory disease.

Viral Pneumonias

Canine Distemper. Canine distemper is an important and ubiquitous infectious disease of dogs, other Canidae, wild Felidae, Mustelidae, and marine mammals throughout the world. It is caused by a Morbillivirus that is antigenically related to the human measles, rinderpest (officially eradicated in 2011), "peste de petit ruminants," and phocine distemper viruses. Canine distemper virus (CDV) is transmitted to susceptible puppies through infected body fluids. The virus invades through the upper respiratory tract and conjunctiva, proliferates in regional lymph nodes, becomes viremic, and in dogs with an inadequate antibody response, infects nearly all body tissues (pantropic), particularly the epithelial cells. Distemper virus hampers the immune response, downregulates cytokine production, and persists for a long time in some tissues. CDV can target the lungs either directly as a viral pneumonia or indirectly by its immunosuppressive effects rendering the lungs susceptible to secondary bacterial and protozoal infections, or as a coinfection with other viruses such as canine adenovirus-2 and canid herpesvirus 1.

Gross lesions in the acute stages include serous to catarrhal to mucopurulent nasopharyngitis and conjunctivitis. The lungs are edematous and have a diffuse interstitial pneumonia (Fig. 9-100) microscopically characterized by necrotizing bronchiolitis, necrosis and exfoliation of pneumonocytes, mild alveolar edema, and, several hours later, thickening of the alveolar walls because of interstitial mononuclear cell infiltrates and hyperplasia of type II pneumonocytes. Secondary infections with *Bordetella bronchiseptica* and mycoplasmas are common and induce life-threatening suppurative bronchopneumonia. The thymus may be small relative to the age of the animal because of viral-induced lymphocytolysis.

Microscopically, eosinophilic inclusions are present in the epithelial cells of many tissues, in the nuclei or cytoplasm, or in both (see Fig. 9-100). They appear early in the bronchiolar epithelium but are most prominent in the epithelium of the lung, stomach, renal pelvis, and urinary bladder, making these tissues good choices for diagnostic examination. Viral inclusions are rarely seen in the later stages of this disease. The suppurative secondary bronchopneumonias often hinder the detection of viral lesions in the lung, particularly because bronchiolar cells containing inclusion bodies exfoliate and mix with the neutrophils recruited by the bacterial infection. Distemper virus antigens can be readily demonstrated in infected cells by the immunoperoxidase technique (see Fig. 9-100), which can also be used in skin biopsies for the antemortem diagnosis of canine distemper.

Distemper virus also has a tendency to affect developing tooth buds and ameloblasts, causing enamel hypoplasia in dogs that recover from infection. Of all distemper lesions, demyelinating encephalomyelitis, which develops late, is the most devastating (see Chapter 14). Sequelae to distemper include the nervous and pneumonic complications mentioned previously and various systemic infections, such as toxoplasmosis and sarcocystosis, because of depressed immunity. Persistent viral infection occurs in some dogs that survive the disease, and they may become carriers and the source of infection for other susceptible animals.

Clinical signs consist of biphasic fever, diarrhea, vomiting, weight loss, mucopurulent oculonasal discharge, coughing, respiratory distress, and possible loss of vision. Weeks later, hyperkeratosis of the foot pads ("hard pad") and the nose are observed, along with nervous signs, including ataxia, paralysis, convulsions, or residual myoclonus (muscle twitches, tremors, and "tics").

Canine Adenovirus Type 2 Infection. CAV-2 infection is a common but transient contagious disease of the respiratory tract of dogs, causing mild fever, oculonasal discharge, coughing, and poor weight gain. The portal of entry is generally by inhalation of infected aerosols followed by viral replication in the surface cells of the upper respiratory tract, mucous cells of the trachea and bronchi, nonciliated bronchiolar epithelial cells, and type II pneumonocytes. Pulmonary lesions are initially those of bronchointerstitial pneumonia, with necrosis and exfoliation of bronchiolar and alveolar epithelium, edema, and, a few days later, proliferation of type II pneumonocytes, mild infiltration of neutrophils and lymphocytes in the alveolar interstitium, and hyperplastic bronchitis and bronchiolitis. Large basophilic intranuclear viral inclusions are typically seen in bronchiolar and alveolar cells (Fig. 9-101). Infection with CAV-2 is clinically mild unless complicated with a secondary bacterial infection or coinfections with other viruses such as distemper virus. Experimental work suggests CAV-2 reinfection may lead to hyperreactive airways, a nonspecific condition in which the bronchial mucosa becomes highly "responsive" to irritation such as that caused by cold air, gases, or cigarette smoke. However, it is not clear if this outcome is true in natural infections.

Canid Herpesvirus 1. Canid herpesvirus 1 (CaHV-1) can cause fatal systemic disease in newborn puppies and is probably a contributing factor in "fading puppy syndrome." Hypothermia has been suggested as a pivotal component in the pathogenesis of fatal infections in puppies. Many dogs are seropositive, suggesting that transient or subclinical infections are more common than realized; the virus remains latent in the trigeminal and other ganglia and can be reactivated after stress, resulting in asymptomatic transmission of CaHV-1 virus to offspring via the placenta, thus resulting in abortion or stillbirths. In puppies, CaHV-1 causes ulcerative tracheitis, interstitial pneumonia (E-Fig. 9-26), and focal necrosis and inflammation in the kidneys, liver, and brain. Eosinophilic intranuclear inclusion bodies occur within epithelial cells in early lesions. CaHV-1 has also been identified as a cause of ulcerative keratoconjunctivitis in older dogs.

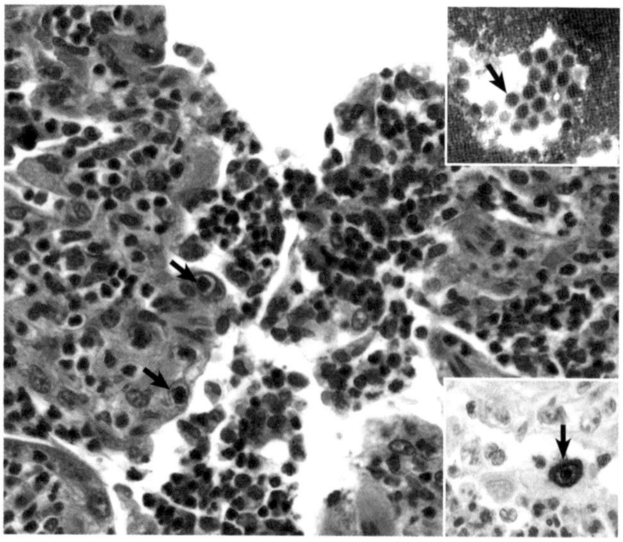

Figure 9-101 **Necrotizing Bronchiolitis, Canine Adenovirus-2, Puppy.** Note necrosis and exfoliation of bronchiolar epithelial cells and the neutrophilic infiltrates in the mucosa and bronchiolar lumen. Large basophilic inclusion bodies are present in nuclei of some bronchiolar cells *(arrows)*. H&E stain. *Inset top right corner,* Paracrystalline arrays of electron dense particles typical of adenovirus *(arrow)* in a transmission electron photomicrograph. Uranyl acetate and lead citrate stain. *Inset, right bottom corner,* Immunopositive staining for CAV-2 antigen *(arrow)*. Immunoperoxidase stain. (From Rodríguez LE, Ramírez-Romero R, Valdez-Nava Y, et al: *Can Vet J* 48:632-634, 2007.)

Canine Influenza (Canine Flu). Canine influenza is an emerging contagious respiratory infection of dogs that was first described in the United States and subsequently in other countries. It has a high morbidity (close to 100%), but the mortality, as with most other influenza infections, is relatively low (less than 8%). This disease, first diagnosed in greyhounds, is caused by a novel influenza-A virus (canine influenza virus or CIV), a mutation from a previously recognized H3N8 strain of equine influenza virus. Dog-to-dog transmission does occur and therefore this infection must be distinguished from other viruses of the canine infectious respiratory disease (CIRD) group. Pulmonary lesions are generally mild and transient, but infected dogs are susceptible to secondary bacterial bronchopneumonia. The most relevant lesions in dogs dying unexpectedly from canine influenza are pleural and pulmonary hemorrhages. Microscopically, there is necrotizing tracheitis, bronchitis, and bronchiolitis with exudation of neutrophils and macrophages. In severe cases, hemorrhagic interstitial or bronchointerstitial pneumonia may be accompanied by vasculitis and thrombosis. Influenza antigen can be demonstrated by immunohistochemistry in airway epithelium and alveolar macrophages. Clinically, dogs with canine influenza are lethargic, inappetent, and hyperthermic and frequently cough and show nasal discharge. These signs resemble those seen in dogs with kennel cough or secondary bacterial pneumonia. In addition, there are confirmed cases of canine influenza caused by the porcine H1N1 presumably transmitted from infected pet owners.

Bacterial Pneumonias. Dogs generally develop bacterial pneumonias when the pulmonary defense mechanisms have been impaired. *Pasteurella multocida, Streptococcus* spp., *Escherichia coli, Klebsiella pneumoniae,* and *Bordetella bronchiseptica* can be involved in pneumonia secondary to distemper or after aspiration of gastric contents (Fig. 9-102 and E-Fig. 9-27). *Streptococcus zooepidemicus* can cause acute and fatal hemorrhagic pleuropneumonia with

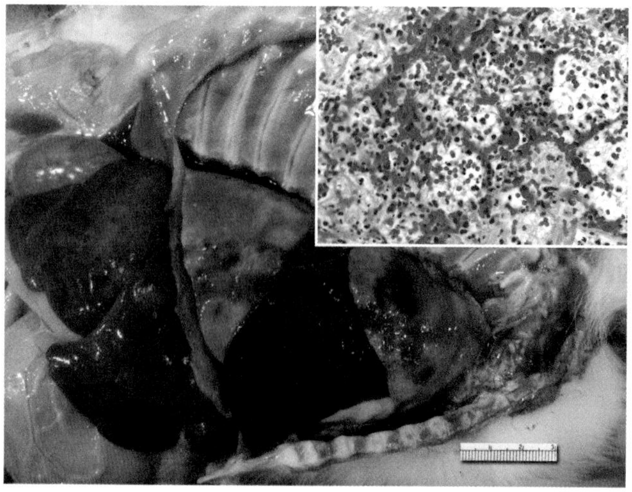

Figure 9-102 **Aspiration Pneumonia, Bronchopneumonia, Right Lung, Dog.** Acute to subacute bronchopneumonia. The right middle lung lobe and portions of the cranial and caudal lung lobes are dark red and consolidated. Aspiration pneumonia starts as an acute necrotizing bronchitis and bronchiolitis caused by aspiration of irritant materials such as gastric acid or a caustic material administered by mouth. Acute lesions caused by caustic damage are hemorrhagic and necrotizing. *Inset,* Alveolar spaces filled with erythrocytes, fibrin, and inflammatory infiltrates. (Courtesy Dr. A. López, Atlantic Veterinary College.)

hemorrhagic pleural effusion in dogs. Death is generally a consequence of severe sepsis and septic shock or from β-hemolytic streptococcal bacteremia causing emboli in the lungs, liver, brain, and lymph nodes. The primary source of the infection cannot be determined in most cases. Dental disease in dogs may be a source of systemic and pulmonary infection, a concept well-recognized in human medicine for many years. The role of mycoplasmas in canine pneumonia is still uncertain because these organisms are frequently isolated from normal nasopharyngeal flora.

Tuberculosis is uncommon in dogs because these animals appear to be quite resistant to infection; most cases occur in immunocompromised dogs or in dogs living with infected human beings. Dogs are susceptible to the infection with *Mycobacterium tuberculosis*, *Mycobacterium bovis*, and *Mycobacterium avium* complex, and therefore canine infection presupposes contact with human or animal tuberculosis. The clinicopathologic manifestation is pulmonary after inhalation or alimentary after oral exposure, but in most cases infection is disseminated to lymph nodes and visceral organs. The gross lesions are multifocal, firm nodules with necrotic centers, most often seen in the lungs, lymph nodes, kidneys, and liver. Diffuse granulomatous pleuritis and pericarditis with copious serofibrinous or sanguineous effusion are common. Microscopically, granulomas are formed by closely packed macrophages but with very little connective tissue.

Mycotic Pneumonias. Mycotic pneumonias are serious diseases seen commonly in animals in some regions. There are two main types: those caused by opportunistic fungi and those caused by a group of fungi associated with systemic "deep" mycoses. All of these fungi affect human beings and most domestic animals but are probably not transmitted between species.

Aspergillosis. Opportunistic fungi, such as *Aspergillus* spp. (particularly *Aspergillus fumigatus*), are important in birds, but in domestic animals, they mainly affect immunosuppressed individuals or those on prolonged antibiotic therapy. The pulmonary lesion is a multifocal, nodular, pyogranulomatous, or granulomatous pneumonia. Microscopically, there is necrosis and infiltrates of neutrophils, macrophages, and lymphocytes, with proliferation of fibroblasts eventually leading to encapsulation of the granuloma. Fungal hyphae are generally visible in the core of the lesion and in the walls of blood vessels.

Systemic Mycoses (Dimorphic Fungal Infections). Systemic (deep) mycoses are caused by *Blastomyces dermatitidis*, *Histoplasma capsulatum*, *Coccidioides immitis*, and *Cryptococcus neoformans*/*Cryptococcus gatti* (see Fig. 9-35). Blastomycosis mainly affects dogs and is discussed here, whereas cryptococcosis is discussed in the section on Pneumonias of Cats. In contrast to other fungi, such as *Aspergillus* spp., organisms of the systemic mycosis group are all primary pathogens of human beings and animals and thus do not necessarily require a preceding immunosuppression to cause disease. These fungi have virulence factors that favor hematogenous dissemination and evasion of immune and phagocytic responses. Systemic dissemination is often exacerbated by the administration of immunosuppressant drugs such as corticosteroids. These fungi are usually detected by cytological evaluation of affected tissues.

Blastomycosis. Blastomycosis occurs in many countries of the North American continent, Africa, the Middle East, and occasionally in Europe. In the United States, it is most prevalent in the Atlantic, St. Lawrence, and Ohio-Mississippi River Valley states, compared with the Mountain-Pacific region. *Blastomyces dermatitidis* is a dimorphic fungus (mycelia-yeast) seen mainly in young dogs and occasionally in cats and horses. This fungus is present in the soil, and inhalation of spores is considered the principal route of infection; thus it most frequently affects outdoor and hunting dogs. From the lung, infection is disseminated hematogenously to other organs, mainly bone, skin, brain, and eyes.

Pulmonary lesions are characterized by multifocal to coalescing pyogranulomatous pneumonia, generally with firm nodules scattered throughout the lungs (Fig. 9-103). Microscopically, nodules are pyogranulomas with numerous macrophages (epithelioid cells), some neutrophils, multinucleated giant cells, and thick-walled yeasts (see Fig. 9-35, C). Yeasts are 5 to 25 μm in diameter and are much better visualized when they are stained with PAS reaction or Gomori's methenamine silver stain. Nodules can also be present in other tissues, chiefly lymph nodes, skin, spleen, liver, kidneys, bones, testes, prostate, and eyes. This fungus can be easily identified in properly prepared and stained transtracheal washes or lymph node aspirates.

Clinical signs can reflect involvement of virtually any body tissue; pulmonary effects include cough, decreased exercise tolerance, and terminal respiratory distress.

Coccidioidomycosis. Coccidioidomycosis (San Joaquin Valley fever), caused by the dimorphic fungus *Coccidioides immitis*, occurs mainly in animals living in arid regions of the southwestern United States, Mexico, and Central and South America. It is a primary respiratory tract (aerogenous) infection commonly seen at slaughterhouses in clinically normal feedlot cattle. In dogs, coccidioidomycosis also has an aerogenous portal of entry and then

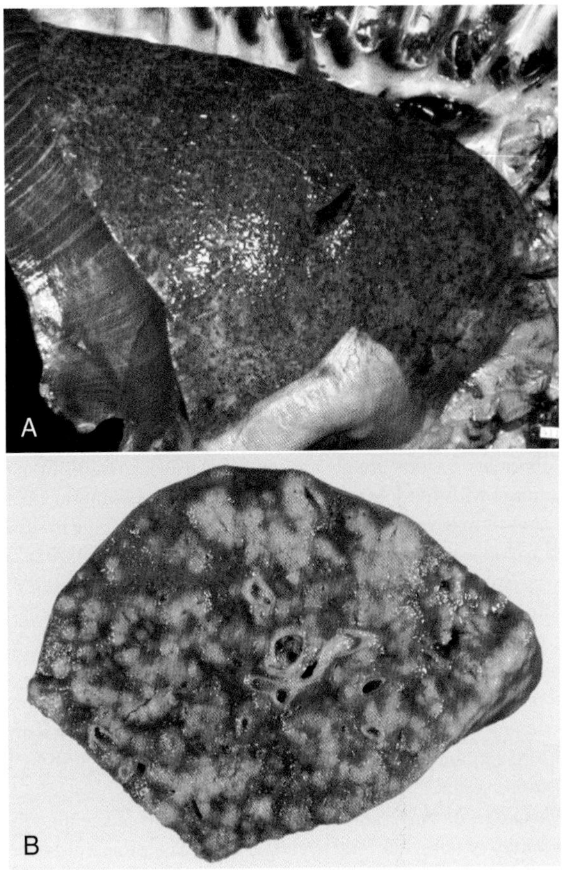

Figure 9-103 Granulomatous Pneumonia, Blastomycosis (*Blastomyces dermatitidis*), Right Lung, Dog. A, The lung contains large numbers of small granulomas distributed throughout all pulmonary lobes. **B,** The cut surface of the lung shows multiple discrete and coalescing gray-white granulomas distributed randomly throughout the lung. (**A** courtesy Ontario Veterinary College. **B** courtesy College of Veterinary Medicine, University of Illinois.)

disseminates systemically to other organs. Clinical signs relate to the location of lesions, so there can be respiratory distress, lameness, generalized lymphadenopathy, or cutaneous lesions, among others.

The lesions caused by *Coccidioides immitis* consist of focal granulomas or pyogranulomas that can have suppurative or caseated centers. The fungal organisms are readily seen in histologic or cytologic preparation as large (10 to 80 μm in diameter), double-walled, and highly refractile spherules containing numerous endospores (see Fig. 9-35, *D*).

Histoplasmosis. Histoplasmosis is a systemic infection that results from inhalation and, in dogs, possibly ingestion of another dimorphic fungus, *Histoplasma capsulatum*. Histoplasmosis occurs sporadically in dogs and human beings and, to a lesser extent, in cats and horses. Bats often eliminate *Histoplasma capsulatum* in the feces, and droppings from bats and birds, particularly pigeons, heavily promote the growth and survival of this fungus in the soil of enzootic areas.

Pulmonary lesions are grossly characterized by variably sized, firm, poorly encapsulated granulomas and, sometimes, more diffuse involvement of the lungs. Microscopically, granulomatous lesions typically have many macrophages filled with small (1 to 3 μm), punctiform, intracytoplasmic, dark oval bodies (yeasts) (see Fig. 9-35, *A*) that are best demonstrated with PAS reaction or Gomori's methenamine silver stain. Similar nodules or diffuse involvement can be present in other tissues, chiefly lymph nodes, spleen, intestine, and liver.

Parasitic Pneumonias

Toxoplasmosis. Toxoplasmosis is a worldwide disease caused by the obligate intracellular, protozoal parasite *Toxoplasma gondii*. Cats and other Felidae are the definitive hosts in which the mature parasite divides sexually in the intestinal mucosa. Human beings, dogs, cats, and many wild mammals can become intermediate hosts after accidental ingestion of fertile oocysts shed in cat feces or ingestion of undercooked or raw meat containing tissue cysts, and fetuses can be infected transplacentally from an infected dam. In most instances, the parasite infects many cells of different tissues and induces an antibody response (seropositive animals) but does not cause clinical disease. Toxoplasmosis is often triggered by immunosuppression, such as that caused by canine distemper virus. Toxoplasmosis is characterized by focal necrosis around the protozoan.

Pulmonary lesions are severe, multifocal necrotizing interstitial pneumonia with notable proliferation of type II pneumonocytes and infiltrates of macrophages and neutrophils. Other lesions in disseminated toxoplasmosis include multifocal necrotizing hepatitis, myocarditis, splenitis, myositis, encephalitis, and ophthalmitis. The parasites appear microscopically as small (3 to 6 μm) basophilic cysts that can be found free in affected tissues or within the cytoplasm of many epithelial cells and macrophages (see E-Fig. 8-8). Similar findings can be seen sporadically in dogs infected with *Neospora caninum* and *Sarcocystis canis*, and immunohistochemistry would be required to differentiate those protozoal organisms from *Toxoplasma gondii*.

Filaroides hirthi. *Filaroides hirthi*, a lungworm of the alveoli and bronchioles of dogs, has long been known as a cause of mild subclinical infection in large colonies of beagle dogs in the United States. However, it can on occasion cause severe and even fatal disease in individual pets, presumably as a result of immunosuppression. Clinical signs may include coughing and terminal respiratory distress. Grossly, the lesions are multifocal subpleural nodules, often with a green hue because of eosinophils, scattered throughout the lungs. Microscopically, these nodules are eosinophilic granulomas arising from the alveolar interstitium associated with larvae or dead worms because little reaction develops to the live adults.

Crenosoma vulpis. *Crenosoma vulpis* is a lungworm seen commonly in foxes and sporadically in dogs with access to the intermediate hosts—slugs and snails. The adult lungworms live in small bronchi and bronchioles in the caudal lobes, causing eosinophilic and catarrhal bronchitis manifested grossly as gray areas of inflammation and atelectasis. In some animals, *Crenosoma vulpis* causes bronchiolar goblet cell metaplasia and mucous obstruction, resulting in lobular atelectasis due to the valve effect of the mucous plug.

Eucoleus aerophilus. *Eucoleus aerophilus* (*Capillaria aerophila*) is a nematode parasite typically found in the trachea and bronchi of wild and domestic carnivores. In some cases, this parasite may also involve the nasal passages and sinuses. Although generally asymptomatic, some dogs cough because of the local irritation caused by the parasites on the tracheal or bronchial mucosa.

Paragonimus spp. *Paragonimus kellicotti* in North America and *Paragonimus westermani* in Asia are generally asymptomatic fluke infections in fish-eating species. The life cycle involves two intermediate hosts, the first a freshwater snail and the second a freshwater crab or crayfish; in North America, cats and dogs acquire infection by eating crayfish. Gross lesions include pleural hemorrhages where the metacercariae migrate into the lungs. Later, multifocal eosinophilic pleuritis, and subpleural cysts up to 7 mm long containing pairs of adult flukes, are found along with eosinophilic granulomas around clusters of eggs. Like many other parasitic pneumonias, lesions and scars are more frequent in the caudal lobes. Pneumothorax can occur if a cyst that communicates with an airway ruptures to the pleural surface.

Other Parasitic Infections. *Angiostrongylus vasorum* and *Dirofilaria immitis* are parasites of the pulmonary arteries and right ventricle and, depending on the stage, can produce different forms of pulmonary lesions. Adult parasites can cause chronic arteritis that leads to pulmonary hypertension, pulmonary arterial thrombosis, interstitial (eosinophilic) granulomatous pneumonia, pulmonary interstitial fibrosis, congestive right-sided cardiac failure, and eventually caudal vena caval syndrome. Other lesions include pleural petechial hemorrhages and, in later stages, diffuse pulmonary hemosiderosis and multifocal pulmonary infarcts. Larvae and eggs also cause alveolar injury, thickening of the alveolar walls with eosinophils and lymphocytes (interstitial pneumonia), and multifocal or coalescing granulomas with giant cells (parasitic granulomas). *Pneumocystis carinii* has been reported as a sporadic cause of chronic interstitial pneumonia in dogs with a compromised immune system (see Pneumonias of Horses; also see Fig. 9-20).

Aspiration Pneumonia. Aspiration pneumonia is an important form of pneumonia that occurs in dogs when vomit or regurgitated materials are aspirated into the lungs, or when drugs or radiographic contrast media are accidentally introduced into the airways (E-Fig. 9-28). As in other animal species, aspiration pneumonia may be unilateral or may more often affect the right cranial lobe (Fig. 9-104). The severity of lesions depends very much on the chemical and microbiologic composition of the aspirated material. In general, aspiration in monogastric animals, particularly in dogs and cats, is more severe because of the low pH of the gastric contents (chemical pneumonitis). In severe cases, dogs and cats die rapidly from septic shock and ARDS (see Fig. 9-63), which is microscopically characterized by diffuse alveolar damage, protein-rich pulmonary edema, neutrophilic alveolitis, and formation of typical hyaline membranes along the alveolar walls (see Fig. 9-104). In animals that survive the acute stages of aspiration, pulmonary lesions progress to bronchopneumonia. Aspiration pneumonia is a common sequela to

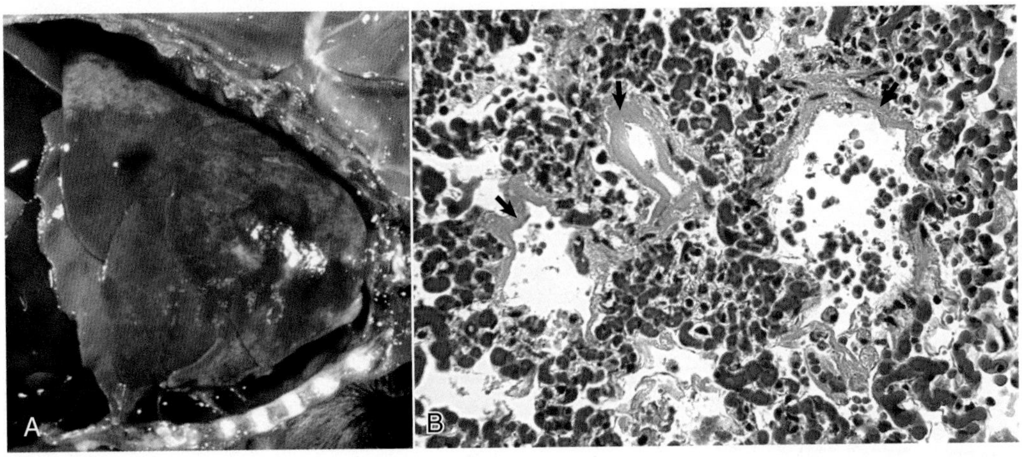

Figure 9-104 **Acute Hemorrhagic Bronchopneumonia, Acute Respiratory Distress Syndrome (ARDS), Lungs, 4-Week-Old Puppy (Also See** Fig. 9-63**). A,** Note that the lungs did not collapse when the thorax was opened (loss of negative pressure) and as a result fill almost the entire thoracic cavity. The cranioventral aspects of the lung are consolidated with hemorrhage. **B,** Alveolar capillary congestion, thick hyaline membranes along the alveolar septa *(arrows)*, and intraalveolar hemorrhage. These microscopic changes are typical of the diffuse alveolar damage seen in lungs with ARDS. H&E stain. (Courtesy Dr. A. López, Atlantic Veterinary College.)

cleft palate, and in dogs with megaesophagus secondary to either myasthenia gravis or persistent right aortic arch. It is also an important complication of general anesthesia or neurologic diseases affecting laryngeal function.

Toxic Pneumonias

Paraquat. Paraquat, a broad-spectrum herbicide widely used in gardening and agriculture, can cause severe and often fatal toxic interstitial pneumonia (pneumonitis) in dogs, cats, human beings, and other species. After ingestion or inhalation, this herbicide selectively accumulates in the lung where paraquat toxic metabolites are produced by Club (Clara) cells. These metabolites promote local release of free radicals in the lung, which causes extensive injury to Club cells and to the blood-air barrier, presumably through lipid peroxidation of type I and II pneumonocytes and alveolar endothelial cells (see Fig. 9-89). Paraquat toxicity has been used experimentally as a model of oxidant-induced alveolar injury and pulmonary fibrosis. Soon after poisoning, the lungs are heavy, edematous, and hemorrhagic because of extensive necrosis of epithelial and endothelial cells in the alveolar walls. The lungs of animals that survive acute paraquat toxicosis are pale, fail to collapse when the thorax is opened, and have interstitial emphysema, bullous emphysema, and occasionally pneumomediastinum. Microscopic findings in the acute and subacute phases include necrosis of type I pneumonocytes, interstitial and alveolar edema, intraalveolar hemorrhages, and proliferation of type II pneumonocytes. In the chronic stages (4 to 8 weeks later), the lesions are typically characterized by severe interstitial and intraalveolar fibrosis.

Uremic Pneumopathy. Uremic pneumonopathy (pneumonitis) is one of the many extrarenal lesions seen in dogs with chronic uremia. Lesions are characterized by a combination of pulmonary edema and calcification of vascular smooth muscle and alveolar basement membranes. In severe cases, alveolar calcification prevents lung collapse when the thorax is opened. In the more advanced cases, the lungs appear diffusely distended, pale red or brown in color, and show a rough pleural surface with rib imprints (see Fig. 9-51). On palpation, the pulmonary parenchyma has a typical "gritty" texture because of mineralization of the alveolar and vascular walls, which are best visualized microscopically by using special stains such as von Kossa (see Fig. 9-51). Because this is not primarily an inflammatory lesion, the term *pneumonitis* should not be used.

Other Pneumonias. *Idiopathic pulmonary fibrosis* is a rare condition of uncertain etiology reported in the West Highland white terrier breed that shares similarities with human and feline idiopathic pulmonary fibrosis. Microscopically, there is diffuse interstitial pneumonia and progressive alveolar fibrosis with capillary obliteration, hyperplasia of type II cells, some of which exhibit cellular atypia, and finally hypertrophy and hyperplasia of smooth muscle. The interstitial fibrosis eventually spills over alveolar spaces causing conspicuous intraalveolar fibrosis.

Pneumonias of Cats

Although upper respiratory tract infections are common and important in cats, pneumonias are uncommon except when there is immunosuppression or aspiration of gastric contents. Viral infections such as feline rhinotracheitis and calicivirus may cause lesions in the lungs, but unless there is secondary invasion by bacteria, they do not usually cause a fatal pneumonia.

Viral Pneumonias

Feline Rhinotracheitis. Feline rhinotracheitis is an important viral disease of cats caused by the ubiquitous felid herpesvirus 1 (FeHV-1). This infection affects primarily young or debilitated cats causing inflammation in the nasal, ocular, and tracheal mucosa and, to a much lesser extent, the lung (see Species-Specific Diseases of the Nasal Cavity and Paranasal Sinuses). When lungs are affected, FeHV-1 causes bronchointerstitial pneumonia with necrosis of bronchiolar and alveolar epithelium, thickening of the alveolar walls, and extensive permeability edema. Eosinophilic intranuclear inclusion bodies may be seen in infected epithelial cells early in infection.

Feline Calicivirus. Feline calicivirus (FCV) causes upper respiratory disease, stomatitis, conjunctivitis, and, to a lesser extent, interstitial pneumonia. Microscopically, affected lungs exhibit the typical pattern of bronchointerstitial pneumonia with necrotizing bronchiolitis, thickening of alveolar walls, occasionally hyaline membranes, hyperplasia of type II pneumonocytes, and macrophages admixed with cellular debris in the alveolar lumens. Because pulmonary lesions are similar to those caused by FeHV-1, isolation or in situ detection is required for final diagnosis.

Feline Infectious Peritonitis. Feline infectious peritonitis (FIP) is caused by FIP virus (FIPV), a mutated form of feline enteric coronavirus (FECV), and is one of a few viral infections of domestic animals that result in pyogranulomatous pneumonia. This disease is microscopically characterized by a vasculitis affecting many tissues and organs (Fig. 9-105).

Other Viral Pneumonias. Other viruses sporadically incriminated in feline interstitial pneumonia are cowpox virus (CPXV) and influenza A H1N1.

Bacterial Pneumonias

Pasteurellae. Bacteria from the nasal flora such as *Pasteurella multocida* and *Pasteurella*-like organisms are occasionally associated with secondary bronchopneumonia in cats (Fig. 9-106). *Pasteurella multocida* also causes otitis media and meningitis, but its role as a respiratory pathogen is mainly associated with pyothorax. Interestingly, there are reports of *Pasteurella multocida* pneumonia in older or immunosuppressed human beings acquired through contact with domestic cats.

Mycoplasmas. Mycoplasmas are often isolated from the lungs of cats with pulmonary lesions but are not definitively established as primary pathogens in feline pneumonias.

Feline Pneumonitis. The term *feline pneumonitis* is a misnomer because the major lesions caused by *Chlamydophila felis* (formerly *Chlamydia psittaci*) are severe conjunctivitis and rhinitis (see Species-Specific Diseases of the Nasal Cavity and Paranasal Sinuses). The elucidation of the importance of feline viral rhinotracheitis and feline calicivirus has removed *Chlamydophila felis* from its previously overstated importance as a lung pathogen.

Tuberculosis. Cats are susceptible to three types of mycobacterial infections: classic tuberculosis, feline leprosy, and atypical mycobacteriosis. Classic tuberculosis in cats is rare and generally caused by *Mycobacterium bovis* and *Mycobacterium microti* but also, to a lesser extent, by *Mycobacterium tuberculosis*. Nosocomial tuberculosis (*Mycobacterium bovis*) in cats has been reported with increased frequency. The usual route of infection for feline tuberculosis is oral, through infected rodents/meat or unpasteurized milk, so the granulomatous lesions are mainly in the intestine and mesenteric lymph nodes where they may disseminate through infected phagocytes to other organs. The solid and noncaseated appearance of tuberculous nodules is grossly similar to that of neoplasms, so they must be differentiated from pulmonary neoplasms (e.g., lymphoma). Classic tuberculosis with dermal lesions in cats should be differentiated from feline leprosy (localized skin granulomas) caused by *Mycobacterium lepraemurium* and other nonculturable species of acid-fast bacilli. Atypical mycobacteriosis is caused by contamination of a skin wound with saprophytic and nonsaprophytic mycobacteria such as those of the *Mycobacterium avium* complex. Advances in PCR techniques have notably reduced the time required for etiologic diagnosis of mycobacteriosis in veterinary diagnostic laboratories.

Mycotic Pneumonias

Cryptococcosis. Cryptococcosis (pulmonary *Cryptococcus neoformans* or *Cryptococcus gatti*) is the most frequent systemic mycosis in cats, and lesions are akin to those discussed in the section on mycotic pneumonias of dogs. It occurs worldwide in all species but is diagnosed most frequently in cats, horses, dogs, and human beings. Some healthy dogs and cats harbor *Cryptococcus* in the nasal cavity and become asymptomatic carriers. Clinical infection may occur in immunocompetent cats and in cats that are immunologically compromised, such as by FeLV, FIV, malnutrition, or corticosteroid treatment. Lesions can occur in nearly any tissue, resulting in a wide

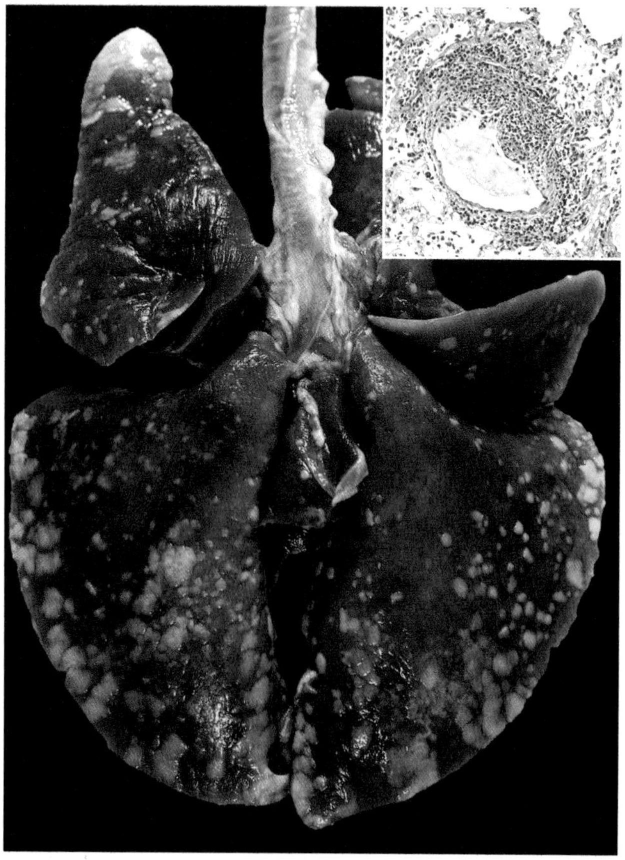

Figure 9-105 Feline Infectious Peritonitis, Granulomatous Pneumonia, Cat. Multifocal to coalescing granulomas scattered throughout all pulmonary lobes. *Inset,* Pulmonary vasculitis with transmural infiltrates of macrophages, neutrophils, and lymphocytes. H&E stain. (Courtesy Facultad de Medicina Veterinaria y Zootecnia, Universidad Nacional Autónoma de México. *Inset* courtesy Dr. A. López, Atlantic Veterinary College.)

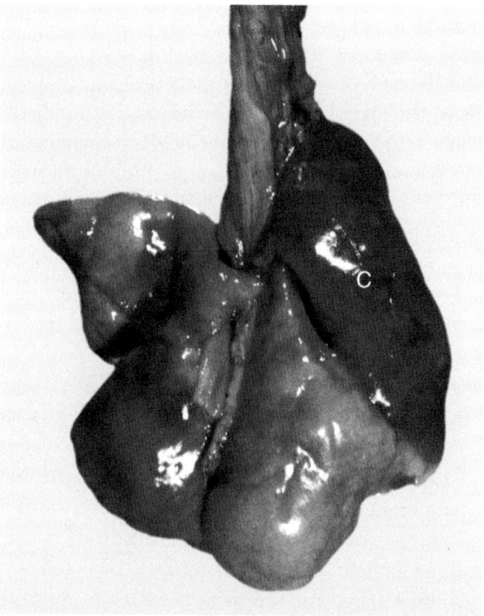

Figure 9-106 Fibrinopurulent Bronchopneumonia, Lungs, 5-Month-Old Kitten with History of Conjunctivitis, Rhinitis, and Bacterial Pneumonia. Cranioventral consolidation (C) of the right lung involves approximately 40% of its parenchyma. The consolidated lung is firm. (Courtesy Dr. S. McBurney, Atlantic Veterinary College.)

variety of clinical signs. However, granulomatous rhinitis, sinusitis, otitis media and interna, pneumonia, ulcerative dermatitis, and meningoencephalitis are most common.

The pulmonary lesion in cryptococcosis is a multifocal granulomatous pneumonia and, like those occurring in other internal organs, they are small, gelatinous, white foci. The gelatinous appearance is due to the broad mucous capsule around the yeast (see Fig. 9-35, *B*). Microscopically, lesions contain great numbers of fungal organisms (4 to 10 μm in diameter without the capsule) and only a few macrophages, lymphocytes, and multinucleated giant cells. This thick polysaccharide capsule does not stain well with H&E, and thus there is a large empty space or halo around the yeast.

Parasitic Pneumonias of Cats

Feline Lungworm. *Aelurostrongylus abstrusus*, known as *feline lungworm*, is a parasite that occurs in cats wherever the necessary slug and snail intermediate hosts are found. It can cause chronic respiratory disease with coughing and weight loss and, sometimes, severe dyspnea and death, particularly if there are secondary bacterial infections. The gross lesions are multifocal, amber, and subpleural granulomatous nodules up to 1 cm in diameter throughout the lungs. On incision, these nodules may contain viscous exudate. Microscopically, the adult parasites, eggs, and coiled larvae are in the bronchioles and alveoli, where they cause catarrhal bronchiolitis, hyperplasia of submucosal glands, and, later, granulomatous alveolitis, alveolar fibrosis, and fibromuscular hyperplasia (Fig. 9-107). During routine examination of feline lungs, it is quite common to find fibromuscular hyperplasia in bronchioles and arterioles in otherwise healthy cats. It was alleged in the past that this fibromuscular hyperplasia was a long-term sequela of subclinical infection with *Aelurostrongylus abstrusus*. However, this view has been challenged; thus the pathogenesis and significance of pulmonary fibromuscular hyperplasia in healthy cats remains uncertain. In severe cases, fibromuscular hyperplasia is grossly visible in the lungs as white subpleural nodules.

Other Parasitic Pneumonias. *Toxoplasma gondii*, *Paragonimus kellicotti*, and *Dirofilaria immitis* can also affect cats (see the section on Parasitic Pneumonias of Dogs). *Cytauxzoon felis* is an apicomplexan hemoparasite that affects domestic and wild Felidae. The organism infects erythrocytes in the erythrocytic stage of disease and multiplies in intravascular macrophages/monocytes, including those in the alveolar capillaries (E-Fig. 9-29), during the leukocytic stage of disease.

Aspiration Pneumonia. Aspiration pneumonias are common in cats as a result of vomiting, regurgitation, dysphagia, or anesthetic complication or after accidental administration of food, oral medicaments, or contrast media into the trachea (iatrogenic). Pulmonary lesions are similar to those described for dogs, and the type of lung lesion depends on the chemical and bacterial composition of the aspirated material (see the section on Aspiration Pneumonia of Dogs).

Other Pneumonias

Feline Idiopathic Pulmonary Fibrosis. Feline idiopathic pulmonary fibrosis is a rare, progressive, and fatal disease of cats of uncertain etiology characterized by multifocal fibrotic nodules subpleurally and randomly in the lung making the pleural surface resemble nodular cirrhosis of the liver (Fig. 9-108). Microscopically, the affected alveolar and peribronchiolar interstitium is thickened by excessive fibrosis, abundant deposition of extracellular matrix, and hypertrophy of smooth muscle. Some investigators suggest an intrinsic cellular defect in type II pneumonocytes as the underlying cause. The alveolar walls are diffusely lined by cuboidal hyperplastic type II pneumonocytes, and the alveolar lumens often contain exfoliated cells and necrotic debris. This feline condition has morphologic features similar to "equine multinodular pulmonary fibrosis" and "cryptogenic pulmonary fibrosis" in human beings.

Fetal and Perinatal Pneumonias

Fetal Pneumonias. Pneumonia is one of the most frequent lesions found in fetuses submitted for postmortem examination, particularly in foals and food-producing animals. Because of autolysis, lack of inflation, and the lungs being at various stages of development, fetal lesions are often missed or misdiagnosed. In the nonaerated fetal lung, the bronchoalveolar spaces are filled with a viscous, locally produced fluid known as *lung fluid* or *lung liquid*. It has been estimated that an ovine fetus produces approximately 2.5 mL of "lung fluid" per kilogram of body weight per hour. In the

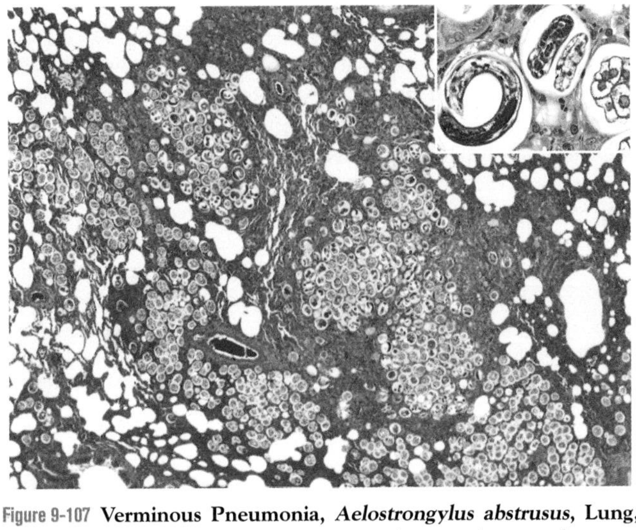

Figure 9-107 **Verminous Pneumonia, *Aelostrongylus abstrusus*, Lung, Cat.** Pulmonary nodules containing numerous larvae and eggs, and interstitial thickening due to fibrosis and smooth muscle hypertrophy of arteries and bronchioles. *Inset*, Coiled *Aelostrongylus* larvae. (Courtesy Dr. D.L. Dungworth and Dr. A. López, Atlantic Veterinary College.)

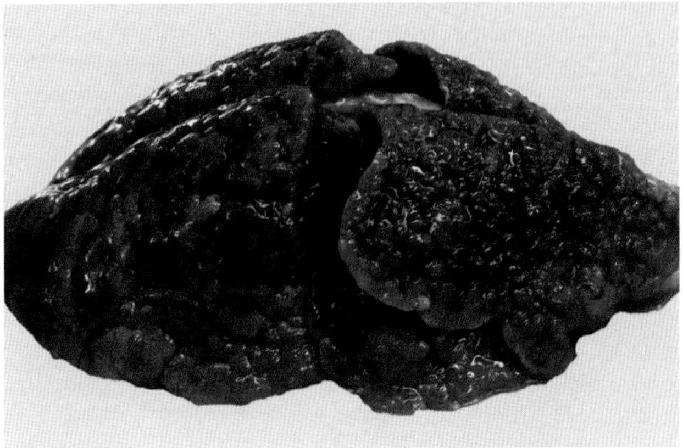

Figure 9-108 **Idiopathic Nodular Pulmonary Fibrosis, Lung, Cat.** The lung contains large numbers of nodules distributed throughout all pulmonary lobes. These nodules are formed by focal areas of fibrosis with retraction of the pulmonary parenchyma admixed with focal areas of pulmonary hyperinflation. This cat had a history of chronic respiratory problems. (Courtesy Facultad de Medicina Veterinaria y Zootecnia, Universidad Nacional Autónoma de México.)

fetus, this fluid normally moves along the tracheobronchial tree, reaching the oropharynx, where a fraction is swallowed into the gastrointestinal tract, and a small portion is released into the amniotic fluid. At the time of birth, the lung fluid is rapidly reabsorbed from the lungs by alveolar absorption and lymphatic drainage.

Aspiration of amniotic fluid contaminated with meconium and bacteria from placentitis is the most common route by which microbial pathogens reach the fetal lungs. This form of pneumonia is secondary to fetal hypoxia and acidosis ("fetal distress"), which cause the fetus to relax the anal sphincter, release meconium into the amniotic fluid, and, in the terminal stages, inspire deeply with open glottis, resulting in the aspiration of contaminated fluid (Fig. 9-109). Gross lesions are only occasionally recognized, but microscopic changes are similar to those of a bronchopneumonia. Microscopically, bronchoalveolar spaces contain variable numbers of neutrophils, macrophages, epidermal squames, and pieces of meconium that appear as bright yellow material because of its bile content. In contrast to postnatal bronchopneumonia, lesions in fetuses are not restricted to the cranioventral aspects of the lungs but typically involve all pulmonary lobes.

In cattle, *Brucella abortus* and *Trueperella* (*Arcanobacterium*) *pyogenes* are two of the most common bacteria isolated from the lungs of aborted fetuses. These bacteria are usually present in large numbers in the amniotic fluid of cows with bacterial placentitis. Inflammation of the placenta interferes with oxygen exchange between fetal and maternal tissue, and the resultant fetal hypoxia induces the fetus to "breathe" with an open glottis and aspirate the amniotic fluid. *Aspergillus* spp. (mycotic abortion) and *Ureaplasma diversum* cause sporadic cases of placentitis, which results in fetal pneumonia and abortion.

In addition to the respiratory route (aspiration), pathogens, such as bacteria and viruses, can also reach the lungs via fetal blood and cause interstitial pneumonia. Listeriosis (*Listeria monocytogenes*), salmonellosis (*Salmonella* spp.), and chlamydiosis (*Chlamydophila abortus* [*C. psittaci*]) are the best known examples of blood-borne diseases that cause fetal pneumonia in farm animals. Gross lesions in the lungs are generally undetected, but microscopic lesions include focal necrotizing interstitial pneumonia and focal necrosis in the liver, spleen, or brain. Fetal bronchointerstitial pneumonia also occurs in some viral abortions, such as those caused by infectious bovine rhinotracheitis (IBR) virus and bovine parainfluenza virus 3 (BPIV-3) in cattle and equine viral rhinopneumonitis (EVR) in horses. Fetal pneumonias in dogs and cats are infrequently described, perhaps because aborted puppies and kittens are rarely submitted for postmortem examination. With advancements in molecular biology techniques, the etiologic diagnosis of abortions and their association with pulmonary fetal lesions is rapidly improving.

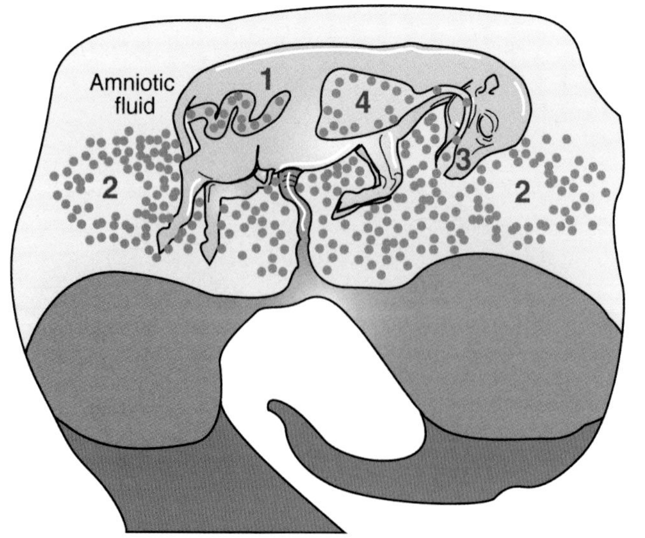

Figure 9-109 **Meconium Aspiration Resulting From Intrauterine Hypoxia.** *1*, Increased peristalsis and relaxation of anal sphincter. *2*, Meconium contamination of amniotic fluid. *3*, Meconium in the oropharynx. *4*, Intrauterine gasping with open glottis causing aspiration of meconium and amniotic fluid into fetal lung. (Redrawn with permission from Dr. J. Martinez-Burnes, Facultad de Medicina Veterinaria y Zootecnia, Universidad Autónoma de Tamaulipas, México.)

Neonatal Pneumonias and Septicemias. These entities are rather common in newborn animals lacking passive immunity because of the lack of either ingestion or absorption of maternal colostrum (failure of passive transfer or hypogammaglobulinemia). In addition to septicemias causing interstitial pneumonia, farm animals with hypogammaglobulinemia can develop bronchopneumonia by inhalation of bacterial pathogens. These include *Histophilus somni* and *Pasteurella multocida* in calves; *Streptococcus* spp. in foals; and *Escherichia coli*, *Listeria monocytogenes*, and *Streptococcus suis* in pigs.

Meconium Aspiration Syndrome. Meconium aspiration syndrome (MAS) is an important but preventable condition in human babies that originates when amniotic fluid contaminated with meconium is aspirated during labor or immediately after birth. The pathogenesis of MAS is basically the same as in those of fetal bronchopneumonia (see Fig. 9-109). Fetal hypoxia, a common event during dystocia or prolonged parturition, causes the fetus to relax the anal sphincter and release meconium into the amniotic fluid. Aspiration of meconium can occur directly from aspirating contaminated amniotic fluid before delivery (respiratory movements with an open glottis) or immediately after delivery when the meconium lodged in the nasopharynx is carried into the lung with the first breath of air. This latter form of aspiration is prevented in delivery rooms by routine suction of the nasopharynx in meconium-stained babies. MAS is well known in human babies, but the occurrence and significance in animals remains largely unknown. MAS has been reported in calves, foals, piglets, and puppies. Although pulmonary lesions are generally mild and transient, aspiration of meconium can be life-threatening for newborn babies and animals because it typically occurs in compromised neonates already suffering from intrauterine hypoxia and acidosis. Neonatal acidosis is known to impair colostrum absorption in calves. Common MAS sequelae are lobular atelectasis, pulmonary hypertension, and possibly airway hyperreactivity.

In the most severe cases of MAS, focal (patchy) atelectasis can be observed grossly in the lung, indicating failure of the lungs to be fully aerated because of the mechanical obstruction and the chemical effect of meconium on pulmonary surfactant (see Fig. 9-52). Microscopically, meconium and keratin exfoliated from skin of the fetus into the amniotic fluid are present in bronchi, bronchioles, and alveoli and accompanied by mild alveolitis characterized by infiltration of leukocytes followed by alveolar macrophages and occasional giant cells (E-Fig. 9-30).

Neoplasms of the Lungs

Lung cancer in animals is rare, unlike in human beings, in which the incidence is alarming and continues to be the number one cause of death due to cancer in Canada, the United States, and Europe. Interestingly, prostatic and breast cancers, so much feared by men and women, are a distant second. To say that cigarette smoking is responsible for this epidemic of lung cancer is unnecessary. Although dogs have been proposed as valuable "sentinels" for environmental hazards, such as exposure to passive smoking, asbestos, dyes, and insecticides, it is not known if the prevalence of canine lung tumors has increased in geographical areas with high contamination. Alterations in genes (oncogenes) and chromosomes and changes in biologically active molecules have been linked to lung cancer in recent years. As with many other forms of cancer, epidemiologic studies indicate that the incidence of pulmonary neoplasms increases with age, but there are still insufficient data to confirm that particular canine or feline breeds have a higher predisposition to spontaneous lung neoplasms.

A standard nomenclature of pulmonary neoplasms in domestic animals is lacking, and as a consequence, multiplicity of names and synonyms occur in the veterinary literature. Some classifications are based on the primary site, whereas others emphasize more the histomorphologic type. The most common types of benign and malignant pulmonary neoplasms in domestic mammals are listed in Box 9-2.

Clinically, the signs of pulmonary neoplasia vary with the degree of invasiveness, the amount of parenchyma involved, and locations of metastases. Signs may be vague, such as cough, lethargy, anorexia, weight loss, and perhaps dyspnea. In addition, paraneoplastic syndromes, such as hypercalcemia, endocrinopathies, and pulmonary hypertrophic osteoarthropathy, have been associated with pulmonary neoplasms.

Primary Neoplasms of the Lungs. Primary neoplasms of the lungs arise from cells normally present in the pulmonary tissue and can be epithelial or mesenchymal, although the latter are rare.

Box 9-2 Classification of Pulmonary Neoplasms

PRIMARY EPITHELIAL ORIGIN

Benign

Papilloma
Adenoma

Malignant

Adenocarcinoma (acinar or papillar)
Squamous cell carcinoma
Adenosquamous carcinoma
Bronchiolar-alveolar carcinoma (this term is being abandoned by some pathologists)
Small cell and large cell carcinomas
Anaplastic (undifferentiated) carcinoma
Carcinoid tumor (pulmonary neuroendocrine tumor)
Ovine (retroviral) pulmonary carcinoma

PRIMARY MESENCHYMAL ORIGIN

Benign

Hemangioma

Malignant

Osteosarcoma, chondrosarcoma
Hemangiosarcoma
Histiocytic sarcoma
Lymphomatoid granulomatosis
Granular cell tumor
Mesothelioma

SECONDARY (METASTATIC) LUNG TUMORS

Any malignant tumor metastatic from another body location (e.g., osteosarcoma in dogs, uterine carcinoma in cows, and malignant melanoma in horses)

Primary benign neoplasms of the lungs, such as pulmonary adenomas, are highly unusual in domestic animals. Most primary neoplasms are malignant and appear as solitary masses of variable size that, with time, can metastasize to other areas of the lungs and to distant organs. It is sometimes difficult on gross and microscopic examination to differentiate primary lung cancer from pulmonary metastasis resulting from malignant neoplasms elsewhere in the body.

It is often difficult to determine the precise topographic origin of a neoplasm within the lungs—for example, whether it originates in the conducting system (bronchogenic carcinoma), transitional system (bronchiolar carcinoma), exchange system (alveolar carcinoma), or bronchial glands (bronchial gland carcinoma). According to the literature, pulmonary carcinomas in animals arise generally from Club (Clara) cells or type II pneumonocytes of the bronchioloalveolar region, in contrast to those in human beings, which are mostly bronchogenic. Tumors located at the hilus generally arise from major bronchi and tend to be a solitary large mass with occasional small metastasis to the periphery of the lung. In contrast, tumors arising from the bronchioloalveolar region are often multicentric with numerous peripheral metastases in the lung parenchyma. Because of histologic architecture and irrespective of the site of origin, many malignant epithelial neoplasms are classified by the all-encompassing term of pulmonary adenocarcinomas.

Dogs and cats are the species most frequently affected with primary pulmonary neoplasms, largely carcinomas, generally in older animals. The mean age for primary lung tumors is 11 years for dogs and 12 years for cats. Pulmonary carcinomas in other domestic animals, except for retrovirus-induced pulmonary carcinoma in sheep, are less common, possibly because fewer farm animals are allowed to reach their natural life span. These neoplasms can be invasive or expansive, vary in color (white, tan, or gray) and texture (soft or firm), and often have areas of necrosis and hemorrhage, which result in a "craterous" or "umbilicate" appearance. This umbilicate appearance is frequently seen in rapidly growing carcinomas in which the center of the tumoral mass undergoes necrosis as a result of ischemia. Some lung neoplasms resemble pulmonary consolidation or large granulomas. Cats with moderately differentiated neoplasms had significantly longer survival time (median, 698 days) than cats with poorly differentiated neoplasms (median, 75 days). Dogs with primary lung neoplasms, grades I, II, and III, had survival times of 790, 251, and 5 days, respectively.

Ovine Pulmonary Adenocarcinoma (Ovine Pulmonary Carcinoma). Ovine pulmonary adenocarcinoma, also known as *pulmonary adenomatosis* and *jaagsiekte* (from the South African Afrikaans word for "driving sickness"), is a transmissible, retrovirus-induced neoplasia of ovine lungs caused by Jaagsiekte sheep retrovirus (JSRV). It occurs in sheep throughout the world, with the notable exception of Australia and New Zealand; its incidence is high in Scotland, South Africa, and Peru and unknown but probably low in North America. This pulmonary carcinoma behaves very much like a chronic pneumonia, and JSRV shares many epidemiologic similarities with the ovine lentivirus responsible for maedi and the retrovirus responsible for enzootic nasal carcinoma in small ruminants. Pulmonary adenomatosis has been transmitted to goats experimentally but is not known to be a spontaneous disease in that species.

Ovine pulmonary adenocarcinoma affects mainly mature sheep but can occasionally affect young stock. Intensive husbandry probably facilitates horizontal transmission by the copious nasal discharge and explains why the disease occurs as devastating epizootics with 5% to 80% mortality when first introduced into a flock. Differential diagnosis between maedi and pulmonary adenomatosis can prove difficult because both diseases often coexist in the same flock or in the same animal. Death is inevitable after several months of the initial onset of respiratory signs, and a specific humoral immune response to JSRV is undetectable in affected sheep.

During the early stages of ovine pulmonary carcinoma, the lungs are enlarged, heavy, and wet and have several firm, gray, variably sized nodules that in some cases can be located in the cranioventral lobes mimicking a bronchopneumonic lesion (Fig. 9-110, *A*). In the later stages, the nodules become confluent, and large segments of both lungs are diffusely, but not symmetrically, infiltrated by neoplastic cells. On cross section, edematous fluid and a copious mucoid secretion are present in the trachea and bronchi (Fig. 9-110, *B*). Microscopically, the nodules consist of cuboidal or columnar epithelial cells lining airways and alveoli and forming papillary or acinar (glandlike) structures (see Fig. 9-110, *A*). Because the cells have been identified ultrastructurally as originating from both type II alveolar epithelial cells and Club (Clara) cells, the neoplasm is considered a "bronchioloalveolar" carcinoma. Sequelae often include secondary bronchopneumonia, abscesses, and fibrous pleural adhesions. Metastases occur to tracheobronchial and mediastinal lymph nodes and, to a lesser extent, to other tissues such as pleura, muscle, liver, and kidneys. Neoplastic cells stain strongly positive for JSRV using immunohistochemistry.

Clinically, ovine pulmonary adenocarcinoma is characterized by a gradual loss of condition, coughing, and respiratory distress, especially after exercise (e.g., herding or "driving"). Appetite and temperature are normal, unless there are secondary bacterial infections. An important differentiating feature from maedi (interstitial pneumonia) can be observed if animals with pulmonary adenomatosis are raised by their hind limbs; copious, thin, mucoid fluid, produced by neoplastic cells in the lungs, pours from the nostrils of some animals.

Carcinoid (Neuroendocrine) Tumor of the Lungs. Carcinoid tumor of the lungs is a neoplasm presumably arising from neuroendocrine cells and is sporadically seen in dogs as multiple, large, firm pulmonary masses close to the mainstem bronchi. It has also been reported in the nasal cavity of horses. Tumor cells are generally polygonal with finely granular, pale, or slightly eosinophilic cytoplasm. Nuclei are small, and mitotic figures are absent or rare.

Granular Cell Tumor. Granular cell tumor is a rare and locally invasive tumor that has been reported mainly in human beings and older horses. The cell origin of this tumor was thought to be the myoblast, but it is currently presumed to be Schwann cells, which are normally present in the bronchovascular bundles of the lung. Microscopically, neoplastic cells are large, polyhedron-shaped with abundant cytoplasm containing numerous acidophilic granules, which are positive for PAS and for S-100 protein using immunohistochemistry. Although this tumor can cause bronchial obstruction and respiratory signs, in most cases, it is an incidental finding in older horses submitted for postmortem examination.

Lymphomatoid Granulomatosis. Lymphomatoid granulomatosis is a rare but interesting pulmonary disease of human beings, dogs, cats, and possibly horses and donkeys characterized by nodules or large solid masses in one or more lung lobes. These frequently metastasize to lymph nodes, kidneys, and liver. Microscopically, tumors are formed by large pleomorphic mononuclear (lymphomatoid) cells with a high mitotic rate and frequent formation of binucleated or multinucleated cells. Tumor cells have a distinct tendency to grow around blood vessels and invade and destroy the vascular walls.

Lymphomatoid granulomatosis has some resemblance to lymphoma and is therefore also referred to as angiocentric lymphoma; phenotypic marking confirms that neoplastic cells are a mixed population of plasma cells, B and T lymphocytes, and histiocytes. Cerebral and cutaneous forms of lymphomatoid granulomatosis have also reported in human beings, dogs, and cats.

Secondary Neoplasms of the Lungs. Secondary neoplasms of the lungs are all malignant by definition because they are the result of metastasis to the lungs from malignant neoplasms elsewhere. Because the pulmonary capillaries are the first filter met by tumor emboli released into the vena cava or pulmonary arteries, secondary neoplasms in the lung are relatively common in comparison to primary ones. Also, secondary tumors can be epithelial or mesenchymal in origin. Common metastatic tumors of epithelial origin are mammary, thyroid (Fig. 9-111), and uterine carcinomas. Tumors of mesenchymal origin are osteosarcoma (Fig. 9-112, *A*); hemangiosarcoma (Fig. 9-112, *B*); malignant melanoma in dogs; lymphoma in cows, pigs, dogs, and cats (Fig. 9-113); and vaccine-associated sarcoma in cats. Usually, secondary pulmonary neoplasms are multiple; scattered throughout all pulmonary lobes (hematogenous dissemination); of variable size; and, according to the growth pattern, can be nodular, diffuse, or radiating (E-Fig. 9-31).

The appearance of metastatic neoplasms differs according to the type of neoplasm. For example, dark red cystic nodules containing blood indicate hemangiosarcoma, dark black solid nodules indicate melanoma, and hard solid nodules (white, yellow, or tan color) with bone spicules indicate osteosarcoma. The gross appearances of

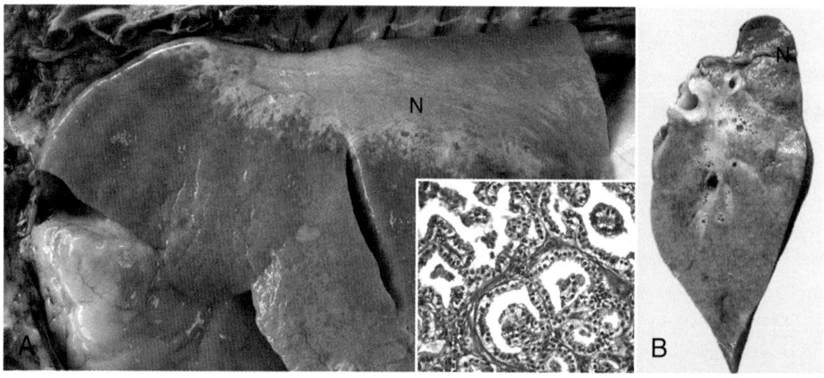

Figure 9-110 **Ovine Pulmonary Carcinoma (Pulmonary Adenomatosis, Jaagsiekte), Lung, 3-Year-Old Sheep. A,** Neoplastic cell infiltration involving the cranial and ventral portions of the lung and mainly sparing the dorsal portions of the caudal lung lobe *(N)*. The affected lung is enlarged and firm. *Inset,* Papillary proliferation of cuboidal epithelial cells (presumed type II pneumonocytes). H&E stain. **B,** Transverse section of the cranial lobe. Note the solid appearance of the ventral portion *(bottom)* of the lung and the frothy fluid (edema) that originates in the alveolar walls. *N,* Normal lung. (Courtesy Dr. M. Heras, Facultad de Veterinaria, Universidad de Zaragoza, Spain.)

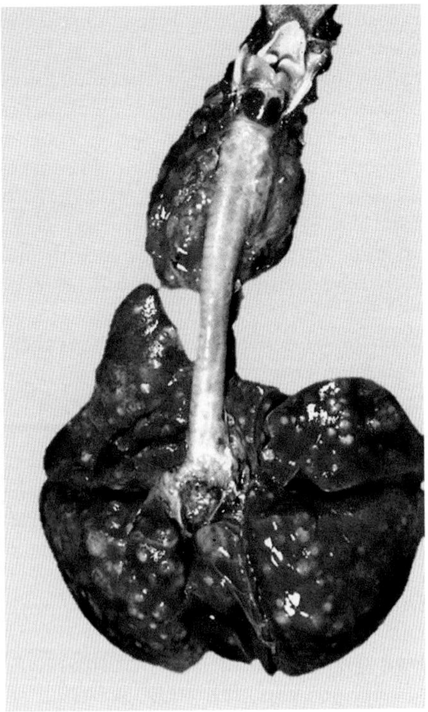

Figure 9-111 **Metastatic Thyroid Carcinoma, Lungs, Adult Dog.** The lungs contain multiple randomly distributed white-pink metastatic nodules, which originated from the enlarged and neoplastic left thyroid gland. (Courtesy Dr. J.M. King, College of Veterinary Medicine, Cornell University.)

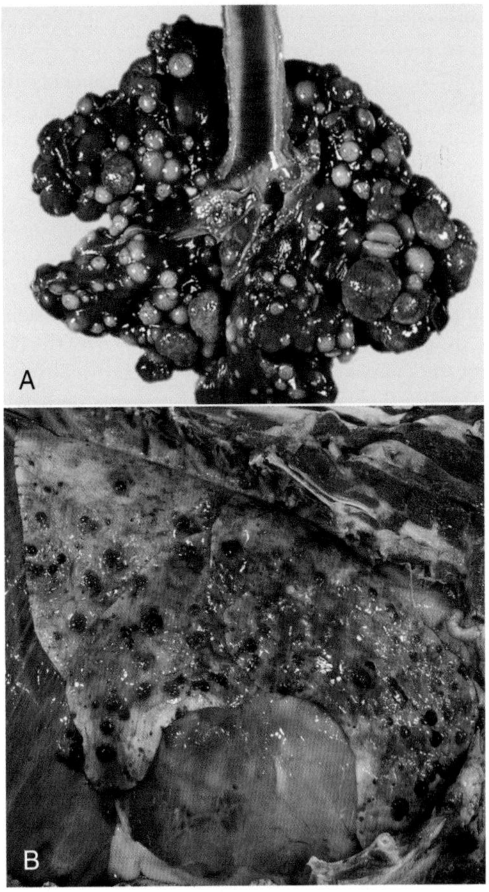

Figure 9-112 **Lung, Metastatic Neoplasms, Dog. A,** Metastatic sarcoma (primary site unknown). Large numbers of gray-white metastatic nodules are randomly distributed throughout all lung lobes. **B,** Metastatic hemangiosarcoma. Note the red to dark red masses throughout the lung parenchyma. If these masses were black, metastatic melanoma would be the likely diagnosis. (**A** courtesy Dr. J.M. King, College of Veterinary Medicine, Cornell University. **B** courtesy Dr. A. Bourque and Dr. A. López, Atlantic Veterinary College.)

metastatic carcinomas are generally similar to the primary neoplasm and sometimes have umbilicated centers. Proper diagnoses of pulmonary neoplasms in live animals require history, clinical signs, radiographs, cytologic analysis of BAL fluid, and, when necessary, a lung biopsy. Identification of a specific lineage of neoplastic cells in biopsy or postmortem specimens is often difficult and requires electron microscopy or immunohistochemical techniques. Electron microscopy allows identification of distinctive cellular components such as osmiophilic lamellar phospholipid nephritic bodies in alveolar type II epithelial cells or melanosomes in melanomas. Immunohistochemical staining is also helpful in identifying tumor cells.

Thoracic Cavity and Pleura

The thoracic wall, diaphragm, and mediastinum are lined by the parietal pleura, which reflects onto the lungs at the hilum and continues as the visceral pleura, covering the entire surface of the lungs, except at the hilus where the bronchi and blood vessels enter. The space between the parietal and visceral pleura (pleural space) is only minimal and under normal conditions contains only traces of clear fluid, which is a lubricant, and a few exfoliated cells. Samples of this fluid are obtained by thoracocentesis, a simple procedure in which a needle is passed into the pleural cavity. Volumetric, biochemical, and cytologic changes in this fluid are routinely used in veterinary diagnostics.

Disorders of the Thoracic Cavity and Pleura

Anomalies[7]

Congenital defects are rare and generally of little clinical significance. Cysts within the mediastinum of dogs and, less often, cats

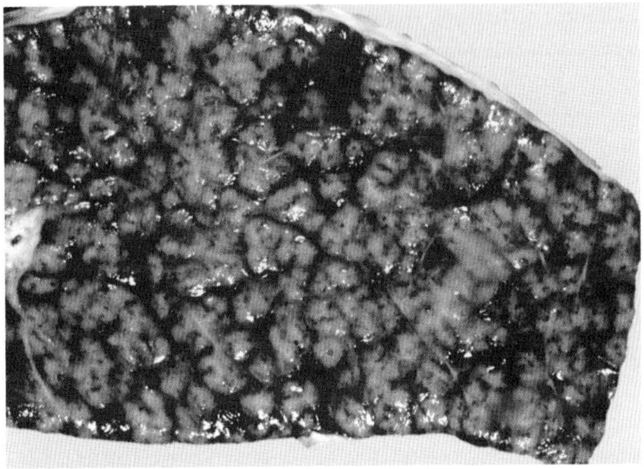

Figure 9-113 **Metastatic Lymphoma (Lymphosarcoma), Lungs, Cut Surface, Cow.** Note the numerous discrete and confluent metastatic nodules with the smooth texture and gray color characteristic of lymphoma. (Courtesy College of Veterinary Medicine, University of Illinois.)

[7]See E-Box 1-1 for potential, suspected, or known genetic disorders.

can be large enough to compromise pulmonary function or mimic neoplasia in thoracic radiographs. These cysts may arise from the thymus (thymic branchial cysts), bronchi (bronchogenic cysts), ectopic thyroid tissue (thyroglossal duct cysts), or from remnants of the branchial pouches, and they are generally lined by epithelium and surrounded by a capsule of stromal tissue. Anomalies of the thoracic duct cause some cases of chylothorax.

Degenerative Disturbances

Pleural Calcification. Pleural calcification is commonly found in dogs and less often in cats with chronic uremia. Lesions appear as linear white streaks in parietal pleura, mainly over the intercostal muscles of the cranial part of the thoracic cavity. The lesions are not functionally significant but indicate a severe underlying renal problem. Vitamin D toxicity (hypervitaminosis D) and ingestion of hypercalcemic substances, such as vitamin D analogs, can also cause calcification of the pleura and other organs.

Pneumothorax. Pneumothorax is the presence of air in the thoracic cavity where there should normally be negative pressure to facilitate inspiration. Human beings have a complete and strong mediastinum so that pneumothorax is generally unilateral and thus not a serious problem. In dogs, the barrier varies, but in general it is not complete, so often some communication exists between left and right sides.

There are two main forms of pneumothorax. In spontaneous (idiopathic) pneumothorax, air leaking into the pleural cavity from the lungs occurs without any known underlying disease or trauma. In secondary pneumothorax, movement of air into the pleural cavity results from underlying pulmonary or thoracic wall disease. The most common causes of secondary pneumothorax in veterinary medicine are penetrating wounds to the thoracic wall, perforated esophagus, iatrogenic trauma to the thorax and lung during a transthoracic lung biopsy or thoracoscopy, tracheal rupture from improper intubation, and rupture of emphysematous bullae or parasitic pulmonary cysts (*Paragonimus* spp.) that communicate with the thoracic cavity. Pneumothorax and pneumomediastinum caused by high air pressure (barotrauma) are also well documented in cats after equipment failure during anesthesia. Clinical signs of pneumothorax include respiratory distress, and the lesion is simply a collapsed, atelectatic lung. The air is readily reabsorbed from the cavity if the site of entry is sealed.

Circulatory and Lymphatic Disturbances

Pleural Effusion. Pleural effusion is a general term used to describe accumulation of any fluid (transudate, modified transudate, exudate, blood, lymph, or chyle) in the thoracic cavity. Cytologic and biochemical evaluations of pleural effusions taken by thoracocentesis are helpful in determining the type of effusion and possible pathogenesis. Based on protein concentration and total numbers of nucleated cells, pleural effusions are cytologically divided into transudates, modified transudates, and exudates.

Hydrothorax. When the fluid is serous, clear, and odorless and fails to coagulate when exposed to air, the condition is referred to as *hydrothorax* (*transudate*). Causes of hydrothorax are the same as those involved in edema formation in other organs: increased hydrostatic pressure (heart failure), decreased oncotic pressure (hypoproteinemia, as in liver disease), alterations in vascular permeability (inflammation), or obstruction of lymph drainage (neoplasia). In cases in which the leakage is corrected, if the fluid is a transudate, it is rapidly reabsorbed. If the fluid persists, it irritates the pleura and causes mesothelial hyperplasia and fibrosis, which thickens the pleura.

In severe cases, the amount of fluid present in the thoracic cavity can be considerable. For instance, a medium-size dog can have 2 L of fluid, and a cow may accumulate 25 L or more. Excessive fluid in the thorax causes compressive atelectasis resulting in respiratory distress (see Fig. 9-54). Hydrothorax is most commonly seen in cattle with right-sided heart failure or cor pulmonale (hydrostatic) (E-Fig. 9-32); dogs with congestive heart failure (hydrostatic), chronic hepatic disease (hepatic hydrothorax) (Fig. 9-114), or nephrotic syndrome (hypoproteinemia); pigs with mulberry heart disease (increased vascular permeability); and horses with African horse sickness (increased vascular permeability).

Hemothorax. Blood in the thoracic cavity is called *hemothorax*, but the term has been used for exudate with a sanguineous component. Causes include rupture of a major blood vessel as a result of severe thoracic trauma (e.g., hit by car); erosion of a vascular wall by malignant cells or inflammation (e.g., aortitis caused by *Spirocerca lupi*); ruptured aortic aneurysms; clotting defects, including coagulopathies; warfarin toxicity; disseminated intravascular coagulation (consumption coagulopathy); and thrombocytopenia. Hemothorax is generally acute and fatal. On gross examination, the thoracic cavity can be filled with blood, and the lungs are partially or completely atelectatic (Fig. 9-115).

Chylothorax. The accumulation of chyle (lymph rich in triglycerides) in the thoracic cavity (Fig. 9-116) is a result of the rupture of major lymph vessels, usually the thoracic duct or the right lymphatic duct. The clinical and pathologic effects of chylothorax are similar to those of the other pleural effusions. Causes include thoracic neoplasia (the most common cause in human beings but a distant second to idiopathic cases in dogs), trauma, congenital lymph vessel anomalies, lymphangitis, dirofilariasis, and iatrogenic rupture of the thoracic duct during surgery. The source of the leakage of chyle is rarely found at necropsy. When the leakage of chyle occurs in the abdominal cavity, the condition is referred to as *chyloabdomen*. Cytologic and biochemical examination of fluid collected by thoracocentesis typically reveals large numbers of lymphocytes, lipid droplets, few neutrophils in chronic cases, and high triglyceride content.

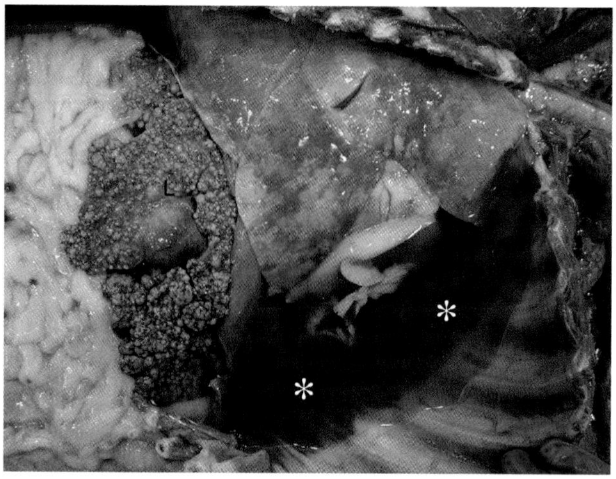

Figure 9-114 **Hydrothorax, Pleural Cavity, 8-Year-Old Dog.** The pleural cavity contains a large amount of deep yellow transudate *(asterisks)* (ventrally). Scattered foci of atelectasis are visible on the surface of the lung. Fluid in the pleural cavity usually compresses the ventral portions of the lung, resulting in a compressive atelectasis. Also note the nodular surface of the cirrhotic liver *(L)*. (Courtesy Dr. S. McBurney and Dr. A. López, Atlantic Veterinary College.)

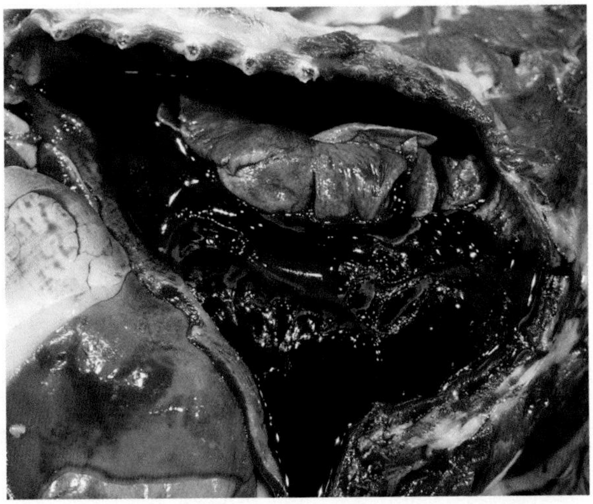

Figure 9-115 **Hemothorax, Right Pleural Cavity, Dog.** The right pleural cavity is filled with a large clot of blood from a ruptured thoracic aortic aneurysm, which caused unexpected death. Canine aortic aneurysms are associated with migration of *Spirocerca lupi* larvae along the aortic wall before their final migration into the wall of the adjacent esophagus. In other cases, like in this dog, the cause remains unknown (idiopathic aortic aneurysm). (Courtesy Dr. L. Gabor and Dr. A. López, Atlantic Veterinary College.)

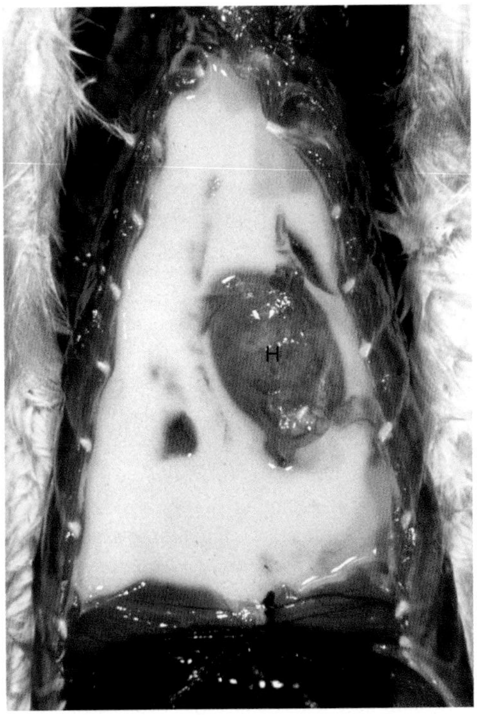

Figure 9-116 **Chylothorax (Cause Unknown), Thoracic (Pleural) Cavity, Mink.** Lymph (chyle) fills both left and right pleural cavities. The heart *(H)* and pericardium are essentially normal because the chyle does not adhere to the outer surface of the pericardial sac, as typically happens with suppurative and fibrinous exudates in the thoracic cavity. (Courtesy Western College of Veterinary Medicine.)

Inflammation of the Pleura

Pleural tissue is readily susceptible to injury caused by direct implantation of an organism through a penetrating thoracic or diaphragmatic wound; by hematogenous dissemination of infectious organisms in septicemias; or by direct extension from an adjacent inflammatory process, such as in fibrinous bronchopneumonia or

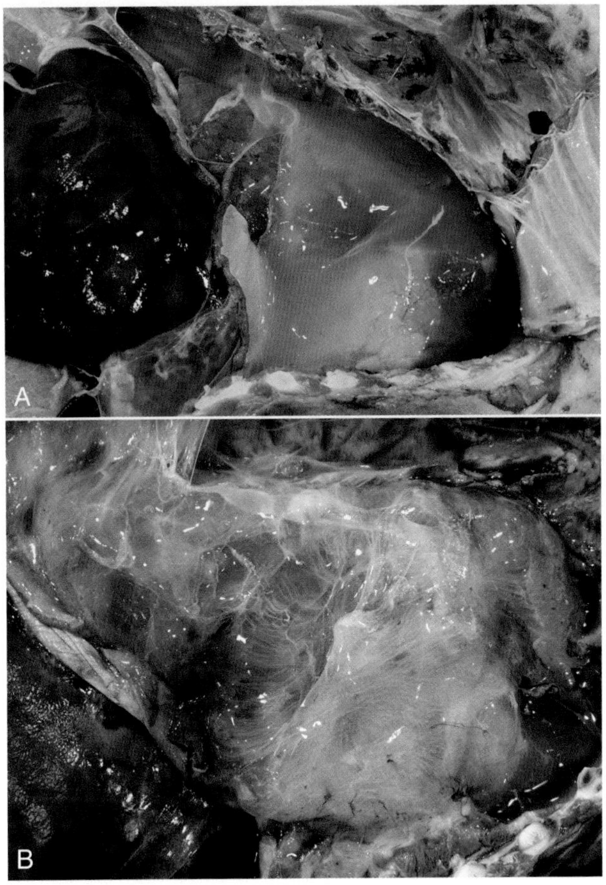

Figure 9-117 **Acute and Chronic Pleuritis, Sheep. A,** A large amount of slightly turbid straw-colored fluid is present in the thorax, and sheets and large clumps of tan-yellow friable material (fibrin and clotted protein) are loosely adhered to the right lung. **B,** The visceral and parietal pleura are covered with a thick layer of immature fibrous connective tissue. (**A** courtesy Dr. S. Martinson, Atlantic Veterinary College. **B** from Muckle A, López A, et al: *Can Vet J* 55:946-949, 2014.)

from a perforated esophagus. Chronic injury typically results in serosal fibrosis and tight adhesions between visceral and parietal pleurae (see Fig. 9-71). When extensive, these adhesions can obliterate the pleural space.

Pleuritis or Pleurisy. Inflammation of the visceral or parietal pleurae is called *pleuritis*, and according to the type of exudate, it can be fibrinous, suppurative, granulomatous, hemorrhagic, or a combination of exudates. Acute fibrinous pleuritis can progress with time to pleural fibrosis (Fig. 9-117). When suppurative pleuritis results in accumulation of purulent exudate in the cavity, the lesion is called *pyothorax* or *thoracic empyema* (Fig. 9-118). Clinically, pleuritis causes considerable pain, and in addition, empyema can result in severe toxemia. Pleural fibrous adhesions (between parietal and visceral pleura) and fibrosis are the most common sequelae of chronic pleuritis and can significantly interfere with inflation of the lungs.

Pleuritis can occur as an extension of pneumonia, particularly in fibrinous bronchopneumonias (pleuropneumonia), or it can occur alone, without pulmonary involvement (Fig. 9-119). Bovine and ovine pneumonic mannheimiosis and porcine and bovine pleuropneumonia are good examples of pleuritis associated with fibrinous bronchopneumonias. Polyserositis in pigs and pleural empyema, particularly in cats and horses, are examples of pleural inflammation in

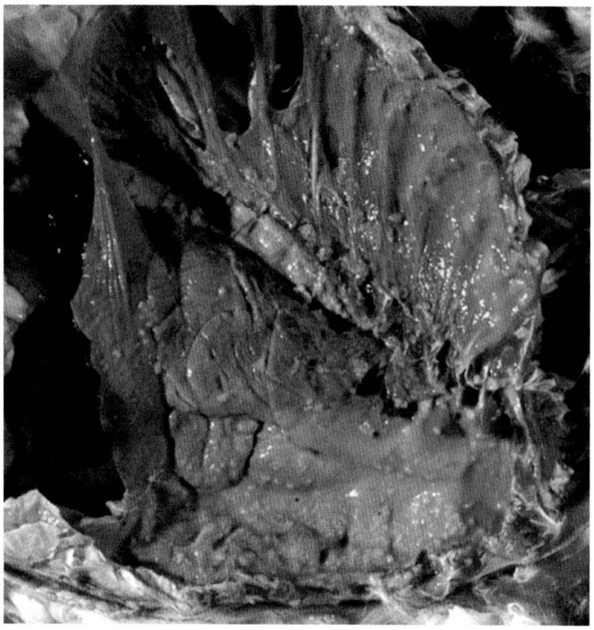

Figure 9-118 **Pyothorax (*Pasteurella multocida*), Right Pleural Cavity, Cat.** Pus in the thoracic cavity is called pyothorax or pleural empyema. Purulent gray-brown exudate also covers the visceral and parietal pleurae. This lesion is also referred to as *suppurative pleuritis*. (Courtesy Dr. A. López, Atlantic Veterinary College.)

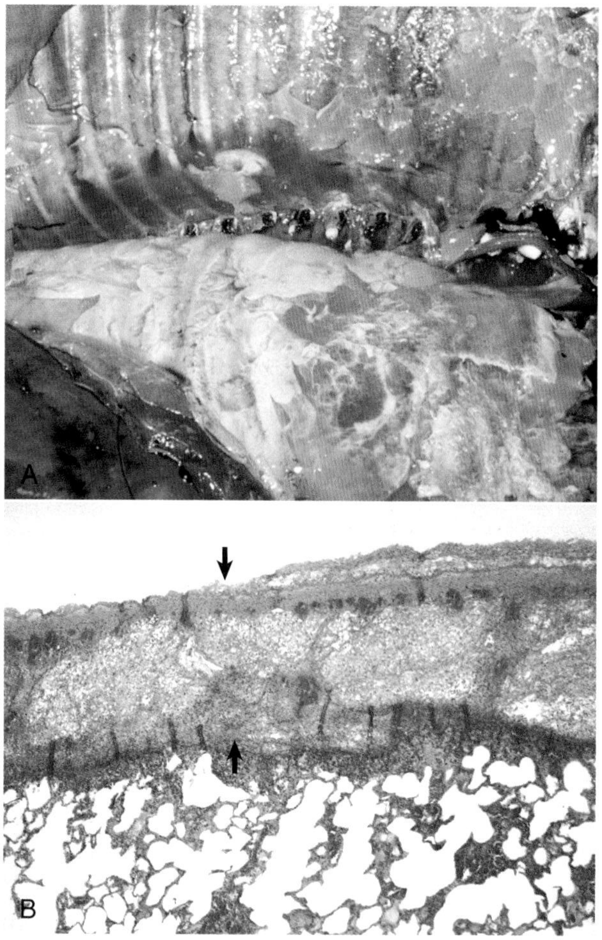

Figure 9-119 **Fibrinous Pleuritis, Right Pleural Cavity, Horse. A,** Large masses of yellow fibrin cover the visceral and parietal pleurae. The lungs are normal. **B,** The visceral pleura is covered by a thick layer of fibrin *(between arrows)*. Subjacent alveoli are essentially normal. H&E stain. (**A** courtesy Dr. A. López, Atlantic Veterinary College. **B** courtesy College of Veterinary Medicine, University of Illinois.)

which involvement of the lungs may not accompany the pleuritis. Pleural inflammation is most frequently caused by bacteria, which cause polyserositis reaching the pleura hematogenously. These bacteria include *Haemophilus parasuis* (Glasser's disease) (see E-Fig. 9-25), *Streptococcus suis*, and some strains of *Pasteurella multocida* in pigs; *Streptococcus equi* ssp. *equi* and *Streptococcus equi* ssp. *zooepidemicus* in horses; *Escherichia coli* in calves; and *Mycoplasma* spp. and *Haemophilus* spp. in sheep and goats. Contamination of pleural surfaces can be the result of extension of a septic process (e.g., puncture wounds of the thoracic wall and, in cattle, traumatic reticulopericarditis) and ruptured pulmonary abscesses (e.g., *Trueperella pyogenes*).

In dogs and cats, bacteria (e.g., *Nocardia*, *Actinomyces*, and *Bacteroides*) can cause pyogranulomatous pleuritis, characterized by accumulation of blood-stained pus ("tomato soup") in the thoracic cavity. This exudate usually contains yellowish flecks called *sulfur granules* (Fig. 9-120), although these are less common in nocardial empyema in cats. Many species of bacteria, such as *Escherichia coli*, *Trueperella pyogenes*, *Pasteurella multocida*, and *Fusobacterium necrophorum*, can be present in pyothorax of dogs and cats. These bacteria occur alone or in mixed infections. The pathogenesis of pleural empyema in cats is still debatable, but bite wounds or penetration of foreign material (migrating grass awns) are likely. Pyogranulomatous pleuritis with empyema occurs occasionally in dogs, presumably associated with inhaled small plant material and penetrating (migrating) grass awns. Because of their physical shape (barbed) and assisted by the respiratory movement, aspirated grass awns can penetrate airways, move through the pulmonary parenchyma, and eventually perforate the visceral pleura causing pyogranulomatous pleuritis.

Cats with the noneffusive ("dry") form of feline infectious peritonitis (FIP) frequently have focal pyogranulomatous pleuritis, in contrast to those with the effusive ("wet") form, in which thoracic involvement is primarily that of a pleural effusion. Cytologic evaluation of the effusion typically shows a low to moderate cellularity with degenerated leukocytes, lymphocytes, macrophages, and mesothelial cells, and a pink granular background as a result of the high protein content.

Pleuritis is also an important problem in horses. *Nocardia* spp. can cause fibrinopurulent pneumonia and pyothorax with characteristic sulfur granules. Although *Mycoplasma felis* can be isolated from the respiratory tract of normal horses, it is also isolated from horses with pleuritis and pleural effusion, particularly during the early stages of infection. The portal of entry of this infection is presumably aerogenous, first to the lung and subsequently to the pleura.

Neoplasms

The pleural surface of the lung is often involved in neoplasms that have metastasized from other organs to the pulmonary parenchyma and ruptured the visceral pleura to seed the pleural cavity. Mesothelioma is the only primary neoplasm of the pleura.

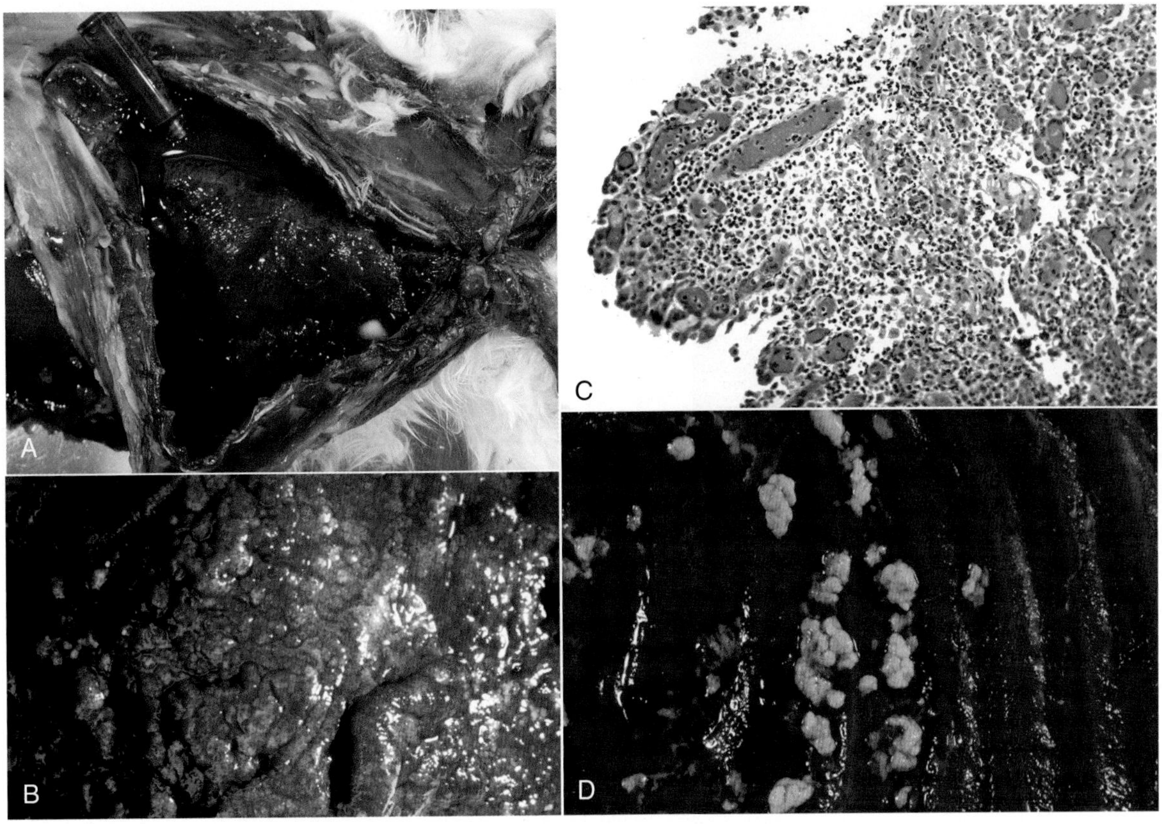

Figure 9-120 **Nocardiosis. A,** Chronic pleuritis (*Nocardia asteroides*), pleural cavity, cat. The pleural cavity is covered with abundant red-brown ("tomato soup") exudate" (syringe). Once considered to be pathognomonic of *Nocardia* spp. infection, it is no longer regarded as being diagnostic of nocardiosis. The fluid contains abundant protein, erythrocytes, granulomatous inflammatory cells, and sulfur granules. **B,** Chronic pleuritis (*Nocardia asteroides*), visceral pleura, dog. The thickened pleura has a granular pink-gray appearance because of granulomatous inflammation and the proliferation of fibrovascular tissue of the pleura. **C,** Chronic pleuritis (*Nocardia asteroides*), dog. The pleura has been thrown up into villous-like projections composed of abundant fibrovascular tissue and granulomatous inflammation. Leakage from the neocapillaries of the fibrovascular tissue is responsible for the hemorrhagic appearance of the pleural exudate. H&E stain. **D,** Chronic pleuritis (*Nocardia asteroides*), thoracic cage, parietal pleura, cat. Large pieces of exudate, which contain yellow sulfur granules, are present on the thickened pleura. (**A** courtesy Dr. F. Marrón-López and Dr. A. López. **B** and **C** courtesy Dr. M.D. McGavin, College of Veterinary Medicine, University of Tennessee. **D** courtesy College of Veterinary Medicine, University of Illinois.)

Primary Neoplasms of the Pleura: Mesothelioma. Mesothelioma is a rare neoplasm of the thoracic, pericardial, and peritoneal mesothelium of human beings that is seen most commonly in calves, in which it can be congenital. In human beings, it has long been associated with inhalation of certain types of asbestos fibers (asbestos mining and ship building) alone or with cigarette smoking as a probable cocarcinogen; no convincing association between the incidence of mesothelioma and exposure to asbestos has been made in domestic animals. In animals, there may be pleural effusion with resulting respiratory distress, cough, and weight loss.

Mesothelioma initially causes a thoracic effusion, but cytologic diagnosis can be difficult because of the morphologic resemblance of malignant and reactive mesothelial cells. During inflammation, mesothelial cells become reactive and not only increase in number but also become pleomorphic and form multinucleated cells that may be cytologically mistaken for those of a carcinoma.

Grossly, mesothelioma appears as multiple, discrete nodules or arborescent, spreading growths on the pleural surface (Fig. 9-121). Microscopically, either the mesothelial covering cells or the supporting tissue can be the predominant malignant component, so the neoplasm can microscopically resemble a carcinoma or a sarcoma. Although considered malignant, mesotheliomas rarely metastasize to distant organs.

Secondary Neoplasms of the Pleura. Secondary tumors may also spread into the visceral and parietal pleura. Thymomas are rare neoplasms that grow in the cranial mediastinum of adult or aged dogs, cats, pigs, cattle, and sheep. Thymomas are composed of thymic epithelium and lymphocytes (see Chapter 13).

Aging Changes of the Respiratory Tract

Old age, both in human beings and in animals, is known to be a risk factor for pulmonary infections, but the precise mechanisms involved in this increased susceptibility are still under investigation. Some studies have shown that in aged individuals the antibacterial properties provided by surfactant proteins, proinflammatory cytokines, and complement are altered.

Pulmonary hyperinflation (often referred to as senile emphysema) has been reported as an age-related change in human and canine lungs. Other age-related changes described in canine lungs include mineralization of bronchial cartilage, pleural and alveolar

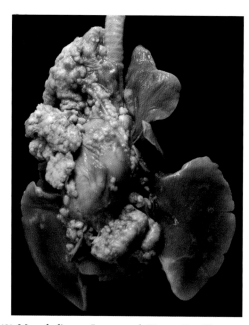

Figure 9-121 **Mesothelioma, Lungs and Heart, Cat.** The tumor *(top left)* has proliferated and extended over the ventral parietal pleurae and pericardium. The pericardial sac was subsequently opened (not shown here), and the epicardium appeared normal, indicating that the tumor, although on the pericardium, had not invaded the pericardial sac to involve the epicardium. (Courtesy Facultad de Medicina Veterinaria y Zootecnia, Universidad Nacional Autónoma de México.)

fibrosis, and heterotopic bone formation (so-called "pulmonary osteomas").

Acknowledgments

We thank all pathologists at the Atlantic Veterinary College, University of Prince Edward Island for providing case material.

Suggested Readings

Suggested Readings are available at www.expertconsult.com.

CHAPTER 10

Cardiovascular System and Lymphatic Vessels[1]

Lisa M. Miller and Arnon Gal

Key Readings Index

Structure

Development of the Heart and Great Vessels

The heart is a conical, muscular organ that in mammals has evolved into a four-chambered pump with four valves. During early fetal development, it is converted from an elongated muscular tube into a C-shaped structure by a process termed *looping* (E-Fig. 10-1). Subsequently, septation occurs to produce the right and left atrial and ventricular chambers and separation of the common truncus arteriosus into the aorta and pulmonary artery, respectively. The heart is interposed as a pump into the vascular system, with the right side supplying the pulmonary circulation and the left side the systemic circulation (E-Fig. 10-2; also see Chapter 2). The vascular system is subdivided into arterial, capillary, venous, and lymphatic segments. The arteries are classified into three types: elastic arteries, muscular arteries, and arterioles. The venous vessels are termed *venules* and *veins*. The lymphatic vasculature includes lymphatic capillaries and lymphatic vessels. Interposed between the arterial and venous segments are the capillary beds. A vascular segment termed the *microcirculation* (systemic capillary beds) includes arterioles, capillaries, and venules and is the major area of exchange between the circulating blood and the peripheral tissue (see E-Fig. 10-2; also see Chapter 2).

Macroscopic Structure

The heart lies within a fibroelastic sac called the *pericardium*, and the wall of the heart is composed of three layers: the epicardium, the myocardium, and the endocardium (Fig. 10-1). Structurally, the heart contains in order of blood flow four major blood vessels (vena cava, pulmonary artery, pulmonary vein, and aorta), four chambers (right atrium/auricle, right ventricle, left atrium/auricle, and left ventricle), and four valves (tricuspid, pulmonic semilunar, mitral, and aortic semilunar) (Fig. 10-2).

Myocardium

The myocardium is the muscular layer of the heart. It consists of cardiac muscle cells (cardiac myocytes [also known as *cardiac rhabdomyocytes*] or cardiomyocytes) arranged in overlapping spiral patterns. These sheets of cells are anchored to the fibrous skeleton of the heart, which surrounds the atrioventricular valves and the origins of the aorta and pulmonary artery. The myocardial thickness is related to the pressure present in each chamber; thus the atria are thin walled and the ventricles are thicker. In adult animals, the thickness of the left ventricular free wall is approximately threefold that of the right ventricle, measured in a transverse section across the middle of the ventricles, because the pressure is greater in the systemic circulation than in the pulmonary circuit.

The arterial supply to the heart is the left and right coronary arteries, which arise from the aorta at the sinus of Valsalva behind the left and right cusps of the aortic valves. The arteries course over the heart in the subepicardium and give off perforating intramyocardial arteries that supply a rich capillary bed throughout the myocardium. Extensive anastomoses occur between the capillaries that tend to run parallel to the elongated cardiac muscle cells. The ratio of the area of capillaries to that of muscle cells is approximately 1 : 1, a fact evident when the myocardium is viewed histologically in cross section. Cardiac myocytes are dependent on oxidative phosphorylation for energy requirements. This requires a constant supply of oxygen delivered by coronary arteries.

Cardiac Conduction System

The heart is a muscular four-chamber pump that simultaneously supplies blood to the pulmonary and systemic circulatory beds (see E-Fig. 10-2). Mechanical pumping is composed of sequential contraction (systole) and relaxation (diastole) that must be preceded by an electrophysiologic process that triggers a coordinated chronologic sequence of electrical events that result in muscle contractions. This electrophysiologic process is made possible by a network of

[1]For a glossary of abbreviations and terms used in this chapter, see E-Glossary 10-1.

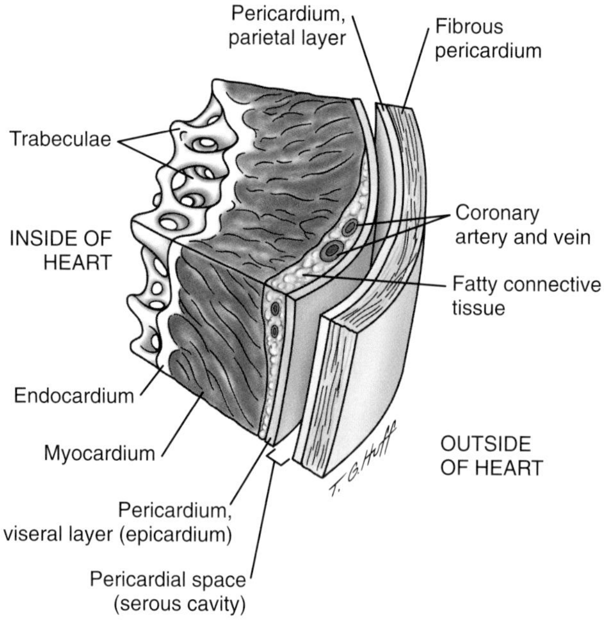

Figure 10-1 **Structure of the Wall of the Heart.**

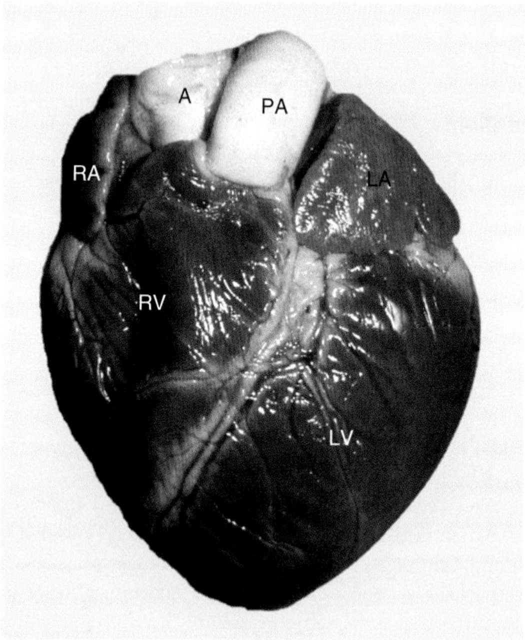

Figure 10-2 **Normal Heart, Pig.** *A*, Aorta; *LA*, left atrium; *LV*, left ventricle; *PA*, pulmonary artery; *RA*, right atrium; *RV*, right ventricle. (Courtesy School of Veterinary Medicine, Purdue University.)

special conducting fibers that are collectively referred to as the *cardiac conduction system*.

The cardiac conduction system is infrequently examined in animals because it is a labor-intensive process. Exceptions are cases with documented electrocardiographic alterations of undetermined origin. Components include (1) the sinoatrial node (SAN) at the junction of the cranial vena cava and the right atrium, (2) the atrioventricular node (AVN) located above the septal leaflet of the tricuspid valve and the atrioventricular (AV) bundle traversing the lower atrial septum onto the dorsal portion of the muscular interventricular septum, and (3) the right and left bundle branches that descend on each side of the muscular interventricular septum and eventually ramify in the ventricular myocardium as the Purkinje fiber network.

The major pacemaker of the cardiac conduction system is the SAN. This disk-shaped structure lies between the wall of the cranial vena cava and the external wall of the right auricular appendage. Four internodal pathways connect the SAN with the AVN. The AVN is present in the wall of the right atrium dorsal to the septal cusp of the tricuspid valve. For the atria to be electrically insulated from the ventricles so that an unwarranted ectopic conduction wave will not activate the ventricles (or vice versa) and disrupt the synchronous events of the cardiac cycle, a fibrous cardiac skeleton composed of a layer of dense collagen (central fibrous body [CFB]), as well as occasional plates of chondroid and osseous metaplasia, separates the atrial from the ventricular myocardium. This skeleton forms two fibrous rings around the AV orifices and the aortic and pulmonic orifices. Conduction fibers arising from the AVN, known as the *bundle of His* or *AV bundle*, pierce through the CFB into the ventricles and continue along the subendocardium of the interventricular septum. The AV bundle then splits into the right and left bundle branches, which further split and ramify into many other smaller branches that blend into the ventricular myocardium. Purkinje fibers constitute the AV bundle and downstream conduction pathways.

Endocardium and Heart Valves

The endocardium is the innermost layer of the heart and lines the chambers and extends over projecting structures such as the valves, chordae tendineae, and papillary muscles. The endocardium of the atria is thicker than that of the ventricles and thus normally appears white to gray on gross examination. The surface of the endocardium is endothelium that lies on a thin layer of vascularized connective tissue; the subendocardial layer contains blood vessels, nerves, and connective tissue. Purkinje fibers are distributed in the subendocardium throughout both ventricles. The heart valves (tricuspid valve [right AV valve], mitral valve [left AV valve], aortic valve, and pulmonary valve) are attached to fibrous rings and have thin avascular cusps. The valves open and close to regulate blood flow through the heart. During embryogenesis, endocardial cushions (mesenchymal tissue covered by endothelium) are precursors of the valve cusps. By remodeling, growth, and elongation, the cushions become thin mature cusps composed of connective tissue with an endothelial covering.

Pericardium and Epicardium

The pericardium, which normally contains a small amount of clear, serous fluid, is composed of an outer fibrous component and an inner serous layer, which form the sac surrounding the heart. The outer component is continuous with the mediastinal pleura. The base of the fibrous pericardium surrounds and blends with the adventitia of the greater arteries and veins exiting and entering the heart. The serous pericardium forms a closed sac surrounding the heart and the roots of the great vessels.

The epicardium (also known as *visceral pericardium*), the outermost layer of the heart, is continuous at the cardiac base with the parietal pericardium. The parietal pericardium is fused with the fibrous pericardium. The entire inner surface of the pericardial cavity is covered by mesothelium. The subepicardial layer is attached to the myocardium and consists of a thin layer of fibrous connective tissue, variable but generally abundant amounts (in well-nourished animals) of adipose tissue, and numerous blood vessels, lymphatic vessels, and nerves.

Blood and Lymphatic Vascular Systems

Blood Vessels. The aorta originates from the left ventricle and provides oxygenated blood to the entire body via arteries. In a tree-like manner, arteries branch and become smaller arterioles as they approach capillary beds (see E-Fig. 10-2; also see Chapter 2). These beds and postcapillary venules provide the site for exchange of oxygen, carbon dioxide, nutrients, and waste. Small venules return the exchanged fluid and blood to larger veins, and eventually the postcava and precava drain into the right atrium. The poorly oxygenated blood enters the pulmonary artery from the right ventricle. Oxygen exchange occurs in the capillaries of the lung, and oxygenated blood is returned to the heart via the pulmonary veins into the left atrium.

Lymphatic Vessels. Lymphatic vessels are thin-walled, endothelial-lined channels that originate near the capillary beds and serve as a drainage system for returning interstitial tissue fluid and inflammatory cells to the blood. Afferent lymphatic vessels drain lymph into regional lymph nodes, which then filter and provide immunologic surveillance of the lymph, its cells, and the foreign matter it contains. The filtered lymph continues into larger efferent lymphatic vessels, which eventually drain into the caval blood via the thoracic duct. Both lymphatic vessels and veins have valves to prevent backflow of fluid. A more complete description can be found in Chapter 2.

Microscopic Structure

Myocardium

The myocardium consists of cardiac muscle cells surrounded by interstitial components that include blood and lymphatic vessels, nerves, and connective tissue cells, such as fibroblasts, histiocytes, mast cells, pericytes, primitive mesenchymal stem cells, and extracellular matrix elements of connective tissue, including collagen fibrils, elastic fibers, and acid mucopolysaccharides. Cardiac muscle cells can be divided into two populations: the contracting myocytes and the specialized fibers of the conduction system. The contracting myocyte is a cross-striated branching fiber of an irregular cylindric shape that measures 60 to 100 μm in length and 10 to 20 μm in diameter, with centrally located, elongated nuclei. Myocytes in young animals are smaller and have less sarcoplasm. Atrial myocytes are smaller than ventricular myocytes. Adjacent myocytes are joined end-to-end by specialized junctions known as *intercalated disks* and less frequently by side-to-side connections termed *lateral junctions*. Multinucleated fibers with nuclei arranged in central rows are frequently seen in hearts of young pigs (Fig. 10-3). The myocytes of old animals commonly have large polyploid nuclei. The cytoplasm (sarcoplasm) of myocytes is largely occupied by the contractile proteins that are highly organized into sarcomeres, the repeating contractile units of the myofibril (see Figs. 15-3 and 15-8). Myofibrils are formed by end-to-end attachment of many sarcomeres. The cross-striated or banded appearance of myocytes is the result of sarcomere organization into A bands composed of myosin in the form of "thick" filaments (12 to 16 nm in diameter), I bands composed of actin in the form of "thin" filaments (5 to 8 nm in diameter), and dense Z bands at the end of each sarcomere. Thick and thin filaments interdigitate and provide the basis for the sliding mechanism of muscle contraction. Myocytes are enclosed by the sarcolemma, which consists of the plasma membrane and the covering basal lamina (external lamina). Other important components of cardiac muscle cells are generally only apparent in electron micrographs and include abundant mitochondria, a highly organized network of intracellular tubules termed the *sarcoplasmic reticulum*, cylindric invaginations of the plasma membrane called *T tubules*, ribosomes, cytoskeletal filaments, glycogen particles, lipid droplets, Golgi complexes, atrial granules (contain atrial natriuretic factor), lysosomes, and residual bodies (E-Fig. 10-3).

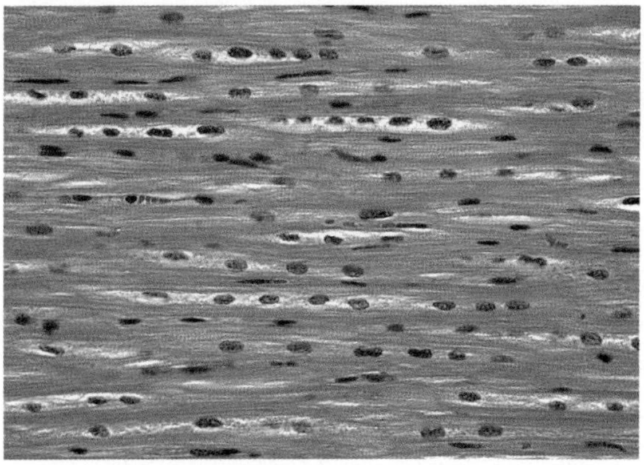

Figure 10-3 Normal Cardiac Muscle. Left ventricular myocardium, longitudinal section, normal young pig. The multiple nuclei in a myocyte are readily seen and evaluated in a longitudinal section. H&E stain. (Courtesy School of Veterinary Medicine, Purdue University.)

Cardiac Conduction System

The morphologic features of the cardiac muscle cells that form specialized conduction tissues, including the SAN, AVN, AV bundle (bundle of His), and bundle branches, vary greatly at different sites and among animal species but generally are thin, branching nodal muscle cells with scarce myofibrils separated by highly vascularized connective tissue (Fig. 10-4; E-Fig. 10-4). Autonomic nerve fibers are contained within the SAN. The Purkinje fibers (cardiac conduction fibers) are distinguished by their large diameters (in horse and ox) and abundant pale eosinophilic sarcoplasm rich in glycogen and poor in myofibrils.

Sinoatrial Node. The SAN is positioned adjacent to the epicardial adipose tissue and is often centered around a branch of the right coronary artery (Fig. 10-4, A). Several large autonomic nervous system ganglions can occasionally be seen clustering in the epicardium adjacent to the node. The SAN lacks discrete structure, and its ill-defined borders merge with the adjacent atrial wall. It structurally consists of a collection of haphazardly oriented myofibers that appear as a pseudosyncytium and are embedded within abundant loose collagenous and elastic connective tissue, with rare cores of epicardially oriented dense collagen fibers (Fig. 10-4, *A1*). The nodal myofibers have discrete cell borders, a moderate amount of wavy sarcoplasm with sparse myofibrils, and an elongated nucleus that contains clumps of coarse chromatin (Fig. 10-4, *A2*).

Atrioventricular Node, Atrioventricular Bundle, and Bundle Branches. The AVN lies within the right atrial subendocardium and consists of a discrete, compact to loose mass of interconnecting myofibers that are often embedded within adipose tissue. A small nodal artery, parasympathetic ganglia, and large myelinated autonomic nerves are often present adjacent to the AVN. The nodal myofibers that have characteristic pale eosinophilic and thin sarcoplasm generally run parallel to each other but occasionally have an interweaving pattern with intervening loose collagen fibers. These myofibers contain a moderate amount of sarcoplasm with abundance of distinct striations and a short oval to elongated nucleus with dispersed chromatin.

The AV bundle (Fig. 10-4, *B*) emerges from the cranial pole of the AVN (Fig. 10-4, *B1*) and pierces through the CFB,

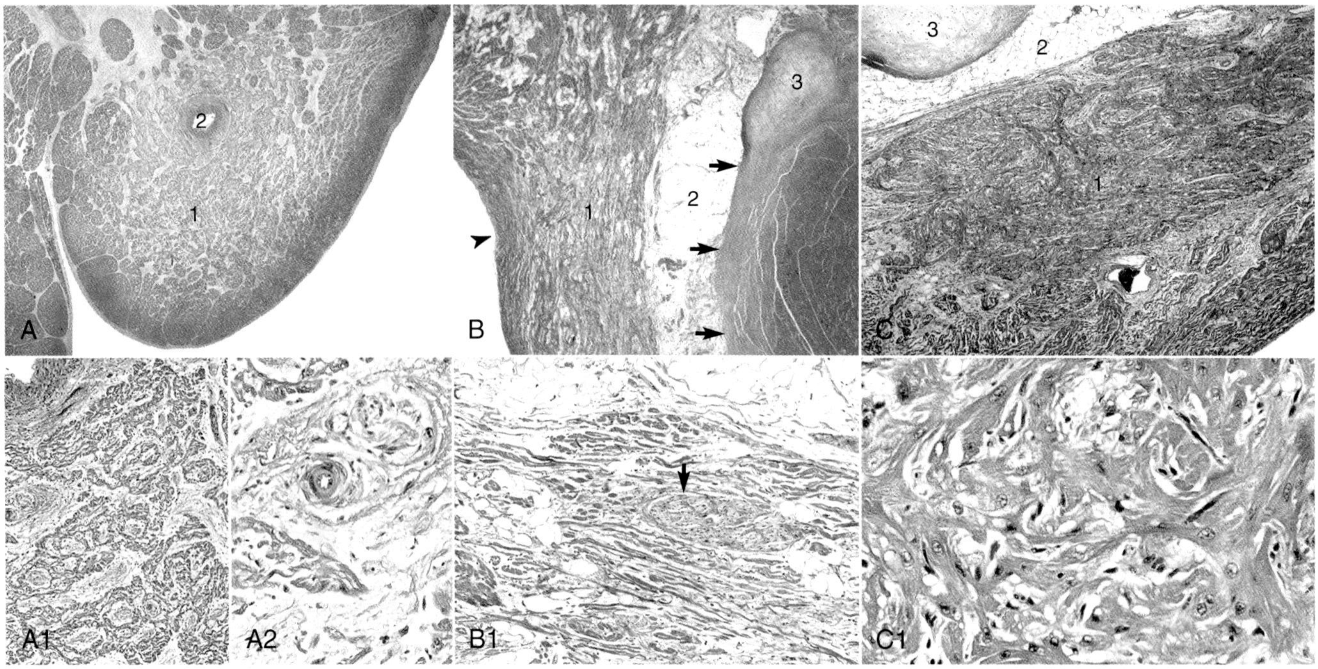

Figure 10-4 **Cardiac Conduction System. A,** Sinoatrial *(SA)* node, foal. The center of the SA node *(1)* contains a nodal artery *(2)*. H&E stain. **A1,** Higher magnification. Haphazardly oriented myofibers are embedded within abundant loose collagenous and elastic connective tissue. H&E stain. **A2,** Higher magnification. Nodal myofibers have discrete cell borders, a moderate amount of wavy sarcoplasm, and an elongated nucleus. H&E stain. **B,** Atrioventricular *(AV)* node, goat. The AV node *(1)* is composed of interconnecting nodal myofibers that are supported by loose collagenous and elastic fibrous stroma. The node is embedded in adipose tissue *(2)*. Note that in this illustration the AV node (1) is a poorly demarcated region (see *B1* for greater detail) that is elongated *(flattened)* from top to bottom and that it and its surrounding adipose tissue are positioned adjacent to the cardiac fibrous skeleton *(arrows)* that has undergone focal chondroid metaplasia *(3)*. The position and overall shape of the AV node in a histologic section is dependent on the plane of section. Endocardium *(arrowhead)*. H&E stain. **B1,** AV node, goat. In this higher magnification of *B*, AV nodal myofibers have a characteristic pale eosinophilic and thin sarcoplasm, with abundance of distinct striations and a short oval to elongated nucleus with dispersed chromatin. An autonomic myelinated nerve is present in the AV node *(arrow)*. H&E stain. **C,** AV bundle, goat. The AV bundle *(1)* travels diagonally through the center of the figure from the lower left to the upper right margins. It is formed by an interweaving pseudosyncytium of cardiac myofibers supported by a loose to dense intervening collagenous stroma (see *C1* for greater detail) and may be surrounded by adipose tissue *(2)*. Cardiac cartilaginous skeleton *(3)*. H&E stain. **C1,** Higher magnification. The AV bundle myofibers of the pseudosyncytium have moderate to large, pale eosinophilic sarcoplasm with prominent striations and large nuclei with fine stippled chromatin. H&E stain. (Courtesy Dr. A. Gal, Institute of Veterinary, Animal and Biomedical Sciences, Massey University; and Dr. J.F. Zachary, College of Veterinary Medicine, University of Illinois.)

approximately at the level of the annuli of the aortic and mitral valves (Fig. 10-4, *B2*), to become the left and right bundle branches. The size of an AV bundle myofiber progressively enlarges, and its cytomorphology transitions from a pale eosinophilic, small and thin (AVN-like morphology) myofiber to a pale eosinophilic, foamy to waxy, large, and somewhat rectangular myofiber that lacks cross-striations (a Purkinje-like cellular morphology) (Fig. 10-4, *C*).

Autonomic Nervous System. The nerve supply to the heart is autonomic and includes sympathetic, parasympathetic, and nonadrenergic noncholinergic innervation. Histologically, large nerves can be seen in the epicardium and adjacent to the coronary blood vessels, whereas special staining techniques are required for demonstration of neural tissue elsewhere. Electron microscopy and immunohistochemistry allow differentiation between sympathetic and parasympathetic nerves that are otherwise indistinguishable with H&E stain. Preganglionic parasympathetic fibers pass to the heart through the cardiac branch of the vagal nerve and synapse with parasympathetic ganglionic neurons. Postganglionic neurons are distributed to the SAN and AVN, as well as to atrial and, to a much lesser extent, ventricular myocardium (however, the ventricular conduction system is well supplied by cholinergic innervation). Postganglionic sympathetic fibers arising from the cervicothoracic and middle cervical ganglia intensely innervate the SAN and AVN and, to a lesser extent, the AV bundle. The atrial endocardium, myocardium, and epicardium are evenly innervated, whereas the ventricles are considerably less innervated, with epicardium more densely populated by neural tissue than the endocardium.

Endocardium and Heart Valves

The endocardium, lining the atrium and ventricles, consists of a continuous endothelium, subendothelium, and subendocardium. The subendothelial layer contains dense irregular fibroblasts intermixed with collagen and elastic fibers and occasional smooth muscle cells. Elastic fibers are abundant within the subendocardium of the atria. The subendocardial layer contains vascular structures, elastic and collagen bands, and fibroblasts and is continuous with the myocardium. Purkinje fibers are located in the subendocardium. The heart valves are poorly vascularized, endocardial folds covered by endothelium. The subendothelial layer is composed of fibroblasts with abundant elastic and collagen fibers. The AV valves (AVVs) consist of a layer of stratum spongiosum and stratum fibrosum. The stratum spongiosum consists of loosely arranged fibroblasts with moderate amounts of collagen and elastin fibers and vascular structures. The stratum fibrosis contains fibroblasts and collagen, which are continuous with the annulus fibrosis and chordae tendineae.

Pericardium and Epicardium

The pericardial sac is composed of parietal and visceral pericardium, both of which are covered by mesothelium. Beneath the visceral mesothelium is a thin layer of fibrous connective tissue, adipocytes, and vascular structures. This organization forms the subepicardium and interdigitates with the myocardium. The parietal pericardium is composed of an inner layer of mesothelium that interdigitates with the dense connective tissue forming the outer pericardial sac.

Blood and Lymphatic Vascular Systems

The overall design of the blood and lymphatic vessels is similar, except that luminal diameter, wall thickness, and the presence of other anatomic features, such as valves, vary between the different segments. The luminal surface of all vessels is lined by longitudinally aligned endothelial cells covering a basal lamina. Vessel walls are divided into three layers or tunics: intima, media, and adventitia. However, some of the layers can be absent or all of the layers can be thinned in some segments of the vascular system, depending on the intravascular pressures. The large elastic arteries such as the aorta have (1) an intima composed of endothelium and subendothelial connective tissue; (2) a very thick tunica media composed of fenestrated elastic laminae with interposed smooth muscle cells and ground substance and bordered internally by the internal elastic lamina and externally by the external elastic lamina; and (3) an outer tunica adventitia layer composed of collagen and elastic fibers and connective tissue cells with penetrating blood vessels, termed the *vasa vasorum*, supplying nutrients to the adventitia and the outer half of the media. In muscular arteries and arterioles, the tunica media is largely composed of smooth muscle cells arranged in a circumferential pattern. Arterioles are the smallest arterial channels and are generally less than 100 μm in diameter and with one to three layers of smooth muscle cells in the tunica media.

Capillaries are 5 to 10 μm in diameter, and their endothelium is one of three types: (1) continuous, (2) fenestrated (as in the endocrine glands), or (3) porous (as in renal glomeruli). The endothelium rests on an external lamina surrounded by pericytes. Pericytes are located abluminally to capillaries and postcapillary venules and because of their location, contractility, and cytoskeletal proteins may play a role in regulating capillary and venular blood flow. Lesions of the endothelium might not be evident by light microscopy, and electron microscopy is required for characterization.

Veins have thin walls in relation to their luminal size compared with those of arteries, in which blood pressure is greater. The adventitia is the thickest layer. Valves are present to prevent retrograde blood flow (i.e., away from the heart).

Lymphatic capillaries lack a basal lamina. Large lymphatic vessels are similar in structure to veins and generally have large lumina, thin walls, and a greater number of intimal valves but contain lymph.

The morphology of large arteries, veins, microvasculature, and lymphatic vessels is described in Chapter 2 and is not discussed further in this chapter.

Necropsy Assessment of Heart and Vascular Structures

For information on this topic, see E-Appendix 10-1 and E-Figs. 10-5 and 10-6 at www.expertconsult.com.

Examination of the Cardiovascular System and Lymphatic Vessels at Necropsy and Tissue Sampling for Histopathologic Evaluation

For information on this topic, see E-Appendix 10-2 and E-Fig. 10-7 at www.expertconsult.com.

Function

The primary function of the cardiovascular and lymphatic systems is to maintain an adequate and steady supply of nutrients to and facilitate the removal of waste products from all organs and tissues of the body. Cardiac myocytes provide the force of contraction; the conduction system and the nervous system control the flow and volume.

Myocardium

The results of normal cardiac function include the maintenance of adequate blood flow, called cardiac output, to peripheral tissues that provide delivery of oxygen and nutrients, the removal of carbon dioxide and other metabolic waste products, the distribution of hormones and other cellular regulators, and the maintenance of adequate thermoregulation and glomerular filtration pressure (urine output). The normal heart has a threefold to fivefold functional reserve capacity, but this capacity can eventually be lost in cardiac disease and the result is impaired function.

Cardiac Conduction System

Cells of the cardiac conduction system are modified cardiac myofibers that are able to spontaneously depolarize, which is also called *autoexcitation*, and function to (1) coordinate the sequence of events required for efficient ventricular filling during diastole and ejection during systole and (2) maintain the pressure in the pulmonary and systemic circuits (see E-Fig. 10-2).

Depolarization of the membrane of these pacemaker cells is due to a transiently increased rapid permeability to sodium ions and a slightly longer lasting increase in permeability to calcium ions that results in their influx into the myofiber sarcoplasm, thus changing the membrane potential (see Chapter 14). As this transient permeability is lost, membranal potassium channels open, and rapid outward potassium flux results in myofiber membranal hyperpolarization (along with sodium and calcium efflux), ultimately bringing the membrane potential back to a "normal" steady state (resting potential). During this period of time (refractory period), the myocyte cannot depolarize again because of a special conformation of membrane sodium channels that is transiently lost with depolarization and regained only with hyperpolarization. Intrinsically, the resting membrane potential of pacemaker cells is more positive than that of contracting cardiomyocytes and slightly more negative than the membrane threshold potential. This difference is due to leakiness of the pacemaker cell membrane to sodium and calcium ions and a steady low-grade influx of these ions.

Once one pacemaker cell depolarizes, a wave of depolarization propagates through the surrounding myocytes because these cells are connected to each other by special membranal pores (gap junctions), which allow for ionic exchange between adjacent cells. The number of gap junctions between cells of the conduction system is therefore a property that affects conduction velocity. Because the heart cycle must be strictly coordinated so that both atria and both ventricles contract and relax at the same time, and atrial contraction occurs simultaneous to the late ventricular relaxation, the depolarization wave has to be conducted fast at certain points along the conduction pathway and slower at others. Therefore, at different anatomic regions along the conduction pathway, the degree of cell-to-cell interaction dictates a slightly different cellular morphology.

When an electric signal (a propagating depolarization front) is generated in the sinoatrial node (SAN) and spreads throughout the atria from cell to cell and eventually reaches the atrioventricular node (AVN), it is also conveyed through the specialized internodal conducting fibers. The conduction in these fibers is approximately three times faster than that of the atrial myofibers. By conveying the signal through these fibers, both atria can contract simultaneously and in a coordinated manner that allows the process of pushing of blood into the ventricles. Correlating with their special fast conducting function, these cells have a Purkinje-like morphology. The conduction velocity is then slowed down when propagating through the AVN. The time it takes to conduct the signal through the AVN and penetrating AV bundles is approximately four times longer than the time it takes for it to be conducted from the SAN to the AVN. This delay in conduction serves to empty the atria from blood before the ventricles start to contract. It also contributes to the unidirectional blood flow between the atria and the ventricles, above and beyond the similar role played by the atrioventricular valves (AVVs).

Finally, the signal is delivered through the AV bundle, bundle branches, and Purkinje fibers in a velocity approximately 150 times faster than that of the AVN. The bundle branches run along the subendocardium of the interventricular septum and free ventricular walls and give rise to Purkinje fibers that supply the myocardium in a subendocardial-to-epicardial direction. This organization allows for a rapid and synchronous contraction of both ventricles at an order that ultimately enables blood to be "squeezed" from apex to base, toward both outflow tracts.

Cardiac myofibers have a unique property of intrinsic coupling of the electrical stimulation with mechanical contraction, which is fundamental for cardiac function. Diastole starts immediately at the end of ventricular contraction, as the cardiac muscle (myocardium) starts to relax. For a brief moment, relaxation leads to a rapid fall in ventricular pressure, without change in ventricular volume as the AVVs are still sealed off (isovolumetric relaxation). Because of the fall in ventricular pressure, the blood that has pooled in the atria during systole, along with incoming blood that constantly flows from systemic and pulmonary veins through the atria, pushes the AVV open and rapidly and passively fills the ventricles (rapid-filling phase). Next, because of the resultant pressure rise in the ventricles, the flow of blood that continues to enter the ventricles through the atria abruptly ends (diastasis phase). The last phase of diastole is active contraction of the atria, which pushes blood into the (now somewhat less compliant) ventricles and further raises their pressure ("atrial kick").

In systole, the myocardium contracts, leading to a rapid increase in intraventricular pressure. Because the aortic and pulmonary valves are shut during diastole, the sudden rise in pressure leads to closure of the AVVs. In this brief period, which is termed *isovolumetric contraction*, the change in ventricular pressure has not led to a change in ventricular volume because the blood had not yet been ejected into the aorta and pulmonary arteries. When the pressure in the ventricles exceeds the pressure in the great arteries, the aortic and pulmonary valves (semilunar valves) open and the ejection of the blood through the right and left side outflow tracts ensues (ejection phase). Simultaneously with the ejection phase, the atria relax, atrial pressure falls, and blood enters the atria and pools within it passively.

An additional level of complexity is brought about by the innervation of the autonomous nervous system (ANS). In general, the ANS influences heart rate (chronotropy), alters the rate of conduction (dromotropy), and controls myocardial contractility (inotropy) and the rate of mechanical relaxation (lusitropy). Parasympathetic postganglionic nerve terminals secrete acetylcholine that affects muscarinic (M2) receptors, whereas sympathetic postganglionic nerve terminals secrete norepinephrine that predominantly acts on the β_1-adrenergic receptors. The latter, when stimulated by catecholamines, lead to a chain of intracellular events that increases calcium influx, increases the magnitude of potassium and chloride repolarization, and shortens the refractory period. Therefore adrenergic agonists are said to be positive chronotropes, inotropes, dromotropes, and lusitropes, whereas parasympathetic agonists have the opposite effects. Heart rate is primarily regulated by opposing effects of adrenergic and cholinergic nerve terminals on the SAN and at the same time by modulation of conduction velocity of the AVN and AV bundle. Physiologically, the force of contraction represents the sum of interactions between myocardial contractility, which is positively modulated by adrenergic nerve terminals that act on β_1 receptors on ventricular myocardial myofibers (positive inotropic effect), and by the volume of blood that is present in the ventricles just before contraction (preload), as well as by the resistance in front of which contraction actually takes place (afterload).

Endocardium and Heart Valves

The endocardium lines the myocardium and contains Purkinje nerve fibers, which transmit a rhythmic action potential throughout the myocardium leading to contraction. The endocardium is lined by endothelial cells, which modulate many aspects of normal hemostasis. In normal states, the endothelial cells are antithrombotic, preventing circulating cells from attaching and thus allowing normal flow of blood through the heart and blood vessels. The endocardium is continuous with the endothelium of blood and lymphatic vessels. Normal flow of blood through the heart depends on functional valves (see Chapter 2). Properly functioning valves serve as one-way valves, allowing blood either to flow from one chamber to another (through AVVs) or to exit from the heart and enter either the pulmonary circulation (pulmonic valve) or the systemic circulation (aortic valve).

Pericardium and Epicardium

The pericardium contains a small amount of serous fluid, which allows frictionless cardiac movement of the mesothelial surfaces of the pericardium and epicardium on each other. The pericardial sac can adapt to changes in the heart size provided adequate time. The pericardium functions to provide a protective environment for cardiac function. Rapid, abnormal filling with blood (hemopericardium), fluid (hydropericardium), or exudate (suppurative pericarditis) can result in compression of the heart (cardiac tamponade), particularly the large veins, right atrium, and right ventricle. Animals can survive without a pericardial sac.

Blood and Lymphatic Vascular Systems

Blood and lymphatic vessels have several important functions. Blood vessels regulate the differential distribution of blood flow to tissues. Blood vessels actively synthesize and secrete vasoactive substances that regulate vascular tone and antithrombotic substances, which maintain the fluidity of the blood. Blood and lymphatic vessels play an important role in transporting and controlling inflammation and thrombosis. Blood and lymphatic vessels also constitute an important pathway for disease dissemination through transport of bacteria and tumor cells to distant sites.

Dysfunction/Responses to Injury

Common pathophysiologic responses of the cardiovascular system to injury are listed in Box 10-1 and shown in E-Fig. 10-8. The key characteristics of these responses are summarized here. The specific diseases that result from these responses are discussed in greater detail in the sections covering diseases that occur in all domestic animal species or that are unique to one species.

Box 10-1 Pathophysiologic Mechanisms of Cardiovascular Dysfunction

- Pump failure: Weak contractility and emptying of chambers, impaired filling of chambers
- Obstruction to forward blood flow: Valvular stenosis, vascular narrowing, systemic or pulmonary hypertension
- Regurgitant blood flow: Volume overload of chamber behind failing affected valve
- Shunted blood flows from congenital defects: Septal defects in heart, shunts between blood vessels
- Rupture of the heart or a major vessel: Cardiac tamponade, massive internal hemorrhage
- Cardiac conduction disorders (arrhythmias): Failure of synchronized cardiac contraction

Dysfunction: Heart Failure

Pathophysiology of Heart Failure

Heart failure is a progressive clinical syndrome in which impaired pumping decreases ventricular ejection and impedes venous return. The heart fails either by decreased blood pumping into the aorta and/or pulmonary artery to maintain arterial pressure (low-output heart failure) or by an inability to adequately empty the venous reservoirs (congestive heart failure) (see Box 10-1). Anamnestic signs of low cardiac output include depression, lethargy, syncope, and hypotension, and those of congestion include ascites, pleural effusion, and pulmonary edema.

Syndromes of Cardiac Failure or Decompensation: Congestive Heart Failure

Congestive heart failure can be right-sided, left-sided, or bilateral and can occur with cardiac dilation and/or hypertrophy (Fig. 10-5). Right-sided congestive heart failure is associated with signs of congestion in the systemic circulation (i.e., ascites and peripheral edema [Figs. 10-6 and 10-7]), whereas left-sided congestive heart failure causes signs of congestion in the pulmonary circulation (i.e., pulmonary edema and dyspnea). In small animals, *pleural effusion* is usually associated with bilateral congestive heart failure.

Heart failure may result from an inability of the heart to eject blood adequately (systolic failure), from inadequate ventricular filling (diastolic failure), or both. The resultant reduction in stroke volume (SV) leads to a decrease in cardiac output (CO) and a decrease in arterial blood pressure.

Indices of Cardiac Function

Arterial blood pressure (ABP) ~ CO × Z (where Z is the *aortic input impedance*) and CO = SV × heart rate (HR). Increases in HR increase CO linearly until a plateau is reached, at which point further increases in HR will decrease CO because of decreased diastolic filling (the Frank-Starling law of the heart). Contractility and the two coupling factors, preload and afterload, primarily determine SV. The latter increases with increases in preload and contractility and decreases in afterload. *Preload* reflects the degree of ventricular filling just before contraction. End diastolic volume (EDV) can estimate preload. The force opposing ventricular ejection is termed *afterload. Aortic input impedance* best describes the opposition that the ventricle encounters at the time of ejection. An increase in afterload communicates itself to the ventricles during systole by increasing wall stress. *Contractility* is a change in the heart's ability to do work when the preload, afterload, and HR are kept constant. Diastolic ventricular filling, ventricular wall motion abnormalities, space-occupying lesions, and arrhythmias also affect SV.

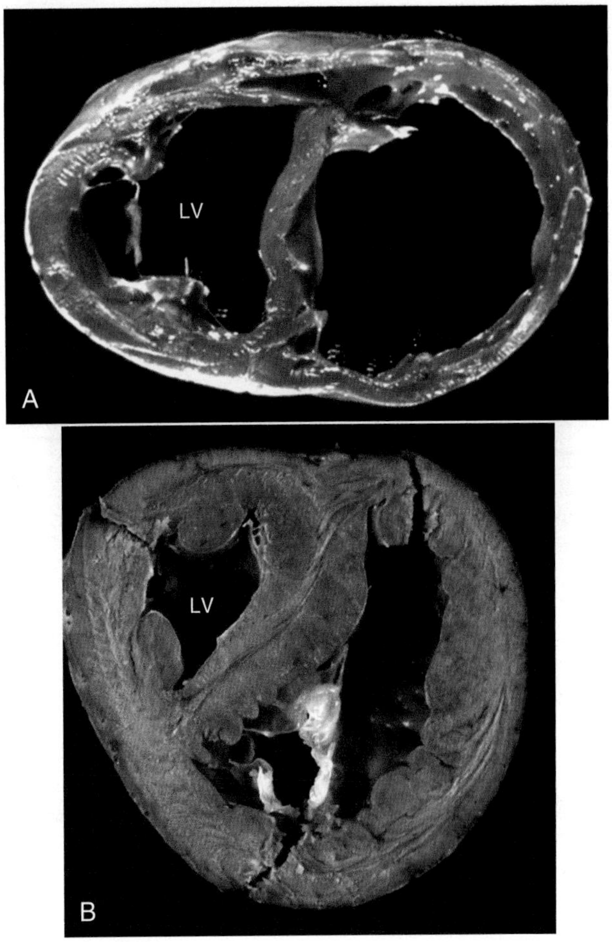

Figure 10-5 **Cardiac Dilation and Hypertrophy, Heart, Transected Ventricles, Dog. A,** Cardiac dilation. Note the thin walls of both dilated ventricles. *LV,* Left ventricle. **B,** Cardiac hypertrophy *(fixed tissue)*. Note that the right ventricular and left ventricular *(LV)* walls are approximately the same thickness, indicating that there is right ventricular hypertrophy. (**A** courtesy Dr. Y. Niyo, College of Veterinary Medicine, Iowa State University; and Noah's Arkive, College of Veterinary Medicine, The University of Georgia. **B** courtesy College of Veterinary Medicine, University of Florida; and Noah's Arkive, College of Veterinary Medicine, The University of Georgia.)

The properties of the arterial system can be described by the total arterial compliance, the peripheral resistance, and the characteristic impedance. *Total arterial compliance* corresponds to the elastic properties of arteries (i.e., aorta) and reflects change in volume from a given change in pressure. *Peripheral resistance* is largely determined by small arteries and arterioles and involves steady (nonpulsatile) flow. *Characteristic impedance* is the opposition to pulsatile flow.

Left ventricular (LV) afterload is increased by an increase in peripheral resistance and characteristic impedance and a decrease in total arterial compliance. Subsequently, the left ventricle ejects into a stiff vasculature, increasing both the energetic cost to maintain blood flow and myocardial oxygen consumption (MVO_2). Characteristic impedance, a property of the proximal aorta, increases whenever the stiffness of the aorta increases or its radius becomes smaller. Peripheral resistance has a greater effect on ventricular performance than does characteristic impedance or compliance.

Systolic and Diastolic Heart Failure

Systolic heart failure is characterized by normal filling of the ventricle and a decrease in the forward stroke volume (SV). The decrease in

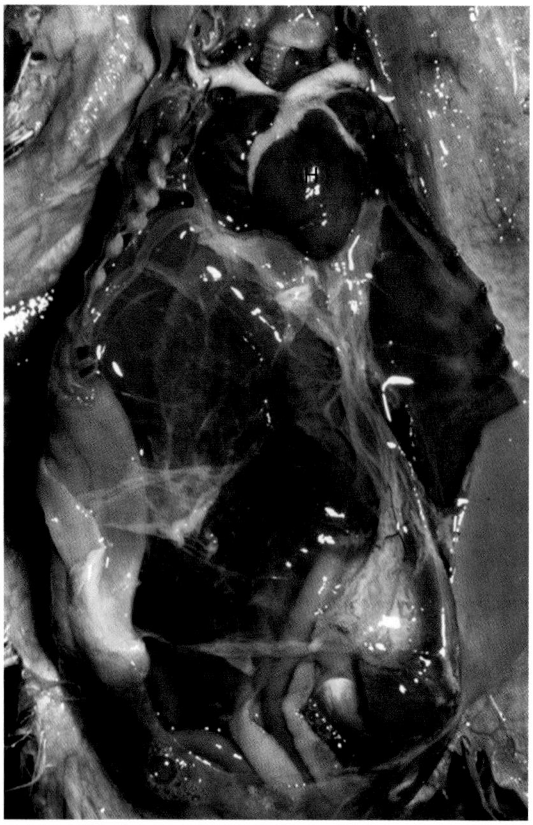

Figure 10-6 **Ascites, Congestive Heart Failure, Furazolidone Cardiotoxicity, Heart and Liver, Duckling.** Note prominent accumulations of serous fluid in the coelomic cavity and fibrin deposits over the surface of the liver. The heart *(H)* is dilated. (Courtesy School of Veterinary Medicine, Purdue University.)

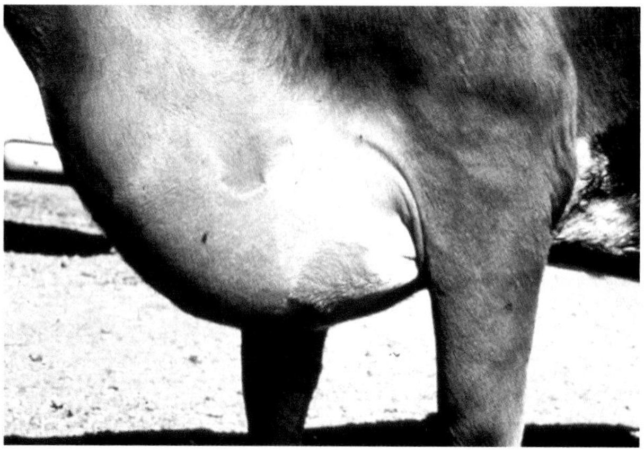

Figure 10-7 **Subcutaneous Edema, High-Altitude Disease with Congestive Heart Failure ("Brisket Disease"), Presternal, Sternal, and Caudal Sternocephalic Regions (Brisket), Cow.** The extensive subcutaneous edema is the result of chronic congestive heart failure. (Courtesy School of Veterinary Medicine, Purdue University.)

Box 10-2 Mechanisms Leading to Systolic Heart Failure

MYOCARDIAL FAILURE
- Dilated cardiomyopathy
- Infectious myocarditis
- Doxorubicin toxicity
- Cardiomyopathy of overload (pressure/volume)
- Myocardial infarcts
- Right ventricular cardiomyopathy

VOLUME OVERLOAD
- Valvular diseases
  - Myxomatous endocardial degeneration
  - Endocarditis
  - Rupture of mitral chordae tendineae
  - Valvular dysplasia
- PDA/VSD/ASD
- Thyrotoxicosis
- Chronic anemia
- Peripheral arteriovenous fistula

PRESSURE OVERLOAD
- Subaortic stenosis
- Pulmonic stenosis
- Systemic hypertension
- Pulmonary hypertension
  - Primary
  - Pulmonary embolism
  - Heartworm disease

ASD, Atrial septal defect; *PDA,* patent ductus arteriosus; *VSD,* ventricular septal defect.

SV may result from a decreased contractility (*myocardial failure*), from a primary increase in ventricular pressure (*pressure overload*), or or from an increase in ventricular volume (*volume overload*) (Box 10-2). Myocardial failure may be primary (e.g., dilated cardiomyopathy) or may occur secondary to chronic volume or pressure overload. The most common causes for pressure overload in domestic animals are subaortic stenosis and hypertension (left-sided congestive heart failure) and heartworm disease (E-Fig. 10-9), pulmonic stenosis (see Fig. 10-32), "brisket disease" ("high-altitude disease") in cattle (see Fig. 10-7), and chronic alveolar emphysema ("heaves") in horses (see Fig. 9-13) (right-sided congestive heart failure). Leaking valves, an abnormal communication between the systemic and pulmonary circulations, or high-output states (e.g., hyperthyroidism) usually result in increased ventricular volume (increased preload). Decrease in contractility lowers the SV, CO, and ABP and negates the heart's ability to compensate for the decrease in CO. *Diastolic heart failure* is characterized by improper filling of ventricles. This dysfunction may be caused by an impaired energy ventricular relaxation, myocardial dysfunction, obstruction to ventricular filling, or pericardial abnormalities (Box 10-3).

Concentric Hypertrophy

In pressure overload states, the increase in resistance to ejected blood leads to compensatory dilation (*concentric hypertrophy*). Chamber dilation in turn helps to overcome the increased resistance and to maintain SV at the expense of MVO_2, which eventually will lead to myocardial failure.

$$\text{LV wall stress} = \text{LV pressure}\frac{\text{LV radius}}{2 \times \text{LV wall thickness}}$$

From the previous equation, it can be depicted that decreased wall stress can be achieved by decreasing LV *radius* and/or by increasing LV *wall thickness*. With a sustained pressure overload, the ventricular muscle adapts by undergoing concentric hypertrophy, which leads to an increase in wall thickness at the expense of a decrease in chamber size (decrease in ventricular radius), thus returning ventricular wall stress toward normal and increasing contractility. The

Box 10-3 Mechanisms Leading to Diastolic Heart Failure

IMPAIRED ENERGY-DEPENDENT VENTRICULAR RELAXATION OR ABNORMAL VENTRICULAR CHAMBER OR MUSCLE PROPERTIES

- Ventricular hypertrophy
  - Hypertrophic cardiomyopathy
  - Subaortic stenosis
  - Pulmonic stenosis
  - Heartworm disease
  - Systemic hypertension
- Dilated cardiomyopathy
- Myocardial infarct
- Restrictive cardiomyopathy

OBSTRUCTION TO VENTRICULAR FILLING AT VEINS, ATRIA, AND ATRIOVENTRICULAR VALVES

- Mitral stenosis
- Tricuspid stenosis
- Intracardiac obstruction by neoplasia
- Cor triatriatum

PERICARDIAL ABNORMALITIES

- Constrictive disease
- Cardiac tamponade

hypertrophied ventricle is prone to ischemia, which leads to fibrosis and an increase in collagen content that interferes with diastolic filling, decreasing preload and SV. Therefore, in the end both systolic and diastolic dysfunction occur.

Eccentric Hypertrophy

In volume overload, the increase in chamber size occurs as a result of the need to accommodate a large ventricular EDV. Dilation of the ventricle by increasing the EDV leads to a lesser increase in wall stress than in pressure overload, and it subsequently results in ventricular *eccentric hypertrophy* in order to normalize wall stress. Volume overload is marked by an eccentric hypertrophy with a mild increase in wall thickness in the face of a large increase in LV radius.

Diastole can be divided into four phases: (1) isovolumic relaxation (aortic valve closure to mitral valve opening), (2) rapid early mitral inflow (rapid filling phase during which most of ventricular filling occurs), (3) diastasis (slow filling phase during which little change occurs in ventricular volume and pressure), and (4) atrial contraction (atrial systole that actively pumps blood to the ventricle). Diastolic ventricular filling takes place during the second through fourth phases. *Relaxation* (phase 1) is a dynamic, *energy-dependent* process. β-Adrenergic stimulation improves relaxation, whereas ischemia, asynchrony of relaxation, an increase in afterload, ventricular hypertrophy, and abnormal calcium fluxes in the myocardial cells *delay relaxation*. Ventricular *compliance* (phases 2 through 4) is the ability of the heart to fill passively. Ventricular compliance is determined by volume, geometry, and the tissue characteristics of the ventricular wall. Ventricular compliance decreases with an increase in filling pressure and intrinsic myocardial stiffness (e.g., infiltrative diseases, fibrosis, and ischemia), with hypertrophy and cardiac tamponade. *Lusitropy* comprises the relaxation and filling phases. Ventricular filling may be affected by several factors, including isovolumic relaxation rate, synchrony between atrial kick and ventricular relaxation, compliance, and atrioventricular pressure gradient. The latter is the driving force for ventricular filling (which is mostly affected by intravascular volume and the degree of vasodilatation). The isovolumic relaxation rate is also an important determinant of early ventricular filling; *adrenergic stimulation* increases the rate of relaxation, improving relaxation to a greater extent than it improves contractility. Tachycardia shortens the duration of the diastasis. Loss of atrial contraction is one reason why dogs with dilated cardiomyopathy or myxomatous valvular degeneration develop heart failure when the atria start to fibrillate.

Asynchronous relaxation (decrease in the uniformity of relaxation) of the left ventricle may be observed in cats with restrictive cardiomyopathy. LV hypertrophy decreases LV compliance and leads to poor diastolic function because of an increase in cardiomyocyte size, collagen formation, and wall thickening. Constrictive pericardial disease or cardiac tamponade impose their mechanical properties on those of the ventricle during the final phases of diastole. Hence, *diastolic dysfunction* results from abnormal relaxation (early diastole), abnormal compliance (early to late diastole), or external constraint by the pericardium (tamponade).

Neuroendocrine Compensatory Mechanisms in Heart Failure

Heart failure results in chronic activation of neuroendocrine compensatory mechanisms to restore and maintain ABP. High-pressure baroreceptors in the aortic arch and carotid sinus, mechanoreceptors in the ventricular myocardium, volume receptors in the atria and great veins, and the juxtaglomerular apparatus in the kidneys can sense alteration in ABP that results from a diminished CO. A reactive neuroendocrine activation decreases parasympathetic drive (immediate and short-lived) and increases sympathetic drive (slow but long-lasting), causing vasoconstriction (increasing arterial impedance) and tachycardia. A decrease in renal blood flow leads to renin-angiotensin-aldosterone system (RAAS) activation, contributing to vasoconstriction and sodium and water retention (increases the circulating volume). To maintain ABP, the cardiovascular system allows the venous pressure to increase and redistributes CO, maintaining blood flow mostly to essential organs. The cardiomyocytes also undergo changes to adapt to ventricular dysfunction, initially by performing extra work (stable hyperfunction) but over a long period these cardiomyocytes die (exhaustion and progressive cardiosclerosis phase). The net effect of neuroendocrine activation is vasoconstriction, sodium and water retention, LV hypertrophy, and coronary and peripheral vessel remodeling.

Role of Catecholamines in the Progression of Heart Failure

Dogs with congestive heart failure have increased norepinephrine (NE) concentrations secondary to NE "spillover" into plasma, and they have decreased uptake by adrenergic nerve endings. Despite the increase in the plasma concentration of NE, there is depletion of NE from the atria and ventricles (secondary to β-adrenoreceptor downregulation), which blunts the response to sympathetic activation. In normal hearts, the ratio of β_1 to β_2 receptors is approximately 80:20, whereas in failing hearts, it approaches 60:40. The decrease in NE stores and the changes in adrenoreceptors lead to a decrease in the contractile response of the myocardial cells and in a positive chronotropic response (increased HR). Chronic adrenergic stimulation also leads to an increase in afterload and MVO_2, development of ventricular arrhythmias, and progression to left ventricular dysfunction.

Role of Baroreceptors in the Progression of Heart Failure

Baroreflex control is altered during congestive heart failure. Normally, an increase in atrial pressure (volume overload) stimulates atrial stretch receptors, inhibits the release of antidiuretic hormone (ADH), decreases sympathetic activity, and increases renal blood flow and the glomerular filtration rate. During congestive heart failure, atrial and arterial receptors have a decreased response to stimulation, and baroreceptor function is impaired. The overall effect is a decrease in parasympathetic activity and subsequent impaired restraint on the SAN, which results in a higher HR and decreased HR variability.

Role of Renin-Angiotensin-Aldosterone System in the Progression of Heart Failure

In congestive heart failure, renin is continuously released in the juxtaglomerular apparatus of the kidneys secondary to the low CO. Consequently, perpetuation of angiotensin II (AGII) effects leads to a vicious cycle that contributes to further declines in ventricular function. These include AGII-mediated increase in afterload, increase in MVO_2, and increase in preload (through a decrease in venous capacity). AGII also stimulates the release of ADH and aldosterone (both contribute to total body water retention); the latter contributes to baroreceptor dysfunction, increased stiffness and decreased compliance of the arterial system, and increased Mg and K excretion. Increases in plasma aldosterone are associated with an inflammatory response that is thought to lead to intramural coronary artery remodeling and fibrosis. AGII stimulates growth factors, promoting remodeling in the vessels and myocardium (reduced NO synthesis or by increasing local angiotensin-converting enzyme breakdown of bradykinin). Consequently, vascular remodeling (i.e., smooth muscle hyperplasia, hypertrophy, and apoptosis) results in structural changes that further decrease the compliance of the arterial system. AGII has a key role in the development of pathologic hypertrophy, exerting cytotoxic effects on the myocardium, causing myocyte necrosis, and contributing to myocardial loss.

Role of Natriuretic Peptides and Nitric Oxide in the Progression of Heart Failure

The natriuretic peptides are counterregulatory hormones involved in volume homeostasis and cardiovascular remodeling, and they promote natriuresis, diuresis, peripheral vasodilatation, and inhibition of the RAAS. They consist of atrial natriuretic peptide (ANP), brain natriuretic peptide (BNP), C-type natriuretic peptide (CNP), dendraspis natriuretic peptides (DNP), and urodilatin. Despite the natriuretic peptides' beneficial effects during congestive heart failure, their release is overridden by the release of agents that cause vasoconstriction and sodium and water retention. NO regulates cardiac function through both vascular-dependent (coronary vessel tone, thrombogenicity, proliferative and inflammatory properties, and cellular cross-talk that supports angiogenesis) and vascular-independent (effects on several aspects of cardiomyocyte contractility, from the fine regulation of excitation-contraction coupling to modulation of autonomic signaling and mitochondrial respiration) effects. Overall, NO may play an important compensatory role in congestive heart failure during resting conditions by antagonizing neuroendocrine vasoconstrictive forces.

Summary of Pathophysiology of Heart Failure

In summary, long-term overload-induced cardiac hypertrophy is accompanied by myocardial cell death and cardiac fibrosis (i.e., cardiomyopathy of overload). The hypertrophied ventricle outstrips its blood supply. The relative decrease in oxygen delivery worsens the increased MVO_2 demand. The ischemia resulting from hypertrophy and stretching beyond certain limits decreases contractile strength and eventually leads to loss of contractile proteins within these cells or loss of these cells. These processes result in atrophy of the affected myocardium and lead to the development of multifocal myocardial fibrosis and atrophy, which consequently interferes with diastolic function. When early interstitial fibrosis progresses to individuation of cardiac myocytes (with progression of hypertrophy), both systolic and diastolic functions are impaired. Therefore congestive heart failure is a progressive and irreversible disease with myocardial cell death and functional myocardial failure that ultimately leads to death. The cycles resulting in progressive left heart failure are detailed in Fig. 10-8.

Cardiac Syncope

Cardiac syncope, an acute expression of cardiac disease, is characterized clinically by collapse, loss of consciousness, and extreme changes in heart rate and blood pressure, and with or without demonstrable lesions. Syncope can be caused by massive myocardial necrosis, ventricular fibrillation, heart block, arrhythmias, and reflex cardiac inhibition (e.g., that associated with high intestinal blockage).

Types of Heart Failure

A wide variety of experimental animal models of heart failure exist (E-Table 10-1). The models have been used to develop an understanding of human cardiac disease.

Clinical Diagnostic Procedures

For information on this topic, see E-Appendix 10-3 at www.expertconsult.com.

Responses to Injury: Myocardium

Common responses of the myocardium to injury are listed in Box 10-4.

Disturbances of Circulation

Hemorrhage: Trauma (Physical Injury). See section on Disorders of Domestic Animals: Myocardium, Disturbances of Circulation, Hemorrhage: Trauma (Physical Injury).

Disturbances of Growth

Myocardial Hypertrophy. See the discussion on hypertrophy in Chapter 1.

Hypertrophy of the myocardium represents an increase in muscle mass, which is the result of an increase in the size of cardiac muscle cells (Fig. 10-9; also see Fig. 10-5, *B* and E-Fig. 10-9). Two anatomic forms of hypertrophy are recognized. Eccentric hypertrophy results in a heart with enlarged ventricular chambers and walls of normal to somewhat decreased thickness. Volume-overload hypertrophy is characterized by new sarcomeres being assembled in series within sarcomeres resulting in increased length of myofibers. In concentric hypertrophy, the heart is characterized by small ventricular chambers and thick walls. Pressure-overload hypertrophy is the result of the formation of new sarcomeres assembled predominantly in parallel to the long axes of cells resulting in an increase in thickness of the myofiber. Some cats with hyperthyroidism have a cardiac hypertrophy that is mediated by enhanced production of myocardial contractile proteins under the influence of increased concentration of circulating thyroid hormones (Fig. 10-10). The hypertrophy is reversible on return to euthyroidism.

Three stages of myocardial hypertrophy are recognizable: (1) initiation, (2) stable hyperfunction, and (3) deterioration of function associated with degeneration of hypertrophied myocytes. Microscopically, in myocardial hypertrophy, the myocytes are enlarged and have large nuclei (Fig. 10-11).

Physiologic Atrophy. Physiologic atrophy of heart muscle may occur in confined animals and also occurs as a result of

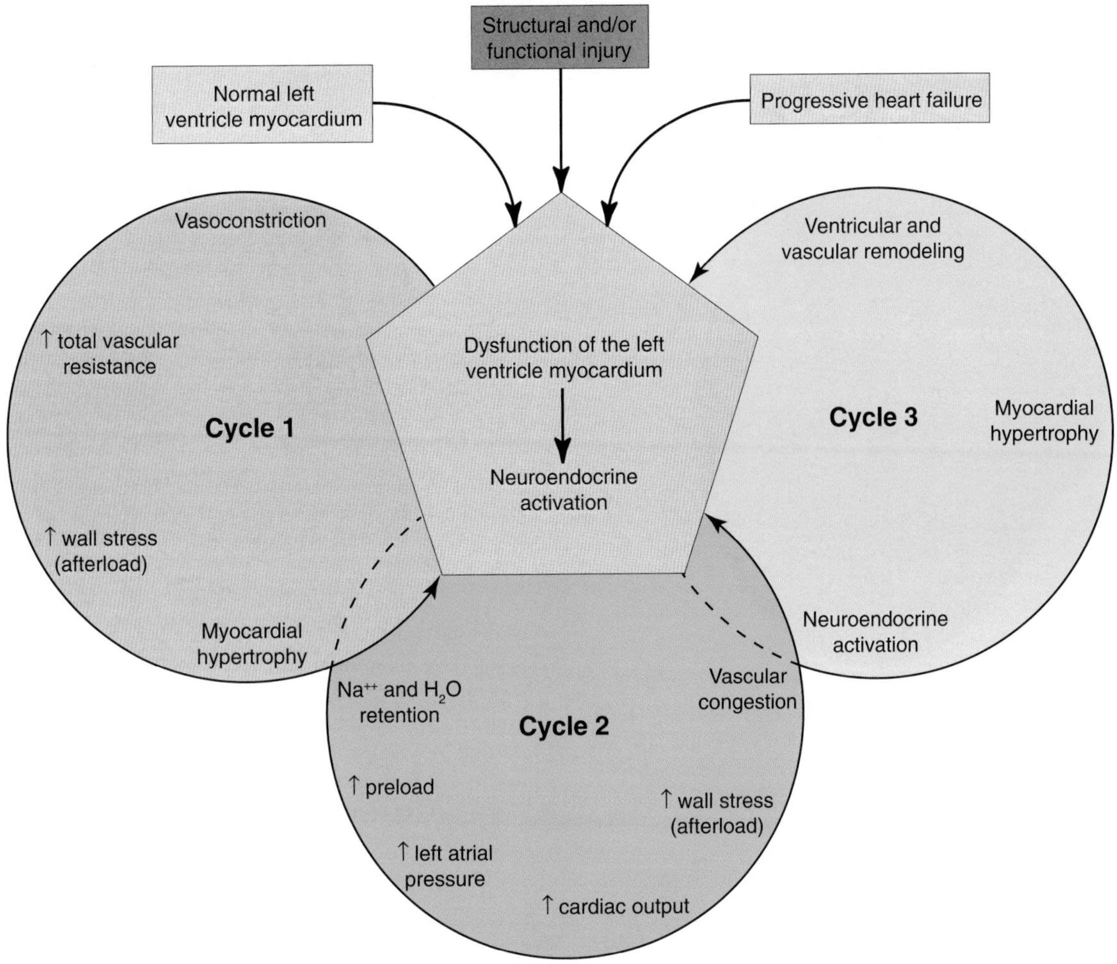

Figure 10-8 Pathophysiology of Left Heart Failure. Pathophysiologic cycles that lead to progressive left heart failure. *Cycle 1:* Increased total vascular resistance increases myocardial wall stress that induces myocardial hypertrophy. *Cycle 2:* Water and sodium retention leads to increased preload and vascular congestion. *Cycle 3:* Neuroendocrine activation leads to myocardial and vascular remodeling. All cycles contribute to further myocardial dysfunction and neuroendocrine activation. (Adapted from Ettinger SJ, Feldman EC: *Textbook of veterinary internal medicine,* ed 6, St. Louis, 2005, Saunders.)

Box 10-4 Responses of the Myocardium to Injury

DISTURBANCES OF CIRCULATION
Hemorrhage
Effusions
Thrombosis and embolism

DISTURBANCES OF GROWTH
Atrophy (dilation)
Hypertrophy
Agenesis (aplasia), hypoplasia, dysplasia (dysgenesis)
Developmental errors, congenital anomalies
Neoplasia (neoplastic transformation)

CELL DEGENERATION AND DEATH
Cell and metabolic dysfunction
Oncotic necrosis
Apoptosis

INFLAMMATION

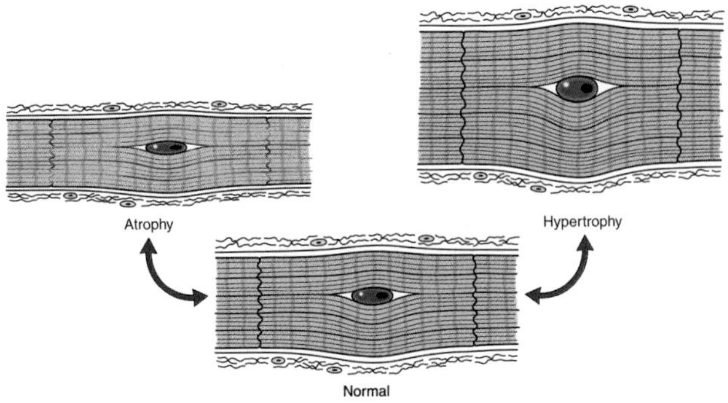

Figure 10-9 Cardiac Muscle Cells. Growth disturbances of atrophy and hypertrophy. (Redrawn with permission from School of Veterinary Medicine, Purdue University.)

decompensation of cardiac myocytes in chronic congestive heart failure (see Fig. 10-5, *A*). Initially, these myocytes respond through hypertrophy with increased contractile force according to the Frank-Starling phenomenon. However, stretching beyond certain limits decreases contractile strength and eventually leads to loss of contractile proteins within these cells or loss of these cells resulting in atrophy of the affected myocardium (see Fig. 10-9).

Neoplastic Transformation. See Chapter 6 for a discussion of the mechanisms involved in neoplastic transformation. Rhabdomyomas and rhabdomyosarcomas are primary tumors that originate from the myocardium in domestic animals. Fibrosarcomas also occur rarely. Numerous types of secondary tumors, such as

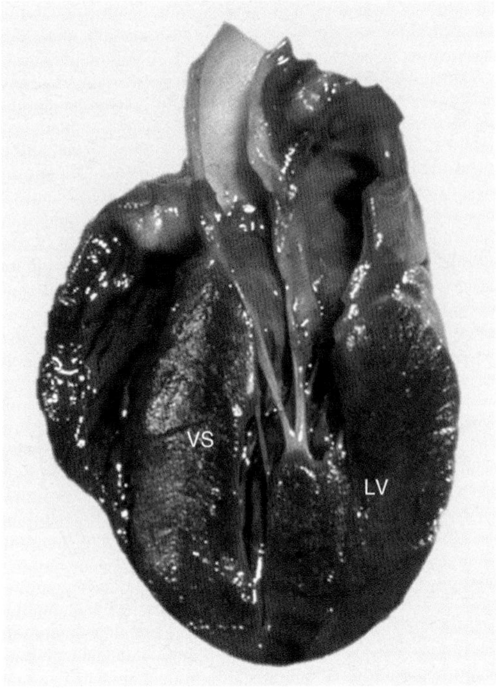

Figure 10-10 **Left Ventricular Hypertrophy, Hyperthyroidism, Heart, Bisected, Cat.** Note prominent thickening of the left ventricular *(LV)* free wall. The ventricular septum *(VS)* is also thickened. (Courtesy School of Veterinary Medicine, Purdue University.)

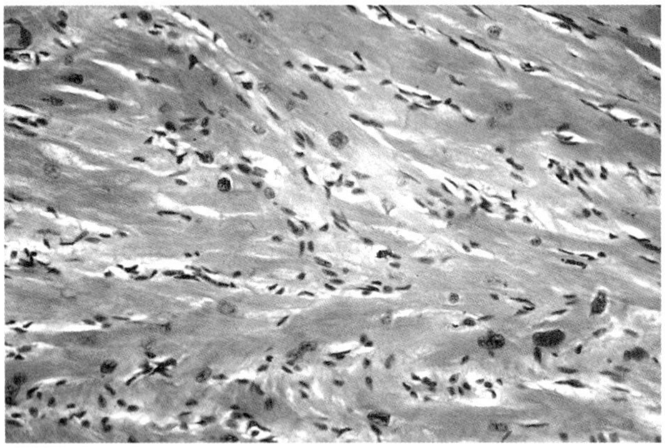

Figure 10-11 **Hypertrophic Cardiomyopathy, Myocyte Hypertrophy, Heart, Myocardium, Cat.** Cardiac myocytes are hypertrophied, and there is an increase in interstitial fibroblasts. H&E stain. (Courtesy School of Veterinary Medicine, Purdue University.)

lymphosarcomas, metastasize to the myocardium and are discussed in this chapter and other chapters of this book. Hemangiosarcomas are tumors of blood vessels of the myocardium of the right atrium and are discussed later.

Cell Degeneration and Death

Sublethal cardiac muscle cell injuries include lipofuscinosis, fatty degeneration, myocytolysis, and vacuolar degeneration (Fig. 10-12; see Chapter 1). Histopathologic study of sections of the myocardium is substantially limited with respect to specific diagnoses and only rarely can an etiologic diagnosis be made from the morphologic alterations. This inadequacy exists because the spectrum of pathologic reactions is limited, and many agents that damage the heart produce similar lesions. Myocardial necrosis can be confused with

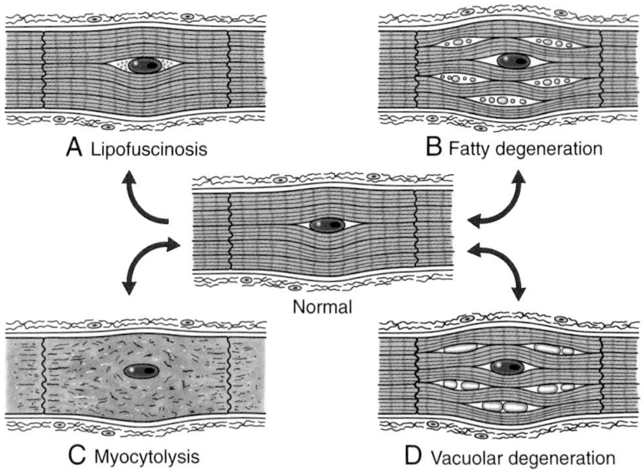

Figure 10-12 **Various Sublethal Cardiac Muscle Cell Injuries. A,** Lipofuscinosis. **B,** Fatty degeneration. **C,** Myocytolysis. **D,** Vacuolar degeneration. (Redrawn with permission from School of Veterinary Medicine, Purdue University.)

myocardial inflammation with secondary necrosis because both lesions have substantial leukocytic infiltration. Some animals that die peracutely from cardiac failure lack detectable microscopic alterations and are presumed to have suffered from an arrhythmic episode resulting in syncope. Hearts with long-standing myocardial damage have foci of fibrosis, regardless of the cause of the loss of myocytes. Correlation between the severity of clinical cardiac disease and the severity of myocardial injury can be poor: A small lesion at a critical site, such as a portion of the conduction system, can be fatal, whereas a widespread myocardial lesion, such as myocarditis, can be asymptomatic.

Cardiac myofibers can respond to toxins in a variety of ways—apoptosis, myofibrillar lysis, and coagulation necrosis are but a few mechanisms that may result from toxic exposure. A long list of toxins are responsible for causing myocardial injury; some of the most frequently observed current examples are ionophore toxicity in horses and ruminants, vitamin E–selenium deficiency in the young of many species, "heart-brain syndrome" of dogs (see Fig. 10-82), anthracycline toxicity in dogs, and gossypol toxicosis in pigs (Box 10-5). In various localized areas throughout the world, numerous deaths in ruminants have resulted from consumption of poisonous plants such as *Acacia georginae* and *Dichapetalum cymosum*.

Cardiotoxicity has emerged as a significant clinical entity in veterinary medicine in recent years with the growing use of antineoplastic drugs in small animal practice and the widespread use of growth promotants in ruminants (see Fig. 10-49). The mechanisms of cardiotoxicities include (1) exaggerated pharmacologic action of drugs acting on cardiovascular tissues, (2) exposure to substances that depress myocardial function, (3) direct injury of cardiac muscle cells by chemicals, and (4) hypersensitivity reactions.

Oncotic Necrosis. Necrosis of cardiac muscle cells is generally followed by leukocytic invasion and phagocytosis of sarcoplasmic debris (Fig. 10-13; also see Figs. 15-13 and 15-14). The end result is persistence of collapsed sarcolemmal "tubes" of basal lamina surrounded by condensed interstitial stroma and vessels. Lesions with severe disruption of the myocardium have residual changes of fibroblastic proliferation and collagen deposition to form scar tissue. Regeneration of cardiac muscle cells generally does not occur, except in less evolved animals, such as amphibians and fish, and in certain inbred mouse strains. The continual contraction of intact cardiac muscle cells impairs the mechanisms for regeneration. Also,

Box 10-5 Causes of Myocardial Necrosis in Animals

NUTRITIONAL DEFICIENCIES

Vitamin E–selenium, potassium, copper, thiamine, magnesium

TOXICITIES

Cobalt, catecholamines, vasodilator antihypertensive drugs, methylxanthines (theobromine, theophylline, caffeine), ionophores (monensin, lasalocid, salinomycin, maduramicin, narasin), vitamin D and calcinogenic plants (*Cestrum diurnum*, *Trisetum flavescens*, *Solanum malacoxylon*, *Solanum torvum*), other poisonous plants (*Acacia georginae*, *Gastrolobium* spp., *Oxylobium* spp., *Dichapetalum cymosum*, *Persea americana*, *Cassia occidentalis*, *Cassia obtusifolia*, *Karwinskia humboldtiana*, *Ateleia glazioviana*, *Eupatorium rugosum*, *Adonis aestivalis*, *Pachystigma pygmaeum*, *Fadogia homblei*, *Pavetta harborii*, *Tetrapterys multiglandulosa*), blister beetles (*Epicauta*), high-erucic-acid rapeseed oil, brominated vegetable oils, gossypol, T-2 mycotoxin, sodium fluoracetate (compound 1080), selenium, uremia

PHYSICAL INJURIES AND SHOCK

Central nervous system lesions and trauma ("heart-brain syndrome"), gastric dilation and volvulus, stress, overexertion, electrical defibrillation, hemorrhagic shock

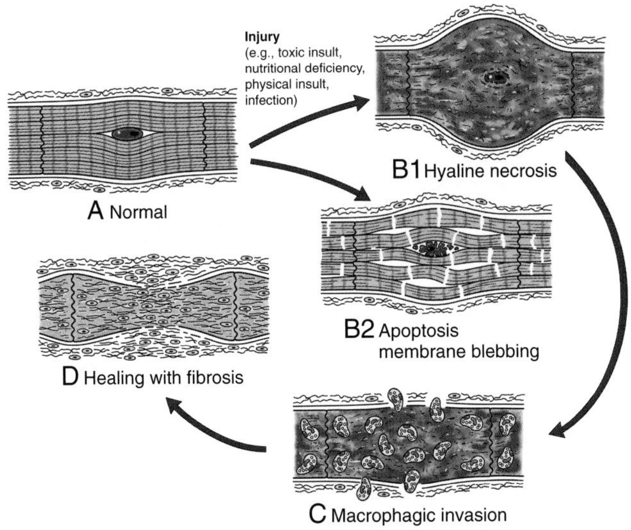

Figure 10-13 Sequential Events in Myocardial Necrosis. **A,** Various injuries lead to **(B1)** hyaline necrosis or **(B2)** apoptosis membrane blebbing. **C,** Healing with phagocytosis of cellular debris by macrophages, and **(D)** subsequent healing with fibrosis, rather than by regeneration. (Redrawn with permission from School of Veterinary Medicine, Purdue University.)

in hearts of neonatal animals and more often in avian hearts, a limited amount of myocyte regeneration has been reported. Hyperplasia of myocytes is a normal component of cardiac growth in fetal development and during the first few weeks of life. Thereafter, proliferation ceases and "normal growth" is the result of hypertrophy until cell size normal for each species is reached. Recent studies indicate that stem cells exist in adult animal and human hearts, and with myocardial injury, these cells may differentiate into cardiac muscle cells. However, the extent of myocyte regeneration is probably minimal.

Apoptosis. Apoptosis (programmed cell death of cardiac myocytes) is increasingly recognized for its role in the development of various myocardial lesions and cardiac diseases (see Chapter 1). These conditions include cardiac development, ischemic injury, several types of experimentally induced heart failure (ischemia-reperfusion, hypoxia, and pressure-overload hypertrophy), and cardiotoxicity. In some cell systems, apoptosis can be triggered by the presence of excessive amounts of oxygen free radicals. Cells dying by apoptosis shrink and form apoptotic bodies. In contrast to cell death by necrosis, apoptosis is not accompanied by an inflammatory reaction and fibrosis.

Fatty Infiltration. Fatty infiltration is the presence of increased numbers of lipocytes interposed between myocardial fibers. The lesion is associated with obesity and age and appears as abundant epicardial and myocardial deposits of adipose tissue. Grossly, the myocardium has irregular layers of adipose tissue infiltrating normal myocardium. The atria and right ventricle are most often affected.

Fatty Degeneration. Fatty degeneration (fatty change) is the accumulation of abundant lipid droplets in the sarcoplasm of myocytes. Microscopically, affected myocytes have numerous variably sized spherical droplets that appear as empty vacuoles in paraffin sections but stain positively for lipids with lipid-soluble stains in frozen sections. This lesion occurs with systemic disorders, such as severe anemia, toxemia, and copper deficiency, but is seen much less often in the heart than in the liver and kidneys (also see Chapter 1).

Hydropic Degeneration. Hydropic degeneration, a distinctive microscopic alteration in cardiac muscle cells, is associated with chronic administration of anthracyclines, a group of antineoplastic drugs. Chronic passive congestion with ascites and cardiac dilation may result (E-Figs. 10-10 and 10-11); see Figs. 10-5, A and 10-6). Affected fibers have extensive vacuolization of sarcoplasm that is initiated by distention of elements of sarcoplasmic reticulum and eventually ends in lysis of contractile material (E-Figs. 10-12 and 10-13).

Hydropic degeneration of cardiac muscle cells may also result from drug-induced injury to mitochondria. Antiretroviral drugs, such as nucleoside reverse transcriptase inhibitors (zidovudine or AZT), are linked to this distinctive lesion. Scattered cardiac muscle cells appear swollen with pale sarcoplasm by light microscopy. Electron microscopy reveals extensive mitochondrial swelling and disruption of cristae with subsequent formation of myelin figures from the membrane debris of damaged mitochondria.

Myofibrillar Degeneration. Myofibrillar degeneration (myocytolysis) represents a distinctive sublethal injury of cardiac muscle cells. Affected fibers have pale eosinophilic sarcoplasm and lack cross-striations. Ultrastructurally, myofibrils have a variable extent of dissolution (myofibrillar lysis). This lesion has been described in furazolidone cardiotoxicity in birds (Fig. 10-14; E-Fig. 10-14) and potassium deficiency in rats.

Lipofuscinosis. Lipofuscinosis (brown atrophy) of the myocardium occurs in aged animals and in animals with severe cachexia, but it also has been described as a hereditary lesion in healthy Ayrshire cattle. Severely affected hearts appear brown and microscopically have clusters of yellow-brown granules at the nuclear poles of myocytes. These granules represent intralysosomal accumulation of membranous and amorphous debris (residual bodies).

Mineralization. Myocardial mineralization (calcium) is a prominent feature in several diseases, such as hereditary calcinosis in mice, cardiomyopathy in hamsters, vitamin E–selenium

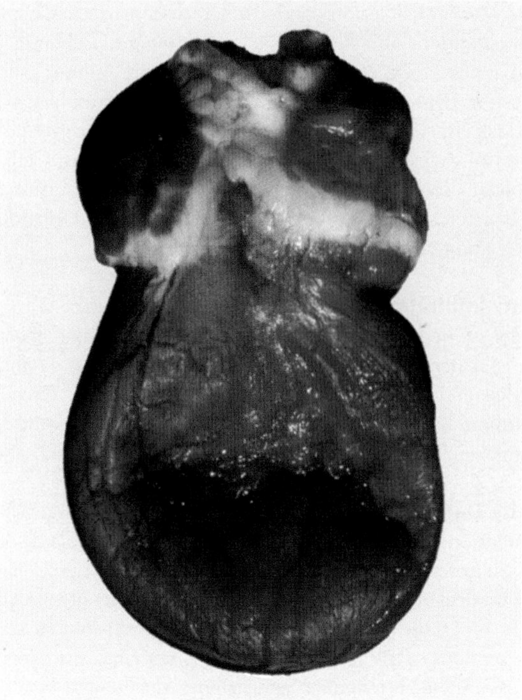

Figure 10-14 **Ventricular Dilation, Furazolidone Cardiotoxicity, Heart, Duckling.** Note that the dilated ventricles have collapsed once the blood was removed. (Courtesy School of Veterinary Medicine, Purdue University.)

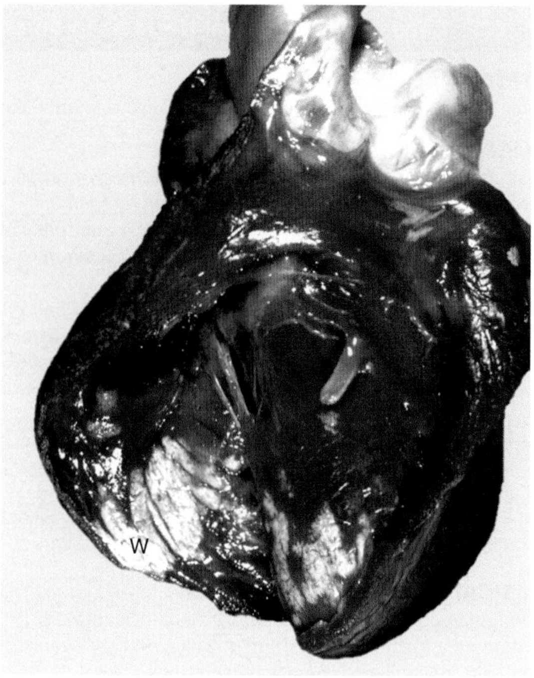

Figure 10-15 **Calcification, Vitamin E–Selenium Deficiency, Myocardial Necrosis, Heart, Right Ventricle, Lamb.** The multiple white *(W)* subendocardial lesions are areas of calcified necrotic cardiac myocytes. (Courtesy Dr. M.D. McGavin, College of Veterinary Medicine, University of Tennessee.)

deficiency in sheep and cattle (Fig. 10-15), vitamin D toxicity in several species, calcinogenic plant toxicosis in cattle ("Manchester wasting disease"), and spontaneous myocardial calcification in aged rats and guinea pigs.

Myocardial Necrosis. Myocardial necrosis can result from a number of causes, including nutritional deficiencies, chemical and plant toxins, ischemia, metabolic disorders, heritable diseases, and physical injuries (see Box 10-5). Grossly, affected areas appear pale initially, and some progress to prominent yellow to white (see Fig. 10-49), dry areas made gritty by dystrophic mineralization. The lesions are focal, multifocal, or diffuse. The most frequent sites of focal lesions are the left ventricular papillary muscles and the subendocardial myocardium, especially when such lesions are related to transient reduction of vascular perfusion. These lesions can be overlooked at necropsy unless multiple incisions are made in the ventricular myocardium. In diseases with diffuse cardiac necrosis, such as white muscle disease of calves and lambs due to vitamin E–selenium deficiency, the discrete white lesions can be readily observed beneath the epicardial and endocardial surfaces (Fig. 10-16).

Microscopically, the appearance depends on the age of the lesions. Fibers in areas of recent necrosis often appear swollen and hypereosinophilic (hyaline necrosis). Striations are indistinct, and nuclei are pyknotic. Necrotic fibers often have scattered basophilic granules (Fig. 10-17) that represent calcified mitochondria and can be confirmed by electron microscopy (E-Fig. 10-15). In a second pattern of necrosis, affected myocytes have a "shredded" appearance because of hypercontraction and the formation of multiple transversely oriented bars of disrupted contractile material (often termed *contraction band necrosis*) (E-Fig. 10-16). A third pattern is seen in necrotic myocytes in large areas of ischemic necrosis (infarcts). These myocytes have features of coagulation necrosis and have relaxed rather than hypercontracted contractile elements.

Within 24 to 48 hours after injury, necrotic areas are infiltrated by inflammatory cells, mainly macrophages and a few neutrophils; these phagocytose and lyse the necrotic cellular debris (E-Fig. 10-17). In early stages of healing of necrosis, it is often difficult to distinguish the lesions from those found in some types of myocarditis (see later discussion). Later, when necrosis has progressed somewhat, lesions consist of persistent stromal tissue (interstitial fibroblasts, collagen, and capillaries) and empty "tubes" of basal laminae formerly occupied by necrotic myocytes (see Chapter 15). The healing phase is characterized by proliferation of connective tissue cells (fibroblasts) (Fig. 10-18) and by deposition of connective tissue products (collagen and elastic tissue and acid mucopolysaccharides). Grossly, these areas with healing of myocardial necrosis appear as white, firm, contracted scars.

The outcome of myocardial necrosis varies, depending on the extent of the damage:

- Many animals die unexpectedly of acute cardiac failure if the myocardial damage is extensive.
- Early deaths from necrosis-related arrhythmias also occur when cardiac conduction is disrupted.
- Some cases eventually develop cardiac decompensation and die with cardiac dilation, scarring, and lesions of chronic congestive failure.

Hearts with minimal damage have only microscopically detectable myocardial fibrosis when death eventually occurs from other diseases.

Inflammation

Myocarditis. The various infectious diseases that cause myocarditis in animals are summarized in Box 10-6. Myocarditis generally

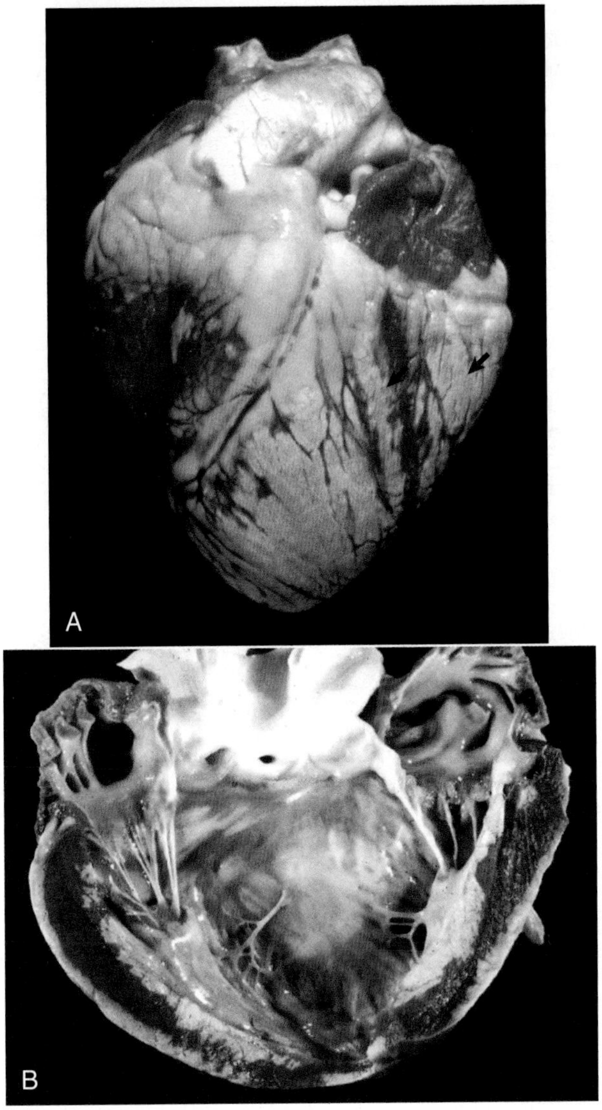

Figure 10-16 Myocardial Necrosis, Vitamin E–Selenium Deficiency, Heart, Left Ventricular Myocardium, Calf. A, Note the prominent white chalky areas of necrosis with mineralization *(arrows)* of the myocardium. **B,** Similar necrosis is subepicardially and subendocardially in the sectioned free walls of the left ventricle and subendocardially in the myocardium of the ventricular septum *(center)*. (**A** courtesy School of Veterinary Medicine, Purdue University. **B** courtesy Dr. P.N. Nation, Animal Pathology Services; and Noah's Arkive, College of Veterinary Medicine, The University of Georgia.)

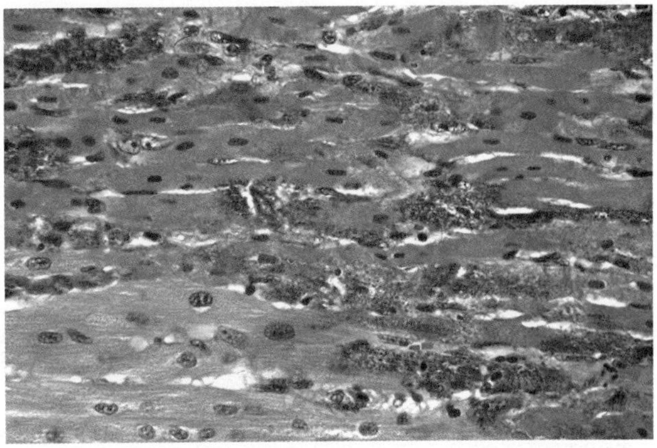

Figure 10-17 Acute Myocardial Necrosis with Mineralization, Minoxidil Cardiotoxicity, Heart, Ventricular Myocardium, Pig. The darker red myocytes are necrotic, and some are mineralized *(purplish areas)*. H&E stain. (Courtesy School of Veterinary Medicine, Purdue University.)

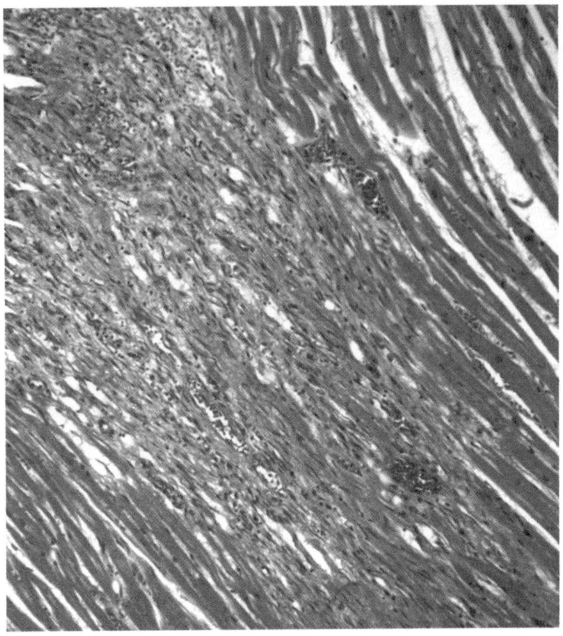

Figure 10-18 Healing, Postmyocardial Necrosis, Heart, Ventricle, Dog. The necrotic myocytes have been removed by phagocytosis by macrophages *(not seen here)*, and the area is now undergoing fibrosis. H&E stain. (Courtesy Dr. J.F. Zachary, College of Veterinary Medicine, University of Illinois.)

is the result of infections spread hematogenously to the myocardium and occurs in various systemic diseases. Infrequently, the heart is the primary location in affected animals and responsible for death. Types of inflammation provoked by infectious agents that produce myocarditis include suppurative, necrotizing, hemorrhagic, lymphocytic, and eosinophilic. Suppurative myocarditis results from localization of pyogenic bacteria in the myocardium (Fig. 10-19) that are trapped in thromboemboli most commonly originating from vegetative valvular endocarditis on the mitral and aortic valves. Septic infarcts with pale, disseminated lesions may be grossly evident in the myocardium. These foci consist of neutrophils and necrotic myocytes that form abscesses.

The pathogenesis and expected outcome of cases of myocarditis remain an important area of research because of the severity of this lesion in cardiac failure in human beings. The sequelae to myocarditis include (1) complete resolution of lesions, (2) scattered residual myocardial scars, or (3) progressive myocardial damage with acute or, in some cases, chronic cardiac failure as secondary dilated (congestive) cardiomyopathy. In experimental studies of myocarditis induced in mice by coxsackie B virus, the severity of myocarditis was influenced by the virulence of the virus and mouse strain and was enhanced by host factors such as young age, male sex, pregnancy, poor nutrition, whole-body ionizing radiation, cold environmental temperatures, alcohol ingestion, exercise, and cortisone administration. Much of the myocardial damage in coxsackie B virus infection is induced by immunologic reactions (with T lymphocyte involvement) rather than by direct viral injury.

Responses to Injury: Cardiac Conduction System

In domestic animals, injury of the cardiac conduction system involves forms of cell degeneration and death, inflammation, and fibrosis. The response to injury of the conduction system is poorly documented because histopathology of the conduction system is labor-intensive and rarely performed. In rare cases in which histopathology and electrocardiographic studies were available, atrial and/or ventricular origin of arrhythmia was associated with inflammation, degeneration, and fibrosis along the cardiac conduction system (Fig. 10-20).

Box 10-6 Diseases that Cause Myocarditis in Animals

VIRAL

Canine parvovirus, encephalomyocarditis, foot-and-mouth disease, pseudorabies, canine distemper, cytomegalovirus, Newcastle disease, avian encephalomyelitis, eastern and western equine encephalomyelitis, West Nile virus

BACTERIAL

Blackleg (*Clostridium chauvoei*), listeriosis (*Listeria monocytogenes*), Tyzzer's disease (*Clostridium piliforme*, formerly *Bacillus piliformis*), necrobacillosis (*Fusobacterium necrophorum*), tuberculosis (*Mycobacterium* spp.), caseous lymphadenitis (*Corynebacterium pseudotuberculosis*), Lyme disease (*Borrelia burgdorferi*), disseminated infections by *Actinobacillus equuli*, *Staphylococcus* sp., *Corynebacterium kutscheri*, *Trueperella* (*Arcanobacter*) *pyogenes*, *Histophilus somni*, *Pseudomonas aeruginosa*, *Streptococcus equi*, and *Streptococcus pneumoniae*

PROTOZOAN

Toxoplasmosis (*Toxoplasma gondii*), sarcocystosis (*Sarcocystis* sp.), neosporosis (*Neospora caninum*), encephalitozoonosis (*Encephalitozoon cuniculi*), trypanosomiasis (Chagas' disease [*Trypanosoma cruzi*]), East Coast fever (*Theileria parva*)

PARASITIC

Cysticercosis (*Cysticercus cellulosae*), trichinosis (*Trichinella spiralis*)

IDIOPATHIC

Eosinophilic myocarditis

Responses to Injury: Endocardium and Heart Valves

Disturbances of Circulation

Hemorrhage. Endocardial hemorrhages are commonly seen and may be the result of trauma or septicemias, especially those with endotoxins, or can occur agonally at death (Fig. 10-21). See the previous sections on the Pericardium and Epicardium and the Myocardium and Box 10-4 and also Chapter 2.

Disturbances of Growth

Valvular Anomalies and Dysplasia. See the discussion on valvular anomalies and dysplasia in the section on Disorders of Domestic Animals, Developmental Errors/Congenital Anomalies: Endocardium and Heart Valves.

Cellular Degeneration and Death

See Chapter 1 for discussion of the causes of cell injury, irreversible cell injury and cell death, and chronic cell injury and cell adaptations.

Myxomatous Valvular Degeneration (Endocardiosis). See the discussion on myxomatous valvular degeneration (endocardiosis) in the section on Disorders of Dogs and Fig. 10-83.

Mineralization. Mineralization of the endocardium is seen with vitamin D toxicity, calcinogenic plant toxicosis in cattle, and calcium phosphorus imbalance, as well as in Johne's disease (Fig. 10-22; see Chapter 7). The endocardium and large elastic arteries are prone to mineralization because of their abundant elastic fibers.

Inflammation

See Chapters 3 and 5 for discussion of the processes and mechanisms of acute and chronic inflammation.

Responses to Injury: Pericardium and Epicardium

Disturbances of Circulation

Hemorrhage. See section on Disorders of Domestic Animals, Disorders of Domestic Animals: Pericardium and Epicardium, Disturbances of Circulation, Hemorrhage.

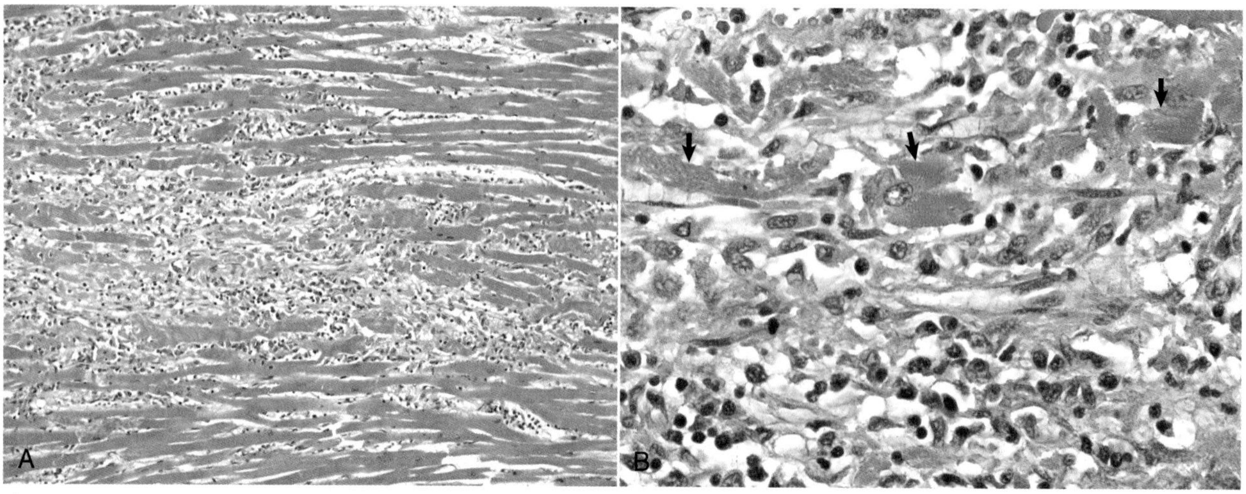

Figure 10-19 **Acute Myocarditis, Horse. A,** The parallel arrays of myofibers are disrupted by acute inflammatory cells, edema fluid, and fibrin. **B,** Higher magnification of **A.** Note the myocardial fiber degeneration and necrosis with loss of cross striations (*arrows*); fragmentation of cardiac rhabdomyocytes (cardiomyocytes); and hypereosinophilia, coagulation, and clumping of the sarcoplasm. Neutrophils are the predominant inflammatory cell in the exudate. H&E stain. (Courtesy Dr. J.F. Zachary, College of Veterinary Medicine, University of Illinois.)

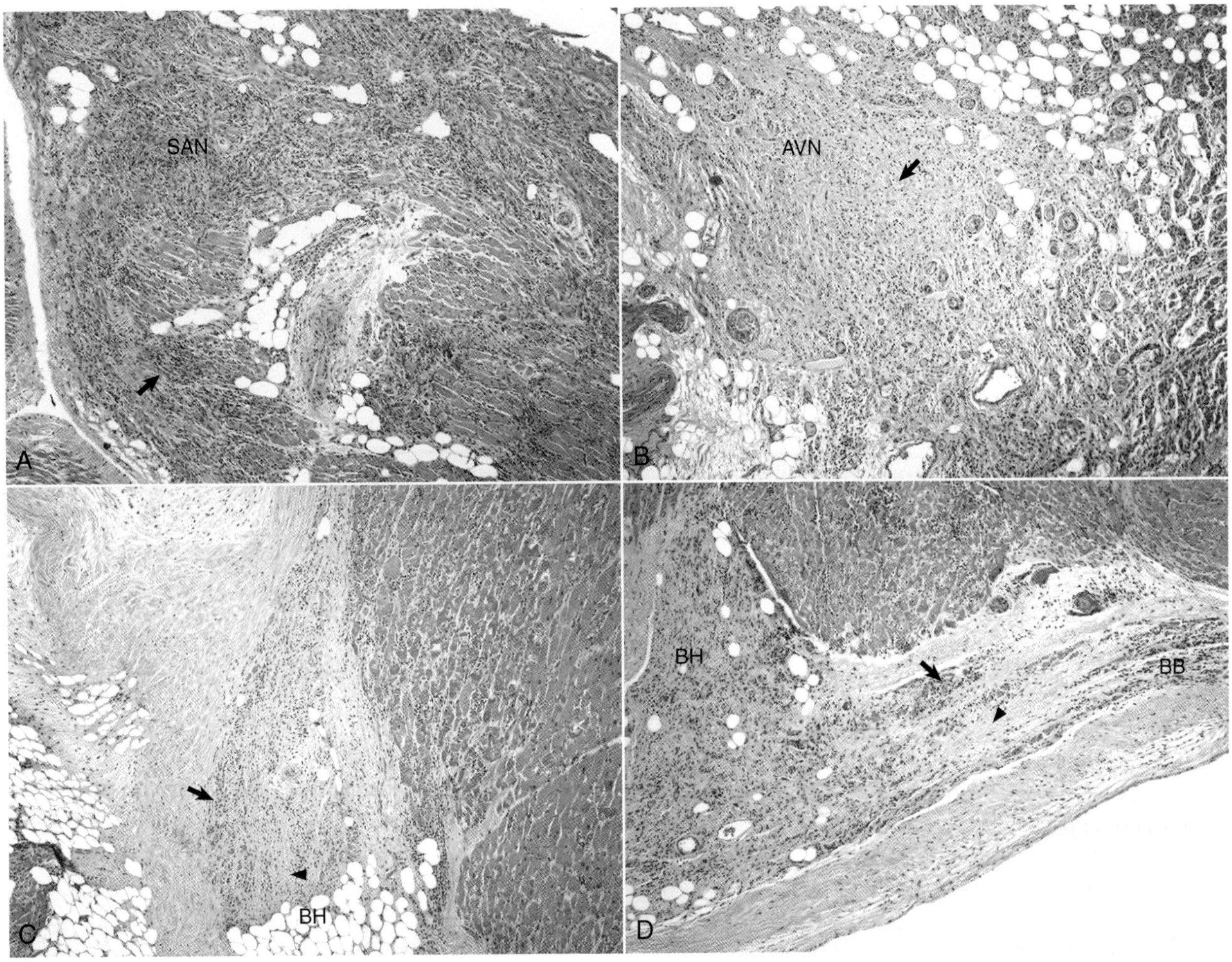

Figure 10-20 Inflammation in the Conduction System From a Dog. A, Sinoatrial node *(SAN)*. Moderate numbers of lymphocytes and plasma cells *(arrow)* multifocally infiltrate the interstitial spaces between cardiomyocytes. H&E stain. **B,** Atrioventricular node *(AVN)*. Small numbers of lymphocytes and plasma cells *(arrow)* multifocally infiltrate the interstitial spaces between cardiomyocytes. H&E stain. **C,** Bundle of His *(BH)*. Small numbers of lymphocytes and plasma cells *(arrow)* multifocally infiltrate the interstitial spaces between cardiomyocytes; fibrous connective tissue *(arrowhead)* multifocally replaces lost cardiomyocytes. H&E stain. **D,** Bundle of His *(BH)* and bundle branch *(BB)*. Small numbers of lymphocytes and plasma cells *(arrow)* multifocally infiltrate the interstitial spaces between cardiomyocytes; fibrous connective tissue *(arrowhead)* multifocally replaces lost cardiomyocytes. H&E stain. (Courtesy Dr. A. Gal, Institute of Veterinary, Animal and Biomedical Sciences, Massey University and Drs. M. Bates and P. Roady, College of Veterinary Medicine, University of Illinois.)

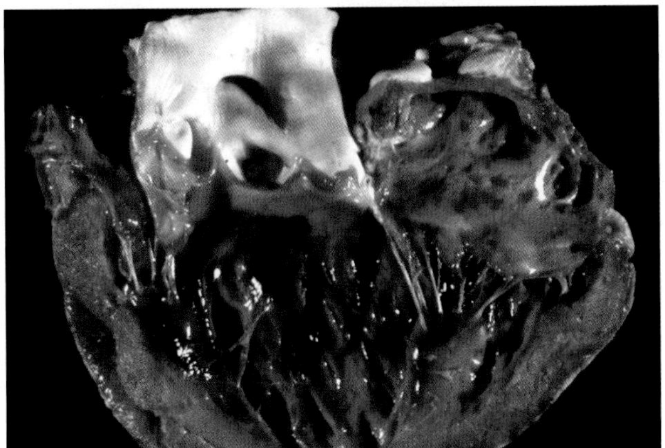

Figure 10-21 Endocardial Suffusive Hemorrhage, Heart, Left Ventricle, Calf. A red to dark-red sheet of suffusive hemorrhage is present in the endocardium of the left ventricle and left atrium. Suffusive hemorrhage is often attributed to severe septicemia, endotoxemia, anoxia, or electrocution. (Courtesy College of Veterinary Medicine, University of Illinois.)

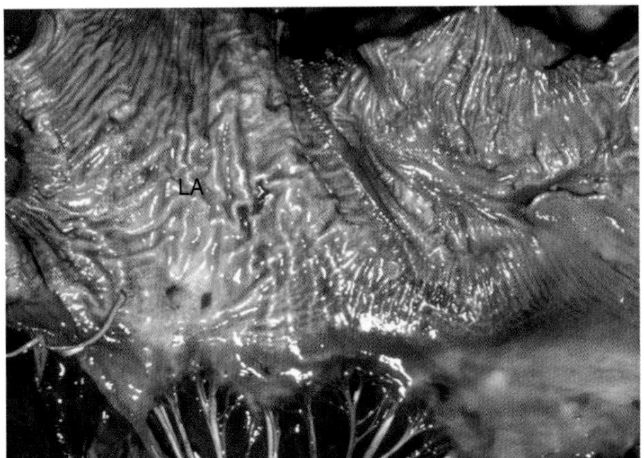

Figure 10-22 Endocardial Mineralization, Johne's Disease, Heart, Left Atrial Endocardium, Cow. The left atrial *(LA)* endocardium is white, thick, and wrinkled from mineralization. (Courtesy School of Veterinary Medicine, Purdue University.)

Effusions. See section on Disorders of Domestic Animals, Disorders of Domestic Animals: Pericardium and Epicardium, Disturbances of Circulation, Hemopericardium and Hydropericardium.

Disturbances of Growth

Anomalies and Dysplasia. See section on Disorders of Domestic Animals, Developmental Errors/Congenital Anomalies.

Serous Atrophy. See section on Disorders of Domestic Animals, Disorders of Domestic Animals: Pericardium and Epicardium, Disturbances of Growth, Serous Atrophy.

Inflammation

Pericarditis. See section on Disorders of Domestic Animals: Pericardium and Epicardium, Inflammation, Pericarditis.

Responses to Injury: Blood and Lymphatic Vascular Systems

The responses of blood and lymphatic vessels to injury involve a complex interaction among the cellular and noncellular elements of the vessel wall and the cellular and noncellular elements of the blood. The key cells of vessels in these reactions are endothelial cells and smooth muscle cells. Endothelial cells are metabolically active and provide a thromboresistant monolayer at the interface of blood and the vessel wall unless damaged. Endothelial cells play an important role in fluid distribution, inflammation, angiogenesis, and hemostasis (see Chapters 2 and 3). Responses of blood vessels to a variety of toxins are listed in E-Box 10-1.

Key functions of endothelial cells include prostacyclin production, macromolecular transport, and recruitment of inflammatory cells. Injury of endothelial cells is followed by separation from the underlying basement membrane and increased permeability to movement of plasma proteins into the subendothelium. Necrosis of endothelium exposes subendothelial collagen and elicits thrombus formation. Endothelial cells at the margin of denuded areas proliferate and re-endothelialize the damaged area. The arterial intima has regional differences in the uptake of macromolecules, as well as other unique structural and functional features that result in lesion-prone areas of the vasculature. Bilirubin staining of the intima results in yellow discoloration in jaundiced animals (Fig. 10-23).

The other major cellular component of vessels involved in reaction to injury is the smooth muscle cell. These cells have important functions, including production of extracellular components, such as collagen, elastin, and proteoglycans; maintenance of vascular tone; monocyte recruitment; lipoprotein metabolism; production of bioactive lipids, such as prostaglandins; and formation of oxygen-free radicals. These functions are regulated by a wide variety of biochemical mediators, such as various growth factors, cytokines, and inflammatory mediators.

Blood Vessels

Disturbances of Circulation

Hemorrhage. Hemorrhage resulting from vascular injury is a frequent lesion of the epicardium, endocardium, and myocardium. Hemorrhages vary in size from petechiae (1- to 2-mm diameter) to ecchymoses (2- to 10-mm diameter) to suffusive (diffuse). Animals dying from septicemia, endotoxemia, anoxia, or electrocution often have prominent epicardial (Fig. 10-24; E-Fig. 10-18 and endocardial (see Fig. 10-21) hemorrhages. Horses dying of any cause usually have agonal hemorrhages on the epicardial and endocardial surfaces. A distinctive example of a specific disease with cardiac hemorrhage is mulberry heart disease, associated with vitamin E–selenium deficiency in growing pigs. In these pigs, hydropericardium accompanies severe myocardial hemorrhage that results in a red, mottled (mulberry-like) appearance of the heart. Also see the previous discussions on disturbances of circulation in the sections on the Pericardium and Epicardium and the Myocardium in the Responses to Injury section.

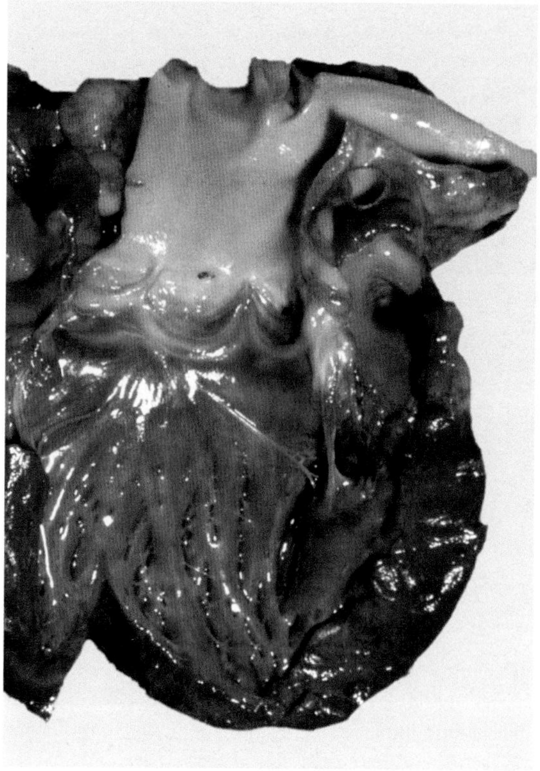

Figure 10-23 **Jaundice, Heart, Aorta, Dog.** Note yellow discoloration of the aortic intima. (Courtesy School of Veterinary Medicine, Purdue University.)

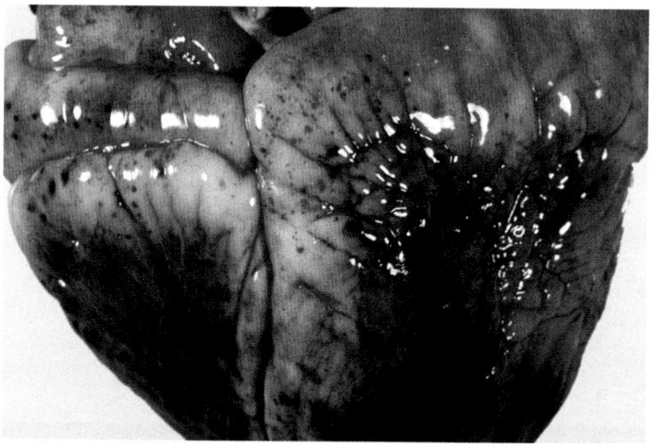

Figure 10-24 **Epicardial Hemorrhage, Petechiae and Ecchymoses, Endotoxemia, Heart, Cow.** Note the epicardial and subepicardial hemorrhages in the fat of the coronary groove (a common site). Petechiae and ecchymoses are often attributable to severe septicemia, endotoxemia, anoxia, or electrocution. In this case, the hemorrhage resulted from injury to the endothelium from endotoxin (component of the cell wall of Gram-negative bacteria). The smaller, pinpoint hemorrhages (1 to 2 mm) are petechiae. The larger hemorrhages (3 to 5 mm) are ecchymoses. (Courtesy Dr. M.D. McGavin, College of Veterinary Medicine, University of Tennessee.)

Effusions. See section on Disorders of Domestic Animals, Disorders of Domestic Animals: Pericardium and Epicardium, Disturbances of Circulation, Hemopericardium and Hydropericardium.

Disturbances of Growth. See Chapter 1 for discussion of the causes of disturbances of cell growth (see cell adaptations).

Anomalies and Dysplasia. See section on Disorders of Domestic Animals, Developmental Errors/Congenital Anomalies.

Hypertrophy. Arterial hypertrophy is a response to sustained increases in pressure or volume loads. Affected vessels are generally muscular arteries, and the increase in wall thickness is predominantly caused by hypertrophy (and, to some degree, hyperplasia) of smooth muscle cells of the tunica media. Muscular pulmonary arteries of cats are frequently affected, and the lesion has been associated with infection by several parasites, including *Aelurostrongylus abstrusus* (the lungworm of cats), *Toxocara* sp., and *Dirofilaria immitis* (Fig. 10-25). However, the lesions often occur in the absence of parasitic infections (Fig. 10-26). Often, no clinical disease is associated with the lesion in cats, but asthmatic signs have been seen in cats with these parasitic infections. Similar hypertrophy of muscular pulmonary arteries occurs in cattle with hypoxia-induced pulmonary arterial vasoconstriction and subsequent pulmonary hypertension associated with right-sided heart failure from exposure to high altitudes (so-called high-altitude disease or "brisket disease") (see section on the stages of myocardial hypertrophy). Also, cardiovascular anomalies that shunt blood left to right in animals result in pulmonary hypertension; these animals may have hypertrophy of the muscular pulmonary arteries, which can result in plexogenic pulmonary arteriopathy. Uterine arteries in pregnant animals are hypertrophic.

Inflammation. See Chapters 3 and 5 for discussion of the processes and mechanisms of acute and chronic inflammation.

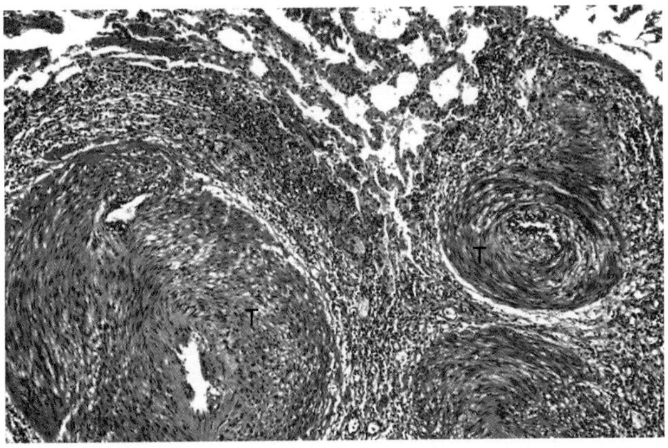

Figure 10-25 Medial Hypertrophy, Periarteritis, Dirofilariasis, Lung, Small Pulmonary Arteries, Cat. Note the massively thickened tunica media *(T)* of the small branches of the pulmonary arteries and their periarterial cuff of chronic inflammatory cells and some eosinophils. H&E stain. (Courtesy School of Veterinary Medicine, Purdue University.)

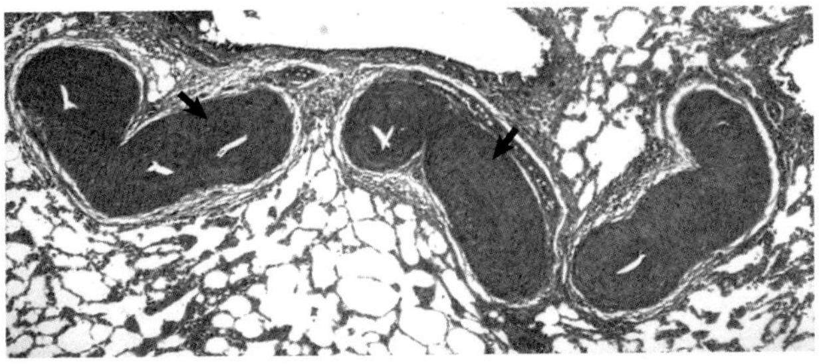

Figure 10-26 Medial Hypertrophy, Lung, Small Pulmonary Arteries, Cat. Proliferation of smooth muscle cells *(arrows)* has resulted in marked thickening of the tunica media. Note luminal narrowing. H&E stain. (Courtesy School of Veterinary Medicine, Purdue University.)

Arteritis and Vasculitis. Arteritis occurs as a feature of many infectious and immune-mediated diseases (Box 10-7). Often, all types of vessels are affected rather than only arteries, and then *vasculitis* or *angiitis* (a term that includes blood and lymphatic vessels) is the term applied to the lesions. The vascular system serves as the major mechanisms for transport of organisms—for example, *Bacillus anthracis*. In inflamed vessels, leukocytes are present within and surrounding the walls, and damage to the vessel wall is evident as fibrin deposits or necrotic endothelial and smooth muscle cells. As a result of endothelial damage, thrombosis, which can result in ischemic injury or infarction in the circulatory field, may be present. Arteritis and vasculitis can develop from endothelial injury caused by either infectious agents or immune-mediated mechanisms or may be caused by local extension of suppurative and necrotizing inflammatory processes in adjacent tissues. Arteritis is a prominent feature of several parasitic diseases.

Systemic infections with phlebitis as a lesion include salmonellosis in several species and feline infectious peritonitis. In pigs with various septicemias, such as salmonellosis and colibacillosis, the gastric fundic mucosa is often severely congested and hemorrhagic because of venous endothelial damage and thrombosis. In severe local infections, such as in metritis or hepatic abscesses, inflammation extends into the walls of adjacent veins and produces phlebitis, with or without thrombosis. Intravenous injections of irritant solutions, injecting solutions into the vascular wall, or intimal trauma produced by indwelling venous catheters result in vascular damage and create an opportunity for localization and proliferation of infectious agents and development of phlebitis and thrombosis (Fig. 10-27). Animals with phlebitis complicated by thrombosis have the additional risk of septic embolism, which can cause endocarditis and pulmonary abscesses or pulmonary infarcts.

Many reportable foreign animal diseases are viral diseases, which are endotheliotropic and result in vasculitis; examples include

Box 10-7 Diseases that Cause Arteritis in Animals

VIRAL

Equine viral arteritis, African horse sickness, equine infectious anemia, equine morbillivirus, malignant catarrhal fever, bovine virus diarrhea, bovine ephemeral fever, bluetongue, hog cholera, African swine fever, feline infectious peritonitis, Aleutian mink disease

BACTERIAL

Bartonella henselae, leptospirosis, Salmonellosis, erysipelas (*Erysipelothrix rhusiopathiae*), *Haemophilus* spp. infections (*Haemophilus suis*, *Haemophilus somnus*, *Haemophilus parasuis*), heartwater (*Ehrlichia ruminantium*), Rocky Mountain spotted fever (*Rickettsia rickettsii*), Lyme disease (*Borrelia burgdorferi*)

MYCOTIC

Phycomycosis, aspergillosis

PARASITIC

Equine strongylosis (*Strongylus vulgaris*), dirofilariasis (*Dirofilaria immitis*), French heartworm (*Angiostrongylus vasorum*), spirocercosis (*Spirocerca lupi*), onchocerciasis, elaeophoriasis (*Elaeophora* sp.), filariasis in primates, aelurostrongylosis

IMMUNE-MEDIATED

Canine systemic lupus erythematosus, rheumatoid arthritis, polyarteritis nodosa, lymphocytic choriomeningitis, drug-induced hypersensitivity

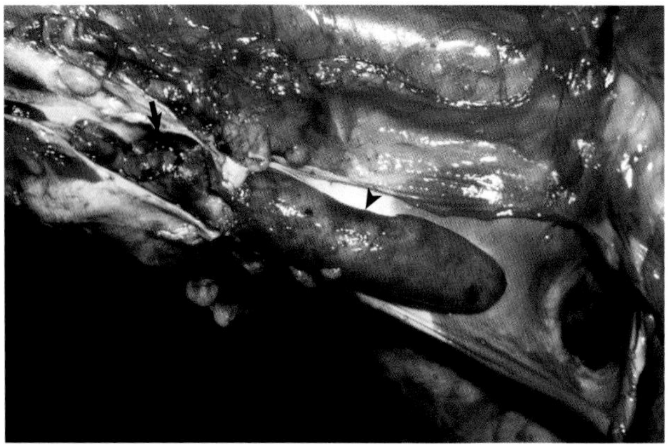

Figure 10-27 **Thrombus (Mural), Jugular Vein (Opened), Dog.** Note the nodular mural thrombus (*left [arrow]*) in the jugular vein. This thrombus likely occurred at a site of venipuncture and a subsequent phlebitis. The smooth-surfaced red-tan thrombus (*right [arrowhead]*) extending toward the heart is a trailing thrombus, a continuation of the mural thrombus. (Courtesy School of Veterinary Medicine, Purdue University.)

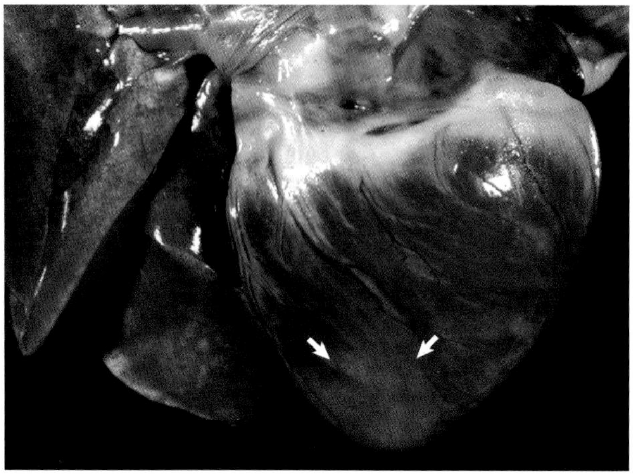

Figure 10-28 **Myocardial Infarction, Heart, Left and Right Ventricles, Dog.** Pale, necrotic, circumscribed areas (*arrows*) are present in the ventricular walls and are most prominent at the apex. (Courtesy Dr. M.D. McGavin, College of Veterinary Medicine, University of Tennessee.)

classic swine fever (hog cholera), African horse sickness, and African swine fever (see the sections on disorders of specific animal species).

Thrombosis and Embolism

Coronary and Other Arteries. Thrombosis or embolism of the coronary arteries can result in myocardial infarction (Fig. 10-28) and cardiac failure. These lesions are much less common in animals than in human beings. Affected animals generally have one of several types of coronary arterial disease, including atherosclerosis, arteriosclerosis, or periarteritis. In atherosclerosis associated with hypothyroidism or diabetes mellitus (discussed previously), severe lesions are present in the extramural (epicardial) coronary arteries of dogs, but this only rarely leads to thrombosis and myocardial infarction. In contrast, severe arteriosclerosis of intramural cardiac arteries in aged dogs can cause small multifocal myocardial infarcts (see Fig. 10-28). Affected dogs often also have myxomatous valvular degeneration (valvular endocardiosis), which is also an age-related disease. Thrombosis of or embolism to other large arteries, such as the interlobular artery of the kidney, can lead to infarction of the tissue supplied by the artery (E-Fig. 10-19; also see Chapter 2).

Box 10-8 Diseases that Cause Lymphangitis in Animals

BACTERIAL

Porcine anthrax (*Bacillus anthracis*), Johne's disease (*Mycobacterium paratuberculosis*), tuberculosis (*Mycobacterium* spp.), actinobacillosis (*Actinobacillus lignieresii*), glanders (farcy) (*Burkholderia mallei*), cutaneous streptothricosis (*Dermatophilus congolensis*), bovine farcy, ulcerative lymphangitis of horses, sporadic lymphangitis of horses, ulcerative lymphangitis (*Corynebacterium pseudotuberculosis*, *Pseudomonas aeruginosa*)

MYCOTIC

Epizootic lymphangitis of horses (*Histoplasma farciminosum*), sporotrichosis (*Sporothrix schenckii*)

PARASITIC

Brugia spp. infection of dogs and cats

Lymphatic Vessels

Inflammation. The endothelial cells lining the lymphatic vessels are subject to the same reactions to injury and inflammation as the vascular system. Inflammation of the lymphatic vessels is called *lymphangitis* and may be seen with specific diseases such as septicemias caused by bacteria like *Salmonella* spp. (Box 10-8). Lymphangitis may be acute, subacute, granulomatous, or chronic resulting in lymphedema. See Chapters 3 and 5, and also see the discussion on Glanders disease and other cutaneous lymphangitides in the section on Disorders of Horses.

Aging

Aging changes are evident in the cardiovascular system. Lipofuscin granules, primarily perinuclear, increase in number with age of cardiac myocytes (see sections on Lipofuscinosis, Cell Degeneration and Death, Disturbances of Growth, and Responses to Injury: Myocardium). Fatty infiltration of the pericardium and myocardium increases with the age of the animal. Hearts from aged sheep often have abundant amounts of adipose tissue, particularly within the right ventricle (see sections on Fatty Degeneration, Cell Degeneration and Death, Disturbances of Growth, and Responses to Injury: Myocardium). Myxomatous valvular disease increases in incidence with age in small breed dogs (see section on Disorders of Dogs; also see Fig. 10-83). Degenerative vascular disease associated with aging includes arteriosclerosis, amyloidosis, and hyaline degeneration of cardiac arteries (see section on Hyaline Degeneration, Fibrinoid Necrosis, and Amyloidosis and section on Disorders of Domestic Animals: Blood and Lymphatic Vascular System). The incidence of neoplastic disease increases with age in the cardiovascular and lymphatic system.

Portals of Entry/Pathways of Spread

Routes used to enter the cardiovascular system and lymphatic vessels are numerous and listed in Box 10-9. Toxic chemicals and pathogenic organisms can enter via ingestion, inhalation, cutaneous contact, trauma, or iatrogenic injection and gain access to the cardiovascular system. Microorganisms and toxins penetrate and enter deeper tissues, dermis, lamina propria, subcutis, or submucosa, triggering an acute inflammatory reaction. All three of the major components of acute inflammation may be responsible for entry of the toxin or organism into the vascular or lymphatic system. The increase in the vascular caliber increasing blood flow increases the number of capillary beds exposed to the agent. Changes in the microvasculature that allow the exit of plasma proteins and leukocytes also increase the entry of an agent. Finally, the increase in leukocytes can result in vascular injury and phagocytosis of material. Organisms that are not diluted, but are denatured by molecules from lysosomes of neutrophils, or restricted in movement by being trapped in fibrin at the site of inflammation can gain entry into the lymphatic vessels, thin-walled capillaries, or venules. Entry into lymphatic vessels allows invading microorganisms to be carried in lymph to draining regional and systemic lymph nodes and eventually via the thoracic duct to the circulatory system. Microorganisms that gain access to veins spread with the circulation and can localize in the lungs. In occurrences in which severe pulmonary inflammation leads to the formation of AV fistulas, microorganisms can gain access to pulmonary veins, be pumped through the left heart, and enter the systemic arterial circulation. The circulatory system can distribute organisms and materials to other organs and tissues (see E-Fig. 10-2; also see Chapter 2).

Myocardium

Pathogens gain entry to the myocardium through the vascular system from the coronary arteries, which provide blood flow to the myocardium. Coronary arteries originate in the sinus of Valsalva at the origin of the aorta and travel in the coronary grooves to the apex of the heart supplying blood to both ventricles. Branches of the coronary arteries bifurcate and send smaller arteries on the outer surface of the heart within the visceral pericardium. These smaller arteries then penetrate the myocardium, becoming arterioles and finally a rich network of capillaries in which there is nearly one vessel adjacent to each cardiac muscle cell. This rich network of capillaries provides an opportunity for bacteria or virus to gain entrance into the myocardium once they have entered the circulatory system. As a result, many bacterial and viral infections may result in myocarditis. Bacteria within fibrin and inflammatory debris loosely attached to affected valves (bacterial valvular endocarditis) may detach and lodge in coronary arteries. This septic emboli damages endothelial cells and initiates acute inflammation resulting in myocarditis. Toxins or toxic by-products can directly damage endothelial cells or diffuse through the endothelium to affect myocardial fibers. In addition, the myocardium is susceptible to direct extension of pathogens located within the endocardium or pericardium.

Box 10-9 Portals of Entry for the Cardiovascular System

PERICARDIUM
Hematogenous dissemination
Foreign body penetration most commonly from reticulum (cattle)
Direct extension from pleural cavity or mediastinum

ENDOCARDIUM
Hematogenous dissemination
Parasitic migration (direct or hematogenous)
Intravenous and intracardiac catheters (long-term placement)
Uremia-induced vascular damage and secondary endocardial ulceration (dog, left atrium)

MYOCARDIUM
Hematogenous dissemination
Embolic dissemination of infective material fragments from vegetative endocarditis lesions into coronary arterial tree
Direct extension from endocardium or pericardium

ARTERIES
Hematogenous dissemination
Local extension of suppurative and necrotizing inflammatory processes
Immune-mediated arterial injury
Parasitic migration

VEINS
Hematogenous dissemination
Local extension of severe inflammatory processes
Intravenous injections and indwelling catheters
Parasitic migration
Immune-mediated venous injury

LYMPHATIC VESSELS
Hematogenous dissemination
Local extension of severe inflammatory processes
Parasitic migration

Endocardium and Heart Valves

The endocardium and the cardiac valves are in direct contact with any pathogen that enters the circulatory system, including parasites, bacterial and viral pathogens, and toxins. The endocardium, especially the left atrial endocardium, is particularly susceptible to toxins resulting from renal failure in the dog.

Epicardium and Pericardium

Bacteria and viruses can enter the pericardial sac via endothelial damage to capillaries on visceral (epicardium) and parietal (pericardium) surfaces. Bacteria can enter by direct penetration. In cattle, foreign bodies exiting the reticulum and penetrating the diaphragm carry bacterial pathogens into the pericardial cavity. Direct entry from bacterial or viral infections in the pleural cavity or mediastinum can also occur.

Blood and Lymphatic Vascular Systems

The circulatory systems are intrinsically susceptible to microbial organisms and toxins because of the primary role of providing oxygen and nutrients to and removing waste from tissues. Hematogenous and lymphogenous dissemination of microbial pathogens and toxins directly exposes the corresponding vasculature to these hazards. Parasitic migration and local extension of an inflammatory process can directly result in entry into the circulatory or lymphatic system and directly damage these tissues.

Defense Mechanisms/Barrier Systems

Defense mechanisms used by the cardiovascular system and lymphatic vessels are listed in Box 10-10. These structures are fortunate

Box 10-10 Defense Mechanisms

CONSTANT BLOOD FLOW
Endocardium, blood and lymphatic vascular components
Endothelium-facilitated barrier systems (see Chapters 2 and 4)

INNATE RESPONSES
Inflammation
Complement
Chemical mediators of inflammation

PHAGOCYTOSIS
Monocyte-macrophage system
Intravascular macrophages
Adaptive immune system

HUMORAL RESPONSES

CELL-MEDIATED RESPONSES

in that most of the components of the innate and humoral immunity are present within the lumen. A review of inflammation (see Chapter 3), immune function (see Chapter 5), and circulatory disturbances (see Chapter 2) is invaluable in understanding the defense mechanisms of the cardiovascular and lymphatic systems. The constant flow of blood and lymph through intact circulatory and lymphatic systems, respectively, provides the surface endothelium of the chambers and vessels with constant exposure to nutrients, plasma proteins such as immunoglobulins, preformed chemical mediators, and circulating leukocytes.

Disorders of Domestic Animals

Developmental Errors/Congenital Anomalies[2]

The complex events involved in the embryologic development of the heart and great vessels allow substantial opportunities for congenital anomalies to develop (see E-Fig. 10-1). The functional significance of these anomalies varies widely. Animals with the most extreme defects are unable to survive in utero, and those with the mildest lesions could have no clinical signs of disease during life. However, animals with defects of intermediate severity are most likely to be presented to a veterinarian because of gradually developing signs of cardiac failure, including poor exercise tolerance, cyanosis, and stunted body growth. Ectopia cordis is a congenital development of the heart at an abnormal site outside of the thoracic cavity. In cattle, cases in healthy adult animals have been described in which the heart was located subcutaneously in the caudoventral neck area. The most frequently observed cardiovascular anomalies in domestic animals are listed in Box 10-11.

Box 10-11 Most Common Cardiovascular Anomalies in Domestic Animal Species

HORSES
Ventricular septal defect
Patent ductus arteriosus
Persistent truncus arteriosus

RUMINANTS (CATTLE, SHEEP, AND GOATS)
Valvular hematomas
Patent foramen ovale
Ventricular septal defect
Transposition of aorta and pulmonary artery

PIGS
Endocardial cushion defects
Dysplasia of the tricuspid valve
Subaortic stenosis

DOGS
Patent ductus arteriosus
Pulmonic stenosis
Subaortic stenosis
Persistent right aortic arch
Ventricular septal defect

CATS
Endocardial cushion defects
Mitral malformation
Ventricular septal defect
Endocardial fibroelastosis
Patent ductus arteriosus

The causes of congenital cardiovascular anomalies are varied. Most animal species have a low background frequency of spontaneous cardiac malformations. In many species, especially in dogs, these defects are heritable and can be attributed to either single or multiple gene effects. Under experimental conditions, cardiovascular congenital defects can be elicited by exposure of pregnant dams to various chemicals and drugs, physical agents, toxins, or nutritional deficiencies. Chemical compounds implicated include thalidomide, ethanol, salicylates, griseofulvin, and cortisone. Prenatal exposure to x-irradiation or fetal hypoxia can induce defects. Maternal nutritional deficiencies of vitamin A, pantothenic acid, riboflavin, or zinc and excess intake of vitamin A, retinoic acid, or copper can result in cardiovascular anomalies in newborn animals. Infectious diseases have been incriminated, but not confirmed, in cardiovascular defects; they include bluetongue infections in sheep, bovine virus diarrhea in cattle, and parvoviral infections in dogs and cats.

Congenital cardiac malformations may be grouped into four large categories according to their pathophysiology: (1) defects that cause volume overload (with subcategories of systemic to pulmonary shunting [left to right shunt] and valvular regurgitation), (2) defects that cause pressure overload, (3) defects that cause cyanosis, and (4) miscellaneous cardiac and vascular defects.

Anomalies in the first category that lead to left to right shunting include patent ductus arteriosus (PDA), ventricular septal defect (VSD), atrial septal defect (ASD), and endocardial cushion defects. In this category, a defect between the right and left cardiac compartments leads to flow of cardiac blood according to a pressure gradient from the left side (systemic circulation, high pressure) to the right side (pulmonic circulation, low pressure). The consequence of blood shunting is overloading of the low-pressured pulmonary circulation, which results in increased volume of blood that enters the left cardiac compartment after returning from the lungs. This in turn leads to eccentric hypertrophy of the left ventricle and atrium to accommodate the increased volume of blood. Anomalies in the first category that lead to valvular regurgitation include mitral and tricuspid dysplasia and aortic and pulmonic insufficiency. The regurgitated blood from the ventricles to the atria leads to progressive atrial dilation and eccentric ventricular dilation.

Anomalies in the second category that cause pressure overload include pulmonic and aortic stenosis and coarctation and interruption of the aorta. In these anomalies, ventricular outflow obstructions result in progressive and chronic increase in intraventricular pressure. The increased intraventricular pressure induces concentric ventricular hypertrophy that eventually results in a diastolic failure.

Anomalies in the third category that cause cyanotic heart disease include tetralogy of Fallot, pulmonary to systemic (right to left) blood shunting (some VSD and PDA), tricuspid atresia/right ventricular hypoplasia, double-outlet right ventricle, transposition of the great vessels, truncus arteriosus, and aorticopulmonary window (see Disorders of Domestic Animals, Developmental Errors/Congenital Anomalies). In these anomalies, nonoxygenated blood from the right cardiac compartment flows to the left compartment or bypasses the left compartment and flows directly into the systemic circulation. This portion of nonoxygenated blood mixes and dilutes the oxygenated blood in the systemic circulation and induces cyanosis in multiple tissues.

Anomalies in the fourth category include peritoneopericardial diaphragmatic hernias (PPDHs), persistent right aortic arch (PRAA), endocardial fibroelastosis, anomalous pulmonary venous return, double aortic arch, retroesophageal left subclavian artery, valvular hematomas, and situs inversus.

[2]See E-Box 10-2 for a list of inherited cardiovascular diseases of animals; E-Box 10-3 for a list of canine breed predilections for congenital cardiac anomalies; and E-Box 1-1 for a list of potential, suspected, or known genetic disorders.

Sites of the major cardiovascular anomalies in the dog are shown in Fig. 10-29.

Developmental Errors/Congenital Anomalies: Myocardium

See the following section on Developmental Errors/Congenital Anomalies: Endocardium and Heart Valves.

Developmental Errors/Congenital Anomalies: Endocardium and Heart Valves

Failure of Closure of Fetal Cardiovascular Shunts

Interventricular Septal Defect. A ventricular septal defect indicates failure of complete development of the interventricular septum and allows the shunting of blood between the ventricles (Fig. 10-30). The defect occurs in many species and more commonly in the upper interventricular septum—below the aortic valves (on the left), proximal to the crista supraventricularis (near the septal tricuspid valve leaflet), or distal to the crista supraventricularis (below the pulmonic valve).

Among breeds of dogs, the greatest frequency has been observed in the English bulldog, English springer spaniel, and West Highland white terrier.

Atrial Septal Defect. An atrial septal defect could represent the failure of closure of the foramen ovale, which is an interatrial septal shunt that allows blood to bypass the lungs of the fetus, or it can be the result of true septal defects at another site because of faulty development of the interatrial septum. Although this defect occurs in all domestic animal species, dog breeds with greatest frequency of this defect are the boxer, Doberman pinscher, and Samoyed.

Tetralogy of Fallot. Tetralogy of Fallot is a complicated cardiac anomaly seen in all animal species with four lesions (Fig. 10-31). The three primary defects are a ventricular septal defect located high in the septum, pulmonic stenosis (see later discussion), and dextroposition of the aorta (see later discussion). The fourth defect, which develops secondarily, is hypertrophy of the right ventricular myocardium. The major pathophysiologic significance in this condition is the increased pressure in the right side that shunts unoxygenated blood from the hypertrophic right side to the underdeveloped left side (systemic circulation) and results in systemic hypoxemia and secondary polycythemia. Cyanosis is often an associated clinical sign. The anomaly is one of the most common cardiac abnormalities seen in hearts of human beings (so-called blue babies). This complex anomaly is inherited in keeshond dogs and is frequent in English bulldogs. In genetic and pathologic studies of keeshond dogs, the basic defect has been determined to be hypoplasia and malpositioning of the conotruncal septum. Wide variability in the severity of the lesions has been observed. The inheritance pattern in keeshonds is a simple autosomal locus with partial penetration in heterozygotes and complete penetrance in homozygotes.

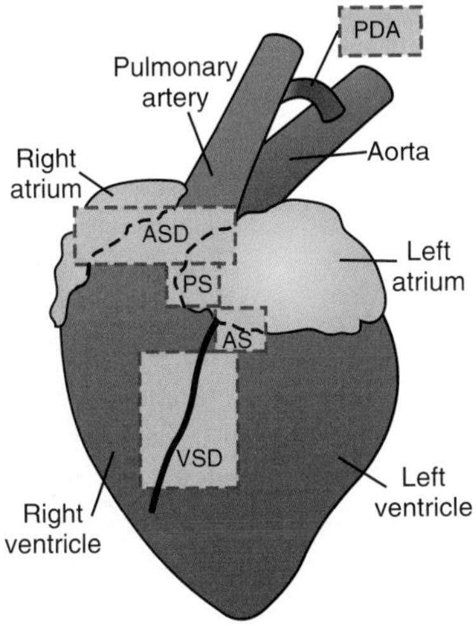

Figure 10-29 Sites of the Major Cardiovascular Anomalies of the Dog. *AS*, Aortic stenosis; *ASD*, atrial septal defect; *PDA*, patent ductus arteriosus; *PS*, pulmonic stenosis; *VSD*, ventricular septal defect. (Redrawn with permission from School of Veterinary Medicine, Purdue University.)

Failure of Normal Valvular Development

Pulmonic Stenosis. Pulmonic stenosis has been recognized as a frequently occurring anomaly in dogs and is inherited in the beagle (Fig. 10-32). Other breeds in which this lesion is frequent are basset hound, boxer, Chihuahua, Chow Chow, cocker spaniel, English bulldog, Labrador retriever, mastiff, Newfoundland, Samoyed, schnauzer, and terrier. Several types of valvular lesions have been described and include formation of a circumferential band of fibrous

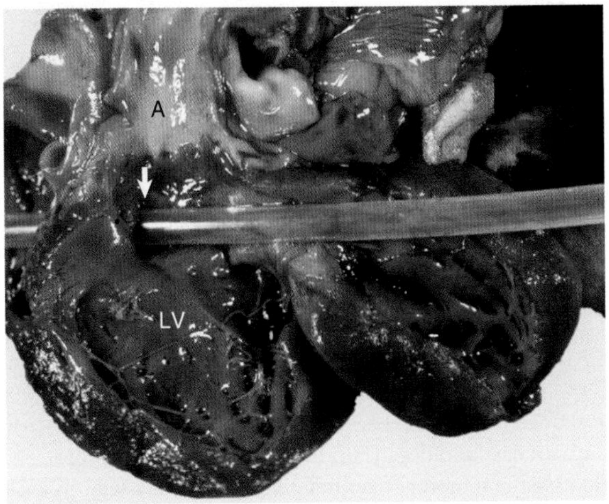

Figure 10-30 Ventricular Septal Defect (High Defect), Heart, Opened Left Side, Calf. Note the large opening in the basal portion of the ventricular septum *(arrow)* immediately below the aortic valve through which the tube has been passed. *A*, Aorta; *LV*, left ventricle. (Courtesy Dr. M.D. McGavin, College of Veterinary Medicine, University of Tennessee.)

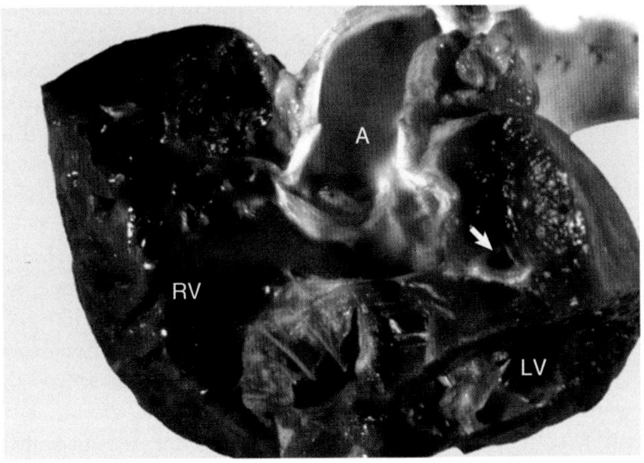

Figure 10-31 Tetralogy of Fallot, Heart, Dissected, Dog. Above the large membranous ventricular septal defect is an overlying, straddling aorta *(A)*. There is also severe pulmonic stenosis *(arrow)* with massive right ventricular hypertrophy. *LV*, Left ventricle; *RV*, right ventricle. (Courtesy School of Veterinary Medicine, Purdue University.)

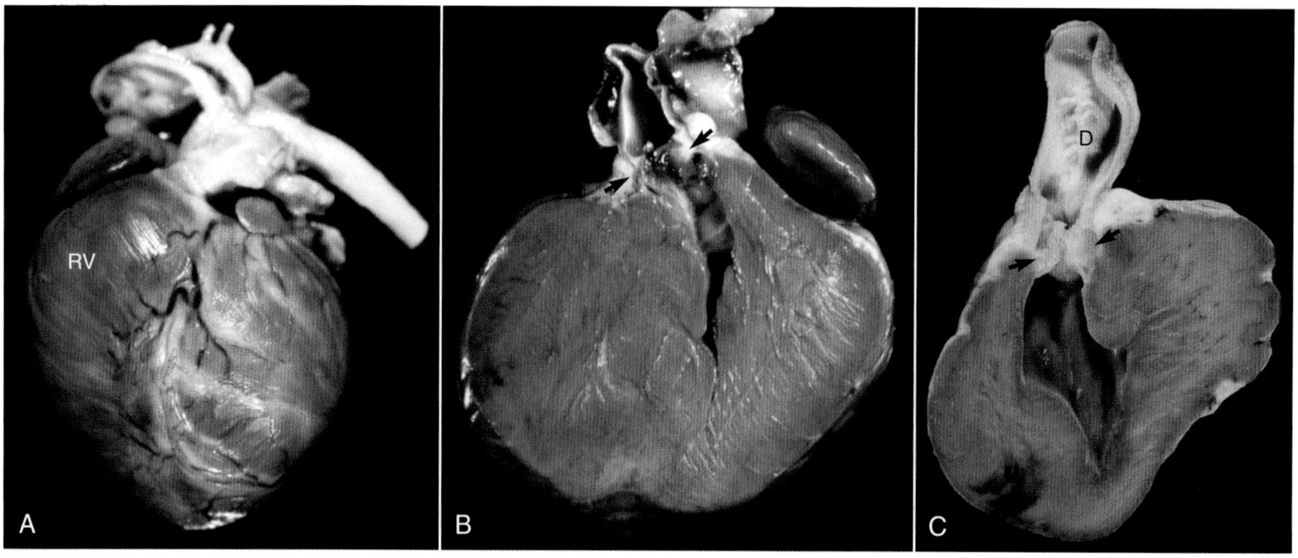

Figure 10-32 **Pulmonic Stenosis, Heart, Pulmonary Artery, Dog. A,** Closed heart, and **B,** sectioned heart. Note the prominent concentric right ventricular *(RV)* hypertrophy resulting from pressure overload. The orifice of the pulmonic valve *(arrows)* is markedly narrowed. **C,** Sectioned heart, there is poststenotic dilation *(D)* of the pulmonary artery with irregular intimal thickenings (jet lesions). (Courtesy Atlantic Veterinary College, University of Prince Edward Island.)

or muscular tissue beneath the valve (subvalvular stenosis) or malformation of the valve (valvular stenosis), with a small central orifice in a dome of thickened valvular tissue. A unique form of subvalvular pulmonic stenosis has been described in English bulldogs and boxers in which an anomalous development of a coronary artery obstructs the right ventricular outflow tract. Notable concentric hypertrophy (see the discussion on hypertrophy in the section on Responses to Injury: Myocardium, Disturbances of Growth) of the right ventricle develops from the resulting pressure overload.

Aortic and Subaortic Stenoses. True stenoses of the aortic valve are uncommon. Subaortic stenosis is a cardiac anomaly frequently observed in pigs and dogs. Subvalvular aortic stenosis is the most common congenital cardiac anomaly of large-breed dogs. Bull terriers and boxers are predisposed, and a genetic basis is present in the Newfoundland dog, in which subvalvular aortic stenosis is inherited in an autosomal dominant pattern. Obstruction of the left ventricular outflow tract (LVOT) results from a raised, partial or complete fibrous ring that arises from the endocardium below the aortic valve and may extend to involve the cranioventral leaflet of the mitral valve and the base of the aortic valve (Fig. 10-33). The lesion is also observed in the German shorthair pointer, golden retriever, Great Dane, Rottweiler, Samoyed, and bull terrier breeds. In clinical cases, the stenosis is produced by the presence of a thick zone of endocardial fibrous tissue that encircles the LVOT below the valve. In mild cases, often subclinical, the lesion is limited to white nodules on the ventricular septum immediately below the valve. Microscopically, the altered endocardial tissue contains loosely arranged elastic fibers, mucopolysaccharide ground substance, and collagen fibers admixed with fibroblasts and chondrocyte-like cells. Other cardiac lesions develop as a result of the altered left ventricular outflow; these include left ventricular concentric hypertrophy, disseminated foci of myocardial necrosis, fibrosis in the inner left ventricular wall, and thickening of the walls of intramyocardial arteries.

Valvular Dysplasias: Endocardial Cushion Defects. Other valvular developmental anomalies include endocardial cushion defects (persistent AV canal and atrioventricular canal defect) in pigs, sheep, and cats; mitral dysplasia in cats and dogs; and tricuspid dysplasia in cats and dogs (Fig. 10-34). Endocardial cushion defects are the most common congenital cardiac anomaly seen in cats.

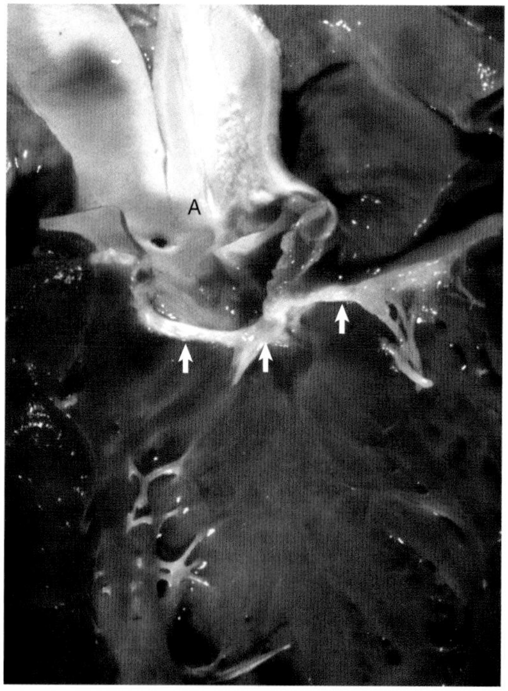

Figure 10-33 **Subaortic Stenosis, Heart, Opened Left Side, Dog.** A thick, white, broad band of fibrous connective tissue *(arrows)* encircles the left ventricular outflow tract below the aortic valve. The force of the blood ejected through the stenotic lesion is responsible for the "jet lesions" in the overlying aorta (A). (Courtesy College of Veterinary Medicine, University of Illinois.)

Tricuspid Valve Dysplasia. Tricuspid valve dysplasia has a genetic basis in the Labrador retriever dog, in which it is an autosomal dominant trait with reduced penetrance that is mapped to chromosome 9. There is a wide spectrum of morphologic abnormalities that may include (1) shortening, rolling, notching, and thickening of

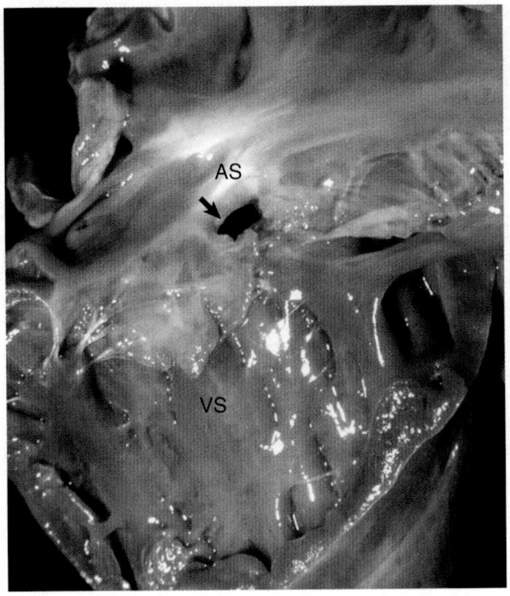

Figure 10-34 Endocardial Cushion Defect and Tricuspid Dysplasia, Heart, Opened Right Side, Pig. The endocardial cushion defect (prominent opening [*arrow*]) can be mistaken as an atrial septal defect but not the location and presence of abnormal valves incorporated in the defect. *AS*, Atrial septum; *VS*, ventricular septum. (Courtesy School of Veterinary Medicine, Purdue University.)

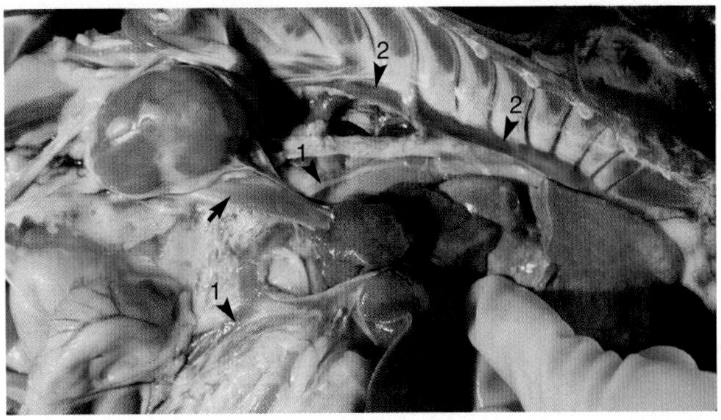

Figure 10-35 Portacaval Shunt, Dog. Note that the branch of the portal vein (*arrowhead 1*) passes under the caudal vena cava (*arrow*) and anastomoses with the azygous vein (*arrowhead 2*). The azygous vein returns the blood to the caudal vena cava near the heart and thus this blood and its ammoniacal and protein metabolites are shunted away from processing to blood urea nitrogen (BUN) in the liver. The liver is normal color but extremely small, which is typical of these types of shunts (see Chapter 8). (Courtesy Dr. M.D. McGavin, College of Veterinary Medicine, University of Tennessee.)

leaflets; (2) incomplete separation of valvular components from the ventricular wall; (3) elongation, shortening, fusion, and thickening of chordae tendineae; (4) direct insertion of the valve edges into a papillary muscle; or (5) atrophy, fusion, and malpositioning of the papillary muscles and chordae tendineae.

Mitral Valve Dysplasia. Mitral valve dysplasia is often associated with other anomalies, such as ASD/VSD and tricuspid valve dysplasia. A similar spectrum of morphological valvular abnormalities is present in mitral valve dysplasia as described previously for tricuspid valve dysplasia. Dysplastic malformations in the atrioventricular valves that result in valvular insufficiency lead to volume overload with resultant atrial dilation and to eccentric ventricular hypertrophy. Dysplastic malformations in the atrioventricular valves that result in valvular stenosis lead to reduced ventricular filling with subsequent low cardiac output (history of syncope, collapse, and hypotension) and increased atrial pressure; in the case of mitral stenosis, increased atrial pressure can lead to pulmonary edema initially and dilation of the right ventricle (right-sided heart failure) from prolonged pulmonary hypertension.

Developmental Errors/Congenital Anomalies: Pericardium and Epicardium

Peritoneopericardial Diaphragmatic Hernias. Peritoneopericardial diaphragmatic hernias (PPDHs) occur in cats and dogs with incomplete development of the diaphragm. PPDHs are rare, but they are the most common congenital pericardial anomaly in cats; Persian and domestic longhair cats were overrepresented in two studies. PPDHs result from defective separation of the developing liver and septum transversum during embryogenesis that allows the peritoneal and pericardial cavities to communicate. Hence, abdominal organs including omental fat may fill the pericardial sac and compress the heart. Parts of the liver are often incarcerated in the pericardial sac and may develop intrahepatic myelolipomas.

Partial/Complete Absence (Agenesis) of the Pericardial Sac. Partial or complete absence of the pericardial sac is an incidental lesion that is rarely found during necropsy and has not been reported to have clinical significance during life. However, there is one report of a dog with a partial tear in the pericardium that was associated with episodes of syncope.

Intrapericardial Cysts. Benign intrapericardial cysts are rare, large fluid-filled masses within the pericardial space that originate from the pericardium and consist of encapsulated and hemorrhagic adipose tissue that possibly originated from congenital entrapment of the omentum or falciform ligament. In other cases, these rare lesions are associated with PPDH.

Developmental Errors/Congenital Anomalies: Blood and Lymphatic Vascular Systems

Blood Vessels

Failure of Closure of Fetal Cardiovascular Shunts

Portacaval Shunts. Portacaval shunts occur in animals, particularly in the dog. The normal flow from the portal vein is diverted, either partially or completely, to the systemic circulation, thus bypassing the liver (Fig. 10-35). Normal hepatic detoxification of portal flow is incomplete and may result in neurologic signs and elevated circulating bile acids. The resulting nervous system syndrome is termed *hepatic encephalopathy*. Specifically, the shunts represent retained fetal vascular structures, as in persistent ductus venosus, or arise from prominent dilation of various portosystemic shunts that normally are quite small vessels. See Chapter 8 on diseases of the liver for further details.

Tetralogy of Fallot. See Disorders of Domestic Animals; Developmental Errors/Congenital Anomalies; Developmental Errors/Congenital Anomalies: Endocardium and Heart Valves, Failure of Closure of Fetal Cardiovascular Shunts, Tetralogy of Fallot.

Patent Ductus Arteriosus. Patent ductus arteriosus is a frequent anomaly in poodle, collie, Pomeranian, Chihuahua, cocker spaniel, English springer spaniel, German shepherd, keeshond, Maltese, Yorkshire terrier, bichon frise, and Shetland sheepdog breeds (Fig. 10-36). In poodles, it is an inherited polygenic trait. Female dogs have a greater incidence. The ductus arteriosus is a fetal communication between the aorta and pulmonary artery that serves to divert blood from the right cardiac chamber to the fetal circulation in order to bypass the collapsed fetal lungs. Following parturition, the smooth

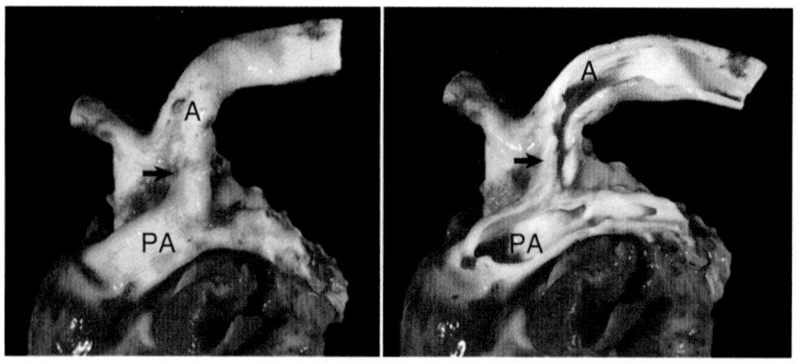

Figure 10-36 Patent Ductus Arteriosus, Heart, Young Dog. Note the prominent ductus arteriosus *(arrow)* between the pulmonary artery *(PA)* and the aorta *(A)* in the undissected *(left)* and dissected vessels *(right)*. (Courtesy Dr. D.D. Harrington, School of Veterinary Medicine, Purdue University; and Noah's Arkive, College of Veterinary Medicine, The University of Georgia.)

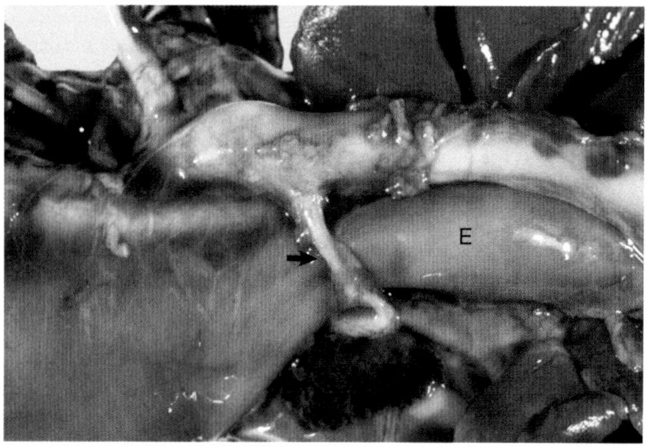

Figure 10-37 Persistent Right Aortic Arch, Ligamentum Arteriosum, Megaesophagus, Calf. During embryogenesis, the aorta was formed from the right aortic arch instead of the left one; thus the aorta is now on the right. For the ligamentum arteriosum *(arrow)* to connect the aorta with the pulmonary artery, it has to pass dorsally over the esophagus and trachea. The ligamentum, together with the aorta and pulmonary artery, form a vascular ring that constricts the esophagus *(E)*, which is dilated cranial to the constriction. (Courtesy Dr. S. Snyder, College of Veterinary Medicine, Colorado State University; and Noah's Arkive, College of Veterinary Medicine, The University of Georgia.)

muscle in the ductus arteriosus contracts, which results in its occlusion within 7 to 10 days after birth in the dog. When this mechanism fails, the ductus arteriosus remains patent and allows for a portion of the blood from the left cardiac chamber to flow from the aorta into the pulmonary artery and results in overcirculation to the lungs, leading to pulmonary hypertension and increased preload to the left ventricle. Grossly, patent ductus arteriosus is a dilated funnel-shaped communication between the descending aorta and the main pulmonary artery. This vascular channel between the pulmonary artery and aorta allows blood to bypass the lungs during fetal life. Normally, the ductus arteriosus is converted to the solid ligamentum arteriosum postnatally.

Malpositioning of Great Vessels

Persistent Right Aortic Arch. Persistent right aortic arch occurs in dogs; German shepherd, Irish setter, and Great Dane dogs are predisposed (Fig. 10-37). This defect arises because the right fourth aortic arch, rather than the normal left fourth aortic arch, develops and ascends on the right side of the midline so that the ligamentum arteriosum forms a vascular ring over the esophagus and trachea. This arrangement eventually results in esophageal obstruction and

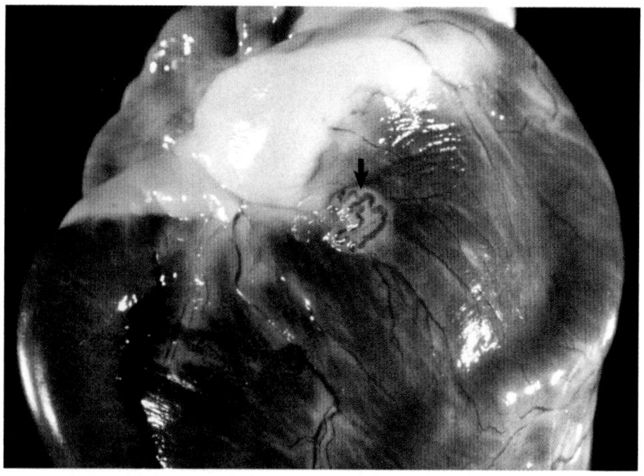

Figure 10-38 Congenital Lymphangiectasia, Epicardium, Young Horse. Note the tortuous appearance of the epicardial lymphatic vessel *(arrow)*. In congenital lymphangiectasia, lymphatic vessels fail to make connections with other vessels or are obstructed because of anomalous development. (Courtesy College of Veterinary Medicine, University of Illinois.)

proximal dilation (megaesophagus), which often results in aspiration pneumonia as the animal matures and consumes solid feed.

Transposition of the Aorta and Pulmonary Artery. Transposition of the aorta and pulmonary artery are severe anomalies, of which there are several types. In complete transposition, the aorta serves as the outflow from the right ventricle and the pulmonary artery is the left ventricle primary outflow. Other congenital anomalies, including ventricular septal defect, often accompany this anomaly.

Truncus Arteriosus. In this lesion, there is a large VSD that allows blood flow between the ventricles and a single large vessel that originates above the VSD. Hypoxemia and cyanosis develop, depending on the amount of mixture of nonoxygenated and oxygenated blood.

Lymphatic Vessels

Lymphangiectasia. Lymphangiectasia is dilation of lymphatic vessels. The cause may be a congenital anomaly (Fig. 10-38) or obstruction of lymph drainage by invading masses of malignant neoplasms or inflammation (Fig. 10-39).

Hereditary Lymphedema. Hereditary lymphedema has been described in dogs, Ayrshire and Angus calves, and pigs. Affected animals have prominent subcutaneous edema that, in calves, often causes severe swelling of the tips of the ears. Interference with lymph drainage results from defective development of the lymphatic vessels that are aplastic or hypoplastic.

Disorders of Domestic Animals: Myocardium

The most common cardiac diseases in horses, ruminants, pigs, dogs, and cats are summarized in Boxes 10-12 and 10-13. The most common locations of major neoplastic diseases in the heart are illustrated in Fig. 10-40. Cardiovascular diseases with known or suspected heritability are listed in E-Boxes 10-2 and 10-3.

Disturbances of Circulation

Hemorrhage: Trauma (Physical Injury). Blunt chest trauma may result in myocardial hemorrhage, which can lead to serious clinical consequences. Tears and rupture of tissue resulting from loss of structural integrity attributable to invasive and destructive properties of neoplasms may result in myocardial hemorrhage. See discussion on hemorrhage in Chapter 2.

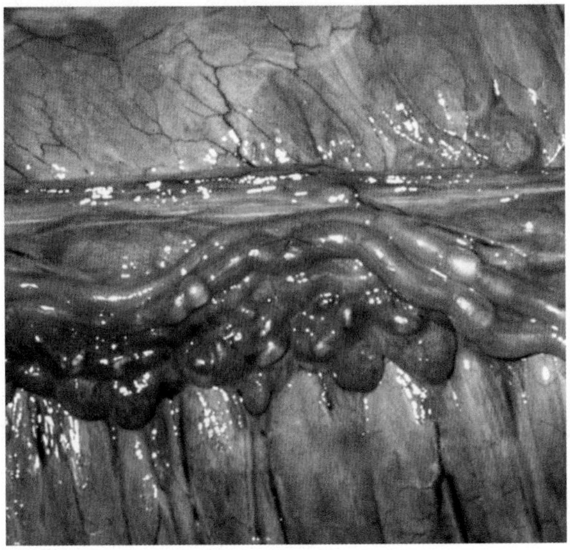

Figure 10-39 **Acquired Lymphangiectasia, Lymphoma (Lymphosarcoma), Mesocolon, Horse.** Note the distended lymphatic vessels on the serosal surface of the large colon, the result of impeded lymph flow through the colic lymph nodes, caused by compression of their cortical and medullary sinuses by proliferating neoplastic lymphocytes. (Courtesy College of Veterinary Medicine, University of Illinois.)

Box 10-12 Most Common Cardiac Diseases of Horses and Production Animals

HORSES

Fibrinous pericarditis
Toxic cardiomyopathy (ionophores, white snakeroot)
Endocardial fibrosis and calcification
Endocarditis

RUMINANTS (CATTLE, SHEEP, AND GOATS)

White muscle disease (vitamin E–selenium deficiency)
Cardiotoxicity (ionophores, gossypol, *Cassia occidentalis*, *Karwinskia humboldtiana*)
Brisket disease (high-altitude disease)
Pericarditis
Endocarditis
Malignant lymphoma

PIGS

Mulberry heart disease (vitamin E–selenium deficiency)
Pericarditis
Endocarditis

Disturbances of Growth

See the discussion on anomalies and dysplasia in the section on Disorders of Domestic Animals, Developmental Errors/Congenital Anomalies: Endocardium and Heart Valves.

Hypertrophy and Atrophy

Cardiomyopathies. Categorization and causes of primary and secondary cardiomyopathies are listed in Box 10-14. These diseases are divided into five morphologic types: hypertrophic, dilated (congestive), restrictive, arrhythmogenic right ventricular, and unclassified cardiomyopathies. Secondary cardiomyopathies (also termed *specific heart muscle diseases*) are generalized myocardial diseases of known cause.

Hypertrophic Cardiomyopathy. Hypertrophic cardiomyopathy (HCM) occurs frequently in cats, especially in young adult to middle-aged males (1 to 3 years old), and is seen infrequently in dogs, usually affecting males of large breeds.

Hypertrophic cardiomyopathy is the most common feline primary myocardial disease, and it occurs frequently in cats (58% to 68% of all cardiomyopathy cases). There is familial heritability in Maine coon, ragdoll, and American shorthaired cats (in which it is transmitted in an autosomal dominant pattern) and breed predisposition in British shorthair, Norwegian forest, Turkish Van, Scottish fold, Bengal, Siberian, and Rex cats. Young adult to middle-aged males (1 to 3 years old) are often affected. Hypertrophic cardiomyopathy is caused by sarcomeric defects in cardiomyocytes, of which two mutations in cardiac myosin-binding protein C (MYBPC) have been identified in Maine coon and ragdoll cats. Altered sarcomeric function ultimately results in myocytes hypertrophy, collagen synthesis, and myocytes disarray (defined as cellular disorientation of cardiomyocytes in which cardiomyocytes are oriented perpendicular or obliquely to each other forming tangled patterns and/or pinwheel configurations). The left ventricle wall progressively thickens (Fig. 10-41), and its lumen narrows (nondilated concentric hypertrophy) (heart weight to body weight ratio of 7.0 ± 0.3 g/kg compared to normal cats' heart weight to body weight ratio of 3.83 ± 0.2 g/kg). In addition, mild right ventricular enlargement is occasionally present. Left ventricular concentric enlargement results in impairment of the left ventricle's ability to relax during diastole (diastolic failure). Increased left ventricular diastolic filling pressure leads to enlargement of the left atrium with subsequent blood backing up to the lungs, resulting in congestive heart failure with pulmonary edema and/or pleural effusion. In a subset of cases, in addition to concentric hypertrophy of the left ventricle, the interventricular septum contains hypertrophied, anteriorly displaced papillary muscles that pull the chordae tendineae and the anterior leaflet of the mitral valve into the left ventricular outflow tract (LVOT), resulting in a dynamic LVOT obstruction during systole (systolic anterior motion [SAM] of the mitral valve). Therefore a unique kissing lesion forms in the LVOT, which has a diagnostic significance

Box 10-13 Most Common Cardiac Diseases in Dogs and Cats

DOGS

Myxomatous valvular degeneration (valvular endocardiosis)
Congenital heart disease
Dilated cardiomyopathy
Hemorrhagic pericardial effusion
Cardiac neoplasia
Dirofilariasis

CATS

Hypertrophic cardiomyopathy
Dilated cardiomyopathy
Hyperthyroidism-associated hypertrophy
Congenital heart disease

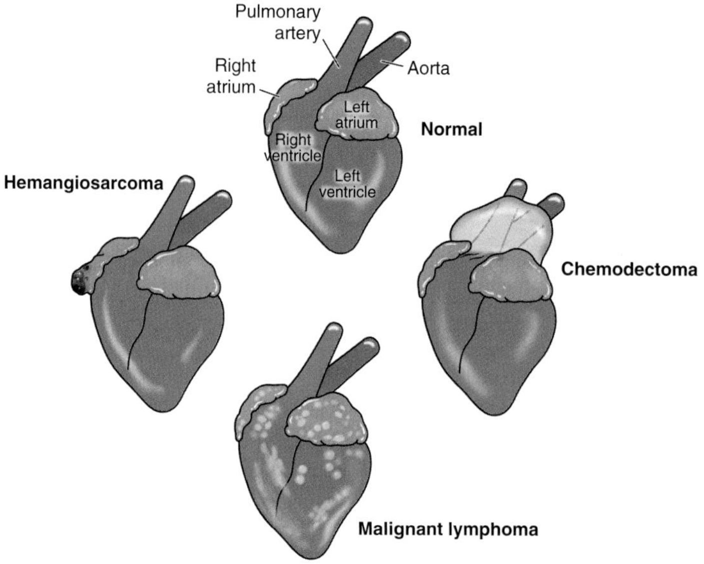

Figure 10-40 **Locations of the Major Cardiac Neoplasms.** (Redrawn with permission from School of Veterinary Medicine, Purdue University.)

Box 10-14 Cardiomyopathies in Animals

PRIMARY CARDIOMYOPATHIES (IDIOPATHIC)

Hypertrophic: Cat, dog, rat, pig
Dilated (congestive): Cat, dog, hamster, turkey, pig, cow, sea otters, sea lions, cynomolgus monkeys
Restrictive: Cat
Arrhythmogenic right ventricular cardiomyopathy: Dog, cat

SECONDARY CARDIOMYOPATHIES (SPECIFIC HEART MUSCLE DISEASES)

Heritable (known or suspected): Hereditary cardiomyopathy of hamsters, mice, rats, turkeys, and cattle; Duchenne's type, X-linked muscular dystrophy of golden retriever dogs with dystrophin deficiency; glycogenoses
Nutritional deficiencies: See list in Box 10-5; other examples include taurine deficiency in cats and foxes
Toxic: See list in Box 10-5; other examples include anthracycline toxicity, furazolidone toxicity, NaCl toxicity
Physical injuries and shock: See list in Box 10-5
Endocrine disorders: Hyperthyroidism, acromegaly (hypersomatotropism), hypothyroidism, glucocorticoid excess, functional pheochromocytoma, diabetes mellitus
Infections: See lists in Boxes 10-6, 10-7, and 10-8
Neoplastic infiltration: Malignant lymphoma
Systemic hypertension in cats and dogs: Spontaneous or associated with chronic renal disease, hyperthyroidism, diabetes mellitus, acromegaly, primary aldosteronism

because it is seen only in this subset of cats with hypertrophic cardiomyopathy. In addition, the systolic obstruction in the LVOT causes further increase in the left ventricular pressure that worsens its hypertrophy. Approximately 10% to 20% of cats with hypertrophic cardiomyopathy have a state of increased coagulability and develop posterior paresis from concurrent thromboembolism of the caudal abdominal aorta ("saddle thrombosis") (see Fig. 10-91). The aortic thrombus is first formed in the stagnant blood flow of the enlarged left atrium and is subsequently launched into the aorta. Some cats with hypertrophic cardiomyopathy die unexpectedly without premonitory clinical signs. Microscopically, the lesions of the myocardium are prominent disarray or disorganizations of myocytes, with interweaving rather than parallel arrangement of fibers (Fig. 10-42). Myocyte hypertrophy, various degenerative alterations in myocytes, and interstitial fibrosis are present. A second common histologic lesion includes remodeling of the coronary microcirculation associated with arteriosclerosis ("small vessel disease"). The lumen of small coronary vessels is severely narrowed due to smooth muscle proliferation and increased connective tissue elements. Replacement fibrosis due to myocardial infarction/necrosis is occasionally found in regions of remodeled coronary arterioles, implying a probable causal relationship (see Figs. 10-41 and 10-42; E-Fig. 10-20).

Idiopathic hypertrophic cardiomyopathy in dogs is an infrequent pathology, unlike in cats. It is defined as inappropriate concentric myocardial hypertrophy of a nondilated left ventricle in the absence of an identifiable stimulus for the hypertrophy. Most reported cases have been in young males (<3 years old), and an inherited basis has been proposed in the pointer dog breed. Hypertrophy of the left ventricle has been reported to be symmetrical (i.e., both left ventricular free wall and interventricular septum) in most dogs. In addition, most dogs had an antemortem diagnosis of dynamic LVOT obstruction. In these dogs, a thickened opaque plaque of connective tissue was present opposite to the anterior mitral valve. These dogs had an abnormally opposing thickened mitral valve leaflet and/or malpositioned papillary muscles, suggesting that hypertrophic cardiomyopathy in these dogs may not be just simply a disease of myocardium. However, at least in one report, myofibers disarray and asymmetrical hypertrophy of the septum has been reported. Secondary changes in medium-sized coronary arteries that have been reported in cats with hypertrophic cardiomyopathy are also present in dogs with hypertrophic cardiomyopathy, and they include tunica intima hyperplasia with hypertrophy and hyaline degeneration of smooth muscle cells in the tunica media.

Dilated (Congestive) Cardiomyopathy. Dilated or congestive cardiomyopathy (DCM) is an important cause of congestive heart failure in cats, dogs, and cattle.

Affected dogs often are males of large breed, such as Doberman pinschers, Portuguese water dogs, Dalmatians, Scottish deerhounds, Irish wolfhounds, Saint Bernards, Afghan hounds, Newfoundland dogs, Old English sheepdogs, Great Danes, and boxers. However, smaller breeds, such as English cocker spaniels and Manchester

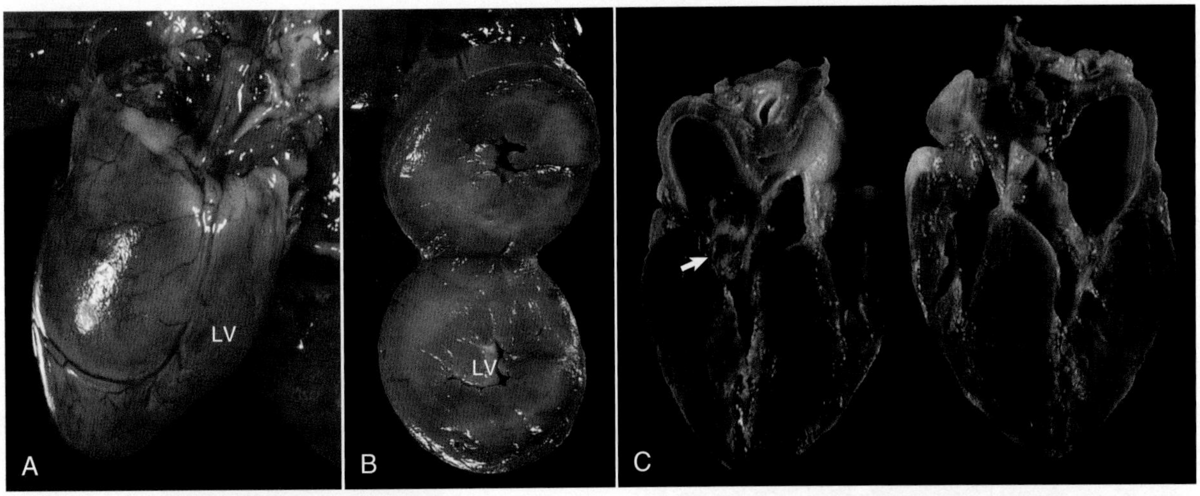

Figure 10-41 **Hypertrophic Cardiomyopathy, Heart, Cats. A,** Note the thickened left ventricular wall *(LV)*. **B,** The thickened left ventricular free wall and septum have markedly reduced the lumen of the left ventricle *(LV)*. **C,** There is severe diffuse concentric hypertrophy of the left ventricular free wall, interventricular septum, and papillary muscles. Left atrial dilation is present and a large thrombus *(arrow)* arises from and extends through the left atrioventricular valve. (**A** and **B** courtesy Dr. W. Crowell, College of Veterinary Medicine, The University of Georgia; and Noah's Arkive, College of Veterinary Medicine, The University of Georgia. **C** courtesy Ettinger SJ, Feldman EC (editors): *Textbook of veterinary internal medicine. Diseases of the dog and cat,* vol 2, ed 7, Philadelphia, 2010, Saunders.)

terriers, may be affected. The disease often has a familial pattern in the affected breeds, and it appears to be inherited as an autosomal recessive mode in the Portuguese water dog breed; as an autosomal dominant mode in the Irish wolfhound, Newfoundland, and Doberman pinscher dog breeds; and likely as an X-linked recessive mode in boxer dogs. At autopsy (syn: necropsy), lesions of congestive heart failure are present and the hearts are rounded because of biventricular dilation (Figs. 10-43 and 10-44), whereas in some cases dilation of the left atrium and ventricle predominates. The ratio between the ventricular wall and chamber diameter is decreased (i.e., eccentric hypertrophy). The circumference of the annulus of the mitral and tricuspid valves is often increased, and the papillary muscles are often flattened and atrophic. Atrioventricular valvular leaflets are occasionally mildly to moderately thickened, and chordae tendineae are thickened and elongated. The dilated cardiac chambers often have a diffusely white, thickened endocardium. Myocardial hypertrophy is best demonstrated by calculating heart weight to body weight ratio. The term hypertrophy implies a pathologic process in which the weight of the organ is increased because of an increase in cell size rather than number. In myocardial eccentric hypertrophy, the sarcomeres are increased in numbers in series (rather than parallel as in concentric hypertrophy). Two histological patterns have been described in dogs with dilated cardiomyopathy. The attenuated wavy fiber type is seen in many giant, large and medium-sized dogs and the fatty infiltration-degenerative type of dilated cardiomyopathy is seen in mainly boxers and Doberman pinschers. Occasionally, there are additional nonspecific findings, such as necrosis, infarcts, fibrosis, vacuolization of myocytes, and hyperplasia of coronary arteries. In the attenuated wavy fiber type, the cardiomyocytes are less than 6 μm in diameter (normal myofiber diameter ranges from 10 to 20 μm) and have a wavy appearance. The myocytes are separated by clear spaces (i.e., edema fluid), and there is minimal to absent cellular infiltrates. The abnormal attenuated wavy fibers are most abundant in the lateral wall of the left ventricle and therefore this site should be sampled when dilated cardiomyopathy is suspected. The sensitivity and specificity of attenuated wavy fibers of the myocardium of dogs for the diagnosis of dilated cardiomyopathy have been shown to be 98% and 100%, respectively. The attenuated wavy fibers form may represent an early pathologic change in the myocardium of dogs with dilated cardiomyopathy because it has been documented in dogs preceding clinical signs of dilated cardiomyopathy. In the fatty infiltration-degenerative type of dilated cardiomyopathy, histopathology consists of myocytolysis, myofiber degeneration, vacuolization, and atrophy along with extensive fibrosis and fatty infiltration that replaces the myofibers. It is proposed that the two histologically distinct forms of idiopathic canine dilated cardiomyopathy reflect different disease processes. Cardiotoxicity leading to chamber dilation similar to DCM (i.e., secondary dilated cardiomyopathy) has been reported secondary to toxic/environmental (e.g., doxorubicin, irradiation, ethanol, cobalt, lead, catecholamines, histamine, and methylxanthines), infectious (e.g., canine parvovirus), and nutritional (taurine and carnitine deficiency) causes.

Idiopathic dilated cardiomyopathy is a rare feline primary myocardial disease with a suggested complex genetic inheritance that results in a systolic heart failure rather than a diastolic heart failure as seen in cats with hypertrophic cardiomyopathy. Most cats develop secondary dilated cardiomyopathy because of nutritional deficiency (taurine), toxicity (doxorubicin), or severe volume overload (severe mitral insufficiency or congenital defects leading to severe left to right shunting) or, rarely, infection with feline panleukopenia virus. The heart globally enlarges through dilation of all chambers (eccentric hypertrophy), and the heart to body weight ratio is increased (5.4 ± 0.3 g/kg vs. 3.83 ± 0.2 g/kg in normal control cats), although the walls of the ventricles are thinned. This is due to addition of sarcomeres in series, rather than in parallel, which leads to a proportional increase in ventricular wall thickness and internal chamber diameter. Hydrothorax, pulmonary congestion, and edema often accompany dilated cardiomyopathy when congestive heart failure ensues. Similar to cats with hypertrophic cardiomyopathy, arterial thromboembolism occasionally accompanies feline dilated cardiomyopathy, unlike in dogs with dilated cardiomyopathy. Cardiac histopathology consists of mild multifocal to severe and diffuse interstitial edema and fibrosis. Myocardiocytes are thinner, attenuated, and wavier than normal, and they often exhibit myocytolysis.

Three forms of bovine dilated cardiomyopathy are dilated cardiomyopathy in cattle of Canadian Holstein origin, cardiomyopathy

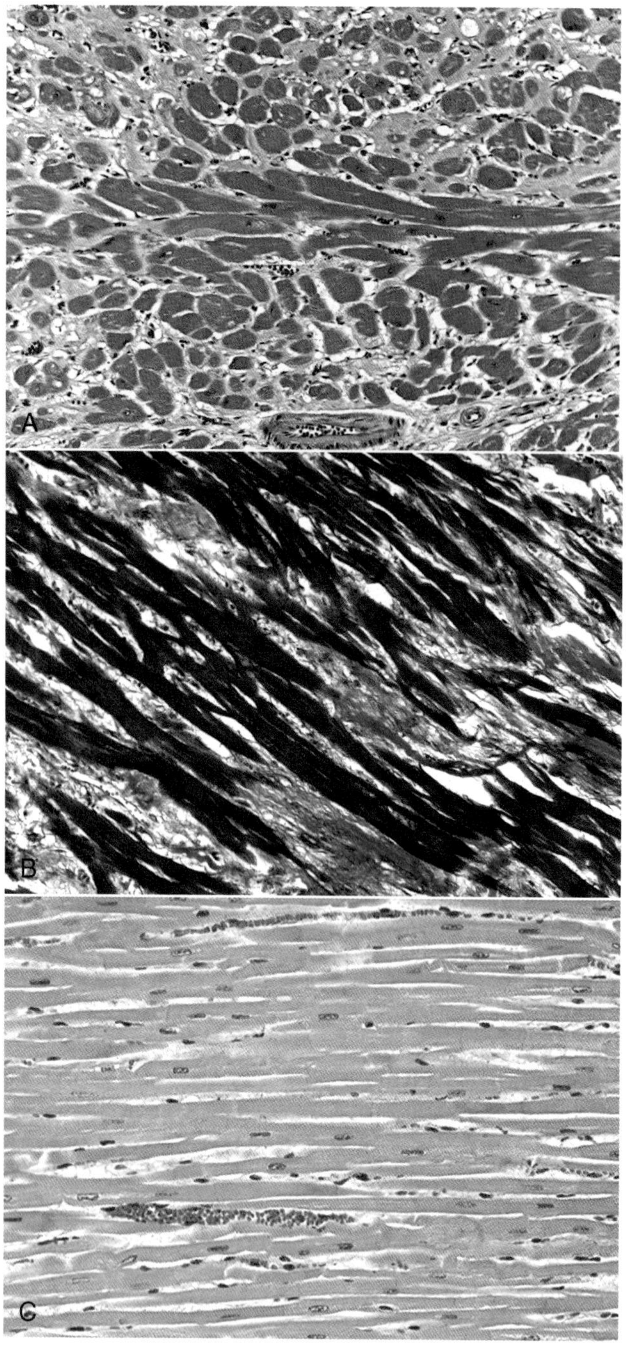

Figure 10-42 **Hypertrophic Cardiomyopathy, Heart, Ventricular Myocardium, Cat. A,** Cardiac myocytes are hypertrophied and in disarray. H&E stain. **B,** Masson's trichrome stain demonstrates abundant amounts of interstitial collagen *(blue)* produced by fibroblasts. **C,** Normal cardiac myocytes arranged in parallel bundles. H&E stain. (**A** and **B** courtesy Atlantic Veterinary College, University of Prince Edward Island. **C** courtesy Dr. L. Borst, College of Veterinary Medicine.)

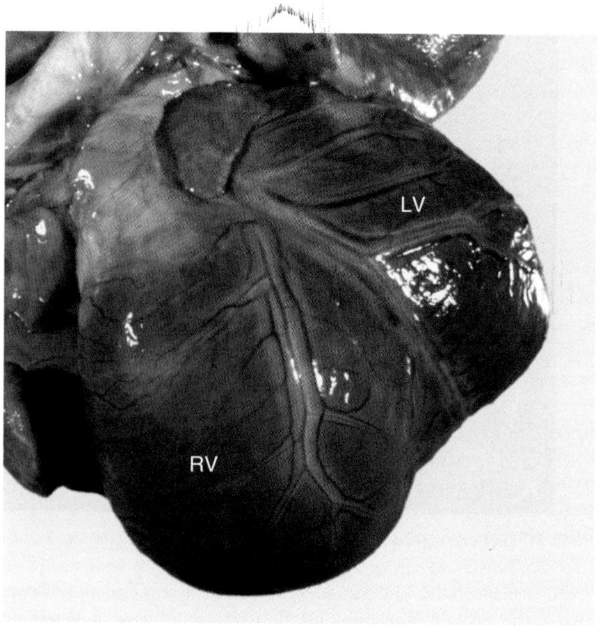

Figure 10-43 **Dilated (Congestive) Cardiomyopathy, Heart, Left Ventricle *(LV)* and Right Ventricle *(RV)*, Dog.** Biventricular dilation has resulted in the heart having a double apex. (Courtesy Dr. T. Boosinger, College of Veterinary Medicine, Auburn University; and Noah's Arkive, College of Veterinary Medicine, The University of Georgia.)

in Japanese black cattle, and congenital cardiomyopathy in Hereford cattle. Cardiomyopathy in cattle of Canadian Holstein origin has been reported in Holsteins, Red Holstein-Friesian, and Red Danish dairy breed; it was first reported in Switzerland for Simmental-Red Holsteins, but is now reported from multiple countries. Breeding studies have indicated an autosomal recessive mode of inheritance. Affected cattle develop congestive heart failure with cardiac dilation. Histopathologic findings are loss of cardiac muscle cells and replacement fibrosis. Japanese black cattle cardiomyopathy occurs in newborn and infant calves. Microscopically, myocardial degeneration and necrosis is marked. A lethal, autosomal recessive gene is suspected. Congenital cardiomyopathy occurs in Poll Hereford cattle in association with wooly haircoat syndrome. Inherited as a lethal autosomal recessive trait, affected calves usually die from congestive heart failure by 12 weeks of age.

Restrictive Cardiomyopathy. Restrictive cardiomyopathy occurs infrequently. Restrictive cardiomyopathy is a functional term rather than disease entity and consists of a spectrum of pathologic phenotype and pathophysiology. The hallmark of restrictive cardiomyopathy is increased stiffness of the myocardium that leads to diastolic heart failure. Stiffness is due to increased myocardial fibrosis and variable infiltration with leukocytes. Sometimes the endocardium is also involved (endomyocardial fibrosis), and it is thought to be a specific subtype of restrictive cardiomyopathy. When the endocardium is involved, there is extreme endocardial thickening secondary to fibrosis and granulation tissue. Restrictive cardiomyopathy in cats can have two types of endocardial changes resultant in impaired vascular filling. In one type, the left ventricular endocardium has diffuse notable fibrosis. Evidence suggests that the fibrotic lesion is preceded by endomyocarditis. The second type results from excessive moderator bands that traverse the left ventricular cavity. Other examples of restrictive cardiomyopathy in animals include endocardial fibrosis in certain strains of aged rats and congenital endocardial fibroelastosis in Burmese cats (Fig. 10-45).

Arrhythmogenic Right Ventricular Cardiomyopathy. Arrhythmogenic right ventricular cardiomyopathy is an important cardiac disease of middle-aged boxer dogs, and rare cases have been reported in cats. Other names for the disease include boxer cardiomyopathy and familial ventricular arrhythmias of boxers. It is inherited as an autosomal dominant trait in boxers, and it is associated with an 8–base pair deletion in the 3′ untranslated region of the Striatin gene on chromosome 17, inhibition of trafficking of Wnt pathway proteins from the endoplasmic reticulum to their proper location within the cell, and potentially with Calstabin2 deficiency. Affected dogs have a high incidence of ventricular arrhythmias with

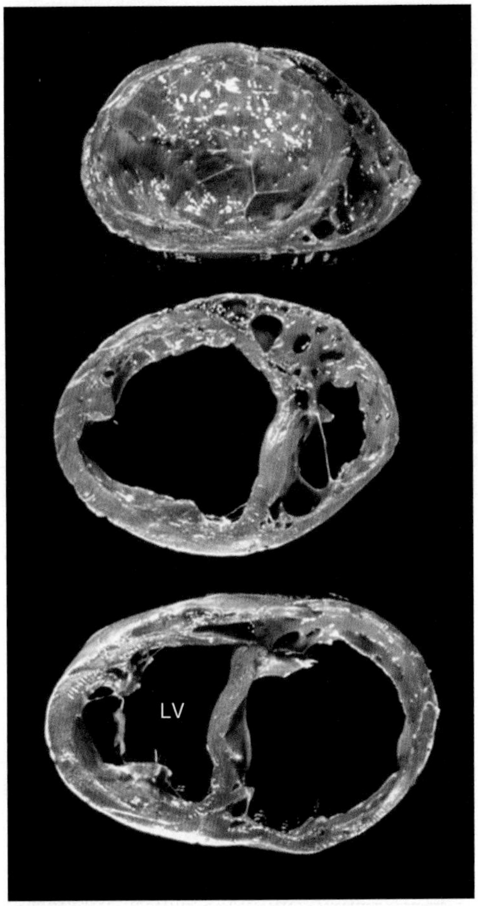

Figure 10-44 Dilated (Congestive) Cardiomyopathy, Heart, Ventricles, Cross Section, Dog. The left ventricle *(LV)* and right ventricle have thin walls, dilated chambers, and white fibrotic endocardium. (Courtesy Dr. Y. Niyo, College of Veterinary Medicine, Iowa State University; and Noah's Arkive, College of Veterinary Medicine, The University of Georgia.)

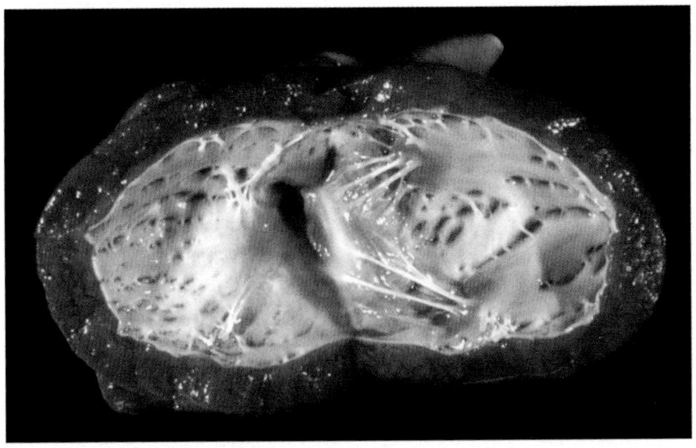

Figure 10-45 Subendocardial Fibroelastosis, Heart, Left Ventricle, Dog. The endocardium is opaque because increased amounts of collagen and elastic fibers were deposited in the subendocardium secondary to turbulence of blood flow within the ventricles. This dog had a persistent ductus arteriosus. This lesion may have a hereditary basis in Burmese cats and is often a sequela to turbulence within ventricles in cardiac disease. (Courtesy College of Veterinary Medicine, University of Illinois.)

predominantly left bundle branch block morphology that originate from the right ventricle, and they often have enlargement of the right ventricular chamber; however, some dogs have normal-sized cardiac chambers, and because of the intermittent nature of the arrhythmia in arrhythmogenic right ventricular cardiomyopathy, they may not have a documented history of ventricular premature complexes on electrocardiogram. Therefore lack of documented arrhythmia and/or enlargement of the right cardiac chamber does not rule out this disease. The distinctive histopathologic findings are similar to those of the disease in human beings and include substantial replacement of right ventricular (RV) cardiac myocytes by adipose or fibrous tissue in a fatty or a fibro-fatty pattern.

It is a rare myocardial disease of cats. Cats have moderate to severe RV eccentric hypertrophy and severe right atrial enlargement with segmental to diffuse wall thinning, and they develop atrial and ventricular arrhythmias from macroreentrant circuits that develop in regions of fibrofatty infiltration.

Unclassified Cardiomyopathy. This is a nebulous category that includes cases with left or bilateral atrial dilation, normal to near normal LV wall thickness, normal systolic function, and diastolic dysfunction. Grossly and histologically, the distinction between restrictive cardiomyopathy and unclassified cardiomyopathy is not apparent unless endomyocardial fibrosis is present. The separation between these two entities can sometimes be made antemortem via echocardiographic evaluation of a restrictive filling pattern on mitral inflow (E and A waves).

Molecular Mechanisms of Hereditary Cardiomyopathies. Our understanding of the molecular mechanisms of the hereditary cardiomyopathies is developing rapidly. In human beings with familial hypertrophic cardiomyopathy inherited in an autosomal dominant manner, a variety of single-gene mutations have been documented. The mutations affect genes that encode sarcomere proteins of cardiac myocytes. Hypertrophic cardiomyopathy-associated altered cardiac proteins include cardiac β-myosin heavy chain, cardiac troponin T and tropomyosin, and myosin-binding protein C. Dilated cardiomyopathy-associated mutated proteins include desmin, mitochondrial proteins, dystropin, titin (titin spans the sarcomere and connects the Z and M restricting the range of sarcomere stretching motion), and a subunit of the surface protein–dystropin-associated glycoproteins. It remains unclear how these mutant proteins result in functional and structural alterations of cardiac muscle cells. However, recent studies suggest hypertrophic cardiomyopathy may arise from defective energy transfer from the mitochondria to the sarcomere. Dilated cardiomyopathy is believed to be associated with abnormalities in the cytoskeletal proteins resulting in abnormal force generation, force transmission, or myocyte signaling. Similar gene mutations and altered proteins were recently discovered in the various heritable cardiomyopathies of animals.

Neoplastic Transformation. Various primary and secondary neoplasms develop either in or near the heart. Primary neoplasms include rhabdomyoma, rhabdomyosarcoma, schwannoma, and hemangiosarcoma. Rhabdomyomas and rhabdomyosarcomas are rare in animals and form white to gray nodules in the myocardium that often project into the cardiac chambers. Congenital rhabdomyomatosis in pigs and guinea pigs is a presumed nonneoplastic hamartoma (i.e., malformation often resembling a neoplasm that is composed of an overgrowth of mature cells and tissues that normally occur in the affected organ). Cardiac rhabdomyomatosis has been reported in cattle, sheep, and dogs. Single or multiple, pale, poorly circumscribed areas are scattered in the myocardium and are composed of large glycogen-laden cells with morphologic features of cardiomyocytes and Purkinje cells.

Malignant lymphoma (lymphosarcoma) is the most common secondary neoplasm occurring in the heart and often causes lesions in the hearts of cattle, which can be severe enough to cause death from cardiac failure. Cardiac lesions may be present in dogs and cats with malignant lymphoma. The neoplastic cell infiltration can be diffuse or nodular and involve the myocardium, endocardium, and pericardium. Lymphomatous tissue appears as white masses that may resemble deposits of fat (Fig. 10-46). Microscopically, extensive infiltrations of neoplastic lymphocytes are present between myocytes (Fig. 10-47). Other neoplasms, such as malignant melanomas, occasionally have metastatic lesions in the heart.

Heart-based tumors are primary neoplasms of extracardiac tissues in dogs and rarely cats. They arise at the base of the heart and can produce vascular obstruction and cardiac failure. The most common neoplasm arising at this location is the aortic body tumor or paraganglioma (chemodectoma), but occasionally ectopic thyroid or parathyroid tissue gives origin to neoplasms in this area. The aortic body is a chemoreceptor organ. In some cases, aortic body tumors become large, white, firm masses that surround and compress the great vessels and atria (Fig. 10-48). Brachycephalic dog breeds are most frequently affected. Microscopically, the neoplastic cells are polyhedral with vacuolated cytoplasm and are supported by a fine connective tissue stroma (see Fig. 12-47).

Cell Degeneration and Death

Myocardial Necrosis and Mineralization. Myocardial necrosis and mineralization can result from a number of causes, including nutritional deficiencies, chemical and plant toxins, ischemia, metabolic disorders, heritable diseases, and physical injuries (see Box 10-5). From this large list of causes of myocardial injury, some of the most frequently observed current examples are ionophore toxicity in horses and ruminants, vitamin E–selenium deficiency in the young of all species, "heart-brain syndrome" of dogs (see Fig. 10-82), anthracycline toxicity in dogs, and gossypol toxicosis in pigs. In various localized areas throughout the world, numerous deaths in ruminants have resulted from consumption of poisonous plants such as *Acacia georginae* and *Dichapetalum cymosum*. The macroscopic lesions are similar regardless of the specific toxin and include pale white to tan areas and linear streaks throughout the myocardium. Microscopic lesions include multifocal myocardial degeneration and necrosis characterized by vacuolation of myocardial cytoplasm; loss of cross-striations; fragmentation of rhabdomyocytes;

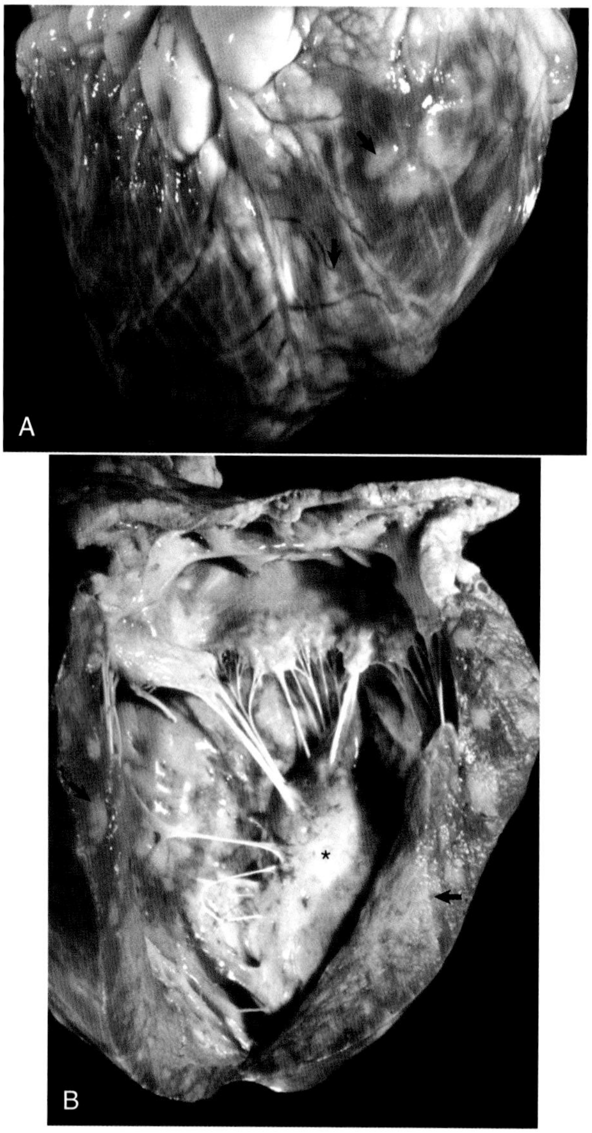

Figure 10-46 **Lymphoma (Lymphosarcoma), Heart, Myocardium, Cow. A,** Sites of infiltrating neoplastic lymphocytes in the ventricular myocardium are evident as numerous white areas and nodules *(arrows)*. **B,** Similar white areas of tumor are visible in the section of the left ventricular wall *(arrows)* and subendocardially (*) in the ventricular septum. (Courtesy College of Veterinary Medicine, University of Illinois.)

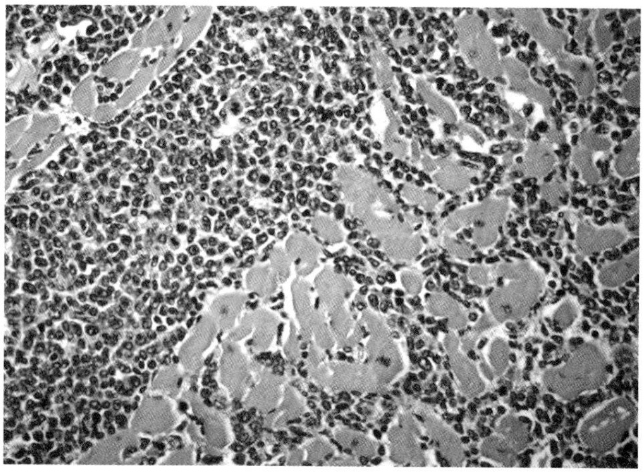

Figure 10-47 **Lymphoma (Lymphosarcoma), Heart, Section of Myocardium, Cow.** Neoplastic lymphocytes have extensively infiltrated between the cardiomyocytes. Extensive infiltration can result in myocyte atrophy and loss. H&E stain. (Courtesy School of Veterinary Medicine, Purdue University.)

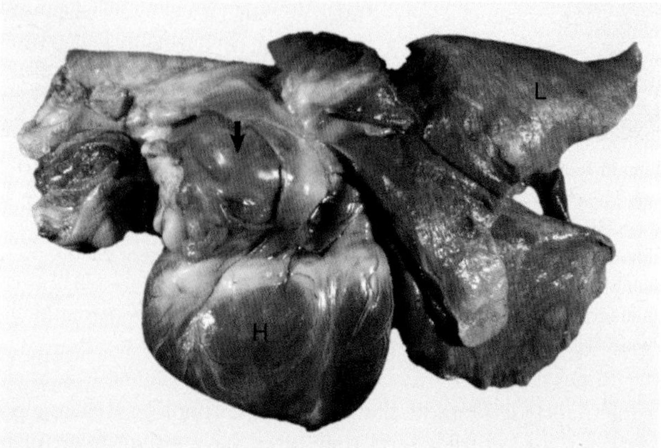

Figure 10-48 **Chemodectoma (Heart Base Tumor), Aortic Body, Dog.** Note the large mass *(arrow)* at the base of the heart *(H)*. *L,* Lungs. (Courtesy College of Veterinary Medicine, University of Illinois.)

hypereosinophilia, coagulation, and clumping of the sarcoplasm; and nuclear pyknosis and karyolysis (Fig. 10-49).

Toxicoses

Ionophore-Induced Myocardial Degeneration. Ionophores (polyether antibiotics), such as monensin, lasalocid, salinomycin, and narasin, are toxic to horses and dogs at extremely low concentrations. They are used as feed additives to increase feed efficiency and weight gain of beef and dairy cattle and to control coccidiosis in poultry. Horses gain access to ionophores when they consume (1) ruminant feed containing ionophores; (2) horse feed accidentally mixed with ionophores; and (3) horse and dog food accidentally contaminated in a mill producing poultry, cattle, horse, and dog feeds. Ionophores cause acute cardiac rhabdomyocyte degeneration and necrosis; this type of injury is discussed in detail in the section on Responses to Injury: Myocardium, Myocardial Necrosis. Ionophores are lipophilic chelating agents that transport cations across phospholipid bilayer membranes and complexes with monovalent cations, such as Na^+ and Ca^+, and cross cell membranes and enter the cell via ion transport systems in exchange for H^+ and K^+ ions. Increases in the concentrations of intracellular Ca^+ and possibly Na^+ are thought to cause cell membrane injury and dysfunction, resulting in mitochondrial swelling and decreased adenosine triphosphate production. In addition, they cause lipid peroxidation of cell membranes leading to loss of cell membrane integrity, fluid and ion shifts, and oncotic necrosis.

Gossypol-Induced Myocardial Degeneration. Gossypol-induced myocardial degeneration can follow the ingestion of cottonseed or cottonseed products that contain excess free gossypol. Gossypol is a potentially toxic pigment in the cotton plant; however, it is toxic only when in a free form (not bound to protein). Gossypol causes myocardial degeneration and necrosis and cardiac conduction failure (see later discussion). The macroscopic and microscopic characteristics of the lesions are in many ways similar to those caused by ionophore-induced and white snakeroot–induced myocardial degeneration in horses. In addition, acute rhabdomyocytic degeneration and necrosis are discussed in detail in the section on Responses to Injury: Myocardium, Myocardial Necrosis and also in Chapter 15. Monogastric animals, particularly pigs and horses, are more sensitive to gossypol-induced myocardial degeneration and necrosis than ruminants. In summary, macroscopic lesions include pale white to tan areas throughout a "flabby" myocardium; microscopic lesions include multifocal myocardial degeneration and necrosis.

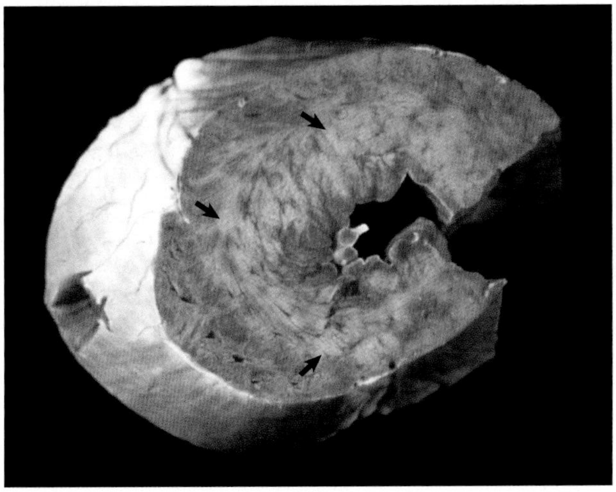

Figure 10-49 Myocardial Necrosis, Acute Monensin Toxicosis, Heart, Cross Section, Left Ventricular Myocardium, Calf. Note the pale, mottled, necrotic areas *(arrows)* distributed throughout the ventricular myocardium. (Courtesy School of Veterinary Medicine, Purdue University.)

Chemotherapeutic Agent-Induced Myocardial Degeneration. Cardiotoxicity has emerged as a significant clinical entity in veterinary medicine in recent years with the growing use of antineoplastic drugs in small animal practice and the widespread use of growth promotants in ruminants (see Fig. 10-49; also see E-Figs. 10-12 and 10-13).

Disorders of Domestic Animals: Cardiac Conduction System

Disturbances of Growth

Neoplastic Transformation

Schwannomas. Schwannomas involve cardiac nerves in cattle and appear as single or multiple white nodules detected as incidental findings at slaughter (see Fig. 14-115).

Cell Degeneration and Death

Conduction system diseases have been described mainly in dogs and horses, probably because clinical cardiac evaluations are done most frequently in these species. Secondary conduction system disorders result from myocardial disease (inflammation, neoplasia, or degeneration) near the conduction system. Specific presumably inherited diseases in dogs include (1) syncope in pug dogs with lesions of the bundle of His; (2) intermittent sinus arrest in deaf Dalmatian dogs, presumably associated with lesions in the sinus node; (3) sinoatrial syncope (sick sinus dysfunction) in female miniature schnauzers, West Highland white terriers, cocker spaniels, and dachshunds; (4) inherited ventricular arrhythmia and sudden unexpected death in German shepherds, and (5) widespread conduction pathology in Alaskan sled dogs that died suddenly and unexpectedly in a race. Other arrhythmias in dogs and horses are atrial fibrillation and heart block. Dogs with atrial fibrillation often have concurrent congestive heart failure and have atrial dilation with AV valve insufficiency, but most horses live a normal or near-normal life span, may respond to cardioversion, and at necropsy have atrial myocardial fibrosis. Heart block of the first degree (delay of impulse through the AV node), second degree (intermittent failure to conduct through the AV node with dropped beats), and third degree (complete) has been associated with myocardial lesions, such as areas of scarring, in horses and dogs. Second-degree heart block is considered to be a normal phenomenon in horses.

Persistent atrial standstill (silent atria, AV myopathy) is a progressive cardiac disease of English springer spaniels and cats characterized by notable atrial dilation and fibrosis.

Atrial fibrillation occurs in cattle in association with right atrial dilation and fibrosis and alterations in the SA mode. Also, sudden (unexpected) cardiac death is described in racehorses with right atrial myocardial fibrosis, fibrosis of the upper ventricular septum, and arteriosclerosis of intramyocardial arteries.

Also see the discussion on the cardiac conduction system in the section on Dysfunction/Responses to Injury; Responses: Cardiac Conduction System.

Inflammation

See the previous section on Cell Degeneration and Death.

Disorders of Domestic Animals: Endocardium and Heart Valves

See the discussion of the endocardium and heart valves in the section on Responses to Injury: Endocardium and Heart Valves. The major types of AV valvular diseases are shown in Fig. 10-50.

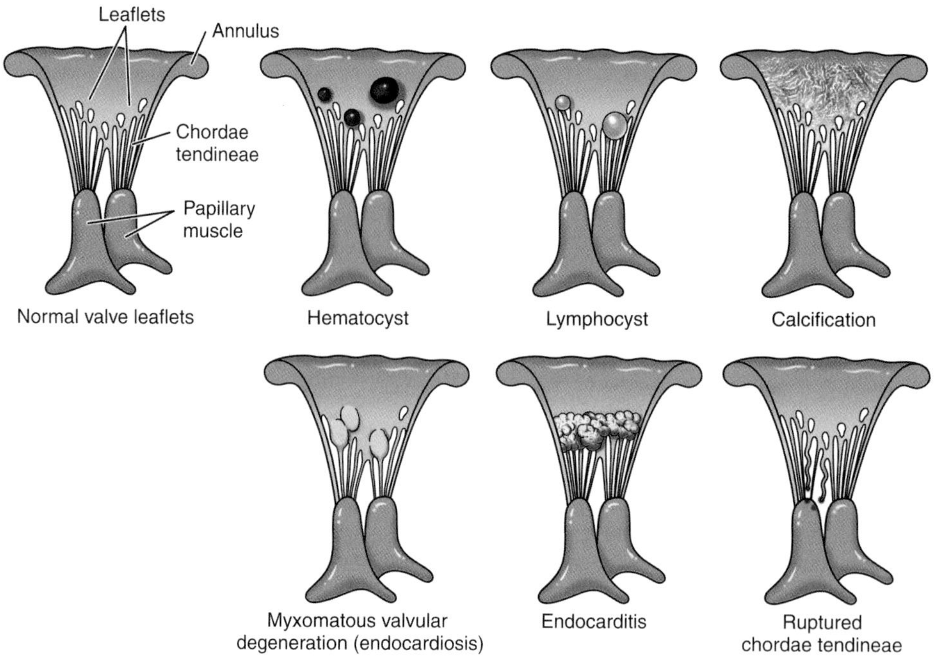

Figure 10-50 **Major Types of Cardiac Atrioventricular Valvular Disease.** (Redrawn with permission from School of Veterinary Medicine, Purdue University.)

Disturbances of Growth

Endocardial Fibroelastosis. Endocardial fibroelastosis in animals was historically recognized as a primary cardiac defect in Burmese and Siamese cats. Affected animals had prominent, white, thickened endocardium, especially of the left ventricle, because of the proliferation of fibroelastic tissue (see Fig. 10-45). Endocardial fibroelastosis is a reaction of the endocardium to hypoxia and often associated with heart disease, which results in dilated cardiac chambers. It is unclear whether this is a true congenital anomaly or a response to left atrial dilation.

Miscellaneous Valvular Anomalies

Valvular Hematomas. Valvular hematomas (hematocysts, valvular telangiectasia) frequently are observed on the AV valves of many species but are common in postnatal ruminants (Fig. 10-51, *A*). These lesions may regress and do not produce any functional abnormalities. Lesions are bulging, blood-filled cysts, several millimeters in diameter, on the AV valves.

Valvular Lymphocysts. Valvular lymphocysts may also occur and appear as yellow serum-filled cysts on the AV valve cusps (Fig. 10-51, *B*).

Cell Degeneration and Death

Ulcerative Endocarditis (Uremic Endocarditis). Uremic endocarditis is most commonly a disorder in dogs that follows acute or repeated episodes of uremia. These episodes cause ulcerative endocarditis (injury of the endothelium) of the left atrium that is resolved via healing characterized by fibrosis, with or without mineralization and chronically dilated atria (Fig. 10-52).

Myxomatous Valvular Degeneration (Valvular Endocardiosis). Degenerative changes in the valves are frequently seen in older dogs, and the process that leads to this lesion is termed *myxomatous valvular degeneration* (valvular endocardiosis). Also see the section on Disorders of Dogs (also see Fig. 10-83).

Endocardial Mineralization. Endocardial mineralization occurs from intake of excessive amounts of vitamin D and from intoxication by calcinogenic plants (*Cestrum diurnum*, *Trisetum flavescens*, *Solanum malacoxylon*, and *Solanum torvum*) that contain vitamin D analogs. These plant-induced syndromes of cattle have been called by different names in various areas of the world, such as “Manchester wasting disease” in Jamaica, “enzootic calcinosis” in Europe, “Naalehu disease” in Hawaii, “enteque seco” in Argentina, and “espichamento” in Brazil. Multiple, large, white, rough, firm plaques of mineralized fibroelastic tissue are present in the endocardium and intima of large elastic arteries. Fibrosis, with or without mineralization, occurs in chronically dilated hearts, in hearts of debilitated cattle with Johne’s disease (Fig. 10-53; also see Fig. 10-22), in dogs with healed lesions of left atrial ulcerative endocarditis associated with a prior uremic episode (see Fig. 10-52), and in the so-called jet lesions produced by the trauma of refluxed blood in valvular insufficiencies.

Inflammation

Vegetative Valvular and Mural Endocarditis. Endocarditis is usually the result of bacterial infections, except for lesions produced by migrating *Strongylus vulgaris* larvae in horses and rarely in mycotic infections. The lesions are often very large by the time of death and are present on the valves (valvular endocarditis), although some lesions originate from the underlying myocardium or extend from the affected valve to the adjacent wall (mural endocarditis). Grossly, the affected valves have large, adhering, friable, yellow-to-gray masses of fibrin termed *vegetations*, which can occlude the valvular orifice (Figs. 10-54, *A*, and 10-55). In chronic lesions, the fibrin deposits are organized by fibrous connective tissue to produce irregular nodular masses termed *verrucae* (wartlike lesions). Microscopically, the lesion consists of accumulated layers of fibrin and numerous embedded bacterial colonies underlain by a zone of infiltrated leukocytes and granulation tissue (see Fig. 10-54, *B*). The relative frequency of valvular involvement with endocarditis in animals is mitral > aortic > tricuspid > pulmonary.

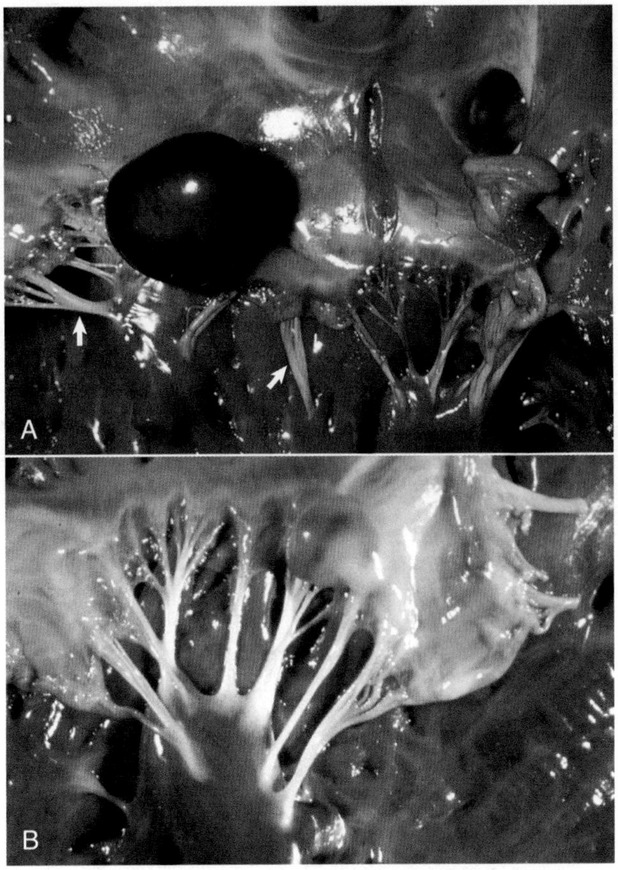

Figure 10-51 Hematocysts and Lymphocysts, Calf. A, Valvular hematocyst, heart, opened left side, mitral valve, postnatal calf. A dark, blood-filled cyst protrudes from a cusp of the mitral valve. *Arrows* indicate chordae tendineae. Hematocysts usually occur in ruminants, do not cause any functional abnormality, and usually regress within a few months of birth. **B,** Valvular lymphocyst, heart. A lymph-filled cyst is on a cusp of the atrioventricular valve. Like hematocysts, lymphocysts usually occur in ruminants, do not cause any functional abnormality, and usually regress within a few months of birth. (**A** courtesy Dr. M.D. McGavin, College of Veterinary Medicine, University of Tennessee. **B** courtesy College of Veterinary Medicine, University of Illinois.)

The pathogenesis of endocarditis is complicated and incompletely understood, but the components of Virchow's triad in thrombogenesis—endothelial injury, turbulence, and hypercoagulability—are involved. Affected animals often have preexisting extracardiac infections, such as gingivitis, mastitis, hepatic abscesses, or dermatitis, resulting in one or more bouts of bacteremia. Turbulent intracardiac blood flow associated with congenital anomalies or the presence of intracardiac and vasculature devices, such as catheters, may contribute to initiation of the lesion. Focal trauma–induced endothelial disruption on the surface of the normally avascular valves allows bacteria to adhere, proliferate, and initiate an inflammatory reaction that results in subsequent deposition of masses of fibrin. Death is the result of cardiac failure from valvular dysfunction or the effects of bacteremia. In some animals, septic emboli lodge in organs such as the heart, synovium, bone, liver, kidneys, and meninges, leading to infarction and/or localized inflammation or abscess formation. See the discussion on vegetative valvular and mural endocarditis in the section on Disorders of Domestic Animals: Endocardium and Heart Valves, Inflammation and also Chapter 3.

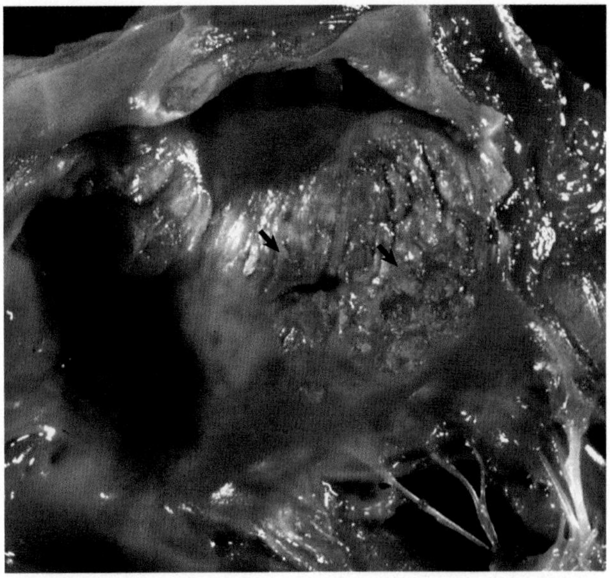

Figure 10-52 Ulcerative Endocarditis (Uremia), Heart, Endocardium of Left Atrium, Dog. Note the white-red, thick, wrinkled area *(arrows)* of endocarditis, mineralization, and fibrous tissue *(scar)* formation caused by uremia in this dog with chronic renal failure. (Courtesy Dr. K. Read, College of Veterinary Medicine, Texas A&M University; and Noah's Arkive, College of Veterinary Medicine, The University of Georgia.)

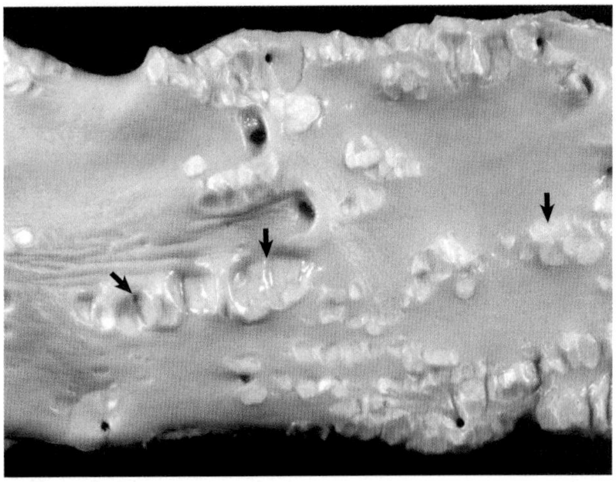

Figure 10-53 Johne's Disease, Arteriosclerosis, Aorta, Cow. Multiple prominent, white, mineralized foci are in the tunica intima and media *(arrows)*. (Courtesy College of Veterinary Medicine, University of Illinois.)

Atrial Thrombosis. Atrial thrombi may occur with valvular or myocardial disease and are the result of hemostatic abnormalities resulting from stasis or turbulence. Endothelial injury, turbulence, and hypercoagulability are involved in the pathogenesis of atrial thrombi.

Disorders of Domestic Animals: Pericardium and Epicardium

Disturbances of Circulation

Hemorrhage. Hemorrhage involving the pericardium and epicardium (see Fig. 10-24; see E-Fig. 10-18) results from stretching, tearing, lacerating, or crushing blood vessels in these structures and may be caused by penetrating wounds (foreign objects, bullets, or

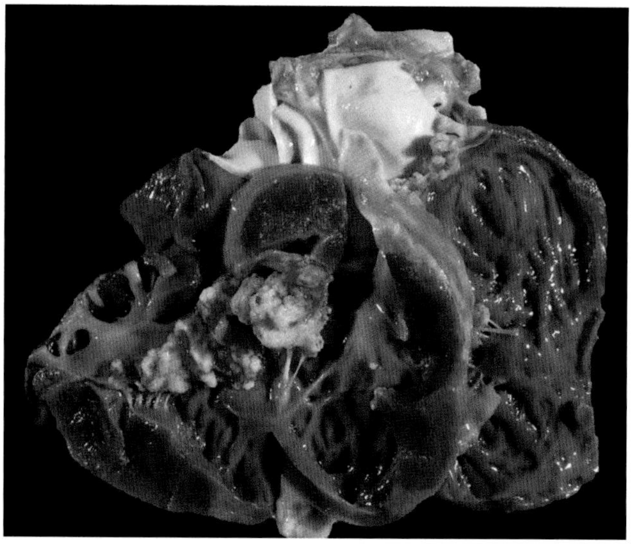

Figure 10-55 **Valvular Endocarditis, *Streptococcus Suis*, Heart Mitral and Pulmonic Valves, Pig.** Note the friable, yellow material adhering to and replacing some of the normal left atrioventricular valve. The left ventricular chamber is dilated due to failure of normal function of the valve (eccentric hypertrophy). (Courtesy Atlantic Veterinary College, University of Prince Edward Island.)

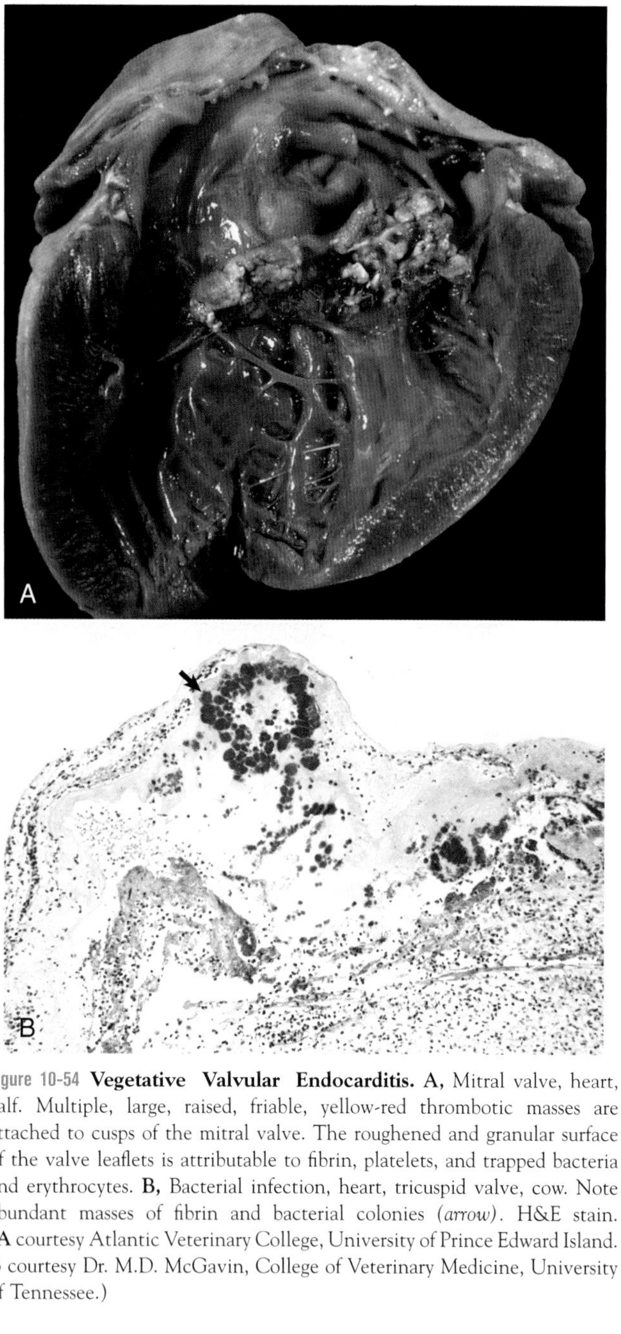

Figure 10-54 **Vegetative Valvular Endocarditis. A,** Mitral valve, heart, calf. Multiple, large, raised, friable, yellow-red thrombotic masses are attached to cusps of the mitral valve. The roughened and granular surface of the valve leaflets is attributable to fibrin, platelets, and trapped bacteria and erythrocytes. **B,** Bacterial infection, heart, tricuspid valve, cow. Note abundant masses of fibrin and bacterial colonies *(arrow)*. H&E stain. (**A** courtesy Atlantic Veterinary College, University of Prince Edward Island. **B** courtesy Dr. M.D. McGavin, College of Veterinary Medicine, University of Tennessee.)

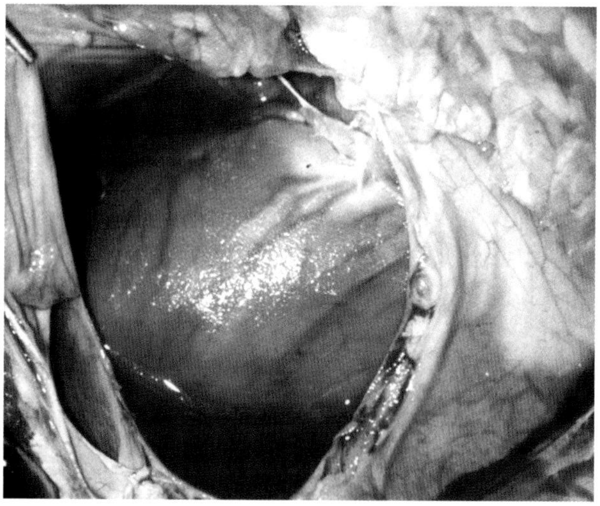

Figure 10-56 **Hydropericardium, Pericardial Sac, Pig.** The thin-walled dilated pericardial sac contains serous fluid that has accumulated secondary to alterations in hydrostatic pressure between the pericardial cavity, circulatory system, and lymphatic system. (Courtesy College of Veterinary Medicine, University of Illinois.)

knives), lacerations from fractured bone, shear forces that stretch and ultimately tear vessels in tissues (blunt force trauma), and tears and rupture of tissue resulting from loss of structural integrity attributable to invasive and destructive properties of neoplasms such as hemangiosarcomas (see Chapters 2 and 6).

Effusions. See the discussions on the mechanisms of edema formation and Figs. 2-6 through 2-10 in Chapter 2 and on the formation of transudates and exudates and Fig. 3-3 in Chapter 3.

Pericardial Dilatation. The pericardium responds to excess fluid in the pericardial space by dilation. However, this outcome requires adequate time to allow adjustments in size. In hemopericardium, blood rapidly fills the pericardial cavity and death often occurs unexpectedly from cardiac tamponade, a condition with compression of the heart caused by blood accumulation leading to reduced cardiac output. Hydropericardium is the accumulation of clear, light yellow, watery, serous fluid (i.e., transudate) in the pericardial sac (Fig. 10-56). In cases associated with vascular injury, a few fibrin strands are present, and the fluid could clot after exposure to air.

Hydropericardium. Hydropericardium occurs in those diseases that have generalized edema (see Fig. 10-56). Thus ascites and hydrothorax often occur concurrently with hydropericardium. Congestive heart failure is an important mechanism of hydropericardium and is usually the result of primary myocardial, valvular, congenital, or neoplastic diseases. Common specific diseases include dilated cardiomyopathy of dogs and cats and "ascites syndrome" of poultry. Hydropericardium can also accompany pulmonary hypertension (e.g., "brisket disease" or "high-altitude disease" of cattle), renal failure, and hypoproteinemia from various chronic debilitating diseases. Hydropericardium can also occur in various systemic diseases with vascular injury, such as septicemia in pigs, "heartwater" (*Cowdria ruminantium* infection) in small ruminants, African horse sickness, and bovine ephemeral fever.

Hydropericardium is the accumulation of clear, light yellow, watery, serous fluid (i.e., transudate) in the pericardial sac (E-Fig. 10-21; also see Fig. 10-56; also see section on Disorders of Domestic Animals). As examples, hydropericardium can occur in animals with (1) hypoproteinemia (decreased colloid osmotic pressure) caused by liver disease or protein-losing nephropathy/enteropathy; (2) heart failure (increased hydrostatic pressure) where there is poor venous return to the heart; and (3) vascular injury, where damage to the barrier function of the vascular wall can result in leakage of small quantities of plasma proteins. In this latter example, a few fibrin strands can be present and the fluid could clot after exposure to air. The pericardial surfaces are smooth and glistening in acute cases, but in chronic cases, the epicardium becomes opaque because of mild fibrous thickening and can appear roughened and granular when there is villous proliferation of fibrous tissue, especially over the atria. The mechanisms involved in these fluid shifts are discussed in Chapters 2 and 3.

Hemopericardium. Hemopericardium is an accumulation of whole blood in the pericardial sac (Figs. 10-57 and 10-58; also see section on Disorders of Domestic Animals). Death often occurs unexpectedly from cardiac tamponade, a condition in which the compression of the heart caused by the accumulation of blood in the pericardial sac leads to reduced cardiac output and poor perfusion of vascular beds in all organ systems. As examples, hemopericardium may be caused by blunt force trauma (impact with an automobile) or from rupture of the wall of the right atrium after invasion by a hemangiosarcoma.

Bleeding into the pericardial sac can result from spontaneous atrial rupture in dogs, atrial rupture in dogs with hemangiosarcoma, rupture of the intrapericardial aorta or pulmonary artery in horses, or as a complication of intracardiac injections (see Figs. 10-57 and 10-58).

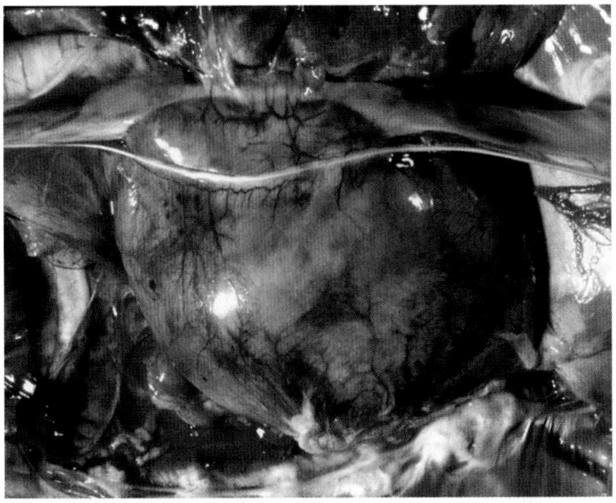

Figure 10-57 **Hemopericardium (Cardiac Tamponade), Right Atrium, Hemangiosarcoma, Heart, Dog.** The pericardium is distended and dark blue because it contains whole blood secondary to rupture of an atrial hemangiosarcoma. Hemopericardium can cause death if it is sudden and is of sufficient volume to compress the heart and thus reduce cardiac output, a condition known as cardiac tamponade. On clinical examination, heart sounds are muffled. (Courtesy College of Veterinary Medicine, University of Illinois.)

Disturbances of Growth

Serous Atrophy. Serous atrophy of fat is readily identified by the gray gelatinous appearance of epicardial fat deposits (Fig. 10-59). Healthy animals normally have abundant white or yellow epicardial fat deposits, especially along the AV junction. Microscopically, lipocytes are atrophic, and edema is present in the interstitial tissue. Serous atrophy of epicardial fat occurs rapidly during anorexia, starvation, or cachexia because fat is catabolized to maintain energy balance.

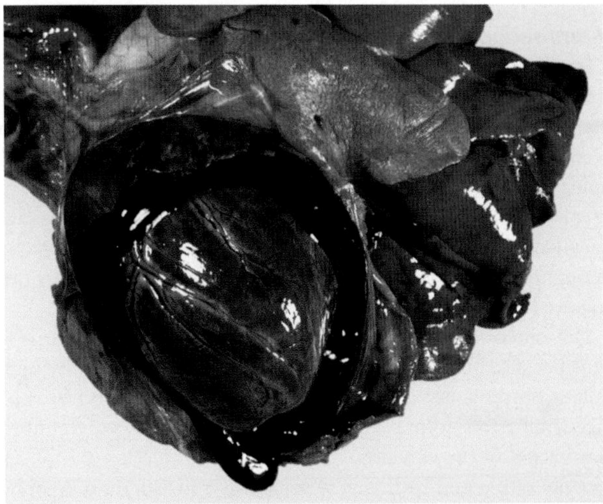

Figure 10-58 **Hemopericardium, Pericardial Sac (Opened), Dog.** The pericardial sac is filled with clotted blood. Hemorrhage into a body cavity results in pooling of coagulated or uncoagulated blood within that cavity. (Courtesy Dr. D.A. Mosier, College of Veterinary Medicine, Kansas State University.)

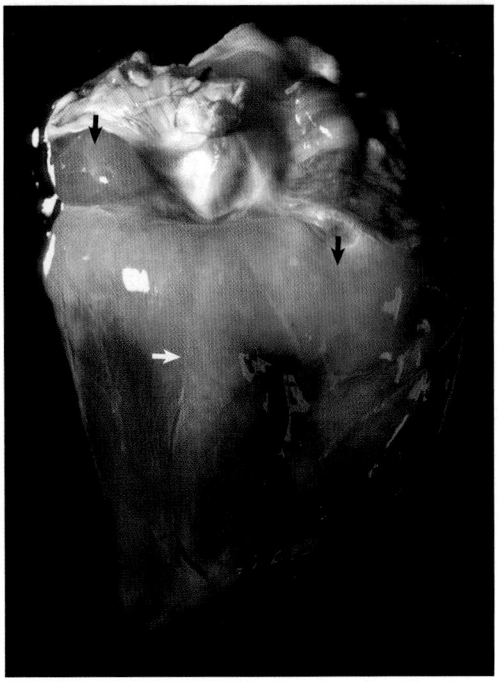

Figure 10-59 **Serous Atrophy of Fat, Heart, Epicardium, Cow.** The epicardial fat deposits are gray and gelatinous *(arrows)*, indicating that fat has been catabolized, for example, as in the early stages of starvation. (Courtesy Dr. M.D. McGavin, College of Veterinary Medicine, University of Tennessee.)

Cell Degeneration and Death

Epicardial Calcification. Epicardial calcification is a feature in hereditary calcinosis in mice and cardiomyopathy in hamsters (E-Fig. 10-22). Myocardial mineralization (discussed later) may be visible on the epicardial surface in vitamin E–selenium deficiency in sheep and cattle, vitamin D toxicity in several species, calcinogenic plant toxicosis in cattle ("Manchester wasting disease"), and spontaneous myocardial calcification in aged rats and guinea pigs.

Gout. Visceral gout has not been reported in domestic animals but does occur in birds and reptiles (E-Fig. 10-23; see Chapter 1).

Inflammation

Pericarditis. Inflammation of the pericardium is frequently seen with bacterial septicemias and typically results in fibrinous pericarditis. Grossly, both the visceral and parietal pericardial surfaces are covered by variable amounts of yellow fibrin deposits, which can result in adherence between the parietal and visceral layers. When the pericardial sac is opened, the attachments are torn away (so-called bread-and-butter heart) (Fig. 10-60). Microscopically, an eosinophilic layer of fibrin with admixed neutrophils lies over a congested epicardium (Fig. 10-61).

The outcome of fibrinous pericarditis varies. Early death is frequent because many of these lesions result from infection by highly virulent bacteria and concurrent septicemia. When survival is prolonged, adhesions form between the pericardial surfaces after fibrous organization of the exudate.

Suppurative pericarditis is seen mainly in cattle as a complication of traumatic reticuloperitonitis ("hardware disease"). Foreign bodies, such as nails or pieces of wire that accumulate in the reticulum, occasionally penetrate the reticular wall and diaphragm, enter the adjacent pericardial sac, and introduce infection. Some affected cattle survive for weeks to months until death ensues from congestive heart failure or septicemia. Grossly, the pericardial surfaces are notably thickened by white, often rough, shaggy-appearing masses of fibrous connective tissue that enclose an accumulation of white to gray, thick, foul-smelling, purulent exudate (Fig. 10-62).

Constrictive pericarditis is a chronic inflammatory lesion of the pericardium accompanied by extensive fibrous proliferation and eventual formation of fibrous adhesions between the surfaces of the visceral and parietal pericardium. The condition is seen in some cases of suppurative pericarditis in cattle and pigs with chronic fibrinous pericarditis. Severe lesions obliterate the pericardial sac and constrict the heart with fibrous tissue and can interfere with cardiac filling and thus cardiac output. Compensatory myocardial hypertrophy can result in diminished ventricular chamber volumes and contribute to the eventual development of heart failure.

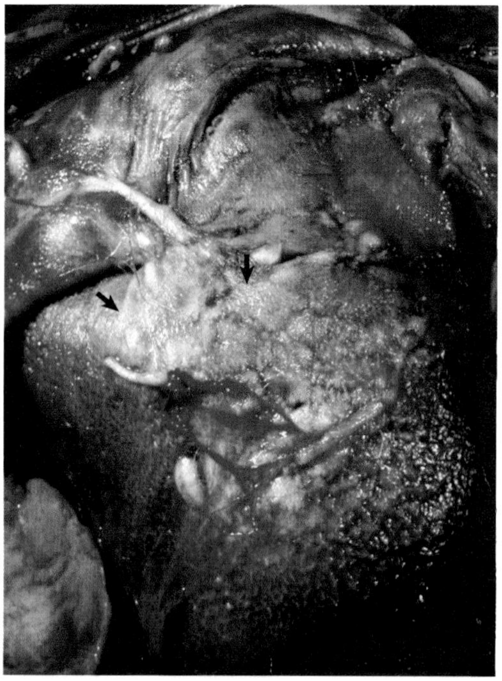

Figure 10-60 Fibrinous Pericarditis, Heart, Epicardium, Horse. The epicardium is covered dorsally by a thick, yellow layer of fibrin *(arrows)* and ventrally by granulation tissue *(finely granular surface)*, thus indicating the chronicity of the inflammatory process. The apposing parietal pericardium (not shown) was also covered with fibrin. This lesion commonly occurs in horses with *Streptococcus equi* subsp. *zooepidemicus* septicemia causing vasculitis. (Courtesy Dr. M.D. McGavin, College of Veterinary Medicine, University of Tennessee.)

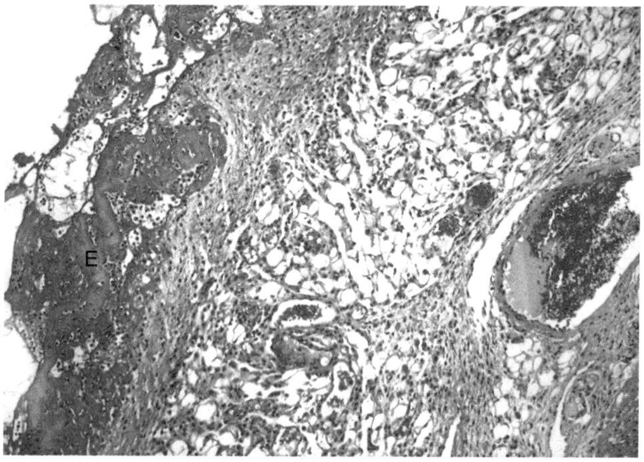

Figure 10-61 Fibrinous Pericarditis, Heart, Epicardium, Pig. Note eosinophilic fibrin deposits *(E)* *(left)* on the epicardial surface. This lesion commonly occurs with septicemias by bacteria that cause vasculitis. H&E stain. (Courtesy School of Veterinary Medicine, Purdue University.)

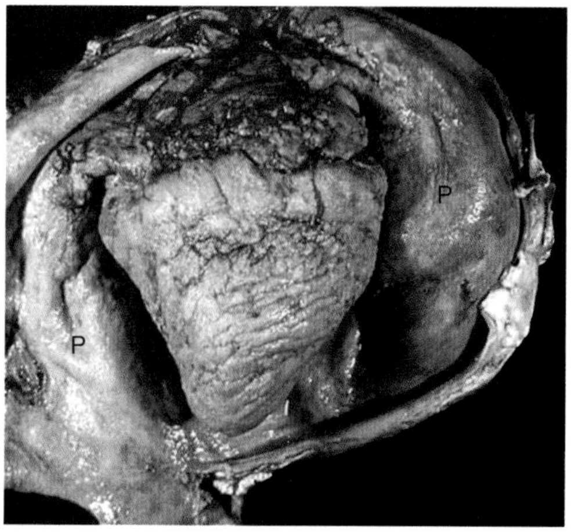

Figure 10-62 Chronic Suppurative (Active) Pericarditis, Traumatic Reticuloperitonitis ("Hardware Disease"), Heart, Pericardial Sac (Opened), Cow. The exposed epicardial and parietal surfaces are notably thickened by fibrous connective tissue and covered by a fibrinopurulent exudate. On clinical examination, heart sounds are muffled. *P,* Reflected parietal pericardium. (Courtesy Dr. J. King, College of Veterinary Medicine, Cornell University.)

Fibrinous Pericarditis. Hematogenous spread of specific organisms may result in fibrinous pericarditis. Mannheimiosis, blackleg, coliform septicemias, contagious bovine pleuropneumonia, sporadic bovine encephalomyelitis, and in utero *Brucella* spp. and *Arcanobacter pyogenesis* fetal septicemias may all produce fibrinous pericarditis. In sheep, Mannheimiosis and streptococcal infections most commonly result in fibrinous pericarditis. Sterile swabs of the pericardial exudates are recommended to identify the causative organism.

Disorders of Domestic Animals: Blood and Lymphatic Vascular Systems

See the discussion on blood and lymphatic vascular systems in the section on Responses to Injury: Blood and Lymphatic Vascular Systems. The major arterial diseases are shown in Fig. 10-63.

Blood Vessels

Disturbances of Circulation

Effusions. See the previous discussion on disturbances of circulation in the sections on Pericardium and Epicardium.

Hemopericardium. See the later discussion on the hemopericardium under Effusions in the section on Disorders of Domestic Animals: Pericardium and Epicardium; Disturbances of Circulation.

Hemothorax and Hemoabdomen. Hemothorax and hemoabdomen arise from spontaneous or traumatic rupture of large arteries or veins or from rupture of aneurysms located in the thoracic or abdominal cavity, respectively. An aneurysm is a localized dilation or outpouching of a thinned and weakened portion of a vessel. Usually, arteries are affected, especially large elastic arteries, but the lesion can also occur in veins. Known causes include copper deficiency in pigs (Fig. 10-64) because copper is necessary for normal development of elastic tissue and damage from infection with *Spirocerca lupi* in dogs or *Strongylus vulgaris* in horses. Most cases are idiopathic. Dissecting aneurysms are infrequent but have been seen in birds, most notably turkeys (Fig. 10-65). They result from disruption of the intima, which allows entry of blood into the media, and this dissects along the wall. Aneurysms can rupture. Usually the consequences are rapidly fatal because rather large arteries typically are involved. See the discussion on effusions in the section on Disorders of Domestic Animals: Pericardium and Epicardium, Disturbances of Circulation, Effusions and also Chapters 3, 7, and 9.

Aortic Rupture and Rupture of Large Arteries. Aortic rupture and rupture of large arteries can be the sequela of severe trauma or occur

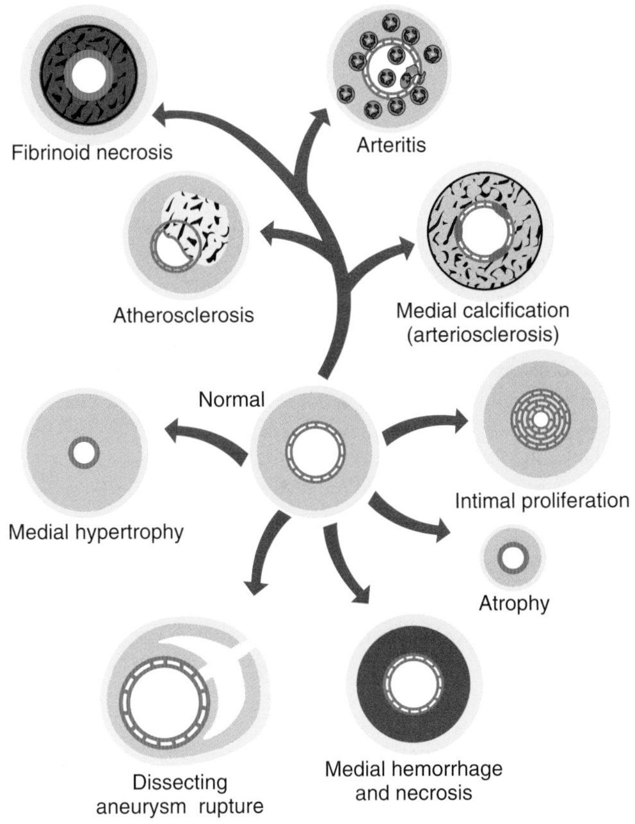

Figure 10-63 **Major Arterial Diseases.** (Redrawn with permission from School of Veterinary Medicine, Purdue University.)

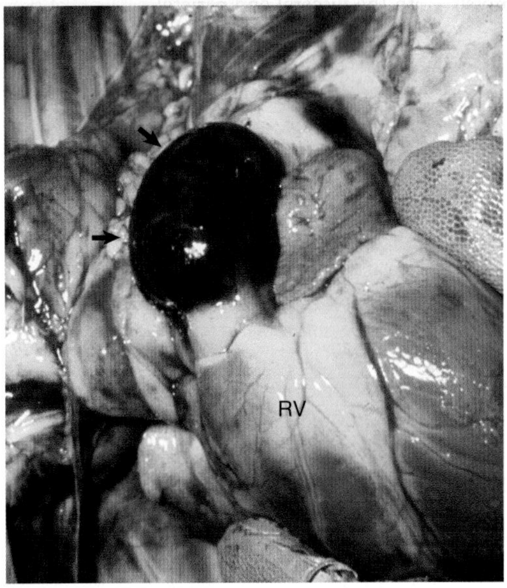

Figure 10-64 **Dissecting Aneurysm, Copper Deficiency, Heart, Pulmonary Artery, Right Ventricle *(RV)*, Pig.** The dark, blood-filled, bulging segment of the wall of the pulmonary artery *(arrows)* has resulted from disruption of elastic fibers. (Courtesy School of Veterinary Medicine, Purdue University.)

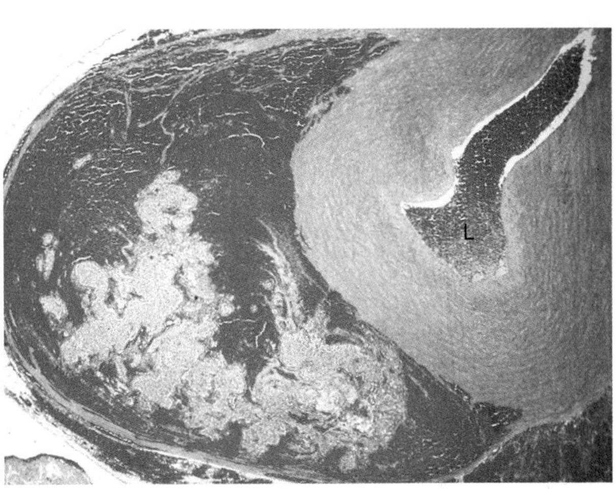

Figure 10-65 **Dissecting Aneurysm, Aorta, Turkey.** Blood has dissected through the tunica media (in a nearby section of the aorta) and in this section has come to lie in the outer layers of the tunica media and adventitia. *L*, Vessel lumen. H&E stain. (Courtesy School of Veterinary Medicine, Purdue University.)

Box 10-15 Most Common Vascular Diseases with Rupture

Aortic rupture: Horse, turkey
Carotid artery rupture: Horse
Thoracic duct rupture: Dog, cat

spontaneously (see Figs. 10-64 and 10-65). Sudden rupture of the ascending aorta or pulmonary artery near the pulmonic valve in horses is associated with notable exertion and severe trauma to the ventral thorax from falling. Death ensues rapidly from cardiac tamponade because the tear is in that portion of the aorta or pulmonary artery within the pericardial sac. In horses, the internal carotid artery can rupture into the adjacent guttural pouch, with subsequent epistaxis. This is a consequence of deep mycotic infection of the guttural pouch. Rupture of the middle uterine artery may occur during parturition in mares and with uterine torsion or prolapse in cows. Aortic rupture, with or without dissection, is an important cause of death in male turkeys. The most common vascular diseases with rupture are listed in Box 10-15.

Gastric Dilation and Volvulus. See the discussion on gastric dilation and volvulus in Chapter 7.

Disturbances of Growth

Neoplastic Transformation

Hemangiosarcoma. Cardiac hemangiosarcoma is an important neoplasm of dogs and can arise either in the heart (primary) or by metastasis (secondary) from sites such as the spleen. This neoplasm is usually seen in the wall of the right atrium and only occasionally involves the right ventricle. The tumor arises from neoplastic transformation of vascular endothelium. Also see Disorders of Dogs, Blood and Lymphatic Vascular Systems, Blood Vessels, Disturbances of Growth, Neoplastic Transformation, Hemangiosarcoma and Hemangioma.

Vascular Melanosis. See the discussion on vascular melanosis in Chapters 1 and 2.

Cell Degeneration and Death. Toxicants that affect vessels are listed in E-Box 10-1.

See Chapter 1. Generalized vascular degenerative diseases in animals are classified into the following three principal groups:

- Arteriosclerosis
- Atherosclerosis
- Arterial medial calcification

Hyaline degeneration, fibrinoid necrosis, and amyloidosis also occur in all animal species.

Arteriosclerosis. Arteriosclerosis is characterized by intimal fibrosis of large elastic arteries, atherosclerosis is characterized by intimal and medial lipid deposits in elastic and muscular arteries, and arterial medial calcification has characteristic mineralization of the walls of elastic and muscular arteries.

Arteriosclerosis is an age-related disease that occurs frequently in many animal species but rarely causes clinical signs. The disease develops as chronic degenerative and proliferative responses in the arterial wall and results in loss of elasticity ("hardening of the arteries") and, less often, luminal narrowing. The abdominal aorta is most frequently affected, but other elastic arteries and peripheral large muscular vessels may be involved. Lesions are often localized around the orifices of arterial branches. Etiologic factors in the development of arteriosclerosis are not well defined, but the significant role of hemodynamic influences is suggested by the frequent involvement at arterial branching sites, in which blood flow is turbulent. Grossly, the lesions are seen as slightly raised, firm, white plaques. Microscopically, initially the intima is thickened by accumulation of mucopolysaccharides and later by the proliferation of smooth muscle cells in the tunica media and fibrous tissue infiltration into the intima. Splitting and fragmentation of the internal elastic lamina are common

Atherosclerosis. Atherosclerosis, the vascular disease of greatest importance in human beings, occurs only infrequently in animals and rarely leads to clinical disease such as infarction of the heart or brain. The principal alteration is accumulation of deposits (atheroma) of lipid, fibrous tissue, and calcium in vessel walls, which eventually results in luminal narrowing. Many studies have established that the pig, rabbit, and chicken are susceptible to the experimental disease produced by the feeding of a high-cholesterol diet; the dog, cat, cow, goat, and rat are resistant. Lesions of the naturally occurring disease have been detected in aged pigs and birds (especially parrots) and in dogs with hypothyroidism and diabetes mellitus that develop an accompanying hypercholesterolemia. Arteries of the heart, mesentery, and kidneys are prominently thickened, firm, and yellow-white (Fig. 10-66, *A*). Microscopically, lipid globules accumulate in the cytoplasm of smooth muscle cells and macrophages, often termed *foam cells*, in the media and intima (see Fig. 10-66, *B* and *C*). Necrosis and fibrosis develop in some arterial lesions. The pathogenesis of atherosclerosis has been extensively studied in human beings. The vascular response-to-injury hypothesis is the current proposed mechanism of injury. The dyslipoproteinemia associated with diabetes or hypothyroidism in the dog results in endothelial injury. A variety of mechanisms, including oxygen free radical production, increase the decay of nitric oxide and decrease its vasodilator activity. The damaged endothelial cell allows lipoproteins to accumulate within the intima, where they are oxidized by free radicals generated by macrophages and endothelial cells. The oxidized products are directly toxic to endothelium and smooth muscle cells. Cellular debris is ingested by macrophages and smooth muscle cells, resulting in the formation of "foam cells." The lesion in dogs differs from that of human beings with respect to the location of lipid, which is abundant throughout the wall of the artery in contrast to human beings, who have lipid accumulation in the tunica intima. The chronic progression of atherosclerosis may result in narrowing of the lumen, ulceration and thrombosis, and hemorrhage or aneurysmal dilation.

Arterial Medial Calcification. Arterial medial calcification is a frequent lesion in animals that often have concurrent endocardial mineralization and involves both elastic and muscular arteries. The causes of arterial medial calcification include calcinogenic plant toxicosis, vitamin D toxicosis, renal insufficiency, and severe debilitation, as seen in cattle with Johne's disease (see Fig. 10-53). Medial calcification occurs spontaneously in horses, rabbits, aged guinea pigs, and in rats with chronic renal disease. Affected arteries, such as the aorta, have a unique gross appearance; they appear as solid, dense, pipelike structures with raised, white, solid intimal plaques (Fig. 10-67). Microscopically, in elastic arteries, prominent basophilic granular mineral deposits are present on elastic fibers of the media, but in muscular arteries, they can form a complete ring of mineralization in the tunica media (Fig. 10-68). Siderocalcinosis (so-called iron rings), the result of deposition of both iron and calcium salts, occurs in the cerebral arteries of aged horses. Lesions in the surrounding brain tissue are generally absent. Siderocalcinosis lesions are considered incidental.

Hyaline Degeneration, Fibrinoid Necrosis, and Amyloidosis. Hyaline degeneration, fibrinoid necrosis, and amyloidosis are vascular lesions of small muscular arteries and arterioles and occur

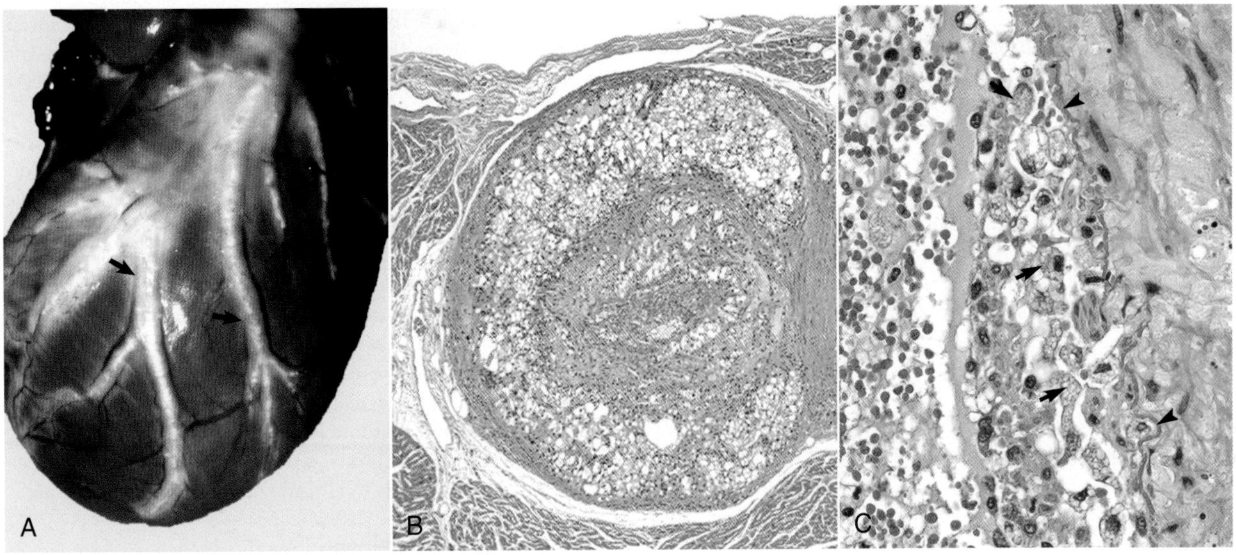

Figure 10-66 Coronary Atherosclerosis, Hypothyroidism, Heart, Left Ventricle, Dog. A, The affected coronary arteries are prominent and cordlike *(arrows)* with thickened walls. The diffuse and focal yellow areas in the walls of the arteries are the sites of atheromatous deposits. **B,** Note the extensive accumulation of lipid-laden (clear vacuoles) macrophages termed "foam cells" throughout the thickened tunica intima and media of this branch of the coronary artery. H&E stain. **C,** Higher magnification of **B.** The tunica intima contains abundant lipid-laden macrophages *(arrows)*. Note the disruption of the endothelium with fibrin on the exposed luminal surface. This condition is highly unstable and is prone to activation of Virchow's triad and the coagulation cascade with the formation of mural thrombi and infarction of myocardium supplied by this artery. The *arrowheads* identify the internal elastic lamina of the tunica intima. H&E stain. (**A** courtesy School of Veterinary Medicine, Purdue University. **B** and **C** courtesy College of Veterinary Medicine, University of Illinois.)

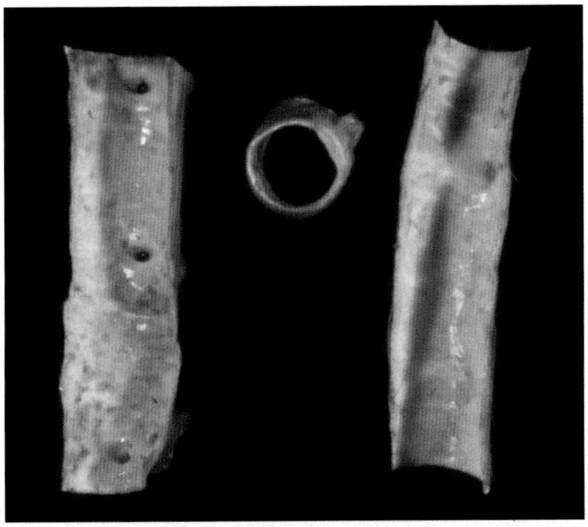

Figure 10-67 Calcification, Vitamin D Toxicosis, Aorta, Rabbit. The aorta is firm and inelastic because of the calcium deposits in the tunica intima and media. (Courtesy School of Veterinary Medicine, Purdue University.)

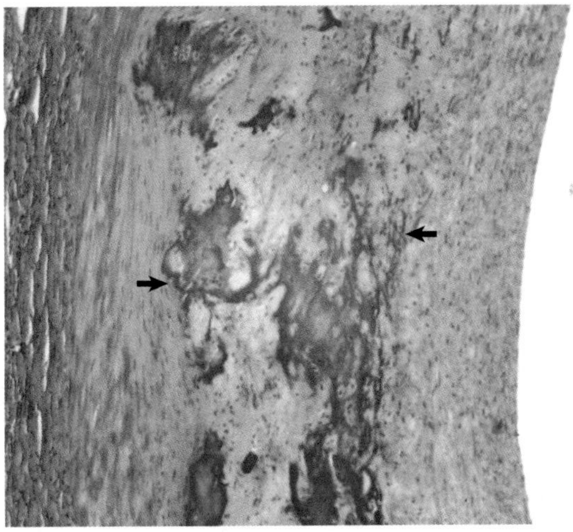

Figure 10-68 Medial Calcification, Aorta, Cow. Note the layer of mineralization *(between arrows)* in the middle of the tunica media. H&E stain. (Courtesy Dr. M.D. McGavin, College of Veterinary Medicine, University of Tennessee.)

in all animal species. These lesions are generally not detected grossly, but in some diseases with fibrinoid necrosis of vessels, hemorrhages and edema are seen in affected organs at necropsy. The microscopic feature shared by these lesions is the formation of a homogeneous eosinophilic zone in the vessel wall (Fig. 10-69; also see Fig. 10-78). Special stains allow differentiation into three types: (1) amyloid confirmed by Congo red and methyl violet; (2) fibrinoid deposits, positive by the periodic acid–Schiff technique; and (3) negative staining of hyaline deposits by these stains. Amyloidosis and hyaline degeneration are often observed in small muscular arteries of the myocardium, lungs, and spleen of old dogs. Lesions in the intramyocardial arteries can cause small foci of myocardial infarction.

Fibrinoid necrosis of arteries is associated with endothelial damage and is characterized by entry and accumulation of serum proteins followed by fibrin polymerization in the vessel wall. These materials form an intensely eosinophilic collar that obliterates cellular detail. This lesion is frequent in many acute degenerative and inflammatory diseases of small arteries and arterioles. Fibrinoid necrosis is seen frequently in dogs with uremia and in dogs with hypertension, although hypertension is an uncommon finding in animals.

Vitamin E–Selenium Deficiency. See the discussion on vitamin E–selenium deficiency in the section on Disorders of Pigs.

Inflammation

Omphalophlebitis ("Navel Ill"). Omphalophlebitis ("navel ill") is inflammation of the umbilical vein that often occurs in neonatal farm animals because of bacterial contamination of the umbilicus immediately after parturition. Bacteria from this site can cause septicemia, suppurative polyarthritis, hepatic abscesses (the umbilical vein drains into the liver), and umbilical abscesses.

Jugular Thrombophlebitis. Jugular thrombophlebitis may be associated with indwelling jugular catheters and is reported to be increased with several concurrent disease conditions, such as hypoproteinemia, salmonellosis, endotoxemia, and large intestinal disease (see Fig. 10-27). The most common diseases with thrombosis and embolism are listed in Box 10-16.

Lymphatic Vessels

Disturbances of Circulation

Effusions

Rupture of the Thoracic Duct. Rupture of the thoracic duct, either as a result of trauma or from spontaneous disruption, causes chylothorax in dogs and cats (see Fig. 9-116). However, many cases of chylothorax occur without injury to the thoracic duct and have been attributed to lesions that interfere with central venous return or produce obstruction of the thoracic duct (right-sided heart failure, neoplasms, granulomas, cranial vena cava thrombosis, or dirofilariasis) or that are idiopathic.

Lymphedema. Lymphedema specifically refers to accumulation of fluid in interstitial space secondary to abnormal lymphatic absorption and should be differentiated from other causes of edema, such as hypoproteinemia, vasculitis, and increased hydrostatic pressure. Lymphatic fluid contains a variable amount of protein that may have an osmotic pressure that allows fluid to be drawn into the interstitial compartment from tissues with a lower osmotic gradient (protein concentration). Lymphedema can be divided into six etiologic categories: overload, inadequate collection, abnormal lymphatic contractility, insufficient lymphatic vessels, lymph node obstruction, and structural defects in lymphatic vessels. Primary lymphedema is caused by aplasia, hypoplasia, or dysplasia of lymphatic ducts, vessels, and/or lymph nodes, whereas secondary lymphedema is an acquired defect due to various disease processes (e.g., neoplasia, radiation, parasites). Primary lymphedema is rare in both dogs and cats, but it is more common in dogs. It can be temporary or permanent, and it usually affects the distal extremities, mainly of the hindlimbs. Secondary lymphedema due to lymphatic filariasis in cats is common in tropical countries and is caused by *Brugia* spp., such as *Brugia malayi* and *Brugia pahangi*. Chronic lymphedema, regardless of its etiology, results in secondary fibrosis, which worsens edema and creates a vicious cycle that leads to chronic progressive lymphedema.

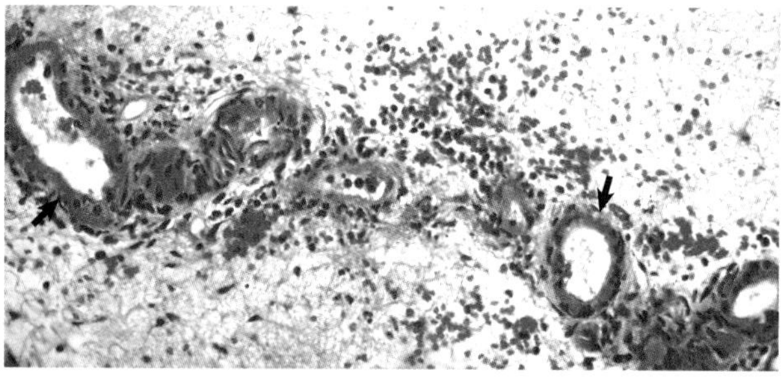

Figure 10-69 **Fibrinoid Necrosis of Small Arteries, Edema Disease, Stomach, Submucosa, Pig.** Note the circumferential eosinophilic (*arrows*) material in the walls of the arterioles and the extensive edema and mild hemorrhage in surrounding submucosa. H&E stain. (Courtesy School of Veterinary Medicine, Purdue University.)

Box 10-16 Most Common Diseases with Thrombosis and/or Embolism in Animals

- Pulmonary thromboembolism: Dogs, cats
- Aortic thromboembolism in cats and dogs with cardiomyopathy: "Saddle" thrombi
- Aortoiliac thrombosis in horses: Verminous or idiopathic
- Verminous arteritis in horses: *Strongylus vulgaris*
- Septic embolism from lesions of vegetative endocarditis
- Fibrocartilaginous emboli: Dogs
- Conditions accompanied by DIC (e.g., hog cholera, ICH, FIP, Gram-negative endotoxemia)
- Thrombosis of caudal vena cava: Cattle

DIC, Disseminated intravascular coagulation; *FIP*, feline infectious peritonitis; *ICH*, infectious canine hepatitis.

Disturbances of Growth. See the discussion on anomalies and dysplasia in the section on Disorders of Domestic Animals, Developmental Errors/Congenital Anomalies: Blood and Lymphatic Vascular Systems.

Neoplastic Transformation. Lymphangioma is a rare benign neoplasm composed of lymphatic channels. Lymphangiosarcoma, the malignant counterpart, occurs more often than the benign neoplasm. Vascular spaces formed by neoplastic lymphatic endothelial cells contain lymph rather than blood. Lymphatic vessels are frequently invaded by primary carcinomas and are a common route of metastasis (see the section on Disorders of Dogs).

Inflammation

Lymphangitis. Lymphangitis is a feature of many diseases (see Box 10-8). The affected vessels are often located in the distal limbs and are thick, cordlike structures (Fig. 10-70). Lymphedema

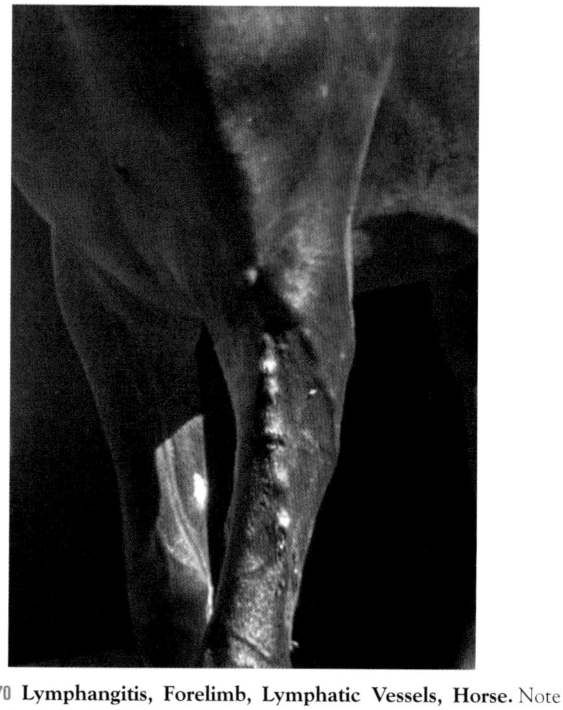

Figure 10-70 **Lymphangitis, Forelimb, Lymphatic Vessels, Horse.** Note the multiple swellings (cordlike) of the afferent lymphatic vessels in the skin. These lymphatic vessels lie in the subcutis and empty into the caudal superficial cervical (prescapular) lymph node. (Courtesy School of Veterinary Medicine, Purdue University.)

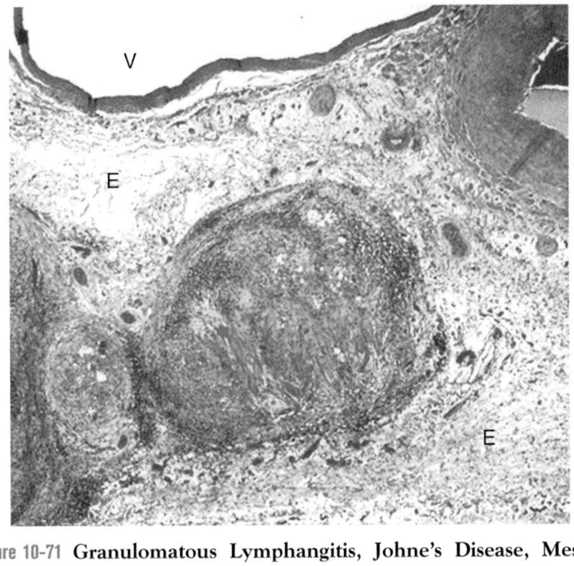

Figure 10-71 **Granulomatous Lymphangitis, Johne's Disease, Mesenteric Lymphatic Vessel, Sheep.** The lymphatic is occluded by a fibrinous thrombus secondary to the destruction of the endothelium by inflammatory cells including macrophages. Early proliferating fibrous tissue and extensive edema *(E)* surround the lymphatic vessel. The adjacent artery *(upper right)* and vein *(V)* are unaffected. H&E stain. (Courtesy School of Veterinary Medicine, Purdue University.)

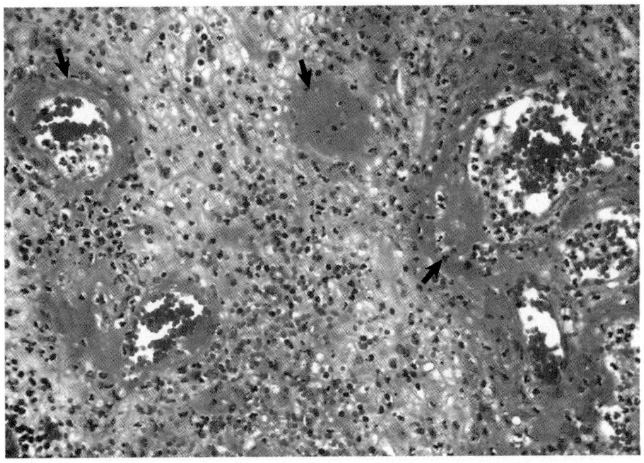

Figure 10-72 **Acute Arteritis, Equine Viral Arteritis, Small Intestine, Submucosa, Horse.** Small arteries have fibrinoid degeneration (circumferential eosinophilic material *[arrows]*) with leukocytic infiltration of the tunica media. The surrounding loose connective tissue is edematous and infiltrated by numerous leukocytes. H&E stain. (Courtesy School of Veterinary Medicine, Purdue University.)

can be present. Nodular suppurative lesions of lymphangitis often ulcerate and discharge pus onto the surface of the skin. In Johne's disease, the mesenteric lymphatic vessels are often prominent because of granulomatous lymphangitis, an extension of the enteric infection producing a granulomatous enteritis and lymphangitis (Fig. 10-71).

Disorders of Horses

Myocardium

Cell Degeneration and Death: Toxicoses

White Snakeroot–Induced Myocardial Degeneration. After ingestion, white snakeroot (*Eupatorium rugosum*) causes myocardial degeneration and necrosis (acute injury) followed by fibrosis (reparative response). Tremetol is the toxic compound in white snakeroot; it becomes toxic after microsomal activation of a precursor compound by cytochrome P450 enzymes in the liver. The mechanism used by tremetol to cause injury is unclear, but dysfunction of mitochondrial oxidative phosphorylation by inhibiting the tricarboxylic acid cycle has been suggested. Acute cardiac rhabdomyocyte degeneration and necrosis are discussed in detail in the section on Responses to Injury: Myocardium, Myocardial Necrosis and also in Chapter 15. Reparative responses are discussed in Chapter 3. Macroscopic lesions include pale white to tan areas and linear streaks throughout the myocardium; microscopic lesions include multifocal myocardial degeneration and necrosis with vacuolation of myocardial cytoplasm; loss of cross-striations; fragmentation of rhabdomyocytes; hypereosinophilia, coagulation, and clumping of the sarcoplasm; and nuclear pyknosis and karyolysis. The pericardium may contain a modified transudate with fibrin.

Ionophore-Induced Myocardial Degeneration. See the discussion on ionophore-induced myocardial degeneration in the section on Disorders of Domestic Animals.

Pericardium and Epicardium

Inflammation

Fibrinous Pericarditis. Hematogenous spread of specific organisms may result in fibrinous pericarditis in the horse. These include *Actinobacillus*, streptococcal, and mycoplasma infections. Sterile swabs of the pericardial exudates are recommended to identify the causative organism. Equine herpesvirus types 1 and 2 and influenza virus infections may result in fibrinous pericarditis. Fibrinous pericarditis has been reported in horses with mare reproductive loss syndrome following exposure to the Eastern tent caterpillars.

Blood and Lymphatic Vascular Systems

Blood Vessels

Inflammation

Equine Viral Arteritis. Equine viral arteritis is a systemic viral infection with a tropism for vascular endothelial cells. In this disease, affected small muscular arteries have lesions of fibrinoid necrosis, extensive edema, and primarily mononuclear infiltration with thrombosis (Fig. 10-72). Grossly, the vascular injury is reflected by hemorrhage and severe edema of the subcutaneous tissues, lymph nodes, and intestinal wall and mesentery accompanied by notable accumulation of serous fluids in body cavities and pulmonary edema.

African Horse Sickness: Subacute Cardiac Form. African horse sickness is an insect-borne (*Culicoides* spp.) viral disease of *Equidae* that is endemic in Africa, the Middle East, India, and Spain. The occurrence is seasonal because the insect vectors thrive in hot, wet conditions. The febrile disease may produce high mortality (up to 95%) and appears in several clinical forms, including the subacute cardiac form described here, as well as an acute respiratory form with massive pulmonary edema. The pathogenesis is initiated by the introduction of the virus by bites of the insect vector. The virus proliferates in local lymph node, and viremia ensues. The virus has a tropism for endothelial cells, monocytes, and macrophages, and increased vascular permeability, edema, hemorrhage, and microthrombosis are produced. The gross lesions are extensive subcutaneous and intermuscular edematous swelling of the head and neck. Massive hydropericardium is present with accompanying epicardial and endocardial ecchymotic hemorrhages. Histopathologically, endothelial degeneration and necrosis occur with the edema. In the myocardium, hemorrhage, edema, and focal myocardial necrosis with inflammatory cell infiltrates are present (see Chapter 4 and Fig. 4-40).

Cranial Mesenteric Arteritis and Thrombosis. Cranial mesenteric arteritis and thrombosis results from fourth-stage larval migration from *Strongylus vulgaris* (Fig. 10-73). Infection of horses by *Strongylus vulgaris* is now less common because of widespread use of highly efficacious antiparasitic drugs. During its larval development, the parasite migrates through the intestinal arteries, and the most severe lesions are generally found in the cranial mesenteric artery near its origin. The affected vessel is enlarged, and its wall is firm and fibrotic. The intimal surface often has an adhering thrombus often admixed with larvae. Microscopically, the affected vessel has extensive infiltration of inflammatory cells and proliferation of fibroblasts throughout the wall. As a consequence, thromboembolism of the intestinal arteries frequently occurs and can produce colic, but the abundant collateral circulation to the equine intestinal tract makes intestinal infarction an unusual event.

Aortoiliac Thrombosis. Aortoiliac thrombosis is characterized by extensive and progressive thrombosis thought to be caused by migration of fourth-stage larval migration from *Strongylus vulgaris*. Aortoiliac thrombosis results in posterior weakness following exercise with recovery following rest. See the previous section on cranial mesenteric arteritis and thrombosis.

Jugular Thrombophlebitis. See the discussion on jugular thrombophlebitis in the section on Disorders of Domestic Animals: Blood and Lymphatic Vessels, Blood Vessels, Inflammation.

Cell Degeneration and Death

Arterial Intimal Calcification. Arterial intimal calcifications (intimal bodies) are distinctively small, mineralized masses within the subendothelium in small muscular arteries and arterioles of horses (E-Fig. 10-24). They have no deleterious effect.

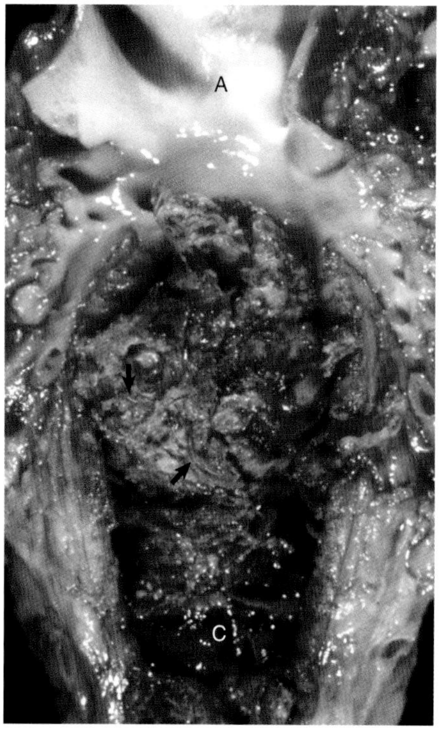

Figure 10-73 **Verminous Arteritis and Mural Thrombosis, Strongylosis, Abdominal Aorta *(A)* and Cranial Mesenteric Artery, Horse.** A pale friable thrombotic mass, in which several *Strongylus vulgaris* larvae *(arrows)* are embedded, is attached to the wall of the cranial mesenteric artery (C). (Courtesy College of Veterinary Medicine, University of Illinois.)

Lymphatic Vessels

Inflammation

Glanders Disease (Farcy): Cutaneous Form. Glanders disease (Farcy) is a contagious disease of horses, donkeys, and mules caused by infection with *Burkholderia (Pseudomonas) mallei*. Once worldwide in distribution, it is now seen in eastern Europe, Asia, and northern Africa. The disease occurs in several clinical forms, and the cutaneous form with involvement of lymphatic vessels is described here. The pathogenesis is initiated by ingestion of contaminated food and water. The organisms enter through the pharynx and are disseminated to the skin hematogenously. The gross lesions of the skin appear as multiple ulcerated nodules that follow infected lymphatic vessels. Most frequent in the limbs, the ulcerated lesions discharge suppurative exudate onto the skin surface. Swollen tortuous cutaneous lymphatic vessels are visible between the ulcerative lesions. Microscopically, the skin nodules represent pyogranulomatous inflammation extending from cutaneous lymphatic vessels with suppurative lymphangitis (see Fig. 4-25).

Miscellaneous Cutaneous Lymphangitides. The cutaneous lesions affecting lymphatic vessels in less common cutaneous lymphangitides are as follows (see Box 10-8):

1. Ulcerative (likely caused by *Corynebacterium pseudotuberculosis* and other cutaneous bacteria)
2. Sporadic (cause unknown)
3. Epizootic lymphangitis (*Histoplasma farciminosum*)
4. Melioidosis (*Burkholderia pseudomallei*)

These lesions mimic those of Glanders disease, and differentiation occurs by impression smears and microbiologic cultures and analyses. The skin of the legs, head, neck, and/or flanks has raised firm nodules (≈1 to 2 cm in diameter), draining nodules, and draining fistulous tracts, often arranged in linear bands (beaded appearance) that follow the flow of lymphatic vessels. These lesions contain or drain pus, which is often thick and white-yellow in color. Microscopically, lesions are characterized by suppurative to pyogranulomatous inflammation. Infectious microorganisms are often present in the exudate (see Fig. 4-25).

Chronic Progressive Lymphedema in Draft Horses. Chronic progressive lymphedema (CPL) occurs in many draft horse breeds and is a debilitating condition. A definitive cause is not known; however, a genetic disorder of elastin metabolism resulting in dysfunction of the lymphatic vessels in the distal extremities with multiple contributing factors including secondary bacterial infections is suspected. The distal limbs are swollen with pitting edema, thickened, scaling skin with exudation, erosions, and ulcerations. Microscopically, dermal lymphatic vessels are markedly dilated within the edematous dermis. In chronic cases, the dermis may become markedly thickened with fibrous connective tissue as a result of the chronic edema. The overlying epidermis may be acanthotic with intraepidermal pustules, erosions, and ulcerations. Folliculitis and deep dermal abscesses may be present. Staining for elastin fibers demonstrates a disorganized and excessive network of elastin fibers within the superficial dermis. Lymphatic vessels within the deep dermis lack normal elastin fibers.

Disorders of Ruminants (Cattle, Sheep, and Goats)

Myocardium

Disturbances of Growth

Dilated Cardiomyopathy. See the discussion on cardiomyopathies in the section on Disorders of Domestic Animals: Myocardium, Disturbances of Growth, Hypertrophy and Atrophy.

Lymphoma (Lymphosarcoma). See the discussion on neoplastic transformation in the section on Disorders of Domestic Animals: Myocardium, Disturbances of Growth.

Inflammation

Blackleg Myocarditis. Hemorrhagic myocarditis occurs together with the hemorrhagic inflammation typically found in skeletal muscle of cattle with blackleg (*Clostridium chauvoei*) (Fig. 10-74). See the discussion on myocarditis in the section on Responses to Injury: Myocardium, Inflammation; sections on disorders of individual animal species; and also Chapter 15.

East Coast Fever (*Theileria parva*). East Coast fever is a tick-transmitted protozoal disease of cattle, sheep, and goats in Africa caused by *Theileria parva*, which causes myocardial necrosis and inflammation (E-Fig. 10-25).

Foot-and-Mouth Disease. Foot-and-mouth disease can cause myocarditis in young lambs and piglets. Focal myocardial necrosis and apoptosis with infiltration of mononuclear inflammatory cells are scattered throughout the myocardium. Myocarditis may precede the typical vesicular lesions (see Chapters 4, 7, and 9).

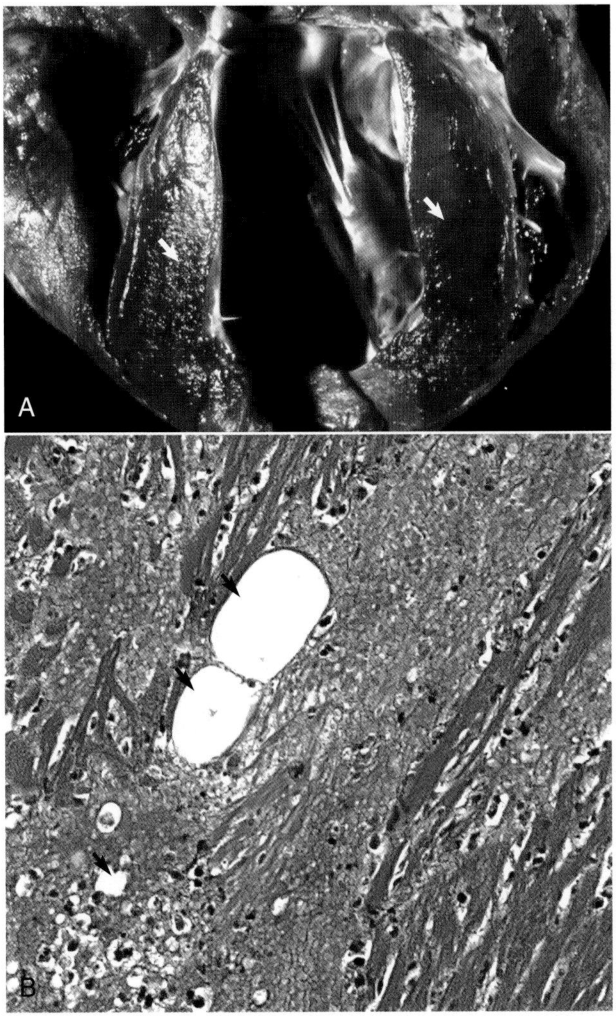

Figure 10-74 **Necrohemorrhagic Myocarditis, "Blackleg," Heart, Steer. A,** Note the area of hemorrhagic myocarditis (*arrows*) in the wall of the ventricular myocardium. This disease is caused by *Clostridium chauvoei*, and lesions are most common in skeletal muscle. **B,** Necrohemorrhagic myocarditis, heart, cow. Note the myocardial necrosis, serocellular interstitial debris, and the clear spaces (*arrows*) representative of gas bubbles. (**A** courtesy Dr. J. Simon, College of Veterinary Medicine, University of Illinois. **B** courtesy Atlantic Veterinary College, University of Prince Edward Island.)

Eosinophilic Myocarditis. Eosinophilic myocarditis and the accumulation of eosinophils in the inflammatory response are the result of some parasitic infections such as sarcocystosis (see Chapter 15).

Cell Degeneration and Death: Toxicoses

Gossypol-Induced Myocardial Degeneration. See the discussion on gossypol-induced myocardial degeneration in Disorders of Domestic Animals: Myocardium, Cell Degeneration and Death, Toxicoses.

Excess Vitamin D and Calcinogenic Plants. See the discussion on mineralization in the section on Disorders of Domestic Animals: Endocardium and Heart Valves, Cell Degeneration and Death, Endocardial Mineralization; in others sections of this chapter; and also Chapters 1 and 15.

Endocardium and Heart Valves

Disturbances of Growth

Valvular Hematomas. Valvular hematomas (hematocysts, valvular telangiectasia) frequently are observed on the AV valves of postnatal ruminants (see Fig. 10-51, *A*). These lesions, which may regress spontaneously by the time the animals are several months of age, do not produce any functional abnormalities. Lesions are bulging, blood-filled cysts, several millimeters in diameter, on the AV valves.

Valvular Lymphocysts. Valvular lymphocysts may also occur and appear as yellow serum-filled cysts on the AV valve cusps (see Fig. 10-51, *B*).

Inflammation

Vegetative Valvular Endocarditis. Endocarditis is usually the result of bacterial infections in which the affected valves have large, adhering, friable, yellow-to-gray masses of fibrin termed *vegetations*, which can largely occlude the valvular orifice (see Fig. 10-54, *A*). Microscopically, the lesion consists of accumulated layers of fibrin and numerous embedded bacterial colonies underlain by a zone of infiltrated leukocytes and granulation tissue (see Fig. 10-54, *B*). See the discussion on vegetative valvular and mural endocarditis in the section on Disorders of Domestic Animals: Endocardium and Heart Valves, Inflammation, and also Chapter 3.

Cell Degeneration and Death

Endocardial Mineralization See the discussion on mineralization in the section on Disorders of Domestic Animals: Endocardium and Heart Valves, Cell Degeneration and Death, Endocardial Mineralization; in others sections of this chapter; and also Chapters 1 and 15.

Pericardium and Epicardium

Inflammation

Fibrinous Pericarditis. Hematogenous spread of specific organisms may result in fibrinous pericarditis. Mannheimiosis, blackleg, coliform septicemias, contagious bovine pleuropneumonia, sporadic bovine encephalomyelitis, and in utero *Brucella* spp. and *Arcanobacter pyogenesis* fetal septicemias may all produce fibrinous pericarditis. In sheep, Mannheimiosis and streptococcal infections most commonly result in fibrinous pericarditis. In goats, *Mycoplasma* *mycoides subspecies mycoides* produces a fibrinous pericarditis. Sterile swabs of the pericardial exudates are recommended to identify the causative organism. See the discussion on pericarditis in Disorders of Domestic Animals: Pericardium and Epicardium, Inflammation and also Chapters 7 and 9.

Suppurative Pericarditis (Traumatic Reticulopericarditis). Suppurative pericarditis is seen mainly in cattle as a complication of traumatic reticuloperitonitis ("hardware disease"). Foreign bodies, such as nails or pieces of wire that accumulate in the reticulum, occasionally penetrate the reticular wall and diaphragm, enter the adjacent pericardial sac, and introduce infection. Some affected cattle survive for weeks to months until death ensues from congestive heart failure and septicemia. Grossly, the pericardial surfaces are notably thickened by white, often rough, shaggy-appearing masses of fibrous connective tissue that enclose an accumulation of white to gray, thick, foul-smelling, purulent exudate (see Fig. 10-62). See the discussion on pericarditis in the section on Epicardium and Pericardium, Disorders of Domestic Animals, and also Chapters 7 and 9.

Blood and Lymphatic Vascular Systems

Blood Vessels

Inflammation: Infectious Diseases

Thrombotic Meningoencephalitis. *Histophilus somni* (formerly *Haemophilus somnus*) causes a systemic vasculitis in cattle resulting in meningoencephalitis. Mural thrombi from local vascular injury rather than thromboemboli from distal sites of vascular injury, such as the lungs, are the major type of thrombus in this disease. Gross lesions in the central nervous system (CNS) are characteristic of infarcts (see Fig. 14-89, *A*). Microscopic lesions are initially vasculitis and vascular necrosis, which are followed by thrombosis and infarction (see Fig. 14-89, *B*). Septic vasculitis, the initial event, is followed by edema and an influx of neutrophils and macrophages in and around vessel walls and adjacent parenchyma. Colonies of small Gram-negative bacilli are frequent in thrombi, in and around affected vessels, and in areas of necrosis. *Histophilus somni* can also cause a necrotizing myocarditis, frequently in the left ventricular papillary myocardium.

Thrombosis of the Caudal Vena Cava. Thrombosis of the caudal vena cava occurs in association with rupture of hepatic abscesses into either the hepatic vein or the caudal vena cava. The hepatic abscess inflammation extends into the adjacent large hepatic veins and results in formation of a septic thrombus in the caudal vena cava. Rupture and release of the contents of the abscess into the lumen can cause multiple septic emboli in the pulmonary capillaries and unexpected death of the affected animal, often preceded by severe hemoptysis.

Foreign Parasitic Diseases. Foreign parasitic diseases important in tropical regions of the world are characterized by the presence of parasites in the lumens of veins. These diseases in cattle and water buffalo include schistosomiasis (blood fluke infection—*Schistosoma* spp.) in which adult parasites are present in the mesenteric and portal veins, and the resulting phlebitis is characterized by intimal proliferation and thrombosis.

Omphalophlebitis ("Navel Ill"). See the discussion on omphalophlebitis ("navel ill") in the section on Disorders of Domestic Animals: Blood and Lymphatic Vascular Systems, Blood Vessels, Inflammation, and also Chapter 8.

Johne's Disease. Lesions of Johne's disease affecting blood and lymphatic vessels and characterized by intimal mineralization and granulomatous lymphangitis, respectively, are discussed in greater detail in Chapters 4, 7, and 13.

Anthrax. Anthrax in herbivores often occurs as an acute febrile highly fatal septicemic disease. Although global in distribution, the disease is enzootic in certain areas. The etiology is *Bacillus anthracis*, a large rod-shaped spore-forming bacterium. The pathogenesis of the disease in affected herbivores is exposure by ingestion of contaminated food (especially bone meal) and water. The organisms produce a variety of lethal toxins that provoke local edema and tissue necrosis and increased vascular permeability associated with lymphangitis and lymphadenitis. Herbivores that die from septicemic anthrax have dark, thick unclotted blood oozing from body orifices. These cases should NOT be subjected to necropsy to avoid massive contamination of the environment by the spores of the organism. Instead, a blood smear should be collected and examined for the presence of the diagnostic bacilli. If a case is necropsied by mistake, the diagnostic findings are massive splenomegaly (so-called blackberry jam spleen), disseminated serosal hemorrhages, and swollen edematous lymph nodes. Microscopic findings (histopathologic evaluation is NOT recommended) include massive numbers of typical large rod-shaped organisms in the blood, congestion, hemorrhage, lymphangitis, and lymphadenitis (see Chapter 4, Fig. 4-23; Chapter 7, Fig. 7-135; and Chapter 13, Fig. 13-57).

Neospora caninum. See the discussion on *Neospora caninum* in Chapter 4.

Malignant Catarrhal Fever. See the discussion on malignant catarrhal fever in Chapter 4.

Bovine Virus Diarrhea. See the discussion on bovine virus diarrhea in Chapters 4 and 7.

Bluetongue. See the discussion on bluetongue in Chapters 4 and 7.

Disorders of Pigs

Myocardium

Cell Degeneration and Death

Mulberry Heart Disease. See the discussion on mulberry heart disease in the next section on Blood and Lymphatic Vascular Systems, Blood Vessels, Cell Degeneration and Death, Dietary Microangiopathy: Mulberry Heart Disease.

Inflammation: Infectious Diseases

Viral Myocarditis

Encephalomyocarditis. Encephalomyocarditis virus is a cardiovirus of the Picornaviridae. The type B strain can affect several species including human beings, but pigs are most often affected. Pigs of any age can be affected. Gross lesions can include multifocal areas of pallor. Multifocal areas of myocardial necrosis with infiltrations of mononuclear inflammatory cells are observed microscopically. Other viruses that can cause myocarditis in pigs include porcine parvovirus and porcine circovirus 2 associated with postweaning multisystemic wasting syndrome.

Endocardium and Heart Valves

Inflammation

Endocarditis. Endocarditis is commonly found in pigs and results from a bacterial septicemia. The most commonly isolated organisms are *Streptococcus* spp. and *Erysipelothrix rhusiopathiae*. Confirmation of the definitive organism requires bacterial isolation. Affected valves have large, adhering, friable, yellow-to-gray masses of fibrin termed *vegetations*, which can largely occlude the valvular orifice (see Fig. 10-54). Microscopically, the lesion consists of accumulated layers of fibrin and numerous embedded bacterial colonies underlain by a zone of infiltrated leukocytes and granulation tissue (see Fig. 10-54, *B*). See the discussion on valvular and mural endocarditis in the section on Inflammation; Disorders of Domestic Animals: Endocardium and Heart Valves, and also Chapter 3.

Pericardium and Epicardium

Inflammation: Infectious Diseases

Fibrinous Pericarditis. Fibrinous pericarditis may accompany Glasser's disease (*Haemophilus parasuis*) (Fig. 10-75), streptococcal infections, enzootic mycoplasma pneumonia, and salmonellosis. Sterile swabs of the pericardial exudates are recommended to identify the causative organism. See the discussion of pericarditis in the section on Disorders of Domestic Animals: Pericardium and Epicardium, Inflammation, and also Chapters 3, 7, and 9.

Porcine Polyserositis (Glasser's Disease, *Streptococcus suis* II). See Fig. 10-75; also see the discussion of edema disease in the next section and in Chapters 4 and 7.

Blood and Lymphatic Vascular Systems

Blood Vessels

Cell Degeneration and Death

Dietary Microangiopathy: Mulberry Heart Disease. Dietary microangiopathy of pigs or "mulberry heart disease" is produced by a deficiency of vitamin E and/or selenium and the resultant effect on the microvasculature, which is characterized by fibrinoid necrosis, and thromboses of small vessels resulting in microhemorrhages. The hemorrhage results in major discoloration of the epicardial surface of the heart, particularly the right atrium said to resemble a mulberry (Figs. 10-76 and 10-77). In addition to the epicardial hemorrhages, hydropericardium often ensues. Massive hemorrhagic hepatic necrosis (hepatosis dietetica) is also produced with vitamin E and/or selenium deficiency (see Fig. 8-74). With either form of the disease, fibrinoid necrosis of small muscular arteries and arterioles is widespread and is accompanied by endothelial damage and fibrin thrombi in capillaries, especially capillaries of the myocardium (Fig. 10-78; E-Fig. 10-26). This complex of vascular lesions has been termed *dietary microangiopathy*.

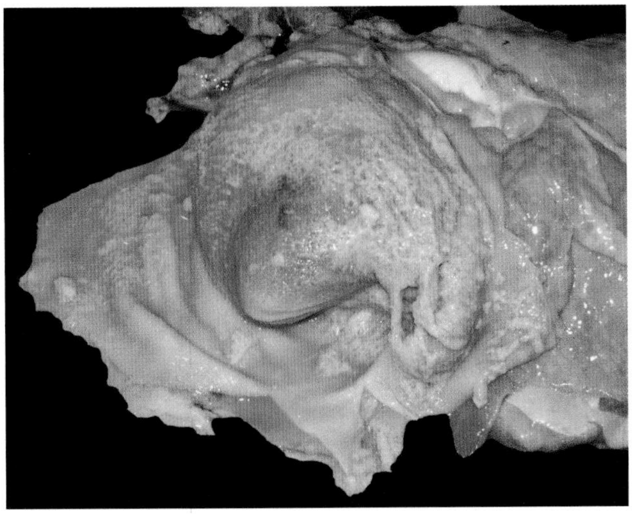

Figure 10-75 Fibrinous Porcine Polyserositis, Glasser's Disease, Pericardium and Epicardium (Pericardial Cavity), Pig. A fibrinous pericarditis is typical of Glasser's disease (*Haemophilus parasuis*). Streptococcal infections, enzootic mycoplasma pneumonia, and salmonellosis can also cause this lesion. (Courtesy Dr. D. Driemeier, Federal University of Rio Grande do Sul, Brazil.)

Fibrinoid Necrosis of Blood Vessels. Fibrinoid necrosis of arteries and veins (see Fig. 10-69) is particularly frequent in pigs and is an important diagnostic feature in cases of vitamin E–selenium deficiency (heart), edema disease (gastric submucosa), cerebrospinal angiopathy, porcine circovirus II vasculopathy, and organic mercury toxicosis (meninges). See the previous section on Dietary Microangiopathy: Mulberry Heart Disease.

Inflammation: Infectious Diseases

Edema Disease (Cerebrospinal Angiopathy). Infections with certain strains of hemolytic *E. coli* produce a cytotoxin that targets vascular endothelium, resulting in fibrinoid necrosis of arterioles and resultant edema. Lesions are often prominent in the arterioles of the gastric submucosa (Fig. 10-79). Vascular changes occurring in the

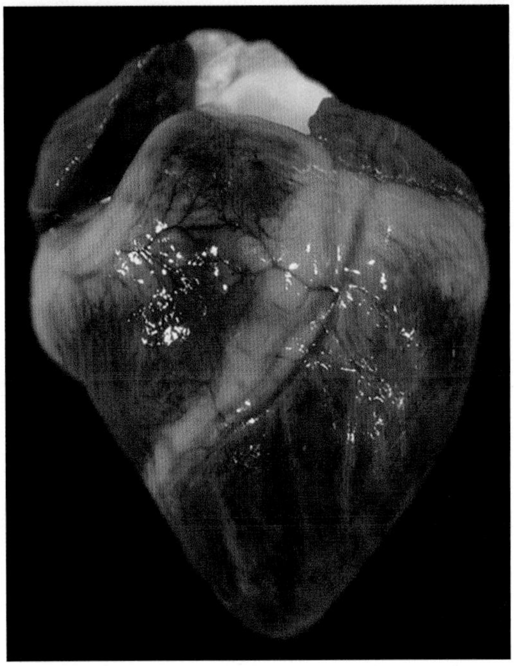

Figure 10-76 "Mulberry Heart Disease," Suffusive Hemorrhage, Epicardium, Right Ventricle, Heart, Pig. Red areas of suffusive hemorrhage ("mulberry-like") are present on the epicardial surface of the right ventricle. (Courtesy Dr. L. Miller, Atlantic Veterinary College.)

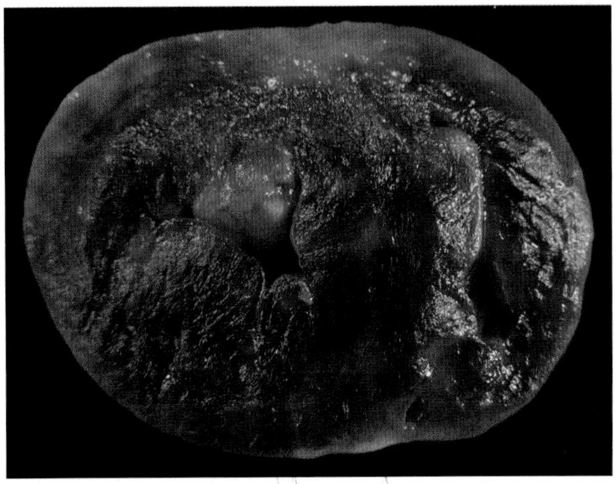

Figure 10-77 "Mulberry Heart Disease," Hemorrhage and Necrosis, Left and Right Ventricular Myocardium, Transverse Section, Pig. Red and pale mottled areas are caused by hemorrhage and necrosis, respectively. (Courtesy Dr. L. Miller, Atlantic Veterinary College.)

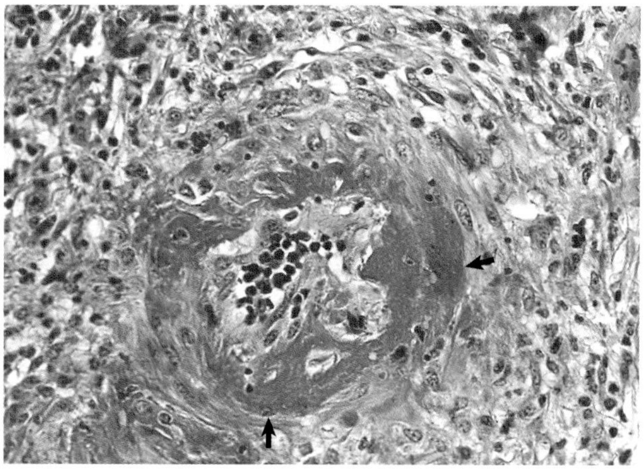

Figure 10-78 **Vitamin E–Selenium Deficiency ("Mulberry Heart Disease"), Fibrinoid Necrosis, Myocardial Arteriole, Heart, Pig.** Note the circumferential eosinophilic deposits *(arrows)* in the wall of the arteriole. H&E stain. (Courtesy Dr. J. Simon, College of Veterinary Medicine, University of Illinois.)

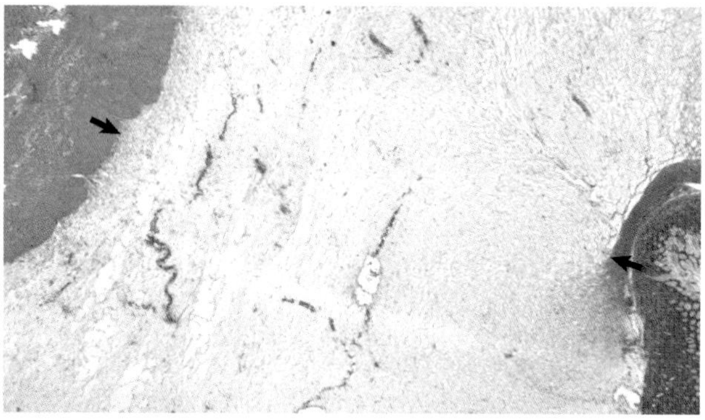

Figure 10-79 **Submucosal Edema, Edema Disease, Stomach, Submucosa, Pig.** The submucosa *(between arrows)* is distended with edema fluid. H&E stain. (Courtesy School of Veterinary Medicine, Purdue University.)

CNS are known as cerebrospinal angiopathy and can produce clinical signs of disease of the nervous system (E-Fig. 10-27; also see Fig. 10-69; Chapters 4, 7, and 11; and Figs. 7-169 and 7-170).

Erysipelosis (Erysipelothrix rhusiopathiae). Cutaneous lesions in erysipelosis are caused by *Erysipelothrix rhusiopathiae* and are the result of bacterial embolization to the skin during sepsis. Lesions consist of square to rhomboidal, firm, raised, pink to dark purple areas (Fig. 10-80; see Fig. 17-70) caused by vasculitis, thrombosis, and ischemia (infarction). The rhomboidal shape likely represents an area of skin supplied by a thrombosed vessel (see Chapter 17).

Porcine Polyserositis (Streptococcus suis II). *Streptococcus suis* II is one of several bacteria that can cause the disease porcine polyserositis. Gross lesions include vasculitis leading to variable quantities of a gray-white friable material (fibrin) on serosal surfaces (fibrinous polyserositis) of the lungs (fibrinous pleuritis), heart (fibrinous pericarditis [see Fig. 10-75]), and abdominal cavity (fibrinous peritonitis). The bacterium gains access to and spreads systemically through the blood vascular system. Lesions suggest this bacterium may have a tropism for vascular endothelial cells of serosae, and bacterial endotoxins may contribute to vascular injury and permeability changes leading to the leakage of fibrinogen and its polymerization to fibrin on serosal surfaces and in some cases to microthrombus formation and disseminated intravascular coagulation (DIC) in other organ systems (see Chapters 4, 7, and 9).

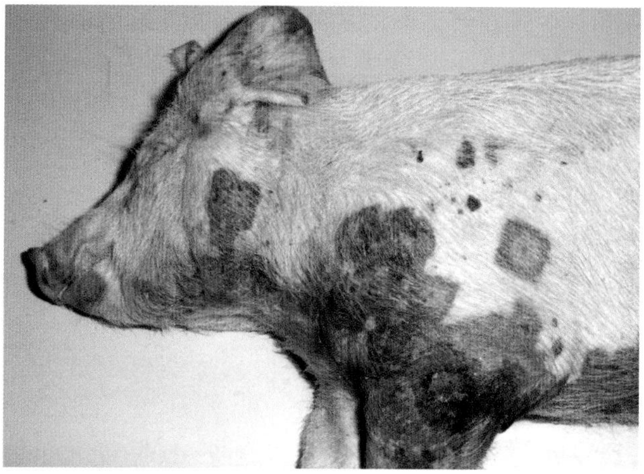

Figure 10-80 **Cutaneous Infarcts, Diamond Skin Disease, *Erysipelothrix Rhusiopathiae* Septicemia, Skin, Pig.** Emboli of *Erysipelothrix rhusiopathiae* have lodged in cutaneous vessels and caused a localized vasculitis, which has resulted in thrombosis followed by ischemia and cutaneous infarction. (Courtesy Dr. M.D. McGavin, College of Veterinary Medicine, University of Tennessee.)

African Swine Fever (Wart Hog Disease, African Pig Disease). African swine fever is a highly contagious febrile hemorrhagic disease of pigs associated with a DNA virus. The clinical and pathologic features are very similar to those of classic swine fever (hog cholera). The disease is enzootic in Africa, and outbreaks have occurred in Europe, South America, and the Caribbean region. The pathogenesis of the disease is via entry in the upper respiratory tract. The virus proliferates in the tonsils and lymph nodes of the head and neck with subsequent viremia and dissemination to the entire body. Transmission to domestic swine is via ingestion of infected tissues of warthogs and bush pigs, which develop an unapparent infection, or by the bite of infected soft ticks (*Ornithodoros moubata*). The distinctive hemorrhagic lesions are attributed to disruption of the clotting mechanism and thrombocytopenia. The gross lesions are characterized by widespread congestion, edema, and hemorrhage. Hemorrhagic visceral lymph nodes and splenomegaly are present along with petechial hemorrhages of the renal cortices, epicardium, and other serosal surfaces. Pulmonary edema and hydrothorax also occur. Microscopically, viral-induced vascular alterations include congestion, hemorrhage, and edema with fibrin microthrombi (E-Fig. 10-28). The virus produces widespread necrosis of lymphocytes and macrophages (see Fig. 4-42).

Hog Cholera/Classic Swine Fever (Swine Fever, Swine Plague, Schweinpest). Hog cholera (also termed *classic swine fever*) is a highly contagious febrile hemorrhagic disease of swine produced by an RNA virus. The disease is enzootic in South America, Central America, Caribbean countries, Asia, and Europe. The pathogenesis of the disease is initiated by inhalation of the virus from direct contact with infected pigs or by ingestion of uncooked infected pork. The virus traverses the oral mucosa, replicates in the tonsils, and initiates viremia. The virus selectively damages endothelial cells, cells of the immune system (lymphoreticular cells and macrophages), and epithelial cells. The characteristic hemorrhagic lesions are associated with increased vascular permeability, thrombocytopenia, and DIC. The gross lesions are characterized by widespread petechial hemorrhages, especially of the renal cortices, urinary bladder, larynx, gastric mucosa, and epicardium with accompanying hemorrhage in lymph nodes and skin. A distinctive finding is hemorrhagic infarction of the spleen and "button ulcers" of the colonic mucosa.

Microscopically, endothelial damage is evident as hydropic degeneration and cellular proliferation. Affected vessels may have fibrinoid necrosis with fibrin deposition in the media and intima. Circulatory alterations include congestion, hemorrhage, thrombosis, and infarction. The brain has a diffuse nonsuppurative encephalitis (see Fig. 4-41).

Porcine Anthrax. See the discussion on anthrax in the section on Disorders of Ruminants (Cattle, Sheep, and Goats), Blood and Lymphatic Vascular Systems, Blood Vessels, and also Chapter 4.

Disorders of Dogs

Myocardium

Disturbances of Growth

Developmental Errors: Congenital Anomalies. See the discussion on anomalies and dysplasia in the section on Disorders of Domestic Animals, Developmental Errors/Congenital Anomalies.

Cardiomyopathies. Also see the discussion on cardiomyopathies in the section on Disorders of Domestic Animals, Disorders of Domestic Animals: Myocardium, Disturbances of Growth, Hypertrophy and Atrophy.

Dilated (Congestive) Cardiomyopathy. Dilated or congestive cardiomyopathy is an important cause of congestive heart failure in dogs. Some affected dogs have low tissue concentrations of taurine, but supplementation has not proved beneficial. Affected dogs often are males of large breeds, such as Doberman pinschers, Portuguese water dogs, Dalmatians, Scottish deerhounds, Irish wolfhounds, Saint Bernards, Afghan hounds, Newfoundland dogs, Old English sheepdogs, Great Danes, and boxers, although smaller breeds, such as English cocker spaniels, may be affected. The disease often has a familial pattern in the affected breeds and appears to be inherited as an autosomal recessive or X-linked recessive trait. At necropsy, lesions of congestive heart failure are present and the hearts are rounded because of biventricular dilation (see Figs. 10-43 and 10-44). The dilated cardiac chambers often have a diffusely white, thickened endocardium. Microscopic and ultrastructural alterations are nonspecific, can be either mild or absent, and may include interstitial fibrosis and fatty infiltration and changes of myocyte degeneration, including the occurrence of so-called attenuated wavy fibers. See the discussion on cardiomyopathies in the section on Disorders of Domestic Animals, Disorders of Domestic Animals: Myocardium, Disturbances of Growth, Hypertrophy and Atrophy.

Cardiac Neoplasms. Cardiac neoplasms comprise primary and secondary (metastatic) tumors. Primary cardiac tumors include hemangiosarcoma (most frequent), thyroid/parathyroid ectopic carcinomas, mesotheliomas, thymomas, granular cell tumor, sarcomas (osteosarcomas, chondrosarcomas, fibrosarcomas/fibromas, rhabdomyosarcomas/rhabdomyoma, neurofibrosarcomas/neurofibroma, and malignant mixed mesenchymal tumor), and chemodectomas (heart-base tumors). Secondary cardiac neoplasms are metastases from distant, primary tumor sites. In a study that included 80 dogs with primary and/or secondary cardiac neoplasms, 36% of dogs had evidence of cardiac metastases.

Inflammation: Infectious Diseases

Canine Parvovirus Myocarditis. Lymphocytic myocarditis is usually a lesion of viral infections and is well illustrated by the lesions of parvoviral myocarditis of puppies. Dogs with parvoviral myocarditis die unexpectedly and have generalized lesions of acute congestive heart failure but lack lesions in the intestine, the primary site of viral damage in approximately 95% of clinical cases. The heart is pale and flabby and has disseminated interstitial lymphocytic infiltrations and scattered myocytes with large, basophilic, intranuclear viral inclusion bodies in dogs that survive fibrosis (Fig. 10-81).

Trypanosoma cruzi. *Trypanosoma cruzi* is the protozoan hemoflagellate that causes American trypanosomiasis (Chagas' disease). The kissing bug (family Reduviidae, subfamily Triatominae) transmits the disease. Infection with *Trypanosoma cruzi* causes fatal chronic myocarditis. Acute disease is characteristic in dogs younger than 1 year of age. Affected dogs develop lymphohistiocytic myocarditis resulting in right-sided congestive heart failure with ascites, lymphadenomegaly, and hepatosplenomegaly. Grossly, the cardiac muscle contains multiple yellow-white myocardial streaks and spots that are often accompanied by hemorrhage. Chronic lymphocytic and plasmacytic myocarditis that leads to right-sided congestive heart failure typically affects older dogs. Grossly, the heart is bilaterally enlarged, thinned and flaccid, and contains fibrous plaques (areas of fibrosis).

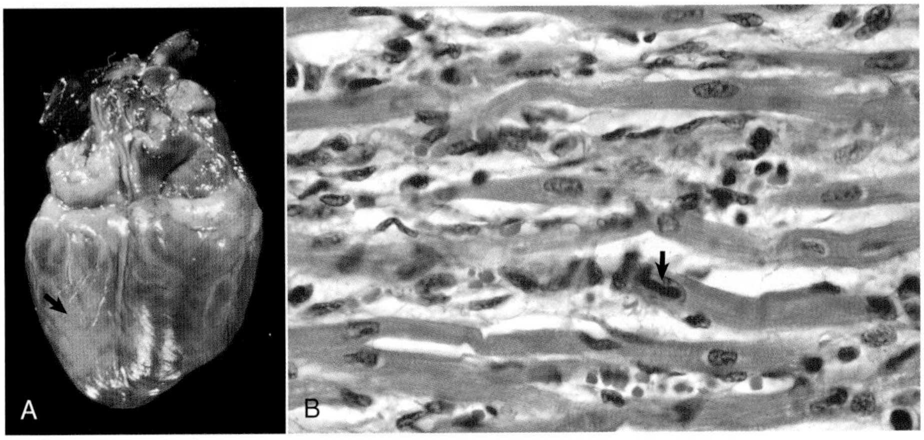

Figure 10-81 **Parvovirus Myocarditis, Heart, Dog. A,** Note the multifocal pale areas *(arrow)* in the ventricular myocardium. **B,** Parvovirus infection, section of myocardium. An intranuclear basophilic inclusion body is in a myocyte *(arrow)*. H&E stain. (**A** courtesy Dr. B. Weeks, College of Veterinary Medicine, Texas A&M University; and Noah's Arkive, College of Veterinary Medicine, The University of Georgia. **B** courtesy School of Veterinary Medicine, Purdue University.)

Cell Degeneration and Death

Neurogenic Cardiomyopathy (Heart-Brain Syndrome). Neurogenic cardiomyopathy (heart-brain syndrome) is a syndrome in dogs characterized by unexpected death 5 to 10 days after diffuse CNS injury (usually hit by car). Affected dogs die of cardiac arrhythmias caused by myocardial degeneration and necrosis. Grossly, the myocardium has numerous discrete and coalescing pale white streaks and/or poorly defined areas of myocardial necrosis—most often involving the papillary muscles of the left ventricle (Fig. 10-82). Neurogenic cardiomyopathy is thought to be caused by overstimulation of the heart by autonomic neurotransmitters and systemic catecholamines released at the time of trauma. It is unknown why there is a 5- to 10-day delay in the development of myocardial necrosis. See Chapter 14 for a discussion of heart-brain syndrome.

Endocardium and Heart Valves

Disturbances of Growth

Valvular Anomalies and Dysplasia. See the discussion on valvular anomalies and dysplasia in the section on Disorders of Domestic Animals, Developmental Errors/Congenital Anomalies: Endocardium and Heart Valves.

Cell Degeneration and Death

Myxomatous Valvular Degeneration (Valvular Endocardiosis). Myxomatous valvular degeneration (valvular endocardiosis) is the most common cardiovascular disease in dogs, and it is the most common cause of congestive heart failure in old dogs. Other names for this disease include endocarditis valvularis chronica fibrosa (nodosa), chronic valvular endocarditis, chronic valvular disease, billowing sail distortion of the mitral valve, endocardiosis, chronic mitral valve fibrosis, senile nodular sclerosis, mucoid degeneration, chronic myxomatous valve disease, and degenerative mitral valve disease. Myxomatous valvular degeneration (MVD) is an age-related cardiac disease of middle-aged to old dogs, especially small, toy, and medium-sized breeds. Males of affected breeds develop the disease at an earlier age than females. MVD appears to have a polygenic inheritance in dachshunds and Cavalier King Charles spaniels. The Cavalier King Charles spaniel breed has a unique susceptibility, with more than 50% prevalence by 4 years of age and 100% prevalence by 10 years of age. Other breeds with high incidence include the cocker spaniel, Lhasa apsos, bichons, Yorkshire terriers, shih tzus, dachshund, poodle, Pomeranian, miniature schnauzer, Chihuahua, fox terrier, Boston terrier, and Pekingese. At autopsies (syn: necropsies) of 3245 dogs, gross lesions occurred on the mitral valve alone (57.3%), mitral and tricuspid valves (26.6%), tricuspid valve alone (7.5%), aortic valve alone (2.1%), pulmonic valve alone (0.4%), and in combinations (6.1%). The lesions in MVD become progressively worse with age. Affected valves are shortened and thickened (nodular), either focal or diffusely, and appear smooth and shiny (Fig. 10-83) rather than rough and granular, as is usual in cases of valvular endocarditis.

MVD is grossly classified into four groups as follows: type 1, a few small discrete nodules in the area of contact that are associated with areas of diffuse opacity in the proximal portion of the valve; type 2, larger nodules that are evident in the area of contact, which tend to coalesce with their neighbors, along with areas of diffuse opacity that may be present; type 3, large nodules that coalesced

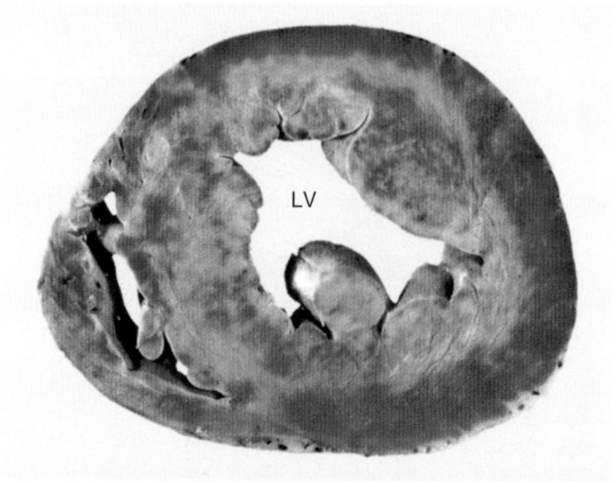

Figure 10-82 **Myocardial Necrosis, "Heart-Brain Syndrome," Heart, Transverse Section of Ventricles, Dog.** Necrotic areas are pale beige to white and are concentrated in the inner half of the wall of the left ventricle (*LV*) and in the ventricular septum. (Courtesy School of Veterinary Medicine, Purdue University.)

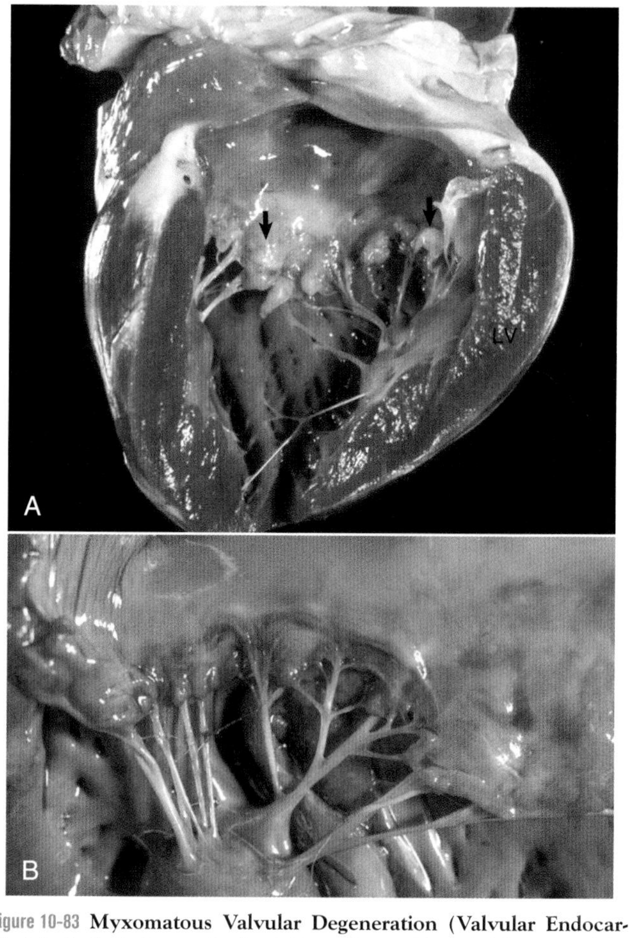

Figure 10-83 **Myxomatous Valvular Degeneration (Valvular Endocardiosis), Left Atrioventricular Valve, Heart, Dog. A,** The cusps of the mitral valve are thickened by white, smooth nodules (*arrows*). *LV*, Left ventricular free wall. **B,** Note the characteristic smooth and shiny (endocardial) surface of the valve and nodules. This differentiates myxomatous valvular degeneration (endocardiosis) from the rough and granular surface of chronic bacterial endocarditis. The pink staining of the valve is caused by postmortem imbibition of hemoglobin. (**A** courtesy Dr. J. Wright, College of Veterinary Medicine, North Carolina State University; and Noah's Arkive, College of Veterinary Medicine, The University of Georgia. **B** courtesy Dr. M.D. McGavin, College of Veterinary Medicine, University of Tennessee.)

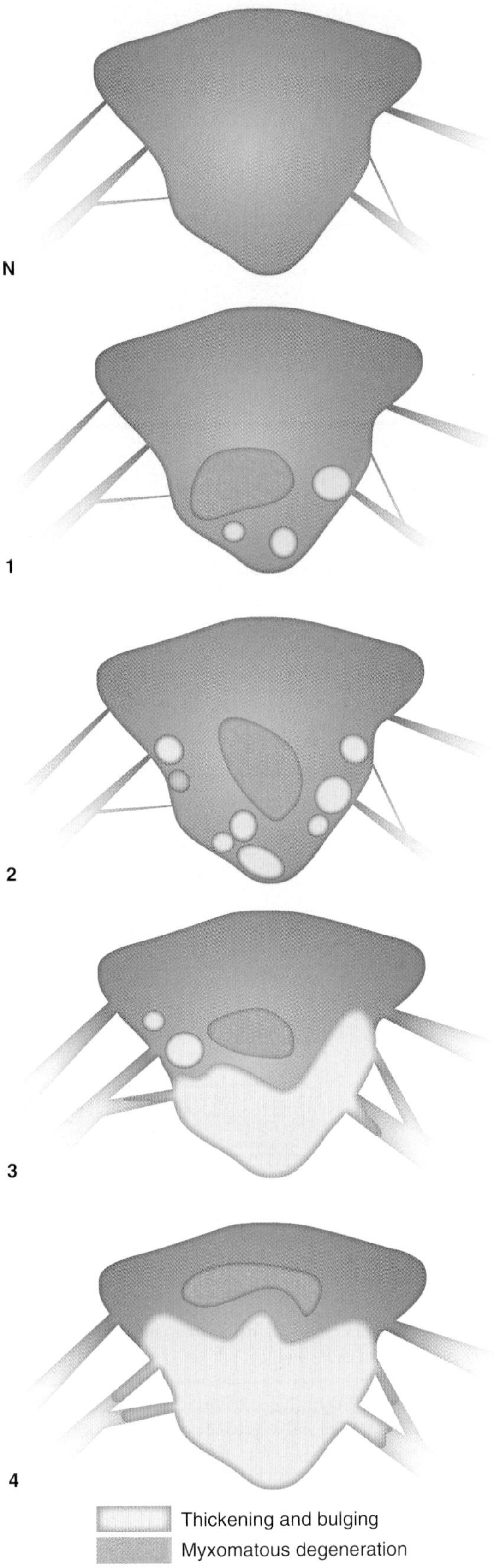

Figure 10-84 Natural Progression of Myxomatous Valvular Disease in the Mitral Leaflet. Myxomatous valvular disease is grossly classified into four groups (1-4). Type 1 has a few discrete nodules (minimal changes); type 2 has larger nodules in contact areas (mild changes); type 3 has large, coalescing nodules forming plaquelike deformities (moderate changes); and type 4 has obvious distortions of the valve (severe changes). The light-colored areas represent areas of nodular or diffuse thickening and ballooning of the valve cusp and proximal chordae tendineae. The dark-colored areas represent areas of diffuse opacity due to accumulation of neutral fat within the spongiosa layer. *N*, Normal valve. (Redrawn from Figure 2 from Borgarelli, M, Buchanan JW: Historical review, epidemiology and natural history of degenerative mitral valve disease, *J Vet Cardiol* 14(1):93-101, 2012.)

into irregular, plaque-like deformities that extend to involve the proximal portions of the chordae tendineae; and type 4, there is gross distortion and "ballooning" of the valve cusp, and the chordae tendinea are thickened proximally (Fig. 10-84). These lesions result in valvular insufficiency with subsequent atrial dilation and development of atrial "jet lesions." The jet lesion is a raised, rough, firm streak of endocardial fibrosis resulting from long-term trauma by a jet of blood leaking through the damaged valve in the closed position. Histologically, the valves are divided into four layers: atrialis, ventricularis, spongiosa, and fibrosa. The atrialis and ventricularis layers face the respective cardiac chambers and consist of endothelium and immediate subendothelial tissue containing fibroblasts, scattered collagen fibers, and a thin layer of elastic fibers. The spongiosa layer is loose connective tissue with interstitial cells and minimal fibers. The fibrosa consists of dense collagen that is continuous with the collagen core of chordae tendineae. Histopathologic lesions in MVD predominate in the distal third of the valve leaflets, and the incidence and severity increase with age. Lesions include progressive expansion of the spongiosa layer and disruption of the fibrosa layer.

Microscopically, the thickened valves have notably increased myofibroblastic proliferation and deposition of acid mucopolysaccharides (Fig. 10-85). It is important not to confuse normal age-related valve thickening in asymptomatic dogs with true pathologic thickening. Therefore a "clinical relevant diagnosis" would be more certain when the mitral valve and chordae tendineae are thickened and/or ruptured or when left heart chambers are enlarged or there are left atrial jet lesions. Severe complications of MVD include occasional rupture of chordae tendineae, occasional splitting or rupture of the left atrial wall that can result in hemopericardium, or acquired atrial septal defects. Frequent accompanying myocardial alterations include arteriosclerosis of intramyocardial arteries and multifocal myocardial necrosis and fibrosis. Progression of MVD is associated with an increase in plasma N-terminal pro-B-type natriuretic peptide concentration and an altered serotonin (5-hydroxytryptamine) signaling pathway.

Inflammation

Endocarditis. Endocarditis is occasionally observed in dogs. Bacterial septicemias result in inflammation of cardiac valves. Bacteria most commonly isolated include *Streptococcus* spp., *Bartonella* spp., and *Escherichia coli*. The mitral valve is most commonly involved and is associated with polyarthritis. Infections with *Bartonellosis* may only have inflammatory changes involving the aortic valve leaflets. *Erysipelothrix tonsillarum* (formally known as *Erysipelothrix* serovar 7) is occasionally isolated. Confirmation of the definitive organism requires bacterial isolation and/or identification by

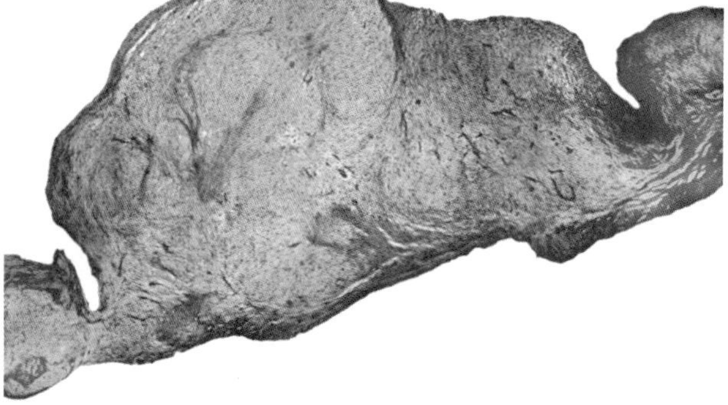

Figure 10-85 **Myxomatous Valvular Degeneration (Valvular Endocardiosis), Cusp of Right Atrioventricular Valve, Heart, Dog.** The valve is thickened and nodular from an increase in myxomatous tissue supported by a fibrous stroma. H&E stain. (Courtesy School of Veterinary Medicine, Purdue University.)

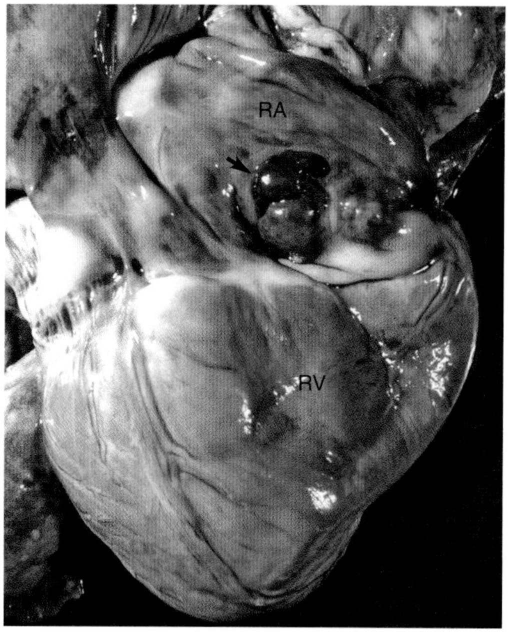

Figure 10-86 **Hemangiosarcoma, Heart, Right Atrium, Dog.** A dark-red hemangiosarcoma protrudes from the wall of the right atrium *(RA)*, a predilection site in the dog for this tumor *(arrow)*. *RV,* Right ventricle. (Courtesy Dr. M.D. McGavin, College of Veterinary Medicine, University of Tennessee.)

molecular tools. See the discussion on vegetative valvular and mural endocarditis in the section on Disorders of Domestic Animals: Endocardium and Heart Valves, Inflammation, and also Chapter 3.

Pericardium and Epicardium

Disturbances of Circulation

Idiopathic Pericardial Effusion (Hemorrhagic Pericardial Effusion). Idiopathic pericardial effusion is one of the most common causes of canine pericardial effusion and accounts for approximately 19% of all canine pericardial effusions. Large or giant breeds, such as the Great Dane, Saint Bernard, Great Pyrenees, German shepherd, and golden retriever, are most often affected. It is a diagnosis of exclusion after all other potential causes (neoplastic, traumatic, infectious, metabolic, cardiac, and coagulopathy) have been ruled out. Idiopathic pericardial effusion can be hemorrhagic or serosanguinous. The pericardium is thickened by diffuse fibrosis; neovascularization; areas of lymphocytic, plasmacytic, and histiocytic infiltrates; and areas of mesothelial hyperplasia alongside regions void of parietal mesothelium. See the discussion on effusions in the section on Disorders of Domestic Animals: Pericardium and Epicardium, Disturbances of Circulation, Effusions, and also Chapters 3, 7, and 9.

Blood and Lymphatic Vascular Systems

Blood Vessels

Disturbances of Growth

Anomalies and Dysplasia. See the discussion on anomalies and dysplasia in the section on Disorders of Domestic Animals, Developmental Errors/Congenital Anomalies.

Neoplastic Transformation

Hemangiosarcoma and Hemangioma. Cardiac hemangiosarcoma (HSA) is an important neoplasm of dogs and can arise either in the heart (primary) or via metastasis (secondary) from primary sites such as the spleen. In a recent study, HSA frequently occurred in older golden retrievers, followed by Maltese dogs and miniature dachshunds. Mass lesions of HSA were found more commonly in the right auricle and right atrium, and the right atrial masses were significantly larger than the right auricular masses, potentially accounting for their higher antemortem detection rate by echocardiography. Grossly, protruding red to red-black blood-containing masses are located on the epicardial surface (Fig. 10-86) and may also protrude into the atrial lumen. Rupture can produce fatal hemopericardium and cardiac tamponade. Microscopically, the neoplasms are composed of scattered, elongated, plump neoplastic endothelial cells, which may or may not form vascular spaces containing blood (Fig. 10-87). Pulmonary metastases are frequent. Immunohistochemistry staining for factor VIII-related antigen or CD31 (an endothelial marker) confirms the tumor cells are endothelial in

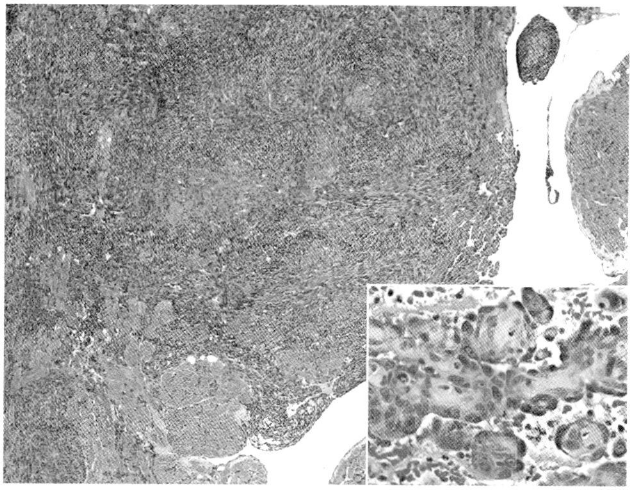

Figure 10-87 **Hemangiosarcoma, Heart, Right Atrium, Dog.** Malignant endothelial cells have invaded the myocardium of the right atrium, thus giving it the bluish granular appearance (cell nuclei) at low magnification. The high magnification *(inset)* shows these endothelial cells with large, round-to-oval nuclei forming poorly delineated and haphazardly arranged vascular channels. These cells can also "pile up" and be arranged in clusters or solid sheets. Mitotic figures can be prominent and numerous (not shown here). A golden-brown pigment (hemosiderin) can form secondary to erythrophagocytosis of damaged or effete erythrocytes (not shown here). H&E stain. (Courtesy Dr. J.F. Zachary, College of Veterinary Medicine, University of Illinois.)

origin. Hemangiomas are benign neoplasms often found in the skin of dogs (Fig. 10-88). These red, blood-filled masses are well circumscribed.

Heart-Base Tumors. See the discussion on cardiac neoplasms in the section on Disorders of Dogs, Myocardium, Disturbances of Growth; on neoplastic transformation in the section on Disorders of Domestic Animals, Blood and Lymphatic Vascular Systems, Blood Vessels, Disturbances of Growth; and also see Fig. 10-48.

Cell Degeneration and Death

Medial Necrosis and Hemorrhage. Medial necrosis and hemorrhage is a distinctive lesion produced in muscular arteries and arterioles of dogs and rats by a wide variety of vasoactive drugs. These vascular lesions, detected during evaluations of new compounds, produce grossly apparent hemorrhage, especially in the epicardium. Microscopically, acute damage is evident as necrosis of smooth muscle cells in the tunica media with surrounding erythrocytes. Healing lesions have fibrosis of the vessel wall and perivascularly.

Segmental Arterial Mediolysis. Segmental arterial mediolysis is a distinctive lesion produced in muscular arteries and arterioles of dogs and rats that most often occurs in the splanchnic muscular and coronary arteries and causes catastrophic hemorrhages. The pathology can be induced experimentally by administration of ractopamine, a synthetic β_2-adrenoceptor agonist to dogs. Exposure to α_1-adrenergic receptor agonists or β_2 agonists induces the release of norepinephrine from the peripheral nervous system. Epinephrine is thought to induce injury at the adventitial medial junction through medial muscle apoptosis. Microscopically, acute damage is evident as necrosis of smooth muscle cells in the tunica media with surrounding erythrocytes. Healing lesions have fibrosis of the vessel wall and perivascularly.

Fibrocartilaginous Embolism. Fibrocartilaginous embolism of the spinal cord vasculature and resultant infarction of the spinal cord supplied or drained by the obstructed blood vessel lead to posterior paresis or paralysis. Affected dogs are typically middle-aged large or giant breeds, but occurrence in young Irish wolfhounds has been reported. The mechanism of formation of the arterial or venous emboli is still unclear, but movement within the spinal vasculature of fibrocartilaginous fragments from degenerated intervertebral disks is generally considered to underlie the presence of these unusual emboli (Fig. 10-89; E-Fig. 10-29).

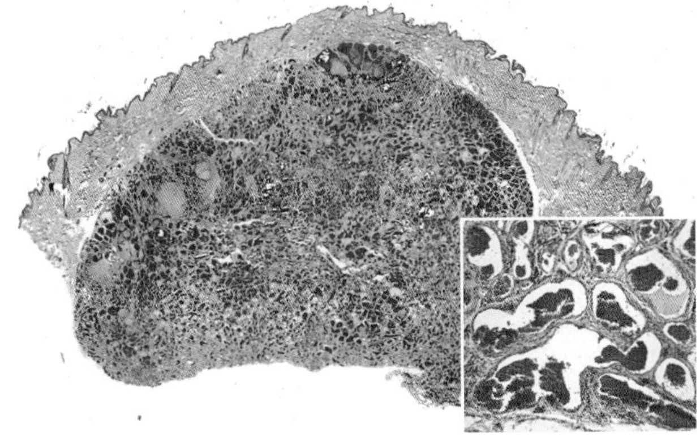

Figure 10-88 **Cutaneous Hemangioma, Skin, Dog.** The subcutis contains a well-demarcated mass formed by vascular channels lined by a single layer of well-differentiated endothelial cells. *Inset,* Higher magnification of the well-differentiated endothelial cells lining the vascular channels. H&E stain. (Courtesy Dr. M.D. McGavin, College of Veterinary Medicine, University of Tennessee.)

Pulmonary Artery Thromboembolism. Pulmonary artery thromboembolism (Fig. 10-90) is often a life-threatening condition and in dogs has an incidence of 0.9% over a 10-year period. A wide variety of predisposing conditions may result in altered blood flow, hypercoagulability, or endothelial damage. These include sepsis, immune-mediated hemolytic anemia, neoplastic disease, protein-losing nephropathy/amyloidosis, disseminated intravascular coagulation, cardiac disease, hyperadrenocorticism, dirofilariasis, and use of intravenous catheters. The thrombus in the pulmonary arteries lyses within a few hours and therefore may be absent at the time of autopsy (syn: necropsy) in approximately 15% of cases, as was indicated by one study. Because of extensive collateral pulmonary arterial circulation, the presence of a large thrombus in the pulmonary artery or its main branches makes a clinically relevant diagnosis of pulmonary artery thromboembolism more certain, unless antemortem ancillary tests such as pulmonary angiography and ventilation/perfusion scanning are strongly supportive of it.

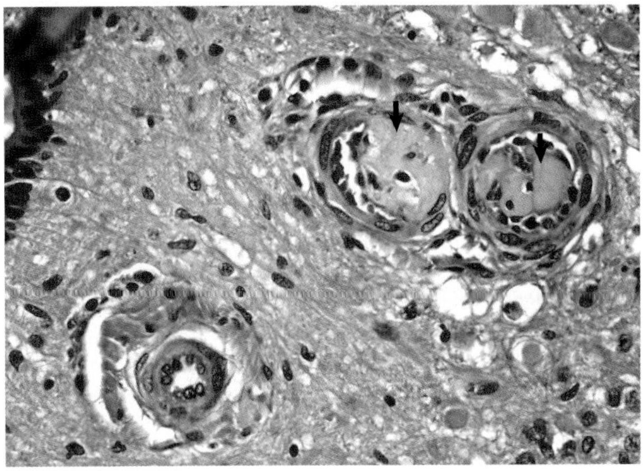

Figure 10-89 **Fibrocartilaginous Emboli, Spinal Cord, Pig.** The basophilic masses *(arrows)* occluding small arteries *(cross sections)* in the spinal cord gray matter adjacent to the central canal *(top left margin)* are fibrocartilaginous emboli. H&E stain. (Courtesy School of Veterinary Medicine, Purdue University.)

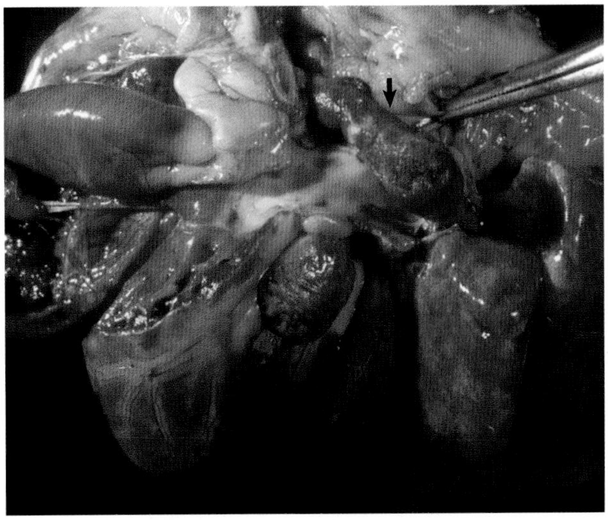

Figure 10-90 **Arterial Thrombus, Pulmonary Artery, Dog.** Arterial thrombi are composed primarily of platelets and fibrin because the rapid flow of blood tends to exclude erythrocytes from the thrombus, and thus arterial thrombi are usually pale beige to gray *(arrow)*. (Courtesy Dr. D.A. Mosier, College of Veterinary Medicine, Kansas State University.)

Arterial Thromboembolism and Thrombosis. Arterial thromboembolism and thrombosis occur in dogs and arise from injury to vascular endothelium, propagated via the coagulation cascade (see Chapter 2). In dogs, the most common site is the aortoiliac trifurcation (Fig. 10-91), in which a thromboembolus extends from the caudal aorta distally to the external and internal iliac arteries. Embolization of the subclavian and brachial arteries also results in lameness of the forelimb, albeit less commonly. Other sites include embolization of the coronary arteries in the heart, renal arteries, and intestinal arteries. Aortoiliac thromboembolism in dogs has been reported with infection by *Spirocerca lupi* and *Blastomyces dermatitides* and in association with various disease conditions, such as protein-losing nephropathy, hypothyroidism, hypercortisolism, diabetes mellitus, and aortic neoplasia.

Thrombosis of the Femoral Artery. Thrombosis of the femoral artery, with resulting partial to complete occlusion, has been reported in Cavalier King Charles spaniels. Affected dogs generally do not develop hindlimb ischemia, in contrast to human patients with this condition, because of extensive collateral circulation and thrombus recanalization. It is a common but clinically insignificant pathology in Cavalier King Charles spaniels that is suspected to result from a probable weakness in the femoral artery wall.

Inflammation

Heartworm Dirofilariasis (Dirofilaria immitis). Dirofilariasis (heartworm disease) may occur in 35% to 45% of dogs and 2% of cats in areas of high infection rates, such as within 150 miles of the Atlantic and Gulf coasts from Texas to New Jersey and along the Mississippi River and its major tributaries. The extent of cardiac alterations is related to the number of adult parasites present. Initially, the parasites accumulate in the pulmonary arteries (Fig. 10-92), and as the numbers increase, they are present in the right ventricle, then in the right atrium, and finally may occupy the vena cavae. Pulmonary hypertension results from vascular blockage and pulmonary vascular lesions produced by the parasites, and right ventricular hypertrophy follows. Right-sided heart failure may eventually develop. The pulmonary arteries containing parasites initially have an infiltration of the intima (termed *endarteritis*) by eosinophils, with subsequent development of an irregular fibromuscular proliferation of the intima visible grossly as a rough granular or shaggy appearance of the luminal surface (see Fig. 10-92; E-Figs. 10-30 and 10-31). Live or dead parasites can be present within these vascular lesions and be accompanied by thromboembolism and pulmonary infarction. The pleura of the caudal lung lobes may contain multifocal areas of hemorrhage, hemosiderosis, and fibrosis. The presence of a massive number of adult worms may result in filling the right heart extending into venae cavae, resulting in venal caval syndrome. This syndrome results in sudden collapse, liver failure, intravascular hemolytic anemia, shock, and death if the adult worms are not removed surgically.

Polyarteritis: "Beagle Pain Syndrome." Polyarteritis is a disease that occurs sporadically in many animal species and is an important disease of aged rats called *polyarteritis nodosa* (E-Fig. 10-32). Many recent reports have described the occurrence of polyarteritis in a disease termed *idiopathic necrotizing polyarteritis* (idiopathic canine polyarteritis, juvenile polyarteritis syndrome) involving multiple arteries, including the coronary and meningeal arteries in dogs, most often pet and laboratory beagle dogs ("beagle pain syndrome"). Clinically, affected dogs typically show recurrent episodes of fever, body weight loss, and occasionally cervical pain manifested by a stilted gait and stiff neck with a hunched body posture. However, some affected dogs do not display clinical signs of disease. The lesions are usually attributed to an immune-mediated vascular injury. Small and medium-sized muscular arteries in a wide variety of organs, including the heart, meninges, epididymis, and thymus, are selectively involved and grossly appear thick and tortuous, have associated focal hemorrhage, and develop aneurysms and thrombosis. Microscopically, the early lesions include fibrinoid necrosis and

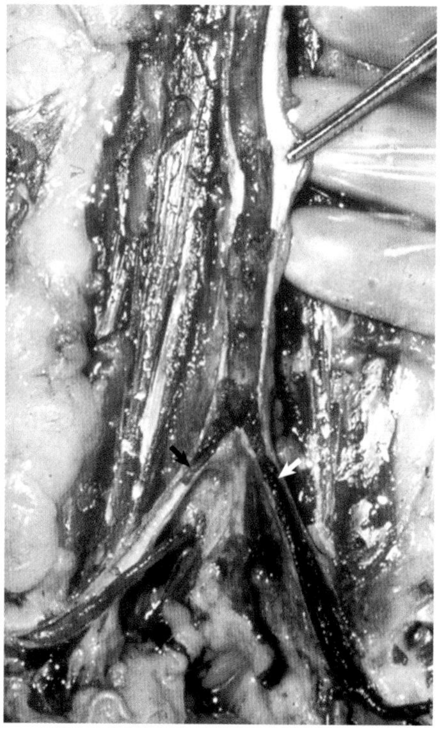

Figure 10-91 **Aortic Thrombosis, Aorta and External Iliac Arteries, Dog.** The tan thrombus occluding the caudal abdominal aorta is a cranial extension of the red saddle thromboembolus at the aortic bifurcation and in the external iliac arteries *(arrows)*. (Courtesy School of Veterinary Medicine, Purdue University.)

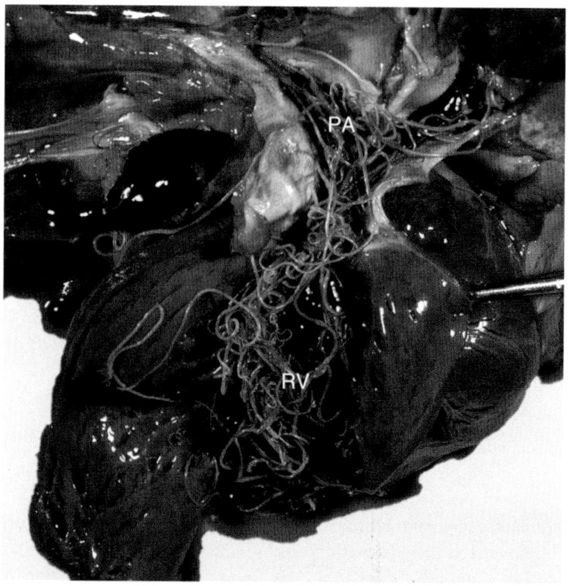

Figure 10-92 **Dirofilariasis, Heart, Opened Right Ventricle, and Pulmonary Artery, Dog.** Numerous adult *Dirofilaria immitis* are present in the right ventricle *(RV)*, right atrium, and pulmonary artery *(PA)*. (Courtesy Dr. M.D. McGavin, College of Veterinary Medicine, University of Tennessee.)

leukocytic invasion of the intima and media (E-Fig. 10-33). In chronic lesions, inflammatory cells and fibrosis involve all layers of the vascular wall.

Lymphatic Vessels

Disturbances of Circulation

Primary Lymphedema. Primary lymphedema is a rare pathology in dogs that often involves the distal hindlimbs, and it results from aplasia/hypoplasia of superficial lymphatic vessels and/or draining lymph nodes of the distal hindlimbs. Antemortem, dogs are being presented with nonpainful pitting edema of the distal hindlimbs. At autopsy (syn: necropsy) there is lymphatic hypoplasia and/or absence of popliteal lymph nodes with distal secondary lymphatic hyperplasia. Marked delay in lymphatic filling in lymphangiography, in lymphoscintigraphy, or in the patent blue violet dye absorption test are antemortem ancillary test results that strongly support the diagnosis of primary lymphedema.

Primary Intestinal Lymphangiectasia. Primary intestinal lymphangiectasia is a rare intestinal pathology of dogs that results in severe protein-losing enteropathy. The Lundehund breed is predisposed. Clinically, dogs are presented for wasting, diarrhea, and ascites. Lacteals in the intestinal villi are fused, blunted, and have markedly distended tips, whereas lymphatic vessels throughout the wall of the intestine, and occasionally mesentery and mesenteric lymph nodes, are distended with milky opaque fluid (i.e., chyle) (see Fig. 7-14). In dogs, the role of obstruction of lymphatic vessels or their structural integrity (i.e., hypoplasia) in the pathogenesis of this disease is still unclear. Secondary intestinal lymphangiectasia is much more common and results from obstruction of lymphatic drainage by inflammation or neoplasia.

Disorders of Cats

Myocardium

Disturbances of Growth

Anomalies and Dysplasia. See the discussion on anomalies and dysplasia in the section on Disorders of Domestic Animals, Developmental Errors/Congenital Anomalies: Myocardium.

Cardiomyopathies. See the discussion on cardiomyopathies in the section on Disorders of Domestic Animals, Disorders of Domestic Animals: Myocardium, Disturbances of Growth, Hypertrophy and Atrophy.

Endocardium and Heart Valves

Disturbances of Growth

Valvular Anomalies and Dysplasia. See the discussion on valvular anomalies and dysplasia in the section on Disorders of Domestic Animals, Developmental Errors/Congenital Anomalies: Endocardium and Heart Valves.

Inflammation

Endomyocarditis. Endomyocarditis is a disease of cats of undetermined cause. The affected areas are thickened and often in the area of the outflow of the left ventricle. Lesions consist of a mixed population of inflammatory cells, which extends into the adjacent myocardium. Chronic lesions have marked, often visible fibrous connective tissue with fewer inflammatory cells within the endocardium.

Pericardium and Epicardium

Disturbances of Circulation

Effusions. See the section on Disorders of Domestic Animals, Disorders of Domestic Animals: Pericardium and Epicardium, Disturbances of Circulation, Hemopericardium and Hydropericardium.

Pericardial Effusions

Hemopericardium. Rodenticide toxicity and systemic consumption of clotting factors from disseminated intravascular coagulation are the most common causes of hemopericardium in cats.

Hydropericardium. Cats develop hydropericardium most commonly from congestive heart failure. Neoplasms, including heart-base tumors, mesotheliomas lymphoma, rhabdomyosarcoma, and fibrosarcoma, can produce hydropericardium. Uremia, through systemic damage to blood vessels, may result in hydropericardium.

Inflammation

Pericarditis. Feline infectious peritonitis (FIP) is a cause of fibrinous pericarditis in cats. The etiological agent is mutated feline enteric corona virus, and in that case pericarditis is a local manifestation of a multisystemic and generalized disease process.

Blood and Lymphatic Vascular Systems

Blood Vessels

Disturbances of Growth

Medial Hypertrophy of Pulmonary Arteries. Medial (tunica media) hypertrophy of pulmonary arteries is a disorder of cats of unknown cause (see Fig. 10-26); however, a response to antigens during nematode infections may be involved.

Inflammation

Pulmonary Artery Thromboembolism. See the discussion on pulmonary artery thromboembolism in the section on Disorders of Dogs.

Arterial Thromboembolism. Arterial thromboembolism (ATE) is defined as obstruction usually followed by infarction of arterial beds by embolic material derived from a thrombus from a distant site and in the presence of intact endothelial surface (to be distinguished from arterial thrombosis). The most common cause of ATE in cats is cardiomyopathy in which a large thrombus is formed in the enlarged left atrium. However, other conditions, such as protein-losing nephropathy/enteropathy, sepsis, DIC, and endocrinopathies, should be considered in the diagnostic workup. The fate of the infarcted area depends on the ability to establish collateral blood flow, thus bypassing the occluded artery. In cats and dogs, the most common site is the aortic trifurcation ("saddle embolus"), and the right subclavian artery is the second most common cause of ATE in cats with cardiomyopathy. Renal, splanchnic, and cerebral circulations can also be affected on occasion. In a saddle embolus, occlusion of limb(s) blood flow results in ischemic neuromyopathy of the limb(s). Grossly, distal limbs below the stifle are most severely affected, and the affected limb is often dark red to blue and edematous due to hemorrhagic ischemic necrosis.

Feline Infectious Peritonitis. Feline infectious peritonitis is a severe viral infection that produces phlebitis in various organs. This lesion appears to result from deposition of immune complexes, which subsequently induce an inflammatory reaction in affected vessels (see Chapters 4, 7, and 11).

Heartworm-Associated Respiratory Disease. *Dirofilaria immitis* infection in cats occasionally results in heartworm-associated respiratory disease. Cats are more susceptible than dogs to infection with *Dirofilaria immitis*, although many do not have adult worms or have only a few (one to four worms). Grossly, there may be a visible shaggy or roughened appearance to the large lobar arteries, especially the right caudal lobar artery. The pulmonary arteries develop villus endarteritis with medial hypertrophy (see Fig. 10-26). Initially, small pulmonary arteries may become embolized and infarcted, leading to small areas of hemorrhage and necrosis in the lung and sudden death in some cats. Many cats that survive this initial phase develop collateral blood supply, but histologically they have multiple small pulmonary arteries with villus endarteritis and multifocal areas with type II pneumocyte hyperplasia, which is indicative of chronic alveolar injury. The most common clinical manifestation is an asthma-like syndrome potentially from inflammatory mediators that are released by numerous eosinophils and other leukocytes that cuff affected small pulmonary arteries.

Foreign Parasitic Diseases. Foreign parasitic diseases important in tropical regions of the world are characterized by the presence of parasites in the lumens of veins and lymphatic vessels. These diseases include infection of cats in South America by *Gurltia paralysans*, infection of cats in tropical regions with *Brugia* spp., and infection of pulmonary vessels by *Dirofilaria immitis*. Cats infected with *Gurltia paralysans* have spinal cord damage from thrombophlebitis in the lumbar veins, associated with the presence of adult parasites in affected vessels. *Brugia* spp. infect lymphatic vessels and lead to secondary lymphedema.

Lymphatic Vessels

Disturbances of Circulation

Lymphedema. See the section on Disorders of Domestic Animals, Disorders of Domestic Animals: Blood and Lymphatic Vascular Systems, Lymphatic Vessels, Disturbances of Circulation, Lymphedema.

Suggested Readings

Suggested Readings are available at www.expertconsult.com.

CHAPTER 11

The Urinary System[1]

Melanie A. Breshears and Anthony W. Confer

Key Readings Index

Kidney[2]

Structure

Mammalian kidneys are paired organs present in the retroperitoneum, ventrolateral and adjacent to the lumbar vertebral bodies and their corresponding transverse processes. These complex organs, which function in excretion, metabolism, secretion, and regulation, are susceptible to disease insults that affect the four major anatomic structures of the kidney: the glomeruli, tubules, interstitium, and vasculature. Because of the limited ways that renal tissue can respond to injury and the limited patterns of injury, in severe and prolonged disease, the endpoint will be similar—chronic renal disease and failure. Interdependence between components of the nephron also are responsible for producing a narrow range of repeatable injury patterns, which students can come to recognize on gross or histologic assessment.

Macroscopically, kidneys are organized functionally and anatomically into lobules. Each lobule represents collections of nephrons separated by the medullary rays. Renal lobules should not be confused with renal lobes. Each lobe is represented by a renal pyramid (Fig. 11-1). Among domestic animals, carnivores and horses have unilobar kidneys. Porcine and bovine kidneys are multilobar, but only bovine kidneys have external lobation (Fig. 11-2). A diffuse fibrous capsule that in normal kidneys can be easily removed from the renal surface covers the kidneys. The renal parenchyma is divided into a cortex and medulla (see Fig. 11-1). The corticomedullary ratio is usually approximately 1 : 2 or 1 : 3 in domestic animals. The ratio varies among species; for example, those adapted to the desert have a far larger medulla and thus a corticomedullary ratio that can approach 1 : 5. Normally the cortex is radially striated and dark red-brown except in mature cats, in which the cortex is often yellow because of the large lipid content of tubular epithelial cells. The renal medulla is pale gray to tan and has a single renal papilla, as in cats; a fused, crestlike papilla (renal medullary crest), as in dogs, sheep, and horses; or multiple renal papillae, as in pigs and cattle. The medulla generally can be subdivided into an outer zone, that portion of the medulla close to the cortex, and an inner zone, that portion closer to the pelvis. Papillae are surrounded by minor calyces that coalesce to form major calyces, which empty into the renal pelvis (Fig. 11-3), where urine collects before entry into the ureters.

Microscopically, for ease of discussion, the kidney (and nephron) can be divided into four structural units: renal corpuscle (glomerulus and Bowman's capsule), tubules, interstitium, and vasculature. The functional unit of the kidney is the nephron, which includes the renal corpuscle and renal tubules (the tubular system includes the proximal convoluted tubules, the loop of Henle, and the distal convoluted tubule). The uriniferous tubule is composed of the nephron and the collecting ducts, which are embryologically distinct from the renal tubules (Fig. 11-4). The uriniferous tubule is embedded structurally in the renal interstitium formed by a meshwork composed of stromal cells such as fibroblasts. The interstitium also contains the renal vasculature, which supplies blood first to the glomerulus and then to the renal tubules.

Glomerulus (Glomerular Tuft, Renal Corpuscle)

Macroscopically, glomeruli are difficult to detect in the normal kidney but can be accentuated by lesions that allow them to be identified on cut section as randomly distributed granular foci or as red dots throughout the cortex (Fig. 11-5). Microscopically, the glomerulus is a complex, convoluted tuft of fenestrated endothelial-lined capillaries held together by a supporting structure of cells in a glycoprotein matrix, the mesangium (see Fig. 11-5). The entire glomerulus is supported by mesangial matrix that is secreted by the mesangial cells, a type of modified pericyte. Mesangial cells are pluripotential mesenchymal cells, which are contractile and phagocytic (see E-Figs. 11-5 and 11-6) and capable of synthesizing

[1]For a glossary of abbreviations and terms used in this chapter, see E-Glossary 11-1.

[2]See E-Appendix 11-1 for methods of examining the kidney.

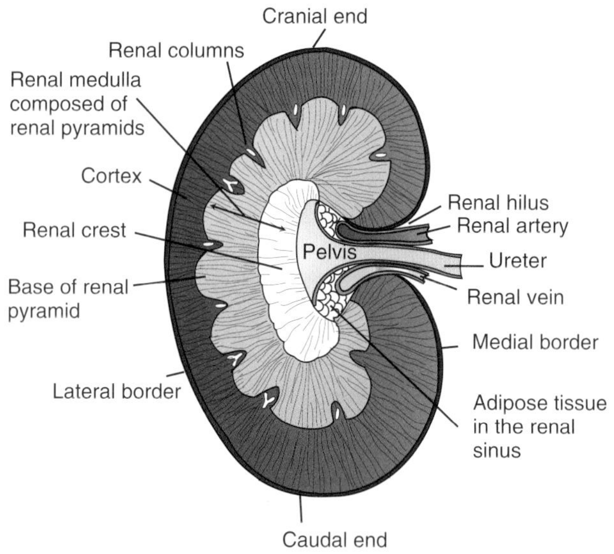

Figure 11-1 **Kidney, Dorsal Section, Dog.** (Based on Schaller O, Constantinescu GM, editors: *Illustrated veterinary anatomical nomenclature*, Stuttgart, Germany, 2007, Enke Verlag.)

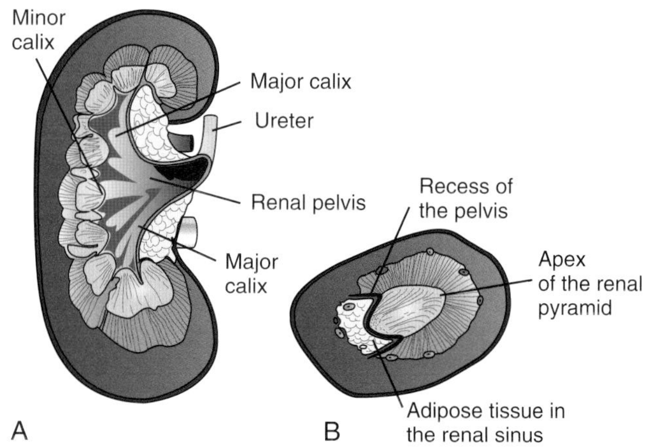

Figure 11-3 **Structure of the Kidney. A,** Dorsal section through hilus, pig. **B,** Transverse section through hilus, dog. (Based on Schaller O, Constantinescu GM, editors: *Illustrated veterinary anatomical nomenclature*, Stuttgart, Germany, 2007, Enke Verlag.)

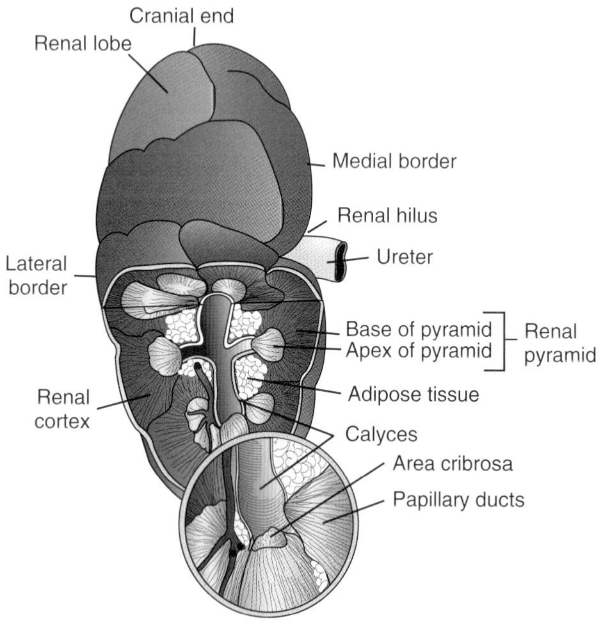

Figure 11-2 **Kidney, Dorsal Surface and Partial Dorsal Section, Cow.** (Based on Schaller O, Constantinescu GM, editors: *Illustrated veterinary anatomical nomenclature*, Stuttgart, Germany, 2007, Enke Verlag.)

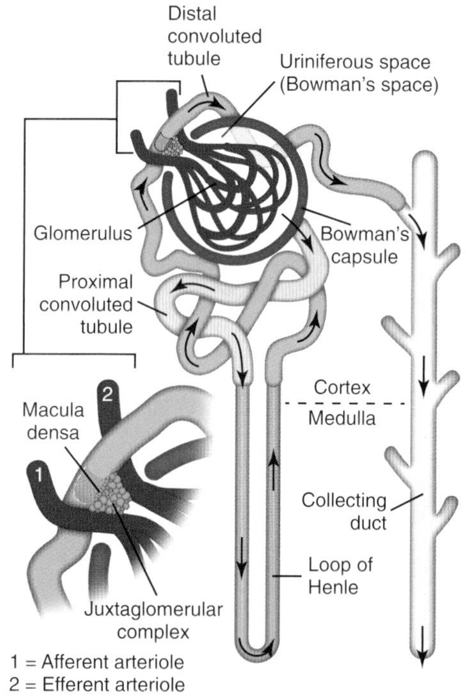

Figure 11-4 **Uriniferous Tubule.** A uriniferous tubule is composed of a nephron and its collecting duct. The nephron is formed by a renal corpuscle and its connecting renal tubules (proximal tubule, loop of Henle, and distal tubule). Bowman's capsule surrounds the glomerulus, and together these structures form the renal corpuscle. (Courtesy Drs. M.A. Breshears and A.W. Confer, Center for Veterinary Health Sciences, Oklahoma State University; and Dr. J.F. Zachary, College of Veterinary Medicine, University of Illinois.)

collagen and mesangial matrix, as well as secreting inflammatory mediators.

Glomerular Filtration Barrier. The glomerular filtration barrier is composed of (1) pedicles of podocytes (visceral epithelium of Bowman's capsule), (2) glomerular basement membrane (GBM) or basal lamina (produced by both endothelial and epithelial cells), and (3) the fenestrated endothelium of glomerular capillaries (Fig. 11-6).

Visceral Epithelium (Podocytes). Visceral epithelial cells (podocytes), aligned on the external surface of the basement membrane, are responsible for synthesis of basement membrane components and have special cytoplasmic processes (foot processes) that are embedded in the lamina rara externa. Negatively charged glycoproteins overlying the endothelial cells and the podocytes

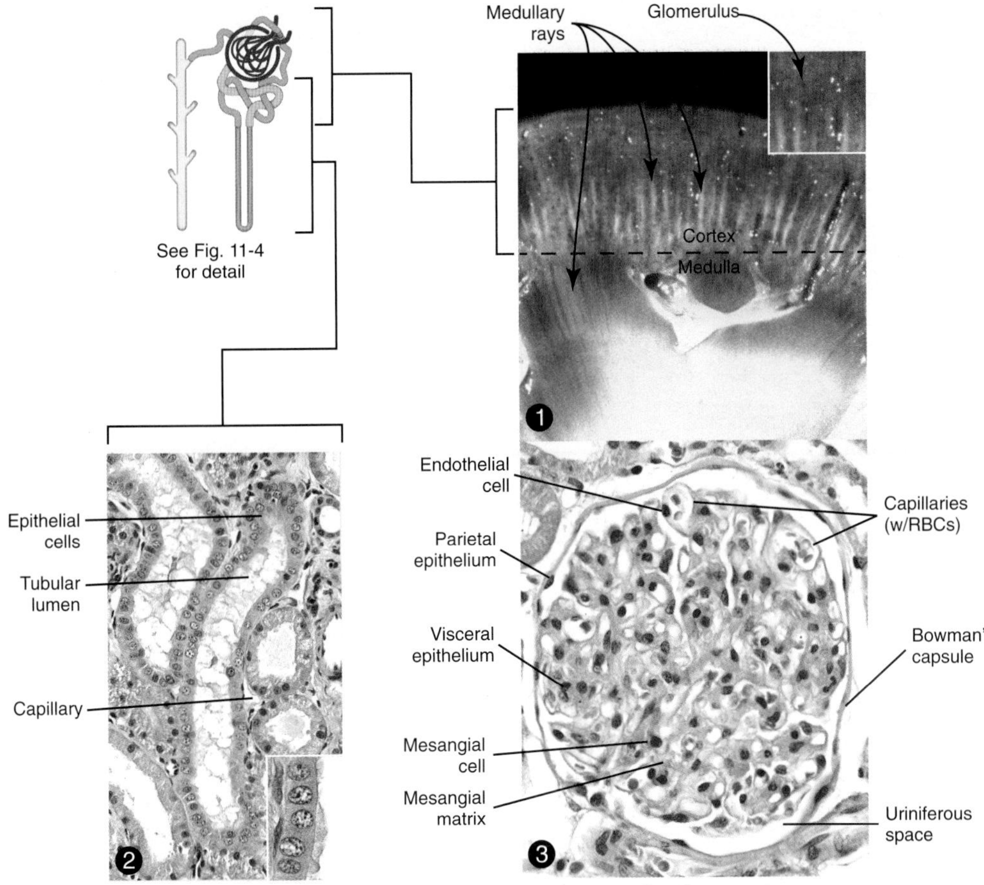

Figure 11-5 Macroscopic and Microscopic Structure of Renal Cortex, Medulla, and Corpuscle. *1*, Medullary rays are grossly visible as radial striations in the deep cortex of the kidney and are composed of collecting tubules and ducts draining nephrons located in the more superficial cortex. Glomeruli are difficult to detect grossly in the normal kidney, but they may appear as red dots (when filled with blood) or white to gray granular foci, especially when accentuated by inflammatory or reparative (healing) glomerular lesions. *2*, Renal tubules. *Inset*, Higher magnification of renal tubular epithelium. *3*, Renal corpuscle. (Courtesy Drs. M.A. Breshears and A.W. Confer, Center for Veterinary Health Sciences, Oklahoma State University; and Dr. J.F. Zachary, College of Veterinary Medicine, University of Illinois.)

contribute to the charge differential of the GBM. Foot processes from adjacent visceral epithelium interdigitate to form filtration slits between them (see Fig. 11-6). Filtration slit diaphragms are composed of nephrin, a cell adhesion molecule of the immunoglobulin superfamily, which controls slit size by its connection to podocyte actin.

Glomerular Basement Membrane (Basal Lamina). The glomerular basement membrane has a thick, dense central layer, the lamina densa, which is covered by thinner, more electron-lucent inner and outer layers, the lamina rara interna and lamina rara externa, respectively (see Fig. 11-6). The basement membrane has a network of type IV collagen, which forms a tetrameric porous infrastructure. Numerous glycoproteins, such as acidic proteoglycans and laminin, together with the collagen fibers form the complete structure of the membrane. The glomerular filtration barrier selectively filters molecules based on size (70 kDa), electrical charge (the more cationic, the more permeable), and capillary pressure. In summary, both size-dependent and charge-dependent filtration is possible because of the porous structure of capillary walls, which is a function of endothelial fenestrations, a basement membrane formed of type IV collagen, basement membrane anionic glycoproteins, and filtration slits of the visceral epithelium.

Glomerular Capillaries. The glomerular capillaries exist between the afferent and efferent arterioles and form the glomerular tuft. Glomerular capillaries interdigitate with the visceral lining of Bowman's space. The capillary endothelium is fenestrated and covered by a complete basal lamina.

Bowman's Capsule

Bowman's capsule is a cup-shaped, membranous sac at the beginning of the nephron that encloses each glomerulus and is separated from the glomerular tuft by the uriniferous space (see Fig. 11-4).

Parietal Epithelium. The capillary tuft (glomerulus) is covered by visceral epithelial cells (podocytes) and is contained within Bowman's capsule that is lined by parietal epithelial cells resembling squamous epithelium (see Figs. 11-5 and 11-6).

Tubules

The renal tubular system (in the order of flow of urine) consists of a proximal tubule, loop of Henle, and distal tubule (see Fig. 11-4). The tubules connect to the renal pelvis at the distal end of the collecting ducts, and the whole structure—including the renal corpuscle, renal tubules, and collecting ducts—is referred to as the *uriniferous tubule* (see Fig. 11-4). The proximal and distal convoluted

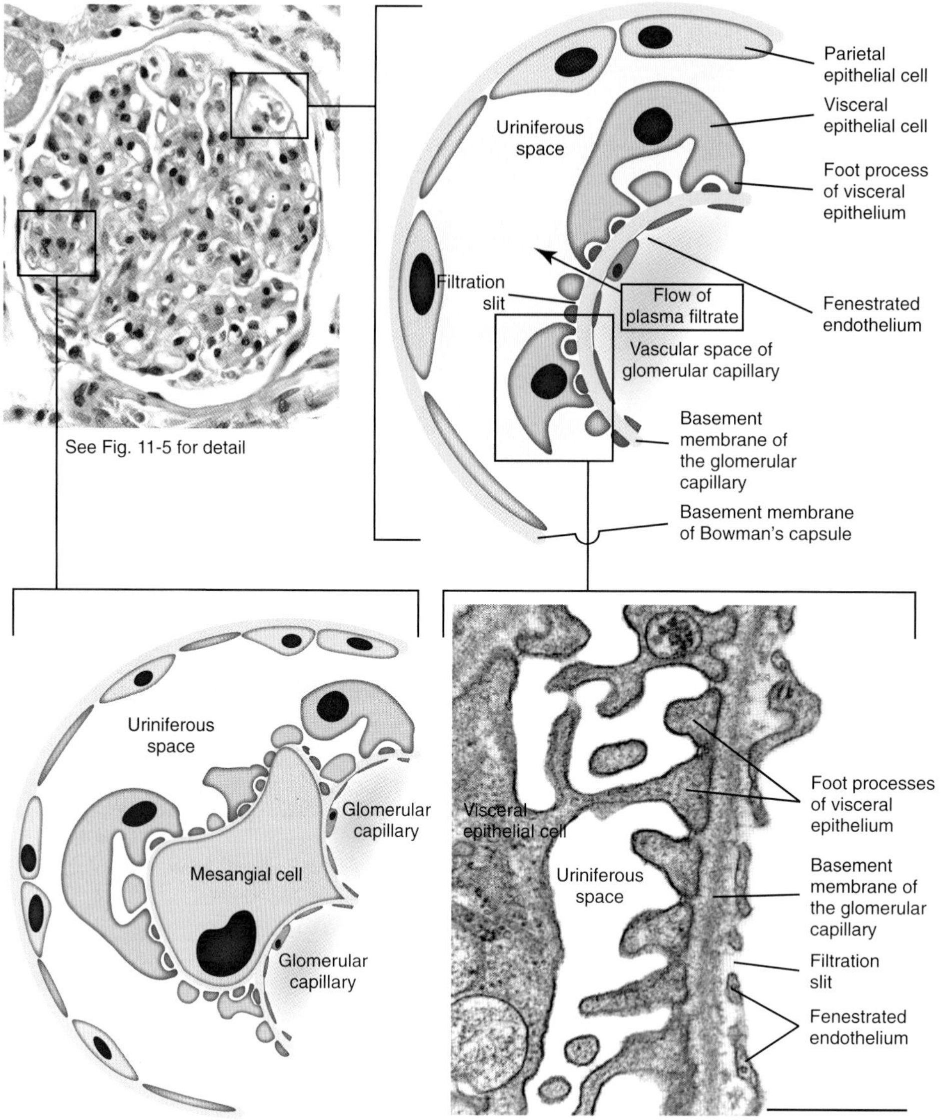

Figure 11-6 **Glomerular Filtration Barrier.** The glomerular filtration barrier is a layer formed by endothelial cells, basement membrane, and visceral epithelial cells (podocytes). Its main function is to filter plasma to maintain ionic and osmotic homeostasis in the blood. The filtration barrier is relatively impermeable to larger macromolecules, such as albumin and hemoglobin, and larger proteins, such as immunoglobulins. However, small and medium-sized solutes (ions), such as sodium and potassium, and other soluble moieties, such as sugar molecules, pass through the barrier as glomerular filtrate, which then travels through the renal tubules and the collecting duct to form urine. Certain molecules within the filtrate, such as sugars, can be resorbed in the tubules and returned to the plasma as needed to maintain homeostasis. In the electron micrograph, note the central electron-dense layer (lamina densa) of the glomerular basement membrane covered by lighter, more electron-lucent inner and outer layers (lamina rara interna and lamina rara externa, respectively). The small spaces visible between foot processes of visceral epithelial cells (podocytes) are filtration slits, through which plasma filtrate passes into the uriniferous space. Scale bar in the electron micrograph (lower right corner) = 500 μm in length. (Courtesy Drs. M.A. Breshears and A.W. Confer, Center for Veterinary Health Sciences, Oklahoma State University; and Dr. J.F. Zachary, College of Veterinary Medicine, University of Illinois. Electron photomicrograph courtesy Dr. A.G. Armien, Diagnostic Ultrastructural Pathology Service, College of Veterinary Medicine, University of Minnesota.)

tubules are linked by the loop of Henle, which is divided into a descending and an ascending limb. The wall of the descending limb and initial portion of the ascending limb is thin (permeable), whereas the cortical portion of the ascending limb is thick (impermeable). Microscopically, the proximal tubule is lined by columnar epithelial cells that have a microvillous (brush) border. This arrangement greatly increases their absorptive surface, and their numerous intracellular mitochondria supply energy for the various secretory and absorptive functions. Distal tubules, collecting tubules, and the loop of Henle are lined by cuboidal epithelial cells that contribute to the concentration of urine by absorptive and secretory activities.

Interstitium

Macroscopically, the interstitium consists of a relatively scant fibrovascular connective tissue stroma, primarily present as a fine reticular meshwork found around and between uriniferous tubules. Microscopically, renal interstitium is composed of fibroblasts, connective tissue, and extracellular matrix that provide most of the interstitial tissue support. Glycosaminoglycans secreted as part of the extracellular matrix (ECM) increase with age and ischemic damage. Cells in the interstitium, particularly in the medulla, are responsible for local production of prostaglandins. Blood vessels, nerves, and lymphatic vessels are present in the renal interstitium.

Vasculature

Macroscopically, knowledge of the normal renal blood supply is important in understanding the pathogenesis and distribution of various renal lesions, especially renal infarcts. Kidneys receive blood primarily through the renal artery. An interlobar artery extends along the boundary of each renal lobe (renal column) and then branches at right angles to form an arcuate artery that runs along the corticomedullary junction (Fig. 11-7). Interlobular arteries branch from the arcuate artery and extend into the cortex. They have no anastomoses, making them susceptible to focal ischemic necrosis (infarct) as in any organ with end arteries.

Microscopically, interlobular arteries have small branches that become afferent glomerular arterioles, which enter the renal corpuscle and subsequently exit at the vascular pole as efferent glomerular arterioles (see Fig. 11-7). Efferent arterioles supply the blood for the extensive network of capillaries that surround the cortical and medullary tubular system of the kidneys, known as the *peritubular capillary network*. The latter surrounds cortical segments of the tubules and then drains into the interlobular vein, arcuate vein, interlobar vein, and ultimately the renal vein. In addition, the vasa recta are formed from the deeper portions of the peritubular capillary network and descend into the medulla and around the lower portions of the loop of Henle before ascending to the cortex and emptying into venous vessels that connect to the interlobular and arcuate veins. The vasa recta parallel the descending and ascending limbs of the loop of Henle and the collecting ducts (see Fig. 11-7). Therefore the blood supply to the tubules depends on passage through the glomerular vessels.

Function

The kidney has the following five basic functions:

- Formation of urine for the purpose of elimination of metabolic wastes.
- Acid-base regulation, predominantly through reclamation of bicarbonate from the glomerular filtrate.
- Conservation of water through reabsorption by the proximal convoluted tubules, the countercurrent mechanism of the loop of Henle, antidiuretic hormone (ADH) activity in the distal tubules, and the urea gradient in the medulla. The tubular system is capable of absorbing up to 99% of the water in the glomerular filtrate.
- Maintenance of normal extracellular potassium ion concentration through passive reabsorption in the proximal tubules and tubular secretion in the distal tubules under the influence of aldosterone.
- Control of endocrine function through three hormonal axes: renin-angiotensin-aldosterone (see Fig. 12-14, A), most important, but also erythropoietin and vitamin D. Erythropoietin, produced in the kidneys in response to reduced oxygen tension, is released into the blood and stimulates bone marrow to produce erythrocytes. Vitamin D is converted in the kidneys to its most active form (1,25-dihydroxycholecalciferol [calcitriol]), which facilitates calcium absorption by the intestine.

Glomerular Basement Membrane

The GBM is structurally adept at separating substances based on size and charge. In addition, the glomerulus is equipped with its own

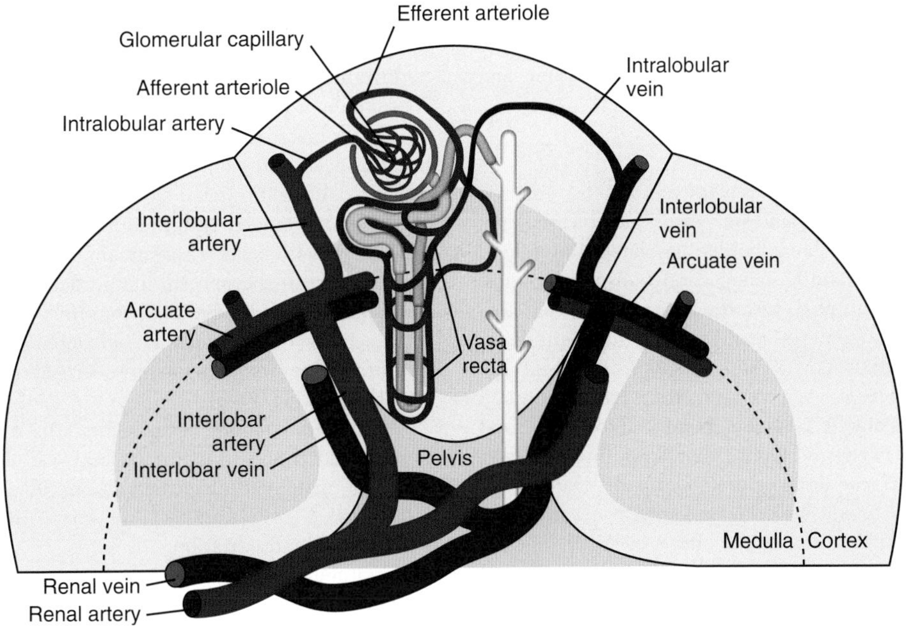

Figure 11-7 Vasculature of the Kidney. The interlobar artery branches at right angles at the corticomedullary junction to give rise to arcuate arteries that in turn branch to form interlobular arteries that extend into the cortex. Interlobular arteries give rise to smaller branches (intralobular arteries), eventually forming glomerular afferent arterioles that enter the glomerular capillary tuft and then exit at the glomerular vascular pole as efferent arterioles. The peritubular capillary network (including vasa recta) is supplied by efferent glomerular arterioles before emptying into the venous system, beginning as intralobular veins and progressing toward interlobular veins, arcuate veins, and interlobar veins before finally draining through the renal vein. (Courtesy Drs. M.A. Breshears and A.W. Confer, Center for Veterinary Health Sciences, Oklahoma State University; and Dr. J.F. Zachary, College of Veterinary Medicine, University of Illinois.)

specialized mesangial cells, a component of the monocyte-macrophage system (see Figs. 11-5 and 11-6; also see E-Figs. 11-5 and 11-6). Both size-dependent and charge-dependent filtration are possible because of the porous structure of capillary walls, which is a function of endothelial fenestrations, laminin, polyanionic proteoglycans, fibronectin, entactin and other glycoproteins, and filtration slits between adjacent visceral epithelium. Thus the normal glomerulus restricts many proteins and charged molecules from being filtered into the uriniferous (Bowman's) space and proximal tubular lumen whereby allowing permeability to water, proteins <70 kDa, and small solutes. The fluid that filters through the glomerulus into the urinary space is called *glomerular filtrate*, and it arises after passage through the glomerular filtration barrier. This ultrafiltrate of plasma (primary urine), which contains water, salts, ions, glucose, and albumin, passes into the uriniferous space and then empties into the proximal convoluted tubule at the urinary pole to traverse through and be acted on by the tubular system.

In addition to the principal glomerular function of plasma filtration, glomerular functions also include regulation of blood pressure by means of secreting vasopressor agents and/or hormones, regulation of peritubular blood flow, regulation of tubular metabolism, and removal of macromolecules from circulation by the glomerular mesangium. Integral to these functions is the juxtaglomerular apparatus, which functions in tubuloglomerular feedback by autoregulating renal blood flow and glomerular filtration rate. The juxtaglomerular apparatus is composed of four components: (1) an afferent arteriole whose smooth muscle is modified to form myoepithelial cells, which are the juxtaglomerular cells that secrete renin; (2) an efferent arteriole; (3) the macula densa; and (4) the extraglomerular mesangium. Renin, produced by cells of the juxtaglomerular apparatus, stimulates the production of angiotensin I from circulating angiotensinogen. The angiotensin-converting enzyme in the macula densa converts angiotensin I to angiotensin II, which then functions to constrict afferent renal arterioles; maintain renal blood pressure; stimulate aldosterone secretion from the adrenal gland, thus increasing sodium (Na^+) reabsorption; and stimulate ADH release (see Fig. 12-14, A). ADH principally increases the permeability of collecting tubules to water and increases the permeability of the medullary region to urea.

Proximal Tubules

A key function of the proximal tubules is to reabsorb Na^+, chloride (Cl^-), potassium (K^+), albumin, glucose, water, and bicarbonate. This is facilitated by luminal brush border, basolateral infoldings, magnesium-dependent Na^+ and K^+ pumps, and transport proteins. The proximal tubule is continuous with the loop of Henle that is in close physiologic and anatomic association with the peritubular capillary network (within the cortex) and the vasa recta (within the medulla). The loop of Henle, via a countercurrent mechanism and Na^+/K^+-adenosine phosphatase (ATPase) pumps, absorbs Na^+ and Cl^- ions, producing a hypotonic filtrate that flows into the next portion of the nephron—the distal convoluted tubule. Here, water is reabsorbed from the tubule into the interstitium because of a solute concentration gradient and by the effects of ADH. The filtrate is further concentrated in the collecting ducts by water and sodium reabsorption by a Na^+/K^+-ATPase pump and additional water reabsorption into the medullary interstitium by a urea gradient. Intercalated cells of the collecting tubule regulate acid-base balance and reabsorb potassium. Thus the final excretory product, urine, is formed.

Renal Failure (Loss of Function). Renal failure occurs when one or more of the functions previously listed are altered. When renal functional capacity is abruptly impaired approximately 75% or more, such that the kidneys fail to carry out their normal metabolic and endocrine functions, acute renal failure can ensue. It is important to remember that the glomerulus, tubules, collecting ducts, and capillary blood supply in each nephron are closely interrelated, both anatomically and functionally. Alterations in tubular structure or function influence glomerular structure and function and vice versa. For example, necrosis or atrophy of renal tubules results in loss of function of the affected nephrons and secondary atrophy of the glomerulus. In addition, because most of the capillary blood supply to tubules is through postglomerular capillaries, a reduction in glomerular blood flow consequently reduces the blood supply to the tubules.

Acute Renal Failure. Acute renal failure can be caused by (1) tubular necrosis from infectious microbes, such as bacteria (*Leptospira* spp., *Escherichia coli*, *Streptococcus* spp., *Staphylococcus* spp., and *Proteus* spp.) or viruses (infectious canine hepatitis virus and canine herpesvirus); (2) obstructive nephropathy from urolithiasis, transitional cell neoplasms of the lower urinary system, or trauma; (3) renal ischemia with tubular necrosis from occlusive vasculitis/vasculopathy caused by bacteria, bacterial toxins, or tumor emboli; (4) tubular necrosis from nephrotoxic drugs, such as aminoglycoside-based antimicrobial drugs or antineoplastic drugs; and/or (5) tubular necrosis from chemicals, such as ethylene glycol and heavy metals.

Functionally, acute renal failure can be caused by prerenal (compromised renal perfusion), intrarenal (compromised kidney function), or postrenal (obstruction of the urinary tract) factors. Prerenal factors include reduced renal blood flow, whether secondary to circulatory collapse (shock, severe hypovolemia) or local obstruction of vascular supply (thrombus or lodgment of embolus). Acute tubular necrosis, a form of intrarenal acute renal failure, induces clinical oliguria (decrease in urine production) or anuria (absence of urine production) by one or several mechanisms. These mechanisms include the following:

- Leakage of tubular ultrafiltrate from damaged tubules across disrupted basement membranes into the renal interstitium
- Intratubular obstruction resulting from sloughed necrotic epithelium

The latter mechanism is less well accepted, but both mechanisms result in decreased glomerular filtration rate.

Prerenal and intrarenal factors are most responsible for episodes of acute renal failure, with prerenal azotemia and ischemic tubular damage actually being a continuum. Postrenal obstructive diseases are discussed in the lower urinary tract section. Intrarenal disease can target tubules by the following three main mechanisms:

- Ascending disease, such as pyelonephritis
- Intraluminal toxic metabolites derived from glomerular filtrate
- Ischemia (Fig. 11-8)

Acute renal failure occurs when the kidney fails to excrete waste products and to maintain fluid and electrolyte homeostasis. The four main pathologic alterations in acute renal failure are as follows:

- Decreased ultrafiltration
- Intratubular obstruction
- Fluid back leak
- Intrarenal vasoconstriction

These alterations can occur after many insults, including the following:

- Decreased renal perfusion
- Decreased glomerular filtration
- Ischemic tubular damage
- Toxic tubular damage

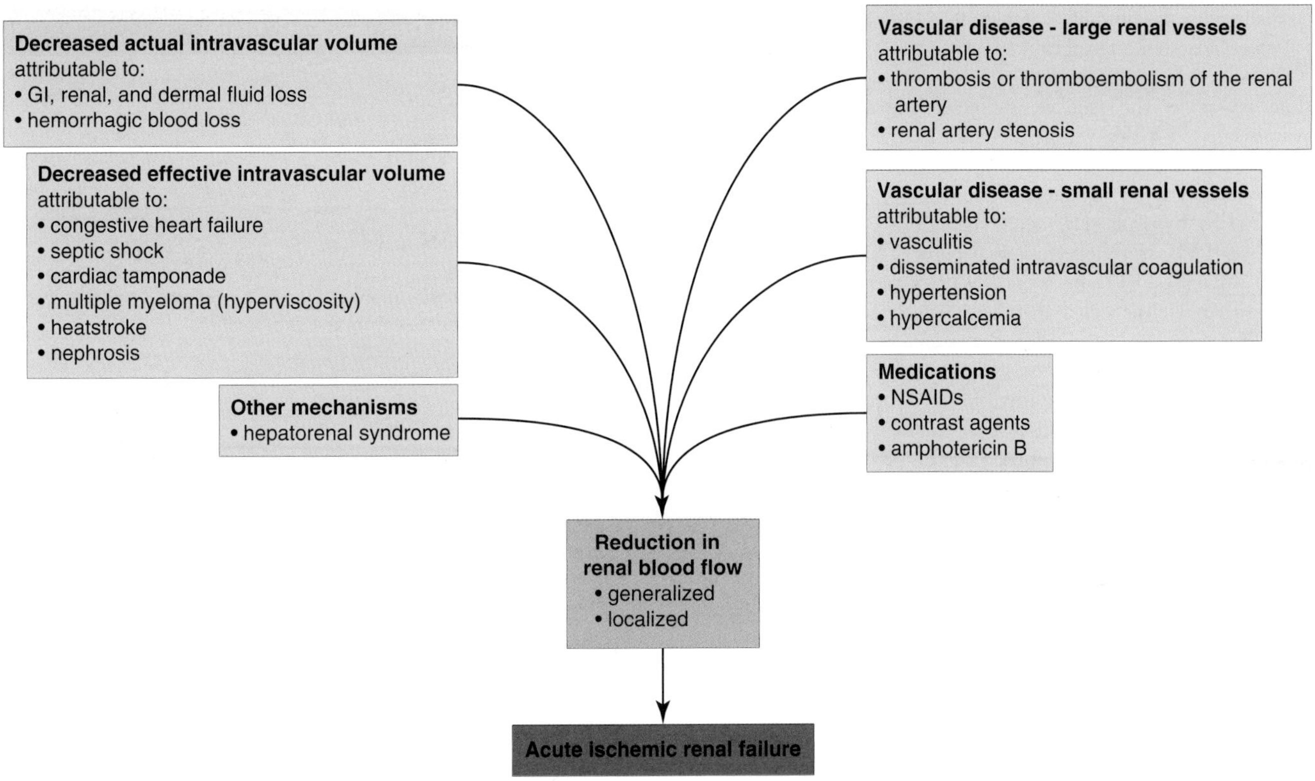

Figure 11-8 **Proposed Mechanisms of Acute Ischemic Renal Failure.** A wide spectrum of clinical conditions can result in a generalized or localized reduction in renal blood flow, thus increasing the likelihood of acute ischemic renal failure. Kidney ischemia and acute renal failure are often the result of a combination of factors. Decreased renal perfusion may be due to hypovolemia, decreased cardiac output, medications that alter blood flow, and vascular disease. (Courtesy Drs. M.A. Breshears and A.W. Confer, Center for Veterinary Health Sciences, Oklahoma State University; and Dr. J.F. Zachary, College of Veterinary Medicine, University of Illinois.)

- Obstructive renal tubular damage
- Tubulointerstitial inflammation, edema, or fibrosis

Animals that die of acute renal failure often do so because of the cardiotoxicity of elevated serum potassium, metabolic acidosis, and/or pulmonary edema. Hyperkalemia results from decreased filtration, decreased tubular secretion, and decreased tubular sodium transport. Cell lysis and the extracellular shift of fluid in acidic environments also contribute to the increased serum potassium concentrations. These alterations are reflected clinically by signs such as oliguria or anuria, vomiting and diarrhea, and ammoniacal-smelling breath, and an array of nonrenal lesions described later and can be detected and monitored with biochemical tests of serum, plasma, and urine for azotemia and uremia.

Azotemia and Uremia. Assays for plasma or serum concentrations of urea, creatinine, and the nitrogenous waste products of protein catabolism are routinely used as indices of diminished renal function. The intravascular increase of these nitrogenous waste products is referred to as *azotemia*. Renal failure can result in the following:

- Intravascular accumulation of other metabolic wastes such as guanidines, phenolic acids, and large-molecular-weight alcohols (e.g., myoinositol)
- Reduced blood pH (metabolic acidosis)
- Alterations in plasma ion concentrations, particularly potassium, calcium, and phosphate
- Hypertension

The result and pathologic manifestations of renal failure are a toxicosis called *uremia*. Uremia can therefore be defined as a syndrome associated with multisystemic lesions and clinical signs because of renal failure. These multisystemic lesions are discussed in greater detail in the section on Kidney and Lower Urinary Tract, Disorders of Domestic Animals.

Chronic Renal Failure. Chronic renal failure usually results from progressive renal disease with loss of nephrons and severe scarring. The pathogenesis of the underlying renal lesion can be unknown and slowly progressive or can be scarring resulting from an acute insult (see Renal Fibrosis [Scarring]). Severely scarred kidneys lack the ability to concentrate urine, resulting in polyuria and polydipsia. Anorexia with chronic progressive weight loss commonly occurs as well as other signs of uremia, such as vomiting and seizures. In the diseased kidney, production of erythropoietin, a stimulant of erythropoietic maturation, is reduced and contributes to nonregenerative anemia, as does uremia-associated increased erythrocytic fragility. Most animals in renal failure have hyperphosphatemia and low to normal calcium concentrations, although variations exist, depending on species and stage of the disease. Alterations in calcium-phosphorus metabolism in the uremic animal are a hallmark of chronic renal failure and result from a complex set of events as outlined in the following:

- When the glomerular filtration rate is chronically reduced to less than 25% of normal, phosphorus is no longer adequately secreted by the kidneys and hyperphosphatemia results.
- Because of the mass law interactions between serum calcium and phosphorus, ionized calcium concentration in serum is reduced as a result of precipitation of calcium and phosphorus.
- Reduced ionized serum calcium concentration stimulates parathyroid hormone (PTH) secretion, causing calcium release from

the readily mobilizable calcium stores in the bone and from osteoclastic bone resorption.

These changes in calcium-phosphorus metabolism are made more severe by the reduced ability of the diseased kidneys to hydroxylate 25-hydroxycholecalciferol to the more active 1,25-dihydroxycholecalciferol (calcitriol), resulting in decreased intestinal absorption of calcium. Calcitriol production is further inhibited by hyperphosphatemia. In addition, calcitriol normally suppresses PTH secretion; therefore reduced calcitriol production further increases PTH secretion. With time, these events lead to parathyroid chief cell hyperplasia (renal secondary hyperparathyroidism), fibrous osteodystrophy (renal osteodystrophy), and soft tissue calcification.

Renal secondary hyperparathyroidism is further thought to perpetuate and enhance renal disease by stimulating nephrocalcinosis (see Fig. 11-25; also see Chapter 12), the process by which renal tubular epithelium is damaged by an increase in intracellular calcium. Calcium is precipitated in mitochondria and in tubular basement membranes. Soft tissue calcification associated with uremia occurs in numerous sites and represents both dystrophic and metastatic calcification. These lesions are discussed in greater detail in the section on Kidney and Lower Urinary Tract, Disorders of Domestic Animals.

Dysfunction/Responses to Injury

The response of the urinary system to injury is the response of each of its components—kidney, ureter, bladder, and urethra—to injury. In addition, components within the kidney, such as the glomeruli, tubules, interstitium, and vasculature, have their own unique responses to injury. Responses to injury are described sequentially in this section and are summarized in Box 11-1.

Box 11-1 Renal Responses to Injury

GLOMERULI
- Acute inflammation
- Endothelial proliferation
- Hypertrophy
- Inclusion bodies
- Necrosis
- Mesangial cell proliferation
- Amyloid deposition
- Glomerular cell proliferation
- Glomerular basement membrane proliferation
- Increased vascular permeability
- Atrophy of the glomerular tuft
- Fibrosis of the glomerular tuft

TUBULES
- Cell degeneration
- Cell necrosis
- Basement membrane rupture
- Basement membrane thickening
- Cell regeneration
- Renal fibrosis

INTERSTITIUM
- Hyperemia
- Edema
- Inflammation
- Fibrosis

VASCULATURE
- Hyperemia and congestion
- Hemorrhage and thrombosis
- Embolic nephritis
- Infarction

Kidney

The functional unit of the kidney is the nephron, and damage to any component of the nephron (renal corpuscle and tubules) results in diminished function and progressive damage to the kidney. Renal disease can be best summarized by dividing it into general tissue responses that affect the primary anatomic components: glomeruli, tubules, interstitium, and vasculature. In the early stages of disease, specific anatomic components may be targeted by specific insults: glomeruli in immune-mediated disease and tubules in toxin-induced necrosis. However, in the more chronic stages of disease, the kidney undergoes changes related to nephron loss that are not specific to the original cause but are considered common end-stage responses to any number of inciting injurious stimuli.

Renal Corpuscle. Primary glomerular damage often occurs as a result of deposition of immune complexes, entrapment of thromboemboli and bacterial emboli, or direct viral or bacterial infection of glomerular components. Such insults are reflected morphologically by necrosis, thickening of membranes, or infiltration of leukocytes, and they are reflected functionally by reduced vascular perfusion. Continued or severe injury can result in chronic changes characterized at first by atrophy and fibrosis of the glomerular tuft (sclerosis) and secondarily by atrophy of renal tubules resulting in loss of function of the entire nephron. Similarly, chronic glomerular changes can result from reduced blood flow or chronic loss of tubular function.

Damage to the glomerular filtration barrier can result from several causes and produce a variety of clinical signs. The major clinical finding of glomerular disease is the leakage of various low-molecular-weight (small molecule size) proteins, such as albumin, into the glomerular filtrate. As a result, large quantities of albumin overload the protein reabsorption capabilities of the proximal convoluted tubular epithelium such that protein-rich glomerular filtrate accumulates in the variably dilated tubular lumina, and protein subsequently appears in the urine. Renal diseases that result in proteinuria are called *protein-losing nephropathies*. Protein-losing nephropathy is one of several causes of severe hypoproteinemia in animals. Prolonged, severe renal protein loss results in hypoproteinemia, reduced plasma colloid osmotic (oncotic) pressure, and loss of antithrombin III. These changes can lead to the *nephrotic syndrome*, which is further characterized by generalized edema, ascites, pleural effusion, and hypercholesterolemia.

The functions of the glomerulus listed in the following are affected by processes that injure it in disease:

- Plasma ultrafiltration
- Blood pressure regulation
- Peritubular blood flow regulation
- Tubular metabolism regulation
- Circulating macromolecule removal

The pathophysiologic mechanisms of glomerular injury from infectious or chemical insults have been summarized by the following three theories:

- Intact nephron hypothesis
- Hyperfiltration hypothesis
- The theory of complex deposition

The intact nephron hypothesis proposes that damage to any portion of the nephron affects the entire nephron function. This is seen when glomerular damage interferes with peritubular blood flow and results in decreased tubular resorption or secretion. Not all nephron damage is irreversible; for example, renal tubular epithelium can regenerate but whole nephrons are not capable of regeneration. Thus the outcomes for the nephrons vary from hypertrophy to repair.

Unlike the intact nephron hypothesis, the hyperfiltration hypothesis helps explain the progressive nature of glomerular disease. Glomerular hyperfiltration is a result of increased hydrostatic pressure that damages delicate glomerular capillaries and in cases of prolonged hypertension produces a sustained deleterious effect on the glomerulus, ultimately resulting in glomerulosclerosis. Increased dietary protein can produce a transient increase in glomerular hyperfiltration and if persistent can result in glomerulosclerosis. There may be a species effect because dogs that undergo experimental hyperfiltration are much less prone to development of progressive glomerular disease than are rats.

The theory of complex deposition is derived from the fact that glomeruli are the primary site for removal of macromolecules (principally immune complex) from the circulation, even when those complexes are in small quantities and nonpathogenic. Complexes may be deposited in subepithelial, subendothelial, or mesangial locations. These immune complexes are capable of triggering a sequence of inflammatory responses including the following:

- Recruitment and localization of inflammatory cells at the site
- Release of inflammatory mediators and enzymes
- Destruction of glomerular structures such as the basement membrane
- Further compromise of nephron function
- Continuing damage by altered transglomerular hyperfiltration and perfusion shifts between nephron populations, so the less affected become overworked and succumb to the same fate

Kidney lesions differ slightly, depending on the duration of the glomerular disease. Acute disease may be identified by pallor of the parenchyma and accentuation of the glomerular tufts as fine red dots. Accompanying petechial hemorrhages may be noted. In the more chronic stage, the kidney can be shrunken and show a fine granularity to the cortical cut section. The capsule may be adherent.

Tubules

Renal tubular epithelial cells can respond to injury by undergoing degeneration, necrosis, apoptosis, and/or atrophy. The basement membrane can respond by rupturing or thickening. Tubular disease occurs as a result of tubular epithelial damage from the following:

- Blood-borne infections
- Ascending infections (intratubular pathogens)
- Direct damage from toxins (intratubular effects)
- Ischemia, infarction

When nephrons are lost because of injury, remaining tubules can undergo compensatory hypertrophy in an attempt to maintain overall renal function, but there is no regeneration of entire nephrons. In many instances of tubular epithelial cell necrosis, particularly as a response to toxins, tubular epithelium has an incredible capacity to regenerate and contribute to restoration of function, providing the tubular basement membrane scaffolding remains intact. Severe damage to or loss of tubular basement membranes, as occurs after ischemic damage, results in necrosis and loss of tubular segments, failure of functional repair, and permanent loss of function of the entire nephron, despite the potential for tubular epithelial hyperplasia.

Atrophy. Tubular atrophy can occur secondary to the following:

- External compression of tubule by a space-occupying mass, neoplasm, or abscess
- Interstitial fibrosis as the end result of ischemia
- Intratubular obstruction and backpressure
- Diminished glomerular perfusion and filtration
- Reduced oxygen tension such as with hypoxia

If the insult to the renal tubules is not lethal and is removed, some forms of acute tubular degeneration are reversible. The success of reparative regeneration is affected by several variables, including severity of degeneration.

Apoptosis. When cells undergo programmed cell death (apoptosis), they do not usually stimulate inflammatory responses. Therefore, if small numbers of tubular epithelium undergo apoptosis, a reepithelization of the tubular epithelial lining is accomplished efficiently by adjacent viable tubular epithelial cells, which by mitotic division fill the epithelial gap. The cells that are lost slough into the lumen to form cellular casts within the lumens of renal tubules.

Acute Tubular Degeneration. More severe generalized loss of tubular epithelial lining cells is repaired by proliferation of the remaining viable epithelial cells over an intact tubular basement membrane to form a low cuboidal rather than a mature columnar epithelial lining. This appears as an ectatic proximal tubule. Restitution of renal function eventually results, despite the presence of replacement low cuboidal epithelium, which is not identical to the tubular lining cell (with microvilli) present before the injury. The exact mechanism of this return to function is not entirely known. The main determinant of this regenerative ability is the viability of tubular basement membranes, which are retained more consistently after toxic rather than ischemic insults.

Tubular Regeneration. Because the regenerative process is reliant on many factors for its success, things often go awry. Examples of adverse outcomes include the following:

- Focal loss of basement membrane scaffolding allows a bulge defect to occur where the regenerative population of proliferating tubular epithelial cells coalesces to form well-differentiated syncytial cells (giant cells) at certain levels of the tubule.
- Regenerative epithelial cells fail to regain all cytoplasmic structural aspects of the original columnar epithelial cells (e.g., microvilli and luminal enzymes) because of a failure to fully differentiate, and thus function may be affected.
- If there is excessive tubular epithelial loss, the potential for regeneration is lost and repair proceeds by replacement fibrosis and scarring.
- Reperfusion is necessary for cell viability following ischemia, but reperfusion injury occurs when activated endothelial cells produce proinflammatory mediators, such as reactive oxygen species, proteolytic enzymes, and cytokines, which result in further renal injury. Evidence indicates that epidermal growth factor secreted by distal convoluted tubules mediates the tubular repair process.

The sequence of events in tubular regeneration after necrosis has been well documented in experimental model systems using mercuric chloride in mice, rats, and rabbits. In that system, morphologic evidence of regeneration of proximal convoluted tubules is seen within 3 days after a toxic dose. At this time, basement membranes are partially covered with low cuboidal to flattened and elongated epithelial cells that are more basophilic than normal because of the increased concentrations of cytoplasmic ribosomes and rough endoplasmic reticulum producing protein for repair. Nuclei are hyperchromatic and mitotic figures are present. Regenerating tubules do not function normally because they lack both a brush border and normal tubular membrane function, and this is evident clinically as polyuria. Normal-appearing tubular epithelium subsequently reappears between 7 and 14 days after toxin exposure. Normal renal structure without residual evidence of tubular damage is restored between 21 and 56 days after exposure to the nephrotoxin. Similar periods for tubular regeneration have been described through sequential renal biopsies from human patients naturally exposed to inorganic mercury and in experimental systems using other nephrotoxins.

Acute Tubular Necrosis. Acute tubular necrosis is the single most important cause of acute renal failure. Acute tubular degeneration and necrosis, often referred to as *nephrosis, lower nephron nephrosis, tubular nephrosis, tubular dysfunction,* or *acute cortical necrosis,* is principally the result of nephrotoxic injury to the renal tubular epithelial cells or ischemia (Box 11-2). This was borne out by a study of cats with renal failure in which 18 of 32 cases were the result of nephrotoxin exposure and 4 of 32 cases were the result of ischemia.

Acute tubular necrosis induces clinical oliguria (decrease in urine production) or anuria (absence of urine production) by one or several mechanisms. These mechanisms include the following:

- Leakage of tubular ultrafiltrate from damaged tubules across disrupted basement membranes into the renal interstitium
- Intratubular obstruction resulting from sloughed necrotic epithelium

The latter mechanism is less well accepted, but both mechanisms result in decreased glomerular filtration rate.

Nephrotoxic Injury. Nephrotoxic injury can be caused by a large group of substances that are called *nephrotoxins*. They preferentially damage kidneys because (1) 20% to 25% of cardiac output goes to the kidney, (2) the substance is filtered into the urine by the glomerulus, and (3) the toxin or its metabolites within the renal tubular lumens are concentrated. Nephrotoxins can do the following:

- Directly damage renal epithelial cells, particularly those of the proximal convoluted tubules, after their intracellular conversion via enzyme pathways to reactive metabolites
- Produce reactive metabolites in the tubular filtrate, which can cause renal tubular epithelial necrosis after reabsorption
- Cause renal tubular epithelial necrosis after diffusion through the intertubular capillary walls and basement membranes into the tubule epithelial cell
- Indirectly stimulate vasoconstriction of the intertubular capillaries, thus causing ischemia, which further compromises renal function
- Result in nephrotoxin-associated ischemia

One of the first events in renal tubular cell damage is altered ion transport at the luminal surface (uptake). This process results in decreased sodium absorption and increased sodium ions in the lumens of the distal tubules, which stimulate the renin-angiotensin mechanism, causing vasoconstriction and reduced blood flow that result in ischemia and tubular cell damage. Nephrotoxins usually do not damage the tubular basement membranes, and if the toxin is removed, regeneration (repair) of tubules can occur in an orderly and expeditious manner. The intact basement membrane acts as a scaffold over which regenerating epithelial cells may slide. Exposure to a variety of nephrotoxins, either from the vasculature (including certain chemicals [glycolaldehyde, glycolic acid, and glyoxylic acid]) or from the tubular lumen (including certain antibiotics [aminoglycosides], pigments [hemoglobin], metals [lead], or chemicals [ethylene glycol–induced calcium oxalate crystals]), or their metabolites cause cells to undergo degeneration followed by necrosis and desquamation into the tubular lumen.

Cell death results from decreased adenosine triphosphate (ATP) production, which is central to many of the secondary metabolic derangements, including calcium ion influx, purine depletion, metabolic acidosis, and generation of oxygen radicals. Increased intracellular calcium is associated with degenerative changes in renal tubular cells, smooth muscle cells, and mesangial cells. Oxygen radicals activate phospholipase, which subsequently increases membrane permeability. Because mitochondrial respiration is disrupted, further cell membrane damage occurs.

Hypoxic or Ischemic Injury (Tubulorrhexis). Notably reduced renal perfusion from any cause can result in tubular necrosis. Severe hypotension associated with shock results in preglomerular vasoconstriction and reduced glomerular filtration. The resulting renal ischemia can produce sublethal tubular cell injury and dysfunction or

Box 11-2 Causes of Ischemic Acute Renal Failure in Small Animals

INTRAVASCULAR VOLUME DEPLETION
Dehydration
Vomiting
Diarrhea
Sequestration or shock
Thermal burns
Blood loss
Trauma
Surgery
Hypoalbuminemia
Hypoadrenocorticism
Hyponatremia (nondilutional)

DECREASED CARDIAC OUTPUT
Congestive heart failure
Low output
Restrictive pericardial disease
Tamponade
Arrhythmia
Positive-pressure ventilation
Prolonged resuscitation after cardiac arrest

INCREASED BLOOD VISCOSITY
Multiple myeloma
Polycythemia (absolute or relative)

ALTERED RENAL AND SYSTEMIC VASCULAR RESISTANCES
Renal vasoconstriction
Circulating catecholamines
Renal sympathetic nervous stimulation
Vasopressin
Angiotensin II
Hypercalcemia
Amphotericin B
Hypothermia
Myoglobinuria
Hemoglobinuria
Systemic vasodilation
Arteriolar or mixed vasodilator therapy
Anaphylaxis
Gaseous anesthesia
Sepsis
Heatstroke

INTERFERENCE WITH RENAL AUTOREGULATION DURING HYPOTENSION
Nonsteroidal antiinflammatory drugs

WARM OR COLD ISCHEMIA

Modified from Chew D, DiBartola S: Diagnosis and pathophysiology of renal disease. In Ettinger SJ, editor: *Textbook of veterinary internal medicine*, ed 7, vol 2, Philadelphia, 2010, Saunders.

cause cell death by necrosis or apoptosis. Following less severe insults and within different portions of the renal tubule, apoptosis may occur in lieu of necrosis. The apoptotic pathway can be triggered by the following:

- Binding of ligands to the tumor necrosis factor (TNF) superfamily
- Deficiency of cellular growth factors
- Imbalance between proapoptotic and antiapoptotic oncogenes
- Alteration of other mediators of apoptotic signaling pathways such as reactive oxygen metabolites, caspases, and ceramide

Proximal tubular epithelium has a microvillous border, which amplifies absorptive surface area and cellular junctional complexes that structurally polarize the cell so that membrane phospholipids and specialized proteins remain in the appropriate domains. The integrity of these cellular structures is critical to absorption and secretion. Early structural changes after ischemic insult include formation of apical blebs, loss of brush border, loss of cellular polarity, disruption of tight junctions, and sloughing of cells, which result in intratubular cast formation (E-Fig. 11-1).

Damage to the cellular cytoskeleton modifies cell polarity, cell-to-cell interactions, and cell-matrix interactions. Initially, ischemic damage modifies cell polarity by disruption of the terminal web and disassembly of the microvillar actin cores. This is followed by conversion of G actin to F actin and its redistribution from the apical cell component to form diffuse aggregates throughout the cytoplasm (E-Figs. 11-2 and 11-3). Cells are attached to each other by junctional complexes, tight junctions, and adherens junctions and to the ECM by integrins. Several mechanisms contribute to tight junction disruption, which is manifested as alteration in cellular permeability and cell polarity. The contributing mechanisms include redistribution of membrane lipids and proteins, such as Na^+/K^+-ATPase, to the apical membrane after alteration of the actin cytoskeleton and redistribution of integrins to the apical cell surface so that cell desquamation occurs. The former results in deranged sodium handling by the proximal tubular cell.

Animals with severe tubular necrosis have accompanying functional derangements of vascular, tubular, and/or glomerular origin. Vascular derangements include the following:

- Afferent arteriolar constriction
- Efferent arteriolar dilation
- Loss of autoregulation of renal blood flow

Prolonged ischemia can produce a paradoxic response of the autoregulatory system, where increased glomerular capillary resistance from tubular fluid stasis results in activation of afferent arteriolar vasoconstriction. Decreased production of or response to vasodilative factors, such as prostaglandin and atrial natriuretic peptide, also contribute. Afferent arteriole vasoconstriction, back leak of fluid, and tubular obstruction account for decreased glomerular filtration rate (GFR) (Fig. 11-9).

Tubuloglomerular feedback is the mechanism by which GFR is matched to the solute load and the solute handling characteristics of the tubules. Because of altered sodium handling, increased concentrations reach the macula densa, and activation of the renin-angiotensin system occurs. This is followed by intrarenal vasoconstriction, particularly affecting outer cortical nephrons, and results in decreased glomerular blood flow, decreased filtration, and reduced formation of urine.

Gross Lesions of Acute Tubular Necrosis. On gross examination, the recognition of acute tubular necrosis is often difficult. Nevertheless, initially the cortex is swollen, pale mahogany to beige, and with a slightly translucent smooth, thinned, capsular surface. The cut surface of the renal cortex bulges and is excessively moist; striations are muted or accentuated by radially oriented opaque, white streaks, presumably related to the stage of the necrosis, with coagulation necrosis being responsible for the white streaks. The medulla is either pale or diffusely congested.

Microscopic Lesions of Acute Tubular Necrosis. The microscopic appearance of kidneys with acute tubular necrosis varies, depending on the following:

- The extent of the tubular necrosis
- The duration of exposure to the damaging agent
- The length of time between the injury and death—in other words, the stage of necrosis or dissolution of necrotic epithelium

Initially, tubular necrosis is randomly distributed in nephrons, but the proximal convoluted tubules are most severely affected because of their high metabolic demands and first line of exposure (Fig. 11-10). Prolonged ischemia can produce necrosis of epithelium of the proximal and distal convoluted tubules, the loops of Henle, and the collecting ducts throughout the cortex and, to a lesser extent, the medulla. Glomeruli are resistant to ischemia and often remain morphologically normal, even when ischemia is prolonged. Initially, proximal tubular epithelium is swollen, and the cytoplasm is vacuolated or granular and intensely eosinophilic, all features indicative of necrosis (Fig. 11-11). In such cells, the nuclear changes are pyknosis, karyorrhexis, or karyolysis. Necrotic tubular epithelium is subsequently sloughed into tubular lumens resulting in dilated, notably hypocellular tubules that contain necrotic cellular debris and hyalinized or granular casts.

A characteristic histologic lesion of ischemic tubular necrosis is possible disruption of the tubular basement membranes, referred to as tubulorrhexis (Fig. 11-12). Tubular repair in these kidneys is imperfect because regenerating epithelial cells do not have their normal scaffolding. Tubules that remain in an affected site are less functional in resorption, can be dilated and lined by flattened epithelium, or are notably atrophic, appearing shrunken with a collapsed lumen lined by flattened epithelium and fail to heal completely by regeneration, resulting in tubular atrophy.

Miscellaneous Responses to Injury of Renal Tubules

Lipofuscinosis. Fine golden granules of brown iron-free pigment with the staining characteristics of lipofuscin ("wear and tear pigment") can accumulate in renal epithelial cells of old cattle and in striated muscle, resulting in lipofuscinosis. Grossly, the renal cortex can have streaks of brown discoloration, but renal function is not affected. Microscopically, the accumulations are noted most prominently within the proximal convoluted epithelial cells. The direct cause is not known, but it is suspected that accumulations result from previous cell membrane breakdown and subsequent storage of end-product in the tubular epithelial cells.

Hydropic Degeneration. Hydropic degeneration and cloudy swelling are traditional names often used to define renal tubular degenerative changes seen during the pathologic process of acute cellular swelling. Acute cellular swelling is a potentially reversible change resulting from cell membrane, sodium/potassium pump, and cell energy breakdown with increased intracellular sodium ions and water. Although rare in the kidney, a severe hydropic degeneration of the proximal convoluted tubules and the ascending loop of Henle has been observed after intravenous administration of hypertonic solutions such as dextrose.

Glycogenic Degeneration. Abundant cytoplasmic vacuolation of tubular epithelium of the outer medulla and inner cortex is seen in dogs and cats with diabetes mellitus. Glycogen can be demonstrated as the accumulating compound within the cells of the ascending limb. Treatment with insulin relieves the deposition. The change is not thought to affect renal function.

Fat. In cats, proximal tubular epithelial cell cytoplasm is usually expanded by accumulations of cytoplasmic lipid resulting in the

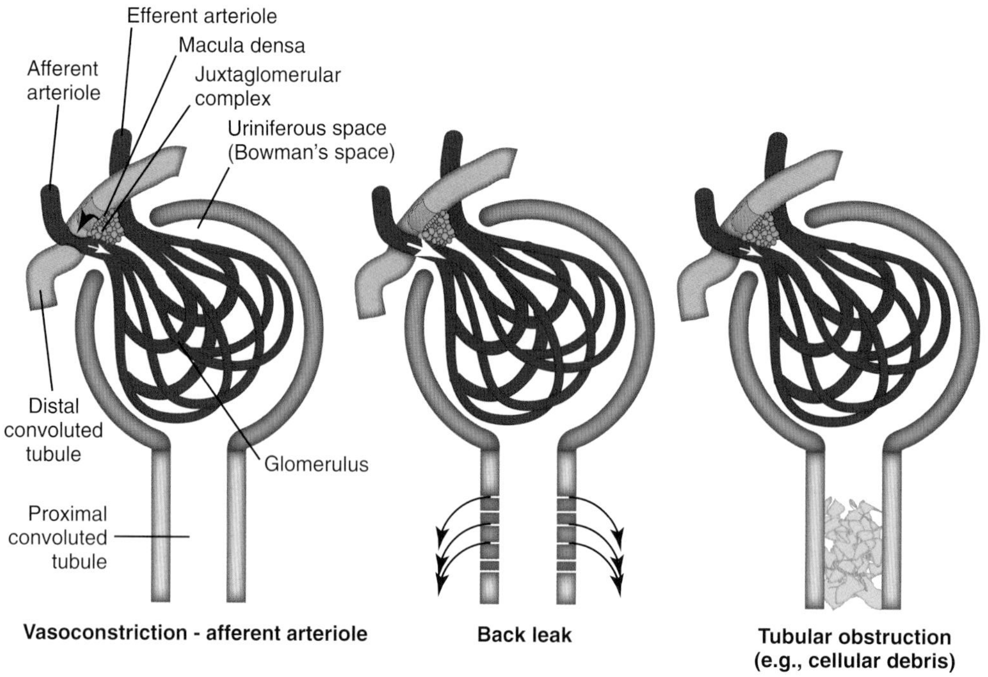

Figure 11-9 **Mechanisms of Decreased Glomerular Filtration Rate (GFR) During Ischemic Acute Renal Failure.** Proposed mechanisms for the decrease in GFR that occurs during ischemic acute renal failure include afferent arteriole vasoconstriction, back leak of glomerular filtrate, and tubular obstruction. All three of these mechanisms relate to ischemia-induced alterations in proximal tubule epithelial cells. Deranged proximal tubule handling of sodium leads to a high delivery of sodium to the macula densa, which in turn causes afferent arteriole vasoconstriction via tubuloglomerular feedback. Afferent arteriole vasoconstriction reduces glomerular capillary pressure and therefore GFR. Altered cell-cell adhesion results in an open tight junction that leads to increased paracellular permeability and subsequent back leak of glomerular filtrate from the tubular lumen into the extracellular space and ultimately into the bloodstream. Disrupted cell-matrix adhesion and abnormal cell-cell adhesion leads to cellular cast formation, which obstructs the tubular lumen and causes increased tubular pressure resulting in diminished or no GFR. (Courtesy Drs. M.A. Breshears and A.W. Confer, Center for Veterinary Health Sciences, Oklahoma State University; and Dr. J.F. Zachary, College of Veterinary Medicine, University of Illinois.)

usual pale, golden color of their kidneys. In dogs, tubular epithelial fat occurs, but it is much less common compared to cats and is usually restricted to the inner cortex. This site is a normal storage location and microscopically is recognized as large clearings within the renal tubular epithelial cells, most prominently in the proximal tubules. There is not thought to be any significant alteration to renal function.

Hemosiderin and Ferritin. Pigment can be present in the renal tubules. The origin of hemosiderin pigment is most likely from degradation of hemoglobin resorbed from the glomerular filtrate by proximal tubular epithelium. However, a history or concurrent lesions of a prior hemolytic crisis are often lacking. In dogs, microscopic granules of hemosiderin are frequent incidental findings in the cytoplasm of proximal convoluted tubular epithelial cells in kidneys that are otherwise normal.

Cloisonné kidneys, which occur in goats, are the result of proximal tubular basement membrane thickening as a result of deposits of ferritin and hemosiderin. Grossly, these kidneys have diffuse, intense, black or brown discoloration of the cortex (Fig. 11-13). The medulla is spared. Although this lesion is striking, renal function is normal.

Other Miscellaneous Tubular Changes. Other causes of incidental tubular changes include the following:

- Vacuolation of renal tubular epithelium in the lysosomal storage diseases, such as feline sphingomyelinosis and ovine GM1 gangliosidosis.
- Intranuclear eosinophilic crystalline pseudoinclusions (so-called crystalloids), which occur in renal tubular epithelium of old dogs. These can be round or rectangular and often greatly distort the nuclei.

Interstitium

Hyperemia. In instances of acute interstitial nephritis, especially those caused by septicemia, there can be an accompanying hyperemia of renal vasculature within the interstitium.

Edema. Similarly, in instances of acute inflammation targeting the interstitium, vascular leakage of high protein fluid (edema) can be the end result. In addition, tubular damage, especially with basement membrane breach, allows for more extensive interstitial edema accumulation.

Inflammatory Infiltrates. Interstitial inflammation is a consistent component of injury to the interstitium, whether acute or chronic, focal or generalized, or suppurative or nonsuppurative. Suppurative interstitial inflammation is typically seen in instances of hematogenous bacteremia. A variety of renal insults result in release of a wide array of cytokines and growth factors that stimulate interstitial inflammation, particularly monocyte infiltration. Fibroblasts often become activated and fibrosis ensues.

Fibrosis. Once interstitial fibroblasts become activated, fibrosis can ensue. Often, at this stage, the underlying or inciting pathogen is not present and thus its role is not determined. Recurrent bouts of fibrosis continue and set up a vicious cycle of loss and scarring so that the result is a common endpoint, known as *end-stage kidney*.

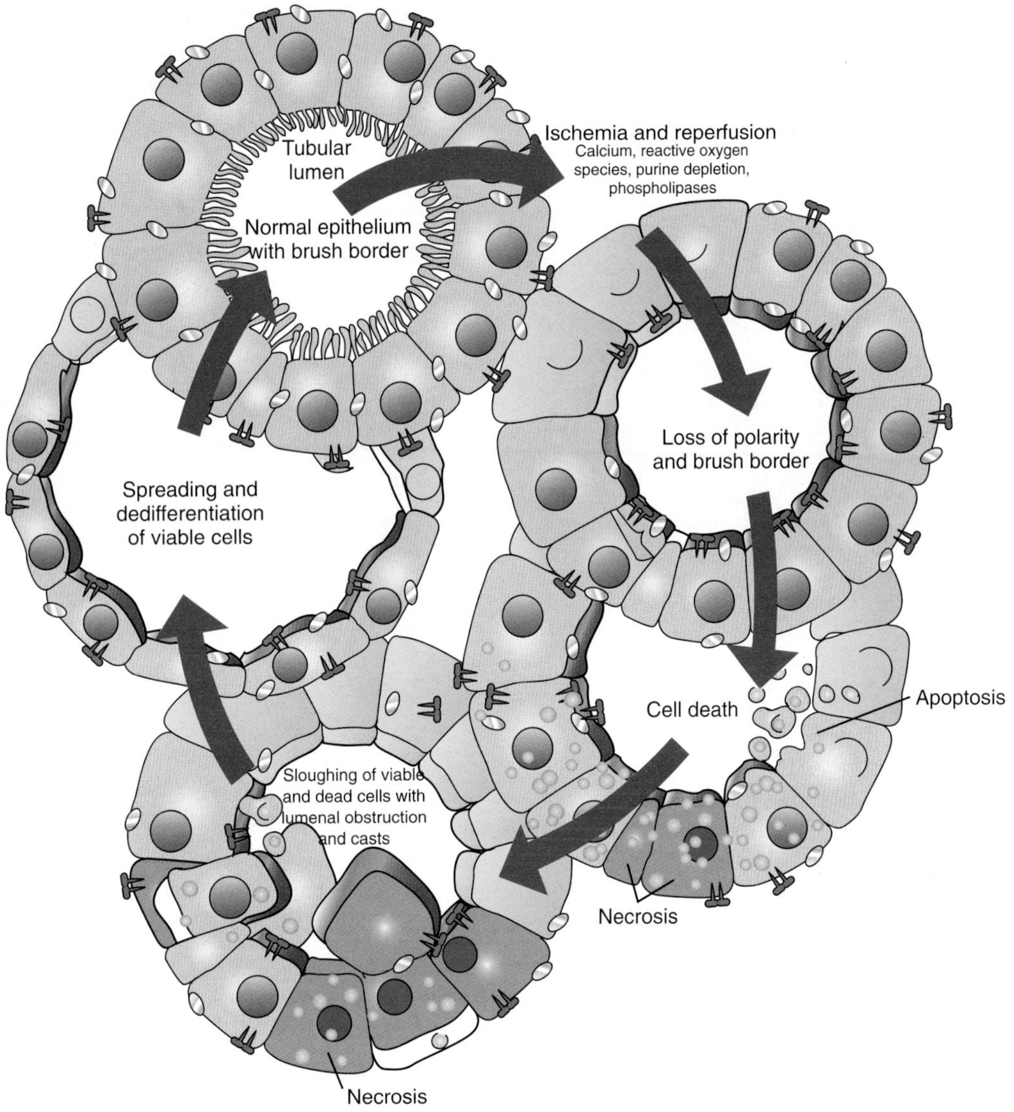

Figure 11-10 **Effects of Ischemia and Reperfusion on Renal Tubules.** After ischemia and reperfusion, morphologic changes occur in the proximal tubules, including loss of the brush border, loss of polarity, and redistribution of integrins and sodium-potassium adenosinetriphosphatase to the apical surface. Calcium, reactive oxygen species, purine depletion, and phospholipases probably have a role in these changes in morphology and polarity and in the subsequent cell death that occurs as a result of necrosis and apoptosis. There is a sloughing of viable and nonviable cells into the tubular lumen, resulting in the formation of casts and luminal obstruction and contributing to the reduction in the glomerular filtration rate. The severely damaged kidney can completely restore its structure and function. Spreading and dedifferentiation of viable cells occur during recovery from ischemic acute renal failure, which duplicates aspects of normal renal development. A variety of growth factors probably contribute to the restoration of a normal tubular epithelium. (Redrawn from Thadhani R, Pascual M, Bonventre JV: *N Engl J Med* 334(22):1448-1460, 1996. Color from Molitoris BA, Finn WF, editors: *Acute renal failure: A companion to Brenner and Rector's the kidney*, Philadelphia, 2001, Saunders.)

Lymphofollicular Inflammation. Lymphofollicular inflammation is the most common response to *Leptospira* infection of the kidney. Severe multinodular lymphocytic inflammatory reaction is confined to the cortex. The reaction subsides slowly and inflammatory cells decrease in numbers and the degree of fibrosis increases. Similarly, with chronic recurrent bouts of pyelonephritis, lymphocyte-rich inflammatory infiltrates are noted within the interstitium.

Interstitial Nephritis. When interstitial inflammation, mounted against the veins, arteries, lymphatic vessels, or connective tissues of kidneys, appears to be a primary lesion, it has traditionally been called *interstitial nephritis* and may have an infectious or noninfectious cause and is acute, subacute, or chronic in its duration. Interstitial nephritis is traditionally associated with a lymphoplasmacytic infiltrate; however, other types of leukocytes can also be present. In many of these diseases, the inflammatory cell infiltrates are visible only microscopically, are not associated with renal failure, and are generally inconsequential (examples are canine ehrlichiosis and equine infectious anemia). When the renal interstitium is the site of moderate to severe, grossly visible, interstitial inflammatory cell infiltrates and fibrosis, renal failure can occur.

The renal interstitium is the fibrovascular stroma that surrounds the nephron and is significantly involved in renal diseases, whether this is of primary interstitial origin as in interstitial nephritis or

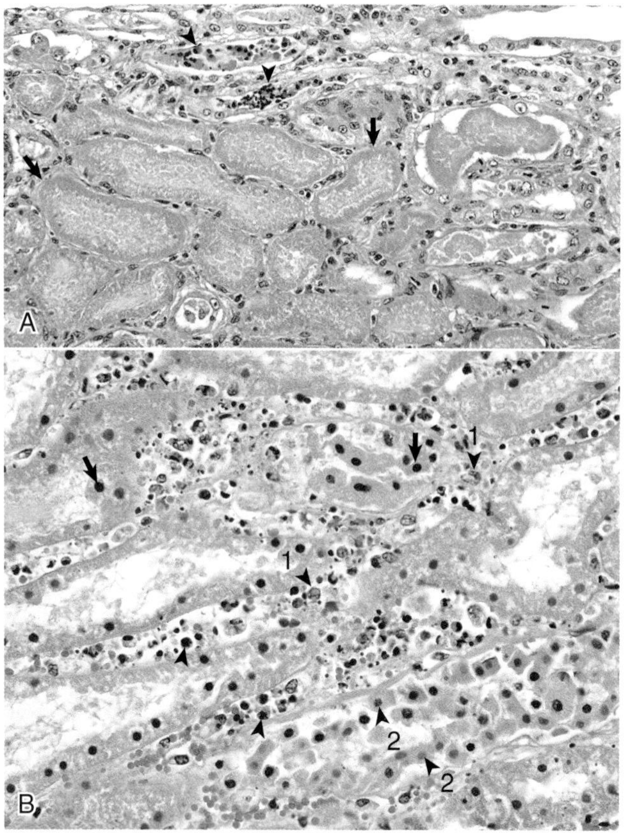

Figure 11-11 **Acute Tubular Necrosis, Kidney, Proximal Tubules, Cat. A,** This lesion is characterized primarily by coagulation necrosis of tubular epithelial cells *(arrows)* and nuclear pyknosis and intratubular nuclear and proteinaceous debris *(arrowheads)*. H&E stain. **B,** This lesion is characterized primarily by nuclear pyknosis *(arrows)*, karyorrhexis *(arrowheads)*, and karyolysis *(arrowheads 1)* with intratubular nuclear and proteinaceous debris and coagulation necrosis with detachment of the epithelium from the tubular basement membrane *(arrowheads 2)*. H&E stain. (Courtesy Dr. J.F. Zachary, College of Veterinary Medicine, University of Illinois.)

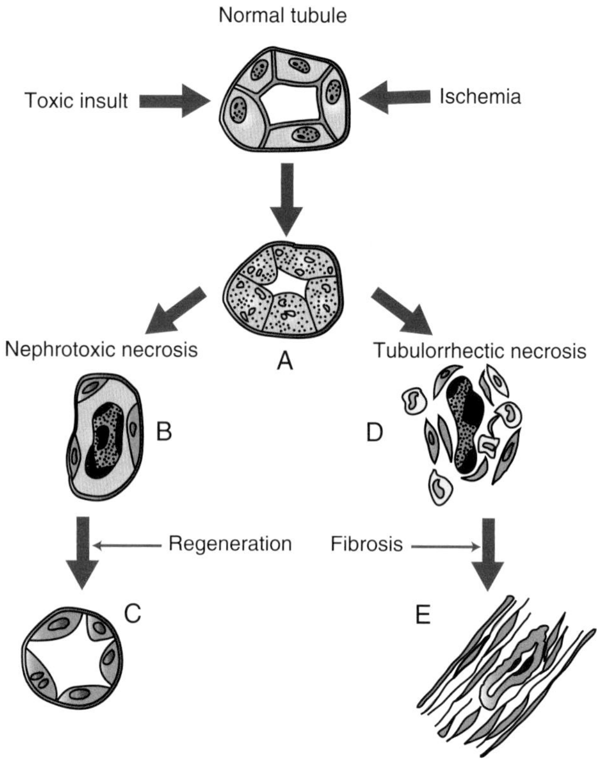

Figure 11-12 **Acute Tubular Necrosis, Kidney, Proximal Tubules.** Acute tubular necrosis results from a nephrotoxin or ischemia. **A,** Both insults cause acute necrosis characterized by cellular swelling, pyknosis, karyorrhexis, and karyolysis. **B,** Subsequent to nephrotoxic necrosis, there is sloughing of necrotic epithelium into the tubular lumina. The basement membranes remain intact and act as a scaffold for **(C)** tubular epithelial regeneration to occur. **D,** Ischemia may result in tubulorrhexis. Necrotic epithelial cells slough into the tubular lumen, the basement membrane is disrupted, macrophages infiltrate, and fibroblasts proliferate. **E,** Fibrosis with tubular atrophy results.

subsequent to tubular damage, when it is referred to as *tubulointerstitial disease*. Interstitial inflammation occurs as the result of ascending urinary tract infections (pyelonephritis), systemically derived infections of tubules and interstitium, toxins, or secondary to injury of tubules or glomeruli. Common acute lesions of the interstitium in response to toxins and tubular necrosis include edema, hemorrhage, and inflammation characterized by infiltration of neutrophils. As lesions become subacute to chronic, neutrophils become less prominent, and in several diseases, infiltrates of macrophages, lymphocytes, and plasma cells predominate. With chronic injury to or after atrophy of nephrons, fibrosis of the interstitium can be severe, resulting in notable reduction in nephron function and accentuation of renal disease.

Tubulointerstitial Nephritis. The term *tubulointerstitial nephritis* has been used to characterize a group of inflammatory diseases that involve the interstitium and tubules. Acute tubulointerstitial disease includes a group of processes, namely inflammation secondary to acute tubular necrosis, whereas chronic tubulointerstitial processes include the progression with time or instances in which the interstitium is the primary target.

Tubulointerstitial nephritis can result from bacterial or viral septicemias, in which these infectious microbes first infect the

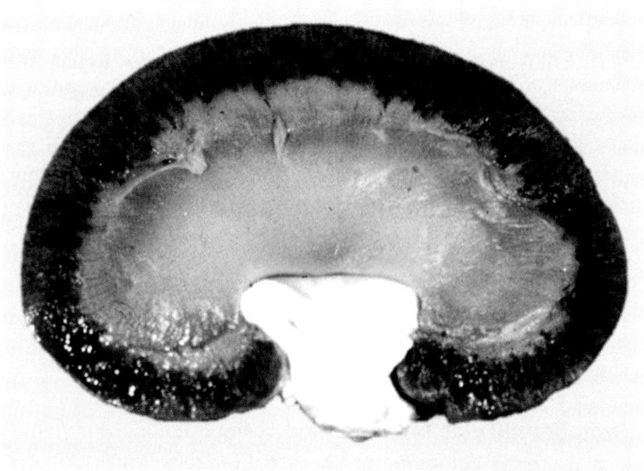

Figure 11-13 **Cloisonné Kidney, Dorsal Section, Goat.** The cortex is diffusely black; the medulla is unaffected. (Courtesy Dr. J. King, College of Veterinary Medicine, Cornell University.)

kidney tubules and damage them, which then incites an inflammatory response in the interstitium (Box 11-3). Acute tubulointerstitial nephritis is characterized by the presence of inflammatory cells (principally neutrophils) within the interstitium and may result from toxicoses or from acute infection with microbes such

Box 11-3 Causes of Interstitial Nephritis

HORSES
Equine viral arteritis

CATTLE
Escherichia coli septicemia, "white-spotted kidney"
Leptospira interrogans serovar *canicola*
Malignant catarrhal fever

SHEEP
Sheeppox

PIGS
Leptospira interrogans serovar *pomona*
Porcine reproductive and respiratory syndrome

DOGS
Leptospira interrogans serovars *canicola*, *icterohaemorrhagiae*, and others
Infectious canine hepatitis virus, recovery phase
Theileria parva

as *Leptospira* (see Fig. 11-66), adenoviruses, lentiviruses, or herpesviruses. Chronic tubulointerstitial nephritis (Fig. 11-14, *A*) is a less well-characterized entity in dogs, but atrophy of tubular segments is a significant feature of this syndrome along with sparse mononuclear cell infiltration, cortical and medullary fibrosis (Fig. 11-14, *B* and *C*), variable degrees of tubular and glomerular atrophy and/or sclerosis, and compromised nephron function.

The pathogenesis of leptospirosis is discussed as an example of acute bacterial tubulointerstitial nephritis, the most well-understood causes of which include numerous serovars of *Leptospira interrogans*; however, *Leptospira kirschneri* and *Leptospira borgpetersenii* serovars are also associated with renal disease (Fig. 11-14, *D*):

- *Leptospira interrogans* serovars *canicola* and *icterohaemorrhagiae* are the most common causes of canine leptospirosis (see the section on Kidney and Lower Urinary Tract, Disorders of Dogs).
- *Leptospira interrogans* serovar *pomona* is the most common cause of the lesion in pigs and less consistently in cattle (see the section on Kidney and Lower Urinary Tract, Disorders of Ruminants (Cattle, Sheep, and Goats)).

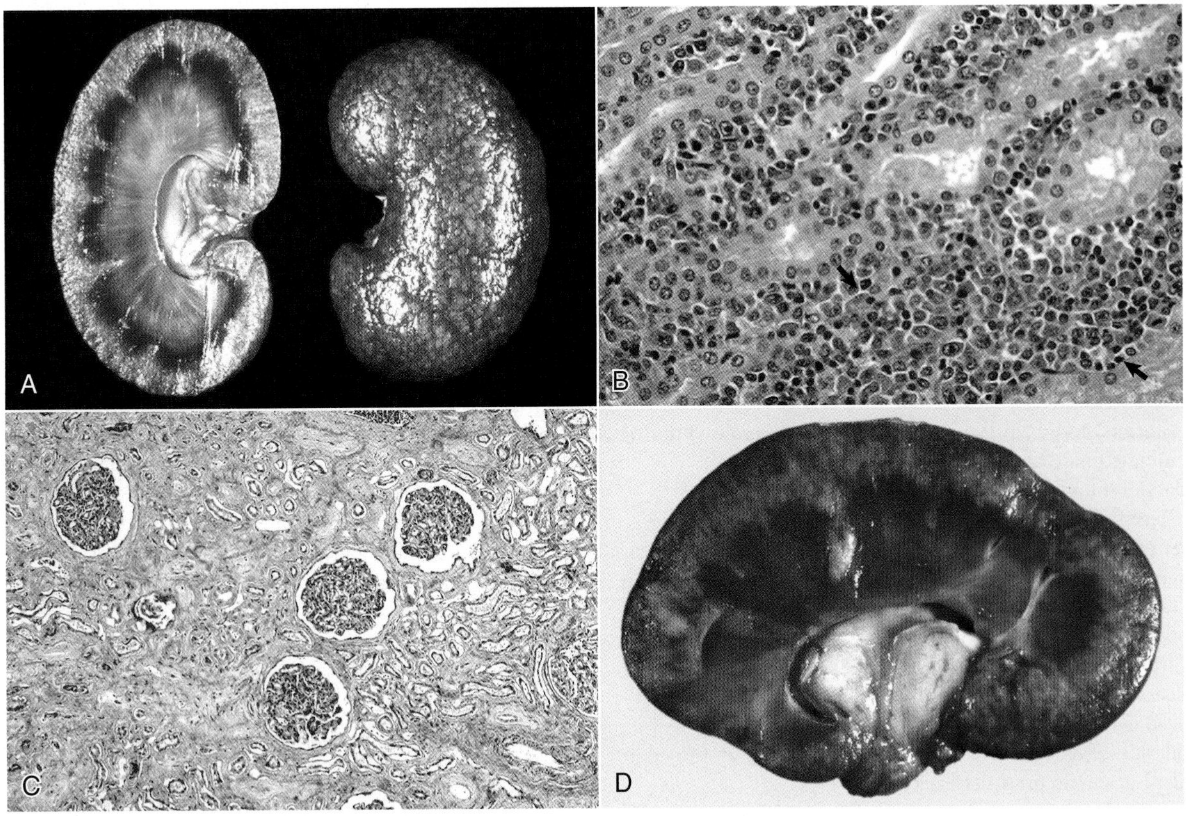

Figure 11-14 **Chronic Tubulointerstitial Nephritis. A,** Kidney, dorsal surface and dorsal section, dog. Note the nodularity of the capsular surface *(right)* from cortical interstitial fibrosis and the reduced width of the cortex (atrophy) *(left)*. **B,** Kidney, dog. Large numbers of lymphocytes and plasma cells expand the interstitium *(arrows)* between renal tubules. H&E stain. **C,** Kidney, exotic zoo animal. This lesion is characterized by cortical and medullary fibrosis, variable degrees of tubular atrophy, and mononuclear cell interstitial infiltrate. Masson trichrome stain. **D,** Leptospirosis, dog. The pale streaks and foci in the cortex, especially near the corticomedullary junction, are chiefly interstitial lymphoplasmacytic infiltrates accompanied by fibrosis. (**A** and **C** courtesy Dr. A. Confer, Center for Veterinary Health Sciences, Oklahoma State University. **B** courtesy Dr. Abdy, College of Veterinary Medicine, The University of Georgia; and Noah's Arkive, College of Veterinary Medicine, The University of Georgia. **D** courtesy Dr. M.D. McGavin, College of Veterinary Medicine, University of Tennessee.)

- *Leptospira kirschneri* serovar *grippotyphosa* and *Leptospira borgpetersenii* serovar *bratislava* have also been associated with renal leptospirosis in several animal species.

Mechanism of Injury of Tubulointerstitial Nephritis. Three theories on the cause of chronic tubulointerstitial nephritis are (1) focal acute interstitial nephritis evolves into the chronic form, (2) it is produced as a secondary manifestation of chronic glomerulonephritis (GN) or chronic pyelonephritis, or (3) it is produced after immune-mediated damage to the renal tubules and interstitium. There are few acute tubulointerstitial diseases to account for the large number of cases of chronic tubulointerstitial nephritis seen in dogs, and thus the first theory cannot account for a high percentage of the cases. As diagnostic techniques improve, some cases of chronic tubulointerstitial nephritis may be reclassified more specifically as either chronic pyelonephritis or secondary to chronic GN.

The mechanism of injury is known in a few instances, most specifically with *Leptospira* infections. After exposure to the organism, leptospiremia occurs and then organisms do the following:

- Localize in the renal interstitial capillaries
- Migrate through vascular endothelium
- Persist in the interstitial spaces
- Migrate via the lateral intercellular junctions of tubular epithelial cells to reach renal tubular lumina
- Associate with epithelial microvilli
- Persist within phagosomes of the epithelial cells of the proximal and distal convoluted tubules
- Induce tubular epithelial cells to undergo degeneration and necrosis as a result of either direct toxic effects of the leptospires or the accompanying interstitial inflammatory reaction

Although neutrophils can be present in tubular lumina, the predominant chronic lesion is an infiltrate of monocytes, macrophages, lymphocytes, and plasma cells in the interstitium (chiefly cortical) (see Fig. 11-14, *D*). In affected dogs, interstitial plasma cells secrete *Leptospira*-specific antibodies. However, the role of those antibodies in pathogenesis or resolution of the lesion is not known.

Another well-documented mechanism for the production of tubulointerstitial nephritis is the immune response that develops secondary to canine adenoviral infection. The sequence of events includes the following:

- Localization of virus in the glomeruli (viral glomerulitis) during the viremic phase of the disease
- Production of a transient immune-complex GN
- Recovery from the acute phase of the disease
- Onset of the systemic immune response
- Disappearance of virus from the glomeruli only to reappear in tubular epithelial cells in various portions of the nephron in basophilic intranuclear viral inclusions
- Persistence of virus in tubular epithelium for weeks to months
- Production of tubular epithelial necrosis as a result of viral-induced cytolysis
- Production of chronic lymphocytic, plasmacytic, and, less commonly, histiocytic interstitial nephritis

Infection with equine arteritis virus or porcine reproductive and respiratory syndrome (PRRS) virus often results in multifocal lymphohistiocytic chronic tubulointerstitial nephritis with interstitial edema. Lesions can involve any area of the cortex but are especially intense in the medulla and at the corticomedullary junction. A severe vasculitis, characterized by fibrinoid necrosis and lymphohistiocytic infiltrates that involve the adventitial and medial layers of cortical and medullary arteries and veins, is present. Virus can be found in endothelium and in macrophages.

Deposition of immune complexes in or interactions between anti-basement membrane antibodies and tubular basement membranes can initiate immune-mediated tubulointerstitial disease in human beings and laboratory animals. Depositions of immunoglobulin (Ig) and complement have rarely been identified in renal tubular basement membranes in domestic animals, but administration of preformed complexes (bovine serum albumin and antibody) to dogs demonstrated that these complexes interacted with proximal renal tubules not glomeruli. Damaged tubules respond with epithelial cell proliferation, basement membrane thickening, and peritubular fibrosis. Currently, the role of immune-mediated mechanisms in tubulointerstitial nephritis in domestic animals is unclear.

Gross Lesions of Tubulointerstitial Nephritis. Gross lesions can be classified as acute, subacute, or chronic; chronic tubulointerstitial nephritis is discussed in more detail later (see the section on Renal Fibrosis). The distribution of lesions can be diffuse as in canine leptospirosis (see Fig. 11-66) or multifocal as in "white-spotted kidneys" of calves as the result of *Escherichia coli* septicemia (see Fig. 11-63), canine herpesvirus infection (see Fig. 11-67), malignant catarrhal fever, or porcine and bovine leptospirosis (see Fig. 11-66). In diffuse tubulointerstitial nephritis, kidneys can be swollen and pale tan with a random gray mottling of the capsular surface. The cut surface bulges; gray infiltrates of varying sizes and intensities obscure the normal radially striated cortical architecture. These renal lesions usually are manifested as coalescing gray foci that are particularly intense in the inner cortex. Focal lesions of tubulointerstitial nephritis are less extensive and composed of more discrete gray areas in the cortex and outer medulla.

Microscopic Lesions of Tubulointerstitial Nephritis. Microscopically, aggregates of lymphocytes, plasma cells, monocytes, and fewer neutrophils are randomly scattered or intensely localized throughout the edematous interstitium. Tubular epithelial cells within severely inflamed areas can be degenerate, necrotic, or both, and profound tubular loss is usually accompanied by eventual replacement fibrosis.

Renal Fibrosis (Scarring). The alternative to regeneration is irreparable damage that results in functional tubular loss when cuboidal epithelium is replaced by nonabsorptive cuboidal or squamous cells or actual physical loss of tubules so that the nephron is lost. This can occur after either an ischemic insult, tubular descruction by infectious microbes, or exposure to a limited number of nephrotoxins. The ultimate result is replacement fibrosis/scarring. This is seen most commonly if the following occur:

- The toxin is not removed.
- The basement membrane does not remain intact.
- Adequate tubular epithelium does not survive destruction by microbes or the toxic dose of a nephrotoxin to allow for complete repair.

Fibrosis with a finely granular pattern can occur subsequent to widespread necrosis of renal tubular epithelium (acute tubular necrosis). An example is oak poisoning of cattle (see Fig. 11-62), in which severe tubular necrosis extends to the level of the renal tubular basement membrane, resulting in leakage of tubular contents. The loss of the continuity of the basement membrane prevents orderly tubular epithelial cell regeneration, which can be followed by interstitial fibrosis. Experimental studies have demonstrated that after severe nephrotoxin-induced tubular epithelial cell injury, the remaining cells undergo accelerated apoptosis resulting in tubular atrophy, interstitial fibroblast proliferation, and eventual fibrosis.

Renal fibrosis is the replacement of renal parenchyma, including tubules, glomeruli, and interstitium, with mature fibrous connective tissue. It can occur as a primary event, but more frequently it is a manifestation of the healing phase of a preexisting tubular or glomerular lesion. It is the common endpoint of all reparative stages and results when conditions are not conducive for healing of the tubular epithelium by regeneration. Regeneration of nephrons as a whole is not possible. Renal fibrosis follows many renal lesions, including primary inflammation of glomeruli (GN), tubules, or interstitial tissue (tubulointerstitial nephritis) (Fig. 11-15) and necrosis of renal tubules. Its severity usually parallels the intensity of the primary renal disease. The mechanisms by which fibrosis is induced are related to destruction and loss of nephron components by inflammatory or, less commonly, noninflammatory processes. T lymphocytes and interleukin-6 (IL-6) play important roles in renal fibrosis. Renal fibrosis is seen commonly following any number of renal insults and includes the following:

- Infarction
- Glomerulonephritis
- Tubulointerstitial disease/chronic pelvic diseases

Renal fibrosis may manifest in a multitude of grossly recognizable forms as described previously. Generally, fibrotic kidneys are recognized grossly by the pale, tan to white, shrunken, pitted, and firm consistency, along with excessive adhesions of the capsule to the underlying cortex. Fibrosis can be diffuse and finely stippled with pinpoint dimpling and granularity on the capsular surface, or it can be coarser as seen by deep and irregularly shaped depressions of the capsular surface in a diffuse, multifocal, or patchy distribution. In addition to these changes of the capsular surface, the cut surface of the cortex is thinned beneath the capsular surface depressions, and these fibrotic areas are pale tan compared with more normal parenchyma.

Microscopically, renal fibrosis is characterized by an increase in interstitial connective tissue and absence of renal tubules or by markedly atrophic nephron components (Fig. 11-16, A). Remaining tubules are usually atrophic and have a reduced luminal diameter or can appear ectatic because they are lined by flattened epithelium, producing an enlarged luminal diameter. A thickened hyalinized basement membrane and a lining of flattened epithelium (squamous or low cuboidal) are also characteristic. Multiple acquired, usually small, cysts can be present throughout the cortex and medulla and can be a result of either dilated Bowman's capsules and associated atrophic glomerular tufts or nephrons whose tubules have segments compressed by connective tissue (Fig. 11-16, B). Even in fibrotic lesions that are not the result of an infectious disease or inflammation, foci of lymphocytes and plasma cells can be seen randomly scattered throughout the interstitium (Fig. 11-16, C). In areas of severe interstitial fibrosis, glomerulosclerosis (as an end-stage of isolated glomeruli) is common. Calcification of vessels, tubular basement membranes, Bowman's capsules, and degenerate tubular epithelium are common in fibrotic kidneys because of alterations in calcium-phosphorus metabolism associated with chronic renal failure.

Renal fibrosis and chronic renal disease are the most frequently recognized renal pathologic processes in mature or aging domestic animals, particularly dogs and cats. When renal fibrosis and loss of nephrons are severe, these lesions can be manifested clinically as chronic renal failure and uremia. One of the most common expressions of this chronic disease is the inability of an animal to concentrate urine, resulting in frequent urination (polyuria) of dilute urine (isosthenuria). Polyuria is accompanied by dehydration and excessive water drinking (polydipsia). Hypoplastic anemia occurs as a result of the kidneys' failure to synthesize and secrete erythropoietin. Fibrous osteodystrophy can develop because of abnormal calcium-phosphorus metabolism and renal secondary hyperparathyroidism.

End-Stage Kidneys. Without careful attention to the pattern of resultant fibrosis, such kidneys are commonly called *end-stage kidneys*; however, fibrosis generally follows a pattern characteristic of the antecedent injury and is described here for tubulointerstitial disease.

A coarser pattern of diffuse renal fibrosis occurs in chronic interstitial nephritis and certain progressive juvenile nephropathies of dogs. Both cortex and medulla can be fibrotic, cortical striations are severely distorted or effaced, and the formation of multiple cortical cysts is common. End-stage kidneys are those referred to as a result of fibrosis, mineralization, sclerotic glomeruli, and foci of hyperplastic and hypertrophic tubules. Progressive interstitial fibrosis is thought to be the final common pathway to chronic renal failure.

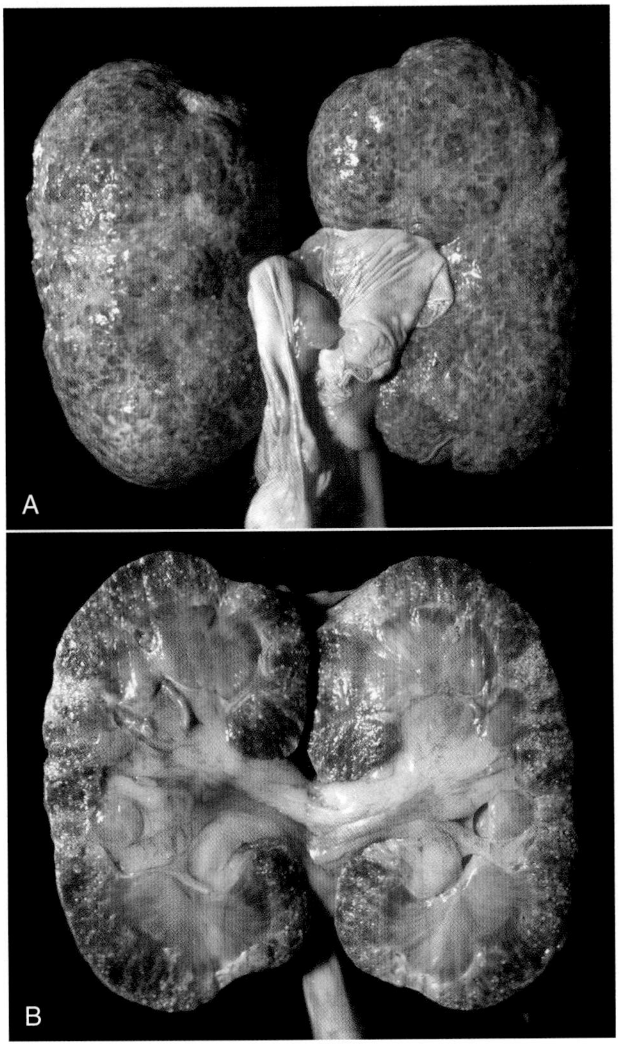

Figure 11-15 **Chronic Interstitial Nephritis, Kidney, Dog. A,** Diffuse interstitial fibrosis is responsible for the fine pitting of the capsular cortical surface, which is stippled red, the result of bands of fibrous tissue *(gray)* surrounding islands of renal cortex. **B,** Dorsal section. The cortex is pitted and granular because of multiple linear and focal scars, and it is also thinner than normal (atrophic). (Courtesy Dr. M.D. McGavin, College of Veterinary Medicine, University of Tennessee.)

Vasculature

Hyperemia and Congestion. Hyperemia refers to an increase in arterial blood flow, and congestion is an increase in venous blood pooling within the vasculature of the kidney. Renal hyperemia is an active process usually secondary to acute renal inflammation.

Renal congestion can be the following:

- Physiologic
- Passive

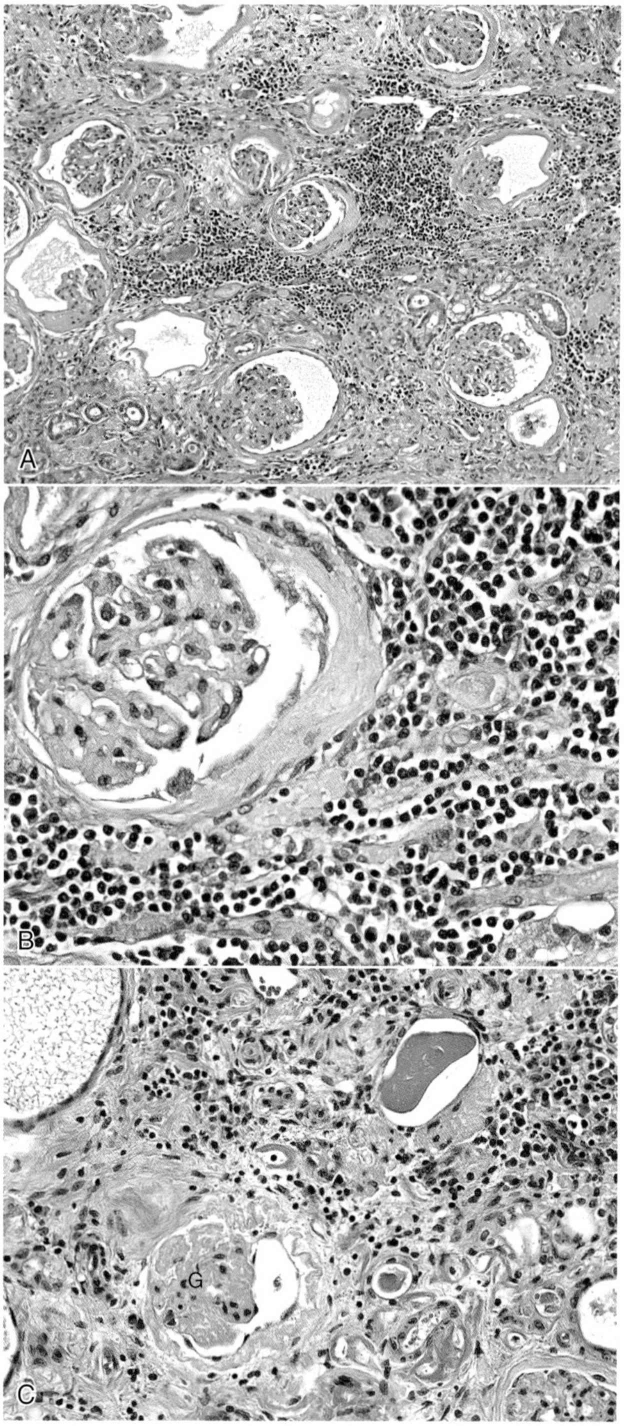

Figure 11-16 Chronic Interstitial Nephritis, Kidney, Dog. A, Dorsal section, cortex. This lesion is characterized by interstitial fibrosis, tubular atrophy, and interstitial inflammatory cell (lymphocytes and plasma cell) infiltration. The renal corpuscles have contracted glomeruli with increased volume of mesangial matrix and thickened Bowman's capsules. H&E stain. **B,** Higher magnification of **A**. H&E stain. **C,** Cortex. Higher magnification showing interstitial fibrosis, lymphocytic inflammatory infiltrates, sclerotic glomerular tufts *(G)*, and ectatic tubules and Bowman's spaces. H&E stain. (**A** and **B** courtesy Dr. J.F. Zachary, College of Veterinary Medicine, University of Illinois. **C** courtesy Dr. M.D. McGavin, College of Veterinary Medicine, University of Tennessee.)

- Secondary to hypovolemic shock
- Secondary to cardiac insufficiency
- Hypostatic

Hyperemic kidneys are darker red than normal, can be perceptibly swollen, and ooze blood from the cut surface. Congested kidneys are dark red and ooze blood from the cut surface as the result of the accumulation of unoxygenated blood in the renal venous system. At autopsy (syn: necropsy), unilateral renal hypostatic congestion is present in animals that die in lateral recumbency, after which the force of gravity pulls the unclotted blood downward. Microscopically, the arterial and venous vessels are distended with blood, and if there has been sufficient time for the blood to clot, serum and blood cells may be present.

Hemorrhage and Thrombosis. Hemorrhage occurs when red blood cells extend beyond the vessel walls. Large intrarenal hemorrhages can result from direct trauma, renal needle biopsy, and systemic bleeding disorders, such as factor VIII deficiency. Subcapsular and renal cortical hemorrhages occur in association with septicemic diseases, vasculitis, vascular necrosis, thromboembolism, and disseminated intravascular coagulation (DIC). Perirenal hemorrhage has been noted with ovine herpesvirus arteritis (malignant catarrhal fever [MCF]) and, of course, blunt abdominal trauma or penetrating projectiles.

Petechial hemorrhages are commonly seen on the surface and throughout the cortex of kidneys from pigs that die of viremia or septicemia caused by diseases such as hog cholera (swine fever), African swine fever, erysipelas (see Fig. 11-64), streptococcal infections, salmonellosis, and other embolic bacterial diseases (e.g., *Actinobacillus* spp.). Renal cortical ecchymotic hemorrhages associated with multifocal tubular and vascular necrosis are salient and diagnostically important lesions of viremia in neonatal puppies infected with herpesvirus. Portions of thrombus that break free from affected heart valves in valvular endocarditis can lodge in the glomeruli or interstitial capillaries in any species.

When DIC causes widespread thrombosis in the glomerular capillaries (Fig. 11-17), the afferent arterioles, and, most important, the interlobular arteries, widespread cortical infarction results and is designated renal cortical necrosis. This lesion is not to be confused with ischemic acute tubular necrosis discussed in this chapter (see the section on Acute Tubular Necrosis). Partial or complete renal cortical necrosis is usually a bilateral lesion that occurs in all animal species, especially as a result of Gram-negative septicemias or endotoxemias, and is related to the following:

- Endotoxin-induced endothelial damage
- Activation of the extrinsic clotting mechanism
- Widespread capillary thrombosis

The lesion can be induced experimentally in animals by two endotoxin injections 24 hours apart and is a manifestation of the generalized Shwartzman reaction. The resulting microthrombosis of vessels throughout the renal cortex results in widespread ischemia and small and large infarcts of coagulation necrosis and hemorrhage. The renal cortex can be diffusely pale with a zone of hyperemia separating the necrotic cortex from the viable medulla, or more often the cortex is a mosaic of large, irregular hemorrhagic areas, resembling hemorrhagic infarcts interspersed with large yellow-gray areas resembling pale infarcts. The necrotic tissue can involve the full width of the cortex or only the outer portion.

Infarction. Renal infarcts are areas of coagulative necrosis that result from the local ischemia of vascular occlusion and usually are due to thromboembolism.

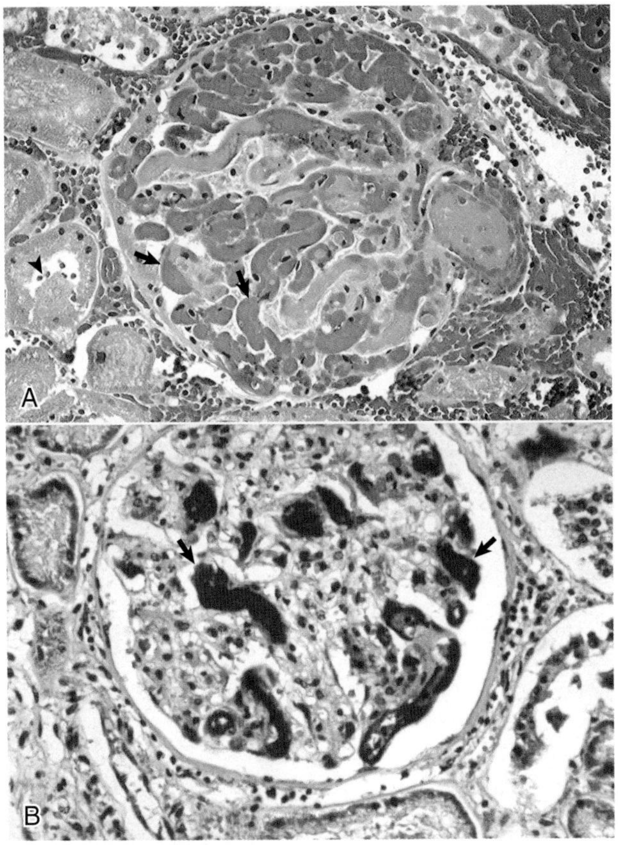

Figure 11-17 **Glomerular Capillary Thrombosis, Kidney, Glomerulus, Dog. A,** Microthrombi. Capillary lumens are occluded by microthrombi *(arrows)* caused by disseminated intravascular coagulation. Adjacent cortical tubular epithelial cells are undergoing coagulation necrosis with nuclei undergoing pyknosis and karyolysis *(arrowhead)*, the result of ischemia from reduced blood flow to the peritubular capillaries, which are downstream from the glomerulus. H&E stain. **B,** Fibrinous microthrombi. A glomerulus similar to the one shown in Fig. 11-23, A, stained to demonstrate fibrinous thrombi *(arrows)*. Fibrin is red. Lendrum-Fraser stain for fibrin. (**A** courtesy Dr. W. Crowell, College of Veterinary Medicine, The University of Georgia; and Noah's Arkive, College of Veterinary Medicine, The University of Georgia. **B** courtesy College of Veterinary Medicine, University of Illinois.)

Renal emboli are derived from the following:

- Thromboemboli
- Mural thrombi on heart valves in valvular endocarditis
- Endarteritis in parasitic diseases such as canine dirofilariasis and equine strongylosis
- Arteriosclerosis in cattle (rare)
- Neoplastic cell emboli
- Bacterial emboli
- Endotoxemia

Because of the high circulating blood volume (20% to 25% of cardiac output) through the kidney, kidneys are common sites of thromboembolism and infarction. Rarely, emboli may occlude the renal artery, causing infarction of the entire kidney. Sometimes, emboli occlude the interlobar/arcuate arteries, causing infarction of triangular (in cross section of the kidney) segments of the cortex and medulla. Most commonly, emboli obstruct smaller vessels (e.g., interlobular arteries), causing infarcts involving only the renal cortex. In general, renal infarction can occur because of thrombosis resulting from endothelial damage of glomerular capillaries associated with a vascular disease (as in Alabama rot in greyhounds; see Fig. 11-37). Renal infarcts in horses can result from emboli lodging in the renal vasculature after mural thrombosis of the aorta, from aortic wall damage caused by migrating larvae of *Strongylus vulgaris*, or from endotoxemia secondary to mucosal damage resulting from colic. Thrombosis and infarction of pulmonary, coronary, splenic, or renal arteries are common in dogs with glomerular amyloidosis, which results in loss of plasma anticoagulants, such as antithrombin III, through damaged glomeruli. Endotoxin-mediated arterial or capillary thromboemboli are a common cause of infarction in association with Gram-negative sepsis, endotoxemia, or endotoxic shock. Septic emboli, particularly those from bacterial valvular endocarditis, caused by *Trueperella pyogenes* in cattle, *Erysipelothrix rhusiopathiae* in pigs, and *Staphylococcus aureus* in small animals, can cause renal infarcts and can progress to microabscesses or granulomas, depending on the microorganism involved.

Grossly, renal infarcts appear red or pale white depending on several factors, including the interval after vascular occlusion (i.e., age of infarct) (Figs. 11-18 and 11-19). Acutely, infarcts are usually wedge-shaped in a cross section of kidney, with the base against the cortical surface and the apex pointing toward the medulla,

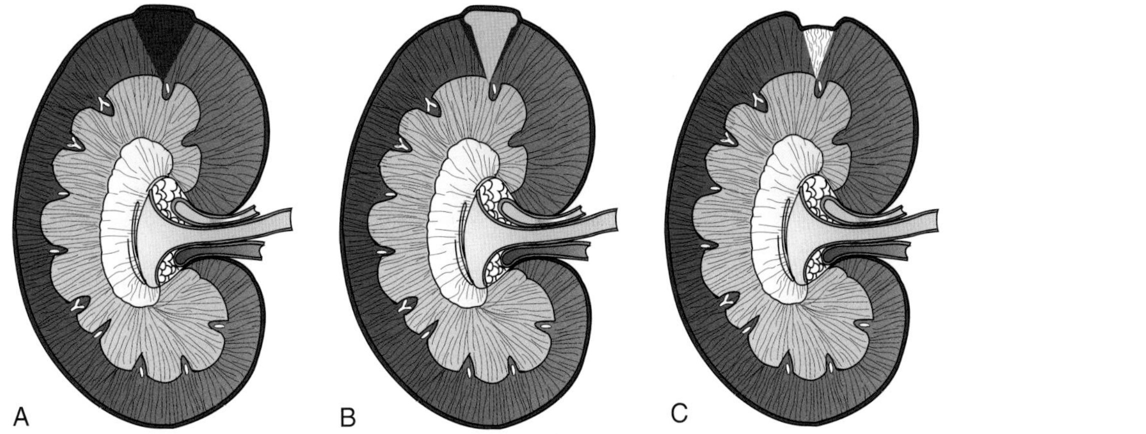

Figure 11-18 **Progression of Renal Infarction.** The normal progression of renal infarcts is outlined. **A** and **B,** Acute renal infarcts. Initially, renal infarcts are swollen and hemorrhagic (**A**). In 2 to 3 days, infarcts become pale (**B**), surrounded by a zone of hyperemia and hemorrhage. **C,** Chronic infarcts are pale, shrunken, and fibrotic, resulting in distortion and depression of the renal contour.

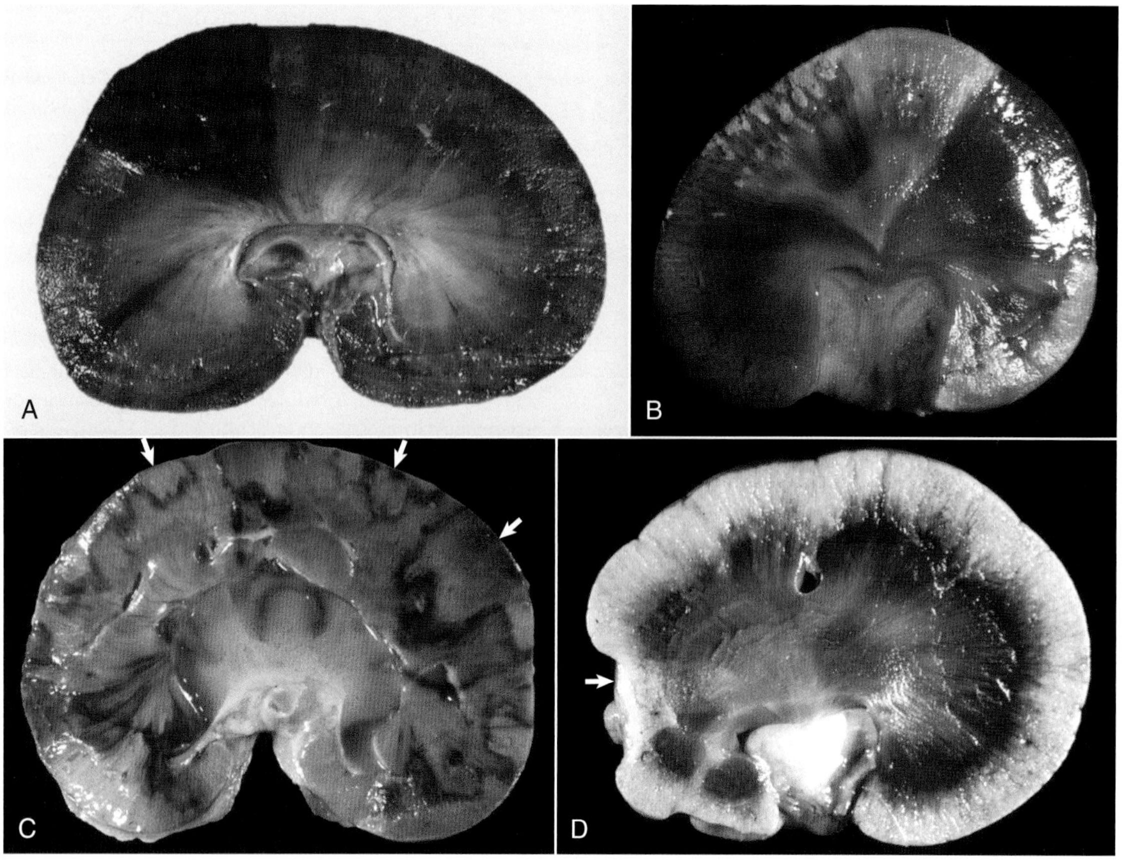

Figure 11-19 **Gross Appearance of Renal Cortical Infarcts with Age, Kidney, Dorsal Sections. A,** Acute (early) hemorrhagic infarct, dog. Focal wedge-shaped area of cortical necrosis. Note how the infarct bulges above the capsular surface due to cell swelling and hemorrhage. **B,** Acute pale infarcts, rabbit. There are two pale white to tan wedge-shaped infarcts *(top, lower right)*. Note how the infarct *(top)* bulges above the capsular surface, indicating cell swelling. **C,** Subacute infarcts, dog. Multiple renal cortical infarcts are pale and surrounded by a red rim of active hyperemia *(arrows)*. The cortical surface of many, but not all, of the infarcts is even with that of the adjacent unaffected cortex, indicating that cell swelling has subsided. **D,** Chronic infarct, cat. A focal pale truncated wedge-shaped scar of fibrous connective tissue has replaced the pole *(arrow)* of the renal cortex. Note that the surface of the infarct is below that of the adjacent normal kidney because of the loss of tissue, fibrosis, and contraction of the fibrous scar. (**A** courtesy Dr. W. Crowell, College of Veterinary Medicine, The University of Georgia; and Noah's Arkive, College of Veterinary Medicine, The University of Georgia. **B** courtesy Dr. M.D. McGavin, College of Veterinary Medicine, University of Tennessee. **C** courtesy Dr. K. Read, College of Veterinary Medicine, Texas A&M University; and Noah's Arkive, College of Veterinary Medicine, The University of Georgia. **D** courtesy Dr. J. Sagartz, College of Veterinary Medicine, The Ohio State University; and Noah's Arkive, College of Veterinary Medicine, The University of Georgia.)

conforming to a zone of cortical parenchyma supplied by the site of the obstruction. From the capsular surface, infarcts are irregular and reflect the red or pale colors of the wedge-shaped infarct seen on cut surface. Occlusion of small interlobular arteries results in infarcts that are initially slightly swollen and red because of hemorrhage (Fig. 11-19, *A*) and later develop a pale yellow-gray center of coagulation necrosis within 2 or 3 days because of lysis of erythrocytes and loss of hemoglobin (Fig. 11-19, *B*). Pale infarcts are usually surrounded by a peripheral red zone of congestion and hemorrhage along with a pale margin because of a surrounding zone of leukocytes (Fig. 11-19, *C*). Although less common, hypoxic renal necrosis as the result of venous occlusion and/or infarction is seen occasionally, and venous infarcts retain their hemorrhagic appearance longer than infarcts resulting from arterial occlusion because of the continued arterial blood flow into the area. Because of the loss of parenchyma, during healing infarcts are depressed below the cortical surface and later become pale and shrunken as a result of fibrosis (Fig. 11-19, *D*).

The scarring that follows infarction is related to several variables, including the size of the ischemic area caused by vascular compromise. Healing is by fibrosis and results in large, deeply depressed wedge-shaped (on cross section of the kidney) scars that involve primarily the cortex but can extend into the medulla. Obstruction of smaller arterioles results in smaller areas of more superficial coagulative necrosis that heal as small-diameter pits in the renal surface, which correspond to pale white, linear scars on the cut surface.

Microscopically, in an acute infarct, nephrons (including tubules, glomeruli, and interstitium) in the central zone of the infarct are necrotic (Fig. 11-20). At the periphery of the infarct, only the proximal tubules, because of their high metabolic rate, are necrotic; the glomeruli tend to be spared. After approximately 2 days, the margin of the necrotic zone contains an inflammatory infiltrate consisting largely of neutrophils and fewer macrophages and lymphocytes. Capillaries adjacent to the necrotic area are notably engorged with blood (hyperemia). Healing of the infarcted area occurs by lysis and phagocytosis of the necrotic tissue and replacement by fibrous connective tissue, which matures to a discrete scar. At autopsy (syn: necropsy), healed scarred areas are visible as pale white to gray contracted depressions from the capsular surface, and they range from linear to broad depending on the size of the acute infarct. *Septic infarcts* are initially hemorrhagic, but because of the

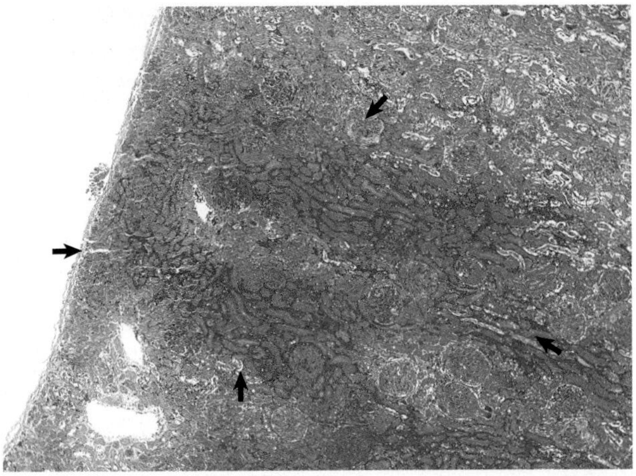

Figure 11-20 **Acute Infarct, Kidney, Cortex, Dog.** Note the acute infarct with a central zone of coagulation necrosis surrounded by a zone of hyperemia and hemorrhage *(arrows)*. H&E stain. (Courtesy Dr. S.J. Newman, College of Veterinary Medicine, University of Tennessee.)

presence of pyogenic bacteria, the necrotic tissue undergoes liquefactive necrosis and the infarcts can eventually develop into abscesses and ultimately into substantial scars. Septic infarcts often fail to respect a solely cortical or medullary pattern of distribution caused by the extensive local inflammation that they generate.

Papillary (Medullary Crest) Necrosis. See the section on Kidney and Lower Urinary Tract, Disorders of Domestic Animals for a discussion of papillary necrosis.

Embolic Nephritis. Acute suppurative glomerulitis, or bacterial (embolic) nephritis, is discussed in the section on Kidney and Lower Urinary Tract, Disorders of Domestic Animals.

Aging of the Kidney

As animals age, they have increased risk of kidney disease; however, aging alone may not cause spontaneous kidney disease, but aging is associated with anatomic and physiologic changes in renal structure, function, and regenerative capacity. After maturity, there begins a slow steady reduction in the number of viable glomeruli with accompanying glomerulosclerosis, atrophic changes in tubules, increased interstitial fibrosis, basement membrane thickening, and reduced renal function. Those changes may be seen incidentally in histologic sections of aged domestic animals, especially dogs and cats. Concurrently, progressive decreased kidney weight and volume and reduced cortical thickness occur. Functionally, with age, glomerular filtration rates slowly decline, hypertension increases, urine concentrating ability declines, and vascular resistance increases. For the average animal, these changes are insidious, may not be obvious at necropsy, and may never lead to renal failure; however, current urinary or systemic disease can accelerate the process.

Portals of Entry/Pathways of Spread

Kidney as a Whole

The urinary system and especially the kidney can be exposed to injurious stimuli and microbes via a number of routes (Box 11-4), including the following:

- Hematogenous
- Ascending from ureter
- Glomerular filtrate
- Direct penetration

Box 11-4 Portals of Entry to the Kidney

ASCENDING FROM URETER
- Extension from lower urinary tract secondary to gastrointestinal content contamination (diarrhea) (females primarily)
- Extension from lower urinary tract secondary to genital tract contamination (pyometra) (females exclusively)
- Extension from lower urinary tract secondary to dermal contamination (perivulvar dermatitis)
  - Targets tubules and interstitium primarily

HEMATOGENOUS
- Localization within corticomedullary vessels
  - Septic–embolic nephritis
  - Nonseptic necrosis with infarction
- Localization within large renal vasculature
  - Massive infarction
- Localization within glomerular tufts
- Localization within interstitial vessels
  - Targets glomeruli, tubules, interstitium, and vasculature

DIRECT PENETRATION
- Activation of products in proximal tubules–necrosis
- Presence of heavy metal–mercury, cadmium
- Crystalline oversaturation
- Direct toxic action–cisplatin
  - Targets tubules

Renal Corpuscle

Hematogenous. The renal cortex has a high rate of blood flow; therefore the sustaining blood supply can provide a portal of hematogenous entry for infectious organisms, which in the kidney can lead to glomerular localization or embolic nephritis.

Tubules

Glomerular Filtrate. Substances secreted into the glomerular filtrate can produce localized trauma to tubular lining cells such as crystalline salt oversaturation (e.g., oxalate crystals). Filtered preformed toxins or metabolized substances processed by the tubular lining epithelium exert their effect principally on the proximal tubular epithelium.

Ascending Injury. Ascension from the exterior via the urethra into the urinary bladder and subsequently from the urinary bladder to the renal pelvis via the ureters (vesicoureteral reflux) can be the source of infectious diseases of the lower urinary tract and kidney. Common etiologic microbes in this process, such as bacteria, may originate from the exterior skin surface and the adjacent orifices of the intestinal or genital tracts.

Hematogenous (Interstitial Capillaries and Vasa Recta). The luminal and abluminal surfaces of epithelial cells lining renal tubules can be exposed to systemic blood-borne (hematogenous) toxins that are secreted via peritubular capillaries into the interstitial and/or luminal fluid, respectively. In addition, some infectious microbes, such as *Leptospira* sp., gain access to the tubules via the interstitial capillaries.

Interstitium

Hematogenous. The interstitium can be entered most successfully by the associated interstitial blood supply, allowing for interstitial localization of blood-borne pathogens, similar to those seen with glomerular blood-borne infections.

Ascending Injury. See previous section on Tubules.

Lymphoid Nodules. Although often present as aggregates or less commonly as nodules, lymphoid infiltrates within the interstitium are not normal; however, small aggregates or nodules are often incidental findings and of unknown cause. Previous insults typically from infectious etiologies, such as *Leptospirosis*, or as a result of ascension secondary to long-standing pyelonephritis can result in larger aggregates and nodules.

Vasculature

As in all visceral organs, the sustaining blood supply can provide a portal of hematogenous entry for infectious organisms, which in the case of the kidney principally leads to arterial localization at one of several gradated sites as follows:

- Localization within large renal vasculature: Massive infarction of the kidney is the result of large-bore renal vessel disease.
- Localization within corticomedullary vessels: In the case of associated bacterial spread, septic embolic nephritis can occur. In those examples in which the embolus is nonseptic, the result is infarctive necrosis.
- Localization within glomerular tufts: In this example, the lesions are localized to the vasculature of the small vessels within the glomerular tuft.
- Localization within interstitial vessels: In this example, the lesions are localized to necrosis of interstitial tissues and tubules.

Defense Mechanisms/Barrier Systems

Defense mechanisms unique to the renal system have evolved to counteract the routes of typical exposure to injurious agents and include those localized to the renal corpuscle, tubules, interstitium, and vasculature (Box 11-5).

Renal Corpuscle

Glomerular Basement Membrane. The most important of these barrier systems is the glomerular filtration membrane (basement membrane or basal lamina) (see Fig. 11-6). The glomerular membrane is structurally adept at separating substances based on size and charge. Both size-dependent and charge-dependent filtration occur because of the porous structure of glomerular capillary walls, which is a function of endothelial fenestrations, a basement membrane formed of type IV collagen, basement membrane anionic glycoproteins, and filtration slits of visceral epithelium. This inherent function of the glomerulus can also protect other regions of the nephron from damage by circulating inflammatory cells and their cytokines, as well as infectious microbes that are present in the systemic circulation (i.e., bacteria in bacteremia).

Glomerular Mesangium. The glomerulus is equipped with its own specialized mesangial cells, a component of the monocyte-macrophage system (see Fig. 11-6), which can remove macromolecules from circulation.

Box 11-5 Renal Defense Mechanisms against Injury and Infectious Microbes

- Barrier system—glomerular basement membrane (GBM)
- Monocyte-macrophage system—glomerular mesangium
- Immune system
  - Innate responses
  - Humoral responses
  - Cellular responses

Tubules

The most effective barrier system associated with the tubules is the tubular basement membrane. Intact basement membranes restrict intraluminal organisms, such as ascending bacteria, from gaining easy access to the interstitium. They also provide the scaffolding for reepithelialization of the tubule, which follows tubular necrosis in association with many toxic principles but not in instances of renal ischemia.

Interstitium

Innate humoral and cellular responses by the immune system contribute to protection of the kidney. Humoral antibodies may protect mucosal surfaces such as those of the renal pelvis and less commonly the tubular epithelial cell lining, especially against insults such as ascending bacterial infections or those accessing the interstitium via interstitial capillaries. Cell infiltrates are typically localized to the interstitial tissues. Lymphocytes and plasma cells within the interstitium provide cell-mediated surveillance against invasive pathogens (i.e., *Leptospira*), and in the case of plasma cells, they can locally produce antibodies.

Vasculature

Intact endothelial lining of the renal vasculature functions as a localized defense mechanism (barrier system) to prevent access by intravascular pathogens, many of which produce toxic by-products (e.g., bacterial endotoxin) that can damage endothelium and allow for localized vasculitis and bacterial colonization. The result is often embolic septic nephritis. Intact endothelium also prevents activation of the clotting cascade and thus reduction in the likelihood of thrombus formation.

Lower Urinary Tract[3]

Structure

The lower urinary tract is the conduit for transport of urinary waste from the kidney to the exterior through paired ureters, the urinary bladder, and the urethra.

Ureters

The ureters enter the bladder wall obliquely and are covered by a mucosal flap, the vesicoureteral valve, which is an important structure because it normally prevents reflux of urine from the bladder into the ureter and renal pelvis. The ureters are lined by transitional epithelium that should normally be smooth and glistening. Microscopically, the ureteral mucosa is folded longitudinally and the underlying tunica muscularis is composed of poorly defined internal and external longitudinal muscle layers with a prominent middle circular muscle layer. Externally, the ureter is surrounded by either adventitia or peritoneal serosa.

Urinary Bladder

At death, the urinary bladder can contract to such a degree that the normal bladder wall appears thick on autopsy (syn: necropsy). The normal mucosa of the urinary bladder should be smooth and glistening. Urine should be clear except in horses, in which it is cloudy because of the normal presence of mucus and crystalline material produced by the branched tubuloalveolar mucous glands in the submucosa of the renal pelvis and proximal ureter. Microscopically, as in other mucous membranes, the lamina propria has small lymphoid follicles, which, after inflammation or antigenic stimulation,

[3]See E-Appendix 11-2 for methods of examining the lower urinary tract.

can be large enough to be seen grossly as discrete, circular, white foci (1 to 2 mm) in the mucosa. Histologically, the bladder is an expanded ureter, lined by pseudostratified transitional epithelium ranging from 3 to 14 cells thick, depending on the species and degree of distention. The urinary bladder wall is composed of poorly defined internal and external longitudinal muscle layers, a prominent middle circular muscle layer, and externally either adventitia or peritoneal serosa.

Urethra

During continence, the bladder is relatively flaccid and the urethra acts as a valve. Microscopically, the urethra is lined by transitional epithelium cranially and stratified squamous epithelium in the caudal segment, immediately cranial to or at the urethral orifice.

Function

Ureters

The function of the ureters is to propel urine from the kidney to the urinary bladder by peristalsis.

Urinary Bladder and Urethra

The urinary bladder stores urine and, in concert with the urethra, expels it. During micturition (urination), contraction of the detrusor muscle (the urinary bladder musculature) pumps urine through the relaxed urethra.

Dysfunction/Responses to Injury

Ureter, Urinary Bladder, and Urethra

Most diseases of the lower urinary tract are related to obstruction of flow or infection. The predominant responses of the lower tubular tract to injury include dilation and pressure necrosis caused by obstruction to the ureter or urethra and inflammation in response to exposure to infectious etiologies. In addition, concentration of excreted urinary substances, such as drug metabolites, pesticides, and other toxins, can damage the surface of the lower urinary system and predispose it to infection, secondary hyperplasia and metaplasia, or neoplastic transformation.

Portals of Entry/Pathways of Spread

Common portals of entry and pathways of spread for infection of the lower urinary tract are shown in Box 11-6.

Box 11-6 Portals of Entry into Lower Urinary System

ASCENDING

Extension from exterior secondary to contamination from the gastrointestinal tract
Extension from exterior secondary to contamination from the genital tract
Extension from exterior secondary to contamination from the skin

DESCENDING

Extension from disease processes that occur within the kidney and renal pelvis

DIRECT EXTENSION OR EXPOSURE FROM THE LUMEN

Accumulation of toxins in the urine during stasis and collection
Urinary tract calculi formation

DIRECT PENETRATION FROM THE ABDOMEN (CYSTOCENTESIS)

Ascending Infection

Extension from the exterior can occur secondary to bacterial contamination from the gastrointestinal tract, the genital tract, or severe bacterial dermatitis and result in damage due to ascension of bacteria. This represents a unique mechanism because the lower urinary tract is a blind-ended tubular system that has only one exit to the exterior (i.e., through the urethra), unlike the intestinal tract, which is a continuous tubular system. This structural arrangement predisposes to bacterial ascension and colonization, especially in females, due to their shorter, easily distensible urethra. In males, risk of ascending infection is decreased but risk of urethral obstruction is increased, due in part to the ureter's narrow diameter and increased length. Bacteria with adhesion capabilities may overcome peristalsis and periodic urine flushing and ascend the ureter to the renal pelvis via a process called vesicoureteral reflux (see Fig. 11-45). Regular and complete emptying of the urinary bladder helps minimize risks of pathologic changes, in contrast to urinary stasis, urine retention, and infrequent urinations, which predispose to ascending disease.

Descending Infection

Extension of disease processes that occur within the kidney and renal pelvis, such as pyelonephritis, may account for spread of inflammation into the lower urinary tract. Aggregates of inflammatory exudate and debris may be seen within the renal pelvis or carried distally by the flow of urine.

Direct Extension or Exposure from the Lumen

When toxic principles are excreted in the urine, they may accumulate to injurious concentrations because urine is stored in the urinary bladder for extended periods. As a result, these agents may injure the mucosa of the lower urinary tract and predispose it to infection, secondary mucosal hyperplasia, or neoplasia. In addition, the presence of a urolith anywhere within the lower urinary tract can result in trauma to the mucosa, with accompanying edema, hemorrhage, ulceration, and, in the most severe cases of obstruction, may lead to rupture caused by pressure necrosis.

Direct Penetration from the Abdomen (Cystocentesis)

Although rare as a portal of entry, it is possible for surface skin bacteria to be transmitted to the urinary bladder lumen through direct penetration of the abdomen after diagnostic procedures such as cystocentesis.

Defense Mechanisms/Barrier Systems

Defense mechanisms unique to the lower urinary system have evolved to counteract the typical forms of injury (Box 11-7). The most notable of these defense mechanisms of the lower urinary tract, which includes the ureters, urinary bladder, and urethra, are as follows:

- The flushing action of urine minimizes risks of bacterial adherence and ascension.
- Peristalsis acts to eliminate bacteria with adhesion capabilities.
- Inhospitable environment for bacterial growth controlled by urine pH and osmolarity.
- Protective urothelial mucus coating.
- Innate immune response.
- Humoral immune response.
- Cellular immune response.

Aging of the Lower Urinary Tract

Age-related changes in the lower urinary tract are not of major significance in domestic veterinary species. Acquired urinary incontinence is a common, long-term sequela of sterilization (spaying) in

Box 11-7 Urinary Tract Defense Mechanisms against Injury and Infectious Microbes

- Urine flow (flushing)
- Peristalsis
- Urine pH and osmolarity
- Urothelial cell protective mucus coat
- Immune system
  - Innate responses
  - Humoral responses
  - Cellular responses

Table 11-1 Nonrenal Lesions of Uremia

Lesion	Mechanism
Pulmonary edema	Increased vascular permeability
Fibrinous pericarditis	Increased vascular permeability
Ulcerative and hemorrhagic gastritis	Ammonia secretion and vascular necrosis
Ulcerative and necrotic stomatitis	Ammonia secretion in saliva and vascular necrosis
Atrial and aortic thrombosis	Endothelial and subendothelial damage
Hypoplastic anemia	Increased erythrocyte fragility and lack of erythropoietin production in the kidney
Soft-tissue mineralization	Altered calcium-phosphorus metabolism (stomach, lungs, pleura, kidneys)
Fibrous osteodystrophy	Altered calcium-phosphorus metabolism
Parathyroid hyperplasia	Altered calcium-phosphorus metabolism

female dogs, but it is more a result of urethral changes associated with sterilization than a result of aging. Sterilization in dogs leads to decreased smooth muscle in the urinary bladder and urethra as well as shorter urethral length, which may impair urethral sphincter function. Additional risk factors for urinary incontinence in dogs include medium to large stature, previous tail docking, and obesity.

Kidney and Lower Urinary Tract

Disorders of Domestic Animals

Nonrenal Lesions of Uremia

Nonrenal lesions of uremia identified clinically or at autopsy (syn: necropsy) are useful indicators of renal failure (Table 11-1). The severity of nonrenal lesions of uremia depends on the length of time that the animal has survived in the uremic state. Therefore, in acute renal failure, nonrenal lesions are few, whereas many lesions can be present in chronic renal failure. During renal failure, numerous so-called "uremic toxins" accumulate in the blood. These toxins fall into three classes: (1) small water-soluble compounds including urea, phosphate, creatinine, and guanidines; (2) medium-sized molecules including fibroblast growth factor-23, β_2-microglobulin, parathyroid hormone, and leptin; and (3) protein-bound compounds including a variety of phenols and indoles. Typically, nonrenal lesions can be attributed to either one of the following mechanisms:

- Endothelial degeneration and necrosis, resulting in vasculitis with secondary thrombosis and infarction in a variety of tissues (i.e., intestinal tract).

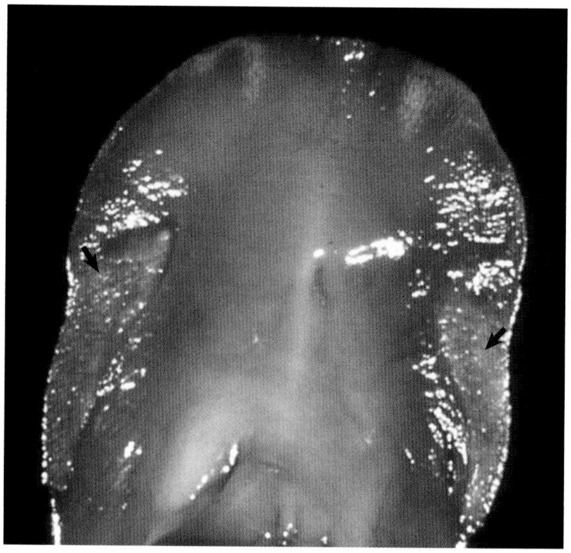

Figure 11-21 **Ulcerative Glossitis, Uremia, Tongue, Ventral Surface, Cat.** Bilaterally symmetrical ulcers *(arrows)* are present on the rostrolateral borders of the ventral surface of the tongue. (Courtesy Dr. M.D. McGavin, College of Veterinary Medicine, University of Tennessee.)

- Caustic injury to epithelium of the oral cavity and stomach, which results in ulcer formation, is secondary to the production of large concentrations of ammonia after splitting of salivary or gastric urea by bacteria.
- Increased erythrocyte fragility and lack of erythropoietin production.
- Altered calcium/phosphorus metabolism (renal secondary hyperparathyroidism).

Systemic nonrenal lesions of uremia include one or more of the following:

- Ulcerative and necrotic glossitis/stomatitis characterized by a brown, foul-smelling, mucoid material adherent to the eroded and ulcerated lingual and oral mucosa. Ulcers are most commonly bilateral (symmetric) and present on the underside of the tongue (Fig. 11-21).
- Ulcerative and hemorrhagic gastritis in dogs and cats (Fig. 11-22), often with secondary midzonal mineralization (Fig. 11-23). Ulcers are not large and often are present along the rugae. The gastric wall can be gritty when cut because of calcification of the inner and middle layers of the mucosa and the submucosal arterioles. This lesion is less commonly seen in horses and cattle, in which intestinal lesions predominate.
- Ulcerative and hemorrhagic colitis in horses and cattle, in which large areas of colonic mucosa are often edematous and dark red because of hemorrhage. The gastrointestinal contents can be bloody and smell of ammonia. Microscopically, coagulative necrosis, hemorrhage, and a neutrophilic infiltrate occur in the intestinal mucosa. Degeneration, necrosis, and mineralization of the arteriolar intima and media are often present in the gastric mucosa and submucosa (Fig. 11-23, *B*).
- Intercostal mineralization/uremic mineralization is characterized, particularly in dogs, by calcification of the subpleural connective tissue of the cranial intercostal spaces (Fig. 11-24). These lesions are white-gray granular pleural thickenings with a horizontal "ladder-like" arrangement. The intercostal muscles are only superficially calcified. Patchy or diffuse pulmonary calcification of the lungs results in their failure to collapse, areas of paleness, and mild to moderate firmness and crunchiness and can

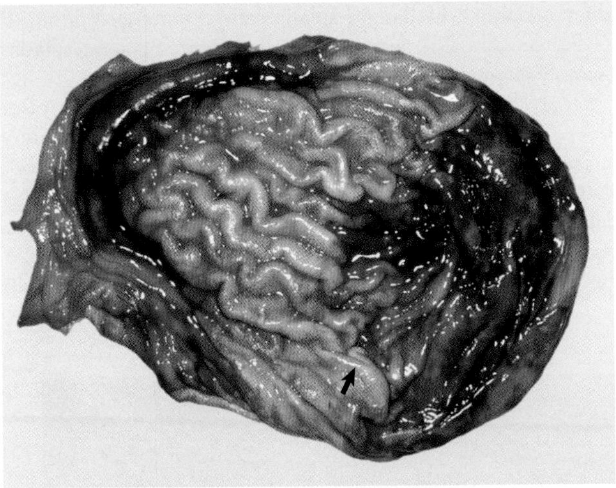

Figure 11-22 **Uremic Gastritis, Stomach, Dog.** Because of uremia, the stomach wall is hemorrhagic *(right)* and the stomach contents may contain blood and mucus (not shown here). Note the edematous mucosal thickening *(arrow)*. (Courtesy Dr. A. Confer, Center for Veterinary Health Sciences, Oklahoma State University.)

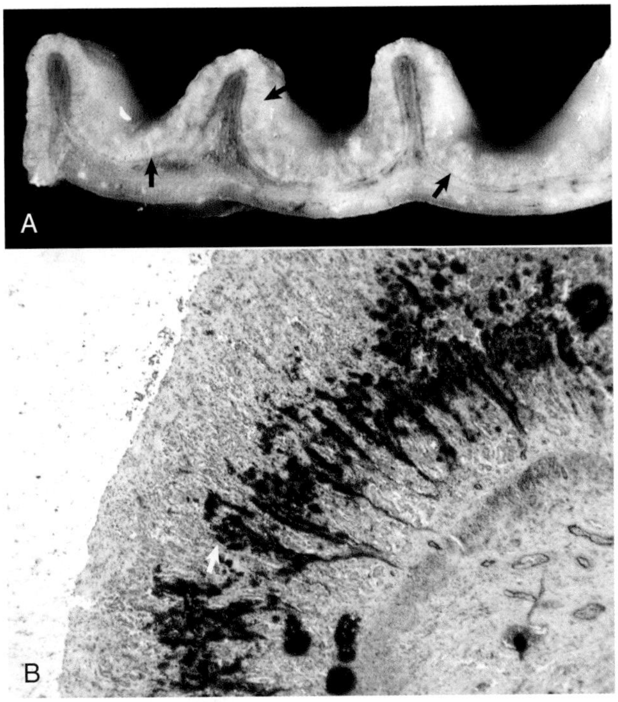

Figure 11-23 **Uremic Gastritis, Stomach, Dog. A,** There is accentuation of the gastric rugae and calcification in the deep mucosa *(arrows)*. **B,** The mucosa has laminar mineralization *(black color)* of gastric glands *(arrow)*, von Kossa stain. (**A** courtesy Dr. J. King, College of Veterinary Medicine, Cornell University. **B** courtesy Dr. M.D. McGavin, College of Veterinary Medicine, University of Tennessee.)

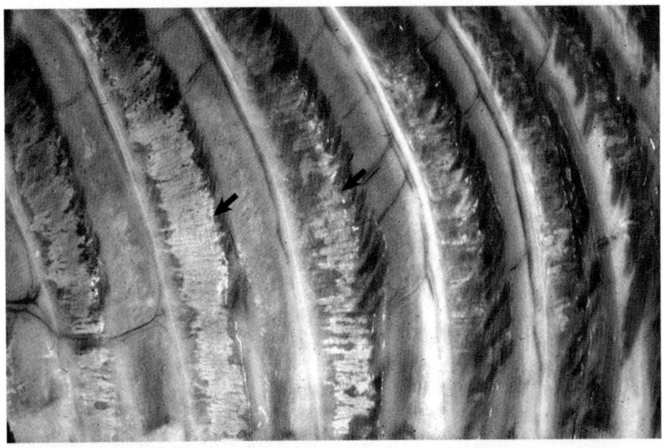

Figure 11-24 **Thoracic Cavity, Parietal Pleura, Cat.** Horizontally oriented streaks *(arrows)* of mineral (intercostal mineralization) are present in the subpleural intercostal connective tissue as a result of chronic uremia. (Courtesy Dr. J. King, College of Veterinary Medicine, Cornell University.)

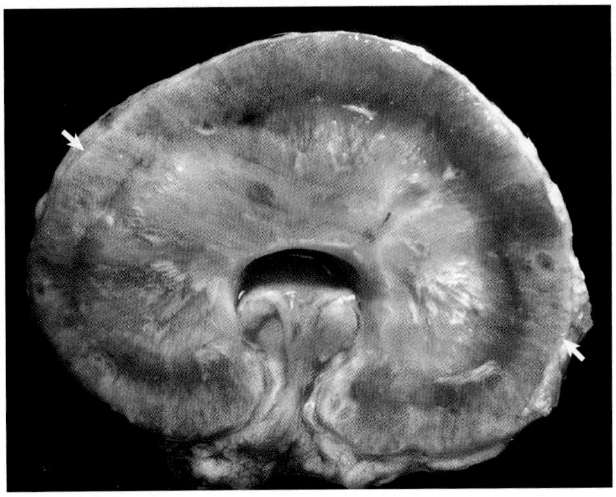

Figure 11-25 **Nephrocalcinosis, Kidney, Dorsal Section, Dog.** Note the white streaks *(arrows)* in the cortex and medulla attributable to mineralization of the interstitium, basement membranes, and tubules. This lesion results from diseases that increase plasma calcium concentrations (e.g., hyperparathyroidism). Renal tubular epithelium is damaged by an increase in intracellular calcium, which is initially precipitated in mitochondria and tubular basement membranes. (Courtesy Dr. M.D. McGavin, College of Veterinary Medicine, University of Tennessee.)

occur occasionally in conjunction with the lesions of uremic pneumonitis and localized emphysema.

- Fibrinous pericarditis is characterized by fine granular deposits of calcium on the epicardium (visceral pericardium).
- Diffuse pulmonary edema is characterized by alveoli that contain fibrin-rich fluid and often a mild infiltrate of macrophages and neutrophils. This lesion is also called *uremic pneumonitis*. The underlying lesion is a vasculitis affecting the alveolar capillaries, which results in increased vascular permeability and high protein effusion.
- Arteritis is characterized macroscopically by finely granular roughened plaques within the left atrial endocardium and less frequently in the proximal aorta and pulmonary trunk. Arteritis in conjunction with loss of the anticoagulant antithrombin III by glomerular leakage is conducive to the formation of large mural thrombi at these sites.
- Nephrocalcinosis (calcification), although usually not visible at autopsy (syn: necropsy), can occur in the damaged kidneys of uremic animals, but it can also occur in vitamin D toxicosis or primary or nutritional hyperparathyroidism (Fig. 11-25). The kidneys can be gritty when cut because of calcification of tubular basement membranes, Bowman's capsules, and necrotic tubular epithelium, especially in the medulla and inner cortex.

Disorders of the Kidney

Developmental Abnormalities

Renal Aplasia, Hypoplasia, and Dysplasia. Renal aplasia (agenesis) is failure of the development of one or both kidneys such that no recognizable renal tissue is present. In these cases, the ureter may be present or absent. If present, the cranial extremity of the ureter begins as a blind pouch. A familial tendency for renal aplasia has been observed in Doberman pinscher and beagle dogs. Because life can be sustained when more than one-fourth of renal function is maintained, unilateral aplasia is compatible with life, if the other kidney is normal. Unilateral aplasia can go unnoticed during life and be recognized at autopsy (syn: necropsy). Bilateral aplasia is obviously incompatible with life and occurs sporadically.

Renal hypoplasia designates incomplete development of the kidneys in a variety of species so that fewer than normal nephrons are present at birth. Renal hypoplasia has been documented as an inherited disease of purebred or crossbred Large White pigs in New Zealand and described in foals of various breeds, as well as in dogs (Fig. 11-26, *A*) and cats (Fig. 11-26, *B*). Hypoplasia can be unilateral (Fig. 11-26, *B*) or bilateral; it is rare and difficult to diagnose subtle

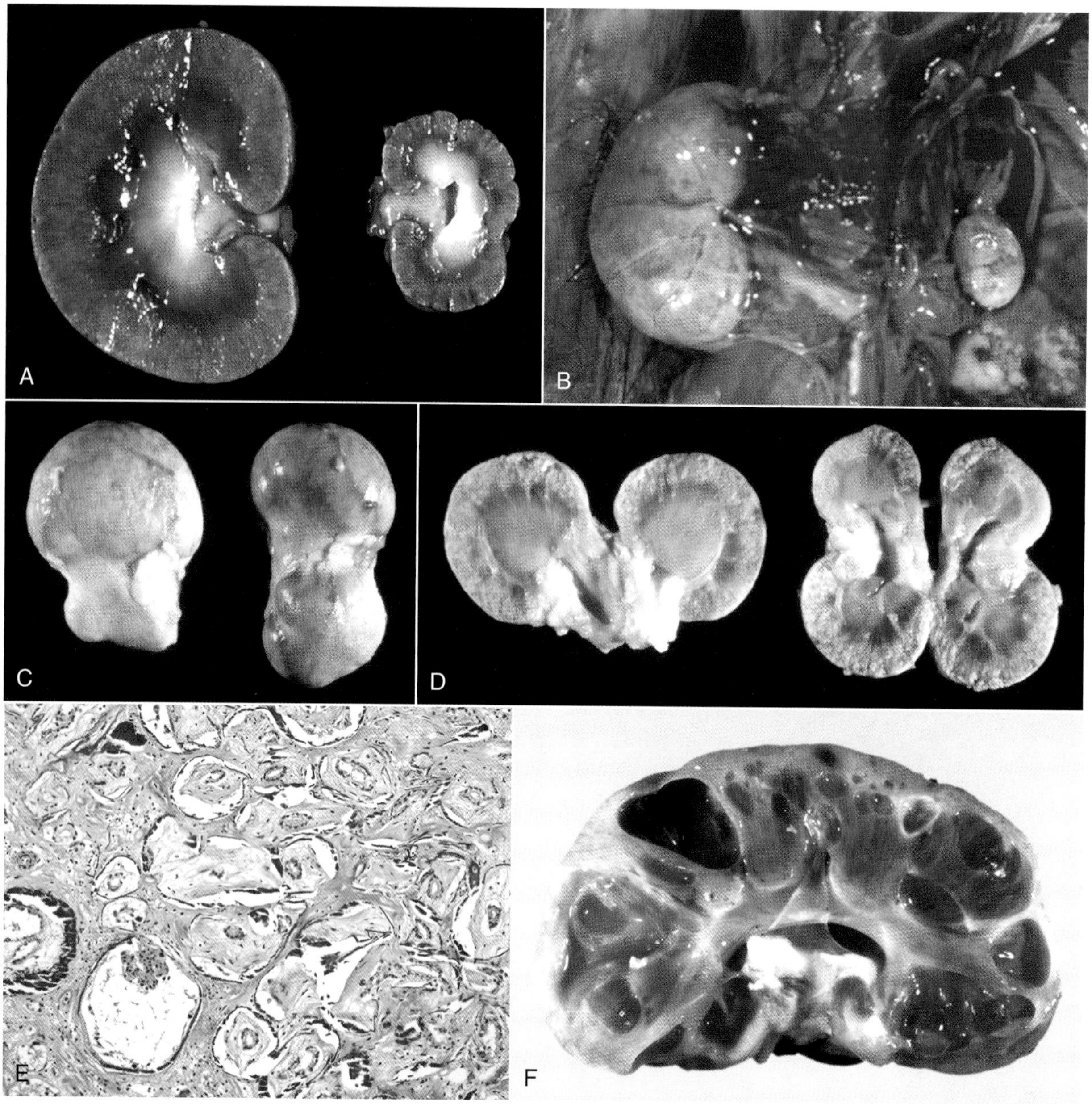

Figure 11-26 **Types of Congenital Developmental Anomalies, Kidney.** A and B, Unilateral hypoplastic kidneys, young dogs. **A,** Dorsal sections. **B,** The grossly affected right kidney is nearly identical in structure to the left kidney but smaller (hypoplasia). **C,** Juvenile progressive nephropathy, young dog. Bilateral abnormally shaped firm kidneys. **D,** Juvenile progressive nephropathy, dorsal sections, dog. Section of the kidneys from **C**. **E,** Juvenile progressive nephropathy, chronic, dog. Note the interstitial fibrosis, tubular atrophy, dilated urinary space, and mineralization. H&E stain. **F,** Polycystic disease, dorsal section, cat. Numerous variably sized tubular cysts are present in the cortex and medulla. The cysts contain clear colorless fluid. This condition is hereditary, and Persian cats are predisposed. (**A** courtesy Dr. B. Weeks, College of Veterinary Medicine, Texas A&M University; and Noah's Arkive, College of Veterinary Medicine, The University of Georgia. **B** courtesy Dr. M. Miller, College of Veterinary Medicine, University of Missouri; and Noah's Arkive, College of Veterinary Medicine, The University of Georgia. **C** and **D** courtesy College of Veterinary Medicine, University of Illinois. **E** courtesy Dr. S.J. Newman, College of Veterinary Medicine, University of Tennessee. **F** courtesy Dr. A. Confer, Center for Veterinary Health Sciences, Oklahoma State University.)

cases grossly or microscopically. In cattle and pigs, the number of renal papillae in the hypoplastic kidney can be compared with those in a normal kidney. Hypoplastic kidneys from pigs and foals have a notable reduction in the number of glomeruli. In foals, for example, 5 to 12 glomeruli are present per low-power field in affected kidneys compared with 30 to 35 glomeruli per low-power field in normal adult kidneys. Unless significant renal mass is compromised by this condition, hypoplasia is clinically silent.

Occasionally, some bovine kidneys are found to have reduced numbers of external lobes, but these kidneys are not hypoplastic and are microscopically and functionally normal; the reduction in external lobes merely represents fusion of the lobes. The shrunken, pitted kidneys in young animals, particularly dogs, are often diagnosed as hypoplastic. However, in most of these cases, these small kidneys are due to the following:

- Renal fibrosis, resulting from renal disease developing at an early age
- Dysplasia
- Progressive juvenile nephropathy

Renal dysplasia is an abnormality of altered structural organization resulting from abnormal differentiation and the presence of structures not normally present in nephrogenesis. Cystic renal dysplasia has been described in sheep and is inherited as an autosomal dominant trait. Renal dysplasia occurs infrequently and, like renal hypoplasia, must be differentiated from renal fibrosis and, in dogs, other forms of progressive juvenile nephropathy. Dysplastic changes can be unilateral or bilateral and can involve much of an affected kidney or occur only as focal lesions. Dysplastic kidneys can be small, misshapen, or both. Microscopically, five primary features of dysplasia are described as follows:

- Asynchronous differentiation of nephrons inappropriate for the age of the animal—aggregates of small hypercellular glomeruli in the cortex
- Persistence of primitive mesenchyme so that the interstitial connective tissue has a myxomatous appearance
- Persistence of metanephric ducts
- Atypical (adenomatoid) tubular epithelium
- The presence of cartilaginous and/or osseous tissue

Interstitial fibrosis, renal cysts, and a few enlarged hypercellular glomeruli (compensatory hypertrophy) are changes seen secondarily to the primary dysplastic changes. The numbers of nephrons, lobules, and calyces are normal. Bilateral renal dysplasia characterized by persistent mesenchyme and atypical tubular development has been described in foals.

Progressive juvenile nephropathy (familial renal disease) of Lhasa apso, shih tzu, golden retriever dogs, and perhaps other canine breeds are likely examples of renal dysplasia (Fig. 11-26, C to E). Asynchronous differentiation is often seen and to a lesser extent several other features of dysplasia. However, until these hereditary lesions of dogs are better characterized, it is probably best to retain the general diagnostic term of progressive juvenile nephropathy (see the section on Kidney and Lower Urinary Tract, Disorders of Dogs).

Ectopic and Fused Kidneys. Ectopic kidneys are misplaced from their normal sublumbar location because of abnormal migration during fetal development. Ectopic kidneys occur most frequently in pigs and dogs and usually involve only one kidney. Ectopic locations often include the pelvic cavity or inguinal position. Although ectopic kidneys are usually structurally and functionally normal, malposition of the ureters predisposes them to obstruction, which results in secondary hydronephrosis. Fused (horseshoe) kidneys result from the fusion of the left and right cranial or left and right caudal poles of the kidneys during nephrogenesis. This fusion results in the appearance of one large kidney with two ureters. The histologic structure and function of the fused kidneys are usually normal.

Renal Cysts. Renal cysts are spherical, thin-walled, variably sized distentions principally of the cortical or medullary renal tubules and are filled with clear, watery fluid. Congenital renal cysts can occur as a primary entity or in cases of renal dysplasia. The pathogenesis of primary renal cysts is not entirely understood. Cysts are likely derived from normal or noncystic segments of the nephron, most commonly the renal tubules, the collecting ducts, and Bowman's (urinary) space. Although genetic mechanisms can be involved in the pathogenesis of renal cysts, experiments with toxic chemicals indicate that genetic predisposition is not a requirement. The following four mechanisms of renal cystic dilation are considered plausible:

- Obstruction of nephrons can cause increased luminal pressure and secondary dilation (called *cystic dilation* when it is well-developed).
- Modifications in ECM and cell-matrix interactions result in weakened tubular basement membranes allowing saccular dilation of tubules.
- Deranged function of renal tubular cilia in genetic polycystic disease resulting in tubular epithelial hyperplasia with production of new basement membranes, increased tubular secretion, and increased intratubular pressure causes development of enlarged, dilated tubules.
- Dedifferentiation of tubular epithelial cells results in loss of polarity of cells with abnormal cell arrangements in tubules, reduced tubular fluid absorption, increased intratubular pressure, and dilation of tubules.

These mechanisms are not mutually exclusive, and several mechanisms often work in concert to create renal cysts.

Cysts range in size from barely visible to several centimeters in diameter. Cysts are usually spherical, delineated by a thin fibrous connective tissue wall lined by flattened epithelium, and filled with clear, watery fluid. The sources of fluid are glomerular filtrate, transepithelial secretions, or both. When viewed from the renal surface, the cyst wall is pale gray, smooth, and translucent. Kidneys can have single or multiple cysts. Congenital solitary or a few incidental cysts can cause no alteration in renal function and are common in pigs and calves. Acquired renal cysts can occur because of renal interstitial fibrosis or other renal diseases that cause intratubular obstruction. These cysts are usually small (1 to 2 mm in diameter) and occur primarily in the cortex.

Polycystic Kidneys. Polycystic kidneys have many cysts that involve numerous nephrons. Congenital polycystic kidneys occur sporadically in many species but can be inherited as an autosomal dominant lesion in pigs and lambs and inherited along with cystic biliary disease in Cairn and West Highland white terriers. The lesion, termed *polycystic kidney disease* (PKD), is inherited as an autosomal dominant trait in families of Persian cats and bull terriers. In addition, PKD is diagnosed sporadically in numerous exotic and domestic animal species. Although less well-characterized in animals than in human beings, this autosomal dominant, high-penetrance, heritable condition is related to mutations in one or more genes (*PKD-1* and/or *PKD-2*) and altered function of the related proteins, principally polycystin-1 and polycystin-2. Manifestation of tubular cysts occurs after mutation of both alleles of these genes, the first of which is a germline mutation, and the second is somatic mutation. Polycystin-1 and polycystin-2 are transmembrane proteins important in cell-to-cell and cell-to-matrix interactions and calcium channeling. In addition, these proteins work together in renal tubular cells and are associated with renal tubular cell cytoplasmic membranes and cilia and are important in renal tubular development, signal transduction, control of cell cycle, and migration. Although the exact mechanisms for cyst formation are not known, polycystin-1 and polycystin-2 mutations modify cilia function, cell proliferation, and migration resulting in tubular epithelial proliferation and increased fluid secretion. In addition, loss of polycystin-1 from its basolateral location may alter critical pathways controlling normal tubulogenesis, thus contributing to cyst formation. Polycystic renal disease with cysts arising from glomeruli has been described in collie puppies. The gross appearance of the cut surface of a polycystic kidney has been described as "Swiss cheese" (Fig. 11-26, *F*). As cysts enlarge, they compress the adjacent parenchyma causing atrophy. When extensive regions of renal parenchyma are polycystic, renal function can be impaired.

Diseases of the Glomerulus

Immune-Mediated Glomerulonephritis. Glomerulonephritis (GN) most often results from immune-mediated mechanisms, most notably after the deposition of soluble immune complexes within the glomeruli and less commonly after the formation of antibodies directed against antigens within the GBM. Antibodies to the basement membrane (anti-GBM disease) bind and damage the glomerulus through fixation of complement and resulting leukocyte infiltration. This mechanism of GN has been well documented in human beings and nonhuman primates but only rarely in other domestic animals. To confirm the diagnosis of anti-GBM disease, Ig and complement (C3) must be demonstrated within glomeruli. Antibodies must be eluted from the kidneys and found to bind to normal GBMs of the appropriate species.

Immune-complex GN (ICGN) occurs most commonly in dogs and cats and is the most common glomerular disease in dogs, accounting for 48% of glomerular diseases in a recent study. ICGN often occurs in association with persistent infections or other diseases that characteristically have a prolonged antigenemia that enhances the formation of soluble immune complexes. ICGN can be associated with specific chronic viral infections, such as feline leukemia virus (FeLV) or feline immunodeficiency virus (FIV); chronic bacterial infections, such as pyometra or pyoderma; chronic parasitism, such as dirofilariasis; autoimmune diseases, such as canine systemic lupus erythematosus; and neoplasia (Box 11-8). In addition to the role of persistent infections, a familial tendency for development of ICGN has been described in a group of related Bernese mountain dogs.

ICGN is initiated by the formation of soluble immune complexes (antigen-antibody complexes) in the presence of antigen-antibody equivalency or slight antigen excess, which then do the following:

- Selectively deposit in the glomerular capillaries
- Stimulate complement fixation with formation of C3a, C5a, and C567, which are chemotactic for neutrophils
- Damage the basement membrane through neutrophil release of proteinases, arachidonic acid metabolites (e.g., thromboxane), and oxidants, particularly oxygen-derived free radicals and hydrogen peroxide
- Continue to damage the glomeruli by the release of biologically active molecules from monocyte infiltrations in the later stages of inflammation (Fig. 11-27, *A*)

Although circulating immune complexes may contribute to this process, antibody binding to endogenous glomerular antigens or entrapped nonspecific antigens is more common. Direct action of C5b to C9 on the glomerular components results in activation of both glomerular epithelial cells and mesangial cells to produce damaging mediators, such as oxidants and proteases.

Many specific factors determine the extent of deposition of soluble immune complexes in the glomerular capillary walls. These include persistence of appropriate quantities of immune complexes in the circulation, glomerular permeability, the size and molecular charge of the soluble complexes, and the strength of the bond between the antigen and antibody (avidity). Small or intermediate complexes are the most damaging because large complexes are removed from circulation through phagocytosis by cells of the monocyte-macrophage system in the liver and spleen. An increase in local glomerular vascular permeability is necessary for immune complexes to leave the microcirculation and deposit in the glomerulus. This process is usually facilitated via vasoactive amine release from mast cells, basophils, or platelets (see Fig. 11-27, *A*). Mast cells or basophils release vasoactive amines because of the interaction of the immune complexes with antigen-specific IgE on the surface of these cells, by stimulation of the mast cells or basophils by cationic proteins released from neutrophils, or by the anaphylatoxin activity of C3a and C5a. Platelet-activating factor (PAF) is released from immune complex–stimulated mast cells, basophils, or macrophages and causes platelets to release vasoactive amines.

Localization of the complexes within the various levels of the basement membrane or in subepithelial locations depends on their molecular charge and avidity. Once small, soluble immune complexes are deposited within the capillary wall, they can become greatly enlarged because of interactions of immune complexes with free antibodies, free antigens, complement components, or other immune complexes.

Box 11-8 Diseases with Immune-Complex Glomerulonephritis

HORSES
Equine infectious anemia
Streptococcus sp.

CATTLE
Bovine viral diarrhea
Trypanosomiasis

SHEEP
Hereditary hypocomplementemia in Finnish Landrace lambs

PIGS
Hog cholera
African swine fever

DOGS
Infectious canine hepatitis
Chronic hepatitis
Chronic bacterial diseases
Endometritis (pyometra)
Pyoderma
Prostatitis
Dirofilariasis
Borreliosis (Lyme disease)
Systemic lupus erythematosus
Polyarteritis
Autoimmune hemolytic anemia
Immune-mediated polyarthritis
Neoplasia–mastocytoma
Hereditary C3 deficiency

CATS
Feline leukemia virus (FeLV) infection
Feline infectious peritonitis (FIP)
Feline immunodeficiency virus (FIV)
Progressive polyarteritis
Neoplasia
Progressive membranous glomerulonephritis (GN)

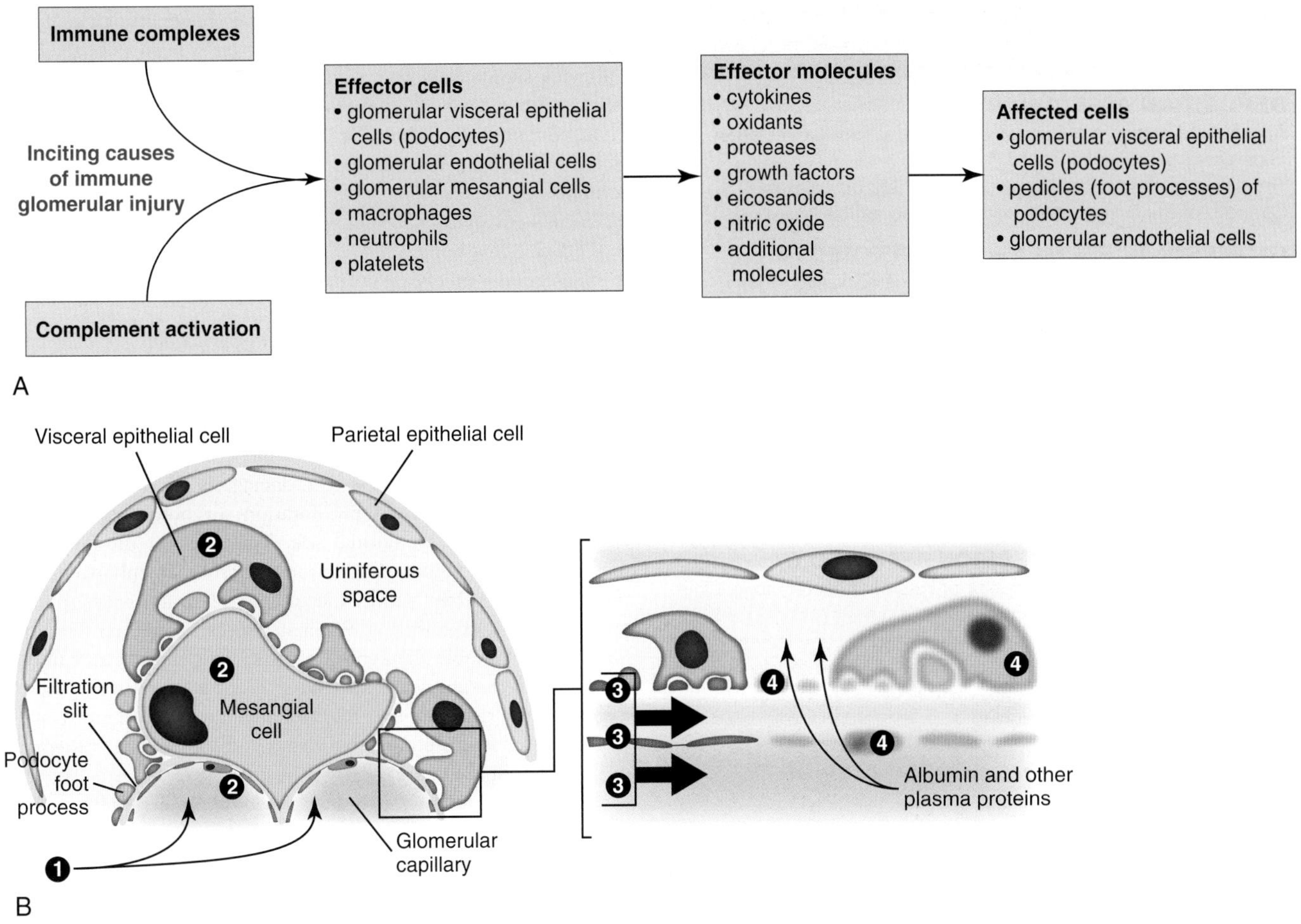

Figure 11-27 Mediators of Immune Glomerular Injury and Epithelial Cell Injury. A, Mediators of immune glomerular injury, including effector cells, molecules, and cells affected or injured. **B,** Visceral epithelial cell (podocyte) injury. The postulated sequence is a consequence of antibodies against epithelial cell antigens, arriving in the circulating blood *(1)* with subsequent activation of effector cells, including podocytes and mesangial cells *(2)*. This leads to liberation of toxins, cytokines, or other effector molecules *(3)* that cause injury of podocytes, podocyte foot processes, and endothelial cells *(4)* with subsequent cell detachment, resulting in protein leakage through the defective glomerular basement membrane and filtration slits. (Courtesy Drs. M.A. Breshears and A.W. Confer, Center for Veterinary Health Sciences, Oklahoma State University; and Dr. J.F. Zachary, College of Veterinary Medicine, University of Illinois.)

After immune-complex deposition, glomerular injury can also occur from the aggregation of platelets and activation of Hageman factor, which results in the formation of fibrin thrombi that produce glomerular ischemia. Furthermore, glomerular epithelial cell and ECM damage can result directly from the terminal membrane attack complex of the activated complement cascade (C5 to C9). This can result in epithelial detachment (causing proteinuria) and GBM thickening subsequent to upregulation of epithelial cell receptors for transforming growth factor (Fig. 11-27, *B*). Cell-mediated cytotoxic responses (from sensitized T lymphocytes) to glomerular antigens or complexes may exacerbate renal lesions. Complexes themselves may modulate the immune response through interaction with receptors on various cells.

Finally, if exposure of the glomerulus to immune complexes is short-lived, as in a transient infection such as infectious canine hepatitis, glomerular immune complexes will be phagocytosed by macrophages or mesangial cells and removed, and the glomerular lesions and clinical signs may resolve. Conversely, continual exposure of glomeruli to soluble immune complexes, such as in persistent viral infections or chronic heartworm disease, can produce progressive glomerular injury, with severe lesions and clinical manifestation of glomerular disease (Box 11-9).

Ultrastructurally, immune complexes either in the GBM or in a subepithelial location appear as electron-dense granular bodies. Complexes that are poorly soluble, fairly large, or of high avidity often enter the mesangium, where they can be phagocytosed by macrophages and appear ultrastructurally as dense granular deposits within the mesangial stroma or within macrophages. Other ultrastructural changes commonly seen are loss, effacement, or fusion of visceral epithelial cell (podocytes) foot processes, cytoplasmic vacuolation, retraction and detachment of visceral epithelium, and infiltrates of neutrophils and monocytes within the mesangium.

A diagnosis of ICGN can be made by immunofluorescent or immunohistochemical demonstration of immunoglobulin and complement components, usually C3, in glomerular tufts. To augment light microscopic findings, transmission electron microscopy can be done to demonstrate typical subepithelial and intramembrane electron-dense deposits, fusion of podocyte foot processes, and intramesangial hypercellularity. In dogs, IgG or IgM are the most common immunoglobulin isotypes demonstrated in ICGN; however, combinations of IgG, IgM, and IgA also occur in the glomeruli of some dogs. In one study, IgA was the only immunoglobulin found in three dogs with ICGN. Both Ig and C3 are usually demonstrated in a granular ("lumpy-bumpy") pattern using immunofluorescent or immunohistochemical techniques (Fig. 11-28; E-Fig. 11-4); however, in anti-GBM disease, as reported in human beings, horses, and a single dog, the antibody deposits have a linear distribution conforming to the basement membranes. It is important to remember that

Box 11-9 Progression of Glomerular Immune-Complex Deposition

DEPOSITION AFFECTED BY

Appropriate quantities of immune complexes in the circulation
Glomerular permeability
The size and molecular charge of the soluble complexes
Strength of the bond between antigen and antibody

GLOMERULAR PERMEABILITY AFFECTED BY

Release of vasoactive amines from mast cells, basophils, or platelets

- Immune complexes interact with antigen-specific immunoglobulin E on surface of mast cells or basophils
- Cationic proteins from neutrophils stimulate release of vasoactive amines from mast cells and basophils
- C3a and C5a cause release of vasoactive amines
- Platelets release vasoactive amines following release of platelet-activating factor from immune-complex stimulated mast cells, basophils, and macrophages

GLOMERULAR PROGRESSION AFFECTED BY

Aggregation of platelets, activation of Hageman factor, fibrin thrombi formation, and glomerular ischemia
Terminal membrane active complex of activated complement cascade damages glomerular epithelial cells and extracellular matrix (ECM) resulting in epithelial cell detachment and basement membrane thickening
Cell-mediated cytotoxic responses from T lymphocytes sensitized to glomerular antigens or complexes may exacerbate renal lesions

fluorescing deposits indicate the presence of immunoglobulin or complement but do not specifically indicate the presence of disease. In addition, immunofluorescence may be negative when all reactive binding sites are occupied, thus complicating diagnosis of this condition.

The diagnosis of preformed ICGN can be confirmed only by demonstrating that the antibodies from the immune complexes, eluted from glomeruli, do not bind to normal glomerular elements and hence represent deposition of preformed circulating complexes. Once this has been done, the ideal situation would be to identify the causative antigen present in the immune complexes. This process is accomplished by eluting antibodies from diseased glomeruli and attempting to identify their specificity for suspected antigens. For example, antibodies eluted from the glomeruli of dogs with GN associated with severe heartworm disease bind to several *Dirofilaria immitis* antigens, including the body wall of adult worms, parasitic uterine fluid, and microfilaria. In most cases of immune-complex GN, the specific causative antigen usually escapes determination. Demonstration of electron-dense deposits in mesangial, subepithelial, or subendothelial locations by electron microscopy is also supportive of the diagnosis of immune-mediated GN.

Gross lesions of acute ICGN are usually subtle. Kidneys are often slightly swollen, have a smooth capsular surface, are of normal color or slightly pale, and have glomeruli that are visible as pinpoint red dots on the cut surface of the cortex (Fig. 11-29). The normal glomeruli of horses are usually visible, so this feature of pinpoint red dots for glomeruli cannot be used for diagnosis in that species. If lesions do not resolve but become subacute to chronic, the renal cortex becomes somewhat shrunken and the capsular surface has a generalized fine granularity. On cut surface, the cortex can be thinned and its surface granular, and glomeruli can appear as pinpoint pale gray dots. With time, more severe scarring can develop throughout the cortex (see the section on Renal Fibrosis).

Microscopically, ICGN has several histopathologic forms. Although various classifications of GN have been published, the following simple classification is well understood among veterinary pathologists. Lesions in glomeruli may be described as membranous or membranoproliferative (Fig. 11-30). Glomerular lesion localization and distribution can be characterized with the following terminology:

- Focal—involving <50% of glomeruli
- Diffuse—involving >50% of glomeruli
- Segmental—involving portions of the glomerular tuft
- Global—involving all of the glomerular tuft
- Hilar—focused primarily near the vascular pole
- Tip—focused primarily near the outer portions of the tuft

Most of the lesions in ICGN are diffuse, but within an individual affected glomerulus, lesions can be either global or segmental. In the more chronic form, a variety of glomerular tuft changes will be noted, depending on whether the damage is related to mesangial proliferation, membranous proliferation, or both. Tufts may be enlarged, shrunken, or normal size depending on the amount of mesangial matrix present. Reduction in cellularity, enhancement of the capillary outlines within the tuft, proliferation of the parietal epithelial cells, expansion of Bowman's space by high protein ultrafiltrate, and variable thickening of Bowman's capsule may also be observed. *Glomerulosclerosis* (see later) is the stage in which there is a reduction in the number of functional glomeruli with replacement by abundant fibrous connective tissue and subsequent obliteration of Bowman's space due to capsular fibrosis.

In addition, in protein-losing glomerulopathies, tubules often contain abundant eosinophilic homogeneous proteinaceous material, and the proximal tubular epithelium often have microscopic eosinophilic intracytoplasmic bodies referred to as *hyaline droplets*, which represent accumulations of intracytoplasmic protein absorbed from the filtrate.

Microscopic details of each type of glomerular disease are discussed in the next sections.

Membranous Glomerulonephritis. Membranous GN is characterized by diffuse glomerular capillary basement membrane thickening without obvious increased cellularity. These thickenings are often most obvious when capillary loops at the periphery of the tuft are examined. Special stains such as periodic–acid Schiff (PAS) or Masson's trichrome can assist in membrane examination. Membrane thickening occurs because of the presence of subepithelial immunoglobulin deposits, as the predominant change (Fig. 11-31; also see Fig. 11-30, *B*). These deposits are separated by protrusions of GBM matrix that eventually encompass these deposits. After removal of the deposited material, cavities are left in the GBM and later these fill with GBM-like material, which results in sclerotic change within the glomerular tuft. This is characterized by increased deposition of positive material (periodic acid–Schiff [PAS]) and a lesser amount of fibrosis. This variation is the most common form of ICGN in cats.

Membranoproliferative Glomerulonephritis. Membranoproliferative GN (mesangioproliferative, mesangiocapillary) is characterized by hypercellularity following proliferation of glomerular endothelial cells, glomerular epithelial cells, and mesangial cells. Concurrently, there is an influx of neutrophils and other leukocytes involving capillary loops and the mesangium with thickening of the capillary basement membrane and mesangium (see Fig. 11-30, C and Fig. 11-31). Sometimes, the hypercellularity is more obvious than membranous thickening, and those cases have traditionally been called "proliferative" glomerulonephritis. More recent classification schemes no longer recognize the "proliferative" glomerulonephritis type, and those cases should more appropriately be considered variants of membranoproliferative GN. Membranoproliferative GN is

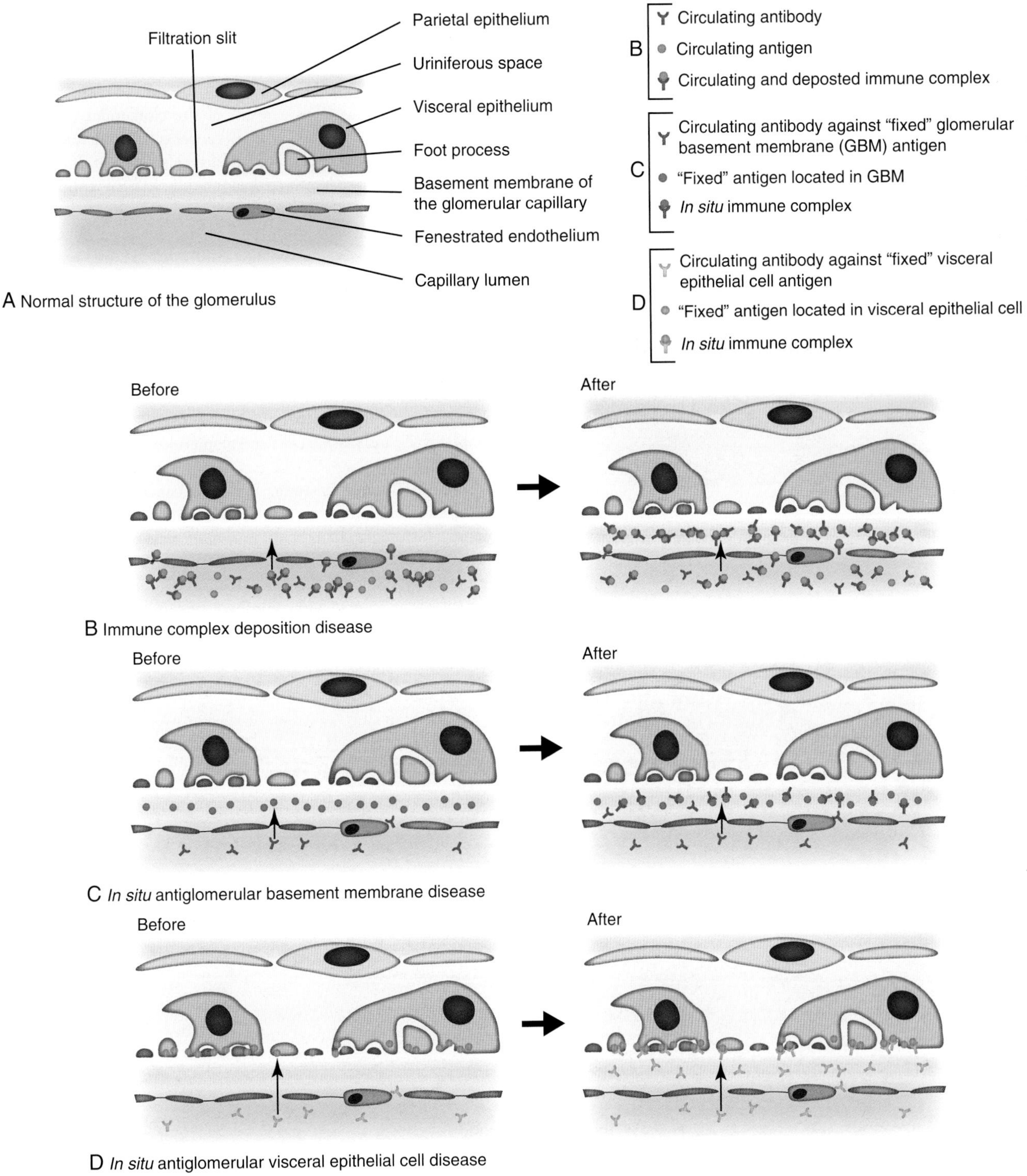

Figure 11-28 **Antibody-Mediated Glomerular Injury. A,** Normal structure of the glomerulus. Antibody-mediated glomerular injury can result either from the deposition of circulating immune complexes **(B)** or from formation of complexes in situ (**C** and **D**). Using immunofluorescence microscopy (not shown here), antiglomerular basement membrane (anti-GBM) disease **(C)** and antiglomerular (visceral epithelial cell) disease **(D)** are characterized by linear patterns of immunofluorescence deposition in glomeruli, whereas deposition of circulating immune complexes in glomeruli is characterized by granular ("lumpy-bumpy") patterns (see E-Fig. 11-4). (Courtesy Drs. M.A. Breshears and A.W. Confer, Center for Veterinary Health Sciences, Oklahoma State University; and Dr. J.F. Zachary, College of Veterinary Medicine, University of Illinois.)

the most common morphologic form of ICGN in the dog. With light microscopy, membranoproliferative GN changes are similar across cases; however, differences can be seen with immunofluorescent and electron microscopy. The latter technique has resulted in subcategorization of human being membranoproliferative GN into types I and II (see Fig. 11-31). Type I lesions, which are typical of those found in domestic animals, are characterized by the presence of subendothelial deposits and a granular pattern after deposition of C3 and lesser quantities of IgG, C1q, and C4. Type I disease appears to be secondary to deposition of circulating immune complexes. Type II is far less common in human beings than type I and is also referred to as *dense deposit disease* because electron-dense material of unknown composition and smaller quantities of C3 form an irregular deposit within the subendothelial space and the lamina densa. Type II disease may be a form of autoimmune disease, but its pathogenesis is not clear.

Several other changes in the glomerulus and Bowman's capsule usually accompany the lesions discussed previously. These changes include adhesions between the epithelial cells of the glomerular tuft and Bowman's capsule (synechiae; singular = synechia); hypertrophy and hyperplasia of the parietal epithelium lining Bowman's capsule; deposition of fibrinogen and fibrinous thrombi in glomerular capillaries, secondary to or as a result of the glomerular damage; and dilated renal tubules filled with homogeneous proteinaceous fluid. An increase in mesangial matrix is often also present. If the damage is mild and the cause is removed, glomeruli can heal without obvious or with minimal residual lesions. However, if the lesion is severe and prolonged, subacute to chronic glomerular changes develop. Bowman's capsule can become thickened, hyalinized, and reduplicated. In severe cases, proliferation of parietal epithelium, an influx of monocytes, and deposition of fibrin can occur within Bowman's capsule, resulting in the formation of a semicircular, hypercellular, intraglomerular lesion known as a *glomerular crescent*. The glomerular crescent can also undergo fibrosis, and if Bowman's capsule ruptures, glomerular fibrosis can become continuous with interstitial fibrosis. Interstitial and periglomerular fibrosis, foci of interstitial lymphocytes, and plasma cells and glomerulosclerosis may be present in chronic GN.

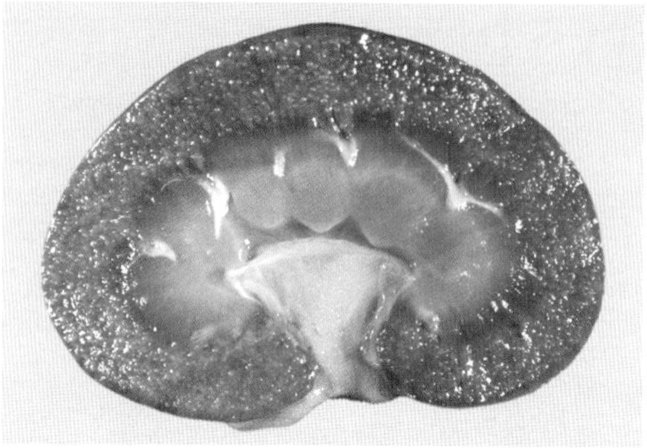

Figure 11-29 **Proliferative Glomerulonephritis (GN), Kidney, Dorsal Section, Dog.** The small, white, round foci in the cortex are enlarged glomeruli. (Courtesy Dr. S.J. Newman, College of Veterinary Medicine, University of Tennessee.)

Minimal Change Disease. In human beings, a common protein-losing glomerulopathy, especially in children, is one in which glomerular histologic changes are minimal or absent, hence the name minimal change disease (MCD). The lesion is characterized ultrastructurally by diffuse effacement of visceral epithelial cell (podocyte) foot processes with minimal or no basement membrane

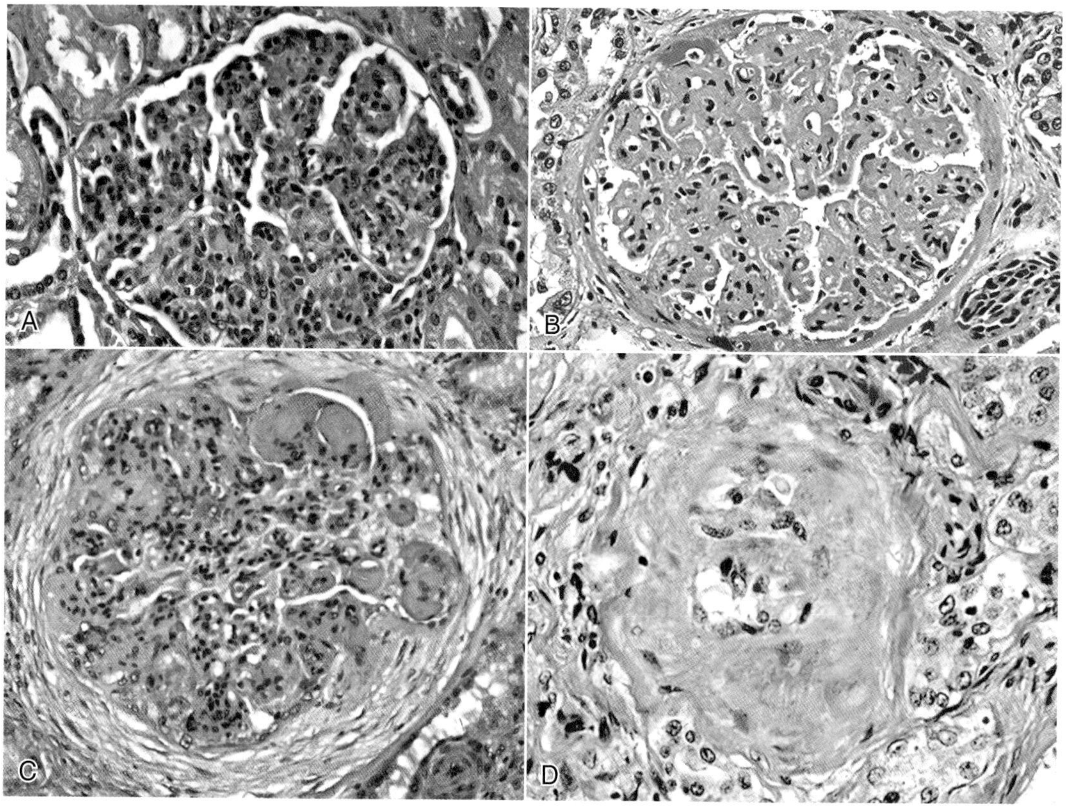

Figure 11-30 **Types of Glomerulonephritis (GN). A,** Proliferative GN, pig. The lesion is characterized principally by hypercellularity of the glomerulus due to increased numbers of mesangial cells. H&E stain. **B,** Membranous GN, dog. The lesion is characterized by generalized hyaline thickening of glomerular capillary basement membranes. It can occur in dogs with dirofilariasis. H&E stain. **C,** Membranoproliferative GN, horse. Membranoproliferative GN has histologic features of both proliferative GN and membranous GN. Abundant periglomerular fibrosis surrounds this hypercellular glomerulus (mesangial cells). Mesangial matrix is prominent in the top-right area of the glomerulus. H&E stain. **D,** Glomerulosclerosis, dog. Note the hypocellularity, shrinkage, and hyalinization due to an increase in fibrous connective tissue and mesangial matrix and almost complete loss of glomerular capillaries. In glomerulosclerosis (the end stage of chronic GN), glomeruli are essentially nonfunctional. H&E stain. (**A** and **C** courtesy Dr. W. Crowell, College of Veterinary Medicine, The University of Georgia; and Noah's Arkive, College of Veterinary Medicine, The University of Georgia. **B** and **D** courtesy Dr. S.J. Newman, College of Veterinary Medicine, University of Tennessee.)

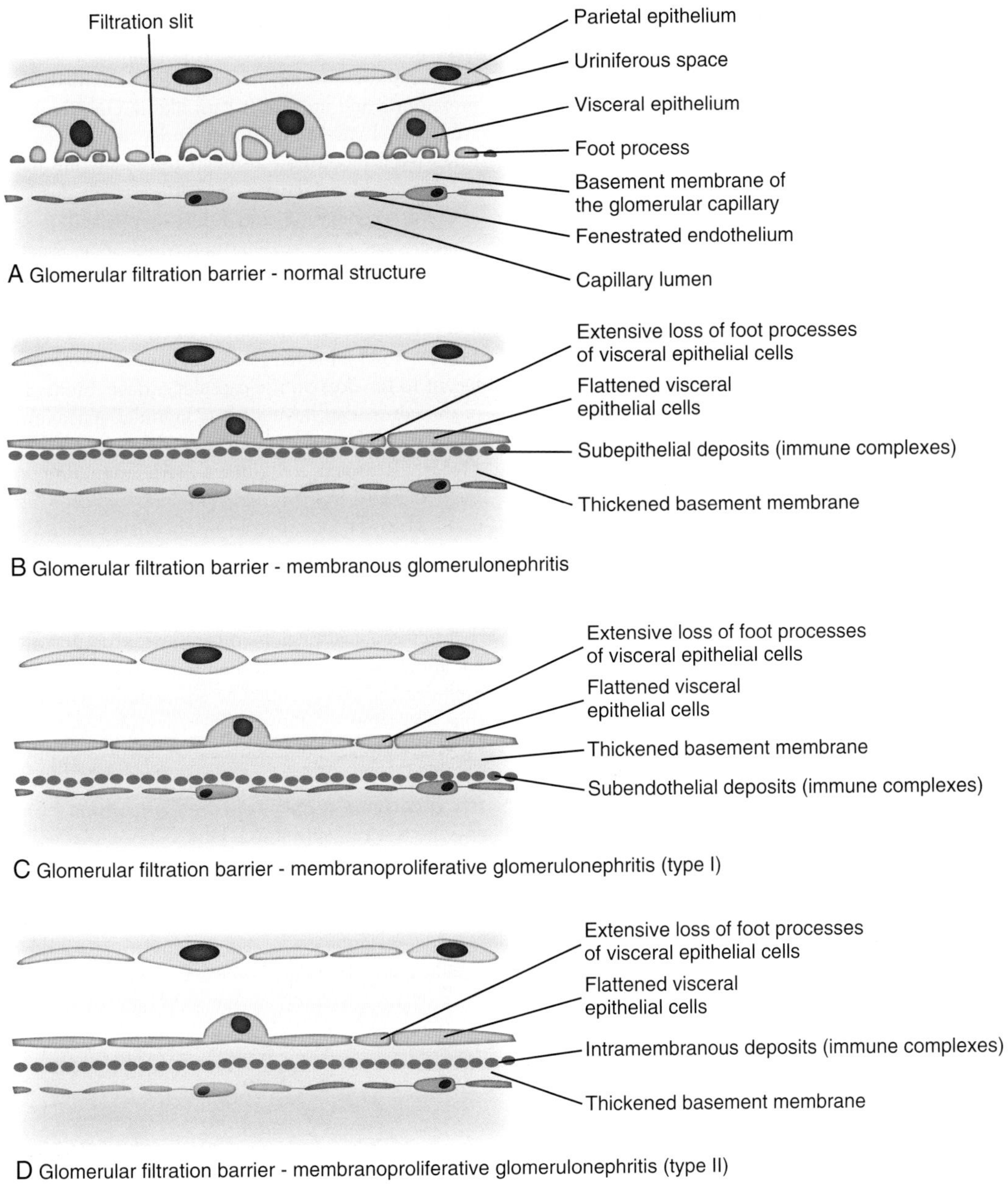

Figure 11-31 Sites of Immune Complex Deposition in the Glomerular Filtration Barrier in the Major Types Glomerulonephritis (GN). **A,** Normal structure of the glomerular filtration barrier. **B,** Membranous glomerulonephritis. Immune complexes are deposited in the basement membrane just beneath the visceral epithelium. **C,** Membranoproliferative glomerulonephritis (type I). Immune complexes are deposited in the basement membrane just beneath the vascular endothelium and lead to a granular pattern in the basement membrane. **D,** Membranoproliferative glomerulonephritis (type II). Immune complexes are deposited in the basement membrane and lead to the irregular deposition of electron-dense material within the lamina densa. Although not shown in this schematic diagram, type I and type II membranoproliferative glomerulonephritis commonly have hypertrophy and hyperplasia (proliferation) of glomerular endothelial cells, epithelial cells, and mesangial cells in response to the immune complexes and the biological processes they induce. Leukocytes (acute inflammation) may also be recruited from the microvasculature into the proliferative response. (Courtesy Drs. M.A. Breshears and A.W. Confer, Center for Veterinary Health Sciences, Oklahoma State University; and Dr. J.F. Zachary, College of Veterinary Medicine, University of Illinois.)

deposits. The cause of MCD is not obvious, but in most cases it is considered to be an immune dysfunction causing visceral epithelial cell damage. In addition, MCD has been correlated with nonsteroidal antiinflammatory drug (NSAID) therapy or treatment with other drugs. MCD has been described in dogs treated with the anti-mast cell tumor drug, masitinib. Histologically, glomeruli are essentially normal; however, ultrastructurally, visceral epithelial cell foot process effacement is diffuse and severe.

Glomerulosclerosis. In chronic GN, severely affected glomeruli shrink and become hyalinized because of an increase in both fibrous connective tissue and mesangial matrix and a loss of glomerular capillaries (Fig. 11-30, *D*). In addition, there is periglomerular fibrosis. These glomeruli are hypocellular and essentially nonfunctional. This process is referred to as *glomerulosclerosis*, and affected glomeruli are sometimes referred to as *obsolescent*. Nomenclature applied to GN for describing the numbers of glomeruli involved and the location of the lesion in the glomerulus can be used to describe glomerulosclerosis. Glomerulosclerosis can be diffuse, involving all glomeruli, or multifocal. In addition, glomerulosclerosis can involve an entire glomerular tuft (global) or only portions of the tuft (segmental), thus appearing as a nodular or segmental hyalinized thickening in affected glomeruli. Because tubules receive their blood supply from the vasa recta, derived from the glomerular efferent arteriole, glomerulosclerosis reduces the blood flow through the vasa recta, thus decreasing oxygen tension in the tubules. The ensuing hypoxia is responsible for tubular epithelial cell death via apoptosis resulting in failure to regenerate to columnar cells. Affected tubules often have reduced diameters and are lined by cuboidal or squamous cells, which lack a brush border and the functions of the normal columnar cells. In addition, chronic proteinuria often accompanies glomerulosclerosis and has been reported to promote tubular epithelial cell loss through apoptosis.

Numerous factors are associated with and accelerate glomerulosclerosis, including the following:

- Unrestricted protein in the diet
- Increased glomerular capillary pressure in the remaining functional glomeruli
- Cytokines from local GN-induced inflammation
- Platelet-derived growth factors (PDGFs)

These factors have the following effects:

- Alter cellular components of the functional glomerular tufts
- Cause hypertension and transglomerular hyperfiltration with resultant damage to endothelium
- Activate mesangial cells to proliferate
- Increase mesangial matrix production
- Accelerate visceral epithelial cell loss, which allows synechiae (i.e., adhesions between visceral and parietal epithelial cell layers in the glomerulus) to form

Glomerulosclerosis is not only the end stage of GN but also can develop in any chronic disease in which severe damage to nephrons or loss of nephron function occurs, including the loss of functional tubules. Mild multifocal glomerulosclerosis of unknown cause is often an incidental finding in aged animals. Glomerulosclerosis has been reported occasionally in animals with hypertension and diabetes mellitus. In these cases, global or nodular eosinophilic glycoprotein material (hyaline material) is deposited in the glomerular mesangium.

Glomerular Amyloidosis. Amyloid, an insoluble fibrillar protein with a β-pleated sheet conformation, is produced after incomplete proteolysis of several soluble amyloidogenic proteins. Amyloid deposits in patients with plasma cell myelomas or other B lymphocyte dyscrasias (called *AL amyloidosis*) are composed of fragments of the light (λ) chains of immunoglobulins. In domestic animals, spontaneously occurring amyloidosis is usually an example of what is called *reactive amyloidosis* (AA amyloidosis). This form of the disease is often associated with chronic inflammatory diseases; the amyloid deposits are composed of fragments of a serum acute-phase reactant protein called *serum amyloid–A* (SAA) protein. Amyloid fibrils from either source are deposited in tissue along with a glycoprotein called *amyloid P component.*

Glomeruli are the most common renal sites for deposition of amyloid in most domestic animal species, although the medullary interstitium is a common site in cats, particularly in Abyssinian breed. Renal amyloidosis commonly occurs in association with other diseases, particularly chronic inflammatory or neoplastic diseases. However, idiopathic renal amyloidosis (i.e., amyloidosis in which an associated disease process is not recognized) is also described in dogs and cats. The underlying pathogenic mechanisms of idiopathic renal amyloidosis are not known. In one study, 23% of dogs that presented with proteinuria had renal amyloidosis. A hereditary predisposition for the development of reactive amyloidosis (AA) has been found in Abyssinian cats and Chinese Shar-Pei dogs. A familial tendency is suspected in Siamese cats, English foxhounds, and beagle dogs. In cattle, renal amyloidosis is nearly always due to chronic systemic infectious disease. Glomerular amyloidosis is responsible for many cases of protein-losing nephropathy in animals that have notable proteinuria and uremia. It can, like ICGN, result in the nephrotic syndrome. Long-standing glomerular amyloidosis results in diminished renal blood flow through the glomeruli and the vasa recta. Such reduced renal vascular perfusion can lead to renal tubular atrophy, degeneration, and diffuse fibrosis and, in severe cases, renal papillary necrosis. Medullary amyloidosis is usually asymptomatic unless it results in papillary necrosis.

Kidneys affected with glomerular amyloidosis are often enlarged and pale and have a smooth to finely granular capsular surface (Fig. 11-32). Amyloid-laden glomeruli may be visible grossly as fine translucent to tan dots on the capsular surface. Similarly, the cut surface of the cortex can have a finely granular appearance with scattered glistening foci, less than 0.5 mm diameter in the cortex (see Fig. 11-32). Treatment of kidneys with an iodine solution, such as Lugol's iodine, in many cases results in red-brown staining of glomeruli, which become purple when treated with dilute sulfuric acid (Fig. 11-33). This technique provides a rapid presumptive diagnosis of renal amyloidosis. Medullary amyloidosis is usually not grossly recognizable.

Microscopically, glomerular amyloid is deposited in both the mesangium and subendothelial locations. Amyloid is relatively acellular and can accumulate segmentally within glomerular tufts; thus a portion of the normal glomerular architecture is replaced by eosinophilic, homogeneous to slightly fibrillar material (Fig. 11-34, *A*). When amyloidosis involves the entire glomerular tuft, the glomerulus is enlarged, capillary lumina become obliterated, and the tuft can appear as a large hypocellular eosinophilic hyaline sphere (Fig. 11-34, *B*). Amyloid can be present in renal tubular basement membranes, and these membranes appear hyalinized and thickened. In addition, in cases of glomerular amyloid deposition, secondary changes may be present in renal tubules, which are usually markedly dilated, have variably atrophic epithelium, and

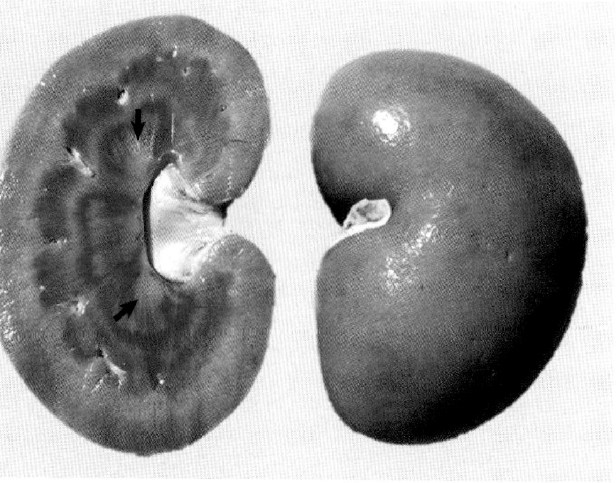

Figure 11-32 **Amyloidosis, Kidney, Dog.** Grossly, kidneys affected by amyloid deposition are diffusely tan, waxy (firm), and of normal size or slightly enlarged. Affected glomeruli are not grossly visible in this specimen, unlike in advanced cases of glomerular amyloidosis or chronic GN. In advanced cases of amyloidosis, glomeruli may be visible as pinpoint, glistening, round, cortical foci. In cats and Shar-Pei dogs, amyloid is deposited in the medullary interstitium, not in the glomeruli. There are also multiple foci of medullary crest necrosis (yellowish-green *[arrows]*). (Courtesy Dr. G.K. Saunders, The Virginia-Maryland Regional College of Veterinary Medicine; and Noah's Arkive, College of Veterinary Medicine, The University of Georgia.)

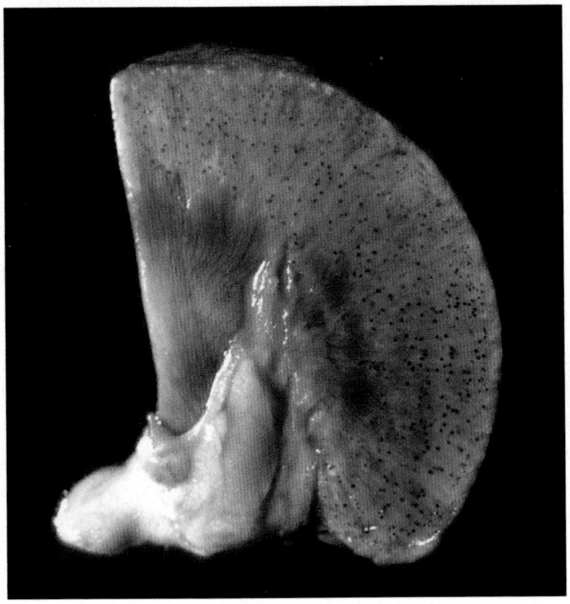

Figure 11-33 Amyloidosis, Kidney, Transverse Section, Dog. On the cut surface of fresh kidney treated with Lugol's iodine followed by dilute sulfuric acid, glomeruli containing amyloid are visible as multiple dark blue dots in the cortex. Lugol's iodine treatment. (Courtesy Dr. M.D. McGavin, College of Veterinary Medicine, University of Tennessee.)

contain proteinaceous and cellular casts. Amyloid is confirmed microscopically by staining with Congo red stain (Fig. 11-34, C). When viewed with polarized light, amyloid has a green birefringence (Fig. 11-34, *D*). Loss of Congo red staining after treatment of a section of affected kidney with potassium permanganate suggests amyloid is AA (i.e., of acute-phase reactant protein origin).

Acute Suppurative Glomerulitis: Bacterial (Embolic) Nephritis. Embolic nephritis, which can also be referred to as *acute suppurative glomerulitis*, is the result of a bacteremia in which bacteria lodge in random glomerular capillaries and to a lesser extent in interstitial capillaries and arterioles causing multiple foci of inflammation (microabscesses) throughout the renal cortex. Although the glomeruli appear targeted, this is really a manifestation of renal vascular disease. A specific example of embolic nephritis is *Actinobacillosis* of foals caused by *Actinobacillus equuli* (Fig. 11-35) (see Disorders of Horses). These foals usually die within a few days of birth and have small abscesses (1 mm or less in diameter) in many visceral organs, especially the renal cortex. Embolic nephritis also occurs commonly in the bacteremia of pigs infected with *Erysipelothrix rhusiopathiae* or sheep and goats infected with *Corynebacterium pseudotuberculosis*. *Trueperella pyogenes* was the most common isolate (26/31) from cases of embolic nephritis in necropsied cattle. *Staphylococcus aureus*, *Mannheimia haemolytica*, and *Streptococcus bovis* were also represented.

Grossly, multifocal, random, raised, 1 mm or less in diameter, tan foci are seen subcapsularly and on the cut surface throughout the

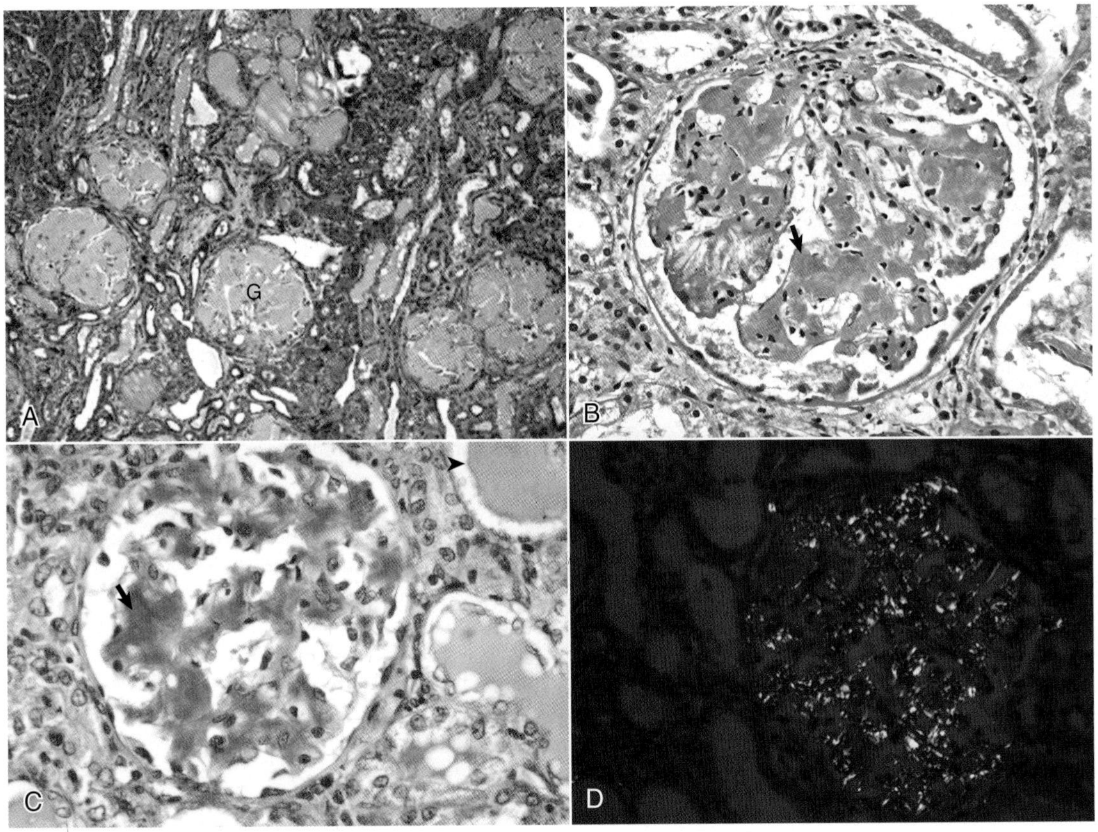

Figure 11-34 Amyloidosis, Glomerulus, Kidney, Dog. A, All glomerular tufts (*G*) are diffusely and notably expanded by amyloid (pale eosinophilic homogeneous deposits), with the result that they are relatively acellular. H&E stain. **B,** Amyloid, the pale eosinophilic homogeneous hyalinized deposits, expands the mesangium of the glomerulus (*arrow*). H&E stain. **C,** Amyloid stains orange with Congo red staining (*arrow*), a technique used to confirm it. Note the proteinaceous casts in tubular lumina (*arrowhead*), a consequence of glomerular damage allowing leakage of proteins into the filtrate (protein-losing nephropathy). Congo red stain. **D,** Congo red–stained amyloid deposits. These deposits have a light-green (often called apple green) birefringence when viewed under polarized light. Polarized light microscopy. (**A** courtesy Dr. B.C. Ward, College of Veterinary Medicine, Mississippi State University; and Noah's Arkive, College of Veterinary Medicine, The University of Georgia. **B** courtesy Dr. S.J. Newman, College of Veterinary Medicine, University of Tennessee. **C** courtesy Dr. M.D. McGavin, College of Veterinary Medicine, University of Tennessee. **D** courtesy Dr. W. Crowell, College of Veterinary Medicine, The University of Georgia; and Noah's Arkive, College of Veterinary Medicine, The University of Georgia.)

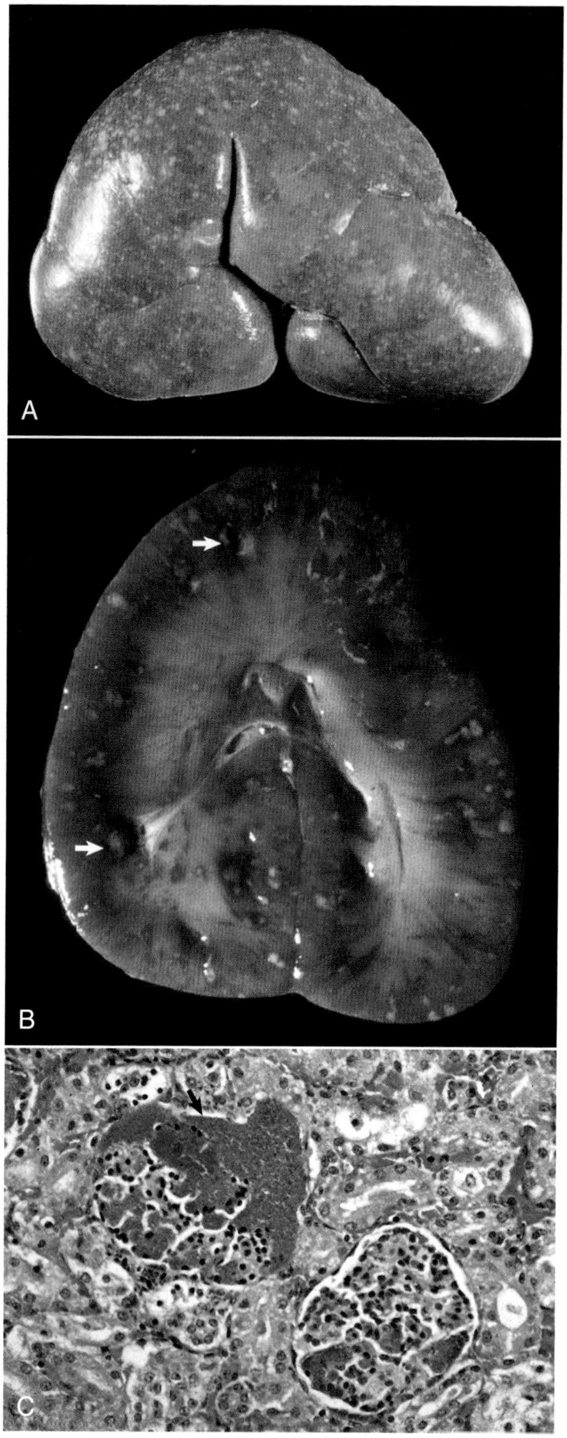

Figure 11-35 **Embolic Nephritis (Suppurative Glomerulitis), Kidney, Horse. A,** Multiple, small pale white necrotic foci and abscesses are present subcapsularly. **B,** Dorsal section. Variably sized abscesses are scattered throughout the cortex *(arrows)*. **C,** Causative bacteria *(arrow)* enter the kidney via the vasculature (bacteremia) and lodge in the capillaries of glomeruli, where they replicate and induce necrosis and inflammation. H&E stain. (**A** courtesy Dr. A. Confer, Center for Veterinary Health Sciences, Oklahoma State University. **B** courtesy Dr. M.D. McGavin, College of Veterinary Medicine, University of Tennessee. **C** courtesy Dr. W. Crowell, College of Veterinary Medicine, The University of Georgia; and Noah's Arkive, College of Veterinary Medicine, The University of Georgia.)

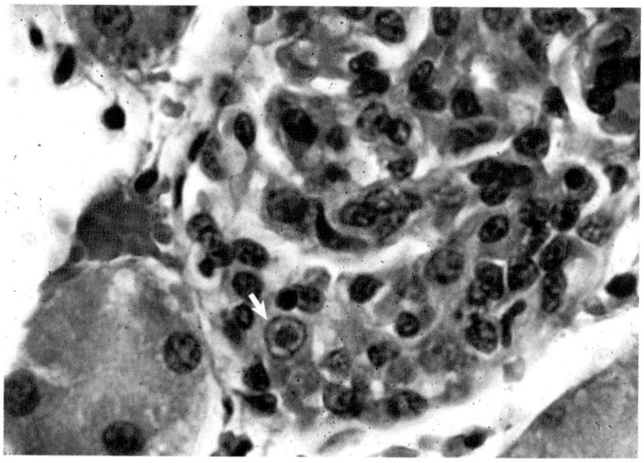

Figure 11-36 **Infectious Canine Hepatitis, Kidney, Cortex, Dog.** Renal glomerular endothelial cells contain intranuclear inclusion bodies *(arrow)*. H&E stain. (Courtesy Dr. W. Crowell, College of Veterinary Medicine, The University of Georgia; and Noah's Arkive, College of Veterinary Medicine, The University of Georgia.)

renal cortex. Microscopically, glomerular capillaries contain numerous bacterial colonies intermixed with necrotic debris and extensive infiltrates of neutrophils that often obliterate the glomerulus. Glomerular or interstitial hemorrhage can occur as well. As with many other inflammatory diseases, if the affected animal survives, the neutrophilic infiltrates either persist as focal residual abscesses or are progressively replaced by increasing numbers of lymphocytes, plasma cells, macrophages, and fibroblasts, ultimately forming coalescing scars.

Viral Glomerulitis. Glomerulitis, caused by a direct viral insult to the glomerulus, occurs in acute systemic viral diseases, such as acute infectious canine hepatitis (Fig. 11-36), equine arteritis virus infection, hog cholera, avian Newcastle disease, and neonatal porcine cytomegalovirus infection. The lesions are mild, usually transient, and result from viral replication in capillary endothelium. Acute viral GN produces the following gross lesions:

- Kidneys are often slightly swollen.
- Renal capsular surface is smooth.
- Kidneys are normal color or pale.
- Glomeruli are visible as pinpoint red dots on the cut surface of the cortex.

Viral-induced intranuclear inclusions are present in glomerular capillary endothelium from viremias of infectious canine hepatitis and cytomegalovirus infections. The inclusions of each disease are similar and are usually large, basophilic to magenta, and either fill the nucleus or are separated from the nuclear membrane by a clear halo. In the other diseases (equine arteritis, hog cholera, maedi-visna, porcine circovirus, and avian Newcastle), viral antigens can be demonstrated in endothelium, epithelium, or mesangial cells by immunofluorescence, immunohistochemistry, or polymerase chain reaction (PCR). In cases of viral glomerulitis, lesions include endothelial hypertrophy, hemorrhages, necrosis of endothelium, and a thickened and edematous mesangium. Clinically, animals are systemically ill from the viral infection, but the glomerular signs are specifically those of a transient proteinuria.

Chemical Glomerulonephritis. Although much less common than the immune-mediated forms of GN, chemically induced glomerular disease occurs in a variety of different ways. Chemicals typically induce glomerular injury by any of the following:

- Direct injury to glomerular epithelial cells
- Direct injury to endothelial cells of the glomerulus

- Altered renal blood flow
- Induction of immunologic reactions and inflammatory responses, which may occur with any of the following:
  - Incorporation of drugs into immune complexes
  - The formation and targeted deposition of antigen-antibody complexes
  - The formation of antinuclear antibodies
  - The formation of anti-GBM antibodies within the glomerular tuft

Puromycin aminonucleoside, adriamycin, and histamine-receptor antagonists all induce proteinuria through targeted damage to glomerular epithelial cells. The immunosuppressive drug, cyclosporine A, alters renal perfusion and ultimately the glomerular filtration rate by damaging glomerular endothelial cells. Numerous foreign substances are capable of producing immune complexes including injectable hyperimmune serum, gold, and D-penicillamine. Procainamide and hydralazine result in production of antinuclear antibodies, and occupational exposure to hydrocarbon solvents can create anti-GBM antibodies. Often, drug-induced lesions lead to irreversible nephron loss and compensatory cellular and functional hypertrophy of other nephrons. The continuing physical loss of nephrons sets up a cycle for an increase in glomerular hypertension and hyperfiltration, which results in glomerulosclerosis, progressive nephron loss, and interstitial fibrosis.

Miscellaneous Glomerular Lesions

Glomerular Lipidosis. Glomerular lipidosis, characterized by small aggregates of lipid-laden, foamy macrophages in glomerular tufts, is an occasional incidental finding in dogs. A similar but more extensive glomerular lipidosis has been described in cats with inherited hyperlipoproteinemia, which is a generalized disease characterized by hyperchylomicronemia, atherosclerosis, and xanthogranulomas in numerous parenchymatous organs, including the kidneys (see the section on Granulomatous Nephritis). Microscopically, glomeruli contain foamy macrophages, characteristic of glomerular lipidosis, as well as increased mesangium and thickened Bowman's capsule.

Glomerular Vasculopathy. An idiopathic renal glomerular and cutaneous vasculopathy was originally described in greyhounds and has since been found in numerous purebred and mixed-breed dogs. The cause of this disease is unknown, but renal lesions are similar to those seen in DIC, thrombotic thrombocytopenic purpura, and hemolytic-uremic syndrome in human beings. At autopsy (syn: necropsy), kidneys from affected dogs are swollen and congested and show cortical petechiae (Fig. 11-37, *A*). Microscopically, numerous glomeruli have segmental or global fibrin thrombi, hemorrhage, and necrosis (Fig. 11-37, *B*). At the glomerular vascular pole, the walls of afferent arterioles have fibrin deposits and foci of necrosis. Affected greyhounds have multifocal erythematous and ulcerated skin lesions and distal limb edema. Variable systemic signs of uremia often accompany the cutaneous lesions.

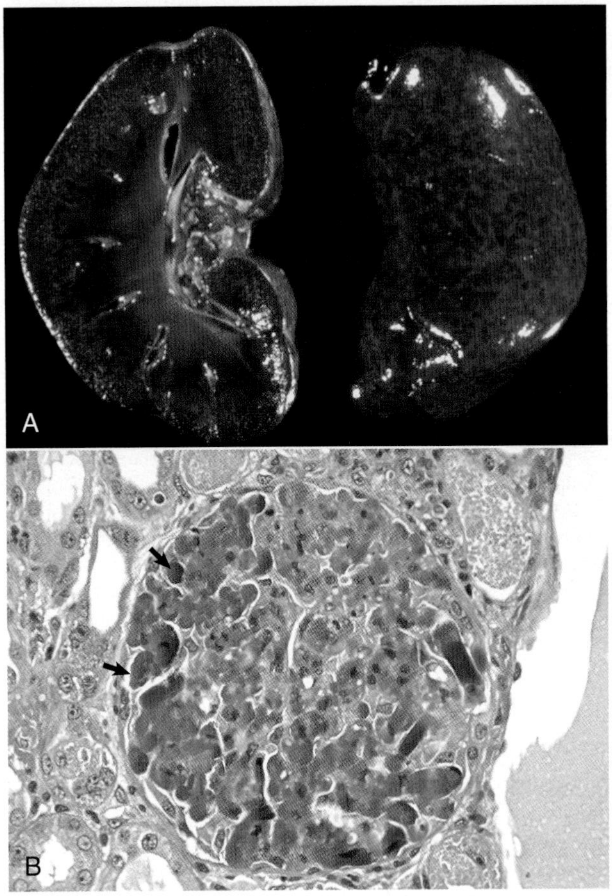

Figure 11-37 **Vasculopathy, Renal (and Cutaneous) Vasculopathy Syndrome, Glomerulus, Kidney, Dog, Greyhound. A,** The fine white dots in the cortex (on both the capsular and cut surfaces) are glomeruli with extensive glomerular capillary thrombosis. **B,** Necrotic glomerular endothelial cells and extensive glomerular capillary thrombosis *(arrows)* are typical of idiopathic glomerular (and cutaneous) vasculopathy syndrome in greyhound dogs. H&E stain. (**A** courtesy Dr. B. Weeks, College of Veterinary Medicine, Texas A&M University; and Noah's Arkive, College of Veterinary Medicine, The University of Georgia. **B** courtesy Dr. B.W. Fenwick, Virginia Tech.)

Diseases of the Tubules

Inherited Abnormalities in Renal Tubular Function. Inherited abnormalities in tubular metabolism, in transport, or in reabsorption of glucose, amino acids, ions, and proteins have been described in dogs. Primary renal glucosuria, an inherited disorder in Norwegian elkhounds and sporadically occurring in other dog breeds, occurs when the capacity of tubular epithelial cells to reabsorb glucose is significantly reduced. Gross and histologic lesions are not seen, because this is a functional disorder. Glucosuria most commonly results from diabetes mellitus, acromegaly, or catecholamine release and predisposes dogs to the following:

- Bacterial infections of the lower urinary tract
- Urinary bladder emphysema, secondary to splitting of glucose molecules by bacteria (principally *Escherichia coli, Clostridium perfringens*, and rarely with *Candida* yeasts), with subsequent release of carbon dioxide (CO_2) into the bladder lumen and absorption of gas into the lymphatic vessels of the bladder (Fig. 11-38)

A hereditary generalized defect in tubular reabsorption similar to the Fanconi syndrome in human beings has been described in Basenji dogs. The underlying tubular defect appears to be abnormal membrane structure of the proximal tubular epithelial cell brush borders because of altered lipid content in the cell membrane. Gross lesions are not identifiable in the early stages. Histopathologic changes in the kidneys are initially minimal, consisting of irregularly sized tubular epithelial cells in the convoluted tubules and loops of Henle. With time, dogs with Fanconi syndrome develop progressive renal insufficiency and associated renal fibrosis. Aminoaciduria, glucosuria, proteinuria, increased phosphaturia, metabolic acidosis, and multiple endocrine abnormalities characterize this disease clinically. Transient acquired forms have been noted in association with copper storage hepatopathy.

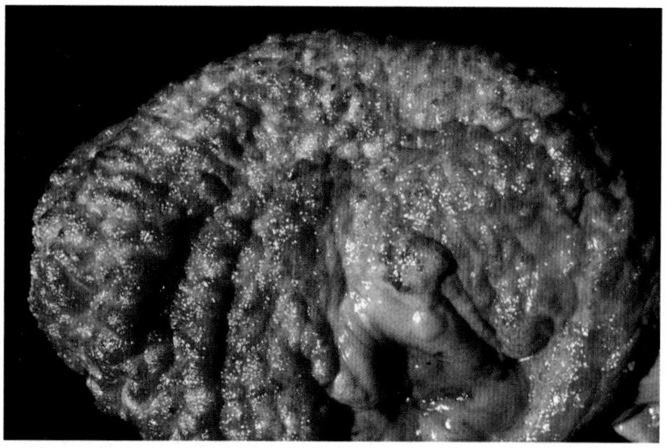

Figure 11-38 **Emphysema, Urinary Bladder Mucosa, Cow.** The multiple "nodules" are mucosal gas bubbles that have expanded the mucosa and are secondary to bacterial infections of the lower urinary tract (principally by *Escherichia coli*, *Clostridium perfringens*, and rarely *Candida* yeasts). Microorganisms split glucose molecules to release CO_2 into the bladder lumen, from where the gas can be absorbed into bladder lymphatic vessels. This animal was injected with calcium borogluconate as a calcium source to treat milk fever. Following intravenous injection, calcium ions readily dissociate from the parent molecule, and the resulting gluconate provides a sugar source for resident urinary bacteria. (Courtesy Dr. M.D. McGavin, College of Veterinary Medicine, University of Tennessee.)

The excretion of large quantities of cystine in the urine (cystinuria) is a sex-linked inherited tubular dysfunction seen occasionally in purebred and mongrel male dogs. It is important because it predisposes affected dogs to calculus formation and obstruction of the lower urinary tract (see the section on Urolithiasis).

Acute Tubular Necrosis. Acute tubular necrosis, as described in the section on tubular response to injury, can be seen following exposure to any of the following nephrotoxins (Box 11-10):

- Pigments
  - Hemoglobin
  - Myoglobin
  - Bile/bilirubin
- Heavy metals
  - Lead
  - Mercury
- Pharmaceutical agents (e.g., chemotherapeutic and antimicrobial agents)
  - Cisplatin
  - Aminoglycosides (see the section on Kidney and Lower Urinary Tract, Disorders of Dogs)
  - Oxytetracycline
  - Amphotericin B
  - Sulfonamides
  - Monensin
- Nonsteroidal antiinflammatory drugs
- Fungal toxins
- Plant toxins
  - Pigweed
  - Oxalate-containing plants
  - Oak tannins
- Antifreeze (ethylene glycol)
- Vitamins and minerals
  - Vitamin D
  - Hypercalcemia
- Bacterial toxins
- Pet food contaminants (see the section on Kidney and Lower Urinary Tract, Disorders of Dogs)
  - Melamine
  - Cyanuric acid
  - Raisins

These nephrotoxins are discussed in greater detail in the next section.

Box 11-10 Common Nephrotoxins of Domestic Animals

HEAVY METALS
Mercury
Lead
Arsenic
Cadmium
Thallium

ANTIBACTERIAL AND ANTIFUNGAL AGENTS
Aminoglycosides
  Gentamicin
  Neomycin
  Kanamycin
  Streptomycin
  Tobramycin
Tetracyclines
Amphotericin B

GROWTH-PROMOTING AGENTS
Monensin

NONSTEROIDAL ANTIINFLAMMATORY DRUGS
Aspirin
Phenylbutazone
Carprofen
Flunixin meglumine
Ibuprofen
Naproxen

FOOD AND FOOD CONTAMINANTS
Grapes or raisins
Melamine
Cyanuric acid

BACTERIAL AND FUNGAL TOXINS
Clostridium perfringens epsilon toxin
Ochratoxin A
Citrinin

PLANTS
Pigweed (*Amaranthus retroflexus*)
Oaks (*Quercus* sp.)
Isotropis sp.
Yellow wood tree (*Terminalia oblongata*)
Lilies (*Zantedeschia* spp., *Lilium* spp., and *Hemerocallis* spp.)

OXALATES
Ethylene glycol (antifreeze)
Halogeton (*Halogeton glomeratus*)
Greasewood (*Sarcobatus vermiculatus*)
Rhubarb (*Rheum rhaponticum*)
Sorrel, dock (*Rumex* sp.)

VITAMIN D
Vitamin D supplements
Calciferol-containing rodenticides
Cestrum diurnum
Solanum sp.
Trisetum sp.

ANTINEOPLASTIC COMPOUNDS
Cisplatin

Nephrotoxic Pigments

Hemoglobinuric Nephrosis. A set of events leading to ischemic tubular necrosis frequently occurs in hypoperfused kidneys complicated by hemoglobinuria. Hemoglobinemia results in hemoglobinuria when the renal threshold for resorption is exceeded. Hemoglobinuria may occur in the following:

- Chronic copper toxicity in sheep
- Leptospirosis or babesiosis in cattle
- Red maple toxicity in horses
- Babesiosis or autoimmune hemolytic anemia in dogs

In these diseases, serum concentrations of hemoglobin are increased. Hemoglobin passes into the glomerular filtrate, producing greatly increased intraluminal concentrations that cause hemoglobinuric nephrosis. Normally, hemoglobin attaches to a carrier haptoglobin for plasma transportation, and the hemoglobin-haptoglobin complex is too big to pass through the glomerular filtration barrier. Hemoglobin is not excreted in the urine until supplies of the carrier molecule are depleted or exceeded and hemoglobin becomes free in the plasma. Hemoglobin is not nephrotoxic itself, and intravenous infusions of hemoglobin into healthy animals produce no recognizable lesions. However, large concentrations of hemoglobin in the glomerular filtrate can increase the tubular necrosis that occurs as a result of renal ischemia. For example, in chronic copper toxicity in sheep, renal ischemia is secondary to hypovolemic shock and severe Heinz body, hemolytic anemia. Therefore hemoglobinuria can have an additive deleterious effect on tubular epithelium already undergoing hypoxia.

At autopsy (syn: necropsy), the renal cortices in severe hemoglobinuria are diffusely stained red-brown to blue-black and have intratubular hemoglobin casts (Fig. 11-39, *A*). Hemoglobin casts appear as a red-black stippling of the capsular surface and continue into the cortex as radially oriented, dark red streaks. The medulla is diffusely dark red or has patchy red streaks. Classically, kidneys from sheep with chronic copper toxicity are diffusely, uniformly, and strikingly blue-black and described as "gunmetal blue." Microscopically, proximal tubular epithelial degeneration and necrosis are severe, and tubular lumens are filled by abundant orange-red granular refractile material, the characteristic appearance of a heme compound (Fig. 11-39, *B*).

Myoglobinuric Nephrosis. Myoglobinuria results from acute and extensive muscle necrosis and occurs in the following:

- Exertional rhabdomyolysis in horses, greyhounds, and wild or exotic animals (see the section on Kidney and Lower Urinary Tract, Disorders of Horses)
- *Cassia* spp. and *Karwinskia* spp. toxicity
- Severe direct trauma to muscle (e.g., traffic accident)

A set of events leading to ischemic tubular necrosis frequently occurs in hypoperfused kidneys complicated by myoglobinuria. In these diseases, serum concentrations of myoglobin are increased, as these products pass into the glomerular filtrate, producing greatly increased intraluminal concentrations that cause myoglobinuric nephrosis. Compared to hemoglobin, myoglobin more freely passes through the glomerular filtration barrier and is excreted in the urine because it does not use a carrier protein for plasma transport and it is a smaller molecule. Myoglobin is not nephrotoxic in itself, and intravenous infusions into healthy animals produce no recognizable lesions. However, large concentrations of myoglobin in the glomerular filtrate can increase the tubular necrosis that occurs as a result of renal ischemia. For example, in rhabdomyolysis in horses, renal ischemia is likely secondary to poor renal perfusion seen in hypovolemic shock. Therefore myoglobinuria can have an additive deleterious effect on tubular epithelium already undergoing ischemic necrosis.

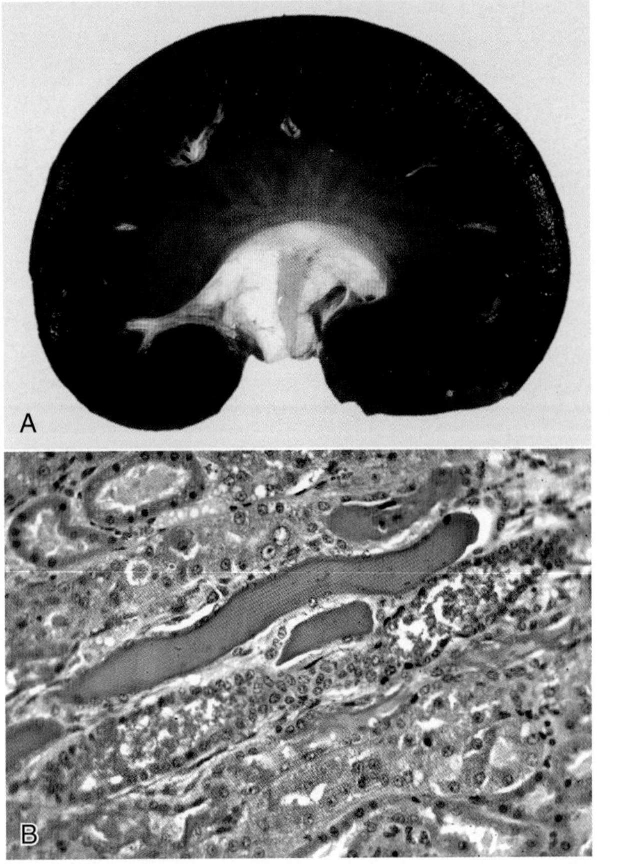

Figure 11-39 Hemoglobinuric Nephrosis, Kidney. A, Dog. Severe diffuse hemoglobin staining of the cortex and medulla is secondary to hemoglobinemia from an acute intravascular hemolytic crisis. Note the yellow staining (jaundice) of the pelvic fat and the intima of cross sections of the arcuate artery at the corticomedullary junction. **B,** Sheep. Several distal tubules contain hyaline and coarsely granular hemoglobin casts that occurred following intravascular hemolysis (hemoglobinemia) from chronic copper toxicosis. H&E stain. (**A** courtesy Dr. A. Confer, Center for Veterinary Health Sciences, Oklahoma State University. **B** courtesy Dr. A.R. Doster, University of Nebraska; and Noah's Arkive, College of Veterinary Medicine, The University of Georgia.)

At necropsy, the renal cortices in myoglobinuria are diffusely stained red-brown to blue-black and have intratubular myoglobin casts, which cannot be differentiated from hemoglobin casts (Fig. 11-40).

Cholemic Nephrosis. Increased serum concentrations of bilirubin, as in young lambs, calves, and foals with immature hepatic conjugating mechanisms, can be associated with proximal tubular cellular swelling, degeneration, and yellow-brown-green pigmentation of the proximal tubular epithelial cells. The term *cholemic nephrosis* has been applied to this lesion; however, its significance is doubtful. Acute tubular necrosis, when seen in association with severe bilirubinemia, the so-called hepatorenal syndrome, probably is not caused by bile acid or bilirubin retention per se but by ischemia from prerenal causes such as constriction of renal vessels related to shock or catecholamine release.

Heavy Metals. Nephrotoxic tubular necrosis is caused by several classes of naturally occurring or synthetic compounds. Inorganic arsenic and certain heavy metals, including inorganic mercury, lead, cadmium, and thallium, are nephrotoxins. Common sources of heavy metals for oral exposure include herbicides (arsenic), old paints (lead), batteries (lead), automobile components (lead),

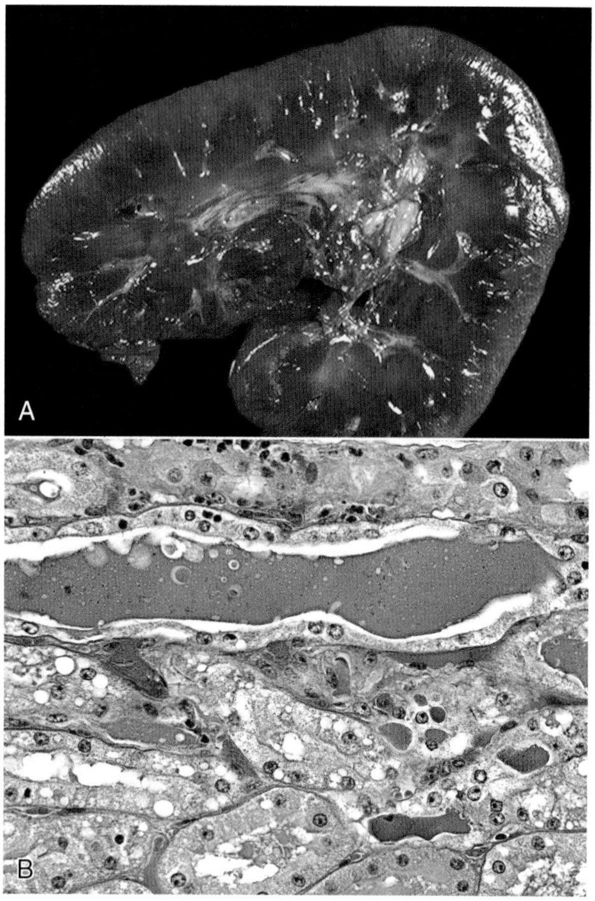

Figure 11-40 **Myoglobinuric Nephrosis, Kidney, Horse. A,** Diffuse myoglobin staining of the cortex and medulla (reddish-brown) is secondary to myoglobinemia from severe rhabdomyolysis. **B,** Myoglobin casts are present in dilated distal tubules, which are lined by flattened epithelial cells. H&E stain. (**A** courtesy Dr. W. Crowell, College of Veterinary Medicine, The University of Georgia; and Noah's Arkive, College of Veterinary Medicine, The University of Georgia. **B** courtesy Dr. J.F. Zachary, College of Veterinary Medicine, University of Illinois.)

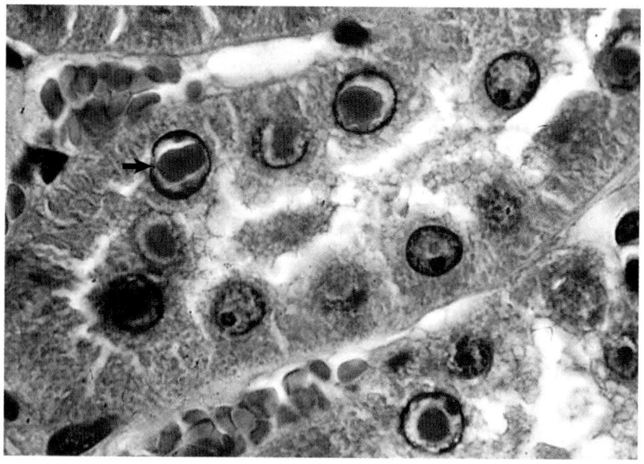

Figure 11-41 **Nephrosis, Lead Toxicosis, Kidney, Cortex, Rat.** Acid-fast intranuclear inclusion bodies *(arrow)* present in the proximal convoluted tubular epithelium are diagnostic of lead poisoning. Acid-fast stain with H&E counterstain. (Courtesy Dr. J. King, College of Veterinary Medicine, Cornell University.)

impure petroleum distillates, and other environmental contaminants. Acute tubular necrosis from mercury is caused by the following:

- Damage to membranes of proximal convoluted tubular epithelial cells.
- Mitochondrial damage produced by these toxins: Damage is often related to the interaction of these metals with protein sulfhydryl groups.

In mercury toxicosis, mercuric ions are in capillary blood and glomerular filtrate and therefore enter the proximal tubular epithelium both from the luminal side and via diffusion from the peritubular side. Mercuric ions concentrate in rough endoplasmic reticulum and cause early tubular changes that include loss of the brush border and dispersion of ribosomes. These changes are followed by mitochondrial swelling and cellular death. In addition, cadmium has been reported to cause cell death in proximal convoluted tubules by apoptosis.

The specific metal involved in toxic tubular injury cannot be identified by the renal lesions alone. The exception is lead toxicity, in which the endothelial and epithelial cells of affected glomeruli and proximal tubules, respectively, sometimes have acid-fast intranuclear inclusions composed of a lead-protein complex (Fig. 11-41).

Pharmaceutical Agents. These agents are nephrotoxic and cause acute tubular necrosis when administered at excessive doses or too frequently. Cisplatin, a platinum-containing cancer chemotherapeutic agent, causes tubular necrosis by the following:

- Direct tubular epithelial damage
- Reducing renal blood flow via vasoconstriction mediated by the renin-angiotensin mechanism

The best-characterized group of nephrotoxic pharmaceutical agents are the aminoglycoside antibiotics (gentamycin, neomycin, etc.). Aminoglycosides concentrate in proximal tubular epithelium lysosomes, Golgi bodies, and endoplasmic reticulum. They reach a threshold, are released into the cytosol, and damage mitochondria causing apoptosis and necrosis. In addition, renal blood flow is reduced, adding a hypoxic component to the toxicity.

Oxytetracycline is occasionally nephrotoxic in cattle and dogs. The mechanism of tubular damage has not been determined, but it is known that large concentrations of tetracycline antibiotics are necessary and are thought to inhibit protein synthesis in tubular epithelial cells.

Amphotericin B, an antifungal polyene antibiotic, is nephrotoxic by vasoconstriction and/or the direct disruption of cellular membranes. This membrane damage interferes with normal cholesterol-lipid interactions and causes potassium ion loss, intracellular hydrogen ion accumulation, acute cellular swelling, and necrosis of proximal and distal tubules. These renal changes are not confined to drug overdose but, rather, can occur in animals given the recommended therapeutic dosage.

Sulfonamide-induced tubular necrosis, a common entity in years past, occurs infrequently today because the presently used sulfonamides have greater solubility than those used in the past. Sulfonamides produce tubular epithelial cell necrosis most readily in dehydrated animals. Crystals form in tubules and cause necrosis of the renal tubular epithelium by direct toxicity and by mechanical damage. Fine granular yellow crystalline deposits can be seen grossly in the medullary tubules of affected animals, but the crystalline deposits are dissolved during fixation in aqueous fixatives such as 10% buffered neutral formalin.

Monensin is an ionophore antibiotic used as a feed additive to control coccidiosis and stimulate weight gains in poultry and cattle. Horses are particularly susceptible to toxicosis with monensin.

Although necrosis of striated muscle is the major lesion, renal tubular degeneration or necrosis occurs concurrently.

Nonsteroidal Antiinflammatory Drugs. Ingestion of nonsteroidal antiinflammatory drugs (NSAIDs), such as phenylbutazone, aspirin, carprofen, flunixin meglumine, ibuprofen, and naproxen, has been associated with acute renal failure in small animals, especially dogs. In horses, NSAID toxicosis is usually associated with nonfatal renal papillary necrosis and mucosal ulceration (see the section on Papillary Necrosis). The mechanism of acute renal failure is related to NSAIDs decreasing the synthesis of renal prostaglandins. Because prostaglandins are responsible for maintaining normal renal blood flow, NSAID administration results in afferent arteriolar constriction that decreases renal perfusion, resulting in acute tubular degeneration and medullary papillary necrosis and acute renal failure. The overall incidence of NSAID-induced renal failure in small animals is low and is seen most commonly in animals that ingest excessive amounts of the drug or have a concomitant disorder such as dehydration, congestive heart failure, or chronic renal disease.

Fungal Toxins. Naturally occurring nephrotoxic mycotoxins can originate from *Aspergillus* sp. and *Penicillium* sp. (e.g., ochratoxin and citrinin). Ochratoxin A is nephrotoxic for monogastric animals, particularly pigs, in which the lesions are tubular degeneration and necrosis. In addition, long-term ingestion results in diffuse renal fibrosis presumably as the result of continual damage to the tubule epithelial cells and thus allowing no time for regeneration.

Plant Toxins. Several species of pigweed, particularly *Amaranthus retroflexus*, can be responsible for acute tubular necrosis and perirenal edema in pigs and cattle. The toxic principle is likely a group of phenolic compounds present in the leaves. Oak toxicosis (*Quercus* spp.) is seen in ruminants after consumption of new leaves or acorns. The toxic principles are tannins and their breakdown products. See the section on Kidney and Lower Urinary Tract, Disorders of Ruminants (Cattle, Sheep, and Goats), Oak Toxicity: Acute Tubular Necrosis (*Quercus* Spp.) for a discussion of tannins. Several nephrotoxic species of lilies (*Lilium* spp., *Zantedeschesia* spp., and *Hemerocallis* spp.) have been associated with acute tubular necrosis in small animals, especially cats. The toxic principle is not known.

Oxalate-induced tubular necrosis occurs in sheep and cattle after ingestion of toxic quantities of oxalates that accumulate in plants of various genera, such as *Halogeton*, *Sarcobatus*, *Rheum*, and *Rumex*. After absorption from the intestine, calcium oxalates precipitate in either vessel lumens or walls or within renal tubules, where they cause obstruction and epithelial cell necrosis. Illness in oxalate poisoning occurs not only because of renal disease but also because of neuromuscular dysfunction, the result of the hypocalcemia produced by chelation of serum calcium by oxalates. An oxalate-induced nephrosis has been described in Tibetan spaniels with an inherited hyperoxaluria. A chronic oxalate nephrosis in ragdoll cats of unknown inheritance and etiology is also reported.

Chemicals

Antifreeze. See the section on Kidney and Lower Urinary Tract, Disorders of Dogs, Ethylene Glycol Intoxication for a discussion of antifreeze as a nephrotoxin.

Vitamins and Minerals

Vitamin D. Vitamin D given as multiple excessive doses (vitamin D intoxication [vitamin D nephropathy]) or by accidental ingestion of calciferol-containing rodenticides can cause nephrosis in dogs and cats. In livestock, chronic ingestion of plants, such as *Cestrum diurnum* in the southern United States or *Solanum* sp. or *Trisetum* sp. in other countries, each of which contains a chemical with vitamin D–like biologic activity, can also cause nephrosis. Ingestion of excessive amounts of vitamin D can induce hypercalcemia. Hypercalcemia results in decreased cAMP formation, which impairs sodium resorption and interferes with ADH receptors. In addition, if the hypercalcemia persists, progressive mineralization of tubular and GBMs occurs (see Fig. 11-25). Development of lesions depends on the length of time between exposure to rodenticides and death or the duration of continued exposure to vitamin D. In acute cases, the kidneys have a smooth capsular surface. Microscopically, tubular epithelium is necrotic and atrophic with a few calcified deposits in the tubules scattered randomly throughout the cortex. In more chronic cases, the surface of the kidney is finely granular as a result of fibrosis. White, chalky deposits can be seen within the cortex. Interstitial fibrosis, tubular dilation, glomerular atrophy, and extensive calcification of tubular basement membranes are seen microscopically.

Interstitial Calcification (Hypercalcemic Nephropathy). Hypercalcemia from a variety of causes results in inactivation of adenyl cyclase with decreased AMP so that sodium transport is impaired in the ascending limb of the loop of Henle, distal tubule, and collecting ducts. Hypercalcemia interferes with ADH receptors in the collecting ducts, resulting in renal diabetes insipidus. Mineralization of the basement membrane and epithelium initially in the outer zone of the medulla and then involving the interstitium, vessels, and glomeruli is seen when hypercalcemia persists. The leading cause of hypercalcemia in dogs and cats is hypercalcemia of malignancy, a paraneoplastic syndrome. PTH-related peptide (PTHrp), a peptide that resembles PTH, results in bone resorption. It is produced most commonly by lymphomas or carcinomas of the apocrine glands of the anal sac. In addition, excess vitamin D either from rodenticides or excess dietary sources (toxic plants) can result in a similar syndrome. Less common causes of hypercalcemia include primary hyperparathyroidism and secondary renal hyperparathyroidism.

Bacterial Toxins. Bacterial toxins, such as the epsilon exotoxin, produced after marked enteric proliferation by *Clostridium perfringens* type D in small ruminants, can result in grossly recognizable bilateral renal lesions termed *pulpy kidney* (Fig. 11-42, A). The pulpy texture of the kidney is due to acute tubular epithelial degeneration and/or necrosis and interstitial edema and hemorrhage (Fig. 11-42, B). Epsilon toxin binds to receptors on distal renal tubular epithelium causing this degeneration. Autolysis can produce similar changes, and this finding should be interpreted with caution, especially with a long post-mortem interval.

Food and Pet Food Contaminants. See the section on Kidney and Lower Urinary Tract, Disorders of Dogs, Toxic Tubulointerstitial Nephritis, Melamine and Cyanuric Acid for a discussion of toxic food and pet food contaminants.

Diseases of the Renal Pelvis

Hydronephrosis. Hydronephrosis refers to dilation of the renal pelvis and accompanying renal atrophy. The cause is partial or complete obstruction of urine outflow causing a progressive increase in pelvic pressure. Obstruction leading to hydronephrosis can be caused by congenital malformations of the ureter, vesicoureteral junction, or urethra or from congenitally malpositioned kidneys with secondary kinking of the ureter. The more common causes of hydronephrosis are as follows:

- Accidental ligation of the ureter
- Ureteral or urethral blockage due to urinary tract calculi (see the section on Lower Urinary Tract)
- Chronic inflammation
- Neoplasia of the ureter, bladder, and urethra
- Neurogenic functional disorders

Hydronephrosis occurs in all domestic animals. Depending on the location of the obstruction, hydronephrosis can be unilateral (ureteral) or bilateral (ureter, bladder trigone, or the urethra).

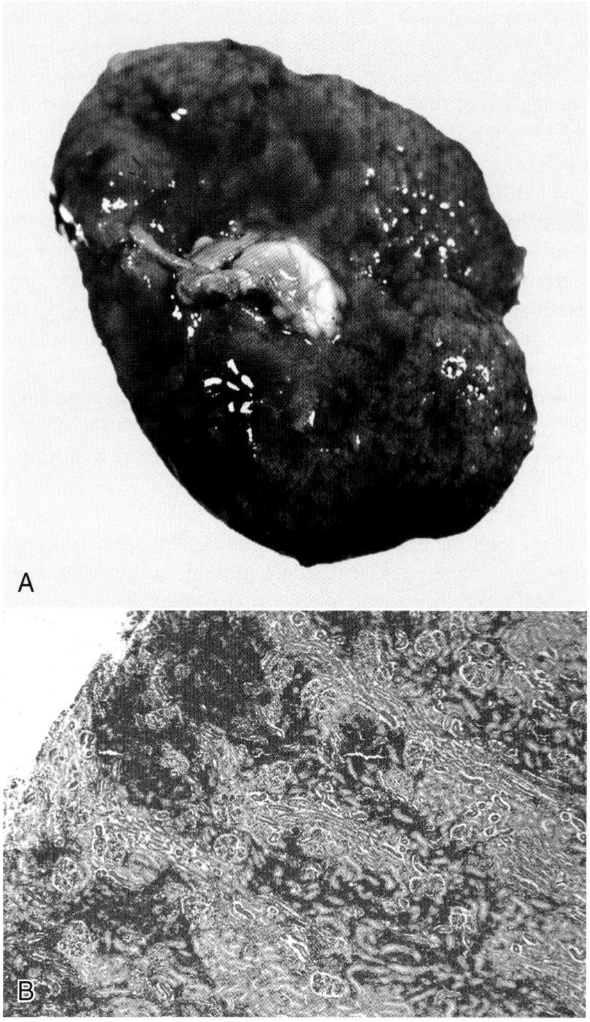

Figure 11-42 **Pulpy Kidney Disease, *Clostridium perfringens* Type D Toxin, Kidney, Lamb. A,** The epsilon exotoxin from an enteric overgrowth of *Clostridium perfringens* type D causes soft, swollen, and pale kidneys, often with hemorrhage, and are termed pulpy kidneys. **B,** The soft pulpy nature of the kidney is the result of acute tubular epithelial cell degeneration and/or necrosis, interstitial edema, and hemorrhage. H&E stain. (**A** courtesy Dr. J. King, College of Veterinary Medicine, Cornell University. **B** courtesy Dr. M.D. McGavin, College of Veterinary Medicine, University of Tennessee.)

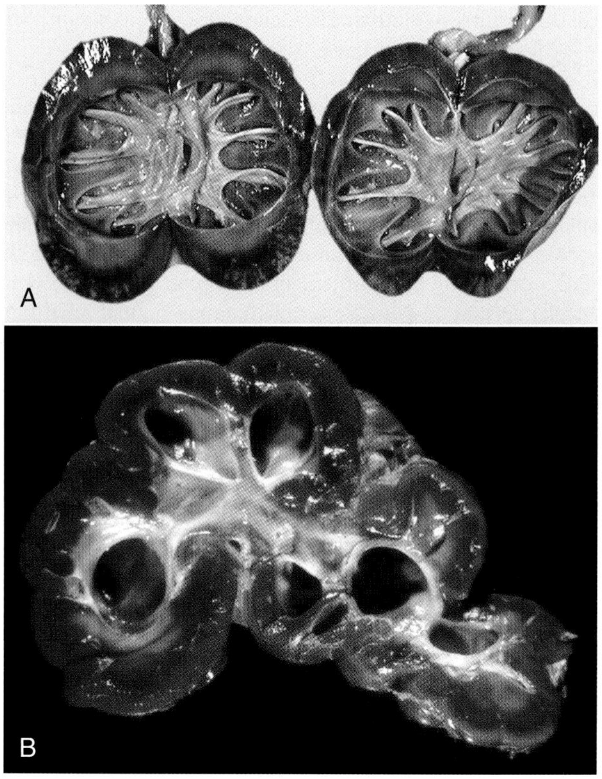

Figure 11-43 **Hydronephrosis, Kidney, Dorsal Section. A,** Sheep. The pelvis of each kidney is markedly dilated. **B,** Cow. Bovine kidneys are lobulated, and each lobule has its own renal papilla surrounded by a calyx, an extension of the pelvis. Thus in early hydronephrosis, each of these calyces is distended, and these distended calyces should not be confused with the cysts of a cystic or polycystic kidney. (**A** courtesy Dr. J. King, College of Veterinary Medicine, Cornell University. **B** courtesy College of Veterinary Medicine, University of Illinois.)

Unilateral hydronephrosis is caused by obstruction of a ureter anywhere throughout its length or at its entrance into the urinary bladder. Bilateral hydronephrosis can be caused by urethral obstruction, bilateral ureteral obstruction, or extensive urinary bladder lesions centered on the trigone. When hydronephrosis is unilateral, pelvic enlargement of the kidney can become extensive, even cystic, before the lesion is recognized clinically. If the obstructive process causes partial or intermittent blockage, bilateral hydronephrosis can become notable because of continual urine production and pooling of urine in the expanding pelvis. When obstruction is complete and bilateral, death as a result of uremia occurs before pelvic enlargement becomes extensive.

When the increase in intrapelvic pressure is substantial and sustained, the following occur:

- Intratubular pressure is increased resulting in microscopic renal tubular dilation.
- Glomeruli remain functional, and even with complete obstruction, glomerular filtration does not stop completely and soon overwhelms tubular reabsorption pathways.
- Much of the glomerular filtrate diffuses into the interstitium, where it is initially removed via lymphatic vessels and veins.
- As intrapelvic pressure increases, the interstitial vessels collapse and renal blood flow is reduced, resulting in hypoxia, tubular atrophy, and, if the pressure increase is continued, interstitial fibrosis.
- The glomeruli have a relatively normal morphologic appearance for a prolonged period, but they eventually become atrophic and sclerotic.

Early changes of hydronephrosis include dilation of the pelvis and calyces and blunting of the renal crest and papillae (Fig. 11-43). When pelvic dilation is progressive, the kidney silhouette is enlarged and rounder than normal, and the cortex and medulla are progressively thinned (Fig. 11-44). Interstitial vascular obstruction from compression produces an expanding front of medullary and later cortical ischemia and necrosis. Continued pelvic dilation causes loss of tubules by degeneration and atrophy, followed by condensation of interstitial connective tissue and fibrosis of the renal parenchyma. In its most advanced form, the hydronephrotic kidney is a thin-walled (2- to 3-mm), fluid-filled sac. This sac is lined by flattened transitional epithelium, which is spared during lesion development. Occasionally, a severely hydronephrotic kidney becomes contaminated by bacteria and the thin-walled sac becomes filled with pus

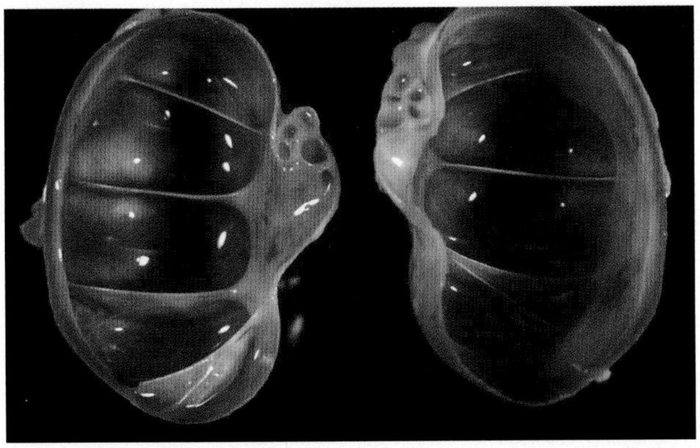

Figure 11-44 **Chronic Hydronephrosis, Kidney, Dorsal Section, Cat.** Advanced hydronephrosis is characterized by loss of medullary tissue and atrophy or even loss of the entire cortex in response to elevated pelvic fluid pressure. Note that this case was so severe that only the renal capsule, which contains clear yellow fluid, remains. (Courtesy Dr. M.D. McGavin, College of Veterinary Medicine, University of Tennessee.)

instead of urine. This lesion, referred to as *pyonephrosis*, is likely the result of blood-borne bacteria lodging in a hydronephrotic kidney.

Pyelonephritis. Bacterial infection of the pelvis with extension into the renal tubules causing concomitant tubulointerstitial inflammation is referred to as *pyelonephritis*. Because of differences in pathogenesis, lesion distribution, and microscopic appearance, pyelonephritis is considered a form of tubulointerstitial nephritis.

Although pyelitis refers to inflammation of the renal pelvis, pyelonephritis is inflammation of both the renal pelvis and the renal parenchyma and is an excellent example of suppurative tubulointerstitial disease. The condition usually originates as an extension of a bacterial infection arising in the lower urinary tract that ascends the ureters to the kidneys and establishes an infection in the pelvis and inner medulla (Fig. 11-45). Therefore anything that predisposes an animal to lower urinary tract infection, such as recent or frequent catheterization, uroliths, or urine stagnation, can potentially result in pyelonephritis. Rarely, pyelonephritis can result from descending bacterial infections, wherein bacterial infection of the kidneys occurs via the hematogenous route (i.e., embolic nephritis). In human pathology, the term *pyelonephritis* is used to include both ascending and descending infections. Ascending infection, however, is by far the most common cause of pyelonephritis in animals.

The pathogenesis of ascending pyelonephritis depends on the abnormal reflux of bacteria-contaminated urine from the lower tract to the renal pelvis and collecting ducts (vesicoureteral reflux). Normally, little vesicoureteral reflux occurs during micturition. Vesicoureteral reflux occurs more readily when pressure is increased within the urinary bladder, as with urethral obstruction. This mechanism has been postulated for end-stage pyelonephritis with mild dysplasia seen in young boxer dogs in Norway. Bacterial infection of the lower urinary tract can enhance vesicoureteral reflux by several other mechanisms as follows:

- When the bladder wall is inflamed (cystitis), the normal competency of the vesicoureteral valve can be compromised because of mucosal thickening due to inflammatory cells and edema. This outcome increases the opportunity for urine to reflux.
- Endotoxin, liberated from Gram-negative bacteria infecting the ureter and bladder, can inhibit normal ureteral peristalsis, increasing reflux.

The urinary tract has a number of protective features in place to help prevent bacterial colonization, including the following:

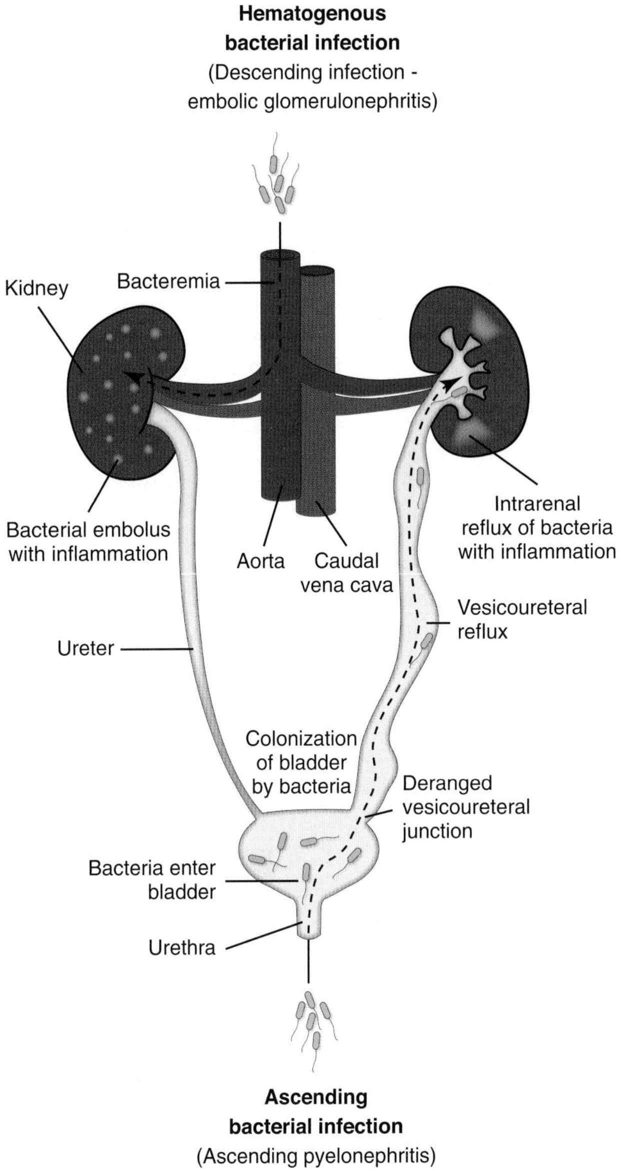

Figure 11-45 **Descending (Hematogenous) and Ascending Bacterial Infections of the Kidney.** Hematogenous (descending) infections of the kidney can result from bacteremia. Common microbes that cause such infections include *Escherichia coli* and *Staphylococcus* spp. The outcome is bacterial emboli in the renal cortex (see Fig. 11-35). Ascending infections result from a combination of urinary bladder infection and vesicoureteral reflux leading to pyelitis and concurrent intrarenal reflux leading to pyelonephritis (see Figs. 11-46 and 11-47). (Courtesy Drs. M.A. Breshears and A.W. Confer, Center for Veterinary Health Sciences, Oklahoma State University; and Dr. J.F. Zachary, College of Veterinary Medicine, University of Illinois.)

- Mucoproteins on the surface urothelial mucosal lining that prohibit bacterial adherence
- Progressive desquamation of superficial urothelial cells to minimize surface colonization
- Goblet cell metaplasia with enhanced mucus production
- Phagocytosis by superficial mucosal urothelial cells
- Bacteria-specific mucosal IgA production can block adhesion and colonization by bacteria

Bacteria that colonize the renal pelvis can readily infect the inner medulla. The medulla is highly susceptible to bacterial infection because of the following:

- A poor blood supply
- High interstitial osmolality and/or osmolarity that inhibits neutrophil function
- Large ammonia concentration that inhibits complement activation

Thus bacteria can infect and ascend collecting ducts, cause tubular epithelial necrosis and hemorrhage, and incite a neutrophilic inflammatory response. Bacterial infection can progressively ascend within tubules and the interstitium until the inflammatory lesions extend from pelvis to capsule. Recurrent or progressive infections can lead to chronic inflammation and scarring.

Because most occurrences of pyelonephritis are ascending infections and because females are more susceptible to lower urinary tract infections, pyelonephritis occurs more frequently in females. *Escherichia coli*, especially uropathogenic strains that produce virulence factors such as α-hemolysin, adhesions, and P fimbria, is one of the most common causes of lower urinary tract disease and pyelonephritis in all domestic animal species. *Proteus* sp., *Klebsiella* sp., *Staphylococcus* sp., *Streptococcus* sp., and *Pseudomonas aeruginosa* are also common causes of lower urinary tract infection and pyelonephritis in all species. *Corynebacterium renale*, *Trueperella pyogenes*, and *Actinobaculum* (*Eubacterium*) *suis* are specifically pathogenic for the lower urinary tract of cattle and pigs, respectively, and are common causes of pyelonephritis. Granulomatous and necrotizing pyelonephritis associated with *Aspergillus* sp. or *Paecilomyces* sp. can occur in rare instances.

A gross diagnosis of pyelonephritis is accomplished by recognizing the existence of pelvic inflammation with extension into the renal parenchyma (Fig. 11-46, *A*). Pyelonephritis can be unilateral, but it is often bilateral and most severe at the renal poles. The pelvic and ureteral mucous membranes can be acutely inflamed, thickened, reddened, roughened, or granular and coated with a thin exudate. The pelvis and ureters can be markedly dilated and have purulent exudate in the lumina (Fig. 11-46, *B*). The medullary crest (papilla) is often ulcerated and necrotic. Renal involvement is notable by irregular, radially oriented, red or gray streaks involving the medulla extending toward and often reaching the renal surface. Occasionally, inflammation extends through the surface of the kidneys to produce patchy areas of subcapsular inflammation.

Microscopically, the most severe acute lesions of pyelonephritis are in the inner medulla. The transitional epithelium is usually focally or diffusely necrotic and sloughed. Necrotic debris, fibrin, neutrophils, and bacterial colonies can be adherent to the denuded surface. Medullary tubules are notably dilated, and their lumina contain neutrophils and bacterial colonies. Focally the tubular epithelium is necrotic. An intense neutrophilic infiltrate is present in the renal interstitium, and it can extend into tubules. Lesions can be accompanied by interstitial hemorrhages and edema (Fig. 11-46, *C*). If obstruction of vasa recta has occurred, coagulative necrosis of the inner medulla (papillary necrosis) can be severe. Similar tubular and interstitial lesions, although less severe, extend radially into the cortical tubules and interstitium. When the lesions become

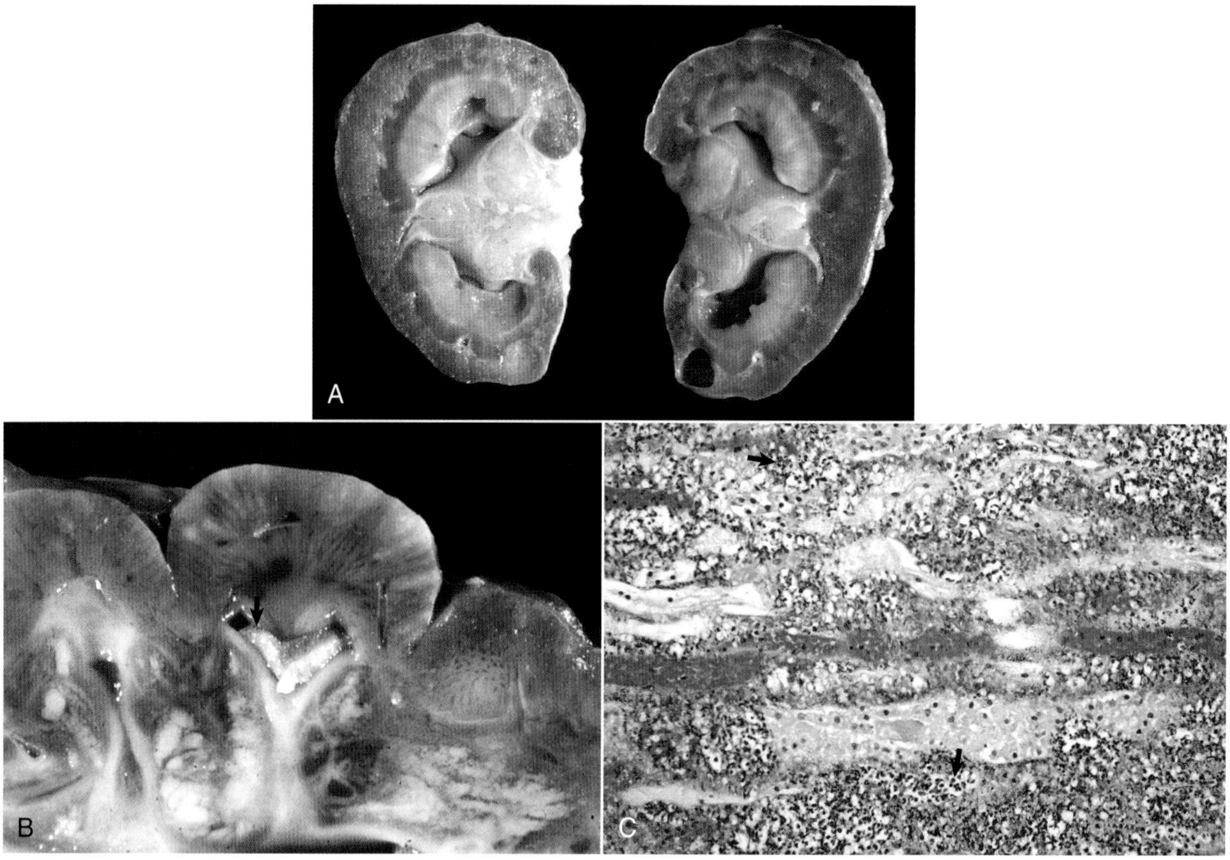

Figure 11-46 **Pyelonephritis, Kidney. A,** Dorsal section, dog. Extensive pelvic inflammation has destroyed areas *(gray-white)* of the inner medulla and extends focally into the outer medulla. **B,** Dorsal section, cow. Renal calyces in the cow contain suppurative exudate *(arrow)*. **C,** Dog. There is both intratubular and interstitial inflammation with tubular necrosis, characterized by infiltrates of principally neutrophils *(arrows)*. H&E stain. (**A** courtesy Dr. M.D. McGavin, College of Veterinary Medicine, University of Tennessee. **B** courtesy Dr. K. Read, College of Veterinary Medicine, Texas A&M University; and Noah's Arkive, College of Veterinary Medicine, The University of Georgia. **C** courtesy Dr. J.F. Zachary, College of Veterinary Medicine, University of Illinois.)

subacute, the severity of the neutrophilic infiltrates diminishes, and lymphocytes, plasma cells, and monocytes infiltrate the interstitium. Chronic lesions have severe fibrosis. If active bacterial infection persists or is untreated, an intense infiltrate of all inflammatory cell types interspersed with tubular necrosis and fibrosis can be seen. All stages of disease progression can occur in a single kidney.

The renal lesions of chronic pyelonephritis, in which an active bacterial infection exists, include most of the elements of acute inflammation described previously and extensive necrosis of the medulla, patchy fibrosis in the outer medulla and cortex, and variable amounts of pelvic inflammatory exudates. Chronic pyelonephritis often produces a grossly visible deformity of the renal parenchyma because of extensive interstitial inflammation and scarring (Fig. 11-47). Fibrosis secondary to the tubulointerstitial inflammation of pyelonephritis follows the pattern of the acute disease (targeting the renal poles) and results in irregularly distributed, patchy scarring that is seen as deeply depressed regions on the renal capsular surface and linear areas extending through both the cortex and the medulla to the pelvis. Such lesions often resemble chronic polar infarcts.

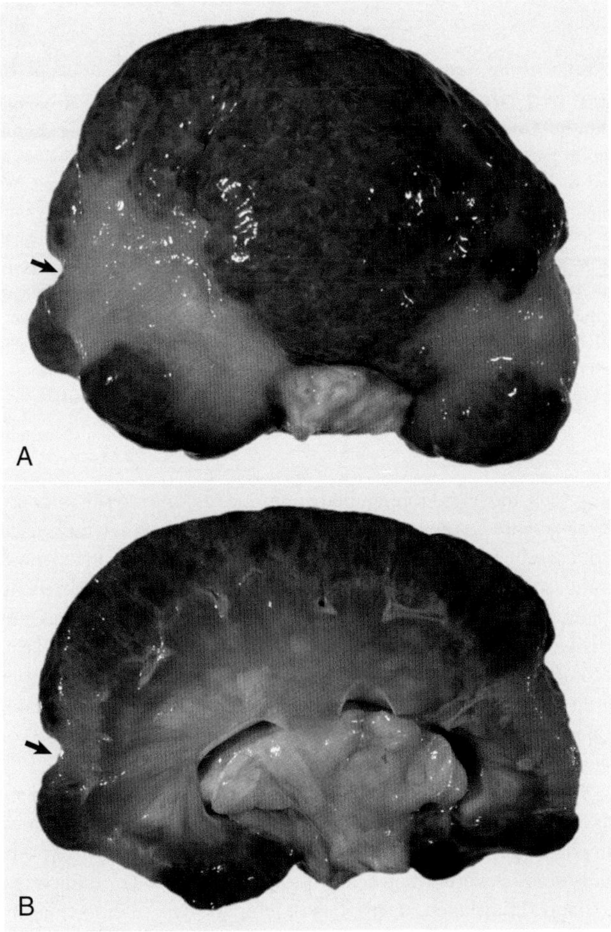

Figure 11-47 Chronic Pyelonephritis, Kidney, Dog. A, Note the two large polar scars visible as large indentations on the capsular surface *(arrow)*. The fine gray spots are regions of chronic inflammatory infiltrates and fibrosis. **B,** Dorsal section. The cortical scars are localized to the renal poles *(arrow)*, but there is a finely stippled pattern of nodularity and fibrosis in the remaining kidney. This polar pattern of scarring suggests previous bouts of pyelonephritis. (Courtesy Dr. A. Confer, Center for Veterinary Health Sciences, Oklahoma State University.)

Papillary (Medullary Crest) Necrosis. Necrosis of the renal papillae, or their counterpart, the medullary crest, is a response of the inner medulla to ischemia. Papillary necrosis can be a primary or secondary lesion. When papillary necrosis occurs as a primary lesion, it can, in some cases, be severe enough to cause clinical disease. This scenario usually occurs in animals treated with NSAIDs, which can result in a clinical disease analogous to analgesic nephropathy in human beings. Primary papillary necrosis occurs quite frequently in horses treated for prolonged periods with phenylbutazone or flunixin meglumine. Additionally in horses, simultaneous treatment with two NSAIDs increases the risk of clinical disease. It is important in dogs and cats because of accidental ingestion of or treatment with ibuprofen, aspirin, or acetaminophen at excessive dosages. Drugs associated with papillary necrosis have been referred to as *papillotoxins*. Medullary interstitial cells are the primary targets of papillotoxins. These cells synthesize prostaglandins, antihypertensive factors, and the glycosaminoglycan matrix of the medullary interstitium. Interstitial cell damage decreases prostaglandin synthesis, which reduces normal blood flow and causes ischemia, increases tubular transport, and modifies the interstitial matrix; the net effect is degenerative changes in tubular epithelial cells in the inner medulla. In addition to its inhibition of prostaglandin biosynthesis, acetaminophen also causes direct oxidative damage to medullary tubular epithelium after covalent binding to the cells, further enhancing necrosis of the renal papillae.

Secondary papillary necrosis results from the following:

- Reduced blood flow in vasa recta
- Glomerular lesions restricting blood flow—amyloid, hyalinization
- Compression of vasa recta—within the medulla
- Interstitial fibrosis—chiefly in the outer medulla, secondary to ischemia (see later discussion)
- Interstitial renal medullary amyloidosis (cats)
- Pyelitis—ascending tubular and interstitial inflammation, edema, and fibrosis
- Compression of renal papilla due to increased intrapelvic pressure secondary to
  - Pelvic calculi
  - Lower urinary tract obstruction
  - Vesicoureteral reflux

Decreased perfusion and compression cause papillary necrosis because the inner medulla is the least well perfused of any zone of the kidneys. Most of the medullary blood supply comes from the cortex after passing through the glomeruli and entering the vasa recta. Because of limited blood flow and high metabolic medullary cellular demand, any lesion or disease process that further reduces medullary blood flow can cause ischemic necrosis (infarction) of the papillae. In addition, the high metabolic demand for cell transport and the maintenance of an ion gradient to enhance urinary concentration makes this area particularly vulnerable. This is most evident after ischemic tubular damage where swollen endothelial and tubular epithelial cells, in conjunction with neutrophil adhesion in small vessels, upset the balance of oxygenation and energy demand by the medullary tubular cells. Medullary blood flow is ultimately balanced through concentrations of vasodilators, such as prostaglandin, nitric oxide, and adenosine, and vasoconstrictors, such as endothelin and angiotensin II.

Typically, acute lesions are irregular, discolored areas of necrotic inner medulla sharply delineated from the surviving medullary tissue (Fig. 11-48). The affected tissue, which initially undergoes coagulation necrosis, is yellow-gray, green, or pink. With time, the necrotic tissue sloughs, resulting in a detached, friable, and discolored tissue fragment in the pelvis. The remaining inner medulla is usually

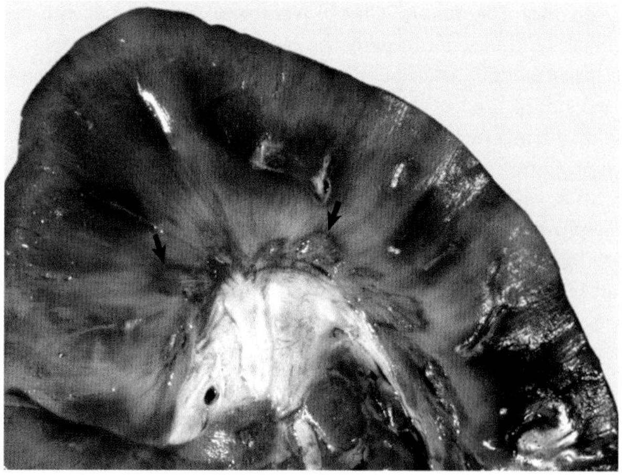

Figure 11-48 **Papillary (Medullary Crest) Necrosis, Chronic Nonsteroidal Antiinflammatory Drug Treatment, Kidney, Dorsal Section, Horse.** Acute coagulation necrosis of the medullary crest and inner medulla (*green areas [arrows]*). There is also hemorrhage of the outer medulla. The term *papillary necrosis* is retained for all animals, although only the pig and cow have distinct renal papillae. In other animals, these have fused to form the medullary crest. (Courtesy Dr. A. Confer, Center for Veterinary Health Sciences, Oklahoma State University.)

attenuated and on cross section is narrowed. Overlying cortex can be somewhat shrunken because of atrophy of some of the nephrons caused by blockage of their tubules in the affected medulla. Small pieces of sloughed necrotic medullary tissue pass inconsequentially into the ureter. However, large pieces can obstruct the ureter, causing hydronephrosis, or form a nidus for precipitation of minerals, resulting in the formation of pelvic or ureteral calculi.

Diseases of the Interstitium

Granulomatous Nephritis. Granulomatous nephritis is an interstitial disease that often accompanies chronic systemic diseases that are characterized by multiple granulomas in various organs. In domestic animals, granulomatous nephritis can be caused by a variety of granuloma-inducing infectious microbes. These can include fungi such as *Aspergillus* sp., *Phycomycetes*, or *Histoplasma capsulatum* (E-Figs. 11-5 and 11-6); algae such as *Prototheca* sp.; parasites (*Toxocara* sp. and *Angiostrongylus vasorum* larvae/eggs); protozoa such as *Encephalitozoon cuniculi*; bacteria such as *Mycobacterium bovis*; and viruses such as feline coronavirus (see Disorders of Cats) and porcine circovirus. Common to each are small, gray-white to tan, granulomatous foci (2 to 5 mm in diameter) or larger nodules (up to 10 cm in diameter) scattered randomly throughout the kidneys, especially the cortex. Foci are often granular and can have calcified, caseous centers. Microscopically, lesions are characterized by central foci of necrosis with variable numbers of neutrophils and are surrounded by epithelioid macrophages, variable degrees of mineral deposits, and possibly giant cells.

In cattle, granulomatous nephritis is part of the multisystemic granulomatous disease caused by hairy vetch (*Vicia villosa*) toxicosis (see the section on Kidney and Lower Urinary Tract, Disorders of Ruminants). Lesions are characterized by multifocal to coalescing cortical granulomas (Fig. 11-49, *A*). Microscopically, infiltrates of monocytes, lymphocytes, plasma cells, eosinophils, and multinucleated giant cells are seen primarily within the interstitium of the renal cortex (Fig. 11-49, *B*).

Migratory *Toxocara canis* larvae can induce small, gray-to-white granulomas (2 to 3 mm) randomly scattered throughout the subcapsular renal cortex of dogs (Fig. 11-50, *A*). Such lesions probably are due to cell-mediated foreign body immune response to the migrating larvae and are composed of aggregates of macrophages, lymphocytes, and eosinophils surrounded by fibroblasts within concentrically arranged fibrous connective tissue (Fig. 11-50, *B*). In recently acquired lesions, nematode larvae can often be seen in the center of these lesions (see Fig. 11-50, *B*). Following death, the larvae become fragmented, and the debris is either phagocytosed and eliminated or, less commonly, retained with a resultant granulomatous response. Lesions heal by fibrosis, leaving a few finely pitted (contracted) foci on the capsular surface.

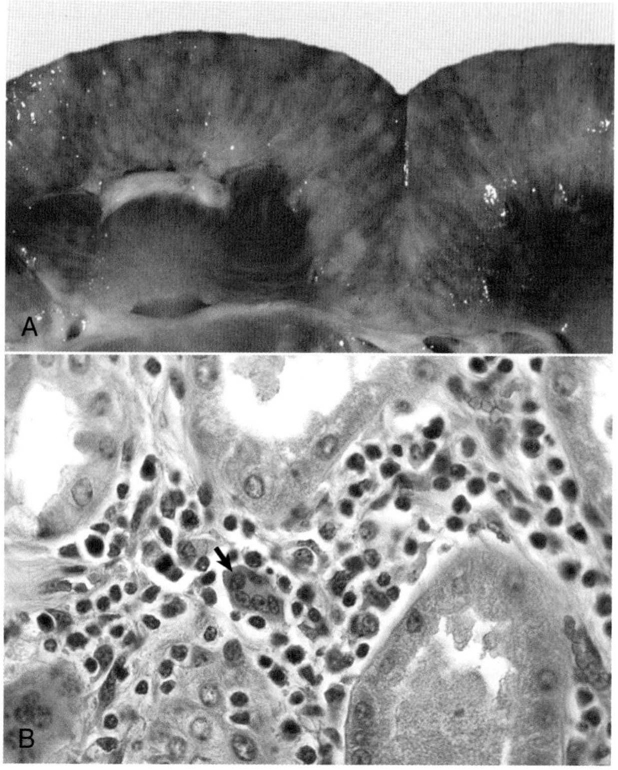

Figure 11-49 **Granulomatous Nephritis, Hairy Vetch Toxicosis, Kidney, Cow. A,** Cortical striations are obliterated by coalescing granulomatous foci associated with hairy vetch toxicosis. **B,** Cortex. Lesions associated with hairy vetch toxicosis are characterized by a mixed cell interstitial inflammatory infiltrate (macrophages, lymphocytes, and occasional multinucleated giant cell [*arrow*]) with renal tubular atrophy. It is specifically known as an unusual type of poisoning because of its ability to induce granulomatous inflammation in addition to the necrosis. The kidney is not the primary organ affected. H&E stain. (**A** courtesy Dr. J. King, College of Veterinary Medicine, Cornell University; and Dr. J. Edwards, College of Veterinary Medicine, Texas A&M University. **B** courtesy Dr. R. Panciera, Center for Veterinary Health Sciences, Oklahoma State University.)

Xanthogranulomas. Cats with inherited hyperlipoproteinemia have xanthogranulomas in various organs, including the kidneys. Similar renal xanthogranulomas can occur in dogs with hypothyroidism and severe atherosclerosis. These lesions are characterized by foamy, lipid-laden macrophages, lymphocytes, plasma cells, and fibrosis interspersed with cleftlike spaces typical of cholesterol deposits (cholesterol clefts).

Renal Interstitial Amyloidosis. Although glomeruli are the most common renal sites for deposition of amyloid in most domestic animal species, deposition can occur in the medullary interstitium (see the section on Amyloidosis). Renal amyloidosis commonly occurs in association with other diseases, particularly chronic inflammatory or neoplastic diseases. However, idiopathic renal

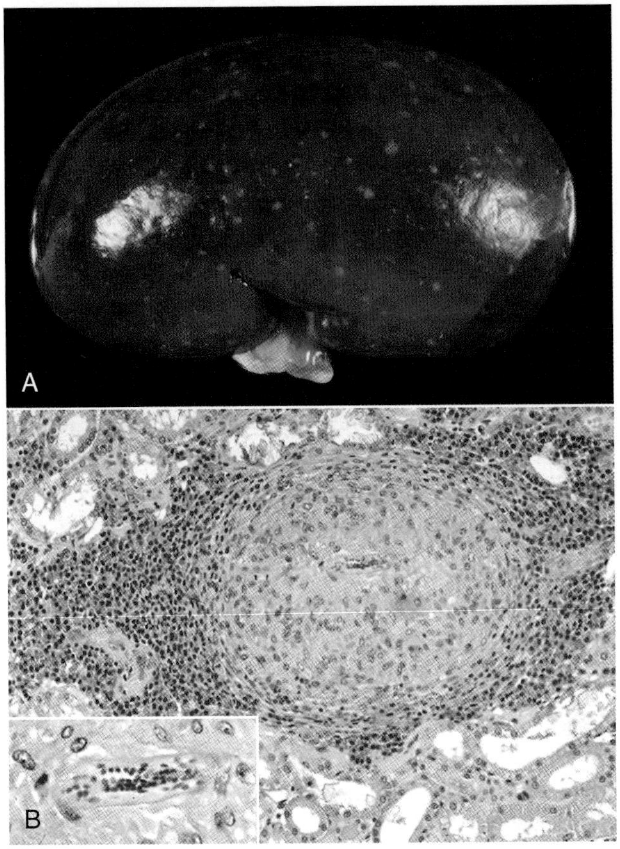

Figure 11-50 **Granulomatous Nephritis, Kidney, Cortex, Dog. A,** Multiple subcapsular, cortical, tan, raised granulomas caused by migrating ascarid larvae. **B,** A mature granuloma composed of a central ascarid larva surrounded by epithelioid macrophages and concentrically arranged fibrous connective tissue and inflammatory cells. H&E stain. *Inset,* Ascarid larva. (Courtesy Dr. W. Crowell, College of Veterinary Medicine, The University of Georgia; and Noah's Arkive, College of Veterinary Medicine, The University of Georgia.)

amyloidosis (i.e., amyloidosis in which an associated disease process is not recognized) is also described in dogs and cats. The underlying pathogenic mechanisms of idiopathic renal amyloidosis are not known. Medullary amyloidosis is usually asymptomatic unless it obstructs blood flow and causes papillary necrosis. A hereditary predisposition for the development of reactive amyloidosis (AA) has been found in Abyssinian cats, and a familial tendency is suspected in Siamese cats. Shar-Pei dogs are one of the most commonly affected canine breeds to have systemic AA amyloidosis, and amyloid often accumulates in the renal medullary interstitium. Shar-Pei amyloidosis is thought to be autosomal recessive in its familial inheritance. Medullary amyloidosis may predispose the dog to various aspects of end-stage renal disease, including interstitial fibrosis, lymphoplasmacytic infiltration, tubular atrophy, tubular dilation, mineralization, deposition of oxalate crystals, glomerular atrophy, and glomerulosclerosis.

Neoplasia. The prevalence of primary renal neoplasms in domestic animals is less than 1% of the total neoplasms reported. They are usually unilateral and can be epithelial, mesenchymal, or embryonal in origin. A study of canine cases revealed carcinomas (49/82), sarcomas (28/82), and nephroblastomas (5/82) with a 4% bilateral involvement. Median survival for carcinomas was 16 months, for sarcomas was 9 months, and for nephroblastoma 6 months. Primary renal tumors are highly malignant and metastatic disease is common (77%). Inappropriate polycythemia is a paraneoplastic condition seen in association with excess erythropoietin production by renal carcinomas and sarcomas.

Epithelial Tumors

Renal Adenomas. Renal adenomas are rare, benign, epithelial neoplasms composed of proliferations of renal cortical epithelial cells, most often reported in dogs, cats, and horses. They are incidental findings at autopsy (syn: necropsy) and are usually small (1 to 3 cm), white-to-yellow, solitary, well-circumscribed, nonencapsulated masses in the cortex. Microscopically, adenomas are composed of solid sheets, tubules, or papillary proliferations of cuboidal epithelial cells of uniform size and have granular eosinophilic cytoplasm and small, round to oval nuclei. Mitotic figures, necrosis, and fibrosis are rare. These incidental tumors are clinically asymptomatic.

Oncocytomas. Oncocytomas are rare benign epithelial tumors that can occur in a variety of tissues. Grossly, renal oncocytomas are tan, homogeneous, well-encapsulated masses. Histologically, oncocytomas are composed of large eosinophilic, granular, round cells with condensed round nuclei. Ultrastructurally, they are characterized by numerous prominent cytoplasmic mitochondria. Their origin in the kidney is speculated to be from the intercalated cells of the collecting ducts. These tumors are clinically asymptomatic.

Renal Carcinomas. Renal carcinomas are the most common primary renal neoplasms and occur most frequently in older dogs. The specific causes of renal adenocarcinomas in human beings are well determined compared with those in animal species, but several mechanisms have been proven in natural animal disease or experimental models, including the following:

- Viruses: Ranid herpesvirus 1 adenocarcinoma (Lucke's tumor) in the kidney of frogs and avian erythroblastosis virus (strain ES4), an oncovirus, induce renal adenocarcinomas in chickens.
- Chemical carcinogens: Several known carcinogens, particularly the nitrosamines, can be causative agents and typically exert their neoplastic influence by direct DNA damage or inhibition of DNA synthesis or repair.
- Autosomal dominant gene mutations in Eker rats: These mutations predispose these rats to bilateral renal cell carcinoma and a variety of other secondary cancers, resembling the human von Hippel-Lindau disease.

Primary renal carcinomas are usually large (up to 20 cm in diameter), spherical to oval, and firm. They often are pale yellow and contain dark areas of hemorrhage and necrosis and foci of cystic degeneration. The masses usually occupy and obliterate one pole of the kidney and grow by expansion, compressing the adjacent normal renal tissue (Fig. 11-51, A and B). Histologic types include papillary, tubular, multilocular cystic, and solid (Fig. 11-51, C). Solid variants can be poorly differentiated and sometimes can be subclassified as clear cell or chromophobe variants if the cytoplasm is clear or vacuolated or granular and eosinophilic, respectively. Metastasis to the lungs, lymph nodes, liver, and adrenal gland occurs frequently, with metastasis reported in 50% to 60% of canine cases.

A variant of the typical renal carcinoma has been seen in German shepherd dogs in conjunction with nodular dermatofibrosis. The lesions are hereditary (autosomal dominant) and consist of multifocal, bilateral, renal cystadenomas or cystadenocarcinomas. Grossly, these tumors resemble the carcinomas described previously, but cysts are more prominent. Neoplastic cells form solid sheets, tubules, or papillary growth patterns within a moderate fibrovascular stroma. Cells are polymorphic ranging from cuboidal and columnar to polyhedral. Clear or granular eosinophilic cytoplasm is usually more atypical and anaplastic than other renal carcinoma variants.

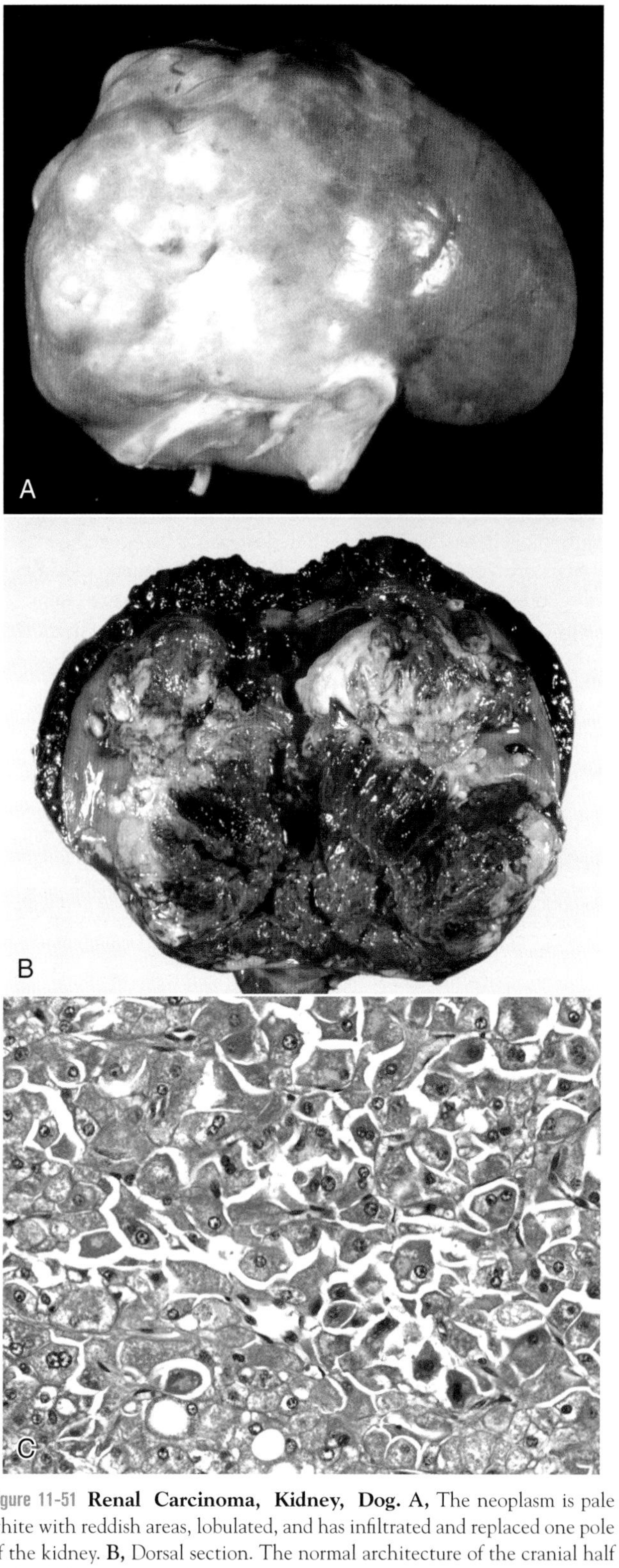

Figure 11-51 **Renal Carcinoma, Kidney, Dog. A,** The neoplasm is pale white with reddish areas, lobulated, and has infiltrated and replaced one pole of the kidney. **B,** Dorsal section. The normal architecture of the cranial half of the kidney has been obliterated by the tumor, which has hemorrhaged caudally into the adjacent kidney and subcapsularly. **C,** The tumor consists of anaplastic renal epithelial cells, typical of the solid, more poorly differentiated variant of renal carcinoma. H&E stain. (**A** and **B** courtesy College of Veterinary Medicine, University of Illinois. **C** courtesy Dr. S.J. Newman, College of Veterinary Medicine, University of Tennessee.)

Nuclei range from small, round, granular, and uniform to large, oval, vesicular, and pleomorphic. Mitotic figures are numerous.

Transitional Cell Papillomas and Carcinomas. Transitional cell papillomas and transitional cell carcinomas arise in the renal pelvis and lower urinary tract and, when large, can obstruct urinary outflow. Renal pelvic transitional cell carcinomas can invade into the kidney and typically carry a poor prognosis. The morphologic features of transitional cell neoplasms are discussed later with the urinary bladder neoplasms (see the section on the Lower Urinary System).

Mesenchymal Tumors. Fibromas, fibrosarcomas, hemangiomas, hemangiosarcomas, renal interstitial cell tumors, and undifferentiated sarcomas can occur in the kidneys. Primary renal sarcomas occur less frequently than primary epithelial tumors and constitute approximately 20% of the primary renal tumors of dogs and cats. Microscopically, fibromas, fibrosarcomas, hemangiomas, and hemangiosarcomas are similar to those in other organs. Undifferentiated sarcomas are often the most common mesenchymal tumor and may require immunohistochemistry to determine with surety that it is a mesenchymal tumor. Renal interstitial cell tumors usually arise at the corticomedullary junction and are similar to fibromas but contain cytoplasmic lipid droplets.

Metastatic Tumors. Carcinomas and sarcomas (metastatic tumors) arising in other organs can metastasize to the kidneys and are characteristically composed of randomly scattered multiple nodules, usually involving both kidneys (Fig. 11-52). Renal lymphoma (lymphosarcoma) occurs with some frequency in cattle and especially cats, particularly as part of generalized or multicentric lymphoma, which is secondary to retrovirus infection. These neoplastic foci appear as single or multiple homogeneous gray-white nodules (Fig. 11-52, *B* and *E*) or as diffuse lymphomatous infiltrates that cause uniform enlargement and pale discoloration of the kidney (Fig. 11-52, *C*). In cats, renal lymphoma must be differentiated histologically from the necrotizing, fibrinous, and granulomatous renal vasculitis of feline infectious peritonitis and less commonly systemic mycoses (Fig. 11-52, *E*). Microscopically, neoplastic lymphocytes form obliterative sheets of cells within the renal parenchyma, unrelated to the vasculature (Fig. 11-52, *F*). Neoplastic lymphocytes have distinct cellular borders, moderate amounts of basophilic cytoplasm, and large round vesicular nuclei with variable prominence to the nucleoli.

Tumors of Embryonal Origin. Nephroblastomas (embryonal nephroma or Wilms tumor) are the most common renal neoplasms of pigs and chickens, in which they are usually recognized as incidental findings at slaughter. They occur in cattle and dogs as well, but less frequently. These neoplasms arise from metanephric blastema and thus occur in young animals, less than 2 years old. It is speculated that neoplasms result from malignant transformation during normal nephrogenesis or from neoplastic transformation of nests of embryonic tissue that persists in the postnatal kidneys. At autopsy (syn: necropsy), nephroblastomas can be solitary or multiple masses that often reach a great size and in which recognizable renal tissue can be difficult to detect. They usually are soft to rubbery and gray with foci of hemorrhage. On a cut surface, they are often lobulated. Because nephroblastomas arise from primitive pluripotential tissue, histologic features vary but are morphologically similar to the developmental stages of embryonic kidneys. Characteristically, three components—including primitive, loose myxomatous mesenchymal tissue interspersed with primitive tubules lined by elongated, deeply staining cells and structures that resemble primitive glomeruli—are present. Nests of cells resembling the metanephric blastema can be present. Nephroblastomas also have mesenchymal components such as cartilage, bone, skeletal muscle, and adipose tissue. Clinically, these tumors can be incidental findings; however,

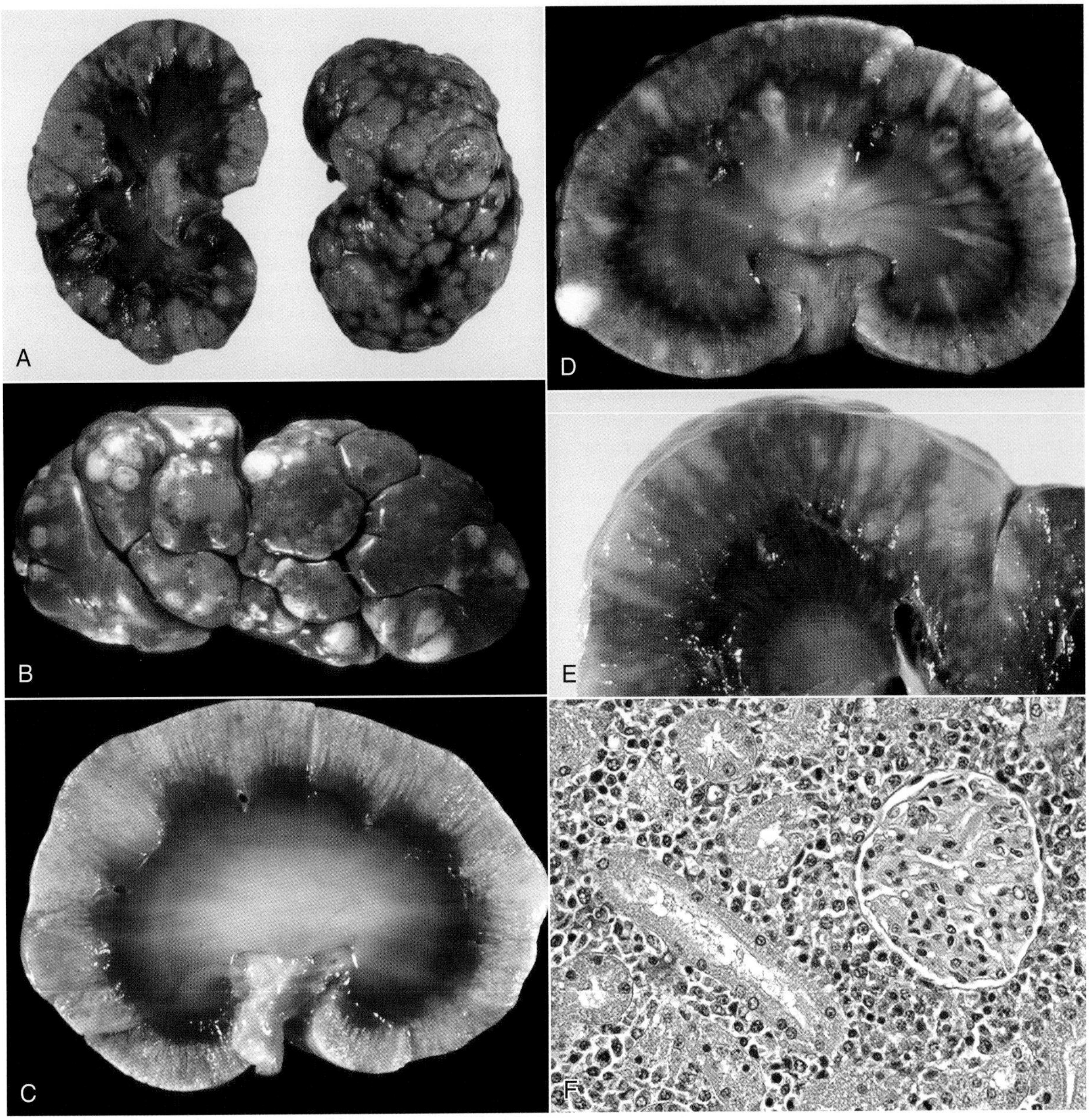

Figure 11-52 **Primary and Metastatic Renal Tumors, Kidney. A,** Metastatic mast cell tumor, dorsal section, dog. Multiple pale tan, raised nodules are randomly scattered throughout the renal cortex. **B,** Lymphoma (lymphosarcoma), cow. Multifocal raised pale white nodules are typical of nodular renal lymphoma. **C,** Lymphoma (lymphosarcoma), dorsal section, cat. Note the pale white areas in the cortex, which bulge from the surface. This lesion can be confused with the granulomatous vasculitis of renal feline infectious peritonitis, thus warranting histologic evaluation. **D,** Systemic cryptococcosis (*Cryptococcus neoformans*), cat. This is not a neoplasm, but the multiple pale, occasionally raised nodules can be confused with the nodular form of lymphoma (**C**), thus requiring histologic examination. **E,** Lymphoma (lymphosarcoma), dorsal section, bovine. Multiple coalescing pale white nodules are present throughout the cortex. **F,** Lymphoma (lymphosarcoma), cow. Neoplastic lymphocytes infiltrate and distend the renal interstitium. H&E stain. (**A** courtesy Dr. A. Confer, Center for Veterinary Health Sciences, Oklahoma State University. **B** courtesy College of Veterinary Medicine, University of Illinois. **C** courtesy Dr. K. Read, College of Veterinary Medicine, Texas A&M University; and Noah's Arkive, College of Veterinary Medicine, The University of Georgia. **D** courtesy Dr. S.J. Newman, College of Veterinary Medicine, University of Tennessee. **E** courtesy Dr. J. King, College of Veterinary Medicine, Cornell University; and Dr. J. Edwards, College of Veterinary Medicine, Texas A&M University. **F** courtesy Dr. J.F. Zachary, College of Veterinary Medicine, University of Illinois.)

in dogs and cats, greater than 50% may metastasize to lymph nodes and visceral organs. In young dogs, a unique spinal cord nephroblastoma has been described. These tumors likely arise from remnants of renal blastema trapped subdurally that grow by expansion and compress the spinal cord.

Disorders of the Lower Urinary Tract

Developmental Anomalies

Aplasia and Hypoplasia. Ureteral aplasia (agenesis) is the lack of formation of a recognizable ureter, and hypoplasia is the presence of a notably small-diameter ureter. Agenesis of the ureters is the result of failure of the ureteral bud to form and may be unilateral or bilateral. Both conditions are rare. If these defects occur alone, disruption of urinary flow from the kidney to the urinary bladder results in obstructive diseases such as hydronephrosis. If these defects occur with concurrent renal aplasia, they are clinically silent if aplasia is unilateral, and incompatible with life if aplasia is bilateral.

Ectopic Ureters. Ectopic ureters are ureters that empty into the urethra, vagina, neck of the bladder, ductus deferens, prostate, or other secondary sex glands rather than terminating normally at the trigone of the bladder. The two possible causes are as follows:

- The ureteral bud arises too far craniad to be incorporated into the urogenital sinus.
- The differential growth of the sinus is abnormal, and the ureter fails to migrate to its usual location.

Ectopic ureters are more subject to obstruction or infection, and thus they predispose animals to pyelitis and pyelonephritis. Ectopic ureters occur most frequently in dogs, and certain breeds, especially the Siberian husky, are at greater risk. Affected animals present clinically with urinary incontinence and consequent urine dribbling.

Patent Urachus. The most common malformation of the urinary bladder is patent urachus (pervious urachus), and it is seen most frequently in foals. This lesion develops when the fetal urachus fails to close, therefore forming a direct channel between the bladder's apex and the umbilicus. As a result, affected animals dribble urine from the umbilicus. The patent urachus is susceptible to infection and abscess formation. Conversely, umbilical inflammation and abscess formation may lead to failure of the urachal remnant and the umbilical arteries and vein to involute, potentially causing a patent urachus. Rupture of the urachus causes uroperitoneum, which must be differentiated from perinatal rupture of the bladder. Occasionally, during urachal closure, the mucosa closes but closure of the bladder musculature is incomplete. When this occurs, a bladder diverticulum (outpouching) at the apex of the bladder can develop. Diverticula of the bladder may also be acquired secondary to partial obstruction of urine outflow and result from pressure changes exerted during normal contractions of the bladder. Urine stasis can occur in the diverticulum, predisposing the animal to cystitis or urinary calculi.

Hydroureter. Hydroureter refers to dilation of the ureter(s) and is most often caused by obstruction of urine outflow due to blockage of the ureter(s) by calculi, chronic inflammation, luminal or intramural neoplasia, or accidental ligation during surgery. Hydroureter can be unilateral or bilateral and is often accompanied by concurrent hydronephrosis (see the previous section on Hydronephrosis). The clinical signs of this condition are related to obstruction.

Urolithiasis (Obstructive Disease). Urolithiasis is the presence of stones or calculi (uroliths) in the urinary collecting system. Uroliths form when familial, congenital, and pathophysiologic factors occur together and cause the precipitation of excretory metabolites in urine into grossly visible stones. These concretions may form anywhere in the urinary collecting system, and although some clearly originate in the lower urinary tract or as microscopic calculi in the renal collecting tubules, the point of development of most is not known. Uroliths may be found in any portion of the lower urinary tract, from the renal pelvis to the urethra, but occur least commonly in the renal pelvis (accounting for 1% to 4% of canine uroliths). The diseases caused by uroliths are among the most important urinary tract problems of domesticated animals, especially cattle, sheep, dogs, and cats, and are of lesser importance in horses and pigs.

Mechanistically, factors that are important either in predisposing to calculus formation or in precipitating disease include the following:

- Urine concentrations of calculus precursor material sufficient to be precipitated
- Unusual metabolism of certain substances, such as uric acid in Dalmatian dogs
- Hereditary defects leading to abnormal processing of substances by the kidney, such as cystine or xanthine
- Abnormally high concentrations of substances in the diet, such as the following:
  - Silicic acid in native pastures (silica calculi)
  - Phosphorus in grain-based rations (struvite calculi)
  - Estrogen in subterranean clover (clover stones containing benzocoumarins; calcium carbonate related to isoflavones)
  - Magnesium in commercial dry cat food
  - Oxalate in oxalate-accumulating plants

Regardless of the type of calculus, factors of variable importance in calculus formation include the following:

- Urinary pH, in terms of its effect on solute excretion and precipitation (oxalates increase at acid pH; struvites and carbonates precipitate at alkaline pH)
- Reduced water intake, in relation to the degree of urine concentration and mineral supersaturation
- Bacterial infection of the lower urinary tract (struvite calculi in dogs)
- Obstruction or structural abnormalities of the lower urinary system
- Foreign bodies (suture, grass awn, catheter, or needle) or a conglomerate of bacterial colonies, exfoliated epithelium, or leukocytes, which can serve as a nidus for precipitation of mineral constituents
- Drug metabolites excreted in the urine (e.g., sulfonamides and tetracyclines)

Supersaturation of urine with the components of stone-forming salts is the essential precursor to initiation of urolith formation (nucleation). Supersaturation may be in the unstable range, in which precipitation occurs spontaneously (homogeneous nucleation), or the metastable range, in which precipitation occurs by epitaxy (one type of crystal grows on the surface of another type; heterogeneous nucleation). In some instances, uroliths may have distinct layers composed of different mineral types. These compound uroliths form when factors promoting precipitation of one mineral type are superseded by factors promoting precipitation of a different type of mineral.

Microscopically apparent crystals are much more common in urine than are grossly visible aggregates of mineral (calculi). Although equine urine is normally supersaturated with calcium carbonate, and crystalluria is normal, horses experience a low prevalence of calculi. In all species, the factors that promote or prevent crystal growth and crystal aggregation are poorly understood. Although it was formerly thought that urinary proteins such as uromodulin (Tamm-Horsfall protein), which make up 5% to 20% or more of some calculi, were initiators of crystal formation, it is now believed that uromodulin and other urinary macromolecules have a role in preventing formation of kidney stones by reducing the aggregation of calcium crystals.

Macroscopically, calculi are grossly visible aggregations of precipitated urinary solutes, principally mineral admixed with urinary proteins and proteinaceous debris. Calculi typically are hard spheres or ovoids, with a central nidus, surrounded by concentric laminae, an outer shell, and surface crystals. Many calculi contain significant quantities of "contaminants" such as calcium oxalates in "silica" calculi; few are relatively pure. Large renal pelvic calculi (nephroliths) classically have a "staghorn" appearance because they take the shape of the renal calyces in animal species that have true calyces (Fig. 11-53). These calculi predispose affected animals to pyelitis and pyelonephritis. Urinary bladder calculi can be single or multiple, variable in size (2 to 10 cm), and sometimes are composed of a fine, sandlike material, which causes cloudy urine (Fig. 11-54).

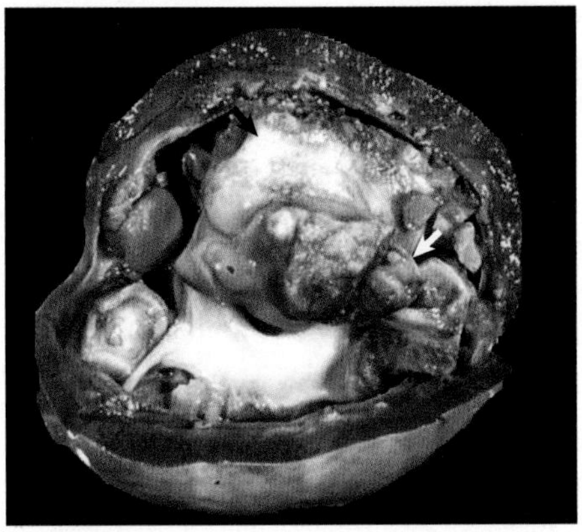

Figure 11-53 **Urolithiasis, Kidney, Dorsal Section, Goat.** A calculus fills and distends the renal pelvis *(arrows)* and has caused pressure atrophy of the medulla. (Courtesy Dr. M.A. Breshears, Center for Veterinary Health Sciences, Oklahoma State University.)

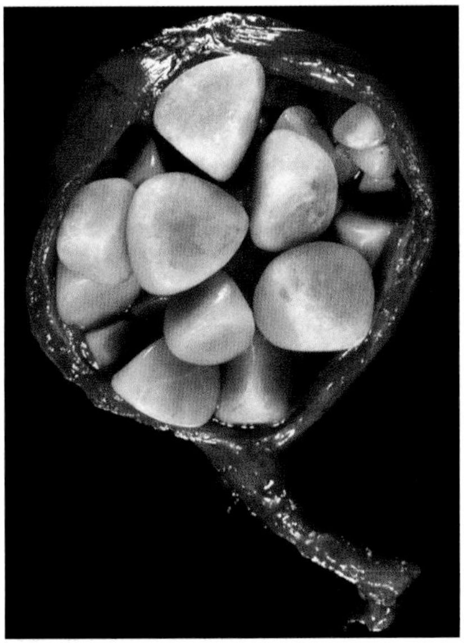

Figure 11-54 **Urolithiasis, Urinary Bladder, Dog.** Multiple smooth calculi are present in the urinary bladder. The bladder wall is diffusely thickened. (Courtesy Dr. A. Confer, Center for Veterinary Health Sciences, Oklahoma State University.)

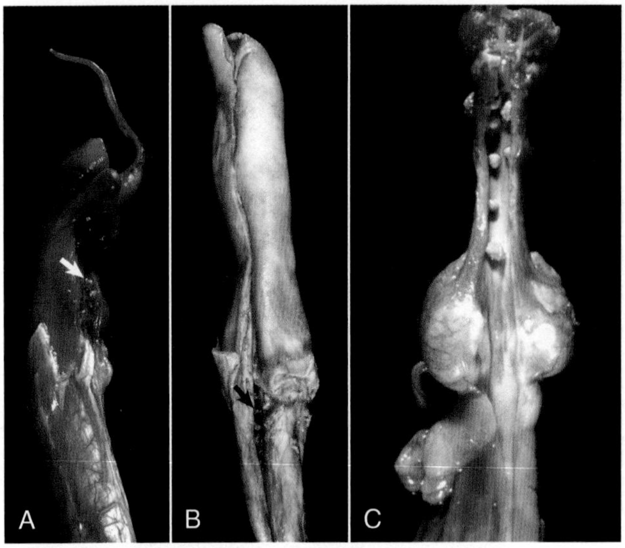

Figure 11-55 **Urolithiasis, Penile Urethra. A,** Sheep. Multiple calculi are present in the penile urethra *(arrow)* and the urethral process (vermiform appendage). **B,** Ventral aspect, dog. Calculi have lodged in the urethra proximal to the caudal end of the os penis *(arrow)*. **C,** Cat. Calculi are present throughout the penile urethra, several just caudal to the external urethral orifice at tip of the penis. (**A** and **B** courtesy Dr. M.D. McGavin, College of Veterinary Medicine, University of Tennessee. **C** courtesy College of Veterinary Medicine, University of Illinois.)

Calculi can have smooth or rough surfaces and may be solid, soft, or friable. Depending on the composition of calculi, their color varies and may be inconsistent, even among calculi of similar composition. The calculi can be white to gray (e.g., struvite and oxalate), yellow (e.g., urate, cystine, benzocoumarin, and xanthine), or brown (e.g., silica, urate, and xanthine), although gross diagnosis of specific mineral type is precluded by variation in appearance and mixed composition.

Small calculi may be voided in the urine, but typically calculi cause urinary obstruction. This is more common in males because of their long and narrow-diameter urethra. The most common sites of lodgment of urethral calculi vary with the animal species. In male cattle, calculi lodge in the urethra at the ischial arch and at the proximal end of the sigmoid flexure; in rams and wethers, the urethral process (vermiform appendage) is the most common site (Fig. 11-55, A); and in dogs, calculi lodge proximal to the base of the os penis (Fig. 11-55, *B*). At the site in which calculi lodge, there is local pressure necrosis, ulceration of the mucosa, and acute hemorrhagic urethritis. Because urethral sites are prone to rupture, hydronephrosis after complete urethral obstruction is less common than with unilateral long-standing ureteral impaction.

In male cats, urethral plugs composed of fine struvite crystals (sand) within abundant rubber-like protein matrix can fill the entire urethra, and they are distinct from calculi, which are composed predominantly of mineral. Either urethral plugs or urethral calculi may be the cause of *feline lower urinary tract disease* (FLUTD) (Fig. 11-55, C). When obstruction or dysuria occurs in females, calculi are usually large and located in the renal pelvis or urinary bladder.

At autopsy (syn: necropsy), animals that have died of urinary obstruction have greatly distended (Fig. 11-56, A), turgid, or ruptured urinary bladders and may have bilaterally dilated ureters and renal pelves. The bladder wall is thin and often has mucosal to transmural ecchymoses or diffuse hemorrhage (Fig. 11-56, *B*). When urine is released from the bladder, because of either rupture or incision at surgery or autopsy (syn: necropsy), the wall of the bladder is flaccid, the mucosa is often dark red and ulcerated, and the urine contains blood clots. Mucosal ulceration, localized lamina propria hemorrhage, and mucosal necrosis are usually present in the ureter, bladder, or urethra adjacent to an obstructive calculus or urethral plug. If the bladder ruptures antemortem, blood clots and fibrin are adhered at the site of rupture, and in some cases there is an acute, localized chemical (urine-induced) peritonitis.

Microscopically, inflammation and hemorrhage are present in the lower urinary tract. Lesions are most severe in cases in which obstruction has been complete. The mucosa is usually ulcerated, and areas of hyperplastic transitional epithelium are interspersed with goblet cells. The lamina propria is usually infiltrated with inflammatory cells. Neutrophils are present at foci of ulceration, and lymphocytes and plasma cells infiltrate perivascularly or uniformly throughout the lamina propria. Hemorrhage is often transmural but is most evident in the mucosa and can cause separation of the smooth muscle bundles. Degeneration and necrosis of smooth muscle occurs in severe cases.

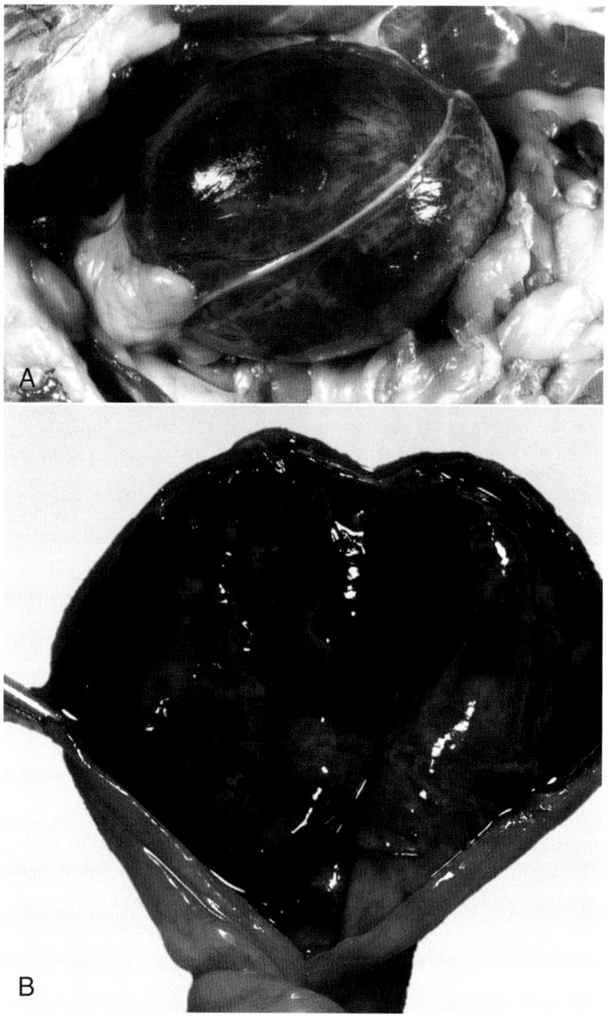

Figure 11-56 Hemorrhagic Urocystitis (Feline Lower Urinary Tract Disease) Urinary Bladder, Cat. A, Obstructive urolithiasis. The bladder is overdistended and turgid as the result of urethral obstruction. Note the serosal and intramuscular ecchymotic and suffusive hemorrhages at the neck and apex of the bladder. **B,** Urolithiasis, acute hemorrhagic cystitis. The severe diffuse transmural hemorrhage throughout the urinary bladder wall is secondary to blockage of the urethra by calculi and distention of the urinary bladder. (Courtesy Dr. M.D. McGavin, College of Veterinary Medicine, University of Tennessee.)

Clinically, urolithiasis can cause urinary obstruction or traumatic injury to the urinary bladder mucosa. Lesions of the urinary bladder are manifested clinically as difficult or painful urination (stranguria; dysuria), with or without grossly apparent hematuria. Small calculi may be voided in the urine, but typically calculi cause urinary obstruction. Dysuria can result from large calculi in the urinary bladder, but urinary tract obstruction with azotemia most commonly occurs because of nearly complete or complete urethral obstruction by small calculi.

Inflammatory Diseases

Acute Cystitis. Inflammation of the urinary bladder (cystitis) is common in domestic animals and may be acute or chronic. Because inflammation of the ureter (ureteritis) or urethra (urethritis) in the absence of cystitis is rare, this discussion focuses on cystitis. The causes of acute cystitis are varied; however, for all animal species, bacterial infection is the most common cause. In health, the bladder is resistant to infection, and contaminating bacteria are quickly eliminated by the flushing action of normal urine flow. Predisposition to urinary tract infection (UTI) occurs when there is stagnation of urine because of urinary tract obstruction, incomplete voiding during urination, or urothelial trauma. Other risk factors for UTI include urinary catheterization, vaginoscopy, vaginitis, urinary incontinence, or recent administration of medications such as antibiotics or corticosteroids. Bacterial cystitis is more common in females because their relatively short urethra provides less of a barrier to ascending infections than the longer, narrower male urethra. In all domestic animal species, the bacterial agent that most commonly causes cystitis is uropathogenic *Escherichia coli* (α-hemolysin–producing strains). Other bacterial pathogens that are important causes of cystis include *Corynebacterium renale* in cattle, *Actinobaculum suis* (*Eubacterium suis*) in pigs, *Enterococcus faecalis* in cats, and *Klebsiella* sp. in horses. In addition, *Proteus* sp., *Streptococcus* sp., and *Staphylococcus* sp. have been isolated from cases of cystitis in several animal species.

Except for the distal urethra, the lower urinary tract is normally free of bacteria. Sterility of the urinary bladder is maintained by normal intermittent voiding of urine and because of the antibacterial properties of urine. These antibacterial properties are attributed to the following:

- The acidic urine of carnivores
- Secretory IgA
- Secreted mucin that inhibits bacterial adhesion
- The high concentration of urea and organic acids
- High urine osmolality

Cystitis occurs when bacteria are able to overcome normal defense mechanisms and adhere to or invade (colonize) the urinary bladder mucosa. Several factors can enhance colonization and predispose animals to cystitis. Bacterial virulence factors, such as the expression of surface molecules that enhance adhesion (e.g., the P and type 1 fimbriae of certain strains of *Escherichia coli* and *Actinobaculum suis* and the pH-dependent adherence by pili of *Corynebacterium renale*) increase the likelihood of bacterial colonization. Other bacterial virulence factors, such as the *Escherichia coli* hemolysin, enhance pathogenicity and help bacteria overcome antibacterial factors of the urinary bladder and urine.

Host factors, such as decreased frequency of urination, incomplete voiding, and urine retention as a result of obstruction or neurogenic causes (e.g., spinal cord disease), often lead to cystitis. Disruption of the urothelium within the urethra or bladder is another factor that increases the risk for bacterial cystitis. Bacterial growth can be enhanced when glucosuria is present, such as in diabetes mellitus. Compromise of the host immune system can also increase susceptibility to bacterial cystitis. Trauma to the mucosa from urinary calculi, faulty catheterization, or other causes can result in mucosal erosion and hemorrhage, which predisposes to bacterial invasion of the lamina propria. Bladder mucosa may also be damaged by excessive ammonia production by urease-producing bacteria, such as *Corynebacterium renale* in cattle and *Actinobaculum suis* in pigs.

Once bacteria gain access to the lamina propria, they cause vascular damage and inflammation. Acute cystitis is often grossly described as hemorrhagic, catarrhal, fibrinopurulent, necrotizing, or ulcerative, and these changes often occur sequentially over time. Vascular damage predisposes to hemorrhage, leakage of fibrin, and, if severe, ischemic necrosis of the bladder. This is often accompanied by mucosal ulceration. Neutrophils are present as a component of vascular damage and in any lesion with accompanying bacterial colonization. In most cases, components of several of these processes are present. The urinary bladder wall often is thickened by edema, an inflammatory cell infiltrate, and is focally or diffusely hemorrhagic. Hemorrhage is most common when obstruction is concurrently present with cystitis or after direct trauma from catheterization. Urine in such cases is described as cloudy, flocculent, foul smelling, and red-tinged. The mucosa can have foci of erosion or ulceration, patches or sheets of adherent exudate and necrotic debris, or adherent blood clots (Fig. 11-57, *A*). *Corynebacterium urealyticum* in dogs and cats and *Corynebacterium matruchotii* in a horse were implicated in a condition known as *encrusted cystitis*, in which plaques and accumulation of sediment predominate. Rarely, surgical debridement in addition to appropriate antimicrobial therapy is required.

Microscopically, acute cystitis is characterized by epithelial denudation with bacterial colonies present on the surface. The lamina propria is markedly edematous and has a diffuse neutrophilic infiltrate. Superficial hyperemia and hemorrhage are usually present (Fig. 11-57, *B*). A mild perivascular leukocytic infiltrate can occur beneath the mucosa and submucosa and also within the tunica muscularis.

Clinically, acute bacterial cystitis results in dysuria, stranguria, and hematuria. An inflammatory sediment is detected on urinalysis, and bacteria can be grown in pure culture from urine samples.

Viral causes of acute cystitis are relatively rare in veterinary medicine. In cats, a cell-associated herpesvirus has been found in some cases of mild cystitis. Hemorrhagic cystitis sometimes occurs in malignant catarrhal fever in cattle and deer and occasionally is the dominant gross feature of the disease.

Acute noninfectious cystitis can result from a variety of chemical causes. Activated metabolites of cyclophosphamide, a drug used to treat neoplastic and immune-mediated diseases of dogs and cats, can cause a sterile hemorrhagic cystitis characterized by mucosal ulceration and hemorrhage. Cantharidin toxicosis in horses results from ingestion of blister beetles (*Epicauta* spp.) in alfalfa hay, and hemorrhagic and erosive or ulcerative cystitis develops from cantharidin excreted through the urinary tract. Chronic ingestion of bracken fern (*Pteridium aquilinum*) by cattle can result in the syndrome of enzootic hematuria, which can manifest as acute urinary bladder hemorrhage, chronic cystitis, or urinary bladder neoplasia.

Chronic Cystitis. Chronic cystitis presents in several different forms based on the pattern and type of inflammatory response. These forms include diffuse, follicular, and polypoid variants. In the diffuse variant of chronic cystitis, the bladder mucosa is irregularly reddened and usually thickened. There is some epithelial desquamation, and the submucosa is heavily infiltrated with mononuclear inflammatory cells accompanied by few neutrophils. In addition, connective tissue of the submucosa is often thickened and the muscularis layer is hypertrophied.

The follicular variant of chronic cystitis is common in dogs and is characterized by multifocal and disseminated, nodular, submucosal lymphoid proliferations that are 1 to 3 mm in diameter, giving the mucosa a cobblestone appearance (follicular cystitis) (Fig. 11-58). This response is particularly common when cystitis occurs concurrently with chronic urolithiasis. A red zone of hyperemia often surrounds these white-gray raised nodules. Microscopically, these raised nodules are aggregates of lymphocytic cells in the superficial lamina propria. Epithelium overlying these foci may be normal or ulcerated and may be accompanied by fibrosis in the lamina propria. Hypertrophy of the tunica muscularis may also be present.

Polypoid masses that characterize chronic polypoid cystitis are seen predominantly in dogs but may occur in any species. They likely develop from inflammatory and hyperplastic responses secondary to chronic irritation, which most often results from persistent bacterial urinary tract infection and/or uroliths. The polyps arising in the bladder mucosa are composed of a core of proliferative connective tissue covered by surface epithelium. Mononuclear inflammatory cells are often present within the connective tissue core. In some cases, eosinophilic inflammation predominates within the core

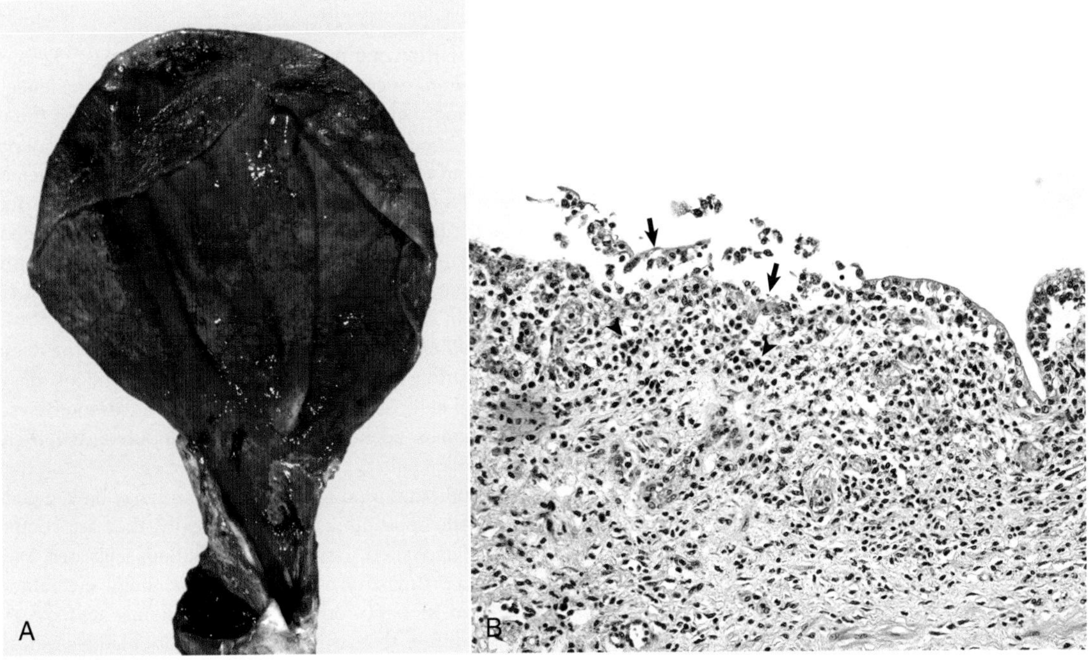

Figure 11-57 Acute Cystitis, Urinary Bladder. A, Mucosal and serosal surfaces, calf. Patchy areas of ulcerated mucosa are interspersed with areas of hemorrhagic mucosa. Note the subserosal hemorrhages *(top)*. **B,** Mucosal surface, dog. The mucosa has been partially denuded of transitional epithelium *(arrows)*. There are mucosal and submucosal infiltrates of neutrophils *(arrowheads)*, which extend into the adjacent tunica muscularis. Note the congested vessels with active hyperemia in the lamina propria. H&E stain. (**A** courtesy Dr. A. Confer, Center for Veterinary Health Sciences, Oklahoma State University. **B** courtesy Dr. J.F. Zachary, College of Veterinary Medicine, University of Illinois.)

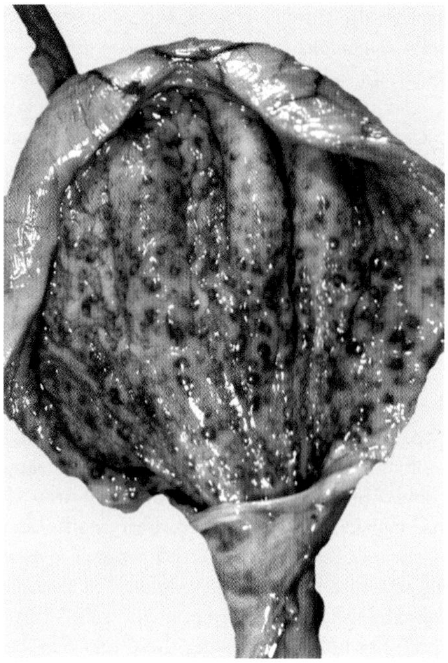

Figure 11-58 Chronic Follicular Cystitis, Urinary Bladder, Mucosal Surface, Dog. Multiple small raised red nodules are present on the mucosal surface. These nodules are foci of hyperplastic lymphoid cells surrounded by hyperemia and hemorrhage. (Courtesy Dr. A. Confer, Center for Veterinary Health Sciences, Oklahoma State University.)

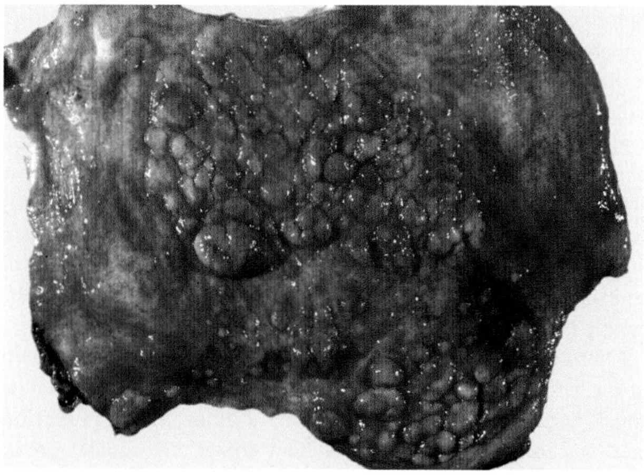

Figure 11-59 Chronic Polypoid Cystitis, Urinary Bladder, Mucosal Surface, Dog. This type of cystitis is characterized by multiple masses composed of proliferative nodules of connective tissue (polyps) mixed with chronic inflammatory cells. (Courtesy Dr. A. Confer, Center for Veterinary Health Sciences, Oklahoma State University.)

of plump spindloid cells composed of fibroblasts and myofibroblasts. Surface epithelium may form nests of hyperplastic transitional epithelial cells in the lamina propria (Brunn's nests) or undergo metaplasia to a mucus-secreting, glandular epithelial type (cystitis glandularis). The resulting polypoid masses, which are composed of inflammation, fibroplasia, and epithelial proliferation, occur most frequently in the cranioventral bladder wall (Fig. 11-59). The masses may be broad-based or pedunculated, ulcerated, or covered by hyperplastic epithelium with goblet cell metaplasia. Chronic polypoid cystitis is often accompanied by clinically evident hematuria.

Toxic Cystitis

Bracken Fern–Induced Hemorrhagic Urocystitis (Enzootic hematuria)

Information on this topic is available at www.expertconsult.com.

Mycotic Cystitis. Mycotic cystitis is occasionally seen in domestic animals when opportunistic fungi, such as *Candida albicans* or *Aspergillus* sp., colonize the urinary bladder mucosa. Such fungal infections usually occur secondary to chronic bacterial cystitis, especially when animals are immunosuppressed or subjected to prolonged antibiotic therapy, which alters the density and diversity of normal bacterial flora. Occasionally, *Blastomyces dermatitidis* can produce lower urinary tract lesions in dogs. The urinary bladder mucosa is usually ulcerated with proliferation of underlying lamina propria; a generalized thickening of the urinary bladder wall is the result of extensive inflammation consisting of neutrophils, lymphocytes, plasma cells, macrophages and edema, and fibrosis.

Neoplasia. Neoplasms of the lower urinary tract occur predominantly in the urinary bladder, and are less common in the urethra and are rare in the ureter. They occur most frequently in dogs, occasionally in cats, and rarely in other species, with the exception of bracken fern–induced bladder neoplasms in cattle. Urinary bladder neoplasms comprise less than 2% of total canine neoplasms. Most occur in older dogs, with a higher frequency in females seen in many studies and with certain breeds, including Scottish terrier, Shetland sheepdog, beagle, and collie, at an increased risk. Multiple factors likely play a role in the development of bladder cancer, but specific risks that have been identified in dogs include the following:

- Topical insecticides
- Exposure to marshes sprayed with chemicals for mosquitoes
- Environments with high industrial activity
- Female gender
- Obesity
- Breed (e.g., Scottish terrier)

Retention of urine in the bladder and longer exposure of mucosal epithelium to carcinogens result in a higher incidence of tumors in the urinary bladder compared to other regions of the urinary tract. Many chemicals, including intermediate components of aniline dyes, aromatic hydrocarbons, and tryptophan metabolites, have been found experimentally or epidemiologically to induce urinary bladder neoplasms. Chemically induced and spontaneous epithelial tumors progress through a series of histologic stages from hyperplasia, squamous metaplasia, papilloma, adenoma, dysplasia, and carcinoma in situ to overt carcinoma.

Epithelial Tumors. Approximately 80% of the neoplasms of the lower urinary tract are epithelial in origin and are classified as transitional cell papillomas, transitional cell carcinomas, squamous cell carcinomas, adenocarcinomas, and undifferentiated carcinomas, as follows:

- Papillomas tend to be multiple and may have a pedunculated or sessile appearance. Microscopically, they are composed of well-differentiated transitional epithelium separated from underlying supporting stroma by an intact basement membrane.
- Transitional (urothelial) cell carcinomas are focal, raised nodules or diffuse thickenings of the urinary bladder wall that are most common in the trigone region of the bladder (Fig. 11-60, A). They are composed of pleomorphic to anaplastic transitional epithelium. Neoplastic transitional cells cover the mucosal surface as irregular layers, readily invade the lamina propria in the form of solid nests and acini, and are found within lymphatic

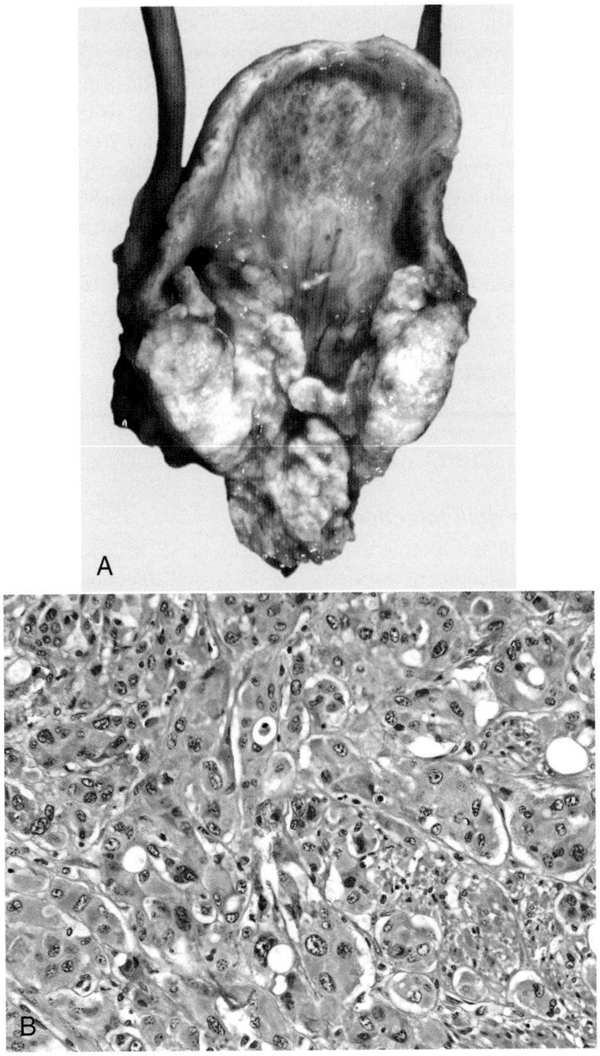

Figure 11-60 **Transitional Cell Carcinoma, Urinary Bladder, Dog. A,** Transitional cell carcinomas are typically adjacent to the trigone (as here), where they can become large enough to obstruct the opening of one or both ureters and result in secondary hydroureter and/or hydronephrosis. **B,** Lamina propria. The tumor is formed by anaplastic cells grouped in small islands and clusters. Nuclei are vesicular with prominent nucleoli, and some nuclei show remarkable anisokaryosis. H&E stain. (**A** courtesy Dr. A. Confer, Center for Veterinary Health Sciences, Oklahoma State University. **B** courtesy Dr. S.J. Newman, College of Veterinary Medicine, University of Tennessee.)

vessels of the submucosal and muscle layers (Fig. 11-60, *B*). Approximately 40% of these neoplasms have metastasized by the time of clinical diagnosis and are present in 50% to 90% of clinically affected dogs at autopsy (syn: necropsy). Lymph nodes and lungs are the most common sites of metastasis; however, more widespread metastasis to other tissues, including bone, is possible. Terriers may be at a slightly elevated risk for transitional carcinoma development, and there has been an association made between occurrence of these tumors and exposure to lawn pesticides. In cats, transitional cell carcinomas are rare but aggressive, and, unlike in dogs, they are more prevalent in males and tend to arise at sites in the bladder distant from the trigone.

- Squamous cell carcinomas and adenocarcinomas comprise a small portion of bladder neoplasms and most likely arise in areas of squamous or glandular metaplasia, respectively. In the bitch, squamous cell carcinomas occur most often in the urethra, which is lined by squamous epithelium in the distal two-thirds. These neoplasms are less likely to metastasize than transitional cell carcinomas. Undifferentiated carcinomas are rare and do not fit into one of the previously mentioned histologic types.

Metastasis of urinary bladder carcinomas is most often first seen in regional lymph nodes adjacent to the aortic bifurcation, including the deep inguinal, medial iliac, and sacral lymph nodes. Other potential sites of metastasis include lungs and kidneys, with metastasis to other parenchymatous organs occurring later.

Mesenchymal Tumors. Mesenchymal tumors, including fibromas, fibrosarcomas, leiomyomas, leiomyosarcomas, rhabdomyosarcomas, lymphomas, hemangiomas, and hemangiosarcomas, comprise fewer than 20% of the neoplasms in the lower urinary tract. Primary fibrosarcomas, leiomyosarcomas, hemangiomas, and hemangiosarcomas are rare. Mesenchymal tumors are classified as follows:

- Leiomyomas arise from smooth muscle of the tunica muscularis and are the most common mesenchymal neoplasms of the lower urinary tract. They may be solitary or multiple and are circumscribed, firm, and pale white to tan masses in the urinary bladder wall. Leiomyomas have the macroscopic consistency and microscopic appearance of normal smooth muscle. Malignant counterparts (leiomyosarcoma) are much rarer, and although they are locally infiltrative, they rarely metastasize.
- Fibromas arise from lamina propria connective tissue and project into the bladder lumen as solitary nodules.
- Lymphoma occasionally infiltrates the wall, not only of the bladder but also of the ureters and renal pelves in cattle, pigs, dogs, and/or cats. Common complications include hydronephrosis and hydroureter.
- Rhabdomyosarcomas are rare but occur in the bladder and urethra of young large breed dogs (younger than age 18 months), suggesting an embryonal origin. The cell of origin is speculated to be embryonic myoblasts from the urogenital ridge. These masses are described as botryoid (grapelike) masses (4 to 18 cm in diameter) that protrude into the bladder lumen. Local invasion and occasional metastasis to lymph nodes characterize the typical behavior. Microscopically, the neoplastic cells form disorganized sheets or lobules in poorly differentiated regions and interlacing streams of fusiform cells in more well-differentiated areas. Microscopic demonstration of cross-striations typical of skeletal muscle or immunohistochemical demonstration of the intermediate filament, desmin, are useful to confirm the diagnosis of rhabdomyosarcoma. Clinical presentation includes hematuria, urinary obstruction, hydroureter, hydronephrosis, and hypertrophic osteopathy.

Disorders of Horses

Embolic Nephritis (Actinobacillus equuli)

Two subspecies of *Actinobacillus equuli* (*A. equuli* subsp. *equuli* and *A. equuli* subsp. *haemolyticus*) are normal inhabitants of the mucous membranes of the alimentary tract. Fecal contamination or extension from oral mucous membranes is the method of inoculation. Umbilical contamination in foals is the most common route of infection resulting in septicemia. Microabscesses occur in a variety of organs, including the liver, adrenal gland, joints, and the kidney, as multifocal random, raised, tan pinpoint foci on the cut surface throughout the renal cortex (see Fig. 11-35, *A* and *B*). Microscopically, glomerular capillaries and to a lesser extent interlobular arterioles contain numerous large bacterial colonies intermixed with necrotic debris and extensive infiltrates of neutrophils that often obliterate the glomerulus (see Fig. 11-35, *C*). If the affected foal survives, the neutrophilic infiltrates will either persist as focal residual abscesses or be progressively replaced by increasing numbers of lymphocytes, plasma cells, macrophages, reactive fibroblasts, and ultimately coalescing scars.

Myoglobinuric Nephrosis (Rhabdomyolysis)

A set of events leading to ischemic tubular necrosis frequently occurs in hypoperfused kidneys complicated by myoglobinuria. In rhabdomyolysis, serum concentrations of myoglobin are increased, as these products pass into the glomerular filtrate, producing greatly increased intraluminal concentrations that cause myoglobinuric nephrosis. Myoglobin does not use a carrier protein for transportation, and because it is a small molecule, it freely passes through the glomerulus and is excreted in the urine. Myoglobin is not nephrotoxic in itself, and intravenous infusions into healthy animals produce no recognizable lesions. However, large concentrations of myoglobin in the glomerular filtrate can increase the tubular necrosis caused by renal ischemia. The mechanism of pigment-induced renal injury is not fully understood, but increased hydroxyl radical formation associated with reduction of ferrous iron compounds and tubular obstruction by myoglobin casts are likely contributing factors.

For example, in equine rhabdomyolysis, renal ischemia is most likely secondary to hypovolemic shock or severe accompanying anemia. Myoglobinuria can have an additive deleterious effect on tubular epithelium already undergoing ischemic necrosis. At autopsy (syn: necropsy), the renal cortices in myoglobinuria are diffusely stained red-brown to blue-black and have intratubular orange-red, refractile myoglobin casts (see Fig. 11-40).

The pathophysiology of this condition is not known; however, exertional rhabdomyolysis is usually the inciting cause. Predisposing and triggering factors are required in this multifactorial disorder, and it typically involves a combination of events, of which exertion is often the main trigger. Possible predisposing factors include carbohydrate overload, local hypoxia, thiamine deficiency, vitamin E and selenium deficiency, metabolic pathway abnormalities, alterations in reproductive hormones, thyroid hormones and cortisol, viruses, electrolyte imbalances, and polysaccharide storage myopathy. Clinical signs tend to occur intermittently during or after exercise and can range from mild to severe. Dark urine occurs when myoglobin level exceeds 40 mg/100 mL. Renal damage may be inconsequential to severe.

Papillary Necrosis

Hypovolemia and dehydration during prolonged or excessive NSAID administration can predispose to papillary necrosis. It is often seen on post-mortem examination in horses with a clinical history of NSAID administration, but rarely does it produce clinical signs.

Necrosis of renal papillae, or in the horse the medullary crest, is a response of the inner medulla to ischemia. Papillary necrosis can be a primary or secondary lesion; however, papillary necrosis occurs as a primary disease in horses treated with NSAIDs. The primary disease occurs quite frequently in horses treated for prolonged periods with phenylbutazone or flunixin meglumine. The medullary interstitial cells are the primary targets for NSAIDs, and interstitial cell damage results in inhibition of cyclooxygenase and decreased prostaglandin synthesis. The resulting reduction in inner medullary blood flow causes ischemia/hypoxia, and it also causes degenerative changes in tubular epithelial cells and ischemic necrosis (infarction) of the medullary crest.

Affected horses also often have ulcers within various areas of the alimentary tract. Usually, clinical cases of NSAID toxicosis present with signs of alimentary tract disease ranging from excessive salivation and inappetence to diarrhea and colic. At autopsy (syn: necropsy), medullary crest necrosis may be present. Acute renal lesions are irregular, discolored areas of necrotic inner medulla sharply delineated from the surviving medullary tissue (see Fig. 11-48). The affected inner medulla is yellow-gray, green, or pink. The cortices may be slightly swollen. With time, the necrotic tissue sloughs, resulting in a detached, friable, and discolored tissue fragment in the pelvis. The remaining inner medulla is usually attenuated and on cross section is narrowed. Overlying cortex can be somewhat shrunken because of atrophy of some of the nephrons caused by blockage of their tubules in the affected medulla.

Patent Urachus

See Kidney and Lower Urinary Tract, Disorders of Domestic Animals, Disorders of the Lower Urinary Tract, Developmental Anomalies, Patent Urachus.

Klossiella equi Infection

Klossiella equi is a sporozoan parasite of the horse, which has various stages of development in the kidney after oral infection. No gross lesions are noted. Various stages of schizogony can be found microscopically in proximal convoluted tubular epithelium and to a lesser extent in glomerular endothelium (Fig. 11-61). Stages of sporogony are present in the epithelial cells of the loop of Henle, but different coccidial stages occur multifocally in affected tubules. Occasionally, however, *Klossiella equi* has been associated with multifocal lesions of mild tubular necrosis and, in the case of tubular rupture, with interstitial infiltrates of lymphocytes and plasma cells. Renal function is typically normal.

Disorders of Ruminants (Cattle, Sheep, and Goats)

Oak Toxicity: Acute Tubular Necrosis (*Quercus* Spp.)

Ruminants develop tubular necrosis after ingestion of leaves, buds, or acorns from oak trees and shrubs (*Quercus* spp.). The toxic substances are metabolites of tannins and include tannic acid, gallic acid, and pyrogallol; however, the mechanism of tubular damage is unknown. Acutely affected cattle often have swollen, pale kidneys that occasionally have cortical petechial hemorrhages (Fig. 11-62). Perirenal edema, which may be hemorrhagic, is a common lesion, and the body cavities contain excessive amounts of a clear fluid. Endothelial cells are a target for the binding of the toxic metabolites, subsequently resulting in vascular leakage. The kidneys are swollen and pale, and they may have fine, often pinpoint hemorrhages on capsular and cortical surfaces. Microscopically, acute proximal tubular necrosis with casts and intratubular hemorrhage are

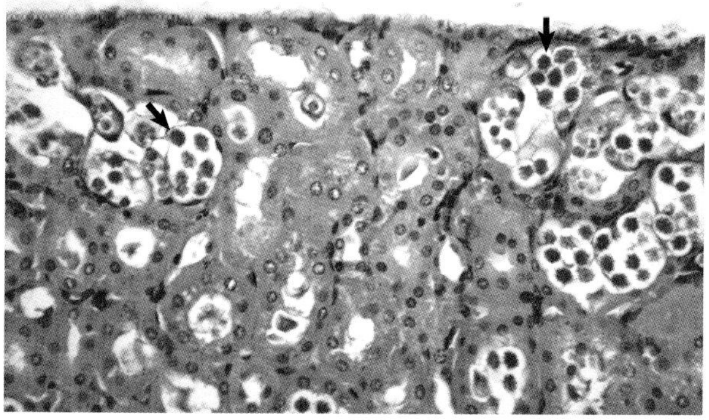

Figure 11-61 ***Klossiella equi* Infection, Kidney, Horse.** Tubular epithelium containing various developmental stages of *Klossiella equi* (*arrows*). H&E stain. (Courtesy Dr. J. Simon, College of Veterinary Medicine, University of Illinois.)

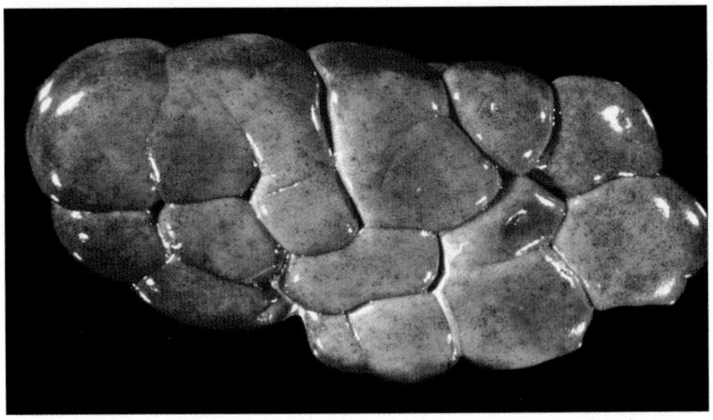

Figure 11-62 **Acute Tubular Necrosis, Oak Toxicity, Kidney, Cow.** Ingestion of leaves, buds, or acorns from oak trees produces cortical petechiation, acute tubular necrosis, and perirenal edema. The toxic principle is a metabolite of oak tannins and causes acute tubular necrosis, which heals by scarring. (Courtesy Dr. K. Read, College of Veterinary Medicine, Texas A&M University; and Noah's Arkive, College of Veterinary Medicine, The University of Georgia.)

characteristic, whereas chronic cases develop chronic interstitial nephritis with the usual changes of fibrosis, atrophy, thinned cortex, and a finely pitted surface.

Pulpy Kidney Disease

Pulpy kidney disease is a unique manifestation of *Clostridium perfringens* type D enterotoxemia in small ruminants, especially sheep. *Clostridium perfringens* epsilon toxin binds to renal tubular epithelial cells and causes selective degeneration of distal tubules. The disease is precipitated by access to excessive starch in the small intestine, which allows for anaerobic bacterial proliferation therein. Hyperglycemia and glucosuria can occasionally be detected. Postmortem interval is critical for assessment of "pulpiness" because these changes resemble autolysis. Classic autopsy (syn: necropsy) lesions are medullary congestion and hemorrhage and also soft to almost liquified (pulpy) cortex (see Fig. 11-42, *A*). Histologic lesions include mild degeneration and necrosis of epithelium of the proximal convoluted tubules with edema, congestion, and interstitial hemorrhage in the renal cortex and congestion of the medulla (see Fig. 11-42, *B*).

Multifocal Lymphoplasmacytic Interstitial Nephritis (Embolic Nephritis; White-Spotted Kidney)

Multifocal interstitial nephritis, or white-spotted kidney, is a well-known example of multifocal lymphoplasmacytic interstitial nephritis in ruminants. It occurs as a result of low-grade, vascular-derived, renal bacterial infection, which likely initially manifested as multiple suppurative foci. In cattle, white-spotted kidneys are seen in calves and are often incidental findings at slaughter or necropsy arising from other systemic causes. *Escherichia coli*, *Salmonella* spp., *Leptospira* spp., and *Brucella* spp. have all been implicated. Usually, by the time the lesion is found, bacteria cannot be cultured from the kidneys. Molecular studies of potential causative microbes of white-spotted kidneys in calves have demonstrated differing findings indicating that the lesion can result from one of several microbes. Lesions can be small to larger, patchy, coalescing areas of pale cortex readily visible from the capsular surface (Fig. 11-63). Histologically, acute lesions, which are rarely seen in cattle, are consistent with neutrophilic embolic nephritis or tubulointerstitial inflammation. Most cases are subacute to chronic and consist of interstitial lymphocytes, plasma cells, and macrophages interspersed with varying numbers of fibroblasts, variable fibrous connective tissue, and atrophic nephron components. Capsular adhesions may be present.

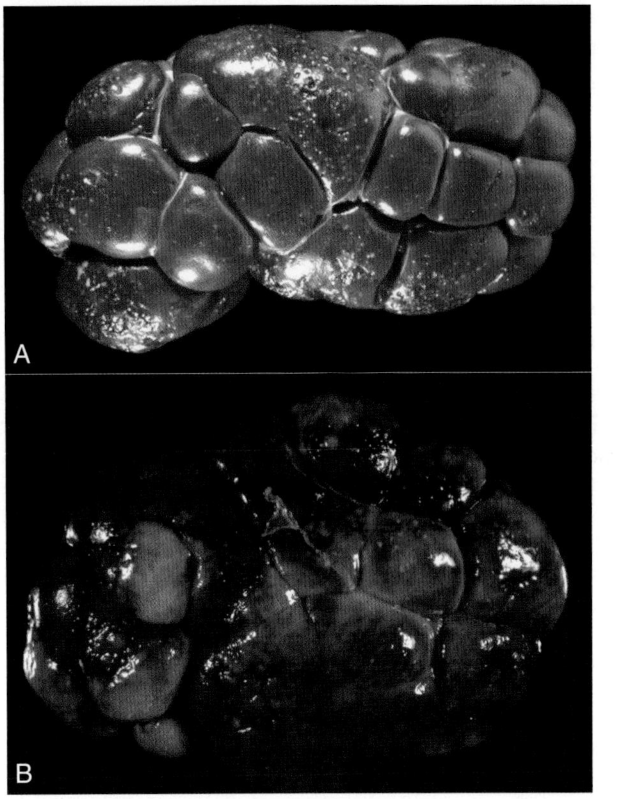

Figure 11-63 **Multifocal Interstitial Nephritis (White-Spotted Kidney).** **A,** Kidney, calf. Multiple pale-yellow to white 2- to 5-mm foci of inflammatory cells (usually neutrophils) are scattered randomly throughout and over the surface of the kidney (as shown here). **B,** Kidney, calf. More severe form of multifocal interstitial nephritis compared to **A**. (**A** courtesy College of Veterinary Medicine, University of Illinois. **B** courtesy Dr. B. Njaa, Center for Veterinary Health Sciences, Oklahoma State University.)

Interstitial Nephritis (Renal Leptospirosis)

In cattle, serovars belonging *to Leptospira interrogans*, *Leptospira kirschneri*, and *Leptospira borgpetersenii* have been associated with carrier status and/or diseases including reproductive failure and abortion, hemolytic anemia and hemoglobinuric nephrosis, and occasionally interstitial nephritis. The pathogenesis of renal leptospirosis was discussed previously as an example of acute bacterial tubulointerstitial nephritis. Although neutrophils can be present in tubular lumina, the predominant chronic lesion is in the interstitium, which becomes infiltrated with monocytes, macrophages, lymphocytes, and plasma cells. Serovars *hardjo*, *pomona*, and *grippotyphosa* are the most commonly implicated in renal infection in cattle. Small ruminants are relatively resistant to infection. Infection with bovine-adapted serovar *hardjo* rarely causes overt dysfunction. Nonadapted serovars create renal lesions from direct damage to the vascular endothelium, hypoxia caused by anemia, tubular epithelial damage from intratubular hemoglobin accumulation, and interstitial nephritis. Lesions range from few to mild interstitial nephritis to diffuse severe lymphocytic interstitial nephritis with fibrosis (see Fig. 11-66).

Chronic interstitial nephritis has mononuclear cell infiltrates, interstitial fibrosis, and generalized tubular atrophy. In the case of exposure to gamma herpesvirus of malignant catarrhal fever, lesions of a chronic interstitial nephritis are characterized by chronic ongoing inflammatory infiltrates composed of lymphocytes and fewer plasma cells within the interstitium accompanied by variable amounts of fibrosis. Occasionally, with this condition, vasculitis can be detected in vessels around which much of the interstitial inflammation occurs and can help differentiate the two microbes.

Hairy Vetch Toxicosis (Vicia Spp.)

Hairy vetch is a legume used throughout regions with extensive farming and can be fed as pasture, hay, or silage. Hairy vetch toxicosis is uncommon and is a unique manifestation of toxic plant ingestion that can result in lesions of eosinophilic and granulomatous inflammation within the kidney, skin, and other viscera. The toxic mechanism is not clearly determined for the visceral disease. It has been postulated that the visceral inflammation is similar to a type IV hypersensitivity reaction and may be caused by plant lectins that serve as haptens (see Chapter 5) or as a complete antigen that sensitizes lymphocytes. Although gross lesions at autopsy (syn: necropsy) can involve multiple organs, the kidney contains multifocal to radiating cortical infiltrates (see Fig. 11-49, *A*). These are often oriented around the vasculature. Histologically, infiltrates are mixed and include monocytes, lymphocytes, plasma cells, multinucleated giant cells, and eosinophils (see Fig. 11-49, *B*). Clinical disease develops several weeks after ingestion of the plant, and dermal manifestation of pruritus is consistently seen concurrently. Mortality can result 10 to 20 days after illness begins, and older Holstein or Angus cattle breeds are the most susceptible. Diagnosis is often made by exclusion.

Pyelonephritis

In cattle, numerous bacteria cause cystitis and pyelonephritis, including *Escherichia coli* and *Trueperella pyogenes*. In addition, *Corynebacterium renale* is an obligate urinary mucosal organism and a potential pathogen in bovine cases because this organism has pili to accommodate mucosal adhesion and to resist shedding from the lower urinary tract. Furthermore, the bacterium produces a urease that hydrolyzes urea, releasing ammonia that causes localized epithelial damage and increased urine pH.

Acute pyelonephritis is uncommon in cattle and often seen as an incidental finding at autopsy (syn: necropsy) (see Fig. 11-46). Subacute to chronic bovine pyelonephritis is a slowly progressive suppurative tubulointerstitial nephritis. The pelvis and calyces are dilated with fluid ranging from turbid urine containing fibrinopurulent clumps to a completely purulent exudate. Bacteria localize in the medulla, and inflammation and medullary necrosis can be so severe that only a thin rim of cortex remains. More commonly, radially distributed interstitial infiltrates with or without fibrosis are present (see Fig. 11-47). As fibrosis progresses, there is contraction of scars that extend from the cortical surface throughout the medulla to the level of the pelvis.

Renal Lymphoma (Lymphosarcoma)

Renal lymphoma can occur in cattle and is one of the most common bovine tumors; however, involvement of the kidney is not as common as it is in feline lymphoma. The cause is bovine leukosis virus (BLV), a retrovirus known to be spread by blood contact between animals. Gross lesions may be seen as diffuse renomegaly or more commonly as multiple poorly defined tan, soft, raised cortical nodules (see Fig. 11-52, *E* and *F*). Peripelvic and periureteral infiltrates are common in cattle and can produce concurrent hydronephrosis. Focal or diffuse infiltrates of neoplastic lymphocytes efface interstitium and/or tubules.

Urolithiasis

In cattle, uroliths result in obstruction most frequently in bulls and castrated males (steers). The urethra narrows in the region of the sigmoid flexure, which is the most commonly affected site. The obstruction can be caused by a large discrete mineral aggregate (urolith) or by accumulation of fine sandlike material within the urethral lumen. Hemorrhage and necrosis of the urethral mucosa typically occurs at the site of urolith lodgment. In more severe cases, leading to subsequent urethral rupture, there can be subcutaneous accumulation of urine in the inguinal area, prepuce, and ventral abdomen (commonly referred to as "water belly").

Silica calculi (75% silica dioxide) are a problem for sheep and cattle grazing native rangeland grasses of western North America. Certain grasses contain as much as 4% to 5% silica; most of the silica is insoluble, except that which is in the cell sap (unpolymerized silicic acid). After absorption, silica is returned to the gut in digestive secretions, such that less than 1% of dietary silica is excreted in urine and up to 60% is resorbed from the filtrate. However, when the volume of urine production is very low, the concentration of silicic acid excretion in urine may reach five times the saturation concentration and precipitation from solution occurs in the presence of proteins or other substances in the urine. Silica calculi are hard, white to dark-brown, radiopaque, often laminated, up to 1-cm-diameter stones and are a major cause of urinary tract obstruction. Silica calculus formation may be reduced to subclinical levels by adding salt to the ration to ensure high water consumption, acidifying the diet, or reducing the dietary calcium to phosphorus ratio.

Struvite calculi are white to gray, chalky, usually smooth, and easily broken. This type of calculus usually forms a gritty sludge within a proteinaceous matrix and develops in feedlot ruminants on cereal-grain rations, particularly those that are pelleted and high in phosphorus. Reduction of the dietary calcium to phosphorus ratio as well as a balance of magnesium, sodium, and potassium in the ration are important in preventing urolith formation.

See the section on Kidney and Lower Urinary Tract, Disorders of Domestic Animals for illustrations.

Enzootic Hematuria

Information on this topic is available at www.expertconsult.com.

Bracken Fern–Induced Neoplasia

Information on this topic is available at www.expertconsult.com.

Amyloidosis

Amyloidosis is a sporadic protein-losing nephropathy of cattle. Chronic diarrhea, poor productivity, and weight loss are common. Amyloid is classified as AA type, which is associated with chronic inflammation, and such conditions are often seen concurrently. AA fibrils are created through abnormal catabolism of serum amyloid A (SAA). On gross examination, kidneys are yellow tan and appear waxy on cut section. Histologic deposition of amyloid occurs in the glomerulus, interstitium, and tubular lumens.

Disorders of Pigs

Glomerulonephritis of Pigs

Although an uncommon entity in pigs, glomerulonephritis (GN) is seen as a sequel to chronic infections with hog cholera, African swine fever, systemic cytomegalovirus, and group A streptococcal abscesses. In addition, inherited forms of membranoproliferative GN in Yorkshire pigs are due to an autosomal recessive deficiency of the complement inhibitory protein factor H. GN and systemic vasculitis can be observed in porcine circovirus 2 infection manifested as porcine dermatitis and nephropathy syndrome. In acute GN, grossly, there is enlargement, pallor, edema, and cortical petechiation of the kidney. Eventually, this process progresses to granular cortical infiltrates and the kidney may appear shrunken and contracted due to cortical fibrosis. Kidney lesions in the acute form of this syndrome are fibrinonecrotizing GN with lymphoplasmacytic tubulointerstitial nephritis and/or granulomatous interstitial nephritis. With prolonged disease, chronic glomerulonephritis may develop. It is thought that this response is an immune-mediated (type III) hypersensitivity response to circovirus and possibly concurrent PRRS viral infection.

Toxic Nephritis

Ingestion of several species of pigweed may cause acute renal failure in pigs. Gross lesions include marked perirenal edema and blood-tinged serous effusions elsewhere in the body. Histologically, swelling and necrosis of the lining epithelial cells, the presence of casts, dilated tubules, and mild interstitial edema are characteristic.

Leptospirosis

Host-adapted *Leptospira* serovars *pomona*, *tarassovi*, and *australis* cause significant disease in pigs. Preferential localization of the organism occurs in the renal proximal tubules and passage to the interstitium results in multifocal interstitial nephritis, similar to that seen in cattle and dogs. Grossly, poorly circumscribed white foci of various shapes and sizes that correspond to infiltrates of lymphocytes, plasma cells, and macrophages in the interstitial tissues are present. In addition, in chronic cases, concurrent interstitial fibrosis occurs.

Urolithiasis

Pigs most commonly have calcium carbonate uroliths formed by calcium phosphate or calcium oxalate. Struvite uroliths occur less frequently. As with other species, obstructive disease and/or rupture can occur at sites of lodgment, which is most commonly seen in castrated males. Neonatal piglets with low nutrient intake after birth may develop uric acid or urate crystals in the kidneys, ureters, and/or urinary bladder as a result of increased purine catabolism.

See the section on Kidney and Lower Urinary Tract, Disorders of Domestic Animals for illustrations.

Kidney Worm

In North America, the kidney worm (*Stephanurus dentatus*) is found most often in adult pigs in southern regions of the United States. The parasite is also a problem in other countries with warm climates. *Stephanurus dentatus* is a strongyloid worm that migrates to the kidney after cycling through the liver. Adult worms normally encyst in perirenal fat; however, some parasites may reside in the kidney. Peripelvic cysts often communicate with the renal pelvis and ureter, and fibrosis and chronic granulation tissue can enclose the parasite. Occasionally, shed nematode eggs are present in the urine sediment.

Erysipelothrix

Erysipelothrix rhusiopathiae is the most common bacterial cause of embolic nephritis in pigs, which can be a renal manifestation of classical diamond skin disease. The organism may spread to the kidney after cutaneous involvement or much more commonly because of bacteremia related to the development of septic valvular endocarditis. Grossly, the disease presents as either glomerular hemorrhages seen as multifocal regions of pinpoint hemorrhage throughout the renal cortex or as multiple foci of tan to white inflammatory infiltrates within the renal interstitium (Fig. 11-64). Histologically, the change described in the former situation is characteristic of septic embolic GN with fibrin and neutrophil aggregates noted within glomerular capillary tufts or as small abscesses within the interstitium.

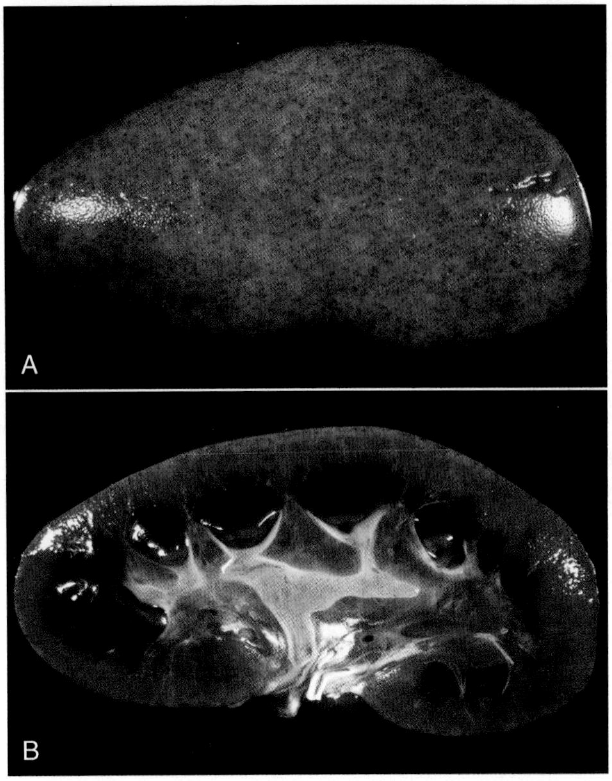

Figure 11-64 Bacterial-Induced Septicemic Renal Cortical Hemorrhages, Erysipelas, Kidney, Pig. A, Petechial hemorrhages caused by septic emboli of *Erysipelothrix rhusiopathiae* are randomly scattered over the capsular surface of the kidney. **B,** Dorsal section. Similar petechiae are present on the cut surface of the renal cortex. (Courtesy Dr. M.D. McGavin, College of Veterinary Medicine, University of Tennessee.)

Disorders of Dogs

Greyhound Vasculopathy

An idiopathic renal glomerular and cutaneous vasculopathy, formerly known as *Alabama rot*, occurs in greyhounds in the United States and the United Kingdom and is a potentially fatal disease of unknown etiology. As the name suggests, it typically affects the skin and kidneys of racing- and training-age greyhounds. Typically, there are multifocal erythematous and/or ulcerated skin lesions, commonly accompanied by distal limb edema as the result of a similar cutaneous vasculitis, with concurrent thrombocytopenia and acute renal insufficiency. The cause of the disease is unknown, but renal lesions are similar to those seen in acute DIC, thrombotic thrombocytopenic purpura, and hemolytic uremic syndrome in human beings. Grossly, kidneys from affected dogs are swollen and congested and show cortical petechiae (see Fig. 11-37, *A*). Microscopically, numerous glomeruli have segmental or global fibrinous thrombi, hemorrhage, and necrosis (see Fig. 11-37, *B*). At the glomerular vascular pole, the walls of afferent arterioles have fibrin deposits and foci of necrosis. In addition, electron microscopy findings indicate that glomerular endothelial damage is an important early event in the pathogenesis of this condition.

Ethylene Glycol Intoxication

Ethylene glycol (antifreeze) ingestion is one of the most common causes of intoxication and acute tubular necrosis in dogs, cats, and occasionally pigs. Ethylene glycol, the major constituent of antifreeze, is readily absorbed from the gastrointestinal tract, and a small percentage is oxidized by hepatic alcohol dehydrogenase to the toxic metabolites glycolaldehyde, glycolic acid, glyoxylate, and oxalate. Ethylene glycol and its toxic metabolic products are filtered by the glomeruli, and acute tubular necrosis is caused by the direct interaction of these toxic metabolites, especially glycolic acid, on tubular epithelium (Fig. 11-65, *A* and *B*). Of particular significance is that large numbers of pale yellow foci of calcium oxalate crystals precipitate in renal tubular lumens, tubular epithelial cells, and the interstitium (Fig. 11-65, *C*). These crystals cause intrarenal obstruction with degeneration and necrosis of tubular epithelium that is postulated to be the direct effect of mechanical damage. With polarized light, the microscopic image is one of large numbers of birefringent, round to pyramidal crystals arranged in rosettes or sheaves within renal tubules, and they are virtually pathognomonic for ethylene glycol ingestion in dogs and cats (Fig. 11-65, *D*).

Acute Tubular Necrosis (Aminoglycosides)

Aminoglycoside antimicrobials, such as gentamicin, neomycin, kanamycin, tobramycin, amikacin, and streptomycin, are nephrotoxic. Relative renal toxicity varies among the different aminoglycoside drugs and correlates with the concentration of the compound in the renal cortex. Neomycin, which is highly nephrotoxic, concentrates to the greatest extent in the renal cortex, whereas streptomycin, the least nephrotoxic, does not concentrate appreciably in the renal cortex. Although gentamicin is intermediate in its nephrotoxicity between neomycin and streptomycin, tubular damage from gentamicin occurs with some frequency because it is a commonly used drug in veterinary medicine.

The susceptibility of animal species to the nephrotoxic effects of these drugs is variable and is related to differences in susceptibility of renal tubules and differences in the rate of excretion or inactivation of the drug among animal species. Aminoglycosides become concentrated in lysosomes, and their toxic effects occur after release of large concentrations of the drugs from these organelles. Toxic concentrations of aminoglycosides produce the following changes:

- Become concentrated in lysosomes
- Subsequently escape from lysosomes to accumulate in the cytoplasm
- Alter tubular cell membrane transport by the inhibition of Na^+/K^+-ATPase, causing an intracellular influx of hydrogen, sodium ions, and water
- Inhibit phospholipase activity so that phospholipids accumulate intracellularly
- Alter mitochondrial function
- Inhibit protein synthesis

These biochemical changes are responsible for the lesions of acute swelling of proximal tubular epithelial cells, mitochondrial swelling, rupture of lysosomes, dilation of endoplasmic reticulum, shedding of the tubular brush border, and cellular death.

Leptospirosis

Dogs are susceptible to several serovars of *Leptospira* spp. Leptospires enter the body through breaches in the mucous membranes, multiply and spread to the kidney, where they persist in the renal tubular cells. Affected dogs may exhibit fever, anorexia, vomiting,

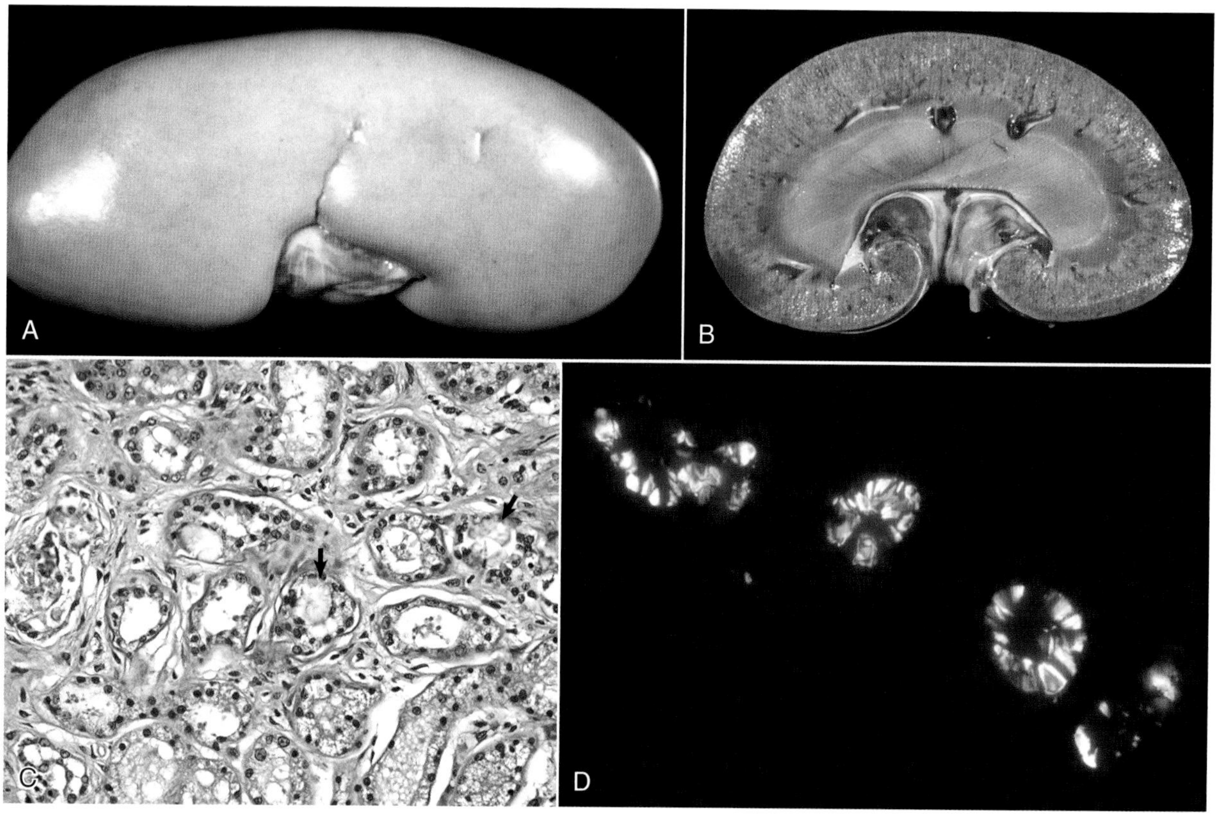

Figure 11-65 **Oxalate Nephrosis, Kidney. A,** Pig. Oxalate nephrosis following ingestion of oxalate-containing plants. The kidney is diffusely pale beige and swollen. **B,** Dorsal section, dog. The cortex is beige and finely mottled due to the deposition of multiple small foci of oxalate crystals in the renal tubules. **C,** Dog. Tubular dilation, necrosis, and early regeneration (increased numbers of epithelial cells lining several tubules). Numerous tubules contain oxalate crystals *(arrows)*, which have dilated the tubules and compressed their epithelium. H&E stain. **D,** Cat. Birefringent radiating sheaves of calcium oxalate crystals in renal tubules. Polarized light. H&E stain. (**A** and **B** courtesy Dr. M.D. McGavin, College of Veterinary Medicine, University of Tennessee. **C** courtesy Dr. S.J. Newman, College of Veterinary Medicine, University of Tennessee. **D** courtesy Dr. J.F. Zachary, College of Veterinary Medicine, University of Illinois.)

dehydration, icterus, muscle pain, and evidence of coagulopathy. In the more chronic infections, fever, anterior uveitis, anorexia, and weight loss are noted. Grossly, multifocal, coalescing inflammatory infiltrates that extend from the cortical medullary junction to the capsular surface are present (Fig. 11-66, *A*). In the more acute stages, in which tubular damage is prominent, there will be neutrophilic infiltrates, but this rapidly changes to lymphocytes and plasma cells (Fig. 11-66, *B*). In more chronic cases, variable amounts of fibrosis and subcapsular scarring occur (Fig. 11-14, *D*). Leptospires may often be identified within the cytoplasm and the lumen of affected tubules when special silver stains or immunohistochemistry are used (Fig. 11-66, *C*).

Infectious Canine Hepatitis

Transient glomerulitis, caused by a direct viral insult to the glomerulus, occurs in acute systemic viral diseases such as acute infectious canine hepatitis. The lesions are mild, usually transient, and result from viral replication in capillary endothelium. Acute viral GN produces the following gross lesions:

- Kidneys are often slightly swollen.
- Renal capsular surface is smooth.
- Kidneys are normal color or pale.
- Glomeruli are visible as pinpoint red dots on the cut surface of the cortex.

Viral-induced intranuclear inclusions are present in glomerular capillary endothelium in cases of infectious canine hepatitis. The inclusions are usually large, basophilic to magenta, and either fill the nucleus or are separated from the nuclear membrane by a clear halo. In cases of viral glomerulitis, lesions include endothelial hypertrophy, hemorrhages, necrosis of endothelium, and a thickened and edematous mesangium. Clinically, animals are systemically ill from the viral infection, but the glomerular signs are specifically those of a transient proteinuria. In addition, in dogs recovering from acute infectious canine hepatitis, lesions of lymphoplasmacytic interstitial nephritis can occur.

Canine Herpesvirus

In puppies younger than 3 to 5 weeks of age, intrauterine or neonatal infections can occur with pathognomonic kidney lesions consisting of petechial and ecchymotic hemorrhages. Typically, there is acute tubular necrosis with hemorrhage and the presence of intraepithelial intranuclear eosinophilic to amphophilic inclusions (Fig. 11-67). Once the puppies are older, typically more than 6 weeks of age, herpesvirus infections fail to induce renal lesions.

Pyelonephritis

Dogs with acute pyelonephritis can exhibit fever, depression, arched back from lumbar or renal pain, polydipsia, and polyuria. The most common causes of bacterial pyelonephritis in order of frequency include infection with *Escherichia coli*, *Staphylococcus aureus*, *Proteus mirabilis*, *Streptococcus* sp., *Klebsiella pneumoniae*, *Pseudomonas aeruginosa*, and *Enterobacter* sp. For the most part, these organisms take advantage of altered lower urinary tract defense mechanisms and ascend from the lower urinary tract to colonize the renal pelvis. Grossly, there can be accumulation of suppurative exudate in the pelvis with variable extension of tan cellular infiltrates from the medulla to variable portions of the overlying cortex (see Fig. 11-46, *A* and *B*). Histologically, there is tubular necrosis and loss with extension of bacterial colonies and variable amounts of neutrophils within tubules and the interstitium (see Fig. 11-46, *C*). In the more chronic forms, neutrophil numbers are reduced and lymphocytes and plasma cells predominate.

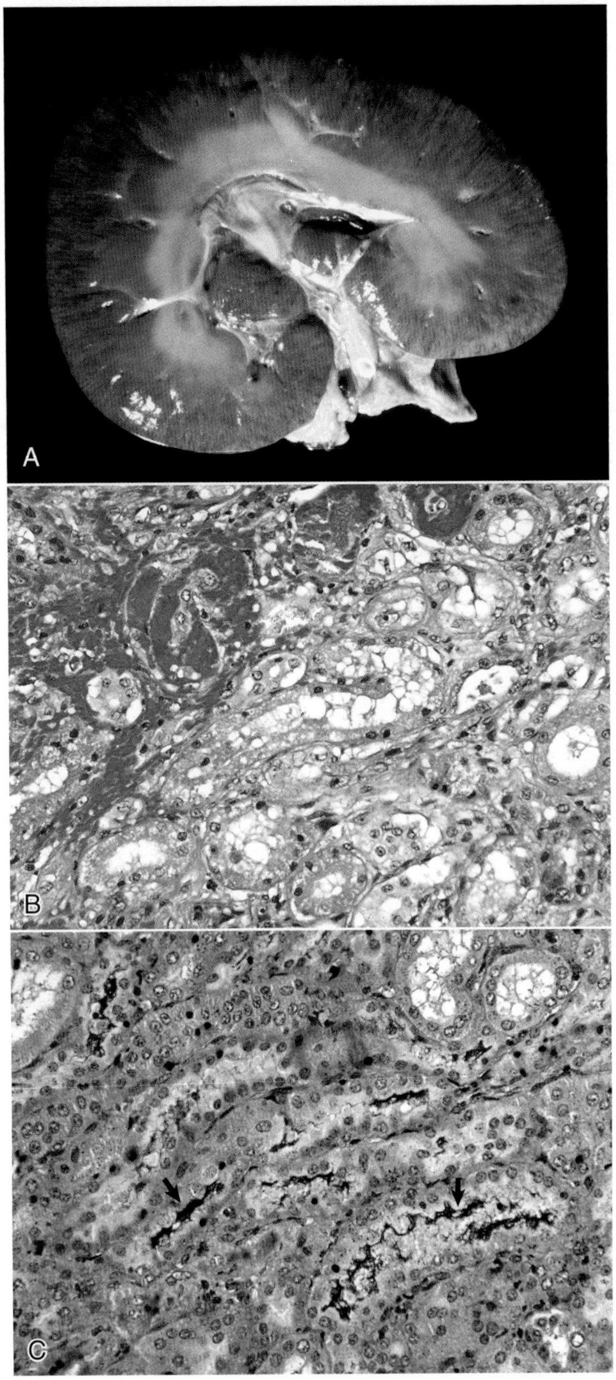

Figure 11-66 Acute Leptospirosis, Kidney. A, Interstitial nephritis, acute leptospira infection, dorsal section, dog. Radiating pale streaks are caused by cortical tubular necrosis and acute interstitial inflammatory infiltrates. The hilar fat and medulla are yellow from jaundice. **B,** Acute tubular necrosis, early regeneration, dog. Note the segments of tubular epithelium devoid of nuclei (coagulation necrosis) *(top left)* and the hemorrhage. At this early stage, there is an almost complete lack of inflammatory cells in the interstitium, but later in the subacute stage of leptospirosis there are interstitial infiltrates of lymphocytes and plasma cells, which tend to be near the corticomedullary junction. H&E stain. **C,** Leptospira, cow. Numerous leptospira *(arrows)* are present in the lumens of tubules. Leptospira colonization of tubule epithelial cells is typical of this bacterium. Warthin Starry silver stain. (**A** and **C** courtesy Dr. M.D. McGavin, College of Veterinary Medicine, University of Tennessee. **B** courtesy Dr. S.J. Newman, College of Veterinary Medicine, University of Tennessee.)

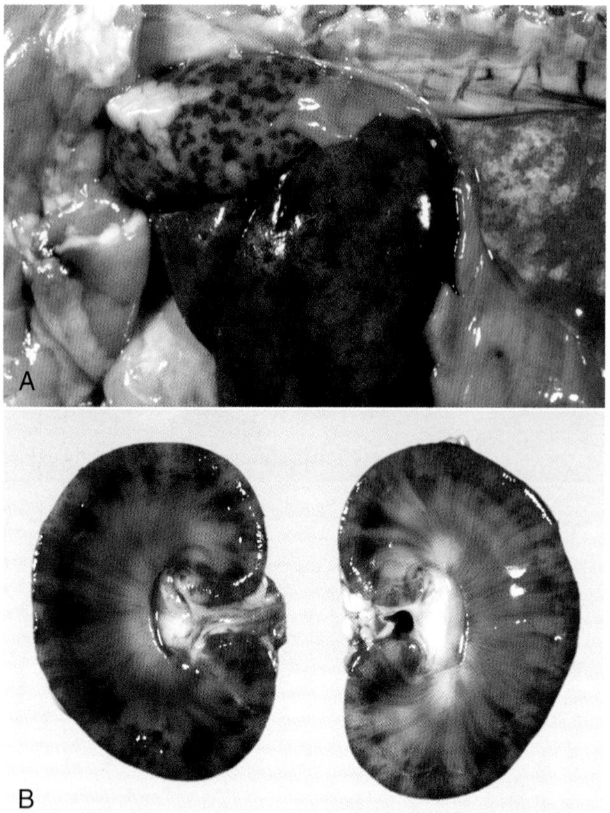

Figure 11-67 **Canine Herpesvirus Nephritis (Canine Herpesvirus Type I), Kidney, Neonatal Puppy. A,** Abdominal viscera. Multifocal renal cortical hemorrhages are grossly characteristic of this disease. **B,** Dorsal sections. Multifocal cortical hemorrhages are due to viral-induced vasculitis with necrosis and secondary hemorrhage. (Courtesy Dr. M.D. McGavin, College of Veterinary Medicine, University of Tennessee.)

Box 11-11 Breeds of Dogs with Progressive Juvenile Nephropathy

- American cocker spaniels
- English cocker spaniels
- Norwegian elkhounds
- Samoyeds
- Doberman pinschers
- Lhasa apsos
- Shih tzus
- Soft-coated Wheaten terriers
- Bull terriers
- Standard poodles
- Alaskan malamutes
- Miniature schnauzers
- German shepherds
- Keeshounds
- Chow Chows
- Weimaraners
- Golden retrievers

Progressive Juvenile Nephropathy

The development of severe bilateral renal fibrosis has been described in young dogs of several breeds and referred to as *progressive juvenile nephropathy* or *familial (hereditary) renal disease*. In many dog breeds, a familial tendency is demonstrated (Box 11-11), but the mode of inheritance has been determined with certainty in only a few dog breeds. In Samoyeds, the lesion is x-linked; in bull terriers, it is autosomal dominant; and in the shih tzu, French mastiff, and English cocker spaniel, the disease appears to have a simple autosomal recessive inheritance.

Progressive juvenile nephropathy is a syndrome in which the morphologic manifestations can be the result of any of several chronic pathologic processes. The main manifestations include the following:

- Type IV collagen defect in the glomerular basement membrane
- Membranoproliferative GN
- Tubular disease of unknown cause with tubular atrophy and interstitial fibrosis
- Renal dysplasia

Gross renal lesions of progressive juvenile nephropathy are variable among affected breeds and among affected dogs within a breed. Generally, kidneys are notably shrunken, pale tan to white, and firm (see Fig. 11-26, *C* and *D*). The renal surface can be diffusely pitted and have a fine granular pattern, particularly in those dogs in which glomerular disease is the primary event. In addition, numerous small cortical cysts may be seen due to dilation of Bowman's capsule and glomerular atrophy. In cases of juvenile nephropathy that are tubular or dysplastic, the renal surface can have patchy, deeply depressed areas of cortical scarring. On the cut surface, the cortex is thin and has linear radial scars. The medulla is usually diffusely fibrotic. Small (1 to 2 mm), variably sized cysts are seen often in the cortex and the medulla.

In the Doberman pinscher, the primary lesion is a glomerulopathy that appears microscopically as a membranoproliferative GN. Later in the clinical course of the disease, the lesions include extensive periglomerular fibrosis, tubular atrophy, and cystic dilation of Bowman's (urinary) space and tubules. In affected Samoyeds and English cocker spaniels, multilamellar splitting of the GBM is caused by inherited abnormalities in basement membrane type IV collagen. These lesions progress to severe glomerulosclerosis.

In Norwegian elkhounds, a tubular disorder of unknown cause has been described and is characterized by progressive tubular atrophy, periglomerular and interstitial fibrosis, and glomerulosclerosis without any indication of a primary glomerular disease.

Progressive juvenile nephropathy has been described in Lhasa apsos, shih tzus, soft-coated Wheaten terriers, Standard poodles, and golden retrievers as a condition resembling renal dysplasia, defined as an abnormality of renal development as a result of anomalous differentiation. Small, shrunken, fetal-like glomeruli composed of small cells with dense nuclei, minimal mesangial tissue, and nonpatent capillaries can be seen interspersed with normal, sclerotic, or hypertrophied glomeruli. Other lesions include marked interstitial fibrosis and tubular dilation. Most of the kidneys have minimal lymphoplasmacellular interstitial cell infiltrates.

Juvenile nephropathy in boxer dogs is characterized by pericapsular and interstitial fibrosis, inflammatory cell infiltration, dilated tubules, sclerotic glomeruli, and dystrophic calcification.

Although variations exist in gross and microscopic lesions (see Fig. 11-26, *E*), as well as in the pathogenesis of progressive nephropathy among the different breeds, a typical case is a dog 4 months to 2 years of age that has polyuria, polydipsia, and uremia. The clinical presentation, gross lesions, and microscopic changes are identical to those of chronic renal disease and renal fibrosis in mature or aging dogs.

Renal Carcinoma

Renal carcinomas are the most common primary renal neoplasms and occur most frequently in older dogs at an incidence of 1.5 in 100,000. The specific causes of renal carcinomas in human beings are well determined compared with those in animal species, and little is specifically known about the pathogenesis of this entity in dogs. These renal neoplasms are usually large (up to 20 cm in diameter), spherical to oval, and firm. They often are pale yellow and contain dark areas of hemorrhage and necrosis and foci of cystic degeneration. The masses usually occupy and obliterate one pole of the kidney and grow by expansion, compressing the adjacent normal renal tissue (see Fig. 11-51). Histologic types include papillary, tubular, and solid (see Fig. 11-51, C), with tubular variants being the most common and solid variants being the most poorly differentiated. Metastasis to the lungs, lymph nodes, liver, and adrenal glands occurs frequently. Renal carcinoma has been associated with paraneoplastic conditions, principally polycythemia. This is because of concurrent overexpression of erythropoietin, which increases bone marrow production of red blood cells.

A variant of the typical renal carcinoma has been seen in German shepherd dogs in conjunction with nodular dermatofibrosis that is inherited as an autosomal dominant trait. The lesions are hereditary and consist of multifocal, bilateral, renal cystadenomas or cystadenocarcinomas. Grossly, these resemble the carcinomas described previously, but cysts are much more prominent. The neoplastic cells form solid sheets, tubules, or papillary growth patterns, and the cells in the carcinomas are more atypical and anaplastic. Cells vary in shape from cuboidal and columnar to polyhedral, vary in size, and have clear or granular eosinophilic cytoplasm. Nuclei range from small, round, granular, and uniform to large, oval, vesicular, and pleomorphic. Mitotic figures are numerous. These neoplasms have a moderate fibrovascular stroma.

Urolithiasis

See the section on Kidney and Lower Urinary Tract, Disorders of Domestic Animals for illustrations and a general discussion of urolithiasis.

Struvite Calculi

Information on this topic is available at www.expertconsult.com.

Calcium Oxalate Calculi

Information on this topic is available at www.expertconsult.com.

Uric Acid and Urate Calculi

Information on this topic is available at www.expertconsult.com.

Xanthine Calculi

Information on this topic is available at www.expertconsult.com.

Cystine Calculi

Information on this topic is available at www.expertconsult.com.

Chronic Cystitis

Several manifestations of chronic cystitis exist in dogs and include those with prominent follicular lymphoid proliferation in the submucosa (follicular cystitis) and those with prominent polypoid epithelial change (polypoid cystitis). Follicular cystitis (see Fig. 11-58) has a grossly recognized cobblestone appearance as a result of the presence of multifocal, disseminated, nodular, submucosal lymphoid proliferations (1 to 3 mm in diameter). This form of cystitis is particularly common in response to chronic urolithiasis. A red zone of hyperemia often surrounds these white-gray lymphoid foci. Microscopically, these raised foci are aggregates of lymphocytic cells in the superficial lamina propria. Epithelium overlying these foci may be normal or ulcerated and may be accompanied by fibrosis in the lamina propria. Hypertrophy of the tunica muscularis may also be present.

Polypoid masses (chronic polypoid cystitis), seen predominantly in dogs, typically develop from inflammatory and hyperplastic responses secondary to chronic irritation, which most often arise from persistent bacterial urinary tract infection or uroliths. The polyps arising in the bladder mucosa are composed of a core of proliferative connective tissue covered by surface epithelium. Mononuclear inflammatory cells are often present within the connective tissue core. Surface epithelium may form nests of hyperplastic transitional epithelial cells in the lamina propria (Brunn's nests) or undergo metaplasia to a mucus-secreting, glandular epithelial type (cystitis glandularis). The resulting polypoid masses, which are composed of inflammation, fibroplasia, and epithelial proliferation, occur most frequently in the cranioventral bladder wall (see Fig. 11-59). The masses may be broad-based or pedunculated, ulcerated, or covered by hyperplastic epithelium with goblet cell metaplasia. Chronic polypoid cystitis is often accompanied by clinically evident hematuria.

Transitional Cell Carcinoma

Transitional cell carcinomas are focal, raised nodules or diffuse thickenings of the urinary bladder wall, most common in the trigone region of the bladder (see Fig. 11-60, A). They are composed of pleomorphic to anaplastic transitional epithelium. Neoplastic transitional cells cover the mucosal surface as irregular layers, readily invade the lamina propria in the form of solid nests and acini, and are found within lymphatic vessels of the submucosa and muscle layers (see Fig. 11-60, *B*). Approximately 40% of these neoplasms have metastasized by the time of clinical diagnosis and are present in 50% to 90% of affected dogs at autopsy (syn: necropsy). Lymph nodes and lungs are the most common sites of metastasis; however, more widespread metastasis to other tissues, including bone, is possible. Terriers may be at a slightly elevated risk for transitional cell carcinoma development, and an association has been made between occurrence of these tumors and exposure to lawn pesticides.

Toxic Tubulointerstitial Nephritis

Melamine and Cyanuric Acid. Relatively recently, pet food contaminated with melamine and cyanuric acid to artificially elevate the dietary protein content produced large-scale outbreaks of renal failure–related mortality in dogs and cats in the United States and Korea. Sick animals had inappetence, vomiting, polyuria, polydipsia, and lethargy. Azotemia was recorded in many affected animals. The unique aspects of this food toxicity outbreak included necrosis that was localized to the distal rather than the proximal tubules. Unique intratubular rough and irregular brown birefringent crystals were noted in the more distal tubular portions of the nephron, and these may have been mistaken for oxalates in some early cases. In contrast, these crystals failed to stain with von Kossa calcium stains or alizarin Red S. A combination of both melamine and cyanuric acid was required to produce the ultimate renal failure in these cases.

Grape Ingestion

Ingestion of grapes or raisins as part of the diet or inadvertently by dogs can lead to a syndrome of acute renal failure and uremia accompanied by vomiting, lethargy, anorexia, and diarrhea. The mechanism for induction of acute proximal renal tubular necrosis is unclear, but tannins, similar to those in oak poisoning, are implicated as a toxic principle in these cases. The gross changes are those of an enlarged pale tan bulging kidney, and the histologic changes are not characteristic but are represented by acute proximal tubular necrosis.

Parasites

The giant kidney worm (*Dioctophyma renale*) is seen infrequently in dogs from temperate and cold countries worldwide. It is endemic in Canada and in northern regions of the United States. Because of a prolonged and complex life cycle, this nematode is seen only in dogs 2 years old or older. The adult nematode is red and cylindric; the females measure 20 to 100 cm long and 4 to 12 mm in diameter, and the males measure 14 to 45 cm long and 4 to 6 mm in diameter. This nematode resides in the renal pelvis where it causes severe hemorrhagic or purulent pyelitis, subsequent ureteral obstruction, and destruction of the renal parenchyma, resulting in a hydronephrotic kidney that appears as a cyst containing the nematode and purulent exudate.

Capillaria plica and *Capillaria feliscati* have been identified infrequently in dogs and cats worldwide. Typically, these nematodes are attached to the renal pelvis, ureter, or bladder of animals of various ages. Microscopically, inflammatory cells infiltrate and focal hemorrhages are associated with sites of attachment in the underlying submucosa. Clinical effects usually are not present, but hematuria and dysuria are produced occasionally.

Disorders of Cats

Granulomatous Nephritis

Cats with feline infectious peritonitis (FIP), particularly the noneffusive (dry) form, often have multifocal pyogranulomatous nephritis, secondary to severe primary vasculitis. The FIP virus is a mutated strain of feline enteric coronavirus that has lost its predilection for enterocytes and replicates in macrophages. The pathogenesis of the granulomatous form of FIP may be a cell-mediated immune response to the FIP virus that is partially effective in containing the virus to a relatively small number of macrophages at focal sites. The immune response causes a granulomatous necrotizing vasculitis and development of renal interstitial pyogranulomas characterized grossly by multiple, large, irregular, and pale gray subcapsular cortical foci (Fig. 11-68, *A*) that are firm and granular on cut surface (Fig. 11-68, *B*). These lesions are somewhat circumscribed and bulge from the capsular surface. They may be misinterpreted as neoplastic infiltrates, such as those associated with renal lymphoma or metastatic neoplasms, which tend not to have such a vascular orientation to the infiltrates. Microscopically, extensive accumulations of macrophages interspersed with lymphocytes, plasma cells, and neutrophils (pyogranulomas) surround foci of necrotizing fibrinoid vasculitis.

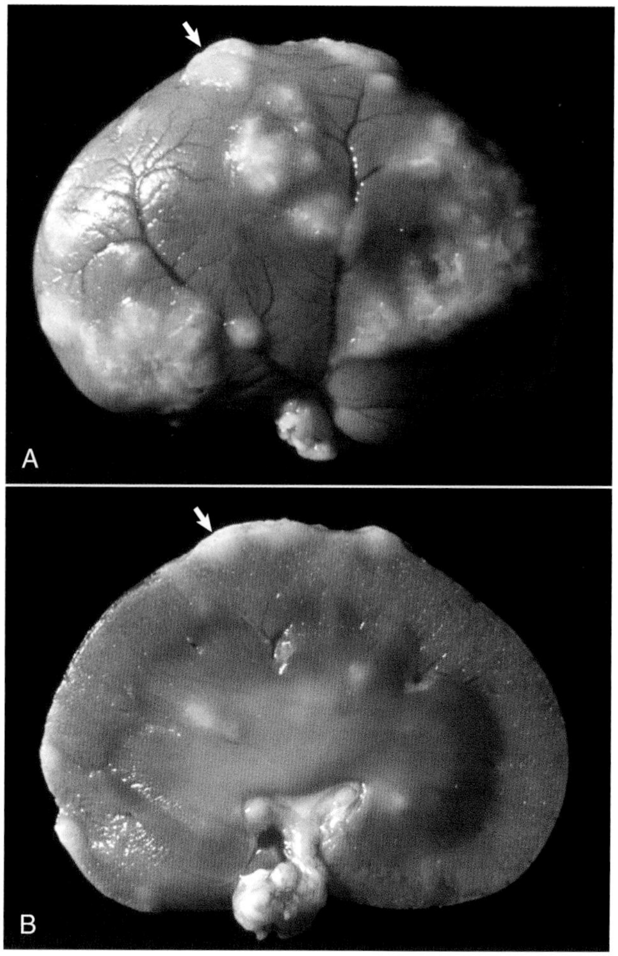

Figure 11-68 **Granulomatous Nephritis, Feline Infectious Peritonitis, Kidney, Cat. A,** Lesions are typical of the noneffusive (dry) form of feline infectious peritonitis. There are multifocal, coalescing white to gray granulomas *(arrow)*, which can be confused with the nodular form of lymphoma (lymphosarcoma), thus warranting histologic examination. **B,** Dorsal section. Multifocal, coalescing white to gray granulomas extend into the cortical parenchyma *(arrow)*. The pathogenesis of this lesion is determined by the effectiveness and/or ineffectiveness of both humoral and cellular immune responses. Depending on the immune response, the pathogenesis can involve a primary immune complex vasculitis (type III hypersensitivity [effusive form]) and/or delayed hypersensitivity response (type IV hypersensitivity [noneffusive form]); thus the lesions are oriented around blood vessels (primarily capillaries and venules) and are granulomatous. (Courtesy Dr. M.D. McGavin, College of Veterinary Medicine, University of Tennessee.)

Renal Lymphoma (Lymphosarcoma)

Lymphoma is one of the most common neoplasms in cats and can affect the kidney as part of a systemic (multicentric) syndrome or may involve the kidney alone. Most affected cats are FeLV positive. The gross appearance of the kidney is that of diffuse renomegaly or multinodular enlargement (see Fig. 11-52). Multiple, white to tan, homogeneous masses of variable sizes are present on capsular surface of the kidney. Occasionally, feline lymphoma can appear as diffuse cortical infiltrates, wherein the kidneys are enlarged, paler than normal, and the subcapsular veins are obscured. Unlike with FIP-induced renal granulomas, the orientation of these neoplastic infiltrates does not typically center on vessels. Histologically, diffuse or nodular infiltrates and/or sheets of neoplastic lymphocytes, especially immunoblastic type, often obliterate normal renal architecture. Immunophenotyping for T or B lymphocyte origin can be performed; however, some feline lymphomas are of a non-B/non-T phenotype and genotype.

Urolithiasis

See the section on Kidney and Lower Urinary Tract, Disorders of Domestic Animals for illustrations and a general discussion of urolithiasis.

Struvite Calculi

Information on this topic is available at www.expertconsult.com.

Calcium Oxalate Calculi

Information on this topic is available at www.expertconsult.com.

Feline Idiopathic Cystitis (Hemorrhagic Urocystitis)

Feline idiopathic cystitis (FIC) is a condition diagnosed in cats that is the most common cause of feline lower urinary tract disease (FLUTD). Feline idiopathic cystitis has also been referred to as "feline interstitial cystitis" because of some commonalities to the condition of a similar name in human beings. In cats, FIC is believed to be the result of complex interactions between the urinary bladder, nervous system, adrenal glands, and environmental factors. Typical clinical signs include dysuria, stranguria, and hematuria. It is a diagnosis of exclusion, made by ruling out the presence of urolithiasis, urethral plugs, trauma or strictures, bacterial cystitis, or urinary tract neoplasia. FIC, as a component of FLUTD, is more common in middle-aged, overweight male cats with indoor housing. Histologic lesions of FIC are nonspecific, but they include submucosal edema, dilation of blood vessels with neutrophil margination, and submucosal hemorrhage. Erosion, ulceration, or thinning of urothelial epithelium is common in chronic cases of FIC. Several other alterations that may reflect the pathogenesis are usually noted in the urinary bladders of affected cats. These changes include an increase in the number of submucosal mast cells, a decrease in the concentration of urothelial glycosaminoglycans, an increase in urothelial permeability, and neurogenic inflammation. It is possible that mast-cell degranulation contributes to inflammation. Decreased glycosaminoglycans may allow urine to penetrate the urothelial barrier and induce submucosal inflammation. Disruption of the tight junctions between urothelial cells results in increased permeability. Neurogenic inflammation may occur after local release of neurotransmitters that results in vasodilation and leakage. Thus potential abnormalities in local, sensory, central, and efferent nervous systems may play a role in this syndrome that arises, at least in part, from complex interactions between the urinary bladder and the nervous system.

Toxic Renal Disease

Melamine and Cyanuric Acid. Cats are similarly affected by melamine/cyanuric acid contamination of pet foods as are dogs (see previous section on Kidney and Lower Urinary Tract, Disorders of Dogs).

Lily Toxicity. Cats are prone to a species-specific toxicity associated with ingestion of leaves or flowers of lily plants. This is often seasonal when Easter lily (*Lilium longiflorum*) plants are purchased and brought into the cat's environment. Day lily (*Hemerocallis* spp.), tiger lily (*Lilium* sp.), Japanese show lily (*Lilium hybridum*), and rubrum lily (*Lilium rubrum*) can all cause renal toxicosis in cats. Vomiting and lethargy within 1 to 5 days of ingestion are common. The toxic ingredient is not known, but renal damage in the form of acute tubular necrosis from exposure seems particularly severe in these cases.

Suggested Readings

Suggested Readings are available at www.expertconsult.com.

CHAPTER 12

Endocrine System[1]

Margaret A. Miller

Key Readings Index

Structure and Function

Endocrine glands release their secretions (hormones) directly into blood vessels; thus, unlike exocrine glands, they do not need (or have) a ductal system. In endocrine signaling (Fig. 12-1), the hormones released into the bloodstream bind to specific receptors on target cells at distant sites. Steroid hormones are lipid-soluble and can cross the plasma membrane of a cell to activate intracellular receptors (e.g., transcription factors that bind nuclear DNA), whereas polypeptide hormones or catecholamines signal through cell surface receptors, such as receptor tyrosine kinases (RTKs).

Major endocrine glands, such as the pituitary gland, thyroid gland, and adrenal glands, are composed of cells of diverse origin, but they function as dedicated endocrine organs. Endocrine tissue can also exist as individual or aggregated endocrine cells within another organ that has other functions, including nonendocrine functions. For example, the pancreatic islets are discrete collections of endocrine cells that form only a small portion of the pancreas. In addition, many organs or tissues that are not generally included in the endocrine system, such as lung, liver, skin, and gastrointestinal tract, contain dispersed endocrine cells. Other cells that might not be considered endocrine at first glance, such as adipocytes, in addition to their principal functions, synthesize and secrete chemicals into the bloodstream with a hormonal effect on distant cells and tissues.

Because endocrine cells require proximity to the vasculature, endocrine tissue, with the exception of thyroid follicles, is generally arranged as cords or packets of cells in scanty fibrous stroma that is well vascularized by sinusoids or capillaries. Ultrastructurally, endocrine cells that synthesize polypeptide hormones or catecholamines have a prominent rough endoplasmic reticulum (ER), a well-developed Golgi apparatus, and cytoplasmic secretory granules (E-Fig. 12-1). At the light microscopic level, the cytoplasm appears eosinophilic and lacy to faintly granular. The secretory granules are variably immunoreactive with antibodies to chromogranins, synaptophysin, and protein gene product (PGP) 9.5, so these immunohistochemical markers can be used to identify so-called "neuroendocrine" cells. In contrast, endocrine cells that synthesize steroid hormones have abundant smooth ER and cytoplasmic lipid bodies that contain cholesterol and other precursor compounds. Histologically, steroid hormone–producing cells have abundant lipid-vacuolated cytoplasm. Somewhat surprisingly and inexplicably, immunohistochemistry for the melanocytic marker, Melan-A, can be used to label cells that produce steroid hormones.

Endocrine glands are subject to all forms of injury and respond by degeneration or cell death, inflammation, vascular disturbances, or disturbances of growth. The endocrine glands are particularly prone to atrophy or proliferation (hyperplasia or neoplasia). These disturbances of growth are often the basis for endocrine dysfunction. Hypofunction of an endocrine gland refers to insufficient production or release of its hormone(s). Primary hypofunction is the result of a biochemical defect in hormone synthesis or the result of either failure of development or destruction of the secretory cells. Hypofunction is considered secondary if the cause occurs outside the hypofunctioning gland; for example, if the pituitary gland fails to release sufficient adrenocorticotrophic hormone, the resultant adrenocortical hypofunction is secondary.

Hyperfunction implies excessive hormone production, and it is considered primary if cells of the endocrine gland autonomously produce and secrete the excess hormone. This result is usually the case in functional neoplasms—that is, neoplasms composed of cells that continue to produce their hormonal products. Hyperfunction is considered secondary if the excessive hormone production is in response to a signal (e.g., one of the pituitary trophic hormones) from outside the hyperfunctioning gland and, as an example, can occur with neoplasms of the pituitary gland that secret a specific type of trophic hormone (see Adenohypophysis [Anterior Pituitary Gland]).

Endocrine dysfunction can also result from (1) failure of target cells to respond to hormones, either through defective receptors or through adenyl cyclase (second messenger system); (2) systemic disease or metabolic disturbances; or (3) administration of exogenous hormones.

Pituitary Gland (Hypophysis)

The pituitary gland (adenohypophysis [anterior pituitary gland] and neurohypophysis [posterior pituitary gland]) is situated ventral to the hypothalamus and just caudal to the optic chiasm (Fig. 12-2).

[1]For a glossary of abbreviations and terms used in this chapter, see E-Glossary 12-1.

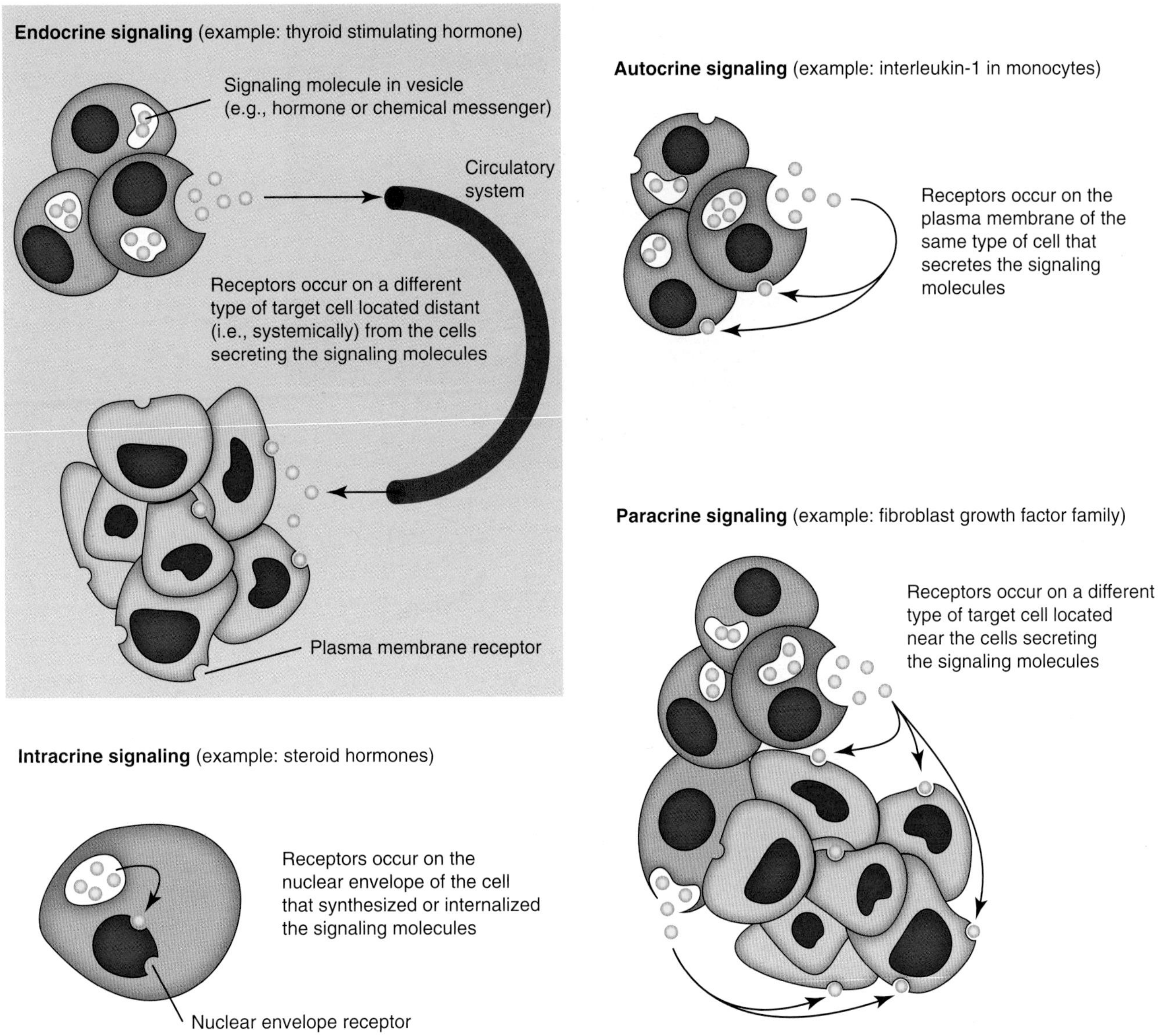
Endocrine signaling (example: thyroid stimulating hormone)
Signaling molecule in vesicle (e.g., hormone or chemical messenger)
Circulatory system
Receptors occur on a different type of target cell located distant (i.e., systemically) from the cells secreting the signaling molecules
Plasma membrane receptor
Autocrine signaling (example: interleukin-1 in monocytes)
Receptors occur on the plasma membrane of the same type of cell that secretes the signaling molecules
Paracrine signaling (example: fibroblast growth factor family)
Receptors occur on a different type of target cell located near the cells secreting the signaling molecules
Intracrine signaling (example: steroid hormones)
Receptors occur on the nuclear envelope of the cell that synthesized or internalized the signaling molecules
Nuclear envelope receptor

Figure 12-1 **Endocrine and Other Cell Signaling Pathways.** In endocrine signaling, hormones are released into the bloodstream and bind to receptors on distant target cells to exert their effect. In intracrine signaling, internalized or self-generated signaling molecules that remain within the cell (e.g., steroid hormones or angiotensin II) act by binding to nuclear receptors of the same cell. In autocrine signaling, secretory products act on the same type of cell that synthesized them. In paracrine signaling, secreted molecules act on neighboring cells. (Courtesy Dr. M.A. Miller, College of Veterinary Medicine, Purdue University; and Dr. J.F. Zachary, College of Veterinary Medicine, University of Illinois.)

Adenohypophysis (Anterior Pituitary Gland)

The adenohypophysis consists of the pars intermedia and the pars distalis. The pars intermedia surrounds the residual Rathke's pouch and separates the pars nervosa (see Neurohypophysis [Posterior Pituitary Gland]) from the pars distalis. Melanotrophs are the predominant cell of the pars intermedia. They synthesize proopiomelanocortin (POMC), which is cleaved first into adrenocorticotrophic hormone (ACTH) and then into α-melanocyte-stimulating hormone (MSH), β-endorphin, and corticotrophin-like intermediate peptide (CLIP), with little ACTH remaining. Melanotrophs do not express glucocorticoid receptors, so generally they do not respond to cortisol concentrations in the peripheral blood. Instead, they are controlled (inhibited) by dopamine released from hypothalamic neurons. The pars intermedia is a common site of hyperplasia and neoplasia in older horses and somewhat less so in dogs, in which pars intermedia cells can produce substantial bioactive ACTH.

The pars distalis (called pars anterior in the horse) consists of cells that produce, store, and release trophic hormones in response to specific releasing hormones or inhibitory factors from the hypothalamus (see Fig. 12-2, C). The hypophyseal trophic hormones act on targeted endocrine cells and cells in other organs and tissues. Importantly, hormone production in response to trophic hormone secretion from the adenohypophysis provides negative feedback in the hypothalamic-pituitary-target organ axis (Fig. 12-3). However, some endocrine glands or cells—for example, thyroid medullary C cells, parathyroid chief cells, and the adrenal medulla—are not under the influence of pituitary trophic hormones and are not regulated by a hypothalamic-hypophyseal-target organ axis.

Historically, trophic hormone–producing cells of the adenohypophysis were classified by their tinctorial characteristics as acidophils, basophils, or chromophobes. The trophic hormones produced by pars distalis cells include adrenocorticotrophic hormone (ACTH) produced by corticotrophs, growth hormone (also known as

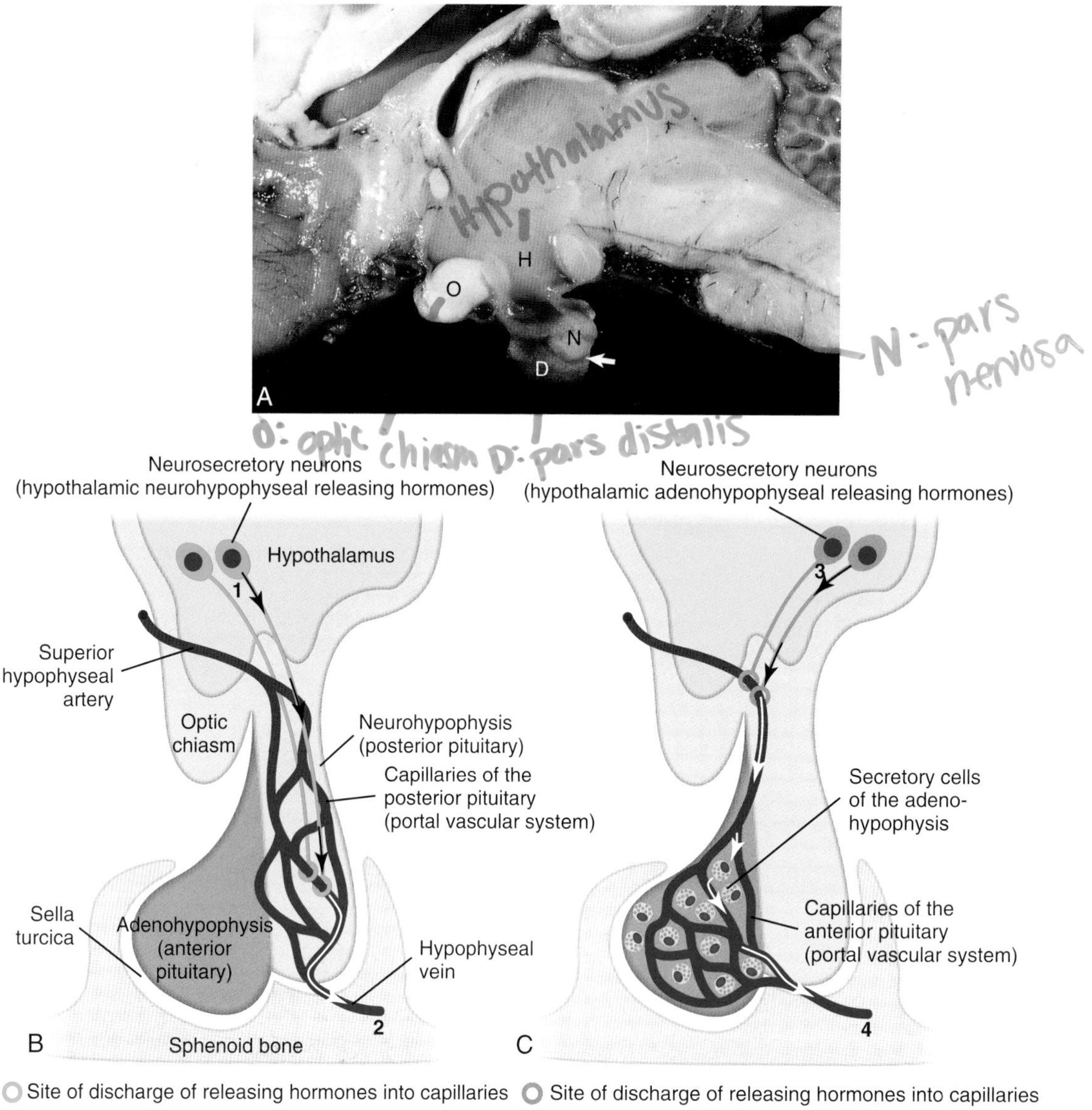

Figure 12-2 Pituitary Gland and Hypothalamus. A, Longitudinal section through the brain of a normal dog, illustrating the close relationship of the pituitary gland to the optic chiasm *(O)* and hypothalamus *(H)*. The pars distalis *(D)* forms a major part of the adenohypophysis (anterior pituitary gland) and completely surrounds the pars nervosa (*N*, posterior pituitary gland). The residual lumen of Rathke's pouch *(arrow)* separates the pars distalis and pars nervosa, and it is surrounded by the pars intermedia. **B,** Schematic of the hypothalamic-pituitary regulatory axis for the neurohypophysis (posterior pituitary gland). Hormones synthesized in supraoptic and paraventricular nuclei of the hypothalamus *(1)* are transported by axons to the neurohypophysis for storage and release into the blood *(2)*. **C,** Schematic of the hypothalamic-pituitary regulatory axis for the adenohypophysis (anterior pituitary gland). Releasing hormones or inhibitory factors synthesized in the hypothalamus *(3)* are transported hematogenously to the adenohypophyseal pars distalis, where they regulate synthesis and secretion of trophic hormones into the hypophyseal portal vasculature *(4)*. (**A** courtesy Dr. C. Capen, College of Veterinary Medicine, The Ohio State University; **B** and **C** courtesy Dr. M.A. Miller, College of Veterinary Medicine, Purdue University; and Dr. J.F. Zachary, College of Veterinary Medicine, University of Illinois.)

somatotrophin) produced by somatotrophs, prolactin produced by lactotrophs, and thyroid-stimulating hormone produced by thyrotrophs. (The gonadotrophic hormones, luteinizing hormone and follicle-stimulating hormone, are addressed in Chapters 18 and 19.) Corticotrophs are typically chromophobes, and somatotrophs are typically acidophils (Fig. 12-4). However, immunohistochemistry, using antibodies against the trophic hormones of interest, is more reliable than histochemical tinctorial characteristics in identifying the trophic hormone produced by a particular cell type in the adenohypophysis. Molecular techniques can be used to detect mRNA in cases in which a cell has the genetic machinery to make a particular trophic hormone but does not (1) produce it in sufficient quantity for immunohistochemical detection or (2) release sufficient bioactive hormone into the circulation for detection by plasma assay.

Each type of trophic hormone–producing cell in the pars distalis is under the control of a specific releasing hormone or factor from the hypothalamus (see Fig. 12-3). These releasing hormones are small peptides synthesized and secreted by hypothalamic neurons and transported by axons to the median eminence at the base of the third ventricle, where they are released into the hypothalamic-hypophyseal portal system. Importantly, the median eminence and the pituitary gland are not encumbered with a blood-brain barrier. Each releasing hormone or factor stimulates the rapid release of secretory granules containing preformed trophic hormone from the

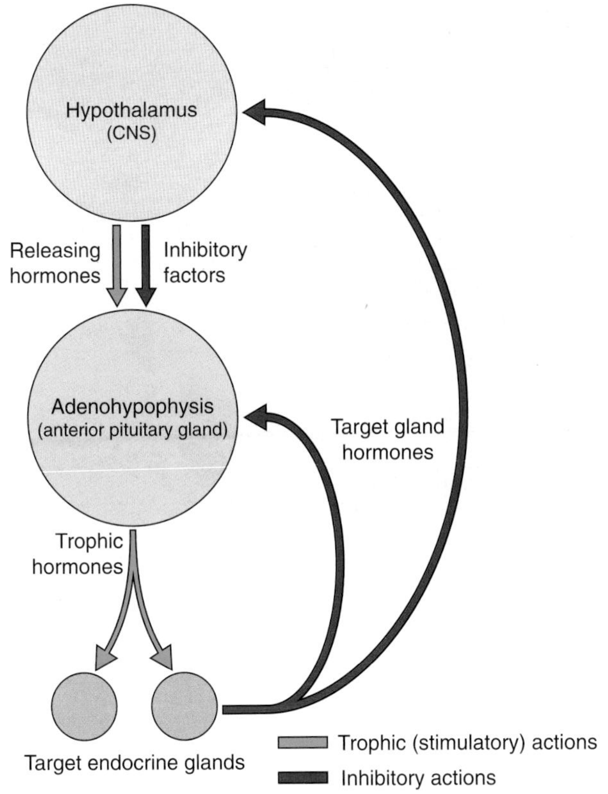

Figure 12-3 **Hypothalamic-Pituitary-Target Gland Axis.** Releasing hormones (or inhibitory factors) produced in the hypothalamus act on the adenohypophysis (anterior pituitary gland) to stimulate (or inhibit) release of trophic hormones. Trophic hormones act on specific endocrine glands, stimulating them in turn to produce hormones that exert their ultimate actions on downstream tissues and also provide negative feedback to the adenohypophysis and hypothalamus. (Courtesy Dr. M.A. Miller, College of Veterinary Medicine, Purdue University; and Dr. J.F. Zachary, College of Veterinary Medicine, University of Illinois.)

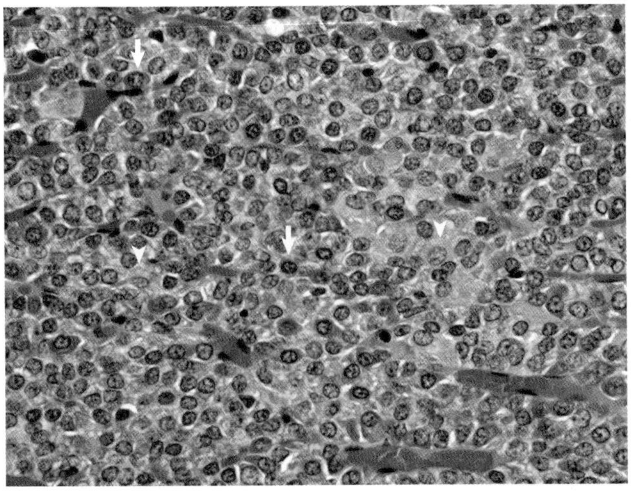

Figure 12-4 **Pars Distalis, Normal Dog.** The pars distalis is composed of acidophils *(arrows)*, basophils (none shown here), and chromophobes *(arrowheads)*. H&E stain. (Courtesy Dr. J.F. Zachary, College of Veterinary Medicine, University of Illinois.)

corresponding adenohypophyseal cells. Corticotrophs, the predominant cell of the pars distalis, respond to corticotrophin-releasing hormone with increased production of proopiomelanocortin (POMC), which undergoes posttranslational proteolysis to form ACTH, β-lipotrophin, and β-endorphin, among other products. Corticotrophs express receptors for glucocorticoids; therefore, they respond to negative feedback from cortisol production by adrenocortical cells.

Neurohypophysis (Posterior Pituitary Gland)

The neurohypophysis contains the pars nervosa, which is connected to the hypothalamus by its infundibular stalk and consists mainly of axonal projections from hypothalamic neurons. Hypothalamic neurons in the supraoptic and paraventricular nuclei synthesize the neurohypophyseal hormones oxytocin and antidiuretic hormone (ADH). These nonapeptide hormones are packaged with a corresponding binding protein into membrane-bound neurosecretory granules and transported by axons to the pars nervosa for storage and secretion into the blood (see Fig. 12-2B).

Thyroid Gland

In most domestic mammals, the thyroid gland has two distinct lobes, connected by a narrow or almost imperceptible isthmus, and is closely associated with the sides of the trachea, just caudal to the larynx. The word *thyroid* comes from the Greek word for shield-like, but among the domestic mammals, the bovine thyroid gland comes closest to a shield shape with its more prominent isthmus and flattened lobes. The porcine thyroid gland lacks distinct lobes and is centered over the ventral aspect of the trachea, closer to the thoracic inlet than to the larynx. The rich vascularity of the thyroid gland colors it red-brown to dark red, so it can be confused with adjacent skeletal muscle at surgery, autopsy (syn: necropsy) (E-Appendix 12-1), or indeed during carcass trimming at the slaughterhouse, where inadvertent inclusion of bovine thyroid gland in ground beef has resulted in elevated blood thyroxine concentrations in those who consumed even well-cooked hamburgers.

The thyroid gland has a unique, among endocrine glands, follicular organization and contains two types of endocrine cells (Fig. 12-5, A and B): (1) follicular cells of endodermal origin that produce the thyroid hormones and (2) parafollicular medullary or C cells of neural crest origin that produce calcitonin. The thyroid gland originates early in gestation from a ventral midline proliferation of endodermal cells between the first and second pharyngeal pouches. Initially, it is connected to the developing tongue by the thyroglossal duct, which mostly disappears later in gestation. Thyroid medullary or C cells are derived from neural crest cells that populate the ultimobranchial body, which fuses with the thyroid gland. Later in gestation, the thyroid gland descends to its adult location near the larynx in most species.

Thyroid Follicular Cells

Cuboidal to columnar thyroid follicular cells are arranged in a single layer around colloid-filled follicles. The follicular cells are equipped for protein (thyroglobulin) production and packaging with their abundant rough endoplasmic reticulum (ER) and well-developed Golgi apparatus. Apical microvilli increase the surface area for interaction with the colloid in the follicular lumen (E-Fig. 12-2).

Thyroid hormone production is regulated through the hypothalamic-pituitary-thyroid axis (Figs. 12-6 and 12-7). Low plasma concentrations of thyroxine (tetraiodothyronine or T_4) and triiodothyronine (T_3) stimulate secretion of thyrotropin-releasing hormone (TRH) by the hypothalamus and thyroid-stimulating hormone (TSH) by pituitary thyrotrophs. When TSH binds with its receptor on follicular cells, the transmembrane receptor associates with G proteins, activating a cAMP-mediated protein kinase signaling cascade that causes hypertrophy and hyperplasia of follicular epithelium (Fig. 12-8, A), and upregulates thyroid hormone production by increasing intracellular calcium concentration and

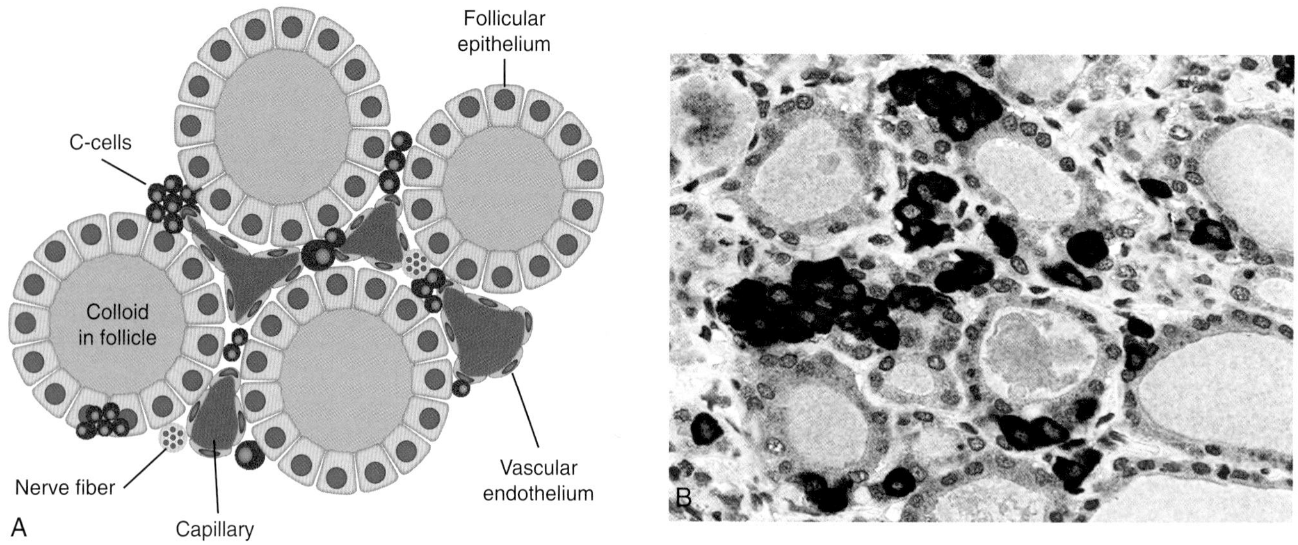

Figure 12-5 **Thyroid Follicular and Parafollicular (Medullary or C) Cells. A,** Colloid-filled follicles are lined by a single layer of follicular epithelium. Individual or clustered C cells are beside the follicular cells or within the thyroid medulla. Note the close proximity of both follicular and C cells to capillaries. **B,** The cytoplasm of medullary C cells, but not that of follicular cells, in a canine thyroid gland is labeled brown (diaminobenzidine chromogen) with immunohistochemistry for calcitonin. (**A** courtesy Dr. M.A. Miller, College of Veterinary Medicine, Purdue University; and Dr. J.F. Zachary, College of Veterinary Medicine, University of Illinois. **B** courtesy Dr. M.A. Miller, College of Veterinary Medicine, Purdue University.)

activating phosphokinase C (PKC). Calcium and PKC synergistically activate the dual oxidase (DUOX) complex in the apical plasma membrane to generate the H_2O_2 needed by thyroid peroxidase as the ultimate electron acceptor.

Thyroxine and triiodothyronine are peptide hormones derived from iodinated thyroglobulin, a glycoprotein with numerous tyrosyl residues (see Fig. 12-7). Thyroglobulin is synthesized in the rough ER of the follicular cell, with glycosylation and packaging in the Golgi apparatus for secretion into the follicle lumen. Iodide from the blood is concentrated in follicular cells by the Na^+/I^- symporter (NIS) in the basolateral plasma membrane and secreted through the apical plasma membrane into the follicular colloid by the Na^+-independent chloride/iodide transporter, pendrin. Human placental trophoblasts have both NIS and pendrin, so they can concentrate iodide from maternal blood, but such transfer would be inefficient with the "anatomic" separation of trophoblasts from maternal blood in the placenta of ruminants, horses, and pigs. The mammary gland also concentrates iodide, making milk another source of iodine for the neonate.

In the follicular lumen, iodide is oxidized by thyroid peroxidase to iodine, which then attaches to tyrosyl residues of thyroglobulin. Two iodinated tyrosyl residues, either monoiodotyrosine (MIT) or diiodotyrosine (DIT), are conjugated to form either T_4 (two DITs) or T_3 (one DIT and one MIT). The concentration of T_3 formed is less than that of T_4. Thyroid peroxidase catalyzes both the iodination of thyroglobulin and the subsequent linking of the iodinated tyrosyl residues to iodothyronines. Under the influence of TSH, the microvilli of follicular cells elongate and form pseudopodia that resorb colloid[2] by endocytosis. The resorbed colloid droplets fuse with lysosomes, where T_4 and T_3 are cleaved from the thyroglobulin molecule by proteases.

The availability of iodine contributes to the regulation of thyroid function. Excess iodide tends to decrease the responsiveness of follicular cells to TSH, reduce iodide trapping from the blood by downregulating the NIS, inhibit oxidation by thyroid peroxidase, and (at high concentration) inhibit thyroid hormone secretion. Depending on the individual animal, however, excess iodine can result in hyperthyroidism or hypothyroidism.

Thyroid hormones act on nearly every cell or tissue in the body with the general effect of increasing the metabolic rate of the targeted cell. Almost all the circulating T_4 and T_3 is bound to thyroxine-binding globulin, transthyretin, or other carrier proteins. At the target cells, most of the free T_4 is deiodinated to T_3, which has much higher affinity for nuclear thyroid hormone receptors. The position of the three iodine molecules in T_3 (3,5,3′-triiodothyronine) is critical because reverse T_3 (3,3′,5′-triiodothyronine), formed in certain disease states such as neonatal protein deficiency, hepatic disease, or renal disease, lacks biologic activity. Elevated circulating T_4 and T_3 concentration suppresses TSH release through negative feedback on the hypothalamus and adenohypophysis, resulting in atrophy of the follicular cells (Fig. 12-8, *B*).

Thyroid C Cells

Thyroid C cells (also known as parafollicular or medullary cells) are the second type of thyroid endocrine cell. The C cells are situated beside follicular cells or within the thyroid medulla (between follicles) and in close proximity to blood vessels (see Fig. 12-5; E-Fig. 12-3). C cells produce *calcitonin*, a polypeptide hormone that is stored in secretory granules. Calcitonin acts to reduce the blood calcium (Ca^{2+}) concentration, and it generally opposes the effects of parathyroid hormone (see Parathyroid Glands). C cells can be distinguished from follicular cells with immunohistochemistry, using antibody to calcitonin (see Fig. 12-5, *B*), or with less specific neuroendocrine markers, such as chromogranin or PGP 9.5.

Unlike thyroid follicular cells, C cells are not under the control of TSH. Instead, they respond to plasma concentration of Ca^{2+}. When blood calcium concentration is low, numerous secretory granules accumulate in quiescent C cells (Fig. 12-9). However, C cells rapidly secrete calcitonin in response to hypercalcemia. Thus, the secretory granules are depleted, and C cells undergo hypertrophy

[2]A proteinaceous fluid containing thyroglobulin in the lumen of the thyroid follicle.

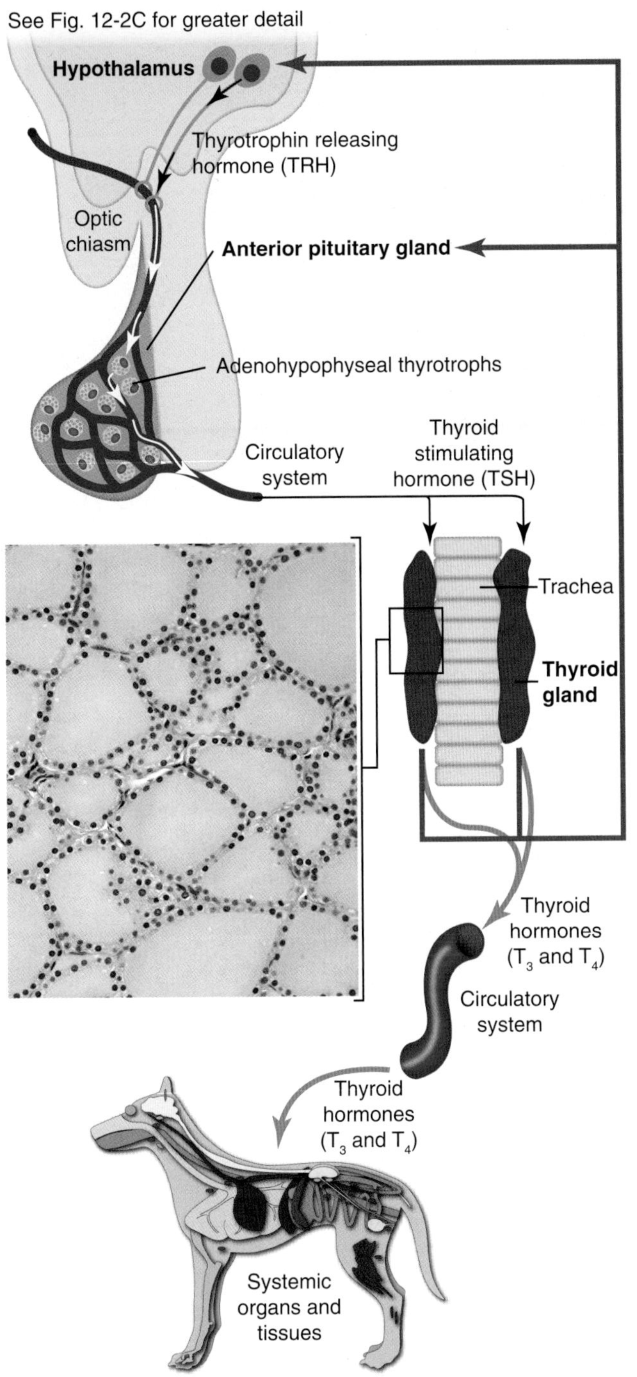

Figure 12-6 **Hypothalamic-Pituitary-Thyroid Axis.** Thyrotropin-releasing hormone *(TRH)*, synthesized and released from hypothalamic neurons, stimulates adenohypophyseal thyrotrophs to release thyroid-stimulating hormone *(TSH)*, which acts on thyroid follicular cells to promote synthesis and secretion of triiodothyronine *(T_3)* and thyroxine *(T_4)* into the circulation. These thyroid hormones have a positive effect *(green arrows)* on development, growth, and metabolism in organs and tissues throughout the body. Thyroid hormones exert negative feedback *(red arrows)* on the anterior pituitary gland and hypothalamus to regulate their own production. (Courtesy Dr. J.F. Zachary, College of Veterinary Medicine, University of Illinois and Dr. M.A. Miller, College of Veterinary Medicine, Purdue University.)

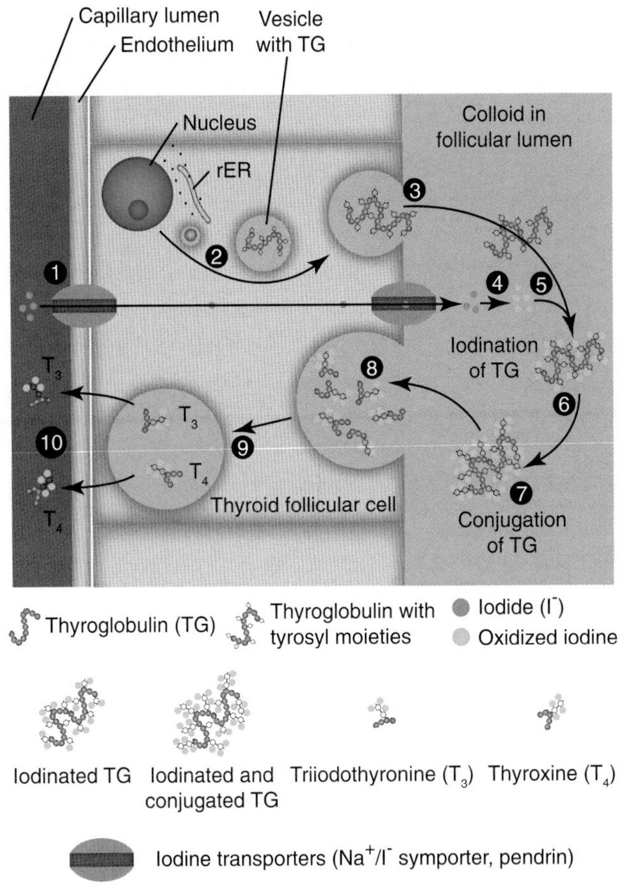

Figure 12-7 **Hormone Synthesis in the Thyroid Follicle.** Blood iodide enters the follicular cell *(1)* through the Na^+/I^- symporter (basolateral plasma membrane) and is transported into the luminal colloid *(right side of drawing)* by pendrin (apical plasma membrane). Thyroglobulin *(TG)* is synthesized from tyrosine and other amino acids in the rough endoplasmic reticulum *(rER)*, glycosylated and packaged into vesicles in the Golgi *(2)*, and secreted into the colloid *(3)*. In the colloid, iodide *(4)* is oxidized to iodine *(5)*, which then attaches to tyrosyl residues of TG *(6)*. Iodinated tyrosyl residues are conjugated *(7)* to form T_4 and T_3 side chains. Colloid that contains conjugated iodinated TG is resorbed into the follicular cell by endocytosis *(8)*. The intracellular colloid droplets fuse with lysosomes where T_4 and T_3 are enzymatically cleaved from thyroglobulin *(9)* and then released into the circulation *(10)*. (Courtesy Dr. M.A. Miller, College of Veterinary Medicine, Purdue University; and Dr. J.F. Zachary, College of Veterinary Medicine, University of Illinois.)

with amplification of rough ER and Golgi. Long-term hypercalcemia causes hyperplasia of C cells.

Calcitonin acts mainly in bone and kidney to downregulate blood calcium concentrations. Calcitonin inhibits resorption of mineral from bone by binding and inhibiting osteoclasts, thereby having the opposite effect of parathyroid hormone (see Parathyroid Glands and Fig. 12-9). In the kidney, however, calcitonin and parathyroid hormone act synergistically to decrease renal tubular reabsorption of phosphorus.

Parathyroid Glands

Most domestic mammals have two pairs of parathyroid glands, so named because of their location beside the thyroid gland. The dog and cat have bilateral external and internal parathyroid glands that truly are beside or within the thyroid gland. The pig has only one pair of parathyroid glands that are located cranial to the thyroid gland, embedded either in the thymus in young pigs or in adipose

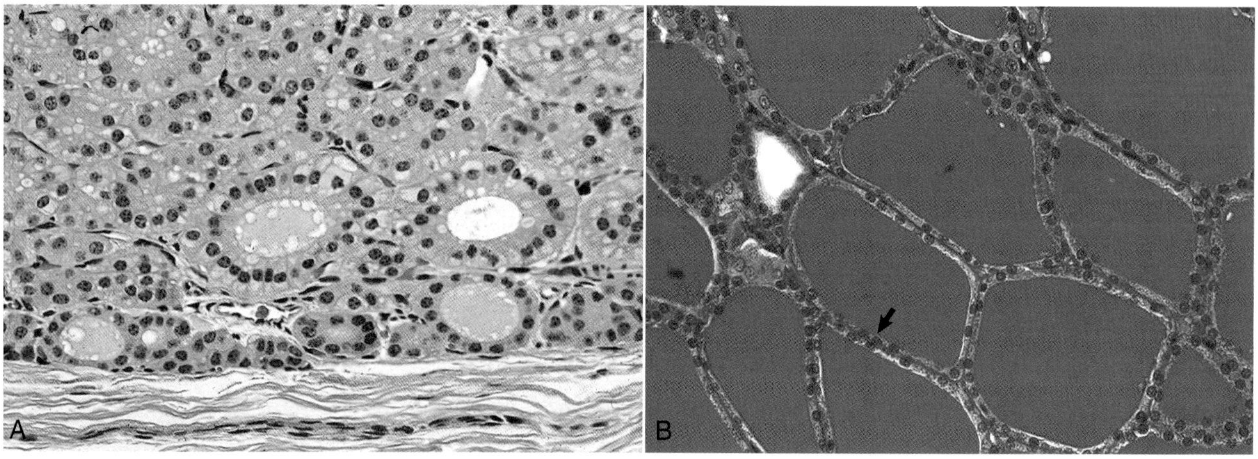

Figure 12-8 **Regulation of Thyroid Follicular Epithelium. A,** Follicular hyperplasia, thyroid gland, horse. Follicular cells under the influence of thyroid-stimulating hormone (TSH) are hypertrophied (tall columnar) and crowded, impinging on the follicular lumen. In follicles with an open lumen, the colloid is pale eosinophilic with resorption vacuoles at the apical surface of follicular cells. H&E stain. **B,** Follicular atrophy, thyroid gland, dog. Thyroid follicular cells *(arrow)* after long-term administration of exogenous thyroxine (T_4)—and therefore minimal secretion of TSH by adenohypophyseal thyrotrophs—are low cuboidal. The follicles are distended with densely stained colloid. Note the lack of apparent resorption vacuoles. Periodic acid–Schiff reaction. (**A** courtesy Dr. B. Harmon, College of Veterinary Medicine, The University of Georgia; and Noah's Arkive, College of Veterinary Medicine, The University of Georgia. **B** courtesy Dr. C. Capen, College of Veterinary Medicine, The Ohio State University.)

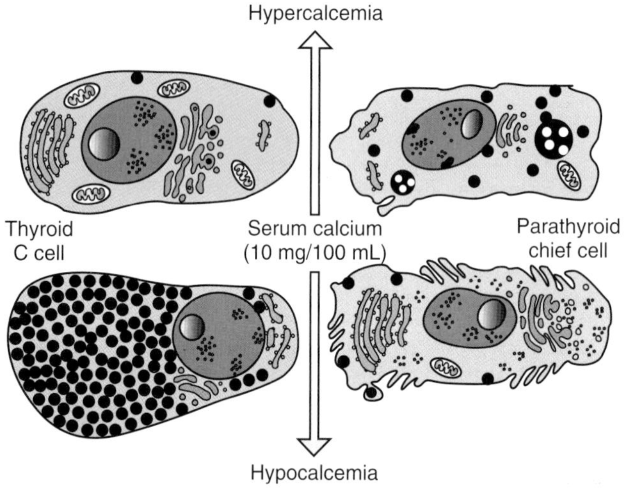

Figure 12-9 **Response of Thyroid C Cells and Parathyroid Chief Cells to Hypercalcemia and Hypocalcemia.** In response to hypocalcemia, C cells become quiescent and accumulate secretory granules, whereas chief cells are nearly degranulated but have hypertrophied rough endoplasmic reticulum and Golgi apparatus for synthesis and packaging of parathyroid hormone. The opposite occurs in response to hypercalcemia—that is, C cells degranulate and undergo hypertrophy, and chief cells return to a quiescent stage. (Redrawn with permission from Dr. C. Capen, College of Veterinary Medicine, The Ohio State University.)

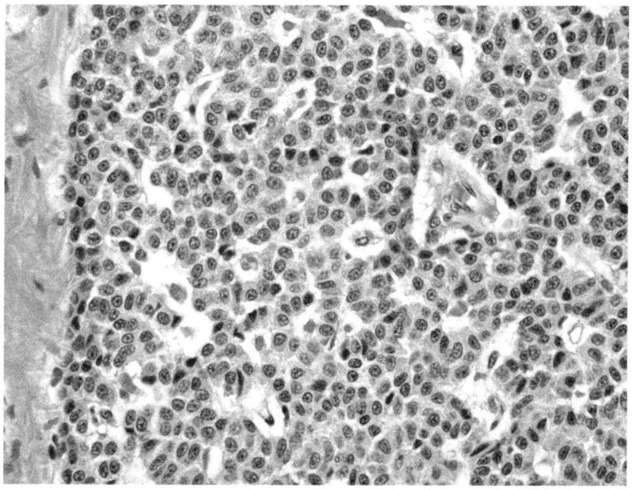

Figure 12-10 **Parathyroid Gland, Normal Dog.** Numerous chief cells are separated and supported by a fine fibrovascular stroma. H&E stain. (Courtesy Dr. J.F. Zachary, College of Veterinary Medicine, University of Illinois.)

tissue in adults. In cattle and sheep, the larger external parathyroid gland is cranial to the thyroid gland in loose connective tissue along the common carotid artery. The smaller internal parathyroid glands are situated on the dorsal and medial surface of the thyroid lobes. In horses, the larger ("lower") parathyroid gland is at a considerable distance from the thyroid gland in the caudal cervical region, whereas the smaller ("upper") parathyroid gland is near the thyroid gland.

The parathyroid glands are composed mainly of cords of chief cells in a fine fibrovascular stroma (Fig. 12-10). Chief cells produce and release parathyroid hormone (PTH) in response to decreased ionized calcium in peripheral blood. They can respond rapidly to changes in blood Ca^{2+} concentration with "bypass secretion"[3] (Fig. 12-11) of newly synthesized PTH. Unneeded PTH is stored in the cytosol as secretory granules. Oxyphil cells, often in clusters, are a second type of parathyroid cell that may be conspicuous by virtue of their more abundant and more eosinophilic cytoplasm (due to numerous hypertrophied mitochondria) but few, if any, secretory granules; their function is poorly understood.

The overall action of PTH is to mobilize calcium into extracellular fluid (Fig. 12-12). In the kidney, PTH acts within minutes to block reabsorption of phosphorus in proximal tubules and to enhance reabsorption of calcium in distal tubules. In bone, PTH activates

[3]Newly synthesized PTH is rapidly released at the plasma membrane from small vesicles into extracellular fluid without interacting with ("bypass") mature secretory granules in the cytosolic storage pool of PTH.

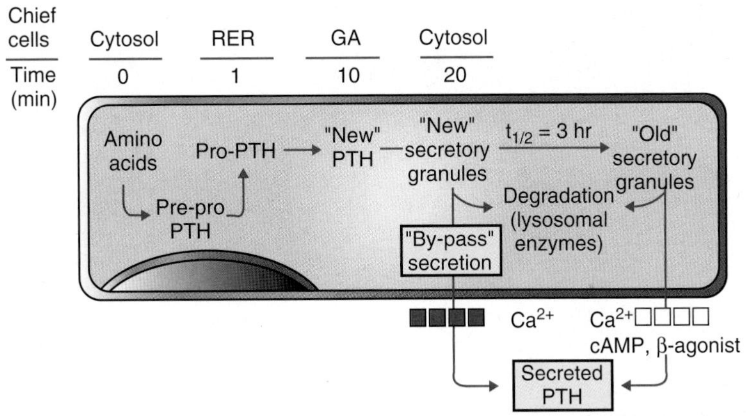

Figure 12-11 Chief Cell Bypass Secretion of Parathyroid Hormone *(PTH)* in Response to Hypocalcemia. Newly synthesized and processed PTH can be released directly into the blood without entering the storage pool of "old" secretory granules. Whereas PTH from the storage pool is mobilized by cyclic adenosine monophosphate *(cAMP)*, β-agonists (e.g., epinephrine, norepinephrine, and isoproterenol), and low blood Ca^{2+} concentration, newly synthesized PTH is secreted only in response to low Ca^{2+} concentration. GA, Golgi apparatus; *RER*, rough endoplasmic reticulum. (Redrawn with permission from Dr. C. Capen, College of Veterinary Medicine, The Ohio State University.)

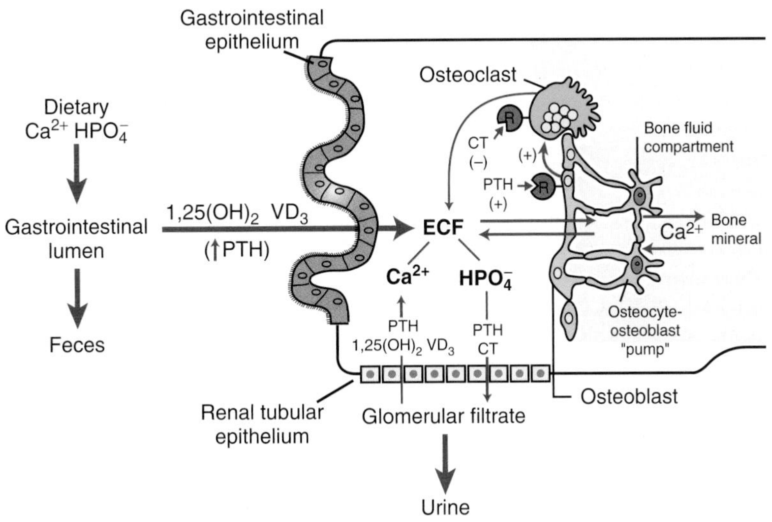

Figure 12-12 Interaction of Parathyroid Hormone *(PTH)*, Calcitonin *(CT)*, and 1,25-Dihydroxycholecalciferol *(1,25-[OH]$_2$ VD$_3$)* in Hormonal Regulation of Calcium and Phosphorus in Extracellular Fluids *(ECF)*. (Redrawn with permission from Dr. C. Capen, College of Veterinary Medicine, The Ohio State University.)

osteoclasts indirectly by binding to its receptor on osteoblasts (see Chapter 16). PTH also promotes absorption of calcium from the intestine.

Calcitonin, PTH, and cholecalciferol act in concert to regulate calcium:phosphorus balance (see Fig. 12-12). From a functional standpoint, vitamin D brings about the retention of sufficient mineral ions for mineralization of bone matrix, whereas PTH maintains the proper calcium:phosphorus ratio in extracellular fluid. Cholecalciferol (vitamin D_3) acts in the small intestine to promote the absorption of calcium from the orad and phosphorus from the aborad mucosa.

Adrenal Gland

The adrenal gland is so-named for its position just craniomedial to the kidney. Although classified anatomically as one gland, the adrenal cortex has mesodermal origin, and adrenocortical cells synthesize steroid hormones (corticosteroids) from cholesterol (E-Fig. 12-4), whereas the adrenal medulla is derived from neural crest ectoderm and its cells produce catecholamines from tyrosine (E-Fig. 12-5). The adrenal medulla is surrounded by the adrenal cortex (Fig. 12-13), so medullary cells are exposed to cortisol-rich blood. This close anatomic association between adrenal cortex and medulla is important because the phenylethanolamine-*N*-methyl transferase that converts norepinephrine to epinephrine is corticosteroid hormone-dependent. Interestingly, ACTH also contributes to catecholamine synthesis by stimulating the activity of two key enzymes: tyrosine hydroxylase and dopamine-β-hydroxylase.

Adrenal Cortex

Adrenocortical cells, especially those of the inner layers (i.e., zonae), have vacuolated, lipid-laden cytoplasm typical of steroid hormone–producing cells; the cytoplasmic lipid imparts a yellowish cast to the cortex. The adrenal cortex is divided into zonae glomerulosa, fasciculata, and reticularis (Fig. 12-14). The zona glomerulosa is the outermost layer, in which cells arranged in arcuate formations produce mineralocorticoids, mainly aldosterone. Aldosterone controls blood pressure and extracellular fluid volume by acting at distal and collecting tubules of the kidney to promote sodium retention

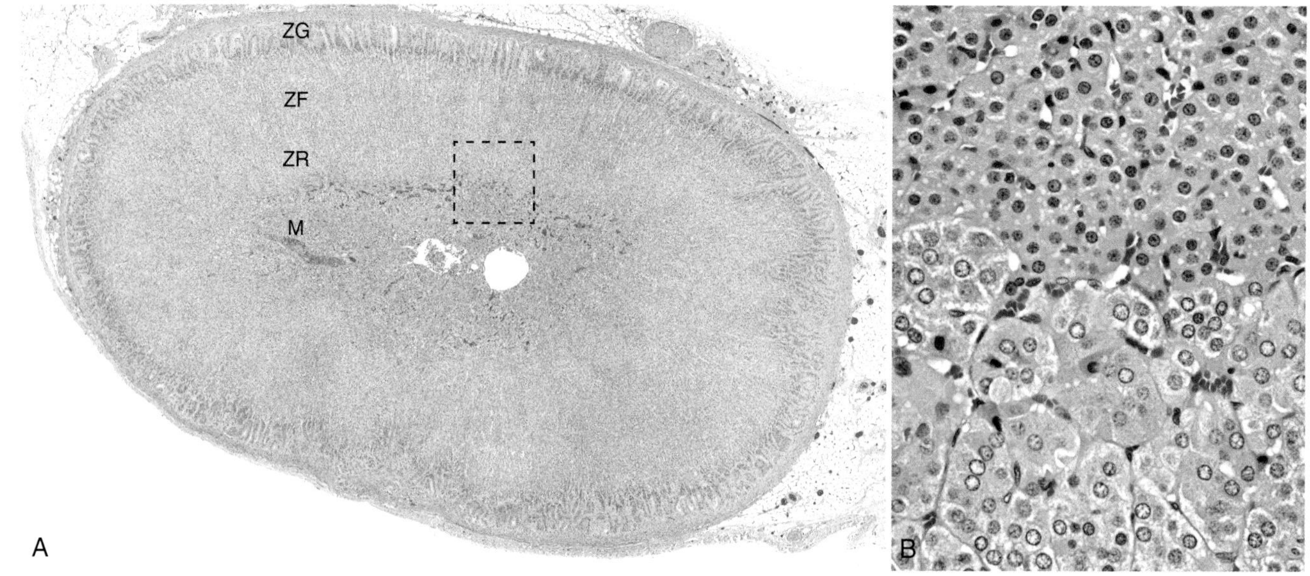

Figure 12-13 **Adrenal Gland, Normal Dog. A,** Cross section of adrenal gland. The cortex surrounds the medulla. Note prominent sinusoidal vasculature at the corticomedullary junction. The *rectangle* outlines an area of the corticomedullary junction like that depicted at higher magnification in Fig. 12-13, *B*. M, Medulla; *ZF*, zona fasciculata; *ZG*, zona glomerulosa; *ZR*, zona reticularis. **B,** Interface between the cortical cells of the zona reticularis *(top)* and the finely granular chromaffin cells of the adrenal medulla *(bottom)*. H&E stain. (**A** courtesy Dr. M.A. Miller, College of Veterinary Medicine, Purdue University. **B** courtesy Dr. J.F. Zachary, College of Veterinary Medicine, University of Illinois.)

and potassium excretion (see Fig. 12-14, *A*). The zona glomerulosa has minimal response to ACTH (in contrast to the inner layers of the adrenal cortex) and is regulated mainly by the renin-angiotensin-aldosterone system with feedback from K^+ concentration in the plasma. Renin, secreted by juxtaglomerular cells of the kidney (see Fig. 11-14) in response to lowered blood pressure (and other factors), converts angiotensinogen to angiotensin I, which in turn is converted in the lung to angiotensin II by angiotensin-converting enzyme (ACE). Angiotensin II raises blood pressure by contracting vascular smooth muscle; it also acts on the zona glomerulosa to stimulate synthesis and release of aldosterone. The zona fasciculata is the middle and largest layer of the cortex. Its cells produce cortisol and other glucocorticoids; thus, it responds to stimulation by ACTH (see Fig. 12-14, *B*) released into the systemic circulation by the adenohypophysis (anterior pituitary gland). Glucocorticoids have diverse actions on many organs and tissues throughout the body, but in general they tend to increase glucose production, decrease lipogenesis, suppress the immune response, and inhibit inflammation and its repair by fibroplasia (E-Fig. 12-6). Cells of the inner adrenocortical layer, the zona reticularis, produce sex hormones (androgens and estrogens), especially in castrated animals, and lower concentrations of glucocorticoid hormones.

Adrenal Medulla

In contrast to the lipid-vacuolated cytoplasm of steroid-producing adrenocortical cells, the chromaffin cells of the adrenal medulla have finely granular amphophilic[4] cytoplasm (see Fig. 12-13, *B*). Adrenal medullary cells produce the catecholamine hormones, norepinephrine and epinephrine, from tyrosine (see E-Fig. 12-5). Most of the epinephrine in circulation, but only a minor portion of circulating norepinephrine, is produced by the adrenal medulla. Epinephrine acts by nonselectively binding adrenergic receptors to exert a variety of effects in most tissues throughout the body. Stress, especially frightening stress that induces the "fight or flight" response, is the major trigger of epinephrine (also known as adrenaline) release. Norepinephrine is a major sympathetic neurotransmitter, with less importance as a hormone.

Pancreatic Islets

The bulk of the pancreas is an exocrine gland (see Chapter 8). The endocrine component is contained in its islets of Langerhans (Fig. 12-15). Pancreatic islet cells have abundant rough ER and well-developed Golgi to produce and package their polypeptide hormones (E-Fig. 12-7). The islets contain a variety of hormone-producing cells, but this chapter is focused on the insulin-secreting β cells, which are confined to pancreatic islets and are the most common islet cell, and the glucagon-secreting α cells. Insulin and glucagon act in concert to control the glucose concentration in extracellular fluid. Insulin is secreted in response to elevated blood glucose and functions to transfer glucose from the blood into cells (especially hepatocytes, adipocytes, and skeletal muscle cells) and to enhance glucose oxidation, glycogenesis, lipogenesis, and formation of ATP and nucleic acids. Glucagon, secreted in response to decreased blood glucose concentration, works in opposition to insulin and promotes glycogenolysis, gluconeogenesis, and lipolysis. Islet α cells, like the other non–β cell types (e.g., somatostatin-secreting δ cells and pancreatic polypeptide-secreting PP cells), are not restricted to pancreatic islets and can be found in other, mainly gastrointestinal, sites.

Pineal Gland

The pineal gland, situated between the cerebral hemispheres just dorsal and caudal to the thalamus, is seldom associated with disease in domestic mammals. The pineal gland is derived from the ependymal lining of the third ventricle in the developing diencephalon and is first observed at 30 to 40 days of gestation in the bovine fetus. Its importance in adult animals lies in its ability to relay information about photoperiod length to the hypothalamic-pituitary axis and thereby regulate circadian rhythm and seasonal reproduction. Pinealocytes secrete several neurotransmitters in addition to the hormone melatonin, a polypeptide derivative of tryptophan, in response to

[4]Stains purple in histologic sections because of affinity for acidic (red) and basic (blue) dyes.

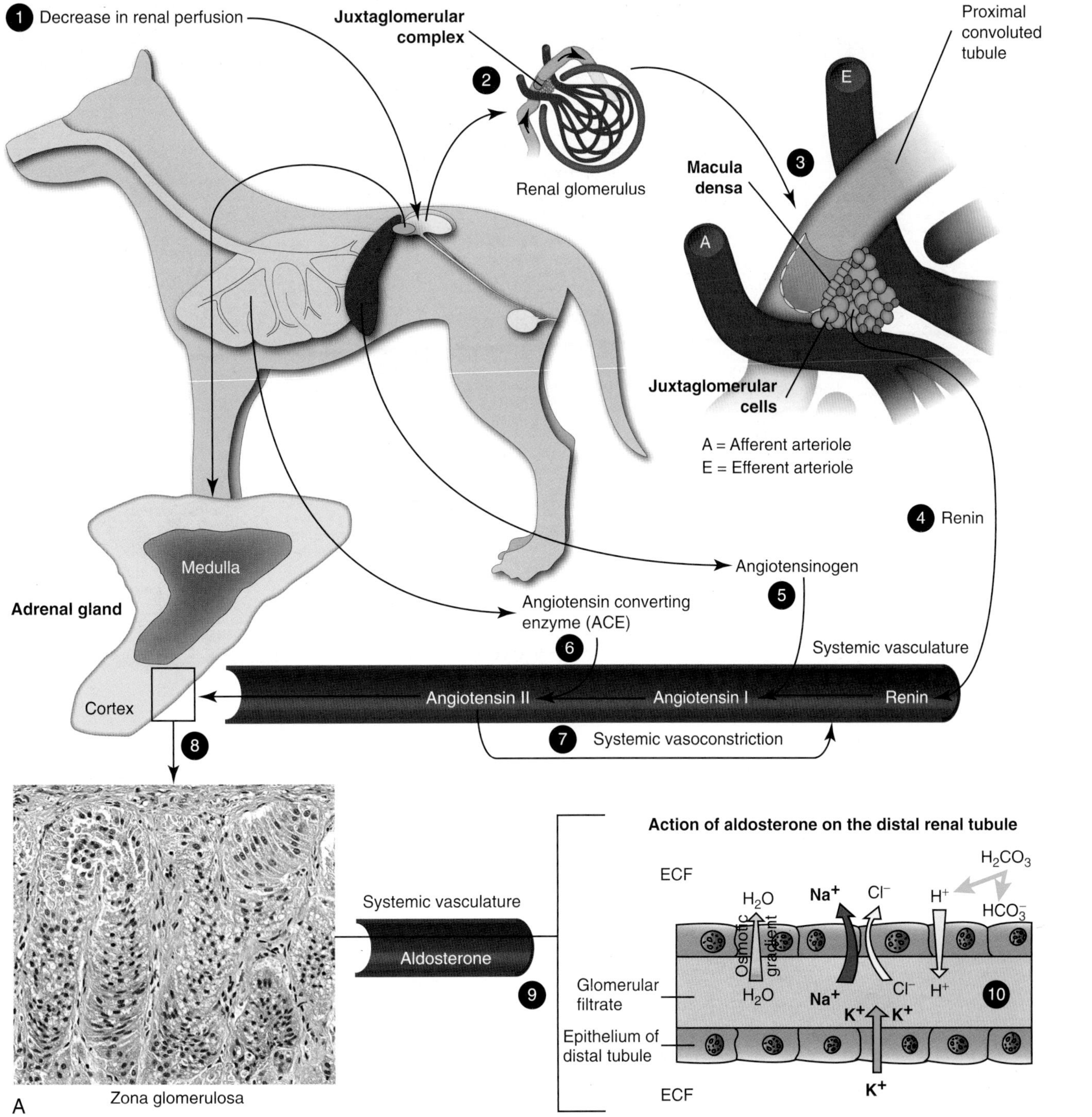

Figure 12-14 **Regulation of Adrenocortical Function. A,** Mineralocorticoid synthesis in the zona glomerulosa (H&E stain) is regulated through the renin-angiotensin-aldosterone system. A decrease in renal perfusion *(1)* activates the juxtaglomerular complex *(2)*. Macula densa cells signal juxtaglomerular cells *(3)* to release renin *(4)* into the systemic vasculature. Renin converts angiotensinogen to angiotensin I *(5)*, which is converted to angiotensin II by angiotensin-converting enzyme *(6)*. Angiotensin II causes vasoconstriction *(7)* and stimulates aldosterone synthesis by adrenocortical cells of the zona glomerulosa *(8)*. Aldosterone acts on renal distal and collecting tubules *(9)* to maintain extracellular fluid volume *(ECF)* by promoting excretion of K^+ and resorption of Na^+.

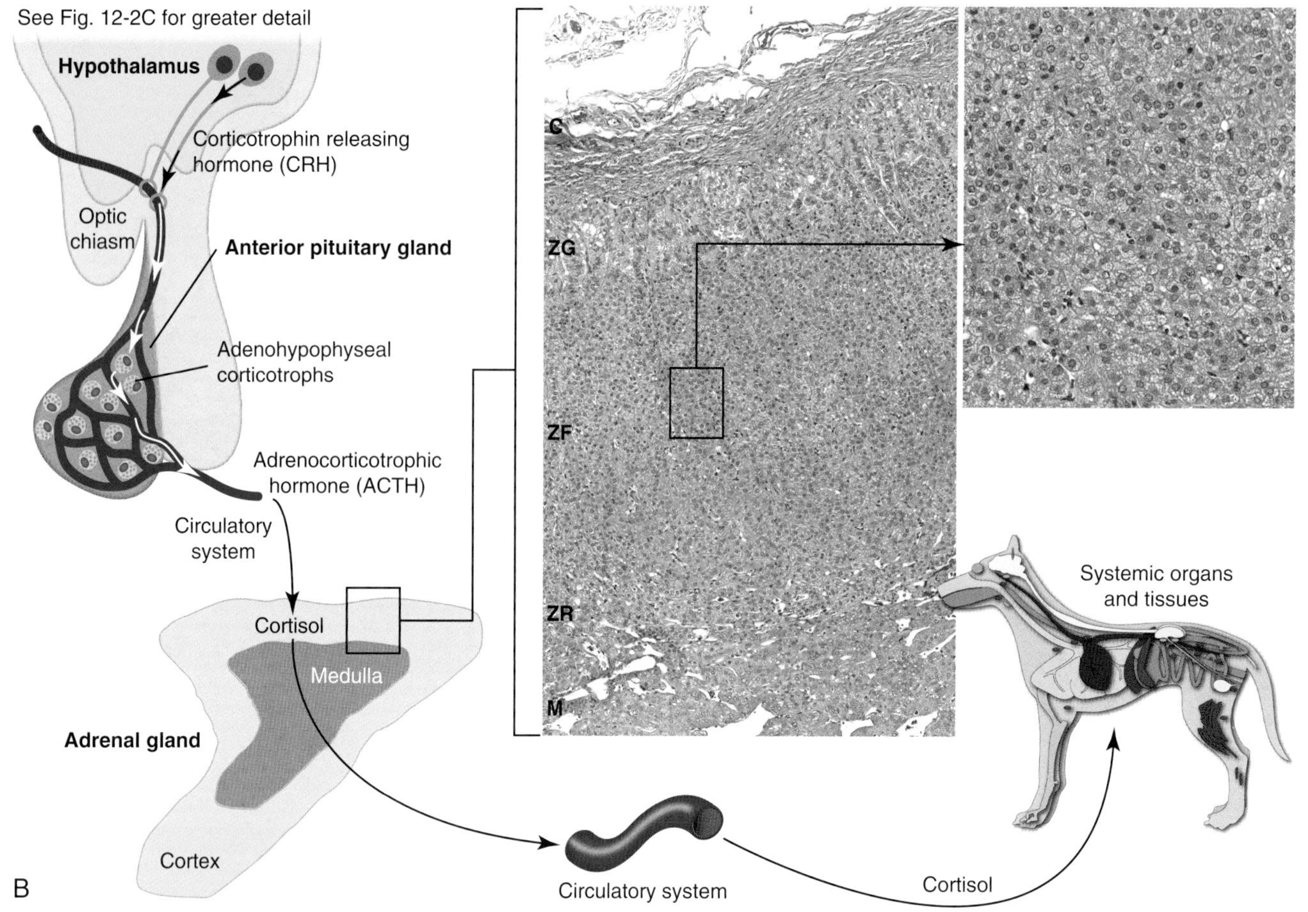

Figure 12-14, cont'd **B,** The three layers of the adrenal cortex, from outer to inner, are the zona glomerulosa *(ZG)*, zona fasciculata *(ZF)*, and zona reticularis *(ZR)*. Glucocorticoid synthesis in the ZF and ZR is regulated through the hypothalamic-pituitary-adrenocortical axis. Corticotrophin-releasing hormone *(CRH)* from the hypothalamus promotes synthesis and release of adrenocorticotrophic hormone *(ACTH)* from the anterior pituitary gland. ACTH acts on the ZF and ZR to increase production and secretion of cortisol and other glucocorticoids. Increased plasma concentration of cortisol provides negative feedback to the adenohypophysis and hypothalamus. Adrenal capsule *(C)* is at *top*; adrenal medulla *(M)* is at *bottom*. H&E stain. (**A** and **B** courtesy Dr. M.A. Miller, College of Veterinary Medicine, Purdue University; and Dr. J.F. Zachary, College of Veterinary Medicine, University of Illinois. Effect of aldosterone on distal nephron redrawn with permission from Dr. C. Capen, College of Veterinary Medicine, The Ohio State University.)

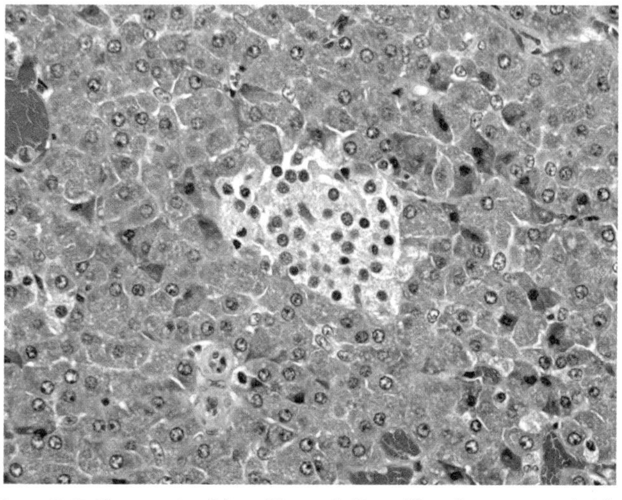

Figure 12-15 **Pancreatic Islet, Normal Dog.** The islet is surrounded by the exocrine pancreas. H&E stain. (Courtesy Dr. J.F. Zachary, College of Veterinary Medicine, University of Illinois.)

decreasing daylight hours. Melatonin binds receptors in the pituitary pars tuberalis and blocks the action of gonadotrophin-releasing hormone on the adenohypophysis. Lengthening of the photoperiod suppresses melatonin secretion, which explains increased reproductive activity in the spring, especially in seasonal breeders such as horses.

Chemoreceptor Organs

Chemoreceptor organs, such as the carotid bodies (near the bifurcation of the carotid arteries) and the aortic body (adjacent to the ascending aorta at the base of the heart), are clusters of glomus cells supported by glia-like cells. The glomus cells have numerous vesicles that contain various neurotransmitters (e.g., dopamine, catecholamines) used to relay their response to hypoxia to the nervous system. Lesions are not commonly encountered in the carotid or aortic bodies of domestic mammals, but the aortic body in particular is an occasional source of neuroendocrine neoplasia, known as chemodectoma, particularly in brachycephalic dogs.

Endocrine Activity in Adipose Tissue

In addition to its metabolic functions of synthesizing fatty acids and storing triglycerides, adipose tissue is a source of chemical compounds that are secreted into the blood and act on distant target cells in the hypothalamus, liver, and skeletal muscle, as examples. This ability qualifies adipocytes as cells capable of endocrine signaling. Two adipokines have particular metabolic importance: leptin and adiponectin. Leptin is involved in appetite suppression and heat generation, and it is proinflammatory. In contrast, adiponectin enhances glucose uptake and metabolism, and it is antiinflammatory. See subsequent sections on Obesity and on the Metabolic Syndrome under Disorders of Horses and Disorders of Pigs.

Dysfunction/Responses to Injury

Pathogenic Mechanisms of Endocrine Diseases

Endocrine organs are subject to all categories of injury, including degeneration and necrosis, vascular disturbances, inflammation from immune-mediated or infectious causes, and disturbances of growth (e.g., atrophy, hyperplasia, or neoplasia). However, the latter category accounts for a disproportionate number of diagnoses. Disturbances of growth (whether atrophic or proliferative) in an endocrine organ can alter its function and have striking effects on distant and diverse target organs. These target organ injuries often account for the clinical presentation and major lesions. For example, cutaneous lesions can reflect hypothyroidism or hyperadrenocorticism; hyperinsulinemia can manifest as seizures.

The clinical signs of endocrine disease reflect hypofunction or hyperfunction. Hypofunction of endocrine tissue usually indicates insufficient production or release of hormone(s); hyperfunction is usually the result of excessive hormone production. Endocrine dysfunction can also result from (1) inability of target cells to respond to hormones, (2) systemic disease or metabolic disturbances, or (3) administration of exogenous hormones.

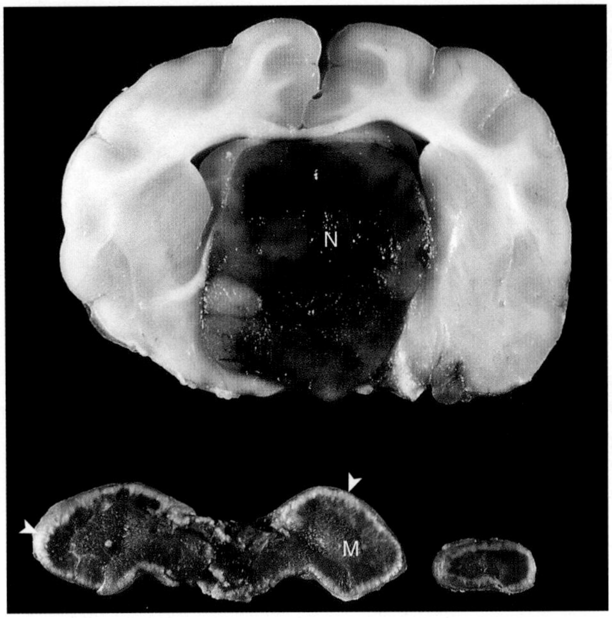

Figure 12-16 Secondary Adrenocortical Hypofunction; Brain with Neoplasm and Left *(Longitudinal Section)* and Right *(Cross Section)* Adrenal Glands, Dog. The neoplasm *(N)*, centered around the third ventricle, has invaded and destroyed the pituitary gland, hypothalamus, and most of the thalamus. Destruction of the adenohypophysis caused a lack of adrenocorticotrophic hormone (ACTH) and other trophic hormones, resulting in bilateral adrenocortical atrophy *(arrowheads)*, especially in the ACTH–dependent zonae fasciculata and reticularis, and (consequently) a relatively more prominent adrenal medulla *(M)*. (Courtesy Dr. C. Capen, College of Veterinary Medicine, The Ohio State University.)

Hypofunction of an Endocrine Gland

Primary Hypofunction. Hypofunction is considered primary if the hormonal deficiency is the result of a biochemical defect in synthesis (e.g., dyshormonogenetic goiter; see Congenital Dyshormonogenetic Goiter) or the result of either failure of glandular development (e.g., from aplasia or hypoplasia) or destruction of the secretory cells of the gland. An example of primary hypofunction caused by anomalous development is canine panhypopituitarism that results from failure of oropharyngeal ectoderm to differentiate into the adenohypophysis (anterior pituitary gland) (see Disorders of Dogs).

Most endocrine organs are susceptible to immune-mediated injury in which autoreactive T lymphocytes and autoantibodies selectively destroy endocrine cells. Unlike immune-mediated diseases, infectious diseases seldom selectively attack a particular endocrine organ; however, endocrine glands, especially the adrenal glands, are vulnerable to inflammation and necrosis in systemic infections and to metastatic neoplasia.

Secondary Hypofunction. Hypofunction is considered secondary if the causative defect or lesion arises outside the hypofunctioning gland. Often, this outcome involves injury of the pituitary gland with resultant trophic hormone deficiency. In other words, primary hypofunction of the pituitary gland causes secondary hypofunction of those endocrine glands that depend on its trophic hormones. In addition to the previously mentioned causes of (primary) pituitary hypofunction, nonfunctional (hormonally inactive) pituitary adenomas or even nearby neoplasms of nonpituitary origin can become large enough to destroy the adenohypophysis (anterior pituitary gland). Because neither the neoplasm nor the residual adenohypophyseal cells would then produce sufficient trophic hormones, atrophy with secondary hypofunction develops in target tissues, such as the adrenal cortex (Fig. 12-16), thyroid follicles, or gonads.

Hyperfunction of an Endocrine Gland

Primary Hyperfunction. In primary hyperfunction, the cells of the affected endocrine gland autonomously (i.e., without dependence on trophic hormone stimulation) synthesize and secrete excess hormone. This outcome is usually the result of a functional (i.e., hormone-producing) neoplasm. Examples and consequences of primary endocrine gland hyperfunction caused by neoplasms are listed in Table 12-1. Although primary neoplasia is the major cause of primary hyperfunction of an endocrine gland, hyperfunction is not the inevitable result of endocrine neoplasia. Nonfunctional endocrine neoplasms (and even once-functional neoplasms that lose their capacity to produce or secrete bioactive hormone) can, as they increase in size, destroy surrounding glandular tissue and result in hypofunction.

Secondary Hyperfunction. In secondary hyperfunction, excessive hormone production is a response to a signal (e.g., a trophic hormone) from outside the hyperfunctioning gland. A common example in dogs and cats is a functional neoplasm of adenohypophyseal (anterior pituitary gland) corticotrophs, in which prolonged and excessive secretion of ACTH causes diffuse adrenocortical hyperplasia of the zonae fasciculata and reticularis (Fig. 12-17) with resulting increased synthesis and secretion of cortisol. Theoretically, secondary hyperplasia and hyperfunction of an endocrine gland should subside when the stimulus of excessive trophic hormone is removed; however, chronic and severe hyperplasia is not always reversible. Endocrine cell proliferation can also be nodular or even

Table 12-1 Primary Hyperfunction of Endocrine Glands

Neoplasia	Hormone	Lesion/Sign
Somatotroph adenoma (pituitary gland)	Growth hormone	Acromegaly
Thyroid follicular cell adenoma	T_4, T_3	↑Basal metabolic rate
C-cell adenoma/carcinoma (thyroid gland)	Calcitonin	Osteosclerosis
Adrenocortical adenoma/carcinoma	Cortisol	Alopecia, polyuria/polydipsia
Pheochromocytoma (adrenal medulla)	Norepinephrine	Hypertension
Parathyroid chief cell adenoma	Parathyroid hormone	Hypercalcemia
Pancreatic β-cell adenoma/carcinoma	Insulin	Hypoglycemia

clonal, rather than diffuse. With long-term trophic hormone stimulation, there seems to be a continuum between focal or nodular hyperplasia and neoplasia.

Secondary hyperfunction can also develop in endocrine glands or cells that are not under the control of pituitary trophic hormones. In renal secondary hyperparathyroidism and nutritional secondary hyperparathyroidism (see Secondary Hyperparathyroidism), the parathyroid glands respond to decreased blood calcium concentrations with hyperplasia and increased production and secretion of PTH.

Hypersecretion of Hormones or Hormone-like Factors by Nonendocrine Neoplasms

Some nonendocrine neoplasms secrete biologically active humoral substances. Most of these hormone-like chemicals produced by neoplastic cells are peptides because nonpeptide hormones (steroids, iodothyronines, or catecholamines) have more complex synthetic pathways. Pseudohyperparathyroidism or humoral hypercalcemia of malignancy is a paraneoplastic syndrome caused by the autonomous hypersecretion of PTH–related peptide (PTHrP) by cancer cells. A well-characterized example is the canine apocrine carcinoma of the anal sac glands (see Disorders of Dogs). PTHrP acts as an agonist of the PTH receptor in target cells (e.g., in bone and kidney), leading to persistent hypercalcemia. Serum PTH concentration is decreased in response to the hypercalcemia, and PTH is not detectable in the neoplastic tissue.

Endocrine Dysfunction Caused by Failure of Target Cell Response

Endocrine dysfunction can be the result of failure of the target organ or tissue to respond to a hormone because of defective cell surface receptors or second messenger systems. For example, downregulation of insulin receptors on target cells (especially adipocytes, hepatocytes, or myocytes) can result in insulin resistance in obese animals.

Iatrogenic Syndromes of Hormone Excess

The administration of exogenous hormones has far-reaching effects on diverse populations of target cells and can result in clinically important functional disturbances. The long-term administration of glucocorticoids, used to treat a variety of conditions, can reproduce most of the abnormalities of spontaneous adrenocortical

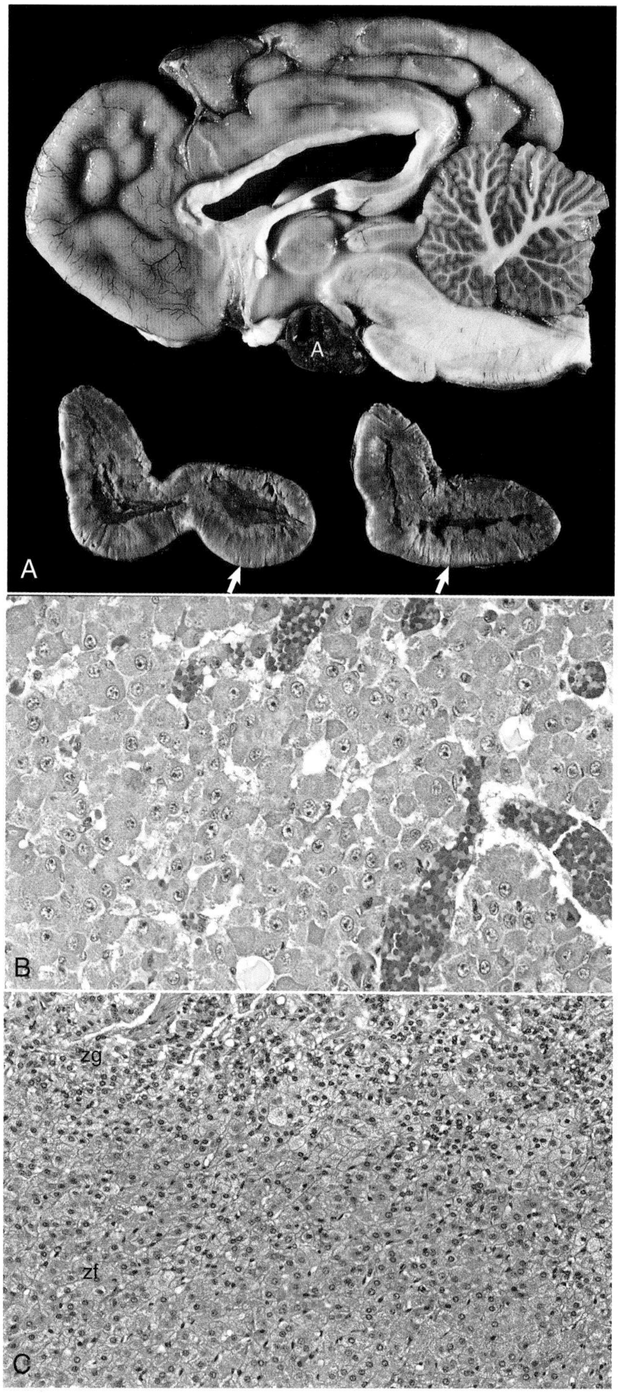

Figure 12-17 **Secondary Adrenocortical Hyperfunction (Pituitary-Dependent Hyperadrenocorticism); Brain, Pituitary Gland and Adrenal Glands, Dog. A,** A functional corticotroph (adrenocorticotrophic hormone [ACTH]-secreting) adenoma *(A)* in the pituitary gland caused diffuse and bilateral adrenocortical hyperplasia *(arrows)* leading to excessive secretion of cortisol (hyperadrenocorticism) by the zonae fasciculata and reticularis. **B,** Adenohypophysis. The corticotroph adenoma consists of a sheet of monotonous chromophobic cells with abundant pale amphophilic cytoplasm. Note the lack of acidophils. H&E stain. **C,** Adrenal cortex. Diffuse adrenocortical hyperplasia. Cells in the zona fasciculata (*zf*) are enlarged with abundant lipid-vacuolated cytoplasm. Zona glomerulosa (*zg*, *top*) is unaffected. H&E stain. (**A** courtesy Dr. C. Capen, College of Veterinary Medicine, The Ohio State University. **B** and **C** courtesy Dr. M.A. Miller, College of Veterinary Medicine, Purdue University.)

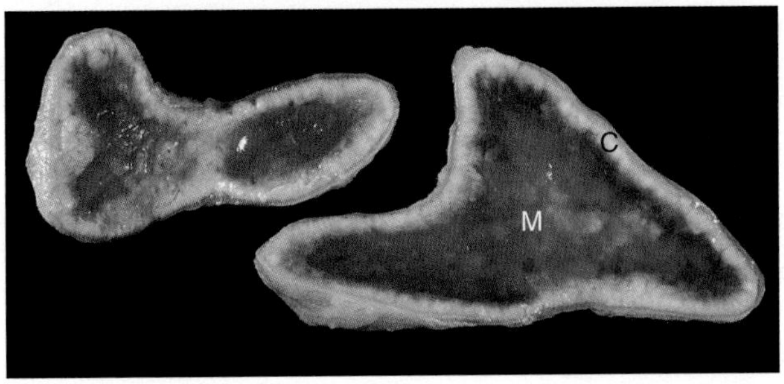

Figure 12-18 **Iatrogenic Hyperadrenocorticism, Left and Right Adrenal Glands, Dog.** Hyperadrenocorticism, caused by long-term administration of exogenous glucocorticosteroids, has resulted in trophic atrophy of the adrenocorticotrophic hormone (ACTH)–dependent zonae fasciculata and reticularis of the adrenal cortex *(C)*. Consequentially, the adrenal medulla *(M)* comprises a relatively greater proportion of the cross-sectional area. (Courtesy Dr. C. Capen, College of Veterinary Medicine, The Ohio State University.)

hyperfunction. However, although naturally occurring adrenocortical hyperfunction is usually the result of a disrupted hypothalamic-pituitary-adrenocortical axis with hyperplasia or neoplasia of endocrine cells, iatrogenic glucocorticoid excess tends to cause profound atrophy of the adrenal cortex (especially in the ACTH-dependent zonae fasciculata and reticularis) via negative feedback through an intact hypothalamic-pituitary-adrenocortical axis (Fig. 12-18). Likewise, long-term administration of exogenous thyroid hormones results in negative feedback on the hypothalamus and on adenohypophyseal (anterior pituitary gland) thyrotrophs with diminished TSH secretion and thyroid follicular atrophy (see Fig. 12-8, *B*).

Exogenous sex hormones can also result in endocrine imbalances. For example, the administration of synthetic progestins, such as medroxyprogesterone acetate (also known as megestrol acetate), can induce mammary hypertrophy and hyperplasia in both male and female cats and dogs (see Chapter 18). Because hyperplastic mammary epithelial cells are an extrapituitary source of growth hormone, some progestin-treated dogs also develop acromegaly (E-Fig. 12-8).

Portals of Entry/Pathways of Spread

Endocrine tissue is well vascularized, so the most common route of entry of a potentially injurious agent—be it microorganisms, leukocytes, trophic hormones, or an exogenous endocrine disruptor—is hematogenous. In addition, inflammation or other disease processes in adjacent tissues can extend to endocrine organs. The pituitary gland, with its neurohypophyseal (posterior pituitary gland) connection to the hypothalamus and third ventricle of the brain and its adenohypophyseal (anterior pituitary gland) origin from the craniopharyngeal duct, is particularly susceptible to extension of inflammation or neoplasia from the brain or from the pharynx.

Defense Mechanisms/Barrier Systems

Because of their ample blood supply, endocrine tissues are subjected to the benefits and potential harm of inflammation and innate and/or adaptive immune responses. The pituitary gland gains some protection from pharyngeal microbiota by its bony encasement in the sella turcica but, at the same time, is more susceptible than the brain to hematogenous insults because of its lack of a blood-brain barrier. In general, because endocrine cells need ready access to the bloodstream in order to secrete their hormones, they are vulnerable to injury by chemical or infectious agents that arrive hematogenously. Most endocrine glands are protected from the external environment by their deep-seated location and from neighboring tissues or body cavities by a thin capsule of fibrous tissue.

Disorders of Domestic Animals[5]

Disorders that are known or thought to have a genetic basis are listed in E-Table 12-1.

Disorders of the Adenohypophysis (Anterior Pituitary Gland)

Developmental Disorders of the Adenohypophysis

Aplasia and Prolonged Gestation. See Disorders of Ruminants (Cattle, Sheep, and Goats).

Pituitary Cysts and Pituitary Dwarfism. See Disorders of Dogs.

Proliferative Disorders of the Adenohypophysis

Hyperplasia and neoplasia are important lesions of the adenohypophysis. Physiologic hyperplasia is the result of stimulation through the hypothalamic-pituitary-target organ axis and tends to affect the trophic hormone–producing cells of interest throughout the adenohypophysis. In contrast, pathologic proliferation tends to be focal or multifocal. Nodular proliferations of cells in the pars distalis or pars intermedia that are multiple and smaller than 1 mm in diameter are classified as hyperplasia. Hyperplastic nodules do not disrupt the reticulin scaffolding of the adenohypophysis, but they can be recognized histologically because the nodule is composed of a monotonous population of one cell type, such as chromophobes (Fig. 12-19, A), instead of the normal mixture of chromophobes and acidophils. Immunohistochemistry can be used to identify the trophic hormone produced. Hyperplastic nodules are seldom large enough to be evident on clinical diagnostic imaging or gross examination; nevertheless, they can secrete excessive bioactive trophic hormones and, thus, be responsible for secondary hyperfunction of the targeted endocrine organs, depending on which trophic hormone is produced.

Adenohypophyseal (anterior pituitary gland) neoplasms are usually solitary and almost always classified as adenomas rather than carcinomas. It is plausible that hyperplastic nodules of adenohypophyseal cells could become clonal or that multiple nodules could coalesce to form an adenoma. Importantly, smaller adenohypophyseal lesions (whether hyperplastic or neoplastic [microadenomas]) are more likely to be functional—that is, to produce and release trophic hormones into the peripheral blood—whereas macroadenomas (Fig. 12-19, *B*) exert their effect mainly through destruction of adjacent pituitary parenchyma, often resulting in insufficient (rather than excessive) trophic hormone(s) or through compression of surrounding tissue, such as optic nerves or overlying hypothalamus. In addition to classifying nonphysiologic pituitary proliferations as hyperplastic nodules, microadenomas, or macroadenomas, it is useful to determine the type of trophic hormone produced by the proliferating cells. In veterinary medicine, this goal is generally accomplished by a combination of biochemical analysis of serum, clinical signs, and/or immunohistochemistry on surgical biopsy or autopsy (syn: necropsy; see E-Appendix 12-1) specimens of affected

[5]Postmortem examination of the endocrine system is discussed in E-Appendix 12-1.

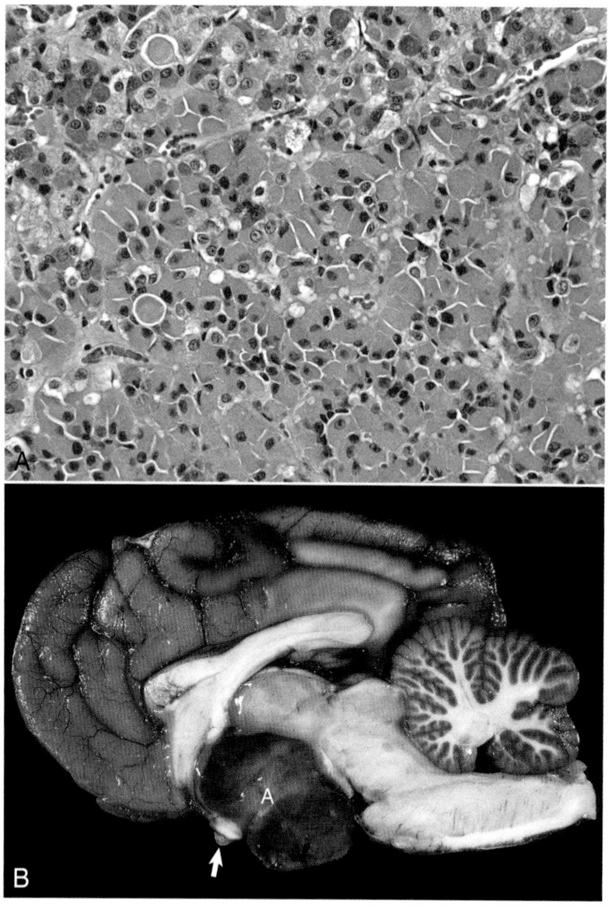

Figure 12-19 **Adenohypophyseal Hyperplasia and Neoplasia, Pituitary Gland. A,** Corticotroph hyperplasia, cat. A hyperplastic nodule (*lower right two-thirds*), less than 1 mm in diameter, is composed of packets of monomorphic chromophobes with abundant amphophilic cytoplasm. Adjacent normal adenohypophyseal tissue (*upper left one-third*) is a mixture of acidophils and (smaller) chromophobes. H&E stain. **B,** Pituitary macroadenoma, dog. The large adenoma (*A*) compresses the brain and optic chiasm (*arrow*). The adenohypophysis (anterior pituitary gland), neurohypophysis (posterior pituitary gland), and hypothalamus have been destroyed by the neoplasm. (**A** courtesy Dr. M.A. Miller, College of Veterinary Medicine, Purdue University. **B** courtesy Dr. C. Capen, College of Veterinary Medicine, The Ohio State University.)

pituitary gland. Immunohistochemical expression of trophic hormone in the cytoplasm of adenohypophyseal cells does not necessarily correlate with increased plasma concentrations of bioactive hormone. In poorly differentiated pituitary neoplasms that do not express detectable immunoreactive hormone, polymerase chain reaction (PCR) testing for mRNA of trophic hormones can be used to determine the cell of origin.

Pituitary Carcinomas. Pituitary carcinomas are exceedingly rare, but that is at least partly due to stringent classification criteria. By convention, to be classified as malignant, a pituitary neoplasm must metastasize, not merely invade, either within the central nervous system or systemically.

Adenomas of the Pars Distalis. Adenomas can arise from any of the trophic hormone–producing cells of the pars distalis. Depending on the cell lineage, the neoplastic cells may produce more than one type of trophic hormone. Of the domestic animal species, pars distalis adenomas are most commonly diagnosed in cats and dogs. Most canine pars distalis adenomas are derived from corticotrophs; feline adenomas are usually derived from corticotrophs or somatotrophs. Pars distalis adenomas that are 1 to 5 mm in diameter are classified as microadenomas; those adenomas that are larger are classified as macroadenomas (see Fig. 12-19, *B*). Somewhat surprisingly, the smaller microadenomas are more likely to secrete bioactive trophic hormone, whereas large macroadenomas tend to have a compressive mass effect[6] rather than a trophic hormone effect. In fact, large pituitary neoplasms are likely to result in decreased trophic hormone secretion with hypopituitarism and atrophy (secondary hypofunction) of the targeted endocrine glands. Histologically, pituitary adenomas are composed of polyhedral or piriform cells that tend to be larger, with more abundant cytoplasm, than nonneoplastic pars distalis cells, but they usually have only mild nuclear atypia and few mitotic figures. Because corticotroph adenomas and somatotroph adenomas are the more common pars distalis neoplasms, they are discussed in the following sections. Neoplasms of thyrotrophs or lactotrophs are less commonly reported in the domestic species.

Corticotroph Adenomas. Functional (ACTH-secreting) corticotroph adenomas are an important cause of canine hyperadrenocorticism (secondary adrenocortical hyperfunction or pituitary-dependent hyperadrenocorticism) and arise in the pars distalis of dogs and cats or, less commonly, in the pars intermedia of dogs. Corticotroph adenomas are rare in the other domestic species. The larger macroadenomas can obliterate most of the pituitary gland, resulting in panhypopituitarism with secondary hypofunction of target endocrine organs, and compress the neurohypophysis, optic chiasm, hypothalamus, and thalamus.

Histologically, corticotroph adenomas of the pars distalis are composed of chromophobic cells arranged in sinusoidal or diffuse patterns (see Fig. 12-17, *B*). The sinusoidal pattern consists of packets of polyhedral neoplastic cells surrounded by thin fibrovascular septa and more elongated neoplastic cells that palisade around sinusoids. In the diffuse pattern, neoplastic cells are arranged in sheets. Neoplastic cells in both patterns are often larger than nonneoplastic chromophobes, with a large hypochromatic nucleus, one or two distinct nucleoli, few mitotic figures, and ample pale eosinophilic to amphophilic cytoplasm with distinct cell boundaries. Secretory granules are numerous but may be inconspicuous or impart only a finely granular pale acidophilic or basophilic appearance to the cytoplasm. Neoplastic cells are immunohistochemically positive for ACTH and may be positive for endorphins. Ultrastructurally, the neoplastic cells have well-developed rough ER and Golgi and numerous small (~170 nm in diameter) dense-core secretory granules.

Somatotroph Adenomas. Somatotroph adenomas have been reported mainly in cats, dogs, and sheep. Hypersecretion of growth hormone (GH), also known as somatotrophin (STH), promotes hepatocellular synthesis and secretion of insulin-like growth factor-1 (IGF-1). Feline somatotroph adenomas are often associated with acromegaly and insulin-resistant diabetes mellitus.

Somatotrophic Hormone (STH)–Producing Tumors. See Disorders of Cats.

Adenomas of the Pars Intermedia. Equine pituitary adenomas (Fig. 12-20) almost always develop in the pars intermedia. In

[6]Compression of normal tissues adjacent to the mass resulting in atrophy and/or necrosis of affected cells and reduced blood supply to the tissue.

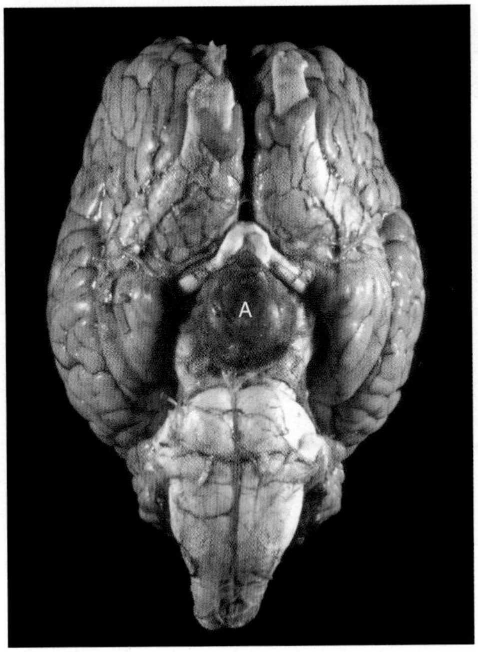

Figure 12-20 Adenoma, Brain, Pituitary Gland, Horse. The pituitary gland is enlarged by an adenoma *(A)* in the pars intermedia. (Courtesy College of Veterinary Medicine, University of Illinois.)

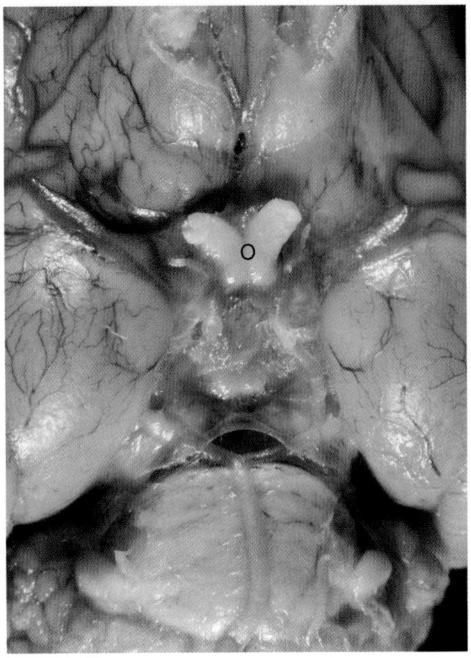

Figure 12-21 Iatrogenic Adenohypophyseal Atrophy, Dog. The adenohypophysis (anterior pituitary gland) in this dog, treated with the somatostatin analog pasireotide for a corticotroph macroadenoma, was so small that it was detectable only histologically. O, Optic chiasm. (Courtesy Dr. D. Bruyette, VCA West Los Angeles Animal Hospital and Dr. M.A. Miller, College of Veterinary Medicine, Purdue University.)

addition, the pars intermedia is the second most common site (after pars distalis) for canine pituitary adenomas, but it is a rare site in the other domestic species. Interestingly, pars intermedia adenomas are practically nonexistent in human beings because the pars intermedia shrinks after fetal life and is only vestigial in adults.

Corticotroph Adenomas. Canine corticotroph adenomas of the pars intermedia tend to be smaller than those in the pars distalis. The presence of colloid-filled follicles interspersed among the chromophobic neoplastic cells serves to distinguish the pars intermedia adenoma from one that originated in the pars distalis. Functional adenomas can result in hyperadrenocorticism; nonfunctional adenomas can cause hypopituitarism or diabetes insipidus secondary to destruction of the neurohypophysis (posterior pituitary gland) or compression of the hypothalamus (i.e., mass effect). Pituitary-dependent hyperadrenocorticism has been documented rarely in cats with corticotroph adenomas of the pars intermedia. Immunohistochemically, the neoplastic cells of pars intermedia corticotroph adenomas typically express both ACTH and α-MSH.

Melanotroph Adenomas. Melanotroph adenomas, derived from cells that produce proopiomelanocortin (POMC)-derived peptides, are the major pituitary neoplasm in horses but are rarely reported in other species.

See Disorders of Horses.

Miscellaneous Disorders of the Adenohypophysis (Anterior Pituitary Gland)

Cellular Atrophy, Degeneration, and Death. Physiologic hypophyseal atrophy is the result of negative feedback from targeted endocrine organs through the hypothalamic-pituitary-target organ axis. This results in selective atrophy of a specific type of trophic hormone–producing cell. For example, increased plasma concentration of thyroxine causes atrophy of thyrotrophs without affecting other adenohypophyseal cells. Therefore, physiologic atrophy seldom causes grossly appreciable shrinkage of the adenohypophysis. In contrast, profound and generalized adenohypophyseal atrophy can be induced by treatment with the somatostatin analogue pasireotide (Fig. 12-21).[7] Injectable pasireotide is used as an alternative to surgical treatment of corticotroph adenomas, and it works by binding somatostatin receptors, which can be overexpressed on neoplastic corticotrophs. Somatostatin is so named because it inhibits the release of growth hormone from adenohypophyseal somatotrophs. In addition to the hypothalamus, other organs and tissues, notably the δ cells of the pancreatic islets, produce somatostatin. Somatostatin inhibits not only the release of growth hormone from somatotrophs but also that of insulin and glucagon from pancreatic islet cells and that of ACTH from corticotrophs.

Hypophyseal degeneration or necrosis can also result from compression by a mass within the pituitary gland or in adjacent tissue (see Fig. 12-16). Alternatively, degeneration can be secondary to vascular disturbances or to inflammation in the pituitary gland (hypophysitis). The term *pituitary apoplexy* is used for acute hemorrhagic infarction of the hypophysis, usually in association with a pituitary neoplasm. This condition is diagnosed mainly in human beings, but it has been reported in dogs.

Inflammation. The pituitary gland can become inflamed as part of a systemic infection, but there are few, if any, infectious agents that target the hypophysis. In a systemic infection, the microbial agent reaches the hypophysis hematogenously. The blood-brain barrier does not protect the hypophysis. Pituitary inflammation, often abscess formation, can also develop as an extension of inflammation from adjacent (e.g., pharyngeal) tissue. Lymphoplasmacytic hypophysitis is thought to be an immune-mediated (probably

[7]Pasireotide is a somatostatin analogue that has a 40-fold increased affinity for somatostatin receptor type 5 (SSTR5). Its trade name is Signifor (Novartis Pharmaceuticals Corporation).

autoimmune) disease and has been described in the canine pituitary gland, but it is less common than similar inflammatory processes in the thyroid or adrenal glands.

Disorders of the Neurohypophysis (Posterior Pituitary Gland)

Diabetes Insipidus

Diabetes insipidus is a form of polyuria caused by an inability to concentrate urine. It is the result of inadequate synthesis and release of antidiuretic hormone (ADH) in the central or hypophyseal form of the disorder or the result of the failure of renal tubular epithelial cells to respond to ADH in the nephrogenic form. In either form, hypotonic urine (with osmolality equivalent to or less than that of plasma) is produced, even in the face of water deprivation. The hypophyseal form of diabetes insipidus can be caused by any process that compresses or destroys the pars nervosa, infundibular stalk, or the supraoptic nucleus (so named for its hypothalamic location just dorsal to the optic chiasm). The hypophyseal form can be distinguished from the nephrogenic form of diabetes insipidus by the ability of the patient to concentrate urine after administration of ADH.

Neoplasms

Most neoplasms of the pars nervosa are extensions of adenohypophyseal (anterior pituitary gland) adenomas. Brain tumors, particularly ependymomas (see Chapter 14) of the third ventricle, also can extend through the infundibular stalk into the pars nervosa. The pituicytoma is a primary neoplasm of the pituicyte, the glial cell of the pars nervosa. The pituicyte is considered a variant of astrocytes and expresses glial fibrillary acidic protein immunohistochemically.

Other Neoplastic Disorders of the Hypophysis

Secondary Neoplasms

Unprotected by the blood-brain barrier, the pituitary gland is vulnerable to metastatic neoplasia. The pars nervosa may be particularly susceptible because of its direct blood supply from the carotid artery. The more common secondary neoplasms of the hypophysis are lymphoma in various species, equine and canine melanoma, and canine thyroid and mammary carcinomas. Secondary neoplasms can also be extensions from adjacent tumors, such as osteosarcoma of the sella turcica or ependymoma of the third ventricle.

Suprasellar Neoplasms

Although most tumors arising in or above the sella turcica (i.e., suprasellar) originate in the pituitary gland, less common suprasellar neoplasms include meningioma, craniopharyngioma, and germ cell tumors. Suprasellar meningiomas resemble those at other locations (see Chapter 14). Whereas pituitary neoplasms are more common in older animals, craniopharyngiomas and germ cell tumors tend to arise in young adult animals.

Craniopharyngiomas (Fig. 12-22, *A* and *B*) are rare epithelial tumors that are thought to be derived from the craniopharyngeal duct and Rathke's pouch remnants. Two histologic patterns are recognized in human beings: the adamantinomatous form, which is more common in childhood and resembles odontogenic tumors such as ameloblastoma, and the squamous (pseudo)papillary form, which occurs mainly in adults and is thought to develop from metaplasia of adenohypophyseal (anterior pituitary gland) cells in the pars tuberalis. Both histologic patterns are recognized in domestic mammals, in which craniopharyngioma has been reported only in dogs and cats, and usually in young animals. The neoplastic tissue consists of nests of polyhedral epithelial cells in fibrous stroma. The neoplastic epithelial cells have eosinophilic cytoplasm, distinct cell borders, and faint intercellular bridges. The cells express cytokeratins immunohistochemically. Tubular formations lined by ciliated cells and goblet cells in some areas of the tumor reflect its association with the craniopharyngeal duct. Reported veterinary cases have

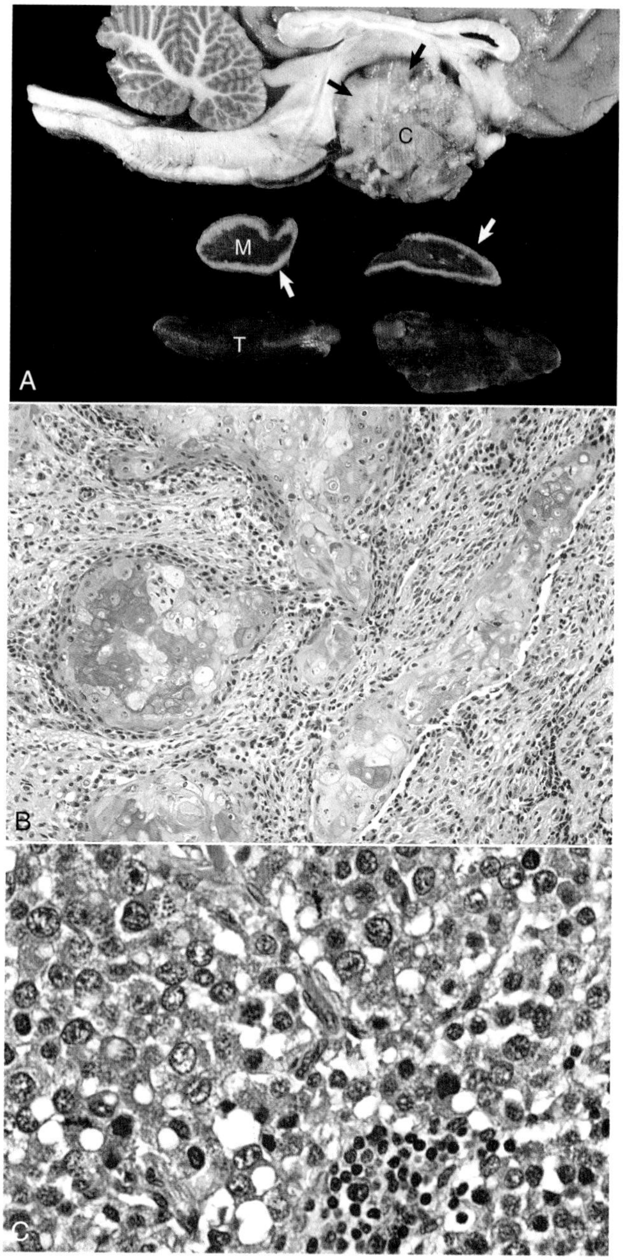

Figure 12-22 **Non-Pituitary Suprasellar Neoplasms, Dogs. A,** Craniopharyngioma *(C)*, left and right adrenal glands and thyroid lobes. The neoplasm has extended dorsally through the hypothalamus and compressed the thalamus *(black arrows)*. Destruction of the pituitary gland resulted in trophic atrophy of the adrenal cortices *(white arrows)*, leaving a prominent medulla *(M)* surrounded by remaining cortical tissue (mainly zona glomerulosa). Thyroid follicles were also atrophied, but colloid involution maintained the overall thyroid *(T)* size within normal limits. **B,** The craniopharyngioma is composed of interconnecting nests of keratinizing epithelial cells in fibrous stroma. H&E stain. **C,** Suprasellar germ cell tumors consist predominantly of seminoma-like germ cells with fewer lipid-laden hepatoid cells and scattered aggregates of small lymphocytes. H&E stain. (**A** courtesy Dr. C. Capen, College of Veterinary Medicine, The Ohio State University. **B** and **C** courtesy Dr. M.A. Miller, College of Veterinary Medicine, Purdue University.)

been expansile or infiltrative, but the mitotic index is typically low. Although malignant craniopharyngioma was diagnosed in two cats, metastasis was not reported.

Suprasellar neoplasms with a population of germ cells, teratomatous features, or immunoreactivity for α-fetoprotein should be classified as suprasellar germ cell tumors (Fig. 12-22, C). Intracranial germ cell tumors have been described only in the suprasellar location and only in dogs of the domestic animal species. These infiltrative neoplasms obliterate the pituitary gland and compress the hypothalamus. The predominant cell type is a germ cell that resembles the neoplastic cells of testicular seminoma. As in seminoma, aggregates of small lymphocytes are commonly scattered through the neoplastic stroma. Suprasellar germ cell tumors also include nests of lipid-laden hepatoid cells and may have scattered tubular formations lined by endodermal cells or other teratomatous features.

Disorders of the Thyroid Gland

Disorders of the thyroid gland are clinically important if they result in thyroid hormone deficiency (hypothyroidism) or excess (hyperthyroidism), or if they produce a mass effect. Other disorders of the thyroid gland may be subclinical and of little importance to the animal.

Developmental Malformations

Ectopic Thyroid Tissue. Ectopic thyroid tissue is usually encountered from the base of the tongue along the path of descent of the developing gland, but it can migrate as far caudally as the diaphragm. In dogs, functional nodules of thyroid tissue are common near the ascending aorta at the base of the heart. Functional ectopic thyroid tissue is a source of hormone production after thyroidectomy. It also can be a site of thyroid carcinoma, mainly in dogs, and usually in a mediastinal location. See Disorders of Dogs, Heart-Base Neoplasms Derived from Ectopic Thyroid Gland Tissue.

Accessory Thyroid Tissue and Thyroglossal Duct Cysts. Accessory thyroid tissue is derived from remnants of the thyroglossal duct. Thyroglossal duct remnants can also form cysts or sinus tracts along the ventral midline of the neck. The cysts that develop near the base of the tongue are typically lined by stratified squamous epithelium, whereas those nearer the thyroid cartilage of the larynx are more likely to be lined by epithelium that resembles that of thyroid follicles. Grossly, the cysts contain watery to mucoid secretions. They seldom exceed 1 cm in diameter, but they can become inflamed, rupture, and form a fistulous tract to the skin. Rarely, thyroglossal duct cysts undergo malignant transformation to carcinoma.

Follicular Hyperplasia and Goiter

The term goiter denotes a nonneoplastic enlargement of the thyroid gland (Fig. 12-23, A) as a result of follicular cell hyperplasia (Fig. 12-23, B; also see Fig. 12-8, A), although follicular hyperplasia does not always cause grossly appreciable enlargement. The causes for follicular hyperplasia include iodine deficiency, iodine excess, goitrogens, and defects in the synthesis of thyroid hormones. Goiter can be diffuse (throughout the gland) or multinodular. Diffuse goiter is typically a compensatory, TSH-induced response to hypothyroidism (decreased plasma concentrations of T_4 and T_3). In contrast, multinodular goiter in old cats (Fig. 12-24, A and B) consists of hyperplastic follicular cells that function autonomously (independent of TSH) with resultant hyperthyroidism. Unaffected follicular cells (those outside the hyperplastic nodules) undergo atrophy because of the low plasma concentration of TSH (Fig. 12-24, C).

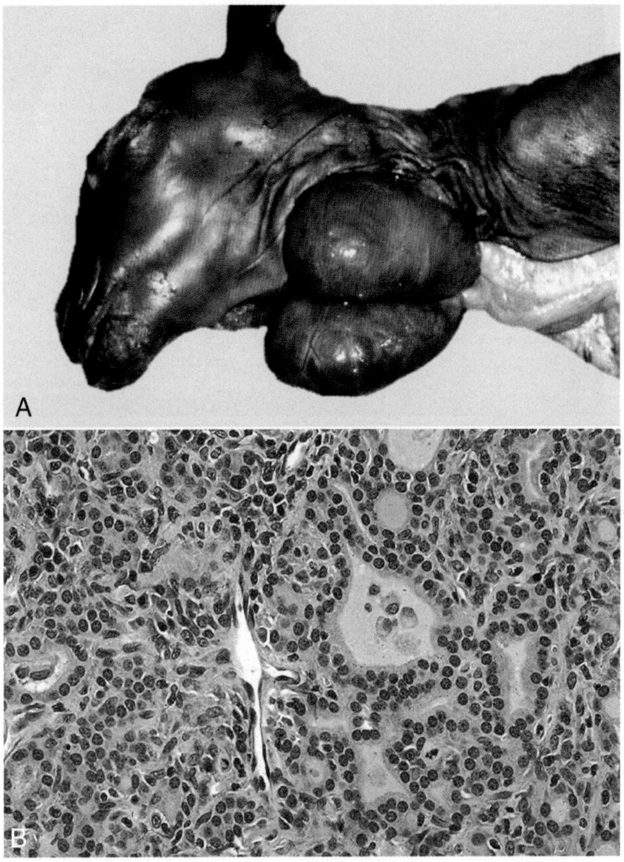

Figure 12-23 Hyperplastic Goiter, Thyroid Gland, Goat. A, Deficiency of maternal dietary iodine during pregnancy resulted in hyperplasia (and hypertrophy) of thyroid follicular cells in this perinatal goat with symmetric enlargement of both lobes (goiter). **B,** Follicular cells are increased in number and size, impinging on the follicular lumen. H&E stain. (**A** courtesy Dr. O. Hedstrom, College of Veterinary Medicine, Oregon State University; and Noah's Arkive, College of Veterinary Medicine, The University of Georgia. **B** courtesy Dr. B. Harmon, College of Veterinary Medicine, The University of Georgia; and Noah's Arkive, College of Veterinary Medicine, The University of Georgia.)

Iodine Deficiency. Iodine deficiency, especially during the fetal and neonatal period when the need for thyroid hormones is greatest, is the major cause of diffuse goiter in certain geographic regions—for example, the Pacific Northwest and the Great Lakes region—especially in horses, cattle, small ruminants, and pigs without dietary iodine supplementation. Without sufficient iodine, deficient synthesis of T_4 and T_3 results in TSH-induced hyperplastic goiter (see Fig. 12-8, A). Grossly, the thyroid gland in hyperplastic goiter is diffusely enlarged and reddened (Fig. 12-25, A; also see Fig. 12-23, A). Histologically, increased vascularity explains the reddening of the gland. Follicles are irregularly enlarged in hyperplastic goiter, but their luminal diameter is diminished because the crowded and hypertrophied (tall columnar) follicular cells form papillary projections into the follicular lumen (E-Fig. 12-9; also see Fig. 12-23, B). Colloid is paler (less eosinophilic) than normal. The periphery of the colloid has a scalloped appearance because of the formation of endocytic resorption vacuoles at the apical surface of the follicular cells (see Fig. 12-8, A). Some hyperplastic follicles may lack apparent colloid or have a collapsed lumen.

Despite a robust response to TSH, many iodine-deficient fetuses and neonates have extrathyroidal lesions, such as myxedema (accumulation of glycosaminoglycans and water in the dermis and

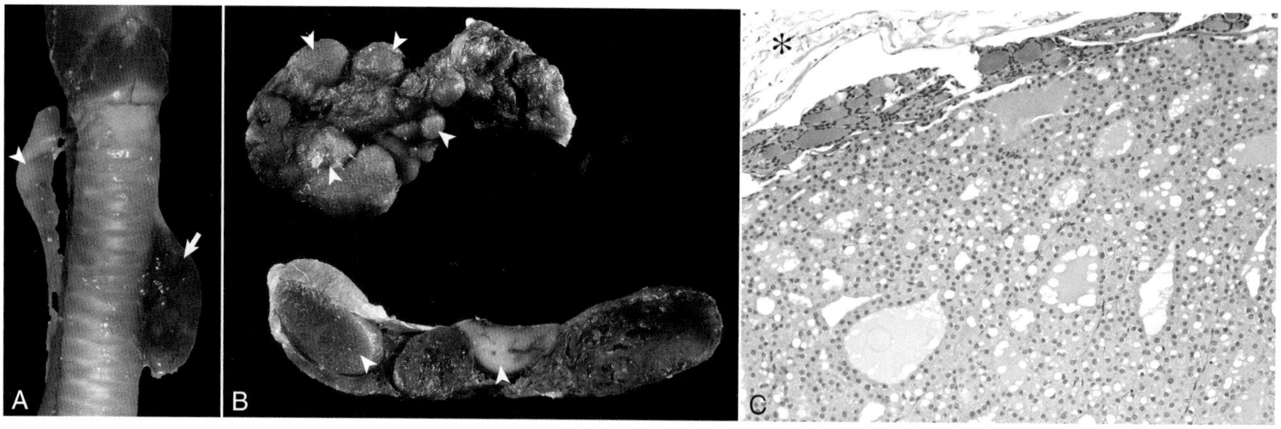

Figure 12-24 **Hyperplasia, Hyperthyroidism, Thyroid Gland, Cats. A,** Larynx, trachea, and thyroid gland. Multinodular hyperplasia in the left *(arrow)* thyroid lobe with atrophy of the right *(arrowhead)* lobe. **B,** Thyroid gland, formalin-fixed. Multinodular follicular hyperplasia *(arrowheads)* involves both thyroid lobes. **C,** Thyroid gland. A hyperplastic nodule is well demarcated from atrophied follicles just beneath the thyroid capsule *(asterisk)*, and it consists of follicles of various diameter, lined by hypertrophied but well-differentiated follicular cells and filled with pale eosinophilic colloid with peripheral resorption vacuoles. H&E stain. (**A** courtesy Dr. M.A. Miller, College of Veterinary Medicine, Purdue University. **B** courtesy Dr. C. Capen, College of Veterinary Medicine, The Ohio State University. **C** courtesy Dr. M.A. Miller, College of Veterinary Medicine, Purdue University.)

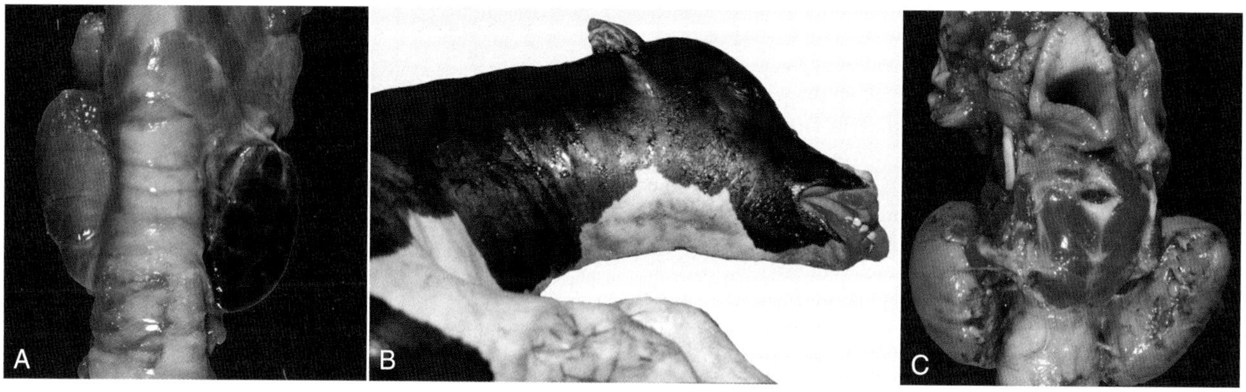

Figure 12-25 **Iodine-Deficiency Goiter in Fetal or Neonatal Animals. A,** Hyperplastic goiter in a foal. Thyroid-stimulating hormone (TSH)–induced follicular cell hyperplasia and increased blood supply impart a deep red color to the enlarged gland. **B,** Near-term bovine fetus with goiter (thyroid gland, not visible), alopecia, and myxedema causing swelling of the soft tissues of the neck. **C,** Colloid goiter in a foal. If iodine deficiency is corrected, hyperplastic goiter undergoes colloid involution. The thyroid gland remains enlarged, but it becomes pale from the accumulation of colloid and the decreased vascularity. (Courtesy Dr. M.A. Miller, College of Veterinary Medicine, Purdue University.)

subcutis) or less hair or wool than expected for the gestational stage, that indicate hypothyroidism (Fig. 12-25, *B*). However, the hypertrophy and hyperplasia of follicular cells does increase their ability to extract available iodide from the blood. Therefore, with correction of the dietary iodine deficiency or with the decreased postnatal demand for thyroid hormones, the hyperplastic thyroid gland may produce sufficient circulating T_4 and T_3 to result in negative feedback on the hypothalamus and hypophysis with diminished TSH secretion. In response to decreased TSH, hyperplastic goiter undergoes involution to colloid goiter (Fig. 12-25, *C*). The thyroid gland remains enlarged, but its color fades from a deep red-brown to pale brown (because of decreased vascularity) and takes on an almost translucent appearance because of the colloid-distended follicles. Histologically, the follicles are distended by intensely stained (eosinophilic or periodic acid–Schiff [PAS]-positive) colloid without the endocytic resorption vacuoles of hyperplastic goiter (see Fig. 12-8, *B*). Although a few papillary projections may remain, the atrophied follicular epithelium becomes low cuboidal. Foals born to mares that grazed endophyte-infected fescue pasture during pregnancy may have thyroid follicular atrophy, low thyroid hormone concentrations, and delayed parturition.

Goitrogens. Goitrogens are compounds, including plants, drugs, and other chemicals, that cause hyperplastic goiter. Marginal iodine deficiency increases the sensitivity of the thyroid gland to goitrogens. Cruciferous plants (genus *Brassica*) are goitrogenic because they contain glucosinolates (sulfur-containing glucosides) that are converted in the intestine to glucose and by-products, such as isothiocyanates, by the enzyme myrosinase derived from the plant or from the intestinal tract. Thiocyanates, perchlorates, and certain other ions compete with iodide for uptake by thyroid follicular cells. Phenobarbital, rifampin, and certain other medicinal compounds are goitrogenic because they increase the degradation of T_4 and T_3.

Somewhat paradoxically, excessive iodine can also be goitrogenic, perhaps by interfering with the proteolysis of colloidal thyroglobulin and thereby inhibiting thyroid hormone secretion. Because iodide is concentrated in the milk, foals of mares fed kelp or seaweed as an iodine supplement are exposed to higher iodide concentrations than their dams and can develop hyperplastic goiter.

Congenital Dyshormonogenetic Goiter. Defective thyroid hormone synthesis (dyshormonogenesis) causes congenital hypothyroidism even when dietary iodine is adequate. Congenital dyshormonogenetic goiter has been linked to genetic defects in thyroglobulin synthesis or in the enzymes thyroid peroxidase or dual oxidase 2 (DUOX2), the oxidase that produces H_2O_2 needed by thyroid peroxidase.

Congenital dyshormonogenetic goiter has been described as an autosomal recessive trait, mainly in sheep (Fig. 12-26) and goats, and rarely in cattle, dogs, and cats. Thyroid peroxidase mutations that result in defective iodide oxidation and organification (binding of iodine to tyrosyl moieties) have been documented in dogs and cats. Ruminants with congenital dyshormonogenetic goiter had defective thyroglobulin synthesis despite normal iodide uptake and organification. Affected animals are born with massive TSH-induced hyperplastic goiter and typically have features of hypothyroidism, such as myxedema, sparse wool or hair, and decreased somatic growth in those that survive the neonatal period.

Multinodular Goiter. Multifocal follicular hyperplasia in geriatric horses or dogs is typically an incidental finding without notable enlargement of the thyroid gland or functional consequences. In contrast, middle-aged to older cats develop multinodular toxic (hyperthyroid) goiter (see Fig. 12-24; also see Disorders of Cats).

Follicular Atrophy

Colloid Goiter. Colloid goiter is the involutional stage of hyperplastic goiter after repletion of dietary iodine in the case of iodine-deficient goiter (see the preceding section) or with diminished need for thyroid hormones as the animal matures. Although the thyroid gland remains enlarged in colloid goiter, the follicular cells have undergone atrophy because of decreased TSH release from adenohypophyseal (anterior pituitary gland) thyrotrophs.

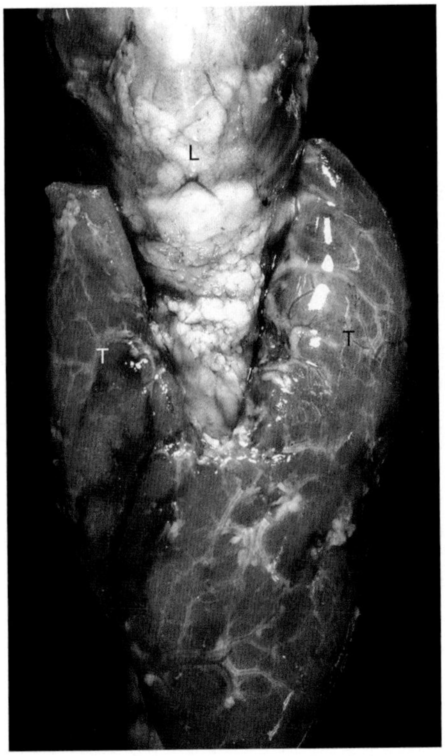

Figure 12-26 **Congenital Dyshormonogenetic Goiter, Thyroid Gland, Lamb.** The symmetrically enlarged thyroid (*T*) lobes are fused at the midline ventral to the larynx (*L*) and trachea. (Courtesy Dr. C. Capen, College of Veterinary Medicine, The Ohio State University.)

Idiopathic Follicular Atrophy. See Disorders of Dogs, Hypothyroidism.

Lymphocytic (Immune-Mediated) Thyroiditis. Autoimmune thyroid disease, with infiltration of the gland by thyroid-reactive lymphocytes, is thought to be triggered by the interaction of genetic and environmental factors (e.g., excessive iodine, infections, pregnancy). In Hashimoto's thyroiditis, considered not only the most common human autoimmune disease but also the most common endocrine disorder, destruction of follicular cells by cytotoxic T lymphocytes leads to thyroid atrophy and hypothyroidism. Histologic features are follicular atrophy with increased interstitial fibrous tissue and lymphocytes with fewer plasma cells and macrophages. The lymphocytes can form lymphoid follicles with germinal centers. Remaining thyroid follicles are lined by so-called Hürthle cells (enlarged follicular cells with granular eosinophilic cytoplasm, a hyperchromatic nucleus, and prominent nucleolus). Hashimoto's thyroiditis is distinct from human Grave's disease, in which autoantibodies bind the TSH receptor on follicular cells, leading to thyroid hyperplasia and hyperthyroidism.

Lymphocytic thyroiditis (Fig. 12-27; E-Fig. 12-10) is the histologic lesion in many cases of canine hypothyroidism. (See Disorders of Dogs, Hypothyroidism.) Lymphocytic thyroiditis with fibrosis has also been reported in a subset of thyroid glands from eastern European horses imported for slaughter in Italy and examined because of macroscopic alterations in their thyroid glands. The authors noted the similarity to Hashimoto's thyroiditis and documented increased thyroglobulin concentration in serum in addition to the presence of antibodies to both thyroglobulin and thyroid peroxidase.

Follicular Neoplasms

Follicular Adenomas. Thyroid follicular cell adenomas are more commonly diagnosed in aged cats than in dogs. In dogs, most thyroid follicular neoplasms are malignant (carcinomas) (see Follicular Carcinomas). Feline follicular adenomas are often functional and result in hyperthyroidism. Macroscopically, adenomas appear as discrete tan to brown nodules that compress adjacent atrophied parenchyma (Fig. 12-28, *A*). Histologically, they resemble nodules of adenomatous hyperplasia with which they may coexist, but they tend to be larger, solitary, and are encapsulated (Fig. 12-28, *B*). Most adenomas have a follicular pattern (Fig. 12-28, *C*). The follicles can be smaller or larger than those in nonneoplastic tissue and have variable colloid production. The neoplastic follicular cells are generally larger than nonneoplastic follicular cells, but mitotic figures are few and the neoplastic tissue can be quite similar in histologic appearance to that of nodular hyperplasia.

Follicular Carcinomas. Thyroid follicular carcinomas are diagnosed mainly in dogs. Thyroid carcinomas (Fig. 12-29; E-Fig. 12-11) can become quite large (thus, they are palpable in most cases) and are typically invasive, with early metastasis, especially to the lungs. Because most follicular carcinomas are nonfunctional, affected animals can develop hypothyroidism when large tumors destroy most of the thyroid gland (i.e., mass effect). Follicular carcinomas can also arise from ectopic thyroid tissue (see Disorders of Dogs). Nuclear atypia and a high mitotic index are histologic features that help to distinguish a well-differentiated follicular carcinoma from an adenoma; however, proof of malignancy requires documentation of invasion of neoplastic cells through the capsule of the thyroid gland. Immunohistochemistry for thyroid transcription factor-1 (TTF-1) and thyroglobulin may be needed to document follicular cell origin in compact (with minimal follicle formation) or poorly

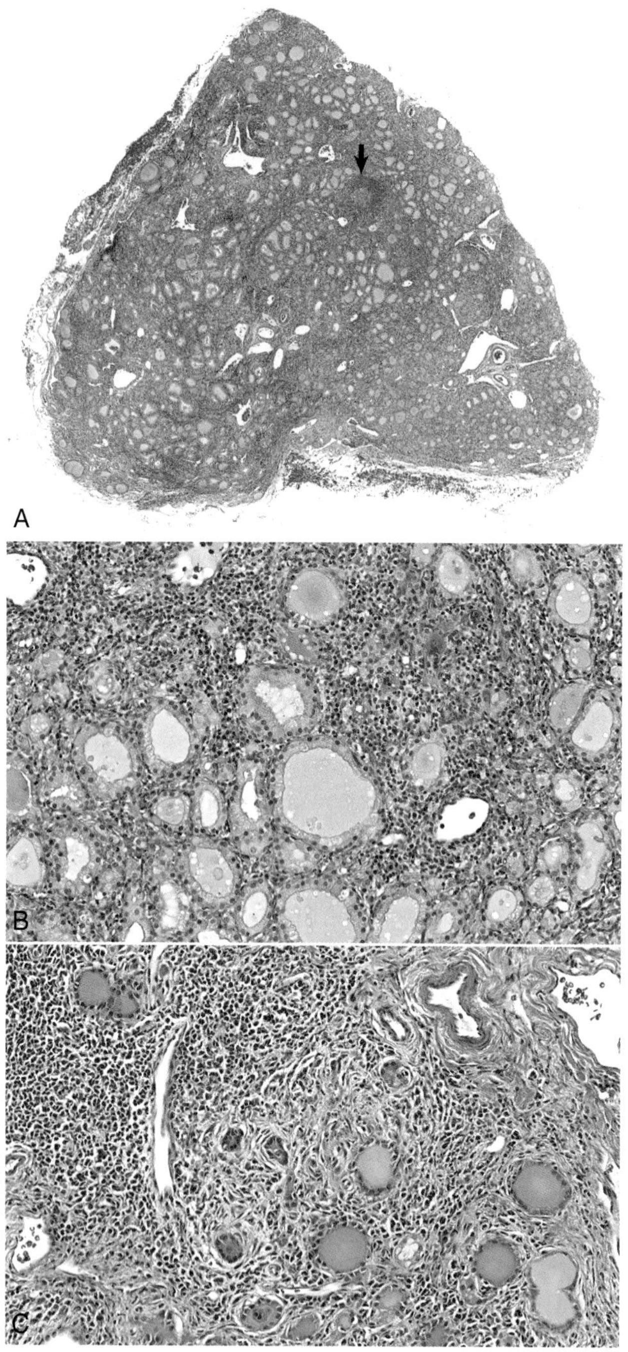

Figure 12-27 Lymphoplasmacytic Thyroiditis, Dog. A, Lymphocytic inflammation can lead to formation of lymphoid follicles *(arrow)* with germinal centers. H&E stain. **B,** Numerous lymphocytes and plasma cells, and few macrophages, are in the interstitium of the thyroid gland. Remaining follicles contain pale colloid with peripheral resorption vacuoles. Follicular cells are columnar. H&E stain. **C,** More chronic lymphoplasmacytic thyroiditis is accompanied by interstitial fibrosis, follicular atrophy, and greater loss of follicles. Remaining follicles have intensely eosinophilic colloid without resorption vacuoles and are lined by low cuboidal cells. H&E stain. (Courtesy Dr. J.A. Ramos-Vara, College of Veterinary Medicine, Purdue University.)

differentiated thyroid carcinomas. Because TTF-1 is also expressed by pulmonary epithelial cells and pulmonary carcinomas, another immunohistochemical marker, paired box gene 8 (Pax8), can be used to distinguish metastatic thyroid carcinomas in the canine lung from primary pulmonary carcinomas. Pax8 is a nuclear protein active in thyroid follicular cell development and in the expression of thyroid-specific genes.

Thyroid Medullary (C-Cell) Proliferative Lesions

Thyroid C-Cell Hyperplasia. Bulls, especially dairy bulls fed a high-calcium diet, are prone to develop C-cell hyperplasia and neoplasia. Physiologic C-cell hyperplasia is an expected response to hypercalcemia and is typically distributed throughout the thyroid gland. Diffuse or multifocal nodular hyperplasia of thyroid C cells also may precede the development of C-cell neoplasms.

Thyroid C-Cell Neoplasms. Thyroid C-cell neoplasms are diagnosed mainly in adult to aged dairy bulls and in aged horses, occasionally in dogs, and infrequently in other species. C-cell neoplasms in bulls are more common with increasing age; affected bulls tend to have increased vertebral bone density. Furthermore, C-cell neoplasms commonly develop concurrently with other endocrine neoplasms, particularly bilateral pheochromocytomas. This arrangement resembles human multiple endocrine neoplasia (MEN) type II syndrome (MEN2), in which C-cell hyperplasia and carcinomas are associated with pheochromocytomas. Mutations in the RET protooncogene result in human MEN2; however, such mutations have not been documented in bulls. In many animal species, amyloid deposits, apparently produced by the neoplastic cells and derived from calcitonin, are found in C-cell adenomas and carcinomas.

C-Cell Adenomas. The C-cell adenoma is the most common equine thyroid tumor and is frequently an incidental finding at autopsy (syn: necropsy; see E-Appendix 12-1) of geriatric horses. These tumors are solitary or multiple, off-white to tan, well-circumscribed nodular masses from a few millimeters to several centimeters in diameter (Fig. 12-30; E-Figs. 12-12 and 12-13). Histologically, C-cell adenomas consist of solid packets of polyhedral cells with few mitotic figures and ample pale amphophilic and faintly granular cytoplasm. Fine fibrovascular septa separate the packets. Entrapment of thyroid follicles can cause confusion with a follicular cell adenoma, but C-cell adenomas are immunohistochemically positive for generic neuroendocrine markers, such as chromogranin and protein gene product 9.5 (PGP 9.5), and specifically for calcitonin. They also express thyroid transcription factor-1, but not thyroglobulin, thus distinguishing themselves from follicular cells.

C-Cell Carcinomas. C-cell carcinomas are invasive tumors that can replace much of the thyroid gland. Whereas C-cell neoplasms in horses are typically benign, those in dogs and bulls are commonly malignant with metastasis to regional lymph nodes (Fig. 12-31; E-Fig. 12-14) or to the lungs. Histologically, the C cells are less well differentiated and associated with more abundant fibrous stroma. C-cell carcinomas in bulls tend to have a more heterogeneous histologic pattern, with hyperplastic nodules of C cells mixed with neoplastic nodules of differentiated C cells as well as areas of primitive ultimobranchial cells and areas with thyroid follicular differentiation.

Disorders of the Parathyroid Glands

Malformations

Parathyroid (Kürsteiner's) Cysts. Cysts (Fig. 12-32) in or immediately adjacent to a parathyroid gland, presumably derived from remnants of the duct that connects the developing gland to the thymus, are relatively common, usually incidental, findings in domestic animal species. The multilocular cysts are lined by ciliated columnar epithelial cells and filled with eosinophilic (proteinaceous) secretion. The cysts vary in diameter, but marked accumulation of inspissated proteinaceous secretion can impart the gross

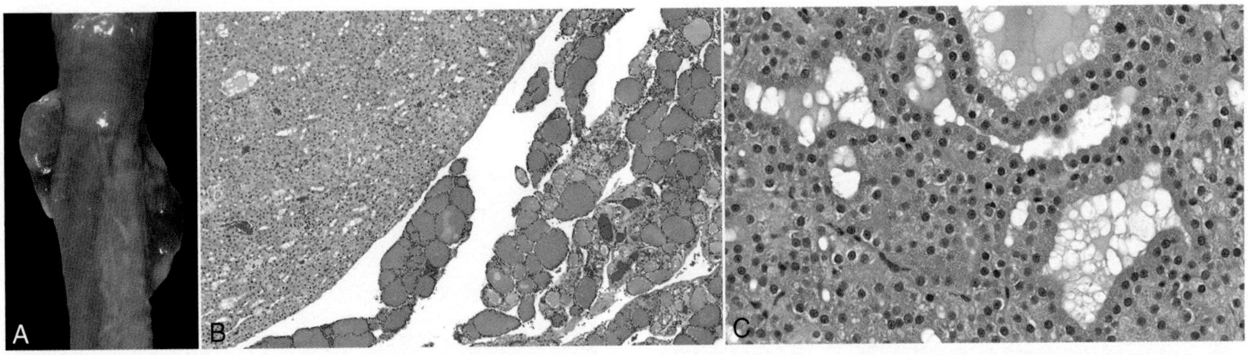

Figure 12-28 **Follicular Adenoma, Thyroid Gland, Hyperthyroid Cats. A,** The left thyroid lobe contains an expansile, pale tan mass that is well demarcated from adjacent parenchyma. Nodules of adenomatous hyperplasia are in the contralateral lobe. **B,** The follicular adenoma *(left)* is thinly encapsulated and well demarcated from adjacent atrophied thyroid gland. H&E stain. **C,** Note increased cell density and size of follicular cells in the adenoma. Follicles are collapsed or filled by pale colloid with numerous resorption vacuoles. H&E stain. (**A** courtesy Dr. J.A. Ramos-Vara, College of Veterinary Medicine, Purdue University. **B** and **C** courtesy Dr. M.A. Miller, College of Veterinary Medicine, Purdue University.)

appearance, on superficial inspection, of an enlarged parathyroid gland.

Chief Cell Atrophy and Hypoparathyroidism

Hypoparathyroidism is the result either of insufficient PTH secretion by parathyroid chief cells or an inability of target cells, mainly in renal tubules and bone, to respond to PTH. Affected animals tend to develop hypocalcemia because of decreased bone resorption and hyperphosphatemia because of increased renal tubular reabsorption (E-Fig. 12-15). Atrophy or destruction of parathyroid chief cells is a major cause of inadequate PTH production and secretion.

In dogs, hypoparathyroidism may be familial in miniature schnauzers and other breeds. Lymphocytic parathyroiditis (E-Fig. 12-16) seems to be less common than lymphocytic inflammation of other endocrine organs, such as thyroid or adrenal glands, but results in chief cell atrophy and loss, and it has been described in dogs as a presumably autoimmune cause of primary hypoparathyroidism. Cats can develop hypoparathyroidism after thyroidectomy (with inadvertent parathyroidectomy) as a treatment for hyperthyroidism. Destruction of parathyroid glands by primary or secondary neoplasms is another uncommon cause of hypoparathyroidism.

Persistent hypercalcemia should, although this is not always the case, cause trophic atrophy of parathyroid chief cells with decreased production of PTH. Trophic atrophy results in shrinkage of all parathyroid glands. Histologically, the atrophied gland has small chief cells with diminished vascularity and a relative increase in stroma.

Chief Cell Proliferation and Hyperparathyroidism

Primary Hyperparathyroidism. Primary hyperparathyroidism is the result of autonomous hypersecretion of PTH by hyperplastic or neoplastic chief cells. Parathyroid (chief cell) adenomas (Fig. 12-33), diagnosed mainly in dogs, are more common than parathyroid carcinomas or primary hyperplasia. Adenomas typically affect only one parathyroid gland with formation of a nodule up to 1 cm in diameter. Microscopically (Fig. 12-33, *B*; E-Figs. 12-17 and 12-18), a parathyroid adenoma is at least partially encapsulated and compresses adjacent parathyroid parenchyma. The neoplastic chief cells have an enlarged nucleus and ample cytoplasm with few mitotic figures. The increase in chief cell size and number compresses the interstitium of the adenoma with a relative decrease in fibrovascular stroma. Adjacent parathyroid tissue and remaining parathyroid glands undergo chief cell atrophy in response to the hypercalcemia of hyperparathyroidism.

Chief cell carcinomas tend to be larger than adenomas with destruction of much of the parathyroid gland and invasion of surrounding tissues. The neoplastic cells may have features of malignancy, such as nuclear atypia and increased mitotic index.

Primary (idiopathic), usually multinodular, hyperplasia of chief cells is also observed in dogs, but it is less common than secondary chief cell hyperplasia (see the following section). The cytologic features of hyperplastic chief cells can resemble those of neoplastic chief cells, but the presence of multiple unencapsulated nodules distinguishes primary hyperplasia from the typically solitary and encapsulated adenoma and from secondary hyperplasia, which tends to be diffuse. Hyperparathyroidism, whether primary or secondary, can result in severe bone resorption and osteopenia (E-Fig. 12-19).

Secondary Hyperparathyroidism. Secondary chief cell hyperplasia is typically diffuse, affecting all parathyroid glands (Fig. 12-34, A), and is usually the result of either a nutritional imbalance of calcium and phosphorus (for responses of bone, see Chapter 16) or chronic renal failure (see Chapter 11). Histologically (Fig. 12-34, *B* and *C*), the chief cells are diffusely hypertrophied and crowded, compressing the fibrovascular stroma and capsule. Dietary imbalances that stimulate chief cell hyperplasia and lead to secondary hyperparathyroidism include insufficient calcium, excessive phosphorus, or cholecalciferol deficiency. Renal disease decreases urinary phosphate excretion resulting in hyperphosphatemia and a corresponding decline in plasma Ca : P ratio. Progressive renal disease also causes decreased production of 1,25-dihydroxyvitamin D_3, which exacerbates the relative hypocalcemia. In long-standing renal failure in human beings and in dogs, the proliferation of parathyroid chief cells can become autonomous (no longer responsive to blood Ca^{2+} concentration) and continue even in the presence of persistent hypercalcemia. Tertiary hyperparathyroidism is the term used for this conversion of secondary hyperparathyroidism to an autonomous state. Although the histologic features are indistinguishable from those of secondary hyperparathyroidism, the diffuse chief cell hyperplasia in all parathyroid glands and the history serve to differentiate tertiary from primary hyperparathyroidism, which is idiopathic and usually results in nodular formation rather than diffuse hyperplasia.

Nutritional Imbalances. The most frequent dietary cause of secondary hyperparathyroidism is excessive phosphorus. Hyperphosphatemia stimulates the parathyroid gland indirectly by reciprocal lowering of the blood calcium concentration. Horses with nutritional secondary hyperparathyroidism usually have been fed grain diets with low-quality roughage. Because bran is often the source of excess phosphorus in equine diets, the disease has been called "bran disease" or "big head." The latter name refers to the hyperostotic

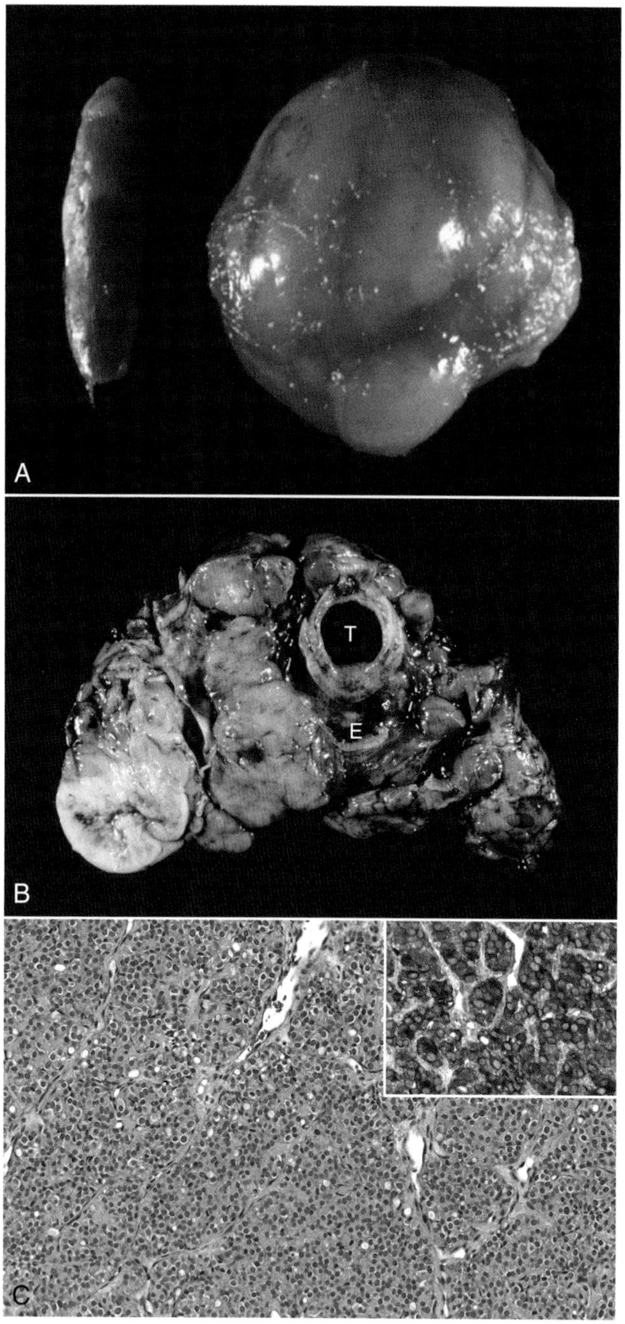

Figure 12-29 **Thyroid Follicular Carcinoma, Dog. A,** A follicular carcinoma has obliterated the right thyroid lobe, but the left lobe is grossly normal. **B,** Cross section through a large follicular carcinoma that has destroyed the entire thyroid gland, surrounded the trachea (*T*) and esophagus (*E*), and invaded adjacent tissue and vasculature. **C,** Neoplastic follicular cells are arranged in compact nests with negligible follicle formation. H&E stain. *Inset,* Immunohistochemical expression of thyroglobulin indicates follicular origin of the neoplastic cells. Immunohistochemistry with diaminobenzidine chromogen. (**A** courtesy Dr. W. Crowell, College of Veterinary Medicine, The University of Georgia; and Noah's Arkive, College of Veterinary Medicine, The University of Georgia. **B** and **C** courtesy Dr. M.A. Miller, College of Veterinary Medicine, Purdue University.)

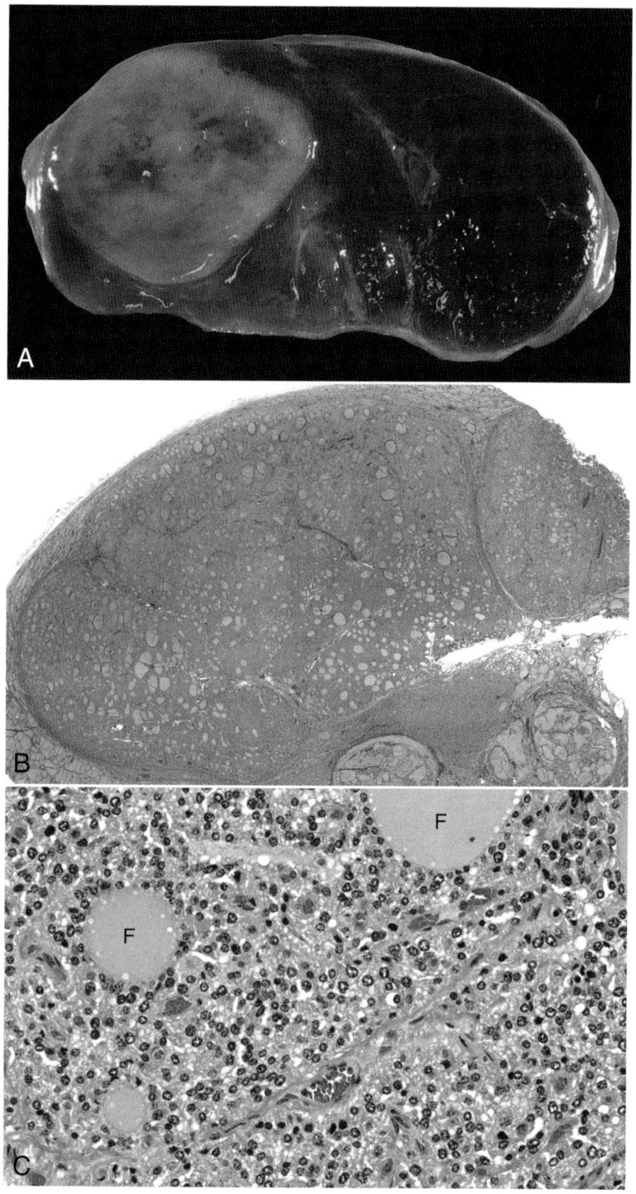

Figure 12-30 **C-Cell Adenoma, Thyroid Gland, Horse. A,** The adenoma is pale gray to pink, thinly encapsulated, and contained within the thyroid gland. **B,** The C-cell adenoma is multinodular but well demarcated from adjacent thyroid parenchyma. H&E stain. **C,** The neoplastic cells are typical neuroendocrine cells, but the presence of entrapped thyroid follicles (*F*) can cause confusion with follicular adenomas. H&E stain. (Courtesy Dr. M.A. Miller, College of Veterinary Medicine, Purdue University.)

fibrous osteodystrophy that is typically most severe in the mandibles and maxillae (see Figs. 16-51 through 16-53. The high-phosphorus diet often has marginal or deficient calcium content, so even though a greater proportion of ingested calcium is absorbed, hypocalcemia develops. The increased PTH secretion acts on renal tubules to increase phosphorus excretion and to decrease calcium loss in the urine. Changes in urinary calcium and phosphorus concentrations are more consistent and diagnostically useful in horses than changes in blood calcium and phosphorus concentrations.

Renal Disease. If renal disease is extensive enough to reduce the glomerular filtration rate, phosphorus is retained and hyperphosphatemia develops. The increased phosphorus concentration causes a reciprocal decline in ionized blood calcium concentration. Chronic renal disease also impairs 1,25-dihydroxyvitamin D_3 (calcitriol) synthesis, thereby diminishing intestinal absorption of calcium. Increased synthesis and secretion of PTH is a response to hyperphosphatemia, hypocalcemia, or low blood concentrations of calcitriol. Diffuse chief cell hyperplasia results in increased size of all parathyroid glands (see Fig. 12-34). The fibrous osteodystrophy

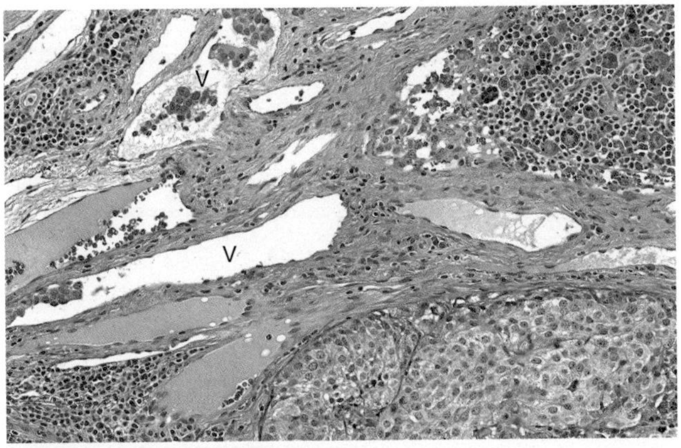

Figure 12-31 Thyroid C-Cell Carcinoma, Dog. This C-cell carcinoma *(lower right)* has invaded the thyroid capsule and its vasculature. Note clusters of neoplastic cells in the lumen of vessels (V). H&E stain. (Courtesy Dr. J.A. Ramos-Vara, College of Veterinary Medicine, Purdue University.)

(see Chapter 16) that develops in chronic renal disease is, as in nutritional secondary hyperparathyroidism, most severe in bones of the skull. Canine mandibles and maxillae may be so severely affected that the dog develops "rubber jaw" (see E-Fig. 16-22).

Pseudohyperparathyroidism: Humoral Hypercalcemia of Malignancy

Pseudohyperparathyroidism is characterized by persistent hypercalcemia without elevated PTH secretion. The source of the excessive calcium is mainly osteoclastic bone resorption, with a lesser contribution from kidneys and the intestinal tract. Malignant neoplasia is the usual cause of pseudohyperparathyroidism, hence the name humoral hypercalcemia of malignancy (HHM). The neoplasms that cause pseudohyperparathyroidism do not arise in the parathyroid glands. In fact, the parathyroid chief cells in affected animals undergo atrophy in physiologic response to the elevated plasma Ca^{2+} concentration. Lymphoma is the most common neoplastic cause of hypercalcemia in dogs and is also associated with hypercalcemia in cats. The pathogenesis of the increased bone resorption in lymphoma has been attributed both to an osteolytic factor released locally by neoplastic cells that invade bone marrow and to the release of a circulating humoral factor (parathyroid hormone-related peptide [PTHrP] and others) by the neoplastic cells. Most dogs with lymphoma and persistent hypercalcemia of malignancy have increased circulating PTHrP concentrations, but less so than in dogs with apocrine carcinomas of the anal sac glands and HHM. The lack of correlation between PTHrP concentration and serum calcium concentration indicates that PTHrP is not the sole humoral factor responsible for osteoclastic bone resorption and development of hypercalcemia. Other substances, such as interleukin-1, tumor necrosis factor, or 1,25-dihydroxycholecalciferol, probably contribute to the hypercalcemia of malignancy in canine lymphoma. In dogs with lymphoma and hypercalcemia, concentrations of parathyroid hormone, which is antigenically distinct from PTHrP, usually are below or within the normal range.

Hypercalcemia often develops in dogs with apocrine carcinoma of the anal sac glands (see Disorders of Dogs and also Chapter 17) because the neoplastic cells secrete PTHrP. Neoplasms that are prone to invade multiple bones, such as multiple myeloma (a neoplasm of plasma cells), can result in hypercalcemia, although this seems to be much less common in domestic animals than it is in human beings. In addition to the osteopenic effect of increased osteoclastic bone resorption (see Chapter 16), the persistent

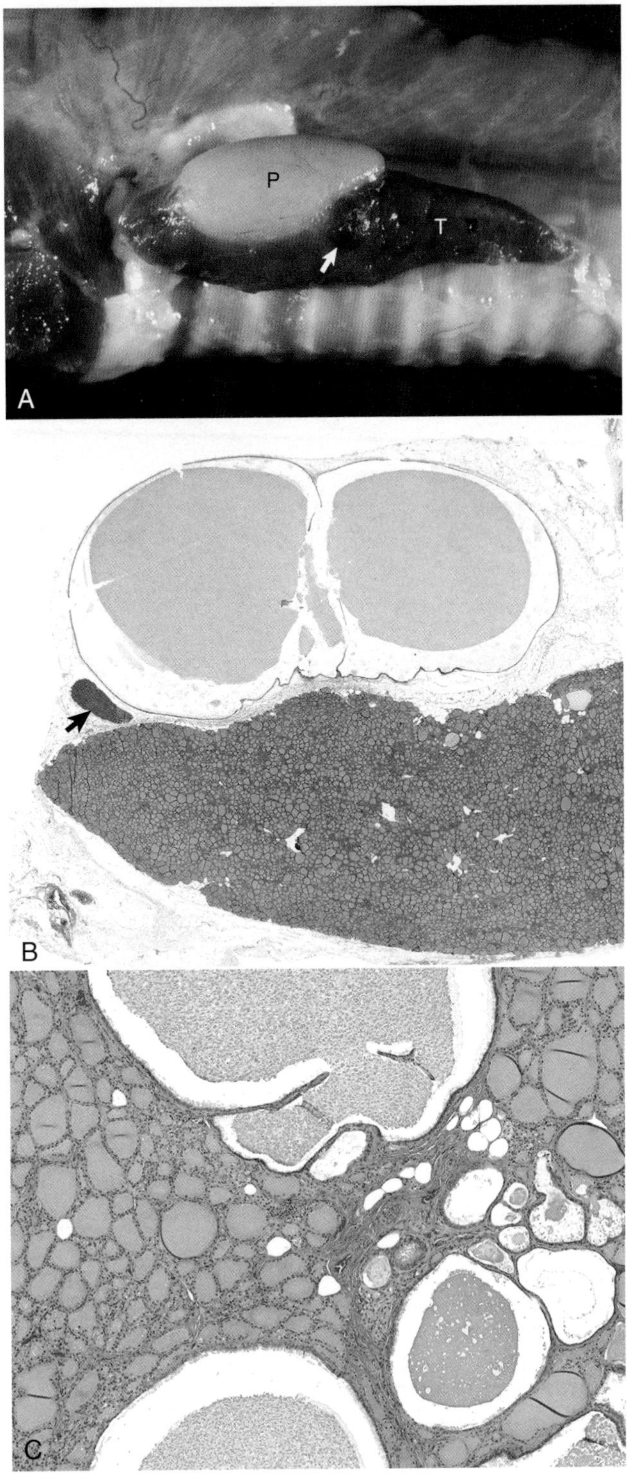

Figure 12-32 Parathyroid Cyst (Kürsteiner's Cyst), Dog. A, The multilocular cyst is derived from the duct that connects embryonic parathyroid-thymic primordia in pharyngeal pouches III and IV. Part of the parathyroid cyst *(P)* is distended with inspissated, opaque secretion; the *arrow* points to a locule with more watery secretion. *T,* Thyroid gland. **B,** A large parathyroid cyst dwarfs the adjacent parathyroid gland *(arrow)*. H&E stain. **C,** Smaller parathyroid cyst locules are scattered through adjacent thyroid interstitium. Their ciliated columnar epithelial lining distinguishes them from thyroid follicles. H&E stain. (**A** courtesy Dr. C. Capen, College of Veterinary Medicine, The Ohio State University. **B** and **C** courtesy Dr. M.A. Miller, College of Veterinary Medicine, Purdue University.)

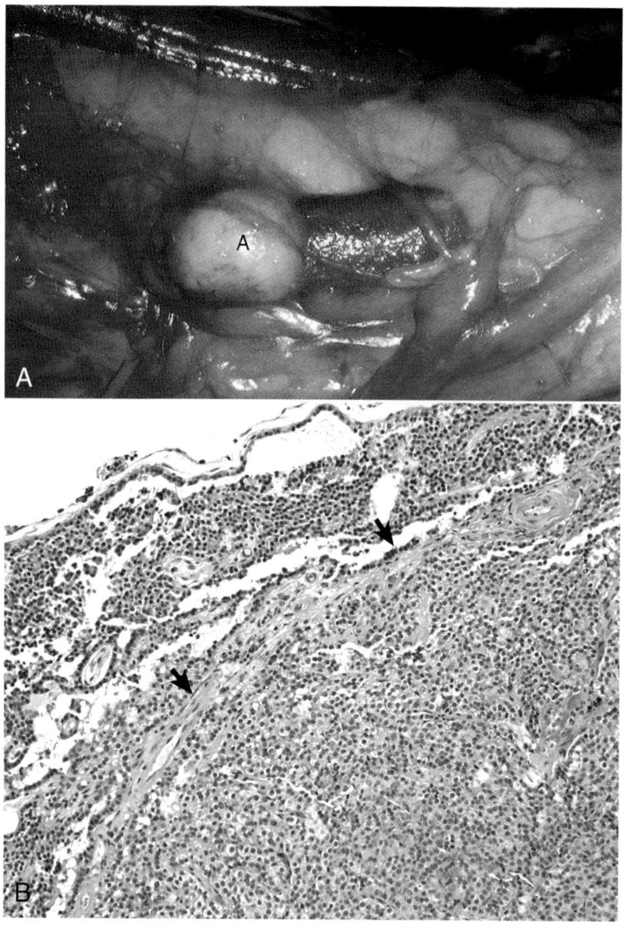

Figure 12-33 **Adenoma, Parathyroid Gland, Dog. A,** The parathyroid adenoma *(A)* forms a discrete nodular mass that is well demarcated from the thyroid gland. **B,** The adenoma consists of packets of hypertrophied chief cells separated by fine fibrovascular septa. A fibrous capsule *(arrows)* separates the adenoma *(lower right)* from adjacent, atrophied parathyroid tissue. H&E stain. (**A** courtesy College of Veterinary Medicine, University of Illinois. **B** courtesy Dr. M.A. Miller, College of Veterinary Medicine, Purdue University.)

hypercalcemia results in calcification of many tissues, especially the kidneys, gastric mucosa, endocardium, pleura, and lungs.

Parturient Hypocalcemia (Parturient Paresis, Milk Fever)

See Disorders of Ruminants (Cattle, Sheep, and Goats).

Disorders of the Adrenal Gland

Disorders of the Adrenal Cortex

Developmental Disorders of the Adrenal Cortex. Maturation of the fetal adrenal gland and the onset of parturition depend on an intact hypothalamic-pituitary-adrenal axis. Therefore, malformations of the brain, especially those that affect the hypothalamic-hypophyseal axis, disrupt adrenal function and can result in prolonged gestation or delayed parturition.

Accessory Adrenal Tissue. Accessory or ectopic adrenocortical tissue is encountered occasionally, usually as an incidental finding, but it can undergo neoplastic transformation. The ectopic tissue is often near the normal site—for example, in perirenal adipose tissue. It also can attach or become embedded in the wall of the reproductive or gastrointestinal tracts.

In many animals, especially horses, the adrenal cortex bulges into the capsule or into the medulla. This anatomic variation is generally

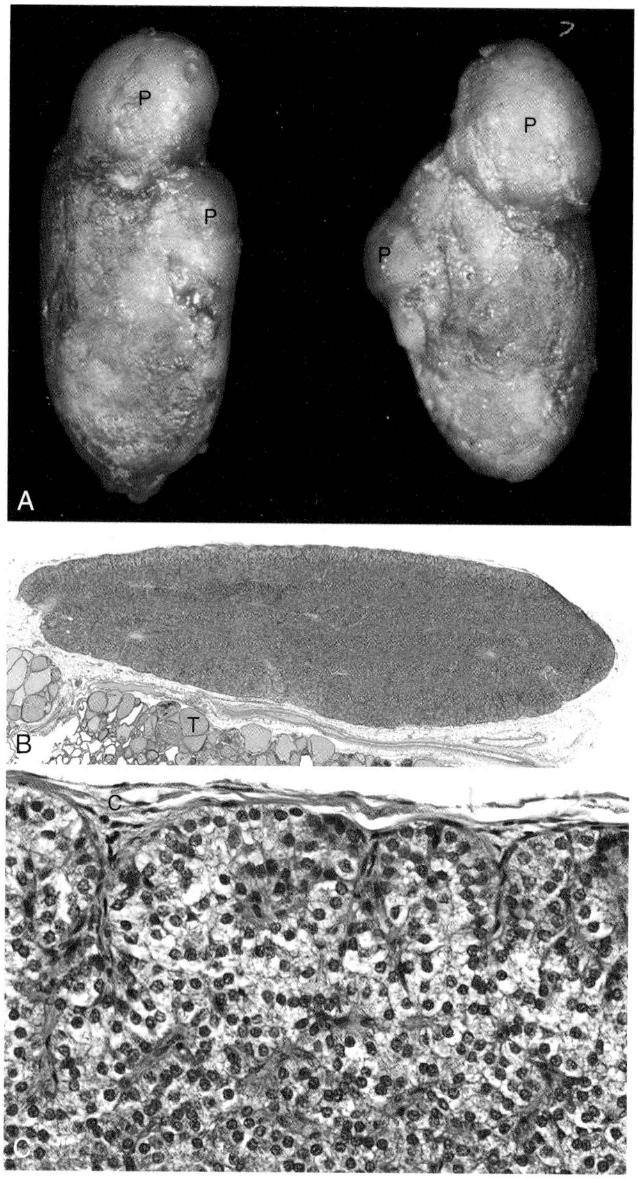

Figure 12-34 **Renal Secondary Hyperparathyroidism, Dog. A,** All four parathyroid glands are enlarged in this dog with chronic renal failure. The size of the thyroid gland is normal. **B,** Hyperplasia of the parathyroid gland in secondary hyperparathyroidism is typically diffuse. *T,* Thyroid gland. H&E stain. **C,** Hyperplastic chief cells are crowded, enlarged with ample cytoplasm, and impinge on the fibrovascular stroma and the parathyroid capsule *(C)*. H&E stain. (**A** courtesy Dr. D.-Y. Cho, College of Veterinary Medicine, Louisiana State University. **B** and **C** courtesy College of Veterinary Medicine, Purdue University.)

of no functional significance and should be distinguished from accessory adrenal tissue (because it is not separated from the adrenal gland) or hyperplastic nodules.

Congenital Adrenal Hyperplasia (Adrenogenital Syndrome). Congenital adrenal hyperplasia is caused by an autosomal recessive defect in one of the genes that encode the various hydroxylases involved in corticosteroid synthesis. The enzyme deficiency generally results in decreased cortisol production (with diversion to androgen synthesis) and, therefore, increased ACTH secretion from adenohypophyseal (anterior pituitary gland) corticotrophs, hence the adrenocortical hyperplasia. The condition is well documented in human beings, in which it is usually due to mutation of the gene for steroid 21-hydroxylase, but is rarely reported in domestic animal species. A case of congenital adrenal hyperplasia in a male cat with gynecomastia and virilization (despite previous castration) was associated with mutation of an 11β-hydroxylase-like gene.

Proliferative Disorders of the Adrenal Cortex

Adrenocortical Hyperplasia. Hyperplasia and hypertrophy of adrenocortical cells is relatively common, especially in older dogs. Adrenocortical hyperplasia can be diffuse (E-Fig. 12-20, *A*; also see Fig. 12-17, A and C) or nodular (Fig. 12-35, A and *B*; E-Fig. 12-20, *B*). Hyperplastic nodules are generally multiple, often paler than adjacent cortical tissue, and seldom larger than a few millimeters in diameter. Histologically (see Fig. 12-35, *B*), the hyperplastic cortical cells typically are in the zonae fasciculata and reticularis, and they resemble their normal counterparts but tend to be larger. The nodules are not encapsulated but tend to be well demarcated. The usual cause of adrenocortical hyperplasia is unregulated hypersecretion of ACTH from hyperplastic or neoplastic adenohypophyseal (anterior pituitary gland) corticotrophs. In dogs with adrenocortical hyperplasia without a proliferative pituitary lesion, it has been proposed that increased hypothalamic catabolism of dopamine (attributed to an age-related increase in monoamine oxidase-β activity) could disrupt negative feedback control in the hypothalamic-pituitary-adrenal axis. Adrenocortical hyperplasia, whether diffuse or nodular, typically results in hyperfunction (hyperadrenocorticism or Cushing's syndrome; Fig. 12-36) with excess production of cortisol. Hyperadrenocorticism affects a variety of tissues or organs, especially the liver (see Fig. 8-73), skin (see Figs. 17-65 and 17-66), and skeletal muscles (see Chapters 8, 15, and 17).

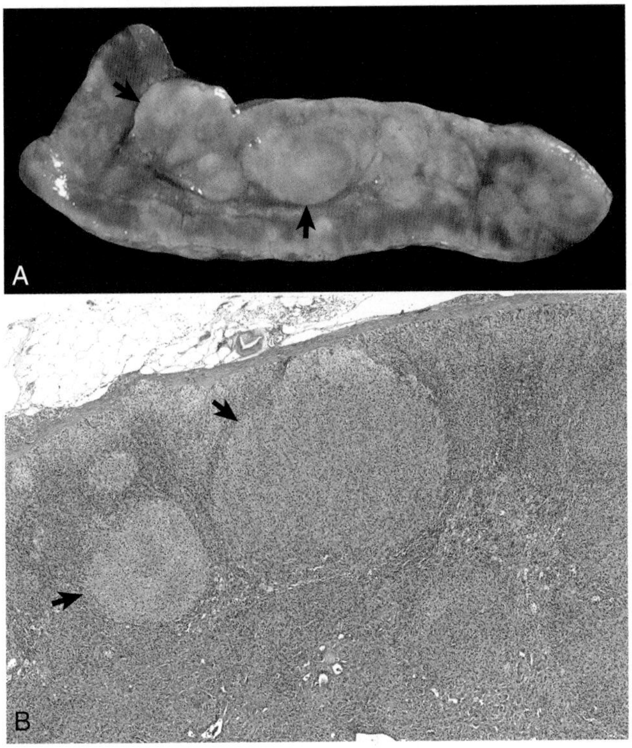

Figure 12-35 Nodular Adrenocortical Hyperplasia, Adrenal Glands, Dog. A, Discrete pale tan nodules *(arrows)* are disseminated through the zonae fasciculata and reticularis. **B,** Hyperplastic nodules *(arrows)* are not encapsulated but are well demarcated from, and consist of cells that are larger and paler than those in, adjacent adrenal cortex. (Courtesy Dr. M.A. Miller, College of Veterinary Medicine, Purdue University.)

Hyperaldosteronism (Conn's Syndrome). See Disorders of Cats.

Adrenocortical Neoplasia

Cortical Adenomas and Carcinomas. Neoplasms of adrenocortical cells can be benign (adenomas) or malignant (carcinomas) and functional or nonfunctional. Although most functional canine adrenocortical neoplasms secrete cortisol, functional neoplasms less commonly arise from aldosterone-secreting cells of the zona glomerulosa (especially in cats) or from estrogen-secreting cells of the zona reticularis (mainly in ferrets [see the following section]). Adrenocortical adenomas (Fig. 12-37, *A*; E-Fig. 12-20, C) typically are well-demarcated, partially encapsulated, solitary and unilateral, yellowish nodules, seldom larger than 2 cm in diameter. Histologically, they are composed of trabeculae or nests of cells that resemble the nonneoplastic cortical cells and usually have numerous cytoplasmic lipid vacuoles. Like other steroid hormone–producing cells, neoplastic adrenocortical cells usually express Melan A. Adrenocortical adenomas are most common in old dogs and cattle, but they also develop in the other domestic animal species.

Adrenocortical carcinomas (Fig. 12-37, *B*; E-Fig. 12-20, *D*) are generally larger than adenomas, are invasive, and can be bilateral. Again, cattle and dogs develop adrenocortical carcinomas more commonly than do the other domestic species. Histologically (Fig. 12-37, C), the neoplastic cells have greater nuclear atypia than their benign counterparts with an increased mitotic index, but the best indicator of malignancy is invasion of the adrenal capsule or vasculature. Bovine adrenocortical carcinomas metastasize most commonly to the lungs; canine adrenocortical carcinomas tend to invade the caudal vena cava and spread to kidney, liver, and lymph nodes.

Secondary Neoplasms of the Adrenal Gland. The adrenal gland, especially at the corticomedullary junction, is a major site for tumor metastases. In one study, the adrenal gland was involved in 15% to 30% of metastatic cancer cases in dogs, cats, horses, and cattle. In animals with adrenal metastases, carcinomas and melanoma were most common in dogs, hemangiosarcoma and melanoma were most common in horses, and lymphoma was most common in cattle and cats. Metastatic neoplasms, if extensive, can result in adrenocortical hypofunction.

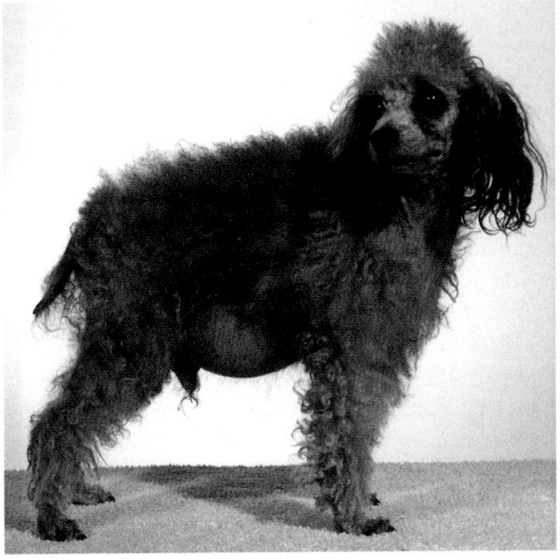

Figure 12-36 Hyperadrenocorticism (Cushing's-Like Disease), Dog. Hyperadrenocorticism after exogenous glucocorticosteroid administration as treatment for idiopathic adrenocortical hyperplasia. Muscle asthenia explains the pendulous abdomen. Alopecia (hair loss) on the abdomen, ventral aspect of the neck, and tail is another feature of hyperadrenocorticism. (Courtesy Dr. C. Capen, College of Veterinary Medicine, The Ohio State University.)

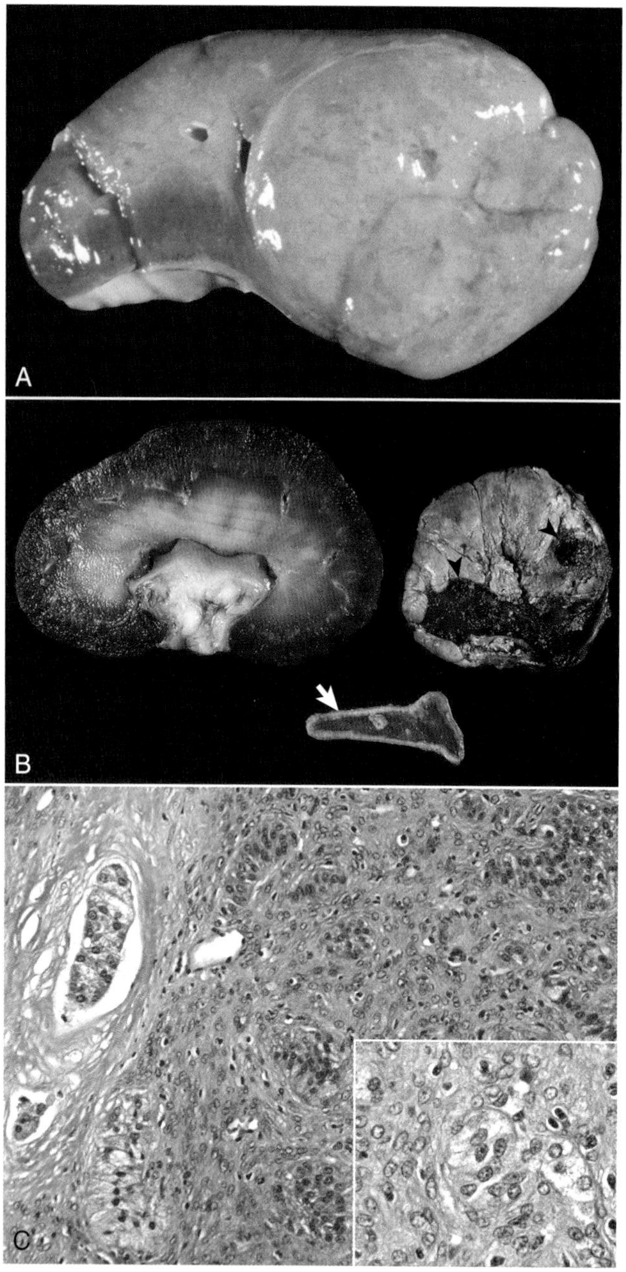

Figure 12-37 **Adrenocortical Neoplasia, Adrenal Glands. A,** Adrenocortical adenoma, ox. The solitary yellow adenoma is thinly encapsulated and contained within the adrenal cortex. **B,** Adrenocortical carcinoma, dog. The adrenal gland *(right)* is mostly replaced by an adrenocortical carcinoma that is almost half the size of the kidney *(left)*. Note coalescing areas of hemorrhage and necrosis *(arrowheads)* in the carcinoma. The contralateral adrenal cortex *(lower center, arrow)* has undergone trophic atrophy of the zonae fasciculata and reticularis. **C,** Adrenocortical carcinoma, dog. The carcinoma *(right)* has invaded the adrenal capsule and its vasculature *(left)*. *Inset,* Cells are haphazardly arranged with variable cellular and nuclear size, typical of malignant neoplasms. H&E stain. (**A** courtesy Dr. J.A. Ramos-Vara, College of Veterinary Medicine, Purdue University. **B** courtesy Dr. C. Capen, College of Veterinary Medicine, The Ohio State University. **C** courtesy Dr. J.F. Zachary, College of Veterinary Medicine, University of Illinois.)

Functional Proliferative Lesions in Ferrets

Information on this topic is available at www.expertconsult.com.

Adrenocortical Atrophy, Degeneration, or Cellular Death. Atrophy of the zonae fasciculata and reticularis is often secondary to insufficient adenohypophyseal (anterior pituitary gland) secretion of ACTH. Iatrogenic causes of atrophy of the zonae fasciculata and reticularis include excessive administration of exogenous glucocorticoids, which causes negative feedback on adenohypophyseal corticotrophs and on hypothalamic corticotrophin-releasing factor, or administration (as treatment for adrenocortical hyperplasia or neoplasia) of *o,p′*-dichlorodiphenyldichloroethane (*o,p′*-DDD; also known as mitotane), which causes lysis of the adrenal cortex.

Primary hypoadrenocorticism (Addison's disease), with insufficient mineralocorticoid and glucocorticoid production (even after administration of exogenous ACTH), generally requires destruction of almost 90% of the adrenal cortex. Although systemic infectious diseases, such as tuberculosis, can destroy the adrenal cortex by means of chronic inflammation and result in hypoadrenocorticism, most human cases in developed countries are considered an autoimmune disease with the enzyme 21-hydroxylase as a major antigenic target of autoantibodies in adrenal cortical cells. The histologic lesion of autoimmune hypoadrenocorticism is lymphoplasmacytic adrenalitis. Lysis of the cortical cells in all three zones (zonae glomerulosa, fasciculata, and reticularis) is attributed mainly to the actions of chemical mediators from T lymphocytes, but humoral immunity probably contributes to the disease. Dogs are the domestic species most commonly affected by primary hypoadrenocorticism (see Disorders of Dogs).

Miscellaneous Disorders of the Adrenal Cortex

Adrenal Inflammation (Adrenalitis). Diffuse lymphoplasmacytic inflammation that is confined to the adrenal cortex suggests an immune-mediated disease in which adrenocortical cells are the target. In addition, the adrenal gland is often inflamed in systemic infections. Cattle with malignant catarrhal fever from ovine herpesvirus-2 infection typically have lymphocytic adrenalitis. Systemic herpesvirus infection in fetuses and neonates of various species is commonly associated with multifocal necrotizing inflammation in the adrenal glands (as well as in other organs). Likewise, granulomatous or suppurative adrenalitis that is part of systemic infection is also typically multifocal. Because adrenocortical cells are not the target in systemic inflammatory diseases, cortical destruction is usually not severe enough to result in functional hypoadrenocorticism.

Vascular Disorders of the Adrenal Gland. The vascular network at the interface between adrenal cortex and medulla is a prime site for thrombosis in disseminated intravascular coagulation and for embolization of infectious microbes or metastatic neoplastic cells. The adrenal gland frequently develops hemorrhages or infarcts in sepsis. Acute adrenal failure due to massive adrenocortical hemorrhage associated with bacterial sepsis is known as Waterhouse-Friderichsen syndrome (Fig. 12-38, E-Fig. 12-21). In addition to bacterial infection, severe stress increases the risk of adrenal hemorrhage, perhaps because elevated ACTH secretion results in increased blood supply to an organ with limited venous drainage.

Disorders of the Adrenal Medulla

Proliferative Lesions

Adrenal Medullary Hyperplasia. Adrenal medullary hyperplasia occurs occasionally in all domestic animal species, but it may be more common in older dairy bulls (E-Fig. 12-22) and horses (Fig. 12-39), especially mares. Adrenal medullary hyperplasia can

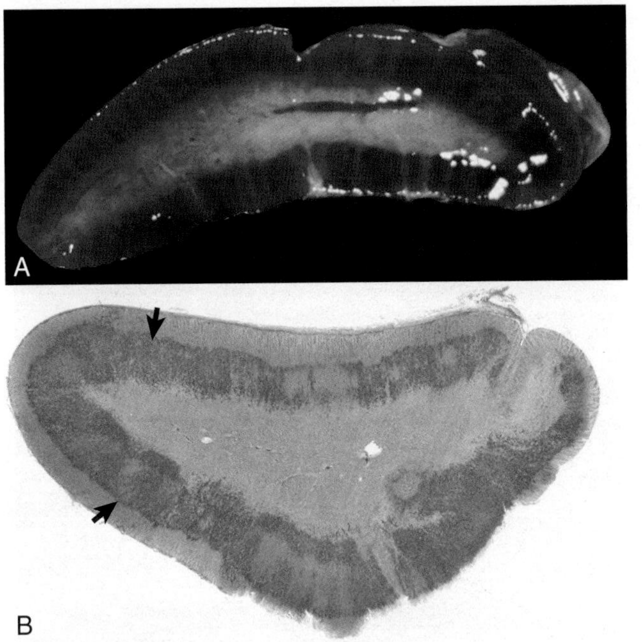

Figure 12-38 **Adrenocortical Hemorrhage (Waterhouse-Friderichsen Syndrome), Adrenal Gland, Foal. A,** Diffuse hemorrhage in the adrenal cortex is common in endotoxic shock. **B,** Subgross photomicrograph of diffuse adrenocortical hemorrhage *(arrows)*. H&E stain. (**A** courtesy Dr. J.A. Ramos-Vara, College of Veterinary Medicine, Purdue University. **B** courtesy College of Veterinary Medicine, University of Illinois.)

be associated with pheochromocytoma (i.e., adrenal medullary neoplasia) or with multiple endocrine neoplasia (MEN) of the adrenal and thyroid medullary cells. Adrenal medullary hyperplasia can be diffuse or nodular. Measurement of adrenal medullary mass or area in cross section is necessary to document diffuse hyperplasia. Hyperplastic nodules typically are multiple, small (microscopic to 5 mm in diameter), and nonencapsulated aggregates of hypertrophied cells with ample cytoplasm that may be less densely granular than that of normal chromaffin cells.

Neoplasms

Pheochromocytomas. Pheochromocytomas (Figs. 12-40 and 12-41) are neoplasms of the chromaffin cells of the adrenal medulla. They occur in all species but are more commonly reported in cattle and dogs. These tumors can be benign or malignant and functional or nonfunctional. Although epinephrine is the predominant catecholamine of the normal adult adrenal medulla, functional pheochromocytomas tend to produce mainly norepinephrine. Excessive catecholamine production by a pheochromocytoma can cause systemic hypertension. Whereas hyperplastic nodules in the adrenal medulla are often multiple, pheochromocytomas are usually solitary but may be present bilaterally. Smaller pheochromocytomas are partially encapsulated red-brown nodules. Histologically (see Fig. 12-40, *B*), the neoplastic tissue consists of packets of neuroendocrine cells separated by fine fibrovascular stroma. The neoplastic cells are polyhedral, tend to be larger than nonneoplastic chromaffin cells, and have ample faintly granular pale amphophilic cytoplasm. The mitotic index varies. The neoplastic cells express generic neuroendocrine markers (e.g., protein gene product 9.5 [PGP 9.5] or chromogranin) immunohistochemically; this immunoreactivity can be useful in distinguishing poorly differentiated pheochromocytomas from adrenocortical carcinomas. Malignant pheochromocytomas tend to be larger than benign tumors, have extensive hemorrhage and necrosis, obliterate the adrenal gland, and invade the vena cava.

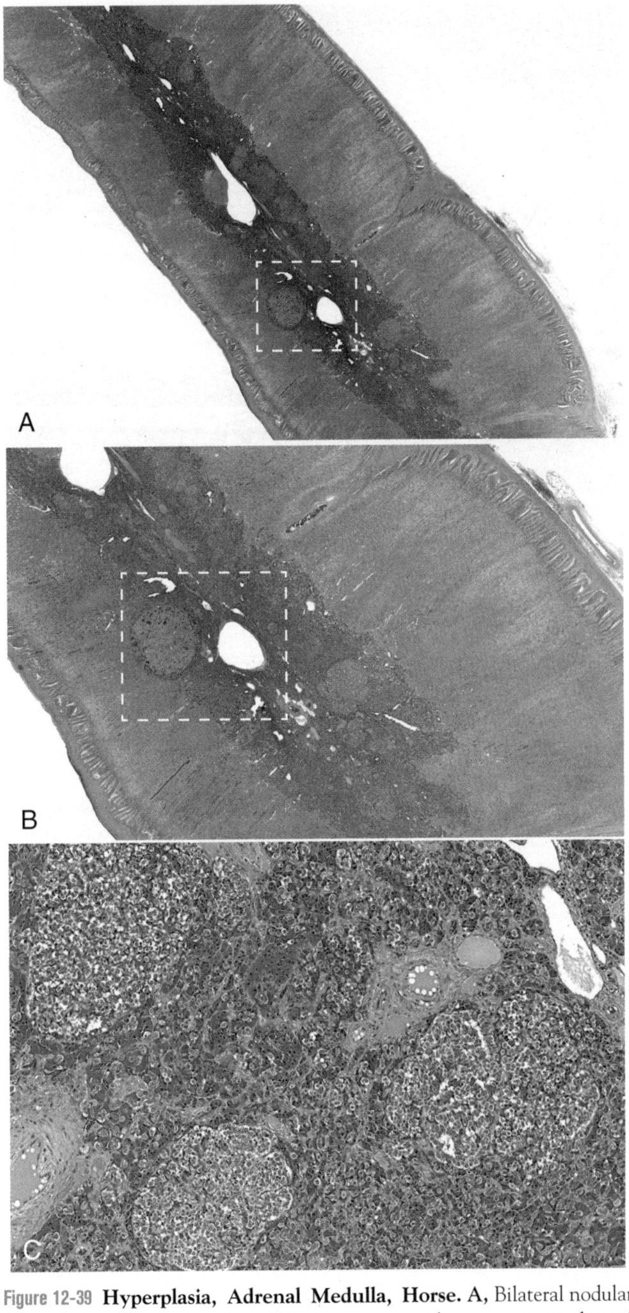

Figure 12-39 **Hyperplasia, Adrenal Medulla, Horse. A,** Bilateral nodular hyperplasia of the adrenal medulla in a mare with concomitant thyroid medullary C-cell hyperplasia and a pituitary pars intermedia adenoma. H&E stain. **B,** Enlargement of **A.** Nodular hyperplasia is shown in areas within rectangles. H&E stain. **C,** The discrete but nonencapsulated nodules consist of cells with more abundant and paler cytoplasm than in adjacent chromaffin cells. H&E stain. (Courtesy Dr. M.A. Miller, College of Veterinary Medicine, Purdue University.)

There is overlap in the histologic features of benign and malignant pheochromocytomas, so proof of malignancy requires invasion through the adrenal capsule (see Fig. 12-41) or distant metastasis. Concurrent pheochromocytoma and thyroid medullary neoplasms may have autosomal dominant inheritance in Guernsey cattle.

Neuroblastomas and Ganglioneuromas. Neuroblastomas are primitive neuroectodermal tumors that can develop in the central or peripheral nervous systems. In the latter, they are frequently located in the adrenal medulla or within sympathetic ganglia. In ganglioneuroma, which can develop in the adrenal medulla or in

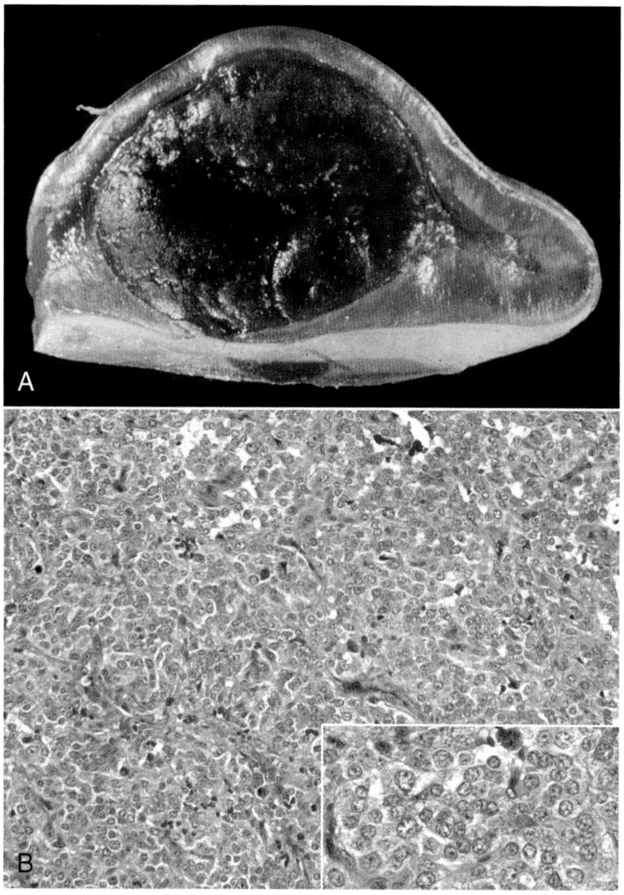

Figure 12-40 **Pheochromocytoma, Adrenal Gland, Horse. A,** A well-demarcated pheochromocytoma is contained within the adrenal medulla. The red-brown neoplastic tissue resembles that of adjacent adrenal medulla in contrast to the pale yellow cast of the adrenal cortex. **B,** Neoplastic chromaffin cells are arranged in poorly demarcated lobules. *Inset,* Higher magnification of the chromaffin cells. There is moderate variation in cellular and nuclear size and shape. H&E stain. (**A** courtesy Dr. B. Weeks, College of Veterinary Medicine, Texas A&M University; and Noah's Arkive, College of Veterinary Medicine, The University of Georgia. **B** courtesy Dr. J.F. Zachary, College of Veterinary Medicine, University of Illinois.)

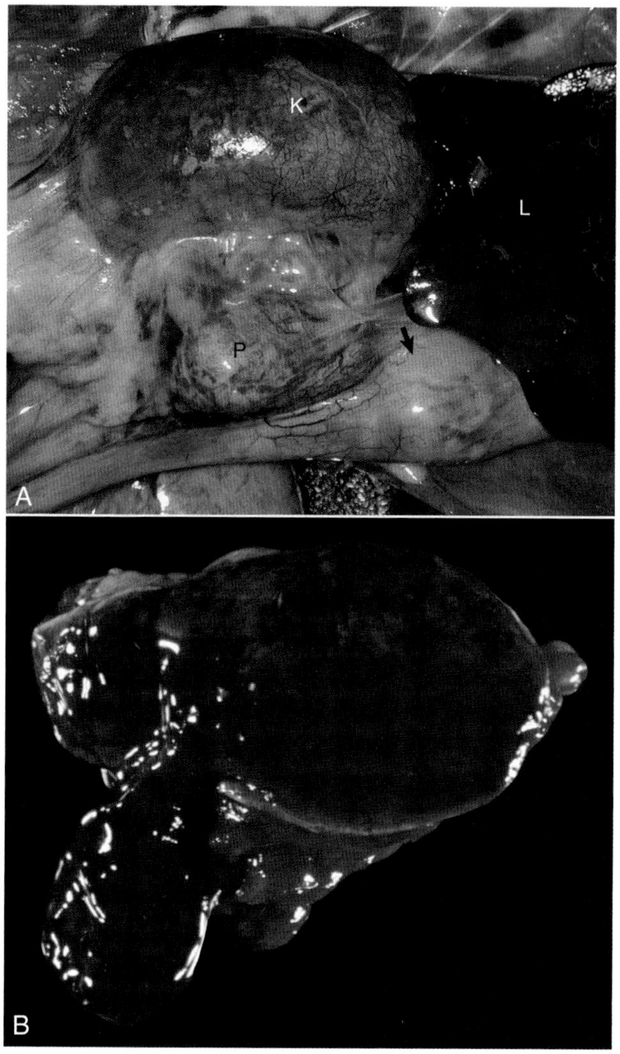

Figure 12-41 **Malignant Pheochromocytoma, Adrenal Gland, Dog. A,** A pheochromocytoma *(P)* has obliterated the adrenal gland and grown into the vena cava *(arrow)*. *K,* Kidney; *L,* Liver. **B,** Adrenal gland cross section. The malignant pheochromocytoma extends through the compressed adrenal cortex and capsule and into adjacent tissue. (**A** courtesy Dr. A. Paulman, College of Veterinary Medicine, University of Illinois. **B** courtesy Dr. M.A. Miller, College of Veterinary Medicine, Purdue University.)

ganglia, the neoplastic cells differentiate into multipolar ganglionic neurons. Thus, the neoplastic tissue consists of neuronal cell bodies and bundles of axons. Adrenal and para-adrenal neuroblastomas and ganglioneuromas resemble their counterparts elsewhere in the nervous system (see Chapter 14).

Disorders of Pancreatic Islet Cells

Hypofunction of Pancreatic Islet Cells

Diabetes Mellitus. Diabetes mellitus, diagnosed mainly in dogs and cats, is the result of a relative or absolute deficiency of insulin production and secretion by islet β cells or of a failure of target cells to respond to insulin. The major metabolic consequence of inadequate insulin activity is decreased movement of glucose into insulin-sensitive cells (particularly hepatocytes, adipocytes, and skeletal myocytes), with a corresponding increase in hepatic glucose production and hyperglycemia. As a functional disorder, diabetes mellitus is not necessarily accompanied by lesions in pancreatic islets. However, microscopic lesions are noted in some cases of diabetes. Aplasia or hypoplasia of pancreatic islets (within normal exocrine pancreatic tissue) has been reported in diabetic puppies. Degeneration (Fig. 12-42, A) or necrosis of pancreatic islets is more common than failure of development as a cause of insulin deficiency. Immune-mediated lymphoplasmacytic inflammation (Fig. 12-42, *B*) can cause selective islet cell destruction. Autoimmune destruction of islet cells is considered the major cause of human type 1 diabetes mellitus. Chronic pancreatitis (Figs. 12-43 and 12-44) indiscriminately destroys both exocrine and endocrine pancreatic tissue.

The inability of target cells to respond adequately to a hormone can be caused by a lack of adenyl cyclase as a second messenger within the cytosol or by an alteration or downregulation of cell-surface receptors. Human type 2 diabetes mellitus is characterized by insulin resistance with insufficient insulin secretion to meet the increased requirement. Hypertrophy or hyperplasia of islet β cells, a response to persistent hyperglycemia, may be detected in insulin-resistant diabetes, but it tends to be a subtle change. Genetic factors predispose to insulin resistance, but obesity is the most common cause of acquired type 2 diabetes. In domestic mammals, insulin-resistant diabetes mellitus, with normal or even elevated blood concentrations of insulin, is most commonly recognized in cats affected

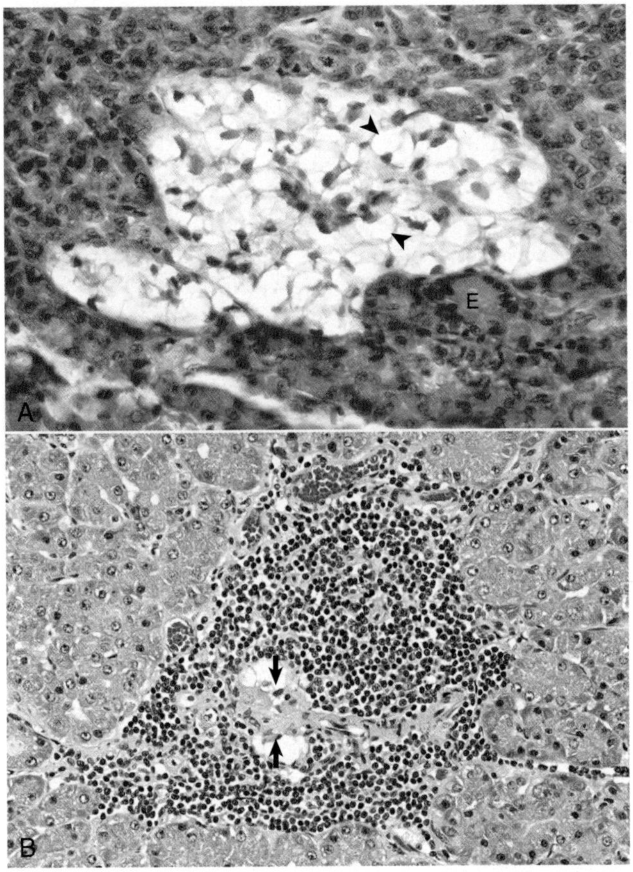

Figure 12-42 Pancreatic Islets, Cat. A, Hydropic degeneration. Discrete unstained vacuoles *(arrowheads)* are in the cytoplasm of β cells. *E,* Exocrine pancreas. H&E stain. **B,** Inflammation. Numerous lymphocytes and plasma cells are in a pancreatic islet. Most of the few remaining islet cells have undergone hydropic degeneration *(arrows)*. H&E stain. (**A** courtesy Dr. C. Capen, College of Veterinary Medicine, The Ohio State University. **B** courtesy Dr. M.A. Miller, College of Veterinary Medicine, Purdue University.)

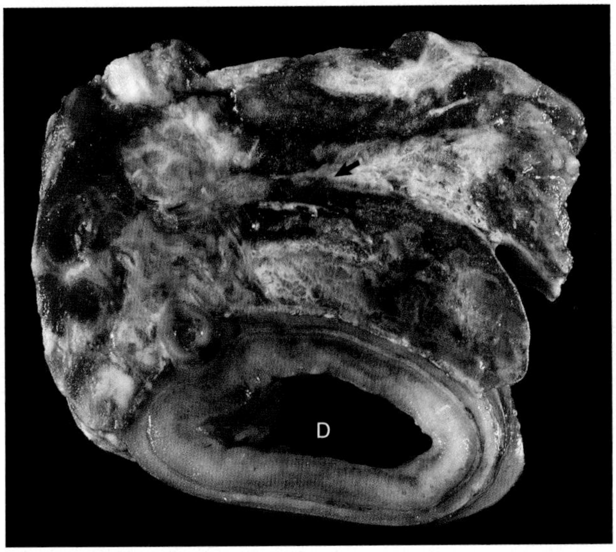

Figure 12-43 Chronic Relapsing Pancreatitis, Pancreas and Duodenum, Cross Section, Dog. The pancreas is multinodular and firm with areas of hemorrhage *(arrow)*, fibrosis, and necrosis. *D,* Duodenum. (Courtesy Dr. C. Capen, College of Veterinary Medicine, The Ohio State University.)

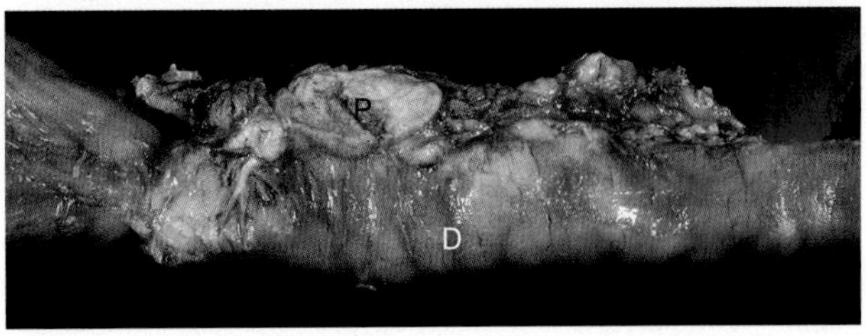

Figure 12-44 Chronic Pancreatitis, Pancreas, Dog. The pancreas *(P)* is markedly atrophied with extensive parenchymal replacement by fibrous tissue in "end-stage" pancreatitis. *D,* Duodenum. (Courtesy Dr. C. Capen, College of Veterinary Medicine, The Ohio State University.)

by obesity or pituitary somatotroph adenomas (see Disorders of Cats). Horses with metabolic syndrome also develop insulin resistance, but they usually do not develop diabetes (see Disorders of Horses).

Often, the lesions of diabetes mellitus are more striking in extrapancreatic organs or tissues than in the pancreatic islets (see Chapters 8, 11, and 21). Although most lesions of diabetes are attributed to insufficient insulin or to insulin resistance, an absolute or relative increase in glucagon secretion can contribute to the disease and its lesions. Increased blood glucagon concentration promotes hepatic gluconeogenesis and fatty acid oxidation, thereby contributing to hyperglycemia and ketoacidosis. Secretion of glucocorticoids, catecholamines, or growth hormone also promotes hyperglycemia.

Diabetes mellitus is an insidious disease with clinical signs that reflect its grave effects on nearly every system in the body. The persistent hyperglycemia and glucosuria lead to polydipsia and polyuria. Diabetic animals have diminished resistance to infection, attributed in part to impaired leukocyte function. Urinary tract infection by glucose-fermenting organisms, such as *Proteus* sp., *Aerobacter aerogenes*, and *Escherichia coli*, results in gas formation in the bladder wall and lumen, making emphysematous cystitis a characteristic lesion of diabetes.

Hepatomegaly in diabetic animals is mainly the result of steatosis (E-Figs. 12-23 and 12-24; also see Figs. 1-29, 8-25, and 8-38). Lipids accumulate in hepatocytes because of increased mobilization of fatty acids and decreased utilization by hepatocytes injured by ketonemia. Cataracts can develop in dogs with poorly controlled diabetes mellitus (E-Fig. 12-25; also see E-Fig. 21-35) because of the sorbitol pathway of glucose metabolism in the lens.

Other extrapancreatic lesions of diabetes mellitus, such as glomerulopathy (see Chapter 11), retinopathy (see Chapter 21), and gangrene, are the result of a microangiopathy (i.e., disorder of the small vessels [capillaries] of organ systems). Other renal lesions include accumulation of glycogen within renal tubular epithelial cells (E-Fig. 12-26). See the sections on Disorders of Dogs and Disorders of Cats.

Hyperfunction of Pancreatic Islet Cells

β-Cell (Insulin-Secreting) Neoplasms (Insulinomas). Islet cell neoplasms (adenomas or carcinomas) are often functional. Most are derived from β cells, but immunohistochemistry for insulin is necessary to document β-cell origin (and many β-cell neoplasms are multihormonal). Neoplasms of β cells develop most commonly in dogs (and in ferrets, in which they are generally benign), but they are also recognized in other domestic species, such as cats and cattle. Unlike other islet cell neoplasms, β-cell neoplasms may be closely associated with amyloid deposition derived from islet amyloid polypeptide (IAPP).

Carcinomas are more common than islet cell adenomas in dogs and often develop in the duodenal (right) lobe of the pancreas. Clinical signs are often neurologic and reflect hypoglycemia, the result of excessive insulin secretion from functional β-cell neoplasms.

Adenomas of β cells are typically solitary, yellow to red, small (<3 cm), spherical nodules of similar consistency to or slightly firmer than surrounding pancreatic parenchyma. Islet cell adenomas are sharply delineated by a thin fibrous capsule (Fig. 12-45). Fine fibrovascular septa subdivide the neoplasm into packets. The neoplastic cells are round to polyhedral with distinct cell borders and pale eosinophilic to amphophilic, faintly granular cytoplasm.

Islet cell carcinomas are typically larger than adenomas and invade adjacent parenchyma (Fig. 12-46), with metastasis to regional lymph nodes and liver or direct extension to the mesentery and omentum. Neoplastic cells of islet cell carcinomas are less uniform in size and shape than those of adenomas, but mitotic figures are usually uncommon. Thus, microscopic evidence of invasiveness or metastasis is the principal criterion of malignancy.

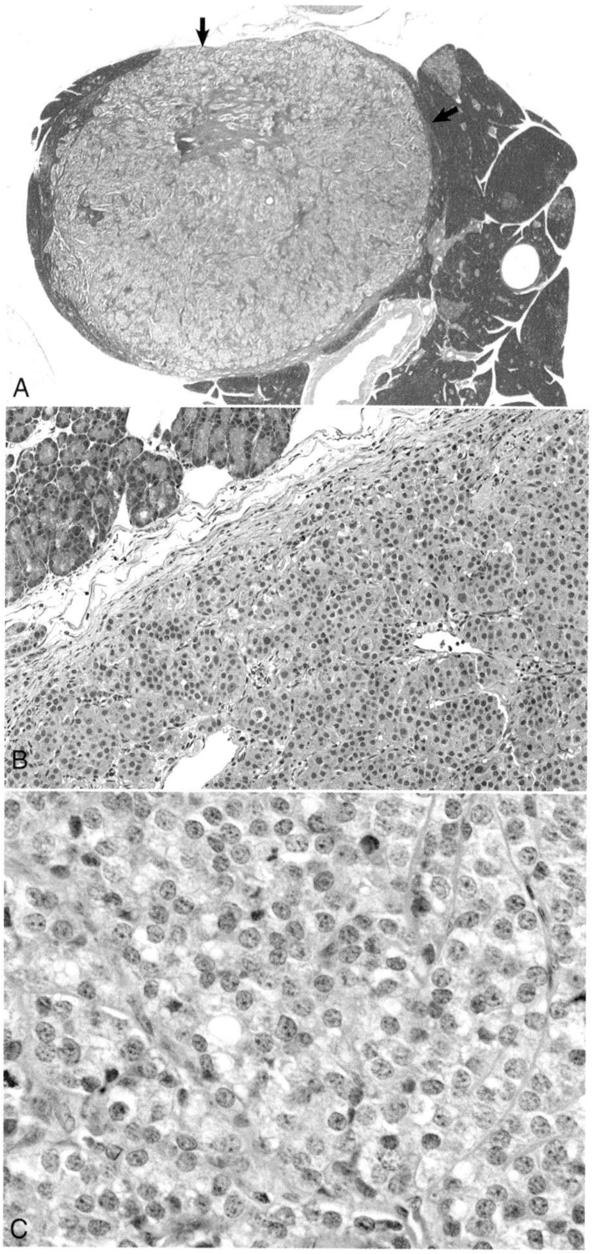

Figure 12-45 **β-Cell Adenoma, Pancreatic Islet, Dog. A,** A solid islet adenoma, surrounded by a thin fibrous capsule, compresses adjacent exocrine pancreas *(arrows)*. H&E stain. **B,** The neoplastic tissue is sharply demarcated from adjacent exocrine pancreas *(upper left corner)*. H&E stain. **C,** The neoplastic β cells are divided into packets by scanty fibrovascular stroma and have abundant finely granular cytoplasm characteristic of neuroendocrine tumors. H&E stain. (**A** courtesy Dr. C. Capen, College of Veterinary Medicine, The Ohio State University. **B** courtesy Dr. J.A. Ramos-Vara, College of Veterinary Medicine, Purdue University. **C** courtesy Dr. J.F. Zachary, College of Veterinary Medicine, University of Illinois.)

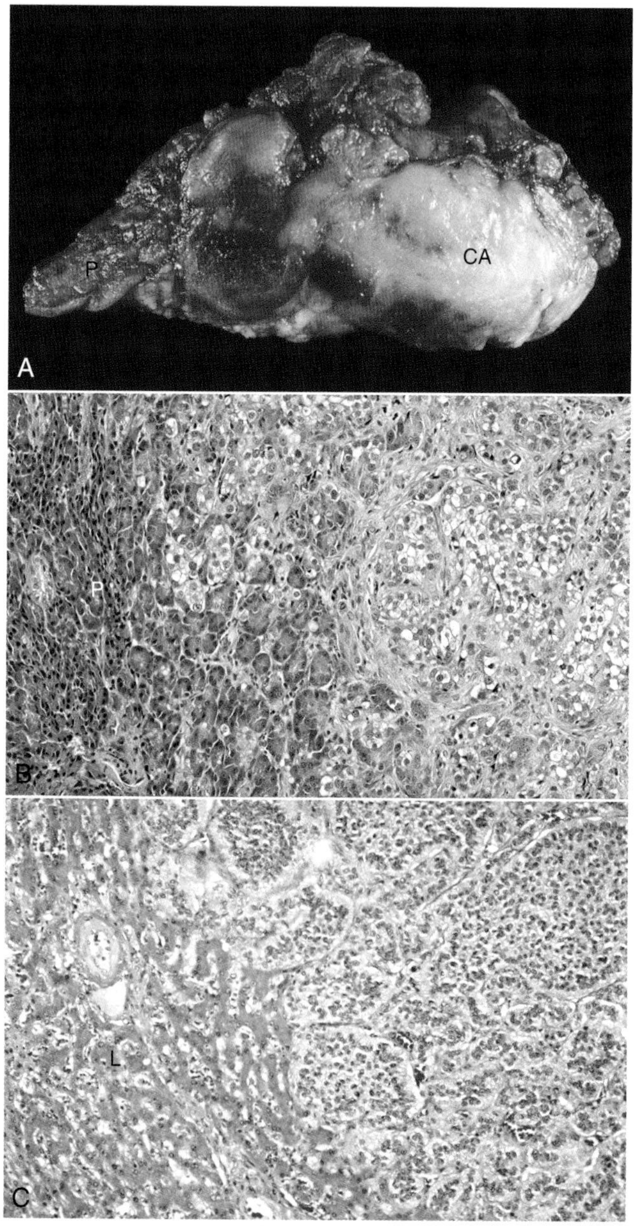

Figure 12-46 **β-Cell Carcinoma, Pancreatic Islet, Dog. A,** The multilobulated carcinoma *(CA)* is interlaced by fibrous tissue and poorly demarcated from adjacent exocrine pancreas *(P)*. **B,** The neoplastic tissue *(right)* has dense fibrous stroma and invades adjacent exocrine pancreas *(P)*. H&E stain. **C,** The β-cell carcinoma *(right)* has metastasized to the liver *(L)*. H&E stain. (**A** courtesy Dr. C. Capen, College of Veterinary Medicine, The Ohio State University. **B** courtesy Dr. M.A. Miller, College of Veterinary Medicine, Purdue University. **C** courtesy Dr. J.F. Zachary, College of Veterinary Medicine, University of Illinois.)

Islet cell neoplasms can be distinguished from pancreatic acinar neoplasms by their typical "neuroendocrine" appearance with packets of cells separated by fine fibrovascular stroma[8] and immunohistochemical reactivity for markers of neuroectodermal origin. Immunohistochemistry with antibody to insulin can be used to confirm β-cell origin.

Non-β Islet Cell Neoplasms. Non-β islet cell neoplasms are rare and include glucagonomas, gastrinomas, and somatostatinomas. Immunohistochemistry for glucagon is necessary to document the origin of an islet cell tumor from α cells. Gastrinomas are sought (but less commonly found) in dogs or cats with Zollinger-Ellison syndrome (hypergastrinemia, hypertrophic or atrophic gastritis, and gastrointestinal ulceration). Gastrin-producing cells are present in fetal and neonatal pancreatic islets but not in the adult pancreas, in which gastrin-producing cells instead are located in the gastric antrum or duodenum. Although gastrin-producing islet cells could dedifferentiate from existing islet cells or be derived from pluripotential nesidioblasts or pancreatic ductular epithelial cells, many human gastrinomas are found in the duodenum; this is also the case for canine gastrinomas. Somatostatinomas have been described in pancreatic islets and in the duodenum. They have also been reported along with gastrinomas as part of multiple endocrine neoplasia (MEN) syndrome in dogs.

Disorders of the Pineal Gland

Inflammation

The pineal gland shares photoreceptor cell–specific proteins with the retina, so it is not surprising that lymphocytic pinealitis occurs concurrently with experimental autoimmune uveoretinitis. Lymphocytic pinealitis has also been described in a horse with recurrent uveitis (see Chapter 21).

Neoplasms

Pineal tumors are exceedingly rare in animals, but they have been reported in a cow, goat, and horse. They are classified as well-differentiated pinealocytomas, anaplastic pinealoblastomas, or mixed tumors. Like other cells of neuroectodermal origin, pinealocytes express synaptophysin immunohistochemically.

Disorders of the Chemoreceptor Organs

Neoplasms

Chemoreceptor organs, especially the carotid body (near the bifurcation of the carotid arteries) and aortic body (near the ascending aorta at the base of the heart), can give rise to neoplasms called chemodectomas or paragangliomas. Aortic body chemodectomas are diagnosed more commonly than those of the carotid body in domestic animals, and they are observed mainly in dogs, especially in the brachycephalic breeds.

Although the cause of aortic and carotid body neoplasms is unknown, a genetic predisposition aggravated by chronic hypoxia could account for the greater risk in brachycephalic breeds, such as the boxer and Boston terrier. Carotid bodies of several mammalian species, including dogs, developed hyperplastic foci when the animals were subjected to the chronic hypoxia of high altitude. Human beings living at high altitudes have 10 times the incidence of chemoreceptor neoplasms as those residing at sea level.

The microscopic features of chemodectomas or paragangliomas are essentially similar, whether they are derived from the carotid or the aortic bodies, but aortic body neoplasms are more common. The neoplastic tissue is lobulated by fibrous trabeculae derived from the capsule and further subdivided into nests by fine fibrovascular septa. Neoplastic cells are aligned along small vessels and are round to polyhedral and closely packed, with pale eosinophilic, finely granular, or faintly vacuolated cytoplasm.

Neoplasms of the Carotid Body. Carotid body chemodectomas are usually unilateral and slow-growing. Benign tumors vary from 1 to 4 cm in diameter and are encapsulated. The bifurcation of the common carotid artery is usually incorporated in the mass, and neoplastic cells are firmly adhered to the tunica adventitia.

Malignant tumors are larger, multinodular, infiltrative, and can invade blood and lymphatic vessels. The external jugular vein and vagus nerve can also be invaded by and/or incorporated into the neoplasm. Metastases to the lungs, lymph nodes, or other organs occur in approximately 30% of the cases of malignant carotid body neoplasms.

Neoplasms of the Aortic Body. Aortic body chemodectomas appear as a solitary mass or multiple nodules near the base of the heart (Fig. 12-47). They vary considerably in size (from 0.5 to 12.5 cm), with malignant tumors usually larger than benign ones. Solitary small tumors are attached to the adventitia of the ascending aorta or embedded in the adipose tissue between the aorta and pulmonic trunk. Larger tumors are multilobular and compress the

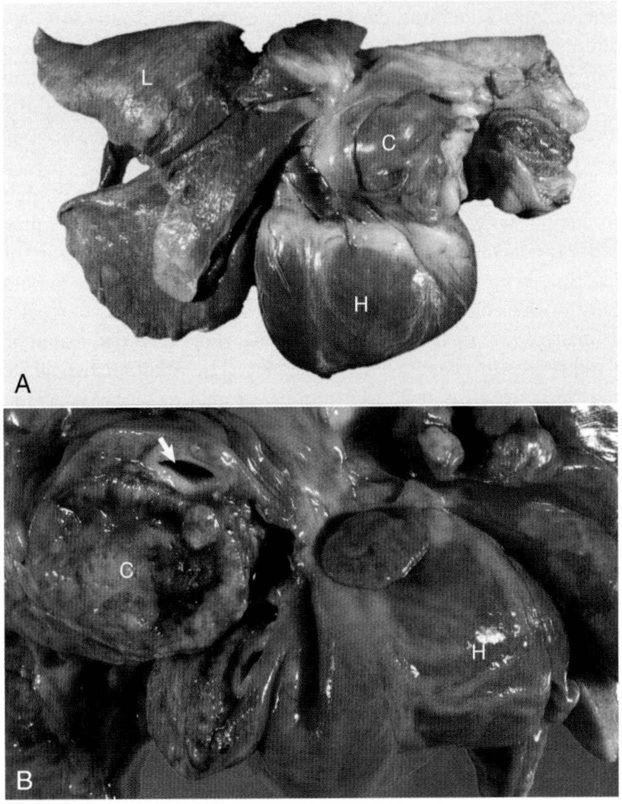

Figure 12-47 **Chemodectoma, Aortic Body, Dog. A,** A chemodectoma (C) is at the base of the heart *(H)*. *L,* Lung. **B,** On cross section, the chemodectoma (C) is closely apposed to the aorta *(arrow)* and encroaches on the right atrium. Metastatic nodules are scattered through the lungs *(upper left)*. *H,* Heart. (**A** courtesy College of Veterinary Medicine, University of Illinois. **B** courtesy Dr. M.A. Miller, College of Veterinary Medicine, Purdue University.)

[8]This cytomorphologic appearance is often referred to in the literature as an "endocrinoid" or "neuroendocrine" pattern or appearance.

atria, displace the trachea, and partially surround the great vessels at the base of the heart. Malignant aortic body neoplasms infiltrate the wall of the pulmonary artery and the cardiac atria. Neoplastic cells often invade blood vessels, but metastases to the lungs or liver are uncommon.

Neoplasms of the aortic bodies in animals are not functional (i.e., they do not secrete excess hormone into the circulation), but as a space-occupying lesion, the larger chemodectomas can lead to cardiac decompensation.

Heart-Base Neoplasms Derived from Ectopic Thyroid Gland Tissue. Adenomas and carcinomas derived from ectopic thyroid tissue account for up to 10% of canine "heart-base" neoplasms. Like chemodectomas, they typically compress or invade cranial mediastinal structures near the base of the heart (Fig. 12-48). Ectopic thyroid neoplasms have a compact cellular (solid) "endocrinoid" pattern that is difficult to distinguish histologically from that of aortic body chemodectomas. Often, primitive follicular structures or colloid-containing follicles can be demonstrated in ectopic thyroid neoplasms, but immunohistochemistry for thyroglobulin or thyroid transcription factor-1 may be necessary to document thyroid origin.

Obesity

Obesity, or the accumulation of excessive adipose tissue, is a complex and major health problem in companion animals, especially dogs and cats. Obese animals are predisposed to a wide variety of diseases affecting many organ systems. Endocrine disorders commonly associated with obesity include decreased glucose tolerance, insulin resistance, diabetes mellitus, dyslipidemia, canine hypothyroidism, and canine pancreatitis. Risk factors for obesity include breed predisposition, neutering, advanced age (of both owner and pet), diet (quantity and quality), and a sedentary lifestyle. Inactive horses that consume high-sugar, high-starch rations are also prone to obesity (see Disorders of Horses, Equine Metabolic Syndrome).

Among ruminants, obesity is of particular concern in high-producing dairy cows, especially during the transition from pregnancy to lactation (see Chapter 8, see Disorders of Ruminants [Cattle, Sheep, and Goats], Ketosis). The spike in glucose requirement at the onset of lactation coincides with a decreased appetite in many cows, so diversion of available glucose to the mammary gland results in negative energy balance. The resultant hypoglycemia decreases insulin concentrations, promoting lipolysis and fat mobilization. Nonesterified fatty acids (NEFA) are cleaved from triglycerides in adipocytes and enter the bloodstream bound to albumin. In homeostasis, the concentration of circulating NEFA is balanced (via reesterification or β-oxidation in the liver) with the demand for glucose; however, the abundant NEFA mobilized by cows with excessive adipose tissue can exceed the metabolic capacity of the liver and thus affected cows develop ketosis. Pregnant sheep and goats, especially if overweight or carrying more than one fetus, are also susceptible to abnormalities of carbohydrate and lipid metabolism.

Obesity is considered an endocrine disease not only for its association with various endocrinopathies but also because white adipose tissue functions as an endocrine organ by synthesizing and secreting adipokines, such as leptin and adiponectin. In fact, maintaining the balance between these opposing adipokines is essential for the prevention of both obesity and insulin resistance. Leptin, the major hormone produced by adipocytes, is critical for appetite suppression and thermogenesis; it is also proinflammatory. Obese animals tend to develop leptin resistance (decreased hypothalamic response to leptin) with compensatory elevation in leptin production.

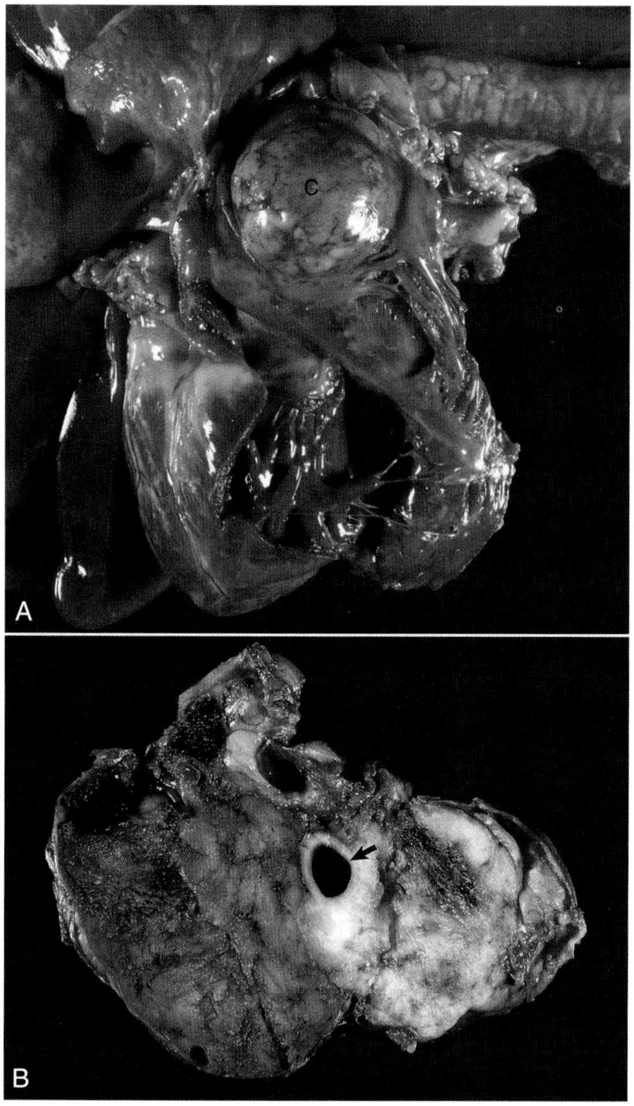

Figure 12-48 **Carcinoma, Ectopic Thyroid Tissue, Cranial Mediastinum, Dog. A,** An ectopic thyroid carcinoma (C) surrounds the aorta and pulmonic trunk, and it bulges against the wall of the right atrium. Distinction of this "heart-base" tumor from an aortic body chemodectoma or other endocrine neoplasm was based on immunohistochemical reactivity for thyroglobulin. **B,** Note the remarkable similarity to chemodectoma (see Fig. 12-47) in the appearance of the neoplastic tissue and its proximity to the aorta *(arrow)*. (**A** courtesy Dr. M.A. Miller, College of Veterinary Medicine, Purdue University. **B** courtesy Dr. C. Capen, College of Veterinary Medicine, The Ohio State University.)

Circulating leptin concentrations rise as the mass of adipose tissue increases. Insulin resistance is correlated with elevated leptin concentration, which at least partially explains the increased risk for diabetes mellitus in obese cats. In contrast to leptin, adiponectin increases insulin sensitivity, enhancing glucose uptake and metabolism, and is antiinflammatory. However, circulating adiponectin concentrations are decreased in obese dogs and cats. Along with the proinflammatory effects of elevated leptin and decreased adiponectin concentration, the number and activity of monocytes and macrophages in adipose tissue increase in obese animals. These leukocytes are the source of cytokines, such as tumor necrosis factor (TNF)-α and interleukin-6. TNF-α, in addition to appetite suppression and proinflammatory effects, decreases insulin sensitivity and promotes lipolysis. Obesity-related insulin resistance and inflammation, through the adipokine imbalance and cytokines of excessive adipose tissue, have far-reaching systemic effects.

Disorders of Horses

Dysfunction of the Pars Intermedia of the Pituitary Gland

Pituitary pars intermedia dysfunction (PPID) is the most commonly diagnosed endocrine disorder of horses. Although it has been called equine Cushing's disease, its pathogenesis is distinct from that of human or canine Cushing's disease. Whereas Cushing's disease reflects an aberration in the hypothalamic-pituitary-adrenal axis control of corticotrophs, pars intermedia melanotrophs do not express glucocorticoid receptors and are controlled instead by dopaminergic inhibition from hypothalamic neurons. Importantly, the adrenal glands of horses with PPID are usually unremarkable—that is, they are free of diffuse or nodular proliferation of cortical cells.

In the normal equine pars intermedia, dopaminergic inhibition is decreased in autumn as the duration of daylight grows shorter. The resultant increased activity of the pars intermedia promotes hair growth and increased volume of adipose tissue deposition in preparation for the winter months. In PPID, pars intermedia dopamine concentrations are decreased year-round, and the melanotrophs, with loss of dopaminergic inhibition, synthesize excessive proopiomelanocortins (POMC) and secrete excessive concentrations of a variety of hormones, especially α-MSH, β-endorphins, corticotrophin-like intermediate peptide (CLIP), and, less so, ACTH. Hypertrichosis (also known as hirsutism [excessively long hair or failure to shed normally in the spring]; Fig. 12-49; E-Fig. 12-27) is considered diagnostic but is not apparent, let alone obvious, in all horses with PPID. Other clinical signs, such as chronic laminitis (inflammation of the hoof lamellae; see Chapter 17), weight loss or abnormal distribution of adipose tissue, and increased susceptibility to infection, are inconsistently present and nonspecific. Hypertrichosis and other clinical signs of PPID may, in part, reflect hypothalamic compression by the space-occupying effect of an enlarged pituitary gland rather than being entirely attributable to overproduction of POMC peptides.

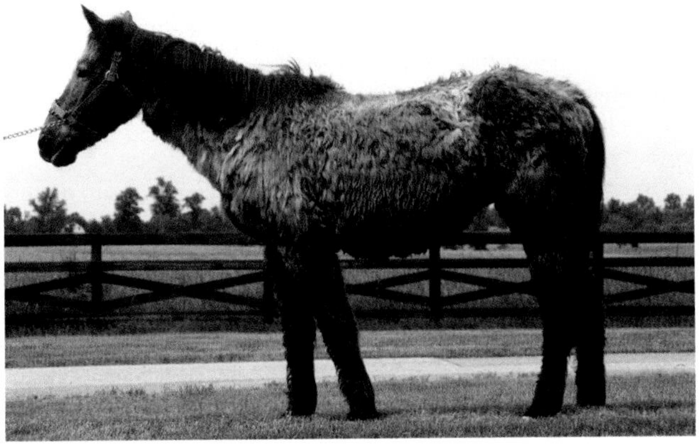

Figure 12-49 **Hypertrichosis (Also Known as Hirsutism), Horse.** Hypertrichosis (excessively long hair or failure to shed in the spring) is attributed to hypothalamic compression by a pituitary pars intermedia adenoma. This horse also has experienced the weight loss that is common with pituitary pars intermedia dysfunction (PPID). (Courtesy Dr. E.M. Green, College of Veterinary Medicine and Biomedical Sciences, Texas A&M University.)

The major risk factor for PPID is advanced age. The pathogenesis may be the result of age-associated oxidative injury of dopaminergic hypothalamic neurons. Focal or multifocal hypertrophy and hyperplasia of the pars intermedia is found at autopsy (syn: necropsy) (see E-Appendix 12-1) in most horses older than 10 years of age and may be accompanied by cyst formation, but these focal lesions are seldom associated with clinical signs of PPID. In contrast, diffuse adenomatous hyperplasia, even without the development of microadenomas or a macroadenoma, can significantly enlarge the pars intermedia and is likely to result in the clinical signs of PPID.

As in the pars distalis, nodules between 1 and 5 mm in diameter are classified as microadenomas (Fig. 12-50, *A*). By definition, macroadenomas (Fig. 12-50, *B*; also see Fig. 12-20) are at least 5 mm (but in horses often are 1 to 3 cm) in diameter. Because microadenomas tend to be multiple, their accumulated mass can reach or exceed that of a macroadenoma. Histologically, equine pars intermedia adenomas form packets of polyhedral to piriform cells separated by thin fibrovascular septa (Fig. 12-50, *C*; E-Fig. 12-28). The neoplastic cells resemble hypertrophied versions of their nonneoplastic counterparts and have variable immunoreactivity for corticotrophin-like intermediate peptide (CLIP), melanocyte-stimulating hormone (MSH), β-endorphin, and β-lipotropin. Although ACTH immunoreactivity is usually detectable, this result is not necessarily bioactive ACTH. Nonfunctional pars intermedia adenomas in horses exert a mass effect with various metabolic abnormalities attributed mainly to compression of the hypophysis and the hypothalamus. Importantly, the pituitary pars nervosa is one of the first tissues to be compressed. Therefore, even a small pars intermedia adenoma can disrupt the hypothalamic-pituitary axis.

Equine Metabolic Syndrome

Physically inactive horses that consume high-energy rations, especially those with a high glycemic index, are susceptible to development of equine metabolic syndrome. Importantly, grass is a major dietary source of sugars. Certain breeds, but especially ponies and miniature horses, are at increased risk. Affected horses are also likely to become obese (or develop regional adiposity; e.g., "cresty neck")[9] with associated increased concentrations of inflammatory mediators and to develop insulin resistance. Insulin resistance is often detected upon screening for hyperinsulinemia as an indicator of equine metabolic syndrome; however, type 2 diabetes mellitus is seldom diagnosed in horses. Hypertriglyceridemia and hyperleptinemia have also been documented in equine metabolic syndrome. Chronic "endocrinopathic" laminitis (see Chapter 17) is a crippling and common complication of equine metabolic syndrome.

Congenital Hypothyroidism-Dysmaturity Syndrome

Particularly in the Pacific Northwest and western Canada, equine perinatal death has been associated with hypothyroidism—possibly the result of maternal iodine deficiency or exposure to excessive nitrate from green forage—and musculoskeletal malformations. The congenital hypothyroidism is thought to cause the associated musculoskeletal malformations, mainly prognathism and (despite normal length or even prolonged gestation) delayed ossification of carpal and tarsal bones with flexural deformities and contracted or ruptured tendons. The thyroid gland in affected foals may not be macroscopically enlarged, but it has histologic features of hyperplasia.

[9]Thickening by fatty infiltration of the dorsal and lateral areas of the neck.

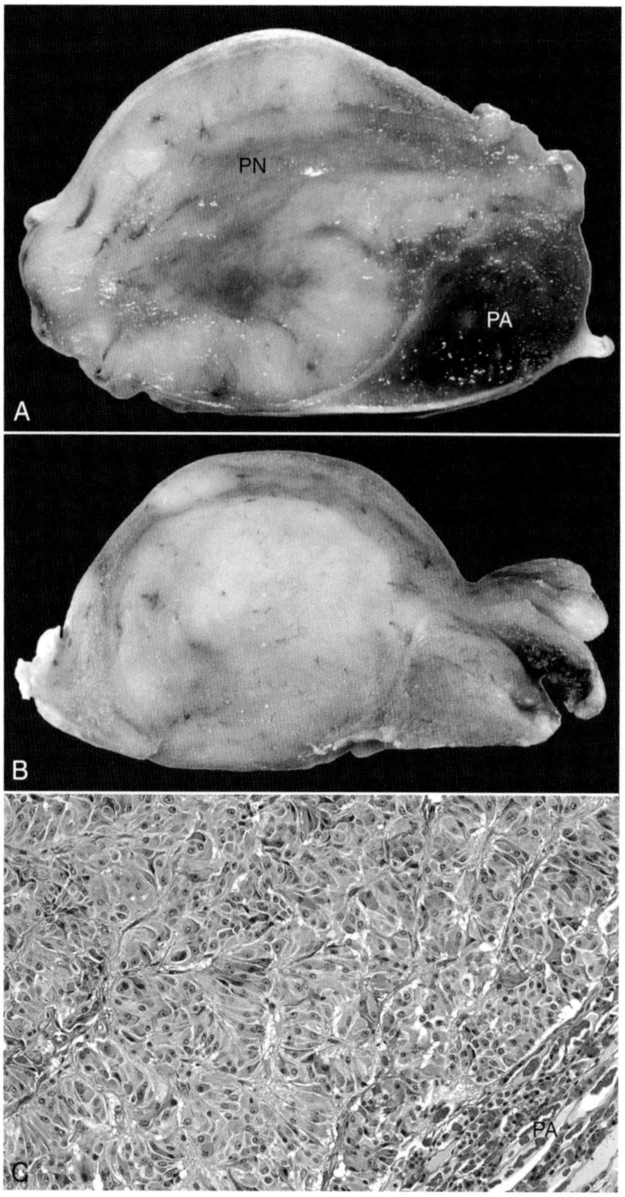

Figure 12-50 **Adenoma, Pituitary Pars Intermedia, Horse. A,** Pituitary gland, sagittal section. Coalescing microadenomas (nodules 1 to 5 mm in diameter) expand the pars intermedia. *PA*, Pars anterior; *PN*, pars nervosa. **B,** Pituitary gland, sagittal section. A macroadenoma, accompanied by several microadenomas, expands the pars intermedia and compresses the pars nervosa and pars anterior. **C,** The melanotroph adenoma consists of hypertrophied polyhedral to pyriform cells with ample pale amphophilic cytoplasm in fine fibrovascular stroma. Note chromophobes and acidophils in the compressed pars anterior (*PA, lower right corner*). H&E stain. (Courtesy Dr. M.A. Miller, College of Veterinary Medicine, Purdue University.)

Lymphocytic (Immune-Mediated) Thyroiditis

See Disorders of Domestic Animals, Disorders of the Thyroid Gland.

Nutritional Hyperparathyroidism

See Disorders of Domestic Animals, Disorders of the Parathyroid Gland.

Pinealitis

See Disorders of Domestic Animals, Disorders of the Pineal Gland.

Disorders of Ruminants (Cattle, Sheep, and Goats)

Adenohypophyseal (Anterior Pituitary Gland) Aplasia and Prolonged Gestation

Studies in sheep and other animals emphasize the importance of the fetal hypothalamic-pituitary-adrenal axis in the initiation of parturition. Corticotrophin-releasing hormone (CRH) from hypothalamic neurons (and from the placenta) stimulates secretion of ACTH from adenohypophyseal corticotrophs, leading to increased cortisol production by the fetal adrenal gland. Both cortisol and CRH stimulate placental prostaglandin production by upregulating cyclooxygenase-2. Induction of placental 17α-hydroxylase by cortisol or PGE_2 promotes the conversion of progesterone to estradiol. The increasing concentration of placental estradiol (and decreasing progesterone concentration) in late gestation provides positive feedback on the hypothalamus and adenohypophysis, stimulating the release of additional ACTH, production of $PGF_{2\alpha}$, and the onset of parturition. Therefore, any injury that disrupts the hypothalamic-pituitary-adrenal axis causes abnormal fetal development and tends to prolong gestation. Aplasia of the adenohypophysis (with normal development of the neurohypophysis [posterior pituitary gland]) is described as a genetic disease in Guernsey and Jersey cattle. The pituitary gland can also fail to develop as a result of hypothalamic malformations (e.g., from ingestion of *Veratrum californicum* by pregnant ewes [see Chapter 18]). Ruminant fetuses with defective adenohypophyseal (anterior pituitary gland) ACTH secretion have subnormal development of the adrenal cortices with inadequate synthesis and secretion of cortisol.

Congenital Dyshormonogenetic Goiter

See Disorders of Domestic Animals, Disorders of the Thyroid Gland.

Thyroid C-Cell (Ultimobranchial) Neoplasms

See Disorders of Domestic Animals, Disorders of the Thyroid Gland.

Parturient Hypocalcemia

Parturient paresis (also known as milk fever and hypocalcemia) in dairy cows is a complex metabolic disorder characterized by the sudden development of hypocalcemia and hypophosphatemia near the onset of parturition and lactation. Biochemical and ultrastructural studies indicate that the parathyroid glands do respond to the hypocalcemia with increased synthesis and secretion of PTH, but bone resorption remains minimal. In small ruminants, especially in dairy goats and ewes, hypocalcemia more commonly develops approximately 2 weeks before or after parturition and coincides with periods of fetal skeletal mineralization or peak lactation, respectively.

Excessive calcium in the ration predisposes dairy cows to parturient hypocalcemia, whereas diets low in calcium or supplemented with vitamin D are protective. Calcium homeostasis in pregnant cows fed a high-calcium diet appears to be maintained principally by intestinal calcium absorption (Fig. 12-51). This greater reliance on intestinal absorption rather than on PTH-stimulated bone resorption could explain the increased risk for development of profound hypocalcemia near parturition in cows fed excessive calcium. Furthermore, the increased secretion of calcitonin in pregnant cows on a high-calcium diet could counteract the effects of PTH on calcium resorption from bone.

Disorders of Pigs

Although pigs are susceptible to goiter for the same reasons as other domestic species, other endocrine disorders are seldom diagnosed in

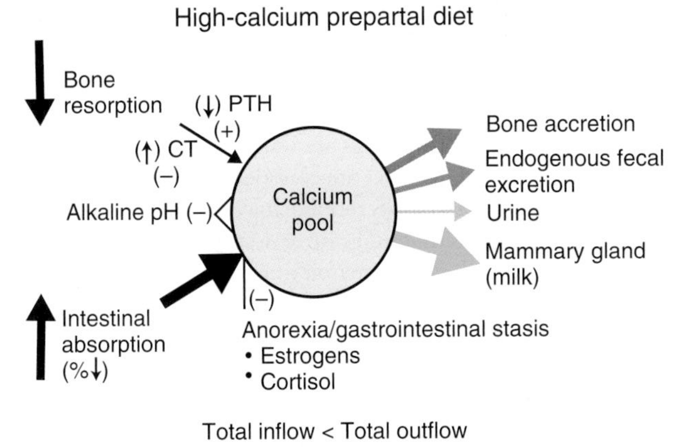

Figure 12-51 **Calcium Homeostasis in Cows Fed a High-Calcium Prepartal Diet.** With high dietary calcium, homeostasis depends mainly on intestinal calcium absorption. The parathyroid glands are inactive, and bone resorption is low. Decreased appetite and gastrointestinal mobility near parturition disrupt the intestinal absorption of calcium into the extracellular fluid calcium pool. Outflow of calcium with the onset of lactation exceeds the rate of inflow into the calcium pool, and cows develop a progressive hypocalcemia and paresis. *CT,* Calcitonin; *PTH,* parathyroid hormone. (Redrawn with permission from Dr. C. Capen, College of Veterinary Medicine, The Ohio State University.)

pigs raised for livestock production (i.e., shortened life span). However, miniature pigs often are sedentary companion animals with unconventional diets and a long life span. Therefore, they are prone to obesity and associated diseases. Importantly, miniature swine also have a different genetic makeup than commercial pigs.

Metabolic Syndrome in Ossabaw Pigs

Information on this topic is available at www.expertconsult.com.

Disorders of Dogs

Pituitary Cysts and Pituitary Dwarfism

Craniopharyngeal duct cysts (Fig. 12-52), lined by respiratory epithelium (pseudostratified columnar epithelium with ciliated cells and goblet cells), are occasionally found near the pars tuberalis and pars distalis of dogs. The cysts fill with mucin but are typically microscopic or less than a few millimeters in diameter, and they do not seem to interfere with pituitary function.

In contrast, Rathke's cleft cysts result from failure of Rathke's pouch ectoderm to differentiate into the adenohypophysis. This progressively enlarging sellar (i.e., within the sella turcica) cyst (Fig. 12-53) is also lined by pseudostratified columnar epithelium with ciliated cells and goblet cells, and it is filled with mucin. However, the accompanying failure of adenohypophyseal (anterior pituitary gland) development results in a deficiency or lack of all trophic hormones and therefore a functional panhypopituitarism. This juvenile panhypopituitarism occurs most frequently as an autosomal recessive disease in German shepherd dogs, but it has also been reported in Spitz, toy pinscher, and Karelian bear dogs. Affected puppies appear normal until approximately 2 months of age, after which subnormal growth, retention of puppy hair coat with progression to hyperpigmentation and bilaterally symmetric alopecia, and lack of primary guard hairs gradually become evident (Fig. 12-54). Adult German shepherd dogs with panhypopituitarism vary from as small as 2 kg in body weight to nearly half normal size, depending on whether the failure of formation of the adenohypophysis is partial or complete. Insulin-like growth factor, which is regulated by somatotrophin (growth hormone), has low activity in dwarf dogs

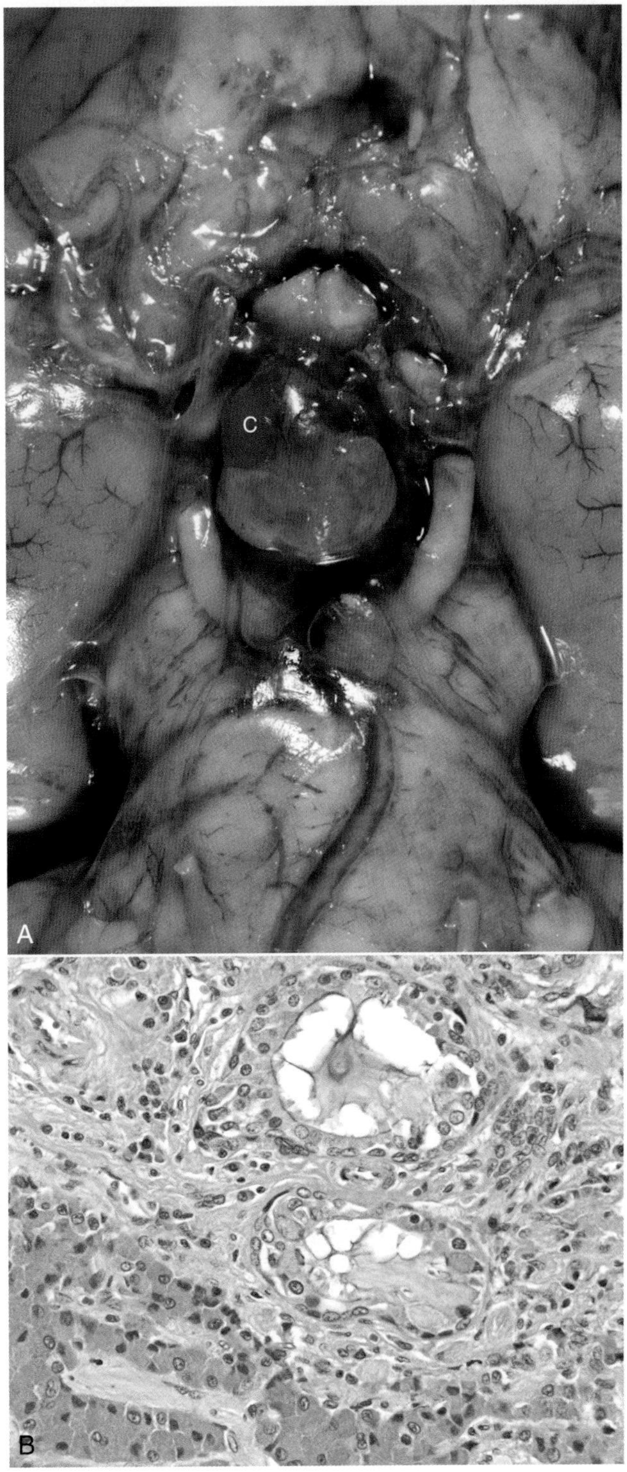

Figure 12-52 **Craniopharyngeal Duct Cysts, Pituitary Gland, Dog.** **A,** A multiloculated, mucus-filled cyst (C) is on the rostroventral aspect of the adenohypophysis. **B,** Microscopic cystic remnants of the craniopharyngeal duct are lined by pseudostratified columnar epithelium with ciliated cells and goblet cells and are surrounded by fibrous tissue. Note unaffected adenohypophysis in the lower left. H&E stain. (Courtesy Dr. M.A. Miller, College of Veterinary Medicine, Purdue University.)

and intermediate concentrations in phenotypically normal ancestors suspected to be heterozygous carriers.

Pituitary Apoplexy

See Disorders of Domestic Animals, Disorders of the Adenohypophysis (Anterior Pituitary Gland).

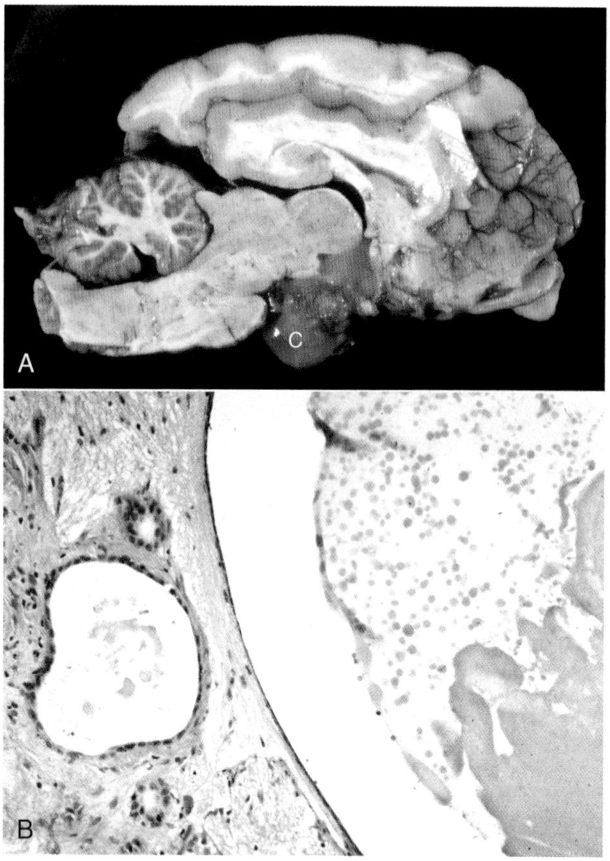

Figure 12-53 **Cystic Rathke's Pouch, Brain, Sagittal Section, Dog.** **A,** A large, multiloculated cyst (*C*) is on the ventral aspect of this brain where the adenohypophysis would normally be located. **B,** The cyst is in the right half of the photomicrograph; the left half of the field consists of disorganized tissue that resembles neurohypophysis with a few ductular structures, but differentiated adenohypophyseal tissue is not recognizable. H&E stain. (Courtesy Dr. J.F. Zachary, College of Veterinary Medicine, University of Illinois.)

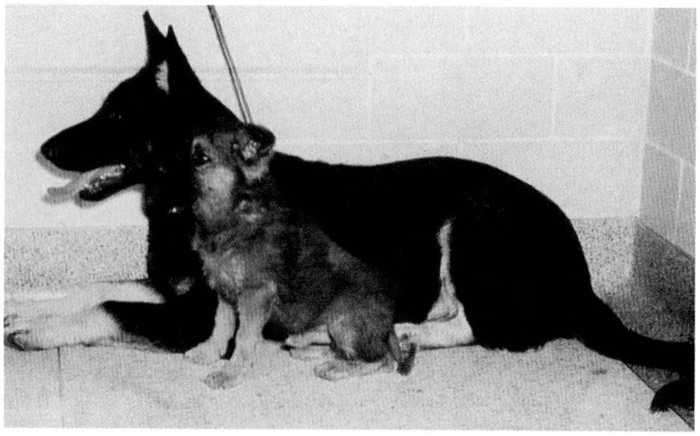

Figure 12-54 **Panhypopituitarism ("Pituitary Dwarfism"), 5-Month-Old German Shepherd and Littermate.** The unaffected littermate weighed 27.3 kg, whereas the dwarf puppy weighed only 4 kg and retained its puppy hair coat. (Courtesy Dr. Jack E. Alexander.)

Craniopharyngioma and Suprasellar Germ Cell Tumors

See Disorders of Domestic Animals, Other Neoplastic Disorders of the Hypophysis, Suprasellar Neoplasms.

Pars Intermedia Adenomas

See Disorders of Domestic Animals, Disorders of the Adenohypophysis (Anterior Pituitary Gland).

Hypothyroidism

Acquired hypothyroidism is the most common canine thyroid disorder. The thyroid lesion in almost all cases of adult-onset hypothyroidism in dogs is follicular atrophy (Fig. 12-55, *A*) or lymphocytic thyroiditis or both. Affected dogs are usually middle-aged or older, and more than 90% of the cases are considered primary, rather than secondary to decreased TSH secretion. However, pituitary macroadenomas or other lesions that infiltrate or destroy the adenohypophysis can result in secondary hypothyroidism, in which the follicles are lined by low cuboidal or flattened epithelial cells and distended by colloid (Fig. 12-55, *B*; also see Fig. 12-8, *B*). Metabolic (hypercholesterolemia is one of the most consistent serum biochemical abnormalities) and dermatologic (E-Fig. 12-29; also see Chapter 17) disturbances are clinical findings that prompt diagnostic testing for hypothyroidism. Hypercholesterolemia from hypothyroidism is one of the few causes of atherosclerosis in dogs (Fig. 12-55, *C*; E-Fig. 12-30; also see Fig. 10-66).

Idiopathic Follicular Atrophy

In idiopathic follicular atrophy, the thyroid gland is shrunken and pale because most of the parenchyma has been lost or replaced by adipose tissue (see Fig. 12-55, *A* and *B*). Although this appearance could be an end stage of autoimmune lymphocytic thyroiditis, inflammation is seldom evident histologically. However, because histology is not part of the diagnostic workup of canine hypothyroidism, the thyroid gland is seldom evaluated until the death of the dog. Furthermore, dogs with a clinical diagnosis of hypothyroidism usually receive hormone replacement therapy, which provides negative feedback on the hypothalamus and hypophysis, lowering circulating TSH concentrations and exacerbating thyroid follicular atrophy. Therefore, knowledge of the progression of idiopathic follicular atrophy is based on histologic evaluation of laboratory dogs, in which early lesions are focal. Affected follicles are small with scanty colloid and tall columnar follicular cells. Subsequently, with the onset of clinical hypothyroidism and thyroid hormone deficiency, atrophy is diffuse and pronounced. The gland consists mainly of adipose tissue with only scattered clusters of recognizable follicles lined by low cuboidal cells.

Lymphocytic Thyroiditis

In lymphocytic thyroiditis (E-Fig. 12-31; also see Fig. 12-27), the interstitium has multifocal or diffuse infiltrates of lymphocytes, plasma cells, and macrophages with at least a relative increase in fibrous tissue. Histologic studies in laboratory beagles indicate an early hypertrophic response of follicular cells to TSH, but usually by the time of histologic examination in clinical cases, most follicles have been destroyed. Because histologic examination is not used for diagnosis, the demonstration of serum autoantibodies to thyroglobulin, T_3, or T_4 can be used (along with measurement of circulating T_3, T_4, and TSH to document hypothyroidism) to infer the presence of lymphocytic thyroiditis. Documentation of thyroglobulin autoantibodies also supports the theory that canine lymphocytic thyroiditis is an autoimmune disease, like Hashimoto's thyroiditis in human beings. In a review of serum biochemical assays for thyroid dysfunction, euthyroid, thyroglobulin autoantibody-positive dogs were younger than hypothyroid, thyroglobulin autoantibody-positive dogs, which in turn were younger than hypothyroid, thyroglobulin autoantibody-negative dogs. These findings indicate the progressive nature of lymphocytic thyroiditis because it is thought that more than 75% of the gland must be destroyed before clinical hypothyroidism ensues. If nearly all follicular tissue is destroyed, then the antigenic stimulation for production of thyroglobulin autoantibodies no longer exists and the lymphocytic inflammation would be

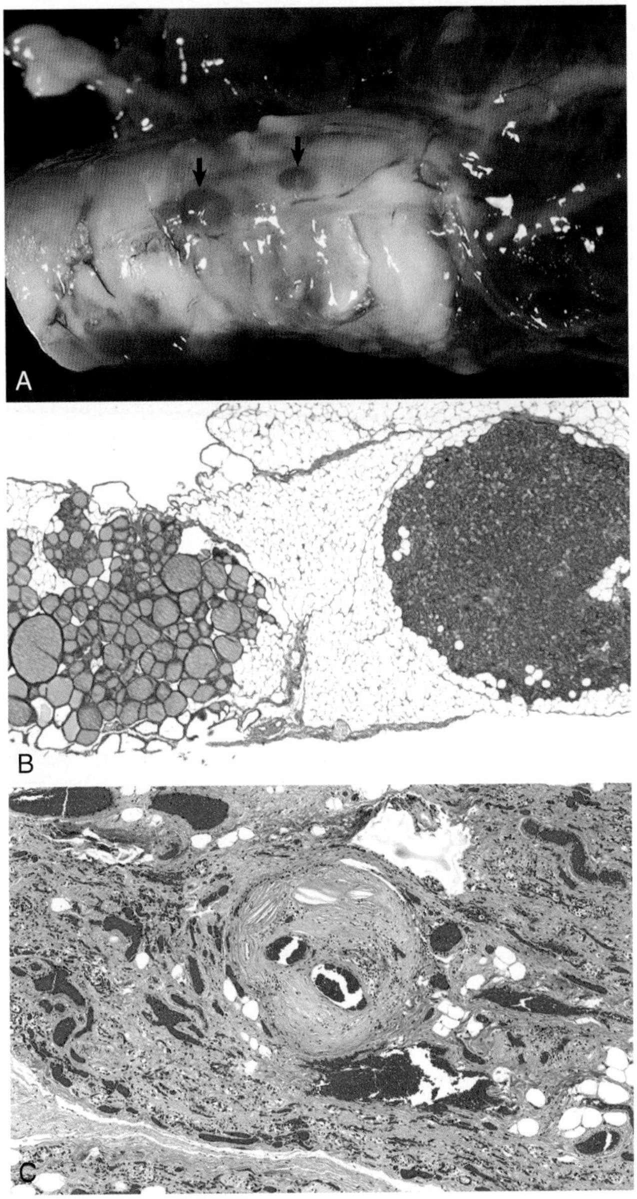

Figure 12-55 Atrophic Thyroid Gland, Dog. A, The shrunken thyroid gland is translucent, pale tan, and barely perceptible. The thyroid atrophy makes the parathyroid glands *(arrows)* appear more prominent. **B,** Thyroid follicles *(left)* are atrophic with low cuboidal epithelium and moderately eosinophilic colloid. Adipose tissue has infiltrated the interstitium. The parathyroid gland *(right)* is of normal size. H&E stain. **C,** Severe atrophy has resulted in collapse of most thyroid follicles and a relative increase in fibrous stroma. Note the sterol clefts of atherosclerosis in a branch of the thyroid artery. H&E stain. (**A** courtesy Dr. W. Crowell, College of Veterinary Medicine, The University of Georgia; and Noah's Arkive, College of Veterinary Medicine, The University of Georgia. **B** courtesy College of Veterinary Medicine, University of Illinois. **C** courtesy Dr. M.A. Miller, College of Veterinary Medicine, Purdue University.)

expected to subside. This result again raises the question of whether idiopathic follicular atrophy, at least in some cases, might be "burnt-out" lymphocytic thyroiditis. Certain breeds or families of dogs, including laboratory beagles, golden and Labrador retrievers, and Doberman pinschers, are at increased risk for hypothyroidism.

Renal Hyperparathyroidism

See Disorders of Domestic Animals, Disorders of the Parathyroid Gland, and Chapter 11.

Apocrine Carcinoma of the Anal Sac Glands

Apocrine carcinomas of the anal sac glands are the most common perianal malignancy in dogs and one of the most common canine causes of hypercalcemia of malignancy. Importantly, approximately half the cases are discovered during rectal palpation, so the serum chemistry finding of hypercalcemia, reported in approximately one-fourth of affected dogs, should prompt a search for this neoplasm. The hypercalcemia is attributed to secretion of parathyroid hormone-related peptide (PTHrP). Circulating concentrations of parathyroid hormone are not increased; in fact, the parathyroid glands are usually atrophied in response to persistent hypercalcemia. In a series of feline cases—the neoplasm is much less common in cats—serum calcium concentration was measured in 5 of 64 cats studied and only 1 cat had borderline hypercalcemia.

Dogs with apocrine carcinoma of the anal sac glands are typically older and usually neutered males or females. Most anal sac gland carcinomas have metastasized to regional lymph nodes by the time of presentation. Grossly, the apocrine carcinomas are firm nodular masses adjacent to one anal sac (Fig. 12-56, *A*; E-Fig. 12-32). Histologically, neoplastic cells are arranged in solid, tubular, or rosette patterns or a combination of patterns (Fig. 12-56, *B* and *C*; E-Figs. 12-33 and 12-34). The neoplastic cells may express neuroendocrine markers, such as chromogranin A or neuron-specific enolase, but expression of these markers does not necessarily correlate with hypercalcemia.

Hyperadrenocorticism (Cushing's Syndrome or Disease)

Hyperadrenocorticism is relatively common in older dogs, increasingly recognized in cats, and rare in other domestic animals. Iatrogenic hyperadrenocorticism is the result of glucocorticoid therapy, which results in decreased ACTH secretion and adrenocortical atrophy. Spontaneous Cushing's syndrome, in contrast, is usually the result of ACTH secretion by hyperplastic or neoplastic adenohypophyseal (anterior pituitary gland) corticotrophs, which causes bilateral, diffuse or multifocal adrenocortical hyperplasia, especially in the zona fasciculata (see Figs. 12-17, *A* and *C*, and 12-35). Functional adrenocortical adenomas or carcinomas (see Fig. 12-37) are a less common cause of canine Cushing's syndrome. Basal plasma cortisol concentration is compared with that after dexamethasone suppression and ACTH stimulation to determine the pathogenesis of hyperadrenocorticism.

Increased gluconeogenesis, lipogenesis, and protein catabolism explain many of the clinical signs and lesions. Atrophy of skeletal muscle results in a pendulous abdomen (see Fig. 12-36). Hepatomegaly is caused by increased deposits of lipid and glycogen (steroid hepatopathy; see Fig. 8-78). Cutaneous lesions develop initially over points of wear (e.g., neck, flanks, or behind the ears) or bony prominences and then spread in a bilaterally symmetric pattern to involve most of the body surface (see Figs. 12-36, 17-74, and 17-75). Cutaneous lesions of hypercortisolism include atrophy of the epidermis and pilosebaceous units, with loss of dermal collagen and elastin. In calcinosis cutis, a characteristic lesion in up to 30% of dogs with hyperadrenocorticism, calcium crystals are deposited along dermal collagen and elastin fibers and can penetrate the atrophic epidermis or follicular epithelium. This cutaneous calcification is probably related to the glyconeogenic and protein catabolic action of cortisol, which results in the molecular rearrangement of collagen and elastin with formation of a matrix that attracts calcium. Calcium can also be deposited in other tissues, such as lungs, skeletal muscle, and stomach.

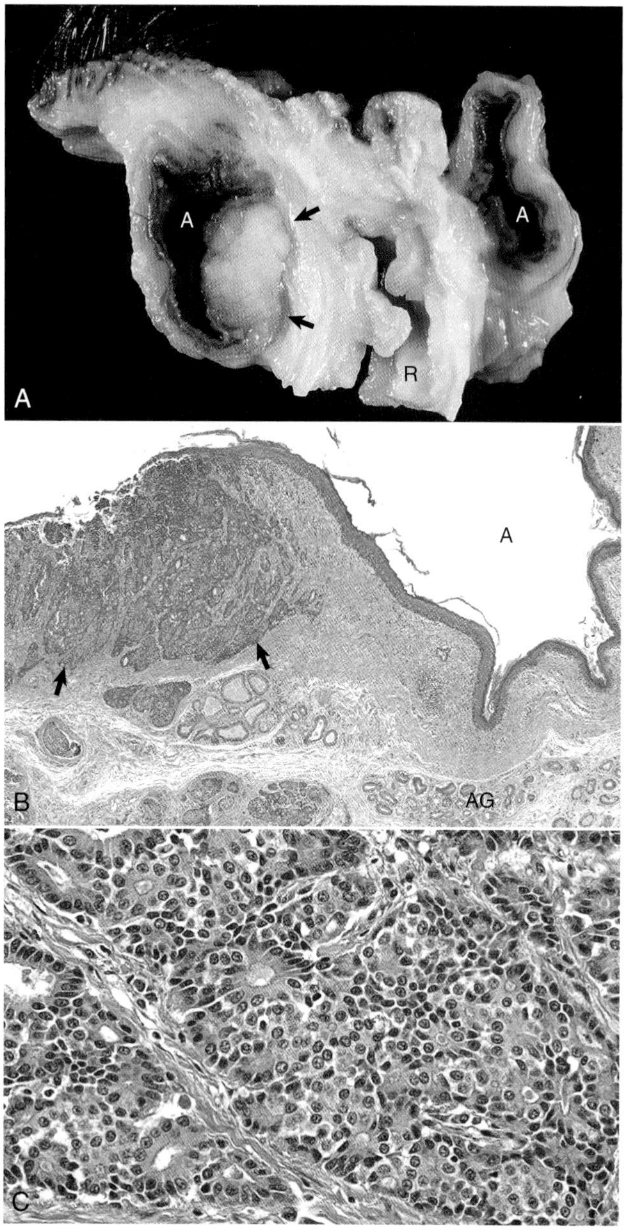

Figure 12-56 **Apocrine Carcinoma of the Anal Sac Glands, Dog. A,** Anus, rectum, and anal sacs, sectioned in the horizontal plane with anus at top. A 1-cm-diameter nodule *(arrows)* protrudes into one anal sac *(left side of figure)*. The other anal sac is normal. *A*, Anal sacs; *R*, rectum. **B,** The invasive apocrine carcinoma *(arrows)* erodes through the stratified squamous epithelium of the anal sac *(A)*. Note nonneoplastic apocrine glands *(AG)* of the anal sac in lower right. H&E stain. **C,** The neoplastic cells form solid nests, acinar or tubular structures, and rosettes. H&E stain. (**A** from Meuten DJ, Cooper BJ, Capen CC, et al: *Vet Pathol* 18:454-471, 1981. **B** and **C** courtesy Dr. M.A. Miller, College of Veterinary Medicine, Purdue University.)

Primary Hypoadrenocorticism

Primary hypoadrenocorticism or canine Addison's disease is a functional disorder that results from insufficient adrenocortical production of mineralocorticoid and glucocorticoid hormones. It is usually attributed to autoimmune destruction of the adrenal cortex. As with many autoimmune disorders, the onset of disease is typically in young adult to middle-aged dogs with slight female predominance, except in breeds with a genetic predilection, such as Portuguese water dogs, bearded collies, and standard poodles. The clinical signs are nonspecific, as are serum biochemical test results. However, the concurrent hyponatremia and hyperkalemia that develop as a result of aldosterone deficiency (see Fig. 12-14, *A*) in most affected dogs supports a diagnosis of Addison's disease. Definitive diagnosis is based on the inability to respond to ACTH stimulation with increased serum cortisol concentration (see Fig. 12-14, *B*) because of inadequate numbers of cortical cells in the zonae fasciculata and reticularis. The histologic lesions of Addison's disease are lymphoplasmacytic adrenalitis and severe lytic destruction of all three layers of the adrenal cortex. The adrenal medulla is not the target of the autoimmunity and is unaffected. In a few dogs, the zona glomerulosa is at least partially spared; these dogs may have normal serum concentrations of sodium and potassium.

In early stages of Addison's disease, lymphocytes (mainly T lymphocytes with fewer B lymphocytes) and plasma cells are distributed diffusely throughout both adrenal cortices, and nearly every cortical cell in the zonae glomerulosa, fasciculata, and reticularis undergoes lytic death. Lipofuscin-laden macrophages accumulate at sites of cortical cell loss. Cortical atrophy is typically diffuse and severe (Fig. 12-57; E-Fig. 12-35); the cortex to medulla area ratio in histologic sections can be well below the 0 percentile for normal dogs of 1.1.[10] Without mineralocorticoid and glucocorticoid replacement therapy, destruction of the adrenal cortices is fatal. However, treated dogs can live with Addison's disease for years. At autopsy (syn: necropsy; see E-Appendix 12-1) of medically managed dogs, the adrenal cortex is collapsed or even histologically undetectable, but it is often free (by then) of appreciable inflammation.

Diabetes Mellitus

Dogs with diabetes mellitus are typically middle-aged to older and often female. Small breeds, such as miniature poodles, dachshunds, and terriers, may be predisposed, but all breeds are susceptible; the disease may be genetic in keeshonds. Certain concurrent diseases, especially hyperadrenocorticism, promote hyperglycemia and decrease insulin sensitivity. Other diabetogenic hormones include growth hormone, which in turn can increase hepatocellular synthesis and secretion of insulin-like growth factor. Dogs can develop insulin resistance, but they are generally not susceptible to type 2 diabetes.

Destruction of islets secondary to chronic relapsing pancreatitis (see Fig. 12-43) or, less commonly, as a result of selective immune-mediated islet cell injury accounts for many cases of canine diabetes mellitus. In chronic relapsing pancreatitis, the pancreas is eventually reduced to a thin fibrous band of nodules (see Fig. 12-44). Histologically, islets can be difficult to find, β cells are reduced in number, and remaining islet cells have vacuolated cytoplasm from glycogen accumulation (E-Fig. 12-36). In immune-mediated injury, lymphocytes and plasma cells are confined to the islets, and β cells are selectively destroyed.

Disorders of Cats

The most commonly encountered endocrine diseases in cats are hyperthyroidism and diabetes mellitus.

Hyperthyroidism

Hyperthyroidism, the result of elevated circulating T_4 and T_3 concentrations, has been recognized in cats since the late 1970s and is

[10]The adrenal cortex to medulla cross-sectional area ratio varies widely, but the median value in dogs without clinical evidence of endocrine dysfunction or histologic adrenal lesions is approximately 2.9; the 0 percentile is 1.1.

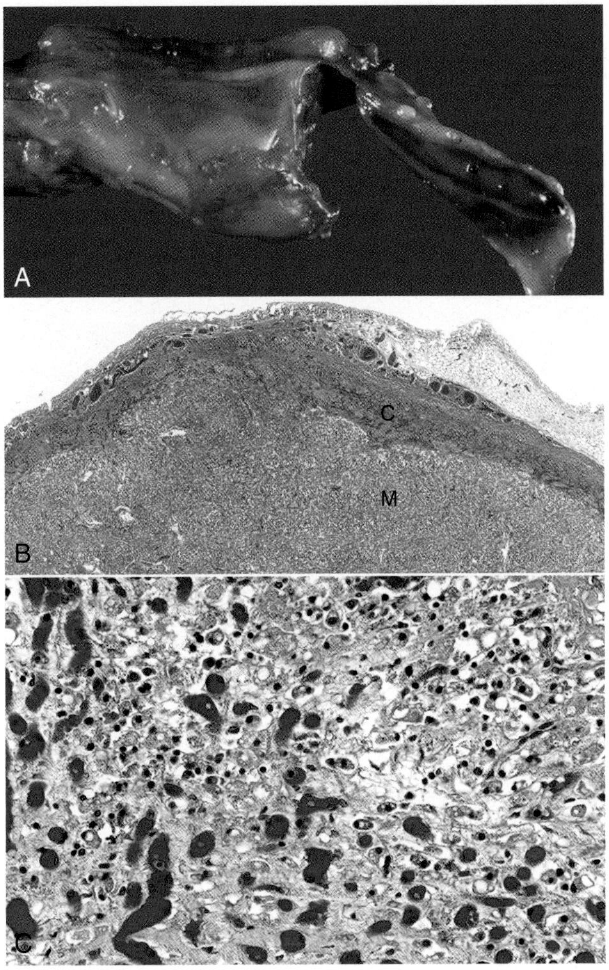

Figure 12-57 **Lymphoplasmacytic Adrenalitis with Adrenocortical Atrophy, Dog. A,** With the severe adrenocortical atrophy, the medulla constitutes the bulk of the cross-sectional area of the adrenal gland. **B,** Severe atrophy of all three layers of the cortex (C) is characteristic of hypoadrenocorticism or canine Addison's disease. M, Medulla. H&E stain. **C,** Nearly all cortical cells have been destroyed, so all that remains of the adrenal cortex is collapsed stroma with lipofuscin-laden macrophages, lymphocytes, and plasma cells. Adrenal capsule is at upper right. H&E stain. (Courtesy Dr. M.A. Miller, College of Veterinary Medicine, Purdue University.)

now one of the two most commonly diagnosed feline endocrinopathies (the other is diabetes mellitus), especially in geriatric cats. The thyroid gland may be palpably enlarged months to years before development of clinical signs. One or both lobes typically contain nodules that are classified histologically as nonencapsulated hyperplastic nodules (multinodular goiter; see Fig. 12-24) or at least partially encapsulated follicular adenomas (see Fig. 12-28). However, distinction between hyperplasia and benign neoplasia in the thyroid gland is difficult, as it is in other endocrine glands, and may have little clinical significance. Less efficient glucuronide and sulfate conjugation and excretion of thyroid hormones in cats explains why cats are more likely than dogs with functional thyroid follicular neoplasms to develop hyperthyroidism.

The histologic appearance (see Figs. 12-24 and 12-28) of nodular thyroid proliferations varies. Some nodules are composed of small follicles with little or no stainable colloid. Other nodules consist of larger, irregularly shaped follicles lined by columnar cells that project into the lumen. Some follicles are involuted and filled with densely eosinophilic colloid. Such variations may reflect alternating periods of hyperplasia and atrophy. Surrounding "normal" thyroid parenchyma undergoes atrophy.

The increased basal metabolic rate in cats with hyperthyroidism results in vague and nonspecific clinical signs. Weight loss despite increased food consumption (polyphagia) in older cats warrants investigation for hyperthyroidism. Hypertrophic cardiomyopathy develops in some hyperthyroid cats (see Chapter 10).

The apparent increase in the incidence of feline hyperthyroidism may reflect in part an increased awareness of the condition and better veterinary care and diagnostic assays for geriatric cats. However, potential risk factors that could explain a true increase in prevalence include a predominantly indoor environment, increased exposure to pesticides and fertilizers, dietary changes (more canned food), and genetics (10-fold risk in non-Siamese breeds). The ability to lower circulating total T_4 concentration and alleviate clinical signs by feeding an iodine-restricted diet suggests that excessive dietary iodine plays a role in the pathogenesis of feline hyperthyroidism.

The pathogenesis of feline hyperthyroidism differs from that of Graves' disease in human beings in that hyperthyroid cats do not have increased circulating autoantibodies to the TSH receptor. However, purified immunoglobulin G (IgG) from hyperthyroid cats does increase ^{3}H-thymidine incorporation into DNA and stimulate follicular cell proliferation, but it does not stimulate intracellular cAMP production. A specific TSH receptor-blocking antibody can inhibit the ^{3}H-thymidine incorporation. These data suggest the presence of increased thyroid growth-stimulating Ig titers in hyperthyroid cats that probably act through the TSH receptor. The feline disease most closely resembles toxic nodular goiter in human beings with mutations in genes encoding either the TSH receptor or $G_{s\alpha}$, a G protein that mediates cAMP-dependent TSH signaling. Mutations in $G_{s\alpha}$ that correspond to the mutations in human beings have been reported in a small group of hyperthyroid cats. In a separate study, all cases of feline follicular hyperplasia and adenomas had immunohistochemical overexpression of the c-ras oncogene. Hyperplastic or neoplastic thyroid tissue from hyperthyroid cats that is transplanted into athymic (nude) mice continues to overproduce T_3 and T_4. Untreated hyperthyroid cats may have hyperphosphatemia of uncertain pathogenesis with reciprocal hypocalcemia and marked elevation in parathyroid hormone concentration. Because both hyperthyroidism and hyperparathyroidism promote bone resorption, their concurrent presence could have clinical implications in terms of bone strength.

Diabetes Mellitus

Feline diabetes mellitus usually resembles type 2 diabetes of human beings with concomitant obesity and insulin resistance. However, pituitary somatotroph adenoma (with secretion of growth hormone) is a less common but important cause of insulin-resistant diabetes in cats. Diabetes mellitus is also a frequent cause of death in cats with hyperadrenocorticism. Burmese cats may have a genetic tendency for deregulated lipid metabolism that predisposes them to geriatric development of insulin-resistant diabetes. In any feline breed, obesity is the major acquired cause for insulin resistance, which is attributed to adipokines (especially leptin) and systemic inflammatory mediators. Although some cats can compensate for insulin resistance with increased insulin synthesis and secretion and do not develop diabetes, obesity is thought not only to increase the metabolic stress on β cells but also to damage them by incompletely understood mechanisms. Proposed causes of damage to pancreatic islet cells include intracellular amylin oligomers and toxic effects of glucose, lipids, reactive oxygen species, and inflammatory cytokines. Among domestic animals, cats are particularly susceptible to islet amyloidosis. Islet β cells co-secrete islet amyloid polypeptide (IAPP or amylin) along with insulin. The IAPP secretion is greater in cats with insulin resistance, and with an amino acid sequence that promotes polymerization, islet amyloidosis (Fig. 12-58) is found in almost all cats with insulin-resistant diabetes. However, because islet amyloidosis is also recognized in cats with normal insulin secretion (and does not alter glucagon secretion by α cells), amyloid deposition per se is not a plausible cause of insulin-resistant diabetes. The toxic oligomer hypothesis proposes that intracellular amylin fibrils could cause β cell death through the misfolded protein response (see Chapter 1).

A major proportion (26% to 32%) of insulin-resistant diabetic cats have hypersomatotropism (excessive secretion of growth hormone from a pituitary somatotroph adenoma or adenomatous hyperplasia). In fact, hypersomatotropism usually results in poorly controlled hyperglycemia because growth hormone decreases insulin sensitivity in target cells. Importantly, the elevated circulating growth hormone concentration causes increased hepatocellular production and secretion of insulin-like growth factor-1 (IGF-1); therefore, IGF-1 serum assay can be used to screen for hypersomatotropism, especially in cats with poorly controlled hyperglycemia.

Hypothyroidism

Primary hypothyroidism is recognized in cats but is not nearly as common as it is in dogs. Most cases of feline hypothyroidism are secondary to treatment for hyperthyroidism (see the previous section).

Hyperadrenocorticism

Adenomas or adenomatous hyperplasia of adenohypophyseal (anterior pituitary gland) corticotrophs results in excess secretion of ACTH. The lesions and clinical signs are similar to those in dogs with corticotroph adenomas. Hyperadrenocorticism is less common in cats than in dogs; usually pituitary-dependent (rather than adrenal-dependent) in cats; and results in decreased insulin sensitivity, increased hepatic gluconeogenesis and glycogenesis, and increased protein catabolism.

Congenital adrenal hyperplasia, attributed to mutation of the CYP11B1 gene that encodes 11β-hydroxylase, has been reported in the cat. 11β-Hydroxylase converts 11-deoxycortisol to cortisol, so defective enzyme activity results in cortisol deficiency and a shift of precursor molecules to androgen production. Inadequate negative feedback on the hypothalamus and pituitary gland causes increased synthesis and secretion of ACTH, hence the adrenocortical hyperplasia.

Hypersomatotropism

Hypersomatotropism or feline acromegaly is the result of an adenoma (Fig. 12-59) or adenomatous hyperplasia (the latter is not visible

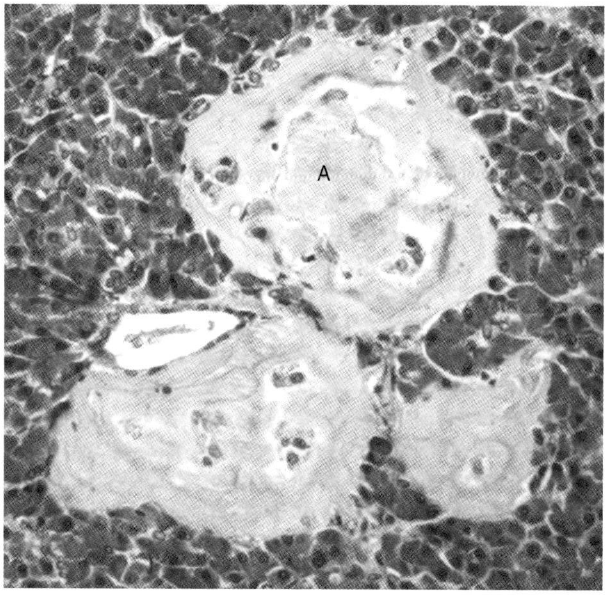

Figure 12-58 **Amyloidosis, Pancreatic Islets, Cat.** Note the deposits of amyloid *(A)* and degeneration and loss of islet cells. H&E stain. (Courtesy College of Veterinary Medicine, University of Illinois.)

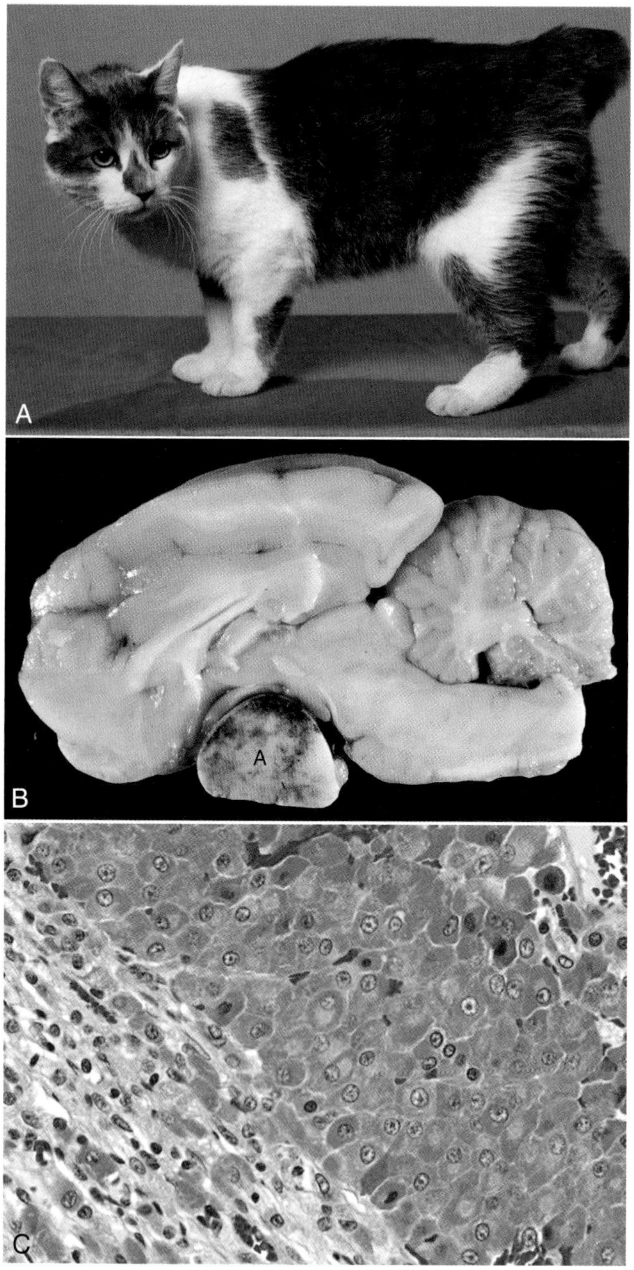

Figure 12-59 **Feline Hypersomatotropism. A,** This cat with a pituitary adenoma had a broad face with mild inferior prognathia and clubbed feet with a plantigrade posture (attributed to diabetic neuropathy). The cat had elevated circulating concentrations of insulin-like growth factor-1 and it had developed insulin-resistant diabetes mellitus. **B,** Brain and pituitary gland, sagittal section. The pituitary mass *(A)* is a somatotroph adenoma. **C,** The somatotroph adenoma *(upper right)* is composed of a densely cellular sheet of hypertrophied acidophils. Note smaller acidophils mixed with chromophobes in the nonneoplastic pars distalis at lower left. H&E stain. (**A** courtesy Dr. J.C. Scott-Moncrieff, College of Veterinary Medicine, Purdue University. **B** and **C** courtesy Dr. M.A. Miller, College of Veterinary Medicine, Purdue University.)

with diagnostic imaging or on gross examination) of adenohypophyseal (anterior pituitary gland) somatotrophs. Proliferation of somatotrophs is more common in cats than in dogs. Somatotrophs are typically acidophils, in contrast to the chromophobic corticotrophs. The excessive secretion of growth hormone promotes growth of soft and bony tissues with decreased insulin sensitivity, increased lipolysis, increased protein synthesis, and increased hepatocellular synthesis and secretion of IGF-1. Growth hormone induces hepatic production of IGF-1 by binding to insulin-dependent hepatocellular growth hormone receptors. Increased IGF-1 concentration not only contributes to the growth of soft and bony tissue by binding to IGF-1 receptors (present on many different types of cells) but also (because IGF-1 is structurally similar to insulin and has weak affinity for insulin receptors) promotes insulin resistance. Cats with hypersomatotropism can develop large stature with broad facial features, inferior prognathism, enlarged feet with plantigrade stance (Fig. 12-59, A), renomegaly, hepatomegaly, and myocardial hypertrophy. Insulin resistance is often severe and results in type 2 diabetes mellitus in many cats with hypersomatotropism. The neoplastic cells resemble those of corticotroph adenomas except that somatotrophs tend to be acidophils, so the neoplastic cells usually have prominent eosinophilic cytoplasmic granules (Fig. 12-59, C). The neoplastic cells are immunohistochemically positive for growth hormone and can also express prolactin. Neoplastic somatotrophs are usually larger than their nonneoplastic counterparts and have numerous secretory granules; however, large neoplastic cells with few cytoplasmic granules or only faintly eosinophilic granules are the predominant cell type in some somatotroph adenomas. Medical management of feline hypersomatotropism with pasireotide, a somatostatin analog, indicates that somatotrophs express somatostatin receptors (see footnote 7).

Hyperaldosteronism

Primary hyperaldosteronism, known in human beings as Conn's disease, is increasingly recognized in cats as the result of adrenocortical carcinoma, adenoma, or hyperplasia. Affected cats are typically older and have systemic hypertension and muscle weakness attributed to hypokalemic polymyopathy. Serum biochemical abnormalities include elevated aldosterone concentration with normal to mild hypernatremia and normal to marked hypokalemia.

Suggested Readings

Suggested Readings are available at www.expertconsult.com.

CHAPTER 13

Bone Marrow, Blood Cells, and the Lymphoid/Lymphatic System[1]

Katie M. Boes and Amy C. Durham

Key Readings Index

Bone Marrow and Blood Cells[2]

Structure and Function

Hematopoiesis, from *haima* (Gr., blood) and *poiein* (Gr., to make), is the production of blood cells, including erythrocytes, leukocytes, and platelets. Also known as *hemopoiesis*, hematopoiesis first occurs in the blood islands of the yolk sac and then transitions to the liver and spleen during gestation. After birth the primary hematopoietic site is the central cavities of bone, termed *bone marrow* (Fig. 13-1). Hematopoiesis occurring elsewhere is called *extramedullary hematopoiesis* (EMH), which is most common in the spleen.

The bone marrow is supported by an anastomosing network of trabecular bone that radiates centrally from the compact bone of the cortex. Trabecular bone is covered by periosteum, consisting of an inner osteogenic layer of endosteal cells, osteoblasts, and osteoclasts, and an outer fibrous layer that anchors the stromal scaffolding of the marrow spaces.

Within the marrow spaces, a network of stromal cells and extracellular matrix provides metabolic and structural support to hematopoietic cells. These stromal cells consist of adipocytes and specialized fibroblasts, called *reticular cells*. The latter provides structural support by producing a fine network of a type of collagen, called *reticulin*, and by extending long cytoplasmic processes around other cells and structures. Both reticulin and cytoplasmic processes are not normally visible with light microscopy but are visible with silver reticulin stains (e.g., Gordon and Sweet's and sometimes with periodic acid–Schiff).

Bone marrow is highly vascularized but does not have lymphatic drainage. Marrow of long bones receives part of its blood supply from the nutrient artery, which enters the bone via the nutrient canal at midshaft. The remaining arterial supply enters the marrow through an anastomosing array of vessels that arise from the periosteal arteries and penetrate the cortical bone. Vessels from the nutrient and periosteal arteries converge and form an interweaving network of venous sinusoids that permeates the marrow. These sinusoids not only deliver nutrients and remove cellular waste but also act as the entry point for hematopoietic cells into blood circulation. Sinusoidal endothelial cells function as a barrier and regulate traffic of chemicals and particles between the intravascular and extravascular spaces. Venous drainage parallels that of the nutrient artery and its extensions.

[1]For a glossary of abbreviations and terms used in this chapter see E-Glossary 13-1.

[2]For tests to evaluate platelet function or immune-mediated thrombocytopenia see E-Appendix 13-1.

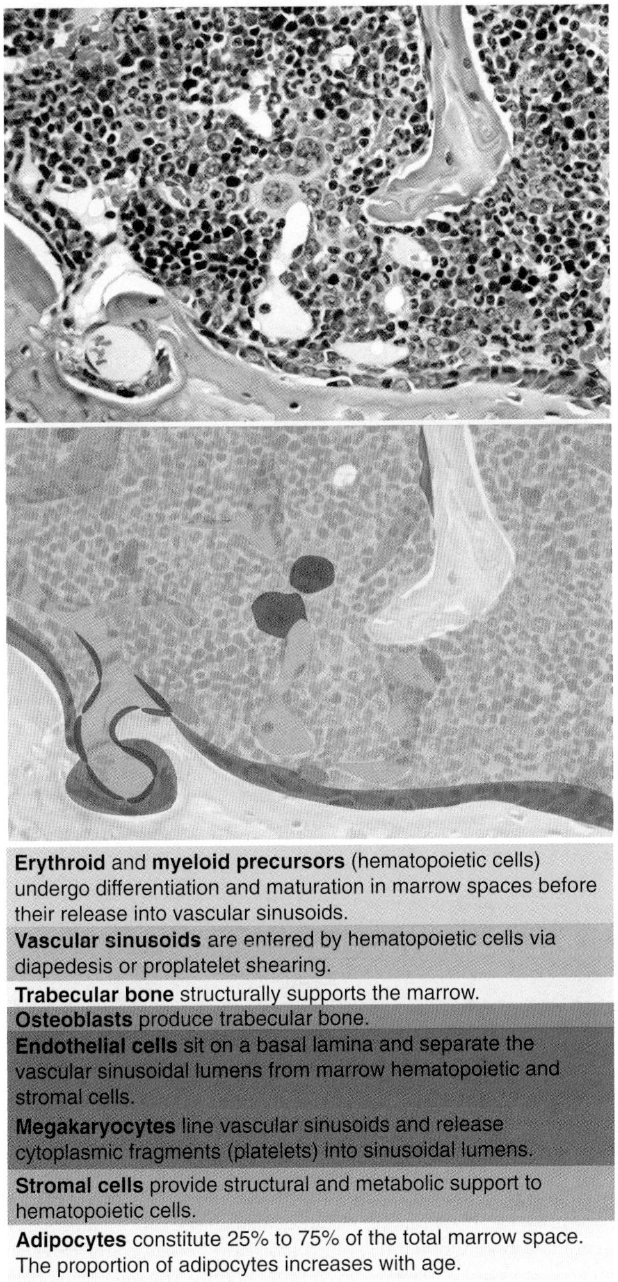
Erythroid and **myeloid precursors** (hematopoietic cells) undergo differentiation and maturation in marrow spaces before their release into vascular sinusoids.
Vascular sinusoids are entered by hematopoietic cells via diapedesis or proplatelet shearing.
Trabecular bone structurally supports the marrow.
Osteoblasts produce trabecular bone.
Endothelial cells sit on a basal lamina and separate the vascular sinusoidal lumens from marrow hematopoietic and stromal cells.
Megakaryocytes line vascular sinusoids and release cytoplasmic fragments (platelets) into sinusoidal lumens.
Stromal cells provide structural and metabolic support to hematopoietic cells.
Adipocytes constitute 25% to 75% of the total marrow space. The proportion of adipocytes increases with age.

Figure 13-1 Structure of Bone Marrow. (Courtesy Dr. K.M. Boes, College of Veterinary Medicine, Virginia Polytechnic Institute and State University; and Dr. J.F. Zachary, College of Veterinary Medicine, University of Illinois.)

Hematopoiesis occurs in the interstitium between the venous sinusoids in the so-called hematopoietic spaces. There is a complex functional interplay among hematopoietic cells with the supporting connective tissue cells, extracellular matrix, and soluble factors, which form the hematopoietic microenvironment. Behavior of hematopoietic cells is influenced by direct cell-to-cell and cell-matrix interactions and by soluble mediators, such as cytokines and hormones that interact with cells and with matrix proteins. Cells localize to specific niches within the hematopoietic microenvironment via adhesion molecules, such as integrins, immunoglobulins, lectins, and other receptors, which recognize ligands on other cells or matrix components. Cells also express receptors for soluble molecules such as chemokines (chemoattractant cytokines) and hormones that influence cell trafficking and metabolism.

Other components of the marrow include myelinated and nonmyelinated nerves, as well as low numbers of resident macrophages, lymphocytes, and plasma cells. Of note, the macrophages play an important role in iron storage and erythrocyte maturation.

The following basic concepts provide a framework for understanding the mechanisms of injury and diseases presented later in the chapter.

- Hematopoietic tissue is highly proliferative. Billions of cells per kilogram of body weight are produced each day.
- Pluripotent hematopoietic *stem cells* are a self-renewing population, giving rise to cells with committed differentiation programs, and are common ancestors of all blood cells. The process of hematopoietic differentiation is shown in Fig. 13-2.
- Hematopoietic cells undergo sequential divisions as they develop, so there are progressively higher numbers of cells as they mature. Cells also continue to mature after they have stopped dividing. Conceptually, it is helpful to consider cells in the bone marrow as belonging to mitotic and postmitotic compartments. Examples of developing hematopoietic cells are shown in Fig. 13-3.
- Mature cells released into the blood circulation have different normal life spans, varying from hours (neutrophils), to days (platelets), to months (erythrocytes), and to years (some lymphocytes).
- The hematopoietic system is under exquisite local and systemic control and responds rapidly and predictably to various stimuli.
- Production and turnover of blood cells are balanced so that numbers are maintained within normal ranges (steady-state kinetics) in healthy individuals.
- Normally the bone marrow releases mostly mature cell types (and very low numbers of cells that are almost fully mature) into the circulation. In response to certain physiologic or pathologic stimuli, however, the bone marrow releases immature cells that are further back in the supply "pipeline."

The composition of the marrow changes with age. The general pattern is that hematopoietic tissue (red marrow) regresses and is replaced with nonhematopoietic tissue, mainly fat (yellow marrow). Thus in newborns and very young animals the bone marrow consists largely of hematopoietically active tissue, with relatively little fat, whereas in geriatric individuals the marrow consists largely of fat. In adults, hematopoiesis occurs primarily in the pelvis, sternum, ribs, vertebrae, and the proximal ends of humeri and femora. Even within these areas of active hematopoiesis, fat may constitute a significant proportion of the marrow volume.

Hematopoiesis

Immature hematopoietic cells can be divided into three stages: stem cells, progenitor cells, and precursor cells. *Hematopoietic stem cells* (HSCs) have the capacity to self-renew, differentiate into mature cells, and repopulate the bone marrow after it is obliterated. *Progenitor cells* and *precursor cells* cannot self-renew; with each cell division, they evolve into more differentiated cells. Later-stage precursors cannot divide. Stem cells and progenitor cells require immunochemical stains for identification, but precursor cells can be identified by their characteristic morphologic features (see Fig. 13-3).

Control of hematopoiesis is complex, with many redundancies, feedback mechanisms, and pathways that overlap with other physiologic and pathologic processes. Many cytokines influence cells of different lineages and stages of differentiation. Primary growth factors for primitive cells are interleukin (IL) 3, produced by T lymphocytes, and stem cell factor, produced by monocytes, macrophages, fibroblasts, endothelial cells, and lymphocytes. Interleukin 7 is an early lymphoid growth factor. Lineage-specific growth factors are discussed in their corresponding sections.

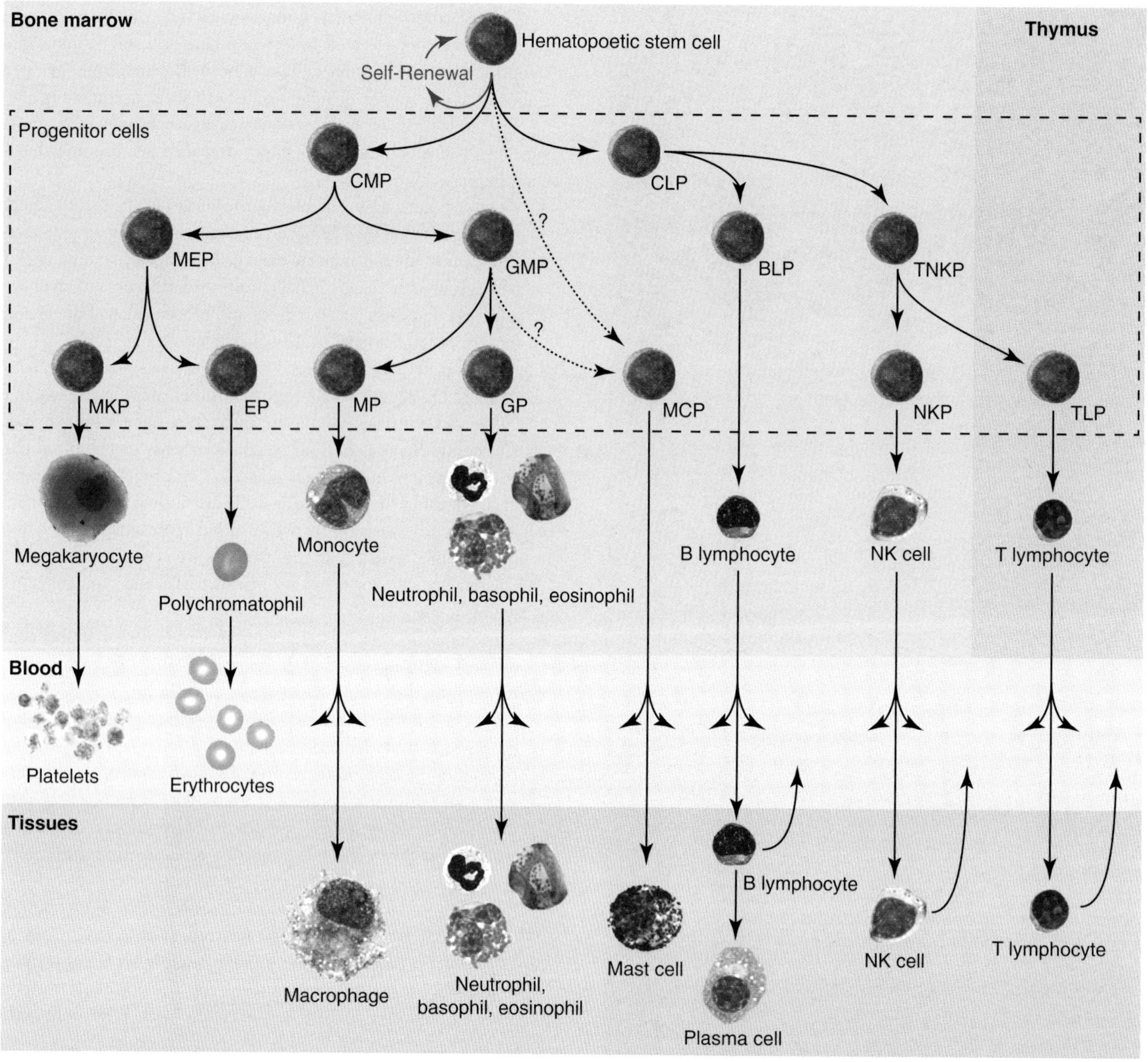

Figure 13-2 **Classic and Spatial Model of Hematopoietic Cell Differentiation, Canine Blood Smears, and Bone Marrow Aspirate.** The bone marrow consists of (1) hematopoietic stem cells, pluripotent cells capable of self-renewal; (2) progenitor cells that evolve into more differentiated cells with each cell division; (3) precursor cells that can be identified by light microscopy (not shown, see Fig. 13-3); and (4) mature hematopoietic cells awaiting release into the blood vasculature. The earliest lineage commitment is to either the common myeloid progenitor (CMP), which produces platelets, erythrocytes, and nonlymphoid leukocytes, or the common lymphoid progenitor (CLP), which differentiates into various lymphocytes and plasma cells. The cell origin of mast cells is unclear, but they may originate from a stem cell or a myeloid progenitor. Megakaryocytes remain in the bone marrow and release cytoplasmic fragments, or platelets, into blood sinusoids. T lymphocyte progenitor (TLP) cells travel from the bone marrow to the thymus during normal T lymphocyte maturation. During homeostasis, platelets and erythrocytes remain in circulation, but the leukocytes leave blood vessels to enter the tissues, where they actively participate in immune responses. In particular, monocytes and B lymphocytes undergo morphologic and immunologic changes to form macrophages and plasma cells, respectively. Macrophages, granulocytes, and mast cells migrate unidirectionally into tissues, but lymphoid cells can recirculate between the blood, tissues, and lymphatic vessels. *BLP*, B lymphocyte progenitor; *EP*, erythroid progenitor; *GMP*, granulocyte-macrophage progenitor; *GP*, granulocyte progenitor; *MCP*, mast cell progenitor; *MKP*, megakaryocyte progenitor; *MEP*, megakaryocyte-erythroid progenitor; *MP*, macrophage progenitor; *NK cell*, natural killer cell; *NKP*, natural killer cell progenitor; *TLP*, T lymphocyte progenitor; *TNKP*, T lymphocyte–natural killer cell progenitor. (Courtesy Dr. K.M. Boes, College of Veterinary Medicine, Virginia Polytechnic Institute and State University; and Dr. J.F. Zachary, College of Veterinary Medicine, University of Illinois.)

Erythropoiesis. *Erythropoiesis*—from *erythros* (Gr., red)—refers to the production of red blood cells, or erythrocytes, whose primary function is gas exchange; oxygen is delivered from the lungs to the tissues, and carbon dioxide is transported from the tissues to the lungs. During maturation, erythroid precursors synthesize a large quantity of a metalloprotein, called *hemoglobin*, to facilitate gas transportation. Erythrocytes have secondary functions, such as blood acid-base buffering.

The dominant regulator of erythropoiesis is a glycoprotein aptly named *erythropoietin* (Epo). Other direct or indirect stimulators of erythropoiesis include interleukins (e.g., IL-3, IL-4, and IL-9), colony-stimulating factors (e.g., granulocyte-macrophage colony-stimulating factor and granulocyte colony-stimulating factor), and hormones (e.g., growth hormone, insulin-like growth factor, testosterone, and thyroid hormone). Epo is synthesized primarily in the kidney and exerts its effects by promoting proliferation and

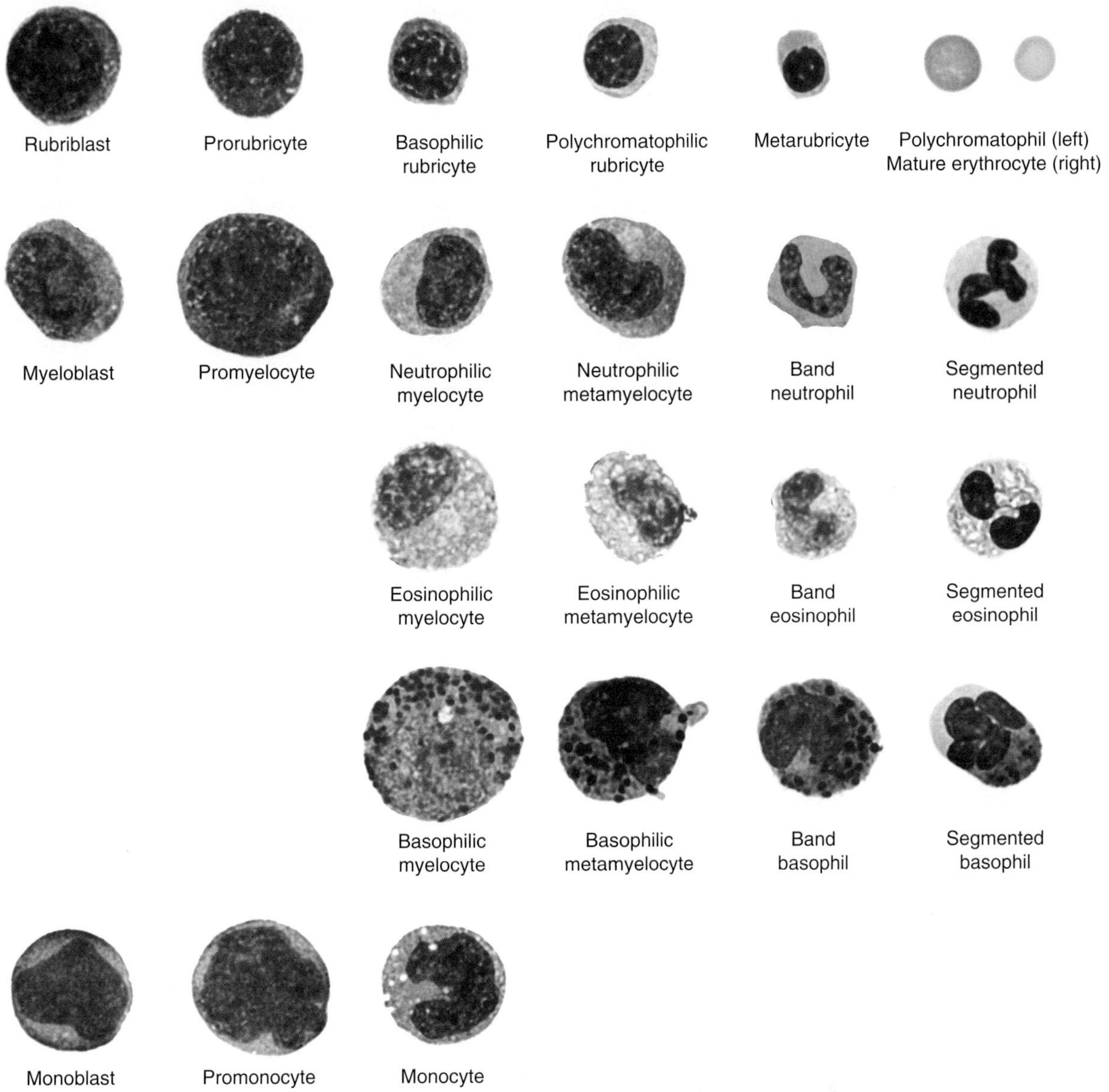

Figure 13-3 **Hematopoietic Cell Morphology, Feline (Erythroid and Granulocyte Lineages) and Canine (Monocyte Lineage) Blood Smears and Bone Marrow Aspirates.** As erythroid cells mature from a rubriblast to a mature erythrocyte, their nuclei become smaller and more condensed. The nucleus is eventually extruded to form a polychromatophil. Erythroid cells also become less basophilic and more eosinophilic as more hemoglobin is produced and as RNA-rich organelles are lost during maturation. (Hemoglobin stains eosinophilic, and RNA stains basophilic with routine Romanowsky's stains.) As granulocytes (e.g., neutrophils, eosinophils, and basophils) mature from a myeloblast to their mature forms, their nuclei become dense and segmented. Granulocytes acquire their secondary or specific granules during the myelocyte stage and can be morphologically differentiated starting at this stage. Neutrophils have neutral-staining secondary granules, eosinophil secondary granules have an affinity for acidic or eosin dyes, and basophil secondary granules have an affinity for basic dyes. Monoblasts differentiate into promonocytes with ruffled nuclear boarders and then into monocytes. (Courtesy Dr. K.M. Boes, College of Veterinary Medicine, Virginia Polytechnic Institute and State University; and Dr. J.F. Zachary, College of Veterinary Medicine, University of Illinois.)

inhibiting apoptosis of developing erythroid cells. The stimulus for increased Epo production is hypoxia.

Within the bone marrow, erythroid precursors surround a central macrophage in specialized niches, termed *erythroblastic islands* (Fig. 13-4). The central macrophage, also known as a nurse cell, anchors the precursors within the island niche, regulates erythroid proliferation and differentiation, transfers iron to the erythroid progenitors for hemoglobin synthesis, and phagocytizes extruded metarubricyte nuclei. Although erythroblastic islands occur throughout the marrow, those with more differentiated erythroid cells neighbor sinusoids, whereas nonadjacent islands contain mostly undifferentiated precursors.

Iron is essential to hemoglobin synthesis and function. It is acquired through the diet and is transported to the bone marrow via the iron transport protein, *transferrin*. Central macrophages either store iron as ferritin or *hemosiderin*, or transfer the iron to erythroid precursors for hemoglobin synthesis. Hemosiderin is identifiable in routinely stained marrow preparations as an intracellular brown pigment. However, Perls's Prussian blue stain is more sensitive and specific for iron detection.

The earliest erythroid precursor identifiable by routine light microscopy is the rubriblast, which undergoes maturational division to produce 8 to 32 progeny cells. Late-stage erythroid precursors, known as *metarubricytes*, extrude their nuclei and become *reticulocytes*, and subsequently mature erythrocytes. The normal transit time from rubriblast to mature erythrocyte is approximately 1 week.

Reticulocytes start maturing in the bone marrow but finish their maturation in the blood circulation and spleen. Horses are an exception in that they do not release reticulocytes into circulation, even in situations of increased demand. Unlike mature erythrocytes, which lack organelles, reticulocytes still contain ribosomes and mitochondria, mainly to support completion of hemoglobin synthesis. These remaining organelles impart a bluish-purple cast (polychromasia) to reticulocytes on routine blood smear examination. The resultant cells are termed *polychromatophils*. Because older reticulocytes do not exhibit polychromasia, more sensitive laboratory techniques must be used for accurate reticulocyte quantification. When a blood sample is incubated with new methylene blue stain, the reticulocytes' ribosomal RNA precipitates to form irregular, dark aggregates (Fig. 13-5). Cats also have a more mature form of reticulocyte, termed punctate reticulocyte, which is stippled when stained with new methylene blue. Punctate reticulocytes indicate prior, not active, regeneration and do not appear polychromatophilic on routine blood smear evaluation.

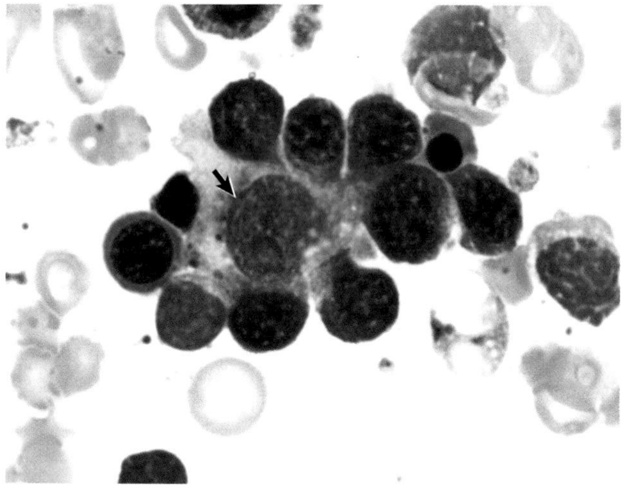

Figure 13-4 **Erythroblastic Island, Canine Splenic Aspirate.** Erythroid precursors surround and adhere to a central macrophage, or nurse cell *(arrow)*, which regulates the erythroid cell's maturation and iron acquisition. (Courtesy Dr. K.M. Boes, College of Veterinary Medicine, Virginia Polytechnic Institute and State University.)

In most mammals, mature erythrocytes have a biconcave disk shape, called a discocyte. Microscopically, these cells are round and eosinophilic with a central area of pallor. However, the central concavity may not be microscopically apparent in species other than the dog. Camelids normally have oval erythrocytes, termed *ovalocytes* or *elliptocytes*, which facilitate better gas exchange at high altitudes. The erythrocytes of some animals are prone to in vitro shape change, including those of cervids, pigs, and some goat breeds (e.g., Angora).

Erythrocyte size during health depends on the species, breed, and age of the animal. In dogs, some breeds have relatively smaller (e.g., Akitas and Shibas) or larger (e.g., some poodles) erythrocytes. Akitas and Shibas also have a high concentration of potassium, unlike erythrocytes in other dogs. Juvenile animals may have larger erythrocytes because of the persistence of fetal erythrocytes, which is followed by a period of relatively smaller cells before reaching adult reference intervals.

Mature mammalian erythrocytes lack nuclei and organelles and are thus incapable of transcription, translation, and oxidative metabolism. However, they do require energy for various functions, including maintenance of shape and deformability, active transport, and prevention of oxidative damage. Red blood cells generate this energy entirely through glycolysis (also known as the Embden-Meyerhof pathway). Except in pigs, glucose enters erythrocytes from the plasma through an insulin-independent, integral membrane glucose transporter.

Within circulation the erythrocyte mean life span varies between species and is related to body weight and metabolic rate: approximately 150 days in horses and cattle, 100 days in dogs, and 70 days in cats. When erythrocytes reach the end of their life span, they are destroyed in a process termed *hemolysis*. Hemolysis may occur within blood vessels (*intravascular hemolysis*) or by sinusoidal macrophages (*extravascular hemolysis*). During intravascular hemolysis, erythrocytes release their contents, mostly hemoglobin, directly into blood. However, during extravascular hemolysis, macrophages phagocytize entire erythrocytes, leaving little or no hemoglobin in the blood. Normal turnover of erythrocytes occurs mainly by extravascular hemolysis within the spleen, and to a lesser extent in other organs such as the liver and bone marrow. The exact controls are not clear, but factors that likely play a role in physiologic hemolysis include the following:

- Exposure of membrane components normally sequestered on the inner leaflet of the erythrocyte membrane, particularly phosphatidylserine.

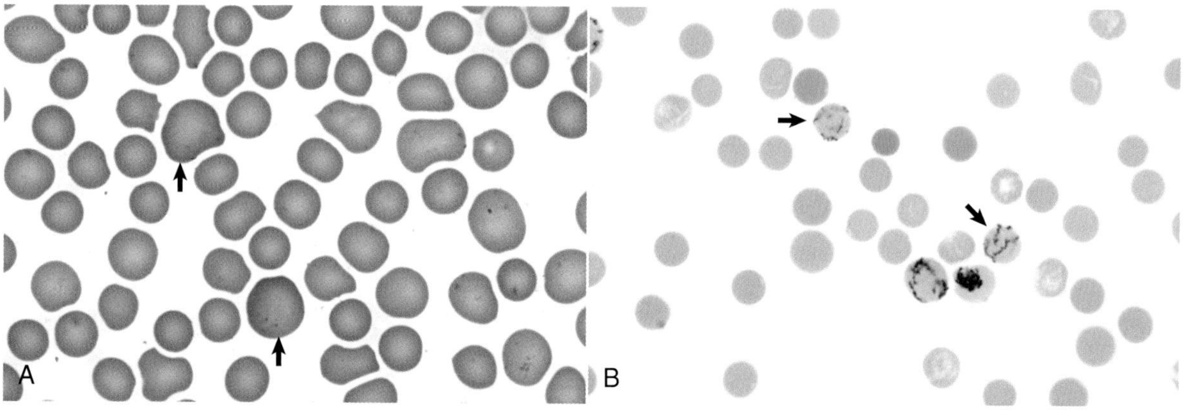

Figure 13-5 **Reticulocytosis, Canine Blood Smears. A,** Reticulocytes *(arrows)* appear polychromatophilic with routine staining. Wright's stain. **B,** Reticulocytes. Precipitated aggregates of RNA are stained blue *(arrows)* with new methylene blue. (Courtesy Dr. M.M. Fry, College of Veterinary Medicine, University of Tennessee.)

- Decreased erythrocyte deformability.
- Binding of immunoglobulin G (IgG) and/or complement to erythrocyte membranes. Complement binding may be secondary clustering of the membrane anion exchange protein, band 3.
- Oxidative damage to erythrocytes.

Macrophages degrade erythrocytes into reusable components, such as iron and amino acids, and the waste product *bilirubin*. Bilirubin is then exported into circulation, where it is transported to the liver by albumin. The liver conjugates and subsequently excretes bilirubin into bile for elimination from the body.

Intravascular hemolysis normally occurs at only extremely low levels. Hemoglobin is a tetramer that, when released from the erythrocyte into the blood, splits into dimers that bind to a plasma protein called *haptoglobin*. The hemoglobin-haptoglobin complex is taken up by hepatocytes and macrophages. This is the major pathway for handling free hemoglobin. However, free hemoglobin may also oxidize to form *methemoglobin*, which dissociates to form metheme and globin. Metheme binds to a plasma protein called *hemopexin*, which is taken up by hepatocytes and macrophages in a similar manner to hemoglobin-haptoglobin complexes. Free heme in the reduced form binds to albumin, from which it is taken up in the liver and converted into bilirubin.

The concentration of circulating erythrocytes typically decreases postnatally and remains below normal adult levels during the period of rapid body growth. The age at which erythrocyte numbers begin to increase and the age at which adult levels are reached vary among species. In dogs, adult values are usually reached between 4 and 6 months of age; in horses, this occurs at approximately 1 year of age.

Granulopoiesis and Monocytopoiesis (Myelopoiesis). *Granulopoiesis* is the production of neutrophils, eosinophils, and basophils, whereas monocyte production is termed *monocytopoiesis*. Granulocytic and monocytic cells are sometimes collectively referenced as myeloid cells. However, the term *myeloid* and the prefix myelo- can be confusing because they have other meanings; they may reference the bone marrow, all nonlymphoid hemic cells (erythrocytes, leukocytes, and megakaryocytes), only granulocytes, or the spinal cord.

The main purpose of granulocytes and monocytes is to migrate to sites of tissue inflammation and function in host defense (see Chapters 3 and 5). Briefly, these cells have key immunologic functions, including phagocytosis and microbicidal activity (neutrophils and monocyte-derived macrophages), parasiticidal activity and participation in allergic reactions (eosinophils and basophils), antigen processing and presentation, and cytokine production (macrophages). Neutrophils are the predominant leukocyte type in blood of most domestic species.

Primary stimulators of granulopoiesis and monocytopoiesis are granulocyte-macrophage colony-stimulating factor and IL-1, IL-3, and IL-6 (granulocytes and monocytes), granulocyte colony-stimulating factor (granulocytes), and macrophage colony-stimulating factor (monocytes). In general, these cytokines are produced by various inflammatory cells, with or without contribution from stromal cells.

The earliest granulocytic precursor identifiable by routine light microscopy is the myeloblast, which undergoes maturational division over 5 days to produce 16 to 32 progeny cells (see Fig. 13-3). These granulocytic precursors are conceptually divided into those stages that can divide, including myeloblasts, promyelocytes, and myelocytes (*proliferation pool*), and those that cannot, including metamyelocytes, and band and segmented forms (*maturation pool*). Within the neutrophil maturation pool is a subpool, termed the *storage pool*, which consists of a reserve of fully mature neutrophils. The size of the storage pool varies by species; it is large in the dog, but small in ruminants. In homeostasis mostly mature segmented granulocytes are released from the marrow into the blood.

The first monocytic precursor identifiable by morphologic features is the monoblast, which develops into promonocytes and subsequently monocytes (see Fig. 13-3). Unlike granulocytes, monocytes do not have a marrow storage pool; they immediately enter venous sinusoids upon maturation. After migrating into the tissues, monocytes undergo morphologic and immunophenotypic maturation into macrophages.

Within blood vessels there are two pools of leukocytes: the *circulating pool* and the *marginating pool*. Circulating cells are free flowing in blood, whereas marginating cells are temporarily adhered to endothelial cells by selectins. In most healthy mammals there are typically equal numbers of neutrophils in the circulating and marginal pools. However, there are threefold more marginal neutrophils relative to circulating neutrophils in cats. Only the circulating leukocyte pool is sampled during phlebotomy. The concentration of myeloid cells in blood depends on the rate of production and release from the bone marrow, the proportions of cells in the circulating and marginating pools, and the rate of migration from the vasculature into tissues.

The fate of neutrophils after they leave the bloodstream in normal conditions (i.e., not in the context of inflammation) is poorly understood. They migrate into the gastrointestinal and respiratory tracts, liver, and spleen and may be lost through mucosal surfaces or undergo apoptosis and be phagocytized by macrophages.

Lymphopoiesis. *Lymphopoiesis*—from *lympha* (Latin, water)—refers to the production of new lymphocytes, including B lymphocytes, T lymphocytes, and natural killer (NK) cells. B lymphocytes primarily produce immunoglobulins, also known as antibodies, and are key effectors of humoral immunity. They are distinguished by the presence of an immunoglobulin receptor complex, termed the B lymphocyte receptor. Plasma cells are terminally differentiated B lymphocytes that produce abundant immunoglobulin. T lymphocytes, effectors of cell-mediated immunity, possess T lymphocyte receptors that bind antigens prepared by antigen-presenting cells. A component of innate immunity, NK cells kill a variety of infected and tumor cells in the absence of prior exposure or priming. Main growth factors for B lymphocytes, T lymphocytes, and NK cells are IL-4, IL-2, and IL-15, respectively.

Lymphocytes are derived from HSCs within the bone marrow. B lymphocyte development occurs in two phases, first in an antigen-independent phase in the bone marrow and ileal Peyer's patches (the site of B lymphocyte development in ruminants), then in an antigen-dependent phase in peripheral lymphoid tissues (such as spleen, lymph nodes, and mucosa-associated lymphoid tissue [MALT]). T lymphocyte progenitors migrate from the bone marrow to the thymus, where they undergo differentiation, selection, and maturation processes before migrating to the peripheral lymphoid tissue as effector cells.

Unlike granulocytes, which circulate only in blood vessels and migrate unidirectionally into target tissues, lymphocytes travel in both blood and lymphatic vessels and continually circulate between blood, tissues, and lymphatic vessels. Also in contrast to nonlymphoid hematopoietic cells, blood lymphocyte concentrations in adult animals are primarily dependent upon extramedullary lymphocyte production and kinetics, and not lymphopoiesis by the marrow.

In healthy nonruminant mammals, lymphocytes are the second most numerous blood leukocyte. According to conventional wisdom, cattle normally have higher numbers of lymphocytes than neutrophils in circulation. However, recent studies suggest that is no longer the case, most likely due to changes in genetics and husbandry. In most species the majority of lymphocytes in blood circulation are T lymphocytes. The concentration of blood lymphocytes decreases with age.

Thrombopoiesis. *Thrombopoiesis*—from *thrombos* (Gr., clot)—refers to the production of platelets, which are small (2 to 4 μm), round to ovoid, anucleate cells within blood vessels. Platelets have a central role in primary hemostasis but also participate in secondary hemostasis (coagulation) and inflammatory pathways (see Chapters 2 and 3).

Thrombopoietin (Tpo) is the primary regulator of thrombopoiesis. The liver and renal tubular epithelial cells constantly produce Tpo, which is then cleared and destroyed by platelets and their precursors. Therefore plasma Tpo concentration is inversely proportional to platelet and platelet precursor mass. If the platelet mass is decreased, less Tpo is cleared, and there is subsequently more free plasma Tpo to stimulate thrombopoiesis.

The earliest morphologically identifiable platelet precursor is the megakaryoblast, which undergoes nuclear reduplications without cell division, termed endomitosis, to form a *megakaryocyte* with 8 to 64 nuclei. As the name suggests, megakaryocytes are very large cells, much larger than any other hematopoietic cell (Fig. 13-6; also see Fig. 13-1). Megakaryocytes neighbor venous sinusoids, extend their cytoplasmic processes into vascular lumens, and shed membrane-bound cytoplasmic fragments (platelets) into blood circulation. Orderly platelet shedding is partially facilitated by β_1-tubulin microtubules within megakaryocytes.

Platelets circulate in a quiescent form and become activated by binding platelet agonists, including thrombin, adenosine diphosphate (ADP), and thromboxane. Platelet activation causes shape change, granule release, and relocation of procoagulant phospholipids and glycoproteins (GPs) to the outer cell membrane. Specific procoagulant actions include release of calcium, von Willebrand factor (vWF), factor V, and fibrinogen, as well as providing phosphatidylserine-rich binding sites for the extrinsic tenase (factors III, VII, and X), intrinsic tenase (factors IX, VIII, and X), and prothrombinase (factors X, V, and II) coagulation complexes. Platelet GP surface receptors include those for binding vWF (GPIb-IX-V), collagen (GPVI), and fibrinogen (GPIIb-IIIa), which facilitate platelet aggregation and adherence to subendothelial collagen. Expansion of surface area and release of granule contents is aided by a network of membrane invaginations known as the open canalicular system. This system is not present in horses, cattle, and camelids.

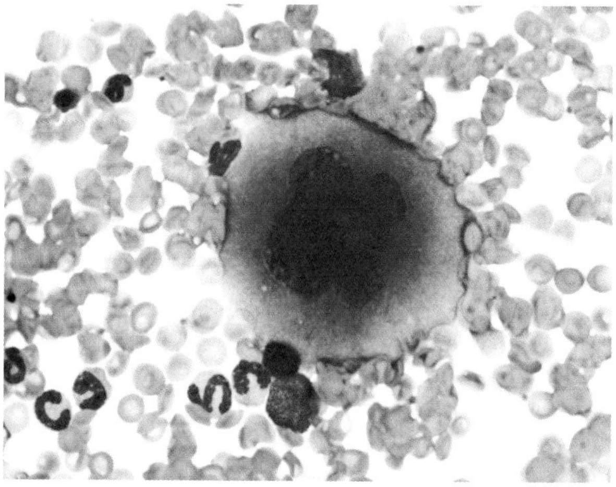

Figure 13-6 **Megakaryocyte, Canine Bone Marrow Aspirate.** Note the cell's very large size, lobulated nucleus, and abundant granular cytoplasm. Wright's stain. (Courtesy Dr. M.M. Fry, College of Veterinary Medicine, University of Tennessee.)

Methods for Examination of the Bone Marrow

Gross and Microscopic Examination

Information on this topic is available at www.expertconsult.com.

Complete Blood Count

Information on this topic is available at www.expertconsult.com.

Additional Tests

Information on this topic is available at www.expertconsult.com.

Hemostasis Testing

Information on this topic is available at www.expertconsult.com.

Dysfunction/Responses to Injury

Bone Marrow

Mechanisms of bone marrow disease are summarized in Box 13-1. Hematopoietic cells' response to injury is dependent upon whether the insult is on the marrow or within extramarrow tissues. In general, marrow-directed injury or disturbances result in production of abnormal hematopoietic cells (*dysplasia*), fewer hematopoietic cells (*hypoplasia*), or a failure of hematopoietic cell development (*aplasia*). Dysplasia, hypoplasia, and aplasia may be specific for one cell line, such as pure red cell aplasia, or affect multiple lineages, as seen with aplastic anemia. Accordingly, decreased blood concentrations of the involved cell types are expected with hypoplasia or aplasia. Erythroid, myeloid, and megakaryocytic hypoplasia or aplasia causes nonregenerative anemia, neutropenia, and thrombocytopenia, respectively. *Bicytopenia* is used to describe decreased blood concentrations of two cell lines, whereas *pancytopenia* indicates decreased blood concentrations of all three cell types. Bicytopenia or pancytopenia may indicate generalized marrow disease, such as occurs with aplastic anemia or marrow malignancies (*leukemia*), necrosis, fibrosis (*myelofibrosis*), or inflammation (*myelitis*). Replacement of hematopoietic tissue within the bone marrow by abnormal tissue, including neoplastic cells, fibrosis, or inflammatory cells, is termed *myelophthisis*.

Box 13-1 Mechanisms of Disease in Bone Marrow and Blood Cells

BONE MARROW
Hypoplasia
Hyperplasia
Dysplasia
Aplasia
Neoplasia
Myelophthisis (fibrosis, metastatic neoplasia)
Necrosis
Inflammation

BLOOD CELLS
Increased destruction
Hemorrhage (especially erythrocytes)
Consumption (platelets)
Neoplasia
Altered distribution
Abnormal function

Insults to extramarrow tissues and cells tend to cause increased production of the involved cell types (*hyperplasia*) with or without dysplasia. Loss of erythrocytes from blood vessels (*hemorrhage*), or premature destruction of erythrocytes (*hemolysis*) causes erythroid hyperplasia. Tissue inflammation may cause neutrophilic, eosinophilic, basophilic, and/or monocytic hyperplasia, depending on the type of inflammation. Megakaryocytic hyperplasia may occur with increased platelet use during hemorrhage or disseminated intravascular coagulation (DIC) or with immune-mediated platelet destruction. Exceptions to these generalizations, such as anemia of chronic disease, iron deficiency anemia, and anemia of renal failure, are discussed in more detail later.

Endothelial cell response to injury specifically within the marrow is poorly characterized, but it is likely similar to that of endothelial cells elsewhere, playing active roles in coagulation and inflammation (see Chapters 2 and 3). However, one potential sign of marrow sinusoidal injury is the presence of circulating nucleated erythrocytes in the absence of erythrocyte regeneration, termed *inappropriate metarubricytosis*. It is proposed that injured marrow endothelial cells allow premature passage of metarubricytes into blood circulation during times of stress. However, a conflicting theory proposes that marrow stress causes decreased metarubricyte attachment to central macrophages, and subsequent release into circulation. Specific causes of marrow injury–induced metarubricytosis include sepsis, hyperthermia, malignancies, hypoxia, and certain drugs and toxins. Inappropriate metarubricytosis may also occur with erythroid dysplasia and splenic disorders.

In addition to a suspected role in inappropriate metarubricytosis, marrow macrophages are integral to altered iron metabolism, including anemia of chronic disease and hemosiderosis. *Anemia of chronic disease* is a mild to moderate nonregenerative anemia observed in animals with a variety of inflammatory and metabolic disorders. This anemia is discussed in more detail later, but briefly, it is primarily a result of iron sequestration within macrophages. *Hemosiderosis* is the excessive accumulation of iron in tissues, typically macrophages. Accumulation of iron in parenchymal organs, leading to organ toxicity, is termed *hemochromatosis*. In animals, iron overload due to blood transfusions or chronic hemolytic anemias may cause marrow hemosiderosis and hemochromatosis.

Myelitis can take different forms. Granulomatous myelitis occurs with systemic fungal infections (e.g., histoplasmosis) or mycobacteriosis. Acute or neutrophilic myelitis may occur with lower-order bacterial infections or those with an immune-mediated component. Dogs and cats with nonregenerative immune-mediated hemolytic anemia (IMHA) often have myelitis, in addition to myelofibrosis and necrosis. The inflammation is evident as fibrin deposition, edema, and multifocal neutrophilic infiltrates; immune-mediated cytopenias may also concurrently occur with bone marrow lymphocytic and/or plasma cell hyperplasia.

Bone marrow necrosis is the necrosis of medullary hematopoietic cells, stromal cells, and stroma in large areas of bone marrow. Potential causes include leukemias, extramarrow malignancies, infection (bovine viral diarrhea virus [BVDV], *Ehrlichia canis*, and feline leukemia virus [FeLV]), sepsis, drugs or toxins (carprofen, chemotherapeutic agents, estrogen, metronidazole, mitotane, and phenobarbital), and irradiation. Direct hematopoietic or stromal cytotoxicity and altered marrow microvasculature (disseminated intravascular coagulation) are proposed pathogeneses. Extensive marrow necrosis results in decreased hematopoiesis and subsequent blood cytopenias, including anemia, neutropenia, and thrombocytopenia. If the animal survives the initial insult, the marrow may recover and resume normal hematopoiesis, or it may undergo scar formation, termed myelofibrosis.

Secondary myelofibrosis is the enhanced deposition of collagen within the marrow by nonneoplastic fibroblasts and reticular cells. Disease pathogenesis is unclear, but there are two leading theories. First, it may represent scar formation after marrow necrosis, as previously presented. And second, high concentrations of growth factors present during times of marrow injury or activation may stimulate fibroblast proliferation. In particular, stimulated megakaryocytes and macrophages produce fibrogenic cytokines, including platelet-derived growth factor, transforming growth factor-β, and epidermal growth factor. Early in disease there is reticulin deposition without reduction of hematopoietic elements. However, fibrous collagen replaces hematopoietic cells with disease progression. Histologic identification of reticulin and collagen fibers can be aided with reticulin silver and Masson's trichrome stains, respectively. In animals, secondary myelofibrosis occurs most commonly with leukemias, extramarrow malignancies, and chronic hemolytic anemias, but many cases are idiopathic. Experimental whole-body gamma irradiation, dietary strontium-90 exposure, and certain drugs and toxins can also induce myelofibrosis.

The responses of marrow adipocytes to systemic and localized disease are under current investigation, especially in relation to energy metabolism, inflammation, and bone trauma. During times of severe energy imbalance, such as cachexia, the marrow may undergo *serous atrophy of fat*, also known as *gelatinous marrow transformation* (E-Fig. 13-1). The pathogenesis of this phenomenon is unknown, but it is characterized by adipocyte atrophy, hematopoietic cell hypoplasia with subsequent cytopenias, and replacement of the marrow with extracellular hyaluronic acid–rich mucopolysaccharides. Positive Alcian blue staining identifies the extracellular material as mucin.

Marrow adipocytes secrete adipose-derived hormones, termed *adipokines*, including leptin and adiponectin. In general, leptin is proinflammatory, prothrombotic, and mitogenic for various cell types, including lymphocytes, hematopoietic progenitors, and leukemic cells. Conversely, adiponectin has antiinflammatory and growth inhibitory properties. During times of inflammation and infection, leptin production is increased.

In response to marrow trauma, such as orthopedic surgery, fat may enter the vasculature, embolize to various tissues, and cause tissue ischemia. The severity of tissue injury caused by *fat embolism* is dependent upon the quantity of fat entering circulation and the tissue's susceptibility to ischemia (see Chapter 2).

Blood Cells

Responses of circulating blood cells to injury include decreased survival (destruction, consumption, or loss), altered distribution, and altered structure or function (see Box 13-1). These responses are not mutually exclusive—for example, altered erythrocyte structure may lead to decreased survival. Often, but not always, these responses result in decreased concentrations of blood cells in circulation.

Abnormal Concentrations of Blood Cells. The concentration of blood cells may be decreased, termed *cytopenia* (from kytos [Gr., hollow vessel] and penia [Gr., poverty]) or increased, designated *cytosis* (from osis [Gr., condition]). A specific blood cell type is denoted as being decreased by using the suffix *-penia* (Table 13-1). A decreased concentration of erythrocytes is the exception and is termed *anemia* (from *a* [Gr., without] and *haima* [Gr., blood]). Decreased concentrations of blood basophils are not recognized in domestic animals because the lower reference interval is typically zero. An increased blood cell type is denoted with the suffix *-osis* or *-philia* (see Table 13-1). Postmortem quantification of blood cell

Table 13-1 Terminology for Increases or Decreases in Hematopoietic Cells in Blood

Cell type	Decreased	Increased
Erythrocytes	Anemia	Erythrocytosis
Reticulocytes	Reticulopenia	Reticulocytosis
Leukocytes	Leukopenia	Leukocytosis
Neutrophils	Neutropenia	Neutrophilia
Lymphocytes	Lymphopenia	Lymphocytosis
Monocytes	Monocytopenia	Monocytosis
Eosinophils	Eosinopenia	Eosinophilia
Basophils	Basopenia	Basophilia
Platelets	Thrombocytopenia	Thrombocytosis

concentrations is not possible due to perimortem coagulation. However, a complete blood count (CBC) with microscopic blood smear evaluation is the foundation for antemortem assessment of blood cells.

Anemia. Anemia causes clinical signs referable to decreased red hemoglobin pigment (e.g., pale mucous membranes), decreased oxygen-carrying capacity (e.g., depression, lethargy, weakness, and exercise tolerance), and decreased blood viscosity (e.g., heart murmur). Recumbency, seizures, syncope, or coma may occur with severe anemia. Anemia is confirmed by identifying a decreased hemoglobin concentration or reduced erythrocyte mass, as measured by the packed-cell volume, hematocrit, or red blood cell concentration.

The three general causes of anemia are blood loss (hemorrhage), red blood cell destruction or lysis (hemolysis), and decreased red blood cell production (erythroid hypoplasia). Classifying anemia as regenerative or nonregenerative is clinically useful because it provides information about the mechanism of disease; regenerative anemia indicates hemorrhage or hemolysis, whereas erythroid hypoplasia or aplasia causes nonregenerative anemia (Table 13-2).

The hallmark of regenerative anemias, except in horses, is *reticulocytosis* (i.e., increased numbers of circulating reticulocytes [immature erythrocytes]), which is evident as *polychromasia* on a routinely stained blood smear (see Fig. 13-5). Reticulocytosis indicates increased bone marrow erythropoiesis (Fig. 13-7) and release of erythrocytes before they are fully mature. Reticulocytosis is an appropriate marrow response to anemia and is often seen with hemorrhage or hemolysis. On a CBC a strong regenerative response may produce an increased mean cell volume (MCV) and decreased mean cell hemoglobin concentration (MCHC) because reticulocytes are larger and have a lower hemoglobin concentration than mature erythrocytes. Horses are an exception to this classification scheme because they do not release reticulocytes into circulation, even with erythroid hyperplasia. Horses with a regenerative response may have an increased MCV and red cell distribution width (an index of variation in cell size). But definitive determination of regeneration in a horse requires demonstration of erythroid hyperplasia via bone marrow examination or an increasing red cell mass over sequential CBCs.

In addition to reticulocytosis there may be increased numbers of nucleated red blood cells (nRBCs) in circulation with erythrocyte regeneration, termed *appropriate metarubricytosis*. When nRBCs are present as part of a regenerative response, they should be in low numbers relative to the numbers of reticulocytes. However, the presence of circulating nRBCs is not in itself definitive evidence of regeneration and may signify dyserythropoiesis (e.g., lead poisoning or bone marrow disease) or splenic dysfunction. These processes should be suspected when nRBCs are increased without reticulocy-

Table 13-2 Causes of Regenerative and Nonregenerative Anemia

Regenerative Anemia	Nonregenerative Anemia
Hemorrhage Trauma Hemostasis defect Neoplasia Gastrointestinal ulceration Parasitism Phlebotomy	Primary bone marrow disease Immune-mediated Infections (e.g., feline leukemia virus) Myelophthisis (e.g., myelitis, leukemia, myelofibrosis) Toxicity (e.g., chemotherapeutic agents, estrogen, bracken fern) Congenital disorders
Hemolysis Immune-mediated Infections (e.g., hemoparasitism) Toxicity (oxidants) Mechanical fragmentation (e.g., disseminated intravascular coagulation) Enzymatic (e.g., bacterial phospholipases) Neoplasia (e.g., hemophagocytic histiocytic sarcoma) Hypophosphatemia Congenital disorders	Extramarrow disease Inflammatory disease Chronic renal failure Liver disease or failure Endocrinopathies (e.g., hypoadrenocorticism, hypothyroidism) Nutritional deficiency (e.g., iron deficiency, vitamin B_{12} deficiency, malnutrition)

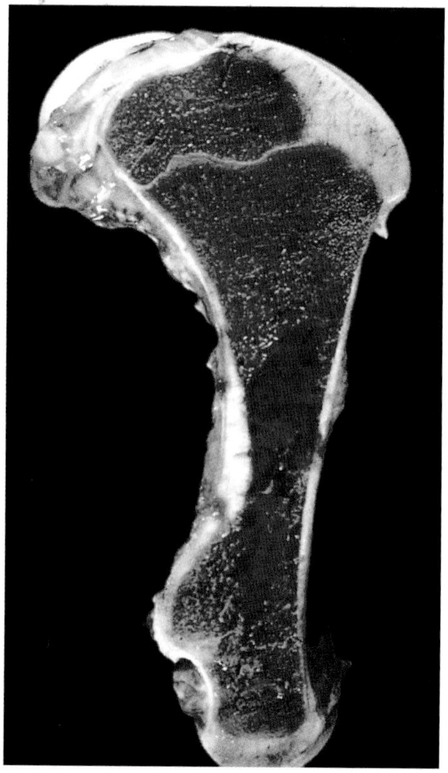

Figure 13-7 **Hemopoietically Active Bone Marrow, Femur, Calf.** Note that the bone marrow has a uniform consistency and is red to dark red. These responses are characteristic of hemopoietically active bone marrow. (Courtesy Dr. Ramos, Autonomous University of Barcelona; and Noah's Arkive, College of Veterinary Medicine, The University of Georgia.)

tosis, or their numbers are high relative to the degree of reticulocytosis, termed *inappropriate metarubricytosis*.

In ruminants, reticulocytosis is often accompanied by basophilic stippling (Fig. 13-8). However, like metarubricytosis, basophilic stippling without reticulocytosis is concerning for lead poisoning or other causes of dyserythropoiesis.

Recall that the stimulus for increased erythropoiesis is increased secretion of Epo in response to tissue hypoxia. Although the action of Epo on erythropoiesis is rapid, evidence of a regenerative response is not immediately apparent in a blood sample. One of the main effects of Epo is to expand the pool of early-stage erythroid precursors, and it takes time for these cells to differentiate to the point where they are released into circulation. In a case of acute hemorrhage or hemolysis, for example, it typically takes 3 to 4 days until reticulocytosis is evident on the CBC and several more days until the regenerative response peaks. The term *preregenerative anemia* is sometimes used to describe anemia with a regenerative response that is impending but not yet apparent on the CBC. Confirming a regenerative response in such cases requires either evidence of erythroid hyperplasia in the bone marrow or emergence of a reticulocytosis on subsequent days.

Hemorrhage results in escape of erythrocytes and other blood components, such as protein, from the vasculature. As a result, a decreased plasma or serum protein concentration, termed *hypoproteinemia*, may be evident on a CBC or chemistry panel. If the hemorrhage is into the gastrointestinal lumen, some of the protein may be resorbed and converted to urea, resulting in an increased urea nitrogen concentration relative to creatinine in plasma. Hemorrhage within the urinary tract may cause red urine with erythrocytes observed in the urine sediment. Causes of hemorrhage include trauma, abnormal hemostasis, certain parasitisms, ulceration, and neoplasia.

Hemorrhage may be acute or chronic, or internal or external. During acute hemorrhage, there are ample iron stores within the body for hemoglobin synthesis and erythrocyte regeneration. However, with chronic external hemorrhage, continued loss of iron may deplete the body's iron stores. As iron stores diminish, so does erythrocyte regeneration, eventually leading to *iron deficiency anemia*. Iron deficiency anemia is either poorly regenerative or nonregenerative and is discussed in more detail later in the chapter. Iron deficiency anemia does not occur with chronic internal hemorrhage, such as into the peritoneal cavity, because iron is not lost from the body and can be reused for erythropoiesis.

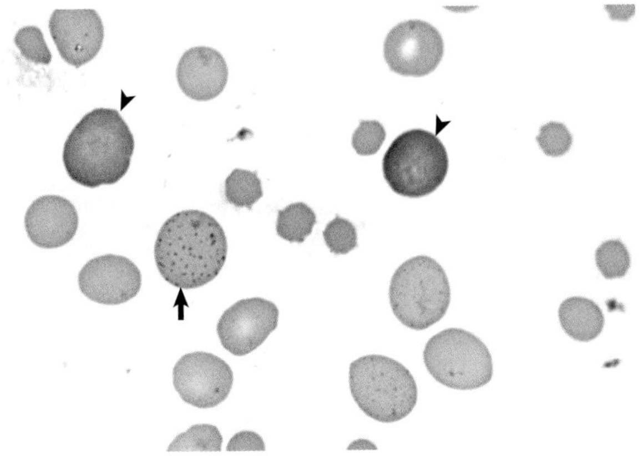

Figure 13-8 Basophilic Stippling and Polychromasia, Bovine Blood Smear. Erythrocytes from this cow with regenerative anemia include several cells with basophilic stippling *(arrow)* and two polychromatophilic cells (reticulocytes) *(arrowheads)*. Wright's stain. (Courtesy Dr. M.M. Fry, College of Veterinary Medicine, University of Tennessee.)

In hemolytic anemia, erythrocytes are destroyed at an increased rate. Whether the mechanism is intravascular or extravascular, or a combination, depends on the specific disease process (specific diseases are discussed later in this chapter). Some clinical indicators of hemolytic anemia and their pathogeneses are summarized in Fig. 13-9 and are further described in the following discussion.

A classic sequela of hemolytic anemias in general is *hyperbilirubinemia*, which is an increase in the plasma bilirubin concentration. Bilirubin is a yellow pigment, which explains why hyperbilirubinemia, if severe enough, causes *icterus*—the grossly visible yellowing of fluid or tissues (Fig. 13-10). Icterus, also known as *jaundice*, is usually detectable when the plasma bilirubin concentration exceeds 2 mg/dL. However, it is important to note that hyperbilirubinemia and icterus are not pathognomonic for hemolysis and may also occur with conditions of impaired bile flow (cholestasis), such as hepatopathy or cholangiopathy.

In addition to icterus, hemolytic anemia often results in splenomegaly (Fig. 13-11), which is secondary to extravascular hemolysis and macrophagic hyperplasia within the spleen, as well as splenic EMH. Splenomegaly may also occur in other conditions, as discussed elsewhere in this chapter.

Intravascular hemolysis is grossly evident as pink-tinged plasma or serum, termed *hemolysis* or *hemoglobinemia*. Hemolysis is not apparent until the concentration of extracellular hemoglobin is greater than approximately 50 mg/dL. Cell-free hemoglobin is scavenged by *haptoglobin* until haptoglobin becomes saturated with hemoglobin at a concentration of approximately 150 mg/dL. When haptoglobin is saturated, any remaining free hemoglobin has a low enough molecular weight to pass through the renal glomerular filter into the urine. This imparts a pink or red discoloration to the urine, called *hemoglobinuria*. Thus extracellular hemoglobin can cause gross discoloration of the plasma, where it is bound to haptoglobin, before becoming grossly visible in urine. The half-life of haptoglobin is markedly decreased when bound to hemoglobin, so when large amounts of haptoglobin-hemoglobin complex are formed, the concentration of haptoglobin in the blood decreases and hemoglobin can pass through the glomerulus at even lower concentrations. Hemoglobinuria is a contributing factor in the renal tubular necrosis (hemoglobinuric nephrosis) that often occurs in cases of acute intravascular hemolysis (see Chapter 11). A similar lesion occurs in the kidneys of individuals with marked muscle damage and resulting myoglobinuria (see Chapters 11 and 15).

Hemoglobinuria cannot be distinguished grossly from hematuria (erythrocytes in the urine) or myoglobinuria (myoglobin in the urine), and all three processes cause a positive reaction for "blood protein" on urine test strips. Comparing the colors of the plasma and the urine may be informative. In contrast to hemoglobin, myoglobin causes gross discoloration of the urine before the plasma is discolored. This is because myoglobin is a low-molecular-weight monomer, freely filtered by the glomerulus, and does not bind plasma proteins to a significant degree. Hematuria can be distinguished from hemoglobinuria on the basis of microscopic examination of urine sediment (i.e., erythrocytes are present in cases of hematuria).

In addition to red plasma and urine, hemoglobinemia may also be identified by increased MCH or MCHC values on a CBC. This is because the hemoglobin concentration is measured by lysing all erythrocytes in the sample and then measuring the total hemoglobin via spectrophotometry. By this method, hemoglobin that originated within or outside of erythrocytes is measured together. However, calculations for MCH and MCHC, which include results for the hemoglobin and red blood cell concentrations, assume that all of

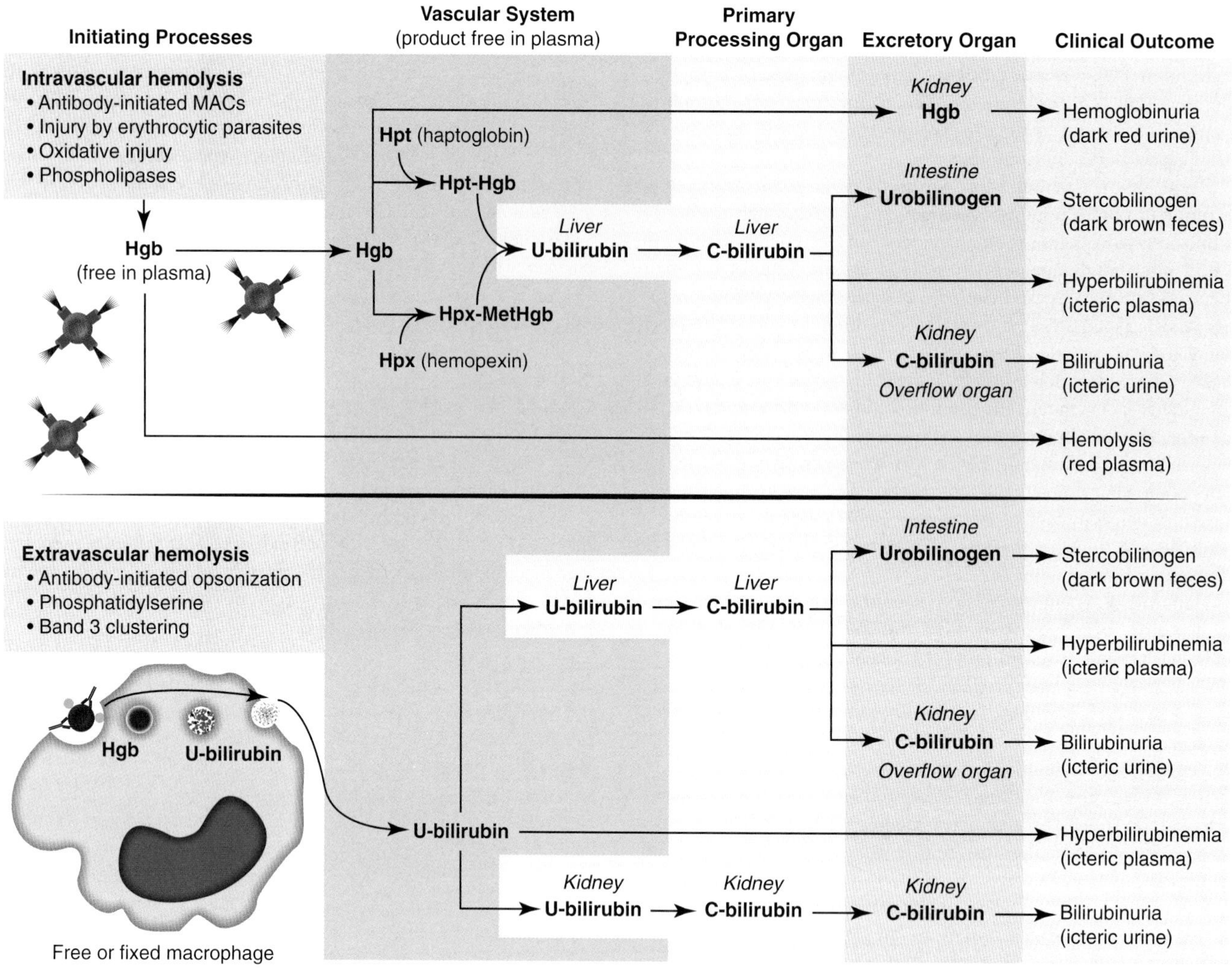

Figure 13-9 Mechanisms of Color Abnormalities of Plasma, Urine, and Feces during Hemolysis. Intravascular hemolysis: Several initiating processes can cause intravascular hemolysis; formation of the complement membrane attack complex is pictured. With intravascular hemolysis, free hemoglobin is release directly into the plasma, where it is scavenged by haptoglobin and hemopexin. When haptoglobin and hemopexin are saturated, the cell-free hemoglobin causes red discoloration of the plasma (hemolysis) and is excreted in the urine (hemoglobinuria; dark red urine). The liver clears haptoglobin-hemoglobin and hemopexin-methemoglobin complexes from plasma and converts hemoglobin to unconjugated bilirubin and then conjugated bilirubin. Conjugated bilirubin is normally excreted in the bile and then converted to urobilinogen (yellow) and subsequently stercobilinogen (dark brown). However, excessive bilirubin will spill over into the plasma, resulting in hyperbilirubinemia, icteric plasma (if severe enough), and urinary excretion of bilirubin (bilirubinuria; icteric urine). **Extravascular hemolysis:** During extravascular hemolysis, erythrocytes are phagocytized by macrophages, which digest erythrocytes, and convert hemoglobin to unconjugated bilirubin. Excessive bilirubin in plasma causes hyperbilirubinemia with or without icteric plasma. Unconjugated bilirubin is processed and excreted by the liver (as previously described) and in dogs, the kidney. *C-bilirubin*, Conjugated bilirubin; *Hgb*, hemoglobin; *Hpt*, haptoglobin; *Hpx*, hemopexin; *MACs*, membrane attack complexes; *MetHgb*, methemoglobin; *U-bilirubin*, unconjugated bilirubin. (Courtesy Dr. K.M. Boes, College of Veterinary Medicine, Virginia Polytechnic Institute and State University; and Dr. J.F. Zachary, College of Veterinary Medicine, University of Illinois.)

the hemoglobin originated within erythrocytes. In the case of hemoglobinemia, the excess extracellular hemoglobin may cause an artifactual increase in the calculated MCH and MCHC. It is important to remember that similar artifactual increases may also occur with lipemia.

Once hemolytic anemia has been identified, the specific cause for hemolysis should be investigated based on signalment, clinical history, and microscopic blood smear evaluation. The most common causes of hemolytic anemia in domestic animals are immune-mediated, infectious, oxidative, and mechanical fragmentation (i.e., microangiopathic) disorders (Table 13-3).

Spherocytosis and autoagglutination are hallmarks of immune-mediated hemolytic anemia, either primary (also known as idiopathic) or secondary to infectious disease, drugs/toxins, or neoplasms. *Spherocytes* form when macrophages (mainly in the spleen) phagocytize part of an erythrocyte plasma membrane bound with autoantibody (Fig. 13-12). The remaining portion of the erythrocyte assumes a spherical shape, thus preserving maximal volume. This change in shape results in decreased deformability of the cells. Erythrocytes must be extremely pliable to traverse the splenic red pulp and sinusoidal walls; spherocytes therefore tend to be retained in the spleen in close association with macrophages with risk for further injury and eventual destruction. In the dog, spherocytes appear smaller than normal and have uniform staining (Fig. 13-13, A), in contrast to normal erythrocytes, which have a region of central pallor imparted by their biconcave shape. This difference in staining between spherocytes and normal erythrocytes is not consistently discernible in many other domestic animals (including horses,

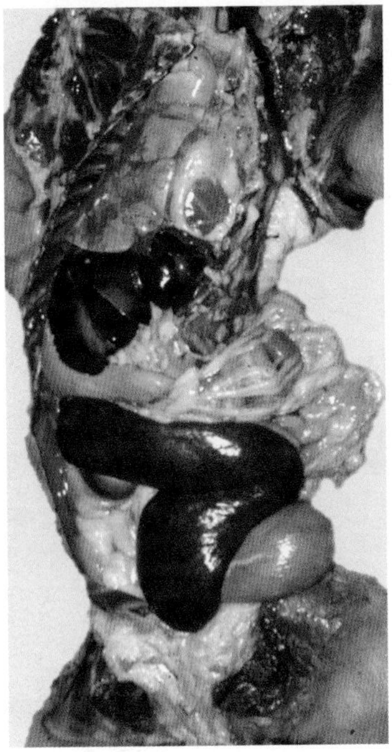

Figure 13-10 **Icterus, Immune-Mediated Hemolytic Anemia, Subcutaneous Fat, Splenomegaly, Spleen, Dog.** The marked yellow discoloration of tissues, most strikingly visible in the subcutaneous fat, is from high concentrations of serum bilirubin produced as a result of the hemolytic anemia. (Courtesy Dr. J.A. Ramos-Vara, College of Veterinary Medicine, Michigan State University; and Noah's Arkive, College of Veterinary Medicine, The University of Georgia.)

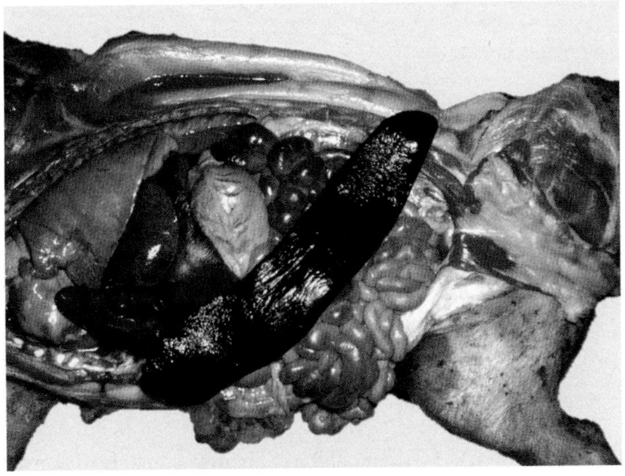

Figure 13-11 **Splenomegaly, Fatal Hemolytic Anemia, *Mycoplasma suis*, Pig.** The spleen is extremely enlarged, meaty, and congested. (Courtesy College of Veterinary Medicine, University of Illinois.)

cattle, and cats), whose erythrocytes differ from those of the dog in that they are smaller and have less pronounced biconcavity and therefore less pronounced central pallor. *Autoagglutination* occurs because of cross-linking of antibodies bound to erythrocytes (see Fig 13-12). Autoagglutination is evident macroscopically as blood with a grainy consistency (see Fig. 13-13, *B*), and microscopically as clusters of erythrocytes (see Fig. 13-13, *C*). Autoagglutination may also result in a falsely increased MCV and decreased red blood cell concentration when clustered cells are mistakenly counted as single cells by automated hematology analyzers. When autoagglutination is present, the packed-cell volume is the most reliable measurement of red blood cell mass.

Ghost cells are ruptured red blood cell membranes devoid of cytoplasmic contents (see Figs. 13-12 and 13-13, *A*). They indicate intravascular hemolysis and may be seen with a variety of hemolytic disorders, including those with immune-mediated, infectious, oxidative, or fragmentation causes. In the case of immune-mediated hemolytic anemia, antibody or complement binds to red blood cell membranes and activates the complement membrane attack complex (see Fig. 13-12). This causes pore formation in the red blood cell membrane and release of cytoplasmic contents into the plasma. Ghost cells are eventually cleared from circulation by phagocytic macrophages, mainly within the spleen.

Oxidative damage to erythrocytes occurs when normal antioxidative pathways that generate reducing agents (such as reduced nicotinamide adenine dinucleotide [NADH], reduced nicotinamide adenine dinucleotide phosphate [NADPH], and reduced glutathione [GSH]) are compromised or overwhelmed, resulting in hemolytic anemia, abnormal hemoglobin function, or both. Hemolysis caused by oxidative damage may be extravascular or intravascular, or a combination. Evidence of oxidative damage to erythrocytes may be apparent on blood smear examination as Heinz bodies or eccentrocytes or on gross examination as methemoglobinemia.

Heinz bodies are foci of denatured globin that interact with the erythrocyte membrane. They are usually subtly evident on routine Wright-stained blood smears as pale circular inclusions or blunt, rounded protrusions of the cell margin but are readily discernible on smears stained with new methylene blue (Fig. 13-14). Cats are particularly susceptible to Heinz body formation and may have low numbers of Heinz bodies normally. There is no unanimity of opinion, but some clinical pathologists believe that the presence of Heinz bodies in up to 10% of all erythrocytes in cats is within normal limits. This predisposition is believed to reflect unique features of the feline erythrocyte, whose hemoglobin has more sulfhydryl groups (preferential sites for oxidative damage) than do erythrocytes of other species and may also have lower intrinsic reducing capacity. It is also possible that the feline spleen does not have as efficient a "pitting" function (splenic structure and function are discussed in more detail later in this chapter).

Eccentrocytes, evident as erythrocytes in which one side of the cell has increased pallor (Fig. 13-15, *A*), are another manifestation of oxidative damage. They form because of cross-linking of

Table 13-3 Four Common Causes of Hemolytic Anemia, and Their Main Hematologic Characteristics

Immune-Mediated	Infectious	Oxidative	Mechanical Fragmentation
Agglutination Spherocytes Ghost cells	Agglutination Spherocytes Ghost cells Hemoparasites	Heinz bodies Eccentrocytes Ghost cells Methemoglobinemia	Schistocytes Acanthocytes Keratocytes Ghost cells

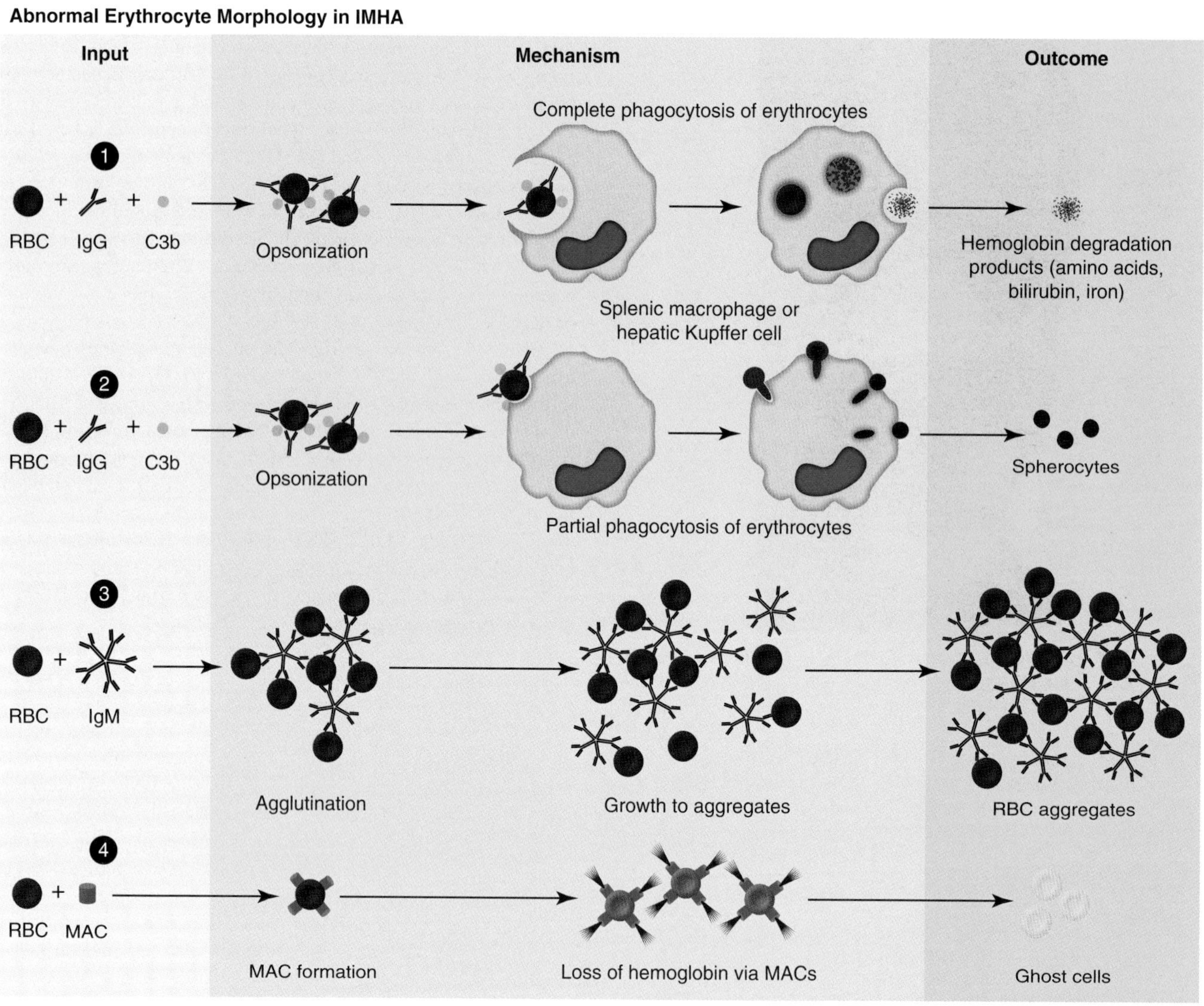

Figure 13-12 **Pathogenesis of Abnormal Erythrocyte Morphologic Changes in Immune-Mediated Hemolytic Anemia.** *1*, Red blood cell (RBC) degradation. Antierythrocyte antibodies bind RBC surface antigens, resulting in RBC opsonization by immunoglobulins (mainly immunoglobulin G [IgG]) and complement (primarily C3b). Immunoglobulin- or C3b-bound RBCs are phagocytized and digested by sinusoidal macrophages. *2*, Spherocytes. Spherocytes form when the membrane of immunoglobulin- or C3b-bound RBCs are phagocytized by macrophages, without removing the entire RBC from circulation. Compared to normal erythrocytes, spherocytes appear smaller, more eosinophilic, and lack central pallor. *3*, RBC aggregation (agglutination). RBC aggregation occurs when antierythrocyte immunoglobulins (immunoglobulin M [IgM] or high concentrations of IgG) bind multiple erythrocytes simultaneously. *4*, Ghost cells. Antierythrocyte antibodies bind RBC surface antigens, resulting in complement activation and formation of the membrane attack complex (MAC). MACs form membrane pores, resulting in rupture of RBCs, and the release of hemoglobin into the circulation. Ghost cells are RBC membrane remnants that lack cytoplasm (hemoglobin). (Courtesy Dr. K.M. Boes, College of Veterinary Medicine, Virginia Polytechnic Institute and State University; and Dr. J.F. Zachary, College of Veterinary Medicine, University of Illinois.)

membrane proteins, with adhesion of opposing areas of the cell's inner membrane leaflet, and displacement of most of the hemoglobin toward the other side. The fused membranes may fragment off of the eccentrocyte, leaving a slightly ruffled border; this cellular morphologic abnormality is called a *pyknocyte* (see Fig. 13-15, *B*).

Oxidative insult may also result in conversion of hemoglobin (iron in the Fe^{2+} state) to *methemoglobin* (iron in the Fe^{3+} state), which is incapable of binding oxygen. Methemoglobin is produced normally in small amounts but reduced back to oxyhemoglobin by the enzyme cytochrome-b_5 reductase (also known as *methemoglobin reductase*). *Methemoglobinemia* results when methemoglobin is produced in excessive amounts (because of oxidative insult) or when the normal pathways for maintaining hemoglobin in the Fe^{2+} state are impaired (as in cytochrome-b_5 reductase deficiency). When present in sufficiently high concentration (approximately 10% of total hemoglobin), methemoglobin imparts a grossly discernible chocolate color to the blood.

By itself, mechanical fragmentation hemolysis tends to cause mild or no anemia. Mechanical fragmentation results from trauma or shearing of erythrocytes within blood vessels. Normal erythrocytes may be flowing through abnormal vasculature, such as with heart valve defects, intravascular fibrin deposition (e.g., disseminated intravascular coagulation), vasculitis, or hemangiosarcoma. Alternatively, the red blood cells may be particularly fragile within normal blood vasculature, as occurs with iron deficiency. In either instance, microscopic evidence of mechanical fragmentation includes the presence of erythrocyte fragments (*schistocytes* [see Fig. 13-15, *C*]), erythrocytes with irregular cytoplasmic projections (*acanthocytes*), erythrocytes with blister-like projections (*keratocytes*), or ghost cells (see Figs. 13-13, *A*, 13-15, *D*, and 13-15, *E*).

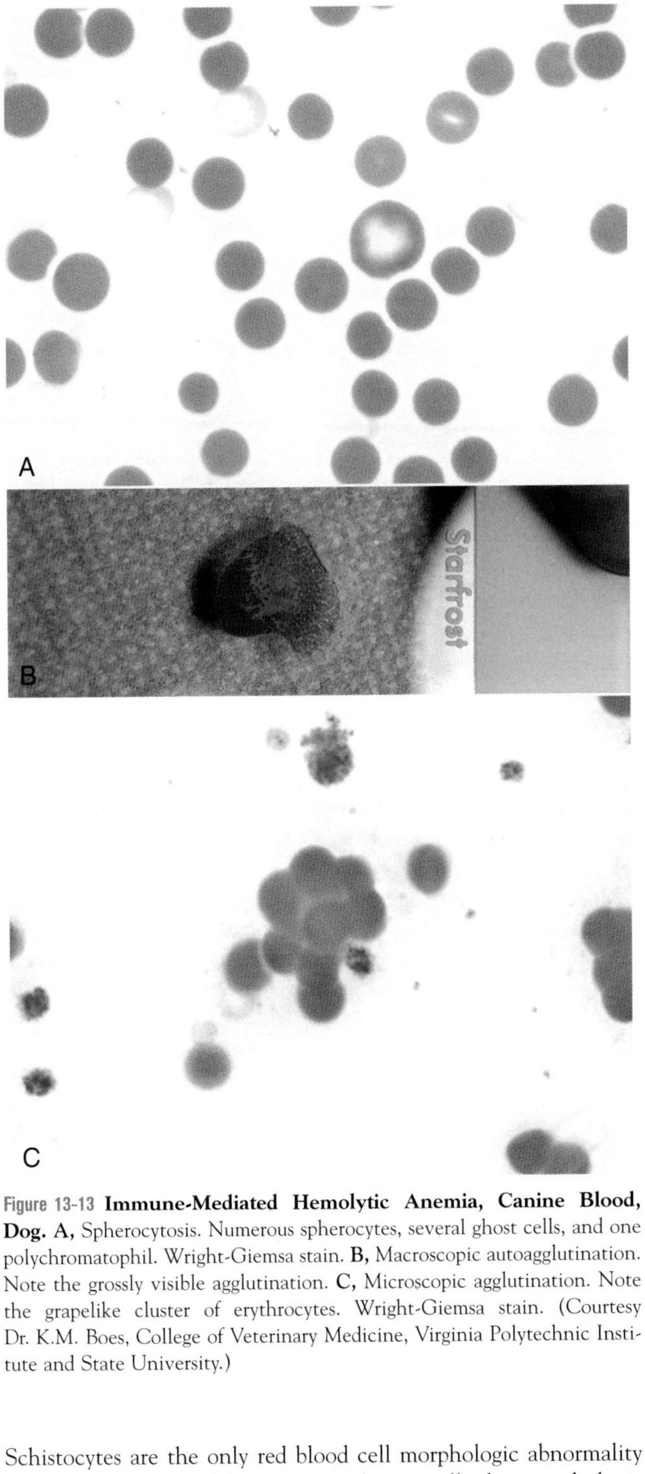

Figure 13-13 **Immune-Mediated Hemolytic Anemia, Canine Blood, Dog. A,** Spherocytosis. Numerous spherocytes, several ghost cells, and one polychromatophil. Wright-Giemsa stain. **B,** Macroscopic autoagglutination. Note the grossly visible agglutination. **C,** Microscopic agglutination. Note the grapelike cluster of erythrocytes. Wright-Giemsa stain. (Courtesy Dr. K.M. Boes, College of Veterinary Medicine, Virginia Polytechnic Institute and State University.)

Schistocytes are the only red blood cell morphologic abnormality specific for mechanical fragmentation because all other morphologic abnormalities can be seen with other disease processes. For example, ghost cells may be observed with other types of hemolysis.

Nonregenerative anemia is characterized by a lack of reticulocytosis on the CBC; however, reticulocytosis does not occur in horses even in the context of regeneration. Most often this is a result of decreased production in the marrow (i.e., erythroid hypoplasia). Erythrocytes circulate for a long time, so anemias caused by decreased production tend to develop slowly.

The most common form of nonregenerative anemia is known as *anemia of inflammation* or *anemia of chronic disease*. In this form of anemia, erythrocytes are decreased in number but are typically normal in size and hemoglobin concentration (so-called normocytic, normochromic anemia). It has long been known that patients with inflammatory or other chronic disease often become anemic, and that this condition results in increased iron stores in the bone marrow. Sequestration of iron may be a bacteriostatic evolutionary adaptation because many bacteria require iron as a cofactor for growth. In recent years, investigators have begun to elucidate the molecular mechanisms underlying anemia of inflammation. *Hepcidin*, an acute phase protein and antimicrobial peptide synthesized in the liver, is a key mediator that limits iron availability. Hepcidin expression increases with inflammation, infection, or iron overload and decreases with anemia or hypoxia. Hepcidin exerts its effects by causing functional iron deficiency. It binds to and causes the degradation of the cell surface iron efflux molecule, ferroportin, thus inhibiting both absorption of dietary iron from the intestinal epithelium and export of iron from macrophages and hepatocytes into the plasma (Fig. 13-16).

Anemia of inflammation involves factors besides decreased iron availability. Inflammatory cytokines are likely to inhibit erythropoiesis by oxidative damage to and triggering apoptosis of developing erythroid cells, by decreasing expression of Epo and stem cell factor, and by decreasing expression of Epo receptors. In addition, experimentally induced sterile inflammation in cats resulted in shortened erythrocyte survival, indicating that anemia of inflammation is likely also a function of increased erythrocyte destruction.

Other causes of decreased erythropoiesis are listed in Table 13-2. Specific examples of diseases causing nonregenerative anemia by these mechanisms are discussed later in this chapter.

Neutropenia. *Neutropenia* refers to a decrease in the concentration of neutrophils in circulating blood. Neutropenia may be caused by decreased production, increased destruction, altered distribution, or a demand for neutrophils in tissues that exceeds the rate of granulopoiesis.

Decreased production is evident on bone marrow examination as granulocytic hypoplasia. This usually results from an insult that affects multiple hematopoietic lineages, such as chemical insult, radiation, neoplasia, infection, or fibrosis, but may also be caused by a process that preferentially targets granulopoiesis. In marked contrast to erythrocytes, neutrophils have a very short life span in circulation. Once released from the bone marrow, a neutrophil is in the bloodstream only for hours before migrating into the tissues. When neutrophil production ceases, a reserve of mature neutrophils in the bone marrow storage pool may be adequate to maintain normal numbers of circulating neutrophils for a few days; however, after the bone marrow storage pool is depleted, neutropenia rapidly ensues.

Immune-mediated neutropenia is a rare but recognized condition in domestic animals. Bone marrow findings range from granulocytic hypoplasia to hyperplasia, depending on where the cells under immune attack are in their differentiation programs. Neutropenia with no evidence of decreased production and in which other causes of neutropenia have been excluded may be a result of destruction of neutrophils before they leave the bone marrow, a condition known as ineffective granulopoiesis. Like other forms of ineffective hematopoiesis, this condition is often presumed to be immune mediated; in cats this condition may occur as a result of infection of hematopoietic cells with FeLV.

As presented in the earlier section on Granulopoiesis and Monocytopoiesis (Myelopoiesis), neutrophils within the blood vasculature are in two compartments: a circulating pool, consisting of those cells flowing freely in the blood, and a marginating pool, consisting of those cells transiently interacting with the endothelial surface. (In reality, neutrophils are constantly shifting between these two pools, but the proportion of cells in either pool normally remains fairly

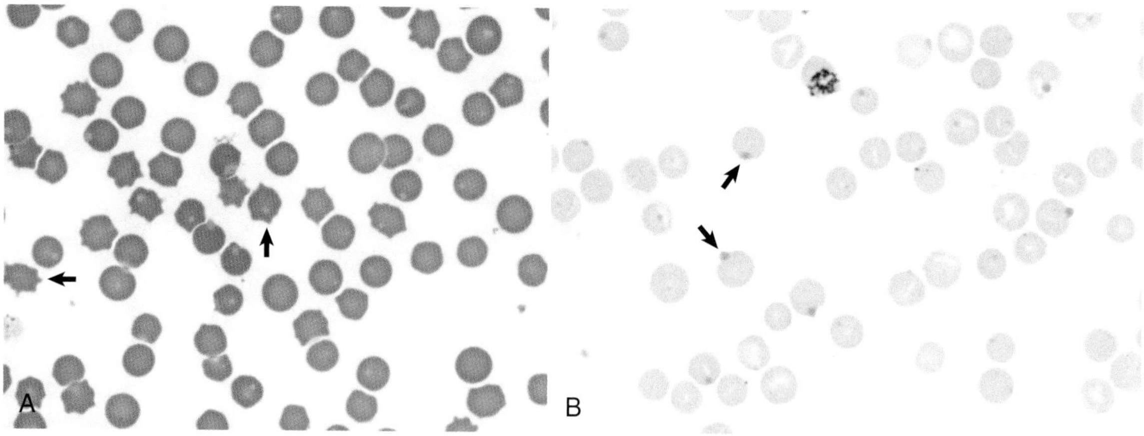

Figure 13-14 **Heinz Bodies, Blood Smears. A,** Feline blood smear. With routine staining, Heinz bodies appear as pale circular intraerythrocytic inclusions that may protrude *(arrows)* from the margin of the cell. Wright's stain. **B,** Canine blood smear. Using a supravital stain, Heinz bodies are blue inclusions *(arrows)* and easier to see. New methylene blue stain. (Courtesy Dr. M.M. Fry, College of Veterinary Medicine, University of Tennessee.)

constant in any given species.) Circulating neutrophils are part of the blood sample collected during routine venipuncture and are thus counted in the CBC, whereas marginating neutrophils are not. *Pseudoneutropenia* refers to the situation in which there is an increased proportion of neutrophils in the marginating pool. This may occur because of decreased blood flow or in response to stimuli, such as endotoxemia, that increase expression of molecules promoting interaction between neutrophils and endothelial cells. This mechanism of neutropenia is rarely observed in clinical practice.

Neutropenia may also result from increased demand for neutrophils in the tissue. How rapidly such a situation develops depends not only on the magnitude of the inflammatory stimulus but also on the reserve of postmitotic neutrophils in the bone marrow. The size of this reserve, or storage pool, is species dependent. In dogs this pool contains the equivalent of 5 days' normal production of neutrophils. Cattle represent the other extreme in that they have a small storage pool and thus are predisposed to becoming neutropenic during times of acute inflammation. Horses and cats are somewhere between the two extremes, closer to cattle and dogs, respectively. It stands to reason that the clinical significance of neutropenia because of a supply and demand imbalance is also species dependent. In dogs, neutropenia as a result of inflammation is an alarming finding because it is evidence of a massive tissue demand for neutrophils that has exhausted the patient's storage pool and is exceeding the rate of granulopoiesis in the bone marrow. However in cows, neutropenia is commonly noted in a wide range of conditions involving acute inflammation and does not necessarily indicate an overwhelming demand.

Eosinopenia/Basopenia. *Eosinopenia* and *basopenia* are decreased concentrations of blood eosinophils and basophils, respectively. In many laboratories, CBC reference values for eosinophils and basophils are as low as zero cells per microliter, precluding detection of eosinopenia or basopenia. When detectable, eosinopenia is often a result of stress (i.e., glucocorticoid mediated).

Monocytopenia. *Monocytopenia* denotes a decreased concentration of monocytes in blood; it is of little to no pathologic significance by itself.

Thrombocytopenia. Thrombocytopenia refers to a decrease in the concentration of circulating platelets. Mechanisms of thrombocytopenia include decreased production, increased destruction, increased consumption, and altered distribution.

Decreased production may occur because of a condition affecting cells of multiple hematopoietic lineages, including megakaryocytes, or because of one specifically depressing thrombopoiesis. In either case, decreased thrombopoiesis is evident as megakaryocytic hypoplasia upon bone marrow examination. General causes of decreased hematopoiesis outlined earlier in the sections on anemia and neutropenia also apply to thrombocytopenia.

Increased platelet destruction due to immune-mediated thrombocytopenia (IMTP) is a fairly common disease in dogs and may also occur in other species. Thrombocytopenia with immune-mediated thrombocytopenia is often severe (e.g., $<10,000$ platelets/μL), resulting in spontaneous multisystemic hemorrhage.

Increased use of platelets occurs with hemorrhage and disseminated intravascular coagulation. Thrombocytopenia secondary to hemorrhage is often mild to moderate, whereas disseminated intravascular coagulation may cause mild to severe thrombocytopenia, often with evidence of mechanical fragmentation hemolysis (e.g., schistocytes). Disseminated intravascular coagulation is a syndrome in which hypercoagulability leads to increased consumption of both platelets and coagulation factors in the plasma, with subsequent hypocoagulability and susceptibility to bleeding. Risk factors for developing disseminated intravascular coagulation include severe inflammation, such as sepsis or pancreatitis, neoplasia, and organ failure.

The spleen normally contains a significant proportion of total platelet mass (up to one-third in some species), and abnormalities involving the spleen may result in changes in the number of circulating platelets. For example, splenic congestion may result in platelet sequestration and thrombocytopenia, and splenic contraction may cause thrombocytosis.

Lymphopenia. *Lymphopenia* refers to a decreased concentration of lymphocytes in blood. It is a common hematologic finding in sick animals. Usually the precise mechanism of lymphopenia is not clear but is often presumed secondary to endogenous glucocorticoid excess that occurs with stress. Excess glucocorticoids, either endogenous or exogenous, cause an altered distribution of lymphocytes; there is increased trafficking of lymphocytes from blood to lymphoid tissue, and decreased egress of lymphocytes from lymphoid tissue to blood. At higher concentrations of glucocorticoids, lymphocytes are destroyed. Other causes of lymphotoxicity include chemotherapeutic agents, radiation therapy, and some infectious agents. Lymphopenia may occur with various mechanisms, including loss of lymphocyte-rich lymphatic fluid (e.g., gastrointestinal disease, repeated drainage of chylous effusions), and disruption of the normal lymphoid tissue architecture because

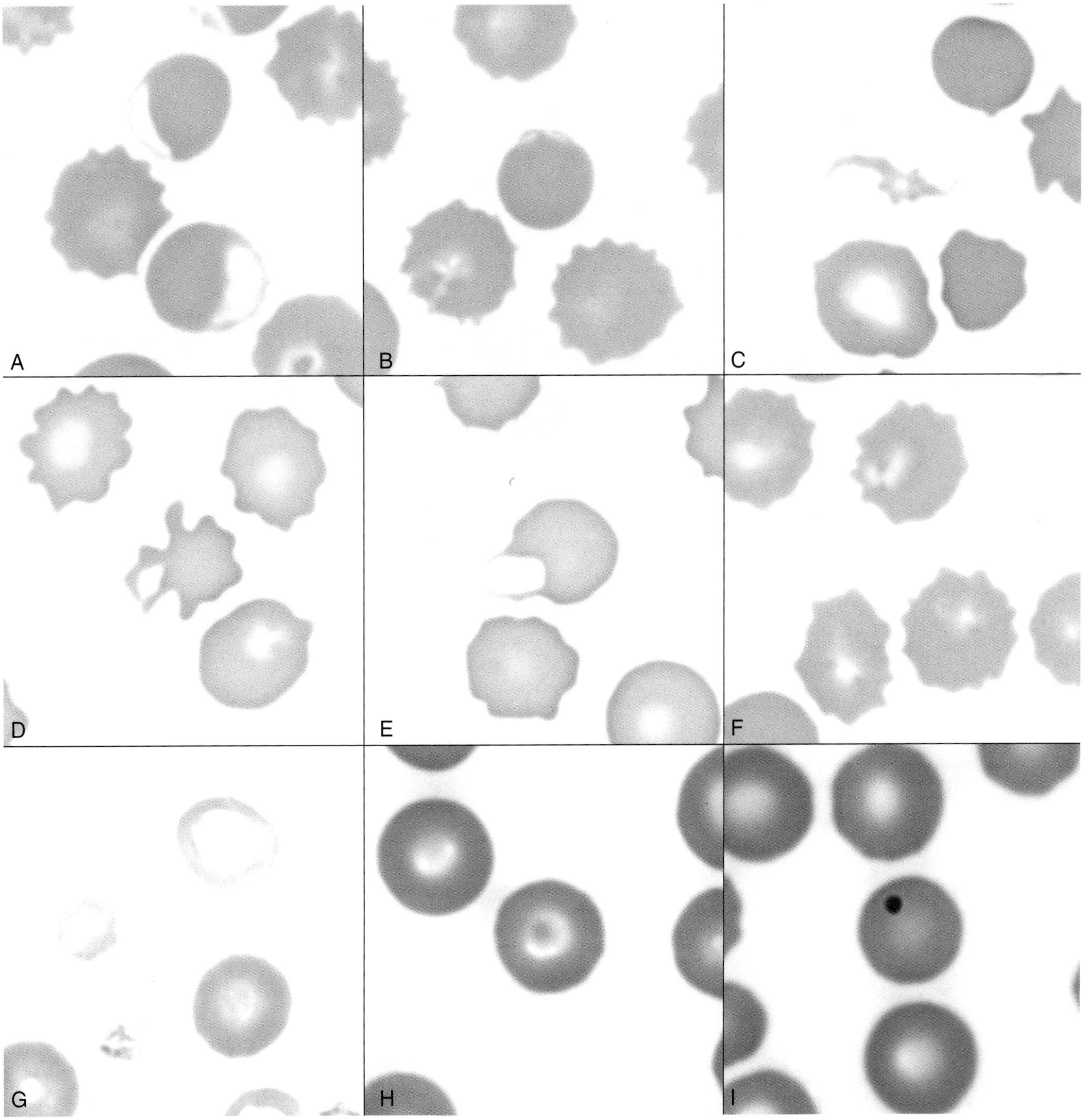

Figure 13-15 Common Erythrocyte Morphologic Abnormalities. A, Blood from a dog that was administered a continuous rate infusion of propofol. The dog developed oxidant-induced hemolytic anemia with eccentrocytes. Wright-Giemsa stain. **B,** Blood from the same dog as in **A,** showing a pyknocyte. Note the spherocyte-like appearance of the pyknocyte, except for a small portion of the red blood cell membrane that is ruffled. Wright-Giemsa stain. **C,** A schistocyte in the blood of a dog with mechanical fragmentation hemolysis from disseminated intravascular coagulation. Wright-Giemsa stain. **D,** Blood from a dog with hemangiosarcoma, showing an acanthocyte. Wright-Giemsa stain. **E,** A keratocyte, exhibiting what appears to be a ruptured "vesicle" in blood from a dog. Wright-Giemsa stain. **F,** Blood from a dog with crenation artifact showing echinocytes. Wright-Giemsa stain. **G,** Blood from a dog with iron deficiency anemia. Note the patient's microcytic and hypochromic cell *(left)* and the normocytic hypochromic cell *(top)*, as well as the normocytic normochromic erythrocyte *(bottom right)* from a recent blood transfusion. Wright-Giemsa stain. **H,** Blood from a dog. The center erythrocyte is a target cell, or codocyte. Wright-Giemsa stain. **I,** Blood from a dog shows a Howell-Jolly body, which is round, deeply basophilic remnant of the erythrocyte's nucleus. Wright-Giemsa stain. (Courtesy Dr. K.M. Boes, College of Veterinary Medicine, Virginia Polytechnic Institute and State University.)

of generalized lymphadenopathy (e.g., lymphoma, blastomycosis). Some hereditary immunodeficiencies, such as severe combined immunodeficiency or thymic aplasia, can cause lymphopenia due to lymphoid aplasia.

Erythrocytosis. An increase in the measured red cell mass above the normal range is known as *erythrocytosis*. The term polycythemia is often used interchangeably with erythrocytosis, but technically and for the purposes of this chapter, polycythemia refers to a specific type of leukemia called *primary erythrocytosis* or *polycythemia vera*.

Causes of erythrocytosis are either relative or absolute. *Relative erythrocytosis* results from a fluid deficit or an altered distribution of erythrocytes within the body (i.e., the body's total erythrocyte mass

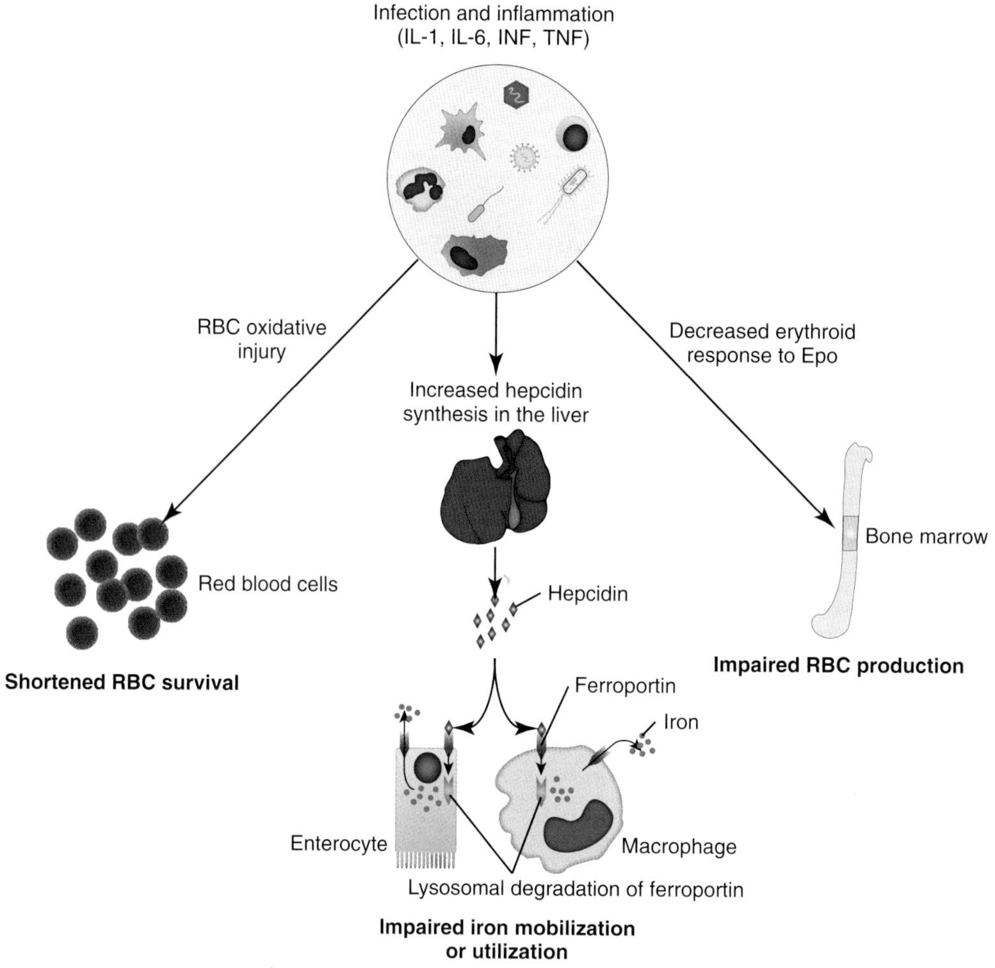

Figure 13-16 **Mechanisms of Anemia in Inflammatory Diseases.** Inflammatory mediators, including interleukin-1 (IL-1), interleukin-6 (IL-6), interferon (INF), and tumor necrosis factor (TNF), cause anemia of inflammatory disease due to oxidative hemolysis, iron sequestration within enterocytes and macrophages, and impaired erythroid responsiveness to erythropoietin (Epo). During homeostasis the membrane transport molecule, ferroportin, transports iron from the cytosol to the extracellular space. The iron is then used for various physiologic processes, including hemoglobin production within bone marrow erythroid precursors. During times of inflammation the liver increases production of hepcidin, which binds ferroportin and causes its internalization and lysosomal degradation. With fewer membrane ferroportin molecules, less iron is absorbed from the diet and mobilized from macrophages. *RBC*, Red blood cell. (Courtesy Dr. K.M. Boes, College of Veterinary Medicine, Virginia Polytechnic Institute and State University; and Dr. J.F. Zachary, College of Veterinary Medicine, University of Illinois.)

is not increased). It occurs most frequently with dehydration, when the decreased proportion of water in the blood results in hemoconcentration. It is observed less frequently with epinephrine-mediated splenic contraction, wherein erythrocytes move from the spleen into peripheral circulation. Erythrocytosis from splenic contraction occurs to the most pronounced degree in horses and cats, especially in young, healthy animals.

Absolute erythrocytosis is a true increase in red blood cell mass due to erythroid neoplasia or hyperplasia and includes causes of primary and secondary erythrocytosis. *Primary erythrocytosis*, or *polycythemia vera*, is a neoplastic proliferation of erythroid cells with a predominance of mature erythrocytes. Diagnosis is based on a marked increase in red cell mass (hematocrit in normally hydrated dogs ranges from 65% to >80%), an absence of hypoxemia, an absence of other tumors, and a normal or decreased plasma Epo concentration.

Secondary erythrocytosis refers to Epo-mediated erythroid hyperplasia causing an increased red blood cell mass. The erythroid hyperplasia may be an appropriate response to chronic hypoxia, such as occurs with right-to-left cardiac shunts or chronic pulmonary disease. Rarely, an Epo-secreting tumor may cause inappropriately elevated levels of Epo in the absence of hypoxia.

Absolute erythrocytosis, whether primary or secondary, causes increased viscosity of the blood, resulting in impaired blood flow and microvasculature distention. Affected individuals are at increased risk for tissue hypoxia, thrombosis, and hemorrhage. Clinical signs of hyperviscosity syndrome may include erythematous mucous membranes (Fig. 13-17), prolonged capillary refill time, prominent scleral vessels, evidence of thrombosis or hemorrhage, and secondary signs related to specific organ systems affected (e.g., neurologic and cardiovascular signs).

Neutrophilia. *Neutrophilia*, an increased blood concentration of neutrophils, occurs in response to a number of different stimuli, which are not mutually exclusive. Major mechanisms of neutrophilia are shown in Fig. 13-18. Understanding the CBC findings characteristic of these responses is an important part of clinical veterinary medicine. Inflammation can result in neutropenia, as discussed earlier, or neutrophilia, as discussed next. However, before moving on to a discussion of inflammatory neutrophilia and the so-called left shift, it is important to mention two other common

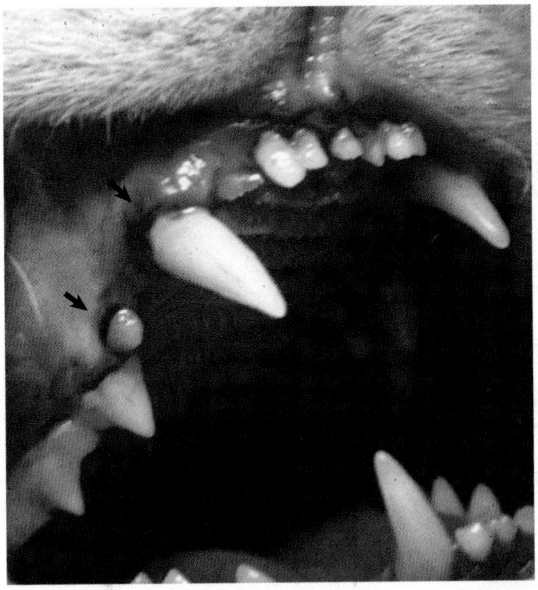

Figure 13-17 **Absolute Erythrocytosis, Hyperviscosity Syndrome, Erythematous Mucous Membranes, Cat.** Erythema of mucous membranes is one of the signs associated with hyperviscosity syndrome. In this case the oral mucous membranes are deeper red *(arrows)* than normal because of an abnormally high concentration of erythrocytes and associated sludging of blood. Hyperviscosity syndrome may also occur as the result of increased plasma immunoglobulin concentration. (Courtesy Dr. C. Patrick Ryan, Veterinary Public Health, Los Angeles Department of Health Services; and Noah's Arkive, College of Veterinary Medicine, The University of Georgia.)

causes of neutrophilia: glucocorticoid excess and epinephrine excess. Less common causes of neutrophilia, such as leukocyte adhesion deficiency and neoplasia, are discussed later in the chapter.

Glucocorticoid excess, either because of endogenous production or exogenous administration, results in a CBC pattern known as the *stress leukogram*, characterized by *mature neutrophilia* (i.e., increased concentration of segmented neutrophils without immature neutrophils) and lymphopenia, with or without monocytosis and eosinopenia. Mechanisms contributing to glucocorticoid-mediated neutrophilia include the following:

- Increased release of mature neutrophils from the bone marrow storage pool
- Decreased margination of neutrophils within the vasculature, with a resulting increase in the circulating pool
- Decreased migration of neutrophils from the bloodstream into tissues

The magnitude of neutrophilia tends to be species dependent, with dogs having the most pronounced response (up to 35,000 cells/μL) and in decreasing order of responsiveness, cats (30,000 cells/μL), horses (20,000 cells/μL), and cattle (15,000 cells/μL) having less marked responses. With long-term glucocorticoid excess, neutrophil numbers tend to normalize, whereas lymphopenia persists.

Epinephrine release results in a different pattern, known as *physiologic leukocytosis* or *excitement leukocytosis*, characterized by mature neutrophilia (like the glucocorticoid response) and lymphocytosis (unlike the glucocorticoid response). This phenomenon is short lived (i.e., <1 hour). Neutrophilia occurs primarily because of a shift of cells from the marginating to the circulating pool. Physiologic leukocytosis is common in cats (especially when they are highly stressed during blood collection) and horses, less common in cattle, and uncommon in dogs.

Of course, neutrophilia may also indicate inflammation, and inflammatory stimuli of varying magnitude and duration produce different patterns of neutrophilia. A classic hematologic finding in patients with increased demand for neutrophils is the presence of immature forms in the blood, known as a *left shift*. Not all inflammatory responses have a left shift, but the presence of a left shift almost always signifies active demand for neutrophils in the tissue. The magnitude of a left shift is assessed by the number of immature cells and their degree of immaturity. The mildest form is characterized by increased numbers of band neutrophils, the immediate predecessor to the segmented neutrophil normally found in circulation. Progressively immature predecessors are seen with increasingly severe inflammation. A left shift is considered orderly if the number of immature neutrophils in circulation decreases as they become progressively immature. The term *degenerative left shift* is sometimes used to describe cases in which the number of immature forms exceeds the number of segmented neutrophils. As with glucocorticoid-mediated neutrophilia, the typical magnitude of neutrophilia caused by inflammation varies by species, with dogs having the most pronounced response.

It might be useful to think of neutrophil kinetics in terms of a producer-consumer model in which the bone marrow is the factory, and the tissues (where the neutrophils eventually go) are the customers. The bone marrow storage pool is the factory inventory, and the neutrophils in the bloodstream are in delivery to the customer. Within the blood vessels, circulating neutrophils are on the highway, and marginating neutrophils are temporarily pulled off to the side of the road. During health, there is an even flow of neutrophils from the factory to the customer. Thus the system is in steady state, and neutrophil numbers remain relatively constant and within the normal range. However, disease states may perturb this system at multiple levels. Decreased granulopoiesis is analogous to a factory working below normal production level. Ineffective granulopoiesis is analogous to goods that are produced at a normal to increased rate but are damaged during manufacturing and never leave the factory. A left shift is analogous to the factory meeting increased customer demand by shipping out unfinished goods. Cases of persistent, established inflammation are characterized by bone marrow granulocytic hyperplasia and mature neutrophilia, analogous to a factory that has had time to adjust to increased demand and is meeting it more efficiently by increasing its output.

Eosinophilia/Basophilia. *Eosinophilia* and *basophilia* are increased concentrations of blood eosinophils and basophils, respectively. They may occur with parasitism, hypersensitivity reactions, paraneoplastic responses (e.g., lymphoma, mast cell neoplasia, or leukemia), and nonparasitic infectious disease. Eosinophilia has also been documented with hypoadrenocorticism and rare idiopathic conditions (e.g., hypereosinophilic syndrome). Most cases of eosinophilia and basophilia are due to eosinophilic and basophilic hyperplasia within the bone marrow in response to inflammatory growth factors. However, cortisol deficiency is thought to cause eosinophilia in dogs with hypoadrenocorticism.

Monocytosis. *Monocytosis* is an increased concentration of monocytes in blood. It most commonly occurs with excessive glucocorticoids or inflammation and uncommonly to rarely with monocytic leukemia, immune-mediated neutropenia, and cyclic hematopoiesis. With excessive endogenous or exogenous glucocorticoids, monocytes shift from the marginating pool to the circulating pool. This stress monocytosis is most common in dogs, less frequent in cats, and rare in horses and cattle. Inflammatory diseases cause monocytosis by cytokine-mediated monocytic hyperplasia in the bone marrow.

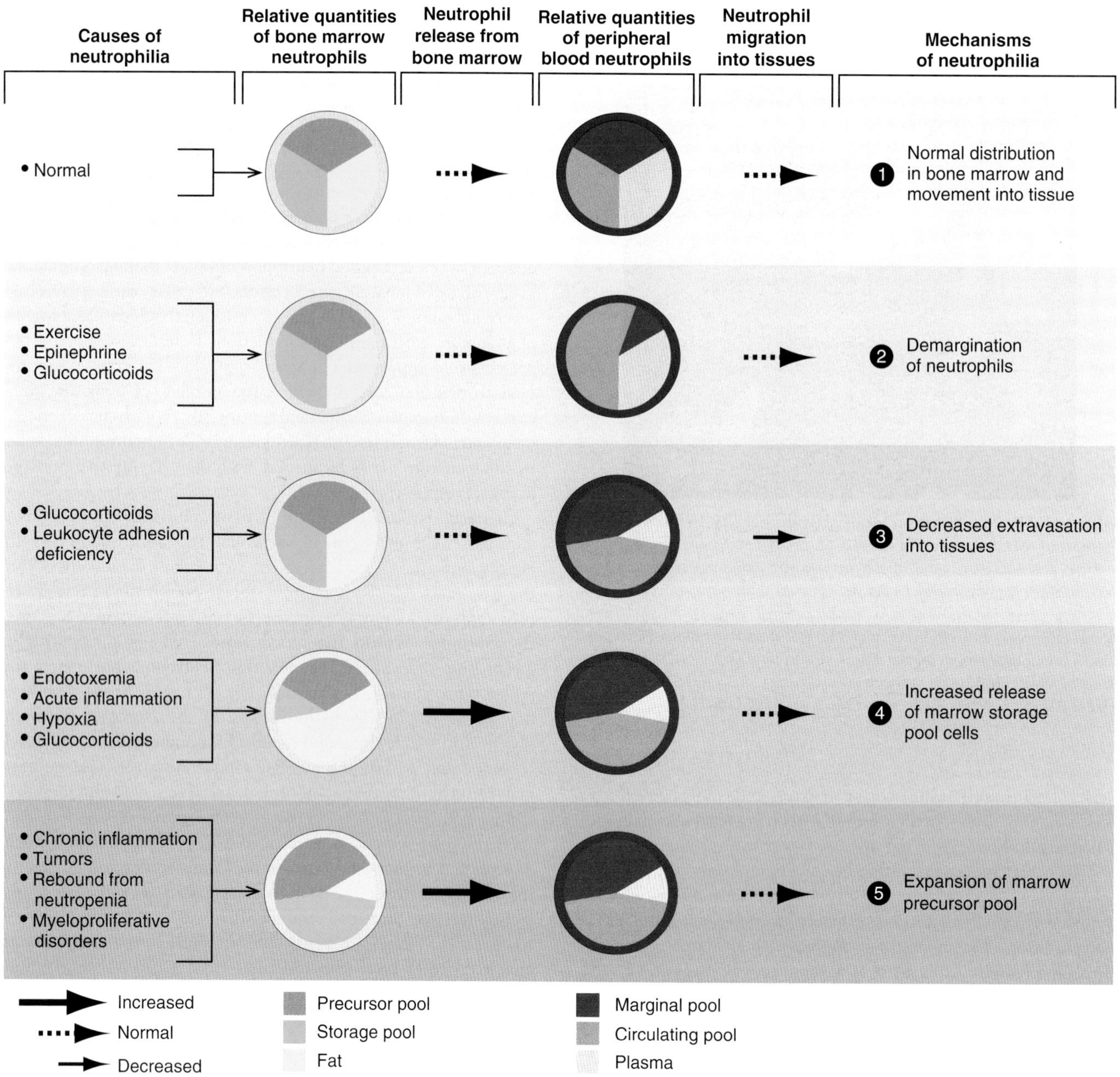

Figure 13-18 **Mechanisms of Neutrophilic Leukocytosis.** *1*, Neutrophils and their precursors are distributed in five pools: a bone marrow precursor pool, which includes mitotically active and inactive immature cells; a bone marrow storage pool, consisting of mitotically inactive mature neutrophils; a peripheral blood marginating pool; a peripheral blood circulating pool; and a tissue pool. The relative size of each pool is represented by the size of its corresponding wedge. The peripheral blood neutrophil count measures only neutrophils within the circulating peripheral blood pool, which can be enlarged by *(2)* increased demargination, *(3)* diminished extravasation into tissue, *(4)* increased release of cells from the marrow storage pool, and *(5)* expansion of the marrow precursor pool. (Courtesy Dr. K.M. Boes, College of Veterinary Medicine, Virginia Polytechnic Institute and State University; and Dr. J.F. Zachary, College of Veterinary Medicine, University of Illinois.)

Thrombocytosis. *Thrombocytosis*, or an increased concentration of platelets in the blood, is a relatively common, nonspecific finding in veterinary patients. In the vast majority of cases, thrombocytosis is reactive—a response to another, often apparently unrelated, disease process. Examples of conditions having reactive thrombocytosis include inflammatory and infectious diseases, iron deficiency, hemorrhage, endocrinopathies, and neoplasia. Factors that may contribute to reactive thrombocytosis include increased plasma concentration of thrombopoietin, inflammatory cytokines (e.g., IL-6), or catecholamines. Thrombocytosis may also occur as part of a regenerative response in patients recovering from thrombocytopenia, as a result of redistribution after splenic contraction, or within the several weeks after splenectomy. In these cases, thrombocytosis is transient. In the case of splenectomy, thrombocytosis may be marked but normalizes after several weeks. Because the body's total platelet mass regulates thrombopoiesis, and a significant portion of the platelet mass is normally in the spleen, it makes sense that splenectomized animals develop thrombocytosis. However, the reason that the number of circulating platelets normalizes in these individuals in the weeks after splenectomy is not clear. There is also a rare form of megakaryocytic leukemia known as essential thrombocythemia, which is characterized by marked thrombocytosis.

Lymphocytosis. *Lymphocytosis* refers to an increase in the concentration of lymphocytes in blood circulation. There are several causes of lymphocytosis, including age, excessive epinephrine, chronic inflammation, hypoadrenocorticism, and lymphoid neoplasia; lymphoid neoplasms are presented later in the chapter. Young animals normally have higher concentrations of lymphocytes than older animals, and normal healthy young animals may have counts that exceed adult reference values. Because this is not pathologic lymphocytosis, but normal physiologic variation, it is often termed *pseudolymphocytosis* of young animals. As discussed earlier in the section on neutrophilia, lymphocytosis is also a feature of epinephrine-mediated physiologic leukocytosis, resulting from redistribution of lymphocytes from the blood marginating pool into the blood circulating pool. Epinephrine-mediated lymphocytosis may be more marked than neutrophilia, particularly in cats (lymphocyte counts of > 20,000/μL are not uncommon). Antigenic stimulation may result in lymphocytosis, which may be marked in rare cases (up to approximately 30,000/μL in dogs and 40,000/μL in cats); however, this is not usually the case, even when there is clear evidence of increased immunologic activity in lymphoid tissues. In cases of antigenic stimulation, it is common for a minority of lymphocytes to have "reactive" morphologic features—larger lymphocytes with more abundant, deeply basophilic cytoplasm and more open chromatin (Fig. 13-19). Just as glucocorticoid excess can cause lymphopenia, glucocorticoid deficiency (hypoadrenocorticism) can cause lymphocytosis, or lack of lymphopenia during conditions of stress that typically result in glucocorticoid-mediated lymphopenia.

A condition known as *persistent lymphocytosis* (PL) occurs in approximately 30% of cattle infected with the bovine leukemia virus (BLV). The condition is defined as an increase in the blood concentration of lymphocytes above the reference interval for at least 3 months. This form of lymphocytosis is a nonneoplastic proliferation (i.e., hyperplasia) of B lymphocytes. In the absence of other disease, cattle with persistent lymphocytosis are asymptomatic. However, cattle infected with BLV, especially those animals with persistent lymphocytosis, are at increased risk for developing B lymphocyte lymphoma.

Secondary Abnormal Structure or Function of Blood Cells. The preceding section focused on abnormalities in the number of blood cells. There are also various acquired and congenital conditions involving abnormal structure or function of blood cells. This section briefly discusses abnormal blood cell structure or function occurring secondary to other underlying disease. Primary disorders of blood cells are discussed later in the chapter in the section on specific diseases.

Morphologic abnormalities detected on routine microscopic examination of blood smears may provide important clues about underlying disease processes. *Poikilocytosis* is a broad term referring to the presence of abnormally shaped erythrocytes in circulation. E-Table 13-1 lists conditions with and mechanisms involved in the formation of a number of specific types of erythrocyte morphologic abnormalities, and Fig. 13-15 shows some examples.

The acquired neutrophil morphologic abnormality known as toxic change (Fig. 13-20) reflects accelerated production of neutrophils as part of the inflammatory response. Features of toxic change include increased cytoplasmic basophilia, the presence of small blue-gray cytoplasmic inclusions known as Döhle bodies (often noted incidentally in cats), and in more severe cases, cytoplasmic vacuolation. Although not causing impaired neutrophil function, toxic change occurs during granulopoiesis and thus is technically a form of dysplasia (e.g., Döhle bodies are foci of aggregated endoplasmic reticulum). Toxic change may accompany any inflammatory response, but in general the more marked the toxic change, the higher the index of suspicion for infection or endotoxemia. Other secondary changes to neutrophils may not be evident morphologically. For example, studies in human beings and dogs have shown that individuals with cancer have abnormal neutrophil function (including phagocytic activity, killing capacity, and oxidative burst activity) before initiation of therapy. The clinical significance of this finding is not clear.

Platelet function disorders, also known as thrombopathies or thrombopathias, may be primary or secondary. Many conditions are known or suspected to cause secondary platelet dysfunction (hypofunction or hyperfunction) by altering platelet adhesion or aggregation or by mechanisms that are not fully understood. Box 13-2 shows underlying conditions having secondary platelet dysfunction.

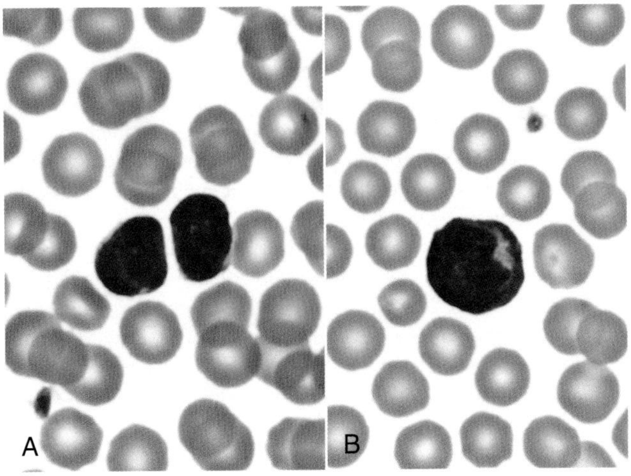

Figure 13-19 **Lymphocytosis (B), Lymphocytes, Canine Blood Smear. A,** Small lymphocytes, the predominant type of lymphocyte in the blood under normal conditions. **B,** A reactive lymphocyte, characterized by mildly increased size and an increased amount of basophilic cytoplasm, from a recently vaccinated 16-week-old dog. Wright's stain. (Courtesy Dr. M.M. Fry, College of Veterinary Medicine, University of Tennessee.)

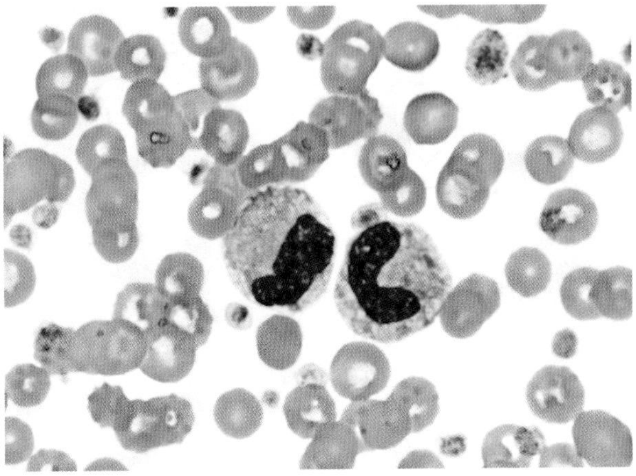

Figure 13-20 **Toxic Change, Neutrophils, Canine Blood Smear.** Two band neutrophils with basophilic, foamy cytoplasm indicate toxic change. This dog also has reactive thrombocytosis. Wright's stain. (Courtesy Dr. M.M. Fry, College of Veterinary Medicine, University of Tennessee.)

Box 13-2 Conditions Known or Suspected to Cause Secondary Platelet Dysfunction in Animals

SECONDARY PLATELET HYPOFUNCTION
Underlying Disease
Uremia
Antiplatelet antibodies (also cause immune-mediated thrombocytopenia)
Infection (BVDV, FeLV)
Hyperglobulinemia
Increased fibrinolytic products
Hypoammonemia
Snake envenomation

Drugs or Other Exogenous Agents
Platelet inhibitors
NSAIDs–irreversible (aspirin) or reversible inhibition of cyclooxygenase
Colloidal plasma expanders (e.g., hydroxyethyl starch)
Other drugs and exogenous agents (many)

SECONDARY PLATELET HYPERFUNCTION
Underlying Disease
Infection (heartworm and RMSF in dogs, FIP, pasteurellosis in cattle)
Inflammation
Neoplasia
Taurine deficiency in cats
Nephrotic syndrome

BVDV, Bovine viral diarrhea virus; *FeLV,* feline leukemia virus; *FIP,* feline infectious peritonitis, *NSAIDs,* nonsteroidal antiinflammatory drugs; *RMSF,* Rocky Mountain spotted fever.

Box 13-3 Portals of Entry into Bone Marrow

BONE MARROW
Hematogenously
Direct penetration (trauma)

Portals of Entry/Pathways of Spread

Invading cells or microorganism gain access to the bone marrow or blood circulation either hematogenously or by trauma. Trauma may be as obvious as a gaping wound or as subtle as the bite of an insect. Portals of entry for the bone marrow are summarized in Box 13-3. Diseases that arise from the bone marrow, such as leukemia, typically spread to other tissues hematogenously.

Defense Mechanisms/Barrier Systems

The bone marrow is encased by a protective shell of cortical bone, and blood supply to the marrow provides access to systemic humoral and cellular defenses. Of course, leukocytes themselves function as an essential part of inflammation and immune function, as discussed briefly in the section on Granulopoiesis and Monocytopoiesis (Myelopoiesis) and in greater detail in Chapters 3 and 5.

Biochemical steps in the glycolytic pathway or linked to it generate antioxidant molecules that enable erythrocytes to withstand oxidative insults throughout their many days in circulation. In addition to producing energy in the form of adenosine triphosphate (ATP), glycolysis generates NADH, which helps convert the oxidized, nonfunctional form of hemoglobin, known as methemoglobin, back to its active, reduced state. Another antioxidant erythrocyte metabolic pathway, the pentose shunt or hexose monophosphate shunt, generates NADPH to help maintain glutathione in the reduced state.

Disorders of Domestic Animals

Aplastic Anemia (Aplastic Pancytopenia)

Aplastic anemia, or more accurately aplastic pancytopenia, is a rare condition characterized by aplasia or severe hypoplasia of all hematopoietic lineages in the bone marrow with resulting cytopenias. The term aplastic anemia is a misnomer because affected cells are not limited to the erythroid lineage.

Many of the conditions reported to cause aplastic anemia do so only rarely or idiosyncratically; more frequently, they cause other hematologic or nonhematologic abnormalities. A partial list of reported causes of aplastic anemia in domestic animals includes the following:

- Chemical agents
  - Antimicrobial agents (dogs, cats)
  - Chemotherapeutic agents (dogs, cats)
  - Phenylbutazone (horses, dogs)
  - Bracken fern (cattle, sheep)
  - Estrogen (dogs)
  - Trichloroethylene (cattle, sheep)
  - Aflatoxin B_1 (horses, cattle, dogs, pigs)
- Infectious agents
  - *Ehrlichia* (Ehrlichiosis [dogs, cats])
  - Parvovirus (dogs, cats)
  - FeLV (cats)
  - Feline immunodeficiency virus (cats)
  - Lentivirus (Equine infectious anemia [horses])
  - Idiopathic (horses, cattle, dogs, cats)

Most of these causes, especially the chemical agents, are directly cytotoxic to HSCs or progenitor cells, resulting in their destruction. However, another proposed mechanism is disruption of normal stem cell function because of mutation or perturbation of hematopoietic cells and/or their microenvironment. This pathogenesis is mostly recognized in retroviral infections.

Aplastic anemia occurs in both acute and chronic forms. Most of the chemical causes result in acute disease. Grossly, affected animals may show signs of multisystemic infection and hemorrhage due to severe neutropenia and thrombocytopenia, respectively. Severe neutropenia typically develops within 1 week of an acute insult to the bone marrow, and severe thrombocytopenia occurs in the second week. This sequence is a result of the circulating life spans of each cell type; in health, neutrophils have a blood half-life of 5 to 10 hours, whereas platelets circulate for 5 to 10 days. The development of signs of anemia, such as pale mucous membranes, is more variable. The presence and severity of anemia depends on how rapidly the marrow recovers from the insult and the erythrocyte life span of the particular species.

Microscopically, bone marrow is hypocellular with markedly reduced hematopoietic cells. Hematopoietic cells are replaced with adipose tissue, and there is a variable inflammatory infiltrate of lymphocytes, plasma cells, and macrophages. In addition, there may be necrosis, hematopoietic cell apoptosis, and an increase in phagocytic macrophages. Fig. 13-21 shows bone marrow aspirates from a dog with pancytopenia from acute 5-fluorouracil toxicosis, before and during recovery.

Congenital Disorders

Many inherited or presumably inherited disorders of blood cells have been recognized in domestic animals, including rare or sporadic cases and conditions that are of questionable clinical relevance. This section and the later sections covering species-specific disorders are

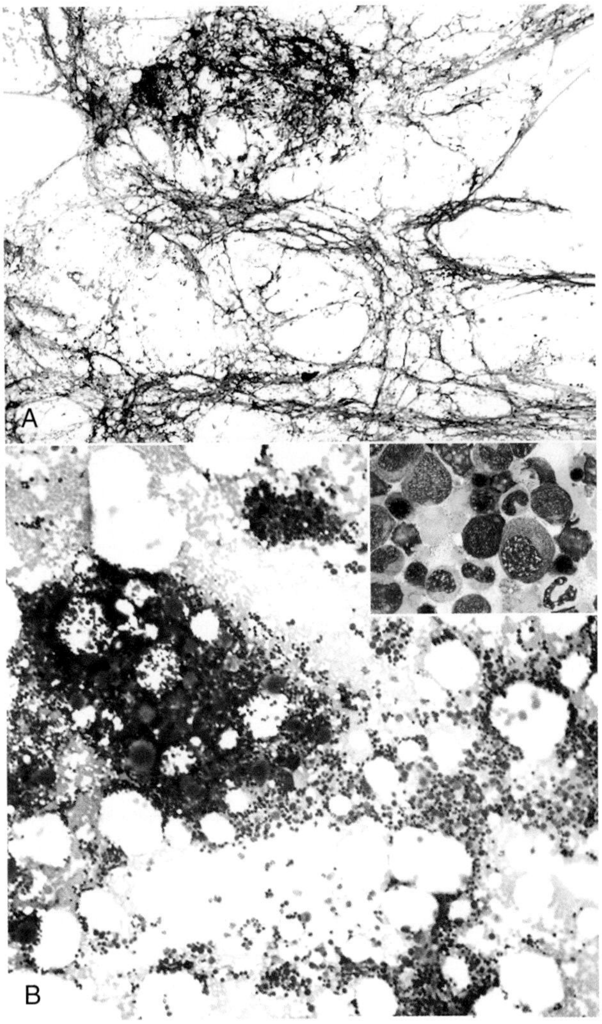

Figure 13-21 Aplastic Anemia, Canine Bone Marrow Aspirate. **A,** Bone marrow aspirate from a dog 8 days after ingestion of a toxic dose of 5-fluorouracil shows stromal cells but a lack of developing blood cells. **B,** Bone marrow aspirate from the same dog 1 week later, after resumption of hematopoiesis. *Inset,* Higher magnification of Figure 13-21, *B,* shows early- and late-stage erythroid and granulocytic precursors. Wright's stain. (Courtesy Dr. M.M. Fry, College of Veterinary Medicine, University of Tennessee.)

not comprehensive but instead focus on the more common, well-characterized, or recently reported conditions.

Erythropoietic Porphyrias. Porphyrias are a group of hereditary disorders in which porphyrins accumulate in the body because of defective heme synthesis. Inherited enzyme defects in hemoglobin synthesis have been identified in Holstein cattle, Siamese cats, and other cattle and cat breeds, resulting in bovine congenital erythropoietic porphyria and feline erythropoietic porphyria, respectively. Accumulation of toxic porphyrins in erythrocytes causes hemolytic anemia, whereas accumulation of porphyrins in tissues and fluids produces discoloration, including red-brown teeth, bones, and urine (see Fig. 1-59). Because of the circulation of the photodynamic porphyrins in blood, these animals have lesions of photosensitization of the nonpigmented skin. All affected tissues, including erythrocytes, exhibit fluorescence with ultraviolet light. Histologically, animals may exhibit perivascular dermatitis, as well as multisystemic porphyrin deposition, hemosiderosis, EMH, and marrow erythroid hyperplasia. Cats may show evidence of renal disease, including hypercellular glomeruli, thickened glomerular and tubular basement membranes, and tubular epithelial lipidosis, degeneration, and necrosis. Other porphyrias have been diagnosed in cattle, pigs, and cats but are not known to cause hemolytic anemia.

Pyruvate Kinase Deficiency. Pyruvate kinase (PK) deficiency is an inherited autosomal recessive condition due to a defective R-type PK isoenzyme that is normally present in high concentrations in mature erythrocytes. To compensate for this deficiency, there is persistence of the M2-type PK isoenzyme, which is less stable than the R-type isoenzyme. The disease is reported in many dog breeds and fewer cat breeds (e.g., Abyssinian, Somali, and domestic shorthair). Erythrocyte PK deficiency results in decreased ATP production and shortened erythrocyte life spans. In dogs the hemolytic anemia is typically chronic, moderate to severe, extravascular, and strongly regenerative. With chronicity, hemolytic anemia causes enhanced intestinal absorption of iron and subsequent hemosiderosis, especially of the liver and bone marrow. Dogs typically die at 1 to 5 years of age of hemochromatosis-induced liver and bone marrow failure. However, cats with PK deficiency typically show no clinical signs, have milder anemia, and do not develop organ failure. Grossly, affected animals have lesions attributed to hemolytic anemia, including splenomegaly, pale mucous membranes, and rarely icterus. Dogs with end-stage disease have cirrhosis, myelofibrosis, and osteosclerosis. Dogs with PK deficiency do not necessarily have the same genetic defect, so mutation-specific DNA-based assays are required. In contrast, a single DNA-based test is available to detect the common mutation affecting Abyssinian, Somali, and domestic shorthair cats.

Cytochrome-b_5 Reductase Deficiency. Deficiency of cytochrome-b_5 reductase (Cb5R, also known as *methemoglobin reductase*), the enzyme that catalyzes the reduction of methemoglobin (Fe^{3+}) to hemoglobin (Fe^{2+}), has been recognized in many dog breeds and in domestic shorthair cats. It is probably an autosomal recessive trait. Affected animals may have cyanotic mucous membranes or exercise intolerance but usually lack anemia and clinical signs of disease. Life expectancies are normal.

Glucose-6-Phosphate Dehydrogenase Deficiency. Deficiency of glucose-6-phosphate dehydrogenase (G6PD), the rate-controlling enzyme of the pentose phosphate pathway (PPP), has been reported in an American saddlebred colt, its dam, and one male dog. The PPP is an antioxidative pathway that generates NADPH, which maintains glutathione in its reduced form (GSH). Therefore in animals with G6PD deficiency, oxidants are not scavenged, and erythrocyte oxidative injury occurs. The colt with G6PD deficiency had severe oxidative hemolytic anemia with eccentrocytes on blood smear evaluation. However, the colt's dam only had eccentrocytes, and showed no hematologic signs of disease.

Leukocyte Adhesion Deficiency. Leukocyte adhesion deficiency (LAD) is a fatal autosomal recessive defect of leukocyte integrins, in particular the β_2 chain (also known as cluster of differentiation [CD] 18 [CD18]). Disease has been recognized in Holstein cattle (known as bovine leukocyte adhesion deficiency [BLAD]) and Irish setter dogs (known as canine leukocyte adhesion deficiency [CLAD]) (see Chapter 3). Without normal expression of this adhesion molecule, leukocytes have severely impaired abilities to migrate from the blood into tissues. As a result, animals with leukocyte adhesion deficiency have marked neutrophilia with nonsuppurative multisystemic infections. Blood neutrophils often have nuclei with greater than five nuclear segments, termed *hypersegmented neutrophils*, due to neutrophil aging within blood vessels (Fig. 13-22). These animals are highly susceptible to infections and usually die at a young age.

Pelger-Huët Anomaly. Pelger-Huët anomaly (PHA) is a condition of hyposegmented granulocytes due to a lamin B receptor mutation. It has been described in dogs, cats, horses, and rabbits, especially in certain breeds. In Australian shepherd dogs the mode of inheritance is autosomal dominant with incomplete penetrance. Most cases of Pelger-Huët anomaly are the heterozygous form and of no clinical significance. However, skeletal abnormalities, stillbirths, and/or early mortality may accompany Pelger-Huët anomaly in rabbits and cats, especially homozygotes. In Pelger-Huët anomaly the nuclei of neutrophils, eosinophils, and basophils fail to segment, resulting in band-shaped, bean-shaped, or round nuclei. Although the nuclear shape is similar to that of an inflammatory left shift, healthy animals with Pelger-Huët anomaly do not have clinical signs or other laboratory findings indicating inflammation. For example, neutrophils in healthy animals with Pelger-Huët anomaly have mature (clumped) chromatin and do not show signs of toxicity (Fig. 13-23). An acquired, reversible condition mimicking Pelger-Huët anomaly, known as *pseudo–Pelger-Huët anomaly*, is occasionally noted in animals with infectious disease, neoplasia, or drug administration.

Chédiak-Higashi Syndrome. Chédiak-Higashi syndrome (CHS) is a rare autosomal recessive defect in the lysosomal trafficking regulator (LYST) protein. The syndrome has been identified in Hereford, Brangus, and Japanese black cattle, Persian cats, and several nondomestic species. The defective LYST protein results in granule fusion in multiple cell types, including granulocytes, platelets, and melanocytes, as well as abnormal cell function. Individuals with Chédiak-Higashi syndrome have severely impaired cellular innate immunity because of neutropenia, impaired leukocyte chemotaxis, and impaired killing by granulocytes and cytotoxic lymphocytes. Platelets lack the dense granules that normally contain key bioactive molecules involved in hemostasis, including platelet agonists, such as ADP and serotonin. In vitro platelet aggregation is severely impaired. As a result, animals with Chédiak-Higashi syndrome exhibit oculocutaneous albinism (due to altered distribution of melanin granules) and are prone to infection and bleeding. Blood smear evaluation reveals granulocytes with large cytoplasmic granules.

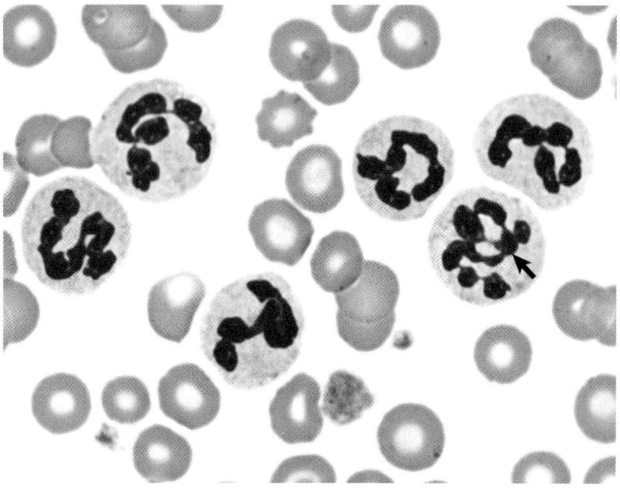

Figure 13-22 **Leukocyte Adhesion Deficiency, Canine Blood Smear.** Neutrophils in animals with leukocyte adhesion deficiency cannot migrate into the tissues, resulting in marked neutrophilia and morphologic signs of aging, such as nuclear hypersegmentation *(arrow)*. Wright-Giemsa stain. (Courtesy Dr. K.M. Boes and Dr. K. Zimmerman, College of Veterinary Medicine, Virginia Polytechnic Institute and State University.)

Glanzmann Thrombasthenia. Glanzmann thrombasthenia (GT) is an inherited platelet function defect caused by a mutated α_{IIb} subunit of the integrin $\alpha_{IIb}\beta_3$ (also known as glycoprotein IIb-IIIa [GPIIb-IIIa]). The disorder has been recognized in Great Pyrenees and otterhound dogs and several horse breeds, including a quarter horse, a standardbred, a thoroughbred-cross, a Peruvian Paso mare, and an Oldenburg filly. The $\alpha_{IIb}\beta_3$ molecule has multiple functions but is best known as a fibrinogen receptor that is essential for normal platelet aggregation. Bleeding tendencies vary widely between affected individuals but mainly occur on mucosal surfaces. The condition is characterized by an in vitro lack of response to all platelet agonists and severely impaired clot retraction (i.e., whole blood samples without anticoagulant often fail to clot). Molecular testing is available to detect diseased or carrier states in dogs and horses.

CalDAG-GEFI Thrombopathia. Calcium diacylglycerol guanine nucleotide exchange factor I (CalDAG-GEFI) is a molecule within the signaling pathway that results in platelet activation in response to platelet agonists. Mutated CalDAG-GEFI has been documented in basset hound, Eskimo spitz, and Landseer dogs, and Simmental cattle. All reported mutations have a bleeding tendency. In vitro platelet aggregation responses to platelet agonists, such as ADP, collagen, and thrombin, are absent or impaired.

von Willebrand Disease

Information on this topic is available at www.expertconsult.com.

Hereditary Coagulation Factor Deficiencies

Information on this topic is available at www.expertconsult.com.

Hereditary γ-Glutamyl Carboxylase Defect

Information on this topic is available at www.expertconsult.com.

Toxicoses

Oxidative Agents. A variety of oxidative toxins cause hemolytic anemia and/or methemoglobinemia in domestic species. More common or well-characterized oxidants are listed here:

- Horses—*Acer rubrum* (red maple)
- Ruminants—*Brassica* spp. (cabbage, kale, and rape), copper

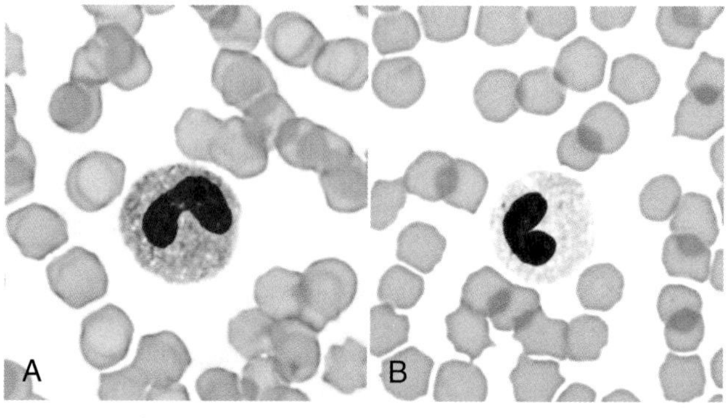

Figure 13-23 **Pelger-Huët Anomaly, Feline Blood Smear.** Eosinophil **(A)** and neutrophil **(B)** have hyposegmented nuclei with mature, condensed chromatin. Wright's stain. (Courtesy Dr. M.M. Fry, College of Veterinary Medicine, University of Tennessee.)

- Dogs—Acetaminophen, propofol, zinc
- Cats—Acetaminophen, propofol, propylene glycol
- All species—*Allium* spp. (chives, garlic, and onions)

In horses, red maple leaves and bark are toxic, especially wilted or dried leaves. The toxic principle is believed to be gallic acid. Plants that contain high concentrations of nitrates, such as cabbage, kale, and rape, may cause oxidative injury to erythrocytes; cattle are more susceptible than sheep and goats. However, sheep are more prone to copper toxicosis relative to other ruminants. The condition occurs in animals that have chronically accumulated large amounts of copper in the liver through the diet. The copper is then acutely released during conditions of stress, such as shipping or starvation. Continuous rate infusions of the anesthetic propofol may cause oxidative hemolytic anemia in dogs and cats, but single or multiple single doses are not expected to cause clinical hemolysis. Zinc toxicosis has been identified in a wide range of animals; however, it is most common in dogs due to their indiscriminate eating habits. Common sources include pennies, batteries, paints, creams, automotive parts, screws, nuts, and coating on galvanized metals. Propylene glycol is an odorless, slightly sweet solvent and moistening agent in many foods, drugs, and tobacco products. Although it is "generally recognized as safe" for animal foods other than for cats by the Food and Drug Administration, it has been banned from cat food since 1996.

Grossly and microscopically, animals show varying signs of oxidative hemolysis and/or methemoglobinemia, as previously presented in the section discussing anemias (see Bone Marrow and Blood Cells, Dysfunction/Responses to Injury, Blood Cells, Abnormal Concentrations of Blood Cells, Anemia). In sheep with copper toxicosis, hemoglobinuric nephrosis, frequently described as gunmetal-colored kidneys with port wine–colored urine, is a classic postmortem lesion.

Snake Envenomation. Hemolytic anemia from snake envenomation has been reported in horses, dogs, and cats. It is most commonly reported with viper and pit viper envenomations, including those from rattlesnakes. Hemolysins within viper venom directly injure erythrocytes, causing intravascular hemolysis. Other mechanisms of hemolysis include the action of phospholipase A_2 on erythrocyte membranes and erythrocyte mechanical fragmentation due to intravascular coagulation and vasculitis. Nonhemolytic lesions depend on the venom's additional components and may include hemorrhage, paralysis, and/or tissue edema, inflammation, and necrosis. On blood smear evaluation, animals with snake envenomation may have ghost cells, spherocytes, and/or echinocytes (see Figs. 13-13 and 13-15).

Avitaminosis K

Information on this topic is available at www.expertconsult.com.

Nutritional and Metabolic Disorders

Severe malnutrition is probably a cause of nonregenerative anemia in all species attributable to combined deficiencies of molecular building blocks, energy, and essential cofactors. By far the most commonly recognized specific deficiency that results in anemia is iron deficiency. Other specific nutritional deficiencies causing anemia in animals are uncommon or rare. Acquired cobalamin (vitamin B_{12}) and folate deficiencies are recognized as causes of anemia in human beings but are rare in animals.

Iron Deficiency Anemia. Iron deficiency is usually not a primary nutritional deficiency but rather occurs secondary to depletion of iron stores via chronic blood loss. The most common route of loss is through the gastrointestinal tract (e.g., neoplasia in older animals or hookworm infection in puppies). Chronic blood loss may also be caused by marked ectoparasitism (e.g., pediculosis in cattle or massive flea burden in kittens and puppies), neoplasia in locations other than the gastrointestinal tract (e.g., cutaneous hemangiosarcoma), coagulation disorders, and repeated phlebotomy of blood donor animals. Rapidly growing nursing animals may be iron deficient when compared with adults because milk is an iron-poor diet. In most cases this has little clinical significance (and in fact is normal). An important exception is piglets with no access to iron, which may cause anemia, failure to thrive, and increased mortality. Neonatal piglets are routinely given parenteral iron for this reason. Copper deficiency can cause iron deficiency in ruminants and may occur because of copper-deficient forage or impaired usage of copper by high dietary molybdenum or sulfate. It is believed that copper deficiency impairs production of ceruloplasmin, a copper-containing enzyme involved in gastrointestinal iron absorption.

Iron deficiency causes anemia by impaired hemoglobin synthesis. Iron is an essential component of hemoglobin, and when it is absent, hemoglobin synthesis is depressed. Because erythrocyte maturation is dependent upon obtaining a critical hemoglobin concentration, maturing erythroid precursors undergo additional cell divisions during iron-deficient states. These additional cell divisions result in small erythrocytes, termed *microcytes* (see Fig. 13-15, G). However, erythrocytes with low hemoglobin concentrations are produced when microcyte formation can no longer compensate for iron deficiency. The classic hematologic picture with iron deficiency anemia is microcytic (i.e., decreased MCV), hypochromic (i.e., decreased MCHC) anemia. Microcytes and *hypochromasia* (see Fig. 13-15, G) may also be discernible on blood smear examination as erythrocytes that are abnormally small and paler-staining, respectively. Early iron deficiency anemia is poorly regenerative, whereas continued hemorrhage and iron loss cause nonregenerative anemia. Additional hematologic changes may include evidence of erythrocyte mechanical fragmentation (e.g., schistocytes) and reactive thrombocytosis.

Hypophosphatemic Hemolytic Anemia. Marked hypophosphatemia is recognized as a cause of intravascular hemolytic anemia in postparturient dairy cows and diabetic animals receiving insulin therapy. In postparturient cows, hypophosphatemia results from increased loss of phosphorus in their milk. Insulin therapy may cause hypophosphatemia by shifting phosphorus from the extracellular space to the intracellular space. In either case, marked hypophosphatemia (e.g., 1 mg/dL in cows, or $\leq$ 1.5 mg/dL in cats) is thought to decrease erythrocyte production of ATP, leading to inadequate energy required for maintenance of membrane and cytoskeletal integrity. An accompanying decrease in reducing capacity and increase in methemoglobin concentration have also been noted in experimental studies of hypophosphatemic hemolytic anemia in dairy cattle, suggesting that oxidative mechanisms may also contribute to anemia. Affected animals are anemic and hemoglobinuric. Gross postmortem findings include pallor, decreased viscosity of the blood, and lesions arising from the underlying metabolic derangement (e.g., discolored pale yellow and swollen liver due to hepatic lipidosis). Renal tubular necrosis and hemoglobin pigment within the tubules is evident microscopically.

Infectious Diseases

This section covers infectious agents within the same genus that are recognized to cause disease in multiple species. Other infectious agents with more limited host specificity (e.g., cytauxzoonosis in cats, feline and equine retroviruses) are covered in later sections on species-specific diseases. Throughout both sections, diseases are organized by taxonomy (protozoal, bacterial and rickettsial, and viral).

Babesiosis (Piroplasmosis). *Babesia* spp. and *Theileria* spp., presented in the next section, are members of the order Piroplasmida, and are generally referenced as *piroplasms*. These organisms are morphologically similar but have different life cycles; *Babesia* spp. are primarily erythrocytic parasites, whereas *Theileria* spp. sequentially parasitize leukocytes and then erythrocytes. Both are protozoan parasites spread by ticks, but other modes of transmission are possible (e.g., biting flies, transplacental, and blood transfusions). Evidence is accumulating that dog fighting also transmits *Babesia gibsoni* infection.

Babesia organisms are typically classified as large (2 to 4 μm) or small (<2 μm) with routine light microscopy (Fig. 13-24). Over 100 *Babesia* species have been identified, some of which are listed here, along with their relative microscopic size in parentheses:

- Horses—*Babesia caballi* (large)
- Cattle—*Babesia bigemina* (large), *Babesia bovis* (small)
- Sheep and goats—*Babesia motasi* (large), *Babesia ovis* (small)
- Dogs—*Babesia canis* (large), *Babesia conradae*, *B. gibsoni* (small)
- Cats—*Babesia cati*, *Babesia felis*, *Babesia herpailuri* (small)

Geographic distributions vary with the species, but most have higher prevalences in tropical and subtropical regions. For example, equine and bovine babesiosis are endemic in parts of Africa, the Middle East, Asia, Central and South America, the Caribbean, and Europe. Both were eradicated from the United States and are now considered exotic diseases in that country. Of the previously mentioned species, only agents of canine babesiosis are thought to be endemic in the United States.

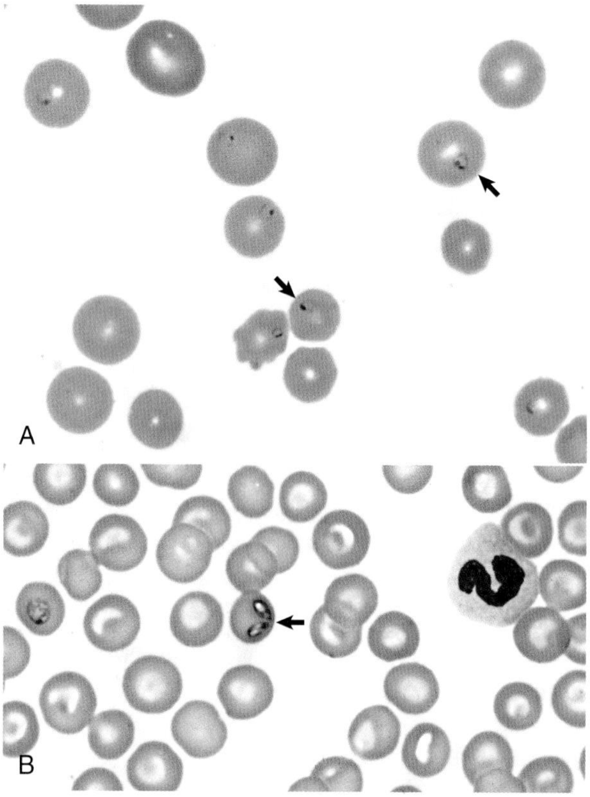

Figure 13-24 Babesiosis, Canine Blood Smear. A, Small form *(arrows)* of Babesia (consistent with *Babesia gibsonii*). **B,** *Babesia canis (arrow)* organisms infecting erythrocytes. Wright's stain. (Courtesy Dr. M.M. Fry, College of Veterinary Medicine, University of Tennessee.)

Babesiosis may cause intravascular and extravascular hemolytic anemia via direct red blood cell injury, the innocent bystander effect, and secondary immune-mediated hemolytic anemia. Infection with highly virulent strains may cause severe multisystemic disease. In these cases, massive immunostimulation and cytokine release cause circulatory disturbances, which may result in shock, induction of the systemic inflammatory response, and multiple organ dysfunction syndromes.

Babesia organisms can usually be detected on a routine blood smear in animals with acute disease. Infected erythrocytes may be more prevalent in capillary blood, so blood smears made from samples taken from the pinna of the ear or the nail bed may increase the likelihood of detecting organisms microscopically. Buffy coat smears also have an enriched population of infected erythrocytes. PCR-based tests are the most sensitive assay for detecting infection in animals with very low levels of parasitemia.

At necropsy, gross lesions are mainly related to hemolysis and include pale mucous membranes, icterus, splenomegaly, dark red or black kidneys, and reddish-brown urine. The cut surface of the congested spleen oozes blood. The gallbladder is usually distended with thick bile. Less common lesions include pulmonary edema, ascites, and congestion, petechiae, and ecchymoses of organs, including the heart and brain. Parasitized erythrocytes are best visualized on impression smears of the kidney, brain, and skeletal muscle.

Microscopic findings in the liver and kidney are typical of a hemolytic crisis and include anemia-induced degeneration, necrosis of periacinar hepatocytes and cholestasis, and hemoglobinuric nephrosis with degeneration of tubular epithelium. Erythroid hyperplasia is present in the bone marrow. In animals that survive the acute disease, there is hemosiderin accumulation in the liver, kidney, spleen, and bone marrow. In chronic cases there is hyperplasia of macrophages in the red pulp of the spleen.

Theileriosis (Piroplasmosis). *Theileria* spp. are tick-borne protozoal organisms that infect many domestic and wild animals worldwide. Numerous *Theileria* spp. have been documented, but only the more economically or regionally important species are mentioned here. Diseases with the greatest economic impact in ruminants are East Coast fever (*Theileria parva* infection) and tropical theileriosis (*Theileria annulata* infection).

- Horses—*Theileria equi* (formerly *Babesia equi*)
- Cattle—*Theileria annulata*, *Theileria buffeli*, *T. parva*
- Sheep and goats—*Theileria lestoquardi* (formerly *Theileria hirci*)

Like babesiosis, theileriosis is generally restricted to tropical and subtropical regions, including parts of Africa, Asia, the Middle East, and Europe. Except for *T. buffeli*, all previously listed species are exotic to the United States.

Infection is characterized by schizonts within lymphocytes or monocytes, and pleomorphic intraerythrocytic piroplasms (merozoites and trophozoites). Within host leukocytes the parasite induces leukocyte cellular division, which expands the parasitized cell population. Infected cells disseminate throughout the lymphoid system via the lymphatic and blood vessels. The infected leukocyte may block capillaries, causing tissue ischemia. Later in infection some schizonts cause leukocyte lysis and release of merozoites. Merozoites then invade and parasitize erythrocytes, causing hemolytic anemia. Possible mechanisms of anemia in theileriosis include invasion of erythroid precursors by merozoite stages and associated erythroid hypoplasia (as occurs with *T. parva* infection), immune-mediated hemolysis, mechanical fragmentation because of vasculitis or microthrombi, enzymatic destruction by proteases, and oxidative damage.

Gross and microscopic lesions are similar to those of babesiosis, except that cattle with East Coast fever tend not to develop hemolytic anemia. In acute East Coast fever, lymph nodes are enlarged, edematous, and hemorrhagic. But with chronic cases they may be shrunken. There is often splenomegaly, hepatomegaly, and hemorrhagic enteritis with white foci of lymphoid infiltrates (pseudoinfarcts) in the liver and kidney. Microscopically, infected leukocytes may block capillaries.

African Trypanosomiasis. Trypanosomes are flagellated protozoa that can infect all domesticated animals. The most important species that cause disease are *Trypanosoma congolense*, *Trypanosoma vivax*, and *Trypanosoma brucei* ssp. *brucei*. Disease is most common in parts of Africa where the biologic vector, the tsetse fly, exists. However, *T. vivax* has spread to Central and South America and the Caribbean, where other biting flies transmit the parasite mechanically. In Africa, cattle are mainly affected due to the feeding preferences of the tsetse fly. African trypanosomiasis must be distinguished from nonpathogenic trypanosomiasis, such as *Trypanosoma theileri* infection in cattle.

Animals become infected when feeding tsetse flies inoculate metacyclic trypanosomes into the skin of animals. The trypanosomes grow for a few days, causing a localized chancre sore, and then sequentially enter the lymph nodes and bloodstream. Trypanosomal organisms do not infect erythrocytes but rather exist as free *trypomastigotes* (i.e., flagellated protozoa with a characteristic undulating membrane) in the blood (Fig. 13-25, *A*) or as *amastigotes* in tissue. The mechanism of anemia is believed to be immune mediated. Cattle with acute trypanosomiasis have significant anemia, which initially is regenerative, but less so with time. The extent of parasitemia is readily apparent with *T. vivax* and *T. theileri* infections because the organisms are present in large numbers in the blood. This is in contrast to *T. congolense*, which localizes within the vasculature of the brain and skeletal muscle. Chronically infected animals often die secondary to poor body condition, immunosuppression, and concurrent infections.

Gross examination of animals with acute disease often reveals generalized lymphadenomegaly, splenomegaly, and petechiae on serosal membranes. An acute hemorrhagic syndrome may occur in cattle, resulting in lesions of severe anemia (e.g., pale mucous membranes) and widespread mucosal and visceral hemorrhages. Main lesions of chronic infections include signs of anemia, lymphadenopathy (e.g., enlarged or atrophied lymph nodes), emaciation, subcutaneous edema, pulmonary edema, increased fluid in body cavities, and serous atrophy of fat.

American Trypanosomiasis (Chagas's Disease). *Trypanosoma cruzi* is the flagellated protozoal agent of American trypanosomiasis. Infections have been reported in more than 100 mammal species in South America, Central America, and the southern United States, but dogs and cats are among the more common domestic hosts.

Infected triatomine insects, or "kissing bugs," defecate as they feed on their mammalian host, releasing infective *T. cruzi* organisms. The parasite then enters the body through mucous membranes or breaks in the skin. Like the other trypanosomes described previously, *T. cruzi* lives in the blood as extracellular trypomastigotes (see Fig. 13-25, *B*) and in the tissues as intracellular amastigotes.

Trypanosoma cruzi primarily causes heart disease. Lesions of acute disease include a pale myocardium, subendocardial and subepicardial hemorrhages, and yellowish-white spots and streaks. There may also be secondary lesions, such as pulmonary edema, ascites, and congestion of the liver, spleen, and kidneys. In chronic disease the heart may be enlarged and flaccid with thin walls. Microscopically, there is often myocarditis and amastigotes within cardiomyocytes.

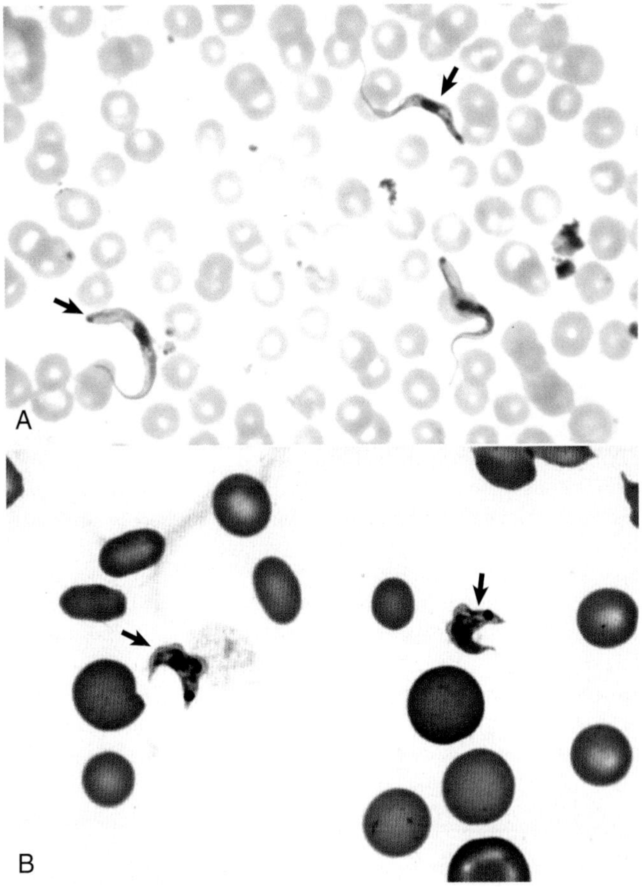

Figure 13-25 Trypanosomiasis, Bovine (A) and Canine (B) Blood Smears. A, The trypomastigote life stage of trypanosomes is a flagellated protozoan *(arrows)* with an undulating membrane, kinetoplast, and nucleus. They may be identified in a wet mount made from the buffy coat portion of the packed cells. **B,** *Trypanosoma cruzi* trypomastigotes from a dog with Chagas's disease. Wright-Giemsa stain. (**A** courtesy Dr. M.D. McGavin, College of Veterinary Medicine, University of Tennessee. **B** courtesy Dr. K.M. Boes, College of Veterinary Medicine, Virginia Polytechnic Institute and State University.)

Anaplasmosis, Ehrlichiosis, Heartwater, and Tick-Borne Fever. Anaplasmosis, ehrlichiosis, heartwater, and tick-borne fever are tick-borne diseases caused by small, pleomorphic, Gram-negative, obligate intracellular bacteria within the order Rickettsiaceae, also colloquially known as *rickettsias*. As a group, rickettsias primarily infect hematopoietic cells and endothelial cells. Rickettsias that predominantly infect endothelial cells (e.g., *Rickettsia rickettsii* [Rocky Mountain spotted fever]), or cause gastrointestinal disease (e.g., *Neorickettsia helminthoeca* [salmon poisoning disease] and *Neorickettsia risticii* [Potomac horse fever]) are discussed elsewhere (see Chapters 4 and 7). Less commonly, transmission may occur via blood transfusions or blood-contaminated medical supplies.

Rickettsias that infect erythrocytes include the following species (the disease name follows in parentheses):

- Cattle—*Anaplasma marginale*, *Anaplasma centrale* (bovine anaplasmosis)
- Sheep and goats—*Anaplasma ovis* (ovine and caprine anaplasmosis, respectively)

Anaplasma marginale and *A. ovis* have worldwide distributions, but *A. centrale* is mostly restricted to South America, Africa, and the Middle East.

Bovine anaplasmosis causes anemia mainly by immune-mediated extravascular hemolysis. The severity of disease in infected animals varies with age. Infected calves under 1 year of age rarely develop clinical disease, whereas cattle 3 years of age or older are more likely to develop severe, potentially fatal, illness. The reason for this discrepancy is not clear. Indian cattle (*Bos indicus*) are more resistant to disease than European cattle (*Bos taurus*). Surviving cattle become chronic carriers (and thus reservoirs for infection of other animals) and develop cyclic bacteremia, which is typically not detectable on blood smears. Splenectomy of carrier animals results in marked bacteremia and acute hemolysis. PCR testing is the most sensitive means of identifying animals with low levels of bacteremia.

Grossly, acute disease causes lesions of acute hemolytic anemia, including pale mucous membranes, low blood viscosity, icterus, splenomegaly, hepatomegaly, and a distended gallbladder. In animals with acute disease it is usually easy to detect *A. marginale* organisms on routine blood smear evaluation (Fig. 13-26) or impression smears from cut sections of the spleen. However, in recovering animals, the organisms may be difficult to find.

Rickettsias that infect leukocytes are broadly divided into those that preferentially infect granulocytes (*Anaplasma phagocytophilum* [previously *Ehrlichia equi*, the agent of human granulocytic ehrlichiosis, and *Ehrlichia phagocytophila*] and *Ehrlichia ewingii*), mononuclear cells (*E. canis* and *Ehrlichia chaffeensis*), or both (*Ehrlichia ruminantium* [previously *Cowdria ruminantium*]). *Anaplasma platys* (previously *Ehrlichia platys*) infects platelets. Some of these agents, such as *A. phagocytophilum* and *E. ruminantium*, are proven to also infect endothelial cells. The rickettsias have variable host ranges, including the domestic hosts listed here (the disease name follows in parentheses):

- Horses—*A. phagocytophilum* (equine granulocytic ehrlichiosis)
- Cattle—*A. phagocytophilum* (tick-borne fever), *E. ruminantium* (heartwater)
- Sheep and goats—*A. phagocytophilum* (tick-borne fever), *E. ruminantium* (heartwater)
- Dogs—*A. phagocytophilum*, *E. ewingii* (canine granulocytic ehrlichiosis [E-Fig. 13-3]); *A. platys* (canine cyclic thrombocytopenia); *E. canis*, *E. chaffeensis* (canine monocytic ehrlichiosis)
- Cats—*A. phagocytophilum*, possibly *E. canis* (feline ehrlichiosis)

Most of these rickettsias have worldwide distributions. However, *E. ewingii* has been reported only in the United States, and *E. ruminantium* is endemic only in parts of Africa and the Caribbean. Although *A. phagocytophilum* has a wide geographic distribution, strain variants are regionally restricted. For example, *A. phagocytophilum* causes disease in ruminants in Europe, but it has not been documented in ruminants in the United States.

Reservoirs of disease vary, depending upon the rickettsial species. Cattle are the reservoir host for *E. ruminantium*, canids are the reservoir host for *A. platys* and *E. canis*, and the other rickettsias have wildlife reservoirs.

Pathogenesis of disease involves endothelial cell, platelet, and leukocyte dysfunction. Those agents that infect endothelial cells cause vasculitis and increased vascular permeability of small blood vessels. If only plasma is lost, then there is hypotension and tissue edema. However, more severe vasculitis causes microvascular hemorrhage with the potential for platelet consumption thrombocytopenia, disseminated intravascular coagulation, and hypotension. Infection of platelets may cause thrombocytopenia by direct platelet lysis, immune-mediated mechanisms, or platelet sequestration within the spleen. Pathogenesis of leukocyte dysfunction is unclear, but may involve sepsis, inhibited leukocyte function, endothelial cell activation, and platelet consumption. Chronic *E. canis* infection may cause aplastic anemia with pancytopenia by an unknown mechanism. Some studies indicate that German shepherd dogs with ehrlichiosis are predisposed to have particularly severe clinical disease. Some breeds of cattle (*Bos taurus*), sheep (merino), and goats (Angora and Saanen) are more susceptible to heartwater.

Upon blood smear evaluation, thrombocytopenia is the most common hematologic abnormality; anemia and neutropenia occur less frequently. In early stages of infection, blood cells may contain morulae, which are clusters of rickettsial organisms within cytoplasmic, membrane-bound vacuoles (Fig. 13-27). Examination of buffy coat smears increases the probability of detecting the organism. Chronic infection may cause lymphocytosis, particularly of granular lymphocytes. *Anaplasma platys* causes recurrent marked thrombocytopenia.

In general, more common gross lesions are splenomegaly, lymphadenomegaly, and pulmonary edema and hemorrhage. More severe cases may also exhibit multisystemic petechiae, ecchymoses, and

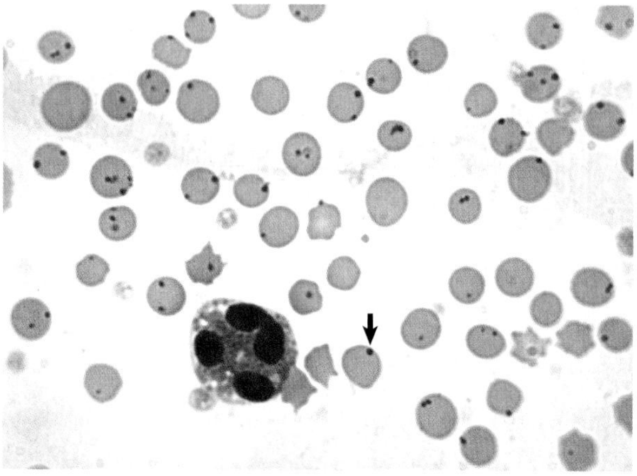

Figure 13-26 Anaplasmosis, Bovine Blood Smear. Note the darkly stained *Anaplasma marginale* organisms *(arrow)*, most of which are located on the edges of the erythrocytes. Anaplasmosis causes anemia mainly by immune-mediated extravascular hemolysis. (Courtesy Dr. J. Simon, College of Veterinary Medicine, University of Illinois.)

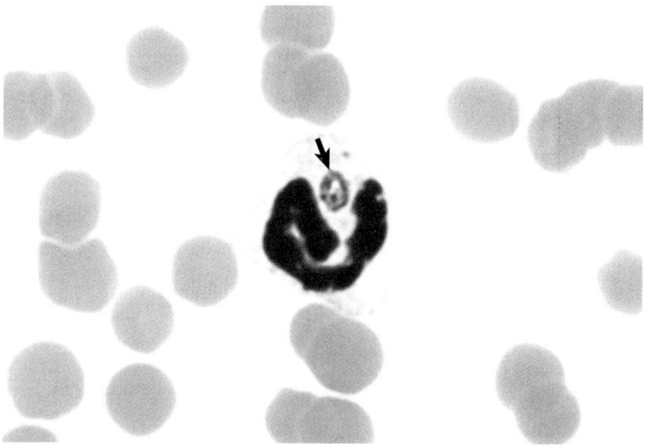

Figure 13-27 Granulocytic Ehrlichiosis, Equine Blood Smear. The neutrophil contains an inclusion *(arrow)* consistent with an *Anaplasma phagocytophilum* morula. Wright-Giemsa stain. (Courtesy Dr. K.M. Boes, College of Veterinary Medicine, Virginia Polytechnic Institute and State University.)

edema, cavitary effusions, and effusive polyarthropathy. Hydropericardium gives heartwater its name but is more consistently found in small ruminants than in cattle. Chronically infected dogs are emaciated. The bone marrow is hyperplastic and red in the acute disease but becomes hypoplastic and pale in dogs with chronic *E. canis* infection. Equine anaplasmosis is often mild but may cause edema and hemorrhages. Disease in cats is rare and poorly documented.

Histologic findings include generalized perivascular plasma cell infiltration, which is most pronounced in animals with chronic disease. Multifocal, nonsuppurative meningoencephalitis, interstitial pneumonia, and glomerulonephritis are present in most dogs with the disease. Rickettsial organisms are difficult to detect histologically; examination of Wright-Giemsa–stained impression smears of lung, liver, lymph nodes, and spleen is a more effective method for detecting the morulae within leukocytes. Heartwater is often diagnosed by observing morulae in endothelial cells of Giemsa-stained squash preparations of brain. Rickettsial diseases are often diagnosed on the basis of serologic testing, but PCR testing is more sensitive.

Clostridial Diseases. Certain *Clostridium* spp. may cause potentially fatal hemolytic anemias in animals; nonhemolytic lesions are presented elsewhere (see Chapters 4, 7, 8, and 19). *Clostridium haemolyticum* and *Clostridium novyi* type D cause the disease in cattle known as bacillary hemoglobinuria. (The phrase "red water" has also been used for this disease and for hemolytic anemias in cattle caused by *Babesia* spp.) Similar naturally occurring disease has been reported in sheep. In cattle the disease is caused by liver fluke (*Fasciola hepatica*) migration in susceptible animals. Ingested clostridial spores may live in Kupffer cells for a long time without causing disease. However, when migrating flukes cause hepatic necrosis, the resulting anaerobic environment stimulates the clostridial organisms to proliferate and elaborate their hemolytic toxins, causing additional hepatic necrosis. The mechanism of hemolysis involves a bacterial β-toxin (phospholipase C or lecithinase), which enzymatically degrades cell membranes, causing acute intravascular hemolysis. Bacillary hemoglobinuria also occurs with liver biopsies in calves.

Clostridium perfringens type A causes intravascular hemolytic anemia in lambs and calves—a condition known as yellow lamb disease, yellows, or enterotoxemic jaundice because of the characteristic icterus. The organism is a normal inhabitant of the gastrointestinal tract in these animals but may proliferate abnormally in response to some diets. *C. perfringens* causes intravascular hemolytic anemia in horses with clostridial abscesses, and clostridial mastitis in ewes. *C. perfringens* type A produces hemolytic α-toxin, which also has phospholipase C activity.

Leptospirosis. Leptospirosis is recognized as a cause of hemolytic anemia in calves, lambs, and pigs. Specific leptospiral organisms that cause hemolytic disease include *Leptospira interrogans* serovars *pomona* and *ictohaemorrhagiae*.

Leptospira organisms are ubiquitous in the environment. Infection occurs percutaneously and via mucosal surfaces and is followed by leptospiremia; organisms then localize preferentially in certain tissues (e.g., kidney, liver, and pregnant uterus). Proposed mechanisms of hemolytic disease include immune-mediated (immunoglobulin M [IgM] cold agglutinin) extravascular hemolysis and enzymatic (phospholipase produced by the organism) intravascular hemolysis. Leptospirosis can also cause many disease manifestations besides hemolysis (e.g., renal failure, liver failure, abortion, and other conditions) that are not discussed here.

In addition to anemia, common findings in animals with leptospirosis-induced hemolysis include hemoglobinuria and icterus. On necropsy, renal tubular necrosis, which occurs in part because of hemoglobinuria (hemoglobinuric nephrosis), may also be present.

Hemotropic Mycoplasmosis (Hemoplasmosis). The term hemotropic mycoplasmas, or hemoplasmas, encompasses a group of bacteria, formerly known as *Haemobartonella* or *Eperythrozoon* spp., that infect erythrocytes of many domestic, laboratory, and wild animals. Hemotropic mycoplasmas affecting common domestic species are as follows:

- Cattle—*Mycoplasma wenyonii*
- Camelids—"*Candidatus* Mycoplasma haemolamae"
- Sheep and goats—*Mycoplasma ovis*
- Pigs—*Mycoplasma suis* (E-Fig. 13-4)
- Dogs—*Mycoplasma haemocanis*, "*Candidatus* Mycoplasma haematoparvum"
- Cats—*Mycoplasma haemofelis*, "*Candidatus* Mycoplasma haemominutum," "*Candidatus* Mycoplasma turicensus"

Like other mycoplasmas, hemoplasmas are small (0.3 to 3 μm in diameter) and lack a cell wall. They are epicellular parasites, residing in indentations and invaginations of red blood cell surfaces. The mode of transmission is poorly understood, but blood-sucking arthropods are believed to play a role; transmission in utero, through biting or fighting, and transfusion of infected blood products are also suspected.

Effects of infection vary from subclinical to fatal anemia, depending on the specific organism, dose, and host susceptibility. Most hemoplasmas are more likely to cause acute illness in individuals that are immunocompromised or have concurrent disease. However, *M. haemofelis* is an exception and tends to cause acute hemolytic anemia in immunocompetent cats. Anemia occurs mainly because of extravascular hemolysis, but intravascular hemolysis also occurs. Although the pathogenic mechanisms are not completely understood, an immune-mediated component is highly probable, as well as direct red blood cell injury by the bacteria and the innocent bystander effect. Hemotropic mycoplasmas induce cold agglutinins in infected individuals, although it is not clear whether these particular antibodies are important in the development of hemolytic anemia.

When detected on routine blood smear evaluation, the organisms are variably shaped (cocci, small rods, or ring forms) and sometimes arranged in short, branching chains (Fig. 13-28). The organisms may also be noted extracellularly, in the background of the blood smear, especially if the smear is made after prolonged storage of the blood in an anticoagulant tube.

In animals dying of acute hemoplasma infection, the gross findings are typical of extravascular hemolysis, with pallor, icterus, splenomegaly, and distended gallbladder (Fig. 13-29). Additional lesions documented in cattle include scrotal and hind limb edema and swelling of the teats. Microscopic lesions in the red pulp of the spleen include congestion, erythrophagocytosis, macrophage hyperplasia, EMH, and increased numbers of plasma cells. Bone marrow has varying degrees of erythroid hyperplasia, depending on the duration of hemolysis.

Immune-Mediated Disorders

Immune-Mediated Hemolytic Anemia. Immune-mediated hemolytic anemia is a condition characterized by increased destruction of erythrocytes because of binding of immunoglobulin to red blood cell surface antigens. It is a common, life-threatening condition in dogs but also has been described in horses, cattle, and cats. Immune-mediated hemolytic anemia may be *idiopathic* (also called

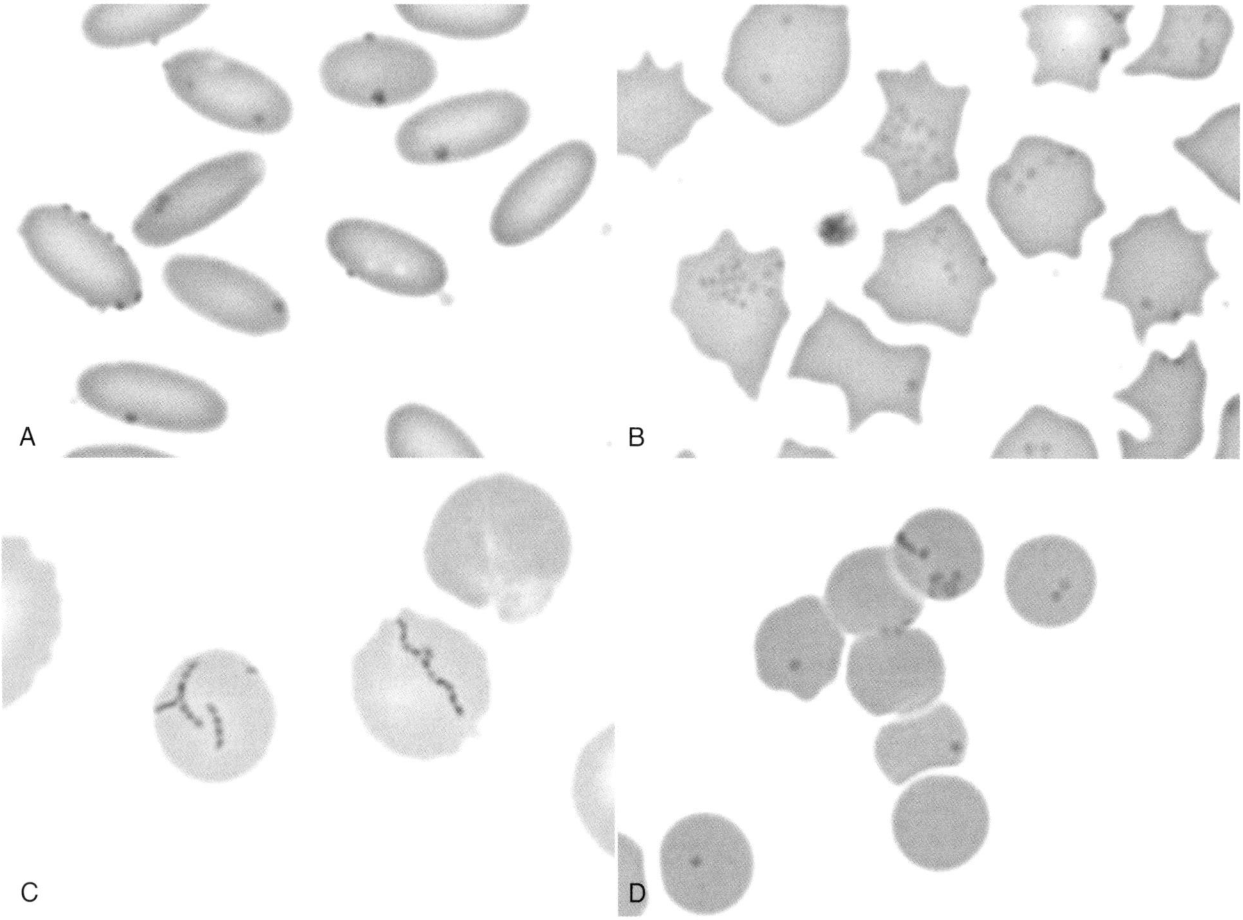

Figure 13-28 **Hemotropic Mycoplasmosis, Alpaca (A), Porcine (B), Canine (C), and Feline (D) Blood Smears.** Blood smears from an alpaca with *Mycoplasma haemolamae* **(A)**, a pig with *Mycoplasma suis* **(B)**, a dog with *Mycoplasma haemocanis* **(C)**, and a cat with *Mycoplasma haemominutum* **(D)** infections. Note the small oval to ring-shaped organisms attached to the surface of the erythrocytes and free in the background of the blood smear. Wright-Giemsa stain. (Courtesy Dr. K.M. Boes, College of Veterinary Medicine, Virginia Polytechnic Institute and State University.)

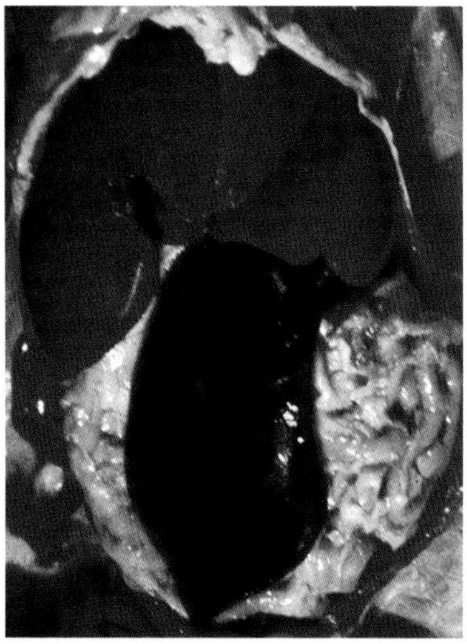

Figure 13-29 ***Mycoplasma haemofelis*, Cat.** Note the splenomegaly, hepatomegaly, and icterus caused by infection of erythrocytes with this hemotropic parasite. Splenomegaly and icterus are the result of increased destruction (extravascular hemolysis) of infected erythrocytes. (Courtesy College of Veterinary Medicine, University of Illinois.)

primary immune-mediated hemolytic anemia or autoimmune hemolytic anemia) or secondary to a known initiator, termed *secondary immune-mediated hemolytic anemia*. Although the cause of idiopathic immune-mediated hemolytic anemia is unknown, certain dog breeds (e.g., cocker spaniels) are predisposed to developing disease, suggesting the possibility of a genetic component. Causes of secondary immune-mediated hemolytic anemia include certain infections (e.g., hemoplasmosis, babesiosis, and theileriosis), drugs (e.g., cephalosporins, penicillin, and sulfonamides), vaccines, and envenomations (e.g., bee stings). Immune-mediated hemolysis directed at nonself antigens, such as in neonatal isoerythrolysis, is presented later.

In most cases of idiopathic immune-mediated hemolytic anemia, the reactive antibody is IgG, and the hemolysis is extravascular (i.e., erythrocytes with surface-bound antibody are phagocytized by macrophages, mainly in the spleen). IgM and/or complement proteins may also contribute to idiopathic immune-mediated hemolytic anemia. Complement factor C3b usually acts as an opsonin that promotes phagocytosis and extravascular hemolysis. However, formation of the complement membrane attack complex on red blood cell surfaces causes intravascular hemolysis; this mechanism more commonly occurs with IgM autoantibodies. Most immunoglobulins implicated in immune-mediated hemolytic anemia are reactive at body temperature (*warm hemagglutinins*). A smaller portion, usually IgM, are more reactive at lower temperatures, causing a condition known as *cold hemagglutinin disease*. This results in ischemic necrosis at anatomic extremities (e.g., tips of the ears), where cooling of the circulation causes autoagglutination of erythrocytes and occlusion of the microvasculature. Typically immune-mediated hemolytic anemia targets mature erythrocytes, causing a marked regenerative response. However, as discussed earlier in the chapter, immune-mediated destruction of immature erythroid cells in the bone marrow may also occur, resulting in nonregenerative anemia.

Pathogenesis of secondary immune-mediated hemolytic anemia is dependent upon the cause. Erythrocytic parasites may cause immune-mediated hemolysis by altering the red blood cell surface and exposing "hidden antigens" that are not recognized as self-antigens by the host's immune system. Alternatively, the immune attack may be directed at the infectious agent, but erythrocytes are nonspecifically destroyed because of their close proximity—this is called the innocent bystander mechanism. Certain drugs, such as penicillin, may cause immune-mediated hemolytic anemia by binding to erythrocyte membranes and forming drug-autoantigen complexes that induce antibody formation, termed *hapten-dependent antibodies*. Other proposed mechanisms include binding of drug-antibody immune complexes to the erythrocyte membrane, or induction of a true autoantibody directed against an erythrocyte antigen.

Hematologic, gross, and histopathologic abnormalities are typical of those of hemolytic anemia, as presented in the earlier section on Bone Marrow and Blood Cells, Dysfunction/Responses to Injury, Blood Cells, Abnormal Concentrations of Blood Cells, Anemia). In brief, there may be spherocytes and autoagglutination on blood smear evaluation, icterus and splenomegaly on gross examination, and EMH, erythrophagocytic macrophages, and hypoxia-induced or thromboemboli-induced tissue necrosis on histopathologic examination. Dogs with immune-mediated hemolytic anemia also frequently develop an inflammatory leukocytosis and coagulation abnormalities (prolonged coagulation times, decreased plasma antithrombin concentration, increased plasma concentration of fibrin degradation products, thrombocytopenia, and disseminated intravascular coagulation). Intravascular hemolysis plays a relatively insignificant role in most cases of immune-mediated hemolytic anemia, but evidence of intravascular hemolysis (e.g., ghost cells, red plasma and urine, dark red kidneys) is noted occasionally, presumably in those cases in which IgM and complement are major mediators of hemolysis.

Neonatal Isoerythrolysis. Neonatal isoerythrolysis (NI) is a form of immune-mediated hemolytic anemia in which colostrum-derived maternal antibodies react against the newborn's erythrocytes. It is common in horses (Fig. 13-30) and has been reported in cattle, cats, and some other domestic and wildlife species. In horses, neonatal isoerythrolysis occurs as a result of immunosensitization of the dam from exposure to an incompatible blood type inherited from the stallion (e.g., transplacental exposure to fetal blood during pregnancy or mixing of maternal and fetal blood during parturition). A previously mismatched blood transfusion produces the same results. Some equine blood groups are more antigenic than others; in particular, types Aa and Qa are very immunogenic in mares. In cattle, neonatal isoerythrolysis has been caused by vaccination with whole blood products or products containing erythrocyte membrane fragments. Neonatal isoerythrolysis has been produced experimentally in dogs, but there are no reports of naturally occurring disease. In cats the recognized form of neonatal isoerythrolysis does not depend on prior maternal immunosensitization but on naturally occurring anti-A antibodies in queens with type B blood. Affected animals are young (hours to days old) with typical gross and microscopic changes of immune-mediated hemolytic anemia.

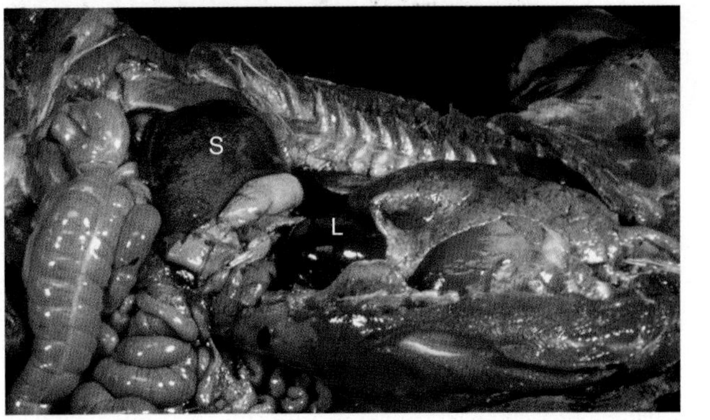

Figure 13-30 Neonatal Isoerythrolysis, Foal. Note the enlarged spleen *(S)* (also liver *[L]*) and icterus. The newborn foal had colostrum-derived maternal antibodies, which reacted against its own erythrocytes. Macrophages in the splenic red pulp remove erythrocytes whose membranes have bound antibody. (Courtesy College of Veterinary Medicine, University of Illinois.)

Pure Red Cell Aplasia. Pure red cell aplasia (PRCA) is a rare bone marrow disorder characterized by absence of erythropoiesis and severe nonregenerative anemia. Primary and secondary forms of pure red cell aplasia have been described in dogs and cats. Primary pure red cell aplasia is apparently caused by immune-mediated destruction of early erythroid progenitor cells, a presumption supported by the response of some patients to immunosuppressive therapy and by the detection of antibodies inhibiting erythroid colony formation in vitro in some dogs. Administration of recombinant human erythropoietin (rhEpo) has been identified as a cause of secondary pure red cell aplasia in dogs, cats, and horses, presumably caused by induction of antibodies against rhEpo that cross-react with endogenous Epo. Experimentation with the use of species-specific recombinant Epo has produced mixed results. Dogs treated with recombinant canine Epo have not developed pure red cell aplasia. However, in experiments reported thus far involving cats treated with recombinant feline Epo, at least some animals have developed pure red cell aplasia. Parvoviral infection has been suggested as a possible cause of secondary pure red cell aplasia in dogs. Infection with FeLV subgroup C causes secondary erythroid aplasia in cats, probably because of infection of early-stage erythroid precursors. Grossly, animals with pure red cell aplasia have pale mucous membranes without indicators of hemolysis (e.g., icterus). Microscopic examination of the bone marrow shows an absence or near absence of erythroid precursors with or without lymphocytosis, plasmacytosis, and myelofibrosis; production of other cell lines (e.g., neutrophils and platelets) is normal or hyperplastic.

Immune-Mediated Neutropenia. Immune-mediated neutropenia is a rare condition that has been reported in horses, dogs, and cats. This disease is characterized by severe neutropenia from immune-mediated destruction of neutrophils or their precursors. The range of causes is presumably similar to that of other immune-mediated cytopenias (e.g., immune-mediated hemolytic anemia, pure red cell aplasia, and immune-mediated thrombocytopenia). Affected animals may have infections, such as dermatitis, conjunctivitis, or vaginitis, which are secondary to marked neutropenia and a compromised innate immune system. Microscopically, there may be neutrophil hyperplasia, maturation arrest, or aplasia in the bone marrow, depending on which neutrophil maturation stage is targeted for destruction. Marrow lymphocytosis and plasmacytosis may be marked (e.g., >60% of nucleated cells). The diagnosis may be supported by flow cytometric detection of immunoglobulin bound to neutrophils but is most often made on the basis of exclusion of other causes of neutropenia and response to immunosuppressive therapy.

Immune-Mediated Thrombocytopenia. Immune-mediated thrombocytopenia (IMTP) is a condition characterized by immune-mediated destruction of platelets. It is a fairly common condition in dogs and is less frequent in horses and cats. The disease is usually idiopathic but may be secondary to infection (e.g., equine infectious anemia and ehrlichiosis), drug administration (e.g., cephalosporins and sulfonamides), neoplasia, and other immune-mediated diseases. When immune-mediated thrombocytopenia occurs together with immune-mediated hemolytic anemia, the condition is called *Evans's syndrome*. The thrombocytopenia is often severe (e.g., < 20,000 platelets/μL), resulting in varying degrees of bleeding tendencies, mainly in skin and mucous membranes. Microscopically, there are multifocal perivascular hemorrhages in multiple tissues, and the bone marrow exhibits megakaryocytic and erythroid hyperplasia. Rarely, immune-mediated destruction of megakaryocytes may cause megakaryocytic hypoplasia, termed *amegakaryocytic thrombocytopenia*.

Neonatal Alloimmune Thrombocytopenia. A form of immune-mediated thrombocytopenia, known as neonatal alloimmune thrombocytopenia, is recognized in neonatal pigs and foals. The pathogenesis of this disease is virtually identical to that of neonatal isoerythrolysis as a cause of anemia: a neonate inheriting paternal platelet antigens absorbs maternal antibodies against these antigens through the colostrum. In principle, a similar situation may occur after platelet-incompatible transfusion of blood or blood products containing platelets. Gross and microscopic changes are similar to those of immune-mediated thrombocytopenia except that the animal is young (e.g., 1 to 3 days).

Inflammatory Disorders

Hemophagocytic Syndrome. Hemophagocytic syndrome is a term used to describe the proliferation of nonneoplastic (i.e., polyclonal), well-differentiated but highly erythrophagic macrophages. The condition is rare but has been recognized in dogs and cats. Unlike hemophagocytic histiocytic sarcoma, which is a neoplastic proliferation of phagocytic macrophages, hemophagocytic syndrome is secondary to an underlying disease, such as neoplasia, infection, or an immune-mediated disorder. The primary disease process causes increased production of stimulatory cytokines, which results in macrophage proliferation and hyperactivation. These activated macrophages phagocytize mature hematopoietic cells and hematopoietic precursors at an enhanced rate, resulting in one or more cytopenias. Affected animals usually have lesions of the primary disease, as well as signs of the anemia (e.g., pale mucous membranes), neutropenia (e.g., bacterial infections), and thrombocytopenia (e.g., petechiae and ecchymoses). Microscopically, phagocytic macrophages are found in high numbers in the bone marrow and commonly in other tissues, including lymph nodes, spleen, and liver. Additional bone marrow findings reported in animals with hemophagocytic syndrome vary widely, ranging from hypoplasia to hyperplasia of cell lines with peripheral cytopenias.

Disseminated Intravascular Coagulation. Disseminated intravascular coagulation is a syndrome characterized by continuous activation of both coagulation and fibrinolytic pathways and is also known as consumptive coagulopathy. It is not a primary disease, but rather a secondary complication of many types of underlying disease, including severe inflammation, organ failure, and neoplasia. It is included in the section on Inflammatory Disorders because the coagulation cascade is closely linked to inflammatory pathways.

Information on this topic, including E-Fig. 13-5, is available at www.expertconsult.com. as well as in Chapter 2.

Hematopoietic Neoplasia

The term hematopoietic neoplasia encompasses a large and diverse group of clonal proliferative disorders of hematopoietic cells. Historically, numerous systems have been used to classify hematopoietic neoplasms in human medicine, some of which have been applied inconsistently to veterinary species (examples include the Kiel classification and National Cancer Institute Working Formulation). The World Health Organization (WHO) classification of hematopoietic neoplasia was first published in 2001 (updated in 2008) and is based on the principles defined in the Revised European-American Classification of Lymphoid Neoplasms (REAL) from the International Lymphoma Study Group. The WHO classification system is considered the first true worldwide consensus on the classification of hematopoietic malignancies and integrates information on tumor topography, cell morphology, immunophenotype, genetic features, and clinical presentation and course. A veterinary reference of the WHO classification system, published in 2002, was later validated in 2011 using the canine model of lymphoma. This project, modeled after the study to validate the system in human beings, yielded an overall accuracy (i.e., agreement on a diagnosis) among pathologists of 83%. Currently this classification system is accepted as the method of choice in both human and veterinary medicine.

The WHO classification broadly categorizes neoplasms primarily according to cell lineage: myeloid, lymphoid, and histiocytic. This distinction is based on the fact that the earliest commitment of a pluripotent HSC is to either a lymphoid or nonlymphoid lineage. Many pathologists and clinicians distinguish leukemias from other hematopoietic neoplasms. *Leukemia* refers to a group of hematopoietic neoplasms that arise from the bone marrow and are present within the blood. Leukemia may be difficult to differentiate from other forms of hematopoietic neoplasms that originate outside of the bone marrow but infiltrate the bone marrow and blood. For simplicity, cases of secondary bone marrow or blood involvement may not be considered leukemia but rather the "leukemic phase" of another primary neoplasm. It is now recognized that certain lymphomas and leukemias are different manifestations of the same disease (e.g., chronic lymphocytic leukemia and small lymphocytic lymphoma), and the designation of lymphoma or leukemia is placed on the tissue with the largest tumor burden.

Based on their degree of differentiation, leukemias are classified as acute or chronic. *Acute leukemias* are poorly differentiated or undifferentiated, meaning that there are high percentages of early progenitor and precursor cells, including lymphoblasts, myeloblasts, monoblasts, erythroblasts, and/or megakaryoblasts. In contrast, well-differentiated cells predominate in *chronic leukemias*. Because well-differentiated cells also predominate with nonneoplastic proliferations, chronic leukemias must be differentiated from reactive processes, such as those cells that occur in chronic and/or granulomatous inflammation. Diagnosis of chronic leukemia is often made by excluding all other causes for the proliferating cell type. For example, causes of relative and secondary erythrocytosis are excluded to be able to diagnose polycythemia vera. Furthermore, the designation of acute or chronic also refers to the disease's clinical course. Acute leukemias tend to have an acute onset of severe and rapidly progressive clinical signs, whereas animals with chronic leukemia typically have indolent, slowly progressive disease. This classification scheme is summarized in Table 13-4. Subcategories exist within each of these groups, as discussed further later.

Diagnostic Techniques Used to Classify Hematopoietic Neoplasms

Information on this topic is available at www.expertconsult.com.

Types of Hematopoietic Neoplasia

This section discusses examples of *myeloid neoplasms*, including myelodysplastic syndrome, myeloid leukemias, and mast cell neoplasms (technically a form of myeloid neoplasia), and *lymphoid neoplasms*, including lymphoid leukemias and multiple myeloma. Other lymphoid neoplasms, such as the numerous subtypes of lymphoma and extramedullary plasmacytomas (EMPs), as well as histiocytic disorders are described in the section on Lymphoid/Lymphatic System, Disorders of Domestic Animals, Neoplasia. Additional discussion of hematopoietic neoplasia occurs in the species-specific sections at the end of this chapter.

Myeloid Neoplasia

Myelodysplastic Syndrome. Myelodysplastic syndrome (MDS) most commonly occurs in dogs and cats and may be caused by FeLV infection in cats. The disease refers to a group of clonal myeloid proliferative disorders with ineffective hematopoiesis in the bone marrow, resulting in cytopenias of more than one cell line. Hematopoietic proliferation in bone marrow with concurrent peripheral blood cytopenias is likely a result of increased apoptosis of neoplastic cells within the bone marrow, before their release into circulation. Clinical illness and death often result from secondary manifestations, such as secondary infections or cachexia, attributable to the effects of cytopenias and/or transformation of the neoplasm into acute myeloid leukemia. Gross lesions are dependent upon the type and severity of the cytopenias. However, essential microscopic findings within the bone marrow are normal or increased cellularity, dysplasia of myeloid cells, and fewer than 20% myeloblasts and "blast equivalents."[3]

Table 13-4 Basic Classification of Leukemias

Leukemia	Basic Diagnostic Criteria
Acute undifferentiated leukemia	• No lineage commitment • ≥20% blasts in bone marrow
Lymphoid leukemia	• Commitment to lymphoid lineage
Acute lymphoblastic leukemia	• ≥20% blasts in bone marrow
Chronic lymphocytic leukemia	• <20% blasts in bone marrow • Predominantly small lymphocytes in blood, often > 100,000/μL
Multiple myeloma	• Increased plasma cells in bone marrow • Osteolysis • Monoclonal gammopathy • Light chain (Bence Jones) proteinuria
Myeloid leukemia	• Commitment to myeloid lineage
Myelodysplastic syndrome	• <20% blasts in bone marrow • Normal or increased marrow cellularity • Peripheral blood cytopenias • Myelodysplasia
Acute myeloid leukemia	• ≥20% blasts in bone marrow
Chronic myeloid leukemia	• <20% blasts in bone marrow • Markedly increased numbers of mature myeloid cells in blood

Acute Myeloid Leukemia. Acute myeloid leukemia (AML) is uncommon in domestic animals but most frequently occurs in dogs and cats. In veterinary species, acute myeloid leukemia is most commonly of neutrophil, monocyte, and/or erythroid origin, with rare reports of eosinophil, basophil, or megakaryocytic lineages. It is caused by FeLV infection in cats. Evaluations of blood smears show many early myeloid precursors, including myeloblasts and blast equivalents (Fig. 13-31, *A*). In dogs the total leukocyte concentration averages approximately 70,000/μL; anemia, neutropenia, and thrombocytopenia commonly occur. Grossly, animals show lesions attributed to anemia, neutropenia, and thrombocytopenia, such as pale mucous membranes, secondary infections, and multisystemic bleeding, respectively. Neoplastic cells often infiltrate tissues, resulting in splenomegaly, hepatomegaly, and lymphadenomegaly. Microscopically, myeloid cells efface (replace) the bone marrow and infiltrate extramedullary tissues, especially lymphoid tissue.

Chronic Myeloid Leukemia. Chronic myeloid leukemia (CML), also called chronic myelogenous leukemia or myeloproliferative neoplasia, is rare in animals. Most reported cases occur in dogs and cats. There are various subclassifications of chronic myeloid leukemia, including excessive production of erythrocytes (polycythemia vera), platelets (essential thrombocythemia), neutrophils (chronic neutrophilic leukemia), monocytes (chronic monocytic leukemia), neutrophils and monocytes (chronic myelomonocytic leukemia), eosinophils (chronic eosinophilic leukemia), or basophils (chronic basophilic leukemia). Complete peripheral blood count analysis often reveals very high concentrations of the neoplastic cells, such as greater than 50,000 to 100,000 leukocytes/μL (see Fig. 13-31, *B*) or 2,000,000 platelets/μL. Cellular morphologic features are often normal, but slight dysplasia may be observed. Later in the disease there may be cytopenias of nonneoplastic cell types.

Animals with polycythemia vera often have red mucous membranes and lesions of *hyperviscosity syndrome*, such as bleeding and dilated, tortuous retinal vessels. Essential thrombocythemia results in multisystemic bleeding due to dysfunctional platelets, or multisystemic infarcts from hyperaggregability and excessive platelets. Chronic myeloid leukemias of leukocytes often result in splenomegaly, hepatomegaly, and lymphadenomegaly because of infiltration by the neoplastic cells. Histologically, the bone marrow shows proliferation of the neoplastic cell type characterized by dysplasia and low numbers (e.g., <20%) of myeloblasts and blast equivalents.

Mast Cell Neoplasia. Mast cell tumors (MCTs) of the skin and other sites are common in animals (see Chapters 6, 7, and 17), but mast cell leukemia is rare. In cats, MCTs are the most common neoplasm in the spleen (E-Fig. 13-6). Mast cells normally are not present in the blood vascular system, but the finding of mast cells in the blood (mastocytemia) is highly suggestive of disseminated mast cell neoplasia (systemic mastocytosis) in cats. However, mastocytemia does not necessarily indicate myeloid neoplasia in dogs. In fact, one study found that the severity of mastocytemia in dogs was frequently higher in animals without MCTs than those with MCTs and that random detection of mast cells in blood smears usually is not the result of underlying MCT.

Granulocytic Sarcoma. Granulocytic sarcoma is a poorly characterized extramedullary proliferation of myeloid precursors, most

[3]"Blast equivalents" include other stages of immature myeloid cells, such as abnormal promyelocytes, monoblasts, promonocytes, erythroblasts, and megakaryoblasts.

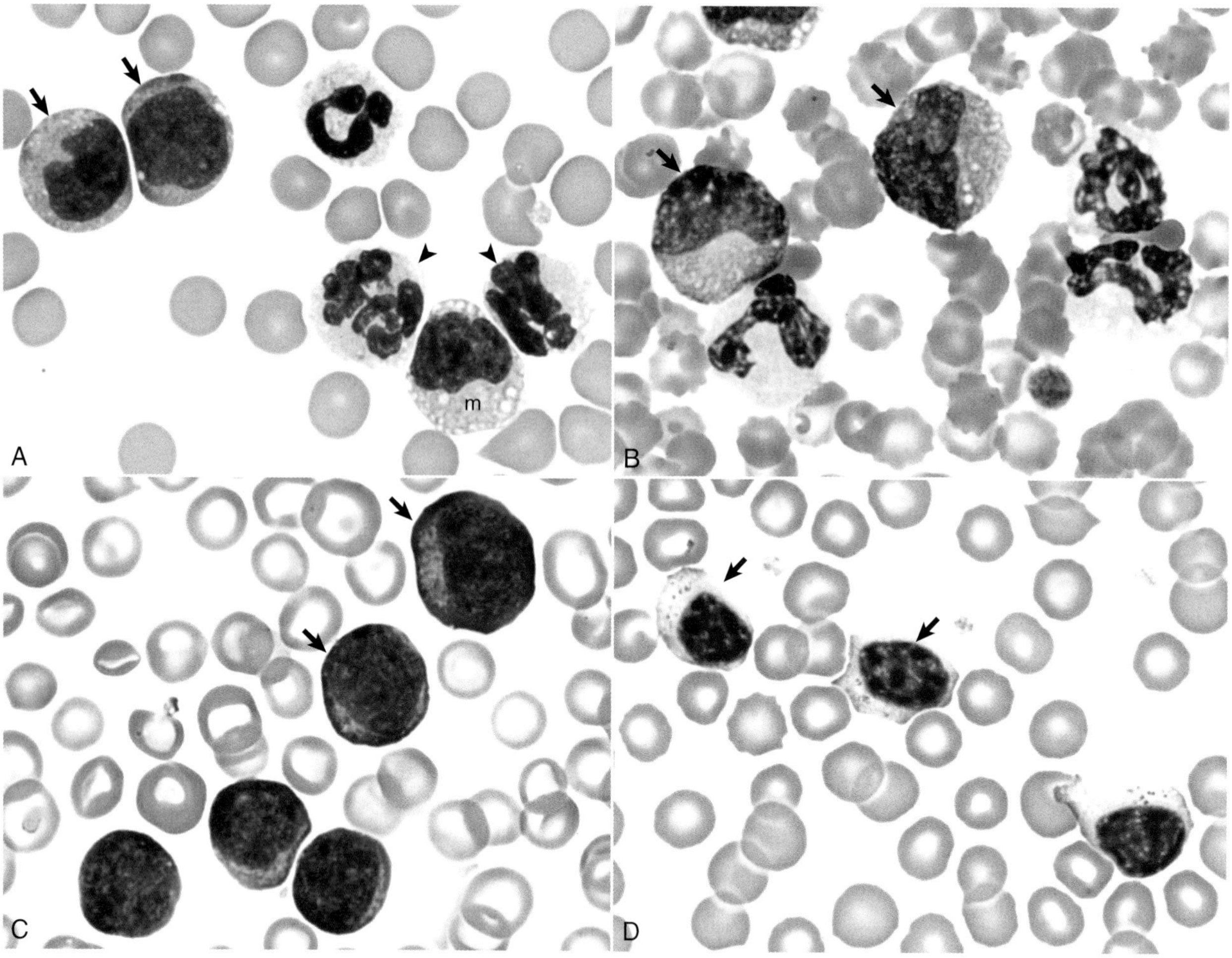

Figure 13-31 **Leukemia, Canine Blood Smears. A,** Acute myeloid leukemia. A dog with acute myelomonocytic leukemia has a marked leukocytosis (52,200 white blood cells/μL) with myeloid blasts *(arrows)* differentiating into dysplastic neutrophils *(arrowheads)* and monocytes *(m)*. Modified Wright's stain. **B,** Chronic myeloid leukemia. A dog with chronic myelomonocytic leukemia *(arrows)* has a marked leukocytosis (138,300 white blood cells/μL) with a predominance of mature neutrophils (105,108/μL) and monocytes (26,277/μL). Wright-Giemsa stain. **C,** Acute lymphoblastic leukemia. Note the large lymphoid cells with immature (fine) chromatin and nucleoli *(arrows)*. The dog also had pancytopenia due to neoplastic myelophthisis. Modified Wright's stain. **D,** Chronic lymphocytic leukemia (CLL). Small lymphocytes predominate in CLL. The neoplastic lymphocytes have clumped chromatin and no to rare nucleoli *(arrows)*. Most canine CLLs are of T lymphocyte origin with a granular phenotype. Modified Wright's stain. (Courtesy Dr. K.M. Boes, College of Veterinary Medicine, Virginia Polytechnic Institute and State University.)

often of eosinophilic or neutrophilic cell lines. Although rare, there are reports of granulocytic sarcoma in dogs, cats, cattle, and pigs, and it may arise in a number of sites, such as lung, intestine, lymph nodes, liver, kidney, skin, and muscle.

Lymphoid Neoplasia

Lymphoid Leukemia

Acute Lymphoblastic Leukemia. Acute lymphoblastic leukemia (ALL) is uncommon in dogs and cats, and rare in horses and cattle. In a recent immunophenotype study of 51 cases of acute lymphoblastic leukemia in dogs, 47 arose from B lymphocytes and 4 arose from double-negative T lymphocytes that were immunonegative for CD4 and CD8 markers. In the blood of animals with acute lymphoblastic leukemia, there are typically many medium to large lymphoid cells with deeply basophilic cytoplasm, reticular to coarse chromatin, and prominent, multiple nucleoli (see Fig. 13-31, C). In affected dogs the mean blood lymphoid concentration is approximately 70,000/μL, but cats with acute lymphoblastic leukemia often have low numbers of neoplastic cells in the circulation. As with animals with acute myeloid leukemia, anemia, neutropenia, and thrombocytopenia commonly occur. Gross and microscopic lesions also are similar to those that occur in cases of acute myeloid leukemia, except that neoplastic cells may differentiate into morphologically identifiable lymphoid cells.

Chronic Lymphocytic Leukemia. Chronic lymphocytic leukemia (CLL) is uncommon in veterinary medicine. It is predominantly a disease of middle-aged to older dogs but is also documented in horses, cattle, and cats. Most canine chronic lymphocytic leukemia cases are of T lymphocyte origin, typically cytotoxic T lymphocytes expressing CD8. In cats the majority of chronic lymphocytic leukemia cases have a T helper lymphocyte immunophenotype. A CBC often shows very high numbers of small lymphocytes with clumped chromatin and scant cytoplasm. Proliferating cytotoxic T lymphocytes frequently contain a few pink cytoplasmic granules when stained with most methanol-based Romanowsky stains (e.g., Wright-Giemsa). However, these granules may not be appreciated with some aqueous-based Romanowsky stains (e.g., Diff-Quik). Although the number of total blood lymphocytes is often greater than 100,000/μL, relatively mild lymphocytosis (e.g., 15,000/μL) has been reported. Seventy-five percent of affected dogs also have anemia, and 15% have thrombocytopenia. Autopsy findings depend on the stage of disease. In advanced cases with marked infiltration of organs with neoplastic cells, there is often uniform splenomegaly, hepatomegaly, and lymphadenomegaly, and the bone marrow is highly cellular (E-Fig. 13-7; see Fig. 13-31, *D*). Other lesions depend on whether there are concurrent cytopenias, such as anemia, neutropenia, and thrombocytopenia, and if the neoplastic cells produce excessive immunoglobulin. Lesions caused by excessive immunoglobulin are further discussed in the section on multiple myeloma. Histologically, the bone marrow is densely cellular with well-differentiated lymphocytes. Small lymphocytes infiltrate and often efface in the architecture of the lymph nodes and spleen. The liver may have dense accumulations of neoplastic cells in the connective tissue around the portal triad.

Plasma Cell Neoplasia. Plasma cell neoplasms are most easily categorized as *myeloma* or *multiple myeloma*, which arises in the bone marrow, and *extramedullary plasmacytoma*, which as the name implies involves sites other than bone; the latter is discussed in the section on Lymphoid/Lymphatic System, Disorders of Domestic Animals: Lymph Nodes, Neoplasia, Plasma Cell Neoplasia.

Multiple Myeloma. Multiple myeloma (MM) is a rare, malignant tumor of plasma cells that arises in the bone marrow and usually secretes large amounts of immunoglobulin. The finding of neoplastic plasma cells in blood samples or smears is rare. Dogs are affected more frequently than other species, but multiple myeloma has also been reported in horses, cattle, cats, and pigs. Diagnosis of multiple myeloma is based on finding a minimum of two or three (opinions vary) of the following abnormalities:

- Markedly increased numbers of plasma cells in the bone marrow (Fig. 13-32, A)
- Monoclonal gammopathy
- Radiographic evidence of osteolysis
- Light chain proteinuria

The classic laboratory finding in patients with multiple myeloma is hyperglobulinemia, which results from the excessive production of immunoglobulin or an immunoglobulin subunit by the neoplastic cells. This homogeneous protein fraction is often called *paraprotein* or M *protein*. Paraproteins produced from the same clone of plasma cells have the same molecular weight and electric charge. Therefore they have the same migration pattern using serum protein electrophoresis, which results in a tall, narrow spike in the globulins region, termed *monoclonal gammopathy* (see Fig. 13-32, *B*). The term gammopathy is used because most immunoglobulins migrate in the γ-region of an electrophoresis gel. However, some immunoglobulins, especially immunoglobulin A (IgA) and IgM, migrate to the β-region. Occasionally, biclonal or other atypical electrophoretic patterns may be seen with multiple myeloma as a result of protein degradation, protein complex formation, binding to other proteins, or when the tumor includes more than one clonal population. It is important to note that monoclonal gammopathy is not specific to multiple myeloma but has also been reported with lymphoma, chronic lymphocytic leukemia, canine ehrlichiosis, and canine leishmaniasis. Definitively distinguishing monoclonal from polyclonal gammopathy requires immunoelectrophoresis or immunofixation using species-specific antibodies recognizing different immunoglobulin subclasses and subunits.

Occasionally, multiple myeloma cells produce only the immunoglobulin light chain. An immunoglobulin monomer consists of two heavy chains and two light chains connected by disulfide bonds. These light chains may deposit in tissues and cause organ dysfunction, especially renal failure. When the light chains form amyloid deposits, the disease is called *amyloid light chain amyloidosis*. But if the light chains deposit as nonamyloid granules, it is termed *light chain deposition disease*. Light chains are low-molecular-weight proteins that pass through the glomerular filter into the urine, wherein they are also known as *Bence Jones proteins*. They tend to not react with urine dipstick protein indicators and are most specifically detected by electrophoresis and immunoprecipitation.

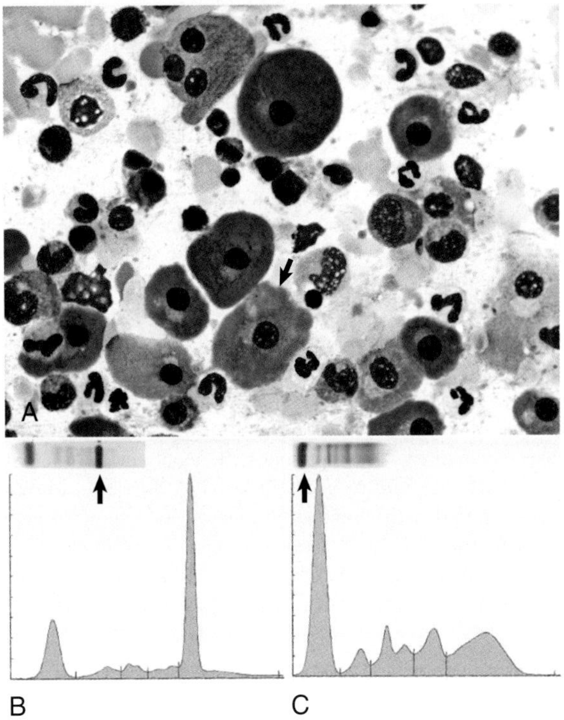

Figure 13-32 **Multiple Myeloma and Monoclonal Gammopathy. A,** Canine bone marrow aspirate. Many of the neoplastic plasma cells in the bone marrow aspirate have pink-tinged cytoplasm *(arrow)*, the result of a high concentration of immunoglobulin. Wright's stain. **B,** Multiple myeloma, cat. Agarose gels and densitometry tracings showing results of serum electrophoresis. The serum has a high concentration of a monoclonal immunoglobulin (the dark band *[arrow]* on the right of the gel, corresponding to the tall peak on the right of the tracing). **C,** Normal cat. Agarose gels and densitometry tracings showing results of serum electrophoresis. The serum has a normal distribution of protein fractions, the most abundant being albumin (the dark band *[arrow]* on the left of the gel, corresponding to the tall peak on the left of the tracing). (**A** courtesy Dr. M.M. Fry, College of Veterinary Medicine, University of Tennessee. **B** and **C** courtesy Dr. S.A. Kania, College of Veterinary Medicine, University of Tennessee.)

In addition to aiding in the diagnosis of multiple myeloma, paraproteins have an important role in pathogenesis of disease. These proteins may inhibit platelet function, increase blood viscosity, deposit in glomerular basement membranes (see Chapter 11; see Figs. 11-27 and 11-28, or precipitate at cool temperatures, which results in bleeding tendencies, hyperviscosity syndrome, glomerulopathies, and cryoglobulinemia, respectively. *Hyperviscosity syndrome* refers to the clinical sequelae of pathologically increased blood viscosity, which are slowed blood flow and loss of laminar flow. Clinical signs include mucosal hemorrhages, visual impairment due to retinopathy, and neurologic signs, such as tremors and abnormal aggressive behavior. *Cryoglobulinemia* is the condition in which proteins, typically IgM, precipitate at temperatures below normal body temperature (cold agglutinins). Precipitation often occurs in blood vessels of the skin and extremities, such as the ears and digits, and results in ischemic necrosis.

In multiple myeloma the neoplastic proliferation of plasma cells results in osteolysis. Work with human cell cultures has shown that osteoclasts support the growth of myeloma cells, and that direct contact between the two cell types increases the myeloma cell proliferation and promotes osteoclast survival. Increased osteoclast activity causes osteolysis, but the exact mechanism is not known. Osteolysis often results in bone pain, lytic bone lesions on radiographs, hypercalcemia, and increased serum alkaline phosphatase activity. Later in disease, osteolysis may cause pathologic fractures.

Morphologically, myeloma cells tend to grow in sheets that displace normal hematopoietic cells in the bone marrow. A proposed diagnostic criterion of multiple myeloma is that plasma cells constitute 30% or more of the nucleated cells in the marrow. Well-differentiated plasma cells are round with abundant basophilic cytoplasm (due to increased rough endoplasmic reticulum) and a perinuclear pale zone (enlarged Golgi apparatus for the production of immunoglobulin); anisocytosis and anisokaryosis are often mild but may be marked. Some plasma cell neoplasms have a bright eosinophilic fringe due to accumulated IgA (see Fig. 13-32, A). Nuclei are round with clumped chromatin and often peripherally placed with the cytoplasm; binucleation and multinucleation are common. Poorly differentiated myeloma cells may lack and/or display less characteristic features. Osteolysis of bone may be present microscopically. Common sites of metastasis include the spleen, liver, lymph nodes, and kidneys.

Disorders of Horses

Congenital Disorders

Flavin Adenine Dinucleotide Deficiency. Flavin adenine dinucleotide (FAD) is a cofactor for cytochrome-b_5 reductase, the enzyme that maintains hemoglobin in its functional reduced state, and for glutathione reductase, an enzyme that also protects erythrocytes from oxidative damage. Reported in a Spanish mustang mare and a Kentucky mountain saddle horse gelding, erythrocyte FAD deficiency is a result of an abnormal riboflavin kinase reaction, which is the first reaction in converting riboflavin to FAD. Clinicopathologic changes include persistent methemoglobinemia of 26% to 46%, eccentrocytosis, a slightly decreased or normal hematocrit, and erythroid hyperplasia in the bone marrow.

Infectious Diseases

Equine Infectious Anemia Virus. Equine infectious anemia virus (EIAV), the agent of *equine infectious anemia*, is a lentivirus that infects cells of the monocyte-macrophage system in horses (also ponies, donkeys, and mules). The virus is mechanically transmitted by biting flies, such as horseflies and deer flies. Less common routes of transmission include blood transfusions, contaminated medical equipment, and transplacentally. Disease may present in acute, subacute, and chronic forms and is potentially fatal. After an acute period of fever, depression, and thrombocytopenia that lasts 1 to 3 days, there is a prolonged period of recurrent fever, thrombocytopenia, and anemia. In most cases, clinical disease subsides within a year, and horses become lifelong carriers and reservoirs of EIAV.

EIAV causes anemia by both immune-mediated hemolysis and decreased erythropoiesis. Hemolysis is typically extravascular but may have an intravascular component during the acute phase. Decreased erythropoiesis may result from direct suppression of early-stage erythroid cells by the virus, as well as anemia of inflammation. Thrombocytopenia likely results from immune-mediated platelet destruction and suppressed platelet production.

Animals dying during hemolytic crises are pale with mucosal hemorrhages and dependent edema. The spleen and liver are enlarged, dark, and turgid, and they and other organs have superficial subcapsular hemorrhages. Petechiae are evident beneath the renal capsule and throughout the cortex and medulla. The bone marrow is dark red as a result of replacement of fat by hematopoietic tissue; the extent of replacement is an indication of the duration of the anemia.

The severity of microscopic lesions is dependent on the chronicity of the disease, and they are most significant in the spleen, liver, and bone marrow. As would be anticipated, microscopic findings of the spleen are predominantly influenced by the number and activity of macrophages, which is a reflection of the duration of the disease and the frequency of hemolytic episodes. Hemosiderin-laden macrophages persist for months to years; therefore large numbers are consistent with chronicity. Kupffer cell hyperplasia with hemosiderin stores and periportal infiltrates of lymphocytes are the most significant changes in the liver. Bone marrow histologic findings vary depending on the duration of the disease. In most animals the marrow is cellular because of the replacement of fat by intense, orderly erythropoiesis. Granulocytes are relatively less numerous, and plasma cells are increased. As in the spleen, hemosiderin-laden macrophages are present in large numbers in chronic cases. Emaciated animals with chronic disease have serous atrophy of fat (see E-Fig. 13-1).

Clinical findings with viremic episodes include fever, depression, icterus, petechial hemorrhages, lymph node enlargement, and dependent edema. Equine infectious anemia infection is diagnosed on the basis of the Coggins test, an agarose gel immunodiffusion test for the presence of the antibody against the virus.

Disorders of Ruminants (Cattle, Sheep, and Goats)

Congenital Disorders

Congenital Dyserythropoiesis in Polled Herefords. A syndrome of congenital dyserythropoiesis and alopecia occurs in polled Hereford calves. The cause and pathogenesis of this often fatal disease are unknown. Early in disease there is hyperkeratosis and alopecia of the muzzle and ears, which progresses to generalized alopecia and hyperkeratotic dermatitis. Histologically, there is orthokeratotic hyperkeratosis with dyskeratosis, as well as erythroid hyperplasia, dysplasia, and maturation arrest in the bone marrow. Ineffective erythropoiesis results in nonregenerative to poorly regenerative anemia.

Erythrocyte Band 3 Deficiency in Japanese Black Cattle. Erythrocyte band 3 is integral membrane protein that connects to the cytoskeleton and aids in erythrocyte stability. A hereditary deficiency of this protein has been identified in Japanese black cattle, resulting in increased erythrocyte fragility, spherocytosis, intravascular hemolytic anemia, and retarded growth. Affected calves show lesions consistent with hemolytic anemia, including pale mucous membranes, icterus, and splenomegaly. Histologically, there are bilirubin accumulations in the liver, and hemosiderin in renal tubules.

Infectious Diseases

Bovine Leukemia Virus. Bovine leukemia virus is discussed in the later section on lymphoma (see Lymphoid/Lymphatic System, Disorders of Domestic Animals: Lymph Nodes, Neoplasia, Lymphoma).

Bovine Viral Diarrhea Virus. BVDV infection may cause thrombocytopenia in cattle, and a thrombocytopenic hemorrhagic syndrome has been specifically caused by type II BVDV infection. Investigations of the mechanism of BVDV-induced thrombocytopenia have resulted in varying, sometimes conflicting, conclusions. More than one study has shown viral antigen within bone marrow megakaryocytes and circulating platelets. Evidence of impaired thrombopoiesis (megakaryocyte necrosis, megakaryocyte pyknosis, and degeneration) and increased thrombopoiesis (megakaryocytic hyperplasia, increased numbers of immature megakaryocytes) in the bone marrow has been reported in type II BVDV–infected animals, including concurrent megakaryocyte necrosis and hyperplasia in some experimental subjects. Calves infected with type II BVDV also have impaired platelet function.

Cattle with the hemorrhagic syndrome are severely thrombocytopenic and neutropenic with multisystemic hemorrhages, particularly of the digestive tract, spleen, gallbladder, urinary bladder, and lymph nodes. Histologic lesions include hemorrhage, epithelial necrosis of enterocytes, intestinal erosions, crypt proliferation with microabscesses, and lymphoid depletion of the gut-associated lymphoid tissue, Peyer's patches, and spleen. Lesions of the bone marrow are variable, as previously described.

Immune-Mediated Disorders

Bovine Neonatal Pancytopenia. Bovine neonatal pancytopenia (BNP) is caused by alloantibodies absorbed from colostrum, resulting in a hemorrhagic syndrome in calves. The syndrome was first recognized in Europe in the early 2000s and has since been experimentally correlated with prior vaccination of affected calves' dams with a commercial BVDV vaccine (Pregsure BVD; Pfizer Animal Health). The vaccine has since been voluntarily recalled from the market. It is thought that vaccination induces alloantibody formation by the dam. The alloantibodies are ingested by the calf and bind to the calf's hematopoietic progenitor cells, resulting in functional compromise of those cells. Acutely affected calves are less than a year of age and have peripheral thrombocytopenia and neutropenia. Death results from thrombocytopenia-induced hemorrhages or neutropenia-induced secondary infections, including pneumonia, enteritis, and septicemia. Within the bone marrow there is erythroid, myeloid, and megakaryocytic hypoplasia.

Disorders of Dogs

Congenital Disorders

Cyclic Hematopoiesis. Cyclic hematopoiesis (also known as lethal gray collie disease) is an autosomal recessive disorder of pluripotent HSCs in gray collie dogs. A defect in the adaptor protein complex (AP3) results in defective intracellular signaling and predictable fluctuations in concentrations of blood cells that occur in 14-day cycles. The pattern is cyclic marked neutropenia, and in a different phase, cyclic reticulocytosis, monocytosis, and thrombocytosis. Production of key cytokines involved in regulation of hematopoiesis is also cyclic. Neutropenia predisposes affected animals to infection, and many die of infectious causes. Affected animals have dilute hair coats and lesions with acute or chronic infectious disease, especially of the lungs, gastrointestinal tract, and kidneys. Dogs older than 30 weeks of age have systemic amyloidosis, which occurs because of cyclic increases in concentration of acute phase proteins during phases of monocytosis.

Phosphofructokinase Deficiency. Inherited autosomal recessive deficiency of the erythrocyte glycolytic enzyme, phosphofructokinase (PFK), is described in English springer spaniel, American cocker spaniel, and mixed-breed dogs. There are three genes encoding PFK enzymes, designated M-PFK in muscle and erythrocytes, L-PFK in liver, and P-PFK in platelets. A point mutation in the gene coding for M-PFK results in an unstable, truncated molecule. Erythrocytes in PFK-deficient dogs have decreased ATP and 2,3-diphosphoglycerate (2,3-DPG) production and increased fragility under alkaline conditions. The disease is characterized by chronic hemolysis with marked reticulocytosis. The marked regenerative response may compensate for the ongoing hemolysis; therefore affected animals are not necessarily anemic. However, acute intravascular hemolytic episodes may occur with hyperventilation-induced alkalemia. Lesions are typical of hemolytic anemia and include pale mucous membranes, icterus, hepatosplenomegaly, and dark red urine with microscopic EMH and marrow erythroid hyperplasia. A single DNA-based test is available to detect the common mutation.

Erythrocyte Structural Abnormalities. Congenital erythrocyte structural abnormalities may occur with abnormal membrane composition or defective proteins within the membrane or cytoskeleton. Some of these morphologic changes occur concurrently with clinical disease, but others do not.

Hereditary stomatocytosis is recognized in Alaskan malamutes, Drentse patrijshonds, and schnauzers. The specific defects are not known, but they are likely different in the various dog breeds. However, all affected dogs have stomatocytes on blood smear evaluation, as identified by their slit-shaped area of central pallor. Erythrocytes also have increased osmotic fragility and decreased survival. Schnauzers are clinically healthy and not anemic but do have reticulocytosis, suggesting that the hemolytic anemia is compensated by erythroid hyperplasia. Mild to marked hemolytic anemia is documented in Alaskan malamutes and Drentse patrijshonds. Alaskan malamutes have concurrent short-limb dwarfism, and Drentse patrijshonds have hypertrophic gastritis and polycystic kidney disease.

Other (presumably heritable) erythrocyte abnormalities in dogs that do not have clinical signs include elliptocytosis caused by band 4.1 deficiency or β-spectrin mutation, and familial macrocytosis and dyshematopoiesis in poodles.

Scott's Syndrome. An inherited thrombopathy resembling Scott's syndrome in human beings, in which platelets lack normal procoagulant activity, has been recognized in a family of German shepherd dogs. The specific defect in these dogs has not been identified on the molecular level but involves impaired expression of phosphatidylserine on the platelet surface. Affected dogs have a mild to moderate clinical bleeding tendency characterized by epistaxis, hyphema, intramuscular hematoma formation, and increased hemorrhage with surgery.

Macrothrombocytopenia. Macrothrombocytopenia is an inherited condition in Cavalier King Charles spaniels in which there are lower than normal concentrations of platelets with enlarged and giant platelets. The condition is caused by defective β_1-tubulin, which results in impaired microtubule assembly. Affected dogs are asymptomatic but may have abnormal platelet aggregation in vitro.

Infectious Diseases

Canine Distemper. Canine distemper virus preferentially infects lymphoid, epithelial, and nervous cells and is presented in greater detail in the lymphoid section. Canine distemper virus may also infect other hematopoietic cells, including erythrocytes, nonlymphoid leukocytes, and platelets (Fig. 13-33), and can cause decreased peripheral blood concentrations of neutrophils, lymphocytes, monocytes, and platelets during viremia. The thrombocytopenia is a result of virus-antibody immune complexes on platelet membranes and direct viral infection of megakaryocytes.

Disorders of Cats

Congenital Disorders

Increased Erythrocyte Osmotic Fragility. A condition characterized by increased erythrocyte osmotic fragility has been described in Abyssinian and Somali cats. The specific defect has

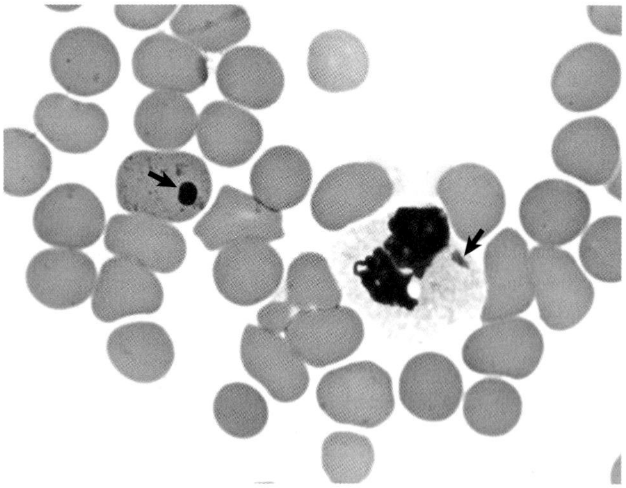

Figure 13-33 **Canine Distemper Viral Inclusions, Canine Blood Smear.** Note the viral inclusions within the erythrocyte and neutrophil *(arrows)*. Inclusions may also be present within other leukocyte types, or rarely, platelets. Diff-Quik stain. (Courtesy Dr. K.M. Boes, College of Veterinary Medicine, Virginia Polytechnic Institute and State University.)

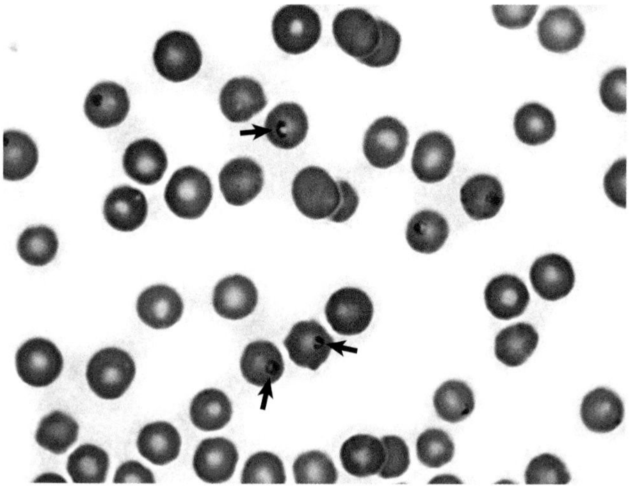

Figure 13-34 **Cytauxzoonosis, Feline Blood Smear.** Erythrocytes parasitized by *Cytauxzoon felis* contain signet ring–shaped inclusions *(arrows)*. (Courtesy Dr. K.M. Boes, College of Veterinary Medicine, Virginia Polytechnic Institute and State University.)

not been identified, but PK deficiency (which has been reported in these breeds) was excluded as the cause. Affected cats have chronic intermittent severe hemolytic anemia and often have other lesions secondary to hemolytic anemia (e.g., splenomegaly and hyperbilirubinemia).

Infectious Diseases

Cytauxzoonosis. Cytauxzoonosis is a severe, often fatal disease of domestic cats caused by the protozoal organism, *Cytauxzoon felis*. Disease is relatively common in the south central United States, particularly during summer months. Bobcats (*Lynx rufus*) and other wild felids are thought to be wildlife reservoirs of disease. *C. felis* is transmitted by a tick vector, *Dermacentor variabilis*, which is probably essential for infectivity of the organism.

Cytauxzoonosis has a schizogenous phase within macrophages throughout the body (especially liver, spleen, lung, lymph nodes, and bone marrow) that causes systemic illness. These schizont-containing macrophages enlarge and accumulate within the walls of veins, eventually causing vessel occlusion, circulatory impairment, and tissue hypoxia. Later in disease, merozoites released from schizonts enter erythrocytes, resulting in an erythrocytic phase of infection. Infected domestic cats often have nonregenerative anemia, but the pathogenesis for the anemia is unclear. However, it likely represents preregenerative hemolytic anemia because erythrocyte phagocytosis is a prominent finding in many organs. Infected cats often also develop neutropenia and thrombocytopenia, which likely result from inflammation and disseminated intravascular coagulation, respectively.

On blood smear evaluation, signet ring–shaped erythrocytic inclusions (piroplasms) may be observed during the erythrocytic phase of disease (Fig. 13-34). These inclusions closely resemble small-form *Babesia* (see Fig. 13-24, *A*) and some *Theileria* organisms. Postmortem examination typically shows pallor, icterus, splenomegaly, enlarged and red lymph nodes, diffuse pulmonary congestion and edema, and multisystemic petechiae and ecchymoses. Vascular obstruction may cause marked distention of abdominal veins. Cavitary effusions are present in some cats. Microscopically, large, schizont-laden macrophages accumulate within venous and sinusoidal lumens and often completely occlude the lumens (Fig. 13-35).

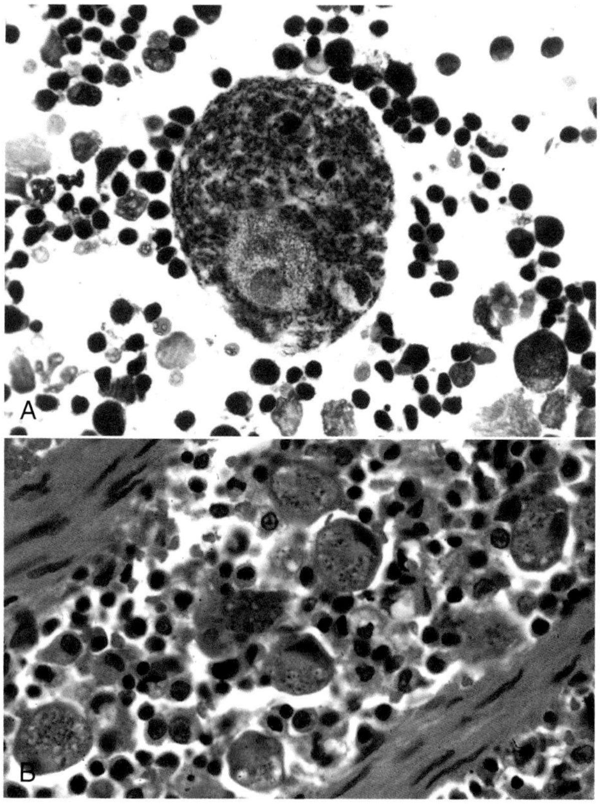

Figure 13-35 **Cytauxzoonosis, Tissue Aspirate (A) and Biopsy (B), Cat. A,** Lymph node aspirate. A large macrophage *(center of figure)* is laden with schizonts of *Cytauxzoon felis*. Wright's stain. **B,** Splenic macrophages are filled with *Cytauxzoon* organisms. H&E stain. (**A** courtesy Dr. D.F. Edwards, College of Veterinary Medicine, University of Tennessee. **B** courtesy Dr. A.R. Doster, University of Nebraska; and Noah's Arkive, College of Veterinary Medicine, The University of Georgia.)

Erythrophagocytosis, thrombosis, and histologic changes of ischemia are common, especially within the spleen, liver, and lungs.

Affected cats typically become acutely ill with fever, pallor, and icterus and usually die within 2 to 3 days. For many years, cytauxzoonosis was considered to be almost always fatal. However, a recent report, in which numerous cats from a subregion of the endemic area in the United States survived infection with an organism with greater than 99% homology to *Cytauxzoon felis*, suggests the emergence of a less virulent strain.

Feline Leukemia Virus. FeLV is an oncogenic, immunosuppressive lentivirus that causes hematologic abnormalities of widely varying types and severity. Manifestations of disease caused by FeLV infection vary depending on dose, viral genetics, and host factors, but normal hematopoiesis is probably suppressed to some degree in all cases.

FeLV infects hematopoietic precursor cells soon after the animal is exposed and continues to replicate in hematopoietic and lymphatic tissue of animals that remain persistently viremic. The virus disrupts normal hematopoiesis by inducing genetic mutations, by other direct effects of the virus on infected hematopoietic cells, or by an altered host immune system. Hematologic changes include dysmyelopoiesis with resultant cytopenias or abnormal cell morphologic features, and neoplastic transformation of hematopoietic cells (leukemia). A notable form of dysplasia is the presence of macrocytic erythrocytes (*macrocytes*) and metarubricytosis in the absence of erythrocyte regeneration (*inappropriate metarubricytosis*). The relatively uncommon subgroup C viruses cause erythroid hypoplasia, probably because of infection of early-stage erythroid precursors. FeLV may be detected in megakaryocytes and platelets in infected cats and may result in platelet abnormalities, including thrombocytopenia, thrombocytosis, increased platelet size, and decreased function. Proposed mechanisms of FeLV-induced thrombocytopenia include direct cytopathic effects, myelophthisis, and immune-mediated destruction. Platelet life span and function have been shown to be decreased in FeLV-positive cats. Persistently viremic cats are immunosuppressed and are prone to developing other diseases, including infectious diseases, bone marrow disorders, and lymphoma.

CBC abnormalities attributed to FeLV infection include various cytopenias, especially nonregenerative anemia, which may be persistent or cyclical. Regenerative anemia may also occur with FeLV infection, often because of coinfection with *M. haemofelis*. Hematopoietic cell dysplasia or neoplasia may also be evident. Grossly, infected cats are often pale, but other lesions are dependent upon the presence of other cytopenias or concurrent disease. Microscopically, the bone marrow is hypocellular, normocellular, or hypercellular. There may be erythroid hypoplasia, erythroid hyperplasia with maturation arrest, or acute leukemia.

Feline Immunodeficiency Virus. Feline immunodeficiency virus (FIV), another feline lentivirus, causes anemia in a minority of infected cats. Immunosuppressive effects of FIV from thymic depletion are discussed elsewhere. It is generally accepted that anemia does not result directly from FIV infection but instead develops because of concurrent disease such as coinfection with FeLV or hemotropic mycoplasma, other infection, or malignancy. The severity and type of anemia in FIV-infected cats depends on the other specific disease processes involved.

Lymphoid/Lymphatic System

The thymus, spleen, lymph nodes, and lymph nodules, including MALT, are classified as part of both the lymphoid and immune systems. The lymphoid system (also known as lymphatic system in some texts) is broadly categorized into primary and secondary lymphoid organs. The main primary lymphoid organs include thymus, bone marrow, and bursa of Fabricius in birds and are the sites at which the B and T lymphocytes proliferate, differentiate, and mature. In mammals, lymphocytes arise from HSCs in the bone marrow, and B lymphocytes continue to develop at this site. Ruminants also have B lymphocyte proliferation and maturation within their Peyer's patches. Progenitor T lymphocytes migrate from bone marrow to mature and undergo selection in the thymus. The spleen, lymph nodes, and lymph nodules are secondary lymphoid organs and are responsible for the immune responses to antigens, such as the production of antibody and cell-mediated immune reactions. At these sites, lymphocytes are activated by antigens and undergo clonal selection, proliferation, and differentiation (see also Chapter 5). In addition, the spleen and lymph nodes contain cells of the monocyte-macrophage system and thus also participate in the phagocytosis of cells and materials.

The bone marrow is described in the first section of this chapter. The remaining primary lymphoid organ, the thymus, is described first in this section, followed by the secondary lymphoid organs: spleen, lymph nodes, and diffuse and nodular lymphatic tissues.

Dissection and Fixation of Lymphoid/Lymphatic Tissues

Errors from selection of inappropriate sampling sites and artifacts from compression and incorrect fixation for histopathologic and immunohistochemical examinations are common in routine veterinary pathologic analysis. The identification and remedies for these problems are discussed in E-Appendix 13-2.

Thymus

Structure and Function

The thymus is essential for the development and function of the immune system, specifically for the differentiation, selection, and maturation of T lymphocytes generated in the bone marrow (see also Chapter 5). The basic arrangement of the thymus in domestic animals consists of paired cervical lobes (left and right), an intermediate lobe at the thoracic inlet, and a thoracic lobe, which may be bilobed. The cervical lobes are positioned ventrolateral to the trachea, adjacent to the carotid arteries, and extend from the intermediate lobe at the thoracic inlet as far cranially as the larynx. The intermediate lobe bridges between the cervical and the thoracic lobe. The right thoracic lobe is usually small or completely absent. The left lobe lies in the ventral aspect of the cranial mediastinum (except in the ruminant, where it is dorsal) and extends caudally as far as the pericardium.

Horse—The cervical lobes in foals are small, and the thoracic lobe constitutes the bulk of the thymus.

Ruminant—The cervical lobes are large. The left and right thoracic lobes are fused and unlike other domestic animals, lie in the dorsal aspect of the cranial mediastinum.

Pig—The cervical lobes are large.

Dog—The cervical lobes regress very early and thus appear absent. The thoracic lobe extends caudally to the pericardium.

Cat—The cervical lobes are small, and the thoracic lobe, which forms the majority of the thymus, extends caudally to the pericardium and molds to its surface.

The thymus is referred to as a lymphoepithelial organ and hence is composed of epithelial and lymphoid tissue. Formed from the endoderm of the third pharyngeal pouch in the fetus, the thymic epithelium is infiltrated by blood vessels from the surrounding mesoderm, resulting in the development of the thymic epithelial reticulum. The lymphocyte population consists of bone marrow–derived progenitor cells, which fill spaces within the epithelial network. A connective tissue capsule surrounds the thymus, and attached thin septa subdivide the tissue into partially separated lobules. Each lobule is composed of a central medulla and surrounding cortex (Fig. 13-36).

The thymic cortex consists mainly of an epithelial reticulum and lymphocytes (Fig. 13-37). The stellate cells of the epithelial reticulum have elongate branching cytoplasmic processes that connect to adjacent epithelial cells through desmosomes, thus forming a supportive network (cytoreticulum). The lymphoid component is composed of differentiating lymphocytes derived from progenitor (also known as precursor) T lymphocytes in the bone marrow. The medulla is composed of similar epithelial reticular cells, many of which are much larger than those in the cortex and have a more obvious epithelial structure. Some of the epithelial reticular cells form thymic corpuscles, also called Hassall's corpuscles, which are distinctive keratinized epithelial structures (see Fig. 13-37). Interdigitating dendritic cells (DCs) are also present within the medulla, but there are far fewer lymphocytes than in the cortex.

The progenitor T lymphocytes released from the bone marrow into the blood enter the thymus in the subcapsular zone of the cortex and begin the differentiation and selection processes, developing into mature naïve T lymphocytes as they traverse the thymic cortex to the medulla. In the cortex, T lymphocytes that recognize self-molecules (major histocompatibility complex [MHC] molecules) but not self-antigens are permitted to mature by a process called *positive selection*. Cells that do not recognize MHC molecules are removed by apoptosis. Those T lymphocytes that recognize both MHC molecules and self-antigens are removed by macrophages at the corticomedullary junction, a process called *negative selection*. Because of the rigid differentiation requirements attributable to MHC restriction and tolerance (positive and negative selection, respectively), only a small fraction (<5%) of the developing T lymphocytes that arrive at the thymus from the bone marrow survive. Mature naïve T lymphocytes exit the thymus through postcapillary venules in the corticomedullary region, enter the circulation, and recirculate through secondary lymphoid tissues, primarily located in the paracortex of lymph nodes and the periarteriolar sheaths of the spleen. In these specialized sites, the mature naïve T lymphocytes are activated upon exposure to their specific antigens and undergo additional phases of development to differentiate into effector and memory cells.

The thymus attains its maximal mass relative to body weight at birth and involutes after sexual maturity; the rate of involution may vary among domestic species. The lymphoid and epithelial components are gradually replaced by loose connective tissue and fat, although remnants remain histologically, even in aged animals.

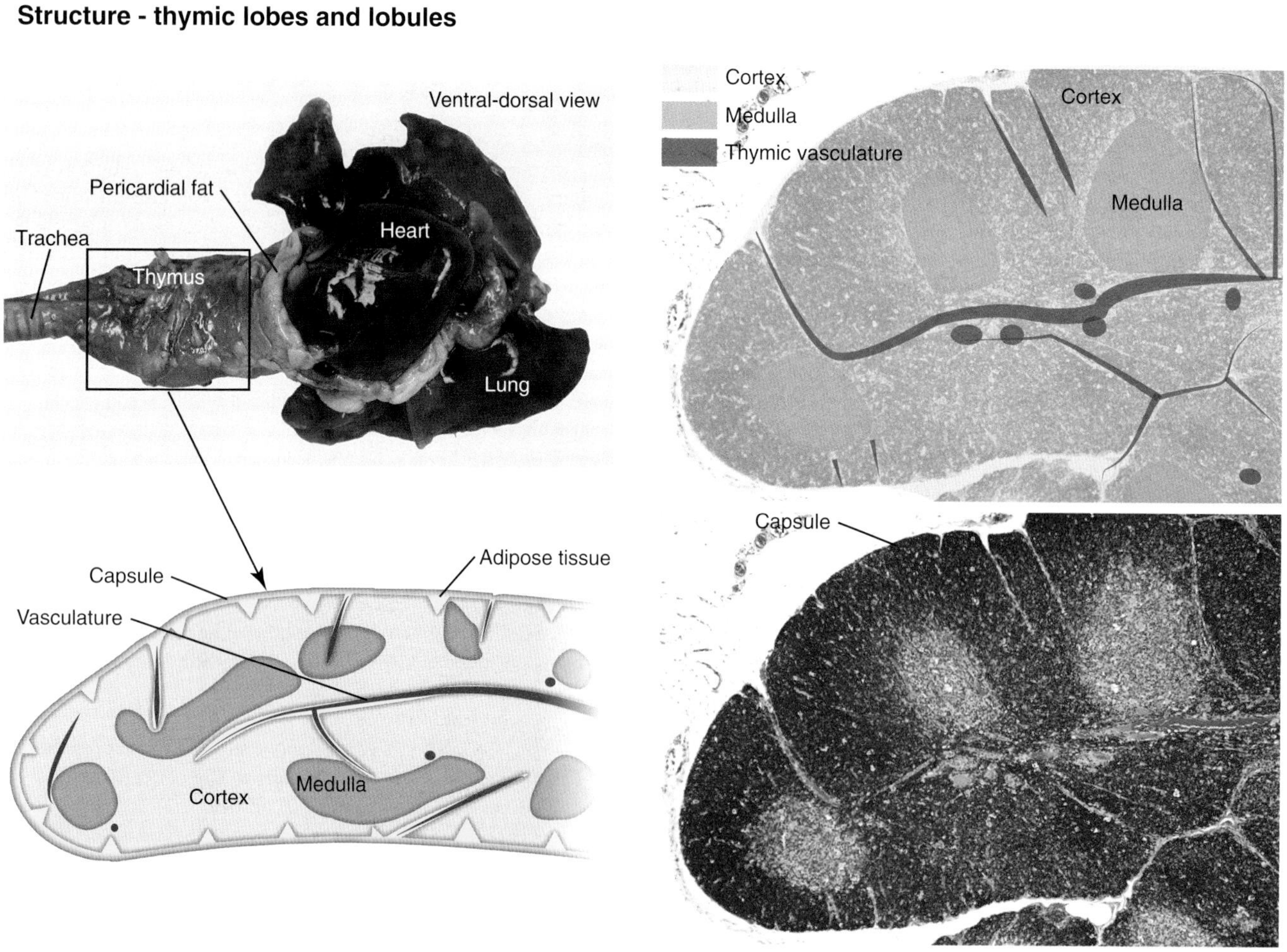

Figure 13-36 **Lobular Organization of the Thymus.** The thymus consists of several incomplete lobules. Each lobule contains an independent outer cortical region, and the central medullary region is shared by adjacent lobules. Trabeculae, extensions of the capsule down to the corticomedullary region, form the boundary of each lobule. The cortex consists of stromal cells, cortical epithelial cells, macrophages, and developing T lymphocytes (thymocytes). Major histocompatibility complex class I and II molecules are present on the surface of the cortical epithelial cells. The characteristic deep blue staining of the cortex in histologic preparation reflects the predominant dense population of T lymphocytes as compared with the less basophilic medulla, which contains a lower number of thymocytes. (Courtesy Dr. A.C. Durham, School of Veterinary Medicine, University of Pennsylvania; and Dr. J.F. Zachary, College of Veterinary Medicine, University of Illinois.)

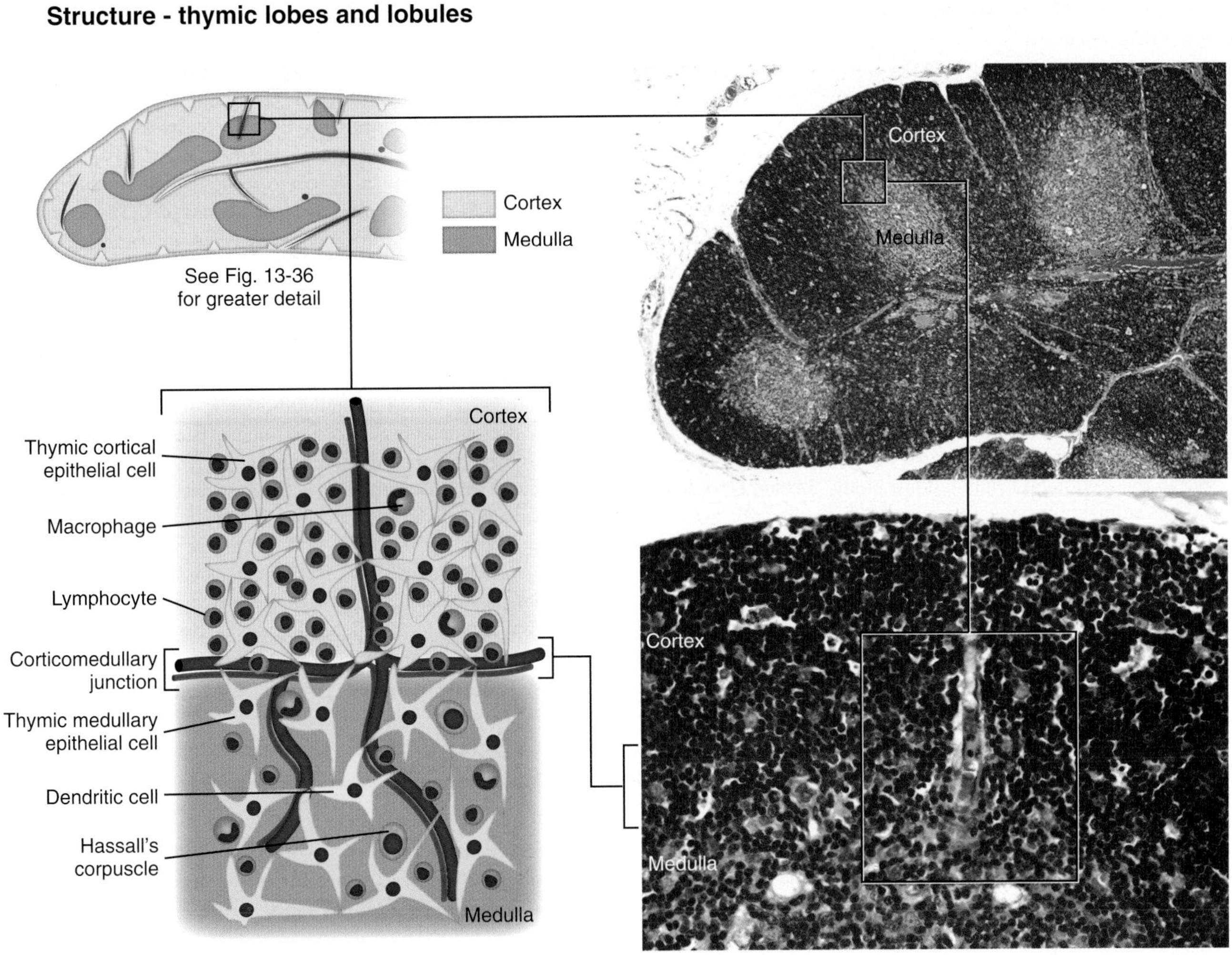

Figure 13-37 **Cell Populations in Lobules of the Thymus.** The functional thymus consists of two cell populations: stromal cells and thymocytes. The stroma consists mainly of epithelial cells present beneath the capsule, lining trabeculae and blood vessels, and forming the supportive network (cytoreticulum) within the cortex and medulla; the medulla also contains Hassall's corpuscles. Macrophages within the cortex and medulla are involved in the removal of apoptotic thymocytes eliminated during clonal selection. (Courtesy Dr. A.C. Durham, School of Veterinary Medicine, University of Pennsylvania and Dr. J.F. Zachary, College of Veterinary Medicine, University of Illinois.)

Box 13-4 Responses of the Thymus to Injury

Lymphoid atrophy (see Box 13-5)
Inflammation—rare
  Infectious agents (e.g., porcine circovirus type 2)
Hemorrhage and hematomas
Neoplasia
  Thymoma
  Lymphoma

Dysfunction/Responses to Injury

The responses of the thymus to injury and causes are listed in Boxes 13-4 and 13-5. The most common change is lymphoid atrophy caused by physical and physiologic stresses, toxins, drugs, and viral infections.

Atrophy. Because the thymus does not contain any lymphopoietic tissue, it depends on the bone marrow for the supply of progenitor T lymphocytes. Thus thymic lymphoid atrophy can be the result of either an inadequate supply of lymphocytes from the bone marrow or lysis of lymphocytes (lymphocytolysis) in the thymus. Thymic

Box 13-5 General Causes of Lymphoid Atrophy in Lymphoid Organs

Lack of antigenic stimulus
Toxins
  For example, halogenated aromatic hydrocarbons, metals (lead, mercury), mycotoxins
Chemotherapeutic agents
  For example, azathioprine, cyclophosphamide, cyclosporin A, corticosteroids
Ionizing radiation (+/–)
  For example, when lymphoid tissue is present within therapeutic field
Viruses
  For example, CDV, canine and feline parvovirus, FIV, BVDV, classic swine fever virus, EHV-1
Malnutrition and Cachexia
Aging

BVDV, Bovine viral diarrhea virus; *CDV,* canine distemper virus; *EHV-1,* equine herpesvirus 1; *FIV,* feline immunodeficiency virus.

atrophy must be differentiated from involution, which normally begins at sexual maturity. This distinction is difficult to make, unless the change is extreme or age-matched control animals are available for comparison.

Inflammation. Inflammation of the thymus is rare. Neutrophils and macrophages are often present within keratinized Hassall's corpuscles during involution and should not be mistaken for a true thymitis. Thymitis has been reported in salmon poisoning disease of dogs (see Chapter 7), epizootic bovine abortion (see Chapter 18), and in pigs infected with porcine circovirus type 2 (PCV2). Necrosis and secondary infiltrates of neutrophils and macrophages may be seen in other infectious diseases (e.g., equine herpesvirus 1 [EHV-1]).

Hemorrhage and Hematomas. Thymic enlargement is often the result of hemorrhage, hematomas, or neoplasia and is discussed further in the section on Lymphoid/Lymphatic System, Disorders of Domestic Animals: Thymus, Disorders of Dogs.

Neoplasia. Primary tumors of the thymus are thymomas, arising from the epithelial component, and lymphomas and are discussed further in the section on Disorders of Domestic Animals: Thymus.

Portals of Entry/Pathways of Spread

The main portal of entry to the thymus is hematogenous. Portals of entry used by microorganisms and other agents and substances to access the lymphatic system are summarized in Box 13-6. These portals include the blood vessels (hematogenous spread by microorganisms free in the plasma or within circulating leukocytes or erythrocytes), afferent lymphatic vessels (lymphatic spread), direct penetration, or through M (for "microfold") cells and DCs in MALT.

Defense Mechanisms/Barrier Systems

Defense mechanisms used by the thymus to protect itself against microorganisms and other agents are the innate and adaptive immune responses, discussed in Chapters 3, 4, and 5. Viruses, bacteria, and particles arriving in the lymph and blood interact with cells of the monocyte-macrophage system through phagocytosis and antigen processing and presentation. Hyperplasia of the macrophages often occurs concurrently. Antigen processing and presentation are followed by an immune response resulting in proliferation of B lymphocytes, plasma cells, and the subsequent production of antibody; proliferation of T lymphocytes may also occur.

Spleen

The relationships between anatomic structures and the different functions of the spleen are complicated. There are also anatomic differences among domestic animal species and confusion about the correct and up-to-date terminology. The following brief discussion aims to define the terms used in this chapter. The term *splenic sinusoid* is used to describe a vascular structure present in the sinusal spleen (also known as sinusoidal spleen); dogs are the only domestic animal with true splenic sinusoids. The term *red pulp vascular spaces* is used (as opposed to "sinus") to describe the vascular spaces in the red pulp of both the nonsinusal and nonsinusoidal spleens of all domestic animals.[4] The other terms used here include *marginal sinus, marginal zone, periarteriolar lymphoid sheath (PALS), periarteriolar macrophage sheath (PAMS), and splenic lymphoid follicles.*

Box 13-6 Portals of Entry into Lymphoid Organs

Thymus	MALT
Hematogenous	Hematogenous
Spleen	Migrating macrophages
Hematogenous	Dendritic cells
Direct penetration	M cells (Peyer's patches)
Lymph node	
Hematogenous	
Afferent lymphatic vessels	

MALT, Mucosa-associated lymphoid tissue.

Structure

The spleen is located in the left cranial hypogastric region of the abdomen, where it is typically suspended in the gastrosplenic ligament between the diaphragm, stomach, and the body wall. The exception is in domestic ruminants, where it is closely adhered to the left dorsolateral aspect of the rumen. The gross shape and size of the spleen vary markedly among domestic animals, but generally it is a flattened, elongated organ. Some species, notably birds, demonstrate seasonal variation in splenic shape and size.

The spleen is covered by a thick capsule composed of smooth muscle and elastic fibers, from which numerous intertwining fibromuscular trabeculae extend into the parenchyma. These trabeculae and reticular cells form a spongelike supportive matrix for the parenchyma of the mammalian spleen in all domestic species. In cattle and horses the three muscular layers of the capsule lie perpendicular to each other, forming a capsule thicker than that of carnivores. Carnivores, small ruminants, and pigs have interwoven smooth muscle within the splenic capsule, and pigs also have abundant elastic fibers within the capsule.

The spleen differs from many other organs in the organization of its parenchyma. Instead of a cortex and medulla, the spleen is divided into two distinct structural and functional components: the red pulp and white pulp (Fig. 13-38). With hematoxylin and eosin (H&E) staining, red pulp appears red-pink because of the abundance of red blood cells, whereas white pulp appears blue-purple because of the heavy concentration of lymphocytes. The *white pulp* consists of splenic follicles, populated by B lymphocytes; the PALS, inhabited by T lymphocytes; and the marginal zone at the periphery of follicles. Macrophages, antigen-presenting cells, and trafficking B and T lymphocytes populate the marginal zone. The radial arteries, branches of the central artery (also known as central arteriole), and capillaries from both red and white pulp drain into the marginal sinus of the marginal zone, although the latter has not been shown to be the case in all species to the same degree (e.g., the cat has a small marginal sinus but a well-developed PAMS) (Figs. 13-39 and 13-40). The *red pulp* consists of cells of the monocyte-macrophage system, PAMS, sinusoids (dogs, rats, and human beings only), red pulp vascular spaces, and associated stromal elements such as reticular cells, fibroblasts, and trabecular myocytes. The labyrinth of the splenic red pulp vascular spaces serves as both a functional and physical filter for circulating blood cells.

The blood circulation of the spleen is particularly suited to enable its functions, namely, (1) filtering and clearing the blood of

[4]There are numerous synonyms and misuse of terms within the literature, which have contributed to the confusion over terminology for *red pulp vascular spaces*. These terms include reticular space, red pulp, splenic cords, sinuses, red pulp sinuses, sinus spaces, pulp spaces, mesh space of the spleen, reticular cell-lined meshwork, interstices of the reticulum network, blood-filled reticular meshwork of the red pulp, chordal spaces, splenic cords, and cords of Billroth. The latter two terms are defined as the red pulp between the sinusoids, which most domestic animals do not have (except the dog). Therefore the term *red pulp vascular spaces* is more appropriate.

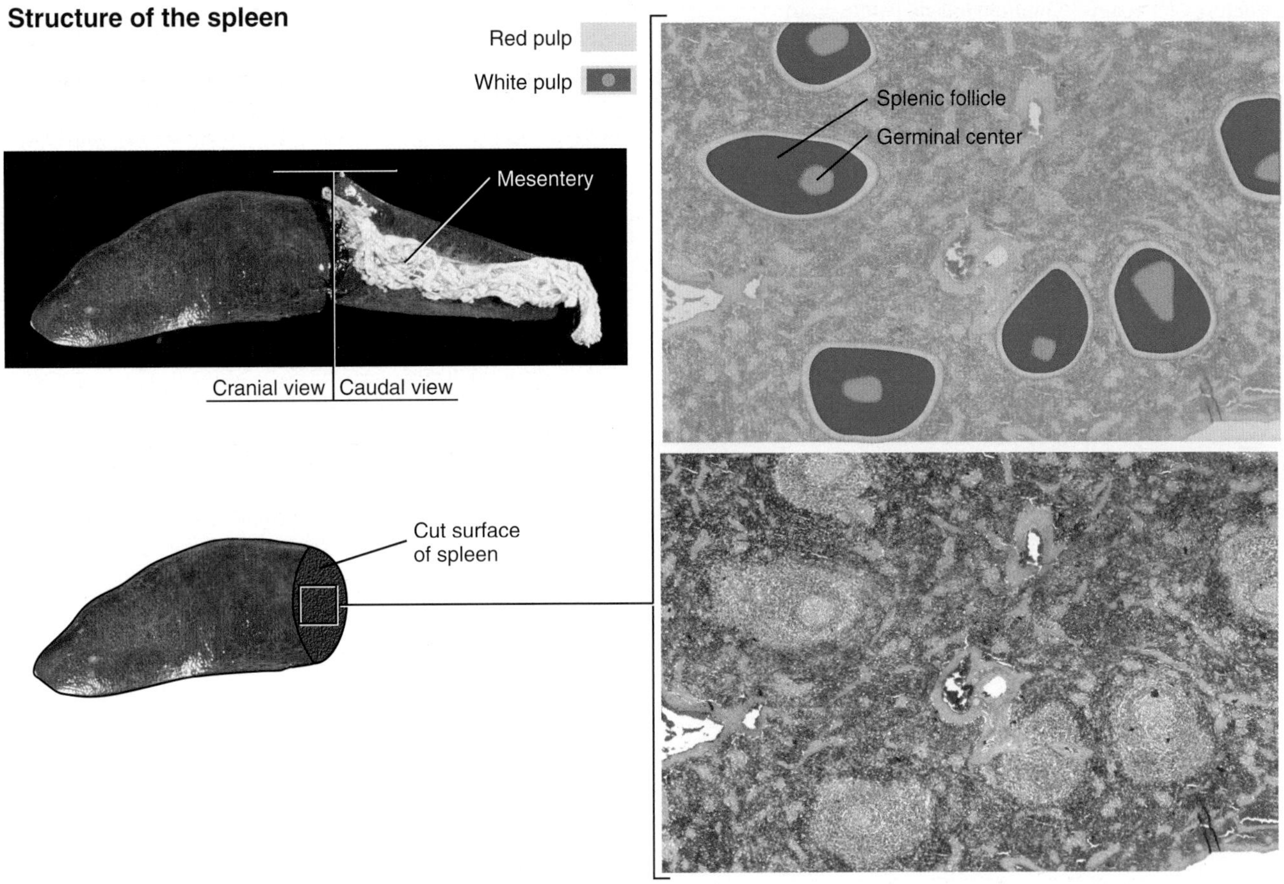

Figure 13-38 **Structure of the Spleen—Red and White Pulp.** The spleen is organized into two distinct components. The *red pulp* consists of cells of the monocyte-macrophage system, periarteriolar macrophage sheaths, sinusoids (dogs, rats and human beings only), red pulp vascular spaces, and associated stromal elements such as reticular cells, fibroblasts and trabecular myocytes. The *white pulp* is composed of splenic follicles (B lymphocytes), periarteriolar sheaths (T lymphocytes), and the marginal zone. (Courtesy Dr. A.C. Durham, School of Veterinary Medicine, University of Pennsylvania; Dr. M.D. McGavin, College of Veterinary Medicine, University of Tennessee; and Dr. J.F. Zachary, College of Veterinary Medicine, University of Illinois.)

particulate matter and senescent cells; (2) transporting recirculating lymphocytes and naïve B and T lymphocytes to the follicle and PALS, respectively, to fulfill their specific immune functions; and (3) storage of blood in some domestic animal species (dog, cat, and horse) (Fig. 13-41). Phagocytosis is particularly effective in the spleen because blood flows through areas within the red pulp that are populated with increased concentrations of macrophages, namely, within the marginal sinuses, in cuffs around the penicillar arteries (PAMS), diffusely on the reticular walls of the red pulp vascular spaces, and along the sinusoids in dogs. Trafficking of naïve and recirculating lymphocytes is facilitated by the proximity of the marginal sinus to the follicular germinal centers and PALS.

Maps of the vascular blood flow in sinusoidal and nonsinusoidal spleens are illustrated in Figures 13-41 to 13-43. The celiac artery is the major branch of the abdominal aorta from which the splenic artery arises. The splenic artery enters the splenic capsule at the hilus, where it branches and enters the fibromuscular trabeculae as trabecular arteries to supply the splenic parenchyma. Trabecular arteries become the central arteries of the white pulp and are surrounded by cuffs of T lymphocytes forming the PALS. The splenic follicles, populated by B lymphocytes, are eccentrically embedded within or just adjacent to the PALS. The central arteries send branches—the radial arteries—to supply the marginal sinus surrounding the splenic follicles. Thus the cells at the circumferences of the follicles are brought into intimate contact with blood-borne antigens and trafficking B and T lymphocytes in the marginal sinus. As a result of this pattern of blood flow, macrophages in the marginal sinus have the first opportunity to phagocytize antigens, bacteria, particles, and other material before macrophages in the sinusoids (in the dog) or in the PAMS and red pulp vascular spaces (all other domestic animals). In the dog the marginal sinus drains into the sinusoids, but in other domestic animals it drains into the red pulp vascular spaces.

The central arteries leave the white pulp, enter the red pulp, and branch into smaller penicillar arterioles. Each arteriole is surrounded by a sheath of macrophages known as periarteriolar macrophage sheaths (PAMS, previously known as ellipsoids), which are notably prominent in pigs, dogs, and cats. In horses, cattle, pigs, and cats the terminal branches of the penicillar arterioles empty into the red pulp vascular spaces lined by reticular cells. Because the red pulp vascular spaces are not lined by endothelium, this type of circulation is known as an *open system*. This system is in contrast to the sinusoidal spleen of the dog (also of the rat and human beings), where the branches of the central artery of the white pulp and vessels from the marginal sinus enter into the sinusoids, which are lined by a discontinuous endothelium, and these empty into splenic venules. This type of circulation is known as a *closed system* because the blood flow is through blood vessels (arterioles, capillaries, sinusoids, and venules), all of which are lined by endothelium. Although circulation in the red pulp is anatomically *open* in nonsinusoidal spleens, under certain conditions (e.g., during splenic contraction) the circulation is functionally closed, and the blood in the red pulp is

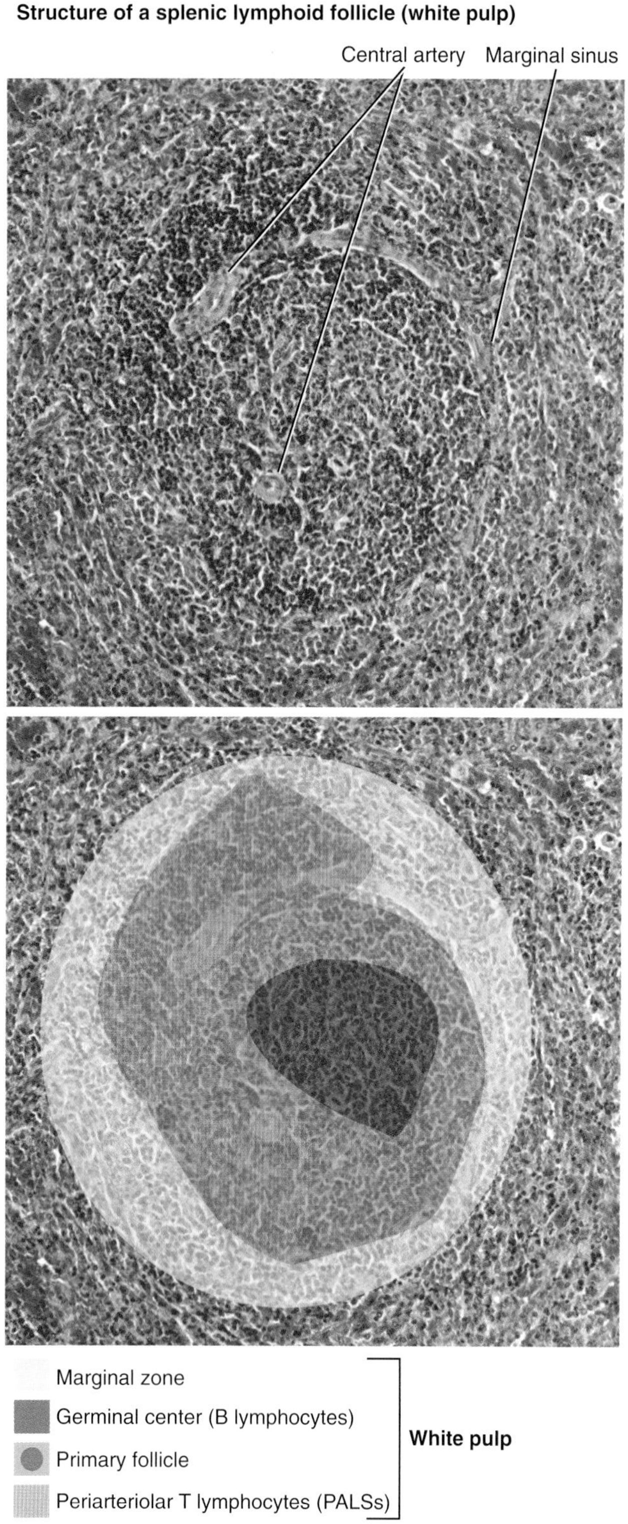

Figure 13-39 **Structure of a Splenic Lymphoid Follicle (White Pulp).** The splenic white pulp is organized into periarteriolar sheaths (PALSs) around central arteries composed mainly of T lymphocytes, splenic follicles primarily composed of B lymphocytes, and the marginal zone, which forms the outer rim of the white pulp nodule. When exposed to antigen, the splenic lymphoid follicles develop germinal centers. (Courtesy Dr. A.C. Durham, School of Veterinary Medicine, University of Pennsylvania; Dr. M.D. McGavin, College of Veterinary Medicine, University of Tennessee; and Dr. J.F. Zachary, College of Veterinary Medicine, University of Illinois.)

diverted into "channels" lined by reticular cells. Because the dog has both sinusoids and red pulp vascular spaces, it has both open and closed splenic circulations, which may allow for both fast and slow flows of blood depending on the physiologic need of the animal. Blood flowing through the sinusoids or red pulp vascular spaces is under the surveillance of macrophages. In dogs the pseudopodia of these perisinusoidal macrophages project into the sinusoidal lumen through the spaces in the discontinuous endothelium. In all domestic animals, blood in the red pulp vascular spaces is under surveillance of macrophages attached to the reticular walls. Blood from the red pulp vascular spaces and sinusoids then drains into the splenic venules, splenic veins, and ultimately into the portal vein, which empties into the liver.

Function

The spleen filters blood and removes foreign particles, bacteria, and erythrocytes that are senescent, have structural membrane abnormalities, or are infected with hemotropic parasites. As a secondary lymphoid organ, its immunologic functions include the activation of macrophages to process and present antigen, the proliferation of B lymphocytes and production of antibody and biologic molecules, and the interaction of T lymphocytes and antigens. In some species the spleen stores significant quantities of blood (Box 13-7). The functions of the spleen are best considered on the basis of the two main components of the spleen: the red and white pulp and the anatomic systems contained within them (monocyte-macrophage system, red pulp vascular spaces, and hematopoiesis in the red pulp, and the B and T lymphocyte systems within the white pulp).

Red Pulp

Monocyte-Macrophage System. Within the red pulp, macrophages are located in the marginal sinus, PAMS, and attached to the reticular walls of the red pulp vascular spaces. In the dog, macrophages are also located perisinusoidally. The supportive reticular network of the red pulp vascular spaces is composed of a fine meshwork of reticular fibers made of type III collagen, on which macrophages are dispersed. Exactly in which of these concentrations of macrophages phagocytosis of blood-borne particles takes place depends upon (1) the sequence in which they are exposed to the incoming blood, (2) the concentration of macrophages in these areas (e.g., the cat marginal sinus is small and thus not a major site of clearance; there is a compensatory increase in PAMS for phagocytosis), and (3) the functions of the macrophages. Some of the macrophages in the marginal sinus and marginal zone are responsible for phagocytosis of particulate matter and others for the trapping and ingestion of antigens and antigen-antibody complexes. Macrophages responsible for phagocytosis of blood-borne foreign material (Fig. 13-44), bacteria, and senescent and/or damaged erythrocytes (e.g., as seen in immune-mediated anemias and infections with hemotropic parasites) are also found in the red pulp. In the dog, sinusoidal macrophages remove entire erythrocytes (erythrophagocytosis), as well as portions of an erythrocyte's membrane and cytoplasmic inclusions, such as nuclear remnants like Heinz bodies, by a process called *pitting*. As such, the presence of large numbers of nuclear remnants in erythrocytes in canine blood smears may indicate malfunction of the sinusoidal system. The normal rate of removal of senescent erythrocytes from the circulating blood does not cause an increase in size of the spleen; however, splenomegaly can be observed when large numbers of defective erythrocytes must be removed, as in cases of severe acute hemolytic anemia. Nonsinusoidal spleens lack the fenestrated endothelium and perisinusoidal macrophages of canine sinusoids that allow for slow processing of red blood cells to determine which are to be returned to the

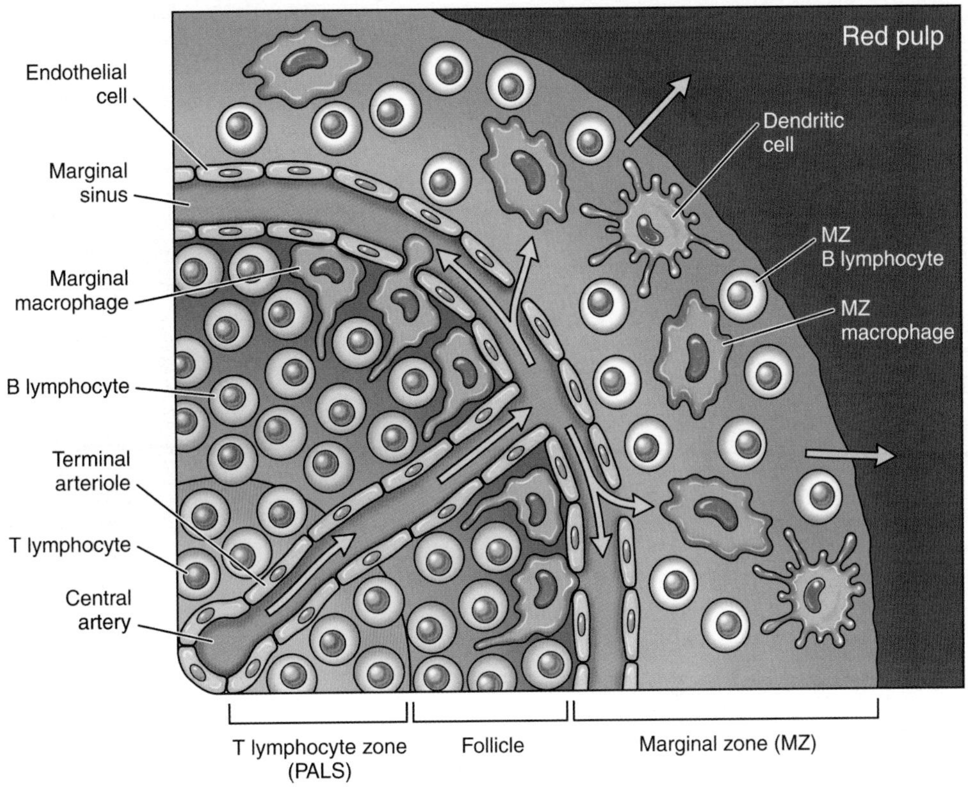

Figure 13-40 **Structure of the Marginal Zone in the Splenic Follicle.** Antigens, bacteria, particles, and other material enter the follicle via the central arteries and reach the marginal sinus, where they are phagocytized by macrophages of the marginal zone. Once captured by these macrophages, blood-borne antigens are processed and presented to the lymphocytes within the white pulp.

circulation, pitted, or phagocytized. Instead, the macrophages of the red pulp perform these functions, and phagocytized cells remain in the red pulp vascular spaces. The location of the primary sites of pitting in nonsinusoidal spleens is unclear, but it is likely that most erythrophagocytosis takes place in the red pulp vascular spaces. The cat's spleen is deficient in pitting, and removal of Heinz bodies is slow; however, some erythrophagocytosis does occur in the marginal sinus.

The macrophages of the sinusoids, marginal sinus, and red pulp vascular spaces are of bone marrow origin. From the bone marrow these cells circulate in the blood as monocytes and migrate into the spleen. Some macrophages are replenished by local proliferation. For example, after phagocytizing large amounts of material from the blood, the macrophages of the PAMS migrate through the wall of the cuff into the adjacent red pulp, denuding the PAMS of macrophages. After 24 hours, local residual macrophages have proliferated to repopulate the PAMS. The fixed macrophages elsewhere in the body, namely, those in connective tissue, lymph nodes (sinus histiocytes), liver (Kupffer cells), lung (pulmonary intravascular macrophages and pulmonary alveolar macrophages), and brain (resident and perivascular microglial cells), are also derived from bone marrow (see Chapters 5, 8, 9, and 14).

Red Pulp Vascular Spaces

Storage or Defense Spleens. Spleens are also classified as either storage or defense spleens, based on whether or not they can store significant volumes of blood. The ability to store blood in the spleen depends on the fibromuscular composition of the splenic capsule and trabeculae. Splenic capsules and trabeculae with a low percentage of smooth muscle and elastic fibers cannot expand and contract and are designated as defense spleens. These are found in rabbits and human beings. The spleens of other domestic animal species have storage and defense functions but are classified as storage spleens because the extensive smooth muscle of the capsule and trabeculae allows the spleen to expand and contract. The spleens of ruminants and pigs are intermediate in their amount of smooth muscle and thus have limited storage capacity. Equine, canine, and feline spleens all have considerable storage and contractile capacity because of their muscular capsule, increased numbers of trabeculae, and the relatively small amount of splenic parenchyma devoted to white pulp. The storage capacity in dogs and horses is remarkable: It has been claimed that the canine spleen can store one-third of the dog's erythrocytes while the animal sleeps and the equine spleen holds one-half of the animal's circulating red cell mass (which is considered advantageous because it reduces the viscosity of the circulating blood). Storage spleens expand and contract quickly under the influence of the autonomic nervous system, via sympathetic and vagal fibers in the trabeculae and reticular walls of the red pulp vascular spaces and other circulatory disruptions, such as hypovolemic and/or cardiogenic shock. Thus storage spleens may be either grossly enlarged and congested or small with a wrinkled surface and a dry parenchyma depending on whether the spleen is congested from stored blood or shrunken from contraction (see Uniform Splenomegaly and Small Spleens).

Hematopoietic Tissue. In the developing fetus the liver is the primary site of hematopoiesis, with the spleen making a minor contribution. Shortly before or after birth, hematopoiesis ceases in the liver and spleen, and the bone marrow becomes the primary hematopoietic organ. Under certain conditions, such as severe demand due to prolonged anemia, splenic hematopoiesis can be reactivated; this outcome is called extramedullary hematopoiesis (EMH). Studies have indicated that splenic EMH in dogs and cats most commonly occurs with degenerative or inflammatory

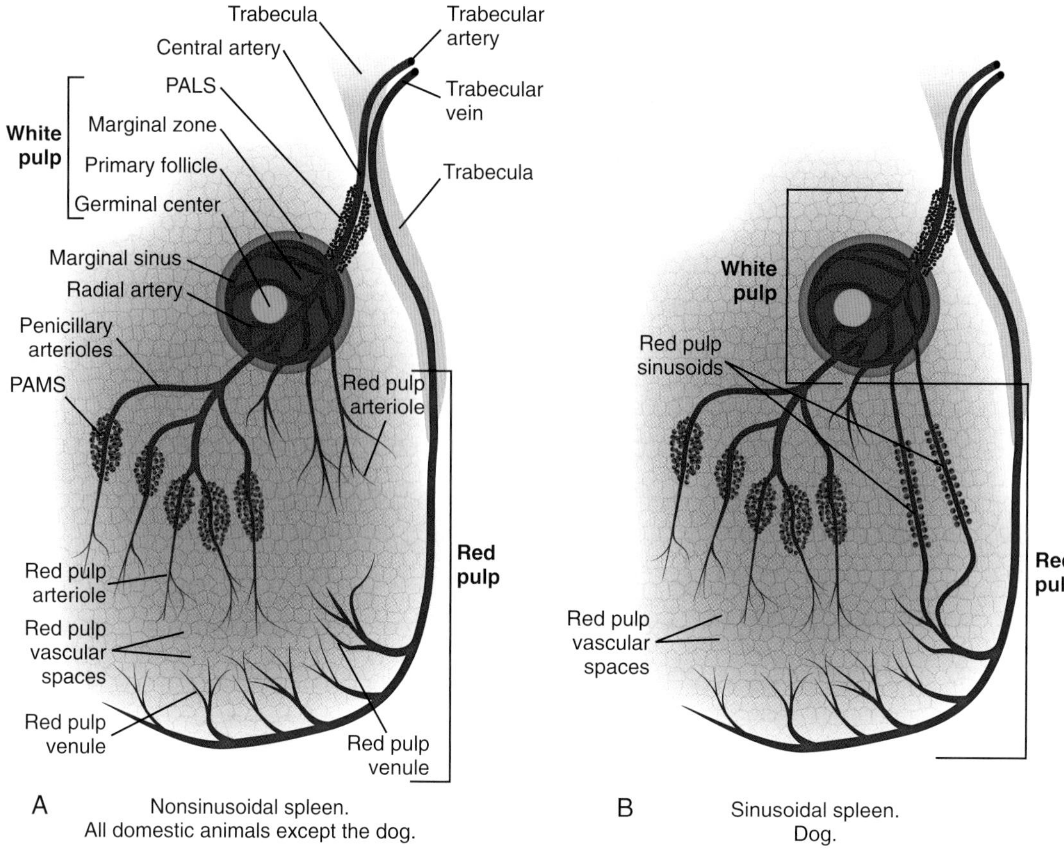

Figure 13-41 **Major Pathways of Blood Flow in Nonsinusoidal and Sinusoidal Spleens. A**, Nonsinusoidal spleen, all domestic animals except the dog. The splenic artery enters at the hilus and divides into arteries, which enter the trabeculae. When a trabecular artery emerges from a trabecula it becomes the central artery and is encased in a periarteriolar lymphoid sheath (PALS), which is composed of T lymphocytes. It then enters the splenic follicle and gives off branches—the radial arteries, which supply the marginal sinus and marginal zone. The central artery emerges from the splenic follicle to enter the red pulp and branches into the penicillary arterioles, which are enclosed in a cuff of macrophages—the periarteriolar macrophage sheath (PAMS). The emerging penicillar arteries branch into arterioles and capillaries that supply the red pulp vascular spaces (see Fig. 13-43). The red pulp vascular spaces also receive blood from capillaries draining from the marginal sinus and drain into the splenic venules and then into the trabecular veins and splenic vein. **B**, Sinusoidal spleen, dog. The blood flow is essentially the same but with the additional feature that arterioles from the marginal sinus drain into the sinusoids and some blood from the red pulp vascular space passes through slits in the sinusoidal wall to enter the sinusoid (see Fig. 13-42). This is the site of pitting and erythrophagocytosis. Note that the major flow in **A** is sequentially past concentrations of macrophages in the marginal sinus, PAMS, and red pulp vascular spaces. In **B** there is the additional route from the marginal zone into the sinusoids. The figure does not illustrate variations in anatomy in the different domestic species such as a small marginal sinus in the cat and large PAMS in the dog, pig, and cattle, or variations in the blood supply, such as the sheathed arteries emptying into the marginal sinus. (Courtesy Dr. A.C. Durham, School of Veterinary Medicine, University of Pennsylvania; Dr. M.D. McGavin, College of Veterinary Medicine, University of Tennessee; and Dr. J.F. Zachary, College of Veterinary Medicine, University of Illinois.)

conditions (e.g., hematomas, thrombosis) and may occur without concomitant hematologic disease (see Uniform Splenomegaly with a Firm Consistency). It is also found in splenic nodular hyperplasia (see Splenic Nodules with a Firm Consistency). In some species, such as the mouse, EMH is a normal function of the adult spleen and not necessarily a response to disease or hypoxic challenge. The splenic red pulp also contains large numbers of monocytes, which function as a reserve for generating tissue macrophages in response to ongoing tissue inflammation in the body.

White Pulp. White pulp consists of PALS, each with a splenic lymphoid follicle surrounded by a marginal zone. Normally these foci of white pulp are so small that they may not be visible on gross examination of a cross section of the spleen. However, if nodules are enlarged either by lymphoid hyperplasia, amyloid deposits, or a neoplastic process (e.g., lymphoma), they can become grossly visible on the cut surface, initially as 0.5- to 1.0-mm white circular foci scattered through the red pulp. In animals with storage spleens, the distention of the red pulp from stored blood separates the foci of white pulp (PALS and lymphoid follicles), making white pulp appear sparser. Splenic white pulp is organized around central arteries in the form of PALS, which are populated primarily by T lymphocytes (see Figs. 13-38, 13-39, and 13-40). Primary splenic follicles are located eccentrically in PALS and are primarily composed of B lymphocytes. When exposed to antigen, the splenic lymphoid follicles develop germinal centers (see Lymphoid/Lymphatic System, Lymph Nodes, Function). Macrophages in the white pulp follicles remove apoptotic B lymphocytes not selected for expansion because of low binding affinity for antigen. Failure of these macrophages to phagocytize has been experimentally correlated with decreased production of growth factors like TGF-β and increased production of inflammatory cytokines that predispose the animal to autoimmune conditions.

The marginal zone surrounds the marginal sinus at the interface of the white and red pulp and consists of macrophages, DCs, and T and B lymphocytes. The blood supply of the marginal sinus is from

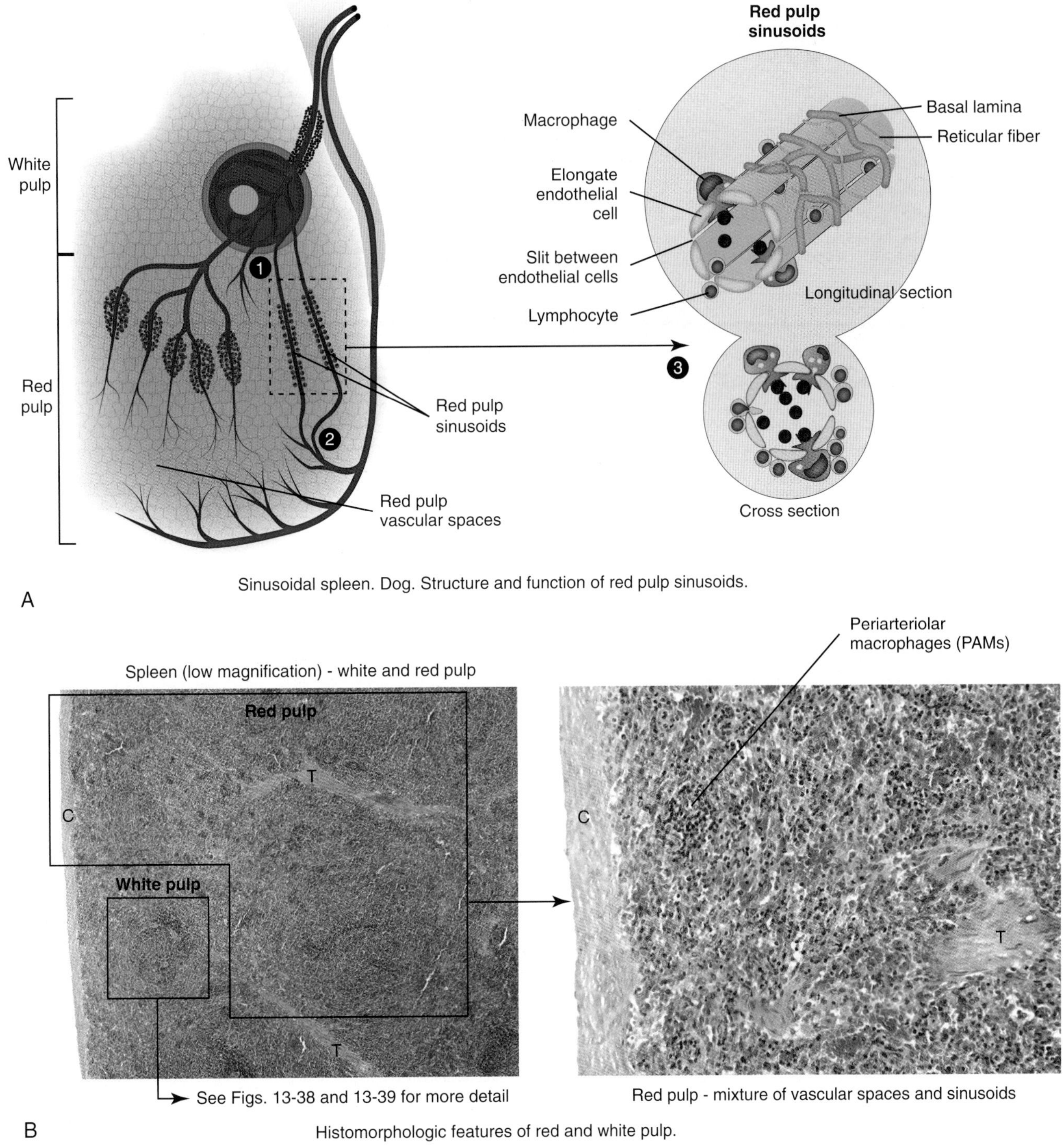

Figure 13-42 Vascular Flow in the Red Pulp of Dogs—Sinusoids. A, Sinusoidal spleen, dog. Structure and function of red pulp sinusoids. *1*, Branches of the central arteries of the white pulp and vessels from the marginal sinus enter into the sinusoids. *2*, Sinusoids are lined by a discontinuous endothelium, and these empty into splenic venules, creating a closed system of circulation. *3*, The red pulp of the dog spleen consists of both sinusoids and red pulp vascular spaces. **B,** Histomorphologic features of red and white pulp. *C*, capsule; *T*, trabeculae. (Courtesy Dr. A.C. Durham, School of Veterinary Medicine, University of Pennsylvania; Dr. M.D. McGavin, College of Veterinary Medicine, University of Tennessee; and Dr. J.F. Zachary, College of Veterinary Medicine, University of Illinois.)

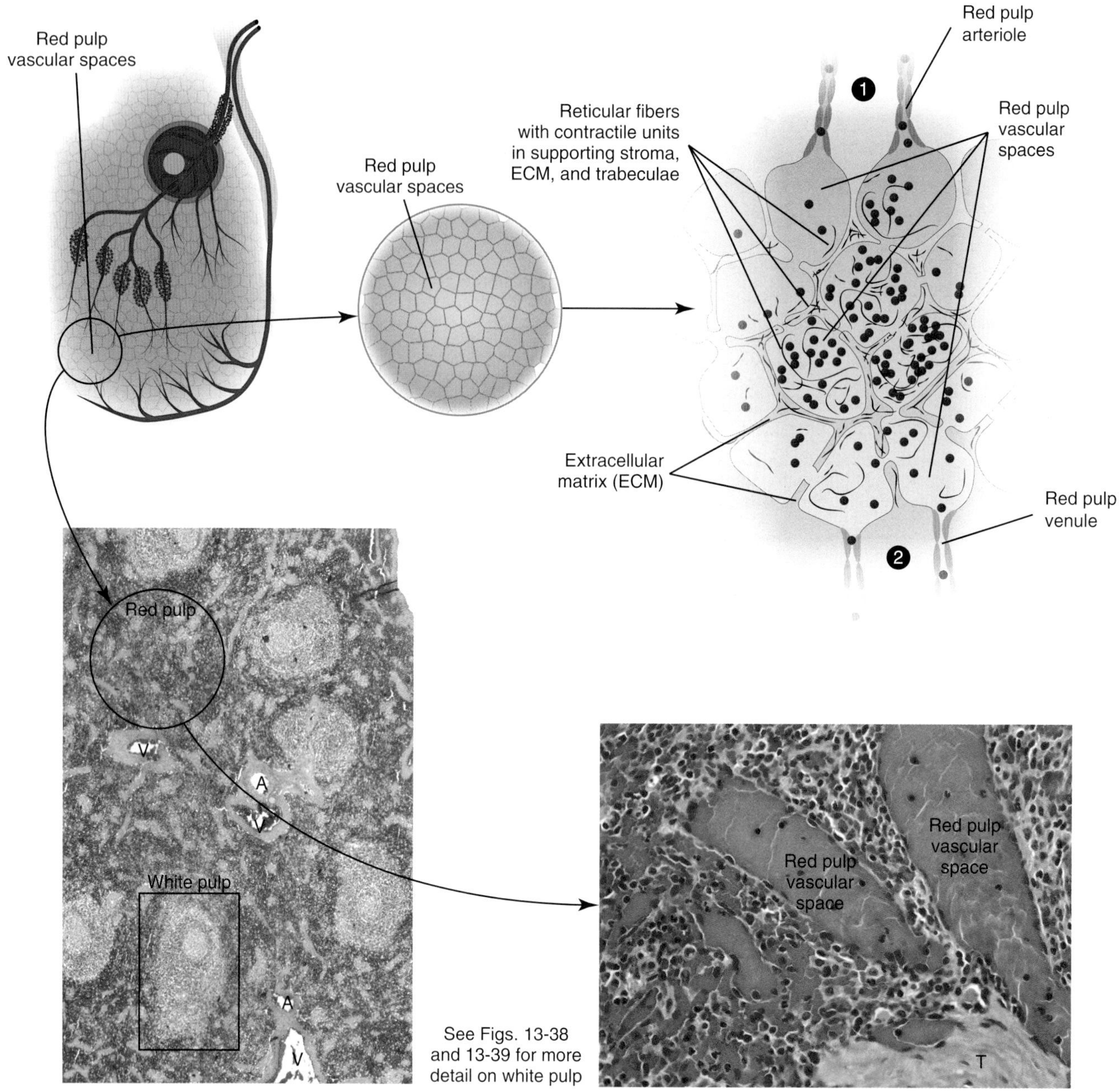

Figure 13-43 **Vascular Flow in the Red Pulp of Domestic Animals—Red Pulp Vascular Spaces.** Red pulp vascular spaces occur in all domestic animals. *1*, Blood travels into red pulp arterioles to enter red pulp vascular spaces in both types of spleens. *2*, Blood leaves red pulp vascular spaces via red pulp venules and the trabecular veins. Red pulp vascular spaces are lined by reticular cells, and macrophages attached to these reticular walls provide constant surveillance of the blood. *A*, Artery; *V*, vein; *T*, trabecula. (Courtesy Dr. A.C. Durham, School of Veterinary Medicine, University of Pennsylvania; Dr. M.D. McGavin, College of Veterinary Medicine, University of Tennessee; and Dr. J.F. Zachary, College of Veterinary Medicine, University of Illinois.)

Box 13-7 Functions of the Spleen

RED PULP
Filtration (Monocyte-Macrophage System)
Removal (phagocytosis) of foreign material and bacteria
Removal of erythrocytes
- Senescent erythrocytes
- Damaged erythrocytes (e.g., immune-mediated anemias)
- Parasitized erythrocytes (e.g., hemotropic parasites)

Storage (Red Pulp Vascular Spaces)
Storage of blood (in *storage spleens*)

Hematopoiesis
Extramedullary hematopoiesis
- Severe demand (e.g., anemias)
- Degenerative/inflammatory conditions without concomitant hematologic disease
- Incidental (e.g., within nodules of hyperplasia)

Monocytes within splenic cords
- Reserve for generating tissue macrophages in response to inflammation

WHITE PULP
Immunologic Functions
PALS, splenic lymphoid follicle
- Lymphocyte transformation and proliferation
- Production of antibodies

Marginal zone
- Homing of circulating lymphocytes in the blood
- Phagocytosis and processing of antigen
- Macrophage activation

PALS, Periarteriolar lymphoid sheath.

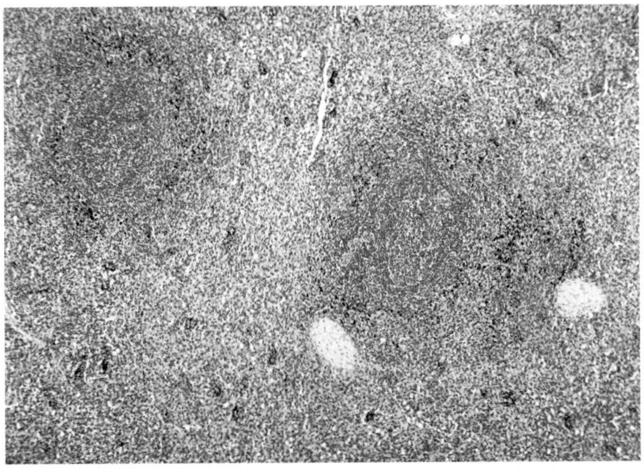

Figure 13-44 **Phagocytosis of Foreign Material by Macrophages of the Splenic Marginal Zone (Calf Injected Intravenously with Micronized Carbon Particles).** Carbon particles *(black pigment)* are present in macrophages of the marginal zone. Macrophages phagocytize blood-borne foreign material, bacteria, viruses, and senescent and/or damaged erythrocytes (as in immune-mediated anemias and infections with hemotropic parasites). Eosin counterstain. (Courtesy Dr. M.D. McGavin, College of Veterinary Medicine, University of Tennessee.)

the radial branches of the central artery, and it serves as the portal of entry into the spleen for recirculating B and T lymphocytes. From here, T lymphocytes migrate to the PALS and B lymphocytes to the germinal centers. Macrophages in the marginal zone capture blood-borne antigens, process them, and present them to the lymphocytes. B lymphocytes that recognize antigens corresponding to their receptors are activated, enter the follicle, and proliferate.

Macrophages in the marginal zone are phenotypically distinct from those in the red pulp. The red pulp macrophages function primarily to filter the blood by phagocytizing particles and by removing senescent or infected erythrocytes and pathogenic bacteria and fungi. Marginal zone macrophages are divided into two types based on their location and the type of cell surface receptors they possess. The first group is positioned toward the periphery of the marginal zone, whereas the second group, the marginal metallophilic macrophages (so called for their silver staining positivity), is at the inner margin of the marginal zone closer to the splenic follicle and PALS. It has been difficult to generate mammalian models that eliminate one of the two classes of marginal zone macrophages, so the degree to which one group specializes in a particular function is not clear. Some marginal zone macrophages actively phagocytize particulate matter or bacteria (e.g., septicemias caused by *Streptococcus pneumoniae, Listeria monocytogenes, Campylobacter jejuni,* or *Bacillus anthracis*) in the blood (see Fig. 13-40). They also play a similar role in limiting the spread of viral infections. Other marginal zone macrophages phagocytize and process antigens. Thus macrophages of the marginal zone serve to bridge the innate and adaptive immune responses by secreting inflammatory cytokines to activate other immune cells and providing receptor-based activation of marginal zone lymphocytes. Studies have shown that a loss of marginal zone macrophages coincides with decreased antigen trapping by resident B lymphocytes of the marginal zone and consequently a decrease in the early IgM response to antigens.

Dysfunction/Responses to Injury

The responses of the spleen to injury (Box 13-8) include acute inflammation, hyperplasia of the monocyte-macrophage system, hyperplasia of lymphoid tissues, atrophy of lymphoid tissues, storage of blood or contraction to expel reserve blood, and neoplasia. These responses are also best considered on the basis of the two main components of the spleen, the red and white pulp, and the anatomic systems associated with each.

Red Pulp

Monocyte-Macrophage System. The distribution and function of macrophages in the spleen is described earlier in the section on Structure and Function. These interactions are complex, and their relationships to both innate and adaptive immunity are areas of intense study (see also Chapter 5). To facilitate filtering, all of the blood in the body passes through the spleen at least once a day, and 5% of the cardiac output goes to the spleen. In dogs, blood flow and transit time depend on whether the spleen is contracted or distended; blood flow is slower in the distended spleen. The extent to which macrophages of the monocyte-macrophage system phagocytize particles depends to a large degree on the sequence in which they receive blood. In most species, macrophages of the marginal sinus are the first to receive blood, and consequently phagocytized particles and bacteria tend to be more concentrated here initially. However, there are differences among domestic animal species; the cat, for instance, has a comparatively small marginal sinus, and thus the PAMS play a larger role in phagocytosis.

The spleen is able to mount a strong response to blood-borne pathogens, which has been demonstrated in several studies. The blood of immunized rabbits injected intravenously with pneumococci cleared 98% of those bacteria within 15 minutes and 100% within an hour. The blood of dogs injected with 1 billion pneumococci per pound of body weight into the splenic artery was cleared of all bacteria in 65 minutes. After splenectomy, blood-borne

Box 13-8 Responses of the Spleen to Injury

RED PULP
Inflammation
Acute inflammation with fibrin and necrosis
Abscesses, microabscesses
Granulomatous inflammation (diffuse, multifocal, focal)

Monocyte-Macrophage System
Hyperplasia
Infectious agents
- Bacteremia/septicemia
- Facultative intracellular pathogens (e.g., *Mycobacterium bovis*)
- Fungi

Chronic hemolytic disease
Chronic splenic congestion

Red Pulp Vascular Spaces
Congestion
Blood storage or expulsion

WHITE PULP
Lymphoid hyperplasia (PALS, splenic lymphoid follicle)
Macrophage hyperplasia (marginal zone)
Atrophy (PALS, splenic lymphoid follicle; see Box 13-5)

NEOPLASIA
Primary
- Lymphoma
- Sarcoma (e.g., hemangiosarcoma, histiocytic sarcoma, leiomyosarcoma)

Metastatic

PALS, Periarteriolar lymphoid sheath.

organisms multiply rapidly and may disseminate widely in the body to cause an overwhelming postsplenectomy infection. Studies have also shown that the phagocytic function of the spleen is critical in the control of plasmodium (causative agent of malaria) in human beings and babesiosis in cattle. If the number of pathogenic bacteria in the circulation exceeds the capacity of the splenic macrophages, as in cases of severe septicemia, it may result in acute splenic congestion (see Uniform Splenomegaly with a Bloody Consistency). This may be followed by inflammation with areas of necrosis, fibrin deposition, and infiltration by neutrophils in bacteremias of pyogenic bacteria. The marginal zone can be the initial site of response to blood-borne antigens and bacteria delivered by the radial branches of the central arteries to the marginal sinus. Similar to the response of the red pulp vascular spaces, the marginal zone can become congested and with time (only hours with highly pathogenic organisms) may contain aggregates of neutrophils and macrophages. Histologically, the congestion and inflammation form a complete or partial concentric ring around the circumference of the splenic nodule (see Anthrax).

Hyperplasia of the red pulp macrophages is also seen in chronic hemolytic diseases, because there is a prolonged need for phagocytosis of erythrocytes. Similarly, chronic splenic congestion, usually the result of portal or splenic vein hypertension, can lead to proliferation of the macrophages present on the walls of the red pulp vascular spaces and results in thickening of the reticular walls between the red pulp vascular spaces. Macrophages in the red pulp also proliferate in response to fungi and facultative intracellular pathogens (e.g., *Mycobacterium bovis*) arriving hematogenously to the spleen. The number of red pulp macrophages may be augmented by monocytes recruited from the blood to form granulomatous inflammation, which may be diffuse or multifocal/focal (e.g., blastomycosis and tuberculosis, respectively).

Red Pulp Vascular Spaces. The main response to injury of the red pulp vascular spaces is congestion (see Uniform Splenomegaly with a Bloody Consistency), as well as the storage of blood or contraction to expel reserve blood.

White Pulp. The responses to injury within the white pulp are most pronounced in the splenic lymphoid follicles. Lymphoid follicular hyperplasia is a response to antigenic stimuli and results in the formation of secondary follicles; marked hyperplasia may be grossly evident. Hyperplasia of splenic lymphoid follicles follows a similar sequence of events and morphologic changes as seen in other secondary lymphoid organs and is discussed in more detail in Lymphoid/Lymphatic System, Lymph Nodes, Dysfunction/Responses to Injury. Similarly, atrophy of splenic lymphoid follicles has similar causes as lymphoid atrophy in other lymphoid organs (see Box 13-5). Briefly, atrophy occurs in response to lack of antigenic stimulation (e.g., from regression after antigenic stimulation has ceased), from the effects of toxins, antineoplastic chemotherapeutic agents, microorganisms, radiation, malnutrition, wasting/cachectic diseases, or aging, or when the bone marrow and thymus fail to supply adequate numbers of B and T lymphocytes, respectively. The follicles are depleted of lymphocytes, and with time, germinal centers and follicles disappear. The amount of the total lymphoid tissue is reduced, and the spleen may be smaller.

The response to injury of the monocyte-macrophage system in the marginal sinus and marginal zone is also phagocytosis and proliferation.

Capsule and Trabeculae. Lesions in the capsule and trabeculae are uncommon and include splenic capsulitis secondary to peritonitis, and complete or partial rupture of the splenic capsule, usually due to trauma.

Portals of Entry/Pathways of Spread

The two main portals of entry to the spleen for infectious agents are hematogenous spread and direct penetration. The splenic capsule is thick, and thus direct penetration is less common. Inflammation from an adjacent peritonitis is unlikely to penetrate the capsule into the splenic parenchyma. Cattle with traumatic reticulitis may have foreign objects migrate into the ventral extremity of the spleen, causing a splenic abscess. Splenic abscesses also develop secondary to perforation of the gastric wall in horses, due to foreign body penetration, gastric ulcers, or gastric inflammation. Portals of entry used by microorganisms and other agents and substances to access the lymphoid/lymphatic system are summarized in Box 13-6.

Defense Mechanisms/Barrier Systems

Defense mechanisms used by the spleen to protect itself against microorganisms and other agents are the innate and adaptive immune responses, discussed in Chapters 3, 4, and 5. Other defense mechanisms are structural in nature to protect against external trauma and include the thick fibrous capsule of the spleen.

Lymph Nodes

Structure

Lymph nodes are soft, pale tan, round, oval or reniform organs with a complex three-dimensional structure. On gross examination of a cross section of lymph nodes, two main areas are visible: an outer rim of cortex and an inner medulla (Fig. 13-45). To understand the pathologic response of the lymph node, it is important to consider its anatomic components and their relationship with antigen processing (Fig. 13-46):

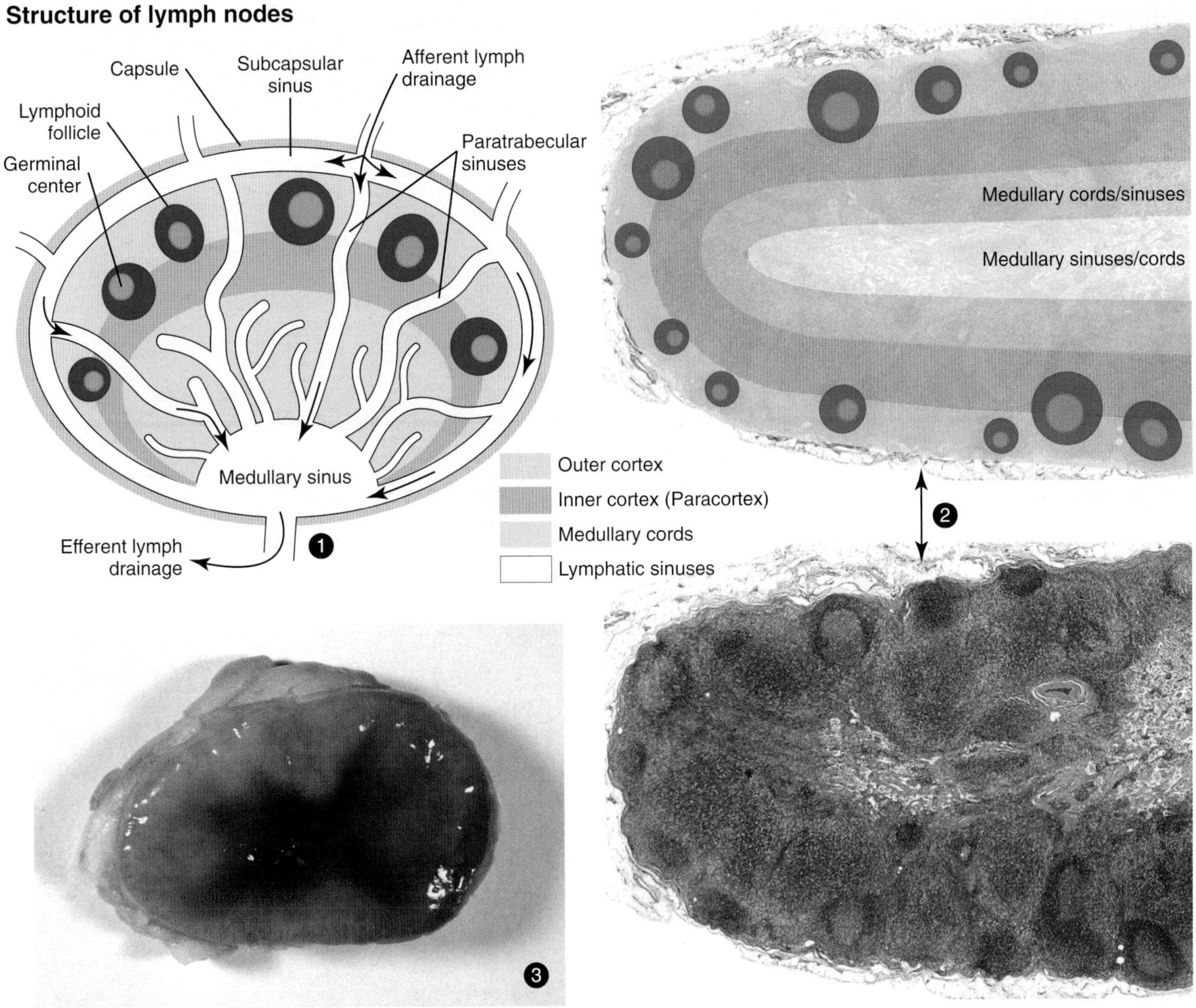

Figure 13-45 **Structure of a Lymph Node.** *1* and *2*, Lymph node architecture consists of an outer cortex composed of lymphoid follicles (B lymphocytes), inner/deep paracortex (T lymphocytes), and medulla (medullary cords and sinus). *Lower right*, Histologic section. H&E stain. *3*, Gross photograph of a lymph node: The cortex (both outer and inner) is pale tan-pink, and the medulla is dark red. (Courtesy Dr. A.C. Durham, School of Veterinary Medicine, University of Pennsylvania; Dr. M.D. McGavin, College of Veterinary Medicine, University of Tennessee; and Dr. J.F. Zachary, College of Veterinary Medicine, University of Illinois.)

- Stroma—Capsule, trabeculae, and reticulum
- Cortex—“Superficial” or “outer” cortex (lymphoid follicles, B lymphocytes)
- Paracortex—“Deep” or “inner” cortex (T lymphocytes)
- Medulla—Medullary sinuses and medullary cords
- Blood vessels—Arteries, arterioles, high endothelial venules (HEVs), efferent veins
- Lymphatic vessels—Lymphatic afferent and efferent vessels; lymphatic sinuses (subcapsular, trabecular, and medullary)
- Monocyte-macrophage system—Sinus histiocytes

Stroma. The lymph node is enclosed by a fibrous capsule penetrated by multiple afferent lymphatic vessels, which empty into the subcapsular sinus (see also Figs. 13-45 and 13-46). At the hilus, efferent lymphatic vessels and veins exit, and arteries enter the node. Fibrous trabeculae extend from the capsule into the parenchyma to provide support to the node and to house vessels and nerves. The lymph node is also supported by a meshwork of fibroblastic reticular cells and fibers. Besides providing structural support, this reticulum helps form a substratum for the migration of lymphocytes and antigen-presenting cells to the follicles and facilitates the interaction with B and T lymphocytes.

Cortex. The outer/superficial cortex contains the lymphoid follicles (also referred to as lymphoid nodules) (see Figs. 13-45 and 13-46). The follicles are designated as *primary* if they consist mainly of small lymphocytes: Mature naïve B lymphocytes expressing receptors for specific antigens exit the bone marrow and circulate through the bloodstream, lymphatic vessels, and secondary lymphoid tissues. On their arrival at lymph nodes, B lymphocytes exit through HEVs in the paracortex and home to a primary follicle (which also contains follicular DCs in addition to the resting B lymphocytes). Lymphoid follicles with germinal centers are designated as *secondary follicles*: B lymphocytes that recognize the antigen for which they are expressing receptors are activated and proliferate to form the secondary lymphoid follicles characterized by prominent germinal centers. Germinal centers are areas with a specialized

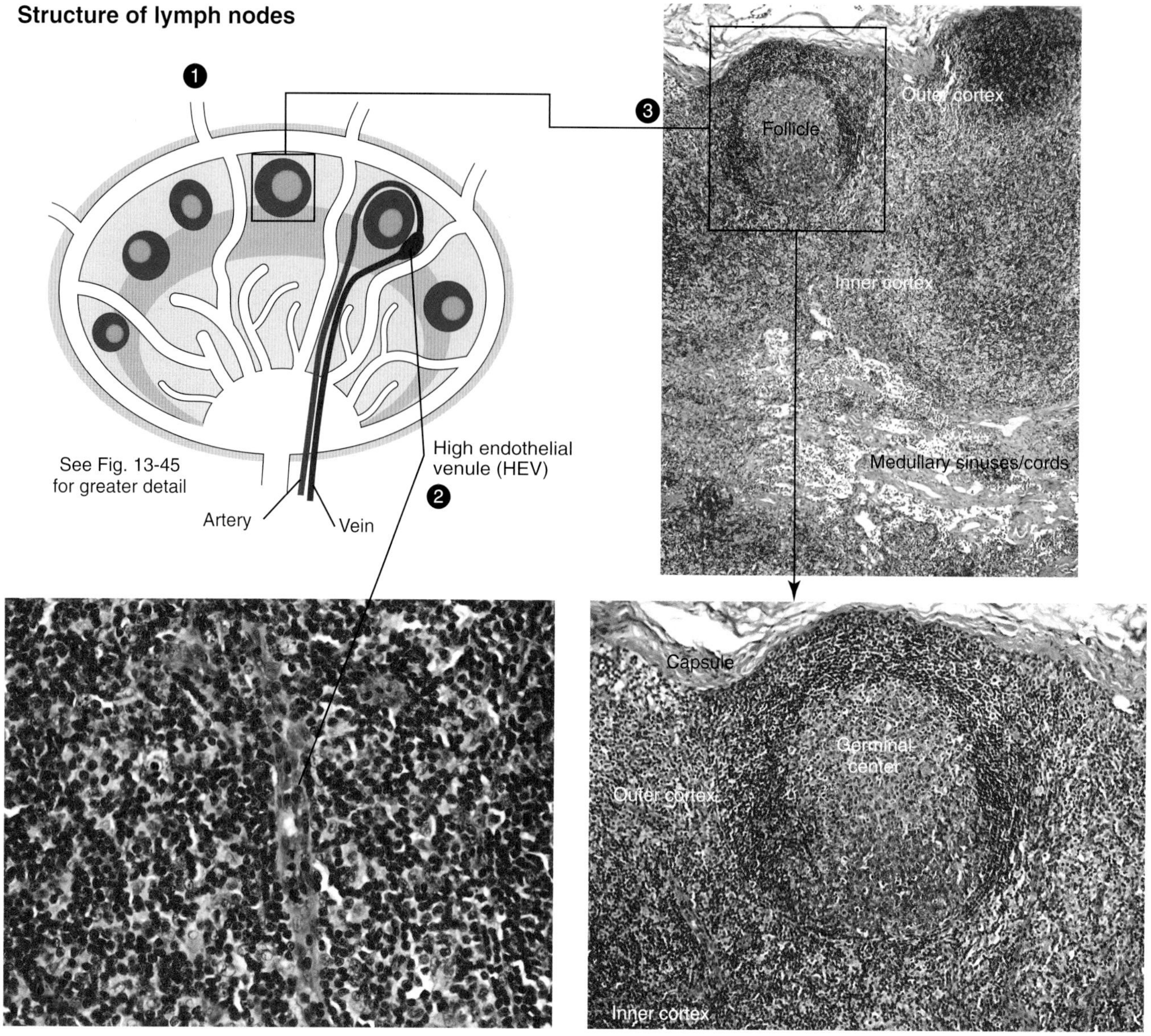

Figure 13-46 Cellular Zones of a Lymph Node. *1,* Antigen arrives in the afferent lymphatic vessels, empties into the subcapsular sinus, and drains into the trabecular and medullary sinuses. *2,* As antigens travel through the sinuses, they are captured and processed by macrophages and dendritic cells (DCs), or antigen-bearing DCs in blood can enter through high endothelial venules (HEVs). B lymphocytes encounter DCs charged with antigen, are activated, and migrate to a primary follicle to initiate germinal center formation, creating secondary follicles. *3 and lower right image,* lymphoid follicles. Germinal centers have a distinct polarity (superficial or *light zone* and a deep *dark zone*), and the mantle cell rim partially encircles the germinal center and is wider over the light pole of the follicle. (Courtesy Dr. A.C. Durham, School of Veterinary Medicine, University of Pennsylvania; Dr. M.D. McGavin, College of Veterinary Medicine, University of Tennessee; and Dr. J.F. Zachary, College of Veterinary Medicine, University of Illinois.)

microenvironment that support the proliferation and further development of B lymphocytes to increase their antigen and functional capacity (see Lymphoid/Lymphatic System, Lymph Nodes, Function). The mantle cell zone surrounds the germinal center and consists of small inactive mature naïve B lymphocytes and a smaller population of T lymphocytes (approximately 10%).

Paracortex. The diffuse lymphoid tissue of the paracortex (also referred to as the deep or inner cortex) consists mainly of T lymphocytes, as well as macrophages and DCs (see Figs. 13-45 and 13-46). This region contains the HEVs through which B and T lymphocytes migrate from the blood into the lymphoid follicles and paracortex, respectively. T and B lymphocytes may also enter the lymph node via the lymphatic vessels.

Medulla. The medulla is composed of medullary cords and medullary sinuses (see Figs. 13-45 and 13-46). The medullary cords contain macrophages, lymphocytes, and plasma cells. In a stimulated node the cords become filled with antibody-secreting plasma cells. The medullary sinuses are lined by fibroblastic reticular cells and contain macrophages ("sinus histiocytes"), which cling to reticular fibers crossing the lumen of the sinus. These macrophages phagocytize foreign material, cellular debris, and bacteria from the incoming lymph.

Vasculature: Blood Vessels, Lymphatic Vessels, and Lymphatic Sinuses. The blood vessels of the lymph node include arteries, arterioles, veins, and postcapillary venules (HEVs) lined by specialized cuboidal endothelium (see Figs. 13-45 and 13-46).

Approximately 90% to 95% of lymphocytes enter lymph nodes through the HEVs, which also play an important role in lymph fluid balance. The lymphatic vasculature consists of afferent lymphatic vessels, which pierce the capsule and drain into the subcapsular sinus. Lymph continues to drain through the trabecular sinuses to the medullary sinuses and finally exits at the hilus via efferent lymphatic vessels.

All lymph nodes receive afferent lymphatic vessels from specific areas of the body. The term *lymphocenter* is often used in veterinary anatomy to describe a lymph node or a group of lymph nodes that is consistently present at the same location and drains from the same region in all species. For example, the popliteal lymph node, caudal to the stifle, drains the distal hind limb. The tracheobronchial nodes (bronchial lymphocenter), located at the tracheal bifurcation, collect lymph from the lungs and send it to the mediastinal nodes or directly to the thoracic duct. Because lymph from a single afferent lymphatic vessel drains into a discrete region of a lymph node, only these regions of the node may be affected by the contents of a single draining lymph vessel (e.g., antigen, infectious organisms, or metastatic neoplasms [Fig. 13-47]).

The lymph node of the pig has a different structure. The afferent lymphatic vessels enter at the hilus instead of around the periphery of the node and empty lymph into the center of the node. The lymph drains to the "subcapsular" sinus (the equivalent of the medullary sinuses of other domestic animals) and then into several efferent lymphatic vessels, which pierce the outer capsule. This reversal of flow is the result of an inverted nodal architecture, with the cortex in the middle of the node surrounded by the medulla at the periphery. Thus a pig lymph node that is draining an area of hemorrhage will have blood accumulate in the periphery (subcapsular) instead of in the center of the node (which may be grossly visible).

Function

The functions of the lymph node are (1) to filter lymph of particulate matter and microorganisms, (2) to facilitate the surveillance and processing of incoming antigens via interactions with B and T lymphocytes, and (3) to produce B lymphocytes and plasma cells. Material arriving in the lymph can be subdivided into free particles and larger molecules, small molecules and free antigens, and antigen within DCs. It is helpful to consider the paths taken by particles, molecules, antigens, and cells arriving at a lymph node. The following account describes the journey of an antigen as it enters a lymph node to trigger an immune response.

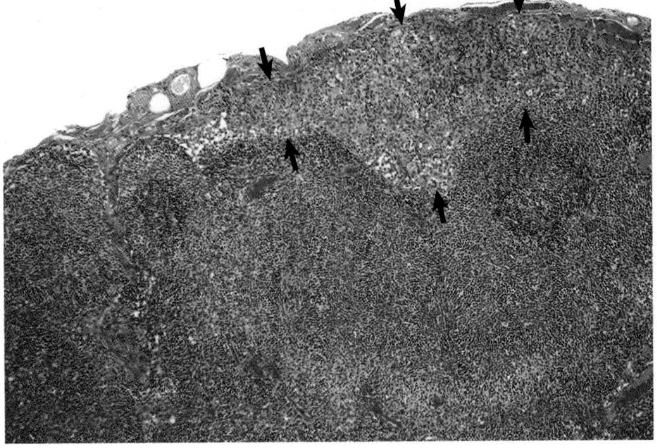

Figure 13-47 **Subcapsular Sinuses with Metastatic Carcinoma, Lymph Node, Dog.** Subcapsular sinuses are sites for embolization, lodgment, invasion, and growth of neoplastic emboli *(arrows)*, most commonly carcinomas. Emboli initially lodge in that portion of the lymph node drained by the branch of the afferent lymphatic vessel draining the site of the primary carcinoma. H&E stain. (Courtesy Dr. A.C. Durham, School of Veterinary Medicine, University of Pennsylvania.)

Antigen in the lymph arriving in the afferent lymphatic vessels empties into the subcapsular sinus. Hydrostatic pressure here is low, and reticular fibers crossing the sinus impede flow, and thus particles tend to settle, which facilitates phagocytosis by the sinus macrophages. Lymph then flows down the trabecular sinuses that line the outer surface of fibrous trabeculae, to the medullary sinus, and eventually exits via efferent vessels. As antigens within the lymph travel through the sinuses, they are captured and processed by macrophages and DCs. Alternatively, DCs charged with antigen can migrate within blood vessels to the node and enter the paracortex via the HEVs. Circulating B lymphocytes also enter across the HEVs, and if they encounter antigen-bearing DCs, there is a local reaction involving the appropriate T helper lymphocytes, B lymphocytes, and DCs. This results in the migration of the activated B lymphocytes to a primary follicle, where they initiate formation of a germinal center.

Germinal centers, upon migration of antigen-activated B lymphocytes, develop a characteristic architecture. Distinct polarity composed of a superficial or *light zone* and a deep *dark zone* is present in cases of antigenic stimulation. The light zone, orientated at the source of antigen, consists mainly of small lymphocytes, called centrocytes, which have moderate amounts of pale eosinophilic cytoplasm. The cells of the dark zone, called centroblasts, are large, densely packed lymphocytes with scant cytoplasm, giving this area a darker appearance on H&E staining. The centroblasts undergo somatic mutations of the variable regions of the immunoglobulin gene, followed by isotype class switching (from IgM to IgG or IgA). During this process most centroblasts undergo apoptosis, and cell fragments are phagocytized by macrophages, which are then termed *tingible (stainable) body macrophages*. The cells that have survived the affinity maturation process are now called centrocytes and along with T lymphocytes and follicular DCs, populate the germinal center light zone. These post–germinal center B lymphocytes leave the follicle as plasma cell precursors (immunoblasts or plasmablasts) and migrate from the cortex to the medullary cords, where they mature and excrete antibody into the efferent lymph. Some of these cells may colonize the region surrounding the mantle cell zone to form a *marginal zone*. Marginal zones are apparent only in situations of prolonged and intense immune stimulation and serve as a reservoir of memory cells. The elliptical mantle cell cuff is wider over the light pole of the follicle, though in instances of strong antigenic stimulation, the cuffs can completely encircle the germinal center.

Dysfunction/Responses to Injury

Responses to injury are listed in Box 13-9, and the responses are discussed on the basis of the following systems: sinus histiocytes of the monocyte-macrophage system, cortex, paracortex, and medulla (medullary sinuses and medullary cords).

Generally, enlarged lymph nodes can be distributed in several different patterns in the body. First, all lymph nodes throughout the body (systemic or generalized) may be enlarged (lymphadenopathy or lymphadenomegaly). This pattern is usually attributed to systemic infectious, inflammatory, or neoplastic processes. If a single lymph node or regional chain of nodes is enlarged, then the area drained by that node should be checked for lesions (e.g., evaluate the oral cavity if the mandibular lymph nodes are enlarged). Thus it is important to know the area drained by specific lymph nodes. Mesenteric lymph nodes are normally larger because of follicular

Box 13-9 Responses of the Lymph Node to Injury

HYPERPLASIA
Sinus histiocytosis (monocyte-macrophage system)
Follicular hyperplasia (B lymphocytes)
Paracortical hyperplasia (T lymphocytes)

ATROPHY
Lymphoid atrophy (see Box 13-5)

INFLAMMATION
Acute or chronic lymphadenitis

NEOPLASIA
Primary (lymphoma)
Metastatic

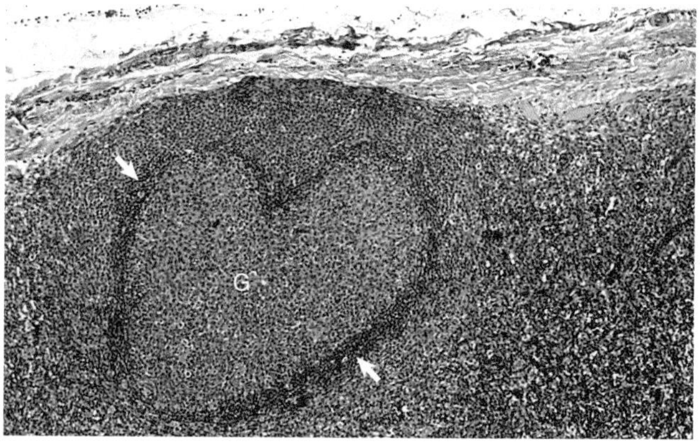

Figure 13-49 **Benign Follicular Hyperplasia, Lymph Node, Dog.** Antigenic stimulation results in a secondary follicle with germinal center formation *(G)*. The centroblasts of the germinal center undergo somatic mutations and isotype class switching, a process during which most centroblasts undergo apoptosis and cell fragments are phagocytized by tingible body macrophages. The cells that have survived the affinity maturation process (centrocytes) leave the germinal center as plasma cell precursors. Some of these cells migrate to the medullary cords, where they mature and excrete antibody into the efferent lymph, whereas others colonize the region surrounding the mantle cell zone to form a *marginal zone*. In instances of strong antigenic stimulation, the mantle cell cuffs can completely encircle the germinal center *(arrows)*. H&E stain. (Courtesy Dr. M.D. McGavin, College of Veterinary Medicine, University of Tennessee.)

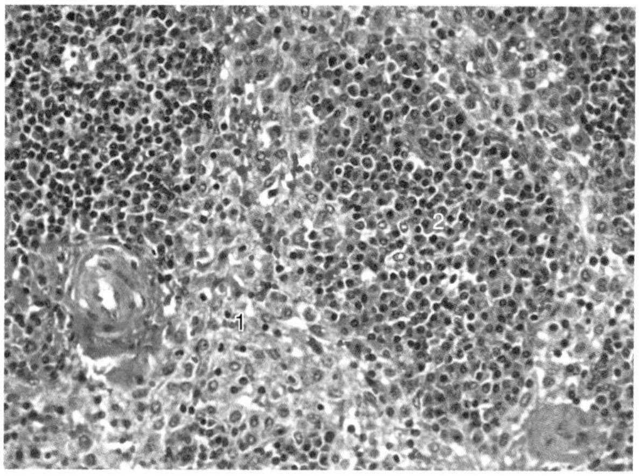

Figure 13-48 **Medullary Sinus Histiocytosis and Medullary Cord Plasmacytosis, Lymph Node, Dog.** *1,* The medullary sinuses are filled with histiocytes (macrophages) in response to drainage of infectious and noninfectious agents in the incoming lymph. *2,* The medullary cords are filled with plasma cells and fewer lymphocytes. Plasma cell precursors are formed in the germinal centers, mature into plasma cells, and migrate to the medullary cords. The presence of large numbers of plasma cells in the medullary cords indicates ongoing production of antibody due to an antigenic stimulus. (Courtesy Dr. M.D. McGavin, College of Veterinary Medicine, University of Tennessee.)

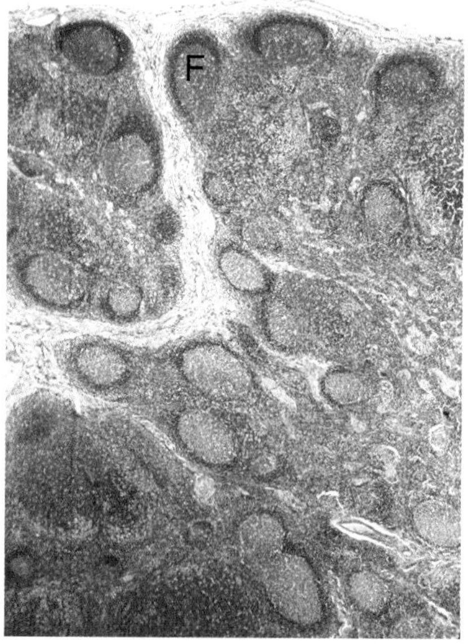

Figure 13-50 **Benign Follicular Hyperplasia, Chronic Demodicosis, Prescapular Lymph Node, Dog.** There is diffuse hyperplasia of the lymphoid follicles *(F)* with prominent and often coalescing germinal centers. H&E stain. (Courtesy Dr. M.D. McGavin, College of Veterinary Medicine, University of Tennessee.)

hyperplasia and sinus histiocytosis, because these nodes continuously receive and respond to barrages of antigens and bacteria from the intestinal tract.

Sinus Histiocytes (Monocyte-Macrophage System). Sinus histiocytes (macrophages) are part of the monocyte-macrophage system and the first line of defense against infectious and noninfectious agents in the incoming lymph. In response to these draining agents, there is hyperplasia of the macrophages ("sinus histiocytosis"), most notable in the medullary sinuses (Fig. 13-48). Leukocytes, often monocytes, may harbor intracellular pathogens (e.g., *Mycobacterium* spp., cell-associated viruses such as parvovirus), arrive in the blood or lymph, infect the lymph node, and then are disseminated throughout the lymphoid tissues of the body via the efferent lymph and circulating blood.

Cortex (Lymphoid Follicles). Follicular hyperplasia of the cortex is discussed in the section Lymphoid/Lymphatic System, Lymph Node, Function. An antigenically stimulated lymph node that is undergoing follicular hyperplasia is enlarged and has a taut capsule, and the cut surface may bulge. Histologically, the follicles contain active germinal centers with antigenic polarity (light and dark zones) (Figs. 13-49 and 13-50; also see Fig. 13-46). Depending on the duration and continued exposure to the antigen, there may also be concomitant paracortical hyperplasia and medullary cord plasmacytosis. Less florid follicular reactions will have smaller separated germinal centers, whereas nodes receiving persistent high levels of antigen stimulation may have coalescing germinal centers (termed "atypical benign follicular hyperplasia"). In such cases of chronic strong antigenemia, the highly reactive nodes may also exhibit colonization of lymphocytes into perinodal fat, and germinal centers may contain irregular lakes of eosinophilic material, known as *follicular hyalinosis*. As the immune response declines, there is follicular lymphoid depletion and the concentration of lymphocytes in the germinal centers is reduced, allowing the underlying follicular stroma (including DCs and macrophages) to become visible. With ongoing lymphocyte depletion, the mantle cell zones are thinned, less populated, and discontinuous. Eventually, residual mantle cells collapse into the follicular stroma, forming clusters of small dark cells within the bed of DCs and macrophages, referred to as *fading follicles*.

Paracortex. Paracortical atrophy may result from a variety of causes, including deficiency in lymphocyte production in the bone marrow, reduced differential selection of lymphocytes in the thymus, or destruction of lymphocytes in the lymph node by viruses, radiation, and toxins directly on the lymphocytes in the lymph node (see Box 13-5). Examination of H&E-stained sections allows evaluation of follicular activity in the cortex and the concentration of plasma cells in the medullary cords, which serve as a reasonable estimate of B lymphocyte activity for comparison.

Paracortical hyperplasia may have a nodular or diffuse appearance depending on which and how many afferent lymphatic vessels are draining antigen. This reaction may precede or be concurrent with the germinal center reaction of follicular hyperplasia. Proliferation of T lymphocytes has been reported in the paracortex (and PALS of the spleen) in malignant catarrhal fever (MCF) in cattle and in pigs with porcine reproductive and respiratory syndrome. PCV2 can cause a diffuse proliferation of macrophages within the paracortex.

Medulla (Medullary Sinuses and Cords). Responses to injury by the medullary sinuses are dilation of the sinuses and proliferation of histiocytes ("sinus histiocytosis"). Sinus macrophages proliferate in response to a wide variety of particulate matter in the lymph, including bacteria and erythrocytes (erythrophagocytosis) draining from a hemorrhagic area (see Lymphoid/Lymphatic System, Disorders of Domestic Animals: Lymph Nodes, Pigmentation of Lymph Nodes). Dilation of the sinuses due to edema occurs with many underlying conditions, including chronic cardiac failure or drainage from an acutely inflamed area. As the inflammation progresses, the sinuses become filled with neutrophils, macrophages, and occasionally fibrin, in addition to the hyperplastic resident sinus histiocytes (see Fig. 13-48). Depending on the intensity of the inflammation, the adjacent parenchyma may become affected (see Lymphoid/Lymphatic System, Disorders of Domestic Animals: Lymph Nodes, Enlarged Lymph Nodes [Lymphadenomegaly], Acute Lymphadenitis).

As pointed out in the section on Lymph Nodes, Function, after activation and proliferation of B lymphocytes in the follicle, the immunoblasts formed there move to and mature in the medullary cords, which as a result are distended with plasma cells that secrete antibody into the efferent lymphatic vessels ("medullary plasmacytosis"). The concentration of medullary plasma cells correlates with the activity of the germinal centers. As the immune response subsides, the number of plasma cells decreases and the medullary cords return to their resting state populated by few lymphocytes and scattered plasma cells.

Portals of Entry/Pathways of Spread

The two main portals of entry to the lymph node for infectious agents and antigens are afferent lymphatic vessels (lymphatic spread) and blood vessels (hematogenous spread). Portals of entry used by microorganisms and other agents and substances to access the lymphoid/lymphatic system are summarized in Box 13-6. Infectious microorganisms, either free within the lymph or within lymphocytes or monocytes, are transported to regional lymph nodes through lymphatic vessels. Agents may escape removal by phagocytosis in one lymph node and be transported via efferent lymphatic vessels to the next lymph node in the chain and cause an inflammatory or immunologic response there. This process can continue serially down a lymph node chain, and if the agent is not removed, it may eventually be transported via the lymphatic vessels to either the cervical or thoracic ducts and then disseminated throughout the body.

Although most pathogens are transported to lymph nodes via afferent lymphatic vessels, bacteria can be transported to lymph nodes hematogenously (free or within leukocytes such as monocytes) in septicemias and bacteremias. Direct penetration of a lymph node is uncommon, because it is protected by a thick fibrous capsule. Occasionally, inflammatory cells or neoplasms can extend directly into nodal parenchyma from adjacent tissues.

Defense Mechanisms/Barrier Systems

Defense mechanisms used by the lymphatic system to protect itself against microorganisms and other agents are the innate and adaptive immune responses, discussed in Chapters 3, 4, and 5. Other defense mechanisms are structural in nature to protect against external trauma and include the thick fibrous capsules of lymph nodes.

Hemal Nodes

Structure and Function

Hemal nodes are small, dark red to brown nodules found most commonly in ruminants, mainly sheep, and have also been reported in horses, primates, and some canids. Their architecture resembles that of a lymph node with lymph follicles and sinuses, except that in the hemal node, sinuses are filled with blood (E-Fig. 13-8). Because erythrophagocytosis can be present, it is presumed that hemal nodes can filter blood and remove senescent erythrocytes, but as their blood supply is small, their functional importance is not clear.

Mucosa-Associated Lymphoid Tissue

Structure and Function

MALT is the initial site for mucosal immunity and is crucial in the protection of mucosal barriers. MALT is composed of both diffuse lymphoid tissues and aggregated lymphoid (also known as lymphatic) nodules, which can be subcategorized based on their anatomic location: (1) bronchus-associated lymphoid tissue (BALT), which is often at the bifurcation of the bronchi and bronchioles; (2) tonsils (pharyngeal and palatine) form a ring of lymphoid tissue at the oropharynx; (3) nasal-, larynx-, and auditory tube–associated lymphoid tissues (NALT, LALT, and ATALT, respectively) within the nasopharyngeal area; (4) gut-associated lymphoid tissue (GALT), which includes Peyer's patches and diffuse lymphoid tissue in the gut wall; (5) conjunctiva-associated lymphoid tissue (CALT); (6) other lymphoid nodules (e.g., genitourinary tract) (Fig. 13-51).

Diffuse lymphoid tissue consists of lymphocytes and DCs within the lamina propria of the mucosa of the alimentary, respiratory, and genitourinary tracts. These cells intercept and process antigens, which then travel to regional lymph nodes to initiate the immune response, leading ultimately to the secretion of IgA, IgG, and IgM.

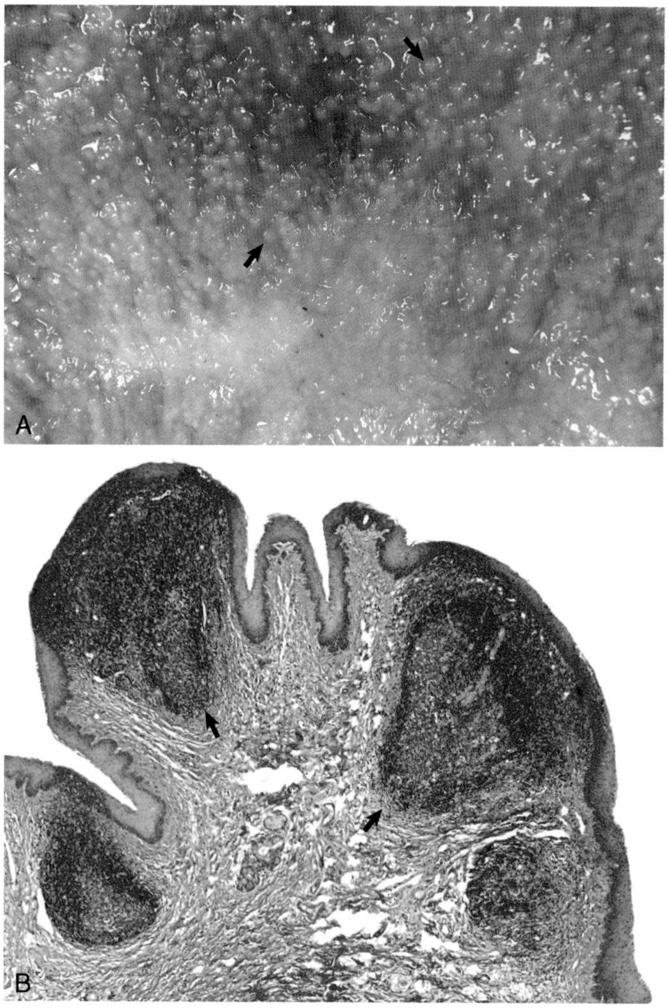

Figure 13-51 **Lymphoid Follicular Hyperplasia, Mucosa-Associated Lymphoid Tissue. A,** The mucosa contains multifocal, slightly raised, soft white nodules *(arrows)*. **B,** Prominent lymphoid follicles *(arrows)* have formed within the submucosa. H& E stain. (Courtesy Dr. A.C. Durham, School of Veterinary Medicine, University of Pennsylvania.)

Solitary lymphoid nodules are localized concentrations of lymphocytes (mainly B lymphocytes) in the mucosa and consist of defined but unencapsulated clusters of small lymphocytes (primary lymphoid nodule). They are usually not grossly visible in the resting or antigenically unstimulated state, but upon antigenic stimulation, they proliferate and form germinal centers and surrounding mantle cell zones (secondary lymphoid nodules).

Aggregated lymphoid nodules consist of groups of lymph nodules, the most notable of which are the tonsils and Peyer's patches. The aggregated lymphoid follicles of the Peyer's patches are most obvious in the ileum. The latter are covered by a specialized epithelium, the follicle-associated epithelium (FAE). The FAE is the interface between the Peyer's patches and the luminal microenvironment and consists of enterocytes and interdigitated M cells. M cells transport (via endocytosis, phagocytosis, pinocytosis, and micropinocytosis) antigens, particles, bacteria, and viruses from the intestinal lumen to the underlying area rich in DCs , which deliver the material to the lymphoid tissue of the Peyer's patches. M cells also express IgA receptors, which allows for the capture and transport of bacteria entrapped by IgA. The proportion of enterocytes and M cells within the FAE is modulated by the luminal bacterial composition. For instance, M cells increase in animals transferred from pathogen-free housing to the normal environment. M cells may also be exploited as a portal for entry by some microbes (see Lymphoid/Lymphatic System, Portals of Entry/Pathways of Spread). Table 13-5 lists the interactions of the MALT with different microorganisms.

Dysfunction/Responses to Injury

The responses of MALT to injury are similar to those of other lymphoid tissues: hyperplasia, atrophy, and inflammation (Box 13-10).

Hyperplasia. Hyperplasia of lymphoid nodules is a response to antigenic stimulation and consists of activation of germinal centers with subsequent production of plasma cells (see Fig. 13-51, *B*). Lymphoid nodule hyperplasia is often present in chronic disease conditions, such as BALT hyperplasia in chronic *Dictyocaulus* spp. (horses, cattle, sheep, and goats) or *Metastrongylus* spp. (pigs) associated bronchitis or bronchiolitis. *Mycoplasma* spp. pneumonias of sheep and pigs display marked BALT hyperplasia that can encircle bronchioles and bronchi ("cuffing pneumonia").

Hyperplastic lymphoid nodules can be so enlarged that they become grossly visible as discrete white plaques or nodules (see Fig. 13-51, *A*). They can be seen in the conjunctiva of the eyelids and the third eyelid in chronic conjunctivitis, the pharyngeal mucosa in chronic pharyngitis, the gastric mucosa in chronic gastritis, and the urinary bladder in chronic cystitis (follicular cystitis). The normal fetus has no detectable BALT, though it may be present in fetuses aborted due to infectious disease.

Atrophy. Atrophy of the diffuse lymphoid tissue and lymphoid nodules has the same causes as atrophy affecting other lymphoid tissues (see Box 13-5) and includes lack of antigenic stimulation, cachexia, malnutrition, aging, viral infections, or failure to be repopulated by B lymphocytes from the bone marrow or T lymphocytes from the thymus. Lymphocytolysis of germinal center lymphocytes of Peyer's patches is a characteristic lesion in BVDV infection in ruminants and canine and feline parvovirus infections ("punched-out Peyer's patches) (see Chapters 4 and 7).

Portals of Entry/Pathways of Spread

The main portals of entry to MALT for infectious agents are hematogenous spread and through migrating macrophages, DCs , and M cells. Pathogenic bacteria such as *Escherichia coli, Yersinia pestis, Mycobacterium avium* ssp. *paratuberculosis* (MAP), *L. monocytogenes, Salmonella* spp., and *Shigella flexneri* can invade the host from the lumen of the intestine through dendritic or M cells. Some viruses (e.g., reovirus) may be transported by M cells. The scrapie prion protein (PrP^{Sc}) may also accumulate in Peyer's patches. Many viruses, such as bovine coronavirus, BVDV, rinderpest virus, malignant catarrhal fever virus, feline panleukopenia virus, and canine parvovirus, cause lymphocyte depletion within the MALT. Portals of entry used by microorganisms and other agents and substances to access the lymphoid system are summarized in Box 13-6.

Defense Mechanisms/Barrier Systems

Defense mechanisms used by MALT to protect itself against microorganisms and other agents are the innate and adaptive immune responses, discussed in Chapters 3, 4, and 5.

Disorders of Domestic Animals: Thymus

Congenital Disorders

Congenital disorders of the thymus are discussed in detail in Chapter 5. Summaries of the gross and microscopic morphologic changes are

Table 13-5 Function of Mucosa-Associated Lymphoid Tissue (MALT) in Viral and Bacterial Diseases in Livestock

Function	Species	Microorganism
TONSILS		
Portal of entry	Sheep and goats	*Chlamydia psittaci*
Initial site of infection	Cattle	BVDV
Early site of infection	Cattle	BHV-1
Site of replication	Pig	Porcine circovirus type 2
		PMWS infection
Carriers (reservoirs)	Horses	*Streptococcus equi* subsp. *zooepidemicus*
	Cattle	*Mannheimia haemolytica*
	Sheep	*Salmonella* spp.
		Pasteurella haemolytica
		Scrapie agent (PrP^{Sc})
	Pigs	*Mycoplasma* spp.
		Streptococcus suis
		Salmonella spp.
		Yersinia pseudotuberculosis
GALT (PEYER'S PATCHES)		
Portal of entry	Cattle	*Brucella abortus*
		Mycobacterium avium ssp. *paratuberculosis*
	Sheep and goats	*Yersinia tuberculosis*

BVDV, Bovine viral diarrhea virus; *BHV-1,* bovine herpesvirus 1; *PMWS,* postweaning multisystemic wasting syndrome.
Data from Liebler-Tenorio EM, Pabst R: *Vet Res* 37:257-280, 2006.

Box 13-10 Responses of Mucosa-Associated Lymphoid Tissue to Injury

Hyperplasia
- Lymphoid hyperplasia with germinal center formation due to antigenic stimulation

Atrophy
- Lymphoid atrophy (see Box 13-5)

Inflammation
- Granulomatous (Johne's disease; see Diseases of Ruminants)

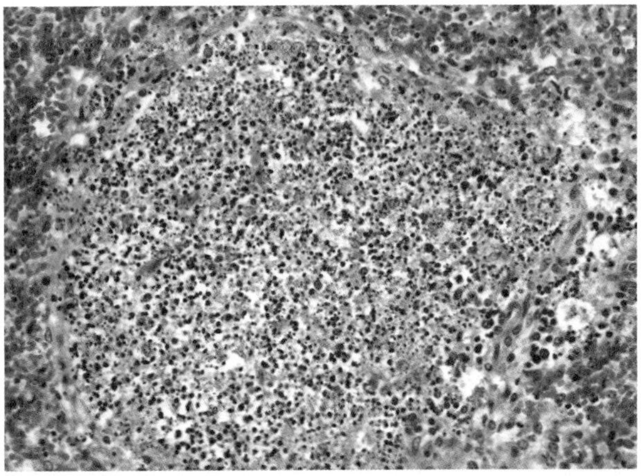

Figure 13-52 Equine Herpesvirus 1, Spleen, Aborted Foal. Most of the splenic follicle is occupied by nuclear debris, the result of lymphocytolysis. NOTE: lymphocytolysis may be caused by other infectious and noninfectious agents (e.g., chemotherapeutic drugs). H&E stain. (Courtesy College of Veterinary Medicine, University of Illinois.)

described in the sections on Disorders of Horses and Disorders of Dogs.

Thymic cysts can be found within the developing and mature thymus and in thymic remnants in the cranial mediastinum. Thymic cysts are often lined by ciliated epithelium and represent developmental remnants of branchial arch epithelium and are usually of no significance.

Inflammatory and Degenerative Disorders

Thymitis is an uncommon lesion and may be seen in PCV2 infection (see Disorders of Pigs and also Chapter 4), enzootic bovine abortion (see Chapter 18), and salmon poisoning disease of dogs (see Chapter 7). Infectious agents more commonly cause thymic atrophy. Variable degrees of acquired immunodeficiency can be also be caused by toxins, chemotherapeutic agents and radiation, malnutrition, aging, and neoplasia. Of infectious agents, viruses most commonly infect and injure lymphoid tissues and include the following: EHV-1 in aborted foals (Fig. 13-52), classic swine fever virus, BVDV, canine distemper virus, canine and feline parvovirus, and FIV; severe thymic lymphoid depletion is an early lesion in FIV-infected kittens.

Environmental toxins, such as halogenated aromatic hydrocarbons (e.g., polychlorinated biphenyls and dibenzodioxins), lead, and mercury have a suppressive effect on the immune system. Halogenated aromatic hydrocarbons cause dysfunction of DCs through several mechanisms that lead to atrophy of the primary and secondary lymphoid organs. Heavy metals, such as lead, mercury and nickel, are immunosuppressive and generally affect the levels of B and T lymphocytes, NK cells, and inflammatory cytokines. Other metals, such as selenium, zinc, and vanadium, may be immunostimulatory at low doses. The immunotoxic mechanisms may differ and include chelation of molecules and effects on protein synthesis, cell membrane integrity, and nucleic acid replication. The toxic effects of mycotoxins such as fumonisins B_1 and B_2 (secondary fungal metabolites produced by members of the genus *Fusarium*) and aflatoxin (produced by *Aspergillus flavus*) include lymphocytolysis in the thymic cortex.

Chemotherapeutic drugs inhibit the cell cycle through various mechanisms, and thus all dividing cells, including lymphocytes, bone marrow cells, and enterocytes, are sensitive to their effects. As such, bone marrow suppression, immunosuppression, and gastrointestinal disturbances are common side effects of anticancer drugs. Purine analogues (e.g., azathioprine) compete with purines in the synthesis of nucleic acids, whereas alkylating agents like cyclophosphamide cross-link DNA and inhibit the replication and activation of lymphocytes. Cyclosporin A specifically inhibits the T lymphocyte signaling pathway by interfering with the transcription of the IL-2 gene. Methotrexate, a folic acid antagonist, blocks the synthesis of thymidine and purine nucleotides. The immunosuppressive effects of some of these agents is desirable for the treatment of immune-mediated disease (e.g., immune-mediated hemolytic anemia) or to prevent allograft rejection after transplantation. Corticosteroids may be given at an immunosuppressive dose, though the degree of suppression is highly variable among species. Local or palliative treatment of cancer may include *radiotherapy (ionizing radiation)* to target and damage the DNA of the neoplastic cells. Although some immunosuppression may be noted, particularly if bone marrow or lymphoid tissue is within the therapeutically irradiated field, mounting evidence suggests that radiotherapy can induce a cascade of proimmunogenic effects that engage the innate and adaptive immune systems to contribute to the destruction of tumor cells.

Malnutrition and cachexia, which may occur with cancer, lead to secondary immunosuppression through several complex metabolic and neurohormonal aberrations. Thymic function may be impaired in young malnourished animals, resulting in a decrease in circulating T lymphocytes and subsequent depletion of T lymphocyte regions of secondary lymphoid organs. Lymphoid atrophy may result from physiologic and emotional stress, which can cause the release of catecholamines and glucocorticoids.

Aging

As part of the general effects of aging in cells (see Chapter 1), all lymphoid organs decrease in size (atrophy) with advancing age. In the case of the thymus this reduction in size occurs normally after sexual maturity and is more appropriately termed *thymic involution*. The term *involution* should be reserved for normal physiologic processes in which an organ either returns to normal size after a period of enlargement (e.g., postpartum uterus) or regresses to a more primitive state (e.g., thymic involution).

Neoplasia

Because the thymus has both lymphoid and epithelial components, neoplasms may arise from either component. Thymic lymphoma arises from the T lymphocytes in the thymus (and very rarely B lymphocytes). It is most often seen in young cats and cattle and less frequently in dogs (Fig. 13-53) (see Hematopoietic Neoplasia). Thymomas arise from the epithelial component and are usually benign neoplasms that occupy the cranial mediastinum of older animals. Histologically, these neoplasms consist of clustered or individualized neoplastic epithelial cells, often outnumbered by nonneoplastic small lymphocytes ("lymphocyte-rich thymoma"). Thymomas are common in goats and often contain large cystic structures. Immune-mediated diseases, including myasthenia gravis and immune-mediated polymyositis, occur with thymomas in dogs, and also rarely in cats. Myasthenia gravis is caused by autoantibodies directed toward the acetylcholine receptors, which lead to destruction of postsynaptic membranes and reduction of acetylcholine receptors at neuromuscular junction. Megaesophagus and aspiration pneumonia are common sequelae to this condition.

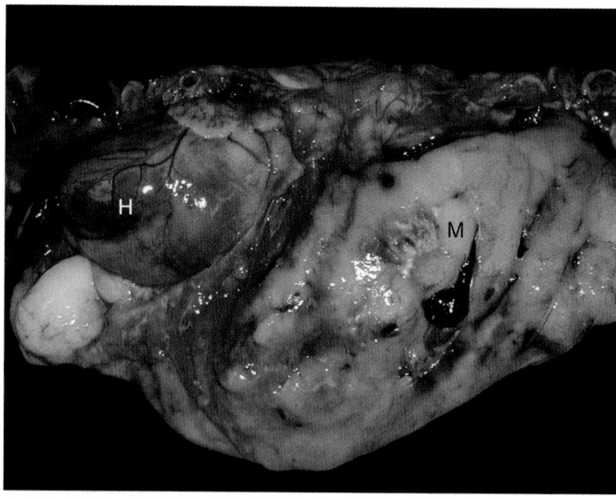

Figure 13-53 **Thymic Lymphoma, Cat.** The large pale tan mass *(M)* fills the cranial mediastinum and caudally displaces the lungs. *H*, Heart. (Courtesy Dr. A.C. Durham, School of Veterinary Medicine, University of Pennsylvania.)

Miscellaneous Disorders

Thymic Hyperplasia. Asymptomatic hyperplasia may occur in juvenile animals in association with immunizations and results in symmetrical increase in the size of the thymus. Autoimmune lymphoid hyperplasia of the thymus has germinal center formation and occurs with myasthenia gravis.

Thymic Hematomas. See Disorders of Dogs.

Disorders of Domestic Animals: Spleen

Congenital Disorders

Asplenia or the failure of a spleen to develop in utero occurs rarely in animals, and the effect on the animal's immune status is uncertain. (Splenic aplasia is present in certain strains of mice, but because these are usually maintained under either germ-free or specific pathogen–free [SPF] conditions, the effect of asplenia cannot be evaluated.) Congenital immunodeficiency diseases are described in detail in Chapter 5, and in the sections on Disorders of Horses and Disorders of Dogs.

Splenomegaly

Gross examination of the spleen involves deciding whether the spleen is enlarged (splenomegaly), normal, or small (see E-Appendix 13-2). Diffuse enlargement of the spleen may be due to congestion (termed bloody spleen) or other infiltrative disease (termed meaty spleen). The cut surface of congested spleens will exude blood, whereas meaty spleens are more firm and do not readily ooze blood. The diseases and disorders having splenomegaly are discussed using the following categories, which list the common causes of uniform splenomegaly (Table 13-6):

- Uniform splenomegaly with a bloody consistency (bloody spleen) (Fig. 13-54, *A*)
- Uniform splenomegaly with a firm consistency (meaty spleen) (see Fig. 13-54, *B*)
- Splenic nodules with a bloody consistency
- Splenic nodules with a firm consistency

Uniform Splenomegaly with a Bloody Consistency–Bloody Spleen. The common causes of a bloody spleen are (1) congestion (due to gastric volvulus with splenic entrapment, splenic volvulus

Table 13-6 Common Causes of Uniform Splenomegaly in Domestic Animals

Species	Congested (Bloody) Spleen	Firm (Meaty) Spleen
Horse	Barbiturate euthanasia or anesthesia Acute septicemia Salmonellosis Acute hemolytic disease EIA	Chronic septicemia Salmonellosis Chronic hemolytic diseases EIA IMHA Hematopoietic neoplasia Lymphoma
Cattle, sheep, and goat	Septicemia Anthrax Salmonellosis Acute hemolytic disease Babesiosis	Chronic septicemia Salmonellosis Chronic hemolytic diseases Babesia Anaplasmosis Trypanosomiasis Hemotropic mycoplasmosis Hematopoietic neoplasia Lymphoma
Pig	Septicemia Salmonellosis Splenic torsion	Chronic septicemias Salmonellosis Erysipelas Chronic hemolytic disease Hemotropic mycoplasmosis Hematopoietic neoplasia Lymphoma
Dog and cat	Barbiturate euthanasia or anesthesia Splenic torsion with GDV (dog)	Chronic hemolytic disease IMHA Chronic infectious disease Histoplasmosis Leishmaniasis Hematopoietic neoplasia Lymphoma Mast cell neoplasia Histiocytic sarcoma Extramedullary hematopoiesis Amyloidosis

EIA, Equine infectious anemia; *GDV,* gastric dilatation and volvulus; *IMHA,* immune-mediated hemolytic anemia.

[all of which compress the splenic vein], and barbiturate euthanasia, anesthesia, or sedation), (2) acute hyperemia (due to septicemia), and (3) acute hemolytic anemia (due to an autoimmune disorder or an infection with a hemotropic parasite).

Congestion

Splenic Torsion. Torsion of the spleen occurs most commonly in pigs and dogs; in dogs this usually involves both spleen and stomach and is seen more often in deep-chested breeds (see Chapter 7). In contrast to ruminants, in which the spleen is firmly attached to the rumen, the spleens of dogs and pigs are attached loosely to the stomach by the gastrosplenic ligament. It is the twisting of the spleen around this ligament that results initially in occlusion of the veins, causing splenic congestion, and later in occlusion of the artery, causing splenic infarction. In dogs the spleen is uniformly and markedly enlarged and may be blue-black from cyanosis. It is often folded back on itself (visceral surface to visceral surface) in the shape of the letter "C." Treatment for this condition is most often splenectomy.

Barbiturate Euthanasia, Anesthesia, or Sedation. Intravenous injection of barbiturates induces acute passive congestion in the spleen due to relaxation of smooth muscle in the capsule and trabeculae. This phenomenon is seen most dramatically at autopsy (syn: necropsy) in horses and dogs that have been euthanized or anesthetized with barbiturates. Grossly, the spleen is extremely enlarged (Fig. 13-55), and the cut surface bulges and oozes copious blood. Because of the splenic distention, the splenic capsule can be fragile and easily ruptured. Histologically, the red pulp is distended by erythrocytes, and the lymphoid tissues of the white pulp are small and widely separated (Fig. 13-56). Electric stunning of pigs at slaughter may result in a large congested spleen; the mechanism is unknown, but it should not be confused with a pathologically congested spleen. Splenic congestion in acute cardiac failure is rarely seen in animals.

Acute Congestion/Hyperemia. Acute septicemias may cause acute hyperemia and concurrent acute congestion of marginal zones and splenic red pulp. Microbes are transported hematogenously to these sites, where they are rapidly phagocytized by macrophages. Enormous numbers of intravenous bacteria can be cleared by the spleen from the blood in 20 to 30 minutes, but when this defensive mechanism is overwhelmed, the outcome is usually fatal. The response of the spleen depends on the duration of the disease. In acutely fatal cases, such as anthrax and fulminating salmonellosis, distention by blood may be the only gross finding. If the animal survives longer, as in swine erysipelas and the less virulent forms of

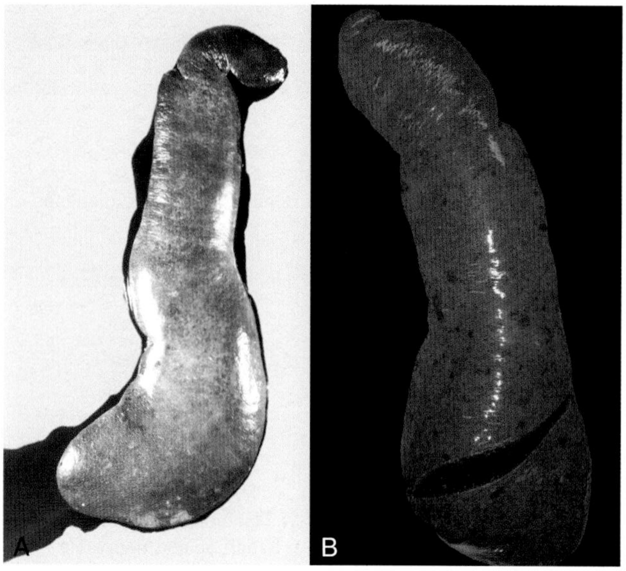

Figure 13-54 **Uniform Splenomegaly. A,** Congested bloody spleen. This condition occurs secondary to compromises in vascular flow into and out of the spleen (e.g., torsion), from intravenous barbiturates (e.g., euthanasia or anesthesia), and from acute hyperemia due to septicemia. **B,** Meaty spleen. This condition may be due to proliferation of macrophages in cases of chronic septicemias, hemolytic diseases, diffuse granulomatous disease, or neoplasia (e.g., lymphoma). (**A** courtesy College of Veterinary Medicine, University of Illinois. **B** courtesy Dr. A.C. Durham, School of Veterinary Medicine, University of Pennsylvania.)

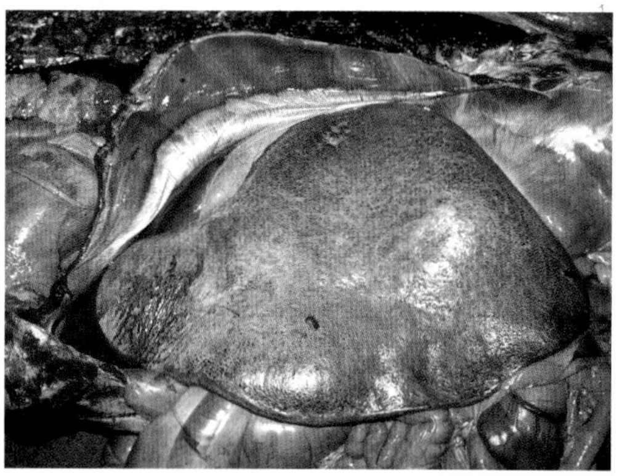

Figure 13-55 **Splenic Congestion From Barbiturate Euthanasia, Horse.** The spleen is enlarged and congested from storage of blood. (Courtesy Dr. M.D. McGavin, College of Veterinary Medicine, University of Tennessee.)

salmonellosis, there may be sufficient time for neutrophils and macrophages to accumulate in the marginal sinuses, marginal zones, and splenic red pulp vascular spaces.

Anthrax. *B. anthracis*, the causative agent of anthrax, is a Gram-positive, large, endospore-forming bacillus, which grows in aerobic to facultative anaerobic environments. Anthrax is primarily a disease of ruminants, especially cattle and sheep (see Chapters 4, 7, 9, and 10). Once the spores are ingested, they replicate locally in the intestinal tract, spread to regional lymph nodes, and then disseminate systemically through the bloodstream, resulting in septicemia. *B. anthracis* produces exotoxins, which degrade endothelial cell membranes and enzyme systems.

Grossly, the spleen is uniformly enlarged and dark red to bluish-black and contains abundant unclotted blood. In peracute cases the

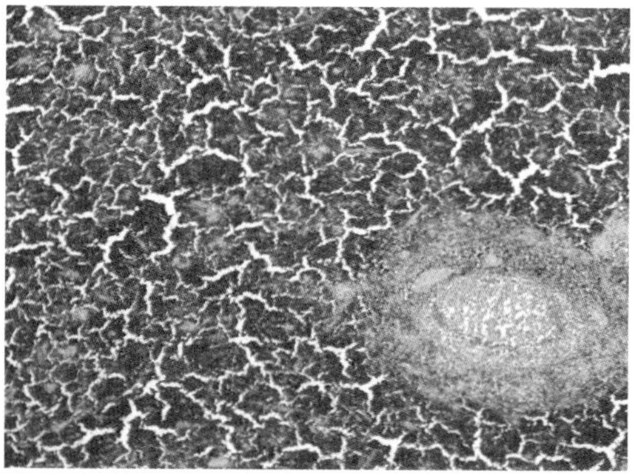

Figure 13-56 **Splenic Congestion From Barbiturate Euthanasia, Dog.** The red pulp vascular spaces are markedly distended by blood. One white pulp splenic follicle is present in the lower right. H&E stain. (Courtesy Dr. M.D. McGavin, College of Veterinary Medicine, University of Tennessee.)

only histologic lesion may be marked congestion of the marginal sinuses and the splenic red pulp vascular spaces. At low magnification, congestion of the marginal sinus may appear as a circumferential red ring around the splenic follicle, and there is marked lymphocytolysis of follicles and PALS. Intravascular free bacilli are noted and may be seen in impression smears of peripheral blood, presumably because death is so rapid from the anthrax toxin that there is insufficient time for phagocytosis to take place. If the animal lives longer, scattered neutrophils are present in the marginal sinuses and red pulp vascular spaces (Fig. 13-57). Anthrax cases are not normally autopsied because exposure to air causes the bacteria to sporulate—anthrax spores are extremely resistant and readily contaminate the environment.

Acute Hemolytic Anemias. Hemolytic diseases, including acute babesiosis, hemolytic crises in equine infectious anemia, and immune-mediated hemolytic anemia, can cause marked splenic congestion. The splenic congestion is due to the process of removal (phagocytosis) and storage of large numbers of sequestered parasitized and/or altered erythrocytes from the circulation. Histologically, there is dilation of the red pulp vascular spaces with erythrocytes and erythrophagocytes. With chronicity there is hyperplasia of the red pulp macrophages, hemosiderosis, and reduced congestion because the number of sequestered diseased erythrocytes is diminished.

Uniform Splenomegaly with a Firm Consistency–Meaty Spleen. The three general categories of conditions leading to uniform splenomegaly with a firm meaty consistency are (1) marked phagocytosis of cells, debris, or foreign agents/material; (2) proliferation or infiltration of cells as occurs in diffuse lymphoid and histiocytic hyperplasia, diffuse granulomatous disease (E-Table 13-2), EMH, and neoplasia; (3) storage of materials in storage diseases or amyloidosis. It is important to recognize that more than one of these processes can occur in the same patient (e.g., dogs with immune-mediated hemolytic anemia may have both marked erythrophagocytosis and EMH). The appearance of the cut surface of a meaty spleen depends on the underlying cause. In diffuse marked lymphoid hyperplasia, large, disseminated, discrete, white, bulging nodules are visible. Spleens with diffuse infiltrative neoplasms, such as lymphoma, are pink–light purple on cut surface.

Phagocytosis and Proliferation of Cells

Diffuse Lymphoid Hyperplasia. Lymphoid hyperplasia has been described in detail in the section on Dysfunction/Responses to Injury. In cases of prolonged antigenic stimulation the lymphoid

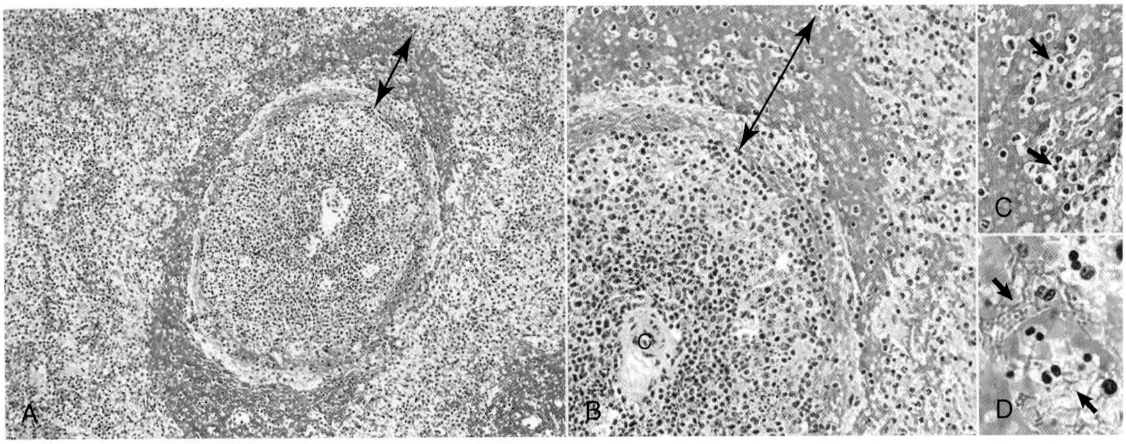

Figure 13-57 **Anthrax, Spleen, Monkey.** (See Fig. 13-40 for schematic illustration of the marginal zone.)**A**, Acute septicemias may cause acute congestion of the marginal zone *(double-headed line)* and then of the red pulp vascular spaces (not shown). **B**, Higher magnification of **A** with marginal zone *(double-headed line)* and central artery *(C)* of the follicle. **C**, Higher magnification of **B** with small aggregates of neutrophils within the marginal zone *(arrows)*. **D**, Higher magnification of **B** with accumulation anthrax bacilli within the marginal zone *(arrows)*. This form produces anthrax toxins, which cause severe tissue injury, resulting in inflammation and cell death. All H&E stain. (Courtesy Dr. J.F. Zachary, College of Veterinary Medicine, University of Illinois. Photographed from slides provided by Toxicology Battelle Columbus to the Wednesday Slide Conference [2003-2004, Conference 13, Case 1], Armed Forces Institute of Pathology, Department of Veterinary Pathology.)

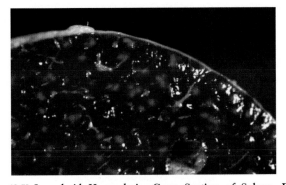

Figure 13-58 **Lymphoid Hyperplasia, Cross Section of Spleen, Dog.** The hyperplastic white pulp follicles are grossly evident as 1 to 3 mm in diameter pale gray-white foci. These structures are not visible in the normal spleen but become enlarged and visible from marked lymphoid hyperplasia. (Courtesy Dr. S. Wolpert, USDA/FSIS; and Noah's Arkive, College of Veterinary Medicine, The University of Georgia.)

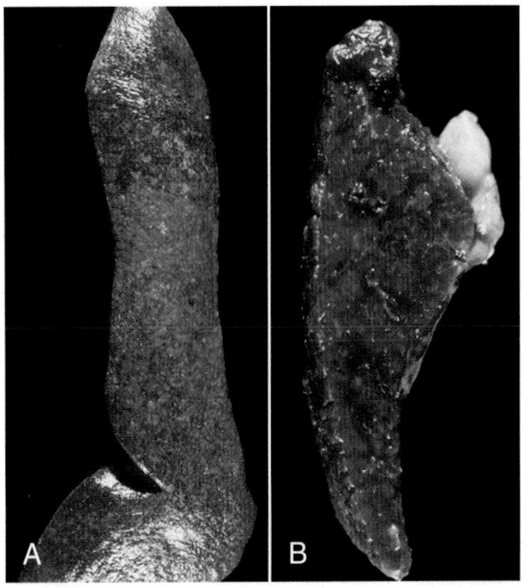

Figure 13-59 **Histoplasmosis, Spleen, Dog. A,** There is uniform splenomegaly with a firm consistency (meaty spleen). **B,** Cross section of spleen. The red pulp has been almost completely replaced by diffuse granulomatous inflammation. (Courtesy Department of Veterinary Biosciences, The Ohio State University; and Noah's Arkive, College of Veterinary Medicine, The University of Georgia.)

follicles throughout the splenic parenchyma can become enlarged and visible on gross examination (Fig. 13-58), leading to diffuse splenomegaly. In contrast to B lymphocyte hyperplasia of the lymphoid follicles, certain diseases (e.g., malignant catarrhal fever in cattle) may lead to T lymphocyte hyperplasia of the PALS.

Diffuse Histiocytic Hyperplasia and Phagocytosis. Splenomegaly from hyperplasia and increased phagocytosis of splenic macrophages is a response to the need to engulf organisms in prolonged bacteremia or parasitemia from hemotropic organisms. Whereas acute hemolytic anemias cause splenomegaly with congestion (*bloody* spleen), with chronicity there is decreased sequestration of diseased erythrocytes and hence less congestion. Therefore in cases of chronic hemolytic disease, splenomegaly is attributed to diffuse proliferation of macrophages, phagocytosis, and concurrent hyperplasia of the white pulp due to ongoing antigenic stimulation. For example, equine infectious anemia has cyclical periods of viremia, with immune-mediated damage to erythrocytes and platelets, and phagocytosis to remove altered erythrocytes and platelets. These cycles result in proliferation of red pulp macrophages, hyperplasia of hematopoietic cells (EMH) to replace those lost, and hyperplasia of lymphocytes in the white pulp.

Diffuse Granulomatous Disease. Chronic infectious diseases may cause a uniformly firm and enlarged spleen, mostly due to macrophage hyperplasia and phagocytosis, diffuse lymphoid hyperplasia, or diffuse granulomatous disease. Diffuse granulomatous diseases (see E-Table 13-2) occur in (1) intracellular facultative bacteria that infect macrophages (e.g., *Mycobacterium* spp., *Brucella* spp., and *Francisella tularensis*); (2) systemic mycoses (e.g., *Blastomyces dermatitidis*, *Histoplasma capsulatum*) (see Lymphoid/Lymphatic System, Disorders of Domestic Animals: Lymph Nodes, Enlarged Lymph Nodes [Lymphadenomegaly]) (Fig. 13-59, *A* and *B*), and (3) protozoal infections that infect macrophages (e.g., *Leishmania* spp.). Some of these organisms may also produce nodular spleens with the formation of discrete to coalescing granulomas (e.g., *M. bovis*) (see Splenic Nodules with a Firm Consistency).

Extramedullary Hematopoiesis. EMH is the development of blood cells in tissues outside the medullary cavity of the bone (E-Fig. 13-9). The formation of single or multiple lineages of hematopoietic cells is often observed in many tissues and commonly in the spleen. The ability of blood cell precursors to home, proliferate, and mature in extramedullary sites relies on the presence of HSCs and pathophysiologic changes in the microenvironment (i.e., extracellular matrix, stroma, and chemokines). In the spleen, HSCs have been found within vessels and adjacent to endothelial cells to form a *vascular niche*; thus splenic EMH occurs in the red pulp, both within the red pulp vascular spaces and sinusoids (of the dog). The predilection for EMH to occur varies among species (for instance, splenic EMH persists throughout adulthood in mice), and the underlying mechanisms are not completely understood, but four major theories to explain the causes of EMH are (1) severe bone marrow failure; (2) myelostimulation; (3) tissue inflammation, injury, and repair; and (4) abnormal chemokine production.

Because splenic EMH is often observed in animals without obvious hematologic abnormalities, tissue inflammation, injury, and repair is the most likely mechanism of EMH in this organ. In dogs and cats EMH occurs most frequently with degenerative and inflammatory disorders, such as lymphoid nodular hyperplasia, hematomas, thrombi, histiocytic hyperplasia, inflammation (e.g., fungal splenitis), and neoplasia. EMH in multiple tissues may be observed in chronic cardiovascular or respiratory conditions, chronic anemia, or chronic suppurative diseases in which there is an excessive tissue demand for neutrophils that exceeds the supply available from the marrow (e.g., canine pyometra).

Primary Neoplasms. Primary neoplastic diseases of the spleen arise from cell populations that normally exist in the spleen and include hematopoietic components, such as lymphocytes, mast cells, and macrophages, and stromal cells, such as fibroblasts, smooth muscle, and endothelium. The primary neoplasms that result in diffuse splenomegaly are the round cell tumors, including lymphoma (Fig. 13-60), leukemia, visceral mast cell tumor, and histiocytic sarcoma. It is important to note that all of these types of neoplasms can produce nodular lesions instead of—*or along with*—a diffusely enlarged spleen. The different types of lymphoma in domestic animals are discussed in the section on Hematopoietic Neoplasia. Secondary neoplasms of the spleen are due to metastatic spread and most often form nodules in the spleen, not a uniform splenomegaly.

Storage of Material

Amyloid. The accumulation of amyloid in the spleen may occur with primary (AL) or secondary (AA) amyloidosis (see Chapters 1 and 5). Rarely, severe amyloid accumulation may cause uniform splenomegaly (Fig. 13-61), in which the spleen is firm, rubbery to waxy, and light brown to orange. Microscopically, amyloid is usually in the splenic follicles, which if large enough, are grossly visible as approximately 2-mm-diameter gray nodules. Amyloid deposition can also be seen within the walls of splenic veins and arterioles. Plasma cells tumors within the spleen may also be associated with amyloid (AL) deposits.

Lysosomal Storage Diseases. Storage diseases are a heterogeneous group of inherited defects in metabolism characterized by accumulation of storage material within the cell (lysosomes). Genetic defects, which result in the absence of an enzyme, the synthesis of a catalytically inactive enzyme, the lack of activator proteins, or a defect in posttranslational processing, can lead to a storage disease. Acquired storage diseases are caused by exogenous toxins, most often plants that inhibit a particular lysosomal enzyme (e.g., swainsonine toxicity due to indolizidine alkaloid found in *Astragalus* and *Oxytropis* plant spp.). Storage diseases typically occur in animals less than 1 year of age. In general, these substrates are lipids and/or carbohydrates that accumulate in the cells, the result of the lack of normal processing within lysosomes. Major categories of stored materials include mucopolysaccharides, sphingolipids, glycolipids, glycoproteins, glycogen, and oligosaccharides. Macrophages are commonly affected by storage diseases, and thus

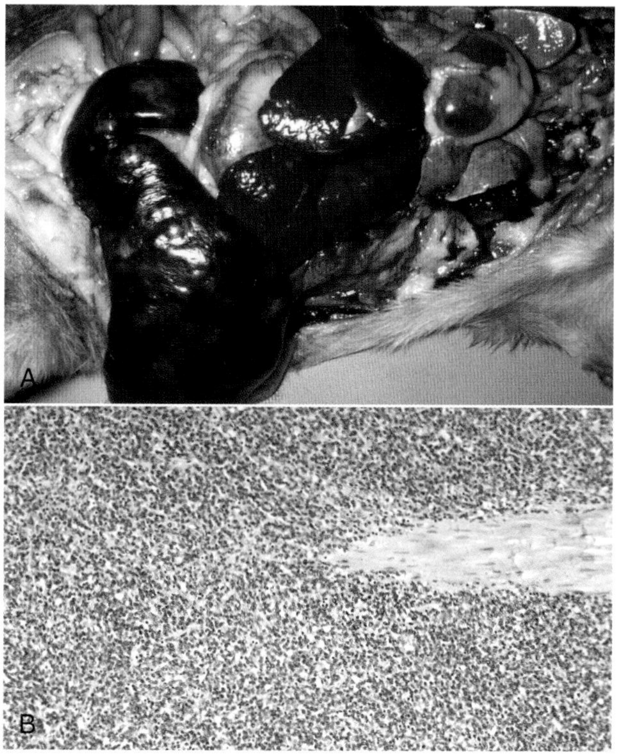

Figure 13-60 **Lymphoma, Spleen and Liver. A,** Dog. There is diffuse splenomegaly and multiple tan splenic nodules. Mild hepatomegaly with an irregular surface corresponds to the neoplastic infiltration into the portal areas. **B,** Cow. The spleen is diffusely infiltrated by neoplastic lymphocytes, which have completely obliterated all normal architecture (absence of the red and white pulp). H&E stain. (**A** courtesy College of Veterinary Medicine, University of Illinois. **B** courtesy Dr. M.D. McGavin, College of Veterinary Medicine, University of Tennessee.)

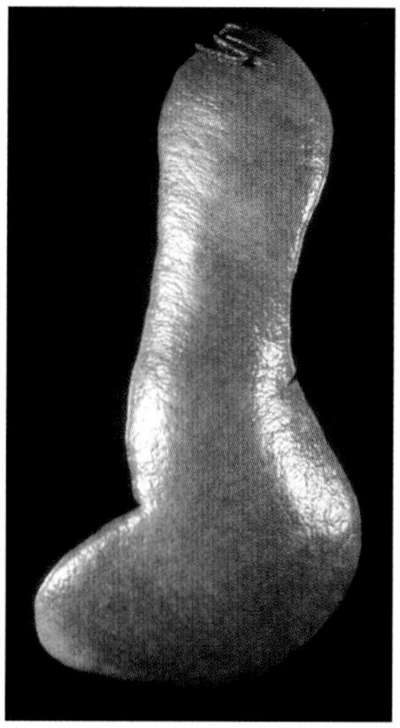

Figure 13-61 **Splenic Amyloid, Dog.** The spleen is enlarged, pale tan, firm, and waxy in this advanced case of amyloidosis. (Courtesy College of Veterinary Medicine, University of Illinois.)

accumulations of macrophages within several organs, including splenic macrophages, Kupffer cells of the liver, and macrophages in the brain are often observed.

Splenic Nodules with a Bloody Consistency. The most common disorders of the spleen with bloody nodules are (1) hematomas, including those induced by nodular hyperplasia or occurring with hemangiosarcoma, (2) incompletely contracted areas of the spleen, (3) acute splenic infarcts, and (4) hemangiosarcomas. The term *nodule* has been applied rather loosely here. In some of these conditions, such as incompletely or irregularly contracted areas of the spleen, the elevated area of the spleen is not as well defined as the term *nodule* would imply.

Hematomas. Bleeding into the red pulp to form a hematoma is confined by the splenic capsule, and produces a red to dark red, soft, bulging, usually solitary mass of varying size (2 to 15 cm in diameter) (Fig. 13-62). Resolution of a splenic hematoma progresses over days to weeks, through the stages of coagulation and breakdown of the blood into a dark red-brown soft mass (Fig. 13-63, *A*), infiltration by macrophages that phagocytize erythrocytes and break down hemoglobin to form hematoidin and hemosiderin (see Fig. 13-63, *B*), and repair leading to fibrosis. On occasion the capsule (splenic capsule and visceral peritoneum) over the hematoma can rupture, resulting in hemoperitoneum, hypovolemic shock, and death.

The origin or cause of many hematomas is unknown. Some are due to trauma, and others may also be induced by splenic nodular hyperplasia. It is postulated that as the splenic follicles become hyperplastic they distort the adjacent marginal zone and marginal sinus, which compromises their drainage into sinusoids and red pulp vascular spaces. The result is an accumulation of pooled blood surrounding the hyperplastic nodule, which leads to hematoma formation. Splenic hematomas can also occur secondary to the rupture of hemangiosarcomas within the spleen.

Incompletely Contracted Areas of the Spleen. Incompletely or irregularly contracted areas of the spleen are caused by failure of the smooth muscle to contract in response to circulatory shock (hypovolemic, cardiogenic, or septic) or sympathetic "fight-or-flight" response, resulting in a lack of splenic evacuation of stored blood. Grossly, incompletely contracted areas are characterized by multiple, variably sized and irregularly shaped, dark red to black, raised, soft, blood-filled "nodules." These areas are usually at the margins of the spleen, and the intervening tissues are depressed and pink-red, corresponding to the contracted portions of red pulp devoid of blood. Incompletely contracted areas may be confused with acute splenic infarcts or hematomas on gross examination.

Acute Splenic Infarcts. Splenic infarcts are wedge-shaped or triangular hemorrhagic lesions that occur primarily at the margins of the spleen. In dogs, splenic infarcts most often occur with hypercoagulable states (e.g., liver disease, renal disease, Cushing's disease), neoplasia, and cardiovascular disease. Splenic vein thrombi may occur in association with traumatic reticulitis, splenic abscesses, portal vein thrombosis, and arterial thrombosis in bovine theileriosis in cattle. Valvular endocarditis may also lead to multiorgan infarcts, including the spleen. Splenic infarcts are common in pigs with classical swine fever.

Acute splenic infarcts may not always be grossly visible in the early stages but develop into discrete, dark red and blood-filled, bulging, wedge-shaped foci with the base toward the splenic capsule (Fig. 13-64, *A*). With chronicity the lesion becomes gray-white and contracted due to fibrosis (see Fig. 13-64, *B*).

Hemangiosarcoma. Hemangiosarcoma is a malignant neoplasm of endothelial cells and is a common primary tumor of the spleen, especially in dogs. Benign splenic hemangiomas are extraordinarily rare. Grossly, hemangiosarcomas may appear as single, multifocal, or coalescing dark red-purple masses and cannot be easily differentiated from a hematoma (Fig. 13-65). On cut surface they are bloody with varying amounts of soft red neoplastic tissue; in more solid areas the neoplasm can be slightly more firm and white-tan. Metastatic spread occurs early in the disease process. Seeding of the peritoneum results in numerous discrete red-black masses throughout the omentum and serosa of abdominal organs, and hematogenous spread to liver and lung are common. Hemangiosarcomas in dogs also occur in the right atrium of the heart, retroperitoneal fat, and skin (dermal and/or subcutaneous) and multiorgan hemangiosarcomas are described in horses, cats, and cattle. Because hemangiosarcomas have often metastasized at the time of initial

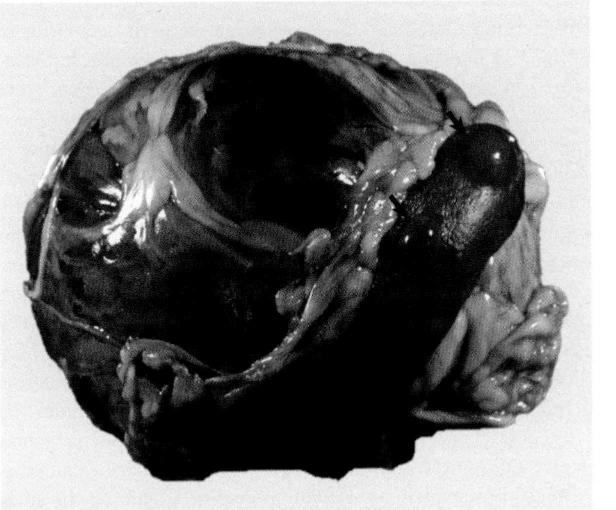

Figure 13-62 Hematoma, Spleen, Dog. The ventral extremity of the spleen has a large hematoma on its visceral surface. Note the two nodules on the dorsal extremity *(arrows)* of splenic nodular hyperplasia, a common site for hematomas to arise. (Courtesy College of Veterinary Medicine, University of Illinois.)

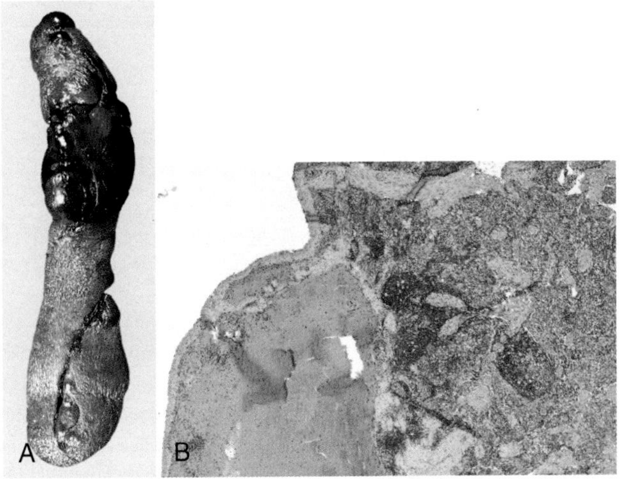

Figure 13-63 Subcapsular Hematoma, Spleen, Dog. A, Note the separation of the splenic capsule from the underlying parenchyma by a mass of blood. **B,** The hematoma is subjacent to the capsule. Hematoidin *(yellow)* or hemosiderin *(brown)* pigments may be seen in or around these lesions as a result of the breakdown of erythrocytes. H&E stain. (Courtesy Dr. M.D. McGavin, College of Veterinary Medicine, University of Tennessee.)

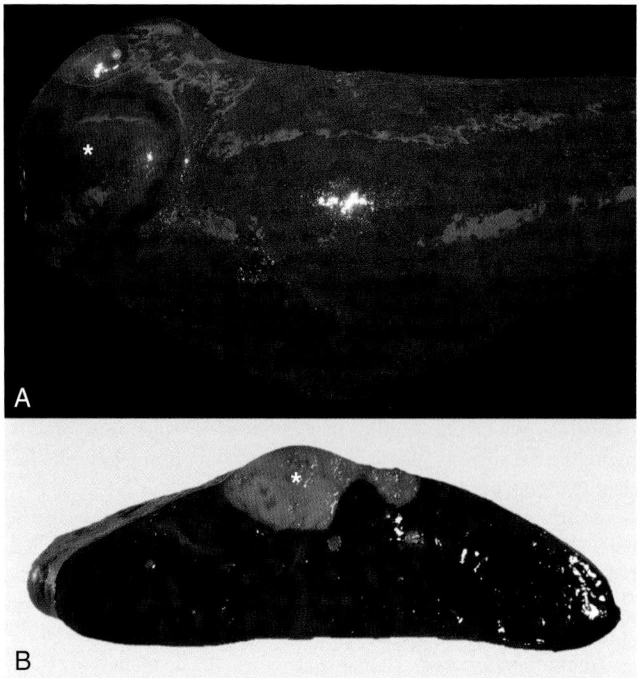

Figure 13-64 Acute and Chronic Splenic Infarcts, Spleen, Dogs. A, Acute splenic infarct *(asterisk)*. Acute infarcts are red-black wedge-shaped foci filled with blood. **B,** Chronic splenic infarct. Chronic infarcts are wedge-shaped *(asterisk)*, pale gray-white, firm, and often contracted due to fibrosis. (**A** courtesy Dr. A.C. Durham, School of Veterinary Medicine, University of Pennsylvania. **B** courtesy Dr. M.D. McGavin, College of Veterinary Medicine, University of Tennessee.)

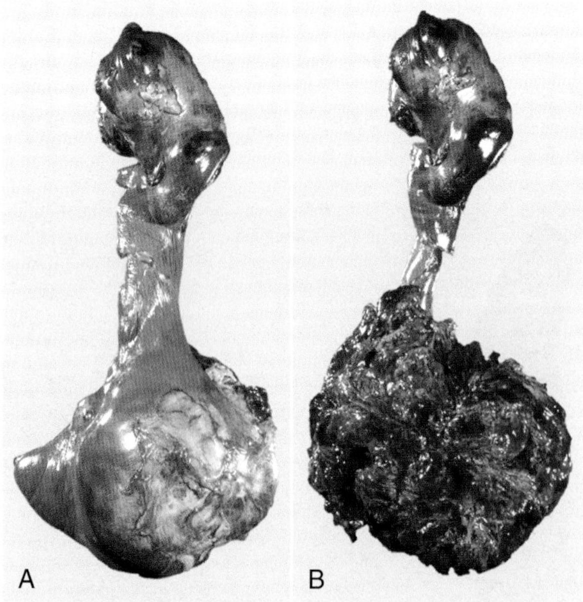

Figure 13-65 Hemangiosarcoma, Spleen, Dog. A, There are multiple neoplastic nodules on the dorsal extremity and a large nodule on the ventral extremity of the spleen. **B,** The ventral mass has been incised to reveal the cut surface of the hemangiosarcoma. (Courtesy Dr. M.D. McGavin, College of Veterinary Medicine, University of Tennessee.)

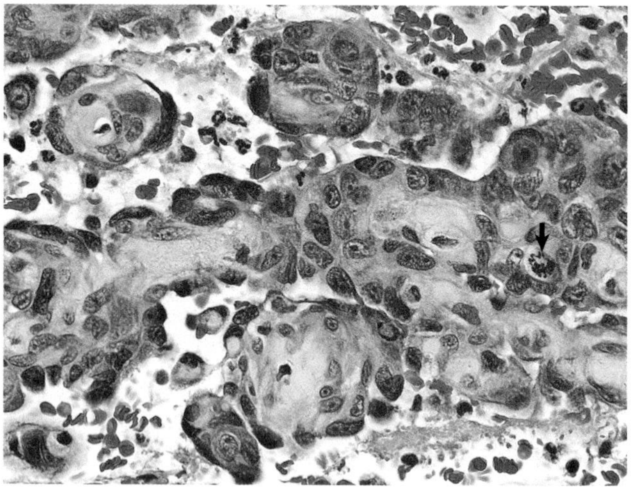

Figure 13-66 Hemangiosarcoma, Spleen, Dog. Neoplastic endothelial cells form haphazardly organized blood-filled vascular channels. Mitotic figure *(arrow)*. H&E stain. (Courtesy Dr. J.F. Zachary, College of Veterinary Medicine, University of Illinois.)

diagnosis, it may be difficult (and futile) to determine the primary site. Histologically, hemangiosarcomas are composed of plump neoplastic endothelial cells, which wrap around stroma to form haphazardly arranged and poorly defined blood-filled vascular spaces (Fig. 13-66).

Splenic Nodules with a Firm Consistency. The most common disorders of the spleen with firm nodules are (1) lymphoid nodular hyperplasia, (2) complex nodular hyperplasia, (3) primary neoplasms, (4) secondary metastatic neoplasms, (5) granulomas, and (6) abscesses.

Lymphoid and Complex Nodular Hyperplasia. See Lymphoid/Lymphatic System, Disorders of Dogs.

Primary Neoplasms. The primary neoplastic diseases of the spleen that result in firm nodules include lymphoma (multiple subtypes), histiocytic sarcoma, leiomyoma, leiomyosarcoma, fibrosarcoma, myelolipomas, liposarcomas, myxosarcomas, undifferentiated pleomorphic sarcomas, solid hemangiosarcomas, and rare reports of primary chondrosarcomas. These locally extensive neoplasms may be solitary or multiple, raised above the capsular surface, but usually confined by the capsular surface. The consistency and cut surface appearance varies depending on the type of neoplasm; spindle cell tumors like leiomyosarcomas and fibrosarcomas will be white and firm, liposarcomas and myelolipomas are soft and bulging, and myxomatous neoplasms are gelatinous. It is important to remember that many round cell neoplasms, such as lymphoma, mast cell tumors, plasma cell tumors, myeloid neoplasms, and histiocytic sarcomas, can form nodules or diffuse splenic enlargement (or both).

Metastatic Neoplasms. Neoplasms that metastasize to the spleen usually result in enlarged nodular spleens (Fig. 13-67) and include any number of sarcomas, carcinomas, or malignant round cell tumors. Metastatic sarcomas can include fibrosarcomas, leiomyosarcomas, chondrosarcomas, and osteosarcomas. Mammary, prostatic, pulmonary, anal sac gland and neuroendocrine carcinomas may metastasize widely to abdominal viscera, including the spleen.

Granulomas and Abscesses. Microorganisms that cause diffuse granulomatous splenitis and uniform splenomegaly may also cause focal to multifocal nodular lesions (e.g., *Mycobacterium* spp., fungal organisms) (see Diffuse Granulomatous Diseases of the Spleen and also Enlarged Lymph Nodes). Although there are a large number of

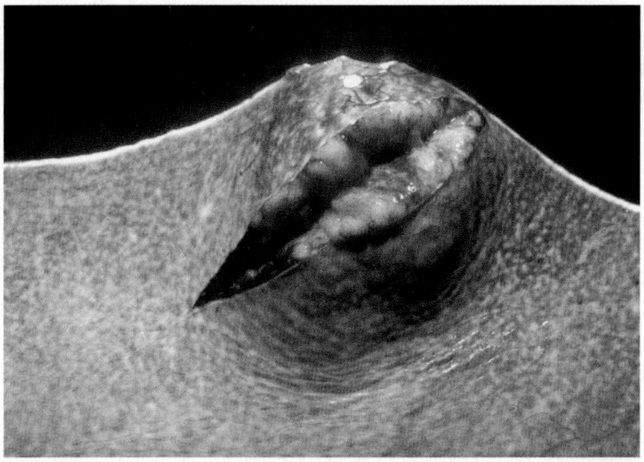

Figure 13-67 **Metastatic Carcinoma, Spleen, Cow.** The firm, lobulated, white mass is an undifferentiated carcinoma, which has metastasized to the spleen. (Courtesy Dr. M.D. McGavin, College of Veterinary Medicine, University of Tennessee.)

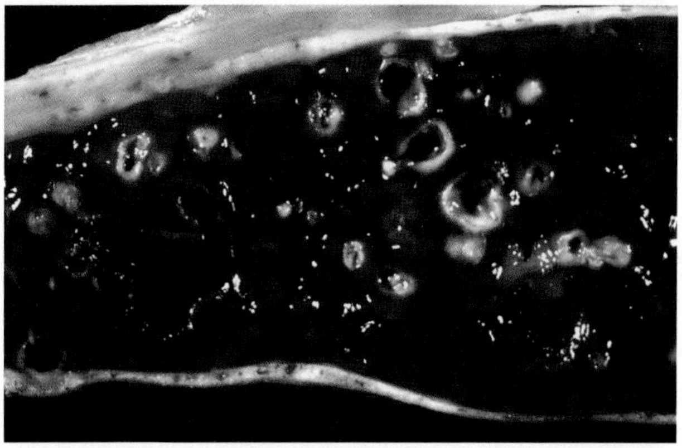

Figure 13-69 **Chronic Multifocal Suppurative Splenitis (Splenic Abscesses), *Trueperella pyogenes*, Spleen, Cow.** Multiple encapsulated yellow-white abscesses are present throughout the parenchyma of the spleen as a result of a previous bacteremia. (Courtesy Department of Veterinary Biosciences, The Ohio State University; and Noah's Arkive, College of Veterinary Medicine, The University of Georgia.)

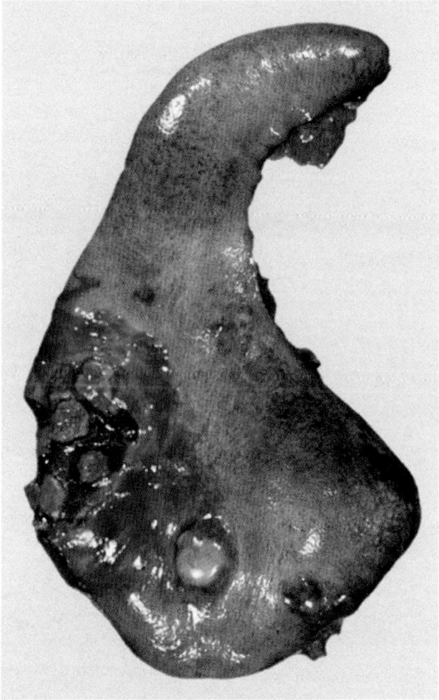

Figure 13-68 **Multiple Subcapsular Splenic Abscesses, *Rhodococcus equi*, Spleen, Horse.** (Courtesy Dr. P. Carbonell, School of Veterinary Science, University of Melbourne.)

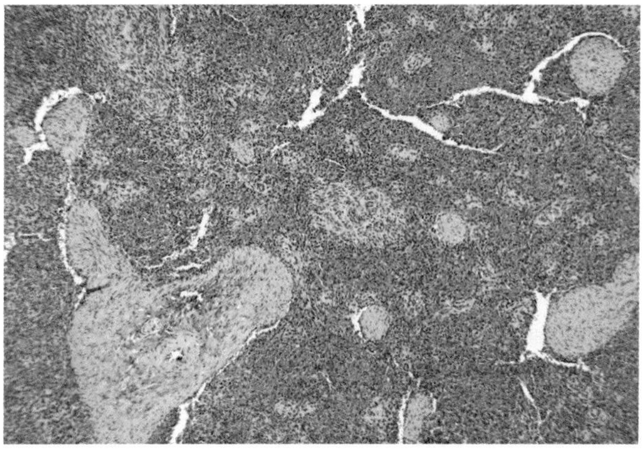

Figure 13-70 **Severe Combined Immunodeficiency Disease, Spleen, Arabian Foal.** There is notable absence of the white pulp (the large pale pink areas are splenic trabeculae). H&E stain. (Courtesy Dr. M.D. McGavin, College of Veterinary Medicine, University of Tennessee.)

diseases and conditions commonly caused by bacteremia (e.g., navel ill, joint ill, chronic respiratory infections, bacterial endocarditis, chronic skin diseases, castration, tail docking, and ear trimming and/or notching), these rarely result in visible splenic abscesses. Pyogranulomas and abscesses in the spleen (multifocal chronic suppurative splenitis) that do develop after septicemia and/or bacteremia are usually caused by pyogenic bacteria such as *Streptococcus* spp., *Rhodococcus equi* (Fig. 13-68), *Trueperella pyogenes* (Fig. 13-69), and *Corynebacterium pseudotuberculosis*. Cats with the wet or dry form of feline infectious peritonitis virus may have nodular pyogranulomatous and lymphoplasmacytic inflammatory foci throughout the spleen. Splenic abscesses due to direct penetration by a migrating foreign body are reported in cattle (from the reticulum) and less commonly in the horse (from the stomach). Perforating gastric ulcers in horses due to *Gasterophilus* and *Habronema* spp. have also reportedly led to adjacent splenic abscesses. Granulomas and abscesses bulge from the capsule and cut surfaces, and the exudate can vary in amount, texture, and color depending on the inciting organism and the age of the lesion.

Small Spleens (Splenic Hypoplasia and Atrophy)

The most common diseases or conditions that have small spleens are (1) developmental anomalies, (2) aging changes, (3) wasting and/or cachectic diseases, and (4) splenic contraction.

Developmental Anomalies

Splenic Hypoplasia. Primary immunodeficiency diseases can result in splenic hypoplasia, as well as small thymuses and lymph nodes (which may be so small as to be grossly undetectable in some diseases). These diseases affect young animals and involve defects in T and/or B lymphocytes (Fig. 13-70). Spleens are exceptionally small, firm, and pale red and lack lymphoid follicles and PALS. These diseases and their pathologic findings are discussed in Chapter 5 and in the sections on Disorders of Horses and Disorders of Dogs.

Congenital Accessory Spleens. Accessory spleens can be either congenital or acquired (see Splenic Rupture). Congenital accessory spleens are termed *splenic choristomas*, which are nodules of normal splenic parenchyma in abnormal locations. These are usually small and may be located in the gastrosplenic ligament, liver, or pancreas (see Fig. 13-74, *B*).

Splenic Fissures. Fissures in the splenic capsule are elongated grooves whose axes run parallel to the borders of the spleen. This developmental defect is seen most commonly in horses but also occurs in other domestic animals and has no pathologic significance. The surface of the fissure is smooth and covered by the normal splenic capsule.

Aging Changes. As part of the general aging change of cells as the body ages, there is reduction in the number of B lymphocytes produced by the bone marrow and decline of naïve T lymphocytes due to age-related thymic involution. Consequently, there is lymphoid atrophy in secondary lymphoid organs. The spleen is small, and its capsule may be wrinkled. Microscopically, the white pulp is atrophied, and splenic follicles, if present, lack germinal centers. Sinuses may also collapse from a reduced amount of blood, possibly because of anemia, which makes the red pulp appear fibrous.

Wasting/Cachectic Diseases. Any chronic disease, such as starvation, systemic neoplasia, and malabsorption syndrome, may produce cachexia. Starvation has a marked effect on the thymus, which results in atrophy of the T lymphocyte areas in the spleen and lymph nodes, which is in part mediated by leptin. B lymphocyte development is also diminished, because B lymphocytes require accessory signals from helper T lymphocytes to undergo somatic hypermutation and immunoglobulin isotype switching.

Splenic Contraction. Contraction of the spleen is a result of contraction of the smooth muscle in the capsule and trabeculae of storage spleens. It can be induced by the activation of the sympathetic "fight-or-flight" response and is seen in patients with heart failure or shock (cardiogenic, hypovolemic, and septic shock) and also occurs in acute splenic rupture that has resulted in massive hemorrhage (hemoabdomen/hemoperitoneum). The contracted spleen is small, its surface is wrinkled, and the cut surface is dry.

Miscellaneous Disorders of the Spleen

Hemosiderosis. Hemosiderin is a form of storage iron derived chiefly from the breakdown of erythrocytes, which normally takes place in the splenic red pulp. Thus some splenic hemosiderosis is to be expected, and the amount varies with the species (it is most extensive in the horse). Excessive amounts of splenic hemosiderin are seen when erythropoiesis is reduced (less demand for iron) or from the rapid destruction of erythrocytes in hemolytic anemias (increased stores of iron), such as those caused by immune-mediated hemolytic anemias or hemotropic parasites. Excess splenic hemosiderin may also occur in conditions such as chronic heart failure or injections of iron dextran or as focal accumulations at the sites of old hematomas, infarcts, or trauma-induced hemorrhages. Hemosiderin is also present in siderofibrotic plaques.

Siderofibrotic Plaques. Siderofibrotic plaques are also known as siderocalcific plaques and Gamna-Gandy bodies. Grossly, they are gray-white to yellowish, firm, dry encrustations on the splenic capsule. Usually they are most extensive along the margins of the spleen but can be elsewhere on the capsule (Fig. 13-71) and sometimes in the parenchyma. With H&E staining these plaques are a multicolored mixture of yellow (hematoidin), golden brown (hemosiderin), purple-blue (hematoxylinophilic calcium mineral), and pink (eosinophilic fibrous tissue) (Fig. 13-72; E-Figs. 13-10 and 13-11). Siderofibrotic plaques are extremely common in aged dogs and

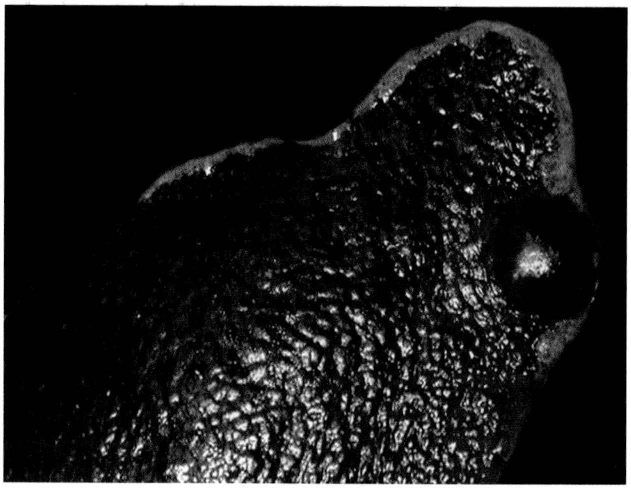

Figure 13-71 **Siderofibrotic Plaques, Spleen, Macroscopic View, Dog.** Siderofibrotic plaque along the margins (golden-brown area) of the spleen; a focal nodule of hyperplasia is also present. Both are common lesions in older dogs. (Courtesy Dr. A.C. Durham, School of Veterinary Medicine, University of Pennsylvania.)

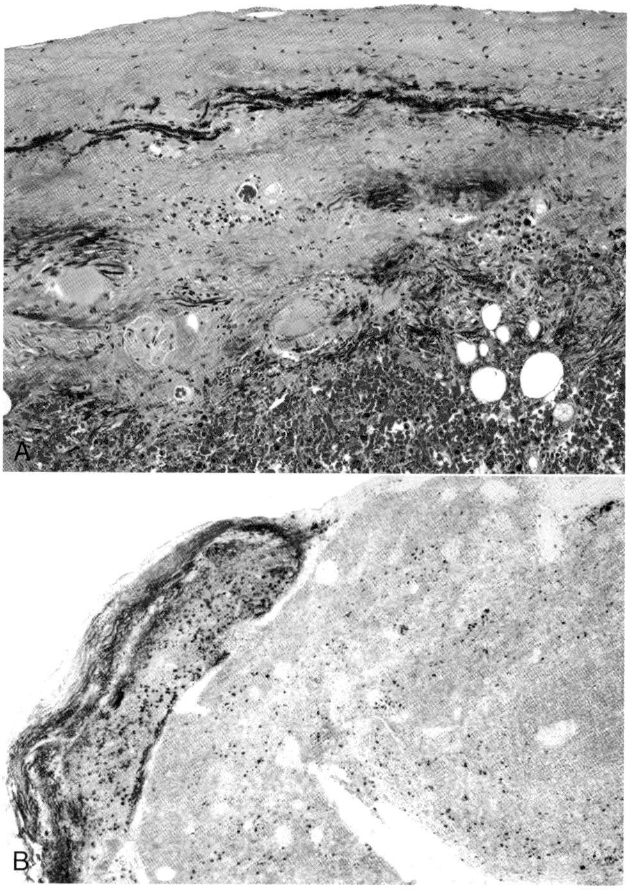

Figure 13-72 **Siderofibrotic Plaques, Spleen, Microscopic View, Dog.** **A,** The thick splenic capsule contains fibrosis connective tissue *(pink)*, linear bands of mineral *(dark purple)*, small lakes of hematoidin pigment *(yellow)*, and hemosiderin-laden macrophages *(brown)*. H&E stain. **B,** The plaque is composed of fibrous connective tissue, hemosiderin *(blue)* and hematoidin *(orange)* pigments, and mineral. Prussian blue reaction. (**A** courtesy Dr. A.C. Durham, School of Veterinary Medicine, University of Pennsylvania. **B** courtesy Dr. M.D. McGavin, College of Veterinary Medicine, University of Tennessee.)

may represent sequelae to previous hemorrhages from trauma to the spleen.

Splenic Rupture. Splenic rupture is most commonly caused by trauma, such as from an automobile accident or being kicked by other animals. Thinning of the capsule from splenomegaly can render the spleen more susceptible to rupture, and this may occur at sites of infarcts, hematomas, hemangiosarcomas, and lymphoma. In acute cases of splenic capsular rupture, the spleen is contracted and dry and the surface wrinkled from the marked blood loss (Fig. 13-73). In more severe cases the spleen may be broken into two or more pieces, and small pieces of splenic parenchyma may be scattered throughout the omentum and peritoneum (sometimes called *splenosis*) (Fig. 13-74, *A*). Clotted blood, fibrin, and omentum may adhere to the surface at the rupture site. If the rupture is not fatal, the spleen heals by fibrosis, and there may be a capsular scar. Occasionally there are two or more separate pieces of spleen adjacent to each other and sometimes joined by scar tissue in the gastrosplenic ligament. The functional capabilities of the small accessory spleens are questionable, although erythrophagocytosis, hemosiderosis, hyperplastic nodules, EMH, and neoplasia can be present in these nodules.

Accessory spleens due to traumatic rupture should be distinguished from peritoneal seeding of hemangiosarcoma and the developmental anomaly splenic choristomas (see Fig. 13-74, *B*), which are nodules of normal splenic parenchyma in abnormal locations (such as liver and pancreas).

Chronic Splenic Infarcts. In the early stage, splenic infarcts are hemorrhagic and may elevate the capsule (see Splenic Nodules with a Bloody Consistency). However, as the lesions age and fibrous connective tissue is laid down, they shrink and become contracted and often depressed below the surface of the adjacent capsule.

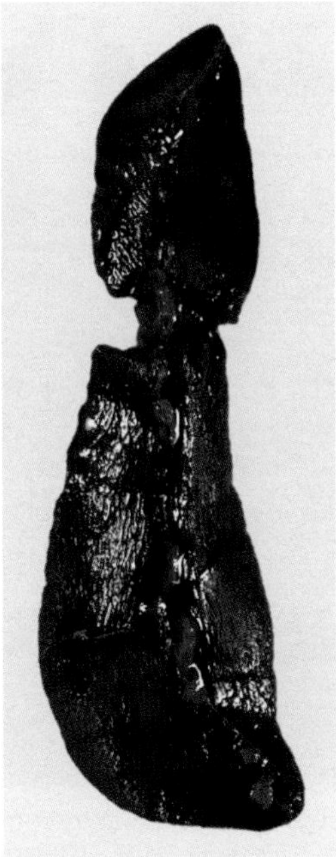

Figure 13-73 **Acute Splenic Rupture, Spleen, Dog.** The spleen has been almost transected by recent trauma. Because of the loss of blood, the spleen is contracted, the surface is wrinkled, and the exposed parenchymal surface is dry. (Courtesy Dr. M.D. McGavin, College of Veterinary Medicine, University of Tennessee.)

Parasitic Cysts. Occasionally, parasitic cystic nodules are present within the spleen. These cysts are intermediate stages of *Echinococcus granulosus* and *Cysticercus tenuicollis* and are seen most commonly in wild animal species.

Disorders of Domestic Animals: Lymph Nodes

Small Lymph Nodes

The diseases or conditions with small lymph nodes are (1) congenital disorders, (2) lack of antigenic stimulation, (3) viral infections, (4) cachexia and malnutrition, (5) aging, and (6) radiation.

Congenital Disorders. Primary immunodeficiency diseases are described in detail in Chapter 5 and in the sections on Disorders of Horses and Disorders of Dogs. Neonatal animals with primary immunodeficiency diseases often have extremely small to undetectable lymph nodes. In dogs and horses with severe combined immunodeficiency disease (SCID), lymphoid tissues, including lymph nodes from affected animals, are often grossly difficult to identify and characterized by an absence of lymphoid follicles. Congenital

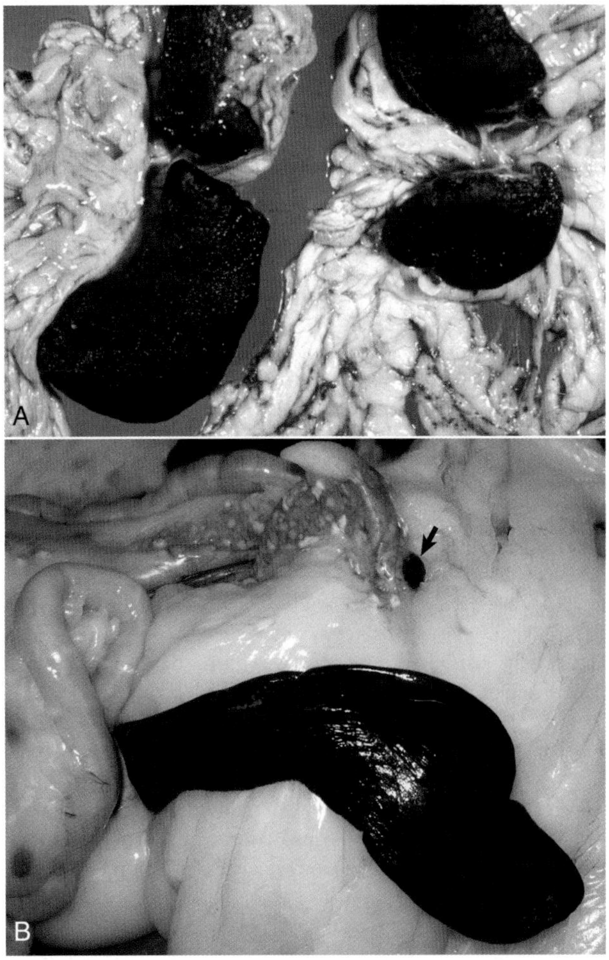

Figure 13-74 **Accessory Spleens and Splenic Choristoma, Dogs. A,** Accessory spleens. The spleen had been broken into several parts, and the rupture sites have healed by fibrosis. These small pieces of spleen (also referred to as daughter or progeny spleens) are found on the gastrosplenic ligament. **B,** Splenic choristomas. These nodules of normal splenic parenchyma are usually small and may be located in the gastrosplenic ligament, liver, or pancreas. Splenic choristoma *(arrow)*. (**A** courtesy Dr. H.B. Gelberg, College of Veterinary Medicine, Oregon State University. **B** courtesy Dr. A.C. Durham, School of Veterinary Medicine, University of Pennsylvania.)

hereditary lymphedema has been reported in certain breeds of cattle and dogs. Grossly, the most severely affected animals have generalized subcutaneous edema (see Fig. 2-10) and effusions. In severe cases the peripheral and mesenteric lymph nodes are hypoplastic and characterized by an absence of follicles. Nodes draining an edematous area may be grossly enlarged from marked sinus edema.

Lack of Antigenic Stimulation. The size of the lymph node depends on the level of phagocytosis and antigenic stimulation; lymph nodes that are not receiving antigenic stimuli (e.g., SPF animals) will be small with low numbers of primary lymphoid follicles and few, if any, secondary follicles or plasma cells in the medullary cords. Conversely, nodes receiving constant antigenic material (such as those draining the oral cavity or intestines) are large with active secondary lymphoid follicles. The number of follicles increases or decreases with changes in the intensity of the antigenic stimuli, and the germinal centers go through a cycle of activation, depletion, and rest, as described previously (see Lymph Nodes, Function). As the antigenic response wanes, germinal centers become depleted of lymphocytes, and lymphoid follicles become smaller.

Viral Infections. Many viral infections of animals target lymphocytes and cause the destruction of lymphoid tissue. Of infectious agents, viruses most commonly infect and injure lymphoid tissues and include the following: EHV-1 in aborted foals, classic swine fever virus, BVDV, canine distemper virus, and canine and feline parvovirus.

Although some viruses destroy lymphoid tissue, others can lead to lymph node hyperplasia (e.g., follicular B lymphocyte hyperplasia in FIV and paracortical T lymphocyte hyperplasia in malignant catarrhal fever virus) or cause neoplasia (e.g., FeLV, BLV, and Marek's disease).

Cachexia and Malnutrition. Malnutrition and cachexia, which occur with cancer, lead to secondary immunosuppression through several complex metabolic and neurohormonal aberrations. Starvation has marked effect on the thymus with resultant atrophy of the T lymphocyte areas in the spleen and lymph nodes and may also affect B lymphocyte development. Lymphoid atrophy may result from physiologic and emotional stress and the concurrent release of catecholamines and glucocorticoids. Glucocorticoids reduce B and T lymphocytes via redistribution of these cells and glucocorticoid-induced apoptosis. T lymphocytes are more sensitive to glucocorticoid-induced apoptosis than are B lymphocytes.

Aging. As part of the general aging change of cells as the body ages, there is reduction in the number of lymphocytes produced by the bone marrow and regressed thymus, and consequently a reduction in the B and T lymphocytes in secondary lymphoid organs, resulting in lymphoid atrophy. Consequently, lymph nodes are small, with loss of B and T lymphocytes and plasma cells in the cortical follicles, paracortex, and medullary cords, respectively.

Radiation. Local or palliative treatment of cancer may include radiotherapy (ionizing radiation) to target and damage the DNA of the neoplastic cells. Although some immunosuppression may be noted, particularly if bone marrow or lymphoid tissues are within the irradiated field, mounting evidence suggests that radiotherapy can induce a cascade of proimmunogenic effects that engage the innate and adaptive immune systems to contribute to the destruction of tumor cells. Fibrosis of tissues within the irradiated field also occurs as mainly a late effect of chronic radiation.

Enlarged Lymph Nodes (Lymphadenomegaly)

Conditions causing lymphadenomegaly include (1) lymphoid hyperplasia (follicular or paracortical), (2) hyperplasia of the sinus histiocytes (monocyte-macrophage system), (3) acute or chronic lymphadenitis, (4) lymphoma, and (5) metastatic neoplasia.

Lymphoid Hyperplasia and Hyperplasia of the Monocyte-Macrophage System. Detailed descriptions of lymphoid follicular hyperplasia, paracortical hyperplasia, and hyperplasia of sinus histiocytes are in the sections on Lymph Nodes, Function, and Lymph Node, Dysfunction/Responses to Injury. Follicular lymphoid hyperplasia can involve large numbers of lymph nodes, as in a systemic disease, or can be localized to a regional lymph node draining an inflamed or antigenically stimulated (e.g., vaccine injection) area.

Acute Lymphadenitis. Lymph nodes draining sites of infection and inflammation may develop acute lymphadenitis (e.g., retropharyngeal lymph nodes draining the nasal cavity with acute rhinitis, tracheobronchial lymph nodes in animals with pneumonia (Fig. 13-75), and mammary [supramammary] lymph nodes in animals with mastitis). Grossly, affected lymph nodes in acute lymphadenitis are red and edematous, have taut capsules, and may have necrotic areas (Fig. 13-76). In some instances the afferent lymphatic vessels may also be inflamed (lymphangitis). The material draining to the regional lymph node may be microorganisms (bacteria, parasites, protozoa, and fungi), inflammatory mediators, or a sterile irritant. In septicemic diseases, such as bovine anthrax, the lymph nodes are markedly congested and the sinuses filled with blood. Examination of these lymph nodes should include culturing for bacteria and the examination of smears and histologic sections for bacteria and fungi. Pyogenic bacteria, such as *Streptococcus equi* ssp. *equi* in horses (Fig. 13-77), *Streptococcus porcinus* in pig, and *Trueperella pyogenes* in cattle and sheep, cause acute suppurative lymphadenitis (see Disorders of Horses and Disorders of Pigs).

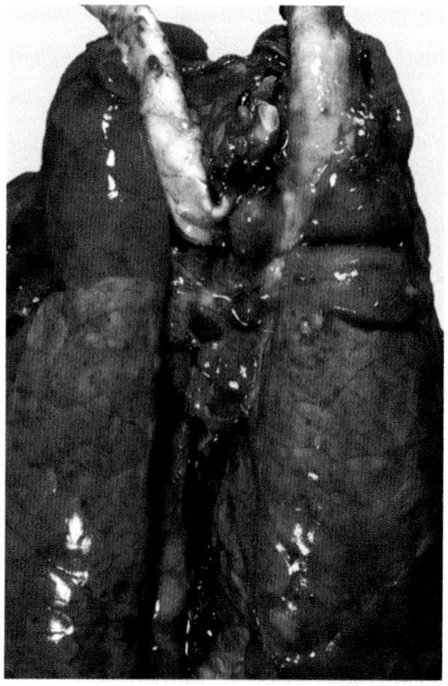

Figure 13-75 **Acute Lymphadenitis, Tracheobronchial Lymph Nodes, Pig.** The tracheobronchial lymph nodes are draining the cranial lung lobes, which are consolidated due to severe pneumonia. The nodes are enlarged and reddened. This appearance is due to the "reversed" anatomic arrangement in the pig lymph node; the blood-filled sinuses are obvious at the surface. (Courtesy Dr. M.D. McGavin, College of Veterinary Medicine, University of Tennessee.)

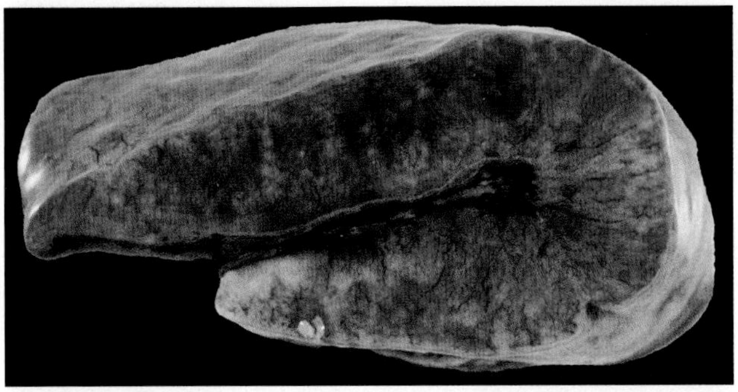

Figure 13-76 Acute Lymphadenitis, Lymph Node, Dog. Acute lymphadenitis usually occurs when a regional lymph node drains a site of inflammation caused by microorganisms and subsequently becomes infected. The lymph node is firm and enlarged with a tense capsule. The cut surface bulges and is wet with blood, edema, and an inflammatory cell infiltrate. (Courtesy Dr. M.D. McGavin, College of Veterinary Medicine, University of Tennessee.)

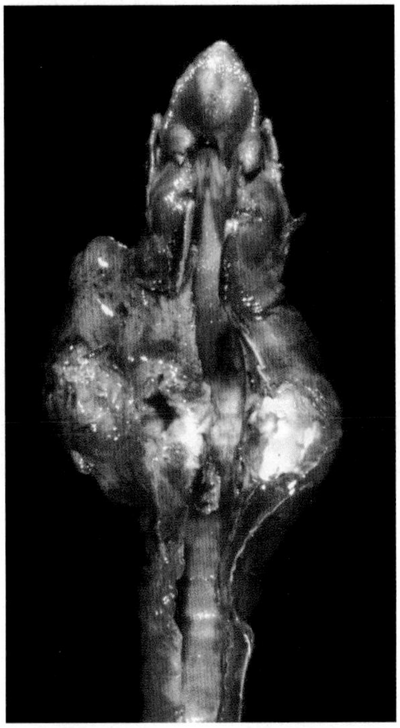

Figure 13-77 Acute Suppurative Lymphadenitis, Equine Strangles (*Streptococcus equi* ssp. *equi*), Dorsal View of Larynx, Left and Right Retropharyngeal Lymph Nodes, Horse. The lymph nodes are grossly distended with suppurative inflammation (pus). (Courtesy College of Veterinary Medicine, University of Illinois.)

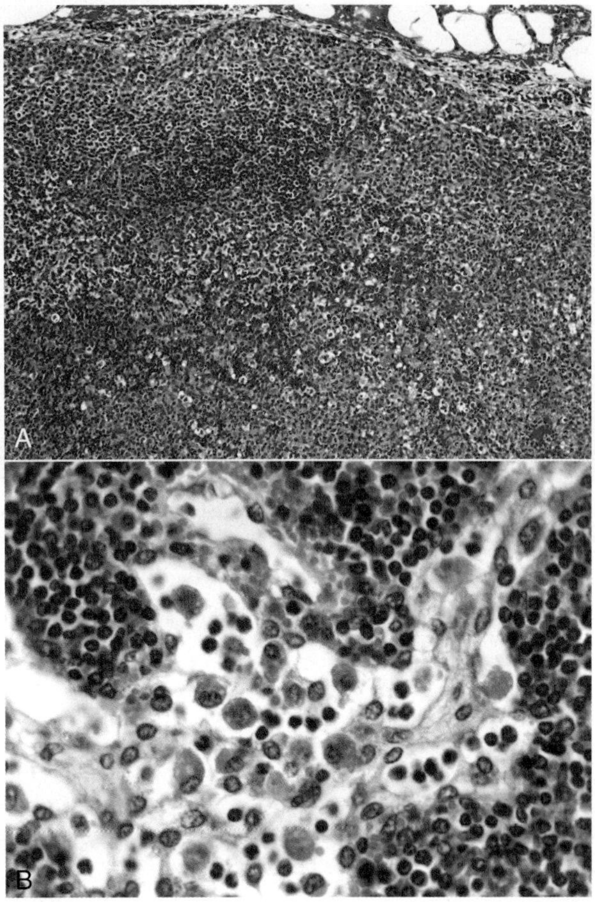

Figure 13-78 Acute Lymphadenitis (Early), Lymph Node, Dog. A, The sinuses and the parenchyma of the cortex and medulla have coalescing foci of neutrophilic inflammation, necrosis, hemorrhage, and fibrin deposition. H&E stain. **B,** The medullary sinus contains numerous macrophages (sinus histiocytosis) and fewer neutrophils. This is the type of early response seen when a lymph node drains an inflamed area. Medullary cords are filled with lymphocytes and plasma cells. H&E stain. (**A** courtesy Dr. A.C. Durham, School of Veterinary Medicine, University of Pennsylvania. **B** courtesy Dr. H.B. Gelberg, College of Veterinary Medicine, Oregon State University.)

Histologically, the subcapsular, trabecular, and medullary sinuses and the parenchyma of the cortex and medulla have focal to coalescing foci of neutrophilic inflammation, necrosis, and fibrin deposition (Fig. 13-78). If inflammation in the lymph node continues for several days or longer, the lymph node is further enlarged by follicular hyperplasia and plasmacytosis of the medullary cords from the expected immune response.

Chronic Lymphadenitis. The types of chronic lymphadenitis include chronic suppurative lymphadenitis, diffuse granulomatous inflammation, and discrete granulomas. In chronic suppurative inflammation, abscesses range in size from small microabscesses to large abscesses that occupy and obliterate the whole node. Recurrent bouts of chronic lymphadenitis (e.g., regional lymph node draining chronic mastitis in cows) lead to fibrosis and lymphoid hyperplasia, in addition to chronic abscesses. The classic example of chronic suppurative lymphadenitis with encapsulated abscesses is caseous lymphadenitis, a disease of sheep and goats caused by *C. pseudotuberculosis* (Figs. 13-79 and 13-80) (also see Disorders of Ruminants). It is also the cause of ulcerative lymphangitis in cattle and horses and pectoral abscesses in horses.

Focal Granulomatous Lymphadenitis. Classic examples of focal to multifocal granulomatous lymphadenitis are *Mycobacterium tuberculosis* complex, which includes *M. bovis* among others. Members of *M. avium* complex cause similar lesions and have been described in a number of species, including dogs, cats, primates, pigs, cattle, sheep, horses, and human beings. Infection may begin by inhalation of aerosol droplets containing the bacilli, which may spread via the lymphatic vessels to regional lymph nodes, resulting in granulomatous lymphangitis and lymphadenitis (Fig. 13-81). Initially lesions in the lymphatic system are confined to the lymphatic vessels (granulomatous lymphangitis) and regional lymph nodes (e.g., the tracheobronchial lymph nodes in the case of pulmonary

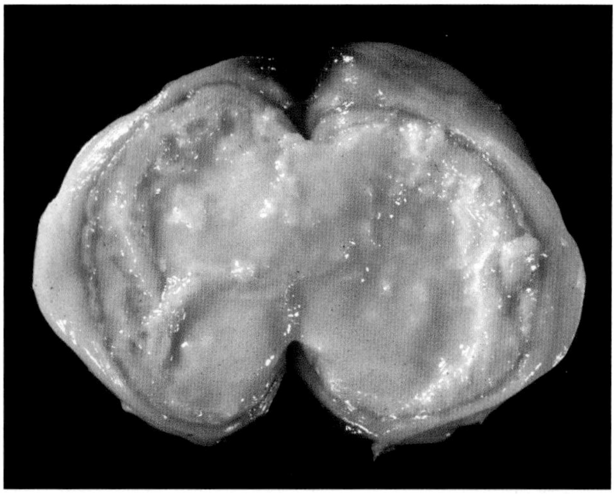

Figure 13-79 **Caseous Lymphadenitis, *Corynebacterium pseudotuberculosis*, Lymph Node, Sheep.** The entire lymph node is replaced by an abscess. This is an early stage of caseous lymphadenitis, before the pus has become inspissated and lamellated. (Courtesy Dr. K. Read, College of Veterinary Medicine, Texas A&M University; and Noah's Arkive, College of Veterinary Medicine, The University of Georgia.)

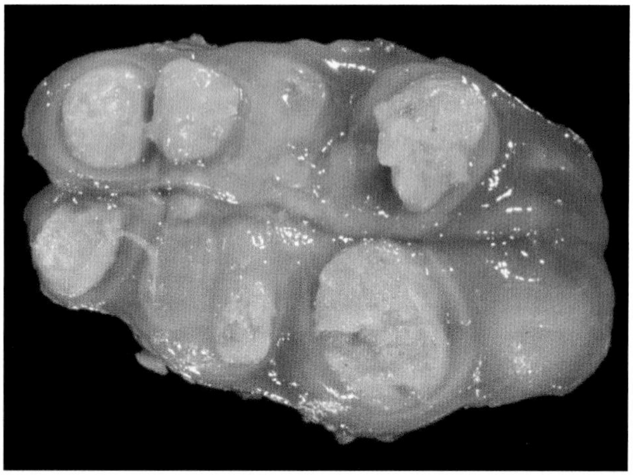

Figure 13-80 **Chronic Caseous Lymphadenitis, *Corynebacterium pseudotuberculosis*, Lymph Node, Sheep.** Three encapsulated chronic abscesses contain yellow-white caseous pus. (Courtesy Dr. W. Crowell, College of Veterinary Medicine, The University of Georgia; and Noah's Arkive, College of Veterinary Medicine, The University of Georgia.)

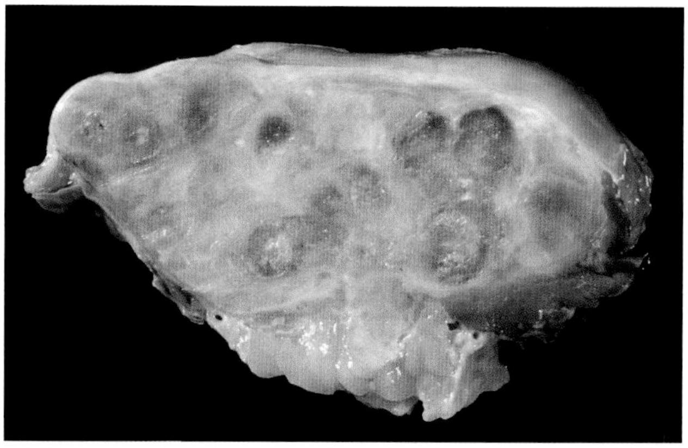

Figure 13-81 **Tuberculosis (*Mycobacterium bovis*), Lymph Node, Ox.** The normal architecture of the lymph node has been completely obliterated by multiple yellow-brown caseating granulomas, typical of M. *bovis* lesions. (Courtesy Dr. M.D. McGavin, College of Veterinary Medicine, University of Tennessee.)

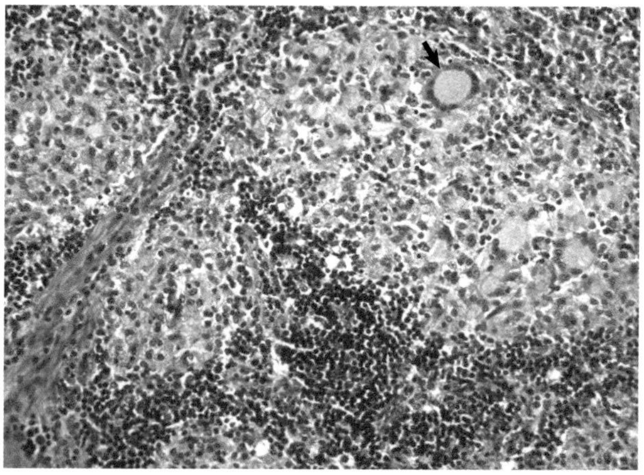

Figure 13-82 **Johne's Disease (*Mycobacterium avium* ssp. *paratuberculosis*), Lymph Node, Ox.** Several noncaseating granulomas *(areas of pallor)* have replaced the normal lymphoid tissue *(blue)*. Note the Langhans giant cell *(arrow)*. H&E stain. (Courtesy College of Veterinary Medicine, University of Illinois.)

tuberculosis), but once disseminated in the lymph or blood, lymph nodes throughout the body will have lesions. Well-organized granulomas consist of a central mass of macrophages with phagocytized mycobacteria, surrounded by epithelioid and foamy macrophages and occasional multinucleated giant cells (Langhans type). These inflammatory nodules are surrounded by a layer of lymphocytes enclosed in a fibrous capsule. Over time the center of the granuloma may undergo caseous necrosis due to the high lipid and protein content of the dead macrophages (see Chapter 3). In bovine Johne's disease the mesenteric lymph nodes draining the infected intestine can have noncaseous granulomas (Fig. 13-82).

Diffuse Granulomatous Lymphadenitis. Coalescing to diffuse granulomatous lymphadenitis is seen in disseminated fungal infections such as blastomycosis, cryptococcosis (E-Fig. 13-12), and histoplasmosis (see Disorders in Dogs). In feline cryptococcosis (most often *Cryptococcus neoformans*), the inflammatory response may be mild due to the thick polysaccharide capsule, which has strong immunomodulatory properties and promotes immune evasion and survival within the host. Therefore the nodal enlargement is due mainly to a large mass of organisms (see E-Fig. 13-12). Pigs with PCV2 infection may have a multifocal to diffuse infiltrate of macrophages and multinucleated giant cells of varying severity (see Disorders of Pigs).

Secondary (Metastatic) Neoplasms. Carcinomas typically metastasize via lymphatic vessels to the regional lymph node. Other common metastatic neoplasms include mast cell tumor and malignant melanoma. Although sarcomas most often metastasize hematogenously, some more aggressive sarcomas (e.g., osteosarcoma) may spread to regional lymph nodes. Histologically, single cells or clusters of neoplastic cells travel via the afferent lymphatic vessels and are deposited in a sinus, usually the subcapsular sinus (see Fig. 13-47). Here the cells proliferate and can ultimately occupy the whole lymph node, as well as drain to the next lymph node in the chain.

Pigmentation of Lymph Nodes

Red discoloration is caused by (1) draining erythrocytes from hemorrhagic or acutely inflamed areas, (2) acute lymphadenitis with hyperemia and/or hemorrhage, (3) acute septicemias with endotoxin-induced vasculitis or disseminated intravascular coagulation, and (4) dependent areas in postmortem hypostatic congestion. Blood in pig lymph nodes is especially obvious due to the inverse anatomy (the equivalent of the medullary sinuses are subcapsular and thus readily visible in the unsectioned node). Initially erythrocytes fill trabecular and medullary sinuses and then rapidly undergo erythrophagocytosis by proliferating sinus macrophages. Hemosiderin deposition occurs within 7 to 10 days in these macrophages, imparting a brown discoloration of the node.

Black discoloration is often present in the tracheobronchial lymph nodes due to draining of carbon pigment (pulmonary anthracosis, see Chapter 9). Black ink from skin tattoos will drain to the regional lymph node. These pigments are usually noted within the medullary sinus macrophages.

Brown discoloration may be due to melanin, parasitic hematin, or hemosiderin. Melanin pigment is seen in animals with chronic dermatitis when melanocytes are damaged and their pigment is released into the dermis and phagocytized by melanomacrophages (pigmentary incontinence) and drained to the regional lymph node. The mandibular lymph nodes often contain numerous melanomacrophages in animals with heavily pigmented oral mucosa, presumably due to chronic low levels of inflammation. This must be distinguished from metastatic malignant melanomas. Lymph nodes draining areas of congenital melanosis may have melanin deposits.

Parasitic hematin pigment is produced by *Fascioloides magna* (cattle) and *Fasciola hepatica* (sheep) in the liver and then transported via the lymphatic vessels to the hepatic lymph nodes.

Hemosiderin, an erythrocyte breakdown product, may form in a hemorrhagic node or arrive in hemosiderophages draining from congested, hemorrhagic, or inflamed areas. Drainage of iron dextran from an intramuscular injection may also cause hemosiderin pigment accumulation within the draining lymph node.

Green discoloration is rare and may be caused by green tattoo ink (often used in black animals); ingestion of blue-green algae, which drain to mesenteric lymph nodes; massive eosinophilic inflammation; and in mutant Corriedale sheep, which have a genetic defect that results in a deficiency in the excretion of bilirubin and phylloerythrin by the liver. The phylloerythrin or a metabolite stains all the tissues of the body a dark green, except for the brain and spinal cord, which are protected by the blood-brain barrier.

Miscellaneous discolorations of lymph nodes may be seen with intravenously injected dyes (e.g., methylene blue or trypan blue) or subcutaneous drug injections. Lymph nodes may be yellow in severely icteric patients. The pigmented strain of MAP (Johne's disease) may impart an orange discoloration in the mesenteric lymph nodes of sheep.

Miscellaneous Lymph Node Disorders

Inclusion Bodies. Many viruses produce inclusion bodies, and some of these occur in lymph nodes. These viruses include EHV-1 in horses, bovine adenovirus, cytomegalic virus in inclusion body rhinitis and PCV2, herpesvirus of pseudorabies in pigs, and rarely parvovirus in dogs and cats.

Emphysema. Emphysema in lymph nodes is a consequence of emphysema in their drainage fields and is seen most frequently in tracheobronchial lymph nodes in bovine interstitial emphysema and in porcine mesenteric lymph nodes in intestinal emphysema (see Chapter 7). The appearance of the lymph node varies with the extent of the emphysema. In severe cases the lymph node is light, puffy, and filled with discrete gas bubbles, and the cut surface may be spongy. Histologically, the sinuses are distended with gas and lined by macrophages and giant cells. This change has been considered a foreign body reaction to the gas bubbles. Macrophages and giant cells are also seen in afferent lymphatic vessels (granulomatous lymphangitis).

Vascular Transformation of Lymph Node Sinus (Nodal Angiomatosis). Vascular transformation of the sinuses is a non-neoplastic reaction to blocked efferent lymphatic vessels or veins. This pressure-induced lesion results in the formation of anastomosing vascular channels and may be confused with a nodal vascular neoplasm. These proliferative but noninvasive masses usually begin in the subcapsular sinuses and may be followed by lymphoid atrophy, erythrophagocytosis/hemosiderosis, and fibrosis. The blockage may be caused by malignant neoplasms of the tissues that the lymph node drains (e.g., thyroid carcinoma with nodal angiomatosis of the mandibular lymph node).

Neoplasia

See section on Bone Marrow, Disorders of Domestic Animals, Hematopoietic Neoplasia for a discussion of the WHO classification of hematopoietic neoplasia that predominantly arise and proliferate within bone marrow. This section will cover neoplasms of lymphoid tissue(s) arising outside of bone marrow.

Lymphoma. The term lymphoma (also known as lymphosarcoma) encompasses a diverse group of malignancies arising in lymphoid tissue(s) outside of bone marrow. Grossly, there may be diffuse to nodular enlargement of one or more lymph nodes (Fig. 13-83), and the cut surface is soft, white, and bulging with loss of normal corticomedullary architecture. There is great variation in the clinical manifestations and cytopathologic features of lymphoma, which underlie the importance of classification to better predict the clinical behavior and outcome. An understanding of lymphocyte maturation is crucial, because the WHO classification of lymphoma postulates a normal cell counterpart for each type of lymphoma (when possible). In other words, lymphoma can arise at any stage in the development/maturation of a lymphocyte—from precursor lymphocytes (B or T lymphoblasts) to mature lymphoid B and T, lymphocytes and NK cells (Table 13-7 and Box 13-11).

Pathologists use gross features, histomorphologic features, immunophenotype (B or T lymphocyte), and clinical characteristics to

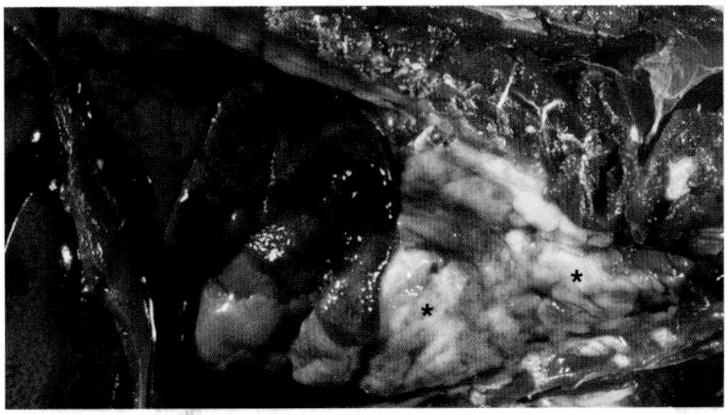

Figure 13-83 **Lymphoma, Cranial Mediastinal Lymph Nodes, Cat.** The cranial mediastinal lymph nodes are grossly enlarged *(asterisks)*, fill the cranial thoracic cavity, and have caudally displaced the lungs and heart. (Courtesy Dr. M.D. McGavin, College of Veterinary Medicine, University of Tennessee.)

Table 13-7 Common Lymphoma Diagnoses in Domestic Animals Using the WHO Classification System

Lymphoma Subtype	Pattern	Cell Size	Grade	Postulated Normal Cell Counterpart	Defining Histopathologic Features
DLBCL	Diffuse	Large	Mid to high	Germinal center or post–germinal center (activated) B lymphocyte	Multiple nucleoli (centroblastic variant) or single central nucleoli (immunoblastic variant)
PTCL	Diffuse	Large	Mid to high	Activated mature T lymphocyte	Nuclei of variable size and shape; eosinophils may be present
Burkitt-like lymphoma	Diffuse	Intermediate	High	Either germinal center or post–germinal center (activated) B lymphocyte	Uniform nuclear size with multiple distinct small nucleoli; numerous tingible body macrophages
T-LBL	Diffuse	Intermediate	High	Naïve T lymphocyte	Dispersed chromatin that obscures nuclear detail
TZL	Nodular	Small to intermediate	Indolent	Activated mature T lymphocyte; paracortical	Abundant clear cytoplasm, sharp shallow nuclear indentations; expansion of paracortex with peripheralization of "fading" follicles
MZL	Nodular	Intermediate	Indolent	Post–germinal center marginal zone B lymphocyte	Prominent single central nucleoli; expansion of marginal zone with encircling of "fading" follicles
TCRLBCL	Nodular/diffuse	Large	Indolent to low	Germinal center B lymphocyte	Large irregularly-shaped nuclei with 1-2 prominent nucleoli; numerous small reactive T lymphocytes
EATCL	Diffuse	Small to intermediate	Low	Intestinal intraepithelial T lymphocytes	Hyperchromatic nuclei with dispersed chromatin

DLBCL, Diffuse large B cell lymphoma; *EATCL,* enteropathy-associated T cell lymphoma; *MZL,* marginal zone lymphoma; *PTCL,* peripheral T cell lymphoma; *TCRLBCL, T* cell–rich large B cell lymphoma; *T-LBL,* T cell lymphoblastic lymphoma; *TZL,* T zone lymphoma, *WHO,* World Health Organization.

Box 13-11 Histologic Classification of Hematopoietic Tumors of the Lymphoid System in Domestic Animals

B LYMPHOCYTE LYMPHOID NEOPLASMS

Precursor B Lymphocyte

B cell lymphoblastic leukemia/lymphoma

Mature B Lymphocyte

- B cell chronic lymphocytic leukemia/lymphoma
- B cell lymphocytic lymphoma intermediate type
- Lymphoplasmacytic
- Follicular lymphomas
  - Mantle cell lymphoma
  - Follicular center cell lymphoma (I, II, III)
  - Nodal marginal zone lymphoma
  - Splenic marginal zone lymphoma
- Extranodal marginal zone lymphoma of MALT
- Hairy cell leukemia
- Plasmacytic tumors
  - Indolent plasmacytoma
  - Anaplastic plasmacytoma
  - Plasma cell myeloma
- Large B cell lymphomas
  - T cell–rich large B cell lymphoma
  - Diffuse large B cell lymphoma
  - Thymic B cell lymphoma
  - Intravascular large B cell lymphoma
- Burkitt-like lymphoma

T LYMPHOCYTE AND NK CELL LYMPHOID NEOPLASMS

Precursor T Lymphocyte

T cell lymphoblastic leukemia/lymphoma

Mature T Cell/NK Lymphocyte

- Large granular lymphoproliferative disorders
  - T cell chronic lymphocytic leukemia
  - T cell LGL lymphoma/leukemia
  - NK cell chronic lymphocytic leukemia
- Cutaneous T cell lymphomas
  - Cutaneous epitheliotropic lymphoma
  - Cutaneous nonepitheliotropic lymphoma
- Extranodal/Peripheral T cell lymphoma
- Adult T cell–like lymphoma/leukemia
- Angioimmunoblastic lymphoma
- Angiotropic lymphoma
- Intestinal T cell lymphoma
- Anaplastic large cell lymphoma

MALT, Mucosa-associated lymphoid tissue; *LGL,* large granular lymphocyte; *NK,* natural killer.

Modified from Valli VE, Jacobs RM, Parodi AL, et al: Histologic classification of hematopoietic tumors of domestic animals. In *World Health Organization international histological classification of tumors in domestic animals,* second series (vol 8), Washington, DC, 2002, Armed Forces Institute of Pathology.

classify lymphomas. The morphologic features used in histopathologic classification are the following:

- Histologic pattern—Nodular or diffuse.
- Cell size—The nuclei of the neoplastic lymphocytes are compared to the diameter of a red blood cell (RBC ≅ 5 μm). Small is less than 1.5 times the diameter of an RBC; intermediate is 1.5 to 2.0 times the diameter of an RBC; large is more than 2.0 times the diameter of an RBC.
- Grade—Mitotic figures are counted in a *single* high-power (400×) field. Indolent is 0 to 1; low is 2 to 5; mid is 6 to 10; high is more than 10.

Although there are numerous subtypes of lymphoma recognized under the WHO system, a detailed discussion of each subtype is outside the scope of this textbook. However, a select number of subtypes are more commonly seen in domestic animals (see Table 13-7) and currently best described in the dog (see Disorders of Dogs, Neoplasms, Lymphomas). The most common types in dogs are large cell lymphomas and include diffuse large B cell lymphoma and peripheral T cell lymphoma. T cell–rich large B cell lymphoma is thought to be a variant of diffuse large B cell lymphoma with a distinctive reactive T lymphocyte infiltrate. Intermediate cell lymphomas include B or T lymphocyte lymphoblastic lymphomas and Burkitt-like lymphoma (both high grade), marginal zone lymphoma, and the intermediate cell variant of T zone lymphomas (both indolent and nodular). Small cell lymphomas most commonly diagnosed in domestic animal species include enteropathy-associated T cell lymphoma, commonly seen in the cat, T zone lymphoma (small cell variant), and small cell lymphoma. Cutaneous lymphomas are most often of T lymphocyte origin and may be epitheliotropic or nonepitheliotropic, and a distinct entity of inflamed T cell lymphoma has been recently described in dogs (see Chapter 17).

Plasma Cell Neoplasia. Plasma cell neoplasms are most easily categorized as *myeloma* or *multiple myeloma*, which arises in the bone marrow, and *extramedullary plasmacytoma*, which as the name implies involves sites other than bone.

Multiple Myeloma. See Bone Marrow and Blood Cells, Disorders of Domestic Animals, Types of Hematopoietic Neoplasia, Plasma Cell Neoplasia.

Extramedullary Plasmacytomas. Extramedullary plasmacytomas are most commonly diagnosed in the skin of dogs (also cats and horses), where they constitute 1.5% of all canine cutaneous tumors (see Chapter 17). The pinnae, lips, digits, and chin are the most commonly affected locations, and most lesions are solitary, though multiple plasmacytomas are infrequently diagnosed. Other tissues affected include the oral cavity, intestine (colorectal in particular), liver, spleen, kidney, lung, and brain; of these, the oral cavity and intestine (colorectal) are involved most often. In one study, extramedullary plasmacytomas represented 5% of all canine oral tumors and 28% of all extramedullary plasmacytomas diagnosed. Most cutaneous extramedullary plasmacytomas are benign, and complete excision is usually curative; oral cavity and colorectal extramedullary plasmacytomas are likely to behave in a similar manner. More aggressive forms may occur at any site.

As with multiple myeloma, the neoplastic cells composing the tumor may vary from well differentiated to pleomorphic, often within the same tumor. The cells often have a characteristic perinuclear Golgi clearing or "halo," and the more pleomorphic cells exhibit karyomegaly and binucleation (Fig. 13-84). Extramedullary plasmacytomas may produce monoclonal immunoglobulins with resulting monoclonal gammopathy. Amyloid deposition (which may mineralize) is also observed in a proportion of cases. Differentiation from other round cell tumors may be aided by immunohistochemistry (MUM1/IRF4 is particularly sensitive and specific for plasma cell neoplasms).

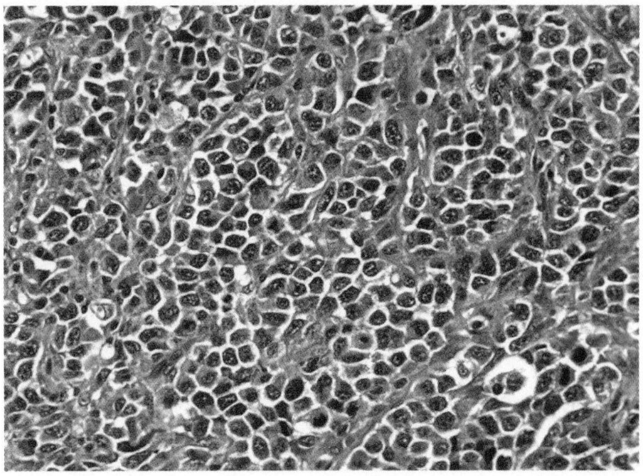

Figure 13-84 **Plasmacytoma (Extramedullary), Oral Cavity, Dog.** Note the moderately well-differentiated plasma cells arranged in small clusters separated by a fibrovascular stroma. H&E stain. (Courtesy College of Veterinary Medicine, University of Illinois.)

Histiocytic Disorders. Histiocytic disorders are frequently diagnosed in dogs and occur less often in cats. Briefly, histiocytes are categorized as macrophages and DCs, the latter of which are subdivided into *Langerhans cells* (LCs), found in skin, gastrointestinal, respiratory, and reproductive epithelia (mucosae), and *interstitial DCs* (iDC), located in perivascular spaces of most organs. The term *interdigitating DCs* describes DCs (either resident or migrating) found in T lymphocyte regions of lymph nodes (paracortex) and spleen (PALS); interdigitating DCs consist of both LCs and iDCs. These lineages can be differentiated using immunohistochemical stains. Histiocytic disorders that are diagnosed in veterinary medicine at this time include the following: canine cutaneous histiocytoma, canine LC histiocytosis, canine cutaneous and systemic histiocytosis, feline pulmonary LC histiocytosis, feline progressive histiocytosis, dendritic cell leukemia in the dog, and histiocytic sarcoma and hemophagocytic histiocytic sarcoma in both dogs and cats.

Lymph node involvement is seen in many of these conditions. Rare reports of regional lymph node metastasis in cases of solitary canine cutaneous histiocytoma have been published. Lymphatic invasion with subsequent regional nodal involvement may be seen in dogs with LC histiocytosis, which is a poor prognostic indicator and likely reflects systemic infiltration. The normal architecture of tracheobronchial lymph nodes is often effaced in cats with pulmonary LC histiocytosis.

Canine reactive histiocytoses are not clonal neoplastic proliferations but likely reflect an immune dysregulation consisting of activated dermal iDCs (and T lymphocytes). They are categorized as *cutaneous histiocytosis* (CH), involving skin and draining lymph nodes, and a more generalized *systemic histiocytosis* (SH), affecting skin and other sites (e.g., lung, liver, bone marrow, spleen, lymph nodes, kidneys, and orbital and nasal tissues).

Histiocytic Sarcoma Complex. Histiocytic sarcomas (HSs) are neoplasms of iDCs and therefore can arise in almost any tissue, frequently the spleen, lung, skin, meninges, lymph nodes, bone marrow, and synovium. Secondary involvement of the liver is common as the disease progresses. This neoplasm is most commonly diagnosed in dogs, and a lower incidence is seen in cats. *Localized histiocytic sarcoma* may be a focal solitary lesion or multiple nodules within a single organ. *Disseminated histiocytic sarcoma* describes lesions that involve distant sites and has replaced the term malignant histiocytosis. Breed predispositions to histiocytic sarcoma complex are seen in Bernese mountain dogs, Rottweilers, golden retrievers, and flat-coated retrievers, though the disease can occur in any breed. Histiocytic sarcoma complex is considered to have a rapid and highly aggressive course, and the clinical signs depend on the particular organ(s) involved.

Grossly, affected organs may be uniformly enlarged and/or contain multiple coalescing white-tan nodules. Tissue architecture is effaced by sheets of pleomorphic round to spindle-shaped cells. There is marked cellular atypia with numerous karyomegalic and multinucleated neoplastic cells (Fig. 13-85).

Hemophagocytic Histiocytic Sarcoma. Hemophagocytic histiocytic sarcoma is seen in dogs and cats and is a neoplasm of macrophages of the spleen and bone marrow. Clinically, dogs present with hemolytic regenerative anemia and thrombocytopenia, thus mimicking Evans's syndrome, though they are Coombs negative. This form of histiocytic sarcoma carries the worst prognosis of the histiocytic sarcomas, which is likely in part related to the severe anemia and coagulopathy. It is characterized by a non–mass forming infiltrate of histiocytes within the bone marrow and splenic red pulp, causing diffuse splenomegaly. The neoplastic cells exhibit marked erythrophagocytosis, but the severe cellular pleomorphism seen in the histiocytic sarcoma complex may be lacking. The neoplastic cells are often intermixed with EMH and plasma cells. Metastasis is frequently to the liver, where the cells concentrate within the sinuses. Tumor emboli within the lung are often present.

Disorders of Domestic Animals: Mucosa-Associated Lymphoid Tissue

MALT is involved in a variety of ways with bacteria and viruses, and these are summarized for large animals in Table 13-5. These interactions include being a portal of entry for pathogens (e.g., *Salmonella* spp., *Yersinia pestis*, MAP, and *L. monocytogenes*); a site of replication for viruses (e.g., BVDV); a site for hematogenous infection (e.g., panleukopenia virus and parvovirus); and a site of gross or microscopic lesions in some viral diseases. Bovine coronavirus, BVDV, rinderpest virus, malignant catarrhal fever virus, feline panleukopenia virus, and canine parvovirus cause lymphocyte depletion within the MALT.

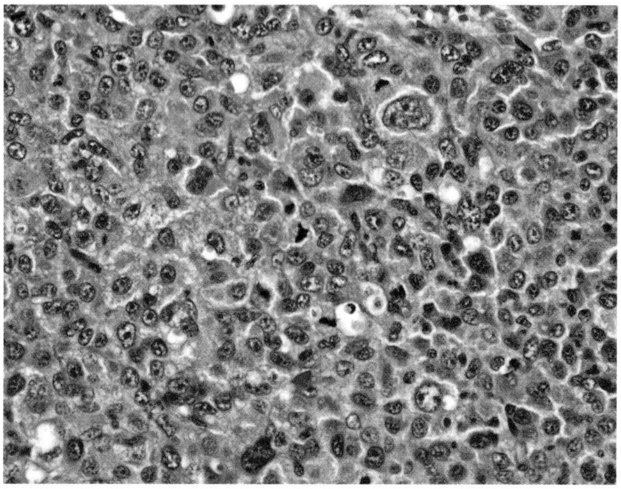

Figure 13-85 **Histiocytic Sarcoma, Spleen, Dog.** The neoplastic cells are markedly pleomorphic with karyomegalic cells, binucleation, and numerous mitotic figures. H&E stain. (Courtesy Dr. A.C. Durham, School of Veterinary Medicine, University of Pennsylvania.)

Disorders of Horses

Severe Combined Immunodeficiency

Severe combined immunodeficiency disease of Arabian foals is an autosomal recessive primary immunodeficiency disorder characterized by the lack of functional T and B lymphocytes caused by a genetic mutation in the gene encoding for DNA-dependent protein kinase catalytic subunit (DNA-PKcs). This enzyme is required for receptor gene rearrangements involved in the maturation of lymphocytes, and the resulting loss of functional T and B lymphocytes leads to a profound susceptibility to infectious diseases. Though normal at birth, these foals develop diarrhea and pneumonia by approximately 10 days of age, often due to adenovirus, *Cryptosporidium parvum*, and *Pneumocystis carinii* infections. Affected foals often die before 5 months of age. Lymph nodes and thymus are small and often grossly undetectable, and the spleen is small and firm due to the absence of white pulp (see Fig. 13-70). The development of genetic tests to identify carriers of the disorder has led to a decrease in the prevalence of severe combined immunodeficiency disease. Recently, severe combined immunodeficiency disease was diagnosed in a single Caspian filly, though the exact genetic defect was not determined. Congenital immunodeficiency diseases are also discussed in detail in Chapter 5.

Strangles

Streptococcus equi ssp. *equi*, the etiologic agent of equine strangles, is inhaled or ingested after direct contact with the discharge from infected horses or from a contaminated environment. The bacteria attach to the tonsils, penetrate into deeper tissues, enter the lymphatic vessels, drain to regional lymph nodes (mandibular, retropharyngeal, and occasionally parotid and cervical lymph nodes), and cause large abscesses (see Fig. 13-77). Retropharyngeal enlargement from abscesses may lead to compression of the pharynx and subsequent respiratory stridor and dysphagia. Abscesses may rupture and discharge pus through a sinus to the skin surface or spread medially into guttural pouches, where residual pus dries and hardens to form chondroids (which serve as a nidus for live bacteria to persist in carrier animals). In up to 20% of these cases, ruptured abscess material may spread via blood or lymph to other organs (metastatic abscess formation, *bastard strangles*), including lung, liver, kidney, synovia, mesenteric and mediastinal lymph nodes, spleen, and occasionally brain. Purpura hemorrhagica, a type III hypersensitivity reaction, may result in necrotizing vasculitis in some horses with repeated natural exposure to *S. equi* ssp. *equi* or after vaccination in horses that have had strangles.

Rhodococcus Equi Infection

The typical manifestation of *R. equi* infection is chronic suppurative bronchopneumonia with abscesses (see Chapter 9). Approximately 50% of foals also develop intestinal lesions characterized by pyogranulomatous ulcerative enterotyphlocolitis, often over Peyer's patches, and pyogranulomatous lymphadenitis of mesenteric and colonic lymph nodes (see Chapter 7; see Fig. 13-68). Large abdominal abscesses may be the only lesion in the abdomen and presumably originate from an infected mesenteric lymph node. The diffuse lymphatic tissue in the lamina propria may contain granulomatous inflammation with the phagocytized bacteria. Mediastinal pyogranulomatous lymphadenitis may compress the trachea, causing respiratory distress. *R. equi* lesions also can develop in the liver, kidney, spleen, or nervous tissue.

Lymphoma

Lymphoma is the most common malignant neoplasm in horses and mostly affects adult animals (mean age 10 to 11 years) with no apparent breed or sex predisposition. The most frequent anatomic locations of equine lymphoma are multicentric, cutaneous, and gastrointestinal tract.

Multicentric lymphoma, defined as involving at least two organs (excluding the regional lymph nodes), is the most common manifestation, followed by skin and gastrointestinal tract types. Solitary locations have been reported in the mediastinum, lymph nodes, ocular/orbital region, brain, spinal cord, oral cavity, and spleen. Of the multicentric lymphomas, the most frequently observed type is T cell–rich large B cell lymphoma (TCRLBCL), reportedly in one study affecting 34% of the cases. Peripheral T cell lymphoma (PTCL) was the second most common, followed by diffuse large B cell lymphoma (DLBCL).

The most common lymphoma type in the gastrointestinal tract is also T cell–rich large B cell lymphoma, followed by enteropathy-associated T cell lymphoma. Cutaneous lymphomas in horses account for up to 3% of all equine skin tumors. T cell–rich large B cell lymphoma is again the most common lymphoma subtype in the skin, representing up to 84% of all cutaneous lymphomas, and most frequently presents clinically as multiple skin masses. Cutaneous T cell lymphoma (CTCL) is the second most common form and arises as smaller solitary nodules. Thoroughbreds may have a higher incidence of cutaneous T cell lymphoma compared to other breeds. Overall, horses with cutaneous T cell–rich large B cell lymphoma appear to have a longer survival time than horses with other types of lymphoma of the skin. Progesterone receptor–positive lymphomas have also been identified in horses, and there is one report of subcutaneous tumor regression following removal of an ovarian granulosa-theca cell tumor. There may be an increased frequency of lymphoma in horses diagnosed with equine herpesvirus 5 (EHV-5, gammaherpesvirus), when compared to healthy horses, although the exact cause-effect role of this observation in lymphomagenesis[5] is not yet known.

Histologically, the hallmark features of T cell–rich large B cell lymphoma include a majority of small (nuclei approximately the size of an RBC), reactive, mature T lymphocytes admixed with a neoplastic population of large B lymphocytes whose nuclei are two to three times the diameter of an equine RBC. These large atypical cells are often binucleated and have prominent eosinophilic nucleoli (Fig. 13-86). The large cells may be observed in mitosis or in necrosis as single cells with retracted cytoplasm and pyknotic nuclei. T cell–rich large B cell lymphoma is often accompanied by the presence of a dense fibrovascular network.

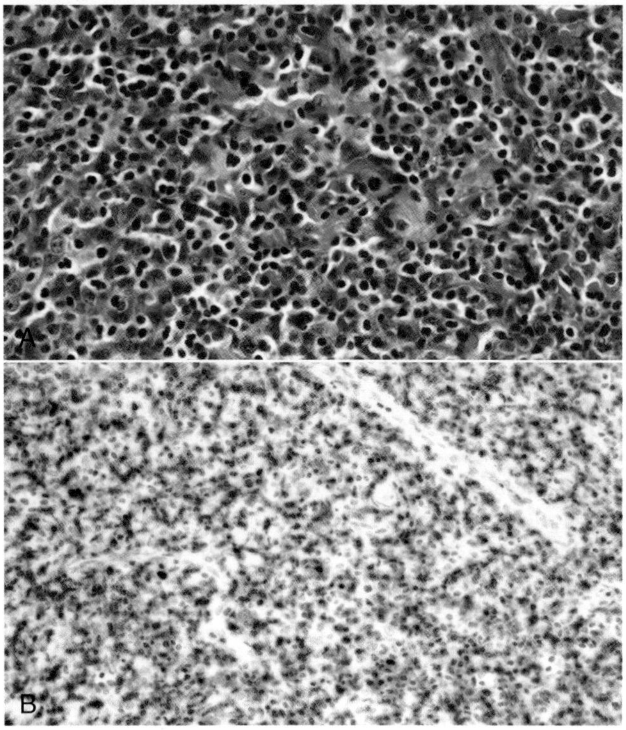

Figure 13-86 T Cell–Rich Large B Cell Lymphoma, Skin, Horse. A, The majority of the cells are small T lymphocytes and are mixed with fewer neoplastic large pleomorphic B lymphocytes. H&E stain. **B,** The small reactive T lymphocytes are strongly CD3 positive. Immunohistochemistry with anti-CD3, hematoxylin counterstain. (Courtesy Dr. A.C. Durham, School of Veterinary Medicine, University of Pennsylvania.)

Disorders of Ruminants (Cattle, Sheep, and Goats)

Johne's Disease

Johne's disease primarily affects domestic and wild ruminants (and rarely pigs and horses) and is due to infection by MAP. The characteristic lesions include granulomatous enteritis usually confined to the ileum, cecum, and proximal colon; lymphangitis; and lymphadenitis of regional lymph nodes (see Fig. 13-82). The bacteria are ingested, engulfed by the M cells overlying Peyer's patches, and then transported to macrophages in the lamina propria and submucosa. Among cattle, sheep, goats, and wild ruminants, there is wide variation in the severity, distribution of lesions, primary inflammatory cell type (lymphocytes, epithelioid macrophages, multinucleated giant cells), and numbers of bacteria within lesions (multibacillary or paucibacillary). Histologically, the architecture of the ileocecal lymph nodes may be partially replaced by aggregates of epithelioid macrophages and multinucleated giant cells, and the remaining nodal tissue contains large secondary follicles with reactive germinal centers. Cattle tend to have noncaseating granulomas, whereas sheep and goats may have granulomas with necrotic caseous centers and mineralization. Variable numbers of acid-fast bacilli are detected within epithelioid macrophages. The intestinal lesions of Johne's disease are described in detail in Chapter 7.

Anthrax

Anthrax is caused by *B. anthracis*, a Gram-positive bacillus found in spore form in soil. Cattle, sheep, and goats become infected when grazing on infected soil, and infection causes fulminant septicemia. The spleen in infected animals is markedly enlarged and congested (see Uniform Splenomegaly with a Bloody Consistency; see also Chapter 4).

Bovine Viral Diarrhea

Bovine viral diarrhea is caused by BVDV, a pestivirus. Cattle are the natural host, but other animals such as alpacas, deer, sheep, and goats are also affected. BVDV preferentially infects cells of the immune system, including macrophages, DCs, and lymphocytes. The associated lesions in lymphoid tissues are severe lymphoid depletion in mesenteric lymph nodes and Peyer's patches, whose intestinal surface may be covered by a fibrinonecrotic membrane. Histologically, there is marked lymphocytolysis and necrosis of germinal centers in Peyer's patches and cortices of lymph nodes. There is thymic atrophy because the thymus is markedly depleted of lymphocytes and may consist of only collapsed stroma and few scattered lymphocytes. BVD is discussed in detail in Chapters 4 and 7.

[5]The growth and development of a lymphoma.

Splenic Abscesses

Splenic abscesses can be the result of bacteremia (see Fig. 13-69) or direct penetration by a foreign body from the reticulum (see Spleen and also Portals of Entry/Pathways of Spread).

Caseous Lymphadenitis

C. pseudotuberculosis is a Gram-positive intracellular bacterium that causes caseous lymphadenitis, a chronic suppurative disease of sheep and goats. The bacterium may enter through skin wounds (e.g., shearing cuts in sheep, tagging, tail docking, or castration), drain to the regional lymph node, and then be disseminated in lymph and circulating blood to external and internal lymph nodes, as well as other internal organs, including lung. External abscesses are most often detected in the "jaw and neck" region, specifically in the mandibular and parotid lymph nodes. On gross examination the abscesses are encapsulated and filled with greenish semifluid pus due to an infiltrate of eosinophils (see Fig. 13-79). Over time the abscesses lose the greenish hue, and contents become inspissated to form the characteristic concentric laminations (see Fig. 13-80); old abscesses may reach a diameter of 4 to 5 cm.

Bovine Lymphoma

Bovine lymphoma is broadly classified into *enzootic* and *sporadic* forms. The enzootic form, called enzootic bovine leukosis (EBL), is caused by BLV, a retrovirus common in cattle. There is a higher prevalence in dairy cattle compared to beef breeds. BLV is transmitted horizontally (e.g., blood, milk/colostrum, saliva) or iatrogenically (e.g., rectal sleeves, instruments/equipment). Following infection, BLV invades and integrates into the genome of infected B lymphocytes, resulting in a polyclonal B lymphocyte lymphocytosis in approximately 30% of cattle. In approximately 1% to 5% of BLV-infected cattle, a single clone will emerge, leading to the development of B lymphocyte leukemia/lymphoma. The average incubation period between infection and development of lymphoma is 7 to 8 years, and this low conversion rate suggests that the latency period may be longer than the life span of most animals (dairy cattle seldom live to the 7- to 8-year peak incidence of lymphoma occurrence). Other contributing variables, such as genetic background, coinfections, and environmental factors, may also play a role in lymphomagenesis. The exact mechanism of BLV-induced tumorigenesis is poorly understood. Recently BLV microRNAs (miRNAs) were identified in preleukemic and malignant B lymphocytes, which showed repression of structural and regulatory gene expression. These findings suggested that miRNAs may play a key role in tumor onset and progression.

Grossly, multiple tissues may be affected in cattle that develop lymphoma, including peripheral lymph nodes (cephalic, cervical, sublumbar) (Fig. 13-87), abdominal lymph nodes, retrobulbar region, abomasum, liver, spleen, heart, urogenital tract, bone marrow, vertebral canal (Fig. 13-88), and spinal cord. One study indicates most of these high-grade lymphomas are diffuse large cell lymphomas (66%), and approximately 20% are intermediate cell lymphomas (Burkitt-like and lymphoblastic lymphomas).

The *sporadic* form of bovine lymphoma is most often of T lymphocyte immunophenotype and has three subcategories: cutaneous, calf, and thymic. There is no known viral cause for the sporadic form, and each subcategory has a much smaller prevalence compared to the enzootic form. Of the three sporadic forms, the cutaneous form seems to be the most common and manifests itself as multiple skin nodules in 1- to 3-year-old cattle. The calf form presents as generalized lymphadenopathy with weight loss, lethargy, and weakness in calves less than 6 months old. The thymic form is reportedly more common in beef cattle, 6 to 24 months of age.

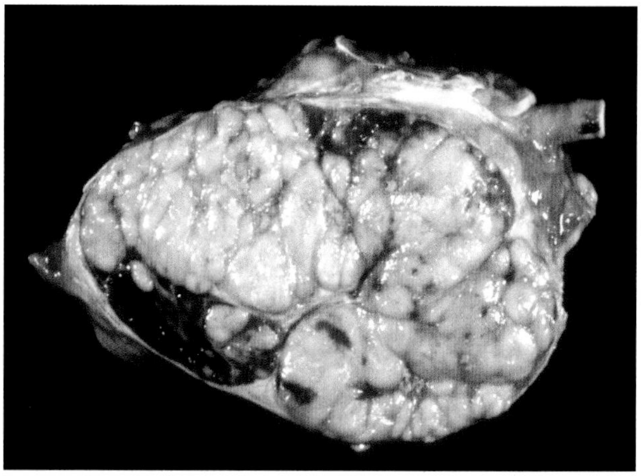

Figure 13-87 **Lymphoma, Bovine Lymph Node.** The normal architecture of lymph node has been replaced by white lobules of neoplastic lymphocytes. (Courtesy College of Veterinary Medicine, University of Illinois.)

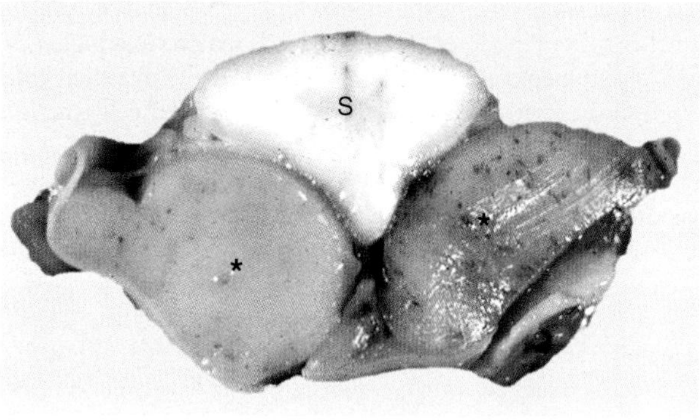

Figure 13-88 **Lymphoma *(Asterisks)*, Vertebral Canal, Epidural Space, Cow.** S, spinal cord. (Courtesy Dr. J.M. King, College of Veterinary Medicine, Cornell University.)

Disorders of Pigs

Postweaning Multisystem Wasting Syndrome

PCV2, a small single-stranded DNA virus, is highly prevalent in the domestic pig population. Several clinical syndromes are attributed to PCV2 infection and collectively termed PCV-associated diseases (PCVADs). These include postweaning multisystemic wasting syndrome (PMWS), porcine respiratory disease complex (PRDC), porcine dermatitis and nephropathy syndrome, and enteric disease (see Chapters 4 and 9).

The major postmortem findings of postweaning multisystemic wasting syndrome are poor body condition, enlarged lymph nodes, and interstitial pneumonia. The lesions of the lymphoid system are commonly observed in the tonsil, spleen, Peyer's patches, and lymph nodes. Some pigs have all lymphoid tissues affected, whereas others may have only one or two affected lymph nodes. The characteristic microscopic lesions are lymphoid depletion of both follicles and paracortex with replacement by histiocytes, mild to severe granulomatous inflammation with multinucleated giant cells, and intrahistiocytic sharply demarcated, spherical, basophilic cytoplasmic inclusion bodies. Necrosis of prominent lymphoid follicles (necrotizing lymphadenitis) is occasionally observed, and PCV2 can be detected within the necrotic regions. The loss of lymphocytes may be due to reduced production in the bone marrow, decreased proliferation in the secondary lymphoid organs, or necrosis of lymphocytes.

Porcine Reproductive and Respiratory Syndrome

Porcine reproductive and respiratory syndrome (PRRS) is caused by an arterivirus and causes two overlapping clinical syndromes: reproductive failure and respiratory disease. The virus is transmitted by contact with body fluids (saliva, mucus, serum, urine, and mammary secretions and from contact with semen during coitus), but often it first colonizes tonsils or upper respiratory tract. The virus has a predilection for lymphoid tissues (spleen, thymus, tonsils, lymph nodes, Peyer's patches). Viral replication takes place in macrophages of the lymphoid tissues and lungs, though porcine reproductive and respiratory syndrome virus antigen is found in resident macrophages in many tissues and may persist in tonsil and lung macrophages. The result of this infection is a reduction in the phagocytic and functional capacity of macrophages of the monocyte-macrophage system. As a consequence, there is reduction in resistance to common bacterial and viral pathogens. Most porcine reproductive and respiratory syndrome–infected pigs are coinfected with one or more pathogens, including *Streptococcus suis* and *Salmonella choleraesuis*. Infection with *Bordetella bronchiseptica* and *Mycoplasma hyopneumoniae* appear to increase the duration and severity of the interstitial pneumonia.

The major lesions are interstitial pneumonia and generalized lymphadenopathy, and tracheobronchial and mediastinal lymph nodes are most commonly affected. Coinfections often complicate the gross and histopathologic changes. Lymph nodes are enlarged, pale tan, occasionally cystic, and firm; some strains of virus also cause nodal hemorrhage. Microscopically, the lesions in the lymph nodes, tonsils, and spleens consist of varying degrees of follicular and paracortical hyperplasia and lymphocyte depletion in follicular germinal centers.

Porcine Jowl Abscess

Streptococcus porcinus causes jowl abscesses in pigs. The bacteria colonize the oral cavity and spread to infect tonsils and regional lymph nodes. The mandibular lymph nodes are the most often affected and have multiple, 1- to 10-cm abscesses; the retropharyngeal and parotid lymph nodes may also be involved (Fig. 13-89). This once-prevalent disease is now rare, presumably due to improvements in husbandry, feeder design, and hygiene. It is occasionally isolated in pigs with bacteremia.

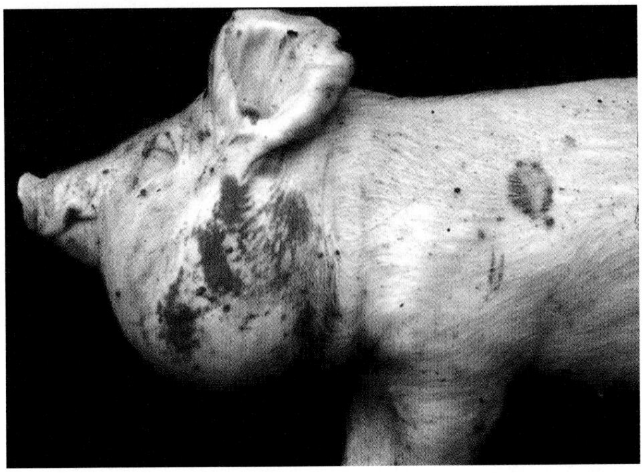

Figure 13-89 Jowl Abscess, Pig. The mandibular lymph nodes are markedly enlarged from a suppurative lymphadenitis caused by *Streptococcus porcinus*. (Courtesy Dr. J.M. King, College of Veterinary Medicine, Cornell University.)

Lymphoma

Lymphoma is the most frequently reported cancer of pigs based on abattoir surveys. Affected pigs are typically less than 1 year of age, and there is no reported breed predisposition, although a hereditary basis is suspected in cases arising in inbred herds. The two main forms of porcine lymphoma are thymic/mediastinal and multicentric; the latter is more common. Spleen, liver, kidney, bone marrow, and lymph nodes are affected in the multicentric form, with visceral lymph nodes reportedly more commonly involved than peripheral nodes. A recent study of lymphoma in 17 pigs found the majority to be multicentric, and subtypes included the following: B lymphoblastic leukemia/lymphoma, follicular lymphoma, diffuse and intestinal large B cell lymphoma, and peripheral T cell lymphoma. One case each of thymic B cell and T cell lymphomas were also described.

Disorders of Dogs

Severe Combined Immunodeficiency Disease

Several types of severe combined immunodeficiency diseases have been described in dogs. A mutation in DNA-PKcs (similar to Arabian horses) with an autosomal recessive mode of inheritance is seen in Jack Russell terriers. An X-linked form of severe combined immunodeficiency disease is well described in basset hounds and is caused by mutations in the common γ-chain (γc) subunit of the receptors for IL-2, IL-4, IL-7, IL-9, IL-15, and IL-21. A similar disease is seen in Cardigan Welsh corgi puppies, though it is an autosomal mode of inheritance in this breed. The mutation inhibits the signal transduction pathways initiated by any of these cytokines, which are critical for the proliferation, differentiation, survival, and function of B and T lymphocytes. Affected dogs have normal numbers of circulating B lymphocytes that are unable to class switch to IgG or IgA and reduced numbers of T lymphocytes, which are nonfunctional due to the inability to express IL receptors. Affected puppies are remarkably susceptible to bacterial and viral infections and rarely survive past 3 to 4 months of age. The thymus of these dogs is small and consists of only small dysplastic lobules with a few of Hassall's corpuscles. Tonsils, lymph nodes, and Peyer's patches are often grossly unidentifiable due to the severe lymphocyte hypoplasia. Congenital immunodeficiency diseases are also discussed in detail in Chapter 5.

Thymic Hematomas

Thymic hemorrhage and hematomas have been reported in dogs and are most often seen in young animals. A variety of causes are described, including ingestion of anticoagulant rodenticides (warfarin, dicumarol, diphacinone, and brodifacoum), dissecting aortic aneurysms, trauma (e.g., automobile accident), and idiopathic/spontaneous. Histologically, hemorrhage variably expands the thymic lobules and septa, and in severe cases the lobular architecture is obscured by hemorrhage. In cases of anticoagulant rodenticide toxicosis, the medulla appears to be the main site of hemorrhage.

Gastrosplenic Volvulus

See Uniform Splenomegaly with a Bloody Consistency (also see Figs. 7-72 and 7-73).

Splenic Hematomas, Incomplete Splenic Contraction, Acute Splenic Infarcts, and Hemangiosarcomas

See the section on Splenic Nodules with a Bloody Consistency for discussion on splenic hematomas (including those induced by nodular hyperplasia or occurring with hemangiosarcoma), incomplete splenic contraction, acute splenic infarcts, and hemangiosarcomas.

Siderofibrotic Plaques, Splenic Rupture, and Accessory Spleens

See the section on Miscellaneous Disorders of the Spleen for discussions on siderofibrotic plaques, splenic rupture, and accessory spleens.

Lymphoid and Complex Splenic Nodular Hyperplasia

Splenic nodular hyperplasia is common in dogs and categorized based on their cellular components as lymphoid nodular hyperplasia or complex nodular hyperplasia. Hematomas may arise within nodules of hyperplasia (see Splenic Nodules with a Bloody Consistency).

Lymphoid (or simple) nodular hyperplasia consists of a focal well-demarcated mass composed of discrete to coalescing aggregates of lymphocytes. The lymphocytes may form follicular structures with germinal centers and/or consist of a mixture of lymphocytes with mantle and marginal zone cell morphologic features. The intervening tissue is often congested and may contain plasma cells, but stroma is not observed (Fig. 13-90; E-Fig. 13-13).

Complex nodular hyperplasia is a focal mass that contains two proliferative components: lymphoid and stroma (E-Fig. 13-14). The lymphoid component resembles lymphoid nodular hyperplasia described above. There is proliferation of the intervening stromal tissues with fibroplasia, smooth muscle hyperplasia, and histiocytic hyperplasia; EMH and plasma cells may also be present.

Splenic Fibrohistiocytic Nodules

It has recently come to light that the entity splenic fibrohistiocytic nodule (SFHN), first described in 1998, is not a single condition, but in fact a complex group of diseases. Our better understanding of the spectrum of diseases once described under the term splenic fibrohistiocytic nodule is due to increasing knowledge of histiocytic disorders and immunochemistry. The original definition of splenic fibrohistiocytic nodule is a nodule characterized by a stromal population of histiocytoid and spindle cells intermixed with lymphocytes. Grading was based on the lymphocyte percentage of the population (e.g., > 70% lymphocytes = grade 1; < 40% lymphocytes = grade 3); dogs with grade 1 splenic fibrohistiocytic nodule had a much better 1-year survival rate, and dogs with grade 3 nodules may develop sarcomas (often malignant fibrous histiocytoma, a now outdated term).

With our increasing knowledge of histiocytic disorders and additional immunohistochemical stains, diseases that likely were encompassed by the term splenic fibrohistiocytic nodule include the following: complex and lymphoid nodular hyperplasia (see earlier), stromal sarcoma, histiocytic sarcoma, marginal zone hyperplasia, marginal zone lymphoma, and diffuse large B cell lymphoma (see Lymphoid/Lymphatic System, Disorders of Domestic Animals: Lymph Nodes, Neoplasia, Lymphoma).

Histoplasmosis

Histoplasma capsulatum can cause a disseminated fungal disease that is widely endemic, particularly in areas with major river valleys and temperate or tropical climates (e.g., midwestern and southern United States). Free-living organisms in the mycelial phase produce macroconidia and microconidia that are inhaled and converted to the yeast phase in the lung. Yeasts are phagocytized and harbored by macrophages of the monocyte-macrophage system. In some dogs the disease is limited to the respiratory tract and causes dyspnea and coughing. However, in most dogs, the disease is disseminated throughout the body, predominantly affecting the liver, spleen, gastrointestinal tract, bone marrow, skin, and eyes; primary gastrointestinal disease is also reported. The clinical signs in cases of disseminated histoplasmosis include wasting, emaciation, fever, respiratory distress, diarrhea with hematochezia or melena, and lameness.

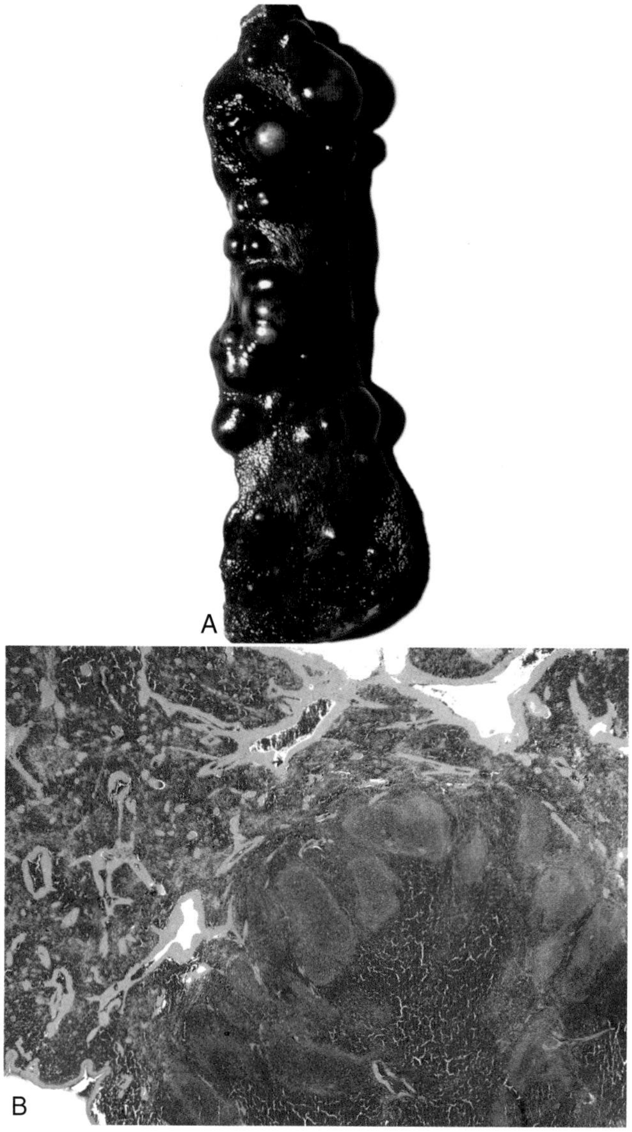

Figure 13-90 Lymphoid (Simple) Splenic Nodular Hyperplasia **A,** Nodular hyperplasia, spleen, dog. **B,** The well-demarcated nodule (lower right of image) is composed of hyperplastic lymphoid follicles, and the intervening tissue is congested. H&E stain. (**A** courtesy Dr. M.D. McGavin, College of Veterinary Medicine, University of Tennessee. **B** courtesy Dr. A.C. Durham, School of Veterinary Medicine, University of Pennsylvania.)

The clinicopathologic changes of disseminated histoplasmosis may include neutrophilia, monocytosis, nonregenerative anemia in chronic infections, changes in total serum protein level, and liver enzyme level elevations with hepatic involvement. The anemia is likely a result of chronic inflammation, *Histoplasma* infection of the bone marrow, and/or intestinal blood loss in dogs with GI disease. Cytologic examination is useful for the diagnosis of histoplasmosis (tracheal wash preparations, aspirates of bone marrow and lymph nodes), where organisms are often visible in macrophages (E-Fig. 13-15).

Grossly, there is hepatosplenomegaly, the intestines are thickened and corrugated, and the lymph nodes are uniformly enlarged (Fig. 13-91) with loss of normal architecture (somewhat similar to

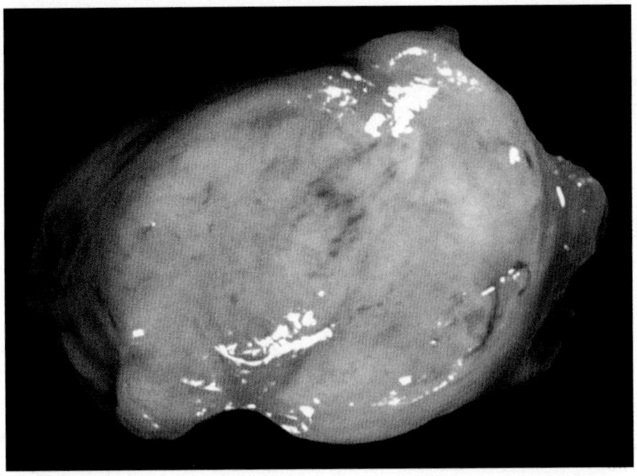

Figure 13-91 Mesenteric Lymph Node, Diffuse Granulomatous Lymphadenitis, Histoplasmosis, Dog. The lymph node is enlarged, the cut surface shows loss of architecture, and the tissue bulges because of the diffuse granulomatous inflammation (see Fig. 13-92). (Courtesy Dr. M.D. McGavin, College of Veterinary Medicine, University of Tennessee.)

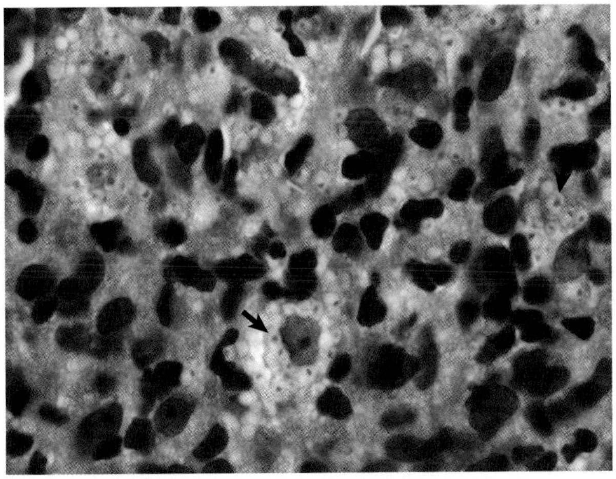

Figure 13-92 Histoplasmosis, Lymph Node, Dog. Diffuse granulomatous lymphadenitis. Macrophages contain the phagocytized *Histoplasma capsulatum* organisms *(arrows)*. H&E stain. (Courtesy Dr. A.C. Durham, School of Veterinary Medicine, University of Pennsylvania.)

lymphoma, though the nodes tend to be more firm in histoplasmosis). Histologically within the node, there is a multifocal to coalescing infiltrate of epithelioid macrophages with intracytoplasmic, small (2 to 4 μm in diameter) yeast organisms with spherical basophilic central bodies surrounded by a clear halo (Fig. 13-92).

Leishmaniasis

Leishmaniasis is a disease of the monocyte-macrophage system caused by protozoa of the genus *Leishmania*. It occurs in dogs and other animals and is endemic in parts of the United States, Europe, Mediterranean, Middle East, Africa, and Central and South America. The protozoa proliferate by binary fission in the gut of the sand fly and become flagellated organisms, which are introduced into mammals by insect bites, where they are phagocytized by macrophages and assume a nonflagellated form. Cutaneous and/or visceral forms of the disease are observed. In the visceral form, dogs are emaciated and have general enlargement of abdominal lymph nodes and hepatosplenomegaly (E-Fig. 13-16). Histologically, the lymph node sinuses and splenic red pulp are filled with macrophages that contain intracytoplasmic, round, 2-μm-diameter organisms with a small kinetoplast. Though there is an initial stage of lymphoid hyperplasia in the spleen and lymph node, subsequent lymphoid atrophy occurs with chronicity. The atrophy is due to impairment of follicular DCs, B lymphocyte migration, and germinal center formation. There may be lymphoid atrophy of the spleen and lymph nodes in severe chronic infections.

Canine Distemper

Canine distemper virus preferentially infects lymphoid, epithelial, and nervous cells (see Chapter 14). Dogs are exposed through contact with oronasal secretions, and the virus infects macrophages within the lymphoid tissue of the tonsil and respiratory tract (including tracheobronchial lymph nodes) and later disseminates to the spleen, lymph nodes, bone marrow, MALT, and hepatic Kupffer cells. The virus causes necrosis of lymphocytes (especially CD4 T lymphocytes) and depression of lymphopoiesis in the bone marrow, leading to severe immunosuppression. Dogs are therefore susceptible to secondary infections, including *Bordetella bronchiseptica*, *Toxoplasma gondii*, *Nocardia*, *Salmonella* spp., and generalized demodicosis.

Canine Parvovirus

Canine parvovirus type 2 (CPV-2) is a highly contagious disease of dogs spread through the fecal-oral route or oronasal exposure to contaminated fomites. The virus has tropism for rapidly dividing cells, and replication begins in the lymphoid tissues of the oropharynx, thymus, and mesenteric lymph nodes and then is disseminated to the small intestinal crypt epithelium. By infecting lymphoid tissues, canine parvovirus type 2 causes immunosuppression directly through lymphocytolysis and indirectly though bone marrow depletion of lymphocyte precursors. There is marked lymphoid atrophy of thymus and follicles of the spleen, lymph nodes, and MALT—particularly of Peyer's patches to produce the classic gross lesion of depressed oval regions of the mucosa (so-called punched-out Peyer's patches).

Neoplasms

Thymomas. See Lymphoid/Lymphatic System, Disorders of Domestic Animals: Thymus, Neoplasia.

Lymphomas. Lymphoma is the most common hematologic malignancy in the dog. Using the WHO classification scheme, several lymphoma subtypes are identified in dogs and clinically range from slow-growing indolent tumors to highly aggressive tumors. Of all domestic animal species, lymphoma is the most extensively studied in dogs. The most common clinical presentation in dogs is generalized lymphadenopathy, with or without clinical signs such as lethargy and inappetence.

The majority of lymphomas in dogs are large cell mid- to high-grade lymphomas, and up to half of all lymphoma cases are subtyped as diffuse large B cell lymphoma. Diffuse large B cell lymphomas are further subdivided into centroblastic or immunoblastic based on nucleolar morphologic features (see Table 13-7 and Box 13-11), although it is unclear if this difference has any prognostic significance. Histologically, lymph node architecture is most often completely effaced by sheets of large neoplastic cells, which may invade through the capsule and colonize the perinodal tissue. These dogs are often treated with chemotherapy and achieve remission. The overall median survival time for dogs with diffuse large B lymphocyte lymphoma is approximately 7 months, although this number varies based on the study and the grade of the tumor (as determined by mitotic figures). Peripheral T cell lymphomas–not otherwise specified are the second most common subtype in dogs. This category includes all T cell lymphomas that do not fit into the other categories (e.g., T zone lymphoma, enteropathy-associated T cell lymphoma, and hepatosplenic T cell lymphoma). Peripheral T cell lymphoma also effaces nodal architecture, and when compared to diffuse large B cell lymphoma, there is more variation in nuclear size and morphologic features. Dogs with this subtype tend to have shorter survival times.

Intermediate cell size, high-grade lymphomas are less common in dogs, and the two most frequently encountered subtypes are lymphoblastic lymphoma (LBL) and Burkitt-like lymphoma (BLL). Lymphoblastic lymphoma may be of B or T lymphocyte origin, though T cell lymphoblastic lymphoma is more common of the two. *It is important to recognize a common misuse of the term "lymphoblast" in lymphoblastic lymphoma—by definition in lymphoblastic lymphoma, lymphoblasts are intermediate-sized cells with a distinct dispersed chromatin pattern, and* not *the large lymphocytes seen in cases of diffuse large B cell lymphoma or peripheral T cell lymphoma*. T lymphocyte lymphoblastic lymphoma is an aggressive disease that is often resistant to treatment. Burkitt-like lymphoma is a high-grade lymphoma of B lymphocytes.

Numerous other subtypes of lymphoma have been reported in dogs, including several forms of cutaneous lymphomas, most often of T lymphocyte origin and epitheliotropic (see Chapter 17). Hepatosplenic T cell lymphoma, thought to be of γ/δ T lymphocyte origin, affects the liver and spleen without significant nodal involvement. Hepatocytotropic T cell lymphoma is a distinct form of lymphoma with tropism for the hepatic cords; clusters or individual neoplastic lymphocytes invade the hepatic cords, without hepatocyte degeneration. Intravascular lymphoma is a proliferation of large neoplastic lymphocytes within blood vessels of many tissues, leading to progressive occlusion and subsequent thromboses and infarcts. This neoplasm does not form an extravascular mass, and neoplastic cells are not found in peripheral blood smears or bone marrow.

Indolent lymphomas constitute up to 29% of all canine lymphomas. Indolent lymphomas in dogs, in descending order of frequency, include T zone lymphoma (TZL), marginal zone lymphoma (MZL), mantle cell lymphoma (MCL), and follicular lymphoma (FL). Mantle cell lymphoma and follicular lymphoma are less commonly diagnosed than T zone lymphoma and marginal zone lymphoma; therefore the reader is referred to the Suggested Readings to learn more on mantle cell lymphoma and follicular lymphoma.

T Zone Lymphoma. T zone lymphoma is the most common indolent lymphoma in dogs (Fig. 13-93). It presents as a solitary or

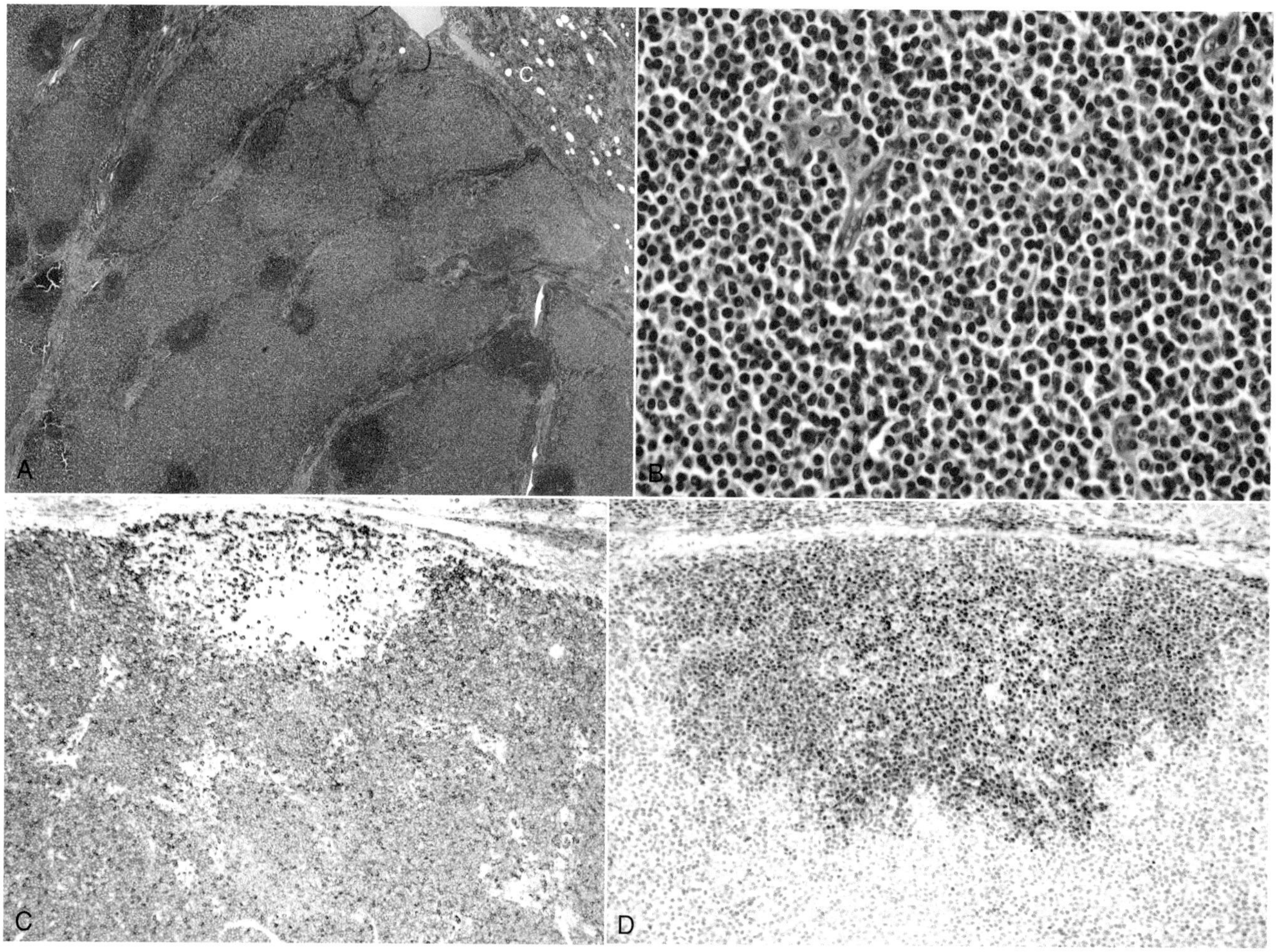

Figure 13-93 **T Zone Lymphoma, Lymph Node, Dog. A**, The characteristic histopathologic architecture is a nodular expansion of the paracortex by neoplastic cells, which push atrophied "fading" cortical follicles against the capsule *(C)* and trabeculae *(interconnected pink bands)*. H&E stain. **B**, The neoplastic cells are small to intermediate in size, and mitotic figures are rare. H&E stain. **C**, The neoplastic cells are T lymphocytes. Immunohistochemistry anti-CD3, hematoxylin counterstain. **D**, The remnants of the "fading" cortical follicles are composed of B lymphocytes. Immunohistochemistry anti-pax5, hematoxylin counterstain. (Courtesy Dr. A.C. Durham, School of Veterinary Medicine, University of Pennsylvania.)

multiple peripheral lymphadenomegaly (often mandibular lymph nodes) in otherwise healthy-appearing dogs. The characteristic histopathologic architecture is a nodular expansion of the paracortex by neoplastic cells, which push atrophied "fading" cortical follicles against the thinned capsule and trabeculae. This unique architectural feature is best highlighted with immunohistochemical stains (often CD3 for T lymphocytes and CD79a, pax5, or CD20 for B lymphocytes). The neoplastic cells are small to intermediate in size with pale eosinophilic cytoplasm and oval nuclei with sharp shallow indentations. Mitotic figures are rare. Dogs with this lymphoma subtype tend to be diagnosed with an advanced stage of the disease, likely because they present clinically healthy, without loss of appetite or activity level. Even so, dogs with T zone lymphoma have a relatively long survival time compared to other lymphomas: reports on median survival time range from 13 to 33 months, and data suggest that dogs who do not receive chemotherapy actually have longer median survival times.

Marginal Zone Lymphoma. Marginal zone lymphoma is an indolent B lymphocyte neoplasm derived from the cells of the marginal zone of lymphoid follicles. Most marginal zone lymphomas (and mantle cell lymphomas) are assumed to originate in the spleen with slow spread to lymph nodes and often present as a mottled white-red smooth spherical splenic mass. Histopathologic assessment of tissue architecture is needed for a diagnosis of marginal zone lymphoma and is characterized by a distinct nodular pattern in which the lighter-staining neoplastic marginal zone cells form a dense cuff around small foci of darkly stained mantle cells (fading follicles). The neoplastic marginal zone lymphocytes are intermediate in size and have a single prominent central nucleolus. Mitotic figures are often rare or absent early on and increase with disease progression.

Differentiating between marginal zone lymphoma and marginal zone hyperplasia (which refers to a proliferation of marginal zone cells and contains a mixture of small and intermediate lymphocytes) is challenging because marginal zone lymphoma arises on the background of marginal zone hyperplasia. Additionally, lymphoid and complex nodular hyperplasia are common in the dog spleen (see Disorders of Dogs), and it is possible that many cases of nodular hyperplasia contain areas of marginal zone lymphoma. Therefore immunophenotyping and molecular clonality are ultimately required for a definitive diagnosis of marginal zone lymphoma. The overall median survival time in dogs with splenic marginal zone lymphoma after splenectomy is approximately 13 months (even longer if it is diagnosed as an incidental finding).

Plasmacytomas. See Disorders of Domestic Animals: Lymph Nodes, Neoplasia, Plasma Cell Neoplasia, Extramedullary Plasmacytomas (see Fig. 13-84).

Disorders of Cats

Feline Panleukopenia (Parvovirus)

Feline panleukopenia, caused by the single-stranded DNA virus feline parvovirus (FPV), is a highly contagious and often lethal disease of cats and other Felidae, as well as other species (including raccoons, ring-tailed cats, foxes, and minks). FPV is transmitted by the fecal-oral route through contact with infected body fluids, feces, or fomites. Following intranasal or oral infection, the virus initially replicates in the macrophages in the lamina propria of the oropharynx and regional lymph nodes, followed by viremia, which distributes the virus throughout the body. Because FPV requires rapidly multiplying cells in the S phase of division for its replication, replication occurs in mitotically active tissues (lymphoid tissue, bone marrow, and intestinal mucosa). By infecting lymphoid tissues, FPV causes immunosuppression directly through lymphocytolysis and indirectly through depletion of lymphocyte precursors in the bone marrow. Consequently there is marked lymphoid atrophy of thymus, spleen, lymph node, and MALT (particularly Peyer's patches).

Mast Cell Tumors

See Bone Marrow and Blood Cells, Disorders of Domestic Animals, Types of Hematopoietic Neoplasia, Myeloid Neoplasia, Mast Cell Neoplasia and see E-Fig. 13-6.

Lymphoma

Lymphoma is the most commonly diagnosed neoplasm in cats, and the incidence is reportedly the highest for any species. Mediastinal or multicentric lymphomas are seen in young, FeLV-infected cats (see Fig. 13-53). With the advent of FeLV vaccine and routine testing, the prevalence of FeLV-associated lymphoma is decreased. Currently the alimentary tract is the most commonly affected site, and typically occurs in cats greater than 10 years of age (Figs. 13-94 and 13-95). Other miscellaneous sites commonly affected are brain, spinal cord, eye, kidney, and nasopharynx.

The retrovirus FeLV has long been recognized as a cause of lymphoma in cats—the risk for lymphoma is increased sixtyfold in infected cats. Before the advent of a vaccine in 1985, approximately 70% of cats (mainly young animals) with lymphoma were FeLV positive. FeLV infects T lymphocytes and can cause myelodysplastic syndrome, acute myeloid leukemias (see Myeloid Neoplasia), and T lymphocyte leukemia/lymphoma. In the latter the mediastinum (thymus, mediastinal, and sternal lymph nodes) is the site most commonly involved, although a multicentric distribution also occurs. Routine FeLV vaccination has led to a significant decrease in the prevalence of FeLV infection, which has resulted in a decrease in the proportion of mediastinal lymphomas.

The risk for developing lymphoma in FIV-infected cats is fivefold to sixfold higher than in uninfected cats. Cats that underwent kidney transplantation and thus received immunosuppressive drug therapy had a similar risk for developing lymphoma. Both FIV-infected and posttransplantation cats predominantly developed extranodal, high-grade, diffuse large B lymphocyte lymphomas. This form is also the most common subtype in human immunodeficiency virus and posttransplantation patients caused by the Epstein-Barr virus (EBV). Therefore it is reasonable to question whether these two groups of immunosuppressed cats may be more prone to infection by a gammaherpesvirus similar to EBV, leading to lymphoma. Recently a novel feline gammaherpesvirus (FcaGHV1) was

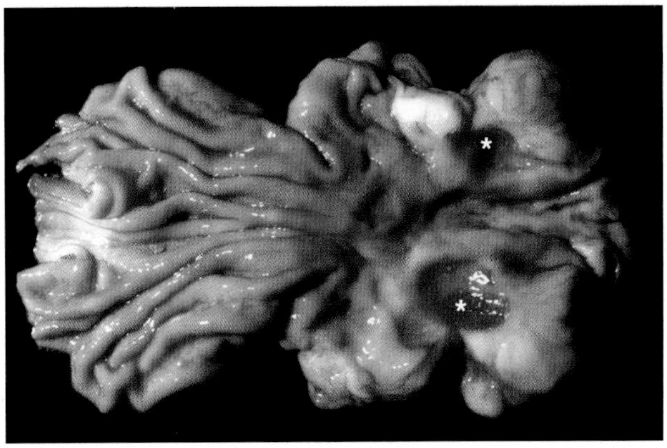

Figure 13-94 **Alimentary Lymphoma, Stomach, Cat.** The stomach mucosa is markedly thickened by the neoplastic cells *(gray-white areas in the right half of the image)*; focal ulcers are also noted *(asterisks)*. (Courtesy Dr. M.D. McGavin, College of Veterinary Medicine, University of Tennessee.)

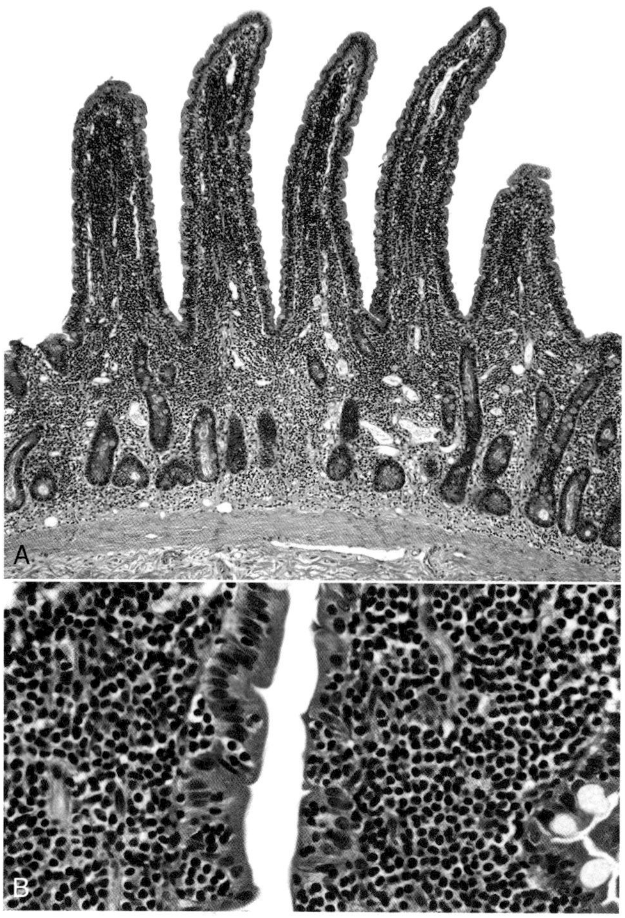

Figure 13-95 **Intestinal Small Cell Lymphoma, Jejunum, Cat.** Enteropathy-associated T cell lymphoma. **A**, The neoplastic cells expand the lamina propria of intestinal villi and submucosa, lifting the crypts from the muscularis mucosa. **B**, Higher magnification of a villus. The neoplastic lymphocytes in the lamina propria are small and often colonize in clusters within the epithelium. H&E stain. (Courtesy Dr. A.C. Durham, School of Veterinary Medicine, University of Pennsylvania.)

discovered in domestic cats with a 16% prevalence in North America, and further studies to investigate its role in lymphomagenesis are needed.

The overall incidence of feline lymphomas has increased, mainly due to an increase in gastrointestinal lymphomas. Mucosal T cell lymphoma, also known as enteropathy-associated T cell lymphoma (EATCL type II), is the most common and arises from diffuse MALT of the small intestine. The neoplastic cells are small (nuclei are equal to the diameter of a feline RBC), mitotic figures are infrequent (low grade), and mucosal and crypt epitheliotropism is common (see Fig. 13-95). A diagnosis of this subtype of lymphoma may be difficult (particularly in endoscopic biopsy samples), because this disease often is multifocal and concurrent with or arises within lymphoplasmacytic inflammatory bowel disease (IBD). The neoplastic lymphocytes are morphologically similar to the inflammatory lymphocytes. Early small cell mucosal T cell lymphomas often require additional diagnostic testing, namely, immunohistochemistry and molecular clonality testing (PCR for antigen receptor rearrangement [PARR]) to confirm a clonal neoplasm.

Transmural T cell lymphomas also occur focally or multifocally in the small intestine of cats (best classified as enteropathy-associated T cell lymphoma type I) and by definition must extend into the submucosa and muscularis. Some tumors invade the serosa and adjacent mesentery. T cell large granular lymphocyte (LGL) lymphoma is often diagnosed, and the intestinal segments orad and aborad to the transmural mass may also have mucosal lymphoma. Gastrointestinal B cell lymphomas are less prevalent in cats but occur in the stomach, jejunum, and ileocecocolic region as transmural lesions. Most are diagnosed as diffuse large B cell lymphomas.

Lymphomas in other sites also occur less frequently in cats. The upper respiratory tract (nasal and/or nasopharyngeal region) is a relatively rare site for lymphoma. However, lymphoma is the most common primary nasal tumor, and diffuse large B cell lymphomas (of immunoblastic type) are the predominant subtype. Both cutaneous (cutaneous T cell lymphoma) and subcutaneous lymphomas (usually large cell lymphomas) are rare. Presumed solitary ocular lymphomas have also been reported.

T cell–rich large B cell lymphoma, also referred to as feline Hodgkin-like lymphoma in some studies, is composed of a mixture of reactive small lymphocytes and large neoplastic B lymphocytes, many of which may be binucleated and/or have prominent nucleoli (thus resembling the Reed-Sternberg cells of human Hodgkin's lymphoma). This disease is typically characterized by a distinctive clinical presentation of an indolent unilateral neoplasm of the cervical lymph nodes, which spreads slowly to adjacent nodes within the chain. However, a proportion of cases may go on to develop into a more aggressive multicentric large to anaplastic B lymphocyte lymphoma that can affect peripheral and central nodes and multiple organs.

Suggested Readings

Suggested Readings are available at www.expertconsult.com.

CHAPTER 14

Nervous System[1]

Andrew D. Miller and James F. Zachary

Key Readings Index

Nervous System

Development of the Adult Nervous System

The vertebrate embryo is formed by three layers of cells—the ectoderm (outermost layer), the mesoderm (middle layer), and the endoderm (innermost layer). Nervous tissues are derived from the ectoderm and eventually form all central nervous system (CNS) and peripheral nervous system (PNS) tissues of the adult animal. In the developing embryo, neurogenesis begins with a locally extensive, elongate proliferation of cells known as the *neural plate*, located along the cranial surface of the neuroectoderm (E-Fig. 14-1). The neural plate is bordered on either side by *neural folds*, which eventually fuse dorsally to form the *neural tube* (i.e., the eventual brain, spinal cord, and ventricular system). Immature neuroepithelial cells that line the neural tube ultimately become the source of neurons, astrocytes, ependymal cells, and oligodendrocytes. Resident microglial cells arise from mesodermal stem cells in the yolk sac that migrate to the neural tube during development, whereas the development and maturation of the brain and spinal cord proceed through a series of coordinated mechanisms characterized by cellular proliferation and subsequent remodeling (e.g., apoptosis) to produce the final morphologic features of the adult brain and spinal cord.

Neuroepithelial cells, which form the spinal cord, reorganize during neurogenesis to produce centrally located gray matter (shaped like a butterfly with paired dorsal and ventral horns) and peripherally enveloping white matter (also see later section on gray and white matter). The white matter tracts of the spinal cord are further subdivided into *funiculi*, which contain variable numbers of ascending axons (i.e., action potential travels in the direction of the brain) and descending axons (i.e., action potential travels in the direction of the cauda equina). *Segmentation* (i.e., formation of the general regions of the brain and spinal cord) and *stratification* (i.e., formation of the lamina of the cerebral cortex) of the neural tube during embryologic development require a great deal more remodeling. Initial expansion of the neural tube results in a developing brain that is segmented into sections called the prosencephalon (forebrain), mesencephalon (midbrain), and rhombencephalon (hindbrain) (E-Box 14-1; E-Fig. 14-2). With further development the brain divides into the five segments: telencephalon, diencephalon (both derived from the prosencephalon), mesencephalon, and the metencephalon and myelencephalon (both derived from the rhombencephalon) (see E-Box 14-1). The telencephalon in the adult animal becomes paired cerebral hemispheres. The diencephalon becomes the thalamus and its associated structures. The mesencephalon gives rise to the corpora quadrigemina (superior and inferior colliculi) and the cerebral peduncles. The pons and cerebellum arise from the metencephalon, and lastly the medulla oblongata arises from the myelencephalon (see E-Fig 14-1). Concurrently, the spinal cord is segmented into cervical, thoracic, lumbar, and sacral sections, which are further subdivided into individual spinal nerves.

The ventricular system develops in parallel with the brain and spinal cord. It originates from the space formed by the closing of the neural folds to form the neural tube and thus gives rise to the lateral ventricles, the third ventricle, the mesencephalic (cerebral) aqueduct, the fourth ventricle, and the central canal of the spinal cord. The dispersal of agents in the cerebrospinal fluid (CSF) to seemingly disparate regions of the CNS is explained by the interconnectedness of the ventricular system.

Following the development and differentiation of the brain into the five segments listed earlier, there is differential growth (i.e., occurs at different extents, rates, and times) in each of these parts of the developing brain. For example, the brainstem (pons and medulla) undergoes marked reorganization to form numerous

[1]For a glossary of abbreviations and terms used in this chapter see E-Glossary 14-1.

specific nuclei that are the source of not only the majority of the cranial nerves, but also a neural relay network for the majority of neural impulses that arise in the prosencephalon (e.g., cerebral hemispheres and thalamus). It is also during this period of embryologic differentiation that stratification occurs within the cerebral cortex resulting in the formation of cerebral lamina. Lamina are distinct topographic layers of neuron cell bodies that have similar functions and innervate specific areas of the body as designated by these similar functions. They serve as topographic maps for specific activities within the CNS such as sensory, motor, and associative functions. Additionally, these activities are spread out into distinct "functional" lamina within lobes within the cerebral cortex, such as the frontal lobe (cognitive functions), parietal lobe (motor and sensory functions), occipital lobe (vision), and the temporal lobe (auditory functions). Lastly, the cerebellum undergoes significant reorganization with the development of multiple integrated layers of neurons, including the granule cell layer, the molecular cell layer, and the Purkinje cell layer.

The adult CNS is arranged to form two basic parts: the gray and white matter (Figs. 14-1 and 14-2). In the CNS, gray matter is found in the cerebral cortex, in the cerebellar cortex and cerebellar nuclei, around the base of the cerebral hemispheres (basal nuclei [often called *basal ganglia*]: caudate nucleus, lentiform nucleus [putamen, globus pallidus], amygdaloid nucleus, claustrum), and throughout the brainstem, often in nuclei. The gray matter is typified by numerous neuronal cell bodies, plus a feltwork of intermingled thinly myelinated axons and dendrites, their synaptic junctions, and processes of oligodendroglia, astrocytes, and microglia. This network of processes and synapses in the gray matter is referred to as the *neuropil*. The white matter consists of well-myelinated axons that arise from neuronal cell bodies in the gray matter and terminate distally in synapses or myoneural junctions, plus oligodendroglia, astrocytes, and microglia. In the cerebral hemispheres, white matter is located centrally, whereas in the brainstem, white matter is intermingled with gray matter (nuclei). In the spinal cord, white matter is located peripherally surrounding the gray matter.

The embryologic development of the PNS is as complex as the CNS and is also dependent on the normal development of the neural tube. A population of *neural crest* cells that form bilaterally in the dorsal regions of the neural tube is the origin of the majority of cells that populate the PNS, such as neurons and Schwann cells. These neural crest cells also migrate peripherally in developing tissues and organ systems within the mesoderm and endoderm to form structures such as spinal ganglia, enteric plexuses, and the adrenal medullas. Neurons of the PNS are divided into afferent and efferent types based on whether they conduct impulses to or from the CNS, respectively. Cell bodies for somatic efferent neurons, such as those in cranial or spinal nerves, are located in nuclei of the brain or the ventral horns of the gray matter of the spinal cord and project ventrolaterally long distances to innervate peripheral tissues, such as skeletal muscle. The cell bodies for somatic afferent neurons are located bilaterally within spinal ganglia (dorsal root ganglia) that are developmentally associated with specific spinal cord segments. The neurogenic control of visceral tissues and organ systems such as the alimentary system is complex; involves at a minimum two neurons, a preganglionic neuron and a postganglionic neuron; and is facilitated by the sympathetic, parasympathetic, and enteric nervous systems (i.e., visceral nervous systems). As a basic rule, for all three visceral nervous systems the preganglionic neuron cell body is located in the intermediate gray matter between the dorsal and ventral horns of the spinal cord or brain nucleus.

As noted earlier, during the development of the CNS a variety of differing cell types populate the brain and spinal cord, including the neurons, glia, ependyma, endothelial cells, pericytes and smooth muscle cells of blood vessels, and various cells in the meninges (Fig. 14-3; Box 14-1). Neurons vary in size, shape, and function, and their cell bodies are organized into functional groups such as nuclei, horns of gray matter in the spinal cord, and cerebral lamina. Neuronal processes called axons and dendrites traverse through the brain and spinal cord, the former often as organized bundles (tracts, fasciculi) forming synapses on cell bodies, dendrites, and axons of other functionally related neurons. It is estimated that there are 1×10^{11} neurons in the human brain. Each neuron makes approximately 10,000 synapses with other neurons; therefore there are approximately 1×10^{15} synapses in the human brain. The neurons maintain a close association with various glial cells, including microglia, astrocytes, and oligodendrocytes. The glia are responsible for helping to maintain CNS homeostasis and play an important role in the immune response and healing. Astrocytes, oligodendrocytes, and ependymal cells are derived from neuroectoderm, whereas microglia, part of the monocyte-macrophage system, are derived from progenitors in the embryonic yolk sac that populate the CNS during development. In the mammalian CNS, glia outnumber neurons 10 to 1. Ependymal cells line the ventricular system, whereas choroid plexus epithelial cells form the outer covering of the choroid plexuses. Lastly, the exterior of the CNS is covered by the meninges. The meninges consist of three layers named, from outermost to innermost layers, the *dura mater*, *arachnoid*, and *pia mater*. The arachnoid and pia enclose the subarachnoid space.

Central Nervous System

Structure[2] and Function

Cells of the Central Nervous System

Neurons. The structure and basic cellular biology of neurons is similar to that of other cells (Fig. 14-4); however, there are, as discussed later, some notable differences. The neuron consists of three structural components: dendrites, a cell body, and a single axon. The length of the axon varies, depending on the function of the neuron. The length of axons of motor or sensory neurons can be 10,000 to 15,000 times the diameter of the neuronal cell body, which results in these axons being several meters in length. The axon terminates in synaptic processes or neuromuscular junctions.

Neuronal cell bodies vary considerably in size and shape, from the large neurons of the lateral vestibular nucleus, Purkinje cell layer of the cerebellum, and the ventral gray matter of the spinal cord to the very small lymphocyte-like granule cells of the cerebellar cortex (Fig. 14-5). Neuronal nuclei tend to be vesicular to spherical in shape, are usually centrally located, and often, particularly in large neurons, tend to contain a prominent central nucleolus. Neurons contain focal arrays of rough endoplasmic reticulum and polysomes, termed *Nissl substance*, that are responsible for the synthesis of proteins involved in many of the neuron's vital cellular processes such as axonal transport. Nissl substance is present in all neurons, regardless of the size of the cell body, but tends to be more prominent in those cells with voluminous cytoplasm such as motor neurons.

Axonal Transport (Axoplasmic Transport). Axonal transport is a cellular mechanism used to move synaptic vesicles, proteins such as neurotransmitters, mitochondria, lipids, and other cell organelles from the neuron cell body through the axon to the synapses and then bring their degradation products back to the cell body.

[2]Postmortem examination of the CNS is discussed in E-Appendix 14-1.

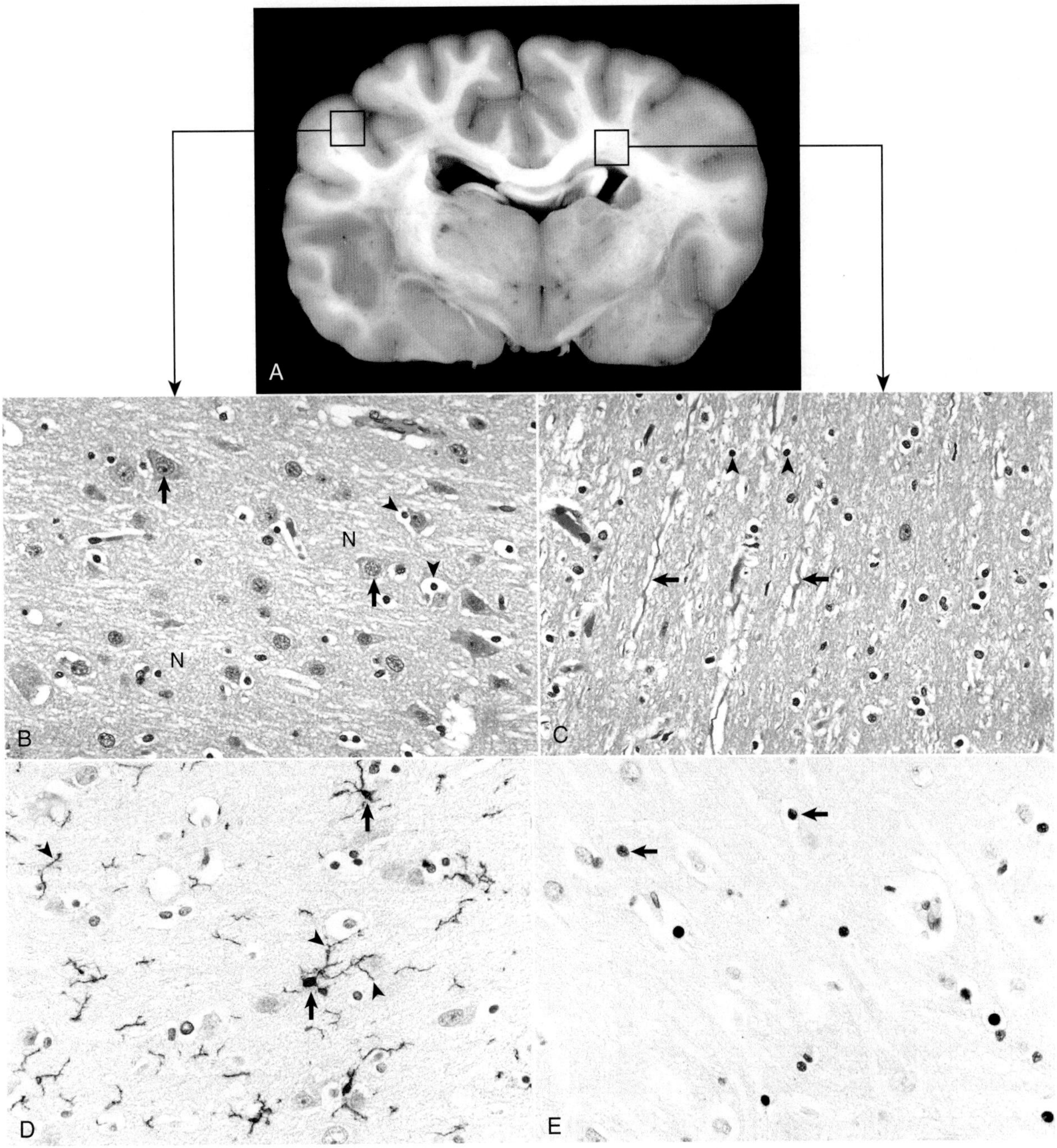

Figure 14-1 **Organization of the Brain, Gray Matter, and White Matter. A,** Transverse section at the level of the thalamus, dog. Gray matter *(darker areas)* of the cerebral cortex lies beneath the leptomeninges on the external surface of the brain, whereas in the thalamus there is a mixture of gray and white matter. Major white matter areas *(light areas)* include corona radiata, centrum semiovale, and corpus callosum of the cerebrum, and internal capsule and optic tracts bordering the lateral and ventral surfaces of the thalamus, respectively. **B,** Gray matter consists primarily of the cell bodies of neurons *(arrows)* and a network of intermingled thinly myelinated axons, dendrites, and glial cell processes. This network is referred to as the neuropil *(N)*. Other components include oligodendroglia *(arrowheads)*, astrocytes, and microglia. H&E stain. **C,** White matter primarily consists of well-myelinated axons *(arrows)* plus oligodendroglia *(arrowheads)* and astrocytes. The clear spaces surrounding large axons are artifacts formed when the lipid components of myelin lamellae are dissolved away by solvents in the process of embedding tissue in paraffin for sectioning. H&E stain. **D,** Immunohistochemical (IHC) stain for ionized calcium binding adapter molecule 1 (Iba1). This IHC stain identifies microglia within a section of brain *(arrows)*. Their ramified processes are similarly highlighted *(arrowheads)*. DAB IHC stain. **E,** IHC stain for Olig2, a transcription factor that is expressed in the nucleus of oligodendrocytes *(arrows)*. DAB IHC stain. (**A, B,** and **C** courtesy Dr. J.F. Zachary, College of Veterinary Medicine, University of Illinois. **D** and **E** courtesy Dr. A.D. Miller, College of Veterinary Medicine, Cornell University.)

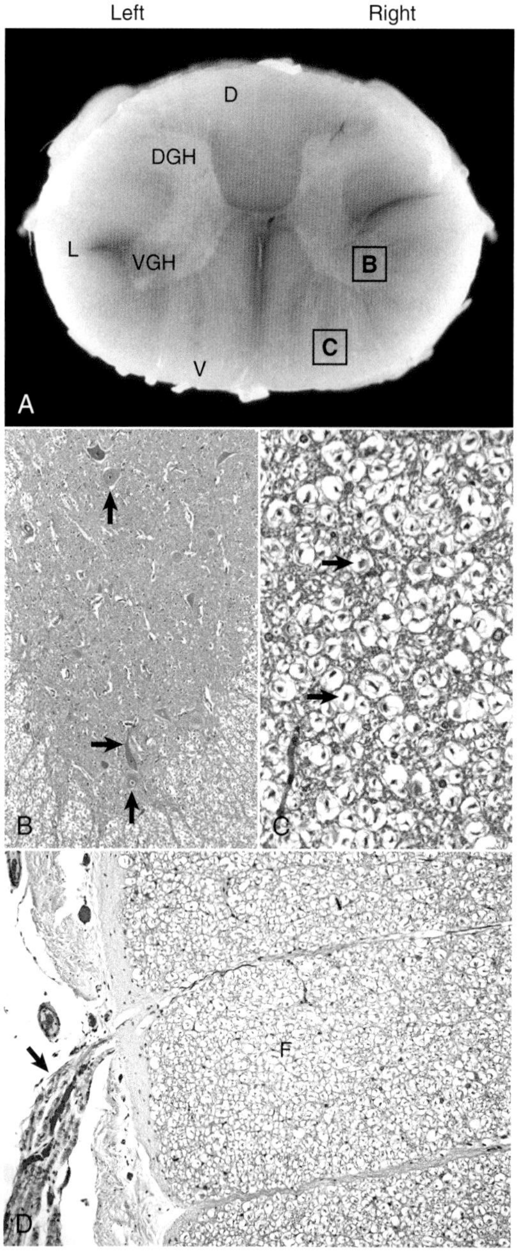

Figure 14-2 Organization of the Spinal Cord, Gray Matter, and White Matter. A, White matter in the spinal cord is located peripherally and divided into dorsal, lateral, and ventral funiculi. As a general rule, dorsal funiculi *(D)* consist of ascending sensory axons, lateral funiculi *(L)* have a mixture of sensory and motor axons, and ventral funiculi consist of descending motor axons *(V)*. Histologically, the right side is a mirror image of the left side. The areas labeled *B* and *C* and contained within the boxes correspond to the areas illustrated in **B** and **C**. **B,** Transverse section of spinal cord, ventral gray horn, horse. The cell bodies of large motor neurons *(arrows)* are those of lower motor neurons, and their axons extend in peripheral nerves to myoneural junctions that innervate skeletal muscle. H&E stain. **C,** Transverse section of spinal cord, ventral funiculus, horse. Because most axons course up and down the length of the spinal cord, in a transverse section, axons *(arrows)* are cut in cross section. They are surrounded by myelin sheaths whose lipid components are dissolved out during the preparation of paraffin-embedded sections, resulting in clear spaces that are an artifact. H&E stain. **D,** Efferent spinal nerve (longitudinal section shown here), transverse section of spinal cord, ventral funiculus, dog. Axons of lower motor neurons leave funiculi *(F)* and assemble as nerve rootlets *(arrow)* eventually forming peripheral nerves that innervate skeletal muscle. H&E stain. *DGH,* Dorsal gray horn; *VGH,* ventral gray horn. (Courtesy Dr. J.F. Zachary, College of Veterinary Medicine, University of Illinois.)

More information on this topic, including E-Figure 14-3, is available at www.expertconsult.com

Membrane Potentials and Transmitter/Receptor Systems. A fundamental activity of neurons is to modulate and effectively transmit chemical and electric signals from one neuron to another via synapses in the CNS or from one neuron to a muscle cell via junctional complexes, myoneural junctions, or motor end plates in the PNS. The process of nerve impulse conduction is made possible by the establishment and maintenance of an electric potential across the cell membrane of the neuron/axon.

More information on this topic, including E-Figure 14-4, is available at www.expertconsult.com.

Astrocytes. The functions of astrocytes in the CNS are regulation, repair, and support, as depicted in Figure 14-6. All regions of the CNS contain astrocytes, and they are derived from pluripotential neuroepithelial progenitor cells during the development of the CNS. Astrocytes are the most numerous cell type in the CNS and have traditionally been classified into two types based on morphologic features. Protoplasmic astrocytes are located primarily in gray matter, whereas fibrous astrocytes occur chiefly in white matter. Microscopically, astrocytes have relatively large vesicular nuclei, indistinct or inapparent nucleoli, and no discernible cytoplasm with routine hematoxylin and eosin (H&E) staining (Fig. 14-7). With suitable histochemical stains, silver impregnation, or immunohistochemical staining for glial fibrillary acidic protein (GFAP [the major intermediate filament in astrocytes]), the cell body and the extensive arborization and interconnections of astrocytic processes can be demonstrated. Processes vary from short and brushlike to long branching processes in protoplasmic and fibrous astrocytes, respectively (Fig. 14-8). Expression of GFAP is the standard immunohistochemical marker for tumors of astrocyte origin and can also be used to qualitatively or quantitatively characterize disorders in which astrocytes are proliferative or reactive. However, caution should be taken when assessing astrocyte numbers and/or the extent of ramification of their processes because GFAP immunoreactivity can be diminished in terminal processes and/or cell bodies, and therefore the total GFAP immunoreactivity in any given section of brain may not be representative of the overall astrocytic response in the disorder.

Functions of Astrocytes

Regulation of the Microenvironment. The microenvironment of the CNS must be under strict control to maintain normal function. Astrocytes are involved in homeostasis of the CNS and regulate ionic and water balance, antioxidant concentrations, uptake and metabolism of neurotransmitters, and metabolism or sequestration of potential neurotoxins, including ammonia, heavy metals, and excitatory amino acid neurotransmitters such as glutamate and aspartate. Structurally, the homeostatic role of astrocytes is illustrated by the morphologic characteristics of the neuropil, where astrocytic processes surround synapses and maintain a microenvironment that is adequate for normal synaptic transmission.

Additionally, interactions between astrocytes, microglia, and neurons orchestrate immune reactions in the brain. In this regard, astrocytes can express major histocompatibility complex (MHC) class I and II antigens, a variety of cytokines and chemokines, and adhesion molecules that modulate inflammatory events in the CNS. Astrocytes also secrete growth factors and extracellular matrix molecules that play a role not only in embryonic development but also in repair of the CNS following injury. In this latter role, astrocytes can fuse with adjacent astrocytes via a variety of gap junctions, and

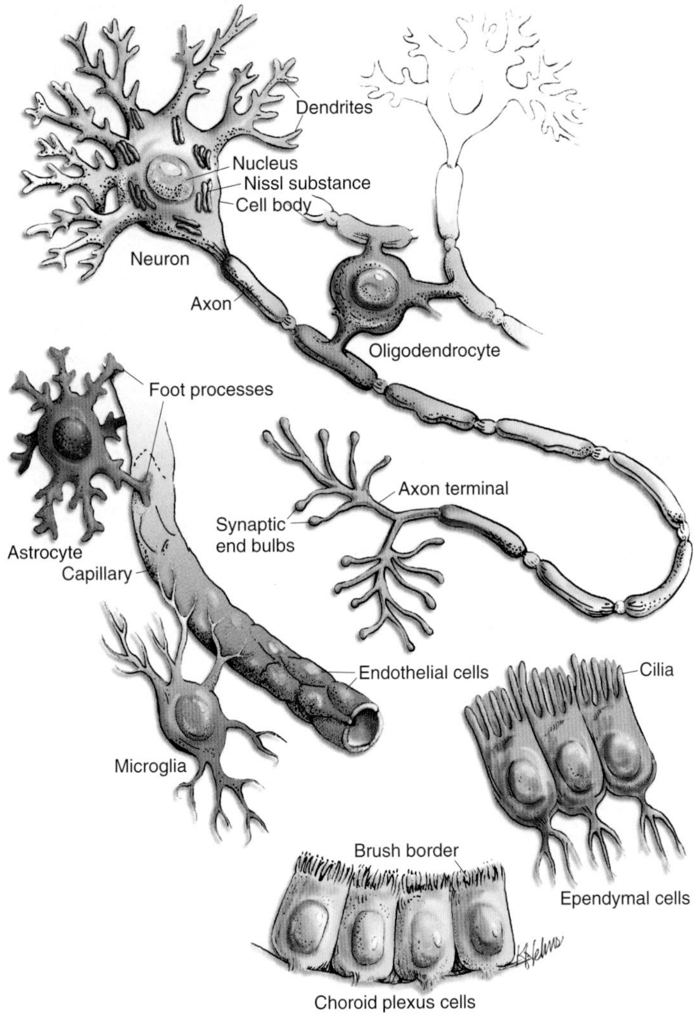

Figure 14-3 **Cell Types in the Central Nervous System Include Neurons, Astrocytes, Oligodendroglia, Microglia, Ependymal Cells, Choroid Plexus Epithelial Cells, and Vascular Endothelial Cells.** (Courtesy Dr. J.F. Zachary, College of Veterinary Medicine, University of Illinois.)

Box 14-1 Cells of the Central Nervous System and Their Primary Functions

NEURONS
Transmission of electric and chemical impulses
Spatial and temporal interpretation of impulses
Inhibitory and stimulatory regulation of impulses

ASTROGLIA (PROTOPLASMIC [TYPE I] AND FIBROUS [TYPE II])
Regulation of extracellular neurotransmitter concentrations and fluid/electrolyte imbalances
Repair of injury by proliferation of astrocytic cellular processes
Support and bundling of functionally related axons traversing through the CNS
Participation in barrier systems
Glia limitans
Blood-brain barrier

OLIGODENDROGLIA
Myelination of axons within the CNS
Proposed neuronal cell body homeostasis within the CNS

EPENDYMA
Movement of CSF through the ventricular system

CHOROID PLEXUS EPITHELIAL CELLS
Secretion of CSF
Barrier function (blood-CSF barrier)

MICROGLIA
Immunosurveillance, immunoregulation, phagocytosis
Monocyte-macrophage system

MENINGES
Arachnoid-CSF barrier
Subarachnoid CSF cushioning of head trauma

ENDOTHELIA
Barrier function (blood-brain barrier)
Selective molecule transport systems

CNS, Central nervous system; *CSF*, cerebrospinal fluid.

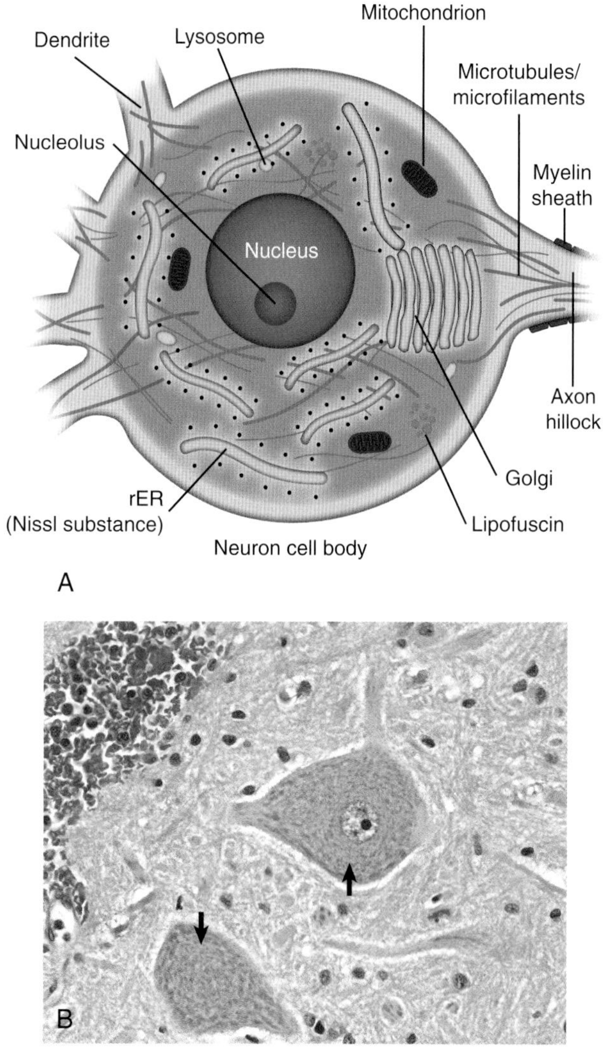

Figure 14-4 **Neuron Structure. A,** Basic cell biology and structure of neurons are similar to other cells in the body. Additionally, neurons have dendritic arborizations and an axon, specializations for the initiation, propagation, and transmission of impulses that underlie the basic function of these cells. **B,** The cytoplasm of the neuronal cell body has blue (basophilic [H&E stain]) granular material (rough endoplasmic reticulum) called Nissl substance *(arrows)*. Nissl substance synthesizes proteins, including precursor neurotransmitter proteins and the structural proteins (neurofilaments), active in maintaining the integrity (length and diameter) of the axon. H&E stain. *rER*, Rough endoplasmic reticulum. (**A** courtesy Dr. A.D. Miller, College of Veterinary Medicine, Cornell University; and Dr. J.F. Zachary, College of Veterinary Medicine, University of Illinois. **B** courtesy Dr. J.F. Zachary, College of Veterinary Medicine, University of Illinois.)

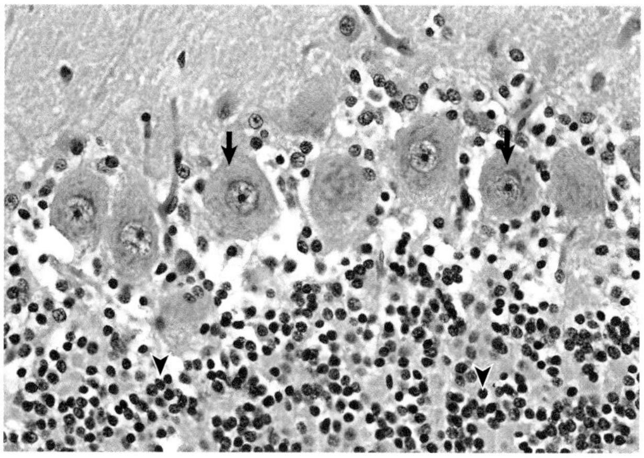

Figure 14-5 **Variations in Neuronal Morphologic Features, Cerebellum, Granule Cells, and Purkinje Neurons, Normal Animal.** The granule cell neurons of the cerebellar cortex *(arrowheads)* are very small basophilic cells that have relatively little demonstrable Nissl substance when compared with Purkinje neurons *(arrows)* and large motor neurons (depicted in Fig. 14-4, *B*). H&E stain. (Courtesy Dr. J.F. Zachary, College of Veterinary Medicine, University of Illinois.)

the coupling of multiple astrocytes together can play an important role in normal CNS function and repair (see next section). The gap junctions between various astrocytes are mediated by *connexins*. Astrocytes also play an integral role in CNS metabolism and can accumulate glycogen that can later be used to sustain neurons, especially during periods of hypoglycemia.

Repair of Injured Nervous Tissue. In the CNS, reparative processes that occur after injury, such as inflammation and necrosis, are chiefly the responsibility of astrocytes. In these reparative processes, astrocytes are analogous to fibroblasts in the rest of the body. Astrocytes do not synthesize collagen fibers, as do fibroblasts. Instead, repair is accomplished by astrocytic swelling and division, and abundant proliferation of astrocytic cell processes containing intermediate filaments composed of GFAP, a process called *astrogliosis*. As an example, neuronal necrosis occurs in some viral diseases of the CNS. When neurons die, the spaces left by the loss of the neuronal cell bodies are filled, and such spaces (<1 mm in diameter) are filled by processes of astrocytes. Larger spaces that form after injury, such as an infarct, are often too large to be filled and therefore exist in the CNS as fluid-filled spaces (cysts) surrounded by a capsule of astrocytic processes. Astrocytes will also attempt to wall off abscesses, but they are not as effective as fibroblasts, and the capsule can be incomplete or weak (Fig. 14-9). In the case of direct extension of bacteria from the meninges or meningeal blood vessels, which contain or are surrounded by fibroblasts, respectively, fibroblasts play a larger role in isolating the inflammatory process.

Structural Support of the Central Nervous System. Structurally, astrocytic processes provide support for other cellular elements and ensheathe and insulate synapses. Astrocytes also provide guidance and support of neuronal migration during development; thus tracts and fasciculi of axons with similar functions are arranged and structurally supported by astrocytic processes. Processes of astrocytes (foot processes) also terminate on blood vessels throughout the CNS, forming a component of the blood-brain barrier. Astrocytes influence the induction of tight junctions between endothelial cells that serve as the structural basis for the blood-brain barrier. A dense meshwork of astrocytic processes also forms the glia limitans beneath the pia mater and is variably prominent in subependymal areas. During CNS development, cells termed *radial glia* provide a scaffold and guidance for migrating neurons. When development is completed, radial glia mature into astrocytes. Some of these radial glia (also known as radial neural stem cells) remain active throughout life in the subventricular zone of the lateral ventricles, where they can repopulate lost populations of glial cells.

Oligodendroglia. There are two types of oligodendroglia: (1) interfascicular oligodendrocytes and (2) satellite oligodendrocytes (satellite cells). The function of interfascicular oligodendroglia is myelination of axons, whereas the function of satellite oligodendroglia is thought to be regulation of the perineuronal microenvironment. Oligodendroglia have been compared with neurons with

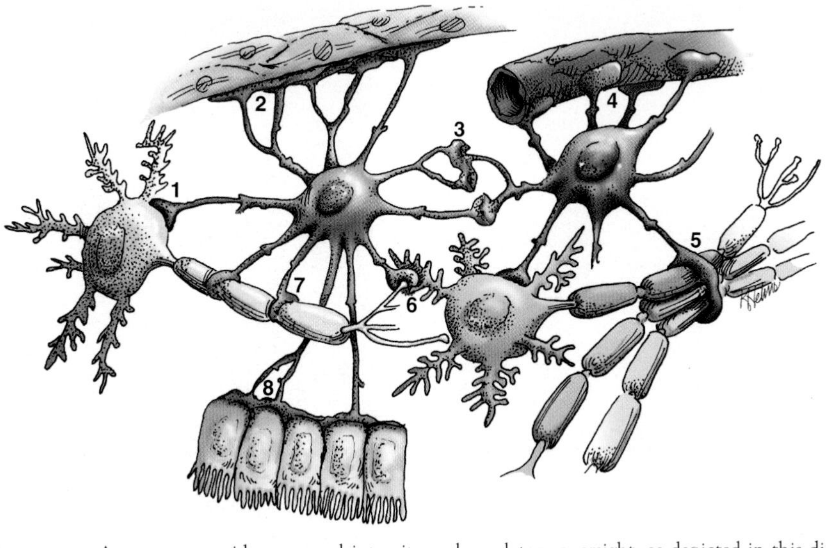

Figure 14-6 **Functions of Astrocytes.** Astrocytes provide structural integrity and regulatory oversight, as depicted in this diagram. They: *1*, monitor and regulate fluid and electrolyte balances within neurons and surrounding extracellular space; *2*, form the glial limitans at the base of the pia mater; *3*, interconnect with other astrocytes to provide a system to monitor and regulate fluid and electrolyte balances throughout the central nervous system (CNS); *4*, participate in the formation and functions of the blood-brain barrier; *5*, participate in the support of axon tracts of functionally related neurons; *6*, monitor for and remove excessive release of neurotransmitters in synapses; *7*, protect and insulate nodes of Ranvier; and *8*, participate in the cerebrospinal fluid–brain barrier. In addition, astrocytes are a reparative (healing) cell after CNS injury with loss of tissue because nervous tissue, per se, is devoid of fibroblasts. Fibroblasts exist in the meninges and around blood vessels. Everywhere else, healing depends on the astrocyte, which responds by increased length, branching, and complexity of cellular processes (astrogliosis). The astrocyte has many functions in the nervous system; one of them is to act in healing to produce a scar in attempts to isolate cavities and abscesses. Fibroblasts may also contribute to the formation of a scar, if this cell type is present, as it is in the leptomeninges. (Courtesy Dr. J.F. Zachary, College of Veterinary Medicine, University of Illinois.)

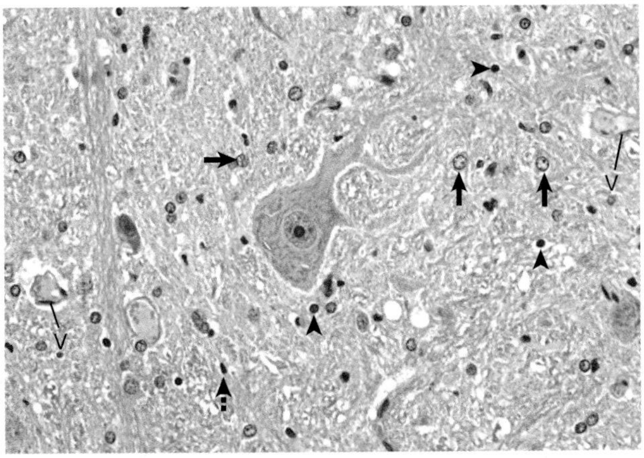

Figure 14-7 **Histologic Features of Glial Cells, Ventral Gray Horn, Spinal Cord, Horse.** A neuronal cell body and its processes are in the center of the illustration. To the inexperienced, identifying specific types of glial cells in H&E-stained histologic sections can be challenging. Astrocytes *(arrows)* have larger vesicular nuclei (dispersed chromatin), and the cell membrane and cytoplasm are rarely seen in nondiseased conditions. Thus these nuclei just seem to "sit" in the midst of the neuropil. The majority of nuclei in the neuropil here are astrocytic. Oligodendroglial cells *(arrowheads)* have smaller and dense round nuclei (condensed chromatin) often surrounded by a clear zone indicative of cell cytoplasm and a cell membrane. Oligodendroglial cells in gray matter are called perineuronal satellite cells; those in white matter are called interfascicular oligodendrocytes. Microglial cells can be difficult to identify in H&E-stained sections of the central nervous system (CNS) but are often identified by their small, dense elongated nuclei *(dashed arrow)*. The light pink homogeneous tissue distributed in large quantities between these cell types is the neuropil. *V*, Blood vessels. H&E stain. (Courtesy Dr. J.F. Zachary, College of Veterinary Medicine, University of Illinois.)

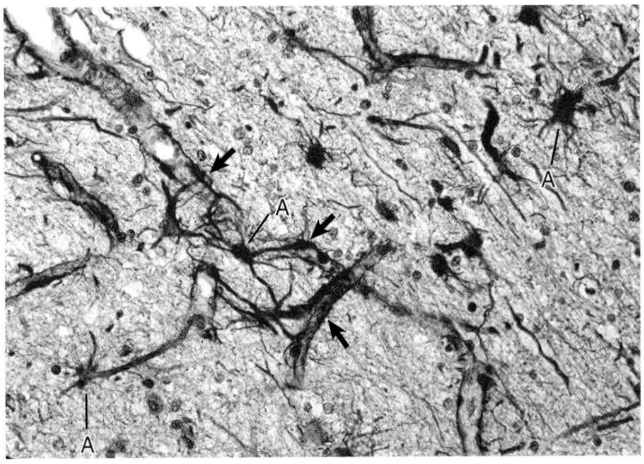

Figure 14-8 **Astrocytic Processes, Brain, Cerebral Cortex, Normal Animal.** Processes of astrocytes arborize extensively throughout the central nervous system *(structures stained purple)*. Note that some of the processes are on the outside of blood capillaries (end feet) *(arrows)*. Holzer's stain. *A*, Cell body of astrocyte. (Courtesy Dr. M.D. McGavin, College of Veterinary Medicine, University of Tennessee.)

regard to their total cell size in that their processes occupy much more space than the cell body. Neurons have very long axons, which account for their size; oligodendroglia have extensive myelin sheaths, which account for their size. In H&E-stained sections, oligodendroglia are often confused with lymphocytes because of the similarity of the morphologic features of their nuclei and cytoplasmic volume. Interfascicular oligodendroglia and perineuronal satellite oligodendroglia are located primarily in white and gray matter

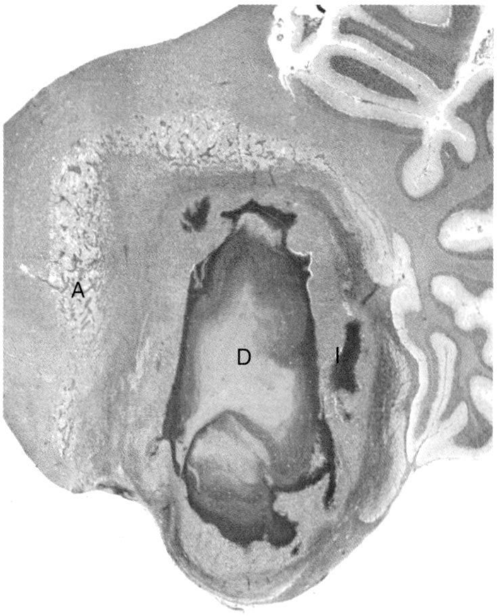

Figure 14-9 **Astrocytic Repair, Bacterial Abscess, Brainstem, Sheep.** The abscess has a central core of necrotic debris *(D)* surrounded by a layer of inflammatory cells *(I)* and a less dense pink-staining zone representing an attempt by astrocytes and fibroblasts to form a capsule *(A)*. This capsule is formed by fibrous tissue on the ventral and right sides, those sides closest to the pia, which contains fibroblasts. A fibrous capsule is absent from the dorsal and left sides of the abscess, adjacent to brain parenchyma. Here, there is no population of resident fibroblasts, and the capsule is formed by astrocytes and their processes, which are often delicate and do not form an effective capsule *(A)*. H&E stain. (Courtesy Dr. J.F. Zachary, College of Veterinary Medicine, University of Illinois.)

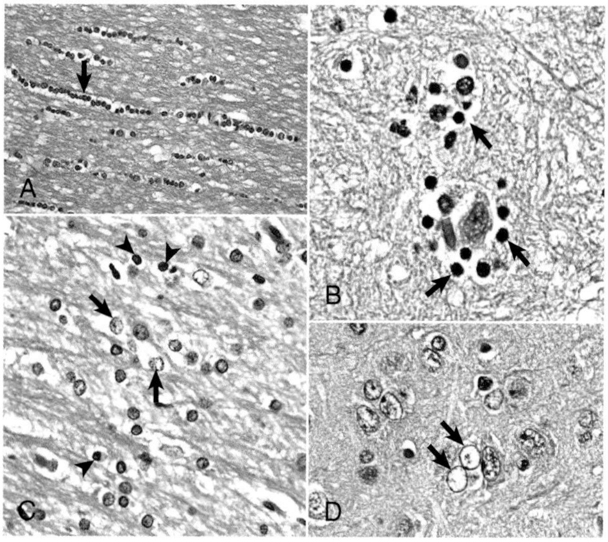

Figure 14-10 **Responses of Glial Cells to Injury in H&E-Stained Central Nervous System (CNS) Sections. A,** White matter. In nondiseased states, oligodendroglia in white matter are often arranged linearly (interfascicular oligodendroglia) *(arrow)* and are responsible for the formation of myelin around axons. In gray matter (not shown; see Fig. 14-17), oligodendroglia are dispersed as individual cells around neuronal cell bodies as perineuronal satellite cells **(B)**. H&E stain. **B,** Gray matter. When neurons are injured or there exists some perturbation of the perineuronal microenvironment, oligodendroglia around neurons can hypertrophy and proliferate in a process referred to as satellitosis. Perineuronal satellite oligodendroglia *(arrows)* surround a small degenerate neuron with condensed chromatin and little cytoplasm. H&E stain. **C,** White matter. Astrocytes *(arrows)* and oligodendroglia *(arrowheads)* have a limited repertoire of responses to injury in the CNS. Astrocytic proliferation can occur but is very difficult to determine in sections stained with H&E. Here, astrocyte nuclei are somewhat enlarged and appear more numerous than expected. H&E stain. **D,** Gray matter. Astrocytes respond to injury in hyperammonemia, such as occurs with hepatic encephalopathy, by forming astrocytes with enlarged, markedly vesicular ("watery"), often elongated nuclei called Alzheimer's type II astrocytes *(arrows)*. This type of astrocyte may occur in pairs that are surrounded by a clear space indicative of cellular swelling. H&E stain. (**A** courtesy Dr. M.D. McGavin, College of Veterinary Medicine, University of Tennessee. **B** to **D** courtesy Dr. J.F. Zachary, College of Veterinary Medicine, University of Illinois.)

of the CNS, respectively (Fig. 14-10); however, interfascicular oligodendroglia can also be found along axons that traverse through the gray matter. The mature, small oligodendrocyte has a spherical, hyperchromatic nucleus (see Figs. 14-7 and 14-10). As with astrocytes, the cell body and processes of this cell do not stain with conventional H&E staining methods and can only be demonstrated following special procedures that include metallic (silver) impregnation and immunohistochemical methods, including CNPase and Olig2.

Most interfascicular oligodendroglia (see Fig. 14-10) are aligned in rows parallel to myelinated axons and are responsible for the formation and maintenance of segments (internodes) of myelin sheaths. One oligodendroglial cell can form as many as 50 different internodes of myelin, each of which can be located on many different axons (Fig. 14-11). Altered function of oligodendroglial cells, as occurs in infectious canine distemper virus (CDV) infection, can cause primary demyelination of these segments, resulting in severe neurologic dysfunction. Oligodendroglia also influence maturation and maintenance of axons and inhibit regeneration of established myelinated axons.

Perineuronal satellite oligodendroglia (see Fig. 14-10) are adjacent to neuronal cell bodies and are also located around blood vessels in the gray matter. They are thought by some investigators to regulate the perineuronal microenvironment and respond to perturbation by proliferation. When the perineuronal microenvironment is altered or neuron cell bodies are injured, perineuronal satellite oligodendroglia, in an attempt to regulate the environmental perturbation, hypertrophy and proliferate in a process referred to as *satellitosis*. However, this term is imprecise as other glial cells can also contribute to sattelitosis. Similarly, alterations in the microenvironment of gray and white matter away from areas surrounding neuron cell bodies result in hypertrophy of oligodendroglia (see Fig. 14-10). It should be noted that in some sections of the normal CNS there are increased numbers of oligodendrocytes that surround neurons, giving a false impression of pathologic satellitosis. This arrangement is especially true for interstitial white matter neurons found in the cerebral cortices.

Microglia. The basic functions of microglia are immunosurveillance, immunoregulation, and reparative (phagocytic) activities after neural cell injury and death. Resident microglia originate from mesodermal stem cells in the yolk sac and enter and populate the CNS during embryonic development and early postnatal life, analogous to the formation of the monocyte-macrophage system in other organs. Microglia can become amoeboid by phagocytosing dead cells and cellular debris during remodeling and maturation of the CNS. Amoeboid cells then enter a quiescent stage and transform into ramified microglia. Ramified microglia constitute up to 20% of the glial cells and are present throughout the mature CNS, serving as sentinels of brain injury. Ramified microglia, also called *resting cells*, are most numerous in perineuronal and perivascular areas and in

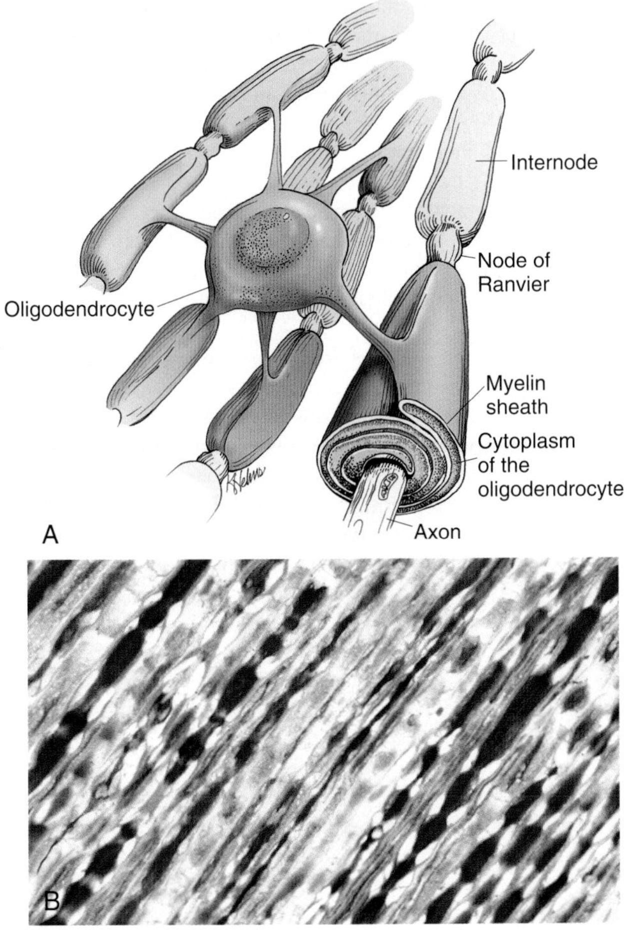

Figure 14-11 **Central Nervous System (CNS) Myelin.** Oligodendroglia myelinate axons within the CNS (also see Fig. 14-3). **A,** As depicted in this illustration, each oligodendrocyte sends out numerous cytoplasmic processes that repetitively encircle (myelinate) the portion of an axon between two nodes of Ranvier (internode) on the same and several different axons. Direct or indirect injury to an oligodendrocyte can result in "demyelination" of those internodes myelinated by that oligodendrocyte. This injury will slow the rate of conduction of an action potential and depending on the site of the lesion, may lead to clinical signs of neural dysfunction (ataxia, proprioception deficits). **B,** CNS nerves, longitudinal section. Axons and their neurofilaments *(brown stain)* and myelin *(red stain)* are demonstrated by this immunohistochemical stain for neurofilament and myelin basic protein. (Courtesy Dr. J.F. Zachary, College of Veterinary Medicine, University of Illinois.)

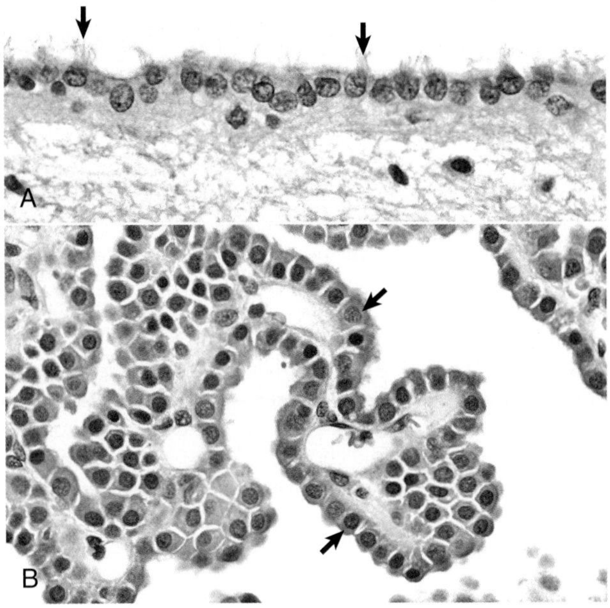

Figure 14-12 **Ependymal and Choroid Plexus Epithelial Cells. A,** Ependymal cells are ciliated *(arrows)* and assist with the flow of cerebrospinal fluid (CSF) through the ventricular system. H&E stain. **B,** Choroid plexus epithelial cells *(arrows)* produce CSF from a brush border (microvilli) on the luminal surface. The surface of the choroid plexus also has cilia that occur singly or more often in groups of three or more on a single cell. H&E stain. (Courtesy Dr. J.F. Zachary, College of Veterinary Medicine, University of Illinois.)

interfascicular locations in white matter. Evidence of pinocytosis in ramified cells suggests some role in maintaining the neural microenvironment. The principal function of microglia is phagocytosis, the initiation of and participation in the innate and adaptive immune responses, and in degenerative and inflammatory diseases of the CNS.

Microscopically, ramified microglia have small, hyperchromatic ovoid-, rod-, or comma-shaped nuclei and no appreciable cytoplasm with routine H&E staining; thus the term *rod cell* is sometimes used to describe them (see Fig. 14-7). With special labeling techniques or metallic impregnation, ramified cells have delicate branching processes. The small hyperchromatic nuclei and nuclear shape distinguish microglia from astrocytes and oligodendroglia. However, microglia are often difficult to identify in H&E-stained sections without some expertise in neuropathology.

Activated microglial cells are not the major source of active macrophages in inflammation of the CNS. Blood monocytes recruited from the circulation account for up to 70% of the macrophages in inflammatory and degenerative diseases of the CNS. These macrophages differentiate from blood monocytes involved in normal "leukocytic trafficking" through the CNS and can be involved in immunologic and phagocytic responses (gitter cells) to disease processes and infectious microbes. These macrophage populations are found mainly in the leptomeninges, choroid plexus, and perivascular areas.

Ependyma (Including Choroid Plexus Epithelial Cells). The basic functions of ependymal cells, which line the ventricular system, are to help move CSF through the ventricular system via movement of their cilia and to regulate the flow of materials between the CNS and the CSF. The ependyma is a single-layered, cuboidal to columnar epithelium that lines the ventricles and mesencephalic aqueduct of the brain and central canal of the spinal cord (Fig. 14-12). This layer of cells is therefore situated between the CSF and nervous tissue. Ependymal cells have cilia that project into the CSF and beat in a coordinated manner in the direction of CSF flow. Other structures, referred to as *circumventricular organs*, which include the choroid plexuses, are covered by highly specialized ependymal cells. The surface of ependymal cells that form the choroid plexus have microvilli (microvillus border) and cilia that occur singly or more often in groups of three or more. The choroid plexus epithelial cells also have specialized tight junctions (zonulae occludens) that are a functional part of the blood-CSF barrier. In contrast to the choroid plexus, junctions between the conventional ependymal cells include gap junctions (transmembrane proteins form a pore, allowing communication between adjacent cells) and zonulae and fasciae adherentes, which permit movement of materials, such as proteins from the CSF, into the extracellular space of the brain. This cellular lining, however, is not a static membrane in that it regulates several processes that involve interaction between the CSF and brain. The functions include regulation of fluid homeostasis between the ventricular cavities and the brain, secretion and absorption of CSF, endocytosis, phagocytosis, and metabolism of substances such as iron resulting from the lysis of erythrocytes after hemorrhage into the ventricular system. Finally, ependymal cells have the structural and enzymatic characteristics necessary for scavenging and detoxifying a wide variety of substances in the CSF.

During embryonic development the medial wall of the lateral ventricle (choroid fissure), the roof of the third ventricle, and the rostral part of the roof of the fourth ventricle consist of a single layer of neuroectoderm that is adherent on its outer surface to the pia mater. This neuroectoderm-pia union forms the tela choroidea, providing an anchor for the choroid plexuses, which is formed by an invagination of this bilayer membrane into the ventricular spaces.

Choroid plexus epithelial cells are modified ependymal cells. The choroid plexus epithelium is a single-layered, cuboidal to columnar epithelium with a microvillus border (see Fig. 14-12). CSF is secreted from the microvillus border. Choroid plexus epithelial cells, along with capillaries and the pia mater, form the choroid plexuses that project into the lateral, third, and fourth ventricles. The basic function of choroid plexuses is to produce the CSF that fills the ventricular system and the subarachnoid space. CSF has two important functions: (1) to act as a "shock absorber" to mitigate the effects of trauma to the brain and spinal cord and (2) to deliver nutrients to and remove wastes from the CNS.

The normal flow pattern of CSF is regulated by an intraventricular biologic pressure gradient in which the pressure created by secretion of CSF exceeds the pressure created by its absorption in arachnoid villi (arachnoid granulations). Arachnoid villi are focal extensions of the arachnoid and subarachnoid space that extend into the dorsal sagittal venous sinus of the brain. CSF is secreted by the choroid plexuses in the lateral, third, and fourth ventricles. It should be noted, however, that fluid from other sources, such as secretion by the ependyma, interstitial fluid of the brain, and ultrafiltrate of the blood, has also been reported to contribute to the formation of CSF. It moves from the lateral ventricles into the third ventricle, from the third ventricle through the mesencephalic aqueduct (aqueduct of Sylvius in human beings), and then to the fourth ventricle. Once in the fourth ventricle, the CSF exits through the two lateral apertures of the fourth ventricle to enter the subarachnoid space. Lateral apertures are the two openings in the caudal medullary velum that forms the roof of the fourth ventricle into the subarachnoid space, one at each side of the cerebellopontine angle. Although the central canal of the spinal cord is connected to the ventricular system at the caudal end of the fourth ventricle, there apparently is little active movement of CSF within the central canal. CSF in the subarachnoid space is reabsorbed by the arachnoid villi in the meninges. Recent evidence indicates that other routes of CSF drainage, in addition to arachnoid granulations, also exist and vary in different species. Venous sinuses, lymphatic drainage, and the cribriform plate appear to play important roles in CSF drainage and the maintenance of normal interventricular CSF pressure. In fact, experimental evidence suggests that the cribriform plate route may be the most important of the four. In human beings the entire volume of CSF is circulated approximately four times a day; however, with aging, the entire volume of CSF circulates less than two times a day.

Meninges. The meninges, which enclose the CNS, consist of three layers: the dura mater (outermost layer), the arachnoid membrane, and the pia mater (innermost layer) (Fig. 14-13). Together, the arachnoid membrane and pia mater are frequently referred to as the *leptomeninges*, *pia-arachnoid layer*, or *pia-arachnoid*. The arachnoid membrane and pia mater are held together by bands of fibrous tissue called *arachnoid trabeculae*. This arrangement forms a compartment called the *subarachnoid space* in which CSF flows and which also contains blood vessels and nerves. The leptomeninges form a protective covering for the CNS and provide an external envelope filled with CSF that provides additional protection.

The dura mater, once referred to as the pachymeninx (thick meninges), is a strong and dense collagenous membrane (Fig. 14-14). In the cranium the dura consists of two layers that are fused with each other. The outer layer serves as the periosteum of the cranial bone, except in the areas of the venous sinuses (surrounded by dura) and falx cerebri, which is the longitudinal layer that extends ventrally between the two cerebral hemispheres. At the level of the foramen magnum, the two layers become separated; the outer layer continues to function as the periosteum of the vertebral (spinal) canal, and the inner layer forms the free dural membrane that surrounds the spinal cord. The inner aspect of dura mater is lined by elongated, flattened mesothelial-like cells. Except in neonates, there is no epidural (extradural) space in the cranial vault as there is in the spinal cord. There can be a "potential" epidural or extradural space in mature animals from hemorrhage caused by trauma.

The arachnoid consists of both the multilayered membrane composed of cells that overlap one another and the trabeculae that join it to the pia. The arachnoid has tight junctions between its cells, although other junctions have also been described. It contains no blood vessels and has an outer smooth surface formed by mesothelial-like cells that abut similar cells in the dura mater. The mesothelium-like surfaces of the dura and arachnoid oppose and slide over each other, analogous to the parietal and visceral surfaces of other serous membranes.

The pia mater is closely adherent to the surface of the brain and spinal cord and is penetrated by a large number of blood vessels that supply the underlying nervous tissue (Fig. 14-15). The pia mater consists of flat, thin, overlapping connective tissue cells (fibroblasts) that are separated from the underlying neural tissue by variable amounts of loose collagen fibers and the glia limitans. In many areas the pia, which lacks a basal lamina, is only one-cell-layer thick and has fenestrations, so that the glia limitans is exposed directly to the subarachnoid space. Pial and arachnoid cells also ensheathe blood vessels, collagen bundles, and nerves that are within or cross the subarachnoid space and also are around arteries that penetrate into the CNS up to 1 to 2 mm in depth. Macrophages including dendritic cells also are present throughout the leptomeninges.

Endothelium. The basic functions of endothelium in the CNS are to line luminal surfaces of blood vessels; form the blood-brain barrier; regulate thrombosis, thrombolysis, and platelet adherence; and maintain a nonthrombogenic boundary between coagulation cascade molecules and luminal surfaces of endothelial cells. Additionally, endothelial cells function as regulatory barriers to small and large molecules crossing the endothelium, and they control the adherence of leukocytes to their luminal surfaces. The endothelial cells of the blood-brain barrier actively transport those molecules that the brain consumes rapidly and in large quantities such as glucose, amino acids, lactate, and ribonucleosides.

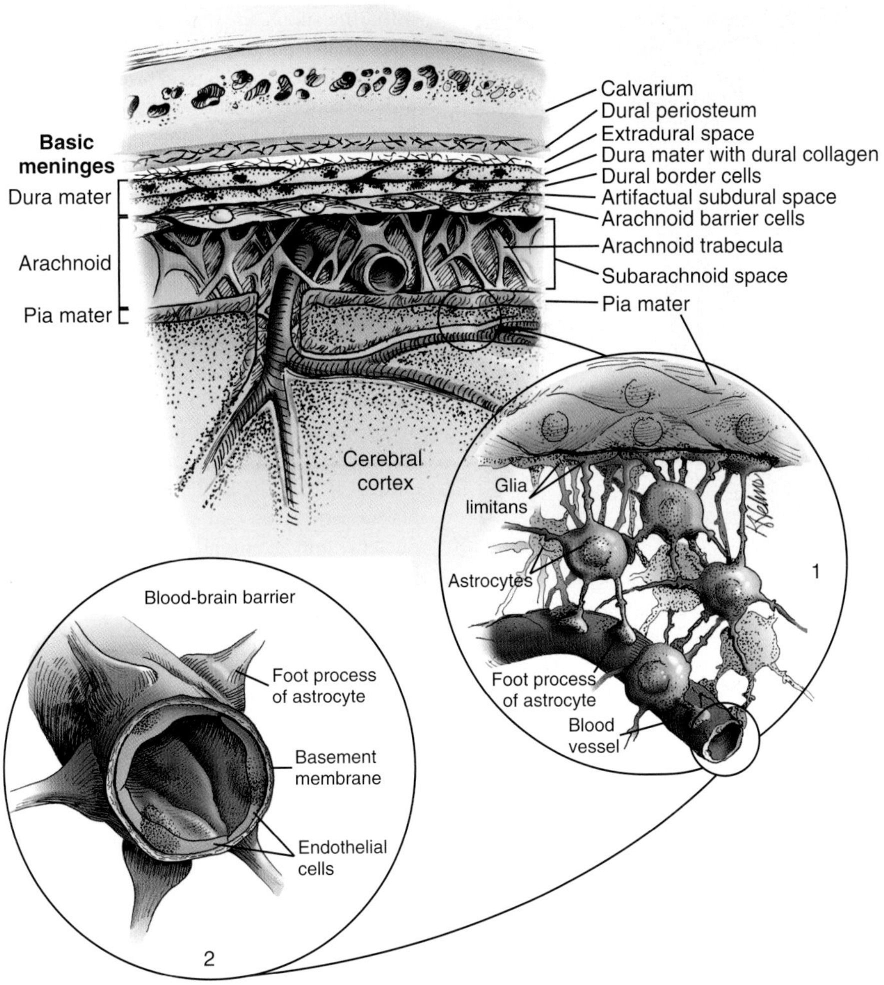

Figure 14-13 **Organization of the Meninges.** The meninges, from outside to inside, are the dura mater, arachnoid mater, and pia mater as illustrated in the diagram. The arachnoid mater and the pia mater form the leptomeninges. These two layers of the leptomeninges also enclose the subarachnoid space, which contains the arteries, veins, and nerves and is filled with cerebrospinal fluid. The pia mater is attached to the surface of the central nervous system (CNS). Astrocytes and their foot processes underlie the pia mater and form the glia limitans *(inset 1)* and surround the endothelial cells that form the blood-brain barrier. As arterioles penetrate the cortex to supply the tissue with blood, they carry the pia and glia limitans with them for 1 to 3 mm until the arteriole structurally becomes a capillary. At this transition site within the cortex, the capillary penetrates the pia and is surrounded by the glia limitans, and the end feet of the astrocytes become part of the blood-brain barrier *(inset 2)*. Components of the blood-brain barrier are capillary endothelial cells, basement membrane, and astrocytic foot processes, but the barrier is formed structurally by tight junctions between endothelial cells and functionally by specialized transport systems in these cells. (Courtesy Dr. J.F. Zachary, College of Veterinary Medicine, University of Illinois.)

Dysfunction/Responses to Injury

Ground Rules for Understanding Injury in the Central Nervous System

Before the responses of the CNS to injury are discussed, some fundamental concepts are reviewed in Box 14-2.

Neurons

Neurons are the most vulnerable cells in the nervous system and probably within the body. They have large requirements for energy to maintain normal metabolism, transport systems, and the formation of cytoskeleton proteins in the axon, which can extend over long distances (>1 m). Because neurons lack adequate intracellular glucose reserves, they are completely dependent for survival on an adequate blood supply to provide glucose. Additionally, neurons are vulnerable to free radical oxidative stresses and have a limited ability to buffer shifts of calcium ions into the cell, which can interfere with oxidative phosphorylation and ATP production, such as occurs with ischemia.

Neurons are especially sensitive to excessive stimulation with excitatory amino acid neurotransmitters called *excitotoxins* (e.g., glutamate and aspartate). These neurotransmitters are also released in a wide variety of neuronal injuries, especially ischemia. Under normal conditions, astrocytic processes surrounding synapses have efficient uptake systems to remove excitotoxins, and neurons are not injured. In excessive quantities, persistent binding of excitotoxins to receptors can lead to neuronal degeneration and death.

The microscopic appearance of the neuronal cell body can vary according to the injury. Characteristic changes of the neuronal cell body are reviewed in Box 14-3.

Neuronal Cell Death. Neurons can die after injury as a result of one of two mechanisms: apoptotic cell death and necrotic cell death. These mechanisms are summarized next and discussed in greater detail in Chapter 1. Both apoptotic and necrotic neuronal cell death can occur concurrently or in temporal or spatial sequences within the nervous system. Although apoptotic and necrotic neuronal death represent different responses of neurons to injury, a

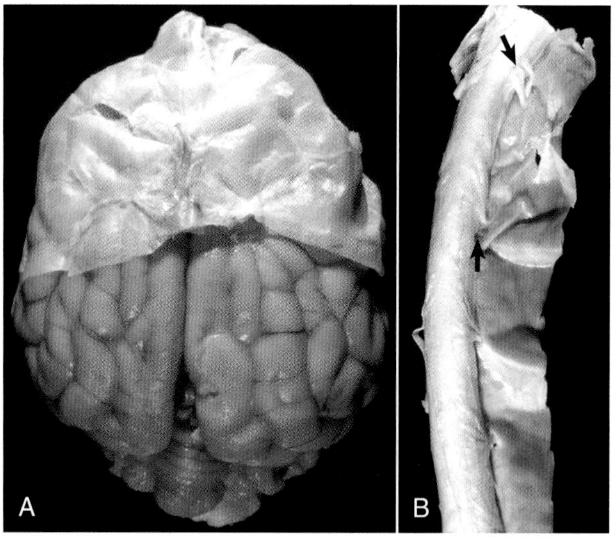

Figure 14-14 **Layers of the Meninges. A,** Brain, dog. The dura matter is a thick opaque layer. Here it covers the rostral (cranial) half of the brain and has been dissected away from the caudal half of the brain to expose the underlying leptomeninges. In old animals the dura mater often fuses with the periosteum of the calvaria, and at necropsy to expose the brain, it is usually removed attached to the calvaria. The leptomeninges are present, but because they are so transparent, they are barely visible on the surface of the caudal half of the brain between gyri. **B,** Spinal cord, horse. The dura mater is the thick opaque layer dissected from and lying to the right of the spinal cord. The leptomeninges (pia-arachnoid layer) are present (but not readily visible in this photograph) on the exposed surface of the spinal cord. Arrows indicate spinal nerve roots. (Courtesy Dr. J.F. Zachary, College of Veterinary Medicine, University of Illinois.)

network of receptors, messenger systems, and mechanisms of cytotoxicity are involved in both apoptotic and necrotic cell death. Factors that determine whether the apoptotic or necrotic pathway is activated include the character on the initiating ligand or injury, type of cell membrane receptors activated, and caspases expressed in response to injury.

Apoptotic Cell Death (Programmed Cell Death). Apoptosis is a single cell-initiated, gene-directed, and self-destructive regulatory mechanism that leads to "programmed" cell death. This mechanism is used (1) during the development of the nervous system to ensure proper migration and orientation of cell layers and removal of excess embryonic cells, (2) to remove "aged" cells (i.e., cell turnover) in organs, and (3) to maintain cell number homeostasis in organ systems that have regenerative capacity (endocrine glands).

Apoptotic neuronal death is characterized by a sequence of cellular degenerative steps that can be identified biochemically and morphologically. After appropriate signals are recognized and interpreted by cell membrane receptors (Fas, tumor necrosis factor [TNF] receptor-1, TNF-related apoptosis-inducing ligand receptors), a family of proteins known as caspases are activated. Caspases cleave cellular substrates that are required for cellular function and include cytoskeleton proteins and nuclear proteins such as DNA repair enzymes. Caspases also activate other degradative enzymes, such as deoxyribonucleases, which cleave nuclear DNA.

The role of apoptotic neuronal death in specific neurologic diseases is discussed in greater detail in subsequent sections. As examples, some viral infections, such as feline panleukopenia virus infection, that occur in utero produce developmental anomalies by initiating apoptosis that leads to faulty differentiation of embryonic granule and Purkinje cell layers. Mild ischemia, excitotoxins, hormones, corticosteroids, and proinflammatory cytokines can similarly induce apoptotic cell death. Rabies virus and Borna disease virus have been linked experimentally to apoptotic neuronal death.

Apoptosis results in characteristic morphologic changes in cells such as shrinkage, cytoplasmic condensation and blebbing, and chromatin clumping and fragmentation (see Figs. 1-13, 1-22, 1-23, and E-Fig. 1-11). As cells continue to shrink, nuclear chromatin is cleaved into smaller units and along with condensed cytoplasm is packaged for removal by macrophages. Inflammation is not induced by apoptotic cell death.

Necrotic Cell Death. Necrosis is a process that usually affects groups of cells in contrast to single isolated cells as observed in apoptosis. It is characterized by the following sequence: hydropic degeneration, swelling of mitochondria, loss of ionic gradient control across the cell membrane, activation of numerous cytoplasmic and lysosomal enzymes, pyknosis and fragmentation of the nucleus, and eventual cell lysis (see Figs 1-12, 1-13, 1-16, and E-Fig. 1-11). Cellular debris associated with necrotic neuronal death elicits an inflammatory response in contrast to apoptotic neuronal death.

Acute Neuronal Necrosis. Acute neuronal necrosis (also sometimes referred to as acidophilic or ischemic necrosis) is a common response to a variety of CNS injuries, such as cerebral ischemia caused by blood loss and hypovolemic shock, vascular thrombosis, and cardiac failure; inflammatory mediators; bacterial toxins; thermal injury; heavy metals; nutritional deficiencies, such as thiamine deficiency; and trauma. Additionally, conditions that reduce ATP generation through oxidative phosphorylation also lead to neuronal degeneration and death. Such conditions include (1) interference with cytochrome oxidase activity in mitochondria caused by cyanide poisoning, (2) competitive inhibition of oxygen uptake in carbon monoxide poisoning, and (3) inadequate availability of glucose for neuronal metabolism in hypoglycemia.

The susceptibility of cells and tissue structures of the CNS to ischemia in decreasing order of susceptibility are neurons, oligodendroglia, astrocytes, microglia, and blood vessels. However, within groups of neurons, some neurons are more sensitive to injury than others. This phenomenon is called *selective neuronal vulnerability*. Purkinje cells; some striatal neurons; neurons of the third, fifth, and sixth cerebral cortical lamina; and hippocampal pyramidal cells have the highest vulnerability. A regional vulnerability of neurons has also been reported (cerebral cortex and striatum > thalamus > brainstem > spinal cord). It is hypothesized that the most vulnerable neurons likely produce the most excitotoxins, such as glutamate, and are the most sensitive to them. Because of the microanatomic arrangement of the cerebral cortex, ischemic neurons often occur in a laminar pattern within the cerebrocortical gray matter. This microanatomic pattern accounts for the laminar lesions observed in thiamine deficiency–induced polioencephalomalacia in ruminants and in other diseases such as salt poisoning in pigs and lead poisoning in ruminants. Immunohistochemical stains for neuronal specific markers (e.g., neuronal nuclei) often delineate a linear pattern of neuronal necrosis better than that observed with an H&E stain and histologic examination.

After the various types of CNS injury, there is an early increase in ATP-dependent release of normally sequestered intracellular calcium ions from altered mitochondria and endoplasmic reticulum. Also during this time, neuronal depolarization potentiates the release of the neuroexcitatory neurotransmitter glutamate. Persistent activation of glutamate receptors of target cells results in a disturbance referred to as excitotoxicity. This altered activity leads

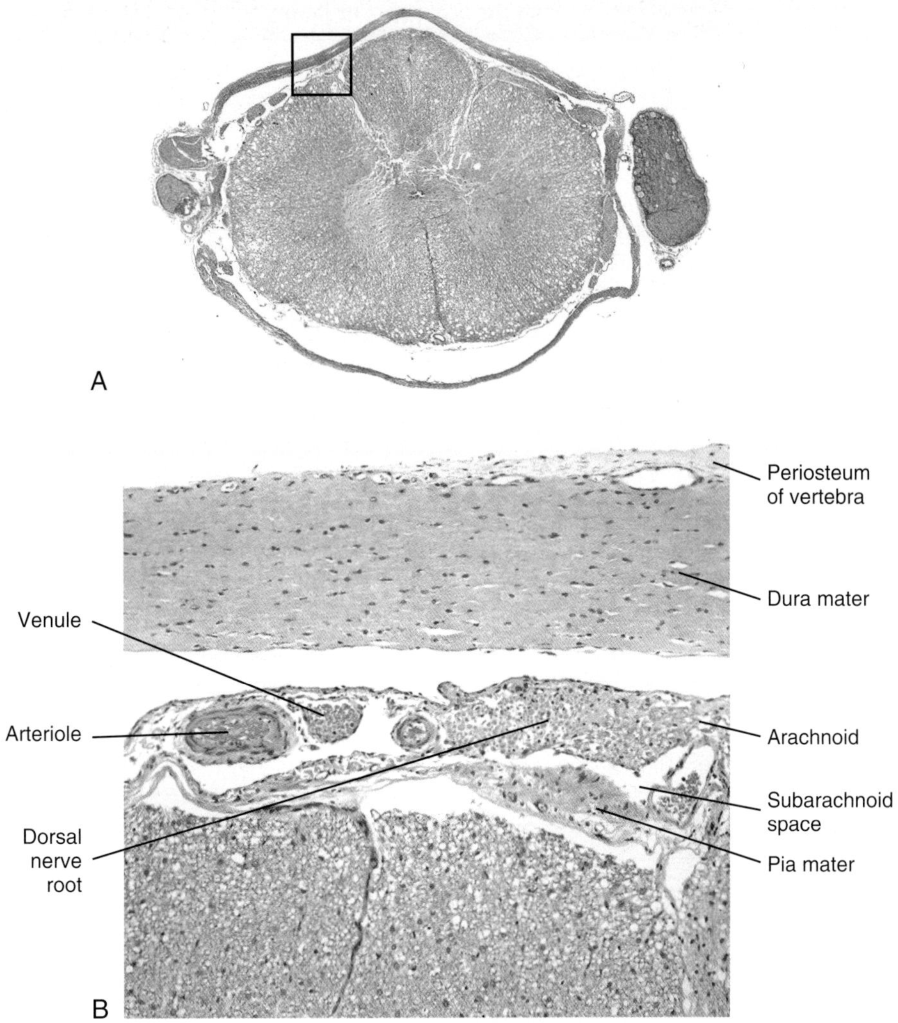

Figure 14-15 Histologic Section of Spinal Cord and Meninges. A, Low magnification of a cross-section of the spinal cord and meninges with spinal nerve rootlets and a dorsal root ganglion from which **B** was selected *(box)*. H&E stain. **B,** The inner surface of the dura mater and the outer surface of the arachnoid mater are covered with mesothelial cells, and the space between them is the subdural space. Blood vessels and nerves of the dorsal and ventral roots traverse in the subarachnoid space. H&E stain. (Courtesy Dr. J.F. Zachary, College of Veterinary Medicine, University of Illinois.)

to a notable influx of extracellular calcium into cells, causing further impairment of mitochondrial function and the generation of reactive oxygen species, such as superoxide, hydrogen peroxide, hydroxyl radicals, and nitric oxide. These reactive oxygen species, exerting their effects especially on lipid-rich cell membranes, can enhance the existing excitotoxicity, cause further influx of calcium into cells as a result of membrane damage, and ultimately result in neuronal dysfunction and death. Additionally, reperfusion of ischemic tissue after the initial ischemic injury can enhance the generation of reactive oxygen metabolites, thus amplifying the tissue damage. Other influencing factors include the temperature of the brain at the time of ischemia, with lower temperatures (as little as 2° C decrease) having a sparing effect and elevated temperatures having an enhanced effect on neuronal injury following ischemia.

Neurons depend on a continuous supply of oxygen to remain viable, and if the supply is interrupted for several minutes, the vulnerable neurons as described previously degenerate. Ischemic cell change can also result from metabolic disturbances other than ischemia, such as in thiamine deficiency and cyanide toxicosis, which interferes with oxygen use. In H&E-stained sections the cytoplasm of the neuronal cell body is shrunken, deeply eosinophilic, and frequently sharply angular to triangular in shape (Fig. 14-16). The nucleus is reduced in size, often triangular, frequently assumes a central position in the cell, and is pyknotic. The nucleolus and Nissl substance are usually not detectable. Ischemia neurons die and are removed either by a process called *neuronophagia,* which is phagocytosis by resident microglial cells and recruited macrophages or by lysis (see Fig. 14-16). After neuronal necrosis there is swelling of perineuronal and perivascular astrocytic processes and eventual replacement of the space left by loss of the neuron cell body by astrocytes and their processes.

Chronic Neuronal Loss (Brain Atrophy). Neuronal death and loss of neurons can occur as a result of progressive disease processes of long duration in the CNS. This loss, termed *simple neuronal atrophy,* is seen with slowly progressive neurologic diseases, such as cerebral cortical atrophy of aging, ceroid-lipofuscinosis, and various manifestations of selective or multisystem neuronal degeneration. Gross lesions are usually not visible, but when cerebrocortical neurons die, there can be atrophy of cerebral gyri, which results in widening of the sulci (Fig. 14-17). Microscopic lesions indicative of an earlier

Box 14-2 Concepts in Understanding Responses of the Central Nervous System to Injury

The cells of the CNS vary in their susceptibility to injury (neurons > oligodendroglia > astrocytes > microglia > blood vessels). Neurons are the most sensitive to injury, whereas glial and other cells are more resistant to injury.

1. Neurons have only small energy stores; therefore they depend on an intact blood flow to supply oxygen and nutrients, particularly glucose. Neurons with the highest metabolic rate, such as some neurons in the cerebral cortex, will die 6 to 10 minutes after the cessation of blood flow after cardiac arrest.
2. There is no regeneration of neurons. The neurons you have now are the ones you were born with; however, their metabolism is dynamic, and metabolites are continually turned over and replaced.
3. If nerve fibers in the CNS are cut by transection of the cord, no or little regeneration of nerve fibers results. Therefore if sufficient motor nerve fibers are cut, there is paralysis; if not, there is a neurologic deficit.
4. If fibers in the PNS are cut, they can regenerate under certain circumstances. This outcome depends on axoplasmic flow, alignment of the proximal and distal portions of the nerve, and the preservation and alignment of the proximal and distal portions of the endoneurial tube (the structure in which the axon lies).
5. Healing in the CNS is different than in the rest of the body. There are few fibroblasts in the CNS, and they are principally found only in the leptomeninges and in the outer few millimeters of the CNS, where they are pulled into the cerebral cortex with blood vessels. Therefore wounds deep in the CNS heal by proliferation of astrocyte processes. Astrocytic processes fill small dead spaces of less than a few millimeters and encapsulate large dead spaces and abscesses. Superficial wounds or wounds that extend through the leptomeninges heal by synthesis and deposition of collagen by fibroblasts (fibrous connective tissue) and by proliferation of astrocytic processes. However, in contrast to the fibroblast, astrocytic processes produce a very poor capsule, which can break down easily.
6. The cranial cavity is nearly filled by the brain, its coverings, and fluids. Therefore many lesions, such as tumors, abscesses, hemorrhages, and hydrocephalus in the brain, produce clinical signs because they are space-occupying lesions, which in neuropathology implies that they cause atrophy or displacement of portions of the brain or cord, depending on the duration of the injury.
7. The blood-brain barrier can exert control over drugs and antibodies and prevent them from entering the intact brain. It is also a barrier to infection and is formed by the tight junctions of the endothelial cells, aided by basement membrane, and the end feet of the astrocytes, which lie on the outside of the capillary.
8. Although the CNS has the ability to resist infection and injury, once the CNS is infected, it has a low degree of resistance when compared with other tissues of the body. Microbes, such as *Cryptococcus neoformans,* which normally would be relatively nonpathogenic in other organs, may produce death if the CNS is infected. This outcome in part is attributable to the complexity of the CNS and the fact that it is the most vital organ in the body. Any disease process will often cause catastrophic results in the CNS, as opposed to tissues such as the lung, liver, and kidney.

CNS, Central nervous system; *PNS,* peripheral nervous system.

Box 14-3 Microscopic Changes That Can Occur in the Neuronal Cell Body

1. Central chromatolysis after axonal injury, degenerative conditions, viral infection, or inherited conditions
2. Ischemic cell change
3. Enlargement of the cell body in lysosomal storage diseases
4. Accumulation of lipofuscin pigment in aging
5. Accumulation of neurofilaments in certain neuronal degenerative diseases
6. Inclusion body formation in certain viral diseases
7. Cytoplasmic vacuolation in spongiform encephalopathies

loss of neurons include diminished numbers of neurons, astrogliosis, and atrophy and loss of neurons in functionally related systems. Loss of neurons over time results in progressively worsening neurologic dysfunction as the afferent and efferent neurons that directly interact with the now dead neuron are similarly affected and eventually degenerate.

Wallerian Degeneration and Central Chromatolysis. Injury to axons of the CNS and PNS can result from a variety of causes such as (1) traumatic transection leading to Wallerian degeneration, (2) compression and crushing, (3) therapeutic neurectomies, (4) nerve stretching injury, and (5) intoxication.

Wallerian Degeneration. In 1850 Dr. Augustus Volney Waller described the pattern of microscopic lesions (necrosis) in axons and myelin sheaths after transection. These changes became what we now refer to as *Wallerian degeneration*. Although Waller described this process in peripheral nerves, the term Wallerian degeneration is also used to describe necrosis that occurs in nerve fibers in the CNS after axons are injured (compressed or severed). Focal damage to a nerve fiber results in decreased or halted axonal transport, which manifests most prominently as segmental swellings in the axon called spheroids (Fig. 14-18). Eventually the axon's myelin degenerates, forming areas of vacuolation into which macrophages infiltrate and digest the now necrotic axonal and myelin debris (forming *digestion chambers*). In the neuronal cell body of the damaged axon, lesions include swelling of the neuronal cell body, peripheral displacement of the nucleus, and dispersion of centrally located Nissl substance (*central chromatolysis*) (Fig. 14-19). It must be stressed that this is only one of several ways in which chromatolysis can develop. Chromatolytic neurons can also be found in a wide variety of neurologic diseases including viral infection and degenerative diseases like equine motor neuron disease. The development of Wallerian degeneration is directly related to the diameter of the axon, with a larger axon undergoing a faster rate of Wallerian degeneration.

More information on this topic, including E-Figure 14-5, is available at www.expertconsult.com.

Macroglia

Astrocytes. Common astrocytic reactions in CNS injury are swelling, hypertrophy, division, and the laying down of intermediate filaments in cell processes. The term astrocytosis means that astrocytes have increased in size and number in response to injury, whereas the term *astrogliosis* (somewhat synonymous with hypertrophy) implies synthesis of intermediate filaments and an increased

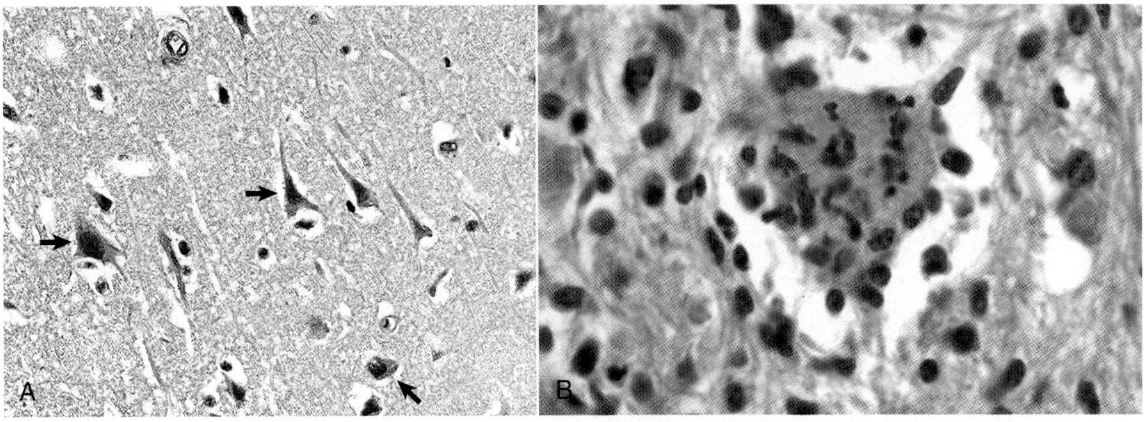

Figure 14-16 Neuronal Necrosis (Acute), So-Called Ischemic Cell Change, Cerebrum, Dog. A, Neuronal ischemia. Neuronal cell bodies of cerebral cortical laminae are red, angular, and shrunken *(arrows)*, and their nuclei are contracted and dense. This lesion can be caused by neuronal ischemia. H&E stain. **B,** Neuronophagia. This necrotic neuron cell body *(center of figure)* is surrounded and infiltrated by macrophages that will phagocytose the cell debris. H&E stain. (**A** courtesy Dr. J.F. Zachary, College of Veterinary Medicine, University of Illinois. **B** courtesy Dr. M.D. McGavin, College of Veterinary Medicine, University of Tennessee.)

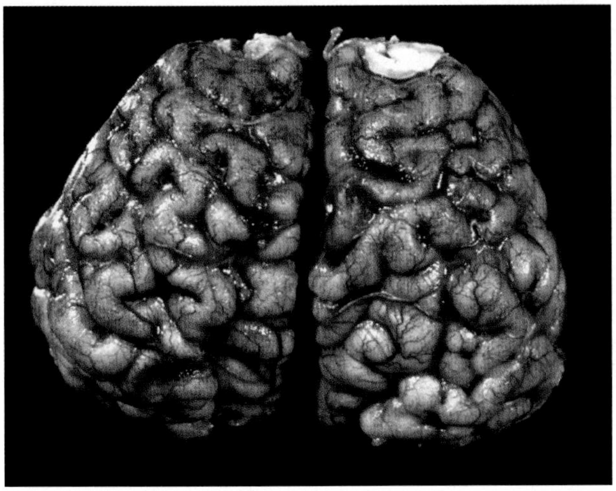

Figure 14-17 Cerebral Cortical Atrophy, Horse. Atrophy is seen with a variety of slowly progressive neurologic diseases in which there is a progressive loss of neurons. These diseases include cerebral cortical atrophy of aging and ceroid-lipofuscinosis. The characteristic gross lesions are narrowing of the cerebral gyri with a consequent widening of the sulci. (Courtesy the Department of Veterinary Biosciences, The Ohio State University.)

length, complexity, and branching of the astrocytic processes. The recognition of these differences is based on histopathologic and immunohistochemical evaluation.

Swelling is an acute response and is reversible, or it may progress with time to hypertrophy. Swollen astrocytes have clear-staining or vacuolated cytoplasm. Astrocytes swell after ischemia because of the increased uptake of sodium, chloride, and potassium ions and water in an effort to maintain homeostasis in the extracellular microenvironment. It is important to remember that such swelling depends on the astrocyte being viable and still having a semipermeable plasma membrane, even though its function may be altered. With progression and if the degree and duration of ischemia are sufficiently severe to result in cell death, the plasma membrane becomes fully permeable, and the cell does not swell but becomes shriveled or shrunken and undergoes disintegration, as described for the ischemic cell change of neurons.

If injury is severe, astrocytic processes fragment and disappear followed by lysis of the cell body. Hypertrophied astrocytes, often referred to as *reactive*, represent a response to a milder and more protracted injury to the CNS. Because of increases in intermediate filaments, mainly GFAP, the cytoplasm becomes apparent along with increased length and branching of the processes with H&E staining. The increase of intermediate filaments and consequently the intensity of GFAP immunohistochemical staining in these cells are so dramatic that some have defined reactive astrocytes on the basis of this change. In protracted degenerative or reparative conditions, astrocytes termed *gemistocytes* can be observed (Fig. 14-20). These cells have eccentric nuclei and abundant pink homogeneous cytoplasm, in contrast to the lack of visible cytoplasm in normal astrocytes, with routine H&E staining. Animals with hepatic and, less commonly, renal encephalopathy can have a unique microscopic lesion in the brain affecting astrocytes of the cerebral cortices. In these types of encephalopathies, astrocytic nuclei tend to be in pairs, triplets, quartets, or more occasionally with prominent central nucleoli and are surrounded by a clear space, which is the edematous cytoplasm. They are called *Alzheimer's type II astrocytes* (see Fig. 14-10, *D*).

Astrocytic proliferation can occur in CNS injury, but in most instances, proliferative capacity is limited. When it occurs, the most dramatic examples are associated with attempts by reactive astrocytes (astrogliosis) to "wall off" abscesses and neoplasms or to fill in cavitated areas that result after lysis of necrotic neurons with the processes of astrocytes. The astrocytes that form regions of astrogliosis are more commonly fibrillary in appearance. In large numbers they may form a *glial scar*, which is a network of interlaced astrocytic processes and provides a loose barrier that separates the injured brain from the more normal adjacent tissue. In this respect the astroglia act to reform a glia limitans around the injured region of the CNS in an effort to restore the blood-brain barrier and reestablish fluid and electrolyte balances.

Oligodendrocytes. Oligodendroglia react to injury by cell swelling, hypertrophy, and degeneration. Both perineuronal and interfascicular oligodendroglia can swell, hypertrophy, and degenerate; however, only oligodendroglia precursor cells can proliferate to replace degenerate cells. The role that perineuronal or satellite oligodendroglia play in normal neuronal function and neuronal

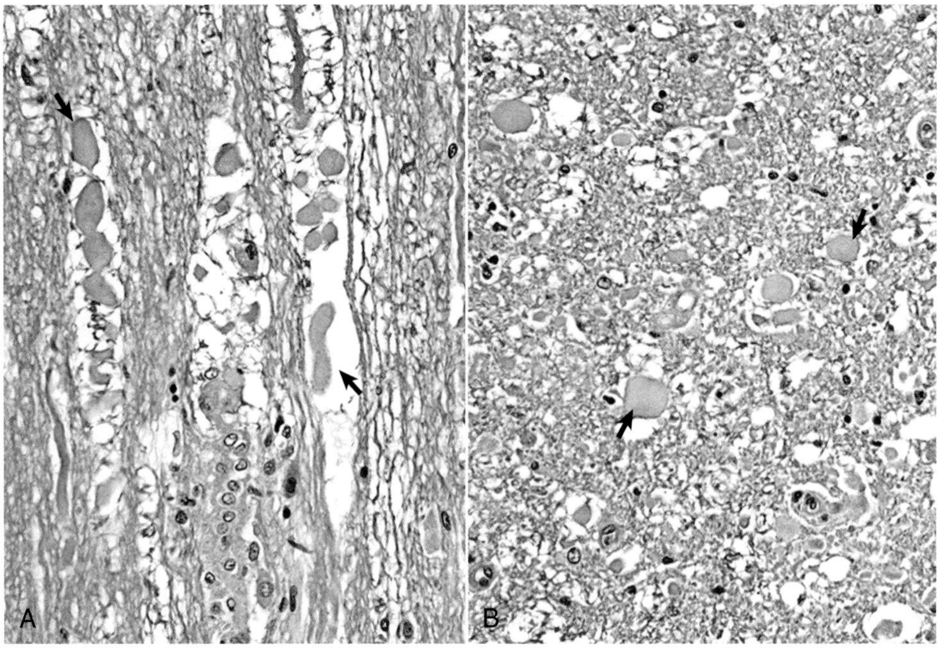

Figure 14-18 **Wallerian Degeneration, Transverse Section of Spinal Cord, Dog. A,** Longitudinal section. Arrows illustrate swollen axons. H&E stain. **B,** Transverse section. Laceration and/or severe compression of myelinated nerves cause a specific sequence of structural and functional changes in the axon and the myelin (distal from the point of injury), referred to as Wallerian degeneration (see E-Fig. 14-5). Axons are initially swollen *(arrows)* and eventually removed by phagocytosis to leave clear spaces, which were once the sites of nerve fibers. The cell bodies of affected neurons usually have central chromatolysis, but are metabolically active in an attempt to regenerate the lost portion of the axon (not shown; see Fig. 14-19). H&E stain. (Courtesy Dr. J.F. Zachary, College of Veterinary Medicine, University of Illinois.)

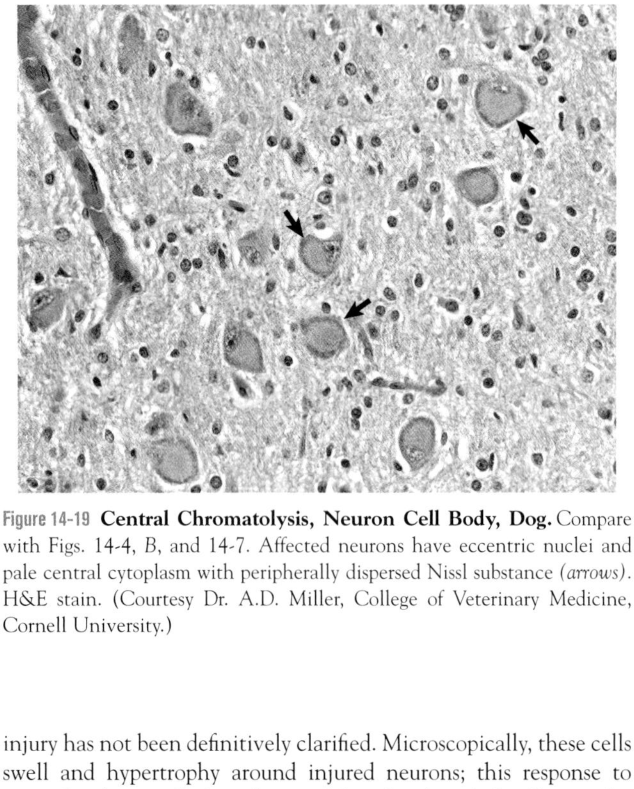

Figure 14-19 **Central Chromatolysis, Neuron Cell Body, Dog.** Compare with Figs. 14-4, *B*, and 14-7. Affected neurons have eccentric nuclei and pale central cytoplasm with peripherally dispersed Nissl substance *(arrows)*. H&E stain. (Courtesy Dr. A.D. Miller, College of Veterinary Medicine, Cornell University.)

injury has not been definitively clarified. Microscopically, these cells swell and hypertrophy around injured neurons; this response to injury has been called *satellitosis*, although other glial cells can also contribute to satellitosis (see Fig. 14-10, *B*).

Degeneration of interfascicular oligodendroglia caused by ischemia, certain viruses, lead toxicity, and autoimmunity can result in selective degeneration of myelin sheaths referred to as *primary demyelination*. Primary demyelination is the loss of myelin around an intact axon and results in the alteration of the conduction velocity of an action potential down the axon, leading to clinical dysfunction (Fig. 14-21). Mechanisms of primary demyelination are summarized in Box 14-4. Protracted or repetitive injury to myelinating cells and their myelin sheaths can lead to irreversible neuronal atrophy. Oligodendroglia precursor cells located in the subventricular zone of the CNS can mature into interfascicular oligodendroglia and can also proliferate in response to noncytocidal injury and become involved in remyelination after primary demyelination.

CNS or PNS injury can also lead to loss of myelin secondary to injury of the axon and its cell body or to death of the neuron. When axons are injured, myelin lamellae forming the internodes are retracted and removed by phagocytosis. In some instances, oligodendroglia or Schwann cells, the myelin-forming cells in the PNS, also degenerate. This form of myelin degeneration is termed *secondary demyelination* and is secondary to axon degeneration or loss (resembles Wallerian degeneration).

Ependymal Cells. Ependymal and choroid plexus epithelial cell responses to injury include atrophy, degeneration, and necrosis. Compression of ependymal cells lining the ventricles followed by atrophy usually occurs in response to enlargement of the ventricles as occurs with hydrocephalus. The cilia and microvilli of affected cells are reduced in number, and there is also a reduction in their cellular organelles such as endoplasmic reticulum and mitochondria. An additional lesion that accompanies ventricular enlargement is stretching and tearing of the ependymal lining. In such instances the resulting areas of ependymal discontinuity result in the subependymal CNS being directly exposed to the CSF. Unfortunately, mammalian ependymal cells do not regenerate and therefore do not repair the denuded areas. After 1 to 2

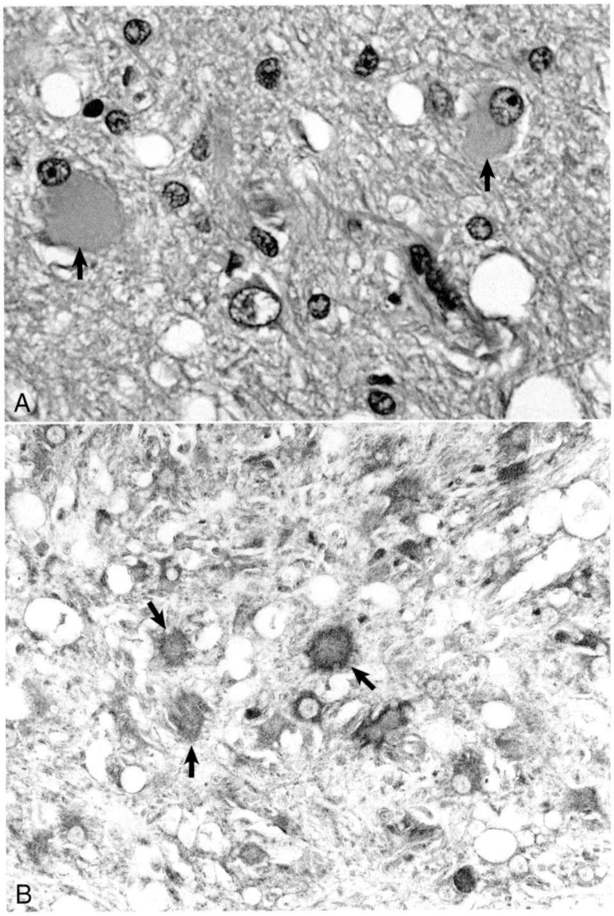

Figure 14-20 **Gemistocytes (Gemistocytic Astrocytes), Cerebrum, Dog. A,** When astrocytes react to injury, initially by hypertrophy and later by the synthesis of increased glial filaments (astrogliosis), the nuclei enlarge and often the cell body, which is not normally visible in H&E-stained sections, will become visible. This type of reactive astrocyte is called a gemistocyte (plump astrocyte) *(arrows)*. They occur in diseases in which there is alteration of intracellular and extracellular fluid balances or injury to the parenchyma, where healing will be by glial scarring (astrogliosis, e.g., to encapsulate a deep abscess or fill in a small area of dead space). H&E stain. **B,** Gemistocytes *(arrows)* are identified by immunohistochemical staining *(brown color)* with antibody to glial fibrillary acid protein. IHC DAB stain. (**A** courtesy Dr. J.F. Zachary, College of Veterinary Medicine, University of Illinois. **B** courtesy Dr. A.D. Miller, College of Veterinary Medicine, Cornell University.)

weeks, astrogliosis, which varies greatly in degree and uniformity, occurs in the exposed areas. Astrogliosis can extend into the ventricular space or be minimal in extent and confined to the periventricular area. Periventricular interstitial edema, myelin loss, and axon loss can ensue.

Inflammation of the ependyma, called *ependymitis*, can also occur following dissemination of microbes, especially bacteria, into the CSF. Microbes most commonly gain entrance to the ependyma via the circulation by lodging in the choroid plexuses, by direct contamination from a rupture of a cerebral abscess into the ventricular system, and by retrograde reflux through the lateral apertures of infected CSF from the subarachnoid space in cases of leptomeningitis. In the case of bacterial infection the suppurative exudate that forms in the CSF can cause obstructive hydrocephalus, although the development of hydrocephalus cannot always be explained solely on the basis of obstruction.

Microglia

Microglia are often the first cells in the CNS to react to injury, and the magnitude of the response is graded to correlate with the severity of damage. The responses of microglia to injury include hypertrophy, hyperplasia, phagocytosis of cellular and myelin debris, and neuronophagia, which is the removal of dead neuronal cell bodies. After injury, microglia progress through a stage of activation, becoming fully immunocompetent reactive cells. These reactive cells readily proliferate, either focally, forming glial nodules (Fig. 14-22), or more diffusely, depending on the nature of the injury. As mentioned, in concert with astrocytes and neurons, microglia help coordinate inflammatory events in the CNS. Resident microglia and blood-derived macrophages express major histocompatibility complex class I and II antigens, serve as antigen-presenting cells, and possess a broad armament of adhesion molecules, cytokines, and chemokines. Once activated, these cells can also produce nitric oxide, reactive oxygen intermediates, and other chemical mediators of inflammation that can damage the CNS if not under strict control. When tissue necrosis occurs, macrophages derived from blood monocytes phagocytose the lipid-laden debris of dead neurons, parenchyma, and glial remnants and accumulate in the damaged CNS. These cells are called *gitter cells* (Fig. 14-23).

Meninges

Pathologic processes that initially involve the meninges, most commonly the leptomeninges, can secondarily invade the CNS because of the close apposition between the two tissues. Conversely, processes that primarily affect the CNS can secondarily affect the meninges, most commonly the leptomeninges.

Meningitis refers to inflammation of the meninges. In common usage the term generally refers to inflammation of the leptomeninges in contrast to inflammation of the dura mater, which is referred to as *pachymeningitis*. Leptomeningitis can be acute, subacute, or chronic and depending on the cause, suppurative, nonsuppurative, or granulomatous, and the exudate and inflammatory cells are chiefly in the subarachnoid space. Besides retrograde axonal transport, as occurs with, for example, *Listeria monocytogenes*, infectious microbes spread to the meninges hematogenously by direct extension or by leukocytic trafficking.

Other meningeal lesions include (1) inflammation of the external periosteal dura after osteomyelitis, formation of extradural abscesses, and skull fracture and involve the inner dura as an extension of leptomeningitis and (2) proliferation of the inner dural mesothelial cells, arachnoid cells, fibroblasts, and cells of the pia mater in response to irritation. Additional lesions likely related to aging or degeneration include formation of cellular nests of meningial cells on the outer surface of the arachnoid membrane, mineralization of the arachnoid membrane, and mineralization plus ossification of the dura mater of the spinal cord. Dural ossification in older dogs, which tends to affect the ventral, cervical, and lumbar dura mater, is most commonly encountered in large breeds, although smaller breeds can be affected. These lesions are of little clinical significance.

Circulatory System

Endothelial Cell (and Blood Vessel) Responses to Injury. Because many of the infectious and neoplastic disease processes demonstrated in this book are spread through the body via the circulatory system, endothelial cells lining blood vessels, especially capillaries, are subject to a variety of injuries. Bacterial hematogenous CNS diseases occur at the interface between the white and gray matter in the cerebral hemispheres. This phenomenon is thought to result from abrupt changes in vascular flow or luminal

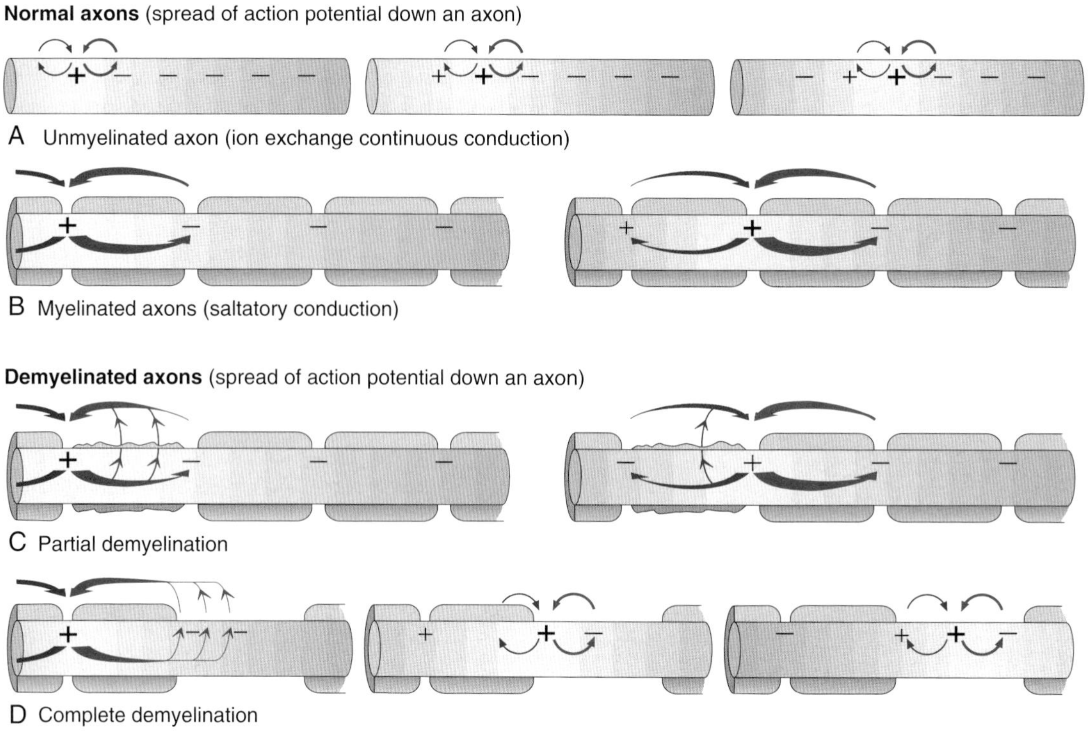

Figure 14-21 **Axonal Action Potential Conduction and the Effect of Demyelination.** The speed of the conduction process is determined by the diameter of the axon and the degree of myelination. As axons increase in diameter, the resistance to ion flow decreases, allowing the action potential to flow faster. In addition, the degree of myelination is directly proportional to the diameter of the axon. Thus the concept that the more myelin the faster the speed of the impulse is true up to the point in which the myelin is normal in thickness. For an axon whose myelin is reduced, conduction of the action potential is slower. Under normal conditions, locomotion is a well-coordinated event that requires precise timing (speed) of impulse conduction to get coordinated movements. If the speed of the action potential is altered by disease, especially demyelination, then the conduction of the action potential will be delayed, and what are normally coordinated movements become uncoordinated. **A,** In unmyelinated axons, action potentials are conducted at a relatively "slower" velocity by the process of ion exchange continuous conduction (see E-Fig. 14-4). **B,** In myelinated axons, action potentials are conducted at a relatively "faster" velocity by a mechanism called saltatory conduction. Optimal function of saltatory conduction is dependent on having the proper degree of myelination of the axon (as determined by axonal diameter) throughout the full length of the axon. **C,** In axons that have lost some but not all of their myelin lamellae from one or more internodes so that there is a "thinner" covering of myelin, the speed of saltatory conduction is reduced because of leakage of the action potential across this thinner myelin sheath, resulting in clinical dysfunction of the nervous system. **D,** In axons that have lost all of their myelin from one or more internodes (complete primary demyelination of the internode), the speed of saltatory conduction is reduced because of the conversion from saltatory conduction to ion exchange continuous conduction in the areas where internodes have lost their myelin. Thus the speed and timing of the action potential is substantially reduced, leading to clinical dysfunction of the nervous system. (Courtesy Dr. J.F. Zachary, College of Veterinary Medicine, University of Illinois.)

diameter of vessels at the interface. These changes may make endothelial cells more susceptible to injury, vasculitis, and thrombosis or predispose the vessels to entrapment of tumor or bacterial emboli.

Endothelial injury can be reversible or nonreversible, resulting in necrosis. Injury resulting in endothelial dysfunction can include the activation and release of vasoactive mediators, such as histamine, leading to local and/or systemic changes in vascular flow, pressure, and permeability. Bacterial products and elicited inflammatory cytokines can directly or indirectly cause vascular inflammation (vasculitis) leading to thrombosis and disseminated intravascular coagulation. Thrombotic meningoencephalitis of cattle caused by the bacterium *Histophilus somni* is an example of this type of injury (see Fig. 14-89). Certain herpesviruses and protozoa can also infect endothelial cells and cause endothelial necrosis with vasculitis, hemorrhage, and thrombosis. Finally, some pathogens, such as angioinvasive fungi, directly invade blood vessels, resulting in necrosis of the endothelium. Vasculitis resulting in thrombosis can cause tissue ischemia, infarction, and vasogenic edema of the affected area of the CNS. A review of endothelial injury can be found in Chapter 2. Angioinvasive fungi are discussed in Chapter 4.

Infarction. Infarction means necrosis of a tissue after obstruction (ischemia) of its arterial blood supply. The rate at which ischemia occurs in the CNS determines the degree of injury that follows. The more rapid the onset of ischemia, the more severe the lesion. However, if the obstruction is sudden, as caused by an embolus, many of the neurons can die within minutes and other components within hours (Fig. 14-24). This outcome also applies to compressive injuries to the CNS that produce a sudden reduction in blood flow, such as can happen with sudden compression in rapidly occurring Hansen type I disk herniation in the dog. If the blood flow through an artery is gradually reduced, for example, because of atherosclerosis, there is often sufficient time for anastomotic vessels to dilate and compensate. Anastomoses of the arteries that penetrate from the ventral and cortical surfaces of the brain are insufficient to prevent infarction after sudden occlusion of one or more of these arteries. If the compression is slow—such as is caused by a slowly developing

Hansen type II disk herniation in a dog or by a slowly growing neoplasm from the exterior, such as meningioma in a cat—adjacent neural tissue will atrophy to accommodate the mass.

Cerebral necrosis, comparable to infarction after vascular occlusion, can also result from other causes, including cessation of cerebral circulation caused by cardiac arrest, sudden hypotension caused by reduced cardiac output, and reduced or absent oxygen in inspired air. Additional causes include altered function of hemoglobin as a result of carbon monoxide poisoning, inhibition of tissue respiration after cyanide poisoning, ingesting toxic substances and poisons, and nutritional deficiencies.

When an artery supplying the CNS is suddenly occluded, blood supply to cells at the center of the infarcted area is rapidly stopped, and if blocked for a sufficient period, all cells die. Neurons at the border of this area continue to receive some blood from unobstructed vessels. It is proposed that the axonal terminals of degenerated ischemic neurons in the center of the infarct release excessive amounts of the neurotransmitter glutamate, causing injury to still-viable neurons in the borders, which increases the extent of the infarct. This process begins after the binding of the neurotransmitter glutamate to receptors on viable neurons in the borders, inducing an abnormal movement of calcium ions into the recipient cells followed by an increase in intracellular calcium ion concentration. This buildup of calcium ions contributes to a multifunctional

Box 14-4 Mechanisms of Primary Demyelination

1. Inherited enzyme defects resulting in formation of abnormal myelin
   Leukodystrophies in human beings and animals
2. Impairment of myelin synthesis and maintenance
   Infection
   Mouse hepatitis virus in mice and progressive multifocal leukoencephalopathy in human beings; in both cases oligodendrocytes are selectively destroyed by viral agents, and myelin cannot be maintained.
   Nutritional
   Lack of maintenance of myelin is due to copper deficiency, malnutrition, vitamin B_{12} deficiency.
   Toxins
   Cyanide poisoning
   Cuprizone toxicity
3. Loss of myelin as a consequence of cytotoxic edema (status spongiosus)
   Hexachlorophene poisoning, usually prolonged edema
4. Destruction of myelin by detergent-like metabolites
   Lysolecithin, a metabolite of phospholipase A (normally present in the nervous system) may destroy myelin.
5. Immunologic destruction of myelin
   Cell mediated
   Experimental allergic encephalitis
   Landry-Guillain-Barré (human beings)
   Coonhound paralysis
   Marek's disease (chickens)
   Various stages of multiple sclerosis in human beings
   Various stages of canine distemper

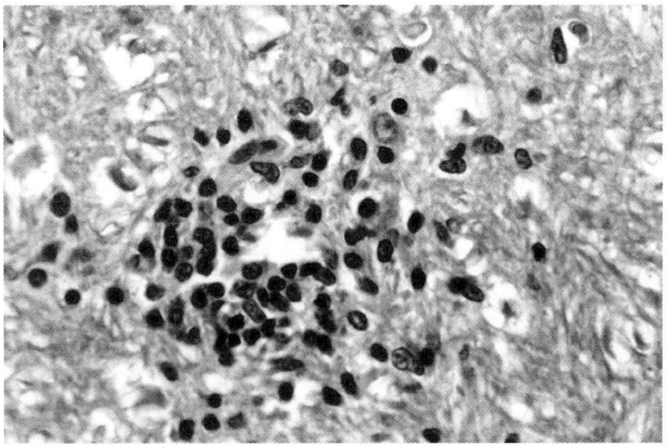

Figure 14-22 Glial Nodule, Brainstem, Dog. These nodules *(center of figure)*, formed by reactive microglial cells and infiltrating macrophages, occur most frequently in viral and protozoal encephalitides. H&E stain. (Courtesy Dr. M.D. McGavin, College of Veterinary Medicine, University of Tennessee.)

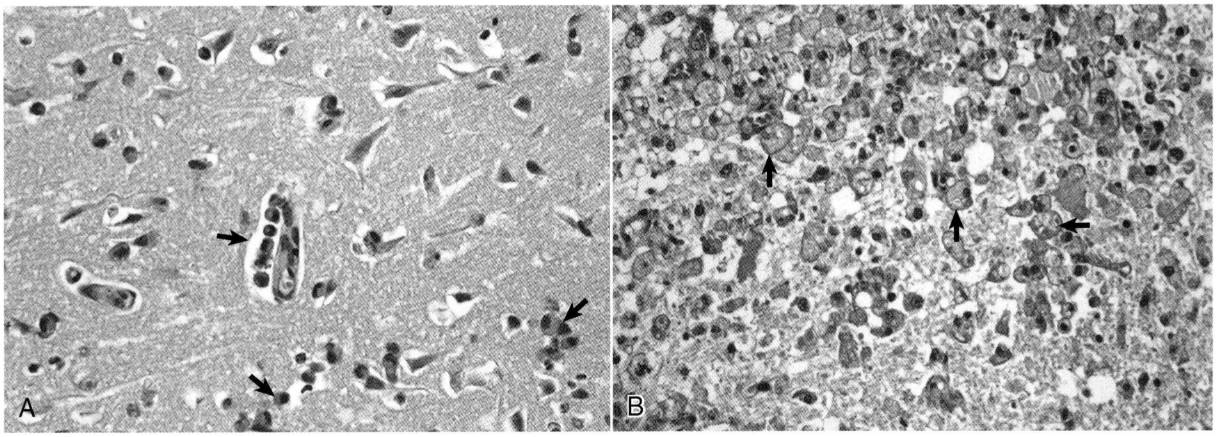

Figure 14-23 Gitter Cells, Cerebrum. A, Early polioencephalomalacia, cow. Note the angular, eosinophilic neurons with pyknotic nuclei (ischemic cell change). Macrophages *(arrows)* in the perivascular space have been recruited from the circulating monocytes. These cells phagocytose cellular debris from the necrotic neurons and the myelin from the nerve fibers undergoing degeneration after the death of their neurons. Microglia also participate in this phagocytic response. Macrophages that have ingested degenerate myelin or other cellular debris have foamy cytoplasm and are termed gitter cells. H&E stain. **B,** Previous region of necrosis, dog. The normal brain parenchyma has liquefied, and the debris has been ingested by macrophages *(arrows)*, which has resulted in the cytoplasm of these cells becoming foamy. They are now designated as gitter cells or, simply, foamy macrophages. H&E stain. (Courtesy Dr. J.F. Zachary, College of Veterinary Medicine, University of Illinois.)

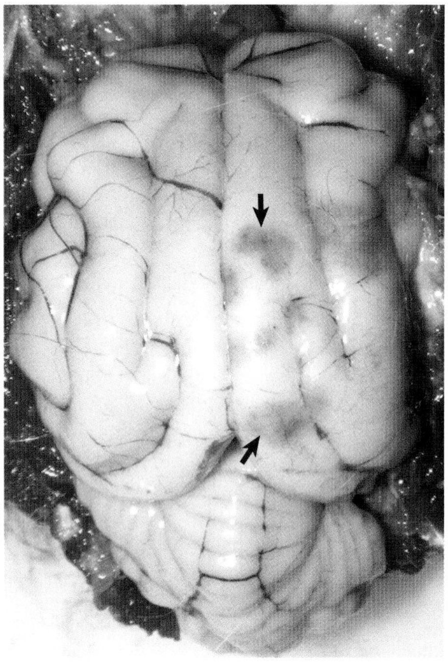

Figure 14-24 **Malacia, Vascular Occlusion, Ischemia, Infarction, Cerebrum, Cat.** Several red-pink foci (*arrows*) are areas of ischemic necrosis secondary to vascular occlusion caused by cerebral metastasis of a bronchoalveolar carcinoma. (Courtesy Drs. C.A. Lichtensteiger and R.A. Doty, College of Veterinary Medicine, University of Illinois.)

cascade that leads to neuronal death. When there is hemorrhage with the infarct, the mechanical injury from the pressure, plus tissue displacement by the hemorrhage, can cause additional damage. See Table 14-1 for the reparative responses associated with the resolution of infarcts.

Although they occur through the same mechanisms, areas of cerebral infarction differ somewhat in gross appearance from infarcts in other tissues (Fig. 14-25). The abundance of lipids and enzymes, plus the relative lack of fibrous connective tissue stroma in the brain and spinal cord, results in the affected areas eventually becoming soft because of liquefaction necrosis. The gross appearance of infarction may also differ according to location. Lesions affecting the gray matter tend to be hemorrhagic, whereas infarction of the white matter is often pale. This difference is probably due in part to the less-dense capillary meshwork in the white matter because vessels supplying the white matter have fewer anastomoses than those of the gray matter. Infarcted tissue goes through a characteristic sequence of changes that can permit a relatively accurate determination of the age of the infarct. An outline of the chronologic events that occur after an ischemic episode that lasts more than 5 to 6 minutes and is followed by resuscitation of an animal is given in Table 14-1. As can be seen, the tissue changes listed in Table 14-1 take different periods of time to develop in the living resuscitated animal after ischemia occurs. Variation in the times that specific lesions occur depends on the extent and duration of the initial ischemic event. Following removal of cellular and myelin debris, the

Table 14-1 Chronologic Sequence of Changes within Infarcted Tissue (in the Living Animal) after an Ischemic Event

Time Following Ischemic Event	Tissue Change
Immediate (seconds)	Cessation of blood flow (ischemia) and accumulation of waste products
Few minutes	Cellular injury and death; necrosis and edema; hemorrhage (especially in gray matter)
20 minutes	First microscopic evidence of neuronal injury (perfusion-fixation)
1-2 hours	First microscopic evidence of neuronal injury (immersion-fixation)
2 hours	Pale staining of infarct microscopically (white matter); swelling of capillary endothelium; increase in size of astrocytic nuclei
3-5 hours	Ischemic cell change in most neurons; swelling of oligodendroglia and astroglia; beginning clasmatodendrosis of astrocytes
6-24 hours	Beginning neutrophilic infiltration; alteration of myelin (pale staining), 8-24 hours; degeneration and decrease of oligodendroglia, 8-24 hours; astrocytic swelling and retraction and fragmentation of processes (clasmatodendrosis), and degeneration*; cytoplasm of astrocytes visible, 8-24 hours*; vascular degeneration and fibrin deposition, 8-24 hours; thrombosis,† 6-24 hours; beginning endothelial proliferation at margin of infarct, 9 hours
8-24 (up to 48) hours	Initial gross detection of infarct unless hemorrhagic; infarct edematous (swollen), soft, pale, or hemorrhagic and demarcated
1-2 days	Swelling of axons and myelin sheaths; prominent neutrophilic infiltration
2 days	Prominent loss of neuroectodermal cells; continued proliferation of endothelial cells; reduced number of neutrophils; beginning increase in mononuclear cells (gitter cells)
3-5 days	Prominent number of mononuclear cells (gitter cells); disappearance of neutrophils; continued endothelial cell proliferation; number of capillaries appear increased; beginning of astrocytic proliferation (often at margin of infarct)
5-7 days	Grossly, swelling of infarct reaches maximum
8-10 days	Reduction in gross swelling of infarct; liquefaction necrosis; prominent number of mononuclear cells (gitter cells); continued endothelial cell proliferation; beginning fibroblastic activity with collagen formation, variable but most prominent in CNS tissue adjacent to the meninges; beginning increase of astroglial fiber production, 5-13 days
3 weeks-6 months	Mononuclear cells decreased; astroglial fiber density increased (especially at margin); astrocytic proliferation reduced; astrocytes return to original appearance; cystic stage of infarct, 2-4 months; vascular network may be present within cyst; endothelial cell proliferation reduced

*The degree of astrocytic injury depends on location (e.g., central or peripheral) of the cells within the infarct.
†Obviously, thrombosis may occur earlier than 6 hours. This is the time when it may initially be prominent.
CNS, Central nervous system.

infarct is repaired by astrocytes. If the infarct is small (<1 mm), it is filled via astrogliosis; if the infarct is larger, it is encapsulated to form a cyst.

Central Nervous System Swelling and Edema

Congestive Brain Swelling. Congestive brain swelling, as distinguished from cerebral edema, partially represents unregulated vasodilation after trauma, and it can cause serious brain damage (even more severe than the primary injury) if not properly controlled. This lesion therefore represents an enlargement of the brain resulting in elevated intracranial pressure caused by the increased diameter of the blood-containing vasculature, whereas edema results in an increased pressure following accumulation of fluid in the interstitium or intracellularly outside the circulation. Acute brain swelling can be localized (usually of lesser significance) when associated with focal lesions or generalized (often serious) when caused by diffuse brain injury. Although rarely seen in domestic animals, one exception to the importance of focal lesions is extracerebral hemorrhage (acute subdural hematoma in human beings), which—though principally involving the surface of one hemisphere—can cause more mass effect (brain swelling) in the underlying cerebral hemisphere than the hematoma itself. In subdural hematomas, blood accumulates between the dura mater and the meninges. Hematomas also occur in the epidural region; however, the subdural variety are usually poorly circumscribed. If the hematoma is removed, the acute brain swelling can progress so rapidly that the brain protrudes (herniates) through the site of the craniotomy.

The more serious forms of diffuse brain injury are associated with generalized acute brain swelling. It is sometimes difficult to determine the relative importance of swelling in affected individuals because initial acute swelling (detectable as soon as 30 minutes after injury in human beings) can be followed after several hours to days by true cerebral edema (as a result of increased vascular permeability), which can be the actual deleterious lesion. Peroxidative injury to blood vessels has been one proposed cause of pathologic vasodilation in the posttraumatic CNS.

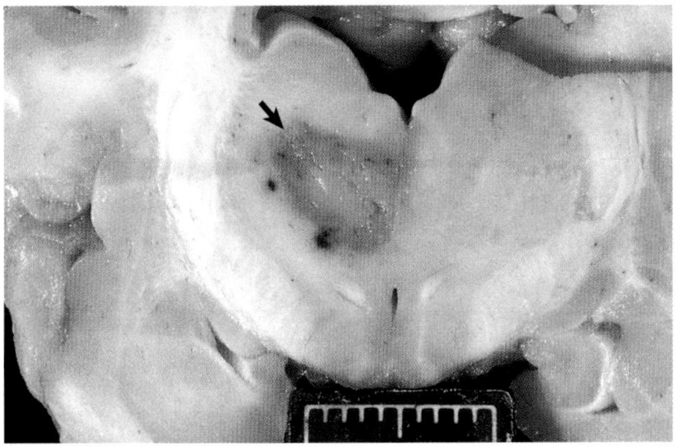

Figure 14-25 Central Nervous System Infarct, Brain, Thalamus, Dog. The pattern of a focal, sharply demarcated region of yellow discoloration and malacia (softening) *(arrow)* in the left central thalamus indicates an infarct. Scale bar = 2 cm. (Courtesy Dr. R. Storts, College of Veterinary Medicine, Texas A&M University.)

Cerebral Edema. The basis of our current understanding of cerebral edema was advanced by Klatzo in 1967 when he proposed two distinct types: (1) cytotoxic edema, or cell swelling, caused by increased intracellular fluid with normal vascular permeability and (2) vasogenic edema, or tissue swelling, caused by increased extracellular fluid resulting from increased vascular permeability (Fig. 14-26). Other types of cerebral edema have been identified as hydrostatic (or interstitial) edema associated with increased hydrostatic pressure of the CSF (resulting from obstructive internal hydrocephalus) and hypo-osmotic edema, which is dependent on development of an abnormal osmotic gradient between the blood and nervous tissue. The types of edema in the CNS are summarized in Table 14-2. It should be emphasized that, depending on the nature of the injury, multiple mechanisms can contribute to edema in the CNS and these distinctions are not always clearly defined or distinct. For continuity, spongiform change and status spongiosus will also be discussed in this section.

Vasogenic Edema. In animals, vasogenic edema is the most common type of edema in the CNS. It occurs following vascular injury often adjacent to inflammatory foci, hematomas, contusions, infarcts, cerebral hypertension, and neoplasms. The underlying mechanism of vasogenic cerebral edema is a breakdown of the

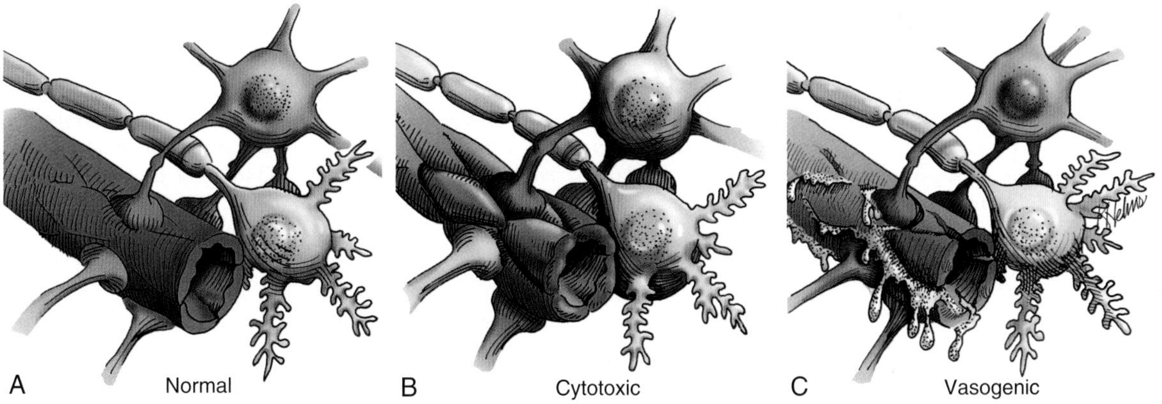

Figure 14-26 Types of Cerebral Edema. A, Normal blood-brain barrier. Endothelial cells are red; astrocytes are beige; neurons are light yellow. **B,** Cytotoxic edema. Cytotoxic edema is characterized by the accumulation of fluid intracellularly (in neurons, astrocytes, oligodendroglia, and endothelial cells) as a result of altered cellular metabolism, often caused by ischemia. The gray and white matter are both affected. The fluid taken up by swollen cells is primarily derived from the extracellular space, which becomes reduced in size and has an increased concentration of extracellular solutes. **C,** Vasogenic edema. This type of edema is seen in acute inflammation, and its basic mechanism is an increase in vascular permeability from the breakdown of the blood-brain barrier. This breakdown allows movement of plasma constituents such as water, ions, and plasma proteins into the extracellular space, particularly that of the white matter. (Courtesy Dr. J.F. Zachary, College of Veterinary Medicine, University of Illinois. Redrawn and modified from an illustration from Leech RW, Shuman RM: *Neuropathology: a summary for students*, Philadelphia, 1982, Harper & Row.)

Table 14-2 Types of Edema in the Central Nervous System

Type of Edema	Cause	Outcome
Cytotoxic	Altered cellular metabolism (often due to ischemia)	Intracellular accumulation of fluid (neurons, glial cells, endothelial cells)
Vasogenic	Vascular injury with breakdown of the blood-brain barrier	Extracellular accumulation of fluid (cerebrocortical white matter)
Hydrostatic (interstitial)	Elevated ventricular hydrostatic pressure (hydrocephalus)	Extracellular accumulation of fluid (periventricular white matter)
Hypo-osmotic	Osmotic imbalances (blood plasma versus extracellular and intracellular microenvironments of the CNS)	Extracellular and intracellular accumulation of fluid (cerebrocortical gray and white matter)

CNS, Central nervous system.

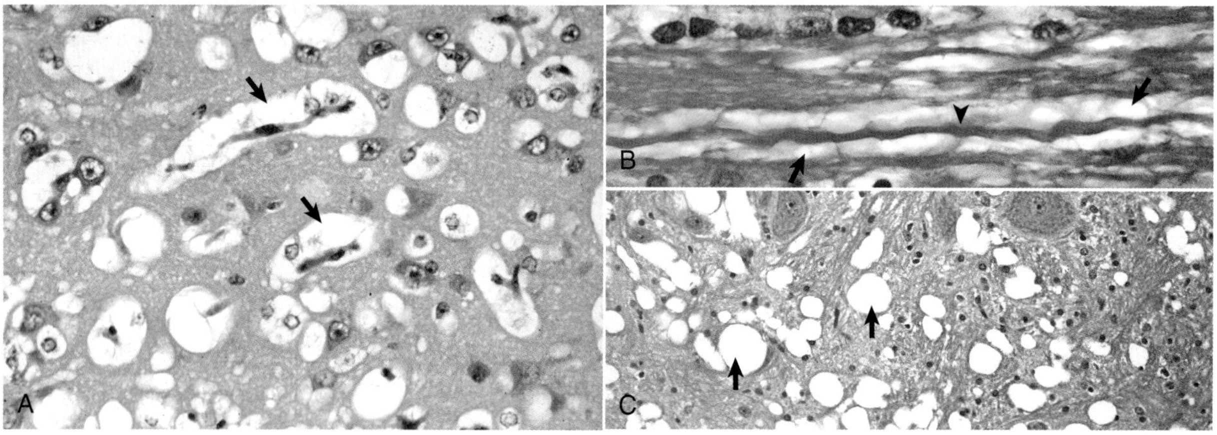

Figure 14-27 **Edema. A,** Vasogenic edema. The perivascular spaces are wide as a result of fluid leakage through the blood-brain barrier *(arrows)* (see Fig. 14-26). A similar change can be seen around neurons. These fluid-filled spaces are often very difficult to differentiate from artifactual spaces caused by shrinkage from fixation and dehydration in the preparation of the paraffin-embedded sections. H&E stain. **B,** Intramyelinic edema. Note the accumulation of edema fluid *(arrows)* between myelin lamellae that surrounds the axon *(arrowhead)*. This lesion was caused by hexachlorophene added to a medicated shampoo. Such products are no longer available for use in veterinary practice. H&E stain. **C,** Edema (spongy change, status spongiosus), hepatic encephalopathy, dog. This lesion is characterized by variably sized fluid-filled spaces within the white matter *(arrows)*. It can develop by several different mechanisms, which include splitting of myelin sheaths, accumulation of extracellular fluid, and swelling of astrocytic and neuronal cellular processes. Such changes can reflect osmotic imbalances as well as a direct toxic effect on cells (cytotoxic edema). H&E stain. (**A** and **C** courtesy Dr. J.F. Zachary, College of Veterinary Medicine, University of Illinois. **B** courtesy Dr. M.D. McGavin, College of Veterinary Medicine, University of Tennessee.)

blood-brain barrier that results in movement of plasma constituents, such as water, ions, and organic osmolytes, and proteins into the perivascular extracellular space, particularly that of the white matter (Fig. 14-27). In addition to extracellular accumulation of fluid, vasogenic edema can also be accompanied by some cellular swelling involving astrocytes. Vasogenic edema with the resulting accumulation of extracellular fluid can cause an increase in intracranial pressure within the CNS. This pressure can also be so severe as to cause neurologic dysfunction and caudal displacement of brain structures such as the parahippocampal gyri and cerebellar vermis (see Figs. 14-59 and 14-60).

Cytotoxic Edema. Cytotoxic edema is characterized by the accumulation of fluid intracellularly in neurons, astrocytes, oligodendroglia, and endothelial cells (called *hydropic degeneration* in other cells of the body) as a result of altered cellular metabolism, often caused by ischemia. Although not all of the cells listed previously may be involved in all cases of cytotoxic edema, affected cells swell within seconds of injury. The mechanism is thought to involve an energy deficit that interferes with normal function of the cell's Na^+/K^+-ATPase pump. Thus the cell cannot maintain homeostasis, which requires the secretion of intracellular sodium, and the elevated concentration of intracellular sodium and presumably other ions, as well as organic osmolytes, is followed by an increased influx of water. The gray and white matter of the brain are both affected, the brain swells, and the sulci and gyri become indistinct and flattened (Fig. 14-28), respectively. The fluid taken up by the swollen cells is primarily derived from the extracellular space, which becomes reduced in size and has an increased concentration of extracellular solutes.

However, for this lesion to be described accurately as cerebral edema, there must be additional fluid movement into the brain and not merely a change of existing fluid from extracellular to intracellular compartments. In practical terms, this is not always the case and can be difficult to determine. The term *cytotoxic edema* has been used rather loosely to refer simply to cellular swelling in many cases. Additional fluid may originate from the circulation by way of the transcapillary fluid exchange or possibly from the CSF, which has extensive diffusional communication with the extracellular fluid of the brain. The blood-brain barrier remains intact during development of this type of edema, so fluid does not enter the brain by a disturbance in vascular permeability. Specific causes of this lesion include hypoxia-ischemia, particularly in the early stages;

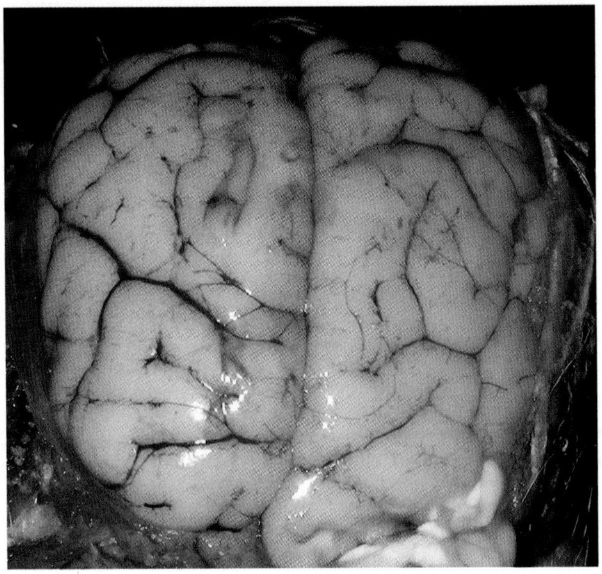

Figure 14-28 Cerebral Edema, Dog. On the dorsal surface, gyri are swollen and flattened and sulci have become less distinct. Accumulation of extracellular fluid has caused the brain to swell, and because space within the cranial vault is limited, the brain has been pressed against the calvaria. In extreme cases, notable brain swelling can cause caudal displacement of the parahippocampal gyri and vermis of the cerebellum (see Figs. 14-59 and 14-60). (Courtesy Drs. C.A. Lichtensteiger and A. Gal, College of Veterinary Medicine, University of Illinois.)

intoxication with metabolic inhibitors, such as 2,4,dinitrophenol, 6-aminonicotinamide, and ouabain; and severe hypothermia.

Interstitial (Hydrostatic) Edema. Interstitial edema is characterized by the accumulation of fluid in the extracellular space of the brain because of elevated ventricular hydrostatic pressure that accompanies hydrocephalus. Fluid moves across the ependyma of the ventricular wall and accumulates extracellularly in the periventricular white matter. Unlike the other forms of cerebral edema that cause swelling of affected CNS tissue, hydrostatic edema causes variable degeneration and loss of the periventricular white matter mostly through primary demyelination accompanied by loss of axons. As the periventricular white matter is reduced in volume, the ventricle expands to fill the void by displacement, thereby exacerbating the hydrocephalus. The blood-brain barrier remains intact in hydrostatic edema.

Hypo-osmotic Edema. Hypo-osmotic edema occurs after overconsumption of water (water intoxication), leading to dilution of the osmolality of the plasma. Under normal conditions the osmolality of CSF and extracellular fluid in the CNS is slightly greater than that of plasma. When the osmolality of plasma is further decreased, water moves from the vasculature into the brain after the osmotic gradient, resulting in osmotic edema. This form of edema accounts for the clinical signs and lesions in osmotic demyelination syndrome and salt poisoning, as discussed later.

Spongiform Change and Status Spongiosus. *Spongiform change* is a term whose exact meaning varies in different scientific disciplines and experimental situations. In this chapter, wherever possible, spongiform change is used to describe morphologic changes in H&E-stained sections that occur primarily in gray matter. These changes are characterized by small clear vacuoles of varied sizes that form in the cytoplasm of neuron cell bodies and proximal dendrites in diseases such as the transmissible spongiform encephalopathies (TSEs) and rabies encephalitis and in the processes of astrocytes that are spatially related to the affected neurons.

Status spongiosus (spongy degeneration) is also a phrase whose exact meaning varies. It is defined as multiple fluid-filled clear spaces in the white matter of H&E-stained sections of the CNS and may be extracellular or intracellular (see Fig. 14-27, C). This lesion results from the accumulation of edema fluid in the white matter secondary to a variety of causes, including cytotoxic edema, vasogenic edema, intramyelinic edema, Wallerian degeneration, and other hypoxic, toxic, and metabolic diseases.

In some instances the term *spongy degeneration* or *spongy change* has been used in the veterinary literature to describe microscopic lesions in a group of diseases of young dogs, cats, and cows characterized by fluid accumulation in white matter. These diseases are discussed in later sections.

Box 14-5 Portals of Entry into the Central Nervous System

DIRECT EXTENSION

Penetrating trauma through the calvaria or vertebral bodies
- Extension of middle and/or inner ear infection
- Extension of a nasal cavity/sinus infection through the cribriform plate or calvaria
- Extension from osteomyelitis

HEMATOGENOUS

Localization within capillary beds of the meninges and parenchyma of the CNS
- Localization within capillary beds of the choroid plexuses and extension into the cerebrospinal fluid

LEUKOCYTE TRAFFICKING

Macrophages or lymphocytes (containing microbes) during their migration through the CNS

RETROGRADE AXONAL TRANSPORT

Transported from the periphery into the CNS by neuronal retrograde axoplasmic flow

CNS, Central nervous system.

Portals of Entry/Pathways of Spread

Disease processes of the CNS enter the brain and spinal cord through one of four principal portals (Box 14-5). These portals are (1) direct extension, (2) hematogenous entry, (3) leukocytic trafficking, and (4) retrograde axonal transport.

Direct Extension

Direct extension is a common portal of entry and includes a wide range of disease processes. Penetrating trauma through the calvaria or vertebrae as a result of a gunshot wound or other forms of trauma can provide a direct portal into the CNS. Disease processes can also extend into the brain and/or spinal cord as a result of (1) a middle and/or inner ear infection (Fig. 14-29), (2) nasal cavity/sinus infection or neoplasia through the cribriform plate or calvaria (Fig. 14-30), or (3) bacterial osteomyelitis or neoplasia of vertebral bodies with extension through the vertebrae into the vertebral canal.

Benign growths of the calvaria and vertebrae, such as osteomas, chondromas, and osteochondromas, often extend into and compress the brain and spinal cord. One specific neoplasm, the multilobular osteochondrosarcoma, has been described as originating from the periosteum of the canine skull and can cause marked compression of the brain. Also, malignant neoplasms adjacent to the cranium or spinal column can cause injury by direct invasion. Some examples

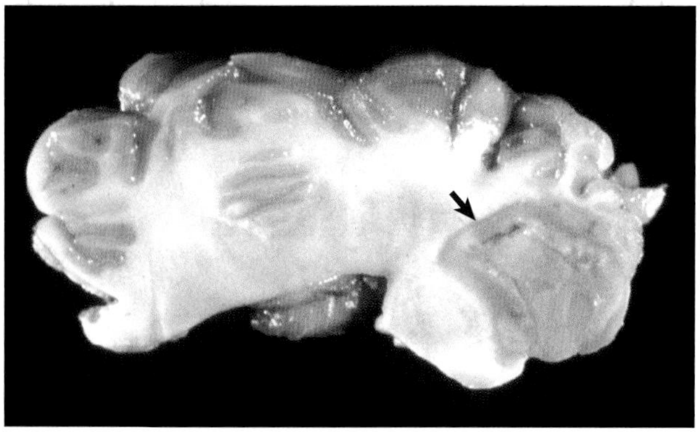

Figure 14-29 Chronic Bacterial Abscess, Leptomeninges of the Cerebellum, Sheep. The abscess *(arrow)*, which resulted from direct extension from an inner ear infection, compresses and distorts the cerebellum. It is walled off from the adjacent cerebellum by a distinct fibrous capsule synthesized by fibroblasts from the adjacent leptomeninges. This abscess likely arose in the leptomeninges of the cerebellum and grew to compress adjacent cerebellum. (Courtesy College of Veterinary Medicine, University of Illinois.)

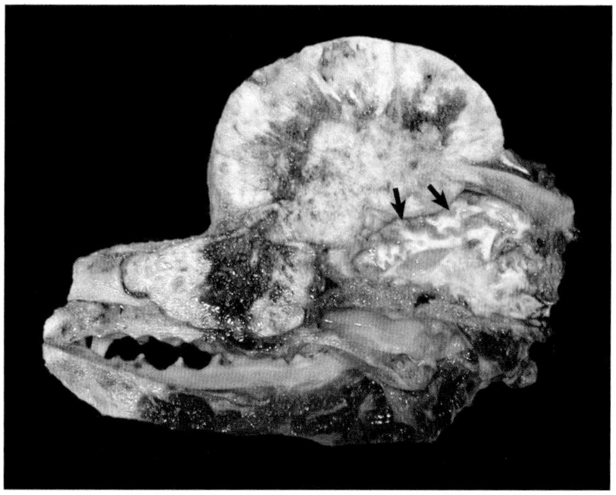

Figure 14-30 Osteochondrosarcoma, Calvaria, Dog. The neoplasm has destroyed and penetrated the calvaria and compressed the cerebral hemispheres *(arrows)*. There is also invasion of frontal sinuses and the nasal cavity. (Courtesy Dr. K. Bailey, College of Veterinary Medicine, University of Illinois.)

include osteosarcoma and fibrosarcoma in the dog. Also, malignant melanoma of the soft palate in the dog and melanoma involving the paravertebral lymph nodes in the horse can compress and invade adjacent CNS tissue. Other examples of direct extension include spinal cord lymphosarcoma in cattle, dogs, horses, and cats; nasal carcinomas in dogs and cats; and peripheral nerve sheath tumors in dogs.

Hematogenous Entry

The most common portal of entry into the CNS is the bloodstream. In neonates, infectious microbes, such as *Escherichia coli*, can enter the blood through the umbilical vein or through the venous system after surgical procedures such as castration. A CNS disease in cows called *thrombotic meningoencephalitis* is caused by *H. somni* bacteremia with localization of bacteria in blood vessels of the brain, which leads to vasculitis, hemorrhage, and thrombosis (see Fig. 14-89). In adult animals, sites of chronic inflammation, such as abscesses, bacterial skin disease, and ear infections, can also serve as sustained sources of bacteria, which can enter the venous system and spread to distant sites through the bloodstream hematogenously.

Capillary beds of the meninges, neuropil, and choroid plexuses are common sites for localization of specific infectious microbes. Such localization patterns may be attributable to receptor-mediated phenomena or vascular flow patterns related to the size of the infectious pathogen. The bloodstream is also a portal of entry into the CNS for metastasizing tumors such as hemangiosarcoma and a variety of carcinomas.

Leukocyte Trafficking

As part of the systemic immunologic surveillance system, macrophages (monocytes) and lymphoid cells continually move in and out of capillary beds in the CNS and thus serve as sentinel cells monitoring for the presence of disease processes within the brain and spinal cord (see Fig. 4-11). As examples, retroviruses, such as feline leukemia virus, and mycotic agents, such as *B. dermatitidis*, have stages of their life cycles within the cytoplasm of lymphocytes or macrophages. During the movement of lymphocytes and macrophages in and out of the CNS, cells infected with such agents are activated to release their infectious contents and infect cells of the CNS.

Retrograde Axonal Transport

Retrograde axonal transport provides a unique portal of entry for viruses such as rabies and the bacterium *L. monocytogenes*. These pathogens replicate in tissues richly innervated with receptors and motor end plates from sensory and motor neurons, respectively, which provide a connection between peripheral infection and the CNS. Retrograde axoplasmic flow is then used to gain entry into the CNS (see E-Fig. 14-3).

Defense Mechanisms/Barrier Systems

Barrier Systems

The CNS has several unique structural and functional barrier systems that serve to protect it from diseases affecting the vascular and ventricular systems and to actively facilitate transfer of necessary molecules, such as glucose, to cells within the CNS.

Blood-Brain Barrier. The blood-brain barrier, formed by vascular endothelial cells, endothelial-derived basement membrane, and foot processes of astrocytes, exists in the capillaries of the CNS (see Fig. 14-13). The most important structural component of the blood-brain barrier is the tight junctions between endothelial cells of cerebral capillaries. By means of the blood-brain barrier the CNS can selectively regulate its extracellular compartment and isolate itself from sudden biochemical changes that may occur in the systemic circulation. In the majority of the CNS, endothelial cells are nonfenestrated and are held together by intercellular tight junctions. These tight junctions actively prevent the movement of protein, hydrophilic molecules, and ions from capillary lumina into the intercellular compartment of the CNS. Endothelial cells also have a transmembrane lipophilic pathway for the diffusion of small lipid molecules and numerous highly selective polarized receptor-mediated transport systems for molecules such as insulin, transferrin, glucose, purines, and amino acids. Finally, endothelial cells express a net negative charge on their abluminal side and at the basement membrane, providing an additional selective mechanism that impedes movement of anionic molecules such as chloride ions across the barrier. Foot processes of astrocytes cover more than 90% percent of the abluminal surface of capillary endothelial cells.

Experimental evidence suggests that secretion of growth factors from astrocytes promotes the formation and maintenance of the blood-brain barrier.

Capillaries in the area postrema, median eminence, neurohypophysis, pineal body, subfornical organ, commissural organ, and supraoptic crest lack tight junctions and are fenestrated; thus the blood-brain barrier is absent at these sites.

Glia Limitans. The CNS is separated from the subarachnoid CSF by the pia mater and the glia limitans (see Fig. 14-13). The glia limitans, which covers the outer surface of the brain and spinal cord and is situated immediately subjacent to the pia mater, consists of astrocytic fibers with many foot processes that form a distinct layer that lies subjacent to the pia mater. In many areas the pia is only one-cell-layer thick and has fenestrations, so that the glia limitans is exposed directly to the subarachnoid space. As arterioles penetrate the cerebral cortex to supply the CNS with blood, they carry the pia mater and surrounding glia limitans with them until the arteriole structurally and functionally becomes a capillary. At the capillary level the pia mater disappears, but the layer of pericapillary astrocytic foot processes remains and serves as a component of the blood-brain barrier. This transition zone occurs at a depth approximately 1 to 3 mm within the cerebral cortex and explains why in cases of meningitis the infiltrate can be observed to track along blood vessels a short distance into the parenchyma without causing actual parenchymal disease.

Blood–Cerebrospinal Fluid Barrier. The blood-CSF barrier is formed by the choroid plexus and the arachnoid. This barrier is formed by tight junctions between apposing surfaces of choroid plexus epithelial cells that cover the choroid plexuses. As noted previously, blood vessels of the choroid plexus are fenestrated. The barrier formed by tight junctions between choroid plexus epithelial cells restricts the movement of molecules that leak from fenestrated capillaries into the extracellular compartment of the choroid plexus and then into the CSF. Similarly, the arachnoid membrane also has tight junctions that prevent the movement of molecules from the blood into the CSF. The arachnoid membrane is generally impermeable to hydrophilic molecules but lacks specialized transport systems, and its role in forming the blood-CSF barrier is largely passive.

Cerebrospinal Fluid–Brain Barrier (Ependymal Barrier). The CNS is separated from ventricular CSF by ependymal epithelial cells and foot processes of astrocytes. Although the ependymal lining does form a cellular barrier of sorts, materials within the ventricular system can without too much difficulty penetrate into the brain. The CSF-brain barrier is far more permeable than the blood-brain barrier.

Innate and Adaptive Immune Responses

Although infectious microbes have developed unique approaches to gain entry into the CNS, the body has also evolved a strong suite of defense mechanisms to protect the CNS against infectious pathogens and disease processes. The skin and mucous membranes of the alimentary, respiratory, and urinary systems provide structural and functional barriers against disease. The inflammatory response, immune system, and monocyte-macrophage system provide a strong local and systemic defense against pathogen replication and disease spread. Finally, barrier systems in the CNS, reviewed in an earlier section, represent structural and functional protection against a wide range of pathogens and toxic injuries. These defense mechanisms are summarized in Box 14-6.

Box 14-6 Defense Mechanisms against Injury and Infectious Microbes in the Central Nervous System

SKIN
Structural and functional (secretions) barrier.

CALVARIA, VERTEBRAE
Structural barrier.

MENINGES, CEREBROSPINAL FLUID
Structural and functional (continuous flow of CSF) barrier.

BARRIER SYSTEMS

Blood-Brain Barrier
Structural and functional barrier formed by vascular endothelium, basement membrane, and astrocytic foot processes. This barrier regulates the movement of agents from the blood to the CNS.

Blood-CSF Barrier
Structural and functional barrier formed by choroid plexuses cells and the arachnoid membrane. This barrier regulates movement of agents from the blood to the CSF.

Glia Limitans
Formed by astrocytic foot processes immediately subjacent to the pia mater. This structure may have some barrier function in preventing movement of microbes from CSF into the CNS through the pia mater.

MICROGLIA, TRAFFICKING MACROPHAGES
Resident and migrating cells that are part of the monocyte-macrophage system.

IMMUNOLOGIC RESPONSES
Innate and adaptive immunologic responses that form the body's overall immune system.

CNS, Central nervous system; *CSF*, cerebrospinal fluid.

Inflammation of the Central Nervous System. Inflammation of the CNS is different from inflammation in other organs because of the presence of the blood-brain barrier. Under normal conditions this barrier provides limited isolation of the CNS from circulating cellular and humoral elements of the immune system. Macrophages (monocytes) and T lymphocytes can penetrate an intact blood-brain barrier and enter the perivascular and subarachnoid spaces, transit these spaces, and return to the circulation in a role of protective immunologic surveillance of the CNS.

It is important to remember that inflammation in the CNS is regulated by a complex system of recognition and adhesion molecules, cytokines, chemokines, and their corresponding receptors (see Chapters 3 and 5). In particular within the CNS, chemokines and their receptors regulate physiologic and pathologic leukocyte trafficking and cellular migration events.

When pathogens use one of the four portals of entry to gain access to the CNS, the inflammatory process that ensues disrupts the blood-brain barrier. Thus, in addition to inflammation, edema and hemorrhage can result. Selectins and integrins in cooperation with chemokines are active in initiating and regulating the acute inflammatory response and the movement of neutrophils across the blood-brain barrier in response to a variety of pathogens. Migration of inflammatory cells within the CNS is poorly understood. Chemotactic gradients are likely established by chemokines that diffuse from sites of production within foci of inflammation. Activated glial cells, including astrocytes and resident microglia, form chemokine networks in areas of inflammation in response to cytokines produced by T lymphocytes that recognize foreign antigens.

Depending on the type of antigen and the pathogenicity of the infectious agent, the inflammatory response resolves (heals) or progresses to a chronic or granulomatous phase with attempts at resolution and clearance of the infectious agent. In the CNS the type of inflammatory response can vary with the cause. A rather simplistic guideline, to which there are always exceptions, that compares the type of inflammation with different causal agents is as follows:

1. Serous to suppurative or purulent responses can be the result of several species of bacteria.
2. Eosinophil responses occur in salt poisoning of pigs and with parasitic larval migration.
3. Lymphocytic, monocytic/macrophage, nonsuppurative, lymphomonocytic, and lymphohistiocytic responses can be caused by viruses and certain protozoa.
4. Granulomatous inflammation can be the result of fungi, certain protozoa, and some higher-order bacteria such as the *Mycobacterium* spp.

Disorders of Domestic Animals

Disorders that occur in many or all animal species are discussed in this section. Disorders of individual animal species are discussed in later sections covering disorders unique to that species.

Malformations[3]

Neural Tube Closure Defects (Dysraphia). *Dysraphia* means an abnormal seam, and these anomalies result from defective interaction of neuroepithelium with adjacent notochordal and mesenchymal cells during closure of the neural tube in the early stages of development. Neuroepithelium is the progenitor cell for neurons and astrocytes, oligodendrocytes, and ependymal cells.

Experimental studies of closure of the neural tube show that it occurs at four distinct locations called *closure initiation sites* in the embryo, and disruption of this process at these sites leads to site-specific dysraphic anomalies. Closure site I contributes to the posterior neuropore (the opening at the posterior end of the embryonic neural canal), whereas closure sites II to IV contribute to the anterior neuropore (the opening at the anterior end of the embryonic neural canal). Anencephaly is caused by a failure of closure sites II or IV; spina bifida is caused by a failure of closure site I. Genes possibly involved in neural tube closure defects include those involved in folate metabolism and transport.

Dysraphic anomalies, also called *neural tube closure defects*, in animals are typified by anencephaly and prosencephalic hypoplasia, cranium bifidum, spina bifida, abnormal spinal cord development (duplication or abnormal cell migration), and syringomyelia.

Anencephaly and Prosencephalic Hypoplasia. *Anencephaly* means an absence of the brain, but in many instances of so-called anencephaly only the rostral part of the brain (cerebral hemispheres) is absent, or very rudimentary, and to varying degrees the brainstem is preserved. Thus this abnormality is best designated prosencephalic hypoplasia. Such anomalies result from an abnormal development of the rostral aspect of the neural tube and failure of their fusion. Although the cause for these anomalies is largely unknown, anencephaly is most commonly reported in calves, where it is accompanied by other defects. It is an extremely rare event in other domestic species. Additionally, anencephaly—after initial cranium bifidum and exencephaly (protrusion of brain not covered by skin or meninges)—has been reported to occur in rat fetuses after exposure of the pregnant dam to excessive concentrations of vitamin A and cyclophosphamide.

Meningoencephalocele and Cranium Bifidum. Cranium bifidum is characterized by a dorsal midline cranial defect through which meningeal and brain tissue can protrude. The protruded material, which forms a sac (-cele), is covered by skin and can be lined by meninges (meningocele) or meninges accompanied by a part of the brain (meningoencephalocele) (Fig. 14-31). Although the sac is readily apparent grossly, diagnosis of the presence or absence of brain tissue typically requires histologic examination. These malformations are hereditary in pigs and cats and are also caused by griseofulvin treatment in pregnant cats during the first week of gestation. They are uncommon and sporadic in other domestic species.

Meningomyelocele and Spina Bifida. Spina bifida is the vertebral counterpart of cranium bifidum. This lesion, which frequently tends to affect the caudal spine, is characterized by a dorsal defect in the closure of one to several vertebral arches that form the dorsal portions of the vertebral canal encasing the spinal cord. The lesion results from a failure of the neural tube and developing vertebral arches to close properly, which may result in herniation of either meninges (meningocele) or meninges and spinal cord (meningomyelocele) through the defect, forming a sac covered with skin. In some cases there is no herniation of the meninges or spinal cord through the defect, and this variation is termed *spina bifida occulta* (Fig. 14-32). In this variation there is an absence of skin over the affected vertebral arches, vertebral musculature is visible, and the dura mater and spinal cord can be seen in the spinal canal.

Spina bifida has been reported in several species, including horses, calves, sheep, dogs (especially English bulldogs), and cats, particularly the Manx breed, in which it is inherited as an autosomal dominant trait. An additional lesion, myeloschisis, also refers to failure of the neural tube to close and is therefore similar to spina bifida, except in its severe form it results from failure of the entire spinal neural tube to close. This lesion is therefore characterized by lack of development of the entire dorsal vertebral column, because

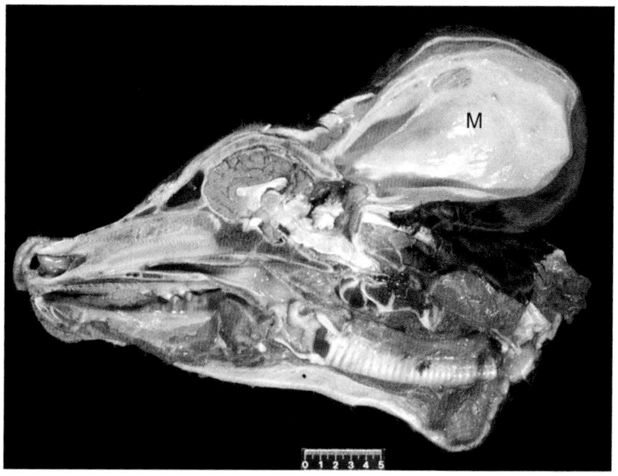

Figure 14-31 **Meningocele (M), Brain, Calf.** A defect in the caudodorsal portion of the skull has allowed the meninges to herniate into a large external pouch covered by skin. The pouch contains fluid and is lined by arachnoid and dura, which are continuous with those surrounding the brain. The cerebellum is small, and the occipital cortex truncated. Scale bar = 5 cm. (Courtesy Dr. R. Storts, College of Veterinary Medicine, Texas A&M University.)

[3]See E-Box 1-1 for a listing of potential, suspected, or known genetic disorders in the nervous system.

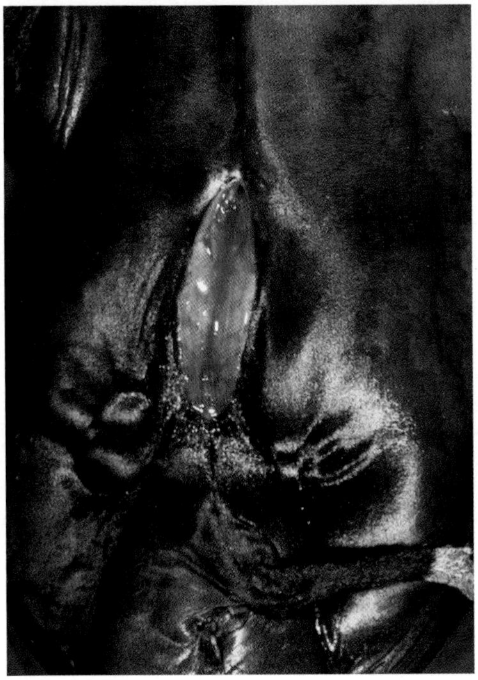

Figure 14-32 **Spina Bifida Occulta, Calf.** There is a cleft in several vertebrae of the dorsal spinal column resulting from defective closure of the neural tube. Although not always the case, note the lack of herniation of the meninges or spinal cord through the defect. The spinal cord is not visible (i.e., occulta) because it is located in the vertebral canal at the deepest ventral extent of the cleft and is covered by edematous muscle. (Courtesy Dr. M.D. McGavin, College of Veterinary Medicine, University of Tennessee.)

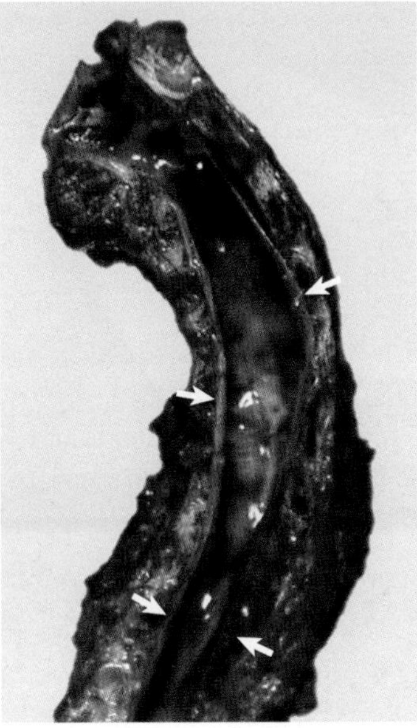

Figure 14-33 **End-Stage Hydromyelia, Spinal Cord, Dog.** The white and gray matter of the spinal cord are missing as a result of compression atrophy from a space-occupying, fluid-filled central canal. The only recognizable remnants of nervous tissue is the dura *(arrows)*. In less severely affected animals, there would be variable dilation of the central canal of the spinal cord with much less severe compression atrophy. (Courtesy College of Veterinary Medicine, University of Tennessee.)

the developing neural tube remained open, unable to fuse and develop normally.

Hydromyelia. Congenital hydromyelia is an abnormal dilation of the central canal of the spinal cord (Fig. 14-33) that leads to the formation of a cavity in which CSF may accumulate. In animals this disorder likely results from infectious or genetic injury that results in damage to ependymal cells lining the canal and the subsequent disruption of the normal flow of CSF and the formation of abnormal CSF pressure gradients within the central canal. As CSF accumulates in the enlarging space, the increased pericanalicular pressure placed on the spinal cord compresses the white and gray matter, leading to loss of white matter and possibly neurons in gray matter. Acquired hydromyelia is rare and is caused by obstruction of the central canal CSF flow. Causes of obstruction include infection, inflammation, and neoplasia.

Clinical signs in young animals with congenital hydromyelia vary, depending on the location and size of the dilation of the central canal in the spinal cord. Signs may include ataxia, urinary incontinence, respiratory difficulty, muscle weakness in front and/or hind limbs, and abnormal proprioceptive reflexes. It can accompany other defects in the spinal cord and has been seen as an abnormality associated with spinal dysraphism in Weimaraner dogs.

Neuronal Migration Disorders

Lissencephaly. Lissencephaly (agyria) and a similar change called *pachygyria* (large, broad gyri) are developmental anomalies that result in part of or the entire cerebrum having smooth surfaces lacking normal gyri and sulci (Fig. 14-34). The cortex is thicker than normal on a transverse section, and the normal laminar pattern of neurons is disrupted. It has been reported most commonly in the Lhasa apso dog, but scattered reports also exist in kittens and lambs.

This lesion is thought to have a genetic basis and results from an arrest of or defect in neuronal migration during development. Recent experimental studies suggest that this migrational disorder is linked to mutations and/or deletions in the doublecortin, filamin-1, LIS1, and reelin genes. These genes control the spatial and temporal expression of proteins in the extracellular microenvironment that subsequently bind to receptors on migrating cells. Patterns of cell membrane binding signals are interpreted by migrating cells and are reflected in their movements by changes in intracellular cytoskeletal reorganization. This process allows cells to migrate to their final destinations within the CNS. Thus alterations in signaling pathways lead to abnormal neuronal migration and CNS anomalies.

The brains of many species, including birds and some laboratory animals, such as rabbits, rats, and mice, lack gyri and sulci; therefore agyria is normal in these species and has no functional significance.

Encephaloclastic Defects

Porencephaly and Hydranencephaly. The formation of fluid-filled cavities in the brain, termed *porencephaly* (small cavities) and *hydranencephaly* (large cavities), usually occurs in utero during gestation. *Porencephaly* refers to a cleft or cyst in the wall of the cerebral hemisphere that typically communicates with the subarachnoid space, but it can also communicate with a lateral ventricle. The cavitation results from destruction of immature neuroblasts whose loss prevents normal development as a result of faulty or aberrant neuroblast migration. Hydranencephaly is considered a severe form of porencephaly and is characterized by cavitation in areas normally occupied by the white matter of the cerebral hemispheres and results from improper development of this part of the cerebrum.

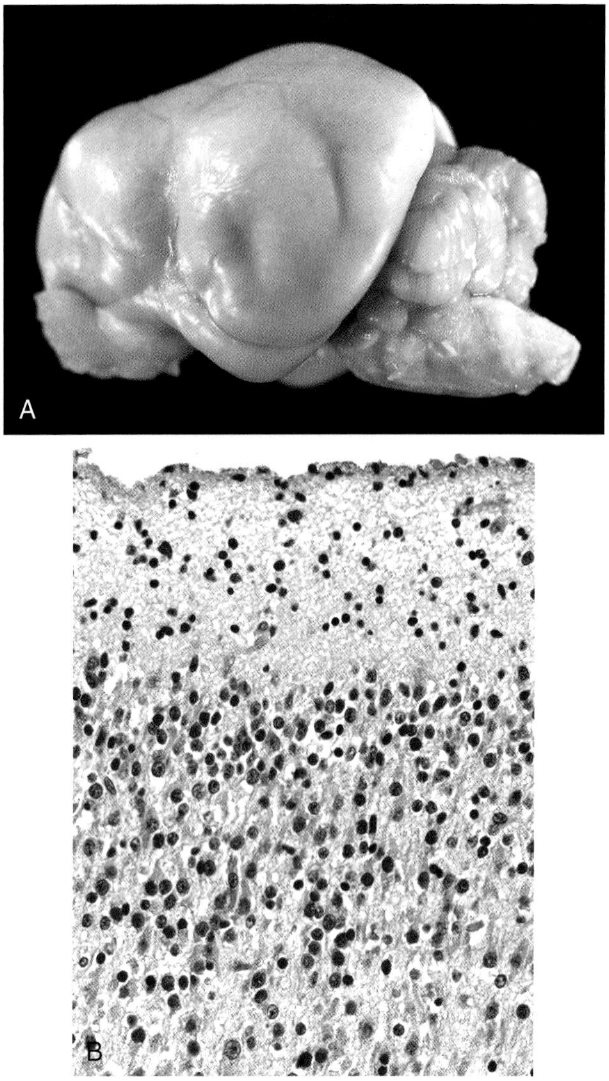

Figure 14-34 **Lissencephaly, Brain, Dog. A,** Note the smooth surfaces of the cerebral hemispheres, which are without gyri and sulci. Gyri and sulci fail to form, possibly from failure of neuronal development and migration. Lissencephaly is an abnormality in domestic animals but is a normal feature in some species, including mice, rats, rabbits, and birds. **B,** The development and migration of neurons have been disrupted such that the cortical gray matter lacks normal lamina formed by neuronal cell bodies. H&E stain. (**A** courtesy Dr. L. Roth, College of Veterinary Medicine, Cornell University. **B** courtesy Dr. R. Mantene, College of Veterinary Medicine, University of Illinois.)

Hydranencephaly is often quite severe, with very little tissue present between the dilated lateral ventricles and the leptomeninges.

Type I and type II porencephaly have been described in human infants, and cases of porencephaly reported in animals can also be categorized using this scheme. Type I porencephaly is caused by vascular injury or vasculitis. Injury, resulting in infarction in the area of the subependymal germinal matrix, results in the formation of a cyst within the focus of dead cells and effete erythrocytes. The germinal matrix is very sensitive to ischemia because of sparse stroma, delicate vasculature, and high metabolism. The initial focus of hemorrhage can grow by centripetal expansion, depending on the severity of hemorrhage and hypoxia, into a cyst of considerable size. Type II porencephaly is caused by injury of neuroblasts in the germinal matrix and the failure of these neuroblasts to migrate within the matrix to form the cerebral cortex. A cyst results from the expansion of the subarachnoid space into the void left by the absence of the cortex.

Type II porencephaly appears to be the form of porencephaly that occurs in domestic animals. Viruses, such as those that cause Akabane, bovine viral diarrhea, blue tongue, border disease, Rift Valley fever, Schmallenberg disease, and Wesselsbron disease, infect and destroy differentiating neuroblasts and neuroglial cells in the developing fetus in utero. Although neuroblasts appear to be the primary target for viral infection in these diseases, additional experimental studies need to be conducted to clarify whether endothelial cells are also infected.

Grossly, porencephaly/hydranencephaly appears as thin-walled fluid-filled cysts of varied sizes in the cerebral hemispheres. Because of the lack of brain substance, the ventricles expand into this space (hydrocephalus ex vacuo), and the ependymal lining remains relatively preserved or may have scattered defects characterized by absent ependyma. The cranium and meninges are generally unaltered. In some cases cerebellar hypoplasia (all or part of the cerebellum) and hypoplasia of the spinal cord may also occur. Microscopically, necrosis of undifferentiated cells, including potential neuroblasts and neuroglia, surrounding a fluid-filled cavity is present in the subventricular zone of the cerebral hemispheres. Degeneration and loss of motor neurons of the ventral horns of the spinal cord may also be observed. This lesion may result in denervation atrophy of limb muscles with a resultant lack of joint movement and arthrogryposis, a persistent congenital flexure or contraction of a joint. Nonsuppurative encephalitis, typified by the accumulation of macrophages, lymphocytes, and plasma cells, also occurs.

Malformations of the Cerebellum

Cerebellar Hypoplasia. In animals the most common causes of cerebellar hypoplasia are parvoviruses (kittens: panleukopenia virus [Fig. 14-35]) and pestiviruses (calves: bovine viral diarrhea virus [Fig. 14-36; E-Fig. 14-6] and piglets: classical swine fever virus). These viruses infect and destroy mitotic cells, primarily the cells of the external granule layer of the cerebellum that are still dividing during the late gestational and early neonatal periods. Necrosis of these cells means they are not available to form the granule layer, and thus the cerebellum is hypoplastic. In calves the cerebellar lesion (cerebellar hypoplasia/atrophy), which follows infection at 150 days of gestation (midtrimester), is considered to involve two processes. One process is typified by early necrosis of the undifferentiated cells in the external granule layer. A second process involves viral-induced vasculitis and ischemia of cerebellar folial white matter.

Grossly, the size of the cerebellum is reduced; the reduction in size varies in severity, depending on the age and developmental stage of the brain when the fetus or neonate is infected.

Microscopically, there is necrosis and loss of the external granule layer and degeneration and loss of Purkinje cells that are postmitotic but immature. Reasons for degeneration of Purkinje cells might include infection by the virus or lack of normal development of the cerebellar cortex. The Purkinje cells can also be malpositioned and located in the molecular layer as a result of the viral-induced alteration in development of the cerebellar cortex. In calves, edema of the folial white matter with focal hemorrhage in the cortex, followed by focal cavitation of the white matter and atrophy, may also be present. These latter lesions are due to ischemia resulting from vasculitis. Leptomeningitis, characterized by accumulation of lymphocytes and plasma cells and occasionally fibroplasia, may cause adhesions between adjacent cerebellar folia and focal obliteration of the subarachnoid space.

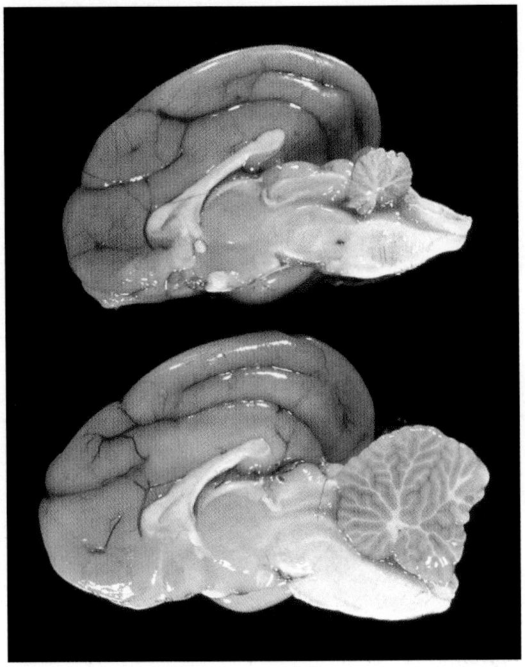

Figure 14-35 **Cerebellar Hypoplasia, Cerebellum, Cat.** In the cat, cerebellar hypoplasia (cerebellar hypoplasia, *top specimen*; normal cat, *bottom specimen*) most commonly is the result of in utero infection with feline panleukopenia virus (parvovirus). The virus infects and causes lysis of dividing cells in the external granule layer (on the outside of the cerebellum in the fetus). Because these cells are no longer available to migrate to form the granule layer, the cerebellum remains small. (Courtesy Dr. Y. Niyo, College of Veterinary Medicine, Iowa State University; and Noah's Arkive, College of Veterinary Medicine, The University of Georgia.)

Malformations of the Spinal Cord

Syringomyelia. Syringomyelia (congenital and acquired forms) is a disorder in which a cavity forms in the spinal cord. The cavity, called a *syrinx*, is not lined by ependyma and is separate from the central canal. The syrinx can extend over several spinal cord segments. The lesion is well known in human beings and has also been described most commonly in calves and also in many breeds of dogs. The syrinx can communicate with the central canal but should not be confused with hydromyelia, which means dilation of the central canal. In instances of communication, the term *syringohydromyelia* should be used. The cavity contains fluid and is unlined, except for varying degrees of mural astrocytosis. Proposed causes include the presence of an anomalous vascular pattern that results in low-grade ischemia, leading to infarction or failure of cells destined for this area to develop in utero trauma in human beings or an infection that causes degeneration and cavitation. An acquired form of syringomyelia is similar to congenital syringomyelia; however, it occurs in older animals. Proposed causes include injury after trauma to the central canal or its vascular supply caused by trauma, infection, or neoplasia that result in degeneration and cavitation of the spinal cord. The presence of syringomyelia and hydromyelia in some animals with vertebral malformations also suggests that local perturbations in CSF flow and pressure may allow for these dilations and cavities to develop.

Although the central canal of the spinal cord is connected to the ventricular system via the fourth ventricle, there apparently is little active movement of CSF within the central canal. Recently it has been hypothesized that there may be alteration of "normal" CSF flow (see the discussion on ependyma in the section on Cells of the Central Nervous System) with redirection of the flow along a pressure gradient into the central canal and into the syrinx. It has also been suggested that pressure differences in the vertebral column cause CSF to continually move into the cyst, resulting in enlargement of the syrinx and additional compressive damage to the spinal cord.

Clinical signs in young dogs and calves with syringomyelia vary, depending on the location and size of the spinal cord lesion. Signs may include ataxia, urinary incontinence, respiratory difficulty, muscle weakness in front and/or hind limbs, and abnormal proprioceptive reflexes.

Hydrocephalus. By far the most common congenital CNS abnormality identified in domestic animals is hydrocephalus. It has a variety of causes, including in utero viral infection, developmental abnormalities in the ependyma or ventricular system, infection and subsequent blockage of the ventricular system, or periventricular parenchymal loss. There appears to be a genetic predisposition in some dog breeds (toy and brachycephalic), but the mechanism of injury has not been as clearly established in domestic animals as it has in human beings.

In laboratory animals, several neonatal in utero experimental viral infections, including mumps virus, reovirus type 1, and parainfluenza virus types 1 and 2, can induce congenital hydrocephalus. In utero infection with panleukopenia virus in cats and parainfluenza virus in dogs can also cause congenital hydrocephalus in affected offspring. Although there are some differences among the different viral infections, the basic lesion is stenosis of the mesencephalic aqueduct that results in the development of noncommunicating hydrocephalus. In the dog, closure of the mesencephalic duct can be incomplete. The virus grows in and causes destruction of ependymal cells lining the ventricular system. The infection is initially accompanied by an inflammation that resolves within 2 weeks.

The notable lesion resulting from this injury to the ependyma of the mesencephalic duct is its occlusion. This end-stage lesion is not the result of an astroglial response or due to the presence of viral antigen. Instead, the original ependyma-lined aqueduct is replaced by focal aggregates of remaining ependymal cells that have separated from the adjacent tissue, which appears normal. The appearance of the final lesion is therefore more suggestive of an agenesis than a viral infection. Infection of adult laboratory animals (mice with influenza viral infection) also can induce mesencephalic duct stenosis resulting in hydrocephalus, but in contrast to neonatal infection, there is a persistent astroglial response in the area of stenosis.

Congenital Hydrocephalus. CSF can accumulate in the ventricular system, the subarachnoid space, or both. The type of hydrocephalus that develops depends on the site of blockage that disrupts normal flow of CSF.

Exactly which portions of the ventricular system will be dilated in hydrocephalus depends on the site of the blockage:

1. Blockage of the interventricular foramen between a lateral and third ventricle leads to unilateral dilation of that lateral ventricle.
2. Blockage of both interventricular foramina leads to bilateral dilation of both lateral ventricles.
3. Blockage of the mesencephalic duct leads to bilateral dilation of the lateral ventricles, the third ventricle, and the segment of the mesencephalic duct proximal to the blockage.
4. Blockage of the lateral apertures of the fourth ventricle leads to bilateral dilation of lateral ventricles, the third ventricle, the mesencephalic duct, and the fourth ventricle.
5. Blockage of reabsorption leads to bilateral dilation of lateral ventricles, the third ventricle, the mesencephalic duct, the fourth ventricle, and the subarachnoid space.

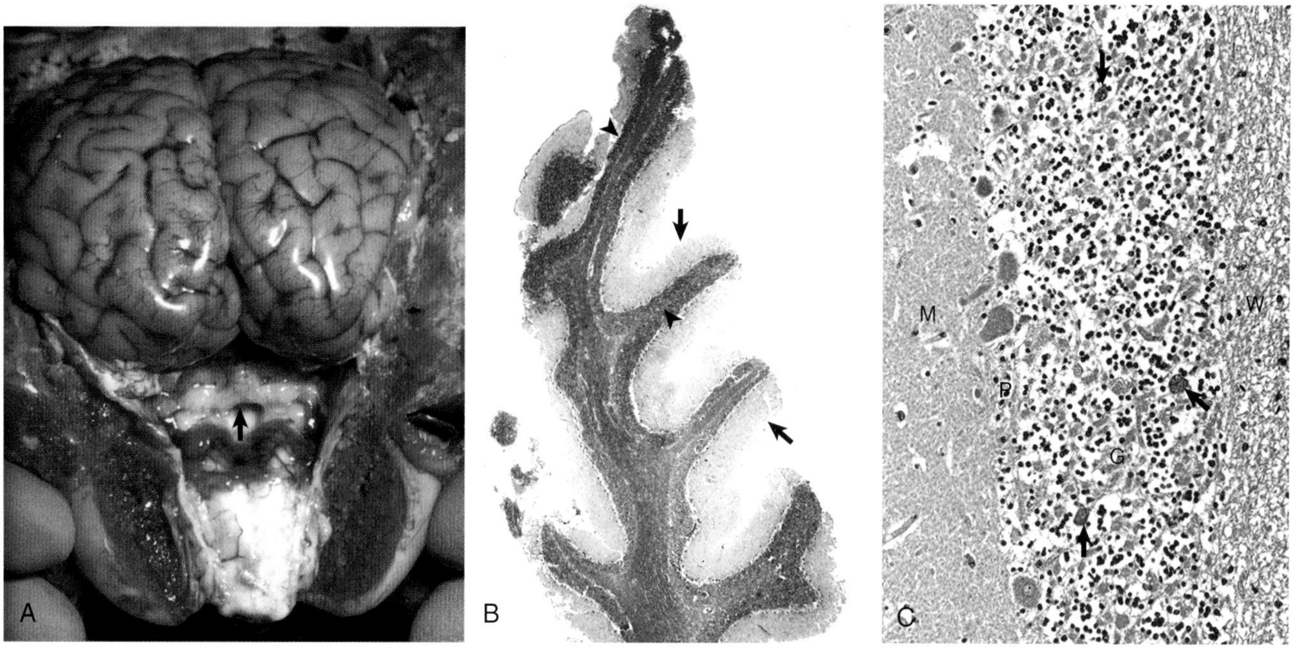

Figure 14-36 **Cerebellar Hypoplasia, Cerebellum, Calf.** In the normal neonatal calf, cells of the external granule layer of the cerebellum migrate to form the granule layer (not shown). Bovine viral diarrhea virus infects and kills mitotic cells of the granule layer of the cerebellum. These cells are still dividing during the late gestational and early neonatal periods in the cat and between 100 to 180 days of gestation in the calf. Necrosis of these cells means they are not available to migrate to form the granule layer, and thus the cerebellum does not obtain full size. Depending on the stage of gestation, injury can also alter development of cells in others ways, including altered patterns of migration, resulting in various other lesions termed dysplasia. **A,** Cerebellar hypoplasia *(arrow)*. In utero infection with bovine viral diarrhea virus (pestivirus) results in cytolysis of dividing germinal cells of the granule layer and vascular impairment secondary to vasculitis of the cerebellum during organogenesis. The severity of the lesion involving the granule cells is at its greatest if dividing cells are infected during the earliest stages of cellular differentiation, and occurs between 100 to 180 days of gestation. **B,** Note the folia of the cerebellum are hypoplastic and dysplastic with a reduced thickness of the molecular layer *(arrows)* and haphazardly organized and thinned granule cell layer *(arrowheads)*. H&E stain. **C,** The molecular layer *(M)* of the cerebellum is reduced in thickness and lacks the normal number of neuronal nuclei. The Purkinje cell layer *(P)* has large gaps between adjacent cells as the result of the loss of neuron cell bodies or the failure of neurons to migrate properly to form this layer. Note the retention of Purkinje cells *(arrows)* in the granule cell layer *(G)*. The granule cell layer has significantly reduced numbers of neurons as shown by the lack of nuclei. H&E stain. *W,* White matter. (**A** courtesy Dr. M.D. McGavin, College of Veterinary Medicine, University of Tennessee. **B** and **C** courtesy Dr. J.F. Zachary, College of Veterinary Medicine, University of Illinois.)

As an example, following blockage of the interventricular foramina, the pressure in the lateral ventricles increases; the ventricles dilate; the ependyma becomes atrophied and focally discontinuous; and because of the pressure gradient, CSF is forced into the periventricular white matter, leading to hydrostatic edema. Hydrostatic edema results in degeneration and atrophy of myelin and axons, and this loss of tissue results in further expansion of the ventricles.

The forms of hydrocephalus are communicating and noncommunicating hydrocephalus. Communicating hydrocephalus, the least common of the two forms, occurs when there is communication of ventricular CSF with the subarachnoid space where the CSF can be in excess. Noncommunicating hydrocephalus results from obstruction within the ventricular system at, or rostral to, the lateral apertures of the fourth ventricle. An area of great vulnerability for obstruction is the mesencephalic aqueduct. Noncommunicating hydrocephalus can also occur without any evidence of obstruction to CSF flow as a result of failure of the reabsorption of CSF.

Another type of hydrocephalus, referred to as *hydrocephalus ex vacuo* (or compensating hydrocephalus), is not usually a congenital abnormality but occurs secondary to absence or loss of cerebral tissue. This type of hydrocephalus can occur in utero from destruction and loss of cerebral tissue surrounding the lateral ventricles (e.g., in hydranencephaly). Hydrocephalus ex vacuo is discussed further in the next section on acquired hydrocephalus.

Gross lesions associated with communicating and noncommunicating congenital hydrocephalus include enlargement (doming) of the cranium if obstruction occurs before the sutures have fused (Fig. 14-37). The bones of the calvaria are extremely thin, and the fontanelles are prominent (Fig. 14-38). In the brain there is prominent enlargement of the ventricular system proximal to the point of obstruction (Fig. 14-39). White matter adjacent to the dilated lateral ventricles is reduced in thickness, although the gray matter can retain a relatively normal appearance. As the hydrocephalus progresses, atrophy with fenestration and cavity formation of the interventricular septum (septum pellucidum), atrophy of the hippocampus in the floor of the lateral ventricles, and flattening of cortical gyri can occur. If the obstruction is abrupt and pressure builds rapidly, the cerebral hemispheres can be displaced caudally, causing herniation of the parahippocampal gyri under the tentorium cerebelli and of the vermis of the cerebellum through the foramen magnum. The resulting coning of the cerebellum can be accompanied by hemorrhage and necrosis of cells in the cerebellar folia as a result of ischemia and infarction. Microscopically the ependyma can become atrophied and focally discontinuous, and there is loss of cells and cell processes in adjacent white matter and variably in the gray matter.

Clinically, congenital hydrocephalus occurs most frequently in brachycephalic or toy breeds such as the Chihuahua, Lhasa apso,

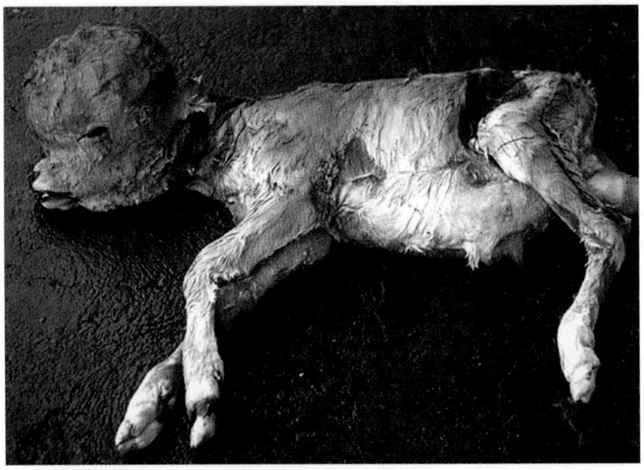

Figure 14-37 Congenital Hydrocephalus, Brain, Calf. Note the symmetrically enlarged and dome-shaped calvaria. The bone of the calvaria is thinned and distorted from pressure from the expanding brain during gestation. (Courtesy Dr. J. King, College of Veterinary Medicine, Cornell University.)

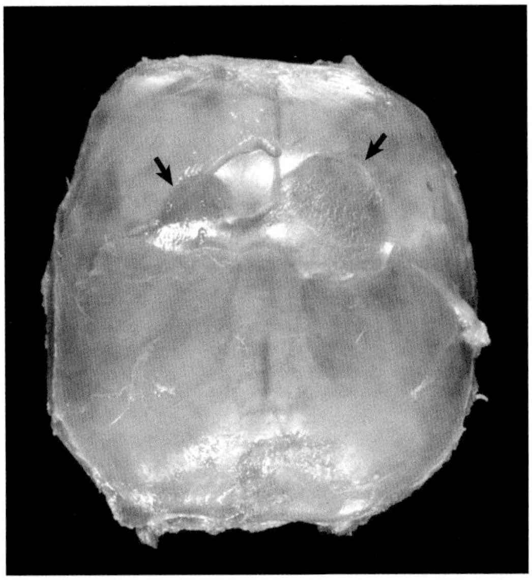

Figure 14-38 Calvaria, View of the Dorsal Surface, Congenital Hydrocephalus, Dog. The bone of the calvaria is thin and the fontanelles *(arrows)* are enlarged. The translucent membrane covering the fontanelles is periosteum. (Courtesy Drs. J. Wright and D. Duncan, College of Veterinary Medicine, North Carolina State University; and Noah's Arkive, College of Veterinary Medicine, The University of Georgia.)

and toy poodle. Clinical signs occur within the first year of life, often before 3 months of age. Behavioral changes are the most common and include poor motor skill development; delay in learned behavior, such as house training; somnolence; dullness; episodic confusion; circling; periodic aggression; and seizures.

Acquired Hydrocephalus. Noncommunicating acquired hydrocephalus has been associated with injury of the ependyma, resulting in obstruction of any of the following: the lateral apertures of the fourth ventricle, the cerebral aqueduct, or the interventricular foramen. Causes of obstruction include compression by cerebral abscesses and neoplasms, and blockages by infectious/inflammatory disease resulting in a ventriculitis and, uncommonly, by cholesteatomas in the choroid plexus of the lateral ventricles of the horse.

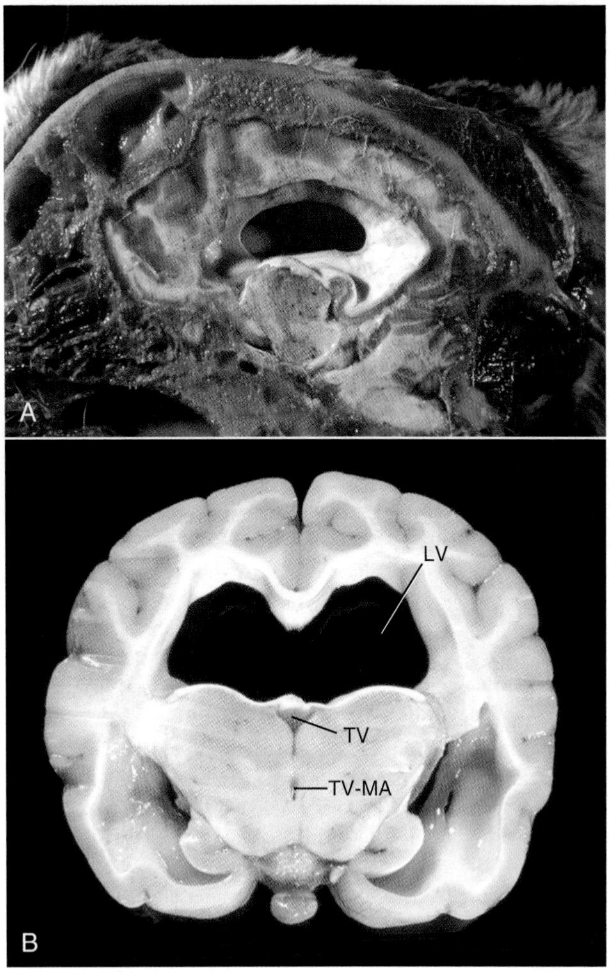

Figure 14-39 Hydrocephalus, Brain, Dog. A, Midsagittal section of the head, third ventricle. Note the dilated third and lateral ventricles and the absence of most of the septum pellucidum between the left and right lateral ventricles. **B,** Junction between parietal and occipital lobes, level of thalamus. Bilateral dilation of lateral ventricles *(LV)* dorsally, and ventrolaterally. The fornix has separated and lies on the flattened floor of the ventricle. Note that the third ventricle *(TV)* and junctional area between the third ventricle and mesencephalic aqueduct *(TV-MA)* are not enlarged and are possibly even reduced in size, suggesting that the obstruction may be at, or rostral to, this plane of section. (**A** courtesy Dr. M.D. McGavin, College of Veterinary Medicine, University of Tennessee. **B** courtesy Dr. R. Storts, College of Veterinary Medicine, Texas A&M University.)

Because the calvaria has now ceased to grow, unlike congenital hydrocephalus, it is of normal size and shape, and its bone is of normal thickness.

A second type of acquired hydrocephalus, referred to as hydrocephalus ex vacuo (or compensating hydrocephalus), usually occurs in the cerebral hemispheres secondary to loss of neural tissue. If there is loss of neurons in the cerebral cortex, as in bovine polioencephalomalacia or other types of laminar cortical necrosis, the axons of these neurons, which normally traverse the white matter of the cerebral hemispheres, will disappear, and there will be atrophy of the cortex from the loss of neuronal cell bodies and of the white matter from the loss of axons. The lateral ventricles will expand into the space once occupied by white matter. This dilation of the lateral ventricles may be bilateral when there has been a loss of white and gray matter from both cerebral hemispheres, or it may be unilateral. If the loss of cortex is localized, as in an infarct, then dilation of the lateral ventricle will not uniformly involve the whole lateral ventricle. Examples of disorders in which hydrocephalus ex vacuo occur include some storage diseases (ceroid-lipofuscinosis in sheep), aging, and postradiation exposure, all of which are associated with cerebral atrophy. There is no evidence of obstruction of the normal flow of CSF in this type of hydrocephalus.

Diseases Caused by Microbes

Bacteria

Brain Abscesses. Cerebral abscesses in animals are relatively uncommon but arise after entry of bacteria into the CNS. This may occur either from direct extension or hematogenously. With direct extension, abscesses occur following penetrating wounds, such as calvarial fractures, or from spread of infection from adjacent tissues, such as the meninges, paranasal sinuses, and internal ear, and through the cribriform plate of the ethmoid (see Fig. 14-29). Diseases that cause bacteremia or septicemia result in infectious microbes being trapped in vascular beds within the CNS and meninges. Abscesses usually arise within gray matter because it receives a disproportionate share of blood flow in the CNS, usually at the gray-white (cortex–subcortical white matter) junction. They exert effects in the CNS by disruption and destruction of tissue and by displacement as space-occupying lesions. If the abscess grows quickly, tissue is more likely to be disrupted and destroyed and in the worst case penetrate the wall of the lateral ventricle and cause a ventriculitis. Bacteria in the CSF may be carried into the subarachnoid space and cause a leptomeningitis. On the other hand, if growth is slow, tissue is more likely to be displaced. Chronic abscesses become encapsulated by either fibrous tissue if they are close to the leptomeninges or by astrocytes away from the meninges. The mechanism of tissue injury is likely a secondary bystander effect related to the actions of the mediators of inflammation and the toxins and other products elaborated from bacteria. Bacteria appear to localize in specific areas of the CNS based on receptor-mediated attachment or because of vascular flow patterns unique to the gray matter–white matter interface of the CNS that allow bacteria to attach to and move through the blood-brain barrier. This latter flow mechanism likely occurs because small blood vessels supplying the cerebrum fail to continue into the white matter and end with their horizontal branches running parallel to the surface of the gyrus within the gray matter at the interface with the white matter. Once within the CNS or meninges, bacteria replicate and elicit an inflammatory response. Lytic enzymes released from lysosomes of neutrophils and other inflammatory cytokines secreted by lymphocytes and macrophages destroy neurons and their processes and disrupt synapses, thus affecting neurotransmission.

Grossly, brain abscesses can be single or multiple, be discrete or coalescing, and have varied sizes (Fig. 14-40). Early in the process, abscesses consist of a white to gray to yellow, thick to granular exudate. The color of the exudate can be influenced by the exuberance of the pyogenic response elicited by the inciting bacteria and by any pigments produced by the bacteria. *Streptococcus* spp., *Staphylococcus* spp., and *Corynebacterium* spp. may produce a pale-yellow to yellow, watery to creamy exudate. Coliforms, such as *E. coli* and *Klebsiella* spp., may produce a white to gray, watery to creamy exudate. *Pseudomonas* spp. may produce a green to bluish-green exudate. The borders of abscesses are often surrounded by a red zone of active hyperemia induced by inflammatory mediators acting on capillary beds.

Brain abscesses can arise in some food animal species from an extension of otitis interna (see Fig. 14-29). These animals often display evidence of facial nerve paralysis, such as a drooping ear. The cerebellopontine angle and adjacent structures are the common locations for such abscesses. In horses, *Streptococcus equi* subsp. *equi* (strangles) can cause brain abscesses via hematogenous spread (Fig. 14-41). Direct penetration may also occur in small ruminants that lack frontal sinuses because of improper dehorning procedures. Brain abscesses are space-occupying lesions and as such can have a devastating effect on brain function. Depending on size and location, compression via mass effect (increased intracranial pressure) of vital structures (nuclei that regulate cardiac and respiratory rhythms) and brain displacements (cerebellar vermis, parahippocampal gyri) are two common sequelae to acute abscesses. Abscesses can occur in the spinal cord as a result of direct extension of bacterial vertebral osteomyelitis through the dura (Fig. 14-42), after tail docking in lambs, and occasionally from hematogenous spread.

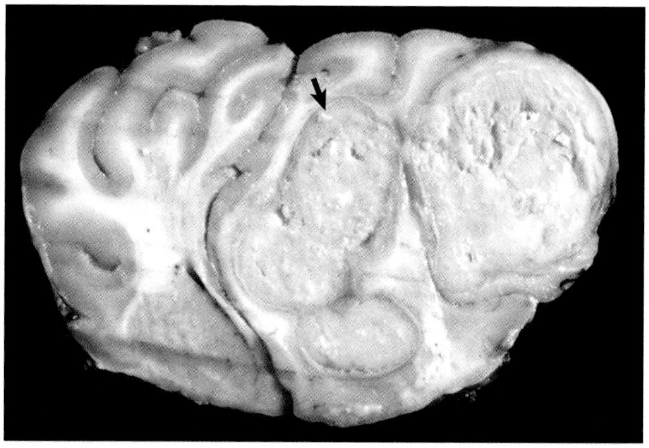

Figure 14-40 Chronic Cerebral Abscesses, Sheep. Abscesses with caseous centers *(arrow)* have replaced most of the right cerebral hemisphere, enlarged it, and displaced the midline to the left. The abscesses are encapsulated by a thick fibrous capsule generated by fibroblasts of the pia and perivascular spaces of the outer cortex. (Courtesy Dr. M.D. McGavin, College of Veterinary Medicine, University of Tennessee.)

Clinically, animals with brain abscesses can show abnormal mental behaviors, ataxia, head tilt, circling, and loss of vision.

Diffuse Encephalitis. Common bacteria have the potential to produce disease in the CNS by hematogenous spread and vasculitis (see the section on Neonatal Septicemia).

Ependymitis and Choroid Plexitis. Infectious microbes, especially pus-forming bacteria, such as the coliform and *Streptococcus* spp., can enter the CNS hematogenously or via direct extension, invade the choroid plexuses, and be released into the CSF, gaining access to ependymal cells lining the ventricular system. Inflammation of the ependyma is called ependymitis, whereas inflammation of the choroid plexus is called choroid plexitis. Gross lesions usually consist of gray-white to yellow-green thick to gelatinous CSF within the ventricular system and choroid plexuses that are granular and gray-white, with areas of active hyperemia and hemorrhage. If the bacteria traverse through the lateral apertures of the fourth ventricle, they can enter and spread throughout the subarachnoid space, possibly inducing suppurative bacterial leptomeningitis. The exudate can also obstruct CSF flow, leading to noncommunicating hydrocephalus. Although most cases are caused by bacteria, cats infected with feline infectious peritonitis (FIP) can develop protein-rich fluid and exudate within the ventricular system that can lead to plugging of the mesencephalic aqueduct with subsequent hydrocephalus. Microscopically, inflammatory cells, especially neutrophils, mixed with fibrin, hemorrhage, and bacteria, can be seen in the exudate.

Meningitis. *Meningitis* refers to inflammation of the meninges (Fig. 14-43). In animals, meningitis is most commonly caused by bacteria such as *E. coli* and *Streptococcus* spp. that traverse to the

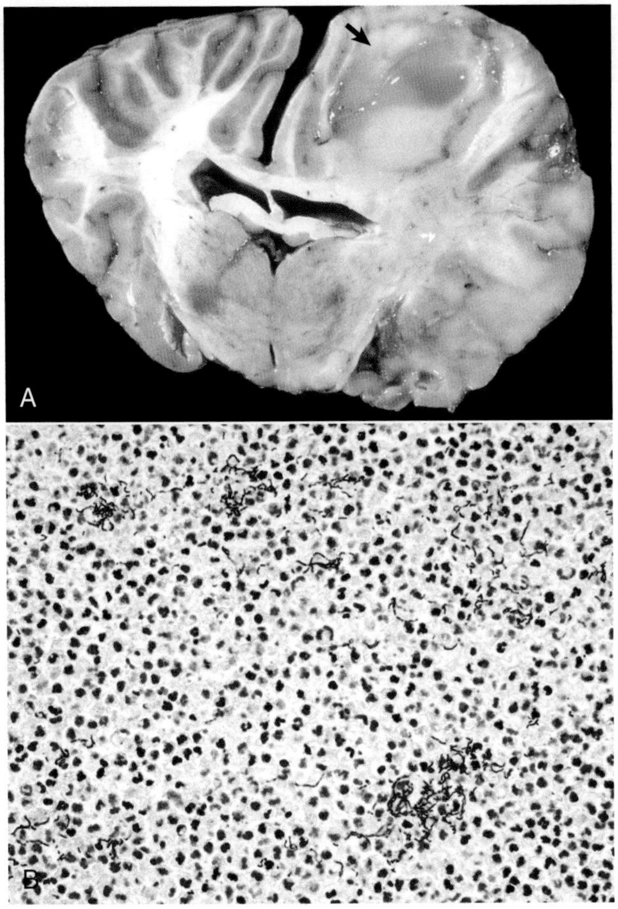

Figure 14-41 Abscess, Right Cerebral Hemisphere, Horse. A, The cerebral cortex contains an abscess *(arrow)* caused by *Streptococcus equi* subsp. *equi* entering the central nervous system via the blood. A fibrous capsule is present on the lateral, medial, and dorsal sides of the abscess (most obvious on the lateral side as a *gray band*). There is no obvious capsule present on the ventral side (i.e., toward the right lateral ventricle). Microscopically, there is a thin glial capsule (astrogliosis). Note also the increased size of the right hemisphere with blurring of the distinction between gray and white matter, an indication of edema. **B,** Chains of Gram-positive *(blue staining)* cocci in the inflammatory exudate from an abscess caused by *Streptococcus equi* subsp. *zooepidemicus*. Gram stain. (**A** courtesy Dr. K. Read, College of Veterinary Medicine, Texas A&M University; and Noah's Arkive, College of Veterinary Medicine, The University of Georgia. **B** courtesy Dr. J.F. Zachary, College of Veterinary Medicine, University of Illinois.)

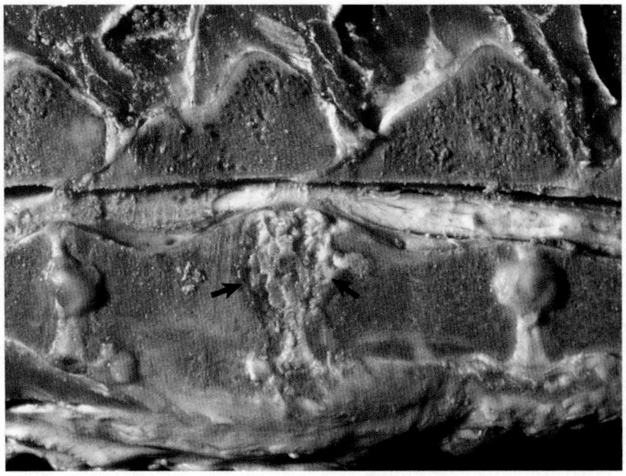

Figure 14-42 Diskospondylitis, Thoracic Spinal Cord, Pig. This type of abscess *(arrows)* is commonly caused by bacterial emboli that lodge in intervertebral disks or in the body of vertebrae causing osteomyelitis, which can extend into intervertebral disks. Large intervertebral abscesses can compress the spinal cord and cause Wallerian degeneration of nerves, mainly in the ventral funiculi but also in other funiculi. In this case, remodeling and proliferation of the vertebral bone secondary to the infection also contributed to the narrowing of the spinal canal and compression of the spinal cord. (Courtesy Dr. M.D. McGavin, College of Veterinary Medicine, University of Tennessee.)

leptomeninges and subarachnoid space hematogenously. Bacteria can also spread to the meninges by direct extension and leukocytic trafficking. In common usage the term meningitis generally refers to inflammation of the leptomeninges (the pia mater, subarachnoid space, and adjacent arachnoid mater) in contrast to inflammation of the dura mater, which is referred to as pachymeningitis. Leptomeningitis can be acute, subacute, or chronic and, depending on the cause, suppurative, eosinophilic, nonsuppurative, or granulomatous. Inflammation of specific parts of the dura mater of the cranial cavity can occur in the external periosteal dura after osteomyelitis, formation of extradural abscesses and pituitary abscesses, and skull fracture and involve the inner dura in association with leptomeningitis. Abscesses of the pituitary fossa occur with some frequency in cattle, including in bulls with nose rings. Bacteria isolated from the cases include *Pasteurella multocida* and *Trueperella pyogenes*. The abscess can result from spread of infection arising in the caudal nasal cavity or sinuses, possibly through direct extension or through the venous circulation. Incision of the pituitary fossa releases a thick, viscous, opaque tan to yellow exudate, which can elevate the dura mater surrounding the fossa. Infection can extend via the infundibular recess of the third ventricle into the ventricular system, resulting in ventriculitis, ependymitis, and empyema. Systemic bacterial infections in neonates are a common cause of acute meningitis (leptomeningitis), which are suppurative and fibrinous. In animals, leptomeningitis secondary to a selective viral infection only of the leptomeninges is very rare and is usually seen in combination with viral-induced encephalitides.

Neonatal Septicemia. Neonatal septicemia typically involves *E. coli*, *Streptococcus* spp., *Salmonella* spp., *Pasteurella* spp., and *Haemophilus* spp. The release of endotoxins and bacterial cell wall components, such as lipopolysaccharide, teichoic acid, and proteoglycans, in the CNS vasculature leads to the secretion of cytokines (TNF, interleukin, platelet-activating factor, prostaglandins, thromboxane, and leukotrienes) from the endothelium and trafficking CNS macrophages, followed by adhesion of neutrophils, injury to the endothelium and blood-brain barrier, and vasculitis resulting initially in brain swelling and brain edema and increased intracranial pressure.

Although there are differences in the diseases caused by these microbes, they tend to produce fibrinopurulent inflammation of membranous tissues (serosal surfaces) of the body. Leptomeninges, choroid plexus, and ependyma of the CNS—as well as sites often preferentially involved in hematogenous spread of bacteria like the synovium, uvea, and the serosal lining of body cavities—can be affected in various combinations. Infections are often acquired perinatally, and onset is usually within a few days of birth up to 2 weeks (Box 14-7). The initial portal of entry can be oral; intrauterine; umbilical; or surgical, via postsurgical procedures such as castration and ear notching; or via the respiratory system, but the bacteria eventually spread to the CNS hematogenously.

Gross CNS lesions are commonly present and include congestion, hemorrhage, and diffuse to focal cloudiness or opacity in the leptomeninges, resulting in a leptomeningitis caused by

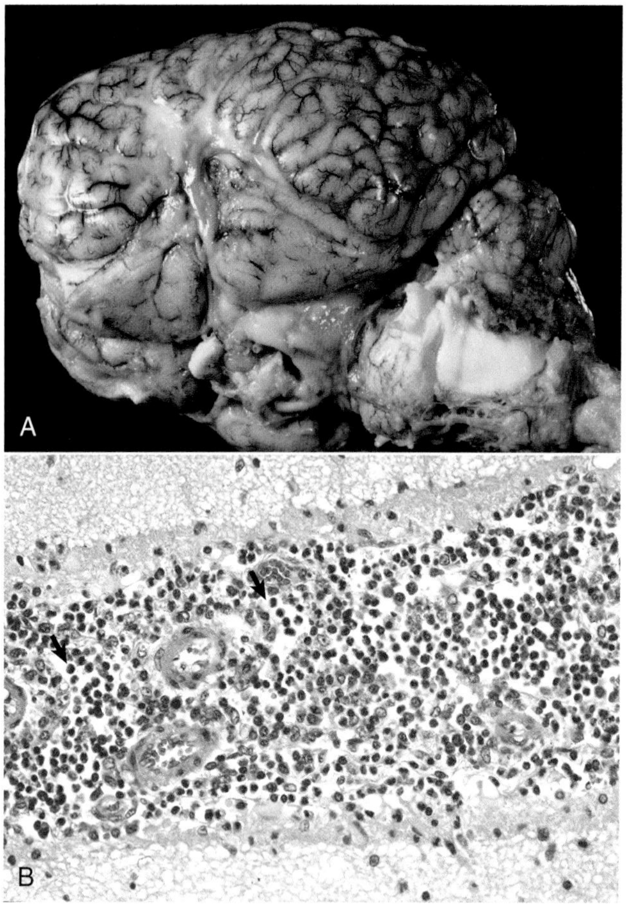

Figure 14-43 **Suppurative Bacterial Meningitis, Cerebral Hemispheres, Horse. A,** Pale yellow-white thick exudate consistent with an infiltrate of neutrophils admixed with bacteria, cellular debris, edema fluid, and fibrin is present in the subarachnoid space on the lateral surface and also in the sulci. Overall the gyri are flattened, indicating brain swelling and compression. **B,** The arachnoid space of the leptomeninges in this sulcus contains a mixture of neutrophils *(arrows)*, other mononuclear inflammatory cells, cellular debris, edema fluid, and fibrin. H&E stain. (**A** courtesy Dr. M.D. McGavin, College of Veterinary Medicine, University of Tennessee. **B** courtesy Dr. J.F. Zachary, College of Veterinary Medicine, University of Illinois.)

Box 14-7 Central Nervous System Bacterial Infections in Young Animals

CALF

Escherichia coli: Leptomeningitis, choroiditis, ependymitis and ventriculitis, synovitis, ophthalmitis, and perioptic neuritis
Pasteurella/Mannheimia spp.: Leptomeningitis, ependymitis and ventriculitis
Streptococcus spp.: Leptomeningitis, synovitis, ophthalmitis

FOAL

Escherichia coli: Leptomeningitis, ventriculitis, polyserositis, synovitis
Streptococcus spp.: Leptomeningitis, polyserositis, synovitis
Salmonella typhimurium: Leptomeningitis, ependymitis and ventriculitis, choroiditis, synovitis

LAMB

Escherichia coli: Leptomeningitis, ependymitis and ventriculitis, peritonitis, synovitis
Pasteurella/Mannheimia spp.: Leptomeningitis

PIG

Escherichia coli: Leptomeningitis, ophthalmitis
Haemophilus parasuis: Leptomeningitis, polyserositis, synovitis
Streptococcus suis type I and II: Leptomeningitis, choroiditis, ependymitis, cranial neuritis, myelitis
Salmonella choleraesuis: Leptomeningitis, ophthalmitis

accumulation of exudates (see Fig. 14-43). The ventricles contain fibrin, usually as a thin layer on the ependymal surface or as a pale coagulum in the CSF of the ventricular lumen, secondary to a choroid plexitis and/or ependymitis.

Microscopic lesions vary according to the microbe. With the exception of *Salmonella* spp., the lesions consist of deposits of fibrin and an infiltration of mainly neutrophils in and around the blood vessels and capillaries of the leptomeninges, choroid plexus, and ependymal or subependymal areas of the brain. The epithelium of the choroid plexus and ependymal lining of the ventricles can be disrupted by cellular degeneration, disorganization, and necrosis, and this inflammation can extend into the adjacent CNS. A vasculitis with thrombosis and hemorrhage can be associated with lesions caused by *E. coli*. Lesions caused by *Salmonella* spp. are not limited to the perinatal period. CNS involvement in salmonellosis is generally limited to foals, calves, and pigs, and in contrast to the infections mentioned earlier, the leukocytic response tends to have a greater proportion of macrophages and lymphocytes, often to the extent that the inflammation is designated histiocytic or granulomatous. This difference presumably reflects the fact that *Salmonella* spp. can be facultative pathogens of the monocyte-macrophage system. As is true in other tissues, vasculitis, thrombosis, necrosis, and hemorrhage often accompany *Salmonella* infections of the CNS. *Haemophilus parasuis*, which causes Glasser's disease, is also a frequent cause of leptomeningitis, polyserositis, and polyarthritis in 8- to 16-week-old pigs. Again, lesions are as previously noted with fibrinopurulent inflammation involving the leptomeninges, serosal linings of body cavities, and joints.

Bacterial infection with CNS and visceral involvement occurs in neonatal pigs and through the weaning period. These diseases are deserving of special mention because of the incidence and stereotyped nature of the infections. Several strains of *Streptococcus suis* are capable of causing disease. Type I strains generally cause disease in suckling pigs ranging in age from 1 to 6 weeks, whereas type II strains affect older pigs 6 to 14 weeks old. Type II strains are recognized as one of the more important serotypes, causing meningitis not only in pigs but also in human beings, particularly those working with pigs or handling porcine tissues. Other serotypes and untyped strains can also cause systemic disease that results in leptomeningitis, choroid plexitis, and ependymitis. Extension to involve cranial nerve roots or the central canal of the cervical spinal cord also occurs. The character of the inflammation is fibrinopurulent, and necrotic foci can be found in brainstem, cerebellum, and anterior spinal cord.

Clinically, affected animals are initially ataxic and then become laterally recumbent with rhythmic paddling of the limbs. As the disease progresses, they may become comatose and die.

Viruses. The viruses causing CNS disease in domestic animals are listed in Table 14-3.

Arboviruses

Japanese Encephalitis. See E-Appendix 14-2.

Louping Ill. See E-Appendix 14-2.

Herpesviruses. Encephalitic herpesviruses, members of the subfamily Alphaherpesvirinae, cause cell injury through (1) necrosis of

Table 14-3 Viruses Causing Central Nervous System Disease in Domestic Animals

Virus Genus	Disease	Type of Injury
Arbovirus	Equine encephalomyelitis	Encephalitis/myelitis/meningitis/vasculitis
	Japanese encephalitis	Encephalitis/myelitis/meningitis
	Louping ill	Encephalitis/myelitis/meningitis
	West Nile viral encephalomyelitis	Encephalitis/myelitis
	Wesselsbron virus	Malformations
Bornavirus	Borna disease	Encephalitis/myelitis
Bunyavirus	Akabane disease	Malformations/encephalitis
	Arthrogryposis hydranencephaly complex (Cache Valley fever)	Malformations/encephalitis
	Rift Valley fever, Schmallenberg virus	Malformations/encephalitis
Coronavirus	Feline infectious peritonitis	Vasculitis/encephalitis/myelitis/meningitis
	Hemagglutinating encephalomyelitis	Encephalitis/myelitis/meningitis/ganglioneuritis
Enterovirus	Enterovirus-induced porcine polioencephalomyelitis	Encephalitis/myelitis
Herpesvirus	Equine herpesvirus 1 myeloencephalopathy	Encephalitis/myelitis/meningitis/vasculitis
	Bovine malignant catarrhal fever	Encephalitis/myelitis/meningitis/vasculitis
	Infectious bovine rhinotracheitis	Encephalitis
	Pseudorabies	Encephalitis/myelitis/meningitis
Lentivirus	Visna	Encephalitis/myelitis/demyelination
	Caprine leukoencephalomyelitis-arthritis	Encephalitis/myelitis/demyelination
Orbivirus	Bluetongue	Malformations/encephalitis
Paramyxovirus	Canine distemper	Demyelination/encephalitis/myelitis
	Old-dog encephalitis	Encephalitis/demyelination/meningitis/vasculitis
Parvovirus	Feline panleukopenia virus	Malformations/meningitis
Pestivirus	Classical swine fever	Malformations/hypomyelination/encephalitis/meningitis/vasculitis
	Bovine viral diarrhea	Malformations/meningitis/dysmyelination
	Border disease	Malformations/hypomyelination
Polyomavirus	Progressive multifocal leukoencephalopathy	Demyelination
Rhabdovirus	Rabies	Encephalitis/myelitis/meningitis/vasculitis/ganglioneuritis

infected neurons and glial cells, (2) necrosis of infected endothelial cells, and (3) secondary effects of inflammation, cytokines, and chemokines. Although necrosis appears to be the principal mechanism for cell injury, recent studies indicate that apoptotic cell death also plays a role.

Neurotropic herpesviruses enter the CNS principally by retrograde axonal transport; however, entry by hematogenous spread via viremia and leukocytic trafficking may occur. These viruses also have a unique survival mechanism that allows them to hide in a latent form in nervous tissue, for example, in trigeminal ganglion of pigs infected with pseudorabies virus. Stress or other factors can activate latent virus, resulting in encephalitis.

Rhabdoviruses

Rabies Encephalitis. Rabies virus (family Rhabdoviridae) is one of the most neurotropic of all viruses infecting mammals. It is generally transmitted by a bite from an infected animal; however, respiratory infection has also been uncommonly reported after exposure to virus in bat caves, accidental human laboratory exposure, and corneal transplants.

The mechanism for spread of rabies virus from the inoculation site to the CNS is illustrated in Figure 14-44. Rabies virus may first replicate locally at the site of inoculation. Infection of and replication in local skeletal muscle myocytes is an important initiating event. The virus then enters peripheral nerve terminals by binding to nicotinic acetylcholine receptors at the neuromuscular junction. The probability is greater that the virus will be taken up by both axon terminals and myocytes after a large inoculation dose. If the virus directly enters peripheral nerve terminals, the incubation period will more likely be short, regardless of whether muscle cells are infected. With progressively lower doses of virus, however, there is a greater possibility that the virus will enter either nerve terminals or myocytes but not both. This situation can result in a short incubation period if the virus directly enters nerve terminals as described previously or could result in a more prolonged incubation period if there was initial infection and retention of virus in myocytes before its release and uptake by nerve terminals.

The virus moves from the periphery to the CNS by fast retrograde axoplasmic transport, apparently via sensory or motor nerves, at a rate of 12 to 100 mm per day. Experimental data suggest that rabies virus phosphoprotein interacts with dynein LC8, a microtubule motor protein used in retrograde axonal transport. With sensory axons the first cell bodies to be encountered after inoculation of a rear leg would be those of spinal ganglia, whose neuronal processes extend to the dorsal horn of the spinal cord. For motor axons the cell bodies of the lower motor neurons in ventral horn gray matter or neuronal cell bodies of the autonomic ganglia are the ones initially infected. It is not known whether viral infection and replication in neurons of dorsal root ganglia are essential for infection of the CNS. The virus then moves into the spinal cord and ascends to the brain using both anterograde and retrograde axoplasmic flow. During the spread of the virus between neurons within the CNS, there is also simultaneous centrifugal movement via anterograde axonal transport of the virus peripherally from the CNS to axons of cranial nerves. This process results in infection of various tissues, including the oral cavity and salivary glands, permitting transmission of the disease in saliva. An additionally important feature of

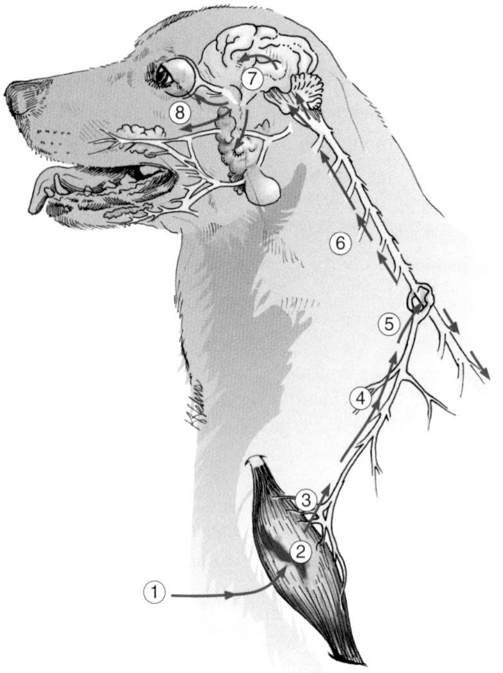

Figure 14-44 **Pathogenesis of Rabies.** After a bite wound, *1*, the rabies virus initially replicates in muscle (can enter peripheral nerves directly), *2*, enters, *3*, and ascends (retrograde axonal transport) the peripheral nerve, *4*, to the dorsal root ganglion, *5*, enters the spinal cord, *6*, and ascends, *7*, to the brain via ascending and descending nerve fiber tracts, infects brain cells, spreads to salivary glands, *8*, and the eye and is excreted in saliva.

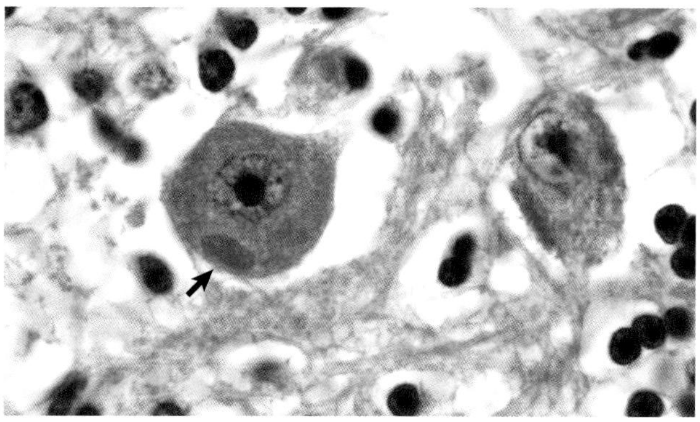

Figure 14-45 **Rabies, Negri Body, Cerebellum, Purkinje Cell, Cow.** A large pale red (eosinophilic) inclusion (Negri body) is present in the cytoplasm of the neuron cell body *(arrow)*. In the cow, Negri bodies are commonly seen in Purkinje cells and in other neurons, such as those of the red nucleus and cerebral cortex. H&E stain. (Courtesy Dr. M.D. McGavin, College of Veterinary Medicine, University of Tennessee.)

rabies is that infection of nervous and nonnervous tissue, such as the salivary glands, occur at the same time, which permits affected animals to have the required aggressive behavior plus passage of the virus into the saliva to facilitate the transmission of the disease.

The results of recent experimental studies have helped clarify the mechanism by which the virus spreads within the CNS. After axoplasmic spread of the virus from an inoculated rear leg to neurons of the associated segments of the spinal cord, rapid spread of infection to the brain occurs via long ascending and descending fiber tracts, bypassing the gray matter of the rostral spinal cord. This early spread of the virus has been suggested to explain how induction of behavioral changes occurs before there is sufficiently severe injury to cause paralysis and allows dissemination of infection before there is time for a notable immune response. Spread of infection within neurons of the CNS occurs via both anterograde and retrograde axoplasmic flow, with corresponding neuron-to-neuron spread by axosomatic-axodendritic and somatoaxonal-dendroaxonal transfer of virus. Transsynaptic spread can occur by budding of developing virions from the neuronal cytoplasm (cell body or dendrite) into a synapsing axon or in the form of bare viral nucleocapsid (ribonucleoprotein-transcriptase complexes) in the absence of a complete virion.

In vivo experimental studies using a laboratory strain of rabies virus showed that the virus caused a downregulation of approximately 90% of genes in the brain at more than fourfold lower levels. Affected genes were those involved in regulation of cell metabolism, protein synthesis, growth, and differentiation. Other experimental studies have shown increased quantities of nitric oxide in brains of rabies-infected animals, suggesting that nitric oxide neurotoxicity may mediate neuronal dysfunction. Finally, the rabies virus has been shown to induce apoptotic cell death of brain neurons in mouse models. The exact mechanism of rabies virus–induced neuronal injury in domestic and wildlife species remains to be fully determined.

Gross lesions of the infected central nervous tissue are often absent but can include hemorrhage, especially in the spinal cord gray matter. Microscopic lesions of the CNS are typically lymphocytic and include a variable leptomeningitis and perivascular cuffing with lymphocytes, macrophages, and plasma cells; microgliosis, which sometimes is prominent; variable, but often not severe, neuronal degeneration; and ganglioneuritis. Emphasis should be given to the fact that infected neurons often are minimally altered morphologically, and in some cases the only lesion noted is intracytoplasmic, acidophilic inclusion bodies, called Negri bodies (Fig. 14-45). Also, dogs are reported to have a tendency to develop a more severe inflammatory reaction than other species, such as the cow, in which little if any inflammation might occur. Nonneural lesions include variable nonsuppurative sialitis accompanied by necrosis and presence of Negri bodies in salivary epithelial cells.

Negri bodies, formed within neurons of the CNS and even in the cranial trigeminal, spinal, and autonomic ganglia, have long been the hallmark of rabies infection, although they are not present in all cases. The inclusions are intracytoplasmic and initially develop as an aggregation of strands of viral nucleocapsid, which rather quickly transforms into an ill-defined granular matrix. Mature rabies virions, which bud from the nearby endoplasmic reticulum, can also be located around the periphery of the matrix. With time the Negri body becomes larger and detectable by light microscopy. Classically in H&E-stained sections the Negri body, which is eosinophilic, has one or more small, light clear areas called *inner bodies* that form as a result of invagination of cytoplasmic components (that include virions) in the matrix of the inclusion. Inclusions that do not possess "inner bodies" have been referred to as Lyssa bodies, but they are actually Negri bodies without cytoplasmic indentation. It should also be noted that both fixed viruses (adapted to the CNS by passage) and street viruses (that produce the naturally occurring disease) produce the same ultrastructural features, but fixed viral strains generally cause severe neuronal degeneration that precludes the development and thus the detection of Negri bodies. Negri bodies also tend to occur more frequently in large neurons such as the pyramidal neurons of the hippocampus (most common in carnivores, like the dog), neurons of the medulla oblongata, and

Purkinje cells of the cerebellum (most common in herbivores, like cattle). The preferred tissues for rabies examination by light microscopy and by florescent antibody technique for virus include hippocampus, cerebellum, medulla, and the trigeminal ganglion. The typical samples submitted for fluorescent antibody staining are the medulla and cerebellum.

A spongiform lesion, indistinguishable qualitatively from the lesion characteristic for several of the spongiform encephalopathies, was described for the first time in 1984 by Charlton. This lesion was initially detected in experimental rabies in skunks and foxes and later in the naturally occurring disease in the skunk, fox, horse, cow, cat, and sheep. The lesion occurs in the neuropil of the thalamus and cerebral cortex most prominently, initially as intracytoplasmic membrane-bound vacuoles in neuronal dendrites and less commonly in axons and astrocytes. The vacuoles enlarge, compress surrounding tissue, and ultimately rupture, forming a tissue space. Although the mechanism responsible for the development of this lesion has not been determined, it is thought to result from an indirect effect of the rabies virus on neural tissue (possibly involving an alteration of neurotransmitter metabolism).

The clinical signs in domestic animals are similar with some differences between species. The clinical disease in the dog has been divided into three phases: prodromal, excitatory, and paralytic. In the prodromal phase, which lasts 2 to 3 days, the animal can have a subtle change in temperament. *Furious rabies* refers to animals in which the excitatory phase is predominant, and *dumb rabies* refers to animals in which the excitatory phase is extremely short or absent and the disease progresses quickly to the paralytic phase. Cattle and carnivores generally have the furious form of rabies, and affected animals are restless and aggressive. Other somewhat unique signs of cattle with rabies include bellowing, general straining, tenesmus, and signs of sexual excitement followed by paralysis and death. Mules, sheep, and pigs usually have the excitatory form of rabies. Horses can have early signs that are atypical for a neurologic disease but terminally tend to have the excitatory form.

When conducting a necropsy on an animal suspected of having rabies, it is important to remember (1) to provide additional protection (double gloves, mask, eye protection, and proper ventilation) for the prosector above those used for routine postmortem examination and (2) to collect the appropriate CNS tissues (hippocampus, cerebellum, and medulla and optionally the spinal cord) for examination by immunofluorescence and sometimes mouse inoculation. The remainder of the brain should be fixed by immersion in 10% neutral buffered formalin for histopathologic examination.

Bornaviruses

Borna Disease. See E-Appendix 14-2.

Fungi and Algae. Infection of the CNS by a variety of fungi and algae has been reported in domestic animals. Most reported cases are typically isolated occurrences and often represent opportunistic infection in immunocompromised individuals. Infections have involved genera such as *Aspergillus*, *Candida*, and *Mucor*; dematiaceous fungi; and the blue-green algae, *Prototheca*. These infections do not have a predilection for the nervous system. Of the systemic fungi, CNS infections have occurred with *Coccidioides immitis*, *Blastomyces dermatitidis*, *Histoplasma capsulatum*, and *Cryptococcus neoformans*, but only *C. neoformans* has a particular affinity for the CNS. These agents reach the CNS by leukocytic trafficking and hematogenous spread from primary sites of infection located in other areas (lung and skin commonly) of the body.

This group of pathogens usually elicits, as characterized by *B. dermatitidis*, a granulomatous to pyogranulomatous inflammatory response (Fig. 14-46). This response can be locally extensive, or distinct granulomas can form in the CNS and meninges. Grossly, CNS lesions consist of moderately well demarcated expansile yellow-brown foci that displace and disrupt normal tissue (Fig. 14-47). Microscopically, the exudate consists of neutrophils, macrophages (epithelioid type), and multinucleated giant cells. The latter two cell types may contain microbes in their cytoplasm. *B. dermatitidis* microbes are broad-based, budding, spherical yeastlike microbes 8 to 25 mm in diameter (Fig. 14-48). The inflammatory response, including cells (granulomatous inflammatory cells) and cytokines, leads to the axonal, neuronal, and myelin disruption observed in these mycotic diseases.

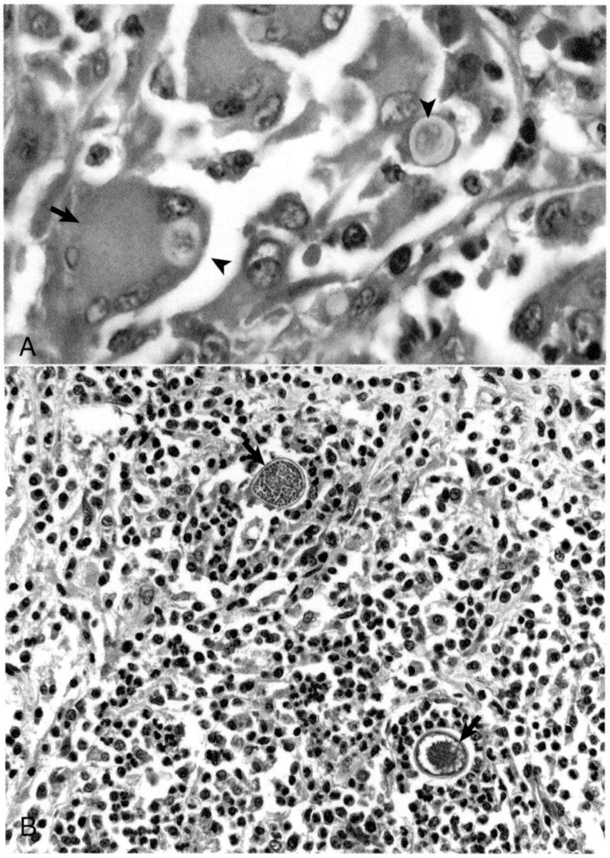

Figure 14-46 **Granulomatous Encephalitis, Brain. A,** Dog. This inflammatory response, consisting of a mixture of macrophages, multinucleated giant cells *(arrow)*, lymphocytes, varying numbers of neutrophils, and occasional plasma cells, is typical of central nervous system infections by fungi and algae. *Blastomyces dermatitidis* microbes are present in the exudate and within macrophages and giant cells *(arrowheads)*. H&E stain. **B,** Alpaca. *Coccidioides immitis*–associated encephalitis. Large numbers of neutrophils and macrophages (pyogranulomatous inflammation) surround sporangia of *C. immitis (arrows)*. H&E stain. (**A** courtesy Dr. J.F. Zachary, College of Veterinary Medicine, University of Illinois. **B** courtesy Dr. A.D. Miller, College of Veterinary Medicine, Cornell University.)

CNS infections with *C. immitis* or *H. capsulatum* elicit an inflammatory response similar to that which occurs in *B. dermatitidis*. In coccidioidomycosis the microbes are extracellular and/or intracellular spherules (20 to 30 mm in diameter) containing endospores (<5 μm in diameter), whereas in histoplasmosis the microbe principally is located intracellularly and is 5 to 6 mm in diameter. The microscopic features of these fungi are compared in Figure 14-48.

***Cryptococcus* spp.** Cryptococcosis, most commonly occurring in cats, dogs, and occasionally horses, is caused by two species

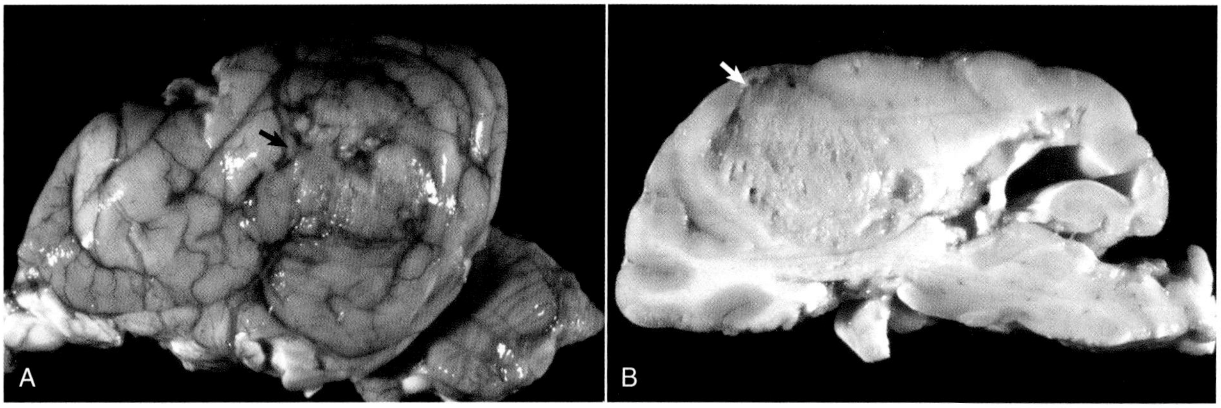

Figure 14-47 Blastomycosis, Cerebrum, Dog. A, The subarachnoid space (leptomeninges) of the left cerebral hemisphere (parietal-temporal lobes) contains a locally extensive focus granuloma caused by *Blastomyces dermatitidis (arrow)* with extension into subjacent cortex. **B,** A parasagittal section of a similar lesion from another dog shows a moderately well demarcated granuloma in the white matter of the frontoparietal cortex *(arrow)*. (Courtesy College of Veterinary Medicine, University of Illinois.)

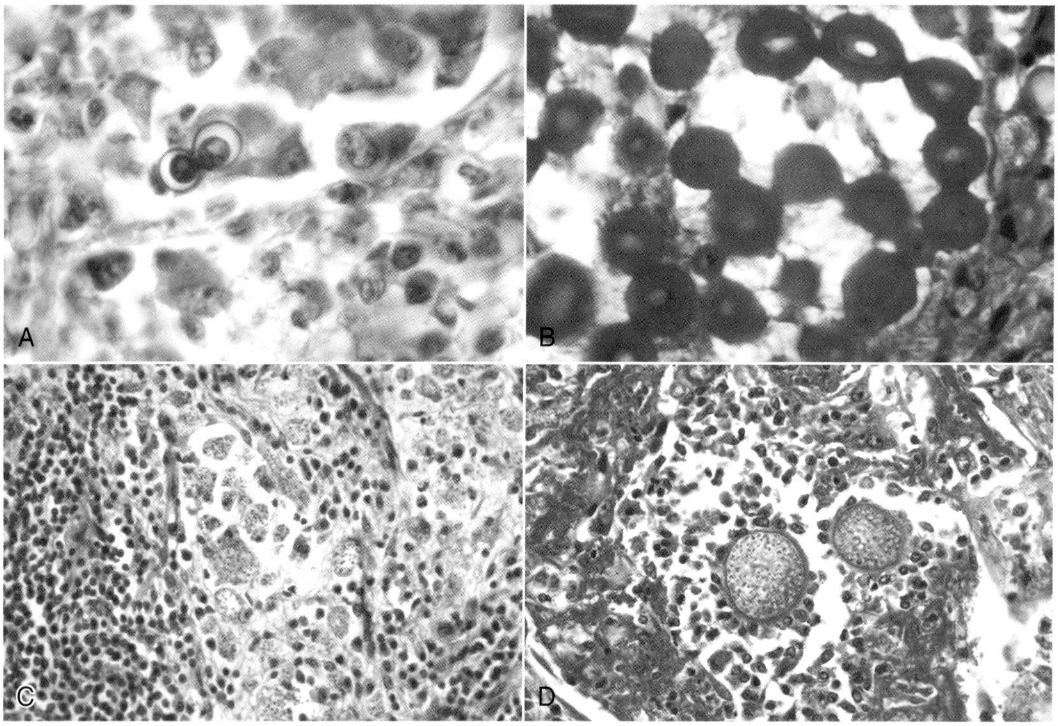

Figure 14-48 Morphologic Features of Fungi That May Infect the Central Nervous System. A, *Blastomyces dermatitidis*, 8 to 25 mm in diameter, broad-based budding spherical yeast-like microbes, intracellular or extracellular location. H&E stain. **B,** *Cryptococcus neoformans*. In this illustration the microbe is surrounded by a mucinous capsule that is stained with Mayer's mucicarmine. The capsule varies in width but can be so thick as to give the microbe an overall diameter of 30 mm. The microbe without its capsule is 5 to 20 mm in diameter. The capsule does not stain with H&E, thus causing the microbe to appear to be surrounded by a clear halo (see Fig. 14-50, A). The microbes are oval to spherical but may be crescentic or cup shaped in routine mucicarmine- and H&E-stained sections. Dehydration that occurs during processing of the tissue to embed it in paraffin causes this shrinkage and distortion. Mayer's mucicarmine stain, aqueous wet mount. **C,** *Histoplasma capsulatum*, located intracellularly, is spherical to elongated, 5 to 6 mm in diameter. H&E stain. **D,** *Coccidioides immitis*, spherules (20 to 30 mm in diameter) containing endospores (<5 mm in diameter), can be intracellular or extracellular. H&E stain. (Courtesy Dr. M.D. McGavin, College of Veterinary Medicine, University of Tennessee.)

of *Cryptococcus*, *C. neoformans* and *Cryptococcus gattii*. These pathogens enter the leptomeninges and subarachnoid space by direct extension through the cribriform plate after a nasal or sinus infection or hematogenously by leukocytic trafficking usually from a pulmonary infection. Leptomeningeal inflammation can also extend along the roots of cranial nerves. *Cryptococcus* spp. secrete a thick mucopolysaccharide capsule that protects the microbe from host defenses. The accumulation of the microbe and its mucopolysaccharide capsule gives the leptomeninges a cloudy to viscous appearance. The leukocytic response can vary from sparse to granulomatous. In some infected cats *Cryptococcus* spp. may be present in large numbers without an inflammatory response. It is unclear whether this absence of inflammation is the result of suppression of the immune response by the microbe or a defect in the cat's immune and/or inflammatory responses to the pathogen.

Two virulence factors have been documented. First, a thick mucopolysaccharide capsule protects the microbe from host defenses. Second, virulent microbes possess a biochemical pathway that can use catecholamines and that consists of a specific transport pathway and the enzyme phenoloxidase with production of a melanin or melanin-like compound through a series of oxidation-reduction reactions. This pathway can help protect the microbe from oxidative damage in the brain. Both virulence factors are important for survival of the microbe in the host. In addition, CSF lacks alternative pathway complement components that bind to the microbe's carbohydrate capsule and facilitate phagocytosis and killing by neutrophils.

Grossly, in CNS tissue and the leptomeninges, multiple small "cysts" with a viscous, gelatinous appearance can be seen (Fig. 14-49). Microscopically, leptomeningeal lesions have a loosely organized, lacy appearance with often myriad cryptococcal microbes and little or no inflammation. This is especially true in the cat as opposed to the dog, where the inflammatory response is often more intense. The leptomeningeal reaction can extend along the roots of cranial nerves. Spread of the CNS infection results in ventriculitis and choroiditis. In CNS tissue, in addition to the presence of the microbe and its capsule, the response can vary from being sparse to a granulomatous inflammation.

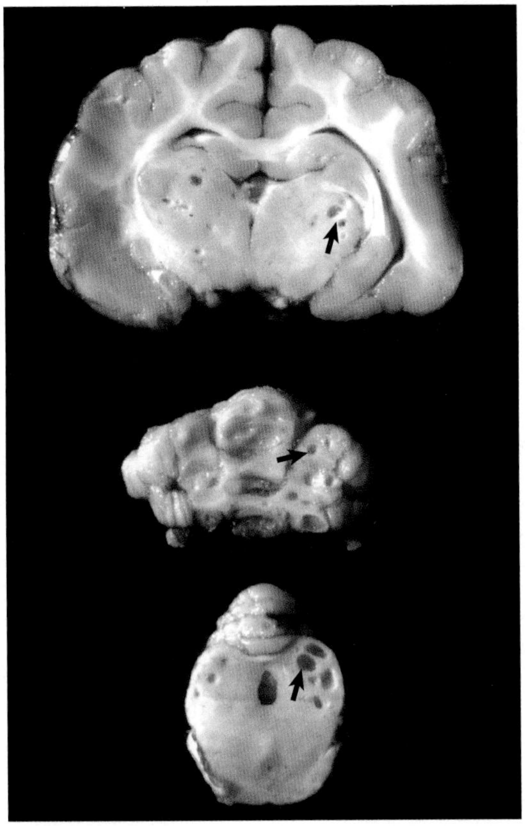

Figure 14-49 Cryptococcosis, Thalamus, Cerebellum, and Mesencephalon, Transverse Sections, Cat. Note the "cavitational" lesions caused by *Cryptococcus neoformans (arrows)*. Although the lesions look like cavities, they are filled with microbes, and the faint gray appearance is caused by the mucinous capsules of numerous cryptococci. *Cryptococcus neoformans* usually induces a granulomatous inflammation in most domestic animals, but in some animals, especially the cat, inflammation is minimal or absent. (Courtesy Dr. M.D. McGavin, College of Veterinary Medicine, University of Tennessee.)

The leukocytic response consists of neutrophils, eosinophils, macrophages, giant cells, and small mononuclear cells, depending on the immune status of the host. Animals with normal immune responses usually clear the infection from nasal cavities, sinuses, and the pulmonary system before its spreads systemically. Resistance to infection is provided by cell-mediated immunity. Immunosuppression of cell-mediated immunity caused by feline immunodeficiency virus and feline leukemia virus in cats and by *Ehrlichia canis* or long-term glucocorticoid therapy in dogs appears to increase susceptibility to cryptococcosis.

The yeast is spherical (2 to 10 mm in diameter), crescentic, or "cup shaped," usually surrounded by a thick nonstaining (H&E stain) capsule (1 to 30 mm in diameter), and reproduces by narrow-based buds (Fig. 14-50, *A*). Special stains, such as periodic acid–Schiff (PAS) and Gomori's methenamine silver, demonstrate the microbes readily, and the capsule can be stained with mucicarmine and Alcian blue (see Fig. 14-50, *B*).

Clinically, the character of neurologic signs varies with the location of the lesions but can include depression, ataxia, seizures, paresis, and blindness.

Opportunistic Fungi. Opportunistic fungi, including those fungi in the Zygomycetes group, such as *Absidia corymbifera, Mucor spp., Rhizomucor pusillus,* and *Rhizopus arrhizus,* and those fungi in the genus *Aspergillus,* such as *Aspergillus niger,* can invade blood vessels (angiotropic) and cause vascular thrombosis and infarcts in the CNS (Fig. 14-51). It must be noted that the term *opportunistic* implies that some form of tissue damage precedes fungal invasion. As an example, necrotizing enterocolitis caused by *Salmonella* spp. in the horse can provide an "open" vascular bed in the lamina propria of the intestinal mucosa that may be invaded by such fungi. Affected animals are often immunocompromised.

Protozoa

Neosporosis. Neosporosis, caused by *Neospora caninum,* has been recognized in a variety of animals, including dogs, cats, cattle, sheep, and horses, as well as laboratory rodents. In horses, neosporosis can also be caused by *Neospora hughesi.* First described in 1988 as a multisystemic infection in the dog, the microbe has an affinity

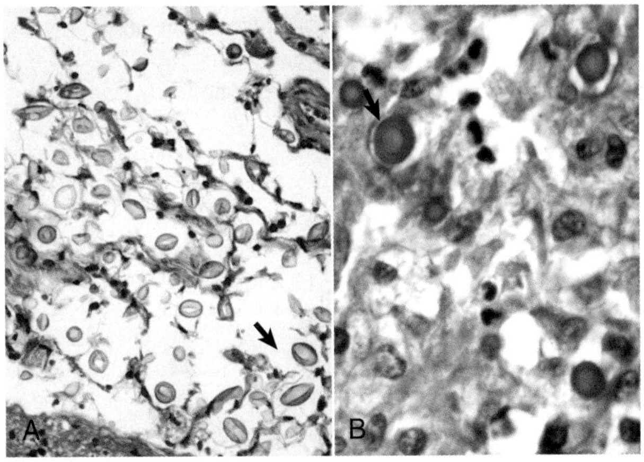

Figure 14-50 Leptomeningeal Cryptococcosis. A, The thick unstained mucinous capsule surrounding the microbe results in the formation of a clear space (halo) in H&E-stained sections *(arrow)*. This feature is useful in identifying the microbe in cytologic preparations and tissue sections. Also see Fig. 14-48, *B*. H&E stain. **B,** The mucinous capsule surrounding the microbe also stains with mucicarmine, providing a simple method to identify the microbe *(arrow)*. Mayer's mucicarmine stain. (Courtesy Dr. J.F. Zachary, College of Veterinary Medicine, University of Illinois.)

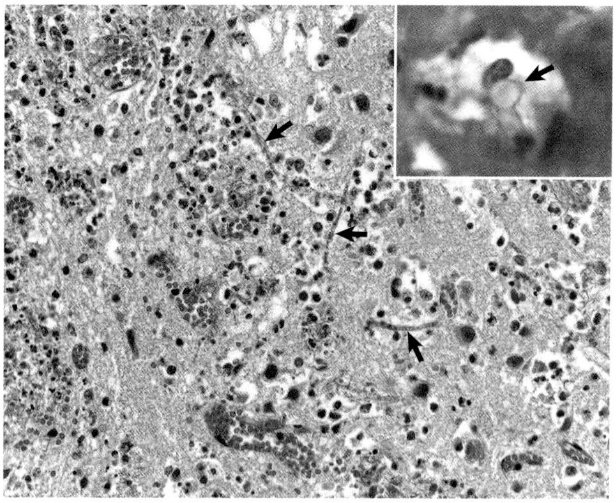

Figure 14-51 **Opportunistic Angioinvasive Fungi.** Fungi such as *Absidia corymbifera*, *Rhizomucor pusillus*, and *Rhizopus arrhizus* and fungi in the genus *Aspergillus*, such as *Aspergillus niger*, can invade blood vessels (angiotropic) and cause vascular necrosis and infarcts in the central nervous system. Note the vasculitis, hemorrhage, and disruption of the vessel and the fungal hyphae in the lumen *(arrows)*. H&E stain. *Inset*, Fungal hyphae in the lumen of a blood vessel *(arrow)*. H&E stain. (Courtesy Dr. A.D. Miller, College of Veterinary Medicine, Cornell University. Inset courtesy Dr. J.F. Zachary, College of Veterinary Medicine, University of Illinois.)

for the nervous system. The dog and its wild relatives, including coyotes and wolves, are the definitive hosts for the microbe, whereas herbivores like cattle are the typical intermediate hosts. Some of the features of the microbe are similar to those of *Toxoplasma gondii*, including division of tachyzoites by endodyogeny and having both proliferative (tachyzoites) and tissue cyst phases. However, *N. caninum* does not develop within a parasitophorous vacuole of a host cell, as does *T. gondii*. This latter feature is evident only with the use of transmission electron microscopy.

Although there are morphologic differences between the microbes (*N. caninum* has a thicker cyst wall), differentiation by light microscopy is unreliable, and electron microscopic examination or immunohistochemical analysis is required. Transmission occurs when the definitive host ingests tissue from an intermediate host that contains *Neospora* cysts. Such tissues include, but are not limited to, fetal membranes and aborted fetal tissues. Transplacental infection can also occur. *N. caninum* can infect a variety of cell types, but outside of the CNS, it appears to have an affinity for cells of the monocyte-macrophage system. The most likely method of spread to the CNS is via leukocytic trafficking.

Neurons and ependymal cells in the CNS, mononuclear cells in the CSF, and cells of blood vessels, including endothelium, intimal connective tissue, and tunica media smooth muscle cells, can harbor microbes. Microbes have also been detected in spinal nerves. Overall the morphologic pattern and character of lesions caused by *Neospora* spp. in the CNS are most consistent with multifocal necrotizing lesions with glial nodules and mixed inflammatory infiltrates. In dogs, lesions caused by *Neospora caninum* appear most frequently in the cerebellum.

Neurologic disease can be divided into two categories: that occurring during postnatal life and that associated with midterm to late-term abortions, the latter a notable problem in dairy cattle. Postnatal syndromes have been observed mainly in young and adult dogs, but horses are also affected. In young dogs, clinical signs are due to an ascending polyradiculoneuritis and polymyositis. In adult dogs, clinical signs are more referable to CNS lesions complicated by polymyositis, myocarditis, and dermatitis.

In horses the pathogen causing neosporosis is *N. hughesi*. Clinical signs resemble those of protozoal myeloencephalitis caused by *Sarcocystis neurona*. Lesions in horses include meningoencephalomyelitis; variable vasculitis and necrosis with microgliosis; and perivascular cuffing by macrophages, multinucleated giant cells, lymphocytes, plasma cells, or neutrophils, most commonly in the gray and white matter of the spinal cord but also in the pons and medulla.

Gross lesions can involve the white and/or gray matter. Peracute gross lesions may include foci of hemorrhage and necrosis distributed in a vascular pattern. Acute lesions have the same pattern of distribution but are on cut surface granular in texture and yellow-brown to gray. In some cases the periventricular white matter may be more affected. Chronic lesions have larger areas of granular yellow-brown to gray discoloration, which often makes white matter indistinguishable from gray matter. Microscopically the lesions and their temporal occurrence are similar to those described for *T. gondii*, including brain lesions that occur in aborted animals. *Neospora* spp. can be identified in tissue sections by H&E stain and immunohistochemical staining methods. Clinical signs are similar to those described for encephalitides induced by *T. gondii*.

Toxoplasmosis. Toxoplasmosis is a disease in cats and other mammalian species caused by the obligate intracellular protozoan, *T. gondii*. Domestic, feral, and wild cats are the definitive hosts of *T. gondii*. Cats acquire *T. gondii* by ingesting infective cysts, oocysts, or tachyzoites when eating infected prey, such as rodents or birds. Ingestion of one of these stages initiates the intraintestinal life cycle, which occurs only in members of the cat family. *T. gondii* replicates and multiplies within epithelial cells of the small intestine and produces oocysts. Oocysts are released into the feces in large numbers for 2 to 3 weeks following initial ingestion of cysts, oocysts, or tachyzoites. When oocysts sporulate, usually within 5 days after passage in the feces, they become infectious for intermediate hosts. Sporulated oocysts are highly resistant and can survive in moist shaded soil or sand for months. Cats are unique in the biology of the microbe, serving as both definitive (intraintestinal life cycle) and intermediate (extraintestinal life cycle) hosts.

T. gondii can infect a wide variety of animals as intermediate hosts (extraintestinal life cycle), including fish, amphibians, reptiles, birds, human beings, and many other mammals. New World monkeys and Australian marsupials are the most susceptible, whereas Old World monkeys, rats, cattle, and horses seem highly resistant.

T. gondii can also parasitize a wide variety of cell types in the intermediate host and can cause lesions in such tissues as the lungs, lymphoid system, liver, heart, skeletal muscle, pancreas, intestine, eyes, and nervous system. After ingestion, bradyzoites from tissue cysts or sporozoites from oocysts enter intestinal epithelia and multiply. There is active penetration of plasma membranes by microbe-secreted lytic products, allowing a portal of entry rather than by uptake via phagocytosis. *T. gondii* can then spread locally, free in lymph or intracellularly in lymphocytes, macrophages, or granulocytes to Peyer's patches and regional lymph nodes. Intracellularly, microbes multiply as tachyzoites within a parasitophorous vacuole by repeated cycles of endodyogeny during the early acute stages of infection. Dissemination to distant organs is via lymph and blood, either as free microbes or intracellularly in lymphocytes, macrophages, or granulocytes via leukocytic trafficking.

With chronicity and an increasing antibody response by the host, tachyzoites of *T. gondii* transform into slow-growing bradyzoites that replicate in cysts within muscle. Infection of the CNS occurs hematogenously; neurons and astrocytes are the eventual target cells. The typical sequence of events in the pathogenesis of the characteristic lesion is similar to that in *S. neurona* infection. In utero infections in animals and human beings can result in CNS infection. In fetal brains, foci of necrosis are most common in the brainstem and induce the formation of microglial nodules. Additionally, foci of necrosis and mineralization occur in the cerebrocortical white matter and are caused by fetal hypoxia and ischemia resulting from severe placentitis, fetal myocardial damage, or initiation of a systemic inflammatory reaction in the fetus. In older more mature individuals, *T. gondii* infections have been associated with immunosuppression such as occurs in concurrent CDV infection and toxoplasmosis. In some cases this could represent activation of latent inactive *T. gondii* cysts (bradyzoites) in neural tissues.

Lysis of infected cells by primed cytotoxic, $CD8^+$ T lymphocytes also could potentially contribute to the tissue damage through the production of cytokines, such as interferon-γ, which can activate microglia and astrocytes to inhibit parasite replication and induce cytotoxic T lymphocytes to kill infected cells. This exuberant inflammatory response and the cytokine cascade that ensues to kill the microbe also causes severe damage to cells in the area of inflammation, especially axons and neurons. Intracellular growth of tachyzoites also has been advanced as a cause of cellular necrosis. The microbe does not produce a cytotoxin.

The blood-brain barrier of the CNS is breached when free microbes or those located intracellularly (leukocytic trafficking) infect endothelial cells of the CNS vasculature, especially capillaries. Gross lesions can involve any area of the CNS without predilection for gray or white matter, may also involve nerve rootlets, and may initially include foci of hemorrhage and necrosis and later, granular, yellow-brown to gray foci. Peracute lesions initially include endothelial cell swelling as the result of infection by tachyzoites and vasculitis with hemorrhagic infarcts followed by vasogenic edema. If the edema is sufficiently severe to cause increased brain volume, the edema can lead to brain displacement and herniation.

Early microscopic lesions include infection of and proliferation within endothelial cells by *T. gondii* tachyzoites. Endothelial injury results in endothelial cell swelling, endothelial cell degeneration, hemorrhage, capillary occlusion, ischemic necrosis, and edema of adjacent tissue. Subsequently tachyzoites invade the CNS, inducing a prominent acute inflammatory response leading to necrosis and hemorrhage often striking in severity. With time the inflammatory response consists of perivascular cuffing of blood vessels within the CNS and leptomeninges by lymphocytes and macrophages. CNS responses to injury consist of microgliosis and astrogliosis; however, these responses are often insufficient to replace the loss of tissue in the cerebral hemispheres, resulting in dilation of the lateral ventricles (hydrocephalus ex vacuo) and the formation of persistent cysts in the tissue. With chronicity and increasing inflammatory and immunologic responses by the host, tachyzoites change to slow-growing bradyzoites that replicate in and form tissue cysts. Polyradiculoneuritis (i.e., inflammation of peripheral nerves, spinal nerve roots, and spinal cord) is also a potential sequela to infection with the microbe. Microbes in lesions can often be identified with an H&E stain, but immunohistochemical evaluation facilitates their detection and identification. Because the infection is systemic, lesions can occur in several other tissues.

Occasionally cysts (bradyzoites) can be observed in "normal" CNS tissue without an inflammatory or tissue lesion. These cysts are likely the result of a previous infection with *T. gondii* that was successfully resolved. Experimental studies have confirmed that administration of corticosteroids and thus immunosuppression increases susceptibility or exacerbates the infection with *T. gondii* or both or may contribute to the reactivation of tissue cysts.

Clinical signs can vary, depending on the age of the animal, species infected, and areas of the CNS involved and may include depression, weakness, incoordination, tremors, circling, paresis, and blindness.

Parasites. As a general concept, lesions resulting from parasitic infestation of the CNS vary in degree of severity and distribution, depending on the parasite and the host response to infection. Gross lesions of hemorrhage and malacia in parasite migratory tracts or space-occupying cysts occur with the various parasitic stages. Microscopically, there is necrosis, hemorrhage, and a leukocytic response, typically with a significant infiltrate of eosinophils. The extent of the host response is often dictated by the degree of trauma and disruption created by the parasite and the level of sensitivity of the host for parasite antigens. This section is not intended to be an extensive review of veterinary parasitology but will cover those parasites most commonly seen in veterinary practice.

Insect Larvae. Among the most common larvae are those of *Oestrus ovis* and *Hypoderma bovis*. The larvae of *O. ovis* develop in the nasal cavity of sheep but can penetrate into the cranial vault through the ethmoid bone. Larvae of *H. bovis* can enter the spinal canal during their migration in the subcutis from the hoof to the dorsal midline in cattle and rarely as an aberrant parasite in the brain of horses. Damage in the CNS caused by *H. bovis* in cattle is typically the result of inflammation directed at the degenerating parasites after anthelmintic treatment. Larvae of *Cuterebra* spp., usually a parasite of rabbits and rodents, can invade the CNS of dogs and cats and cause extensive meningeal or parenchymal lesions depending on the location through which it migrates (see the section on Feline Ischemic Encephalopathy).

Cestodes. *Coenurus cerebralis*, the larval form of the dog tapeworm *Taenia multiceps*, most commonly infests sheep and occasionally other ruminants. The larval form reaches the CNS hematogenously and then cause damage during migration and encystation, forming space-occupying lesions. In this disease the initial larval migration is associated with severe necrosis, and inflammation with larvae is often present. Another form of the parasite, in which there is an encysted "bladder," causes extensive compression of the parenchyma and associated atrophy. The parasite produces a neurologic disease known as gid. Another parasite for which human beings are the definitive host is *Taenia solium*, with pigs being the intermediate host. The larval stage, *Cysticercus cellulosae*, generally develops in muscle of the pig but can also occur in the meninges and brain, resulting in a disease called "cysticercosis." Involvement of the CNS has been termed "neurocysticercosis."

Initially, viable cysticerci become "trapped" within capillaries of the CNS, but they do not apparently elicit an inflammatory response. At some point the host responds immunologically and the cyst becomes denser, collapses inwardly, and disintegrates to eventually become calcified debris in a focus of inflammation. The inflammatory response has humoral and cellular components. Antibodies of the immunoglobulin G family are directed against the cyst; however, cysts are likely killed by mediators released from eosinophils, which are attracted to the site by mediators released from lymphoid cells in the inflammatory exudate. For undetermined reasons, in "susceptible" animals viable cysts can become established and grow slowly for years. Viable cysticerci can cause asymptomatic infection by actively evading and suppressing the immune response of the host. These cysts cause vasogenic edema and increased intracranial pressure related to behavior as "space-occupying" masses.

Gross lesions are usually seen in the cerebral hemispheres, commonly at the interface of gray and white matter in a hematogenous pattern. Cysts can also be found in the cerebellum, medulla, ventricles, subarachnoid space, and the spinal cord. There are usually no gross changes in the CNS surrounding the cysts. Cysts are round to oval and of varied sizes and number, many of which can be large and visible up to centimeters in diameter. They have a translucent cyst wall and contain a thick, clear fluid. Within the fluid is a scolex, visible as a small 2- to 3-mm nodule. Microscopically, there is little or no inflammation or tissue injury surrounding the cysts, except for compression and edema.

Nematodes (Cerebrospinal Nematodiasis). Aberrant migration of larval stages of nematode parasites into and through the CNS is called cerebrospinal nematodiasis. Important causes of cerebrospinal nematodiasis include *Parelaphostrongylus tenuis* (ruminants, camelids), *Strongylus vulgaris* (horse), *Elaphostrongylus rangiferi* (small ruminants), *Toxocara canis* (dogs), and *Baylisascaris procyonis* (many species including dogs, primates, rabbits, and birds). They gain access to the CNS hematogenously and actively enter the CNS by crossing the blood vessel wall through their locomotive processes. Nematodes cause damage in the cerebromedullary area of the brain and/or spinal cord either from aberrant migration in the definitive host or migration in an aberrant host (Table 14-4; Fig. 14-52). Greater CNS damage is often created by the migration of the parasites in an aberrant host.

Macroscopic lesions of nematode larval migration often appear as linear or serpentine tracts of necrosis and/or hemorrhage in the tissue. Migration results in endothelial injury, vasculitis, and thrombosis, which may result in vascular occlusion and infarction. Larvae can often be found in histologic sections, and they induce a mononuclear cell inflammatory exudate, including abundant eosinophils (Fig. 14-53).

Halicephalobus gingivalis is a free-living rhabditiform nematode that can infest the nasal cavity, CNS, and kidneys of the horse. The life cycle, pathogenesis, and route of infection of *Halicephalobus gingivalis* are poorly understood. It has been proposed that the CNS is infected hematogenously in a manner similar to that described for cerebrospinal nematodiasis and that larvae penetrate skin and mucous membranes in recumbent horses with subsequent invasion of sinuses and/or blood vessels. In the CNS, microscopic lesions are prominently associated with blood vessels along which the parasite apparently migrates.

Table 14-4 Nematodes Causing Central Nervous System Disease in Domestic Animals

Parasite	Normal Host	Aberrant Host
NEMATODE MIGRATION IN ABERRANT HOST		
Angiostrongylus cantonensis	Rat	Dog
Baylisascaris procyonis	Raccoon	Dog
Elaphostrongylus rangiferi	Reindeer	Sheep, goat
Parelaphostrongylus tenuis	Deer	Sheep, goat
Setaria digitate	Cattle	Sheep, goat, horse
ABERRANT NEMATODE MIGRATION IN NORMAL HOST		
Angiostrongylus vasorum	Dog (coyote)	
Dirofilaria immitis	Dog (cat)	
Stephanurus dentatus	Pig	
Strongylus spp.	Horse	

Prions

Transmissible Spongiform Encephalopathies. Ovine spongiform encephalopathy (scrapie), bovine spongiform encephalopathy (BSE), and human spongiform encephalopathies are classified within a group of diseases called *transmissible spongiform encephalopathies*. Table 14-5 lists the known transmissible spongiform encephalopathies in animals and human beings. These diseases are caused by proteinaceous infectious particles (prions) that (1) are composed of an abnormal isoform of a normal cellular protein, the prion protein (PrP^C [a 27- to 30-kD polypeptide]), designated PrP^{Sc} and (2) resist inactivation by procedures that degrade nucleic acids and proteins (i.e., heat, ultraviolet irradiation, and strong enzymes). PrP^C is expressed throughout the body and is the product of a highly

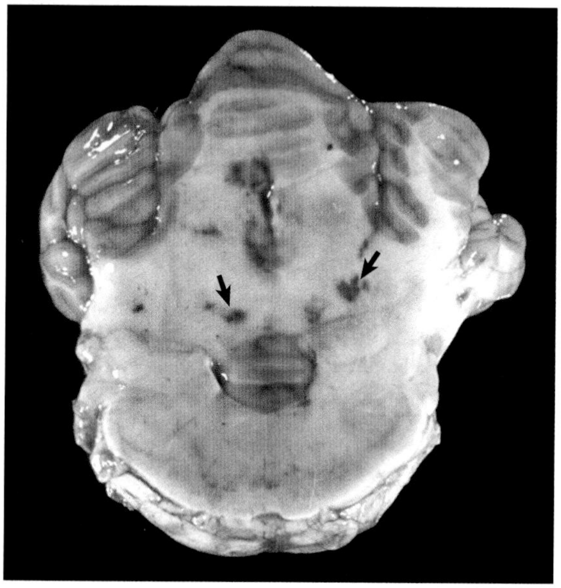

Figure 14-52 **Cerebrospinal Nematodiasis, Brain, Cerebellum, and Medulla at the Level of the Pons, Horse.** *Strongylus vulgaris* migration. Several small foci of hemorrhage and necrosis in the cerebellar white matter are sites of larval migration *(arrows)*. (Courtesy Dr. R. Storts, College of Veterinary Medicine, Texas A&M University.)

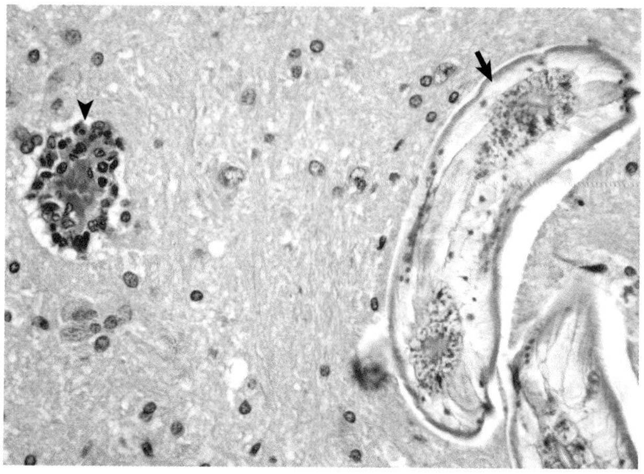

Figure 14-53 **Cerebrospinal Nematodiasis, Central Nervous System (CNS), Rabbit.** Migration of *Baylisascaris procyonis (arrow)* in the CNS elicits a perivascular lymphomonocytic inflammatory response mixed with eosinophils *(arrowhead)* and results in direct injury to blood vessels, axons, and dendrites. H&E stain. (Courtesy Dr. J.F. Zachary, College of Veterinary Medicine, University of Illinois.)

Table 14-5 Transmissible Spongiform Encephalopathies (i.e., Prion Diseases)

Disease	Natural Host(s)	Prion	Pathogenic PrP Isoform
ANIMALS			
Ovine spongiform encephalopathy (scrapie)	Sheep, goats	Scrapie prion	$OvPrP^{Sc}$
Bovine spongiform encephalopathy (BSE)	Cows	BSE prion	$BoPrP^{Sc}$
Feline spongiform encephalopathy (FSE)	Cats	FSE prion	$FePrP^{Sc}$
Chronic wasting disease (CWD)	Mule deer, elk, black-tailed deer, white-tailed deer, mink	CWD prion	$MdePrP^{Sc}$
Transmissible mink encephalopathy (TME)		TME prion	$MkPrP^{Sc}$
Exotic ungulate encephalopathy (EUE)	Nyala, greater kudu, oryx	EUE prion	$UngPrP^{Sc}$
HUMAN BEINGS			
Kuru	Human beings	Kuru prion	$HuPrP^{Sc}$
Creutzfeldt-Jakob disease (CJD)	Human beings	CJD prion	$HuPrP^{Sc}$
Variant Creutzfeldt-Jakob disease (VCJD)	Human beings	VCJD prion	$HuPrP^{Sc}$
Gerstmann-Sträussler-Scheinker syndrome (GSS)	Human beings	GSS prion	$HuPrP^{Sc}$
Fatal familial insomnia (FFI)	Human beings	FFI prion	$HuPrP^{Sc}$

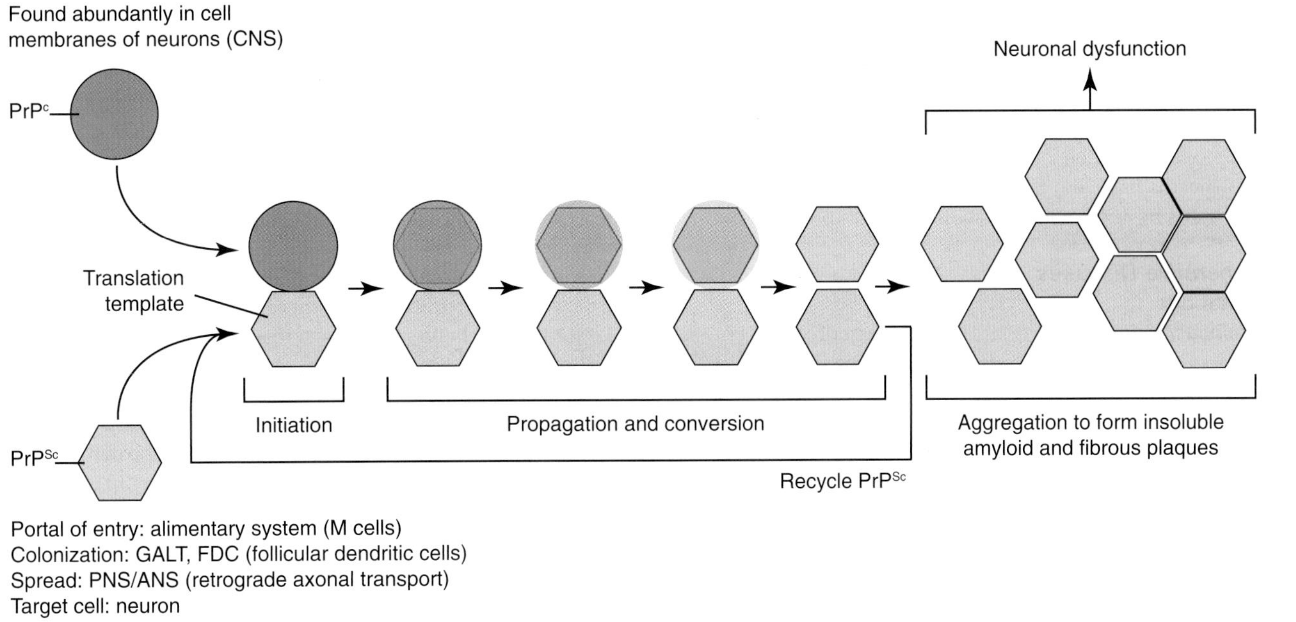

Figure 14-54 Prion Protein. In prion diseases (spongiform encephalopathies), PrP (PrP^C), a normal neuronal protein, is converted to an abnormal β-pleated sheet isoform (PrP^{Sc}) through the interaction of PrP^{Sc} with PrP^C. *ANS*, Autonomic nervous system; *CNS*, central nervous system; *GALT*, gut-associated lymphoid tissue; *PNS*, peripheral nervous system. (Courtesy Dr. A.D. Miller, College of Veterinary Medicine, Cornell University; and Dr. J.F. Zachary, College of Veterinary Medicine, University of Illinois.)

conserved gene found in microbes as diverse as fruit flies and human beings. The "Sc" superscript is derived from the word "scrapie" because scrapie is the prototype prion disease.

Although the mechanism by which PrP^{Sc} forms has not been completely explained, a posttranslational modification of PrP^C has been proposed (Fig. 14-54). This mechanism proposes that PrP^{Sc} acts as a template on which PrP^C undergoes a conformational change (is refolded) by a process facilitated by another protein (referred to as protein X), whereby the α-helical content of PrP^C diminishes and the amount of β-sheet increases, resulting in the formation of PrP^{Sc}. The features of a specific PrP^{Sc} are determined by the animal in which it is formed. When PrP^{Sc} of one species is inoculated into a different species, the recipient is less readily infected and generally has a prolonged incubation period. This resistance to infection is referred to as the species barrier.

Spongiform encephalopathies occur through horizontal transmission (feeding rendered cattle CNS tissue to cattle) or through an inherited mutation of the normal human prion gene. In animals the primary route of infection appears to be through horizontal transmission. For chronic wasting disease, horizontal transmission is surprisingly effective, and prions can be readily transmitted in saliva, blood, and urine. It has been proposed that prions ingested in infective feedstuffs enter the body through the intestine. Prions cross the intestinal wall at Peyer's patches and are phagocytosed and transported to other lymph nodes by leukocytic trafficking. Prions replicate in lymphocytes and macrophages of the lymphoid system before gaining access to the blood. The autonomic nervous system is important in delivering the prions to the CNS and neurons; however, the exact mechanisms of spread remain to be elucidated. Eventually neurons accumulate sufficient PrP^{Sc} to alter the normal function (it can take years), and neurologic signs are observed.

Prion diseases are fatal. The adaptive immune system does not recognize prions as foreign; therefore no immunologic protection develops. How the accumulation of PrP^{Sc} causes neurodegeneration and neuron loss in prion diseases is not clear; however, astrocyte and microglial cell activation and apoptosis appear to be likely components of the pathway leading to neuronal injury.

No gross lesions of the nervous system are detectable in animals with spongiform encephalopathies. Microscopic lesions in scrapie-infected sheep and goats are limited to the CNS and are most commonly present in the diencephalon, brainstem, and cerebellum (cortex and deep nuclei), with variable lesions in the corpus striatum and spinal cord. Except for some minor changes, the cerebral cortex is essentially unaffected.

The type of neuronal degeneration can vary and commonly is characterized by shrinkage with increased basophilia and cytoplasmic vacuolation (Fig. 14-55, *A*), although other changes, such as central chromatolysis and ischemic cell change, variably occur. Astrocytosis in affected areas of the brain, including the cerebellar cortex, can be severe (see Fig. 14-55, *B*). There has been speculation whether the astrocytic reaction is a primary or a secondary response. An abnormal protein (prion amyloid protein) first accumulates in astroglial cells in the brain during scrapie infection, which could mean that this cell is the primary site of replication. The spongiform change tends to affect the gray matter, and greater severity of this lesion has been associated with long incubation periods. The lesion in the gray matter is the result of dilation of neuronal processes, but vacuolation of neuronal and astroglial perikarya, swelling of astrocytic processes, dilation of the periaxonal space, and splitting of myelin sheaths have also been reported. Finally, the disease is not accompanied by any notable inflammation within the CNS.

Degenerative Diseases

Metabolic

Aminoacidopathies. Two diseases characterized by errors of amino acid metabolism have been described in neonatal calves. One disease, maple syrup urine disease (MSUD), occurs in young polled Hereford and Hereford calves. The second disease, bovine citrullinemia, which was originally described in Australia, occurs in neonatal Friesian calves.

Maple syrup urine disease is caused by an inherited defect in the branched-chain α-ketoacid enzyme decarboxylase and results in a deficiency of this enzyme, which is necessary to metabolize the branched-chain amino acids leucine, isoleucine, and valine. These amino acids are essential and must be obtained from protein in the diet. After consumption, proteins are digested, and the amino acids are released to be used to generate energy and for other metabolic processes. In maple syrup urine disease there is a mutation in one or more of the genes that regulate this degradation process; therefore abnormal metabolites and ketoacids accumulate to toxic levels and cause disease. Urine has a sweet odor attributable to a derivative of isoleucine resembling the smell of maple syrup. In human infants the disease is confirmed biochemically by finding elevated concentrations of leucine, isoleucine, and valine in the blood.

Gross lesions are not typically present. Microscopically, marked spongiosis, caused by vacuolation of myelin sheaths, is present throughout the neuraxis. The spongiosis affects both gray and white matter. Lesions are often most notable in areas, such as the brainstem, in which there is an intermingling of gray and white matter.

Affected calves may be normal at birth. Within a few days, depression, dullness, and weakness progress to recumbency and opisthotonus.

Bovine citrullinemia is a rare inborn error of metabolism of the urea cycle that results in a pronounced accumulation of citrulline and ammonia in the body fluids because of a failure of the normal synthesis of arginosuccinic acid by the enzyme arginosuccinate synthetase. In human infants the disease is confirmed biochemically by finding elevated concentrations of citrulline in the blood. The cerebral lesions have also been suspected to result from the hyperammonemia or possibly some defect in excitatory neurotransmitter metabolism. However, the pathogenesis of the disease in calves remains unsettled.

Grossly, brains are normal and have normal weights. Livers are pale yellow. Microscopically, there is fatty change in the liver. Lesions in the brain are characterized by mild to moderate diffuse astroglial swelling in the cerebral cortex. Perivascular, perineuronal, and periglial spaces are typically expanded by edema.

Calves are normal at birth. Within a few days a severe generalized CNS disorder develops characterized by apparent blindness, depression, and tremors that rapidly progress to seizures, coma, and death within a few hours.

Cerebral Cortical Atrophy. Brain atrophy caused by the loss of neurons in the cerebral cortex can occur in all animal species and is most commonly associated with chronic degenerative conditions

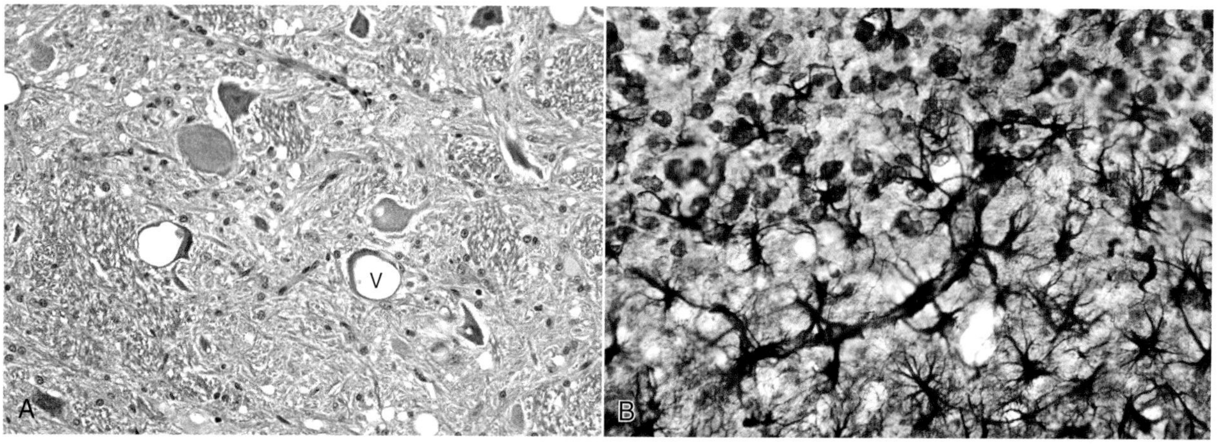

Figure 14-55 Spongiform Encephalopathy (Scrapie), Brain, Motor Neurons, Sheep. A, Neuronal cell bodies contain one or more discrete and/or coalescing clear vacuoles (*V*). There are no inflammatory cells in this disease. Similar spongiosis is evident in the neuropil. H&E stain. **B,** Scrapie, experimental, brain, cerebellum, mouse. The cerebellar granule cells are at the top of the figure. There is notable hypertrophy and proliferation (astrocytosis) of astrocytes and their fibers (astrogliosis) (*black branching fibers*). Some of the processes (running diagonally across the illustration) end, as is normal for astrocytes, on the walls of capillaries. Cajal's gold sublimate stain for astrocytes. (**A** courtesy Dr. D. Gould, College of Veterinary Medicine and Biomedical Sciences, Colorado State University; and Dr. M. McAllister, College of Veterinary Medicine, University of Illinois. **B** courtesy Dr. W.J. Hadlow.)

of the CNS in which neuronal dysfunction and eventual loss occurs. An example of cortical atrophy is seen in cerebral ceroid-lipofuscinosis, a storage disorder that occurs in many different species. Atrophy most frequently involves the cerebral hemispheres, especially the cortex. The cerebral hemispheres are increased in firmness and often have a tan color (lipofuscin), gyri are thinned, and the sulci widened. Microscopically, there is loss of neuron cell bodies in cortical laminae without inflammation. Astrogliosis in response to neuronal loss is also observed, as is an increased prominence of the adventitial layer of blood vessels.

Channelopathies. Channelopathies are a newly emerging group of inherited neuromuscular diseases of human beings that affect the excitability of membranes of neurons and skeletal myocytes. These diseases result from mutations in genes encoding ion channel proteins that regulate calcium, sodium, and chloride channels and acetylcholine receptors. In human beings, neurologic diseases, such as epilepsy and migraine headaches, have been attributed to channelopathies. In veterinary neurology, channelopathies will likely be shown in the future to be the underlying mechanism for epilepsy and other primary neuronal degenerations; however, investigation into this type of neurologic disorder is still in its infancy in veterinary medicine. Examples of this type of disorder are the recent demonstration of mutated cyclic nucleotide-gated ion channels in several dog breeds with vision disorders.

Degenerative Leukomyelopathies. Degenerative leukomyelopathies are a heterogeneous group of familial, likely inherited, and acquired diseases that have been described in dogs, cows, and horses. Although there is no universal agreement, the degenerative leukomyelopathies described here are best characterized as axonal degenerations with spheroid formation predominantly within spinal cord white matter and secondary changes in myelin sheaths and myelin loss. In dogs, familial or inherited diseases include degenerative axonopathy of Ibizan hounds, axonopathy in Labrador retrievers, and axonopathy in Jack Russell and smooth fox terriers. A disease in Rottweilers (see the section on Primary Cerebellar Neuronal Degeneration in the section on Dogs and the section on Cats) is another disorder with spinal cord white matter involvement that is familial and inherited. An acquired disease, hound ataxia, has been described in the United Kingdom and Ireland in harriers, beagles, and foxhounds. Hound ataxia may represent a nutritional disorder in hunting dogs fed paunch (tripe). Degenerative leukomyelopathies in cattle can be inherited as an autosomal recessive trait or have a familial predisposition. Leukomyelopathies have been reported in Murray Grey, Holstein-Friesian, and in certain lines of Brown Swiss cattle.

Gross lesions are usually not observed. Microscopically, lesions in the white matter of the spinal cord are bilaterally symmetric and consist of axonal degeneration with formation of spheroids, loss of axons, and secondary myelin degradation. Depending on the species or breed affected, lesions can involve any of the funiculi. Spinocerebellar tracts in the dorsolateral aspects of the lateral and septomarginal areas of ventral funiculi are commonly affected, as is the fasciculus gracilis in the dorsal funiculus. Severe involvement of the dorsal spinocerebellar tracts can extend into the caudal brainstem and via caudal cerebellar peduncles to the cerebellar cortex and Purkinje cells. In some species and breeds, there can also be involvement of additional specific brainstem structures.

Age of onset varies with the familial or inherited disorders. Paresis, ataxia, and dysmetria are the predominant clinical signs.

Epileptic Brain Damage. Brain damage caused by prolonged (usually > 30 minutes) convulsive seizures (status epilepticus) is not widely recognized; however, it has been described secondary to either malformative lesions or tumors in the CNS. In human beings and experimental animals, brain damage resulting from status epilepticus is well documented. One study reported a relatively high incidence of brain lesions in dogs caused by status epilepticus. In this study, acute brain damage was widespread and corresponded well with areas of the brain prone to hypoxic-ischemic injury such as the cerebral cortex, pyriform cortex, basal nuclei, and hippocampus.

The cause of neuronal injury with prolonged convulsive seizures is debatable. It remains unclear if necrosis, apoptosis, or a combination of these two mechanisms causes neuronal injury in status epilepticus. During seizures there is an increased metabolic demand for glucose and oxygen by neurons; however, cerebral blood flow increases during seizures so that the amount of glucose and oxygen available for neurons to generate energy remains adequate, at least during earlier stages. Acute neuronal necrosis still occurs even when cerebral blood flow, oxygenation, body temperature, and other metabolic parameters are maintained within normal limits in experimental animals with status epilepticus.

Excitotoxic injury caused by accumulation of neurotoxic amino acid neurotransmitters, such as glutamate, during the extreme neuronal activity occurring in status epilepticus, is an attractive explanation for neuronal necrosis. Excitotoxicity would account for both the selective vulnerability of certain brain areas and the character of the lesions. Status epilepticus induced experimentally in rats with kainic acid, an excitatory amino acid receptor agonist, has been shown to cause primarily neuronal necrosis and some characteristics of apoptosis. Other experimental studies have suggested that astrocytes produce clusterin during status epilepticus. Clusterin (dimeric acidic glycoprotein), a sulfated glycoprotein, initiates apoptosis when expressed in cells in elevated concentrations. It is proposed that clusterin secreted by astrocytes during status epilepticus is actively endocytosed by hippocampal neurons, and these neurons die by an apoptotic mechanism. The exact mechanism of neuronal injury remains to be proved. There is some evidence that the mature brain is more prone to injury induced by status epilepticus than the immature brain.

Gross lesions, if present, usually consist of widened and flattened gyri and narrow indistinct sulci caused by cerebral edema. Acute neuronal ischemic cell change and astrocytic swelling are observed microscopically. In experimental animals with status epilepticus, neuronal degeneration is observed within 30 minutes and neuronal necrosis within 60 minutes.

Hepatic Encephalopathy. Acute and chronic liver failure, as well as hepatic atrophy associated with congenital or acquired vascular shunts, often results in hepatic encephalopathy and disordered neurotransmission because of the accumulation of toxic substances, principally ammonia, in the systemic circulation and thus the CNS. Ammonia is formed in the gastrointestinal tract by bacterial degradation of amines, amino acids, purines, and urea from proteins consumed in the diet. In healthy animals, ammonia is detoxified in the liver by conversion to urea by the ornithine citrulline arginine urea cycle. Urea is far less toxic than ammonia and is excreted in the urine. Ammonia has several neurotoxic effects such as (1) changing the transit of amino acids, water, and electrolytes across the neuronal cell membranes and (2) inhibiting the generation of both excitatory and inhibitory postsynaptic potentials in neurons. Ammonia and other toxic metabolites also (1) cause increased permeability of the blood-brain barrier, leading to vasogenic edema, and (2) alter osmoregulation within the CNS. These mechanisms likely led to the spongy change (status spongiosus) characteristic of the disease microscopically. Because astrocytes play an important role in regulating fluid and electrolyte balances in the CNS and are the primary cell type having lesions

(Alzheimer's type II astrocytes) in hepatic encephalopathy, it is not surprising that alterations in osmoregulation are a component of the pathogenesis of the disease. Astrocytes also contain high concentrations of glutamine synthetase, an enzyme that breaks ammonia into glutamine. Recent research indicates that glutamine, although a normal breakdown product, may actually have deleterious effects on astrocytes and may be one of the main contributors to astrocyte dysfunction noted in hyperammonemic states. Ammonia and other toxic metabolites likely also affect oligodendroglia. Finally, it has been proposed that alterations in the blood-brain barrier may facilitate passage of neurotoxins such as short-chain fatty acids, mercaptans, false (pseudo-) neurotransmitters (tyramine, octopamine, and β-phenylethanolamine), ammonia, and GABA into the CNS, leading to neuronal dysfunction. A similar condition, termed renal encephalopathy, has been described in dogs, ruminants, and horses. It is likely related to high concentrations of ammonia or ammonia-metabolites in the circulation because of inadequate renal clearance caused by severe glomerular or tubular injury.

In all species except the horse, lesions of hepatic encephalopathy are of two types: spongy change and formation of Alzheimer's type II astrocytes (see Fig. 14-10, *D*). Spongy change can be present throughout the neuraxis but typically involves areas of confluence or intermingling of gray and white. It is bilateral and symmetric in distribution. These areas include the deep cerebrocortical gray-white matter interface where the peripheral fibers that radiate from the corona radiata are found, basal nuclei and adjacent internal capsule, reticular areas throughout the brainstem, and deep cerebellar nuclei. The spongy change is due to intramyelinic edema, causing splitting and vacuolation of myelin sheaths. Spongy change can be produced experimentally by ammonia infusion and is reversible. Alzheimer's type II astrocytic change is a subtle alteration that has been reported in all domestic animals and is the only CNS change observed in horses with hepatic failure. Alzheimer's type II astrocytes are found in gray matter and have enlarged vesicular nuclei with peripheral chromatin, glycogen deposits, and demonstrable nucleoli or nucleolar-type bodies. They often occur in diads, triplets, or clusters of even high numbers. Immunohistochemical staining for GFAP is typically weak or absent, possibly indicating a toxic effect on astrocytes.

Clinically, affected animals show CNS signs such as seizures, ataxia, depressed mentation, walking aimlessly, and head pressing.

Mitochondrial Encephalopathies. In human beings, various encephalopathic and myopathic syndromes caused by point mutations in mitochondrial DNA affecting tRNA genes are grouped under the acronyms MELAS (mitochondrial encephalopathy, lactic acidosis, strokelike episodes) and MERRF (myoclonic epilepsy with ragged red fibers). The various human syndromes include Leigh's disease (subacute necrotizing encephalomyelopathy), Kearns-Sayre syndrome, and Leber's hereditary optic atrophy.

Diseases that might be classified as mitochondrial encephalopathies are not well characterized in animals. Despite this caveat, the diseases reported in the Australian cattle dogs, English springer spaniel dogs, and a Jack Russell terrier, as well as in Limousin and Simmental cattle and New Zealand South Hampshire sheep, could represent mitochondrial disorders. Table 14-6 summarizes the salient features of the diseases. Characteristics of these diseases in both human beings and animals are symmetric bilateral involvement of the neuraxis and lesions typified by status spongiosus (edema of cerebral white matter) with variable progression to cavitation or necrosis. The CNS is highly dependent on oxidative metabolism and is therefore the most severely affected organ in mitochondrial disorders. Mitochondria isolated from affected human patients have impaired oxygen consumption and reduced respiratory chain enzyme complex activity.

Notably excluded from this list is the Alaskan husky, a breed that has a well-characterized encephalopathy that is morphologically similar to Leigh's disease in human beings. However, recent research has failed to reveal mutations in mitochondrial genes but rather has found an association between a mutation in the thiamine transporter 2 gene (*SLC19A3*) and the development of the disease. In this disease, bilaterally symmetric foci of encephalomalacia are often found in the thalamus, caudate, pons, medulla oblongata, and along the gray-white matter border of the cerebral cortices. The histologic lesions are typified by an abundance of astrocytes, some of which can be highly bizarre and vacuolated. The disease is included in this section because it can be considered a secondary mitochondrial disease, rather than a primary mitochondrial dysfunction.

Primary Neuronal Degeneration. Primary neuronal degeneration that occurs in many or all animal species is discussed in this section. Disorders of individual animal species are discussed in sections covering disorders unique to that species.

The term *primary neuronal degeneration* encompasses three groups of diseases affecting specific regions of the CNS in a temporally and

Table 14-6 Possible Mitochondrial Encephalopathies in Animals

Animal	Age of Onset (months)	Clinical Signs	Primary Lesions
Cattle dog	5 to 12	Seizures, behavioral abnormalities followed by locomotor signs	Spongiosis and cavitation in cerebellum, brainstem nuclei, and spinal gray matter
English springer spaniel	15 to 16	Ataxia, disorientation, visual deficits	Status spongiosus in accessory olivary nucleus; axon loss and gliosis in optic nerve and tracts
Jack Russell terrier	2.5	Ataxia, hypermetria, and deafness	Neuronal degeneration and mineralization of the medulla oblongata, vestibulocochlear nerve, choroid plexus, and granule cell layer of the cerebellum
Limousin cattle	1 to 4	Locomotor signs, aggressive behavior, blindness	Spongiosis, cavitation in cerebral and cerebellar white matter, brainstem nuclei, optic chiasm
Simmental cattle	5 to 12	Ataxia, behavioral changes	Spongiosis and necrosis in internal capsule, caudate nucleus, putamen, brainstem nuclei, spinal gray matter

spatially stereotyped manner and are characterized by degeneration, necrosis, and loss of specific populations of functionally linked neurons. Box 14-8 gives an overview of these diseases. The first group includes the multisystem neuronal degenerations, which are diseases that affect populations of functionally related neurons in the basal ganglia, brainstem, and cerebellum. The second group includes the primary cerebellar neuronal degenerations, which are diseases that affect populations of neurons restricted to the cerebellum and cerebellar roof nuclei. The third group includes primary spinal cord degenerations, which are diseases associated with axonal swellings (axonal spheroids) in the neuraxis termed neuroaxonal dystrophies. Another term used to denote some of these diseases in the biomedical literature and veterinary textbooks is *abiotrophy*; this term was introduced by Gowers in 1902. The term literally means lack of ("a") a vital ("bios") nutrition ("trophy") required to sustain the life of a tissue. For discussion of the primary neuronal degeneration affecting individual animal species, see sections covering disorders specific for the species.

Box 14-8 Multisystem Neuronal Degenerations and Brainstem/Spinal Syndromes in Domestic Animals

MULTISYSTEM NEURONAL DEGENERATIONS

Canine: Kerry blue terrier, red-haired cocker spaniel, Cairn terrier

PRIMARY CEREBELLAR DEGENERATION

Neonatal Syndromes

Canine: Beagle, Samoyed, Irish setter
Ovine: Welsh mountain, Corriedale
Bovine: Hereford, Hereford cross, Ayrshire

Postnatal Syndromes

Canine: Airedale, German shepherd, Gordon setter, rough-coated collie, border collie, Finnish terrier, Bernese mountain dog, Bern running dog, Labrador retriever, golden retriever, cocker spaniel, Cairn terrier, Great Dane
Bovine: Holstein-Friesian, Hereford cross, Angus
Equine: Arabian, Arabian cross, Gotland pony
Ovine: Merino
Porcine: Yorkshire

MITOCHONDRIAL ENCEPHALOPATHY (ENCEPHALOMYOPATHY)

Canine: English springer spaniel, Alaskan husky, Australian cattle dog, English setter dog, Jack Russell terrier
Bovine: Simmental, Limousin
Sheep: New Zealand South Hampshire

SPONGY DEGENERATION

Canine: Labrador retriever, Saluki, silky terrier, Samoyed
Bovine: Jersey, shorthorn, Angus-shorthorn, Hereford
Feline: Egyptian Mau

BRAINSTEM AND SPINAL SYNDROMES

Neuroaxonal Dystrophy

Canine: Border collie, Chihuahua, Rottweiler
Feline: Domestic
Equine: Morgan
Ovine: Suffolk

Motor Neuron Disease–Spinal Cord

Canine: Brittany spaniel, Swedish Lapland, English pointer, Rottweiler, German shepherd, sheepdog, collie, pug, dachshund, fox terrier
Feline: Siamese
Bovine: Brown Swiss, Hereford (shaker calf syndrome)
Equine: Various breeds (not believed hereditary)
Porcine: Hampshire, Yorkshire

Degenerative Leukomyelopathies (Spinal Cord–White Matter)

Canine: German shepherd, Afghan hound, Kooikerhondje, Labrador retriever, Ibizan hound, harrier, beagle, foxhound, Rottweiler, smooth fox terrier, Jack Russell terrier
Bovine: Brown Swiss, Holstein-Friesian, Murray Grey
Equine: Various breeds (see vitamin E deficiency)

Multisystem Neuronal Degeneration. Multisystem neuronal degeneration is discussed in sections covering disorders unique to individual animal species.

Primary Cerebellar Neuronal Degeneration. Depending on the degree of maturation of the cerebellum and related systems at the time of birth in the various species, clinical signs in animals with the neonatal syndromes can be manifest in the immediate postnatal period (bovine, ovine) or can be delayed until the time of ambulation (canine). Hereditary transmission is known or suspected in some instances. Lesions vary among affected species and breeds but overall include degeneration or absence of Purkinje cells, proximal swelling of Purkinje cell axons, variable loss of granule cells, cortical astrogliosis, and degeneration of nuclei in the cerebellar medulla.

Animals with postnatal cerebellar syndromes are normal at birth or at the time of ambulation. Onset of ataxia with various other clinical signs referable to cerebellar disease begins weeks, months, or even years after a period of apparently normal development. Initial clinical signs are often subtle. Progression of the signs can be slow or rapid, relentless, or with static periods. Some individuals reach a stage without further progression of signs, but this is not typical of the syndrome in most animals.

Grossly, the cerebellum can be normal or reduced in size and atrophic. Microscopically, lesions are analogous to those that occur in the neonatal syndromes with loss of Purkinje cells, variable neuronal depletion in the granule layer, and astrogliosis in the molecular layer. Fusiform swellings of proximal Purkinje cell axons are found in the rough-coated collie and the Yorkshire pig. In the rough-coated collie and Merino sheep, lesions occur in other areas of the neuraxis. In these syndromes, degeneration and loss of neurons in the deep cerebellar and other nuclei are accompanied by axonal degeneration in the cerebellum, brainstem, and spinal cord. Loss of spinal ventral horn motor neurons has been noted in the rough-coated collie. An autosomal recessive mode of inheritance is suspected or documented in several of the diseases. For individual disorders, see sections covering disorders of individual animal species.

For discussion of the primary cerebellar neuronal degeneration affecting individual animal species, see sections covering disorders specific for the species.

Neuroaxonal Dystrophy. Diseases associated with axonal swellings (axonal spheroids) have been termed *neuroaxonal dystrophy*. Diseases include those putatively associated with vitamin E deficiency or that have been interpreted as an aging change (see the section on Degenerative Diseases). Included here are diseases with a species and breed association and onset relatively early in life, generally before 1 year of age but varying between 4 weeks and 3 years. A hereditary basis is often suspected or proved. Neuroaxonal dystrophies have been described in many animal species; however, they seem to be most common in dogs and horses. Neuroaxonal dystrophies of the horse are discussed in the section covering disorders unique to that species.

Dystrophy is defined as a disorder arising from defective or faulty nutrition of a cell, tissue, or organ, and the term is most commonly applied to muscle diseases. In this usage it applies to neurons and their axons (neuroaxonal). Lesions differ in severity and distribution, but are characterized by prominent axonal swellings in various nuclei (often sensory) in the brainstem, cerebellum, and spinal cord. Loss of cerebellar Purkinje and granule cells have been reported in Rottweilers and cats and the loss of brainstem neurons in cats. In the Morgan horse the axonal swellings are associated with vacuolation.

Neuroaxonal dystrophies are often characterized clinically by severe and often profound muscular weakness and widespread muscle atrophy. Sporadic cases in older adult animals also occur of unknown cause or suspected extraneous influence. Clinical signs vary but include gait abnormalities, dysmetria or hypermetria, proprioceptive disturbance, ataxia, or other cerebellar signs.

Motor Neuron Diseases. Motor neuron diseases have been described predominately in dogs, cats, cows, horses, and pigs. Degeneration and loss of motor neurons in the ventral horns of the spinal cord and variable axonal degeneration in the ventral spinal nerve rootlets and peripheral nerves characterize the lesions in motor neuron diseases. In some of the motor neuron diseases there is prominent swelling of ventral horn neuronal cell bodies or axons, or both, associated with marked accumulation of neurofilaments. This accumulation is presumably caused by posttranslational protein modification and impairment of neurofilament protein transport. Degeneration in some diseases is not strictly limited to motor neurons of the spinal cord or to motor neurons in general. Other sites of involvement are motor or sensory nuclei, or both, in the brainstem and white matter tracts in the spinal cord.

In horses, lesions in motor neurons are analogous to those already described. The disease affects various breeds, no definitive familial association or age predilections are known, and an inherited basis is not suspected. Generalized weakness, muscle atrophy, and weight loss progress over 1 to several months.

In calves a disease known as *shaker calf syndrome* in horned Hereford calves can be only loosely termed a motor neuron disease. There is marked accumulation of neurofilaments within neurons of the central, peripheral, and autonomic nervous systems. All segments of the spinal cord are severely affected. Neurons and neuronal processes in ventral horns, intermediolateral nucleus, Clarke's column, and substantia gelatinosa are swollen and distended. Wallerian degeneration occurs in ventral nerve rootlets and white matter of the spinal cord. Brainstem lesions are less prominent. Swollen cerebellar Purkinje cells and neuronal degeneration in the lateral geniculate body and frontal cortex are reported. The disorder occurs in newborn calves and is characterized clinically by tremulous shaking of the head, body, and tail.

Nutritional

Vitamin B_1 (Thiamine) Deficiency. Thiamine pyrodiphosphate is the active form of thiamine. It is a critical cofactor for several thiamine-dependent enzymes involved in carbohydrate metabolism, and brain damage is thought to be related to a decline in thiamine-dependent enzymes, energy deprivation, and oxidative stress with the abnormal metabolism of free radicals in neurons. These enzymes are also important in the synthesis of several cell constituents, including neurotransmitters. Thiamine deficiency has been associated with neurologic disease in carnivores (Chastek's paralysis), human beings (Wernicke's encephalopathy), and ruminants. For discussion of nutritional diseases affecting individual animal species, see sections covering disorders specific for the species.

Vitamin A Deficiency. See the section on the PNS and Chapter 21.

Box 14-9 Other Toxicities Involving the Nervous System

CHEMICALS

Heavy metals: Cadmium, manganese, mercury, tin (trimethyltin), zinc
Hexacarbons: n-Hexane, others
Pesticides: Carbaryl, bromethalin, chlorinated hydrocarbons
Drugs: Nitrofurazones, ivermectin, levamisole, metronidazole

PLANTS

Cycads, *Chrysocoma tenuifolia*, *Helichrysum* spp., *Solanum* spp. (*dimidiatum*, *fastigiatum*, *kwebense*), sorghum, *Stypandra* spp.

MYCOTOXINS

Acremonium, *Aspergillus*, *Claviceps*, fumonisin, *Penicillium*

Toxicoses. Space constraints do not allow a comprehensive discussion of all toxicities affecting the nervous system. Box 14-9 is a partial listing of poisons with the potential to cause CNS injury and neurologic illness. Some of these, such as mercury, have in the past caused high morbidity and mortality in isolated outbreaks. An example is the 1956 Minamata Bay incident in Japan of human beings eating fish containing high concentrations of methylmercury. Methylmercury accumulates in the aquatic food chain, and thus the highest concentrations exist in predatory fish at the top of the food chain. In human beings and animals with methylmercury toxicosis, neuronal cell bodies of the cerebral cortex and cerebellum die through a mechanism suggested to be apoptosis; however, microtubule dysfunction, oxidative stress, alterations of calcium homeostasis, and the potentiation of glutaminergic excitotoxicity may be involved. The potential remains for serious neurologic illnesses and death from these intoxications, and the interested reader is referred to more comprehensive reference sources. In this chapter, discussion of toxicities is limited to those conditions most likely to be encountered in veterinary practice.

Chemicals. Chemically induced distal axonopathies have been classified by functional alterations affecting motor or sensory neurons, location of injury within the nerve (distal, proximal), or by the type of nerve affected (cranial or spinal). Because of the large number and wide use of chemicals in commerce, there exists an extensive list of experimental studies describing toxic axonopathies and neuropathies. Their complete discussion is outside the scope of this chapter.

Chemicals used in agricultural, industrial, and pharmaceutical commerce can injure nerves by interfering with axoplasmic flow. Such chemicals include acrylamide (polymerizing agent to strengthen paper), carbon disulfide (fat solvent, used for extraction of oil from oil-bearing fruit such as olives), triorthocresyl phosphate (high-performance lubricants in airplane engines), halomethane (refrigerants), methylene chloride (extraction agents, paint solvents, and degreasing agents), carbon tetrachloride (solvents), and butane (fuel source).

Acrylamide causes a unique distal axonopathy (dying-back axonopathy) primarily affecting axons of the PNS (less commonly the CNS) in which there is accumulation of neurofilaments within affected axons. Axonal spheroids are thought to be related to alteration of axonal transport resulting from phosphorylation of neurofilaments and their abnormal rearrangement within the axon. This "dying-back" axonopathy is microscopically characterized by degeneration of axons starting at or near synapses and proceeding toward the neuronal cell body. The most distal axonal projections are furthest from the cell body and thus cannot be maintained. Thus they are most vulnerable to functional alterations; however, it is unclear whether this degeneration is caused by energy deficits, lack of antioxidants, or physical obstruction of axoplasmic flow. Axonal degeneration is followed by secondary demyelination.

Certain types of toxic and biochemical injury to axons result in a stereotypic pattern of morphologic change that affects either distal or proximal segments of the axon and results in the formation of segmental axonal spheroids. Based on the location of the spheroids, such diseases are divided into one of two groups, either diseases affecting axons a distance away from their cell bodies (distal axonopathies) or diseases affecting axons near their cell bodies (proximal axonopathies).

Axonal spheroid formation and subsequent axonal degeneration are caused by alterations in axoplasmic flow and by alterations of anterograde or retrograde flow, depending on the nature of the injury resulting in the accumulation and/or rearrangement of cytoskeletal proteins. The histologic lesion common to these two types of axonopathies is the formation of axonal spheroids with subsequent degeneration of the axon and secondary demyelination, which is a process that in many ways resembles the lesions described for Wallerian degeneration. Axonal spheroids are common to a variety of neuronal derangements; therefore distal and proximal axonopathies must be differentiated from other diseases that cause spheroids such as the compressive axonopathies.

Distal and proximal axonopathies have been further subdivided by some scientific disciplines into groups based on whether initial axonal lesions progress in an anterograde or retrograde direction. The terminology and classification schemes, although useful to some, are outside the scope of this chapter and are often confusing. The occurrence of secondary anterograde or retrograde lesions is discussed in the context of some of the diseases presented next.

Organophosphates. Organophosphates are divided into two groups according to their use, mode of action, and type of toxicity. The first group, organophosphate esters, used as pesticides (parathion, malathion, diazinon, carbaryl, or aldicarb), fungicides, herbicides, or rodenticides, cause acute toxicity by inhibiting cholinesterase either directly or indirectly and allowing acetylcholine to accumulate at synaptic (nerve-nerve junctions) or myoneural junctions (nerve-muscle junctions), resulting in persistent depolarization. In acute organophosphate toxicosis, clinical effects vary but are manifested in the following:

1. Parasympathetic nervous system, leading to salivation, lacrimation, urination, defecation, bradycardia, and pupillary constriction
2. Skeletal muscular system, resulting in muscle fasciculations followed by weakness and muscle paralysis (i.e., death is due primarily to respiratory failure)
3. CNS, leading to anxiety, restlessness, hyperactivity, anorexia, and generalized seizures (i.e., observed in dogs and cats but uncommon in cattle)

Gross and microscopic lesions in the nervous system are absent, and those in other tissues are nonspecific.

The second group causes chronic toxicosis and is the most common cause of chemically induced distal axonopathy in veterinary medicine. This group of organophosphates includes the cresyl and related compounds such as triorthocresyl phosphate used in hydraulic fluids, lubricants, flame retardants, and plasticizers. The triaryl phosphate group of compounds used as high-temperature lubricants is toxic for several species of animals and human beings.

Chronic exposure (delayed neuropathy) to certain organophosphate pesticides and herbicides (trichlorphon, merphos, triorthocresyl phosphate, leptophos, parathion, malathion, and diazinon) causes delayed neurotoxicity unrelated to cholinesterase inhibition as seen in acute organophosphate toxicosis. The type of axonal injury caused by these chemicals follows the stereotypic process of morphologic changes described previously and occurs approximately 10 to 14 days after exposure. Organophosphorus compounds causing delayed neurotoxicity inhibit the activity of an enzyme referred to as *neuropathy target esterase*. The function of the enzyme in the PNS and CNS is not fully understood.

Phosphorylation of the enzyme by the toxic compound is proposed to interfere with its normal function, resulting in axonal injury. Other studies have shown that organophosphates causing delayed neurotoxicity interact with Ca^{2+} or calmodulin kinase II, an enzyme responsible for phosphorylation of cytoskeletal proteins, such as microtubules, neurofilaments, and microtubule-associated protein-2, resulting in disassembly and accumulation of these proteins in the distal portions of axons, producing axonal swelling and degeneration.

No specific gross lesions are present in chemically induced distal axonopathies. Microscopically, there is retrograde degeneration beginning in the distal part of axons, especially those with a larger diameter. Affected areas in the spinal cord include dorsal funiculi, spinocerebellar tracts in lateral funiculi, and ventromedial aspects of the ventral funiculi. Central chromatolysis of cell bodies of affected nerves has occurred.

Clinically, signs of toxicity are usually delayed 1 to 2 weeks after exposure. Young animals, because of their ability to compensate for the neurologic deficits, tend to be less seriously affected, whereas recovery is slow and incomplete in adults. Susceptible animals include cats, domestic and exotic ruminants, chickens, pheasants, and ducks. Small laboratory animals, dogs, and some nonhuman primates are less sensitive. Clinical signs are those of combined sensory and motor neuropathy and spinal cord damage, such as proprioceptive deficits expected by damage to the spinocerebellar nucleus and tract, as well as the fasciculus gracilis.

Selenium. An acute paralytic syndrome termed *bilateral poliomyelomalacia* has been observed in feeder pigs associated with the inadvertent inclusion of toxic amounts of selenium (selenium-enriched yeast, sodium selenite, or sodium selenate) in pig rations. The pathogenesis of the lesions is not proved but could involve an induced nicotinamide or niacin deficiency. Experimentally, 6-aminonicotinamide, a gliotoxin and antagonist of the vitamin, causes lesions analogous to those seen in the natural porcine disease.

Grossly, bilateral (symmetric) areas of softening and yellow discoloration occur in the ventral spinal gray matter of the cervical and lumbar intumescences. Microscopically, acute lesions consist progressively of neuronal chromatolysis, neuronal necrosis, neuronal loss, microcavitation, and glial necrosis. As would be expected, these changes are subsequently followed by astrogliosis and the accumulation of gitter cells. Prominent capillaries are typical. Wallerian degeneration occurs in ventral spinal nerve rootlets of those cord segments whose ventral gray horn motor neurons have been destroyed. Identical lesions have been observed in the brainstem.

Clinically, affected pigs are alert, rest in sternal recumbency, and squeal loudly when disturbed. They eventually progress to quadriplegia with flaccid paralysis of the rear limbs. Cutaneous manifestations of the toxicity also occur and include rough hair coats, partial alopecia, and separation and sloughing of the hoofs. Historically, a similar ovine bilateral symmetric poliomyelomalacia has been reported from Africa, but an association with selenium toxicity was not made.

Sodium Chloride. Sodium chloride toxicity, also known as *sodium ion toxicosis*, *water deprivation syndrome*, or *salt poisoning*, occurs primarily in pigs, poultry, and occasionally in ruminants, dogs, horses, nonhuman primates, and sheep. The disease occurs after overconsumption of sodium chloride in rations or supplements and can be complicated by limited availability of drinking water, resulting in severe dehydration. A similar sequence of events can occur with simple water restriction of sufficient duration to allow compensation by the brain's adaptive response to chronic hypernatremia (hyperosmolarity). Sodium chloride toxicity is due to hyperosmolarity (hypernatremia) caused by excessive intake of sodium salts or severe dehydration followed by rehydration and a "rapid" hypernatremic to normonatremic or hyponatremic shift.

During the initial hypernatremic phase the brain "shrinks" because of the osmotic loss of water. An influx of sodium, potassium, and chloride ions into the brain, beginning within minutes after the osmotic loss of water, is an acute adaptive response to equalize the sodium imbalance. Maintenance of a normal ionic balance in the brain is critical, however, for normal function, and although a new ionic equilibrium is established, this acute response alone cannot compensate for severe or prolonged hypernatremia.

A second, more delayed adaptive response of the brain is an influx or endogenous production of organic osmolytes, such as certain amino acids, polyols, and methylamines, to equalize the osmotic imbalance created by hypernatremia. This response requires hours or days to establish a new osmotic equilibrium. When animals are given free access to fresh water, an acute hypernatremic to hyponatremic shift occurs. Within minutes the brain attempts to offset this osmotic imbalance by eliminating sodium, potassium, and chloride ions by actively transporting these ions into the vasculature. This early response cannot, however, offset the osmotic stress created by the increased organic osmolytes in the brain. As a result of the osmotic gradient created by the elevated organic osmolytes, water enters the brain with subsequent brain swelling.

Grossly, lesions are inconsistent, but include cerebral and leptomeningeal congestion and edema. Zones of cerebrocortical laminar necrosis can be detected in transverse slices of fixed brain. Microscopically, cerebrocortical neuronal necrosis, often laminar, is accompanied by astrocytic swelling. In pigs, leptomeninges and perivascular spaces can have an infiltrate of eosinophils, and with longer survival, an influx of macrophages occurs, depending on the extent of necrosis (Fig. 14-56). The leptomeningeal and perivascular infiltrate of eosinophils is an inconsistent finding and can be a nonspecific finding in various porcine encephalitic disorders. However, when it occurs in conjunction with laminar cortical necrosis, it is indicative of salt toxicity in this species. Pallor of subcortical white matter is indicative of edema, and prominence of small cortical blood vessels is due to congestion and swelling of endothelial cell nuclei. In ruminants, arteriolar degeneration with a transmural neutrophilic infiltrate, cerebellar Purkinje cell necrosis, and edema of basal nuclei, thalamus, and midbrain have been observed.

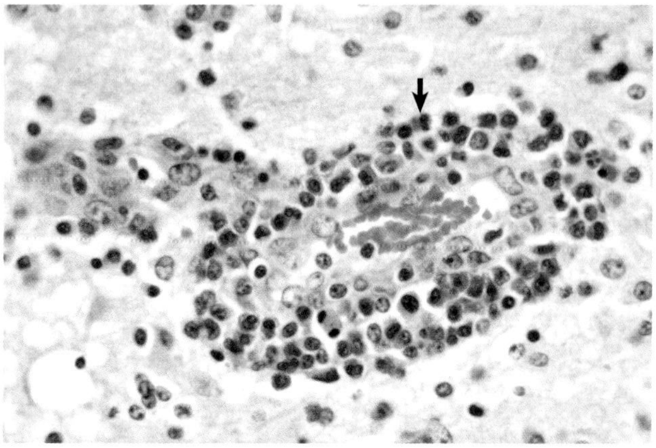

Figure 14-56 **Eosinophilic Meningoencephalitis, Cerebral Cortex, Gray Matter, Pig.** Note the accumulation of eosinophils *(arrow)* in the perivascular space. This response is characteristic of the lesions of hypo-osmotic edema caused by water deprivation or excessive consumption of sodium salts. The surrounding neuropil is edematous. H&E stain. (Courtesy Dr. M.D. McGavin, College of Veterinary Medicine, University of Tennessee.)

Clinical signs include inappetence and dehydration early followed by heading pressing, incoordination, blindness, circling, paddling, and convulsions. Animals are often found dead in their pasture or pen.

Metals

Arsenic. Toxicity caused by ingestion or cutaneous absorption can occur with inorganic and organic arsenicals and can affect multiple organs, including the nervous system. Inorganic compounds are predominantly herbicides or pesticides, whereas organic arsenicals (e.g., arsanilic acid) have been used as feed additives in the pig and poultry industries as growth promoters and to control enteric diseases.

Poisoning with inorganic arsenicals is an acute enteric disease with hepatic and renal manifestations, but neurologic signs can occur. Probably because of the nature of the organic compounds and the manner of their use, there is greater potential for neurotoxicity. Arsanilic acid has a greater tendency to cause peripheral and optic nerve and tract damage, whereas 3-nitro compounds tend to affect the spinal cord more severely.

Gross lesions are not present. Microscopically, lesions in cranial and peripheral nerves and spinal cord consist of axonal degeneration and fragmentation of myelin sheaths. In the spinal cord after 3-nitro poisoning, lesions are found chronologically in the cervical and thoracic cord followed by lesions in the lumbar cord. Spinocerebellar tracts and dorsal funiculi are predominantly affected. The distribution of lesions suggests that the distal segments of long ascending fiber tracts can be preferentially injured. Inorganic arsenicals inhibit sulfhydryl enzyme systems and disrupt cellular metabolism. The exact mode of action of organic arsenicals is unknown.

In pigs clinical signs include blindness resulting from damage to optic nerves and tracts and incoordination, paresis, and paralysis related to spinal cord and peripheral nerve lesions.

Lead. Lead poisoning has occurred in a variety of animals, but with the increased awareness of the potential for toxicity and environmental contamination and current regulations, such as reduced concentrations in paint and unleaded gasoline, poisoning is uncommon and if it occurs is most common in cattle. Potential sources include discarded car batteries and old flaking or peeling lead paint in barns and farm buildings.

Depending on the quantity absorbed, poisoning can be peracute with no gross or microscopic lesions, acute, subacute, or chronic. In peracute or acute cases, contents of the upper digestive tract, such as fragments of battery plates or flakes of paint, could indicate the possibility of lead poisoning. Lead poisoning can affect many tissues and organs, including CNS, PNS, liver, kidneys, gastrointestinal tract, bone marrow, blood vessels, and organs of the reproductive and endocrine systems. In horses grazing lead-contaminated pastures, a cranial neuropathy with laryngeal and facial paralysis has been described.

Lead poisoning in cattle and other species is via the oral route or less commonly via the respiratory system or skin (inorganic lead). Lead can damage the brain through a variety of mechanisms. Direct toxic effects on neurons, astrocytes, and cerebral endothelial cells occur by disrupting metabolic pathways and altering the function of dopaminergic, cholinergic, and glutaminergic neurotransmitter systems. Lead crosses the blood-brain barrier rapidly using a cationic transporter, concentrates in the brain because of its ability to substitute for calcium ions in the pump, and enters astrocytes and neurons by voltage-sensitive cell membrane calcium channels. Lead disrupts calcium homeostasis, causing the accumulation of calcium in lead-exposed cells, and induces mitochondrial release of calcium, leading to apoptotic cell death. Astrocytes contain metallothionein and can sequester potentially toxic metals in the CNS, thus protecting more vulnerable neurons from the toxic effects of lead. However, astrocytes may also be sensitive to the toxic effects of lead, leading to functional deficits such as in the uptake, transport, and metabolism of neurotransmitters. Transplacental (human beings and sheep) and neonatal lead exposure can result in delayed brain maturation and biochemical abnormalities.

Gross lesions in the CNS are usually absent. When present, they can resemble those present in polioencephalomalacia of cattle, but this is uncommon. In general, gross lesions, if present, are distributed in a laminar pattern and include meningeal and cerebrovascular congestion, brain swelling with flattening of gyri, or hemorrhage. With longer survival times, there may be foci of cerebrocortical malacia (softening), cavitation, and laminar necrosis followed by cerebral cortical atrophy, widened sulci, narrowed gyri, and loss of white matter.

Microscopically, lesions in peracute cases are absent. In acute cases, congestion, astrocytic swelling, status spongiosus, and microvascular prominence caused by endothelial hypertrophy are present, and often ischemic neuronal cell change is characteristically confined to the tips of cerebrocortical gyri. For most cases in cattle, only a few necrotic neurons at gyral tips and minimal astrocytic swelling, vascular prominence, and congestion can be found. With longer survival times, cerebrocortical lesions progress to laminar necrosis, accumulations of macrophages, or liquefactive necrosis, although the last is rare. Because of their similarities, lesions of lead encephalopathy in ruminants must be differentiated from those of thiamine deficiency–associated polioencephalomalacia and sulfur-related polioencephalomalacia.

Lesions in dogs resemble those in cattle, but vascular damage is more obvious and consistent. Vascular lesions can progress to mural hyalinization, necrosis, and thrombosis. Other lesions include neuronal necrosis in the cerebral cortex, hippocampus, and cerebellum (Purkinje cells), myelin destruction in cerebrocortical white matter, and a peripheral neuropathy.

Clinically, affected cows are often found down or dead in the pasture. If clinical signs are present, they range initially from depression, inappetence, and diarrhea to teeth grinding (bruxism), circling, head pressing, incoordination, and blindness later. In small animals, especially dogs, clinical signs include ataxia, tremors, clonic-tonic seizures, blindness, and deafness.

Bromethalin. Bromethalin, a highly lipophilic (i.e., high fat concentration in the brain) nonanticoagulant rodenticide, kills rodents, such as moles and voles, and domestic animals (predominantly dogs and cats secondary to accidental exposure) by uncoupling oxidative phosphorylation in mitochondria of neural cells. As a result, there is a decrease in ATP synthesis and dysfunction of ATP-dependent Na^+ and K^+ ion channel pumps. This outcome results in the accumulation of Na^+ (and water) in neural cells and thus cytotoxic cerebral edema (see the section on Cerebral Edema [Permeability Changes]), leading to increased intracranial pressure and injury of neurons and their myelinated axons. Lesions, in addition to cerebral edema, include intramyelinic edema, myelin splitting, and axonal swelling, which all manifest as white matter spongiosis. Poisoned animals are usually depressed, have convulsions, varying degrees of ataxia, paresis, and paralysis, and may die.

Organotins. Excessive exposure to organotins, such as triethyltin (stabilizer, catalyst, wood and textile preservative, fungicide, bactericide, and insecticide), causes cytotoxic edema principally affecting myelin sheaths of oligodendroglial cells in the white matter. Experimental studies have shown that triethyltin selectively damages myelin sheaths and causes a decrease in potassium concentrations in the white matter with a concurrent increase in intracellular water content. The blood-brain barrier is not affected. The mechanism of injury is thought to be uncoupling of oxidative phosphorylation and inhibition of mitochondrial ATPase activity within cell membranes. Loss of Na^+/K^+-dependent ATPase activity in cell membranes of myelin lamellae leads to the formation of intramyelinic edema.

Gross lesions, if present, consist of an enlarged brain and spinal cord. Because of compression against the cranium, an affected brain has flattened gyri and shallow indistinct sulci. Microscopically, fluid accumulates between myelin layers and leads to splitting of the myelin lamellae and the formation of intramyelinic spaces.

Microbial Toxins

Botulism. See the section on Peripheral Nervous System.

Tetanus. Tetanus is a spastic paralytic disease caused by the neurotoxin called *tetanospasmin* produced by *Clostridium tetani*. Similar to *Clostridium botulinum*, the bacterium is a ubiquitous Gram-positive spore-forming anaerobe commonly found in soil. Tetanospasmin is synthesized in anaerobic wounds and first binds at myoneural junctions and/or sensory receptors. It is transported via retrograde axoplasmic flow within the axon and across synaptic junctions until it reaches the CNS (see Fig. 4-28). In the CNS the toxin is transferred across synapses until it becomes fixed to gangliosides in the presynaptic inhibitory motor neuron. Tetanospasmin blocks the release of inhibitory neurotransmitters such as glycine and GABA. Inhibitory neurotransmitters act to dampen the actions of excitatory nerve impulses from upper motor neurons that are imposed on lower motor neurons. If these impulses cannot be dampened by normal inhibitory mechanisms, the generalized muscular spasms characteristic of tetanus ensue. Tetanospasmin appears to act by selective cleavage of a protein component of synaptic vesicles, thus preventing the release of neurotransmitters by the cells. Once toxin is bound to synapses, the administration of antitoxin is useless.

This disease is most common in horses but may also occur in lambs castrated in areas contaminated with spores of *C. tetani*. Tetanus also has been reported in cows, pigs, dogs, and cats. Except for the anaerobic wound, there are no macroscopic and microscopic tissue lesions in tetanus. Infected horses initially show signs of colic and muscle stiffness involving muscle groups of the lips, nostrils, ears, jaw (lockjaw), and tail. Horses are hyperesthetic and rapidly have a spastic and tetanic paralytic syndrome develop.

Plant Toxins

***Astragalus*, *Oxytropis*, and *Swainsona* Poisoning.** *Astragalus*, *Oxytropis*, and *Swainsona* represent three genera of plants with species that are toxic to livestock. As many as 300 species of *Astragalus* grow in North America, and the genus is the largest of any legume family in this part of the world. Three categories of toxicity can be observed with *Astragalus*, depending on the mechanism or manner of toxicity: nitro-containing, selenium-accumulating, and poisoning of the locoweed type. Only the last is discussed here. Locoweed poisoning, or locoism, is associated with ingestion of certain species of *Astragalus* and *Oxytropis* in North America and *Swainsona* in Australia. The toxic principles have been termed *locoine* and *swainsonine*, respectively.

The mechanism of toxicity has been clarified by the isolation of the indolizidine alkaloids swainsonine and swainsonine N-oxide from *Astragalus lentiginosus*. Recent discoveries have pinpointed the fungal endophyte *Undifilum oxytropis* as the ultimate source of swainsonine. The swainsonine compounds inhibit lysosomal α-mannosidase, thus inducing an acquired α-mannosidosis that mimics the inherited storage disease mannosidosis. Mannosidases are glycoside-hydrolyzing enzymes that are found in the Golgi, lysosomes, and cytoplasm of all mammalian cells. Analyses of tissue from animals poisoned with swainsonine have shown that swainsonine is present in all tissue; however, neurons; epithelial cells in organ systems, such as the liver; and macrophages of the monocyte-macrophage system of the spleen and lymph nodes are commonly affected. Therefore, as occurs in the inherited storage disease (mannosidosis), acquired swainsonine-induced storage diseases affect similar cells throughout the body. Additionally, swainsonine interferes with normal synthesis of glycoproteins containing asparagine-linked complex oligosaccharides. Swainsonine also inhibits Golgi mannosidase II, an effect not recognized in the inherited disorder.

There are no specific gross lesions in acquired swainsonine-induced storage diseases. Microscopically, lesions involve neuronal cell bodies throughout the neuraxis and autonomic ganglia and are analogous to the inherited lysosomal storage diseases.

Microscopically, neuron cell bodies are swollen, and nuclei are sometimes displaced to the periphery of the cell body. The cytoplasm appears foamy or finely vacuolated. The material that accumulates in the cytoplasm does not stain for lipid. Irregular fusiform enlargements, called *meganeurites*, occur in the proximal axon segment, and aberrant synapses form. With time, lesions include distal axonal degeneration and neuronal necrosis with mineralization. The presence of cytoplasmic lesions in other cells of the CNS, such as astrocytes, depends on the degree to which α-mannosidase is expressed in individual cell populations. Astrocytes are hydropic or swollen, but their appearance is less dramatic and diagnostic when compared with changes in neurons. Macrophages recruited from the bloodstream to phagocytose debris and mannose released from dead neurons also are affected by swainsonine. Microgliosis and neuronophagia are present but inconspicuous.

Similar to the swelling and vacuolation of neurons, this process also occurs in cells throughout the body, including hepatocytes, exocrine pancreatic cells, renal tubular epithelium, endocrine organs (thyroid, parathyroid, and adrenal glands), circulating leukocytes, and cells of the monocyte-macrophage system in liver, spleen, and lymph nodes. Ingestion of the plants of these species by females during gestation can also result in abortion or birth of weak neonates that have similar lesions.

Cattle, sheep, and horses are generally affected. Toxicity is usually insidious, and clinical signs are not observed until after the plants have been grazed on for 14 to 60 days. Clinical signs include poor condition, depression, head pressing, incoordination, stumbling, circling, blindness, recumbency, and paddling.

Miscellaneous Conditions

Meningeal Melanosis (Congenital). The leptomeninges of animals and human beings with heavily pigmented skin, especially black-faced sheep and black-skinned pigs, can have melanin (Fig. 14-57). The extent and degree of pigment deposition varies dramatically from animal to animal. Similar pigment deposits can be found in other areas of the body, including the pleurae, uterine caruncles, liver, and respiratory and alimentary systems' mucous membranes. Congenital meningeal melanosis produces no clinical impairment in affected animals and is an expected, normal finding.

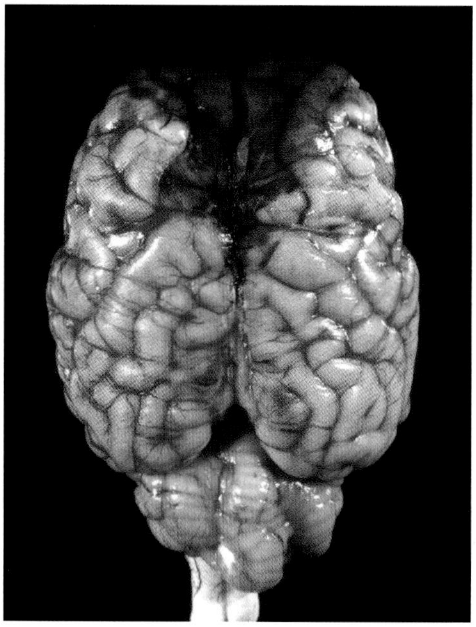

Figure 14-57 **Melanosis, Leptomeninges (Pia-Arachnoid Mater), Sheep.** Note the black pigmentation of the leptomeninges overlying the olfactory poles and dorsal aspect of the frontal lobe. Meningeal melanosis is a normal finding in black-faced sheep and other animals with heavily pigmented skin. (Courtesy Dr. D. Morton, College of Veterinary Medicine, University of Illinois.)

Circulatory Disturbances

Many diseases of the CNS in veterinary medicine result from injury to the circulatory system and vascular endothelium. Vascular diseases of the CNS can result from inflammation/infection, either as a component of a systemic disease process or from extension of inflammatory meningeal or cerebral disease. The incidence of cerebrovascular diseases analogous to those in human beings, including trauma, is low in animals, and neurologic manifestations associated with these diseases are uncommon. Arteriosclerosis ("hardening" of arteries) can be categorized as lipid (atherosclerosis) or nonlipid arteriosclerosis with the latter including arterial fibrosis, mineralization, and amyloid deposition (see Chapter 10).

Atherosclerosis. Atherosclerosis is reported in a variety of animals, including nonhuman primates, pigs, dogs, and several avian species. Older pigs are most commonly and severely affected. Occasional older dogs with chronic hypothyroidism or diabetes mellitus can have severe atherosclerosis. The pathogenesis of atherosclerosis and atherosclerotic plaque formation is most well understood in human beings, and the results of experimental studies may have some application to understanding atherosclerosis in domestic animals.

Atherosclerotic plaques arise from a complex and partially understood interaction among endothelium, smooth muscle cells, platelets, T lymphocytes, and monocytes. Endothelial injury induced by oxidized low-density lipoprotein (LDL) cholesterol results in vascular inflammation of the tunica intima. Monocytes migrate into the intima of the vessel wall to phagocytose LDL cholesterol. This process results in the formation of foam cells characteristic of early atherosclerosis (fatty streak). In addition, activated macrophages produce factors that also injure the endothelium. LDL cholesterol concentrations in foam cells and smooth muscle cells often exceed the antioxidant properties of normal endothelium. Oxidized LDL leads to additional metabolic changes that foster a procoagulant microenvironment and enhanced platelet-mediated thrombus formation, and initiates a cascade of events leading to the lesions associated with the development of mature atherosclerotic plaques (fibrous plaques with a cap [lipid-laden macrophages walled off by connective tissue]). The location of atherosclerotic plaques in the circulatory system depends on fluid shear stresses and their interaction with injured vascular endothelium. Atherosclerotic plaques characteristically occur in areas of vessel branching or areas where blood undergoes a sudden change in velocity and/or direction of flow.

Although atherosclerotic plaques can reach sizes large enough to significantly reduce blood flow to regions of the brain, the stability of the plaques determines the seriousness of the disease. A stable plaque is characterized by an excess of smooth muscle cells with few lipid-containing macrophages. An unstable plaque is characterized by a large lipid-rich core with abundant lipid-containing macrophages, thin fibrous cap, and inflammation. Rupture of unstable plaques can lead to vascular thrombosis or thromboembolism and infarction of areas supplied by these vessels in the CNS.

Grossly, vessels that can be involved include the aorta and its major branches, extramural coronary arteries, renal arteries, and cerebral arteries. Affected arteries are rigid, irregularly thickened, and white to yellow-white (atheromatous plaques) (Fig. 14-58, *A*). Arterial lumina are narrowed or almost obliterated, but there is usually no appreciable ulceration, thrombosis, or hemorrhage (see Fig. 14-58, *B*). Intimal thickening in intracranial arteries often contains less lipid, and these arteries have a greater tendency for fibrosclerosis than other vessels. In arteries within the brain there is collagenous adventitial or transmural thickening. The arterial lesions can be associated with hemorrhage or infarcts involving basal nuclei, fornix, internal and external capsules, hippocampus, and thalamus.

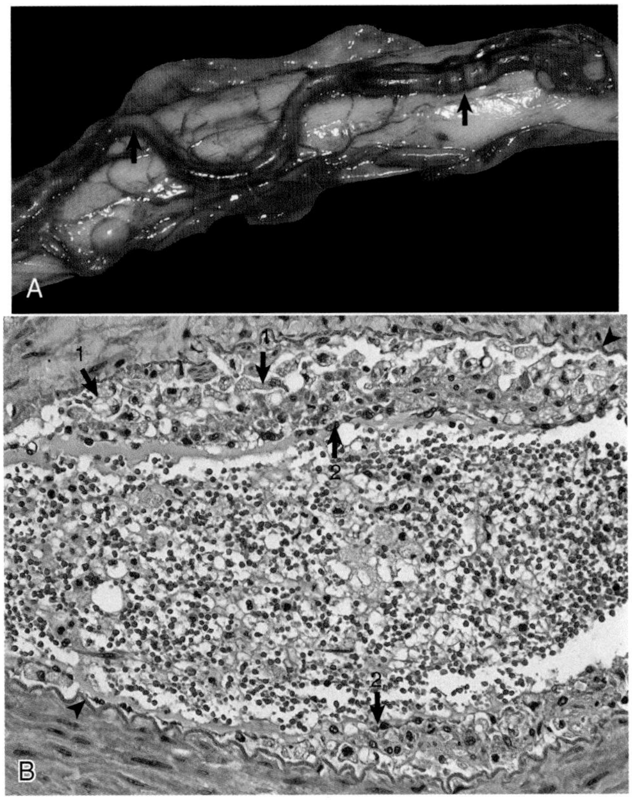

Figure 14-58 Atherosclerosis, Ventral Spinal Artery, Spinal Cord, Ventral Surface, Dog. A, The ventral spinal artery is segmentally yellow, thickened, and beaded in appearance from atheroma *(arrows)*. This dog had long-standing hypothyroidism. **B,** The tunica intima contains numerous foamy (lipid-laden) macrophages *(arrows 1)*. *Arrowheads,* Internal elastic lamina; *arrows 2,* endothelium. H&E stain. (**A** courtesy Dr. J. Hammond, Pieper Memorial Veterinary Center. **B** courtesy Dr. J.F. Zachary, College of Veterinary Medicine, University of Illinois.)

In the dog, lesions most commonly involve cerebral, coronary, and renal arteries and are most severe in the intima and media. Hemorrhage, ischemia, and infarction of the cerebral cortex are uncommon but can occur. Infarctive changes associated with presumptive hypothyroidism-associated atherosclerosis have been identified in dogs by magnetic resonance imaging examinations. Many of these lesions resolve with treatment of the underlying endocrinopathy with minimal residual CNS lesions.

Cerebral Edema (Permeability Changes). The causes and mechanisms of cerebral edema are presented in the section on vasogenic, cytotoxic, and interstitial edema. Cerebral edema has also been associated with "water intoxication," which can result from an increased body hydration caused by (1) excessive, faulty intravenous hydration; (2) compulsive drinking caused by abnormal mental function; or (3) altered antidiuretic hormone secretion. The increased body hydration produces a hypotonic (hypo-osmolar) plasma, with subsequent development of an osmotic gradient between the hypotonic plasma and the relatively hypertonic state of the normal cerebral tissue. Fluid moves from the plasma into the brain. In this type of edema the blood-brain barrier remains intact. If it did not, the change in plasma osmolarity would soon be transmitted to the brain tissue (through vascular leakage) and would abolish the necessary osmotic gradient. Fluid accumulation occurs primarily intracellularly but can also be present extracellularly. In addition, typically a pronounced increase occurs in the rate of formation of CSF originating from the choroid plexus and the extracellular fluid of the brain.

The gross lesions that accompany cerebral edema are the result of enlargement of an organ in an enclosed, limited space; the degree of swelling obviously determines the type and extent of lesions that develop. In evaluating lesions it is particularly important initially to examine the brain and spinal cord in the fresh state and in situ.

Microscopically, in contrast to some other tissues, such as the lungs, the extracellular fluid associated with vasogenic edema fluid is often not detectable, except in instances of marked vascular injury. When the extracellular space-occupying fluid cannot be identified, only its effects (separation of the cells and their processes causing reduced staining intensity) can be recognized. Additionally, after prolonged vasogenic edema the lesions include hypertrophy and hyperplasia of astrocytes, activation of microglia, and demyelination. Cytotoxic edema is characterized by cellular swelling, including swelling of astrocytes.

Because of compression against the cranium, an affected brain has flattened gyri and shallow sulci, and it can shift in position. If the edema is confined to one side, the displacement is unilateral, which can be associated with herniation of the cingulated gyrus under the falx cerebri; the extent of the unilateral intracerebral enlargement can be best appreciated after the examination of transverse sections. Diffuse swelling usually causes a caudal shifting that can result in herniation of the brain (parahippocampal gyri of temporal lobes) beneath the tentorium cerebelli (Fig. 14-59) or herniation of the cerebellar vermis through the foramen magnum, resulting in "coning" of the vermis (Fig. 14-60). On a cut surface the white matter is most often affected (frequently with the vasogenic type of edema, which is the most common). It is swollen and soft, has a damp appearance, and is light yellow in the fresh, unfixed state.

Ischemic Myelopathy (Fibrocartilaginous Embolic Myelopathy). Fibrocartilaginous embolic myelopathy has been described in almost all domestic species but it most commonly occurs in the dog. Herniation of fibrocartilage from the intervertebral disk into the vasculature, forming occlusive emboli, is the known cause, but the route taken by fibrocartilaginous material into the vessels of the spinal cord is uncertain. It has been suggested that trauma to the nucleus pulposus causes it to fragment and that the pressure of trauma forces small fragments into damaged veins, venous plexuses, or small arterioles. The ventral spinal artery and vein and their tributaries are commonly affected, presumably due to their proximity to the extruded disk material. Larger breed dogs are more frequently affected than chondrodystrophic breeds.

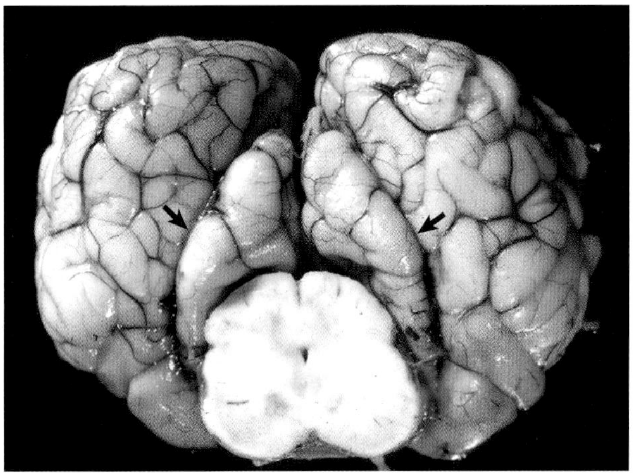

Figure 14-59 **Gyral Herniation, Parahippocampal Gyri, Brain, Transverse Section, Caudal Face, at Level of the Rostral Colliculi and Crus Cerebri, Horse.** The caudal displacement of the parahippocampal gyri *(arrows)* was caused by a sudden swelling of the brain (increase in intracranial pressure) from severe cerebral blunt force trauma to the head. The other cerebral gyri are swollen and flattened, and sulci are indistinct (cerebral edema). (Courtesy Dr. M.D. McGavin, College of Veterinary Medicine, University of Tennessee.)

The gross lesion is an acute focal infarct involving cervical or lumbar spinal cord most commonly, but any portion can be affected (Fig. 14-61). Microscopically, emboli histochemically identical to the fibrocartilage of the nucleus pulposus of intervertebral disks occlude meningeal or CNS arteries or veins, or both, in affected areas (Fig. 14-62). Clinically, there is a sudden onset of spinal cord deficits, sometimes with cerebral involvement, in certain species. In dogs, larger breeds are more commonly affected. The disease occurs in young and old animals. One study reported that 60% of confirmed cases of canine ischemic myelopathy had a history of trauma or exercise.

Nonlipid Vascular Changes. Arterial fibrosis occurs more frequently in older animals and has been described in dogs and horses. In the dog, fibrosis of the intima, media, or adventitia occurs with some frequency in cerebrospinal vessels of all types and caliber. Fibrous thickening of the adventitia of small meningeal and CNS arteries can be accompanied by variable degrees of extension of fibrosis into other layers of the vessel wall. A preferential site is the choroid plexus, where hyalinization and perivascular/vascular thickening is a common finding in older animals. In old horses a similar pattern of fibrosis occurs in vessels, and the adventitia may be preferentially affected. Amyloid deposits in meningeal and cerebral vessels are reported in older dogs and other animals. Mineralization (deposition of calcium or iron salts) of cerebral blood vessels occurs in the brains of several species but is especially common in adult horses. Vessels of the internal capsule, globus pallidus, cerebellar dentate nucleus, and infrequently the hippocampus are preferentially affected in horses, cattle, and less commonly, dogs. Meningeal vessels in old cats, old horses, and cattle and vessels of the choroid plexus in old cats are other sites of vascular mineralization. Almost always these areas of vascular mineralization should be considered incidental findings and are unlikely to be associated with clinical signs. Overt ischemic damage is rarely associated with these nonlipomatous vascular lesions in any species; therefore clinical signs are not seen with this lesion.

Lysosomal Storage Diseases

Dysfunction of lysosome-mediated degradation of products (substrates) of normal cellular metabolism results in diseases referred to as *lysosomal storage diseases*. These substrates cannot be degraded by

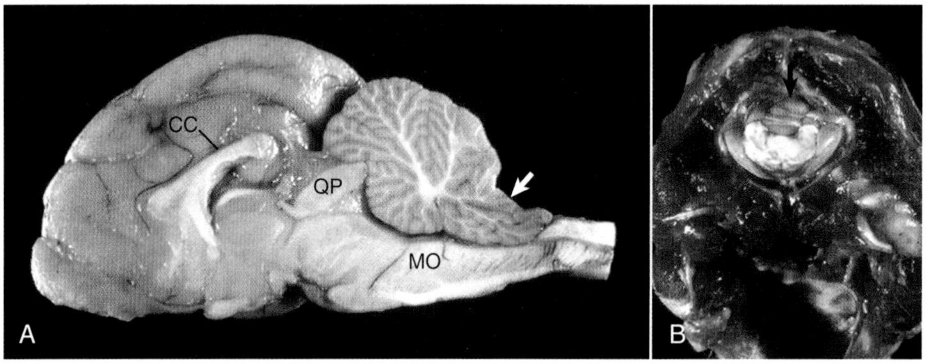

Figure 14-60 **Coning of the Cerebellar Vermis, Brain, Cat. A,** Sagittal section. Coning of the cerebellum. The caudal cerebellar vermis has been displaced caudally through the foramen magnum; note the notch on the dorsal surface *(arrow)*. This result has compressed the medulla oblongata *(MO)*, which can cause death from compression of the respiratory center. Note the elevation of the corpus callosum *(CC)* and focal compression of the rostral cerebellar vermis by the tectum (quadrigeminal plate) *(QP)*. **B,** Coning of the cerebellum through the foramen magnum, caudal view through the foramen magnum. Note that in this case not only has the cerebellar vermis *(arrow)* been displaced caudally, but also the medulla. The caudal cerebellar peduncles have been displaced caudally as far as the foramen magnum. (**A** courtesy Dr. D. Cho, College of Veterinary Medicine, Louisiana State University; and Noah's Arkive, College of Veterinary Medicine, The University of Georgia. **B** courtesy College of Veterinary Medicine, University of Illinois.)

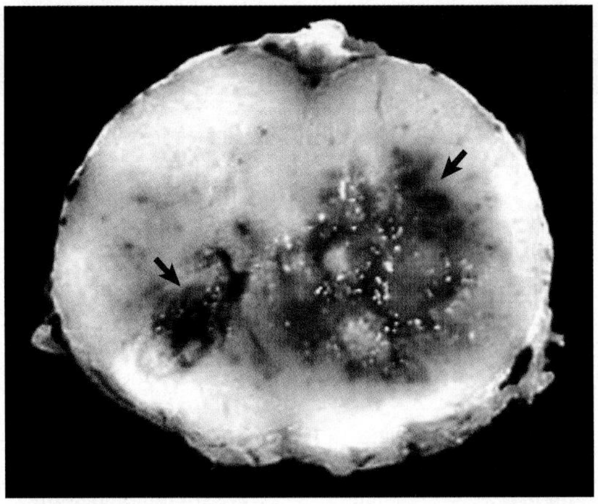

Figure 14-61 Spinal Cord Infarction (Ischemic Necrosis), Dog. The yellow-brown region of necrosis *(arrows)* in the right lateral and ventral funiculi was the result of fibrocartilaginous emboli that occluded branches of the ventral spinal artery and obstructed blood flow. (Courtesy Dr. J. Edwards, College of Veterinary Medicine, Texas A&M University; and Dr. J. King, College of Veterinary Medicine, Cornell University.)

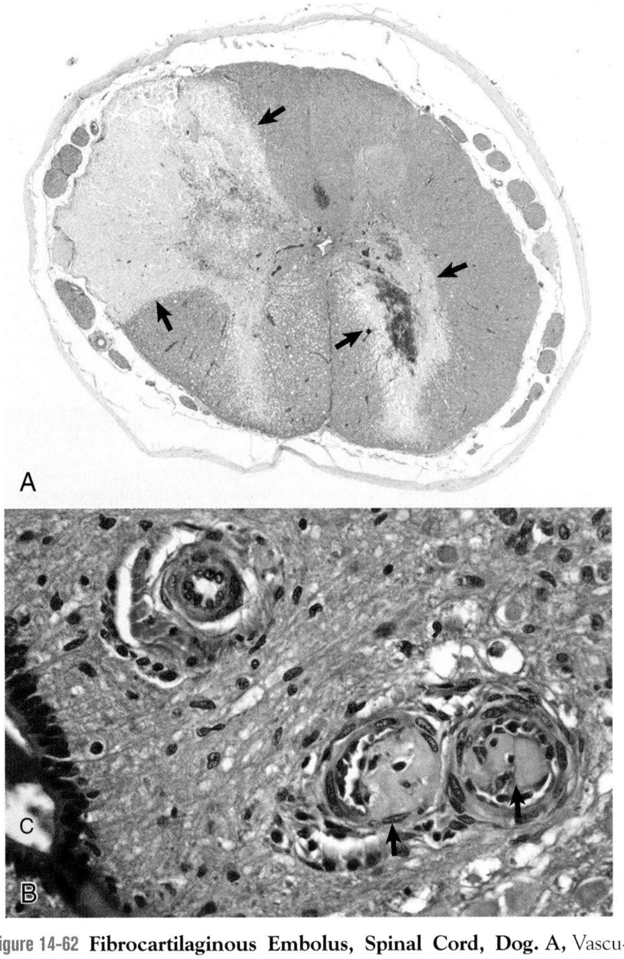

Figure 14-62 Fibrocartilaginous Embolus, Spinal Cord, Dog. A, Vascular occlusion and infarction. Fibrocartilaginous emboli have obstructed the dorsolateral artery *(top left)* and branches of the ventral spinal artery to the right ventral gray horn and adjacent white matter, causing infarction *(arrows)*. H&E stain. **B,** Fibrocartilaginous emboli in arterioles *(arrows)*. C, Central canal. H&E stain. (**A** courtesy Dr. M.D. McGavin, College of Veterinary Medicine, University of Tennessee. **B** courtesy Dr. J. Van Vleet, College of Veterinary Medicine, Purdue University.)

lysosomes, and the accumulated substrate eventually results in death of the affected cells.

Cell death is the end point of a chronic and progressive process of substrate accumulation that interferes with cellular biochemical processes and transport systems. When neurons or myelinating cells die, they release their accumulated substrate into adjacent tissue. Macrophages are recruited from the bloodstream as monocytes, and they phagocytose cellular debris and unprocessed substrate released from dead cells. Macrophages, however, have the same genetic defect and thus also accumulate substrate in their lysosomes. Although less vulnerable to the effects of substrate accumulation, macrophages eventually die, and their released substrate is phagocytosed by additional macrophages recruited from the blood.

Lipid storage diseases, such as globoid cell leukodystrophy, are covered in more detail later. Features of some selected lysosomal storage diseases of animals are provided in Table 14-7.

Lysosomal storage diseases were originally thought to develop exclusively because of mutations that result in a reduction in lysosomal enzyme synthesis. More recently, however, it has become clear that there are other defects such as the following:

1. Synthesis of catalytically inactive proteins that resemble normal active enzymes
2. Defects in posttranslational processing (glycosylation, phosphorylation, addition of fatty acids in the Golgi) of the enzyme, which results in it being misdirected to sites (extracellular) other than to lysosomes
3. Lack of enzyme activator (an enzyme that normally increases the rate of an enzyme-catalyzed reaction) or protector protein (facilitates repair and refolding of stress-damaged proteins)
4. Lack of substrate activator protein required to assist with the hydrolysis of substrate
5. Lack of transport protein required for elimination of digested material from lysosomes

Characterization of lysosomal disorders has therefore been broadened to include involvement of any protein that is essential for normal lysosomal function

The best-known diseases are characterized by accumulation of the substrate or substrate precursors and sometimes even by the absence of a critical metabolic product for normal lysosomal function. As a general principle, cell swelling and cytoplasmic vacuolation occur because of the accumulation of unprocessed substrate in the lysosomes; therefore differences in the size and appearance of cells (neurons versus hepatocytes) depend on the availability of the substrate (carbohydrate or lipid) in the organ system. Many lipids and glycolipids are unique to the nervous system; thus when there is a lysosomal defect, neural cells often accumulate in the substrate.

Examples of lysosomal storage diseases that affect human beings and animals are the gangliosidoses. With few exceptions, these diseases are inherited in an autosomal recessive pattern. They are also often gene-dose dependent and correspondingly, recessive homozygotes manifest the disease, whereas heterozygotes are phenotypically and functionally normal, but the affected enzyme's activity is reduced by approximately 50% of normal. The age of onset of clinical signs and the severity of the disease process can vary among the different diseases because the deficiency of the involved enzyme is not always the same. If the gene defect is such that the mutant enzyme is not synthesized at all, there is an early onset of a severe disease. Conversely, if there is some residual synthesis of the deficient enzyme, later onset and a milder form of the disease result because partial catabolism of the accumulated substrate permits a longer period of time before the lysosomes are so distended with substrate that they cause loss of cell function.

Table 14-7 Classification of Selected Lysosomal Storage Diseases That Involve the Central Nervous System of Animals

Disease	Storage Product	Deficient Enzyme	Species	Breed
GM_1 gangliosidosis	GM_1 ganglioside	β-Galactosidase	Bovine	Holstein-Friesian
			Canine	Beagle, English springer spaniel, Portuguese water dog, Alaskan huskies
			Feline	Siamese, domestic shorthair
			Ovine	Suffolk, Coopworth-Romney
GM_2 gangliosidosis	GM_2 ganglioside	β-Hexosaminidase	Canine	German shorthair pointer, Japanese spaniel
			Feline	Domestic shorthair, Korat
			Porcine	Yorkshire
Globoid cell leukodystrophy (Krabbe's-like disease)	Galactosylceramide (galactocerebroside) and galactosylsphingosine (psychosine)	Galactosylceramidase (galactocerebroside β-galactosidase)	Canine	West Highland terrier Cairn terrier, miniature poodle, bluetick hound, beagle, Pomeranian
			Feline	Domestic shorthair, domestic longhair
			Ovine	Polled Dorset
α-Mannosidosis	Mannose-containing oligosaccharide	α-Mannosidase	Bovine	Angus, Murray Grey, Galloway
			Feline	Persian, domestic shorthair
β-Mannosidosis	Mannose-containing oligosaccharide	β-Mannosidase	Caprine	Nubian
			Bovine	Salers
Mucopolysaccharidosis	Different glycosaminoglycans	Several different enzyme deficiencies	Canine	Plott hound (type I, Hurler's disease), miniature pinscher (type VI, Maroteaux-Lamy disease) German shepherd (type VII, Sly disease)
			Feline	Domestic shorthair (type I, Hurler's disease) Domestic shorthair, Siamese (type VI, Maroteaux-Lamy disease) Domestic shorthair (type VII, Sly disease)
			Caprine	Nubian (type III, Sanfilippo's disease)
Ceroid-lipofuscinosis	Subunit c of mitochondrial ATPase	Prelysosomal defect?	Canine	English setter, border collie, Tibetan terrier
			Ovine	South Hampshire
			Bovine	Devon
	Sphingolipid	Palmitoyl protein thioesterase	Canine	Miniature schnauzer
	Activating proteins A and D		Ovine	Swedish Landrace
	Unknown	Unknown	Canine	Chihuahua, cocker spaniel, Saluki, terrier-cross, blue heeler, Yugoslavian shepherd, Dalmatian, Australian cattle dog, golden retriever, dachshund, corgi
			Ovine	Rambouillet
			Bovine	Beefmaster
			Feline	Siamese, domestic shorthair
Niemann-Pick type c disease	Primarily ganglioside in neurons	Unknown	Feline	Domestic shorthair
			Canine	Boxer

ATPase, Adenosine triphosphatase.

Gross lesions of the CNS vary among the different types of lysosomal storage diseases. Brain atrophy occurs with globoid cell leukodystrophy in latter stages of the diseases because of the loss of myelin. Brain atrophy is also seen with ceroid-lipofuscinosis but is not prominent in other lysosomal storage diseases, although brains of animals with gangliosidoses can have a firm, rubbery consistency. Microscopically, affected neurons often have a foamy, finely vacuolated, or granular cytoplasm, which is a reflection of the degree to which the stored material is removed during histologic processing (Fig. 14-63). The specific features of the stored material can be best appreciated by ultrastructural examination.

Ceroid-lipofuscinosis is a lysosomal storage disease characterized by abnormal sphingolipid (lipopigments) metabolism that occurs in cats, dogs, cattle, and sheep. Its lysosomal dysfunction has not been clearly identified, but experimental studies have shown alterations in the activity of palmitoyl-protein thioesterase and concentration of acid protease. The disease resembles other lysosomal storage diseases in that it can have a recessive mode of inheritance, but it is dissimilar in that it has no gene-dose effect. Brain atrophy occurs with ceroid-lipofuscinosis in later stages of the diseases (in sheep) (see Fig. 14-17). The atrophy, which most frequently involves the cerebral cortex but also sometimes the cerebellum, can result in a 50% reduction in brain weight. The cerebral hemispheres are increased in firmness and often have a tan color, whereas the gyri are thinned and the sulci widened, a clear indication of cerebrocortical atrophy. Microscopically, the cytoplasm of affected neurons has an eosinophilic granular material (with H&E staining) and a decrease in the number of neurons. Reactive astrogliosis is prominent, and microgliosis may also be observed.

Globoid Cell Leukodystrophy. As discussed previously, lysosomal storage generally refers to a cellular alteration in which an increased amount of substrate material, which normally is degraded, accumulates within lysosomes, often eventually resulting in cell death. These diseases have a hereditary basis, occur in young animals, and are transmitted in an autosomal recessive pattern. Features of some selected lysosomal storage diseases of animals are given in Table 14-7.

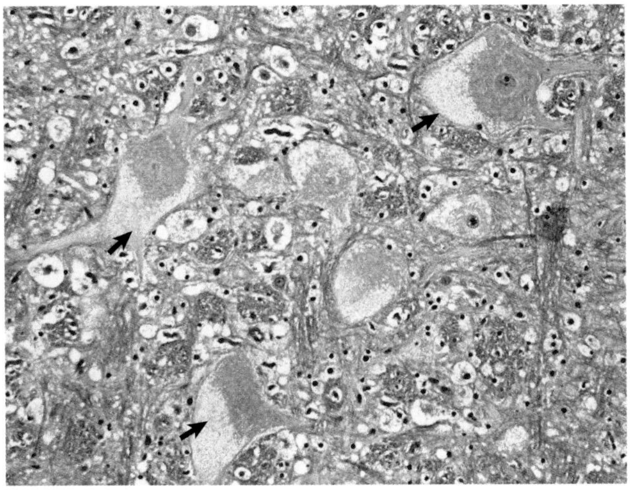

Figure 14-63 **Glycogen/Carbohydrate (Lysosomal) Storage Disease, Brainstem, Neuron Cell Bodies, Cat.** Note the enlargement of the neuron cell bodies, displacement of nuclei, and accumulation of unprocessed substrate in the cytoplasm of the neuronal cell bodies *(arrows)* giving the appearance of "foamy" cytoplasm. H&E stain. (Courtesy Dr. J.F. Zachary, College of Veterinary Medicine, University of Illinois.)

Globoid cell leukodystrophy, a sphingolipidosis, is a lysosomal storage disease; its principal lesion is primary demyelination involving oligodendrocytes of the CNS and Schwann cells of the PNS. The disease, which has an autosomal recessive inheritance in the Cairn and West Highland white terrier, is generally seen in younger animals, often younger than 1 year old. It has also been described in beagles, miniature poodles, basset hounds, Pomeranians, bluetick hounds, and domestic short- and long-haired cats.

Mechanistically, the proposed sequence of events in this disease includes (1) early "normal" myelination that progresses up to a certain stage; (2) disruption of normal myelin turnover because of deficient galactosylceramidase activity; (3) degeneration and necrosis of myelinating cells because of the accumulation of psychosine; (4) primary demyelination; (5) recruitment of phagocytes, both resident microglia and trafficking blood monocytes; and (6) infiltration of macrophages, which become globoid cells after phagocytosing myelin byproducts into the nervous tissue. The last-named changes occur in response to the demyelination and unmetabolized galactocerebroside.

Affected oligodendroglia and Schwann cells are deficient in the lysosomal hydrolase, galactosylceramide β-galactosidase (GALC), which is responsible for degradation of galactosylsphingosine (psychosine) and galactosylceramide (galactocerebroside). Psychosine is highly toxic, and because it is not degraded, it has been hypothesized that it accumulates during the disease and causes direct injury to oligodendrocytes and Schwann cells, possibly through an apoptotic mechanism of cell death, in part, mediated by psychosine-induced production of cytokines and inducible nitric oxide synthase.

In globoid cell leukodystrophy the composition of myelin is not qualitatively abnormal. Galactosylceramide is highly concentrated in myelin but is nearly absent in systemic organs except for the kidney. Peak synthesis and turnover of galactosylceramide coincides with the peak period of myelin formation and turnover during the first year of life. GALC activity also increases in relation to the galactosylceramide peak. Myelination continues at a slower rate as animals mature, and in an adult myelin formation is stable with minimal turnover.

A deficiency in GALC activity results in the accumulation of galactosylceramide, especially during the early phase of myelin maturation and turnover, and in the formation of globoid cells discussed later. Psychosine also accumulates, leading to rapid and massive degeneration of oligodendroglia and Schwann cells, extensive myelinolysis, and reduction in myelination.

Gross lesions of the CNS are characterized by a gray discoloration of the white matter, especially of the centrum semiovale of the cerebral hemispheres and white matter of the spinal cord (Fig. 14-64). The lesion in the spinal cord tends to start in the peripheral white matter and spread inward. Microscopically, such areas have pronounced loss of myelin (Fig. 14-65, *A*) and prominent globoid cells containing galactocerebroside that can be demonstrated with a periodic acid–Schiff stain (Fig. 14-65, *B*; E-Fig. 14-7). Peripheral nerves are also affected, and lesions are typified by primary demyelination and secondary axonal degeneration. Small sensory branches of peripheral nerves are useful sites to take biopsies to make diagnoses (see Fig. 14-112).

Clinically, affected animals are ataxic and have limb weakness and tremors that progress to paralysis and muscular atrophy. Poor vision or blindness may also occur.

Disease Processes Affecting Myelin Formation and Maintenance

Hypomyelination and Dysmyelination. Disorders of myelin formation include hypomyelinogenesis (hypomyelination) and

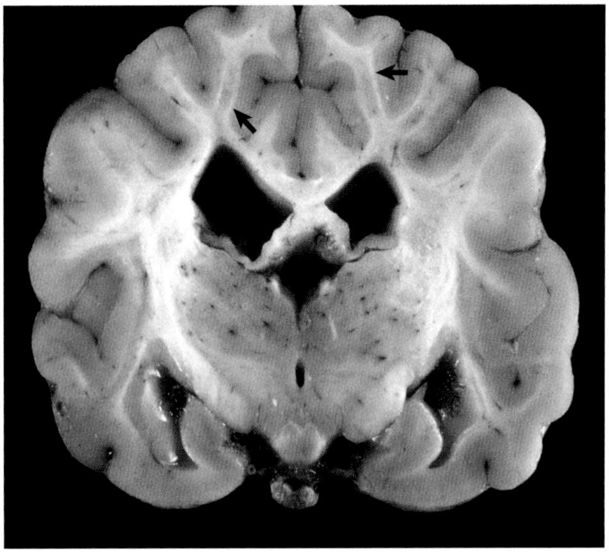

Figure 14-64 **Lipid Storage Disease, Globoid Cell Leukodystrophy, Brain, Transverse Section at the Level of the Mammillary Body, Dog.** The white matter, especially of the gyri, has an off-white to light gray appearance *(arrows)*. Macrophages (globoid cells) derived from blood monocytes (also enzymatically deficient in β-galactocerebrosidase) accumulate in white matter to phagocytose galactocerebroside and oligodendroglial debris secondary to the toxic effects of galactosylsphingosine (psychosine) on oligodendroglia (and in the peripheral nervous system Schwann cells). There is also bilateral hydrocephalus of the lateral ventricles, presumably hydrocephalus ex vacuo, as a result of the loss of neurons and their axons. (Courtesy Dr. H.B. Gelberg, College of Veterinary Medicine, Oregon State University.)

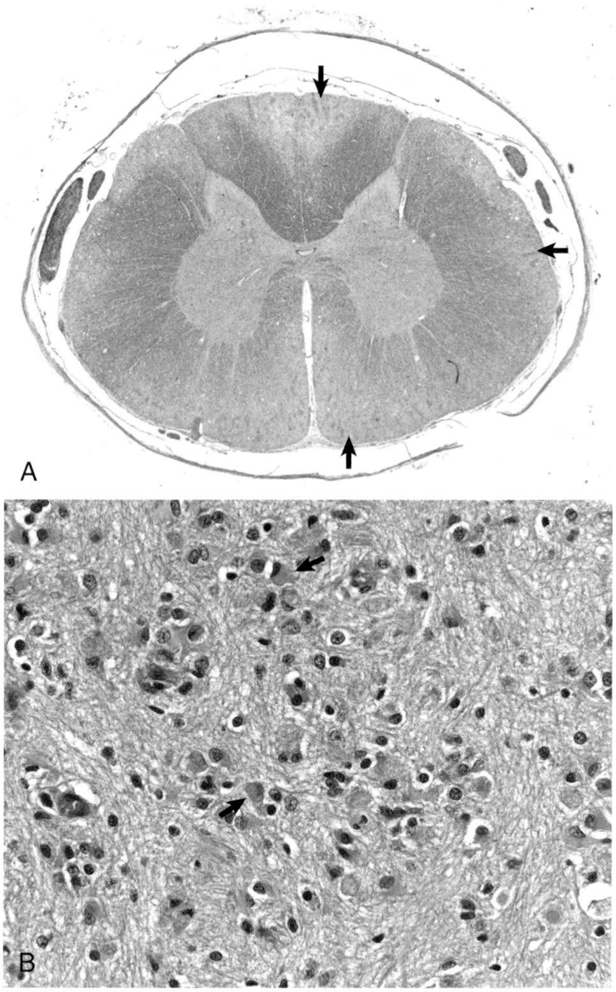

Figure 14-65 **Globoid Cell Leukodystrophy, Dog. A,** Spinal cord. This section of spinal cord has been stained with Luxol fast blue, a histochemical reaction that stains myelin blue. Note the loss of myelin from the periphery of the cord, where axons are heavily myelinated *(arrows)*, the first area to be affected. Luxol fast blue stain with a nuclear fast red counterstain. **B,** Early stage of the disease. The white matter contains globoid cells (macrophages) that are characterized by abundant eosinophilic cytoplasm and an eccentric nucleus *(arrows)*. The number and size of macrophages increase over the time course of the disease due to progressive loss of myelin. H&E stain. (**A** courtesy Dr. M.D. McGavin, College of Veterinary Medicine, University of Tennessee; **B** courtesy Dr. A.D. Miller, College of Veterinary Medicine, Cornell University.)

dysmyelination. Hypomyelinogenesis is a process in which there is underdevelopment of myelin. Dysmyelination refers to the formation of biochemically defective myelin. Hypomyelinogenesis and dysmyelination most often occur in the early postnatal period and have similar clinical and pathologic features. There are some differences in the lesions and the mechanisms by which they develop. Some of these diseases in domestic animals are outlined in Table 14-8.

Hypomyelinogenesis

Diseases Caused by Viruses. Classical swine fever (hog cholera) virus, a pestivirus, can be teratogenic in the porcine fetus. The best-known neural defects resulting from fetal infection are hypomyelinogenesis and cerebellar hypoplasia, although other lesions of the CNS, such as microencephaly and nonneural tissue, have been reported. The mechanism of lesion development has not been definitively determined, but a persistent infection that results in inhibition of cell division and function of selected tissues has been proposed.

Border disease viral infection (also a pestiviral infection) is capable of inducing maldevelopment in the CNS and nonneural tissues (skeleton) of lambs and goats after natural infection of the dam during pregnancy. One of the characteristic lesions in the CNS is hypomyelinogenesis, primarily affecting the white matter of the cerebrum and cerebellum. Grossly, it may be difficult to distinguish between white and gray matter in transverse sections of cerebrum and cerebellum. The brain and spinal cords from affected lambs may be smaller when compared with unaffected lambs. The PNS is unaffected. Hypomyelinogenesis may be related to a viral-induced decrease of myelin-associated glycoprotein, myelin basic protein, and activity of nucleotide phosphodiesterase in oligodendroglia. Other lesions detected in lambs include early inflammation, porencephaly-hydranencephaly, cerebellar malformation including hypoplasia, microencephaly, and reduction in diameter of the spinal cord.

Globoid Cell Leukodystrophy. See the earlier section on Lysosomal Storage Diseases.

Spongy Degeneration (Status Spongiosus). Spongy degeneration is a group of diseases of young animals characterized by a moth-eaten appearance (referred to here as *status spongiosus*) that primarily occurs in the white matter of the CNS but also extends into the gray matter. Status spongiosus is a somewhat nonspecific term and can develop by several different mechanisms. It includes a variety of lesions, such as splitting of lamella forming myelin sheaths (characteristic of the diseases discussed here), accumulation of extracellular fluid (extracellular cerebral edema; see section on Central Nervous System Swelling and Edema) swelling of cellular processes (astrocytic, neuronal), and Wallerian degeneration at a later stage

Table 14-8 Hypomyelinogenesis and Dysmyelination in Animals

Species	Breed	Disease Designation	Genetic Cause	Infectious Cause	Metabolic Cause
Bovine	All breeds	Bovine virus diarrhea (dysmyelination)		Bovine virus diarrhea (pestivirus)	
	Charolais	Progressive ataxia	Suspected		
Ovine	All breeds	Border disease (hypomyelinogenesis-dysmyelination)		Border disease virus (pestivirus)	
Porcine	Landrace	Congenital tremor (myelin agenesia)	Sex-linked recessive		
	Saddleback	Congenital tremor	Autosomal recessive		
	Chester-white	Myoclonia congenita	Autosomal recessive	Suspected	
	All breeds	Congenital tremor (dysmyelinogenesis and cerebellar hypoplasia)		Classic swine fever (pestivirus)	
	All breeds	Congenital tremor (dysmyelinogenesis)		Unknown virus suspected	
	All breeds	Congenital ataxia and tremor (hypomyelinogenesis and cerebellar hypoplasia)			Trichlorfon (acaricide)
Canine	Dalmatian	Hypomyelinogenesis			
	Chow Chow	Dysmyelination	Suspected		
	Springer spaniel	Shaking pups (hypomyelination)	Sex-linked recessive		
	Samoyed	Tremor (hypomyelination)	Suspected		
	Lurcher	Tremor syndrome (hypomyelination)			
	Weimaraner	Hypomyelination	Suspected		

when the necrotic myelin and axons have been phagocytosed and the spaces once occupied by these structures are empty.

Gross brain lesions reported for spongy degeneration range from no gross lesions to swelling, edema, and pallor of the white matter, and dilation of the ventricles. Microscopically, the lesion is characterized by variably sized empty spaces within the white matter. Ultrastructurally, with spongy degeneration and some other disease processes characterized by status spongiosus, there is splitting or separation of the myelin sheath at the intraperiod line with the formation of large intramyelinic spaces. In some cases, myelin formation is deficient.

Some species and breeds affected with spongy degeneration include the canine (Labrador retriever, Saluki, silky terrier, Samoyed), feline (Egyptian Mau), and bovine (Jersey, shorthorn, Angus shorthorn, Hereford), and an autosomal recessive mode of transmission has been proposed for some forms of this disorder. A unique form of the spongy degeneration also occurs in a group of metabolic inherited diseases called *aminoacidopathies*.

The term *spongiform change* should not be confused with spongy degeneration. Spongiform change is characterized by small clear vacuoles of varied sizes that form in the cytoplasm of neuron cell bodies and proximal dendrites in diseases, such as the transmissible spongiform encephalopathies and rabies encephalitis, and in the processes of astrocytes that are spatially related to the affected neurons.

Demyelination. Demyelination, which means degeneration and loss of myelin already formed, can be divided into primary and secondary types. *Primary demyelination* refers to a disease process in which the myelin sheath is selectively affected, with the axon remaining essentially intact. *Secondary demyelination*, a designation criticized by some, refers to "secondary" degeneration of myelin after "primary" injury to and loss of the axon, as in Wallerian degeneration, and is not a selective injury of the myelin sheath.

Injury to oligodendroglia that results in myelin sheath breakdown or direct injury to myelin sheaths causes the release of lipids and other myelin components into the extracellular space. These materials readily activate microglial cells and attract blood monocytes, which phagocytose myelin debris.

Metabolic Causes

Osmotic Demyelination Syndrome. In human beings, osmotic demyelination syndrome is termed *central* or *extrapontine myelinolysis*. The disorder was first reported in 1959, and the majority of cases were in severely malnourished alcoholics. Since then the disorder has been observed in a variety of clinical disease states. A major risk factor is chronic hyponatremia treated in hospitals by the administration of intravenous saline solution. The disease has been experimentally reproduced in dogs and laboratory rodents by inducing hyponatremia, allowing a period of stabilization (3 to 4 days is sufficient), and then administering saline-containing fluids.

Cases of osmotic demyelination syndrome are rarely reported in the veterinary literature. Several of the cases had Addison's disease with treatment consisting of intravenous administration of fluids containing normal saline solution to correct the hyponatremia typical of hypoadrenocorticism. The reported rates of correction were 22 mmol/L in 24 hours and 16.4 mmol/L in 24 hours. All of these rates of correction exceed the limits established for human beings and are consistent with human cases of the syndrome. Osmotic demyelination syndrome has also been reported in a cat and may have been due to poor nutrition.

The pathogenesis of osmotic demyelination syndrome is thought to be opposite to that occurring with salt poisoning (i.e., a hyponatremic to hypernatremic shift after saline administration). Lesions occur in areas of the brain in which there is a confluence or intermingling of gray and white matter. Rapid (within 24 to 48 hours) correction of chronic hyponatremia from an established equilibrium exceeds the adaptive responses of the brain, resulting in myelin destruction. The exact mechanism of demyelination is not known. It is proposed that osmotic imbalance and water shifts induce osmotic stress in the CNS that results in myelin destruction.

In contrast to human beings, gross lesions in dogs are either not apparent or subtle. Slight softening and discoloration has been observed in affected brain regions. Microscopically, lesions can be limited to the reticular formation at the level of the pons or can be extensive, affecting cerebellar folia, midbrain, thalamus, basal nuclei, and at the interface of the corona radiata and cerebrocortical gray matter. In affected areas the white matter is pale in routine H&E-stained sections and is heavily infiltrated with foamy macrophages. Special stains (Luxol fast blue for myelin) confirm acute myelin destruction and accumulation of myelin debris in macrophages. As is typical of strictly demyelinating lesions, axons are well preserved.

Circulatory and Physical Disturbances. Physical compression of CNS tissue that results from various causes, usually chronic, can also induce demyelination. Some possible mechanisms include compression of myelin sheaths and oligodendroglia, interference with circulation resulting in CNS ischemia, and disease processes resulting in the accumulation of extracellular fluid.

It is well known that vasogenic and hydrostatic edema caused by inflammation, neoplasia, trauma, and obstructive hydrocephalus can cause degeneration of myelin sheaths. The underlying mechanisms for this injury are multiple and include creation of a hypoxic-anoxic environment, degeneration of oligodendroglia, and alteration in stability of the myelin sheath, permitting entrance of injurious proteolytic enzymes from the surrounding environment.

Diseases Caused by Microbes.

Progressive Multifocal Leukoencephalopathy. See Table 14-3.

Immune-Mediated Diseases. In veterinary medicine, naturally occurring immune-mediated demyelination in domestic animals is rare, and other than canine polyradiculoneuritis (coonhound paralysis), it is usually only suspected rather than proved. These diseases are mostly known to occur in human beings as sequelae to postinfectious and postvaccinal events. They result in primary demyelination of the CNS. Autoimmune diseases of the CNS are mechanistically either a type II hypersensitivity (antibody-mediated) or a type IV (cell-mediated) hypersensitivity, and T lymphocytes and macrophage-derived cytokines play contributory roles.

Autoimmune injury to oligodendroglia in the CNS arising from aberrant cellular and/or humoral immune responses can result from one of the following four proposed mechanisms:

1. Molecular mimicry: The CNS has antigens that are similar or identical to those expressed by certain pathogens (virus or bacterium). The normal inflammatory and immunologic responses to these pathogens result in the expression of antibodies that cross-react with "antigens" normally expressed by CNS cells.
2. Abrogation of immune tolerance: The CNS is an "immune privileged" organ (like the eye). The immune system therefore does not recognize CNS antigens as innate antigens, and if they are exposed to the immune system after inflammation or trauma, an autoimmune response can ensue. Injury, physical or otherwise, to blood vessels within the CNS can cause the release of "sequestered antigens" into the bloodstream, leading to an autoimmune response.
3. Genetic factors: Functions of the immune system that are strictly regulated genetically may be under the control of abnormal inherited genes or altered normal genes that regulate immune responses to CNS antigens and thus increase the susceptibility to autoimmune diseases.
4. Stress factors: Environmental stresses mediated through the CNS can depress the functions of the immune system, leading to the formation of autoantibodies.

The mechanism of myelin breakdown in immune-mediated demyelination is not clearly understood. The initial step is thought to be exposure of antigens in myelin basic protein of the major dense line of myelin lamellae after injury. Myelin proteins are substrates for calpain, a calcium-activated neutral proteinase. Calpain has been implicated in several autoimmune diseases and may play an important role in CNS demyelination. Exposed antigens are then recognized by the immune system, and experimental studies suggest that lesions result from a complex interaction between inflammatory cells and their mediators and lamellae of myelinating cells. T lymphocytes, some B lymphocytes, and activated macrophages (recruited monocytes) and microglia cells, adhesion molecules, cytokines, chemokines, and their receptors have been demonstrated in the lesions. This interaction results in primary demyelination.

Gross lesions are usually not present but can include a gray-to-yellow discoloration of white matter. Microscopically, lesions are best observed in white matter and are characterized by vacuolation of myelin and the presence of lymphocytes, macrophages, and plasma cells. Myelin sheaths degenerate from injury caused by (1) inflammatory mediators and (2) direct actions of macrophages on lamellae. Myelin lamellae separate as a result of intramyelinic edema, fragment, and are phagocytosed by macrophages.

The best-known model of immune-mediated demyelination is an experimental model referred to as *experimental allergic encephalomyelitis* (EAE). Experimental allergic encephalomyelitis is produced by inducing a hypersensitivity to myelin or more specifically, to myelin basic protein. If appropriate laboratory animals are inoculated with white matter or myelin basic protein (suspended in complete Freund's adjuvant), they become paralyzed after 2 to 3 weeks. Lesions are characterized by perivascular (perivenular) demyelination accompanied by accumulation of lymphocytes and macrophages.

A similar process, referred to as *postvaccinal encephalomyelitis*, occurred occasionally in human beings when human rabies vaccine contained CNS tissue. The incidence decreased after 1957 when duck embryo rabies vaccine came into use. In some cases with mild clinical signs, recovery was complete, and axons were remyelinated after immune-mediated demyelination.

A third situation in which this type of demyelination occurs follows infection with certain viruses in human beings (rubeola virus) and animals (e.g., influenza virus). These diseases, which are rare and designated as postinfectious encephalomyelitis, are also characterized by development of lesions in the CNS comparable to those of experimental allergic encephalomyelitis.

Traumatic Injury

Traumatic injury of the CNS is caused by physical insults such as compression, stretching, and/or laceration of neurons/axons. When the brain and spinal cord collide with the bony ridges lining the cranial vault and the bony wall of the vertebral canal, respectively, or when axial, rotational, and angular forces (Fig. 14-66) are applied to neurons and axons during trauma, the force of impact and sudden acceleration of neurons and axons, both within the CNS and in the adjacent cranial and spinal nerves, can cause them to compress, twist, stretch, and tear. Concurrently, the same type of forces can injure blood vessels in the CNS and leptomeninges and may result in small hemorrhages or hematomas within the parenchyma of the brain and in the leptomeninges (subarachnoid space) (Fig. 14-67).

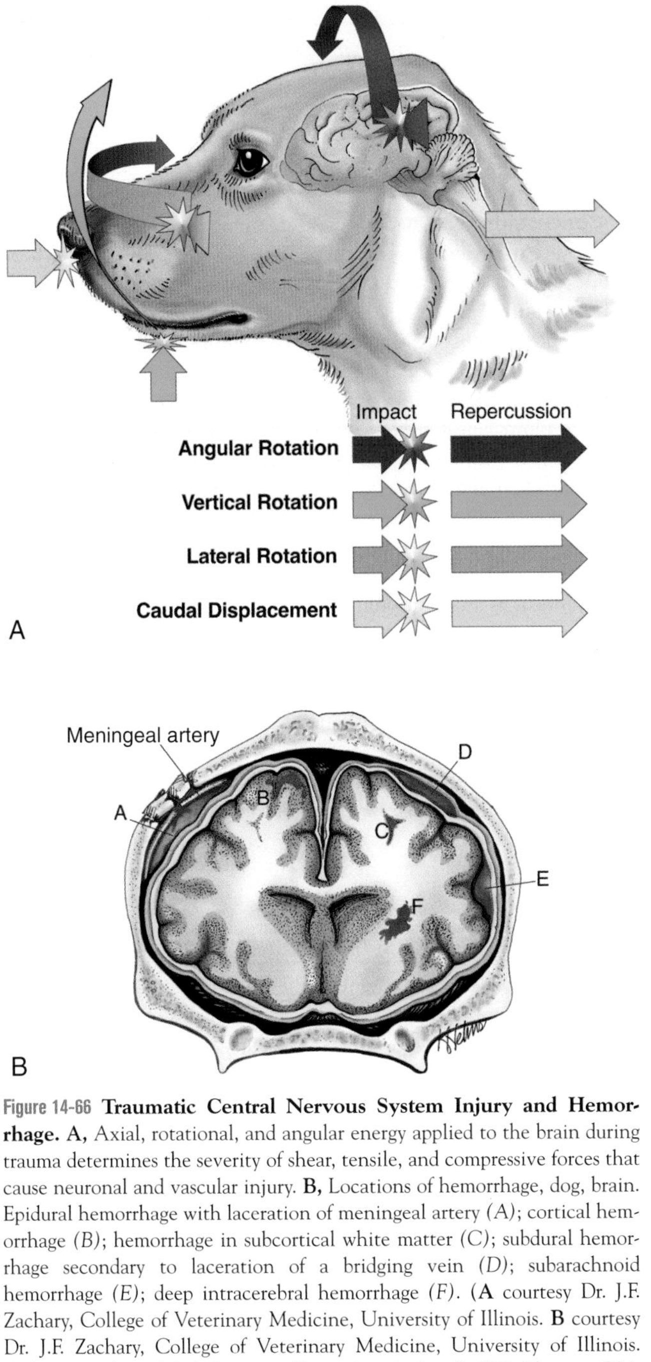

Figure 14-66 Traumatic Central Nervous System Injury and Hemorrhage. A, Axial, rotational, and angular energy applied to the brain during trauma determines the severity of shear, tensile, and compressive forces that cause neuronal and vascular injury. **B,** Locations of hemorrhage, dog, brain. Epidural hemorrhage with laceration of meningeal artery *(A)*; cortical hemorrhage *(B)*; hemorrhage in subcortical white matter *(C)*; subdural hemorrhage secondary to laceration of a bridging vein *(D)*; subarachnoid hemorrhage *(E)*; deep intracerebral hemorrhage *(F)*. (**A** courtesy Dr. J.F. Zachary, College of Veterinary Medicine, University of Illinois. **B** courtesy Dr. J.F. Zachary, College of Veterinary Medicine, University of Illinois. Redrawn and modified from an illustration in Leech RW, Shuman RM: *Neuropathology: a summary for students*, Philadelphia, 1982, Harper & Row.)

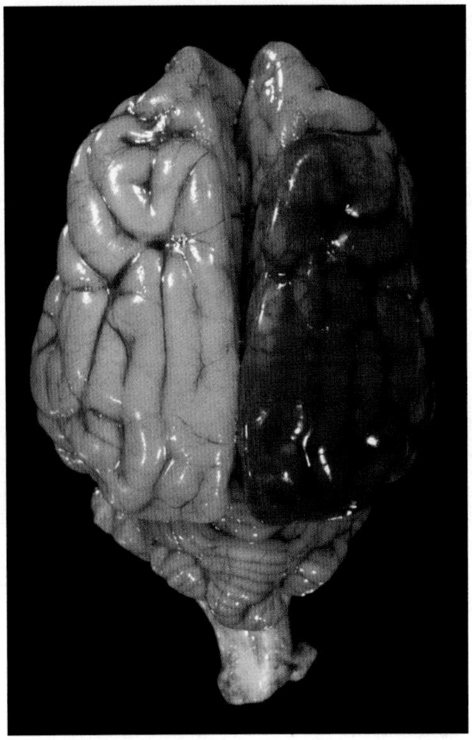

Figure 14-67 Leptomeningeal (Subarachnoid) Hemorrhage, Brain, Right Cerebral Hemisphere, Dog. (Courtesy Dr. R. Storts, College of Veterinary Medicine, Texas A&M University.)

Diffuse brain injury (often present in concussion) is caused by acceleration/deceleration forces applied to many areas of the CNS rather than in one specific location. Diffuse brain injury involves neuronal processes, cell bodies, transmitter mechanisms, and macroglial cells and blood vessels. The most severe injury to axons appears to be at the gray matter–white matter junction. A variant of diffuse brain injury is diffuse axonal injury in which axons of large myelinated nerve fibers are injured by shearing forces. In diffuse brain and axonal injury, mechanical deformation results in physical disruption of cell membranes and cytoskeleton and increased membrane permeability, resulting in major ionic fluxes in and out of the cell. Such changes can lead to excessive release of glutamate, excitotoxicity and cell death, free radical formation, apoptosis, and delayed inflammatory responses. The end result can be Wallerian degeneration.

In general, trauma of the CNS in animals occurs less frequently than in human beings. Animals are not exposed as frequently to potentially trauma-causing situations (e.g., automobile travel) as are human beings, and there are anatomic differences (see later), including a quadruped posture, which increases stability and helps protect the brains of animals.

Among animals, trauma to the brain is probably most frequently caused in dogs as a result of automobile-induced injury and in cats from falls from significant heights (high-rise apartment buildings, balconies, and roofs). Even after falling from considerable heights, cats often have remarkably minor injury to the CNS. Other examples include fracture of the spinal column or cranium of jumping horses and fractious animals, such as horses and ruminants, during excitement and restraint.

Predisposition to cerebral trauma is also influenced by anatomic differences. The percentage of brain mass in relation to skull size is much less in domestic animals than in primates, and in the bovine and porcine species the cranial cavity is additionally protected dorsally by prominent frontal sinuses. Birth trauma, which can be important in human beings, is essentially insignificant in animals because in the latter, the shoulders and particularly the pelvis, rather than the head, are likely to be compressed in the birth canal. Exceptions to this generalization include brachycephalic breeds of dogs. Several factors also influence the susceptibility of the spinal cord to trauma. The amount of space between the spinal cord and the wall of the vertebral canal is very important in determining the degree of injury after edema or compression with disk herniation. This space is greater in the cervical area of the dog than at the thoracolumbar level. Thus disk herniation at the latter area is more likely to result in severe spinal cord injury.

Functional factors also play an important role in brain injury. The brain of a freely movable head is much more susceptible to injury than one that is fixed in place. The increased susceptibility of the former has been attributed to the ability of the cranium (the bone) and its contents (the brain) to impact each other after nonpenetrating trauma. This interaction occurs because the brain does not completely fill the cranial cavity, thus resulting in a very short distance (or space) between brain and bone.

The type and location of the lesion (contusion and/or hemorrhage) depends on the location of the point of contact and the direction of the blow, relative to the head. If the blow is directly on the back or front of the head, the head and brain will move straight forward or backward, respectively (see Fig. 14-66, axial force). If the blow is horizontal to the top of the head or horizontal to the rostral portion, the head will rotate on the atlantooccipital axis (angularly and rotationally, respectively). In the case of an axial blow to the back of the head (an animal falling onto the back of its head), the head and thus the cranial vault will accelerate faster than the brain, which will lag behind, and the caudal aspect of the vault may move forward and contact the caudal aspect of the cerebral hemispheres, usually the occipital cortex. In the case of an animal falling onto the back of its head, the head will accelerate abruptly and the momentum will carry the brain caudally, where it may strike the inside of the caudal brain in the cranial vault. A vertical blow delivered directly down onto the dorsal surface of the head will have the same type of result on the dorsal aspect of the cerebral hemispheres as the blow to the back of the head. It is more common, from the same blows described previously, to see hemorrhage, usually subarachnoid, on the opposite side of the point of impact with the brain. For example, a vertical blow to the top of the head causes hemorrhage of the ventral surface of the medulla and cerebral hemispheres. Thus after an impact on a stationary, freely movable head, the bone of the cranial vault will move on the stationary brain and injure it (coup injury) and on the opposite side the nerves and blood vessels will be stretched, possibly resulting in nerve damage and hemorrhage (contrecoup injury). In addition, the mass and velocity of the object striking the head are important. Trauma after impact of a relatively large blunt object can create notable head movement and a large-impact injury, whereas a small object, such as a bullet moving at a high rate of speed, can cause less head movement and a smaller but deeper area of direct tissue damage. In summary, the basic concept is the transfer of kinetic energy by the striking object to the head. A large blunt object will cause the head to accelerate without deforming it; a smaller object, such as a bullet, will penetrate.

Factors involved in the protection of the brain include the rigidity of the cranium (depending on age), the round shape of the dorsum of the skull, the structure of the parietal, occipital, and temporal cranial bones (two layers of compact bone separated by spongy bone referred to as diploë), cranial sutures, sinuses, ridges in the floor of the cranial cavity, meninges, and CSF. The spinal cord is enclosed and protected by the vertebral column, which is surrounded by soft adipose tissue and muscle. Other structures that help protect the spinal cord by absorbing shock are the intervertebral disks and the cancellous bone of the vertebrae. Vertebral ligaments maintain the alignment of the vertebral column; denticulate ligaments support the spinal cord in the middle of the vertebral canal, and the meninges, particularly the CSF, cushions trauma.

Clinically, animals with CNS trauma have signs referable to the area injured, brain, or spinal cord. With brain trauma, signs can vary widely and range from unconsciousness lasting a few seconds followed by complete recovery and return to normal function to depression, abnormal behaviors such as disorientation and irritability, semiconsciousness with responsiveness only to noxious stimuli, and unconsciousness with no response to any stimulus. With spinal cord trauma, signs vary, depending on the severity of the injury and the rate of onset. Paralysis results from severance of the cord or ruptured disks. Paresis and ataxia result from less severe injury.

Concussion. Concussion is often thought of as a clinical designation of temporary loss of consciousness with recovery after head injury. As in human beings, a movable head is much more susceptible to trauma than a fixed, supported one. Application of an appropriate concussive trauma to the mobile head of an animal results in a reversible cerebral dysfunction that lasts for a matter of seconds or at most a few minutes and is usually reversible, with stronger blows causing more severe injury and even death.

Concussive injuries of the diffuse type also occur in animals, but there are some differences between animals and human beings. For example, it is difficult to produce severe concussion in animals because the margin between the force of a stunning blow and one causing fatal injury is very small. The smaller the brain, the less vulnerable it is to rotational forces and the larger are the forces necessary to cause concussion. It should be noted, however, that concussion, particularly when there is rapid recovery from unconsciousness, can occur more frequently than appreciated in animals because the clinical signs may not be recognized.

Diffuse brain injury does not usually cause gross lesions. Microscopic lesions detected in animals include diffuse axonal injury characterized by axonal degeneration, and this may be followed by Wallerian degeneration. Damage to neurons ranges from central chromatolysis to death and neuronal loss. The more severe forms of diffuse brain injury can also have generalized acute brain swelling caused by unregulated vasodilation, which can be followed after some time by cerebral edema.

Spinal concussion is the term applied to the immediate and temporary loss of function that sometimes follows severe direct blows to the spinal column. Loss of function usually affects the long tracts/bundles of nerve fibers (funiculi), but usually there is no demonstrable external change in the vertebrae or spinal cord. As with cerebral concussion, there is often only a temporary functional disability of the cord after injury, but if the trauma is more severe, permanent neurologic deficits can result.

Contusion. *Contusion* means bruising, which is generally associated with rupture of blood vessels, and in the cerebrum, this injury results in grossly detectable lesions, such as hemorrhage, which can, like concussion, result in unconsciousness and even death. The factors that cause concussion and contusion can occur together in the same animal. Lesions can be superficial (cerebral gyri) or more central (brainstem), and there can be concurrent skull fractures.

Although hemorrhage is the most common lesion, contusion of the brain can also result in tearing of CNS tissue. Tearing results in tissue necrosis and neuronal loss. Two designations are used to identify the location of contusive injury. A coup contusion is located at the impact site, and a contrecoup contusion at a location on the opposite side of the brain. When the two lesions occur together (coup-contrecoup or contrecoup-coup), the first term indicates the site of most severe injury. Box 14-10 summarizes the pathogenesis of coup-contrecoup contusion.

Many investigations have been made to determine the mechanisms involved in the development of contusive lesions, and the kinetics are complicated and still not completely resolved. Factors considered to be significant include the ability of the head to move freely, the occurrence of a rotational movement of the brain over

Box 14-10 Pathogenesis of Coup-Contrecoup Contusion

CONDITIONS INVOLVED IN COUP-CONTRECOUP CONTUSION

1. Head freely movable.
2. Head accelerated rapidly (by being struck by a broad object, such as an automobile) or decelerated rapidly (head strikes pavement after a fall from a standing position).
3. Because the brain does not fill the cranial vault, it may lag behind the movement of the cranium when the head is accelerated or decelerated rapidly.
4. As a result, the inside of the cranial vault may strike the stationary brain at the point of impact (coup injury), or the lesion may occur on the opposite side (contrecoup), either from the stretching and tearing of vessels at that site or by the brain being struck by the inside of the cranial vault on the opposite side when there is reduced amount of cerebrospinal fluid buffer present.

rough surfaces on the inside of the cranial vault, and the development within the cranial cavity of positive and negative pressures and gravitational forces. The basic results of the different types of blows to the heads of animals have been discussed previously, and it is interesting to compare these with the lesions in human beings. Several neuropathologic principles have been generally accepted regarding craniocerebral contusive trauma in human beings, as follows:

1. A blow to the stationary (but freely movable) head produces a cerebrocortical coup contusion beneath the point of cranial impact, but with rare exceptions causes no cerebrocortical contrecoup contusion opposite the point of cranial impact. This outcome is not always true of animals, in which a blow to the dorsum of the head from a flat object, such as a spade, causes marked subarachnoid hemorrhage on the ventral surface (contrecoup).
2. An impact of a moving head (moving before impact, as in a fall from a standing position) against a firm or unyielding surface causes a cerebrocortical contrecoup contusion opposite the point of cranial collision (often at the poles and inferior surfaces of the frontal and temporal lobes), but with rare exceptions there is no contusion beneath the point of impact. In contrast, horses that fall backward and land on their backs and strike the occiput often have subarachnoid hemorrhage over the occipital poles of the cerebral hemispheres.
3. Falls from great heights and crushing of the head between a strong external force and unyielding surface are generally not associated with the occurrence of contrecoup lesions.

Dawson and coworkers proposed a mechanism for both contrecoup and coup injury of the human brain that also addressed the specific deficiencies of mechanisms that have been advanced by others. An example explaining the mechanism of contrecoup injury states that when a person falls backward from a standing position because of loss of balance, the gravitational torque acting on the body causes downward acceleration of the head in excess of the acceleration as a result of gravity. Under these circumstances the brain lags toward the trailing anterior surface of the cranium before impact (causing displacement of the protective CSF layer between the brain and skull) and permits compressive stress to develop at this site, although impact occurs at the opposite side of the head. Because dissipation of the CSF at the anterior (contrecoup) site allows compressive stress to be focal at this contrecoup site and because of the shearing stress generated, injury occurs. In addition, a relative rotational gliding motion between the brain and skull is produced when the impact suddenly stops the skull's motion and rotation, thus creating an additive shearing stress because the fluid lubrication necessary to facilitate gliding of the brain over the cranial surface is reduced. The concentration of this rotational shearing stress is likely to occur beneath the frontal and temporal lobes because of the rough surface of the skull that exists in this location. In contrast to contrecoup injury, coup contusions occur infrequently in this type of fall. In such situations the brain lags away from the impact site, which results in a thickening of the protective CSF layer between the brain and skull immediately beneath the point of impact, which helps explain the absence of coup injury in primates and human beings in typical moving head trauma.

Coup injury in human beings can occur when a stationary but freely movable head is impacted. In this type of trauma there is neither brain lag nor disproportionate distribution of CSF before impact, which accounts for the typical absence of contrecoup contusions. With regard to falls from great heights, the dynamics involving rotation of the body about a fixed point of ground contact associated with a fall from a standing position do not occur. Because gravity produces no torque on a freely falling object, no angular acceleration of the body is produced; therefore such a fall is a true free-fall state that is associated with an absence of brain lag. For this reason, contrecoup lesions occur infrequently with this type of trauma. One point should be emphasized with regard to the evaluation of coup and contrecoup cortical contusions just described. Displacement of bone associated with skull fracture can contuse the subjacent brain, regardless of the resting or moving status of the head, and such fracture-contusions have nothing to do with the coup-contrecoup mechanisms described. Also, even though the basic mechanisms discussed earlier apply to human beings, they should also be considered when evaluating cerebral contusions of domestic animals, but the situation in human brains is made far more complex because of the numerous wide bony ridges that project into the cranial vault.

Evaluation of spinal cord trauma should include examination not only of the spinal cord but also of the vertebral column and spinal nerve roots. Injuries to the spinal cord can involve concussion, contusion, hemorrhage, laceration, transection, and compression secondary to vertebral trauma and fracture. Contusion in the spinal cord is characterized by vascular tears, hemorrhage, and necrosis. Tears are generally focal and grossly visible. Contusion can occur without fracture of the vertebral column, with fracture, and with fracture plus dislocation of the spinal column. The latter combination can result in tearing and transection of the spinal cord.

In the acute phase of spinal cord trauma, contusions are microscopically identified by regions of perivascular hemorrhage. This lesion occurs rapidly and over time progresses to include blood diffusing into adjacent cortical tissue, where, if enough time lapses, reactive astrocytes and infiltration of macrophages occur. If allowed to heal, a region of gliosis and hemosiderin pigment is commonly found in these regions.

Central Nervous System Hemorrhage. Although hemorrhage and hematomas in animal brains can be caused by a wide variety of injuries, trauma to the head is the most common cause. (Box 14-11 lists common causes of brain hemorrhage.)

After trauma to the head, hemorrhages can develop in the epidural, subdural, and subarachnoid locations, under the pia mater (subpial), and in the brain (see Fig. 14-66, *B*). Hemorrhage can be diffuse (see Fig. 14-67) or focal (e.g., hematomas) (Fig. 14-68). Such hemorrhages can result from sliding of the brain over bony ridges

Box 14-11 Common Causes of Hemorrhage in Animal Brains

Vasculitis (such as *Histophilus somni* infection; angioinvasive fungal infections)
Damage to endothelium lining blood vessels (by the virus of canine infectious hepatitis, by septicemia or endotoxemia, by immune complexes, or by parasite larval migration)
Trauma
Contusion
- Coup lesion
- Contrecoup lesion

Penetrating wounds

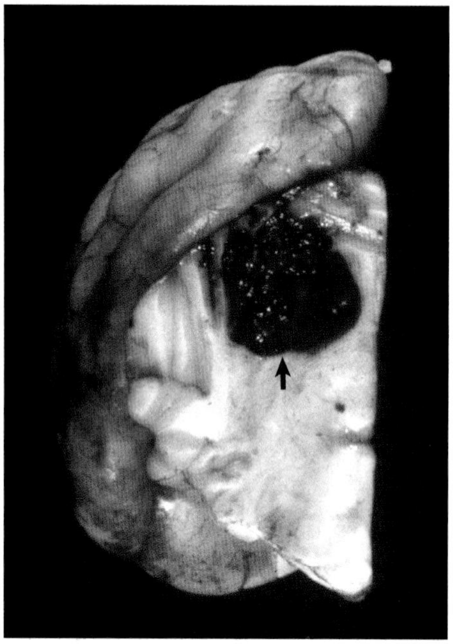

Figure 14-68 Hematoma, Cerebellum, Transverse Section, Dog. Traumatic injury to the head resulted in hemorrhage and the formation of a hematoma *(arrow)* from shear, tensile, compressive axial, rotational, and angular forces. (Courtesy Dr. H.B. Gelberg, College of Veterinary Medicine, Oregon State University.)

within the cranium, with resultant stretching and tearing of blood vessels and tissue, after the cutting and penetration of bone fragments from skull fracture. Cerebral epidural hemorrhage, which is not commonly described in animals, has been reported in the horse, especially jumpers, resulting from falls while working. Epidural hemorrhage does not usually occur because the dura is tightly adhered to the inner surface of the calvaria and there is no epidural space. In trauma causing skull fractures, bleeding from local blood vessels can separate the dura from the calvaria, forming a hematoma in the dural space.

Subdural hemorrhage, which is an extravasation of blood between the dura mater and the cortex, occurs in dogs and cats. It is rare and usually diffuse and does not commonly organize into focal hematomas as seen in human beings, where they can be life threatening from compression and herniation of the brain. Subarachnoid and intracerebral hemorrhages are most common in all species after head injury (Fig. 14-69). Hemorrhage can result from injury to the brain with or without a fractured cranium by the mechanisms given

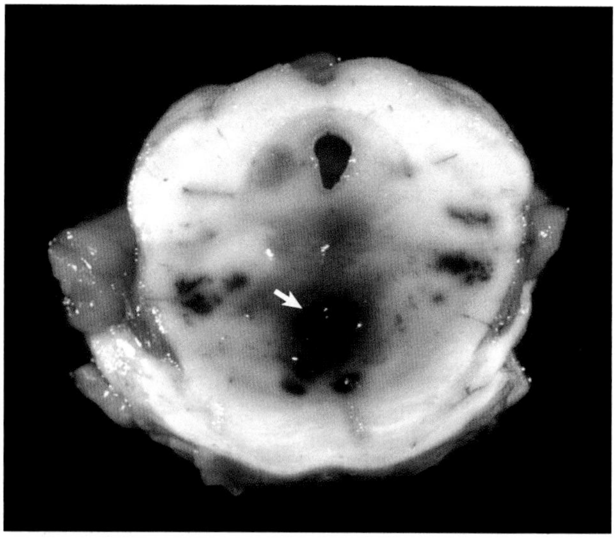

Figure 14-69 "Duret" Hemorrhages, Brainstem, Transverse Section at the Level of the Mesencephalon. Note the multiple hemorrhages in the ventral mesencephalon *(arrow)*. These hemorrhages are the result of twisting of the brainstem on a longitudinal axis from rotational and axial forces. (Courtesy Dr. M.D. McGavin, College of Veterinary Medicine, University of Tennessee.)

previously and also from penetrating objects (bullets and stab wounds).

The same types of hemorrhage that affect the brain (epidural [rare], subdural [rare], and parenchymal) also occur in the spinal cord and its meninges. Causes are similar to those for the brain.

Hematomyelia (Hemorrhagic Myelomalacia). Traumatic injury to the spinal cord can cause stretching and tearing of blood vessels, usually arterioles, within the gray matter, resulting in hematomyelia. Hematomyelia is also particularly associated with severe type I disk herniation. If larger vessels are torn, blood pressure can force blood into the gray matter. This outcome results in the formation of a dissecting blood-filled cavity ascending and/or descending initially within the gray matter of the spinal cord. This lesion, which is characterized by a softening to semiliquefaction (myelomalacia) and hemorrhage of the tissue, can develop within 12 to 24 hours after injury and can progress both cranially and caudally from the original site of trauma. As the cavity extends cranially, the hemorrhage at the original site also extends into the white matter and can transect the spinal cord. If this lesion extends to the fifth cervical cord segment, the phrenic nerves to the diaphragm will be denervated and respiratory paralysis will result. Bleeding continues until pressure in the blood-filled cavity is equal to the vascular pressure or until bleeding ceases because of hemostasis in the vessel. Hemorrhage can also result from bleeding in arteriovenous malformations within the spinal cord. Hematomyelia is characterized by neurologic deficits consistent with a sudden onset of ascending or descending flaccid paralysis and sensory abnormalities.

Compressive Injury. Diseases resulting in compressive injury can affect the brain, spinal cord, or both concurrently. In the brain, diseases, such as neoplasia, reticulosis, canine granulomatous meningoencephalitis, and chronic cerebral abscesses, can compress adjacent nervous tissue. In the spinal cord, compression can be intramedullary (within the spinal cord) or extramedullary (outside the spinal cord). Causes of intramedullary compression include hemorrhages, neoplasms such as nephroblastoma of the young dog, and chronic expansile inflammatory diseases. Extramedullary compression can be caused by intervertebral disk herniation in the dog; cervical stenotic myelopathy (wobbler syndrome) in the horse and dog; vertebral fracture and dislocation; neoplasms of the meninges, such as the meningioma; nerve rootlets, such as nerve sheath tumors; or tumor metastasis, such as lymphosarcoma. Finally, developmental anomalies of bone, such as atlantooccipital malformation, and vertebral deformities with hemivertebrae, such as scoliosis, lordosis, and kyphosis (Fig. 14-70), can result in compression of the spinal cord.

Compression of CNS tissue causes neuronal dysfunction by impeding normal anterograde and retrograde axoplasmic flow in axons (see E-Fig. 14-3). In addition, compression of nerves may result in reduced blood flow to nerves and thus also contribute to neuronal dysfunction. Mild compression can result in partial blockage of slow axoplasmic flow and gradual accumulation of neurofilaments and microtubules, which results in mild enlargement of the axon proximal to the compression site and atrophy of the axon distal to the compression. Eventually, with a long period of time of complete blockage, the distal axon is lost.

Brain Displacements. See the discussion of cerebral edema (permeability changes) in the section on Central Nervous System Swelling and Edema.

Cervical Stenotic Myelopathy. Cervical stenotic myelopathy, or wobbler syndrome, is characterized by stenosis of the cervical vertebral canal, which causes compressive trauma to the cervical spinal cord (Fig. 14-71). This disease occurs primarily in young rapidly growing large breeds of horses and dogs. Reports indicate that the disease is not caused by a straightforward mechanism but apparently involves several factors (multifactorial disease). For example, stallions that have a genetic predisposition for rapid growth and large body size are reported to be at greater risk for developing the disease. Oversupplementation with protein, vitamins, and minerals used to promote rapid growth may also be another environmental factor in developing cervical stenotic myelopathy.

Gross and microscopic lesions of the CNS in cervical stenotic myelopathy are similar to the lesions in intervertebral disk herniation. The severity depends on the speed and degree to which the compression is applied and the specific area of the cord that is involved. Central nervous tissue can tolerate a considerable degree of compression if it is applied slowly. Rapid compression can lead to quickly developing hypoxia-ischemia, necrosis, and direct damage to compressed axons. Lesions detected include a spectrum of changes characterized by axonal injury and disruption of myelin sheaths, resulting in Wallerian degeneration and necrosis of the gray or white matter or of both. Lesions can be visible grossly from the exterior but are more commonly seen on cross section of the spinal cord.

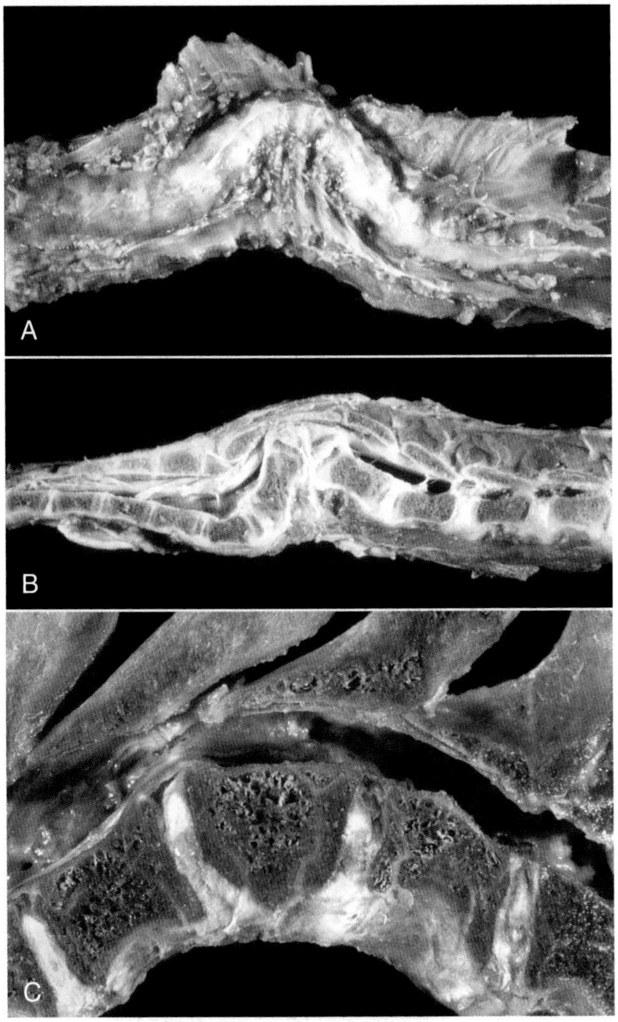

Figure 14-70 Vertebral Abnormalities, Vertebral Column. A, Scoliosis, thoracic vertebrae, ventrodorsal view, sheep. Lateral deviation of the spinal column. **B,** Kyphosis, thoracolumbar vertebrae, lateral view, sheep. Dorsal deviation of several vertebrae and a wedge-shaped vertebra (hemivertebra; C) have resulted in compression of the spinal cord. **C,** Hemivertebra, lumbar vertebrae, dog. Note that the craniodorsal portion of the body of the hemivertebra has protruded into the vertebral canal. (**A** and **B** courtesy College of Veterinary Medicine, University of Illinois. **C** courtesy Department of Veterinary Biosciences, The Ohio State University.)

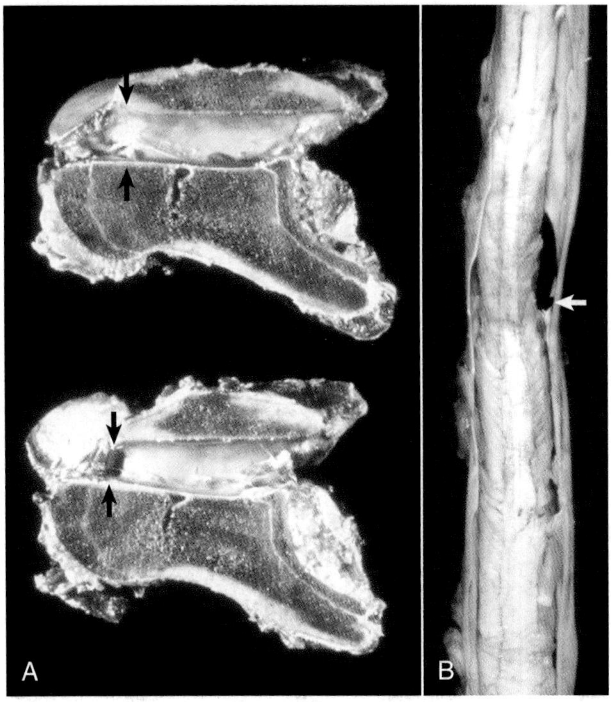

Figure 14-71 Cervical Stenotic Myelopathy. A, Cervical static stenosis, vertebral column, sagittal section, sixth cervical vertebra, horse. The vertebra on the bottom is stenotic *(arrows)* and will compress the spinal cord. The vertebra on the top is normal *(arrows)*. **B,** Cervical vertebral instability, spinal cord, fifth cervical segment, dog. Note the narrowing of the spinal cord at the site of compression *(arrow)*. (Courtesy College of Veterinary Medicine, University of Illinois.)

Microscopically, particularly at the site of injury, there is initial swelling of axons followed after several days by loss of architecture of the CNS as a result of necrosis and a beginning accumulation of gitter cells that have phagocytosed the lipid-rich tissue debris. Eventually the necrotic area is cleared and a cystic space is formed, which is surrounded by varying degrees of astrocytosis and astrogliosis, although not usually prominent unless there is severe destruction. Rostral and caudal to this location, the lesion is primarily one of Wallerian degeneration in the white matter, and the pattern of lesion development seen depends on the level of the spinal cord that is examined relative to the site of compression. At the site of injury, all parts of the white and gray matter of the spinal cord are affected and often necrotic, if the compressive force is sufficient. Rostral to this site, white matter degeneration is generally limited to the ascending tracts in the dorsal funiculi and the superficial portions of the dorsolateral part of the lateral funiculi. Caudal to the area of injury, degeneration is limited to the descending tracts in the ventral funiculi, and the more central portions of the lateral funiculi. It should also be noted that (1) a lesion may occur at the point of compression because of ischemia, but a lesion can also occur on the opposite side of the compression also because of ischemia that results from compression of the tissue against bone on that side, and (2) Wallerian degeneration can be observed in distal segments of affected axons far from the point of compression within the spinal cord. In the former case, compressive forces can be transferred through the spinal cord to axons and blood vessels away from the contact point, whereas in the latter example, degeneration of the distal axon segments can extend for a length of centimeters to meters away from the point of contact.

Cervical stenotic myelopathy has been known for many years to affect horses and more recently has been recognized in the large dog breeds. The disease in the horse has been referred to by several designations: the wobbler syndrome, wobbles, equine incoordination, and more recently, cervical stenotic myelopathy. The disease has been described in many horse breeds.

Cervical stenotic myelopathy in the horse has been divided into two syndromes: cervical static stenosis and cervical vertebral instability (dynamic stenosis). Cervical static stenosis commonly affects horses 1 to 4 years of age. The spinal cord is compressed at C5 through C7 as the result of an acquired dorsal or dorsolateral narrowing of the spinal canal (see Fig. 14-71). The stenosis is due to formation of bone that requires time to develop. The compressive effect with this type of stenosis is present regardless of head position. The second form of cervical stenotic myelopathy (cervical vertebral instability [dynamic stenosis]) occurs in horses ranging in age from 8 to 18 months and is characterized by a narrowing of the spinal canal during flexion of the neck, primarily at C3 through C5 vertebrae.

A disease process with many similarities to that in the horse also affects the dog. It has been known as wobbler syndrome, vertebral instability, vertebral subluxation, and cervical spondylolisthesis. The disease has been most frequently described in the Great Dane and Doberman pinscher breeds but has also been reported in the Saint Bernard, Irish setter, fox terrier, basset hound, Rhodesian ridgeback, and Old English sheepdog. Dogs can have signs develop between 8 months and 1 year of age, with a range of 1 month to 9 years. Great Danes tend to have lesions develop at a young age (8 months to 1 year), whereas Doberman pinschers are generally older, often more than 1 year of age. The vertebral and associated spinal cord lesions in the dog have been reported to most often involve the caudal cervical area from C5 through C7 vertebrae. An exception is the basset hound, in which C3 is affected.

Tumors. In the brain, diseases, such as neoplasia, cause compression of adjacent nervous tissue. Compression of CNS tissue causes neuronal dysfunction by impeding normal anterograde and retrograde axoplasmic flow in axons (see the later discussion of specific types of CNS tumors).

Leptomeningeal Hemorrhage. Physical trauma to the CNS compresses, twists, and stretches blood vessels until they are torn. Such injury results in bleeding and leptomeningeal (subarachnoid) hemorrhage (see Fig. 14-67). In the spinal cord, laceration of a large artery or vein can result in prolonged bleeding that ascends or descends the leptomeninges, causing neurologic dysfunction on examination compatible with ascending or descending neurologic deficits in spinal nerve roots.

Tumors

Neoplasms of the CNS in domestic animals occur most frequently in dogs, and at frequency and variety similar to human beings. These tumors share many gross and histologic features with their human counterparts. In human neuropathology, brain tumors are typically graded according the World Health Organization classification of tumors of the CNS (2007). This human grading scheme is being increasingly applied to brain tumors of domestic animals, most notably the dog; however, its usefulness and applicability in animal species needs to be established. The majority of neoplasms described have been in dogs and cats, and a large portion of these tumors occur in the older population. The intention in discussing CNS neoplasms in this chapter is to present a brief overview of the more common or better-known neoplasms that occur in animals and is not meant to be all-inclusive. The location and characteristics of the primary and common secondary (metastatic) tumors of the nervous system are summarized in Table 14-9. Clinical signs in animals with intracranial tumors (e.g., gliomas, choroid plexus tumors) vary, depending on the location of the tumor in the CNS, but can include behavioral changes, ataxia, tetraparesis, seizures, circling, and abnormal cranial nerve and proprioceptive reflexes. The average age of affected dogs ranges from 6 to 12 years, and certain dog breeds are predisposed including brachycephalic breeds (e.g., boxer, Boston terrier) and golden retrievers.

Embryonal or Primitive Neoplasms. Considering the complexities of brain development and the fact that astrocytes and oligodendrocytes arise from common stem cells early in development, it should not be surprising that some neoplasms arising in the CNS have multiple lines of differentiation as indicated by immunohistochemical analysis. One such neoplasm is the rare primitive neuroectodermal tumor. These tumors have been described sporadically in cattle, horses, and dogs. They are found most commonly in young animals and are considered aggressive biologically. Histologic features include poorly differentiated embryonal cells with Homer Wright rosettes and a relatively high mitotic rate. Immunohistochemical staining for specific markers confirms multiple lines of differentiation such as neuronal, astrocytic, and oligodendroglial. Typically, one cell type dominates, most commonly neuronal.

Other uncommon embryonal tumors include medulloblastoma, ependymoblastoma, and malignant rhabdoid tumor. Like primitive neuroectodermal tumors, medulloblastomas are most common in young animals. They have been reported in horses, cattle, pigs, dogs, and cats and arise in the cerebellum, usually in close proximity to the vermis, and invade into adjacent structures. The cell of origin for the medulloblastoma has not been definitely determined. It has been proposed that the neoplasm arises from primitive cells originating in the neuroepithelial roof of the fourth ventricle that give rise

Table 14-9 Primary Tumors of the Nervous System

Cell of Origin	Tumor Type	Location	Species Affected	Gross Appearance
CNS				
Embryonal cell	Medulloblastoma	Cerebellum (WM&GM)	Dog, cow, cat, pig (young animals)	Well-circumscribed, soft, gray to pink expansile mass (usually does not have hemorrhage, cysts, or necrosis).
Oligodendroglia	Oligodendroglioma	Cerebrum, brainstem, interventricular septum (WM&GM)	Dog, cat, cow	Well-demarcated, gray to pink-red, soft or gelatinous expansile mass, usually with areas of hemorrhage.
Astroglia	Astrocytoma	Pyriform lobe, cerebral hemispheres, thalamus-hypothalamus, midbrain, cerebellum, spinal cord (WM&GM)	Dog, cat, cow	Poorly demarcated, firm, gray-white when well differentiated; anaplastic neoplasms are moderately to well-demarcated, soft and friable (usually with areas of necrosis, hemorrhage, edema, and cavitation).
Ependyma	Ependymoma	Ventricular system (lateral; less commonly, third and fourth), central canal of the spinal cord	Dog, cat, cow, horse	Poorly to moderately to well-demarcated, soft and gray-white, invasive, destructive gelatinous expansile mass (usually with areas of hemorrhage and cavitation).
Choroid plexus epithelium	Choroid plexus tumor	Ventricular system (fourth; less commonly, third and lateral)	Dog, horse, cow	Well-demarcated, granular to papillary, gray-white to red, expansile mass.
Microglia	Microgliomatosis	Cerebrum, brainstem	Dog	Poorly demarcated, gray-white, infiltrative mass (may have perivascular pattern).
Endothelium	Hemangiosarcoma	Cerebrum, brainstem	Dog	Well-demarcated, invasive red to dark red, expansile mass.
Arachnoid cells	Meningioma	Meningeal surface of the CNS (convexity and lateral surfaces of the cerebral hemispheres, tentorium cerebelli, flax cerebri, ventral brainstem, spinal cord)	Cat, dog, horse, cow, sheep	Well-demarcated, variable shapes, firm, encapsulated, and gray-white to soft, red-brown or gray, expansile masses (usually with areas of hemorrhage and necrosis).
PNS				
Schwann cells (other supportive cells)	Peripheral nerve sheath tumor*	Cranial nerves, spinal nerves (brachial plexus)	Dog, cow, cat	Firm or soft (gelatinous), white or gray, nodular masses.

*Other names for this tumor type include schwannoma, neurofibroma, and neurilemmoma.
CNS, Central nervous system; *PNS,* peripheral nervous system; *WM&GM,* white matter and gray matter.

to the external granule cell layer. Medulloblastomas are well circumscribed, soft, gray to pink masses and usually do not cause hemorrhage and/or necrosis or form cysts. Their expansile growth can compress the fourth ventricle and cause obstructive hydrocephalus and can also infiltrate adjacent structures, including the leptomeninges, and metastasize throughout the ventricular system. Histologic features, including Homer Wright rosettes and a high mitotic rate, are similar to those occurring in other embryonal tumors described in the veterinary literature; however, the neoplastic cells are typically small and round with variably elongate nuclei and ill-defined cytoplasm. Ependymoblastomas and rhabdoid tumors are extremely rare embryonal tumors that have been only sporadically reported and have not been adequately described in the veterinary literature.

Astrocytomas. Astrocytomas have been morphologically classified based on their degree of differentiation (histologic features in H&E-stained sections) and include the following three types: diffuse astrocytomas, anaplastic astrocytomas, and glioblastoma multiforme. The degree of differentiation refers to how closely astrocytes forming the tumor resemble normal astrocytes within the CNS. Diffuse astrocytomas tend to have the most well differentiated astrocytes, whereas glioblastoma multiforme has the most poorly differentiated astrocytes. All of these tumors are malignant; however, the degree of malignancy is often inversely related to the degree of differentiation.

Astrocytomas have been reported most commonly in dogs (10% to 15% incidence) and cats, and rarely in horses, cattle, and pigs. Brachycephalic breeds, such as Boston terriers and boxers, and dogs

5 to 11 years of age are most commonly affected. Common sites include the cerebral hemispheres, especially the temporal and pyriform lobes, thalamus-hypothalamus, midbrain, and less frequently, the cerebellum and spinal cord.

Astrocytomas often displace normal tissue; however, their gross appearance often depends on their rate of growth and degree of differentiation (Fig. 14-72). Slow-growing, well-differentiated astrocytomas (less malignant) are usually difficult to distinguish from normal tissue and are rather solid or firm and gray-white. Rapidly growing, poorly differentiated astrocytomas are more malignant and easier to discern because they have areas of necrosis, hemorrhage, cavitation, and edema.

Microscopically, the more well-differentiated diffuse astrocytomas consist of a uniform cell type that is typically loosely organized. Cell size varies, and distinct ramifying cytoplasmic processes can be observed. Nuclei vary in size and shape and contain more chromatin than normal astrocytes. Cells tend to be arranged around and along blood vessels. The boundary between neoplastic and normal tissue is indistinct. Well-differentiated diffuse astrocytomas occur as pilocytic and gemistocytic variants, both of which recapitulate the histologic features of the astrocyte phenotype described earlier.

Conversely, anaplastic astrocytomas and glioblastoma multiforme have increased cellular pleomorphism, a high mitotic rate, and areas of necrosis. Glioblastoma multiforme is characterized by glomeruloid-like vascular proliferation and serpiginous tracts of necrosis that are often lined by neoplastic cells (pseudopalisading). Foci of oligodendroglial differentiation can be observed in these tumors. Grossly, hemorrhage is commonly observed in glioblastoma multiforme and can be a useful diagnostic feature.

Increasing use of immunohistochemical markers for glial cells and indicators of cellular proliferation can undoubtedly enhance the specificity and prognostic significance of the diagnosis of different glial cell neoplasms in animals. The most reliable marker for astrocytomas is GFAP, although vimentin has proved useful in some cases. Recent studies have also indicated that immunoreactivity for insulin-like growth factor–binding protein 2, epidermal growth factor receptor, and platelet-derived growth factor receptor-α may eventually become reliable markers for canine glioblastomas.

Oligodendrogliomas. Neoplasms composed of oligodendrocytes occur most commonly in the dog, but cases have been reported in cats, horses, and cattle. The reported incidence varies; some reports indicate oligodendrogliomas as the most common neuroectodermal neoplasm (5% to 12% incidence), whereas others place it second to astroglial neoplasms. As with astrocytomas in dogs, there is a predilection for brachycephalic breeds (Boston terriers, boxers, and bulldogs), and the age range is the same as for astrocytomas (5 to 11 years of age). Neoplasms occur in all areas of the cerebrum and brainstem, especially in close proximity to the lateral ventricles (Fig. 14-73; E-Fig. 14-8). Neoplasms tend to extend to meningeal and ventricular surfaces, and dissemination via the CSF and the ventricular system to distant brain sites can be a common finding.

Grossly, the typical oligodendroglioma is a well-demarcated mass of variable size that is characteristically gray to pink-red and soft to gelatinous with areas of hemorrhage. In larger tumors the central area may be cystic. Microscopically, the neoplasms are composed of densely packed cells. Nuclei are round, centrally located, and hyperchromatic. The cells are often surrounded by a halo (so-called honeycomb effect), which is an artifactual retraction of the cytoplasm caused by delayed fixation. Other patterns of growth include cells arranged in rows, especially peripherally in the mass, or in semicircles. Mitoses are generally infrequent. Other changes include mucoid degeneration (accounting for the gelatinous appearance seen grossly), edema, cavitation, and rarely mineralization. Extensive necrosis is uncommon, except in higher-grade variants (i.e., more anaplastic morphologic changes) of the tumor, where serpiginous tracts of necrosis, nuclear atypia, glomeruloid-like vascular proliferation, and high mitotic rate are commonly encountered. Immunohistochemical identification of neoplastic oligodendrocytes can be aided by the use of CNPase and Olig1/Olig2; however, these markers are not 100% specific for the identification of neoplastic oligodendrocytes, and routine histologic examination remains the standard by which to diagnose these tumors.

Oligoastrocytomas. Mixed gliomas (i.e., oligoastrocytomas) are characterized by atypical populations of neoplastic oligodendroglia and astrocytes. These tumors are uncommon in veterinary

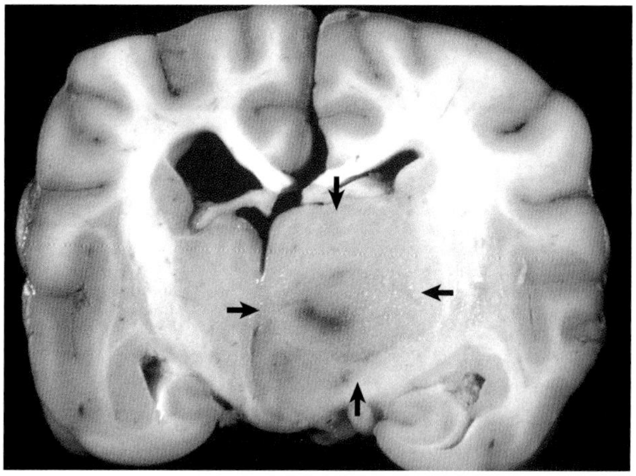

Figure 14-72 **Astrocytoma, Brain, Transverse Section at the Level of the Thalamus, Dog.** The deep ventromedial area (thalamus/hypothalamus) of the right hemisphere *(arrows)* contains a poorly demarcated, nonencapsulated, expansile mass, which is a space-occupying lesion that has displaced the midline to the left and compressed the right lateral ventricle. The left lateral ventricle is mildly dilated, most likely from compression of the interventricular foramen. (Courtesy Dr. M.D. McGavin, College of Veterinary Medicine, University of Tennessee.)

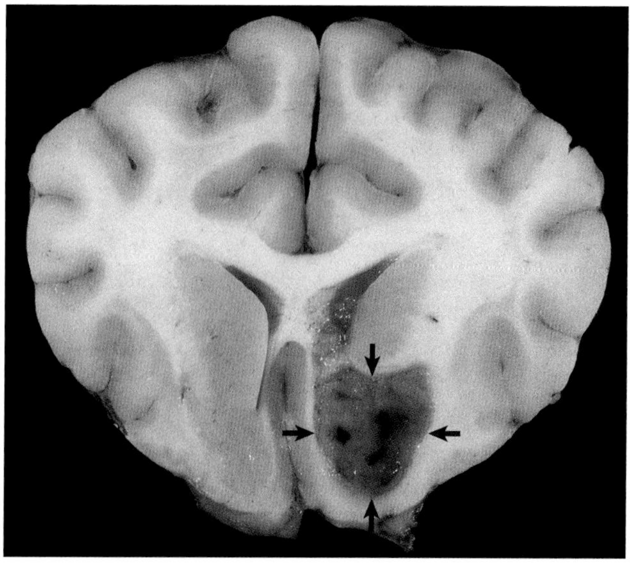

Figure 14-73 **Oligodendroglioma, Brain, Cerebrum, Transverse Section.** The tumor *(arrows)* is arising in the ventral cerebral cortex. It is well demarcated, gray, and gelatinous. (Courtesy Drs. A. de Lahunta and A.D. Miller, Cornell University College of Veterinary Medicine, Cornell University.)

medicine with most cases reported in the dog. Although foci of oligodendroglioma and astrocytoma differentiation can be seen in astrocytomas and oligodendrogliomas, respectively, to be diagnosed as a mixed glioma, the proportion of each cell population in the tumor needs to be greater than 30%. Histologic features are similar to those described earlier in the sections covering astrocytomas and oligodendrogliomas. The degree of necrosis, mitotic activity, and microvascular proliferation vary based on the anaplastic grade of the tumor.

Gliomatosis Cerebri. Gliomatosis cerebri is a widely infiltrating glioma that is uncommonly encountered in veterinary medicine with most reports confined to the dog. Gross lesions are typically not present, unless the diffusely infiltrating cells coalesce to form a distinct "mass lesion." The cells, which infiltrate the CNS, are elongate with a prominent nuclear chromatin pattern and scant cytoplasm. They do not have any topographic perivascular orientation. Mitoses can be common and typically increase in number directly correlated to the anaplastic grade of the tumor. An astrocytic origin for the majority of these tumors is suspected, and neoplastic cells can stain positive by immunohistochemical reaction for GFAP. However, some of these tumors are negative for GFAP, suggesting either a different cell of origin (i.e., microglia) or the possibility that the mass consists of dedifferentiated astrocytes that are not expressing GFAP. Rarely oligodendroglial tumors can have a similar pattern of spread.

Ependymomas. Ependymomas are one of the less frequently occurring neoplasms in dogs, cats, cattle, and horses. Some reports on the dog indicate a higher frequency in brachycephalic breeds. Ependymomas usually involve the lateral or less commonly, mesencephalic aqueduct, third, and fourth ventricles. They also occur in the central canal of the spinal cord. The neoplasm can be observed within the ventricular system and anywhere along the subarachnoid space, likely attributable to local metastasis via the CSF. Noncommunicating hydrocephalus may result from obstruction of CSF flow within the ventricular system.

Grossly, ependymomas are usually large expansile intraventricular masses with generally well-demarcated margins (Fig. 14-74). The neoplasm is soft and gray-white to red, depending on blood content, and has a smooth cut surface in dogs. In cats the cut surface can have a granular texture. In some ependymomas the cut surface may have gelatinous consistency and be cavitated. More aggressive tumors show invasion into the normal tissue at its margins. Microscopically, ependymomas are highly cellular and well vascularized. Cells have hyperchromic, round-to-oval nuclei with scant or undetectable cytoplasm. Cells form perivascular rosettes (pseudorosettes) with nuclear polarity away from the vessel wall. Cells are also arranged in sheets and bands. The mitotic rate is variable. Hemorrhage, cystic degeneration, and capillary proliferation occur. Higher-grade tumors display invasive growth, frequent mitoses, and anaplasia. Currently no reliable specific immunohistochemical markers for ependymomas exist; however, GFAP immunoreactivity can be observed, especially in the pseudorosettes where the anuclear areas are GFAP positive. Cytokeratin immunoreactivity has a patchy pattern of distribution.

Choroid Plexus Tumors. Choroid plexus tumors (papillomas and carcinomas) occur most commonly in the dog but have been reported in horses and cattle. In the dog they are reported to be 5% to 10% of all primary brain tumors, and there is a breed predilection reported for golden retrievers. The age at clinical presentation varies widely, but it is usually seen in middle-aged to older dogs. In the dog the neoplasm occurs most frequently in the fourth ventricle, but it also can be located in the third and lateral ventricles.

Grossly, the neoplasm is a well-defined, expansive, granular to papillary growth located within the ventricular system that is gray-white to red and compresses the adjacent nervous tissue (Fig. 14-75). Noncommunicating hydrocephalus may result from obstruction of CSF flow within the ventricular system. Microscopically, these neoplasms generally resemble the choroid plexus and are characterized by an arborizing vascular connective tissue stroma that is covered with a cuboidal to columnar epithelial layer. Mitoses are not typically present in the benign form. A more malignant variety, choroid plexus carcinoma, is characterized by invasiveness, increased mitoses, additional occurrence of solid tumor growth, and a tendency to metastasize within the ventricular system or into the subarachnoid space (carcinomatosis), where implantation in the

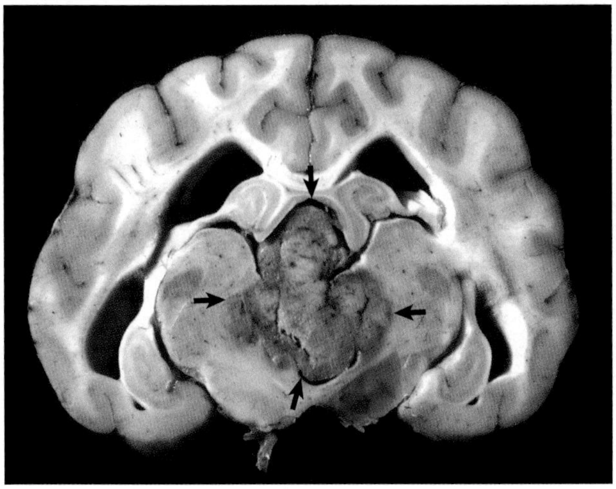

Figure 14-74 **Ependymoma, Brain, Transverse Section at the Level of the Hippocampus, Dog.** The third ventricle contains a moderately well demarcated expansile mass *(arrows)* that has invaded normal tissue ventral to it. Moderate hydrocephalus is present in both lateral ventricles from blockage of the third ventricle. (Courtesy Dr. M.D. McGavin, College of Veterinary Medicine, University of Tennessee.)

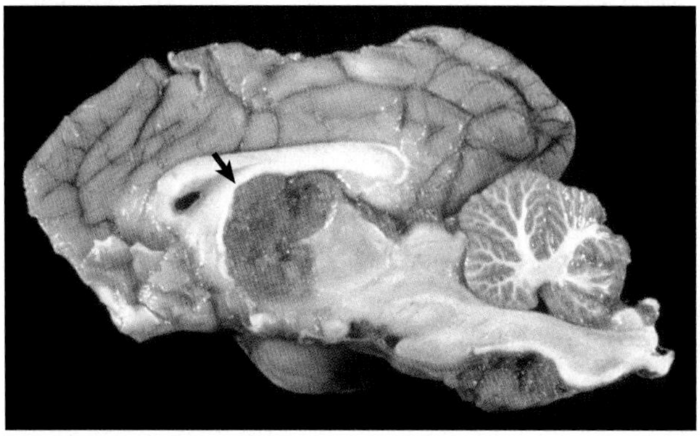

Figure 14-75 **Choroid Plexus Tumor (Carcinoma), Brain, Sagittal Section, Dog.** The third ventricle contains an expansile mass *(arrow)* that has invaded the normal tissue ventral to it. The mass ventral to the medulla *(right)* may be a metastasis arising from tumor cells that entered the third ventricle and then spread in the cerebrospinal fluid caudally, through the mesencephalic duct, into the fourth ventricle, and out through a lateral aperture into the subarachnoid space. (Courtesy Dr. Y. Niyo, College of Veterinary Medicine, Iowa State University; and Noah's Arkive, College of Veterinary Medicine, The University of Georgia.)

ependyma or meninges, respectively, occurs. Immunohistochemical identification with cytokeratin and E-cadherin can be useful. Patchy GFAP immunoreactivity is also reported.

Meningiomas. Meningiomas are the most common neoplasm of the CNS in dogs and cats, and there are rare reports in horses and ruminants. The majority of meningiomas occur in dogs between 7 and 14 years of age and in cats 10 years old or older. Sites of occurrence in the dog include the basal area of the brain, the area over the convexity of the cerebral hemispheres, the cerebellum-tentorium area, the lateral surface of the brain, the falx cerebri, and the surface of the spinal cord. Retrobulbar involvement (originating from the optic nerve sheath) also occurs. In the cat the neoplasm uniquely occurs in the tela choroidea of the third ventricle (E-Fig. 14-9) but also occurs over the cerebral hemispheres, along the falx cerebri, over the cerebellum and tentorium, and rarely at the base of the brain. Occurrence in the meninges of the spinal cord is not common. Meningiomas arise from the arachnoid cell layer, which is on the external surface of the arachnoid membrane. These cells cover the surface of the arachnoid layer that opposes the surface layer of the dura mater, and thus these tumors project into the subdural space and often compress or invade the underlying CNS parenchyma.

Grossly, neoplasms in the dog are solitary and vary in size. The neoplasms are well defined, spherical, lobulated, lenticular, or plaquelike in shape; firm; encapsulated; and gray-white (Fig. 14-76). Sometimes on the cut surface there are soft, red, brown, or gray areas of hemorrhage and necrosis. Because these neoplasms grow slowly, they cause pressure atrophy of the adjacent nervous tissue. Meningiomas can be invasive, and sometimes there is hyperostosis of the overlying bone. In the cat, meningiomas vary in size from barely detectable to 2 cm in diameter. Cats can develop more than one neoplasm over the cerebrum, and meningiomas can also be incidental, old-age findings. Other characteristics are comparable with those described in the dog.

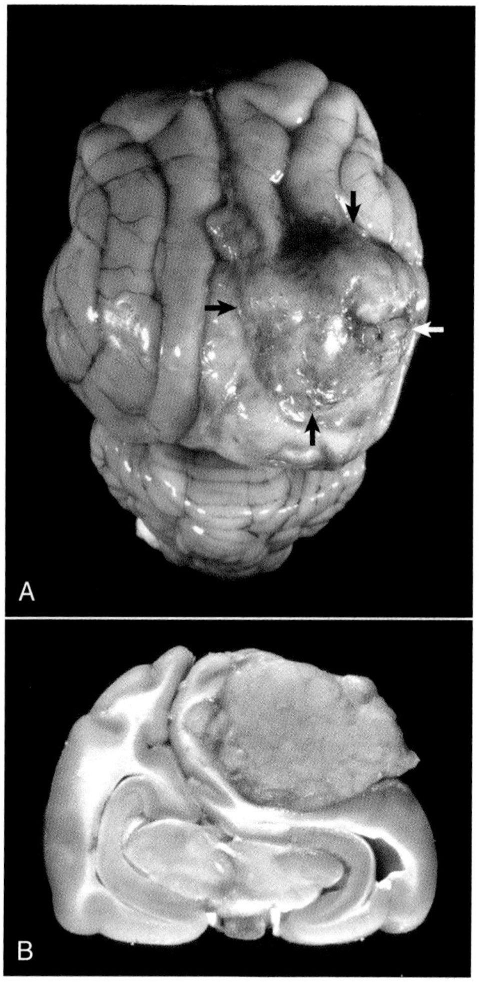

Figure 14-76 **Meningioma, Brain, Cat. A,** On the surface of the right parietal cortex is a mass *(arrows)* that has compressed and distorted the adjacent parenchyma. It is a space-occupying lesion that has displaced the midline (cerebral longitudinal fissure) to the left. **B,** Transverse section at the level of the hippocampus of the brain depicted in **A**. The tumor has compressed the right cerebral hemisphere, and this has resulted in the midline being displaced to the left with compression of the left cerebral hemisphere. The meningioma does not invade the brain and can be "shelled" out at necropsy or surgery. (Courtesy College of Veterinary Medicine, University of Illinois.)

Microscopically, several patterns of neoplastic cells can occur, and more than one pattern can be present in a given neoplasm. Based on their cytomorphologic features, the majority of these tumors can be subtyped as follows: (1) transitional; (2) meningothelial; (3) psammomatous; (4) fibrous; (5) atypical; or (6) malignant. The transitional, meningothelial, psammomatous, fibrous, and atypical subtypes appear to be the most common in the dog. In the cat, almost all meningiomas have features that are more typical of the meningothelial or transitional type with psammoma bodies being a common feature. Other less common subtypes include angiomatous, chordoid, microcystic, malignant, and papillary. Although cytomorphologic features of all subtypes are beyond the scope of this chapter, general features of the most common subtypes are mentioned here. The transitional subtype is composed of nests of polygonal to spindle cells arranged in whorls. The meningothelial variant is composed of cellular sheets lacking distinct morphologic characteristics, whereas the fibrous variant is composed of interlacing bundles of spindle cells. The psammomatous variant is characterized by a predominance of mineral concretions (psammoma bodies). Typically in these variants the neoplastic cells have large cell bodies with abundant cytoplasm, ill-defined cell boundaries, and elongated, oval, open-faced nuclei with peripherally located chromatin. The number of cells making up a whorl can vary from a few to many. Additional microscopic lesions include hemorrhage, foci of necrosis, and infiltrates of neutrophils. Whereas necrosis is an indication of a poorer prognosis in human beings, it is common in canine variants of meningioma, and its significance in tumor progression is unknown. Invasive growth occurs but is less common than growth by expansion. Currently, immunohistochemical staining is not as advanced in veterinary medicine as it is in the diagnosis of meningiomas in human beings; however, vimentin can be useful.

Hemangiosarcoma. Primary hemangiosarcoma of the CNS is a rare neoplasm arising from endothelial cells. The disease is most common in dogs but can occur in all domestic species. The neoplasm is a solitary expansile red to dark red mass within the cerebral cortex. Its color and bloody consistency are helpful in differentiating it from a primary or metastatic melanoma. Most hemangiosarcomas found in the CNS are from metastases.

Hematopoietic Tumors

Lymphoma. A variety of hematopoietic tumors affect the CNS, both as primary and as metastatic neoplasms. The most common of these tumors is lymphoma. Primary CNS lymphoma occurs in all domestic animal species but is most common in the dog and the cat. In the cow it can occur as part of a manifestation of bovine leukosis virus–associated lymphoma; however, this tumor more commonly presents as an extradural white to yellow lobulated compressive mass in the spinal canal. Primary lymphoma in the dog and the cat has no sites of predilection and can involve adjacent organs, including the pineal gland and the pituitary gland. They are composed of dense sheets of neoplastic lymphocytes that typically have a high mitotic rate and many regions of single cell to confluent necrosis. The primary cell type may be a T or B lymphocyte. Identification of the cell type requires immunohistochemical analysis; CD3 (T lymphocyte) and CD79a/CD20/Pax5 (B lymphocyte) are the markers most commonly used to classify these tumors.

An uncommon variant of CNS lymphoma is intravascular lymphoma. This variant occurs almost exclusively in the dog. Histologically, it presents as dense aggregates of neoplastic lymphocytes that fill meningeal and parenchymal blood vessels. Thus these tumors are often associated with the formation of thrombi and infarction of local tissues. Neoplastic infiltration into the parenchyma apparently only occurs with rupture of the affected vessels. Presumably, these neoplastic lymphocytes lack appropriate migration signals or receptors needed to cross the blood-brain barrier. These tumors typically have a B lymphocyte origin in dogs, which contrasts to the more typical T lymphocyte phenotype in human beings.

Histiocytic Sarcoma. Histiocytic sarcoma is another hematopoietic neoplasm that can present either as a primary CNS tumor or as part of disseminated disease. The primary tumor typically presents as a meningeal mass that compresses and less commonly invades the underlying neuroparenchyma. Although certain breed predilections are reported for this (including Bernese mountain dog and Pembroke Welsh corgi), many breeds have been reported to develop this disease. Histologically, these tumors are composed of neoplastic round cells that often have reniform nuclei. Multinucleated cells are common, and the mitotic index is often quite high. These tumors can be further identified through a variety of immunohistochemical stains, including CD18 and Iba1.

Other Hematopoietic Tumors. Other hematopoietic tumors, including extramedullary plasmacytomas, have been reported rarely in the CNS; however, these tumors represent a very small fraction of the primary hematopoietic tumors of the CNS.

Metastatic Tumors. Hematogenously metastasizing neoplasms occur and affect the brain more often than the spinal cord. The species in which metastasis has been most commonly reported is the dog; the next most frequent is the cat. Of the metastasizing carcinomas, mammary gland carcinoma in the dog has been reported to occur most frequently, although others, especially nasal carcinoma due to local metastasis, have been described. Hemangiosarcoma is one of the most common metastasizing sarcomas in the dog and the most common metastasizing tumor to the brain. Metastases of many other sarcomas, including lymphosarcoma, fibrosarcoma, and malignant melanoma, have also been reported. In the CNS, metastatic hemangiosarcomas appear to have predilection for the gray matter–white matter interface (Fig. 14-77). In the cat the neoplasms that metastasize to the CNS include the mammary gland carcinoma (Fig. 14-78) and lymphosarcoma.

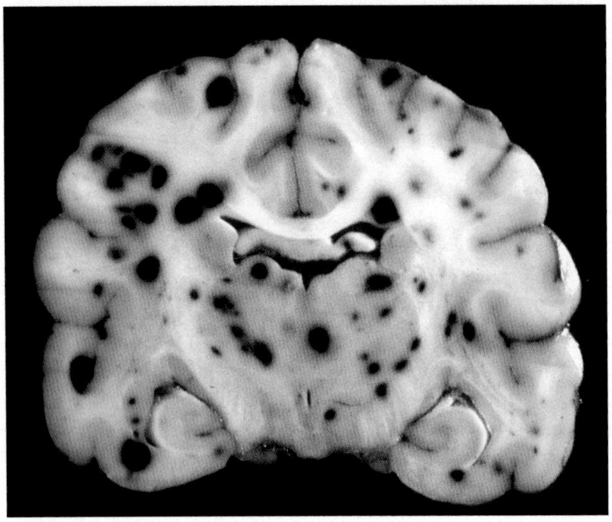

Figure 14-77 **Hemangiosarcoma, Metastatic, Brain, Formalin-Fixed, Transverse Section at the Level of the Thalamus, Dog.** Note the prominent hematogenous metastases, which appear as black nodules of various sizes distributed throughout the brain, sometimes at the gray matter–white matter interface. In an unfixed (fresh) specimen the nodules would be red to dark red. Black nodules in a fresh specimen would be consistent with metastatic melanoma. (Courtesy Dr. M.D. McGavin, College of Veterinary Medicine, University of Tennessee.)

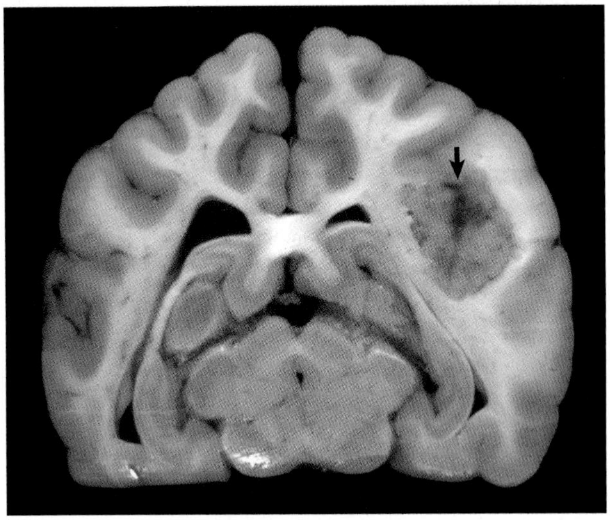

Figure 14-78 **Mammary Carcinoma, Metastatic, Brain, Transverse Section at the Level of the Hippocampus, Dog.** The right cerebral hemisphere contains a well-demarcated mass *(arrow)*, which has caused enlargement of the right cerebral hemisphere and compression of the right lateral ventricle. The left lateral ventricle is slightly dilated, probably because of pressure on the interventricular foramen. (Courtesy Drs. F. Moore and J. Carpenter, Angell Memorial Animal Hospital; and Noah's Arkive, College of Veterinary Medicine, The University of Georgia.)

Aging Changes

Throughout this chapter, specific disorders have been correlated with aging because they occur in older animals and include, as examples, cerebral cortical atrophy of aging, hydrocephalus ex vacuo, the accumulation of lipofuscin pigment in neurons, and some forms of neuroaxonal dystrophy. Their relationship to behavioral changes is unclear. More recently, suspected aging changes in the nervous system of dogs and cats (i.e., senility of advanced age or "dementia") have been correlated with behavioral changes such as deficiencies in learning and memory, as well as loss of other "normal routine" and long-established behavioral patterns. This collection of clinical signs in dogs has been termed canine cognitive dysfunction (CCD) and has been compared, in some respects, to Alzheimer's disease in human beings. Senile plaques and cerebrovascular amyloidosis have been described in the brains of aged dogs and are thought to result in structural and functional alterations in chemical pathways leading to cognitive dysfunction.

Disorders of Horses

Disorders that occur in many or all animal species are discussed in the section on Disorders of Domestic Animals.

Diseases Caused by Microbes

Viruses

Arboviruses

Equine Encephalomyelitis. Eastern equine encephalomyelitis (EEE), western equine encephalomyelitis (WEE), and Venezuelan equine encephalomyelitis (VEE) viruses are members of the family Togaviridae, genus *Alphavirus*. The primary target cell for infection and injury is the neuron; however, these viruses can cause vasculitis followed by thrombosis. After inoculation (by mosquito) the hematogenously circulating virus initially infects several tissues, including endothelial cells of local blood vessels, tissues of the lymphoreticular system (also known as monocyte-macrophage system), muscle, and connective tissue. In lymphoid tissue and bone marrow this infection may cause cellular depletion, necrosis, or both. A second viremia results in hematogenous infection of the CNS. Experimental evidence suggests that the virus replicates in endothelial cells before entering the nervous system and infecting neurons and to a lesser extent glia. There is also evidence that viruses of this group (notably Venezuelan equine encephalomyelitis) can cause alterations in the metabolism of neurotransmitters in the CNS and that these alterations are responsible for some of the clinical signs.

Recent experimental evidence from in vivo and in vitro models of Venezuelan equine encephalomyelitis suggests that the virus causes upregulation of multiple proinflammatory genes, including inducible nitric oxide synthase and TNF-α. This upregulation, occurring principally in astrocytes, affected other glial cells and influenced neuronal survival. In addition to these mediators of innate immune responses, apoptotic cell death also contributes to neurodegeneration after virus infection.

In the CNS, all three viruses induce a polioencephalomyelitis that has similar characteristics, but there are some differences. Overall, gross lesions are uncommon and nonspecific. They can include cerebral hyperemia, edema, petechiation, focal necrosis, and increased CSF in the subarachnoid space. Gross lesions, although not often present, are usually found in gray matter, which is appreciated best in the spinal cord (Fig. 14-79). Microscopic lesions are most prominent in the gray matter of the brain and spinal cord and are characterized by perivascular cuffing with lymphocytes, macrophages, and neutrophils; variable neutrophilic infiltration of the gray matter; microgliosis; neuronal degeneration; focal cerebrocortical necrosis; perivascular edema and hemorrhage; necrotizing vasculitis; thrombosis; choroiditis; and leptomeningitis. Neutrophils are detectable during the early stages (2 days) of clinical eastern equine encephalomyelitis and Venezuelan equine encephalomyelitis. Vasculitis, thrombosis, and cerebrocortical necrosis are particularly evident in Venezuelan equine encephalomyelitis, but also in eastern equine encephalomyelitis. No lesions are detected in the trigeminal ganglion.

Infection of horses with eastern equine encephalomyelitis, western equine encephalomyelitis, and Venezuelan equine encephalomyelitis viruses produces a range of progressive clinical maladies, including fever, rapid heart rate, anorexia, depression, muscle weakness, and behavioral changes, such as dementia, aggression, head pressing, wall leaning, circling, blindness, and paralysis of facial muscles. Eastern equine encephalomyelitis has also been reported in cattle, sheep, camelids, and pigs.

West Nile Viral Encephalomyelitis. West Nile virus (WNV), a mosquito-borne virus (family Flaviviridae, genus *Flavivirus*) that causes acute polioencephalomyelitis primarily in human beings, birds, and horses, is most commonly transmitted via a bird-mosquito cycle. In 2002, West Nile virus infection was diagnosed in 47,000 horses in 40 states in the United States, and it was estimated that more than 4500 horses died after infection. It remains an important cause of viral encephalitis in horses, and the disease is ubiquitous in the lower 48 states of the United States.

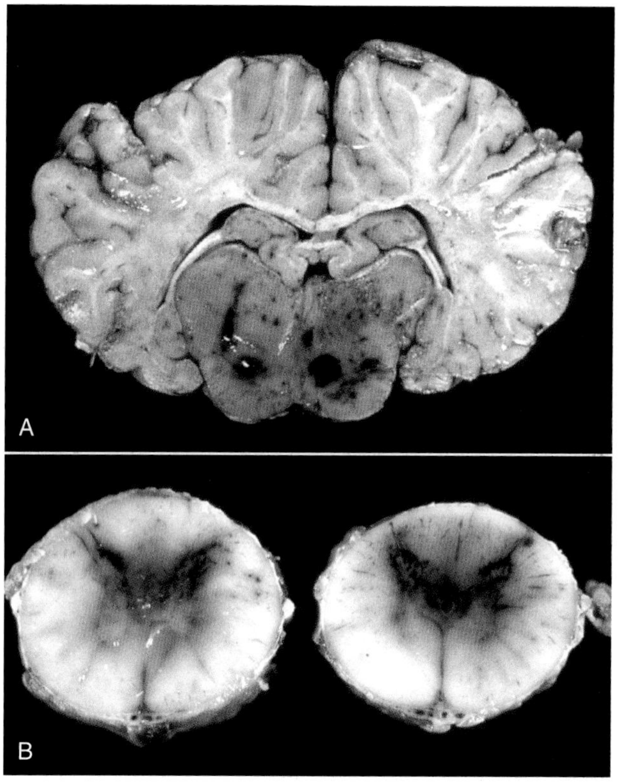

Figure 14-79 **Hemorrhagic Encephalitis and Myelitis, Eastern Equine Polioencephalomyelitis, Brainstem and Spinal Cord, Horse. A,** Brain, transverse section at the level of the hippocampus, horse. The gray matter of the brainstem has dark red to black discoloration as a result of congestion and hemorrhage. The lesion is the result of viral infection, which has an affinity for neurons; this virus also causes vascular necrosis followed by thrombosis, but this is not common. **B,** Spinal cord, horse. Note the red to brown discoloration of the gray matter in the dorsal and ventral horns (caused by congestion and hemorrhage). The lesion is the result of viral infection that has an affinity for neurons; however, this virus can also cause vascular necrosis followed by thrombosis. (Courtesy College of Veterinary Medicine, University of Florida; and Noah's Arkive, College of Veterinary Medicine, The University of Georgia.)

The virus passes freely through a variety of wild-songbird populations with members of the Corvidae (crow family) and American robins playing important roles in the propagation and dissemination of the virus. Additionally, a variety of *Culex* mosquitoes disseminates the virus among animal populations. Birds develop a fulminate viremia with viral spread to all organs, whereas horses, representing a dead-end species for the virus, only have infections of the CNS.

The pathogenesis of West Nile virus encephalomyelitis remains to be fully elucidated; however, it is likely to be similar to the mechanism described previously for equine encephalomyelitis viruses. The primary target cell for infection and injury is the neuron; microglial cells are also affected. Gross lesions of West Nile viral infection in horses usually involve the gray matter and include hyperemia and petechiation to prominent hemorrhage with prevalent involvement of the lower brainstem and ventral horns of the thoracolumbar spinal cord. Gross lesions of hemorrhage are more likely to occur with West Nile virus than with the three equine encephalitides (eastern equine encephalomyelitis, western equine encephalomyelitis, Venezuelan equine encephalomyelitis). Microscopic lesions in birds and horses that have died of the disease are characterized by a polioencephalomyelitis and hemorrhage of the CNS that can vary in degree of severity. The inflammation is predominately mononuclear; however, neutrophils can be detected in some cases. Lesions outside of the nervous system in affected horses do not occur. Clinical signs of the equine West Nile viral infection include variable fever, depression, ataxia, weakness to paralysis of the hind limbs, tetraplegia, convulsions, coma, and death.

Herpesviruses

Equine Herpesvirus 1 Myeloencephalopathy. Equine herpesvirus 1 (EHV-1) (an alphaherpesvirus) is an important cause of equine abortion and perinatal foal infection and death, in addition to myeloencephalitis. EHV-1 can also cause rhinopneumonitis. EHV-1 does not appear to be neurotropic, which is in contrast to some herpesvirus encephalitides of other species in which the virus replicates in neurons (herpes simplex viral infection in the human, infectious bovine rhinotracheitis viral infection in calves, and pseudorabies viral infection in pigs). In addition to vasculitis being the principal lesion, the infection in the horse also differs somewhat from most other herpetic infections of the CNS in being primarily a disease of the adult, although young animals can be affected.

Equine herpesvirus myeloencephalopathy begins with inhalation of the EHV-1. The virus infects epithelial cells of the nasopharynx and spreads to local lymphoreticular tissue, where it infects lymphocytes and macrophages (monocytes). Through trafficking by monocytes, EHV-1 is transferred to endothelial cells of the CNS. The virus, which is endotheliotropic, even though infection of neurons and astrocytes can occur, localizes in small arteries and capillaries of the CNS and some other tissues after direct spread from the circulating infected cells. Inflammation of endothelial cells then results in vasculitis, leading to thrombosis and infarction of the neural tissue supplied by the thrombosed vessel. Latent infection of the trigeminal ganglion and lymphoid tissues can also occur. Although viral infection can be identified in neurons, the virus is not neurovirulent and has no effect on neural cells; thus the gross and histologic lesions noted in this disease are entirely related to vasculitis.

The characteristic lesion in the CNS caused by EHV-1 infection is a vasculitis affecting endothelial cells of small blood vessels with thrombosis and resulting in focal CNS necrosis (infarction). Lesions occur in both the gray and white matter of the spinal cord, medulla oblongata, mesencephalon, diencephalon, and cerebral cortex (Fig. 14-80, A). The endothelium appears to be the initial site of involvement (see Fig. 14-80, *B*), with the subsequent intimal and medial degeneration resulting in hemorrhage, thrombosis, extravasation of plasma proteins into the perivascular space, axonal swelling with ballooning of the myelin sheath and degeneration of the cell body, and variable mononuclear cell cuffing. Other lesions include cerebrospinal ganglioneuritis and vasculitis in nonneural tissues, including the endometrium, nasal cavity, lungs, uvea of the eye, hypophysis, and skeletal muscle. Inclusion bodies are not observed in CNS lesions.

The neurologic form of EHV-1 infection has a worldwide distribution and affects other Equidae, including zebras in addition to the horse, but appears to be relatively uncommon when compared with the incidence of abortion and upper respiratory tract disease caused by EHV-1. The neurologic disease may accompany or follow outbreaks of respiratory disease or abortion. An outbreak of epizootic acute encephalitis in Thomson's gazelle (*Gazella thomsoni*) was reported in 1997 from a zoologic garden in Japan. That disease resembled equine herpesvirus encephalitis, and the virus, named *gazelle herpesvirus 1*, was serologically related to EHV-1 and had a strong tropism for endothelium.

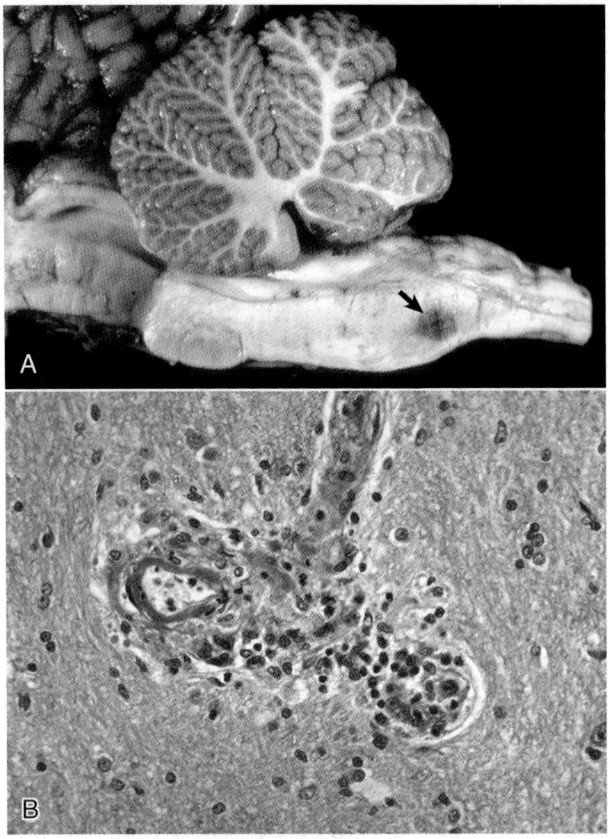

Figure 14-80 **Equine Herpesvirus 1 Myeloencephalopathy, Brain, Midsagittal Section. A,** Hemorrhage, brainstem, horse. Focal or multifocal areas of hemorrhage and/or necrosis *(arrow)* are characteristic of equine herpesvirus encephalitis but also occur in equine arteritis virus encephalitis, cerebrospinal nematodiasis, and equine protozoal encephalomyelitis (*Sarcocystis neurona*). **B,** Vasculitis and hemorrhage, brainstem, horse. Vasculitis is the primary lesion. The virus localizes in small arteries, venules, and capillaries of the central nervous system, resulting in vasculitis and fibrinoid necrosis, which at times leads to thrombosis and focal infarction of the brain and spinal cord. H&E stain. (**A** courtesy College of Veterinary Medicine, University of Illinois. **B** courtesy Dr. J. Simon, College of Veterinary Medicine, University of Illinois.)

Protozoa

Equine Protozoal Encephalomyelitis (Sarcocystosis). Equine protozoal encephalomyelitis is a disease in horses caused by *Sarcocystis neurona*. The microbe enters the body through ingestion of sporocysts, but how the parasite enters the CNS is unclear. Experimental studies suggest that ingested sporocysts multiply in visceral tissue, perhaps the intestine, and then are transported to the CNS probably via leukocytic trafficking. In the CNS the typical sequence of events in the pathogenesis of the characteristic lesion is thought to be (1) leukocytic trafficking with focal parasitic activation and replication, (2) marked inflammation, (3) edema, and (4) pronounced tissue destruction affecting both white and gray matter.

Gross lesions can occur throughout the neuraxis but are more common in the spinal cord, particularly the cervical and lumbar intumescences, than in the brain. In the brain, lesions are most commonly seen in the brainstem. When gross lesions are present, they consist of discolored necrotic foci, often with hemorrhages of varied sizes that are located randomly throughout the white or gray matter (Fig. 14-81).

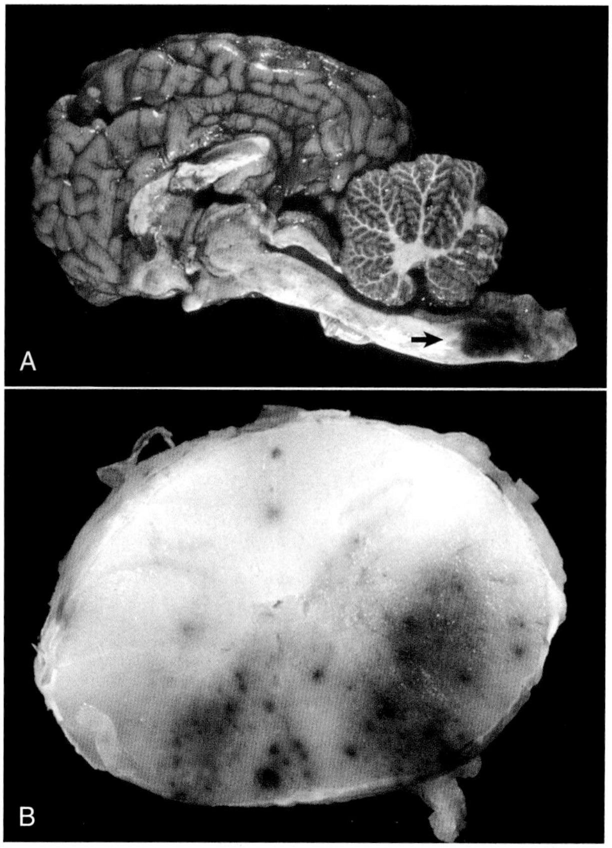

Figure 14-81 **Protozoal Encephalomyelitis, Brain, Sagittal Section, Horse. A,** Note the large focus of hemorrhage and necrosis *(arrow)* in the caudal medulla caused by *Sarcocystis neurona.* **B,** Lumbar spinal cord, transverse section. Myelitis due to *S. neurona* infection. Prominent focal hemorrhage and necrosis are present in the right lateral funiculus and in the right and left ventral funiculi. (**A** courtesy College of Veterinary Medicine, University of Illinois. **B** courtesy Dr. R. Storts, College of Veterinary Medicine, Texas A&M University.)

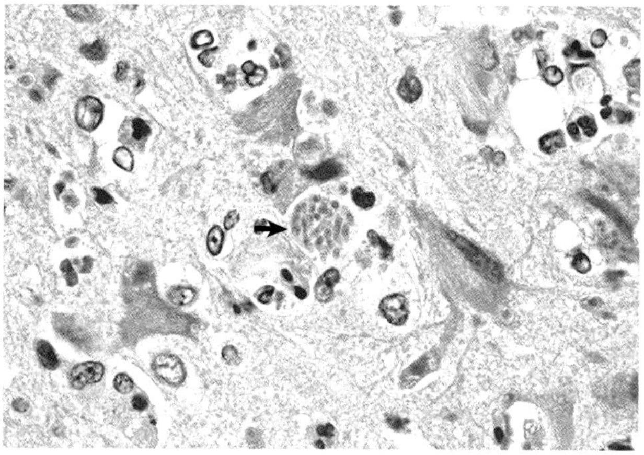

Figure 14-82 ***Sarcocystis Neurona,* Brain, Horse.** *S. neurona* is a small, crescent-shaped to round protozoan microbe found in neurons, endothelial cells, and microglial cells. The microbes can be arranged in nonencysted aggregates *(arrow)* or rosettes intracellularly and in central nervous system tissue often with a mixed leukocytic cellular inflammatory response of varied severity. Microbes can be difficult to detect in histologic sections. H&E stain. (Courtesy Dr. J. Simon, College of Veterinary Medicine, University of Illinois.)

Microscopic lesions occur in both the white and gray matter and include necrosis, hemorrhage, and accumulations of lymphocytes, macrophages, neutrophils, eosinophils, and variable numbers of multinucleated giant cells in perivascular areas and the neuropil, or less commonly, the leptomeninges and the axonal swelling. Gemistocytic astrocytosis can be prominent. In lesions, *S. neurona* is small and crescent shaped to round, has a well-defined nucleus, and is often arranged in aggregates or rosettes (Fig. 14-82). Microbes can be difficult to detect but occur intracellularly in neurons, giant cells, neutrophils, or macrophages or occur extracellularly in cysts within the neuropil. *S. neurona* is not typically seen in vascular endothelial cells, a common site for other members of this genus.

S. neurona can be propagated in tissue culture where it develops in the host cell cytoplasm. It divides by endopolygeny, with development of schizonts containing merozoites arranged in rosettes around a prominent residual body. The schizont stage of the microbe differs from those of the genera *Toxoplasma, Isospora, Eimeria, Besnoitia, Hammondia,* and *Neospora* because the merozoites lack rhoptries but resemble the schizont stage of other members of *Sarcocystis* spp. and of the *Frenkelia* genus. Studies have shown that the opossum represents the definitive host and avian species represent the intermediate host, providing a reservoir for infection of the horse.

Sarcocystis spp. infection in nonequine species involves microbes similar to *S. neurona.* Such microbes have been associated with encephalomyelitis in cattle, sheep, cats, and dogs, as well as raccoons, but such infections are sporadic. Lesions and microbes have additionally been seen in the CNS of infected bovine fetuses and consist of multifocal glial nodules with or without microbes. Rare cases of equine protozoal myelitis have occurred concurrently with *Neospora hughesi* or *N. caninum.*

Clinical infection typically occurs in young adult horses, and signs depend on the area of the CNS parasitized. Signs can include depression, behavioral changes, seizures, gait abnormalities, ataxia, facial nerve paralysis, head tilt, paralysis of the tongue, urinary incontinence, dysphagia, atrophy of masseter and/or temporal muscles, and atrophy of the quadriceps and/or gluteal muscles.

Degenerative Diseases

Metabolic

Equine Degenerative Myeloencephalopathy and Neuroaxonal Dystrophy. Equine degenerative myeloencephalopathy has been reported in a variety of purebred and mixed-breed horses, and a similar disease exists in zebras. To date the exact mechanism by which the disease develops is unknown; however, a genetic component likely underlies many of the cases. For cases in which a genetic basis cannot be determined, and for cases in which a genetic basis is known, the primary predisposing factor is dietary insufficiency of vitamin E. In some horses with low plasma concentrations of vitamin E, supplementation with vitamin E has resulted in clinical improvement of the horse. Additionally, the use of vitamin E supplementation in rations on farms with a high incidence of degenerative myeloencephalopathy has reduced the occurrence of the disease. A hereditary predisposition for equine degenerative myeloencephalopathy has not been excluded, but identifying a specific mechanism has so far been elusive.

In horses with degenerative myeloencephalopathy, lesions are microscopic. Axonal degeneration in the spinal cord is the most notable lesion, is bilateral, and can affect all funiculi, although lesions predominate in the sensory axons. Dorsal spinocerebellar tracts in lateral funiculi and septomarginal areas of the ventral funiculus are often severely affected. Myelin loss occurs secondary to the axonal degeneration. Depending on duration of clinical illness, astrogliosis occurs and is often most prominent in the region adjacent to the glia limitans. Another less dramatic lesion in affected horses is the formation of eosinophilic spheroids (Fig. 14-83). In horses, spheroids have been described in the nucleus gracilis, medial and lateral cuneate nuclei of the terminal brainstem, and thoracic nucleus of the spinal cord. Spheroids represent a focal eosinophilic swelling in the course of an axon that can be somewhat homogeneous, laminated, or granular. The swellings are filled with amorphous debris, membranous profiles, and effete organelles.

Neuroaxonal dystrophy has been reported in several horse breeds, most commonly the Morgan and Haflinger breeds. Lesions consist of spheroids in brainstem nuclei as previously noted, but the severe axonal degeneration does not occur in the spinal cord. The cause of axonal spheroids and dystrophic axons in equine degenerative myeloencephalopathy and neuroaxonal dystrophy is unclear; however, alteration of axoplasmic flow is suspected. Immunohistochemical analyses have shown that spheroids and dystrophic axons contain elevated quantities of proteins involved in movement, docking, and fusion of synaptic vesicles to plasma membranes. These findings suggest that disruption of axoplasmic flow plays a role in the pathogenesis of dystrophic axons in equine degenerative myeloencephalopathy and neuroaxonal dystrophy.

Clinically, equine degenerative myeloencephalopathy and neuroaxonal dystrophies typically occur in young horses. The onset is insidious, and clinical signs are symmetric with spasticity, ataxia, and paresis of the limbs.

Primary Neuronal Degeneration

Primary Cerebellar Neuronal Degeneration. Equine cerebellar abiotrophy, a primary cerebellar neuronal degeneration, occurs in Arabian or part-Arabian foals and Swedish Gotland ponies. The disease is inherited in an autosomal recessive pattern; however, the underlying pathologic mechanism for Purkinje cell loss remains elusive. Altered expression of MUTYH, a DNA-repair enzyme, has been shown in some affected horses. Grossly, the cerebellum may be slightly reduced in size and retracted from the overlying calvaria. Microscopically, early in the disease course Purkinje cells and their proximal axons are swollen (Fig. 14-84). With time there is loss of Purkinje cells and neurons of the granule layer. Clinical signs appear between the time of birth and 9 months of age and include head tremors, ataxia, and spasticity.

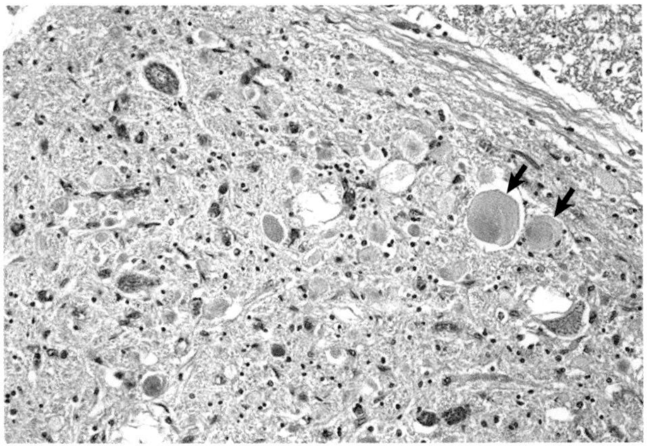

Figure 14-83 **Axonal Spheroids and Dystrophic Axons, Degenerative Myeloencephalopathy, Spinal Cord, Dorsal Gray Horn, Horse.** Axons of the thoracic nucleus are swollen, rounded, and pale pink (axonal spheroids, which are accumulations of neurofilaments and effete organelles) *(arrows)*. Attributed to vitamin E deficiency, through which vitamin E functions as an antioxidant, protecting cells from free radical–mediated injury. H&E stain. (Courtesy Dr. J.F. Zachary, College of Veterinary Medicine, University of Illinois.)

Nutritional

Vitamin E Deficiency. See the previous section on Equine Degenerative Myeloencephalopathy and Neuroaxonal Dystrophy.

Toxicoses

Microbial Toxins

Leukoencephalomalacia. Ingestion of moldy feed composed of corn or corn by-products contaminated with the fungus *Fusarium moniliforme* causes an acute fatal neurologic disease in horses called *leukoencephalomalacia*. The primary toxin isolated from *F. moniliforme* has been named *fumonisin* B_1, although other fumonisins have been extracted. Based on the character and progression of lesions, vascular damage has been inferred as the primary injury; however, fumonisins can also disrupt sphingolipid metabolism via the inhibition of ceramide synthase. Sphingolipids are bioactive compounds that participate in the regulation of cell growth, differentiation, metabolic functions, and apoptotic cell death. In addition, fumonisins are associated with lipid peroxidation of cells and cellular membranes, inhibit synthesis of macromolecules and DNA, and may enhance production of TNF-α by macrophages.

Gross lesions involve the white matter of the frontal and parietal lobes of the cerebral hemispheres most commonly, but cases with involvement of major white matter tracts in the brainstem and deep cerebellar white matter have occurred (Fig. 14-85). As a result of the white matter damage, including edema, brain swelling is marked with flattening of cerebrocortical gyri. The lesions are often bilateral but not symmetric, are unequal in severity, and can be quite extensive. The characteristic gross lesion at the time of death is malacia and liquefaction of the affected white matter due predominantly to the breakdown of lipids accompanied by hemorrhage. The reason white matter, including subcortical white matter, is principally involved—whereas the cerebral cortical gray matter is spared—is thought to be related to a unique vulnerability of the blood vessels in the white matter. The mechanism for this selective vulnerability is unknown.

Microscopically, the affected white matter is liquefied, and the parenchyma is disrupted by accumulation of pink-staining proteinaceous fluid with scattered neutrophils, lymphocytes, macrophages, and rarely eosinophils (see Fig. 14-85, C). The border of the lesion is surrounded by diffuse or perivascular edema, perivascular hemorrhage, and blood vessels with small leukocytic cuffs. In the acute

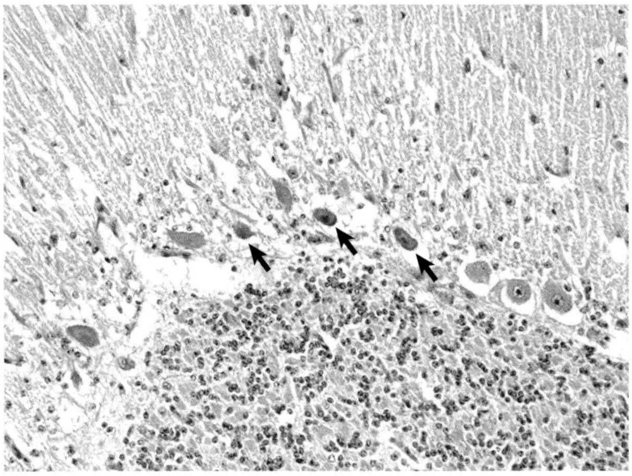

Figure 14-84 **Equine Cerebellar Degeneration, Cerebellum, Horse.** Purkinje cells in the cerebellum are undergoing necrosis with shrunken cell bodies and nuclear pyknosis *(arrows)*. H&E stain. (Courtesy Dr. J.F. Zachary, College of Veterinary Medicine, University of Illinois.)

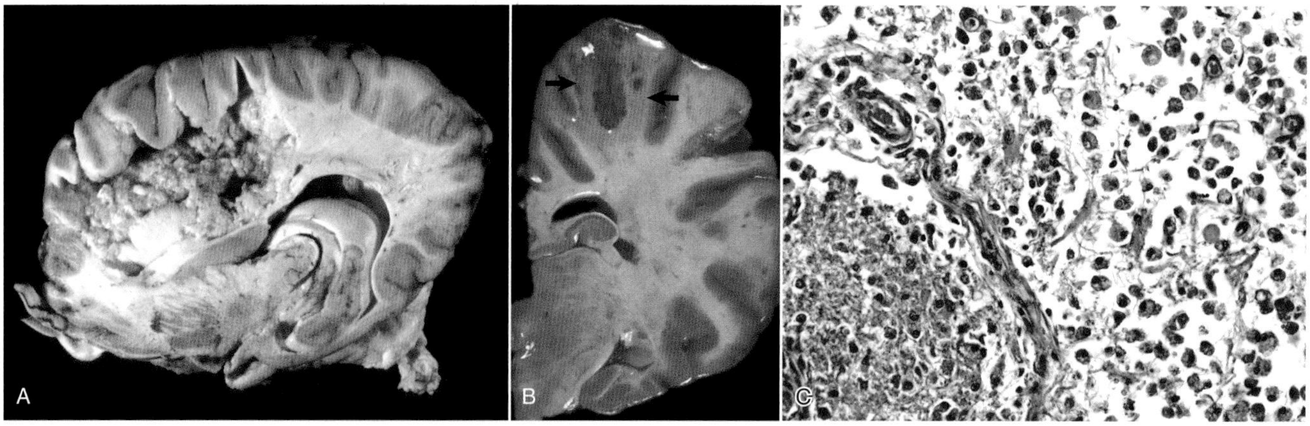

Figure 14-85 **Leukoencephalomalacia, Brain, Horse. A,** Sagittal section. The white matter of the frontal and parietal lobes is necrotic (malacia). The gray matter is not affected. This disease is caused by the toxin fumonisin B_1 produced by the fungus *Fusarium moniliforme*, which grows in damaged feed grains. Note that this case demonstrates the extent and distribution of liquefactive necrosis in the white matter in this disease. A more typical presentation is shown in **B. B,** Transverse section. The white matter of the three cerebral gyri located at the top of the illustration has areas of yellow gelatinous softening *(arrows)* and hemorrhage. Because of the absence of cavitation (liquefactive necrosis), the age of this lesion is likely less than the lesion depicted in **C. C,** Note the severe injury of the white matter. Myelinated axons are fragmented, and myelin debris is abundant. Numerous macrophages are present in the space previously occupied by myelinated axons, and they are phagocytosing the cellular debris. H&E stain. (**A** courtesy Dr. J. Simon, College of Veterinary Medicine, University of Illinois. **B** courtesy Dr. W. Crowell, College of Veterinary Medicine, University of Georgia; and Noah's Arkive, College of Veterinary Medicine, The University of Georgia. **C** courtesy Dr. W. Haschek-Hock, College of Veterinary Medicine, University of Illinois.)

phase especially, blood vessel walls are degenerate or necrotic, and some are infiltrated with neutrophils, plasma cells, and eosinophils. Although not often detected, thrombosis occurs. Less characteristic changes include edema and perivascular cuffing in the leptomeninges and neuronal necrosis in deeper layers of the overlying gray matter near the affected white matter.

Leukoencephalomalacia can also be associated with hepatotoxicity, or hepatotoxicity can be the sole manifestation. Additionally, other animals, including pigs, are susceptible, but clinical disease and lesions generally reflect pulmonary, hepatic, or renal injury. Clinical signs can include depression, somnolence, head pressing, aimless wandering, blindness, or seizures. Rapid progression of these clinical signs followed by death is typical, ranging from 1 to 10 days after onset.

Plant Toxins

Centaurea spp. Poisoning. Horses grazing *Centaurea solstitialis* (yellow star thistle) or *Centaurea repens* (Russian knapweed) develop a disorder known as *nigropallidal encephalomalacia*. This disease is similar to Parkinson's disease in human beings and has been proposed as a model for experimental studies; however, the equine disease is not associated with abnormal cytoplasmic accumulation of α-synuclein as seen in Parkinson's disease. The specific cause of the syndrome is not proved. A sesquiterpene lactone isolated from *C. repens* termed *repin* could provide a basis for the neurotoxicity. Cytotoxicity in cell culture was associated with depletion of glutathione (a major antioxidant), an increase in reactive oxygen species, and evidence of membrane damage in PC12 cells (a pheochromocytoma cell line) and mouse astrocytes. High concentrations of monoamine oxidase involved in dopamine metabolism normally found in the dopaminergic strionigral tract (i.e., striatum and substantia nigra [regulate balance and movement]) could render these areas of the brain more susceptible to oxidative damage caused by repin. The mechanism is unknown. Repin is also reported to inhibit dopamine release in the rat striatum, potentially contributing to the clinical manifestations of the disorder.

Gross brain lesions are sharply demarcated foci of yellow discoloration and malacia in the globus pallidus (pallidal) and substantia nigra (nigro) (Fig. 14-86). Lesions are usually bilateral and vary in severity; however, unilateral lesions also occur. Microscopically, necrosis with loss of neurons is the primary lesion; however, axons, glia, and blood vessels also are necrotic. The debris is phagocytosed by macrophages recruited into the lesion from the bloodstream.

Grazing the plants for 1 month or longer during the hot summer months when other forage is dried and unpalatable can cause clinical disease. Affected horses are somnolent, have persistent chewing movements, and have difficulty in prehension of feed and drinking water. With clinical evaluation, lip and tongue paralysis with reduced jaw tone are commonly recognized early in the disorder. Death generally is due to emaciation and starvation.

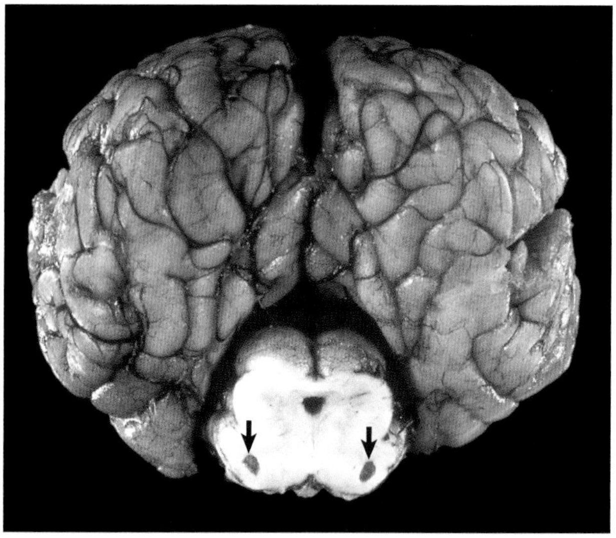

Figure 14-86 **Equine Nigropallidal Encephalomalacia, Brain, Transverse Section Through the Midbrain at the Level of the Rostral Colliculi, Horse.** This lesion is caused by yellow star thistle poisoning. Note the symmetrically cavitated (malacia) lesions in the substantia nigra *(arrows)*, resulting from necrosis and phagocytosis by gitter cells. (Courtesy Dr. L. Lowenstine, School of Veterinary Medicine, University of California-Davis; and Noah's Arkive, College of Veterinary Medicine, The University of Georgia.)

Miscellaneous Conditions. For discussion of miscellaneous conditions affecting individual animal species, see sections covering diseases specific for the species.

Cholesteatomas. Cholesteatomas, also called *cholesterol granulomas,* form in choroid plexuses of the ventricles in horses typically as an aging change, although rarely these granulomas can form in young horses. These masses are usually incidental, but if they grow large enough and occlude the flow of CSF, acquired hydrocephalus can result. Cholesteatomas are tan to yellow-brown firm masses with a smooth often glistening surface (Fig. 14-87). Occasionally the masses are mineralized. This lesion is thought to result from edema and minor, but repeated hemorrhages within the choroid plexuses, which result in cholesterol deposits. These deposits elicit a foreign body inflammatory reaction (foreign body granuloma) in the choroid plexus.

Circulatory Disturbances

Peripartum Asphyxia Syndrome. Peripartum asphyxia syndrome (dummy foal, neonatal maladjustment syndrome, or barker foal) is attributed to impairment of normal umbilical blood flow between the mare and foal during parturition, resulting in decreased vascular flow to the brain. Causes usually are those related to interruption of umbilical blood flow, such as a twisted or pinched umbilical cord as occurs in a dystocia or premature separation of the placenta, possibly caused by endophyte fescue toxicity.

In the early stages of the syndrome, hemorrhages are often widespread in nervous tissue, and cerebral gyri are edematous and swollen. If the foal survives for several days or longer, laminar cortical necrosis may occur. Microscopically, initial lesions consist of laminar cortical edema and neuronal necrosis, followed by gitter cell accumulation and phagocytosis of cellular debris. Ischemic neuronal injury can be found throughout the neuraxis.

Clinical signs in foals with peripartum asphyxia syndrome include barking like dogs, seizures, aimless wandering, absence of a suckling reflex, and loss of affinity for the mare. Affected foals are usually normal for the first 12 to 24 hours and then decline rapidly as neuronal necrosis ensues.

Postanesthetic Myelopathy. A hemorrhagic myelopathy has been reported in young horses secondary to general anesthesia in which the animals are placed in dorsal recumbency. Following surgery, they are typically unable to stand. Grossly, there is marked hemorrhage throughout the gray matter of the spinal cord and acute neuronal necrosis, histologically. Presumably the lesion develops secondary to the weight of the animal blocking normal venous drainage from the vertebral sinuses leading to an infarctive lesion in the spinal cord.

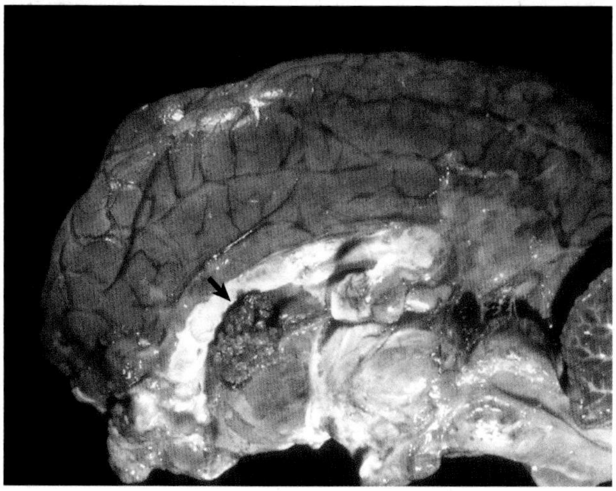

Figure 14-87 Cholesterol Granuloma (Cholesteatoma), Brain, Sagittal Section, Horse. The choroid plexus of the lateral ventricle contains an expansile mass consisting chiefly of cholesterol and a granulomatous inflammatory response *(arrow)*. (Courtesy College of Veterinary Medicine, University of Illinois.)

Disorders of Ruminants (Cattle, Sheep, and Goats)

Disorders that occur in many or all animal species are discussed in the section on Disorders of Domestic Animals.

Diseases Caused by Microbes

Bacteria

Listeriosis. Listeriosis, a bacterial disease with particular affinity for the CNS, is seen mainly in domestic ruminants. *L. monocytogenes,* a facultative intracellular Gram-positive bacterium, invades through the mucosa of the oral cavity and into sensory and motor branches of the trigeminal nerve. Other cranial nerve branches that innervate the oral cavity and pharynx may also be involved. The invasion through the mucosa is facilitated by trauma to the mucosa, thereby allowing the pathogen to gain access to the underlying tissues and nerve endings. The bacteria migrate via sensory axons using retrograde axonal transport to the trigeminal ganglion and then into the brainstem or via motor axons directly to the midbrain and medulla (motor neurons—nucleus of cranial nerve V). The infection can then spread rostrally and caudally to other areas of the CNS. These sites are likely the result of direct extension of infection because *L. monocytogenes* is a motile bacterium that spreads from cell to cell in its replicative phase.

The mechanism of tissue injury is not completely defined; however, injury to neurons and axons is likely a secondary bystander effect related to inflammation. A correlation between the degree of cell-mediated immunity and severity of brain damage suggests that immunologic injury may also occur. The microbe produces multiple virulence factors, including a hemolysin (listeriolysin), which is required for intracellular multiplication, and internalin, which internalizes E-cadherin, thereby allowing the infection to spread beyond localized regions.

Once bacteria enter the CNS, recent experimental studies suggest that *L. monocytogenes* can directly infect neurons, glia cells, and macrophages recruited in the inflammatory exudate. The bacteria spread from cell to cell using a secreted phospholipase that cleaves a variety of phospholipids, including sphingomyelin (a component of myelin) and phospholipids in cell membranes (see Fig. 4-30). Axonal injury and neuronal death are likely attributable to inflammatory processes, especially to the action of listeriolysin and lipases.

Gross lesions are usually absent, but leptomeningeal opacity, foci of yellow-brown discoloration (0.1 to 0.2 mm in diameter in the area of the nuclei of cranial nerves V and VIII), hemorrhage, necrosis in the terminal brainstem, and cloudy CSF can all be observed. Microscopically, a meningoencephalitis centered on the pons and medulla and involving both gray and white matter is characteristic (Fig. 14-88). The lesions, however, can extend from the diencephalon to the caudal medulla or cranial cervical spinal cord. Small, early lesions consist of loose clusters of microglial cells. With time, these lesions enlarge and contain variable numbers of neutrophils (see Fig. 14-88, *B*). Later in the process, microabscesses form, and neutrophils are the principal inflammatory cell. Although uncommon, some microabscesses contain macrophages as the principal cell type. Necrosis and accumulation of gitter cells can be prominent in some cases. Numerous Gram-positive bacilli can be detected in some lesions (see Fig. 14-88, C). Leptomeningitis is regularly present and

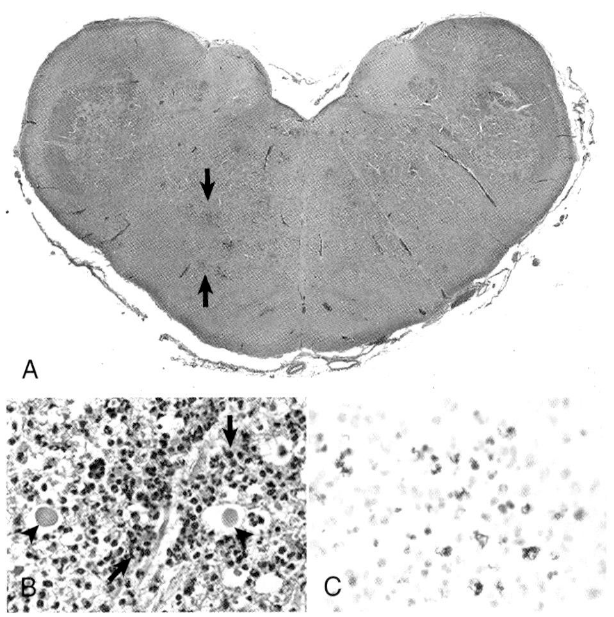

Figure 14-88 Listeriosis, Medulla, Cow. A, Microabscesses. Note the areas of faint blue discoloration in this subgross magnification of the medulla *(arrows)*. The less well defined blue areas are aggregates of neutrophils (microabscesses), and the blue linear lesions are perivascular cuffs. *Listeria monocytogenes*, the causative agent, uses retrograde axonal transport via the cranial nerves to enter the central nervous system and localize in the medulla (brainstem) and proximal cervical spinal cord. The lesion is rarely visible on gross observation. H&E stain. **B,** Early microabscesses *(arrows)* and inflammation are the result of inflammatory mediators that have injured axons *(arrowheads)* and will lead to Wallerian degeneration, seen here at the stage of swollen eosinophilic axons. H&E stain. **C,** *L. monocytogenes*, which is Gram-positive *(blue coccobacilli)*, can sometimes be detected in microabscesses in a histologic section stained with a Gram stain. Gram stain. (Courtesy Dr. M.D. McGavin, College of Veterinary Medicine, University of Tennessee.)

is often severe, and the exudate is composed predominantly of mononuclear cells (macrophages, lymphocytes, plasma cells) with fewer neutrophils. Cranial ganglioneuritis involving the trigeminal nerve and ganglion is often present. Vasculitis may occur in cases of cerebral listeriosis.

Listeriosis presents in three disease forms: meningoencephalitis, abortion and stillbirth, and septicemia. The last commonly develops in young animals, possibly from an in utero infection. The encephalitic and reproductive forms of the disease rarely occur together in an individual animal or in the same flock or herd. Infections in human beings also occur. Clinical signs in meningoencephalitic listeriosis are related to lesions in the brainstem and include dullness, torticollis, circling, unilateral facial paralysis, and drooling caused by pharyngeal paralysis. Signs of cranial nerve dysfunction occur because of inflammation in the brainstem. Death usually occurs within a few days after the initial signs and is preceded by recumbency and paddling of the limbs. Silage is the most common source of infection. If silage is contaminated with soil containing *L. monocytogenes* and is improperly prepared and stored (pH > 5.4), the microbe can multiply.

Thrombotic Meningoencephalitis. *H. somni*, a small Gram-negative bacillus, causes septicemia in cattle with variable clinical presentations, including pneumonia, polyarthritis, myocarditis, abortion, and meningoencephalitis. The disease is most prevalent in feedlot cattle but can occur in other situations. All manifestations, particularly meningoencephalitis, tend to be sporadic with single to multiple animals in a herd affected. The CNS form of the disease has been termed *thrombotic meningoencephalitis*, previously referred to as *thromboembolic meningoencephalitis*. Mural thrombi from local vascular injury rather than thromboemboli from distal sites of vascular injury, such as the lungs, are the major type of thrombus in this disease.

The pathogenesis of *H. somni* infection is not completely understood. Many cattle harbor the microbe in the upper digestive tract without evidence of disease, but under some circumstances it invades to cause severe clinical infection. The mechanism(s) of invasion into the bloodstream is not definitely known, but the respiratory tract is the initial site of bacterial replication followed by hematogenous spread to the CNS. The bacterium produces profound damage to endothelial cells, from which the majority of its thrombotic lesions develop. One of the primary bacterial virulence factors, lipooligosaccharide, has been shown in experimental studies to cause apoptosis of endothelial cells. This mechanism likely contributes to the profound damage of endothelial cells occurring with this disease. Once endothelial cells are damaged, thrombosis occurs, and tissues dependent on the obstructed blood vessel undergo infarction and necrosis.

Gross lesions in the CNS are irregularly sized foci of hemorrhage and necrosis scattered randomly and visible both externally and on cut surfaces (Fig. 14-89). Lesions are most frequent in the cerebrum, commonly at the cortical gray matter–white matter interface. The location of the lesion may reflect a change in the diameter and flow patterns of blood vessels, allowing bacteria to preferentially damage these areas. The spinal cord can also be affected. Other lesions include brain swelling caused by edema and leptomeningitis with cloudiness of the CSF.

Microscopic lesions in all organs, including the CNS, consist of a marked vasculitis and vascular necrosis, which are followed by thrombosis and infarction. The vasculitis is associated with regional edema and infiltration of neutrophils and macrophages in and around the affected blood vessel. Colonies of small Gram-negative bacilli can be found in the thrombi, affected blood vessels, and in the infarcted tissue.

Clinically, affected cows are initially ataxic and circle, head press, and appear blind. As the disease progresses, they may have convulsions, become comatose, and die.

Viruses

Herpesviruses

Bovine Malignant Catarrhal Fever. Malignant catarrhal fever is usually a sporadic highly fatal disease of cattle and other ruminants, including deer, buffalo, and antelope, and can involve several animals in a herd. The disease has a worldwide distribution, and the clinicopathologic features do not differ significantly from one part of the world to another. The primary target tissues are the vasculature, lymphoid organs, and epithelium (particularly of the respiratory and gastrointestinal tracts), but the kidneys, liver, eyes, joints, and CNS can also be affected. The virus appears to be transferred between lymphoid tissue/cells and endothelial cells via leukocytic trafficking in T lymphocytes. Two general types of the disease occur, the sheep-associated and wildebeest-derived forms, although several other less common causes of the disease have also been described. The causative agents involved belong to the herpesvirus subfamily Gammaherpesvirinae. The disease occurring outside Africa, caused by ovine herpesvirus 2, often involves close contact of presumed "carrier" sheep with susceptible ruminants. The disease has recently been reported in musk ox (*Ovibos moschatus*), Nubian ibex (*Capra nubiana*), and gemsbok (*Oryx gazella*). In Africa and occasionally in wildlife facilities outside the continent, the source of the infection

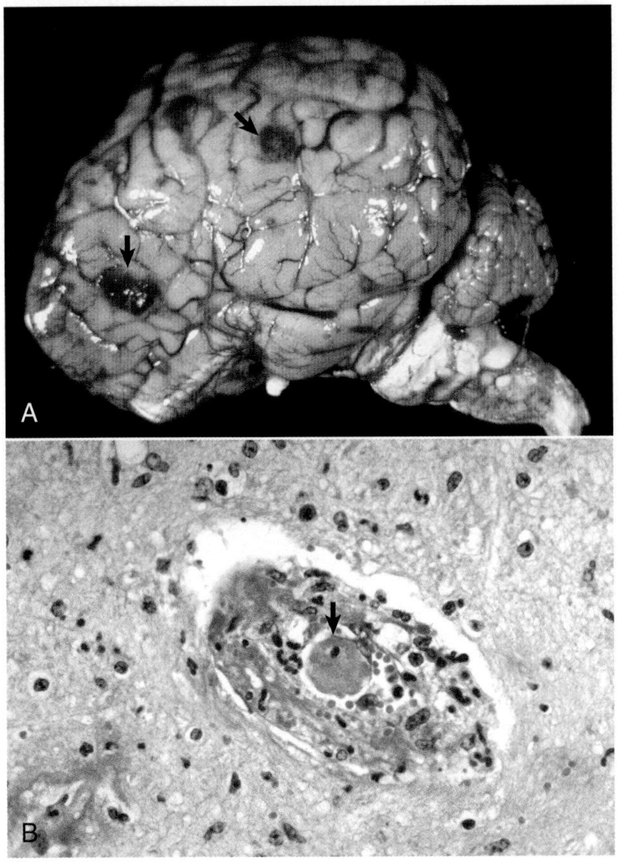

Figure 14-89 Thrombotic Meningoencephalitis, Cerebrum, Steer. A, On the surface of the cerebral cortex *(arrows)* are several red-brown lesions. These lesions are areas of necrosis, hemorrhage, and inflammation secondary to vasculitis and thrombosis caused by *Histophilus somni*. Such septic infarcts are distributed randomly (hematogenous portal of entry) throughout the central nervous system, including the spinal cord. The lesions depicted here are unusually severe. **B,** A thrombus *(arrow)* is present in the vascular lumen. Note the acute inflammatory response, edema, fibrinogenesis, and hemorrhage in the vessel wall. H&E stain. (**A** courtesy Dr. H. Leipold, College of Veterinary Medicine, Kansas State University. **B** courtesy Dr. M.D. McGavin, College of Veterinary Medicine, University of Tennessee.)

(designated *Alcelaphine herpesvirus 1*) is the wildebeest. Two other antigenically related viruses, which apparently do not cause natural disease, include Alcelaphine herpesvirus 2 and Hippotraginae herpesvirus 1, which have been isolated from African hartebeest and roan antelope, respectively. It is generally accepted that cattle and other susceptible ruminants contract the disease in nature after respiratory or oral infection during association with carrier sheep (presumed) and wildebeest, particularly at the time of parturition. A cell-mediated and cytotoxic lymphocytic process has been proposed as involved in the development of the necrotizing vasculitis.

Gross lesions of the CNS include active hyperemia and cloudiness of the leptomeninges caused by nonsuppurative meningoencephalomyelitis and vasculitis. Lymphocytic perivascular cuffing and varying degrees of necrotizing vasculitis occur in the leptomeninges and in all parts of the brain and occasionally in the spinal cord, with the white matter most consistently involved. Other lesions in the affected CNS include variable neuronal degeneration, microgliosis, choroiditis, necrosis of ependymal cells, and ganglioneuritis. Clinical signs referable to CNS infection may include trembling, shivering, ataxia, and nystagmus.

Bovine Alphaherpesvirus Meningoencephalitis. Although bovine herpesvirus 1 (BHV-1) occasionally causes a nonsuppurative meningoencephalitis, primarily in young cattle, two variants of BHV-1 isolated in Argentina and Australia (referred to as BHV-1, subtypes 3a and 3b, respectively) and more recently BHV-5 (isolated in South America, mainly Argentina and Brazil) have a particular tropism for the CNS. Recent evidence suggests that BHV-5 uses an intranasal route to infect and replicate in the nasal mucosa and then enters the CNS by retrograde axonal transport predominantly through olfactory nerves.

Gross lesions in the CNS are nonspecific and include meningeal congestion, petechiation, hemorrhage, and malacia in the frontal and olfactory cortices. Microscopic lesions consist of dense perivascular infiltrates of lymphocytes, plasma cells, and macrophages accompanied by neuronal degeneration, vasculitis, necrosis, and presence of intranuclear acidophilic inclusions in neurons and astrocytes. Trigeminal ganglia, where the virus remains latent, often have some degree of ganglioneuritis, satellitosis, and Nageotte nodule formation.

Clinically, outbreaks of disease occur in young cattle ranging in age from 5 to 18 months. Lesions can also involve the eyes (conjunctivitis) and tissues of the reproductive, alimentary, and integumentary systems in addition to the nervous system.

Bunyaviruses

Schmallenberg Virus. Schmallenberg virus causes fetal malformations in ruminants. It is an emergent orthobunyavirus that was first detected in Germany in 2011 before spreading widely throughout Europe. This virus appears to be a novel viral infection whose origin continues to be elusive. Evidence for a reemergent virus as a cause was not found when this novel virus was compared to older, stored samples that had similar pathologic findings. The virus is in the Bunyaviridae family and the *Orthobunyavirus* genus. The life cycle of the virus remains poorly characterized; however, it is believed to be similar to other members of the Bunyaviridae family. The virus is likely transmitted by a variety of *Culicoides* spp. (i.e., biting midges) vectors.

Adult sheep, cattle, and goats can develop fever, diarrhea, and reduced milk production associated with viral infection; however, the most important lesions are observed in fetuses secondary to circulating viremia and viral replication in the developing fetus. Similar to other members of the Bunyaviridae family like Akabane virus and Aino virus, fetal malformations are the primary manifestation of in utero infection with the virus. Gross lesions include congenital malformations of the fetus such as torticollis, ankyloses, arthrogryposis, brachygnathia inferior, hydranencephaly, porencephaly, and cerebral/cerebellar hypoplasia. The skull can be domed. Microscopically, affected CNS tissue has lymphocytic and histiocytic perivascular inflammation in the gray and white matter as well as overlying meninges. Inflammation occurs in animals that survive early gestational infection. Sporadic glial nodules can be found, most commonly in the mesencephalon and hippocampus. Diffuse gliosis consisting of increased numbers of astrocytes and microglia is also a consistent finding. Clinical signs in animals born alive include ataxia and behavioral abnormalities.

Other Bunyavirus Diseases. Akabane disease, arthrogryposis hydranencephaly complex (Cache Valley fever), and Rift Valley fever are additional diseases caused by members of the Bunyaviridae family. These insect vector–transmitted viruses have a shared tropism for fetal tissues and cause congenital malformations and encephalitis.

Lentiviruses

Visna. Visna, which means wasting in Icelandic, is a slowly progressive, transmissible disease of sheep. The disease is caused by a distinct viral strain of the ovine maedi-visna virus (MVV) complex, a lentivirus within the family Retroviridae. A different strain of the same virus causes a lymphocytic interstitial pneumonia referred to as *maedi*.

Visna is a persistent viral disease in which the elimination of the virus does not occur. Similar to other lentiviruses, the virus is cell associated, can undergo antigenic drift (see Chapter 4), and replicates slowly (hence lentivirus, from the Latin "lente," meaning slow). Although the visna virus and other lentiviruses can infect promonocytes and monocytes in the bone marrow and blood, viral replication is restricted in these cells, where it remains as proviral DNA until their maturation and differentiation to macrophages. Primary viral replication occurs in cells of monocyte-macrophage-microglial lineage. Thus visna virus enters the CNS by way of leukocytic trafficking of virus-infected macrophages. Visna virus can also be present in oligodendrocytes and astrocytes located in foci of demyelination. Recent studies suggest the virus can also infect and productively replicate in endothelial cells. This mechanism may provide an additional route for viral entry into the CNS and the potential for alterations of the blood-brain barrier.

Although gross lesions are not frequently observed, they may occur in areas of prominent inflammation, where they appear as yellow-tan areas. Early microscopic lesions primarily affect the gray and white matter subjacent to the ependyma of the ventricular system of the brain and central canal of the spinal cord. These lesions are characterized by a nonsuppurative encephalomyelitis accompanied by pleocytosis, variable edema, CNS necrosis, astrocytosis, choroiditis, and nonsuppurative leptomeningitis. Degeneration of myelin sheaths also occurs at this time but is often accompanied by axonal degeneration, suggesting that it could be a secondary lesion, such as in Wallerian degeneration. Oligodendroglial and neuron injury and necrotic cell death are attributable to cytokines and other toxic factors secreted by inflammatory cells and glial cells. Recent in vitro studies suggest that caspase activation leading to apoptotic cell death may play a role in visna.

The primary demyelination that occurs during the late stages of the disease process (6 months to 8 years after infection) has been proposed to result from oligodendroglial cell infection. The main sources of excreted virus are the udder and lungs (as cell-associated virus), and transmission occurs most readily between the dam and lamb via the milk and between confined individuals, probably via respiratory secretions. MVV has also been detected in semen of infected rams. It is important to emphasize that no profound immune deficiency occurs with MVV infections, as is the case for immunodeficiency lentiviral infections that infect $CD4^+$ T lymphocytes. Nonetheless, secondary infections can still significantly accompany MVV infection.

In addition to pneumonia, MVVs can also cause mastitis, arthritis (uncommonly of the carpus or hind limb joints), and a mesangial glomerulitis. Irrespective of the target organ, the lesions are to be regarded as chronic and lymphoproliferative, in contrast to the well-known immunodeficiency infections caused by human immunodeficiency virus 1, simian immunodeficiency virus, and feline immunodeficiency virus.

Viral strain differences and breed of sheep can influence the lesions that develop. For example, the visna form of the disease does not commonly occur in ovine breeds of North America, although some degree of visna-like lesions can be seen with maedi. Visna originally was described in Iceland, but sheep with similar lesions of the CNS have been detected in the Netherlands, Kenya, the United States, and Canada. CNS signs include an abnormal hind limb gait that progresses to incoordination and rear limb paresis over a period of weeks or months.

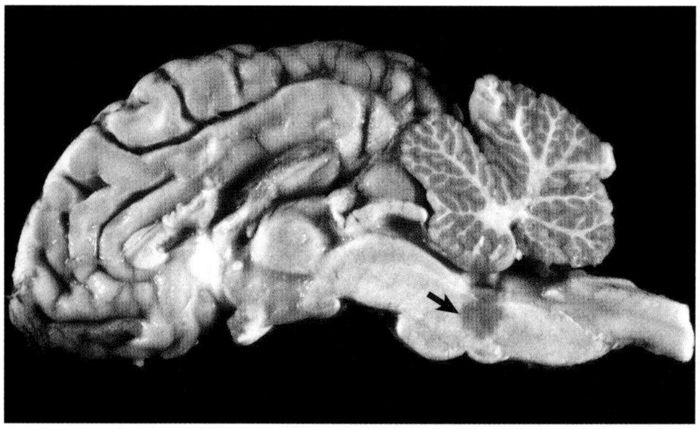

Figure 14-90 **Leukoencephalitis, Caprine Retrovirus-Induced Encephalitis, Brainstem, Goat.** A focal area of the brainstem *(arrow)* is yellow-brown and was found, microscopically, to be infiltrated by lymphocytes, plasma cells, and histiocytes. A similar lesion commonly occurs in the spinal cord. (Courtesy Dr. H.E. Whiteley, College of Veterinary Medicine, University of Illinois.)

Caprine Leukoencephalomyelitis. Caprine leukoencephalomyelitis was first described in the United States and has since been recognized in other parts of the world. The infection can be readily transmitted by colostrum and milk after birth, or by direct contact. A close relationship exists between the MVV of sheep and the causative agent of caprine leukoencephalomyelitis, caprine arthritis encephalitis (CAE) virus. As with MVV infection of sheep, caprine arthritis encephalitis viral infection is also a lymphoproliferative disease with a tropism for the macrophage, which acts as a carrier for the virus.

Gross lesions in the nervous system include tan- to salmon-colored foci of necrosis and inflammation that can occasionally be detected in the brain (Fig. 14-90) and most prominently in the spinal cord. Microscopic lesions of the nervous system are similar to those of visna (nonsuppurative encephalomyelitis) but can be more severe with caprine arthritis encephalitis. Nonneural lesions include interstitial pneumonia of moderate severity in some affected kids. Such lungs fail to collapse completely and are mottled red or blue. As discussed under visna, the mechanism of infection and cell death appear similar.

The pattern of disease in caprine arthritis encephalitis is age dependent. Neurologic manifestations are usually seen in young kids 2 to 4 months of age, but unlike visna in sheep, there is a more rapid progression and signs progressing to quadriplegia develop within weeks to months. As with visna, affected goats have pleocytosis. In adult goats the primary target tissue is the synovium of the joints, and animals that survive the initial infection have lymphoproliferative synovitis and arthritis develop. Pneumonia, lymphocytic mastitis, and encephalomyelitis also occur in adult animals.

Chlamydia

Sporadic Bovine Encephalomyelitis. See E-Appendix 14-2.

Prions. See the section on Disorders of Domestic Animals for additional discussion of prions.

Bovine Spongiform Encephalopathy. Bovine spongiform encephalopathy was originally identified in the United Kingdom in 1986 but likely existed there as early as April 1985. Through the end of 2003, more than 183,000 cows from more than 35,000 herds were reported with BSE. With regard to the origins of BSE, epidemiologic evidence indicates that the disease was caused initially (during the early 1980s) by the feeding of rations containing meat and bone meal supplements that were contaminated with the scrapie agent. Countries that have reported cases of BSE or are considered to have a substantial risk to have animals with BSE include Albania, Austria, Belgium, Bosnia-Herzegovina, Bulgaria, Canada, Croatia, Czech Republic, Denmark, Yugoslavia, Finland, France, Germany, Greece, Hungary, Ireland, Israel, Italy, Japan, Liechtenstein, Luxembourg, Macedonia, the Netherlands, Norway, Oman, Poland, Portugal, Romania, Slovak Republic, Slovenia, Spain, Sweden, Switzerland, the United States, and the United Kingdom (Great Britain, including Northern Ireland and the Falkland Islands). Since the number of affected animals peaked in the 1990s and early 2000s, the number of animals affected yearly has diminished to only small numbers (<6/year).

In December 2003, BSE was confirmed in a single dairy cow from a herd in Washington State. This cow was apparently imported into the United States 2 to 3 years earlier from a farm in northern Alberta, Canada, which was the source of the positive BSE case in Canada confirmed in May 2003. In 2004, additional cases of BSE likely linked to a common source were reported in Washington State, Oregon, and Canada, and in June 2005 a cow tested positive for BSE in Texas.

Signs that accompany BSE include changes in behavior such as nervousness or aggressiveness, abnormal posture, abnormal gait, incoordination, difficulty in rising, decreased milk production, and loss of body weight despite continued appetite. Clinically, affected cattle deteriorate until they either die or require euthanasia. This clinical period usually ranges from 2 weeks to 6 months. All cases of the disease in cattle have occurred in adult animals, with an age range of 3 to 11 years, but most animals have clinical signs develop between 3 and 5 years of age.

The National Veterinary Services Laboratory (Animal and Plant Health Inspection Service [APHIS]) of the U.S. Department of Agriculture has developed and implemented through local and regional veterinary diagnostic laboratories procedures for sampling, preparing, and submitting brains for BSE analysis. Space limitations prevent describing these procedures. They can be obtained through APHIS or a diagnostic laboratory. Dead or sick animals that display neurologic signs and are suspected of being potential BSE candidates are tested using immunohistochemical analysis, Western blot analysis, or enzyme-linked immunosorbent assay (ELISA) to identify PrP^{Sc} in brain tissue. Genetically valuable animals that may be exported or have their embryos or DNA saved for future use and are from transmissible spongiform encephalopathy risk groups can be tested for PrP^{Sc}. Immunohistochemical analysis for PrP^{Sc} of samples obtained (i.e., under anesthesia) from biopsies of tonsil, rectal lymphoid tissue, and lymphoid tissue of the third eyelid can be performed ante mortem.

Ovine Spongiform Encephalopathy (Scrapie). Scrapie is best known as a degenerative disease that affects the CNS of sheep and was first recognized in Great Britain and other countries of western Europe more than 250 years ago. The disease, which is currently reported throughout the world except for Australia and New Zealand, also occurs naturally in the domestic goat. The name is derived from the characteristic clinical signs of pruritus, which often results in loss of wool in sheep. The disease progresses inexorably with early signs of subtle change in behavior or temperament followed by scratching and rubbing against fixed objects because of the pruritus. Additional signs include incoordination, weight loss (despite retention of appetite), biting of the feet and limbs, lip smacking, gait abnormalities, trembling (when suddenly stressed), recumbency, and eventually death after 1 to 6 months or longer.

Much of our current understanding of the pathogenesis of the natural infection of scrapie in Suffolk sheep has been advanced by Dr. William Hadlow and coworkers. It should be noted that Dr. Hadlow is a veterinary pathologist and diplomate of the American College of Veterinary Pathologists, who first recognized and reported the similarity between scrapie and kuru of human beings. This important contribution led to the current understanding of the transmissible spongiform encephalopathies and a Nobel Prize for the medical scientist (Dr. D. Gajdusek) who originally investigated kuru in the South Pacific.

Degenerative Diseases

Metabolic

Primary Neuronal Degeneration

Primary Cerebellar Neuronal Degeneration. Primary cerebellar neuronal degeneration has been reported to occur in Merino and Charolais lambs, Holstein-Friesian calves, and Angus calves. An autosomal recessive mode of inheritance is suspected or documented in several of the diseases, but the mechanism of injury is unclear. Grossly, the cerebellum can be normal or reduced in size and atrophic. Microscopically, lesions may include loss of Purkinje cells, variable neuronal depletion in the granule layer, fusiform swellings of proximal Purkinje cell axons, and astrogliosis in the molecular layer.

Animals with postnatal primary cerebellar neuronal degeneration are normal at birth or at the time of ambulation. Onset of ataxia with various other clinical signs referable to cerebellar disease begins weeks or months after a period of apparently normal development. Initial clinical signs are often subtle. Progression of the signs can be slow or rapid, relentless, or with static periods. Some individuals reach a stage without further progression of signs, but this is not typical of the syndrome in most animals.

Nutritional

Vitamin B_1 (Thiamine) Deficiency

Thiamine Deficiency in Ruminants. Thiamine deficiency in cattle, sheep, and less commonly, goats, has been termed *polioencephalomalacia*. Rumen microbes are able to synthesize thiamine, and therefore only very young ruminants, whose rumens have not yet been populated by thiamine-producing microbes, should be susceptible to thiamine deficiency. Hence conclusive evidence of an absolute thiamine deficiency as the sole cause of polioencephalomalacia in ruminants has been elusive. Evidence or theories linking thiamine with the ruminant disorder include the following:

1. Clinical response to thiamine injection in some individuals.
2. Decreases in ruminal thiamine or overgrowth of thiaminase-producing microbes such as *Bacillus thiaminolyticus*.
3. Ingestion of thiaminase-containing plants such as bracken fern.
4. Production of inactive thiamine analogues.
5. Decreased absorption or increased fecal excretion of thiamine.
6. Sulfur toxicosis can result in identical lesions through the process of sulfite cleaving thiamine.

Gross lesions, if present, are limited primarily to the cerebral cortex. Initially, 2 days after onset, the surface of the brain can be swollen (cerebral edema) as indicated by flattening of cerebrocortical gyri and narrow sulci. In rare cases with more severe brain swelling, brain displacement with herniation of the parahippocampal gyri beneath the tentorium cerebelli and the vermis of the cerebellum into the foramen magnum can occur. By 4 days after onset, yellow discoloration of the cerebrocortical gray matter occurs (Fig. 14-91), and it is at this time that autofluorescence (see later for more detail) is seen when the brain is examined under 365-nm ultraviolet light (Fig. 14-92). Eight to 10 days after onset, edematous separation and necrosis involving the middle to deep lamina or gray matter–white matter interface may be appreciable (Fig. 14-93). In advanced cases with prolonged survival, areas of marked atrophy of cerebral gyri with an attenuated or absent gray matter zone are covered by meninges (Fig. 14-94).

Microscopically, the earliest lesions are laminar cortical necrosis and astrocytic swelling. Laminar cortical necrosis is characterized by neuronal necrosis (ischemic change), with a laminar pattern of edema in the cerebral cortex. Neurons in the middle to deep lamina of the parietal and occipital lobes of the cerebral cortex are preferentially affected (Fig. 14-95, A). In the early stages or in mild cases, lesions can be limited to the depths of cerebrocortical sulci, but generally there is involvement of entire gyri that may be confluent over extensive areas of the cortex. After 4 to 5 days, neuronal necrosis and edema are more severe, and there is an early influx of blood monocytes that mature into tissue macrophages and become gitter cells as they phagocytose necrotic debris. Macrophages and gitter cells are observed most commonly in perivascular and perineuronal spaces and in the pia arachnoid (see Fig. 14-23, A). After 8 to 10 days, necrosis and edema have resulted in laminar separation (at the gray matter–white matter interface) in which there are prominent accumulations of macrophages (see Fig. 14-95, *B*).

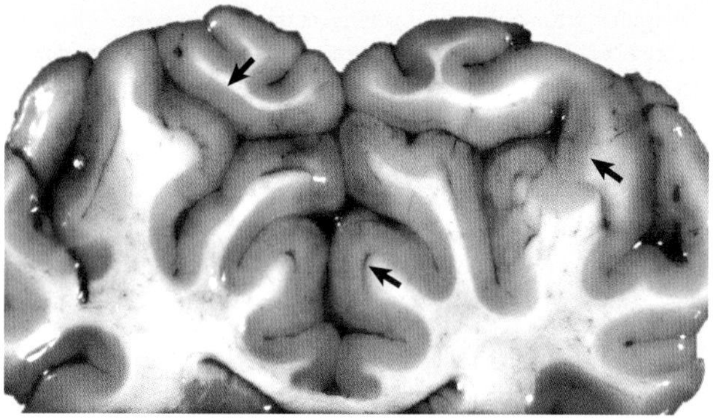

Figure 14-91 **Acute Polioencephalomalacia, Cerebral Cortex, Cross-Sectional View, Cow.** Gyri are yellow and swollen *(arrows)*. The cause of this yellow color is unknown but has been shown experimentally not to be caused by ceroid-lipofuscin pigments. Changes involving the sulci and gyri in acute polioencephalomalacia are shown in Figure 14-93. (Courtesy Dr. L. Roth, College of Veterinary Medicine, Cornell University.)

Lesions that accompany the necrosis include vascular prominence caused by endothelial cell and perithelial cell hypertrophy and hyperplasia, congestion, and a minimal, if any, influx of neutrophils. Bilaterally symmetric focal lesions, similar to those seen in carnivores, occur in the thalamus and midbrain or colliculi and rarely in other brainstem structures. Animals that survive can have cerebral atrophy and develop hydrocephalus ex vacuo and have been known to live 1 to 2 years. It should be noted that laminar cortical necrosis can be caused by a variety of metabolic abnormalities. In ruminants, in addition to thiamine deficiency, water deprivation–sodium ion toxicosis, and lead poisoning can cause polioencephalomalacia and laminar cortical necrosis.

When exposed to ultraviolet light (365-nm wavelength), the brains of affected ruminants may have autofluorescent bands of necrotic cerebral cortex. Autofluorescence is likely secondary to the accumulation of autofluorescent substances in degenerating neurons that seem to be localized to mitochondria. The belief that ceroid-lipofuscin pigments are the cause of the autofluorescence is still unproven. An association between mitochondria and autofluorescence has also been shown in the neuronal ceroid lipofuscinoses (Batten's disease, ceroid-lipofuscin storage diseases). These diseases are characterized by the accumulation of an autofluorescent (365-nm ultraviolet light), intracytoplasmic storage material in CNS neurons composed mostly of subunit c of mitochondrial ATP synthase.

Clinically, the disease is seen most commonly in cattle 6 to 18 months of age fed concentrated rations. In sheep, most cases occur in younger age groups (2 to 7 months). Clinical signs in cattle and small ruminants may include depression, stupor, ataxia, head pressing, apparent cortical blindness, opisthotonos, convulsions, and recumbency with paddling and then death. If animals survive or respond to therapy, clinical signs can persist.

Polioencephalomalacia commonly occurs in cattle fed rations rich in carbohydrates with little roughage and is also associated with clinical or subclinical acidosis that may precipitate changes in rumen microflora. The disorder also occurs in association with other dietary factors, including cobalt deficiency, molasses- and urea-based diets, and diets high in elemental sulfur and sulfates and sulfides, some of which are not specifically associated with thiamine deficiency.

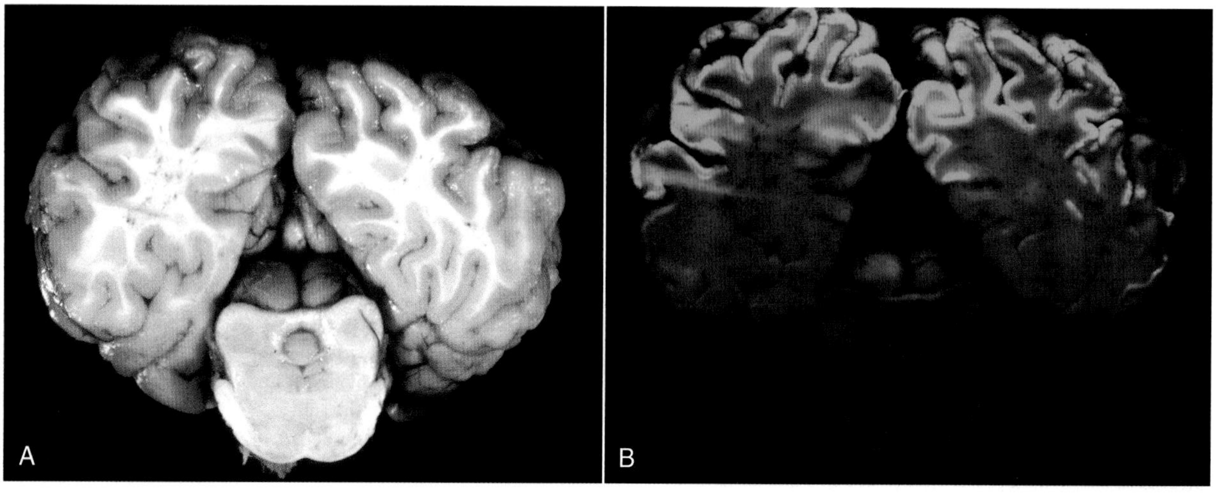

Figure 14-92 **Acute Polioencephalomalacia, Brain, Cerebral Hemispheres and Midbrain, Steer. A,** Compare the relative lack of gross lesions with those revealed by ultraviolet (UV) light in **B**. **B,** Bilaterally symmetric laminar pattern of apple-green autofluorescence (from mitochondrial derivatives) involving the full thickness of the cortex indicates areas of necrosis in the gray matter. Although not shown here, the colliculi were also autofluorescent. The cerebrum is exposed to 365-nm UV light from a Wood's lamp. Similar results can be obtained with fixed (preserved) brain. (Courtesy Dr. P.N. Bochsler, School of Veterinary Medicine, University of Wisconsin-Madison.)

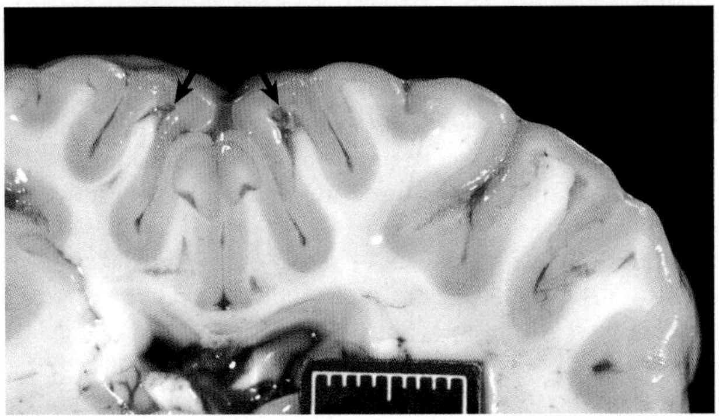

Figure 14-93 Acute cerebrocortical polioencephalomalacia, thiamine deficiency, brain, parietal lobe, level of thalamus, goat. Note the liquefactive necrosis with varying degrees of tissue separation *(arrows)* in the deep cortex. Scale bar = 2 cm. (Courtesy Dr. R. Storts, College of Veterinary Medicine, Texas A&M University.)

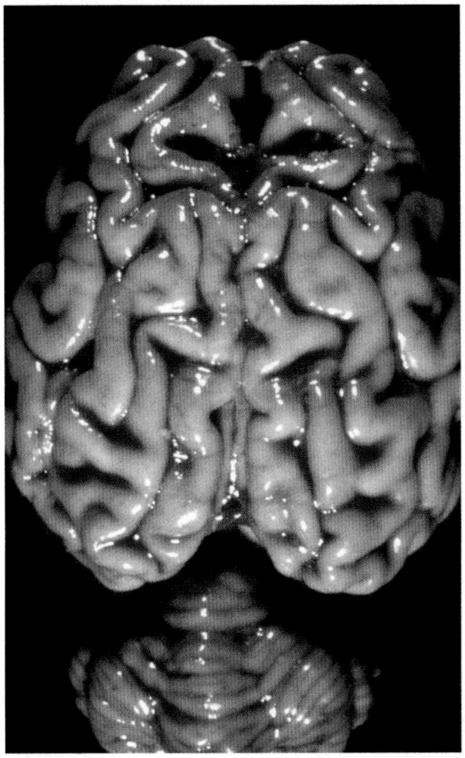

Figure 14-94 **Chronic Cerebral Cortical Atrophy, Brain, Cow.** Gyri are atrophic and narrow with widened sulci. In this case the loss of cerebral cortex was caused by thiamine deficiency several years previously. (Courtesy College of Veterinary Medicine, University of Illinois.)

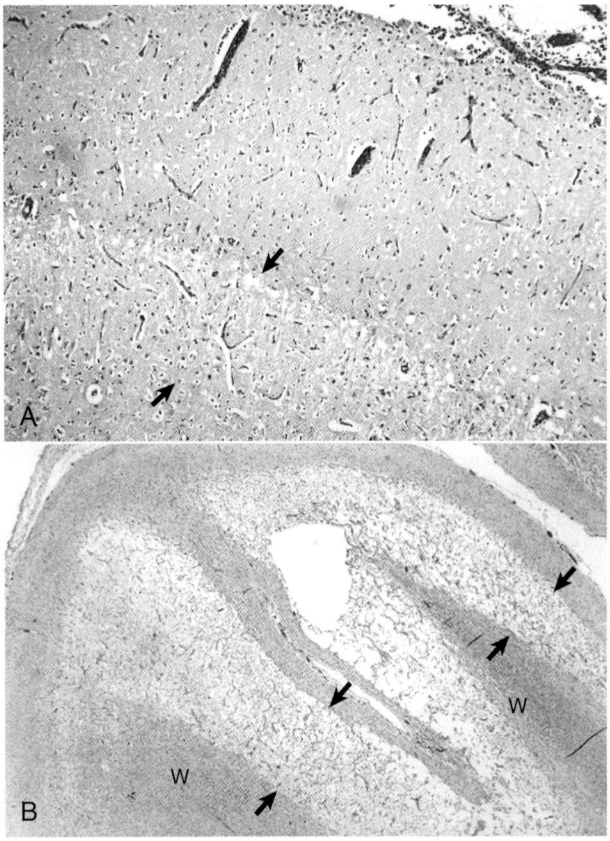

Figure 14-95 **Polioencephalomalacia, Cerebral Cortex, Cross-Sectional View, Cow. A,** Acute stage. Note the zone of edema and acute neuronal necrosis affecting lamina 4-6 *(area between arrows)* of the cerebral cortex. Monocytes can be seen in the pia-arachnoid layer and subarachnoid space *(upper right)* in response to neuronal injury and the need to phagocytose cellular debris. Monocytes will also rapidly appear in perivascular spaces of blood vessels in the area of laminar edema and neuronal necrosis. H&E stain. **B,** Chronic stage. Areas of microcavitation in the deep cortical laminae next to the subcortical white matter are poorly stained *(area between arrows)* when compared with those of the normal superficial cortex *(left)*. *W,* White matter. H&E stain. (**A** courtesy Dr. W. Haschek-Hock, College of Veterinary Medicine, University of Illinois. **B** courtesy Dr. J.F. Zachary, College of Veterinary Medicine, University of Illinois.)

There has been considerable interest in the relationship of high dietary sulfur to polioencephalomalacia. All sources of sulfur, including formulated rations, plants rich in sulfur (*Kochia scoparia*), and high concentrations of sulfur in the drinking water, are additive. Total dietary intake should not exceed 0.3% to 0.4%. The exact mechanism to explain sulfur-induced polioencephalomalacia in ruminants has not been proved but most likely involves interference with cytochrome oxidases thereby distrupting the mitochondrial respiratory chain.

Copper Deficiency. Swayback and enzootic ataxia are descriptive terms used to describe the disease related to copper deficiency in lambs and kid goats. Swayback refers to the congenital form of the disease, whereas in enzootic ataxia, onset is delayed for up to 6 months after birth. Although copper deficiency is involved, the pathogenesis is likely complex and involves interplay with other metals, including zinc, iron, and molybdenum. Lesions occur in the cerebrum, brainstem, and spinal cord in the congenital form, but only in the brainstem and spinal cord in cases with a postnatal onset.

Additionally, deficiency of copper can affect wool, hair growth, and pigmentation; musculoskeletal development; and integrity of connective tissue. Copper deficiency can be primarily the result of copper-deficient soils and inadequate intake from forage or secondary from defective absorption because of interactions between copper, molybdenum, zinc, cadmium, or inorganic sulfates. Copper is a component of several enzyme systems, including cytochrome and lysyl oxidases, such as mitochondrial cytochrome-c oxidase; dopamine β-monooxygenase; peptidylglycine α-amidating monooxygenase; tyrosinase; and superoxide dismutase and the protein ceruloplasmin. These enzyme systems are essential for energy generation by mitochondria in the brain, regulating oxidative stress, catecholamine synthesis, and the modification of peptide neurotransmitters.

The pathogenesis of the lesions that occur in swayback and enzootic ataxia is poorly understood. It has been suggested that cerebral lesions result from loss of embryonic cells at the same stage of brain development as occurs in porencephaly and hydranencephaly after in utero viral infection or dysgenesis caused by a biochemical disturbance. Biochemical disturbances could also account for the axonal/neuronal degeneration in the brainstem and spinal cord. Altered function of the mitochondrial enzyme cytochrome oxidase leading to energy failure could play a role in cerebral dysgenesis and axonal and ultimately neuronal degeneration.

More intriguing is the possible involvement of the enzyme copper-zinc superoxide dismutase. A mutation in this enzyme is present in approximately 20% of human beings with familial amyotrophic lateral sclerosis and in some individuals with the sporadic form of the disease. This human disorder, which is classified as a motor neuron disease, has a much later onset, and the mutation results in a "gain of function" of the enzyme rather than lack of function as might be present in copper deficiency. Neurofilament accumulation in brainstem and spinal ventral horn neurons and fiber tract degeneration (corticospinal in human beings versus spinocerebellar in lambs and kids with copper deficiency) are similar. Drawing a relevant association between these diseases of human beings and abnormal function of superoxide dismutase in swayback and enzootic ataxia in animals is premature at this time, however. It is also possible that the cortical white matter degeneration and brainstem or spinal lesions arise from different mechanisms.

Grossly, approximately 50% of congenitally affected lambs and rarely kids have bilateral cerebrocortical lesions. Externally the cerebral cortex can be focally soft and fluctuant or collapsed. These foci correspond to areas of rarefaction, which have either a gelatinous consistency or cystic cavities filled with clear serous fluid, in the white matter of the corona radiata and centrum semiovale. Microscopically, a variable astrogliosis is associated with the degeneration of white matter, but the cavities lack a capsule of glial fibers. Myelin degradation and an influx of macrophages are minimal. Delicate neuronal and astroglial processes traverse the cavities. Neuronal necrosis in cortical gray matter overlying these white matter lesions is sometimes observed.

Microscopic lesions in the brainstem and spinal cord in both the congenital (swayback) and delayed-onset (enzootic ataxia) forms of copper deficiency are similar in lambs and kids, and they affect both gray and white matter. Large multipolar neurons of the brainstem reticular formation, certain brainstem nuclei—such as the red and vestibular nuclei—and the ventral, lateral, and less commonly, dorsal horns of the spinal cord are affected. Neuronal cell bodies lack stainable Nissl substance (chromatolysis). The cytoplasm is variably dense, pink, and homogeneous to fibrillar as a result of the accumulation of neurofilaments, and nuclei are often displaced to an eccentric position against the cell membrane. The extent of neuronal necrosis varies. Lesions in the white matter of the spinal cord consist of bilateral areas of pallor in the dorsolateral aspects of the lateral funiculi (corresponding roughly to the spinocerebellar tracts) and also in the ventral funiculi adjacent to the ventral median fissure. The pallor of the white matter is due to degeneration of myelinated axons. Involvement of the medial (septomarginal) aspect of the dorsal funiculi is infrequent. In the terminal brainstem, lesions are similar but have a somewhat scattered distribution. The spinocerebellar tracts extending into the middle cerebellar peduncles are affected. Astrogliosis is usually mild. Definitive microscopic lesions in the cerebellum and ventral spinal nerve rootlets and peripheral nerves are usually lacking in lambs but can be frequent in kids. Changes in Purkinje cells are analogous to those already noted in neurons in other areas. Additionally, ectopic Purkinje cells and thinning of the granule cell layer occur. Bergmann glial cell processes in the molecular layer undergo hypertrophy. Lesions in ventral spinal nerve rootlets and peripheral nerve are caused by axonal degeneration secondary to injury of motor neurons in the ventral gray horns.

Clinically, CNS disease as a result of copper deficiency in animals is mainly a disorder of sheep and goats and can be present at birth (swayback in lambs, rarely kids), or onset can be delayed up to 6 months (enzootic ataxia in lambs and kids). Swayback occurs in newborn lambs from ewes with inadequate dietary copper intake. Affected lambs can be born dead, weak, or unable to stand. If mobile, they are ataxic. Enzootic ataxia is characterized by ataxia.

Toxicoses

Microbial Toxins

Clostridium perfringens Type D Encephalopathy (Pulpy Kidney Disease, Overeating Disease). *Clostridium perfringens* type D enterotoxemia, associated with epsilon toxin production, is a disease of sheep, goats, and cattle, but only sheep commonly exhibit the neurologic manifestations of the disease. Brain damage is due to vascular injury and breakdown of the blood-brain barrier. Binding of epsilon toxin to endothelial cell surface receptors results in opening of tight junctions, disturbed transport processes, increased vascular permeability that results in vasogenic edema, swelling of astrocytic foot processes, and ultimately necrosis caused by hypoxic-ischemic mechanisms. Some of the effects of epsilon toxin can be mediated by an adenyl cyclase–cyclic adenosine monophosphate (cAMP) system.

Gross lesions are absent in some peracute cases but when present, consist initially of bilaterally symmetric foci of malacia, leading to yellow-gray to red foci with malacia and cavitation (Fig. 14-96, *A*). Lesions can be found in the internal capsule, basal nuclei, thalamus, hippocampus, rostral colliculus and substantia nigra, pons, corona radiata of frontal cortex, and cerebellar peduncles, especially the middle peduncle. Lesions in other tissue consist of pulmonary congestion and edema, serous pericardial effusion, petechiation, and soft (pulpy) kidneys (see Fig. 11-42).

Microscopically, the CNS lesion in acute cases is vasogenic edema secondary to vascular injury. The fluid in perivascular spaces is frequently protein rich and eosinophilic. Walls of arterioles can be hyalinized, and endothelial cell nuclei swollen and vesicular (see Fig. 14-96, *B*). Vasogenic edema, which is interstitial in location, gives a light or pink-staining, spongy appearance to the CNS parenchyma. Both gray matter and white matter are affected. Pericapillary hemorrhage and acute necrosis of neurons and macroglia occur. Other changes occur with longer survival and include axonal swelling, accumulation of neutrophils and foamy macrophages (see Fig. 14-96, *B* and *C*), vascular prominence caused by perithelial-endothelial nuclear enlargement or swelling, lymphocytic perivascular cuffing, and liquefactive necrosis.

Sheep of all ages, except newborns, are susceptible; incidence peaks between 3 and 10 weeks of age and in feeder lambs shortly after arrival at a feedlot. Resistance of newborns can be related to lack in the gut of pancreatic proteolytic enzymes necessary for activation of the epsilon toxin, and to trypsin inhibitors in colostrum. Lambs are typically in good condition and are found dead.

Disorders of Pigs

Disorders that occur in many or all animal species are discussed in the section on Disorders of Domestic Animals.

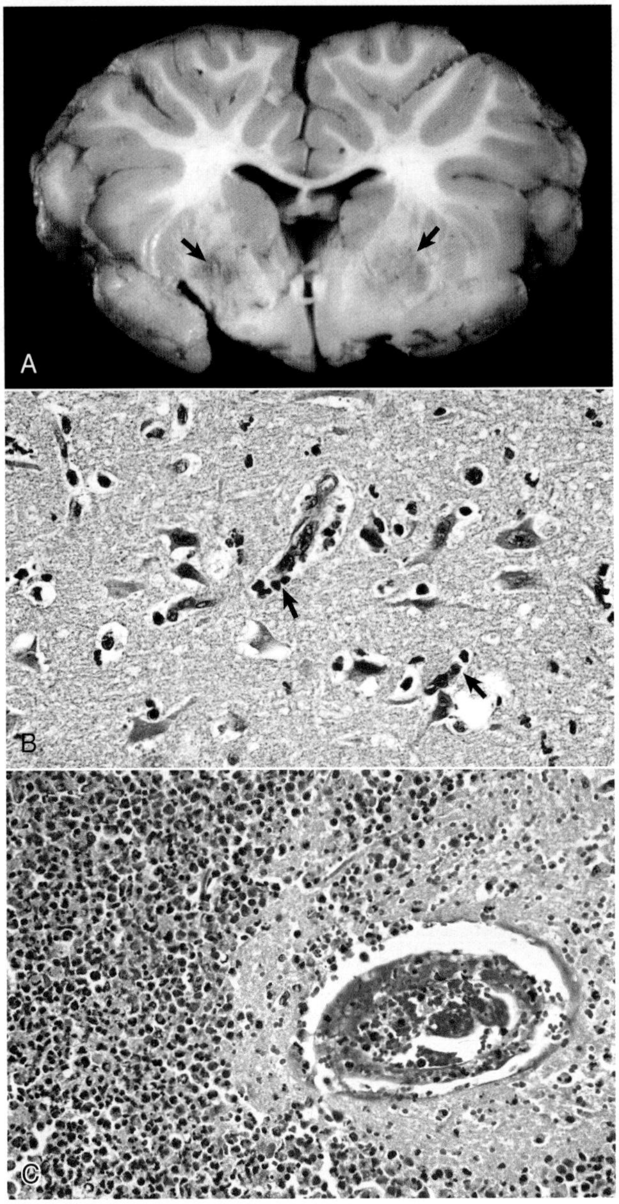

Figure 14-96 Focal Symmetric Encephalomalacia, Brain, Transverse Section at the Level of the Basal Nuclei and Rostral Thalamus, Sheep. A, There are bilateral discoloration and malacia *(arrows)* in a portion of the basal nuclei. These lesions are caused by an enterotoxin produced by *Clostridium perfringens* type D. **B,** Early stage. Note the acute neuronal necrosis *(red neurons)* with perivascular and perineuronal edema. Inflammatory cells *(arrows)*, including neutrophils and macrophages, are beginning to appear in the perivascular space and will migrate to the necrotic neurons and phagocytose the debris. H&E stain. **C,** Later stage. Microscopically, the walls of arterioles can be hyalinized and endothelial cell nuclei swollen and vesicular (not shown here) with perivascular leakage of proteinaceous fluid. Pericapillary hemorrhage and acute necrosis of neurons and macroglia can occur. With longer survival, as seen here, lesions include destruction of neuropil, accumulation of neutrophils and foamy macrophages, and lymphocytic perivascular cuffing. In this case the inflammatory response is pronounced and would not be considered typical of this disease. H&E stain. (**A** courtesy Dr. D. Cho, College of Veterinary Medicine, Louisiana State University; and Noah's Arkive, College of Veterinary Medicine, The University of Georgia. **B** courtesy Dr. B.E. Walling, College of Veterinary Medicine, University of Illinois. **C** courtesy Dr. J. Simon, College of Veterinary Medicine, University of Illinois.)

Diseases Caused by Microbes

Viruses

Enteroviruses

Enterovirus-Induced Porcine Polioencephalomyelitis. See E-Appendix 14-2.

Coronaviruses

Hemagglutinating Encephalomyelitis. See E-Appendix 14-2.

Herpesviruses

Pseudorabies. Pseudorabies virus (*suid herpesvirus 1*), an alphaherpesvirus, causes encephalitis primarily in pigs; although a wide variety of domestic and wild animals are also susceptible. The ingestion of infected pig meat is the traditional source of infection in domestic dogs and cats. The disease is also known as *Aujeszky's disease* and "mad itch" and is not zoonotic. Pseudorabies is not related to rabies but was named because its clinical signs sometimes resemble those seen with rabies. The disease in susceptible species other than pigs is generally fatal. Although pigs—particularly young, suckling piglets—can die from infection, most mature pigs remain persistently infected and act as latent carriers.

The route of natural infection in pigs is intranasal, pharyngeal, tonsillar, or pulmonary by direct contact or aerosolization, followed by reproduction of virus in epithelial cells of the upper respiratory tract. The virus then travels to the tonsil and local lymph nodes by way of the lymph vessels. After replication in the nasopharynx, virus invades sensory nerve endings and is then transported in axoplasm via the trigeminal ganglion and olfactory bulb to the brain. The virus has also been reported to be capable of spreading transsynaptically. Recent studies have additionally shown that some strains produce lesions in the gastrointestinal tract and myenteric plexuses, suggesting that infection might spread from the intestinal mucosa to the CNS via autonomic nerves. In latently infected pigs the oronasal epithelium can be recurrently infected by virus spreading from the nervous system, followed by its excretion in oronasal fluid. The virus can also spread hematogenously, although in low titer, to other tissues of the body. As an example, it can cause placenta disease in pregnant sows and is an important cause of fetal maceration and mummification in the pig. Cellular attachment, entry, and cell-to-cell spread of the virus are mediated by glycoprotein projections that extend from the surface of the viral particle.

Gross lesions in pigs occur in several nonneural tissues, including organs of the respiratory system, lymphoid system, digestive tract, and reproductive tract. Focal tissue necrosis also occurs in the liver, spleen, and adrenal glands, particularly in young suckling pigs, and mortality can be high. Evidence of facial pruritus is a common sequela to infection, although the actual incidence varies considerably. The CNS is free of gross lesions except for nonspecific leptomeningeal congestion. Microscopic lesions in pigs are characterized by a nonsuppurative meningoencephalomyelitis with trigeminal ganglioneuritis. Injury to CNS tissue can be marked, with neuronal degeneration and necrosis. Intranuclear amphophilic inclusion bodies are not commonly detected in pigs but can be present in neurons and astrocytes. In cattle, sheep, dogs, and cats, the pathogenesis involving axonal spread to the CNS is comparable to that of pigs, with lesions that include nonsuppurative encephalomyelitis accompanied by ganglioneuritis and intraneuronal inclusion bodies

Pestiviruses

Classical Swine Fever (Hog Cholera). See E-Appendix 14-2 and Chapters 4 and 10.

Degenerative Diseases

Toxicoses

Microbial Toxins

Edema Disease (Enterotoxemic Colibacillosis). Edema disease is a disorder of rapidly growing, healthy feeder pigs being fed a high-energy ration. The disease is caused by strains of *E. coli* producing a Shiga-like toxin, which is similar to toxins produced by *Shigella dysenteriae* and is designated Shiga-like toxin type IIe. Serotypes O138, O139, and O140 seem to be most commonly reported. This toxin causes necrosis of smooth muscle cells in small arteries and arterioles and a reduction focally in the degree of circulation to the CNS parenchyma, leading to infarction manifested grossly as malacia in the CNS. Glycolipid cell surface receptors on endothelial cells, globotriaosylceramide or globotetraosylceramide, are binding sites for the toxin, and their presence confers susceptibility to the disease. Binding of the toxin to these receptors can initiate a chain of inflammatory and immunologic reactions that lead to vascular damage.

The basic lesion is an angiopathy that leads to edematous and hypoxic-ischemic injury in a variety of tissue, including the brain. Grossly, edema is present in the subcutis often prominent in the palpebrae, cardiac region of the gastric submucosa, gallbladder, colonic mesentery, mesenteric lymph nodes, larynx, and lungs, and serous effusions occur in the thoracic cavity and pericardial sac (see Figs. 7-169 and 7-170). Congestion and sometimes hemorrhage also occur. The characteristic gross lesions in the brain are usually bilaterally symmetric foci of necrosis in the caudal medulla, but they can extend rostrally as far as the basal nuclei. The lesions are yellow-gray, soft, and slightly depressed.

The primary microscopic lesion, a degenerative angiopathy/vascular necrosis, is noted most frequently and is most severe in the caudal medulla to the diencephalon and in cerebral and cerebellar meninges (see Fig. 10-69). Cerebral, cerebellar, and spinal blood vessels are also affected. Initially, perivascular edema results from early vascular injury. Edema is followed by necrosis of medial smooth muscle cells, deposition of fibrinoid material, and accumulation of macrophages and lymphocytes in the adventitia; however, inflammation is not a primary process in this disease. Although endothelial cells and their nuclei become swollen and vesicular, this layer generally remains intact, and consequently thrombosis is not a feature. Lesions associated with the angiopathy include pallor and spongiosis of the CNS parenchyma caused by vasogenic edema and necrosis of neurons and glia. An influx of macrophages into the necrotic lesions can be observed in chronic lesions.

Pigs are usually 4 to 8 weeks of age, but younger and older pigs can be affected. Clinically, affected animals are initially ataxic and then become laterally recumbent with rhythmic paddling of the limbs. As the disease progresses, they may become comatose and die. Most pigs die within 24 hours; however, pigs that survive for several days typically develop CNS lesions (see Table 14-1).

Disorders of Dogs

Disorders that occur in many or all animal species are discussed in the section on Disorders of Domestic Animals.

Diseases Caused by Microbes

Viruses

Morbillivirus

Canine Distemper. Canine distemper is one of the most important viral diseases of the canine species. It is caused by a *Morbillivirus* (family Paramyxoviridae) and has a worldwide distribution. Morbilliviruses other than CDV include measles virus, rinderpest virus, peste-des-petits-ruminants virus, phocine distemper virus of seals, and dolphin and porpoise morbilliviruses. The virus is pantropic and has a particular affinity for lymphoid and epithelial tissues (lung, gastrointestinal tract, urinary tract, skin) and the CNS (including the optic nerve). In the CNS there is demyelination without any substantial amount of inflammation.

Dr. Brian Summers (formerly of Cornell University, College of Veterinary Medicine) has commented on the sequence of events in CDV infection based on his studies of its pathogenesis. CDV is spread between dogs by aerosol transmission. The virus is trapped in the mucosa of the nasal turbinates (centrifugal turbulence), infects local macrophages, and is spread by macrophages (leukocytic trafficking) to regional lymph nodes (retropharyngeal). CDV replicates in these regional lymph nodes, and replication is followed by a primary viremia that infects systemic lymph nodes, spleen, and the thymus approximately 48 hours after exposure. With infection of the lymphoid system, immunosuppression can occur, resulting in secondary bacterial infections, such as conjunctivitis, rhinitis, and bronchopneumonia, which are commonly seen in CDV infections.

Four to 6 days after the primary viremia, a secondary viremia occurs largely via leukocytic trafficking. CDV spreads from cells of the lymphoid system to infect the CNS and epithelial cells of the respiratory mucosa, urinary bladder mucosa, and gastrointestinal tract. In the CNS, trafficking leukocytes form perivascular cuffs, and from these cells CDV is disseminated throughout the CNS. It should be noted that the degree of inflammation in the CNS at this stage is minimal.

Under laboratory conditions the severity of the disease and the cell populations and areas infected in the CNS depend on the (1) age of the dog, (2) strain of CDV, and (3) kinetics of the antiviral immune response. Virtually all cells of the CNS, including those in the meninges, choroid plexus, neurons, and glia, are susceptible to infection, but oligodendrocytes are novel in that the infection in these cells is usually defective (incomplete). In dogs infected experimentally with the A75-17 strain of CDV, isolated from a dog with CDV in 1975, approximately one-third of the dogs died from encephalomyelitis and the effects attributable to severe immunosuppression. One-third of infected dogs developed a timely systemic immune response, and the CNS disease was quickly resolved and they recovered. Finally, one-third of the dogs infected with CDV developed a subacute to chronic inflammatory/demyelinating disease of the white matter with some gray matter involvement because of a delayed and deficient immune response.

The encephalomyelitis of canine distemper is initiated after viral entry into the CNS, perhaps 1 week after exposure to CDV. Leukocytic trafficking spreads CDV to the gray and white matter of the CNS and to epithelial cells and macrophages of the choroid plexuses. The virus is shed from choroid plexus epithelial and ependymal cells into the CSF in infected macrophages. It is disseminated throughout the ventricular system, infects ependymal cells lining the ventricular system, and then spreads locally to infect astrocytes and microglia. Periventricular white matter lesions, especially those surrounding the fourth ventricle, are the result of this sequence of events.

By 25 days after exposure, CDV-infected leukocytes in the perivascular cuffs have disappeared; however, lesions in the white matter consist of periventricular foci of myelin degeneration and swollen astrocytes. CDV infects astrocytes, microglia, and other cells. Microglia and recruited blood monocytes phagocytose myelin fragments.

Inflammatory mediators released from lymphocytes, microglial cells, and trafficking macrophages result in expansion of the initial lesions. These inflammatory mediators may cause necrosis of cells and cell processes in the focus but do not result in a "selective" demyelinating process affecting axons. The characteristic white matter vacuolation (intramyelinic edema) seen in H&E-stained sections of CDV-infected CNS is apparently caused by a direct effect of the virus on oligodendrocytes, because it appears in the earliest white matter lesions before they have acquired an "inflammatory" character—a dense infiltrate of lymphocytes, monocytes, and plasma cells.

Gross lesions characteristically occur in the cerebellum (medullary area, folial white matter, and subpial white matter) and cerebellar peduncles (with both white matter and sometimes gray matter involvement of the pons). Lesions also occur in medulla oblongata (particularly in the subependymal area of the fourth ventricle), rostral medullary vellum, cerebrum (both white matter and gray matter), optic nerves, optic tracts, spinal cord, and meninges.

Microscopically, in addition to demyelination there is status spongiosus, astrocytic hypertrophy and hyperplasia with focal and variable syncytial cell formation, reduced numbers of oligodendroglia, and variable neuronal degeneration (Fig. 14-97, *A*). Inclusion bodies (cytoplasmic, nuclear, or both) are detectable, particularly in astrocytes, which are important target cells for the distemper virus, but also in ependymal cells and occasionally in neurons (Fig. 14-97, *B*). The earliest evidence of myelin injury is a ballooning change resulting from a split in the myelin sheath or more degenerative changes, including axonal swelling. This lesion is also variably associated with astroglial and microglial proliferation. This initial injury of the myelin sheath, which has been suggested to be a result of perturbed astrocytic function after viral infection, is followed by a progressive removal of compact myelin sheaths by phagocytic microglial cells that infiltrate the myelin lamellae and variable axonal necrosis.

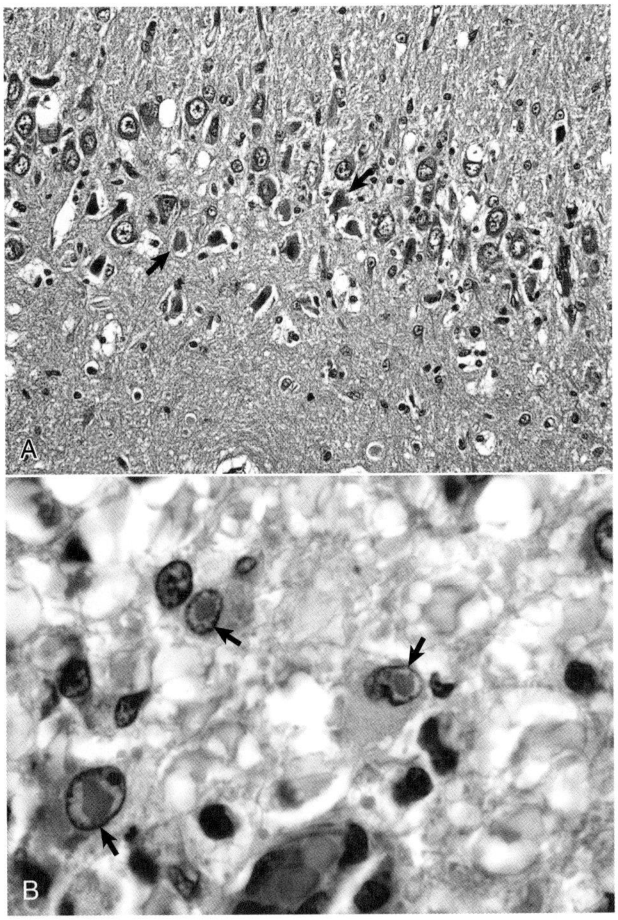

Figure 14-97 Canine Distemper, Dog. A, Acute polioencephalomyelitis. Hippocampus. Note the necrotic neurons *(arrows)* and edema of the dentate gyrus. Low numbers of mononuclear inflammatory cells are present. H&E stain. **B,** Inclusion bodies, brain, midbrain periventricular white matter, dog. Distinct acidophilic *(red)* intranuclear inclusion bodies *(arrows)* are present in astrocytes and some gemistocytes. Similar inclusions can be observed in the cytoplasm of epithelial cells throughout the body (bladder epithelium, respiratory epithelium, gastric epithelium). H&E stain. (**A** courtesy Dr. W. Haschek-Hock, College of Veterinary Medicine, University of Illinois. **B** courtesy Dr. M.D. McGavin, College of Veterinary Medicine, University of Tennessee.)

A late stage of demyelination, which is a reflection of an affected animal's improved immune status, is more pronounced and is characterized by nonsuppurative inflammation (perivascular cuffing, leptomeningitis, and choroiditis) and also can be accompanied by tissue degeneration and accumulation of gitter cells.

In addition to the dog, animals of the families Ailuridae (red panda), Canidae (fox, wolf), Hyaenidae (hyena), Mustelidae (ferret, mink), Procyonidae (raccoon, panda), Ursidae (bear), Viverridae (civet, mongoose), and Felidae (exotic felids including lions, tigers, and leopards) are susceptible to canine distemper viral infection. Additionally, canine distemper has recently been reported in javelinas (collared peccaries) of the family Tayassuidae in the United States.

Neurologic signs in all affected species include convulsions, myoclonus, tremor, disturbances in voluntary movement, circling, hyperesthesia, paralysis, and blindness.

Old-Dog Encephalitis. Old-dog encephalitis is thought to arise from long-term persistent infection of the CNS with a defective form of CDV. This pathogenesis has been demonstrated in experimental infections with the CDV. Although the virus has the same general polypeptide composition and contains all of the major viral proteins as the one causing conventional distemper, some differences among peptides have been reported. The mechanisms involved in development of lesions are not known; however, they result in a proliferation of nonsuppurative inflammatory cells.

Lesions are primarily in the cerebral hemispheres and brainstem. Microscopic lesions are characterized primarily by demyelination with disseminated, nonsuppurative encephalitis with variable, sometimes prominent, lymphoplasmacytic perivascular cuffing, microgliosis, astrogliosis, and variable leptomeningitis and neuronal degeneration. Nuclear and cytoplasmic inclusions, positive for distemper viral antigen, have been detected in neurons and astrocytes in the cerebral cortex, thalamus, and brainstem but in contrast to distemper, not in the cerebellum.

Old-dog encephalitis is a rare condition occurring in mature adult dogs. Clinical signs include depression, circling, head pressing, visual deficits, seizures, and muscle fasciculations.

Degenerative Diseases

Metabolic

Aging-Related Degenerative Myelopathy (German Shepherd Myelopathy). A degenerative myelopathy is most commonly seen in the German shepherd, but a similar condition has been described in other predominatly large canine breeds (Belgium shepherd, Old English sheepdog, Rhodesian ridgeback, Weimaraner, Pembroke Welsh corgi, and Great Pyrenees). Based on its prevalence in German shepherds, it has been suggested that there is a genetic "aging" predisposition in this breed. Altered suppressor lymphocyte activity has been noted in affected dogs, but the relevance to the CNS disease is unknown. Some investigators have reported low vitamin E concentrations and suggested oxidative stress injury; others have found elevated concentrations of acetylcholinesterase in CSF. The cause of this disorder remains to be discovered.

Gross lesions in the CNS are not present in dogs with age-related degenerative myelopathy; however, atrophy of caudal axial and appendicular muscles occurs. Microscopic lesions are most notable in the thoracic spinal cord and can be diffuse or multifocal. Dorsal aspects of the lateral and ventromedial areas of ventral funiculi can be more severely affected, but lesions can be diffuse in all funiculi. Lesions consist predominantly of ballooning and degeneration of myelin sheaths accompanied by axonal degeneration and loss. Degeneration of dorsal nerve rootlets and peripheral nerves, loss of neuron cell bodies in spinal gray matter, and involvement of brainstem nuclei are also described.

Clinically, affected dogs are usually older than 8 years, but the disease has occurred as early as 5 years of age. They have progressive ataxia referable to the thoracolumbar spinal cord and muscle weakness.

Primary Neuronal Degeneration

Multisystem Neuronal Degeneration

Progressive Neuronal Abiotrophy of Kerry Blue Terriers. Progressive neuronal abiotrophy of Kerry blue terriers (hereditary striatonigral and cerebello-olivary degeneration of Kerry blue terriers) is a well-characterized example of a disease with multisystem neuronal degeneration. The disease has an autosomal recessive inheritance pattern and affects connected neural systems, including basal nuclei and the substantia nigra (i.e., striatonigral) and the cerebellar cortex and caudal olivary nucleus (cerebello-olivary).

The pathogenesis is unknown, but an excitotoxic mechanism associated with abnormalities in the glutaminergic corticostriatal and in the granule–Purkinje cell neurotransmitter systems is proposed. The caudate nucleus and cerebellar cortex are believed to be the primary sites of involvement, whereas lesions in the olivary nucleus and substantia nigra represent transsynaptic degeneration.

Gross lesions are a slight reduction in size of the cerebellum and narrowing of cerebellar folia (Fig. 14-98). In more advanced stages, small foci of softening and discoloration occur in the caudal olivary nucleus and substantia nigra (Fig. 14-99). Lesions in the caudate nucleus initially consist of vague areas of pallor that progress to marked malacia and cavitation. There can be similar involvement of the putamen at this advanced stage. Microscopic lesions in chronologic order are degeneration and loss of cerebellar Purkinje and granule cells, followed by neuronal loss in the caudal olivary nucleus, caudate nucleus, putamen, and substantia nigra. Astrogliosis occurs in later stages and is especially prominent in the cerebellar molecular layer. The caudate nucleus and putamen are eventually reduced to microcystic cavities bisected by a few nerve and glial fibers.

Affected dogs typically start to develop clinical signs in the first 2 to 5 months of age. Clinical signs include rear limb ataxia, intention tremors, hypermetria of front and rear limbs, and atrophy of appendicular and epaxial muscles, presumably from disuse.

Multisystem Neuronal Degeneration of the Red-Coated English Cocker Spaniel. Multisystem neuronal degeneration of the red-coated English cocker spaniel is suspected of being inherited. The pathogenesis is unknown. Bilaterally symmetric diffuse nerve cell loss, astrogliosis, and axonal swellings occur in several nuclei, including septal nuclei, globus pallidus, subthalamic nuclei, substantia nigra, tectum, medial geniculate bodies, and cerebellar and vestibular nuclei. Central cerebellar white matter, corpus callosum, thalamic striae, and subcortical (particularly subcallosal gyri) white matter involvement also are noted. White matter lesions consist of axonal spheroids, intense astrogliosis, subtle myelin loss, and perivascular accumulation of macrophages. Clinical signs occur during the first year of life and consist of progressive ataxia and behavioral changes.

Multisystemic Neuronal Degeneration of the Cairn Terrier. Multisystemic neuronal degeneration of the Cairn terrier has features of an inherited disorder. The pathogenesis is unknown. Widespread neuronal chromatolysis affecting multiple neuronal systems is observed in the CNS and PNS. Affected areas include brainstem sensory and motor nuclei, cerebellar nuclei, ventral and dorsal gray columns of the spinal cord, and various ganglia. Other lesions include degeneration in lateral and ventral spinal funiculi, necrosis of substantia gelatinosa and adjacent white matter most notable in caudal thoracic and cranial lumbar segments, and degeneration in dorsal and ventral spinal nerve rootlets and peripheral nerves. Clinical signs occur usually by 5 months of age, and there is onset of progressive cerebellar ataxia, spastic paresis, and collapse.

Primary Cerebellar Neuronal Degeneration. Primary cerebellar neuronal degenerations (referred to as abiotrophies) occur in many breeds of dogs, including American Staffordshire terriers, Australian

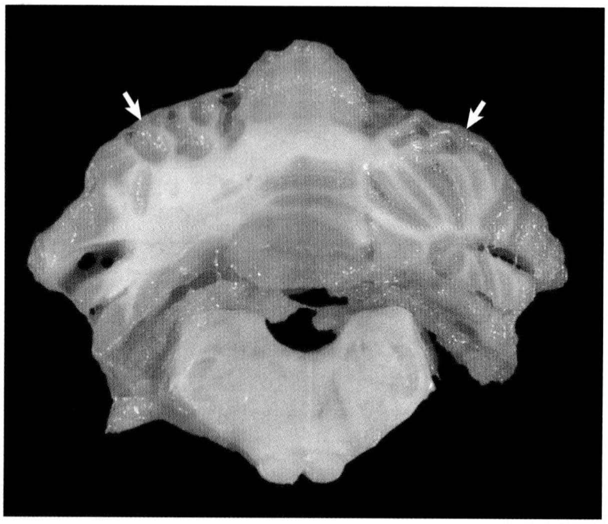

Figure 14-98 **Striatonigral and Cerebello-Olivary Degeneration, Brain, Cerebellum, Kerry Blue Terrier.** Marked atrophy and thinning of folia of dorsal cerebellum *(arrows)* has resulted in increased width of sulci. (Courtesy Drs. D. Montgomery and R. Storts, College of Veterinary Medicine, Texas A&M University.)

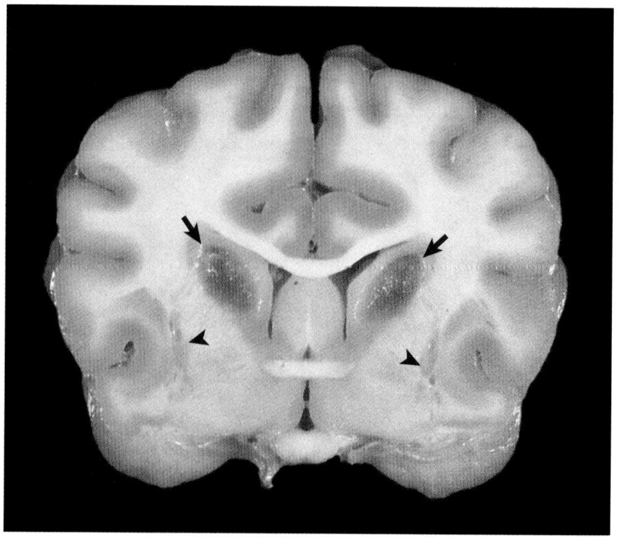

Figure 14-99 **Striatonigral and Cerebello-Olivary Degeneration, Brain, Rostral Parietal Lobe, at Level of Optic Chiasm, Kerry Blue Terrier.** Note malacia (softening), microscopically due to microcavitation and loss of neurons, in caudate nuclei *(arrows)* and putamen *(arrowheads)*. (Courtesy Drs. D. Montgomery and R. Storts, College of Veterinary Medicine, Texas A&M University; and *Vet Pathol* 20:143-159, 1983.)

kelpie, Italian hound, border collie, Brittany spaniel, beagle, Portuguese podengo, and Scottish terriers. This list is not inclusive and serves only to provide a few examples. Although most common in young animals of the breeds listed, cerebellar degeneration in the American Staffordshire terrier and Brittany spaniel occurs later in life. An autosomal recessive mode of inheritance is suspected or documented in several of the diseases. Grossly, the cerebellum can be normal or reduced in size and atrophic. Microscopically, the distribution and characteristics of lesions vary, depending on the breed and species of animal affected. A detailed discussion of the microscopic lesions for each breed and species is outside the scope of this chapter; however, lesions may include a combination of the following changes: loss of Purkinje cells and neurons of the granule layer, astrogliosis, fusiform swelling of proximal Purkinje cell axons, and axonal degeneration in the cerebellum, brainstem, and spinal cord.

Neuronal Vacuolation and Spinocerebellar Degeneration. A syndrome causing neuronal vacuolation and spinocerebellar degeneration has been reported most commonly in Rottweiler dogs as well as sporadically in boxers and mixed-breed dogs. The cause of this disease has not been determined but appears to have a hereditary basis. Apoptotic cell death is apparently not involved in neuronal degeneration. No gross lesions are observed in the brain, but atrophy of the dorsal cricoarytenoid muscles of the larynx has been seen. Microscopic lesions are characterized by spongiform change affecting neuron cell bodies and the neuropil. The cytoplasm of neurons of the cerebellar nuclei and nuclei of the extrapyramidal system contain one or more clear vacuoles (1 to 45 μm in diameter). Similar vacuoles are found in neurons in dorsal nerve root ganglia, myenteric plexuses, and other ganglia of the autonomic nervous system. Purkinje cells are also vacuolated, and in terminal stages of the disease there is degeneration with segmental Purkinje cell loss.

Clinical signs, seen as early as 6 weeks (commonly between 3 and 8 months of age in both sexes), include generalized weakness, ataxia, proprioceptive deficits, and paresis that progress in severity over the course of the disease.

Nutritional

Vitamin B_1 (Thiamine) Deficiency

Thiamine Deficiency in Carnivores. In monogastric carnivores and human beings the relationship between neurologic disease and thiamine deficiency is firmly established, and lesions in these species are similar. In carnivores (dog, cat, mink, and fox), there is an absolute dietary requirement for vitamin B_1. Dietary factors, such as the ingestion of fish containing thiaminase, deficient diets, or diets in which the vitamin has been destroyed by other means such as heating, can all lead to thiamine deficiency.

Gross and microscopic lesions are bilaterally symmetric and commonly involve the midlaminae of the cerebral cortex, with the occipital and temporal cortices most consistently affected. Additionally, a variety of brainstem nuclei are affected, with the caudal colliculus being the most common (Fig. 14-100). Lesions consist of neuronal vacuolation accompanied by neuronal degeneration and necrosis with variable hemorrhage, vascular proliferation, and astrogliosis, the latter of which is time dependent. If the degree of necrosis is severe enough, accumulation of gitter cells is a common sequela. Clinical signs in carnivores may include a combination of the following: anorexia, vomiting, depression, wide-based stance, ataxia, spastic paresis, circling, seizures, muscle weakness, recumbency, opisthotonus, coma, or death.

Miscellaneous Conditions

Dural Ossification. Dural ossification (ossifying pachymeningitis and dural osseous metaplasia) is a metaplastic aging change of

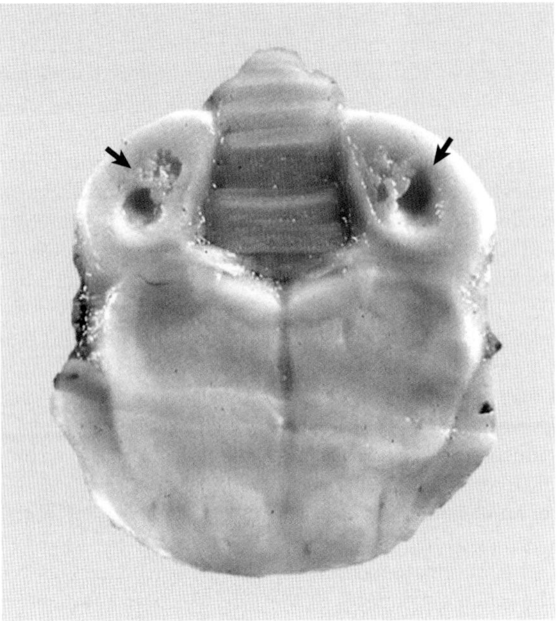

Figure 14-100 **Thiamine Deficiency Encephalopathy, Midbrain, Caudal Colliculi, Dog.** In the dog, lesions of thiamine deficiency encephalopathy are generally restricted to the brainstem. Note the symmetrically cavitated (malacic) lesions in the caudal colliculi *(arrows)* resulting from neuronal necrosis. (Courtesy Dr. J. Edwards, College of Veterinary Medicine, Texas A&M University; and Dr. J. King, College of Veterinary Medicine, Cornell University.)

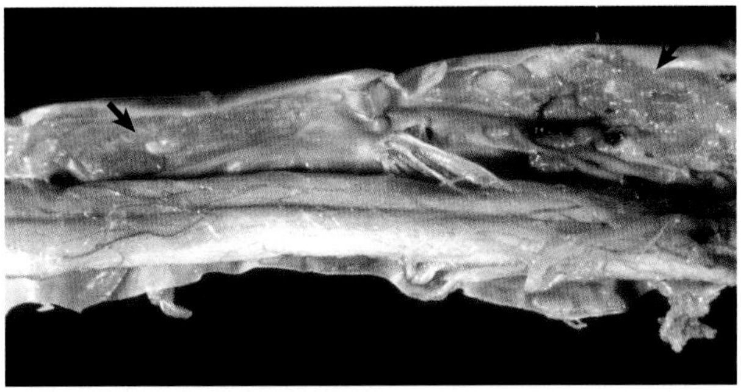

Figure 14-101 **Osseous Metaplasia, Dura Mater, Dog.** Also called *ossifying pachymeningitis* and *dural ossification*, the dura mater contains well-differentiated bone and bone marrow *(arrows)*. With movement of the vertebrae, the metaplastic bone can impinge on nerve roots and cause pain in large breed dogs. (Courtesy College of Veterinary Medicine, University of Illinois.)

predominantly large breed dogs. Grossly, the dura of the cervical and lumbar enlargements of the spinal cord has reddish-brown plaques that histologically are composed of bone, adipose tissue, and hematopoietic cells. These plaques typically recapitulate the normal bone marrow (Fig. 14-101). Thoracolumbar pain in affected dogs is thought to arise after flexion/extension of the spinal column as a result of compression of either the spinal cord or the spinal nerve roots; however, they are generally viewed as incidental, age-associated lesions.

Inherited Necrotizing Myelopathy of Afghan Hounds. Inherited necrotizing myelopathy of Afghan hounds has an autosomal recessive inheritance. A similar disease has been reported in Dutch Kooikerhondje dogs, but the relative degrees of axonal degeneration versus demyelination have not been adequately described.

Topographically, gross lesions are consistently observed in the midthoracic segments, with extension to the midcervical and midlumbar segments in the most severe cases. Gross lesions include softening and cavitation of the affected segments. Lesions are bilateral and symmetric regardless of the region affected. In the thoracic segments the ventral funiculi are most severely affected, although lesions can be found circumferentially around the spinal cord white matter. In the cervical and lumbar segments, the lesions tend to be focused either in the dorsal or ventral horns. Histologically, in severe lesions there is destruction of white matter, with an influx of macrophages accompanied by myelin degradation, glial cell loss, and vascular proliferation. The gray matter and the fasciculus proprius are typically spared in this disease. Neuronal cell bodies in spinal cord gray matter and ventral spinal nerve rootlets are similarly unaffected.

Clinical signs begin between 3 and 13 months of age and progress rapidly to paraplegia or tetraplegia within 1 to 3 weeks.

Leptomeningeal Fibrosis. Aging dogs have varying degrees of leptomeningeal fibrosis involving the recesses of the cerebral sulci (Fig. 14-102). This lesion is not present in the leptomeninges covering the outermost surfaces of the gyri. This latter feature can be useful in differentiating meningeal fibrosis from suppurative meningitis. In cases of suppurative meningitis, exudate accumulates over the entire surface of the gyri.

Granulomatous Meningoencephalitis. Granulomatous meningoencephalitis (GME) is one of two important idiopathic encephalitides of the dog, the second one being necrotizing encephalitis, of which there are two variants (see later). Granulomatous meningoencephalitis occurs most commonly in young to middle-aged small breed dogs, including poodles and various terrier breeds. No sex predilection is known, although some studies are skewed slightly toward female. Clinical signs in cases with brain lesions are variable and include behavioral changes and circling. Spinal cord lesions can result in paresis and ataxia.

When present, gross lesions consist of gray-white to red, expansive areas within the white matter of the brain and brainstem (Fig. 14-103, *A*). Lesions can have irregular, well-defined margins and a gelatinous or rubbery consistency or appear granular. There are two different distribution patterns of the disease, a disseminated form and a focal form. The focal form is most commonly seen in the thalamus and brainstem. Histologically, this disease causes distinct perivascular cuffs composed almost entirely of lymphocytes and macrophages with scattered numbers of plasma cells and neutrophils. These cuffs are almost entirely restricted to the white matter. The proportion of lymphocytes and macrophages can vary in affected foci. Macrophages are commonly epithelioid, and in chronic cases there is abundant deposition of reticulin and collagen in the affected perivascular regions (see Fig. 14-103, *B*). The inflammatory lesion in granulomatous meningoencephalitis is predominantly $CD3^+$ lymphocytes and perivascular accumulations of $CD163^+$ macrophages. This observation has led to the suggestion that the underlying mechanism of the disease process is a T lymphocyte–mediated delayed-type hypersensitivity of an organ-specific autoimmune disease. Regardless, the cause of granulomatous meningoencephalitis has remained enigmatic, and various attempts to consistently isolate pathogens from affected dogs have proved fruitless.

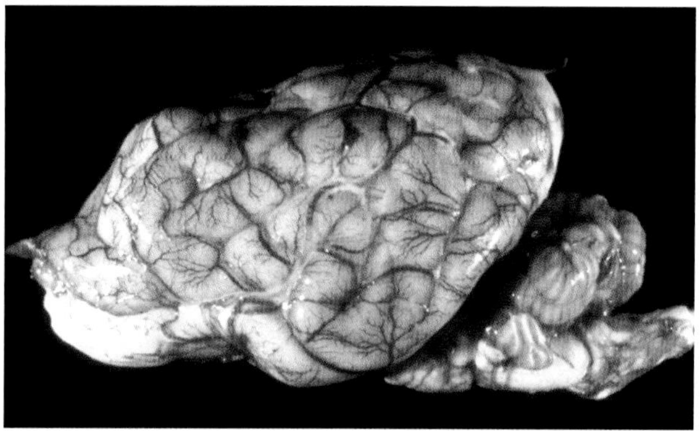

Figure 14-102 **Meningeal Fibrosis, Leptomeninges (Pia-Arachnoid Mater), Dog.** In old dogs the leptomeninges can have areas of fibrosis (*white areas around blood vessels in sulci*), particularly in the sulci. This lesion must not be confused with acute leptomeningitis and accumulation of exudate in the leptomeninges and subarachnoid space. In the latter the exudate extends into the sulci and also covers the gyri (see Fig. 14-43, *A*). (Courtesy College of Veterinary Medicine, University of Illinois.)

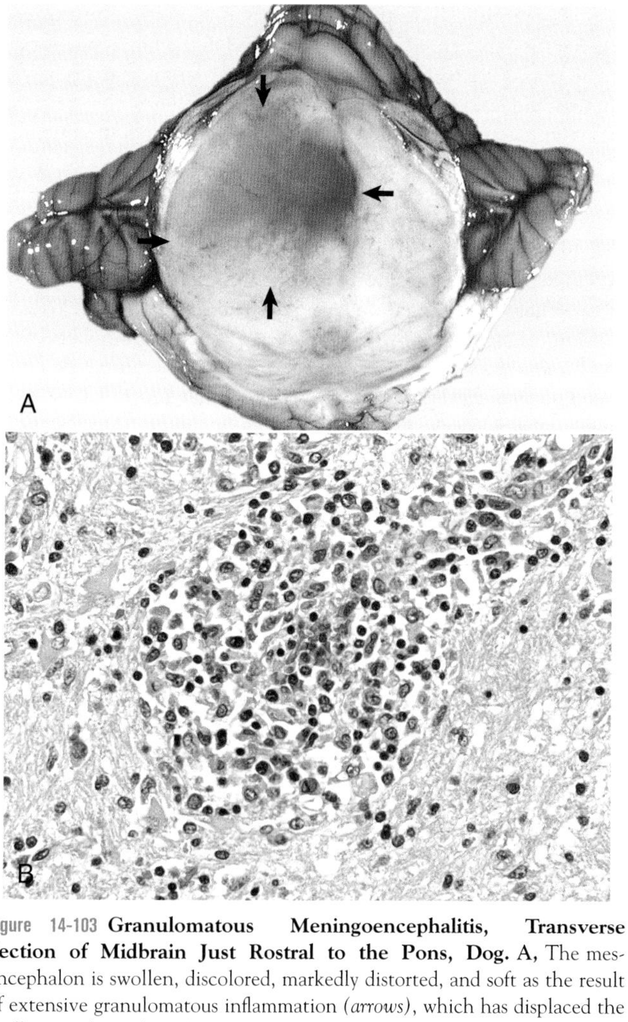

Figure 14-103 **Granulomatous Meningoencephalitis, Transverse Section of Midbrain Just Rostral to the Pons, Dog. A,** The mesencephalon is swollen, discolored, markedly distorted, and soft as the result of extensive granulomatous inflammation (*arrows*), which has displaced the midline to the right. The mesencephalic aqueduct is also compressed and distorted. **B,** Note the accumulation of granulomatous inflammatory cells in the perivascular space. Such layers of cells expand over time and compress adjacent neural tissue, resulting in Wallerian-like degeneration of affected myelinated axons and atrophy of affected neuron cell bodies. H&E. (**A** courtesy Dr. J. Edwards, College of Veterinary Medicine, Texas A&M University; and Dr. J. King, College of Veterinary Medicine, Cornell University. **B** courtesy Dr. J.F. Zachary, College of Veterinary Medicine, University of Illinois.)

Necrotizing Encephalitis. Necrotizing encephalitis, a second important idiopathic encephalitis of the dog, has two variants, necrotizing meningoencephalitis (NME) and necrotizing leukoencephalitis (NLE). Necrotizing meningoencephalitis is a disease that is almost always restricted to small breed dogs like the pug, shih tzu, and Maltese terrier. It was once referred to as pug-dog encephalitis before it was recognized in a wide variety of small breed dogs. Grossly, this disease appears as bilateral foci of malacia and discoloration of the cerebral hemispheres. Histologically, this gross lesion corresponds to regions of meningoencephalitis in which the inflammation is typically robust, nonsuppurative, and associated with marked gliosis. Unlike in cases of granulomatous meningoencephalitis, spinal cord involvement is uncommon. The second disease is known as necrotizing leukoencephalitis. This disease predominates in the white matter. It is most commonly seen in Yorkshire terriers, although sporadic reports exist in other small breed dogs. Gross lesions consist of prominent bilateral cavitation and necrosis of the cerebral white matter. Histologically, there is robust nonsuppurative inflammation accompanied by gliosis, cavitation, edema, and gitter cell infiltration. The etiopathogenesis of both diseases is unknown, and whether they represent a continuum of the same disease or distinct diseases is still debated. Populations of lymphocytes and macrophages as determined by experimental analysis are similar in the two variants. Clinical signs in both variants are typically nonspecific and can involve a variety of prosencephalic processes such as behavior, processing of sensory and associative information, and the initiation of voluntary movement.

Traumatic Injury

Intervertebral Disk Disease. Although the anatomy of vertebrae and intervertebral disks is similar in dogs and human beings, there are notable differences in the anatomy of the spinal cord and spinal nerve roots that result in differences between the two species in clinical signs caused by herniated disks. Disk herniations in human beings commonly occur laterally, rather than dorsally as in dogs, contributing to the differences in clinical presentations (i.e., lateral herniations compress spinal nerve rootlets, whereas dorsal compression in dogs impinges on the spinal cord directly). In human beings the spinal cord terminates at the level of the second lumbar vertebra. Spinal nerve roots forming the cauda equina traverse the remaining lumbar and sacral vertebrae before they exit the spinal canal to innervate structures. In dogs the spinal cord terminates at the level of the sixth lumbar vertebra, and nerve roots forming the cauda equina traverse the remaining lumbar, sacral, and coccygeal vertebrae before they exit the spinal canal to innervate structures. Therefore in human beings, disk disease involving the caudal lumbar vertebrae (caudal to L2) results in compression of spinal nerve roots that innervate limbs and are reflected clinically in a condition known as *sciatica* that is defined as referred pain in the sciatic nerve. In dogs, herniated disks in the lumbar vertebra primarily compress the spinal cord and under certain circumstances spinal nerves. Dogs thus present clinically with different neurologic signs.

Differences in clinical signs between dogs and human beings caused by herniated disks arise not only from anatomic differences discussed previously, but also from postural differences and the application of shear and stress forces applied to the vertebrae and intervertebral disks. Human beings, with bipedal locomotion and erect posture, dissipate the forces of walking (also running) by transferring these forces from the legs up the vertebral column to the lumbar vertebrae (i.e., first in line to absorb and dissipate forces). In addition, lumbar vertebrae are not stabilized by the rib cage, and thus lumbar vertebrae must also absorb rotational forces (i.e., twisting forces) of motion. Therefore lumbar vertebrae are the primary sites for disk herniation in human beings; however, because of the anatomy discussed earlier, herniated disks compress nerve roots and not the spinal cord. This arrangement results in pain but rarely leg paralysis.

Dogs, having quadrupedal locomotion and horizontal posture, normally dissipate the forces of walking by transferring these forces up the limbs at right angles to the vertebral column and spinal cord. However, when a dog jumps with downward motion, as an example, from a chair to the floor, the force is directed down the vertebral column and results in greater "end on" compression of disks and increased likelihood of herniation. Additionally, thoracic vertebrae are fixed in place by the ribs, and lumbar vertebrae can rotate freely around the axial skeleton. This arrangement directs the impact of stress and shear forces to the thoracolumbar vertebrae and is a primary site of disk herniation and spinal cord compression. In dogs, because the spinal cord is compressed, paralysis of the rear limbs results.

Intervertebral disk disease occurs in the canine species, particularly dogs of the chondrodystrophic breeds typified by the dachshund and Pekingese (Fig. 14-104). Contiguous vertebrae are held together by the annulus fibrosus of intervertebral disks and dorsal and ventral longitudinal ligaments. This anatomic arrangement results in the spinal canal being properly aligned in an axial plane, so the spinal cord can traverse through the space without compression. Extradural space surrounding the cervical, cranial thoracic, and caudal lumbar spinal cord is sufficient to allow for the accumulation of herniated disk material without substantial compression of the spinal cord. In contrast, there is little extradural space surrounding the thoracolumbar spinal cord; this is the site most likely to have clinically significant disk herniation. As a result in dogs, thoracolumbar disk herniation is often more debilitating than cervical disk herniation.

Degeneration of intervertebral disks in chondrodystrophic breeds of dogs is a genetically programmed metaplastic change of the nucleus pulposus, resulting in peripheral to central replacement of the nucleus pulposus with cartilage. It begins as early as 6 months of age, progresses rapidly, and results in the loss of elasticity of the nucleus pulposus. The loss of elasticity places additional mechanical stress forces on the annulus fibrosus, which itself is experiencing degenerative changes similar to those occurring in the nucleus pulposus. The annulus fibrosus is thinnest and thus weakest at its point of contact with the spinal canal. If the annulus fibrosus is ruptured after stress forces placed on the disk by movement, such as jumping downward from a chair, fragments of the nucleus pulposus can be released into the spinal canal (Hansen type I herniation). If the annulus fibrosus ruptures dorsally, fragments compress the ventral funiculi of the spinal cord. If the annulus fibrosus ruptures dorsolaterally to laterally, fragments compress the ventral funiculi, lateral funiculi, and/or spinal nerve roots. Degeneration of intervertebral disks in nonchondrodystrophic breeds of dogs is an aging change of the nucleus pulposus resulting from fibrous metaplasia. This change causes a gradual loss of elasticity of the nucleus pulposus, which may be noticed clinically by 8 to 10 years of age. The gradual loss of elasticity places mechanical stress forces on the annulus fibrosus and results in its protrusion into and compression of the spinal canal (Hansen type II herniation).

Disk herniation causes injury to the CNS by several mechanisms. As discussed previously, the primary injury is caused by the physical trauma of compression and the resulting Wallerian degeneration of affected axons. Additionally, disk material can compress the vascular supply to a spinal cord segment, resulting in ischemia, neuronal excitotoxicity, and necrosis. Type I herniation causes the most severe spinal cord damage because there is insufficient time for the spinal cord to compensate and for collateral circulation to develop, as may occur in type II herniation.

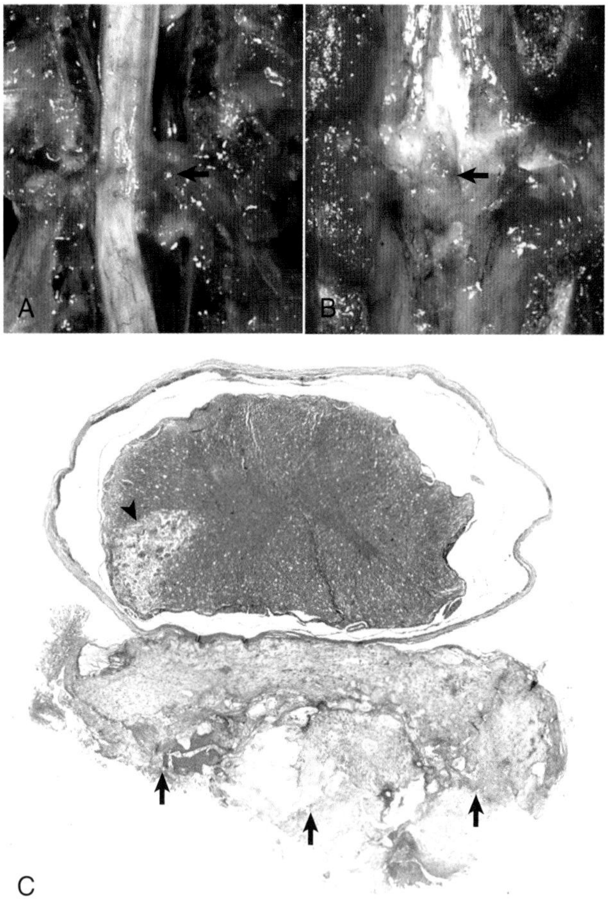

Figure 14-104 **Intervertebral Disk Disease, Dog. A,** Disk rupture (herniated intervertebral disk), spinal cord compression. Disk material compresses the spinal cord *(arrow)* resulting in Wallerian degeneration. **B,** Vertebral column, lumbar vertebrae. Herniated intervertebral disk *(arrow)* protrudes into the vertebral canal. **C,** Herniated intervertebral disk, spinal cord. The disk material *(arrows)* lies in the epidural space, touches the dura mater, and compresses the overlying spinal cord. An area of necrosis, possibly caused by infarction, is present in the ventral area of the left lateral funiculus *(arrowhead)*. The multiple small holes in all funiculi are the sites of lost nerves as the result of spinal cord compression, which caused Wallerian degeneration. H&E stain. (Courtesy Dr. M.D. McGavin, College of Veterinary Medicine, University of Tennessee.)

Aging Changes

See Disorders of Domestic Animals, Aging Changes.

Canine cognitive dysfunction has been compared to Alzheimer's disease in human beings. Senile plaques and cerebrovascular amyloidosis have been described in the brains of aged dogs and are thought to result in structural and functional alterations in chemical pathways, leading to cognitive dysfunction.

Disorders of Cats

Disorders that occur in many or all animal species are discussed in the section on Disorders of Domestic Animals.

Diseases Caused by Microbes

Viruses

Coronaviruses

Feline Infectious Peritonitis. Feline infectious peritonitis, which is caused by a coronavirus and has a worldwide distribution, is mainly a disease of domestic cats, although wild felids can be affected. A similar virus has recently been recognized in ferrets and can cause similar lesions in the CNS. There are two recognized feline coronaviruses: feline enteric coronavirus (FECV) and feline infectious peritonitis virus (FIPV), which cause FECV and feline infectious peritonitis infections, respectively. The viruses for each infection are antigenically and morphologically indistinguishable and are currently considered to represent avirulent (FECV) and virulent (FIPV) strains of the same basic feline coronavirus. After ingestion, FECV infects and replicates in epithelial cells of the intestine and usually is an insignificant infection, although severe intestinal disease can occur. Recent research suggests that a mutation in the gene for the furin cleavage site of a spike protein (a structural glycoprotein) in the FECV viral envelope gives the virus the ability to mutate to FIPV and replicate in monocytes/macrophages, use leukocyte trafficking (see Chapter 4) by these cells to spread systemically, and cause lesions characteristic of feline infectious peritonitis in other organ systems.

FIPV enters the susceptible cat primarily by ingestion of contaminated saliva or feces, although transmission by direct inoculation (e.g., cat bites, licking open wounds) and in utero (rarely) have been reported. After infection the virus replicates in macrophages that spread the virus to the liver, serosal surfaces, uvea, the meninges, and ependyma of the brain and spinal cord.

After dissemination of the virus in the body, the development of disease depends on the type and degree of immunity that develops. Virus containment with resistance to disease occurs following development of a strong cell-mediated immunity. Humoral immunity by itself is not protective and can actually enhance development of the effusive form of feline infectious peritonitis (wet form) by two proposed mechanisms. The first involves the development of virus-antibody-complement complexes that particularly accumulate in the same areas as infected macrophages around small blood vessels, resulting in inflammation and subsequent vascular injury (type III hypersensitivity) accompanied by effusion of large amounts of fluid. The second mechanism involves a process referred to as antibody-dependent enhancement (demonstrated to occur experimentally), which involves uptake of virus-antibody-complement complexes by macrophages followed by significant viral replication. The heavily infected macrophages, frequently perivascularly oriented, release cytokines that result in alteration of endothelial junctional complexes that leads to leakage of substantial amounts of fluid.

Noneffusive feline infectious peritonitis (i.e., dry form), in comparison, is thought to occur when partial cell-mediated immunity (type IV hypersensitivity) develops and represents an intermediate stage between nonprotective humoral immunity alone and protective cellular immunity. Support for this mechanism is the fact that cats that develop the noneffusive form of feline infectious peritonitis after experimental infection usually have a preceding and transient bout of effusive-type disease. In addition, there is evidence to support the theory that cats recovered from feline infectious peritonitis are immune by a process of "infection immunity" or "premunition." Once these cats no longer retain such infections, they seem to also lose protective (cell-mediated) immunity and are in fact more sensitive to a subsequent challenge exposure because of the presence of humoral antibody.

The basic lesion in effusive and noneffusive feline infectious peritonitis is a pyogranulomatous inflammation, leading to vasculitis followed by an inconsistent vascular necrosis resulting in infarction. Unlike the majority of immune-mediated vasculitides in human medicine, feline infectious peritonitis shows preferential involvement of small- and medium-sized veins. The phlebitis that occurs is associated with activated, virally infected monocytes as they egress from the blood vessel to become macrophages. The effusive form is typified by serositis, accumulation of fluid in the abdominal and thoracic cavities, with varying degrees of severity of inflammation. Lesions of the noneffusive form more frequently result in leptomeningitis, chorioependymitis, focal encephalomyelitis, and ophthalmitis, although involvement of the kidneys, hepatic and mesenteric lymph nodes, and less frequently, serosa and other abdominal viscera can occur. In the CNS, pyogranulomatous vasculitis tends to affect blood vessels of (1) the leptomeninges, especially in sulci and near their entrance into subjacent CNS tissue and around the circle of Willis (Fig. 14-105), and (2) the periventricular white matter, especially around the fourth ventricle (Fig. 14-106). The uvea, retina, and optic nerve sheath are also commonly involved in feline infectious peritonitis.

Feline infectious peritonitis generally occurs sporadically in cats of all ages, but it is most common in younger cats between the ages of 3 months and 3 years and can be clinically significant because it can result in death. The disease manifests itself in effusive (wet) or noneffusive (dry) forms. Clinical signs caused by involvement of blood vessels in the CNS can include behavioral changes, dullness, coma, paresis, ataxia, paralysis, and seizures.

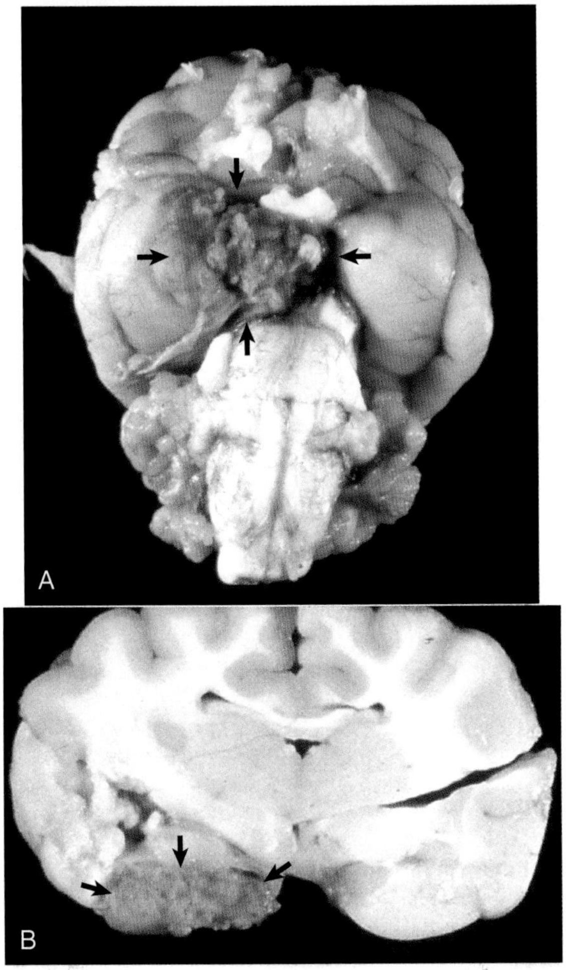

Figure 14-105 Pyogranulomatous Vasculitis, Feline Infectious Peritonitis, Cat. A, Ventral brain, cerebral vasculature of the circle of Willis. A white-yellow pyogranulomatous inflammation distorts and obscures the blood vessels. Lesions are attributed to viral induced inflammation that targets vessel walls *(arrows)*. The character of the inflammatory response can vary from an exudate with accumulation of serous fluid and fibrin mixed with neutrophils and histiocytes to a reaction that is more pyogranulomatous, and in which commonly there are lymphocytes and plasma cells. The severity and magnitude of the lesion depicted here is much more dramatic than usual. **B,** A cross-sectional view of **A**. The pyogranuloma *(arrows)* is principally in the subarachnoid space and has compressed the adjacent cerebral cortex. (**A** and **B** courtesy Dr. J. Sundberg, College of Veterinary Medicine, University of Illinois.)

Degenerative Diseases

Primary Neuronal Degeneration

Primary Cerebellar Neuronal Degeneration. A discussion of primary cerebellar neuronal degeneration in dogs and cats is in the previous section on Disorders of Dogs.

Circulatory Disturbances

Feline Ischemic Encephalopathy. Feline ischemic encephalopathy is associated with aberrant cerebrospinal migration of *Cuterebra* fly larvae that enter the brain via the nasal cavity. A vascular-mediated vasospasm of the middle cerebral artery, resulting from hemorrhage or a toxin elaborated by the parasite, is the most likely mechanism behind the vascular lesions. Acute vascular lesions are uncommonly noted; however, the chronic inflammatory lesions are typical for the disease.

The gross lesions of acute disease are predominantly unilateral and occur in the white and gray matter of the cerebral hemispheres, usually in the area supplied by the middle cerebral artery (Fig. 14-107). The necrosis can be multifocal or involve up to two-thirds of one hemisphere. Hemorrhages can occur in the CNS or leptomeninges. In chronic cases, cerebral atrophy, most severe adjacent to the middle cerebral artery of the affected hemisphere, is most typical. Microscopically, lesions include vasculitis, thrombosis,

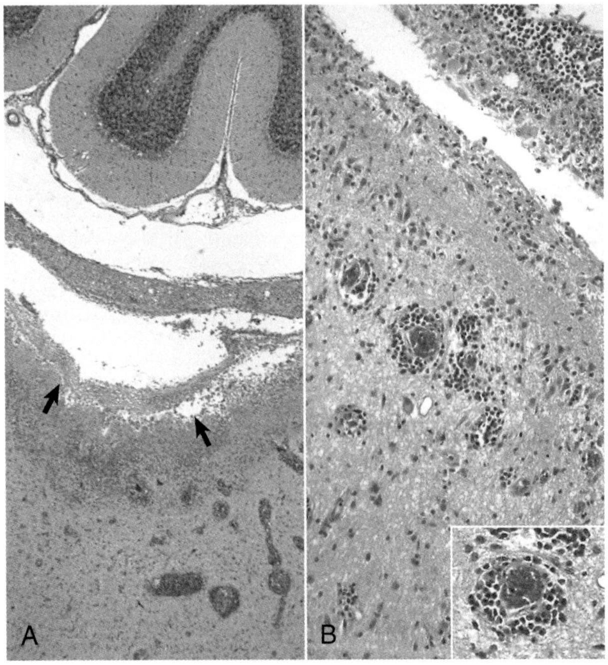

Figure 14-106 Pyogranulomatous Vasculitis, Feline Infectious Peritonitis (FIP), Cat. A, Periventricular white matter *(arrows)* beneath the fourth ventricle (between the medullary vellum and medulla). The pyogranulomatous inflammation that occurs with FIP causes vascular and perivascular injury, vasogenic edema, and parenchymal disruption. H&E stain. **B,** A higher magnification of **A**. Ventriculitis and ependymitis are evident. Note the prominent perivascular cuffs of small mononuclear cells and macrophages. H&E stain. *Inset,* Higher magnification of **B**. H&E stain. (Courtesy Dr. J.F. Zachary, College of Veterinary Medicine, University of Illinois.)

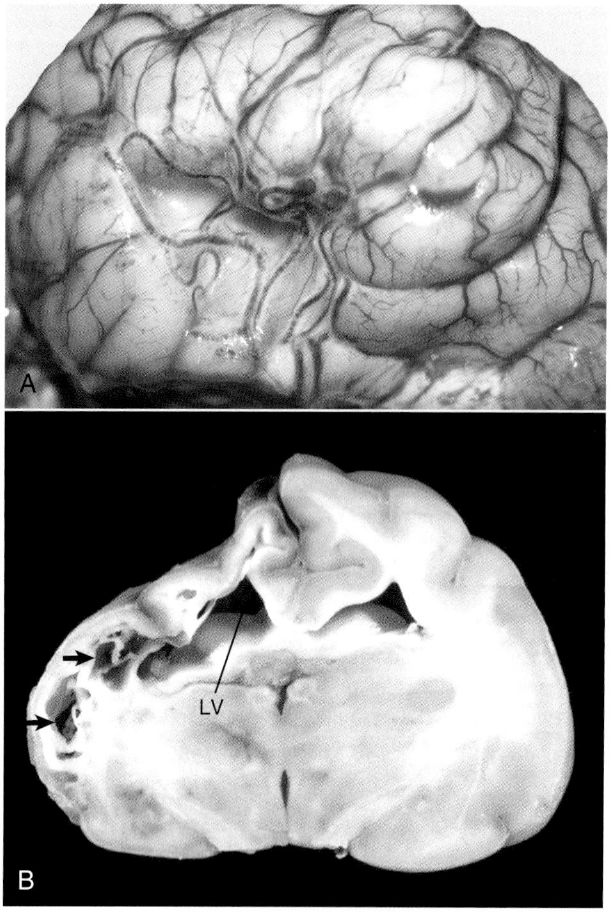

Figure 14-107 **Feline Ischemic Encephalopathy, Brain. A,** Lateral view of a collapsed area of the cerebral cortex. Note the torturous pattern of the vascular supply, likely a component of the reparative response to ischemic injury. **B,** Transverse section at the junction between the left parietal and occipital lobes, level of thalamus, cat. Chronic feline ischemic encephalopathy with unilateral cerebral degeneration-atrophy. The dorsolateral aspect of the left cerebral hemisphere has undergone necrosis, followed by cyst formation and collapse after phagocytic removal of the necrotic debris. Cystic spaces *(arrows)* have placed the previously existing parenchyma and the left lateral ventricle *(LV)* has expanded into the area of lost tissue (hydrocephalus ex vacuo). (**A** courtesy Drs. V. Hsiao and A. Gillen, College of Veterinary Medicine, University of Illinois. **B** courtesy Dr. R. Storts, College of Veterinary Medicine, Texas A&M University.)

ischemia, and infarction, and the cerebral cortical lesions follow the sequence of changes for infarction listed in Table 14-1.

Feline ischemic encephalopathy has a peracute to acute onset and affects cats of any age. Clinical signs usually reflect unilateral cerebral involvement. The disease most often occurs in the summer months and is accompanied by signs that can include depression, mild ataxia, seizures, behavioral changes, and blindness.

Peripheral Nervous System

Structure and Function

The PNS is typically divided into three parts: the sensorimotor division, the autonomic division, and the enteric division. The sensorimotor division is formed by sensory neurons (afferent components of cranial and spinal nerves, sensory receptors, and cranial and spinal ganglia) and motor neurons (efferent components of cranial and spinal nerves and lower motor neurons) that innervate skeletal muscle via myoneural junctions (Fig. 14-108). The autonomic and enteric divisions consist of networks of afferent and efferent nerves and their ganglia (Meissner's [submucosal] and Auerbach's [myenteric] plexuses) that regulate, as examples, the contractility and relaxation of smooth muscle of the vascular and alimentary (peristalsis) systems and glandular secretions via sympathetic and parasympathetic fibers. Afferent and efferent nerve fibers of the autonomic and enteric divisions are carried in the afferent and efferent branches of the sensorimotor division (cranial and spinal nerves).

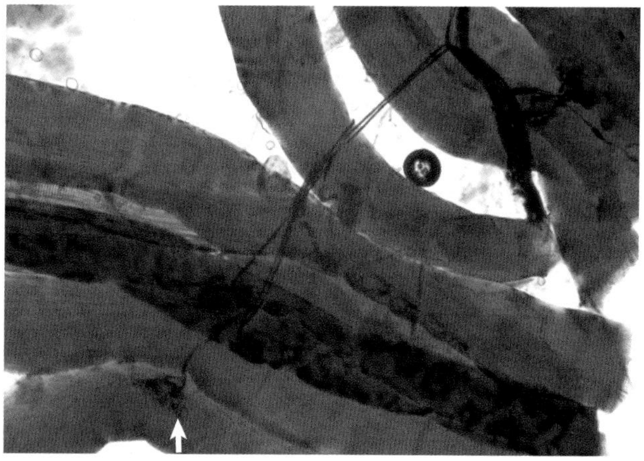

Figure 14-108 **Myoneural Junctions.** Peripheral nerve with terminal axons ending at myoneural junctions on muscle fibers *(arrow)*. Dissected and glycerol-mounted muscle fibers. (Courtesy Dr. M.D. McGavin, College of Veterinary Medicine, University of Tennessee.)

Peripheral nerves are composed of groups of axons, both myelinated and nonmyelinated, and of varying caliber (Fig. 14-109). As with the CNS, conspicuous components of axons are neurofilaments and microtubules. Neurofilaments provide structural support; microtubules are intimately involved in bidirectional axoplasmic flow of structural components, nutrients, and trophic factors to and from the cell body required for maintenance of the axons and neuronal integrity. Transport from the neuron cell body to the distal axon (anterograde flow) occurs at fast (400 mm per day or approximately 0.25 mm per minute) and slow (1 to 4 mm per day) rates. Retrograde transport from the distal axon to the cell body progresses at a rate of 200 mm per day (approximately 0.125 mm per minute) (see E-Fig. 14-3).

Supporting cells in the PNS include Schwann cells and fibroblasts of the endoneurium and the satellite cells (Schwann cell–like cells) of the dorsal root ganglion. Schwann cells surround both myelinated and nonmyelinated axons and are responsible for formation of the myelin sheaths (see Fig. 14-109). In contrast to the CNS, where one oligodendroglial cell can send out numerous processes to myelinate many different axonal internodes of several different axons, one Schwann cell myelinates one internode of one axon. As a result, the entire length of an axon in the PNS is myelinated by many individual Schwann cells.

Although Schwann cells do not appear to play a role in axon guidance during formation of the PNS, these cells are necessary for maintenance of axons and secrete neurotrophic factors that play a role in regeneration. Axons are grouped into fascicles with surrounding loosely organized tissue fibrils and specialized endoneurial fibroblastic cells with phagocytic capabilities (see Fig. 14-109). When an axon is damaged so badly as to cause Wallerian degeneration, removal of the debris is by these putative endogenous phagocytic cells, augmented by an influx of blood monocytes. Mast cells and small blood vessels also are present among the nerve fibers.

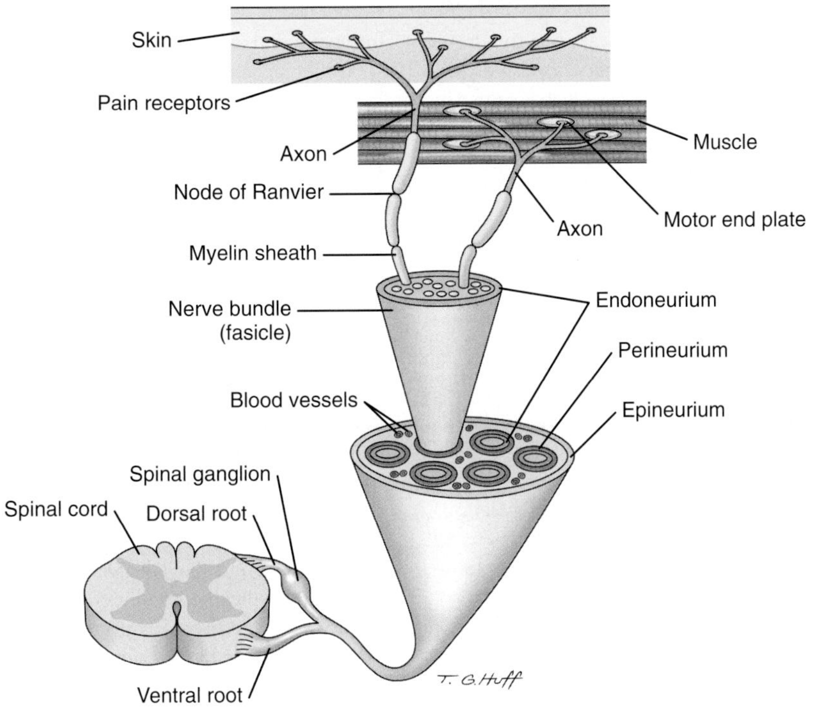

Figure 14-109 **Organization of a Peripheral Nerve, and Sensory and Motor Branches and Their Coverings.**

Depending on species and anatomic location, endothelial cells of endoneurial blood vessels can be joined by tight junctions, preventing free passage of some macromolecules and providing an incomplete blood-nerve barrier. Collagen bundles and modified fibroblastic cells, termed perineurial cells, form the perineurium that ensheathes individual nerve fascicles. The perineurium contributes some barrier properties by preventing the free diffusion of macromolecules into the nerve fascicles. The fibrous epineurium is continuous with the dura mater as a peripheral nerve joins the CNS and encloses groups of nerve fascicles. The epineurium contains fibroblasts, mast cells, and adipocytes, the latter probably providing some protection to the nerve. Satellite cells are found in dorsal root ganglia within the matrix formed by the endoneurium that envelops cell bodies of peripheral nerves. They function in a supportive, nonmyelinating role, much like perineuronal oligodendroglia in the CNS.

The autonomic and enteric divisions of the PNS function primarily to transmit impulses from the CNS to peripheral organs (efferent nerves) that regulate (involuntary control) the function of these organ systems (heart, vascular system, visceral smooth muscle, and exocrine and endocrine glands). These effects include but are not limited to the rate and force of contraction and relaxation in smooth (visceral organs and blood vessels) and striated muscle (heart). Afferent nerves, which transmit from the periphery to the CNS, mediate visceral sensation and vasomotor and respiratory reflexes through baroreceptors and chemoreceptors in the carotid sinus and aortic arch. Autonomic and enteric functions are regulated in the medulla, pons, and hypothalamus of the CNS.

The autonomic division has two structural and functional components: the sympathetic and parasympathetic systems. These systems usually have opposing effects on innervated organ systems. The parasympathetic system acts, for example, to lessen the effects of increased vasoconstriction (smooth muscle) and contractility (heart rate) exerted by the sympathetic system.

The enteric division of the PNS system exerts effects on digestive processes, such as motility, secretion, and absorption, and blood flow. The main components of the enteric nervous system are myenteric plexuses (Auerbach's plexuses), located between the longitudinal and circular layers of muscle, and submucosal plexuses (Meissner's plexuses) that innervate esophageal and intestinal smooth muscle. Injury to these plexuses can lead to dysautonomias, which are discussed in a later section.

Dysfunction/Responses to Injury

See Central Nervous System, Dysfunction/Responses to Injury

Responses of the Axon to Injury

See a discussion on Wallerian degeneration and central chromatolysis in the section on Responses of Neurons to Injury in the section on the CNS.

Portals of Entry/Pathways of Spread

See Central Nervous System, Portals of Entry/Pathways of Spread

Defense Mechanisms/Barrier Systems

Blood-Nerve Barrier

The blood-nerve barrier regulates the free movement of certain substances from the blood to the endoneurium of peripheral nerves. Barrier properties are conferred by tight junctions between endothelial cells of the capillaries of the endoneurium and perineurium and by selective transport systems in the endothelial cells.

Disorders of Domestic Animals

Peripheral Neuronopathies and Myelinopathies

Many disorders affecting the CNS are also manifested in lesions in the PNS, either (1) because of damage to neuron cell bodies of lower motor neurons residing in the CNS or (2) because the PNS is equally vulnerable to the disease. An example in the first case is lysosomal storage diseases, in which substrate accumulates in cell bodies of lower motor neurons. Cell death and axonal degeneration of the PNS are the end points of a chronic and progressive process of substrate accumulation that interferes with cellular biochemical processes and transport systems. In the second case, substrate also accumulates in cell bodies of sensory neurons located in the dorsal root ganglion of the PNS, resulting in cell death and axonal degeneration. Despite this caveat, there are certain diseases that primarily affect the PNS. Depending on whether the lesion is in a sensory or motor nerve or both, diseases of the PNS can manifest clinically as motor disturbance, sensory deprivation, or a combination of motor and sensory alterations. Space constraints do not allow an exhaustive coverage of disorders of the PNS. Many of the reported disorders seem to represent isolated occurrences in a specific breed. This section covers the major types of PNS diseases with reference to specific disorders for illustrative purposes.

Congenital/Hereditary/Familial Diseases

Primary Sensory Neuropathies. Primary sensory neuropathies included here are the hereditary, familial, and breed- or species-associated syndromes reported in a variety of domestic animals that result in degeneration of PNS sensory neurons (dorsal root ganglion) or axons innervating the limbs. Two examples of primary sensory neuropathies have been described in English pointers and long-haired dachshunds. In pointer dogs the onset is 2 to 12 months of age with signs of self-mutilation and insensitivity to pain resulting in neuro-pododermatitis or acral mutilation syndrome (Fig. 14-110). Additional signs can include ataxia, loss of conscious proprioception, and patellar hyporeflexia. In dachshunds a sensory neuropathy is manifested shortly after birth by ataxia and alterations in the function of the autonomic division of the PNS, such as urinary incontinence and digestive disturbances. Lesions in pointer dogs consist of small dorsal root ganglia with neuronal loss and replacement by satellite cells (Nageotte nodules) and mild reduction in size of dorsal nerve rootlets because of degeneration and loss of myelinated and nonmyelinated axons with the presence of cell bands of Büngner (indicative of attempts at remyelination). In dachshunds, lesions are a distal axonopathy with loss of large myelinated and unmyelinated axons. Lesions can occur in the vagus nerve.

Other degenerative distal axonopathies of the PNS have also been reported in Birman cats and in dog breeds, including Bouvier des Flandres, Siberian huskies and crossbreeds, boxer dogs (sensory axonopathy), Rottweilers (sensory axonopathy), dachshunds (sensory axonopathy), Dobermans (dancing Doberman disease is thought to be a primary myopathy), German shepherds (giant axonal neuropathy), and Dalmatians. They may have a genetic basis and be inherited.

A noninherited form of sensory neuropathy also occurs in dogs and is associated with ganglioradiculitis. Although many viruses, including pseudorabies virus and rabies virus, can cause inflammation in the spinal ganglia, this specific sensory neuropathy appears not to be associated with a viral infection. Gross lesions in affected animals often reveal a zone of pallor in the dorsal funiculus corresponding to Wallerian degeneration secondary to severe inflammation within the dorsal root ganglia. The inflammation is often associated with Nageotte nodule formation, neuronal loss and degeneration, and some degree of nonspecific gliosis. The inflammation is also typically mononuclear (i.e., the character of the inflammatory cells involved), raising the possibility that this form of ganglioradiculitis has an autoimmune basis.

In all forms of sensory neuropathy, animals are usually young (birth to 15 months of age) and show signs of ataxia, muscle weakness (paresis and tetraparesis) followed by muscle atrophy, proprioceptive deficits, urinary incontinence, and digestive disturbances (enteric division involvement).

Dysautonomias

Hereditary Dysautonomias. Dysautonomia is a degeneration of neurons in the ganglia of the enteric division of the PNS that has been reported in dogs, cats (Key-Gaskell syndrome), a llama, sheep, cattle, and horses. The cause is unknown, and a hereditary basis is suspected in some cases. A toxic cause has been postulated in the cat. Lesions recently reported in sheep with abomasal emptying defect resemble those reported in dysautonomic diseases of human beings and other animals.

Lesions are observed in peripheral and enteric (autonomic) ganglia and vary from neuronal chromatolysis and nuclear pyknosis in more acute cases to loss of neurons and proliferation of satellite cells in cases with longer duration (Fig. 14-111). Minimal to mild leukocytic infiltrates occur, but the lesions are not overtly

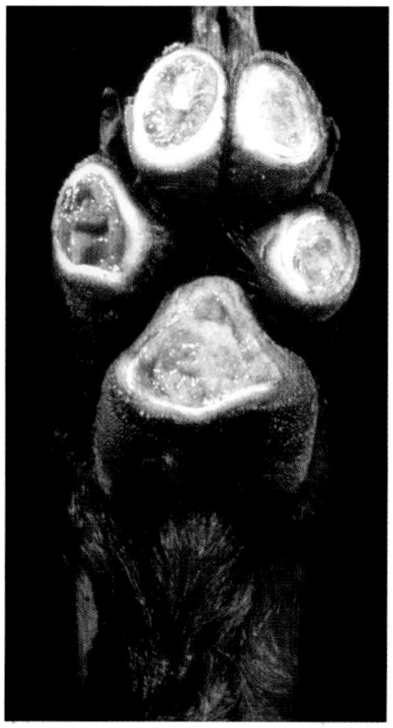

Figure 14-110 **Neuro-Pododermatitis (Acral Mutilation Syndrome), Dog.** This disorder, a primary sensory peripheral neuronopathy with self-mutilation and insensitivity to pain, is caused by the absence of (or small) dorsal root ganglia, reduction in size of dorsal nerve rootlets, and degeneration and loss of myelinated and nonmyelinated sensory axons. This dog wore off its footpads when placed on a concrete run. Satellite cell proliferation is commonly present in other large autonomic ganglia (i.e., celiac ganglion). (Courtesy College of Veterinary Medicine, University of Illinois.)

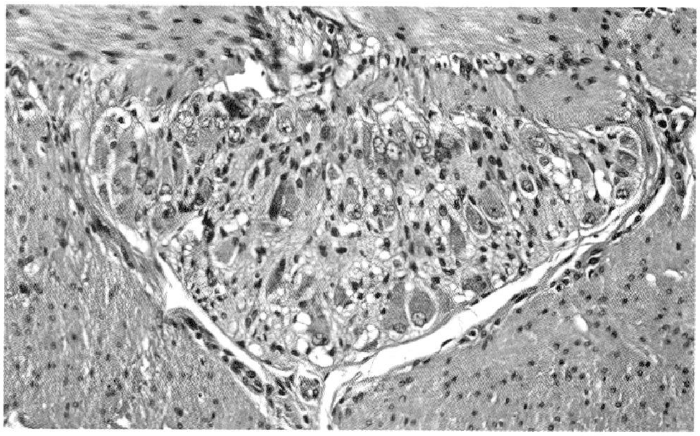

Figure 14-111 **Dysautonomia, Submucosal (Auerbach's) Plexus, Dog.** Neuronal central chromatolysis, nuclear pyknosis, and loss of neurons are the characteristic histologic features of enteric dysautonomia. H&E stain. (Courtesy Dr. J.F. Zachary, College of Veterinary Medicine, University of Illinois.)

inflammatory. In cats and dogs, clinical signs are varied and include gastrointestinal disturbances, urinary incontinence, mydriasis, unresponsive pupils, bradycardia, and other signs associated with autonomic dysfunction.

Acquired Dysautonomias

Equine Grass Sickness (Equine Dysautonomia). Equine grass sickness (equine dysautonomia) is discussed in the later section on Disorders of Horses.

Peritonitis-Induced Dysautonomias. Degeneration of autonomic neurons in the myenteric and submucosal ganglion (plexuses) can occur in animals with peritonitis. The degree of neuronal degeneration appears to be related to the severity and type of inflammatory response in the peritoneal cavity and the ability of inflammatory mediators and other potentially toxic molecules to reach the ganglia by diffusion or hematogenously. Degeneration does not appear to progress to neuronal cell death if the peritonitis is resolved. Affected neurons have vesicular nuclei that are two to three times normal size (see Fig. 14-111). Nissl substance is also displaced (central chromatolysis). Nerve fiber bundles are edematous, and supporting cells can be remarkably hyperplastic and compress adjacent supporting stroma.

This lesion is thought to arise from inflammatory cytokine-mediated injury to autonomic neurons, and this may cause alterations of intestinal motility. It appears that the morphologic changes observed in autonomic and enteric neuron cell bodies are reversible with resolution of the peritonitis. Whether the neuronal lesion results from diffusion or hematogenous or retrograde axonal transport of cytokines to the ganglion from the site of inflammation remains to be proved.

This lesion is likely the cause of paralytic ileus seen with peritonitis.

Hypomyelination/Dysmyelination Diseases. In contrast to the CNS, congenital and postnatal disorders of myelin formation are rare in the PNS but have been described in dogs, calves, and a cat. These disorders are thought to have a genetic predisposition and to be inherited. In dogs, hypomyelination has been described in golden retrievers with onset at approximately 7 weeks of age. Clinical signs include a peculiar hopping gait, depressed spinal reflexes, and circumduction of the limbs while walking. Lesions in peripheral nerves include thin myelin sheaths, increased numbers of Schwann cells, neurolemma cells with abnormally increased cytoplasmic volume, and no evidence of active demyelination or effective remyelination. The lesions are believed to involve a defect in Schwann cells or an abnormal axon–Schwann cell interaction.

In calves a myelinopathic peripheral neuropathy has been described in Santa Gertrudis–Brahman crossbreeds. Microscopically, lesions were present in the vagus nerves, somatic peripheral nerves of the brachial plexuses, and the sciatic nerves. Dorsal and ventral spinal nerve roots also had similar lesions. There was "sausage-shaped" thickening of the myelin sheaths as a result of excess myelin arranged about the axons or as irregularly folded myelin sheaths not surrounding axons. Onset of clinical signs was at 6 to 10 months of age. Clinical signs were dysphagia, abnormal rumination with bloat, and a weak shuffling gait. Congenital hypomyelination has also been described in a 2-month-old Dorset lamb with tremors and incoordination.

Demyelination Diseases. A variety of injuries similar to those described in the CNS can cause primary demyelination in the PNS. Specific demyelinating diseases are covered in the next sections. In response to injury, Schwann cells can proliferate to restore the myelin sheaths, often forming longitudinal columns along the course of a degenerated axon termed *Büngner's bands*. Remyelination results in internodes that are shorter than the internodes of adjacent normal myelinated axons, and this change is used microscopically to detect areas of remyelination in peripheral nerves. Another lesion that occurs with repeated episodes of demyelination is proliferation of Schwann cell processes forming concentric whirls, called *onion bulbs* that surround the axon.

Coyotillosis. Another cause of primary demyelination is the shrub coyotillo *(Karwinskia humboldtiana)* affecting mainly small ruminants in the semidesert areas of the southwestern United States. Seeds in the fruit contain polyphenolic compounds that are toxic when ingested. Four toxic compounds have been isolated, including a substance called *karwinol* A that induces primary demyelination of peripheral nerves. Based on electron microscopic evaluation of lesions, the damage appears to be due directly to axonal injury caused by consolidation of neurofilaments and margination of microtubules.

Endocrine Diseases. Endocrine disorders, such as hypothyroidism, hyperadrenocorticism, and diabetes mellitus, can affect the PNS. The lesions of these neuropathies are not well characterized and can include evidence of primary demyelination, remyelination, and axonal degeneration. Distal portions of the axon are commonly affected. The extent to which demyelination or axonal degeneration is the primary lesion remains to be determined. From a clinical standpoint, it may be difficult to distinguish neurologic signs from those signs attributed to hormonal-influenced injury of myofibers. Clinical signs can be caused by sensory and motor deficits.

Nutritional Diseases

Vitamin A, Vitamin D, and Riboflavin Deficiencies. Nutritional axonopathies are relatively uncommon and are chiefly caused by vitamin A and some of the B vitamin deficiencies. Vitamin A deficiency results indirectly in peripheral neuropathy by affecting bone growth and remodeling. In neonatal calves the neuropathy is due to narrowing of the optic foramina caused by continued bone deposition with decreased resorption resulting in compression of the optic nerves, Wallerian degeneration, and blindness. B vitamin deficiencies are primarily diseases of pigs and poultry. In pigs, deficiency of pantothenic acid (B-complex vitamin, vitamin B_5) causes a sensory neuropathy with axonal degeneration, demyelination, and chromatolysis and neuron loss in the dorsal root ganglia, resulting in proprioceptive deficits, goose-stepping, and dysmetria. The exact sequence of events in pantothenic acid–deficiency neuropathy is controversial because one study in pigs described initial lesions in the axon, whereas a second study described initial lesions in the cell body. Riboflavin deficiency in poultry, named *curled-toe paralysis*, is primarily a demyelinating neuropathy. Peripheral nerves are swollen because of endoneurial edema, and there is subsequent demyelination with mild axonal degeneration.

Vitamin E Deficiency

Equine Motor Neuron Disease. Equine motor neuron disease is discussed in the later section on Disorders of Horses.

Toxic Diseases

Chemicals. Toxic diseases resulting from chemicals are discussed in greater detail in the section on the CNS. Examples of chemical toxins causing distal axonal degeneration are the vinca alkaloids, vincristine and colchicine, both causing disassembly of microtubules and inhibiting axoplasmic flow. Paclitaxel (Taxol), an alkaloid from the western yew *(Taxus brevifolia)*, promotes the assembly of and stabilizes microtubules but also causes an axonopathy. An outbreak of distal polyneuropathy has been reported in cats fed commercial diets contaminated with the ionophore salinomycin, which is used as a coccidiostatic drug in poultry and growth promoter in cows. There was acute onset of lameness and paralysis affecting the hind limbs that progressed to the forelimbs. Demyelination of peripheral nerves followed the axonal degeneration. Some toxins seem to cause different patterns of injury in the CNS and PNS. For example, in the CNS, lead is noted to cause neuronal necrosis, whereas in the PNS, demyelination, preferentially affecting Schwann cells, is prominent in some species.

Other Toxic Neuropathies. A number of toxins can affect the PNS, with or without damage in the CNS. The initial toxic effects can be at the level of the neuron cell body, the axon, or the myelin sheaths. Examples of toxins targeting neuronal cell bodies are organomercurial compounds such as methylmercury and the cancer chemotherapeutic agent doxorubicin. Methylmercury is particularly toxic because it directly alters biochemical reactions. Although methylmercury poisoning can result from ingestion of water or forage contaminated with industrial discharge, in animals the consumption of fish containing excessive concentrations of methylmercury is the most likely source of the toxin. Fish accumulate methylmercury in their muscle as a result of a "normal" environmental process called *biomethylation*. Biomethylation converts elemental mercury to methylmercury, which is ingested in the diet of fish. In mercury poisoning, sensory neuron cell bodies of the dorsal root ganglion are preferentially involved, and the motor neurons are spared, whereas with doxorubicin, both dorsal root ganglion and autonomic cell bodies are affected. Experimental studies suggest that neuronal cell death is caused by apoptosis of neuronal cell bodies resulting in axonal and Wallerian degeneration.

Autoimmune Diseases

Neuromuscular Junction Diseases

Myasthenia Gravis. Myasthenia gravis is a disorder of neuromuscular impulse transmission at myoneural junctions and results in flaccid paralysis of skeletal muscle. The disease can be caused by an autoimmune mechanism (acquired) or result from inherited genetic abnormalities (congenital). In autoimmune myasthenia gravis the antibody binds to acetylcholine receptors (type II hypersensitivity) on postsynaptic muscle membranes. This interaction results in distortion of receptors and blocks binding of the receptors with acetylcholine. Acquired myasthenia gravis often occurs concurrently with thymic abnormalities such as thymoma and thymic hyperplasia. Because the thymus is responsible for immunologic self-tolerance, thymic abnormalities leading to induced alterations in tolerance have been suggested as the mechanism for developing an antibody response against acetylcholine receptors.

Congenital myasthenia gravis is caused by a genetically determined deficiency in the number of acetylcholine receptors expressed in motor end plates.

There are no gross or microscopic lesions in the PNS or CNS caused by myasthenia gravis. Clinical signs and lesions are the result of impairment of skeletal and esophageal muscles and muscle weakness followed by muscle atrophy.

Diseases Caused by Microbes

Bacteria

Botulism. Botulism is characterized by a flaccid paralysis caused by the neurotoxin of *Clostridium botulinum* type A, B, or C in North America and type D in South Africa. The bacterium is a ubiquitous Gram-positive spore-forming anaerobe commonly found in soil. This disease most commonly occurs in horses in North America and cows in South Africa. In North America, type B is most prevalent along the Mid-Atlantic states to Kentucky, whereas type A often predominates in the western United States. However, recent literature suggests that type A may be more prevalent along the Mid-Atlantic states that previously recognized. Different forms of botulism affect foals and adult horses. Toxicoinfectious botulism occurs in foals. Foals contract the disease by ingesting soil contaminated with clostridial spores.

In adult horses, poisoning after ingestion of toxin-contaminated forage and less commonly wound botulism occur. Adult horses contract the disease principally through the ingestion of preformed toxin in contaminated feeds, usually haylage that is prepared and stored improperly. Less commonly, adult horses contract the disease through tissue injury and an anaerobic environment, such as hoof abscesses and skin wounds. Spores of *C. botulinum* are either carried into wounds by nails or other contaminated foreign objects or into gastric ulcers by ingestion of contaminated soil. In either case the spores germinate only in necrotic tissue that has an anaerobic environment. The bacteria replicate and produce exotoxin, which is absorbed through the capillary endothelium and enters the bloodstream. In adult horses that ingest contaminated feeds, the toxin is absorbed from the alimentary system and enters the bloodstream.

Other than the wound where the bacteria replicates, the toxin of *C. botulinum* causes no macroscopic and microscopic tissue lesions. Once botulinum toxin is in the bloodstream, it enters myoneural junctions and binds to receptors on presynaptic terminals of peripheral cholinergic synapses (see Fig. 4-28). The toxin is then internalized into vesicles, translocated to the cytosol, and then mediates the proteolysis of components of the calcium-induced exocytosis apparatus, thus interfering with acetylcholine release. Inhibition (blockage) of the release of acetylcholine results in flaccid paralysis of muscles innervated by cholinergic cranial and spinal nerves, but there is no impairment of adrenergic or sensory nerves.

Clinically, affected horses have progressive paralysis of the muscles of the limbs, mandible, larynx/pharynx, upper eyelid, tongue, and tail. Death is usually caused by flaccid paralysis of the diaphragm, resulting in respiratory failure. Blockage of acetylcholine release at presynaptic cholinergic terminals is permanent. Improvement occurs only when axons develop (sprout) new terminals to replace those damaged by botulinum toxin.

Viruses and Protozoa. Inflammation of the PNS can occur in conjunction with viruses such as herpesvirus and rabies. Neuritis of the cauda equina in horses and dogs is primarily an inflammatory disorder with secondary demyelination. The cause of the neuritis in the horse is unknown, and attempts to consistently recover infectious microbes from affected animals have proven fruitless. These so-called cases of cauda equina neuritis (also known as polyneuritis equi) are often granulomatous with multinucleate giant cells and degenerative changes in the nerves and ganglia. Cranial nerve ganglia can be similarly affected. Polyradiculoneuritis and to a lesser extent ganglionitis occur in toxoplasmosis and neosporosis. The vomiting in pigs infected with hemagglutinating encephalomyelitis virus is presumed to result from altered function of the vagal nucleus and its ganglion and gastric intramural autonomic plexuses.

Lysosomal Storage Diseases

Globoid Cell Leukodystrophy. Peripheral nerves are also affected in globoid cell leukodystrophy, and lesions are typified by primary demyelination followed by axonal degeneration. Small sensory branches of peripheral nerves are useful sites for biopsies to make the diagnoses (Fig. 14-112). Gross lesions are not evident; however, microscopically, such areas have pronounced loss of myelin and abundant globoid cells (activated blood monocytes).

Other lysosomal storage diseases known to affect the PNS include α-L-fucosidosis (nerve enlargement due to macrophage

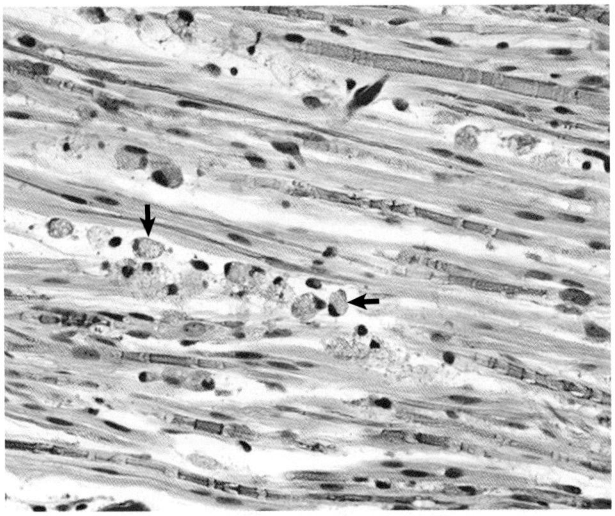

Figure 14-112 **Globoid Cell Leukodystrophy, Small Branch of a Peripheral Sensory Nerve, Dog.** Primary demyelination, secondary axonal degeneration, and globoid cells *(arrows)* between the nerve fibers (also see Figs. 14-64 to 14-65). H&E stain. (Courtesy Dr. J.F. Zachary, College of Veterinary Medicine, University of Illinois.)

infiltration); α- and β-mannosidosis (vacuolated Schwann cells), and gangliosidoses (vacuoles in neurons with demyelination).

Traumatic Injury

Trauma to peripheral nerves (lower motor or sensory) is relatively common in animals and can result from lacerations, violent stretching and tearing, or compression or contusion. Reaction patterns after PNS injury are analogous to those in the CNS, but peripheral nerves have a greater capacity for repair. Three patterns of lesions in the PNS have been described. Mild injury that leaves the axon intact (neurapraxia) can result in temporary conduction block, but total recovery of function is possible. More severe damage that destroys the axon but leaves the connective tissue framework intact (axonotmesis) results in Wallerian degeneration distal to the point of injury, but the potential for regeneration and reinnervation is good. Finally, severance of the nerve with destruction of the supporting framework (neurotmesis) results in Wallerian degeneration distal to the injury with the potential for regeneration but little chance of normal reinnervation. Destruction of the supporting framework results in fibrosis between the proximal and distal ends of the nerve and this gap may be large depending on the severity of the injury. Fibrous tissue can obstruct the regenerating proximal axon from reaching the distal supporting framework of the axon. If the regenerative response is exuberant but unproductive, a "potentially" palpable bulbous-like growth can form at the severed stump of the proximal axon called a "neuroma." The pattern of Wallerian degeneration and the reaction of the neuronal cell body to damage of its axon are described in an earlier section.

Recurrent Laryngeal Paralysis. Recurrent laryngeal paralysis is discussed in the later section on Disorders of Horses.

Neurogenic Cardiomyopathy (Brain-Heart Syndrome). Neurogenic cardiomyopathy, or brain-heart syndrome, is discussed in the later section on Disorders of Dogs.

Neurogenic Shock. Neurogenic shock is caused by an alteration in the function of the autonomic nervous system and its regulation of muscle tone in systemic blood vascular beds (Fig. 14-113).

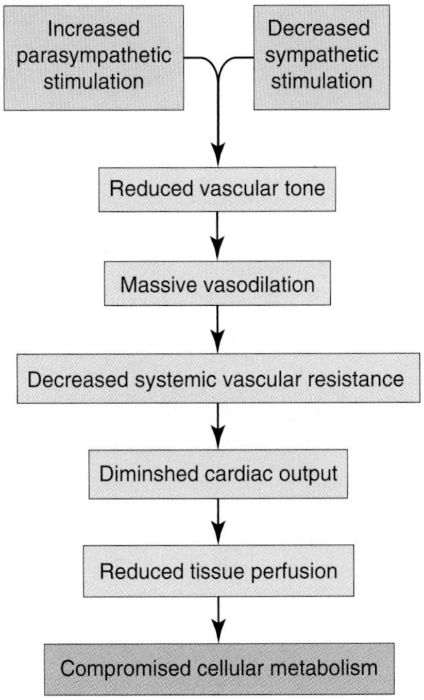

Figure 14-113 **Mechanism of Neurogenic Shock.** (Courtesy Dr. A.D. Miller, College of Veterinary Medicine, Cornell University; and Dr. J.F. Zachary, College of Veterinary Medicine, University of Illinois.)

The onset of neurogenic shock usually coincides with traumatic injury to the CNS; however, the factors that determine whether it occurs are poorly understood. It is thought to be caused by massive discharge of the autonomic nervous system. After trauma there is immediate vasoconstriction of vascular smooth muscle. Vasoconstriction is shortly followed by vasodilation, expanded circulatory volume, and a reduction in blood pressure leading to shock. Brain-heart syndrome in veterinary medicine is likely a manifestation of neurogenic shock and vasoconstriction of arterioles leading to myocardial necrosis.

Tumors

The objective of this section is not to be all encompassing regarding neoplasms of the PNS but to review one of the best-known examples of how neoplasia can involve this system. Although tumors of the PNS are often lumped into categories of either benign or malignant nerve sheath tumors, pathologists currently recognize three distinct types of nerve sheath tumors: Schwannomas, perineuriomas, and neurofibromas. Schwannomas and perineuriomas are derived from Schwann cells and perineurial cells respectively, whereas neurofibromas include elements derived from Schwann cells and fibroblasts. Malignant tumors show more anaplastic cytoarchitectural features and aggressive growth into adjacent normal tissue. Nerve sheath tumors occur in both cranial (Fig. 14-114) and spinal nerves (Fig. 14-115) of the PNS. Currently there are no reliable immunohistochemical markers for these tumors.

Schwannomas of animals have been most recognized in the dog and less commonly in the cat, horse, and cow. In the dog the neoplasm most commonly affects the cranial (fifth) or spinal nerve roots (posterior cervical–anterior thoracic roots of the brachial plexus and their extensions and roots at the thoracic and lumbar levels). Although true schwannomas of the dermal soft tissues have been reported, there should always be careful consideration of other soft tissue sarcomas that can have similar morphologic features.

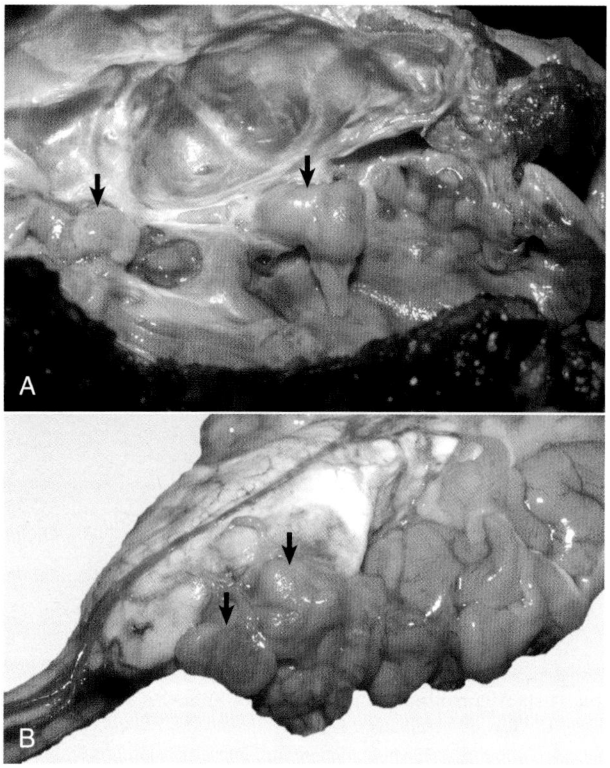

Figure 14-114 **Nerve Sheath Tumors. A,** Inner surface of the cranial vault, cranial nerves, dog. These tumors are usually lobulated, well-defined, tan, solitary to multiple masses that arise from the coverings of a cranial or spinal nerve *(arrows)*. In the central nervous system, the trigeminal nerve is usually affected, and the masseter and temporalis muscles innervated by it may atrophy. Tumors compress the nerves, causing wallerian degeneration. **B,** Brain from dog in **A**. Peripheral nerve sheath tumors *(arrows)*. (**A** and **B** courtesy Dr. J.F. Zachary, College of Veterinary Medicine, University of Illinois.)

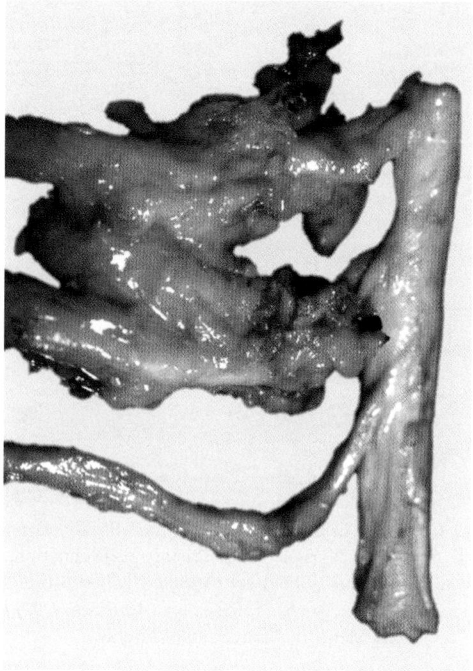

Figure 14-115 **Nerve Sheath Tumor, Spinal Nerve, Cow.** These tumors are similar to those described in Figure 14-114 and occur most commonly in cows and dogs. Although schwannoma has been proposed as the best term to classify these tumors, the term *nerve sheath tumor* groups all morphologic diagnoses under a common umbrella. (Courtesy College of Veterinary Medicine, University of Illinois.)

Grossly, schwannomas are nodular or varicose thickenings along nerve trunks or nerve roots. They can be firm or soft (gelatinous) and white or gray. Schwannomas of the spinal cord nerve roots can remain inside the dura mater or extend through a vertebral foramen to the exterior.

Histologically, schwannomas are composed entirely of neoplastic Schwann cells and are typically composed of two morphologic patterns, known as *Antoni type* A and *type* B, that occur in variable proportions within the neoplasm. Antoni A tissue is cellular and consists of monomorphic sheets, fascicles, and whorls of spindle-shaped Schwann cells. These cells have poorly defined eosinophilic cytoplasm and pointed basophilic nuclei and are present in a collagenous stroma of variable extent. The nuclei of these cells are commonly arranged in rows, between which are parallel arrays (stacks) of their cytoplasmic processes, and this arrangement is called a *Verocay body*. Antoni B areas are also composed of Schwann cells, but their cytoplasm is inconspicuous, and their nuclei appear to be suspended in a copious myxoid, often microcystic, matrix. Other histologic findings include hyalinized stroma and the absence of nerve fibers. These tumors can reliably be stained immunohistochemically with antibodies to laminin or type IV collagen that highlight the basal lamina produced by the neoplastic Schwann cells. S-100 immunoreactivity is typically diffuse throughout the neoplasm.

Neurofibromas consist of Schwann cells, perineurial cells, and fibroblasts. This type of tumor is not common in domestic animals. However, a unique form occurs in the cow as part of a benign neurofibromatosis syndrome in which it occurs most commonly in mature animals, although the lesion has also been reported in young calves and involves the cranial eighth nerve, brachial plexus, and intercostal nerves. Additionally, autonomic nerves of the liver, heart, mediastinum, and thorax can be affected. The skin can be infrequently involved. Some microscopic features of the neurofibroma include elongated spindle cells with poorly defined pale eosinophilic, tapering wavy or buckled nuclei, and numerous small nerve fibers (which are not present in schwannomas). Presence of mast cells is also reported. These neoplastic components are situated in a variably prominent fibromyxoid to myxoid matrix (myxoid neurofibroma), although another variant of the neoplasm contains prominent collagen (collagenous neurofibroma). Neurofibromas have far less immunoreactivity for either laminin or S-100, with the latter staining the Schwann cell component, but not the other cell types.

The last nerve sheath tumor is the perineurioma. It usually behaves as a benign neoplasm. It is a very rare variant of nerve sheath tumors in domestic animals, with only rare reports in the dog. It consists of tight, concentric whorls of perineurial cells that surround a central axon. Immunohistochemical stains for neurofilament proteins often highlight the central axon, whereas stains like laminin highlight the spindle cell population.

All of the aforementioned neoplasms can undergo malignant transformation and are then referred to as malignant nerve sheath tumors. They typically invade surrounding structures or can, based on location, invade or surround the spinal cord.

Disorders of Horses

Peripheral Neuropathies

Congenital/Hereditary/Familial Diseases

Colonic Agangliosis. Colonic agangliosis (lethal white foal syndrome) is a disorder involving development of the enteric division of the PNS and is analogous to Hirschsprung's disease in infants. This disease occurs most commonly in foals of American paint horses with overo markings. Affected foals have white or nearly white skin color. Specific information on these skin marking patterns can be obtained from the American Paint Horse Association. The gene, which results in the "colonic agangliosis" phenotype being expressed, is inherited as a homozygous dominant.

Mutations in the endothelin-B receptor gene have been detected in affected horses and in some patients with Hirschsprung's disease. Both glial-derived neurotrophic factor and endothelin-3 are required for normal development of the enteric nervous system and enteric ganglia. It is proposed that glial-derived neurotrophic factor is required for proliferation and differentiation of neuronal precursor cells destined to populate the gut. Endothelin-3 might modulate these effects by inhibiting differentiation, thus allowing sufficient time for precursor cells to migrate and populate the intestinal wall in a cranial to caudal progression before they differentiate to form enteric ganglia.

The lumen of the large intestine is often small or narrowed in affected animals. Microscopically, the myenteric and submucosal enteric ganglia are absent, and the areas affected vary but can extend anywhere between the ileum and distal large colon. Affected foals die within days after birth from functional blockage of the ileum and/or colon because of the lack of innervation and thus normal gut motility.

Toxic Diseases

Acquired Dysautonomias

Equine Grass Sickness (Equine Dysautonomia). Equine dysautonomia is a disease that affects the postganglionic sympathetic and parasympathetic neurons and is most commonly reported in the United Kingdom and a variety of European countries. In addition, prevertebral and paravertebral ganglia are commonly affected, as are cranial nerve nuclei of the brainstem. The lesions consist of neuronal chromatolysis followed by degeneration and loss of lower motor neurons of the general visceral efferent nuclei of cranial nerves III and X and the general somatic efferent nuclei of cranial nerves III, V, VII, and XII. It has been suggested that equine dysautonomia should be classified as a multisystem disease. Clinically, injury of neurons results in dysphagia, reflux esophagitis, and gut stasis (colic).

Although the cause is unknown, oxidative stress, fungal toxins, changes in weather, and exposure to *C. botulinum* type C have been proposed. Pasture grasses stressed by rapid growth or sudden cold weather can have reduced concentrations of antioxidants and increased concentrations of glutamate and aspartate (excitotoxic amino acids) and the neurotoxin malonate. It has been proposed that ingestion of high concentrations of these compounds either directly (excitotoxicity-apoptotic cell death) or indirectly (nitric oxide toxicity) induces neuronal injury within the autonomic nervous system, resulting in alimentary system dysfunction. Because mycotoxins were suspected as a cause of equine grass sickness, studies conducted to investigate this hypothesis demonstrated high levels of *Fusarium* spp. fungi in pastures from confirmed cases of grass sickness. The significance of these fungi in the pathogenesis of grass sickness is unclear. Current research is focused on the role that *C. botulinum* type C plays in the development of the disease. Higher levels of immunoglobulin A against *C. botulinum* type C1 neurotoxin have been reported in acute cases. Historical evidence also suggests that use of *C. botulinum* vaccination may prevent some aspects of the disease.

There are no gross lesions in the PNS, except potentially for lesions related to paralytic ileus (i.e., distended gastrointestinal tract, impacted large intestine, esophagitis due to reflux); however, microscopically and principally in the small intestine (ileum), the cell bodies of neurons in ganglia of the autonomic and enteric divisions of the PNS are chromatolytic, have displaced and pyknotic nuclei, are swollen and vacuolated, and with time there is neuronal loss and satellite cell proliferation in affected ganglia. Interstitial cells of Cajal are also reduced in number. Equine dysautonomia affects horses, ponies, and donkeys primarily between the ages of 2 and 7 years old. The disorder occurs principally between the months of April and July. Injury to enteric neurons results clinically in acute to chronic dysphagia and gut stasis (colic). The only way to diagnose equine grass sickness ante mortem is by taking a biopsy of the small intestine during surgery.

Nutritional Diseases

Deficiencies

Equine Motor Neuron Disease. Equine motor neuron disease resembles amyotrophic lateral sclerosis in human beings. Because vitamin E concentrations are very low in affected horses, this and other dietary antioxidant deficiencies have been suggested as a possible factor in the mechanism of equine motor neuron disease. Thus dietary factors, especially the long-term absence (>1 year) of green feeds with high vitamin E concentrations, have been implicated in the pathogenesis of the disease. Vitamin E supplementation may be useful in treating this disease if detected and treated early in its course.

Neural injury in equine motor neuron disease involves the cell bodies and axons of lower motor neurons (ventral horn cells, cranial nerves). Microscopically, cell bodies are swollen, have chromatolysis, and contain spheroids. As the disease progresses, the cell bodies become shrunken and degenerate and are removed by neuronophagia. When the cell bodies are lost, the resulting empty neuronal space can be replaced by astrogliosis. The axons of affected lower motor neurons have lesions consistent with Wallerian degeneration. Abundant amounts of lipofuscin are often found in neurons and endothelial cells.

The injury in lower motor neurons has been attributed to an oxidative stress mechanism because vitamin E is an antioxidant that offsets the harmful effects of free radicals and reactive oxygen species that can cause membrane lipid peroxidation. However, it is not linked to a mutation in the equine Cu/Zn superoxide dismutase gene. This gene regulates the production of the enzyme superoxide dismutase, whose function is to convert free radicals and reactive oxygen species (highly toxic to cells) to hydrogen peroxide (much less toxic to cells). The enzyme catalase is used to convert hydrogen peroxide to water and oxygen molecules. The muscle lesion in equine motor neuron disease is atrophy of type I myofibers secondary to loss of type 1 lower motor neurons.

Clinically, equine motor neuron disease is characterized by progressive degeneration and loss of lower motor neurons resulting in muscle atrophy, weight loss, difficulty standing, and muscle fasciculation

Vitamin E Deficiency

Equine Degenerative Myeloencephalopathy. Equine degenerative myeloencephalopathy is discussed in the section on Disorders of Horses in the section on the CNS.

Traumatic Injury

Recurrent Laryngeal Paralysis. Laryngeal paralysis (roarer syndrome) is caused by axonal injury to the left recurrent laryngeal nerve, which results in neurogenic atrophy of the left dorsal, lateral, and transverse cricoarytenoid muscles and consequently dysfunction of the larynx and laryngeal folds (see Fig. 15-16). The cricoarytenoid dorsalis muscle is the main abductor muscle of the larynx, which keeps the arytenoid cartilages in a lateral position. The possible causes of this axonopathy are multiple, and there may be different causes for different age groups of animals and different forms of the disease. Known causes include (1) transection of the axon by extension of inflammation from the guttural pouches because the nerve runs through the pouch within a connective tissue fold and (2) other trauma to the nerve. There is also some evidence that laryngeal paralysis may be inherited in younger horses. Currently a genetic age-onset abnormality of axoplasmic flow appears to be the most likely cause in horses in which trauma and inflammation can be excluded as causes.

Affected horses have disabilities of performance and a characteristic and diagnostic "roaring" sound with inspiration. Laryngeal hemiplegia can affect the right or left dorsal cricoarytenoid muscles; however, 95% of cases involve the left side. The cause of this specificity is unclear. Some have suggested it is related to the long course of the left recurrent laryngeal, which extends down into the chest and loops under the arch of the aorta to return to the larynx, but this hypothesis is weakened by the fact that the axonal injury is distal to where the nerve innervates the larynx. Curiously, studies have shown that other long nerves in the horse can also show degenerative changes, which may indicate that this disorder is a polyneuropathy, rather than a specific disease of the recurrent laryngeal nerve.

Gross lesions can vary from being recognizable to being inapparent. Microscopically, the lesion is Wallerian degeneration. Affected nerves are often shrunken with loss of axons and myelin, and Büngner's bands can be plentiful. Laryngeal hemiparesis is primarily a disease of large horse breeds between the ages of 2 and 7 years old.

Disorders of Dogs

Peripheral Neuropathies

Congenital/Hereditary/Familial Diseases

Dysautonomias. A discussion on hereditary dysautonomias can be found in the section on Peripheral Nervous System, Disorders of Domestic Animals.

Miscellaneous Neuropathies

Canine Inherited Hypertrophic Polyneuropathy. Canine inherited hypertrophic polyneuropathy is a familial disorder in Tibetan mastiffs. The primary defect is in the Schwann cells, but the pathogenesis is undetermined. There are no gross lesions in the PNS. Microscopic lesions consist of demyelination with onion bulb formation. The Schwann cell's cytoplasm is distended by accumulations of actin filaments. Axonal degeneration occurs but is mild. Clinical signs in canine inherited hypertrophic polyneuropathy begin at 7 to 10 weeks of age. They include pelvic limb muscle weakness, depressed spinal reflexes, and muscle atrophy that later progress to involve forelimbs and eventually cause recumbency. Neuropathies with primary developmental demyelination have also been reported in Alaskan malamutes and in beagle–basset hound crosses. A hypertrophic polyneuropathy has rarely been reported in unrelated domestic cats with onset at approximately 1 year of age.

Toxic Diseases

Dysautonomias

Acquired Dysautonomias

Peritonitis-Induced Dysautonomias. Peritonitis-induced dysautonomias are discussed in the section on Peripheral Nervous System, Disorders of Domestic Animals.

Miscellaneous Neuropathies

Acute Idiopathic Polyneuritis. Acute idiopathic polyneuritis (coonhound paralysis) is an acute, fulminating polyradiculoneuritis with ascending paralysis that occurs in dogs after the bite or scratch of a raccoon. By definition, polyradiculitis refers to disease or injury involving multiple cranial or spinal nerve roots, whereas polyradiculoneuritis refers to disease or injury involving multiple cranial or spinal nerve roots and their corresponding peripheral nerves.

Coonhound paralysis has been compared with Guillain-Barré syndrome. This human syndrome typically follows a viral illness, vaccination, or some other antecedent disease that results in an autoimmune response resulting in primary demyelination of cranial and spinal rootlets and nerves and delayed conduction of action potentials down the axon. Humoral and cell-mediated components are suspected to be involved in the autoimmune response.

Coonhound paralysis, like Guillain-Barré syndrome, is believed to represent an autoimmune primary demyelination. Despite the lack of close association of macrophages with the degenerating myelin and axons early in the development of the lesions, secretion of TNF-α by these cells could explain both the demyelination and axonal degeneration.

Acute idiopathic polyneuritis has been reported in dogs without an association with raccoons and also occurs rarely in cats, suggesting multiple factors might be involved in this type of nerve damage. Lesions in coonhound paralysis are most severe in ventral spinal nerve rootlets and progressively diminish distally in the peripheral nerve. Involvement of dorsal spinal nerve rootlets and ganglia is not constant and relatively minor. Lesions in the ventral nerve rootlets consist of segmental demyelination with a variable influx of neutrophils, depending on the acuteness and severity of clinical signs, along with lymphocytes, plasma cells, and macrophages (Fig. 14-116). Axonal degeneration is a common sequela. Evidence of remyelination with Büngner's bands and axonal sprouting occur during the recovery phase, but the effectiveness of the latter to establish continuity of the nerve rootlet and thus reinnervation of muscle is limited.

A chronic polyradiculoneuritis with infiltrations of lymphocytes, plasma cells, or macrophages; demyelination; and variable axonal

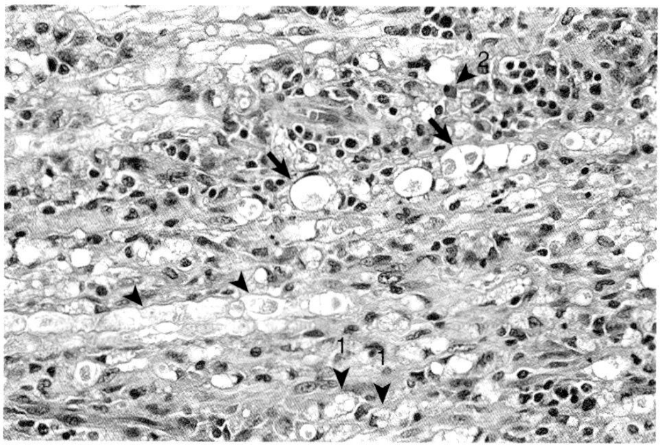

Figure 14-116 **Polyradiculoneuritis, Coonhound Paralysis, Peripheral Nerve, Dog.** This disease results from an autoimmune response leading to primary demyelination of cranial and spinal rootlets and nerves. Myelin sheaths in this peripheral nerve are distended and fragmented along their length *(arrowheads)* and have been infiltrated by a mixed population of inflammatory cells consisting of lymphocytes, macrophages *(1)*, and plasma cells *(2)*. Enlarged spaces in the myelin sheath, termed *digestion chambers (arrows)*, which form in response to inflammatory and degradative processes, contain myelin debris and macrophages (not shown in this example). Axonal degeneration can occur secondary to primary demyelination. H&E stain. (Courtesy Drs. R.A. Doty, J.J. Andrews, and J.F. Zachary, College of Veterinary Medicine, University of Illinois.)

degeneration in cranial and spinal nerve rootlets and cranial nerves is also reported in dogs and cats. With repeated episodes of demyelination, onion bulbs can be apparent. Both sensory and motor nerves can be involved with sensory disturbances and muscle atrophy.

Clinically, affected dogs have signs of coonhound paralysis that develop 1 to 2 weeks after exposure to raccoon saliva. Initial signs of hyperesthesia, weakness, and ataxia are replaced in 1 to 2 days by tetraparesis and/or tetraparalysis that may last from weeks to months. Dogs can die from respiratory paralysis. Recovery is common, but the paralysis can be prolonged in dogs with extensive muscular atrophy.

Traumatic Injury

Neurogenic Cardiomyopathy (Brain-Heart Syndrome). Neurogenic cardiomyopathy is a syndrome in dogs characterized by unexpected death 5 to 10 days after diffuse CNS injury (usually hit by car). Affected dogs die of cardiac arrhythmias caused by myocardial degeneration. Grossly, the myocardium has numerous discrete and coalescing pale white streaks and/or poorly defined areas of necrosis. Neurogenic cardiomyopathy is thought to be caused by overstimulation of the heart by autonomic neurotransmitters and systemic catecholamines released at the time of trauma. It is unknown why there is a 5- to 10-day delay in the development of myocardial necrosis.

Suggested Readings

Suggested Readings are available at www.expertconsult.com.

CHAPTER 15

Skeletal Muscle[1]

Beth A. Valentine

Key Readings Index

Structure

Normal Skeletal Muscle

Understanding the normal structure and function of muscle, including gross, histologic, biochemical, physiologic, electrophysiologic, and ultrastructural features, is critical to understanding muscle disease.

Structure of Myofibers

Structural and physiologic features of skeletal muscle determine much of its response to injury. Although muscle cells are frequently called muscle *fibers* or *myofibers*, they are in fact multinucleated cells of considerable length, which in some animals may approach 1 m. Myonuclei are located peripherally in the cylindrical myofiber (Fig. 15-1) and direct the physiologic processes of the cellular constituents in their area through a process known as *nuclear domains*. This anatomic arrangement allows segments of the cell to react independently of other portions of the cell. Myonuclei are considered terminally differentiated, with little or no capacity for mitosis and thus for regeneration.

Associated with myofibers are the satellite cells, also known as *resting myoblasts* (E-Fig. 15-1). These cells are distributed along the length of the myofiber, between the plasma membrane (sarcolemma) and the basal lamina. Satellite cells in skeletal muscle are very different from cells of the same name found within the peripheral nervous system. Muscle satellite cells are fully capable of dividing, fusing, and reforming mature myofibers. Thus, under favorable conditions, muscle cells (myofibers) are able to fully restore themselves after damage. Recent studies have found that pluripotent cells derived from bone marrow can also contribute to skeletal muscle repair, albeit only to a very small degree.

Each myofiber is surrounded by a basal lamina and outside of this by the endomysium, a thin layer of connective tissue containing capillaries. Myofibers are organized into fascicles surrounded by the perimysium, a slightly more robust layer of connective tissue (E-Fig. 15-2). Entire muscles are encased in the epimysium, a protective fascia that merges with the muscle tendon. This connective tissue framework is not inert but in fact forms an integral part of the contractile function of muscle by storing and relaying force generated by myofiber contraction.

Ultrastructural examination reveals that skeletal muscle is a highly and rigidly organized tissue, with what are perhaps the most highly structured cells in the body. Each myofiber is composed of many closely packed myofibrils containing actin and myosin filaments. The striations visible with light microscopy (Fig. 15-2) represent the sarcomeric arrangement of muscle cells, in which actin and myosin filaments attached to transverse Z bands form the framework, and other organelles and intracytoplasmic materials are interspersed within this framework (Fig. 15-3). The endoplasmic reticulum of myofibers is called the *sarcoplasmic reticulum* and is modified to contain terminal cisternae that sequester the calcium ions necessary to initiate actin and myosin interaction and thus contraction. Sarcolemmal invaginations that traverse the cell, the T (for transverse) tubules, allow rapid dispersion of a sarcolemmal action potential to all portions of the myofiber. The terminal cisternae of two adjacent sarcomeres and the T tubule form what is called the *triad* (Fig. 15-3, A).

Neuromuscular junctions can only be visualized using electron microscopy or other specialized procedures (Fig. 15-4). Neuromuscular junctions occur only in specific zones within the muscle, usually forming an irregular circumferential "band" midway between myofiber origin and insertion.

Types of Myofibers

Mammalian muscles are composed of muscle fibers of different contractile properties. A common classification of these fibers is based on three major physiologic features: (1) rates of contraction (fast or slow), (2) rates of fatigue (fast or slow), and (3) types of metabolism (oxidative, glycolytic, or mixed). These physiologic differences form the basis of histochemical methods that demonstrate fiber types. There are several fiber-type classifications. Classification of fibers into type 1, type 2A, and type 2B (Table 15-1) has proved to have practical application in muscle pathology. It is the classification used in this text. Type 1 fibers are rich in mitochondria, rely heavily on oxidative metabolism, and are slow-contracting and slow-fatiguing.

[1]For a glossary of abbreviations and terms used in this chapter, see E-Glossary 15-1.

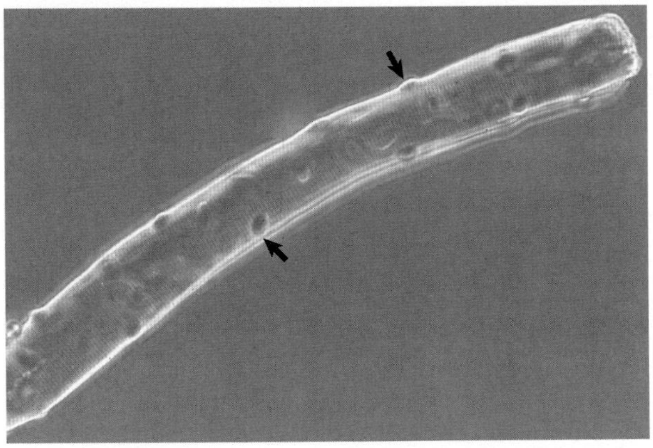

Figure 15-1 **Skeletal Muscle, Isolated Intact Myofiber.** Note the multiple peripherally located nuclei *(arrows)*. Phase contrast microscopy. (Courtesy Dr. B.A. Valentine, College of Veterinary Medicine, Oregon State University.)

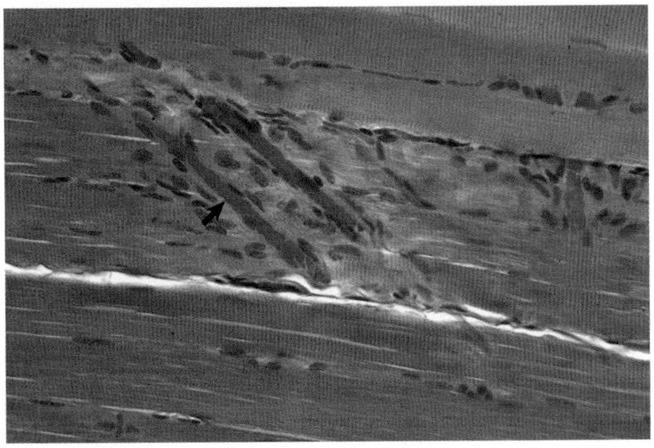

Figure 15-2 **Skeletal Muscle, Longitudinal Section, Normal Mammalian Muscle, Cytoarchitectural Characteristics.** Note the peripherally located myofiber nuclei and cross-striations on the muscle fibers. The cross-striations correspond to the A bands *(dark lines)* and I bands *(light lines)* in the transmission electron micrograph of Fig. 15-3, *B*. Myofibers are surrounded by an extensive capillary network *(arrow)*. H&E stain. (Courtesy Dr. M.D. McGavin, College of Veterinary Medicine, University of Tennessee.)

Type 2 fibers have fewer mitochondria and are glycolytic, fast-contracting, and more easily fatigable. In most species, type 2 fibers can be subdivided into type 2A and type 2B. Type 2B fibers are the fast-contracting, fast-fatiguing, glycolytic fibers that depend on glycogen for their energy supply. Type 2A fibers are mixed oxidative-glycolytic and therefore, although fast-contracting, are also slow-fatiguing. Thus type 2A fibers are "intermediate" in the concentration of mitochondria, fat, and glycogen between type 1 and type 2B.

Most muscles contain both type 1 and type 2 fibers, and these can be demonstrated by the myosin adenosine triphosphatase (ATPase) reaction (Fig. 15-5, *A*). Notice that the different fiber types are normally intermingled, forming what is called a mosaic pattern of fiber types. In most mature muscles, the staining pattern of the ATPase reaction reverses when sections are preincubated in an acid rather than an alkaline solution. There are examples of both patterns in the illustrations in this section. Acid preincubation can also be used to distinguish type 2A and type 2B fibers (Fig. 15-5, *B*). Regenerating fibers, classified as type 2C fibers, stain darkly in both acid and alkaline preparations, which is a distinguishing feature. In most species, oxidative enzyme reactions to demonstrate mitochondria also demonstrate fiber types to some degree (Fig. 15-6, *A*). Fiber typing can also be done by utilizing immunohistochemical procedures to identify specific myosin isoforms.

The percentage of each fiber type varies from muscle to muscle (Fig. 15-7). Type 1 fibers (slow-contracting, slow-fatiguing, and oxidative) are plentiful in those muscles in which the main function is slow, prolonged activity, such as those that maintain posture. Type 1 predominant postural muscles are most often located deep in the limb. Within the same muscle, the percentage of type 1 fibers often increases in the deeper portions. Muscles that contract quickly and for short periods of time, such as those designed for sprinting, contain more type 2B fibers. Only rarely are muscles composed of only one fiber type (e.g., the ovine vastus intermedius is type 1). Athletic training causes some type 2B fibers to be converted to 2A. There are also variations within breeds and differences in the same muscle in different species. For example, the dog has no type 2B purely glycolytic fibers; all canine fibers have strong oxidative capacity (see Fig. 15-6, *B*).

Innervation and Motor Units

The axons of the peripheral nerve trunks contain terminal branches that innervate multiple myofibers. The terminal branches form synapses with the myofibers at the neuromuscular junction. The myofibers innervated by a single axon form a motor unit, all fibers of which will contract simultaneously after stimulation. Different muscles have different sized motor units that relate to their function. For example, extraocular muscle function does not call for forceful contraction but, rather, for many fine movements to smoothly move the globe. Therefore these muscles have very small motor units, with only a small number of myofibers (1 to 4) innervated by each axon. In contrast, the quadriceps muscle is not designed for fine movement but instead is designed for generation of force; therefore motor units are quite large, with many myofibers (100 to 150 or more) innervated by a single axon.

Function

Skeletal muscle has many functions in the body. Some obvious and major functions are maintaining posture and enabling movement, including locomotion. The rhythmic contraction of the respiratory muscles (the intercostal muscles and the diaphragm) is essential for life. In addition, muscles play a major role in whole body homeostasis and are involved in glucose metabolism and maintenance of body temperature. On a purely esthetic level, muscle contributes to pleasing body contours.

The function of skeletal muscle is intimately related to the function of the peripheral nervous system. The physiologic attributes of a muscle fiber—its rate of contraction and type of metabolism (oxidative, anaerobic, or mixed)—are determined not by the muscle cell itself but by the motor neuron responsible for its innervation (Fig. 15-8). This fact is significant in evaluating histologic changes in muscle fibers. It is possible to divide changes in muscle fibers into two major classes: neuropathic and myopathic. Neuropathic changes are those that are determined by the effect or the absence of the nerve supply (e.g., atrophy after denervation). The term *myopathy* should be reserved for those muscle diseases in which the primary change takes place in the muscle cell, not in the interstitial tissue and not secondary to effects from the nerve supply. The term *neuromuscular disease* encompasses disorders involving lower motor neurons, peripheral nerves, neuromuscular junctions, and muscles.

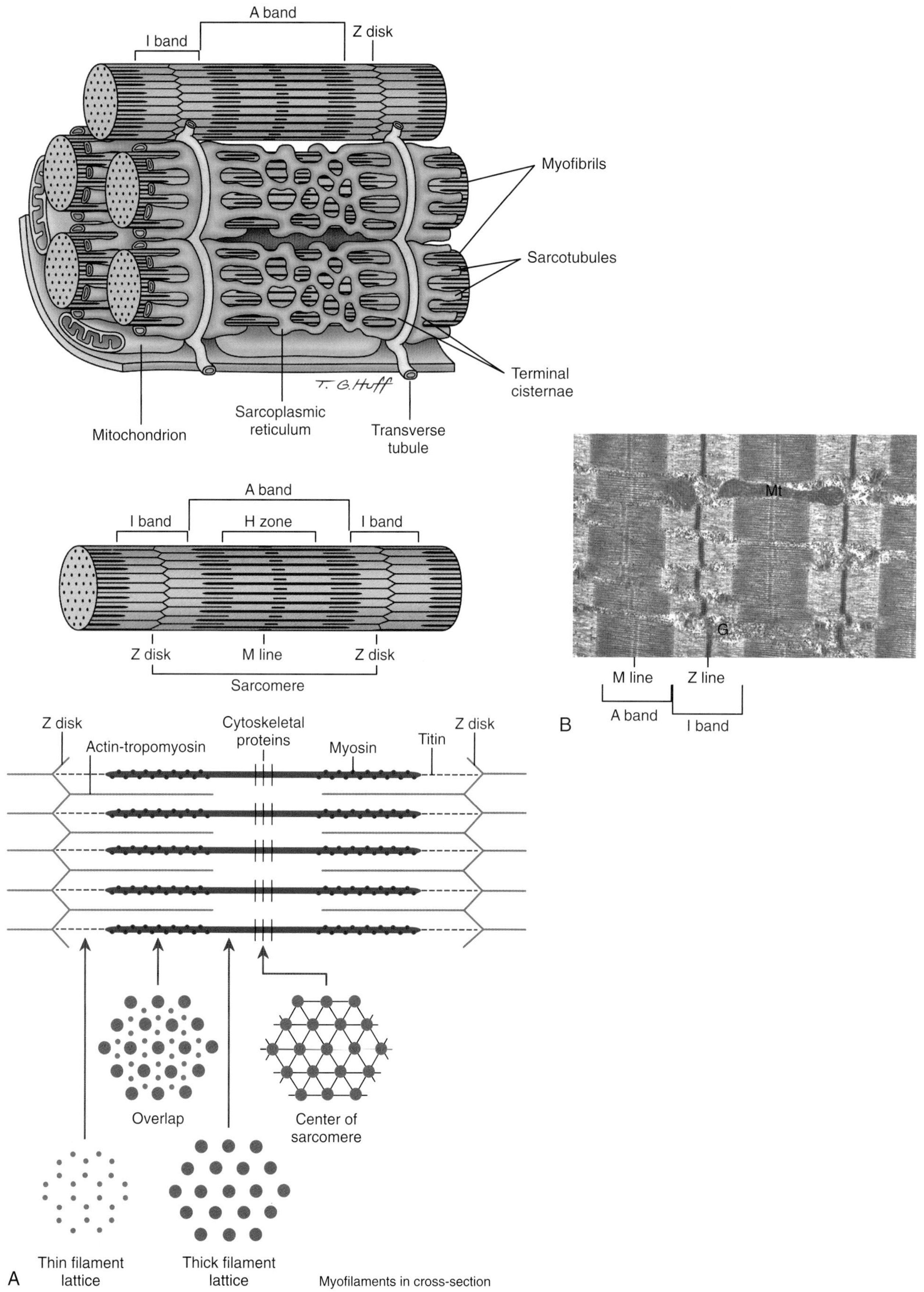

Figure 15-3 Myofiber Structure. A, Schematic diagram of skeletal muscle illustrating the sarcomeric arrangement of myofilaments that form myofibrils, cytoskeletal proteins, and interspersed organelles. **B,** Skeletal muscle, longitudinal section, mammalian skeletal muscle. Sarcomeres are defined by Z lines, thick myosin filaments form A bands, and thin actin filaments form I bands. Bisecting the A bands are dense M lines with adjacent clear H zones. Elongate mitochondria (*Mt*) and granular glycogen (*G*) are interspersed between the myofibrils. TEM. Uranyl acetate and lead citrate stain. (**B** courtesy Dr. B.A. Valentine, College of Veterinary Medicine, Oregon State University.)

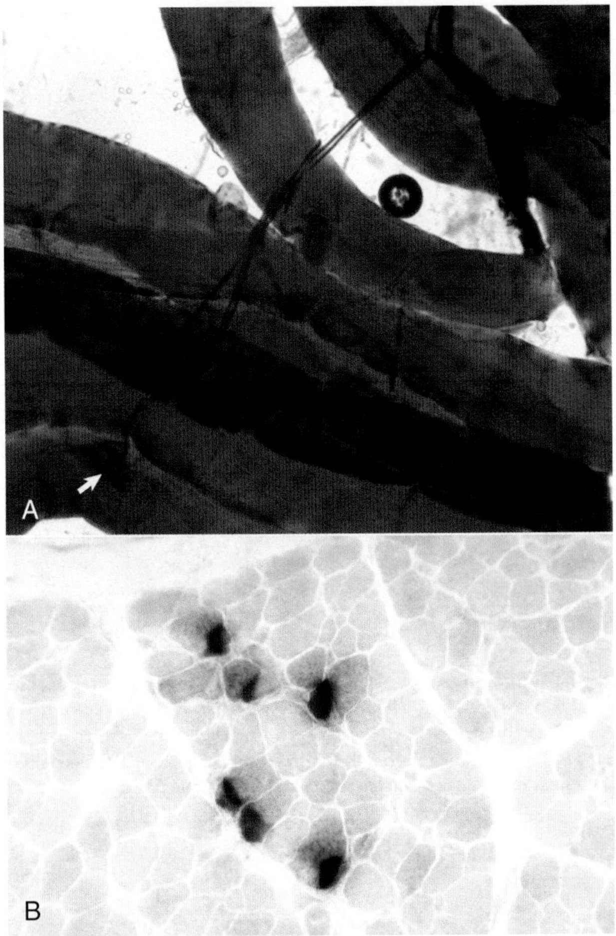

Figure 15-4 **Neuromuscular Junctions. A,** An intramuscular nerve *(top right)* has given off axons, which terminate on a myofiber at a neuromuscular junction *(arrow)*. Teased preparation, silver impregnation method. **B,** Neuromuscular junctions, transverse section through the center region of normal mammalian muscle. The neuromuscular junctions *(red-brown stain)* form a cluster. Nonspecific esterase stain, frozen section. (**A** courtesy Dr. M.D. McGavin, College of Veterinary Medicine, University of Tennessee. **B** courtesy Dr. B.A. Valentine, College of Veterinary Medicine, Oregon State University.)

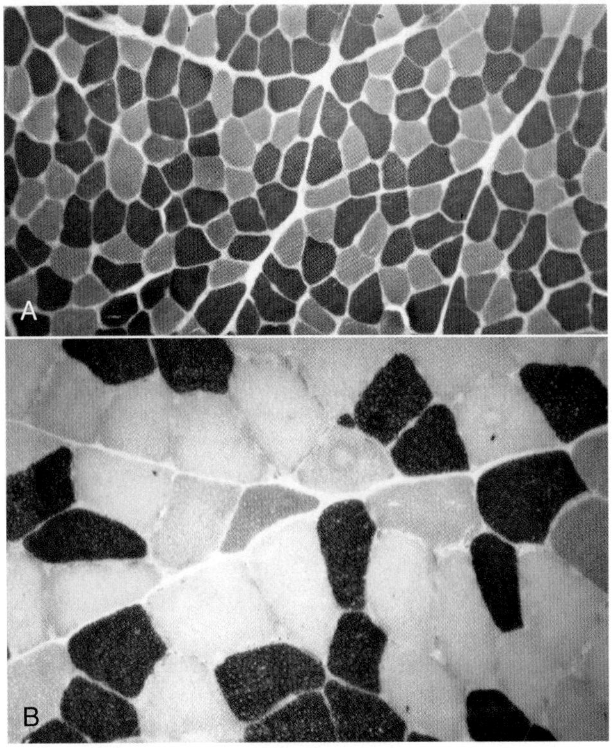

Figure 15-5 **Muscle Fiber Typing, Myofibrillar Adenosine Triphosphatase (ATPase) Reaction, Normal Skeletal Muscle, Transverse Section. A,** Dog. Type 1 *(light)* and type 2 *(dark)* fibers are arranged in a mosaic pattern. Frozen section, ATPase pH 10.0. **B,** Horse. Acid preincubation allows differentiation of three fiber types: type 1 *(dark)*, type 2A *(light)*, and type 2B *(intermediate = gray)*. Frozen section, ATPase 4.35. (Courtesy Dr. B.A. Valentine, College of Veterinary Medicine, Oregon State University.)

Table 15-1 Skeletal Muscle Fiber Types

Fiber Type	Physiologic Characteristics	Morphologic Characteristics
1	Slow twitch, oxidative, fatigue resistant, "red muscle," aerobic	High mitochondrial content, high fat content, low glycogen content
2A	Fast twitch, oxidative and glycolytic, fatigue resistant	Intermediate mitochondria, fat, and glycogen content
2B	Fast twitch, fatigue sensitive, glycolytic, "white muscle," anaerobic	Low mitochondrial and fat content, high glycogen content

Metabolism and Ionic Homeostasis

Myofibers require a great deal of energy in the form of adenosine triphosphate (ATP) to generate force and movement. Type 1 oxidative and type 2A oxidative-glycolytic fibers use aerobic metabolism of glucose, stored in the muscle as glycogen, and fat. Type 2B glycolytic fibers rely primarily on anaerobic metabolism of glycogen for energy. Inherent or acquired metabolic defects that reduce skeletal muscle energy production can result in severe muscle dysfunction. A commonly encountered postmortem change, rigor mortis, illustrates the importance of ATP generation within skeletal muscle. The muscle contractile apparatus is still active immediately after death. ATP is necessary for the release of actin from myosin, the interaction that results in the sliding of myofilaments and contraction of muscle. After death, the absence of adequate ATP production causes the muscle fibers to undergo sustained contraction, which is known as *rigor mortis*. Rigor mortis eventually disappears because of muscle structural breakdown caused by autolysis or putrefaction (bacterial decomposition). The period of time for onset and release of rigor mortis varies, depending on physiologic (glycogen stores at the time of death) and environmental factors such as the environmental temperature (see Chapter 1).

Skeletal muscle is also excitable tissue, similar to that of the nervous system. Maintenance of proper ionic gradients across the sarcolemma is essential for initiation of the action potential. Internal ionic gradients, especially of calcium ions, are critical for initiation and termination of contraction. Alterations of ionic fluxes across the sarcolemma, or within the sarcoplasmic reticulum, can have a serious negative impact on myofiber function.

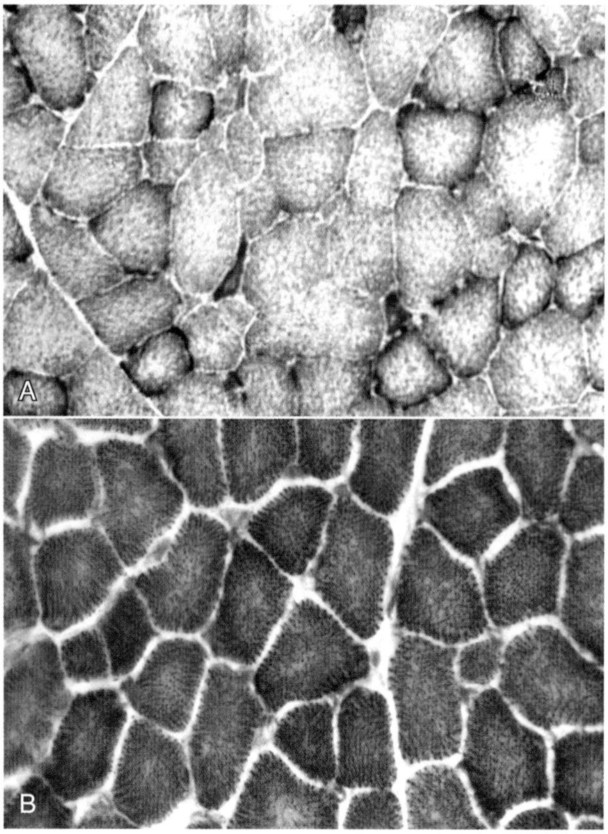

Figure 15-6 **Mitochondria, NADH Reaction *(Blue Stained)*, Skeletal Myocytes, Normal Skeletal Muscle, Transverse Section. A,** Horse. Type 1 fibers contain the most mitochondria, type 2B the least, and mitochondrial content of type 2A fibers is intermediate between type 1 and type 2B. Frozen section, NADH reaction. **B,** Dog. All fiber types have a similar mitochondrial content; therefore this reaction cannot be used to identify different types of myofibers in canine muscle. Frozen section, NADH reaction. (Courtesy Dr. B.A. Valentine, College of Veterinary Medicine, Oregon State University.)

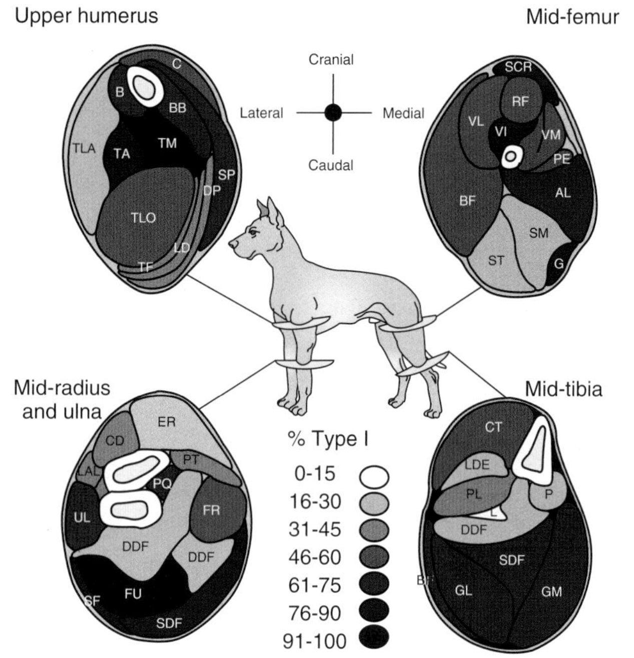

Figure 15-7 **Percentage of Type 1 and Type 2 Myofibers in Limb Muscles in the Dog.** There is a wide variation from muscle to muscle. Deeply located muscles have the most type 1 myofibers, indicative of their function in maintaining posture. (Redrawn from Armstrong RB, Sauber CW, Seeherman HJ, Taylor CR: *Am J Anat* 163:87-98, 1987.)

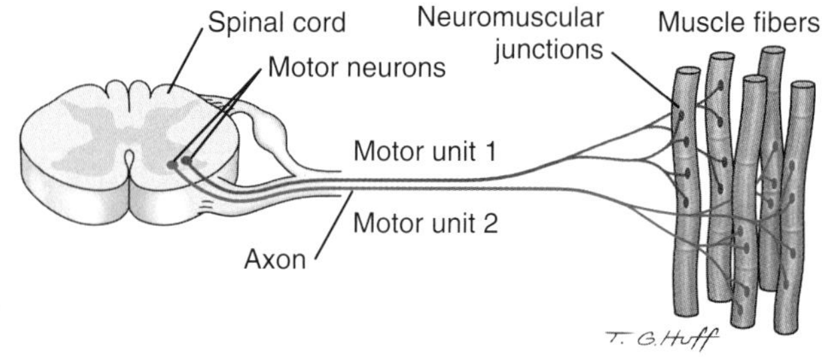

Figure 15-8 **Motor Units of a Muscle.** Motor neuron cell bodies within the ventral horn of the spinal cord give rise to axons that often travel long distances (meters) and eventually branch to innervate multiple skeletal muscle fibers at neuromuscular junctions.

Examination of Muscle: Clinical, Gross, and Microscopic

The decision to closely examine muscle, either by a biopsy or at necropsy, relies on recognition of indicators of neuromuscular dysfunction. A summary of clinical signs of muscle disease is provided in Box 15-1.

Box 15-1 Clinical Signs of Muscle Disease

Muscle atrophy	Muscle spasm
Muscle hypertrophy	Abnormal gait
Muscle swelling	Esophageal dysfunction (dogs, cats, camelids)
Weakness	

Clinical Findings

Information on this topic is available at www.expertconsult.com.

Clinicopathologic Findings

Information on this topic is available at www.expertconsult.com.

Electromyography

Information on this topic is available at www.expertconsult.com.

Methods of Gross and Microscopic Examination of Muscle

A variety of examination techniques are often necessary to best appreciate changes occurring in muscle.

Gross Examination of Muscle

Gross examination includes evaluation of changes in size (atrophied, hypertrophied, or normal), color, and texture. The gross pathologic appearance of skeletal muscle can be quite deceiving. What appear to be mild changes in muscle on gross examination often can be severe on microscopic examination, and what appear to be severe changes on gross examination can turn out to be artifact. Subjective evaluation of size can be highly unreliable unless control muscles (e.g., from normal animals or from the opposite sides) are available for weighing and measuring.

Color changes are common. The intensity of the red color of muscle varies, depending on the type of muscle, the age and species

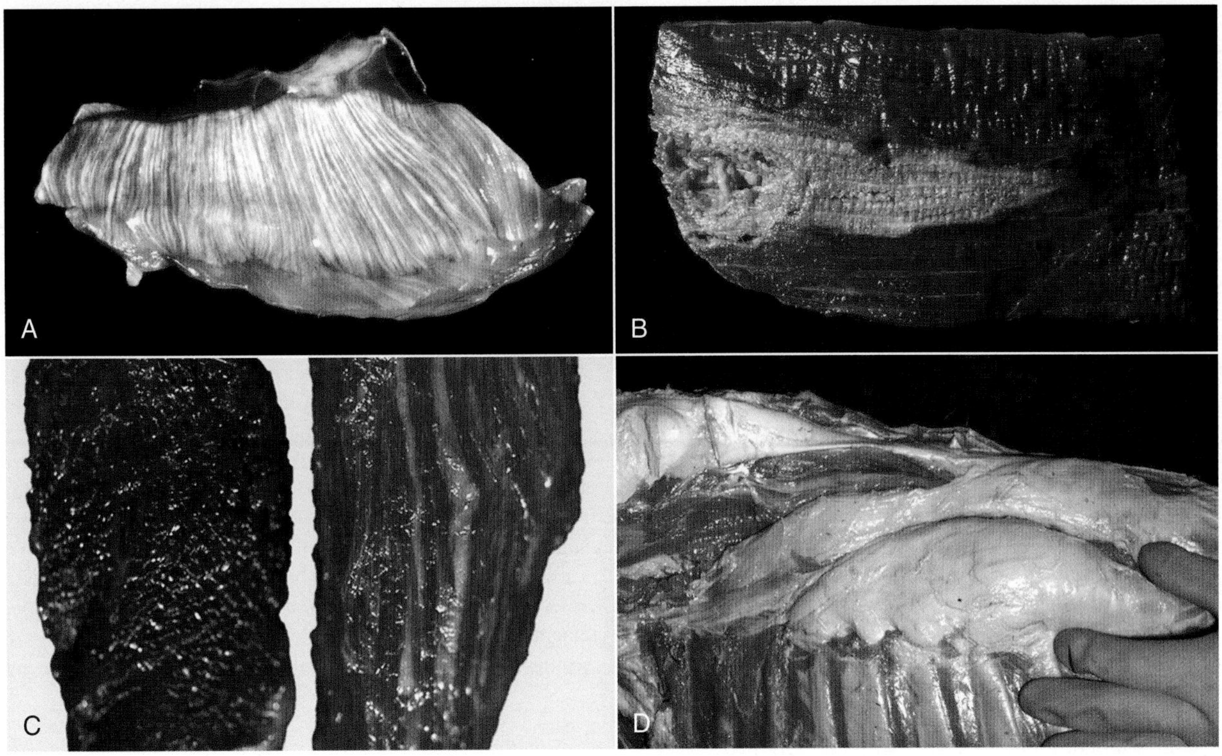

Figure 15-9 Pathologic Changes Resulting in Pale Skeletal Muscle. A, Pale streaks, necrosis and mineralization, degenerative myopathy, canine X-linked muscular dystrophy, diaphragm *(left side)*, dog. **B,** Localized pallor, necrosis, injection site of an irritant substance, semitendinosus muscle, cow. The irritant was injected just under the perimysium and caused necrosis and disruption of the myofibers. Some irritant seeped down between the fascicles to cause necrosis, but the fascicles of myofibers are still in place. **C,** Overall pale muscle with pale streaks from collagen and fat infiltration, denervation atrophy, equine motor neuron disease, horse. Equine motor neuron disease muscle *(right)* compared with normal muscle *(left)*. **D,** Enlargement and pallor, steatosis, longissimus muscles, neonatal calf. The majority of the muscles have been replaced by fat. (**A** courtesy Dr. B.A. Valentine, College of Veterinary Medicine, Oregon State University. **B** and **D** courtesy Dr. M.D. McGavin, College of Veterinary Medicine, University of Tennessee. **C** courtesy Dr. A. de Lahunta, College of Veterinary Medicine, Cornell University.)

of animal, and the extent of blood perfusion. Pale muscle can indicate necrosis (Fig. 15-9, *A* and *B*; see Figs. 15-25; 15-33, *A*; 15-35, *A*; and 15-39) or denervation (Fig. 15-9, *C*; see Fig. 15-36) but is also common in young animals and anemic animals. Pale streaking of muscle most often reflects myofiber necrosis and mineralization (see Fig. 15-9, *A* and *B*) or infiltration by collagen or fat (see Fig. 15-9, *C* and *D*), and it is one of the more reliable indicators of gross pathologic changes. Muscle parasites can be grossly visible as discrete, round to oval, pale and slightly firm zones (see Figs. 15-40 and 15-41, *A*). Dark red mottling of skeletal muscle can indicate congestion, hemorrhage, hemorrhagic necrosis (see Figs. 15-31, *A*, and 15-37), inflammation, or myoglobin staining after massive muscle damage (see Fig. 15-35, *A*) or can simply reflect vascular stasis (hypostatic congestion) after death. Hemorrhagic streaks within the diaphragm often accompany death caused by acute exsanguination. A green discoloration can indicate either eosinophilic inflammation (Fig. 15-10) or severe putrefaction. Lipofuscin accumulation in old animals, especially cattle, can cause a tan-brown discoloration of muscle. Black discoloration of the fascia occurs in calves with melanosis as an incidental finding and in older gray horses with metastasis of dermal melanoma to muscle fascia.

Evaluation of texture is also important. Severely thickened and often calcified fascia occurs in cats with fibrodysplasia ossificans progressiva. Fat infiltration or necrosis can result in abnormally soft muscle. Decreased or increased muscle tone can be caused by denervation. Decreased tone can also occur as a result of a lack of muscle conditioning or postmortem autolysis.

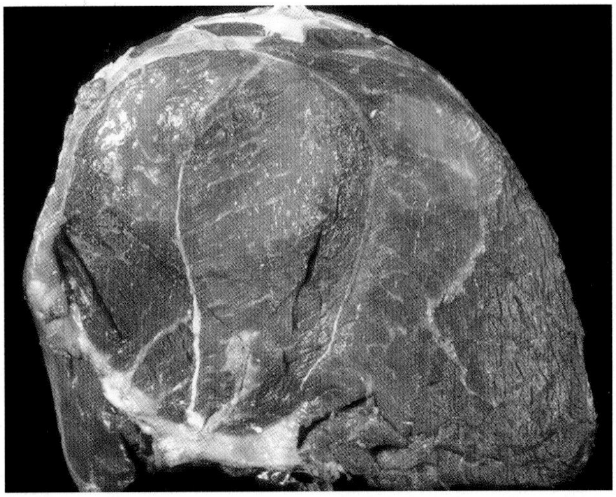

Figure 15-10 Bovine Eosinophilic Myositis, Gluteal Muscles, Cow. Green discoloration of the muscle is due to inflammation that has abundant eosinophils. The inflammation is attributed to degenerating *Sarcocystis* spp. For histopathologic findings, see Fig. 15-38. (Courtesy Dr. M.D. McGavin, College of Veterinary Medicine, University of Tennessee.)

Careful microscopic examination of multiple muscles is often required to detect lesions. In cases of suspected neuromuscular disease, multiple muscle samples should include active muscle (tongue, diaphragm, intercostals, and masticatory muscles), proximal muscle (lateral triceps, biceps femoris, semimembranosus, semitendinosus, and gluteal), and distal muscle (extensor carpi radialis and cranial tibial). For purposes of a biopsy, certain muscles (e.g., lateral triceps, biceps femoris, cranial tibial, semimembranosus, and semitendinosus) are easier to sample because of their parallel myofiber orientation. The ideal samples will also vary, depending on the suspected disorder, such as a type 1 predominant postural muscle for diagnosis of equine motor neuron disease, a type 2 predominant locomotory muscle for diagnosis of equine polysaccharide storage myopathy (EPSSM), and temporal or masseter muscle for diagnosis of masticatory myositis in dogs and masseter myopathy in horses. Short fibers, such as those in the intercostal muscle, are preferred for physiologic studies in which intact muscle fibers are necessary and for studies of neuromuscular junction zones.

Sampling of Muscle for Examination

Information on this topic is available at www.expertconsult.com.

Microscopic Examination

Information on this topic is available at www.expertconsult.com.

Enzyme Histochemistry and Immunohistochemistry

Information on this topic is available at www.expertconsult.com.

Electron Microscopy

Information on this topic is available at www.expertconsult.com.

Other Methods of Evaluation

Information on this topic is available at www.expertconsult.com.

Dysfunction/Responses to Injury

It is often said that the range of response of muscle to injury is limited, consisting primarily of necrosis and regeneration. Actually, muscle is a remarkably adaptive tissue, with a wide range of response to physiologic and pathologic conditions. Myofibers can add or delete sarcomeres to cause elongation or shortening of the entire muscle. In addition to necrosis and regeneration, myofibers can atrophy and hypertrophy, they can split, they can undergo a variety of cytoarchitectural alterations, and they can completely alter their physiologic functions when undergoing fiber-type conversion. To describe muscle response to injury as stereotypical does not do justice to this inherent plasticity. What is true, though, is that it is frequently not possible to determine the cause of muscle injury based on gross or histologic lesions alone. Supplementary tests and clinical histories are often essential.

Necrosis and Regeneration

Myofiber necrosis can accompany a variety of disorders. Because of their multinucleate nature, myofibers often undergo segmental necrosis, with involvement of only one or several contiguous segments within the cell. Global necrosis of the entire length of the myofiber occurs only under severe duress, such as extreme pressure to the entire muscle causing crush injury, or widespread ischemia because of pressure on, or thromboembolism of, a large artery.

Necrotic portions of myofibers have several different histologic appearances. The earliest change is often segmental hypercontraction, resulting in segments of slightly larger diameter that are slightly darker staining ("large dark fibers") that are best seen on transverse sections (Fig. 15-11, *A*). On longitudinal sections, "twisting" or "curling" of affected fibers is often seen. But similar changes occur as an artifactual change in improperly handled samples. The cytoplasm of fully necrotic portions of the fiber is often homogeneously eosinophilic and pale (hyaline degeneration), with loss of the normal cytoplasmic striations and the adjacent muscle nucleus. The affected cytoplasm then becomes floccular or granular as that portion of the myofiber starts to fragment (Fig. 15-11, *B*; see Fig. 15-14, *B*).

Increased intracellular calcium is a common trigger of necrosis in all cells, and myofibers contain a high level of calcium ions stored in the sarcoplasmic reticulum. Therefore myofibers may be particularly sensitive to calcium-induced necrosis, either as a result of damage to the sarcolemma, causing influx of extracellular calcium, or from damage to the sarcoplasmic reticulum, releasing intracellular stores of calcium. Small wonder then that necrotic myofibers are often prone to overt mineralization. Overtly mineralized myofibers appear as chalky white streaks on gross examination (see Fig. 15-9, *A*) and as basophilic granular to crystalline material within myofibers on histologic examination. Large deposits of mineral can induce a foreign body granulomatous response. Although the presence or absence of myofiber mineralization has sometimes been used as a diagnostic aid, the circumstances under which a necrotic myofiber segment can become mineralized are so diverse that myofiber

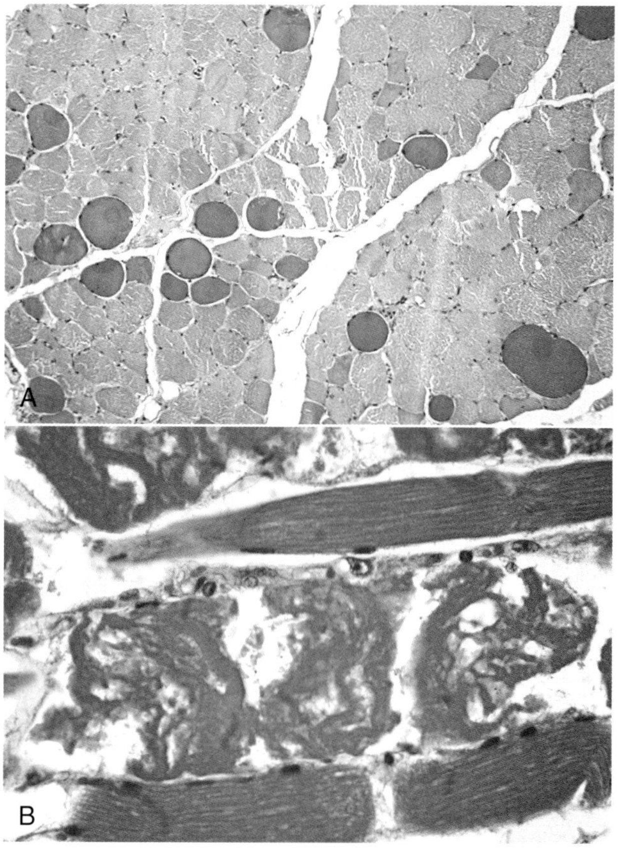

Figure 15-11 **Myofiber Necrosis, Skeletal Muscle. A,** Hypercontraction, transverse section. Large, deeply stained fibers (*large dark red fibers*) are hypercontracted segments of a myofiber, the initial stage of necrosis. Note the rounded outline of these myofibers compared with the polygonal outlines of normal myofibers. Formalin fixation, H&E stain. **B,** Segmental necrosis, monensin toxicosis, longitudinal section, horse. Segments of the myofibers have undergone hypercontraction (*center of figure*), and the remaining cytoplasm is fragmented. Formalin fixation, H&E stain. (Courtesy Dr. M.D. McGavin, College of Veterinary Medicine, University of Tennessee.)

mineralization must be considered a nonspecific response, indicative only of myofiber necrosis. Myofiber mineralization can be confirmed with histochemical stains, such as alizarin red S and von Kossa. Histochemical staining for calcium in frozen sections also detects increased intracytoplasmic calcium in damaged myofibers that are not overtly necrotic or mineralized (Fig. 15-12, *A*).

Provided there is still an adequate blood supply, macrophages derived from transformation of blood monocytes rapidly infiltrate areas of myofiber necrosis (Fig. 15-12, *B*). Macrophages are able to traverse the basal lamina and rapidly clear cytoplasmic debris (Fig. 15-13, *A*). Other leukocytes, including neutrophils, eosinophils, and lymphocytes, can also be recruited to sites of extensive myonecrosis, presumably because of various cytokines released from damaged muscle. The infiltration of macrophages and other cells into areas of damaged muscle to clear away necrotic myofibers does not in any way constitute a form of myositis.

Because myonuclei are unable to divide, regeneration of muscle relies on satellite cell activation. Muscle satellite cells are resistant to many of the insults that result in myofiber necrosis, and activation of satellite cells is triggered by necrosis of adjacent segments of that myofiber. Therefore, as macrophages are clearing cytoplasmic debris, satellite cells are becoming activated and begin to divide in preparation for regeneration of the affected myofiber segment. If the myofiber basal lamina is still intact, it will leave an empty cylindrical space known as a *sarcolemmal tube*. This name is clearly a misnomer, dating from the days when the term *sarcolemma* was applied to the

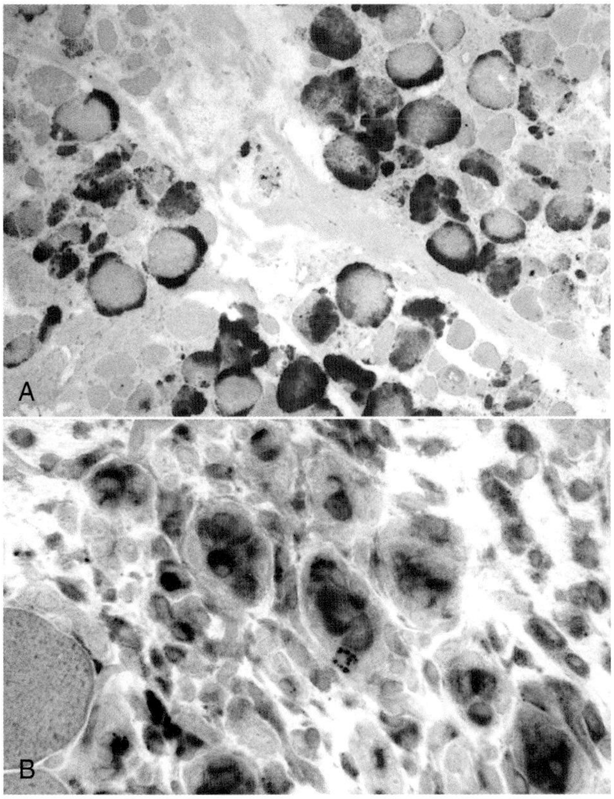

Figure 15-12 Myofiber Necrosis, Skeletal Muscle, Transverse Section. A, There has been a massive influx of calcium *(stained red-orange)* into acutely necrotic fibers. Frozen section, alizarin red S stain. **B,** Macrophages with red-brown staining cytoplasm invading necrotic myofibers. Portions of intact fibers are in the lower left. Frozen section, nonspecific esterase stain. (**A** courtesy Dr. B.A. Valentine, College of Veterinary Medicine, Oregon State University. **B** courtesy Dr. B.J. Cooper, College of Veterinary Medicine, Oregon State University.)

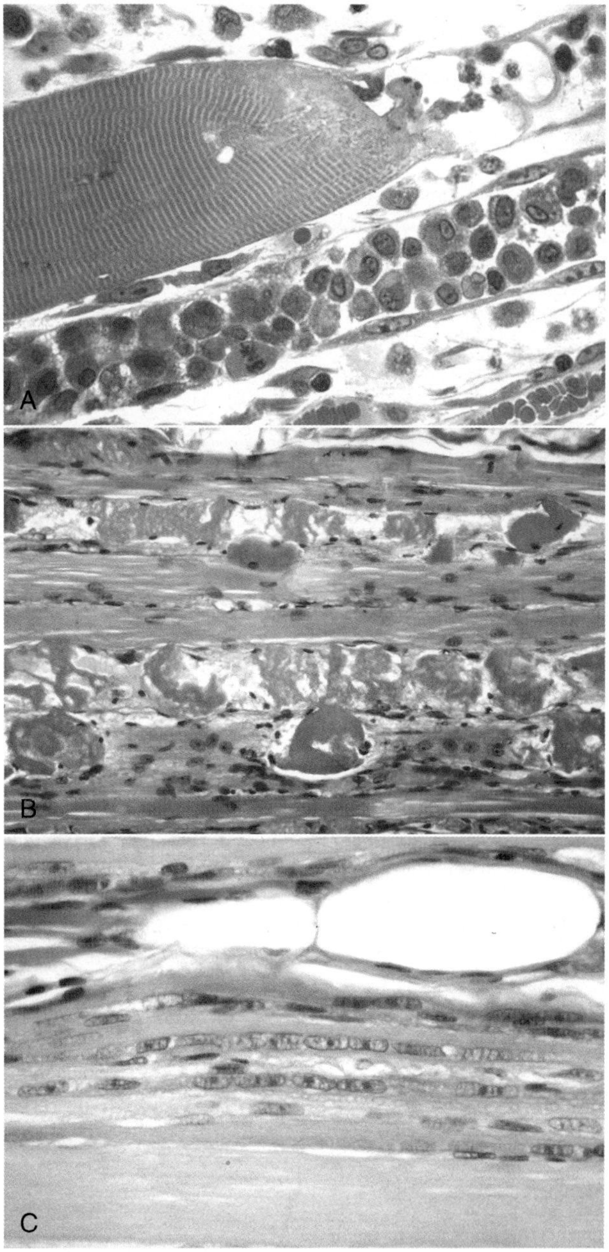

Figure 15-13 Segmental Necrosis and Regeneration. A, Monophasic segmental coagulation necrosis, skeletal muscle, longitudinal section of two myofibers. A segment of the upper fiber *(right)* and all the visible portion of the lower fiber have undergone necrosis, and macrophages have invaded through the intact basal lamina and cleared the cytoplasmic debris. Satellite cells on the inner surface of the basal lamina of the lower fiber are activated, and one *(lower left side)* is in mitosis. One-micron-thick plastic-embedded section, H&E stain. **B,** Polyphasic injury, segmental coagulation necrosis and regeneration of myofibers, muscle, longitudinal section. Between each of the foci of coagulation necrosis in the lowest myofiber is a segment of small-diameter faintly basophilic cytoplasm lacking cross-striations, in which there is an internal chain of euchromatic nuclei. This is a late stage of regeneration. Formalin fixation, H&E stain. **C,** Monophasic injury, late-stage regeneration, skeletal muscle, longitudinal section. The regenerating segment of the myofiber consists of myotubes, which have small diameters, with slightly basophilic cytoplasm and internal rows of large euchromatic nuclei. Formalin fixation, H&E stain. (**A** courtesy Dr. A. Kelly, University of Pennsylvania. **B** courtesy Dr. B.A. Valentine, College of Veterinary Medicine, Oregon State University. **C** courtesy Dr. B.J. Cooper, College of Veterinary Medicine, Oregon State University.)

tube formed by the basal lamina that remains after segmental myofiber necrosis. Clearly what is now termed the sarcolemma (plasmalemma) of necrotic fiber segments is lost, but this is a misnomer that is firmly entrenched. The important concept to remember is that, if intact, the basal lamina forms a cylindrical scaffold to guide proliferating myoblasts and to keep fibroblasts out. Satellite cells may be seen undergoing mitosis, at which stage they are known as *activated myoblasts*, on the inner surface of this tube (see Fig. 15-13, *A*). Within hours, proliferating myoblasts will fuse end-to-end to form myotubes (Fig. 15-13, *B* and C), and within days the myotube produces thick and thin filaments and undergoes maturation to a myofiber, reestablishing myofiber integrity. If the basal lamina is ruptured, myotubes are said to be able to bridge gaps of 2 to 4 mm and larger ones heal by fibrosis (see later discussion). The process of myofiber regeneration recapitulates embryologic development of skeletal muscle and is depicted schematically in Fig. 15-14. A percentage of dividing satellite cells do not fuse with the forming myotube but instead become new satellite cells capable of future regeneration.

In summary, the success of muscle regeneration depends on (1) the presence of an intact basal lamina and (2) the availability of viable satellite cells. The stages of successful muscle regeneration are summarized in Box 15-2.

Thus myofibers undergoing segmental necrosis in which the basal lamina is preserved, as in metabolic, nutritional, and toxic myopathies, regenerate very successfully. However, when large areas of satellite cells are killed (e.g., by heat, intense inflammation, or infarction), the situation is very different. In this case, a return to normal is not possible, and healing is chiefly by fibrosis.

If the insult to the muscle is sufficient to disrupt the myofiber basal lamina but not enough to damage the satellite cells, regeneration attempts are ineffective. Because the basal lamina is not intact, there is no tube to guide the myoblasts proliferating from each end. Myoblast proliferation under these conditions results in formation of so-called muscle giant cells (Fig. 15-15). Thus the presence of muscle giant cells indicates that conditions for regeneration have not been optimal and occurs after destructive lesions, such as those caused by trauma that transects myofibers, infarction, and intramuscular bacterial infection or injection of irritants. Muscle giant cells are often accompanied by fibrosis, which will unite the ends of the damaged myofibers. This also occurs in muscle damaged by invasive or metastatic sclerosing carcinomas. Cytokines released from damaged muscle fibers contribute to the signaling pathways that initiate macrophage infiltration and regeneration, but they also contribute to interstitial fibroblast activation. Collagen is inelastic, and thus large areas of fibrosis inevitably reduce the ability of the muscle to contract and to stretch. Fibrosis within locomotory muscles often results in obvious alteration of the gait.

Because segmental necrosis and regeneration are such a common result of a wide variety of insults (e.g., overexertion, selenium deficiency, and toxic injury), a histologic diagnosis of segmental necrosis is often not helpful in determining the cause of the disease. Pathologic classification of lesions according to distribution (i.e., focal, multifocal, locally extensive, and diffuse) and duration (i.e., acute, subacute, and chronic) has proven to be extremely useful in determining the possible causes of segmental muscle necrosis. Pathologic classification of degenerative myopathies is enhanced by use of the terms *monophasic necrosis* and *polyphasic necrosis*. Monophasic lesions are of the same duration, indicative of a single insult. Polyphasic lesions indicate an ongoing degenerative process. Thus a focal monophasic lesion could be the result of a single traumatic incident such as an intramuscular injection (see Fig. 15-9, *B*). A multifocal monophasic lesion could represent a single episode of overly strenuous exercise (exertional myopathy) or a toxin being ingested on one occasion (e.g., a horse eating one dose of monensin; see Figs. 15-11, *B*, and 15-33, *B*). However, if the insult is repeated or ongoing, such as occurs in muscular dystrophy (see Fig. 15-44), selenium deficiency, or continuous feeding of a toxin, then new lesions (segmental necrosis) will form at the same time that regeneration is taking place; in other words, it will be a multifocal and polyphasic disease (see Fig. 15-11, *B*). Using this approach, it is sometimes possible to rule out a diagnosis (e.g., muscular dystrophy and selenium deficiency myopathy are typically polyphasic), but this is not an invariable rule. For example, in livestock with borderline concentrations of selenium, a sudden stress can cause a monophasic necrosis.

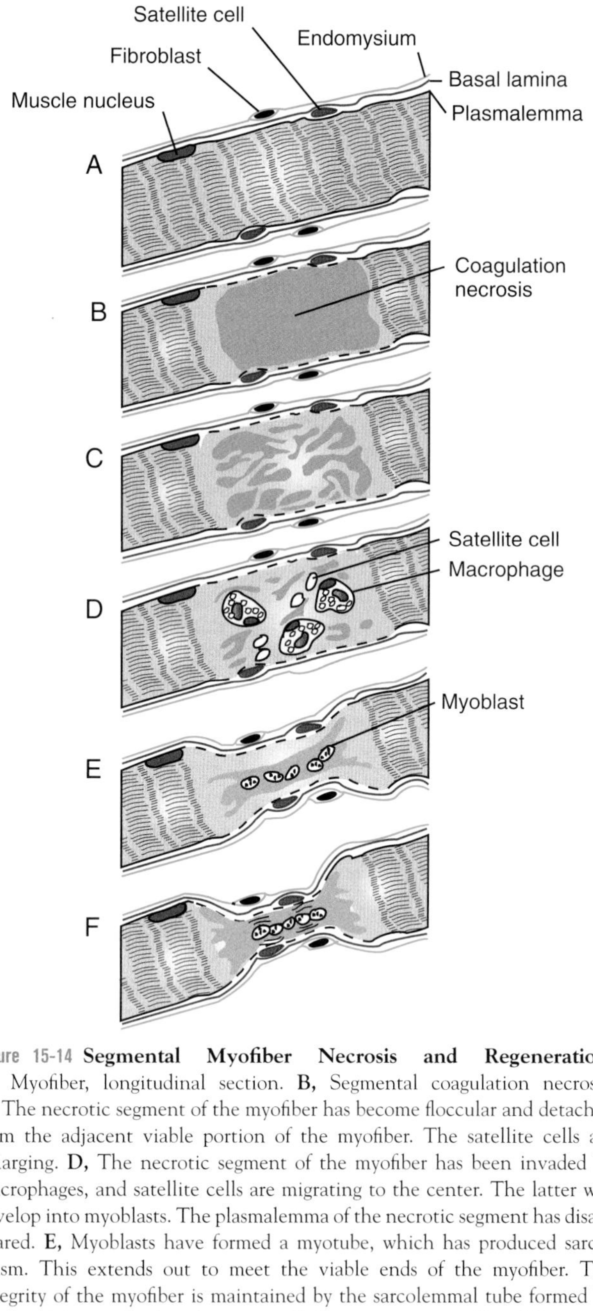

Figure 15-14 **Segmental Myofiber Necrosis and Regeneration. A,** Myofiber, longitudinal section. **B,** Segmental coagulation necrosis. **C,** The necrotic segment of the myofiber has become floccular and detached from the adjacent viable portion of the myofiber. The satellite cells are enlarging. **D,** The necrotic segment of the myofiber has been invaded by macrophages, and satellite cells are migrating to the center. The latter will develop into myoblasts. The plasmalemma of the necrotic segment has disappeared. **E,** Myoblasts have formed a myotube, which has produced sarcoplasm. This extends out to meet the viable ends of the myofiber. The integrity of the myofiber is maintained by the sarcolemmal tube formed by the basal lamina and endomysium. **F,** Regenerating myofiber. There is a reduction in myofiber diameter with central rowing of nuclei. There is early formation of sarcomeres (cross-striations), and the plasmalemma has re-formed. Such fibers stain basophilically with H&E. (Redrawn with permission from Dr. M.D. McGavin, College of Veterinary Medicine, University of Tennessee.)

Box 15-2 Stages of Muscle Regeneration Under Optimal Conditions

Muscle nuclei disappear from the necrotic segment and the sarcoplasm becomes hyalinized (eosinophilic, amorphous, and homogeneous) because of the loss of normal myofibrillar structure (see Fig. 15-15, *B*). The necrotic portion may separate from the adjacent viable myofiber (see Fig. 15-12, *B*; Fig. 15-14, *A* and *B*; and Fig. 15-15, *C*).

Within 24 to 48 hours, monocytes emigrate from capillaries, become macrophages, and enter the necrotic portion of the myofiber (see Fig. 15-13, *B*; Fig. 15-14, *A*; and Fig. 15-15, *D*). Concurrently, the satellite cells, located between the basal lamina and the sarcolemma, begin to enlarge (see Fig. 15-14, *A*; and Fig. 15-15, *C* and *D*), become vesicular with prominent nucleoli, and then undergo mitosis to become myoblasts.

Myoblasts migrate from the periphery to the center of the sarcolemmal tube, admixed with macrophages (see Fig. 15-15, *D*).

Macrophages lyse and phagocytose necrotic debris and form a clear space in the sarcolemmal tube, and the shape and integrity of the sarcolemmal tube are maintained by the basal lamina (see Fig. 15-14, *A*).

Myoblasts fuse with one another to form myotubes, which are thin, elongated muscle cells with a row of central, closely spaced nuclei. Developing myotubes send out cytoplasmic processes in both directions within the sarcolemmal tube (see Fig. 15-15, *E*). When the processes contact each other or a viable portion of the original muscle fiber, they fuse. The regenerating fiber is characterized by (1) basophilia as a result of increased RNA content; (2) internal nuclei, often in rows, that have differentiated to myonuclei; (3) a lack of striations; and (4) a smaller than normal diameter (see Fig. 15-14, *B* and *C*, and Fig. 15-15, *F*).

The fiber grows and differentiates. Its diameter increases, the sarcoplasm loses its basophilia, and longitudinal and cross-striations appear, indicating the formation of sarcomeres.

In most species, within several days, the muscle nuclei of regenerating fibers move to their normal position at the periphery of the fiber, just under the sarcolemma.

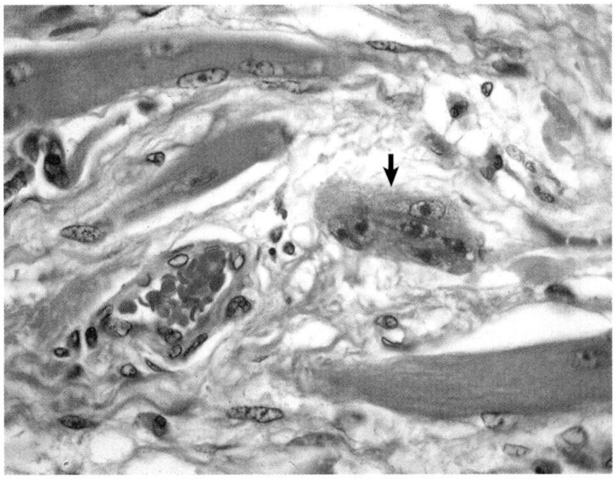

Figure 15-15 **Ineffectual Regeneration.** Large, bizarre multinucleate muscle giant cells *(arrow)* are indicative of regeneration in an area in which the myofiber's basal lamina has been damaged. Because the wall of the "myotube" of basal lamina is not intact, regenerating sarcoplasm exudes through the defect, and in cross section this appears as a "muscle giant cell." Formalin fixation, H&E stain. (Courtesy Dr. M.D. McGavin, College of Veterinary Medicine, University of Tennessee; and Noah's Arkive, College of Veterinary Medicine, The University of Georgia.)

The term *rhabdomyolysis* is often encountered, particularly in the clinical arena, and especially in association with exercise-induced muscle injury (exertional rhabdomyolysis) in human beings, horses, and dogs. Technically, *rhabdomyolysis* simply means necrosis (lysis) of striated muscle. Rhabdomyolysis generally indicates the presence of a severe degenerative myopathy with a large degree of myofiber necrosis (see Fig. 15-35). In horses, the term *exertional rhabdomyolysis* has become firmly entrenched as a clinical entity in which exercise-induced muscle injury is the presenting sign. The term *recurrent exertional rhabdomyolysis* is often employed in cases in which repeated bouts of exercise-induced muscle damage have been documented.

Alteration in Myofiber Size

The normal myofiber diameter will vary, depending on fiber type, the muscle examined, the species, and the age of the animal. In some species (e.g., horse, cat, and human beings), there are three distinct populations based on diameter: Type 1 fibers are the smallest, type 2B fibers are the largest, and type 2A fibers are intermediate in size. Different sizes in diameters are in part a reflection of the oxidative needs of the fibers; oxygen diffuses more readily into the interior of small-diameter fibers. In the dog, all fiber types are oxidative, and fiber-type diameter is much more uniform. A histogram generated from morphometric analysis of fiber diameters will reveal the characteristics of individual muscles in various species. Not surprisingly, this type of detailed information is more readily available for human patients than for animals. Even without morphometric analysis, however, a pathologist experienced in examination of muscle can often determine whether there is a normal fiber-size distribution (based on fiber diameter in transverse section) or whether there is an increase in fiber-size variation. The finding of increased fiber-size variation suggests that something is wrong but in itself does not give any indication of cause. Increased fiber-size variation can be a result of fiber atrophy, fiber hypertrophy, or both and is considered part of the spectrum of changes included in the term *chronic myopathic change* (Box 15-3).

Atrophy

The term *atrophy* is used to imply either a reduction in the volume of the muscle as a whole or a reduction in the diameter of a myofiber. In the early stages of atrophy, it may be difficult or impossible to detect loss of muscle mass by gross observation, and morphometric evaluation of myofiber diameters may be required. Several cellular physiologic processes can be activated to result in muscle atrophy. These include induction of lysosomal action to result in autophagy of cytoplasmic components, apoptosis (programmed cell death), and activation of the cytoplasmic ubiquitin-proteosomal machinery. Lysosomal activation is prominent in denervation atrophy and is the basis for the positive reaction of denervated fibers in alkaline phosphatase and nonspecific esterase preparations. The causes of muscle fiber atrophy include physiologic and metabolic processes and denervation. In most instances, muscle atrophy is reversible provided the cause is corrected. The type of fiber undergoing atrophy varies, depending on the cause; therefore fiber typing is often required for

Box 15-3 Findings Associated with Chronic Myopathic Change

Excessive fiber-size (diameter) variation	Other cytoarchitectural changes
Internal nuclei	Fibrosis
Fiber splitting	Fat infiltration

Box 15-4 Fiber Types Affected in Different Types of Muscle Atrophy

Denervation: Type 1 and type 2 fibers; reinnervation leads to altered fiber-type patterns (fiber-type grouping)
Disuse: Predominantly type 2 fibers; may vary, depending on the species and cause
Endocrine disease: Predominantly type 2 fibers; associated with hypothyroidism and hypercortisolism
Malnutrition, cachexia, and senility: Predominantly type 2 fibers
Congenital myopathy: Often predominantly type 1 fibers

a definitive diagnosis. Interestingly, type 2 fibers are the most likely to atrophy under a variety of circumstances (Box 15-4). Signaling molecules involved in muscle atrophy include tumor necrosis factor-α (TNF-α) and interleukin (IL)-1 and IL-6.

Physiologic Muscle Atrophy. Decrease in myofiber diameter and therefore in the overall muscle mass is a physiologic response to lack of use (disuse atrophy), cachexia, and aging. Type 2 fibers are preferentially affected (E-Fig. 15-4). Disuse atrophy occurs relatively slowly, and only in muscles not undergoing normal contraction, as is caused by severe lameness or in muscles of a limb that is splinted or enclosed in a cast. The degree of disuse atrophy will be variable, but typically it is not as severe as the atrophy of cachexia or denervation (see later discussion). Disuse atrophy is often asymmetric. Muscle atrophy caused by cachexia can be profound, especially in cases of cancer cachexia in which increased circulating levels of TNF alter the muscle metabolism, favoring catabolic processes rather than anabolic processes. Cachexia also develops relatively slowly and causes symmetric muscle atrophy. Starvation, malnutrition, neoplasia, and chronic renal and cardiac diseases are possible causes of cachexia.

Atrophy Caused by Endocrine Disease. Preferential atrophy of type 2 fibers causing symmetric muscle atrophy also occurs because of various endocrine disorders. The most common are hypothyroidism and hypercortisolism in dogs. Aging horses with pituitary dysfunction or tumors (leading to equine Cushing's syndrome) often develop type 2 muscle fiber atrophy. Myofibers contain a high concentration of surface receptors for several hormones, and atrophy caused by endocrine disease reflects the intimate interrelationship between the endocrine and the muscular systems.

Denervation Atrophy. Denervation atrophy, also known by the misnomer *neurogenic atrophy*, is not uncommon in veterinary medicine. Maintenance of normal myofiber diameter depends on trophic factors generated by an intact associated nerve. Loss of neural input results in rapid muscle atrophy, and more than half the muscle mass of a completely denervated muscle can be lost in a few weeks. This trophic effect is not dependent on contractile activity because denervation atrophy is not a feature of neuromuscular junction disorders such as botulism and myasthenia gravis. In these disorders, there is a failure of neuromuscular transmission, but the nerve to the muscle is intact; therefore the muscle is technically still innervated. Generalized neuropathies or neuronopathies, such as equine motor neuron disease, result in widespread and symmetric muscle atrophy. More commonly, however, only select nerve damage is present, resulting in asymmetric muscle atrophy. One example is equine laryngeal hemiplegia (roaring) secondary to damage to the left recurrent laryngeal nerve (Fig. 15-16). Note that purely demyelinating disorders of peripheral nerves can cause profound neuromuscular dysfunction, but axons are still intact. Associated myofibers are not technically denervated and therefore do not undergo denervation atrophy.

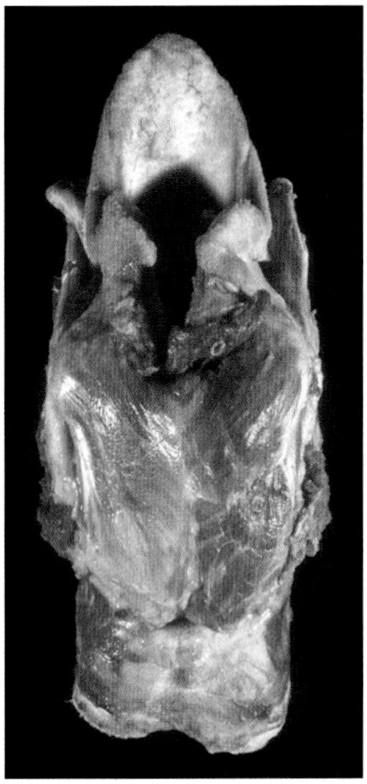

Figure 15-16 **Denervation Muscle Atrophy, Left Cricoarytenoideus Dorsalis Muscle, Larynx, Dorsal Surface, Horse.** Note the unilateral *(left side)* atrophy and pale gray to white discoloration of the muscle. This horse had a peripheral neuropathy, which led to laryngeal hemiplegia. (Courtesy Dr. J.F. Zachary, College of Veterinary Medicine, University of Illinois.)

After denervation, fibers become progressively smaller in diameter as peripheral myofibrils disintegrate. If an atrophic fiber is surrounded by normal fibers, it will be pressed into an angular shape, called an angular atrophied fiber. The angular atrophied fibers of denervation atrophy most often occur either singly or in small contiguous groups (small group atrophy) (Fig. 15-17, *A*). In more severe denervating conditions, in which many fibers within muscle fascicles are undergoing denervation atrophy, there are no normal fibers to cause compression and angularity, and affected fibers occur as larger groups of small-diameter, rounded fibers (large group atrophy; Fig. 15-17, *B*). Although myofibrils disappear rapidly, muscle nuclei do not do so at the same rate, and therefore denervation atrophy is often associated with a notably increased concentration of myonuclei. The breakdown of glycogen in the myofiber is an early change in denervation atrophy, and therefore denervated fibers stain faintly or not at all with the PAS reaction.

A histologic diagnosis of denervation atrophy may be suspected, based on the characteristic features of routinely processed muscles, but is most reliably documented with histochemistry or immunohistochemistry to detect fiber types. The loss of a nerve fiber to a muscle results in atrophy of all myofibers innervated by that nerve. Because of the intermingling of motor units forming a mosaic pattern of fiber types, myofibers undergoing denervation atrophy are scattered in a section of muscle. Because the motor neuron determines the histochemical myofiber type and because denervating diseases typically involve both type 1 and type 2 neurons or nerves, atrophy of both type 1 and type 2 myofibers in muscle fasciculi is the hallmark of denervation atrophy (Fig. 15-18, *A*).

In denervation atrophy, histologic examination of the intramuscular nerves is warranted because it may reveal axonal degeneration

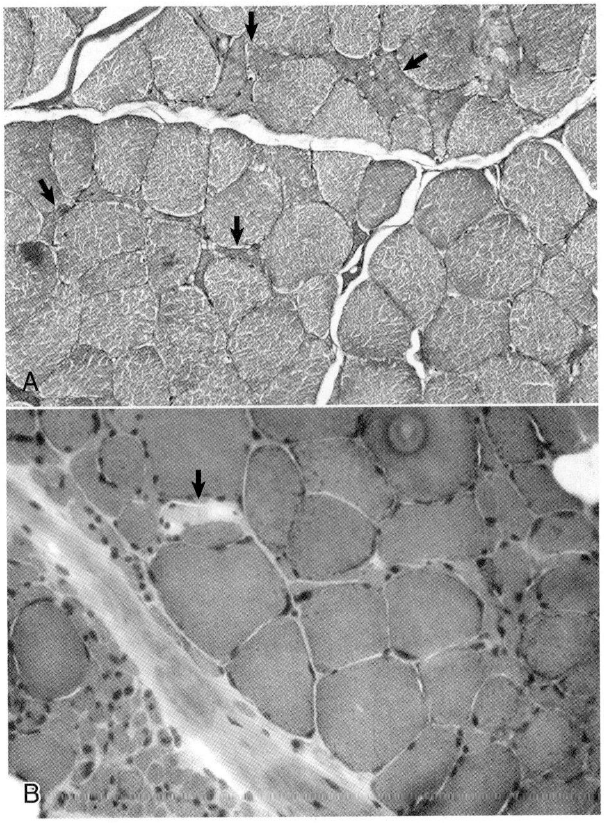

Figure 15-17 **Denervation Atrophy, Transverse Sections.** Both sections are from horses with equine motor neuron disease. **A,** In relatively mild denervation, severely atrophied and angular fibers form small contiguous clusters indicative of small group atrophy (*arrows*). Formalin fixation, Masson trichrome stain. **B,** In severe denervation, entire fascicles of fibers undergo rounded atrophy characteristic of large group atrophy (*lower left*). Small group atrophy and admixed fiber hypertrophy are also present. A single pale stained fiber (*arrow*) is undergoing acute necrosis. There is also mild endomysial and perimysial fibrosis and mild fat infiltration (*empty vacuoles in the upper right and lower left*). Frozen section, modified Gomori's trichrome stain. (Courtesy Dr. B.A. Valentine, College of Veterinary Medicine, Oregon State University.)

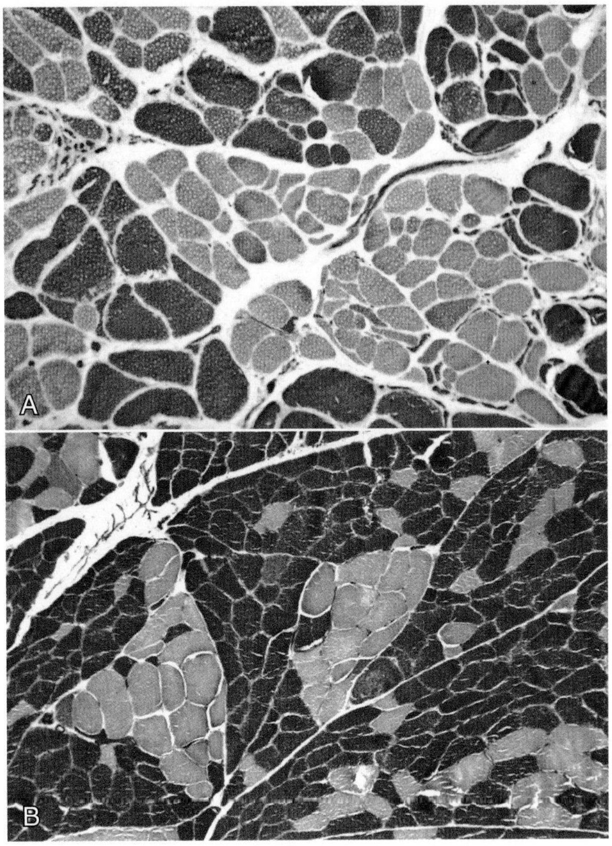

Figure 15-18 **Denervation Atrophy and Reinnervation, Skeletal Muscle, Transverse Sections. A,** Fiber typing reveals angular atrophy of both type 1 (*light*) and type 2 (*dark*) fibers, characteristic of denervation atrophy. In this case, there is also a loss of the normal mosaic pattern of fiber types, with groups of type 1 and of type 2 fibers indicative of reinnervation. This section is from a horse with laryngeal hemiplegia. Frozen section, ATPase pH 10.0. **B,** Fiber-type grouping in a dog indicative of denervation and reinnervation secondary to corticosteroid therapy. There is a loss of the normal mosaic pattern of fiber types, with grouping of type 1 (*light*) and type 2 (*dark*) fibers. The lack of angular atrophied fibers indicates that active denervation is not occurring at this time. Frozen section, ATPase pH 9.8. (**A** courtesy Dr. B.A. Valentine, College of Veterinary Medicine, Oregon State University. **B** courtesy Dr. M.D. McGavin, College of Veterinary Medicine, University of Tennessee.)

or loss of myelinated fibers. Masson trichrome stain can be useful here because it will differentiate myelin (red) from collagen (blue). If the nerve damage does not incapacitate the animal and the muscle can still be used (e.g., in locomotion), the remaining innervated myofibers often undergo notable hypertrophy because of increased workload. Often, the hypertrophied fibers in chronic denervation are type 1. Even without fiber typing, a pattern of severe small or large group atrophy (see Fig.15-17, *A*), especially if associated with notable fiber hypertrophy (see Fig. 15-17, *B*), is strongly suggestive of denervation atrophy. A finding of damage in an associated peripheral nerve is definitive.

Under many circumstances, denervated muscle fibers can be reinnervated by subterminal sprouting of axons from adjacent normal nerves. Reinnervation results in return to normal myofiber diameter, but reinnervation is often from sprouts of a different type of nerve. Because muscle fiber type is a function of the motor neuron, the newly innervated myofiber takes on the fiber type determined by that neuron. This process results in a loss of the normal arrangement of type 1 and type 2 myofibers and the formation of groups of the same fiber type adjacent to each other, called *fiber-type grouping* (see Fig. 15-18). Thus fiber-type grouping is the hallmark of denervation followed by reinnervation. What appears to be fiber-type grouping can also occur because of fiber-type conversion (most often to type 1 fibers) in chronic myopathic conditions. Careful evaluation of the structure and function of peripheral nerves helps distinguish neuropathic from myopathic changes. If previously reinnervated fibers are denervated again, the pattern includes large groups of atrophied fibers of a single fiber type, a process known as *type-specific group atrophy*. Type-specific group atrophy is far less common in animals than in human beings. Fiber-type grouping and type-specific group atrophy can only be detected by methods that distinguish fiber types. Changes occurring as a result of denervation and reinnervation are illustrated in Fig. 15-19.

Atrophy Caused by Congenital Myopathy. Congenital myopathy in children is often associated with selective type 1 fiber atrophy. This finding is less common in the congenital myopathies identified thus far in animals. Selective type 1 atrophy is, however, a feature of feline nemaline myopathy, an animal model of congenital nemaline myopathy in children.

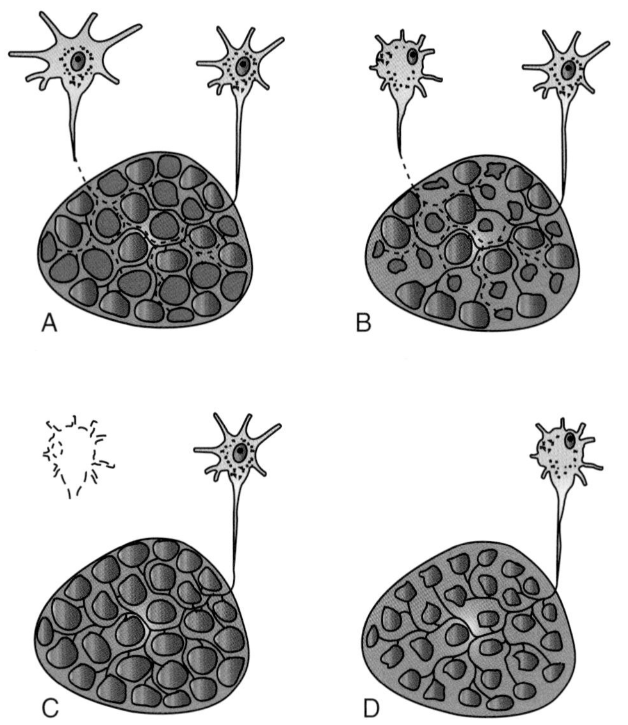

Figure 15-19 **Motor Units Undergoing Denervation and Reinnervation. A,** Terminal axon branches innervate multiple myofibers, and myofiber type is determined by the electrical activity of the type of neuron innervating the myofiber. Normally the terminal axons of the motor units are intermingled, with the result that the differently stained myofiber types form a mosaic pattern. **B,** If a neuron (or axon) is damaged, the axon will undergo Wallerian degeneration, and the myofibers in that motor unit will undergo denervation atrophy. Small group atrophy is illustrated here. **C,** Axonal sprouts from a healthy neuron can reinnervate affected fibers and cause restoration of their normal diameter. The myofibers will assume the fiber type of the new motor unit, which often causes fiber-type conversion, leading to fiber-type grouping. **D,** If neuronal (or axonal) damage is progressive, denervation atrophy of large groups of fibers of a single type can occur, known as type-specific group atrophy. This type of atrophy is less common in animals than in human beings. (Redrawn with permission from Dr. B.A. Valentine, College of Veterinary Medicine, Oregon State University.)

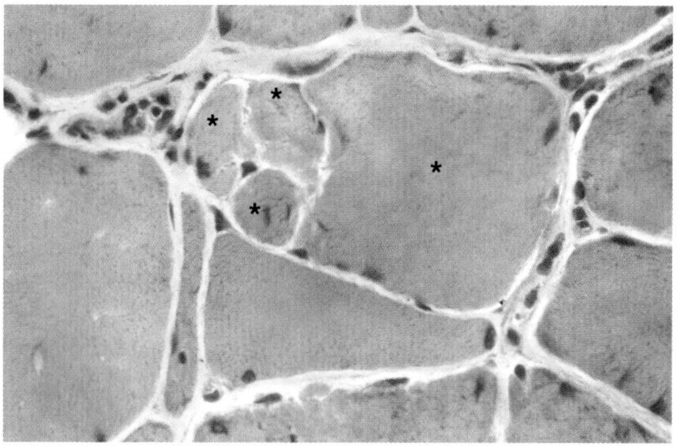

Figure 15-20 **Fiber Splitting of Hypertrophied Myofibers, Nemaline Myopathy, Skeletal Muscle, Transverse Section, Cat.** Sarcolemmal ingrowth into the myofiber has resulted in multiple partitions with the formation of four myofibers *(asterisks)*; however, all myofibers are enclosed by one basal lamina. Frozen section, modified Gomori's trichrome stain. (Courtesy Dr. B.A. Valentine, College of Veterinary Medicine, Oregon State University.)

Hypertrophy

Myofibers increase in diameter by the addition of myofilaments. Physiologic hypertrophy is the normal process of myofiber enlargement that occurs with exercise conditioning. Compensatory hypertrophy occurs because of pathologic conditions that (1) decrease the number of functional myofibers and therefore increase the load on remaining fibers or (2) interfere with normal cellular metabolic or other physiologic processes. Compensatory myofiber hypertrophy is therefore considered a relatively nonspecific response to a variety of insults. Fibers undergoing compensatory hypertrophy can enlarge to more than 100 μm in diameter (normal is less than approximately 60 to 70 μm). Fiber hypertrophy often accompanies fiber atrophy, which contributes to increased fiber-size variation in various myopathic and neuropathic conditions.

Compensatory hypertrophy can occur because of a decrease in the number of functional myofibers. Thus, in a partially denervated muscle, the remaining innervated fibers hypertrophy (see Fig. 15-17, *B*), presumably as a result of increased workload. Pathologically, hypertrophied fibers have less oxygen diffusion from interstitial capillaries to internal portions of the myofiber because of the increase in the distance from the capillary to the internal portions of the myofibers, which can lead to myofiber damage. Mechanical overloading of hypertrophied muscle fibers is also possible. For example, overloading of hypertrophied fibers can result in segmental necrosis of the hypertrophied fibers (see Fig. 15-17, *B*), or fibers can undergo longitudinal fiber splitting to generate one or more smaller-diameter "fibers," all contained within the same basal lamina (Fig. 15-20). Serial sections of areas of fiber splitting generally reveal that splits do not extend the entire length of the myofiber. Fiber splitting is considered a form of cytoarchitectural alteration (see later discussion). Insulin-like growth factor 1 (IGF-1) is an important molecular signal involved in skeletal muscle hypertrophy. Genetic inactivation of the regulatory gene myostatin results in muscle hypertrophy caused by an increase in the number of myofibers.

Cytoarchitectural Changes

In addition to fiber splitting, a variety of other cytoarchitectural changes can occur within myofibers. Some are degenerative, the result of an insult that damages the myofiber but does not culminate in myofiber necrosis. Others reflect underlying ultrastructural alterations that may be either pathologic or compensatory in nature. The functional significance of many of the myofiber cytoarchitectural changes is not known.

Vacuolar Change

Vacuolar change is a common cytoplasmic alteration. In formalin-fixed paraffin-embedded sections or in any sample subjected to less than ideal handling, true vacuolar change can be very difficult to distinguish from artifacts. Vacuoles can be an early manifestation of processes leading to necrosis, they can reflect underlying sarcotubular dilation as occurs in many myotonic conditions (see later discussion), and they can be caused by abnormal storage of carbohydrate or lipid, or they can reflect underlying myofibrillar abnormalities. Additional studies are often necessary to determine the nature of the vacuoles. When severe, such as in glycogen storage diseases, the term *vacuolar myopathy* is often employed.

Internal Nuclei

Myonuclei of mature myofibers in domestic animals are normally found peripherally, just beneath the sarcolemma. Nuclei located one nuclear diameter or more from the sarcolemma are known as *internal*

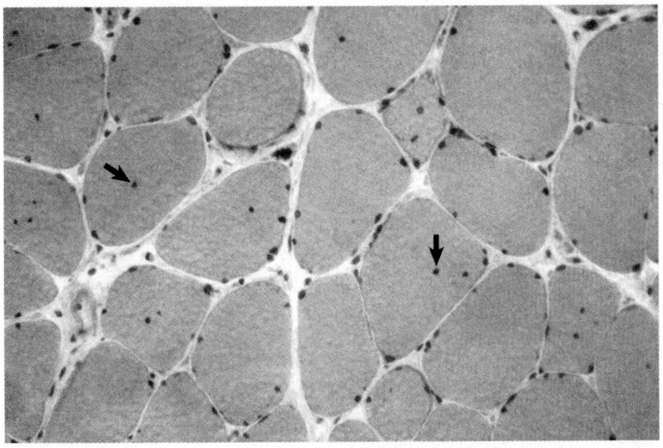

Figure 15-21 Chronic Myopathic Change, Medial Triceps Muscle, Horse. The variation in myofiber diameter and the presence of one or more internal nuclei in most myofibers *(arrows)* are indicative of a chronic myopathic change. Frozen section, H&E stain. (Courtesy Dr. B.A. Valentine, College of Veterinary Medicine, Oregon State University.)

nuclei. (NOTE: The previously used term *central nuclei* is considered incorrect because few abnormally placed nuclei are exactly centrally located.) Internal nuclei are rare in normal mammalian muscle, but a small percentage can be found normally in avian and reptilian species. Rows of internal nuclei in small-diameter, slightly basophilic myofibers are characteristic of the myotubular stage of regeneration (see Fig. 15-13, *B* and *C*). In most species, myonuclei return to the normal peripheral location early in regeneration, within days of myotube formation. Rodents are the exception. In rodents, internal nuclei are retained after regeneration, which, in these species, provides a handy marker for identification of fibers that have undergone necrosis and regeneration. In other mammalian species, the presence of internal nuclei in normal or hypertrophied fibers is a nonspecific finding indicative of chronic myopathic change (Fig. 15-21; see Box 15-3). In hypertrophied fibers, the migration of myonuclei to the internal portion of the myofiber can precede the sarcolemmal infolding that creates longitudinal fiber splitting.

Whorled and Ring Fibers

The cytoarchitectural rearrangements resulting in whorled and ring fibers are best appreciated in transverse sections. Whorled fibers contain spirals of cytoplasm with internally located nuclei. Whorled fibers can be seen in areas of chronic denervation and also in areas in which myofiber necrosis with incomplete regeneration has occurred. Ring fibers (also known as *ringbinden*) contain a peripheral rim of sarcomeres oriented perpendicular to their normal orientation, resulting in peripheral radiating striations. Ring fibers are visible with many stains, both in frozen sections and in routinely processed sections. In either frozen or routine sections, they are best visualized in sections stained with PAS (Fig. 15-22, *A*) or iron hematoxylin. In human beings, ring fibers are common in a specific form of inherited muscular dystrophy known as *myotonic dystrophy*, but they are also seen in other myopathic and in neuropathic conditions and therefore are not specific for myotonic dystrophy. Similarly, there is no animal disorder in which ring fibers are specific, and these fibers can be seen in a variety of myopathic and neuropathic conditions such as ovine congenital muscular dystrophy. The presence of ring fibers can only be considered a chronic myopathic change. For example, numerous ring fibers were found in muscle from the contralateral weight-bearing limb from a horse with longstanding, non–weight-bearing foreleg lameness.

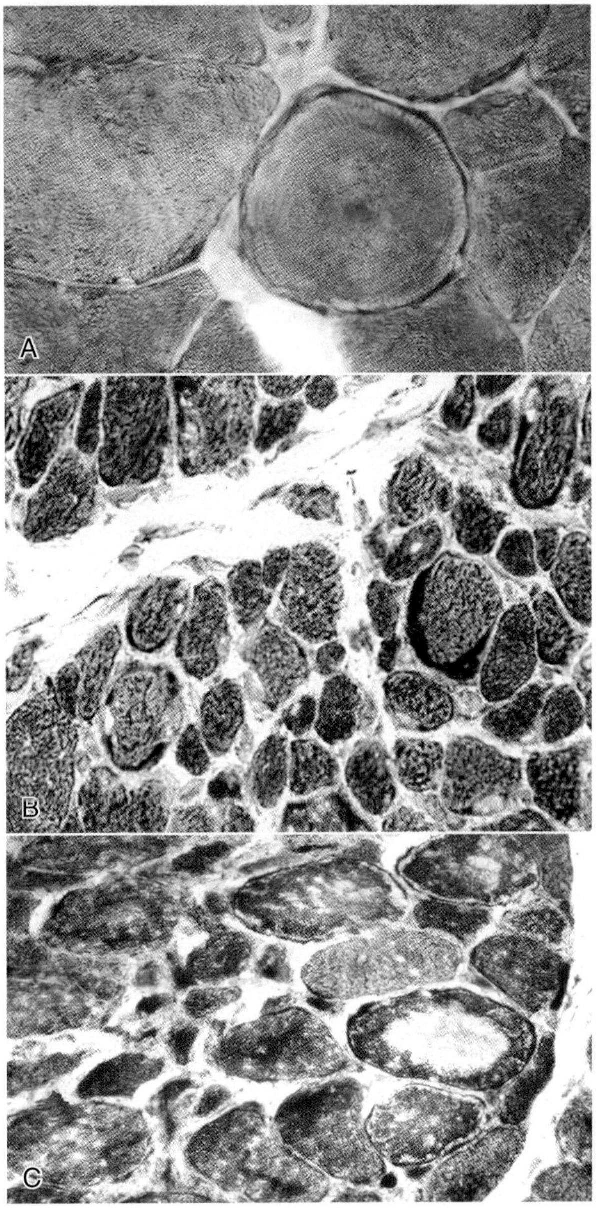

Figure 15-22 Cytoarchitectural Changes, Skeletal Muscle, Transverse Sections. A, Ring fiber, extensor carpi radialis muscle, horse. A ring fiber *(center right)* is characterized by a peripheral rim of sarcomeres, arranged circumferentially around a myofiber and with their length at right angles to the long axis of the myofiber. Frozen section, PAS reaction. **B,** Irregular mitochondrial distribution with peripheral aggregates of blue staining mitochondria, Labrador centronuclear myopathy, temporalis muscle, dog. Frozen section, NADH reaction. **C,** Irregularity of mitochondrial *(blue-stained)* distribution and "moth-eaten" fibers, polyneuropathy, dog. Fibers containing pale zones are characteristic of moth-eaten fibers. Frozen section, NADH reaction. (Courtesy Dr. B.A. Valentine, College of Veterinary Medicine, Oregon State University.)

Other Cytoarchitectural Changes

Many other cytoarchitectural changes reflect alterations in mitochondrial density or integrity and are best appreciated on examination of frozen sections, in which mitochondria can be visualized, or on ultrastructural examination. The presence of peripheral aggregates of mitochondria, which stain red with modified Gomori's trichrome stain, form the basis of "ragged red" fibers. Ragged red fibers are a hallmark of mitochondrial myopathy in human beings. In animals, however, ragged red fibers are common in various myopathic conditions and also occur in normal dog and horse muscle. Mitochondrial abnormalities are also detected by oxidative enzyme reactions such as NADH (Fig. 15-22, *B* and *C*) and SDH in frozen sections. Nemaline rods, formed by expansions of the Z-line material, stain purple to red with modified Gomori's trichrome stain in frozen sections. These rods can also be seen in animals with other myopathic conditions. Moth-eaten fibers contain multiple pale zones because of loss of mitochondrial oxidative enzyme activity on frozen sections and occur in denervating disorders and in myopathic conditions (Fig. 15-22, *C*). Sarcoplasmic masses are pale-staining zones usually at the periphery of myofibers but occasionally central. These can be seen in H&E-stained muscle sections and appear as light blue areas with few or no myofibrils. Ultrastructurally they often contain disarrayed myofilaments with or without degenerate mitochondria. Other less commonly encountered alterations in animal muscle are pale central cores visible with mitochondrial stains, tubular aggregates composed of sarcotubular membranes, and target fibers in which mitochondrial oxidative enzyme reactions reveal central clear zones surrounded by a thin rim of highly reactive cytoplasm. Other less commonly encountered alterations in H&E-stained sections of animal muscle are pale central cores. As demonstrated in sections stained by mitochondrial oxidative enzyme reaction (e.g., SDH), these are of three types: (1) cores rich in mitochondria and similar to the peripheral sarcoplasmic masses described previously, (2) target fibers so designated because of a pale center surrounded by a rim of densely staining mitochondria, and (3) aggregates of sarcotubular membranes that do not stain with mitochondrial stains.

Chronic Myopathic Change

Evaluation of abnormal skeletal muscle often reveals chronic myopathic change, which includes alterations in myofiber diameter, cytoarchitectural alterations, and interstitial fibrosis and fat infiltration (see Box 15-3). Chronic myopathic change accompanies a variety of myopathic and neuropathic conditions. In particularly severe cases, a definitive cause may not be identified. Chronic inflammation or denervation and chronic degenerative myopathy resulting in repeated bouts of myonecrosis and regeneration often cause diffuse endomysial and perimysial fibrosis (see Figs. 15-17, *B*, and 15-47, *B*). Interstitial infiltration of muscle by mature adipocytes is less common than fibrosis and occurs most commonly in chronically denervated muscle (see Fig. 15-17, *B*), particularly neonatal muscle that lacks appropriate innervation (Fig. 15-23). Fat infiltration can also occur because of severe chronic degenerative myopathy. A chronically damaged or denervated muscle that develops profound fibrosis and/or fat infiltration can be grossly enlarged, despite atrophy or loss of myofibers—a condition known as *pseudohypertrophy* (see Fig. 15-9, *D*).

Aging

Aging changes in skeletal muscle are well documented in human beings but less well documented in domestic animals. The term *sarcopenia* refers to generalized reduction in muscle mass, strength, and function related to aging, in the absence of underlying disease. In contrast, *cachexia* is generalized muscle atrophy caused by underlying disease or malnutrition. Changes in mitochondrial function and progressive denervation are implicated as possible causes of sarcopenia in aging human beings. Aged animals often exhibit mild to severe muscle atrophy. To what degree this atrophy in animals is due strictly to age-related changes rather than to underlying chronic organ dysfunction (e.g., renal failure, cardiac disease, and neoplasia) is most often unknown. Sarcopenia and cachexia can occur concurrently in aged animals and people. Old cattle can accumulate lipofuscin within skeletal muscle, which can cause a tan-brown discoloration, but there is no apparent clinical significance to this change.

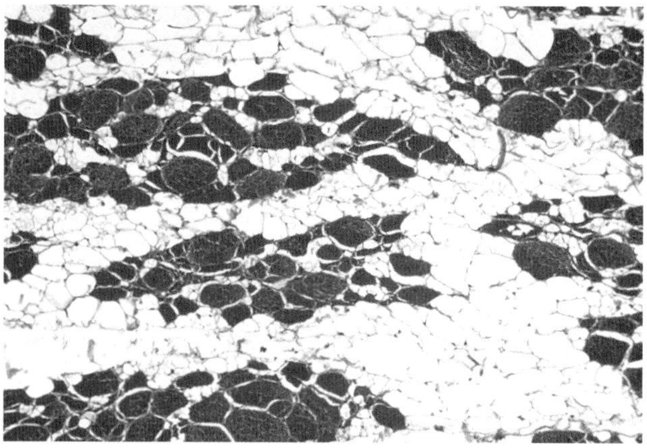

Figure 15-23 **Lipomatosis (Steatosis), Calf.** Lost myocytes have been replaced by mature adipocytes *(clear [nonstaining] areas)*. Islands of remaining myofibers have groups of angular atrophied fibers admixed with hypertrophied fibers, suggestive of denervation atrophy. Formalin fixation, H&E stain. (Courtesy Dr. M.D. McGavin, College of Veterinary Medicine, University of Tennessee.)

Box 15-5 Portals of Entry and Pathways of Spread Into the Muscular System

DIRECT

- Penetrating wounds
- Intramuscular injections
- Bone fracture causing trauma to adjacent muscle
- External pressure causing crush injury

HEMATOGENOUS

- Blood-borne pathogens, toxins, autoantibodies, and immune complexes
- Cytotoxic lymphocytes causing immune-mediated damage
- Other inflammatory cells

Portals of Entry/Pathways of Spread

Portals of entry and pathways of spread are summarized in Box 15-5. Injury to muscle can occur secondary to trauma or infection. Muscle lying superficially can be damaged by penetrating wounds, including those created by intramuscular injections (Fig. 15-24; see also Fig. 15-9, *B*), which can also allow entry of infectious agents. Muscles located deeply are often injured after bone fracture. Crush injuries from external forces cause extensive muscle damage, and excessive tension can cause muscle tearing. Muscles are endowed with an extensive vascular network that can allow entry of blood-borne pathogens, immune complexes, antibodies and toxins, and inflammatory cells.

Other routes by which muscle can become dysfunctional are summarized in Box 15-6. Some muscular disorders are genetically determined. Inherited or acquired dysfunction of motor neurons or nerves causes muscle injury in the form of atrophy. Toxins or an altered endocrine or electrolyte status can affect muscle, and physiologic damage can be caused by exhaustive or overexuberant exercise.

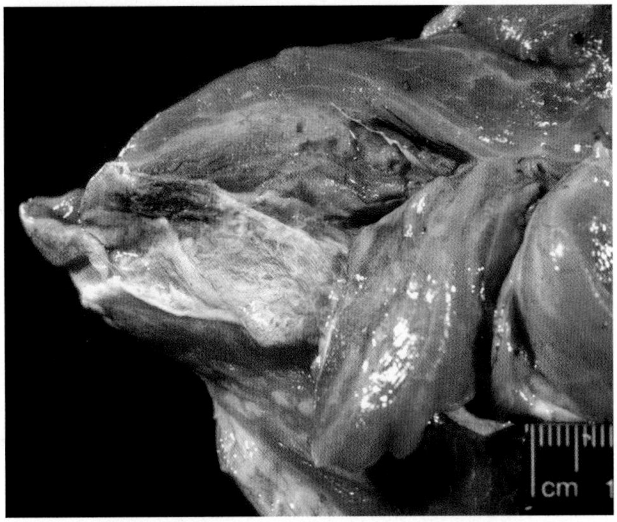

Figure 15-24 **Inflammation and Myofiber Necrosis, Injection Site, Muscles, Lateral Thigh, Cow.** Necrotic muscle has been stained green by the injected material, which has spread distally down the fascial plane between the two muscles from the original injection site *(top right)*. (Courtesy Dr. M.D. McGavin, College of Veterinary Medicine, University of Tennessee.)

Box 15-6 Other Causes of Muscle Dysfunction

PHYSIOLOGIC
Excessive muscle tension causing muscle rupture
Exercise-induced damage to myofibers
Loss of innervation
Loss of blood supply
Endocrine and electrolyte abnormalities

GENETIC
Inborn errors of metabolism
Genetic defects of myofiber structural components
Developmental defects

NUTRITIONAL/TOXIC
Deficiency of selenium and/or vitamin E
Toxic plants or plant products
Feed additives (ionophores)
Other toxins (e.g., some snake venoms)

Defense Mechanisms/Barrier Systems

Defense mechanisms and barrier systems are summarized in Box 15-7. The thick encircling fascia (epimysium) of many muscles provides some protection from penetrating injuries and from extension of adjacent infection. This fascia can, however, also contribute to injury under circumstances that lead to increased intramuscular pressure causing hypoxia (compartment syndrome). Tissue macrophages are not typically found in normal muscle but are recruited rapidly from circulating monocytes in the vasculature. Macrophages can cross even an intact basal lamina and effectively clear debris from damaged portions of myofibers, allowing for rapid restoration of the myocyte through satellite cell activation. Neutrophils and other inflammatory cells are also recruited from the bloodstream in response to injury or infection. The extensive vascular network of muscle includes extensive collateral circulatory pathways that render muscle relatively resistant to ischemic damage caused by thrombosis or thromboembolism. Despite the high vascular density of muscle, metastasis of neoplasms to muscle is quite rare. There is evidence that the capillary endothelium of skeletal muscle is inherently resistant to neoplastic cell adhesion and invasion.

Box 15-7 Defense Mechanisms and Barrier Systems of Skeletal Muscle

SKIN, SUBCUTIS, AND FASCIA
Form structural barriers to protect against external injury

VASCULATURE
Collateral circulation to protect against ischemia
Recruitment of monocytes that become tissue macrophages
Recruitment of neutrophils and other inflammatory cells
Capillary endothelium resistant to tumor metastasis

IMMUNOLOGIC RESPONSES
Innate humoral and cellular immunologic responses

OTHER
Adequate tissue antioxidant concentrations
Physiologic adaptation (e.g., hypertrophy, fiber type alteration)
Regenerative capacity of myofibers

Disorders of Domestic Animals

Types of Muscle Disease

Classification of muscle diseases based on lesions alone is not very satisfactory, and many classifications are based on cause (e.g., toxic myopathy or nutritional myopathy). An example of such a classification is given in Table 15-2. Myopathic conditions can be inherited or acquired. Inherited disorders can affect muscle metabolism or myofiber structure. Acquired muscle disease in livestock is often associated with nutritional deficiency or with ingestion of myotoxins, whereas acquired muscle disease in the dog is most often caused by immune-mediated inflammatory conditions. Other causes of acquired myopathies include ischemia, infectious agents, hormonal or electrolyte abnormalities, and trauma. There are also many neuropathic conditions that result in denervation atrophy (see peripheral nerve discussion). More information on most of the disorders described in this section can also be found under the appropriate species heading or in E-Appendix 15-1.

Degenerative

Degenerative myopathies are those resulting in segmental or global myofiber necrosis in which inflammatory cells are not the cause of the myofiber damage.

Disturbance of Circulation. Given the numerous capillary anastomosis and rich collateral circulation of skeletal muscle, only disorders that result in occlusion of a major artery or that cause widespread intramuscular vascular damage will result in myofiber necrosis (Box 15-8). Vascular occlusion of a major artery, most often aortoiliac thrombosis, occurs most commonly in cats (thromboembolism) and horses (mural thrombosis). Intramuscular vascular damage occurs in many species, and there are a variety of causes.

The basic factor in determining the effect of ischemia on muscle is the differential susceptibility of the various cells forming the muscle as a whole. Myofibers are the most sensitive, satellite cells less sensitive, and fibroblasts the least sensitive to anoxia. Thus obstruction of the blood supply to an area of muscle leads first to myofiber necrosis, then to the death of satellite cells, and finally to the death of all cells, including the stromal cells. The size of skeletal muscle infarcts depends on the size of the vessel obstructed and the

Table 15-2 Classification of Muscle Disease

Classification	Cause or Type of Disorder
Degenerative	Ischemia Nutritional Toxic Exertional Traumatic
Inflammatory	Bacterial Viral Parasitic Immune-mediated
Congenital and/or inherited	Anatomic defects Muscular dystrophy Congenital myopathy Myotonia Metabolic Malignant hyperthermia
Endocrine	Hypothyroidism Hypercortisolism
Electrolyte	Hypokalemia Hypernatremia Other electrolyte imbalances
Neuropathic	Peripheral neuropathy Motor neuronopathy
Neuromuscular junction disorders	Myasthenia gravis Botulism Tick paralysis
Neoplasia	Primary tumors (rhabdomyoma, rhabdomyosarcoma) Secondary tumors (hemangiosarcoma, fibrosarcoma, infiltrative lipoma, other tumor phenotypes) Metastatic tumors

Box 15-8 Causes of Muscle Ischemia

Occlusion of a major blood vessel
External pressure on a muscle
Swelling of a muscle in a nonexpandable compartment ("compartment syndrome")
Vasculitis/vasculopathy

duration of blockage. Because of the numerous anastomoses, blockage of capillaries causes less severe ischemia but can result in segmental myofiber necrosis, which is usually multifocal and if the cause is ongoing, polyphasic, with regenerating and necrotic myofibers. However, when larger arteries are blocked, whole areas of muscle, including the satellite cells, are killed, resulting in a monophasic necrosis and healing by fibrosis. Ischemia can also cause peripheral nerve damage and neuropathy, leading to denervation atrophy of intact myofibers.

Increased intramuscular pressure can occur in a recumbent animal of sufficient weight after a prolonged period of recumbency, because of either disease or general anesthesia. Myofiber necrosis caused by recumbency can occur because of (1) decreased blood flow as a result of compression of major arteries, (2) reperfusion injury causing massive calcium influx into muscle cells when the animal moves or is moved and the compression relieved, (3) increased intramuscular pressure causing compartment syndrome (see later definition), or (4) any combination of these factors. Localized myonecrosis caused by recumbency is common in horses, cattle, and pigs; occurs only in large breeds of dogs; and is virtually unheard of in cats. In downer cows, the weight of the body of the animal in sternal recumbency can cause ischemia of the pectoral muscles and of any muscles of the forelimbs or hind limbs that are tucked under the body. Ewes in advanced pregnancy with twins or triplets can develop an ischemic necrosis of the internal abdominal oblique muscle, which can lead to muscle rupture. Plaster casts or bandages that are too tight can put external pressure on muscles, leading to ischemia. The duration of ischemia determines the severity of necrosis and the success of regeneration (see the section on Necrosis and Regeneration). Postanesthetic myopathy is a monophasic, multifocal necrosis. In the downer cow, the lesions are multifocal to locally extensive (Fig. 15-25) and, depending on the duration since the onset of recumbency, can be either monophasic or polyphasic.

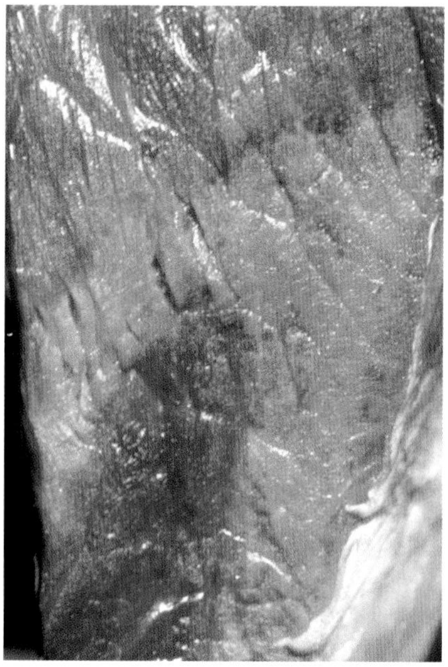

Figure 15-25 **Ischemic Necrosis, Downer Cow Syndrome, Pectoral Muscle, Cow.** Increased intramuscular pressure during prolonged periods of recumbency has resulted in localized muscle pallor (lighter-colored areas of muscle) from myofiber necrosis secondary to decreased blood flow caused by compression of arteries. (Courtesy Dr. M.D. McGavin, College of Veterinary Medicine, University of Tennessee.)

Any severe insult, whether it be ischemia caused by recumbency or another myodegenerative disorder that causes myonecrosis within a muscle covered by a tight and nonexpansible fascia, can result in ischemic injury because early in the necrosis, there is increased intramuscular pressure. The resulting compromise of blood circulation leads to ischemic myodegeneration, which is known as *compartment syndrome*. The phenomenon of compartment syndrome is best illustrated in the anterior tibial muscle of human beings after strenuous exercise. This condition is believed to be a consequence of swelling of the anterior tibial muscle, which is surrounded anteriorly by the inelastic anterior fascial sheath and posteriorly by the tibia. Swelling impedes blood supply, resulting in ischemia. A similar phenomenon occurs in muscles surrounded by tight fascia in animals, particularly horses. Horses that are recumbent because of general anesthesia can develop compartment syndrome affecting gluteal or lateral triceps muscles. Horses can also develop compartment syndrome in gluteal muscles because of exertional rhabdomyolysis and in temporal and masseter muscles because of selenium deficiency. Compartment syndrome is also possible in the temporal and masseter muscles of dogs with masticatory myositis.

Damage to intramuscular blood vessels will also cause myofiber necrosis. Vasculitis can cause areas of muscle damage (e.g., in horses with immune-mediated purpura hemorrhagica because of *Streptococcus equi* infection [see Fig. 15-32] and in pigs with erysipelas). Viral diseases that target blood vessels of many organs, such as bluetongue in sheep, can also affect muscle. Exotoxins produced by clostridial organisms cause myositis and severe localized vascular damage, leading to hemorrhage and myofiber necrosis. The familial myopathy of Gelbvieh cattle is characterized by fibrinoid necrosis of intramuscular blood vessels and associated myonecrosis.

Nutritional Deficiency. Myofibers are particularly sensitive to nutritional deficiencies that result in the loss of antioxidant defense mechanisms. Nutritional myopathies are most common in livestock, including cattle, horses, sheep, and goats (Table 15-3). Although nutritional myopathy of livestock is often referred to as *selenium/vitamin E deficiency*, in the vast majority of cases, it is deficiency of selenium that is the cause of myofiber degeneration. The trace mineral selenium is a vital component of the glutathione peroxidase system, which helps to protect cells from oxidative injury. The high oxygen requirement combined with contractile activity makes striated muscle, both skeletal and cardiac, particularly sensitive to oxidative injury. Neonatal animals, which rely on stores of selenium accumulated during gestation, are most frequently affected. Affected muscle is pale as a result of necrosis (see Fig. 15-39), thus the common name *white muscle disease*. As should be evident from the previous discussion, a gross observation of pale muscle is not specific for necrosis caused by nutritional deficiency; therefore the term *nutritional myopathy* is much preferred.

Toxic Myopathies. Livestock are the animals most prone to develop a degenerative myopathy from the ingestion of a toxin (see Table 15-3). Myotoxins can be present in plants in pastures or hay and in plants or plant products in processed feed. Examples of toxic plants and plant products include *Cassia* (coffee senna), *Karwinskia* (coyotillo), *Eupatorium* (white snakeroot), *Acer negundo* (box elder tree) seeds, and gossypol present in cottonseed. Clinical signs are weakness, often leading to recumbency, and are accompanied by a moderate to severe increase in serum muscle enzyme concentrations. Gross and histologic findings of multifocal necrosis that can be either monophasic or polyphasic are typical. Diagnosis is based on identification of causative plants within feed, pasture, or stomach contents or, when available, detection of toxic compounds in stomach content or liver.

Ionophore antibiotics, such as monensin, lasalocid, maduramicin, and narasin, are often added to ruminant feeds to enhance growth. Ionophores form lipid-soluble dipolar reversible complexes with cations and allow movement of cations across cell membranes, often against the concentration gradient. This causes a disruption of ionic equilibrium that can be detrimental, especially to excitable tissue such as the nervous system, heart, and skeletal muscle. Ionophore toxicity results in calcium overload and death of skeletal (see Figs. 15-11, *B*, and 15-33) and cardiac muscle. Most domestic ruminants are quite tolerant of moderate ionophore levels, but toxicity occurs at very high levels. Most cases of ionophore toxicity involve the ingestion of monensin. The LD_{50} (the dose at which 50% of animals die) of monensin in cattle is 50 to 80 mg/kg, and the LD_{50} for sheep and goats is 12 to 24 mg/kg. Horses are exquisitely sensitive to ionophores and even very low levels are toxic, with an LD_{50} for monensin of only 2 to 3 mg/kg of body weight.

Exertional Myopathies. The ionic and physical events associated with myofiber contraction can under certain circumstances predispose a myofiber to necrosis. Exercise-induced myonecrosis, which can be massive, can occur because of simple overexertion. This outcome is well known in the capture and restraint of nondomesticated species, a syndrome known as *capture myopathy*. More often, however, exercise-induced myofiber damage occurs in animals with preexisting conditions such as selenium deficiency, muscular dystrophy, severe electrolyte depletion, or glycogen storage disease. The term *exertional rhabdomyolysis* (also known as *exertional myopathy*, *azoturia*, *setfast*, *blackwater*, *Monday morning disease*, and *tying up*) has long been applied to a syndrome recognized in horses (see Fig. 15-35). Only recently have underlying myopathic conditions been identified as the most common predisposing cause of equine exertional rhabdomyolysis (see Disorders of Horses). A similar disorder affects working dogs such as racing sled dogs and greyhounds, the cause of which is still unclear.

Trauma. External trauma to muscle includes crush injury, lacerations and surgical incisions, tearing caused by excessive stretching or exercise, burns, gunshot and arrow wounds, and certain injections. Some of these result in complete or partial rupture of a large muscle. The diaphragm is the most common muscle to rupture and in dogs and cats is most often the result of a sudden increase in intraabdominal pressure such as from being hit by a car. In horses, diaphragmatic rupture is thought to occur most often during falls in which the pressure of the abdominal viscera causes diaphragmatic damage. A partial rupture of a muscle results in a tear in the fascial sheath, through which the muscle can herniate during contraction. In racing greyhounds, spontaneous rupture of muscles, such as the longissimus, quadriceps, biceps femoris, gracilis, triceps brachii, and gastrocnemius, can occur during strenuous exercise. In horses, damage to the origin of the gastrocnemius muscle has been linked to overexertion during exercise or while struggling to rise. Tearing of muscle fibers occurs in the adductor muscles of the hind limbs of cattle doing the "splits" (sudden bilateral abduction) on a slippery floor. Because there is often extensive disruption of the myofibers'

Table 15-3 Nutritional and Toxic Myopathies

Disorder	Species Affected	Cause
Nutritional myopathy	Horses, cattle, sheep, goats, camelids, pigs	Selenium or (less commonly) vitamin E deficiency
Ionophore toxicity	Horses, cattle, sheep, goats, pigs	Monensin, other ionophores used as feed additives
Plant toxicity	Horses, cattle, sheep, goats, pigs	*Cassia occidentalis*, other toxic plants; gossypol in cottonseed products
Pasture-associated myopathy (United Kingdom, Midwestern United States)	Horses	Box elder tree *(Acer negundo)* toxicity

basal laminae, most of the healing is accomplished by fibrosis. If muscle trauma is accompanied by fractures of bones and the animal moves the limb, further trauma by laceration by sharp bone fragments can result.

An abnormal response to localized muscle trauma is thought to be a possible underlying cause of two uncommon reactions of muscle: myositis ossificans and musculoaponeurotic fibromatosis. The term *myositis ossificans* is a misnomer, because the lesion does not involve inflammation, but it has attained the status of acceptance by common usage. Myositis ossificans is a focal lesion usually confined to a single muscle and has been seen in horses, dogs, and human beings. The lesion is essentially a focal zone of fibrosis with osseous metaplasia, often with a zonal pattern. The central zone contains proliferating undifferentiated cells and fibroblasts; the middle one, osteoblasts depositing osteoid and immature bone; and the outer one, trabecular bone, which may be being remodeled by osteoclasts. These lesions can cause pain and lameness, which are often cured by surgical excision. A connective tissue disorder in cats, fibrodysplasia ossificans progressiva, has been inappropriately called *myositis ossificans*. Musculoaponeurotic fibromatosis has so far been described only in horses and human beings. It is a progressive intramuscular fibromatosis that has also been called a *desmoid tumor*. Musculoaponeurotic fibromatosis is not, however, considered to be a true neoplastic process. Progressive dissecting intramuscular fibrosis accompanied by myofiber atrophy are the characteristic features. In most cases, the extent of intramuscular involvement makes surgical excision impossible, although wide excision of early lesions has proved to be curative.

Inflammatory Myopathies (Myositis, Myositides [Plural])

In addition to the misnomer "myositis ossificans," the term *myositis* has been inappropriately applied to various other veterinary disorders, such as exertional and nutritional myopathy, in the horse. These two disorders are degenerative myopathies, not inflammatory myopathies. It is vitally important to distinguish between a true myositis and a degenerative myopathy in which there is a secondary inflammatory response. In the normal response to the myofiber necrosis, the necrotic segment is infiltrated by macrophages recruited from the circulating monocyte population (see Figs. 15-12, B, and 15-13 A), which phagocytose the cellular debris. Severe acute necrotizing myopathy can also be accompanied by a certain degree of infiltrating lymphocytes, plasma cells, neutrophils, and eosinophils. Cytokines released from damaged muscle fibers are likely to recruit a variety of inflammatory cells under various circumstances, but these cells are not involved in causing the muscle cell damage. True myositis occurs only when inflammatory cells are directly responsible for initiating and maintaining myofiber injury and when inflammation is directed at the myofibers and not at the stroma. In some cases, it may take careful evaluation of the overall tissue changes, an understanding of the probable underlying cause, and years of experience with muscle pathology to differentiate a florid cellular response with macrophages on a "cleanup" mission from true inflammation. Lymphocytic myositis must also be distinguished from lymphoma involving skeletal muscle (see the section on Neoplasia).

Bacterial. Bacterial infections of muscle are not uncommon, particularly in livestock. Bacteria can cause suppurative and necrotizing, suppurative and fibrosing, hemorrhagic, or granulomatous lesions (Table 15-4). Bacterial infection can be introduced by direct penetration (wounds or injections), hematogenously, or by spread from an adjacent cellulitis, fasciitis, tendonitis, arthritis, or osteomyelitis (see the section on Portals of Entry).

Table 15-4 Bacterial Causes of Myositis and Neuromuscular Junction Disease

Infectious Agent	Species Affected
Clostridium spp. causing myositis (e.g., *Cl. septicum*, *Cl. chauvoei*, *Cl. sordellii*, *Cl. novyi*)	Horses, cattle, sheep, goats, pigs
Clostridium botulinum causing neuromuscular junction disease	Horses, cattle, sheep, goats, dogs
Pyogenic bacteria causing myositis (e.g., *Trueperella* [*Arcanobacterium*] *pyogenes*, *Corynebacterium pseudotuberculosis*)	Horses, cattle, sheep, goats, pigs, cats
Bacteria causing fibrosing and granulomatous myositis (e.g., *Actinomyces bovis*, *Actinobacillus lignieresii*)	Cattle, sheep, goats, pigs

Various clostridial species, particularly *Clostridium perfringens*, *Clostridium chauvoei*, *Clostridium septicum*, and *Clostridium novyi*, can elaborate toxins that damage myofibers and intramuscular vasculature, resulting in hemorrhagic myonecrosis (see Figs. 15-31 and 15-37). Toxemia is typical and often lethal. *Clostridial myositis* is most common in cattle and horses. *Clostridial myositis* has also been called *gas gangrene* and *malignant edema* in horses and *blackleg* in cattle.

Pyogenic bacteria introduced into a muscle usually cause localized suppuration and myofiber necrosis. This may resolve completely or become localized to form an abscess. In some cases, the infection can spread down the fascial planes (see Fig. 15-24). For example, a nonsterile intramuscular injection into the gluteal muscles of cattle can cause an infection that extends down the fascial planes of the muscles of the femur and tibia and erupts to the surface through a sinus proximal to the tarsus. Although the majority of inflammation involves fascial planes, some bacteria extend into and cause necrosis of adjacent muscle fasciculi. *Streptococcus zooepidemicus* (horses), *Trueperella* (*Arcanobacterium*) *pyogenes* (cattle and sheep), and *Corynebacterium pseudotuberculosis* (horses, sheep, and goats) are common causes of muscle abscesses. After bite wounds from other cats, cats can develop cellulitis caused by *Pasteurella multocida* that extends into the adjacent muscle.

Bacteria causing single or multiple granulomas (focal or multifocal granulomatous myositis) are relatively uncommon. Most such lesions are caused by *Mycobacterium bovis* (tuberculosis), usually in cattle and pigs, but this disease is rare in North America.

Chronic fibrosing nodular myositis of the tongue musculature in cattle is the result of infection with *Actinobacillus lignieresii* (wooden tongue) or *Actinomyces bovis* (the agent causing lumpy jaw). A similar lesion caused by *Staphylococcus aureus* is known as *botryomycosis* and is most commonly seen in horses and pigs. It is most often wound related and can occur at a variety of sites. Histologically, actinobacillosis, actinomycosis, and botryomycosis are similar in that the lesions are encapsulated inflammatory lesions containing a central focus of "radiating clubs" of amorphous eosinophilic material associated with bacteria and neutrophils (Splendore-Hoeppli reaction). Neutrophils admixed with macrophages (pyogranulomatous inflammation) can also be seen. Gram-stained tissue can be used to differentiate between the clusters of Gram-positive cocci in *Staphylococcus* infection, the Gram-positive bacilli causing actinomycosis (*Actinomyces bovis*), and the Gram-negative bacilli causing actinobacillosis (*Actinobacillus lignieresii*).

Viral. Relatively few of these are recognized in veterinary medicine. Spontaneous ones are listed in Table 15-5. Gross lesions may or may not be visible and, if present, are small, poorly defined foci or streaks. Muscle lesions induced by viruses are either infarcts secondary to a vasculitis, as seen in bluetongue in sheep, or multifocal necrosis, presumably because of a direct effect of the virus on the myofibers.

Parasitic. Parasitic infections of the skeletal muscles of domestic animals are not uncommon and include protozoal organisms and nematodes. The most important ones are listed in Table 15-6 and are discussed under the appropriate species heading. Most parasitic diseases have little pathologic or economic importance, with the exceptions of *Neospora caninum*, *Hepatozoon americanum*, and *Trypanosoma cruzi* in dogs and *Trichinella spiralis* in pigs.

As the name *Sarcocystis* suggests, intramyofiber protozoal cysts caused by *Sarcocystis* spp. are a common finding. This protozoal organism is a stage in the life cycle of an intestinal coccidium of carnivores that uses birds, reptiles, rodents, pigs, and herbivores as an intermediate host. Ingestion of oocysts by an intermediate host releases sporozoites that penetrate through the intestinal wall, enter blood vessels, and are hematogenously disseminated and invade tissue, including muscle. This parasite rarely causes clinical disease and is therefore most often considered an incidental finding. *Sarcocystis* infection of muscle is seen most often in horses, cattle, and small ruminants and occasionally in cats. Because they are intracellular, cysts are protected from the host's defense mechanisms; thus there is no inflammatory response (Fig. 15-26).

Immune-Mediated. Immunologically induced myositis, not associated with vascular injury, has been recognized primarily in the dog. Rarely, immune-mediated myositis occurs in cats and horses. Infiltrating lymphocytes, most often cytotoxic T lymphocytes, are the cause of myofiber injury. Although cytotoxic T lymphocytes are the effector cells causing myofiber damage, the inflammatory infiltrate is a mixture of lymphocyte types. The characteristic histologic pattern of immune-mediated myositis is an interstitial and perivascular lymphocytic infiltration (Fig. 15-27, A; see also Fig. 15-47), often with invasion of intact myofibers by lymphocytes (Fig. 15-27, B). A variety of forms of immune-mediated myositis occur in the dog and can be localized to specific muscles, presumably because of unique myosin isoforms within those muscles. These are listed in Table 15-7. Acquired myasthenia gravis is also an immune-mediated disease and is included in this table for completeness, but this is a disorder causing damage to the neuromuscular junction rather than to myofibers. In cats, feline immunodeficiency virus infection is a cause of immune-mediated myositis. In horses, lesions consistent with immune-mediated myositis are occasionally found after exposure to *Streptococcus equi* ssp. *equi* or infection with equine influenza virus. Note that small perivascular and interstitial infiltrates of lymphocytes, with no apparent myofiber damage, are a frequent incidental finding in equine muscle.

Immune-mediated vasculitis resulting in muscle injury occurs in horses and is known as *purpura hemorrhagica*. Purpura hemorrhagica has been classically associated with *Streptococcus equi* ssp. *equi*, but other bacteria, such as *Corynebacterium pseudotuberculosis*, can also cause purpura hemorrhagica.

Table 15-5 Viral Myopathies

	RNA VIRUSES	
Disease	**Family**	**Causal Agent**
Porcine encephalomyelitis	Picornaviridae	Enterovirus
Foot-and-mouth disease	Picornaviridae	Aphthovirus
Bluetongue	Reoviridae	Orbivirus
Akabane disease	Bunyaviridae	Akabane virus

Table 15-6 Parasitic Myopathies

Infectious Agent	Type of agent	Species Affected
Sarcocystis spp.	Protozoan	Horses, cattle, sheep, goats, camelids, pigs
Trichinella spiralis	Nematode	Pigs
Neospora caninum	Protozoan	Dogs, fetal cattle
Trypanosoma cruzi	Protozoan	Dogs
Cysticercus spp.	Cestode (larval form)	Cattle, sheep, goats, pigs
Nematode larval migrans	Nematode	Dogs
Hepatozoon americanum	Protozoan	Dogs

Congenital and Inherited Disorders

Muscle is subject to numerous hereditary, congenital, and neonatal defects (E-Box 15-1). Muscular disorders that are apparent at birth are congenital, but they may or may not be inherited. Inherited disorders can manifest at birth or soon thereafter, or they may not be apparent for many years. Molecular biologic studies and development of molecular genetic tests have greatly enhanced our understanding of several muscular disorders of animals and the ability to detect affected and carrier animals.

Anatomic Defects. Anatomic defects in skeletal muscle are apparent at birth or soon thereafter. These defects can be either genetic or acquired and result from either abnormal in utero muscle development or abnormal innervation.

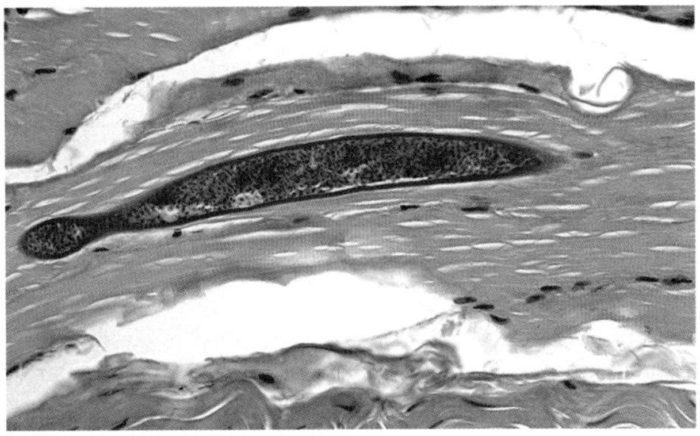

Figure 15-26 **Sarcocystosis, Skeletal Muscle, Longitudinal Section, Cow.** The horizontally elongate encysted intramyofiber protozoan *(dark purple structure)* is characteristic of *Sarcocystis* spp. There is no associated inflammation. These parasites are common in the muscles of many species of domestic animals and are usually an incidental finding. Formalin fixation, H&E stain. (Courtesy Dr. M.D. McGavin, College of Veterinary Medicine, University of Tennessee.)

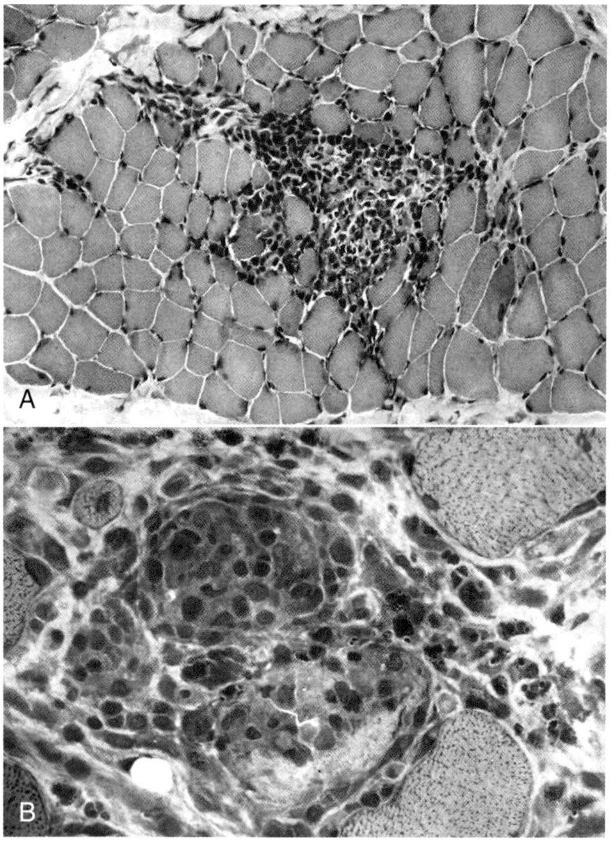

Figure 15-27 **Immune-Mediated Myositis, Canine Polymyositis, Skeletal Muscle, Transverse Sections, Dog. A,** There is a dense interstitial infiltrate of primarily mononuclear inflammatory cells. Frozen section, H&E stain. **B,** Note the interstitial infiltrate of mononuclear inflammatory cells and mononuclear cells that have invaded intact myofibers causing myofiber necrosis. Frozen section, modified Gomori's trichrome stain. (**A** and **B** courtesy Dr. B.J. Cooper, College of Veterinary Medicine, Oregon State University.)

Table 15-7 Immune-Mediated Muscle Disorders

Disorder	Species Affected
Purpura hemorrhagica	Horses
Viral-associated	Horses, cats
Polymyositis	Dogs, horses (rare)
Masticatory myositis	Dogs
Extraocular muscle myositis	Dogs
Acquired myasthenia gravis	Dogs, cats

Innervation Defects. Congenital defects in the lower motor neuron system, involving motor neurons or peripheral nerves, result in severe alteration of myofiber development. Denervation occurring in fetal and neonatal animals can result in very complex muscle lesions because of the importance of innervation in myofiber development and maturation. Depending on the nature of the nervous system defect, muscular lesions can reflect failure of innervation, denervation of previously innervated fibers, or a combination of both. The most common example of this is arthrogryposis in cattle and sheep in which in utero infection or toxin ingestion causes nervous system lesions that lead to failure of innervation or to denervation of skeletal muscle. In addition, a disorder thought to have a genetic basis has been reported in black Angus cattle and results in failure of innervation of skeletal muscle. Failure of innervation or severe denervation injury in utero most often result in failure of the myofibers to develop and their subsequent replacement by adipose tissue (fatty infiltration). This outcome can be severe in affected muscle and may be the basis for some cases of congenital muscular steatosis in livestock (see Figs. 15-9, *D*, and 15-23).

Genetic Defects. Congenital muscular hyperplasia (double muscling) is a genetic disease causing a congenital anatomic skeletal muscle defect (increased number of myofibers) in cattle, dogs, and children. This disorder is caused by defects in the myostatin gene, which controls in utero muscle development. There is more information on this disease in E-Appendix 15-1. With continued selective breeding and advancement in molecular biologic techniques, it is likely that other genetic defects affecting muscle structure may occur or be recognized.

Failure of Normal Development. In addition to failure of myofiber maturation caused by innervation defects, inherent myofibrillar developmental defects can occur. This is exemplified by myofibrillar hypoplasia causing splay leg in neonatal pigs. A similar condition has been reported in a calf.

Congenital defects in the diaphragmatic muscle (diaphragmatic hernia) can occur in all species but are most well documented in dogs and rabbits. A genetic basis with a multifactorial inheritance is suspected. Clinical signs of respiratory distress caused by herniation of abdominal viscera into the thoracic cavity generally occur at or soon after birth. Defects in the left dorsolateral and central portions of the diaphragm because of failure of closure of the left pleuroperitoneal canal are most common.

Muscular Dystrophy. The term *muscular dystrophy* has been grossly misused in the veterinary literature. Using the definition applied to human beings, muscular dystrophy should only be applied to inherited, progressive, degenerative primary diseases of the myofiber characterized histologically by ongoing myofiber necrosis and regeneration (polyphasic necrosis). Several types of muscular dystrophy occur in human beings and animals. The enormous recent advances in genetic and molecular characterization of muscle diseases have resulted in defining their exact genetic defects, such as those in the dystrophin gene responsible for Duchenne's muscular dystrophy and trinucleotide repeat sequences in myotonic dystrophy, and in the reclassification of others. Similarly, reevaluation of some inherited disorders previously classified as muscular dystrophy, such as muscular dystrophy in sheep and cattle, suggests that they would be better classified as progressive congenital myopathies.

Congenital Myopathies. Those inherited disorders of muscle that do not qualify as anatomic defects, muscular dystrophy, myotonia, or a metabolic myopathy (see later discussion) are classified as congenital myopathies. These include structural defects leading to abnormal myofiber cytoarchitecture. In some cases, the defective gene is known, whereas the cause of others remains undetermined.

Myotonia (Channelopathies). Myotonia is defined as the inability of skeletal muscle fibers to relax, resulting in spasmodic contraction. Various inherited myotonic conditions have been recognized in human beings and animals for many years. Only recently has the basis for many of these myopathies been determined. Most have been found to be related to inherited defects resulting in abnormal ion channel function. Maintenance of ionic equilibrium and control of the ionic fluxes of excitable tissue, such as muscle, are critical to normal muscle functioning. A variety of sarcolemmal ion channels exist that control fluxes of ions such as sodium, potassium, chloride, and calcium. Defective sodium or chloride channels most often result in myotonia.

Metabolic Myopathies. Inherited disorders of muscle metabolism (see E-Box 15-1) are characterized by reduced muscle cell energy production. Clinical signs include exercise intolerance, exercise-induced muscle cramps, and rhabdomyolysis (acute segmental myofiber necrosis). Metabolic defects can involve glycogen metabolism, fatty acid metabolism, or mitochondrial function. Metabolic disorders often cause increased blood lactate after exercise. Inheritance patterns vary. Glycolytic, glycogenolytic, and nonmitochondrial DNA–encoded enzyme defects are generally inherited in an autosomal recessive manner. Defects involving mitochondrial DNA–encoded enzymes are inherited through the dam because all mitochondria are contributed by the oocyte.

The pathways of glycolysis and glycogenolysis are complex, involving a cascade of enzymatic reactions. Deficiency of a glycolytic or glycogenolytic enzyme leads to accumulation of glycogen and in some cases glycogen-related proteoglycans. There are many different types of glycogen storage diseases, and their categorization is dependent on which enzyme is deficient. Of the types of glycogenoses recognized in human beings, five types (II, III, IV, V, and VII) cause glycogen accumulation in muscle. Of the glycogenoses affecting muscle, only types II (acid maltase deficiency), IV (glycogen branching enzyme deficiency), V (myophosphorylase deficiency), and VII (phosphofructokinase deficiency) have so far been recognized in animals. Storage diseases in which glycogen accumulates in muscle have been described in horses, cattle, sheep, dogs, and cats.

Inherited lipid storage myopathies have not yet been described in animals, although dogs appear to have a predilection for development of neuromuscular weakness because of acquired lipid storage myopathy with concurrent reduction in skeletal muscle carnitine activity. Mitochondrial myopathies are rarely recognized in animals, perhaps because of the difficulty in confirming mitochondrial defects. A few such disorders have been described in dogs, and a mitochondrial myopathy has been reported in one Arabian horse. Mitochondrial disorders may affect only muscle, or muscle involvement may be part of an encephalomyopathic condition.

Malignant Hyperthermia. Malignant hyperthermia (MH) is a condition characterized by unregulated release of calcium from the sarcoplasmic reticulum, leading to excessive myofiber contraction that generates heat, resulting in a severe increase in body temperature. MH is often fatal. In human beings, pigs, horses, and dogs, a congenital defect in the sarcoplasmic reticulum calcium-release channel, the ryanodine receptor, causes dysregulation of excitation-contraction coupling leading to MH. Episodes in affected individuals can be triggered by general anesthetic agents, especially halothane, or by stress, thus the name *porcine stress syndrome* for the disorder in pigs (see Fig. 15-42).

An MH-like condition can also occur because of other myopathic conditions, especially those that result in uncoupling of mitochondrial oxidative phosphorylation from the electron transport chain. Inherently uncoupled mitochondria within brown fat are the physiologic basis for production of heat during breakdown of this fat in neonates, and pathologically uncoupled or loosely coupled mitochondria in muscle as a result of an underlying myopathy release energy as heat.

Gross and microscopic lesions are described in the discussion on the disorder in the section on Disorders of Pigs.

Endocrine and Electrolyte Abnormalities

Various endocrinologic abnormalities can result in myopathic conditions (Table 15-8). The most common are hypercortisolism and hypothyroidism in dogs. In horses, pituitary hyperfunction resulting in Cushing's disease also causes muscle disease. In most cases of endocrine myopathy, the end result is myofiber atrophy, particularly of type 2 fibers. A unique syndrome of muscle hypertrophy and pseudomyotonia occurs in dogs associated with hypercortisolism. Endocrine myopathies can also be complicated by the fact that endocrinopathy can also cause pathologic changes in peripheral nerves, leading to a mixture of myopathic (type 2 fiber atrophy) and neuropathic changes (denervation atrophy and alteration in fiber-type pattern) within muscle. Denervation followed by reinnervation leading to fiber-type grouping can be seen in dogs with chronic hypercortisolism (see Fig. 15-18, *B*) and hypothyroidism.

Table 15-8 Myopathies Caused by Endocrine and Electrolyte Abnormalities

Disorder	Species Affected
Hypothyroidism	Dogs
Hypercortisolism	Dogs
Hypokalemia	Cattle, cats
Hypophosphatemia	Cattle
Hypernatremia	Cats
Hypocalcemia	Cattle
Hypothalamic/pituitary dysfunction	Horses

Normal electrolyte status is vital to normal skeletal muscle function. Hypocalcemia, hypokalemia, hypernatremia, and hypophosphatemia can cause profound skeletal muscle weakness, sometimes associated with myofiber necrosis, in various species.

Neuropathic and Neuromuscular Junction Disorders

Dysfunction of the lower motor neurons, peripheral nerves, or neuromuscular junction can have profound effects on muscle function.

Neuropathic Disorders. There are many peripheral nerve disorders and a few motor neuron disorders that can lead to denervation atrophy of muscle in animals. These can be inherited or acquired. Long nerves, such as the sciatic and left recurrent laryngeal nerves, appear to be particularly sensitive to development of acquired neuropathy. Many of the peripheral nerve disorders of animals are discussed in Chapter 14. Characteristic features of denervation atrophy are described in the section on Dysfunction/Responses to Injury, Alterations in Myofiber Size, Atrophy.

Neuromuscular Junction Disorders. The neuromuscular junction is a modification of the postsynaptic myofiber membrane. At the neuromuscular junction, the membrane is folded to increase surface area and is studded with specialized ion channels known as *acetylcholine receptors*. After arrival of an action potential at the distal end of a motor nerve, the terminal axons release acetylcholine, which diffuses across the synaptic space to bind to the acetylcholine receptors. Binding opens these channels, leading to sodium influx, which initiates the skeletal muscle action potential that culminates in muscle contraction. Acetylcholine is rapidly degraded by acetylcholinesterase released from the postsynaptic membrane, which prevents continued stimulation and thus contraction of the muscle fiber.

Disorders that impair the ability of nerve impulses to travel across the neuromuscular junction have profound effects on skeletal muscle function. Technically, however, the myofibers are still innervated, so denervation atrophy does not occur and no light microscopic abnormalities in the muscle or nerve are present. Various neurotoxins (i.e., in snake and spider venom and in curare-containing plants) and drugs can affect the neuromuscular junction, but the most common neuromuscular junction disorders affecting animals are myasthenia gravis, botulism, and tick paralysis.

Myasthenia Gravis. Myasthenia gravis can be either acquired or congenital. Acquired myasthenia gravis is an immune-mediated disorder caused by circulating autoantibodies against skeletal muscle acetylcholine receptors (Fig. 15-28). Binding of these antibodies to the acetylcholine receptor on the postsynaptic membrane leads to a severe decrease in the number of functional receptors. The mechanisms by which antibodies damage these receptors are (1) direct damage to the neuromuscular junction, which may be visible with electron microscopy as simplification of the folding of the membrane, and (2) formation of cross-linked antibodies leading to receptor internalization. Sufficient functional acetylcholine receptors are present to initially allow normal neuromuscular transmission, but if there is sustained muscular activity the decrease in the number of available receptors leads to progressive weakness and collapse. Therefore acquired myasthenia gravis results in episodic collapse, and repetitive nerve stimulation causes a characteristic rapid decrease in amplitude of the muscle compound motor action potential. Diagnosis of myasthenia gravis can also be made after intravenous injection of cholinesterase inhibitors such as edrophonium chloride (Tensilon, ICN Pharmaceuticals, Costa Mesa, CA) in collapsed animals. The reduction in cholinesterase activity leads to more active acetylcholine being available within the synapse and rapid, although transient, restoration of skeletal muscle contraction. Detection of autoantibodies to acetylcholine receptors in the blood confirms the diagnosis of acquired myasthenia gravis.

The origin of the autoantibodies causing myasthenia gravis is not always known, but there is a strong link between thymic abnormalities and development of myasthenia gravis in both human beings and animals. Specialized cells within the thymic medulla, known as *myoid cells*, express skeletal muscle proteins, including those of the acetylcholine receptor. It is thought that these cells participate in development of self-tolerance. Abnormalities of the thymus, most commonly thymoma in animals and thymic follicular hyperplasia in human beings, can lead to loss of self-tolerance to acetylcholine receptors. In such cases, removal of the abnormal thymus can result in restoration of normal neuromuscular junction activity. When thymic abnormalities are not present, treatment with long-acting anticholinesterase agents and in some cases immunosuppressive agents, such as corticosteroids, is necessary.

Congenital myasthenia gravis is an inherited disorder that is much less common than acquired myasthenia gravis. To date it has been described only in human beings, dogs, and cats. Animals with congenital myasthenia gravis are born with defective neuromuscular junctions that often have a decreased membrane surface area, best visualized with electron microscopy, and as a consequence an inherently reduced acetylcholine receptor density. Such animals may be normal at birth because there are sufficient functional acetylcholine receptors to support muscle contraction in a neonate. However, with rapid postnatal growth, clinical signs of profound, sustained, and progressive weakness occur as a consequence of insufficient functional receptors to support the function of growing muscles.

Botulism. Botulism is a neuromuscular disorder caused by the exotoxin of the bacterium *Clostridium botulinum*. Botulinum toxin is considered one of the deadliest of the known toxins. Botulism is characterized by profound generalized flaccid paralysis. Seven serologically distinct but structurally similar forms of botulinum toxin are designated A, B, C, D, E, F, and G. Sensitivity to these toxin types varies among different species. Dogs are most sensitive to type C toxin, ruminants to types C and D, and horses to types B and C.

Botulinum toxin consists of a light chain and a heavy chain linked by a disulfide bond. Binding of botulinum toxin to receptors on the presynaptic terminals of peripheral nerves is followed by endocytosis of the toxin. Within the endocytotic vesicle of the terminal nerve, the disulfide bond is cleaved, and the released light chain is translocated into the axonal cytoplasm (see Fig. 4-27). Botulinum toxin light chains are metalloproteinases. Numerous proteins are involved in the release of acetylcholine from presynaptic vesicles, and botulinum toxin blocks release of acetylcholine by irreversible enzymatic cleavage of one or more of these proteins. Different forms of botulinum toxin affect different proteins, but the end result is the same. Active neuromuscular junctions are the most

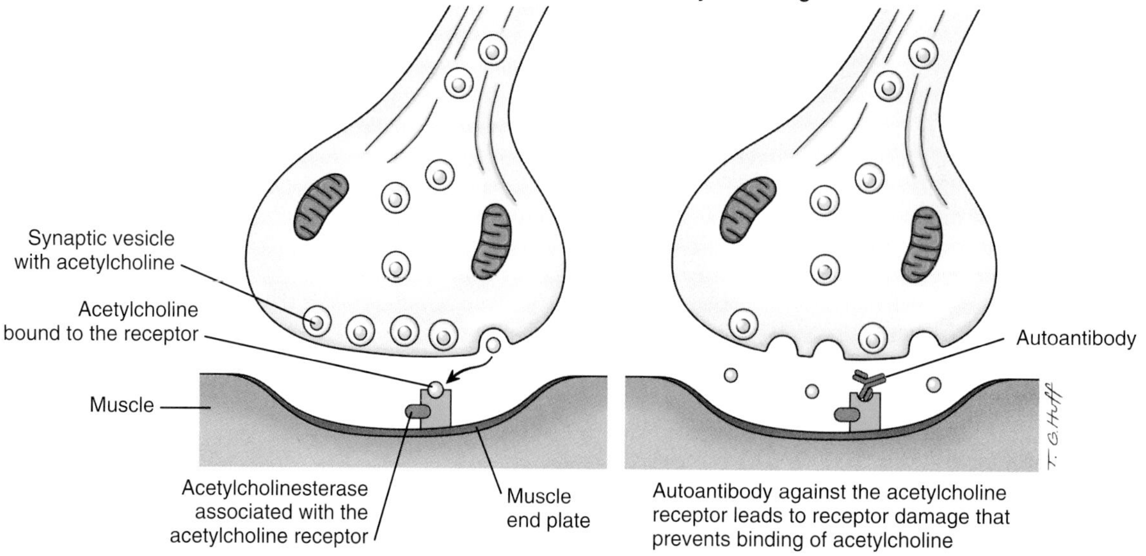

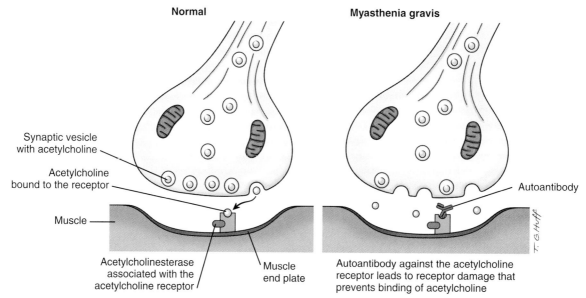

Figure 15-28 **Pathogenesis of Acquired (Immune-Mediated) Myasthenia Gravis.** Myoneural junction in normal muscle *(left panel)*. When acetylcholine binds to acetylcholine receptors, a signal from the receptor opens ligand-gated sodium channels in the muscle cell membrane leading to contraction. Myoneural junction in myasthenia gravis *(right panel)*. Autoantibody directed against acetylcholine receptors causes receptor injury and blocks the binding of acetylcholine to the receptor, resulting in episodic weakness and collapse.

sensitive, which has led to the use of low concentrations of locally injected botulinum toxin as a treatment for localized muscular disorders resulting in spasm.

Clostridium botulinum spores are commonly present in the gastrointestinal tract of animals and in the soil. Under favorable anaerobic and alkalinic conditions, these spores become active, with resultant toxin production. Botulism can occur because of ingestion of preformed toxin, such as in feed contaminated by dead rodents or soil-borne organisms, or from toxin produced by *Clostridium botulinum* organisms within the gastrointestinal tract or superficial wounds (Box 15-9). Dogs and cats are the species most likely to ingest dead rodents containing botulinum toxin and are quite resistant to developing botulism. In veterinary medicine, horses are the most sensitive to botulinum toxin. Death of horses, most often the result of respiratory muscle paralysis, can result from exposure to only very small amounts of botulinum toxin. The damage to presynaptic axon terminals is irreversible, and recovery from botulism occurs only after terminal axon sprouting and reestablishment of new functioning synapses.

Tick Paralysis. *Dermacentor* and *Ixodes* ticks can elaborate a toxin that also blocks release of acetylcholine from axon terminals. Tick paralysis is seen most often in dogs and children. Recovery after tick removal can be rapid (within 24 to 48 hours), indicating that the mechanism of toxin action in tick paralysis does not result in irreversible presynaptic damage and thus is different from that of botulinum toxin.

Neoplasia

Neoplasms involving skeletal muscle are most often those that arise within the muscle or its supporting structures or that invade muscle from adjacent tissue. Neoplasms metastatic to muscle are rare.

Primary Muscle Tumors. Tumors with striated muscle differentiation are thought to arise from intramuscular pluripotential stem cells rather than from satellite cells. These tumors are uncommon and are either benign (rhabdomyoma) or malignant (rhabdomyosarcoma [Fig. 15-29]). Primary intramuscular tumors can also arise from fibrous tissue, vasculature, or neural elements. The most common tumor to arise from muscle-supporting structures is hemangiosarcoma.

Rhabdomyoma and Rhabdomyosarcoma. Tumors of striated muscle that occur at sites other than within muscle are rhabdomyomas of the heart or lung and botryoid rhabdomyosarcomas of the urinary bladder; these are not discussed in this section. Rhabdomyoma and rhabdomyosarcoma arising within skeletal muscle are most common in the dog, followed by the horse and cat. Morphologic variants include round cell, spindle cell, and mixed round and spindle cell, reflecting the developmental stages of skeletal muscle. Historically, diagnosis of tumors of skeletal muscle has relied on identification of cross-striations indicative of sarcomeric differentiation. Cross-striations are most often seen in elongated multinucleate cells known as *strap cells* (Fig. 15-29, C) and in ovoid cells known as *racquet cells*. They are most easily recognized after staining with phosphotungstic acid hematoxylin (PTAH) stain, but the search for cross-striations can be extremely frustrating and often unrewarding. These days, the diagnosis of tumors of skeletal muscle origin relies primarily on results of immunohistochemical examination using

Box 15-9 Portals of Entry–Equine Botulism

Gastrointestinal colonization of ingesta: Foals up to 6 months of age
Ingestion of preformed botulinum toxin: Adults, usually from rodent carcasses in hay or concentrated feed, or environmental contamination
Wound contamination: Adults, deep wounds, uncommon

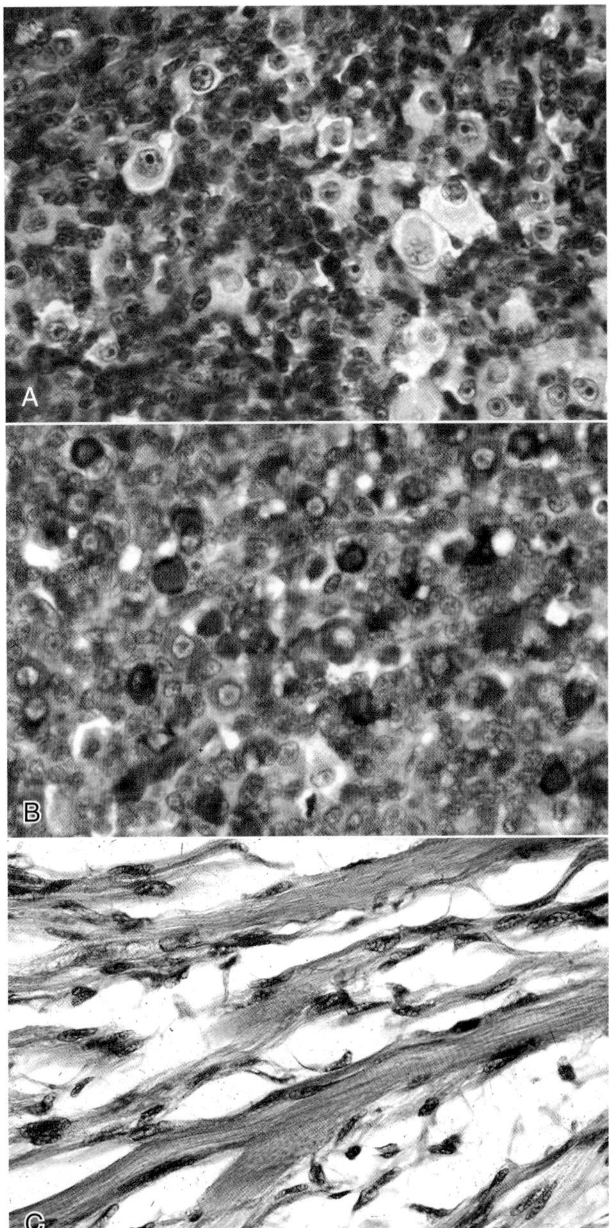

Figure 15-29 **Rhabdomyosarcoma. A,** Skeletal muscle, cat. An admixture of small round basophilic cells with a lesser number of larger round cells with prominent eosinophilic cytoplasm is characteristic of embryonal rhabdomyosarcoma. Nuclei are central and euchromatic, most often with a single large nucleolus. H&E stain. **B,** Immunostaining reaction of the same rhabdomyosarcoma as depicted in **A,** showing intense cytoplasmic expression of desmin in many tumor cells, indicative of muscle origin (skeletal, cardiac, or smooth). These cells also express myoglobin and sarcomeric actin (not shown), which differentiates skeletal muscle tumors from smooth muscle tumors. Immunoperoxidase reaction for desmin. **C,** Botryoid rhabdomyosarcoma, urinary bladder, large breed dog. Cross-striations, characteristic of a well-differentiated rhabdomyosarcoma, are present in the elongated multinucleate tumor cells. H&E stain. (Courtesy Dr. B.A. Valentine, College of Veterinary Medicine, Oregon State University.)

antibodies for muscle-specific proteins. Muscle actin and desmin are expressed by smooth and skeletal muscle tumors, but myoglobin, sarcomeric actin, myogenin, and MyoD1 are specific for skeletal muscle. Evidence of muscle differentiation, such as primitive myofilaments and Z-band structures, can also be detected by electron microscopy.

Rhabdomyoma is most often a round cell tumor and occurs most commonly in the larynx of adult dogs. The youngest reported age is 2 years. Tumors are generally smooth and nodular, pink, and unencapsulated. Histologic features are closely packed plump round cells that have central euchromatic nuclei, generally with a single prominent nucleus, and abundant vacuolated to granular eosinophilic cytoplasm. A small number of multinucleate and elongate strap cells can also be seen. Mitoses are rare, and evidence of invasion is uncommon.

Similar to the situation in human beings, rhabdomyosarcomas in animals most often occur at a young age and are most common in the neck or oral cavity, especially in the tongue. These tumors are pink and fleshy, and they often have prominent local invasion. The most common and most distinctive form of rhabdomyosarcoma in animals is embryonal rhabdomyosarcoma, composed of primitive round cells with prominent euchromatic nuclei, a single prominent nucleolus, and either indistinct or prominent eosinophilic cytoplasm ("rhabdomyoblasts"; see Fig. 15-29, *A* and *B*). Rhabdomyosarcoma can also contain elongate multinucleate strap cells (see Fig. 15-29, *C*) and ovoid racquet cells. Cellular and nuclear pleomorphism is common, as is mitotic activity. These tumors are locally invasive and frequently metastasize, although too few cases have been studied to document any pattern of metastasis.

Hemangiosarcoma. Malignant vascular neoplasms (hemangiosarcoma) arising within muscle are most common in the horse and dog (Fig. 15-30). Clinical signs include swelling within a muscle, often with associated lameness. Cytologic preparations frequently reveal only peripheral blood, which is suggestive of a hematoma. Pathologic diagnosis can be difficult if multiple sites within the lesion are not sampled, because the amount of hemorrhage often far exceeds the area composed of proliferating neoplastic endothelial cells. Intramuscular hemangiosarcoma has a high incidence of metastasis, often to the lungs.

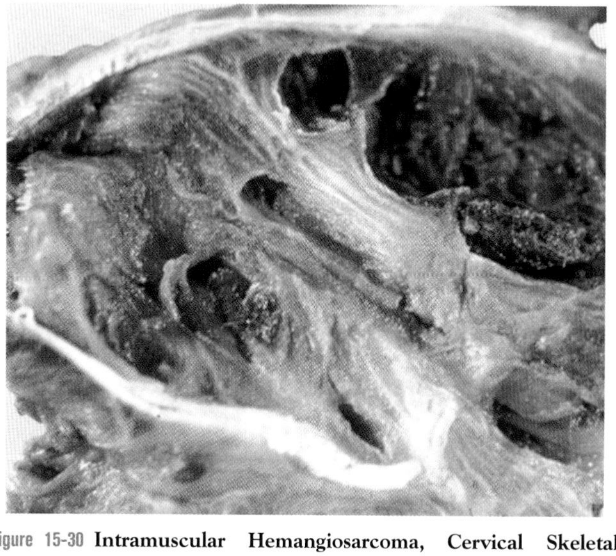

Figure 15-30 **Intramuscular Hemangiosarcoma, Cervical Skeletal Muscle, Horse.** Multiple irregular zones of cavitated *(upper right)* to solid tumor with hemorrhage have replaced normal muscle. Formalin-fixed specimen. (Courtesy Dr. A. de Lahunta, College of Veterinary Medicine, Cornell University.)

Other Tumors Involving Skeletal Muscle. A variant of lipoma, known as infiltrative lipoma, is often located in skeletal muscle. Characteristic gross pathologic and histopathologic findings are mature adipocytes invading skeletal muscle. This tumor is most common in the dog but has also been reported in young horses. Wide excision is the treatment of choice because this tumor recurs as a result of local invasion, but it does not metastasize.

Infiltration of skeletal muscle by neoplastic lymphocytes is not uncommon. Neoplastic lymphocytic infiltrates surround myofibers and can cause myofiber atrophy. These cells do not invade myofibers, however, and myonecrosis is rare. This helps to distinguish intramuscular lymphoma from lymphocytic myositis. Careful examination of infiltrating neoplastic cells typically reveals a relatively monomorphic population of lymphocytes, which may be atypical in appearance. Immunohistochemistry to confirm a single infiltrating cell type is also useful.

Vaccine-associated sarcoma in the muscle of the cat can arise within an intramuscular vaccination site or extend into underlying skeletal muscle from a subcutaneous injection site. Occasionally, mast cell tumors and carcinomas exhibit prominent skeletal muscle invasion. Melanoma arising in the skin of older gray horses often metastasizes to muscle fascia and may exhibit some extension into the muscle itself. Intramuscular metastasis of tumors is rare (see the section on Defense Mechanisms). Intramuscular metastasis of carcinoma, particularly prostatic, and of hemangiosarcoma can occur in dogs. When carcinomas with areas of sclerosis involve muscle, either by extension or by metastasis, the muscle basement membrane of adjacent myofibers is typically destroyed, often resulting in bizarre multinucleate cells representing attempts at muscle regeneration (see Fig. 15-15). These bizarre cells should not be misidentified as tumor cells.

Disorders of Domestic Animals by Species

Adequate muscle function is essential for the survival of any species. Many domestic animals have been selectively bred for improved musculature for meat production, performance, or appearance. Therefore muscle disease in animals can have a significant economic impact. In some cases, it is selection pressure imposed by human beings that has resulted in development and perpetuation of various myopathic conditions in animals. It is likely that continued selection for what appears to be a phenotypically desirable trait will lead to the recognition of new genetic mutations and myopathic conditions in the future.

It is interesting to compare the effects of muscular disorders that affect human beings and animals. The four-footed stance of animals allows for greater stability, which can allow an animal to remain ambulatory for some time, when a similarly affected person would be confined to a wheelchair. However, disorders that result in recumbency, even if it is transitory, can be devastating in livestock. It is much more difficult to nurse a large animal through a period of recumbency than it would be for a hospitalized human or small animal.

The most common and important muscle disorders of animals are discussed by species because this is the way diseases are considered clinically. The same disease may occur in different species. Details of less common muscle disorders are presented in E-Appendix 15-1.

Disorders of Horses

There is perhaps no other domestic animal species for which optimal muscle development and function is so critical as the horse. Selective breeding for better muscling has occurred in virtually all horse and pony breeds. The ability of such selection pressure to perpetuate equine muscle mutations is exemplified by the relatively recent occurrence of hyperkalemic periodic paralysis (HYPP), in which a muscle mutation results in visually appealing increased muscle bulk and definition. Unfortunately, as noted in the discussion of HYPP later, such mutations do not often result in improved muscle function.

Bacterial and Parasitic Myopathies

Infection by various bacterial organisms and clostridial toxins can cause myopathy in the horse. Protozoa (*Sarcocystis* spp.) are common incidental findings in equine muscle, but *Sarcocystis*-induced muscle damage resulting in clinical signs of muscle disease is rare.

Clostridial Myositis (Malignant Edema; Gas Gangrene). Clostridial myositis in the horse is an often fatal disorder caused by infection by various toxin-producing clostridial species, which are large Gram-positive anaerobic bacilli. *Clostridium septicum* is the most common cause of clostridial myositis in horses, but *Clostridium perfringens* types A to E, *Clostridium chauvoei*, *Clostridium novyi*, and *Clostridium fallax* can also cause infection. Infection can involve more than one clostridial species. *Clostridium* spp. are ubiquitous organisms that form spores within the soil and within the gastrointestinal tract. Unlike cattle, in which nonpenetrating trauma can cause muscle bruising and anaerobic conditions that activate clostridial spores already in the muscle, clostridial myositis in horses is virtually always secondary to a penetrating wound. Most often, this is an injection site of a nonantibiotic substance, but infection of sites of puncture wounds and of perivascular leakage of irritants in intravenously administered compounds are also possible. It is also possible that clostridial bacteria entering the blood from an injured gastrointestinal tract can colonize damaged muscle. This is one possible explanation for the frequent occurrence of signs of colic before development of clostridial myositis at the site of intramuscular injection of medications such as flunixin meglumine that cause localized muscle damage. Under anaerobic conditions, clostridia proliferate and produce toxins that damage blood vessels, resulting in hemorrhage and edema, and cause necrosis of adjacent muscle fibers.

Clinical signs are acute onset of heat, swelling, and pain within a muscle group and adjacent fascia, with concurrent fever, depression, dehydration, and anorexia. If sufficient muscle necrosis is present, serum CK and AST concentrations may be mildly to moderately increased. Death from toxemia and/or septicemia often occurs within 48 hours. Affected muscle and adjacent fascia are swollen and often hemorrhagic, with edema, suppurative inflammation, and necrosis; gas may also be present (Fig. 15-31). Vasculitis is not seen. Gram-positive bacilli characteristic of *Clostridium* spp. are generally demonstrable within affected tissue.

The diagnosis can be made with reasonable certainty based on typical historic, gross pathologic, cytologic, and histopathologic findings. *Clostridium* spp. can also be identified by culture under anaerobic conditions or by a fluorescent antibody test. Treatment must be initiated rapidly and includes surgical incisions into affected muscle to allow drainage and oxygenation, antibiotic therapy, and supportive care.

Botulism. Technically, this disease is a neuromuscular junction disorder and is included in this section for convenience. Botulism is caused by *Clostridium botulinum* toxin and is often not associated with *Clostridium botulinum* infection. The portals of entry of botulinum toxin in horses are summarized in Box 15-9. *Clostridium botulinum* bacteria are found as spores within the gastrointestinal tract of many mammals, and spores are common in the soil. Preformed

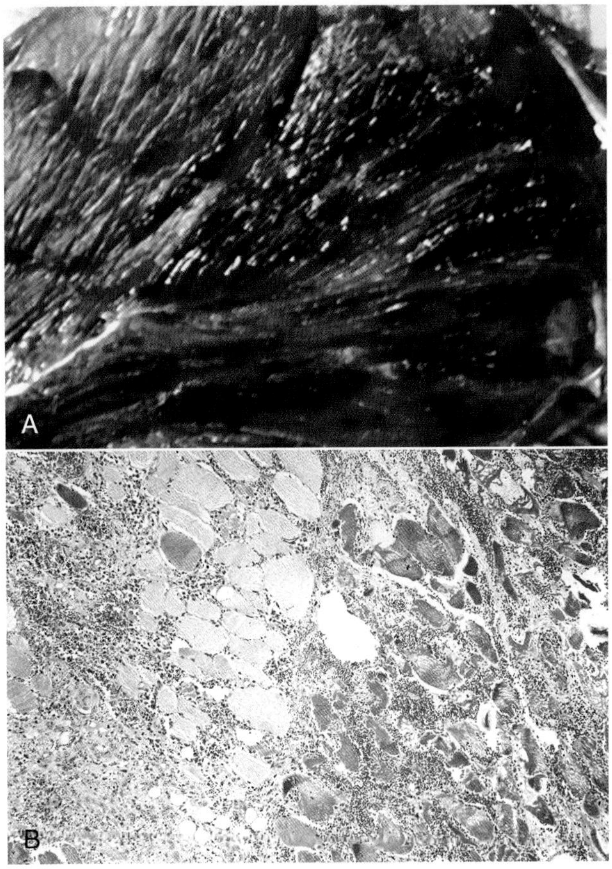

Figure 15-31 **Clostridial Myositis, Malignant Edema, Horse. A,** *Clostridium septicum* is the most common cause of clostridial myositis in horses. Affected muscle *(shown here)* and adjacent fascia *(not shown here)* are swollen and often hemorrhagic. **B,** Interstitial edema, hemorrhage, and inflammatory cells surround numerous swollen and fragmented necrotic myofibers. Formalin fixation, H&E stain. (Courtesy Dr. B.A. Valentine, College of Veterinary Medicine, Oregon State University.)

toxin within contaminated feed or soil is the most common cause of botulism in adult horses. However, in foals, usually between 1 week and 6 months of age, ingestion of *Clostridium botulinum* spores can lead to proliferation of toxin-producing *Clostridium botulinum* within the intestinal tract, resulting in toxicoinfectious botulism (shaker foals). Wound infection is an uncommon cause of botulism in horses.

The pathogenesis of botulism has been previously discussed in the section on Neuropathic and Neuromuscular Junction Disorders. Irreversible binding of toxin to presynaptic nerve terminals and blockage of acetylcholine release lead to the profound generalized flaccid paralysis that is the hallmark of botulism. Clinical signs are acute and progress rapidly, generally resulting in recumbency. Dysphagia and tongue weakness are common findings that help to distinguish botulism from other neuromuscular diseases causing recumbency. Serum concentrations of CK and AST are within normal limits (indicating the absence of damage to myofibers) or are possibly slightly increased as a result of ischemic myopathy secondary to recumbency (see later discussion).

No specific gross or histopathologic lesions are present in horses dying with botulism, although aspiration pneumonia caused by dysphagia can occur. Muscle fibers are intact unless recumbency has compromised their blood supply, causing ischemia and localized myofiber necrosis.

Evaluation of stomach contents or contaminated feed may reveal the presence of toxin. However, horses are exquisitely sensitive to botulinum toxin, and because only a small concentration of the toxin may be present in an affected horse, available tests may not detect such a low concentration of toxin. In most equine cases, the diagnosis is made based on the clinical history after elimination of other possible causes of profound muscular weakness. Affected animals should be treated with polyvalent botulinum antitoxin to prevent further binding of toxin. Recovery occurs after terminal axon sprouting and reestablishment of functional neuromuscular junctions. Vaccination with botulinum toxoid is an effective preventive measure.

Corynebacterium pseudotuberculosis (Pigeon Fever). Intramuscular abscesses caused by *Corynebacterium pseudotuberculosis* occur almost exclusively in horses in arid regions of the western United States and Brazil. *Corynebacterium pseudotuberculosis* is a Gram-positive pleomorphic facultative anaerobic bacillus present within the soil. It can enter muscle via penetrating wounds, including injection sites. The biotype most common in horses is different from that which affects sheep and goats because it is unable to reduce nitrates to nitrites. The high lipid content of the bacterial cell wall contributes to the survival of *Corynebacterium pseudotuberculosis* within macrophages. Bacterial exotoxins, such as phospholipase D, contribute to vascular damage and inhibition of neutrophil function. Equine infections occur most frequently during the fall and early winter, and a higher incidence of the disease is often seen after rainy winters. Infections are most common in the pectoral musculature, but other locations are possible. Affected muscles are swollen and edematous and contain variably sized zones of localized suppurative inflammation. Fever is common. The causative agent is readily isolated from affected tissue and can be seen in aspirates from intramuscular abscesses. Treatment is generally curative and includes antibiotic therapy and establishment of drainage of abscesses. Rarely, infection with *Corynebacterium pseudotuberculosis* in horses leads to immune-mediated vasculitis (purpura hemorrhagica; see next section).

Streptococcal-Associated Myopathies. Two distinct degenerative myopathies are associated with infection or exposure of the horse to *Streptococcus equi* ssp. *equi*. One, known as *purpura hemorrhagica*, has been recognized for many years. The other, known as *streptococcal-associated rhabdomyolysis and muscle atrophy*, has only recently been recognized.

Purpura Hemorrhagica. In this disease, muscle damage is not caused by the direct infection of the muscles but, rather, by an immune response to the bacterial pathogen. *Streptococcus equi* is the most common cause of purpura hemorrhagica in horses, but *Corynebacterium pseudotuberculosis* and possibly other bacteria can also cause purpura hemorrhagica. In cases caused by *Streptococcus equi*, circulating immune complexes composed of immunoglobulin A (IgA) antibodies and streptococcal M antigen deposit in the walls of small vessels. This leads to vasculitis and vascular wall necrosis (Fig. 15-32), with resultant hemorrhage and infarction of myofibers. It is also possible that antibodies to streptococcal M protein cross-react with skeletal and cardiac muscle myosins to cause direct injury.

Signs of myopathy often accompany systemic signs of poststreptococcal purpura in horses (i.e., depression, fever, dependent edema, petechiae or ecchymoses, leukocytosis, increased serum fibrinogen, and anemia), but myopathy can also be the primary presenting disease process. Affected horses are weak, may have a short-strided gait, and can become recumbent. Myoglobinuria and very high increases in serum concentrations of CK and AST are common.

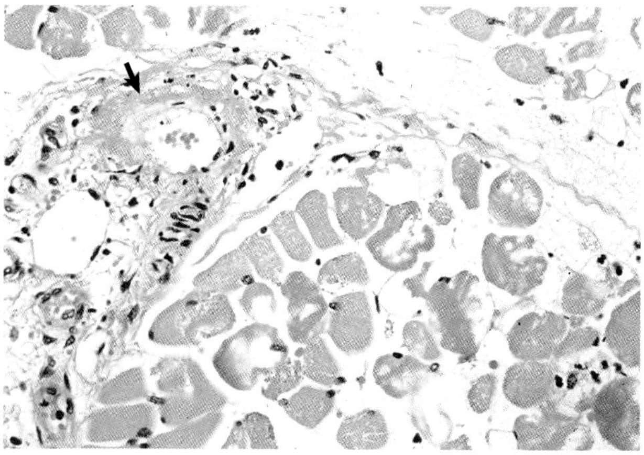

Figure 15-32 **Intramuscular Vasculitis, Purpura Hemorrhagica, Skeletal Muscle, Transverse Section, Horse.** In the wall of the blood vessel *(arrow)* is a band of circumferential fibrinoid necrosis containing nuclear debris. Many of the adjacent myofibers are necrotic *(center to lower right areas)*. Some of these myofibers are fragmented, and a small number contain fine basophilic deposits of mineral. Formalin fixation, H&E stain. (Courtesy Dr. B.A. Valentine, College of Veterinary Medicine, Oregon State University.)

Multiple muscles are involved (as opposed to the locally extensive lesion of clostridial myositis), and affected muscles contain multifocal to locally extensive hemorrhage and edema that dissects between necrotic muscle fibers and muscle fasciculi. Gross pathologic findings are similar to those seen in clostridial myositis (see Fig. 15-31, A), but lesions do not contain gas bubbles. Vascular injury (leukocytoclastic vasculitis and fibrinoid necrosis of blood vessels; see Fig. 15-32) is seen on microscopic examination and is the diagnostic feature.

Diagnosis is based on a history of exposure of the horse to *Streptococcus equi* and the typical clinical, clinicopathologic, and histopathologic findings. Because this is an immune-complex disorder, histopathology, cytology, and bacterial cultures of affected muscle do not reveal *Streptococcus equi*. This bacterium or other causative bacteria may be cultured from other affected tissues, especially lymph nodes or guttural pouch. A high serum titer to *Streptococcus equi* M protein is strongly supportive of a diagnosis of streptococcal-associated purpura hemorrhagica. Treatment includes corticosteroid therapy and supportive care, but horses frequently succumb to other sequelae of systemic vasculitis, such as gastrointestinal infarcts.

Streptococcal-Associated Rhabdomyolysis and Muscle Atrophy. A syndrome of severe acute rhabdomyolysis resulting in profound rapidly progressive generalized loss of muscle mass has also been seen in horses with clinical infection by *Streptococcus equi* or in horses that have been exposed to this bacterium but that did not develop obvious clinical signs of infection. This syndrome occurs most frequently in young to young adult quarter horses, but young horses of other breeds can also be affected. Clinically recognizable muscle atrophy is often most evident in paraspinal and gluteal muscles. Some cases have microscopic evidence of concurrent EPSSM (see the section on Inherited or Congenital Myopathies), which may be a predisposing factor. In others, nonsuppurative perivascular and interstitial inflammation has been detected, and the proposed mechanism is immune-mediated damage caused by cross-reaction of streptococcal antibodies with muscle proteins. Affected horses do not show typical signs of purpura hemorrhagica but often have very high serum concentrations of CK (often greater than 100,000 units per liter) and AST (often greater than 10,000 units per liter). Affected horses may respond to corticosteroid therapy.

Most will recover, but recurrence after subsequent exposure to *Streptococcus equi* is possible.

Protozoal Myopathy. Protozoa (*Sarcocystis* spp.) are common incidental findings in equine skeletal and cardiac muscles. Because the protozoa are in cysts within the myofiber itself and thus are protected from the body's surveillance, there is no inflammatory response. Massive infection by *Sarcocystis fayeri* is suspected of causing a degenerative myopathy in horses, but this is rare. Rarely, localized thickening of the tongue has been found in horses with granulomatous myositis, the result of sarcocystis organisms within tongue musculature. The cause of the intense inflammation apparently incited by protozoa in these rare cases is unknown.

Ear Tick–Associated Muscle Spasms. Episodic muscle spasms of various muscle groups can occur in horses with ear ticks (*Otobius megnini*). The mechanism is not known. Dimpling of affected muscles after percussion can be seen, but myotonic discharges are not found with electromyography. Treatment for ear ticks results in rapid recovery.

Nutritional and Toxic Myopathies

Nutritional deficiency, most often of selenium, and various toxins are relatively common causes of degenerative myopathy in the horse.

Nutritional Myopathy. Foals (most commonly up to 2 weeks of age) and young adult horses are most susceptible to nutritional myopathy because of a deficiency of the antioxidants selenium or (less commonly) vitamin E. In severely selenium-deficient areas, such as the Pacific Northwest, selenium deficiency myopathy can occur in horses of any age. Normally the selenium present in the soil is taken up by growing plants. In many areas, the soil is selenium deficient, and selenium supplements to the animal's ration must be provided. Vitamin E deficiency occurs in horses that eat marginal- to poor-quality grass hay and have little or no access to pasture and no supplemental vitamin E. Oxidative injury to actively contracting muscle fibers occurs as a result of a lack of antioxidant activity.

Affected foals are most likely to be those born to selenium-deficient mares. Foals have generalized weakness, which may be present at birth or become apparent soon after birth. Affected foals may become recumbent but are generally bright and alert. They often continue to suckle if bottle fed, but weakness of the tongue and pharyngeal muscles can lead to weak suckling.

Affected adult horses are most often stabled horses fed only selenium-deficient hay, with clinical disease being seen most commonly in the late winter or early spring. In the Pacific Northwest, selenium deficiency myopathy can occur in adult horses fed only pasture or hay, and it can occur at any time of year. Affected adult horses often show preferential involvement of the temporal and masseter muscles (the condition is sometimes inappropriately termed *maxillary myositis* or *masseter myositis*) with swelling and stiffness of these muscles and impaired mastication. Involvement of pharyngeal muscle results in dysphagia and involvement of the tongue results in impaired prehension of food, which can be mistaken for botulism. In more chronic cases, bilaterally symmetric atrophy of the masseter muscles may be evident, which can be mistaken for atrophy secondary to protozoal myeloencephalitis. Careful examination of these horses often reveals generalized weakness, evident as a stiff, short-strided gait. Severely affected horses can have an acute onset of recumbency that mimics neurologic disease.

Serum concentrations of CK and AST are generally mildly to moderately increased, although extremely high concentrations can be seen in severely affected foals and horses. Concentric needle EMG of affected muscles results in abnormal spontaneous activity (positive sharp waves, fibrillations, and myotonic bursts).

Muscles of affected horses appear pale (hence the common name white muscle disease), often in a patchy distribution (see Fig. 15-39). The most severely affected muscles are those that have the highest workload (e.g., cervical muscles in foals used during suckling and "bumping" the udder, proximal limb muscles, tongue, and masticatory muscles). The gross appearance depends on the extent of the necrosis and the stage. In early stages, yellow and white streaks are present, and later pale, chalk white streaks often appear. Horses with impaired swallowing can have cranioventral aspiration pneumonia. Severely selenium-deficient foals and horses also have pale areas of necrosis within the myocardium, especially the left ventricular wall and septum, which are areas that have a high workload. The stage of the necrosis depends on the age of the lesions. In foals with severe, acute myopathy leading to death or euthanasia, lesions are at the stage of massive muscle necrosis and mineralization with minimal macrophage infiltration (monophasic). In animals that have lived longer (i.e., subacute cases), the lesions are polyphasic, and active necrosis, macrophage infiltration, and regeneration are present. Although type 1 fibers may be more likely to develop necrosis because of nutritional myopathy, in severely affected muscles almost all fiber types are affected. In cases with myocardial involvement, myocardiocyte necrosis and mineralization are present. If the animal survives, the necrotic myocardiocytes are replaced by fibrovascular connective tissue that matures to form a scar.

A provisional diagnosis of nutritional myopathy is based on typical history, increases in serum concentrations of CK and AST, and characteristic gross and histopathologic findings. The diagnosis is confirmed by detecting deficient concentrations of selenium or vitamin E in blood of live animals or in liver samples obtained at necropsy. If horses live long enough, myofiber regeneration can restore the muscles to normal. This disorder in foals can be prevented by supplementing the ration of mares with selenium during gestation. Foals born in selenium-deficient areas can also be given injectable vitamin E and selenium soon after birth. Young adult horses should be given sufficient dietary vitamin E and selenium. Treatment with selenium and vitamin E after the onset of clinical signs is far less effective than prevention.

Ionophore Toxicity. The pathogenesis of ionophore toxicity is discussed in the section on Toxic Myopathies. Horses are exquisitely sensitive to ionophores and succumb to very small doses. Ionophores may be present as contaminants within horse feed, or the horse may be accidentally fed ionophore-containing feeds intended for other domestic animals.

Most of the available literature relates to monensin toxicity, but the effects of other ionophores should be similar. In acute monensin toxicity, death occurs because of shock and cardiovascular collapse, and no specific lesions are seen on postmortem examination within the first 48 hours, although these may be stained diffusely pink by myoglobin. If the horse survives 3 to 4 days, affected skeletal and cardiac muscles often contain pale streaks (Fig. 15-33, *A*) and, microscopically, cardiac muscle necrosis and segmental necrosis of skeletal muscle is present (Fig. 15-33, *B*; see Fig. 15-11, *B*), with concurrent increases in serum concentrations of CK and AST, which may be severe. Given the profound sensitivity of horses to ionophores, ionophore toxicity in horses is typically the result of a single dose and thus the lesion is a monophasic multifocal process. This helps to differentiate ionophore toxicity from nutritional

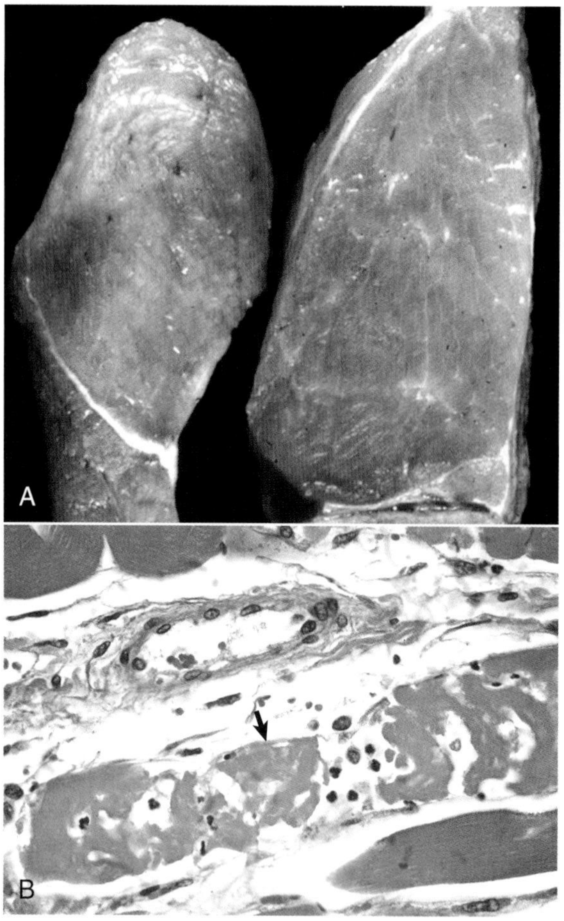

Figure 15-33 **Ionophore Toxicity, Monensin, Skeletal Muscle. A,** Necrosis. The pale white to gray foci are areas of necrotic myofibers. Myocardium will often contain similar lesions. **B,** Segmental myofiber necrosis (2 days old), longitudinal section, horse. The segment of myofiber *(arrow)* visible here is necrotic, fragmented, and infiltrated by macrophages and neutrophils. Note the intact basal lamina and endomysium on both sides of the myofiber, which will contain the regenerating myofiber and thus facilitate resolution. Ionophore toxicity results in calcium overload and death of skeletal (also cardiac) myocytes. Formalin fixation, H&E stain. (**A** courtesy Dr. J. Wright, College of Veterinary Medicine, North Carolina State University; and Noah's Arkive, College of Veterinary Medicine, The University of Georgia. **B** courtesy Dr. M.D. McGavin, College of Veterinary Medicine, University of Tennessee.)

myopathy, which is often polyphasic. Both type 1 and type 2 fibers are affected. If the horse survives, necrosis is followed by myofiber regeneration, which can restore the muscles to normal, but necrotic myocardiocytes are replaced by fibrosis because of the lack of significant regeneration by myocardiocytes. Horses dying at 14 days after ionophore exposure often have normal skeletal muscles and extensive myocardial fibrosis. Acute cardiac failure and death because of myocardial scarring can occur months to years after apparent clinical recovery from ionophore exposure.

Diagnosis is based on a history that includes both ingestion of ionophores and the presence of the characteristic gross or histopathologic findings. Analysis of feed or stomach contents for ionophores is definitive. Treatment for ionophore-intoxicated horses is supportive because there is no specific therapy.

Plant Toxicities. A number of toxic plants are known to cause muscle necrosis in horses (see also Toxic Myopathies). These include *Cassia occidentalis* (coffee senna) and *Thermopsis* spp. Most plant-associated toxicities in horses are associated with plants growing in pastures or in baled hay. Necrosis is most often polyphasic, indicating a prolonged period of ingestion. Cardiac myonecrosis may or may not also be present. In the United Kingdom and less commonly in the Midwestern United States, a syndrome of pasture-associated myonecrosis caused by ingestion of the toxin hypoglycin A, contained within seeds of *Acer negundo* (box elder) trees, occurs in horses. This disorder has also been called *atypical myoglobinuria.*

Inherited or Congenital Myopathies and Myotonic Disorders

Hyperkalemic Periodic Paralysis. Hyperkalemic periodic paralysis (HYPP) is a myotonic disorder that affects horses whose ancestry traces back to a quarter-horse stallion named *Impressive.* Affected horses generally have remarkably well-defined muscle groups, which has led to their popularity for showing in halter. The disease is inherited as an autosomal dominant disease; therefore affected horses can be either heterozygotes or homozygotes. Homozygous foals often have a distinctive laryngeal muscle dysfunction that results in laryngospasm and labored breathing. Most homozygous horses do not survive; if they do, they are invalids.

The underlying defect in HYPP is a point mutation in the gene encoding the α subunit of the skeletal muscle sodium channel. This defect causes abnormal (delayed) inactivation of sodium channel activity, resulting in membrane instability and continuous muscle fiber electrical activity, which is reflected in EMG findings (see later discussion). The pathogenesis of clinical signs of HYPP is complex and not entirely understood, either in horses or in human beings with a similar disorder. Affected heterozygotes have a mosaic of abnormal and normal sodium channels, and resting muscle membrane potentials are typically lower than normal. This leads to an increased likelihood of electrical generation of a prolonged muscle action potential, resulting in transient myotonia. When abnormal sodium channels are activated, the response to the resulting abnormally increased intracellular sodium is release of potassium into the extracellular space and bloodstream, resulting in hyperkalemia. Hyperkalemia is not, however, a consistent finding. Feeding of high-potassium feeds, such as alfalfa products or feeds with added molasses, can precipitate clinical signs of HYPP, possibly by activating abnormal sodium channels. Another potential consequence of prolonged activation of abnormal sodium channels is inactivation of normal sodium channels, resulting in flaccid paralysis and collapse. This result would explain the typical signs seen during episodes, which include transient muscle spasm (myotonia), with protrusion of the third eyelid, followed by generalized flaccid paralysis. Decreased muscle temperature, as can occur as a result of a chilling rain, can precipitate episodic collapse in HYPP horses, possibly by decreasing the activity of the muscle sodium-potassium exchanger (the Na-K ATPase), an important means by which affected muscle compensates for abnormal sodium channel activity. Postanesthetic recumbency and anesthesia-associated hyperthermia have also been seen in HYPP horses. Affected horses can appear normal for many years, can have multiple episodes of collapse, or can die acutely. Serum concentrations of CK and AST are generally normal. Abnormal ionic fluxes occur at all times in affected horses, and concentric needle EMG between paralytic episodes reveals characteristic persistent myotonic bursts.

There are no gross pathologic findings in horses with hyperkalemic periodic paralysis other than gross prominent muscling. Skeletal muscle dysfunction in HYPP horses is due to abnormal ionic fluxes that can lead to spasms and weakness; therefore affected skeletal muscle is generally histologically normal. In some cases, scattered intracytoplasmic vacuoles (vacuolar myopathy) can be present in type 2 fibers. The characteristic pathologic finding of HYPP is only evident at the ultrastructural level, where dilated terminal cisternae of the sarcoplasmic reticulum are found.

Diagnosis can be made with reasonable certainty based on characteristic clinical signs (muscle spasms often leading to flaccid paralysis) and clinicopathologic findings (hyperkalemia) in a horse of Impressive line breeding. Myotonic bursts with concentric needle EMG are also diagnostic. The simplest and most reliable test, however, is a DNA-based test performed on peripheral white blood cells or, as described more recently, on cells obtained from the base of pulled mane or tail hairs. Treatment consists of feeding a low-potassium diet, which means avoiding alfalfa products and molasses. A low-potassium diet can be successful in controlling signs in many cases. More severe cases can be treated with the diuretic acetazolamide, which causes increased urinary excretion of potassium. Acute episodes can be treated with intravenous dextrose or insulin or oral sugar solutions such as sugar syrup. Administration of glucose to stimulate insulin secretion, or of insulin itself, aids in alleviating signs by helping drive the intracellular movement of potassium along with glucose.

Equine Polysaccharide Storage Myopathy. Equine polysaccharide storage myopathy (EPSSM) is a myopathy most commonly recognized in quarter horse, warm blood, Arabian, Morgan, pony of the Americas, and draft-related breeds. It also occurs in many other horse and pony breeds, including miniature horses. Surveys of equine muscle samples have revealed an astonishingly high incidence of approximately 66% in all draft-related horses and approximately 30% in all light horses. Not all affected horses exhibit obvious clinical signs of muscle dysfunction. This disorder is inherited as an autosomal dominant trait.

In contrast to other glycogenoses affecting skeletal muscle, to date no abnormality in the glycolytic or glycogenolytic pathways in skeletal muscle has been identified, making this equine disorder unique, but an underlying carbohydrate metabolic disorder is still suspected. Affected horses appear to have a more rapid intramuscular uptake of blood glucose than controls, although the exact mechanism for this phenomenon is still unknown. A point mutation in the skeletal muscle glycogen synthase 1 (GYS1) gene has been associated with some, but not all, cases of EPSSM. A DNA test for this mutation is available, and horses with GYS1 mutations are sometimes classified as EPSSM type 1. Abnormal accumulation of intracytoplasmic glycogen (confirmed by being PAS-positive, amylase-sensitive) within type 2 fibers is the histologic finding. In severe cases, aggregates of abnormal glycogen are eventually ubiquitinated, resulting in amylase-resistant inclusions composed of glycogen and filamentous protein. Certain breeds, such as quarter horse and draft-related breeds, seem to be most prone to the development of amylase-resistant inclusions, whereas glycogen aggregates are more common in other breeds. The explanation for this difference is as yet unknown, although breeds prone to developing amylase-resistant inclusions are also those breeds most likely to have the GYS1 mutation.

Clinical signs are variable, but all are thought to be caused by insufficient energy production by affected muscle fibers. Abnormal myofiber function caused by architectural alteration secondary to intramyofiber deposition of complex polysaccharide is also a possible mechanism, but the excellent response to therapy, even in horses with severe intramyofiber inclusions of accumulated polysaccharide, suggests that this is less significant than is altered energy metabolism. Recurrent exertional rhabdomyolysis (see later discussion) is a commonly recognized sign, but unexplained pelvic limb lameness is even more common than clinical rhabdomyolysis. Affected horses can also have a stiff gait, symmetric muscle atrophy, back soreness, muscle cramping resulting in abnormal hind limb flexion characteristic of shivers, and bilateral pelvic limb or generalized weakness. In draft horses, sudden onset of spontaneous recumbency or postanesthetic recumbency because of myopathy can occur. Serum concentrations of CK and AST are markedly increased after episodes of exertional rhabdomyolysis but may be only mildly to moderately increased in affected horses after exercise or onset of recumbency. Normal serum concentrations of CK and AST in affected horses are thought to indicate that the muscle dysfunction is not accompanied by overt myonecrosis. Concentric needle EMG may reveal abnormal spontaneous activity (scattered positive sharp waves and fibrillations).

In severe cases, in which horses have died or been euthanatized because of rhabdomyolysis or recumbency, muscles may be pale pink or diffusely red-tinged (myoglobin staining), which can be mistaken for autolysis. Multifocal pale zones may be present (see Fig. 15-35, *A*). In draft horses and sporadically in horses of other breeds, chronic myopathy can result in overall reduction in muscle mass. Muscles in severely affected draft horses can also be of normal size but may contain pale streaks where myofibers have been replaced by fat. The most severely affected muscles are those of the proximal hind limb (especially gluteal, semimembranosus, and semitendinosus muscles) and epaxial muscles of the back (e.g., longissimus), although any of the large "power" muscle groups, including pectoral and shoulder girdle muscles, can be affected. Swollen, dark kidneys (pigmentary nephrosis) caused by myoglobinuria can be seen in horses dying with severe rhabdomyolysis. The extent of overt myofiber necrosis is extremely variable; massive necrosis or regeneration can be seen after severe rhabdomyolysis, whereas only minimal scattered necrotic fibers may be seen in recumbent horses. Lesions are monophasic if there has been only a single bout of exertional rhabdomyolysis, or they are polyphasic if there have been repeated bouts of less severe exercise-induced injury. Abnormal polysaccharide is always present, but fiber necrosis is uncommon in muscle biopsy samples taken from affected horses while they are clinically normal.

The characteristic histologic finding is aggregates of intracytoplasmic material that stain positively with the PAS reaction for glycogen (Fig. 15-34, *A*). In severe cases, multiple pale intracytoplasmic inclusions are also present in H&E stained sections (Fig. 15-34, *B*). These inclusions are PAS-positive (Fig. 15-34, *C*) and resist digestion by amylase and are thus not glycogen. Terms used to describe this amylase-resistant material include *amylopectin*, *polyglucosan*, and *complex polysaccharide*. In chronic cases, myofibers also have chronic myopathic change (atrophy, hypertrophy, or internal nuclei), and fat replacement of myofibers after myofiber loss can occur in severely affected cases.

At this time, the detection of the GYS1 mutation provides a definitive diagnosis of EPSSM, but this test is not very sensitive. The most sensitive test for diagnosis of EPSSM depends on finding characteristic histopathologic changes in muscle samples of horses with appropriate clinical signs. Gluteal, semimembranosus, or semitendinosus muscle samples are preferred, although changes in longissimus muscle are also found, especially in horses with back pain. A presumptive diagnosis of EPSSM can be made based on characteristic clinical findings in a predisposed breed. Treatment has relied on altering the diet to minimize starch and sugar intake (less than 15% of total daily calories) and maximize fat intake (at least 20% to 25% of total daily calories from fat). Grains and sweet feeds are replaced by high-fiber, low-starch, low-sugar feeds, with added fat in the form of vegetable oil, powdered fat, or high-fat rice bran supplements. Providing the horse with regular exercise and as much time

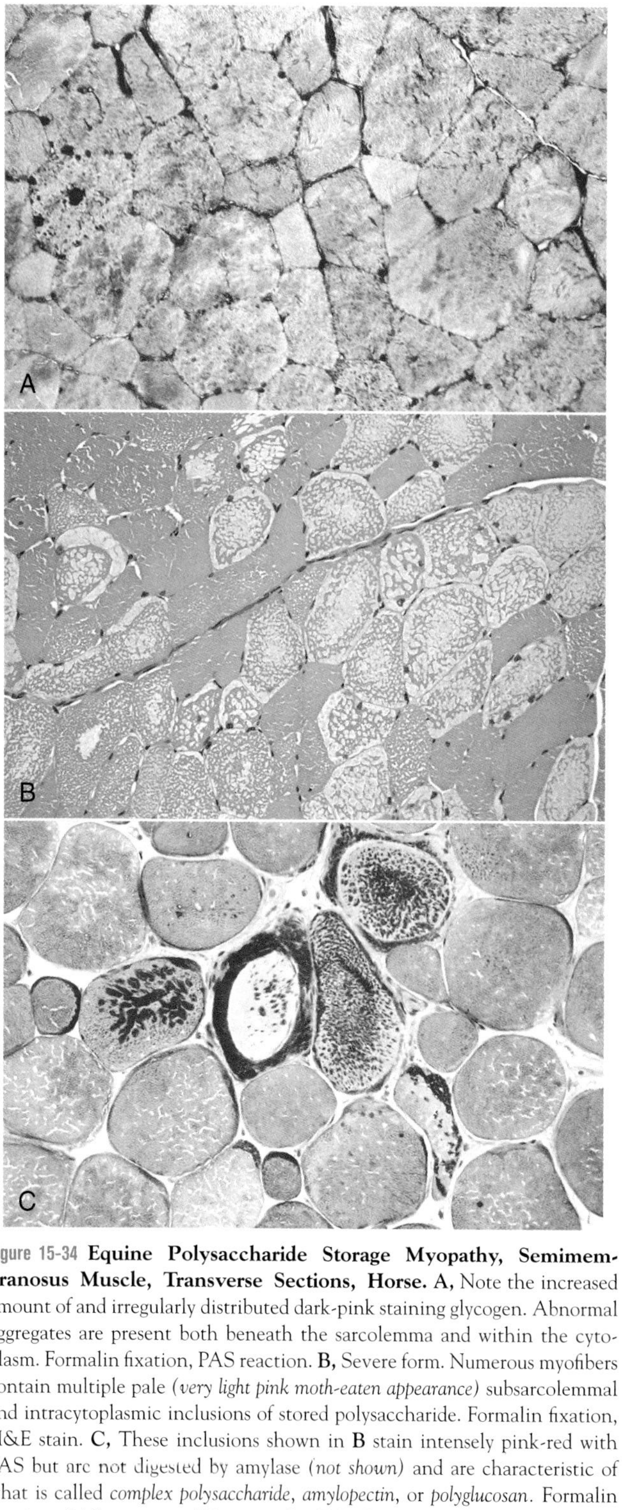

Figure 15-34 **Equine Polysaccharide Storage Myopathy, Semimembranosus Muscle, Transverse Sections, Horse. A,** Note the increased amount of and irregularly distributed dark-pink staining glycogen. Abnormal aggregates are present both beneath the sarcolemma and within the cytoplasm. Formalin fixation, PAS reaction. **B,** Severe form. Numerous myofibers contain multiple pale *(very light pink moth-eaten appearance)* subsarcolemmal and intracytoplasmic inclusions of stored polysaccharide. Formalin fixation, H&E stain. **C,** These inclusions shown in **B** stain intensely pink-red with PAS but are not digested by amylase *(not shown)* and are characteristic of what is called *complex polysaccharide*, *amylopectin*, or *polyglucosan*. Formalin fixation, PAS reaction. (Courtesy Dr. B.J. Cooper, College of Veterinary Medicine, Oregon State University.)

as possible in a pasture or paddock are also important. Treatment is very successful in most cases.

Glycogen Brancher Enzyme Deficiency. Glycogen brancher enzyme (GBE) deficiency, or glycogenosis type IV, is a disorder caused by a congenital lack of a glycogenic enzyme, GBE, and is an emerging disease in quarter horses and American paint horses. It is inherited as an autosomal recessive trait. Affected foals may be aborted, stillborn, or weak at birth or can have contracted tendons, rhabdomyolysis, or cardiac failure at an early age. The consequence of GBE deficiency is the accumulation of long unbranched chains of glucose within cells that leads to abnormal glycogen formation and intramyofiber deposits. These molecules would normally be converted into glycogen in the presence of GBE in the final step in the formation of glycogen. There are no specific gross pathologic findings. Pulmonary edema may be found in foals that die from cardiac failure. Characteristic histologic findings are round hyaline inclusions resembling amylopectin (polyglucosan bodies) within skeletal and cardiac myocytes, especially Purkinje fibers, and to a lesser degree within hepatocytes. Unlike glycogen, inclusions are PAS-positive and resistant to amylase digestion. As with other carbohydrate metabolic defects, a lack of energy production by affected fibers is thought to underlie cellular dysfunction. Disruption of cytoarchitecture caused by amylopectin deposition may also contribute. Analysis of peripheral blood or skeletal muscle for GBE activity identifies affected animals with severely reduced GBE activity and carriers in which GBE activity is moderately reduced. A DNA test to detect carriers and affected horses using pulled mane or tail hairs is now available. There is no treatment for this disorder.

Myotonia and Mitochondrial Myopathy. A myotonic disorder occurs occasionally in horses, and a mitochondrial myopathy has been described in an Arabian horse. These disorders are discussed in more detail in E-Appendix 15-1.

Other Equine Myopathies

Exertional Rhabdomyolysis. Equine exertional rhabdomyolysis (tying up, azoturia, Monday morning disease, setfast, and blackwater) is characterized clinically by sudden onset of stiff gait, reluctance to move, swelling of affected muscle groups (especially gluteal), sweating, and other signs of pain and discomfort. Serum concentrations of CK and AST are often markedly increased. Signs may appear during or immediately after exercise, but only rarely is exertional rhabdomyolysis associated with exhaustive exercise. In severely affected horses, even minimal exercise, such as walking out of a stall, can cause clinical signs. High grain feeding and lack of regular exercise have been recognized to be factors leading to exercise-induced muscle injury for many years. Previous theories regarding the pathogenesis of equine exertional rhabdomyolysis include development of muscle lactic acidosis, vitamin E and/or selenium deficiency, hypothyroidism, and systemic electrolyte abnormalities. Only recently have studies concluded that lactic acidosis is not a finding in horses with exertional rhabdomyolysis, that hypothyroid horses show no signs of degenerative myopathy, and that electrolyte abnormalities as a primary cause of equine exertional rhabdomyolysis are rare. It is still thought that vitamin E or selenium deficiency can exacerbate signs of exertional rhabdomyolysis in predisposed horses, but neither vitamin E nor selenium deficiency is considered a primary cause. Recent studies have found that affected horses typically have an underlying myopathy, most often equine polysaccharide storage myopathy (EPSSM). There is evidence that recurrent exertional rhabdomyolysis in thoroughbreds is the result of abnormal calcium homeostasis within skeletal muscle, although some affected thoroughbreds have been found to have EPSSM. Because muscle necrosis per se is not painful and does not cause muscle swelling, it is suspected that other factors play a role in this disorder in the horse. These factors include oxidative injury to muscle membranes occurring secondary to segmental necrosis and the subsequent production of oxygen-derived free radical compounds and vascular compromise resulting in ischemia (i.e., compartment syndrome when muscle damage occurs in a muscle with a tight and relatively nonexpandable fascia such as the gluteal and longissimus muscles). Oxidative injury may explain the perceived benefit of supplemental vitamin E and selenium to affected horses.

Gross findings are similar to those described for equine polysaccharide storage myopathy (EPSSM)—that is, initially areas of muscle that are pale pink or diffusely red-tinged (Fig. 15-35, *A*). Histologic findings are localized or widespread muscle fiber necrosis (Fig. 15-35, *B*), followed by the usual sequence of events: macrophage infiltration and regeneration. Affected fibers are primarily type 2 fibers. Lesions can be either monophasic or polyphasic.

Diagnosis is based on typical clinical signs and clinicopathologic evidence of muscle injury (increased activity of CK or AST). Treatment for an acute episode includes nonsteroidal antiinflammatory agents, acepromazine, and rest. Careful evaluation of the patient for evidence of renal damage ([pigmentary] myoglobinuric nephrosis) because of myoglobin released from damaged muscle is indicated. Long-term treatment and prevention include correction of any concurrent electrolyte, mineral, or vitamin deficiencies and, most important, a change in diet to one that is high in fat and fiber and low in starch and sugar, as described for horses with EPSSM (see the section on Inherited or Congenital Myopathies). Thoroughbreds with recurrent exertional rhabdomyolysis caused by suspected underlying skeletal muscle calcium-handling abnormalities also respond well to this type of diet.

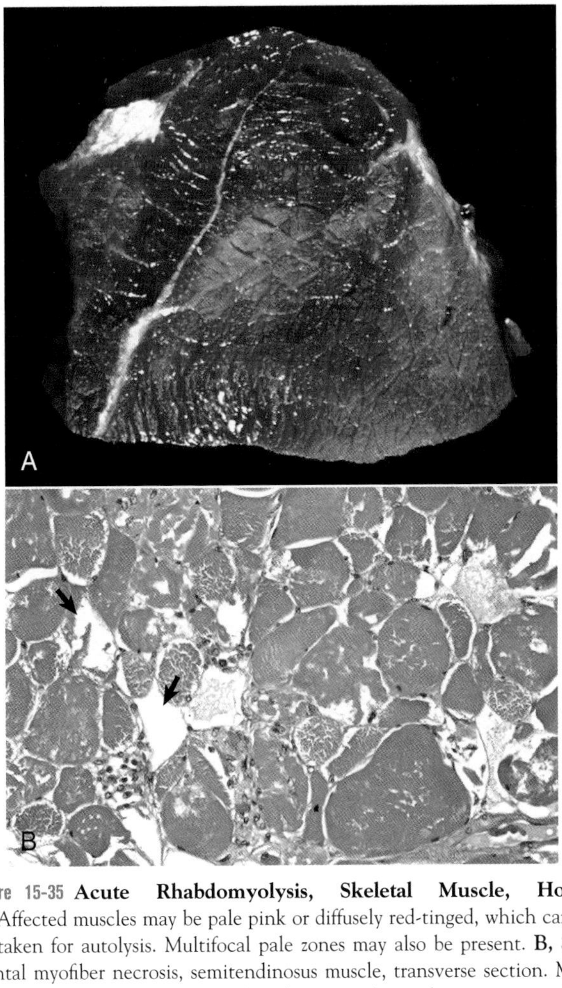

Figure 15-35 Acute Rhabdomyolysis, Skeletal Muscle, Horse. **A,** Affected muscles may be pale pink or diffusely red-tinged, which can be mistaken for autolysis. Multifocal pale zones may also be present. **B,** Segmental myofiber necrosis, semitendinosus muscle, transverse section. Most of the myocytes are necrotic and at the stage of coagulation necrosis. In a few myofibers, necrosis is at a later stage and the necrotic sarcoplasm has lysed, leaving empty sarcolemmal tubes *(arrows)*. A couple of necrotic myofibers are at an even later stage and contain a small number of macrophages. Formalin fixation, H&E stain. (**A** courtesy Dr. W. Crowell, College of Veterinary Medicine, The University of Georgia; and Noah's Arkive, College of Veterinary Medicine, The University of Georgia. **B** courtesy Dr. B.J. Cooper, College of Veterinary Medicine, Oregon State University.)

Malignant Hyperthermia. In horses, malignant hyperthermia (MH) can occur during general anesthesia. Hyperthermia can also occur during recovery from anesthesia, which is sometimes called *hypermetabolism* to distinguish it from true MH. A genetic defect in the skeletal muscle ryanodine receptor, similar to that in MH in human beings, dogs, and pigs, has been identified in some horses with MH triggered by anesthetic agents. A genetic test for the MH mutation is available. Some horses affected with a hyperthermia-like syndrome during anesthesia or during recovery from anesthesia have hyperkalemic periodic paralysis (HYPP) or equine polysaccharide storage myopathy (EPSSM), but in some cases the exact cause of the hyperthermia is not clear. It is likely that, as is similar to hyperthermia in human beings, a variety of underlying myopathies, especially those that result in uncoupling of mitochondria within skeletal myocytes (see the section on Malignant Hyperthermia), can predispose animals to anesthesia-associated hyperthermia. Studies of muscle from horses with exertional rhabdomyolysis have detected loosely coupled mitochondria, which could predispose them to MH–like episodes. The extent of overt muscle fiber necrosis caused by hyperthermia varies but is often severe.

Ischemic Myopathy. In addition to vascular damage resulting from clostridial toxins or immune-mediated vasculitis, ischemic myopathy of pectoral and limb muscle can be seen in recumbent horses as the result of pressure interfering with vascular perfusion. Once the horse is moved or is standing, reperfusion injury can occur. Development of compartment syndrome can contribute to ischemic injury (see the section on Disturbance of Circulation). Ischemic myopathy of the abdominal muscles can be seen after prolonged pressure from being supported in a sling. In these cases, affected muscles generally show degenerative or regenerative changes that are all at about the same stage (monophasic necrosis). Concurrent necrosis and regeneration (polyphasic necrosis) can also be seen in horses that are in a sling or recumbent for an extended period of time such as for several days. Recovery depends on the extent of the ischemic area and the ability of the muscle to regenerate (i.e., depending on whether the basal lamina is intact and whether satellite cells have become necrotic from ischemia).

Transient pelvic limb muscle ischemia as the result of aortoiliac mural thrombosis occurs in horses. The cause of the thrombosis is unknown, although it has been attributed to migration of strongyle larvae through the aortic wall, damaging the intima. Typically the thrombus is not occlusive, and clinical signs of pelvic limb dysfunction occur only during or after strenuous exercise, such as racing. A short-stride gait and a decreased surface temperature of the distal portion of the affected limb during episodes are characteristic. Because the ischemia is transient, pathologic studies are few. But overt myofiber necrosis is thought to be minimal, and recovery is typically rapid. Surgery to remove the thrombus can be curative.

Postanesthetic Myopathy. Degenerative myopathy can occur in horses undergoing prolonged recumbency during general anesthesia. In some cases, muscle damage may be the result of ischemia from systemic hypotension leading to muscle hypoxia or from pressure caused by the weight of large muscle masses during recumbency, especially when adequate padding has not been provided. Underlying myopathy of various types also predisposes to postanesthetic myopathy. In ischemic damage, the location of the lesions depends on the position of the horse during anesthesia. In dorsal recumbency, the gluteal and the longissimus muscles are ischemic; in lateral recumbency, the triceps brachii, pectoralis, deltoideus, and brachiocephalicus muscles of the leg under the body become ischemic. The basic mechanism is that the pressure in the muscle exceeds the perfusion pressure in the capillaries. The use of adequate padding under the recumbent horse and the maintenance of normal blood pressure during anesthesia have greatly reduced the incidence of postanesthetic myopathy from muscle ischemia in horses. These days, underlying myopathy, particularly equine polysaccharide storage myopathy (EPSSM), appears to be the most common cause of postanesthetic myopathy in horses.

Endocrine Myopathies. Although hypothyroidism is often suggested to be a cause of muscle dysfunction in the horse, studies of experimentally thyroidectomized horses have failed to support hypothyroidism as a cause of equine myopathy. Pituitary hyperfunction caused by adenoma or hyperplasia in older horses, causing equine Cushing's disease, is the most common equine endocrine disorder causing muscle atrophy (preferentially of type 2 fibers) and weakness. The characteristic pot-bellied appearance of affected horses is thought to be secondary to abdominal muscle weakness.

Denervating Diseases

Localized or generalized muscle dysfunction can be caused by disorders affecting motor neurons or peripheral nerves. Several syndromes of peripheral nerve dysfunction are recognized in the horse.

Peripheral Neuropathy. Injury to the motor nerves in a peripheral nerve results in localized muscle atrophy and dysfunction of those myofibers innervated by those nerves. Damage to the suprascapular nerve results in unilateral scapular muscle (supraspinatus and infraspinatus) atrophy, and the clinical condition is known as sweeney. In working draft horses, this nerve can be compressed by a poorly fitted harness collar. In nonharness horses, trauma is the most common cause. Traumatic injury to the radial nerve or axillary plexus is also relatively common in horses.

Stringhalt is a sporadic pelvic limb neuropathy characterized by an exaggerated flexion of one or both hind limbs. It can be caused by trauma to the hind leg, ingestion of plant toxins, or can be of unknown cause. Outbreaks of stringhalt in pastured horses in Australia and New Zealand are the result of ingestion of *Hypochoeris radicata* and related species, also known as flatweed, false dandelion, and hairy cat's ear. Lesions of denervation atrophy are found in the distal lateral digital extensor muscle, and surgical removal of this muscle is one method of correction. *Hypochoeris radicata* grows prolifically in the Pacific Northwest, and a similar syndrome of plant-induced stringhalt is said to occur there, but evidence to support this hypothesis has been difficult to find. Feeding trials at Oregon State University have failed to reproduce the syndrome.

Fibrotic myopathy is a condition most often attributed to hamstring (semitendinosus, semimembranosus, and biceps femoris) muscle trauma, but pelvic limb neuropathy as a result of trauma or unknown causes can also cause fibrotic myopathy. Fibrotic myopathy causes a restriction of the forward swing of the affected pelvic limb. Gross examination often reveals pale, firm muscle caused by collagen deposition. When fibrotic myopathy is actually the result of neuropathy, affected muscle shows characteristic microscopic lesions of chronic denervation atrophy.

Laryngeal hemiplegia is a well-documented condition in horses in which degeneration of nerve fibers within the left recurrent laryngeal nerve results in unilateral laryngeal muscle denervation atrophy (see Fig. 15-16) and laryngeal dysfunction. Affected horses often make a characteristic respiratory noise during exercise, hence the name *roaring*. There are many possible causes of injury to the left recurrent laryngeal nerve, including extension of infections from the guttural pouches or tumors in that area, lead toxicity, and direct trauma. Most cases, however, are considered idiopathic. Although the exact cause of idiopathic laryngeal hemiplegia in horses is not known, the fact that it occurs only in tall, long-necked horses, and virtually never in ponies, suggests that whatever the mechanism of injury, very long nerves (particularly the very long left recurrent laryngeal nerve of tall long-necked horses) are predisposed.

Lead intoxication can also cause generalized peripheral neuropathy resulting in muscle atrophy and weakness mimicking equine motor neuron disease (see later discussion). Polyneuritis equi (neuritis of the cauda equina) and peripheral nerve lymphoma also cause denervation atrophy in horses. Polyneuritis equi most often involves the caudal nerve roots and facial nerves, and lymphoma has been found affecting multiple nerve roots or selectively involving the facial nerve.

Motor Neuronopathy. Damage to motor neurons in the nuclei of the brainstem or in the ventral horns of the spinal cord will result in Wallerian degeneration of peripheral nerves. In the horse, protozoal myeloencephalitis caused by *Sarcocystis neurona* is a common cause of unilateral denervation atrophy, usually of facial or gluteal musculature because of preferential damage to cranial nerve nuclei in the brainstem or motor neurons of the lumbosacral intumescence. Affected horses often also have Wallerian degeneration in spinal cord white matter and exhibit ataxia and proprioceptive deficits.

Equine motor neuron disease occurs as the result of severe and prolonged vitamin E deficiency, which leads to motor neuron degeneration. Clinical signs are sudden onset of rapid muscle wasting, weakness, trembling, and increased time spent in recumbency. Type 1 motor neurons and muscles are preferentially affected, supporting the proposed pathogenesis of oxidative injury to motor neurons secondary to vitamin E deficiency. The severe denervation atrophy occurring in postural muscles (medial head of the triceps, vastus intermedius, and sacrocaudalis dorsalis medialis) in horses with motor neuron disease often results in a remarkable pale yellow-tan color (Fig. 15-36; see Fig. 15-9, C) and gelatinous texture of the affected muscle. Severely affected horses may become persistently recumbent, leading to death or euthanasia. In some cases, high-dose vitamin E supplementation (10,000 IU or more per day) can halt the progression of the disorder, and affected horses on vitamin E therapy can even develop some compensatory muscle hypertrophy and regain muscle mass. There is little or no evidence of reinnervation in this disorder, and affected horses are considered disabled for life.

Disorders of Cattle

Although cattle have not been selected for muscle performance, many breeds have been selected for meat quality. This process has led to selection for at least one genetic disorder. Disorders affecting muscle can have a profound economic effect on the cattle industry.

Bacterial and Parasitic Myopathies

Clostridial Myositis (Blackleg). Clostridial myositis (blackleg), due to *Clostridium chauvoei*, is an extremely economically important disease that is most common in beef cattle. It can also occur in dairy cattle, especially those housed in free-stall barns where jostling and muscle bruising are possible. *Clostridium chauvoei* is a spore-forming, Gram-positive anaerobic bacillus. Its spores are ubiquitous in the soil and manure, and after ingestion they are

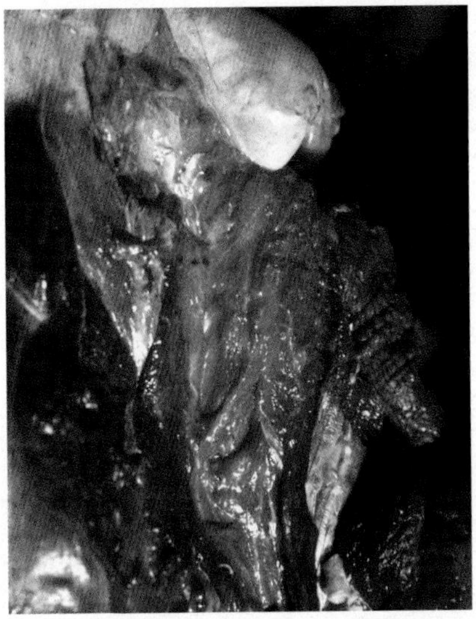

Figure 15-36 **Denervation Atrophy, Equine Motor Neuron Disease, Medial Triceps Muscle, Horse.** The medial triceps muscle *(center, top to bottom)*, a type 1 predominant postural muscle deep in the foreleg, is diffusely pale tan and gelatinous in appearance because of severe denervation atrophy. The adjacent muscles (*left* and *right*) have a normal appearance *(dark red)*. (Courtesy Dr. B.A. Valentine, College of Veterinary Medicine, Oregon State University. For histopathologic findings, see Fig. 15-18.)

capable of crossing the intestinal mucosa, entering the bloodstream, and being carried to skeletal muscles. The spores lie dormant until localized trauma to the muscle, which in cattle is most often caused by bruising during handling in a chute or from trauma in a crowded feedlot, results in muscle damage and localized hypoxia and anoxia. The resultant anaerobic conditions allow the spores to activate and the bacteria to proliferate and produce toxins that cause capillary damage with resultant hemorrhage, edema, and necrosis of adjacent myofibers.

The most common presentation is acute death. Signs before death are referable to toxemia; to the heat, swelling, crepitus, and dysfunction of the affected muscle group; and to fever. Serum concentrations of CK and AST are typically increased. Locally extensive hemorrhage and edema, often with crepitus caused by gas bubbles, are seen in affected muscles and in overlying fascia and subcutaneous tissue. Necrotic muscle fibers appear dark red to red-black. Lesions are either wet and exudative (early lesions) or dry (later lesions) (Fig. 15-37, A). A characteristic odor of rancid butter from butyric acid is typical. Cardiac muscle can also be involved. In other parts of the body, hemorrhages and edema can occur from the toxemia. Affected carcasses autolyze rapidly, likely because of the effects of clostridial toxins on tissue and of high body temperature before death. Histologically, locally extensive areas of muscle fibers undergoing coagulation necrosis and fragmentation are seen, as are interstitial edema and hemorrhage. Overt vasculitis is not seen. Gas bubbles are typical. Gram-positive bacilli whose appearance is compatible with that of *Clostridium chauvoei* may be demonstrable within affected muscle (Fig. 15-37, C).

Isolation of *Clostridium chauvoei* on anaerobic media or visualization by fluorescent antibody techniques are useful for the diagnosis of blackleg but are confirmatory only if typical gross and histopathologic lesions are present because dormant spores of *Clostridium chauvoei* can be found in normal muscle. The vaccination history and evaluation of husbandry practices are also important; unvaccinated or inadequately vaccinated (i.e., vaccinations not up to date) animals in situations in which muscle trauma is possible are most at risk. There is generally no effective treatment for cattle with blackleg, and death occurs rapidly. Prevention is the best approach. Vaccination against clostridial toxins and maintenance of a safe environment are critical.

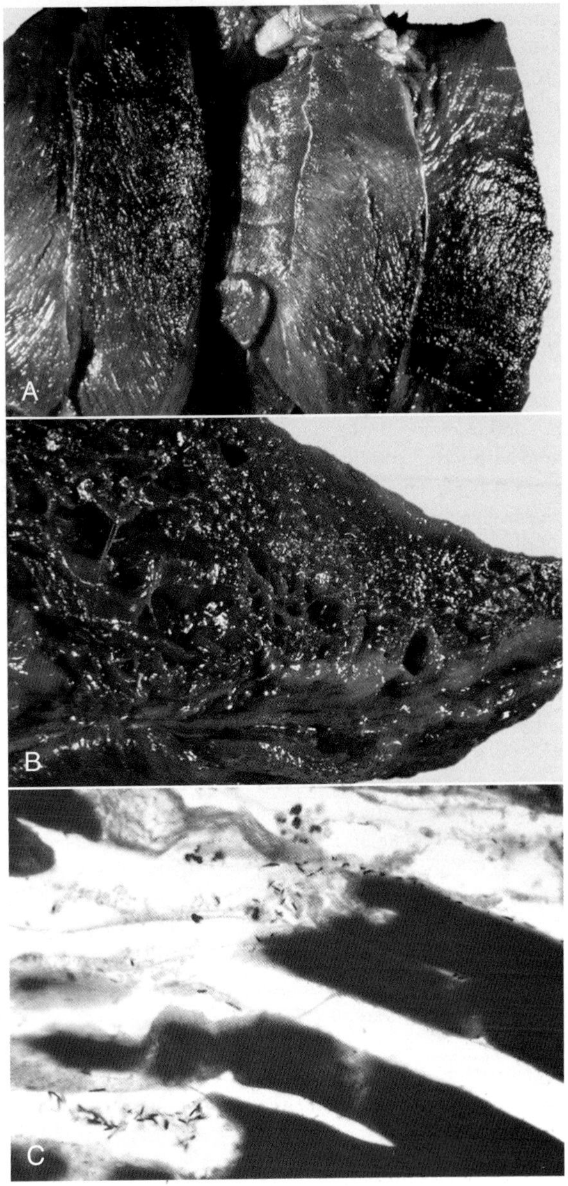

Figure 15-37 **Blackleg, Hemorrhagic-Necrotizing Myositis (*Clostridium Chauvoei*), Thigh Muscle, Cow. A,** The dark red areas are caused by hemorrhagic necrosis of the affected muscle. These lesions are characteristic of blackleg. **B,** *Clostridium chauvoei* can also produce substantial quantities of gas within infected tissues as shown here by the numerous ("pseudocystic") spaces within hemorrhagic and necrotic muscle. **C,** Gram-positive bacilli *(blue-stained rods)* are present in the affected tissue. Formalin fixation, Gram stain. (**A** courtesy Dr. B.A. Valentine, College of Veterinary Medicine, Oregon State University. **B** and **C** courtesy Dr. M.D. McGavin, College of Veterinary Medicine, University of Tennessee.)

Botulism. Botulism caused by ingestion of *Clostridium botulinum* toxin from contaminated feed or soil occurs in cattle, and clinical signs of flaccid paralysis and pathogenesis are similar to those in the adult horse. Cattle are most susceptible to type C and D botulinum toxins, and herd outbreaks are possible. Cattle, however, are much more resistant to botulism than are horses. Botulinum toxin, most often from animal cadavers such as mice or rats, within silage, haylage, or hay is the most common cause of outbreaks of botulism in cattle. Abnormal eating habits (pica) can result in ingestion of *Clostridium botulinum* toxin from the soil or carrion. Botulism in cattle is usually fatal.

Pyogenic Bacteria. Cattle are prone to develop abscesses and cellulitis (fasciitis) from infections with pyogenic bacteria, most commonly *Trueperella* (*Arcanobacterium*) *pyogenes*. Abscesses in muscle occur most commonly in the hind leg. Swelling and lameness of the affected limb caused by widespread necrotizing cellulitis and myositis are seen.

Trueperella (*Arcanobacterium*) *pyogenes* is a ubiquitous bacterium that can infect muscle by two routes: by direct contamination of wounds and injection sites and hematogenously. The bacterium can be found within the reproductive tract of cows and within the rumen wall, and it has been speculated that *Trueperella* (*Arcanobacterium*) *pyogenes* from a transient bacteremia after parturition or from disruption of the rumen wall can result in colonization of damaged muscle. Lesions vary, depending on the virulence of the bacteria and the age of the lesions. They vary in extent from encapsulated intramuscular abscesses adjacent to the site of injection to a diffuse purulent cellulitis extending down the tissue and fascial planes (see Fig. 15-24). The cellulitis may be so severe as to involve much of the musculature of the affected limb. When abscesses are present, the gross appearance is of an encapsulated mass filled with thick, yellow-green, foul-smelling pus. In cases of cellulitis, pus dissects along fascial planes outside the muscle and between perimysial sheaths within muscles. Inflammation extends into the adjacent myofibers, resulting in myonecrosis and subsequent replacement by fibrous tissue. The greenish color of the exudate is distinctive, and small Gram-positive pleomorphic bacteria are often seen within tissue sections or cytologic preparations. *Trueperella* (*Arcanobacterium*) *pyogenes* is readily isolated on aerobic culture.

Actinobacillus lignieresii (Wooden Tongue). Infection of oral tissue, particularly of the tongue musculature (see Figs. 7-26 and 7-27), by *Actinobacillus lignieresii* results in a severe chronic granulomatous to pyogranulomatous and fibrosing myositis. Infection occurs through oral wounds or by penetrating plant fragments. Affected cattle have difficulty prehending and swallowing and often have excessive salivation. Histologic features include marked fibrosis caused by tissue destruction and chronicity and foci of inflammation containing eosinophilic material ("radiating clubs") and characteristic Gram-negative bacilli. Aggressive antibiotic therapy can be curative.

Actinomyces bovis (Lumpy Jaw). *Actinomyces bovis* frequently involves bones of the jaw, causing chronic granulomatous to pyogranulomatous and fibrosing osteomyelitis (see Fig. 16-58). Occasionally *Actinomyces bovis* involves the musculature of the tongue, causing gross and histologic lesions similar to those caused by *Actinobacillus lignieresii*. Gram stain reveals Gram-positive bacilli, which distinguishes this lesion from the Gram-negative *Actinobacillus lignieresii* infection.

Protozoal Myopathies. *Sarcocystis* spp. forming intracytoplasmic cysts (see Fig. 15-26) is a common incidental finding that may even be grossly visible as nodules within skeletal and cardiac myofibers of cattle (see Fig. 15-40). Massive infection may result in fever, anorexia, and progressive wasting, but this is uncommon. More often, *Sarcocystis* infection is diagnosed as an incidental finding at necropsy or during meat inspection at slaughter. If the cyst wall breaks down, a focus of myofiber necrosis and later granulomatous inflammation result.

Eosinophilic myositis is a disease of cattle thought to be a relatively uncommon manifestation of *Sarcocystis* infection that may involve hypersensitivity. There is overt green discoloration (see Fig. 15-10) of affected muscles caused by the massive infiltration of eosinophils (Fig. 15-38, *A* and *B*). This is accompanied by myofiber necrosis and, in chronic cases, fibrosis. Fragments of degenerating intralesional protozoa can sometimes be found (Fig. 15-38, *C*).

Neospora caninum can also infect cattle. Adults have no clinical disease, but infection of the fetus can cause multifocal nonsuppurative inflammation of skeletal muscle and heart and brain.

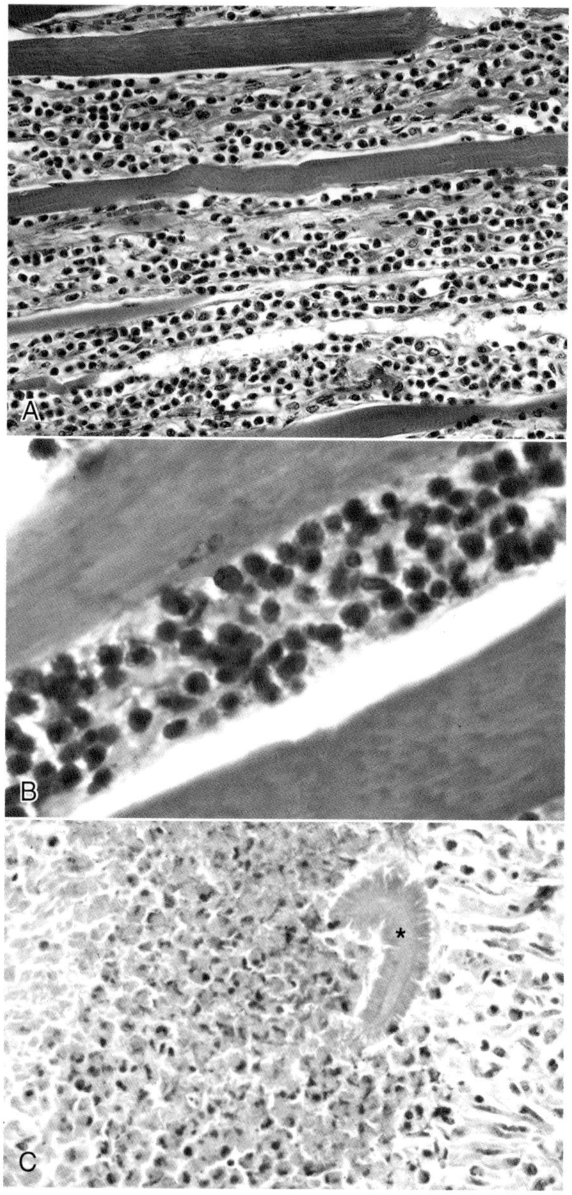

Figure 15-38 **Bovine Eosinophilic Myositis, Skeletal Muscle, Longitudinal Section, Cow. A,** Dense interstitial infiltrate of eosinophils has separated the muscle fibers, some of which are atrophic. Formalin fixation, H&E stain. **B,** Higher magnification demonstrating the large population of eosinophils in the inflammatory exudate. Formalin fixation, H&E stain. **C,** Degenerate *Sarcocystis* organism *(asterisk)* surrounded by degenerate eosinophils. Formalin fixation, H&E stain. (**A** courtesy Dr. M.D. McGavin, College of Veterinary Medicine, University of Tennessee; and Noah's Arkive, College of Veterinary Medicine, The University of Georgia. **B** courtesy Dr. M.D. McGavin, College of Veterinary Medicine, University of Tennessee. **C** courtesy Dr. R. Bildfell, College of Veterinary Medicine, Oregon State University.)

Nutritional and Toxic Myopathies

Nutritional Myopathy. Similar to horses, calves and young cattle are susceptible to nutritional myopathy caused by a selenium or (less commonly) vitamin E deficiency. But the profound involvement of temporal and masseter muscles ("maxillary myositis") that can occur in horses is not seen in cattle. In the latter species, the postural muscles and muscles of locomotion are most commonly affected. Muscles of affected calves appear pale pink to white, often in a patchy distribution and in cervical muscles used during suckling and "bumping" the udder. The gross appearance depends on the extent of the necrosis and the stage of the lesion. In early stages, yellow and white streaks are present, and later pale, chalk white streaks from calcification often appear, thus the common name *white muscle disease* (Fig. 15-39). Confirmation of the diagnosis is based on blood or liver analysis for selenium and vitamin E.

Plant Toxicities. *Cassia occidentalis* (coffee senna, coffee weed) is the most common cause of degenerative myopathy in cattle as the result of plant toxicity. This plant grows throughout the southeastern United States. Pale areas within skeletal muscle, with lesser involvement of cardiac muscle, are caused by myofiber necrosis, generally with minimal to no mineralization. Other plant toxicities are discussed in the toxic myopathies section.

Ionophore Toxicity. The pathogenesis of ionophore toxicity is discussed in the toxic myopathy section. Ionophore toxicity in cattle is seen only with overdoses because of improper feed mixing. Anorexia, diarrhea, and weakness are the primary clinical signs. Serum concentrations of CK and AST are often extremely high (e.g., CK greater than 50,000 U/L and AST greater than 5000 U/L). Pale areas within skeletal and cardiac muscle are due to myofiber necrosis. In animals that survive, regeneration will restore the skeletal muscle completely, but cardiac lesions heal by fibrosis.

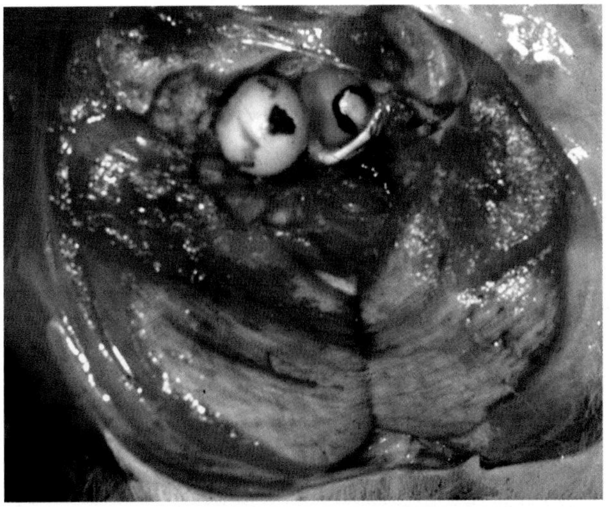

Figure 15-39 **Nutritional Myopathy (White Muscle Disease), Skeletal Muscles of the Caudal Thigh, Sagittal Section, Calf.** In this early stage, affected muscles have yellow and white streaks, often in a patchy distribution. These streaks are areas of necrotic myofibers. Later as the necrotic myofibers calcify, white streaks (chalky texture, mineralization) are visible grossly. (Courtesy Dr. G.K. Saunders, Virginia-Maryland Regional College of Veterinary Medicine; and Noah's Arkive, College of Veterinary Medicine, The University of Georgia.)

Congenital or Inherited Disorders

Steatosis. Steatosis in cattle, sometimes called *lipomatosis*, is most often recognized as an incidental finding at necropsy or at slaughter. This disorder is thought to be the result of defective in utero muscle development, in which large areas of myofibers are replaced by adipocytes. An inherited basis has not been established. Lesions can be symmetric or asymmetric, with the most severely affected muscles being those of the back and loin (longissimus muscles; see Fig. 15-9, *D*). The most severely affected muscles are composed entirely of fat, whereas less severely affected muscles appear streaked because of partial replacement by fat. Histologically, the space normally occupied by myofibers is filled with mature adipocytes. In utero denervation or failure of innervation results in a similar muscle lesion (see Fig. 15-23), and careful evaluation of the peripheral nerves and spinal cord is indicated.

Diagnosis is readily made on gross examination and can be confirmed by histologic examination, specifically in frozen sections stained with Oil Red O or Sudan black for fat. Because this condition is usually not diagnosed during life and the loss of myofibers is irreversible, treatment is neither necessary nor possible.

Other Bovine Congenital or Inherited Myopathies and Neuronopathies. Congenital muscular hyperplasia ("double muscling") resulting from defects in the myostatin gene occurs in a variety of cattle breeds. An unusual multisystemic disease with characteristic necrotizing vasculopathy occurs in young Gelbvieh cattle. Glycogenosis type II (acid maltase deficiency) has been recognized in shorthorn and Brahman cattle, and glycogenosis type V (myophosphorylase deficiency) occurs in Charolais cattle. An inherited motor neuron degenerative disease occurs in Brown Swiss cattle. These disorders are discussed in more detail in E-Appendix 15-1.

Electrolyte Abnormalities

Hypokalemic Myopathy. Decreased potassium interferes with normal muscle cell function and can lead to muscle weakness and myofiber necrosis. Type 2 fibers are preferentially affected. The pathogenesis of hypokalemic myopathy is not clear, but myofiber necrosis may be the end result of either decreased myofiber energy production or focal ischemia secondary to vasoconstriction. Hypokalemia can also interfere with normal cardiac conduction, and atrial fibrillation is common. Hypokalemia in cattle can be the result of anorexia. A history of ketosis occurring within a month of parturition is common. Glucocorticoids with high mineralocorticoid activity, such as isoflupredone acetate used to treat ketosis, are a recognized cause of hypokalemic myopathy in cattle. Activation of glucose transport into cells by intravenously administered glucose or insulin also causes intracellular movement of potassium and can result in hypokalemia. No specific findings are present at postmortem examination, although ischemic necrosis secondary to recumbency can be seen in muscles of the hind limbs (see later discussion). Lesions of multifocal polyphasic myofiber necrosis and vacuolated myofibers (vacuolar degeneration) are present in all muscles, including those not involved in weight-bearing, and are indicative of myodegeneration as a direct effect of hypokalemia.

Affected cows are profoundly weak and become recumbent and unable to support the weight of their heads. Serum concentration of potassium is below normal (<2.3 mEq/L), and CK and AST levels are moderately high (CK up to approximately 25,000 U/L and AST up to approximately 2000 U/L). The diagnosis is based on typical historic and clinical findings and a low serum potassium concentration. Intravenous and oral supplementation with potassium salts and supportive therapy may result in recovery in some cases, but this disorder is often fatal.

Other Electrolyte Abnormalities. Both hypocalcemia and hypophosphatemia can result in profound muscle weakness and recumbency in cattle. In hypocalcemia, weakness is primarily the result of disruption of neuromuscular transmission. Significant changes are not seen in affected muscles, although ischemic necrosis can occur secondary to recumbency (see later discussion). Diagnosis relies on clinical findings and identification of abnormally low serum calcium or phosphorus concentrations. Treatment includes correction of the electrolyte defect by intravenous administration of the appropriate electrolyte-containing fluids, supportive care, and correction of any dietary abnormalities that may predispose to electrolyte problems.

Ischemic Myopathy

Ischemic muscle necrosis caused by recumbency is common in cattle. The muscular lesion is similar to that seen in other species, but in cattle, prolonged sternal recumbency is more common than lateral recumbency, and pectoral muscles and muscles of limbs tucked under the body or splayed out limbs are most prone to injury (see Fig. 15-25).

Disorders of Sheep and Goats

Selection pressures and economic consequences of muscle disorders similar to those in beef cattle exist in small ruminants raised for meat. In goats, selection for an interesting mutant has resulted in perpetuation of myotonia.

Bacterial and Parasitic Myopathies

Clostridial Myositis (Blackleg). Clostridial myositis (blackleg) occurs occasionally in sheep and goats and is similar to the disease in cattle.

Botulism. Botulism can occur in small ruminants, but, as in cattle, it is rare.

Protozoal Myopathy. Intracytoplasmic cysts of *Sarcocystis* spp. are commonly found within skeletal and cardiac muscle fibers of sheep and goats as an incidental finding, similar to findings in muscle and heart of cattle. Eosinophilic myositis as a result of sarcocystosis is rare in sheep and is not recognized in goats. In camelids, massive infection with *Sarcocystis* can occur (Fig. 15-40), especially in animals imported from South America where sarcocystosis is common. In rare cases, *Sarcocystis* infection in camelids is associated with widespread eosinophilic myositis.

Nutritional and Toxic Myopathies

Degenerative myopathy caused by nutritional deficiency or toxin ingestion is relatively common in many small ruminant species. The nonselective eating habits of goats make them particularly likely to ingest poisonous plants.

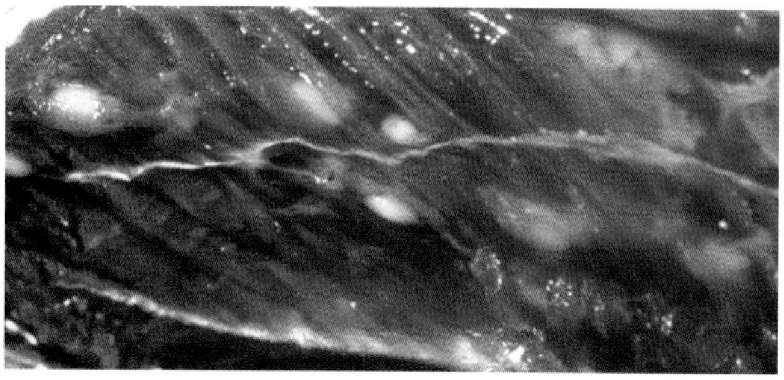

Figure 15-40 **Sarcocystosis, Skeletal Muscle, Alpaca.** Multiple pale gray-white nodules within the muscle indicate the location of *Sarcocystis* cysts. (Courtesy Dr. B.A. Valentine, College of Veterinary Medicine, Oregon State University.)

Nutritional Myopathy. Young goats and sheep are susceptible to degenerative myopathy associated with selenium or, less commonly, vitamin E deficiency. A similar disorder occurs rarely in young camelids. The disease in these species is similar to the disease in young cattle.

Toxic Myopathies. Sheep and goats are susceptible to plant and ionophore toxicities, similar to those in cattle. In goats, ingestion of honey mesquite (*Prosopis glandulosa*) causes degeneration of the motor nucleus of the trigeminal nerve, resulting in denervation atrophy of the muscles of mastication, and consequent inability to adequately chew feed, leading to progressive emaciation.

Congenital or Inherited Myopathies

Myotonia in Goats. Myotonia in the goat is inherited as an autosomal dominant trait, and the variable clinical severity is attributable to increased severity in homozygotes compared with heterozygotes. The genetic defect affects the skeletal muscle chloride channel, resulting in decreased chloride conductance and associated ionic instability of the sarcolemma. Starting at approximately 2 weeks of age, affected goats develop severe muscle spasms in response to sudden voluntary effort, for example, when startled by the blowing of a locomotive's horn. Episodes of myotonia can last from 5 to 20 seconds and are characterized by generalized stiffness and adoption of a "sawhorse" stance. Goats often fall over. Sustained dimpling of muscle occurs after percussion. Serum concentrations of CK and AST are normal. Concentric needle EMG reveals the characteristic waxing and waning ("dive bomber") spontaneous activity of myotonia. There are no gross pathologic findings. Histologically, muscle fibers in affected goats may show moderate hypertrophy. But characteristic abnormalities are revealed only with ultrastructural examination in which dilated and proliferated T tubules and terminal cisternae of sarcoplasmic reticulum are seen. Diagnosis is based on characteristic clinical signs and EMG findings. There is no treatment for this disorder, and it is rarely fatal. Affected animals are actually prized by collectors of so-called fainting goats. If nothing else, housing for these animals is simplified because fencing need not be nearly as high as that required for normal goats.

Other Inherited Myopathies. An inherited myopathy (ovine muscular dystrophy) in Merino sheep and an inherited glycogen storage myopathy have been identified in sheep in Australia. These disorders are discussed in more detail in E-Appendix 15-1.

Megaesophagus in Camelids

The tunica muscularis of the esophagus of camelids contains a large amount of skeletal muscle, and adult llamas and alpacas are prone to develop abnormal motility and dilation of the esophagus (megaesophagus). Affected animals often lose body condition and exhibit abnormal rumination of feed boluses. Histopathologic findings of angular atrophy of type 1 and type 2 fibers in the esophagus of affected older llamas suggest that this disorder is an acquired denervating disease, but further studies are necessary. Megaesophagus in alpacas occurs in young animals, and to date no diagnostic muscular lesions have been detected.

Disorders of Pigs

The economic impact of muscle disease in pigs is profound. The high percentage of pigs with the genetic defect that predisposes to malignant hyperthermia is another example of selection pressure leading to skeletal muscle genetic mutations.

Bacterial and Parasitic Myopathies

Clostridial Myositis (Malignant Edema). Pigs occasionally develop clostridial myositis (usually *Clostridium septicum*), particularly at sites of intramuscular injection. The resulting disease is similar to that seen in cattle, sheep, and goats, although heart involvement appears to be rare.

Pyogenic Bacteria. Abscesses within muscles and their fascia as a result of infection by pyogenic bacteria, such as *Trueperella* (*Arcanobacterium*) *pyogenes*, are common in pigs and are similar to those in cattle.

Trichinosis. Infection of pigs by the nematode parasite *Trichinella spiralis* is of major economic importance to the porcine industry and poses a serious health hazard to human beings. Pigs infected with *Trichinella spiralis* show no clinical signs.

The adult nematode resides in the mucosa of the small intestine. Larvae penetrate the intestinal mucosa and enter the bloodstream, through which they gain access to the muscle. Larvae invade and encyst within myocytes. Encysted larvae are typically not visible on gross examination, although dead larvae can calcify and be visible as 0.5- to 1-mm white nodules (Fig. 15-41, A). Active muscles, such as the tongue, masseter, diaphragm, and intercostal, laryngeal, and extraocular muscles, are preferentially affected. Focal inflammation consisting of eosinophils, neutrophils, and lymphocytes occurs associated with invasion of the muscle by *Trichinella* larvae. After cyst formation, the larvae are protected from the host's immune response and inflammation is minimal to absent (Fig. 15-41, B).

Diagnosis is based on identification of the characteristic nematode larvae encysted within muscle fibers. In those cases in which the larvae have died and calcified, a presumptive diagnosis of trichinosis can still be made.

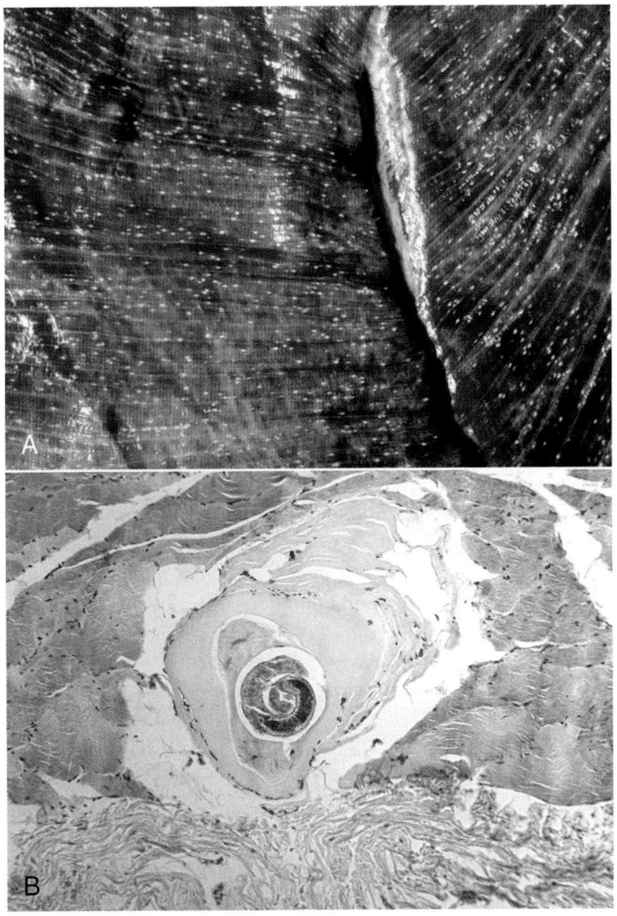

Figure 15-41 Trichinosis, Encysted Larvae, Diaphragm, Bear. A, Encysted larvae of *Trichinella spiralis* appear as pale elongated gray-white foci in the muscle. **B,** Encysted larvae *(center)* of *Trichinella spiralis* incite minimal inflammation until they die. Formalin fixation, H&E stain. (Courtesy Dr. M.D. McGavin, College of Veterinary Medicine, University of Tennessee.)

Protozoal Myopathies. Intracytoplasmic cysts of *Sarcocystis* spp. are not common in pigs but can occasionally be found in the skeletal and cardiac muscle fibers as an incidental finding. Eosinophilic myocarditis has been reported after experimental infection.

Nutritional and Toxic Myopathies

Nutritional Myopathy. Young pigs are susceptible to degenerative myopathy caused by selenium or vitamin E deficiency, and the pathologic changes are similar to those seen in calves. A distinctive clinical disorder seen in very young Vietnamese pot-bellied pigs, in which affected piglets have a short, stilted gait and tend to stand on their toes, is thought to be related to selenium or vitamin E deficiency. Histologically, there is multifocal polyphasic myofiber necrosis. Affected piglets appear to recover spontaneously.

Toxic Myopathies. Pigs are susceptible to poisoning by *Cassia occidentalis* and develop segmental necrosis of myofibers, especially in the diaphragm. Monensin toxicity results in segmental necrosis of skeletal muscle and necrosis of cardiac muscle, particularly of the atria. The pathogenesis of ionophore toxicity is discussed in the previous section on Toxic Myopathies. Gossypol present in cottonseed products is toxic to pigs when these products are fed at 10% or more of the ration and causes skeletal and cardiac muscle necrosis, as well as lesions in the liver and lung.

Congenital and Inherited Myopathies

Myofibrillar Hypoplasia (Splay Leg). Myofibrillar hypoplasia (splay leg) is a congenital disorder that affects young piglets and results in splaying of the limbs laterally (abduction). Affected animals propel themselves by pushing against the ground with the pelvic limbs. This posture results in progressive flattening of the sternum. Although delayed myofibril development has been suggested, the histopathologic findings are inconclusive because similarly poorly developed myofibers can be seen in normal littermates. Affected piglets can recover with treatment, which includes the use of a harness that partially supports their bodies, holds their legs under their bodies, and encourages locomotion. Providing affected pigs with a nonslip floor is also important.

Steatosis. Pigs can have large areas of muscle replaced by mature adipose tissue, similar to that described in cattle.

Malignant Hyperthermia (Porcine Stress Syndrome; Pale Soft Exudative Pork). MH (porcine stress syndrome, pale soft exudative pork) affects several strains of pigs, most commonly those with unpigmented hair coats. A similar syndrome occurs in Vietnamese pot-bellied pigs. Incidence varies but can be very high within certain herds. The disease in pigs is an accurate animal model of the disease in human beings and is an important cause of economic losses in the pig industry. Susceptibility to MH is inherited as an autosomal recessive trait. The genetic defect results in abnormal activity of the skeletal muscle ryanodine receptor. The ryanodine receptor is a calcium release channel located in the sarcoplasmic reticulum terminal cisternal membrane that links the T tubule to the sarcoplasmic reticulum during excitation-contraction coupling. Uncontrolled intracytoplasmic calcium release because of abnormal ryanodine receptor activity leads to excessive contraction with resultant heat production. Clinical disease occurs only in pigs homozygous for the defect, although human heterozygotes can also be susceptible to hyperthermic episodes after halothane anesthesia. It is suspected that this defect originated more than 50 years ago in a foundation animal and resulted in offspring with increased muscling and reduced body fat. Affected pigs are clinically normal until an episode of hyperthermia is triggered by a precipitating factor such as halothane anesthesia or stress. Episodes consist of severe muscle rigidity and dramatically increased body temperature. Severe cases progress rapidly to death. Serum concentrations of CK and AST are markedly increased during episodes.

In animals dying during a hyperthermic episode, affected muscles are pale, moist, and swollen and appear "cooked" (Fig. 15-42), thus the common name "pale, soft, exudative pork." Muscles of the shoulder, back, and thigh are preferentially affected. Affected fibers are either hypercontracted or, if the animal has survived for some hours, are undergoing coagulation necrosis. Histopathologic findings in susceptible pigs sampled during clinically normal periods include chronic myopathic change (fiber-size variation, internal nuclei) and rare necrotic fibers.

This disorder is most commonly diagnosed in pigs dying acutely and is made based on the clinical history of a precipitating stress and on the characteristic gross and histopathologic findings. Given that the precise defect is known, genetic testing allows for identification of carrier and affected animals. Avoidance of precipitating stress factors in susceptible pigs and removal of carrier and affected animals from the breeding stock reduce the incidence of this disorder.

Ischemic Myopathy

Large pigs are susceptible to ischemic myopathy secondary to recumbency, resulting in ischemic necrosis similar to that seen in horses and cattle. The proximal limb muscles are most susceptible.

Disorders of Dogs

Selection pressures for a certain type of muscular development are far less frequent in dogs than in livestock. A few disorders, such as myotonia, have been suggested to occur more often in dogs originally bred for meat, but this is pure speculation. The canine genome may have genes prone to new mutations, similar to human beings, leading to genetic disorders, such as X-linked muscular dystrophy. In general, the impact of muscular disorders in dogs is much less than in livestock. Dogs with muscular weakness can still make good house pets.

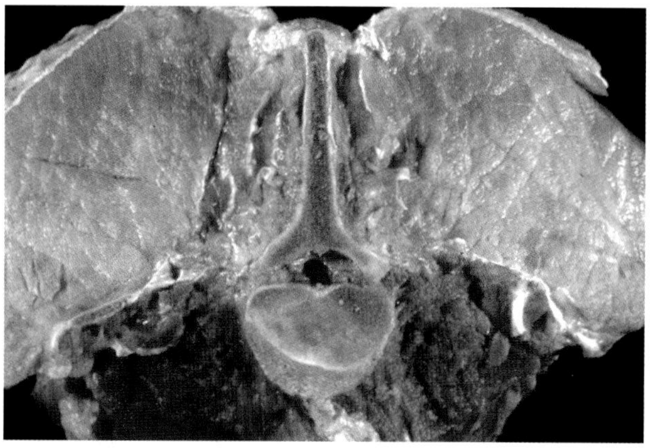

Figure 15-42 **Malignant Hyperthermia (Porcine Stress Syndrome, Pale Soft Exudative Pork), Lumbar Epispinal Muscles, Transverse Section, Pig.** The affected muscles are pale pink, moist, and swollen and have a "cooked" pork appearance ("parboiled"). (Courtesy Dr. J. Wright, College of Veterinary Medicine, North Carolina State University; and Noah's Arkive, College of Veterinary Medicine, The University of Georgia.)

Parasitic Myopathies

Protozoal Myopathy. The parasitic diseases affecting skeletal muscle in the dog are primarily caused by protozoal organisms, of which *Neospora caninum* is the most important. It is now suspected that early reports of myositis and radiculoneuritis attributed to *Toxoplasma gondii* in young dogs were actually the result of *Neospora caninum* infections. *Neospora caninum* is often transmitted in utero, and evidence suggests that affected bitches are chronic carriers of the organism. Both the peripheral nervous system and the skeletal muscle are invaded by organisms. Ventral spinal roots are preferentially involved, and damage results in denervation atrophy of muscles. Signs of progressive neuromuscular weakness, most profound in the pelvic limbs, begin in affected pups several weeks of age. Marked muscle atrophy of the pelvic limb muscles occurs rapidly, and fixation of pelvic limb joints occurs as a result of denervation of muscle in an actively growing limb. Serum concentrations of CK and AST may be slightly increased. Concentric needle EMG reveals dense, sustained spontaneous activity (fibrillations and positive sharp waves) consistent with denervation.

Pelvic limb muscles are severely atrophied, firm, and pale. Fixation of the pelvic limb joints persists after anesthesia or death. Scattered foci of mixed inflammation with associated segmental myofiber necrosis are often seen within skeletal muscle, and characteristic intracytoplasmic protozoal cysts may be present.

Neospora caninum infection should be suspected based on characteristic progressive neuromuscular dysfunction in a young growing pup. Infection of older dogs is also possible but is uncommon. The finding of a mixed inflammatory-neuropathic lesion within affected skeletal muscle should prompt a search for protozoa, although these are often present in small numbers and may not be seen. Serologic tests can detect antibodies to *Neospora caninum*, and antibodies are available for immunohistochemical studies of paraffin-embedded, formalin-fixed tissue. Antiprotozoal treatment may kill the organisms, but denervation atrophy and pelvic limb fixation will persist.

Hepatozoon americanum and *Trypanosoma cruzi* are other protozoal organisms that can affect canine skeletal muscle. These parasitic diseases are discussed in more detail in E-Appendix 15-1.

Other Parasites. Rarely, cysts of *Trichinella spiralis* are found as an incidental finding in canine muscle.

Congenital or Inherited Myopathies

X-Linked Muscular Dystrophy (Duchenne's Type). X-linked muscular dystrophy (Duchenne's type) has been confirmed or suspected in several breeds of dogs, including Irish terrier, golden retriever, Labrador retriever, miniature schnauzer, Rottweiler, Dalmatian, Shetland sheepdog, Samoyed, Pembroke Welsh corgi, Japanese spitz, and Alaskan malamute. This canine disorder is homologous to Duchenne's muscular dystrophy of human beings and involves defects in the dystrophin gene, which codes for a membrane-associated cytoskeletal protein present in skeletal and cardiac muscle. The absence of dystrophin renders skeletal muscle fibers susceptible to repeated bouts of necrosis and regeneration. Necrosis of cardiac myocytes also occurs and is followed by replacement with connective tissue, resulting in a progressive cardiomyopathy. This disorder is inherited as an X-linked recessive trait, affecting approximately 50% of males born to a female carrier. Experimentally, affected females have been produced from breeding of an affected male to a carrier female. It is suspected that new mutations in the canine dystrophin gene may be relatively common, as is the case in human beings. Therefore this disorder could occur in any breed, including crossbreeds. There is variable severity of clinical disease even within littermates, and small breed dogs are often less severely affected than are large breed dogs.

Severely affected pups develop a rapidly progressive weakness and die within the first few days of life. In less severely affected dogs, clinical signs are a stiff, short-strided gait and exercise intolerance beginning at 8 to 12 weeks of age, followed by progressive weakness and muscle atrophy. Development of a degree of joint contracture and splaying of the distal limbs is typical (Fig. 15-43). Weakness of the tongue, jaw, and pharyngeal muscles results in difficulty with prehension and swallowing of food, and affected dogs often drool excessively. Involvement of skeletal muscle within the esophagus can result in megaesophagus, which can cause regurgitation, and aspiration pneumonia. Markedly increased concentrations of serum CK, AST, and ALT are characteristic, even before the onset of obvious clinical disease. Concentric needle EMG reveals remarkable spontaneous activity in the form of pseudomyotonic bursts. Muscles do not dimple with percussion.

In pups dying within the first few days of life, the thin superficial muscles of the shoulder, neck, and pelvic limbs (trapezius, brachiocephalicus, deltoid, and sartorius) and the diaphragm have pale yellow-to-white streaks throughout (see Fig. 15-9, A). Death in these cases is thought to be caused by respiratory failure related to severe diaphragmatic myonecrosis. In animals with clinical disease beginning at 8 to 12 weeks, pale streaks within muscle are much less evident, although affected muscles often appear diffusely pale and may be fibrotic. All skeletal muscles, with the exception of the extraocular muscles, appear to be affected to varying degrees. Overt myofiber necrosis is most severe in earlier stages of the disorder and typically affects small clusters of contiguous myofibers. Scattered large, darkly stained myofibers ("large dark fibers") in the early stages of hypercontraction and segmental necrosis are common (see Fig. 15-11, A). Regeneration of affected segments occurs rapidly, and characteristically both myofiber necrosis and fiber regeneration are present within the same section (i.e., the lesion is a multifocal polyphasic necrosis) (Fig. 15-44). Scattered mineralized fibers can also be found. With time, ongoing necrosis and regeneration are less common, and endomysial fibrosis occurs. Chronically affected muscles can have remarkable fibrosis, infiltration by adipocytes, and other chronic myopathic changes. Fiber-type conversion can also be seen as a chronic myopathic change.

In all dogs 6 months of age or older, multifocal pale yellow to white zones will be present within the heart, predominantly involving the subepicardial region of the left ventricular wall, the papillary muscles, and the ventricular septum. Histologically, necrosis, mineralization, and progressive dissecting myocardial fibrosis are found. Death in older animals is the result of either progressive cardiac failure or aspiration pneumonia secondary to dysphagia, although affected dogs may survive for many years.

The diagnosis should be suspected based on characteristic clinical findings in a young male dog but must be confirmed by muscle biopsy and analysis of muscle for dystrophin. The absence of dystrophin in muscle fibers of affected dogs can be confirmed using immunohistochemical staining on frozen sections (Fig. 15-45) or by Western blot analysis. There is no treatment for this disorder.

Carrier females show no clinical signs, but scattered necrotic and regenerating fibers and moderate increases in serum CK and AST are common in young carriers. At birth, dystrophin in carriers is expressed as a mosaic pattern in individual cardiac and skeletal myofibers (Fig. 15-45, C). Because they are multinucleate, skeletal myofibers are able to eventually upregulate and translocate dystrophin to restore this protein to those segments where it is missing throughout the entire myofiber. Fiber necrosis is therefore rare in older carriers. Cardiac muscle, however, remains mosaic for life. Foci

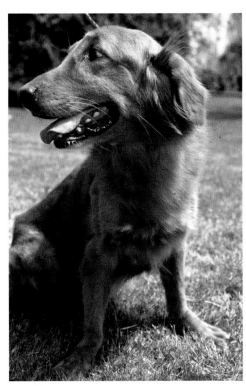

Figure 15-43 **Canine Muscular Dystrophy, X-Linked Muscular Dystrophy, Adult Golden Retriever.** Note the diffuse muscle wasting and splaying (outward rotation) of the forelimbs. (Courtesy Dr. B.A. Valentine, College of Veterinary Medicine, Oregon State University.)

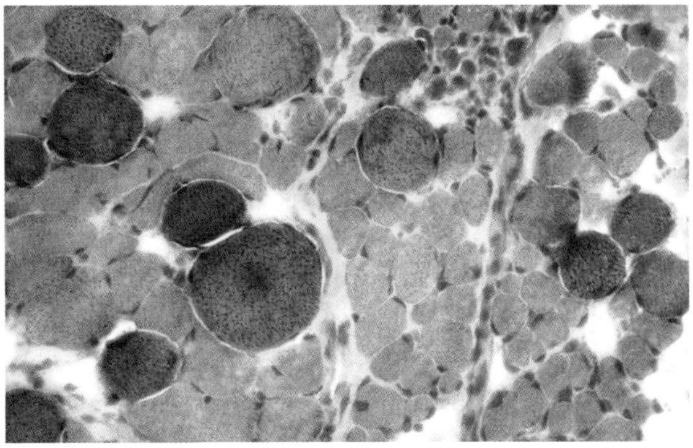

Figure 15-44 **Canine Muscular Dystrophy, X-Linked Muscular Dystrophy, Biceps Femoris Muscle, Transverse Section, Dog.** The numerous large dark blue staining fibers *(left)* are undergoing acute necrosis, and the cluster of small-diameter fibers with large prominent nuclei *(top right)* are regenerating. The presence of both necrotic and regenerating fibers is indicative of polyphasic necrosis. Frozen section, modified Gomori's trichrome stain. (Courtesy Dr. B.A. Valentine, College of Veterinary Medicine, Oregon State University.)

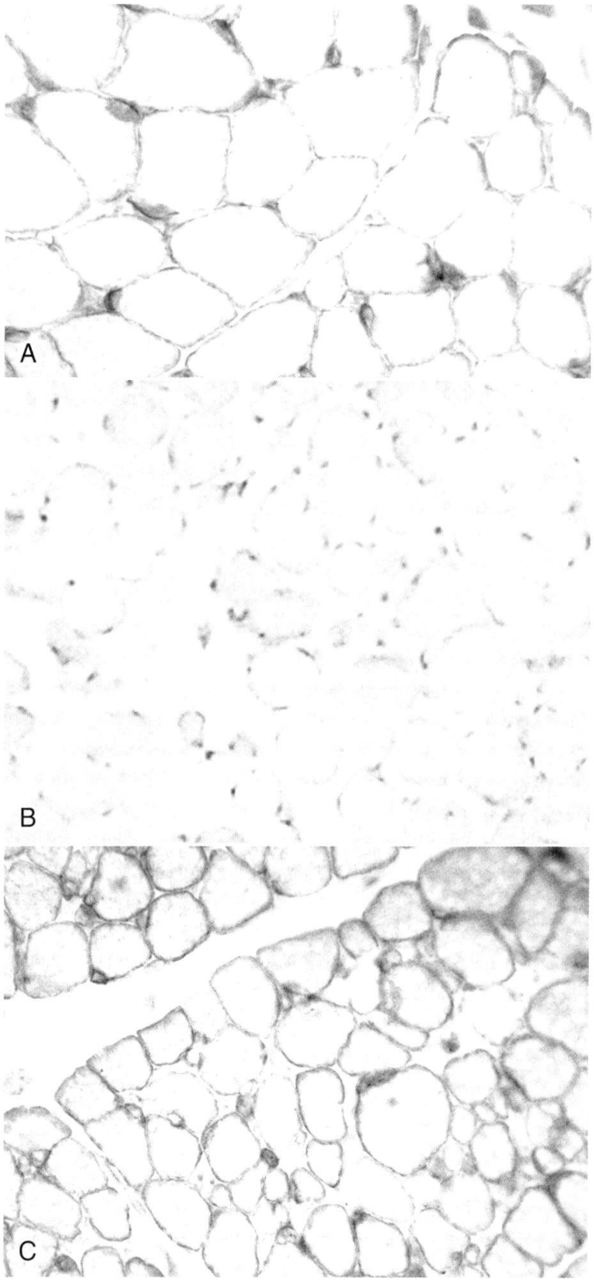

Figure 15-45 Dystrophin Localization *(Brown Stain)* in Transverse Sections of Canine Muscle, Immunostain for Dystrophin, Skeletal Muscle. A, Normal dog. Note that the dystrophin is localized at the sarcolemma. Frozen section, immunoperoxidase reaction for dystrophin. **B,** X-linked muscular dystrophy, dog. Dystrophin is completely absent. Frozen section, immunoperoxidase reaction for dystrophin. **C,** X-linked muscular dystrophy carrier, young carrier female dog. Note the mosaic pattern in which some fibers contain normal dystrophin and others completely lack dystrophin. Frozen section, immunoperoxidase reaction for dystrophin. (Courtesy Dr. B.J. Cooper, College of Veterinary Medicine, Oregon State University.)

of necrosis and development of fibrosis occurs in the cardiac muscle of carrier females, but to date, none have developed overt cardiac failure. Any female dog producing affected pups is a carrier, and approximately half of all of her female offspring will also be carriers. Carrier females can also be identified by either dystrophin or DNA analysis and should be spayed.

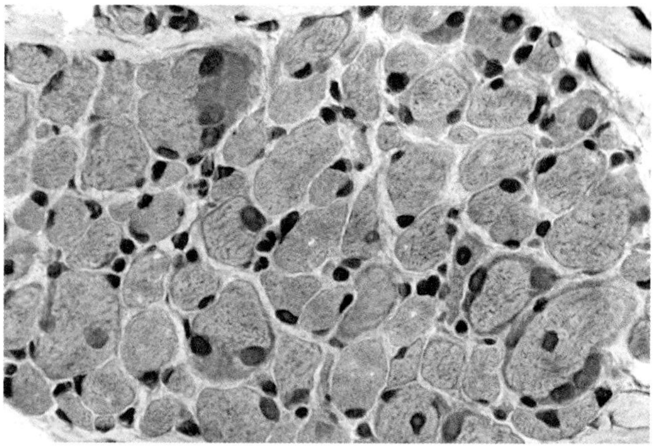

Figure 15-46 Labrador Retriever Centronuclear Myopathy, Skeletal Muscle, Transverse Section, Labrador Retriever Dog. There is excessive fiber-size variation, and some fibers contain one or rarely two internal nuclei. Nuclei are abnormally large. Frozen section, H&E stain. (Courtesy Dr. B.A. Valentine, College of Veterinary Medicine, Oregon State University.)

Other Canine Muscular Dystrophies. Dystrophin has been found to be associated with a series of dystrophin-associated proteins, forming a membrane complex. The genes for many of these proteins are autosomally inherited; therefore not all canine muscular dystrophies are X-linked disorders. Autosomal recessive inheritance of dystrophin-associated gene defects leading to muscular dystrophy is common in human beings, and defects in dystrophin complex proteins leading to non-Duchenne's type muscular dystrophy have also been identified in various breeds of dogs. These are discussed in more detail in E-Appendix 15-1.

Labrador Retriever Centronuclear Myopathy. Labrador retriever centronuclear myopathy is inherited as an autosomal recessive trait. Affected dogs occur within the working or sporting breed lines rather than the show dog lines. Studies suggest similarity to inherited centronuclear myopathy of human beings, and a genetic test to detect carrier and affected dogs has been developed. Affected Labrador retrievers develop signs of neuromuscular weakness within the first 6 months of life. Exercise intolerance leads to collapse during prolonged exercise, and episodes of collapse can also be elicited by exposure to cold. Loss of triceps and patellar reflexes is characteristic. Affected dogs usually do not develop normal muscle mass. Concentric needle EMG reveals intense and abnormal spontaneous activity with normal motor nerve conduction velocities. Serum concentrations of CK and AST are often normal, although they can be mildly to moderately increased. Megaesophagus can be present.

The only specific abnormalities seen at necropsy are generalized poor muscling and possibly megaesophagus. On histologic examination, affected dogs have remarkable myopathic changes characterized by clusters of atrophic myofibers, myofiber hypertrophy, and internal nuclei (Fig. 15-46). Abnormal mitochondrial distribution, often with peripheral mitochondrial aggregates (identified as ragged red fibers in frozen sections stained with modified Gomori's trichrome stain), can also be seen (see Fig. 15-22, *B*). Segmental necrosis and regeneration are rare; therefore this disorder does not qualify as a muscular dystrophy. The initial reports described this disorder as a type 2 deficiency myopathy, but further studies have shown that fiber-type proportions vary remarkably between muscles and between dogs, although an increase in type 1 fibers (type 1 fiber predominance) is often seen. Alteration of the normal mosaic pattern of myofiber types is also seen. There is fiber-type grouping, usually considered a neuropathic change, despite the absence of peripheral nerve lesions. These changes are thought to reflect fiber-type conversion unassociated with denervation.

Based on the clinical findings, the diagnosis may be suspected but should be confirmed by genetic testing. There is no treatment for the disorder, although the disease is nonprogressive after 6 months to 1 year of age, and affected animals can still be kept as pets. Dogs producing affected pups should not be rebred.

Congenital Myotonia. Myotonia is seen most commonly in the Chow Chow dog, miniature schnauzer, and Staffordshire terrier. Autosomal recessive inheritance has been confirmed in the miniature schnauzer, and available evidence supports similar inheritance in the Chow Chow. The underlying cellular defect in miniature schnauzers is decreased chloride conduction, and a similar defect is suspected in Chow Chow dogs. Affected pups can begin to show signs of a stiff gait as early as 6 weeks of age. The signs progress for several months and then stabilize with variable severity. Affected dogs move with splayed, stiff thoracic limbs and often a "bunny hop" gait in the pelvic limbs. Signs are most severe on initiation of movement and improve with continued exercise. But affected dogs are never clinically normal. During severe episodes, dogs can fall over, and laryngospasm can result in transient dyspnea and even cyanosis. The musculature becomes remarkably hypertrophied, and sustained muscle dimpling occurs after percussion. Characteristic waxing and waning ("dive bomber") myotonic bursts are found with concentric needle EMG. Serum concentrations of CK and AST are normal or mildly increased.

Overall muscle hypertrophy, with prominently defined muscle groups, is the only finding on postmortem examination. In early stages of the disease, muscle appears relatively normal on histologic examination. With time, myofiber hypertrophy and myofiber atrophy of both type 1 and type 2 fibers and rare scattered segmental necrosis or regeneration are seen. Fibrosis is mild to inapparent.

Diagnosis is based on clinical signs and can be confirmed by concentric needle EMG or by examination of a muscle biopsy. Molecular testing is available to detect carrier and affected miniature schnauzers. Therapeutic agents that act to stabilize excitable cell membranes, such as quinidine, procainamide, and phenytoin, can relieve some of the signs of myotonia.

Swimmer Pups. Swimmer pups are clinically similar to piglets with splay leg. Affected pups cannot adduct the limbs beneath their bodies and develop a characteristic "swimming" gait and, because of the weight of the body, progressive dorsoventral flattening of the sternum and thoracic wall. Although this syndrome can occur in pups with neuromuscular disease of any sort that leads to weakness, it is more commonly associated with overfeeding leading to excess body weight. Affected overfed pups often recover completely after reduction in total daily milk intake, provision of a nonslippery floor surface, and development of harnesses and physical therapy to encourage them to bring their legs underneath their bodies and walk. In pups that die or are euthanized, sternal flattening and abnormal lateral deviation of the limbs are consistent necropsy findings. Histopathologic abnormalities in muscle vary, depending on the cause (e.g., myofiber necrosis and regeneration in pups with muscular dystrophy, and denervation atrophy in denervating disease) and are absent in pups in which this disorder simply reflects overfeeding.

Endocrine Myopathies

Hypothyroidism. Because of its role in muscle metabolism, decreased thyroid hormone often results in skeletal myofiber weakness and atrophy. Hypothyroidism can also cause a peripheral neuropathy, and damage to motor nerves can cause denervation atrophy and contribute to the neuromuscular weakness. Signs of neuromuscular dysfunction caused by hypothyroidism are extremely varied and include generalized weakness, muscle atrophy, laryngeal paralysis, and megaesophagus. EMG studies are often normal; abnormal spontaneous activity and decreased motor nerve conduction velocities can be found if there is concurrent peripheral neuropathy. Serum concentrations of CK and AST are generally normal. Other systemic manifestations of hypothyroidism may or may not be present.

At necropsy, overall muscle atrophy can be seen. Thyroid glands are often bilaterally atrophied, and megaesophagus can be present. Symmetric alopecia (endocrine dermatopathy) can also be seen. Type 2 myofibers are preferentially atrophied. Axonal degeneration can occur in peripheral nerves and, because of denervation, can lead to angular atrophy of both type 1 and type 2 fibers and to fiber-type grouping as a result of reinnervation.

Diagnosis is suspected on the basis of clinical findings and selective type 2 atrophy or evidence of denervation or reinnervation in affected muscles, but it should be confirmed by evaluation of thyroid function. In many cases, replacement thyroid hormone improves the signs of neuromuscular weakness.

Hypercortisolism. Hypercortisolism can occur because of either increased adrenocortical cortisol production or administration of exogenous corticosteroids. Clinical findings of neuromuscular weakness can be very similar to those in hypothyroidism. A unique manifestation of hypercortisolism in some dogs is development of a remarkably stiff, stilted pelvic limb gait, with increased bulk and tone of proximal thigh muscles (Cushingoid pseudomyotonia). The cause of Cushingoid pseudomyotonia is not known, although induction of sarcolemmal ionic instability is postulated. Concentric needle EMG of these muscles reveals myotonic bursts that do not wax and wane (pseudomyotonic activity). Muscles do not dimple after percussion. Other systemic signs of hypercortisolism, such as symmetric muscle atrophy and alopecia, can also be present. Serum concentrations of CK and AST are normal. Adrenal glands have bilateral cortical atrophy caused by exogenous corticosteroid administration or bilateral hypertrophy caused by stimulation secondary to pituitary neoplasia. Adrenal cortical neoplasia causes enlargement of the affected gland and atrophy of the contralateral gland. Findings in affected muscle and peripheral nerves are similar to those seen in hypothyroid myopathy (i.e., selective type 2 fiber atrophy), and evidence of axonal degeneration in peripheral nerves, type 1 and type 2 fiber atrophy indicative of denervation atrophy, and fiber-type grouping reflecting reinnervation are possible (see Fig. 15-18, *B*).

Diagnosis is suspected on the basis of clinical and histopathologic findings but should be confirmed by evaluation of adrenocortical function and total serum cortisol. Cessation of exogenous corticosteroids, removal of adrenal neoplasms, or chemical destruction of hyperplastic adrenal cortical tissue results in improvement in muscle mass and strength, although signs of pseudomyotonia may persist.

Immune-Mediated Myopathies

Polymyositis. Polymyositis is the result of immune-mediated inflammation that attacks components of the skeletal myofibers and results in myofiber necrosis (Fig. 15-47; also see Fig. 15-27 and Table 15-8). The immunologic injury can be directed against skeletal muscle only or can be part of a more generalized immune-mediated disease such as systemic lupus erythematosus. Polymyositis can also occur in dogs with thymoma. This inflammatory myopathy can have an acute and rapidly progressive course or an insidious onset of muscle atrophy and generalized weakness. Muscles throughout the body are affected, but atrophy of temporal and masseter muscles may be most obvious, mimicking the appearance of dogs with masticatory myositis (see later discussion). Esophageal muscle involvement can lead to esophageal fibrosis and esophageal dysfunction, including megaesophagus. Respiratory muscle involvement can occur and, if severe, will cause respiratory distress. Pain on palpation of muscles is rare. Serum concentrations of CK, AST, and ALT can be increased, but in chronic cases these concentrations can also be within normal limits. Concentric needle EMG often reveals scattered foci of abnormal spontaneous activity, and motor nerve conduction velocities are normal.

At necropsy, overall muscle atrophy may be the only finding. Aspiration pneumonia can occur secondary to megaesophagus. Histologic findings within affected muscles are extremely variable. In acute, fulminating cases, the muscle sections are filled with inflammatory cells, predominantly lymphocytes (Fig. 15-47, *A*), although interstitial eosinophils and neutrophils can also be present. The degree of myofiber necrosis is variable. Necrotic fibers in early stages are surrounded by lymphocytes that can be seen to invade intact myofibers (see Fig. 15-27, *B*). Similar to human polymyositis, $CD8^+$ cytotoxic/suppressor T lymphocytes are the primary infiltrating cells. Necrosis is followed by regeneration, but basal lamina damage is common and results in some degree of healing by fibrosis. In more chronic and insidious cases, the only lesion consists of scattered lymphocytes in the interstitial tissue adjacent to myofibers, with a variable degree of fibrosis and chronic myopathic change (Fig. 15-47, *B*). Sampling multiple muscles for histopathologic examination is recommended.

Polymyositis should be suspected based on the clinical findings, but identification of characteristic changes within muscle sections is often necessary to confirm the diagnosis. A positive circulating antinuclear antibody titer (ANA) is useful but is not always present. Treatment with immunosuppressive drugs, such as corticosteroids, can be curative, but affected animals may require lifelong therapy.

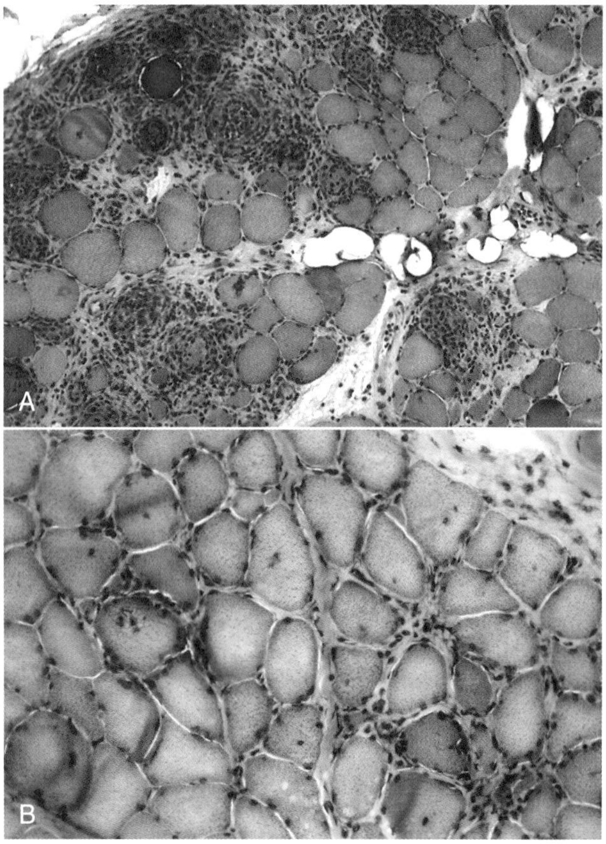

Figure 15-47 **Canine Polymyositis, Skeletal Muscle, Transverse Section, Dog. A,** Acute polymyositis. Dense interstitial and intramyofiber mononuclear inflammatory cell infiltrates are associated with myofiber necrosis. Frozen section, H&E stain. **B,** Chronic polymyositis. At this stage, there are only scattered interstitial mononuclear inflammatory cell infiltrates, scattered degenerate fibers, and chronic myopathic change (excessive fiber-size variation, internal nuclei, endomysial fibrosis). Frozen section, H&E stain. (**A** courtesy Dr. L. Fuhrer, Clinic Vétérinaire de St. Avertin, France. **B** courtesy Dr. B.A. Valentine, College of Veterinary Medicine, Oregon State University.)

Masticatory Myositis (Eosinophilic Myositis; Atrophic Myositis). The type 2 myofibers in the masticatory muscles of the dog contain a unique myosin isoform (type 2M myosin). Occasionally, antibodies to this myosin form, and the result is an inflammatory myopathy confined to the temporalis and masseter muscles. Severe, acute cases display bilaterally symmetric swelling of, and pain in, those muscles and an inability to fully open the jaw. Affected dogs can have difficulty prehending food. More chronic or insidious cases have bilaterally symmetric atrophy of the temporal and masseter muscles (Fig. 15-48 and Table 15-8) and decreased jaw mobility. Pain may or may not be evident at this stage. Concentric needle EMG often reveals foci of spontaneous activity in active cases but can be normal in more chronic cases. Serum concentrations of CK and AST are normal or only mildly increased.

Severely atrophied muscles often contain pale streaks. The degree and nature of the inflammation are variable. In acute cases, infiltrates of lymphocytes and plasma cells, similar to those in polymyositis, are present. But, in contrast to canine polymyositis, the infiltrating cells in masticatory myositis are primarily B lymphocytes. There can also be numerous eosinophils, and these can be the predominant cell type. Neutrophils are much less common. Inflammation is associated with myofiber necrosis. Regeneration can restore myofibers, but because the basal lamina is often damaged, healing by fibrosis is common. The presence of fibrosis is an important prognostic indicator because fibrosis is an irreversible change.

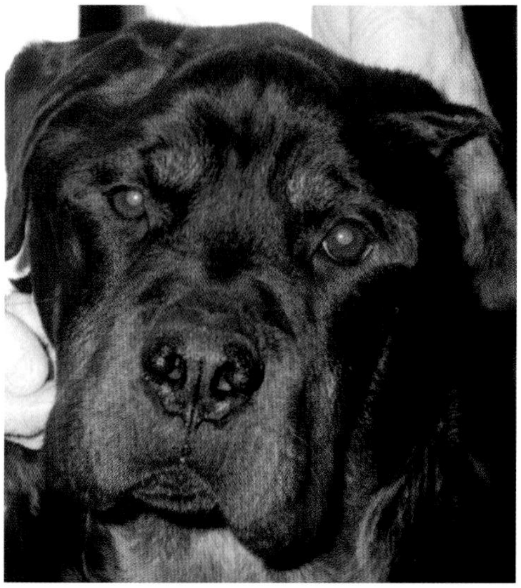

Figure 15-48 **Chronic Masticatory Myositis, Skeletal Muscle, Dog.** Note the severe atrophy of the temporalis and masseter muscles. (Courtesy Dr. W. Hornbuckle, College of Veterinary Medicine, Cornell University.)

The diagnosis is suggested on the basis of characteristic clinical findings. Masticatory myositis must be differentiated from polymyositis, which can also have severe involvement of the temporal and masseter muscles. Serologic testing to detect anti–type 2M myosin antibodies specific to masticatory muscle myositis is available, and serum from affected dogs will bind to type 2M fibers (Fig. 15-49). EMG and histopathologic evaluation of multiple muscles can also help to differentiate these two disorders. Treatment with immunosuppressive doses of corticosteroids generally alleviates pain and results in increased mobility of the jaw and an increase in muscle mass. Some degree of atrophy and loss of complete jaw mobility can persist. A single course of corticosteroids can be curative; however, some cases require extended therapy.

Extraocular Muscle Myositis. An immune-mediated attack directed specifically at extraocular muscles is the suspected cause of this disorder. Acute onset of bilateral exophthalmos is seen (see Table 15-8). Affected dogs are usually younger than 2 years of age, and golden retriever dogs appear to be predisposed. Serum concentrations of CK and AST are generally normal.

The extraocular muscles, with the exception of the retractor bulbi muscle, are swollen and pale yellow. A predominantly lymphocytic inflammation resulting in myofiber necrosis and regeneration is seen. Because it is difficult to obtain a biopsy sample of the extraocular muscles, diagnosis is generally based on typical clinical findings. Corticosteroid therapy is effective, but episodes can recur.

Disorders of the Neuromuscular Junction

Myasthenia Gravis. The pathogenesis of myasthenia gravis is discussed in the section on neuropathic and neuromuscular junction disorders (see Fig. 15-28). In most cases, myasthenia gravis is an acquired disease, with circulating antibodies directed at the acetylcholine receptors of the neuromuscular junction. An inherited predisposition to development of acquired myasthenia gravis has been reported in Newfoundland dogs. In some cases, onset of myasthenia gravis occurs because of thymoma or, less commonly, thymic hyperplasia. Myasthenia gravis associated with hypothyroidism also occurs in dogs but is rare. Congenital myasthenia gravis is due to abnormal development of the neuromuscular junction and is inherited as an autosomal recessive trait in Jack Russell terriers, smooth fox terriers, and springer spaniels. Congenital myasthenia gravis also occurs in smooth-haired miniature dachshunds. Typical signs of acquired disease are episodic collapse in an adult dog, with normal gait and strength after rest. Clinical signs can, however, be variable. The canine esophagus contains a large percentage of skeletal muscle throughout the length of the tunica muscularis; therefore megaesophagus is common in dogs with myasthenia gravis and may be the only presenting sign. This differs from human beings, in which only the proximal one-third of the esophageal muscularis is completely skeletal muscle and the lower third is completely smooth muscle. In some cases, mild weakness persists between episodes. Clinical signs of congenital myasthenia gravis appear at an early age (6 to 8 weeks of age) and in most affected breeds are progressive and typically quite severe. Affected dachshunds, however, appear to recover by 6 months of age. Repetitive motor nerve stimulation reveals an initial sharp decremental response, followed by relatively uniform amplitude potentials. Serum concentrations of CK and AST are normal.

No findings are evident at postmortem examination unless megaesophagus, thymic abnormalities, or thyroid abnormalities are present, and no abnormalities in muscle are seen on light microscopic examination. Ultrastructural abnormalities of the neuromuscular junctions (simplification of the postsynaptic membrane) may be present.

Diagnosis is suspected on the basis of typical clinical findings and results of repetitive nerve stimulation. In patients with acquired myasthenia gravis, dramatic transient improvement in muscle strength after administration of intravenous acetylcholinesterase inhibitors such as edrophonium (Tensilon) is seen, and the diagnosis is confirmed by identification of circulating antibodies to skeletal muscle acetylcholine receptors. In cases of acquired myasthenia gravis, the presence of a thymic abnormality should be determined because removal of a thymoma or of a hyperplastic thymus results in resolution of clinical signs. In other cases, long-acting acetylcholinesterase inhibitor therapy, sometimes combined with corticosteroid therapy, is often beneficial. There is no effective treatment for congenital myasthenia gravis.

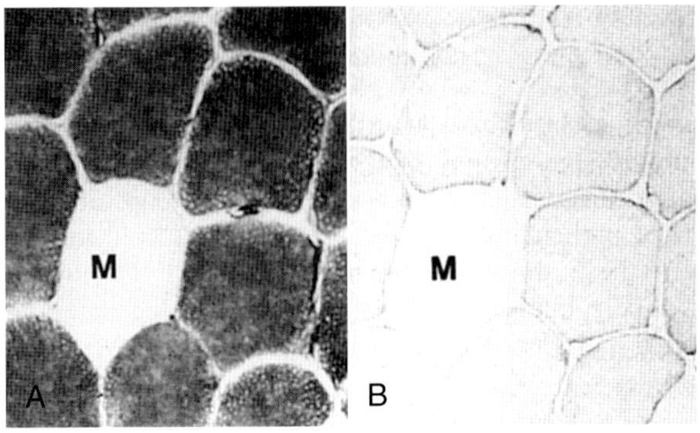

Figure 15-49 Canine Masticatory Myositis, Skeletal Muscle, Temporalis Muscle, Transverse Sections, Normal Dog. A, A single type 1 fiber (*light staining,* M) surrounded by type 2 fibers (*dark staining*). Frozen section, ATPase pH 9.8. **B,** After incubation with serum from a dog with masticatory myositis, type 2 fibers stain positively because of binding of anti–type 2M myosin antibodies from the affected dog. Notice that the type 1 fiber (M) is unstained. Frozen section, staphylococcal protein A-peroxidase. (Courtesy Dr. G.D. Shelton, University of California, San Diego.)

Tick Paralysis. In a dog with flaccid tetraparesis, a diagnosis of tick paralysis should be considered along with polyradiculoneuritis (coonhound paralysis; see Chapter 14) and botulism. Clinical signs of tick paralysis appear 5 to 7 days after infestation with causative *Dermacentor* or *Ixodes* ticks. Initial clinical signs are pelvic limb weakness, with progression to recumbency within 48 to 72 hours. Cranial nerve function is normal. Clinical signs of tick paralysis are very similar to those of coonhound paralysis (see Chapter 14). Treatment for tick infestation can result in recovery within a few days, although death from respiratory muscle paralysis is still possible.

Botulism. Botulism occurs in dogs, resulting in rapid onset of flaccid tetraparesis, but is rare. Reported cases of canine botulism are most often the result of types C and D of *Clostridium botulinum* neurotoxins. Diagnosis is often presumptive, based on a failure to identify other causes of diffuse neuromuscular weakness and, with luck, a history of consumption of a rotted carcass. Recovery has been reported in dogs with botulism, although many cases are fatal.

Other Canine Myopathies

Exertional Rhabdomyolysis. Massive acute rhabdomyolysis associated with exertion occurs in racing greyhounds and sled dogs. Muscles of the back (longissimus) and thigh (gluteal) are most often affected and may be severely swollen. Predisposing factors are not clear, but in sled dogs a change to a very high-fat diet has resulted in a decrease in exercise-induced muscle injury.

Malignant Hyperthermia. Malignant hyperthermia (MH) occurs sporadically in dogs, and breeding studies indicate an autosomal dominant inheritance. The cause has been determined to be a genetic defect in the muscle ryanodine receptor, which is also the cause of MH in pigs and human beings. MH-like episodes can also occur in any dog after ingestion of hops used for brewing beer.

Other Breed-Specific Myopathies. A number of breed-specific myopathies have been reported in the dog, including dermatomyositis in collies and Shetland sheepdogs; mitochondrial myopathy in Old English sheepdogs and other breeds; central core myopathy in Great Danes; exercise-induced collapse in Labrador retrievers; and myopathy of Bouvier des Flandres dogs, English springer spaniels, and Rottweilers. Myoclonus and intramuscular Lafora-like bodies occur in wirehaired miniature dachshunds. These are discussed in more detail in E-Appendix 15-1.

Idiopathic Masticatory Muscle Atrophy

Dogs can develop a progressive atrophy of temporal and masseter muscles that is not associated with pain or difficulty opening the jaw or prehending food. Examination of affected muscle from these dogs reveals mild generalized atrophy of myofibers, but there is no evidence of inflammation, degeneration, fibrosis, or denervation. The cause is not known, and there is no treatment.

Denervating Diseases

There are numerous causes of inherited and acquired peripheral nerve disorders causing axonal damage and resultant denervation in dogs (see Chapter 14). Motor neuron disease is most often inherited, as in the Brittany spaniel and Rottweiler. Such disorders cause symmetric atrophy of affected muscles. Neoplasms arising in peripheral nerves (nerve sheath neoplasms) cause compression of the nerve resulting in Wallerian degeneration, leading to progressive gait abnormalities and ultimately denervation atrophy of muscles of the affected limb.

Disorders of Cats

Relatively few muscular disorders have thus far been identified in cats. This may in part be the result of low performance expectations of the average house cat. It is entirely possible that there are many cats lying around with muscular disorders that have as yet gone unrecognized.

Inherited or Congenital Myopathies

X-Linked Muscular Dystrophy (Duchenne's Type). Dystrophic cats lack the muscle cytoskeletal protein dystrophin, which is also the cause of Duchenne's dystrophy in boys and X-linked muscle dystrophy in the dog. Affected cats develop a progressive, persistent, stiff gait associated with marked muscular hypertrophy. The cause of the remarkable muscular hypertrophy seen in affected cats, as opposed to the muscle atrophy seen in the dog and in human beings, and the pseudohypertrophy as a result of fat infiltration into affected muscle that can occur in human beings, is not known. Age of onset is from a few months to 21 months of age. Affected cats have difficulty grooming, jumping, and lying down. Concentric needle EMG reveals dense and sustained abnormal spontaneous activity, similar to findings in the dystrophic dog. Serum concentrations of CK, AST, and ALT are elevated, typically to very high levels. Affected cats can die under anesthesia or after restraint or sedation because of an MH-like syndrome.

At necropsy, all muscles are severely hypertrophied and may contain pale areas. Focal pale or chalky areas within the myocardium are typically found. Histologically, muscles show a range of changes. Concurrent segmental myonecrosis and myofiber regeneration (polyphasic necrosis) are characteristic. Chronic myopathic changes, found in older animals, include severe myofiber hypertrophy, myofiber atrophy, internal nuclei, and mild to moderate endomysial fibrosis. Myocardial lesions consist of multifocal necrosis and mineralization of cardiac myofibers and fibrosis, primarily in the left ventricular free wall, papillary muscles, and septum. Affected cats may have a relatively normal life span, although unexpected death during anesthesia or forced restraint is common. The exact cause of this is unclear.

The diagnosis is suspected on the basis of characteristic clinical, clinicopathologic, and histopathologic findings in a young male cat. Confirmation relies on assay of muscle samples for dystrophin or on immunohistochemical staining for dystrophin in frozen sections.

Other Feline Inherited or Congenital Myopathies. A form of autosomal recessively inherited muscular dystrophy due to deficiency of the dystrophin complex protein α-dystroglycan occurs in Sphinx and Devon rex cats. Glycogenosis type IV (GBE defect) affecting skeletal muscle is seen as an inherited disorder in Norwegian Forest cats. A histologically similar condition occurs occasionally in other breeds. Feline nemaline myopathy is a rare congenital myopathy in the cat. These disorders are discussed in more detail in E-Appendix 15-1.

Myopathies Caused by Electrolyte Abnormalities (Hypokalemia and Hypernatremia)

Similar to cattle, cats with severe electrolyte abnormalities can show signs of neuromuscular weakness that can be caused by degenerative myopathy. Although degenerative myopathy has been reported secondary to increased blood sodium concentrations (hypernatremia), hypokalemic myopathy occurs far more frequently.

The cause of the weakness and myofiber necrosis associated with electrolyte abnormalities is complex and involves abnormal skeletal muscle energy metabolism and possible ischemia because of vasoconstriction. Hypokalemia (serum potassium concentration less than 3.5 mEq/L) can occur because of decreased dietary intake or increased urinary excretion of potassium. In cats, hypokalemia is often a consequence of chronic renal disease. A genetic defect in the nephron causing renal potassium loss has been linked to periodic hypokalemic myopathy in Burmese related cats. Hypokalemia can also occur secondary to gastrointestinal disease or inappropriate fluid therapy. Hyperthyroidism has been associated with development of hypokalemic myopathy in cats. Hypernatremic myopathy is less common but has been reported in a 7-month-old cat with hydrocephalus and transient hypopituitarism.

Affected cats show severe generalized weakness, with notable ventroflexion of the neck. Concentric needle EMG often demonstrates foci of abnormal spontaneous activity. Serum concentrations of CK, AST, and ALT are often increased, sometimes severely. Clinically diagnosed cases of hypokalemia and hypernatremia can be confirmed by determining if the serum potassium is low or the serum sodium is high, respectively.

No specific gross pathologic findings are present except in cats with hypokalemia as a result of chronic renal disease, in which the kidneys are small and fibrotic. In hypokalemic myopathy, myofiber necrosis and regeneration of variable severity are present concurrently (polyphasic necrosis). Chronic renal disease is commonly due to chronic interstitial nephritis. No abnormalities were detected in a muscle biopsy from a cat with hypernatremic myopathy, although the mildly increased serum concentration of CK and the abnormal EMG suggest mild and perhaps transient myofiber necrosis and regeneration.

Diagnosis is based on characteristic clinical findings of weakness and concurrent hypokalemia or hypernatremia. Treatment of affected cats has been very successful. Immediate fluid therapy is used to correct the electrolyte abnormality, followed by diet change to maintain normal electrolyte concentrations. If there is an underlying hyperthyroidism, this should also be treated.

Immune-Mediated Disorders

An immune-mediated myositis has been described in cats infected with feline immunodeficiency virus (FIV). Serum concentration of CK is moderately increased, but clinical signs of muscle dysfunction are not apparent. Infiltration of muscle by $CD8^+$ lymphocytes, similar to human immunodeficiency virus (HIV)-associated polymyositis, is characteristic.

Disorders of the Neuromuscular Junction

Myasthenia Gravis. Feline acquired and congenital myasthenia gravis are similar to these disorders in the dog but occur less commonly.

Botulism. Although theoretically possible, confirmed or highly suspicious cases of botulism in cats have not been reported. This result likely reflects both an inherent resistance to botulinum toxin and the typical feline fastidious appetite.

Denervating Diseases

Disorders affecting peripheral motor nerves are much less common in cats compared to dogs. A chronic relapsing polyneuritis primarily affecting ventral spinal roots has been seen in young adult cats, which can cause denervation atrophy in affected muscles. Diabetes mellitus can also result in peripheral neuropathy in cats.

Suggested Readings

Suggested Readings are available at www.expertconsult.com.

CHAPTER 16

Bones, Joints, Tendons, and Ligaments[1]

Erik J. Olson and Cathy S. Carlson

Key Readings Index

The skeleton consists of bones and joints and their supporting structures and is responsible for supporting and protecting the body and enabling movement initiated by the nervous system and facilitated by muscles. The skeleton can be divided into the axial skeleton (head, vertebrae, ribs, and sternum) and the appendicular skeleton (thoracic and pelvic limbs). Information on the methods for postmortem examination and evaluation of the skeleton is available in E-Appendix 16-1, which can be found at www.expertconsult.com.

Structure and Function

Bone

Bone at the Cellular Level

Structure and function can be discussed at the organ, tissue, and cellular levels. In this section, normal structure and function are briefly reviewed, beginning at the cellular level and including bone matrix and mineral. Cells directly involved with the structural integrity of bone include osteoblasts, osteocytes, and osteoclasts (Box 16-1).

Osteoblasts are cells on any bone surface (periosteal, endosteal, trabecular, and intracortical) that produce bone matrix (osteoid), initiate the mineralization of this matrix (deposition of hydroxyapatite), and seemingly paradoxically initiate the resorption of this matrix by osteoclasts. Osteoblasts are derived from mesenchymal stem cells. Active osteoblasts are plump (Figs. 16-1 and 16-2; E-Fig. 16-1), with abundant basophilic cytoplasm that is rich in rough endoplasmic reticulum and contains prominent Golgi apparatus and numerous mitochondria (E-Fig. 16-2). Inactive osteoblasts are disk-shaped with little cytoplasm because fewer organelles are needed for matrix synthesis and secretion (E-Figs. 16-3 and 16-4). Osteoblasts likely interact with osteocytes to assist in fine control of calcium homeostasis and detection of mechanical use and microscopic damage to bone, as discussed later. Indirect measurements of osteoblast activity are reflected in blood concentrations of the bone-specific isoform of alkaline phosphatase, an enzyme on the cell membrane of osteoblasts, and the noncollagenous protein, osteocalcin, that is secreted by osteoblasts and is present in bone matrix. Both are thought to have roles in mineralization and calcium ion homeostasis.

Osteocytes are osteoblasts that have been surrounded by mineralized bone matrix (E-Fig. 16-5; also see Fig. 16-2) and are the most numerous and longest living of the bone cell types. They occupy small spaces in the bone called *lacunae* (singular: lacuna) and make contact with osteoblasts and other osteocytes by means of long cytoplasmic processes that pass through thin tunnels in the bone called *canaliculi* (singular: canaliculus). Under conditions of extreme stress to calcium homeostasis, osteocytes might have the ability to resorb perilacunar mineral and matrix, thus enlarging the lacuna (osteocytic osteolysis). This process apparently is rare and likely does not contribute significantly to development of osseous lesions. Osteocytes also retain a limited capacity to form bone and are exquisitely sensitive to mechanical strain in the form of shear stress. Other functions of osteocytes are somewhat speculative and are presented later in osteoblast-osteocyte interactions.

Osteoclasts are multinucleated cells that are derived from hematopoietic stem cells of the monocyte-macrophage series and are responsible for bone resorption (Fig. 16-3). They have abundant eosinophilic cytoplasm and a specialized brush border along the margin of the cell that is adjacent to the bone surface that is being resorbed (E-Figs. 16-6 and 16-7). For osteoclasts to resorb bone, they must gain access to the bone surface that is usually covered by osteoblasts, and they must attach to the mineralized surface by transmembrane receptors in their sealing zones. The transmembrane receptors bind to specific ligands in the matrix that likely reside in noncollagenous proteins; however, osteoclasts are not able to bind to unmineralized bone matrix even though it contains these same ligands. Once bound to the matrix, the osteoclast resorbs bone in two stages. First, the mineral is dissolved by secretion of hydrogen ions through a proton pump located in the brush border. These

[1]For a glossary of abbreviations and terms used in this chapter, see E-Glossary 16-1.

Box 16-1 Bone Cell Function

Osteoblasts: Cells of stromal stem cell origin that reside on the surface of bone and form bone matrix, initiate bone mineralization, and initiate bone resorption (by signaling to osteoclasts) in response to physiologic stimuli
Osteocytes: Osteoblasts that have become encased in bone matrix. These cells detect changes in stress (force applied to the bone) and strain (structural deformation in response to the force) in the bone and signal these changes to osteoblasts to either form bone or initiate resorption; may mobilize calcium from the bone through osteocytic osteolysis
Osteoclasts: Cells formed by the fusion of cells of the monocyte-macrophage cell line; function is to resorb mineralized bone matrix

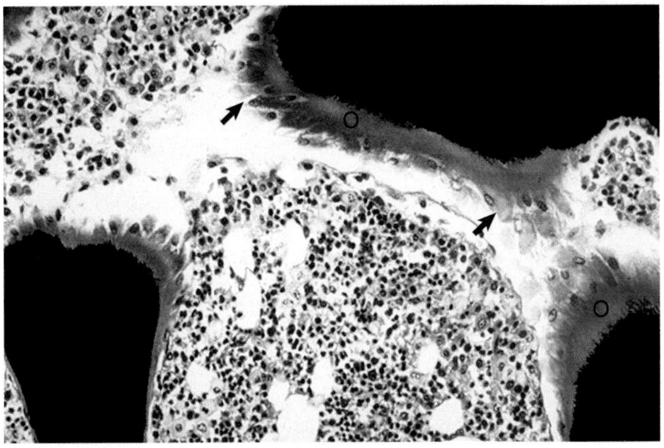

Figure 16-1 Osteoblasts and Osteoid, Long Bone, Cynomolgus Macaque. Prominent cuboidal (active) osteoblasts *(arrows)* line the trabecular surfaces. Mineralized trabecular bone is *black*; unmineralized bone matrix (osteoid *[O]*) is present *(light blue)* between mineralized bone and osteoblasts. Hematopoietic marrow is present between trabeculae. Von Kossa tetrachrome stain. (Courtesy Dr. C.S. Carlson and Dr. E.J. Olson, College of Veterinary Medicine, University of Minnesota.)

hydrogen ions are derived from carbonic acid produced within the osteoclast from water and carbon dioxide by the enzyme carbonic anhydrase. Second, the collagen of the matrix is cleaved into polypeptide fragments by cysteine proteinases, metalloproteinases, and cathepsins, particularly cathepsin K, released from the numerous lysosomes in the osteoclast and secreted through the brush border. The concavity in the bone created by the resorbed bone matrix is called a *Howship's lacuna*, or a resorption lacuna. Physiologically, osteoclast activation is controlled by osteoblasts and bone marrow stromal cells (see later discussion of interactions). Calcitonin is a systemic inhibitor of osteoclasts. Osteoclasts have receptors for calcitonin and respond to this hormone by involuting their brush border and detaching from the bone surface. The activity of osteoclasts can be indirectly measured by determining serum concentrations of collagen degradation products (pyridinoline and deoxypyridinoline cross-links) or tartrate-resistant acid phosphatase (TRAP) activity. TRAP is a glycosylated monomeric metalloenzyme that is highly expressed by osteoclasts. TRAP staining also may be used as a histochemical marker of osteoclasts in histologic sections (E-Fig. 16-8).

Osteoblast-osteocyte interactions are apparent from their connections to each other by thin, tortuous, cytoplasmic processes. This network of osteoblasts and osteocytes forms a functional membrane

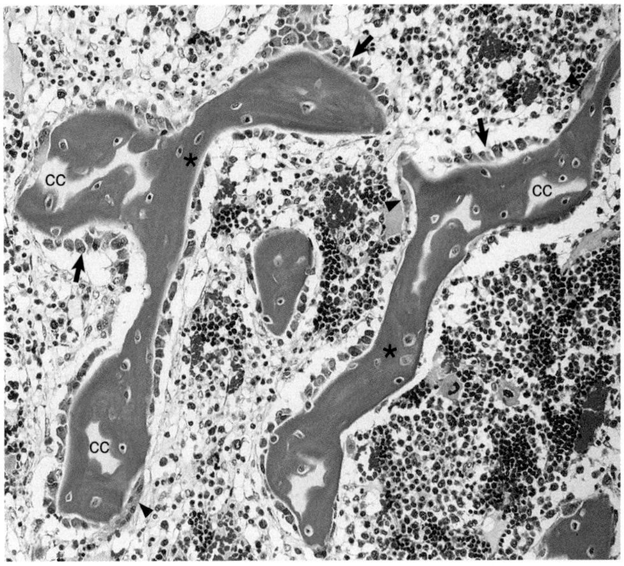

Figure 16-2 Osteoblasts, Osteocytes, and Osteoclasts, Femoral Head, Immature Pig. Active osteoblasts *(arrows)* on the trabecular surface; osteocytes are embedded in bone matrix *(asterisks)*; multinucleated osteoclasts *(arrowheads)*. Areas of retained calcified cartilage (cc) are present within and hematopoietic marrow is present between bone trabeculae in this young animal. H&E stain. (Courtesy Dr. C.S. Carlson and Dr. E.J. Olson, College of Veterinary Medicine, University of Minnesota.)

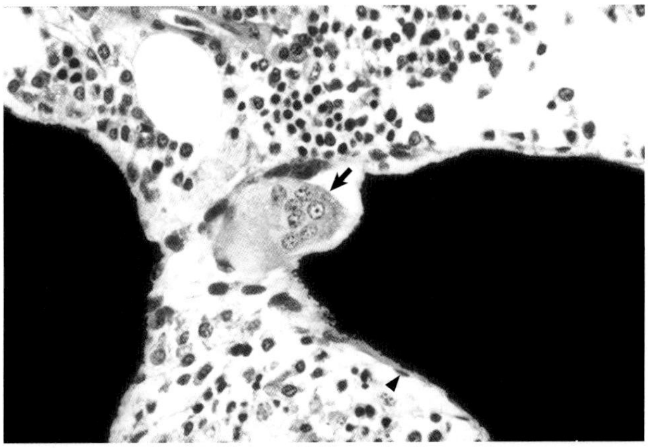

Figure 16-3 Osteoclast and Quiescent Osteoblast, Long Bone, Cynomolgus Macaque. A large multinucleated cell (osteoclast) *(arrow)* is present within a scalloped cavity of resorbed bone known as a *Howship's* (or erosion/resorption) *lacuna*. Quiescent osteoblast *(arrowhead)*. Von Kossa tetrachrome stain. (Courtesy Dr. C.S. Carlson and Dr. E.J. Olson, College of Veterinary Medicine, University of Minnesota.)

that separates the extracellular fluid bathing bone surfaces from the general extracellular fluid and can regulate the flow of calcium and phosphate ions to and from the bone fluid compartment (E-Fig. 16-9). Because of the large surface area of perilacunar and canalicular bone available for rapid ion exchange, significant amounts of calcium can be shifted from the bone fluid compartment to the extracellular fluid compartment without structural changes within the bone. In addition, this network allows osteocytes to detect alterations in the fluid flow within the bone extracellular fluid compartment. It is thought that such flow contributes to electric currents called *streaming potentials*. Changes in these streaming potentials caused by altered stress and strain on the bone or disruption of these potentials by microcracks (minuscule fractures within the bone visible only microscopically) might be detected by osteocytes with subsequent signaling to the overlying osteoblasts to initiate bone formation or resorption. Osteocytes also are capable of secreting *sclerostin*, a protein that inhibits bone formation by osteoblasts. During bone modeling (change of shape in response to normal growth, altered mechanical use, or disease), sclerostin may keep bone-lining cells in a quiescent state and may therefore prevent activation of osteoblasts and bone formation. Sclerostin also has been shown to decrease the life span of osteoblasts by stimulating apoptosis.

In modeling, bone surfaces (periosteal, endosteal, intracortical, and trabecular) can go directly from resting to either formation or resorption, depending on the stimulus. In modeling, bone resorption and formation occur independently on separate surfaces/anatomic locations (i.e., they are not directly coupled). This process allows the shape or size of bone to change, enables the medullary cavity to enlarge, and allows the overall shape of the bone to be maintained while it is growing. Modeling is in contrast to remodeling, in which resorption must precede formation to keep bone mass and shape constant (see later discussion).

Osteoclast-osteoblast/stromal cell interactions are required for physiologic resorption of bone. The bone surface is protected from osteoclastic resorption by a continuous layer of osteoblasts and also by a very thin layer of unmineralized bone matrix normally present beneath resting osteoblasts (lamina limitans) (see E-Fig. 16-2). For parathyroid hormone (PTH) to initiate bone resorption, receptors on the osteoblast bind PTH. The binding of PTH to osteoblasts signals them to retract and secrete collagenases, which erode the unmineralized layer of matrix and allow osteoclasts access to a mineralized bone surface. More recently, it has been determined that human being osteoclasts express PTH and can respond directly to PTH. In addition, osteoblasts and bone marrow stromal cells that are activated by binding PTH and in response to a variety of other bone-resorbing stimuli (1,25-dihydroxyvitamin D_3; interleukin [IL]-1, IL-6, and IL-11; tumor necrosis factor-α [TNF-α]; prostaglandin E_2 [PGE_2]; and glucocorticoids) express or secrete receptor activator for nuclear factor κ B ligand (RANKL), also called *osteoclast differentiation factor* (ODF). RANKL binds to the RANK receptor on osteoclasts and activates the resorption process. Recent evidence indicates that osteocytes also express RANKL and have been shown to regulate osteoclasts during bone remodeling. Osteoblasts and bone marrow stromal cells also can secrete osteoprotegerin (OPG), a RANK homolog that works by binding to RANKL, thus blocking the RANK-RANKL interaction and inhibiting the differentiation of osteoclast precursors into mature osteoclasts. OPG expression can be stimulated by transforming growth factor-β (TGF-β). Therefore osteoblasts and stromal cells have the ability to both up- and down-regulate osteoclastic bone resorption (Fig. 16-4). In conditions of inflammation and necrosis, inflammatory mediators, such as IL-1 and TNF-α, can stimulate osteoclasts directly, causing bone resorption independent of the presence of viable osteoblasts.

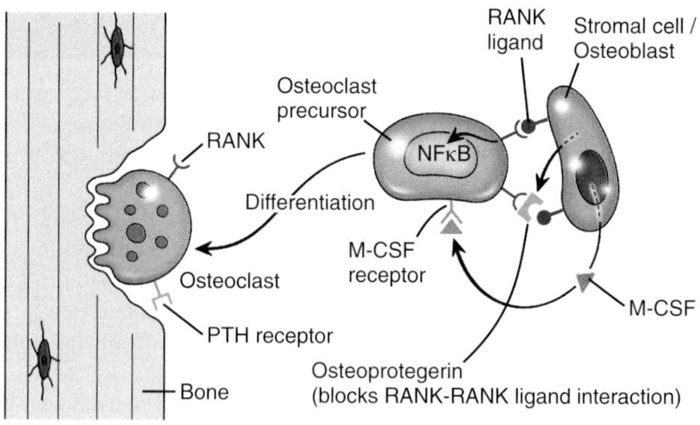

Figure 16-4 **Interaction between Stromal Cells/Osteoblasts and Osteoclast/Osteoclast Precursors.** M-CSF produced by stromal cells/osteoblasts binds to a receptor on osteoclast precursors to enhance their differentiation to mature osteoclasts. Stromal cells/osteoblasts are also involved in the activation of osteoclasts through production of RANK ligand, which binds to the RANK receptor on the osteoclast and its precursors. This process results in the differentiation of osteoclast precursors to mature osteoclasts and the activation of mature osteoclasts, allowing them to dissolve and resorb bone tissue (osteoclasis). Conversely, osteoblasts and stromal cells can inhibit the activation of osteoclasts by secreting osteoprotegerin, which can bind to RANK ligand and block its binding to RANK receptor. PTH receptors on osteoblasts (not shown) bind PTH to initiate and signal these cells to retract from the bone surface and secrete collagenases. Osteoclasts also have been shown to express PTH receptors allowing them to respond directly to PTH. *M-CSF,* Macrophage colony-stimulating factor; *NFκB*, nuclear factor κB; *PTH*, parathyroid hormone.

Bone at the Organic Matrix and Mineral Level

The mineralized matrix of bone provides the organ's strength. Bone organic matrix consists of type I collagen and "ground substance" (the noncollagenous extracellular matrix that includes water, proteoglycans, glycosaminoglycans, noncollagenous proteins, and lipids). Type I collagen polymers are secreted by osteoblasts and assembled into fibrils that are embedded in the ground substance and then mineralized. The fundamental unit of the type I collagen molecule (known as *tropocollagen*) is composed of three intertwined amino acid chains, unique to which is the hydroxylated form of the amino acid proline (hydroxyproline). Type I collagen molecules have extensive cross-linkages among the amino acid chains within the molecule and between adjacent molecules. Collagen molecules are deposited in rows with a gap between each molecule and with the rows staggered so that the molecules overlap by one-quarter of their length. This specific packing of the collagen molecules and the cross-linkages contribute to the strength and insolubility of the fibrous component of the bone matrix. Other than in rapidly deposited bone (i.e., woven bone found in the embryonic skeleton or in pathologic conditions such as fracture repair, in which the collagen fibers are arranged haphazardly), collagen fibers in bone are arranged in parallel lamellae (singular: lamella) and the tissue is called *lamellar bone*. In cortical (compact) bone, lamellae are arranged concentrically (E-Fig. 16-10). In trabecular bone, the lamellae usually are arranged parallel with the bone surface. The collagen content of bone and its lamellar arrangement give bone its strength and flexibility. The ground substance of bone, which also is synthesized by osteoblasts, consists of noncollagenous proteins, proteoglycans, and lipids. Many of the noncollagenous proteins are cytokines that are capable of influencing bone cell activity and may play pivotal roles in controlling the extent of bone formation and resorption in normal remodeling and in disease (Fig. 16-5). Also, among the noncollagenous proteins are enzymes that can function in the degradation of collagen (e.g., matrix metalloproteinases) and can destroy inhibitors of mineralization (e.g., pyrophosphates). Other noncollagenous proteins in the matrix can function as adhesion molecules and help bind cells to cells, cells to matrix, and mineral to matrix. Examples of these are osteonectin and osteocalcin. The role of proteoglycans in bone matrix is uncertain; however, there is evidence that they influence bone cell differentiation and proliferative activity. Lipids may assist in binding calcium to cell membranes and in promoting calcification.

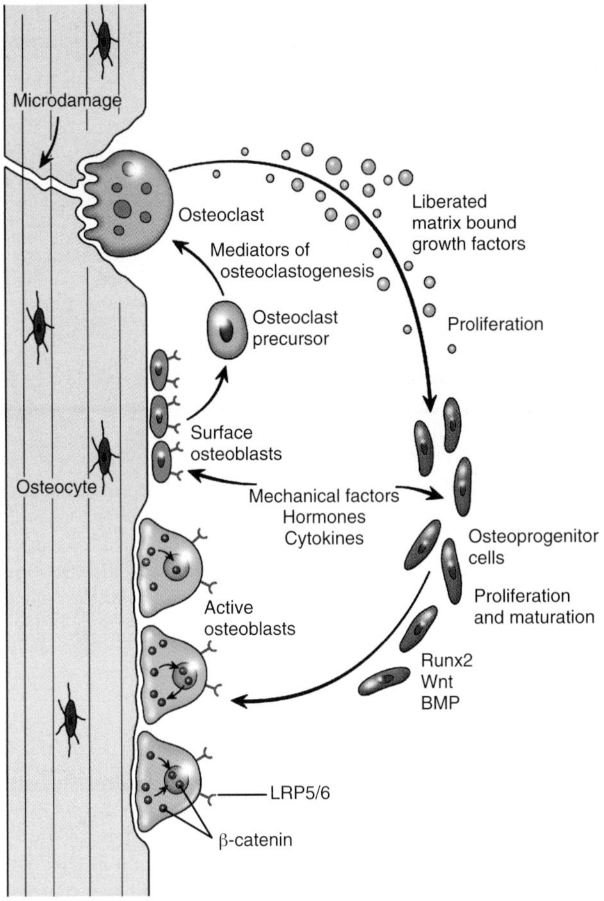

Figure 16-5 **Relationship between Osteoclasts, Osteoblasts, and Growth Factors.** Osteoclasts are able to liberate and activate growth factors from the matrix that are stimulatory to osteoblast progenitor cells, allowing them to proliferate and differentiate to mature osteoblasts, which may stimulate osteoclast differentiation and activation as described in Fig. 16-4. The result is a "coupling" of the process of osteoclastic bone lysis with subsequent bone formation.

Bone mineral is in the form of a crystal called *hydroxyapatite*. Fully mineralized bone comprises approximately 65% of the bone by weight and consists in part of calcium, phosphorus, carbonate, magnesium, sodium, manganese, zinc, copper, and fluoride. The mineral content gives bone its hardness. The production of osteoid (unmineralized organic matrix) by osteoblasts is followed by a period of maturation, after which mineral is deposited in exchange for water. Mineralization in woven bone is initiated within cytoplasmic blebs (matrix vesicles) of osteoblasts in the osteoid (see E-Fig. 16-2). Initiation of mineralization involves concentrating calcium, phosphorus, and other elements in these matrix vesicles to a level that causes precipitation of the mineral in the form of amorphous (not yet crystalline) hydroxyapatite. Matrix vesicles contain phospholipids and enzymes such as alkaline phosphatase and adenosine triphosphatase in their membranes. It is speculated that the membrane phospholipids attract calcium and phosphorus to the surface of the vesicle and that the alkaline phosphatase and adenosine triphosphatase enzymes might function in the pumping of these ions into the cell against a concentration gradient.

On reaching a critical mass, the amorphous mineral becomes crystalline. The crystalline hydroxyapatite pierces the lipid membrane of the matrix vesicle and extends to the gaps (holes) between collagen molecules. It is within these holes that the mineral crystals are first deposited in collagen. For the mineralization to spread beyond these gaps between the collagen molecules, it is necessary for naturally occurring inhibitors of mineralization, such as inorganic pyrophosphate, in the matrix to be destroyed. Inorganic pyrophosphates are normal by-products of cellular metabolism and are deposited in unmineralized matrix by osteoblasts. The phosphatase enzymes described previously on the matrix vesicles have the ability to cleave these inorganic pyrophosphates and, in doing so, destroy these inhibitors. Once the gaps are filled with mineral and the inhibitors of mineralization are destroyed, the process continues so that eventually the surfaces of collagen fibers, as well as spaces between collagen fibers, are mineralized. Initiation of mineralization in lamellar bone might not require matrix vesicles because glycoproteins, such as sialoprotein and osteonectin, can act as the nidus for the mineralization process.

Bone as a Tissue

In the cortex and subjacent to articular cartilage (subchondral bone), bone is organized into osteons (also called *Haversian systems*), which are cylinders of concentric layers of lamellae that are oriented parallel to the longitudinal axis of the bone and contain centrally located vessels and nerves (Fig. 16-6). The bone between the osteons is called *interstitial lamellae*. Layers of bone oriented parallel to the internal and external circumference of the bone (beneath the endosteal and periosteal surfaces) are called *circumferential lamellae*. The osteonal system provides channels for the vascular supply to the cortex and also acts as tightly bound cables, giving the cortical bone strength and limited flexibility. This osteonal system also might be important in limiting propagation of microcracks in bone by diverting cracks along cement lines, which are collagen-poor, proteoglycan-rich seams between adjacent remodeling and/or modeling units (see later discussion). In hematoxylin and eosin (H&E)-stained histologic sections of decalcified bone, cement lines appear as basophilic lines.

In contrast to the dense compact bone of the cortex and the subchondral bone plates, the bone in the medullary cavity is in the form of anastomosing plates or rods and is called *cancellous*, *trabecular*, or *spongy bone* (see Figs. 16-6 and 16-8). The orientation of the trabeculae usually reflects adaptation (modeling) to mechanical stresses applied to the bone. This is readily apparent when examining the trabeculae in the femoral neck, which are oriented in lines and arcs that are perpendicular to the stress applied and are thicker and more numerous on the ventral aspect (side of compression) compared with the dorsal aspect (side of tension). The lamellae within a trabecula usually are arranged parallel to the surface of the trabecula and are not arranged into tubes or osteons, as they are in cortical bone.

In most species, bone undergoes a low but constant process called *remodeling* in which old bone is resorbed and replaced by new bone. Remodeling is a tightly coordinated event that includes synchronized activities of multiple cellular participants to ensure that bone resorption and formation occur sequentially at the same anatomic location to preserve bone mass. The basal level of this remodeling activity (number of sites in the skeleton being remodeled at any one time) is likely "programmed" for each species. The number of active remodeling sites, however, can be markedly increased or decreased in response to altered mechanical use (see later discussion). This turnover of old bone to new bone allows for the repair of accumulated microscopic injury in the bone (microfractures). In normal bone remodeling, slightly less bone is replaced than removed, leaving a small negative net change in bone mass with each remodeling cycle and explaining in part the reduced bone mass in aged animals. Furthermore, in disease states, such as

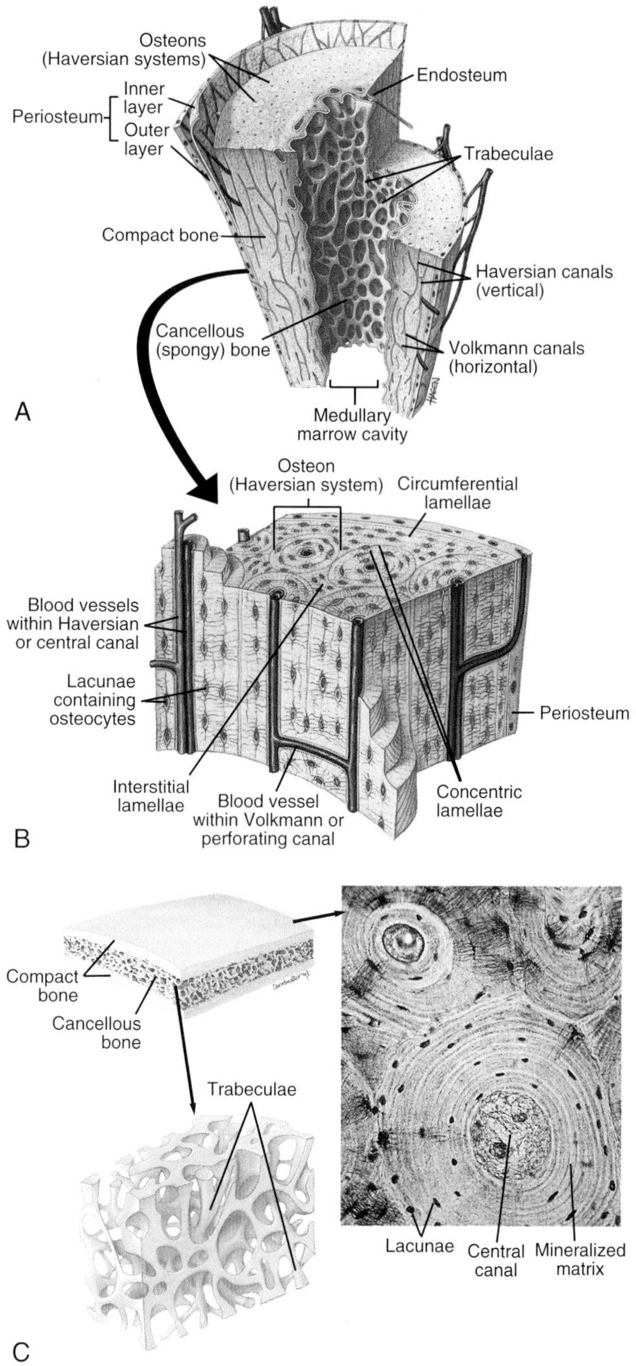

Figure 16-6 **Structure of Compact and Cancellous Bone. A,** Longitudinal section of a long bone showing both cancellous and compact bone. **B,** Magnified view of compact bone. **C,** Section of a flat bone. Outer layers of compact bone surround centrally located cancellous bone. Fine structure of compact and cancellous bone is shown at a higher magnification. (From Thibodeau GA, Patton KT: *Anatomy and physiology*, ed 6, St. Louis, 2007, Mosby.)

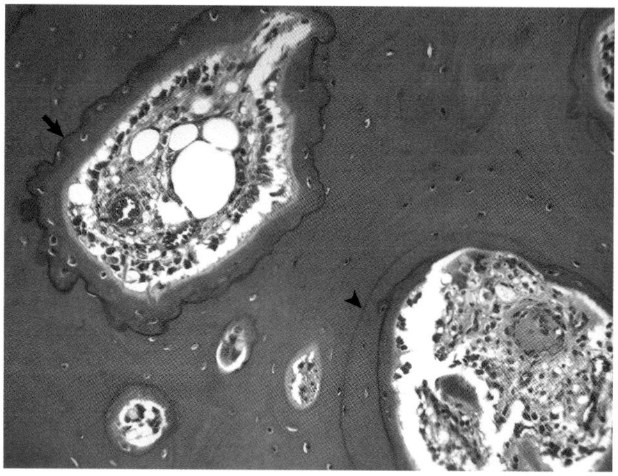

Figure 16-7 **Remodeling in Compact Subchondral Bone Adjacent to a Joint with Bacterial Infection, Bone, Horse.** Resting cement lines appear as basophilic smooth lines indicating where formation has temporarily stopped *(arrowhead)*. Reversal lines are scalloped basophilic lines *(arrow)* indicating where bone resorption stopped and was followed by formation. H&E stain. (Courtesy Dr. S.E. Weisbrode, College of Veterinary Medicine, The Ohio State University.)

hyperparathyroidism, resorption is often increased and formation decreased, leaving a significant net negative bone balance. Interestingly, in small, short-lived animals, such as the mouse and rat, cortical bone is not remodeled.

The remodeling unit of cortical bone is called the *osteon*, whereas the remodeling unit of trabecular bone is called the *basic structural unit*. The shape of the osteon is cylindrical; however, the basic structural unit has the contour of a shallow trench filled with parallel lamellae. The time required from initiation to completion of these remodeling units (from initiation of bone removal by osteoclasts to complete filling of the defect by osteoblasts), regardless of the type of bone, is estimated to be 3 to 4 months in human beings. Basophilic cement lines that mark the limit of previous resorptive activity are usually somewhat scalloped, following the contours of the Howship's lacunae created by osteoclasts, and are called *reversal lines* (where resorption stopped and the process was reversed by formation) (Fig. 16-7). Cement lines also can occur when osteoblast formation ceases and subsequently resumes, and these are called *"resting lines"* and are usually smooth, following the contour of the overlying surface.

Bone as an Organ

Individual bones of the skeleton vary in their manner of formation, growth, structure, and function. Flat bones of the skull develop by the process of intramembranous ossification, in which mesenchymal cells differentiate into osteoblasts and produce bone directly, in the absence of a preexisting cartilage model. In contrast, most bones develop from cartilaginous models by the process of endochondral ossification, in which cartilage is invaded by blood vessels, undergoes mineralization, and forms primary (diaphyseal) and secondary (epiphyseal) centers of ossification. Bones forming by endochondral ossification, such as the long bones of the appendicular skeleton and the vertebral bodies, are divided anatomically into epiphyses, metaphyseal growth plates (physes), metaphyses, and diaphyses (Fig. 16-8).

Blood Supply to Bone

Developmentally, long bones are first apparent as a mesenchymal condensation that then differentiates to hyaline cartilage (Fig. 16-9). Osteogenic cells (stem cells) differentiate into osteoblasts, which secrete bone matrix onto the periphery of the diaphysis, forming a bony periosteal collar. The central area of the shaft then mineralizes and becomes vascularized, forming the primary center of ossification. At a later stage of development, the ends of the growing long bones mineralize centrally and become vascularized, forming

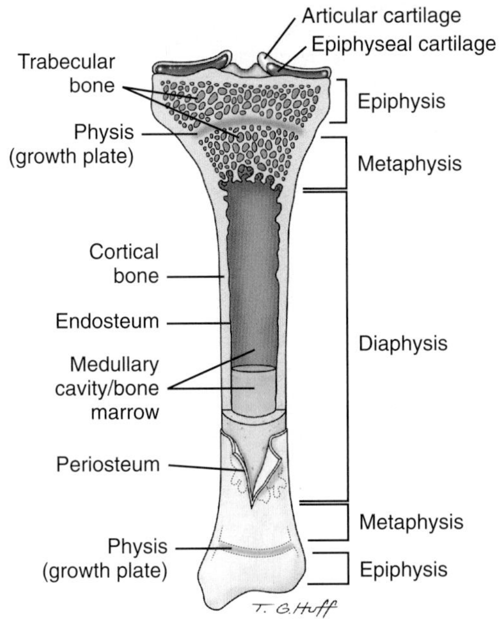

Figure 16-8 **Longitudinal Section of Long Bone (Tibia) Showing Trabecular (Cancellous) and Compact (Cortical) Bone and Names of the Regions of Bone.**

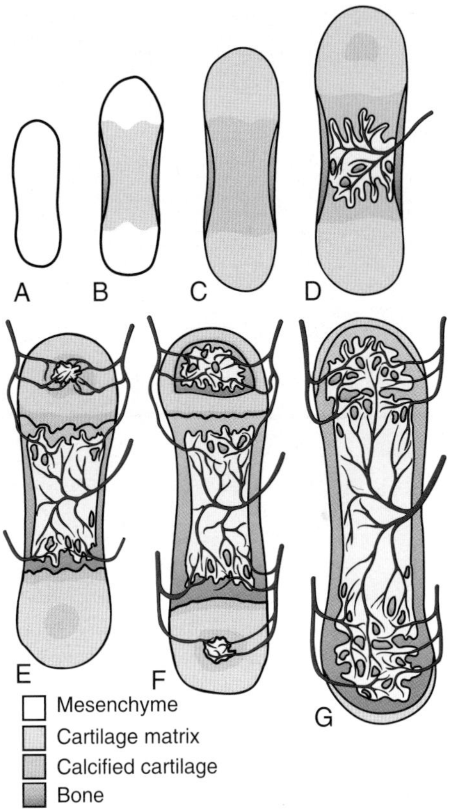

Figure 16-9 **Correlation of Long Bone Development and Vascularization.** The primitive mesenchyme that makes up the skeletal primordia contains no blood vessels **(A)**. This mesenchyme condenses and undergoes central mineralization; a bony collar forms in the periosteum of the diaphysis **(B and C)**. The nutrient artery enters the mineralized cartilaginous tissue in the diaphysis, bringing osteogenic and osteoclast precursors and enabling endochondral ossification to occur (primary center of ossification) **(D)**. Similarly, the epiphyseal arteries bring these cells to the secondary centers of ossification in the epiphyses (located at the ends of the growing long bones) **(E)**. Extensive anastomoses develop as the bone continues to develop and as the subarticular growth cartilage is replaced by bone and the growth plates close **(F and G)**. Cartilage canal vessels, arising from the perichondrium and entering the epiphyseal cartilage present at the ends of the growing long bones, are not shown in this diagram but are present prior to the development of the secondary centers of ossification and persist for a variable time frame afterwards, depending on site and species. (Redrawn from Banks WJ: *Applied veterinary histology*, ed 3, St. Louis, 1993, Mosby.)

the secondary centers of ossification. The growth plate (physis) forms between the primary and secondary centers of ossification and is composed of epiphyseal (growth) cartilage that is responsible for longitudinal growth. Epiphyseal cartilage also is present at the ends of the growing long bones, subjacent to the articular cartilage, and is responsible for forming the shape of these structures. Arterial blood from the systemic circulation enters bones through nutrient, metaphyseal, periosteal, and epiphyseal arteries (see Fig. 16-9). Nutrient arteries penetrate the diaphyseal cortex through a nutrient foramen covered by strong, protective fascial attachments; once within the medulla, these arteries divide into proximal and distal intramedullary branches. Other arteries penetrating the cortex are the proximal and distal metaphyseal arteries, which are smaller and more numerous than the nutrient arteries. They penetrate the cortex and anastomose with the terminal branches of the nutrient arteries in the medullary cavity, protecting against infarction in case of obstruction of a nutrient artery.

Small periosteal arteries also pass through the diaphyseal cortex at sites of fascial attachment and can supply one-quarter to one-third of the outer cortex. The remainder of the cortex is supplied by the nutrient artery and its anastomotic branches. This blood flow is centrifugal (from medulla to periosteum) because of greater pressures in the intramedullary vessels. The chondrocytes of the physis nearest the epiphysis are supplied by epiphyseal arteries, whereas the chondrocytes of the physis nearest the metaphysis are supplied by branches of metaphyseal and nutrient arteries. As capillaries from these vessels approach the metaphyseal side of the physis, they make abrupt turns (loops), which are sites of predisposition to bacterial embolization in neonatal sepsis, sometimes resulting in osteomyelitis.

Bone Growth

Bone grows in length by interstitial growth within the metaphyseal growth plates (physes) (Fig. 16-10). The calcified longitudinal septa of the growth plates serve as struts on which bone is deposited, a process called *endochondral ossification*. The metaphyseal growth plate is divided into a reserve or resting zone, a proliferative zone, a hypertrophic zone, and a calcifying zone (see Fig. 16-10). The resting or reserve zone serves as a source of cells for the proliferating zone in which cells multiply, accumulate glycogen, produce matrix, and become arranged in longitudinal columns. In the hypertrophic zone, the chondrocyte volume expands and the chondrocytes secrete macromolecules that modify the matrix to allow capillary invasion and initiate matrix mineralization. The overall lengthening of the bone is due both to chondrocyte proliferation and hypertrophy; recent experimental evidence indicates that the latter is more important to this process. Calcification begins in the longitudinal septa of cartilaginous matrix between columns of chondrocytes. Although the majority of the terminal hypertrophic/calcifying chondrocytes appear to undergo apoptosis, these cells also are capable of undergoing transformation to osteoblasts. Matrix vesicles derived from chondrocytes (analogous to those described previously for mineralization of bone) form in the calcifying zone and initiate the mineralization process. The processes of mineralization and vascular invasion of the growth plate are codependent events. To supply

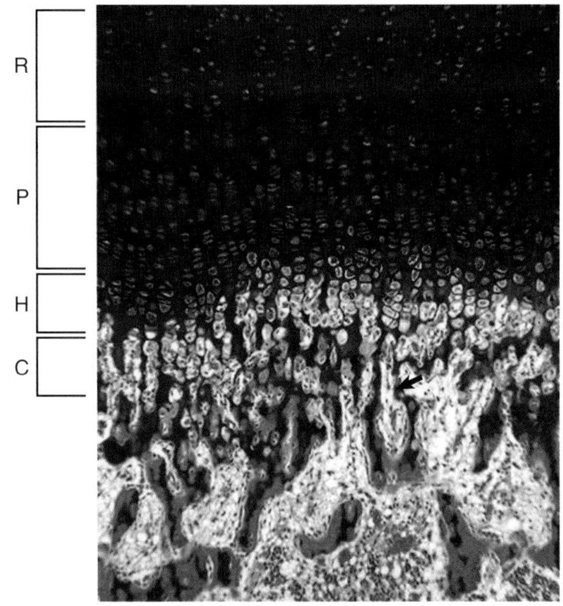

Figure 16-10 **Growth Plate (Physis), Long Bone, Immature Dog.** Resting *(R)*, proliferating *(P)*, hypertrophic *(H)*, and calcifying *(C)* zones of the growth plate are visible. Apoptotic chondrocytes are released from their lacunae by invading vessels and chondroclasts, leaving only the longitudinal septa *(arrow)* as a template on which bone will be deposited to form a primary trabecula. H&E stain. (Courtesy Dr. S.E. Weisbrode, College of Veterinary Medicine, The Ohio State University.)

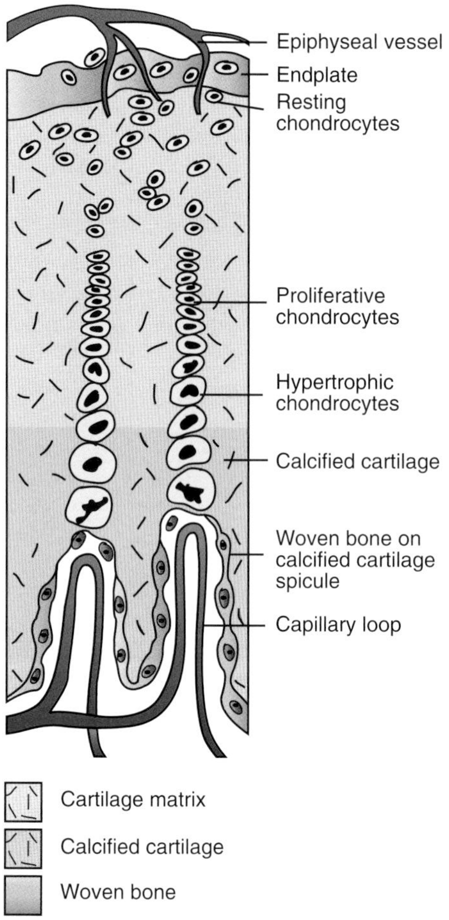

Figure 16-11 **Major Blood Supply to the Physis.** Branches of the epiphyseal artery supply the resting zones of the growth plate. Branches of the metaphyseal artery form capillary loops at the metaphyseal side of the physis where endochondral ossification is occurring. (Redrawn from Banks WJ: *Applied veterinary histology,* ed 3, St. Louis, 1993, Mosby.)

salts for the mineralization, a nearby blood supply is necessary. Vascular invasion, a critical step in endochondral ossification, does not take place in mammalian growth plates unless there is mineralization of the longitudinal septum. Blood vessels from the metaphysis invade into the advancing growth plate, providing an entryway for osteoblasts that form bone on the cartilage spicules (Fig. 16-11). The chondro-osseous junction in the metaphysis is a fragile lattice of bone-covered spicules of calcified cartilage (primary spongiosa). As the growth plate advances and elongates the metaphysis, the more mature trabeculae deeper in the metaphysis become fewer and thicker (secondary spongiosa) and are composed primarily of bone with only residual fragments of cartilage.

Growth plates (physes) are thickest when growth is most rapid; as growth slows, the growth plate becomes thin and "closes" (becomes replaced by bone) at skeletal maturity. The age at which a growth plate closes varies, depending on site, species, and sex. For example, the physes of vertebrae usually remain open longer than the physes of the long bones. Androgens and estrogens play a major role in determining the time of growth plate closure, and early castration results in delayed growth plate closure with subsequent increased length of bones compared with intact individuals.

Growth of the epiphysis contributes both to the overall length of the bone and to the shape of the ends of the bone. This is accomplished by endochondral ossification at the articular-epiphyseal cartilage complex (AECC). The AECC is composed of permanent articular cartilage, as well as a subjacent temporary growth/epiphyseal cartilage that is vascularized and contains the same zones as the growth plate (Fig. 16-12). In the mature individual, endochondral ossification no longer occurs at the AECC. Although the articular cartilage remains throughout life, the epiphyseal cartilage is completely replaced by bone once growth has ceased (Fig. 16-13). Bone grows in width by intramembranous bone formation. Except for articular surfaces (including the ends of the vertebral bodies), the surfaces of bones are covered by periosteum. This covering is a thin membrane that is loosely attached to underlying bone except at heavy fascial attachments on bony prominences and at tendon insertions, where its attachments are strong and are associated with large vessels penetrating the underlying bone. Microscopically, the periosteum is composed of an outer fibrous layer that provides structural support and an inner osteogenic or cambium layer that is capable of forming normal lamellar appositional bone on the cortex of growing bones (Fig. 16-14). The cambium layer also is capable of forming woven bone, known as *periosteal new bone*, in response to injury. The periosteum is well supplied with lymph vessels and with fine myelinated and nonmyelinated nerve fibers that account for the intense pain that occurs with periosteal injury.

The periosteum covering the physis is called the *perichondral ring*. The perichondral ring adds new cartilage to the periphery of the physis, enabling it to expand in width as the animal grows. The metaphyseal cortex immediately adjacent to the perichondral ring is normally very thin in the growing bone because its surfaces are the sites of very active osteoclastic bone resorption. Structurally, this area is the weakest part of the bone.

Joints

Joints (articulations) join skeletal structures, provide for movement, and in some cases have shock-absorbing functions. This section of the chapter is primarily devoted to synovial joints, also called *movable* or *diarthrodial joints*.

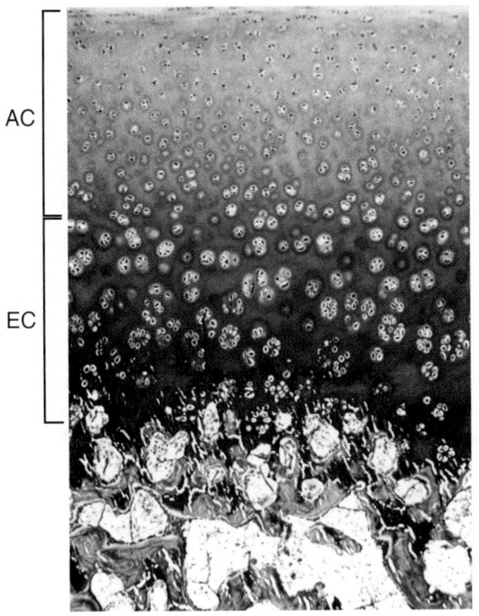

Figure 16-12 Articular-Epiphyseal Cartilage Complex *(AECC)*, Long Bone, Immature Pig. The AECC is composed of a layer of articular cartilage *(AC)* and a subjacent layer of growth (epiphyseal) cartilage *(EC)*. The growth cartilage is present only in immature individuals, and it often contains cartilage canal vessels (not shown); its structure and function are similar to those of the physis. Compare with Fig. 16-13. Toluidine blue stain. (Courtesy Dr. C.S. Carlson, College of Veterinary Medicine, University of Minnesota.)

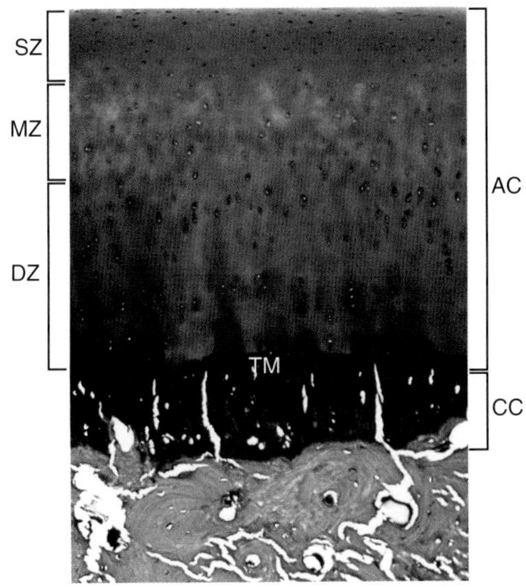

Figure 16-13 Articular Cartilage, Long Bone, Adult Dog. The articular cartilage is present throughout life and contains superficial, middle, and deep zones; however, the epiphyseal cartilage is absent in adults. In adults, endochondral ossification has ceased and the tidemark *(TM)* delimits the boundary between the uncalcified articular cartilage *(AC)* and the calcified cartilage *(CC)*. Compare with Fig. 16-12. *SZ*, Superficial zone; *MZ*, middle zone; *DZ*, deep zone. Toluidine blue stain. (Courtesy Dr. C.S. Carlson, College of Veterinary Medicine, University of Minnesota.)

Synovial joints occur in both the axial and the appendicular skeleton. These joints allow for a variable degree of movement, and anatomically, they are composed of two bone ends joined together by a fibrous capsule and ligaments. The inner surface of the articular capsule is lined by a synovial membrane, and the bone ends are covered by articular cartilage. The joint space contains synovial

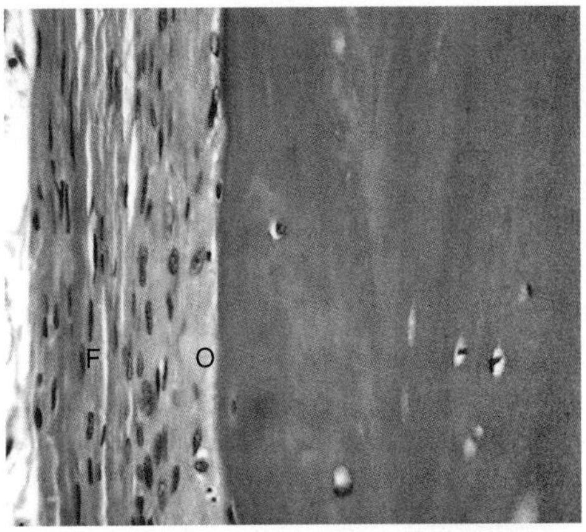

Figure 16-14 Periosteum, Bone, Dog. The outer fibrous layer *(F)* and inner osteogenic layer *(O)* line the periosteal surface. The osteogenic layer is able to rapidly deposit woven bone as a nonspecific response to injury. H&E stain. (Courtesy Dr. S.E. Weisbrode, College of Veterinary Medicine, The Ohio State University.)

fluid, and fibrocartilaginous menisci or disks are present at some sites (e.g., femorotibial and temporomandibular joints). Synovial joints operate with very low coefficients of friction and are self-lubricating. Articular cartilage serves as the bearing substance and subchondral bone as the supporting material. Articular cartilage functions to minimize friction created by movement to transmit mechanical forces to underlying bone and to maximize the contact area of the joint under load. Joints receive and absorb energy of impact. Both articular cartilage and subchondral bone deform under pressure, but it is the subchondral bone that has the most significant force-attenuating properties.

Articular Cartilage

Articular (hyaline) cartilage is normally a white to blue-white material with a smooth, moist surface. Cartilage thickness is greatest in the young and at sites of maximal weight bearing. Thinning and yellow discoloration occur in old age. At its margins, articular cartilage merges with a periosteal surface that is lined by fibrous tissue contiguous with the synovial membrane. Synovial fossae are normal depressions on non–weight-bearing articular cartilage surfaces (Fig. 16-15) that develop bilaterally in the larger appendicular joints of the horse, pig, and ruminant. These fossae are usually not present at birth but are fully formed by skeletal maturity. The function of synovial fossae is not known; however, they are significant because they are often mistaken for lesions. Adult articular cartilage contains no nerves or blood or lymph vessels, and its nutrients are obtained by diffusion from synovial fluid and to a lesser extent from subchondral vessels. In the immature skeleton, articular cartilage overlies the temporary growth cartilage of the epiphysis (epiphyseal cartilage) (see Fig. 16-12). The epiphyseal cartilage is highly dependent on a network of blood vessels that originate from the perichondrium and the subchondral bone. Similar to the physis, it undergoes endochondral ossification and thereby contributes to the growth/development of the epiphysis. At skeletal maturity, the epiphyseal cartilage has been entirely replaced by bone, and the only joint cartilage remaining is the adult articular cartilage, which includes a thin subjacent zone of calcified cartilage. In skeletally mature individuals, the junction between the noncalcified articular cartilage and the deeper calcified cartilage forms a thin basophilic line in H&E stained sections called the *tidemark* (see Fig. 16-13). As animals age, multiple tidemarks can be formed, indicating an advance (thickening) of the calcified layer of articular cartilage and thinning of the overlying

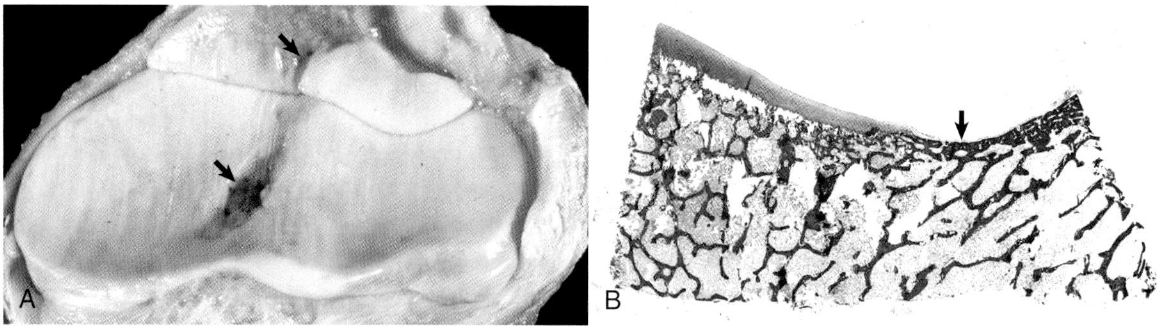

Figure 16-15 **Synovial Fossa, Joint, Radius and Ulna, Bone, Proximal End, Adult Horse. A,** Synovial fossae are depressions in the cartilage on the non–weight-bearing surfaces of the sagittal ridge of the radius and in the semilunar notch of the ulna *(arrows)*. The parallel linear grooves apparent on the weight-bearing surface (articular cartilage) of the radius are the result of degenerative joint disease. **B,** Histologically, the surface of the synovial fossa is covered by a thin fibrous membrane *(arrow)* rather than articular cartilage. H&E stain. (Courtesy Dr. S.E. Weisbrode, College of Veterinary Medicine, The Ohio State University.)

noncalcified articular cartilage. The calcified cartilage serves to anchor articular cartilage to subchondral bone and limits the diffusion of substances between bone and cartilage.

Articular cartilage is 70% to 80% water by weight. It is a viscoelastic, hydrated fiber-reinforced gel that contains chondrocytes, collagen fibers (mostly type II), noncollagenous proteins, and proteoglycan aggregates. The largest proteoglycan in articular cartilage is aggrecan, which is composed of the immensely long, nonpolysulfated glycosaminoglycan, hyaluronan, to which core proteins are attached in a perpendicular arrangement like bristles on a brush. Similarly, smaller, negatively charged polysulfated glycosaminoglycans (chondroitin sulfate and keratan sulfate) are attached to the core proteins. The large content of negatively charged polysaccharide chains in the aggrecan aggregate is responsible for the extremely high osmotic swelling pressure of cartilage. The swelling pressure provided by aggrecan is counteracted by the resistance of the intact type II collagen fibers, giving cartilage its characteristic properties of being able to resist compressive forces and having a high tensile strength. Collagen fibers are arranged in arcades so that the tops of the arcades are parallel to the articular surface, and the sides are perpendicular to the surface and parallel with the radial or intermediate zone of chondrocytes. Functionally, the superficial zone of articular cartilage resists shearing forces, the middle zone functions in shock absorption, and the calcified deep zone of cartilage serves to attach articular cartilage to the subchondral bone by its irregular (and therefore interlocking) interfaces. Scanning electron microscopy reveals that the surface of articular cartilage is not smooth but, rather, contains numerous depressions that can serve as reservoirs for synovial fluid.

Articular cartilage contains a single population of cells called *chondrocytes* that are responsible for the production, maintenance, and turnover of intercellular substances. In routine histologic sections, chondrocytes appear to be present within lacunae. However, although the lacunae within which osteocytes reside contain fluid spaces, the apparent lacunae of chondrocytes have been clearly demonstrated to be the result of shrinkage artifact. In fact, the chondrocyte cell membrane is in direct contact with the pericellular matrix and contains surface receptors for matrix components (e.g., hyaluronan).

Normal matrix turnover is enzymatic and this process is balanced by enzyme inhibitors. Proteases capable of degrading aggrecans are called *aggrecanases* and are members of the ADAM (A Disintegrin And Metalloprotease) protein family, whereas proteases capable of breaking the peptide bonds in collagen are called *collagenases*. Damage to the matrix occurs if there is increased destruction or decreased synthesis of matrix components. It is important to remember that compared with bone that normally renews itself by remodeling, articular cartilage has extremely poor regenerative capabilities; damaged articular cartilage repairs through the replacement of hyaline cartilage with fibrocartilage. Although there is evidence for proteoglycan synthesis in normal articular cartilage, the turnover of cells and type II collagen occurs at an extremely low rate. Correspondingly, the cellularity of articular cartilage declines with age and the life span of individual chondrocytes is thought to be long.

Articular Capsule/Synovium/Synovial Fluid

The articular capsule consists of outer fibrous and inner synovial tissue layers. The outer layer is a heavy sheath that contributes to joint stability and, at its insertion, attaches to bone at the margins of the joint, thereby enclosing a segment of bone of variable length within the joint cavity. It is well supplied with blood vessels and nerve endings. The inner synovial tissue layer is called the *synovial membrane* and covers all the inner surfaces of the joints except for the surface of the articular cartilage. The synovial membrane is normally very thin, lacks a basement membrane, and is barely visible grossly. In fact, collection of normal synovial membrane for histologic evaluation is best done immediately after opening the joint because it quickly retracts and becomes difficult to locate. The inner surface of the synovial membrane may be flat or may contain tiny projections (villi). Synovial intimal or lining cells, one to four cells thick, form a discontinuous surface layer and include two cell types: (1) A cells, which are macrophages that are responsible for the removal of microbes and the debris resulting from normal wear and tear in the joint (Fig. 16-16; E-Fig. 16-11), and (2) B cells, which are fibroblast-like cells that produce synovial fluid. These cell types are not distinguishable from each other in routine histological sections. Normal synovial fluid contains hyaluronic acid, lubricin (a water-soluble glycoprotein), proteinases, and collagenase and is clear, colorless to pale yellow, and viscous. In addition to lubricating the joint surfaces, it supplies oxygen and nutrients to and removes carbon dioxide and metabolic wastes from the chondrocytes in articular cartilage. The synovial subintima can be classified according to the type of tissue that predominates (areolar, adipose, or fibrous), and it contains blood and lymph vessels that supply and drain the intraarticular structures. Adipose tissue sometimes accumulates in the deep layers of the synovium, forming fat pads that serve as soft cushions in joint cavities (e.g., the infrapatellar fat body of the stifle joint).

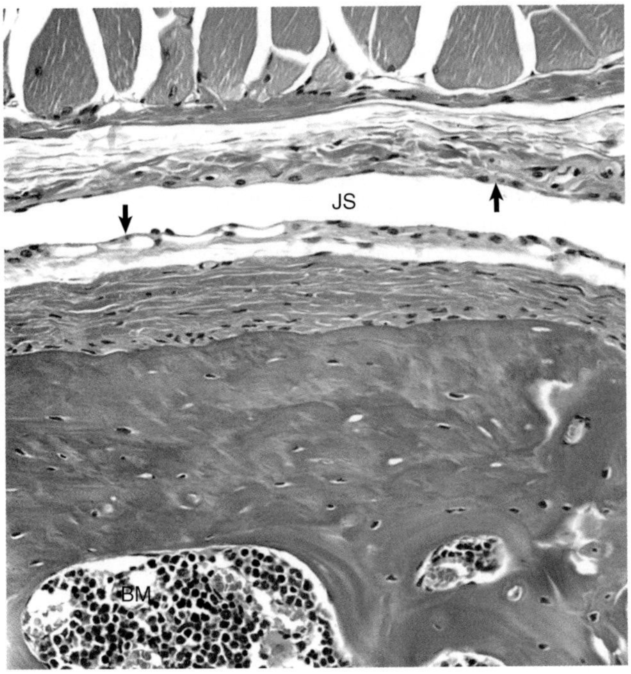

Figure 16-16 **Synovial Membrane, Stifle Joint, Mouse.** The normal synovial membrane *(arrows)* encloses an optically clear joint space *(JS)* and consists of an incomplete layer of histiocytes (phagocytic cells) and fibrocytes with subjacent loose fibrous and/or fibrofatty tissue. *BM*, Bone marrow. H&E stain. (Courtesy Dr. C.S. Carlson and Dr. E.J. Olson, College of Veterinary Medicine, University of Minnesota.)

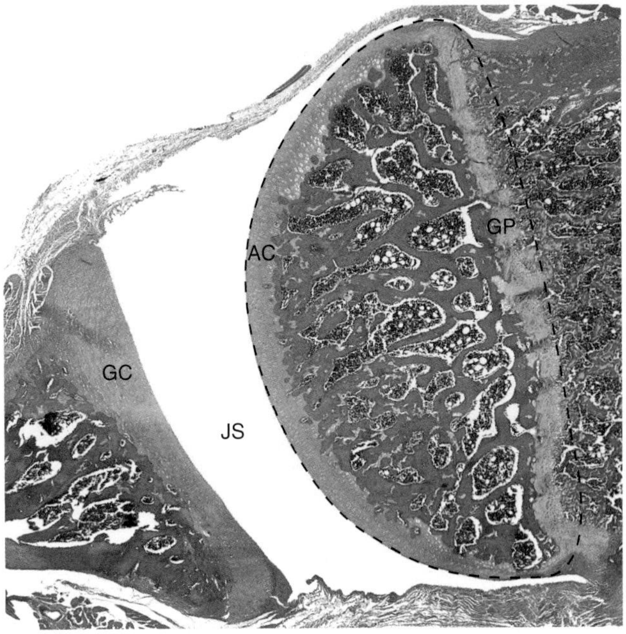

Figure 16-17 **Shoulder Joint, Rat.** Glenoid cavity (*GC*), articular cartilage (*AC*) of humeral head *(dashed line ellipsoid)*, secondary center of ossification lies between the articular cartilage and the growth plate (*GP*). *JS*, Joint space. H&E stain. (Courtesy Dr. C.S. Carlson and Dr. E.J. Olson, College of Veterinary Medicine, University of Minnesota.)

Joint lubrication depends on the microscopic roughness, elasticity, and hydration of articular cartilage and on the presence of hyaluronic acid and lubricin in synovial fluid. The lubricating properties of lubricin depend on its ability to bind to articular cartilage, where it retains a protective layer of water molecules. In contrast, hyaluronic acid, the molecule that makes synovial fluid viscous, has largely been excluded as a lubricant of the cartilage-on-cartilage bearing and instead lubricates the site of surface contact between synovium and cartilage. When pressure is applied to the joint, such as during weight bearing, the articular surface is supplied with pressurized fluid that carries most of the load. Synovial fluid is combined with water that is released from the underlying cartilage when pressure is applied during weight bearing. When the load is removed, the water returns to the cartilage because of the hydrophilic properties of proteoglycans. This flushing of fluid in and out of the articular cartilage enables nutrients to enter cartilage from the synovial fluid and waste products to be removed.

Subchondral Bone

The subchondral bone has a variable morphological appearance depending on the maturity of the individual. In immature individuals, it is composed of fine interconnecting trabeculae that contain a large calcified cartilage component and is the result of replacement of epiphyseal cartilage by bone through the process of endochondral ossification (see Fig. 16-12). In mature individuals, it is composed of interconnecting bone trabeculae located immediately subjacent to the calcified cartilage zone that is known as the subchondral bone plate (see Fig. 16-13). In both cases, it acts to support the overlying cartilage and dissipate concussive forces to the peripheral cortical bone (Fig. 16-17; E-Fig. 16-12). The thickness of the subchondral bone plate varies in proportion to the degree of weight bearing. Increased subchondral bone thickness is a common pathological finding in osteoarthritis. In larger animals (nonrodent species), subchondral bone often is composed of compact osteonal bone rather than trabecular bone.

Tendons and Ligaments

A tendon is a unit of musculoskeletal tissue that transmits force from muscle to bone. Morphologically, tendons are similar to ligaments and fascia; however, ligaments join bone to bone, and fascia connects muscle to muscle. The musculotendinous unit is composed predominantly of parallel arrays of closely packed collagen fibers and rod- or spindle-shaped fibroblast-like cells (tenocytes) within a well-ordered extracellular matrix (Fig. 16-18). Collagen fibrils are bundled into large fibers that are evident throughout the tendon and are visible under light microscopy as a crimped or a sinusoidal pattern that facilitates a 1% to 3% elongation of the tendon. This elongation of the individual fibers serves to buffer the tendon from sudden mechanical loading. Water represents approximately 55% of the weight of tendon, is present mainly in the extracellular matrix, and is believed to reduce friction, facilitating the gliding of fibrils in response to mechanical loading. The major fibrillar component of tendon is type I collagen, which constitutes approximately 80% of the dry weight, whereas type III collagen is present in the endotenon (connective tissue binding together groups of collagen fibers into fascicles) and epitenon (exterior sheath of connective tissue that surrounds groups of fascicles). The remainder of the tendon components include elastin, proteoglycans, and inorganic components. Collagen is synthesized by the tenocytes and constitutes the basic structural unit of tendon. The collagen polypeptides form a triple helix, which self-assembles into collagen fibrils with intermolecular cross-links that form between adjacent helices. The collagen polypeptides and the ensuing triple helix are synthesized inside the cell, secreted into the extracellular matrix, and assembled into the microfibrillar units that constitute the collagen fibers. This step is promoted by a specialized enzyme called *lysyl oxidase*, which promotes cross-link formation—a process involving placement of stable

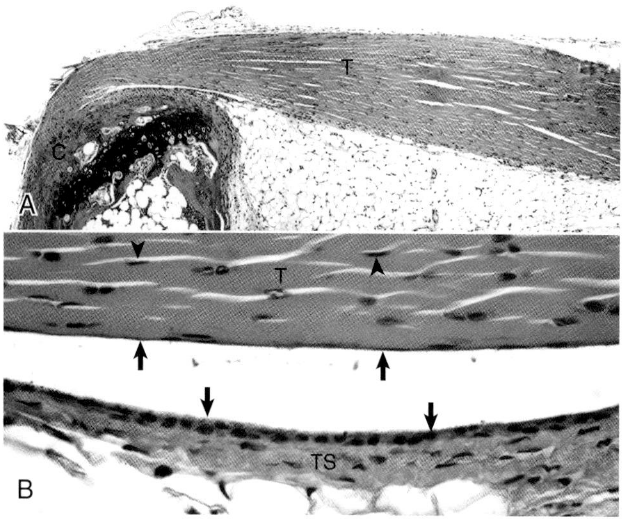

Figure 16-18 **Tendon, Joint, Mouse. A,** Gastrocnemius tendon *(T)*. The tendon is composed of parallel arrays of closely packed collagen fibers and low numbers of fibroblast-like cells called *tenocytes* (see higher magnification in **B**; *arrowheads*). The tendon is covered by flattened synoviocytes (see higher magnification in **B**), so it may glide smoothly over the synoviocytes of the tendon sheath. C, Calcaneus insertion. H&E stain. **B,** Higher magnification of tendon sheath. The enveloping structure enclosing the tendon is the tendon sheath *(TS)*, and it is lined by synoviocytes *(arrows)*. *T*, Gastrocnemius tendon. H&E stain. (Courtesy Dr. J.F. Zachary, College of Veterinary Medicine, University of Illinois.)

cross-links within and between the molecules. Cross-link formation is the critical step that gives collagen fibers their strength. Tendon is stronger per unit area than muscle, and its tensile strength equals that of bone, although it is flexible and slightly extensible. The parallel arrangement of tendon collagen fibers resists tension so that contractile energy is not lost during transmission from muscle to bone. The mechanical properties of tendons depend on the collagen fiber diameter and orientation; however, the proteoglycan components of tendons also are important to the mechanical properties. Whereas the collagen fibrils allow tendons to resist tensile stress, the proteoglycans allow them to resist compressive stress.

Skeletal ligaments are defined as dense bands of collagenous tissue that span a joint and then become anchored to the bone at either end. They vary in size, shape, orientation, and location. Their bony attachments are called *insertions*. Biochemically, ligaments are approximately two-thirds water and one-third solid. Type I collagen accounts for 85% of the collagen (other collagen types include III, V, VI, XI, and XIV), and the collagens account for approximately 75% of the dry weight, with the balance being made up by proteoglycans, elastin, and other proteins. While the ligament appears as a single structure, during joint movement some fibers appear to tighten or loosen depending on the bone positions and the forces that are applied, confirming the complexity of these structures. Histologically, ligaments are composed of fibroblasts that are surrounded by matrix. The fibroblasts are responsible for matrix synthesis and are relatively few in number, representing a small percentage of the total ligament volume. Recent studies have indicated that normal ligament cells may communicate by means of prominent cytoplasmic extensions that extend for long distances and connect to cytoplasmic extensions from adjacent cells, thus forming an elaborate three-dimensional architecture. Gap junctions have also been detected in association with these cell connections, raising the possibility of cell-to-cell communication and the potential to coordinate cellular and metabolic responses throughout the tissue. Ligament microstructure reveals collagen bundles aligned along the long axis of the ligament and displaying an underlying "waviness" or crimp along the length, similar to that present in tendon. Crimp is thought to play a biomechanical role, possibly relating to the ligament's loading state with increased loading likely resulting in some areas of the ligament uncrimping, allowing the ligament to elongate without sustaining damage.

One of the main functions of ligaments is mechanical because they passively stabilize joints and help guide those joints through their normal range of motion when a tensile load is applied. Another function of ligaments relates to their viscoelastic behavior in helping provide joint homeostasis. Ligaments "load relax," which means that loads/stresses decrease within the ligament if they are pulled to constant deformations. A third function of ligaments is their role in joint proprioception. In joints such as the stifle, proprioception is provided principally by joint, muscle, and cutaneous receptors. When ligaments are strained, they invoke neurologic feedback signals that then activate muscular contraction, which appears to play a role in joint position sense.

Tendons and ligaments attach to bone in a similar manner, through osteotendinous or osteoligamentous junctions, respectively. These junctions are known as *entheses* and are distinguished as fibrous and fibrocartilaginous according to the type of tissue present at the attachment site. At fibrous entheses, the tendon or ligament attaches either directly to the bone or indirectly to it via the periosteum. Fibrocartilaginous entheses are sites in which chondrogenesis has occurred and commonly contain four tissue types: dense fibrous connective tissue, uncalcified fibrocartilage, calcified fibrocartilage, and bone.

Dysfunction/Responses to Injury

Bone

Mechanical forces that can affect bone are both internal and external. Internal forces associated with extremes in work or exercise can influence modeling or remodeling (see previous discussion) and occasionally cause fracture (failure of the bone). External forces (trauma) are more commonly associated with damage to the periosteal surface or fracture of the cortex and/or trabecular bone.

Hormonal agents, particularly calcitriol and PTH, enter the bone by the bloodstream as described previously. Infectious agents are discussed later in the section on Inflammation of Bone.

Defense against mechanical forces includes the structure of the bone and the bone's ability to model and remodel to adapt to chronic changes in forces applied to it. The dense bone of the cortex enables the bone to resist most external forces. The formation of osteons and cement lines in the cortex (primary remodeling) facilitates dissipation of microcracks and bending of the bone in response to stress.

Defense against hormonal agents that are capable of resorbing bone include the protective covering on mineralized surfaces by the lamina limitans and osteoblasts. In addition, hormonal signaling to resorb bone is done through the osteoblast, which has the ability to modulate the resorption signal. Defense against infectious agents is discussed later in the section on Disorders of Domestic Animals, Bone, Inflammation. The hard tissue of bone can be likened to the rings in a tree that leave clues to the history embedded in its hard structure. Interpreting these clues requires understanding the ways in which bone uniquely responds to injury (Box 16-2).

Disruption of endochondral ossification can alter the appearance of the primary spongiosa. Examples of this are growth arrest lines and the growth retardation lattice. Growth arrest lines can be seen

Box 16-2 Bone-Specific Reactions to Injury

- Disruption of endochondral ossification affects metaphyseal trabeculae and may decrease the rate of bone elongation.
- Bone changes its shape to adapt to damage and abnormal use.
- Bone alters its mass in response to systemic disease and altered use.
- Newly formed bone is woven rather than lamellar.
- Injured periosteum often responds by forming bone.

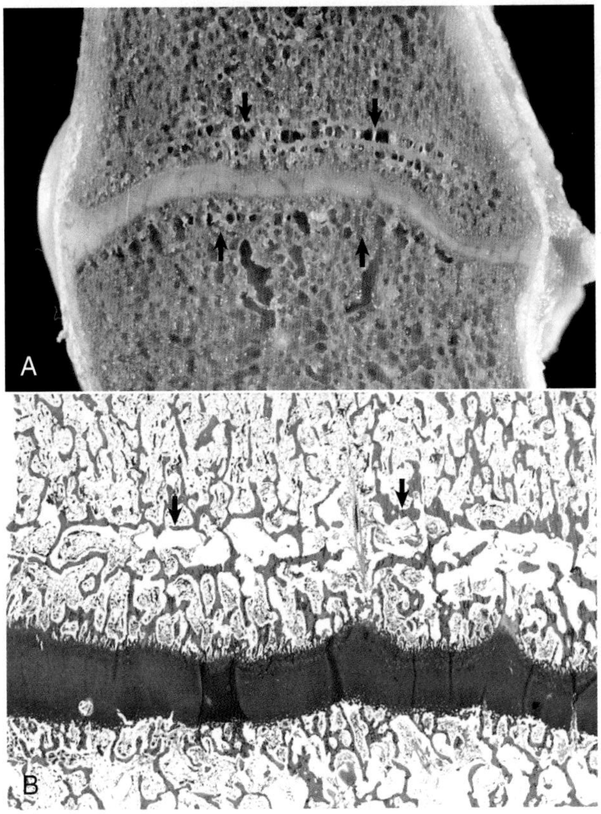

Figure 16-19 Growth Arrest Lines, Long Bone, Metaphysis, Immature Zebra. Gross (**A**) and microscopic (**B**) appearance of growth arrest lines. The zebra was ill from a bacterial renal infection and became anorexic. The animal made a brief clinical recovery before euthanasia. The period of inappetence is responsible for the parallel horizontal lines of bone in the metaphysis (growth arrest lines; *arrows* in both A and B). These lines are the result of transverse (horizontal) orientation of the trabeculae during the period of slowed growth. H&E stain. (Courtesy Dr. S.E. Weisbrode, College of Veterinary Medicine, The Ohio State University.)

in conditions such as debilitating disease or malnutrition, in which multiple nutrient deficiencies are present. The growth plate becomes narrow (growth is impaired), and the metaphyseal face of the plate can be sealed by a layer of bone as a result of transverse trabeculation (trabecular bone forming parallel versus perpendicular to the long axis of the bone), immediately subjacent to the growth plate. If endochondral ossification resumes, this layer of bone becomes separated from the physis and becomes located more distally in the metaphysis. The resulting bony trabeculae that are oriented parallel to the growth plate can be seen grossly and radiographically and are called *growth arrest lines* (Fig. 16-19, A and B).

A growth retardation lattice results from acquired impairment of osteoclastic resorption of bone within the primary spongiosa, which elongates because of continued endochondral ossification. This process results in a dense band of vertically oriented trabecular bone subjacent to the growth plate that is called a *growth retardation lattice* (Fig. 16-20). The band is apparent because there is impairment of the normal modeling process that resorbs many primary trabeculae completely and converts the remaining ones into progressively fewer but thicker structures. Diseases that cause growth retardation lattices include canine distemper and bovine viral diarrhea, in which viral infection of osteoclasts results in defects in cell function, resulting in reduced bone resorption. Similarly, toxic damage to osteoclasts, such as in lead poisoning, can cause a growth retardation lattice ("lead line"). Abnormal retention of primary trabeculae also can be seen with congenital defects in the function of osteoclasts (see later discussion of osteopetrosis). The phrase *growth retardation lattice* is perpetuated here because it is in common use; however, it is important to understand that the lesion is caused by a failure in modeling of the trabeculae rather than by a reduction in longitudinal growth. Weakening or destruction of the matrix of the physeal cartilage, such as occurs in animals with hypervitaminosis A and with manganese deficiency, can lead to premature closure of growth plates. If the entire plate is affected, no further longitudinal growth is possible. If closure is focal, such as can be seen subsequent to localized inflammation or traumatic damage to vessels, the remainder of the growth plate continues to undergo endochondral ossification, resulting in an angular limb deformity.

Osteochondrosis is an important example of a disease caused by disruption of endochondral ossification and is discussed later under disorders of endochondral ossification.

The ability of bone to change its shape and size (modeling) to accommodate altered mechanical use, as can occur in hip dysplasia as an example, is called *Wolff's law* (Fig. 16-21). Tension and compression are important mechanical factors that affect bone modeling, with *formation* favored at sites of compression and *resorption* favored at sites of tension. In addition, trabecular bone aligns along lines of stress. The ways in which bone cells detect altered mechanical use are not precisely known but likely include input from a variety of signals, including stretch receptors on bone cells, streaming potentials, and piezoelectrical activity. Streaming potentials are electrical currents in bone that are detected by the osteocyte-osteoblast network and are caused by fluid fluxes through canalicular spaces. Piezoelectrical activity refers to the production of electrical currents in bone as a result of deformation of collagen fibers and mineral crystals. Electrical currents can affect cell function (bone formation and resorption) and thus influence bone modeling. Bone mass can be altered to accommodate mechanical use. Normal mechanical use suppresses programmed bone resorptive activity and is required for maintenance of bone mass. Decreased mechanical use reduces this inhibition (allowing resorption to proceed) and also suppresses bone formation. The net effect of decreased mechanical use (e.g., casting of a long bone) therefore is a reduced amount of bone as a result of increased resorption and decreased formation (Fig. 16-22). In contrast, increased mechanical use suppresses bone resorption and allows bone mass to increase (Fig. 16-23; E-Fig. 16-13). Chronic suppression of remodeling, however, could result in retention of aged bone and lead to accumulated microcracks, which in turn could override the suppression and stimulate remodeling in these regions.

Woven bone is newly formed, hypercellular bone that is deposited in reaction to injury. Although woven bone is normally present in immature individuals, the presence of woven bone in the adult skeleton is considered to be pathologic. The collagen fibers in woven bone are irregularly/randomly arranged rather than being oriented in a lamellar pattern, a change that is best appreciated using polarized light microscopy (Fig. 16-24). In addition, osteocytes are larger

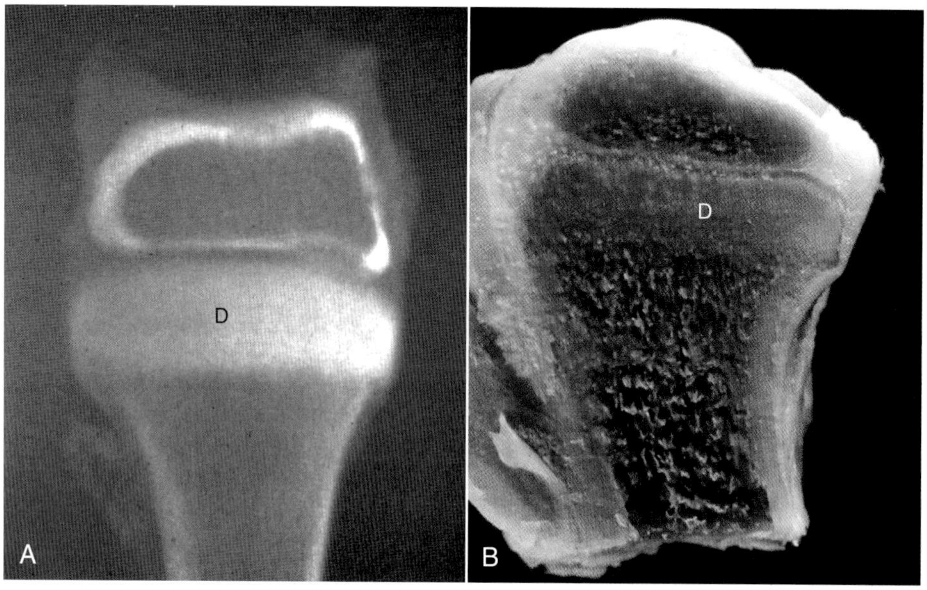

Figure 16-20 **Growth Retardation Lattice, Bone, Radius, Distal End, Dog.** Radiograph (A) and longitudinal section (B) of a growth retardation lattice. The increased bone density *(D)* of the metaphysis represents failure of osteoclasts to resorb unnecessary primary trabeculae. In this case, the failure of osteoclastic resorption was caused by canine distemper virus infection of osteoclasts. (Courtesy Dr. S.E. Weisbrode, College of Veterinary Medicine, The Ohio State University.)

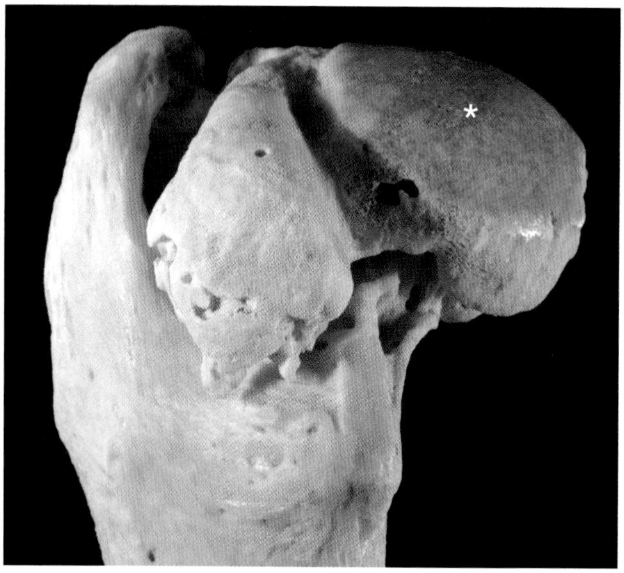

Figure 16-21 **Hip Dysplasia, Bone, Femoral Head and Neck, Dog.** The femoral head *(asterisk)* is severely flattened and periosteal new bone and coalescing osteophytes have formed a massively thickened femoral neck. Macerated specimen. (Courtesy Dr. E.J. Olson, College of Veterinary Medicine, University of Minnesota.)

and more numerous per unit area than in lamellar bone, and there is no preferred orientation to their lacunae versus in lamellar bone in which the alignment of the elliptical lacunae is parallel to the lamellae. Over time, woven bone remodels into lamellar bone.

The periosteum is programmed to respond to injury by producing woven bone, which usually is oriented perpendicularly to the long axis of the cortex. Although nodular periosteal new bone is sometimes referred to as *osteophytes*, the use of this term should be restricted to periarticular new bone that occurs in response to joint injury/instability. Reactive periosteal woven bone may be admixed with hyaline cartilage and sometimes is composed predominantly of cartilage. The extent to which cartilage is produced by the periosteum is thought to be a result of the available oxygen. When oxygen tension is low, cartilage proliferation may predominate; however, when oxygen tension is normal, there may be no cartilage present. Cartilage produced in such circumstances can eventually undergo endochondral ossification. In addition, woven bone produced by the periosteum may be remodeled to lamellar bone or may be removed by osteoclastic resorption. In addition to producing woven bone in response to injury, the periosteum also is capable of producing lamellar bone during slower stages of appositional growth of the diaphysis, and this bone also is subject to osteoclastic resorption. During growth, the regions of the cutback zone of the metaphysis, in which the bone diameter is reduced from a larger diameter at the physis to the narrower diameter of the diaphysis, exhibit marked osteoclastic bone resorption at the periosteal bone surface. Infectious inflammation of the periosteum also can lead to marked osteoclastic bone resorption at the periosteal bone surface.

Joints

Articular Cartilage

Although articular cartilage contains metabolically active cells, it has a limited response to injury and minimal capacity for repair that is largely due to its lack of a blood supply. Superficial cartilage defects (cartilage erosions) that do not extend to the level of the subchondral bone persist for long periods with few or no histologic changes. Clusters or clones of chondrocytes (evidence of local chondrocyte replication in response to injury) may be present, particularly along the margins of the defect, but are ineffective in filling it. Progression of the lesion, with matrix degeneration and eventual loss of the remaining articular cartilage, may occur over time, particularly if thickened (sclerotic) subchondral bone is present subjacent to the defect. In contrast, if a cartilaginous defect extends into subchondral bone (cartilage ulceration), allowing mesenchymal cells in the bone marrow access to the defect, it is quickly filled with vascular fibrous tissue that often undergoes metaplasia to fibrocartilage but rarely, if ever, to hyaline cartilage. Formation

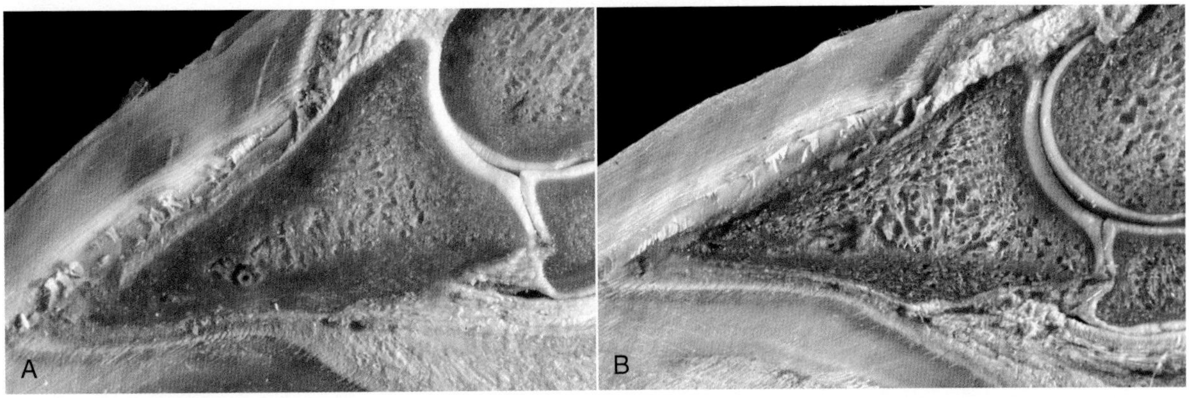

Figure 16-22 **Bone, Third Phalanx, Rear Legs, Foal.** The left leg was in a cast for 2 months to repair an avulsion of gluteal muscles from their insertions. **A,** Normal right third phalanx. **B,** Left third phalanx. There is pronounced disuse osteopenia (atrophy) compared with the right third phalanx shown in **A.** The increase in resorption and decrease in formation associated with disuse has resulted in marked porosity of the cortical and subchondral bone. The cortex now has the appearance of trabecular bone (trabeculation of the cortex). (Courtesy Dr. S.E. Weisbrode, College of Veterinary Medicine, The Ohio State University.)

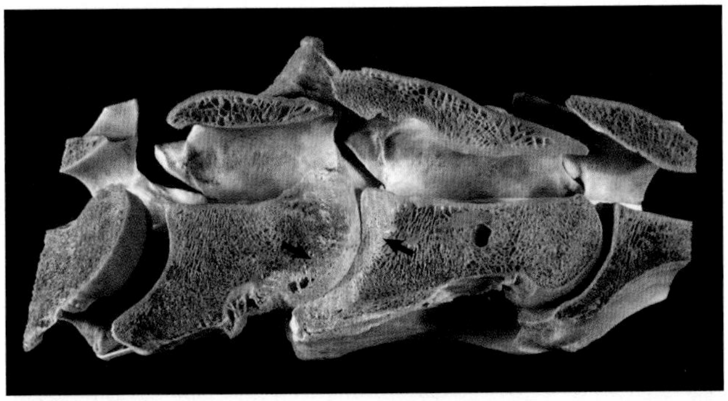

Figure 16-23 **Osteosclerosis, Intervertebral Disk Disease, Bone, Vertebrae, Horse.** Osteosclerosis (increased bone per unit of area) is evident in the two vertebrae (C6-C7, cervical) in the center of the vertebral column image. The cancellous bone of the medullary cavities has been obliterated by newly formed compact bone *(arrows)*. The osteosclerosis is in response to increased mechanical stress in the bodies of the vertebrae as a result of degeneration and loss of the intervertebral disks between these vertebrae. Macerated specimen. (Courtesy Dr. C.S. Carlson, Dr. E.J. Olson, and Dr. M.C. Speltz, College of Veterinary Medicine, University of Minnesota.)

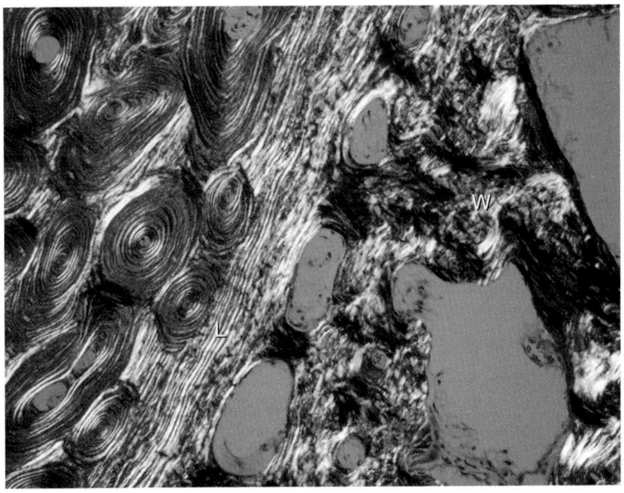

Figure 16-24 **Cancellous and Woven Bone, Dog, Hypertrophic Osteopathy, Polarized Microscopy.** Preexisting lamellar bone *(L)* and newly formed periosteal woven bone *(W)*. The woven bone exhibits a disorganized orientation of collagen fibers compared with the adjacent lamellar bone, in which the collagen fibers are arranged in parallel layers. H&E stain; polarized light micrograph. (Courtesy Dr. C.S. Carlson and Dr. E.J. Olson, College of Veterinary Medicine, University of Minnesota.)

of fibrocartilage can be hastened in full-thickness cartilaginous defects by exercise or prolonged passive motion. Because articular cartilage is aneural and avascular, injury to articular cartilage is not painful unless the synovium or subchondral bone is involved. Although it does not participate directly in the inflammatory response, articular cartilage is very much affected by inflammation in the synovium, subchondral bone, or subarticular growth (vascularized) cartilage of the epiphysis in young animals. Given that alternating compression and release of normal weight bearing facilitates the diffusion of fluid with nutrients into the articular cartilage and fluid with metabolic waste products out of articular cartilage, it follows that constant compression or lack of weight bearing leads to atrophy (thinning) of articular cartilage.

Sterile injury to cartilage can be a consequence of trauma, joint instability, or lubrication failure because of changes in synovial fluid, synovial membrane, or incongruity in joint surfaces. Destruction of articular cartilage in response to sterile injury and infectious inflammation is mediated by a combination of enzymatic digestion of matrix and failure of matrix production when chondrocytes become degenerate or necrotic. These changes can be initiated by damage to the cartilage directly or may occur indirectly, secondary to lesions in the synovium.

Matrix metalloproteinases are enzymes capable of matrix digestion; they are normal constituents of the matrix, but they are present in an inactive form. Matrix metalloproteinases can be broadly categorized as gelatinases, collagenases, and stromelysins. Collagenases are most capable of digestion of collagen fibers; gelatinases digest type I collagen and basement membrane collagens but are less effective against type II collagen of cartilage. Stromelysins destroy noncollagenous proteins. Matrix metalloproteinases can be activated by products of degenerating or reactive chondrocytes and inflammatory cells. In addition, tissue inhibitors of metalloproteinases (TIMPs) are present in the matrix, acting as a control on the destructive effects of activated metalloproteinases. As mentioned previously, proteases capable of degrading aggrecans are called aggrecanases and are members of the ADAM protein family. The loss of proteoglycans from cartilage alters the hydraulic permeability of the cartilage, thereby interfering with joint lubrication and leading to further mechanically induced injury to the cartilage. The loss of proteoglycans, with subsequent inadequate lubrication of the articular surface, leads to disruption of collagen fibers on the surface of articular cartilage. Grossly, the surfaces of affected areas of cartilage are yellow-brown and have a dull, slightly roughened appearance. As more proteoglycans are lost, the collagen fibers condense and fray (fibrillation) with multiple clefts and/or fissures forming along the vertical axis of the arcades of collagen fibers (Figs. 16-25 and 16-26). The vertical axis of the collagen fibers in these arcades is perpendicular to the plane of movement of the joint. Fibrillation is accompanied by loss of surface cartilage (erosion) and eventual thinning of the articular cartilage. Necrosis of chondrocytes results in hypocellularity of the remaining cartilage. In response to the fibrillation, erosion, and necrosis of chondrocytes, remaining chondrocytes can undergo regenerative hyperplasia (cluster or clone formation), but the ability of chondrocytes in the adult to repair the damaged tissue is ineffective. Loss of articular cartilage can become complete (ulceration), resulting in exposure of subchondral bone, which typically is eburnated (thickened/sclerotic; from the Latin word for ivory) and is characterized grossly by a polished appearance due to direct bone-on-bone contact (Fig. 16-27).

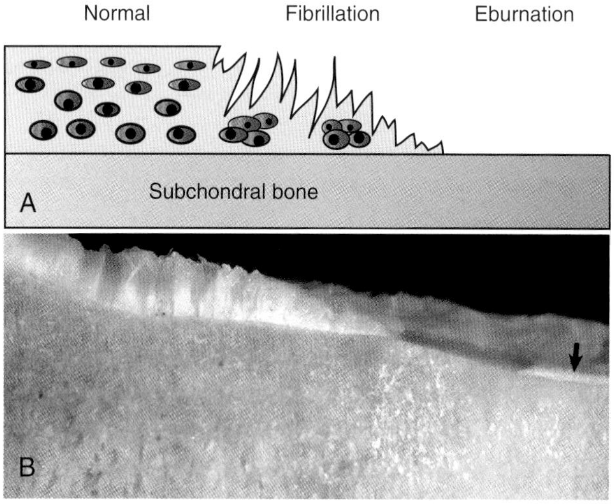

Figure 16-25 Fibrillation. A, Schematic diagram showing the structural changes that characterize fibrillation and loss of articular cartilage as well as eburnation of subchondral bone. In the area of eburnation, the cartilage is missing, and the exposed subchondral bone has increased density. **B,** Fibrillation and ulceration of articular cartilage, degenerative joint disease, proximal tibia, sagittal section, bull. To the left, the cartilage is frayed (fibrillation), and its surface has the appearance of a shag rug. To the right of the fibrillated region is an ulcer (full-thickness loss of articular cartilage). The cartilage to the right of the ulcer is very thin, indicating erosion *(arrow)*. (**B** courtesy Dr. S.E. Weisbrode, College of Veterinary Medicine, The Ohio State University.)

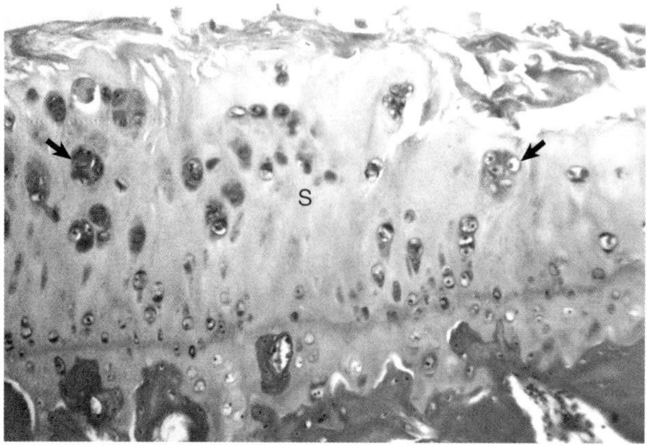

Figure 16-26 Degenerative Joint Disease, Hip Dysplasia, Femoral Head, Articular Cartilage, Dog. The superficial cartilage *(S)* is fibrillated, hypocellular, and contains clusters of chondrocytes *(arrows)* representing ineffectual attempts at repair. H&E stain. (Courtesy Dr. S.E. Weisbrode, College of Veterinary Medicine, The Ohio State University.)

Articular Capsule/Synovium/Synovial Fluid

Intraarticular prostaglandins, nitric oxide, TNF-α, IL-1, and neurotransmitters—such as substance P, among other cytokines and chemokines—are increased in degenerative and inflammatory joint disease. Prostaglandins and nitric oxide inhibit proteoglycan synthesis in synovium and chondrocytes; this reduction in proteoglycan content can lead to degeneration and loss of the cartilage (see previous discussion). IL-1 and TNF-α are cytokines secreted by activated macrophages (synovial type A cells or subintimal macrophages); they promote secretion of prostaglandins, nitric oxide, and neutral

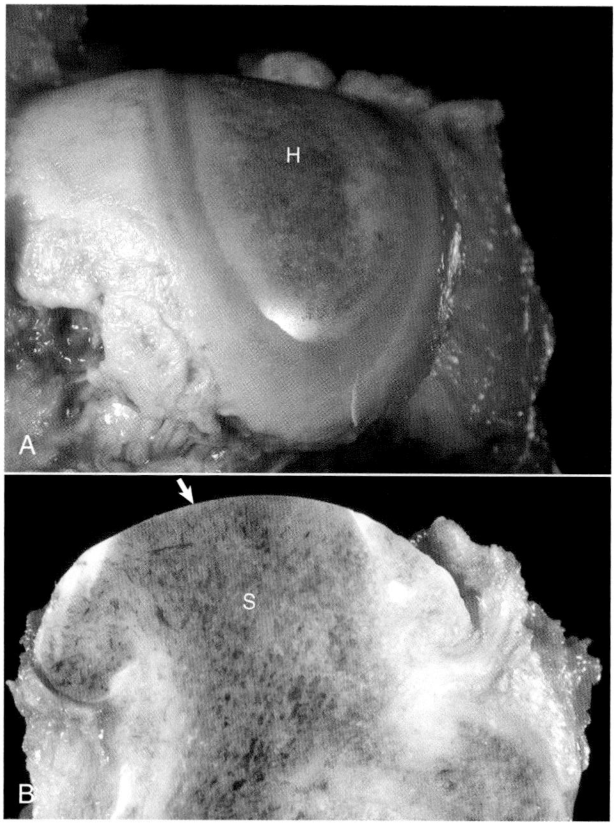

Figure 16-27 Degenerative Joint Disease, (A) Humeral Head with Eburnation, Tiger; (B) Hip Dysplasia, Femoral Head with Eburnation, Dog. A, Extensive loss of articular cartilage with thickening (sclerosis) of subchondral bone (eburnation) such that the humeral head *(H)* in the affected area has become smooth and shiny. **B,** The femoral head viewed in a sagittal plane. The head is flattened and ulcerated. The ulcerated region appears darker *(arrow)* because of congestion of blood vessels in the marrow spaces of the subchondral bone *(S)*. The zone of attachment of the round ligament to the head of the femur has been destroyed. (**A** courtesy Dr. A. Wuenschmann, College of Veterinary Medicine, University of Minnesota. **B** courtesy Dr. S.E. Weisbrode, College of Veterinary Medicine, The Ohio State University.)

proteases from synovial fibroblasts and chondrocytes. Increasing concentrations of these agents decrease matrix synthesis and increase matrix destruction. Cytokines and growth factors that have anabolic effects on cartilage include IL-6, TGF-β, and insulin-like growth factor (IGF).

Lysosomal enzymes (collagenase, cathepsins, elastase, and arylsulfatase) and neutral proteases, which are capable of degrading proteoglycans or collagen, can be derived from inflammatory cells, synovial lining cells, and chondrocytes.

The synovial membrane commonly responds to injury by villous hypertrophy and hyperplasia (Fig. 16-28), hypertrophy and hyperplasia of synoviocytes, and pannus formation (see later discussion). Villous hypertrophy/hyperplasia occurs with or without synovitis. The proportions of A (macrophages) and B (fibroblast-like) cells in the synovium also can change in various disease processes. Fragments of articular cartilage can adhere to the synovium, where they are surrounded by macrophages and giant cells. Larger pieces of detached cartilage (as in *osteochondrosis dissecans*) can float free and survive as chondral or osteochondral fragments (sometimes referred to as "joint mice") that continue to remain viable through nutrient supply from synovial fluid.

Inflammatory cell infiltrates (see the discussion on infectious and noninfectious arthritis in the section on Inflammatory Lesions) in the synovial membrane can impair fluid drainage from the joint and can cause joint fluid to lose some of its lubricating properties as the result of degradation of hyaluronic acid by the superoxide-generating systems of neutrophils.

Pannus can develop in association with chronic infectious fibrinous synovitis and with some immune-mediated diseases; the classic example is rheumatoid arthritis. Pannus is a fibrovascular and histiocytic tissue (also called an *inflammatory granulation tissue*) that arises from the synovial membrane and spreads as a membrane over articular cartilage (Figs. 16-29 and 16-30). In the pannus, tissue histiocytes and monocytes of bone marrow origin transform into macrophages and they, along with the collagenases from fibroblasts, cause lysis and destruction of the underlying cartilage (Fig. 16-31). In time, if both opposing cartilaginous surfaces are involved, the fibrous tissue can unite the surfaces, causing fibrous ankylosis (fusion of the joint). In some cases of immune-mediated arthritis, pannus is present in the subchondral bone marrow (bone marrow pannus), as well as in the synovium, and may penetrate into the overlying articular cartilage.

Sterile degenerative changes in articular cartilage are often accompanied by the formation of periarticular osteophytes (Fig. 16-32; E-Fig. 16-14) and by some degree of secondary synovial inflammation and hyperplasia. The synovitis is characterized by the presence of variable numbers of plasma cells, lymphocytes, and macrophages in the synovial subintima (beneath the layers of synoviocytes) and by hyperplasia and hypertrophy of synovial lining cells. The pathogenesis of this synovitis is not known but is suspected to result, at least partially, from the presence of degenerate cartilage debris within the joint. The pathogenesis of osteophytes also is

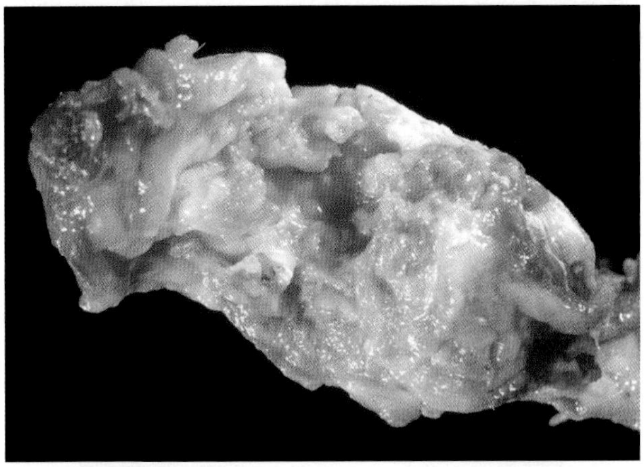

Figure 16-29 Pannus, Rheumatoid-Like Arthritis, Proximal Radius and Ulna, Dog. Fibrovascular granulation tissue (pannus) covers all articular surfaces. Also see Figs. 16-30 and 16-31. (Courtesy Dr. S.E. Weisbrode, College of Veterinary Medicine, The Ohio State University.)

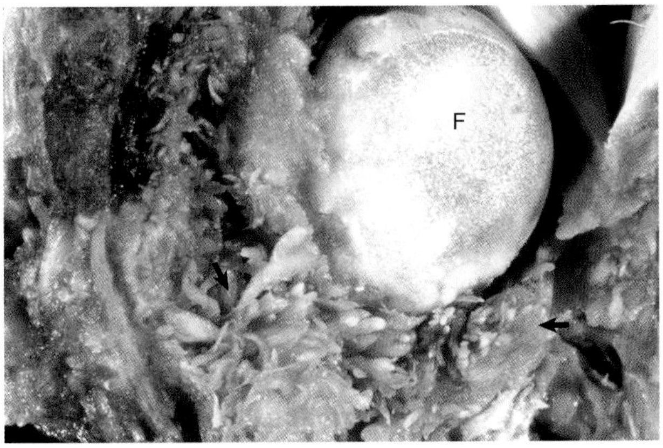

Figure 16-28 Synovial Villous Hyperplasia, Hip Dysplasia, Coxofemoral Joint, Articular Capsule, and Femoral Head, Dog. There is marked villous synovial hyperplasia *(arrows)*. The femoral head *(F)* has extensive loss of articular cartilage with thickening of subchondral bone that has become smooth and shiny. The extent of the proliferation is unusually severe for hip dysplasia. Microscopically, villous synovial hyperplasia is routinely accompanied by variable lymphoplasmacytic inflammation that is independent of the cause of the articular damage. (Courtesy Dr. S.E. Weisbrode, College of Veterinary Medicine, The Ohio State University.)

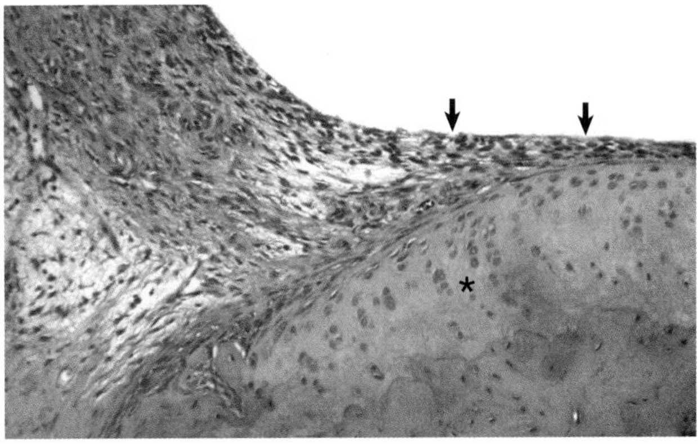

Figure 16-30 Pannus, Rheumatoid-Like Arthritis (Experimentally Induced), Distal Articular Cartilage, Tibia, Rat. The experimentally induced rheumatoid-like arthritis was produced by injecting Freund's adjuvant and *Mycobacterium butyricum* into the subcutis at the base of the tail. The pathogenesis of "adjuvant arthritis" is uncertain, other than it appears to be T lymphocyte mediated. Macrophages and other chronic (mononuclear) inflammatory cells may also be present in some forms of pannus (not shown here). Here, fibrovascular repair tissue (pannus) is seen arising from the synovium *(left)* and growing onto the surface of the articular cartilage *(arrows)*, which is relatively undamaged at this stage of the disease. H&E stain. *Asterisk*, articular cartilage. (Courtesy Dr. S.E. Weisbrode, College of Veterinary Medicine, The Ohio State University.)

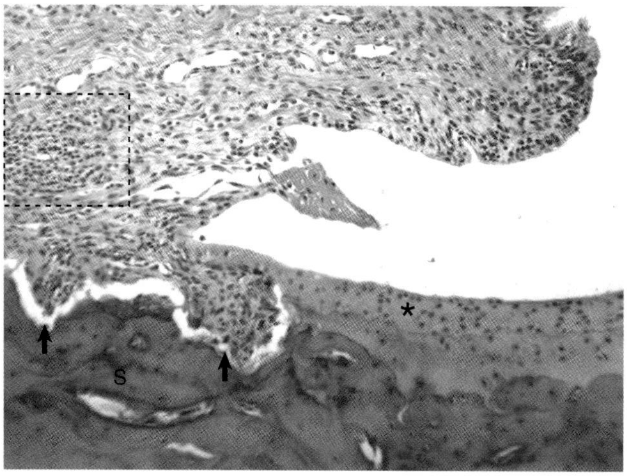

Figure 16-31 **Pannus, Rheumatoid-Like Arthritis (Experimentally Induced), Articular Cartilage, Distal Tibia, Rat.** Pannus originating from the synovium *(left)* is invading and destroying the articular cartilage *(arrows)* and subchondral bone (S). Macrophages and other chronic (mononuclear) inflammatory cells are present in the pannus (box with dashed lines). H&E stain. *Asterisk*, articular cartilage. (Courtesy Dr. S.E. Weisbrode, College of Veterinary Medicine, The Ohio State University.)

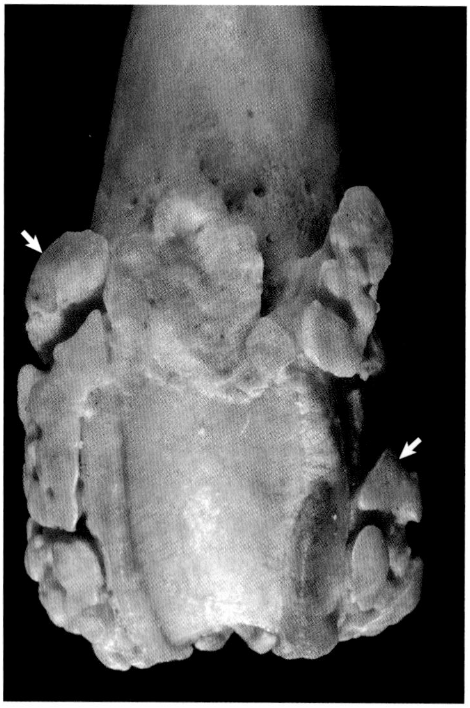

Figure 16-32 **Osteophytes, Degenerative Joint Disease, Distal Femur, Dog.** Note the large number of osteophytes *(arrows)* along the lateral and medial margins of the trochlear ridges. Macerated specimen. (Courtesy Dr. E.J. Olson, College of Veterinary Medicine, University of Minnesota.)

unclear. They can arise from mesenchymal cells with chondro-osseous potential within the synovial membrane at the junction of the synovial membrane with the perichondrium/periosteum, just peripheral to the articular cartilage, or on the surface of the bone where the articular capsule and the periosteum merge. Osteophytes do not grow continuously, but once formed, they persist as multiple periarticular spurs of bone. These spurs can be confined within the joint cavity if they arise from the perichondrium or can be protrusions from the periosteal surface of the bone if they arise from the insertion site of the joint capsule with the periosteum. Osteophytes can result from mechanical instability within the joint, causing stretching or tearing of the insertions of the articular capsule or ligaments, or they can form from stimulation by cytokines such as TGF-β that are released from reactive or degenerating mesenchymal cells within the joint.

Because of their antiinflammatory effects, glucocorticoids often are therapeutically injected into joints. Although the usual result is decreased pain and inflammation, glucocorticoid injection sometimes is followed by a rapid progression of degenerative changes within the joint that is designated "steroid arthropathy." These degenerative changes relate to the antianabolic effects of glucocorticoids on chondrocytes, in which synthesis of cartilaginous matrix is reduced, proteoglycans are depleted, repair is retarded, and the mechanical strength of cartilage is reduced.

Subchondral Bone

With the loss of matrix proteoglycans in degenerate articular cartilage, a greater component of concussive forces is transmitted to the subchondral bone. The bone responds to the increased mechanical use by decreasing resorption and increasing formation, resulting in a net increase in amount of bone per unit area (increased subchondral bone density or subchondral sclerosis). If the cartilage ulcerates to the level of the bone and the joint is still being used, the surface of the dense subchondral bone can become smooth and shiny (eburnation) (see Fig. 16-27, A). There is interest in the possible role subchondral bone might play in initiating cartilage damage in degenerative joint disease, as some studies have reported an increase in subchondral bone thickness/density before the development of articular cartilage lesions. Some believe that this dense bone is less effective in dissipating normal concussive forces and causes some of the impact to be deflected back into the articular cartilage, causing injury to the chondrocytes.

Tendons and Ligaments

The site where ligament or tendon attaches to bone is known as an *enthesis* but is also called an *insertion site* or an *osteotendinous* or *osteoligamentous junction*. Entheses are vulnerable to acute or overuse injuries in sports as the result of stress concentration at the hard-soft tissue interface. Abnormal bony proliferations located in these regions are termed *enthesophytes*.

The initial stage of repair of tendons and ligaments involves formation of scar tissue to provide continuity at the injury site. For tendons in particular, mobility must be maintained during healing to prevent or at least decrease the formation of adhesions and to increase strength. The sequence of repair includes three phases: (1) tissue inflammation, (2) cell and matrix proliferation, and (3) remodeling and maturation. The inflammatory stage usually involves the formation of a hematoma, which activates the release of chemotactic factors, including TGF-β, IGF-1, platelet-derived growth factor (PDGF), and basic fibroblast growth factor (bFGF). Inflammatory cells are attracted from the surrounding tissues to engulf and resorb the clot, cellular debris, and foreign material. Fibroblasts are recruited to the site to begin to synthesize components of the extracellular matrix, and angiogenic factors that are released during this phase initiate the formation of a vascular network. During the cell proliferation phase, recruitment and proliferation of fibroblasts continues because these cells are responsible for the synthesis of collagens, proteoglycans, and other extracellular matrix components, which initially are arranged randomly. At this point in the repair process, the extracellular matrix is composed largely of type III collagen. At the end of the proliferative stage, the repair tissue is highly cellular and contains relatively large amounts of water and an abundance of extracellular matrix components. The remodeling stage begins 6 to 8 weeks after injury and is characterized by a decrease in cellularity, reduced matrix synthesis, a decrease in type III collagen, and an increase in type I collagen synthesis. The type I collagen fibers are organized longitudinally along the tendon axis and are responsible for the mechanical strength of the regenerating tissue. Despite multiple ongoing phases of remodeling, the repair tissue never achieves the characteristics of normal tendon.

Portals of Entry/Pathways of Spread

Bone

Infectious agents can enter bone directly through the periosteum and cortex or through the vasculature. Agents can gain access through the periosteum by means of trauma that may or may not break the bone or by extension from adjacent inflammation, as in periodontal tissue (e.g., periodontitis progressing to mandibular or maxillary osteomyelitis) or the middle ear (otitis media extending into the bone, resulting in osteomyelitis of the tympanic bulla). Blood vessels gain access to the marrow cavity of the diaphysis and metaphysis through the nutrient foramen. The primary blood supply of the epiphysis in young animals is the epiphyseal artery, multiple branches of which arborize into the growth plate, providing vascularization of the proliferative zone (see Figs. 16-9 and 16-11). Blood-borne bacterial infection of bone in the perinatal animal may originate from the umbilicus (e.g., omphalitis/omphalophlebitis/omphaloarteritis) or, more commonly, by the oral-pharyngeal route. In theory, hematogenous osteomyelitis can begin in any capillary bed in bone in which viable bacteria localize. In practice, it occurs most commonly in young animals and is localized typically at the zone of vascular invasion on the metaphyseal side of the growth plate (Figs. 16-33 and 16-34, *A*) or immediately subjacent to the articular-epiphyseal cartilage complex (AECC) (Fig. 16-34, *B*; E-Fig. 16-15), where capillaries in both sites make sharp bends to join medullary veins (Fig. 16-35). In these locations, bacterial localization is apparently facilitated by slow flow and turbulence of blood, a lower phagocytic capacity, and a discontinuous endothelial lining. In addition, no vascular anastomoses are located in this region; therefore thrombosis of these capillaries results in bone infarction that is a predisposing factor for bacterial localization. From this nidus, the inflammation can extend into other structures, including the overlying joint cavity for AECC lesions (see Fig. 16-34, *B*) and the epiphysis, periosteum, or joint cavity for physeal lesions (Fig. 16-36; also see Fig. 16-35).

Joints

Microbial and other agents enter the joints via hematogenous spread (Fig. 16-37). For example, neonatal bacteremia secondary to omphalitis or oral-intestinal entry commonly leads to polyarthritis. Bacteria can also reach the joint by direct inoculation, as in a puncture

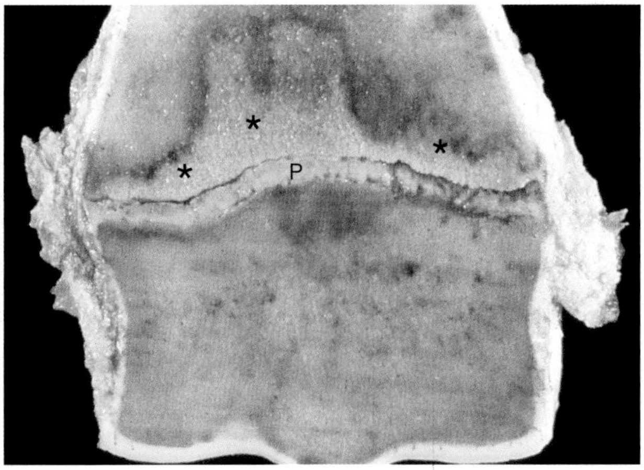

Figure 16-33 Embolic (Suppurative) Osteomyelitis and Physitis, Bone, Distal Radius, Foal. The pale region in the metaphysis *(asterisks)* extending upward to the top middle border of the illustration represents suppurative inflammation and necrosis. It is bordered by a red rim of active hyperemia. A fissure (the linear space along the metaphyseal margin of the physis [*P*]) and the porosity *(darker regions within the growth plate, right)* are the result of bone lysis (primary trabeculae) and destruction of cartilage canal blood vessels in the growth plate, respectively, caused by the infection. (Courtesy Dr. S.E. Weisbrode, College of Veterinary Medicine, The Ohio State University.)

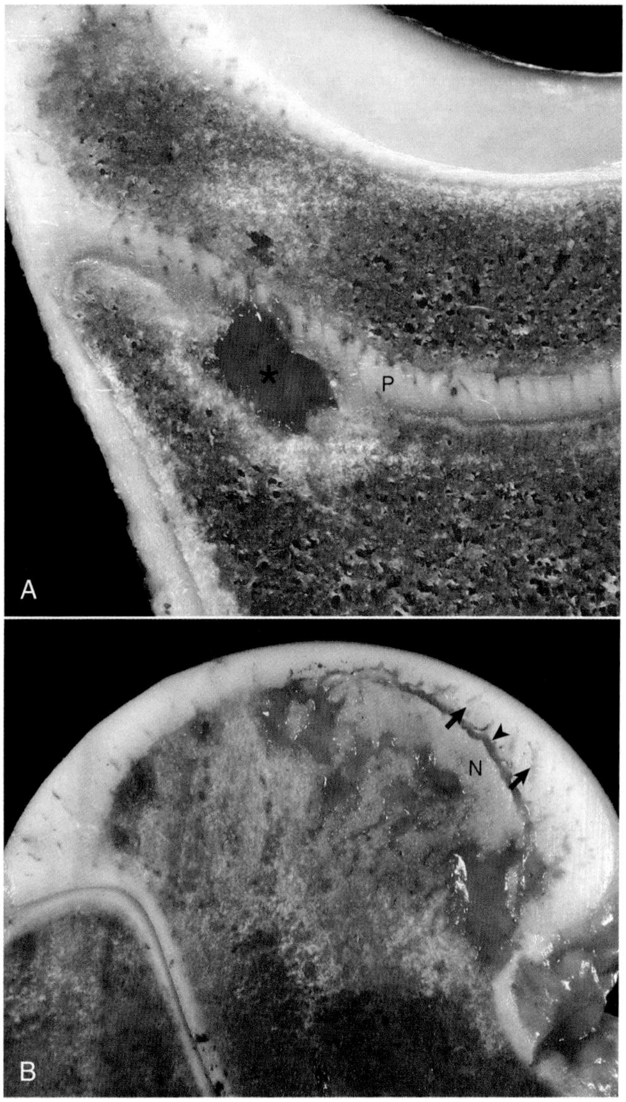

Figure 16-34 Embolic (Suppurative) Osteomyelitis, Bone, Horse, (A) Distal Tibial Physis, (B) Talus. A, Localized area of infection and bone lysis *(asterisk)* within physis and proximal metaphysis. *P,* Physis. **B,** Suppurative osteomyelitis has extended from its site of origin in the cancellous bone into the articular-epiphyseal cartilage complex (AECC) via cartilage canal vessels *(arrows)*. The affected bone contains multiple cavities, is separated by a cleft *(arrowhead)* from the overlying cartilage, and is pale and opaque (necrosis [*N*]). (Courtesy Dr. A. Wuenschmann, College of Veterinary Medicine, University of Minnesota.)

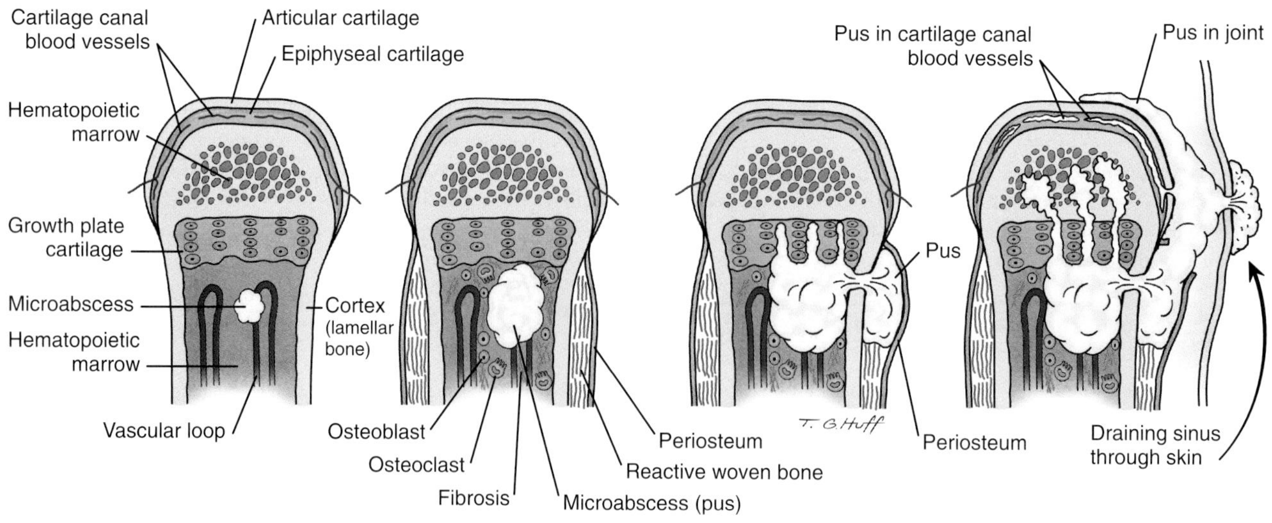

Figure 16-35 Patterns of Spread of Embolic Osteomyelitis From the Physis. Capillary loops in the metaphyseal side of the physis serve as a predilection site for septic emboli to lodge (**A**). Lysis of metaphyseal bone and growth plate cartilage secondary to inflammation may cause mechanical instability, to which the periosteum responds by producing reactive bone (**B**). Lysis of the cortex at its thinnest point (the metaphyseal cut back zone) may lead to extension of inflammation/pus into the periosteum (periostitis), perichondrium and cartilage canal vessels, or into the joint (arthritis) (**C** and **D**).

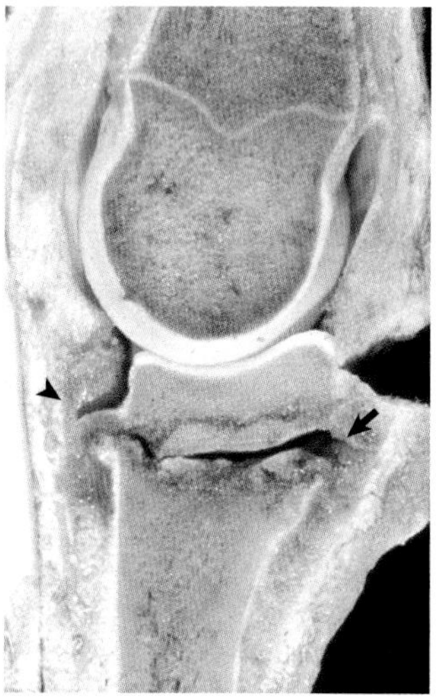

Figure 16-36 Embolic Bacterial Physitis, Osteomyelitis, Periostitis, Proximal First Phalanx and Arthritis, Metacarpal-Phalangeal Joint, Horse. Bacterial inflammation has destroyed the physis *(arrow)* and has extended into the periosteum and joint cavity *(left [arrowhead])*. (Courtesy Dr. S.E. Weisbrode, College of Veterinary Medicine, The Ohio State University.)

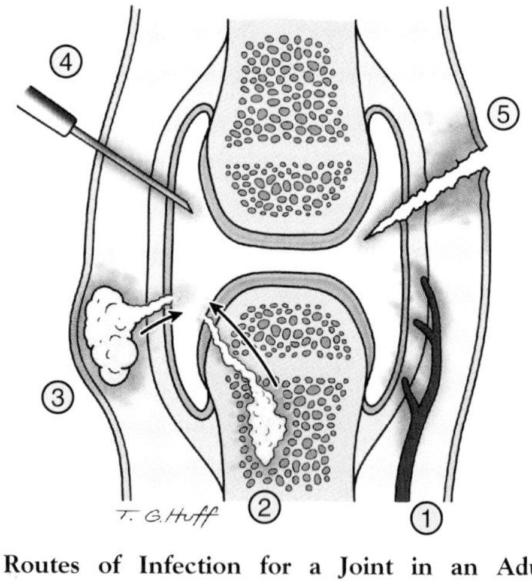

Figure 16-37 Routes of Infection for a Joint in an Adult. *1*, The hematogenous route. *2*, Extension from osteomyelitis. *3*, Spread from an adjacent soft tissue infection. *4*, Iatragenic (diagnostic or therapeutic procedures). *5*, Penetrating damage from puncture wound or incision (e.g., during surgery).

wound, by extension from adjacent periarticular soft tissues, or by extension from adjacent bone.

Tendons/Ligaments

Infection of tendons and ligaments usually requires a sharp force injury or puncture wound because of the dense connective tissue covering of the tendon (epitenon) or ligament (epiligamentum). Less commonly, there may be extension of infection from infected skin or from an adjacent joint. The sequelae of bacterial infection of tendons and ligaments most often include adhesions and accompanying loss of function.

Defense Mechanisms/Barrier Systems

Bone

The defense against infectious agents is no different in bone than in other tissues. However, the consequences of an inflammatory response can greatly affect the structure and function of bone. Many soluble inflammatory mediators can increase both bone formation and resorption, resulting in varying degrees of reactive bone formation and bone lysis. The exudate associated with some acute infections in the medullary cavity can increase the pressure in this region and cause compression of the nutrient artery, resulting in ischemic necrosis. If resorbed cortical bone is replaced by fibrous repair tissue, the bone can become unstable.

For more detailed information on inflammation, infectious agents, and immune defense mechanisms, see Chapters 3, 4, and 5, respectively.

Joints

The cellular and humoral defenses against infectious agents are no different in the joint from those in other tissues. However, because articular cartilage has such limited ability to regenerate, progression to degenerative joint disease could occur following inflammation that either destroys the ability of synovium to provide nutrients and synovial fluid to the cartilage or destroys areas of the cartilage.

For more detailed information on inflammation, infectious agents, and immune defense mechanisms, see Chapters 3, 4, and 5, respectively.

Tendons/Ligaments

The cellular and humoral defenses against infectious agents are no different in tendons and ligaments from those in other tissues.

For more detailed information on inflammation, infectious agents, and immune defense mechanisms, see Chapters 3, 4, and 5, respectively.

Disorders of Domestic Animals[2]

Bone

Abnormalities of Growth and Development

Disorders of Bone Resorption

Osteopetrosis. Osteopetrosis is a heterogeneous group of conditions that is characterized by an increase in bone density due to a failure in bone resorption by osteoclasts. Although bone mineral density is increased, the bones usually are more fragile than normal. Pathologic fractures (abnormal bone that fractures with minimal trauma; see further discussion in the section on fracture repair) are reported in animals that survive birth, although most affected animals are stillborn. Although trabecular bone accumulates in epiphyses, metaphyses, and diaphyses, there is a reduction in cortical bone quantity and quality due to a failure of bone modeling at this site, which likely is the explanation for the fractures that are seen in these animals. The disease occurs in human beings and in multiple animal species, including dogs, cats, sheep, horses (Peruvian Paso breed), cattle (Angus, Herefords, and Belgian Blue), rats, and several strains of mice. Osteopetrosis can be caused by mutations that impair the generation or the function of osteoclasts. Although most forms are inherited, some are associated with infectious agents (*in utero* bovine viral diarrhea virus [BVDV] or feline leukemia virus [FeLV] infections; avian leukosis virus), and these are termed "infectious forms of osteopetrosis." In severe forms of osteopetrosis, the insufficient bone marrow cavity is unable to support hematopoiesis, resulting in thrombocytopenia, anemia, and susceptibility to infections. Neurological complications (including blindness) may occur secondary to bony compression of the brainstem and/or cranial nerves. Other features of the disease may include brachygnathia inferior, impacted molar teeth, and deformed cranial vaults.

Because osteoclasts arise from the hematopoietic precursors, bone marrow transplantation (in which normal donor marrow components are injected) is curative for some types of osteopetrosis in human beings due to repopulation by normal osteoclast precursors.

Growth plate: There are no primary lesions in the growth plate in osteopetrosis.

Trabecular bone: Although osteoclasts may be numerous, these cells are unable to resorb and shape (model) the primary trabeculae (Fig. 16-38; E-Fig. 16-16). As a result, spicules of bone with central cores of calcified cartilage fill the medullary cavity. Affected bones are dense and have little or no medullary cavity.

Cortical bone: Cortical bone lesions in osteopetrosis are not reported consistently but can range from the cortex being too thin to it being inadequately compacted in animals that have plexiform (laminar) cortical bone growth (e.g., rapidly growing large animals such as sheep and cattle).

Disorders of Bone Formation

Osteogenesis Imperfecta. Osteogenesis imperfecta (OI) is a heterogeneous group of heritable connective tissue disorders that is characterized clinically in its most severe form by bone fractures (due to osteopenia; bone density that is lower than normal peak density), joint laxity (defective composition of tendons), dental abnormalities including fractured teeth (defective dentin), and blue sclerae (due to reduced thickness of this tissue). It is the most common heritable connective tissue disorder in human beings and has been described in the veterinary literature in multiple species, including calves, lambs, kittens, puppies, and mice. Many cases of OI (estimated 90% of cases in human and veterinary medicine) are associated with mutations in COL1A1 or COL1A2, which are genes that encode the pro-α_1 or pro-α_2 chains of type 1 procollagen. For example, the 1A1 mutation has been described in golden retrievers and the 1A2 mutation has been described in beagles. Genes coding for enzymes responsible for posttranslational modification of collagen are mutated less commonly. Mild forms of the disease, caused by inactivation of an allele of one of the genes, result in reduced amounts of normal collagen. Conversely, mutations causing substitutions in critical amino acids necessary for collagen helix formation and cross-linking can result in production of normal amounts of structurally inferior collagen. Interestingly, the clinical manifestations of these mutations are usually limited to the bone, teeth, and eyes, even though type I collagen is also the major structural collagen in skin. Exceptions include some forms of Ehlers-Danlos syndrome that are associated with COL1A1 mutations and have skin changes. A mutation in the SERPINH1 gene has been reported in OI in dachshund dogs. SERPINH1, also known as heat shock protein 47 (Hsp47), is an endoplasmic reticulum resident procollagen–specific molecular chaperone that is essential for the proper assembly of the triple helical procollagen molecules, which eventually are transported across the Golgi apparatus to the extracellular space.

Growth plate: Growth plates are not affected in osteogenesis imperfecta (primary collagen of hyaline cartilage is type II collagen).

Trabecular bone: In severe cases, there is greatly reduced trabecular bone without evidence of marked osteoclasis or proliferation of fibrous tissue, as would be expected in severe cases of fibrous osteodystrophy (see later discussion). Osteoblasts may appear normal or small. In some cases, the amount of bone and its microscopic appearance are normal, but there is evidence of fractures. These fractures may occur *in utero* and are recognized at birth by callus formation. Bone fragility in cases in which bone morphology and mass are normal is likely to be caused by errors in helix formation or cross-linking of tropocollagen molecules. Affected individuals may become osteopenic with age, possibly as a result of decreased mechanical use because of bone pain from fractures.

Cortical bone: There is a delay in the compaction of cortical bone. During normal development, species-dependent spaces of

[2]Examples of known or suspected genetic disorders are listed in E-Box 1-1.

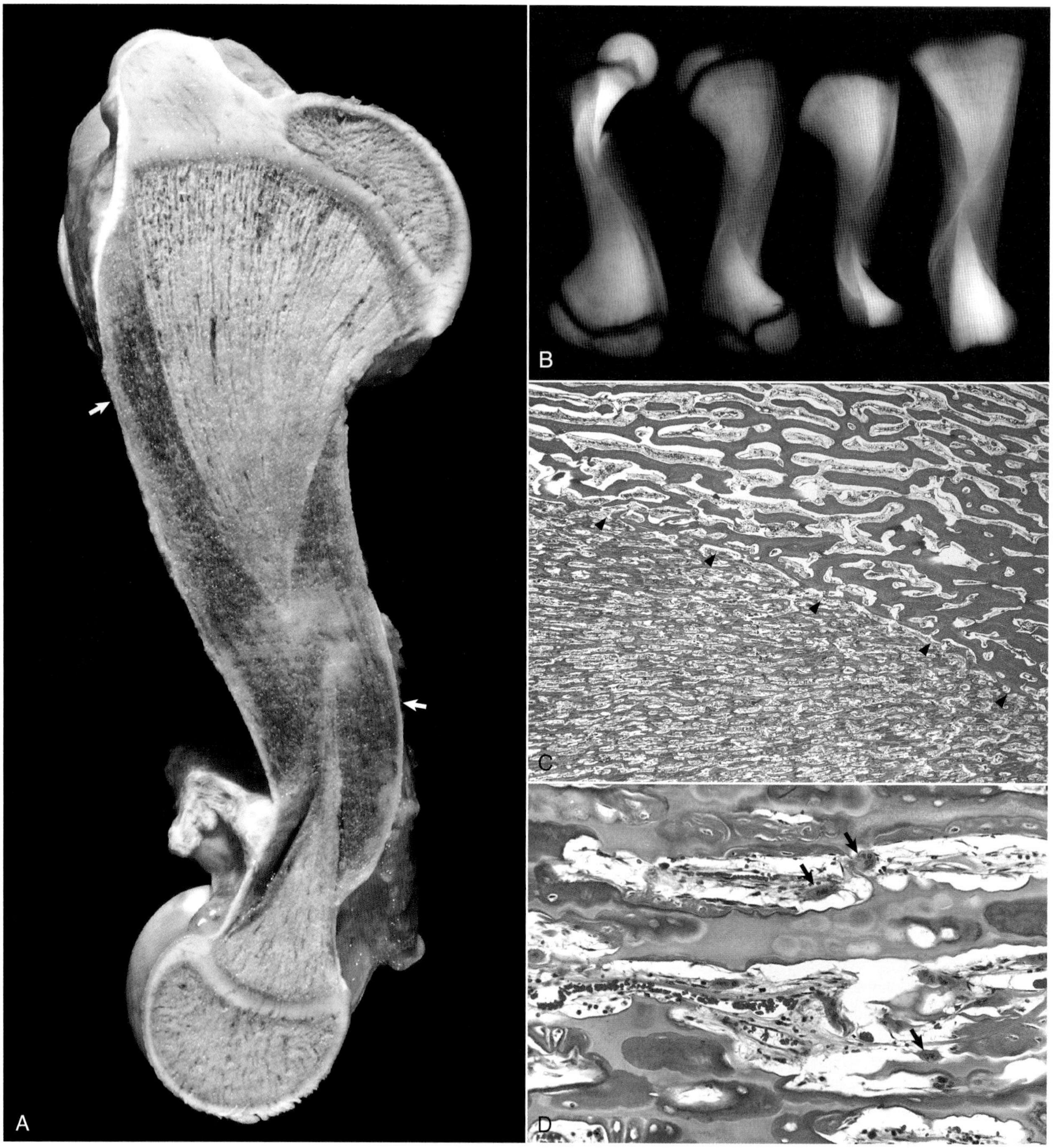

Figure 16-38 **Osteopetrosis, Bone, Foal (Peruvian Paso). A,** Longitudinal section of humerus. The primary trabeculae are retained and fill the entire medullary cavity forming a triangular shape. Although the overall amount of bone is increased, the cortices are thin *(arrows)*. **B,** Radiographs of multiple long bones exhibiting the triangular-shaped radiodensities within the metaphyses and diaphysis as demonstrated grossly in **A**. **C,** Histological section showing the transition *(arrowheads)* from trabeculated cortical bone *(upper half of image)* to retained small bony trabeculae containing numerous cartilaginous cores *(lower half of image)*. H&E stain. **D,** Osteoclasts *(arrows)* increased in number, but ineffective in resorbing retained bone. The pale basophilic areas of matrix represent retained cartilaginous cores. H&E stain. (Courtesy Dr. C.S. Carlson, Dr. E.J. Olson, and Dr. N.A. Robinson, College of Veterinary Medicine, University of Minnesota.)

varying size and contour remain between trabeculae of woven bone in the developing cortex. The filling of these spaces by bone to solidify the cortex is called *compaction*. The cortices in osteogenesis imperfecta may be composed of woven bone containing large vascular spaces that remain empty. If the animal survives, these vascular spaces may eventually fill in with bone to form compact cortical bone.

Teeth: Teeth may be structurally normal other than the presence of fractures or may be pink because of visibility of the dental pulp through the thin crown. Dental fractures also may be present. Histologically, the dentin tubules are short, tortuous, and sometimes absent. The disorganization of the dentin is a qualitative change that allows confirmation of the diagnosis without requiring an age-matched control animal.

Disorders of Bone Modeling

Congenital Cortical Hyperostosis. See Disorders of Pigs.

Craniomandibular Osteopathy. See Disorders of Dogs.

Disorders of Endochondral Ossification

Chondrodysplasias. Chondrodysplasias are hereditary disorders of bone growth that occur as a result of primary lesions in growth cartilage. Growth cartilage is present in the physis (responsible for longitudinal bone growth) and the epiphyseal cartilage of the articular-epiphyseal cartilage complex (AECC; growth cartilage at the ends of growing long bones; responsible for development of epiphysis), both of which are replaced by bone in the adult individual. Chondrodysplasias can result in disproportionate dwarfism. Affected animals usually are short-legged with normal-sized heads because the bones of the calvarium (but not the maxilla and mandible) arise from intramembranous, rather than by endochondral, ossification. Primordial dwarfism, in which the limbs are proportional to body length, is not classified as a chondrodysplasia and may occur secondary to underlying endocrine disease (pituitary dwarfism) or malnutrition but also may be genetically determined (e.g., by selective pressure to reduce the size of popular dog breeds). Both types of dwarfism are represented by distinct breeds. For example, dachshund, Pekingese, and basset hounds are examples of chondrodysplastic dwarfs, and miniature poodles, miniature schnauzers, and miniature pinschers are examples of primordial dwarfs.

The mechanisms of chondrodysplasias in animals are becoming better understood through genetic studies and often involve inherited errors in genes that control chondrogenesis. In human beings, the most common dwarfism is called *achondroplasia* (a misnomer because growth cartilage is present). The condition is inherited as an autosomal dominant trait caused by a single point mutation in the fibroblast growth factor receptor 3 (FGFR3) gene, which is a negative regulator of bone growth. This mutation results in constant activation of this receptor causing downregulation of chondrocyte proliferation. Conversely, spider lamb chondrodysplasia, which occurs in Suffolk and Hampshire sheep, is the result of a single base change in the tyrosine kinase II domain of FGFR3, which removes the FGFR3-induced inhibition of chondrocyte proliferation and results in elongation of the limbs and the presence of multiple secondary centers of ossification in the epiphyses (Fig. 16-39). This unusual type of chondrodysplasia also has been reported in mice. Recently, the genetic mutation for the chondrodysplasia typifying the commonly recognized chondrodysplastic canine breeds, including dachshunds, Pekingese, and basset hounds, has been identified as a conserved fibroblast growth factor 4 (FGF4) retrogene on canine chromosome 18 that likely arose before the division of early dogs into modern breeds. Atypical expression of the FGF4 transcript in the chondrocytes may cause inappropriate activation of one or more of the FGF receptors, such as FGFR3.

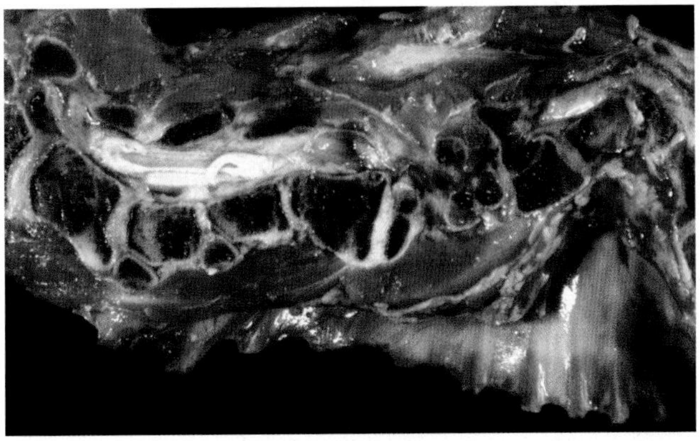

Figure 16-39 Spider Lamb Chondrodysplasia, Thoracic Spine, Longitudinal Section, Suffolk Lamb. The vertebral column has multiple, disorganized ossification centers resulting in variation of the size, shape, and orientation of the vertebrae. (Courtesy Dr. C.S. Carlson, College of Veterinary Medicine, University of Minnesota.)

Skeletal dysplasias have also been reported in animals with inherited lysosomal storage diseases such as mucopolysaccharidosis and gangliosidosis. In these individuals, chondrocytes may be vaculated due to cytoplasmic retention of glycosaminoglycans and lipid. It is likely that chondrocyte function is altered, adversely affecting the process of endochondral ossification, as epiphyseal cartilage and cartilage canals in the AECC are reported to be retained in at least one feline model of gangliosidosis and the shape of the epiphyses in these animals is markedly altered.

Growth plate: Growth plate widths can be normal or reduced depending on the specific disease. Likewise, chondrocytes can be arranged in columns or markedly disorganized. The cartilage matrix also may have a normal appearance or may be rarefied (less compact or dense, characterized by reduced staining intensity).

Trabecular bone: Trabeculae in the primary and secondary spongiosa may be thickened and irregular and may exhibit lateral bridging between trabeculae. Cartilage cores may be larger than normal and may be retained in the secondary spongiosa. These changes may vary greatly, depending on the type of chondrodysplasia.

Cortical bone: Lesions in cortical bone are variable and are reflected primarily by grossly apparent abnormalities in shape or size. Histologically, this tissue usually has a normal appearance.

Osteochondrosis Latens and Manifesta. The osteochondroses consist of a heterogeneous group of lesions involving the growth cartilage of young animals and are characterized by focal or multifocal failure (or delay) of endochondral ossification. The sites where these lesions occur are the metaphyseal growth plate and the epiphyseal cartilage of the articular-epiphyseal cartilage complex (AECC). The lesions are common, often occur with bilateral symmetry, and represent an important orthopedic entity that has a number of different clinical manifestations in pigs, dogs, horses, cattle, and poultry. The hallmark of the uncomplicated gross lesions of osteochondrosis is focal retention of growth cartilage because of its failure to become calcified and replaced by bone (a failure of endochondral ossification). In the growth plate, this is the result of an accumulation of viable hypertrophic chondrocytes, whereas in the AECC it results from an area of necrosis of epiphyseal cartilage.

The etiology of osteochondrosis appears to be multifactorial, with genetics, rapid growth rate, vascular factors, and trauma all being implicated. Trauma is the most widely proposed etiology in both human beings and animals; however, its most likely role is as a final insult to compromised epiphyseal cartilage rather than as an initiating factor in the development of early lesions. Rapid growth and nutritional factors also are cited. Although osteochondrosis occurs during the period of rapid growth and is most common in species that grow rapidly, most experimental work has failed to document rapid growth as a cause of the disease. In addition, little evidence is available to indicate that the lesions of osteochondrosis result from a specific nutritional deficiency. Copper deficiency, perhaps induced by excess dietary zinc, produces lysis of the AECC and formation of thin flaps of cartilage in thoroughbred suckling foals; however, the distribution of these lesions and their extent and severity distinguish them from the multifocal failure of endochondral ossification that is the hallmark of osteochondrosis.

Experimental work in pigs and horses has demonstrated that a defect (unknown cause) in vascular supply to growth cartilage, resulting in localized areas of ischemic necrosis, is important in the initiation of subclinical lesions. Although articular cartilage is avascular throughout life, subarticular epiphyseal cartilage of the AECC and growth plate cartilage both are highly vascularized tissues and depend on a vascular supply for viability (Fig. 16-40; E-Fig. 16-17). The blood vessels supplying growth cartilage run in channels that are termed *cartilage canals*. Both growth plate and epiphyseal (growth) cartilage are temporary, by definition. As endochondral ossification proceeds during growth, the epiphyseal cartilage gradually becomes reduced in volume and requires the nutritional support of fewer vascular channels, until it becomes entirely avascular and eventually is completely replaced by bone. It is during the time frame in which the epiphyseal cartilage is supplied by blood vessels that subclinical lesions of osteochondrosis occur. This time frame varies, based on site, age, and species, which likely explains, along with biomechanical factors, why different species have different predilection sites for the development of osteochondrosis. Detailed studies in pigs and horses have revealed that subclinical lesions occur within the first few weeks of life in some predilection sites. The finding of extensive areas of necrosis of epiphyseal cartilage in 2-week-old foals suggests that the underlying lesion may, in some cases, even occur *in utero* or soon after birth. Although the nature of the insult to the vessel(s) is unclear, the site of the injury appears to be localized to the chondro-osseous junction, and the timing of its occurrence corresponds with the formation of vascular anastomoses between vessels in epiphyseal cartilage and vessels in the subchondral bone as the ossification front reaches the vessels that are present in the epiphyseal cartilage. The result is a well-demarcated area of necrosis of epiphyseal cartilage that is centered on necrotic blood vessels, visible only microscopically, and termed *osteochondrosis latens* (Fig. 16-41). When the ossification front of the secondary center of ossification reaches the area of necrosis, failure of endochondral ossification occurs, resulting in an area of retained necrotic epiphyseal cartilage that is visible grossly and radiographically. The lesion at this stage is termed *osteochondrosis manifesta* (Fig. 16-42; E-Fig. 16-18). This lesion is highly vulnerable to traumatic clefting through the area of necrosis and extending into the overlying articular cartilage, at which point it is termed *osteochondrosis dissecans* (Fig. 16-43; E-Fig. 16-19). It may also result from normal physiologic pressure. Once clefting through the articular cartilage occurs and subchondral bone is exposed, the lesion is highly painful and results in clinical signs of lameness. In the majority of cases, however, cleft formation does not occur, and the subclinical lesions heal. In these cases, the necrotic epiphyseal cartilage becomes surrounded by the advancing ossification front, as adjacent viable epiphyseal cartilage undergoes endochondral ossification. Over

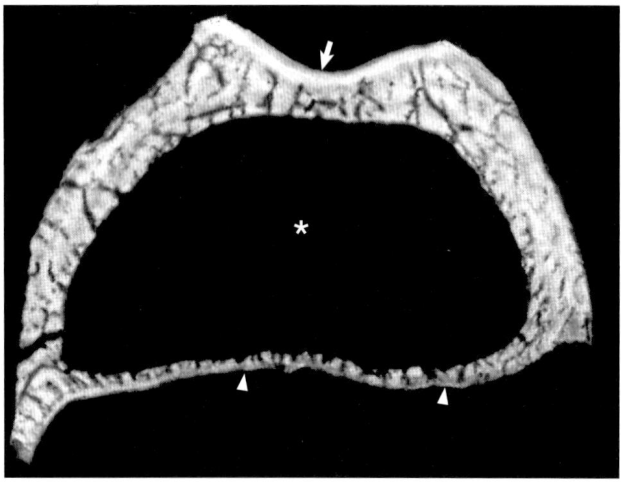

Figure 16-40 **MRI Image Using Susceptibility Weighted Imaging, Distal Femur, Coronal Section, Immature Pig.** Avascular articular cartilage of femoral trochlea *(arrow)*; cartilage canal vessels indicated by black lines; secondary center of ossification *(asterisk)*; physis *(arrowheads)*. (Courtesy Dr. C.S. Carlson and Dr. F. Tóth, College of Veterinary Medicine, University of Minnesota.)

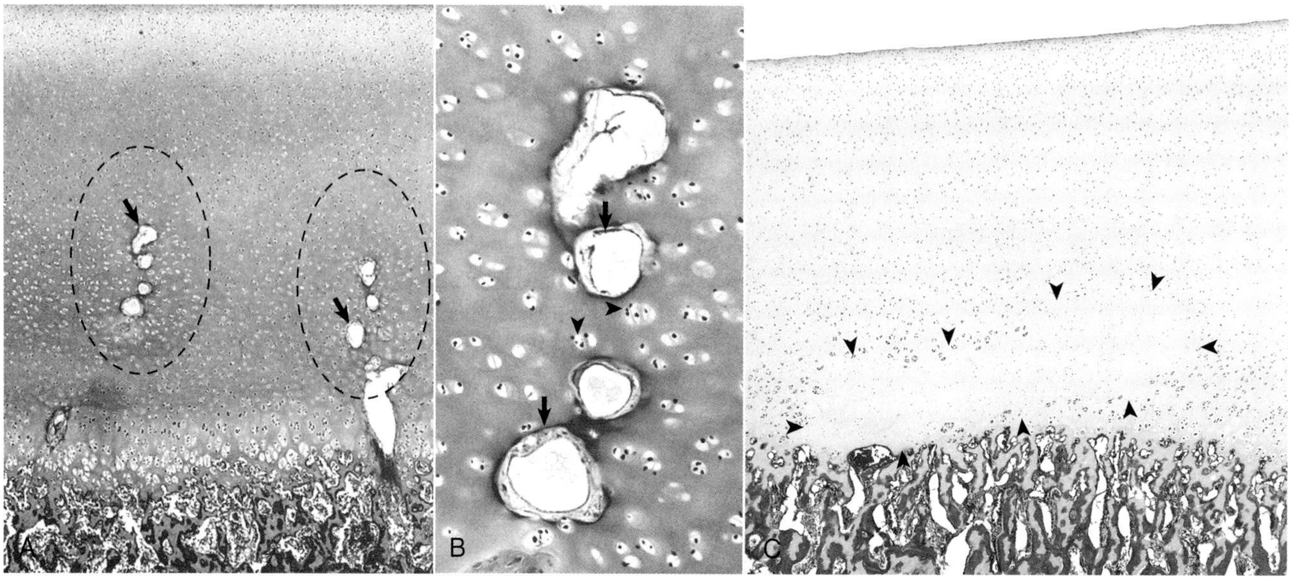

Figure 16-41 **Osteochondrosis Latens, Lateral Femoral Condyle, 12-Week-Old Pig. A,** Locally extensive area of chondronecrosis *(within ellipses)* within the epiphyseal cartilage of the articular-epiphyseal cartilage complex (AECC), centered on necrotic cartilage canal blood vessels *(arrows)*. Neither the overlying articular cartilage nor the subjacent subchondral bone is involved at this stage of the disease. H&E stain. **B,** Higher magnification of **A** showing necrotic cartilage canal blood vessels *(arrows)* and necrotic chondrocytes *(arrowheads)*. **C,** Low-magnification image of osteochondrosis latens lesion *(arrowheads)* confined to epiphyseal cartilage and composed of necrotic cartilage. H&E stain. (Courtesy Dr. C.S. Carlson, College of Veterinary Medicine, University of Minnesota.)

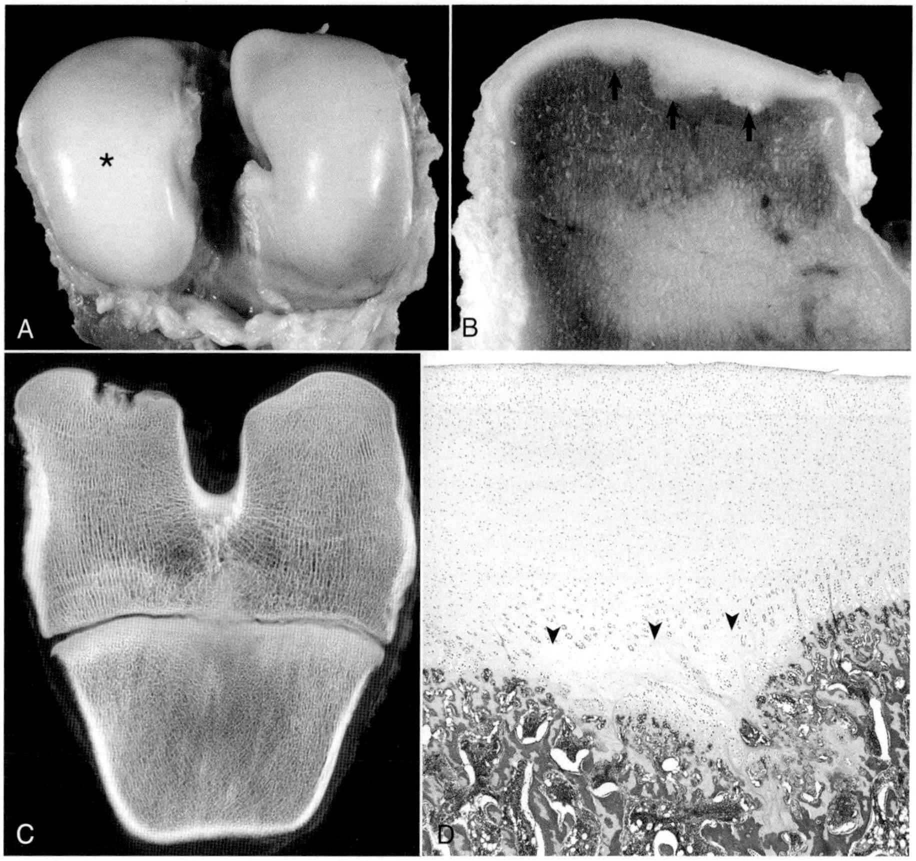

Figure 16-42 **Osteochondrosis Manifesta, Bone, Distal Femur, Immature Pig. A,** Femoral condyles (with medial femoral condyle on the left *[asterisk]*) showing no articular cartilage surface abnormalities. **B,** Coronal slab section through medial femoral condyle showing intact articular surface and areas of retained cartilage *(arrows)* typical of locally extensive delay of endochondral ossification (osteochondrosis manifesta). **C,** Faxitron radiograph of 3-mm-thick coronal slab section showing focal area of radiolucency typical of osteochondrosis manifesta lesion involving the medial femoral condyle (same animal/anatomic site as in **A** and **B**). **D,** Locally extensive area of chondronecrosis in epiphyseal cartilage resulting in delayed endochondral ossification (osteochondrosis manifesta); upper limit of lesion demarcated by *arrowheads*. H&E stain. (Courtesy Dr. C.S. Carlson and Dr. E.J. Olson, College of Veterinary Medicine, University of Minnesota.)

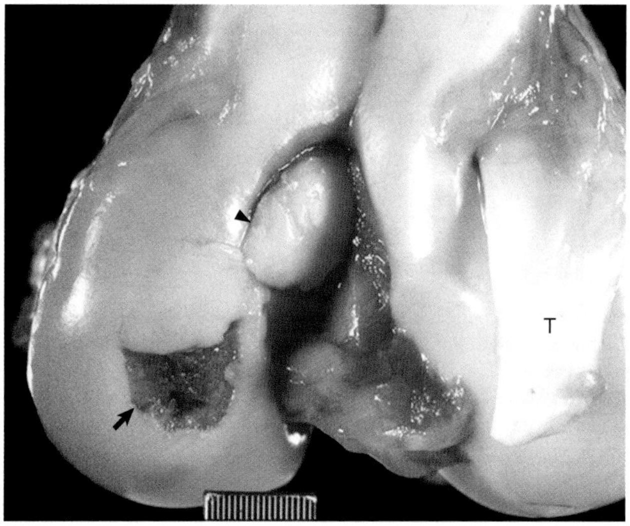

Figure 16-43 **Osteochondrosis Dissecans, Bone, Articular Cartilage, Femur, Distal End, Pig.** A chondro-osseous fragment *(arrowhead)* has detached from the underlying bone *(arrow)* of the medial femoral condyle and is displaced to the intercondylar area within the joint; long digital extensor tendon *(T)*. (Courtesy Dr. C.S. Carlson and Dr. E.J. Olson, College of Veterinary Medicine, University of Minnesota.)

time, the area of necrotic cartilage gradually diminishes in size and eventually becomes completely replaced by bone. In horses, particularly in the medial femoral condyle (weight-bearing location), evidence strongly supports the theory that some of these early lesions of osteochondrosis develop into subchondral bone cysts.

Physeal lesions of osteochondrosis also are likely to have a vascular etiology but are characterized by multifocal areas of retained, viable, hypertrophic chondrocytes. If these involve an extensive area of the growth plate, the growth plate may fracture, either partially or completely, resulting in a variety of clinical sequelae including angular limb deformities.

Growth plate and articular-epiphyseal cartilage complex (AECC): Lesions of osteochondrosis are not recognized grossly until they result in a focal failure of endochondral ossification, at which time they are composed of a well-demarcated wedge of retained cartilage involving the epiphyseal cartilage at the AECC (osteochondrosis manifesta) or physis (physeal osteochondrosis). Often, there is considerable reaction of the underlying marrow spaces, including increased numbers of osteoblasts, osteoclasts, and fibroblasts. Predilection sites for both clinical and subclinical lesions include the AECC of the distal femur (especially the medial femoral condyle) and humerus (condyles and head) of pigs; the distal femur (medial condyle and both trochlear ridges), distal tibia (cranial intermediate ridge and medial malleolus), talus (trochlear ridges), and articular processes of the cervical vertebrae of horses; the humerus (humeral head and medial humeral condyle), distal femur (both condyles), and talus (medial and lateral trochlear ridges) of dogs; the talus (medial and lateral trochlear ridges) and distal femur (both trochlear ridges) of cattle; and the proximal tibia of rapidly growing birds.

Osteochondrosis latens lesions are only recognized histologically in the AECC and occur as well-demarcated areas of necrosis of epiphyseal cartilage, usually adjacent to or surrounding one or more necrotic cartilage canal blood vessels (see Fig. 16-41). The overlying articular cartilage and subjacent subchondral bone are not affected at this stage of the disease. Osteochondrosis manifesta lesions also are composed of necrotic epiphyseal cartilage, but at this point of the disease, the ossification front has reached and partially surrounded the area of necrosis so that it is grossly visible (see Fig. 16-42). Lesions of physeal osteochondrosis, in contrast to those occurring in the AECC, are composed of columns of retained, viable, hypertrophic chondrocytes without evidence of mineralization or vascular invasion.

Trabecular bone: In lesions of osteochondrosis latens, trabecular bone is normal. Osteochondrosis manifesta lesions, however, include direct contact of the subchondral bone with an area of necrotic cartilage. Marked myelofibrosis and bony remodeling, with formation of locally extensive areas of woven bone, are nearly always present; however, inflammatory cells are rarely a feature of the lesion. A closely similar bony reaction is seen in lesions of physeal osteochondrosis. In both sites, cleft formation may occur at the junction of the retained cartilage and the underlying bone or within the necrotic cartilage (see the following section on Osteochondrosis Dissecans).

Cortical bone: Lesions in cortical bone are not expected at any stage of osteochondrosis of the AECC complex or physis.

Osteochondrosis Dissecans. *Osteochondrosis dissecans* (OCD) is the name given to osteochondrosis at the AECC that forms clefts in the necrotic cartilage with subsequent fracture of the overlying articular cartilage (Fig. 16-44; also see Fig. 16-43; E-Fig. 16-20; also see E-Fig. 16-19). The result is a cartilaginous or osteochondral flap, depending on whether bone is present within the lesion. This may change with the duration of the lesion because cartilaginous flaps that have a blood supply will ossify over time. OCD can be accompanied by pain, joint effusion, and nonspecific secondary lymphoplasmacytic synovitis. Free-floating chondral or osteochondral fragments occasionally interfere with mechanical movement of the joint. Common sites of OCD are the same as those of osteochondrosis manifesta (see the previous section). The disease is extremely common in young breeding pigs and is a significant cause of lameness in this species. Although less common in horses and dogs, it is also an important cause of lameness in these species. The articular cartilage defect in OCD has poor healing capabilities, and such joints commonly develop some degree of degenerative joint disease. Surgical removal of the flap reduces the long-term clinical consequences; however, the defect repairs by the formation of fibrocartilage, which provides suboptimal biomechanical properties to the joint surface compared with articular cartilage.

For the development of OCD, clefts must develop in the necrotic epiphyseal cartilage of the AECC, usually at the stage of osteochondrosis manifesta (see Fig. 16-42). Cleft formation can cause mechanical instability and lead to separations within cartilage or between cartilage and the underlying bone. External pressure, most commonly due to normal physiologic activity, can cause the cleft to extend through the overlying articular cartilage, resulting in the formation of a flap (see Figs. 16-43 and 16-44). At this stage of the disease, the affected animal may exhibit lameness.

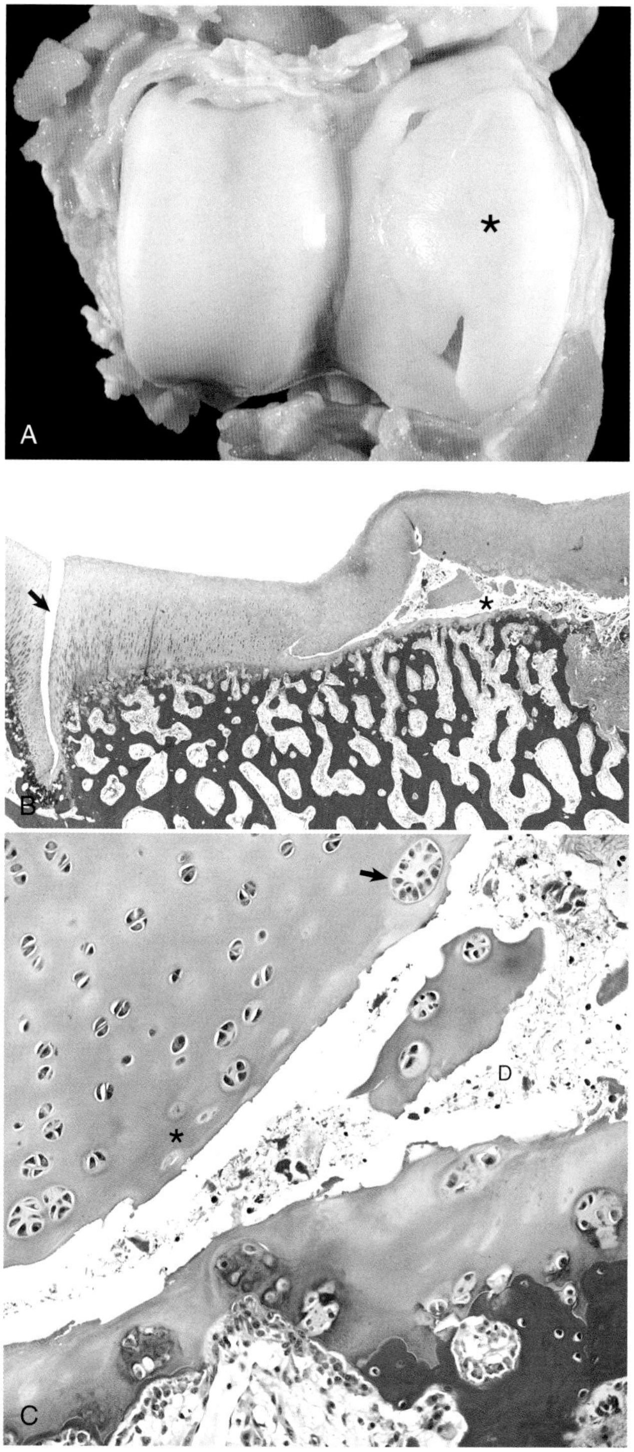

Figure 16-44 **Osteochondrosis Dissecans of the Articular-Epiphyseal Cartilage Complex (AECC), Bone, Humerus, Distal End, Immature Pig. A,** Partially detached cartilage fragment *(asterisk)* involving almost the entire trochlea (medial aspect). **B,** Partially detached cartilage flap (involving the right half of the figure) subjacent to which are cartilage fragments and bone dust *(asterisk)*; synovial fossa *(arrow)* separates medial from lateral aspect of the distal humerus. H&E stain. **C,** High-magnification image of cleft; necrotic chondrocytes *(asterisk)*; chondrocyte cluster/clone *(arrow)*; bone dust *(D)*. H&E stain. (Courtesy Dr. C.S. Carlson and Dr. E.J. Olson, College of Veterinary Medicine, University of Minnesota.)

Cartilage flap formation involving extensive areas of multiple joints can develop in horses without predisposing lesions of osteochondrosis latens or manifesta. In these cases, articular cartilage of normal thickness can be peeled from the subjacent bone because of fissuring in the deeper layers of the AECC. Such lesions have been seen in foals that have licked fences with zinc-based white paint. The pathogenesis of the lesion is thought to involve copper deficiency induced by the zinc excess (zinc blocks the absorption of copper from the gastrointestinal tract). Copper is a required cofactor for enzymes that facilitate cross-linkages between tropocollagen molecules; however, these foals do not appear to have a generalized collagen dysplasia. The extensive distribution of the articular lesions distinguishes them from OCD, which occurs multifocally in species-dependent predilection sites.

Growth plate and AECC: The growth plate is not involved in OCD. The lesion in the AECC includes a locally extensive area of fibroplasia, neovascularization, and bony remodeling at the chondro-osseous junction. Even in the most chronic lesions, variably sized areas of necrosis (usually a thin margin) of epiphyseal cartilage often can be identified at the chondro-osseous junction or along the deep surface of the articular cartilage. The articular cartilage may be morphologically normal, other than the presence of a fissure that extends from the necrotic zone of epiphyseal cartilage to the articular surface. In cases in which the cartilage fragment has been displaced, all or part of the AECC is replaced by an area of cartilage ulceration that overlies reactive and fibrotic subchondral bone.

Trabecular bone: The severity of changes in trabecular bone of the epiphysis reflects the extent of the cleft formation. Marked myelofibrosis, locally extensive osteopenia, and formation of reactive woven bone are expected at the base of the flap.

Cortical bone: Lesions in cortical bone are not expected with OCD.

Epiphysiolysis. Epiphysiolysis is the separation of the epiphysis from the metaphysis as the result of the formation of a horizontal fissure through an abnormal physis. The condition is most common in pigs and dogs, but it is also reported in calves, lambs, and foals. In market-weight pigs and in young gilts, the femoral head may be involved, whereas in sows, separation of the ischial tuberosity (site of insertion of semimembranosus, semitendinosus, and biceps femoris muscles) at its growth plate (often bilaterally) is a common cause of caudal weakness and inability to stand and often occurs at parturition. In dogs, the process of epiphysiolysis can affect the anconeal process of the ulna, resulting in a condition known as *ununited anconeal process*. This may occur as one aspect of a condition known as the *elbow dysplasia syndrome*, which includes one or more of the following: OCD of the medial humeral condyle, fragmentation of the medial coronoid process, and ununited anconeal process. Elbow incongruity (shortening of the ulna relative to the radius secondary to lesions in the distal ulnar growth plate) is recognized as the major cause for the manifestations of elbow dysplasia. Because these lesions have primarily been studied in their chronic stages, the nature of the initial lesion is unclear; however, it is strongly suspected that they occur secondary to an extensive area, or to multifocal coalescing areas, of physeal osteochondrosis.

A similar disease, known as *physeal dysplasia with slipped capital femoral epiphysis*, is described in young cats, most commonly in overweight castrated males. The growth plates in these cats are widened and appear to remain open longer than expected. Histologically, the growth plates have a disorganized appearance in which chondrocytes are present in clusters, rather than columns, and are separated by variable amounts of extracellular matrix. It has been hypothesized that this dysplastic lesion may be present in all growth plates in affected animals, but fractures occur only in sites (e.g., femoral head) where shear forces occur during weight bearing. Transphyseal fractures occurring secondary to this condition are distinguished from traumatic fractures histologically by the presence of irregular clusters of chondrocytes separated by abundant extracellular matrix on both the epiphyseal and metaphyseal sides of the physeal cleavage site versus retention of the linear arrangement of chondrocytes on both sides of the growth plate (traumatic fracture). Osteochondrosis is rarely reported in cats, and the histologic changes in affected and contralateral growth plates are more characteristic of a physeal dysplasia (a diffuse process that affects the entire physis) than of osteochondrosis (focal to multifocal physeal lesions) in this species.

Several types of underlying conditions may result in partial closure of the physis, causing an angular limb deformity in the affected limb. This condition is most common in horses, in which it usually occurs secondary to lesions of physeal osteochondrosis. Other causes include trauma and inflammation of the growth plate and/or primary trabeculae.

Growth plate: Grossly there is a horizontal fissure/fracture through the physis with complete or partial separation of the epiphysis from the metaphysis. In cats, the remaining physeal cartilage is dysplastic, as described previously (disorganized arrangement of chondrocytes with separation by variable amounts of extracellular matrix). In fissures occurring secondary to osteochondrosis, the remaining physeal cartilage on the metaphyseal side of the growth plate contains areas of delayed endochondral ossification. The chronicity of the lesions (with accompanying secondary changes) complicates their interpretation.

Trabecular bone: The response to trabecular bone in epiphysiolysis is characteristic of a reaction to trauma and fracture and includes myelofibrosis, proliferation of reactive woven bone, and the presence of variable amounts of hemorrhage and fibrin.

Cortical bone: There are no primary changes in cortical bone with this condition; any lesions that develop would be secondary to altered mechanical use.

Cervical Vertebral Myelopathy. Cervical vertebral stenotic myelopathy, sometimes called "Wobbler syndrome," is a neurologic disease of horses and dogs (usually giant breeds) that occurs secondary to static or dynamic compression of the spinal cord by abnormally developed cervical vertebrae. This compression can be constant as the result of an anatomic stenosis of the spinal/vertebral canal, termed *cervical vertebral static stenosis* (CVS), or may occur only during movement (usually flexion), which is termed *cervical vertebral instability* (CVI). CVS involves the less mobile caudal cervical vertebrae, mainly C5-C6 and C6-C7, and most commonly affects older horses (usually 1 to 4 years old). In contrast, the spinal cord lesions of CVI are centered on the more mobile cranial cervical vertebrae, primarily at C3-C4 and C4-C5, in younger horses (6 to 15 months of age). In both syndromes, anatomic localization of the lesion by neurologic examination, myelography, or computed tomography is very helpful to the pathologist. In thoroughbred and standardbred horses and in dogs, the static compression is usually the result of a grossly appreciable narrowing of the spinal canal from caudal to cranial within a single vertebral body that almost certainly occurs during development (Fig. 16-45; E-Fig. 16-21). In adult quarter horses, localized hyperplasia and fibrocartilaginous metaplasia of the ligamentum flavum (the ligament between the dorsal lamina), likely occurring secondary to chronic mechanical irritation and/or trauma, can protrude into the spinal canal causing static compression of the spinal cord and closely similar clinical signs.

The lesions associated with dynamic compression of the spinal cord are more variable and less definitive because identical lesions often are present in asymptomatic animals. In horses, the most

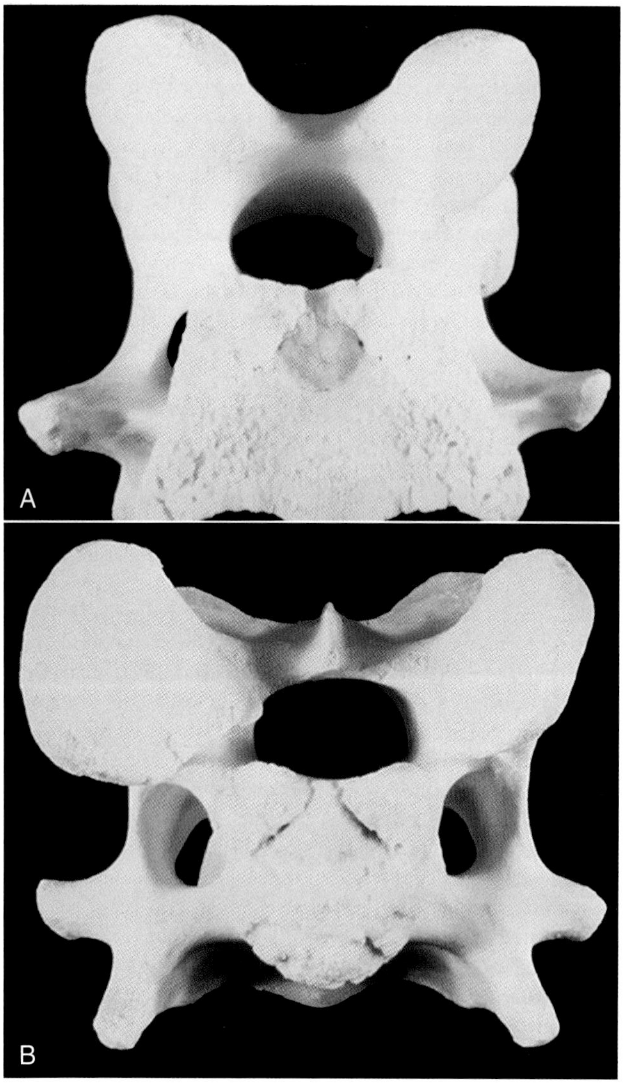

Figure 16-45 **Static Stenosis, Bone, Cervical Vertebra, Macerated Specimen, Horse. A,** Caudal aspect. **B,** Cranial aspect. Note the narrowing of the spinal canal from caudal to cranial. (Courtesy University of Minnesota Veterinary Diagnostic Laboratory Archives.)

common lesions are those of osteochondrosis (see previous discussion) of the cervical facets. Osteochondrosis can cause abnormal and asymmetrical development of the facets or abnormally large cranial vertebral epiphyses. With either lesion, the dorsal aspect of the vertebral body may compress the ventral aspect of the spinal cord during flexion, causing transient ischemia. Such compression may initially cause functional deficits without lesions in the spinal cord but also may progress to produce notable Wallerian degeneration. The frequency of osteochondrosis of the cervical vertebrae in clinically normal horses is the same as in horses with clinical signs of CVI; however, the severity is worse in the latter cases. In addition, the frequency and severity of osteochondrosis lesions in the appendicular skeleton are greater in horses with clinical signs of CVI, further supporting the hypothesis that osteochondrosis may be an important underlying cause for this condition.

Metabolic Bone Diseases

Metabolic bone diseases are systemic skeletal diseases that are generally of nutritional, endocrine, or toxic origin (Table 16-1; E-Table 16-1) and occur in both growing and adult skeletons. Metabolic bone diseases are often called *osteodystrophies*, which is a general term that implies defective bone formation. The classic metabolic osteodystrophies are osteoporosis, fibrous osteodystrophy, rickets, and osteomalacia. These terms imply specific pathologic lesions, but these lesions may occur due to multiple different causes. In addition, different osteodystrophies can coexist in the same skeleton. In fact, most nutritional deficiencies in domestic animals are multiple, relatively mild, and do not produce the "classical" lesions that occur under experimental conditions.

Osteoporosis. Osteoporosis is a disease in which bone fractures occur secondary to a reduction in bone density or mass (Fig. 16-46). The bone present, although reduced in amount, is normally mineralized. When there is reduced bone mass but no clinical disease (fractures), the term *osteopenia* is more appropriate; however, once fractures occur, the disease is called *osteoporosis*. In senile osteoporosis in human beings, in addition to decreased bone density, the turnover rate of bone is reduced, allowing microcracks (small cracks in the bone visible only microscopically) to accumulate. These microcracks, superimposed on the reduced bone mass, make bones more brittle than would be predicted from the reduced mass alone. In growing animals, osteoporosis is potentially reversible; however, in adults the loss of trabecular bone is generally considered to be permanent. Although osteoporosis affects both cortical and trabecular bone, the loss of trabecular bone occurs earlier because of its higher surface area, which creates a greater opportunity for osteoclastic bone resorption. Although the thickness and density of cortical bone generally determine bone strength, trabecular bone contributes significantly to bone strength in some locations, including the femoral neck, vertebral bodies, and distal radius in human beings, thus explaining why osteoporotic fractures occur most commonly in these locations. Causes of osteopenia include calcium deficiency, starvation, physical inactivity, hypogonadism, and chronic glucocorticoid administration. Calcium deficiency can result in hypocalcemia, which is compensated for by increased PTH output resulting in increased bone resorption. Starvation and malnutrition can result in arrested growth and osteoporosis, largely because of reduced bone formation resulting from deficiencies of protein and mineral. Reduced physical activity (disuse or immobilization osteoporosis) causes increased bone resorption and decreased bone formation. This loss of bone from disuse might be mediated through changes in piezoelectrical activity, streaming potentials, and stretch receptors that are able to detect decreased mechanical use of the skeleton. Loss of bone mass associated with long-term paralysis or immobilization is not necessarily progressive; rather, the skeleton stabilizes at a new (reduced) level. Postmenopausal osteoporosis is a common and important disease in human beings and occurs primarily due to declining concentrations of estrogens. Osteopenia associated with reduced estrogens from ovarian atrophy or ovariectomy appears to be greatest in animals with estrous cycles that extend throughout the year (e.g., rat, pig, and primate), rather than being seasonal.

Growth plate: Lesions in the growth plate are not expected in osteoporosis unless the disease is related to pituitary dysfunction or protein calorie malnutrition, in which case the growth plate would be reduced in thickness.

Trabecular bone: Trabeculae become thinner, decrease in number, and develop full-thickness perforations due to osteoclastic resorption that result in loss of trabecular continuity. With time, the normal structure of trabecular bone (anastomosing plates) is replaced by smaller, more widely spaced trabeculae that do not interconnect but are separated by marrow spaces. The loss of trabecular continuity results in reduced ability of the trabeculae to withstand stress.

Table 16-1 Metabolic Bone Disease

Disease	Characteristics	Causes
Osteoporosis	Reduced bone mass: porous, thin, and fragile bones	Protein calorie malnutrition, immobilization, dietary calcium deficiency, glucocorticoid excess, estrogen or androgen deficiency and advanced age
Osteomalacia (adult animals)	Decreased bone mineralization (accumulation of osteoid): soft bones	Vitamin D deficiency, phosphorus deficiency
Rickets (growing animals)	Decreased bone mineralization (accumulation of osteoid): soft bones; thickened hypertrophic zone of growth plate (failure of endochondral ossification)	Vitamin D deficiency, phosphorus deficiency
Fibrous osteodystrophy	Decreased bone mass and increased pliability of bone due to resorption and replacement by fibro-osseous tissue	Hyperparathyroidism 1. Primary: functional chief cell adenoma of parathyroid gland 2. Paraneoplastic: parathyroid hormone–related protein (and possibly also interleukin-1 [IL-1] and transforming growth factors α and β [TGF-α and TGF-β]) secreted from neoplasms such as adenocarcinoma of apocrine glands of anal sac 3. Secondary nutritional: from diets low in calcium and high in phosphorus 4. Secondary renal: from failure of the kidney to secrete phosphorus and reduced synthesis of 1,25-dihydroxyvitamin D

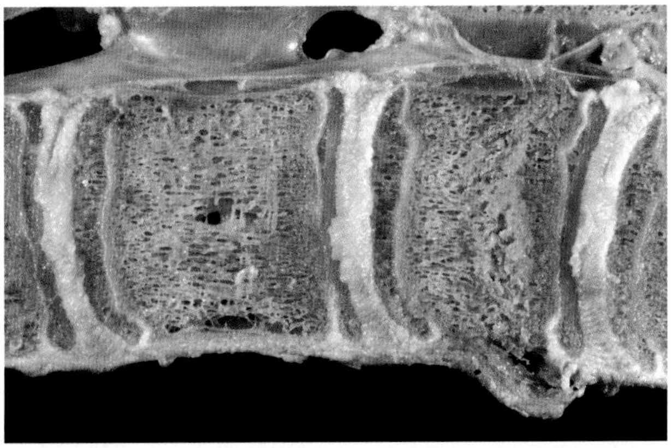

Figure 16-46 **Osteoporosis, Bone, Two Cervical Vertebrae, Sagittal Section, Horse.** Note the markedly thin cortices, particularly dorsally. The thickness of trabeculae also has been reduced, but this is difficult to appreciate grossly. The vertebra to the right has a compression fracture, causing shortening of the length of the vertebral body between the growth plates and fracture of the ventral cortex. The marrow has been flushed from the specimen in order to illustrate the bone changes. (Courtesy Dr. S.E. Weisbrode, College of Veterinary Medicine, The Ohio State University.)

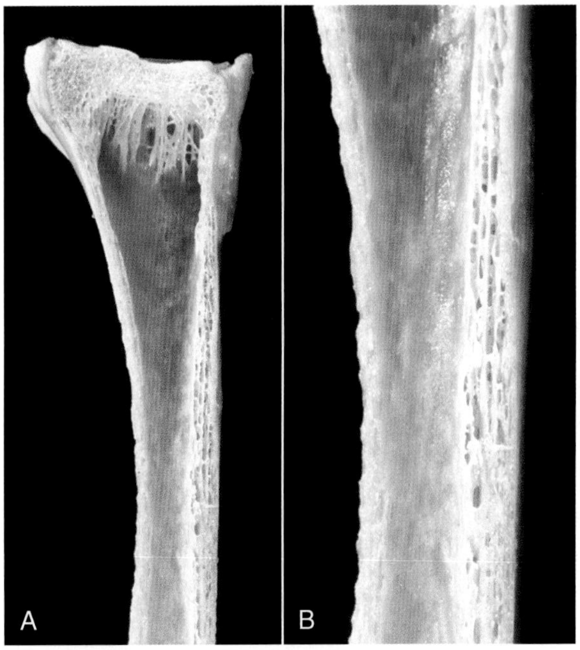

Figure 16-47 **Osteopenia, Bone, Metatarsal, Sheep. A,** There is marked reduction in the number and length of metaphyseal trabeculae. **B,** The cranial cortex *(right)* is markedly porous (trabeculated), and the caudal cortex *(left)* is thin. The marrow has been flushed from the specimen. (Courtesy Dr. S.E. Weisbrode, College of Veterinary Medicine, The Ohio State University.)

Cortical bone: Cortical bone becomes thin due to osteoclastic resorption on the endosteal surface, with corresponding enlargement of the medullary cavity. The porosity of the cortex also increases because of increased osteoclastic resorption within the cortical vascular spaces and Haversian systems and/or decreased osteoblastic activity. With increased time or severity of disease (osteopenia), the resulting tissue may more closely resemble trabecular bone than cortical bone (Fig. 16-47). In severe cases, loss of cortical bone results in an increased susceptibility to fracture.

Rickets and Osteomalacia. Failure of mineralization with subsequent bone deformities and fractures is called *rickets* in the growing skeleton and *osteomalacia* (soft bone) in the adult. Rickets is a disease of bone and epiphyseal (growth) cartilage in immature animals, whereas osteomalacia is a disease of adults in which the lesions are confined to bone. Affected animals have bone pain, pathologic fractures, and deformities such as kyphosis and scoliosis.

The most common causes of rickets and osteomalacia are deficiencies of vitamin D or phosphorus. However, both disorders can occur in chronic renal disease and in chronic fluorosis. Dietary phosphorus deficiency is not common but can occur in herbivores grazing on phosphorus-deficient pastures. Phosphorus-deficient animals often have reduced feed intake, are unthrifty, and have impaired reproductive performance. Due to the common addition of this vitamin to commercial feed, vitamin D deficiency is rare in domestic animals other than in New World primates (in which vitamin D_2 appears to be less active than vitamin D_3) and "sun-basking" reptiles (when housed indoors). In addition, animals exposed to adequate sunlight should be able to synthesize vitamin D if their kidneys are normal. Although calcium deficiency is not commonly considered to be a cause of rickets in animals (other than birds), studies in human beings provide evidence that some cases of rickets may be attributable to extremely low dietary calcium intake in the presence of adequate vitamin D intake, particularly in infants and younger children (versus adolescents). In addition, low dietary calcium is known to exacerbate the development of vitamin D deficiency rickets in children. The mechanisms of this phenomenon are not known; however, it has been shown that knockout mice with no receptors for vitamin D develop rickets that can be corrected by feeding a high-calcium diet.

Growth plate: The growth plates in rickets are diffusely but irregularly thickened because of failure of cartilage matrix mineralization and endochondral ossification (Fig. 16-48). This lesion may be evident in the costochondral junctions as prominent, nodular thickenings that historically have been called *rachitic rosary* due to the resemblance to a string of prayer beads. This thickening is apparent grossly as retained epiphyseal cartilage. Microscopically, the columns of chondrocytes in the growth plate may appear somewhat disorganized. In mammals, there is an increased number of chondrocytes in the zone of hypertrophy compared with normal, and this increase may be marked. It is uncertain if the disorganization of chondrocytes in vitamin D–deficiency rickets is caused by a primary effect of a lack of vitamin D metabolites (specifically, 24,25-dihydroxyvitamin D) or to a mechanical consequence of the failure of endochondral ossification. Because of the inadequate absorption of calcium, the rachitic growth plate does not undergo mineralization. In mammals, when mineralization of the cartilage matrix does not occur, blood vessels with accompanying chondroclasts do not invade the physis and the process of endochondral ossification does not proceed.

Trabecular bone: Grossly and radiographically, the metaphyses are "flared" in rickets because of failure of bone and cartilage removal in the cutback zones (see Fig. 16-48). Poorly mineralized matrices cannot be resorbed because osteoclasts cannot bind to an unmineralized matrix (see previous discussion). Microscopically, the surfaces of trabecular bone in rickets and osteomalacia contain excessive amounts of osteoid (unmineralized matrix) (Fig. 16-49). Because osteoclasts are not able to adhere to or resorb osteoid, bone modeling and remodeling is impaired. Hypocalcemia can develop concurrently with vitamin D deficiency, and lesions of secondary hyperparathyroidism (fibrous osteodystrophy [see later discussion]) also can develop.

Cortical bone: Grossly, cortical bone can appear normal or the softened bone can be deformed by weight bearing. In severe cases, the bones are so soft that they can be cut with a knife. Microscopically, many endocortical and trabecular surfaces in the cortex contain wide seams of unmineralized osteoid. Osteomalacic bone is susceptible to accumulation of microcracks because of the impaired remodeling and modeling secondary to the inability of osteoclasts to bind to surfaces covered by osteoid.

Fibrous Osteodystrophy. Fibrous osteodystrophy is the name given to the skeletal lesions that result from primary hyperparathyroidism, secondary hyperparathyroidism, and pseudohyperparathyroidism (also known as humoral hypercalcemia of malignancy). These disorders are characterized by increased, widespread osteoclastic resorption of bone and replacement by primitive fibro-osseous tissue, which results in a weakened bone structure. Sequelae include lameness, pathologic fractures, and deformities. As described previously, osteoblasts—but not osteoclasts—have receptors for PTH and respond by upregulating production of RANKL and downregulating secretion of OPG. Bone marrow stromal cells also have receptors for PTH, and when the hormone is expressed constantly at high levels,

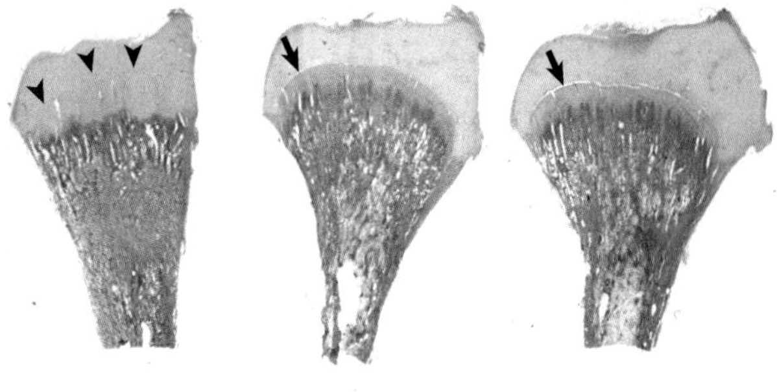

Figure 16-48 **Vitamin D Deficiency (Experimental), Bone, Tibia, Chicken.** Left specimen: rachitic tibia; middle and right specimens: normal chicken and a chicken fed a vitamin D–deficient diet supplemented with calcitriol. The latter two specimens appear normal and are indistinguishable from each other. The growth plate in the rachitic bird is thickened. The *arrowheads* indicate the junction between the growth plate and the epiphyseal cartilage. The metaphysis has not undergone modeling ("cutback"). In the normal-appearing bones, notice the tapering of the metaphysis ("cutback" zone) and the thickness of the growth plate. In these normal chickens, the cleft *(arrows)* separating the growth plate from the epiphyseal cartilage is an artifact. There is no ossification center present in the epiphysis, which is normal for young broilers. H&E stain. (Courtesy Dr. L. Nagode.)

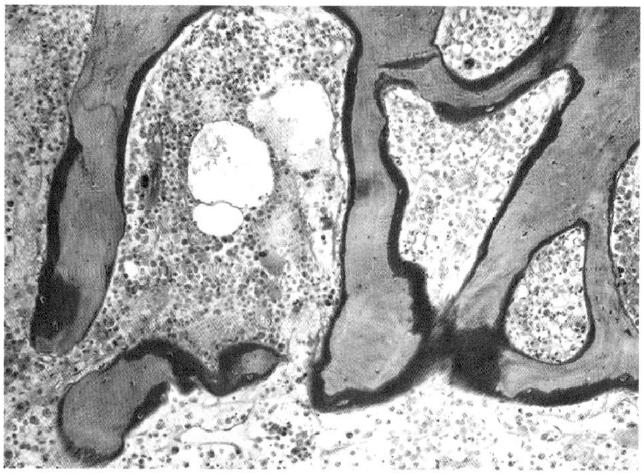

Figure 16-49 **Osteomalacia, Bone, Cross Section, Metaphysis, Trabeculae, Human Being.** This person had osteomalacia secondary to malabsorption of fat-soluble vitamins (including vitamin D) associated with gastrectomy. This section was not demineralized and was stained to show the difference between osteoid *(red)* and fully mineralized bone *(blue-green)*. Normally, no more than 10% of trabecular surfaces should be covered by osteoid seams; however, in this case almost all surfaces are covered by osteoid. Goldner's trichrome stain. (Courtesy Dr. S.E. Weisbrode, College of Veterinary Medicine, The Ohio State University.)

these cells differentiate into fibroblasts. Paradoxically, intermittent (versus continuous) dosing of PTH has the opposite effect on bone (increased number of osteoblasts and increased bone formation) and is used clinically in human beings for the treatment of osteoporosis.

In domestic animals, primary hyperparathyroidism, which includes functional parathyroid adenoma, parathyroid carcinoma, and idiopathic bilateral parathyroid hyperplasia, is rare. Secondary hyperparathyroidism is more common and can be either nutritional or renal in origin. Nutritional hyperparathyroidism is caused by dietary factors that tend to decrease the concentration of serum ionized calcium, to which the parathyroid glands respond by increasing output of PTH. Nutritional hyperparathyroidism is most common in young, growing animals that are fed rations that are deficient in calcium and have a relative excess of phosphorus. Unsupplemented cereal grain rations fed to pigs, all-meat diets fed to dogs and cats, and bran fed to horses are examples of low-calcium, high-phosphorus diets that can cause secondary nutritional hyperparathyroidism and, eventually, fibrous osteodystrophy. Increased concentrations of dietary phosphorus are important in the evolution of fibrous osteodystrophy, perhaps by interfering with the intestinal absorption of calcium. Pseudohyperparathyroidism is also known as humoral hypercalcemia of malignancy and is discussed in Chapter 12.

Growth plate: No lesions are expected in the growth plate or AECC.

Trabecular bone: Trabeculae are replaced by irregular spicules of woven bone that are separated by variable amounts of fibrous connective tissue and are accompanied by numerous osteoclasts. Osteoblastic proliferation can be marked but is ineffectual in that little osteoid is produced. Proliferation of fibrous tissue in the marrow space is usually marked but may be subtle in early stages, consisting of only two or three layers of fibroblasts between the bone lining cells and the marrow space (Fig. 16-50; tunneling resorption). In severe cases, the marrow cavity is filled with fibrous tissue.

Cortical bone: Bone resorption and replacement by fibrous tissue can be so extensive that the bone becomes pliable (E-Fig. 16-22). Clinically and at postmortem examination, severely affected bones can be bent at a right angle without fracture. This outcome, when it affects the mandible, has been called *rubber jaw*. Osteoclastic resorption begins on the endocortical bone surface, but any vascular spaces within the bone can undergo marked enlargement by osteoclastic resorption and replacement by fibrous tissue. In advanced disease, the entire width of the cortex may be replaced by reactive woven bone and fibrous tissue. The proliferation of fibrous tissue may be so exuberant that the external dimension of the bone is increased (Figs. 16-51, 16-52, and 16-53). This lesion is most common in the maxilla and mandible and may reflect the response of the weakened bone to the intense mechanical stress of mastication.

Renal Secondary Hyperparathyroidism (Renal Osteodystrophy). See Disorders of Dogs.

Inflammation

Infectious Inflammation. Inflammation of bone is termed *osteitis*. *Periostitis* is the appropriate term if the periosteum is involved, and *osteomyelitis* is the appropriate term if the medullary cavity (and bone marrow) of the bone is involved (Table 16-2). These conditions generally occur together and may be life threatening, requiring early diagnosis and vigorous treatment. They often involve the simultaneous necrosis and removal of bone and the compensatory production of new bone, occurring over a prolonged period of time. Infectious inflammation of bone in animals is usually caused by bacteria. Hematogenous bacterial osteomyelitis is uncommon in dogs and cats, but it is common in neonatal foals and animals used for food and fiber production. A wide range of Gram-positive and Gram-negative bacteria is responsible for hematogenous osteomyelitis in calves and foals. *Trueperella* (formerly known as *Arcanobacterium*) *pyogenes* and other pyogenic bacteria (e.g., *Streptococcus* spp. and *Staphylococcus* spp.) and *Salmonella* spp., *Escherichia coli*, and other coliforms are among the most common microbes that cause hematogenous osteomyelitis. *Staphylococcus intermedius* is the most common cause of hematogenous osteomyelitis in dogs.

Diskospondylitis ("spondyl" = spine/vertebral body) refers to an infection (inflammation) of the intervertebral disk with concurrent osteomyelitis of contiguous vertebrae (see Fig. 16-78). Hematogenous spread of bacteria (similar list as those described previously for osteomyelitis as well as *Brucella canis*) is one of the most common

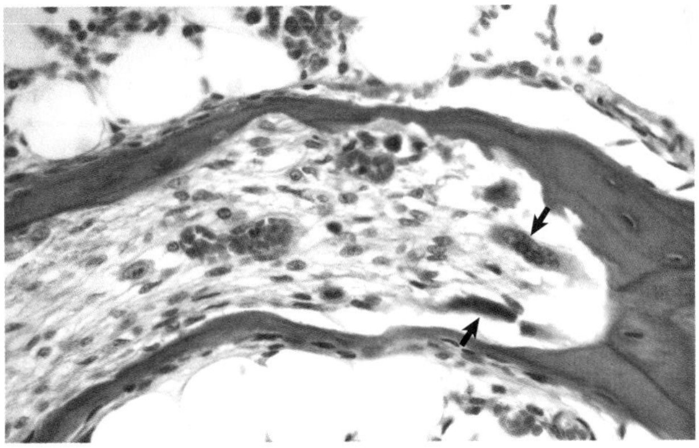

Figure 16-50 Tunneling Resorption (Within a Trabecula), Fibrous Osteodystrophy, Bone, Longitudinal Section, Dog. Osteoclasts (*arrows*) have resorbed the central portion of the trabecula, and this tissue is being replaced by fibrous tissue rather than bone. H&E stain. (Courtesy Dr. S.E. Weisbrode, College of Veterinary Medicine, The Ohio State University.)

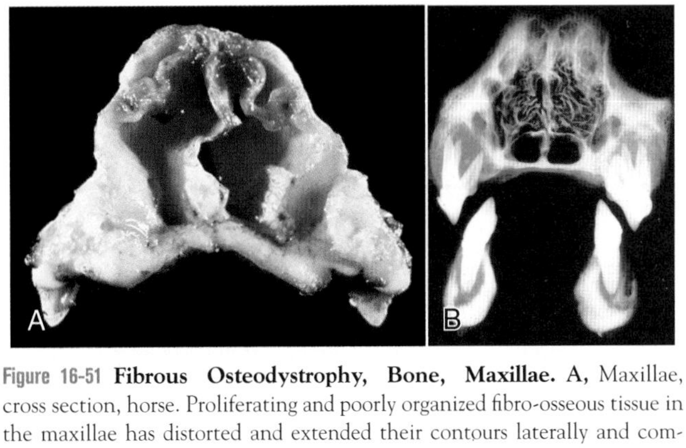

Figure 16-51 Fibrous Osteodystrophy, Bone, Maxillae. A, Maxillae, cross section, horse. Proliferating and poorly organized fibro-osseous tissue in the maxillae has distorted and extended their contours laterally and compressed the nasal cavity medially. Note the absence of normal bone. **B,** Radiograph, renal fibrous osteodystrophy, dog. Note the reduced bone density (radiodensity) of the proliferative woven bone and fibrous tissue that has replaced the preexisting maxillary bones. Postmortem transverse slab section. (**A** courtesy Dr. W. Crowell, College of Veterinary Medicine, The University of Georgia; and Noah's Arkive, College of Veterinary Medicine, The University of Georgia. **B** courtesy Dr. S.E. Weisbrode, College of Veterinary Medicine, The Ohio State University.)

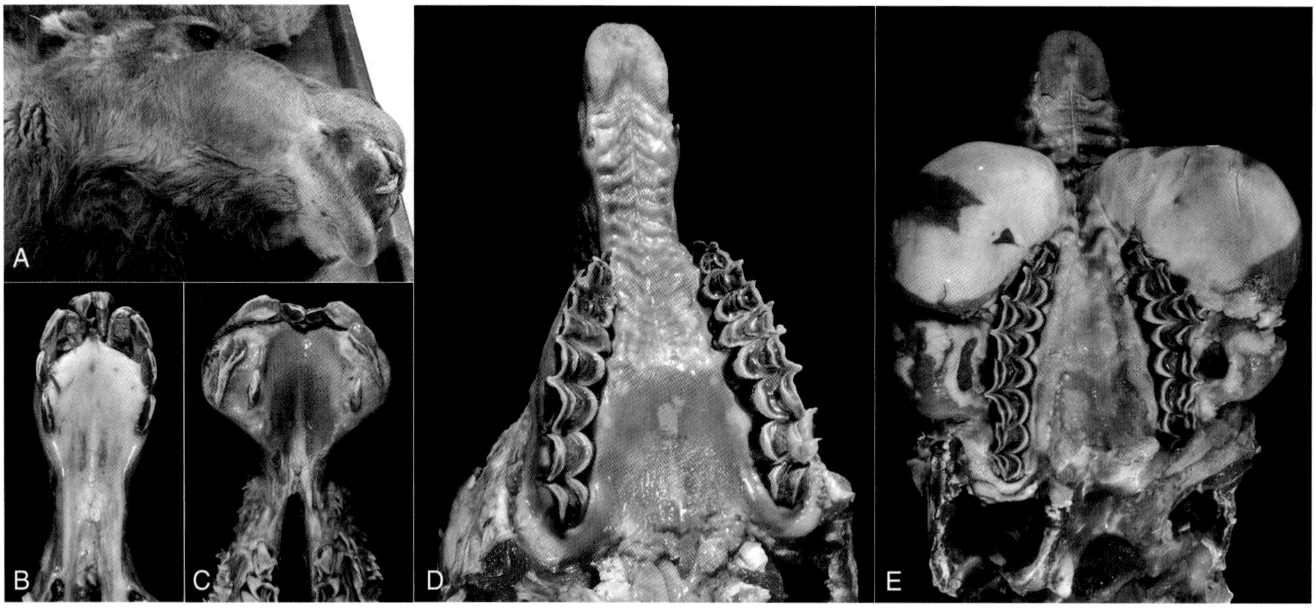

Figure 16-52 **Fibrous Osteodystrophy, Bone, Maxillae and Mandibles, Dromedary Camel. A,** Swollen maxillae and mandible of affected camel with displaced mandibular incisor teeth, right lateral aspect. **B,** Dorsoventral view of mandible of unaffected camel. **C**, Dorsoventral view of affected rostral mandible showing fibro-osseous proliferation and displaced incisor teeth. **D,** Ventrodorsal view of unaffected rostral maxillae. **E,** Ventrodorsal view of affected maxillae showing marked locally extensive enlargement. (**A, C,** and **E** courtesy Dr. A.G. Armién, Dr. E.J. Olson, and Dr. N.A. Robinson, College of Veterinary Medicine, University of Minnesota. **B** and **D** courtesy Dr. J.A. Dykstra and Dr. A. Wuenschmann, College of Veterinary Medicine, University of Minnesota.)

Table 16-2 Lesions of Inflammatory Joint Disease

Time/Exudate	Synovial Fluid	Synovial Membrane	Articular Cartilage
Acute suppurative	Reduced viscosity Neutrophils	Hyperemia Edema	No lesions
Subacute suppurative	Reduced viscosity Neutrophils	Hyperplasia Lymphoplasmacytic inflammation	Usually no lesions
Chronic suppurative	Reduced viscosity Neutrophils	Hyperplasia Lymphoplasmacytic inflammation Fibrosis	Erosion Ulceration
Acute fibrinous	Reduced viscosity Fibrin	Hyperemia Edema	No lesions
Subacute fibrinous	Reduced viscosity Fibrin	Hyperplasia Lymphoplasmacytic inflammation	Usually no lesions
Chronic fibrinous	Reduced viscosity Fibrin	Hyperemia Lymphoplasmacytic inflammation Fibrin Pannus	Erosion Ulceration Pannus

causes. Vertebral infections caused by grass awn migration are often associated with mixed bacterial infections.

Fungi, viruses, and protozoa also can cause bony lesions. Mycotic agents, such as *Coccidioides immitis* and *Blastomyces dermatitidis*, frequently spread hematogenously to bone to produce (pyo-)granulomatous osteomyelitis, accompanied by bone lysis and irregular new bone formation. The viruses of hog cholera (classical swine fever; pestivirus) and infectious canine hepatitis (canine adenovirus type 1 [CAV-1]) can cause endothelial damage, resulting in metaphyseal hemorrhage, necrosis, and acute inflammation. Osseous localization of the canine distemper virus injures osteoclasts, resulting in disrupted metaphyseal modeling and producing a growth retardation lattice (described previously). A variant of the feline leukemia virus (FeLV) has been associated with myelosclerosis (increased density of medullary bone) in cats; however, neither canine distemper virus nor feline leukemia virus causes inflammation of bone. Canine hepatozoonosis caused by *Hepatozoon americanum* (an apicomplexan protozoal organism) is an emerging tick-borne disease of dogs in North America. In addition to the characteristic skeletal and cardiac myositis, there is disseminated periosteal new bone formation (proliferation) in many affected dogs. It is thought that cytokines elaborated by the animal in response to the infection are involved, and the bone lesions have been attributed to periosteal stimulation by humoral factors rather than local ones.

Growth plate: Epiphyseal cartilage (Fig. 16-54) (cartilage of the epiphysis that has yet to undergo endochondral ossification) and

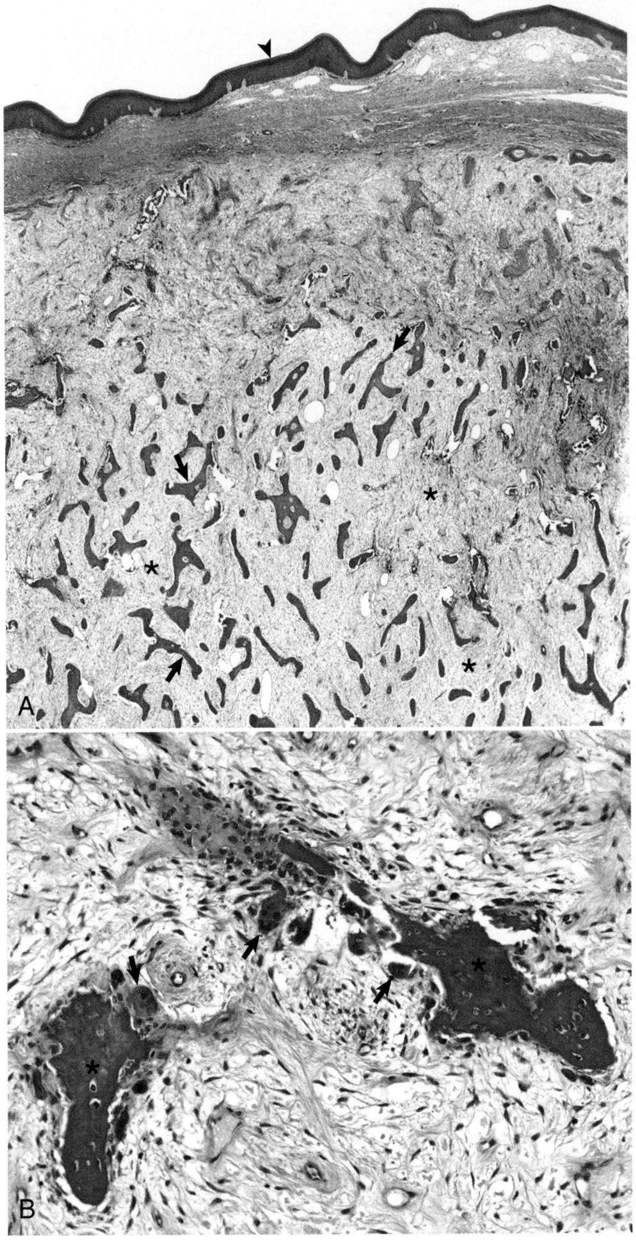

Figure 16-53 Fibrous Osteodystrophy, Bone, Maxilla, Dromedary Camel. A, Multiple small bony trabeculae *(arrows)* separated by loose fibrous connective tissue *(asterisks)* that fills marrow spaces. Oral mucosa *(arrowhead)* lines the upper surface of the tissue. **B,** Primitive new bone formation *(asterisks)* accompanied by numerous osteoclasts *(arrows)* within resorption/erosion lacunae and surrounded by loose fibrovascular connective tissue. (Courtesy Dr. C.S. Carlson and Dr. E.J. Olson, College of Veterinary Medicine, University of Minnesota.)

physeal cartilage can be eroded by invasion of inflammation from adjacent bone or may undergo direct bacterial embolization via cartilage canal blood vessels or metaphyseal vessels at sites of endochondral ossification (see the section on Portals of Entry). Growth cartilage may appear thickened secondary to osteomyelitis because of disruption of endochondral ossification by the inflammatory process and the resulting failure to replace cartilage with bone. In growing animals, articular cartilage can undergo lysis by extension of osteomyelitis from the subjacent epiphyseal cartilage of the AECC, a lesion that may be mistaken for primary arthritis (see Fig. 16-34).

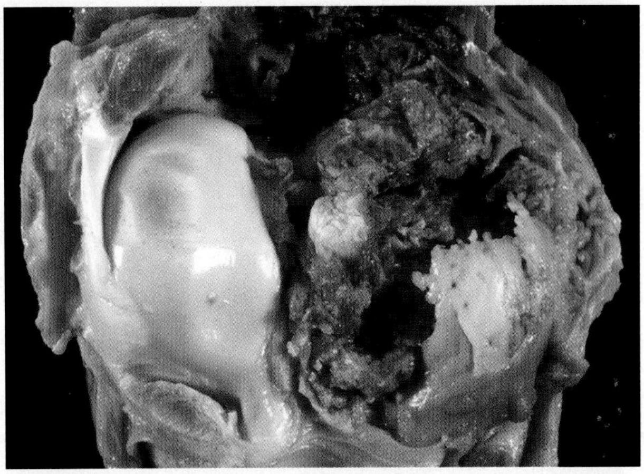

Figure 16-54 Embolic (Suppurative) Epiphysitis, Bone, Distal Femur, Foal. Bacterial emboli in the articular-epiphyseal cartilage complex (AECC) have produced suppurative inflammation that has destroyed both the subchondral bone and the overlying articular cartilage of the right condyle. (Courtesy Dr. S.E. Weisbrode, College of Veterinary Medicine, The Ohio State University.)

Trabecular bone: The composition of the exudate in metaphyseal osteomyelitis is determined by the infectious agent and typically is purulent in bacterial infections in domestic animals. Exudate in the medullary cavity increases the intramedullary pressure and can cause compression of blood vessels resulting in thrombosis and infarction of intramedullary fat, hematopoietic marrow, and bone. In areas of inflammation, bone resorption is mediated primarily by osteoclasts that are stimulated by prostaglandins and cytokines released by local tissue and inflammatory cells. Reduced blood flow through large vessels also promotes osteoclastic bone resorption, possibly by altering electrostatic charges in bone. Proteolytic enzymes released by inflammatory cells and activation of matrix metalloproteinases by the acidic environment of inflammation also assist in resorbing matrix. Lack of drainage and persistence of the offending agent in areas of necrotic bone account for the chronicity of the process, which may continue for years. Inflammation in the medullary cavity also may penetrate into and through cortical bone and undermine the periosteum, where it can further disrupt the blood supply to the bone at the nutrient foramen and nutrient canal.

Cortical bone: The lesions involving cortical bone that occur with infectious osteomyelitis may vary based on the route of entry of the organism and the nature of the exudates. Bone lysis is expected with suppurative inflammation and is subperiosteal for bacteria induced traumatically via the periosteum and endosteal in cases of embolic osteomyelitis. Lysis within the cortex begins within existing vascular channels and can occur with either route of entry. Periostitis can develop by direct inoculation from trauma (e.g., puncture wounds) or by centrifugal spread of inflammation from the marrow cavity and through the cortex. Chronic bacterial periostitis is characterized by multiple coalescing pockets of exudate and areas of irregular periosteal new bone formation and cortical lysis. A classical example of this entity is mandibular or maxillary osteomyelitis occurring secondary to infection with *Actinomyces bovis*, also known as "lumpy jaw" (Fig. 16-55). Additional sequelae of osteomyelitis include extension of inflammation to adjacent bone, hematogenous spread to other bones and to soft tissues, pathologic fractures, and development of sinus tracts that penetrate cortical bone and drain to the exterior (Fig. 16-56). Occasionally, fragments of dead bone become isolated from their blood supply and surrounded by exudate (*bone sequestrum*; plural, *sequestra*). Sequestra can form when bone

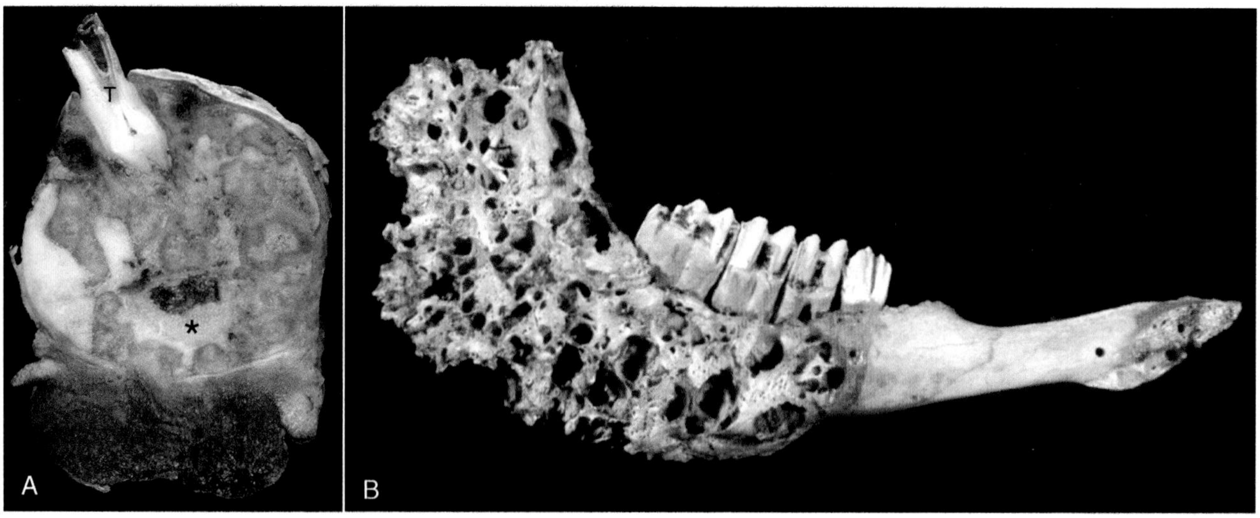

Figure 16-55 **Chronic Pyogranulomatous Osteomyelitis, Actinomycosis (*Actinomyces bovis*), Maxilla, "Lumpy Jaw," Cow. A,** Transverse section of the maxilla. The nodules apparent within the mass in the maxilla represent pockets of pyogranulomatous inflammation that are surrounded by fibrous tissue and woven bone *(asterisk)*; tooth *(T)*. **B,** Macerated and bleached specimen of the mandible. Note the spicules of woven bone radiating from the mandible. Within the spaces formed by this reactive bone were nodules of pyogranulomatous inflammation and colonies of *Actinomyces bovis*. (**A** courtesy University of Minnesota Veterinary Diagnostic Laboratory Archive. **B** courtesy Dr. S.E. Weisbrode, College of Veterinary Medicine, The Ohio State University.)

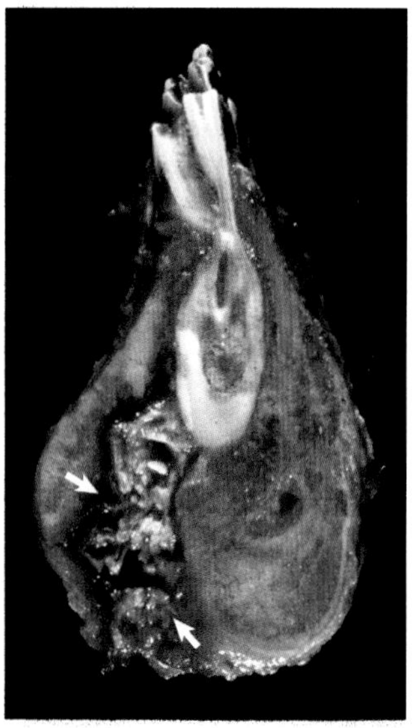

Figure 16-56 **Chronic Suppurative Osteomyelitis, Bone, Mandible, Transverse Section, Sheep.** Chronic suppurative osteomyelitis has caused a fistulous tract *(arrows)* that penetrates through the full dorsoventral thickness of the mandible. This lesion likely began as a periodontal bacterial infection. (Courtesy Dr. S.E. Weisbrode, College of Veterinary Medicine, The Ohio State University.)

fragments are contaminated at the site of a compound fracture, when the fragments at a fracture site become infected hematogenously, or when fragments of necrotic bone become isolated (and thus avascular) in osteomyelitis (Fig. 16-57). These sequestra and associated exudates can become surrounded by a dense collar of reactive bone, which is termed the *involucrum*. Extracellular matrix is not living tissue; therefore it cannot be resorbed in an area in which the cells (bone or marrow) are necrotic. For this reason, relatively large sequestra can persist for long periods of time and may interfere with repair. Grossly, they often become pale and chalky and lack the glistening appearance of normal bone (see Fig. 16-57).

Noninfectious Inflammation

Metaphyseal Osteopathy. See Disorders of Dogs.

Panosteitis. See Disorders of Dogs.

Aseptic Necrosis

Aseptic necrosis of bone in human beings occurs in a variety of clinical conditions, including occlusive vascular disease (bone infarction), hyperadrenocorticism, fat embolism, nitrogenous embolism, sickle cell anemia, and intramedullary neoplasms, all of which likely result in arterial or venous infarction of the bone (Table 16-3). In domestic animals, aseptic necrosis of bone has been associated with intramedullary neoplasms and various nonneoplastic lesions, which likely result in decreased venous outflow from the bone and increased bone marrow pressure. The long-term use of corticosteroids in human beings has been associated with necrosis of the femoral head in adults, and this lesion has been reproduced experimentally in several animal species (e.g., mice and rabbits).

The gross appearance of necrotic bone varies with the extent of the affected area and the response of the body to it. Microscopically, the hallmark of bone necrosis is cell death and loss of osteocytes from their lacunae, which must be distinguished from similar changes that may occur secondary to over decalcification of the sample.

After an episode of ischemia leading to infarction, the cellular elements of the marrow lose their differential staining, and circular spaces (pooled lipid) develop within a few days. If the region of dead bone remains avascular, the coagulated tissue and mineralized matrix can persist for some time. Dead osteocytes elicit little reaction; their nuclei become pyknotic, but their disappearance from lacunae is slow and might not be complete for 2 to 4 weeks.

Reaction to and repair of necrotic bone requires revascularization that is associated with infiltration of macrophages and invasion by fibrous tissue that advances from the margins of the lesion. The bone marrow might eventually regenerate entirely, or a scar might form and remain. The necrotic matrix remains fully mineralized and might even "hypermineralize" because of calcification of the dead osteocytes and their lacunae. This mineralization is only possible if

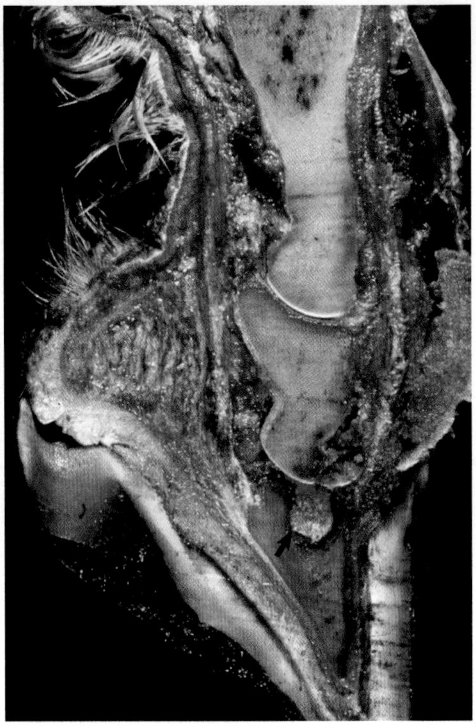

Figure 16-57 **Suppurative Periostitis and Osteomyelitis, Phalanges, Horse.** Trauma to the dorsal aspect of the hoof inoculated bacteria into the subcutis, causing suppurative cellulitis and periostitis and, subsequently, cortical osteolysis of the dorsal aspect of the distal first phalanx and the entire dorsal surface of the second phalanx. From there, the infection spread to the distal interphalangeal joint and then to the third phalanx, where it caused suppurative osteomyelitis, loss of articular cartilage, and formation of a sequestrum in the proximal portion of the third phalanx (*arrow*). The viable tissue immediately adjacent to the sequestrum is not different from that which is more distant, implying that in this case an involucrum (reactive bone surrounding the exudate around a sequestrum) was not formed. (Courtesy Dr. S.E. Weisbrode, College of Veterinary Medicine, The Ohio State University.)

there is vascularization that brings additional calcium to the region. Dead bone is slowly removed by osteoclasts. The resorption of necrotic bone with simultaneous replacement by new bone is termed *creeping substitution*. The process is slow and often incomplete. Small areas of bone necrosis might not be detected clinically or radiographically.

Growth plate: Ischemic necrosis of metaphyseal bone and bone marrow can result in retained growth cartilage. The metaphyseal necrosis would not directly affect the zones of proliferative and hypertrophic chondrocytes; however, the physeal thickness would increase because the conversion of epiphyseal cartilage to bone by endochondral ossification at the chondro-osseous junction would be impaired. Ischemic necrosis of the epiphysis could result in premature closure of the growth plate because of the death of the proliferating chondrocytes, which depend on the epiphyseal blood vessels. Endochondral ossification would continue normally if the metaphyseal blood supply was not affected, and the growth plate would close because of failure to generate new proliferating zone chondrocytes.

Trabecular bone: In the femoral heads of young, small and miniature breed dogs, aseptic necrosis of the femoral head is associated with clinical signs because of the collapse of the articular cartilage as a result of resorption of the necrotic subchondral bone (Legg-Calvé-Perthes disease) that occurs late in the course of the disease. Apparently the initial infarction is asymptomatic (Fig. 16-58; E-Fig. 16-23). The cause of the infarction is usually not determined, but it might be caused by venous compression or increased pressure within the articular cavity. This pressure can result in increased intraosseous pressure and bone necrosis. In clinical cases of aseptic necrosis, the dead bone is not replaced by creeping substitution but is ultimately resorbed and replaced by fibrous tissue. The fibrous tissue does not provide adequate support for the articular cartilage, and the femoral head collapses. In stages preceding complete resorption, it is common, in revascularized necrotic medullary bone, for reactive new bone to be deposited on trabeculae of necrotic bone (Fig. 16-59). This "sandwich" of central dead bone covered by viable reactive woven bone can persist for months and may give (along with osteocyte mineralization described previously) the affected region a radiodense appearance. Ultimately, in clinical cases of aseptic necrosis of the femoral head, even these foci of new bone formed over dead bone are resorbed and replaced by fibrous tissue.

Cortical bone: Large areas of necrotic cortical bone have a dry, chalky gross appearance and the periosteum can be removed easily. These areas can remain as subclinical lesions for years. The formation of sequestra almost always requires inflammation; sequestra formation after sterile necrosis of bone is unusual.

Proliferative and Neoplastic Lesions

Surprisingly, bone, as a tissue, offers little resistance to an expanding or invading neoplasm, and many skeletal neoplasms are accompanied by bone resorption as well as new bone formation. Pain, hypercalcemia, increased serum alkaline phosphatase activity, pathologic fracture, and distant metastases are other possible manifestations of a skeletal neoplasm. New bone formation occurs, at least in part, in response to mechanical stress on a weakened cortex and is prominent in neoplasms that have a marked fibrous stroma. Neoplasms with little stroma, such as plasma cell myeloma and lymphoma, are associated with minimal reactive bone formation, even though bone may be destroyed by marked bone lysis. Tumor-associated bone destruction is largely accomplished by osteoclasts, but prostaglandins, cytokines, acid metabolic by-products, and lytic enzymes released by inflammatory or neoplastic cells can also be responsible for local bone resorption and formation. Hypercalcemia, a result in part of bone resorption induced by release of bone-resorbing factors from extraskeletal neoplasms, is well documented and is termed *humoral hypercalcemia of malignancy* (HHM). The best-known examples in animals occur in dogs secondary to adenocarcinoma of the apocrine glands of the anal sac and T cell lymphoma, in which the neoplastic cells produce parathyroid hormone-related protein (PTHrP). Other tumors include myeloma, leiomyosarcoma, and squamous cell carcinoma (especially in horses); other humoral effectors of HHM include IL-1, TGF-α, and TGF-β.

Nonneoplastic Proliferative and Cystic Lesions. The nonneoplastic proliferative and cystic lesions considered here vary widely in their cause, structure, and ultimate effect on the host. Reactive bone formation, sometimes exuberant, can occur in fracture repair, chronic osteomyelitis, and degenerative joint disease in the form of periarticular osteophytes. An *exostosis* is a nodular, benign, bony growth projecting outward from the surface of a bone. An *osteophyte* is a similar growth that occurs at the margins of a diarthrodial (movable) joint. An *enthesophyte* is the ossification of a tendon or ligament (forming abnormal bony projections) at the point of its insertion into the bone. In addition to bone, these proliferations may include variable amounts of cartilage. The bone component can be woven and/or lamellar, depending on rate of growth and duration of lesion. The term *hyperostosis* usually is used to indicate that the diameter of the bone has increased and implies

Table 16-3 Necrosis of Bone

Cause/Duration of Necrosis	Lesion	Clinical Significance
Acute aseptic (ischemic) necrosis	Death of bone cells and marrow; bone structure intact.	Can be clinically silent.
Chronic aseptic (ischemic) necrosis	1. If no revascularization, dead bone can remain intact structurally for a long time but will accumulate microcracks. 2. If revascularization takes place, dead bone can be resorbed slowly and replaced by new bone. 3. If revascularization takes place, dead bone may be resorbed slowly and NOT be replaced by bone but by fibrous tissue.	1. Can remain clinically silent, but risk of microcrack progressing to complete clinical fracture increases with time and mechanical use. 2. Can remain clinically silent from initiation of lesion to completion of repair. 3. Can cause structural failure and collapse of the bone (e.g., chronic idiopathic necrosis of the femoral head).
Acute septic necrosis	Exudate, usually suppurative, forms at junction of dead bone and viable tissue with subsequent bone lysis and reactive bone formation.	Pain caused by cytokines from the inflammation and pressure in marrow cavity and periosteum.
Chronic septic necrosis	1. If the focus of dead bone is relatively small, it can be completely resorbed by the inflammatory process and osteoclastic bone lysis; there can be marked modeling of bone, usually with resorption predominating and replacement by fibrous tissue; in some cases, excess formation can occur. 2. If the focus of dead bone is relatively large, it can be sequestered (sequestrum) by a peripheral wall of reactive fibrous tissue or reactive bone (involucrum).	Pain caused by cytokines and pressure in marrow cavity and periosteum; draining tracts can form; strength of the bone can be weakened because of resorption, or its function can be affected by exuberant new bone formation.

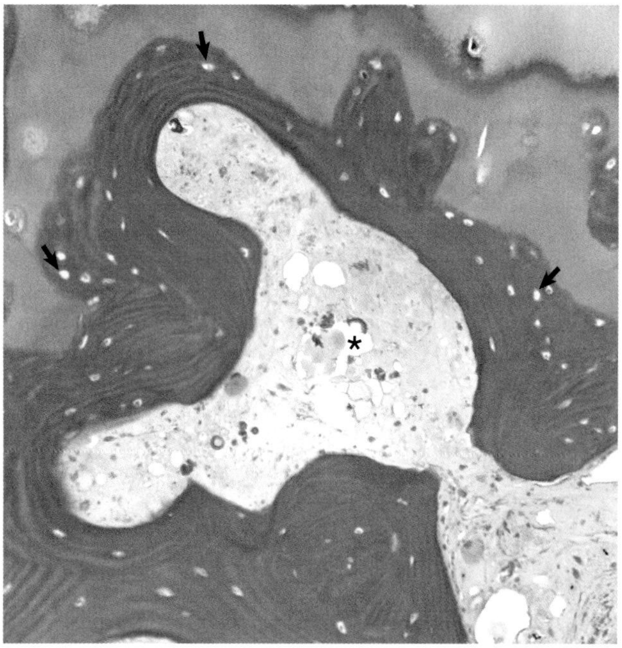

Figure 16-58 **Bone Necrosis (Chronic Osteochondrosis Dissecans Lesion), Femur, Distal End, Adult Human Being.** Osteocyte necrosis represented by empty osteocyte lacunae *(arrows)*; marrow spaces filled with necrotic cellular debris *(asterisk)*. H&E stain. (Courtesy Dr. C.S. Carlson and Dr. E.J. Olson, College of Veterinary Medicine, University of Minnesota.)

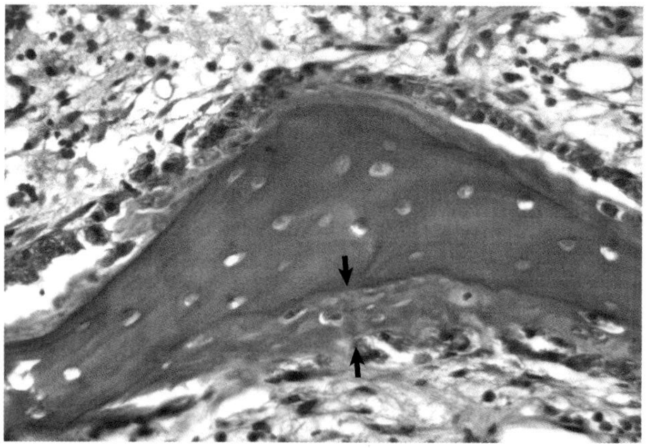

Figure 16-59 **Revascularization, Ischemic Necrosis (Experimentally Induced), 1-Month Duration, Femoral Head, Epiphyseal (Cancellous) Bone, Pig.** Reactive woven bone *(between arrows)* has been deposited on the surface of the necrotic bone in which lacunae are empty or contain pale eosinophilic nuclear remnants. Fibrovascular repair tissue in the marrow surrounds the bone. H&E stain. (Courtesy Dr. S.E. Weisbrode, College of Veterinary Medicine, The Ohio State University.)

more uniform thickening on the periosteal surface rather than the nodular appearance of an osteophyte or exostosis. An *enostosis* is a bony growth within the medullary cavity, usually originating from the cortical-endosteal surface, and can result in obliteration of the medullary cavity. These are nonneoplastic proliferative lesions in which growth is seldom continuous. Some exostoses can remodel (e.g., an osteophyte may become indistinguishable from the preexisting bone over time, and its presence is only recognizable by a change in shape of the affected area), and some regress. Nonneoplastic proliferative lesions can be mistaken for skeletal neoplasia, particularly in small biopsy specimens. Conversely, a malignancy may be missed when small superficial biopsies contain only nonneoplastic reactive bone that is present adjacent to the tumor. These statements serve to highlight the problem of making a morphologic diagnosis from a small biopsy specimen, without the benefit of a clinical history, radiographic findings, and other laboratory data. One must also remember that more than one process might be active at any one site (e.g., osteosarcoma might be complicated by fracture repair or by osteomyelitis).

Hypertrophic Osteopathy (Hypertrophic Pulmonary Osteopathy). Hypertrophic osteopathy occurs in human beings (known as Marie's disease; hypertrophic pulmonary osteoarthropathy) and a variety of domestic animal species, with dogs being the most commonly affected. The disease is characterized by progressive, often bilateral, periosteal, new bone formation in the diaphyseal and metaphyseal regions, particularly of the distal limbs, that occurs as a secondary reaction to a primary space-occupying lesion (Figs. 16-60 and 16-61; E-Fig. 16-24). The earliest bony involvement (radiographic evidence) often includes the abaxial aspects of the second and fifth metacarpal and/or metatarsal bones. The word "pulmonary" is sometimes included because most cases occur in association with intrathoracic neoplasms (as a paraneoplastic syndrome) or inflammation. Other, less commonly associated lesions or agents include endocarditis, heartworms, rhabdomyosarcoma of the urinary bladder in young giant-breed dogs, right-to-left shunting patent ductus arteriosus (PDA) in dogs, and ovarian neoplasms in the horse. Although the association between the pulmonary lesions and the proliferation of new periosteal bone on the extremities is not clear, it has been postulated that pulmonary lesions lead to reflex vasomotor changes (mediated by the vagus nerve; stimulation of afferent visceral nerves) and to increased blood flow (and angiogenesis) to the extremities resulting in proliferation of connective tissue and periosteum. Evidence to support this theory includes the observation that the bony lesions regress after the primary lesion is removed, as well as after vagotomy. In addition, lesions similar to hypertrophic osteopathy can be reproduced in dogs by creating shunts that allow blood to bypass the pulmonary circulation, thereby increasing the stroke volume of the left side of the heart, leading to increased blood flow to peripheral tissues. Increased arterial pressure, hyperemia, and edema of the periosteum lead to thickening first by fibrous tissue and later by new bone formation.

Recent human medical literature highlights the potential role of vascular endothelial growth factor (VEGF) and platelet-derived growth factor (PDGF) in peripheral vascular beds in stimulating local fibrovascular proliferation, edema, and eventual ossification.

Osteochondromas. Osteochondromas (multiple cartilaginous exostoses) reflect a defect in skeletal development (lesions appear soon after birth) rather than being true neoplasms and are confirmed to have a hereditary etiology in human beings and horses. A hereditary basis has been suggested in dogs as well. Osteochondromas project from bony surfaces as eccentric masses that are located adjacent to physes. They arise from long bones, ribs, vertebrae, scapulae, and bones of the pelvis, and they may be numerous (Fig. 16-62; E-Fig. 16-25) Osteochondromas in dogs and horses do not occur on bones of intramembranous origin (e.g., skull). Microscopically, they have an outer cap of hyaline cartilage that undergoes orderly endochondral ossification to give rise to trabecular bone that forms the base of the lesion (Fig. 16-62, C). The medullary cavity of the osteochondroma usually communicates with the medullary cavity of the underlying bone because the cortex of the underlying bone at this site has not completely developed. Normally, growth ceases at skeletal maturity when the cartilage cap is replaced by bone. Although the origin of osteochondromas is not clear, some arise secondary to a defect in the perichondral ring as peripheral areas of physeal cartilage that are separated and removed from the growth plate during longitudinal growth. Clinically, their importance is threefold: They might interfere mechanically with the action of tendons or ligaments, they can act as space-occupying masses that protrude into the vertebral canal and cause spinal cord compression, and they can undergo malignant transformation and give rise to chondrosarcomas or osteosarcomas. Osteochondromas in cats are

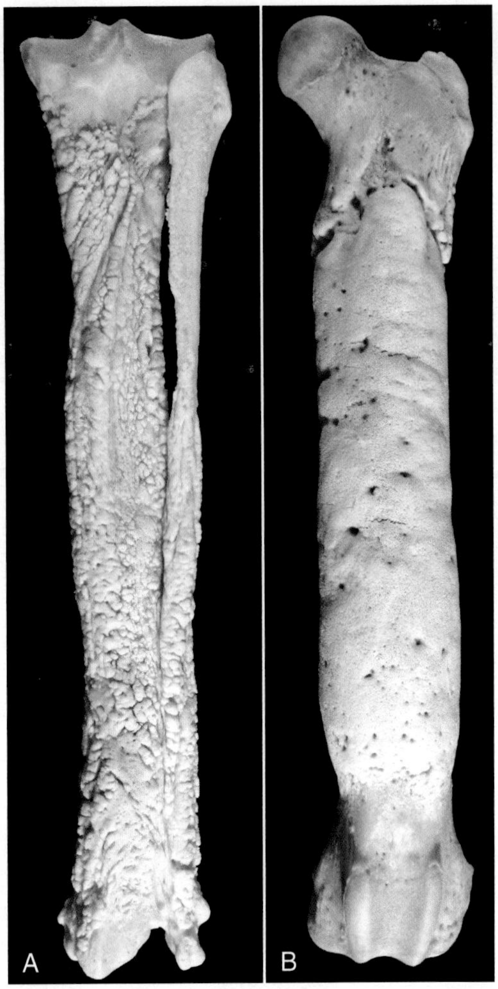

Figure 16-60 **Hypertrophic Osteopathy, Bone, Dog. A,** Tibia and fibula. Marked periosteal proliferation of woven bone has resulted in the surfaces of both bones being irregularly roughened/thickened. **B,** Femur. In this specimen, which exhibits diffuse severe diaphyseal periosteal new bone proliferation, chronicity of disease has resulted in remodeling and a smooth exterior surface. **A** and **B,** Epiphyses are relatively spared. Macerated specimens. (Courtesy Dr. E.J. Olson, College of Veterinary Medicine, University of Minnesota.)

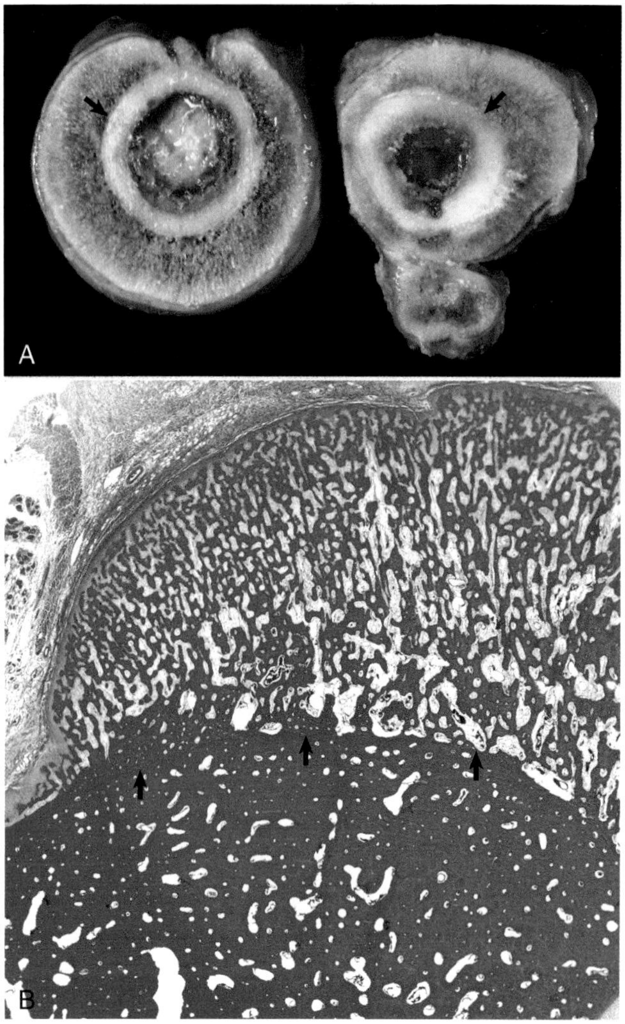

Figure 16-61 **Hypertrophic Osteopathy, Bone, Dog. A,** Cross section of femur *(left)* and tibia/fibula *(right)*. Preexisting cortices *(arrows)* surrounded by a halo of periosteal new bone. **B,** Transition *(arrows)* from preexisting lamellar bone *(lower half of image)* to periosteal new/woven bone *(upper half of image)*. H&E stain. (**A** courtesy Dr. I. Matise and Dr. J. Paulin, College of Veterinary Medicine, University of Minnesota. **B** courtesy Dr. C.S. Carlson and Dr. E.J. Olson, College of Veterinary Medicine, University of Minnesota.)

different in that they develop in mature animals, less commonly affect long bones, do not exhibit orderly endochondral ossification, and might be of viral origin; however, like those in horses and dogs, osteochondromas in cats may undergo malignant neoplastic transformation. The term *osteochondroma* is not recommended for cartilaginous osteophytes that have undergone central endochondral ossification. As will be discussed regarding callus formation in the section on Fracture Repair, the osteogenic tissue (cambium layer) of the periosteum can form hyaline cartilage instead of bone when the oxygen tension of the tissue is low.

Fibrous Dysplasia. Fibrous dysplasia is an uncommon focal to multifocal, lytic, intraosseous lesion that has been found at various sites (skull, mandible, and long bones) in young animals of a variety of species. Typically, preexisting bone, either cancellous or cortical, is replaced by an expanding mass of fibro-osseous tissue that can weaken the cortex and enlarge the external contour of the bone. The lesion is firm, often contains mineralized areas, and may contain multiple cysts filled with sanguineous fluid. Microscopically, the lesion is composed of well-differentiated fibrous tissue containing trabeculae of woven bone that are relatively regularly spaced and sized. Osteoblasts are not recognizable on trabecular surfaces, which is a feature that helps to distinguish this lesion from ossifying fibroma. In human beings, fibrous dysplasia is recognized as a genetic disorder and is associated with a missense mutation in the *GNAS1* gene.

Bone Cysts. Bone cysts are classified as subchondral, simple, or aneurysmal. Radiographically, all appear as well-demarcated lucent areas without evidence of aggressive growth. Subchondral cysts are sequelae to osteochondrosis and degenerative joint disease. Subchondral bone cysts caused by osteochondrosis represent failure of endochondral ossification with either subsequent necrosis and cavitation of retained growth cartilage (pseudocyst; not separated from surrounding tissue by a distinct lining) or dilation of cartilage canal blood vessels within the area of necrosis (true cysts; separated from surrounding tissue by endothelial lining). These are most common in the medial femoral condyle in young horses (1 to 3 years of age) and also may be identified in older horses. Subchondral cysts secondary to degenerative joint disease represent herniation of synovial fluid into the subchondral bone through fissures in degenerated articular cartilage. These herniations become lined by a synovial-like membrane, and the lysis of bone occurs by osteoclasis, secondary either to pressure or to cytokines released from the expanding cyst. Trauma to intact articular cartilage also is proposed as an etiology because cystic lesions have been reproduced experimentally by incising the articular cartilage to the level of the subchondral bone.

Simple bone cysts can contain clear, colorless, serum-like fluid or serosanguineous fluid. The wall of the cyst is composed of variably dense fibrous tissue and woven to lamellar bone. The bone located peripheral to the cyst undergoes modeling to accommodate the expansile growth of the cyst. Simple bone cysts may be difficult to distinguish from fibrous dysplasias, depending on the biopsy sample and radiographic and clinical information that is available.

Aneurysmal bone cysts contain spaces that are filled with blood or serosanguineous fluid and are not usually lined by endothelium. Tissue adjacent to the spaces can vary from well-differentiated fibrous or fibro-osseous tissue to pronounced proliferation of undifferentiated mesenchymal cells admixed with osteoclast-like multinucleated giant cells. Hemorrhage and hemosiderosis are frequent. The cause of simple and aneurysmal bone cysts is unknown; however, they could be consequences of ischemic necrosis, hemorrhage, or congenital or acquired vascular malformations. Caution should be exercised in the interpretation of microscopic lesions in biopsy specimens of cysts, and these lesions should be correlated with the radiographic appearance to rule out cystic cavitation in a neoplasm.

Primary Neoplasms. There are many types of primary neoplasms involving the canine skeleton, the most common being composed of cells that form bone (osteoma/osteosarcoma), cartilage (chondroma/chondrosarcoma), or fibrous connective tissue (fibroma/fibrosarcoma) (Table 16-4). The histopathologic diagnosis of skeletal neoplasia in domestic animals often involves evaluation of needle, trephine, or wedge biopsies. Bone biopsy samples usually are small relative to the size of the neoplasm, and the most easily accessible tissue often is reactive periosteal tissue that is located exterior to the neoplasm. Therefore it is important that the pathologist incorporate the radiographic and clinical findings in the interpretation of the sample. Cases in which there are radiographically aggressive lesions that have an effect on bone mass are usually associated with malignancy or inflammation; therefore, if the microscopic findings from these cases indicate the presence of a benign lesion and/

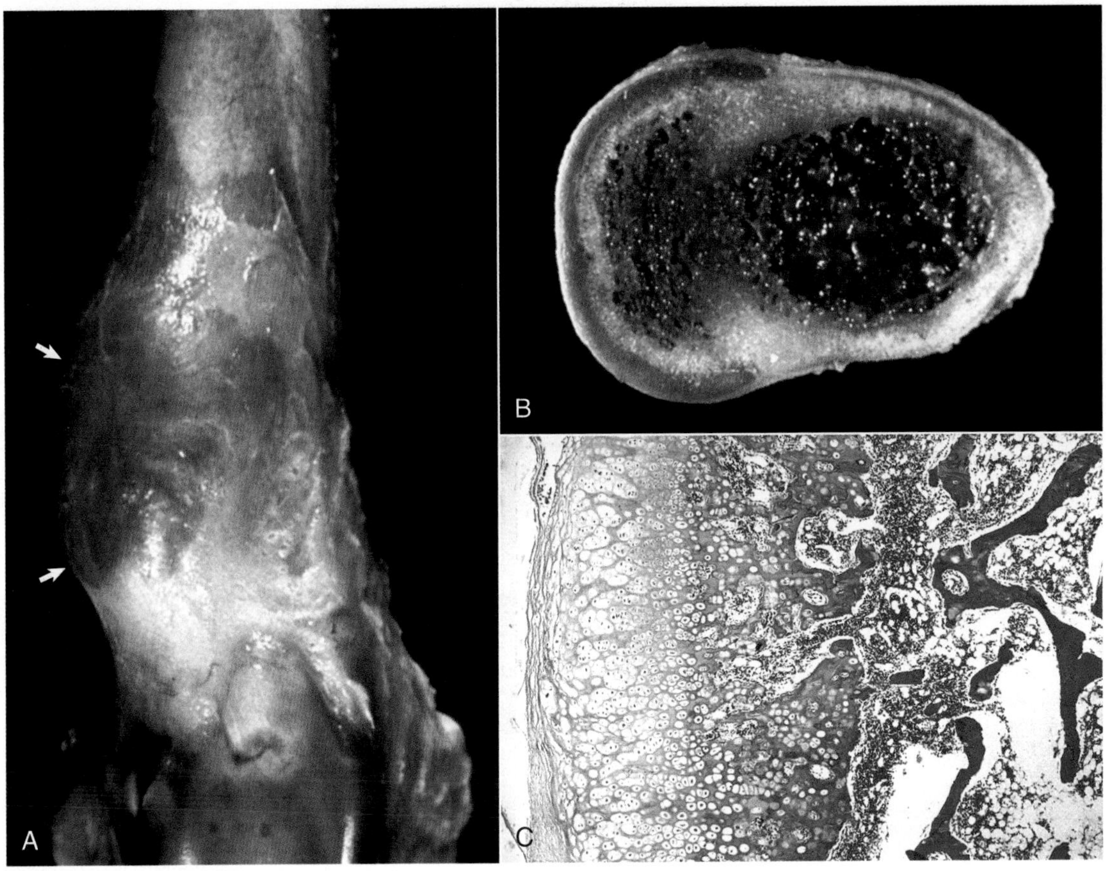

Figure 16-62 **Osteochondroma (Cartilaginous Exostosis), Bone, Distal Femoral Metaphysis, Dog. A,** A plateau-like mass *(left; arrows)* protrudes from the metaphyseal cortex. **B,** On cross section, the mass *(left)* has a cartilage cap. **C,** Histologically, the cartilage cap *(left third of image)* is undergoing endochondral ossification, similar to that which occurs in an articular-epiphyseal cartilage complex. H&E stain. (Courtesy Dr. S.E. Weisbrode, College of Veterinary Medicine, The Ohio State University.)

Table 16-4 Primary Skeletal Neoplasms of the Dog

Name	Cell of Origin	Incidence	Primary Site	Biologic Behavior
Osteoma	Osteoblast	Rare	Flat bones	Benign
Osteosarcoma	Osteoblast	Common	Predominantly metaphyses of larger appendicular bones	Highly malignant with metastases early in clinical course
Chondroma	Chondroblast/chondrocyte	Rare	Flat bones	Benign
Chondrosarcoma	Chondroblast/chondrocyte	Relatively rare	Ribs, sternum, nasal cavity	Metastases not common and late in clinical course
Fibroma	Fibroblast			Not commonly recognized as a primary tumor of bone
Fibrosarcoma	Fibroblast	Relatively rare	Diaphysis of bones of appendicular skeleton	Metastasizes relatively late in clinical course

or provide no explanation for the radiographic changes, it may be necessary to examine additional tissue to reconcile these differences.

Ossifying Fibromas. Ossifying fibromas are uncommon masses in the maxillae and mandibles of horses and cattle. In their early stages, these are intramedullary neoplasms; however, although considered benign, they destroy adjacent cortical and trabecular bone by expansile growth. Microscopically, they are composed of well-differentiated fibrous tissue with scattered spicules of woven bone covered by osteoblasts.

Fibrosarcomas. Fibrosarcomas are malignancies of fibroblasts that produce collagenous connective tissue but do not directly produce bone or cartilage. Microscopically the matrix of fibrosarcomas should not mineralize or entrap cells in lacunae as occurs in normal and neoplastic bone and cartilage, and the cells often are arranged in a whorling or interlacing pattern. Central fibrosarcomas arise from fibrous tissue within the medullary cavity, whereas periosteal fibrosarcomas arise from periosteal connective tissue. Central fibrosarcomas must be distinguished grossly and microscopically from osteosarcoma. In general, central fibrosarcomas grow more slowly, are accompanied by less formation of reactive new bone, are slower to metastasize, and produce a smaller tissue mass than osteosarcomas. Grossly, fibrosarcomas are gray-white, fill part of the medullary cavity, and replace cancellous and cortical bone.

Chondromas. Chondromas are benign neoplasms of hyaline cartilage. They are very rare neoplasms of dogs, cats, and sheep and often arise from flat bones; those arising in the medullary cavity are termed *enchondromas*. Cartilaginous neoplasms in the skeleton do not arise from articular cartilage, most likely because of its low mitotic potential and avascularity. Because they usually occur in adult animals, which do not possess growth cartilage, the cell of origin is presumed to be a stromal cell with chondrogenic potential. Chondromas are multilobulated and have a blue-white appearance on cut surface. They tend to enlarge slowly, but progressively, and can cause thinning of adjacent bone. Microscopically, they are composed of multiple lobules of well-differentiated hyaline cartilage that may include areas of endochondral ossification. Chondromas may be very difficult to distinguish from low-grade, well-differentiated chondrosarcomas; distinguishing between these two tumor types may require clinical information.

Chondrosarcomas. Chondrosarcomas are malignant neoplasms in which the neoplastic cells produce cartilaginous matrix but not osteoid or bone. Chondrosarcomas arise most frequently in the flat bones of the skeleton and occur most commonly in mature, large-breed dogs and in sheep (Figs. 16-63 and 16-64). In dogs, the major sites of origin are the nasal bones, ribs, and pelvis; in sheep, they arise from the ribs and sternum. Most chondrosarcomas arise in the medullary cavity and destroy preexisting bone. Given time, they become large, lobulated neoplasms with a gray or blue-white cut surface. Grossly, some neoplasms are gelatinous, and some contain large areas of hemorrhage and necrosis. Microscopically (Fig. 16-65), the range of differentiation of neoplastic cells is wide: Some neoplasms (grade I chondrosarcomas) are well differentiated, lack mitotic figures, and are difficult to distinguish from chondroma. Grade II chondrosarcomas are composed of pleomorphic chondrocytes, contain low to moderate numbers of mitotic figures, and contain no undifferentiated areas. Grade III chondrosarcomas exhibit marked nuclear atypia, numerous mitotic figures, and contain areas of undifferentiated sarcoma. Some chondrosarcomas are composed primarily of primitive mesenchymal tissue and contain abundant basophilic interstitial mucin and rare foci of chondroid differentiation (mesenchymal chondrosarcoma). Nonneoplastic bone can be present as the result of endochondral ossification of the malignant cartilage; however, the presence of malignant osteoblasts in close association with foci/areas of osteoid supports a diagnosis of osteosarcoma, even in tumors in which the majority of the tissue present is cartilaginous. Chondrosarcomas have a longer clinical course, grow more slowly, and develop metastases later than osteosarcomas. Metastases are usually pulmonary via the venous system, without metastasis to the regional or bronchial lymph nodes.

Osteomas. Osteomas are uncommon benign neoplasms more often recognized in horses and cattle that usually arise from bones that form by intramembranous ossification, usually occurring on the head as a single, dense mass that projects from the surface of the bone (Fig. 16-66). They do not invade or destroy adjacent bone; their growth is slow and progressive but not necessarily continuous. Microscopically, osteomas are covered by periosteum and are composed of cancellous bone; trabeculae are lined by well-differentiated

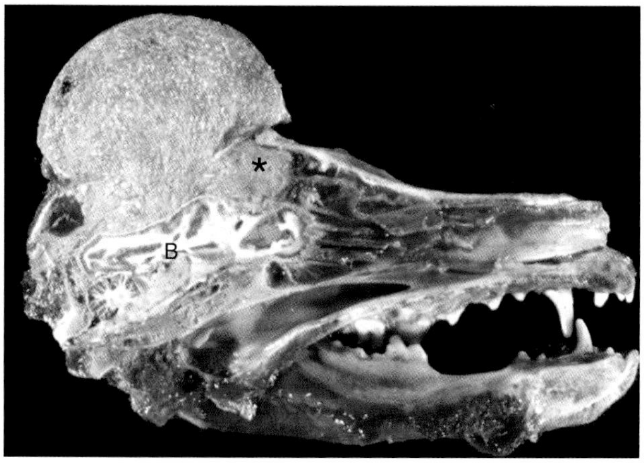

Figure 16-64 **Chondrosarcoma, Bone, Calvarium, Dog.** A chondrosarcoma protrudes dorsally from the skull, compresses the underlying brain *(B)*, and has invaded the frontal sinus *(asterisk)*. The widespread white foci within the mass represent areas of mineralization. (Courtesy Dr. K. Read, College of Veterinary Medicine, Texas A&M University; and Noah's Arkive, College of Veterinary Medicine, The University of Georgia.)

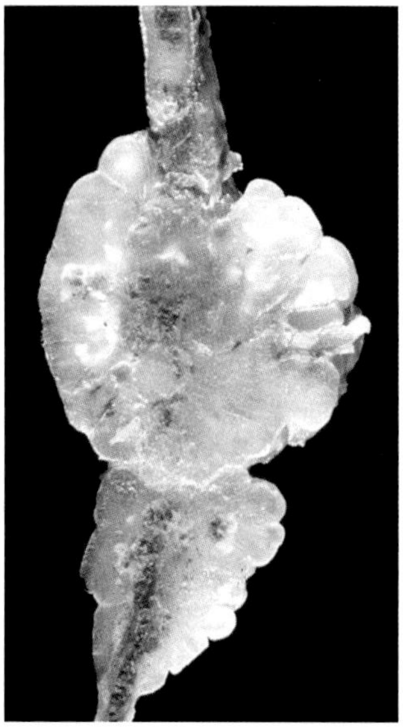

Figure 16-63 **Chondrosarcoma, Bone, Rib, Cat.** A chondrosarcoma arising in a rib has destroyed and replaced the normal bone structure. (Courtesy Dr. S.E. Weisbrode, College of Veterinary Medicine, The Ohio State University.)

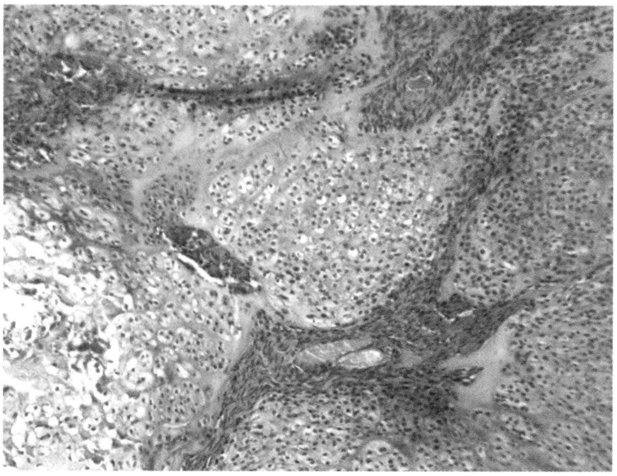

Figure 16-65 **Chondrosarcoma, Bone, Dog.** Chondrocyte lacunae are prominent in well-differentiated regions *(left)* but are less apparent in the more poorly differentiated regions *(lower right)*. (Courtesy Dr. S.E. Weisbrode, College of Veterinary Medicine, The Ohio State University.)

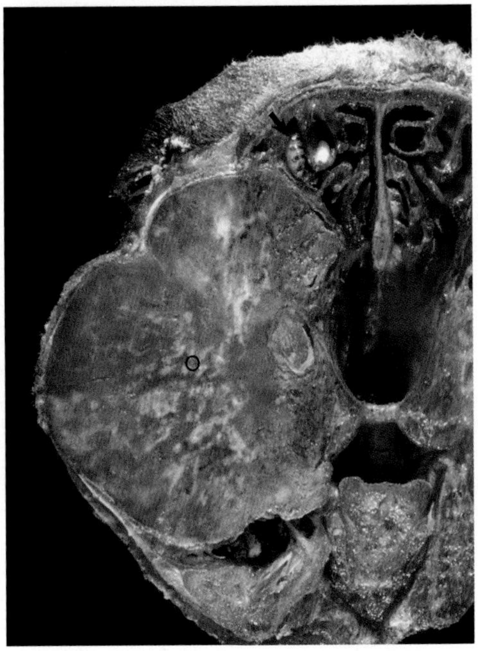

Figure 16-66 **Osteoma, Bone, Maxilla and Maxillary Sinus, Sheep.** The osteoma *(O)* has proliferated and formed a dome-shaped mass above the normal contour of the maxilla and has compressed the maxillary sinus. Grossly, this mass was diffusely hard; histologically, it was composed of closely spaced trabeculae lined by well-differentiated osteoblasts. An *Oestrus ovis* larva *(arrow)* is present in the nasal cavity. (Courtesy Dr. S.E. Weisbrode, College of Veterinary Medicine, The Ohio State University.)

osteoblasts and osteoclasts. The intertrabecular spaces contain delicate fibrous tissue, adipocytes, and hematopoietic tissue.

Osteosarcomas. Osteosarcomas are malignant neoplasms, the cell of origin (mesenchymal stem cell, osteoblast, or even osteocyte) of which has not yet been conclusively determined, although it must have or acquire the potential to produce osteoid (the unmineralized, organic component of the bone matrix). These tumors are common neoplasms in dogs and cats, in which they comprise approximately 80% and 50%, respectively, of all primary bone neoplasms; however, they are rare in other domestic animals. Osteosarcomas typically occur in mature dogs of the large and giant breeds and arise most commonly in the metaphyses.

Predilection sites include the weight-bearing regions of the long bones (especially proximal humerus and distal radius; also femur, distal ulna, and proximal tibia) (Figs. 16-67 and 16-68; E-Fig. 16-26); however, osteosarcomas also can occur in ribs, vertebrae, bones of the head, and various other parts of the skeleton (Fig. 16-69; E-Fig. 16-27). Rarely, they arise in soft tissue/visceral organs (*extraskeletal osteosarcoma*). Growth of the neoplasm is often rapid, aggressively locally invasive, and painful. Except for those tumors arising in the axial skeleton and particularly the head, early hematogenous pulmonary metastasis is common. Metastasis also may be widespread, involving soft tissues, as well as other bones. Osteosarcoma also occurs in small breed dogs but less commonly than in the large and giant breeds, representing less than 50% of all skeletal neoplasms. Osteosarcomas in small dogs frequently affect the axial skeleton, with no apparent predilection for the radius, and tend to have a better prognosis than osteosarcomas occurring in the large and giant breeds.

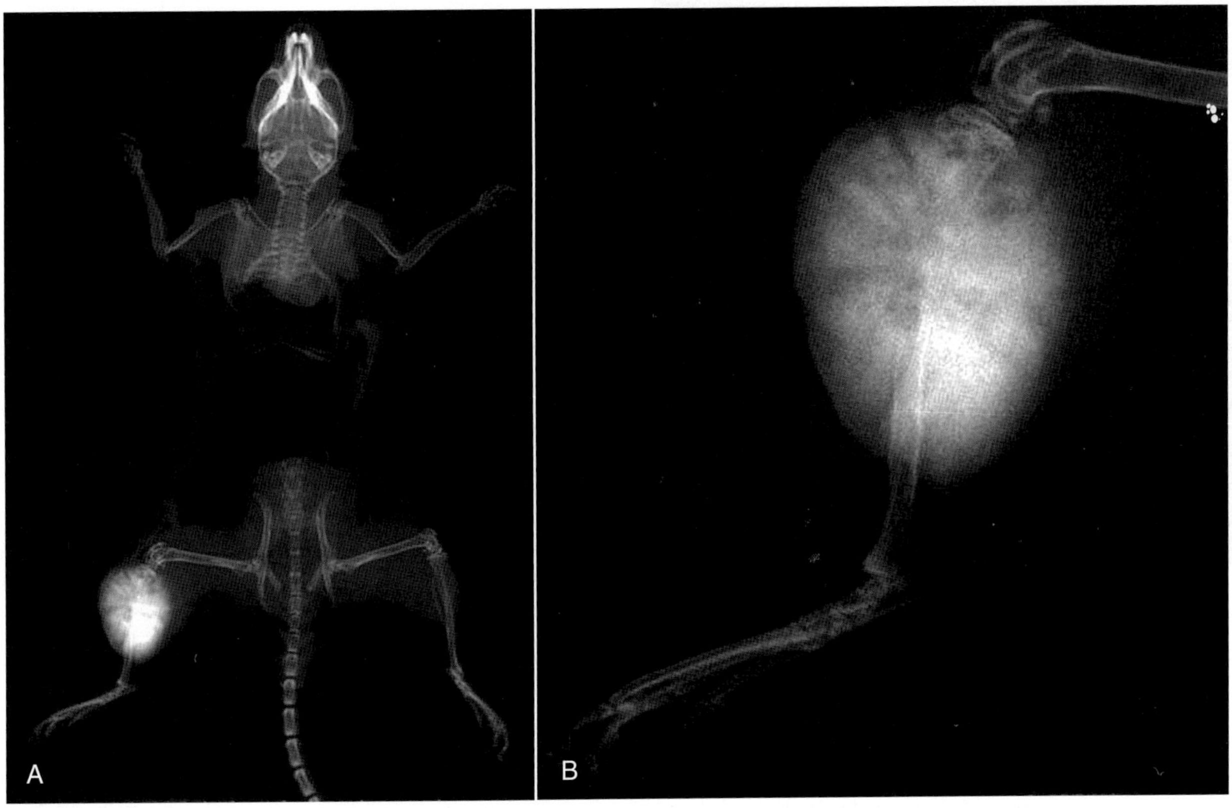

Figure 16-67 **Osteosarcoma, Bone, Tibia/Fibula, Mouse. A,** Postmortem whole body radiograph demonstrating focal neoplasm involving the tibia/fibula *(left)*; the radiolucent areas in the thorax and abdomen are the result of tissue removal prior to radiography. **B,** Higher magnification illustrating proliferation of neoplastic and reactive bone and destruction of preexisting bone. (Courtesy Dr. C.S. Carlson, College of Veterinary Medicine, University of Minnesota.)

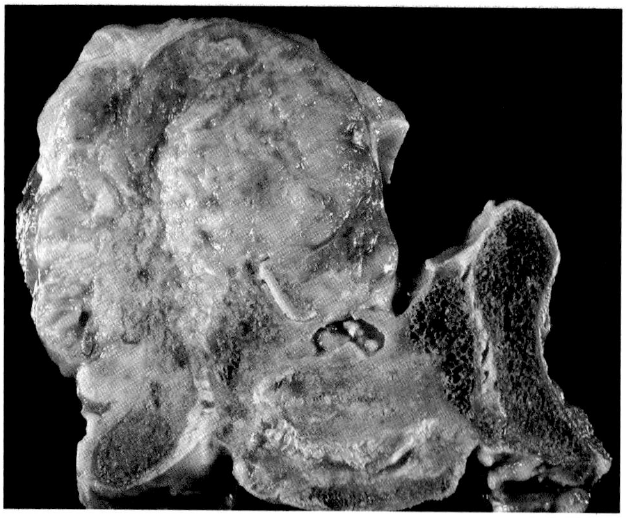

Figure 16-68 **Osteosarcoma, Bone, Pelvis, Dog.** Mass involving the pelvis and expanding the majority of the pelvis (including the wing of the ilium *[left side]*) The mass has grown by expansion into the adjacent soft tissues and invasion of the vertebra. (Courtesy Dr. A. Wuenschmann, College of Veterinary Medicine, University of Minnesota.)

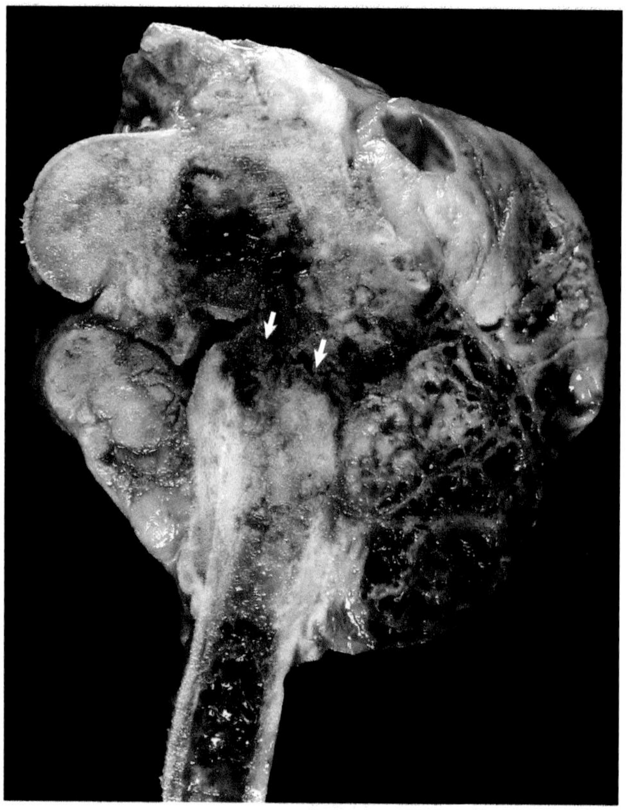

Figure 16-69 **Osteosarcoma, Bone, Humerus, Proximal End, Dog.** Osteosarcoma has lysed preexisting bone and formed a large mass of neoplastic bone; multiple cystic cavities are present (hemorrhage and necrosis); possible pathologic fracture *(arrows)*. (Courtesy Dr. A. Wuenschmann, College of Veterinary Medicine, University of Minnesota.)

Osteosarcomas can be classified as simple (bone formed in a collagenous matrix), compound (both bone and cartilage are present), or pleomorphic (anaplastic, with only small islands of osteoid present). Classification has also been based on cell type and activity (osteoblastic, chondroblastic, or fibroblastic), radiographic appearance (lytic, sclerotic, or mixed), or site of origin (central/intraosseous, juxtacortical, or periosteal). An uncommon form of osteosarcoma is the telangiectatic type that grossly resembles hemangiosarcoma and is composed of osteoblasts, osteoid, and large cystic, blood-filled cavities lined by malignant osteoblasts. Another uncommon form of osteosarcoma is the giant cell type, which resembles nonproductive osteoblastic osteosarcoma except for areas in which tumor giant cells predominate. This form of osteosarcoma must be differentiated from the malignant primary giant cell tumor of bone, which is a very rare neoplasm in animals, characterized by large numbers of multinucleated giant cells that resemble osteoclasts that are closely associated with neoplastic mononuclear clear cells. Because there may be a great deal of heterogeneity within an individual tumor, classifying osteosarcomas may be difficult and is not recommended when the diagnosis is based solely on a small biopsy sample.

Central (intraosseous) osteosarcomas have a gray-white gross appearance and contain variable amounts of mineralized bone. Large, pale areas surrounded by zones of hemorrhage (areas of infarction) and irregular, randomly located areas of hemorrhage are common in rapidly growing intramedullary neoplasms. Neoplastic tissue tends to fill the medullary cavity locally and can extend proximally and distally but typically does not penetrate articular cartilage and therefore does not invade the joint space. Cortical bone is usually destroyed, and neoplastic cells penetrate and undermine the periosteum and can extend outwardly as an irregular lobulated mass (E-Fig. 16-28). Destruction of cortical bone is accompanied by varying amounts of reactive (nonneoplastic) periosteal bone, which may be differentiated from tumor bone microscopically by its regular appearance and well-differentiated lining osteoblasts. Variable amounts of woven bone or osteoid are produced by the neoplastic osteoblasts; in fact, bone/osteoid production by the tumor cells is the hallmark lesion of this neoplasm (Figs. 16-70 and 16-71; E-Fig. 16-29). Bone formation by the malignant cells can be abundant and widespread, or it can be minimal, as occurs in anaplastic or fibroblastic osteosarcomas that are composed of sheets of poorly differentiated mesenchymal cells or fibroblastic tissue with minimal evidence of bone formation.

Periosteal osteosarcomas also have an aggressive behavior and invade into the medullary cavity from the periphery. As with central or intraosseous osteosarcomas, periosteal osteosarcomas cause bone lysis and reactive bone formation in addition to production of neoplastic bone. At the time of presentation, it is often impossible to determine if the osteosarcoma originated from the periosteum or the medullary cavity. Rarely, osteosarcomas are also juxtacortical (parosteal) in origin. These neoplasms arise within the periosteum and form an expansive mass that adheres to and surrounds but does not invade the underlying cortex. Invasion of the shaft and metastasis can occur with parosteal osteosarcomas, but these are late events; therefore early en bloc excision might effect a cure. Although parosteal osteosarcomas are very rare, it is important to distinguish them from periosteal osteosarcomas because of their more favorable prognosis.

Multiple skeletal osteosarcomas (polyostotic; involving multiple bones) occur in human beings and dogs, and these may represent a primary neoplasm that has metastasized to bone or may have a multicentric origin. The bony lesions have a random distribution, and pulmonary metastases are likely to be present. Although the cause of naturally occurring osteosarcomas is largely unknown in both human beings and domestic animals, it is known that osteosarcomas can develop in association with or subsequent to other conditions at the same bony site, including infarction, fracture, and the presence of orthopedic metallic implants. Several inciting or

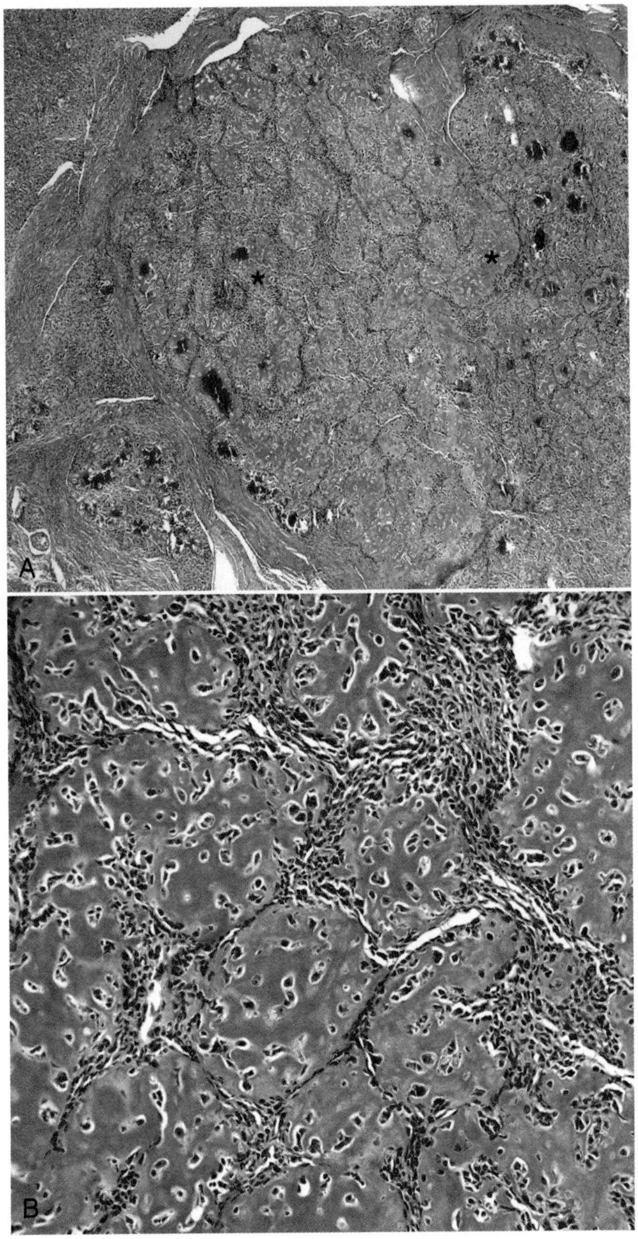

Figure 16-70 Osteosarcoma, Bone, Dog. A, Islands of eosinophilic osteoid *(asterisks)*, some with central mineralization *(dark purple)*, are being produced by aggregates of malignant osteoblasts. **B,** At higher magnification, malignant osteoblasts surround and invest osteoid *(eosinophilic areas)*. Mineralization is not apparent in this field. H&E stain. (Courtesy Dr. C.S. Carlson and Dr. E.J. Olson, College of Veterinary Medicine, University of Minnesota.)

causal factors have been proposed for development of fracture- or implant-associated sarcoma, including chronic infection and inflammation, local tissue reaction to the implant, corrosion of the implant and the resultant effects of corrosion products on local tissue, delayed bone healing, and decreased vascularity of the fractured bone. Osteosarcomas of viral origin are reported in mice and esophageal osteosarcomas are reported to occur subsequent to *Spirocerca lupi* infection in dogs.

A unique form of skeletal neoplasia occurs in the skull of dogs and is awkwardly called a *multilobular tumor of bone* (referred to as *chondroma rodens* in the older literature). These tumors are single, nodular, smooth-contoured, immovable masses that occur on the flat bones of the skull (bones formed by intramembranous

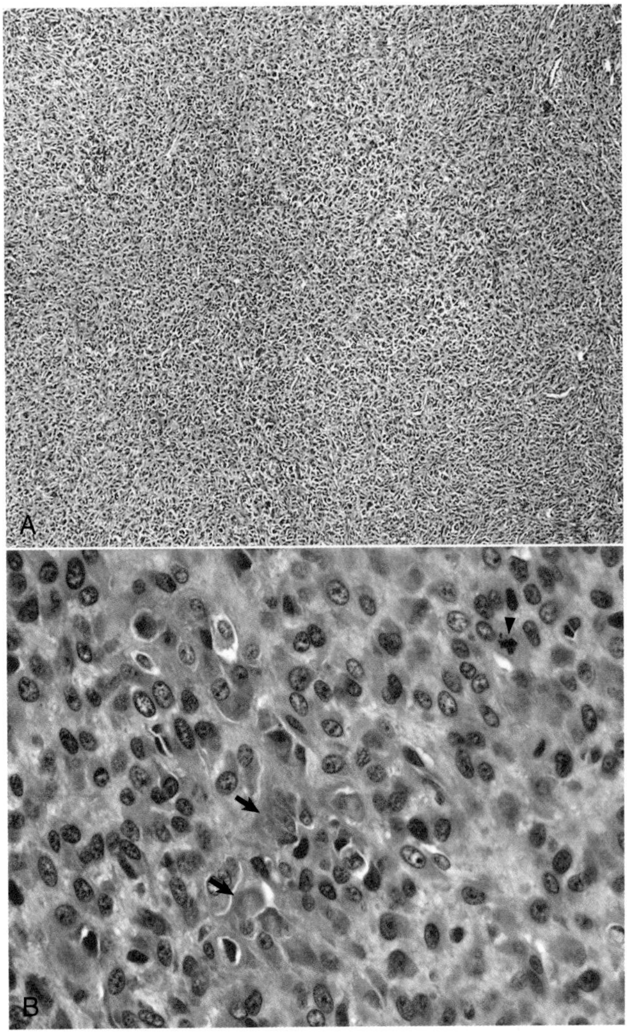

Figure 16-71 Osteosarcoma, Bone, Dog. A, An example of osteosarcoma with very little osteoid production. **B,** At higher magnification, the tumor cells exhibit atypia, mitotic figures are present *(arrowhead)*, and osteoid is recognizable *(arrows)*; compare with Figure 16-70, *B*. H&E stain. (Courtesy Dr. C.S. Carlson and Dr. E.J. Olson, College of Veterinary Medicine, University of Minnesota.)

ossification) and the hard palate. Neoplastic tissue is firm, and the cut surface is composed of multiple, gray, partially mineralized lobules separated by fibrous tissue. These neoplasms are slow growing and locally invasive and may compress and invade the brain. They metastasize to the lungs late in the clinical course; however, the metastases are frequently small and clinically silent. Histologically, these tumors consist of multiple lobules, each having centrally located cartilage or bone that is surrounded by plump mesenchymal cells that blend into well-differentiated interlobular fibrous tissue.

Various other neoplasms, such as liposarcomas, giant cell tumors, and hemangiomas/hemangiosarcomas, can arise in bone, and neoplasms such as lymphomas and plasma cell myelomas can involve the bone marrow and surrounding bone.

Secondary Neoplasms. At autopsy, 60% of human cancer patients have skeletal metastases. These metastases are predominantly in red (hematopoietic) bone marrow, in which the vascular sinusoidal system is apparently predisposed to trap circulating malignant cells. The true incidence of skeletal metastasis in animals is unknown, and estimates might be artificially low because early euthanasia shortens the course of the disease and because bone scanning and other types of clinical imaging techniques are done less often than in human beings. Metastatic neoplasms in bone can be associated with pain, hypercalcemia, lysis of bone, pathologic fracture, and reactive new bone formation. Rib shafts, vertebral bodies, and humeral and femoral metaphyses (proximal appendicular skeleton) are common sites of metastatic neoplasms in dogs, and these most commonly involve carcinomas. The most common sites of the primary tumors are the same as those in human carcinomas (mammary gland, liver, lung, and prostate). In cats, skeletal metastases are rare but, when present, appear to involve the distal appendicular skeleton. Clinically silent pulmonary carcinomas in cats are reported to metastasize to the digits, particularly the third phalanx, causing destruction of the nail bed epithelium and sloughing of the claw.

In approximately 50% of the carcinomas that are identified in the proximal appendicular skeleton in the dog, there is no clinical evidence of a primary tumor, nor is one located at postmortem, raising the possibility that these are primary intraosseous carcinomas. Primary intraosseous carcinomas are reported in the mandible and maxilla of human beings but are uncommon and are nearly always diagnosed as squamous cell carcinomas, some of which have features indicating an odontogenic origin.

Fracture Repair

Bone fractures are a common occurrence; therefore it is important to understand how and why fractures heal and, more important, why they sometimes do not heal. Fractures can be classified as *traumatic* (normal bone broken by excessive force) or *pathologic* (an abnormal bone broken by minimal trauma or by normal weight bearing). Osteopenia, osteomyelitis, and bone neoplasia are examples of lesions that can weaken a bone and predispose it to pathologic fracture.

Growth plate: The Salter-Harris classification of growth plate fractures has been widely accepted and can be readily found in texts on clinical orthopedics. This classification scheme involves up to nine different types; however, the first five types (I to V) are considered to be the most common. Fractures that involve only the growth plate (Salter-Harris I = fracture through the growth plate) and/or the primary bone trabeculae (II = fracture through growth plate and metaphysis) usually heal with few or no complications. Fractures that cross the growth plate (III = fracture through growth plate and epiphysis; and IV = fracture through growth plate, epiphysis, and metaphysis) or crush the growth plate (V) have the potential to heal with secondary growth abnormalities. Fractures that crush or cross the growth plate may irreversibly injure chondrocytes of the reserve (resting) cell layer of the growth plate or damage the branch of the epiphyseal artery that nourishes these cells. Loss of reserve cells can result in premature closure of the growth plate in these regions, potentially leading to angular limb deformities.

Trabecular bone: Fractures of trabeculae without external deformation of the cortex are called *infractions*. Inflammation and/or necrosis of bone often are predisposing factors.

Cortical bone: Fractures of cortical bone can be classified in many ways: *closed* or *simple*, if the skin is unbroken; *open* or *compound*, if the skin is broken and the bone is exposed to the external environment; *comminuted*, if the bone has been shattered into multiple small fragments; *avulsed/avulsion*, if the fracture was caused by the traction of a ligament at its insertion onto bone; *greenstick*, if one cortex of the bone is broken and the other cortex is intact so that there is no separation or displacement of the fracture site; *transverse/spiral/oblique*, depending on the orientation of the fracture line; and *compression/impacted/impaction*, in which bone fragments are compressed together.

Table 16-5 Stable Fracture Repair

Time	Tissue at Repair Site	Stability
Immediate	Hematoma	Unstable
24-48 hours	Undifferentiated mesenchymal cells and neovascularization	Unstable
36 hours	Earliest woven bone	Unstable
4-6 weeks	Primary callus of woven bone and possibly hyaline cartilage	Stable
Months to years	Modeling of woven bone into lamellar bone	Stable

Stable fracture repair means that the fracture ends have been immobilized to give relative clinical stability (not necessarily weight-bearing ability) but have not been rigidly fixed surgically (Table 16-5). The events that normally occur in the healing of a closed stable fracture of cortical bone are summarized here; however, the reader should understand that this description represents a summary of a complex process that is subject to a great deal of variation. At the time of fracture, the periosteum is torn, bone fragments are displaced, soft tissue is traumatized, and bleeding occurs to form a hematoma (Fig. 16-72). Because of impaired blood flow and the presence of isolated bone fragments, bone and marrow tissue adjacent to the fracture sites can (and often does, at least to some extent) undergo necrosis. The hematoma and tissue necrosis can be important in subsequent callus formation. Growth factors are released by macrophages and platelets in the blood clot and by the proliferating osteogenic tissue, and even from the dead bone through the lysis and acidification of the matrix. These growth factors (bone morphogenetic proteins [BMPs], TGF-β, and PDGFs, among others) are important in stimulating proliferation of repair tissue (woven bone). Undifferentiated mesenchymal cells having osteogenic potential, along with proliferating blood vessels, begin to penetrate the hematoma from the periphery in 24 to 48 hours. The mesenchymal cells are derived from the periosteum, endosteum, stem cells in the medullary cavity, and possibly from metaplasia of endothelial cells. These mesenchymal cells proliferate in the hematoma to form a loose collagenous tissue that, combined with neovascularization, has been called *granulation tissue*; however, this is misleading because the ultimate outcome of granulation tissue is fibrous tissue, whereas the mesenchymal cells in the early stages of fracture healing have the potential to undergo metaplasia to cartilage and bone. Woven bone is visible microscopically as early as 36 hours, and regenerating nerve fibers are visible in the hematoma as early as 3 days after the fracture has occurred.

The term *callus* refers to a disorganized meshwork of woven bone that forms after a fracture. It can be external (formed by the periosteum) or internal (formed between the ends of the fragments and in the medullary cavity or endosteum). This "primary" callus should bridge the gap, encircle the fracture site, and stabilize the area (Fig. 16-73). In time, woven bone at the fracture site is replaced by stronger, mature lamellar bone ("secondary" callus). Depending on the mechanical forces acting at the site, the callus can eventually be reduced in size by osteoclasts until the normal shape of the bone is restored. This process, however, might take years to complete, depending on multiple variables, including anatomic location, age, and activity level.

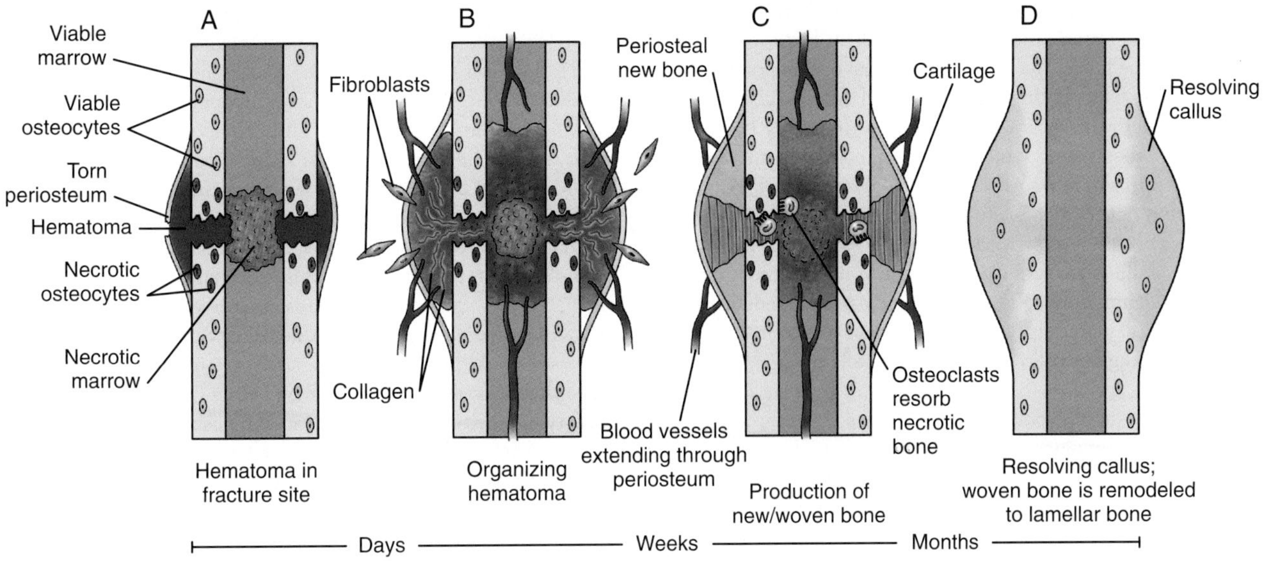

Figure 16-72 Temporal Course of Callus Formation and Fracture Repair. A, At the time of fracture, the periosteum is torn, followed by necrosis of osteocytes near the site of the fracture, hematoma formation, and necrosis of adjacent bone marrow. **B,** Over a period of days, the hematoma organizes through neovascularization and the production of collagen by fibroblasts. **C,** Over a period of weeks, the necrotic bone is resorbed by osteoclasts, cartilage forms centrally within the callus, and periosteal new bone becomes evident. **D,** Over a period of months, the cartilage and periosteal new bone are replaced by lamellar bone. Eventually, the bone is restored to its original shape (not shown).

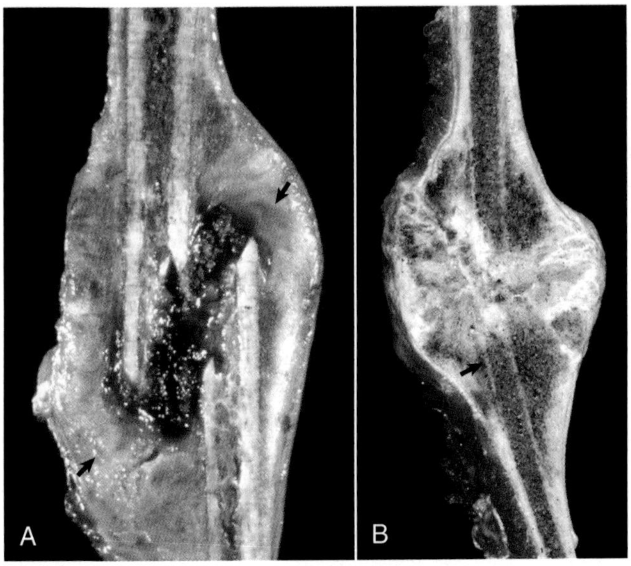

Figure 16-73 Fractures, Stable and Unstable, Bone, Rib. A, Unstable fracture. The fractured edges of the rib are improperly aligned, and there is abundant external callus composed of cartilage and bone *(arrows)*; also present are areas of fibrous tissue admixed with hemorrhage. Fibrous tissue is produced in regions of tension in an unstable fracture. **B,** Stable fracture. The fractured edges of the rib are adequately aligned, and the fracture is stabilized by abundant cartilaginous callus that is partially replaced by new bone. Note the location of the original cortex (*arrow* indicates original periosteal surface). (**A** courtesy College of Veterinary Medicine, University of Illinois. **B** courtesy Dr. F.A. Leighton, College of Veterinary Medicine, University of Saskatchewan; and Noah's Arkive, College of Veterinary Medicine, The University of Georgia.)

A callus often contains hyaline cartilage, the amount of which reflects the adequacy of the blood supply, as less than optimal oxygen supply promotes mesenchymal stem cells to differentiate into chondroblasts rather than osteoblasts. Cartilage does not provide as strong a callus as woven bone; however, it will eventually undergo endochondral ossification and therefore ultimately contribute to the formation of the bony callus.

Rigid fracture repair is usually a result of surgical intervention that involves the application of devices to keep the bone ends in contact or in very close proximity for stability during the repair process. Ideally (but rarely achieved across an entire fracture), contact healing occurs in which the fractured ends are touching each other and there is no instability. Under these conditions, healing is by direct osteonal bridging of the fracture site (E-Fig. 16-30). Osteoclasts forming channels for new osteons will cross the fracture line, and the new osteons will unite the bone without formation of a callus. If a gap less than 1 mm is present between the bone ends, bone cells will migrate from the fracture ends and form lamellar bone at a right angle to the fracture line. This will eventually model into osteonal bone parallel to the long axis of the bone. In rigid fractures with gaps greater than 1 mm, woven bone fills the gap and must be modeled into osteonal bone (E-Fig. 16-31).

The most common complications of fracture healing are inadequate blood supply, instability, and infection. If the blood supply is less than optimal, hyaline cartilage will form; if blood supply is disrupted to the point of anoxia, necrosis will occur. Mechanical tension and compression at the fracture site also influence the reparative process because excessive movement and tension favor the development of fibrous tissue. Mature fibrous tissue is not desirable; it does not stabilize the fracture and, unlike cartilage, does not act as a template for bone formation. Excessive fibrous tissue between bone ends in a fracture might result in a nonunion. With time, the bony ends of the nonunion can become smooth and move in a pocket of fibrous tissue and cartilage to form a false joint or *pseudoarthrosis*. Other factors that can interfere with the normal repair process include malnutrition and the interposition of large fragments of necrotic bone, muscle, or other soft tissue that might lead to delayed union or nonunion. Fractures heal more slowly in aged animals likely because of decreased hematopoietic marrow and its constituent stromal stem cells.

There are several complications of fracture repair specifically associated with metallic implants used in fracture stabilization.

Metallic devices that are too large deprive the bone of normal mechanical forces (stress shielding) and result in bone loss (disuse atrophy). Intramedullary fixation devices have the potential to damage the blood supply. Implanted material (metal, plastics, and bone cement) often is separated from the surrounding bone by a thin layer of fibrous tissue, sometimes accompanied by metaplastic cartilage that forms in response to operative trauma, implant mobility, or corrosion of the implant. In addition, the implant surface can be a nidus for bacterial growth, and the admixture of bacteria with amorphous host fluid can form a biofilm that is resistant to antibiotics and host inflammatory cells. Microscopic particulate debris from implanted fixation materials ("wear debris") can elicit a macrophage or multinucleated giant cell response. These inflammatory cells can release cytokines and growth factors that result in bone resorption and deterioration at the bone-implant surface, causing loosening and failure of the implant. Neoplasia thought to be induced by metallic fracture fixation devices has been reported rarely in human and veterinary literature and is usually secondary to chronic osteomyelitis but also thought to be related to the presence of metallic fragments that are shed from the implants. The mechanism by which chronic osteomyelitis could be a predisposing factor for development of osteosarcoma is not known with certainty. Generally, it is believed that any lesion that causes cell proliferation (as would be expected in chronic osteomyelitis and also in osteotomies/surgical "cutting" of bone) can increase the chance of cancer-causing spontaneous DNA damage by, for example, free radicals.

Pulmonary embolization of marrow fat from the trauma of the fracture or from trauma associated with repair of the fracture can cause severe clinical disease in human beings. Although the frequency of fat embolization secondary to trauma to the bone marrow appears to be relatively common in human beings and dogs, the clinical consequences of such embolization are relatively rare. Experimentally, fat embolization can be created readily in dogs by reaming the medullary cavity, followed by pressurization. Interestingly, fat released from the marrow cavity in dogs by reaming is greater from intact bones than from fractured bones because of decompression of the marrow cavity by the fracture in the latter.

Joints

The joints, or junctions between the bones, can be classified as those that allow essentially no movement (fibrous joint or synarthrosis [e.g., sutures between the bones of the skull]), those that allow limited movement (cartilaginous joint or amphiarthrosis [e.g., intervertebral joints]), and joints that are freely movable (synovial joint or diarthrosis [e.g., stifle joint]). The guide for postmortem examination of the joints is presented in E-Appendix 16-1.

Abnormalities of Growth and Development

Arthrogryposis. See Disorders of Ruminants (Cattle, Sheep, and Goats).

Hip Dysplasia. See Disorders of Dogs.

Inflammatory Lesions

The term *synovitis* is restricted to inflammation of the synovium, whereas the term *arthritis* implies that lesions also are present in articular cartilage. Although arthritis is characterized by the presence of inflammatory cells in the synovial membrane, the nature of the inflammatory process is often reflected best in the volume and character of the exudate in the joint fluid. In general, it is useful to classify joint diseases as inflammatory (e.g., rheumatoid arthritis) or noninflammatory (e.g., osteoarthritis, better termed *osteoarthrosis*), although some degree of inflammation may be present in noninflammatory joint disease. Arthritis also can be classified by cause (bacterial, viral, sterile immune-mediated, or urate deposits of gout), duration (acute, subacute, or chronic), or the nature of the exudate produced (serous, fibrinous, suppurative, or lymphoplasmacytic). The term *arthropathy* is all-encompassing and refers to any joint disease. Like osteomyelitis, arthritis can be a serious threat to the well-being of an animal by causing pain and leading to permanent deformity. Chronicity can be the result of an inability of the animal to remove the causative agent or substance, repeated trauma, persistence of bacterial cell wall material, or ongoing immune-mediated inflammation. If there is extensive damage to cartilage or synovium, even if the cause of the primary inflammation is cleared, the joint could progress to degenerative joint disease. In fact, end-stage rheumatoid arthritis in human beings (the prototype of inflammatory arthritis) may be indistinguishable from end-stage osteoarthritis (considered by most to be a noninflammatory condition). Injury to intraarticular structures can be the result of the offending agent or substance, inflammation, proteolytic enzymes released from cells of cartilage or synovial tissues, activation of latent matrix metalloproteinases, or failure of degenerating or necrotic chondrocytes to maintain the proteoglycan content of the matrix. Mediators of inflammation that contribute to joint injury include prostaglandins, cytokines, leukotrienes, lysosomal enzymes, free radicals, nitric oxide, neuropeptides, and products of the activated coagulation, kinin, complement, and fibrinolytic systems in synovial fluid.

Infectious Arthritis. Neonatal bacteremia secondary to omphalitis or oral-intestinal entry commonly leads to polyarthritis in lambs, calves, piglets, and foals. Although less common, bacteria can also reach the joint by direct inoculation (as in a puncture wound), by direct extension from periarticular soft tissue, or by extension from adjacent bone. Bacterial osteomyelitis can extend through the cortex at the metaphysis into the joint (see Figs. 16-35 to 16-37) (especially in young animals in which the cortex at this site is thin or incomplete). Alternatively, epiphyseal osteomyelitis can lyse directly through articular cartilage (see Fig. 16-54). Bacterial arthritis is not common in dogs or cats. In a retrospective study in a university veterinary hospital, most cases of bacterial arthritis in dogs involved the stifle and occurred as surgical complications.

The lesions of infectious arthritis may be very similar regardless of the inciting agent; therefore the lesions in the next section are presented by time frame and whether the initial exudates are primarily neutrophilic (suppurative arthritis) or fibrinous (fibrinous arthritis) (see Table 16-2 and Fig. 16-74).

Articular cartilage: The response of cartilage to inflammation depends on the nature and severity of the exudates. In acute inflammation, independent of the nature of the initial exudate, the articular cartilage is grossly and microscopically normal. In subacute suppurative or fibrinous arthritis, cartilage may be thinned due to lysis and erosion (see previous discussion) of collagenous matrix by the enzymes in the exudates, activation of matrix metalloproteinases, and collapse of the cartilage as a result of a loss and failure to replace the water-binding proteoglycans by the degenerate or necrotic chondrocytes. In chronic suppurative arthritis, extensive cartilage erosion and ulceration is expected. In chronic fibrinous arthritis, cartilage ulceration may occur but not as consistently as with chronic suppurative arthritis. Pannus formation also may occur in chronic fibrinous arthritis, resulting in cartilage erosion and ulceration, but is unusual with chronic suppurative arthritis. In chronic infectious arthritis in which there is no acute exudate in the joint, cartilage loss might be mild and occurs secondary to low-grade lymphoplasmacytic synovitis (see later discussion).

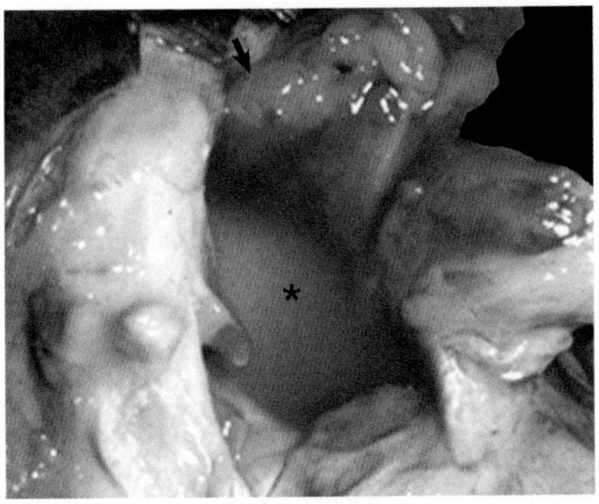

Figure 16-74 **Serofibrinous Arthritis, Tibiotarsal Joint, Foal.** Opened joint reveals increased amounts of cloudy, yellow synovial fluid *(asterisk)* characteristic of serofibrinous arthritis of nonspecific cause; synovial proliferation *(arrow)* indicates some degree of chronicity. (Courtesy University of Minnesota Veterinary Diagnostic Laboratory Archive.)

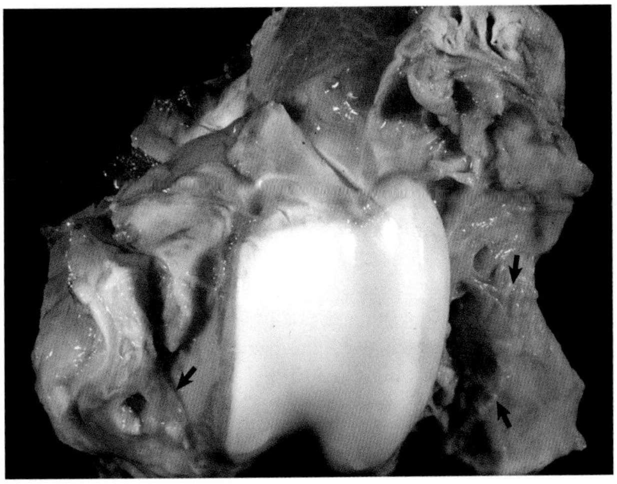

Figure 16-75 **Acute Fibrinous Arthritis, Bone, Tibial-Tarsal Joint (Hock), Calf.** The joint space is distended by layers of yellowish-brown fibrin that coat the synovial surface *(arrows)* of the joint capsule; articular cartilage is white and glistening. (Courtesy Dr. C.S. Patton, College of Veterinary Medicine, University of Tennessee.)

Articular capsule/synovium/synovial fluid: In acute suppurative and fibrinous arthritis, the synovial fluid is usually reduced in viscosity because of a combination of enzymatic digestion of the glycosaminoglycans and dilution of the synovial fluid with edema fluid. The fluid may be turbid due to the presence of neutrophils and strands of fibrin and may be reddened due to mild hemorrhage. Exudate in the synovial fluid can be extensive in acute lesions (Fig. 16-75), whereas the synovial membrane may appear only slightly hyperemic and edematous, even microscopically. Therefore, in acute arthritis, evaluation of synovial fluid may be much more informative than evaluation of synovial membrane; however, to increase the likelihood of a correct diagnosis, it may be prudent to culture both sites and to evaluate the synovial membrane histologically. In acute fibrinous or suppurative bacterial arthritis that has been treated effectively with antibiotics, the lesions may resolve without residual defects.

In subacute suppurative and fibrinous arthritis and subacute infectious arthritis in which there was no acute exudation into the joint, the synovium is expected to contain lymphoplasmacytic inflammation and exhibit variable hyperplasia of synovial lining cells, regardless of the cause (Fig. 16-76). The lymphoplasmacytic inflammation reflects the immunogenicity of the infectious agent. The synovial cell hyperplasia is a nonspecific response but presumably is an attempt to increase production of synovial fluid. In subacute (and chronic) suppurative and fibrinous arthritis, it is uncommon to find significant numbers of neutrophils and fibrin deposits, respectively, in the synovial membrane because they are expected to exude from the membrane and enter the joint space.

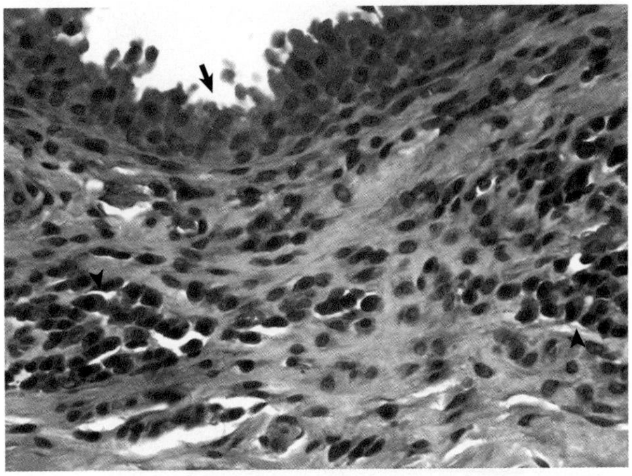

Figure 16-76 **Subacute Synovitis, Joint Capsule, Dog.** There is marked synovial cell hyperplasia *(arrow)* and infiltration of lymphocytes and plasma cells into the synovial subintima *(arrowheads)*. H&E stain. (Courtesy Dr. S.E. Weisbrode, College of Veterinary Medicine, The Ohio State University.)

In chronic suppurative arthritis, granulation tissue with pronounced lymphoplasmacytic inflammation can replace the synovial membrane and there can be notable fibrosis of the articular capsule. If fibrinous arthritis persists and if deposits of fibrin are extensive, they may be replaced by fibrous tissue, leading to restricted articular movement. Fibrinous arthritis (e.g., caused by *Erysipelothrix rhusiopathiae* and *Mycoplasma* sp. [see later discussion]) of long duration is often accompanied by pronounced villous hypertrophy/hyperplasia, lymphoplasmacytic synovitis and pannus formation, and progressive destruction of cartilage (Fig. 16-77). In both chronic fibrinous arthritis and chronic suppurative arthritis, fibrin and suppurative exudate (pus) continue to be produced and are present in the joint space in active (bacteria is still present) lesions. Fibrous ankylosis (rigidity/fusion) of joints can occur in severe chronic cases of either fibrinous or suppurative arthritis.

Subchondral bone: Subchondral bone is affected only secondarily in infectious arthritis. In chronic suppurative arthritis, the exudates can erode the overlying cartilage and extend into the subchondral bone plate (Fig. 16-78). If there is severe chronic lameness, the subchondral bone may undergo disuse atrophy and become osteopenic.

Bacterial Arthritis. Many different bacteria cause arthritis in animals. The duration of bacterial arthritis is variable; some organisms are rapidly removed and synovitis is short-lived. In other instances, bacteria can persist, and the inflammatory process can become chronic but remain active. The extent and mechanism of cartilage destruction differ somewhat depending on the nature of the exudates. In turn, the nature of the exudates can depend on the infectious agent involved. Generally, fibrinous inflammation is expected more often with Gram-negative bacteria, whereas suppurative arthritis is expected more often with Gram-positive bacteria. The exudates in the joint in acute stages of infection with

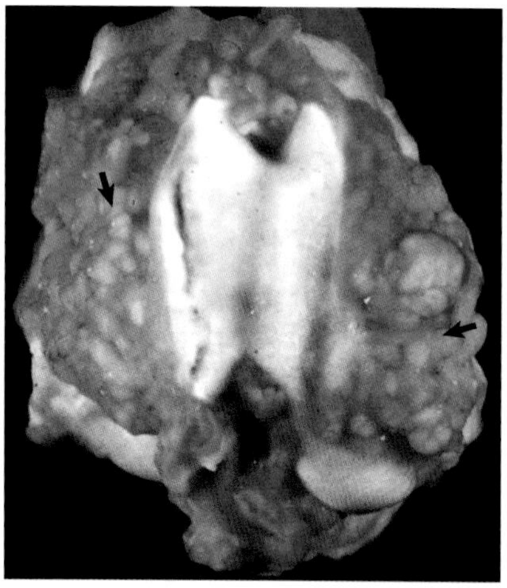

Figure 16-77 **Chronic Fibrinous (Active) Synovitis, Erysipelas, Stifle Joint, Pig.** A chronic arthritis caused by *Erysipelothrix rhusiopathiae* has resulted in villous hypertrophy *(arrows)* of the synovial membrane. The tips of some villi are hemorrhagic and necrotic. (Courtesy Dr. D. Harrington, College of Veterinary Medicine, Purdue University; and Noah's Arkive, College of Veterinary Medicine, The University of Georgia.)

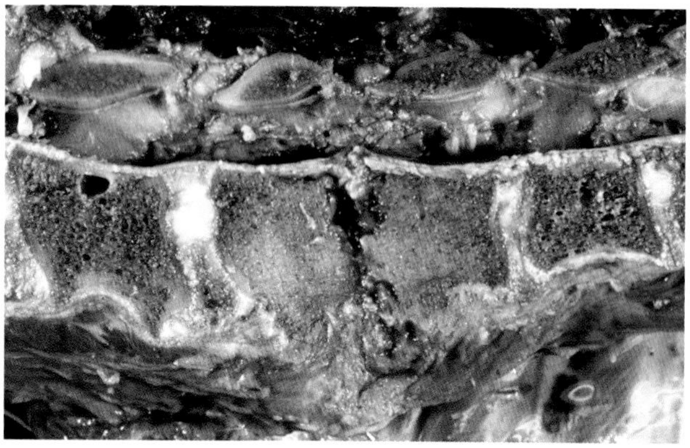

Figure 16-78 **Suppurative Diskospondylitis, Joint, Intervertebral Disk, Dog.** Chronic marked suppurative diskospondylitis (inflammation of the intervertebral disk and adjacent vertebrae) with marked lysis *(center of image)* of the disk and cortices, epiphyses, and metaphyses of the adjacent vertebrae. (Courtesy Dr. S.E. Weisbrode, College of Veterinary Medicine, The Ohio State University.)

Gram-positive bacteria, however, can be primarily fibrinous but become suppurative with time. An example of chronic fibrinous arthritis occurs in pigs in which the cause is *Erysipelothrix rhusiopathiae* septicemia. This is a notable exception to the previous generality about fibrinous inflammation being caused by Gram-negative bacteria. *Erysipelothrix rhusiopathiae*, a Gram-positive bacterial organism, causes a fibrinous arthritis that does not become suppurative with time. Survivors may have lesions secondary to localization of *Erysipelothrix rhusiopathiae* in the skin, synovial joints, valvular endocardium, or intervertebral disks. Chronic painful polyarthritis is a common sequela. *Trueperella* (formerly *Arcanobacterium*) *pyogenes* is a common cause of suppurative arthritis in cattle and pigs. *Escherichia coli* and streptococci initially cause septicemia in neonatal calves and piglets before localizing in joints, meninges, and, sometimes, serosal surfaces. The synovitis often is acutely serofibrinous, becoming more suppurative with time. *Haemophilus parasuis* causes Glässer's disease in pigs 8 to 16 weeks of age. Lesions consist of fibrinous polyserositis, polyarthritis, and meningitis. Acute serofibrinous polyarthritis is seen frequently in cattle dying of thrombotic meningoencephalitis caused by *Histophilus somni* (formerly *Haemophilus somnus*).

Borrelia burgdorferi, a spirochete, is the tick-borne cause of Lyme disease (borreliosis). Arthritis occurs with Lyme disease in dogs, cattle, and horses and affects single or multiple joints. In experimental studies in dogs, lameness developed in approximately half of the infected animals 2 months or longer after infection. In the acute stages of the disease, the exudate is a combination of fibrinous and suppurative (fibrinosuppurative) inflammation. In the chronic stages, pannus (usually a sequela to fibrinous arthritis) and chronic suppurative inflammation can be seen.

Mycoplasma Arthritis. Generally, the lesions of arthritis caused by *Mycoplasma* sp. are similar to those described previously for bacteria causing fibrinous arthritis. Multiple joints usually are involved, indicative of a hematogenous route of infection. *Mycoplasma hyorhinis* causes fibrinous polyarthritis and polyserositis in weanling pigs, and *Mycoplasma hyosynoviae* causes fibrinous polyarthritis in pigs older than 3 months of age. It is not certain how these mycoplasmas/-ata gain access to the circulation and, ultimately, the joints; however, the route is likely oral-pharyngeal/pulmonary facilitated by stress or concurrent respiratory disease, as both agents are commonly isolated from nasal and pharyngeal regions in asymptomatic individuals.

Mycoplasma bovis causes fibrinous to pyogranulomatous polyarthritis in feedlot cattle, and the disease is characterized by lameness and swelling of the large synovial joints of the limbs, which can contain large volumes of serofibrinous to frankly suppurative exudate. *Mycoplasma bovis* likely gains access to joints through a hematogenous route, possibly secondary to mycoplasma pneumonia or mastitis.

Viral Arthritis. Reoviral arthritis in chickens was the first viral arthritis to be discovered, and it has been followed by the discovery of reoviral arthritis in turkeys. Although it was hoped that a viral etiology also would be demonstrated in idiopathic arthritides such as rheumatoid arthritis, viral arthritis does not appear to be a significant, or even recognized, disease in domestic mammals other than in goats. The caprine arthritis-encephalitis (CAE) virus (a lentiviral retrovirus) causes chronic fibrinous arthritis in older goats. The disease is characterized by debilitating lameness, carpal hygromas (fluid-filled sac on the affected joints), and distention of the larger synovial joints. Chronic cases exhibit lymphoplasmacytic synovitis, synovial villous hypertrophy/hyperplasia, and pannus formation typical of chronic fibrinous arthritis. An additional lesion that is peculiar to chronic cases of this disease is necrosis and mineralization of synovial villi that may give the membrane a chalky white appearance.

Noninfectious Arthritis. Noninfectious arthritis includes specific joint diseases that have inflammation as the initiating event but are known to be sterile. These disorders are often classified as erosive or nonerosive, depending on whether or not the articular cartilage is involved. Three examples of sterile erosive arthritis follow. These diseases often are chronic, sometimes lasting for months, because they can be very difficult to control medically (e.g., with antiinflammatory and immunomodulatory agents).

Rheumatoid Arthritis. See Disorders of Dogs.

Reactive Arthritis. *Reactive arthritis* is the name given to a sterile erosive oligoarthritis (affecting a small number of joints) of uncertain pathogenesis. This condition is rarely reported in domestic animals but is a recognized problem in primate research colonies as occurring subsequent to diarrheal disease and is likely to be underdiagnosed in other species. Reactive arthritis is defined clinically as sterile inflammation in joints that occurs subsequent to infectious inflammation in other organ systems—usually intestinal and urogenital in human beings and usually caused by bacteria such as *Yersinia*, *Salmonella*, *Campylobacter*, and *Shigella*. Several hypotheses have been presented that are not mutually exclusive, including cross-reactivity (molecular mimicry) between bacterial heat-shock proteins and articular glycosaminoglycans, inexplicable homing of sensitized gut lymphocytes to joints, and unexplained localization of antigenic bacterial peptidoglycans in joints.

Postinfectious Sterile Arthritis. Postinfectious sterile arthritis is suspected to represent the immune reaction to antigenic breakdown products of bacterial cell walls that can remain sequestered in a joint after a confirmed bacterial infection within the joint. A description of the lesions occurring in all three types of erosive, noninfectious arthritis follows.

Articular cartilage: Cartilage erosion that is clearly related to the presence of pannus is expected at the subacute phases of disease and is later followed by ulceration that may be extensive.

Articular capsule/synovium/synovial fluid: Grossly, the lesions in advanced cases consist of marked villous hypertrophy/hyperplasia of the synovial membrane, pannus formation that may appear as a velvet-like layer overlying the subchondral bone, periarticular osteophytes, and, in some cases, fibrous ankylosis of affected joints. Microscopically, the alterations in the joint include hypertrophy/hyperplasia of synovial lining cells and infiltration of the synovium by large numbers of plasma cells and lymphocytes. In addition, necrotic foci, fibrinous exudate, and infiltrating neutrophils may be present. The synovial fluid contains large numbers of neutrophils.

Subchondral bone: Particularly in cases of active disease in which there is pannus formation, subchondral bone exhibits lytic changes. Secondary osteoarthritis may be present in chronic disease and may result in subchondral bone sclerosis.

Nonerosive Noninfectious Arthritis. Nonerosive noninfectious arthritis has been best described in the dog. Most cases are idiopathic symmetric oligoarthritides, but they can be associated with concurrent sterile immune-mediated diseases such as steroid responsive meningitis/arteritis, neoplasia, infectious inflammation in other organ systems (nonerosive reactive arthritis), and systemic lupus erythematosus (SLE). Dogs with SLE may also have dermatitis, anemia, thrombocytopenia, polymyositis, and glomerulonephritis. It is not clear why nonerosive noninfectious arthritis, which is thought to be mediated by synoviotropic immune complexes, does not result in articular destruction, as occurs in rheumatoid arthritis.

Articular cartilage: Articular cartilage lesions are not expected in nonerosive arthritis, even in chronic cases.

Articular capsule/synovium/synovial fluid: Villous hypertrophy/hyperplasia can be minimal to marked, with variable neutrophilic and lymphoplasmacytic synovitis. Pannus formation does not occur; the exudate in the synovial fluid in chronic nonerosive arthritis is neutrophilic.

Subchondral bone: Subchondral bone lesions are not expected in nonerosive arthritis.

In sterile inflammatory joint disease, a definitive diagnosis is often not possible. It should be remembered that response to antibiotics does not confirm that a process was a result of infectious agents. Antibiotics that reduce Gram-positive bacteria in the intestine may allow coliform overgrowth and increased lipopolysaccharide (LPS) production. Increased intestinal absorption of LPS is associated with decreased clinical signs in autoimmune arthritis, possibly by downregulation of the immune system or by establishing a more rigorous immunologic recognition of self.

Crystal Deposition Disease. Crystal deposition disease is characterized by deposits of minerals, such as urates, calcium phosphates, and calcium pyrophosphates, in articular cartilage and/or the soft tissue of joints. Clinical disease caused by crystal deposition is rare in domestic mammals. Species that lack the enzyme uricase (certain nonhuman primates, birds, and reptiles), an enzyme that promotes the oxidation of uric acid to allantoin, may experience excessive accumulation of uric acid in the bloodstream. Crystal-induced synovitis with secondary degeneration of articular cartilage occurs when urate crystals are deposited in and around joints, a condition known as *gout*. Deposits of urate, called *tophi*, incite a granulomatous inflammation and can appear grossly as white caseous material. Joint disease involving one or multiple joints also has been reported in young dogs resulting from deposition of calcium and phosphorus in different forms (calcium pyrophosphate deposition disease [CPDD; formerly known as pseudogout] and calcium phosphate deposition disease) in the soft tissue of the synovium, articular capsule, and adjacent ligaments. Underlying metabolic disease in this condition is not recognized. Intraarticular crystal deposition disease is perhaps the most common of the crystal deposition diseases but usually is clinically silent. This condition is usually caused by calcium pyrophosphate deposition and may occur in locations in horses and dogs that are subjected to increased mechanical use (scapulohumeral joint of racing dogs and metacarpophalangeal and metatarsophalangeal joints of horses). The crystal deposition is initiated around the chondrocytes and can be seen grossly as bright white gritty foci. The significance of the deposition is uncertain, but it might play a role in the progression of degenerative joint disease.

Degenerative Joint Disease

Degenerative joint disease (osteoarthritis, osteoarthrosis), recognized since antiquity, is a destructive disease of synovial joints that occurs in all animals with a bony skeleton (Table 16-6). It can be monoarticular (affecting a single joint) or polyarticular (affecting multiple joints), can occur in immature or mature animals, and can be symptomatic or clinically silent. Affected animals have variable degrees of joint enlargement and deformity, pain, and articular malfunction. The etiopathogenesis of degenerative joint disease is incompletely understood, and it is likely that the term encompasses a variety of diseases that have a common end stage (E-Fig. 16-32). Initial changes can be the result of traumatic injury to articular cartilage; inflammation of the synovium; increased stiffness of the subchondral bone; or abnormalities in conformation, joint stability, and congruence of joint surfaces. The number one risk factor for degenerative joint disease in human beings is age, although the disease is not considered to be an inevitable consequence of aging. Most cases in human beings are primary (no identifiable cause); however, most cases in animals appear to be secondary, with osteochondrosis being an important predisposing factor in those species having a high prevalence of this disease.

The initial biochemical change in articular cartilage in degenerative joint disease is loss of proteoglycan aggregates. In the early stages of degeneration, this loss of proteoglycans is associated with an increase in water content in the cartilage matrix that causes swelling of the tissue. This may seem contradictory because proteoglycans in normal cartilage play a critical role in binding water. The explanation is not clear; however, the increased water in the matrix in early degenerative joint disease is not bound normally to the proteoglycans and does not contribute to the normal lubrication and flushing of nutrients and waste products. In addition, core proteins of proteoglycan aggregates are susceptible to the action of neutral proteoglycanases, which are increased in early degenerative joint disease. In electron micrographs, the findings in early degenerative joint disease include focal loss of the amorphous layer covering the surface of the articular cartilage and fraying of the superficial

Table 16-6 Degenerative Joint Disease

Name of Stage	Gross Appearance	Microscopic Lesion
Early degeneration	Normal; articular cartilage may be somewhat softened on palpation	Mild increase in thickness of articular cartilage; decreased proteoglycan content apparent with histochemical stains for sulfated polysaccharides (e.g., toluidine blue and safranin O)
Mild	May appear normal; articular cartilage may contain superficial erosions and may have normal or reduced thickness	Degenerative changes involving superficial articular cartilage, including chondrocyte degeneration/death and superficial fibrillation
Moderate	Articular cartilage contains locally extensive areas of fibrillation (frayed appearance)	Loss of articular cartilage integrity, with fibrillation and loss of tissue extending into middle and deep zones; this change may be accompanied by a mild synovitis, locally extensive increased thickness of subchondral bone, and the presence of periarticular osteophytes
Chronic	Full thickness loss of articular cartilage with exposure of the subchondral bone, which is thickened; the surface of the thickened subchondral bone may be smooth (eburnation); osteophytes may be grossly visible and joint capsule is thickened	Loss of cartilage to the level of the subchondral bone; subchondral bone may be severely thickened; periarticular osteophytes are often present; subchondral cysts may be present; synovium exhibits chronic inflammation and fibrosis

collagen fibers. Continued proteoglycan loss interferes with joint lubrication and allows collagen fibers to collapse along lines perpendicular to the joint surface because of the loss of the hydrated gel of proteoglycans and water that normally keeps the fibers separated.

Synovitis in degenerative joint disease is generally mild and occurs secondary to release of inflammatory mediators by injured chondrocytes and from synovial macrophages that have phagocytosed cartilaginous breakdown products.

Articular cartilage: Lesions often are topographically variable within a joint. The loss of proteoglycans and improper binding of water (actual increase in water content) causes the articular cartilage to become soft (*chondromalacia*). In hinge-type joints, linear grooves often are present in the articular cartilage, particularly in horses (see Fig. 16-15). Histologically, these represent linear depressions in the cartilage associated with scattered necrotic chondrocytes and localized loss of proteoglycan. The pathogenesis of these grooves is uncertain, but they might represent sequelae to jetties of synovial fluid secondary to incongruities of the joint surfaces. Alternatively, these may appear on an opposite joint surface to a lesion such as a chip fracture, in which case direct mechanical injury is more likely. Chondromalacia is followed by abnormal wearing of the cartilage and loss of superficial articular cartilage (early erosion). As the lesions progress, erosions becomes deeper (cartilage becomes thinner) and grossly apparent fraying of collagen fibers along their radial arrangement can be seen (*fibrillation* [see Figs. 16-25 and 16-26]). This outcome can be appreciated grossly as a roughened, opaque articular surface, often with discoloration of the cartilage to yellow or brown. Advanced lesions can have notable loss of cartilage to the level of the calcified layer and subchondral bone (*ulceration* [see Fig. 16-27]).

Articular capsule/synovium/synovial fluid: Synovitis characterized by villous hypertrophy, hyperplasia of synoviocytes, and infiltration of lymphocytes, plasma cells, and macrophages is usually present in chronic cases, but the magnitude of the inflammation is considerably less than that occurring in inflammatory arthritides. The synovial fluid does not contain exudates and is clear and colorless but might have reduced viscosity because of increased plasma filtrate relative to glycosaminoglycans in the synovial fluid and increased degradation of glycosaminoglycans by enzymes released by the inflamed synovium. Fibrosis of the articular capsule caused by instability of the joint or release of cytokines, such as TGF-β, might contribute, along with osteophytosis and joint incongruity, to the joint stiffness and limited range of motion seen in advanced degenerative joint disease.

Subchondral bone: In advanced disease, sclerosis of subchondral bone, which may be severe, is a consistent finding. Some investigators consider a mild increase in subchondral bone thickness to be an early lesion of degenerative joint disease, possibly preceding articular cartilage damage. If the articular cartilage is ulcerated and the joint remains in use, the exposed subchondral bone may develop a smooth, polished appearance (eburnation). Marginal (periarticular) osteophytes form, particularly with joint instability, and there can be pronounced modeling of the epiphyseal and metaphyseal bone because of altered mechanical use. Joint fusion, caused by a combination of bony or fibrous bridging (ankylosis) of the joint space, may occur (E-Fig. 16-33). Subchondral bone cysts, cavities in the subchondral bone with a synovial-like lining and peripheral osteoclastic bone lysis and fibrosis, may be present, particularly in severe cases. Presumably, these cysts arise secondary to fissures in the overlying cartilage or eburnated bone that allow synovial fluid to be forced into the subchondral bone. These cysts appear to be more common in human beings than in domestic animals, possibly the result of the longer duration of the disease in human beings. The Hartley guinea pig spontaneously develops degenerative joint disease in the stifle joints before 1 year of age. Subchondral cysts are present in the proximal tibial articular surface, and in this model, they appear to be invaginations of synovial membranes surrounding the cruciate ligaments as they insert into the subchondral bone.

Degeneration of Intervertebral Disks

Degeneration of the intervertebral disks is an age-related phenomenon in many species. In general, loss of water and proteoglycans, reduced cellularity, and an increase in collagen content of the nucleus pulposus occur so that the distinction between the nucleus pulposus and the annulus fibrosus is obscured. Grossly, the central part of the degenerated disk is yellow-brown and is composed of friable fibrocartilaginous material (Fig. 16-79). These degenerative changes are likely caused by various metabolic and mechanical insults that lead to a breakdown of proteoglycan aggregates in the nucleus pulposus and to degenerative changes in the annulus

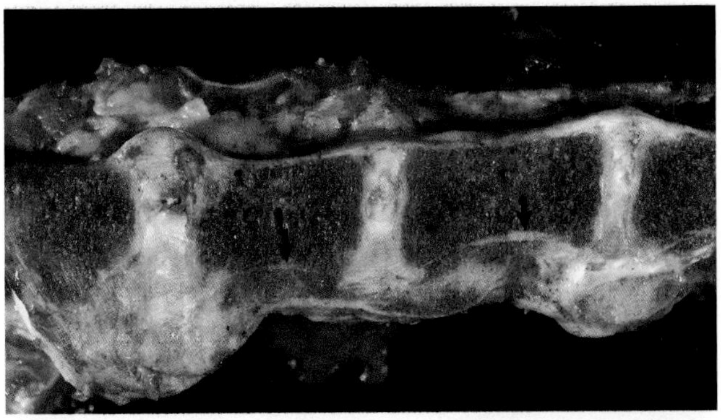

Figure 16-79 **Ankylosing Spondylosis and Intervertebral Disk Disease, Lumbar Spine, Dog.** The bony proliferation (ventrally) has bridged the intervertebral spaces between the adjacent vertebrae and caused fusion (ankylosis) of several joints; proliferative new bone is present ventral to the preexisting vertebral cortical surface *(arrows)*. Intervertebral disks are discolored (mottled yellow-green) and exhibit variable dorsal protrusion into the spinal canal. (Courtesy Dr. M.S. Bouljihad and Dr. N.A. Robinson, College of Veterinary Medicine, University of Minnesota.)

fibrosus. Both rotational and compressive types of movement may further injure the annulus fibrosus. Changes in structure of the nucleus pulposus, together with a weakened annulus, often lead to concentric and radial tears or fissures in the annulus that allow bulging or herniation of the nucleus pulposus material (Fig. 16-80). Herniation usually occurs dorsally in domestic animals due, in part, to the fact that the annulus fibrosus is thinner dorsally than ventrally. In human beings (rarely in domestic animals), disk material can be extruded through the end plate into the vertebral body, producing a lesion known as a *Schmorl's node*.

In chondrodystrophic breeds of dogs, such as the dachshund, chondroid metaplasia of the nucleus pulposus is followed by calcification during the first year of life. These alterations can result in disk prolapse, with total rupture of the annulus fibrosus and often rapid or acute extrusion of disk material into the vertebral canal at sites of mechanical stress such as the cervical and thoracolumbar vertebrae (Hansen type I herniation) (Fig. 16-81 and E-Fig. 16-34; also see Fig. 16-80).

Senile degenerative disk disease is independent of breed in the dog and also occurs in pigs and horses. These lesions are characterized by progressive dehydration and collagenization of the nucleus pulposus and degeneration of the annulus fibrosus. The lesions develop slowly and calcification is rare. Prolapse of the disk is secondary to partial rupture of the annulus fibrosus and is characterized by bulging of the dorsal surface of the disk into the vertebral canal (Hansen type II herniation) (Fig. 16-82; also see Fig. 16-80). Prolapse or herniation can be dorsal (spinal cord compression) or lateral (spinal nerve compression and entrapment). Because each intervertebral joint is a three-joint complex (intervertebral joint and two facet joints), the reduced disk thickness that follows degeneration and dehydration allows overriding of articular facets and some degree of joint instability. These changes contribute to the development of degenerative disease and enlargement of articular facets, which may cause impingement on spinal nerves and even compression of the spinal canal because the medial aspect of these facets is adjacent to the intervertebral foramen. Degeneration of intervertebral disks (often in the ventral annulus fibrosus, leading to stretching of the ventral longitudinal ligament) and the ensuing intervertebral joint instability can result in the development of periosteal new bone formation on the ventral (most commonly), lateral, or dorsal surfaces of the vertebrae. This is termed *spondylosis*; occurs in many

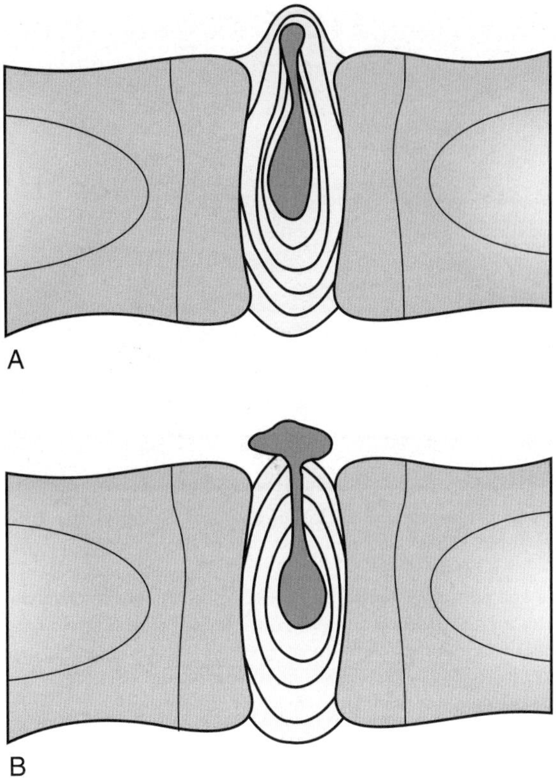

Figure 16-80 **Stages of Prolapse of the Nucleus Pulposus in Intervertebral Disk Disease. A,** Prolapse of the nucleus pulposus may be secondary to partial rupture of the annulus fibrosus (Hansen type II). **B,** Complete rupture of the annulus fibrosus allows extrusion of the nucleus pulposus into the vertebral canal (Hansen type I).

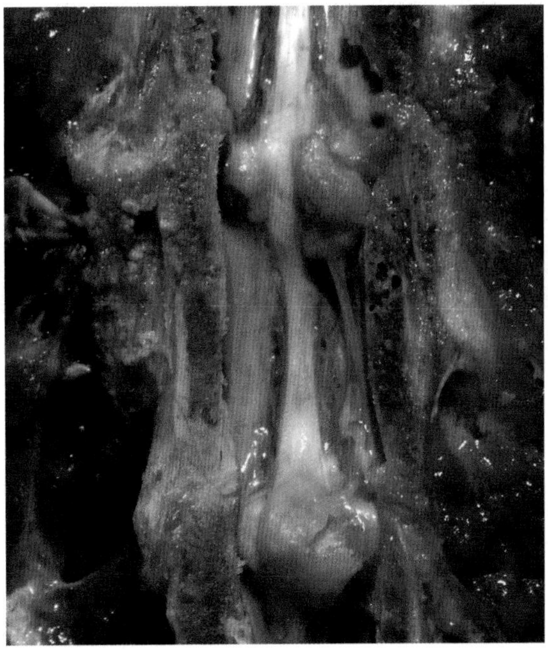

Figure 16-81 **Intervertebral Disk Disease, Degenerate Intervertebral Disk, Prolapsed Disk, Intervertebral Joint, Dog.** The dorsal arches and spinal cord have been removed to demonstrate two sites in which there is dorsal extrusion of intervertebral disk material into the spinal canal. (Courtesy Dr. M.D. Chalkley and Dr. E.J. Olson, College of Veterinary Medicine, University of Minnesota.)

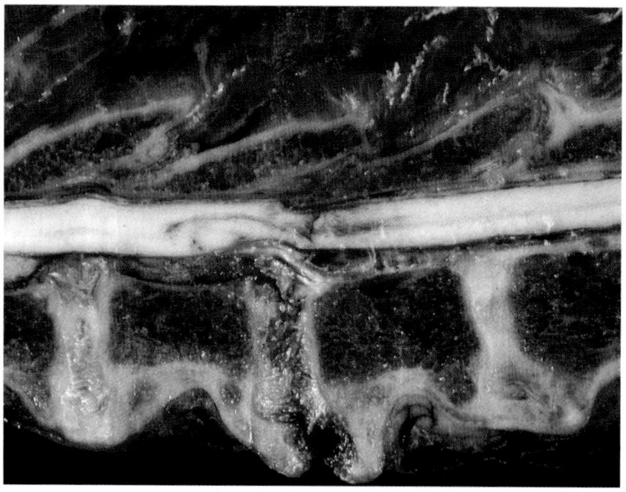

Figure 16-82 **Intervertebral Disk Disease and Spondylosis, Intervertebral Joint, Dog.** Longitudinal section of thoracic vertebrae showing three adjacent intervertebral disks, all exhibiting varying degrees of degeneration and associated ventral spondylosis. The central intervertebral disk has extruded into the overlying spinal canal causing compression and hemorrhage of the spinal cord. A fractured spondylosis lesion is present ventrally and may have contributed to local instability. (Courtesy Dr. A.G. Armién, College of Veterinary Medicine, University of Minnesota.)

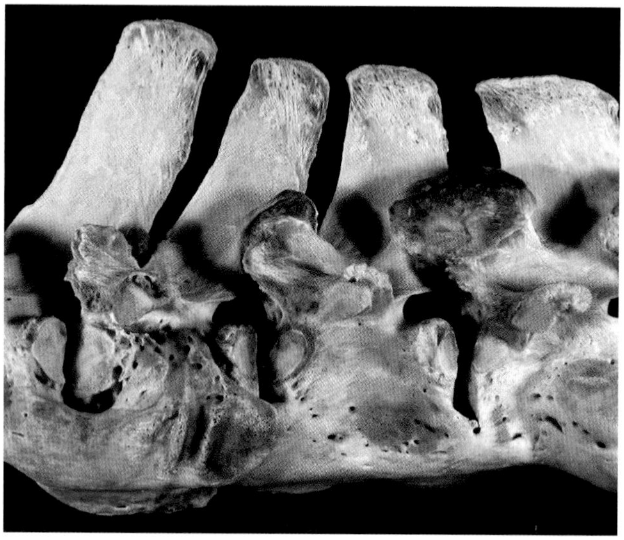

Figure 16-83 **Ankylosing Spondylosis, Thoracic Spine, Moose.** Marked ventral and lateral periosteal proliferation in this severe case of ankylosing spondylosis has resulted in bony bridging of adjacent vertebral bodies. Macerated specimen. (Courtesy Dr. E.J. Olson and Dr. A. Wuenschmann, College of Veterinary Medicine, University of Minnesota.)

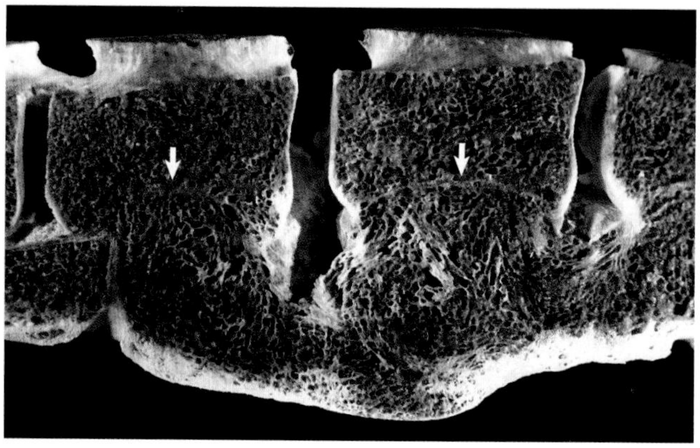

Figure 16-84 **Ankylosing Spondylosis, Spine, Dog.** Mid-longitudinal section of vertebral column demonstrating marked bony proliferation forming a bony bridge between adjacent vertebral bodies; preexisting ventral margins of vertebral bodies *(arrows)*. Macerated specimen. (Courtesy Dr. B.A. Goupil, Dr. E.J. Olson, and Dr. A. Wuenschmann, College of Veterinary Medicine, University of Minnesota.)

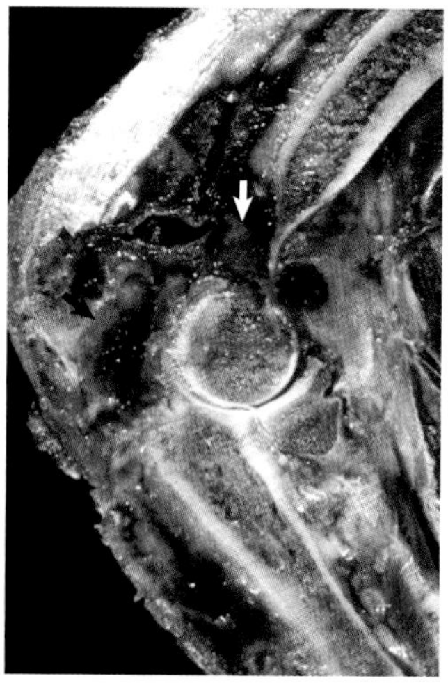

Figure 16-85 **Synovial Cell Sarcoma, Joint, Elbow, Dog.** Synovial cell sarcoma presenting as a tan and hemorrhagic mass within the joint has invaded into the distal humeral condyle *(white arrow)* and caused pronounced lysis of the proximal ulna *(black arrow)*. (Courtesy Dr. S.E. Weisbrode, College of Veterinary Medicine, The Ohio State University.)

species, including dogs, cattle, pigs, and horses; and may lead to bony fusion (ankylosis) of several adjacent intervertebral joints (Figs. 16-83 and 16-84; also see Fig. 16-82 and E-Fig. 16-34; also see E-Fig. 16-33).

Neoplasms

Primary neoplasms within joints arise from the synovial membrane and are considered to be malignant, but they vary notably in their metastatic potential. These tumors are uncommon in dogs and very rare in other species. Two different malignancies of the synovium are recognized. One is derived from histiocytes and is called a *histiocytic sarcoma*. As the name implies, these cells have a histiocytic phenotype; atypia is sometimes extreme with bizarre mitotic figures and pronounced pleomorphism. Histiocytic sarcomas have a high probability of distant metastasis.

Synovial cell sarcoma is the term given to a malignancy of synovial fibrocyte origin (Fig. 16-85). These tumors are more common in joints but may also occur in synovia of tendon sheaths. The malignant cells comprising synovial cell sarcoma are immunonegative for histiocytic cell markers (e.g., CD18) and immunopositive for mesenchymal markers (vimentin); inexplicably, a small percentage are immunopositive for epithelial markers (cytokeratins). Such epithelial cell expression is not found in the synovia of normal joints. Synovial cell sarcomas have a moderate to low chance of distant metastasis. Some fibrocytic cell tumors in the synovium have notable myxomatous metaplasia and have been called *myxomas*. Myxomas sometimes exhibit infiltrative behavior, including invasion of bone, and are considered low-grade malignancies but do not appear to have metastatic potential.

Articular cartilage: Articular cartilage is usually not affected other than secondarily as a result of a loss of subchondral bone support caused by invasion by the tumor.

Articular capsule/synovium/synovial fluid: Grossly, the synovium can be markedly and asymmetrically thickened by the presence of a gray to tan mass; myxomas have a gelatinous appearance. Microscopically, synovial sarcomas have the appearance of a moderate- to low-grade fibrosarcoma, with little collagen production. Myxomas are characterized by the presence of multiple myxomatous islands.

Subchondral bone: Radiographically, all three tumor types may exhibit evidence of invasion into subchondral and periosteal bone, usually on both sides of the joint space and ranging from minimal to extensive. However, this bone invasion can be subtle and often is not apparent on gross examination.

Tendons and Ligaments

Of the 33 million musculoskeletal injuries reported in the United States in human beings each year, roughly 50% involve injuries to the soft tissue, including tendons and ligaments. These injuries also are common in veterinary medicine, particularly in dogs and horses. Traumatic injuries may result in either partial or complete ligament or tendon discontinuities. Aging changes that occur in tendons/ligaments, including chondroid metaplasia, ischemia, and local fibroblastic proliferations, may make them more susceptible to traumatic injury, although these changes often are present in animals with intact tendons/ligaments.

Degeneration and rupture of the cranial cruciate ligament is a common cause of lameness in some large breed dogs. Cranial cruciate ligament rupture can lead to severe degenerative joint disease. The pathogenesis is not well understood but appears to require the presence of synovial inflammation and is likely complicated by genetic and conformational factors. It is uncertain if the pathogenesis of the synovitis associated with this disease is the same or different from the pathogenesis of the synovitis seen in degenerative joint disease (see previous section) of other causes. The degenerative changes in the ruptured ligament consist of a variable degree of coagulation necrosis and loss of fibroblasts, chondroid metaplasia of some of the remaining fibroblasts, and loss of the normal crimp of the collagen fibers (see previous section).

Neoplasms

A lesion termed *localized nodular tenosynovitis* has been diagnosed occasionally in dogs and may actually be better characterized as a benign neoplasm. Histologically, the lesion has cleft-like spaces lined by synoviocytes and proliferating fibrous connective tissue. Variable numbers of multinucleated giant cells, hemosiderin-laden macrophages, and mononuclear inflammatory cells also are present. Some nodules contain a spindle cell population, resembling fibroma. Lesions containing increased numbers of multinucleated giant cells may fall under the category of benign giant cell tumor but may simply be a variant of localized nodular tenosynovitis. Similarly, fibromas arising from the mesenchyme of the paratenon have been described in horses, but these may actually be sclerotic variants of localized nodular tenosynovitis. Regardless of the histologic subtype, these lesions are slow growing, lack malignant change, and are not reported to metastasize. Malignant tumors originating in tendons and ligaments are rare.

Disorders of Horses

For disorders occurring in two or more species of animals, see the section on Disorders of Domestic Animals.

Bone

See Disorders of Domestic Animals.

Joints

See Disorders of Domestic Animals.

Tendons and Ligaments

See Disorders of Domestic Animals.

Disorders of Ruminants (Cattle, Sheep, and Goats)

For disorders occurring in two or more species of animals, see the section on Disorders of Domestic Animals.

Bone

Disorders of Endochondral Ossification

Chondrodysplasias (Spider Lamb Syndrome [see Fig. 16-39]**).** See Disorders of Domestic Animals, Bone, Abnormalities of Growth and Development, Disorders of Endochondral Ossification, Chondrodysplasias.

Joints

See Disorders of Domestic Animals.

Abnormalities of Growth and Development

Arthrogryposis. Arthrogryposis refers to the congenital contracture of one or more joints, a condition that usually occurs with bilateral symmetry. The cause of arthrogryposis is often not established when it occurs sporadically. However, the pathogenesis is well established in outbreaks involving damage to the fetal central nervous system (CNS) with intrauterine viral infections (e.g., Akabane virus [Bunyaviridae] and bluetongue virus [Reoviridae]) in cattle and sheep. In other cases, CNS lesions that are clearly hereditary occur, affecting significant numbers of offspring after introduction of a new sire. Regardless of cause, the CNS lesions likely result in some degree of fetal paralysis. It is known that maternal intoxication with certain alkaloids (coniine in poison hemlock and anagyrine in lupine plants) results in fetal paralysis. Lack of fetal motion during a critical window of development results in arthrogryposis, and this has been well documented experimentally. In arthrogryposis occurring secondary to lack of fetal motion *in utero*, the joints are morphologically normal. In rare circumstances, articular malformation results in incongruous joint surfaces.

Articular cartilage: Articular cartilage is usually normal, but subtle malformations can be present.

Articular capsule/synovium/synovial fluid: Articular capsule/synovium/synovial fluid is without gross lesions other than the lack of flexibility.

Subchondral bone: Subchondral bone is usually normal.

Tendons and Ligaments

See Disorders of Domestic Animals.

Disorders of Pigs

For disorders occurring in two or more species of animals, see the section on Disorders of Domestic Animals.

Bone

Abnormalities of Growth and Development

Disorders of Modeling

Congenital Cortical Hyperostosis. Congenital cortical hyperostosis is an autosomal recessive hereditary disease of newborn pigs that is characterized by abnormal periosteal bone formation involving the major long bones. One or several limbs may be affected. The pathophysiology of the bone lesions is not understood.

Growth plate: Growth plates are not involved.

Trabecular bone: Trabecular bone is not involved.

Cortical bone: The subperiosteal cortex is normal; however, trabeculae of woven bone, oriented perpendicularly to the long axis of the cortex, radiate outward from its periphery. These trabeculae arise from the cambium layer of the periosteum and, other than extent of the change, are typical of the nonspecific reaction of the periosteum to injury described previously.

Joints

See Disorders of Domestic Animals.

Tendons and Ligaments

See Disorders of Domestic Animals.

Disorders of Dogs

For disorders occurring in two or more species of animals, see the section on Disorders of Domestic Animals.

Bone

Abnormalities of Growth and Development

Disorders of Modeling

Craniomandibular Osteopathy. Craniomandibular osteopathy, also known as *lion jaw*, typically occurs as an autosomal recessive condition in West Highland white terriers; however, similar lesions have been reported as isolated occurrences in other breeds and also have been associated with a leukocyte adhesion molecule deficiency (CLAD) in a colony of Irish setter pups that had concurrent metaphyseal osteopathy (see the discussion of noninfectious inflammation of bone in the section on Disorders of Domestic Animals, Bone, Inflammation).

Lesions are bilaterally symmetric, resulting in diffuse, irregular thickening of the mandible(s), occipital and temporal bones, and, occasionally, other bones of the skull (Fig. 16-86). The tympanic bullae are often severely affected. Less commonly, the disease can affect the appendicular skeleton. The disease often becomes apparent at 4 to 7 months of age and can regress. For affected dogs, mastication is painful and difficult, and the muscles of the skull become atrophic from disuse. The etiopathogenesis of this disease is unknown. A similar self-limiting disease has recently been reported in the calvaria of young bullmastiff dogs (calvarial hyperostotic syndrome [CHS]).

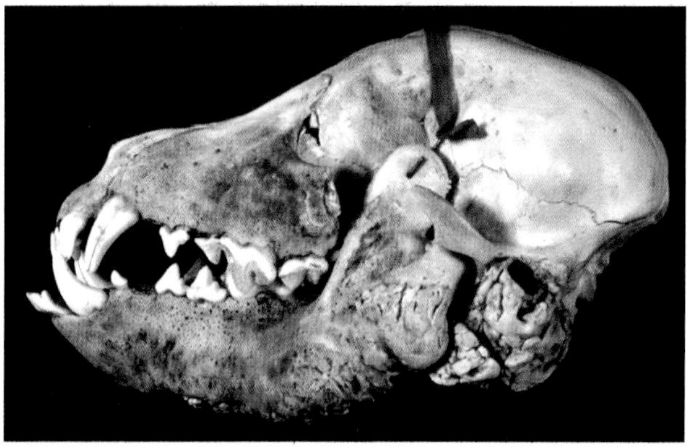

Figure 16-86 **Craniomandibular Osteopathy, Bone, Skull, Dog (West Highland White Terrier).** Extensive periosteal new bone formation on the lateral surfaces of the body and ramus of the mandible, caudolateral maxilla, bulla tympanica, and occipital condyle. Macerated and bleached specimen. (Courtesy Dr. H. Leipold, College of Veterinary Medicine, Kansas State University.)

Growth plate: Growth plates are not involved.

Trabecular bone: In the medullary cavities of the bones of the skull and jaw, trabeculae become osteosclerotic (increased bone per unit area) because of proliferation of woven bone by the osteoblasts of the endosteum with subsequent modeling and remodeling (see next discussion on cortical bone).

Cortical bone: In the skull and jaw, the cortices are thickened because of proliferation of periosteal woven bone. Characteristic of the disease is rapid disorganized modeling and remodeling, causing a mosaic of reversal cement lines with regions of lamellar bone adjacent to regions of woven bone.

Disorders of Endochondral Ossification

Chondrodysplasias. See Disorders of Domestic Animals, Bone, Abnormalities of Growth and Development, Disorders of Endochondral Ossification, Chondrodysplasias.

Metabolic Diseases

Renal Osteodystrophy. Renal osteodystrophy is a general term that refers to the skeletal lesions that develop secondary to chronic, severe renal disease. In human beings, this can include osteomalacia and fibrous osteodystrophy, either as separate diseases or in combination. Although fibrous osteodystrophy is the most common consequence of chronic renal disease in animals, particularly in dogs, this sometimes also is complicated by osteomalacia. Clinical signs of the disease include bone pain (lameness) and loss of teeth and deformity of the maxilla or mandible as the result of osteoclastic resorption of bone and replacement by fibro-osseous tissue. Renal osteodystrophy has a complex pathogenesis that likely depends on both the extent and nature of the renal disease and the availability of dietary vitamin D. Loss of glomerular function, inability to excrete phosphate, inadequate renal production of 1,25-dihydroxyvitamin D (calcitriol), and acidosis are central to its development. As the glomerular filtration rate falls in chronic renal disease, hyperphosphatemia develops, stimulating PTH synthesis and secretion. Hyperphosphatemia also suppresses the renal hydroxylation of inactive 25-hydroxyvitamin D to 1,25-dihydroxyvitamin D (calcitriol). Hypocalcemia develops primarily from decreased intestinal calcium absorption because of low serum calcitriol levels. Low serum calcitriol levels, hypocalcemia, and hyperphosphatemia have all been demonstrated to independently promote PTH synthesis and secretion. If serum levels of PTH remain elevated, fibrous osteodystrophy develops. The reduced production of 1,25-dihydroxyvitamin D by the diseased kidneys together with impaired mineralization because of the acidosis of uremia explain the development of osteomalacia.

Inflammation

Noninfectious Inflammation

Metaphyseal Osteopathy. Metaphyseal osteopathy, previously termed *hypertrophic osteodystrophy* (HOD), is a disease of young (usually 3 to 6 months of age), growing dogs of the large and giant breeds that results in severe pain that is localized to the metaphyses of the long bones. The distal radius and ulna are most severely affected; bones distal to the tarsus and carpus are usually spared. Both names, unfortunately, are misleading because the initial lesion is a suppurative and fibrinous osteomyelitis of the trabecular bone of the metaphysis, which is replaced in the chronic stages of the disease by the formation of abundant periosteal new bone. Remissions/exacerbations may occur over weeks to months, but most cases resolve completely if the pain can be managed successfully. The cause and pathogenesis are unknown; although the initial lesion is inflammatory, infectious agents have not been isolated. There are reports of metaphyseal osteopathy in litters of Weimaraners, in which granulocytopathies have been suspected, and in littermates of Irish setters, in which canine leukocyte adhesion deficiency (CLAD) was confirmed. The lack of CD18 expression on the neutrophil surface in the affected Irish setters results in the failure of neutrophils to marginate or extravasate, as well as a failure of these cells to phagocytose by CD18. Affected dogs have an underlying genetic defect that is expressed clinically to various degrees, ranging from normal to the development of severe, repeated infections. Interestingly, 75% to 85% of these dogs developed metaphyseal osteopathy by 10 to 12 weeks of age, and hematopoietic stem cell transplants led to resolution of all lesions. Based on these findings, it is possible that neutrophil entrapment at the chondro-osseous junction in the metaphysis (same location that is predisposed to the development of osteomyelitis in young animals; see the section on Portals of Entry) results in autoinflammation and necrosis, with the periosteal proliferation occurring as a secondary event. Clinically, metaphyseal osteopathy is characterized by lameness, fever, and swollen, painful metaphyses in multiple long bones.

Growth plate: Lesions in the growth plate are not expected in metaphyseal osteopathy.

Trabecular bone: Lesions are usually bilaterally symmetric. Radiographically, alternating metaphyseal zones of increased lucency and increased density are present parallel to the physes, resulting in a "double physis line" (Fig. 16-87, A and B). Microscopically, the lucent areas represent fibrinosuppurative inflammation and necrosis of the metaphyseal marrow and bone (Fig. 16-87, C). The death of osteoblasts results in primary trabeculae that are not reinforced by apposition of bone matrix. These trabeculae collapse and fracture without external distortion of the bone (infractions) and appear radiographically as relatively dense regions.

Cortical bone: The inflammation can extend from the medulla through the cutback zone into the periosteum. This periosteal inflammation, along with mechanical instability caused by the metaphyseal infractions, can cause striking metaphyseal periosteal new bone formation in chronic cases.

Panosteitis. Panosteitis (also known as eosinophilic panosteitis) is another canine bone disease with an unfortunate name because the lesion is neither inflammatory nor eosinophilic. The cause is unknown, and the disease is almost always self-limiting and thus is rarely seen at necropsy. It occurs in growing (commonly large breed) dogs, usually at 5 to 12 months of age, which present with painful limbs. German shepherd dogs appear to be predisposed. Morphologic studies are few because the disease is easily recognized clinically and resolves spontaneously so that biopsy evaluation is rarely necessary. Radiographically, the lesions are recognized as increased densities in the medullary cavity in the diaphysis, usually beginning near the nutrient foramen; these can also be present in the periosteum. The increased densities are the result of proliferation of well-differentiated woven bone and fibrous tissue. No inflammation is present. The cause of the lameness is presumed to be pressure on nerves by the proliferating woven bone both within the medullary cavity and on the periosteum.

Joints

Abnormalities of Growth and Development

Luxating Patella. A *luxation* is a complete dislocation of a joint, and a *subluxation* is a partial dislocation of a joint. Patellar luxations are inherited as a polygenic trait and occur commonly in dogs (especially small breeds) and less commonly in horses. Most are associated with developmental anatomic defects, such as hypoplasia of one or both trochlear ridges.

Hip Dysplasia. Hip dysplasia in dogs is a major orthopedic problem and occurs most commonly in large and giant breeds. It is inherited as a complex polygenic trait; gene expression in individuals may be modified by environmental factors, including weight and exercise. Dogs on restricted caloric intake have a significantly delayed time of onset of both hip dysplasia and degenerative joint disease. Many different theories regarding the etiopathogenesis have been advanced, but most agree that it is a biomechanical disease in which joint laxity of the hip (instability) is one of the essential early findings, eventually resulting in chronic subluxation and severe secondary degenerative joint disease with marked modeling of the acetabulum and femoral head and neck. The lesions are not present

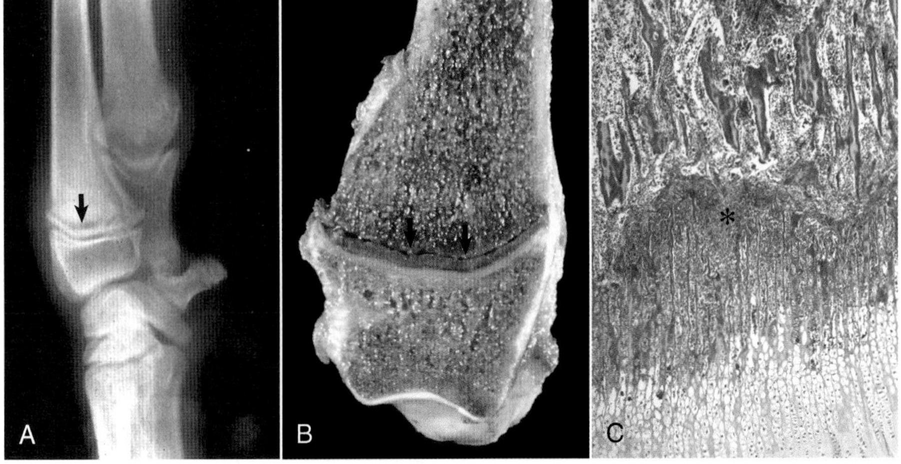

Figure 16-87 Metaphyseal Osteopathy, Bone, Distal Radius, Dog. A, Radiograph. The radiolucent line in the metaphysis *(arrow)*, parallel with growth plate, is characteristic of metaphyseal osteopathy. **B,** Grossly, this line appears to be a fracture *(arrows)* within the metaphysis. **C,** Histologically, this line is a hypercellular band *(asterisk)* of neutrophils between the primary and secondary trabeculae. (Courtesy Dr. S.E. Weisbrode, College of Veterinary Medicine, The Ohio State University.)

at birth but can be well advanced by 1 year of age. The earliest radiographic lesion is delayed ossification of the craniodorsal acetabular rim, which may be identified as early as 7 weeks of age in severely affected individuals.

Hip dysplasia also occurs as an inherited disease (recessive, sex-limited) in bulls of certain beef breeds, including Herefords. Affected animals have shallow acetabula and joint laxity and instability, which lead to degenerative joint disease early in life.

Articular cartilage: In the advanced disease, there is notable erosion and ulceration of articular cartilage of both the femoral head and acetabulum.

Articular capsule/synovium/synovial fluid: In advanced disease, the articular capsule is distended and thickened, sometimes containing areas of osseous and chondroid metaplasia, and synovial fluid is increased in amount. The round ligament of the femoral head may be ruptured.

Subchondral bone: In advanced disease, the dorsal rim of the acetabulum flattens and becomes shallow and wide. Subsequent to ulceration of cartilage of the femoral head, there is eburnation of underlying bone and formation of periarticular osteophytes on both the proximal femur and the acetabulum (see Fig. 16-21).

Inflammatory Lesions

Noninfectious Arthritis

Rheumatoid Arthritis. Rheumatoid arthritis in dogs is an uncommon, chronic, sterile, erosive polyarthritis that resembles the disease in human beings. The cause is unknown in both species, although it is clear that the process is immune mediated (humoral and cell-mediated immunity). Antibodies (rheumatoid factor) of the immunoglobulin (Ig) G (IgG) or IgM classes are produced in response to an unknown stimulus. Factors that may be involved include alterations in the steric configuration of IgG, persistent bacterial cell wall components that cross-react with normal proteoglycans, anticollagen antibodies, and defective suppressor T lymphocyte activity. Neutrophils that are activated by phagocytosis of immune complexes release lysosomal enzymes, which sustain the inflammatory reaction and injure intraarticular structures. In addition to inflammatory mediators and their effects on synovium and cartilage, rheumatoid arthritis characteristically includes exuberant pannus formation (see Figs. 16-29 and 16-30). Fibroblasts in pannus can enzymatically degrade cartilage. In addition, pannus may act as a physical barrier between the synovial fluid and the cartilage to prevent the delivery of nutrients to the chondrocytes. Antibodies against normal and altered articular cartilage collagen are present in human cases of rheumatoid arthritis and might be important mediators of the ongoing joint inflammation and injury that occur in this disease. In dogs, rheumatoid arthritis is characterized clinically by progressive lameness involving primarily the distal joints of the limbs (carpal, tarsal, and phalangeal joints).

Degeneration of Intervertebral Disks

See Disorders of Domestic Animals, Joints, Degeneration of Intervertebral Disks.

Tendons and Ligaments

See Disorders of Domestic Animals.

Disorders of Cats

For disorders occurring in two or more species of animals, see the section on Disorders of Domestic Animals.

Bone

See Disorders of Domestic Animals.

Joints

See Disorders of Domestic Animals.

Tendons and Ligaments

See Disorders of Domestic Animals.

Aging

Bone Aging. Aging changes of bone have been well characterized in human beings and include both quantitative and qualitative changes (alterations in the dynamics of bone cell populations, changes in bone architecture, accumulation of microfractures, localized disparity in the concentration of deposited minerals, changes in crystalline properties of mineral deposits, and changes in the protein content of matrix material). The net result of these changes is a loss of bone architecture, density, and strength.

Tendons and Ligaments Aging. Aging changes in tendons and ligaments that have been documented in human beings include poorly characterized vascular and compositional changes that alter their mechanotransduction, biology, healing capacity, and biomechanical function.

Summary. Aging changes in bone, tendons, and ligaments of domestic animals are presumed to be similar to those reported in human beings but are much less well documented due in part to the fact that most domestic animals are reproductively active throughout the majority of their life span and do not experience the dramatic reduction in sex hormones that occurs, for example, in postmenopausal women. Age is an important risk factor in many of the degenerative orthopedic diseases in domestic animals, including but not limited to osteoarthritis, intervertebral disk disease, tendon/ligament rupture, and spondylosis.

Suggested Readings

Suggested Readings are available at www.expertconsult.com.

CHAPTER 17

The Integument[1]

Ann M. Hargis and Sherry Myers

Key Readings Index

Structure

The skin is the largest organ in the body and has haired and hairless portions (Figs. 17-1 and 17-2). It consists of epidermis, dermis, subcutis, and adnexa (hair follicles and sebaceous, sweat, and other glands). The histologic structure varies greatly by anatomic site and among different species of animals. The haired skin is thickest over the dorsal aspect of the body and on the lateral aspect of the limbs and is thinnest on the ventral aspect of the body and the medial aspect of the thighs. Haired skin has a thinner epidermis, whereas nonhaired skin of the nose and pawpads has a thicker epidermis (see Figs. 17-1 and 17-2). The skin of large animals is generally thicker than the skin of small animals. The subcutis, consisting of lobules of adipose tissue and fascia, connects the more superficial layers (epidermis and dermis) with the underlying fascia and musculature.

Epidermis

The epidermis is divided into layers based on the morphologic features of the keratinocyte, the major cell type of the epidermis. The epidermis of haired skin consists of four basic layers: stratum corneum, stratum granulosum, stratum spinosum, and stratum basale (Fig. 17-3). The epidermis of hairless skin has an additional layer, the stratum lucidum, which is located between the stratum granulosum and stratum corneum (see Fig. 17-2). Keratinocytes originate from germinal cells in the stratum basale of the epidermis, ascend through the layers of the epidermis, changing in appearance and other characteristics in each layer until they reach the stratum corneum as fully cornified, dead corneocytes. Keratinocytes are continuously shed from the stratum corneum. The transit time for a keratinocyte from the stratum basale to shed in the stratum corneum is approximately 1 month, although this time can be accelerated in some disorders such as primary seborrhea characterized clinically by scaling.

The outermost layer of the epidermis is the stratum corneum, which consists of many sheets of flattened, cornified cells termed corneocytes. Keratin is an intracellular fibrous protein that is in part responsible for the toughness of the epidermis, enabling the epidermis to form a protective barrier. The next layer is the stratum granulosum, which consists of cells containing basophilic keratohyalin granules. In nonhaired skin the stratum corneum and stratum granulosum are separated by an additional layer of compacted, fully cornified cells, the stratum lucidum (see Fig. 17-2), best seen in the pawpad. This layer has a translucent appearance due to the presence of eleidin, a protein similar to keratin, but with different staining affinity. Deep to the stratum granulosum is the stratum spinosum, a layer of polyhedral-shaped cells attached to one another by desmosomes. During fixation and processing for microscopic examination, the cells of the stratum spinosum contract, except for the desmosomal attachments. These attachment sites create the appearance of "spines" or intercellular bridges, leading to the name of this layer. The visibility of the intercellular bridges is enhanced when there is intercellular edema of the epidermis. The stratum spinosum in haired areas is thicker in horses, cattle, and pigs and is thinner in dogs and cats. The innermost layer of the epidermis is the germinal layer, or stratum basale, which consists of a single layer of cuboidal cells resting on a basement membrane. Intermixed within the basal cell layer are melanocytes, Langerhans cells, and Merkel cells.

Melanocytes, embryologically derived from neural crest cells, are also present in lower layers of the stratum spinosum and produce melanin pigment, giving skin and hair their color. Melanocytic granules are transferred to and become distributed in keratinocytes as a caplike cluster of granules between the nucleus and the external surface of the skin to help protect the nucleus from UV light–induced injury. Langerhans cells are bone marrow–derived cells of monocyte-macrophage lineage that process and present antigen to sensitized T lymphocytes, thereby modulating immunologic responses of the skin. Langerhans cells are present in the basal, spinous, and granular layers of the epidermis but have a preference for a suprabasal position. Merkel cells are located in the basal layer, attach to keratinocytes via desmosomal junctions, and express keratin proteins 8, 18, 19, and 20. Merkel cells are located in haired and hairless skin, particularly in regions of the body with high tactile

[1]For a glossary of abbreviations and terms used in this chapter see E-Glossary 17-1.

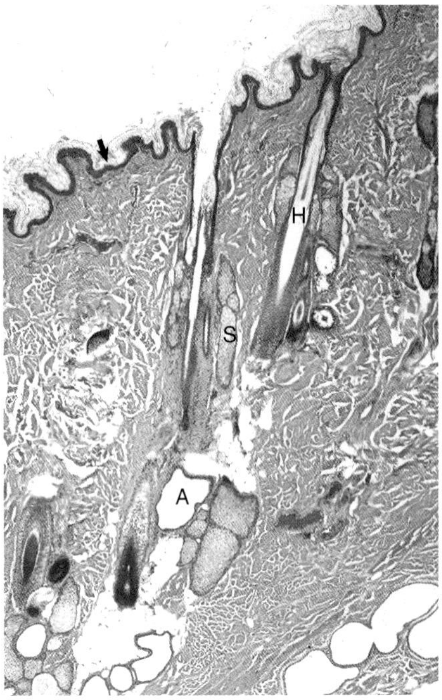

Figure 17-1 **Normal Skin, Haired, Thorax, Dog.** The epidermis *(arrow)* in haired skin has an undulating surface but lacks rete pegs (ridges or processes). The epidermis in haired skin has fewer nucleated cell layers than the epidermis in nonhaired (hairless) skin such as that on the nose and pawpads (see Fig. 17-2); thus it is referred to as "thin" skin. Hair follicles *(H)*, apocrine glands *(A)*, and sebaceous glands *(S)* are present. Rete peg formation is not required because the hair follicles strengthen the attachment between the epidermis and dermis. The haired skin is thickest over the dorsal aspect of the body and on the lateral aspect of the limbs, and it is thinnest on the ventral aspect of the body and the medial aspect of the thighs. H&E stain. (Courtesy Dr. Ann M. Hargis, DermatoDiagnostics.)

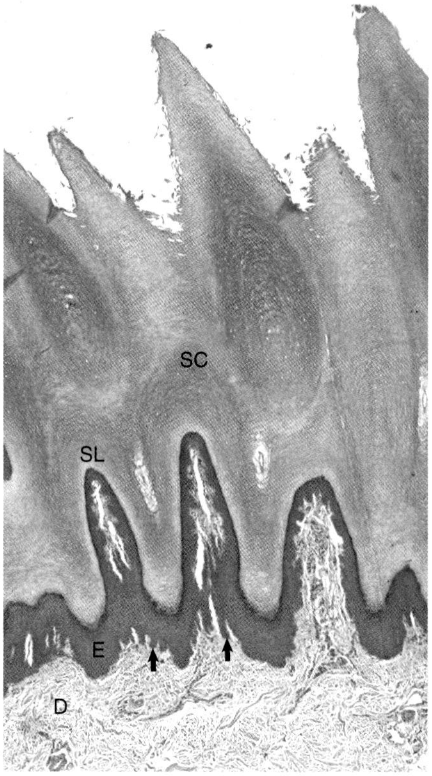

Figure 17-2 **Normal Skin, Hairless, Pawpad, Dog.** The epidermis *(E)* in hairless (nonhaired) skin has more nucleated cell layers, a thicker stratum corneum, and an additional layer termed the stratum lucidum *(SL)*, than the epidermis in haired skin; thus it is referred to as "thick" skin. Note the dense zone of compact stratum corneum *(SC)* over the surface. The epidermal pegs *(arrows)* and dermal papillae in the superficial dermis *(D)* interdigitate and thus strengthen the attachment between the epidermis and dermis. Also note that in the pawpad of the dog, the contour of the cornified surface follows the epidermal contour and thus is papillated. H&E stain. (Courtesy Dr. Ann M. Hargis, DermatoDiagnostics.)

sensitivity (digits and lips), and in the outer portion of hair follicles. When Merkel cells are associated with an axon, they form a Merkel cell–neurite complex and function as a slowly adapting mechanoreceptor. The specialized areas of the skin containing these Merkel cell–neurite complexes are known as *tylotrich pads* (hair disks, tactile pads). The axon associated with the Merkel cell is myelinated but near the epidermis, the myelin sheath is lost, and the nerve fibers terminate at the basal aspect of the Merkel cell. Merkel cells have granules that contain chemical mediators (metenkephalin, vasoactive intestinal peptide, chromogranin A, acetylcholine, calcitonin gene-related peptide, neuron-specific enolase, and synaptophysin). In addition to functioning as mechanoreceptors, Merkel cells may also influence keratinocyte proliferation, stimulate and maintain hair follicle stem cells, and alter blood flow and sweat production. The origin of Merkel cells is thought to be a primitive epidermal stem cell.

Basement Membrane Zone

The epidermis and dermis are separated by a basement membrane. In hairless areas, such as the pawpads and nasal planum, this junction is irregular because of epidermal projections (e.g., rete pegs/also known as rete ridges or rete processes) that interdigitate with dermal papillae, thus strengthening the dermal-epidermal attachment by providing resistance to shearing. In densely haired areas the junction is smoother and has an undulating appearance because the dermal-epidermal attachment is strengthened by the hair follicles. The more sparsely haired skin of pigs has more dermal-epidermal interdigitations (rete pegs) and fewer hair follicles. The basement membrane zone is composed of hemidesmosomes of basal cells (i.e., keratin intermediate filaments and attachment plaques), the lamina lucida (cell membrane, subdesmosomal dense plate, and anchoring filaments), and the lamina densa (i.e., type IV collagen), which also serve to anchor the epidermis to dermis (Fig. 17-4). The importance of the basement membrane in anchoring function is noted in some immune-mediated diseases in which antibodies target, bind, and ultimately damage a component in the basement membrane and result in the formation of bullae (see the discussion on reactions characterized grossly by vesicles or bullae as the primary lesion and histologically by vesicles or bullae within the basement membrane [bullous dermatoses] in the section on Selected Autoimmune Reactions). The basement membrane zone also serves as a scaffold for migration of epidermal cells in wound healing and as an initial barrier to invasion of the dermis by neoplastic cells originating in the epidermis.

Dermis

The dermis (corium) consists of collagen and elastic fibers in a glycosaminoglycan ground substance, and it supports hair follicles, glands, vessels, and nerves. By convention the dermis is generally subdivided into superficial and deep layers that blend together without a clear line of demarcation. The superficial dermis conforms to the contour of the epidermis and generally supports the upper

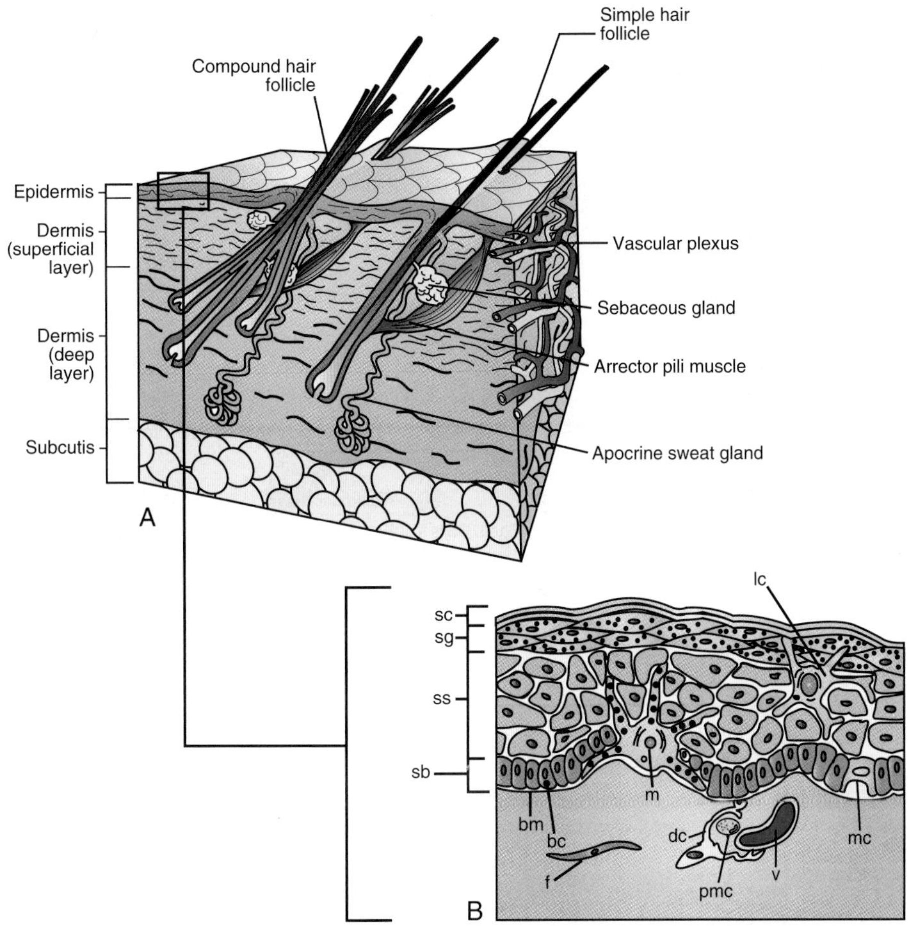

Figure 17-3 Structure of the Skin. A, The skin is composed of epidermis, dermis, and subcutis, with hair follicles, sebaceous glands, apocrine glands, and arrector pili muscles. The vascular plexuses, superficial, middle, and deep, are illustrated on the right side. **B,** This projection of the epidermis demonstrates the progressive upward maturation of basal cells *(bc)* in the stratum basale *(sb)* through the stratum spinosum *(ss)*, stratum granulosum *(sg)*, and stratum corneum *(sc)*. Melanocytes *(m)*, midepidermal dendritic Langerhans cells *(lc)*, and Merkel cells *(mc)* are also present. The subjacent dermis contains small vessels *(v)*, fibroblasts *(f)*, perivascular mast cells *(pmc)*, and dendrocytes *(dc)*, potentially important in dermal immunity and repair. (Revised and redrawn from Dellman DH, Brown EM: *Textbook of veterinary histology*, ed 3, Philadelphia, 1987, Lea and Febiger; and Gawkrodger DJ: *Dermatology: an illustrated colour text*, ed 2, New York, 1997, Churchill Livingstone.)

portion of the hair follicle and sebaceous glands. It is composed of fine collagen fibers and is thicker in the skin of horses and cattle than in the skin of dogs and cats. The deep dermis supports the lower portion of the hair follicle and apocrine glands and is composed of collagen bundles larger than those in the superficial dermis. Smooth muscle fibers of the arrector pili muscle attach the connective tissue sheath of the hair follicle to the epidermis and are responsible for causing the hair to stand erect. Skeletal muscle fibers from the cutaneous muscle extend into the lower dermis and are responsible for voluntary skin movement. Mast cells, lymphocytes, plasma cells, macrophages, and rarely eosinophils and neutrophils can be found in normal dermis. These cells are bone marrow–derived cells and arrive via the blood vascular system; thus they are typically concentrated around small superficial blood vessels.

Vessels and Nerves

Cutaneous arteries give rise to three vascular plexuses: deep, middle, and superficial (see Fig. 17-3). The deep plexus supplies the subcutis and deep portions of follicles and apocrine glands; the middle plexus supplies the sebaceous glands, midportion of follicles, and arrector pili muscles; and the superficial plexus supplies the superficial portions of follicles and epidermis. Lymph capillaries arise in the superficial dermis and connect with a subcutaneous plexus. The lymph vessels then converge to form larger channels that eventually reach peripheral lymph nodes.

The skin is an important sensory organ containing millions of microscopic nerve endings that perceive itch (pruritus), pain, temperature, pressure, and touch (Fig. 17-5). The nerve endings consist of Meissner's corpuscles, Pacini's or pacinian corpuscles, free sensory nerve endings, and mucocutaneous end organs (similar to Meissner's corpuscles but located in mucocutaneous skin). These nerve endings are minute, and the free sensory nerve endings are so delicate that they require special staining techniques, such as silver impregnation, to be visualized microscopically. The sensations of itch, pain, touch, temperature, and displacement of body hair are detected by the free sensory nerve endings. Itching, a form of mild pain that promotes the desire to scratch, is one of the most common reasons animals are presented to veterinarians. The sensations of pressure and touch are detected by Meissner's and Pacini's corpuscles. Sensations detected by free sensory nerve endings and by the corpuscles are transmitted to the spinal cord via the dorsal root ganglia. Sensory fibers to facial skin are supplied by the trigeminal nerve. Motor fibers (adrenergic and cholinergic) are supplied by the sympathetic component of the autonomic nervous system (see Fig. 17-5). Adrenergic fibers travel from the spinal cord through postganglionic fibers in peripheral nerves and arborize into plexuses that innervate blood

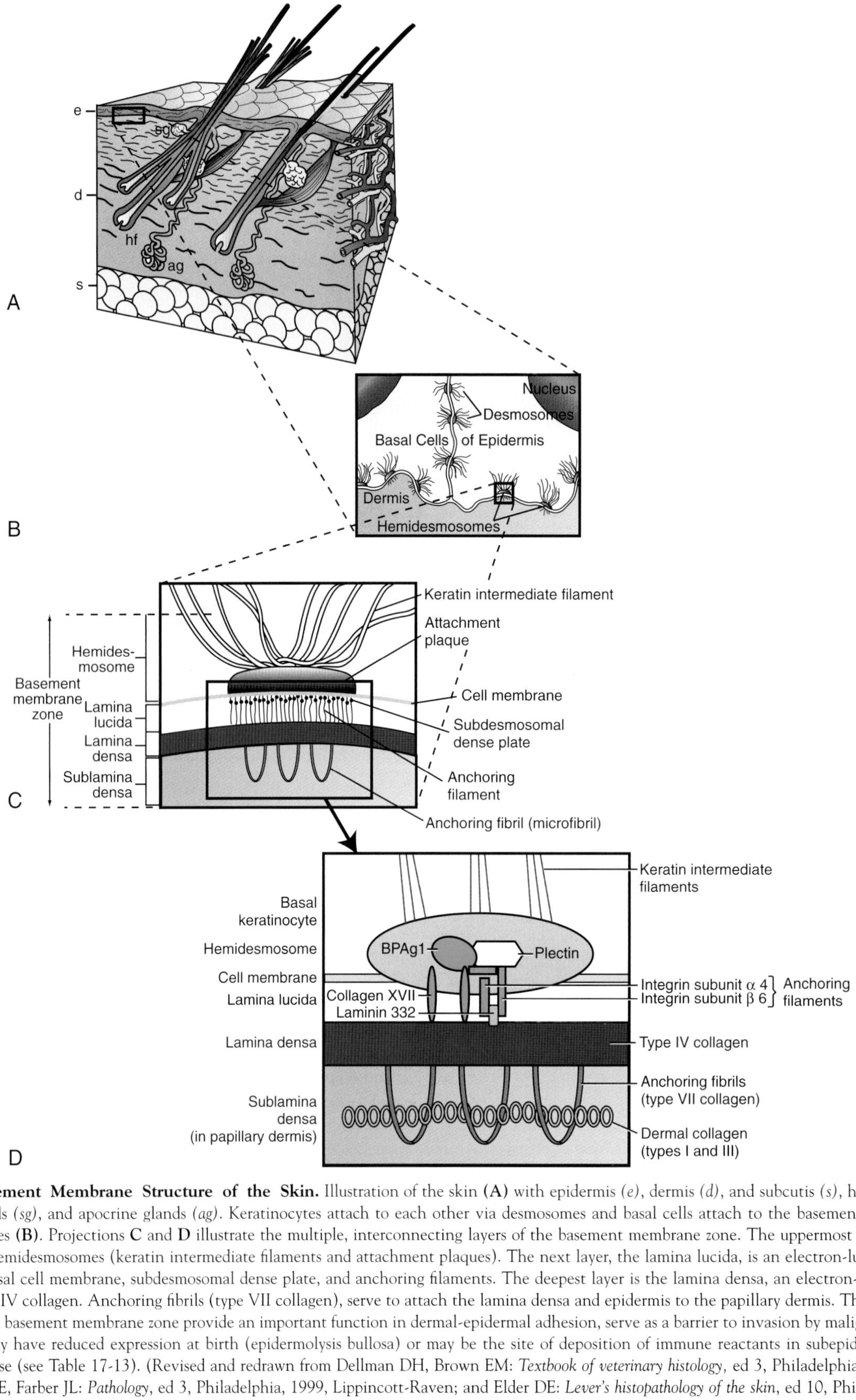

Figure 17-4 **Basement Membrane Structure of the Skin.** Illustration of the skin **(A)** with epidermis *(e)*, dermis *(d)*, and subcutis *(s)*, hair follicles *(hf)*, sebaceous glands *(sg)*, and apocrine glands *(ag)*. Keratinocytes attach to each other via desmosomes and basal cells attach to the basement membrane via hemidesmosomes **(B)**. Projections **C** and **D** illustrate the multiple, interconnecting layers of the basement membrane zone. The uppermost layer consists of the basal cell hemidesmosomes (keratin intermediate filaments and attachment plaques). The next layer, the lamina lucida, is an electron-lucent zone composed of the basal cell membrane, subdesmosomal dense plate, and anchoring filaments. The deepest layer is the lamina densa, an electron-dense zone that consists of type IV collagen. Anchoring fibrils (type VII collagen), serve to attach the lamina densa and epidermis to the papillary dermis. The interconnecting layers of the basement membrane zone provide an important function in dermal-epidermal adhesion, serve as a barrier to invasion by malignant epidermal tumors, and may have reduced expression at birth (epidermolysis bullosa) or may be the site of deposition of immune reactants in subepidermal blistering cutaneous disease (see Table 17-13). (Revised and redrawn from Dellman DH, Brown EM: *Textbook of veterinary histology*, ed 3, Philadelphia, 1987, Lea and Febiger; Rubin E, Farber JL: *Pathology*, ed 3, Philadelphia, 1999, Lippincott-Raven; and Elder DE: *Lever's histopathology of the skin*, ed 10, Philadelphia, 2009, Lippincott Williams & Wilkins.)

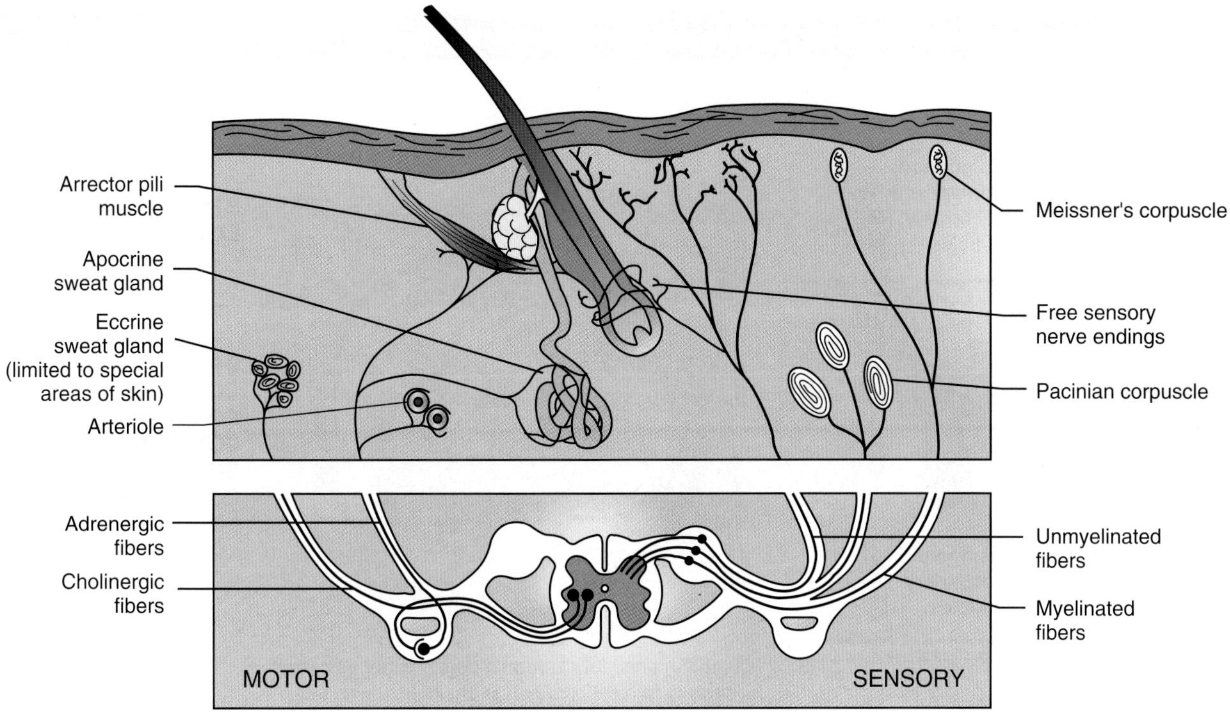

Figure 17-5 **Cutaneous Innervation.** Cutaneous nerve endings transmit sensations of itch (pruritus), pain, temperature, pressure, and touch via dorsal root ganglia to the central nervous system. Motor fibers in skin are supplied by the autonomic nervous system. Adrenergic fibers activate arterioles, arrector pili muscles, and apocrine sweat glands; cholinergic fibers stimulate eccrine sweat glands. (Adapted from Moschella SL, Pillsbury DM, Hurley JH Jr: *Dermatology*, ed 2, Philadelphia, 1975, WB Saunders.)

vessels, arrector pili muscles, and apocrine sweat glands. Stimulation by these adrenergic fibers causes vasoconstriction and piloerection (raising of the hair shafts). Cholinergic fibers travel from the spinal cord and arborize into plexuses that innervate the eccrine sweat glands. In the haired skin, equine sweat glands are considered to be the epitrichial (apocrine) type, where the duct opens into the follicular canal near the skin surface, but less commonly the duct may open in a depression near the follicle opening or directly on the skin surface. As in human beings, sweating in the horse is important in thermoregulation. However, the precise mechanisms that control sweating in the horse are unknown. The horse has a rich supply of vessels and nerves around sweat glands. It appears that equine sweat gland secretion is controlled by an interaction among neural, humoral, and paracrine factors. The only other domestic animal in which apocrine gland secretion is thought to play a thermoregulatory role is cattle, but sweating is not typically clinically visible except in horses. Dogs and cats lack eccrine glands in haired skin; however, cholinergic and to a lesser degree adrenergic fiber stimulation in dogs and cats causes sweating of the eccrine glands of pawpads at times of excitement or agitation.

Subcutis (Panniculus, Hypodermis)

The subcutis attaches the dermis to subjacent muscle or bone (with some regional exceptions where the subcutis may be absent such as involving the lip, cheek, eyelid, external ear, and anus) and consists of adipose tissue and collagenous and elastic fibers, which provide flexibility. Adipose tissue insulates against temperature variation and in the case of pawpads, serves in shock absorption. Adipose tissue also stores calories as triglycerides. In addition, there is recent evidence that fat cells secrete via autocrine, paracrine, and endocrine mechanisms a variety of cytokines, chemokines, and hormone-like factors such as adiponectin, leptin, resistin, tumor necrosis factor-α (TNF-α), interleukin 6 (IL-6), and acute phase proteins. These factors have been called adipokines and are thought to play a role in metabolism, and some may also contribute to adverse events associated with obesity.

Adnexa

Hair Follicles

Structure

Types of Hair Follicles. Hair follicles are classified into several types, primary or secondary, and simple or compound (Table 17-1). Primary hair follicles are large and produce primary hairs or guard hairs. They have a hair bulb located deeply in the dermis or subcutis, a sebaceous and apocrine gland, and an arrector pili muscle. Secondary hair follicles are generally smaller than primary follicles and produce secondary hairs (also called undercoat hairs or wool fibers). They have a hair bulb located superficially in the dermis, may have a sebaceous gland but lack an apocrine gland and arrector pili muscle. Simple hair follicles have a single hair shaft that emerges from the follicle opening through the epidermis, and may be either a primary or secondary type of follicle. In contrast, compound hair follicles have multiple hair shafts, either one primary and more numerous secondary hairs, or multiple secondary hairs only, that emerge from one follicle opening through the epidermis (see Table 17-1). The follicles forming a compound follicle each have their own lower segment, and they are joined at the level of the sebaceous duct to form a single common opening to the skin surface.

Tactile hairs include sinus and tylotrich hairs that function as mechanoreceptors (i.e., touch receptors). Sinus hairs, also termed whiskers or vibrissae, arise in simple follicles with a blood-filled sinus located between the inner and outer layers of the dermal sheath. Sinus hairs generally occur on the nose, above the eyes, on the lips and throat, and, in cats, on the palmar aspect of the carpus. Tylotrich hairs also arise in simple follicles and are scattered among the regular

Table 17-1 Morphologic Characteristics of Simple and Compound Hair Follicles

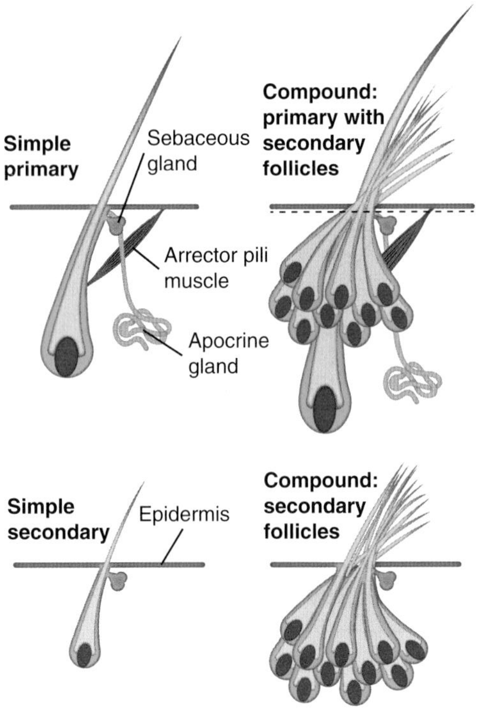

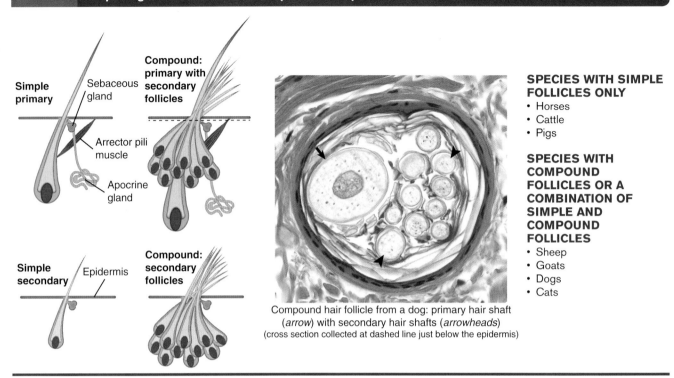

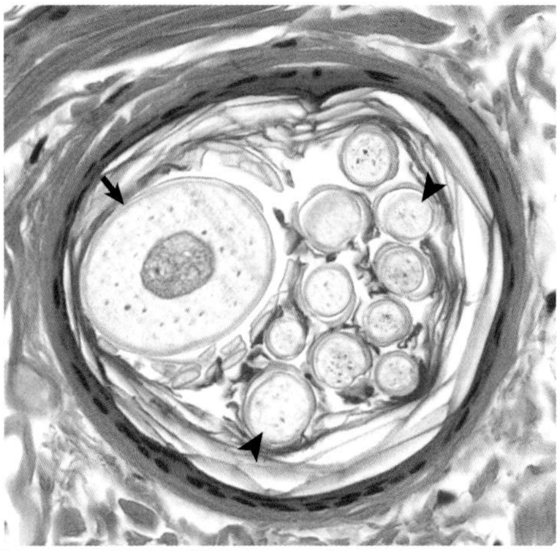
Compound hair follicle from a dog: primary hair shaft (*arrow*) with secondary hair shafts (*arrowheads*)
(cross section collected at dashed line just below the epidermis)

SPECIES WITH SIMPLE FOLLICLES ONLY
- Horses
- Cattle
- Pigs

SPECIES WITH COMPOUND FOLLICLES OR A COMBINATION OF SIMPLE AND COMPOUND FOLLICLES
- Sheep
- Goats
- Dogs
- Cats

Inset courtesy Dr. A.M. Hargis, DermatoDiagnostics; Dr. S. Myers, Prairie Diagnostic Services; and Dr. J.F. Zachary, College of Veterinary Medicine, University of Illinois.)

body hairs. Each tylotrich hair is associated with a tylotrich pad, and together they function as mechanoreceptors.

Structural Subdivisions within Hair Follicles. Fully developed hair follicles are traditionally subdivided into three anatomic segments: superficial, middle, and deep. The superficial segment, or infundibulum, extends from the follicular opening on the surface of the epidermis to the level where the sebaceous duct enters the follicle. The cells of the infundibulum are identical to and continuous with those of the epidermis. They keratinize slowly and form a granular cell layer before cornifying (through a process termed infundibular cornification). The middle segment, or isthmus, is quite short and extends from the level of sebaceous duct to the attachment of the arrector pili muscle. The cells of the follicular isthmus keratinize without forming a granular cell layer before cornifying (through a process termed trichilemmal cornification). The deep, or inferior, segment consists of the follicle below the attachment of the arrector pili muscle and includes the hair bulb, which consists of the hair matrix cells that partially enclose the follicular papilla, also called the dermal papilla. Two patterns of keratinization with cornification occur in the inferior portion of the follicle. One form is hair matrix (trichogenic) cornification, which occurs abruptly (does not form a granular layer), retains the nuclear outlines of keratinocytes, and produces the cortex of the hair shaft. The other form is inner root sheath cornification, which is compact and opaque and consists of Henle's and Huxley's layers, which contain red, trichohyalin granules. Cornification of viable keratinocytes is first recognized in an area termed *Adamson's fringe*, the upper margin of the keratogenous zone located between the mitotically active hair bulb and the hair shaft.

Depth of Hair Follicles/Hair Bulbs. The depth of follicles/hair bulbs varies among species. In horses and cattle the anagen hair bulbs (growing hair bulbs) are in the mid-dermis, whereas in dogs and cats the anagen hair bulbs of primary follicles are at the dermal-subcutaneous junction. In all species the bases of telogen follicles (resting follicles) are more superficially located than the bases of anagen follicles.

Development of Hair Follicles and Hair Shafts. The postnatal hair follicle and hair shaft form by proliferation and differentiation of the hair matrix cells of the hair bulb into various layers of the follicle wall, and subsequent keratinization with cornification centrally to form the hair shaft. Briefly, during the anagen stage of the hair cycle, the hair matrix cells in the hair bulb proliferate and differentiate to form multiple distinct, concentric cell layers or "sleeves" that eventually form the hair follicle wall (Table 17-2). The structure of the follicle wall from the inside out includes the hair shaft, the inner root sheath (IRS), the companion layer, the outer root sheath (ORS), the basement membrane, and the connective tissue sheath (CTS). The most centrally located hair matrix cells of the hair bulb form the hair shaft. If melanocytes are present in the hair bulb, melanin is transferred to the hair matrix cells that form the cortex and medulla of the hair shaft. As the cells that form the hair cortex cornify, they harden and die and are pushed upward toward the skin surface as the hair matrix cells in the hair bulb continue to proliferate, and a hair shaft is produced. Keratin proteins constitute the majority of the hair shaft and are stabilized mostly by disulfide bonds. These strong bonds link the keratin proteins together and confer durability and strength to the hair shaft. The hair cuticle also provides durability to the hair shaft via sulfur-rich keratinocyte-associated proteins and hydrophobicity to the hair surface via long-chain fatty acids. The cells of the hair cuticle flatten and resemble scales as they emerge from the hair bulb. Similar to the cells that form the hair cortex, as the cuticle cells cornify, they can no longer

Table 17-2 Structure and Function of Components of Hair Bulb

Function of Mesenchymal and Melanocytic Components

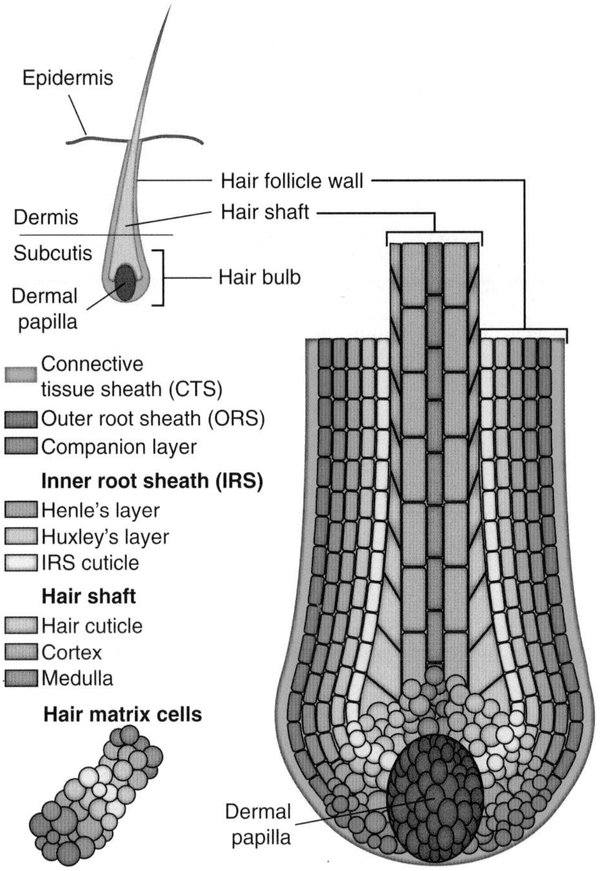

Melanocytes (not illustrated for simplicity) are present in pigmented hair bulbs. Their function is to produce and transfer melanin to hair matrix keratinocytes to produce a pigmented hair.

Mesenchymal components:

Connective tissue sheath (CTS), collagen and stromal cells that rest on a basement membrane; provides physical support and may be a reservoir for mesenchymal stem cells.

Dermal papilla regulates hair follicle growth, thought to be reservoir of stem cells.

Cell Layers	Select Functions of Cell Layers
Outer root sheath (ORS)	Storage area for hair follicle stem cells Cytoplasmic glycogen may serve as source of energy for the hair bulb and follicular cornification
Companion layer*	Thought to serve as slippage plane to allow the IRS with attached hair to move upward in the follicle while the ORS remains stationary
Inner root sheath (IRS) Henle's layer Huxley's layer Inner root sheath cuticle	Provides hair with surface shape and features and protects the developing hair IRS cuticle anchors to hair cuticle so both move upward together during growth Degraded at the level of the sebaceous gland by proteases and is sloughed as the hair emerges from the follicle
Hair shaft Cuticle Cortex Medulla Cuticle provides durability via sulfur-rich keratinocyte-associated proteins and hydrophobicity via long-chain fatty acids Medulla is not always present, and its function is unclear	The keratinocytes of the hair cortex synthesize, deposit, and assemble the keratin intermediate filaments and keratin-associated proteins that constitute the majority of the hair. These proteins are stabilized by formation of disulfide bonds and form the hair shaft, which, unlike the IRS, is resistant to proteolysis by sebaceous gland secretions
Hair matrix cells	Produce cell layers of the hair follicle including the hair shaft

*Companion layer thought by some to be a part of ORS, by others to be a part of the IRS, and most recently thought to represent a separate layer.
Inset courtesy Dr. A.M. Hargis, DermatoDiagnostics; Dr. S. Myers, Prairie Diagnostic Services; and Dr. J.F. Zachary, College of Veterinary Medicine, University of Illinois. Revised and redrawn from: Schneider MR, Schmidt-Ullrich R, Paus R, Curr Biol. 2009 Feb 10;19(3):R132-42.

function and also die. Some, but not all, hair shafts contain a medulla, the function of which is not completely understood. The medulla is usually absent in secondary hairs.

The IRS extends from the hair bulb to the follicular isthmus. It differentiates into three layers and has a variety of functions (see Table 17-2). The hair shaft and IRS are securely anchored together by the interlocking of cuticle cells, so that during growth the hair shaft and IRS move upward though the follicle concurrently. The IRS gives the hair shaft its surface shape and features and serves as a rigid protective covering around the developing hair. The keratin proteins of the IRS and of the hair cortex are of different composition. The proteins of the IRS are degraded by proteases from the sebaceous gland, but those of the hair shaft are not degraded, thus allowing the hair shaft to emerge as an independent structure from the follicular opening.

The companion layer (see Table 17-2), located between the IRS and ORS, is tightly anchored to the IRS, but not to the ORS. It is thought to act as a slippage plane against which the IRS and hair shaft can move upward during hair growth, whereas the ORS remains stationary. The ORS extends from the hair bulb the entire length of the follicle and is continuous with the outer aspect of the sebaceous gland and with the overlying epidermis. The ORS also serves as a storage area for hair follicle stem cells. In addition, in the zone of the hair follicle where cornification occurs (the upper margin of the keratogenous zone, Adamson's fringe), the ORS cells have glycogen-rich cytoplasm that probably serves as a source of energy for the proliferative activities of the hair bulb and follicular cornification. The connective tissue sheath and its basement membrane provide physical support for the hair follicle, and the sheath may be a reservoir for mesenchymal stem cells.

Species Differences

Horses. Horses have simple hair follicles, both primary and secondary types, which are evenly distributed throughout the skin.

Ruminants (Cattle, Sheep, and Goats). Cattle have simple hair follicles, both primary and secondary types, which are distributed throughout the skin in subtle groups of three. Goats have primary follicles in groups of three, and each group usually has three to six secondary follicles. Compound follicles in goats are composed of secondary follicles. Hair follicles in sheep have been studied extensively because of the commercial importance in wool production. Sheep have mostly simple follicles in sparsely haired regions, including the face, distal legs, and pinnae, and mostly compound follicles in the densely covered wool-growing areas. The typical follicle group has 3 primary follicles and 15 to 16 secondary follicles. The compound follicles in sheep consist of multiple secondary follicles that originate in the region of the sebaceous gland by branching from an original secondary follicle. Selective breeding has substantially increased the number of secondary follicles in fine-wooled or medium-wooled sheep and goats.

Pigs. Pigs have sparse hair coats composed mostly of widely spaced simple primary follicles that occur in groups of two to four with the groups bordered by dense connective tissue.

Dogs and Cats. Dogs and cats have mostly compound follicles that are arranged in groups of one to six. The groups most often consist of three primary follicles associated with a greater number of smaller secondary follicles (see Table 17-1). There is breed variation in the number of secondary follicles with some breeds such as German shepherd dogs having more secondary follicles than short-coat breeds such as terriers. Cats have more secondary follicles (10 to 20) compared to dogs (2 to 15). Primary hair shafts may emerge independently through a single opening, whereas secondary hairs generally emerge through a common opening. The three larger primary follicles within a follicular group are located closer to the head, whereas the smaller secondary follicles are located caudal to the primary follicles (Fig. 17-6). Within the follicular group the secondary follicles also become progressively smaller toward the caudal aspect (i.e., the tail) of the animal. This pattern of follicular group structure together with the slanted orientation of the hair shafts results in a hair coat that covers the surface of the epidermis smoothly with guard hairs on top of the finer undercoat.

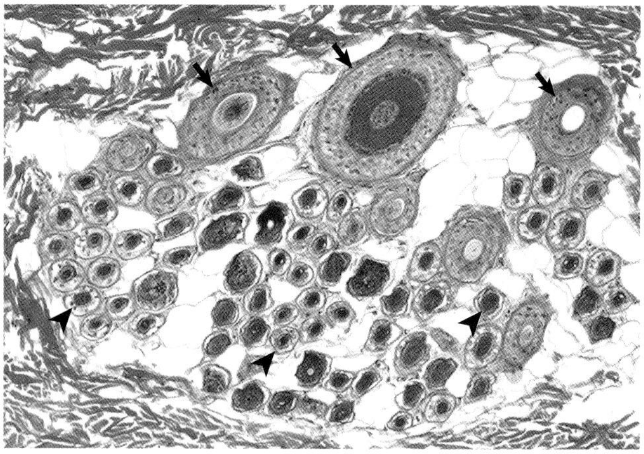

Figure 17-6 **Hair Follicle Group, Skin, Dog.** Horizontal section of hair follicle group from skin of a dog. The three large primary follicles (*arrows*) are located toward the head of the dog. The smaller secondary follicles (*arrowheads*) are located caudal to the primary follicles. The secondary follicles become progressively smaller toward the caudal portion of the body. H&E stain. (Courtesy Dr. Ann M. Hargis, DermatoDiagnostics.)

Growth and Distribution of Hair. During embryologic morphogenesis of the skin, hair follicles develop from a downgrowth of epidermis into the dermis and subcutis. They populate specific areas of the skin in varying densities and, with rare exceptions, no new hair follicles form thereafter. The distribution and type of hair follicles vary among different species, breeds, and individual animals. In general, the hair coat of animals is usually densest on the dorsal and lateral aspects of the body and sparsest on the ventrum. Hair follicles generally grow obliquely, at an angle of 30 to 60 degrees, with respect to the surface of the epidermis so that the hair shafts generally slant caudally and ventrally on the animal to create a more water repellant and aerodynamic hair coat.

Hair Cycle. In post-natal life, hair follicles that develop during morphogenesis enter stages of growth and regression termed the hair cycle (Fig. 17-7). The reason that hair growth occurs in cycles is not clear, but the hair cycle may permit the animal to: (1) control the length of body hair in different anatomic sites, (2) shed fur to clean the body surface, (3) adapt and change hair coat in response to changing environment (winter to summer) or social conditions, or (4) protect against malignant transformation that might occur in a rapidly dividing tissue.

During the stages of the hair cycle, the infundibular and isthmus portions of the follicle are permanent because they remain structurally the same and do not visibly change. In contrast, the lower portion of the follicle below the isthmus regresses and is reconstructed during each cycle. The hair follicle stages include hair growth, regression, quiescence, shedding or loss of the hair shaft, and latency (Box 17-1 and see Fig. 17-7). In the anagen stage of the hair cycle, mitotic activity and growth occur. The catagen stage is an apoptosis-driven regressing stage during which cellular proliferation ceases and the hair follicle cells are lost via programmed cell death. The hair follicle then enters a resting or relatively quiescent stage, telogen, after which mitotic activity and new hair production resumes. The kenogen stage refers to follicles that have lost their hair shaft and that remain empty for an indefinite period of time before anagen is reinitiated. This stage also has been referred to as "hairless telogen." In many hair loss disorders in domestic animals, increased numbers of kenogen follicles are evident histologically. Exogen is the stage in which the old hair shaft is shed. Exogen occurs independent of the hair cycle stage but often follows telogen.

All hairs of the body proceed through the hair cycle, but the duration of the cycle, duration of individual stages, and the length of hair shafts produced vary among animals and specific anatomic sites. In human scalp hair, each hair follicle has its own inherent rhythm, and thus hair cycles are asynchronous. Anagen is the longest stage of the cycle, and as a result human scalp hair grows almost constantly. In contrast, hair follicle growth occurs synchronously in many other mammals, resulting in periodic loss or shedding of the hair coat. Most mammals have a telogen-based hair cycle in which the hair shafts grow to a genetically predetermined length after which the follicle enters a prolonged stage of inactivity (telogen) and the hair shaft remains firmly attached to the follicle. The telogen-based hair cycle likely has an advantage in the conservation of protein and energy required for hair synthesis. There are exceptions to this general rule because some animals have continuously growing hair similar to scalp hair in human beings

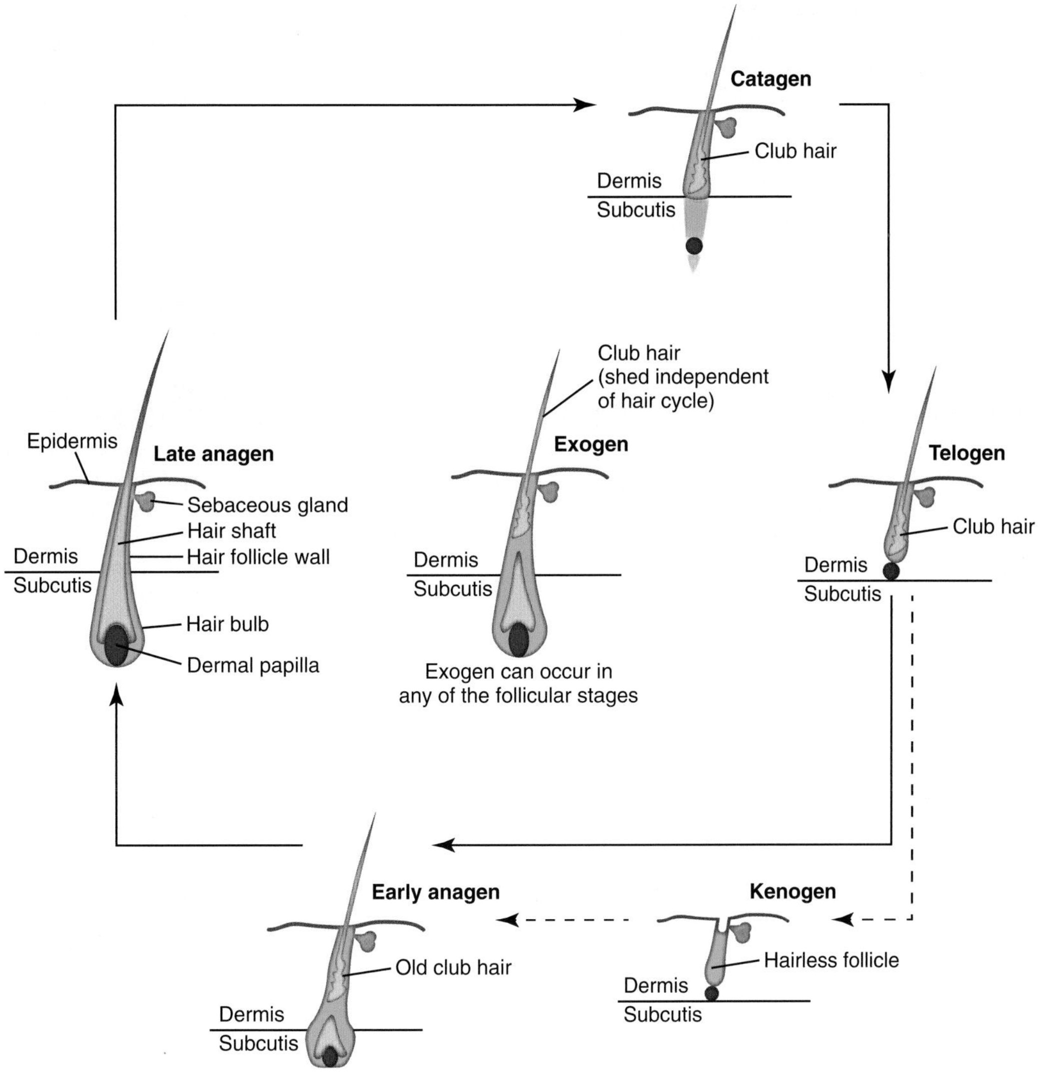

Figure 17-7 The Hair Cycle. Anagen is the growth stage. During early anagen the secondary germ grows down to enclose the dermal papilla (follicular papilla), and a new hair bulb forms. The old club hair remains in the upper portion of the hair follicle. Hair is produced by mitosis of the hair matrix cells covering the apex of the dermal papilla. By late anagen the club hair has usually shed and the new hair has emerged from the follicular opening. Catagen is the regression stage. A constriction occurs at the hair bulb, and the hair shaft above this becomes a "club hair." The follicle wall of the club hair becomes thick and corrugated. Telogen is referred to as the resting or quiescent stage in which the follicle is the shortest and dermal papilla is small and located at the base of the follicle. Exogen refers to the shedding of the old hair shaft, which can occur in different stages of the cycle (e.g., anagen, telogen) depending on type of hair and species. Kenogen refers to hair follicles that have lost their hair shaft and remain empty for an indefinite time before anagen is reinitiated. This stage also has been referred to as "hairless telogen." Note the location of the horizontal line on the diagram indicates the location of the hair bulb relative to the dermal-subcutaneous junction. The anagen and exogen hair bulbs are located deeper than the catagen, telogen, and kenogen hair bulbs. (Courtesy Dr. A.M. Hargis, DermatoDiagnostics; Dr. S. Myers, Prairie Diagnostic Services; and Dr. J.F. Zachary, College of Veterinary Medicine, University of Illinois.)

Box 17-1 Stages of Hair Follicles

Structure	Function/Outcome
Anagen hair follicle	Growing hair follicle
Catagen hair follicle	Regressing hair follicle
Telogen hair follicle	Quiescent (resting) hair follicle
Exogen hair follicle	Shedding of hair from hair follicle
Kenogen hair follicle	Latent (hairless) hair follicle

(predominant anagen hair cycle) such as the mane and tail hairs of horses, the fleece of Romney sheep, and hair in poodle dogs.

The cyclic growth of hair is directed by stem cells in the hair follicle and by biologic factors from the dermal papilla via complex, incompletely understood signaling pathways. The ability to regenerate a portion of the body is unique to hair follicles. The mechanisms that govern stem cells and the intrinsic signaling pathways that control the regeneration of follicles are under active investigation to provide insight into ways to use stem cells to regenerate damaged hair follicles, epidermis, and other tissues. Hair follicle stem cells have been studied most extensively in human beings and mouse models, and more recently in dogs. The hair follicle stem cells are located in the area of the ORS in the isthmus region of the follicle. The stem cells in the ORS give rise to a second population of stem cells, termed the secondary germ, located directly above the dermal papilla of the telogen follicle. During late telogen–early anagen the secondary germ cells, in response to signals from the dermal papilla, become activated, proliferate, and surround the dermal papilla, initiating the anagen growth phase of the cycle.

The stem cells in the ORS also become activated but proliferate later and more slowly (within anagen) probably to sustain hair follicle growth throughout the anagen phase. In addition to hair follicle stem cells, melanocyte stem cells also reside in the ORS and the secondary germ. During fetal development the melanocyte stem cells migrate from the neural crest and colonize the developing follicle. The melanocyte stem cells and the hair follicle stem cells are activated concurrently during anagen. The melanocyte stem cells provide the hair bulb with mature melanocytes that produce and transfer melanin to hair matrix cells and result in the formation of a pigmented hair shaft.

Extrinsic factors are also important in governing the hair cycle and growth. For example, nutrition and health status have a significant influence on hair growth and quality. Hair is largely composed of protein, thus diets low in protein or disease states associated with severe protein loss, such as protein-losing enteropathy (see Chapter 7) result in poor-quality hair coat. Also, in disease states, cuticle formation can be defective, resulting in a dull or dry hair coat. Hair growth responds to photoperiods and to a lesser extent to ambient temperatures. Photoperiod effects act via the hypothalamus, pituitary, and pineal gland, which secrete tropic hormones, such as melatonin, prolactin, and the gonadal, thyroid, and adrenal hormones, that influence hair growth. Some hormones, such as thyroid and growth hormone, stimulate hair growth, whereas excessive concentrations of estrogen or glucocorticoids suppress hair growth. Intrinsic and extrinsic factors also interact. For example, cells in the dermal papilla (mesenchymal in origin) that mediate growth-stimulating signals to hair matrix cells are thought to be the primary target cells that respond to these tropic hormones.

Arrector Pili Muscles

The arrector pili are smooth muscle bundles that are oriented almost perpendicularly to the wall of the follicle and are well developed on the back of animals, especially dogs. On one side the arrector pili muscle connects to the basement membrane of the epidermis, and on the other side inserts in the connective tissue sheath at the junction of the middle and inferior portion of the hair follicle. Muscle contraction causes erection of hairs and expression of the contents of sebaceous glands.

Sweat Glands

There are two basic types of sweat glands: apocrine glands and eccrine glands. Apocrine glands are located throughout haired areas of skin in domestic animals and are tubular- or saccular-coiled glands (see Fig. 17-3). The ducts of the apocrine glands open in the superficial portion of the hair follicle; thus these glands are also called epitrichial glands. The glands are lined by secretory cuboidal to low columnar epithelium surrounded by contractile myoepithelial cells. Other apocrine glands include glands of the external ear canal and eyelids of domestic animals, the interdigital glands of small ruminants, the mental organ of pigs, and the anal sac glands of dogs and cats. Eccrine glands are merocrine in secretion. The ducts of eccrine glands, in contrast to apocrine glands, open directly onto the epidermal surface; thus eccrine glands are also called atrichial glands. They are tubular glands lined by cuboidal epithelium surrounded by myoepithelium and are confined mainly to the frog region of ungulates, nasolabial region of ruminants and pigs, the carpus of pigs, and pawpads of dogs and cats.

Sebaceous Glands

Sebaceous glands are simple, branched, or compound alveolar glands that undergo holocrine secretion, with ducts opening into hair follicles except at some mucocutaneous junctions where the glands open on the surface of the skin (e.g., meibomian gland, also known as tarsal gland). Well-developed sebaceous glands are found in the preputial glands of horses; the infraorbital, inguinal, and interdigital regions of sheep; the base of the horn of goats; the supracaudal gland of the base of the tail of dogs and cats; the anal sac glands of cats; and the submental organ of the chin of cats.

Specialized Structures[2]

Anal sacs are specialized cutaneous structures that are especially prone to develop lesions. Anal sacs are bilateral diverticula located between internal and external anal sphincter muscles in dogs and cats and have ducts that open onto the anus at the level of the anocutaneous junction. Ducts and sacs are lined by stratified squamous epithelium. In dogs the wall has only apocrine glands, but in cats the sac wall has sebaceous and apocrine glands. The anal sacs can become distended with secretory products, rupture after trauma, and cause bacterial infection and chronic inflammation (foreign body reaction) in contiguous tissues. Carcinomas of the apocrine gland of the anal sac in dogs are often associated with tumor cell production of parathyroid hormone–related protein (PTH-rP) and humoral hypercalcemia of malignancy.

Hepatoid (i.e., circumanal or perianal) glands occur most commonly in the skin around the anus and are also present in skin near the prepuce, tail, flank, and groin. These glands are modified sebaceous glands that have nonpatent ducts and are composed of peripheral reserve cells that surround lobules of differentiated cells resembling hepatocytes, resulting in the name "hepatoid" glands. Adenomas of the perianal glands in male dogs are often testosterone dependent.

Hooves of horses consist of the wall, sole, and frog. The hoof wall comprises three structurally distinct cornified layers, which from the outside in include the stratum externum, stratum medium, and stratum internum. The stratum externum is a thin flaky cornified layer that arises from the germinal cells (basal cells) of the epidermis of the periople (an area of modified skin above the coronary band of the hoof). Toward the back of the foot the periople expands to form a broad cornified area or bulb (heel) supported by corium (dermis). The stratum medium consists of tubular and intertubular horn (the hard cornified component, stratum corneum) that arises from the basal cells of the epidermis lining the coronary band, or *coronet*, and is the thickest layer of the hoof wall and the main load support structure of the equine foot. The coronary epidermis is supported by the coronary dermis, which forms long papillae that extend into the epidermis and that are oriented parallel to the outer surface of the hoof wall. The coronary basal cells at the distal tip and along the sides of the dermal papillae form the tubular horn (or horn tubules), which also are parallel to the outer hoof wall. In cross section, the tubular horn may be circular, oval, or wedge shaped and consists centrally of a loosely arranged medullary area bordered by three layers of tightly or more loosely coiled cortical cells. The coiled (or springlike) pattern of tubular horn helps reduce compressive forces of the hoof. The coronary basal cells of the interpapillary dermis form the intertubular horn, which surrounds the tubular horn. The stratum internum (stratum lamellatum) of the inner hoof wall is present from the deep edge of the coronary region to the sole. It is a complex structure composed of approximately 600 parallel,

[2]Structurally, the mammary gland (mamma[e]) is part of the skin; however, because of historical traditions in the practice of veterinary pathology, these materials are found in Chapter 18, Female Reproductive System and Mammae.

cornified primary epidermal lamellae that extend inward (toward the distal phalanx) from the stratum medium in which they are firmly incorporated or fused. Each primary epidermal lamella has approximately 150 to 200 outwardly radiating secondary epidermal lamellae, the dermal side of which orients toward the distal phalanx. The secondary epidermal lamellae consist of a central core of partially cornified spinous layer cells that attach at their apical surface to the sides of the primary epidermal lamellae, and a single layer of basal cells that attach to the subjacent secondary dermal lamellae via hemidesmosomes in the basement membrane (see Fig. 17-4). The primary and secondary epidermal lamellae interdigitate with the primary and secondary dermal lamellae, providing a large surface area to the inner hoof wall. The blood vessels that nourish the epidermal cells are located in the dermal lamellae. On one side of the basement membrane the epidermal cells of the epidermal lamellae are firmly attached, and on the other side of the basement membrane the collagen fibers of the lamina densa and sublamina densa are tightly interwoven with the tendon-like connective tissue that is firmly attached to the parietal surface of the distal phalanx, thereby anchoring the inner hoof wall to the dermis that covers the distal phalanx. In this way the epidermal and dermal lamellae serve as the suspensory apparatus of the distal phalanx, and if the attachment of the epidermal and dermal lamellae fails, the shearing forces of body weight and movement can result in the separation of the distal phalanx from the inner hoof wall, which can lead to the painful condition of laminitis (also called laminopathy in some instances) most often seen in horses and cattle (see section on Cutaneous Manifestations of Systemic Disorders, Laminitis). The sole consists of epidermis that interdigitates with its supportive dermis, which blends with the periosteum of the distal surface of the distal phalanx. The sole epidermis forms the tubular and intertubular horn of the sole, the surface of which is loosely attached and can be easily removed as small flakes. At the junction of the sole epidermis and stratum lamellatum, the lamellar epidermis is redirected (changes orientation) toward the distal aspect of the foot, and the horn of the stratum lamellatum joins and interconnects with the tubular and intertubular horn of the sole epidermis. The horn from the lamellar epidermis has a different degree of compactness and orientation, which provides a different shade of color, and has been termed the *white line* or *white zone*. The color difference allows the hoof wall to be visually distinguished from the sole. The frog consists of tubular and intertubular horn that is softer than the horn of the sole and wall of the hoof, and that is supported by dermis that blends with the digital cushion, a wedge-shaped mass of collagen, elastic tissue, and adipose tissue that serves to help absorb the impact of walking and running. Eccrine (atrichial) glands are also present in the frog.

The chestnuts and ergots of the horse are considered to be vestiges of the first, second, and fourth digits. Chestnuts are located in the supracarpal and tarsal area on the medial surface of the limbs, and the ergot is located at the flexion of the fetlocks (metacarpophalangeal articulation). Chestnuts and ergots are histologically similar, and each consists of a thick layer of tubular and intertubular horn covering thick cellular layers of the epidermis. The rete pegs are long and interdigitate with long dermal papillae.

The hooves of ruminants and pigs are cloven or divided into two parts, each of which consists of a wall, sole, and prominent bulb (also called the heel). The histologic characteristics of the wall and sole are similar to those of the horse; however, the interdigitating lamellae are smaller and less well developed, and only primary lamellae are present. Instead of a frog, ruminants and pigs have a prominent bulb lined by soft, thin cornified epidermis that is continuous with the skin and forms a large part of the distal hoof surface.

The claws of dogs and cats shield the distal phalanx and consist of a wall (i.e., dorsal and lateral) and sole (i.e., distal), both of which are stratified squamous cornifying epidermis. The epidermis of the wall produces a hard, cornified layer (stratum corneum), whereas the epidermis of the sole produces a softer, flakier stratum corneum. The dermis of the claw consists of dense collagen, elastic tissue, and blood vessels that can bleed profusely if the claw is trimmed too short. The claw fold is a fold of skin that covers the wall laterally and dorsally for a short distance.

The digital pads of dogs and cats have a thick epidermis composed of all layers, including the stratum lucidum. The surface is covered by compacted layers of stratum corneum and is smooth in the cat; however, in the dog the surface is covered by conical papillae that conform to the outline of the epidermal surface (see Fig. 17-2). The epidermis and dermis interdigitate via rete pegs and dermal papillae, thus providing resistance to shear forces. Eccrine (atrichial) glands are present in the dermis and the adipose tissue. Lobules of adipose tissue that act as a cushion are subdivided by collagenous stroma and elastic tissue.

Function

Hair provides a variety of functions for animals, including thermal regulation, physical protection, sensory perception, and social interaction, and serves as a mechanism of camouflage (Box 17-2). The skin is not only the largest organ in the body, but one of the most important. Without the skin, terrestrial mammalian life could not exist. The skin prevents significant loss of fluid and electrolytes (e.g., the stratum corneum barrier), protects against physical and chemical injury (e.g., the stratum corneum barrier, keratin filaments, desmosomal and hemidesmosomal junctions, collagen, and elastic fibers), participates in temperature and blood pressure regulation (e.g., the hair coat, sweat glands, and vascular supply), produces vitamin D (e.g., ultraviolet [UV] light photolysis of dehydrocholesterol), serves as a sensory organ (e.g., tactile hairs, Merkel cells, and nerves), and stores fat, water, vitamins, carbohydrates, protein, and other nutrients (e.g., subcutaneous fat). Absorption, although not a primary function, also occurs. In addition, the keratinocyte, a major source of cytokines and antimicrobial peptides, is now considered to be an integral part of the innate and adaptive immune systems protecting against microbial injury and participating in inflammation and tissue repair.

Dysfunction/Responses to Injury

A Primer to Histologic Patterns Characterizing Responses to Injury

A number of "new" terms commonly used to classify diseases of the skin are used throughout this chapter. For convenience and to provide quick reference, these terms are listed online in E-Glossary

Box 17-2 Functions of the Skin

- Provides a protective barrier against fluid loss, microbiologic agents, chemicals, and physical injury
- Regulates temperature and blood pressure
- Produces vitamin D
- Functions as a sensory organ
- Stores nutrients
- Absorptive surface
- Participates in innate and adaptive immunity and inflammation and repair

17-1. Although there are many new terms to learn, it should be realized that the system used to form these terms is similar to that used for other anatomic systems. Basically, prefixes and suffixes are added to word roots to create specific terms that define the pathology of the skin. For example, the prefix "epi" (meaning on or above) combined with the word root "dermat(o)" (referring to skin) creates the word "epidermis," which simply means the portion of the skin above the dermis. Likewise, the term hypodermis refers to the portion of the skin below the dermis, also called the subcutis or panniculus. Suffixes are used in the same way. For example, the suffix "itis" (meaning inflammation) combined with the word root "dermat(o)" forms the word "dermatitis," which simply means inflammation of the skin. Similarly, terms referring to inflammation predominantly within the epidermis, follicles, or the panniculus are epidermitis, folliculitis, and panniculitis, respectively. The suffix "osis" refers to a disease process, often noninflammatory. Thus combining dermat(o) and osis forms the word "dermatosis," which means any disease of the skin, especially one not characterized by inflammation. The term "dermatoses" is the plural of dermatosis and thus typically means noninflammatory skin diseases. However, the term "dermatoses" is also used less specifically to refer to a group of skin disorders of a variety of types, such as immune-mediated dermatoses.

Numerous endogenous and exogenous factors can potentially cause injury of the skin (Fig. 17-8). Determining a definitive diagnosis of a skin disorder often depends on obtaining a complete history, including age, breed, and sex of the animal; conducting a thorough physical examination, paying particular attention to the distribution of skin lesions; and performing additional diagnostic tests, such as skin scrapings, surface cytologic examination, a complete blood cell count, serum chemistry panel, fecal examination (e.g., for hookworm parasite ova), skin biopsy sampling, and microbiologic cultures. Results from cutaneous biopsy sampling are often useful and can be necessary to establish a definitive diagnosis for skin diseases. Although the skin has a limited range of responses to injury, the distribution and types of inflammatory cells in the lesion often represent a recognizable pattern that can be used to (1) formulate a list of specific etiologic agents that could cause the lesion or (2) suggest categories of disease with similar lesions and a common pathogenesis. Algorithms (i.e., a set of directions for accomplishing some task that has a recognizable end point) have been developed for the recognition of histopathologic patterns in veterinary dermatopathology (Table 17-3). Recognition of patterns, both clinically and histologically, can facilitate differential diagnoses of skin disease (Table 17-4). Patterns of responses to injury are illustrated by changes in the epidermis, dermis, adnexa, and panniculus and are discussed in the next sections.

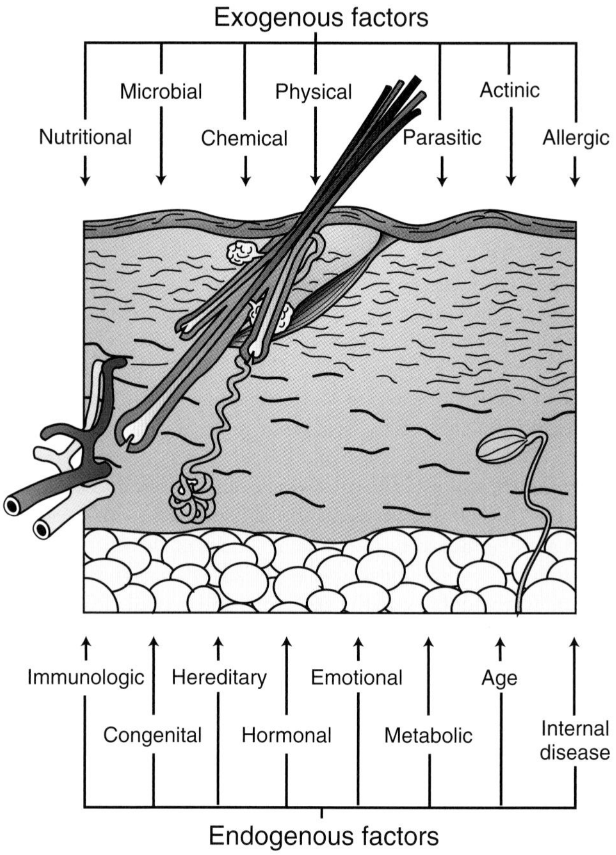

Figure 17-8 **Examples of Exogenous and Endogenous Factors That Influence the Skin.** A myriad of exogenous and endogenous factors influence the gross and microscopic appearance of the skin. Because the skin can respond to these factors in only a limited number of ways, different skin disorders may have a similar histologic appearance. Identification of the cause of a skin disorder therefore often requires not only histopathologic evaluation but also history, including clinical lesion distribution, appearance, duration, location, past medications, and other clinical data. (Revised and redrawn from Dellman DH, Brown EM: *Textbook of veterinary histology*, ed 3, Philadelphia, 1987, Lea and Febiger.)

Responses of the Epidermis to Injury

Alterations in Epidermal Growth or Differentiation. The basal cells (i.e., basal epidermal cells) in their postmitotic state migrate outward from the basal layer, eventually forming the cornified layers (stratum corneum) of the epidermis. In the normal epidermis, balance is established between the rate of proliferation of the basal cells (germinal cells) and the rate of loss of differentiated cells (corneocytes) from the surface, resulting in the constant thickness of the epidermis and each of the layers. The orderly proliferation, differentiation, and cornification of epidermal cells is regulated by cytokines (e.g., epidermal growth factor, fibroblast growth factors [FGFs], insulin-like growth factors [ILGFs], interleukins, and TNF), hormones (e.g., cortisol and vitamin D_3), and nutritional factors such as protein, zinc, copper, fatty acids, vitamin A, and B vitamins. The cytokines that regulate keratinocyte growth and differentiation are produced by a variety of cell types in the skin, including endothelial cells, leukocytes, fibroblasts, and keratinocytes. Thus keratinocytes also have a self-regulatory role (i.e., autocrine) in their growth and differentiation, and inflammatory cells, among others, can influence keratinocyte growth and differentiation.

Disorders of Cornification. Disorders of cornification (i.e., alterations in the formation of the stratum corneum) can be primary, such as occurs in primary seborrhea, but more often are secondary to a variety of factors such as inflammation, surface trauma, environmental conditions (e.g., low humidity), or metabolic or nutritional disorders. A disorder of cornification called hyperkeratosis is characterized by an increase in the thickness of the stratum corneum. There are two forms of hyperkeratosis, orthokeratotic and parakeratotic hyperkeratosis, which are distinguished by the completeness of the cornification process and whether the keratinocytes ultimately lose or retain their nucleus. In orthokeratotic hyperkeratosis (also referred to as hyperkeratosis), the keratinocytes undergo complete cornification and thus lose their nucleus to become anuclear, whereas in parakeratotic hyperkeratosis (also referred to as parakeratosis), the keratinocytes undergo only partial or incomplete cornification and thus retain their nucleus. Subtypes of hyperkeratosis include basket weave (exaggerated undulating pattern of layers of

Table 17-3 Examples of Pattern Diagnosis in the Skin

Component of Skin	Reaction to Injury	Pattern	Disease Examples
Epidermis	Prominent hyperkeratosis	Hyperkeratotic diseases of the epidermis	Primary seborrhea Ichthyosis Vitamin A deficiency Callus
Dermis	Interface inflammation	Interface dermatitis	Lupus erythematosus Dermatomyositis
Follicle	Inflammation of the follicular lumen	Luminal folliculitis	Infection with staphylococci, dermatophytes
Panniculus (subcutis)	Predominantly neutrophilic inflammation	Neutrophilic panniculitis	Abscess Feline pansteatitis (early)

A pattern consists of two parts: a component of the skin (e.g., epidermis) + a histologic reaction of that component to injury (e.g., hyperkeratosis) = pattern (hyperkeratotic diseases of the epidermis).

Table 17-4 Differential Diagnoses of Selected Patterns That Can Be Recognized Clinically and Histologically

PATTERN	Pustules Crusts (epidermal)	Vesicles Bullae (epidermal to subepidermal)	Necrosis or ulceration (epidermal)	Scaling or other hyperkeratotic lesions* (epidermal)	Nodules ± draining sinuses (dermal and pannicular)	Alopecia (adnexal)	Hypopigmentation or depigmentation (epidermal)
DISORDERS	Superficial bacterial infection Pemphigus foliaceus and panepidermal pustular pemphigus Dermatophilosis Exudative epidermitis Subcorneal pustular dermatosis Pawpads* Pemphigus foliaceus Superficial necrolytic dermatitis Lupus erythematosus	Pemphigus vulgaris Paraneoplastic pemphigus Lupus erythematosus Dermatomyositis Subepidermal bullous dermatoses Drug reactions Chemical and thermal burns Photosensitization Viral diseases	Vasculitis/infarction Chemical and thermal burns Superficial necrolytic dermatitis Erythema multiforme Stevens-Johnson syndrome Toxic epidermal necrolysis Ergot/fescue grass toxicity Frostbite Feline indolent ulcer Feline ulcerative dermatitis syndrome Vesicular cutaneous lupus erythematosus Self-trauma Epitheliogenesis imperfecta	Primary seborrhea Ichthyosis Zinc-responsive dermatosis Sebaceous adenitis Ear margin seborrhea Vitamin A responsive dermatosis Feline exfoliative dermatitis with and without thymoma Callus Cutaneous horn Solar (actinic) dermatosis	Masses caused by deep infections with bacteria, fungi, algae, *Pythium,* migratory parasites (e.g., abscesses, actinomycosis, feline leprosy, mycetoma, blastomycosis, pythiosis, habronemiasis) "Sterile" nodular inflammation (e.g., foreign body reactions, histiocytosis, sterile pyogranuloma, xanthoma, venomous bites, injection site reactions, eosinophilic granulomas) Panniculitis/steatitis Neoplasms	Folliculitis: infectious/noninfectious Postinflammatory and posttraumatic Endocrine alopecia Cyclic, idiopathic and seasonal alopecias Telogen effluvium Anagen effluvium Prolonged alopecia postclipping Follicular dysplasia Congenital alopecia and hypotrichosis Feline psychogenic alopecia Poor nutrition with protein deficiency Feline pancreatic paraneoplastic alopecia	Vitiligo Uveodermatologic syndrome Lupus erythematosus Copper deficiency Alopecia areata (healing stage) Inherited disorders (Chédiak-Higashi syndrome, Maltese and other coat color dilutions) Waardenburg-like syndrome Piebaldism Albinism Cyclic hematopoiesis Contact with rubber

Some of these disorders could be placed in different patterns. For instance, disorders characterized by vesicles or bullae may develop into an ulcerative pattern after the vesicles or bullae rupture.

*Hyperkeratotic disorders may also affect the nasal planum and pawpads; see Box 17-16.

the normal stratum corneum), compact (compacted layers of basket weave stratum corneum), and laminated (layers of stratum corneum that are more even and linear, and less undulating). Both parakeratosis and hyperkeratosis are common nonspecific responses to chronic stimuli (e.g., superficial trauma, inflammation, or sun exposure) and also occur as primary lesions. For example, hyperkeratosis is a feature of the cornification disorder, primary seborrhea, of the cocker spaniel (Fig. 17-9), ichthyosis, and vitamin A deficiency. Diffuse parakeratosis is a feature of zinc-responsive dermatosis and superficial necrolytic dermatitis (hepatocutaneous syndrome) (Fig. 17-10). Hyperkeratosis and parakeratosis can be accompanied by alterations in the thickness of the granular cell layer (stratum granulosum). Generally hyperkeratosis is associated with an increased thickness of the granular cell layer (hypergranulosis), and parakeratosis is associated with a decreased thickness of the granular cell layer (hypogranulosis).

Epidermal Hyperplasia. Epidermal hyperplasia is an alteration in epidermal growth or differentiation characterized by an increase in the number of cells within the epidermis, most often within the stratum spinosum, and is also referred to as acanthosis. Hyperplasia is a response common to a variety of stimuli, often chronic, and occurs in a variety of types, including regular, irregular, papillated, and pseudocarcinomatous (pseudoepitheliomatous) (Fig. 17-11). Some forms of epidermal hyperplasia (regular, irregular, and pseudocarcinomatous) can develop in sequence. In early stages of epidermal hyperplasia, the dermal-epidermal interface is mildly undulating, but as the hyperplasia progresses, there often is an elongation of the rete pegs that extend into the dermis and interdigitate with dermal papillae, and that can be regular or irregular. In regular epidermal hyperplasia the rete pegs are approximately evenly sized and shaped, whereas in irregular epidermal hyperplasia the rete pegs are less uniform. Pseudocarcinomatous hyperplasia is a chronic and late stage of epidermal hyperplasia that develops after milder forms (regular or irregular). It refers to marked hyperplasia of the epidermis, resulting in many branching and anastomosing epidermal projections (rete pegs) that deeply interdigitate with dermal collagen fibers. Mitotic figures can be numerous in proliferating basal cells, but in contrast to squamous cell carcinoma, the keratinocytes

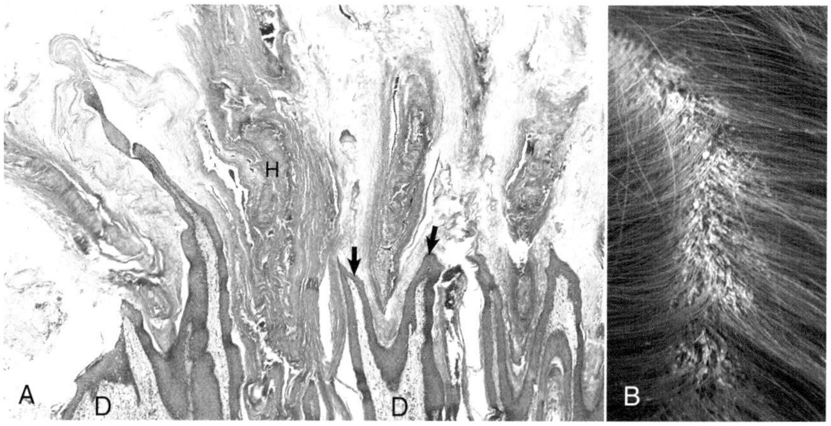

Figure 17-9 **Primary Idiopathic Seborrhea, Skin, Haired, Dog. A,** Note the marked orthokeratotic hyperkeratosis *(H)*. The stratum corneum within the hair follicles is increased in quantity; extends through the follicular openings to the external skin surface, where it surrounds hair shafts above the epidermal surface forming "hair casts"; and distends follicular openings *(arrows)*, creating a papillomatous appearance in the epidermis. *D*, Dermis. H&E stain. **B,** Hair is parted to reveal excessive scaling and keratin casts that are adhered to the hair shafts near their base, the result of orthokeratotic hyperkeratosis. (Courtesy Dr. A.M. Hargis, DermatoDiagnostics.)

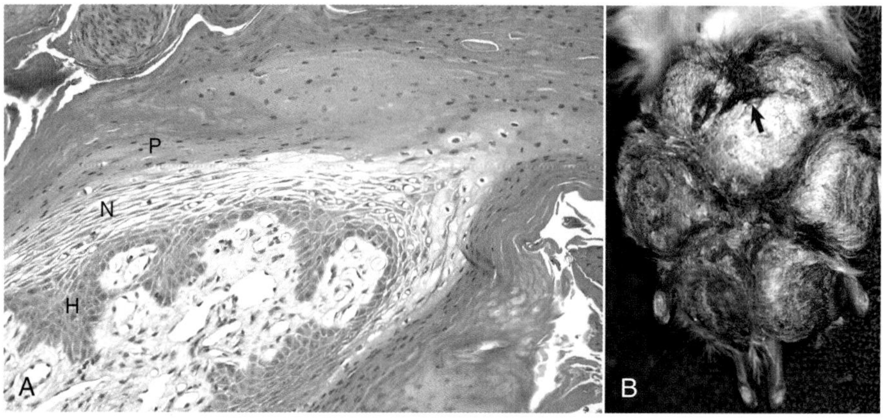

Figure 17-10 **Superficial Necrolytic Dermatitis, Skin, Dog. A,** Nuclei of the thickened stratum corneum have been retained (parakeratotic hyperkeratosis [parakeratosis]). The epidermis has a trilaminar pattern (red, white, and blue) created by three layers: (1) parakeratotic layer *(P)*, (2) subparakeratotic edema/necrolytic layer *(N)*, and (3) deep epidermal hyperplastic layer *(H)*. The pathogenesis of superficial necrolytic dermatitis is not completely understood but is speculated in most cases to be the result of an underlying systemic disease (such as severe liver disease or diabetes mellitus) that interferes with the normal nutrient metabolism needed to form a healthy epidermis. H&E stain. **B,** Pawpad. Note the fissure *(arrow)* and crusts. The crusting is largely a result of the parakeratosis. Secondary infections by bacteria, yeast, and fungi can also contribute to the formation of crusts by causing fluid, leukocytes, and other cellular debris to accumulate on the surface. (Courtesy Dr. A.M. Hargis, DermatoDiagnostics.)

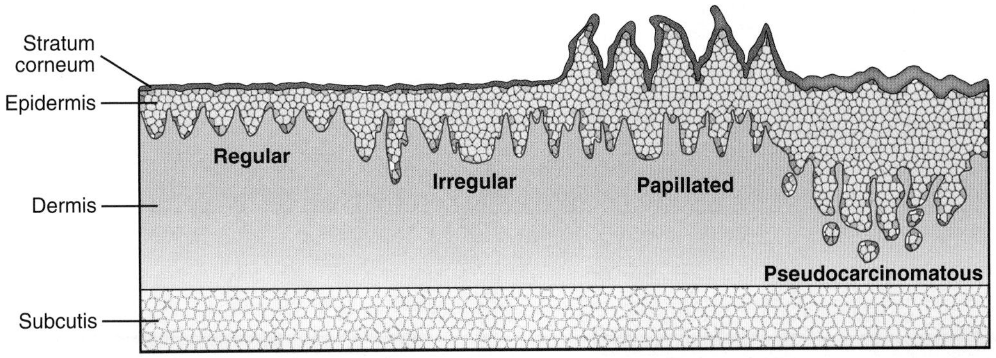

Figure 17-11 **Patterns of Epidermal Hyperplasia.** Epidermal hyperplasia is an increase in the number of cells within the epidermis and is the result of a variety of chronic insults; thus it is often considered a nonspecific finding. The four forms of epidermal hyperplasia, regular, irregular, papillated, and pseudocarcinomatous, are illustrated with an intact basement membrane *(red line)*. Each form of epidermal hyperplasia may develop independent of the others, although some forms may develop in sequence. Epidermal hyperplasia does not penetrate or breach the basement membrane, which is an important distinguishing feature from invasive carcinoma. (Courtesy Dr. S. Myers, Prairie Diagnostic Services; and Dr. J.F. Zachary, College of Veterinary Medicine, University of Illinois.)

maintain normal polarity, are not atypical, and do not penetrate the basement membrane. Pseudocarcinomatous hyperplasia develops subsequent to chronic injury, as seen with chronic dermal suppurative or granulomatous dermal inflammation or at the edges of persistent, nonhealing ulcers. Psoriasiform epidermal hyperplasia is an exaggerated type of regular epidermal hyperplasia in which the epidermis forms elongated rete pegs that are of similar length and width and that interdigitate with similarly elongated dermal papillae. This type of hyperplasia has very regular or uniform histologic appearance and is a feature of certain disease syndromes, such as psoriasiform lichenoid dermatitis of the springer spaniel and porcine juvenile pustular psoriasiform dermatitis (pityriasis rosea). Papillated epidermal hyperplasia is a unique form of epidermal hyperplasia in which fingerlike (papillary) projections of epidermis develop above the skin surface; it is a feature of some papillomas, hamartomas, and calluses and occasionally develops in response to cyclosporine drug therapy in dogs.

Apoptosis. Apoptosis refers to programmed cell death (see Chapter 1 for mechanisms of development), an important, normal physiologic process that contributes to embryologic development, wound healing, the removal of damaged cells, and adult tissue homeostasis and remodeling and is responsible for regression of the lower segment of the hair follicle during the catagen stage of the hair cycle. Apoptosis is tightly regulated because too little or too much may lead to pathologic processes. Neoplasia may develop when there is increased proliferation and inadequate apoptosis-driven removal of DNA-damaged cells. In contrast, the presence of numerous apoptotic keratinocytes is a feature of some immune-mediated diseases such as erythema multiforme (Fig. 17-12) and more rare conditions, including toxic epidermal necrolysis and graft-versus-host disease. Apoptotic cells typically condense and fragment into small bodies that are phagocytosed by adjacent parenchymal cells or tissue macrophages. However, keratinocytes, in contrast to other cells in the body, contain tonofilaments that provide structure and some rigidity to the cell. Thus the fragmentation into small bodies is less complete in apoptotic keratinocytes than other cells in the body. This is particularly so for keratinocytes that have accumulated more filaments through the process of maturation in the epidermis. The terms *dyskeratosis* or *filamentous degeneration* have been used to describe these keratinocytes. The fragmented (apoptotic) bodies in dyskeratotic keratinocytes are usually larger than in other cells, and they tend to resist phagocytosis. Dyskeratotic keratinocytes are separated from adjacent keratinocytes and have a pyknotic nucleus and brightly eosinophilic cytoplasm. Apoptosis differs significantly from necrosis, in which cell lysis liberates cellular contents into the extracellular space and elicits an inflammatory response. The development of an acute inflammatory response is prevented in apoptosis through phagocytosis of apoptotic keratinocytes, by adjacent keratinocytes, before their cellular disintegration.

Necrosis. Necrosis refers to the death of cells and is characterized by nuclear pyknosis (shrunken and dense nucleus), karyorrhexis (nuclear membrane rupture with fragmentation and release of contents), or karyolysis (complete dissolution of the nucleus with loss of chromatin material), organelle swelling, cell membrane rupture, and release of cytoplasmic elements into the extracellular space accompanied by an acute inflammatory response. Causes of epidermal necrosis include physical injury (lacerations, thermal burns), chemical injury (irritant contact dermatitis), and injury as a result of ischemia and infarction (vasculitis, thromboembolism). Necrosis of the epidermis can result in erosion (partial-thickness loss of an area of epidermis) or ulceration (full-thickness loss of epidermis and a portion of the dermis and sometimes deeper tissue).

Dysplasia. Dysplasia is defined as abnormal development of tissues or organs. The term is used in two different situations: (1) in association with a congenital or inherited abnormality of development and (2) in association with an abnormality in maturation of cells within a tissue (e.g., preneoplastic). In this second situation, it refers to an alteration in size, shape, and organization of adult cells (keratinocytes). Dysplasia is a stage of abnormal development that precedes the formation of a noninvasive (in situ) carcinoma. This is the stage of carcinoma that occurs before the abnormal epidermal cells penetrate the basement membrane. The histologic features of dysplasia include lost stratification of keratinocytes, variation in cell and nuclear size, increase in number of mitoses, and large hyperchromatic nuclei.

Epidermal Atrophy. Atrophy is a decrease in the number and size of the cells within the epidermis and occurs as a consequence of sublethal cell injury. Cutaneous atrophy can affect the epidermis, follicles, sebaceous glands, and dermal collagen and occurs in

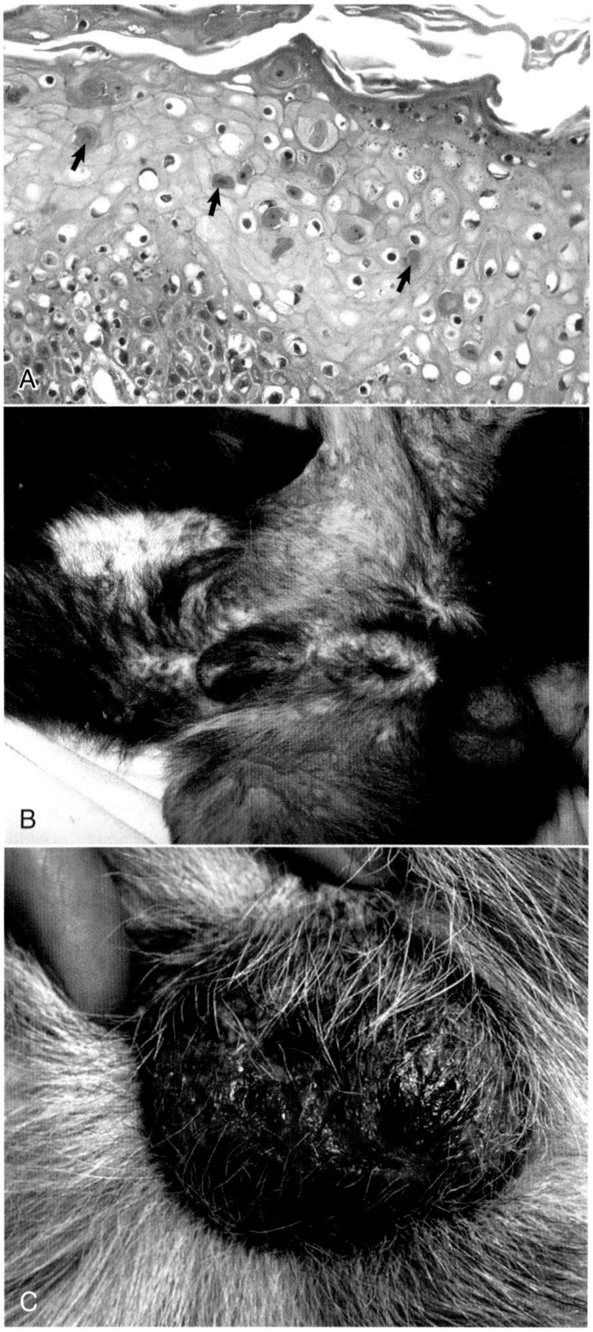

Figure 17-12 Erythema Multiforme, Skin, Dog. A, Apoptotic keratinocytes *(arrows)* are present in multiple layers of the epidermis. The increased staining intensity of apoptotic keratinocytes is a result of condensation of cytoplasmic organelles and nuclei. H&E stain. **B,** Skin of abdomen, inguinal region, and scrotum. Note the circular and linear erosions. The clinical lesions resulting from apoptotic keratinocytes depend on the prevalence and location of the apoptotic cells in the epidermal strata. Numerous deeply located apoptotic keratinocytes can lead to partial- or full-thickness loss of the epidermis, resulting in erosions and ulcers. **C,** Scrotum, erythema, ulceration, and crusting are present. Crusts form because the ulceration (injury) results in the release of inflammatory mediators, leading to the accumulation of fluid and cellular exudate that covers and dries on the ulcerated surface. (**A** courtesy Dr. A.M. Hargis, DermatoDiagnostics. **B** courtesy Clinical Dermatology Service, College of Veterinary Medicine, University of Florida. **C** courtesy Dr. A. Werner, Valley Veterinary Specialty Service.)

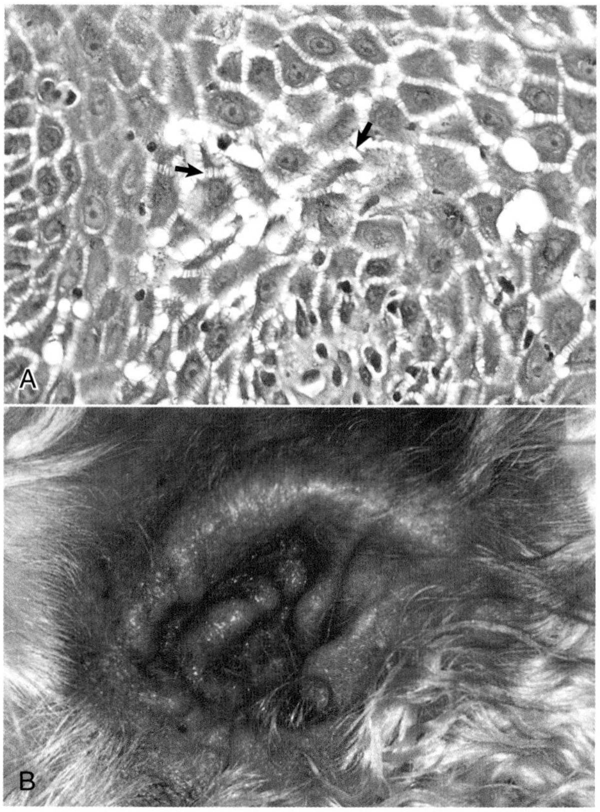

Figure 17-13 Edema, Skin, Dog. A, Intercellular epidermal edema. The epidermis appears "spongy" and the "spines" between keratinocytes *(arrows)* are accentuated from edema that widens the intercellular spaces. The keratinocytes remain connected to each other via desmosomal attachment sites (see Fig. 17-4). H&E stain. **B,** Acute allergic otitis, ear. The skin surface appears moist and glistening from dermal and epidermal edema, and there is erythema from dermal congestion (hyperemia). (**A** courtesy Dr. A.M. Hargis, DermatoDiagnostics. **B** courtesy Dr. D. Duclos, Animal Skin and Allergy Clinic.)

response to hormonal imbalances, such as hyperadrenocorticism in dogs and cats, partial ischemia, and severe malnutrition and may also develop as a consequence of aging.

Alterations in Epidermal Fluid Balance and Cellular Adhesion

Edema and Intracellular Fluid Accumulation. Edema refers to fluid accumulation between cells. Intercellular edema of the epidermis is called spongiosis because as the intercellular space expands with fluid, the epidermis develops a "spongy" appearance (Fig. 17-13). The term "spongiosis" is used in other chapters of this book to describe responses to injury that are unique to other tissues or organ systems, and in those circumstances the term "spongiosis" has different meanings. Severe intercellular edema of the epidermis results in the formation of spongiotic vesicles, which are variably sized clefts or spaces in the epidermis. The spongiotic vesicles often blend with intercellular spaces that are also widened but to a lesser degree; thus intercellular bridges are often prominent between keratinocytes bordering spongiotic vesicles. Spongiosis is common in epidermal inflammation (epidermitis) caused by staphylococci or *Malassezia* sp.

Intracellular fluid accumulation results in cytoplasmic swelling of keratinocytes, and if the swelling is severe, the swollen keratinocytes can burst, forming microvesicles supported by the walls of the ruptured cells. This type of epidermal damage is termed *reticular degeneration*. Intracellular fluid accumulation limited to the basal layer of the epidermis is termed *hydropic* or *vacuolar degeneration* and can result in the formation of intrabasilar vesicles. Hydropic degeneration is a consequence of damage to basal keratinocytes when the basal keratinocytes cannot maintain normal homeostasis, and fluid accumulates within the cells (Fig. 17-14). Rapid cytoplasmic swelling leads to cell membrane rupture and organelle breakdown typical of cell necrosis and is referred to as *oncosis*. Examples of diseases commonly resulting in hydropic degeneration include lupus erythematosus, dermatomyositis, and drug eruptions. Ballooning degeneration, a form of intracellular fluid accumulation of keratinocytes in more superficial layers of the epidermis, such as the stratum spinosum, is characterized by swollen cells losing their intercellular attachments. This type of degeneration can result in the formation of a fluid-filled vesicle. Viruses that infect cells of the epidermis, such as the pox and parapox viruses, can cause lysis of cytoplasmic keratin and a buildup of excessive fluid, resulting in ballooning degeneration (see section on Pathologic Reactions of the Entire Cutaneous Unit).

Acantholysis. Acantholysis is the disruption of intercellular junctions (desmosomes) between keratinocytes of the epidermis. The process is initiated by damage to transmembrane glycoproteins belonging to the cadherin family of adhesion molecules and leads to splitting of the extracellular core of the desmosomes. Subsequently the desmosomal plaques dissolve, and intermediate filaments retract to the perinuclear region of the keratinocytes. Acantholysis occurs with immune-mediated injury, as seen in pemphigus (type II cytotoxic hypersensitivity), with release of exfoliative toxins by staphylococci as seen in superficial pyoderma, and uncommonly with some *Trichophyton* sp. infections, presumably because of secretion of proteases by the fungi. The microscopic lesions vary with the location of acantholysis within the various layers of the epidermis. In pemphigus foliaceus (PF), acantholysis occurs in the subcorneal epidermis, resulting in release of free-floating keratinocytes in subcorneal vesicles and pustules (Fig. 17-15). In pemphigus vulgaris (PV), acantholysis occurs in the epidermis, just above the basal layer, resulting in the separation of the upper epidermis from the basal cells (which are often referred to as a row of tombstones) attached to the dermis via the basement membane (Fig. 17-16). Fluid accumulating between the separated layers of the epidermis forms vesicles of varied sizes and shapes.

Vesicles. Vesicles are fluid-filled cavities within or beneath the epidermis (Fig. 17-17). If the cavity is less than 1 cm in diameter, it is called a vesicle; if it is greater than 1 cm in diameter, it is called a bulla (pl. bullae). Vesicles can develop in any layer of the epidermis or beneath the epidermis and can form as the result of acantholysis, epidermal or dermal edema, degeneration of basal cells and keratinocytes, or other processes, such as immune-mediated targeting of components of the basement membrane, or frictional trauma and burns that damage proteins and lead to a lack of cohesion between the epidermal cells or between the epidermis and dermis, resulting in the accumulation of fluid within a cavity. The location of vesicles or bullae within the layers of the epidermis is suggestive of certain diseases. For instance, intraepidermal vesicles can occur in viral infections, subcorneal vesicles in pemphigus foliaceus, panepidermal vesicles in panepidermal pustular pemphigus, suprabasilar vesicles in pemphigus vulgaris, and subepidermal vesicles in bullous pemphigoid or thermal burns (Fig. 17-18 and see Fig. 17-17).

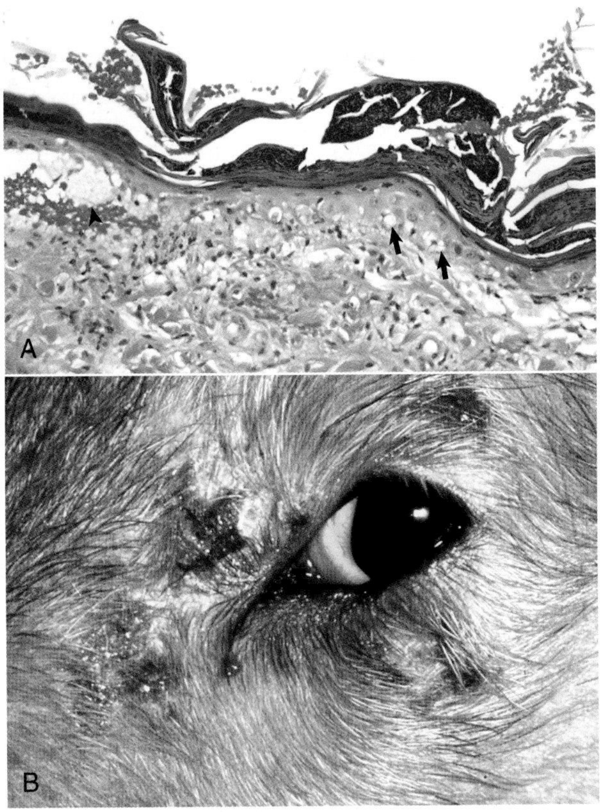

Figure 17-14 Hydropic Degeneration, Skin, Dog. A, Note vacuolization of the cells of the basal layer *(arrows)*. The vacuolated basal cells have resulted in a cleft *(arrowhead)* between the epidermis and dermis. A few lymphocytes are also present in the superficial dermis and lower layers of the epidermis. H&E stain. **B,** Dermatomyositis, periocular. Erythema, depigmentation, erosion, and crusting are the result of injury to basal cells. The vacuolar degeneration of basal cells weakens the dermal-epidermal attachment and results in formation of vesicles, erosions, and ulcers. In addition, inflammatory mediators are released, resulting in fluid and cellular exudate, which dry on the surface and form crusts. (Courtesy Dr. A.M. Hargis, DermatoDiagnostics.)

Inflammatory Lesions of the Epidermis. Acute inflammation of the epidermis actually begins in the dermis with active hyperemia, edema, and migration of leukocytes, often neutrophils (see Inflammatory Disorders of the Dermis). The edema fluid arises from dilated venules and can move intercellularly through the epidermis, widening the intercellular spaces and causing spongiosis (see Fig. 17-13). In thermal burns of the skin, larger quantities of fluid accumulate within or below the epidermis, forming vesicles (see Fig. 17-18); the fluid reaching the epidermal surface dries to form a largely acellular crust. The leukocytes (often neutrophils in acute inflammation) migrate from the superficial dermal vessels, through the superficial dermis, and into the intercellular spaces of the deep and then superficial layers of the epidermis. The aggregation of migrating leukocytes in the epidermis is termed exocytosis. Exocytosis of leukocytes is common in inflammation and is usually accompanied by spongiosis. If the inflammation progresses, the migrating leukocytes form pustules within the epidermis or the stratum corneum. Pustules usually dry rapidly and become crusts (Fig. 17-19). The type of leukocyte recruited into the epidermis is influenced by complex interactions of cytokines involved in the pathogenesis of the disease and can be useful in classifying and ultimately diagnosing the disease. For instance, intraepidermal eosinophils can be seen in association with ectoparasite bites. Lymphocytic infiltrates into the epidermis are often seen with immune-mediated diseases such as lupus erythematosus. Malignant lymphoma that predominantly affects the epidermis is also characterized by intraepidermal lymphocytes. Erythrocytes can also be present in the epidermis, usually

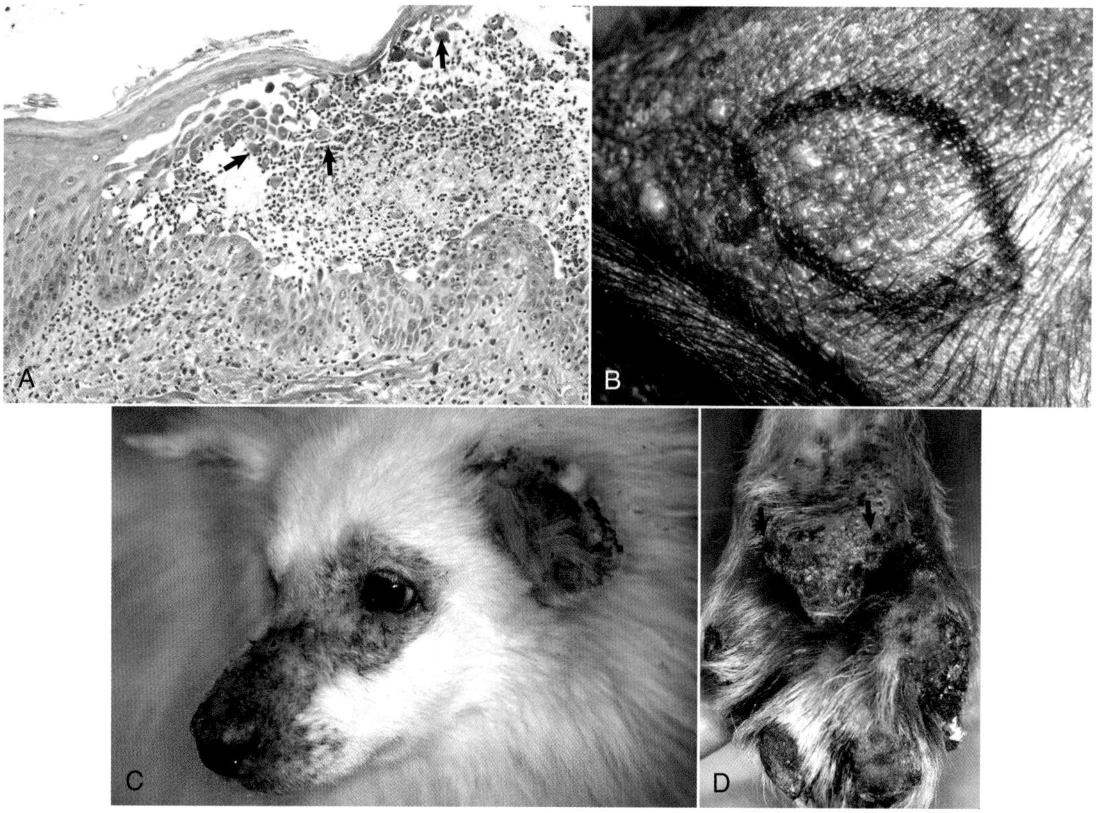

Figure 17-15 **Pemphigus Foliaceus, Skin. A,** Horse. Pustules in pemphigus foliaceus are located in the superficial epidermis, such as this subcorneal pustule that contains neutrophils and numerous acantholytic cells, which are epidermal cells separated from each other as a result of the loss of desmosomal attachments. Acantholytic cells may shed as individual cells *(arrows)* or in clusters. The roof of the pustule is the stratum corneum, and the base of the pustule is the stratum spinosum. Superficial pustules can rupture to form erosions and crusts. Forceful clipping or scrubbing of the surface of the pustule can lead to rupture and thus can make the sample nondiagnostic. H&E stain. **B,** Inguinal region, dog. Multiple pustules (circumscribed accumulations of pus in the epidermis visible as irregularly ovoid, slightly elevated yellowish tan areas) are present in the sparsely haired skin of the inguinal region. The skin within the black ellipse has been injected with local anesthetic in preparation for biopsy sampling. **C,** Face, dog. Erythema, alopecia, focal erosion, crusting, and depigmentation are present on medial surface of the pinnae, periocular skin, and dorsum of the muzzle and the nasal planum. Crusts develop as the result of upward growth of the epidermis and disruption of pustules. Erosions develop as the result of loss of stratum corneum and pustular exudate, which exposes the stratum spinosum. Depigmentation can result from inflammation and damage to pigment-containing epidermal cells. **D,** Pawpad, dog (same dog as in **C**). Erosions *(arrows)*, depigmentation, and crusts are present, and typically affect all pawpads. (**A** courtesy Dr. P.E. Ginn, College of Veterinary Medicine, University of Florida. **B** courtesy Dr. D. Duclos, Animal Skin and Allergy Clinic. **C** and **D** courtesy Dr. A.M. Hargis, DermatoDiagnostics.)

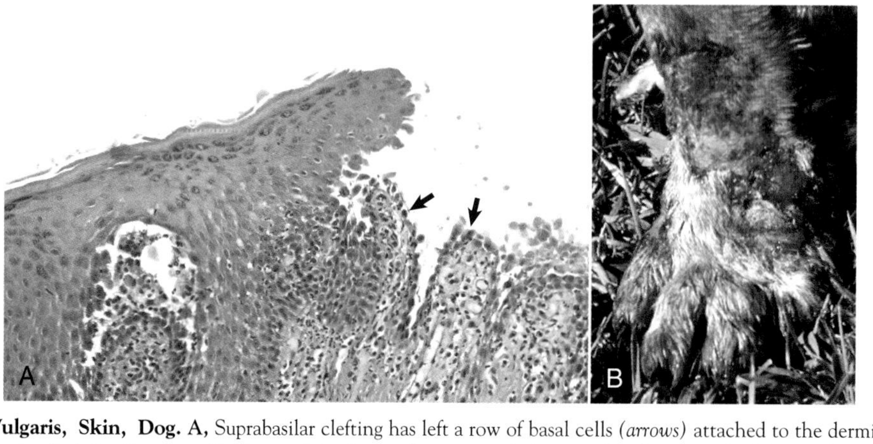

Figure 17-16 **Pemphigus Vulgaris, Skin, Dog. A,** Suprabasilar clefting has left a row of basal cells *(arrows)* attached to the dermis via the basement membrane. The single row of basal cells is fragile and easily damaged, leading to formation of ulcers, with subsequent fluid loss and secondary bacterial infection. H&E stain. **B,** Leg. Note the erythema and large confluent areas of ulceration. In contrast to pemphigus foliaceus (more commonly characterized by vesicopustules, erosions, and crusts), pemphigus vulgaris is characterized by larger, more confluent ulcers because the acantholysis in pemphigus vulgaris occurs deeper in the epidermis and the vesicles rapidly progress to ulcers. (**A** courtesy Dr. A.M. Hargis, DermatoDiagnostics. **B** courtesy Dr. A. Mundell, Animal Dermatology Service.)

associated with trauma, or circulatory disturbances, such as marked vasodilation and vasculitis.

Pustules. Pustules (microabscesses) are accumulations of inflammatory cells (pus) within the epidermis (see Fig. 17-15). Epidermal pustules vary in inflammatory cell content and location in the epidermis, depending on the pathogenesis of the disease. The pustules of superficial bacterial infections generally contain degenerate neutrophils and coccoid bacteria and are often located beneath the stratum corneum (subcorneal). In ectoparasitic hypersensitivity, pemphigus foliaceus, and feline eosinophilic plaque, the pustules can be filled with eosinophils. Small pustules containing neoplastic lymphocytes (Pautrier's microabscesses) are present in epitheliotropic lymphoma.

Crusts. Crusts are composed of dried fluid and cellular debris (i.e., dried exudates) located on the epidermal surface; thus crusts are indicative of a previous exudative process. Crusts are not specifically diagnostic but can hold the key to diagnosis in some diseases. For example, in dermatophilosis, the most diagnostic portion of the skin sample is the crust, which is multilaminated (or stratified) and contains the Gram-positive, branching coccoid organism *Dermatophilus congolensis*. Similarly, crusts formed through aging of pustules in pemphigus foliaceus are multilaminated because of numerous episodes of pustular eruption, and the crusts frequently contain numerous acantholytic cells. Crusts can also contain hair shafts infected with spores and hyphae of dermatophytes.

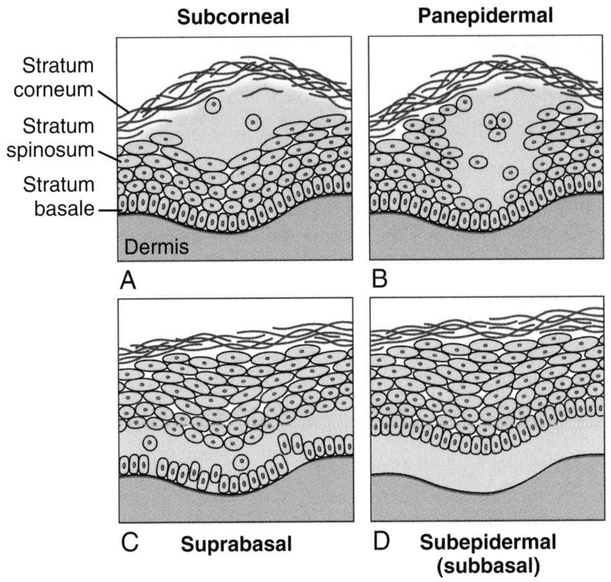

Figure 17-17 Locations of the Types of Vesicles That Form in the Skin. A, Subcorneal vesicle (as in impetigo or pemphigus foliaceus) is located between the stratum corneum and the superficial layers of the stratum spinosum. **B,** Panepidermal vesicle (as in panepidermal pustular pemphigus in the dog) extends through multiple levels of the stratum spinosum, and the stratum corneum may form the roof of the vesicle. **C,** In a suprabasal vesicle, a portion of the epidermis (stratum spinosum) forms the roof (as in pemphigus vulgaris). **D,** In a subepidermal vesicle, the entire epidermis separates from the dermis and forms the roof (as in bullous pemphigoid). The roof of the vesicle may be missing in biopsy specimens.

Alterations in Epidermal Pigmentation. Pigmentary alterations include hyperpigmentation, hypopigmentation, and pigmentary incontinence. Melanin is produced by melanocytes located in the basal and lower spinous layers of the epidermis, in the ORS and hair matrix of follicles, and perivascularly in the dermis. Melanocytes have surface receptors for hormones, such as melanocyte-stimulating hormone, and these hormones regulate melanogenesis. Other factors that influence the amount of melanin pigment in skin and hair are genes, age, temperature, and inflammation.

Hyperpigmentation. Hyperpigmentation results from an increased production of melanin from existing melanocytes or an increase in the number of melanocytes. An example of hyperpigmentation caused by an increased number of melanocytes is a lentigo, a rare localized nonneoplastic proliferation of melanocytes confined to the epidermis and resulting in formation of a black macular circumscribed lesion that is usually less than 1 cm in diameter. Most hyperpigmentation of the epidermis results from increased production of melanin from existing melanocytes. Possible mechanisms of increased melanin production include increases in the rate of production of melanosomes (i.e., granules within melanocytes that contain tyrosinase and synthesize melanin), in melanosome size, and in rates of melanosome transfer to keratinocytes and increased survival of melanosomes in keratinocytes. Examples of epidermal hyperpigmentation by increased production of melanin include chronic inflammatory diseases (most common cause), such as chronic allergic dermatitis, and endocrine dermatoses, such as

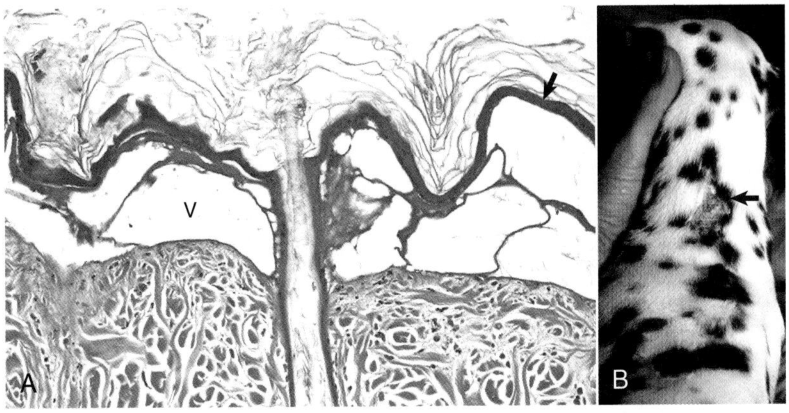

Figure 17-18 Thermal Burn, Full-Thickness (Third-Degree) Skin, Dog. A, There is necrosis of the epidermis *(arrow)*, follicular infundibulum, and dermis that is indicated by the diffuse deep acidophilic stain uptake, a lack of cellular detail, and an absence of nuclei. Because of increased capillary permeability, fluid has accumulated between the dermis and epidermis, forming vesicles *(V)*. H&E stain. **B,** The dry necrotic skin is the site of the burn *(arrow)*. (From Hargis AM, Lewis TP: Full thickness cutaneous burn in black haired skin on the dorsum of the body of a Dalmatian puppy, *Vet Dermatol* 10:69-83, 1991.)

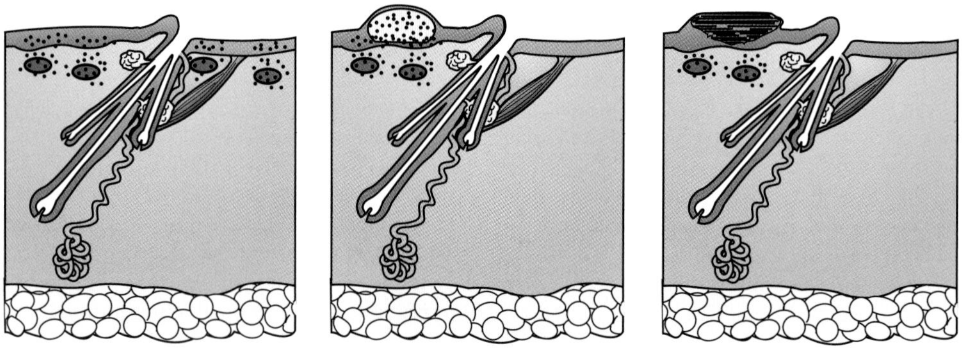

Figure 17-19 **Inflammatory Patterns of the Epidermis. A,** Leukocytes *(black dots)* migrate from the perivascular dermis into the epidermis, a process called exocytosis. **B,** Leukocytes migrate into the epidermis and accumulate to form a pustule. **C,** The pustule dries to form a crust. (Redrawn from Dr. A.M. Hargis, DermatoDiagnostics; and Dr. P.E. Ginn, College of Veterinary Medicine, University of Florida.)

hyperadrenocorticism. Hyperpigmentation secondary to inflammation is thought to result from release of melanocyte-stimulating factors from keratinocytes. It is thought that these factors are present in normal epidermis, but that their level or activity is increased in response to stimulation or keratinocyte stress.

Hypopigmentation. Hypopigmentation can be congenital or hereditary and develops because of a lack of melanocytes, failure of melanocytes to produce melanin, or failure of transfer of melanin to epidermal cells. Hypopigmentation can also be acquired via a loss of existing melanin or melanocytes (depigmentation). Because copper is a component of tyrosinase, production of melanin pigment depends on copper, and copper deficiency can result in reduced pigmentation. In addition to providing color to the skin, hair, and eyes, melanocytes are also important in the inner ear where they function to control ion transport necessary for the function of the inner ear. Thus animals without melanocytes in the inner ear are often deaf.

Pigmentary Incontinence. Pigmentary incontinence refers to the loss of melanin pigment from the basal layer of the epidermis or ORS or bulb of the hair follicles caused by damage to the cells of the basal layer or of the follicular components and the accumulation of the pigment in macrophages in the upper dermis or perifollicular regions, respectively. Basal layer pigmentary incontinence can be a nonspecific lesion associated with inflammation; however, it is also seen with diseases that specifically damage basal cells or melanocytes such as lupus erythematosus or vitiligo. Perifollicular pigmentary incontinence occurs in diseases in which inflammation targets the follicular wall, such as demodicosis, or when there is abnormal growth or development of hair follicles, such as in some types of follicular dysplasia. Leukotrichia and leukoderma (Fig. 17-20) refer to decreased pigmentation of hair and skin, respectively.

Responses of the Dermis to Injury

Alterations in Growth, Development, or Tissue Maintenance

Dermal Atrophy. Dermal atrophy results from a decrease in the quantity of collagen fibrils and fibroblasts in the dermis and leads to a decrease in the thickness of the dermis noted clinically by thin, translucent skin with more visible vasculature. The principal causes of dermal atrophy in domestic animals are catabolic diseases associated with protein degradation, such as hyperadrenocorticism (particularly in dogs and cats), and starvation. In cats with hyperadrenocorticism, collagen loss is sufficient to increase fragility of the skin, which tears with normal handling. Severe dermal atrophy can also be caused by repeated topical application of glucocorticoids.

Fibrosis. Fibrosis (fibroplasia) develops in response to various injuries, particularly ulceration of the epidermis. It consists of proliferation of fibroblasts and newly formed collagen fibrils (extracellular matrix). In the early stage of fibroplasia (called granulation tissue), the long axis of the fibroblasts and collagen fibrils are parallel to the surface of the skin and are oriented perpendicular to vertically aligned proliferative vessels. Clinically, the capillaries are seen on the surface as minute red dots that create a "granular" appearance, thus the name "granulation tissue." Microscopically, the orientation pattern provides a "latticework" appearance to the tissue (Fig. 17-21). Fibrosis refers to the gradual deposition and maturation of collagen to form a scar. During fibrosis, collagen production increases and fibroblast and capillary numbers decrease, resulting in less cellular dense collagen oriented in thick hyaline bundles in parallel arrangement (e.g., a scar), which grossly appear white and glistening.

Collagen Dysplasia. Collagen dysplasia is generally an inherited abnormality of collagen that results in decreased tensile strength and an increased ability of the skin to stretch beyond normal limits. Because the tensile strength is reduced, even minor trauma can cause the skin to tear. Healing results in formation of scars. Microscopic features vary among the different types of collagen dysplasia disorders and may include collagen bundles that vary in size and shape and consist of tangled fibers with an abnormal organizational pattern; however, in some of these disorders the skin has no detectable microscopic alterations.

Solar Elastosis. Solar elastosis is caused by chronic exposure of the skin to the UV spectrum of sunlight. UV radiation (UVR) consists of UVA (400 to 315 nm), UVB (315 to 280 nm), and UVC (280 to 100 nm). As sunlight passes through the atmosphere, the UVC and approximately 90% of UVB are absorbed. The UVA spectrum is less influenced by the atmosphere, so most UVR reaching the surface of the earth is UVA and a small amount of UVB. UVB penetrates into the epidermis and superficial dermis and is the portion of UV light most damaging to the skin. UVA penetrates deeper into the dermis, but its role in causing cutaneous injury is less well understood. Both UVB and UVA are thought to contribute to photoaging and carcinogenesis. The amount of UVR reaching the skin is dependent on a variety of host and environmental factors that can greatly influence the geographic incidence and anatomic locations of solar damage.

Environmental factors include quantity of ozone, smog, and cloud cover that tend to absorb and scatter some of the UV rays.

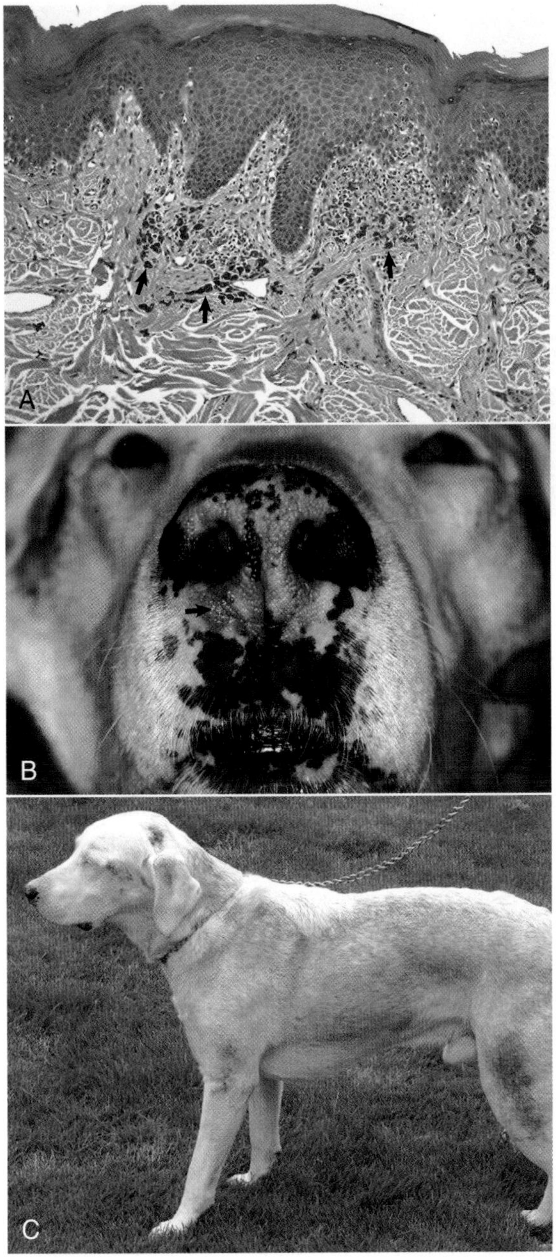

Figure 17-20 **Leukoderma, Skin, Dog. A,** Injury to the epidermal pigment-containing cells (predominantly melanocytes) has caused loss of melanin pigment in the epidermis (leukoderma). The pigment from the damaged melanocytes has been phagocytosed by dermal macrophages (pigmentary incontinence) *(arrows)*. Mild to moderate lymphocytic inflammation is present along the epidermal dermal interface. H&E stain. **B,** Nose and lips. Areas of the normally black skin of the planum nasale and lips have been partially *(bluish gray)* or totally *(pink)* depigmented. The bluish-gray areas are in the process of becoming depigmented. Biopsy samples should be collected from the bluish-gray areas *(arrow)* to identify active inflammation and diagnostic lesions. Biopsy samples from black skin or from already totally depigmented skin will likely only show normal-appearing black or nonpigmented skin, respectively, with no evidence of inflammation. **C,** Leukotrichia, body. This dog is the same one depicted in **B**. He was a black Labrador retriever mix. More than 90% of the black hair coat became white (leukotrichia). Biopsy samples from white-haired areas may be normal because the inflammatory event that caused the pigment loss is likely gone by the time nonpigmented hair shafts emerge from the hair follicles. (**A** courtesy Dr. A.M. Hargis, DermatoDiagnostics. **B** and **C** courtesy Dr. D. Duclos, Animal Skin and Allergy Clinic.)

Altitude and latitude are also very important. The atmosphere at high altitude is thinner, so there is less oxygen and particulate matter to absorb and scatter the UV rays. Latitude is also critically important. The incidence of sunlight-induced cancer is estimated to double for every 265 miles closer to the equator that human beings reside. At high latitudes the path of sunlight through the ozone layer is longer than at lower latitudes, so the ozone absorbs more of the harmful UV light. The path of sunlight through the ozone layer is also one of the reasons that sunlight has more damaging UV rays in summer months and at midday. Increased wind velocity has also been shown to have an enhancing influence on damaging effects of UV light on the skin. Local environmental factors can influence the quantity of UV light reaching an animal's skin. Such factors include availability of shelter from sunlight in the form of trees, shade panels, or indoor housing, and color of the ground material (lightly colored sand) that can increase exposure to UV light through reflection. Host factors include quantity of hair, degree of pigmentation, thickness of stratum corneum, and other difficult-to-define genetic factors. Therefore solar damage is more prevalent in high-altitude, low-latitude parts of the world and in animals residing outside for long periods of time. Lesions generally develop in poorly haired and lightly pigmented sites. Solar elastosis develops in the superficial dermis of chronically sun-exposed skin, and consists of increased numbers of thick, interwoven, basophilic fibers with the staining characteristics of elastin (thus the name "solar elastosis"). In the nonpigmented abdominal skin of dogs, solar elastosis may develop intermixed with or below a linear band of dermal scarring parallel to the epidermal surface (laminar fibrosis). The pathogenesis of the development of solar elastosis is complex and not fully understood and may vary with species. Current evidence involving studies in human beings and mouse models supports the view that a majority of the elastotic material (elastin, fibrillin, and glycosaminoglycans) is newly formed as the result of altered function of sun-damaged fibroblasts, but that degradation of preexisting dermal matrix proteins, including elastin and also most likely collagen, seems to be involved as well. Solar elastosis is less prominent in the skin of domestic animals than in human beings but is often prominent in lightly pigmented, poorly haired sun-exposed skin and eyelids of horses and in the lower eyelids of Hereford cattle residing in sunny locations.

Degenerative Collagen Disorders of the Dermis. The term collagen degeneration has been used to refer to an altered histologic appearance of collagen fibers in hematoxylin and eosin (H&E)-stained sections, whereby there is brightly eosinophilic granular to amorphous material bordering the fibers and somewhat obscuring the fiber detail. The collagen fibers and bordering eosinophilic material have also been referred to as flame figures, due in part to the irregular, sometimes radiating edges and brightly eosinophilic staining intensity. Electron microscopic studies in cats and human beings indicate that the collagen fibers can be disrupted, but they are not "degenerate." Instead, the brightly eosinophilic granular and amorphous material consists of aggregates of many eosinophils and eosinophil granules that border slightly disrupted but otherwise normal collagen fibers. These flame figures are seen in conditions in which eosinophils are prominent, including reactions to insect bites, mast cell tumors, and eosinophilic granulomas (collagenolytic granulomas) (Fig. 17-22). Collagen lysis refers to dissolution of collagen fibrils morphologically consisting of amorphous, lightly eosinophilic material lacking fibrillar detail. Collagen lysis is likely a secondary event caused by proteolytic enzymes released by a variety of cells, including eosinophils (collagenase) and neutrophils (collagenolytic proteinase, collagenase).

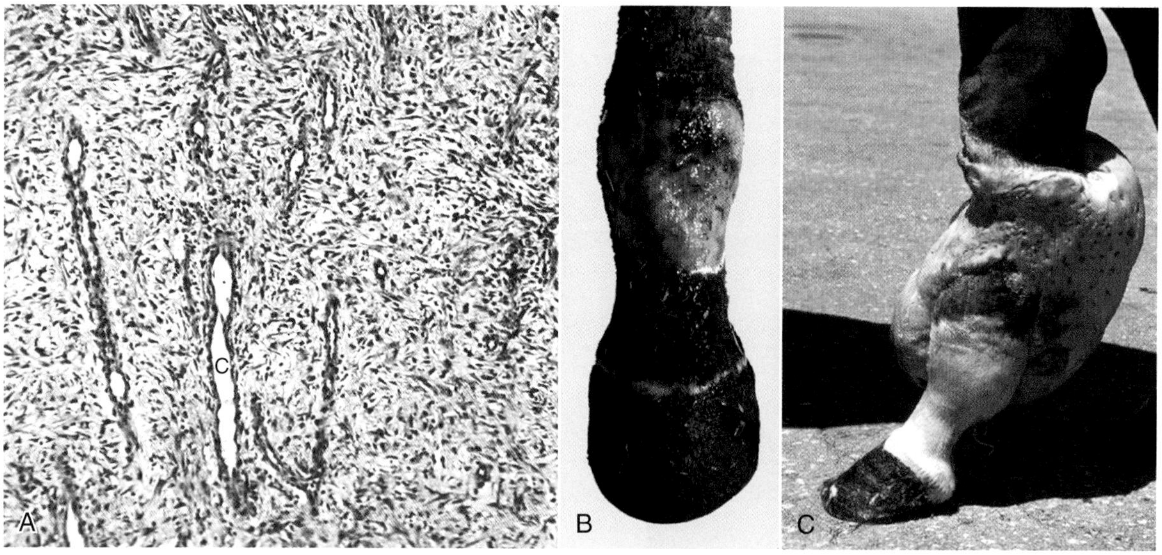

Figure 17-21 **Granulation Tissue, Skin, Horse. A,** Note vertically oriented capillaries (C) and horizontally oriented fibroblasts and a few collagen fibers providing a "latticework" appearance to the granulation tissue. **B,** Leg. Note ulcerated area filled with granulation tissue. **C,** Exuberant granulation tissue, leg. Granulation tissue is a normal component of wound healing. However, excessive or exuberant granulation tissue can develop as a pathologic process. This condition occurs, especially in horses, when an ulcer fails to become reepithelialized. Although this process is commonly called "exuberant granulation tissue," at the stage depicted in this photograph, most of the granulation tissue has been converted to fibrous connective tissue. (Courtesy Dr. M.D. McGavin, College of Veterinary Medicine, University of Tennessee.)

Disorders Characterized by Abnormal Deposits in the Dermis

Amyloid. Amyloid is an abnormal proteinaceous substance that can be deposited in a localized site in the body (organ limited) or can be "systemic," in which multiple organs are involved. In the systemic form, amyloid deposition can be the result of a primary abnormality of plasma cells (primary amyloidosis), in which case the amyloid is derived from components of immunoglobulin light chains (AL amyloid), or as a result of chronic inflammatory conditions (secondary amyloidosis), in which case the amyloid is derived from serum amyloid-associated protein (SAA protein), an acute phase reactant produced by the body in response to inflammation. Cutaneous amyloid deposition can occur in association with systemic amyloidosis, but visceral involvement is more common and clinically important. Cutaneous deposition of amyloid is rare but is seen in horses, dogs, and cats. In horses it can occur in association with secondary systemic amyloidosis or in a localized (organ-limited) form. In organ-limited amyloidosis the skin and/or upper respiratory tract are typically involved, the condition is not associated with recognized triggering causes, and the amyloid is produced from immunoglobulin light chains (AL amyloid). Clinical lesions vary from papules and plaques to nodules that usually are covered by a normal hair coat. Similar nodules can also develop in the respiratory mucosa and regional lymph nodes. Histologic lesions include nodular to diffuse granulomatous dermatitis and panniculitis with deposition of amyloid, an eosinophilic hyaline material. Cutaneous deposition of amyloid in dogs and cats is usually the localized type and is seen in association with extramedullary plasma cell tumors (AL amyloid). However, cutaneous deposition of amyloid in dogs also can be triggered by a monoclonal gammopathy (AL amyloid). Clinical and histologic lesions reflect the triggering disease.

Mucin. Mucin (glycosaminoglycan [GAG]), a normal component of the ground substance of the dermis, consists of protein bound to hyaluronic acid and can be deposited in increased quantity in focal areas or diffusely. Because hyaluronic acid has a great affinity for binding water, the skin in cases of mucin deposition (mucinosis) has a thick, puffy appearance. In cases of severe mucinosis, the skin, when pricked with a needle, can exude mucin (a stringy fluid material). In histologic sections, much of the water is lost, and mucin appears as fine amphophilic granules or fibrils that separate dermal collagen. Examples of disorders with dermal mucin deposition are termed myxedema in hypothyroidism and mucinosis (hereditary cutaneous hyaluronosis) in the Chinese Shar-Pei dog.

Calcium Deposits. Mineralization is a general term for the deposition of insoluble, inorganic minerals in the cutaneous tissue and usually consists of calcium in combination with phosphate or carbonate. Because the mineral most often deposited is calcium, the terms mineralization and calcification are often used interchangeably. Mineralization can occur in four basic forms: (1) dystrophic, (2) metastatic, (3) idiopathic, and (4) iatrogenic. Mineralization can also occur in tissues that have been traumatized, which may encompass more than one of these pathogenic mechanisms. Dystrophic mineralization occurs as a result of injury or degeneration of cellular and extracellular components of the skin, with normal serum calcium concentrations, and without abnormalities in calcium metabolism. Examples include deposition of mineral in granulomas and calcinosis cutis seen in some cases of hyperadrenocorticism. In metastatic mineralization the calcium deposits develop without preceding tissue injury or degeneration and in association with hypercalcemia, usually the result of abnormal metabolism of calcium, phosphorus, or vitamin D. Examples include deposition of calcium salts in soft tissues in chronic renal disease and in poisoning with cholecalciferol (vitamin D_3). Mitochondria have a high affinity for calcium and phosphate and participate in both dystrophic and metastatic calcification by concentrating intracellular calcium and phosphate to concentrations that allow crystallization. Mechanisms leading to calcium deposition in dystrophic mineralization involve reduced pH of injured tissue, the influx of calcium into injured cells, and then into mitochondria. Metastatic calcification may be the result of increased extracellular calcium concentrations and the failure of the cell's normal ability to strictly regulate intracellular calcium with resultant accumulation within mitochondria.

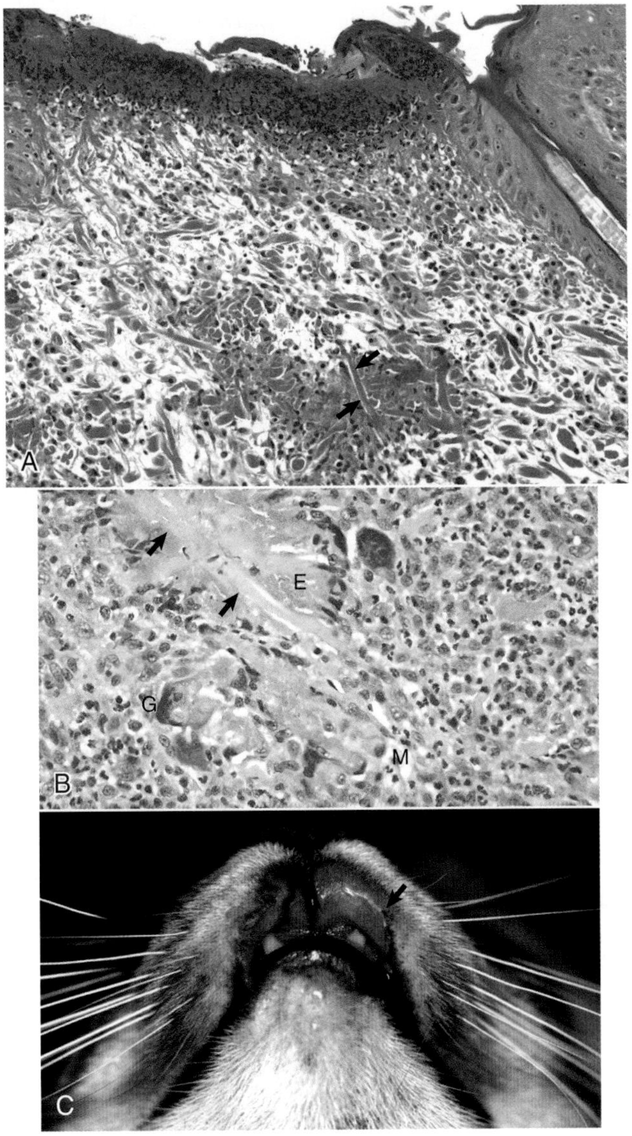

Figure 17-22 Eosinophilic Granuloma, Skin of Lip, Cat. A, Ulcerated skin (left) with fragmented collagen *(arrows)* is bordered by degranulated eosinophils. H&E stain. **B,** Fragmented collagen *(arrows)* is bordered by a row of macrophages *(M)*, multinucleated giant cells *(G)*, and degranulated eosinophils *(E)*, somewhat resembling a flame ("flame figure"). H&E stain. **C,** Upper lip. Bilateral ulcers are present on the upper lips, but the ulcer on the right side of the photograph is more extensive *(arrow)*. (Courtesy Dr. A.M. Hargis, DermatoDiagnostics.)

Mineralization can affect individual or groups of collagen fibers, resulting in increased basophilia and fragmentation of fibers in H&E-stained sections. The causes of idiopathic mineralization are not known; it occurs in the absence of tissue injury or abnormalities in calcium or phosphorus metabolism. Calcinosis circumscripta is a form of tissue mineralization in which calcium is deposited as amorphous nodular aggregates in the soft tissues of the tongue and in the subcutis of the pawpads of dogs. The pathogenesis is not defined, but some cases are considered idiopathic, whereas others may be the result of tissue trauma. Calcium deposits can elicit a granulomatous inflammatory response, a foreign-body reaction to the deposits. Iatrogenic mineralization develops via direct exposure to calcium salts such as occurs with topical exposure to calcium chloride deicing solutions.

Inflammatory Disorders of the Dermis. Dermatitis is inflammation of the dermis. Acute dermatitis begins with active hyperemia (increased blood flow), edema, and migration of leukocytes and results from release of cytokines and other mediators of acute inflammation (see Chapter 3). Active hyperemia is caused by vasodilation of arterioles, which causes increased blood flow at reduced velocity to capillary beds and postcapillary venules. Edema is caused by increased vascular permeability. Fluid leaves vessels mostly through widened interendothelial cell junctions. With a mild increase in vascular permeability, the edema fluid is clear (serous) because there are very few plasma proteins in the fluid. With increasing vascular permeability or endothelial cell injury, larger protein molecules, such as fibrinogen, escape from vessels, and the edema fluid becomes more eosinophilic and amorphous to fibrillar (fibrinous). The next step in acute dermatitis is migration of leukocytes from vessels into the perivascular dermis. The slowing of the blood flow and the endothelial cell expression of adhesion molecules that bind circulating leukocytes permit the migration of leukocytes in acute inflammation. The slowing of the blood flow allows leukocytes to move from the center of the vessel, where blood flow is fastest, to the margin, where they contact and attach to the activated endothelial cells.

After attaching to activated endothelial cells, leukocytes migrate between the endothelial cells into the perivascular dermis. The type of leukocyte that migrates and the sequence of cellular influx depend on activation of different adhesion molecules and chemotactic factors in the different phases of inflammation. In many types of acute inflammation, neutrophils are one of the first cells to arrive. Neutrophils predominate in the first 6 to 24 hours of injury and are generally replaced by macrophages in 24 to 48 hours. This sequence of cellular exudation can vary. For example, in reactions mediated by immunoglobulin E (IgE) cross-linking, such as type I hypersensitivity responses, mast cells (located in the perivascular dermis) are stimulated to release contents of granules (occurs in seconds) and synthesize and release inflammatory mediators (prostaglandins, leukotrienes, and cytokines), resulting in the influx of eosinophils, basophils, $CD4^+$ T helper type 2 (T_H2) lymphocytes, and macrophages. Mast cell degranulation and T_H2 lymphocyte activation cause eosinophils to accumulate in large numbers. Thus eosinophils often constitute the majority of leukocytes in inflammatory reactions against parasites and other allergic reactions.

Acute dermatitis typically results in one of four outcomes. First, there can be complete resolution, which occurs when the inciting stimulus has short duration and there is little tissue damage that is completely repaired. Second, an abscess can form, which occurs with pus-producing (pyogenic) bacterial infections. Third, healing occurs by replacement of the injured area by fibrous connective tissue (e.g., scarring), which occurs when there is significant tissue destruction (such as a deep burn) in which the parenchymal tissues are lost and thus cannot regenerate. Fourth, there is progression of acute dermatitis to chronic dermatitis.

Chronic dermatitis is inflammation of the skin that lasts weeks or months. Histologic features of chronic dermatitis include accumulation of macrophages, lymphocytes, and plasma cells; tissue destruction in part caused by the inflammatory cells; and a reparative host response of fibrosis and angiogenesis. Chronic dermatitis is usually caused by persistent infections often associated with delayed hypersensitivity and the formation of granulomas (e.g., *Mycobacteria* sp.), presence of foreign material in the skin (e.g., embedded suture), or autoimmune reactions in which self-antigens provoke an ongoing immunologic inflammatory response against host tissue (e.g., lupus erythematosus). Macrophages are a key cell in chronic dermatitis. They arise from monocytes in the peripheral blood and mature to macrophages whose primary function is phagocytosis. Macrophages also become activated by a variety of chemical mediators, including the cytokine interferon-γ (IFN-γ) secreted by sensitized T lymphocytes. When activated, macrophages also secrete many mediators of tissue injury (toxic oxygen metabolites, proteases, and coagulation factors) that contribute to chronic inflammation and fibrosis (growth factors, angiogenesis factors, and collagenases). The presence of lymphocytes and plasma cells in chronic inflammation is indicative of a host immune response.

The inflammatory milieu in the progression of acute and chronic dermatitis can be further complicated by other superimposed factors, notably physical injury from self-trauma, secondary bacterial infection of traumatized surface, injury from insect bites attracted by odor or exudate, and moderation by the host immune response or therapy. Thus dermal inflammatory responses to different stimuli often have overlapping histologic features, providing a diagnostic challenge for the dermatopathologist. Even so, the distribution of leukocytes often evolves into recognizable patterns that, when combined with the inflammatory cell type and other morphologic changes, suggest a group of differential diagnoses or the cause or pathogenesis of a specific disease (see Tables 17-3 and 17-4). Dermal patterns of inflammation that have been used in histologic diagnosis include perivascular dermatitis, vasculitis, interface dermatitis (inflammation affecting the basilar epidermis and superficial dermis that often obscures the dermal-epidermal interface), nodular to diffuse dermatitis with infectious agents, and nodular to diffuse dermatitis without infectious agents (Fig. 17-23). For example, perivascular dermatitis with eosinophils is suggestive of hypersensitivity associated with parasites or other antigens; interface dermatitis with lymphocytes is suggestive of an immune response directed toward epidermal cells, such as lupus erythematosus or erythema multiforme; and nodular dermatitis with macrophages (granulomatous dermatitis) indicates a persistent stimulus, such as infection with acid-fast bacteria or fungi. Thus patterns of inflammation combined with cellular composition of infiltrates are useful in microscopic diagnosis.

Responses of the Adnexa to Injury

The term adnexa refer to appendages or adjunct parts, which in the skin includes hair follicles and glands. The major clinical and histologic changes involve the hair follicles, and thus follicular lesions are emphasized in the next discussion.

Alterations in Maintenance, Growth, and Development

Atrophy. Atrophy refers to gradual reduction (involution) in size and can be physiologic or pathologic. Physiologic atrophy is related to the normal progression of the hair follicle cycle (i.e., the hair cycle stages of transition [catagen], rest [telogen], shed [exogen], and latency [kenogen]). Pathologic atrophy occurs when the degree of atrophy is greater than that expected for a given stage of the hair cycle and may involve a greater frequency and duration of kenogen. Causes of follicular atrophy include hormonal abnormalities,

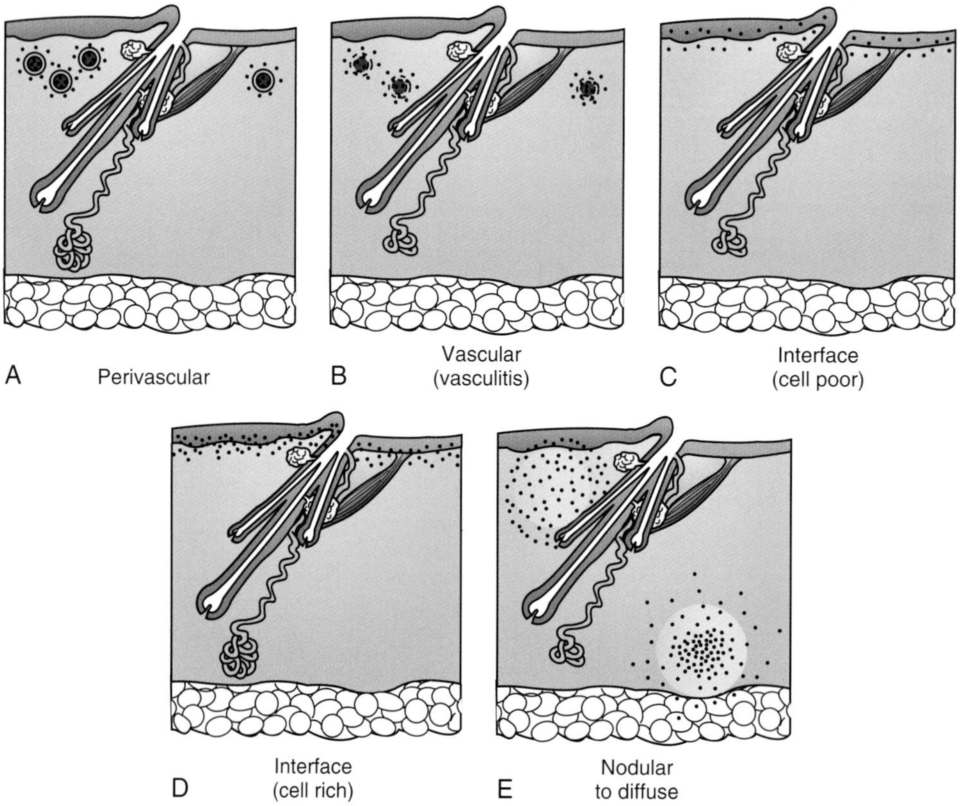

Figure 17-23 Inflammatory Patterns of the Dermis. A, Perivascular: Leukocytes *(black dots)* migrate from the dermal vessels into the perivascular dermis. This is the least specific pattern because all inflammatory patterns are at one stage, perivascular. **B,** Vascular (vasculitis): Leukocytes target the vessel wall, resulting in necrosis, inflammation, leakage of fibrin and red blood cells, and if severe, thrombosis and infarction. **C,** Interface, cell poor: Mild, often lymphocytic, inflammation located along the dermal-epidermal interface with vacuolar or apoptotic degeneration of basal cells. **D,** Interface, cell rich: Dense band of inflammation along the dermal-epidermal interface, obscuring the basilar layer of the epidermis, and with vacuolar or apoptotic degeneration of basal cells. **E,** Nodular to diffuse with or without microorganisms. Inflammation, typically granulomatous to pyogranulomatous, which partially effaces the architecture of the dermis may be associated with infectious agents or may be sterile. (Redrawn from Dr. A.M. Hargis, DermatoDiagnostics; and Dr. P.E. Ginn, College of Veterinary Medicine, University of Florida.)

nutritional abnormalities, inadequacy of blood supply, inflammation, and general state of health, including stressful events or systemic illness. Some types of pathologic atrophy can be reversed when the underlying cause is corrected. Damage to germinal epithelial cells can result in destruction or total loss of the adnexa with replacement by a scar. Examples include extensive inflammation and disruption of the follicle (folliculitis and furunculosis) and bordering glands and dermis that destroys a significant portion of the adnexal germinal epithelium, thermal burns sufficiently deep to involve the adnexa and dermal vessels, thrombosis causing infarction (i.e., diamond skin disease in pigs), and severe physical trauma such as lacerations that remove components of the skin, including adnexa.

Hypertrophy. Hypertrophy is an increase in the unit size of a structure or an individual cell. Follicular hypertrophy, which results in follicles that are longer and wider than normal for the site, develops secondary to repeated surface trauma such as in acral lick dermatitis. Hyperplasia is an increase in the number of cells in a structure. Enlargement of adnexa, a common response to injury, usually involves both hypertrophy and hyperplasia and is observed in follicles and sebaceous and apocrine glands associated with chronic allergic dermatitis.

Abnormalities of Hair Cycle Stages. Abnormalities of hair cycle stages occur when there is disruption in the normal progression from the anagen, catagen, telogen, exogen, and kenogen stages of the hair cycle (see Fig. 17-7). Clinical and histopathologic lesions can vary. Telogen effluvium is associated with a sudden noticeable shedding of the hair coat (telogen hairs) that may result in a bilateral, patchy to more diffuse alopecia. In domestic animals no scientific studies regarding cause or pathogenesis have been performed. Anecdotal reports usually associate the condition with a past episode of systemic illness or severe stress such as high fever, pregnancy and lactation, or anesthesia and surgery. The illness or stressful event is thought to cause synchronization of the hair cycle leading to many of the hair follicles eventually entering anagen simultaneously with subsequent sudden loss of telogen hairs. It is unclear if there are differences in telogen effluvium between animals with an anagen-dominant hair cycle (as occurs in animals with continuously growing hair coats such as poodles) versus a telogen-dominant hair cycle (as occurs in most domestic animals). In most cases the hair loss typically does not develop until several weeks or months after the systemic illness or stress, and it eventually resolves as the new hair shafts emerge from the follicles and the new hair coat becomes visible. Diagnosis is usually made clinically with the history of rapid, often widespread hair loss after a systemic illness or severe stress. Examination of epilated hair shafts reveals telogen hair bulb (usually straight, rough surfaced, club or spear shaped, and without pigment). Most clinical cases have biopsy samples collected during the late stages (during the stage of excessive shedding), when the majority of follicles are in the anagen stage of the hair cycle (recovery stage). Histopathologic evaluation is most useful in ruling out other disorders that may also cause alopecia.

Anagen effluvium has been studied the most in human beings and is associated with sudden hair loss that occurs within days of insult to the anagen hair follicle that impairs its mitotic or metabolic activity. The hair loss is usually associated with chemotherapeutic agents used to treat cancer, especially combination drugs at higher doses. Damage to the hair matrix cells of the follicle can result in failure to produce a hair shaft or production of a narrow fragile hair shaft susceptible to breakage. Examination of the affected hair shaft reveals a fracture at a narrowed area. Histopathologic lesions include apoptosis and fragmented nuclei of hair matrix cells of the anagen hair bulbs. Anagen effluvium has been reported in animals that have had fever, infectious disease, metabolic disease, or antimitotic drugs. However, as many animals have telogen-based hair cycles with fewer hair follicles in the anagen stage of growth, the degree and pattern of hair loss in anagen effluvium are variable, and animals with anagen-dominant cycles (such as poodles) may be predisposed to this side effect. Diagnosis is usually made based on history of drug therapy or illness, examination of affected hairs, in conjunction with sudden onset of alopecia. Histopathologic evaluation is rarely performed.

Other animals with hair cycle abnormalities have gradual but progressive loss of hair shafts associated with an arrested hair cycle such as the endocrine disease termed hyperadrenocorticism.

Follicular Dysplasia. Follicular dysplasia refers to incomplete or abnormal development of the structure of follicles and hair shafts that ultimately leads to alopecia. Structure refers to the permanent physical structure of the hair follicle in contrast to temporary changes that may occur cyclically. Follicular dysplasia is usually an inherited abnormality of the hair follicles in which there is production of defective hair shafts, failure to maintain hair within follicles, or failure of hair growth. Follicular dysplasia may be congenital (present at birth) or tardive (later onset in life). Different types of follicular dysplasia syndromes are described in animals, but most are poorly characterized. Clinical features include reduced, absent, or poor-quality hair coat. Microscopic features vary but include abnormal keratinocytes in the hair matrix or abnormally formed components of the follicular wall. In contrast to the follicular dysplasia syndromes that are not associated with coat color, the color-linked follicular dysplasia syndromes such as color mutant alopecia (color dilution follicular dysplasia, color dilute alopecia) and black (dark) hair follicular dysplasia (Fig. 17-24) have more obvious microscopic lesions in which melanin pigment abnormalities serve as a marker for the dysplasia. These pigment abnormalities include abnormally clumped melanin pigment granules in keratinocytes and melanocytes in the epidermis and hair bulb; melanin pigment clumps that are of irregular size, shape, and distribution in hair shafts that may cause the hair to weaken and break above the epidermal surface;

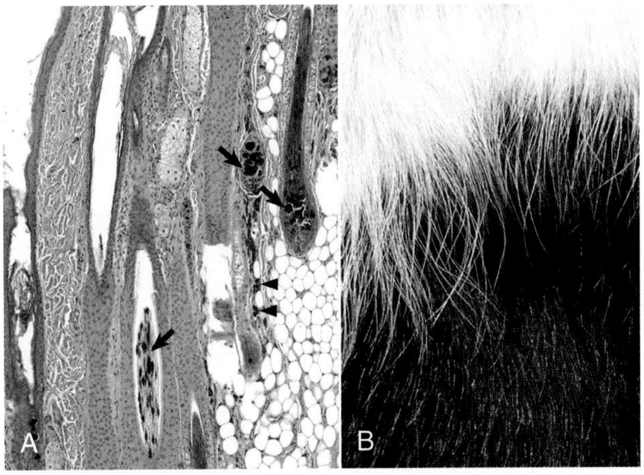

Figure 17-24 **Black (Dark) Hair Follicular Dysplasia, Skin, Dog. A,** Melanin pigment granules in hair shafts and hair matrix cells are large and variably sized, shaped, and distributed *(arrows)*. Perifollicular macrophages *(arrowheads)* that are most prominent near hair bulbs have phagocytosed melanin pigment presumably released from damaged hair matrix cells. H&E stain. **B,** The hair coat is normal in white-haired areas. Alopecia affects black-haired areas only but is difficult to recognize from a distance because the skin in affected areas is also black. (**A** courtesy Dr. A.M. Hargis, DermatoDiagnostics. **B** from Hargis AM, Brignac MM, Al-Bagdadi FAK, et al: Black hair follicular dysplasia in black and white Saluki dogs: differentiation from color mutant alopecia in the Doberman pinscher by microscopic examination of hairs, *Vet Dermatol* 2:69-83, 1991.)

and perifollicular melanophages that are most prominent near hair bulbs and that have phagocytosed melanin pigment presumably spilled from damaged hair matrix cells. The pathogenesis of the abnormal hair coat appears to involve weakened hair shafts that break at areas of aberrantly large pigment deposits, abnormal cuticle development, and possibly abnormal hair shaft development caused by damaged hair matrix cells. The dysplastic follicles may also become atrophic with time, contributing to the alopecia.

It should be noted that not all dogs that have coat color dilution have concurrent follicular dysplasia because the prevalence of follicular dysplasia varies among breeds with dilute coat colors. The propensity to develop follicular dysplasia is high in some breeds with coat color dilution such as the Doberman. For example, it is estimated that follicular dysplasia develops in approximately 93% of blue and 75% of fawn Dobermans.

Sebaceous Gland Dysplasia. Abnormal development of sebaceous glands is rare, is presumed to be genetic in origin, and has been reported in dogs and cats. The pathogenesis is unknown. Histologically, in early stages there are increased numbers of small epithelial reserve cells compared with mature sebaceous gland cells. The number of mature sebaceous gland cells may be reduced, cytoplasmic vacuolization may be irregular, and the orderly differentiation of reserve cells to mature cells is lost or absent. In the late stage there is subtotal atrophy, in which only a few reserve cells and a few mature sebaceous gland cells remain. Clinical lesions consist of adherent scales, poor hair coat, and progressive alopecia. The poor hair coat and alopecia are presumed to be the result of follicular atrophy and dysplasia that develop after or secondary to the sebaceous gland lesions.

Adnexal Inflammatory Disorders

Folliculitis. Folliculitis, inflammation of the hair follicle, affects most domestic animals. It is histologically classified according to the affected component of the hair follicle, the type of leukocytes in the inflammatory infiltrate, and the severity of the inflammation (Fig. 17-25). The types of follicular inflammation include perifolliculitis, mural folliculitis, luminal folliculitis, and inflammation of the hair bulb (bulbitis). The inflammation of hair follicles begins in the perifollicular blood vessels with the same hemodynamic, permeability, and leukocytic changes that constitute dermal inflammation. Leukocytes migrate from perifollicular blood vessels to the dermis, resulting in perifolliculitis (inflammation around but not involving the hair follicle). Perifolliculitis is not specific for any category of disease but is an initial event in the development of folliculitis. Perifolliculitis also often coincides with folliculitis of a variety of causes. The perifollicular inflammatory cells then migrate into the follicular wall, resulting in mural folliculitis (inflammation limited to the wall of the follicle). Depending on the cause of the inflammatory process, the leukocytes can remain localized to the follicular wall or can progress into the follicular lumen.

Mural. In mural folliculitis, leukocytes remain largely confined to the follicular wall. Mural folliculitis is further subdivided by the location, type, or severity of involvement of the follicular wall such as interface (outer aspect of the follicular wall), infiltrative (more

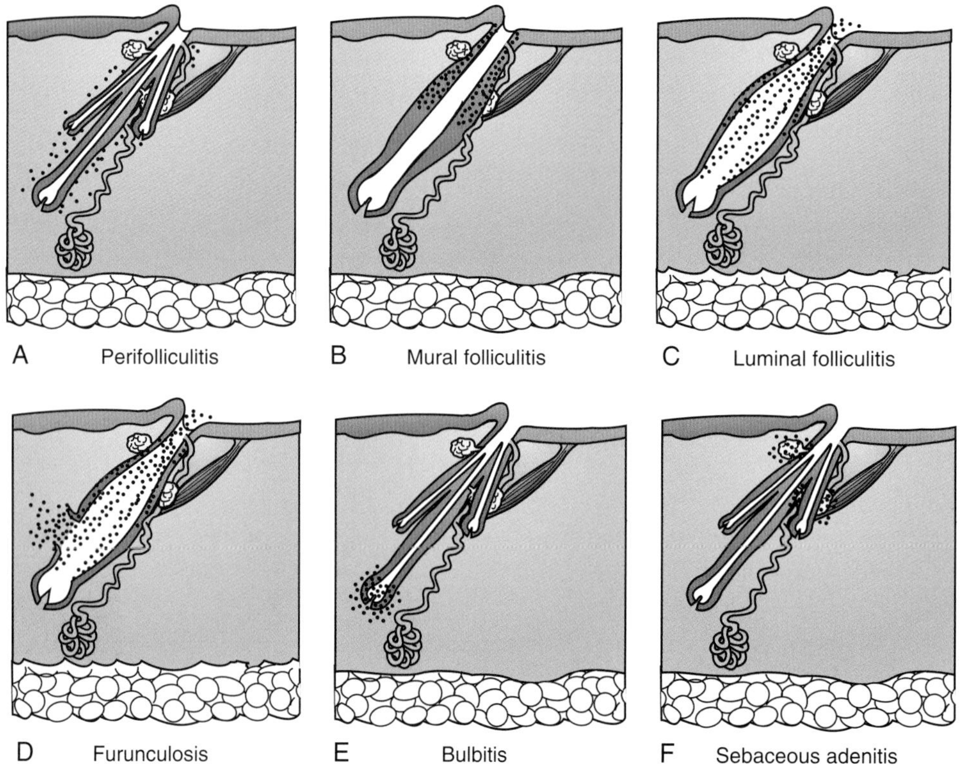

Figure 17-25 **Inflammatory Patterns of the Adnexa. A,** Perifollicular: Leukocytes *(black dots)* migrate from the dermal vessels near follicles into the perifollicular dermis. **B,** Mural folliculitis: Inflammation targets the follicular wall. There are subtypes of mural folliculitis that vary with level of involvement (superficial versus inferior), type of inflammation (pustular versus necrotizing), and the degree or severity of penetration into the follicular wall (interface versus infiltrative). **C,** Luminal folliculitis: Inflammatory exudate is present in the follicular lumen, and inflammation also usually involves the wall, often a response to follicular infection. **D,** Furunculosis: Disruption of the follicular wall, resulting in release of luminal contents into the bordering dermis. **E,** Bulbitis: Inflammation targeting the inferior segment or hair bulb of the hair follicle. **F,** Sebaceous adenitis: Inflammation targeting the sebaceous glands. For simplicity, a simple hair follicle is illustrated in parts **B, C,** and **D.** (Redrawn from Dr. A.M. Hargis, DermatoDiagnostics; and Dr. P.E. Ginn, College of Veterinary Medicine, University of Florida.)

infiltration into the follicular wall), pustular (presence of pustules in the follicular wall), or necrotizing (necrosis and disruption of the follicular wall). The subtype of mural folliculitis can provide insight into the pathogenesis of folliculitis (e.g., disease process). For example, pustular mural folliculitis is a feature of pemphigus foliaceus, and interface mural folliculitis is a feature of demodicosis (Fig. 17-26).

Bulbitis. Bulbitis refers to inflammation directed to the deepest portion of the hair follicle, the hair bulb. Alopecia areata is a specific example of bulbitis that develops in horses, cattle, dogs, and cats. Inflammation and subsequent damage to the hair matrix cells in the growing hair bulb ultimately result in alopecia. Although alopecia areata is recognized as an immune-mediated disorder, its precise etiopathogenesis is uncertain. In horses and dogs, antifollicular cell-mediated immunity and humoral immunity may participate. In some cases of alopecia areata, the hair bulb melanocyte also may be a target. Microscopic lesions consist of lymphocytic infiltrates within and around growing (anagen) hair bulbs up to the level of the isthmus. The cellular infiltrates within the hair bulb are mostly cytotoxic $CD8^+$ lymphocytes and $CD1^+$ antigen-presenting dendritic cells, whereas $CD4^+$ lymphocytes dominate the peribulbar T lymphocyte infiltrate. The role of circulating autoantibodies that target trichohyalin, hair keratins, and other components of the hair follicle remain unresolved; however, their appearance before the onset of clinically apparent alopecia in many cases of alopecia areata suggests these autoantibodies are not simply produced as a secondary response to hair follicle damage. The inflammation associated with the anagen hair bulb is thought to disrupt the function of the follicles, which subsequently enter the catagen and then telogen stages of the hair cycle. Alopecia areata can spontaneously resolve, but the newly growing hairs can be white instead of pigmented, probably as a result of damage to melanocytes in the hair bulb. In some instances the inflammation disappears, but the hair matrix cells do not fully recover, and instead follicles develop abnormal shapes or contours

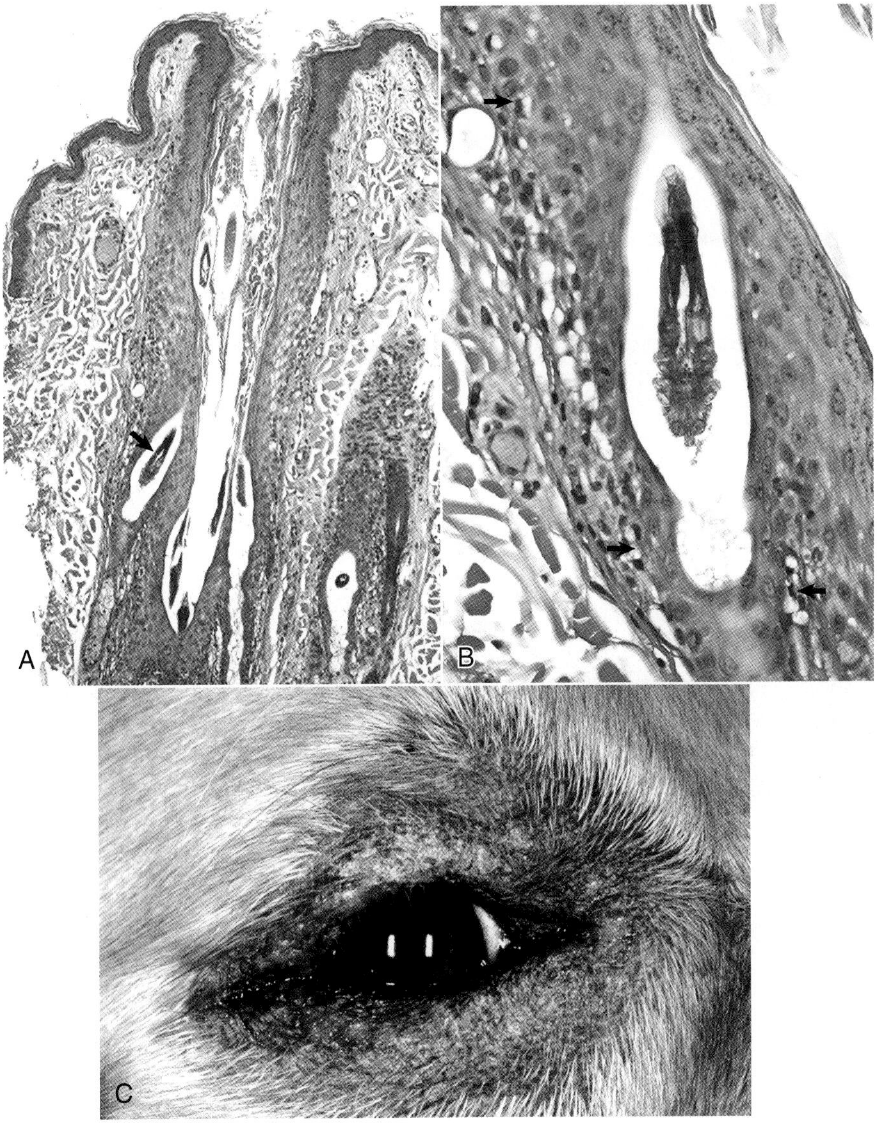

Figure 17-26 **Demodicosis, Skin, Dog. A,** Note mites deep in the follicle lumens *(arrow)* and also inflammation in the outer wall of the follicle (interface mural folliculitis) and in the perifollicular dermis (perifolliculitis). H&E stain. **B,** Note the mite in the follicular lumen. A few lymphocytes border the follicular wall, and there is mild vacuolar degeneration of basal cells *(arrows)* (lymphocytic interface mural folliculitis) of the follicular wall. H&E stain. **C,** Localized demodicosis, periocular. Skin is alopecic and lichenified, with mottled hyperpigmentation and hypopigmentation that are likely caused by inflammation, initiated by an immune response to mite infestation and possibly secondary bacterial infection, that results in damage and sometimes disruption of the follicular wall (furunculosis). (Courtesy Dr. A.M. Hargis, DermatoDiagnostics.)

and produce defective hair shafts. In the past these noninflamed but abnormal hair follicles and hair shafts were mistakenly thought to represent a primary form of follicular dysplasia, but it is now realized that these abnormal follicles are the result of previous hair bulb inflammation and hair matrix cells that do not fully recover function.

Luminal. Luminal folliculitis refers to inflammation predominantly involving the lumen and usually the wall of the follicle. It develops when leukocytes migrate from the wall into the lumen because they are attracted by various intraluminal stimuli, such as a follicular infection with bacteria (staphylococci), dermatophytes (*Microsporum*, *Trichophyton*), or infestation with parasites (*Demodex*, *Pelodera*) (Fig. 17-27). The inflammation can weaken the follicular wall, leading to rupture, known as *furunculosis* (Fig. 17-28), and release of follicular contents into the dermis. There are other causes of furunculosis, including trauma to the surface of the skin resulting in epidermal hyperplasia at the opening of the follicle, plugging of the follicle by stratum corneum, and accumulation of follicular contents, including glandular secretions (comedo formation). The gradual accumulation of this luminal material can cause distention of the follicle and thinning of the follicular wall, leading to rupture. Regardless of the cause of furunculosis, the presence of hair fragments, keratin proteins, sebum, and possible infectious agents in the dermis leads to a suppurative inflammatory response that progresses to more long-standing chronic pyogranulomatous inflammation and scarring. Perifolliculitis, luminal folliculitis, and furunculosis often follow in sequence (Fig. 17-29). The inflammation can resolve with appropriate therapy, can extend into the deep dermis and panniculus, and/or can form sinuses that drain to the surface of the skin and are difficult to resolve. Severe inflammation can lead to complete destruction of adnexal units and replacement by scar tissue that diminishes the likelihood of hair regrowth and complete recovery by the skin.

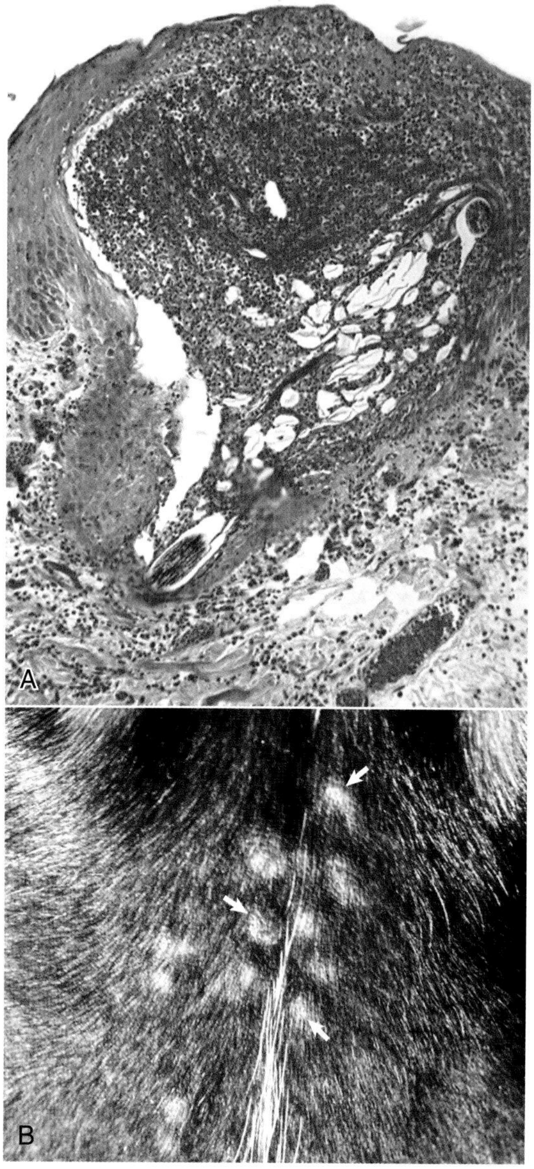

Figure 17-27 **Luminal Folliculitis, Skin, Haired, Dog. A,** The hair follicle lumen is distended with inflammatory cells (mostly neutrophils). H&E stain. **B,** Multiple alopecic papules *(arrows)* are caused by perifollicular inflammation, congestion and edema, and hair follicles distended with exudate. (**A** courtesy Dr. M.D. McGavin, College of Veterinary Medicine, University of Tennessee. **B** courtesy Dr. A.M. Hargis, DermatoDiagnostics.)

Sebaceous Adenitis. Sebaceous adenitis is a specific inflammatory reaction of unknown cause that targets sebaceous glands and results in alopecia and epidermal and follicular hyperkeratosis. It is largely a disease of dogs (Fig. 17-30) but rarely is seen in horses and cats. Early histologic lesions are characterized by accumulations of lymphocytes around sebaceous ducts or glands. Fully developed lesions consist of lymphocytes, neutrophils, and macrophages that efface sebaceous glands. Chronic lesions have total loss of sebaceous glands (atrophy), scarring, epidermal and follicular hyperkeratosis, and follicular atrophy. The inflammation of sebaceous glands is thought to be the result of a cell-mediated immune response, but the pathogenesis of alopecia and scaling is incompletely understood. Sebaceous gland inflammation also can occur secondary to folliculitis, demodicosis, uveodermatologic syndrome, or leishmaniasis, in which the inflammation primarily targets other areas of the skin (follicles, epidermal cells, or dermis) and involves the neighboring sebaceous glands because of their proximity to the inflammation.

Hidradenitis. Hidradenitis, which is inflammation of apocrine glands, has rarely been studied in detail in domestic animals. Suppurative hidradenitis has been described in dogs in which most cases developed in conjunction with staphylococcal folliculitis and furunculosis, either affecting the same or other follicular units. It is speculated, because of the physical connection between the apocrine gland and hair follicle in dogs, that suppurative hidradenitis is most often an extension of hair follicle infection and is the result of the bacteria that cause the folliculitis. There are no clinical signs that are unique to or suggest the presence of hidradenitis other than the association with follicular bacterial infection. Histologically, dogs with hidradenitis associated with bacterial folliculitis and furunculosis have suppurative inflammation of the apocrine gland and surrounding dermis.

Responses of the Vessels to Injury

Vasculitis, inflammation of vessels (see Fig. 17-23, *B*) in which the vessels are the primary target of injury, can be the result of infection by microbes, immunologic injury, toxins, photodynamic chemicals, UV light, or disseminated intravascular coagulation (DIC) or can be idiopathic. The species most commonly presenting with vasculitis are the horse and the dog, and most cases are idiopathic in that a specific cause cannot be determined. Histologic diagnosis of vasculitis is often challenging because it is difficult to differentiate between vessels taking part in inflammation simply by providing a conduit for inflammatory cells to reach a site of injury in the epidermis or dermis or vessels that are destroyed by their proximity to

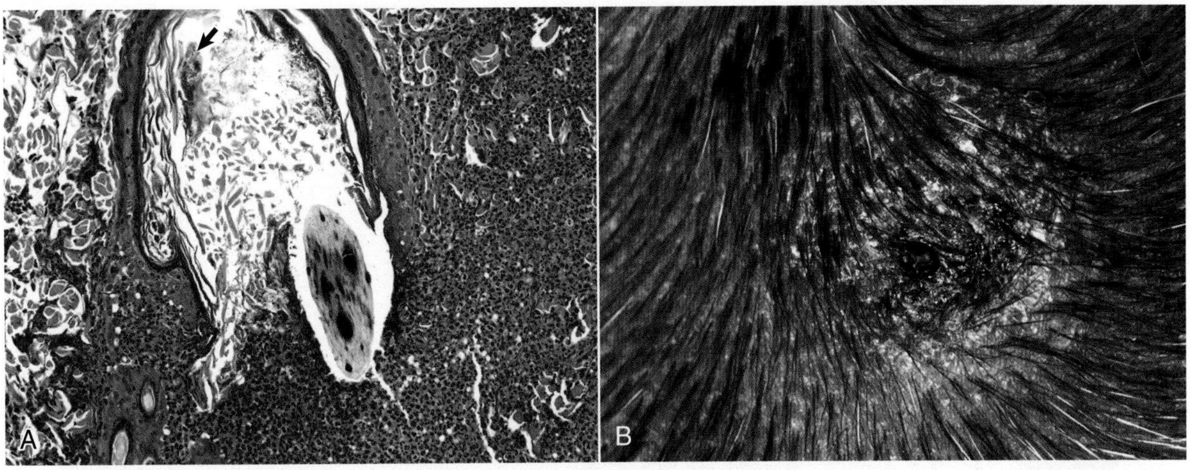

Figure 17-28 **Folliculitis and Furunculosis, Skin, Haired, Dog. A,** The wall of the follicle is disrupted, resulting in the release of follicular contents (a hair shaft, stratum corneum of the follicle, and exudate) into the dermis. The follicular lumen also contains numerous coccoid bacteria *(arrow)*. Note that the hair shaft has variably sized and shaped melanin pigment granules, indicating that this dog also has coat color dilution, which may increase susceptibility to folliculitis. H&E stain. **B,** A circular area of erythema, scaling, and crusting *(center of image)* is caused by follicular inflammation and rupture (furunculosis). The exudate in the perifollicular dermis has extended into the surrounding dermis and onto the skin surface through a draining sinus, and dried to form a crust. (Courtesy Dr. A.M. Hargis, DermatoDiagnostics.)

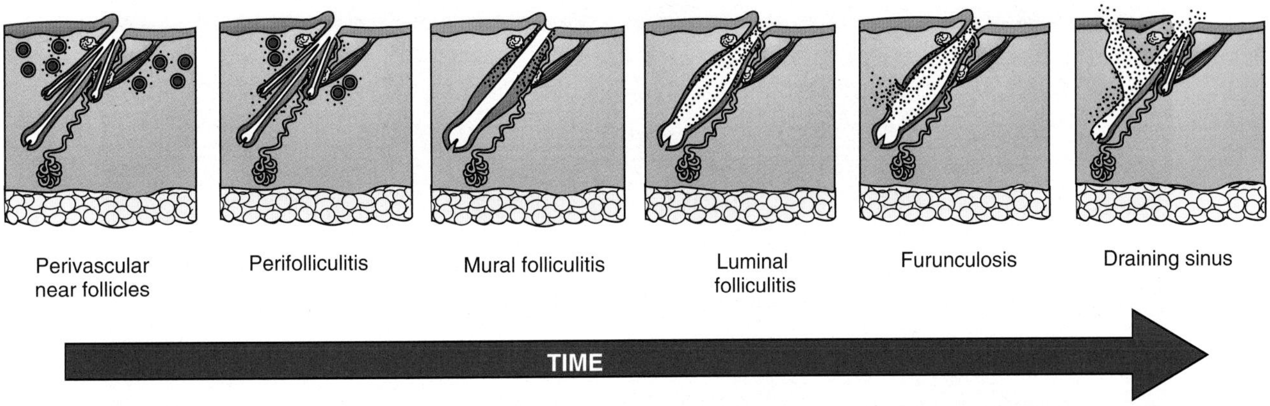

Figure 17-29 **Progression of Folliculitis.** Inflammation begins with migration of leukocytes *(black dots)* from perifollicular dermal vessels into the perifollicular dermis (perifolliculitis). Inflammation progresses to involve the follicular wall (mural folliculitis) and then the lumen (luminal folliculitis). If the inflammation continues, the follicular wall is weakened and ruptures, and follicular contents are released into the dermis (furunculosis). The inflammation can extend into the deep dermis and panniculus and/or form sinuses that drain to the surface of the skin. For simplicity, a simple hair follicle is illustrated in some frames. (Redrawn from Dr. A.M. Hargis, DermatoDiagnostics; and Dr. P.E. Ginn, College of Veterinary Medicine, University of Florida.)

surrounding inflammation that is severe and those vessels that are actually the target of injury. Also, the type of inflammatory cell that participates in the vasculitis reaction can vary more with the age of the vascular lesion than with the type of disease process inciting the stimulus. Histologic lesions in vasculitis include damage to the vessel wall such as the presence of few necrotic cells or foci of fibrinoid necrosis, mural infiltrates of leukocytes, and intramural or perivascular edema, hemorrhage, or fibrin exudation. Vascular injury leads to the clinical lesions of edema and hemorrhage and, if severe, can include ischemic necrosis and cutaneous infarction. Ulceration with or without sloughing of the skin can occur. Sustained partial ischemia can lead to atrophic changes in the components of the skin. Classic examples include immune-complex deposition in vessel walls (systemic lupus erythematosus and equine purpura hemorrhagica), vasculitis and ischemic dermatopathy associated with subcutaneous rabies vaccination, infection with an endotheliotropic organism (*Rickettsia rickettsii*), and septicemia with bacterial embolism and infarction in pigs (*Erysipelothrix rhusiopathiae*).

Responses of the Panniculus to Injury

Panniculitis. Panniculitis, inflammation of the subcutaneous adipose tissue, affects most domestic animals and can be caused by infectious agents (bacteria, fungi), immune-mediated disorders (systemic lupus erythematosus), physical injury (trauma, injection of irritant material, foreign bodies), nutritional disorders (vitamin E deficiency), or pancreatic disease (pancreatitis, pancreatic carcinoma) or can be of undetermined cause (idiopathic). Panniculitis can be primary or secondary. In primary panniculitis the

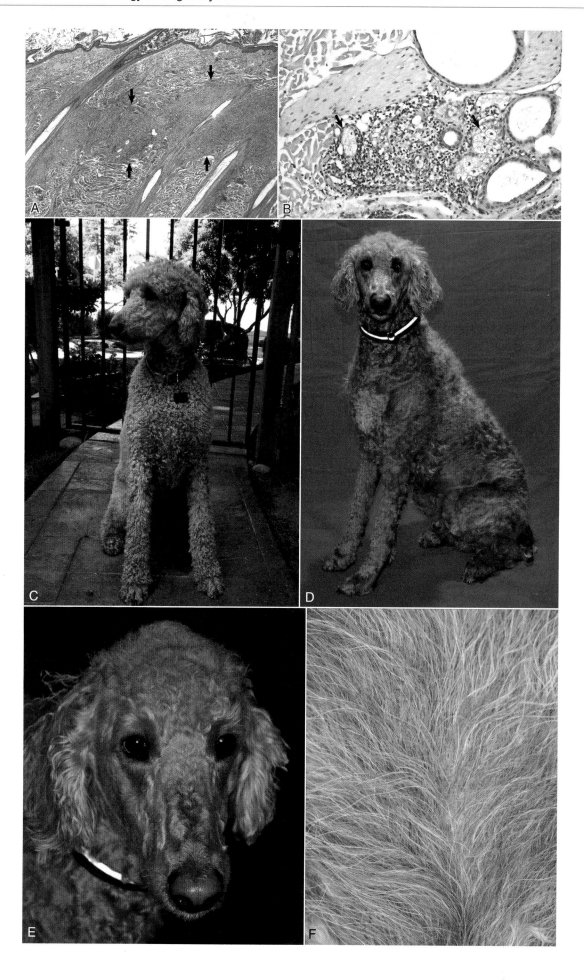

Figure 17-30 Sebaceous Adenitis, Skin, Haired, Dog. A, The inflammation in this fully developed sebaceous adenitis lesion forms a band of inflammatory cells parallel to the epidermis at the level of the sebaceous glands *(arrows)*, which are absent. Epidermal and infundibular hyperkeratosis are present. H&E stain. **B,** The inflammation in this early or mild sebaceous adenitis lesion is beginning to efface the sebaceous glands. A few sebaceous glands are visible within the area of inflammation *(arrows)*. H&E stain. **C,** Normal curly hair coat before development of sebaceous adenitis (face and paws are more closely clipped). **D** to **F,** Hair coat after development of sebaceous adenitis. Much of the hair coat of the entire body gradually shed. The poodle was treated with therapy, some of the hairs regrew, but the hair coat that remains is thinner than normal, and the hair shafts are darker, straighter, and coarser. The skin of the dorsal lumbar area is visible through the hair coat **(F)**. (**A** to **C** courtesy Dr. A.M. Hargis, DermatoDiagnostics. **D** to **F** courtesy Dr. D. Duclos, Animal Skin and Allergy Clinic.)

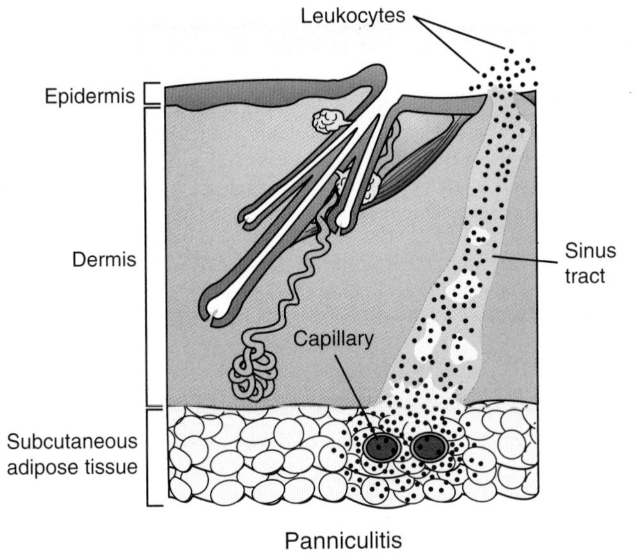

Figure 17-31 Inflammation of the Panniculus. Note the leukocytic inflammation *(black dots)* in the subcutaneous adipose tissue (panniculitis). In addition to spreading locally, the inflammation can form a sinus tract through the dermis and epidermis to the surface. The exudate can have an oily composition as a result of the fat content of the panniculus that is liberated following injury and forced via physical pressure applied locally to the skin to the surface of the skin through the sinus tract. (Redrawn from Dr. A.M. Hargis, DermatoDiagnostics; and Dr. P.E. Ginn, College of Veterinary Medicine, University of Florida.)

subcutaneous adipose tissue is the target of the disease process (Fig. 17-31). An example of primary panniculitis is feline pansteatitis, which occurs in cats fed diets high in polyunsaturated fatty acids and low in antioxidants, such as vitamin E. Lack of vitamin E leads to oxidation of lipids (free radical–induced membrane lipid peroxidation) of the subcutaneous adipose tissue, inciting a pyogranulomatous inflammatory response. In secondary panniculitis the subcutis is affected by inflammation primarily involving the contiguous dermis; the inflammation extends down into the subcutis. For example, deep bacterial folliculitis with furunculosis can lead to a secondary panniculitis, as can a penetrating wound contaminated with microbial agents or a foreign body. Animals with panniculitis clinically have palpable nodules that can ulcerate and drain an oily or hemorrhagic material (see Fig. 17-31). Lesions are most often on the trunk and proximal limbs and can be solitary or multifocal. Solitary lesions may be cured by excision, whereas multiple lesions may resolve with specific therapy or result in scar formation. In animals, panniculitis is subdivided based on cell type and presence or absence of microorganisms into the following basic categories: predominantly neutrophilic, predominantly lymphocytic, predominantly granulomatous to pyogranulomatous with infectious agents, predominantly granulomatous to pyogranulomatous without infectious agents, and fibrosing.

Pathologic Reactions of the Entire Cutaneous Unit

Skin diseases uncommonly affect just one component of the skin (e.g., only the epidermis or only the lumens of hair follicles). More often, multiple components of the skin are involved in the disease process. In addition, lesions evolve through different stages; some lesions can resolve, and there can be secondary lesions, such as self-induced trauma, complicating the initial lesions. Therefore multiple biopsy samples collected from different areas of the skin are often necessary to help illustrate the range of lesions necessary to reach a diagnosis. Multiple biopsy samples provide a more representative picture of the disease process than a single biopsy sample could. Even so, evaluation of multiple biopsy samples does not always lead to a specific diagnosis, but the pattern of lesions identified often suggests categories of disease and rules out other differential diagnoses.

The involvement of multiple components of the skin in a disease process can be illustrated by a poxvirus infection (Fig. 17-32). When a poxvirus invades the epidermis, the virus replicates in the cells of the stratum spinosum and causes cytoplasmic swelling (ballooning degeneration) and rupture (reticular degeneration) of some of the epidermal cells. Cytoplasmic viral inclusions form in some cells. Cellular constituents released from damaged epidermal cells act as chemical mediators of the acute inflammatory response and are chemotactic for leukocytes. These chemical mediators and chemotactic factors (1) increase blood flow to the site of viral invasion by dilation of arterioles, (2) cause margination of leukocytes in capillaries and postcapillary venules in the dermis, (3) increase vascular permeability (dermal edema), and (4) cause migration of leukocytes out of vessels into the tissue, creating the formation of macular lesions. The epidermal degeneration, dermal edema, and perivascular inflammation can progress to exudative lesions. Ballooning and reticular degeneration of keratinocytes result in the formation of intraepidermal vesicles. Leukocytes in perivascular sites under the influence of inflammatory mediators from the epidermis migrate to the epidermis and enter the vesicle to form pustules. Some poxviruses also cause epidermal hyperplasia by stimulating host cell DNA synthesis, presumably by a viral gene product similar to epidermal growth factor, resulting in pseudocarcinomatous hyperplasia. The pustule enlarges and eventually ruptures, releasing the exudates onto the skin surface. The exudates dry and form a crust (scab). The primary lesions of vesicles and pustules are fragile and often transient, lasting only hours, and so are difficult to identify and collect in biopsy samples. The secondary lesions of crusting and scarring are typical lesions at clinical presentation because they are more long-standing, but these older (late stage) lesions are less

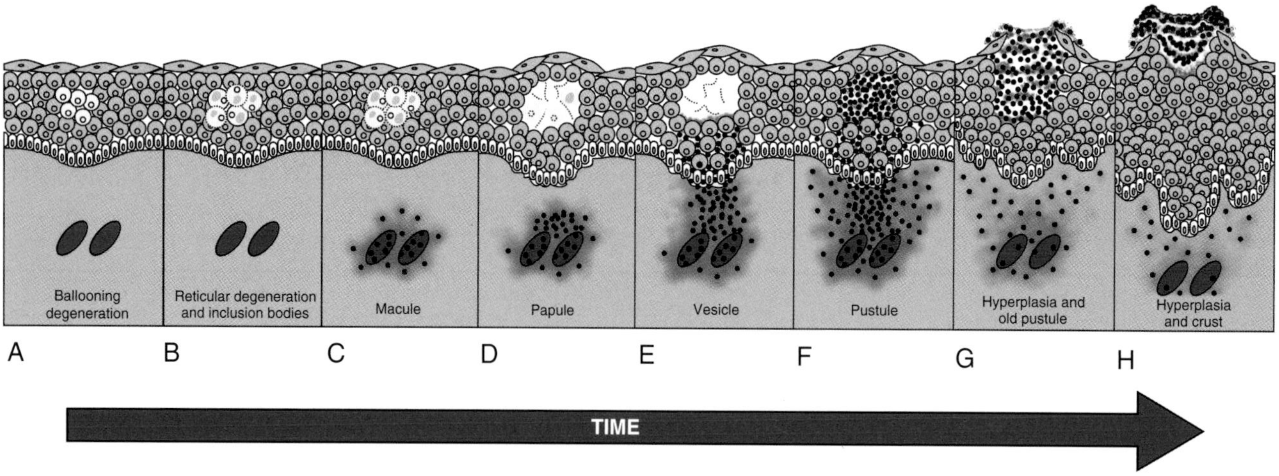

Figure 17-32 **Development of a Poxvirus Lesion Over Time. A,** Ballooning degeneration of keratinocytes. **B,** Reticular degeneration of keratinocytes with cytoplasmic viral inclusion bodies shown in pale gray. Both **A** and **B** are subclinical stages. **C,** Congestion, edema (illustrated in darker pink color images **C** to **H**), margination, and migration of leukocytes *(black dots)* form the macule stage. **D,** Continued epidermal reticular degeneration, epidermal hyperplasia (acanthosis), dermal edema, and perivascular inflammation form the papule stage. **E,** The vesicle stage develops by coalescing areas of reticular degeneration (disrupted swollen keratinocytes). **F,** Inflammatory cells migrate and fluid (illustrated in darker pink color in images **C** to **H**) extends from the dermal vessels into the vesicle, and the inflammatory cells and fluid accumulate in the vesicle to form the pustule stage. **G,** The epidermis begins to proliferate and becomes more acanthotic, and the old pustule is moved toward the epidermal surface. **H,** Epidermal hyperplasia progresses with the formation of elongated dermal-epidermal interdigitations, and the old pustule ruptures to form a crust. Larger pustules can be umbilicated or create a more irregular papillary epidermal surface, and result in scarring. (Redrawn from Dr. A.M. Hargis, DermatoDiagnostics; and Dr. P.E. Ginn, College of Veterinary Medicine, University of Florida.)

diagnostic histologically. In this way, multiple components of the skin participate in the development of the lesions and are responsible for the clinical stages of macule, papule, vesicle, pustule, crust, and scar.

Hypersensitivity and Autoimmune Reactions–Mechanisms of Tissue Damage

Diseases associated with excessive or aberrant immunologic responses are classified as either hypersensitivity (allergy) or autoimmune. Hypersensitivity is a mild to severe reaction that develops in response to normally harmless foreign compounds, including antiserum, pollen, and insect venoms. In contrast, autoimmune diseases develop when antibodies or T lymphocytes react against self-antigens when mechanisms of self-tolerance fail. Typically the immune system randomly generates millions of lymphocytes that can each respond to a different foreign protein and subsequently also removes any lymphocytes that may also respond to a self-antigen. Failure to remove or cull lymphocytes that respond to self-antigens may result in autoimmune disease. Autoimmune disease in this section is a general term referring to a spectrum of diseases in which autoimmune mechanisms appear to participate in lesion production. Four basic immune reactions, types I, II, III, and IV, mediate the tissue damage in both hypersensitivity and autoimmune diseases (Table 17-5). Most cutaneous hypersensitivity reactions are mediated by either type I or type IV reactions, or by a combination of one or more of the four reactions. In contrast, most autoimmune reactions tend to be mediated by type II or III reactions, although more than one mechanism can be involved. Hypersensitivity reactions are common in horses and dogs, less common in cats, and uncommon in food animals. Autoimmune diseases with cutaneous manifestations are uncommon in domestic animals, accounting for 1% to 2% of dermatoses in most species. Of the cutaneous autoimmune disorders, pemphigus foliaceus is the most prevalent, followed in incidence by discoid and systemic lupus erythematosus. In domestic animals, certain breeds of horses, dogs, and cats seem to be predisposed to develop particular autoimmune diseases.

Type I Reactions

Type I reactions are mediated by preformed or newly synthesized pharmacologically active substances released by mast cells and basophils after reaction between foreign antigen and specific antibody (usually IgE) bound to high-affinity IgE receptors on the membrane of the mast cells or basophils (see Table 17-5). Preformed substances released from mast cells include histamine, factors chemotactic for eosinophils and neutrophils, prostaglandins, serine esterases, and TNF-α. Substances synthesized on mast cell stimulation include leukotrienes, cytokines, and platelet-activating factor. Type I hypersensitivity can be systemic (anaphylaxis), localized to the skin, or both. In the skin the reaction results clinically in pruritic, circumscribed wheals with raised, erythematous borders. The reaction occurs in two phases, immediate (15 to 30 minutes) and late (6 to 12 hours), and is generally referred to as an immediate hypersensitivity reaction. The eosinophil products, major basic protein and eosinophil cationic protein, are toxic to epithelial cells and contribute to tissue damage in the late phase reaction. The production of IgE is genetically controlled, and therefore inherited predispositions to type I hypersensitivity occur. Cutaneous type I hypersensitivity reactions include atopic dermatitis (most common), urticaria, angioedema, hypersensitivity resulting from bites of flies such as *Culicoides* sp. and mites such as *Sarcoptes* sp., the presence of gastrointestinal parasites, and ingested dietary components (e.g., proteins, grains, preservatives). This type of reaction is characterized microscopically by mast cell degranulation, capillary dilation, edema, and infiltrates of eosinophils.

Type II Reactions

Type II reactions, also called *cytotoxic reactions*, depend on IgG or IgM antibodies formed against either normal or altered cell membrane antigens. The reaction engages Fc receptor and

Table 17-5 Mechanisms of Tissue Damage in Cutaneous Hypersensitivity or Autoimmune Diseases

There are four types of cutaneous hypersensitivity reactions (type I, II, III, IV) that cause tissue damage by immunologic mechanisms. Types I, II, and III are mediated by antibodies and are distinguished by the type of antigen and class of antibody involved. Type I responses are mediated by IgE bound to the high-affinity IgE receptor on the surface of mast cells. Binding of foreign (exogenous) antigen to IgE cross-links these receptors, inducing mast-cell activation. Type II responses are mediated by IgG or IgM directed to antigens bound to the surface of the cell or part of cell membrane. The reaction can engage Fc receptor and complement-mediated effector mechanisms. Type III responses are mediated by IgG or IgM directed against soluble antigens, and the tissue damage is caused by responses triggered by immune complexes. Type IV hypersensitivity reactions are mediated by T lymphocytes and can be subdivided into three groups. In the first group, tissue damage is caused by $CD4^+$ T_H1 lymphocytes directed to soluble antigen bound to MHC II and that release cytokines, including IFN-γ, resulting in an inflammatory response via macrophage activation. In the second, damage is caused by activation by $CD4^+$ T_H2 (helper) lymphocytes directed to soluble antigen bound to MHC II and that release IL-4 and IL-5, resulting in an inflammatory response in which eosinophils predominate. In the third, damage is caused by cytotoxic T lymphocytes ($CD8^+$) directed to cell-associated antigen bound to MHC I.

	Type I	Type II	Type III	Type IV		
Immune reactant	IgE	IgG or IgM	IgG or IgM	$CD4^+$ lymphocyte, T_H1 type	$CD4^+$ lymphocyte, T_H2 type (T helper)	$CD8^+$ cytotoxic lymphocyte
Time frame	15-30 min	Minutes to hours	3-10 hr	48-72 hr	48-72 hr	48-72 hr
Antigen	Exogenous antigen	Antigen is bound to surface of cell or is a part of the cell membrane	Soluble antigen, endogenous or exogenous	Soluble antigen bound to MHC II–injected into skin	Soluble antigen bound to MHC II	Cell-associated antigen bound to MHC I
(Examples)	(Pollens, molds, insect salivary antigens)	(Desmosomal or hemidesmosomal proteins)	(DNA, histones, ribosomes) (*Streptococcus equi*)	(Tuberculin)	(Atopic dermatitis: mites, pollens)	(Contact antigen or self-antigen)
Effector mechanism	Mast cell activation	FcR^+ cells (macrophages, NK cells) complement	FcR^+ cells complement	Macrophage activation	Eosinophil activation	Cytotoxicity
Examples of hypersensitivity	Atopic dermatitis, urticaria, anaphylaxis	Pemphigus, pemphigoid	Systemic lupus erythematosus; Purpura in *S. equi* infection	Diagnosis of infections by *Mycobacteria* spp. and systemic fungal infections	Atopic dermatitis	Contact hypersensitivity; Graft-versus-host disease

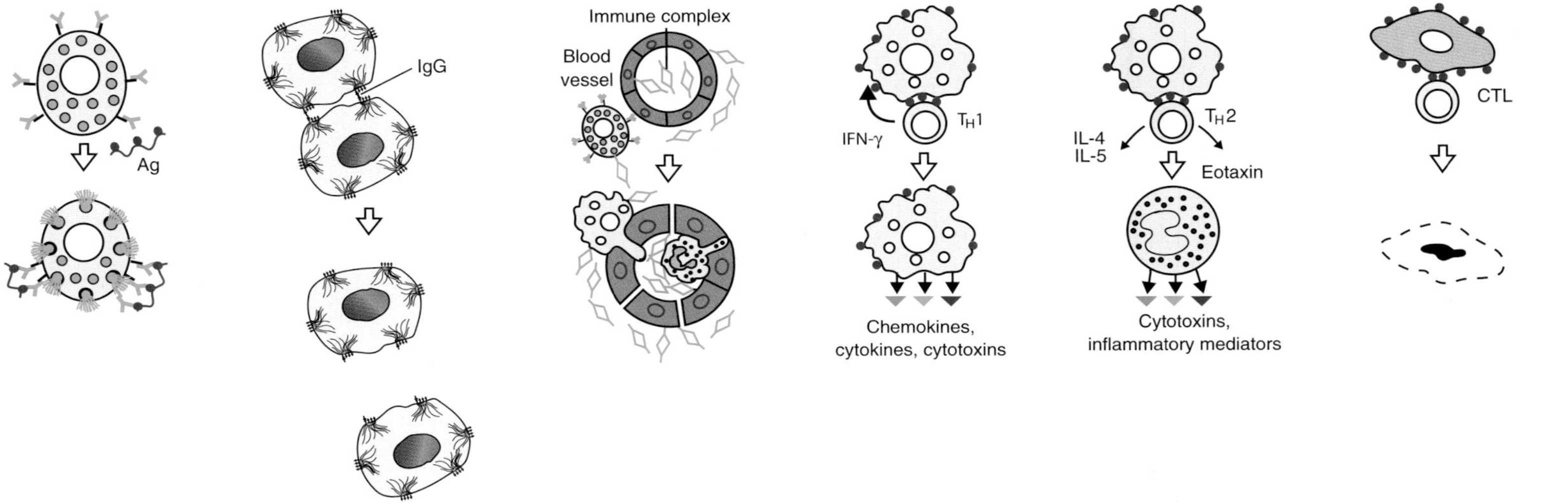

FcR, Fragment crystallizable protein receptor; *IFN-γ,* interferon-γ; *Ig,* immunoglobulin; *IL,* interleukin; *MHC,* major histocompatibility complex; *NK,* natural killer.
Modified from Janeway CA, Travers P, Walport M, et al: *Immunobiology: the immune system in health and disease,* ed 5, New York, 2001, Garland Publishing.

complement-mediated effector mechanisms. Cell damage occurs by complement-mediated lysis, antibody-dependent cell-mediated cytotoxicity, or antibody-directed cellular dysfunction (see Table 17-5). The first two mechanisms are most common in type II reactions affecting the skin. Examples include deposition of autoantibody to desmoglein 1, desmocollin 1, or desmoglein 3, transmembrane proteins found in desmosomes that provide physical connections between keratinocytes and are present in pemphigus (uncommon), and autoantibody to bullous pemphigoid antigen 2 (also called collagen XVII), a 180-kD hemidesmosomal transmembrane molecule in bullous pemphigoid (rare). The lesions vary with the location of the target antigen. In pemphigus foliaceus, desmosomal damage leads to formation of superficial epidermal vesicles that rapidly become pustules and crusts, whereas in bullous pemphigoid the deeper hemidesmosomal damage leads to formation of subepidermal vesicles that rapidly become ulcers.

Type III Reactions

Type III reactions are mediated by soluble immune complexes mostly of the IgG class formed in the circulation or in tissues. The antigen can be exogenous (e.g., bacterial) or endogenous (organ specific as in systemic lupus erythematosus). Immune complexes are often deposited in vessel walls and result in complement fixation and in the generation of cytokines and leukotactic factors, leading to vasculitis (see Table 17-5). Tissue damage results from lysosomal enzymes released from neutrophils, activation of complement and coagulation systems, platelet aggregation, and free oxygen radicals. Immune-complex vasculitis is believed responsible for the purpura seen in infections in horses with *Streptococcus equi* and is responsible for some of the lesions of systemic lupus erythematosus. Clinical lesions associated with immune-complex vascular damage include hemorrhages and edema with serum exudation. In severe cases, vascular damage leads to ischemic necrosis and ulceration of the skin. Microscopic lesions consist of the vascular wall disrupted by neutrophils (neutrophilic vasculitis), perivascular edema, hemorrhage, and fibrin exudation.

Type IV Reactions (T Lymphocyte–Mediated Reactions)

Type IV reactions are mediated by antigen-specific effector T lymphocytes. These include sensitized $CD4^+$ lymphocytes (T_H1 or T_H2) or $CD8^+$ lymphocytes (cytotoxic T lymphocytes) (see Table 17-5). The reaction mediated by sensitized $CD4^+$ T_H1 lymphocytes develops after contact with a specific persistent or nondegradable antigen (such as tuberculin), causing the release of cytokines and recruitment of other lymphocytes and macrophages. The reaction largely depends on IFN-γ or other cytokines, including IL-2. IFN-γ activates macrophages that work to eliminate the targeted antigen. In reactions mediated by $CD4^+$ T_H2 lymphocytes (T-helper lymphocytes), contact with soluble antigen bound to major histocompatibility complex class II (MHC II) results in inflammatory responses in which eosinophils predominate. This type of reaction is believed to participate in the pathogenesis of atopic dermatitis. In the cytotoxic reaction the $CD8^+$ T lymphocytes kill the targeted host cell directly. This is the mechanism of damage in allergic contact dermatitis associated with antigens such as poison ivy and can also participate in graft-versus-host disease. Type IV reactions take many hours to develop and are initiated by antigens bound to host cell major histocompatibility molecules. Type IV reactions mediated by $CD4^+$ T_H1 lymphocytes are used in the diagnosis of diseases such as tuberculosis, histoplasmosis, and coccidioidomycosis. The skin reaction typically develops 24 to 48 hours after exposure to the specific antigen and consists of perivascular mononuclear cell accumulations and dermal edema.

Combination Reactions

The strict categorization of hypersensitivity reactions is an oversimplification. Categories and lesions can overlap, and there are species differences. Hypersensitivity to fleas, ticks, *Staphylococcus* sp., hormones, and drugs are mediated by a combination of types I, II, III, or IV reactions. Therefore histopathologic examination may provide the general category of inflammatory reaction pattern and rule out other disease processes but may not lead to a diagnosis of the specific type of hypersensitivity present.

Regeneration and Repair

Information on this topic is available at www.expertconsult.com.

Healing of Wounds with Opposed Edges

Information on this topic is available at www.expertconsult.com.

Healing of Wounds with Separated Edges

Information on this topic is available at www.expertconsult.com.

Aging Changes

There are two basic causes or types of cutaneous aging, the first is called intrinsic (or natural) aging and is controlled by the animal's genome and specific genes (life span of telomeres [see Chapter 1). Genetic disorders in human beings, including progeria (*LMNA* gene mutation) and wrinkly skin syndrome (mutations in *PYCR1* gene), that accelerate the process of aging are included in this category. The second type of aging is called extrinsic aging and is caused by external or outside factors such as chronic exposure to the sun (UV light), mechanical trauma, diet, and others that are less well understood.

The effects of aging on the skin are manifested by a loss of normal structure and function such as the loss of barrier systems, collagen and elastin, lipids, sebaceous and sweat gland secretions, cutaneous microvasculature, reparative and regenerative capacity (wound healing), and nerve sensory function. These occur together with thinning of the skin, reduced strength and resiliency of the skin, thinning and graying of the hair, and increased prevalence of neoplastic transformation.

Chronologic aging of the skin in domestic animals has not been seriously investigated but is likely similar to some aspects of aging reported in human beings and experimental laboratory animals. Aging changes are perhaps more obvious in those domestic animal species that share a close relationship with their human caretakers, live out their natural lives, and thus age alongside human beings. Disease outcomes of aging in domestic animals are discussed later and illustrated in Box 17-3. The more clinically obvious aging changes in the skin of domestic animals include neoplastic transformation and thinning and graying of the hair. With few exceptions, most cutaneous tumors, benign or malignant, develop in mature adult to older animals. In human beings, many age-related changes in the skin, including the development of selected neoplasms, arise via the extrinsic mechanism of chronic environmental exposure to UV light from the sun. Although the same is true for the sparsely haired and sparsely pigmented skin of domestic animals, such as the skin around the eyes, nose, lips, genitalia, or on the ventral abdomen, chronic sun exposure poses less of a problem for most domestic animals due to the usual protection of the hair coat. For further discussion, see the section on Solar (Actinic) Dermatosis, Keratosis, and Neoplasia.

The overt visibility of the hair coat and regenerative nature of the hair follicles may explain why thinning and graying of the hair, common to many species, are notable features of aging. Thinning and graying of hair with age have been studied most extensively in

Box 17-3 Aging Changes in the Skin of Domestic Animals

DOMESTIC ANIMALS IN GENERAL

Increased incidence of neoplasia and solar dermatosis

HORSES

Gross Change

Graying of hair on face around muzzle and eyes and sometimes other anatomic locations
Genetic breed-related hair coat graying and melanoma formation
Dull, dry hair coat
Loss of dorsal muscle mass, resulting in "swayback"
Depressed grooves above eyes
Excessively long, curly hair coat or failure to shed; related to pars intermedia pituitary gland tumor as seen in aged horses
Reduced or absent stratum externum of hoof wall

DOGS

Gross Change

Graying of hair on face around muzzle and eyes, sometimes also other anatomic locations
Dull, dry hair coat, sometimes with hair coat thinning
Alopecia and callus formation over pressure points
Nodular sebaceous gland hyperplasia
Nasodigital hyperkeratosis
Brittle and malformed claws

Histopathologic Change

Hyperkeratosis of epidermis and hair follicles
Atrophy of the epidermis
Increased numbers of telogen and kenogen follicles
Mineralization of hair follicle basement membrane
Reduced cellularity plus degeneration of collagen bundles
Occasional reduction or degeneration of elastic fibers
Cystic apocrine glands (apocrine cystomatosis) may be senile degenerative change

CATS

Gross Change

Thick, brittle, sometimes overgrown claws
Hair matting, skin odor, and inflammation (less frequent or effective grooming)
Thinner, less elastic skin, more prone to infection and with reduced blood circulation

Histopathologic Change

Variable epidermal and follicular hyperkeratosis
Atrophic follicles (occasional)
Granular, fragmented collagen fibers (occasional)
Sebaceous glands atrophied and vacuolated (occasional)
Arrector pili muscle may appear fragmented and more vacuolated and eosinophilic than normal (occasional)
Cystic ceruminous glands (ceruminous cystomatosis) may be senile change in some cats

human beings and mouse models. Although similar hair coat changes occur in aged domestic animals, little has been investigated or published regarding these changes, which may in part be due to the perceived irrelevance of these changes in animals compared with human beings, or that most domestic animals are unlikely to be a good model for the human condition due to the differences in the type of hair follicles (e.g., compound versus simple), the length of the hair cycle (telogen based versus anagen based), and stronger seasonal and nutritional influences on the hair cycle and the hair coat in animals.

The mechanisms of hair graying are incompletely understood. Perhaps the most relevant and most studied time sequence of hair graying occurs in human beings, in whom the regeneration of an intact hair follicle pigmentary unit, which is formed from the pigment-producing melanocytes anchored to the basement membrane above the dermal papilla and the hair shaft–producing keratinocytes in the hair bulb, occurs optimally only during the first 10 hair cycles, or until approximately 40 years of age. Thereafter there is gradual reduction in the melanin pigment production of each hair follicle, resulting in the growth of gray and white hair shafts, suggesting an age and genetically regulated exhaustion of the pigment production potential of each individual hair follicle. This biologic process appears to be associated with the loss of melanocytes in the hair bulb and loss of the melanocyte stem cells in the isthmus region of the ORS. The endogenous oxidative stress that develops from the hydroxylation of tyrosine and the oxidation of dihydroxyphenylalanine (DOPA) to form melanin may to contribute to the reduction of pigment by causing selective premature aging and apoptosis of melanocytes. In addition, studies using aged human hair follicles and transgenic mice have shown loss of maintenance of melanocytic stem cells, which may involve premature differentiation of stem cells or activation of a senescence program. If stem cells differentiate prematurely, they lose the ability to retain their stem cell capabilities. Other factors that may damage melanocyte stem cells include reduced or inefficient antioxidant systems and oxidative stress from exogenous sources such as inflammation, UV light, psychoemotional stress, and others. Ionizing radiation, experimentally in mice, also has been shown to cause irreparable DNA damage that eliminates renewal of melanocyte stem cells. Oxidative injury, in particular a high degree of endogenous oxidative stress from melanin pigment production, may play a more important role in human beings, who have an anagen-based hair cycle with a long growing phase resulting in production of long and often heavily pigmented hair shafts. In contrast, many domestic animals have a telogen-based hair cycle and thus shorter lengths of hair, which theoretically should result in less oxidative damage to the follicular melanin unit following melanin production and may explain why there is less extensive and less generalized graying of the hair coat of aged animals. Alternatively, animals may have more efficient or enhanced antioxidant systems or may be less susceptible to the various causes of melanocyte or melanocytic stem cell damage. For example, in horses and dogs, the two domestic species in which age-related hair coat graying are reported, the graying occurs predominantly on the face around the muzzle and eyes, although scattered gray hairs are also noted in other anatomic areas of the body. A genetic component may play a role in hair graying in dogs because certain breeds (e.g., German shepherd dogs, Irish setters, Labrador retrievers, golden retrievers) are more likely to develop gray muzzle and chin hairs at a relatively younger age.

The mechanisms underlying hair loss in aging individuals are not clearly understood but may involve progression to a telogen-based hair cycle in addition to senescent hair loss that may be related to reduction of hair follicle epithelial stem cells associated with reduced renewal, premature differentiation, apoptosis, or cellular senescence. Age-related hair loss in human beings is thought to result from a defective hair cycle that causes a shortened anagen (or growth) stage, increased ratio of telogen to anagen follicles, and persistence of telogen follicles. Studies in mice also have shown the duration of the telogen stage increases with each hair cycle, and the entire hair cycle slows considerably with aging. Similarly, it is generally believed that the hair cycle of many animals becomes increasingly telogenic with age. Interestingly, similar changes to those described in human beings and mice have been observed in some aging dogs with anagen-based hair cycles, such as poodles. These changes histologically include a gradual increase in the number of telogen stage hair follicles with age, and the hair coats of some of these aged poodles become less dense over time. However, because most dogs and other mammals have a telogen-based hair cycle and there are seasonal influences associated with the hair cycle, it is difficult to clinically or histologically assess an insidious prolongation of the telogen stage of the cycle in most domestic species. Nevertheless, prolongation of the telogen phase with aging could theoretically result in the presence of older, more worn hair shafts similar to what is observed in some hair cycle arrest disorders (such as endocrine-based alopecia). In fact, aged horses and dogs tend to have a dull, dryer hair coat, which could be associated with prolongation of telogen. Although a telogen-based hair coat may be of lesser quality, telogen stage follicles with retained hair shaft may be the most beneficial for the aging animal because it is thought to be the most energy efficient hair follicle stage (does not require protein production to form a hair shaft), and the inactive telogen bulb that lacks the mitotic activity may also reduce the risk for malignant transformation.

Portals of Entry/Pathways of Spread

Normal intact skin has many natural defenses and barriers that render it impenetrable to most organisms and protect the body from a variety of insults that include pressure, friction, mild mechanical trauma, temperature extremes, UV light exposure, and chemical absorption (see Defense Mechanisms/Barrier Systems).

In order to initiate disease, most infectious agents must first gain entrance into the body via routes termed *portals of entry* (Fig. 17-33). The skin becomes an efficient portal of entry for microorganisms only when the barrier is first damaged by trauma; excessive moisture, heat, or cold; or disruption of the normal flora of the integument; however, a few pathogens, such as hookworm and *Cuterebra* larvae, are able to penetrate intact normally functioning skin. Some organisms may also use more than one portal; for example, *Cuterebra* larvae also gain entrance via ingestion during grooming by the host, or they can migrate over skin to natural body openings such as the nares, where they can more easily penetrate a less defensive barrier, the mucosa. Dermatophytes are able to colonize the nonviable cornified structures such as hair, claws, and the stratum corneum and cause disease without ever entering living tissue. Clinical disease, or dermatophytosis, results from the host's reaction to the organism and its by-products. A number of microorganisms (e.g., *Staphylococcus pseudintermedius*, *Streptococcus* sp., *Corynebacterium pseudotuberculosis*, *Pasteurella* sp., *Proteus* sp., *Pseudomonas* sp., and *Escherichia coli*) gain entrance to the body by entering through natural pores, such as hair follicles or glands with ducts that traverse the epidermis, or by the parenteral route, which includes all types of breaks in the skin, including injections, insect bites, and other types of wounds. Organisms that are able to inhabit hair follicles, such as mites or bacteria, gain entry to the body when the wall of the follicle is ruptured, leading to emptying of follicular contents into the dermis. Similarly, rupture of glands or ducts can lead to entry for some of those microorganisms. Once in the dermis, infectious agents can stimulate a robust host immune response or possibly spread to other areas of the body by gaining entry to the bloodstream or traveling to regional and distant lymph nodes via lymph flow.

Intact skin with its waterproof barrier provides some protection against weak acids and alkali substances and water-soluble compounds, but certain lipid-soluble compounds can be absorbed directly through intact skin as can some artificially engineered gases developed for chemical warfare. UVR can damage the skin by direct exposure if the body's natural defenses, such as the hair coat and melanin pigments, are not present or are inadequate. The lesions of solar (actinic) dermatosis (see section on Disorders of Physical, Radiation, or Chemical Injury; Solar (Actinic) Dermatosis, Keratosis, and Neoplasia) typify the effects of chronic exposure to UVR. In addition to solar dermatosis, squamous cell carcinomas, hemangiomas, and hemangiosarcomas have an increased tendency to develop in skin chronically damaged by UVR. Cutaneous melanomas also have been reported in UVR-exposed Angora goats. Doberman pinscher dogs with autosomal recessive oculocutaneous albinism also develop melanomas in the skin, lips, eyelids, and iris, but the melanomas develop in sun-exposed and non–sun-exposed sites, so the role of UV light in tumor induction in these dogs is unclear.

The dermal capillaries can be a portal of entry to the skin via the hematogenous route. Embolization of infectious agents, such as bacteria (*E. rhusiopathiae* [diamond skin disease]) or fungi (systemic infection with *Blastomyces dermatitidis*), can damage the skin via this route during hematogenous dissemination. Tumor cells (hemangiosarcoma) can also embolize to the skin and lead to metastatic tumor foci or possible cutaneous infarction. The hematogenous route to the skin is also one of the most common delivery systems for drugs (adverse cutaneous reactions to the administration of trimethoprim-potentiated sulfonamides; photosensitization dermatitis that occurs with phenothiazine ingestion) and toxins (gangrenous ergotism caused by the mycotoxin of *Claviceps purpurea*).

Rarely, an infectious agent that is neurotropic can migrate from a ganglion along sensory nerves via axonal flow to the skin and cause dermatitis. An example is reactivation of feline herpesvirus 1 (FHV-1) infection that results in feline herpesvirus dermatitis. The skin can also be secondarily infected or traumatized or damaged by extension of pathologic processes affecting adjacent tissues or support structures such as bone, muscle, lymph nodes, or glands (locally invasive mammary gland carcinoma resulting in cutaneous ulceration).

Defense Mechanisms/Barrier Systems

The skin is a complex organ composed of many integrated components that are structurally and functionally designed to protect the host. Host defenses against injury principally consist of three broad mechanisms: (1) physical defense, (2) immunologic defense, and (3) repair mechanisms. The most critical defense is the barrier derived from the more superficial layers of the skin, which include the stratum corneum, epidermis, basement membrane, and superficial dermis. Without these outer layers of the skin, animals cannot survive (consider, for example, the deleterious effects of extensive burns and ulcerative immune-mediated diseases such as pemphigus vulgaris). One of the most important cells in the skin is the keratinocyte that terminally differentiates to form the stratum corneum, the outermost barrier of the skin. Keratinocytes produce keratin filaments, desmosomes, and hemidesmosomes, providing structural integrity to the cytoplasm and an interconnecting network that anchors the keratinocytes to each other and the basement membrane. Keratinocytes produce cytokines (including IL-1, IL-6, IL-8, IL-3, TNF-α, colony-stimulating factors) and growth factors (including transforming growth factor-α [TGF-α], TGF-β, platelet-derived growth factor [PDGF], FGF), thus participating in innate and adaptive immunity and in the communication between the two. Keratinocytes also dissolve desmosomes and hemidesmosomes and form actin filaments so they can migrate to cover skin wounds and then proliferate to regenerate the wounded skin. Keratinocytes thus not

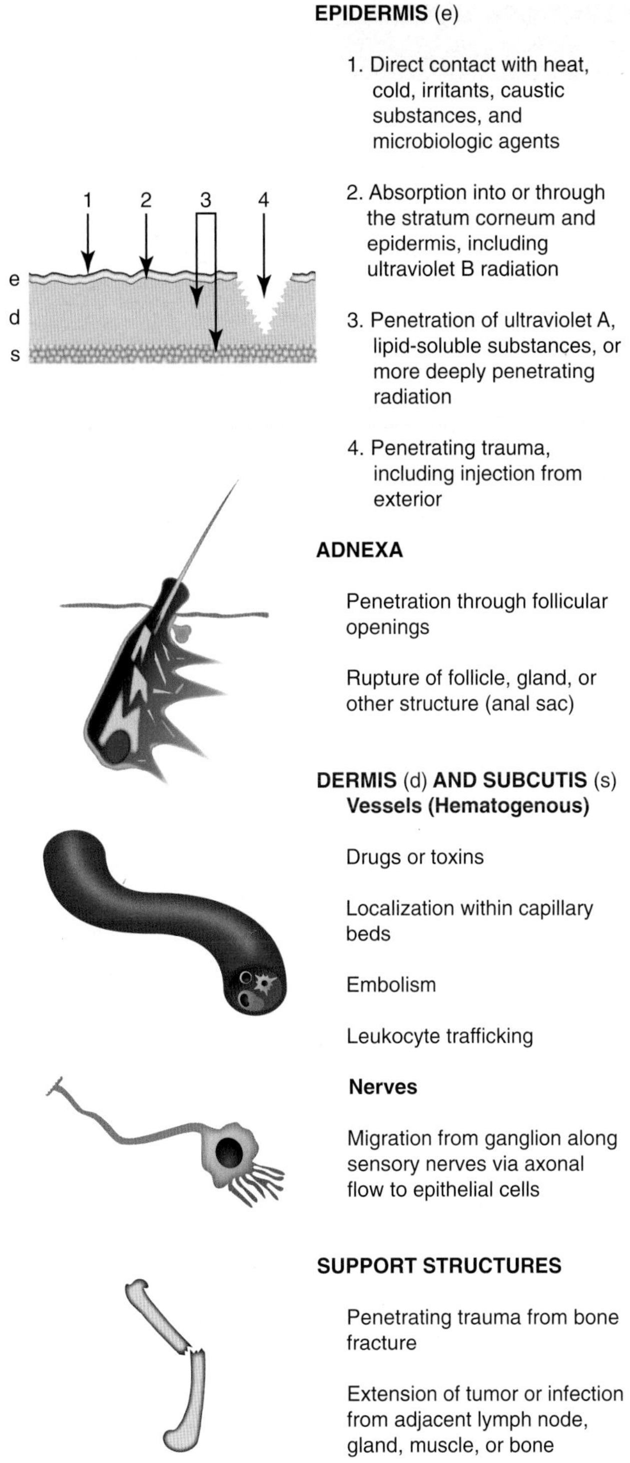
EPIDERMIS (e)
1. Direct contact with heat, cold, irritants, caustic substances, and microbiologic agents
2. Absorption into or through the stratum corneum and epidermis, including ultraviolet B radiation
3. Penetration of ultraviolet A, lipid-soluble substances, or more deeply penetrating radiation
4. Penetrating trauma, including injection from exterior
1
2
3
4
e
d
s
ADNEXA
Penetration through follicular openings
Rupture of follicle, gland, or other structure (anal sac)
DERMIS (d) AND SUBCUTIS (s)
Vessels (Hematogenous)
Drugs or toxins
Localization within capillary beds
Embolism
Leukocyte trafficking
Nerves
Migration from ganglion along sensory nerves via axonal flow to epithelial cells
SUPPORT STRUCTURES
Penetrating trauma from bone fracture
Extension of tumor or infection from adjacent lymph node, gland, muscle, or bone

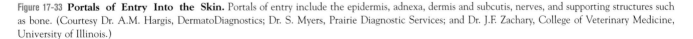

Figure 17-33 Portals of Entry Into the Skin. Portals of entry include the epidermis, adnexa, dermis and subcutis, nerves, and supporting structures such as bone. (Courtesy Dr. A.M. Hargis, DermatoDiagnostics; Dr. S. Myers, Prairie Diagnostic Services; and Dr. J.F. Zachary, College of Veterinary Medicine, University of Illinois.)

only orchestrate the activities of the skin but also serve as many members of the orchestra.

Physical Defense Mechanisms

Barrier Systems

Barriers of the skin against physical injury are listed in Box 17-4. The hair coat, particularly the long dense hair coat of some dogs and cats, serves as a physical barrier to temperature extremes, UVR, and minor trauma. Tail hairs of horses can also be used to swat at insects and thus reduce insect bite–related injury. The hair coat also sheds water as a result of the lipids provided by sebaceous gland secretion. Vibrissae, or tactile hairs, and sensory neurons provide awareness of the physical environment, allowing the animal to make appropriate reactions for survival such as reflex responses to heat and other noxious stimuli. Claws, especially on cats, serve as quite an effective barrier against predators by providing traction for

Box 17-4 Host Defense Mechanisms against Injury: Physical Defense Mechanisms

BARRIER FUNCTIONS

Hair coat: Physical and thermal
Tactile hairs and neurons: Sensory
Claws, horns, hooves: Physical
Stratum corneum: Barrier function
Adnexal glandular secretions: Barrier function
Apocrine gland secretion (sweating in horses and cattle): Defense against excessive heat
Melanin: Defense against ultraviolet radiation, camouflage
Basement membrane zone: Filter to macromolecules, barrier to invasion of neoplastic epidermal cells, anchor epidermis to dermis
Panniculus: Barrier to temperature extremes

RESISTANCE TO MECHANICAL FORCES

Hair follicles and dermal-epidermal interdigitations: Anchor epidermis to dermis
Stratum corneum: Corneocyte, corneocyte envelope, and intercellular lipid adhesion
Desmosomes and hemidesmosomes: Intercellular and basement membrane adhesion
Basement membrane: Anchors epidermis to dermis
Collagen and elastic tissue: Resilience, strength, and support of adnexa and dermal structures
Panniculus: Shock absorption, facilitates movement, anchors dermis to fascia

climbing and serve as weapons to be used against aggressors. Hooves and claws may also function as "shields" that cover and protect underlying bone from trauma or fracture. Hooves, soles, and pawpads also permit ambulation over surfaces that are rough or uneven, or hot or cold. The planum nasale of dogs has a thick stratum corneum that provides additional protection against minor trauma.

The stratum corneum is an exceedingly important component of the barrier, imparting protection from the exterior and preventing water loss from the interior. The stratum corneum is composed largely of keratins, a family of proteins called *intermediate filaments*. Keratin proteins are the major structural proteins of the skin, hair, and claws. The stratum corneum is considered to be the "bricks and mortar" of the barrier. The bricks are the flattened cornified cells (corneocytes) with their resistant cell envelopes and keratin microfibrils, and the mortar consists of intercorneocyte lipids.

The bricks are formed at the level of the stratum granulosum when the keratinocytes are transformed into the flattened corneocytes. The transformation occurs when (1) the nucleus is digested, (2) the keratin intermediate filaments aggregate into microfibrils oriented parallel to the skin surface, (3) the lipids are released into the intercellular space, and (4) the cell membrane is converted into a resilient cell envelope consisting of cross-linked protein with lipids covalently bound to its surface. Filaggrin (which is an acronym for filament-aggregating protein) from the keratohyalin granules in the stratum granulosum plays a significant role in formation of the bricks by participating in the aggregation of keratin filaments into tight bundles. The keratin intermediate filaments and filaggrin compose 80% to 90% of the protein mass of the epidermis. Later filaggrin is digested by proteolytic enzymes to produce components of amino acids that form the "natural moisturizing factor" of the stratum corneum, which serves to help maintain hydration, flexibility, and orderly desquamation that preserve the epidermal barrier. Concurrent with the aggregation of the keratin filaments, the resistant cornified envelope is transformed from the water-permeable phospholipid cell membrane of the keratinocyte when the membrane-bound enzymes (e.g., transglutaminases) cross-link proteins from the keratohyalin granules (e.g., loricrin) and the cytoplasm (e.g., involucrin) in isopeptide bonds. Other proteins (including trichohyalin and small proline-rich proteins) are similarly cross-linked, and eventually the entire cell membrane consists of cross-linked proteins. The proteins of the cornified envelope compose 7% to 10% of the protein mass of the epidermis. The corneocytes are joined together by desmosomes that are modified from those joining keratinocytes in lower layers of the epidermis by the addition of a protein called corneodesmosin. These stratum corneum desmosomes are referred to as *corneodesmosomes*.

The mortar is formed when lipids, from the lamellar bodies in the stratum granulosum, are released into the intercellular space. These intercorneocyte lipids (glycosyl ceramides, cholesterol, cholesterol esters, and long-chain fatty acids) are hydrophobic and prevent transepidermal water loss. Lamellar bodies have other important functions: (1) they provide enzymes that generate ceramides and free fatty acids that are incorporated into the lipid membranes; (2) they provide proteases and antiproteases that regulate digestion of corneodesmosomes and shedding of cornified cells to the exterior; and (3) they secrete antimicrobial peptides, including defensins, into the intercellular compartment of the stratum corneum. The lipid component of the stratum corneum surrounds the protein component to which it is covalently bound and provides adhesion of the cornified cells (i.e., bricks) to the intercellular lipids (i.e., mortar). Layers of the corneocytes and their corneocyte envelope (i.e., bricks) and intercellular lipids (i.e., mortar) form a tough and resilient protective barrier. The keratinocyte and sebum-derived lipids help make the stratum corneum water repellant.

Other barrier functions of the skin include defense against antioxidant injury provided by vitamin E in sebaceous gland secretion and defense against UV light provided by the hair coat and also by melanin pigment in keratinocytes. The cap of melanin pigment over the nucleus scatters and absorbs UV light rays and protects against UV light–induced injury to DNA. The basement membrane zone serves as an initial barrier to invasion of the dermis by neoplastic epidermal cells. The panniculus serves as insulation against temperature extremes, and secretion from apocrine glands (sweating) in cattle and horses provides defense against excessive heat.

Resistance to Mechanical Forces

Anatomic features of the skin that provide resistance to physical injury are listed in Box 17-4. Hair follicles help anchor the epidermis to the dermis, as do dermal-epidermal interdigitations; thus these interdigitations are most numerous in nasal planum and pawpad, where hair follicles are absent and resistance to shearing force is necessary. Host defense against mechanical injury is also provided by the tightly bundled keratin filaments of the corneocyte, the resilience of the cornified envelope, the adhesion of the cornified envelope and intercellular lipids, and the corneodesmosomes. In addition, the keratinocytes contain keratin filaments and form desmosomal junctions with adjacent cells (see Fig. 17-4). The keratin filaments perform a structural role (i.e., cytoskeletal) in the cells, and the desmosomes promote adhesion of epidermal cells and resistance to mechanical stresses. The basement membrane anchors the epidermis to the dermis via hemidesmosomes, providing structural integrity against trauma. Dermal collagen and elastic tissue provide resilience and tensile strength to the skin and support for the vessels, nerves, and adnexa. The panniculus protects against surface trauma by providing some shock absorption (e.g., pawpads), by facilitating movement, and by anchoring the dermis to fascia. Thus the various components of the epidermis, dermis, adnexa, and panniculus provide a flexible and strong interconnecting framework to protect the host against mechanical injury.

Immunologic Defense Mechanisms

Innate Immunity

Information on this topic, including E-Table 17-1 and E-Fig. 17-1, is available at www.expertconsult.com.

Acquired (Adaptive) Immunity

Information on this topic, including E-Table 17-2, is available at www.expertconsult.com.

Disease Example of Barrier Dysfunction

Atopic dermatitis serves as an example of a common disease associated with impaired function of the epidermal barrier and immunity. It is a multifactorial, chronic and relapsing, often severely pruritic skin disease that affects human beings, horses, dogs, and cats. It can cause severe discomfort, including sleeplessness from pruritus, and is associated with secondary skin infections. Although the etiopathogenesis of atopic dermatitis has been studied most extensively in human beings, many similarities with the human disease have been identified in atopic dogs. Advances in the knowledge of canine atopic dermatitis have occurred through the recent development and validation of animal models of the disease; these models have allowed more in-depth investigative studies in dogs and more precise comparisons of the disease between human beings and dogs. Atopic dermatitis is a common problem in dogs; the prevalence varies with survey, but it is estimated to affect up to 27% of the population in the United States (Fig. 17-34). It is also a common human disease estimated to affect 10% to 20% of children. Similarities of the disease in human beings and dogs include young age of onset; genetic inheritance; similar clinical lesion distribution; similar histopathologic lesions, including infiltration of IgE^+ $CD1c^+$ dendritic cells; dry skin with increased transepidermal water loss; decreased stratum corneum ceramides (lipids); decreased epidermal filaggrin (in some subsets of dogs); increased colonization of surface staphylococci; positive atopy patch test; increased IgE-specific responses most commonly directed against environmental allergens; in acute disease T_H2-dominated immune responses; and in chronic disease a switch from T_H2 to T_H1 immune responses. A major difference in the disease is that children with atopic dermatitis often develop asthma and allergic rhinitis, whereas dogs affected with atopic dermatitis do not; the reason for this difference is currently unknown.

Atopic dermatitis in human beings is a multifactorial, heterogeneous genetic disease that arises in association with environmental factors. Defects in three groups of genes important in epidermal barrier function in atopic human beings have suggested that in most cases alterations in the epidermal barrier contribute to the development of atopic dermatitis and may represent the primary event. The type and degree of genetic defect plus interaction with environmental factors appear to influence the severity or probability of developing the disease. A defective epidermal barrier facilitates penetration of allergens though the skin, as well as the interaction of the allergens with the local antigen-presenting and immune effector cells (E-Fig. 17-2). Changes in genes encoding for structural proteins (especially filaggrin), epidermal proteases, and protease inhibitors have been identified in human beings with atopic dermatitis. These defects serve to reduce stratum corneum hydration and increase transepidermal water loss, increase cleavage of corneodesmosome junctions, reduce lamellar body secretion and thus stratum corneum lipids, increase pH, and reduce antimicrobial properties of the stratum corneum. These alterations to the barrier favor population by pathogenic versus nonpathogenic bacteria and sustain allergen entrance through the barrier. The allergens are phagocytosed by dendritic cells, which present the allergen to T_H lymphocytes and recruit other $CD4^+$ T lymphocytes to the site. The activated dendritic cells and the cytokines produced by the $CD4^+$ T lymphocyte (particularly IL-4) lead to switching from a T_H1 to T_H2 response (in early lesions) and release of proinflammatory cytokines and production of IgE, which in the presence of allergen activates mast cells. In atopic dermatitis there is a complex interaction between the immune system and the nervous system that can promote the sensation of itch. For example, at least one of the T_H2 proinflammatory cytokines, IL-31, binds to receptors on neurons to stimulate itch; thus it significantly contributes to pruritus, a hallmark of atopic

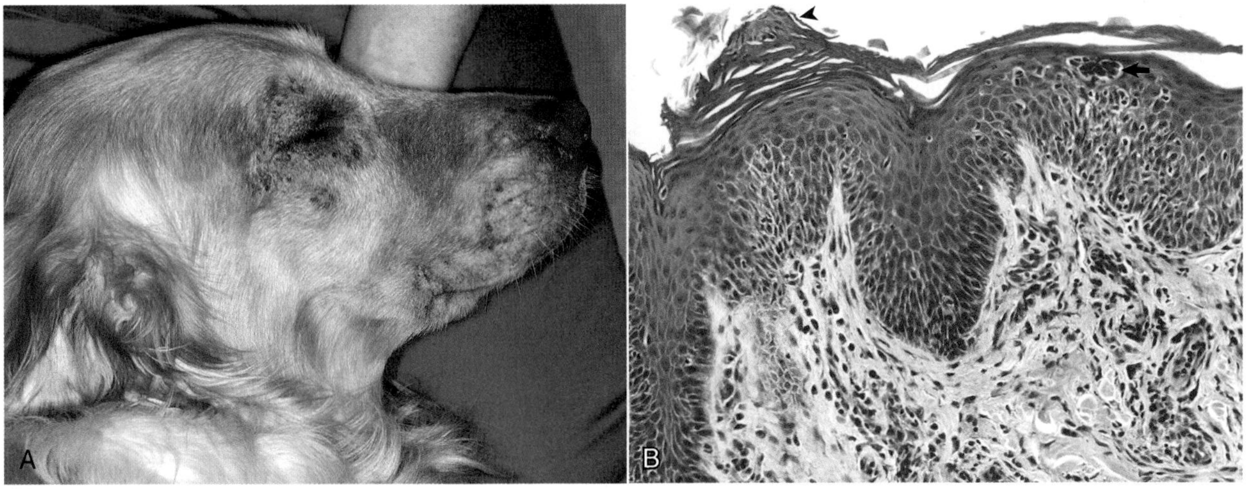

Figure 17-34 **Atopic Dermatitis, Skin, Dog. A,** This golden retriever has erythema, alopecia, and erosions affecting the skin around the eye and muzzle. The lesions are caused by self-trauma from rubbing and scratching as a result of pruritus. **B,** Photomicrograph from experimentally induced lesion of atopic dermatitis in the skin of a dog. The epidermis has acanthosis, mild spongiosis, a few lymphocytes, and clustered Langerhans cells *(arrow)*. Focal parakeratosis *(arrowhead)* is secondary to spongiosis. The superficial dermis contains a mild perivascular infiltrate of small lymphocytes, plasma cells, mast cells, and fibroblasts. H&E stain. (**A** courtesy Dr. D. Duclos, Animal Skin and Allergy Clinic. **B** courtesy Dr. T. Olivry, College of Veterinary Medicine, North Carolina State University.)

dermatitis. Other itch-promoting inflammatory mediators such as neurotrophins or neuroactive peptides also contribute. Langerhans cells also contribute in early lesions because they prime naïve T lymphocytes into the T_H2 type (with high IL-4 production). IL-4 may also be produced by mast cells, basophils, or eosinophils. Exogenous factors also contribute. For example, proteases from house dust mites can facilitate cleavage of corneodesmosomes and additionally contribute to epidermal barrier damage. The resulting inflammation causes pruritus, which stimulates scratching, further damaging the epidermal barrier (and keratinocytes, resulting in release of additional proinflammatory cytokines, including IL-1), and creating a vicious cycle that perpetuates the disease and that is difficult to control. Secondary infections with *Staphylococci* and *Malassezia* also contribute because proteins from these infections more readily pass through the impaired epidermal barrier and can result in development of IgE-mediated bacterial and yeast hypersensitivity. Approximately 25% of human beings with severe atopic dermatitis have IgE antibody directed toward self-proteins. These antibodies may develop after intracellular proteins from keratinocytes are released when the keratinocytes are damaged by scratching. These keratinocyte proteins may mimic microbial structure and induce IgE autoantibodies that further perpetuate the disease. In summary, atopic dermatitis is a complex, multifactorial, heterogeneous disease in which altered epidermal barrier function appears to contribute to the pathogenesis by facilitating penetration of allergens though the skin, as well as the interaction of the allergens with the local antigen-presenting and immune effector cells. It serves as an example of the importance of the epidermal barrier in protecting the host against injury from allergens, microbial infections, and autoreactive disorders.

Definitions of Clinical Terms

Knowledge of the clinical appearance of skin lesions, distribution of lesions, and correlation between the gross and histologic lesions is often critical in formulating differential and final diagnoses. In skin diseases the clinical lesions represent the gross lesions and are typically examined by a practitioner, not the pathologist; thus the practitioner essentially serves as the eyes for the pathologist. It is therefore important for the practitioner to develop the ability to accurately recognize clinical lesion morphologic features and translate that information to the pathologist. To facilitate this process, Table 17-6 is provided to illustrate the morphologic characteristics of the various clinical lesions and provide examples of the disease processes in which those lesions occur.

Techniques for Skin Biopsy Sampling

Important tips for biopsy sampling of the skin are listed in Table 17-7. Biopsy do's and don'ts are listed in Boxes 17-5 and 17-6, respectively.

When to Collect Biopsy Samples

Knowing when to collect biopsy samples helps obtain the most diagnostic samples; facilitates obtaining samples early so acute, serious, or neoplastic disorders are diagnosed quickly; and prevents the frustration and economic loss when samples are inappropriately collected, such as when concurrent therapy might alter diagnostic lesions, when lesions are in a quiescent stage and might not be diagnostic, and when clinical dermatologic evaluation would have been a better method of achieving a diagnosis. Knowing when biopsy is not the best course of action is equally important. Biopsy should not be viewed as a substitute, or equivalent option, for referral to a veterinary dermatology specialist. If in regional proximity, referral to a veterinary dermatology specialist may be recommended before and instead of collecting biopsy samples. Biopsy sampling is recommended when the following are present:

1. The therapy for the skin disorder is associated with significant side effects (to confirm the clinical diagnosis before starting therapy).
2. A nodular lesion, ulcer, or nonhealing wound might represent a tumor (so that surgical excision of the tumor can be performed as early as possible).
3. Lesions develop suddenly, are severe, or are unusual (to help identify a serious disease so that therapy can be instituted early).
4. Lesions develop during the course of therapy (to identify a potential adverse reaction to drug therapy).
5. Lesions are active and before use of therapy that might alter the histologic appearance of the lesions, and there are multiple clinical differential diagnoses, and the thorough clinical dermatologic examination does not differentiate the conditions.
6. A skin disorder fails to respond to apparently appropriate therapy, or the disorder responds to therapy but recurs when therapy is stopped (to establish the correct diagnosis, or evaluate for predisposing factors). Recall that antiinflammatory therapy can alter lesions.

Site Selection

Multiple cutaneous sites representative of the range of lesions should be selected for biopsy. Fully developed nontreated primary lesions, such as macules, papules, pustules, nodules, neoplasms, vesicles, and wheals, are often the most useful for diagnosis (see Table 17-6). However, primary lesions may not be present at the time the animal is examined, so secondary lesions, such as scales, crusts, ulcers, comedones, or scars then need to be sampled and evaluated (see Table 17-6). These secondary lesions can be diagnostic or contribute substantially to the diagnosis when multiple cutaneous sites are selected for biopsy. One of the most useful secondary lesions is the crust because acantholytic cells from drying pustules in pemphigus foliaceus and organisms, such as *D. congolensis* or dermatophytes, may be identified in crusts, providing the information necessary for diagnosis. Also, the margin of a chronic ulcer may represent a squamous cell carcinoma, or the scale at the edge of an epidermal collarette (i.e., peripherally expanding ring of epidermal scales) may represent superficial spreading pyoderma, thus providing the key to diagnosis.

Methods

Excisional biopsy samples (entire lesions) are recommended for large pustules or vesicles that can be damaged by use of a smaller punch biopsy instrument. Deeper excisional biopsy samples are generally necessary for diagnosis of lesions, such as panniculitis, that are deep to the epidermis and dermis. Digital amputation can be required, particularly in dogs, for the diagnosis of claw bed lesions. Electrocautery or laser should not be used for small biopsy samples because the samples can be damaged and rendered nondiagnostic. Tissue forceps (small toothed) should grasp, if at all, only one nonaffected margin, preferably in the subcutis.

Site Preparation

Generally the skin at a punch biopsy site should not be surgically prepared because the procedure may remove a diagnostic portion of the sample. Gentle clipping of hair is acceptable, and surgical preparation of the skin is acceptable for an excisional biopsy of lesions deep to the epidermis. For collection of biopsy samples in areas of alopecia, drawing a line with a fine-tipped permanent marking pen in the direction of the hair coat helps laboratory personnel orient

Text continued on p. 1055

Table 17-6 Definition and Morphologic Features of Primary and Secondary Skin Lesions

Lesion Definition	Drawing	Clinical Photograph
CALLUS* Thick, firm, hyperkeratotic, hairless plaque with increased skin folds, wrinkles, or fissures. In haired skin, follicular plugging and comedones also may develop Example: Trauma over bony prominence such as elbow, sternum, or side of digit	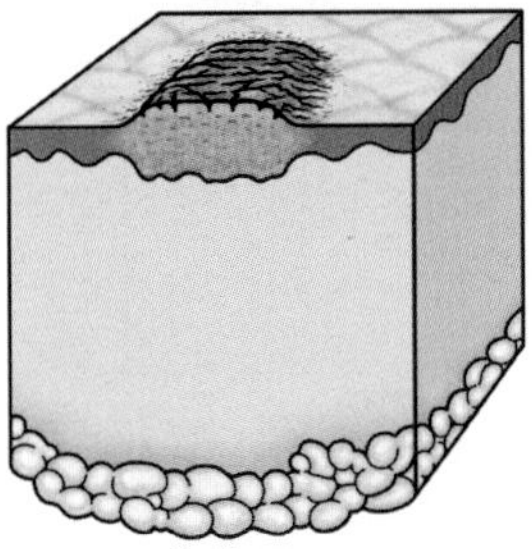 Callus	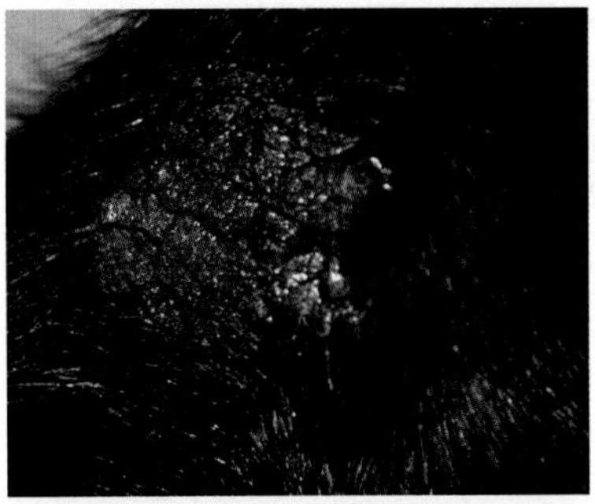
COMEDO (pl. COMEDONES)† Plug of stratum corneum and sebum within the lumen of a hair follicle that leads to follicular distention. The material on the surface of the clinical image has been expressed, for illustrative purposes, from several comedones (*arrows*). Examples: Canine solar (actinic) dermatosis, chin acne, Schnauzer comedo syndrome, hyperadrenocorticism, canine palmar and plantar interdigital cysts	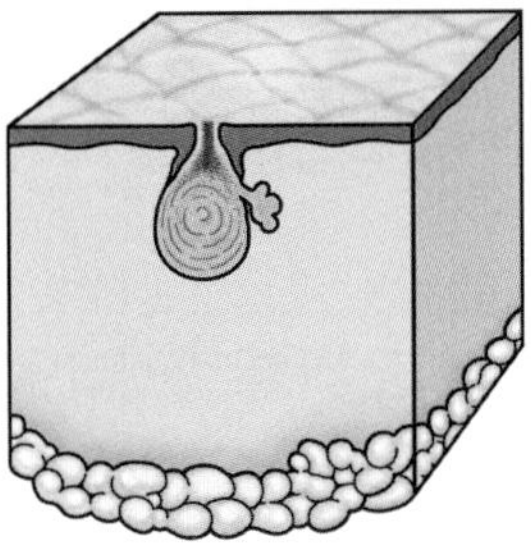 Comedo	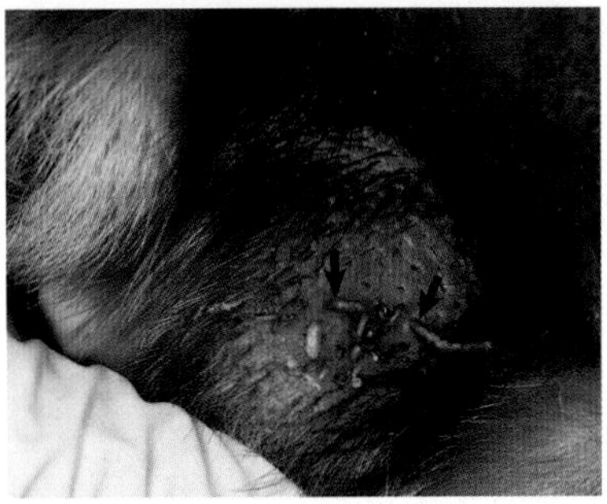
CRUST‡ Dried exudate composed of various components, including fluid, blood, pustular debris, scale, or microorganisms on the skin surface Example: Chronic stage of pustular disease such as staphylococcal infection or pemphigus foliaceus	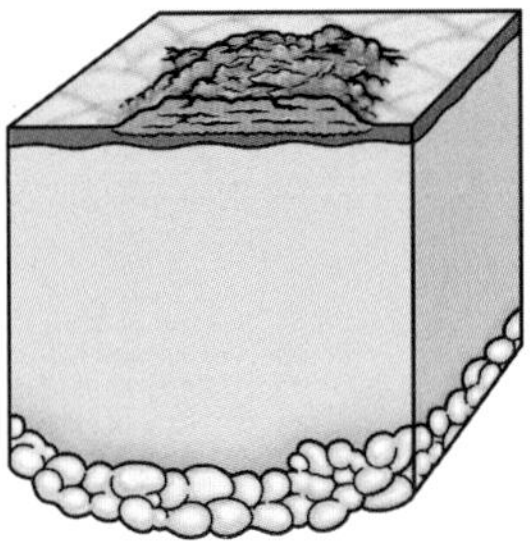 Crust	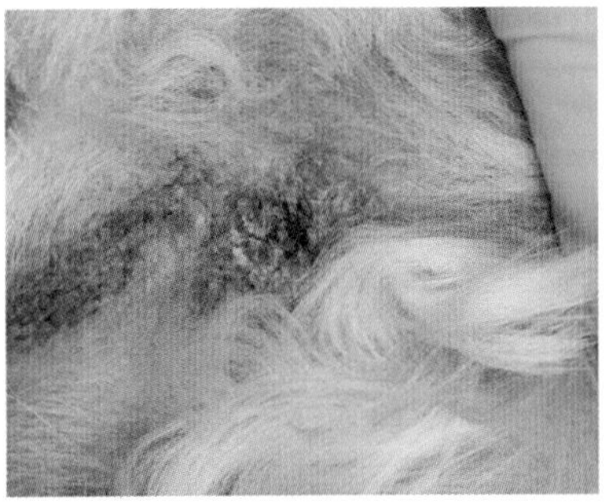
CYST Cavity lined by epithelium and filled with liquid or semisolid material and located in the dermis or subcutis; may communicate with surface via a pore. Examples: Follicular cyst, dermoid cyst, apocrine gland cyst	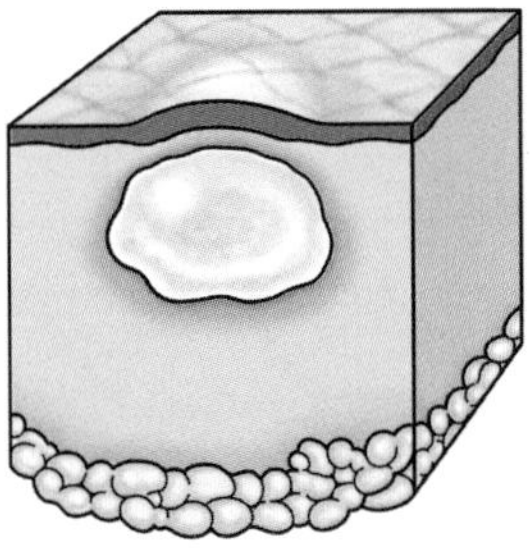 Cyst	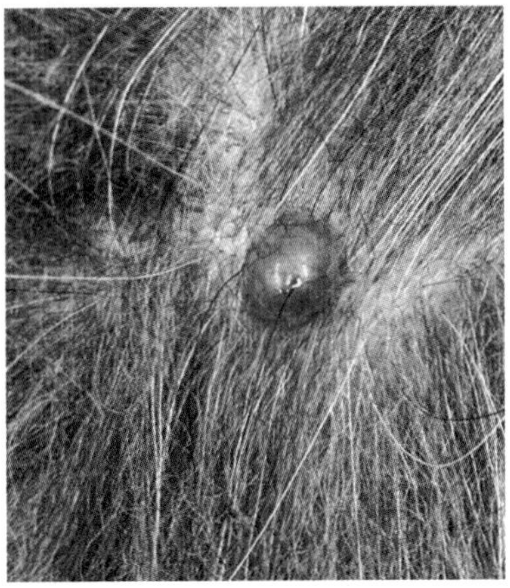

Continued

Table 17-6 Definition and Morphologic Features of Primary and Secondary Skin Lesions–cont'd

Lesion Definition	Drawing	Clinical Photograph
EPIDERMAL COLLARETTE A thin layer of scale that expands peripherally and forms a ring *(arrows)* Examples: Superficial bacterial infection, insect bite, fungal infection	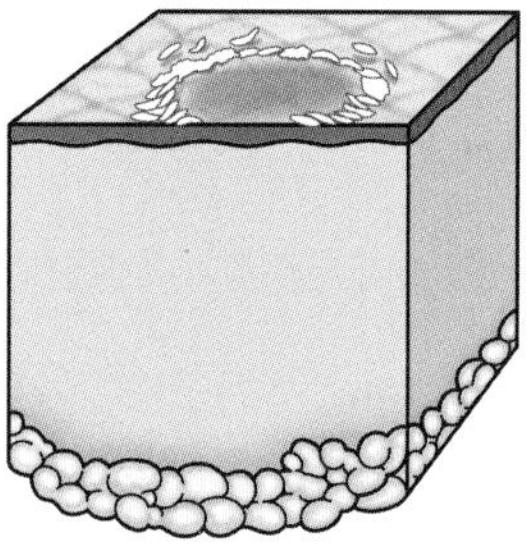 Epidermal collarette	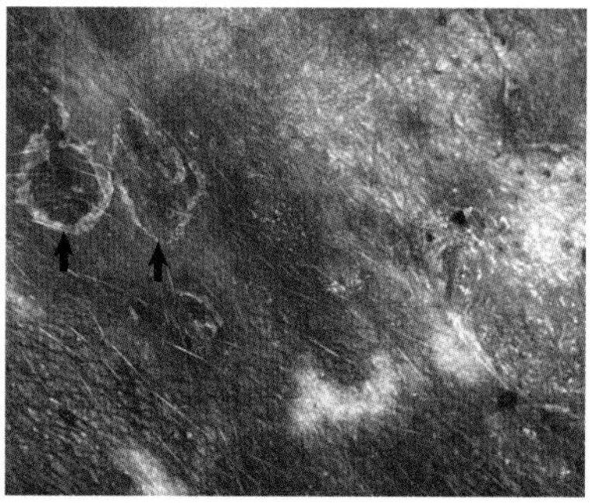
EROSION Partial-thickness loss of epidermis resulting in shallow, moist, glistening depression *(arrows)* Examples: Secondary to vesicle or pustule rupture or secondary to surface trauma	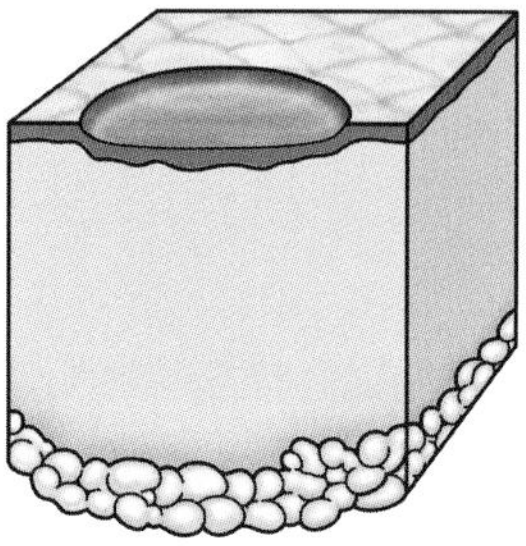 Erosion	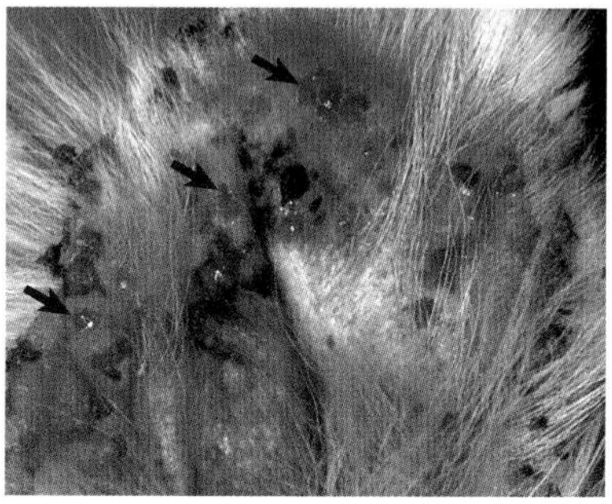
EXCORIATION[‡] Shallow, vertically oriented linear break in skin surface (epidermis) *(arrows)* Example: Abrasion or scratch	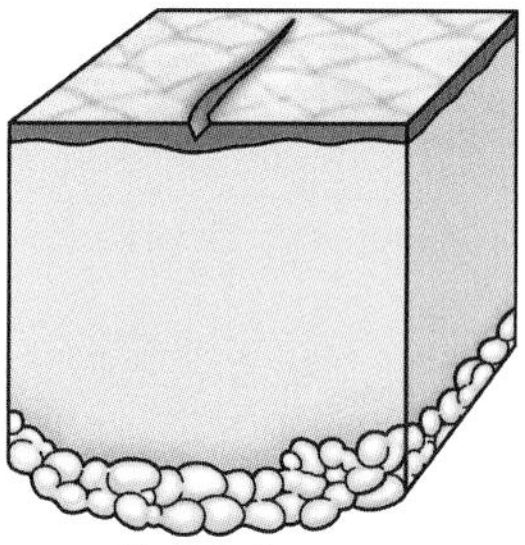 Excoriation	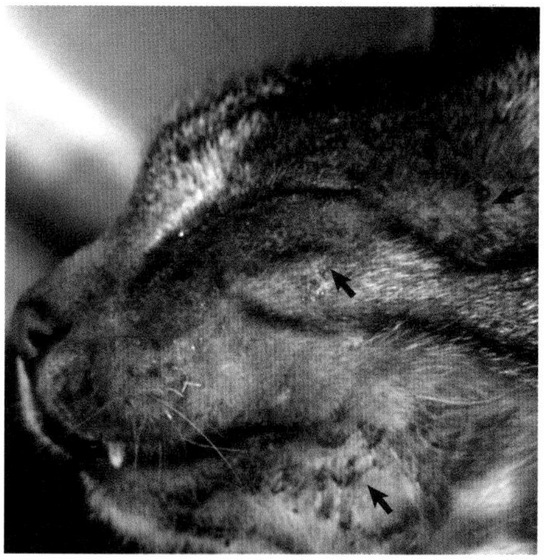
FISSURE Deep, vertically oriented linear cleft or break *(arrow)* from the epidermis into the dermis Examples: Pawpad fissure seen in pemphigus foliaceus, superficial necrolytic dermatitis, or digital hyperkeratosis	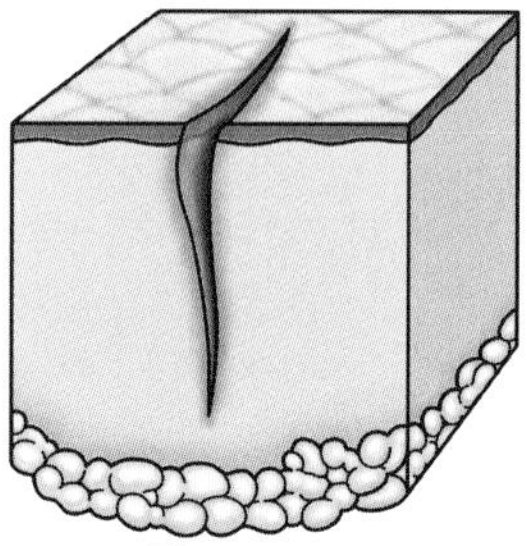 Fissure	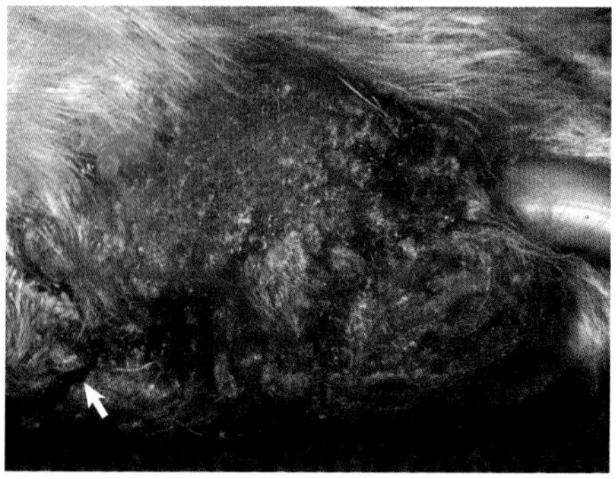

Table 17-6 Definition and Morphologic Features of Primary and Secondary Skin Lesions–cont'd

Lesion Definition	Drawing	Clinical Photograph
LICHENIFICATION[§] Rough, thickened epidermis secondary to persistent rubbing, scratching, or irritation; may have increased pigmentation Example: Chronic dermatitis	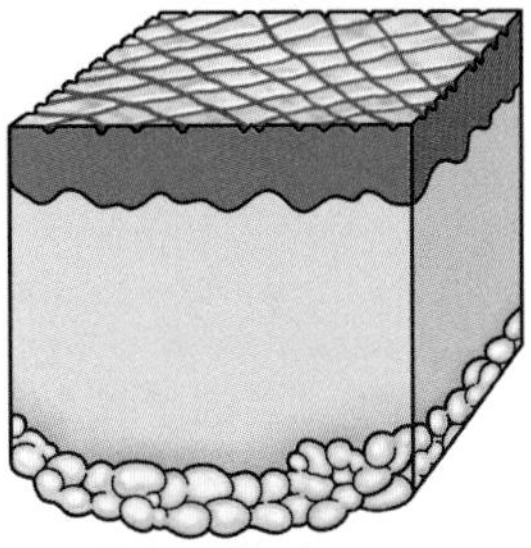 Lichenification	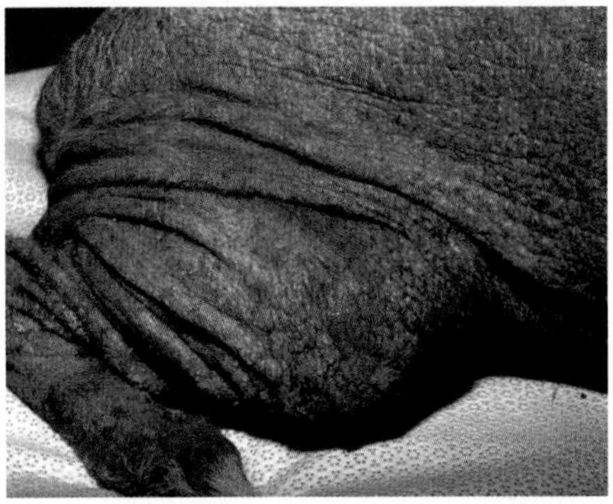
MACULE Flat, circumscribed, nonpalpable area that is a change in the color of the skin, < 1 cm in diameter Examples: Hemorrhage, lentigo, vitiligo	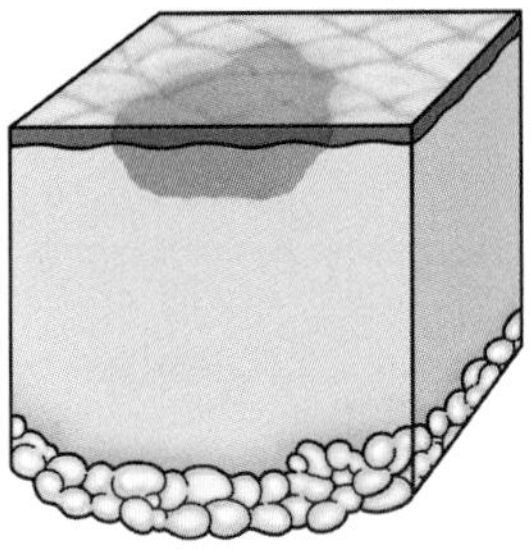 Macule	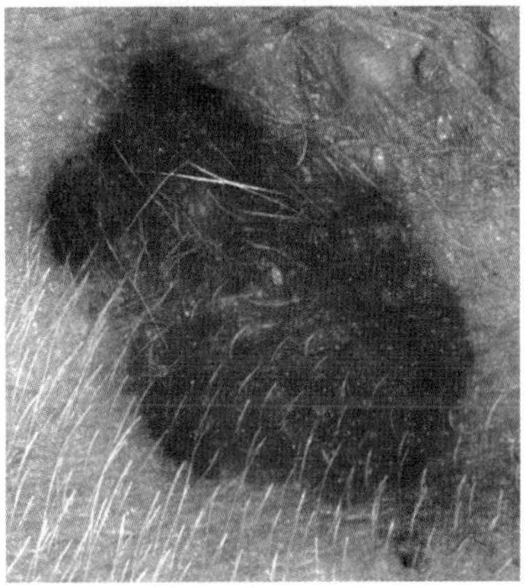
NEOPLASM[‡] "An abnormal mass of tissue, the growth of which exceeds and is uncoordinated with that of normal tissue and persists in the same excessive manner after cessation of the stimuli, which evoked the change"[‖] Examples: Lipoma, mast cell tumor, squamous cell carcinoma	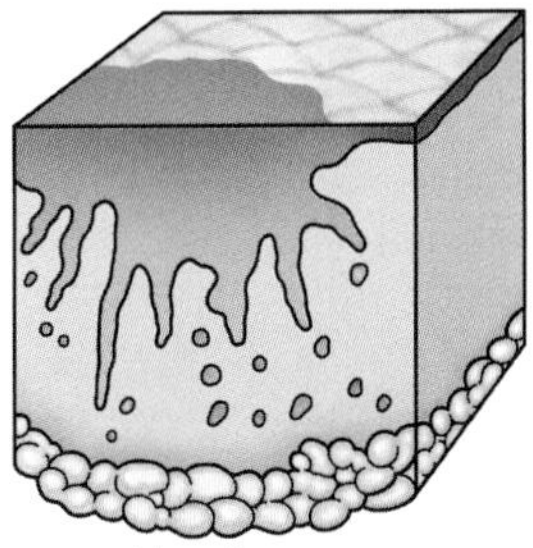 Neoplasm	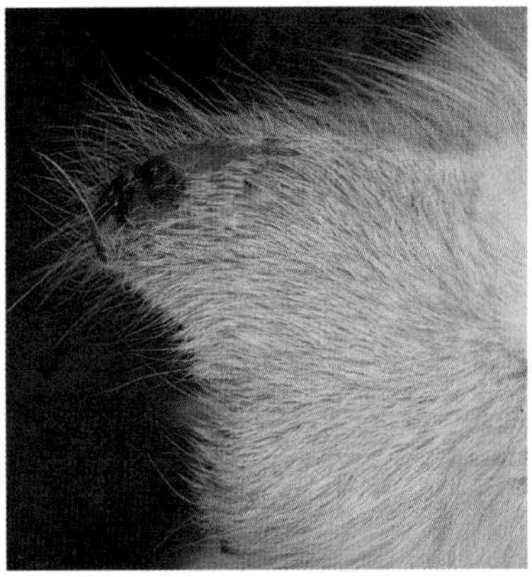
NODULE[¶] Elevated, often firm, circumscribed, solid palpable lesion ≥1 cm in diameter. Often located in dermis or subcutis Examples: Bacterial or fungal infection, infectious or sterile granuloma	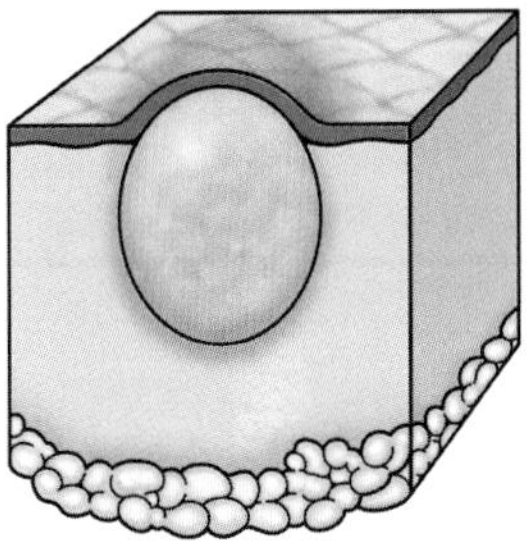 Nodule	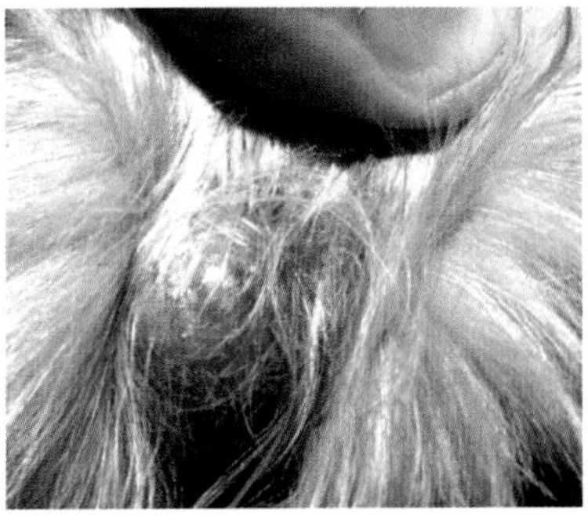

Continued

Table 17-6 Definition and Morphologic Features of Primary and Secondary Skin Lesions—cont'd

Lesion Definition	Drawing	Clinical Photograph
PAPULE Elevated, firm, palpable, circumscribed area < 1 cm in diameter *(arrows),* but may occur grouped together, may coalesce to form a plaque Examples: Insect bite, papilloma, superficial folliculitis	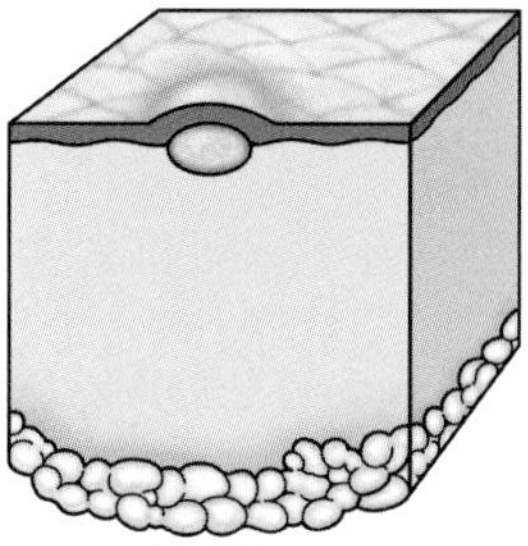 Papule	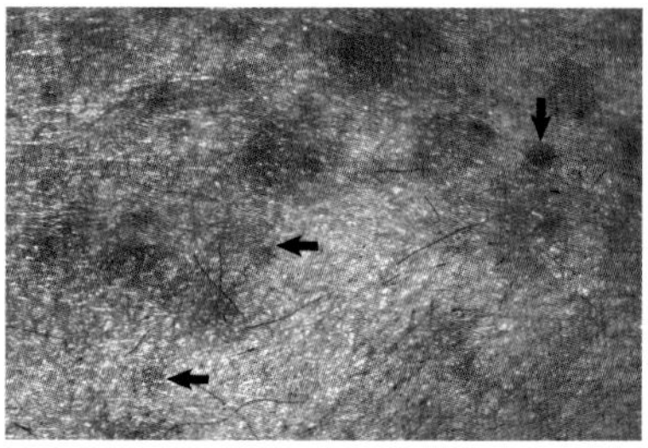
PLAQUE Elevated, usually firm, flat-topped, circumscribed, palpable lesion ≥ 1 cm in diameter, may coalesce to form a larger lesion Examples: Calcinosis cutis, reactive histiocytosis, eosinophilic plaque	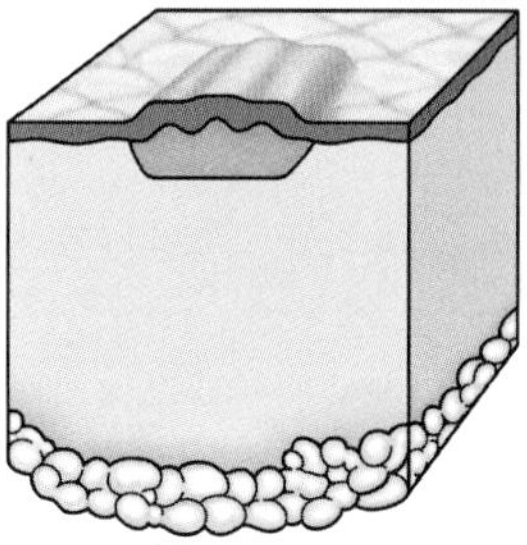 Plaque	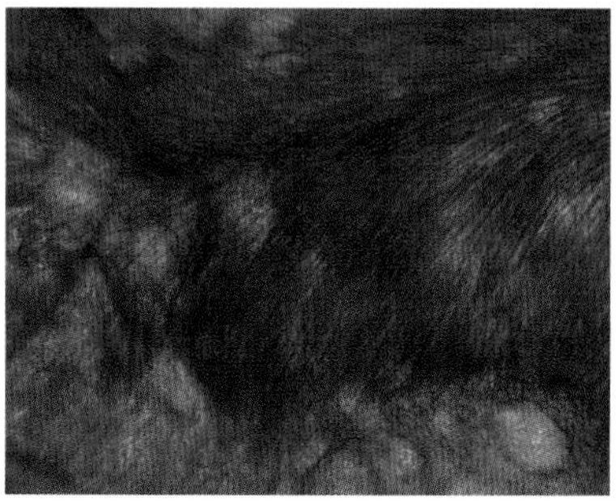
PUSTULE, EPIDERMAL[‡] Circumscribed raised superficial accumulation of purulent fluid within the epidermis *(arrow)* Examples: Bacterial infection, pemphigus foliaceus	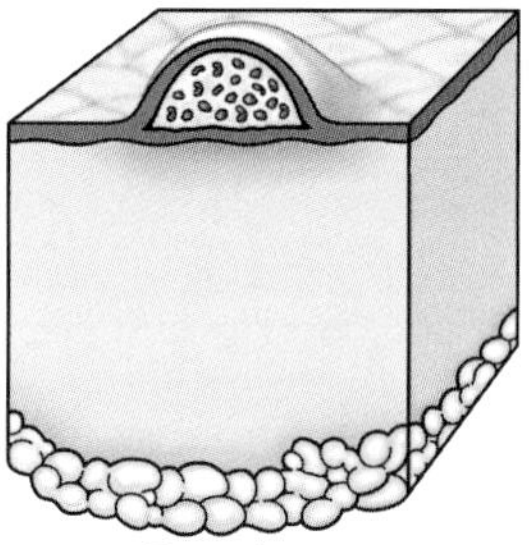 Pustule	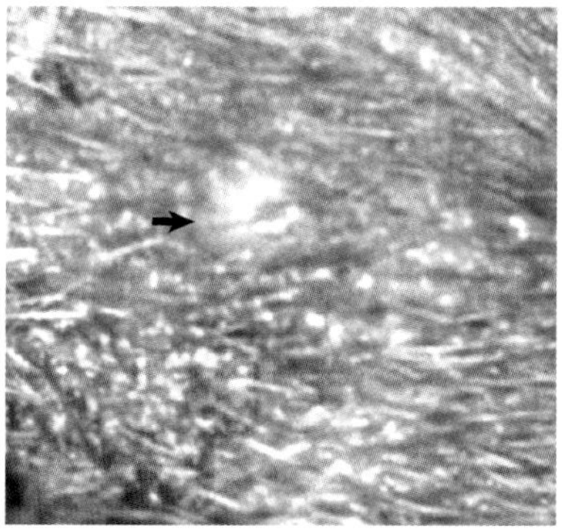
SCALE Sheets of cornified cells that horizontally split and separate from underlying epidermis as irregular, thick or thin, dry or oily fragments, may adhere to hairs. Variations include silvery, powdery, greasy, gritty, and polygonal Examples: Cornification disorders, sebaceous adenitis, ichthyosis	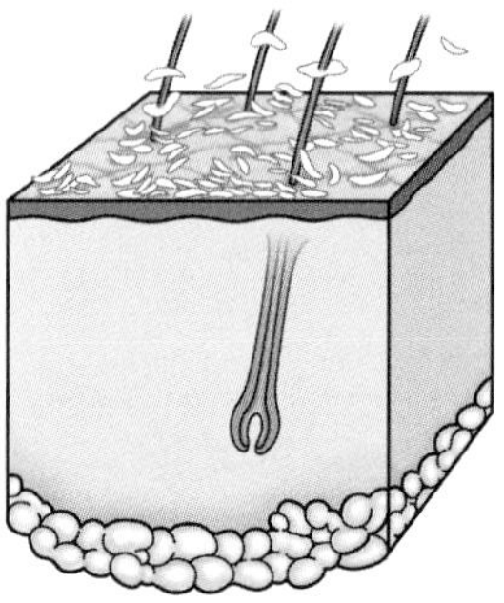 Scale	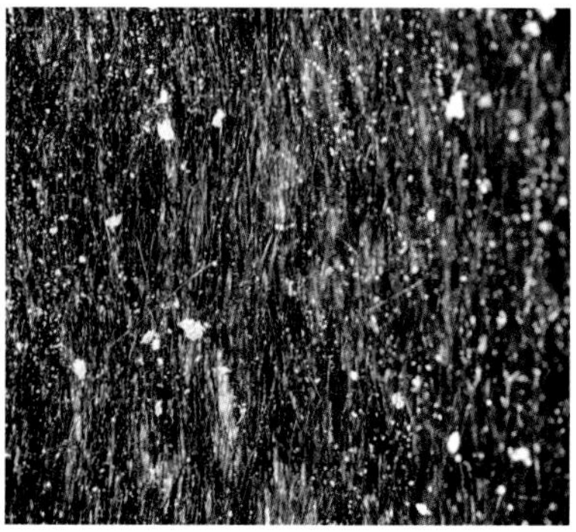

Table 17-6 Definition and Morphologic Features of Primary and Secondary Skin Lesions–cont'd

Lesion Definition	Drawing	Clinical Photograph
SCAR Thin to thick fibrous tissue that replaces normal skin following injury or laceration to the dermis; hair regrowth may not occur Examples: Healed wound, surgical scar	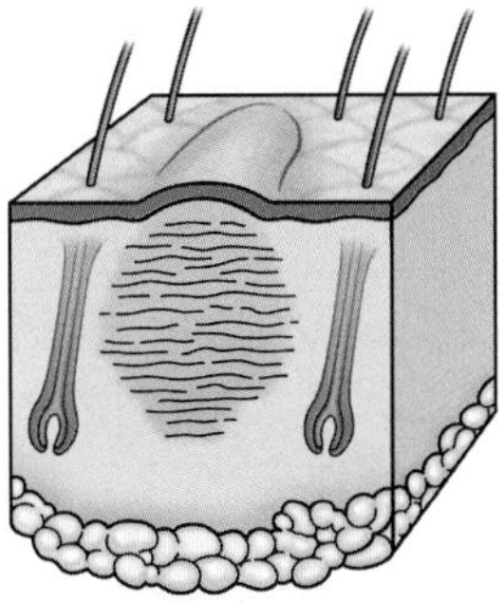 Scar	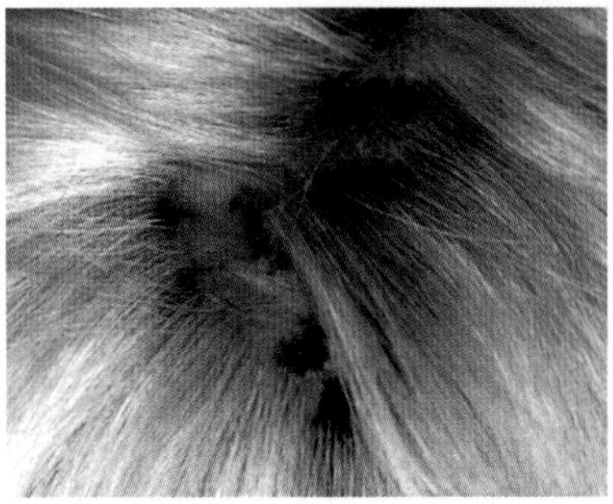
ULCER‡ Full-thickness loss of epidermis and basement membrane, and at least a portion of the dermis with depression of the exposed surface. May extend into deeper tissue Examples: Ischemic lesions resulting from vasculitis, indolent ulcer, feline herpesvirus dermatitis, feline ulcerative dermatitis syndrome	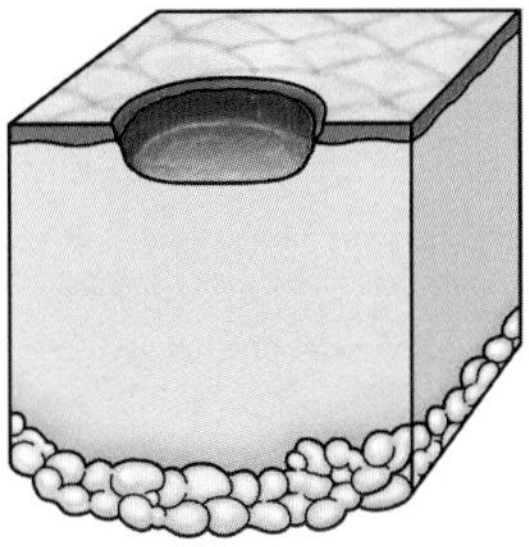 Ulcer	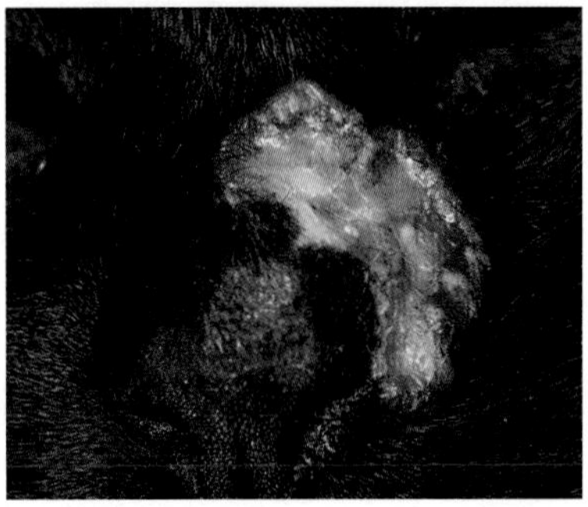
VESICLE AND BULLA** Elevated, circumscribed, horizontal, fluid-filled lesions differentiated by size. Fluid may be clear, tan, or red (hemorrhagic) Vesicle: < 1 cm in diameter Bulla: ≥ 1 cm in diameter *(arrows)* Examples: Burn, viral infection, immune-mediated diseases such as bullous pemphigoid	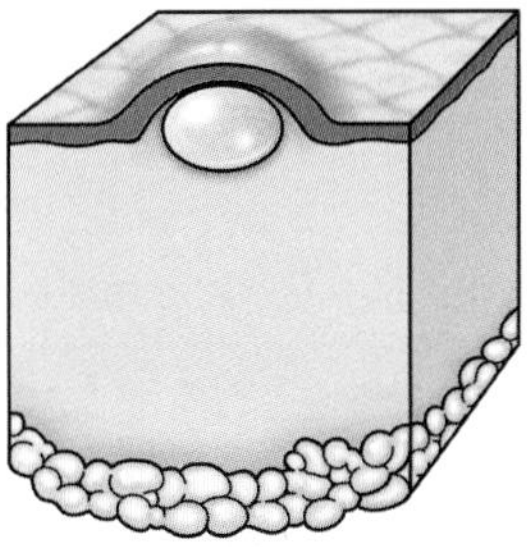 Vesicle	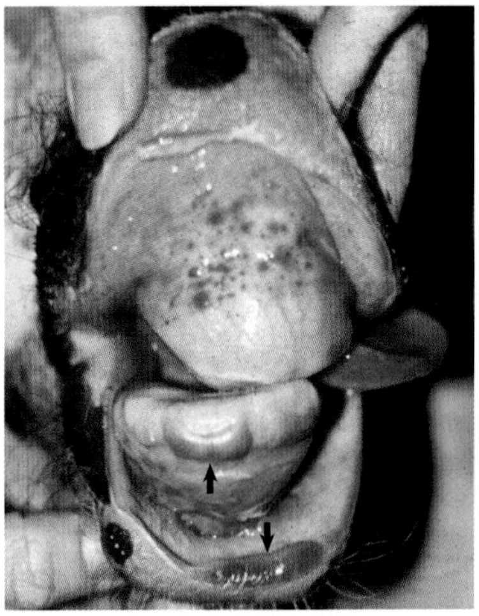

Continued

Table 17-6 Definition and Morphologic Features of Primary and Secondary Skin Lesions–cont'd

Lesion Definition	Drawing	Clinical Photograph
WHEAL‡ Elevated, irregular-shaped area of dermal edema; solid, usually transient, often pale centrally with an erythematous rim *(arrows)* Examples: Insect bites, urticaria, allergic reaction	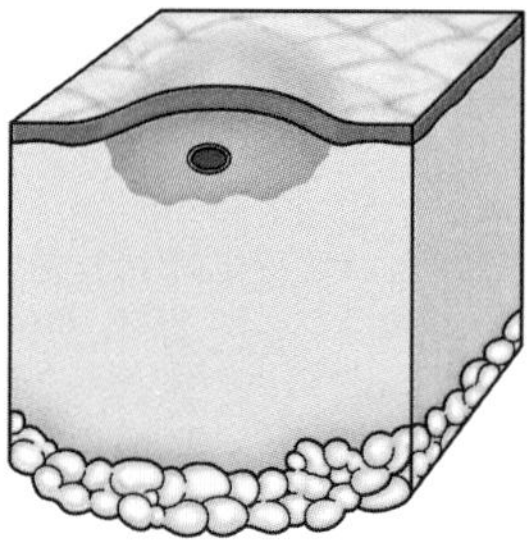 Wheal	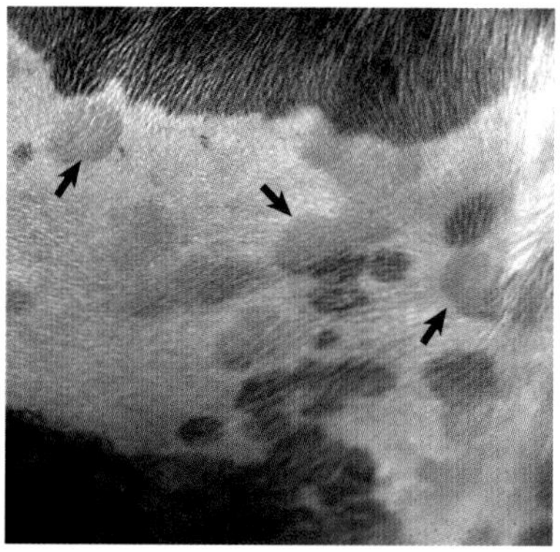

All clinical photographs courtesy Dr. A.M. Hargis, DermatoDiagnostics, unless otherwise noted.
*Courtesy Washington Animal Disease Diagnostic Laboratory.
†Courtesy Dr. D. Duclos, Animal Skin and Allergy Clinic; and Duclos DD, Hargis AM, Hanley PW: *Vet Dermatol* 19:134-141, 2008.
‡Courtesy Dr. D. Duclos, Animal Skin and Allergy Clinic.
§Courtesy Dr. H. Power, Dermatology for Animals.
‖From Willis RA: *Pathology of tumors,* Philadelphia, 1948, FA Davis.
¶Courtesy Dr. A. Mundell, Animal Dermatology Service.
**Courtesy Dr. P.E. Ginn, College of Veterinary Medicine, University of Florida; and Ginn PE, Hillier A, Lester GD: *Vet Dermatol* 9:249-256, 1998.

Table 17-7 Biopsy Sampling Tips

Preparation	Very gently clip or scissor if necessary. Do not surgically prepare the site if sampling lesions in epidermis or dermis. Caveat: Can surgically prepare site for excision of lesions deep in the subcutis or to remove large nodular mass such as a neoplasm.
Lesions	Collect multiple samples representative of the range of lesions. If crusting is significant, collect crust, wrap in lens paper, and place in formalin. For alopecic conditions: Collect samples from the most alopecic areas; draw a line on the sample in the direction of the hair coat. For ulcers or depigmenting lesions (junction important): Use incisional or excisional method or use an 8-mm biopsy punch instrument, and draw a line on the sample perpendicular to the junction between lesion and normal skin.
Punch samples	Use 6- or 8-mm punch instruments for haired skin. Use 4-mm punch for periocular skin, pawpads, or nasal planum.
Incisional and excisional samples	Use incisional or excisional methods if smaller punch would damage large pustule or vesicle. Gently place thin incisional or excisional samples, subcutis side down, on a piece of cardboard; let adhere for approximately 30 seconds, then place in formalin (prevents warping). NOTE: Do not let sample dehydrate. For lesions in the panniculus, use incisional or excisional method to ensure that the sample is of sufficient size and depth for diagnosis.
Fixation	Fix samples in 10% buffered formalin with 10 times the volume of formalin for the volume of samples. For diagnosis of autoimmune skin disease or tumors, begin with standard histopathologic evaluation; selected immunohistochemical stains can usually be done later on the formalin-fixed samples if desired.
Important finale	Submit a history with differential diagnoses or specific conditions you would like to rule out.

Box 17-5 Biopsy Sampling Do's

Consider whether referral to a veterinary dermatologist may be a better option than biopsy sampling.
Be gentle.
Biopsy early.
Collect multiple samples representative of the range of lesions.
Include crusts (additional crust may be peeled from lesions and immersed in formalin with biopsy samples).
Biopsy before using antiinflammatory therapy.
Use the correct biopsy procedure for the type of lesion.
Promptly immerse samples in formalin.
Label samples from different areas.
Prevent samples from temperature extremes during shipping.
Submit a history and photographs if available.

Box 17-6 Biopsy Sampling Don'ts

Don't surgically prepare the site if lesions are in the epidermis or dermis.
Don't use electrocautery or laser for small biopsy samples.
Don't grasp the punch biopsy samples or lesion areas of larger samples with a tissue forceps.
Don't use a biopsy instrument that is too small (4 mm is the minimum useful diameter).

the sample (Fig. 17-35, *A*). In the laboratory the sample is cut along the line so that the hair follicles are oriented longitudinally (see Fig. 17-35, *B*). If the line is not drawn on the sample, the sample might be cut so that the follicles are in cross or tangential section rather than longitudinal section (see Fig. 17-35, C), which reduces histologic value of the sample when evaluating for follicular disease. For collection of ulcers, depigmented lesions, or other lesions in which the junction between normal and affected skin is critical to diagnosis, use of incisional or excisional samples collected from affected skin and contiguous normal skin is often preferable. However, a large (8-mm) biopsy punch instrument can be used to collect the junction between normal and affected skin if a line with a fine-tipped permanent marking pen is drawn perpendicular to the junction between the normal and affected tissue before sample collection (Fig. 17-36). The line instructs laboratory personnel how to trim the sample to ensure that the critical areas are present for dermatopathologic evaluation. For lesions suspected of being invasive tumors, complete excision of the mass, including a 3-cm margin of clinically normal skin around all borders, is recommended (Fig. 17-37).

Fixation

Punch biopsy specimens should be placed in 10 times the volume of 10% neutral buffered formalin (NBF). To prevent warping in the fixative, thin excisional biopsy specimens should be gently attached to a flat object, such as a piece of cardboard or tongue depressor, and permitted to dry for 20 to 30 seconds. Twenty to 30 seconds is all that is necessary for the sample to adhere to the flat object. The specimen and flat object are then immediately immersed in formalin. Care should be taken not to let the sample become dehydrated (i.e., remain unfixed for longer than 20 to 30 seconds), which could damage the morphologic features of small samples and the lesions. In cold climates during winter months, punch biopsy samples should be placed in 10% NBF, fixed overnight, and then transferred into 70% alcohol for shipment to reduce the chance of freezing of specimens during transport.

History

Accurate histopathologic diagnosis and interpretation require knowledge of the gross features of the lesions. Therefore it is essential to include with biopsy samples the following information: (1) age, breed, and sex of the animal; (2) location, gross appearance, and duration of the lesions; (3) presence or absence of lesion symmetry (i.e., the distribution on the patient); and (4) presence or absence of pruritus affecting the animal (Box 17-7). Clinical information, including results of laboratory evaluations (i.e., hemogram, serum biochemical analysis, urinalysis); results of skin cultures, scrapings, or cytologic evaluation; current medications; and response to therapy, should be included along with a list of clinical differential diagnoses. History can be critical to reaching a diagnosis. For example, presence of luminal and mural folliculitis with no apparent follicular infectious agents in H&E-stained sections in conjunction with the history of lack of response to appropriate antibiotic therapy would suggest to the pathologist that a fungal stain to evaluate for occult dermatophyte infection should be performed. Without the history of lack of response to appropriate antibiotic therapy, the folliculitis pattern could easily be presumed to be of bacterial origin, and a fungal infection may be overlooked.

Ancillary Procedures

Other diagnostic procedures can supplement information gained from histologic examination of biopsy samples. These procedures include aspiration of pustule contents or exudates for cytologic evaluation, performing touch imprints of the cut surface of suspected neoplastic or infectious lesions for cytologic evaluation, aseptically

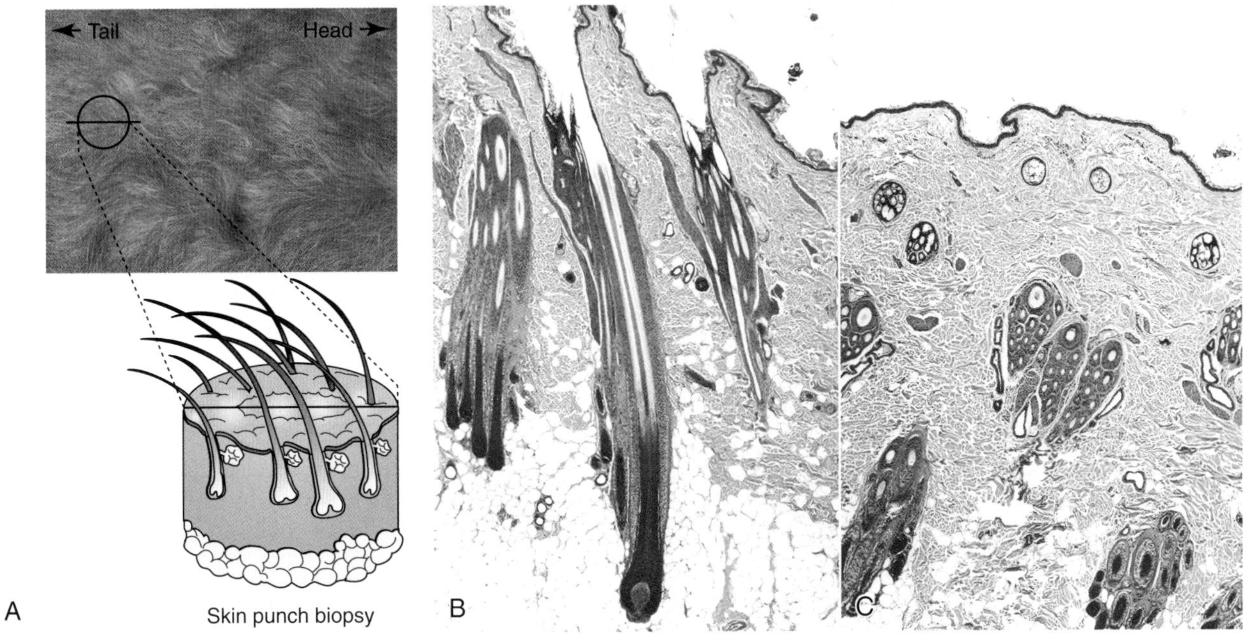

Figure 17-35 Sampling of the Skin for Histopathologic Evaluation, Haired, Dog. A, Clinical photograph of hair on dorsal thorax that illustrates an example of a biopsy sample *(circle)* with a line drawn in the direction of the hair coat. The line directs laboratory personnel to cut and embed the sample parallel to the hair follicles. The result is that hair follicles are visualized along their entire length, which is critical to the histologic evaluation for causes of alopecia. For simplicity, simple secondary follicles are used in this illustration. **B,** Longitudinal section of skin trimmed parallel to the hair follicles. Note that the hair follicles are cut longitudinally so that their full length is visible. H&E stain. **C,** Nonlongitudinal (horizontal) section of skin. Note that the hair follicles are cut in tangential or cross section and that only partial sections of each follicle are present for examination, which reduces the ability to evaluate follicular morphologic features or hair cycle abnormalities. H&E stain. (**B** and **C** courtesy Dr. A.M. Hargis, DermatoDiagnostics.)

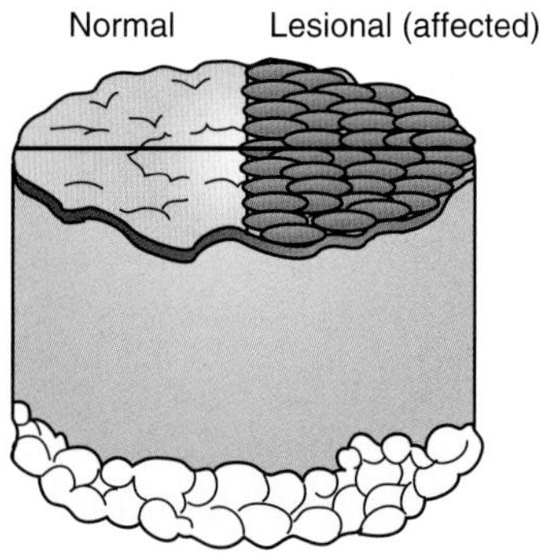

Figure 17-36 **Collecting the Junction of a Lesion and Normal Skin.** When collecting the junction of a lesion and normal skin for the evaluation of ulcers or depigmenting lesions using a large punch biopsy instrument (8 mm), it is necessary to draw a line on the sample from normal into affected skin to direct laboratory personnel to cut and embed the sample so that the junction between the normal and affected skin is present for microscopic examination. Without this line, the sample could be cut at a right angle to the desired line and thus miss the junction between normal and affected skin essential for histologic examination of the area most likely to have diagnostic changes.

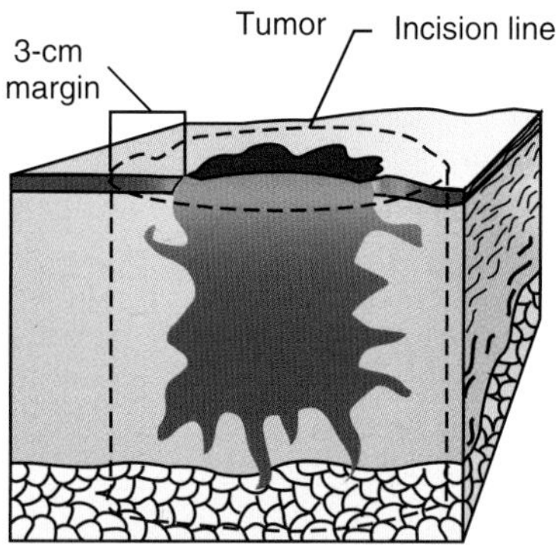

Figure 17-37 **Excisional Sampling.** If possible, 3-cm margins should be collected if the nodule is suspected of being an invasive neoplasm. This facilitates examination of the margins for completeness of excision.

Box 17-7 What Constitutes a History?

Age, breed, sex
Lesion distribution
Lesion appearance, severity, and duration
Influence of specific and/or recent therapy that could change lesions
Other clinical problems
Abnormalities in blood work or urinalysis results
Fecal examination results
Differential diagnoses (important)

collecting a tissue sample for microbiologic culture, and collecting biopsy samples of suspected immune-mediated diseases or poorly differentiated tumors for immunostaining. Cytologic evaluation is a potentially more rapid and sensitive test for detection of infectious agents than histopathologic evaluation, and early diagnosis via cytologic evaluation may help guide further testing or therapy. Use of immunostaining for identification of cell surface or cytoplasmic proteins (to aid in diagnosis of tumors) or for identification of immunoglobulin, complement, or other antigens (to aid in the diagnosis of immune-mediated skin disease, such as pemphigus) can be helpful in some cases. The formalin-fixed tissue submitted for histopathologic evaluation also can be used for most routine immunohistochemical procedures, because most use immunoperoxidase staining rather than immunofluorescence (IF).

Unfortunately, immunostaining techniques for immune-mediated skin diseases can give false-positive or false-negative results; thus they must be done in conjunction with standard histopathologic evaluation. For autoimmune diseases, should IF evaluation be desired, specimens can be fixed in Michel's medium, which preserves immunoglobulin and complement. If immunohistochemical (immunoperoxidase) staining is desired, formalin-fixed samples are used; however, for best results, samples should not remain in formalin longer than 48 hours. Prolonged fixation in formalin results in cross-linking of proteins and false-negative results. For autoimmune disease, newer techniques that detect more specific antigens, such as desmoglein (transmembrane glycoproteins found in desmosomes that provide physical connections between keratinocytes), use of "salt-split" skin sections (a technique used in immunostaining of the skin in which sodium chloride splits the epidermis from the dermis through the lamina lucida, allowing better differentiation of subepidermal bullous dermatoses), use of better substrates for indirect immunostaining, and use of immunoblotting and enzyme-linked immunosorbent assay (ELISA) techniques may improve diagnostic accuracy of immune-mediated skin diseases in the future.

Identification of cell surface or cytoplasmic proteins can help identify the cell type in poorly differentiated tumors (Table 17-8). However, there can be anomalous expression of proteins in some tumors (e.g., anomalous expression of cytokeratin in melanoma); thus evaluation of a series (panel) of antibodies is preferred because the pattern of staining with a panel of antibodies is more reliable than staining with one or two antibodies. In addition, some laboratories also offer "prognosis panels" for some tumors (e.g., mast cell tumors and melanomas), which may help direct therapy. Formalin-fixed specimens are acceptable for most procedures, but for others, fresh or frozen specimens are better. Discussion with a pathologist is recommended regarding when to use immunostaining procedures.

Disorders of Domestic Animals

Congenital and Hereditary Disorders

The terms congenital and hereditary are not synonymous. Congenital lesions develop in the fetus (in utero), are present at birth, and have a variety of causes. An example is hypotrichosis in the fetus associated with maternal dietary iodine deficiency. Inherited conditions are transmitted genetically and are not always manifested phenotypically in utero or at birth but may develop later in life. An example is sebaceous adenitis, which may not develop until 1 to 2 years of age or later. E-Box 17-2 lists selected cutaneous inherited diseases in animals (also see E-Box 1-1). There are many other diseases (e.g., cutaneous and renal glomerular vasculopathy in greyhounds, atopic dermatitis in selected breeds) that may also be inherited, but the mode of inheritance has not been documented.

Congenital Alopecia and Hypotrichosis

Congenital alopecia or atrichia (absence of hair from skin where hair is usually present) and hypotrichosis (less than the normal amount of hair) have been reported in most species of domestic animals. In most instances, congenital hypotrichosis is a hereditary condition caused by spontaneous genetic mutations affecting genes responsible for or influencing the normal development and/or maintenance of hair follicles or other components of the skin. In most cases the exact mutation has not been identified. In some of these

Table 17-8 Examples of Antibodies to Cell Surface or Cytoplasmic Proteins That May Differentiate Tumors with Similar Histologic Appearance

Tumor Type	Antibodies	
	VIMENTIN	**PANCYTOKERATIN**
Carcinoma	–	+
Sarcoma	+	–
	CYTOKERATIN 5/6	**CYTOKERATIN 8**
Squamous cell carcinoma	+	–
Sweat gland carcinoma	–	+
	α-SMOOTH-MUSCLE ACTIN	**GFAP**
Neurofibrosarcoma	–	+
Leiomyosarcoma	+	–
	CYTOKERATIN	**FACTOR VIII RELATED ANTIGEN**
Carcinoma	+	–
Epithelioid hemangiosarcoma	–	+
	CD3	**CD79A**
B lymphocyte lymphoma	–	+
T lymphocyte lymphoma	+	–

GFAP, Glial fibrillary acidic protein; *CD,* cluster of differentiation.

animals the alopecia or hypotrichosis has been recognized as standard for the breed (e.g., Mexican hairless pig, Chinese crested dog, Mexican hairless dog, and sphynx cat), and the mutation is purposefully propagated. The congenital alopecia and hypotrichosis syndromes have been considered to be forms of congenital follicular dysplasia because there is an abnormal development of the hair follicles. Animals with congenital hereditary hypotrichosis can have defects in other body systems, including brachygnathism (abnormal smallness of the mandible) and dental, thymic, and genital abnormalities. When the condition involves the hair follicles plus adnexal glands and teeth, which all arise from the ectoderm, the condition is also termed ectodermal dysplasia. In addition to health problems created by oral, dental, or thymic defects (inability to efficiently chew or graze and immune deficiency that can lead to death), animals with hypotrichosis are more susceptible to sunburn, temperature extremes, and bacterial and fungal infections. The degree, location, and age of onset of hairlessness or hypotrichosis vary. Hair that is present is usually abnormally coarse or fine and easily broken or epilated. Morphologic changes in the skin and hair follicles vary from species to species, most likely representing differences in mutations. A useful example is congenital hypotrichosis with anodontia in German Holstein calves (Fig. 17-38). In this condition, hypotrichosis, lack of most teeth, and complete absence of eccrine nasolabial glands is inherited as a monogenic X-linked recessive trait. Because the condition affects the hair follicles, some adnexal glands, and teeth, it is also classified as an ectodermal dysplasia. The condition varies in severity, with some calves more affected than others. Affected calves have reduced numbers of hairs per surface area in various anatomic locations (especially head, pinnae, neck, back, and tail), and also have reduced length and numbers of eyelashes and vibrissae. The alopecia and hypotrichosis are most severe in newborn calves because the number of fine hairs increases with age. There are no defects in the horns, endocrine glands, genital organs, or other internal organs. Histologically, hair follicles and adnexal glands are absent in the skin on the back of the ears. Hair follicle density is often reduced in other areas. When present, hair bulbs are small and poorly developed. In some areas the apocrine glands are reduced in quantity, and eccrine nasolabial glands are absent.

Especially for purposes of herd health management and disease prevention, it is important to differentiate the congenital inherited alopecia and hypotrichosis disorders from the nongenetic congenital alopecic disorders. The latter includes congenital hypotrichosis caused by maternal iodine deficiency in foals, calves, lambs, and pigs; in utero infection with bovine virus diarrhea or hog cholera virus; and defects in other systems such as adenohypophyseal hypoplasia in some breeds of cattle (Table 17-9). Differential diagnosis of these conditions is usually made by a combination of clinical or gross examination (e.g., thyroid glands, pituitary gland, or dental abnormalities), microscopic examination (e.g., presence of absence of hair follicles or other adnexa), and in some instances evaluation for infectious agents (e.g., immunohistochemical evaluation of hair follicles for bovine virus diarrhea virus in calf skin). For best results in microscopic evaluations, it is important to collect skin samples from the most alopecic areas as well as the most haired areas in similar anatomic locations on the body if possible and to submit the samples in separate and labeled containers.

Collagen Dysplasia

Collagen dysplasia (cutaneous asthenia, hyperelastosis cutis, dermatosparaxis, Ehlers-Danlos–like syndrome) occurs in most domestic animals and comprises a clinically, genetically, and biochemically heterogeneous group of diseases that are rare. In each, skin tears easily and is hyperextensible and loose, but the severity of these lesions varies among species. Specific enzyme defects affecting collagen synthesis or processing are the cause of most collagen dysplasia syndromes. Abnormal synthesis or processing of collagen leads to structurally abnormal dermal collagen that has decreased tensile strength. The cause of some collagen dysplasia syndromes has not been established. Gross lesions consist of cutaneous hyperextensibility and laxity (Fig. 17-39), seromas or hematomas, frequent skin wounds that result even from normal handling and activity, and numerous scars, which are the result of previous tearing of the dermal connective tissues. Microscopic features vary among the different types of collagen dysplasia syndromes, and in some the skin is histologically normal. If microscopic lesions are present, the collagen bundles can vary in size and shape, can be separated by wide spaces, have laminar splits in various levels of the dermis, or have a haphazard arrangement. Electron microscopy or biochemical analyses are sometimes required to make a definitive diagnosis.

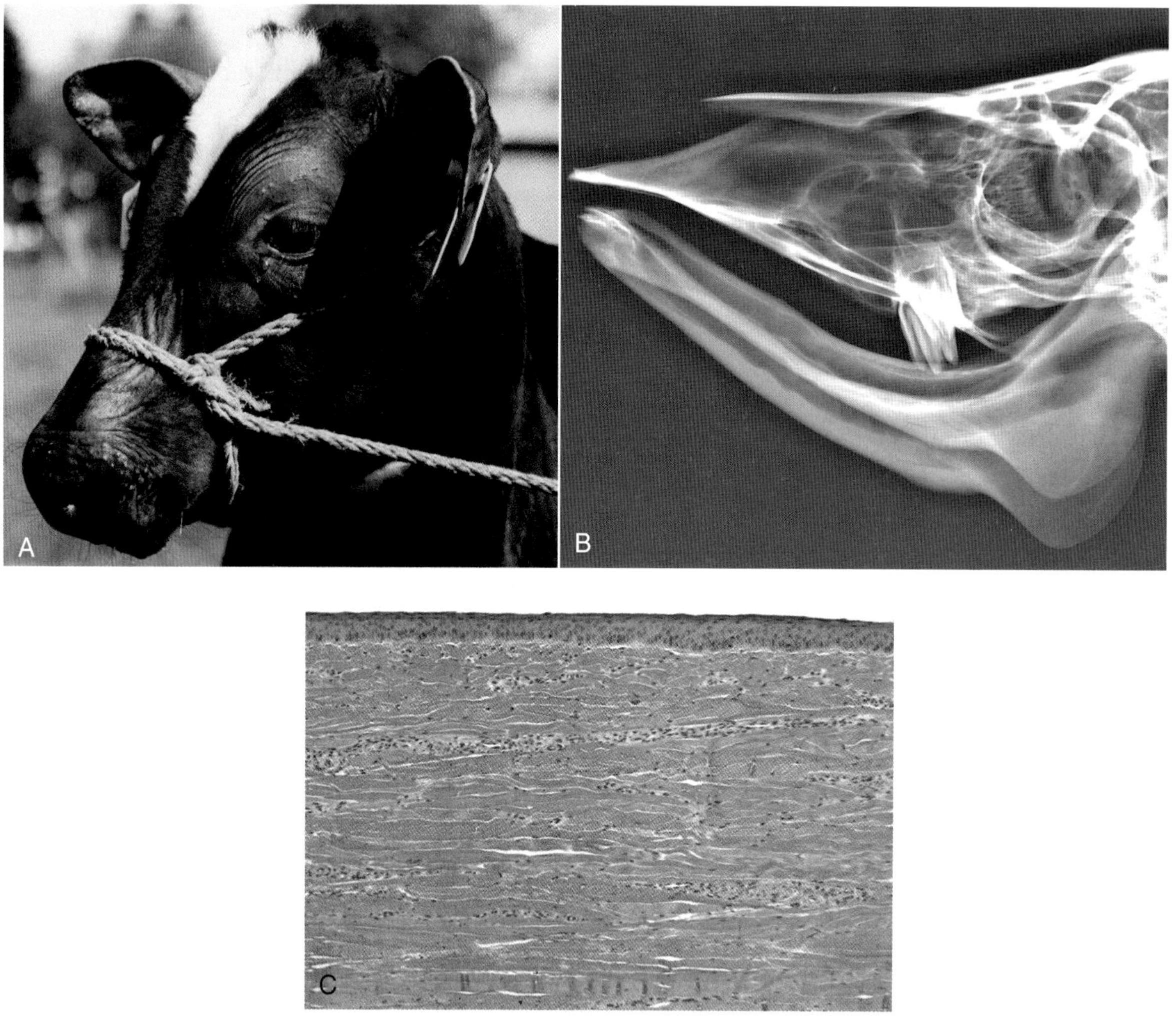

Figure 17-38 **Congenital Hypotrichosis with Anodontia, Calf. A,** The hair coat is sparse and short. Eyelashes and tactile hairs are also sparse and very short. The tail switch (not in this photograph) was approximately one-third the normal length. **B,** Radiograph, skull. Note that most of the teeth are missing (i.e., anodontia). When congenital hypotrichosis involves the hair follicles plus adnexal glands and teeth, which all arise from the ectoderm, the condition is also termed *ectodermal dysplasia*. **C,** Affected skin. Note the lack of hair follicles and other adnexa. Animals with hypotrichosis are susceptible to extremes of temperature, and the skin is more likely to sustain traumatic injury and secondary infection because of the lack of the protective hair coat. Absence of sweat glands may complicate the ability of affected animals (horses and cattle with ectodermal dysplasia) to thermoregulate. H&E stain. (**A** courtesy Professor T. Leeb, Institute of Animal Breeding, School of Veterinary Medicine Hannover; and Drogemuller C, Kuiper H, Peters M, et al: *Vet Dermatol* 13:6;307-313, 2002. **B** courtesy Professor T. Leeb, Institute of Animal Breeding, School of Veterinary Medicine Hannover; and T. Prax. **C** courtesy Dr. F. Seeliger, Department of Pathology, Tieraerztliche Hochschule Hannover.)

Although rare, one of the more common of the collagen dysplasia syndromes, hereditary equine regional dermal asthenia (HERDA), is an autosomal recessive disease that occurs in young quarter horses and horses of quarter horse ancestry. This syndrome is caused by a genetic mutation on equine chromosome 1 in equine cyclophilin B, and a genetic test is available for diagnosis. It has been shown that affected horses have altered cyclophilin B–protein interactions, and that collagen folding is affected, presumably leading to the clinical lesions, which tend to develop in the skin of the dorsal trunk when young horses begin saddle training, initially suggesting that the collagen defect was only regionally present. However, other areas of the body can develop lesions, and additional studies have indicated that the collagen abnormality is uniformly present in skin of affected horses, but that other factors such as trauma, heat, or UV light–associated injury may influence lesion development. Although internal organ collagen dysfunction has not been noted, affected horses may have hyperextensible joints, weaker tendons and ligaments, an increased risk for developing osteoarthritis, and a higher-than-expected incidence of corneal ulcers. Clinical lesions usually develop within the first 2 years of life and include cutaneous swellings (seromas and or hematomas), open wounds or sloughing skin, loose easily stretched skin that does not return to original position, scars, and white hairs (possibly associated with follicular damage during dermal tearing). Histologic lesions are most obvious in the deep dermis and consist of thin and short collagen fibers arranged in clusters separated by clear spaces sometimes accompanied by granulation tissue and fibrosis, presumably from previous injury, but lesions are subtle and may be inconclusive. It is important to include deep dermis in biopsy samples, because samples from more superficial areas (such as samples of skin from seromas, hematomas, or wounds) may only include superficial dermis above the pathologic dermal separation and thus may be nondiagnostic. Ultrastructural evaluation fails to consistently differentiate between control and affected samples and is thus considered insensitive. Therefore definitive diagnosis rests with genetic testing.

Table 17-9 Categories, Causes, and Age of Onset of Hypotrichosis and Alopecia

Category	Cause	Age of Onset	Species
Congenital hypotrichosis or alopecia	Usually inherited, may be accompanied by odontogenic, thymic, genital, or other defects that influence neonatal viability; can be classified as congenital follicular dysplasia syndromes	Usually present at birth or within the first month of life	Mostly calves; less often piglets, puppies, kittens; rarely foals
	Maternal dietary influences (e.g., iodine deficiency)	Present at birth	Calves, piglets, lambs, foals
	Secondary to other defects (adenohypophyseal hypoplasia)	Present at birth	Guernsey and Jersey calves
	In utero infection with bovine virus diarrhea or hog cholera virus	Present at birth	Calves, pigs
Tardive structural follicular dysplasia	Usually inherited	Months to years after birth	Dogs, cattle, horses
Acquired pattern alopecia (follicular miniaturization)	Unknown, genetic predisposition suspected	Young, 6 months to a year	Dogs
Hair cycle disorders of endocrine origin (endocrine disorders)*	Abnormal function of pituitary, thyroid, or adrenal glands, or gonads; or exposure to exogenous hormones (iatrogenic systemic or topical administration, or accidental topical exposure to creams used on human skin)	Develops in young adults to aged	Predominantly dogs
Hair cycle disorders of nonendocrine origin	Factors that influence hair growth such as therapy with antimitotic drugs (chemotherapy); stress, fever, illness (telogen effluvium); close clipping, especially of plush-coated breeds of dogs (prolonged alopecia postclipping†); or unknown cause (alopecia X)	Typically adults	Any species, often dogs Plush-coated breeds of dogs: prolonged alopecia postclipping and alopecia X
Inflammatory conditions or trauma	Follicular infection Posttraumatic and inflammatory Sebaceous adenitis Alopecia areata Traction alopecia	Any age	Any species; dogs most frequently affected with follicular infection and sebaceous adenitis
Excessive grooming	Hypersensitivity reactions, psychogenic causes, occasionally feline hyperthyroidism	Any age, but older with hyperthyroidism	Most often affects cats
Nutrition	Severe protein or protein-calorie nutrition	Any age, especially young or pregnant	Any species
Neoplasia	Paraneoplastic: internal malignancy, often of pancreas	Aged	Cats
	Direct involvement of epidermis, dermis, or adnexa (e.g., lymphoma)	Usually adult to aged	Dogs, cats
Seasonal alopecia Unknown cause	Seasonal alopecia in horses	Horses, straight or curly hair coat	Horses
	Idiopathic winter alopecia in cattle	Young adult, often bulls	Beef cattle
	Idiopathic (cyclic, seasonal) flank alopecia in dogs	Dogs	Dogs

*Endocrine:

1. Clinically manifested endocrine disease in cats is usually caused by hyperadrenocorticism in which marked dermal atrophy leads to tearing of the skin with normal handling procedures. Alopecia can be a feature, but skin fragility is a more significant problem.
2. Clinically manifested endocrine disease in horses is usually caused by hyperadrenocorticism and is typified paradoxically by hypertrichosis rather than alopecia (possibly because of production of adrenal androgens, other hormones, or pressure of the pituitary on thermoregulatory areas of the hypothalamus).

†Prolonged alopecia postclipping: The pathogenesis of this condition is undetermined, but because hair regrowth may take a year or more, an arrest in the hair cycle is suspected.

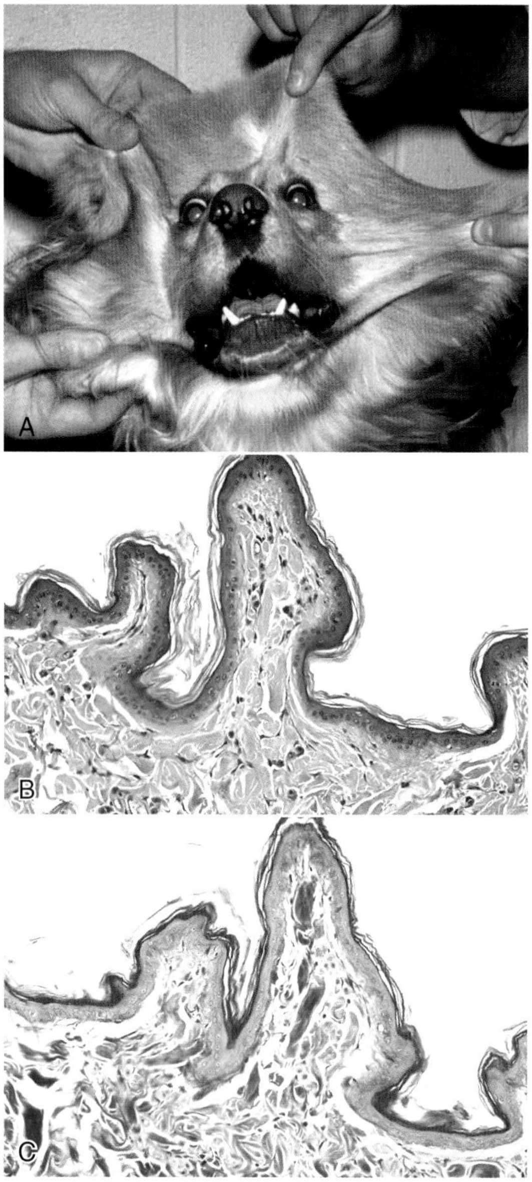

Figure 17-39 **Collagen Dysplasia, Skin, Dog. A,** The skin is hyperextensible. In this dog, the skin can be stretched more than the skin of a normal dog. **B,** The collagen bundles are irregular in size and shape and are arranged haphazardly. The abnormally formed collagen is responsible for the hyperextensibility of the skin, which predisposes to tearing with normal handling and activity. H&E stain. **C,** Deeper level (step section) of the sample shown in **B.** Collagen bundles are stained blue. The variation in diameter and shape of the collagen bundles and their haphazard arrangement is accentuated with this stain. Masson's trichrome stain. (**A** courtesy Dr. B. Baker, Washington State University. **B** and **C** courtesy Dr. A.M. Hargis, DermatoDiagnostics.)

Collagen dysplasia syndromes other than HERDA have developed in various other breeds of horses, including the quarter horse, and in particular, warmbloods. Unlike HERDA, however, lesions develop in young foals, there is more generalized clinical lesion distribution, and the genetic test for HERDA, when performed, has been negative, indicating that more that one type of collagen dysplasia disorder is present in horses.

Lymphedema

Chronic Progressive Lymphedema of Draft Horses. Chronic progressive lymphedema is a disabling disorder of the peripheral lymphatic system that has been described in a variety of breeds of draft horses. Early clinical lesions consist of skin thickening, pitting edema, and scaling that progress to more moderate and extensive areas of permanent thickening (fibrosis) with skin folding and nodules, scaling, ulceration, exudation, and enlarged leg diameter. The lesions are often hidden by the long hair coat, so they may be inapparent until they have become more chronic and extensive. Bacteria and parasites often secondarily infect lymphedematous skin, and the inflammation associated with the secondary infections further aggravates the lymphedema, eventually leading to mechanical impairment, lameness, and sometimes euthanasia. The cause and pathogenesis of this condition are not fully understood but are thought to be multifactorial with an underlying genetic component (see Chapter 10).

Congenital Lymphedema. Congenital lymphedema, also a disorder of the peripheral lymphatic system, has been reported in cattle, pigs, dogs, and cat. The onset of lesions is usually at birth or within the first few months of life. Clinical lesions consist of generalized or regional swellings that vary in severity depending on the species. The condition is often inherited (see Chapter 10).

Epidermolysis Bullosa (Red Foot Disease)

Epidermolysis bullosa refers to a group of mechanobullous diseases resulting in development of cutaneous blisters (bullae) in response to minor mechanical trauma. Blisters develop as a result of poor cohesion of the epidermis and dermis as a result of structural defects at the basement membrane zone. The structural defects are the result of mutations in genes responsible for the synthesis of a variety of structural components of this anatomic region of the skin and include abnormalities in keratin intermediate filaments, proteins associated with hemidesmosomes, and anchoring fibrils such as type VII collagen. The diseases vary in mode of inheritance, clinical manifestations, and anatomic location of the blisters. Animals affected with the diseases usually die because of their inability to obtain nourishment, loss of fluid and protein, and secondary infection leading to bacteremia. Epidermolysis bullosa has been reported in horses, cattle, sheep, dogs, and cats. Lesions can be present at birth or develop shortly thereafter and are located where epithelial surfaces are subjected to minor mechanical trauma, such as oral mucosa, lips, and extremities, and can include sloughing of claws, hooves, or pawpads. Shearing forces that normally cause no problem are sufficient to cause injury in these animals. Microscopic lesions are those of an epidermal vesicular disease in which vesicles form in different locations (subepidermal, dermal-epidermal junction, or intraepidermal), depending on the specific disease. The vesicles progress to ulcers or if secondarily infected, become pustules. As healing occurs, the reepithelialization causes sloughing of the dried exudates over the ulcer, and the pustules dry to form crusts.

Epitheliogenesis Imperfecta (Aplasia Cutis)

Epitheliogenesis imperfecta results from the failure of the stratified squamous epithelium of skin, adnexa, and/or oral mucosa to develop completely. The disease varies in severity and has been reported in most domestic species. It is the result of inherited genetic mutations in some species, but inheritance is not proved in other species. Additional information regarding the pathogenesis is not known. Without the protective covering of the stratified squamous epithelium, the underlying tissue is easily traumatized, can become infected, and bacteremia can develop. Grossly, lesions consist of sharply demarcated areas devoid of the epidermis and adnexa or mucosa, exposing the underlying red, moist dermis or submucosa. Lesions are located most often on the face, extremities, or mucous

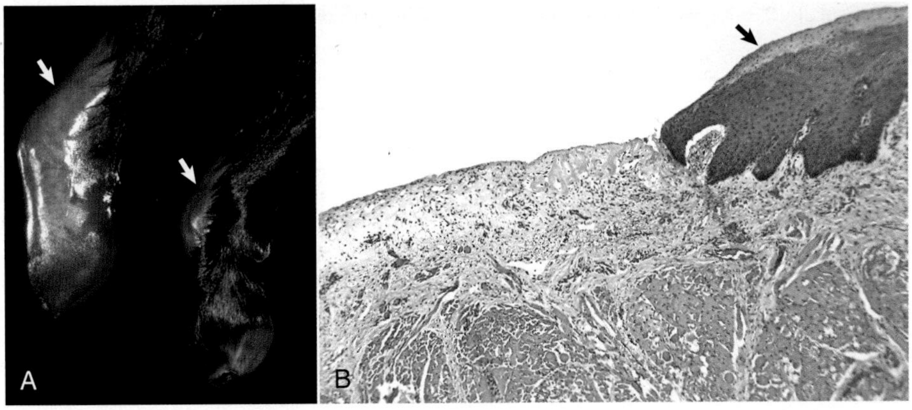

Figure 17-40 Epitheliogenesis Imperfecta, Calf. A, Skin. Areas of epidermis over the extremities are missing *(arrows)*. This condition is the result of inherited genetic mutations in some species, but inheritance is not proven in other species. **B,** Oral mucosa. Junction of normal and affected mucous membrane. Epithelium is present on the right (normal area) *(arrow)* but is abruptly missing on the left. The lack of germinal epithelium results in the failure of the epidermis, adnexa, or mucosae to develop completely. Skin, adnexa, and oral mucosa can be affected in this disease. (Courtesy Dr. M.D. McGavin, College of Veterinary Medicine, University of Tennessee.)

membranes and can be small (1 cm) or involve extensive regions such as the entire distal limb (Fig. 17-40). Small lesions can heal with scarring and not interfere with life. With extensive involvement the entire skin can be affected, including hooves, ears, lips, and eyelids, and may result in abortion of the affected fetus. Animals born alive with extensive lesions usually die from infection or dehydration and electrolyte abnormalities from extensive fluid loss through nonepithelialized surfaces.

Congenital Hypertrichosis

See Disorders of Ruminants (Cattle, Sheep, and Goats).

Dermatosis Vegetans

See Disorders of Pigs.

Disorders of Physical, Radiation, or Chemical Injury

Solar (Actinic) Injury

The majority of ultraviolet radiation (UVR) reaching the surface of the earth is UVA and a small amount of UVB (see Responses of the Dermis to Injury, Alterations in Growth, Development, or Tissue Maintenance, Solar Elastosis). UVB penetrates into the epidermis and superficial dermis and is the portion of UV light most damaging to the skin because it is absorbed by and damages DNA. UVA penetrates deeper into the dermis but is less efficient in causing DNA damage because it is not significantly absorbed by native DNA. However, UVA can act indirectly by causing secondary photoreactions of existing UVB-induced DNA damage or alternatively damage DNA via indirect photosensitizing reactions. For example, if photodynamic chemicals are present in the skin, they can chemically react with the longer wavelengths (UVA and sometimes visible light), thus releasing energy and leading to the formation of reactive oxygen intermediates that initiate a chain of reactions resulting in cutaneous damage (photosensitization, phototoxicity).

Solar (Actinic) Dermatosis, Keratosis, and Neoplasia. The damage to skin by UV light can be acute (sunburn) or chronic (solar dermatosis, neoplasia). An early transient erythema may be caused by the heating effect of the light rays and possibly by photochemical changes. The later developing erythema is called "sunburn erythema," and the skin is warm, tender, and swollen. The pathogenesis of sunburn erythema may involve diffusion of inflammatory mediators, such as cytokines, from radiation-damaged keratinocytes, or from direct damage to endothelial cells of superficial dermal capillaries by UV light. Chronic sun exposure, particularly to UVB, causes damage primarily in the epidermis leading to the development of neoplasia. The damage occurs in three broad categories, as follows:

1. One of the most detrimental changes occurs when UVB radiation contacts the nucleus and causes the formation of "photoproducts," which are abnormal covalent or single bonds between two adjacent pyrimidine bases in a strand of DNA. The two major UVB-induced photoproducts are pyrimidine dimers (covalent bonds between two thymine or two cytosine bases) and 6-4 photoproducts (single bond bridging carbon 4 in one cytosine and carbon 6, either in a cytosine or a thymine). These photoproducts form in keratinocyte DNA (and also in DNA of Langerhans cells and dermal dendritic cells). The damage can be easily and accurately repaired before the cell undergoes mitosis by the nucleotide excision repair enzyme system that removes the damaged area and synthesizes a new strand of DNA. However, if the cell undergoes mitosis before the damage is repaired, a gap in the DNA strand is left at the location of the photoproduct. The gap is repaired by a postreplication repair method that is thought to be error prone and may lead to mutations and the development of neoplasms. Factors that irritate the skin and increase the rate of cell division increase the number of cells repaired by the postreplication repair method and therefore can enhance development of neoplasms.
2. Chronic exposure to UVB radiation also causes damage to DNA in the form of mutations to tumor-suppressor genes, in particular to the p53 gene. Normally, UVR-induced DNA damage causes keratinocyte induction of the p53 gene, which leads to cell cycle arrest, thus allowing the UVR-caused DNA damage to be corrected by the nucleotide excision repair system before the cell undergoes mitosis, and a functional p53 gene also facilitates apoptosis (programmed cell death) of cells with excessive unrepaired damaged DNA so that those defective cells are removed. The p53 gene mutations develop when UVR-induced photoproducts are not repaired before keratinocyte mitosis. The photoproducts form small structural abnormalities in the DNA strand that can result in faulty base paring (i.e., mutations) during replication. The mutations are characterized by the replacement of a cytosine with a thymine (C to T) or double-base

changes in which a cytosine dimer is replaced by two nondimerized thymine bases (CC to TT). Although p53 gene mutations occur in a variety of tumors, those mutations caused by UVR (the C to T or CC to TT mutations) are unique and do not occur with other types of DNA damage or in tumors unassociated with UVR; thus they are termed signature mutations.

3. UVB causes immunosuppression by depressing host cell-mediated immune reactions that normally serve to eliminate or destroy mutated proliferating cells. A variety of mechanisms contribute and involve UVB-damaged keratinocytes, Langerhans cells, dendritic cells, and others. Mechanisms include release of immunosuppressive cytokines such as IL-10 and IL-4, reduction in the number of Langerhans cells (antigen-presenting cells), a switch in Langerhans cell antigen presentation from T_H1 lymphocytes (involved in immune response against tumors) to T_H2 lymphocytes (which release immunosuppressive cytokines), induction of suppressor T lymphocytes, and release of cytokines and other biologic response modifiers that downregulate the immune response.

Other factors may also contribute to the development of solar-associated squamous cell carcinomas. For example, papillomaviruses recently have been identified in mucosal and cutaneous in situ and invasive squamous cell carcinomas, including invasive squamous cell carcinomas arising in sun-exposed skin in cats. However, it is currently not known if the papillomavirus identified within the tumor is merely infecting the tumor or if the virus could have a role in tumor induction. Some papilloma viral gene products have been shown to bind p53 tumor-suppressor gene protein products in cervical squamous cell carcinomas in women, leading to disruption of the cell cycle regulation.

The lesions of sun-induced injury occur in all domestic animals. In horses, lesions occur on the eyelids and nose and around the prepuce. The eyelids of Hereford cattle are also prone to development of lesions. In lightly colored dairy goats, lesions can develop on the lateral aspects of the udder and teats. Lightly pigmented young pigs are also susceptible to more acute solar injury, and the pinnae and tip of the tail can slough if injury is severe. In dogs, lesions develop most commonly in nonpigmented, sparsely haired skin of the ventral abdominal, inguinal, and perianal areas (Fig. 17-41). In cats, gross lesions occur where there is little or no hair and little pigment, particularly on external ear tips, eyelids, nose, and lips, and are most severe in white cats. Grossly, lesions begin as

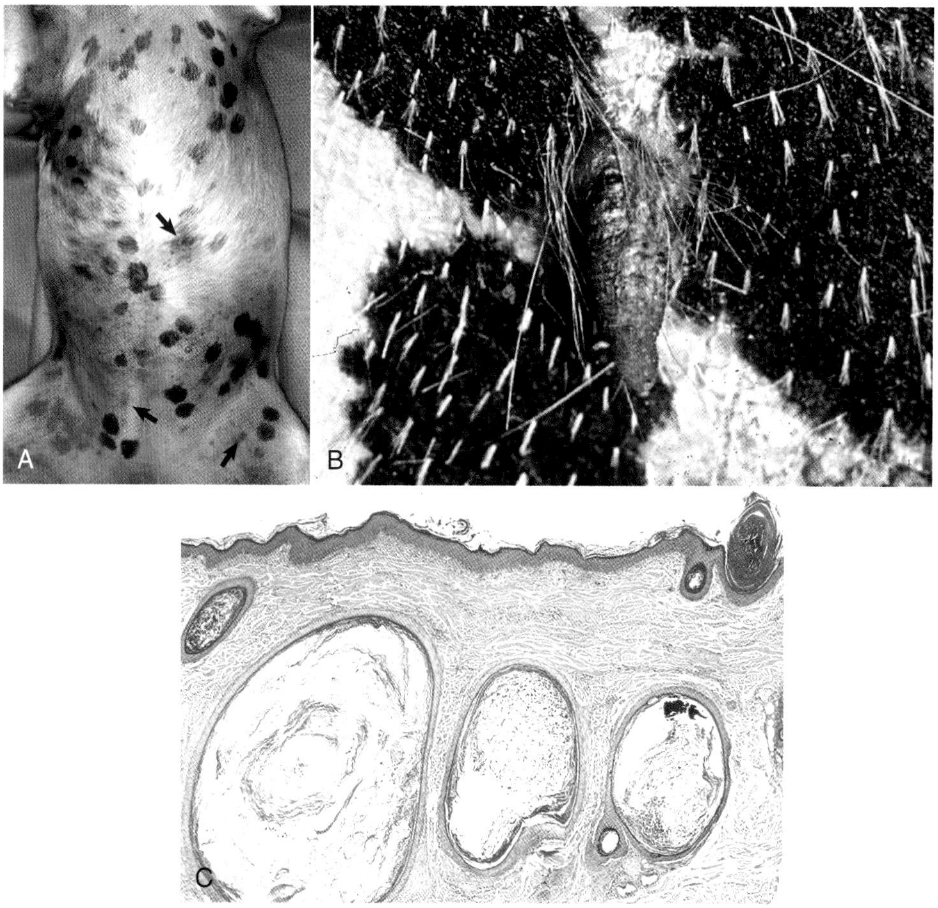

Figure 17-41 **Solar Dermatosis, Skin, Dog. A,** Ventral abdomen and thorax. The nonpigmented and lightly pigmented spots are affected, but the densely pigmented black spots are clinically unaffected. The nonpigmented and sparsely haired skin is erythematous, has comedones and crusts, and is palpably thickened. Comedones can rupture (furunculosis), releasing follicular contents that cause a foreign body inflammatory response and secondary bacterial infection *(arrows)*. Clinically, the inflammation is prominent (erythema and furuncles) and can be misinterpreted as primary. Clinically, the distribution pattern of affected nonpigmented sparsely haired skin and unaffected haired or pigmented skin is supportive of the diagnosis of solar dermatosis. **B,** Ventral abdomen. Solar dermatosis with a solar (actinic) keratosis that has formed a cutaneous horn. Cutaneous horns are keratoses formed from multiple layers of compacted stratum corneum. They may arise from benign or malignant lesions in the epidermis (solar actinic keratosis, squamous cell carcinoma) or adnexa (infundibular keratinizing acanthoma). **C,** The epidermis is thickened by acanthosis, and three comedones (follicular distention and hyperkeratosis) are present. If comedones rupture, a large amount of endogenous foreign material (stratum corneum, hair shafts, and sebum) is released into the dermis, causing a foreign body inflammatory response. Bacteria are also released and cause a secondary bacterial infection. H&E stain. (Courtesy Dr. A.M. Hargis, DermatoDiagnostics.)

erythema, scaling, and crusting. After years of exposure the skin becomes wrinkled and thickened secondary to epidermal hyperplasia, hyperkeratosis, fibrosis, and in some species, elastosis. One or more papular or plaquelike foci covered with thick scale (hyperkeratosis) known as *solar (actinic) keratoses* may develop, some of which progress to invasive squamous cell carcinoma. Occasionally the hyperkeratosis is dense and compact and resembles a "horn" (see Fig. 17-41, *B*). Hemangiomas and hemangiosarcomas have developed in the nonpigmented conjunctiva of horses and dogs and in the dermis of sparsely pigmented and sparsely haired skin of dogs, and a few goats and cats. The cutaneous hemangiomas and hemangiosarcomas are often seen on the abdomen and flanks of dogs that spend time resting in the sun. The difference in type of neoplasm can be a result, in part, of thickness of the epidermis, which influences the depth of penetration of the UV rays. UV light may also play a role in the development of melanomas in goats. Melanomas also develop in the skin, lips, eyelids, and iris in Doberman pinscher dogs with autosomal recessive oculocutaneous albinism. However, the melanomas develop in sun-exposed and non–sun-exposed sites, so the role of UV light in tumor induction in these dogs is unclear.

Microscopically, in early UV-induced injury, the number of apoptotic cells (sunburn cells) scattered in the epidermis can be so numerous as to form a band of these cells along with intercellular edema, vacuolation of keratinocytes, and loss of the granular cell layer. By 72 hours, hyperkeratosis, parakeratosis, and acanthosis are present along with dermal lesions of hyperemia, edema, perivascular mononuclear infiltrates, capillary endothelial cell swelling, and hemorrhage. Hyperkeratosis, parakeratosis, and acanthosis can persist. Comedones (hair follicles dilated with a plug of follicular stratum corneum and sebum) develop in some dogs (see Fig. 17-41, *C*). Affected follicles are often surrounded by a thin layer of fibrosis. In dogs, superficial dermal vessels may have hyalinized or sclerotic walls, and endothelial cells may be missing (solar vasculopathy). In some animals and in some anatomic locations, elastic tissue and collagen are damaged by solar radiation, and the dermis may be thickened by a zone of fibrosis parallel to the epidermal surface (laminar dermal fibrosis). Solar elastosis characterized by deposits of wavy basophilic elastin fibers in the superficial dermis is often present in horses and sometimes dogs. With continued UV exposure, solar keratoses develop. The epidermal surface is thickened by compact hyperkeratosis or parakeratosis. The acanthotic epidermis has atypical keratinocytes starting in the basal layer and progressing into the spinous layer. Keratinocytes are irregularly stratified and irregularly sized and shaped. Nuclei are large and often vary in size. Nucleoli may be large. There may be increased mitoses and apoptotic keratinocytes. The keratinocytes may form downward proliferations, usually as short buds, but occasionally as branching and anastomosing epidermal pegs. However, in solar keratoses the basement membrane remains intact. Invasive squamous cell carcinoma can develop in the site of solar keratoses when atypical keratinocytes breach the basement membrane and invade the contiguous dermis and, less often, subcutis. In some instances the atypical keratinocytes invade lymphatic channels and can metastasize to lymph nodes, lungs, and can more widely disseminate.

Photosensitization. Photosensitization is a disorder caused by long-wavelength UV (UVA), or less frequently by visible light, absorbed by a photodynamic chemical in the skin or by a complex of a photodynamic molecule and a biologic substrate. This process results in a release of energy that produces reactive oxygen molecules, including free radicals. Generation of reactive oxygen molecules leads to mast cell degranulation and the production of inflammatory mediators, which causes damage to cell membranes, nucleic acids, proteins, and organelles. The photodynamic agent usually enters the dermis via the systemic circulation. However, direct contact and absorption of some photodynamic agents, such as occurs in phytophotodermatitis, can result in localized contact photosensitization, and although most cases occur in nonpigmented sun-exposed skin, uncommonly, sun-exposed darkly pigmented skin can be affected.

Photosensitization can occur in several forms. Type I or primary photosensitization is often caused by ingestion of preformed photodynamic substances contained in a variety of plants; thus herbivores are most commonly affected. The plants causing photosensitization usually contain helianthrone or furocoumarin pigments. The helianthrone pigments are red fluorescent pigments such as hypericin (found in *Hypericum perforatum* [St. John's wort]) and fagopyrin (found in *Fagopyrum esculentum* [buckwheat]). Photosensitization attributed to furocoumarin pigments is caused by the presence of psoralens, photodynamic agents found in a variety of plants, including *Cymopterus watsonii* (spring parsley), *Ammi majus* (bishop's weed), and *Thamnosma texana* (Dutchman's breeches). Furocoumarin pigments also form phytoalexins, a group of compounds formed in plants in response to fungal infection or other injury and that inhibit or destroy the invading agent. The phytoalexins formed in fungus-infected parsnips and celery have caused phytophotodermatitis when they are absorbed into the skin and react with UV light.

Primary photosensitization can also occur with the administration of drugs such as phenothiazine, which is converted to a photoreactive metabolite in the intestinal tract. This metabolite is usually converted to a nonphotoreactive compound in the liver by mixed-function oxidases, but occasionally either the reactive metabolite bypasses the liver or mixed-function oxidase activity in the liver is compromised or insufficient and the reactive metabolite reaches the skin.

Type II photosensitization develops because of abnormal porphyrin metabolism, leading to the blood and tissue accumulation of photodynamic agents. These diseases usually are inherited as an enzyme deficiency, resulting in abnormal synthesis of photodynamic agents, including uroporphyrin and coproporphyrin. Examples include bovine congenital porphyria and bovine erythropoietic (hematopoietic) protoporphyria. Photosensitization caused by abnormal porphyrin metabolism has also been reported in pigs and cats.

Type III or hepatogenous photosensitization is caused by impaired capacity of the liver to excrete phylloerythrin, which is formed in the alimentary tract from the breakdown of chlorophyll. This is the most common type of photosensitization and occurs most commonly in herbivores, but any animal with generalized hepatic disease on a chlorophyll-rich diet that is exposed to sufficient solar radiation can develop hepatogenous photosensitization. Hepatogenous photosensitization occurs secondary to primary hepatocellular damage, inherited hepatic defects, or bile duct obstruction. Toxic plants, including but not limited to *Lantana camara* (lantana) and *Tribulis terrestris* (puncture vine), and mycotoxins, such as sporidesmin, are the most common cause of this type of photosensitization. Other plants that cause hepatic damage (such as those that contain pyrrolizidine alkaloids) can also contribute to the development of hepatogenous photosensitization.

Most forms of photosensitization cause lesions that are located on areas of the body with nonpigmented skin and hair and on parts of the body exposed to the sun such as the face, nose, and distal extremities in horses. In cattle, lesions occur in white-haired areas and on the teats, udder, perineum, and nose. In sheep with heavy fleeces, lesions occur on the pinnae, eyelids, face, nose, and coronary band, but in shorn sheep, lesions can occur on the back. Sheep can have extensive edema of the head, prompting terms that are synonyms: "swelled head" and "facial eczema." Onset of lesions may take only hours and initially include erythema and edema, followed by blisters, exudation, necrosis, and sloughing of necrotic tissue. The microscopic lesions consist of coagulative necrosis of the epidermis and possibly hair follicle, adnexal glands, and superficial dermis. Subepidermal vesiculation can occur. Endothelial cells of the superficial, middle, and deep dermal vessels are swollen and necrotic, and fibrinoid degeneration and thrombosis can result in edema; infarction; sloughing of the epidermis, dermis, and adnexa; and secondary bacterial infection.

Ionizing Radiation Injury

Advances in the treatment of cancer in companion animals have made the possibility of radiation-induced skin injury more likely. Ionizing radiation consists of electromagnetic radiation (x-rays, γ-rays) and particulate radiation (e.g., electrons, neutrons, protons) and is most damaging to highly proliferative cells, such as those of the anagen hair matrix, but epidermal basal cells and vascular endothelial cells are also affected. Available radiation modalities offer differing degrees of tissue penetration and thus differing potential for tissue injury. Some forms of radiotherapy penetrate deeper tissues while sparing the skin, and others are more concentrated in the superficial tissues or are preferentially absorbed by specific tissues. The type of radiation therapy and the source, dose, intensity, and duration of exposure dictate the range of possible side effects. Ionizing photons disrupt chemical bonds in cells, leading to injury or cell death. Some cells are not lethally damaged but sustain DNA damage to the extent that replication and/or replacement are not possible. The effects of radiation damage can be divided into acute and chronic forms.

Acute radiation injury to the skin is a result of damage to rapidly dividing cells. Damage is self-limiting, and recovery is associated with rapid cell turnover. Clinical lesions of radiation dermatitis appear 2 to 4 weeks after exposure. Initially there is erythema, pain, edema, and heat, followed several weeks later by dry or moist desquamation depending on the degree of injury. Histologically, the lesions resemble a second-degree burn, with suprabasilar or subepidermal bullae formation, dermal edema with fibrin exudation, and a marked leukocytic infiltrate. Reepithelialization occurs over a period of 10 to 60 days. The damage sustained to germinal cells of hair follicles and sebaceous glands leads to alopecia within 2 to 4 weeks after exposure. Hair regrowth follows over the next several months, but damage to sebaceous glands is not reversible and leads to permanent scaling manifesting histologically as hyperkeratosis. The chronic lesions of radiation injury are evident months to years after treatment and are primarily the result of damage to the microvasculature. Chronic changes include pigmentary alterations (hyperpigmentation with lower doses and hypopigmentation with higher doses), leukotrichia (depigmentation of hair shafts because of loss of follicular melanocytes), dermal scarring, epidermal atrophy, and ulceration. The epidermis is thin, friable, and in some areas hyperplastic and can become neoplastic. Squamous cell carcinomas can develop in some sites of severe radiation damage because of sublethal DNA damage. Chronic nonhealing exudative ulcers can develop, but granulation tissue does not form. The dermis is fibrotic with atypical fibroblasts, telangiectasia, and possibly deep arteriolar changes. Endothelial swelling, necrosis, and thrombosis lead to occlusion and excessive endothelial proliferation, which, when combined with the effects of vascular leakage, leads to vascular collapse. This condition of progressive vessel abnormalities is referred to as *obliterative endarteritis* and is known to form a "histohematic" (tissue-blood) barrier to surrounding tissue, leading to continued anoxia and nutrient shortage.

Chemical Injury

Chemical injuries to the skin can result from local application directly onto the skin or from absorption of chemicals via the gastrointestinal tract and subsequent distribution to the skin. For a chemical to cause injury via local application, it must penetrate the hair and protective epidermal layers. Penetration is enhanced by physical damage to the stratum corneum, especially that caused by excessive moisture. Chemical injuries of the skin include contact irritant dermatitis (local application), systemically distributed chemicals, such as arsenic, mercury, thallium, iodine, and organochlorines and organobromines, and poisonings by fungal-contaminated plants and plants containing selenium, mimosine, and trichothecenes. Externally applied agents that produce irritant contact dermatitis induce cutaneous damage by altering the water-holding capacity of the epidermis or by penetrating the epidermis and directly damaging cells. Systemically absorbed and distributed chemical agents cause lesions by a wide variety of mechanisms, some of which are not known. An example is toxicity caused by systemic absorption of some organochlorine and organobromine compounds, such as highly chlorinated naphthalenes, which were used as additives in lubricants for farm machinery such as feed pelleting equipment. As a result, highly chlorinated naphthalenes were frequent feed contaminants. Toxicosis occurred most commonly in cattle, the most susceptible species, and was known as X-disease or bovine hyperkeratosis. Fortunately, this toxicosis is largely historically interesting, because highly chlorinated naphthalenes have not been used in machinery lubricants since the 1950s. Lesions of chlorinated naphthalene toxicity are the result of the interference of the conversion of carotene to vitamin A and result in vitamin A deficiency. Vitamin A is necessary for normal differentiation of stratified squamous epithelium. Clinical lesions consist of alopecia and lichenified, fissured plaques of scale that spare only the legs. Histologic lesions consist of marked hyperkeratosis of the epidermis and follicles. Squamous metaplasia of the epithelial lining of the glands and ducts of the liver, pancreas, kidneys, and reproductive tract also develop.

Irritant Contact Dermatitis. There are two forms of contact dermatitis. One form is allergic contact dermatitis, which is immunologically mediated and requires prior exposure (sensitization) to the offending agent in a hypersensitive individual (see the discussion on allergic contact dermatitis in the section on Selected Hypersensitivity Reactions). The other form is irritant contact dermatitis, most cases of which are nonimmunologic in origin, and are instead caused by direct contact with substances such as acids, alkalis, soaps, detergents, body fluids (urine or diarrhea scald), wound secretions, some plants, and some topical medications. These substances overwhelm the protective mechanisms of the skin and directly injure cells. It is important to realize that the two types of contact dermatitis can produce very similar histologic lesions, thus differentiation between immune-mediated and irritant contact dermatitis largely depends on history, clinical signs, and anatomic distribution of the lesions. Horses develop lesions on the nose, ventrum, lower limbs, and where riding tack contacts the body, and on the perineum and caudal aspect of the rear legs. In dogs and cats, lesions of irritant contact dermatitis develop on the glabrous (sparsely haired) skin of the abdomen, axillae, flanks, interdigital spaces, perianal area, ventral tail, ventral chest, legs, eyelids, and feet. Grossly, erythematous patches, papules, and rarely, vesicles develop, but self-inflicted trauma can lead to ulcers and crusts. Microscopically, lesions consist of spongiotic dermatitis, neutrophilic vesicopustules, and superficial dermal perivascular neutrophilic inflammation. Chronic lesions consist of epidermal hyperplasia, hyperkeratosis, sometimes confluent parakeratosis, and superficial perivascular inflammation. Lesions can be obscured by self-inflicted trauma, making histologic diagnosis difficult. Corrosive substances (strong acids or alkalis) can cause epidermal necrosis.

Injection Site Reactions. Injections of vaccines or therapeutic drugs into the subcutis can incite a local and persistent (chronic) immunologic response resulting in granulomatous nodules that are palpable. There are no reported histologic descriptions of the acute or subacute inflammatory responses to such injected materials. Histologic changes represented by these chronic post-injection site nodules consist of a localized area of deep dermal or subcutaneous necrosis containing foreign material bordered by macrophages and multinucleated giant cells with a peripheral zone of lymphocytes and variable numbers of plasma cells and eosinophils (foreign body granuloma). Macrophages usually contain amphophilic granular foreign material. Lymphoid follicular development at the margins of these lesions can be extensive. Although many injection site lesions heal without serious consequences, in some cats there is a causal relationship with injections and development of sarcomas such as fibrosarcomas, myxosarcomas, osteosarcomas, rhabdomyosarcomas, chondrosarcomas, and histiocytic sarcomas. The injected substance, inflammation, and eventual fibroblastic proliferation are thought to be important factors predisposing some cats to sarcoma formation. It is speculated that during tissue repair, fibroblasts or myofibroblasts at the injection site are stimulated, and this response, in combination with other factors such as oncogene alterations or unidentified carcinogens, leads to malignant transformation of cells. Tumor development can take months to years, with eventual neoplastic transformation of mesenchymal cells. Any type of vaccine, other injectable materials, microchips, nonabsorbable suture, or other trauma has the potential to contribute to sarcoma formation. It is currently unknown how to identify cats that are at risk for the development of these types of sarcomas. Uncommonly fibrosarcomas have developed in dogs in cutaneous sites of presumed previous vaccination.

In small, often soft-coated, breeds of dogs, especially poodles, subcutaneous injection of killed rabies vaccine can result in localized lymphoplasmacytic panniculitis, subtle vasculitis, and localized ischemia leading to severe follicular atrophy in overlying dermis (Fig. 17-42) that is clinically apparent as a focal area of alopecia and hyperpigmentation. Immunofluorescence staining has identified rabies antigen in the vessels and cells of the hair follicles. A low-grade, immune-mediated vasculitis with resultant tissue hypoxia leading to the atrophic changes in the adnexa has been suggested as the pathogenesis. Vascular lesions are characterized by hyalinization of the vessel wall, lack of endothelial cells, intramural karyorrhectic debris, and perivascular lymphocytic infiltrates. Rarely, small numbers of lymphocytes are found within the walls of affected vessels.

Injection site eosinophilic granulomas with necrotic centers have been reported to occur in horses 1 to 3 days after injections of various substances using silicone-coated needles. The reaction is suspected to be a form of delayed hypersensitivity.

Snake and Spider Bites (Envenomations). The families Elapidae (coral snake) and Viperidae (rattlesnake, water moccasin, and copperhead) contain the majority of the poisonous snakes in the United States. The genera *Latrodectus* (e.g., black widow) and *Loxosceles* (e.g., brown recluse) are the most common venomous spiders causing cutaneous injury. Effects depend on composition of the venom, individual victim response, anatomic location of the envenomation, and specific characteristics of the offending snake or spider, which can be influenced by season of the year, geographic location, time since last inflicted bite or sting, depth of injury, and so forth. Different species of animals respond differently to the same venom.

Spider bites occur most often on the face and legs. The brown recluse spider (*Loxosceles reclusa*) is the spider most known to induce dermal necrosis, although there are a number of others. Brown recluse venom contains numerous enzymes, including lipase, hyaluronidase, and sphingomyelinase-D, which degrade tissue. A blister with a surrounding pale halo and more peripheral erythema characterizes initial reactions documented in human beings and some experimental animals. Necrosis and eschar formation occur within 5 to 7 days. Ulceration can be extensive. Histologically, there is hemorrhage and edema, neutrophilic vasculitis, and arterial wall necrosis. The epidermis and dermis undergo infarction, which can extend into the subcutis and underlying muscle. Panniculitis can be present. Eventually there is dermal scarring and replacement of the subcutis and muscle by hypocellular connective tissue. Brown recluse spider bites in human beings can also lead to massive hemolysis. Differentials include other venomous bites, vasculitis, slough

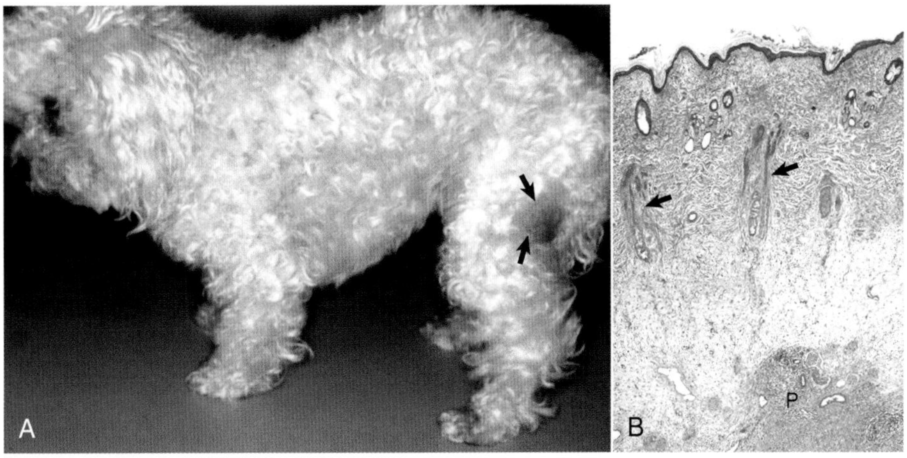

Figure 17-42 Localized Alopecia Associated with Subcutaneous Rabies Vaccination, Skin, Haired, Dog. A, This type of alopecia *(arrows)* generally develops 3 to 6 months after vaccination and is the result of partial ischemia. **B,** Note panniculitis *(P)* with lymphocytes, plasma cells, and histiocytes that has resulted from subcutaneous injection of killed rabies vaccine. Small, atrophic hair follicles *(arrows)* are in the dermis. H&E stain. (**A** courtesy Dr. L. Schmeitzel, College of Veterinary Medicine, University of Tennessee. **B** courtesy Dr. A.M. Hargis, DermatoDiagnostics.)

caused by iatrogenic injection of irritating substances, thermal burns, necrotizing fasciitis or other cutaneous infection, septic embolization, or trauma. Some putative spider bites (and possibly wasp and bee stings) in the dog develop as acute, painful, swollen areas on the dorsal or lateral nose that histologically consist of severe eosinophilic folliculitis and furunculosis (see the discussion on eosinophilic furunculosis of the face in dogs in the section on Disorders Characterized by Infiltrates of Eosinophils and Plasma Cells, Disorders of Dogs), leading to the theory that these lesions are probably caused by hypersensitivity reactions to injected venom.

Snakebites are common in the horse and dog and to a lesser degree in cats and most often inflicted on the head or legs. Snake venom contains various enzymes, proteins, peptides, and kinins. Of the five genera of venomous snakes in the United States, crotaline venom (rattlesnake, copperhead, cottonmouth, and others) contains the highest concentration of proteolytic enzymes. Snakebite envenomation produces pain, edema, and erythema that, if severe, are followed by necrosis and sloughing of tissue, and sometimes death of the animal. Variable systemic effects occur, including paralysis, coagulation disturbances, shock, increased capillary permeability, myocardial damage, rhabdomyolysis, and renal failure.

Selenium. Selenium poisoning is caused by an overdose of a selenium supplement or ingestion of seleniferous plants that have accumulated toxic concentrations of selenium. Some plants selectively accumulate selenium, regardless of soil selenium content. These selective accumulators (obligate accumulators; e.g., *Astragalus*, *Stanleya*) require selenium for growth, generally are not palatable, and are eaten only when other plants are unavailable. Many other plants (facultative accumulators; e.g., *Aster*, *Atriplex*) do not require selenium for growth but will accumulate toxic concentrations of selenium if grown in soil with high selenium concentrations. These facultative accumulator plants are commonly eaten by livestock and more often are the cause of poisoning. The mechanism by which selenium is thought to exert its effects on the integument and appendages is through its competitive replacement of sulfur, which modifies the structure of keratin, a sulfur-containing molecule. Replacement of sulfur by selenium in other molecules can also contribute to toxicity. Acute or chronic selenium poisoning has developed in most domestic animals, although susceptibility to selenium poisoning varies with species, dosage, diet, rate of consumption, chemical form, and other factors. In acute poisonings, signs relate to involvement of multiple organ systems. Chronic selenium toxicity usually develops in livestock (horses, cattle, and sheep) consuming seleniferous forages. It occurs worldwide but is more frequent in Nebraska, Wyoming, and the Dakotas in the United States and in areas of western Canada. Animals with chronic selenium intoxication are emaciated, have poor-quality hair coat, and have partial alopecia. Horses lose the long hair of the mane and tail, develop hoof deformities, and shed the hooves.

Vetch Toxicosis and Vetchlike Diseases. Vetch toxicosis is most commonly seen as a syndrome characterized by dermatitis, conjunctivitis, diarrhea, and granulomatous inflammation of many organs. It occurs in cattle and to a lesser extent in horses after consumption of vetch-containing pastures. Hairy vetch (*Vicia villosa* Roth) is a cultivated legume used as pasture, hay, and silage in most of the United States and other countries. Toxicity from vetch seeds is known to be a result of the presence of prussic acid. The cause of the granulomatous inflammation in this syndrome remains unclear. One proposed pathogenesis is that ingestion of vetch or another substance leads to antigen formation in the form of a hapten or a complete antigen that sensitizes lymphocytes and evokes the cell-mediated immune response upon repeat exposure.

Initial lesions in cattle consist of a rough coat with papules and crusts affecting the skin of the udder, teats, escutcheon (back of udder and perineum), and neck, followed by involvement of the trunk, face, and limbs. The skin becomes alopecic, lichenified, and less pliable. Marked pruritus leads to excoriations from self-induced trauma. The dermis has perivascular to diffuse infiltrates of monocytes, lymphocytes, plasma cells, multinucleated giant cells, and eosinophils. There is marked hyperkeratosis and dermal and epidermal edema.

The clinical syndrome begins 2 or more weeks after consumption and consists of pruritic dermatitis, diarrhea (possibly bloody), and wasting. Morbidity is low, and mortality is high. Holstein and Angus cattle and cattle 3 years or older are more often affected. Death in cattle occurs approximately 10 to 20 days after illness begins. At autopsy (syn: necropsy), yellow nodular infiltrates of mononuclear leukocytes are seen that disrupt the architecture of a wide range of organs but are most severe in myocardium, kidney, lymph nodes, thyroid, and adrenal glands. In cattle, other species of *Vicia* and additional compounds are capable of inducing disease indistinguishable from vetch toxicity. These include feed additives such as di-ureido isobutane and citrus pulp.

Hairy vetch toxicosis in horses resembles that in cattle, except for the infrequent finding of eosinophils in the infiltrate and lack of heart involvement. Conditions very similar to vetch toxicosis also have been reported in horses with no vetch exposure. These cases have been variably referred to as *equine sarcoidosis; equine idiopathic, generalized, or systemic granulomatous disease;* or *equine histiocytic disease/dermatitis* (see Nodular Granulomatous Inflammatory Disorders without Microorganisms, Equine Sarcoidosis). These idiopathic conditions in the horse are fairly indistinguishable and are a differential diagnosis for hairy vetch toxicosis.

The diagnosis of vetch toxicity or vetchlike disease is a diagnosis by exclusion. It is made after review of the herd history, the character and distribution of the lesions, and ruling out other causes of granulomatous inflammation such as infectious agents.

Ergot and Tall Fescue Grass. See Disorders of Ruminants (Cattle, Sheep, and Goats).

Physical Injury

Acral Lick Dermatitis. See Disorders of Dogs.

Pyotraumatic Dermatitis (Acute Moist Dermatitis, "Hot Spots"). See Disorders of Dogs.

Feline Ulcerative Dermatitis Syndrome. See Disorders of Cats.

Callus. A callus is a raised, irregular, patch of thickened skin that develops because of friction, usually over pressure points on bony prominences or on the sternum (see Table 17-6). Callosities can develop in all domestic animals but are particularly common in pigs and giant breed dogs kept on concrete or other hard flooring without adequate bedding. Secondary folliculitis, furunculosis, and ulceration can develop. Microscopically, the epidermis and follicular infundibulum are thickened by hyperkeratosis and acanthosis. Regular epidermal hyperplasia (rete peg and papillary dermal interdigitation) also occurs. Comedones are present in some lesions. The follicular openings can be widened by excessive keratin. Dilated follicles can rupture (furunculosis), releasing bacteria, keratin proteins, and sebum, resulting in secondary pyoderma and an endogenous foreign body inflammatory response to released follicular contents (callus pyoderma).

Intertrigo (Skin Fold Dermatitis). Intertrigo is superficial dermatitis occurring on apposed skin surfaces. It occurs in cows with large pendulous udders and develops between the udder and the medial thigh (udder-thigh dermatitis). Intertrigo also occurs in dogs in the skin of the facial fold (brachycephalic breeds), lower lip fold (breeds with large lips such as the Saint Bernard), body fold (Shar-Pei breed), vulvar fold (obese female dogs with a small vulva), and tail fold (dogs with corkscrew tails such as English bulldogs) (Fig. 17-43). The cause and pathogenesis involve the presence of closely apposed skin surfaces, frictional trauma between the skin surfaces, accumulated moisture (from tears, saliva, cutaneous glandular secretions, urine, or water after drinking, swimming, or bathing), and bacterial infection. The moisture and frictional trauma predispose to bacterial or yeast overgrowth and subsequent infection. Early gross lesions of intertriginous dermatitis typically consist initially of erythema and edema. Later, pustules, ulcers, and crusts can develop. Late lesions in cows can be severe, with occasional sloughing of skin and subcutis. Microscopically, in early stages there is congestion and edema with early perivascular inflammation that progresses to a more diffuse band of inflammation in the superficial dermis, parallel to the epidermis, but often sparing the dermal-epidermal junction. Inflammatory cells include plasma cells, fewer lymphocytes, neutrophils, and macrophages. In more severe cases there can be exocytosis of neutrophils into the epidermis, epidermal pustules, crusts, ulcers, and in cows, necrosis that leads to sloughing of tissue. If the cause is corrected, early and mild chronic lesions heal without scarring (most cases). However, when there is ulceration or necrosis and sloughing of tissue (minority of cases), lesions heal by second intention with the formation of granulation tissue, wound contraction, and scarring.

Temperature Extremes

Information on this topic is available at www.expertconsult.com.

Microbial and Parasitic Disorders

Cutaneous infections develop when there is disruption in the defense mechanisms of the skin (see section on Defense Mechanisms/Barrier Systems). Predisposing factors to skin infections involve compromised epidermal barrier integrity caused by friction, trauma, excessive moisture, dirt, matted hair, chemical irritants, freezing or burning, irradiation, and parasitic infestation. Suppressed immune function resulting from inadequate nutrition, therapy with glucocorticoids, and other acquired or inherited immunologic abnormalities can also contribute to increased susceptibility to microbial and parasitic infections. Infectious agents enter the body via their specific portal of entry (see Portals of Entry/Pathways of Spread), which includes traversing the epidermal surface, entering via hair follicles or the ducts of glands, and migrating via nerves or sometimes via the hematogenous route.

Viral Infections

Poxviruses. See Disorders of Horses, Disorders of Ruminants (Cattle, Sheep, and Goats), and Disorders of Pigs for species-specific poxviruses.

Poxviruses are DNA viruses that infect most domestic, wild, and laboratory animals and birds (Table 17-10). Dogs and cats are rarely infected with poxviruses, although infection with a parapoxvirus (contagious ecthyma of sheep) has been reported in dogs, and cutaneous infection with a poxvirus of the *Orthopoxvirus* genus (cowpox in cattle) has been reported in cats and rarely dogs in Europe. There are rare anecdotal reports of poxvirus infection in the skin of cats in North America, but with the exception of one case, the poxvirus or viruses involved have not been characterized. In the single case in which the virus was identified, polymerase chain reaction (PCR) and gene sequencing identified raccoonpox, an orthopoxvirus, in

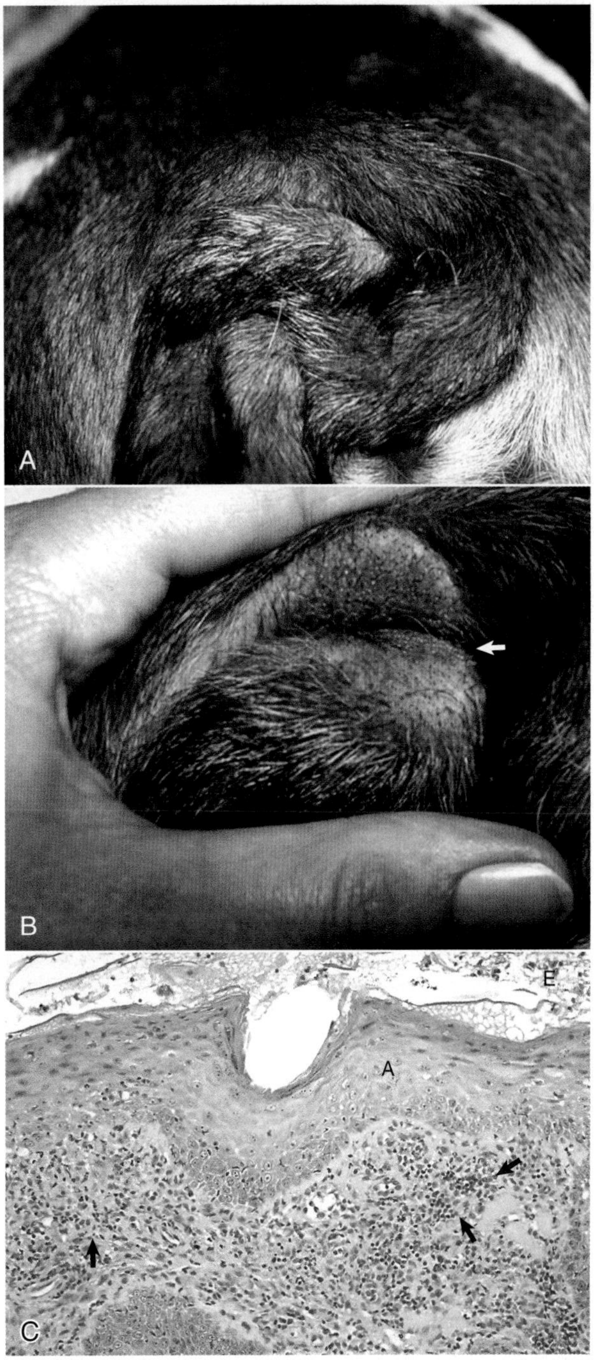

Figure 17-43 **Intertriginous Inflammation (Screw Tail), Skin, Tail, Dog. A,** "Screw tail," English bulldog. Excessive skin folds around the tail cause friction and moisture accumulation, predisposing to bacterial growth. **B,** Intertriginous pyoderma, English bulldog. The skin fold *(arrow)* of the dog depicted in **A** has been opened to expose the erythema, hyperpigmentation, and lichenification. **C,** Intertriginous dermatitis. The epidermis is acanthotic *(A)* and partially covered by fluid debris and cellular exudate *(E)*, and there is perivascular and interstitial inflammation composed of numerous plasma cells and fewer lymphocytes and neutrophils in the dermis *(arrows)*. H&E stain. (**A** and **B** courtesy Dr. A. Werner, Valley Veterinary Specialty Service. **C** courtesy Dr. A.M. Hargis, DermatoDiagnostics.)

Table 17-10 Viral Infections of the Skin

Virus	Diseases	Species Affected	Distribution
Parapoxvirus	Contagious ecthyma	Sheep, goats, cattle; rarely dogs	Cutaneous
	Papular stomatitis	Cattle	
	Pseudocowpox	Milking cows; zoonotic	
Orthopoxvirus	Cowpox	Many species, including cats and rarely dogs in Europe	Cutaneous
Molluscipoxvirus	Molluscum contagiosum	Horses, rarely dogs	Cutaneous
Capripoxvirus	Sheeppox	Sheep	Systemic
	Goatpox	Goats	
	Lumpy skin disease	Cattle	
Suipoxvirus	Swinepox	Pigs	Cutaneous
Unclassified poxvirus	Ulcerative dermatosis of sheep	Sheep	Cutaneous
Equine herpesvirus 2	Granulomatous dermatitis	Horse	Cutaneous
Equine herpesvirus 5	Pustular dermatitis face		Rare single case reports
Bovine herpesvirus 2 (dermatotropic)	Bovine ulcerative mammillitis (bovine herpes mammillitis)	Cattle	Cutaneous
	Pseudo–lumpy skin disease		
Bovine herpesvirus 4 (dermatotropic)	Bovine herpes mammary pustular dermatitis	Cattle	Cutaneous
Ovine herpesvirus 2	Malignant catarrhal fever	Cattle	Cutaneous, oral, systemic
Feline herpesvirus 1	Feline herpesvirus dermatitis	Cats	Cutaneous, oral, ocular, upper respiratory
Papillomavirus	Papilloma, wart	All species	Cutaneous, oral, mucocutaneous
Papillomavirus*	Viral plaques	Horse, dog, cat	Cutaneous, medial pinnae in horse
Papillomavirus*	Bowenoid in situ carcinoma (multicentric carcinoma in situ, Bowen's disease)	Cat, less in dog	Cutaneous
Papillomavirus*	In situ and invasive squamous cell carcinoma	Horse	Genital/penile
		Dog, cat	Cutaneous
Papillomavirus*	Fibropapilloma	Cattle	Cutaneous, genital
Papillomavirus*	Sarcoid (fibropapilloma)	Horse, cat	Cutaneous
Picornavirus	Foot-and-mouth disease	Ruminants, pigs	Oral, cutaneous
Picornavirus	Swine vesicular disease	Pigs	Oral, cutaneous
Rhabdovirus	Vesicular stomatitis	Horses, cattle, pigs	Oral, cutaneous
Calicivirus	Vesicular exanthema	Pigs	Oral, cutaneous
Calicivirus	Feline calicivirus	Cats	Oral, cutaneous, systemic
Parvovirus	Porcine parvovirus	Piglets	Oral, cutaneous
Parvovirus	Canine parvovirus 2	Puppies	Oral, cutaneous
Retrovirus	Feline leukemia virus	Cats	Secondary skin infections; cutaneous horns with feline leukemia virus
	Feline immunodeficiency virus		
Coronavirus, mutated	Feline infectious peritonitis with rare concurrent dermatitis	Cats	Cutaneous disease rare; associated with systemic disease

*Because papillomaviruses can be found in normal skin as well as inflamed skin of a variety of different causes, simply identifying papillomaviruses in lesional tissue of proliferative lesions such as viral plaques, sarcoids, and squamous cell carcinomas does not prove papillomavirus is the cause of the lesions.

the skin lesions. There are major differences between different poxviruses and in the range of species they infect; some are species specific and others are zoonotic. Many poxviruses of animals, such as the contagious ecthyma parapoxvirus, can cause skin lesions in human beings.

Poxviruses induce lesions by a variety of mechanisms. Lesions develop secondary to poxviral invasion of epidermis, by ischemic necrosis caused by vascular injury, and by stimulation of host cell DNA, resulting in epidermal hyperplasia (see Fig. 17-32). Hyperplasia may be explained by a gene, present in several poxviruses, including molluscipoxvirus (the cause of molluscum contagiosum), whose product has significant homology with epidermal growth factor. Poxviruses also encode for functions that may counteract host defenses. These include genes related to those encoding the serpins (a superfamily of related proteins important in regulating serine protease enzymes that mediate kinin, complement, fibrinolytic, and coagulation pathways) and genes encoding antiinterferon activities. The severity of poxviral infection varies, depending on whether the infection is localized (cutaneous) or systemic and whether there are secondary infections.

The sequence of the cutaneous lesions is macule, papule, vesicle (varies in severity), umbilicated pustule, crust, and scar (see Fig. 17-32). Histologically, pox lesions begin as keratinocyte cytoplasmic swelling and vacuolation, usually first affecting the cells of the outer stratum spinosum. Rupture of the damaged keratinocytes produces multiloculated vesicles, so-called reticular degeneration. The early dermal lesions include congestion, edema, vascular dilation, a perivascular mononuclear cell infiltrate, and a variable neutrophilic infiltrate. Neutrophils migrate into the epidermis and aggregate in vesicles to form microabscesses. Large intraepidermal pustules can form and sometimes extend into the superficial dermis. There is usually marked epidermal hyperplasia and sometimes pseudocarcinomatous hyperplasia of the adjacent epidermis. This contributes to the raised border of the umbilicated pustule. Rupture or drying of the pustule produces a crust, often colonized on its surface by bacteria. Poxvirus lesions often contain characteristic intracytoplasmic eosinophilic inclusion bodies. These are single or multiple and of varying size and duration. The inclusions are primarily composed of proteins. Sheeppox and goatpox are the most pathogenic poxviruses, and infection causes significant mortality, especially in young animals as a result of systemic disease. Sheeppox and goatpox do not occur in the United States or Canada.

Herpesviruses. Herpesviruses are DNA viruses that only occasionally produce cutaneous lesions (see Table 17-10). Cutaneous lesions have rarely been reported in nondermatotropic herpesvirus infections, such as infectious bovine rhinotracheitis (bovine herpesvirus 1) and equine coital exanthema (equine herpesvirus 3), and in cats with FHV-1 infection. Two dermatotropic herpesvirus infections with economic importance are bovine herpesvirus 2 and bovine herpesvirus 4. Herpesviruses can be latent, with inactive virus persisting in tissue such as the trigeminal nerve ganglia. It is speculated that up to 80% of adult cats recovered from FHV-1 infection as kittens or young cats have latent FHV-1 infections. During times of stress the virus is reactivated, and lesions can recur. Herpesviruses infect epithelial cells and replicate in the nucleus, leading to lysis of nuclear contents. As immature viral particles enter the cytoplasm, there is degeneration of cytoplasmic organelles, accumulation of cytoplasmic lipid, and precipitation of protein. Death of keratinocytes leads to spread of virus to neighboring cells, leading to rapid necrosis of focally extensive areas of the epidermis. Gross lesions consist of vesicles that rupture to form ulcers that are then covered by crusts. Microscopic lesions in herpesvirus infections depend on the stage, but early degenerative changes include ballooning and reticular degeneration, the sequelae of degeneration of epidermal cells and acantholysis. Syncytial cells may be seen. Intranuclear inclusions develop, but because of rapidly developing necrosis may not be found except at the margins of ulcers. The appearance of the viral inclusions varies with the specific herpesvirus. Some herpesviruses produce large, hyaline amphophilic inclusions that fill the nucleus (FHV-1), whereas others (dermatotropic bovine herpesvirus 2) produce typical Cowdry type A inclusions, which are also intranuclear but smaller and eosinophilic.

Bovine Herpesvirus 2 and Bovine Herpesvirus 4. See Disorders of Ruminants (Cattle, Sheep, and Goats).

Feline Herpesvirus Dermatitis. See Disorders of Cats.

Papillomaviruses. Papillomaviruses are typically species- and site-specific pathogens that infect the squamous epithelium and may infect fibroblasts, and that cause benign proliferative masses and less commonly malignant tumors. As more precise methods of papillomavirus identification have been developed, including in situ hybridization, PCR, and DNA sequencing, increasing numbers of papillomaviruses and papillomavirus-associated lesions have been identified. Papillomavirus may infect squamous epithelium and fibroblasts; however, with the rare exception of bovine papillomavirus 2, reproduction occurs exclusively in keratinocyte nuclei, and complete virions are produced only in squamous epithelium. It has recently been shown that bovine papillomavirus 2 can replicate in other epithelia such as transitional epithelium of bladder and chorionic epithelium of placenta, and possibly also in lymphocytes. Papillomaviruses gain access through defects in the epithelium and enter the basal layer epithelial cells. Once in the cell, there are three possible outcomes: (1) the virus can remain within the basal cell nucleus outside of the chromosomes in a circular DNA episome where the virus replicates synchronously with the host cell, causing a latent infection without morphologic changes in keratinocytes; (2) as the basal cells mature, the virus can convert from latent to productive infection with the formation of complete infectious virions and with morphologic changes recognized as viral cytopathologic changes, including epithelial hyperplasia, keratinocytes with clear cytoplasm and pyknotic nuclei, and sometimes with cytoplasmic or intranuclear inclusion bodies; or (3) the virus can become integrated into the genome of the host cell, resulting in malignant transformation and the morphologic changes of neoplasia. Malignant transformation occurs because the viral genes that remain after integration into the host cell are those associated with cellular regulation. These viral genes promote keratinocyte cell growth by inactivating tumor-suppressor proteins such as p53 and pRb. These events lead to uncontrolled cell proliferation, inability to repair DNA damage, and eventual malignant transformation.

All domestic animals are affected by one or more papillomaviruses (see Table 17-10), and some cross-species infections have been detected, particularly with the bovine papillomaviruses, and there are rare reports of human papillomavirus infections in cats. The specific type or types of papillomaviruses involved in some infections have yet to be determined. Papillomavirus infections cause diverse clinical and histologic lesions, including papillomas, viral plaques, and fibropapillomas, including sarcoids. Papillomavirus DNA has also been identified within in situ and invasive squamous cell carcinomas in animals. However, because papillomaviruses can be found in normal skin as well as inflamed skin of a variety of different causes, simply identifying papillomaviruses in lesional tissue of some of the proliferative lesions such as viral plaques, sarcoids, and squamous cell carcinomas, does not prove papillomavirus is the cause of the lesions. Therefore further work is necessary to prove a cause-and-effect relationship for some of these presumptive papillomavirus-associated lesions.

A common type of cutaneous papillomavirus infection (papilloma, wart) consists of clinical lesions that may be exophytic (proliferating to the exterior) (Fig. 17-44) or endophytic (inverted) papilliferous benign masses. Other papillomas may be flat, plaquelike lesions that lack the prominent papilliferous projections. Histologically, stratified squamous epithelium is covered by thickened orthokeratotic or parakeratotic stratum corneum, is acanthotic, and in the exophytic and endophytic papillomas, has elongated dermal-epidermal interdigitations that project outwardly or inwardly, depending on the type. In some papillomas, keratinocytes, especially of the upper stratum spinosum, are swollen, have clear cytoplasm or a perinuclear halo, and a pyknotic nucleus; these keratinocytes are termed *koilocytes* (meaning hollow or concave). Keratohyalin granules are often large and irregular. Also, pale basophilic intranuclear inclusion bodies, located in degenerating cells in the outer layers of the stratum spinosum and granulosum in which virion production is taking place, occur in some but not all papillomas. Many papillomas spontaneously regress, and in regressing stages, there is reduced epidermal hyperplasia, increased proliferation of fibroblasts, deposition of collagen, and infiltration of T lymphocytes at the dermal-epidermal interface and in the epithelium. Some papillomas, such as those on the genitalia or concave pinnae (also called ear papillomas or aural plaques) of horses and some affecting the teats of cattle, often do not regress.

Viral plaques have been described in dogs and cats. Canine pigmented viral plaques are associated with papillomavirus infection

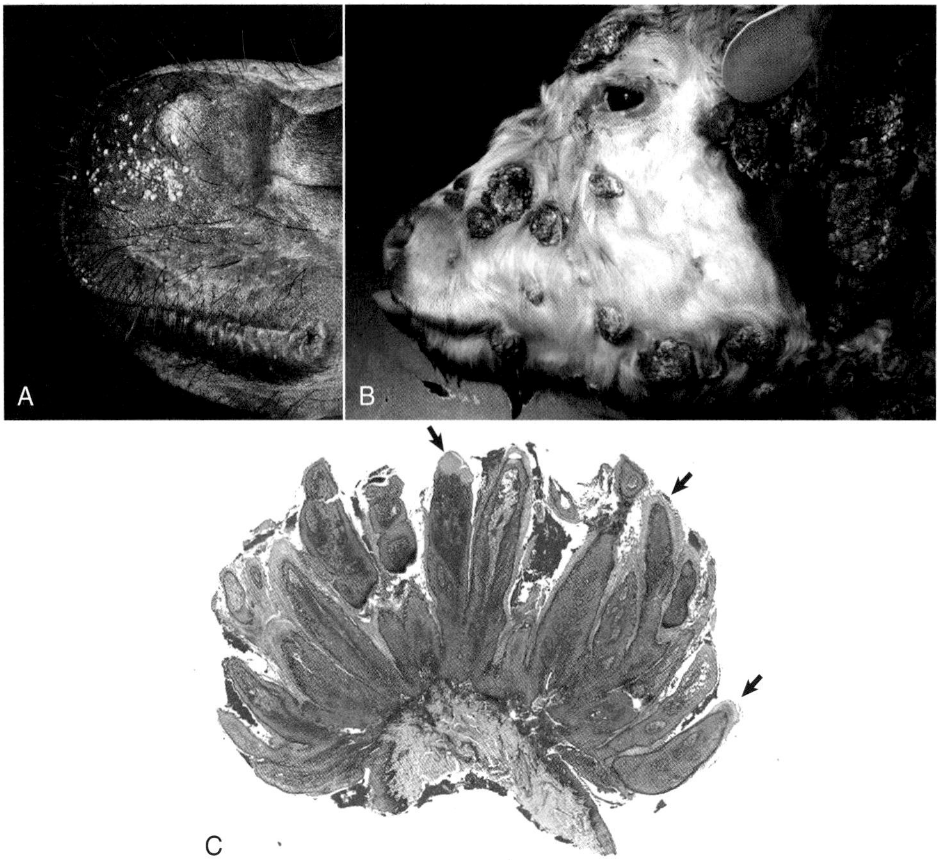

Figure 17-44 **Cutaneous Papillomas, Skin. A,** Chin, horse. Note multiple, small, verrucous papillomas arising in the skin. **B,** Head, cow. Note multiple, irregular, alopecic, verrucous papillomas. **C,** The papillary projections *(arrows)*, often called fronds, are composed of hyperkeratotic epidermis covering a collagenous core. H&E stain. (**A** courtesy Dr. D. Duclos, Animal Skin and Allergy Clinic. **B** and **C** courtesy Dr. M.D. McGavin, College of Veterinary Medicine, University of Tennessee.)

in certain breeds of dogs (miniature schnauzers, pugs, and Shar-Peis) or in other breeds of dogs that are immunosuppressed. Numerous novel papillomaviruses have been detected in some of these plaques. Clinical lesions occur most commonly on the ventral abdomen, groin, ventral thorax, or neck and consist of variably irregular, pigmented macules, or plaques. Histologically, the lesions are sharply demarcated, hyperkeratotic foci, or plaques with pigmented, acanthotic epidermis, and large keratohyalin granules. Canine viral plaques do not regress, are slowly progressive, and occasionally develop into a squamous cell carcinoma. Feline viral plaques are usually multiple, ovoid, slightly raised pigmented or nonpigmented, and slightly scaly and rough plaques less than 8 mm in greatest dimension. Papillomaviruses have been detected in the lesions, and feline papillomavirus 2 is the virus most often identified, suggesting this papillomavirus is the likely etiologic agent. Histologically, there is an abrupt transition between normal epithelium and the plaque, which consists of epidermis thickened by hyperkeratosis, hypergranulosis, and acanthosis. Keratohyalin granules may be enlarged, and koilocytes (keratinocytes with clear cytoplasm and pyknotic nuclei) and cytoplasmic pseudoinclusions may be present. Malignant transformation commonly occurs; lesions resemble the bowenoid in situ carcinoma (see next paragraph).

Papillomavirus infection also has been implicated in the development of another syndrome in cats and less often in dogs termed *multicentric squamous cell carcinoma in situ* (bowenoid in situ carcinoma, Bowen's disease). Although not all the factors contributing to lesion formation have been documented, papillomavirus DNA has been identified in these lesions in cats, suggesting a nonproductive infection promotes the epithelial hyperplasia characteristic of this disease. The papillomaviruses identified in some of these lesions have homology with human papillomaviruses, but feline papillomavirus 2 is thought to be the most likely and most common etiologic agent. Multicentric squamous cell carcinoma in situ clinically consists of sharply demarcated single, or more often multiple, scaly verrucous or irregular plaquelike lesions 0.5 to 3.0 cm in diameter that may develop in pigmented or nonpigmented skin. Histologically, the epidermis and follicular infundibulum are thickened by proliferation of basal keratinocytes that tend to stream together, providing a "windblown" appearance to the epidermis. Nuclei are often varied in size with hyperchromatic nuclei, large nucleoli, and numerous mitoses, some of which are located above the basal layer. The basement membrane, at the time of histologic examination, is intact. Most lesions remain as "in situ" carcinomas indefinitely, but an occasional lesion has progressed to invasive basal cell carcinoma or invasive squamous cell carcinoma.

Some types of papillomaviruses, particularly bovine papillomaviruses 1 and 2, can infect fibroblasts and cause fibropapillomas, flat, verrucous, or nodular masses in which the proliferation of dermal fibroblasts is the prominent feature, often surpassing that of the epidermal hyperplasia (Fig. 17-45). Fibropapillomas occur in horses, mules, donkeys, cattle, sheep, and cats. These lesions in horses are called *sarcoids*, which are thought to represent a nonproductive infection by bovine papillomaviruses 1 and 2. Equine sarcoids are locally aggressive, nonmetastatic fibroblastic skin tumors of horses,

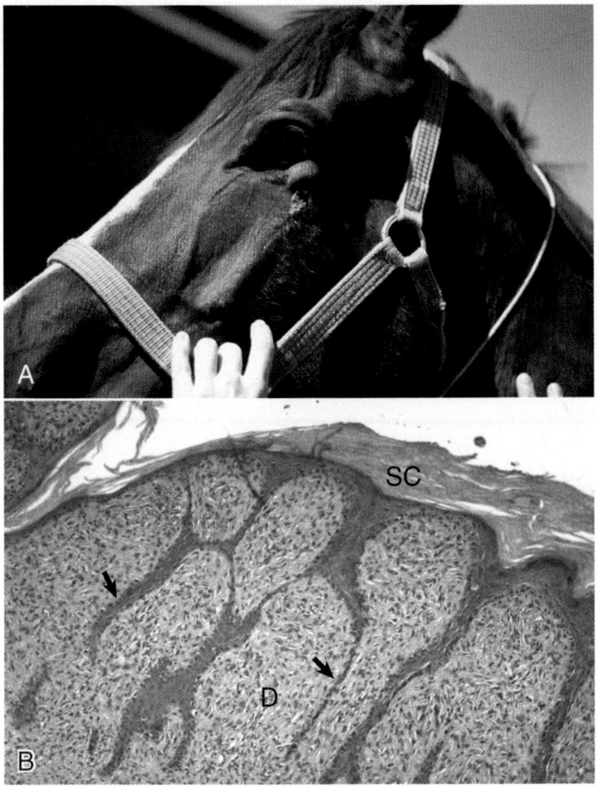

Figure 17-45 Sarcoid, Skin, Horse. A, Equine sarcoid, face. The irregular multinodular mass is present on the ventrolateral periocular skin, especially below the eye. **B,** Sarcoid. The sarcoid consists of an epidermal and dermal component. The hyperplastic epidermis is covered by thick compact stratum corneum *(SC)* and has thin rete pegs that extend into the dermis *(arrows)*. The dermis *(D)* is thickened by proliferating fibroblasts and collagen. H&E stain. (**A** courtesy Dr. H. Power, Dermatology for Animals. **B** courtesy Dr. P.E. Ginn, College of Veterinary Medicine, University of Florida.)

mules, and donkeys. They are the most common skin tumor of horses, accounting for 35% to 90% of tumors in numerous surveys, and occur in any breed, sex, or age. Young adult horses 3 to 6 years of age are most commonly affected. Although sarcoids do not metastasize and typically are not life-threatening lesions, they compromise the value of horses because of their infectious and progressive nature, and depending on their anatomic location, can compromise the use of the horse. Sarcoids frequently develop in areas subjected to trauma or at sites of wounds that occurred 3 to 6 months previously, and they develop anywhere but are most common on the head, legs, and ventral trunk. They can be single or multiple. Sarcoids are clinically subclassified as occult, verrucous, nodular, fibroblastic, mixed, or a more aggressive type (called malignant or malevolent). The occult form consists of a slow-growing, slightly thickened area of skin with slight surface roughening and alopecia that remains static for a long period. The verrucous type is usually a slow-growing, small wartlike growth, often measuring less than 6 cm in diameter, with a dry, irregular (verrucous) surface and variable alopecia. Nodular sarcoids are firm dermal or subcutaneous, often circumscribed masses with a nonulcerated surface. The fibroblastic type of sarcoid (referred to as "proud flesh sarcoid") usually has a raised ulcerated surface prone to hemorrhage and resembles exuberant granulation tissue. The mixed sarcoid has more than one clinical form and is often seen in long-standing lesions or those subject to repeated trauma. The mixed sarcoids can become more clinically aggressive as more fibroblastic transformation occurs. The "malignant or malevolent" sarcoid is deeply invasive and aggressive. The slower growing, less aggressive forms of sarcoid can become more proliferative and aggressive if traumatized, including the trauma of biopsy sampling, and can transform into a more aggressive clinical form. Therefore it is usually recommended before considering biopsy sampling, that a treatment plan be established if the diagnosis of equine sarcoid is confirmed histologically. No treatment protocol has been universally effective, so it is not possible to ensure that the lesion will remain harmless or can be successfully treated.

Histologically, sarcoids are typically biphasic tumors composed of both epidermal and dermal components; however, the epidermal component may be minimal or absent in some tumors, especially those with extensive ulceration. When the epidermis is intact, hyperkeratosis, parakeratosis, and acanthosis with thin rete pegs extending deep into the dermis are common features. The dermal component consists of fibroblasts and collagen in various proportions. The fibroblasts have plump nuclei, and nucleoli may be prominent. The mitotic index is usually low. Fibroblasts at the dermal-epidermal junction are frequently oriented perpendicular to the basement membrane in a "picket fence" pattern, which is a distinctive histologic feature seen in most sarcoids. The cells are arranged in whorls, interlacing bundles, or haphazard arrays of variable density. Tumor margins are typically indistinct, and adequacy of excision is frequently difficult to determine histologically. Spontaneous remission is uncommon. The tumors are characterized by a high rate of recurrence, up to 50%, after surgical excision alone, and additional therapies (e.g., cryotherapy, chemotherapy, immunotherapy, and others) are often recommended or necessary in an attempt to prevent recurrence. Feline fibropapillomas (also called *sarcoids*) are similar morphologically to the equine lesion and also likely represent a nonproductive infection with a papillomavirus resulting from a cross-species infection by a bovine papillomavirus. Affected cats often live in rural areas and have had exposure to cattle. Bovine fibropapillomas are caused by bovine papilloma virus 1 (teats, penis) or bovine papillomavirus 2 (head, neck, shoulder, legs, and teats) and occur in young animals. The lesions generally spontaneously regress within 1 to 12 months.

Papillomaviruses, some as yet to be identified by type, have been found in equine, canine, and feline invasive squamous cell carcinoma. However, the presence of the virus in the tumors does not allow differentiation between actual induction of the tumor and mere infection of the tumor. Further work to characterize the types of papillomaviruses and the role the viruses play in epidermal hyperplasia and neoplasia is necessary.

Other Viruses

Information on this topic is available at www.expertconsult.com.

Bacterial Infections

The portals for entry of bacteria into the skin include pores (follicular openings), hematogenous spread, or direct entry through damaged skin. Cutaneous bacterial infections vary in location (e.g., epidermis, dermis, subcutis, adnexa, or systemic), morphologic characteristics (e.g., pyogenic, granulomatous, or necrotizing), distribution (e.g., focal, multifocal, regional, mucocutaneous, haired skin, or interdigital), and severity (e.g., mild and asymptomatic to severe with systemic signs). The variation is caused by the specific organism involved, predisposing or coexisting factors, and host-immune response. The so-called superficial and deep bacterial infections are frequently pus-producing infections (pyogenic) and are thus referred to as pyodermas. In contrast, bacterial granulomas are characterized by an abundance of macrophages and are usually caused by traumatic implantation of bacteria that generally are saprophytes of low virulence. Systemic bacterial infections or localized infection with toxin-producing bacteria are often most severe because of vascular damage or the presence of endotoxins or exotoxins that have systemic consequences. The most common bacterial infections of the skin are listed in Box 17-8.

Bacterial skin disease is seen much more frequently in dogs than other domestic species, possibly the result of the thin stratum corneum with small amount of lipids, lack of a protective lipid seal at opening of the canine hair follicles, and the relatively high pH of canine skin. Until recently *Staphylococcus intermedius* had been considered the cause of most cases of pyoderma in dogs. However, recent molecular studies involving multilocus gene sequencing have revealed that bacterial isolates phenotypically consistent with *S. intermedius* consist of three separate species (considered to be the *S. intermedius* group), which include *S. intermedius*, *S. pseudintermedius*, and *Staphylococcus delphini*. *S. pseudintermedius* is now considered to be responsible for most cases of pyoderma in dogs, which presents most often as inflammation of the superficial segment of the hair follicle. Coagulase-positive staphylococci are also the most common bacteria isolated from pyoderma in horses (*Staphylococcus aureus*, *S. intermedius*), in cattle and sheep (*S. aureus*), and in goats (*S. aureus*). Molecular studies will likely be required to identify the species involved in some of these infections, particularly those of the *S. intermedius* group. *Staphylococcus hyicus* causes exudative epidermitis in piglets and has been associated with superficial pyoderma in several other species. Many other bacteria can cause skin infections. *D. congolensis* is responsible for superficial pyoderma in many species. Many Gram-negative bacteria are opportunistic pathogens that can invade already diseased or compromised skin.

Staphylococci, especially in dogs, but also in other domestic animals, including horses, have become increasingly resistant to a variety of antibiotics (methicillin-resistant and multidrug resistant), which has led to a limited range of treatment options, resulting in increased morbidity, mortality, and cost of therapy. In addition, concern is developing regarding potential transmission of antimicrobial-resistant strains of bacteria from animals to human beings and vice versa. Therefore it is important to recognize bacterial infections early and manage them appropriately to avoid increasing the prevalence of antimicrobial-resistant strains of bacteria that adversely affect animal and human health and to which treatment options are becoming limited.

Box 17-8 Cutaneous Bacterial Infections

SUPERFICIAL PYODERMAS

- Superficial pustular dermatitis (impetigo)
- Exudative epidermitis
- Canine superficial pyoderma (superficial spreading pyoderma)
- Mucocutaneous pyoderma
- Dermatophilosis
- Ovine fleece rot
- Superficial folliculitis (see bacterial folliculitis and furunculosis below)

DEEP PYODERMAS

- Bacterial folliculitis and furunculosis
- Abscesses
- Cellulitis

BACTERIAL GRANULOMATOUS DERMATITIS

- Mycobacterial granulomas
- Granulomas caused by nonfilamentous bacteria
  - *Staphylococcus* spp.
  - *Streptococcus* spp.
  - *Pseudomonas aeruginosa*
  - *Actinobacillus lignieresii*
  - *Proteus* spp.
- Filamentous bacterial granulomas
  - *Nocardia* spp.
  - *Actinomyces* spp.
  - *Streptomyces* spp.
  - *Actinomadura* spp.

SYSTEMIC OR TOXIC REACTIONS

- *Erysipelothrix rhusiopathiae*
- Systemic salmonellosis, pasteurellosis, *Escherichia coli* infection
- Canine toxic shock syndrome
- Clostridial dermatitis

BACTERIAL DIGITAL INFECTIONS OF HORSES AND RUMINANTS

- Proliferative pododermatitis (horse)
- Necrotizing pododermatitis (horse)
- Papillomatous digital dermatitis (cattle)
- Necrobacillosis of the foot (cattle and sheep)
- Contagious foot rot (cattle and sheep)
- Contagious ovine digital dermatitis (sheep)

Superficial Bacterial Infections (Superficial Pyodermas). Superficial bacterial infections (superficial pyodermas) involve the epidermis and the upper infundibulum of hair follicles, usually heal without scarring, and usually do not involve the regional lymph nodes. Gross lesions include erythema, alopecia, papules, pustules, crusts, and peripheral expanding rings of scale also called "epidermal collarettes" (see Table 17-6). The early microscopic feature of superficial bacterial infection that involves the epidermis is intraepidermal pustular dermatitis. The intraepidermal pustules are fragile and can rupture, leading to crust and superficial scale formation. The major microscopic feature of superficial bacterial infection that involves the follicles is superficial suppurative luminal folliculitis. The cellular infiltrate in and around hair follicles plus dermal congestion and edema correspond to the clinically evident papules and follicularly oriented pustules. Follicular injury leads to alopecia. Although Gram-positive cocci, such as *Staphylococcus* spp., are usually the cause of the superficial bacterial infections, the bacteria are not always demonstrable histologically, but their presence is often suspected when pustular or luminal exudates contain poorly preserved neutrophils. Predisposing factors, such as allergy, seborrhea, and immune deficiency, and other causes of follicular inflammation or dysfunction often play a role. Superficial bacterial folliculitis is discussed in the section on Superficial and Deep Bacterial Folliculitis and Furunculosis and Deep Pyoderma.

Superficial Pustular Dermatitis. Superficial pustular dermatitis, typically caused by staphylococci, encompasses several syndromes, including impetigo in a variety of animal species, exudative epidermitis in pigs (see Disorders of Pigs), and superficial pyoderma in dogs (see Disorders of Dogs). Pathogenicity may correlate with various proteins and toxins produced by the bacteria and thought to act as virulence factors. One of the factors that has come under recent scrutiny includes the exfoliative toxins. These toxins have been isolated from strains of *S. aureus* in human beings with impetigo, an acute contagious superficial bacterial skin infection that usually affects children and is characterized by vesicles and pustules that form yellowish crusts. In addition, similar exfoliative toxins have been identified as a source of another skin condition usually affecting infants and children, termed staphylococcal scalded-skin syndrome, that is typified by generalized blisters and superficial exfoliation of the stratum corneum. In impetigo and staphylococcal scalded-skin syndrome, the exfoliative toxins produced by virulent forms of *S. aureus* cause the loss of adhesion of keratinocytes in the superficial epidermis. These toxins are glutamate-specific serine proteases that cleave a single peptide bond in desmoglein 1, present in the extracellular protein core of the desmosome. The separation of these superficial keratinocytes results in intraepidermal splitting and initiation of lesion development in these infections. In impetigo the *S. aureus* that produces exfoliative toxins can be isolated from the intact pustules. In contrast, in staphylococcal scalded-skin syndrome, cultures from intact vesicles usually are negative for exotoxin-producing *S. aureus*, and it appears that the exfoliative toxins are produced in a distant area of infection and reach the skin via the bloodstream (a process called toxemia). Investigative studies in two domestic species (pigs and dogs) suggest that a similar pathogenic mechanism involving exfoliative toxins may play a role in development of superficial pustular dermatitis caused by staphylococci. For example, it has been shown that *S. hyicus*, which causes exudative epidermitis in piglets, produces an exfoliative toxin that can cleave pig desmoglein 1 and produce cutaneous exfoliation similar to that in pigs with exudative epidermitis. Similarly, an exfoliative toxin isolated from strains of *S. pseudintermedius* from dogs with pyoderma has caused cutaneous exfoliation when injected into the skin of dogs. In addition, the exfoliative toxin gene has been identified in *S. pseudintermedius* isolated from skin, wound, and ear infections in dogs, suggesting a role for the toxin in pathogenicity. Although the exfoliative toxins in canine pyoderma have not been fully characterized, these findings suggest that some strains of *Staphylococcus* spp. in dogs and *S. hyicus* in pigs may cause superficial bacterial infections via a pathologic mechanism involving exfoliative toxins. Further studies are necessary to determine if exfoliative toxins or other virulence factors contribute to the development of superficial pyoderma in other species.

Impetigo. Impetigo is observed most commonly in cows, ewes, does, and dogs and is usually caused by coagulase-positive *Staphylococcus* sp. Predisposing factors, such as cutaneous abrasions, viral infections, increased moisture, and poor nutrition, may contribute. Lesions of impetigo in cows, does, and ewes occur predominantly on the ventral abdomen, perineum, medial thigh, vulva, ventral tail, teats, and udder. In dogs, lesions are largely in nonhaired ventral skin. Prepubescent puppies are usually healthy otherwise, but older dogs with impetigo often have underlying disease, including immunosuppression associated with hyperadrenocorticism. Gross lesions consist of nonfollicular pustules that develop into crusts. The microscopic lesion is a nonfollicular neutrophilic subcorneal pustule. In bullous impetigo, a more severe condition occurring in older dogs with underlying disease, the lesions are large interfollicular flaccid pustules (bullae) that when ruptured lead to more extensive loss of the superficial epidermis. Acantholytic cells may be present in the pustules, probably the result of the cleavage of desmoglein 1 by the exfoliative toxin, thus requiring differentiation between impetigo and pemphigus foliaceus (see Fig. 17-15). The presence of coccoid bacteria within intact pustules can help provide support for a bacterial origin of the lesions. Perivascular to interstitial neutrophilic to mixed mononuclear dermal inflammation is present.

Dermatophilosis (Streptothricosis). Dermatophilosis, caused by *D. congolensis*, is characterized by crusty cutaneous lesions (Fig. 17-46) and occurs in horses, cattle, and sheep more often than goats, pigs, dogs, or cats. The bacterium is transmitted by carrier animals and is more common in tropical and subtropical climates and during wet weather, thus the layman's term rain rot. Lesions tend to develop on the dorsum of the back and distal extremities and after epidermal irritation from ectoparasites, trauma, or prolonged wetting of the skin, hair, or wool, which allows penetration of the damaged epidermis by the *Dermatophilus* "zoospore." The organism also synthesizes various products, including enzymes such as proteases, keratinases, and ceramidase, that may have a role in virulence and pathogenesis.

When *D. congolensis* overcomes the barriers of the skin, the invasive filamentous form grows by subdividing longitudinally and transversely in the ORS of the hair follicle and superficial epidermis (see Fig. 17-46). These bacteria stimulate an acute inflammatory

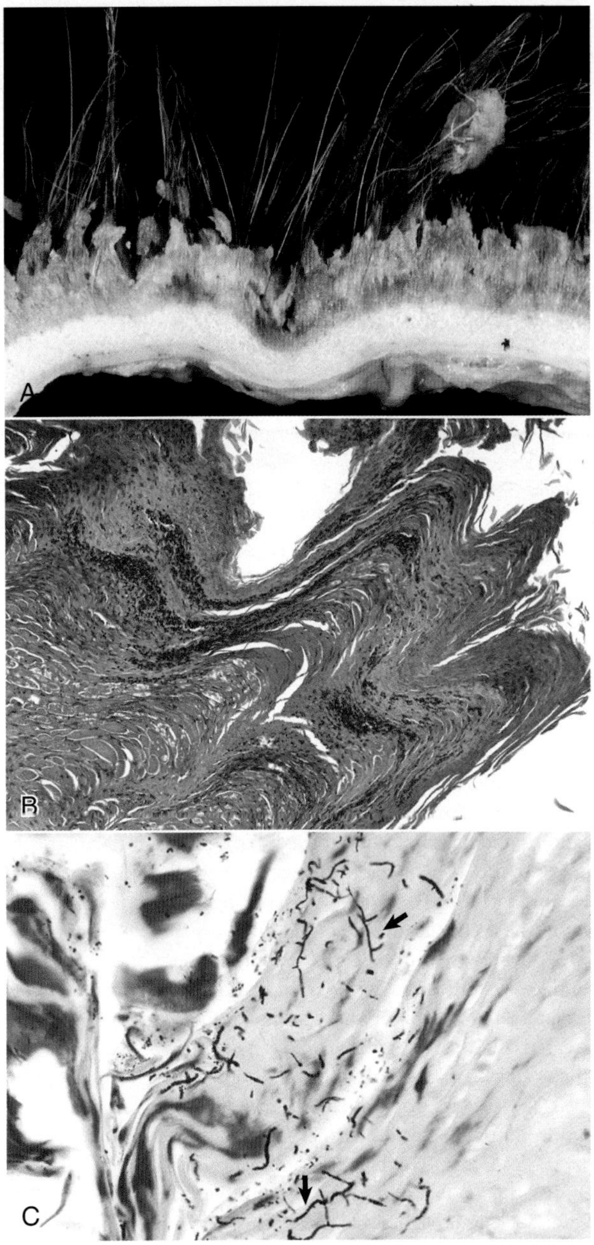

Figure 17-46 ***Dermatophilus Congolensis* Infection, Skin, Haired, Cow. A,** The hair is matted by a thick crust composed of dried exudate, stratum corneum, and bacteria. **B,** The crust is stratified and formed of alternating layers of hyperkeratotic/parakeratotic stratum corneum, proteinaceous fluid, and degenerate neutrophils. H&E stain. **C,** The stratum corneum contains Gram-positive bacteria *(arrows)* that subdivide longitudinally and transversely and can result in filaments that have a "railroad track" (not evident here) or "branched" appearance. Brown and Brenn stain. (**A** courtesy Dr. F. Lozano-Alarcon. **B** courtesy Dr. M.D. McGavin, College of Veterinary Medicine, University of Tennessee. **C** courtesy Dr. A.M. Hargis, DermatoDiagnostics.)

response in which neutrophils migrate from superficial vessels into the dermis and through the epidermis to form intraepidermal microabscesses. The inflammation inhibits further penetration of the bacterium into the dermis. However, residual bacterial organisms subsequently invade the newly regenerated epidermis. Thus repeated cycles of bacterial growth, inflammation, and epidermal regeneration result in the formation of the stratified pustular crusts. Grossly, lesions consist of papules, pustules, and thick crusts that can coalesce and mat the hair or wool (see Fig. 17-46). The microscopic lesions consist of hyperplastic superficial perivascular dermatitis with stratified crusts of alternating layers of stratum corneum, proteinaceous fluid, and neutrophils covering the skin surface. Samples of crusts obtained by biopsy are necessary to identify organisms and make a definitive diagnosis. Human infections have been reported after contact with affected animals, so dermatophilosis may be considered a potential zoonosis.

Ovine Fleece Rot. See Disorders of Ruminants (Cattle, Sheep, and Goats).

Exudative Epidermitis of Pigs (Greasy Pig Disease). See Disorders of Pigs.

Canine Superficial Spreading Pyoderma. See Disorders of Dogs.

Mucocutaneous Pyoderma. See Disorders of Dogs.

Superficial and Deep Bacterial Folliculitis and Furunculosis and Deep Pyoderma (Table 17-11). Numerous bacteria, including *Staphylococcus* sp., *Streptococcus* sp., *C. pseudotuberculosis*, *Pasteurella* sp., *Proteus* sp., *Pseudomonas* sp., and *E. coli* can cause folliculitis and furunculosis, but staphylococcal bacteria are the most commonly involved. Bacteria typically enter the skin via hair follicles, and infections can be superficial or deep. Superficial infections involve the follicular infundibulum but can spread to involve the deeper portions of the follicle (the infundibulum and below). Mild to moderate folliculitis without hair follicle rupture can resolve completely with appropriate antimicrobial therapy. However, untreated or severe folliculitis can progress to involve deeper aspects of the follicle and result in follicular distention with rupture (furunculosis) and release of follicular contents (hair, sebum, bacteria, keratin proteins) into the dermis and sometimes subcutis, resulting in deep pyoderma. The bacteria proliferate in the deep dermis and subcutis and can reach draining lymph nodes. Draining sinuses can develop because of the bacterial infection and a foreign body response to extruded follicular contents. Thus in deep bacterial folliculitis and furunculosis (deep pyoderma), the infection and severe inflammation spread into the surrounding dermis and subcutis, resulting in the need for intensive long-term treatment and increasing the potential for systemic infection and local scarring. Deep bacterial infections of hair follicles often have predisposing causes, such as immune suppression, demodicosis (dogs), or disorders associated with follicular hyperkeratosis (callus or comedo formation), and also originate as a sequel to superficial bacterial folliculitis. Staphylococcal folliculitis and furunculosis develop most commonly in the dog (see Figs. 17-27 and 17-28), frequently affect the horse, sheep, and goat, but are uncommon in the cow, pig, and cat. Deep bacterial infections are less common than superficial infections and develop most frequently in dogs.

In horses, lesions develop most commonly in association with tack, especially on the skin of the saddle area, the tail, or the caudal aspect of the pastern (proximal interphalangeal articulation) or fetlock (metacarpophalangeal articulation). Staphylococcal folliculitis and furunculosis of the pastern or fetlock may involve one or more legs and is a differential diagnosis for the multifactorial syndrome of equine pastern dermatitis (see Disorders of Horses, Equine Pastern Dermatitis). Early thorough clinical evaluation and sometimes microbiologic or histopathologic evaluation may be required to differentiate staphylococcal folliculitis affecting the skin of the pastern from equine pastern dermatitis and other conditions that may affect the skin of the pastern area.

In adult sheep, lesions develop on the face, especially around the eyes, or on the limbs or teats. In otherwise healthy lambs, mild lesions develop most commonly on the lips and perineum and usually spontaneously regress. In goats the face, pinnae, distal limbs, and glabrous areas of the udder, ventral abdomen, medial thighs, and perineum are most commonly affected.

In dogs, lesions are localized or generalized and develop on the dorsal nose, pressure points, interdigital areas, and chin. Other cutaneous areas can also be affected, especially if predisposing conditions (e.g., follicular dysplasia, cornification disorders, or demodicosis) are present. Deep pyoderma of adult German shepherd dogs (German shepherd folliculitis, furunculosis, and cellulitis) is a unique deep pyoderma with an apparent genetic predisposition. Lesions are located on the dorsal lumbosacral, ventral abdominal, and thigh areas. Hypersensitivity to the bites of fleas or alterations in immune or neutrophil function have been proposed as predisposing causes, but most of these potential causes have been discounted. Deep folliculitis and furunculosis, especially on the cheek area or neck of some large-breed dogs (golden and Labrador retriever, Saint Bernard, and Newfoundland), can clinically resemble superficial pyotraumatic dermatitis (acute moist dermatitis), belying the deep nature of the lesions.

Postgrooming furunculosis is an uncommon but acute, severe, and painful form of furunculosis in the dog that is believed to be associated with grooming. A variety of bacteria have been cultured from lesions, including *S. pseudintermedius*, *Pseudomonas aeruginosa*, *E. coli*, and *Proteus* sp.

Grossly the lesions of superficial folliculitis include papules, crusted papules, pustules, epidermal collarettes, and alopecia. Hair follicle involvement by pustules may be difficult to appreciate macroscopically. Multifocal to coalescing patches of alopecia resulting in a "moth-eaten" appearance to the hair coat may be the only visible lesions of superficial bacterial folliculitis, especially in short-coated breeds of dog. Deep folliculitis can have similar lesions plus hemorrhagic bullae, nodules, and draining sinuses. The microscopic patterns include superficial or deep luminal folliculitis, pyogranulomatous furunculosis, draining sinuses, and occasionally panniculitis. Microscopic lesions include suppurative luminal folliculitis with follicular distention often in conjunction with furunculosis. Pyogranulomatous dermatitis in response to release of follicular contents is often severe and may efface the dermal architecture, extend into the deep dermis and panniculus, and form sinuses that drain to the surface. Scarring can lead to loss of adnexal structures and permanent alopecia localized to affected skin.

Subcutaneous Abscesses. Subcutaneous abscesses are localized collections of purulent exudate located within the dermis and subcutis. Abscesses are common in cats because of the frequency of bacterial contamination of puncture wounds. Abscesses also are common in large animals. In addition to puncture wounds, other predisposing causes include foreign bodies, injections, and shearing and clipping wounds. Granulation tissue or mature fibrous connective tissue borders the exudate. Subcutaneous abscesses frequently rupture and drain spontaneously, and heal by scarring. A wide variety of bacteria can cause subcutaneous abscesses. Commonly isolated bacteria include *Pasteurella multocida* (dog and cat bite wounds), *C. pseudotuberculosis* (horses, sheep, and goats), and *Trueperella (Arcanobacterium) pyogenes* (cattle, sheep, goats, pigs). Other

Table 17-11 Bacterial Folliculitis and Furunculosis

Organisms	Predisposing Causes	Portal of Entry	Clinical Lesions	Histologic Lesions	Anatomic Locations	Species
Staphylococcus sp. are most frequently involved Others: *Streptococcus* sp. *Corynebacterium pseudotuberculosis* *Pasteurella* sp. *Proteus* sp. *Pseudomonas* sp. *Escherichia coli*	**Superficial folliculitis:** Allergy Seborrhea Parasitic infestations Hormonal factors Local irritants Matted hair coats **Deep folliculitis:** Sequel to superficial bacterial folliculitis Immune suppression Stresses (large animals) Demodicosis (dogs) Follicular hyperkeratosis (callus or comedones) Irritation from tack (horses) Increased environmental temperature and moisture (horse) **Pastern* folliculitis (horses):** Excessive moisture, trauma, contact dermatitis, mite infestation	Hair follicle openings	**Superficial folliculitis:** Papules, crusted papules, pustules, epidermal collarettes, and alopecia **Deep folliculitis:** Same as superficial folliculitis plus hemorrhagic bullae, nodules, and draining sinuses	**Superficial:** Superficial luminal folliculitis **Deep:** Superficial and deep suppurative luminal folliculitis with follicular distention often in conjunction with furunculosis Pyogranulomatous dermatitis in response to release of follicular contents Sinuses that drain to the surface Scarring with loss of adnexa and permanent alopecia localized to affected skin	Dorsal nose, pressure points, interdigital areas, chin, and can be generalized	Dog; common
					Area covered by tack, especially the skin of the saddle area, the tail, or on the caudal aspect of the pastern* or fetlock†	Horse; frequent
					Face, pinnae, distal limbs, and glabrous areas of the udder, ventral abdomen, medial thighs, and perineum	Goat; frequent
					Adult sheep: face, especially around the eyes, ears, base of horns, limbs, or teats Lambs: mild lesions most commonly on the lips and perineum; usually spontaneously regress	Sheep; frequent
					Tail, perineum; less often scrotum and face	Cattle, more in young bulls; uncommon
					Piglets younger than 8 weeks: generalized body hindquarters, abdomen, chest Young growing piglets: facial lesions related to sharp canine teeth	Piglets; uncommon
					Crusted papular eruption indistinguishable from miliary dermatitis, anywhere, including head and neck	Cat; rare

*Pastern (proximal interphalangeal articulation).
†Fetlock (metacarpophalangeal articulation).

frequently isolated bacteria include β-hemolytic streptococci, *Fusobacterium* sp., *Peptostreptococcus* sp., *Bacteroides* sp., *Staphylococcus* sp., and *Clostridium* sp. Less often, abscesses can develop from a noninfectious cause such as injection of sterile material.

Cellulitis. Bacterial cellulitis, in contrast to an abscess, is a poorly delineated suppurative bacterial infection of the dermis and subcutis that dissects and spreads through surrounding soft tissues. The affected skin is often swollen, erythematous, and warm and may become devitalized and slough. The bacteria can cause a foul odor and some, such as *Clostridium* sp., can produce subcutaneous gas bubbles (subcutaneous emphysema). Cellulitis may be accompanied by fever and enlargement of regional lymph nodes. Histologic lesions consist of poorly delineated areas of purulent to pyogranulomatous inflammation that may include hemorrhage, necrosis, and thrombosis. Bacteria may be visible histologically. As with subcutaneous abscesses, the source of the infection is usually a penetrating wound in the area of infection. A variety of bacteria, including those found in subcutaneous abscesses, can cause cellulitis. A rare but particularly severe subtype of cellulitis, termed necrotizing fasciitis, has been described most often in the dog in association with *Streptococcus canis* infection (see later discussion of infection with toxin-producing bacteria).

Bacterial Granulomatous Dermatitis (Bacterial Granulomas). Bacterial granulomatous dermatitis is usually caused by traumatic implantation of bacteria, which are generally saprophytes of low virulence. Causative organisms usually stimulate a strong cell-mediated immune response by persisting as an antigen in the tissue. Grossly, lesions are slowly progressive, nodular or diffuse, and can ulcerate and drain through the surface of the skin via sinuses. Microscopic lesions consist of mixed populations of inflammatory cells, especially macrophages; thus lesions are granulomatous to pyogranulomatous. Multinucleated giant cells and caseous necrosis are present in some lesions. Causal agents can be present in macrophages, exudate, or in clear spaces or fat vacuoles within tissue but are often in such low numbers that they are difficult to identify in histologic sections.

Mycobacterial Granulomas. Mycobacterial organisms produce granulomatous to pyogranulomatous dermatitis and panniculitis in many species of animals, particularly cats and less frequently in other species including horses, cattle, and dogs. The majority of mycobacteria are intracellular pathogens that are able to persist in tissue by entering macrophages. Many are able to survive and replicate within the macrophages by inhibiting fusion with lysosomes. Tissue destruction results from persistence of antigen in the tissue and a cell-mediated inflammatory response. Infection occurs with obligate pathogens that require a vertebrate host to multiply and saprophytes in the environment that occasionally cause opportunistic infections. Infection occurs with the tuberculosis group considered to be obligate pathogens (*Mycobacterium tuberculosis*, *Mycobacterium bovis*, *Mycobacterium microti*), the leprosy group considered to be obligate pathogens (*Mycobacterium lepraemurium*), and the opportunistic group considered to be saprophytes or facultative pathogens (subdivided based on growth rate and pigment production). Rapid-growing opportunistic organisms (*Mycobacterium fortuitum*, *Mycobacterium smegmatis*, *Mycobacterium chelonae*, *Mycobacterium abscessus*, and *Mycobacterium thermoresistibile*) and slow-growing opportunistic organisms (*Mycobacterium avium-intracellulare* complex, *Mycobacterium kansasii*, and *Mycobacterium ulcerans*) are inhabitants of soil, water, and decomposing vegetation, and infection tends to occur via wound contamination or traumatic implantation. To avoid confusion in terminology, by convention, infections caused by *M. tuberculosis* and *M. bovis* are referred to as tuberculosis. In contrast, infections caused by other mycobacterial agents are referred to as mycobacteriosis, which is sometimes further defined by the group of agents involved (e.g., atypical, opportunistic, or avian).

Mycobacterial infection is more common with the rapidly growing opportunistic mycobacteria (also called *atypical mycobacteria*), and infections are more common in cats, in which lesions are characterized by recurrent nodules, with draining sinuses frequently located in the dermis and subcutis of the inguinal area. The microscopic lesions are characterized by pyogranulomatous inflammation. Organisms are more often found extracellularly in vacuoles sometimes lined by neutrophils (Fig. 17-47). Infections with the slow-growing, opportunistic mycobacteria are more commonly disseminated (not limited to the skin) and resemble those caused by *M. tuberculosis*.

In cattle, cutaneous infections with opportunistic mycobacterial organisms, historically called *skin tuberculosis*, occur as single or multiple nodules 1 to 8 cm in diameter in the dermis and subcutis, particularly of the lower legs. But lesions can spread to the thighs,

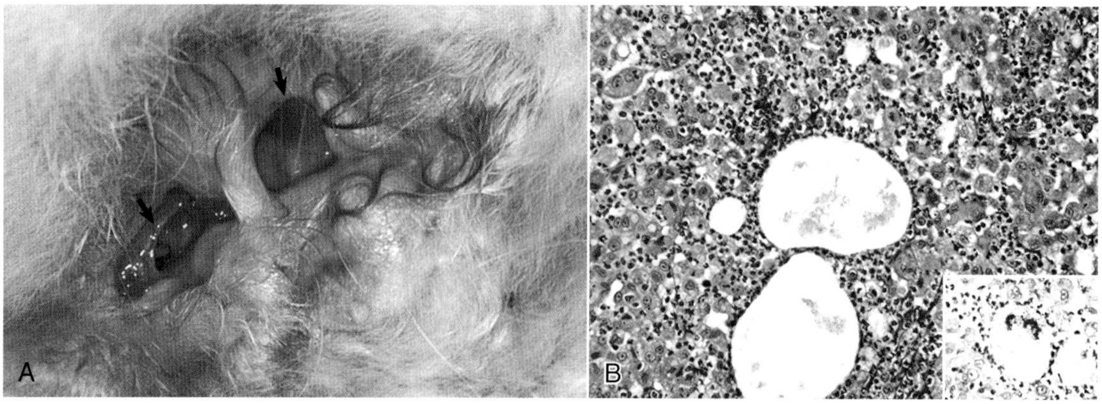

Figure 17-47 **Atypical Mycobacteriosis (Opportunistic Mycobacterial Infection), Rapidly Growing *Mycobacterium* sp., Pyogranulomatous Panniculitis, Skin, Abdomen, Cat. A,** Note the draining sinuses *(arrows)* that overlie areas of nodular inflammation in the dermis and panniculus. **B,** Note pyogranulomatous inflammation (neutrophils and macrophages) surrounding a vacuole containing colonies of bacteria. In atypical *Mycobacterium* sp. infections of this type, the mycobacterial organisms are extracellular. H&E stain. *Inset,* Pyogranulomatous inflammation with a vacuole containing colonies of acid-fast bacilli that are stained red. Fite's method for acid-fast organisms. (**A** courtesy Dr. D. Duclos, Animal Skin and Allergy Clinic. **B** and Inset courtesy Dr. P.E. Ginn, College of Veterinary Medicine, University of Florida.)

proximal forelimbs, shoulders, and abdomen through skin lymphatics. The skin of the udder is sometimes involved. The lymph nodes are unaffected. The causative organisms are thought to be saprophytic atypical mycobacteria that probably enter through cutaneous abrasions. In most of these infections, the specific mycobacteria have not been identified by culture, but M. *kansasii* has been identified in a few cases. A more appropriate name for this condition is *bovine cutaneous opportunistic mycobacteriosis*. Clinical lesions are either firm or fluctuant nodules connected by thin cords of tissue that represent inflamed lymphatic channels (lymphangitis). The firm nodules consist of pyogranulomatous inflammation with fibrosis and sometimes mineralization. The fluctuant nodules are thick-walled abscesses that can ulcerate, rupture, and drain thick, tan exudate. Small lesions can spontaneously resolve, but larger lesions are persistent. This disease became apparent during the time of intense tuberculosis eradication efforts because infection with these opportunistic mycobacterial organisms can cause false-positive reactions to bovine tuberculin tests. Bovine cutaneous opportunistic mycobacteriosis is much less commonly identified now, partly because the prevalence of and thus testing for bovine tuberculosis has been reduced.

Feline leprosy (see Disorders of Cats), caused by M. *lepraemurium* and probably other mycobacterial organisms (see later discussion) develops in cats living in cold, wet areas of the world, including the northwestern United States and Canada.

Rarely, a nodular granulomatous dermatitis caused by acid-fast bacilli develops on the head, dorsal pinnae, or other distal extremities in dogs, often with short hair coats (canine leproid granuloma syndrome). Saprophytic mycobacterial organisms transmitted via the bites of flies are thought to be the cause of the syndrome. The dogs are healthy otherwise, and cultures are negative.

Cutaneous infections caused by M. *tuberculosis* and M. *bovis* are rare; alimentary and pulmonary infections are more common, but skin infections can develop alone or in combination with disseminated infection. Tentative diagnosis of mycobacterial infections is made by considering the animal species affected, clinical lesion appearance and location, and cytologic or histopathologic detection of acid-fast bacilli. In the past, culture was required for definitive identification of the organism involved. The acid-fast bacilli can be rare in tissue sections, especially with the saprophytic opportunistic agents, and some organisms, such as those in feline leprosy and canine leproid granuloma syndrome, are exceedingly difficult to grow on culture media; thus diagnosis is challenging. Fortunately, the need for cultural identification is being reduced by use of immunohistochemical evaluation and PCR techniques that can identify the organisms or their genetic material in tissue and can be completed within a few days. The use of genetic techniques is enhancing studies of mycobacterial diseases in human beings and animals. It is likely that taxonomy of mycobacterial diseases will be refined, based on the use of the genetic techniques.

Bacterial Granulomatous Dermatitis Caused by Other Bacteria. Botryomycosis is a term for a granulomatous dermatitis caused by nonfilamentous bacteria, typically *Staphylococcus* spp., *Streptococcus* spp., *P. aeruginosa*, *Actinobacillus lignieresii*, and *Proteus* spp. In botryomycosis, these bacteria form small yellow "sulfur" granules, which consist of centrally located bacterial colonies surrounded by radiating club-shaped bodies of homogeneous eosinophilic material termed Splendore-Hoeppli material (see Fig. 7-51). This material is considered to be antigen-antibody complexes, tissue debris, and fibrin. Clinically, the lesions are progressive nodular masses located in cutaneous or subcutaneous areas that are composed of granulomatous inflammation with the embedded bacterial colonies bordered by the Splendore-Hoeppli material. Histologic differential diagnoses of botryomycosis include infections with filamentous bacteria that cause similar nodular masses (actinomycotic mycetomas) and nodular masses caused by fungi (eumycotic mycetomas).

Filamentous bacteria also cause bacterial granulomatous dermatitis with granules bordered by Splendore-Hoeppli material and are differentiated from botryomycosis by Gram staining and culture. The bacteria are introduced through traumatic injury; are Gram-positive, filamentous, and branching; and include various species of *Nocardia* and *Actinomyces*. Other actinomycetes (e.g., *Actinomadura*, *Streptomyces*) can also contribute. The granules contain mycelial filaments that are 1 μm or less in diameter. *Nocardia* spp. have a limited tendency to clump together; thus they typically do not form granules. The clinical lesions are progressive nodular cutaneous and subcutaneous masses, often with draining sinuses, which can extend into and involve underlying bone. These nodular masses are called *actinomycotic mycetomas*. Histologic lesions are nodular areas of granulomatous inflammation with abundant fibrosis and embedded bacterial colonies bordered by Splendore-Hoeppli material. Histologic differential diagnoses include botryomycosis and mycetomas caused by fungi (see the discussion of eumycotic mycetomas in the Subcutaneous Mycoses). A classic example of actinomycotic mycetoma in cattle is the so-called lumpy jaw, wherein the infection begins via traumatic implantation of *Actinomyces bovis* into the mandibular mucosa (rather than skin), which progresses to involve mandibular bone (see Chapter 16).

Skin Lesions Secondary to Systemic Bacterial Infections or Infection with Toxin-Producing Bacteria. Systemic bacterial infections can cause skin lesions in animals by bacterial embolization to the skin during sepsis, toxin production, direct infection of vascular endothelial cells, or precipitation of immune-complex disease. In some infections, more than one mechanism is involved. Lesions often reflect vascular damage, specifically vasculitis and thrombosis. Cutaneous lesions caused by *E. rhusiopathiae* (erysipelas) and septicemic salmonellosis are discussed under Disorders of Pigs.

Toxic Shock Syndromes. Recently conditions that resemble toxic shock syndrome in human beings have been described rarely in dogs and more rarely in other domestic species. In human beings, toxic shock syndrome is an acute febrile illness that results in hypotension, shock, an extensive cutaneous rash, and involvement of three or more visceral organ systems. The pathogenesis involves the release of bacterial exotoxins (e.g., toxic shock syndrome toxin 1 and enterotoxins) produced by certain strains of *S. aureus* that usually cause minor or occult infections. The exotoxins act as superantigens and thus do not need to be processed by antigen-presenting cells to cause T lymphocyte activation. As a result, substantial numbers of T lymphocytes are activated in a short period of time, subsequently causing release of proinflammatory cytokines, including TNF-α, IL-2, IL-1, and INF-γ, which are thought to cause the tissue damage and signs of toxic shock syndrome. Less commonly, group A streptococci are the cause of toxic shock syndrome. However, in contrast to the minor or occult infections associated with *S. aureus* toxic shock syndrome, the streptococcal toxic shock syndrome is usually associated with bacteremia and severe necrotizing fasciitis (inflammation of the subcutaneous fat and fascial planes). The involved streptococci produce pyrogenic exotoxin A, which has similarities to toxic shock syndrome toxin 1 and is thought to contribute to the development of the syndrome.

As in human beings, two types of toxic shock–like syndrome occur in dogs. In one, *S. canis* is usually the cause of a severe localized infection in the skin or another site (e.g., lung or urogenital tract) with presumed release of bacterial toxins that cause severe secondary systemic shock. Clinically, the skin lesion, termed *necrotizing fasciitis*, is painful, hot, and swollen, and pain is disproportionately severe relative to the size of the lesion. The subcutaneous fat, fascia, and overlying skin can become necrotic and can slough. The swelling is caused by necrosis of fat and exudate accumulating between the fascial planes (fasciitis and/or cellulitis). Histologic lesions include edema, hemorrhage, necrosis, suppurative inflammation, and thrombosis. Occasionally vasculitis and colonies of cocci are seen. The condition can rapidly lead to sepsis, multiorgan failure, and death if not treated early and aggressively. Fever or shocklike symptoms are present. With the exception of the area with necrotizing fasciitis, the skin is not otherwise affected. The diagnosis of necrotizing fasciitis is clinical and consists of severe pain disproportionate to degree of skin lesions, necrotic fascia, lack of bleeding from fascia, and lack of resistance of fascia to blunt dissection during surgery.

The second type of toxic shock–like syndrome has been described in dogs without concurrent necrotizing fasciitis. This syndrome has distinct clinical and histologic similarities to the staphylococcal toxic shock syndrome in human beings, but the site of infection and production of exotoxin have not yet been documented. The dogs are depressed, febrile, and anorectic. The clinical skin lesions include generalized macular erythema predominantly involving the head, trunk, and legs. Some dogs also have edema of the limbs. Vesicles or pustules are seen in some dogs and can progress to crusts. Ulcers may be seen in advanced lesions. The histologic lesions are identical to those seen in the human staphylococcal toxic shock syndrome. The dogs have superficial to mid-dermal perivascular to periadnexal and interstitial neutrophilic to mixed cellular dermatitis with dermal congestion, edema, and sometimes hemorrhage. A unique feature is the presence of apoptotic keratinocytes in multiple layers of the epidermis and superficial hair follicles bordered by neutrophils or occasional eosinophils. Superficial epidermal pustules and crusts may be seen. Apoptosis may become confluent, resulting in full-thickness necrosis and ulceration of the epidermis. The syndrome can be fatal without early therapy with appropriate antibiotics.

Cutaneous Anthrax. Anthrax is caused by *Bacillus anthracis*, a Gram-positive, spore-forming bacterium. The mechanism of injury is acute coagulative necrosis of cells caused by bacterial toxins. Spores germinate into vegetative bacteria that develop a capsule and produce a deadly three-part exotoxin (AB toxin) that acts on cell membranes to cause vascular injury, edema, hemorrhage, thrombosis, and infarction (see Chapter 4). The capsule is a major virulence factor, the primary role of which is to establish infection. It does this by protecting the bacterium against various host bactericidal factors and phagocytosis, or if phagocytosed, against phagocyte-mediated killing. Once infection is established, anthrax toxins are produced. Anthrax toxins have three antigenic components that individually lack significant biologic activity, but when two or three of these components are combined together, the new grouping becomes highly potent.

In general the outcome of exposure to the anthrax bacterium depends on the susceptibility of the host to infection and toxins, virulence of the organism, infective dose, and route or site of infection. In natural infections of domestic animals, ruminants are considered the most susceptible animal followed by horses and pigs; dogs and cats are considered quite resistant. In domestic animals, anthrax infections occur in gastrointestinal (see Chapter 7), respiratory (see Chapter 9), and cutaneous forms. Most infections are gastrointestinal, and the usual route of infection is ingestion of soil, food, water, or animal byproducts that contain infective material (spores or vegetative bacteria). Respiratory anthrax is rare but can result from inhalation of dust contaminated with spores. Cutaneous lesions may develop secondary to gastrointestinal or respiratory systemic infections or as a primary disease that begins in the skin (cutaneous anthrax). The cutaneous lesions that develop secondary to gastrointestinal or respiratory anthrax result from systemic vascular damage and include extensive edematous swellings and hemorrhages that occur in dependent areas of the neck, ventral thorax and abdomen, perineum, external genitalia, and shoulders in more susceptible species such as ruminants and horses, and in face and neck regions of less susceptible species such as pigs and carnivores.

Cutaneous anthrax, in contrast to the other forms, results from the introduction of infective material via penetrating mechanical injury of the skin through abrasions, wounds from grass seeds, or biting flies. Horses appear to be particularly susceptible to anthrax infections introduced by biting flies. Cutaneous anthrax may develop in conjunction with outbreaks of gastrointestinal or respiratory anthrax because during outbreaks, vegetative bacteria from exudates or blood of sick or dead animals contaminate the environment and form spores. Spores (or the vegetative form) serve as an available source of infective material that may contact wounds or be transferred by biting flies. Damage to the skin is thought to be important in initiating cutaneous anthrax, which appears clinically in two basic patterns: (1) edematous swellings (horses, cattle, sheep) or (2) rarely as discrete, necrotic areas termed "carbuncles" that resemble the more typical lesions of cutaneous anthrax in human beings (cattle, rarely dogs). In domestic animals, edematous swellings in the skin may therefore develop secondary to systemic disease or from primary skin infection. Because the route of infection is not always established, the pathogenesis and significance of cutaneous lesions of anthrax in domestic animals are not always clear. However, in cattle, both edematous swellings and carbuncles of the skin have developed in immunized animals when the herd's resistance to anthrax is waning. Carbuncles also have been reported in the jowl area of dogs, a species considered to have some natural resistance to anthrax. In this example the anthrax bacillus may have been introduced into the skin during ingestion of blood containing the anthrax bacillus. Thus cutaneous carbuncles appear to develop in animals that have cutaneous contact with the anthrax spore or bacillus, and that have partial immunity to anthrax, either natural immunity or that provided via vaccination. In addition, carbuncles in cattle, when present in conjunction with edematous swellings, may help clinically to differentiate cutaneous anthrax from other diseases that cause edematous swellings in this species.

Support for the hypothesis that damage to the skin facilitates cutaneous infection comes from experimental murine models of anthrax that revealed spores have limited ability to penetrate nonlesional skin, and that damage to the epidermis results in more intense infections. Damage to the epidermis appears to increase susceptibility of infection of hair follicle contents and residual epidermis, although direct dermal invasion can also occur. Subsequent invasion and proliferation of the organism in the hair follicles and epidermis is thought to facilitate the development of deeper infections.

In contrast to domestic animals, cutaneous anthrax is the most common form of the disease in human beings and accounts for over 95% of cases. Most human infections result from cutaneous contact with infective material from sick or dead animals or animal by-products. In naturally occurring cutaneous anthrax in human beings, the initial lesion is a pruritic papule that arises 3 to 5 days after infection. Edema is often extensive during early stages of the development of the lesion. The papule progresses to a hemorrhagic vesicle that ruptures and undergoes central necrosis and drying, resulting in a dark eschar (hard crust) with peripheral erythema, termed a carbuncle. The eschar dries and sloughs over a period of 1 to 2 weeks. Histopathologic evaluation of the eschar reveals an ulcer covered by necrotic debris that replaces the epidermis and superficial dermis. The subjacent dermis and subcutis are markedly edematous with vasculitis, hemorrhage, and variable numbers of mixed leukocytes. Large rods typical of the anthrax bacillus may be identified.

The diagnosis of anthrax is generally made in animals with systemic disease, living or dead, when typical organisms are found in impression smears of hemorrhagic exudates from orifices or from blood obtained from a peripheral vein. Bacteria collected from a peripheral vein are less likely to be damaged by putrefaction. Animals suspected of having died from anthrax should not be autopsied (syn: necropsied) to avoid contamination of the environment with bacteria that rapidly form spores in favorable environmental conditions. Anthrax spores are extremely resilient and are a source of infection for animals and human beings.

Toxin-Producing Bacterial Infections from Direct Extension. Bacterial infections can also develop from direct extension of infections of deeper tissue, such as clostridial myositis and cellulitis. *Clostridium novyi* can cause severe cellulitis, toxemia, and death in young rams whose heads have been traumatized by butting during the breeding season. Spores in the soil gain entrance through cutaneous lacerations at the base of the horns, germinate, produce toxins (including α-toxin), and result in cellulitis and toxemia. *C. novyi* α-toxin causes loss of integrity of vascular endothelium with resulting severe local, painful edema, hypotension, organ failure, and death. Swelling of the head and neck result in the common term *big head* or *swelled head*. *Clostridium chauvoei* is a secondary invader of wounds, where spores can germinate, proliferate, and produce necrotizing and hemolytic exotoxins leading to extensive necrosis of the skin and underlying tissue (gas gangrene).

Infection with *Rickettsia rickettsii*. Rocky Mountain spotted fever, the most important rickettsial disease associated with cutaneous lesions, is caused by *R. rickettsii*, an organism that infects endothelial cells. This organism is transmitted by ticks, mainly *Dermacentor andersoni* and *Dermacentor variabilis*. The disease is seasonal, corresponding with the increased activity of ticks and contact with ticks. In addition to systemic signs, affected dogs have cutaneous, ocular, genital, and oral erythema with petechiae, edema, necrosis, and ulceration as a result of the direct endothelial cell damage and vasculitis caused by the rickettsia.

Bacterial Pododermatitis–Digital Infections of Horses and Ruminants (Cattle, Sheep, and Goats) (Table 17-12)

Proliferative Pododermatitis (Canker). See Disorders of Horses.

Necrotizing Pododermatitis (Thrush). See Disorders of Horses.

Papillomatous Digital Dermatitis. See Disorders of Ruminants (Cattle, Sheep, and Goats).

Necrobacillosis of Cattle. See Disorders of Ruminants (Cattle, Sheep, and Goats).

Contagious Foot Rot. See Disorders of Ruminants (Cattle, Sheep, and Goats).

Necrobacillosis of Sheep. See Disorders of Ruminants (Cattle, Sheep, and Goats).

Contagious Ovine Digital Dermatitis. See Disorders of Ruminants (Cattle, Sheep, and Goats).

Fungal (Mycotic) Infections

Mycotic infections have been classified into four basic categories: superficial, cutaneous, subcutaneous, and systemic (Box 17-9). Ability to mount an inflammatory response is paramount to clearing the infection. Mycotic infections tend to occur more often in animals with compromised resistance because of debilitating systemic diseases, such as diabetes mellitus or neoplasia, or in animals treated with glucocorticoids or other immunosuppressive agents or with long-term, broad-spectrum antibiotics.

Superficial Mycoses. Superficial mycoses are infections restricted to the stratum corneum or hair with minimal or no dermal reaction. Piedra is a rare superficial mycosis caused by *Trichosporon* spp. and has been reported in horses and dogs. Lesions consist of minute swellings restricted to the extrafollicular portion of the hair shaft.

Cutaneous Mycoses. Cutaneous mycoses (also included as superficial mycoses by some authors) are infections of cornified tissue, including hair, claws, and epidermis. The fungi are usually restricted to the cornified layers and only very rarely are found in the dermis or subcutis, but tissue destruction and host response can be extensive. Infections in animals include dermatophytosis, cutaneous candidiasis, and *Malassezia* dermatitis.

Dermatophytoses. Dermatophytoses are fungal infections of the skin, hair, and claws of animals caused by taxonomically related fungi known as dermatophytes. Pathogenic genera include *Epidermophyton*, *Microsporum*, and *Trichophyton*. Dermatophytosis occurs worldwide, is the most important cutaneous (superficial) mycosis, and is common in human beings and animals, especially cats. Superficial and cutaneous mycoses (dermatophytosis) are acquired by contact with infected animals or by contact with infective material such as shed scales or hair in the environment or on fomites (e.g., combs, brushes, clippers, equine tack). Dermatophytes are able to colonize the cornified structures (hair, claws) and the stratum corneum and cause disease without ever entering living tissue. Clinical disease in a dermatophyte infection is the result of the host's reaction to the organism and its by-products. Dermatophytes are more contagious than other fungal infections, are more common in hot, humid environments, and young animals are more susceptible than adults. Animals kept in overcrowded, dirty, or damp areas and those with inadequate nutrition, or those that are immunosuppressed, are also more susceptible. It is thought that cell-mediated immune response is the principal means of resolving the infection. Fungal species that more commonly infect domestic animals are included in the genera *Microsporum* and *Trichophyton*. *Epidermophyton* is adapted to human beings (anthropophilic) and rarely infects animals. Zoophilic dermatophytes (e.g., *Microsporum canis* and *Trichophyton mentagrophytes*) are primary animal pathogens but can infect human beings. *M. canis* is so well adapted, especially in long-haired, purebred cats that inapparent infections occur. Yorkshire terriers and Persian and Himalayan cats appear to be predisposed to *M. canis* dermatophytosis. The source of *M. canis* infections is usually an infected cat. *Trichophyton* spp. infections are usually acquired by contact with reservoir hosts, which in the case of *T. mentagrophytes* are rodents or their immediate environment. Geophilic dermatophytes (e.g., *Microsporum gypseum*) occur in the soil as saprophytes but under favorable conditions can infect human beings and animals if the integrity of the skin is broken or the host immune system is compromised.

Dermatophytes invade cornified tissues (stratum corneum, hair shafts, and claws) by producing proteolytic enzymes (e.g., keratinase, elastase, and collagenase), which help them penetrate the cornified surface and hair cuticle, but other factors such as mechanical injury and increased humidity may facilitate penetration. Arthrospores are the typical infective portion of the organism and form by segmentation and fragmentation of fungal hyphae. They adhere strongly to keratin and germinate within hours of contact with the skin and invade the cornified tissue, and as a result, infection of the hair

Table 17-12 Digital Bacterial Infections of Horses and Ruminants

Species	Disorder	Predisposing Factors	Contributing Bacteria	Severity	Contagious
Horse	Proliferative pododermatitis (canker)	Moisture, unclean environment	*Bacteroides* sp., *Fusobacterium necrophorum*, *Treponema* spp., Possible bovine papillomaviruses	Lameness, can be severe	No
Horse	Necrotizing pododermatitis (thrush)	Moisture, impacted manure, mud, hoof conformation	*F. necrophorum*	Severe lameness, foul discharge, loss and deformity of frog, infection of deeper tissues	No
Cattle	Papillomatous digital dermatitis (foot warts; hairy heel warts)	Prolonged wet conditions	Probably *Treponema* sp. Possibly *Serpens* spp.	Moderate to severe lameness	Yes
Cattle	Necrobacillosis of the foot (foul-in-the-foot, interdigital phlegmon, interdigital necrobacillosis)	Trauma, moisture	*F. necrophorum*, *Prevotella melaninogenica*	Can be severe with cellulitis involving tendons, joints, and bone	No
Cattle	Contagious foot rot (benign foot rot, stable foot rot, interdigital dermatitis)	Trauma and moisture	*Dichelobacter nodosus* *F. necrophorum* Other bacteria	Usually mild; similar to benign foot rot in sheep	Yes
Sheep	Contagious foot rot, virulent form	Moisture and trauma	*D. nodosus* strains plus *F. necrophorum* and other bacteria	Severe; virulent strains of *D. nodosus* produce more proteolytic enzymes	Yes
	Contagious foot rot, benign form	Moisture and trauma	*D. nodosus* strains plus *F. necrophorum* and other bacteria	Mild; less virulent strains of *D. nodosus* produce fewer proteolytic enzymes and are less pathogenic	Yes
	Necrobacillosis of the foot				
	I. Ovine interdigital dermatitis		*F. necrophorum* Other bacteria but no *D. nodosus*	Clinically similar to benign foot rot	No
	II. Foot abscesses A. Heel abscesses (infective bulbar necrosis) B. Toe abscesses (lamellar abscesses)	Wet seasons Heavy adult sheep	*F. necrophorum* *Trueperella (Arcanobacterium) pyogenes*	Can cause severe lameness with permanent foot deformity	No
Sheep	Contagious ovine digital dermatitis (CODD)	Moisture and trauma	*Treponema* spp. Role of other bacteria, including *D. nodosus* and *F. necrophorum*, is uncertain	Severe lameness, pain, with possible sloughing of hoof wall	Yes

shaft does not progress below the zone where cornification occurs (keratogenous zone; see the section on development of hair follicles and hair shafts). The products elaborated by the dermatophytes cause dermal irritation and damage to the epidermis. The fungal products and cytokines released from damaged keratinocytes result in epidermal hyperplasia (hyperkeratosis, parakeratosis, and acanthosis) and dermal inflammation. Inflammatory cells arrive via the superficial vessels (superficial perivascular dermatitis) and subsequently migrate through the epidermal layers (exocytosis) to the invaded cornified layers, forming intracorneal microabscesses. Exocytosis of inflammatory cells into follicular walls and lumens results in mural and luminal folliculitis and if the follicular wall is destroyed, in furunculosis. Bacterial infection increases the severity of the folliculitis and furunculosis. Gross and microscopic lesions are highly variable and range from an asymptomatic infection to an eruptive nodular mass (kerion), to deep granulomatous nodular dermal and subcutaneous masses containing distorted fungal hyphae (pseudomycetoma), to discolored, malformed, friable, broken, or sloughed claws (onychomycosis).

Gross lesions in haired skin are often circular or irregularly shaped, scaly to crusty patches of alopecia (Fig. 17-48), which can coalesce to involve large portions of the body. Fungi tend to die in areas of inflammation in the center of lesions but are viable at the periphery, thus giving rise to the peripheral red ring and the term *ringworm*. Hair loss is caused by breakage of hair shafts and loss of hair shafts from inflamed follicles. Follicular papules and pustules can be present. In animals with severe furunculosis, the inflammation can extend into the deep dermis and subcutis, leading to draining sinuses. Microscopic patterns include perifolliculitis, luminal folliculitis, or furunculosis and epidermal hyperplasia with intracorneal microabscesses. In many lesions, septate hyphae or spores are present in hair shafts and in the stratum corneum of the epidermis or follicles (see Fig. 17-48, *B*). Culture and evaluation of macroconidia from the cultured mycelial surface identify the organism involved. Although infections in many animals spontaneously resolve in 3 months, specific therapy is often recommended for affected animals to decrease infective material (scales and hairs) shed into the environment.

Candidiasis. Candidiasis is a yeast infection caused by *Candida* sp., normal inhabitants of the skin and gastrointestinal tract (see Figs. 7-7 and 7-8). Infection occurs when host resistance is compromised. Infections with *Candida* sp. are rare in domestic animals and usually occur on mucous membranes and at mucocutaneous junctions. Gross lesions consist of exudative and pustular to ulcerative inflammation of the lips (cheilitis), oral mucosa (stomatitis), and external ear canal (otitis externa). Microscopic lesions consist of spongiotic neutrophilic pustular inflammation, parakeratosis, and ulceration with exudation. The yeast organisms are present in the superficial exudates. Culture identifies the organism involved.

Malassezia Dermatitis. *Malassezia* infections are seen most commonly in dogs and cats and are usually caused by *Malassezia pachydermatis* (*Pityrosporum canis*), a lipophilic, but non–lipid-dependent yeast that is considered to be a commensal organism in dogs and cats and can be isolated from the normal external canal, skin, anal sacs, and mucosal surfaces. *M. pachydermatis* lives in the stratum corneum and becomes a pathogen when predisposing factors alter host cutaneous microenvironment, epidermal barrier, or immune system. These include increased heat and humidity,

Box 17-9 Cutaneous Fungal Infections

SUPERFICIAL (LIMITED TO HAIR OR STRATUM CORNEUM)

Piedra
- *Trichosporon* spp.

CUTANEOUS (LIMITED TO HAIR, STRATUM CORNEUM, CLAWS)

Dermatophytes
- *Microsporum canis*
- *Microsporum gypseum*
- *Trichophyton mentagrophytes*

Candida spp.
Malassezia spp.

SUBCUTANEOUS (USUALLY LIMITED TO CUTANEOUS AND SUBCUTANEOUS TISSUE, SOMETIMES LYMPHATICS)

Eumycotic mycetoma
- *Curvularia geniculata*
- *Madurella* spp.
- *Acremonium* spp.
- *Pseudallescheria* spp.

Dermatophyte pseudomycetoma
Phaeohyphomycosis
Hyalohyphomycosis
Sporotrichosis
Entomophthoromycosis (zygomycosis)
Oomycosis (pythiosis and lagenidiosis)

SYSTEMIC (USUALLY PULMONARY PORTAL OF ENTRY, BUT SKIN DISEASE ALSO CAN DEVELOP AFTER PUNCTURE OR OTHER INJURY TO SKIN)

Blastomycosis
Coccidioidomycosis
Cryptococcosis
Histoplasmosis

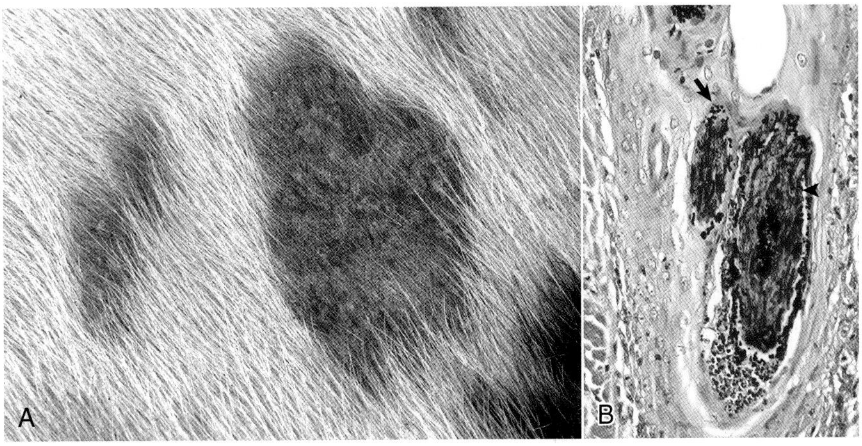

Figure 17-48 Dermatophytosis, Folliculitis, Skin, Haired. A, Dermatophytosis, presumed to be *Trichophyton verrucosum*, cow. Note irregularly ovoid, hairless dark brown areas with mild surface crusting. **B,** Dermatophyte infection presumed to be *Microsporum canis*, involving hair follicle, dog. Note the spores *(arrow)* along periphery and the hyphae *(arrowhead)* within hair shaft are stained black. The hair loss is caused by breakage of hair shafts and mural and luminal folliculitis, which interfere with production of new hairs and cause increased loss of old hairs. Gomori's methenamine silver nitrate–H&E counterstain. (**A** courtesy Dr. H.D. Liggitt, University of Washington. **B** courtesy Dr. A.M. Hargis, DermatoDiagnostics.)

alterations in the amount of composition of surface lipids in response to changes in hormones, cornification disorders, nutritional disturbances, the presence of allergic skin disease such as atopic dermatitis, or disorders associated with immune compromise such as feline immunodeficiency virus (FIV) or paraneoplastic dermatoses in cats. Some dog breeds (basset hounds, West Highland white terrier, cocker spaniels, and others) and cat breeds (sphynx, Devon rex) appear to be predisposed to infection.

Malassezia dermatitis is much more common in dogs than cats and is most often found in dogs with concurrent dermatoses, especially hypersensitivity dermatitis or staphylococcal bacterial folliculitis. M. *pachydermatis* is thought to have a symbiotic relationship with staphylococci, both organisms producing mutually beneficial factors that facilitate their growth. Lesions can be regional (ventral neck, interdigital, otic, perianal, paronychial, or intertriginous) or more generalized (Fig. 17-49). Grossly, the lesions are erythematous, alopecic, often lichenified, and may be hyperpigmented. The lesional surface is often greasy and may be malodorous. Affected claws and paronychial hairs may have red-brown discoloration. Lesions are variably pruritic. Because M. *pachydermatis* does not invade below the stratum corneum, it is likely that animals with intense pruritus associated with *Malassezia* dermatitis have a hypersensitivity reaction to yeast products or antigens. Microscopic lesions consist of hyperkeratosis, focal parakeratosis, variable spongiotic pustular dermatitis, lymphocytic exocytosis, acanthosis, perivascular and interstitial mixed cellular dermatitis, and the presence of M. *pachydermatis* within the surface keratin. Lesions associated with the concurrent disease may also be present.

In otherwise healthy cats, *Malassezia* dermatitis may be regional and seen in association with chin acne, facial dermatitis, or otitis externa. In otherwise healthy cats bred for congenital hairlessness (e.g., sphynx, Devon rex), *Malassezia* spp. (often M. *pachydermatis*) are also commonly found in association with varying degrees of dark brown, greasy exudate on the claws, claw fold, palmar and plantar interdigital areas, axillae, groin, and sometimes ears. These breeds of cats also frequently develop a more generalized greasy dermatitis in which *Malassezia* spp. (often M. *pachydermatis*) are isolated from multiple skin sites. In contrast, more generalized dermatitis in association with *Malassezia* spp. in cats without congenital hairlessness suggests the concurrent presence of underlying systemic disease such as feline pancreatic paraneoplastic alopecia, feline exfoliative dermatitis with or without thymoma, diabetes mellitus, and FIV infection.

Because surface scale and *Malassezia* spp. can be lost during tissue processing, cytologic evaluation is often a more reliable method of detecting and enumerating yeasts, and culture is rarely needed. Because *Malassezia* spp. can be identified in normal skin and because they may be seen in association with other disease processes, the role of *Malassezia* spp. in causing or contributing to the skin disease must be interpreted in regard to clinical findings and may ultimately rest with response to treatment.

Subcutaneous Mycoses. Subcutaneous mycoses are caused by fungi that, after traumatic implantation, invade cutaneous and subcutaneous tissue. Some infections remain localized, but others spread to the lymph vessels. Diseases in this category include eumycotic mycetomas, dermatophyte pseudomycetoma, subcutaneous phaeohyphomycosis, subcutaneous hyalohyphomycosis, sporotrichosis, subcutaneous entomophthoromycosis, and oomycosis (pythiosis and lagenidiosis, not true fungi). The gross appearance of subcutaneous mycoses and deep granulomatous infections caused by bacteria are similar, usually one or more ulcerative nodules, sometimes with draining sinuses. Microscopically the lesions of subcutaneous mycoses consist of nodular to coalescing, suppurative, pyogranulomatous, or granulomatous inflammation. Culture identifies the organism involved; however, some fungi, especially those that are considered "dimorphic," meaning they grow as molds at room temperature and yeast at human body temperature, can be dangerous to culture in routine microbiology laboratory settings because the mycelial phase is infective to human beings. Examples of dimorphic fungi include some species in the genera *Sporothrix*, *Histoplasma*, *Blastomyces*, and *Coccidioides*. If these organisms are suspected clinically, laboratory personnel should be notified when cultures are submitted.

Eumycotic Mycetomas. Eumycotic mycetomas develop most often in horses and dogs and are rare fungal infections resulting in progressive cutaneous and subcutaneous nodular enlargements of granulomatous inflammation that can have draining sinuses and that resemble botryomycosis and actinomycotic mycetomas. The portal of entry is through traumatic injury into the dermis or subcutis, and most of the fungi involved in these infections are saprophytes. *Curvularia geniculata* is the most commonly isolated fungus

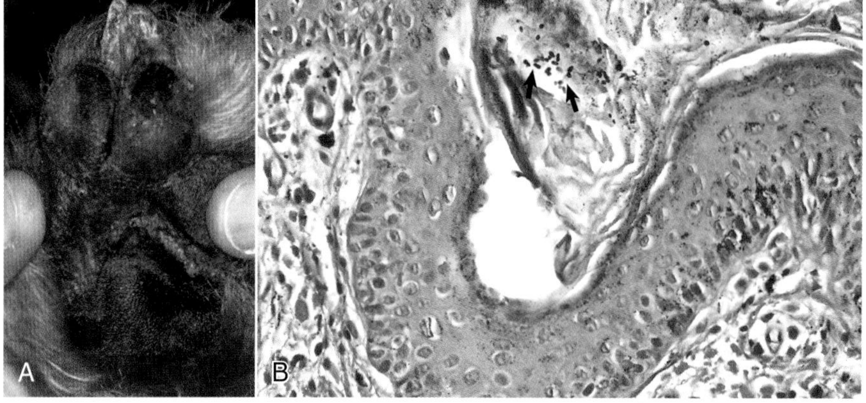

Figure 17-49 **Interdigital Dermatitis (*Malassezia pachydermatis*), Skin, Dog. A,** In this dog with atopic dermatitis, the interdigital skin is erythematous, moist, and mildly lichenified, indicating chronicity. **B,** Haired skin. Stratum corneum contains numerous M. *pachydermatis* yeast *(arrows)*, which are bilobed ("peanut" shaped) and stained black. The dermis is mildly edematous—note the mild separation of the collagen bundles by nonstaining to lightly amphophilic extracellular fluid. Gomori's methenamine silver stain–H&E counterstain. (**A** courtesy Dr. D. Duclos, Animal Skin and Allergy Clinic. **B** courtesy Dr. A.M. Hargis, DermatoDiagnostics.)

in animals; other fungal genera include *Madurella*, *Acremonium*, and *Pseudallescheria*. Histologic lesions are nodular masses of granulomatous inflammation with fibrosis and exudate in which there are embedded granules composed of masses of septate, branching fungal hyphae measuring 2 to 4 μm in diameter. The granules vary in size, shape, color, and texture and are bordered by Splendore-Hoeppli material. Culture identifies the organism involved.

Dermatophytic Pseudomycetoma. See Disorders of Cats.

Phaeohyphomycosis. Phaeohyphomycosis is a mycotic infection caused by species of pigmented fungi (dematiaceous) of a variety of genera that have dark-walled, septate hyphae. Genera include *Alternaria*, *Drechslera*, *Exophiala*, *Phialophora*, and others. These fungi are plant pathogens, soil saprophytes, or in some instances, normal flora that enter the skin at sites of trauma. Most of these infections remain localized to the skin and subcutaneous tissue, but they can spread to other tissue via lymphatic drainage in immunocompromised hosts. Grossly, lesions consist of alopecic or haired cutaneous nodules that can ulcerate and drain (Fig. 17-50). Microscopically, lesions consist of foci of granulomatous, pyogranulomatous, or lymphocyte-rich granulomatous inflammation containing pigmented fungal organisms. Culture is necessary for specific identification of the fungus involved. Subcutaneous phaeohyphomycosis occurs in horses, cattle, cats, and rarely dogs. Hyalohyphomycosis (paecilomycosis) is similar to phaeohyphomycosis except that the fungal hyphae in tissue are nonpigmented (nondematiaceous). Organisms include *Pseudallescheria* sp., *Acremonium* sp., *Fusarium* sp., *Paecilomyces* sp., and *Geotrichum* sp.

Sporotrichosis. Sporotrichosis, caused by the *Sporothrix schenckii* complex, is an uncommon mycosis that occurs in cutaneous, cutaneolymphatic, and disseminated forms in horses, mules, cattle, cats, and dogs. The medically important species in the *S. schenckii* complex are *Sporothrix brasiliensis*, *S. schenckii*, *Sporothrix globosa*, and *Sporothrix luriei*. The most important species in North America is *S. schenckii*, a saprophytic dimorphic fungus found in moist organic debris, and entry into the body is by traumatic implantation. Ulcerated cutaneous nodules and draining sinuses develop at the site of inoculation and along lymph vessels (lymphangitis), but visceral dissemination is uncommon. Deep dermal to subcutaneous pyogranulomatous inflammation develops. Organisms are ovoid to elongate (cigar-shaped) bodies, which are often sparsely distributed and difficult to find in histologic sections but may be detected in cytologic preparations. Immunohistochemical evaluation or culture or both may be required to document infection. The exudate containing organisms is infectious to human beings if introduced into cutaneous wounds.

Oomycosis (Pythiosis and Lagenidiosis). Oomycosis refers to dermal and subcutaneous infection by *Pythium insidiosum* or *Lagenidium* sp., which are both aquatic dimorphic water molds and members of the class Oomycetes. Pythiosis most often affects the skin of the limbs and trunk of horses, cattle, dogs, and cats. Lagenidiosis has been reported only in dogs. Many infections develop in conjunction with exposure to free-standing water. Contamination of minor skin wounds is thought to be necessary for infection to occur. Infections are more common in tropical or subtropical climates, including the Gulf coast of the United States, and are characterized clinically by erythematous, sometimes necrotizing, nodular lesions that ulcerate and drain (Fig. 17-51). There can be extensive tissue destruction by inflammation and necrosis. A unique gross feature of pythiosis in the horse is the presence of yellow, friable fragments of necrotic tissue and hyphae, which can be dislodged from the lesions. Pythiosis in the dog is a rapidly progressive, debilitating, and often fatal disease seen most often in young, large-breed dogs. Although cutaneous pythiosis is most common, gastric pythiosis also occurs in dogs of this same signalment. Lagenidiosis in the dog is also a very aggressive disease, and dogs may have lesions in organs other than the skin and lymph nodes. Histologically, hyphae or hyphal-like structures are in areas of eosinophilic to pyogranulomatous dermal or subcutaneous inflammation. Organisms may not be readily visible in H&E-stained sections; thus special stains, such as Gomori's methenamine silver stain, may be required to identify the organisms. Although pythiosis and lagenidiosis have hyphal morphologic features similar to fungi, they are aquatic water molds and do not respond to antifungal therapy; thus they need to be differentiated from fungi, especially entomophthoromycosis (zygomycosis; see discussion in the next section). Definitive diagnosis of pythiosis can be made by serologic testing (ELISA), culture, or molecular diagnosis using PCR, but for culture, specific specimen handling and culture techniques are required. Diagnosis of lagenidiosis is made by culture of fresh tissue followed by ribosomal RNA (rRNA) gene sequencing.

Entomophthoromycosis (Zygomycosis). Entomophthoromycosis refers to dermal and subcutaneous infections caused by *Basidiobolus* sp. and *Conidiobolus* sp., which are saprophytic fungi that gain entry to the body by inhalation or traumatic implantation by wounds or insects. Most *Basidiobolus* sp. infections have been reported in the horse. Infections with *Conidiobolus* sp. have been reported in horses,

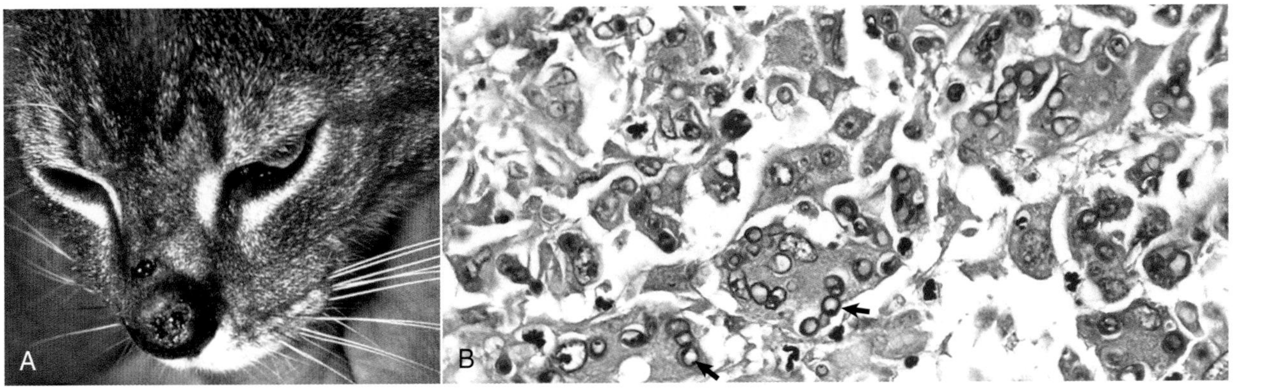

Figure 17-50 Cutaneous Opportunistic Fungal Infection, Phaeohyphomycosis, Granulomatous Dermatitis, Skin, Cat. A, Infection of nasal planum and dorsum of muzzle. There is nodular ulcerative and granulomatous dermatitis affecting the planum nasale. An ulcer is on the dorsum of the muzzle. **B,** Granulomatous dermatitis. The macrophages contain yeastlike pigmented (dematiaceous) fungi *(arrows)* that indicate this is phaeohyphomycosis. The pigment distinguishes phaeohyphomycosis from hyalohyphomycosis. Fungal culture was not performed in this case. H&E stain. (**A** courtesy Dr. A. Werner, Valley Veterinary Specialty Service. **B** courtesy Dr. A.M. Hargis, DermatoDiagnostics.)

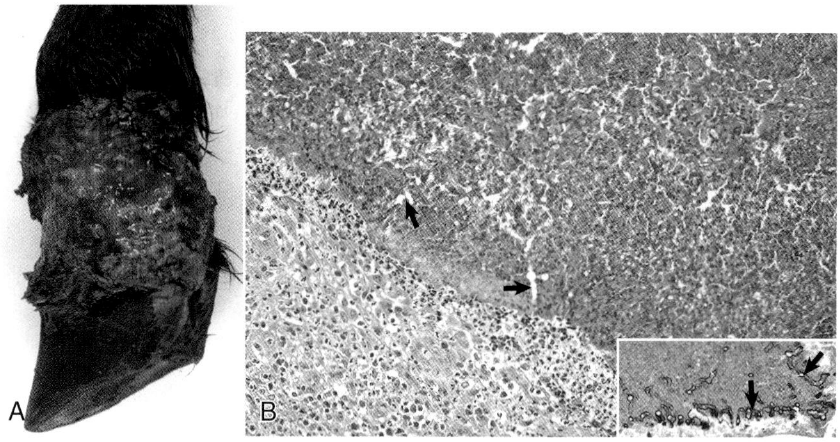

Figure 17-51 **Cutaneous Pythiosis, *Pythium insidiosum*, Skin, Horse. A,** Distal leg. Infection with *P. insidiosum* results in severe, locally extensive, ulcerative dermatitis with multiple coalescing exudative nodules. Necrotic tissue and inflammatory debris exude from the ulcerated surface. **B,** Note margin of necrotic debris *(top right half of figure)* and granulomatous and eosinophilic dermatitis *(bottom left corner of figure)*. Hyphal-like structures of *P. insidiosum* have poor stain uptake with H&E but may be visible as irregular unstained or clear hyphal-like spaces embedded within the necrotic debris *(arrows)*. H&E stain. *Inset,* Numerous *P. insidiosum* organisms stained black *(arrows)*. Gomori's methenamine silver stain. (**A** courtesy University of Florida Clinical Dermatology Service. **B** and Inset courtesy Dr. P.E. Ginn, College of Veterinary Medicine, University of Florida.)

llamas, sheep, and dogs. Systemic dissemination of *Conidiobolus* sp. has developed in the sheep and dog. As in oomycosis, infections are more common in tropical or subtropical climates. Clinical and histologic features are similar to those of oomycosis. Differentiation between entomophthoromycosis and oomycosis requires culture (pythiosis, entomophthoromycosis, lagenidiosis), PCR or ELISA (pythiosis), or rRNA gene sequencing following culture (lagenidiosis) and is therapeutically important because infections with Zygomycetes (true fungi) can be responsive to antifungal treatment, whereas infections with Oomycetes are not.

Systemic Mycoses. The respiratory tract, especially the lung, is almost invariably the primary portal of entry and infection in the systemic mycoses, but cutaneous and subcutaneous infections can occur as part of the disseminated disease or by direct implantation of fungi by trauma. Systemic mycoses include *Blastomyces dermatitidis, Coccidioides immitis, Cryptococcus neoformans*, and *Histoplasma capsulatum*. Infections with these fungi can occur in animals with apparently normal immune function but are more extensive in immunocompromised animals. Grossly, one or more nodular areas in the skin can ulcerate and have draining sinuses. Histopathologically, there are nodular areas of granulomatous or pyogranulomatous inflammation in the dermis and possibly subcutis. *C. neoformans* can cause a granulomatous response, but generally the inflammation is less severe than with the other fungi. The cryptococcal organisms have a mucinous capsule that does not stain with H&E. When inflammation is mild, the capsules of the numerous organisms in a lesion give the tissues a multicystic appearance microscopically. Cytologic or microscopic examination is required for diagnosis. The morphologic features of the organisms (including mucicarmine-positive capsule of *C. neoformans*) are usually sufficient for diagnosis; however, culture may be needed in cases when capsule formation is minimal. There are morphologic overlaps between the systemic mycoses, and cultures may be needed to confirm any of these infections when organisms are in low number. See the section on subcutaneous mycoses regarding precautions when submitting cultures for dimorphic fungi.

Algal Infections

Information on this topic is available at www.expertconsult.com.

Parasitic Infections

Ectoparasites include mites and ticks (which have eight legs as adults), and lice, fleas, and flies (which have six legs as adults) (Box 17-10). The presence of these ectoparasites is called an infestation. Endoparasites causing cutaneous lesions include nematodes, trematodes, and protozoa, and their presence is called an infection. Parasites cause a number of untoward effects, including damage to hides and predisposition to secondary infection. Arthropod parasites (jointed limbs) also serve as vectors of bacterial, spirochetal, helminthic, rickettsial, protozoal, and viral infections. The cutaneous reaction to parasites varies with parasite number, location, feeding habits, and host immune response. The cutaneous reaction is often mediated in part by immune mechanisms (hypersensitivity). Diagnosis of parasitic infestations and infections requires identification of the specific parasite involved, and this may not be possible with skin biopsy evaluation alone. The only mites that are routinely expected to appear in skin biopsy samples of domestic animals are *Demodex* spp.

Mites. Mite infestations can cause serious cutaneous lesions in domestic animals and economic loss in food animals. Mite infestations are rare in horses, except for *Chorioptes* sp., which produce dermatitis of distal limbs in heavy breeds. Cattle can be infested with a variety of mites, including *Sarcoptes*, *Psoroptes*, and *Chorioptes*, which are reportable diseases in the United States. Sheep in the United States are free of mite infestation except for *Demodex* sp. Mite infestations can also cause serious cutaneous diseases in dogs (*Demodex canis*, *Sarcoptes scabiei*, *Otodectes cynotis*), cats (*Demodex cati*, *Demodex gatoi*, *O. cynotis*, *Notoedres cati*), and pigs (*S. scabiei*). In *S. scabiei* infestation, mites can be difficult to find, except for infestation of the skin of the external ears of pigs.

Most species of *Demodex* mites live their entire life cycle in the lumens of hair follicles or sebaceous glands as part of the normal fauna of the skin of most mammals. It is only when the normal equilibrium between the host and the parasite is changed to favor proliferation of the mite that skin lesions of demodectic mange are produced. Thus identification of large numbers of adult mites or an increased number of immature mites in skin scrapings or biopsy samples is required for diagnosis of demodicosis. Demodicosis is

Box 17-10 Cutaneous Parasitic Infestations and Infections

MITES
Demodex sp.
Sarcoptes sp.
Notoedres sp.
Otodectes sp.
Psoroptes sp.
Chorioptes sp.
Cheyletiella sp.
Psorergates sp.
Neotrombicula and *Eutrombicula* spp.

TICKS
Argasid (soft)
Ixodid (hard)

LICE
Mallophaga (biting)
Anoplura (blood sucking)

FLEAS
Ctenocephalides felis and *Ctenocephalides canis*

FLIES
Adult fly bites
Horn fly, stable fly, horsefly, deerfly, blackfly, biting gnats, mosquitoes, sheep ked *(Melophagus ovinus)*
Myiasis
Calliphoridae, Sarcophagidae, *Cuterebra* sp., *Hypoderma* sp., screwworm, *Dermatobia* sp.

HELMINTHS
Larvae
Hookworms, *Habronema* sp., *Pelodera* sp., *Necator* sp., *Strongyloides* sp., *Gnathostoma* sp., *Bunostomum* sp.

Filarial
Onchocerca sp., *Stephanofilaria* sp., *Elaeophora* sp., *Parafilaria* sp., *Suifilaria* sp., *Dirofilaria* sp., *Acanthocheilonema* sp.

PROTOZOA
Leishmania sp.
Rarely other genera

caused by host-specific mites; it is a major problem in dogs but is uncommon in other animals.

Demodicosis. Demodectic mange is rare in the horse. *Demodex caballi* is commonly present in pilosebaceous units of eyelids and muzzle, generally without producing lesions. In contrast, *Demodex equi* is distributed over the body. Clinical lesions are rare, but when present, develop on the face, neck, shoulders, or forelimbs and consist of localized to diffuse alopecia and scaling or of papules, nodules, and pustules.

Demodicosis in cattle (*Demodex bovis*, *Demodex tauri*, and *Demodex ghanaensis*) and goats (*Demodex caprae)* is of little clinical significance, but extensive infection can damage hides by development of multifocal nodules in the skin of shoulders, neck, and face or in a more generalized distribution. Nodules correspond to follicular cysts that are filled with mites and keratinaceous material. Rupture of the cysts leads to severe granulomatous dermatitis and damage to the hide.

Sheep have two species of mites. *Demodex ovis* is located in hair follicles or sebaceous glands distributed over the body and can cause alopecia, erythema, scaling, pustules, and matted fleece. Lesions develop on the face, neck, shoulders, and back, but the ears, limbs, and coronary bands can also be affected. *Demodex aries* is located in sebaceous glands of the vulva, prepuce, and nostrils and can cause papular, rarely pustular, or nodular lesions.

Demodex phylloides of pigs causes scale-covered papules progressing to nodules that are filled with keratinaceous debris and mites and that damage the hide. Lesions develop in the ventral body skin, eyelids, and snout.

Demodicosis is one of the most common skin disorders of dogs in North America. Several different demodectic mites have been identified in dogs, *D. canis* (most common), *Demodex injai* (rare), and *Demodex cornei* (rare), a short-bodied mite. *D. canis* and *D. injai* live in hair follicles and can be found in sebaceous glands. *D. cornei* is found on the skin surface. Mixed infections with *D. canis* and *D. injai* and *D. canis* and *D. cornei* have been reported. *D. injai* has been associated with generalized demodicosis and a clinically greasy hair coat. *D. cornei* has been associated with generalized and localized demodicosis. Most cases of canine demodicosis are caused by *D. canis*, and occur in two clinical forms, localized and generalized, both of which are more common in juvenile dogs. Transmission from mother to offspring occurs via close skin contact, as occurs during suckling. Purebred dogs of many breeds are predisposed to infestation, suggesting an inherited basis for the disease related to a primary deficit in cell-mediated immunity. Research studies suggest the defect is one of T lymphocyte helper dysfunction, resulting in damage by cytotoxic T lymphocytes. Active lesions of demodicosis result in lymphocytic mural folliculitis with lymphocyte-mediated damage to the keratinocytes of the follicular wall. It is speculated that follicular keratinocytes express altered self-antigens or *Demodex* antigens, which leads to immune-mediated destruction of the follicular wall. Secondary immunodeficiency, caused by T lymphocyte suppression, is also associated with demodicosis, particularly if a secondary *S. pseudintermedius* infection is present. The secondary immunodeficiency improves as the demodicosis resolves. Results of studies conflict as to whether the secondary immunodeficiency is caused by the accompanying bacterial infection or the mite infestation. Demodicosis occurs in adult dogs with underlying metabolic disorders (hypothyroidism, hyperadrenocorticism) or that are given drugs (glucocorticoids or cytotoxic drugs) that can compromise the immune system. Idiopathic cases also occur.

Gross lesions of localized demodicosis in the dog consist of one to several small scaly, erythematous, alopecic, areas on the face or forelegs (see Fig. 17-26). Canine generalized demodicosis usually involves large areas of the body; lesions consist of larger coalescing patches of erythema, alopecia, comedones, scales, and crusts. The early microscopic lesions include epidermal hyperkeratosis, perifolliculitis, and lymphocytic interface mural folliculitis, including mild degeneration of follicular basal cells, follicular pigmentary incontinence, and intraluminal mites (see Fig. 17-26). Follicles can become plugged with large numbers of mites, keratin, and sebum. Secondary bacterial infection leads to neutrophilic folliculitis that in conjunction with mite proliferation and follicular hyperkeratosis progresses to follicular rupture. Mites, bacteria, keratin, and sebum spill into the dermis, stimulating a granulomatous to pyogranulomatous dermatitis. Perifollicular granulomas with portions of mites are often seen. Gross lesions in dogs with severe secondary bacterial infection include papules, pustules, edema, and draining sinuses. In severe demodicosis, inflammation and organisms spread into the subcutis, and lymphadenitis and septicemia can develop. Severe chronic lesions consist of dermal fibrosis with effacement of adnexal structures.

In cats, demodicosis is rare and is typically caused by two species of mites, one (*D. cati*) lives in follicles and sebaceous glands, and the other (*D. gatoi*) resides on the skin surface within the stratum corneum. A third species of demodectic mite in the cat (*Demodex* sp. unnamed) resembles, but is larger than, *D. gatoi*, but the significance of this mite has not been determined. Unless the immune response is compromised, lesions associated with *D. cati* are usually localized to the chin, eyelids, head, or neck. When the immune response is compromised, as in feline retroviral infections, generalized lesions of erythema, scaling, alopecia, pustules, and crusts develop. Histologically, cats with *D. cati* have epidermal and follicular hyperkeratosis and follicular atrophy. Inflammation is minimal. The most common sign associated with the presence of *D. gatoi* is pruritus, resulting in excessive grooming and symmetric alopecia. *D. gatoi* is contagious between cats, and there is an asymptomatic carrier state.

Scabies. Scabies is caused by *S. scabiei*. This highly contagious and zoonotic mite is the most important ectoparasite of pigs, is common in dogs, and is uncommon to rare in horses, cattle, sheep, goats, and cats. The mites burrow in tunnels in the stratum corneum and cause intense pruritus principally as a result of hypersensitivity reactions, although irritation from secretions also plays a role. Lesions begin on the external ears, head, and neck and can become generalized. Early gross lesions include erythematous macules, papules, crusts, and excoriations. Chronic lesions are scaly, lichenified, and hairless (Fig. 17-52). Microscopically, early lesions consist of superficial perivascular dermatitis with eosinophils, mast cells, and lymphocytes. Mild focal spongiosis can be seen. Small parakeratotic crusts can develop as spongiotic lesions age. Chronic lesions are associated with epidermal acanthosis with marked rete peg formation, compact hyperkeratosis, parakeratosis, crusting, and perivascular dermatitis with eosinophils, mast cells, and lymphocytes. In areas of excoriation, neutrophils—and with time, dermal scarring—may be evident. Mites, mite eggs, or feces may be found in tunnels in the stratum corneum (see Fig. 17-52, *B*) but are not commonly seen in tissue sections because of small numbers of mites; thus microscopic examination of skin scrapings is usually required for diagnosis.

Notoedric Mites. Notoedric mite infestation is caused by *N. cati*. This mite infests cats, rabbits, and occasionally foxes, dogs, and human beings. It is a rare but highly contagious pruritic disease characterized initially by an erythematous papular rash followed by scales, crusts, and alopecia, and when chronic, with lichenification. Lesions begin on the neck and pinnae and extend to the head, face, and paw and can become generalized. Microscopic lesions consist of a hyperplastic, perivascular eosinophilic dermatitis with mild spongiosis and crusts. In cats, mites are readily found in the stratum corneum in tissue sections or in skin scrapings.

Otodectic Mites. Otodectic mite infestation caused by *O. cynotis* occurs in the external ear canals of dogs and cats and occasionally can be present on other parts of the body. The mite lives on the skin surface and can be seen by direct visualization. Because *Otodectes* mites can be present in areas of the body other than ears, it is important to differentiate them from *Sarcoptes* and *Notoedres* mites, which can be identified in microscopically examined skin scrapings or sometimes in tissue sections.

Psoroptic Mites. Psoroptic mite infestation in horses, cattle, sheep, goats, rabbits, and other animals is caused by several species of host-specific mites. *Psoroptes cuniculi* live on the surface of the skin, feeding on lipids and later on serous and hemorrhagic crusts that exude from the traumatized skin. It infests the external ear canals of horses, sheep, goats, and rabbits. *Psoroptes equi* infests the base of the mane and tail and skin under the forelock of horses. *Psoroptes ovis* causes serious disease in cattle and sheep, producing parasitic lesions of thickened skin and dry scales and crusts that begin on the withers and spread because of persistent self-inflicted trauma. In sheep, psoroptic mite infestation is called sheep scab. Lesions develop on the withers and sides. The wooled areas are chiefly involved with crusts that become adherent to the matted fleece and in time expand and coalesce. Damage is the result of self-inflicted trauma, caused by the pruritus associated with irritation and hypersensitivity reactions. The microscopic lesion is a spongiotic, hyperplastic, hyperkeratotic, or exudative superficial perivascular dermatitis with eosinophils. Self-trauma leads to erosions, ulcers, and exudation of serum and leukocytes. No cases of *P. ovis* have been reported in sheep in the United States since 1970.

Chorioptic Mange. Chorioptic mange, caused by *Chorioptes bovis*, affects cattle, horses, goats, and in some countries, sheep. The mite is not host specific. Mites on the skin surface cause irritation

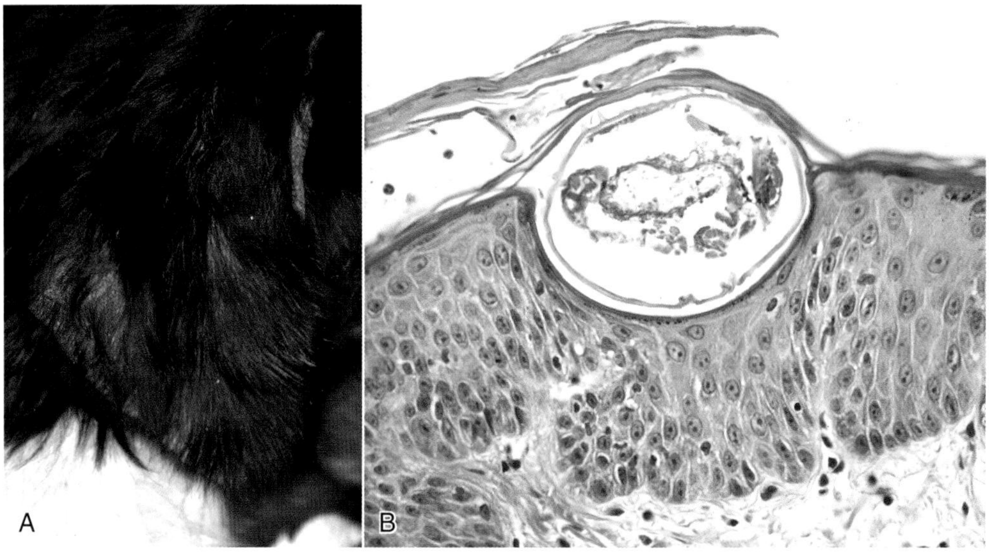

Figure 17-52 ***Sarcoptes scabiei* Infestation, Skin, Dog. A,** Ear. Note the alopecia, erythema, and scaling along the margin of the ear. **B,** Note the section of a mite in a tunnel within the stratum corneum. The epidermal hyperkeratosis, acanthosis, and rete peg formation are in response to both the mite itself and also to self-trauma caused by intense pruritus. H&E stain. (**A** courtesy Dr. A.M. Hargis, DermatoDiagnostics. **B** courtesy Dr. M.D. McGavin, College of Veterinary Medicine, University of Tennessee.)

and pruritus leading to self-trauma and the gross lesions of erythematous, papular, crusted, scaly, hairless, thickened skin on the lower hind limbs, scrotum, tail, perineum, udder, and thigh of cattle; lower limbs and tail of horses; scrotum and lower hind limbs of sheep; and lower limbs, hindquarters, and the abdomen of goats. Microscopic lesions are similar to those seen in other surface-dwelling mite infestations.

Cheyletiellosis

Information on this topic is available at www.expertconsult.com.

Psorergatic (Psorobic) Mites

Information on this topic is available at www.expertconsult.com.

Trombiculiasis

Information on this topic is available at www.expertconsult.com.

Ticks. Ticks comprise two families, Ixodidae (hard ticks that have a scutum, a hard chitinous plate on the anterior dorsal surface) and Argasidae (soft ticks that lack the scutum). Most of the pathogenic ticks are in the family Ixodidae. An exception is *Otobius megnini*, the spinose ear tick, which is parasitic to all domestic animals and causes severe otitis externa. Heavy tick infestations, particularly by adult argasid ticks that engorge repeatedly, can cause anemia. As obligate blood-sucking ectoparasites, ticks also serve as vectors for many potentially severe blood-borne diseases, including, but not limited to, Rocky Mountain spotted fever, borreliosis, babesiosis, anaplasmosis, and ehrlichiosis. Tick bites also cause direct damage to the skin at the site of attachment, which predisposes to secondary bacterial infection leading to abscesses or septicemia and to myiasis. Adverse reactions to ticks depend in part on the content of salivary secretions. Tick saliva has been shown to contain factors that are antihemostatic, antiinflammatory, and immunosuppressive. These factors are thought to facilitate feeding and the transmission of tick-borne diseases. In addition, salivary secretions of several species of ixodid ticks (e.g., *Dermacentor andersoni* and *Dermacentor variabilis* in North America) contain neurotoxins that can cause an acute ascending lower motor neuron paralysis of the host. If the tick is removed, symptoms disappear rapidly.

The severity and type of local cutaneous reactions vary not only with salivary secretions but also with host resistance and whether tick-bone illness is concurrent. In experimental studies it has been shown that in nonsensitized hosts the inflammatory response to tick mouthparts embedded deeply in the dermis develops in the immediate site of the bite, is composed largely of neutrophils, and is minor even approximately 2 days after the tick attaches. In contrast, previously sensitized hosts develop more rapid and intense local reactions (as early as 1 hour after attachment). Cutaneous lesions are present a greater distance from the site of attachment, and basophils, eosinophils, and neutrophils are present in the epidermis and dermis. Cutaneous basophil hypersensitivity, a form of delayed-type hypersensitivity, plays an important role in immunity to ticks.

In naturally occurring cases, gross lesions include red papules that progress to circular erythematous areas up to 2 cm in diameter. Lesions progress to foci of necrosis, erosions, ulcers, crusts, and in some animals, nodules. Lesions heal with scarring and alopecia. Histologic lesions include congestion, edema, and sometimes hemorrhage with an intradermal cavity below which the tick mouthparts may be present. Inflammation consists of perivascular to diffuse accumulations of neutrophils, eosinophils, and basophils, although basophils may be difficult to identify histologically. Later-developing lesions include epidermal and dermal necrosis, the granulocytic leukocytes of more acute lesions plus accumulations of lymphocytes and macrophages at the margin of the necrotic dermis. In a vertical section of skin (from epidermis to panniculus), these lesions can be triangular with the apex at the panniculus. Some lesions comprise granulomas (arthropod bite granulomas) in which the inflammatory cells efface the tissue architecture and lymphoid follicles form.

Lice. Pediculosis is infestation with lice and is caused by two orders of lice: Mallophaga (biting lice) and Anoplura (blood-sucking lice). Infestations are relatively host specific, are spread by direct contact, and are relatively easy to control because the life cycle takes place entirely on the host. Pediculosis occurs more commonly in winter, when temperatures are cooler, the wool or hair coat is longer, animals are congregated, and the plane of nutrition is lower. Thus heavy infestations are usually an indication of underlying problems, such as overcrowding, poor sanitation, or poor nutrition. Generally pediculosis is not a significant threat to the host, and animals with low infestations may not have clinical signs or lesions. Most problems are related to skin irritation and resultant pruritus. However, the Anoplura have piercing mouthparts and suck blood; thus heavy infestations can cause anemia. In addition, *Haematopinus suis*, a sucking louse that parasitizes pigs, is economically important because the lice transmit *Mycoplasma* (*Eperythrozoon*) *suis* and the viruses of swinepox and African swine fever. The Mallophaga cause less severe signs because they feed on epithelial cellular debris. Primary lesions caused by lice are few, and most are secondary to scratching, rubbing, or biting. The cause of the pruritus is not known but is thought to be a result of more than mechanical irritation alone. Gross lesions consist of papules, crusts, excoriations, and self-induced damage to hair and wool. Lice and eggs are visible on hair or wool. Animals infested with sucking lice can be anemic. Weight loss and reduced production of milk can result from the constant irritation associated with some infestations.

Fleas. Flea infestation is principally a problem in dogs and cats. *Ctenocephalides felis* is the most common flea causing infestation, and it also transmits *Dipylidium caninum*. Infestation can occur with *Ctenocephalides canis* and less commonly with fleas that parasitize other mammals and birds. Fleas can cause severe skin irritation because of frequent biting and release of enzymes, anticoagulants, and histamine-like substances; hypersensitivity reactions to saliva; and secondary host-inflicted trauma from scratching and biting. Severe infestations can cause blood loss (anemia), especially in puppies, kittens, or small debilitated adults. Lesions occur over the dorsal lumbosacral region (Fig. 17-53), caudomedial thighs, ventral abdomen, flanks, and the neck area in cats and consist of multiple red papules and secondary excoriations (see the section on Insect Bite Hypersensitivity).

Flies. Cutaneous reactions caused by fly bites range from minor to severe and are caused by bites from adult flies and myiasis by larvae. Reactions to the bites of flies vary and include irritation, anemia, direct toxicity, and hypersensitivity. Biting flies include *Haematobia irritans* (horn fly), *Stomoxys calcitrans* (stable fly), and horseflies, deerflies, blackflies, biting gnats, mosquitoes, and the sheep ked (*Melophagus ovinus*), which is a common wingless fly that sucks blood. Lesions of biting flies are due to local irritation and include wheals and papules centered around a puncture wound that can bleed. Such lesions can persist with hair loss, scales, hemorrhagic crusts, erythema, and secondary excoriations because of self-inflicted trauma, especially if the animals are hypersensitive to the bites. Such hypersensitivity occurs with *Culicoides* sp. in horses (Queensland itch, sweet itch; see the discussion on *Culicoides* hypersensitivity in the section on Selected Hypersensitivity Reactions) and mosquitoes in cats (see the discussion on mosquito

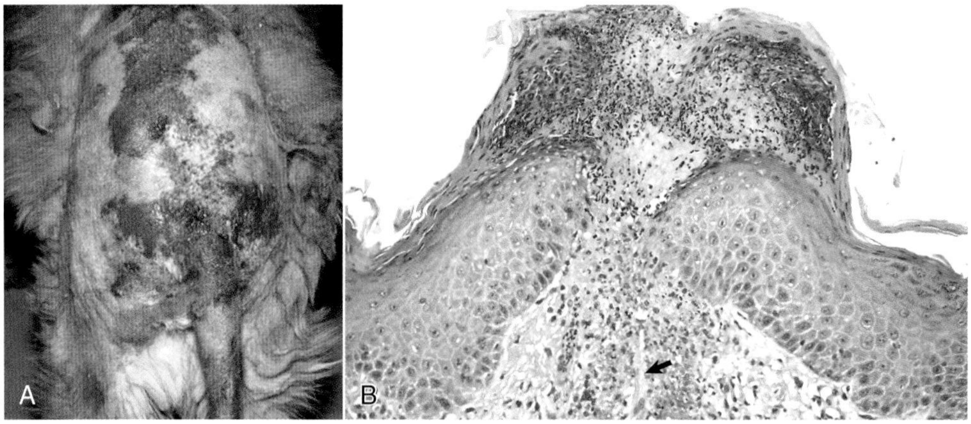

Figure 17-53 **Insect Bite Hypersensitivity, Skin, Acute Moist Dermatitis (Pyotraumatic Dermatitis), Dog. A,** Flea bite hypersensitivity. The hair has been clipped to allow better visualization of the lesions. Hypersensitivity reactions to insect bites can be pruritic and initiate scratching and result in acute moist dermatitis. Self-inflicted trauma is largely the source of the erosion, moist exudation, and crusting in the skin of this dog affected with flea bite hypersensitivity. **B,** Insect bite. The serocellular crust on the epidermal surface covers a defect in epidermis, beneath which in the dermis is a vertical zone of necrosis *(arrow)* infiltrated by eosinophils. H&E stain. (**A** courtesy Dr. B. Baker, Washington State University. **B** courtesy Dr. A.M. Hargis, DermatoDiagnostics.)

bite hypersensitivity in cats in the section on Disorders of Cats). Microscopic lesions associated with fly bites vary, depending on the fly involved. Dermal hemorrhage and edema with a central area of epidermal necrosis are early lesions seen with bites of some flies. Hemorrhagic crust covers areas of necrosis, and perivascular neutrophilic, eosinophilic, and mixed mononuclear inflammation can be seen. Intraepidermal eosinophils, including eosinophilic pustules, are sometimes identified, and eosinophilic folliculitis and furunculosis can be present in reactions to mosquito bites. Epidermal hyperplasia, hyperkeratosis, parakeratosis, and crusting are associated with self-trauma.

Myiasis is infestation of tissues by the larvae of dipterous flies (flies with two wings or winglike appendages) and is a disease of neglect. Lesions develop in skin kept moist and soiled by urine, feces, or body secretions. Flies are attracted by the odor of such areas. Sheep, largely with ovine fleece rot (see section on Bacterial Infections, Disorders of Ruminants [Cattle, Sheep, and Goats]) are most commonly affected. In myiasis caused by blowflies (Calliphoridae) and flesh flies (Sarcophagidae), eggs are deposited in wounds or on soiled hair or wool. Gross lesions consist of matted hair or wool and multiple irregular cutaneous holes or ulcers with an offensive odor. Secretion of proteolytic enzymes by larvae causes lesions to spread. Death can result from septicemia or toxemia.

In *Cuterebra* myiasis, eggs of *Cuterebra* sp. are deposited on stones or vegetation near the burrows of rabbits and rodents, the natural hosts. Less often, cats or dogs become infested. The eggs hatch to first-stage larvae on the vegetation, and when the host contacts the vegetation, larvae attach to the hair coat and move to the skin. Once on the skin, larvae move to natural body openings such as the nares, where they penetrate the mucosa. Other portals of entry are direct penetration of the skin or ingestion by the host during grooming. The larvae migrate to the subcutis, produce a cystlike subcutaneous nodule in which the larvae mature and cut a hole in the skin for respiration. The larvae feed on tissue debris. Wounds heal slowly after larvae are removed or released, but secondary bacterial infection can develop.

In *Hypoderma* myiasis, larvae of *Hypoderma lineatum* and *Hypoderma bovis* penetrate the skin of the legs of cattle and less frequently horses and migrate proximally in the subcutis of the leg. The larvae can be found in many areas of the body. After weeks to months, first-stage larvae reach the esophagus (*H. lineatum*) or vertebral canal (*H. bovis*), where they develop into second-stage larvae. These second-stage larvae then migrate to the subcutis of the back, become established in subcutaneous nodules similar to those of *Cuterebra* sp. with an opening for respiration, and mature to third-stage larvae (Fig. 17-54). Microscopically, these larvae are located in a cavity filled with fibrin, blood, and a few eosinophils and bordered by granulation tissue containing clusters of eosinophils.

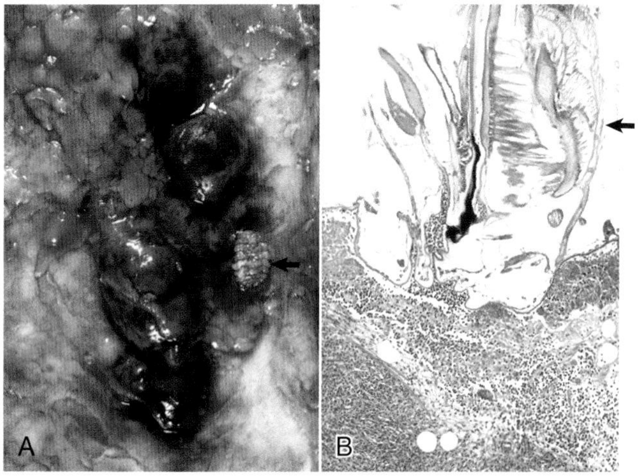

Figure 17-54 **Myiasis, Skin, Subcutis. A,** *Hypoderma* myiasis, *Hypoderma* sp. larva, cow. Multiple hemorrhagic nodules each contain a single larva. One nodule *(right)* has been incised to expose a larva *(arrow)*. **B,** *Cuterebra* myiasis, *Cuterebra* sp. larva, dog. Note a portion of a subcutaneous cystic nodule that contains a segment of a larva *(arrow)*. The subcutaneous inflammation is largely composed of eosinophils. A few lipid vacuoles in the exudate *(clear circular structures)* are remnants of the subcutaneous fat. H&E stain. (Courtesy Dr. A.M. Hargis, DermatoDiagnostics.)

Screwworm myiasis is caused by two species of Diptera larvae, *Cochliomyia hominivorax* (Coquerel), the New World screwworm, and *Chrysomyia bezziana* (Villeneuve), the Old World screwworm. *C. hominivorax* occurs in tropical and semitropical regions of the Western Hemisphere, including Central and South America and some Caribbean islands. It has been eradicated in the United States, Mexico, and Panama. *C. bezziana* (Villeneuve) is found in tropical and semitropical regions of the Eastern Hemisphere, including

Africa, India, and southern Asia. Screwworm flies deposit eggs in wounds or near mucocutaneous junctions of living animals. The eggs develop into first-stage larvae that burrow into tissue head-downwards in a screwlike fashion using sharp, pointed mouth hooks that tear living tissue. Larvae feed on tissues liquefied by secretions of proteolytic enzymes. Screwworm myiasis is an important disease in domestic and wild animals because the larvae develop only in living tissue and thus destroy viable tissue. Grossly, malodorous wounds contain larvae, shreds of tissue, and copious amounts of reddish-brown fluid. Once an animal is infested, death is almost inevitable unless the larvae are removed. Screwworm myiasis is a reportable disease in some countries, including the United States. When it is necessary to differentiate screwworm myiasis from cutaneous myiasis caused by other flies, larvae can be preserved in 70% alcohol and submitted for identification.

Larvae of the tropical warble fly or human botfly, *Dermatobia hominis*, cause cutaneous myiasis in human beings and numerous species of mammals, most commonly and importantly in cattle in South and Central America. It has been suggested that they surpass all other cuterebrines in terms of economic and public health importance. Adult *D. hominis* attaches its eggs to the legs of other insects that then transport the eggs to the mammalian hosts. This unique egg dispersal strategy is responsible for the more generalized host range of *D. hominis* compared with other botfly species. While the insects feed, the eggs are deposited on the skin, hatch into larvae, and quickly penetrate the skin of the host mammal. The larvae grow in subcutaneous nodules sometimes referred to as "warbles," which are similar to those of *Cuterebra* sp., with an opening on the skin surface for respiration, after which they leave the nodule and drop to the ground to complete their life cycle. Individual cattle may be infested by thousands of larvae. *Dermatobia* myiasis is of economic importance because it predisposes the skin to myiasis by other flies, results in losses from cattle mortality or renders the animal as unfit for slaughter, and causes condemnation of hides.

Helminths. Cutaneous infections with helminths are generally not life threatening but can be unsightly and irritating in companion animals and cause hide damage in food animals. Infections are caused by migration of helminth larvae, which live in noncutaneous sites as adults, or by filarial infections (filarial dermatitis), in which adults or microfilaria spend some time in the skin or subcutis. Causes of filarial dermatitis include *Onchocerca* sp., *Stephanofilaria* sp., *Elaeophora* sp., *Parafilaria* sp., *Suifilaria* sp., and rarely *Dirofilaria* sp. or *Acanthocheilonema* sp.

Helminth Larval Migrans

Cutaneous Habronemiasis. See Disorders of Horses.

Hookworm Dermatitis. See Disorders of Dogs.

Filarial Dermatitis. See sections on Disorders of Horses and Disorders of Ruminants (Cattle, Sheep, and Goats).

Protozoa

Information on this topic is available at www.expertconsult.com.

Immunologic Skin Diseases

Mechanisms of Tissue Damage in Hypersensitivity and Autoimmune Reactions

For a detailed description of mechanisms, see section on Hypersensitivity and Autoimmune Reactions—Mechanisms of Tissue Damage.

Selected Hypersensitivity Reactions

Urticaria and Angioedema. Urticaria (hives) and angioedema occur most commonly in horses and dogs and consist of multifocal or localized areas of edema. In urticaria the edema involves the superficial dermis, whereas in angioedema the edema involves the deep dermis and subcutis. There are immunologic (foods, drugs, antisera, insect stings, plants such as stinging nettle, and exposure to chemicals) and nonimmunologic (pressure, sunlight, heat, cold, exercise, and stress) stimuli. Immunologic mechanisms involve type I and type III hypersensitivity reactions. Pruritus is not always present, particularly in the horse. A unique form of urticaria has been described in Jersey and Guernsey cattle because of a type I hypersensitivity reaction to casein in their milk. Urticarial lesions are wheals that typically arise suddenly and remain a few hours, although chronic urticaria (lasting weeks or longer) has been described. In sensitive animals, particularly short-haired dogs or purebred horses, pressure applied to the skin can result in linear urticarial lesions called dermographism. In some animals, serum oozes from the wheals matting the hair coat. Angioedema is a localized or generalized area of extensive deep dermal and subcutaneous edema. Histologic lesions in urticaria and angioedema are subtle and consist of vascular dilation and edema with or without perivascular eosinophilic to mixed mononuclear dermatitis and can be overlooked because the edema fluid may be removed during tissue processing. Occasionally the intercellular epidermal edema (spongiosis) progresses to epidermal vesicles, serum exudation, and serous crusting. The prognosis is generally favorable. Fatalities are rare and probably due to anaphylaxis or associated angioedema involving the respiratory passages.

Atopic Dermatitis (Atopy, Allergic Inhalant Dermatitis). Atopic dermatitis is defined as a genetically predisposed inflammatory and pruritic allergic skin disease with characteristic clinical features associated most commonly with IgE antibodies to environmental allergens. It is an example of a type I hypersensitivity reaction, although type IV mechanisms also participate. The skin is the major target organ in horses, dogs, and cats. There is increasing evidence that the major route of allergen exposure is percutaneous and that epidermal barrier dysfunction contributes to the development of atopic dermatitis. A discussion of the pathogenesis of atopic dermatitis can be found in the section on Disease Example of Barrier Dysfunction.

The predominant clinical sign of atopic dermatitis is pruritus. Horses can have pruritus of the head, pinnae, ventrum, legs, and tail head, or recurrent urticaria. Pruritus causes horses to bite themselves, rub against objects, stomp their feet, and switch their tails. In dogs, pruritus is often manifested as face rubbing (see Fig. 17-34), ear scratching, and paw licking. Severely affected dogs may be restless, may not be able to sleep, and may lose weight because of frequent or persistent scratching. Pruritus may affect the face, distal extremities, ears, and ventrum or may be generalized. Pruritus of the distal extremities and otitis externa are frequent features of dogs with atopic dermatitis. Clinical signs of feline atopic dermatitis vary and include pruritus of the face, neck, or ears or generalized pruritus manifested as self-induced trauma or alopecia. In general, atopic dermatitis is considered a disorder without the presence of primary cutaneous lesions. In horses, urticaria may accompany pruritus. In some dogs, papular, macular, or plaquelike eruptions have been reported. Multifocal crusted papules termed "miliary dermatitis," eosinophilic granuloma complex, and symmetric alopecia are often features of feline atopic dermatitis but are not specific to feline atopic dermatitis because they may be seen in other allergic conditions as well. Most cutaneous lesions are secondary, the result of self-inflicted trauma such as excoriations, erythema, and alopecia. More chronic lesions include lichenification and hyperpigmentation. Microscopic lesions have been studied most in affected dogs, and lesions collected from nontraumatized skin consist of superficial perivascular accumulations of lymphocytes, mast cells, variable numbers of eosinophils, and cells with a histiocytic morphologic appearance. Immunohistochemical evaluation of atopic dog skin has revealed that the lymphocytes are T lymphocytes and the cells with the histiocytic appearance are dendritic antigen-presenting cells. The epidermis is hyperplastic, and sometimes epidermal intercellular edema (spongiosis) progresses to small foci of parakeratosis (see Fig. 17-34, *B*). Uncommonly, intraepidermal eosinophils and subcorneal eosinophil microabscesses have been observed in affected dogs. Lesions of self-trauma, such as excoriations, and secondary infections with staphylococci and *Malassezia* sp. with the accompanying perivascular inflammation and exocytosis of leukocytes into the epidermis, sometimes associated with epidermal or follicular pustules, can mask mild lesions of atopic dermatitis. The inflammation in horses and cats is often deeper than in dogs and consists of perivascular dermatitis with eosinophils as the predominant inflammatory cells. Horses and cats with atopic dermatitis may also develop eosinophilic folliculitis or eosinophilic granulomas. There is no definitive test for atopic dermatitis, so diagnosis is often based on history, clinical signs, physical examination, and ruling out other pruritic diseases with similar presentation (e.g., hypersensitivity to parasites or food). Histopathologic evaluation can be useful in a supportive capacity. Intradermal skin testing and serologic evaluations for elevated levels of allergen-specific IgE are not diagnostic tests but may be considered if immunotherapy is planned.

Insect Bite Hypersensitivity

Culicoides Hypersensitivity. *Culicoides* hypersensitivity in horses is a common worldwide pruritic dermatitis, caused principally by type I and type IV hypersensitivity reactions to salivary antigens from bites of *Culicoides* sp. Signs can be seasonal or nonseasonal depending on climate and thus the prevalence of *Culicoides*. Signs usually develop in horses more than 2 years of age that reside in geographic areas in which *Culicoides* live, and signs usually worsen with age. Gross lesions depend on the stage of disease and severity of pruritus. Initial lesions are papules. Later-developing lesions are pustules and nodules. Self-trauma can cause excoriations, erosions, and sometimes ulcers, crusts, alopecia, and lichenification. Common sites are the tail base, withers, and head. Microscopic lesions include superficial and usually deep perivascular dermatitis with numerous eosinophils. Some horses also have eosinophilic folliculitis, intraepidermal pustules, crusts, erosions or ulcers, and eosinophilic granulomas. Older lesions are nonspecific and consist of epidermal hyperplasia, hyperkeratosis, cellular crusts, and dermal fibrosis, usually the result of ulceration or folliculitis and furunculosis.

Flea Bite Hypersensitivity. Flea bite hypersensitivity is the most common hypersensitivity dermatitis in dogs and cats. It is mediated by type I and type IV reactions, including cutaneous basophil hypersensitivity. Flea bite hypersensitivity is pruritic. In dogs, cutaneous lesions occur principally along the dorsal lumbosacral area (see Fig. 17-53), ventral abdomen, caudomedial aspects of the thighs, and flanks. In cats, lesions occur around the neck but can be generalized, especially in highly sensitive animals. Secondary lesions are caused by self-inflicted trauma. Grossly, there is a papular dermatitis with secondary excoriations. Chronic lesions include lichenification, which is nonspecific (see Table 17-6), and some dogs develop multiple firm alopecic nodules (fibropruritic nodules) in the dorsal lumbosacral area. Microscopically, flea bite hypersensitivity in dogs consists of superficial perivascular dermal accumulations of mast cells, basophils, eosinophils, lymphocytes, and histiocytes. Occasionally, small foci of epidermal necrosis and eosinophils called nibbles are seen, which strongly suggest flea bite hypersensitivity. Fibropruritic nodules consist of a core of coarse thick collagen bundles covered by a hyperplastic epidermis; the end result of chronic inflammation associated with flea bites. In cats, the inflammatory lesions are in the superficial and deep perivascular dermis, and eosinophilic folliculitis and furunculosis also can be a feature. The overlying epidermis is often acanthotic.

Mosquito Bite Hypersensitivity in Cats. See Disorders of Cats.

Allergic Contact Dermatitis. Allergic contact dermatitis, an example of a type IV hypersensitivity reaction, is primarily the result of contact with chemicals such as aniline dyes in carpets, plant resins, chemicals in shampoos and medications, and historically to plastics in food dishes. These chemical substances contain low-molecular-weight haptens that require binding to cell-associated proteins before they are recognized by cytotoxic T lymphocytes ($CD8^+$). Lesions develop on reexposure to the antigen. The lesions are pruritic, result in self-inflicted trauma, vary in severity, and, importantly, are located in regions in contact with the antigen, typically in areas of glabrous (smooth and bare or hairless) skin unless the antigen is a liquid or aerosol. Grossly, lesions consist of erythema, papules with or without vesicles, and exudates that develop into crusts. Chronic lesions are nonspecific and consist of lichenification, hyperpigmentation, and alopecia. Early microscopic lesions are spongiotic superficial perivascular dermatitis with lymphocytes, macrophages, and usually, infrequent eosinophils. However, some lesions have many perivascular eosinophils and eosinophilic epidermal pustules. More chronic lesions, often those identified in biopsy samples, are nonspecific and consist of acanthosis and foci of parakeratotic cellular crusts. Lesions associated with self-induced trauma can also be seen. The location of lesions to contact sites typically affecting poorly haired skin is important diagnostically, because the histologic lesions of allergic contact dermatitis can be present in other types of skin allergy.

Hypersensitivity Reactions to Drugs. Hypersensitivity reactions to drugs are uncommon in dogs and cats, are rare in other domestic animals, and can result from any of the four types of hypersensitivity reactions. The drugs most commonly associated with hypersensitivity reactions include penicillins and trimethoprim-potentiated sulfonamides, but many drugs can cause a hypersensitivity reaction. Gross and microscopic lesions vary greatly. Microscopic lesions have different histopathologic patterns and include perivascular dermatitis, interface dermatitis, epidermal necrosis, vasculitis, vesiculopustular dermatitis, cytotoxic dermatitis, perforating folliculitis (i.e., furunculosis), or panniculitis. The presence of more than one histologic pattern may strongly suggest a hypersensitivity response to a drug.

Selected Autoimmune Reactions

Reactions Characterized Grossly by Vesicles or Bullae as the Primary Lesion and Histologically by Acantholysis. Pemphigus represents a complex group of diseases clinically characterized by transient vesicles or bullae and histologically by acantholysis (Table 17-13). A variety of factors appear to predispose to development of some cases of pemphigus in human beings, including genetic influences, drug intake, viral infections, UVR, emotional stress, and others. In dogs and cats, drug administration has been shown to contribute to some cases of pemphigus, and a few breeds of dogs appear predisposed to developing pemphigus, suggesting that genetic factors may contribute in some dogs. The pemphigus group of diseases is caused by a type II response thought to involve autoantibodies produced against desmosomal proteins (e.g., desmogleins, desmocollins, and plakins), but autoantibodies to nondesmosomal

Table 17-13 Immune-Mediated Dermatoses in Which Vesicles or Bullae Form within or below the Epidermis or Mucosal Epithelium

Disorder	Species	Relative Prevalence	Clinical Distribution	Antigen(s) if Known	Location of Vesicle or Bulla
Pemphigus foliaceus (PF)*	Horse Goat Dog Cat	Common, but rare in goat	Skin	Dog: Dsc 1 Dsg 1	Subcorneal
PF subtype*	Dog	Uncommon	Skin, largely facial	Not defined immunologically	Panepidermal
Pemphigus vulgaris (PV)*	Horse Dog Cat	Rare	Mucosal or mucocutaneous types	Dog: Dsg 3 (mucosal) Dog, horse[‡]: Dsg 3 + Dsg 1 (mucocutaneous)	Suprabasilar
Paraneoplastic pemphigus (PNP)*	Dog Cat	Rare, one putative case in cat	Oral, skin, mucocutaneous	Dsg 3, envoplakin, periplakin, desmoplakins	Suprabasilar
Acquired junctional epidermolysis bullosa (AJEB)[†]	Dog	Rare	Oral, skin	Laminin-332	Lower lamina lucida
Bullous pemphigoid (BP)[†]	Horse Pig Dog Cat	Rare, but seen in multiple species	Skin, mucosae, mucocutaneous, Pigs: skin only	Collagen XVII	Upper lamina lucida
Bullous subtype of systemic lupus erythematosus[†]	Dog	Bullous subtype rare	Oral, skin, mucocutaneous	Collagen VII and nuclear antigens	Sublamina densa in anchoring fibrils
Epidermolysis bullosa acquisita (EBA)[†]	Dog	Rare, but one of the most common AISBDs in dogs	Oral, mucocutaneous junctions, skin, areas of trauma	CollagenVII	Sublamina densa in anchoring fibrils
Linear IgA bullous dermatosis (LAD)[†]	Dog	Rare	Oral, skin of face and extremities	Processed extracellular form of collagen XVII	Upper lamina lucida
Mixed AISBD[†]	Dog	Rare	Skin and mucosae	Collagen VII Laminin-332	Sublamina densa and/or lower lamina lucida
Mucous membrane pemphigoid (MMP)[†]	Dog Cat	Rare, but one of the more common AISBDs in dogs	Mostly mucosae, mucocutaneous junctions	Dog and cat: Collagen XVII Laminin-332 Dog: BPAG 1	Lamina lucida

*Vesicles or bullae form within the epidermis or mucosal epithelium.
[†]Vesicles or bullae form below the epidermis or mucosal epithelium.
[‡]Horse, likely Dsg 1 antigen.
AISBD, Autoimmune subepidermal bullous dermatosis; *BPAG,* bullous pemphigoid antigen; *Dsc,* desmocollin; *Dsg,* desmoglein; *PF subtype,* panepidermal pustular pemphigus.

proteins may also play a role. Traditionally the most important protein antigens thought to contribute in various species are desmoglein 1 and desmoglein 3, and recently desmocollin 1 in dogs. Desmosomes are the sites where cells of the stratum spinosum attach to each other, and during fixation and processing for microscopic examination, the cells of the stratum spinosum contract, except for the desmosomal attachments, which provide the appearance of "spines" or intercellular bridges (see the discussion in the section on Structure, Epidermis). These desmosomal protein antigens are found in various stratified squamous epithelia, including skin, mucocutaneous junctions, oral mucosa, esophagus, and vagina. Damage to desmosomes is thought to result in acantholysis, leading to the formation of vesicles or bullae within varying levels of the epidermis and mucosal epithelia according to the location of the target antigen. Antibodies to more than one of the desmosomal proteins have been identified in affected human beings and dogs, and differences in the specific desmosomal protein or proteins targeted may contribute to some of the morphologic variations in clinical and histologic disease. The pathogenesis of acantholysis is not fully understood and is an active area of investigation. However, the autoantibodies to desmogleins are considered pathogenic because they induce acantholysis when injected into neonatal mice and also cause keratinocyte disassociation in cell culture. There are multiple theories of how autoantibodies cause acantholysis, which may not be mutually exclusive. One theory suggests that the antibodies cause steric hindrance of the desmoglein adhesion site, interfering directly with adhesion. Another theory suggests that antibody binding to desmosomes triggers intracellular signaling pathways that cause disruption of desmosomes and loss of intercellular cohesion by inducing separation of the desmosomal plaque from the intermediate filament cytoskeleton and/or interfering with desmosome turnover. Another relatively recent theory, the multiple hit hypothesis, was developed in part due to discrepancies in correlation of autodesmoglein antibodies alone with type and severity of clinical disease in affected human beings, together with the discovery of other antigens that can be targeted by pemphigus autoimmunity, including not only the desmosomal cadherins, but other adhesion molecules, cell membrane receptors, and mitochondrial proteins. Some of the autoantibodies to nondesmosomal antigens involved in cell adhesion (including the keratinocyte acetylcholine receptors) have induced pemphigus-like lesions when injected into neonatal mice, suggesting that these other autoantibodies contribute to acantholysis in some forms of pemphigus. The multiple hit hypothesis proposes that acantholysis in pemphigus is caused by the synergistic and cumulative effect of autoantibodies targeting keratinocyte cell membrane antigens of different kinds that include molecules that regulate cell shape and adhesion (e.g., acetylcholine receptors) and molecules that mediate cell-to-cell adhesion (e.g., desmosomal cadherins), and that the severity of disease depends on the ratio of different kinds of autoantibodies in each case. Future research may clarify the pathogenesis of acantholysis in pemphigus disorders and lead to more specific therapies.

Pemphigus Foliaceus. Pemphigus foliaceus is the most common and milder form of pemphigus and in domestic animals has been reported in the horse, goat, dog, and cat. The disease develops spontaneously and in dogs and cats, as an adverse reaction to drug therapy. In human beings, pemphigus foliaceus autoantibodies recognize the desmosomal protein, desmoglein 1, which is expressed predominantly in the upper layers of the epidermis. This expression pattern of desmoglein 1 in conjunction with expression patterns of other intercellular adhesion molecules and signaling pathways appears to play a role in location of the vesicles and the anatomic distribution pattern of lesions. Antibodies targeting desmoglein 1 cause cutaneous, rather than oral, lesions, and the acantholytic process occurs at a superficial level in the epidermis, producing clinical lesions that are typically exfoliative (Fig. 17-55). Pemphigus foliaceus in animals is thought to be similar to that in human beings. In fact, autoantibodies to desmoglein 1 have been identified in the serum of a small percentage of dogs with pemphigus foliaceus. However, autoantibodies to desmocollin 1, a desmosomal protein also located in the superficial epidermis, have been identified in the sera of a larger population of dogs with pemphigus foliaceus; thus desmocollin-1 is now thought to be a major autoantigen in canine pemphigus foliaceus. Thus it appears that pemphigus foliaceus is immunologically heterogeneous and that autoantibodies, including those directed toward desmosomal proteins, contribute to the pathogenesis of canine pemphigus foliaceus. Autoantibodies involved in the development of pemphigus foliaceus have not been studied in horses, goats, or cats.

The gross lesions are similar in all species. The primary lesions consist of transient vesicles that rapidly become pustules, which can be localized to specific areas of the skin (nose, pinnae, periocular skin, pawpads, claw beds, and coronary bands) or can be more generalized and symmetric. The pustules are in the superficial epidermis, covered by only a small amount of stratum corneum or a few epidermal cells. Because the pustules are fragile, they quickly rupture from minor mechanical pressure on the surface, and this leads to secondary crusts, scales, alopecia, and superficial erosions

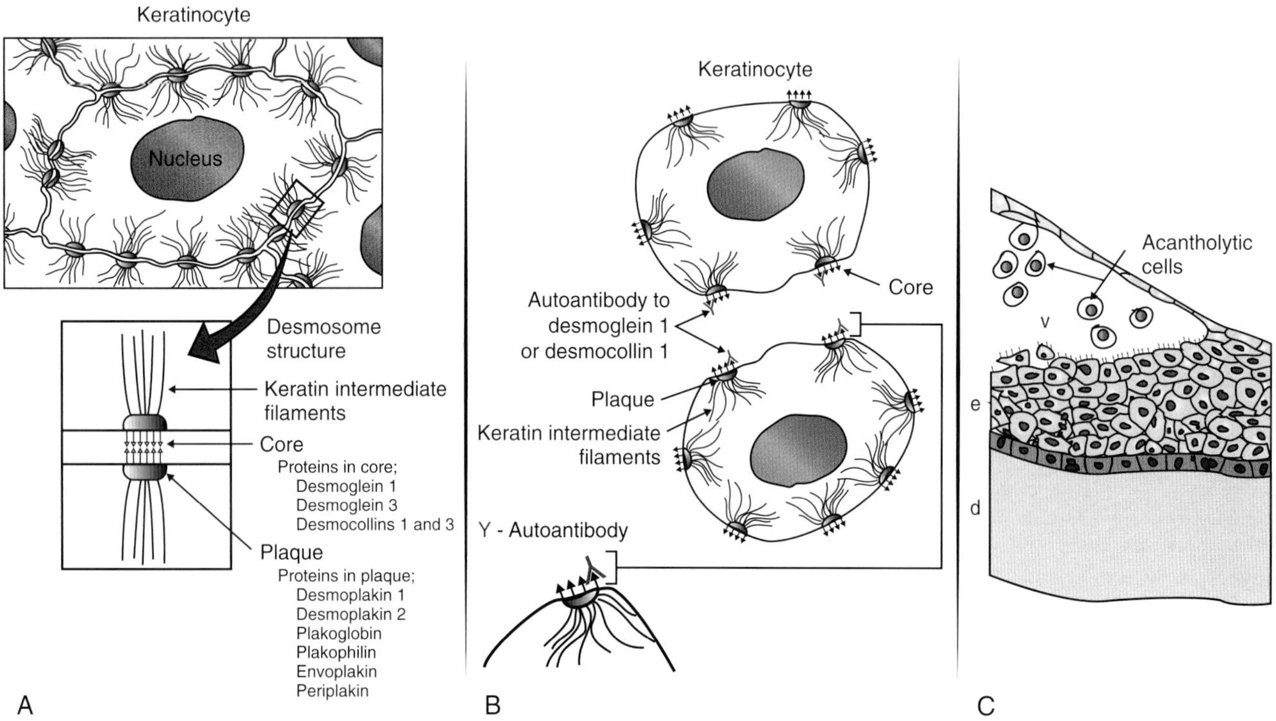

Figure 17-55 **Development of Acantholysis in Pemphigus Foliaceus.** Pemphigus foliaceus develops in association with antibodies to desmosomal proteins that are expressed predominantly in the upper keratinocyte layers. The major pemphigus foliaceus antigens, desmoglein 1 (in human beings) and desmocollin 1 (in dogs), are glycoproteins in the extracellular core of the desmosome. **A,** Desmosomes provide physical connections between keratinocytes and consist of keratin intermediate filaments, an intracytoplasmic attachment plaque region in which the intermediate filaments insert, and an extracellular core region. **B,** Acantholysis in pemphigus foliaceus is thought to be initiated when autoantibodies bind to antigens that are important in cell-to-cell adhesion (also called cadherins), particularly desmoglein 1 or desmocollin 1. Although autoantibodies have been demonstrated in the sera of affected individuals, the precise mechanisms that ultimately result in acantholysis are incompletely understood. **C,** A superficial intraepidermal vesicle containing acantholytic (exfoliated) keratinocytes is the result of lost desmosomal attachments between keratinocytes in the upper layers of the epidermis and sometimes hair follicles. *d,* Dermis; *e,* epidermis; *v,* vesicle. (Revised and redrawn from Rubin E, Farber JL: *Pathology*, ed 3, Philadelphia, 1999, Lippincott-Raven; and Lin MS, Mascaro JM Jr, Liu Z, et al: *Clin Exp Immunol* 107(suppl 1):9-15, 1997.)

(see Fig. 17-15). In horses, lesions often begin on the face or distal extremities or can be localized to the coronary bands. Most horses have multifocal to generalized crusting, scaling, and alopecia of the face, neck, trunk, and extremities. Some horses have been depressed and lethargic. In goats, pustules, crusts, scales, and alopecia develop on the face, abdomen, limbs, perineum, and tail, and in females, udder and teats. In most dogs, lesions are bilateral and symmetric and appear first on the dorsal muzzle, planum nasale, periocular skin, and ears. Pawpads are frequently involved, and claws may be affected and may slough. In more than half the cases, lesions become generalized. Mucosal lesions are rarely seen in dogs with pemphigus foliaceus. Pruritus is present in approximately one-fourth of affected dogs. Systemic signs (anorexia, depression, fever, and weight loss) usually are seen in dogs with more generalized and erosive lesions. In the cat, lesions are similar to those in the dog and occur on the face, ears, and feet and consist of erosions and crusts, because pustules are exceptionally transient. Skin around the nipples may be affected. Pustular exudate and crusting may be seen in the skin of the claw folds. In any species, the lesions can become generalized.

Microscopically, lesions in all species are similar. Subcorneal and intragranular acantholysis result in the formation of very transient "vesicles" (in animals the vesicle stage is not a major clinical feature as it is in human beings because the vesicle stage in animals very rapidly progresses to the pustular stage). Pustules contain neutrophils, less often eosinophils, and acantholytic keratinocytes. The acantholytic keratinocytes may "cling" to the roof of the pustules or may lift from the base of pustules, and occur in clusters. In dogs, cells resembling apoptotic keratinocytes have been noted, but their significance is unknown. Pustules are often large, broad, and extensive and bridge multiple follicles. The pustules may affect the follicular infundibulum. Pustules progress to crusts. In the horse, subcorneal or intragranular pustules are observed, but in the dog, pustules may occur in the stratum spinosum. Crusts should be included in the biopsy sample, especially if well-developed pustules are no longer present because laminated crusts with acantholytic cells can help establish the histologic diagnosis. The laminated crusts are composed of multiple layers of dried pustules, one on top of the other, which result from previous episodes of vesicle and pustule formation at the site. The dermis contains perivascular to interstitial accumulations of mixed inflammatory cells. Eosinophils are the predominant inflammatory cell in approximately one-third of the canine and equine cases. Deposition of IgG at intercellular bridges in all layers of the suprabasilar epidermis or in the superficial epidermis demonstrated by IF or immunohistochemistry (IHC) is a feature of pemphigus foliaceus but is not specific for pemphigus foliaceus. With immunostaining there are frequent false-negative results (poor lesion selection or prior glucocorticoid or immunosuppressive therapy) and false-positive results (chronic skin lesions with plasma cells and secondary immunoglobulin diffusion into the epidermis); thus immunostaining must be interpreted carefully and in conjunction with clinical and histologic findings. Newer techniques that detect more specific antigens, such as desmocollin or desmoglein, and use of better substrates for indirect immunostaining may improve diagnostic accuracy of superficial forms of pemphigus in the future.

Pemphigus Vulgaris. Pemphigus vulgaris (PV) is a very severe form of pemphigus and has been reported in the horse, dog, and cat (see Table 17-13). In the horse and dog, autoantibodies are formed against desmoglein 3, one of the prominent desmosomal proteins involved in adhesion of basal cells of the epidermis and mucosae. In addition, autoantibodies to other proteins involved in intercellular adhesion have been reported in some dogs with pemphigus vulgaris (including desmoglein 1) and were thought to contribute in one horse with pemphigus vulgaris (desmoglein 1). It is thought that the distribution patterns of desmoglein 3 in conjunction with desmoglein 1 in skin and oral mucosa in combination with antibodies to other proteins involved in intercellular adhesion result in vesicular lesions deep in the epidermis, oral mucosa, or both. Thus some forms of pemphigus vulgaris largely affect the oral mucosa (mucosal-dominant pemphigus vulgaris), whereas others affect the skin and oral mucosa (mucocutaneous pemphigus vulgaris). The deep vesicular lesions lead to formation of vesicles or secondary erosions and ulcers in the oral mucosa, at mucocutaneous junctions, and/or skin subject to mechanical stress such as in the axilla or groin. Animals can be febrile, depressed, and anorectic and have leukocytosis. Drooling is often a presenting complaint, because involvement of the oral mucosa is almost always present. Microscopic lesions consist of separation of keratinocytes of the lower epidermis owing to loss of intercellular attachments. However, basal cell keratinocytes remain attached to the basement membrane, resulting in a suprabasilar vesicle leaving a row of basal cells attached to the basement membrane ("row of tombstones") (see Fig. 17-16). There usually is accompanying superficial perivascular to interface mixed inflammation. Direct IF or IHC reveal immunoglobulin and sometimes complement in the intercellular epidermis. Indirect IF has revealed circulating antikeratinocyte antibodies, typically toward desmoglein 3.

Paraneoplastic Pemphigus. Paraneoplastic pemphigus (PNP) is a rare, aggressive form of pemphigus, often but not always associated with solid or hematopoietic neoplasms (see Table 17-13). Paraneoplastic pemphigus has been documented in human beings, dogs, and a putative case in one cat. Cutaneous lesions can precede detection of the neoplastic process and are resistant to treatment. Lesions consist of severe mucosal and mucocutaneous blisters and erosions. Histologically, lesions have a combined or blended pattern of erythema multiforme (a form of cytotoxic dermatitis) together with suprabasilar acantholysis resembling pemphigus vulgaris. Lymphohistiocytic cell–rich interface dermatitis with apoptosis of keratinocytes is present. In addition, lymphocytes border apoptotic keratinocytes (this is often called lymphocytic satellitosis). The pathomechanism for paraneoplastic pemphigus is unknown. Labeling of intercellular bridges is detected by IHC or IF. In human beings with paraneoplastic pemphigus serum autoantibodies targeting multiple cutaneous antigens, including desmoglein 3, desmoplakins, bullous pemphigoid antigens, envoplakin, periplakin, and others, have been reported. Similarly in paraneoplastic pemphigus–affected dogs, autoantibodies to envoplakin, periplakin, desmoglein 3, and desmoplakins have been reported; thus paraneoplastic pemphigus in dogs appears similar to paraneoplastic pemphigus in human beings and likely has an immunologic basis.

Pemphigus Subtypes. Subtypes of pemphigus include pemphigus erythematosus, pemphigus vegetans, and "facially prominent" pemphigus foliaceus. Pemphigus erythematosus occurs in dogs and cats and is considered to be a variant of pemphigus foliaceus with a facial lesion distribution. Currently, there is insufficient clinical, histologic, immunologic, or prognostic evidence to clearly separate pemphigus erythematosus from facially predominant pemphigus foliaceus.

Pemphigus vegetans has very rarely been reported in dogs. Original designations of pemphigus vegetans in dogs were based on similarities to pemphigus vegetans in human beings, a mucocutaneous condition in which pustules evolve into hyperplastic verrucous (vegetative) cutaneous lesions in conjunction with mucosal suprabasilar acantholysis as seen in pemphigus vulgaris. Antibodies to desmoglein 3 are identified in human patients, and sometimes, circulating autoantibodies to other proteins involved in intercellular adhesion have been identified. Some of the dogs diagnosed with pemphigus vegetans have not had oral lesions. In another dog with lesions suggestive of pemphigus vegetans, antibodies to desmoglein 1 rather than desmoglein 3 were identified; thus the rare cases of pemphigus vegetans diagnosed in dogs to date are not directly comparable to those in the human.

Panepidermal pustular pemphigus (PPP) refers to a form of pemphigus in the dog that has some of the features of pemphigus foliaceus, pemphigus vegetans, and pemphigus erythematosus. It appears to represent a variant of pemphigus foliaceus. The term was originally developed when a facially predominant form of pemphigus foliaceus was identified in Akitas, Chow Chows, and a few other breeds of dogs, and there appeared to be a need to reconsider the classification of pemphigus subtypes. The principal diagnostic feature used to distinguish dogs with panepidermal pustular pemphigus from those with pemphigus foliaceus is based solely on histopathologic evaluation: the presence of acantholytic cell–containing pustules that span all layers of the epidermis and the follicular infundibular ORS (e.g., pustules located in deeper epidermis than typical for pemphigus foliaceus [see Fig. 17-17, *B*]). An explanation for the difference in pustule depth may simply reflect the regional variation in various antigens targeted by autoantibodies in different anatomic locations of canine skin. For example, it has been shown that desmoglein 1 can be identified on keratinocytes in all layers of the epidermis in skin from the dorsal muzzle, pinna, and pawpads, whereas desmoglein 1 is detected only in the upper layers of the epidermis in skin from the shoulder, groin, or abdomen. Thus the difference in desmoglein expression could influence pustule location. Further classification of subtypes of pemphigus requires in-depth studies, including immunopathology, as well as the results of therapeutic trials.

Reactions Characterized Grossly by Vesicles or Bullae as the Primary Lesion and Histologically by Vesicles or Bullae within the Basement Membrane (Bullous Dermatoses). Bullous dermatoses are a rare group of autoimmune disorders clinically typified by vesicles or bullae in the skin and often oral mucosa, are caused by autoantibodies directed toward one or more antigens within the basement membrane zone, and are collectively termed "autoimmune subepidermal blistering dermatoses" (AISBDs) (see the discussion in the section on Structure, Basement Membrane Zone, and see Table 17-13). The autoimmune subepidermal blistering dermatoses should be differentiated from the inherited/congenital bullous dermatoses (see section on Disorders of Domestic Animals, Congenital and Hereditary Disorders, Epidermolysis Bullosa [Red Foot Disease]), and from adverse reactions to drug therapy. Much of what is known about the autoimmune subepidermal blistering dermatoses has been borrowed from the human literature, where these diseases are classified based on clinical, histologic, and immunologic features that identify target antigens and autoantibodies. In domestic animals, due to the rarity of these diseases and difficulty and cost of producing stable recombinant antigens, in-depth immunologic classifications are typically limited to research laboratories and have been performed mostly in dogs; however, a few autoimmune subepidermal blistering dermatoses have been identified in the horse, pig, and cat. In the veterinary setting, diagnosis of these diseases is largely based on information obtained from previous research studies that have documented breed predispositions, clinical lesion distribution patterns, and histologic features that help identify lesions consistent with autoimmune subepidermal blistering dermatoses, and that rule out other diseases that can cause vesicles or bullae (e.g., vesicular cutaneous lupus erythematosus, dermatomyositis, and pemphigus vulgaris). Prognosis of the autoimmune subepidermal blistering dermatoses is difficult to predict due to their rarity and the fact that immunologic studies have allowed more definitive diagnosis only in the past 15 years. However, reports indicate that for dogs treated with appropriate combination therapy, there may be complete remission during therapy, and there may be sustained remission after medication withdrawal in some cases. In domestic animals the autoimmune subepidermal blistering dermatoses include acquired junctional epidermolysis bullosa (dog), bullous pemphigoid (horse, pig, dog, cat), bullous systemic lupus erythematosus (dog), epidermolysis bullosa acquisita (dog), linear IgA bullous dermatosis (dog), mixed autoimmune subepidermal blistering dermatoses (dogs), and mucous membrane pemphigoid (dog, cat). In the dog, the species in which most autoimmune subepidermal blistering dermatoses have been documented, approximately 50% of the cases are mucous membrane pemphigoid, approximately 25% are epidermolysis bullosa acquisita, less than 10% are bullous pemphigoid, and the other disorders constitute the remainder. The basic features of subepidermal bullous dermatoses are listed in Table 17-13. Bullous pemphigoid is described in the next section because it affects a wider range of species than the other autoimmune subepidermal blistering dermatoses.

Bullous Pemphigoid. Bullous pemphigoid (BP) is caused by autoantibodies directed against hemidesmosomal proteins. In human beings the autoantibodies are directed toward bullous pemphigoid antigen 1e (BPAG1e), a 230-kD intercellular antigen, and type XVII collagen (also called BPAG2), a 180-kD hemidesmosomal transmembrane molecule. In animals, type XVII collagen has been identified as the major antigen. Bullous pemphigoid has been reported in the horse, Yucatan minipig, dog, and cat. The pathogenesis of vesicle formation is thought to involve a type II immunologic response in which autoantibody binds to the target antigen, and complement activation develops (see Table 17-5). This leads to mast cell degranulation, recruitment and activation of neutrophils and eosinophils, and release of a variety of proteolytic enzymes that result in loss of cell-to-matrix adhesion and in subepidermal vesiculation. It is also possible that autoantibodies might interfere directly with target antigen function or activate cellular signaling and induction of proinflammatory cytokines. Clinical lesions are similar between species and consist of vesicles, erosions, ulcers, and crusts. The location and severity of clinical lesions vary. In horses, lesions are severe and associated with systemic signs; involve the oral mucosa, the squamous lining of the esophagus, and the stomach in some cases; and are generalized in the skin (Fig. 17-56). In Yucatan minipigs, lesions are usually limited to the skin of the back and rump. Dogs are usually mildly affected and have cutaneous lesions in the skin of the abdomen and axillae, concave pinnae, or mucocutaneous junctions. Oral lesions occur in approximately half the dogs. Cats usually have few lesions limited to the face and oral mucosa. Separation of the hemidesmosomes of the basal layer cells from the upper lamina lucida of the basement membrane leads to the microscopic lesions of vesicles and bullae, often with eosinophils and neutrophils in the superficial dermis or within the subepidermal vesicles. Lesions in dogs and pigs have more inflammatory cells than those in horses and cats. Direct IF staining most commonly reveals IgG and in some dogs complement, linearly distributed at the dermoepidermal junction. Evaluation of salt-split epithelial substrates with indirect IF reveals staining on the epithelial side of the artificial split, helping to differentiate bullous pemphigoid from epidermolysis bullosa acquisita, in which staining is located in the sublamina densa or dermal side of the artificial split. The presence of eosinophils is considered to be suggestive of bullous pemphigoid.

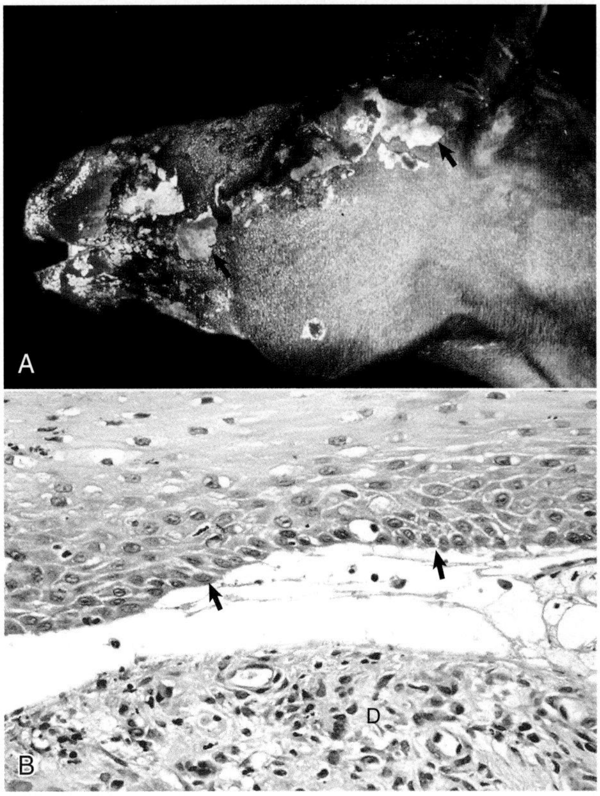

Figure 17-56 **Bullous Pemphigoid-Like Dermatitis, Skin. A,** Bullous pemphigoid-like dermatitis, face, horse. Severe ulceration and hemorrhage are present in the skin, especially lateral to and above the eye, on the nose, and on the chin. Both cutaneous and mucocutaneous sites of the body lined by stratified squamous epithelium were affected. The epidermis had separated easily from the underlying dermis, leading to the formation of vesicles, bullae, and areas of ulceration *(arrows)*. **B,** Subepidermal bullous dermatosis, dog. Note subepidermal vesicle formed when the intact epidermis, including the stratum basale *(arrows)* separated from the dermis *(D)*. The resultant cleft contains a small amount of fibrin and cellular debris. H&E stain. (**A** courtesy Dr. S. Terrell, College of Veterinary Medicine, University of Florida. **B** courtesy Dr. A.M. Hargis, DermatoDiagnostics.)

Reactions Characterized by Depigmentation, Pleomorphic Erythematous Eruptions, Erosion and Ulceration, or Scale/ Crusts and Comedones, and Histologically by Basal Cell or Keratinocyte Degeneration (Cytotoxic Dermatitis). Interface dermatitis, more recently referred to as *cytotoxic* dermatitis, is a histologic pattern of inflammation that affects the dermal-epidermal junction (interface), and that is importantly associated with damage to basal cells (see Fig. 17-14) or in some instances, more superficially located keratinocytes. Basal cells are damaged by oncosis (hydropic or vacuolar degeneration) or apoptosis (shrunken cells due to programed cell death), whereas damage to more superficial keratinocytes is typically due to apoptosis (see Fig. 17-12). The inflammation can be sparse and referred to as cell poor, or dense and referred to as cell rich. This type of dermatitis is referred to as *cytotoxic* because the pathogenesis in part involves T lymphocyte–mediated cytotoxicity of epidermal basal cells or keratinocytes. The clinical features of this histologic reaction pattern are quite variable, the cause of which is not completely understood; however, the location of the apoptotic keratinocytes correlates to a degree with the clinical lesions. For example, if the apoptosis or cellular damage is more prevalent in the basal layer of the epidermis, depigmentation, erosions, and ulceration result from loss of basal layer keratinocytes and melanocytes. In contrast, if apoptosis is more prevalent in the superficial layers of the epidermis and/or hair follicles, hyperkeratosis and parakeratosis result in the clinical features of thick scale/crust and comedones.

Lupus Erythematosus Syndromes. Systemic lupus erythematosus (systemic lupus erythematosus) is a multiorgan disease of dogs and rarely cats and horses. Factors involved in development include genetic predisposition, viral infections, hormones, and UV light. Systemic lupus erythematosus is a disease of immune dysregulation, with abnormalities in both cellular and humoral immunity, including defective T lymphocyte suppressor function and cytokine dysregulation. The defective T lymphocyte suppression function may be caused by anti–T lymphocyte antibodies or a primary suppressor T lymphocyte deficiency. The defective T lymphocyte suppression function results in B lymphocyte hyperactivity and in the formation of autoantibodies to a variety of membrane and soluble antigens, including nucleic acids. Antibodies are also directed to organ-specific antigens, clotting factors, and cells (e.g., erythrocytes, leukocytes, and platelets). The antinuclear antibody titer should be positive. Although the autoantibodies can damage tissue, the principal mechanism of injury in systemic lupus erythematosus occurs via antigen-antibody binding (i.e., immune-complex formation), and deposition of the antigen-antibody complexes in a variety of tissues, including skin. The deposition of these immune complexes, which in the skin occurs at the basement membrane and in the walls of dermal blood vessels, results in a type III hypersensitivity response. Lesions are intensified by exposure to UV light. The enhanced damage may occur via UV-induced expression of nuclear antigens on the keratinocyte surface, autoantibody binding to the newly expressed antigens with resultant keratinocyte damage, and release of keratinocyte cytokines (e.g., IL-1, IL-6, and TNF-α). UV light may also act by inducing the expression of adhesion molecules, thus facilitating trafficking of leukocytes to the epidermis. Systemic signs are variable but can include polyarthritis, myositis, fever, anemia, proteinuria (from glomerulonephritis), and thrombocytopenia.

Cutaneous lesions are highly variable, can be localized or generalized, but commonly involve the face, pinnae, and distal extremities. Lesions consist of erythema, depigmentation, alopecia, scaling, crusting, and ulceration. Stomatitis or panniculitis can be present. Microscopic lesions include lymphohistiocytic interface dermatitis with basal cell apoptosis, pigmentary incontinence, and the presence of subepidermal vacuolization. The basal cell degeneration and subepidermal vacuolization can lead to formation of subepidermal vesicles, which can rapidly ulcerate and crust. Basement membrane thickening caused by accumulation of immune complexes and immune-complex vasculitis of small dermal vessels can also be seen.

Discoid lupus erythematosus (DLE), also called *localized or chronic cutaneous lupus erythematosus (CCLE)* and *photosensitive nasal dermatitis*, is seen most commonly in the dog but is rare in the horse. Historically, discoid lupus erythematosus has been considered to be a mild variant of systemic lupus erythematosus in which there is no involvement of other organ systems and the antinuclear antibody titer is negative. Clinical lesions of discoid lupus erythematosus consist of depigmentation, erythema, scaling, erosion, ulceration, and crusting and generally occur in the skin of the nasal planum, dorsal surface of the nose, and less commonly, the pinnae, lips, periocular region, and rarely in the oral mucosa. The nasal planum may lose the normal surface architecture and become atrophic, scarred, and bleed easily when traumatized. Discoid lupus erythematosus can be exacerbated by sunlight. Microscopic lesions include accumulations of lymphocytes and plasma cells at the dermal-epidermal interface. In early cases the infiltrate can be sparse, but in some cases the lymphocytes and plasma cells are arranged in a dense bandlike pattern that obscures the dermal-epidermal interface. In addition, there are apoptotic basal cells resulting in loss of epidermal pigment that is phagocytosed by dermal macrophages (pigmentary incontinence). As with systemic lupus erythematosus , the basal cell degeneration can, in more severe cases, lead to subepidermal vesicles, loss of the epidermis, and ulceration and crusting. The major differential diagnosis of DLE includes mucocutaneous pyoderma (see section on Superficial Bacterial Infections, Diseases of Dogs), which is differentiated from DLE by the succesful treatment of mucocutaneous pyoderma with antibiotic therapy.

Mucocutaneous lupus erythematosus (MCLE) in dogs is a newly described disorder thought to be a variant of DLE. The condition most often affects German shepherd dogs between 4 and 8 years of age, but other breeds and ages of dogs may be affected. Female dogs are overrepresented. As with DLE, clinical signs suggestive of SLE are absent. Gross lesions occur most commonly in genital, perigenital, anal, and perianal regions, but may also affect periocular, perioral, and perinasal regions and consist of symmetrical, well-demarcated erosions and ulcers, often accompanied by erythema, crusting, and hyperpigmentation. Microscopic lesions are consistent with those described for cutaneous lupus erythematosus, but are often patchy and secondarily infected with bacteria. Focal basement membrane deposition of IgG is the most common immunologic finding. Several disorders require differentiation from MCLE. They include:

1. Mucocutaneous pyoderma, which is differentiated by its complete response to antibiotic therapy and lack of prominent erosions or ulcers
2. Mucous membrane pemphigoid (see Reactions Characterized Grossly by Vesicles or Bullae as the Primary Lesion and Histologically by Vesicles or Bullae within the Basement Membrane (Bullous Dermatoses), which is differentiated by the usual significant oral involvement and presence of vesicles and scars in mucous membrane pemphigoid
3. Erythema multiforme (see section on Erythema Multiforme, Stevens-Johnson Syndrome, and Toxic Epidermal Necrolysis), which is differentiated by the presence of skin lesions in other, nonmucocutaneous sites in erythema multiforme
4. Discoid lupus erythematosus, which is differentiated by the usual restriction of lesions to the skin of the face in DLE.

Exfoliative cutaneous lupus erythematosus was formerly known as *lupoid dermatosis of the German short-haired pointer*. Lesions develop in German short-haired pointers between 3 months and 3 years of age. Clinical lesions consist of scaling and crusting first seen on the face, ears, and back. Lesions then become generalized. The lesions persist but wax and wane. Fever and lymphadenopathy can be present. Rarely there is a positive antinuclear antibody titer. Histologic lesions consist of lymphocytic interface dermatitis with hydropic degeneration of basal cells and apoptosis of keratinocytes. Interface inflammation also affects the basal cells of follicles and sebaceous glands, resulting in sebaceous gland atrophy.

Vesicular cutaneous lupus erythematosus is a disorder formerly known as *ulcerative dermatosis of the collie and Shetland sheepdog*. Lesions develop in middle-aged to older dogs. The Shetland sheepdog, rough collie, and border collie appear predisposed to lesion development. Dogs with this form of lupus have a negative antinuclear antibody titer, but some have antibodies to extractable (soluble) nuclear antigens (e.g., Ro/SSA and La/SSB). Clinical lesions develop most commonly in the groin and axillary areas but may also occur in the mucocutaneous junctions around eyes, mouth, external genitalia, and anus. Lesions consist of vesicles and bullae that progress to ulcers. Lesions can be cyclic and worsen in association with estrus. Lesions also tend to occur in spring and summer; season plus location in less-haired areas has suggested a possible role for sunlight in the pathogenesis of lesions. Histologic lesions include interface lymphocytic dermatitis with hydropic degeneration of basal cells, keratinocyte apoptosis, and extensive vesicles and bullae at the dermal-epidermal junction that progress to ulcers. Mixed inflammation is present in ulcerated lesions, and subepidermal fibrosis may be extensive.

Lupus panniculitis is a rare manifestation of lupus erythematosus and is seen in dogs. Clinical lesions consist of nodules occurring predominantly in the subcutis of the trunk and proximal aspects of the legs. Histologic lesions consist of nodular masses of lymphoplasmacytic and histiocytic inflammation, often with fat necrosis. Vasculitis can also be present. In addition, there may be apoptotic basal cell degeneration, pigmentary incontinence, and thickening of the basement membrane.

Immunostaining in cases of lupus erythematosus may reveal the presence of immunoglobulin and sometimes complement or both at the basement membrane.

Erythema Multiforme, Stevens-Johnson Syndrome, and Toxic Epidermal Necrolysis. Erythema multiforme (EM), Stevens-Johnson syndrome (SJS), and toxic epidermal necrolysis (TEN) are uncommon to rare conditions affecting the skin and sometimes mucous membranes. They have been reported in human beings, horses, cattle, pigs, dogs, and cats. They have been studied most extensively in the human and less so in the dog. Until recently the conditions were considered to represent different expressions or severity of the same clinical disease with erythema multiforme at the mild end and toxic epidermal necrolysis at the severe end of the spectrum. However, in-depth studies scrutinizing the character and extent of clinical and histologic lesions in correlation with the clinical history have prompted a modification. Currently erythema multiforme in human beings is considered to be a separate entity with approximately 90% of cases associated with herpesvirus infection, and now called herpes-associated erythema multiforme (HAEM), but only viral fragments, such as DNA polymerase, and not complete virions are detected in erythema multiforme lesions and thus herpes-associated erythema multiforme is not a productive or active viral infection. Less commonly erythema multiforme in human beings is associated with other infections or is drug associated. In contrast, Stevens-Johnson syndrome and toxic epidermal necrolysis most often represent adverse reactions to drug therapy. Classification of erythema multiforme, Stevens-Johnson syndrome, and toxic epidermal necrolysis in animals is controversial. The results of one multicenter study aimed at better defining these conditions in dogs suggested that although Stevens-Johnson syndrome and toxic epidermal necrolysis were likely to be associated with drug exposure, erythema multiforme was not. A variety of causes for animal erythema multiforme have been proposed, but are usually not proven. These include infections, neoplasia, and adverse responses to dietary substances, drugs, or vaccinations. Virus infections have been implicated as a possible cause of erythema multiforme in animals, including herpesviruses (horses, pigs, cats) and parvovirus (dogs), but these infections either are not proven definitively as a specific cause or they differ from herpes-associated erythema multiforme by being active or productive infections. Most cases of animal erythema multiforme remain idiopathic. Drugs (sulfonamides, cephalexin, levamisole, and others) appear to be the main cause of Stevens-Johnson syndrome and toxic epidermal necrolysis in animals, but drug causation is not usually proven because of the unwillingness to purposely reexpose a patient to the suspected offending drug. However, a new disease-specific algorithm, termed Assessment of Drug Causality in Epidermal Necrolysis, has been validated in human beings with Stevens-Johnson syndrome/toxic epidermal necrolysis. It has been used in a few dogs and shows promise in helping determine if a drug may have contributed to development of toxic epidermal necrolysis lesions. The pathogenesis in erythema multiforme, as well as Stevens-Johnson syndrome and toxic epidermal necrolysis, is thought to involve a misdirected cell-mediated (type IV) immune response against antigens (foreign peptides that are components of infectious agents, drugs, or others) expressed on the surface of keratinocytes. The main effector cells are the cytotoxic T lymphocyte ($CD8^+$ lymphocyte) (see Table 17-5) and natural killer lymphocytes that recognize and bind to the foreign peptide–MHC I complex on the surface of keratinocytes, resulting in apoptosis. In erythema multiforme the apoptosis of keratinocytes is typically patchy and associated with lymphocyte-mediated direct cytotoxicity, which contrasts to Stevens-Johnson syndrome and toxic epidermal necrolysis, where apoptosis is usually more extensive and in some areas may be confluent. The pathogenesis for the more extensive apoptosis in Stevens-Johnson syndrome and toxic epidermal necrolysis is unclear, but the number of inflammatory cells in affected human beings is considered too few to cause such widespread keratinocyte apoptosis. Soluble mediators, such as granulysin released by cytotoxic T lymphocytes and natural killer lymphocytes, and perforin and Fas ligand are considered responsible for the widespread keratinocyte death. The role of soluble mediators in the pathogenesis of Stevens-Johnson syndrome and toxic epidermal necrolysis in animals is unknown.

In animals, erythema multiforme has been studied most extensively in dogs and is initially characterized clinically by polymorphous papules, macules, or plaques that are distributed bilaterally and may coalesce and form circular areas of erythema with firm borders. Although some early lesions of erythema multiforme may resemble urticaria, in contrast to true urticaria, erythema multiforme lesions are not transient. The erythema disappears centrally, producing target-like lesions that are most common on the trunk, axillae, and groin but may be seen on the inner pinnae, footpads, and mucocutaneous junctions. The erythematous areas may progress to vesicles, erosions, ulcers, serpiginous erythematous lesions (see Fig. 17-12), or thick, scaly, or crusted plaques. Erythema multiforme can occur in minor or major forms, depending on the extent of clinical involvement. In erythema multiforme minor, usually either mucosal surfaces are not involved or lesions are restricted to one site. In contrast, more extensive mucous membrane and cutaneous involvement are seen in erythema multiforme major, referred to as *Stevens-Johnson syndrome* (SJS) by some authors, in which clinical lesions may be more extensive, hemorrhagic, vesiculobullous, and ulcerative. Erythema multiforme may have a mild, self-limiting clinical course, and lesions may resolve, especially if the triggering factor is identified and removed. However, especially in dogs and unlike most cases of herpes-associated erythema multiforme in people, the clinical course tends to be chronic or relapsing and may last for years. Systemic signs have been described and are more likely to occur in more severe cases (e.g., erythema multiforme major or Stevens-Johnson syndrome). Histologically, individual keratinocytes in all layers of the epidermis undergo apoptosis (see Fig. 17-12) and are surrounded by lymphocytes (lymphocytic satellitosis). Apoptotic keratinocytes can coalesce, leading to the clinically visible erosions and possibly ulcers. There are perivascular mononuclear cells in the dermis with minor obscuring of the dermal-epidermal interface.

In animals, toxic epidermal necrolysis is seen principally in dogs and cats, is a much more serious condition than erythema multiforme, and may overlap in the spectrum of gross and histologic lesions with Stevens-Johnson syndrome. Both Stevens-Johnson syndrome and toxic epidermal necrolysis are considered clinical emergencies with a high mortality rate in all species. Toxic epidermal necrolysis in particular is a life-threatening disorder that begins clinically as widespread, irregularly shaped, erythematous or purpuric (purple or red, due to hemorrhage) macules and patches that rapidly progress into painful confluent erosions. The epidermis detaches easily (necrolysis means separation of tissue due to necrosis) and forms large areas of translucent sheets that peel from the dermis. Lesions are often present on the face, medial pinnae, and mucocutaneous junctions (especially periocular and perilabial) but can be more widespread. Interdigital skin can be affected, and pawpad involvement is reported in some cases. Histologically, lesions resemble those in erythema multiforme and Stevens-Johnson syndrome with apoptotic keratinocytes in all levels of the epidermis or mucosa, usually accompanied by lymphocytes (lymphocytic satellitosis), but the number and location of apoptotic cells can vary. Full-thickness coagulative necrosis of the epidermis is also a feature. Hair follicles, particularly the follicular infundibulum, are similarly affected. Dermal inflammation in the acute lesions may be minimal and only present in small areas. When present, lymphocytes are at the dermal-epidermal interface and in the superficial perivascular dermis. The coagulative necrosis lesions in toxic epidermal necrolysis are distinguished from thermal burns by the lack of dermal necrosis in toxic epidermal necrolysis. The diagnosis of erythema multiforme, Stevens-Johnson syndrome, and toxic epidermal necrolysis requires both clinical and histologic findings because although there are some histologic differences, those differences may be subtle or evade detection in individual cases for various reasons that include low sample number or sample ulceration. Thus these conditions cannot be reliably differentiated by histopathologic evaluation alone. The presence of systemic signs and the extent of clinical involvement that includes the presence or absence of mucosal lesions are paramount. Similarly, there are other conditions in which keratinocyte apoptosis is present in multiple layers of the epidermis that may require differentiation from some cases of erythema multiforme, Stevens-Johnson syndrome, and toxic epidermal necrolysis. These include graft-versus-host disease in which bone marrow transplantation has occurred (usually experimentally), exfoliative dermatitis in cats with and without thymoma (see section on Disorders of Cats, Paraneoplastic Syndromes), and proliferative, lymphocytic, infundibular mural folliculitis and dermatitis with prominent follicular apoptosis and parakeratotic casts in dogs (see section on Disorders of Dogs).

Feline Exfoliative Dermatitis with or without Thymoma.

See Disorders of Cats, Paraneoplastic Syndromes.

Proliferative, Lymphocytic, Infundibular Mural Folliculitis and Dermatitis with Prominent Follicular Apoptosis and Parakeratotic Casts. See Disorders of Dogs.

Reactions Characterized Grossly by Hemorrhage, Edema, Necrosis, Ulceration, Infarction, or by Alopecia and Scarring and Histologically by Vasculitis or Thrombosis. The histologic diagnosis of cutaneous vasculitis is challenging because it can be difficult to distinguish between inflammatory cells targeting a vessel from inflammatory cells simply migrating through a vessel en route to an area of inflammation elsewhere in the epidermis or dermis. Disproportionate numbers of inflammatory cells in the vessel wall in comparison to the surrounding dermis suggest the vessel is a target of the inflammation. Vasculitis can be primary or secondary to systemic processes such as drug ingestion (e.g., sulfonamides), connective tissue disease (e.g., systemic lupus erythematosus), infections (e.g., *R. rickettsii*, *E. rhusiopathiae*), or it may be incidental to a local process such as ulceration or a thermal burn. In many instances the cause of the vasculitis is unknown (idiopathic). Two principal mechanisms are thought to contribute to the pathogenesis of vasculitis; these are direct invasion of vessels by infectious agents (e.g., *Rickettsia*, herpesvirus) and immune-mediated mechanisms (e.g., allergic, antibody-mediated cytotoxic, immune complex, or cell mediated). The type of inflammatory cell may suggest the pathogenesis. For example, eosinophils may predominate in allergic reactions (arthropod bites or collagenolytic granulomas), neutrophils may predominate in immunologic reactions associated with immune complex deposition (lupus erythematosus, some drug reactions), and lymphocytes may predominate in cell-mediated immune responses (malignant catarrhal fever). However, the cell type may simply reflect stage of disease rather than the mechanism, and in many cases the cellularity is mixed. In animals, type III hypersensitivity reactions (immune complex–mediated processes) are thought to contribute to many cases of immunologic vasculitis, but it is likely that multiple immunologic mechanisms contribute. Evidence for the role of immune complex deposition is derived from experimental studies (Arthus phenomenon and serum sickness) and from identification of immune complexes in serum and tissues in patients with vasculitis caused by infectious agents and hypersensitivity reactions to drugs. Thus infectious agents can contribute to immune complex–mediated vasculitis. The immune complexes can form in the circulation, in the vessel wall, or both.

Small arterioles, capillaries, and postcapillary venules are the most commonly affected vessels. Involvement of the deep vascular plexuses suggests a systemic component is contributing to the vasculitis. Clinical lesions include edema and hemorrhage and in severe cases in which thrombosis can develop, ischemic necrosis and infarction. Ulceration and sometimes sloughing of the skin can occur. In some cases, partial ischemia leading to alopecia and scarring are the main features. Histologic lesions may include the presence of variable numbers of intramural inflammatory cells, intramural or perivascular edema, hemorrhage, or fibrin exudation. Necrosis and fibrin exudation (fibrinoid necrosis) can occur but are rarely seen in small animals. Thrombosis may develop. There is often significant overlap in the clinical and histologic lesions of vasculitis, depending on the severity and stage of disease at the time lesions are examined. Vasculitis is most common in horses and dogs and is rare in cattle, sheep, pigs, and cats.

Cold Agglutinin Disease

Information on this topic is available at www.expertconsult.com.

Vasculitis in Horses

Purpura Hemorrhagica. See Disorders of Horses.

Pastern Leukocytoclastic Vasculitis. See Disorders of Horses.

Vasculitis in Ruminants. See Disorders of Ruminants (Cattle, Sheep, and Goats).

Vasculitis in Pigs. See Disorders of Pigs.

Vasculitis in Dogs. See Disorders of Dogs.

Vasculitis in Cats. See Disorders of Cats.

Disorders with Alopecia or Hypotrichosis (see Table 17-9)

Hair cycle disorders of endocrine origin are due to imbalances in hormones and generally are manifested as nonpruritic, bilaterally symmetric alopecia or hypotrichosis. The remainder of the hair coat is dull, dry, easily epilated, and fails to regrow after clipping. The epidermis is often hyperpigmented or scaly. These lesions are referred to as endocrine alopecia. In disorders associated with alterations in sex hormones, the alopecia often begins in the perineal and genital areas and can extend cranially. However, it is not uncommon for a cutaneous endocrine disorder to have asymmetric alopecia and epidermal hyperpigmentation along with secondary pyoderma or seborrhea. Microscopically, uncomplicated endocrine disorders of the skin consist of normal, atrophic, or hyperplastic epidermis; epidermal hyperkeratosis and increased epidermal pigmentation; follicular infundibular hyperkeratosis and increased trichilemmal cornification; reduced numbers of growing (anagen) follicles; increased numbers of resting (telogen) hair follicles, which may vary with breed; and increased numbers of follicles that lack hair shafts and may also be atrophic (kenogen follicles, also called hairless telogen follicles). Although these general features, including increased numbers of kenogen follicles, support the diagnosis of an endocrinopathic dermatosis, they are not usually diagnostic for a specific endocrine disorder. Also, inflammation caused by secondary seborrhea or pyoderma or previous glucocorticoid therapy for concurrent allergic dermatitis frequently complicates the microscopic changes. Selected clinical and histologic features of individual endocrine disorders (e.g., clinical evidence of epidermal, dermal, and muscle atrophy and histologic evidence of mineral deposition in the case of hyperglucocorticoidism) in conjunction with medication history and clinical testing are used to establish a more definitive diagnosis. Cutaneous endocrine disorders are more common in dogs than in horses, ruminants, or cats.

Hair Cycle Disorders of Endocrine Origin (Cutaneous Endocrine Disorders)

Hypothyroidism. See Disorders of Dogs.

Hyperadrenocorticism. See Disorders of Dogs.

Pituitary Dysfunction in the Horse. See Disorders of Horses.

Hyperestrogenism. See Disorders of Dogs.

Hypersomatotropism. See Disorders of Dogs.

Hyposomatotropism. See Disorders of Dogs.

Hair Cycle Disorders of Nonendocrine Origin

Prolonged Alopecia Postclipping. See Disorders of Dogs.

Alopecia X. See Disorders of Dogs.

Telogen Effluvium and Anagen Effluvium. See Responses of the Adnexa to Injury, Abnormalities of Hair Cycle Stages.

Alopecia Related to Chemotherapy. See Disorders of Dogs.

Alopecic Disorders Associated with Normal Follicles

Excessive grooming, particularly in cats, can result in symmetric alopecia or hypotrichosis that clinically resembles endocrine dermatoses. Excessive grooming can be the result of pruritus (usually associated with cutaneous hypersensitivity reactions) or allegedly from psychogenic problems such as boredom or stress (feline psychogenic alopecia). Excessive grooming has also been reported in feline hyperthyroidism. Thus it is important to determine if the alopecia or hypotrichosis is the result of excessive grooming and if so, what the underlying stimulus is.

Feline Psychogenic Alopecia. See Disorders of Cats.

Alopecia Caused by Hypersensitivity Reactions in the Cat. See Disorders of Cats.

Disorders Associated with Dysplastic Follicles

Follicular Dysplasia Syndromes. Follicular dysplasia syndromes, defined as incomplete or abnormal development of the structure of follicles and hair shafts, comprise a group of generally poorly characterized disorders recognized most commonly in dogs (Box 17-11) but occasionally in horses, cattle, and cats. Structure refers to the permanent physical structure of the hair follicle in contrast to temporary changes that may occur cyclically. The conditions can be congenital (present at birth; see the section on Disorders of Domestic Animals, Congenital and Hereditary Disorders) or tardive (develop months to years after birth) (see Table 17-9). Clinical lesions are alopecia or hypotrichosis, and consequently in animals that develop tardive structural follicular dysplasia, there may be clinical resemblance to the endocrine disorders. The microscopic features help to differentiate syndromes of follicular dysplasia from the endocrine dermatoses. Color-associated follicular dysplasia is discussed in the section on Responses of the Adnexa to Injury, Follicular Dysplasia.

Other Conditions Associated with Alopecia

Seasonal or Cyclic Alopecia. Alopecia apparently associated with seasonal change occurs in horses, cattle, and dogs. Little is known about the cause or pathogenesis of seasonal alopecia in horses because most reports are anecdotal, but it has been reported in four different situations. Icelandic horses in Austria developed recurrent areas of hair loss and scaling at the base of the ears, ocular lateral canthus, dorsal neck, and occasionally cranial shoulder. The hair loss developed in November, resolved in May or June, and recurred in November. The horses were otherwise healthy. Histopathologic evaluation of affected skin revealed the follicles were in a regressing stage of the hair cycle and dermal inflammation was minimal. Although the nutrient content of the feed (hay and silage in this case) was normal, supplements with vitamins, iodine, cobalt, and selenium prevented recurrence. In another situation, different horses developed alopecia in the spring or early summer with resolution in fall or early winter. Lesions were limited to the skin of the face. Two additional situations of excessive hair loss have been reported in association with spring shedding in horses with straight hair coats and some horses with curly hair coats. In horses with straight hair coats, lesions developed on the face, shoulder, and rump. In curly-haired horses the trunk and sometimes the mane and tail areas are affected. After the excessive shedding (hair loss to the degree of alopecia) the hair coats regrew normally. Histopathologic evaluation is not described.

Idiopathic winter alopecia develops in otherwise healthy adult beef cattle in well-managed herds located in western Canada. Thorough clinical evaluations, skin scrapings, and biopsy samples have not identified a cause. The only clinical lesion is alopecia, which occurs most commonly on the dorsal midline but may develop in any site. Multiple animals in the herd develop alopecia, but bulls are affected more often than cows. Alopecia develops during late winter and early spring and spontaneously resolves in late spring or early summer. Timing of skin biopsy in affected cattle often coincides with a resolving phase of the alopecia and, as such, reveals a predominance of growing hair follicles, but no other lesions. Skin biopsy can be used to rule out other causes of alopecia but is not diagnostic. Clinical history and evaluations to rule out other conditions are also required for diagnosis.

Idiopathic (also called cyclic or seasonal) flank alopecia develops more commonly in dogs living in northern latitudes. The cause of this condition is not known, but changes in the photoperiod and thus melatonin released from the pineal gland might play a role. Many breeds are affected, but English bulldogs, boxers, and Airedale terriers are among the more commonly affected breeds. Alopecia develops fairly rapidly, seasonally or cyclically in the skin of the flank (Fig. 17-57). Alopecia usually has a bilaterally symmetric pattern, but there may be variation in severity from one side to another, and alopecia may also involve more cranial areas of the skin such as the shoulder. There may be patches of unaffected (fully haired) skin located within alopecic areas. Hyperpigmentation usually accompanies alopecia. Histopathologic evaluation of the most alopecic areas in the relatively early stages of the disease reveals follicles in the telogen stage of the hair cycle, generally without hair shafts (hairless telogen/kenogen), and follicles markedly dilated by hyperkeratosis. The follicular hyperkeratosis also distends the openings of secondary follicles as they enter the primary follicle, giving the follicles the distorted appearance of an upside-down "footprint" (see Fig. 17-57). The portions of the primary and secondary follicles below the infundibulum may be present in irregular wavy configurations. Biopsy samples collected late in the clinical course of disease or in the stage just before hair growth resumes have numerous anagen follicles, which indicates hair regrowth should be forthcoming. The condition, as the name suggests, is often transient but can be recurrent.

Acquired Pattern Alopecia (Pattern Baldness). See Disorders of Dogs.

Alopecia Related to Trauma. Traction alopecia in dogs and posttraumatic alopecia in cats are presumed a result of interference with the local blood supply to follicles and adjacent skin. Traction alopecia develops in long-haired breeds of dogs in which rubber bands or other devices are used repeatedly or continuously to apply tension to the hair. Lesions usually occur on the top of the head or on the ears, the location where the traction devices are usually applied. Posttraumatic alopecia has been reported in cats that have suffered traumatic pelvic fracture. Alopecic lesions develop on the lower or caudal back several weeks after the fracture. The gross lesion in both conditions is alopecia, which is long term and generally permanent. Histologically, in both traction alopecia and posttraumatic alopecia, follicles are in hairless telogen, are atrophic, and may be partially or completely lost and replaced by dermal fibrosis. Adnexal glands are also usually atrophic and may be absent. In traction alopecia some follicles may contain damaged hair shafts (malacic hairs) or melanin pigment debris, indicating previous

Box 17-11 Selected Tardive* Structural† Follicular Dysplasia Syndromes

- Color dilution alopecia (color mutant alopecia)—many breeds of dogs, a few cattle with hair coat color dilution and with alopecia developing in color-diluted haired areas
- Black (dark) hair follicular dysplasia—many breeds of dogs with solid, bicolored or tricolored hair coats, and with alopecia restricted to black (dark)-haired areas
- Follicular dysplasia of Weimaraner (may be a variant of color dilution alopecia)
- Follicular dysplasia of Siberian husky and Alaskan malamute
- Follicular dysplasia of Doberman pinschers (black or red), miniature pinschers, Manchester terriers, with nondiluted hair coat color
- Follicular dysplasia of Irish water spaniels, Portuguese water dogs, curly-coated retrievers
- Follicular dysplasia of other breeds of dogs—insufficiently characterized

*Having clinical signs that develop slowly or that appear late in development.

†Structural refers to the permanent physical structure of the hair follicle in contrast to temporary changes that may occur cyclically.

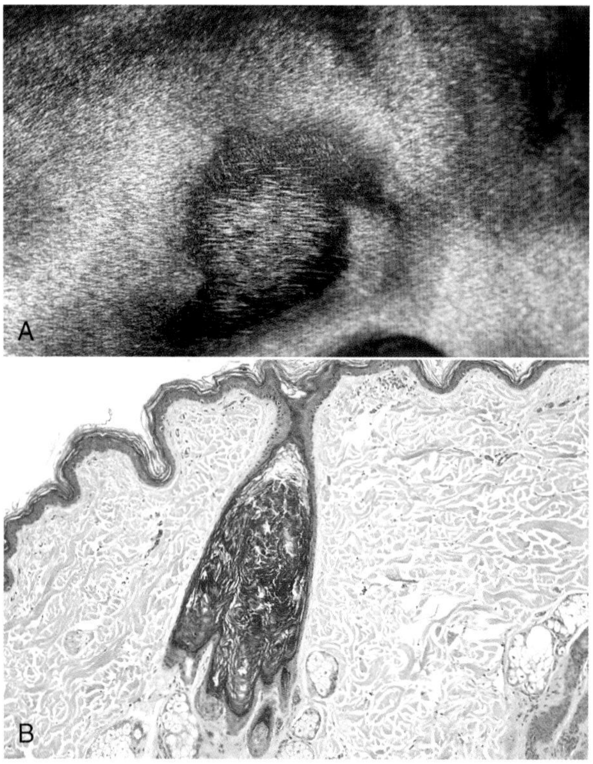

Figure 17-57 **Idiopathic (Cyclic or Seasonal) Flank Alopecia, Skin, Dog. A,** Alopecia and hyperpigmentation are present in the skin of the flank of an otherwise healthy boxer dog. The breed of dog, location of the alopecia, and often seasonal or cyclic nature of the condition suggest that idioipathic (cyclic or seasonal) flank alopecia is a likely diagnosis. Spontaneous hair regrowth in the central area of alopecia *(brown area within hyperpigmented zone)* indicates that lesions are resolving. **B,** Histopathologic examination of a "classic" or relatively early stage lesion illustrates a distorted follicle with dilations at the infundibular base that resembles an upside-down "footprint." This histologic feature, in conjunction with clinical history of cyclic or seasonal lesions in the flank region in the predisposed breeds, supports the diagnosis of this condition. H&E stain. (**A** courtesy Dr. D. Duclos, Animal Skin and Allergy Clinic. **B** courtesy Dr. A.M. Hargis, DermatoDiagnostics.)

traction and fracture of hairs. In posttraumatic alopecia, the shearing force is severe and abrupt and results in degeneration of pannicular adipose tissue and more extensive dermal and superficial subcutaneous scarring.

Disorders Related to Nutrient Imbalances, Deficiencies, or Altered Metabolism

Malnutrition

Information on this topic is available at www.expertconsult.com.

Protein-Calorie Malnutrition

Information on this topic is available at www.expertconsult.com.

Zinc Deficiency

Zinc deficiency occurs chiefly in pigs and dogs and is of less importance in ruminants. It results from diets containing high concentration of phytic acid (binds zinc), low concentration of zinc, or high concentration of calcium (reduces absorption of zinc) or from inherited defective absorption or metabolism. In cattle, sheep, and goats, cutaneous lesions include alopecia, scaling, and crusting of the skin of the face, ears, neck, distal extremities, pressure points, and mucocutaneous junctions. In uncomplicated cases, microscopic lesions consist of parakeratosis and sometimes hyperkeratosis.

Dietary Zinc Deficiency in Ruminants. See Disorders of Ruminants (Cattle, Sheep, and Goats).

Hereditary Zinc Deficiency in Calves and Goats. See Disorders of Ruminants (Cattle, Sheep, and Goats).

Zinc Deficiency in Pigs. See Disorders of Pigs.

Canine Zinc-Responsive Dermatosis. See Disorders of Dogs.

Lethal Acrodermatitis of Bull Terriers. See Disorders of Dogs.

Copper Deficiency

Information on this topic is available at www.expertconsult.com.

Vitamin E Deficiency

See Disorders of Cats.

Vitamin A–Responsive Dermatosis

See Disorders of Dogs.

Disorders of Epidermal Growth or Differentiation

Predominant Epidermal Hyperkeratosis (Scale)

Primary Idiopathic Seborrhea. Primary idiopathic seborrhea is a disorder of epidermal hyperproliferation that results in increased production of corneocytes and visible scale. It occurs most commonly in dogs and less commonly in horses and cats. Most experimental work has been performed in cocker spaniels. The pathogenesis of the disease involves hyperproliferation of the epidermis, hair follicle infundibulum, and sebaceous glands. The basal cell labeling indices are three or four times higher in cocker spaniels with seborrhea than in normal dogs. The hyperproliferation results in reduction in the epidermal turnover time to approximately one-third (e.g., from 22 days to 8 days in the cocker spaniel). In the cocker spaniel the disorder appears to be the result of a primary cellular defect in the keratinocyte, because the epidermal cells remain hyperproliferative when grown in culture and after being grafted onto the dermis of normal dogs. However, the molecular basis of the defect has not been studied. In seborrhea, quantitative studies on sebum production have not been performed, but it is known that there is a relative increase in free fatty acids and a relative decrease in diester waxes on the surface of the seborrheic skin of various breeds. In addition, there is a change from nonpathogenic resident bacteria to pathogenic, coagulase-positive staphylococci. Clinically, two forms of seborrhea have been described, a dry form (seborrhea sicca), with dry skin and white-to-gray scales that exfoliate (see Fig. 17-9), and a greasy form (seborrhea oleosa), with scaling and excessive brown to yellow lipids that adhere to the surface of the skin and hair. An animal can have seborrhea sicca in some areas of the body and seborrhea oleosa in others. Microscopic lesions include marked hyperkeratosis of the epidermis and follicular infundibulum. The epidermis has a papillary appearance caused by widening of follicular ostia by the follicular hyperkeratosis (see Fig. 17-9). Comedones (follicles dilated with a plug of follicular stratum corneum and sebum) are present in some animals. At the edges of follicular ostia, foci of parakeratosis form over a spongiotic epidermis containing a few scattered leukocytes. The superficial dermis is congested and edematous.

Ichthyosis. The ichthyoses are a heterogeneous group of inherited skin disorders seen principally in cattle and dogs (see E-Box 17-2). In severe forms of ichthyosis the skin is thickened by marked scaling and can crack into plates resembling fish scales; thus the disease is named "ichthys" from the Greek word meaning fish. Recently advances in molecular diagnosis have improved the understanding of the defects in some of these disorders. In human beings, most of the ichthyoses are associated with defects in the epidermal barrier, including the intercellular lipid layers, cornified envelope, and keratin proteins. These defects result in increased production of stratum corneum (scaling) characteristic of the disease and can result in an increased prevalence of secondary infections. Recently, molecular defects similar to those in the human ichthyoses have been identified as a cause of some forms of ichthyoses in cattle and dogs.

In cattle, two forms of the disease have been described; both are thought to have an autosomal recessive mode of inheritance. One (ichthyosis fetalis) is lethal, and most calves are stillborn or die within days of birth. Ichthyosis fetalis markedly resembles harlequin ichthyosis in human infants. Defects in a gene (*ABCA12*, a member of the adenosine triphosphate [ATP]-binding cassette family) have been identified as a cause of harlequin ichthyosis. The *ABCA12* gene is involved in the production of a protein necessary for lipid transfer in lamellar granules, a process required for formation of intercellular lipid layers and epidermal barrier structure and function. Because of barrier dysfunction, infants with harlequin ichthyosis develop excessive loss of fluids (dehydration) and life-threatening infections in the first few weeks of life. A loss of functional ABCA12 protein disrupts the normal development of the epidermis, resulting in the hard, thick scales characteristic of harlequin ichthyosis. Recently a mutation in *ABCA12* has been identified in Chianina cattle, one of the breeds of cattle known to develop ichthyosis fetalis, confirming the similarity of the genetic defect for the disease in cattle and human beings. Grossly, thick cornified plaques separated by fissures cover the skin in affected calves. Fissuring of the skin can lead to exudation of protein and secondary bacterial and fungal infections that often lead to death or euthanasia. The ears may be small, and there may be eversion of the eyelids, lips, and other mucocutaneous junctional areas. Microscopically, the epidermis is thickened by marked compact hyperkeratosis with variable parakeratosis. The follicular infundibulum is also affected, and stratum corneum surrounds entrapped hairs. In the less severe form of ichthyosis in cattle (ichthyosis congenita), the molecular defect has not been identified. Lesions may be mild at birth and progress with age. The skin becomes thickened, folded, and covered by plate-like scales separated by shallow fissures in which hairs are entrapped. More severe lesions are seen where hair is shorter, particularly on the limbs, abdomen, and nose. Microscopically, the epidermal surface is wrinkled, variably thickened by acanthosis, and covered by prominent laminated orthokeratotic hyperkeratosis.

Ichthyosis in dogs is usually divided into two basic subtypes, epidermolytic and nonepidermolytic, based on the presence or absence of vacuolization of the keratinocytes of the superficial stratum spinosum and granulosum in conjunction with hyperkeratosis. The molecular basis of canine ichthyosis rarely has been investigated; however, recently transglutaminase 1–deficient recessive lamellar ichthyosis, an autosomal recessive inherited disorder in Jack Russell terrier dogs, has been described. The disease is nonepidermolytic and resembles lamellar ichthyosis in human beings, which is associated with defects in the cornified cell envelope and is caused by mutations in the transglutaminase 1 gene. Transglutaminases catalyze cross-linking of proteins that form the cornified envelope. Clinical lesions in Jack Russell terriers include generalized adherent and loosely attached scales, as well as large, adherent white or tan scales in sparsely haired skin (Fig. 17-58). Pawpads are moderately hyperkeratotic, and claws are soft. Secondary infection with coccoid bacteria and yeast are common, likely the result of the epidermal barrier defect. Histologic lesions consist of laminated to compact hyperkeratosis of the epidermis and follicular infundibulum without epidermolysis. Secondary infections result in inflammation. Ultrastructurally, many layers of corneocytes are present. Corneocytes have irregular margins and linear or oval lamellar inclusions and in comparison to control animals, thin or less prominent cornified envelopes.

Perhaps the most common form of nonepidermolytic hyperkeratosis in dogs occurs in young, otherwise healthy golden retrievers. The mode of inheritance is autosomal recessive, and the genetic defect is due to a mutation in the PNPLA1 gene. The protein encoded by this gene belongs to the patatin-like phospholipase (PNPLA) family, and is important in lipid metabolism. A genetic test is available that can detect carriers (heterozygous for the mutation) as well as affected dogs (homozygous for the mutation). PNPLA1 is important in formation of the epidermal lipid barrier. Clinical lesions vary in severity and consist of large flat scales on the surface of the skin and within the hair coat. Pawpads and nasal planum are not affected. Histologic lesions consist of mild to

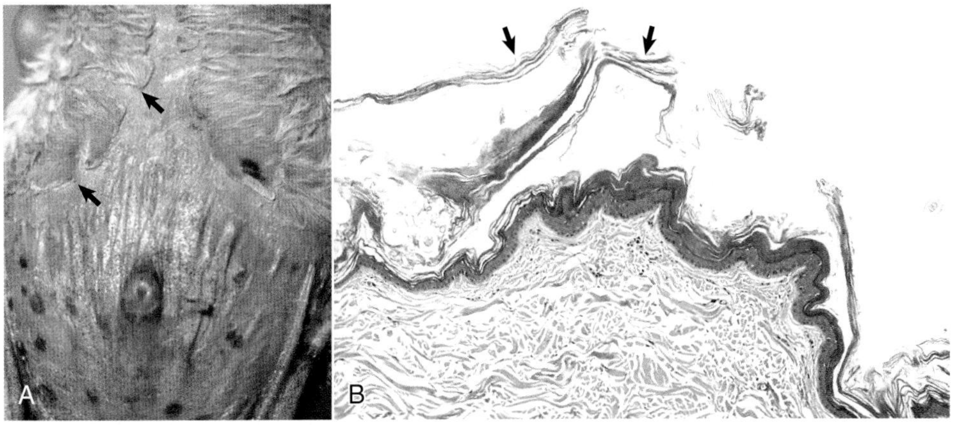

Figure 17-58 Ichthyosis, Skin, Dog. A, Abdomen. The skin is covered with adherent plates of scale *(arrows)*, and the skin surface is wrinkled. **B,** Compact hyperkeratosis is present. Plates of stratum corneum are separating from each other and are lifting off the surface *(arrows)*. H&E stain. (**A** courtesy Dr. D. Lewis, College of Veterinary Medicine, University of Florida. **B** courtesy Dr. A.M. Hargis, DermatoDiagnostics.)

moderate compact orthokeratotic hyperkeratosis without epidermal acanthosis, epidermolysis, or dermal inflammation. Ultrastructurally, affected dogs have more cohesive corneocytes and more numerous corneodesmosomes, suggesting that the disorder may be caused by delayed degradation of corneodesmosomes.

The molecular basis of an autosomal recessive inherited form of epidermolytic hyperkeratosis recently has been described in Norfolk terrier dogs that have a mutation in the gene that encodes for keratin 10 (*KRT10*). Similar histologic lesions have been seen in a few other breeds of dogs (Fig. 17-59). This condition is similar to epidermolytic hyperkeratosis in human beings, caused by defects in keratin proteins 1 and 10. Keratin intermediate filaments are important structural proteins in the epidermis, and defects can be associated with irregular keratin filament aggregation and loss of strength, resulting in disruption of keratinocytes, especially in association with trauma. In Norfolk terrier dogs the clinical lesions include scaling and epidermal fragility, and the superficial epidermis can slough after mild mechanical trauma. Pigmented scaling, especially in intertriginous areas, is present. Pawpads, claws, and hair are normal. Histologically, there is papillary epidermal hyperplasia with minimal to moderate hyperkeratosis, large keratohyalin granules, and disruption (epidermolysis) and clefting of granular cell keratinocytes (see Fig. 17-59). Ultrastructurally, keratinocytes in the upper stratum spinosum and granulosum have a reduction of tonofilaments and abnormal filament aggregation.

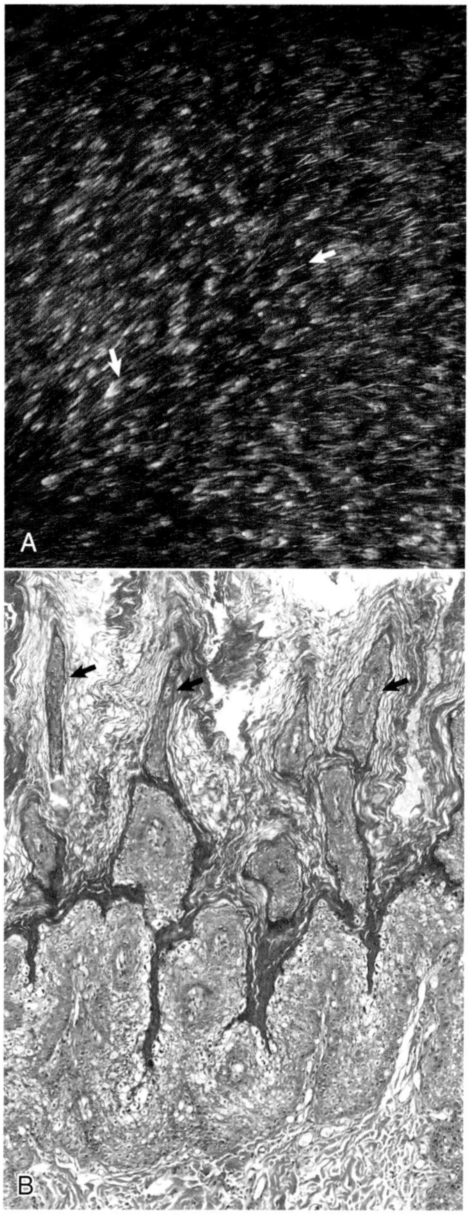

Figure 17-59 Epidermolytic Hyperkeratosis, Skin, Dog. A, Lateral thorax of Rhodesian ridgeback. There are fronds of keratin adherent to hairs (*arrows*). **B,** Papillary epidermal hyperplasia with disruption and clefting of the granular layer and large keratohyalin granules. The papillary hyperplasia with epidermal papillae and hyperkeratosis (*arrows*) contribute to the accumulation of keratin attached to the hairs in this breed of dog. H&E stain. (Courtesy Dr. A.M. Hargis, DermatoDiagnostics.)

Sebaceous Adenitis. Sebaceous adenitis, inflammation of sebaceous glands, occurs most commonly in dogs, rarely is seen in cats, and has been reported in one horse. Two basic types of clinical appearances of sebaceous adenitis have been reported in the dog and include the type seen in long-coated breeds and the type seen in short-coated breeds, but due to the distinctly different clinical presentation of lesions in the short-haired breeds of dogs, it has been suggested that sebaceous adenitis in these breeds is a separate entity. More commonly affected long-haired breeds include the standard poodle, Akita, English springer spaniel, Havanese, German shepherd, and Samoyed, but many other breeds may be affected. More commonly affected short-haired breeds include the vizsla, miniature pinscher, beagle, and dachshund. The cause and pathogenesis are uncertain, but an inherited component of the disease is proposed for the standard poodle and Akita. Immunohistologic studies have shown a predominance of antigen-presenting dendritic cells and T lymphocytes in areas of sebaceous gland inflammation, suggesting a cell-mediated immunopathogenesis. Clinical lesion severity and location vary between breeds of dogs, but in long-haired breeds, scaling with formation of fronds of keratin adherent to hair shafts (follicular casts) and a progressively poor, dry, brittle hair coat are consistently present. Hair loss often begins in more cranial and dorsal regions, but the tail may be severely affected in some cases. The hair coat may become lighter or darker, and in poodles hairs that develop after disease onset are wavy or straight rather than tightly curled (see Fig. 17-30). Secondary bacterial folliculitis and otitis externa commonly develop. In the short-haired breeds of dogs, clinical lesions develop on the trunk and occasionally face and consist of focal, firm plaques and nodules with alopecia and adherent scale that may expand and coalesce. Hair casts may be present, but secondary bacterial folliculitis is rare. In some instances edematous swellings of the face or severe pinnal ulceration may develop, which are not a feature of the disease in long-haired breeds and suggest the short-haired form of sebaceous adenitis is a different entity. Cats have multifocal, circular areas of hair loss, scaling, crusting, and follicular keratin casts that begin on the head, pinnae, and neck and spread caudally. Progressive patches of nonpruritic scaling, crusting, alopecia, and leukoderma are reported in the horse. The reason scaling and alopecia develop in association with loss of sebaceous glands is speculative. Microscopic lesions include lymphocytes, neutrophils, and macrophages that efface sebaceous glands and sometimes form microscopic granulomas (see Fig. 17-30), and in some dogs, extensive orthokeratotic hyperkeratosis. Chronically affected dogs have no remaining sebaceous glands, but mild residual inflammation and fibrosis are present in the perifollicular dermis near the isthmus (site normally occupied by sebaceous glands). Sebaceous gland inflammation or loss can occur in other conditions such as folliculitis, demodicosis, uveodermatologic syndrome, or leishmaniasis, in which the inflammation primarily targets other areas of the skin (follicles, epidermal cells, or dermis) and involves the neighboring sebaceous glands because of their proximity to the inflammation. Thus these conditions are histologic differential diagnoses for sebaceous adenitis predominantly in dogs.

Hyperkeratosis of Nasal Planum or Pawpads in Dogs. See Disorders of Dogs.

Predominant Follicular Hyperkeratosis (Comedones)

Comedones (see Table 17-6) occur in numerous skin disorders, including those associated with surface trauma (callus, solar dermatosis), endocrine dermatosis (especially hyperadrenocorticism), nutritional or inherited disorders of cornification (primary seborrhea, vitamin A–responsive dermatosis), and in some disorders associated with follicular infection (especially demodicosis). In addition, comedones are prominent in three conditions wherein the comedones are considered a major feature of the disease.

Schnauzer Comedo Syndrome. See Disorders of Dogs.

Canine Interdigital Palmar and Plantar Comedones and Follicular Cysts. See Disorders of Dogs.

Acne. Feline acne develops in the skin of the chin, lower lip, and less commonly upper lip. Cats of a variety of ages, sexes, and coat lengths are affected. The cause and pathogenesis are unclear, but defects in follicular cornification and poor grooming habits have been suggested. Gross lesions consist of comedones that can progress to papules, crusts, nodules, and diffuse swelling. Histologic lesions begin as mild follicular hyperkeratosis and progress to comedones, which can become secondarily infected by bacteria, result in folliculitis, follicular rupture (furunculosis), and localized to diffuse dermatitis, panniculitis, and cellulitis. *M. pachydermatis* may contribute to cases of chin acne that are refractory to therapy.

Canine acne is a chronic disorder that develops in the skin of the chin and lips of young dogs, usually with short hair coats. The cause of the disorder is not known, but a follicular cornification disorder has not been definitively documented. Early lesions consist of follicular papules and comedones that with time enlarge to nodules that can ulcerate and drain. Histologically, early lesions consist of moderate to marked follicular hyperkeratosis (the papules and comedones) and later of folliculitis, furunculosis, and draining sinuses (the nodular, ulcerated, and draining lesions).

Predominant Epidermal Hyperplasia (Lichenification or Crusts)

Equine Coronary Band Dystrophy. See Disorders of Horses.

Porcine Juvenile Pustular Psoriasiform Dermatitis (Pityriasis Rosea). See Disorders of Pigs.

Secondary Seborrhea. Secondary seborrhea is not a primary disorder of cornification; however, it clinically resembles the primary cornification disorders (dry exfoliative or greasy adherent scales) and thus needs to be differentiated from them. Secondary seborrhea is common and is caused by a variety of unrelated cutaneous disorders such as allergy; ectoparasitism; bacterial, demodectic, and fungal infections; dietary deficiency; endocrine disease; and internal diseases. The lesions of secondary seborrhea resolve completely if the underlying disease is eliminated. Microscopic changes include epidermal and follicular hyperkeratosis with or without parakeratosis plus the lesions associated with the underlying disease.

Disorders of Pigmentation

Melanocytes produce melanin pigments that are responsible for the coloration of the hair, skin, and eyes and play an important role in photoprotection. In addition, melanocytes are also present in the inner ear, where they function to control ion transport and the function of the inner ear, and the absence of melanocytes can result in deafness. Melanin is synthesized by melanocytes, which are dendritic cells originating as melanoblasts in the neural crest. Melanoblasts develop in the neural crest and migrate to peripheral sites, including the basal and lower spinous layers of the epidermis, hair follicles, and dermis. Melanoblasts differentiate into melanocytes and synthesize melanosomes and melanin. Tyrosinase, a copper-containing enzyme, plays a critical role in the synthesis of melanin. Genetic mutations affecting any of the steps in the formation of melanin can lead to hereditary hypopigmentation. Many types of exogenous influences, such as inflammation, UVR, endocrinopathies, autoimmune diseases, and nutritional status, can affect melanocytes in the skin, resulting in acquired hypopigmentation or hyperpigmentation.

Hypopigmentation

Disorders associated with reduced pigment can (1) be inherited or acquired, (2) involve skin or hair, (3) be generalized or localized, or (4) be idiopathic or linked with other diseases. Reduction in pigmentation of the skin is leukoderma and of the hair is leukotrichia. Leukoderma and leukotrichia can occur independently. They can result from a decrease in melanin (hypomelanosis), a complete absence of melanin (amelanosis), or from a loss of existing melanin (depigmentation). These events result either from an absence of the pigment-synthesizing melanocytes or from a failure of melanocytes to produce normal amounts of melanin or to transfer it to adjacent keratinocytes. Because copper is a component of tyrosinase, production of melanin pigment depends on copper; thus copper deficiency can result in reduced pigmentation.

Inherited Hypopigmentation. Hereditary hypopigmentation can be divided into hypomelanocytic/amelanocytic hypomelanosis, characterized by a reduction in or absence of melanocytes in affected areas, and hypomelanotic/amelanotic hypomelanosis, in which melanocytes are present but defective. Hypopigmentation can be localized, focally extensive, or generalized. Mutations that cause hypopigmentation can interfere with melanocytes at specific points in their development and function leading to specific syndromes, including: (1) melanoblast migrations (Waardenburg syndrome, piebaldism), (2) melanin synthesis in the melanosome (oculocutaneous albinism), (3) melanosome formation within melanocytes (Chédiak-Higashi syndrome), and (4) mature melanosome transfer to the tips of the dendrites (Griscelli syndrome in human beings as has been suggested for color-associated follicular dysplasia in Münsterländer dogs and possibly other dog breeds). Failure of melanocytes to migrate, differentiate, and survive can result in deafness, and thus animals with Waardenburg-like syndrome or piebaldism may be deaf.

Syndromes analogous to the human Waardenburg syndromes have been reported in horses, dogs, and cats. In this hypomelanocytic disorder, there is failure of melanoblasts to migrate from the neural crest to the skin, eye, and inner ear or failure to survive in those locations. Affected animals typically have white coats and blue or heterochromatic irides and are deaf. In dogs this syndrome has been described in breeds such as the Dalmatian, bull terrier, Sealyham terrier, collie, and Great Dane. In horses and dogs the condition is inherited as an autosomal dominant trait with incomplete penetrance. In the cat the inheritance is autosomal dominant with complete penetrance for the loss of pigmentation and an incomplete penetrance for the inner ear degeneration.

Overo lethal white foal syndrome, analogous to human Waardenburg syndrome type 4 (Hirschsprung's disease), has been reported in American paint horses in which white foals from the breeding of two overo spotted paint horses are born with aganglionic colons. The condition has autosomal recessive inheritance and is the result of a genetic mutation in the endothelin signaling pathway, which is critical for correct development and migration of neural crest cells. Neural crest cells give rise to melanocytes and enteric neurons. These foals develop colic from greatly distended colons and die or are euthanized shortly after birth.

Piebaldism is also a form of genetic hypomelanocytic hypomelanosis resulting in multifocal white patches in which there is an absence of melanocytes because of either a congenital failure of melanoblasts to migrate from the neural crest to the skin or their inability to survive and proliferate in the skin. Piebaldism has been seen in many species, including horses, cattle, dogs such as the Dalmatian, and cats.

The various forms of albinism are examples of hypomelanotic hypomelanosis. In albino animals and human beings, melanocytes are present and normally distributed but are defective in function and fail to synthesize melanin. The extent of the biochemical defect varies, so that albinism covers a spectrum from amelanosis, oculocutaneous albinism, through graded pigmentary dilution. Oculocutaneous albinisms and pigment dilutions are inherited as autosomal recessive traits associated with a variety of gene mutations. A partial gene deletion of *SLC45A2* has been reported to cause oculocutaneous albinism in Doberman pinscher dogs that develop melanomas in the skin, lips, eyelids, and iris.

Chédiak-Higashi syndrome in human beings; Hereford, Brangus, and Japanese black cattle; Persian cats; and various other animal species is an example of partial albinism and is inherited as an autosomal recessive trait. Although melanin is produced, there is a mutation of the beige gene, which plays a major role in generating cellular organelles. This results in a membrane defect leading to the formation of giant melanosomes that are transferred with difficulty to the keratinocytes. The clumping of these giant melanosomes produces the color dilution effect. Chédiak-Higashi syndrome is discussed with the hematopoietic system (see Chapter 13).

Cyclic hematopoiesis (cyclic neutropenia), a lethal hereditary disease of collie dogs, is caused by a mutation in the canine *AP3B1* gene, which results in decreased neutrophil elastase enzymatic activity. This is an autosomal recessive genetic disorder with a pleiotropic effect on coat color dilution. Affected dogs are silver-gray. The abnormal hair pigmentation results from the diminished formation of melanin from its precursor tyrosine rather than from pigment clumping. The normal collie coat color is partially restored in animals receiving bone marrow transplants to correct cyclic hematopoiesis. The hematologic aspects of this disease are considered in the discussion on the hematopoietic system in Chapter 13.

Coat color dilution has been reported in many species. It occurs in many breeds of horses, cattle, dogs, and cats but is particularly common in Siamese cats. Clumping of large melanin granules in hair shafts and hair matrix cells is responsible for the pale coat coloration. Similarly clumped melanin granules occur in epidermal melanocytes. In cats, dilute coat color is thought to be a result of an autosomal recessive trait (Maltese dilution) due to a single-base deletion in melanophilin. One or more mutations within or near the melanophilin gene are also responsible for the coat color dilution in dogs.

Acquired Hypopigmentation. Acquired hypopigmentation follows damage to the epidermal melanin unit by various insults, including trauma, inflammation, radiation, contactants, endocrinopathies, infections, nutritional deficiencies, and neoplasia. In general the severity of the injury determines whether an insult will result in hypopigmentation or hyperpigmentation. Mild injury results in pigmentary incontinence and epidermal hypopigmentation from death of melanin-containing keratinocytes. However, hyperpigmentation can occur, possibly from release of melanocyte-stimulating factors from surviving keratinocytes and subsequent increase in production of melanosomes. It is thought that these factors are present in normal epidermis, but their level or activity is increased in response to stimulation or keratinocyte stress. In contrast, severe injury results in the death of melanocytes, which do not regenerate, and thus there is no repigmentation.

Vitiligo is a hypomelanocytic hypomelanosis of human beings and animals that is characterized by gradually expanding pale macules that are often symmetric or segmental in distribution. The immediate cause of vitiligo is the destruction of melanocytes. Theories regarding the pathogenesis of this disease include autoimmune destruction of melanocytes, a neurogenic theory involving release of a neurochemical from peripheral nerves that inhibits melanogenesis, a self-destruction theory that involves failure of protection of melanocytes against the toxic effects of melanin precursors, or a combination of factors. Vitiligo has been described in horses, cattle, dogs, and cats. The condition is best characterized in Belgian Tervuren dogs. The depigmentation in this breed occurs chiefly on the pigmented skin and mucous membranes of the face and mouth in young adult dogs. Histologic examination of affected skin reveals epidermis devoid of both pigment granules and DOPA-positive cells. Electron microscopy confirms the lack of melanocytes in the lesions, their place being taken by Langerhans or indeterminate dendritic cells.

Uveodermatologic syndrome (Vogt-Koyanagi-Harada [VKH]–like syndrome) is a rare syndrome of histiocytic interface dermatitis and granulomatous uveitis in dogs, particularly Akitas, Chow Chows, Samoyeds, Alaskan malamutes, and Siberian huskies. The strong breed associations suggest there is an inherited basis for this disease. In fact, in the Akita, specific dog leukocyte antigen (DLA) class II gene alleles appear to predispose to the development of this disease. The pathogenesis is thought to involve an immune-mediated attack against melanin or melanocytes, particularly a T helper lymphocyte cell-mediated immune attack against melanocyte antigens, but humoral immune responses may also play a role. Ocular lesions usually develop before cutaneous lesions and are more important because they may lead to blindness. Clinical lesions consist of symmetric patchy to diffuse depigmentation of the skin of the nose, lips, eyelids, scrotum or vulva, anal skin, ears, and pawpads. Lesions are occasionally more widespread. Leukotrichia of adjacent hair can be present. Uncommonly, lesions are more severe and consist of erosion, ulceration, and crusting. Fully developed histologic lesions are cell-rich interface inflammation, primarily of histiocytic cells containing melanin pigment (pigmentary incontinence). The inflammation occurs parallel to the epidermal surface but usually does not obscure the interface and may extend around adnexa. Basal cell degeneration is uncommon.

Cutaneous depigmentation in horses and dogs can result from contact with rubber. The monobenzene ether of hydroquinone, a common ingredient in rubber, inhibits melanogenesis. In horses, lesions result from contact with equipment such as rubber bit guards, crupper straps, or with feed buckets (lips, buttocks, and face). In dogs, lesions result from contact with rubber dishes or toys (lips or nose).

In dogs, hypopigmentation can occur in immune-mediated diseases targeting the dermal-epidermal interface, such as lupus erythematosus and dermatomyositis, and in association with neoplastic conditions, such as epitheliotropic lymphoma (mycosis fungoides). The hypopigmentation develops from injury and subsequent loss of the melanin-containing keratinocytes or melanocytes. Leukotrichia (depigmentation of hair) can be seen in the healing stage of alopecia areata, an immune-mediated condition characterized clinically by alopecia and microscopically by lymphocytic inflammation of the hair bulb.

Hyperpigmentation

Primary Hyperpigmentation

Hyperplastic (Lentigo) or Neoplastic (Melanoma) Lesions. See E-Table 17-3 and Box 17-12.

Acanthosis Nigricans. See Disorders of Dogs.

Secondary Hyperpigmentation. Hyperpigmentation can result from a wide range of stimuli, including inflammation, trauma, metabolic disorders, drug therapy (e.g., doxorubicin), subtotal injury to basal layer cells from irradiation, moderate heat, or immune-mediated disorders, and some conditions for which the cause is unknown (alopecia X). Consequently, hyperpigmentation is seen in all species with epidermal melanin pigment. Hypermelanosis results from an increased rate of melanosome production, an increase in melanosome size, or an increase in the degree of melanization of the melanosome. It is usually associated with an accelerated melanocyte turnover with an increased number of melanosomes.

Miscellaneous Skin Disorders

Disorders Characterized by Infiltrates of Eosinophils or Plasma Cells

Disorders characterized by infiltrates of eosinophils or plasma cells are listed in Box 17-13. In addition to the syndromes discussed herein, eosinophils are often a prominent feature of hypersensitivity or parasitic dermatoses, especially in cats and horses, and are also often a feature in feline herpesvirus dermatitis.

Eosinophilic Plaques. See Disorders of Cats.

Eosinophilic Granulomas (Collagenolytic Granulomas). Eosinophilic and granulomatous lesions with brightly eosinophilic, granular to amorphous material bordering collagen fibers and somewhat obscuring the fiber detail (flame figures) occur in horses, dogs, and cats. The causes of these syndromes are poorly understood. The tinctorial change can develop in any lesion with large numbers of eosinophils such as reactions to parasites, foreign bodies (including hair), or in mast cell tumors and in some cases of cutaneous lymphoma. Eosinophils congregate and degranulate near collagen bundles, causing the tinctorial change. Eosinophil degranulation results in release of a wide range of toxic granule proteins (e.g., major basic protein), enzymes (peroxidase, collagenase), cytokines (IL-3, IL-5, granulocyte-macrophage colony-stimulating factor [GM-CSF]), chemokines (IL-8), and lipid mediators (leukotrienes and platelet-activating factor) augmenting an inflammatory response. Gross lesions include papules, nodules, plaques (sometimes linear), and ulcers in the skin (see Fig. 17-22). Nodular or ulcerated lesions can also develop in the oral mucosa of dogs and cats and in the pawpads of cats. Microscopically, nodular dermatitis (or stomatitis) consists of an inflammatory response with a prominence of eosinophils, flame figures, and macrophages, some of which are multinucleated (see Fig. 17-22). Collagen lysis develops in some lesions, likely a secondary event caused by the proteolytic enzymes (e.g., collagenase). Some indolent ulcers on the upper lip of cats have areas of flame figures and granulomatous inflammation and are considered to be eosinophilic granulomas.

Eosinophilic Furunculosis of the Face in Dogs. See Disorders of Dogs.

Hypereosinophilic Syndromes with Systemic Signs or Lesions

Multisystemic Eosinophilic Epitheliotropic Disease in the Horse. See Disorders of Horses.

Feline Hypereosinophilic Syndrome. See Disorders of Cats.

Eosinophilic Dermatitis with Edema in the Dog. See Disorders of Dogs.

Plasma Cell Pododermatitis. See Disorders of Cats.

Nodular Granulomatous Inflammatory Disorders without Microorganisms

Nodular granulomatous inflammatory disorders without microorganisms are listed in Box 17-14. The diseases in this category have traditionally been considered to be sterile because no microorganisms have been identified by microscopic examination, including with special stains or IHC for organisms, by electron microscopic examination, by cultures, or by cytologic evaluation for organisms. However, newer techniques, including PCR that detects minute amounts of DNA, suggest the potential for microbial participation in the pathogenesis of some of these seemingly sterile inflammatory disorders, especially in human beings. It is possible, for instance, for an abnormal immune response to an as yet unidentified microbial antigen to initiate a macrophage-dominated inflammatory response. Defective downregulation of the immune response to the organism could lead to a persistent granulomatous inflammatory process. Currently this issue remains unresolved, but as more of these lesions are probed for microbial agents, a better understanding of these so-called sterile inflammatory disorders will hopefully develop. It is considered important, when possible, to use newer techniques such as PCR in these cases before considering them to be sterile.

Juvenile Sterile Granulomatous Dermatitis and Lymphadenitis (Juvenile Cellulitis, Juvenile Pyoderma, Puppy Strangles). See Disorders of Dogs.

Idiopathic Sterile Granuloma and Pyogranuloma (Sterile Pyogranuloma Syndrome). Idiopathic sterile granuloma and pyogranuloma, or sterile pyogranuloma syndrome, are seen most commonly in dogs and rarely horses and cats, are of unknown cause, and are characterized grossly by single or multifocal papules, plaques, or nodules most commonly in the skin of the head and extremities. Early microscopic lesions include periadnexal to coalescing nodular accumulations of leukocytes predominantly consisting of macrophages (histiocytes), neutrophils, and lymphocytes. Organized granulomas and pyogranulomas are present. Older lesions can efface adnexa and extend into the subcutis. Neither microorganisms nor foreign material are found microscopically, and cultures and cytologic evaluation for organisms are negative. The lesions must be differentiated from those of the infectious granulomatous disorders and reactive histiocytosis in dogs.

Canine Reactive Histiocytosis. See Disorders of Dogs.

Canine Langerhans Cell Histiocytosis. See Disorders of Dogs.

Text continued on p. 1111

Box 17-12 Examples of Tumors of the Skin

ECTODERMAL TUMORS

Trichoblastoma

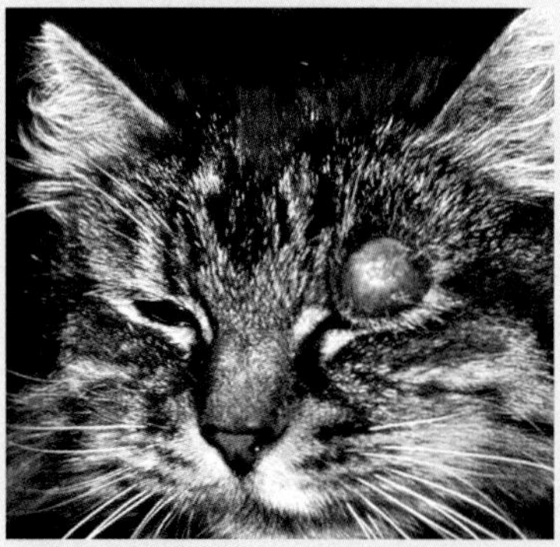

Trichoblastoma, skin, upper eyelid and dorsal to eye, cat. The tumor is circumscribed, raised, and sparsely haired. The tumor and bordering skin can be easily moved from side to side above the deeper tissue because the tumor has not invaded underlying tissue.*

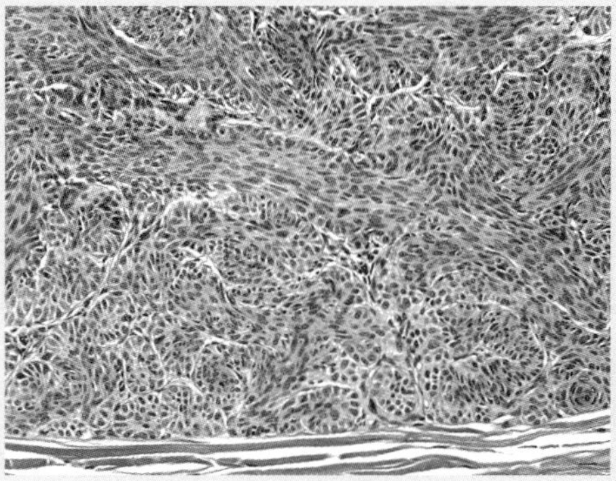

Trichoblastoma, skin, cat. A circumscribed tumor of presumed primitive hair germ origin arranged in irregular aggregates. Some of the trichoblasts are elongate (spindle-shaped), a feature of some trichoblastomas in cats. H&E stain.†

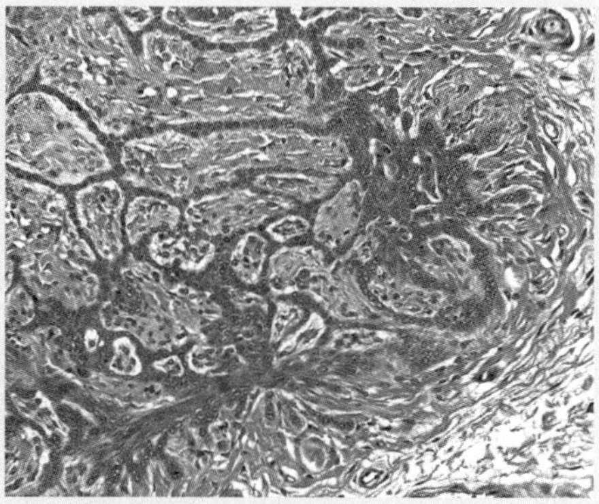

Trichoblastoma skin, dog. Note ribbon (medusoid) pattern produced by the proliferating basal cells. This pattern is one of several patterns (ribbon, trabecular, granular cell, spindle cell) typical of trichoblastomas in dogs. H&E stain.‡

Infundibular Keratinizing Acanthoma

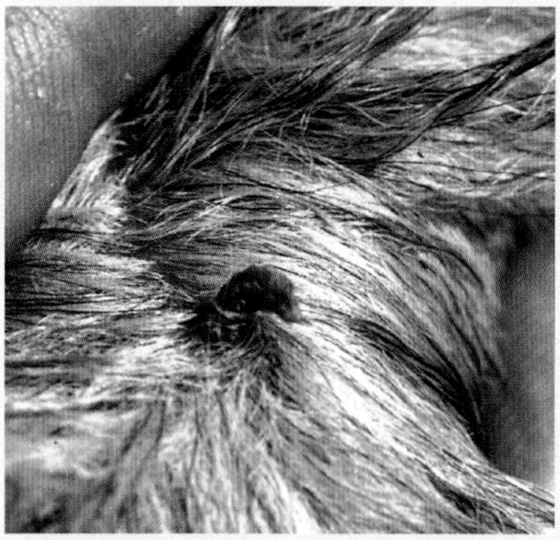

Infundibular keratinizing acanthoma (intracutaneous cornifying epithelioma, keratoacanthoma), skin, dog. Note horny growth (cutaneous horn) projecting from surface of the tumor. Cutaneous horns can arise from a variety of benign or malignant epidermal lesions (viral papilloma, solar keratosis; see Fig. 17-41, *B*, squamous cell carcinoma) or adnexal lesions, especially infundibular keratinizing acanthomas.§

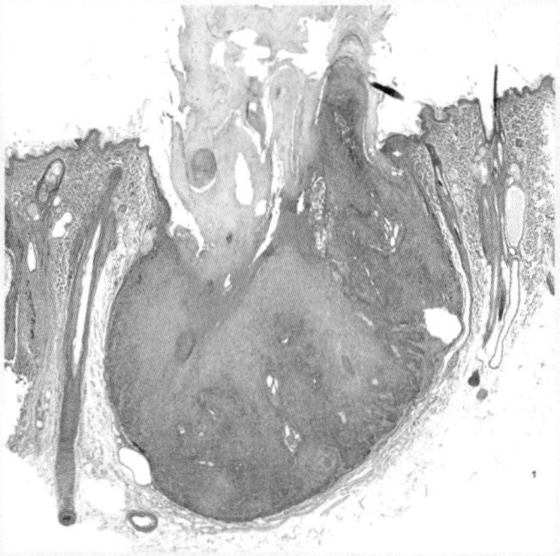

Infundibular keratinizing acanthoma, skin, dog. Note the circumscribed tumor located in the dermis and subcutis. The tumor consists of irregularly sized lobules of stratified squamous cornifying epithelium supported by a small quantity of collagenous stroma. The tumor is often "cystic" and contains laminations of stratum corneum, which can extend through the epidermal surface and form a "cutaneous horn." The epithelium forming the lobules of the tumor blends with the overlying epidermis. H&E stain.

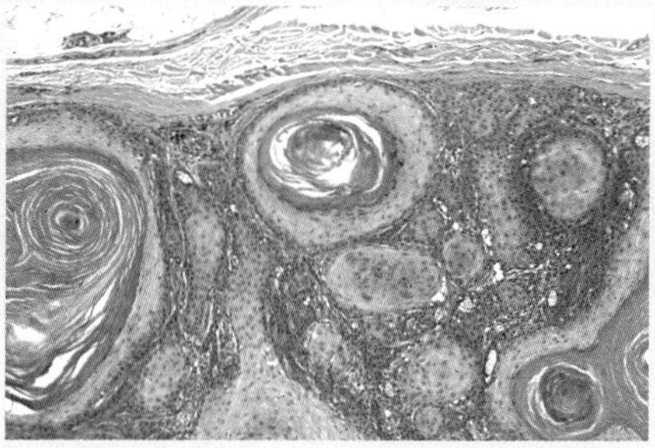

Infundibular keratinizing acanthoma, skin, dog. Infundibular keratinizing acanthoma, skin, higher magnification of wall of the tumor. The lobules border concentric laminations of stratum corneum and are supported by scant mucinous stroma. These tumors resemble squamous cell carcinoma but have a circumscribed, noninvasive border. H&E stain.

Box 17-12 Examples of Tumors of the Skin–cont'd

Sebaceous Gland Adenoma

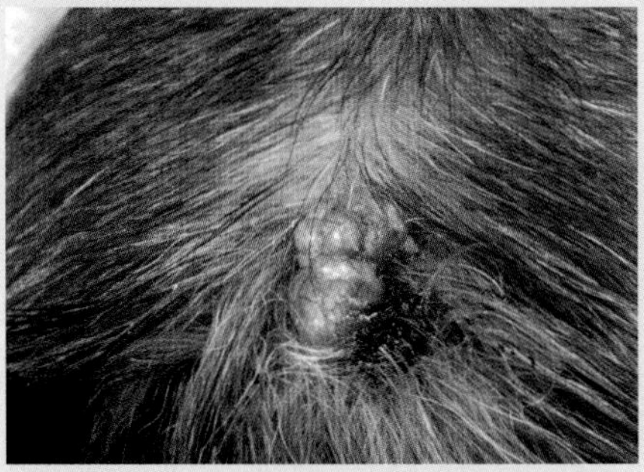

Sebaceous gland adenoma, skin, dog. This common tumor of sebaceous glands often protrudes above the epidermal surface. The tumors are hairless, greasy, and may be shiny due to the sebaceous gland secretion.

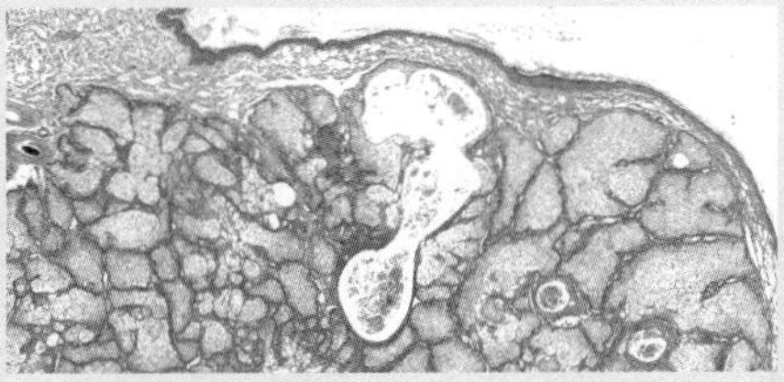

Sebaceous gland adenoma, skin, dog. Lobules of well-differentiated sebaceous glands are present in the dermis and cause polypoid elevation of the overlying epidermis. A duct with sebaceous secretion is also present. H&E stain.

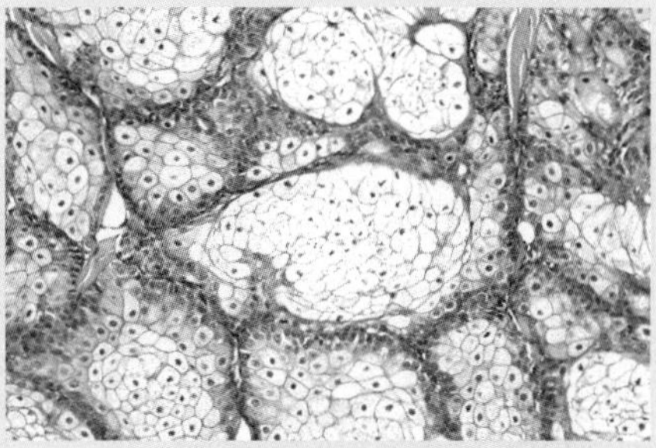

Sebaceous gland adenoma, skin, dog. Note the close resemblance of the lobules of tumor cells to those of nonneoplastic sebaceous glands, a feature suggesting benign behavior. H&E stain.

Squamous Cell Carcinoma

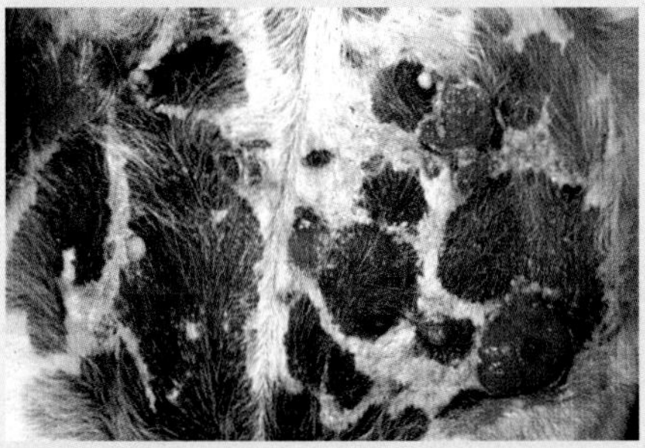

Squamous cell carcinomas, skin, abdomen, dog. Note multiple ulcerated squamous cell carcinomas in nonpigmented, sparsely haired abdominal skin. These are solar-induced squamous cell carcinomas that developed in a beagle dog living outdoors in a high-altitude region where the level of UV light from the sun is increased.

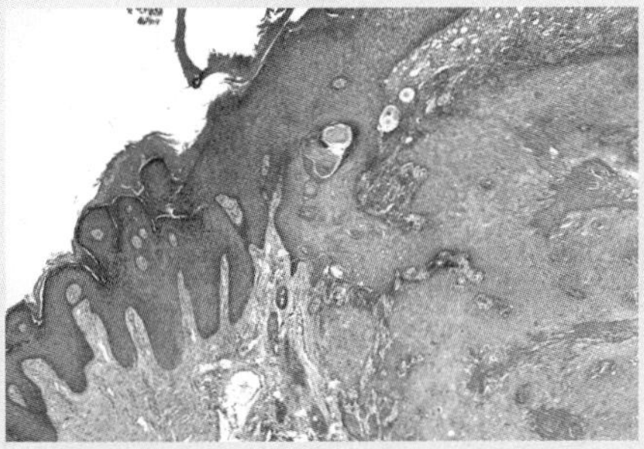

Squamous cell carcinoma, skin, dog. Neoplastic cells that have arisen from the epidermis *(above center)* have invaded the dermis and formed irregular islands of cells with squamous differentiation. H&E stain.†

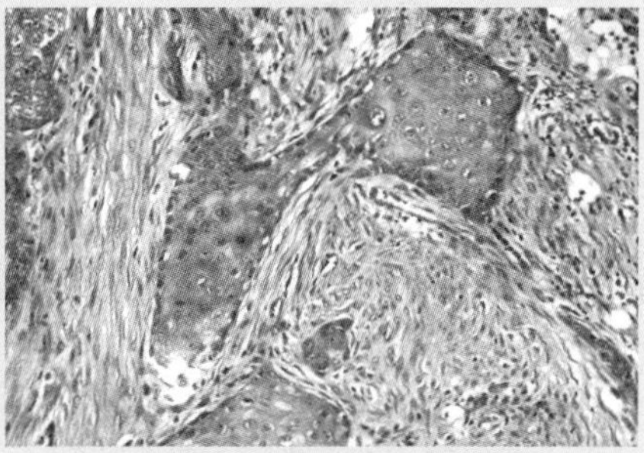

Squamous cell carcinoma, skin, dog. Islands of neoplastic cells with squamous differentiation have invaded the dermis and are surrounded by proliferating fibroblasts and collagen (desmoplasia). H&E stain.†

MESODERMAL TUMORS

Cutaneous Histiocytoma

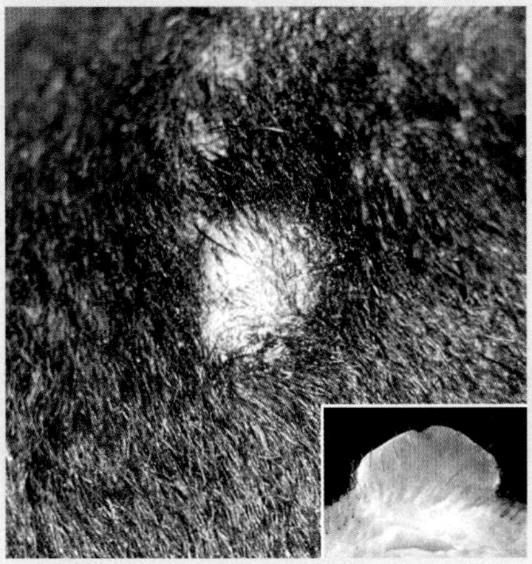

Cutaneous histiocytoma, skin, nose, dog. Circular raised alopecic tan nodule is present. Cutaneous histiocytomas frequently spontaneously regress. *Inset,* Section of cutaneous histiocytoma illustrating the nonencapsulated, solid dermal mass protruding above the epidermal surface.

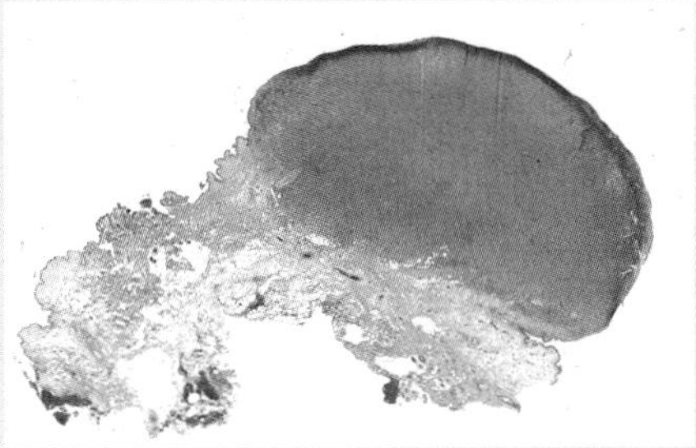

Cutaneous histiocytoma, skin, dog. The histiocytoma elevates the epidermal surface and consists of a solid mass of histiocytic cells. H&E stain.†

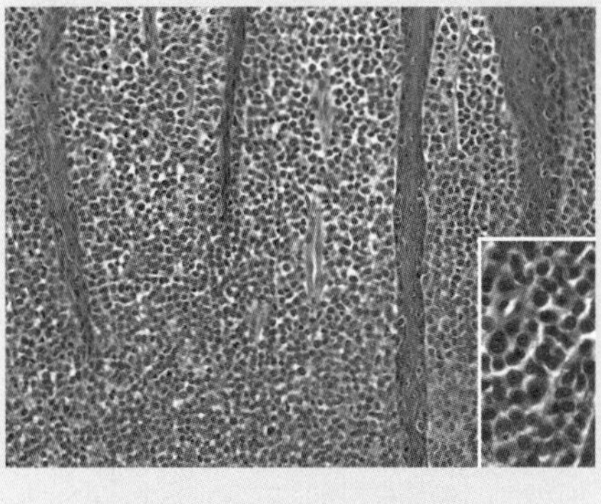

Cutaneous histiocytoma, skin, dog. Note the polyhedral to round cells in the dermis and the elongated down-growth of the epidermis (epidermal pegs) into the histiocytoma (a common feature of these tumors). *Inset,* Higher magnification of the histiocytic cells. H&E stain.

Continued

Box 17-12 Examples of Tumors of the Skin–cont'd

Cutaneous Lymphoma

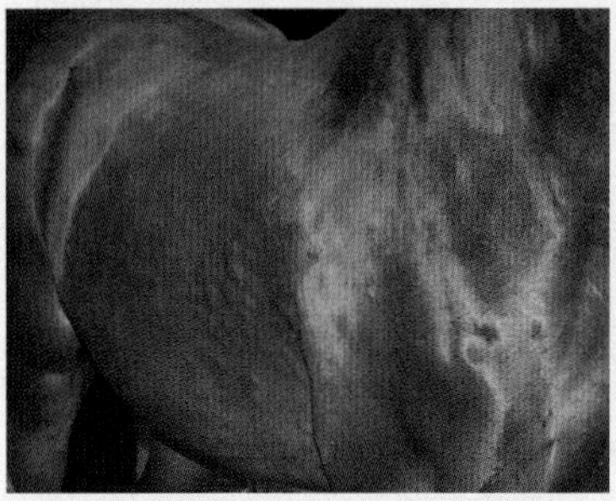

Cutaneous lymphoma, skin, neck, and lateral thorax, horse. Note the nodules that are masses of neoplastic lymphocytes and infiltrating nonneoplastic lymphocytes in the dermis, causing elevation of overlying epidermis.‖

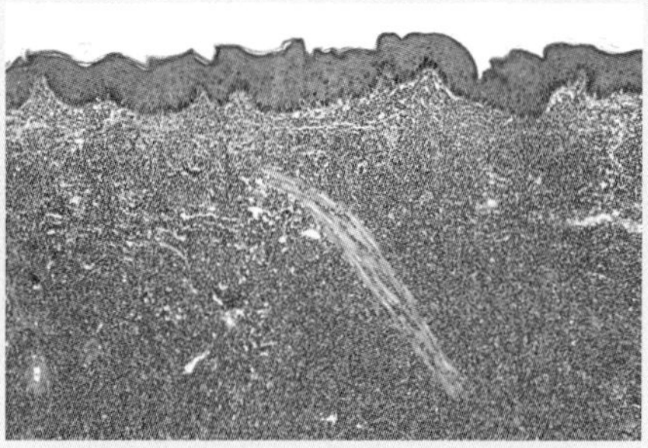

Cutaneous lymphoma, skin, horse. Sheets of neoplastic lymphocytes and infiltrating nonneoplastic lymphocytes have obliterated the normal dermal architecture except for an arrector pili muscle *(center)*. The overlying epidermis is normal. H&E stain.

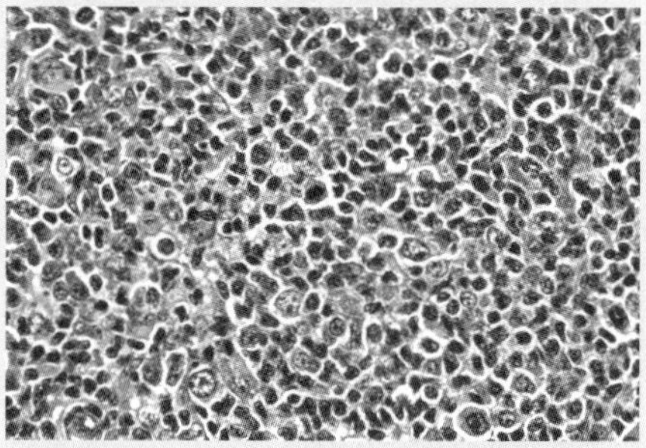

Cutaneous lymphoma, skin, horse. Note the population of different-appearing lymphoid cells. Some resemble normal lymphocytes and are small and well differentiated, whereas others are large and pleomorphic with vesicular nuclei and prominent nucleoli. Immunohistochemical and genetic studies of many cases of cutaneous lymphoma in the horse have demonstrated that the small well-differentiated lymphocytes are nonneoplastic T lymphocytes, whereas the large pleomorphic lymphocytes are neoplastic B lymphocytes. It is speculated that the neoplastic B lymphocytes produce cytokines that lead to infiltrates of nonneoplastic T lymphocytes and sometimes other leukocytes. Cutaneous lymphoma in the horse with these morphologic features and immunophenotype is referred to as a T lymphocyte–rich large B lymphocyte lymphoma subtype. H&E stain.

Epitheliotropic Lymphoma

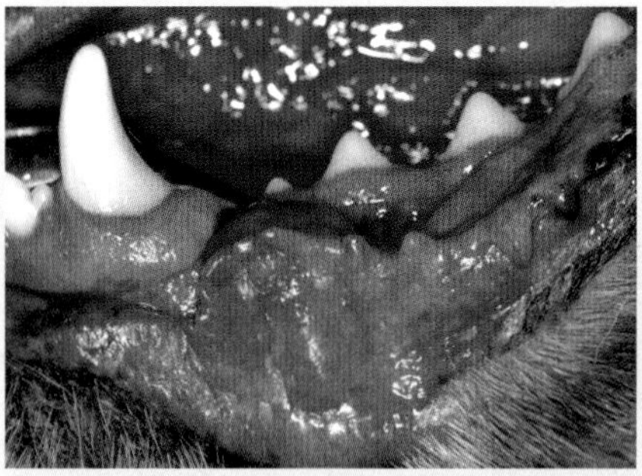

Epitheliotropic lymphoma, skin of lip and oral mucosa, dog. Note swelling, erythema, and depigmentation. Lymphocytes invade the epithelium and can cause depigmentation by displacing and damaging pigment-containing epithelial cells and resident melanocytes of the basal region of the mucosa or epidermis. Because of the involvement of the oral mucosa and mucocutaneous junctions and the presence of depigmentation and sometimes erosions, epitheliotropic lymphoma can be clinically confused with immune-mediated diseases such as systemic lupus erythematosus.

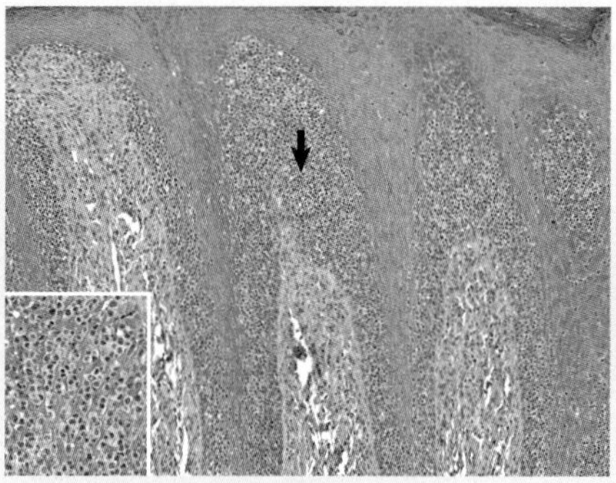

Epitheliotropic lymphoma, skin, pawpad, dog. In this case, neoplastic lymphocytes are located predominantly in the lower layers of the epidermis *(arrow)*. *Inset,* Higher magnification of the neoplastic lymphocytes in the epidermis. Some of the lymphocytes are clustered together, forming microabscesses (Pautrier's microabscesses). H&E stain.

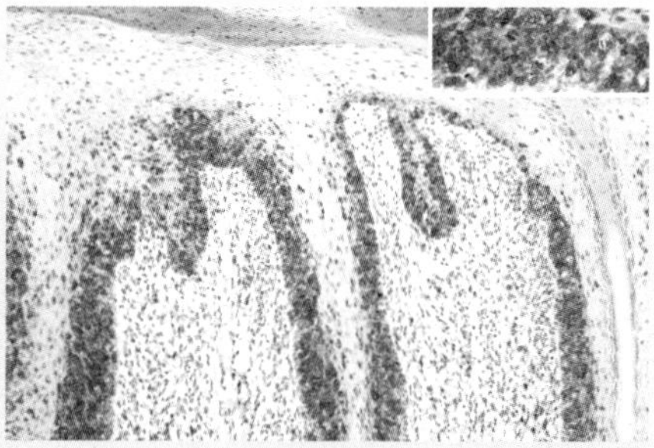

Epitheliotropic lymphoma, skin, pawpad, dog. Neoplastic lymphocytes are located predominantly in the lower layers of the epidermis and are labeled for CD3 *(brown stain in this case)*, indicating that they are T lymphocytes. *Inset,* Higher magnification of the malignant lymphocytes in the epidermis. Immunohistochemical stain for $CD3^+$ lymphocytes.

Box 17-12 Examples of Tumors of the Skin–cont'd

Mast Cell Tumor

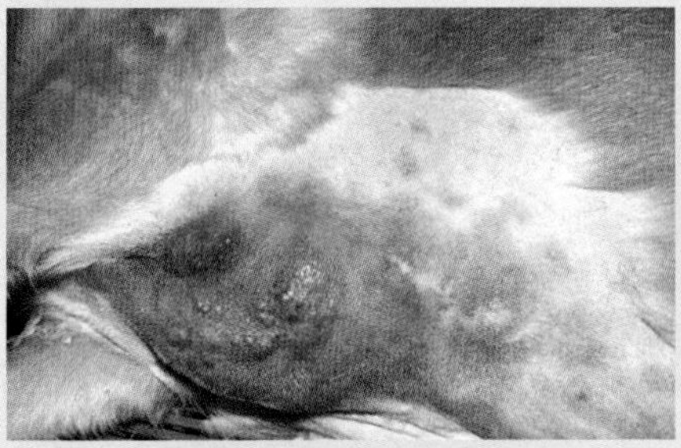

Mast cell tumor, skin, ventral thorax, dog. Note the irregular nodular and erythematous masses. Mast cell tumors in dogs can clinically resemble areas of inflammation because mast cells can degranulate and release inflammatory mediators (e.g., histamine, factors chemotactic for eosinophils and neutrophils, prostaglandins, serine esterases, and TNF-α) causing the inflammatory response.[||]

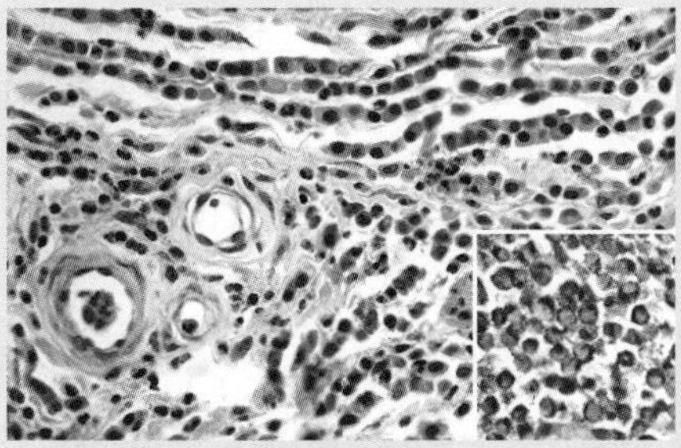

Mast cell tumor, skin, dog. The dermis is infiltrated by well-differentiated neoplastic mast cells with abundant gray to blue, finely granular cytoplasm and centrally located nuclei. H&E stain. *Inset,* Mast cells stained to illustrate metachromatic granules. In some cases it can be difficult to differentiate round cell tumors such as histiocytomas, lymphomas, plasma cell tumors, and mast cell tumors from each other. Demonstration of metachromatic cytoplasmic granules is an indicator of the presence of mast cells. Metachromasia means that the tissue or cellular component stains a color different from that of the staining dye because of a chemical reaction between the dye and the tissue component. For example, mast cell granules stain purple with the blue dye toluidine blue. Toluidine blue stain.[†]

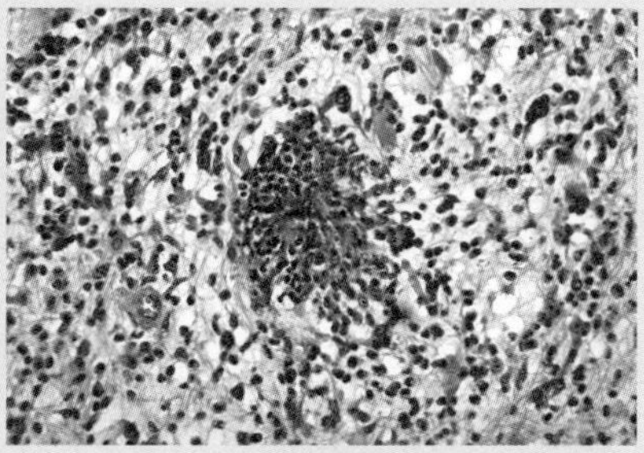

Mast cell tumor, skin, dog. Mast cell tumor with degranulated eosinophils that border a collagen fiber. The collagen fibers and bordering eosinophilic material have been referred to as *flame figures* in part because of their irregular, sometimes radiating, edges and brightly eosinophilic staining intensity. H&E stain.[†]

Fibrosarcoma

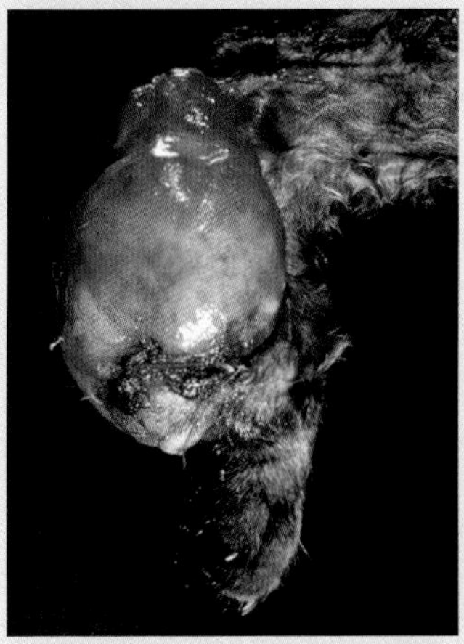

Fibrosarcoma, skin, leg, cat. The tumor has enlarged to such a degree that it has caused ulceration of the epidermis. Fibrosarcomas are locally invasive and difficult to excise completely. Limb amputation is an option for fibrosarcomas located on distal extremities.

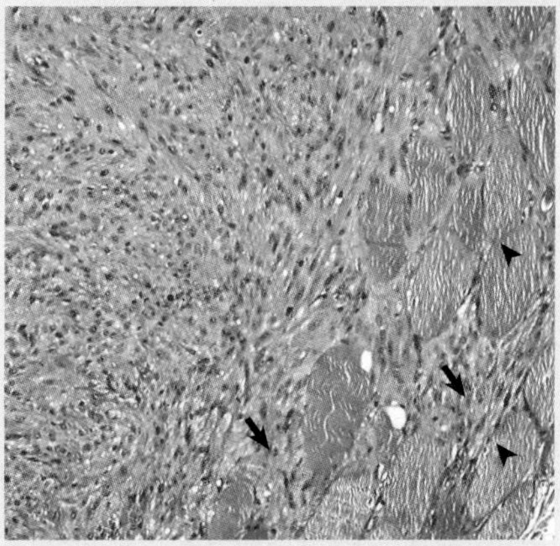

Fibrosarcoma, skin, cat. Cells of the fibrosarcoma *(arrows)* have infiltrated between skeletal muscle fibers *(arrowheads)*. H&E stain.

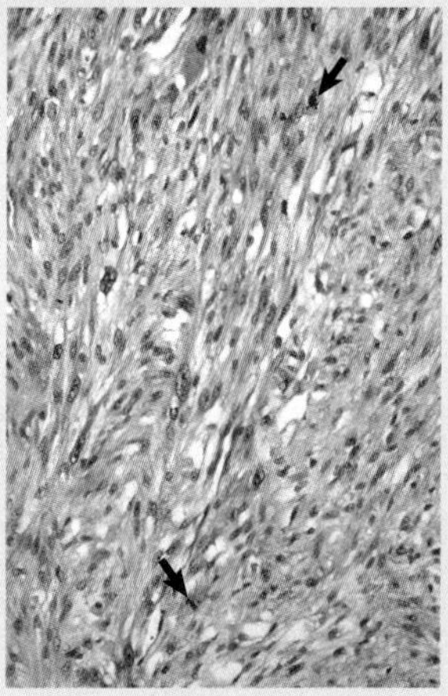

Fibrosarcoma, skin, cat. Note haphazardly arranged intersecting bundles of anaplastic spindle-shaped neoplastic cells within a collagenous stroma. Anaplastic cells are pleomorphic in that they vary in cell size and shape and have a large, vesicular nucleus with increased size and number of nucleoli. Numerous mitotic figures are also present *(arrows)*. H&E stain.[†]

Continued

Box 17-12 Examples of Tumors of the Skin–cont'd

Hemangioma

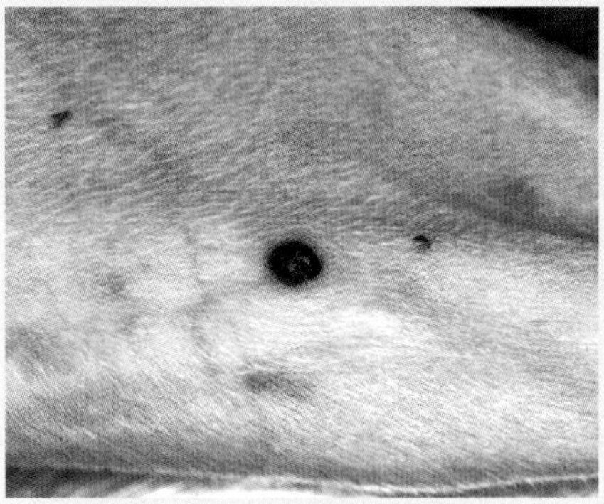

Hemangioma, skin, hind leg, dog. Note raised red to dark red circumscribed mass in nonpigmented and sparsely haired skin.

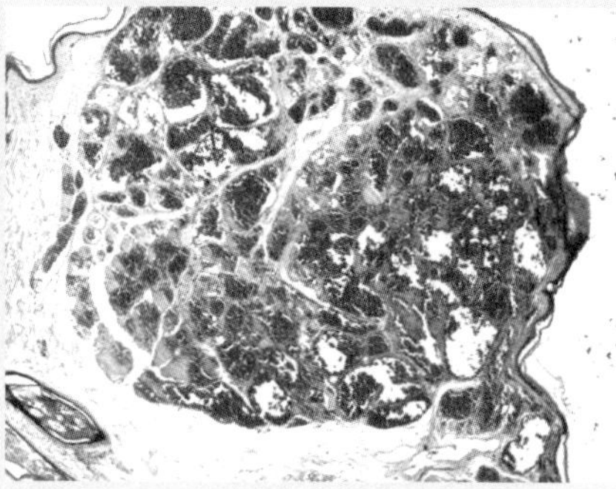

Hemangioma, skin, dog. Well-defined mass of proliferative, blood-filled, vascular channels in the dermis has elevated the epidermis. H&E stain.

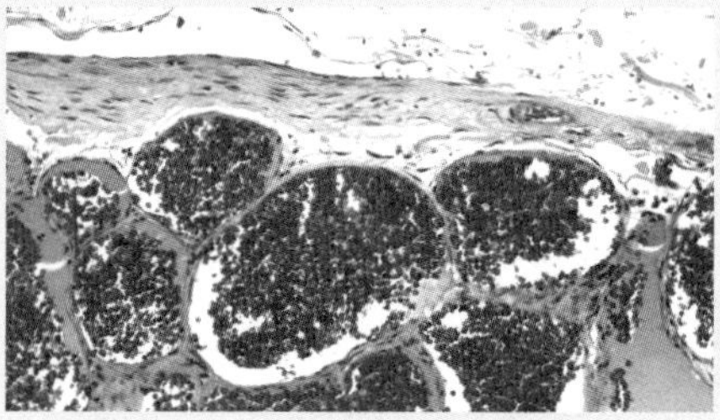

Hemangioma, skin, dog. The dermis is expanded by a circumscribed mass of blood-filled vascular channels lined by well-differentiated endothelial cells. The flattened well-differentiated endothelial cells form a single uniform layer. H&E stain.[†]

Hemangiosarcomas

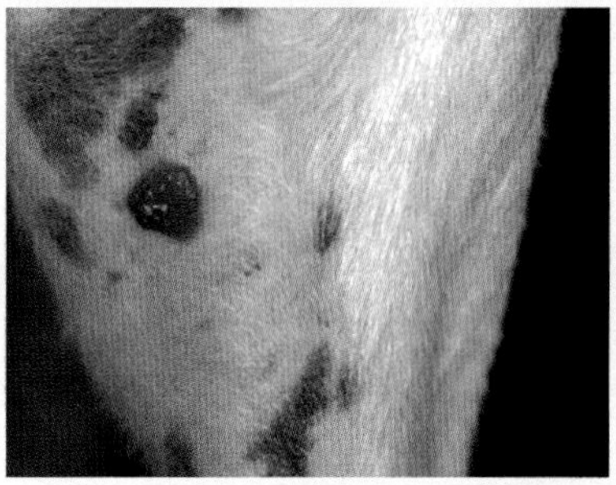

Hemangiosarcoma, skin, dog. Note multiple raised red masses in nonpigmented and sparsely haired skin of whippet.

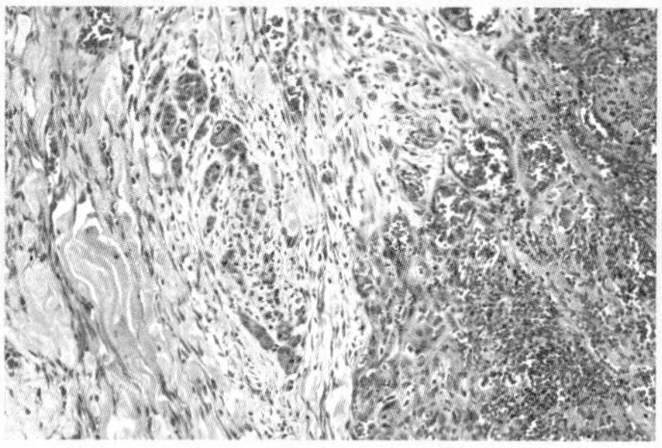

Hemangiosarcoma, skin, dog. Note poorly demarcated margin between tumor (mostly on the *right*) and normal tissue (mostly on the *left*). H&E stain.

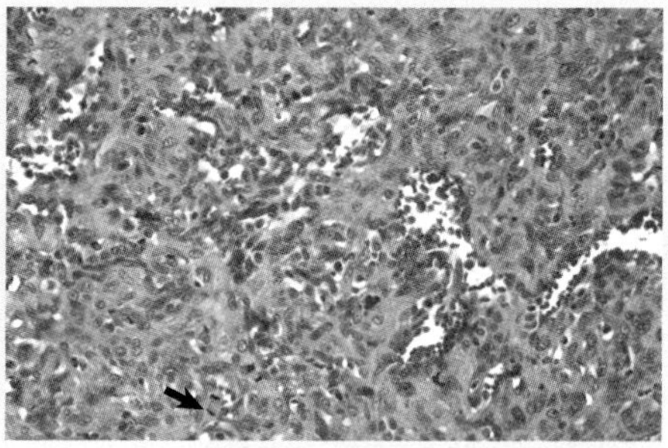

Hemangiosarcoma, skin, dog. The dermis is effaced by highly irregular vascular channels lined by plump, hyperchromatic endothelial cells with numerous mitotic figures *(arrow)*. H&E stain.[†]

MELANOCYTIC TUMORS
Melanocytoma and Melanoma

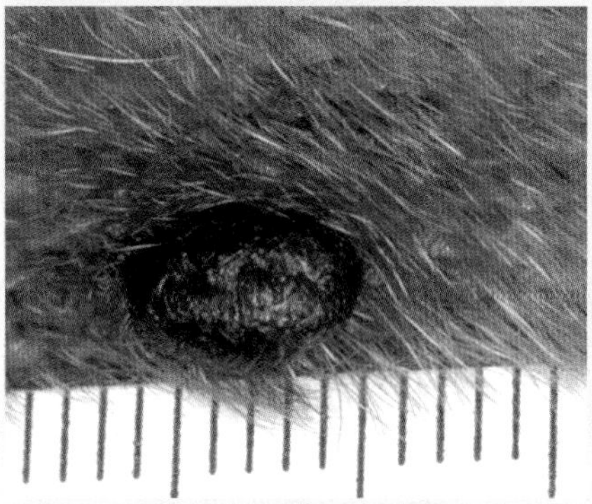

Melanocytoma, skin, dog. Note raised pigmented brown to black hairless mass.[‖]

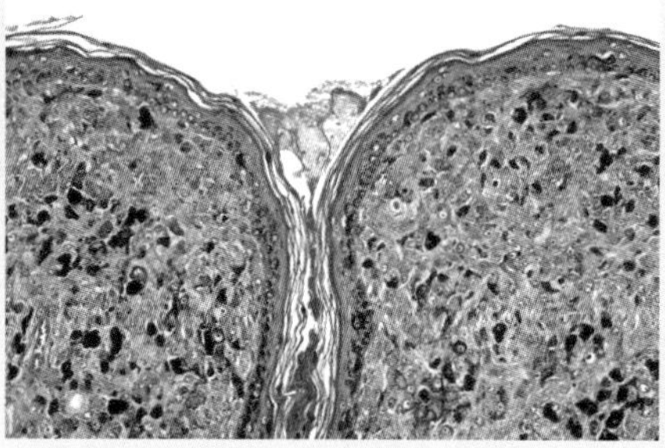

Melanocytoma, skin, dog. The dermis is diffusely infiltrated by sheets of variably pigmented melanocytes, which have prominent nucleoli and moderate variation in the size of cells and nuclei. H&E stain.[†]

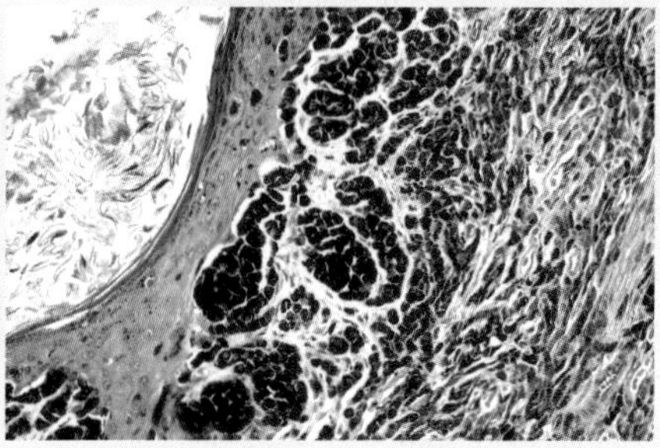

Melanoma, skin, dog. Note clusters of pigmented melanocytes within the epidermis. This is called *junctional activity* and is a feature of melanocytic tumors. H&E stain.[†]

All photographs courtesy Dr. Ann M. Hargis, DermatoDiagnostics, unless otherwise noted.
*Courtesy Dr. P. Ihrke, College of Veterinary Medicine, University of California-Davis.
[†]Courtesy Dr. P.E. Ginn, College of Veterinary Medicine, University of Florida.
[‡]Courtesy Dr. M.D. McGavin, College of Veterinary Medicine, University of Tennessee.
[§]Courtesy Dr. H. Power, Dermatology for Animals.
[‖]Courtesy Dr. D. Duclos, Animal Skin and Allergy Clinic.
CD3, Cluster of differentiation 3; H&E, hematoxylin and eosin; TNF-α, tumor necrosis factor-α; UV, ultraviolet.

Box 17-13 Disorders Characterized by Infiltrates of Eosinophils or Plasma Cells

Hypersensitivity and parasitic dermatitis
Eosinophilic granulomas in horses, dogs, and cats
Eosinophilic furunculosis of the face in dogs
Eosinophilic plaques in cats
Hypereosinophilia syndromes with systemic signs or lesions
- Multisystemic eosinophilic epitheliotropic disease in horses
- Eosinophilic dermatitis with edema in dogs
- Feline hypereosinophilic syndrome

Feline plasma cell pododermatitis
Feline herpesvirus dermatitis

Box 17-14 Nodular Granulomatous Inflammatory Disorders without Microorganisms

Equine sarcoidosis
Juvenile sterile granulomatous dermatitis and lymphadenitis
Sterile pyogranuloma syndrome (idiopathic sterile granuloma and pyogranuloma)
Idiopathic sterile nodular panniculitis
Canine reactive histiocytosis
Canine Langerhans cell histiocytosis
Feline progressive histiocytosis
Xanthoma (xanthogranuloma)
Feline pansteatitis (nutritional)

Feline Progressive Histiocytosis. See Disorders of Cats.

Idiopathic Sterile Nodular Panniculitis. Idiopathic sterile nodular panniculitis develops in dogs, cats, and rarely horses. These lesions are of unknown cause and are characterized grossly by single or multifocal plaques or nodules in the subcutis and occasionally deep dermis of any anatomic site. Lesions can rupture and drain; thus they involve the dermis secondarily. Microscopic lesions consist of discrete, coalescing, or diffuse accumulations of macrophages (histiocytes), neutrophils, lymphocytes, and occasionally other leukocytes. The lesions must be differentiated from those of the infectious granulomatous disorders, sterile pyogranuloma syndrome, and reactive histiocytosis in dogs.

Xanthomas (Xanthogranulomas). Xanthomas are rare, usually multifocal, light tan to yellow papules, plaques, or nodules located in the skin of cats and more rarely horses and dogs. The lesions take their name from the Greek "xanthos," meaning yellow. Some xanthomas are associated with abnormalities in triglyceride or cholesterol metabolism and are thus seen in animals with hereditary defects in lipid metabolism or with metabolic disorders such as diabetes mellitus, hypothyroidism, or hyperadrenocorticism. Histologically, xanthomas associated with abnormalities in triglyceride or cholesterol metabolism consist of sheets of macrophages filled with foamy cytoplasm, scattered giant cells, and interstitial areas of granular to amorphous lipid material and cholesterol clefts. The lipids in the lesions impart a yellow to tan color to the clinical lesions, which is responsible for the name. Rarely, xanthogranulomas also have developed in apparently healthy cats and dogs.

Disorders of the Claw or Claw Bed of Dogs and Cats

A variety of terms are used to define diseases of the claw or claw bed. Onychitis refers to inflammation somewhere in the claw unit, onychodystrophy (onychodysplasia) to abnormal formation of the claw, onychomadesis to sloughing of claws, and paronychia to inflammation of the skin of the claw fold. Paronychia and disorders of multiple claws on multiple feet can occur in association with disease processes that also affect the skin, including infections (e.g., bacterial, fungal, parasitic), immune-mediated disorders (e.g., pemphigus, lupus erythematosus, bullous dermatoses), and systemic disease processes (e.g., hyperadrenocorticism, disseminated intravascular coagulation). However, diseases that affect only the claws are uncommon to rare. One exception is physical trauma to the claws, which is one of the more common causes of claw disease in dogs and cats. Lesions are usually asymmetric and limited to one or just a few claws but can affect all claws in dogs that, for example, have run excessively on hard surfaces or gravel.

Lupoid onychitis (also called lupoid onychodystrophy) is probably the most common cause of onychomadesis that leads to onychodystrophy of multiple claws involving multiple feet in dogs. The condition affects many breeds of dogs of varying ages, and the dogs are healthy otherwise. History includes pain manifested as lameness and sudden loss of one or more claws on multiple paws, eventually involving all claws on all paws. There is partial regrowth of misshapen, friable claws that continue to slough. Paronychia is usually absent. Diagnosis can require amputation of the distal phalanx and the adjacent skin proximal to the claw fold for histopathologic evaluation. Histologic lesions are more prominent on the dorsal aspect of the claw and claw bed skin and include interface lymphoplasmacytic inflammation with basal cell vacuolation and apoptosis and pigmentary incontinence. Secondary bacterial infection and osteomyelitis can develop. However, the histopathologic lesions may represent a nonspecific or stereotypic reaction pattern of the claw, so clinical history as well as other diagnostic tests may be required for diagnosis. Idiopathic onychodystrophy has also been described in dogs and is differentiated from lupoid onychitis by lack of onychomadesis preceding onychodystrophy.

Cutaneous Manifestations of Systemic Disorders

Laminitis

The term *laminitis* technically refers to inflammation of the lamellar (laminar) structures of the hoof, but laminitis is a complex multifactorial syndrome that ultimately results in damage to the lamellae, and thus the suspensory apparatus of the distal phalanx, and in which lamellar inflammation may not always significantly contribute to the pathogenesis of the disease, at least initially. The lamellar region of the hoof consists of primary and secondary epidermal and dermal lamellae that interdigitate to form a significant component of the support system of the foot (see Adnexa, Specialized Structures) (Fig. 17-60). Laminitis can be seen in any hoofed animal (ungulate) but in domestic animals is of greatest importance in horses and cattle. Clinical signs of laminitis may vary from mild to severe; typically include pain that is manifested as abnormal stance, lameness, and reluctance to move; and may lead to euthanasia.

In horses, laminitis traditionally is considered to progress through a series of stages, including developmental (prodromal, preclinical), acute, subacute, and chronic. The developmental stage occurs between the initial causative insult and the first appearance of acute lameness. The acute stage begins with the first appearance of acute lameness and lasts up to 72 hours without physical or radiographic evidence of mechanical collapse of the foot, or alternatively, the acute stage may terminate abruptly with digital collapse and thus proceed directly to the chronic stage. If there is no physical or radiographic evidence of digital collapse after 72 hours of acute lameness onset, the subacute stage begins and lasts a minimum of 8 to 12 weeks, but it may have a more protracted course depending

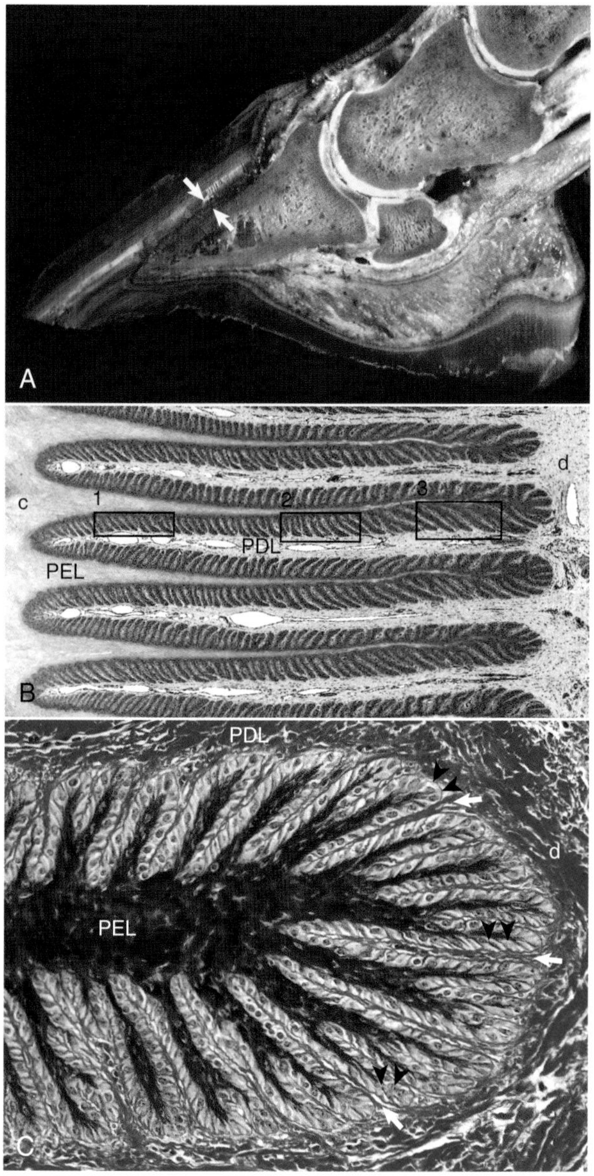

Figure 17-60 **Normal Foot, Horse. A,** Normal foot, midsagittal section. Note that the parietal surface of the distal phalanx is parallel to the epidermal lamellae of the inner surface of the hoof wall *(arrows)*. No space is visible at this junction or at the junction of the distal surface of the distal phalanx and the internal surface of the hoof. **B,** Photomicrograph of normal primary and secondary epidermal and dermal lamellae of equine hoof. Primary epidermal lamella *(PEL)*; primary dermal lamella *(PDL)*; secondary epidermal and dermal lamellae in region closest to hoof wall *(1)*, middle region *(2)*, and region closest to the distal phalanx *(3)*; dermis (corium) in region closest to the distal phalanx *(d)*; epidermal stratum corneum in region closest to the hoof wall (c). H&E stain. **C,** High-magnification photomicrograph of normal lamellae of equine hoof in the region closest to the distal phalanx. The collagen of the primary dermal lamellae *(PDL)* and the secondary dermal lamellae *(arrows)* stains blue, whereas the stratum corneum of the primary epidermal lamella *(PEL)* and the partially cornified core of the secondary epidermal lamellae stain red. A single primary epidermal lamella (one of approximately 600) is illustrated. Each primary epidermal lamella has approximately 150 to 200 outwardly radiating secondary epidermal lamellae the dermal side of which orient toward the distal phalanx. The secondary lamellar epidermal cells *(arrowheads)* are attached via hemidesmosomes to the basement membranes at the dermal/epidermal interface. The large number of interdigitating epidermal and dermal lamellae creates a large surface area for the inner hoof wall, which together with the strong hemidesmosomal attachments between the secondary epidermal and dermal lamellae (and ultimately the parietal surface of the distal phalanx) serves as the suspensory apparatus of the foot. Masson's trichrome stain. (**A** courtesy Dr. P.E. Ginn, College of Veterinary Medicine, University of Florida. **B** and **C** courtesy Professor C. Pollitt and Dr. A. van Eps, School of Veterinary Science, The University of Queensland.)

on disease severity. In severe laminitis (Fig. 17-61), rotation can occur as early as 24 hours after the appearance of lameness. Chronic laminitis (also called *founder*) refers to the stage of laminitis associated with radiographic or physical evidence of rotational or vertical displacement of the distal phalanx relative to the hoof wall (Fig. 17-62). In addition to the four traditionally recognized stages of laminitis, recent research suggests there is a subclinical form or stage of laminitis, in which repeated episodes of lamellar injury occur before the onset of easily recognizable pain or lameness, but gross lesions may be apparent in hooves of the subclinically affected animals, indicating lamellar injury has occurred (Fig. 17-63).

There are four broad categories of naturally occurring laminitis in horses (Table 17-14): (1) sepsis-related or inflammatory laminitis, which is often associated with systemic disease such as carbohydrate overload, endotoxemia, septicemia, retained placenta, septic endometritis, enterocolitis, pleuropneumonia, or contact with black walnut (*Juglans nigra*) shavings; (2) endocrinopathic laminitis (or laminopathy), which is considered to arise from hormonal imbalances such as insulin resistance (including pasture-related laminitis and equine metabolic syndrome), pars intermedia pituitary dysfunction, or administration of glucocorticoids; (3) supporting or contralateral limb laminitis (or laminopathy), which develops in the foot of the contralateral limb in horses with severe unilateral lameness that persists for more than several weeks and is due to excessive weight bearing on the contralateral limb; and (4) traumatic laminitis or "road founder," which occurs in association with intense training and the excessive contusion of repeated foot trauma.

In sepsis-related or inflammatory laminitis, bacterial toxins or other factors associated with changes in large intestinal microflora after carbohydrate overload or septic conditions gain access to the systemic circulation, and this form of laminitis tends to be temporally closely related to the inciting systemic disease. Various theories have been proposed to help explain how the hoof's lamellar structure is initially damaged by these factors, but none has been proven, some are controversial, and more than one mechanism may contribute. The vascular theory suggests that there are abnormalities in the hoof blood flow, including increased capillary pressure (which causes increased tissue pressure and edema), flow in arteriovenous

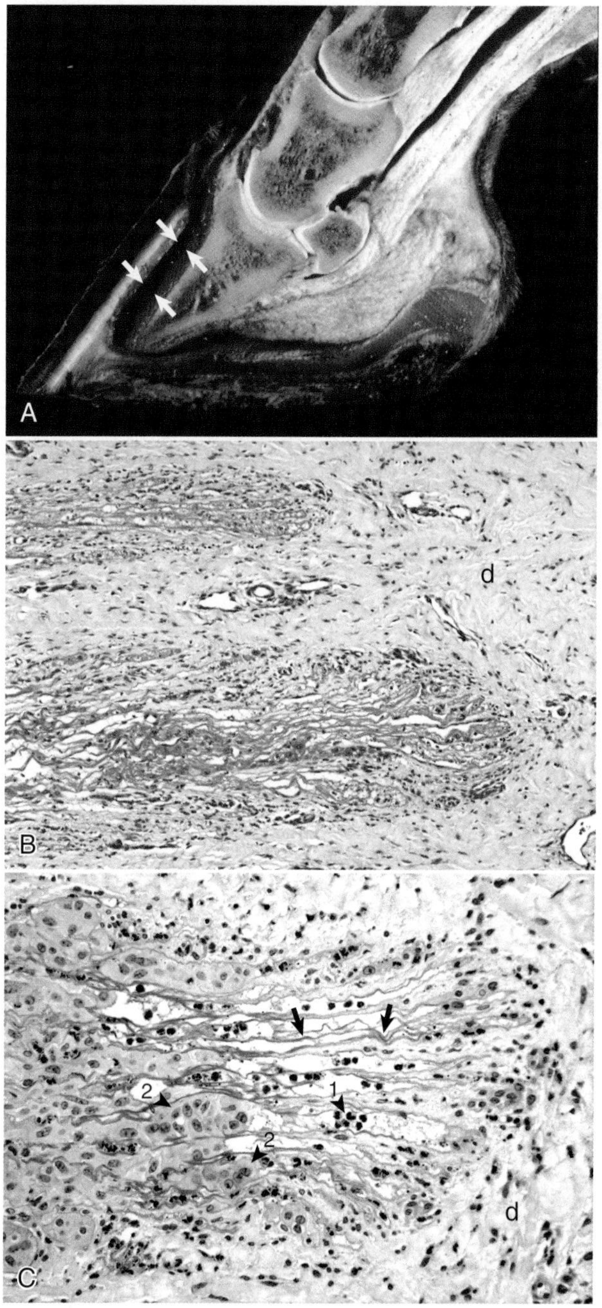

Figure 17-61 **Severe Laminitis with Lamellar Separation, Horse. A,** Severe laminitis with lamellar separation and loss, foot, midsagittal section. Note that the parietal surface of the distal phalanx has separated from the inner surface of the hoof wall *(arrows)*, leaving a large gap due to complete separation of the lamellae (a degloving injury), a feature that may be seen in severe septic inflammatory laminitis. The tip of the distal phalanx has sunk distally toward the sole, crushing the solear corium (a cause of intractable pain and distress). **B,** Photomicrograph of severe inflammatory laminitis in a horse. The lesions were sufficiently severe to result in euthanasia. There is neutrophilic inflammation with extensive loss of secondary epidermal lamellae and lysis and separation of the basement membrane shown here in the lamellar region closest to the distal phalanx. The epidermal stratum corneum to the left (closest to the hoof wall) is not shown in this image. H&E stain. **C,** Higher magnification illustrating displaced secondary epidermal lamellae *(arrowheads 2)* after separating from the basement membrane *(arrows)*. There is loss of normal shape and arrangement of remaining epidermal cells *(arrowheads 2)*. Inflammatory cells are present *(arrowhead 1)*. The epidermal stratum corneum to the left (closest to the hoof wall) is not shown in this image. PAS stain. *d,* dermis (corium). (**A** courtesy College of Veterinary Medicine, University of Illinois. **B** and **C** courtesy Professor Chris Pollitt and Dr. Andrew van Eps, School of Veterinary Science, The University of Queensland.)

anastomoses, and venoconstriction, which deprive the lamellae of oxygen/nutrients and can lead to ischemia. The enzymatic theory suggests that enzymes such as matrix metalloproteinases (MMPs) (especially MMP-2 and MMP-9) located in neutrophils and other tissues, including epidermis, may play a role because these enzymes have been shown to contribute to the separation of the lamellar epidermal cells from the basement membrane; however, new evidence indicates that these enzymes are either present in the inactive form or become activated hours after basement membrane degradation, so MMP-2 and MMP-9 may not be as important as originally thought. The role of other enzymes, including other MMPs and proteins, including proteoglycans, is under investigation. The inflammatory theory suggests that in the early stages of laminitis local digital cytokine (IL-1β, IL-6, and IL-8) and adhesion molecule (intercellular adhesion molecule 1 and E-selectin) gene expression is associated with infiltration of leukocytes into lamellar tissue, and the leukocytes create inflammation and tissue damage.

The endocrinopathic form of laminitis is the most common in horses and ponies, and the term laminopathy has been used for this form of laminitis because inflammation is not considered an early primary feature of lesion development. This form of laminitis is often associated with a slow onset of disease, is recurrent and difficult to treat, and research suggests that it is associated with repeated episodes of subclinical laminitis that occur before onset of clinically recognizable pain. Horses and ponies with metabolic/endocrinopathic abnormalities are at increased risk for developing laminitis, and hyperinsulinemia appears to play a key role. The reasons for this are unclear, but it has been shown that laminitis can be induced in healthy ponies by maintaining superphysiologic circulating concentrations of insulin. Thus it has been hypothesized

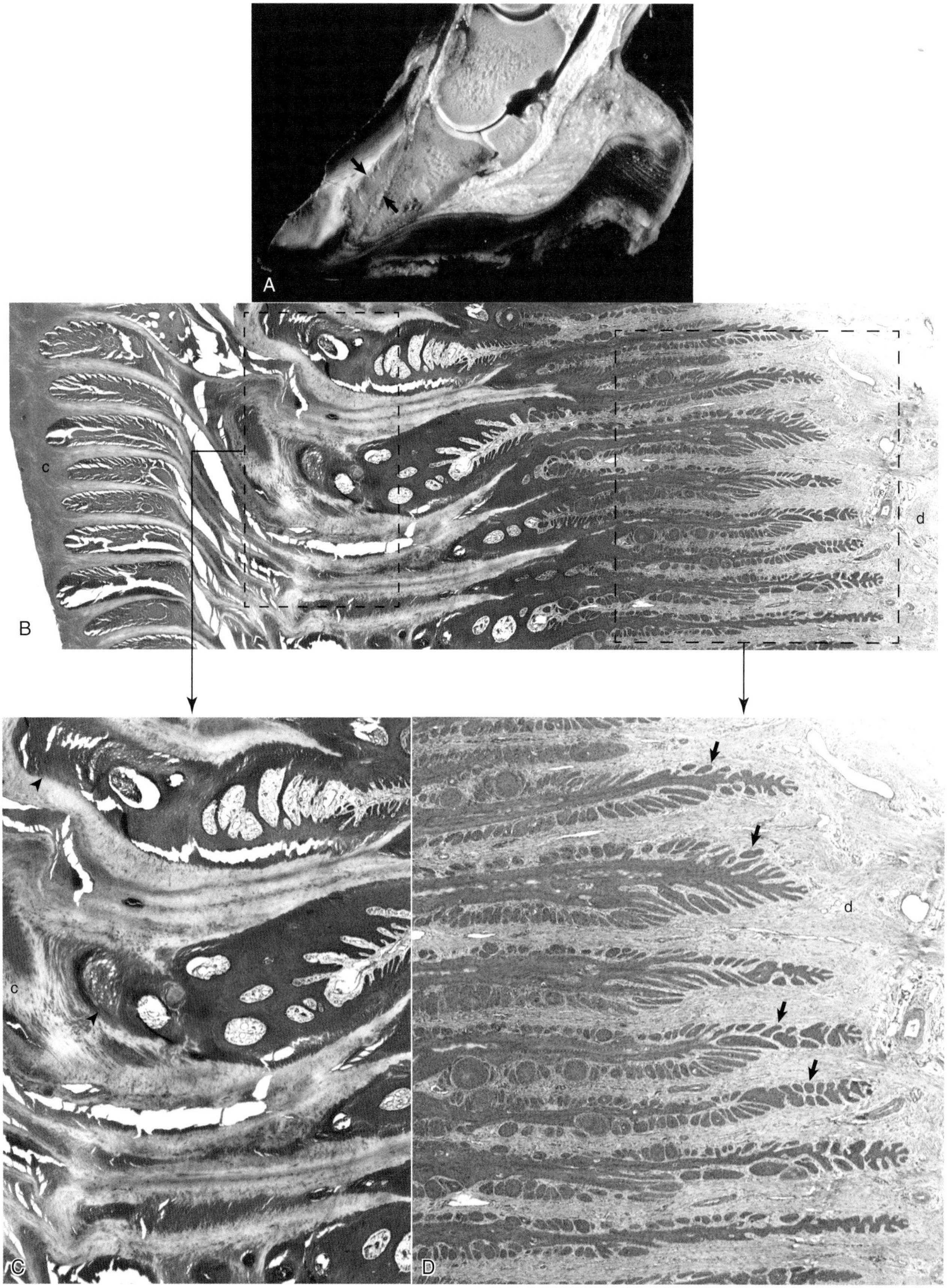
A
B
c
d
C
c
D
d

Figure 17-62 Severe Chronic Laminitis, Horse. A, Severe chronic laminitis, foot, midsagittal section. There is a wide space filled with abnormally cornified epidermal lamellae (*arrows*) between the parietal surface of the distal phalanx and the inner surface of the hoof wall. The tip of the distal phalanx has rotated distally toward the sole. The external surface of the sole horn has been altered, and the weight-bearing capacity of the foot compromised, leading to a turning up and irregular wear of the toe region, and thickening of the sole horn of the heel. **B** to **D,** Photomicrograph of chronic laminitis after carbohydrate overload. The primary epidermal lamellae are elongated **(B)**, and columns of abnormally cornified epidermal cells surround the primary dermal lamellae in the region closest to the hoof wall (*arrowheads*, **C**). With time this mass of abnormal stratum corneum enlarges, which reduces the structural integrity of the foot and complicates recovery. Some of the secondary epidermal lamellae that appear as islands (*arrows*, **D**) have been shown by serial section analysis to be isolated from the primary epidermal lamellae. Isolated islands of secondary epidermal lamellae may develop when basal cells that survive acute injury reconstruct basement membrane but are enclosed by it before they are able to reattach to the primary epidermal lamellae. *c*, epidermal stratum corneum in region closest to the hoof wall; *d*, dermis (corium) in region closest to the distal phalanx. (**A** courtesy Dr. T. Boosinger, College of Veterinary Medicine, Auburn University; and Noah's Arkive, College of Veterinary Medicine, The University of Georgia. **B** to **D** courtesy Professor C. Pollitt and Dr. A. van Eps, School of Veterinary Science, The University of Queensland.)

that laminitis can be triggered in an insulin-resistant horse or pony by conditions that further increase insulin resistance or hyperinsulinemia (e.g., diets high in carbohydrates, overfeeding, or administration of glucocorticoids).

For contralateral or supporting limb laminitis, also referred to as laminopathy, little is known about the early lesions. It occurs in less than 20% of at-risk adult horses, weeks to months after the injury or infection that caused the primary (or first) leg lameness. It is typically a localized disease process, not usually associated with a systemic disease, and the resulting lamellar injury is typically restricted to the overloaded foot. The mechanism of damage is hypothesized to involve load-associated compression of the vasculature in the lamellae, which may lead to poor lamellar blood flow with subsequent platelet activation and microthrombus formation, resulting in lamellar ischemia. Other factors such as secondary inflammation and enzymatic activation may occur. In addition, other as yet unknown factors that may be specific to an individual horse, may also contribute.

There are few detailed studies regarding traumatic laminitis. Historical reports indicate that excessive mechanical overload may directly lead to failure of the suspensory apparatus of the distal phalanx and traumatic lamellar damage.

Recent research also suggests there are interconnecting links between these various forms of laminitis, so they probably are not mutually exclusive, and more than one form of laminitis may be present concurrently in an affected animal. For example, a pony with obesity and insulin resistance that may have endocrinopathic laminitis may develop septic endometritis, which may contribute to sepsis-related lamellar inflammation, or a horse with sepsis-related lamellar inflammation may be forced to place excessive weight on one limb and may develop supporting limb laminitis.

Diagnosis of laminitis is based principally on clinical, radiographic, and gross findings. Histopathologic studies on naturally occurring laminitis are uncommon, and detailed histologic evaluations often have been performed in association with the various experimental models of laminitis to help advance understanding of the pathogenesis of the disease syndrome in an attempt to identify more specific therapeutic and preventative strategies. These experimental models include the carbohydrate overload models (starch overload, oligofructose overload), the black walnut extract model, and the insulin-induced model. The models have advanced the knowledge of the pathophysiology of laminitis, but they also have generated many new, and as yet, unanswered questions.

Gross findings of the external foot in acute laminitis can be minimal. Swelling or edema of the coronary band can be seen. Extravasation of serum through the skin above the coronary band is indicative of severe acute laminitis. In chronic laminitis, common gross lesions include circumferential hoof rings (ridges, founder rings, divergent hoof rings) that are wider at the heel (see Fig. 17-63, A), altered foot shape, separation of the wall from the epidermis at the coronet, depression of the coronary band, a flattened sole, and in some cases, penetration of the distal phalanx through the sole. In horses, laminitis may affect one or more feet, but the front feet are most commonly affected, presumably due to increased weight bearing (in the standing horse, the body mass is divided between fore and hind limbs in an approximate ratio of 60 : 40). Gross evaluation of the external foot in horses or ponies at risk for the development of laminitis is considered an important strategy in prevention of some cases of laminitis, particularly the endocrinopathic form. For instance, the presence of divergent hoof rings (see Fig. 17-63, A) in a horse or pony before the onset of clinically recognizable foot pain, suggests the presence of subclinical lamellar injury, which may allow for earlier implementation of management strategies to slow or prevent further lamellar injury.

In the carbohydrate overload and black walnut extract models, histologic lesions in acute laminitis include loss of normal shape and arrangement of lamellar basal and parabasal cells, and lysis and separation of the basement membrane. In addition, leukocytes are present in the developmental stage of the black walnut extract model and in the acute stage of the carbohydrate models and precede significant histologic changes, which suggests that leukocyte infiltration occurs early and may be a cause of basement membrane separation and structural failure of the foot (see Fig. 17-61, *B* and *C* for an example of histologic lesions in acute laminitis). Histologic lesions 7 days after induction of laminitis in the carbohydrate overload model include significant alterations in the lamellar architecture. Lamellar basal cells that survive acute injury reconstruct basement membrane but are enclosed by it before they are able to reattach to the primary epidermal lamellae. This results in secondary epidermal lamellae that are irregularly sized and shaped and often separated from the primary epidermal lamellae. These changes reduce the surface area of dermal-epidermal interdigitations and weaken the suspensory apparatus of the distal phalanx. In addition, the primary epidermal lamellae elongate. In some instances, columns of abnormally cornified epidermal cells may surround the primary dermal lamellae in the region closest to the hoof wall. With time these mounds of abnormal stratum corneum enlarge, which reduces the structural integrity of the foot and thus complicates recovery. Histologic lesions in chronic naturally occurring endocrinopathic laminitis with hyperinsulinemia occur predominantly in lamellar regions closest to the hoof wall and include epidermal hyperplasia and apoptosis, and fusion and partial replacement of lamellar tissue by increased quantities of abnormal stratum corneum that may contain nuclear debris and pools of proteinaceous fluid. These lesions result

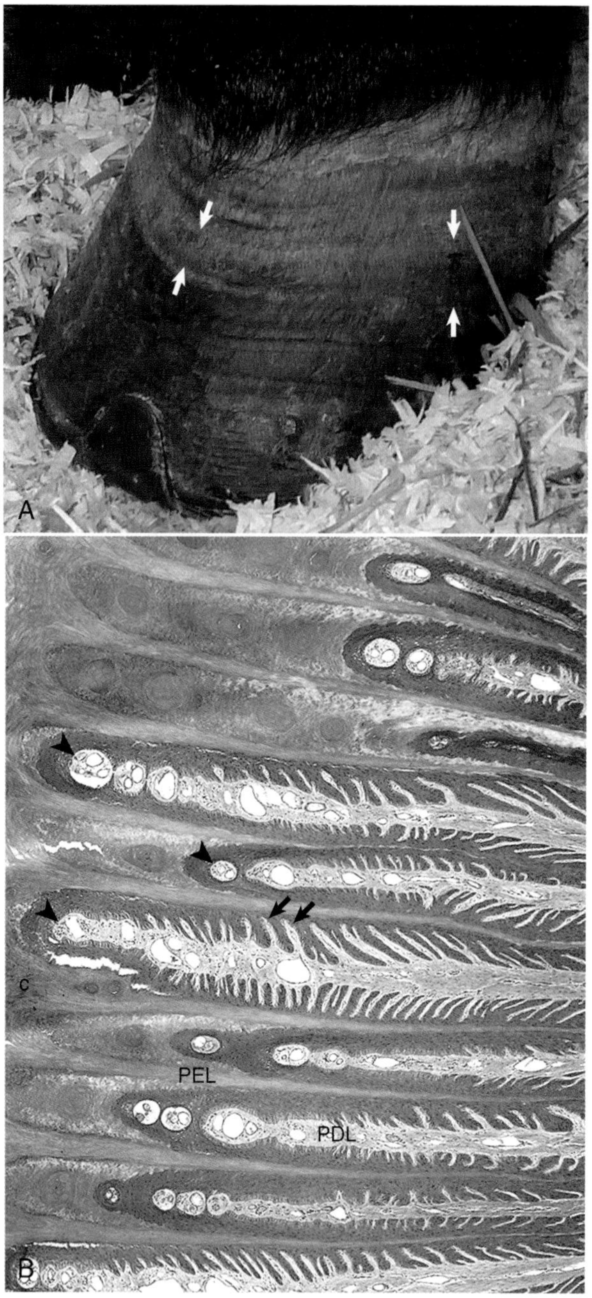

Figure 17-63 Endocrinopathic Laminitis, Horse. A, Chronic, naturally occurring endocrinopathic laminitis, hoof. Note divergent (nonconcentric) hoof rings *(arrows)* on outer hoof wall of a horse with elevated basal insulin level, a form of endocrinopathic laminitis. Divergent hoof rings indicate the presence of damage to the hoof wall and may be evident before clinically detectable lameness. The hoof rings are wider at the heel. **B,** Photomicrograph from the mid-sagittal hoof wall of a horse that had chronic naturally occurring endocrinopathic laminitis and elevated basal insulin level. The highly irregular lamellar-horn margin in the region close to the hoof wall is illustrated. The irregular length of the primary dermal lamellae *(arrowheads)* occurs because of the bridging of dermal lamellar tissue by abnormal columns of degenerate and keratinized epidermal cells that form excessive stratum corneum. The result is an irregular border between the cornified zone of the inner hoof wall and the lamellar tissue. The severity of this change varies within and between affected animals. H&E stain. *Arrows,* Secondary dermal lamellae; *PDL,* primary dermal lamella; *PEL,* primary epidermal lamella; epidermal stratum corneum in the region closest to the hoof wall *(c)*. (**A** and **B** courtesy Karikoski NP, McGowan CM, Singer ER, et al: Pathology of natural cases of equine endocrinopathic laminitis association with hyperinsulinemia, *Vet Pathol* 52(5):945-956, 2015.)

in an irregular border between the cornified zone of the inner hoof wall and the lamellar tissue (see Fig. 17-63, *B*). Acute separation may develop, often between epidermal and dermal lamellae but sometimes between primary epidermal and secondary epidermal lamellae. Primary and secondary epidermal lamellae also elongate. The most frequent change in the region closest to the distal phalanx is tapering of the epidermal lamellae. Minimal inflammation is noted, and basement membrane failure is not extensive in this form of laminitis.

A sequel of progression into chronic laminitis that may develop in some instances is irregular hyperplasia and abnormal stratum corneum production of the epidermal lamellae that form a triangular-shaped mass called the lamellar thickening or lamellar wedge. The lamellar wedge is located between inner hoof wall and the proliferating lamellar epidermis and is evident in sagittal sections of the affected feet. The lamellar wedge forms subsequent to displacement of the distal phalanx and is associated with remodeling of this phalanx. The appearance of the lamellar wedge varies with disease severity, duration, and therapeutic interventions. Histologically the lamellar wedge consists of variable quantities of proliferative epidermis, abnormal stratum corneum, and sometimes resolving fluid accumulation and hemorrhage. Also present in chronic laminitis are changes in the distal phalanx, including increased porosity of cortical bone due to osteoclastic resorption that exceeds osteoblastic proliferation. Edema, proliferation of small-caliber blood vessels, inflammation, and proliferation of a fibromyxoid matrix may develop within the medullary spaces of the bone. The deep digital flexor tendon may develop neovascularization and fibroplasia associated with osteoclasis and bone modeling at the insertion to the distal phalanx.

Laminitis in cattle occurs in dairy and beef cattle, and unlike horses, the rear feet are more commonly involved, which may be due to the fact that the outside digits (claws) of the cow's rear legs bear the burden of the continuously changing weight load. Descriptions include four different stages of laminitis: acute, subacute, chronic, and subclinical. Acute laminitis is not common and is associated with diseases such as metritis, mastitis, or accidental consumption of large quantities of grain and is often an individual animal problem. Subacute laminitis occurs in beef bulls on feeding trials and feeder calves fed diets rich in carbohydrates. Thus acute and subacute laminitis are likely associated with systemic disease, including carbohydrate-induced gastrointestinal disease (ruminal acidosis), and subsequent release into the systemic circulation of inflammatory mediators that may affect the lamellae. A model of acute bovine laminitis confirms the association between dietary carbohydrate (oligofructose) overload and development of laminitis. Acute and subacute laminitis are associated with digital pain, and the claws may be warm with marked digital pulse. The histopathologic features of the more acute forms of laminitis in cattle have been studied using a carbohydrate overload model, in which it has been shown that early lesions are stretching of lamellae, dermal edema, hemorrhage, and basal cell morphologic changes, with white blood cells in the dermis and basement membrane detachment.

The most common form of laminitis in cattle has been described in dairy cows around the time of calving, and lameness may not be evident initially, so this form of laminitis has been referred to as *subclinical laminitis*. However, the role of inflammation and involvement of the lamellae in each case are unclear in this form of disease, and thus the etiopathogenesis of subclinical laminitis in dairy cattle is controversial. Multiple complex factors, including intense management systems, contribute to the development of this form of the disease. These factors include: (1) diet or nutrition such as vitamins (biotin) and minerals that influence the quality of the stratum

Table 17-14 Equine Laminitis, Types, Animals Affected, Time Course, Proposed Pathogeneses, and Experimental Models

Laminitis Type	Associated Diseases	Horses Affected	Time Course*	Proposed Pathogenesis
Sepsis-related laminitis (inflammatory laminitis)	Carbohydrate overload Endotoxemia Septicemia Septic endometritis Retained placenta Enterocolitis Pleuropneumonia Contact with black walnut shavings	Any age of horse that is likely to develop the associated disease condition	Acute, temporally related to systemic disease Subacute form may occur if systemic disease is less severe and lamellar damage is mild and subtotal	Inflammatory toxins in systemic circulation associated with changes in large intestinal microflora after carbohydrate overload, or septic conditions may alter hoof blood flow leading to endothelial and vascular dysfunction, extracellular matrix degradation, and lamellar leukocyte infiltration that precedes separation of epidermis from basement membrane. Experimental models include oligofructose and starch overload, and black walnut–induced models.
Endocrinopathic laminitis Laminopathy is an alternative term because inflammation is not considered an early primary feature Most common form of laminitis	Metabolic syndrome[†]: Obesity (major risk factor) Insulin resistance Hyperinsulinemia Pars intermedia pituitary dysfunction: Hyperadrenocorticism Glucocorticoid administration	Metabolic syndrome: young to middle-aged horses and ponies Often when pastures are lush with abundant nonstructural carbohydrates Pars intermedia pituitary dysfunction: aged horses (50%-80% of horses with this condition have laminitis)	Slow onset Recurrent Repeated episodes of subclinical laminitis before first onset of clinical signs	Mechanism of lesion development in hyperinsulinemia is unknown. Inflammation does not appear to be a major feature. Vascular alteration may contribute. Hyperinsulinemia, vascular endothelial dysfunction, and a proinflammatory state associated with metabolic syndromes may act individually or collectively to lower the threshold for laminitis development when other factors such as intestinal fermentation of carbohydrates in pasture forage invoke a systemic inflammatory response and/or alter digital blood flow. Glucocorticoids may increase plasma insulin level or may act by catabolic effect on basement membrane or by contributing to vasoconstriction. Models include insulin-induced and possibly glucocorticoid-induced laminitis.
Contralateral limb or supporting limb laminitis Laminopathy is an alternative term because inflammation may not be an early primary feature	Unilateral lameness causing increased weight bearing on opposite limb May affect contralateral hindlimb or contralateral forelimb Not usually associated with systemic disease	Less than 20% of at-risk horses Adults Rarely yearlings or foals Heavier horses may be predisposed Horses with more severe and longer duration of first leg injury	Weeks to months after increased weight bearing associated with the first leg lameness When develops, there is often severe, extensive, and catastrophic lamellar separation, extending circumferentially around entire hoof wall No detailed studies	Cyclic loading and unloading of the foot is integral in maintaining adequate perfusion of the digital lamellae, and it is hypothesized that reduction in the frequency of this cyclic loading predisposes and potentially initiates this form of laminitis. Possible load-induced vascular compromise also leads to platelet activation, microthrombi, and possible secondary activation of enzymatic and inflammatory mediators; lack of glucose delivery may participate. Mechanical overload of suspensory apparatus of distal phalanx may be secondary event. Individual horse factors such as coexisting systemic inflammation or hyperinsulinemia, or stress- or pain-related hypercortisolemia with insulin resistance.
Traumatic laminitis (Historical term, "road founder")	Intense training or repeated foot trauma	Overworked horses or high-intensity work in sports horses	Associated with overwork, but no detailed studies	Excessive mechanical overload of hooves leads to failure of the suspensory apparatus of distal phalanx and traumatic lamellar damage.

*Each form may progress to the chronic stage of laminitis.
[†]Some consider pasture-associated laminitis to be a form of equine metabolic syndrome. Ponies appear to be particularly predisposed to metabolic syndrome and endocrinopathic laminitis.

corneum (horn), or factors associated with increased carbohydrate intake that may contribute to subacute ruminal acidosis; (2) hormonal changes at calving that alter the resilience of the feet to external stresses; (3) traumatic injury due to reduced digital cushion thickness, or increased trauma or wear on the sole due to maintenance of cattle on hard surfaces with inadequate time spent lying down; and (4) genetic predisposition. For example, it has been shown in dairy cattle that diets with a large proportion of rapidly fermentable carbohydrates and insufficient quantity and quality of fiber increase the prevalence of laminitis, possibly by influencing rumen metabolism that allows toxins or inflammatory mediators to enter the systemic circulation. Dairy cows housed on hard (concrete) flooring as opposed to rubber mats and cows that are unable to lie down and rest sufficiently have a higher prevalence of laminitis, possibly due to increased hoof trauma. In addition, the suspensory apparatus of cattle is less well developed than that of the horse, so the digital cushion (a structure consisting of adipose tissue under the distal phalanx) supports a greater amount of the body weight. Dairy cattle with a thinner digital cushion have a greater prevalence of lameness and conditions traditionally associated with subclinical laminitis such as ulcers of the sole, suggesting that these lesions are related to contusions within the hoof. Thus the pathogenesis of lesions in subclinical laminitis is multifactorial and may vary in individual animals depending on the degree of or type of contribution of the various nutritional, hormonal, mechanical, and genetic factors. Clinical lesions in affected dairy cattle before the onset of lameness include hemorrhage in the sole and white line (see the section on Structure, Specialized Structures), and yellow discoloration and softening of the sole horn. These lesions in dairy cows are thought to predispose to other foot conditions such as ulceration of the sole, white line separation and fissuring, and subsolar abscesses that can be the main causes of lameness in this form of laminitis in dairy cattle.

If damage in the hoof in acute, subacute, or subclinical laminitis is subtotal, partial recovery may occur, but damaged lamellae, and possibly adjacent support structures, are less able to recover during repeat episodes of laminitis, and thus chronic laminitis may ensue. Chronic laminitis is associated with deformation of the claws, which become flattened and broad, with a concave and furrowed dorsal wall due to disruption and loss of integrity of the lamellae and displacement of the distal phalanx.

Cutaneous Paraneoplastic Syndromes

Cutaneous paraneoplastic syndromes are rare dermatoses that occur in association with internal malignancies (Box 17-15). Confirmation of a dermatosis as a paraneoplastic syndrome requires strict adherence to established clinical, histopathologic, and in some instances, immunologic criteria. Conditions meeting these criteria currently recognized in animals include paraneoplastic pemphigus (discussed in the section on Selected Autoimmune Reactions); paraneoplastic alopecia and internal malignancies in the cat; exfoliative dermatosis and thymoma in the cat, dog, and rabbit; and superficial necrolytic dermatitis in the dog and cat. Dermatofibrosis in the dog, pancreatic panniculitis, and multisystemic eosinophilic disease in the horse have also been associated with underlying neoplasia; however, they have not yet been proved to be true paraneoplastic syndromes. This list does not include the endocrine dermatoses associated with functional tumors of endocrine organs. Many other syndromes are documented in human beings, and it is likely more will be documented in animals in the future. The refractory nature of these syndromes and their significance as an indicator of systemic disease underscores the importance of their recognition.

Box 17-15 Principal Cutaneous Paraneoplastic Syndromes

- Superficial necrolytic dermatitis
- Pancreatic panniculitis (necrotizing panniculitis)
- Nodular dermatofibrosis and renal or uterine tumors in dogs
- Paraneoplastic pemphigus
- Feline pancreatic paraneoplastic alopecia
- Feline exfoliative dermatitis with or without thymoma

Feline Pancreatic Paraneoplastic Alopecia. See Disorders of Cats.

Feline Exfoliative Dermatitis with or without Thymoma. See Disorders of Cats.

Superficial Necrolytic Dermatitis (Diabetic Dermatopathy, Hepatocutaneous Syndrome, Necrolytic Migratory Erythema, Metabolic Epidermal Necrosis). See Disorders of Dogs.

Pancreatic Panniculitis (Necrotizing Panniculitis). See Disorders of Dogs.

Nodular Dermatofibrosis and Renal Disease in the Dog. See Disorders of Dogs.

Paraneoplastic Pemphigus. See the discussion on paraneoplastic pemphigus in the section on Selected Autoimmune Reactions.

Cutaneous Neoplasia

The skin is a common site of neoplastic growth in most animals; the neoplasms are of ectodermal, mesodermal, and melanocytic origin (see Box 17-12). Ectodermal neoplasms of the epidermis and adnexa are most often benign with the exception of the neoplasms of the apocrine sweat glands, apocrine glands of the anal sac, and neoplasms of the surface epidermis (squamous cell carcinomas).

Benign neoplasms do not metastasize or invade adjacent tissue. In general, benign neoplasms are circumscribed, grow by expansion, and are composed of well-differentiated cells that closely resemble the cells or tissue of origin (see Box 17-12). Malignant neoplasms are locally invasive and often metastasize. They are more often composed of anaplastic cells with a high mitotic index that no longer resemble the cells of origin. Anaplastic cells are pleomorphic (vary in cell size and shape) and typically have a large, vesicular nucleus with increased size and number of nucleoli (see Box 17-12). Malignant cells develop surface alterations such as altered antigenicity, decreased numbers or altered location of receptors for adjacent cells, and increased receptors for components of the extracellular matrix. Changes such as these allow malignant cells to detach from the primary site of tumor growth, move through tissues, and in some cases delay or escape detection by the host's immune system. A specific example is the loss of E-cadherins (proteins responsible for epithelial cell-to-cell attachment) by some types of carcinomas. E-cadherins are partially responsible for the "contact inhibition" that leads to density control and inhibits uncontrolled proliferation of epithelial cells.

Neoplasms of the skin develop secondary to the same basic molecular drivers that lead to the development of neoplasms of any tissue. The neoplastic transformation of a cell is the end result of a series of events that cause damage to the cell's DNA. Most agents that are known to be carcinogenic target and damage DNA. Solar radiation, x-radiation, viral infections, and continued trauma are important contributors to neoplastic transformation of components of the skin. Continued trauma contributes to tumor development by increasing cell turnover, which in turn increases the possibility of mutations. Not all factors that contribute to the development of cutaneous neoplasms are known.

Four categories of genes encode for a large number of proteins responsible for regulation of cellular proliferation and differentiation. These categories are the tumor-suppressor genes, the proto-oncogenes, genes that regulate apoptosis, and genes that regulate DNA repair. Damage to these genes results in gain- or loss-of-function defects in proteins such as growth factors, growth factor receptors, signal-transducing proteins, cell cycle regulators, and nuclear transcription factors. The majority of malignant neoplasms have evidence of damage (mutation) of multiple genes within these categories. Mutations are often accumulated by cells in a stepwise manner that imparts increasing degrees of malignant potential. These molecular changes are known to correlate with morphologic changes and the clinical behavior of some neoplasms. For example, it is known that squamous cell carcinomas often develop in a stepwise manner and progress through several recognizable stages: hyperplasia (increased number of cells; no cellular atypia or tissue disorganization) → dysplasia (increased mitoses, cellular atypia, and tissue disorganization consisting of loss of polarity) → carcinoma in situ (increased tissue disorganization, mitoses, anaplastic nuclei, but no invasion of underlying basement membrane) → invasive squamous cell carcinoma (disruption of the basement membrane with dermal invasion by anaplastic carcinoma cells).

The progression of the disease from hyperplasia to an invasive carcinoma represents a series of molecular events whereby the population of cells harbors an increasing number of damaged genes (mutations) belonging to the four categories of genes listed. This series of changes takes place over long periods of time, often years, before a tumor reaches full malignant potential. Many of the genetic mutations are neutral (or passenger) mutations; however, others are considered to be "driver" mutations because they guide and sustain the selection and propagation of a malignant clone (malignant cells that arise from an individual parent cell with the genetic mutations). Under the influence of the driver mutations, clonal populations of malignant cells gain selection advantage over other cells and also gain control of various interactions with the tumor microenvironment, an essential part of tumor physiology, structure, and function that includes many nontumor cells and components such as endothelial cells, mesenchymal cells, immune cells, inflammatory cells, and extracellular matrix. The complex interactions of tumor cells and their adjacent microenvironment contribute to tumor growth and metastasis and are currently being investigated in an attempt to identify more effective anticancer therapies.

Most cutaneous neoplasms are primary because the skin is an uncommon to rare site for metastasis; however, the skin can be the site of secondary tumor growth. Examples include mammary gland neoplasms that invade into adjacent skin, feline pulmonary bronchogenic carcinomas that metastasize to multiple digits of the feet, and canine visceral hemangiosarcomas that can metastasize to the skin. E-Tables 17-3 to 17-6 provide a list of the salient features of the common neoplastic-like lesions and neoplastic lesions in domestic animals.

Disorders of Horses

For disorders occurring in two or more species of animals, see the section on Disorders of Domestic Animals.

Viral Infections

Poxviruses

For more mechanistic detail, see the section on Disorders of Domestic Animals, Microbial and Parasitic Disorders, Viral Infections, Poxviruses.

Molluscum Contagiosum (Molluscipoxvirus)

Information on this topic is available at www.expertconsult.com.

Bacterial Infections

Proliferative Pododermatitis (Canker)

Proliferative pododermatitis in horses, also known as canker (see Table 17-12), is a painful, proliferative, and inflammatory condition of the hoof. The cause of proliferative pododermatitis in the horse is unknown, but the disease appears to be polymicrobial in nature. The condition has been associated with the presence of a variety of Gram-positive and Gram-negative bacteria and in some cases with tissue colonization of *Treponema* spp. spirochetes. *Bacteroides* sp. and *Fusobacterium necrophorum* have been isolated in some cases. Recently, bovine papillomaviruses 1 and 2 have been detected in affected tissue via PCR-based techniques, but it is not known if these viruses have a causative role. The pathogenesis of lesion formation is not yet known, but moisture and unclean environments often predispose to the condition. It most often affects the rear feet of draft horses but can affect any foot or multiple feet of any breed of horse and even those kept in dry, clean environments. Initial lesions consist of a focal raised pink lesion resembling granulation tissue that bleeds easily and is surrounded by a gray or brown zone located in the frog. This lesion will progress to excessive, soft, white filiform papillomatous-like proliferations emanating from the frog, bars, sole, and sometimes hoof wall of the affected foot. Some cases will be foul smelling and have surface collections of caseous white exudate. Microscopically, areas of marked papillary epidermal hyperplasia associated with hyperkeratosis and neutrophilic infiltrates of the epidermis are present. The outer stratum spinosum may have areas of marked ballooning degeneration. The dermis contains superficial neutrophilic to lymphoplasmacytic infiltrates. A mixed population of Gram-positive and Gram-negative bacteria can be identified on the surface epidermis, but the organisms are not consistently associated with the areas of inflammation. In some cases, spirochetes have been identified within the proliferative epidermis.

Necrotizing Pododermatitis (Thrush)

Necrotizing pododermatitis of the horse (see Table 17-12), commonly known as thrush, is a painful, necrotizing condition of the frog and central and lateral sulci of the hoof. It is caused by the anaerobic bacterium, *F. necrophorum*. Trapping of moist and bacterial-ridden materials such as manure and mud leads to softening of the tissue of the frog and allows bacterial colonization. The condition most often affects the hind feet but can affect all hooves. Initial lesions consist of black discoloration and softening of the frog accompanied by a very foul odor. Over time the black discoloring and softening spread to involve deeper tissues and more areas of the frog. The lesions consist of foul-smelling black exudate and loss of frog tissue. In chronic severe cases the distal limb can be swollen and the frog becomes spongy and ragged, easily shreds, and can bleed. There can be long-term atrophy of the frog as tissue disintegration occurs. Gross characteristics are usually diagnostic, but microscopic lesions consist of degeneration, necrosis, and suppurative inflammation of the frog epidermis and sometimes of deeper tissues. Bacterial colonization of the tissues is usually present.

Bacterial Granulomatous Dermatitis (Bacterial Granulomas)

Mycobacterial Granuloma. See the section on Disorders of Domestic Animals, Microbial and Parasitic Disorders, Bacterial Infections, Bacterial Granulomatous Dermatitis (Bacterial Granulomas), Mycobacterial Granulomas.

Parasitic Infections

Helminth Larval Migrans

Cutaneous Habronemiasis. Cutaneous habronemiasis (summer sores) occurs in horses and is caused by infection with the larvae of *Habronema* sp. or *Draschia* sp. deposited on the skin by house or stable flies. Larval deposition and lesions occur on parts of the body where the skin is either traumatized, such as the legs, or moist and soft, such as the prepuce and medial canthus of the eye (Fig. 17-64). Larvae are unable to penetrate normal skin, but fly bites cause sufficient damage to allow larval penetration. Grossly, single or multiple, proliferative, ulcerated red to brown, nodular masses are present that on section have small, yellow to white, gritty foci. The microscopic lesion is a nodular dermatitis with eosinophils, epithelioid macrophages, and sometimes, giant cells bordering larvae or necrotic debris (see Fig. 17-64). Granulation tissue infiltrated by neutrophils is present on the ulcerated surface.

Filarial Dermatitis

Onchocerciasis is a filarial dermatitis principally affecting horses. Adult parasites are located in nodules in connective tissue and can be asymptomatic. Microfilariae are located in the dermis, particularly of the ventral midline, and are the source of the major lesions. Intermediate hosts, such as the Simuliidae (blackflies, gnats) and Ceratopogonidae (biting midges), transmit the microfilariae. Not all horses with microfilariae have clinical signs or lesions. In those horses with cutaneous inflammation attributed to microfilariae, dead or dying microfilariae induce the most intense inflammation, and inflammation can be enhanced by microfilaricidal therapy.

Differences in lesion severity between horses may reflect different degrees of hypersensitivity to microfilariae, different degrees of hypersensitivity to the bites of intermediate hosts, or possibly other factors. Recent evidence in human filarial disease has revealed that the acute inflammatory response in two important diseases, elephantiasis and river blindness, may largely be a result of the endosymbiotic bacteria *(Wolbachia)* harbored within the filarial parasites and released into the blood by living parasites or following death or damage of the adults or microfilariae. The inflammatory stimulus is thought to be induced by proinflammatory and chemotactic cytokines and depends on PRRs known to contribute to innate immunity. *Wolbachia* organisms have been identified in a number of filarial parasites in animals, including *Onchocerca gutturosa*, *Onchocerca lienalis*, *Onchocerca cervicalis*, *Onchocerca ochengi*, *Dirofilaria immitis*, and *Dirofilaria repens*. *O. ochengi* in cattle has been studied as a model of human onchocerciasis in which it has been shown that selective antibiotic therapy against *Wolbachia* results in reduced numbers of *Wolbachia* sp., reduced numbers of adult *O. ochengi*, and reduced numbers of microfilaria. These findings indicate that *Wolbachia* organisms have an important symbiotic relationship with *O. ochengi* (as well as many other filarial parasites) and may represent a new target against filarial and microfilarial parasites.

In equine onchocerciasis, clinical lesions related to microfilariae develop on the head, neck, medial forelimbs, ventral thorax, and abdomen and consist of patchy to diffuse alopecia, erythema, scaling, crusting, and pigmentary changes. Some horses have a characteristic, variably pigmented, circular area of dermatitis on the forehead. Keratitis, conjunctivitis, and uveitis are observed in some horses. Microscopic cutaneous lesions vary from none to superficial and deep perivascular to interstitial dermatitis with eosinophils, lymphocytes, and microfilariae. Fibrosis is seen in older lesions.

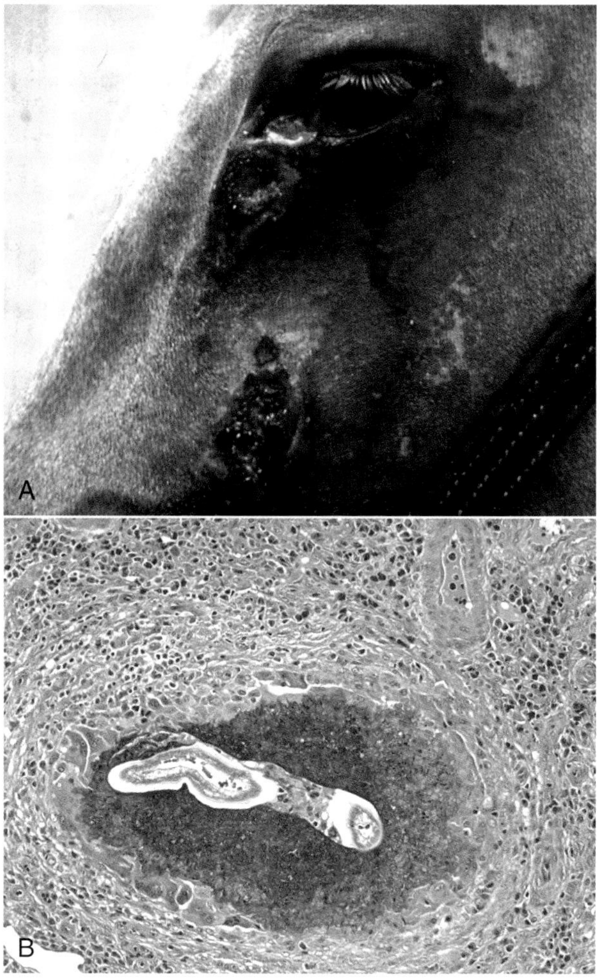

Figure 17-64 **Cutaneous Habronemiasis, *Habronema* sp., Skin, Horse.** **A,** Face. Multiple coalescing nodular granulomatous and ulcerated areas are present on the skin of the medial canthus, skin immediately ventral to the eye, and the skin of the lateral surface of the face. Lesions of cutaneous habronemiasis develop in areas of the skin that are traumatized (often the legs) or in soft moist skin (around the genitalia or eyes). In this case, moisture from ocular secretion (tears) may have predisposed to bites of house or stable flies, with subsequent emergence and migration of *Habronema* sp. larvae into the dermis. **B,** Note sections of larvae within necrotic eosinophilic debris bordered by macrophages and mixed inflammation, including eosinophils. H&E stain. (**A** courtesy Dr. V. Fadok, College of Veterinary Medicine, University of Florida. **B** courtesy Dr. P.E. Ginn, College of Veterinary Medicine, University of Florida.)

Immunologic Skin Diseases Resulting from Autoimmune Reactions

Vasculitis

Purpura Hemorrhagica. Purpura (from the Latin meaning purple) are red or purple macules or patches caused by hemorrhage in the skin or mucous membranes. Purpura hemorrhagica in the horse occasionally develops as a sequel to *Streptococcus equi* infection, often involving the respiratory tract with abscessation in an internal site. Less commonly purpura hemorrhagica is seen subsequent to other infections or vaccinations. Affected horses may be febrile, anorectic, depressed, and reluctant to move. Lymph nodes may rupture and drain to the exterior. The clinical lesions of subcutaneous edema and petechial and sometimes ecchymotic hemorrhages of the skin and mucous membranes develop as a consequence of immune-complex vasculitis, which may also affect vessels of other organs such as the gastrointestinal tract. There may be serum exudation of distal extremities. Severely edematous skin may ooze serum and become necrotic and slough. Microscopic lesions consist of vascular wall disruption by neutrophils (neutrophilic vasculitis), perivascular edema, hemorrhage, and fibrin exudation.

Pastern Leukocytoclastic Vasculitis. Pastern leukocytoclastic vasculitis may represent a photoenhanced dermatosis; however, the cause and pathogenesis are unknown. Sun exposure appears to trigger lesion development in some horses, but lesions do not always resolve with removal from sun exposure. The disease is not considered a form of photosensitization because liver function is normal and exposure to photosensitizing chemicals has not been documented. Lesions typically develop in the white-haired legs, but rarely, similar lesions occur in legs covered with dark hair. Lesions initially consist of well-demarcated erythematous, moist, and crusted areas. More chronic lesions consist of plaques of epidermal acanthosis, hyperkeratosis, and crusting. Microscopically, lesions occur in small, thin-walled vessels of superficial dermal papillae. Early changes include vessel wall degeneration or necrosis and thrombosis. There is controversy regarding the presence of inflammation and true vasculitis. Although leukocytoclasia of neutrophils is described, the failure to demonstrate active vasculitis in many cases leads some veterinary dermatologists and pathologists to the preference of the term *vasculopathy*. Chronic changes include thickening and hyalinization of vessel walls. Epidermal changes include degeneration and hyperplasia, depending on stage of the disease. There may be mixed perivascular inflammation.

Hair Cycle Disorders of Endocrine Origin (Cutaneous Endocrine Disorders)

Hirsutism (Pituitary Dysfunction)

Tumors of the pars intermedia of the pituitary gland occur in older horses and can reach a large size, destroy the pituitary gland, and cause hypopituitarism and diabetes insipidus. The clinical signs in horses with pars intermedia pituitary tumors (polyphagia, polydipsia, polyuria, increased sweating, and an excessively long and thick hair coat) are largely mediated through dysfunction of the hypothalamus or neurohypophysis caused by an underlying expanding pituitary tumor. The long hair coat, also called *hypertrichosis* or *hirsutism*, is the result of failure to seasonally shed; cyclic shedding is mediated through the hypothalamus. Some tumors of the pars intermedia are functional and result in production of pro-opiomelanocortin (POMC), which is processed into high concentrations of various pars intermedia–derived peptides, including corticotropin-like intermediate lobe peptide, melanocyte-stimulating hormone, and β-endorphin, and much smaller concentrations of adrenocorticotropin. The combination of hypothalamic dysfunction and differential expression of pars intermedia–derived peptides over that of adrenocorticotropin results in a unique syndrome of hyperpituitarism in horses that differs from functional pituitary tumors in dogs and cats, which usually are associated with high concentrations of adrenocorticotropin. Some horses with large pituitary tumors also develop insulin-resistant hyperglycemia, which may be the result of down-regulation of insulin receptors secondary to chronic polyphagia and hyperinsulinemia. Insulin resistance is associated with an increased prevalence of laminitis.

Predominant Epidermal Hyperplasia (Lichenification or Crusts) Resulting from Disorders of Epidermal Growth or Differentiation

Equine Coronary Band Dystrophy

Equine coronary band dystrophy is a condition of unknown etiology and pathogenesis. Clinically, the coronary band (coronary border of hoof) is thickened, crusty, and scaly. Cracks and fissures can lead to lameness. The chestnuts and ergots (cornified protuberances considered to be vestiges of the first, second, and fourth digits) are similarly affected and can be ulcerated. Usually all four limbs are affected; however, the lesion may not involve the entire coronary band. Histologically, the epidermis of affected areas has marked papillary epidermal hyperplasia (see Fig. 17-11) and marked orthohyperkeratosis to parakeratotic hyperkeratosis. In some areas there is ballooning degeneration of keratinocytes. Dermal inflammation is minimal unless secondary infection is present. The diagnosis is made by ruling out the various differential diagnoses, including pemphigus foliaceus, hepatocutaneous syndrome, bacterial or fungal infection, selenium toxicosis, mite infestation, and eosinophilic exfoliative dermatitis. The condition is chronic and treatment palliative. Although the condition affects adult horses of any breed, draft breeds are considered predisposed.

Disorders Characterized by Infiltrates of Eosinophils or Plasma Cells

See Disorders of Domestic Animals, Miscellaneous Skin Disorders, Disorders Characterized by Infiltrates of Eosinophils or Plasma Cells.

Eosinophilic Granulomas (Collagenolytic Granulomas)

See Disorders of Domestic Animals, Miscellaneous Skin Disorders, Disorders Characterized by Infiltrates of Eosinophils or Plasma Cells, Eosinophilic Granulomas (Collagenolytic Granulomas).

Hypereosinophilic Syndromes with Systemic Signs or Lesions

Multisystemic Eosinophilic Epitheliotropic Disease in the Horse. Multisystemic eosinophilic epitheliotropic disease is a generalized, exfoliative dermatitis of horses that is of unknown etiology; however, one case report documents the coexistence of an intestinal T lymphocyte lymphoma and postulates a role for tumor cell overproduction of IL-5, a powerful eosinophilopoietin. Initial cutaneous lesions include dry scales and serous exudates of the epithelium of the skin of the head, coronary bands, and oral mucosa. The lesions progress to generalized excoriations with ulceration and alopecia. Secondary infections are common. Histologically, there is superficial and deep, perivascular to interstitial, eosinophilic lymphoplasmacytic, and sometimes granulomatous dermatitis with irregular epidermal hyperplasia and orthokeratotic and parakeratotic hyperkeratosis. Eosinophils, lymphocytes, and apoptotic keratinocytes can be prominent in the epidermis, and eosinophilic folliculitis, furunculosis, and flame figures are occasionally seen. The dermatitis is accompanied by a similar inflammatory response with fibrosis in other organs, including the alimentary tract, pancreas, liver, uterus, and bronchial epithelium. Clinically, most affected horses lose weight, become progressively debilitated, and either die naturally or are euthanized.

Nodular Granulomatous Inflammatory Disorders without Microorganisms

Equine Sarcoidosis

Equine sarcoidosis (equine idiopathic, generalized, or systemic granulomatous disease; equine histiocytic disease/dermatitis) is a rare disorder usually with exfoliative dermatitis, wasting, and granulomatous inflammation in multiple organ systems, although occasional cases limited to the skin have been reported. The cause and pathogenesis are unknown, but an immunologic reaction to a component of an infectious agent or allergen is hypothesized. A variety of breeds of horses, usually over 3 years of age, have been affected. Although some studies report mares are overrepresented, others report geldings are more often affected. Dermatitis usually begins as scaling, crusting, and alopecia on the face and trunk, or legs and progresses to multifocal or generalized exfoliative dermatitis. Cutaneous nodules are rare, and lymph nodes may be enlarged. Although skin may appear to be the only organ affected, most horses progress to more systemic involvement, including many viscera, central nervous system (CNS), and bone, clinically manifested by weight loss, ventral edema, fever, and signs associated with visceral organ dysfunction. Prognosis varies because many horses experience progressive dermatitis and wasting over the course of weeks to months and eventually are euthanized; however, there are reports of positive response to therapy especially if initiated early in the course of the disease, and spontaneous recovery has been reported. Horses with few isolated lesions limited to the skin are usually otherwise healthy. Histopathologic lesions include nodular to diffuse granulomatous inflammation with multinucleated giant cells intermixed with small numbers of lymphocytes, plasma cells, and neutrophils. Electron microscopy, animal inoculation studies, IF, and immunohistochemistry have been negative for microorganisms. Diagnosis is made by histopathologic evaluation, ruling out infectious agents that can also cause granulomatous dermatitis, and evaluation of history for dietary exposure to toxins such as hairy vetch (*Vicia* sp.).

Miscellaneous Disorders of Unknown or Complex Origin

Equine Pastern Dermatitis

Equine pastern dermatitis (also known as grease heel, scratches, or grapes) is a complex syndrome in which secondary staphylococcal folliculitis is common and complicates the diagnosis. There may be a genetic predisposition, which includes a long hair coat on the pastern area as often occurs in draft horses. Other predisposing factors are numerous and include excessive moisture, trauma, and contact dermatitis. Also, many other conditions affect the pastern skin in horses, including immune-mediated diseases (pemphigus foliaceus, vasculitis, or photosensitization), other infections (dermatophilosis, dermatophytosis), chronic progressive lymphedema of draft horses, and mite infestation (*Chorioptes* sp.). Equine pastern dermatitis occurs in male or female adult horses of a variety of breeds, is usually bilateral, and most commonly affects the caudal aspect of the hind legs, but lesions may progress to involve the cranial aspect of the legs, and front legs may also be affected. Early clinical lesions include edema, erythema, and scaling, which rapidly progress to exudation, matting of hair, and crusting. Ulcers may be present. Chronic lesions are thickened and fissured skin, are often painful, and may result in lameness. Diagnosis is facilitated by obtaining a complete history and performing thorough physical, dermatologic, microbiologic, and histopathologic evaluations early in the course of disease. Histopathologic lesions vary with stage of disease and severity, and histopathologic evaluation is most helpful in ruling out other conditions that affect pastern skin. In severe chronic lesions, initiating causes may not be identifiable, and histologic lesions are often nonspecific and consist of ulceration, crusting, and scarring, with mixed inflammatory infiltrates.

Disorders of Ruminants (Cattle, Sheep, and Goats)

For disorders occurring in two or more species of animals, see the section on Disorders of Domestic Animals.

Congenital and Hereditary Disorders

Congenital Hypertrichosis

Congenital hypertrichosis refers to excessive growth of hair, which can be congenital or hereditary. Congenital hypertrichosis has developed in fetal lambs secondary to hyperthermia in pregnant ewes living in areas of high environmental temperature. In addition to the hypertrichosis, the lambs are small, and few survive the first 2 months of life.

In utero border disease virus infection of fetal lambs results in an abnormally hairy fleece at birth, muscle tremors, defective myelination of the brain and spinal cord, abnormalities of body conformation, poor growth, and reduced viability. The fleece abnormalities and the muscle tremors result in the name hairy shaker disease. Fleece abnormalities are noted only in fine- and medium-wooled (smooth-coated) breeds. Fetal infection before 80 days of gestation results in an initial phase of retardation of follicular growth, followed by an extended period of rapid growth of primary follicles. The altered growth rate of follicles results in production of larger, more heavily medullated primary hairs, and the clinical appearance of the "hairy" fleece. The exact mechanism controlling the exaggerated growth of primary follicles is unknown. It has been speculated that reduction in number of the later developing secondary fibers could be the result of impaired nutrition because of placentitis. Microscopically, primary follicles and hairs are enlarged, and the number of the secondary follicles and wool fibers is reduced (see the discussion on hair follicles in the section on Structure and also Fig. 17-6). Diagnosis can be confirmed in affected lambs by histopathologic evaluation of the CNS with immunohistochemical staining for the virus, by viral isolation using precolostral serum or buffy coat, by viral antigen detection ELISA using ethylenediaminetetraacetic acid (EDTA) or heparinized blood, and by reverse transcription PCR (RT-PCR) of clinical specimens.

Disorders of Physical, Radiation, or Chemical Injury

Ergot Poisoning—Chemical Injury

Ergot poisoning is caused by the ingestion of toxic alkaloids produced by the fungus *Claviceps purpurea*. This fungus infects the seed heads of grasses and grains. The alkaloids, particularly ergotamine, cause direct stimulation of adrenergic nerves supplying arteriolar smooth muscle, resulting in marked peripheral arteriolar vasoconstriction and damage to capillary endothelium. Arteriolar spasm and damage to capillary endothelium lead to thrombosis and ischemic necrosis (infarction) of tissue. Cold temperatures increase the severity of the lesions. The species most commonly poisoned are cattle fed contaminated grain or cattle grazing pastures infected with the alkaloid-producing fungus. Lesions develop after approximately 1 week of consumption and begin as swelling and redness of the extremities, particularly the hind legs. Lesions begin at the coronary bands and extend to the fetlocks (metatarsophalangeal joints). The feet may become necrotic, with viable and nonviable tissue separated by a distinct line (dry gangrene). The front feet and tips of ears, teats, and tail can be affected and in severe cases can slough.

Tall Fescue Grass Ingestion—Chemical Injury

Lesions identical to those of ergot poisoning occur after the ingestion of tall fescue grass, a common pasture plant, infected by the endophytic fungus *Neotyphodium coenophialum* (formerly

Acremonium coenophialum). Lesions develop approximately 2 weeks after ingestion of the toxic plant and consist of necrosis (dry gangrene) of distal extremities. The ergot alkaloids, particularly ergovaline, are responsible for toxicity and act as peripheral vasoconstrictors.

Vetch Toxicosis and Vetch-like Diseases—Chemical Injury

See the section on Disorders of Domestic Animals; Disorders of Physical, Radiation, or Chemical Injury; Chemical Injury.

Viral Infections

Poxviruses

For more mechanistic detail, see the section on Disorders of Domestic Animals, Microbial and Parasitic Disorders, Viral Infections, Poxviruses.

Cowpox. Cowpox virus infections occur rarely in cattle in the United Kingdom and other areas of Europe. There is increasing evidence that small wild rodents (i.e., mice, squirrels, voles) serve as a reservoir for infection and that cattle, cats, and rarely other mammals become infected through contact with the wild rodents. Cutaneous infections in cattle usually develop on the teats and udder of cows and on the muzzle of suckling calves. Lesions follow the typical sequence of cutaneous poxviral infections. For cowpox infections in the cat, see the section on Disorders of Cats.

Bovine Papular Stomatitis. Bovine papular stomatitis virus is distributed worldwide, and although it causes disease more commonly in cattle more than 2 years old, disease can occur at any age and in any breed. Lesions occur on the muzzle, nostrils, lips, and mouth, and cows with suckling calves can develop teat and udder lesions. The development and appearance of the lesions are similar to pseudocowpox, with resolution of lesions in days to weeks. A chronic form has been described in which exudative necrotic dermatitis involves the trunk, as well as the mouth, and in which the animals died in 4 to 6 weeks. Transmission to human beings induces lesions identical to "milker's nodule" caused by *Pseudocowpox virus* infection. The histologic appearance of lesions is typical of other poxviral infections.

Capripoxviral Diseases. Capripoxviruses are the cause of sheeppox and goatpox. These viruses cause significant economic losses in countries where they are endemic, and the geographic distribution of these viruses is expanding. Sheeppox and goatpox are present in Africa, Asia, the Middle East, and most of the Indian subcontinent, where, despite attempts at vaccination, capripoxvirus is responsible for cycles of epidemic disease followed by periods of endemic maintenance with low morbidity. The disease is exotic to the Americas, Australia, and New Zealand. Although eradication measures eliminated the disease from Britain in the mid-nineteenth century, these measures have only recently been successful in eastern European countries. The diseases capripoxviruses cause lead to constraints on international trade of livestock and related products and can prevent the importation of new breeds of sheep or goats into endemic areas because fatality rates can be very high in nonindigenous breeds. Capripoxviruses are highly contagious and spread by the respiratory tract in times of close contact and mechanically by insect vectors and fomites. Virus is shed in saliva, conjunctival secretions, milk, urine, and feces, as well as in skin lesions and scabs. Vaccination of susceptible animals for sheeppox and goatpox provides lifelong immunity. The viruses share a high percentage of homology at the nucleotide and amino acid concentrations but are distinguishable phylogenetically using PCR–restriction fragment length polymorphism (PCR-RFLP) techniques. These viruses are also considered potential agents of agroterrorism.

Sheeppox. Sheeppox is caused by the sheeppox virus and is the most serious of the pox diseases of domestic animals. Sheeppox causes extensive economic loss through high mortality; reduced meat, milk, or wool yields; commercial inhibitions from quarantine requirements; and the cost of disease prevention programs.

Transmission of infection is by direct contact with diseased sheep or indirect contact via contaminated environment. Sheeppox virus is resistant to desiccation and remains viable for up to 2 months on wool or 6 months in dried crust. There are breed differences in disease susceptibility. Fine-wooled Merino sheep are particularly sensitive, whereas breeds native to endemic areas, such as Algerian sheep, are comparatively resistant. Sheeppox occurs in all ages of sheep with high morbidity and mortality as high as 50%, but the disease is most severe in lambs, with mortality reaching 80% to 100%. A high level of background immunity, such as occurs in endemic areas of Kenya, is associated with low mortality, even in the young.

Sheeppox is a systemic disease. Infection is usually by the respiratory route but may occur through skin abrasions. The incubation period varies from 4 to 21 days and is followed by a leukocyte-associated viremia. The virus localizes in many organs, including the skin, where the virus concentration is highest 10 to 14 days after infection. The initial clinical signs are fever, lacrimation, drooling, serous nasal discharge, and hyperesthesia. Skin lesions develop in 1 to 2 days and have a predilection for the sparsely wooled areas and typically involve eyelids, cheeks, nostrils, vulva, udder, scrotum, prepuce, ventral surface of the tail, and medial thigh. There is usually a concurrent superficial lymphadenopathy.

The macroscopic lesions follow the typical pattern for pox infections. Erythematous macules progress to papules, which may be firm. Sheeppox lesions have a variably prominent vesicular stage. The pustule stage is characterized by the formation of a thin crust. In severely affected animals the lesions coalesce and form areas of edema, hemorrhage, necrosis, and induration, involving all layers of the skin and subcutis (Fig. 17-65). These areas correspond to the development of vasculitis described later with microscopic lesions (see Fig. 17-65, *B*). Highly susceptible animals often develop hemorrhagic mucosal papules early in the course of the disease, and ulcerative lesions in the gastrointestinal and respiratory tracts develop later. Approximately one-third of animals develop multiple pulmonary lesions that constitute foci of pulmonary consolidation. The kidneys have multifocal, circular, and fleshy nodules throughout the renal cortices.

Healing of the skin lesions is slow, taking up to 6 weeks, and a scar may remain. In the milder form of the disease, seen in endemic areas, the full range of pox lesions does not develop. Instead, epidermal proliferation produces papules covered by scale-crust, which heal with desquamation in a few days. Such lesions often occur on the ventral surface of the tail.

Sheeppox lesions have the typical microscopic poxviral epithelial lesions, including intracytoplasmic inclusion bodies. The lesions affect both surface epidermis and hair follicles. There are also marked dermal lesions reflecting the systemic route of cutaneous involvement and possibly implicating immune-mediated lesions in addition to those caused by direct viral damage. The initial dermal lesions, corresponding to the macroscopic erythematous macule, are marked edema, hyperemia, and neutrophilic exocytosis. During the papular stage, large numbers of mononuclear cells accumulate in the increasingly edematous dermis. These mononuclear cells are called *sheeppox cells* and are characteristic of the disease. The nuclei of sheeppox cells are vacuolated and have marginated chromatin. The

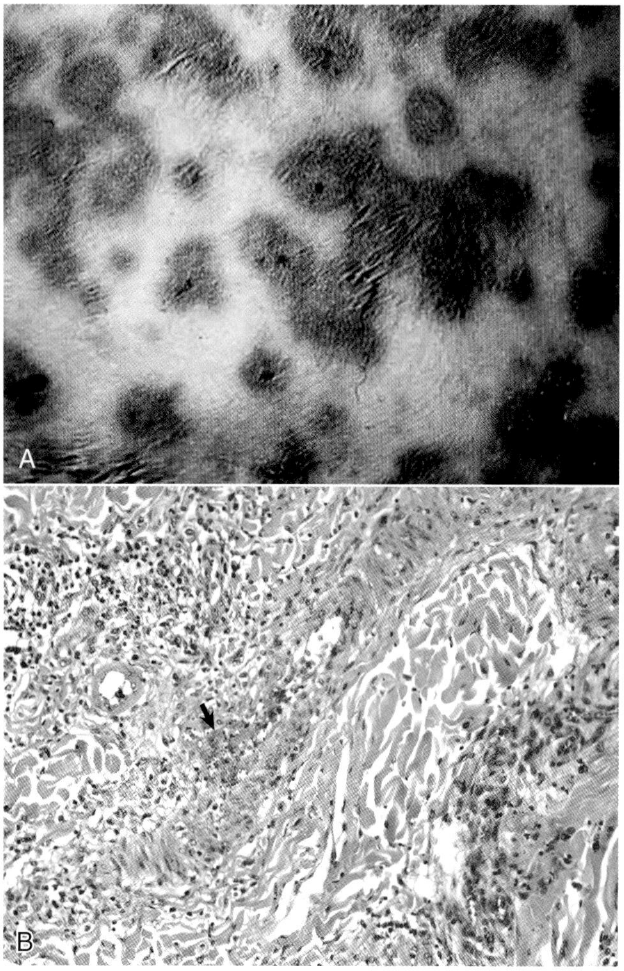

Figure 17-65 Sheeppox (Capripoxvirus), Skin, Lamb. A, The clinical lesions are multifocal coalescing macules and plaques that are indurated, hemorrhagic, and necrotic, likely a result of vasculitis. **B,** Note necrosis of vessel wall with fibrin deposition, red blood cells, and neutrophils and lymphocytes in the bordering dermis (vasculitis) *(arrow)*. H&E stain. (**A** courtesy *Foreign animal diseases*, ed 7, 2008, United States Animal Health Association. **B** courtesy Dr. A.M. Hargis, DermatoDiagnostics. Photographed from slides provided by Division of Animal Medicine, Animal Technology Institute Taiwan. From AFIP WSC October 8, 2008, Conference 5, Case III.)

vacuolated cytoplasm contains single, occasionally multiple, eosinophilic intracytoplasmic inclusion bodies. Sheeppox cells are virus-infected monocytes, macrophages, and fibroblasts, but not endothelial cells. Approximately 10 days after infection and corresponding with the most prominent epithelial lesions and peak of skin infectivity, severe necrotizing vasculitis develops in arterioles and postcapillary venules (see Fig. 17-65, *B*). Virus particles have not been identified in endothelial cells, and the vasculitis may be the result of immune-complex deposition. Ischemic necrosis of the dermis and overlying epidermis follows. The pulmonary lesions are proliferative alveolitis and bronchiolitis with focal areas of caseous necrosis. Alveolar septal cells contain intracytoplasmic inclusion bodies. Additional histologic lesions, characterized by the accumulation of sheeppox cells, may involve heart, kidney, liver, adrenal gland, thyroid gland, and pancreas.

The course and outcome of sheeppox depend not only on the usual host-virus relationship but also on the nature and location of secondary infections. The virus itself may cause death during the febrile, eruptive phase of the disease. Secondary bacterial infection and even septicemia and pneumonia can be the cause of death. Animals are also susceptible to fly strike.

Goatpox. Goatpox, caused by goatpox virus, occurs in the previously described geographic distribution, and a benign form of goatpox occurs in California and Sweden. The clinical signs of goatpox vary in different geographic areas. The disease is generally milder than sheeppox with a low mortality rate (5%), although generalized eruption with mortality rates approaching 100% may occur, with a course of disease similar to that of sheeppox infections in sheep. The cutaneous lesions have a predilection for the same areas as for sheeppox. In nursing kids, lesions may appear on the buccal mucosa or anterior nares. In animals with higher levels of resistance, the lesions may be confined to the udder, teats, inner aspects of thighs, or ventral surface of the tail.

Contagious Ecthyma. Contagious ecthyma (contagious pustular dermatitis, orf, sore mouth) is a common localized cutaneous infection of young sheep and goats caused by a parapoxvirus with worldwide distribution. Less commonly, human beings, cattle, wild ungulates, and dogs are infected. Morbidity in lambs is usually high, and although mortality is usually low, it can approach 15% in lambs. Lesions are initiated by abrasions; however, recent work has shown that active virus infection relies on proliferating keratinocytes that are in response to the cutaneous injury as opposed to the cutaneous injury itself. Cutaneous abrasions are typically acquired from pasture grasses or forage; begin at the commissures of the mouth and spread to the lips (Fig. 17-66), oral mucosa, eyelids, and feet; and are susceptible to secondary bacterial infection. In contrast to other poxviruses, the orf virus infection is typically limited to the skin and does not have a systemic phase to the infection, which may explain why an antibody response is not particularly important or effective for immunity to infection. This contrasts to many other poxvirus infections, which also gain entrance through skin, but their spread to other organs can occur and be partly controlled by antibody response. The orf virus may persist for long periods of time in the environment from infected material such as shed scabs, which is important because past natural infection does not confer immunity to reinfection. Unlike other poxviruses for which attenuated vaccines can be used to protect against infection, protection against contagious ecthyma is best provided by use of fully virulent vaccines, which may result in outbreaks of disease caused by the vaccine. Lambs can transfer the virus to the teats of ewes, and the lesions can spread to the skin of the udder. Contagious ecthyma is economically important as the result of weight loss in lambs that are reluctant to eat because of the pain associated with oral and perioral lesions. Pathogenesis of lesion formation and gross and microscopic features are consistent with the typical cutaneous poxvirus lesions (see previous discussion and see Fig. 17-32), except that the vesicle stage is very brief, the ulcer and crust stage persists and is clinically prominent, and the epidermis is markedly hyperplastic. Viral inclusion bodies are often not identified histologically because they are only briefly detectable during the earliest stages of infection.

Herpesviruses

For more mechanistic detail, see the section on Disorders of Domestic Animals, Microbial and Parasitic Disorders, Viral Infections, Herpesviruses.

Bovine Herpesvirus 2. Bovine herpesvirus 2, a dermatotropic virus (Allerton virus), can cause generalized disease (pseudo–lumpy skin disease) or as seen in the United States, localized infection of the teat called *bovine ulcerative mammillitis* (bovine herpes

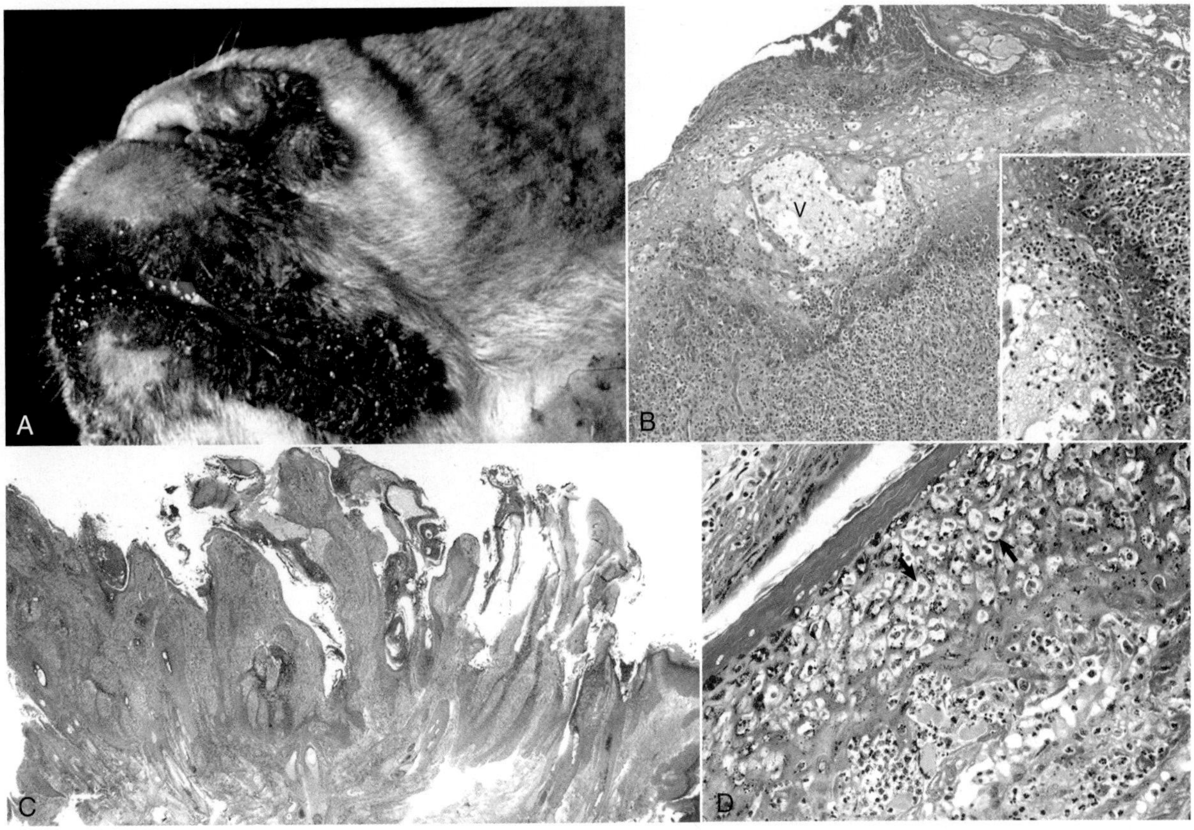

Figure 17-66 **Contagious Ecthyma (Contagious Pustular Dermatitis, Orf, Sore Mouth, or Scabby Mouth), Skin, Lamb. A,** Note crusts around nose and lips. These lesions are the late stage of the disease, are formed after rupture of vesicles and pustules, and are responsible for the common name scabby mouth. Blood may be incorporated into crusts following severe exudation and inflammation that can damage vessel walls secondarily. The blood may contribute to the darkly colored crusts as seen in **A. B,** Note the epidermal hyperplasia (acanthosis), ballooning degeneration, vesicle *(V)*, and neutrophils accumulating in the vesicle, which subsequently results in the formation of a pustule. Free red blood cells are present in the epidermis to the left of the vesicle. Epidermal hyperplasia, upward movement of the pustule, and rupture of the vesicle or pustule contribute to crust formation as seen in **A**. *Inset*, Higher magnification of a portion of the vesicle. H&E stain. **C,** Marked hyperplasia of the epidermis and follicular infundibula results in a papillary appearance of the surface that is further accentuated by mounds and columns of exudative crust overlying the congested and inflamed dermal papillae. H&E. **D,** Segment of ballooning degeneration of keratinocytes in the stratum granulosum near the edge of a lesion. Affected keratinocytes are swollen with pale eosinophilic cytoplasm (ballooning degeneration). The keratohyalin granules are peripheralized, but the nucleus remains in the center of the keratinocyte. One or more large, acidophilic cytoplasmic viral inclusion bodies typical of parapoxvirus infection *(arrows)* are present. H&E stain. (**A** courtesy Dr. M.D. McGavin, College of Veterinary Medicine, University of Tennessee. **B** courtesy Dr. A.M. Hargis, DermatoDiagnostics. **C** and **D** courtesy Dr. S. Myers, Prairie Diagnostic Services.)

mammillitis). Mammillitis is inflammation of the teat or nipple. Localized infection occurs more commonly in lactating dairy cows but can develop in beef cows, pregnant heifers, and suckling calves. Trauma is implicated in the pathogenesis because normal skin is resistant to viral penetration. The pathogenesis of lesion formation is discussed earlier. Bovine ulcerative mammillitis is economically important because of decreased milk production and secondary bacterial mastitis. Lesions develop on the teats and skin of the nearby udder or occasionally the perineum. Suckling calves develop lesions on the muzzle (nose).

Bovine Herpesvirus 4. Bovine herpesvirus 4 (bovine herpes mammary pustular dermatitis) causes a similar but milder disease than the localized form of bovine herpesvirus 2.

Bacterial Infections

Ovine Fleece Rot (Superficial Bacterial Infection [Superficial Pyoderma])

Ovine fleece rot is a superficial bacterial dermatitis usually caused by excessive moisture (usually in the form of rain) that penetrates the fleece (wool), wets the skin, and causes proliferation of *Pseudomonas* spp. Approximately 1 week of continual wetting is usually sufficient to cause marked proliferation of the bacteria on the skin and in the fleece. This is followed by an acute inflammatory response with serum exudation and matting of the fleece. The fleece is also discolored because of production of pigments (chromogens) by the *Pseudomonas* bacteria and has a rotten odor. The condition may be complicated by other concurrent microbial infections such as dermatophilosis. Microscopic lesions include epidermal pustular dermatitis and superficial folliculitis. Ovine fleece rot is important economically because the malodor attracts flies, predisposing to myiasis (infestation of tissue by the larvae of dipterous flies), and the value of the affected wool is reduced.

Bacterial Granulomatous Dermatitis (Bacterial Granulomas)

Mycobacterial Granuloma. See Disorders of Domestic Animals, Microbial and Parasitic Disorders, Bacterial Infections, Bacterial Granulomatous Dermatitis (Bacterial Granulomas), Mycobacterial Granulomas.

Papillomatous Digital Dermatitis (Bacterial Pododermatitis)

Papillomatous digital dermatitis (see Table 17-12), also known as *foot warts* or *hairy heel warts*, is a painful, contagious dermatitis of the feet primarily of high-production dairy cattle. It occurs worldwide. The cause of papillomatous digital dermatitis is multifactorial and likely involves genetic predisposition, management conditions that allow the feet of cattle to remain wet for prolonged periods of time without access to air, in combination with multiple species of bacteria, including spirochetes belonging to the genus *Treponema* playing a predominant role. Papillomatous digital dermatitis most commonly affects the skin proximal and adjacent to the interdigital space at the caudal (plantar) aspect of the hind feet. Early gross lesions are well-circumscribed, round to oval, red plaques up to 6 cm in diameter with a moist granular surface prone to bleeding and with a very strong, pungent odor. Lesions are partially to completely alopecic and can be bordered by hypertrophied hairs two to three times longer than normal. Early microscopic lesions are largely limited to the epidermis, with minimal dermal involvement mostly consisting of minimal perivascular inflammation. Epidermal lesions consist of hyperplasia with foci of erosion, necrosis, ballooning degeneration, and microabscesses. Mixed bacteria can be present in the outer necrotic debris, but only spirochetes are present in the deeper viable epidermis. The lesions become progressively more proliferative and less painful with time. Mature lesions are irregular wartlike growths or filamentous papillae that measure 0.5 to 1.0 mm in diameter and 1 mm to 3 cm in length and are pale yellow, gray, or brown. Histologically the older lesions are composed of frondlike projections or plaques of markedly hyperplastic epidermis with parakeratosis and hyperkeratosis. Foci of necrosis and hemorrhage, ballooning degeneration, and aggregates of neutrophils are scattered throughout the hyperplastic epidermis (Fig. 17-67). At this later stage, inflammation is more intense in the dermis, and plasma cells can be numerous. Lesions are painful, forcing the animal to shift its weight to the toe of the affected foot, which results in a smooth contour to the toe (clubbing) and atrophy of the bulbs of the heels.

Papillomatous digital dermatitis is economically important because it frequently causes moderate to severe lameness that results in weight loss, decreased milk production, and poor reproductive performance. The vast majority of cases are in dairy cows, but the infection has also been reported in beef cattle. Although the disease occurs in cattle of all ages, the highest incidence appears to be in replacement dairy heifers.

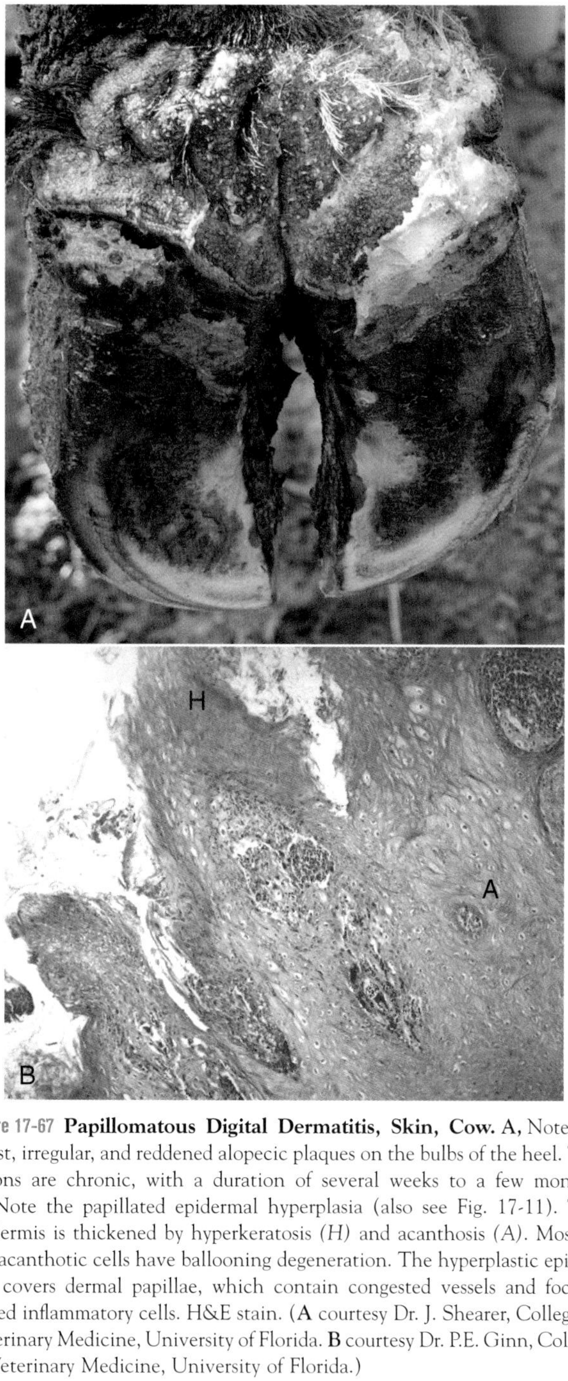

Figure 17-67 **Papillomatous Digital Dermatitis, Skin, Cow. A,** Note the moist, irregular, and reddened alopecic plaques on the bulbs of the heel. The lesions are chronic, with a duration of several weeks to a few months. **B,** Note the papillated epidermal hyperplasia (also see Fig. 17-11). The epidermis is thickened by hyperkeratosis *(H)* and acanthosis *(A)*. Most of the acanthotic cells have ballooning degeneration. The hyperplastic epidermis covers dermal papillae, which contain congested vessels and foci of mixed inflammatory cells. H&E stain. (**A** courtesy Dr. J. Shearer, College of Veterinary Medicine, University of Florida. **B** courtesy Dr. P.E. Ginn, College of Veterinary Medicine, University of Florida.)

Necrobacillosis of Cattle (Bacterial Pododermatitis)

Necrobacillosis (foul-in-the-foot, interdigital phlegmon, interdigital necrobacillosis, foot rot) (see Table 17-12) of cattle is an infection originating in the interdigital skin that is caused by *F. necrophorum* and *Prevotella melaninogenica* (formerly *Bacteroides melaninogenicus*). Predisposing factors include interdigital trauma in combination with increased moisture, heat, and poor housing conditions that allow contact with manure and urine. *F. necrophorum* and *P. melaninogenica* are rumen microbes, are passed through the gastrointestinal tract, and thus readily contaminate the environment. *F. necrophorum* produces an exotoxin (leukotoxin) that causes necrosis and damages leukocytes. The infection usually involves both digits of a single foot in adult cattle, but several feet may be involved in calves. The disease progresses rapidly and is associated with a malodor. Early lesions are swelling and erythema of the soft tissues of the interdigital space and coronary band. The leukotoxin causes necrosis and exudation, which can progress to cellulitis that may extend into the deeper structures of the foot such as the distal phalanx, distal sesamoid bone, distal interphalangeal joint, and tendons. Extensive necrosis can lead to sloughing of affected tissue. The infection causes extreme pain and lameness, and affected individuals may have fever and anorexia. Diagnosis is usually made by clinical examination of the affected foot because clinical lesions and malodor are usually sufficient to provide diagnosis.

Contagious Foot Rot, Benign Foot Rot in Cattle (Bacterial Pododermatitis)

Contagious foot rot (benign foot rot, stable foot rot, interdigital dermatitis) (see Table 17-12) is a slowly progressive, low-grade infection of the interdigital skin that is seen most commonly in intense dairy productions with poor hygiene. Moisture and trauma damage the interdigital epidermis and allow entrance of mixed bacterial populations of which the obligate anaerobic bacteria *Dichelobacter nodosus* is considered to be the most important. Other bacteria, including *F. necrophorum*, may contribute. The infection is spread from infected to uninfected cows through the environment. The bacteria invade the epidermis but usually do not penetrate the dermis and may progress to erosions and ulcers that cause discomfort. Exudate may ooze from the commissures of the interdigital space and dry to form a crust. Diagnosis is usually made by clinical examination. The major differential diagnosis is papillomatous digital dermatitis.

Contagious Foot Rot in Sheep (Bacterial Pododermatitis)

Contagious foot rot in sheep (see Table 17-12) is a serious, economically important disease occurring in most sheep-producing countries. The infection is caused by the Gram-negative anaerobe *D. nodosus*. Depending on climatic and host factors, and the virulence of the bacterial strain, lesions vary from mild interdigital dermatitis (benign foot rot) to severe separation of the horn of the hoof (virulent foot rot). The major virulence factors of *D. nodosus* are type IV fimbria (short fine appendages surrounding the bacterial cell that allow colonization of epidermis) and extracellular proteases that degrade tissue. The virulent form is caused by more virulent *D. nodosus* that produces significantly more proteolytic enzymes (proteases including elastase), allowing more bacterial penetration of the epidermis. The proteases in the virulent form also tend to be more heat stable. Virulent foot rot is more persistent (and can last for more than 1 year if not treated), affects a high percentage of sheep, affects more than one foot, and can result in death of sheep because of emaciation as a result of severe pain and reluctance to graze. Early lesions of virulent foot rot begin in the interdigital axial (inner) region, affect both digits, and consist of red, moist, and swollen eroded skin. The infection spreads to the epidermal matrix of the hoof and results in a malodorous exudate that separates the horn from the interdigital skin. Lesions progress to the bulb (heel) and sole, and finally to the abaxial (outer) surfaces of the hoof wall. The germinal epidermis is not destroyed, and although regeneration is attempted, the new horn is destroyed. In chronic infections, hooves can become long and misshapen. Benign foot rot in sheep is mild, confined to interdigital skin, and can have slight separation of the horn of the heel. The hoof can overgrow. Diagnosis of foot rot in sheep is often made by clinical evaluation of the flock and lesion severity and examination of smears or cultures for *D. nodosus*. However, culture and typing, as for other fastidious anaerobes, is difficult and laborious, is not widely offered in diagnostic laboratories, and culture alone may not distinguish between virulent and nonvirulent strains. More recently PCR testing has been developed that detects and differentiates virulent and nonvirulent strains of *D. nodosus*.

Necrobacillosis of Sheep (Bacterial Pododermatitis)

Necrobacillosis of the foot in sheep includes ovine interdigital dermatitis and foot abscesses (see Table 17-12). Ovine interdigital dermatitis is an acute necrotizing dermatitis that is clinically similar to benign foot rot. Both benign foot rot and ovine interdigital dermatitis have been termed "foot scald." Ovine interdigital dermatitis can be differentiated from foot rot by the failure to demonstrate *D. nodosus* in smears or cultures of exudate, or with PCR from ovine interdigital dermatitis cases, but these differentiating tests are not always performed. Conditions similar to benign foot rot and ovine interdigital dermatitis occur in goats. In sheep, foot abscesses affect the heel (infective bulbar necrosis) or toe (lamellar abscesses). Foot abscesses are more common in wet seasons and in heavy adult sheep. In addition to *F. necrophorum*, *Trueperella pyogenes* (*Arcanobacterium pyogenes*) may be isolated from the lesions.

Contagious Ovine Digital Dermatitis (Bacterial Pododermatitis)

Contagious ovine digital dermatitis (CODD) (see Table 17-12) is a severe infection of the ovine hoof reported in the United Kingdom, with initial reports occurring in 1997. The disease has spread widely in the sheep population and is of major animal welfare concern. It most commonly affects one foot, but multiple digits may be affected, and 80% of affected sheep are lame. The cause of this form of digital dermatitis in sheep is not yet completely defined but thought to be polymicrobial, with spirochetes belonging to the genus *Treponema*, including *Treponema* sp. phylogenetically identical to those associated with bovine digital dermatitis, frequently isolated from affected sheep. *D. nodosus* and *F. necrophorum* have also been isolated from affected sheep, but their role in the pathogenesis of the disease is uncertain. The condition differs from typical contagious foot rot in sheep in that the lesions have an acute onset, are more severe, and are characterized by ulcerative lesions of the coronary band and hoof wall in some cases (contagious foot rot lesions affect the heel and interdigital region). Select systemic antibiotic therapy improves likelihood of recovery and reduces the rate of new infection development. The pathogenesis of lesion formation is not yet known. Early gross lesions consist of ulcers at the coronary band and progress to loosening, and possible shedding, of the hoof wall or capsule. Interdigital lesions are not reported. Microscopic lesions have not been described.

Parasitic Infections

Filarial Dermatitis

Stephanofilariasis, a filarial dermatitis of cattle, buffalo, and goats, is transmitted by flies and caused by six species of parasites of the genus *Stephanofilaria*. Each species of *Stephanofilaria* causes lesions in a different body location. Cutaneous lesions are caused by a reaction to the parasites free in the dermis, to the bites of the flies serving as the vector, and self-inflicted trauma. *Stephanofilaria stilesi* occurs in cattle in the United States and causes lesions along the ventral midline that consist initially of small (1 cm) circular patches with moist erect hairs, foci of epidermal hemorrhage, and serum exudation. Such foci expand and coalesce into a large area covered by crusts, which, on healing, consist of thickened hairless plaques as large as 25 cm in diameter (Fig. 17-68). Microscopic lesions consist of superficial and deep perivascular dermatitis with eosinophils, epidermal hyperkeratosis, parakeratosis, acanthosis with spongiosis, eosinophilic microabscesses, and crusts, and adult parasites and microfilaria can be seen. In addition, adult parasites and microfilaria also can be identified in deep skin scrapings that are macerated in isotonic saline solution and examined microscopically.

Immunologic Skin Disease Resulting from Autoimmune Reactions

Vasculitis

Vasculitis is rare in cattle. It is seen with malignant catarrhal fever (see Chapters 4 and 7). Capripoxvirus causing lumpy skin disease in cattle causes damage to endothelial cells, resulting in vasculitis that is central to the pathogenesis of lesions in this condition. Systemic infection with *Salmonella dublin* can also cause gangrene of the distal extremities, tail, and pinnae as a result of venous thrombosis related to endotoxins.

Vasculitis in sheep and goats is also rare and is seen as part of systemic capripoxvirus infections (see section on Viral Infections).

Zinc Deficiency

Dietary Zinc Deficiency in Ruminants

Information on this topic is available at www.expertconsult.com.

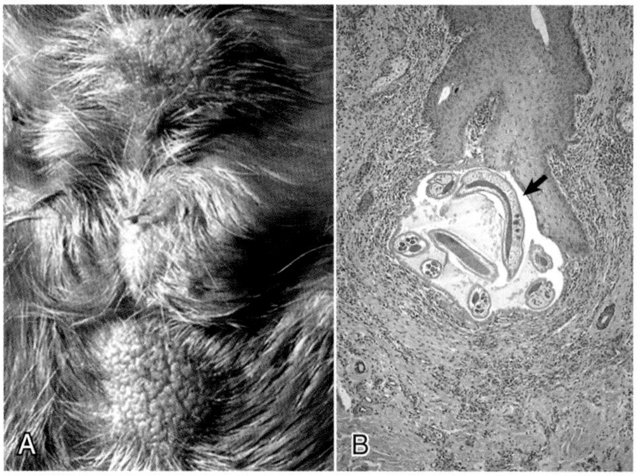

Figure 17-68 ***Stephanofilaria* Dermatitis, *Stephanofilaria stilesi*, Skin, Cow. A,** Ventral abdomen. Note the thickened plaquelike area of alopecia and lichenification. **B,** Note longitudinal and cross sections of adult nematode. The adult nematodes usually live in a cystlike space at the base of a hair follicle *(arrow)* and can destroy follicles. Note the marked infiltrate of mixed inflammatory cells around the cystic space and base of the follicle (perifolliculitis). The follicle has a hyperplastic and irregular wall. H&E stain. (**A** courtesy Dr. M.D. McGavin, College of Veterinary Medicine, University of Tennessee. **B** courtesy Dr. P.E. Ginn, College of Veterinary Medicine, University of Florida.)

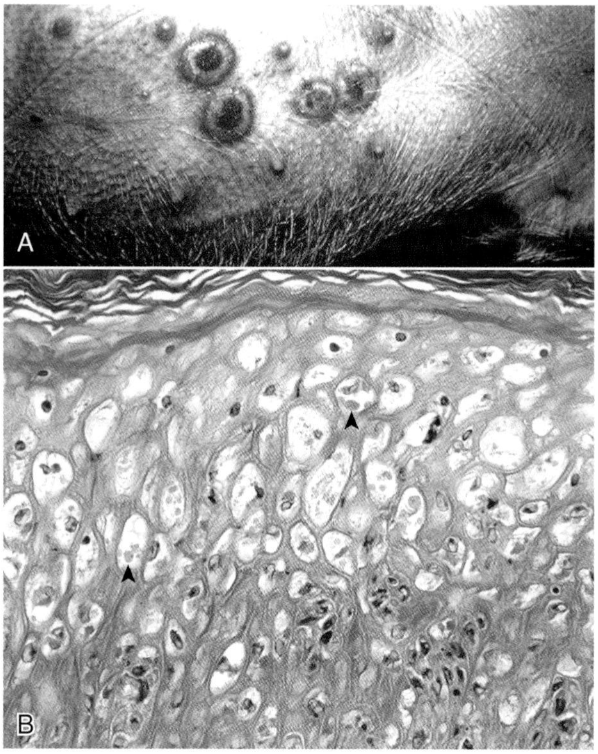

Figure 17-69 **Swinepox, Skin, Piglet. A,** Note the four umbilicated pustules in the abdominal skin. **B,** Note keratinocytes with ballooning degeneration and eosinophilic cytoplasmic viral inclusion bodies *(arrowheads)*. Ballooning degeneration develops before vesicle formation. H&E stain. (**A** courtesy Dr. M.D. McGavin, College of Veterinary Medicine, University of Tennessee. **B** courtesy Dr. A.M. Hargis, DermatoDiagnostics. Photographed from slides provided by Department of Veterinary Pathology, Western College of Veterinary Medicine, University of Saskatchewan. From AFIP WSC January 21, 1998, Conference 15, Case IV.)

Hereditary Zinc Deficiency in Calves and Goats

Information on this topic is available at www.expertconsult.com.

Disorders of Pigs

For disorders occurring in two or more species of animals, see the section on Disorders of Domestic Animals.

Congenital and Hereditary Disorders

Dermatosis Vegetans

Dermatosis vegetans is an inherited disorder of young pigs characterized by vegetating skin lesions, hoof malformation, and giant cell pneumonia. The condition is a simple autosomal recessive trait of Landrace pigs. The pathogenesis of lesion formation is unknown. Skin lesions can be present at birth but might not develop until 2 to 3 months of age. Lesions begin as erythematous papules on the ventral abdomen and medial aspect of the thighs and possibly the sides and back. The papules enlarge peripherally to form plaques with a depressed center filled with gray to brown-black granular brittle material. Each crusty plaque is sharply demarcated from normal skin by a hyperemic raised border. As lesions spread peripherally, they coalesce to form extensive horny, papilloma-like areas covered by black crusts. Hoof lesions, if they occur, are always present at birth. Usually all digits, including accessory digits, on more than one limb are affected. The coronary region is markedly swollen and erythematous, and a yellow-brown greasy material covers the skin. The wall of the hoof is thickened by ridges and furrows parallel to the coronary band. Histologically, fully developed cutaneous lesions have marked orthokeratotic and parakeratotic hyperkeratosis, prominent irregular epidermal hyperplasia, intercellular edema, and intraepidermal pustules and microabscesses containing eosinophils and neutrophils. Affected piglets frequently die of secondary infection when skin lesions reach the typical papilloma-like stage (5 to 8 weeks of age) either from entrance of bacteria from skin lesions or a bacterial pneumonia complicating the giant cell pneumonia characteristic of this disease. Skin lesions begin to resolve if the pig survives.

Viral Infections

Poxviruses

For more mechanistic detail, see the section on Disorders of Domestic Animals, Microbial and Parasitic Disorders, Viral Infections, Poxviruses.

Swinepox. Pox lesions in pigs are caused by the host-specific poxvirus *Suipoxvirus* (swinepox). Normally swinepox is transmitted by contact, although transplacental infection has not been ruled out. The sucking louse *Haematopinus suis* often acts as a mechanical vector and assists infection by causing skin trauma. The virus persists in dried crusts from infected animals. The pathogenesis of lesion formation and morphologic features of the gross and histologic lesions are consistent with the typical pox infection. The gross lesions typically affect the ventral and lateral abdomen, lateral thorax, and medial foreleg and thigh. Occasionally lesions on the dorsum predominate. Lesions can be generalized and rarely involve the oral mucosa, pharynx, esophagus, stomach, trachea, and bronchi. The erythematous papules usually transform into umbilicated pustules without a significant vesicular stage (Fig. 17-69). The inflammatory crust eventually sheds to leave a white scar. The disease occurs worldwide and is endemic to areas of intensive production of pigs. The disease affects young, growing piglets and is mild with very low mortality.

Bacterial Infections (Superficial Bacterial Infections [Superficial Pyodermas])

For more mechanistic detail, see the section on Disorders of Domestic Animals, Microbial and Parasitic Disorders, Bacterial Infections, Superficial Bacterial Infections (Superficial Pyodermas), Superficial Pustular Dermatitis.

Exudative Epidermitis of Pigs (Greasy Pig Disease)

Exudative epidermitis, usually caused by *S. hyicus*, is an acute, often fatal, dermatitis of neonatal piglets, but a mild disease in older piglets. Predisposing factors include cutaneous lacerations and poor nutrition. In piglets, brownish exudates develop around the eyes, pinnae, snout, chin, and medial legs and spread to the ventral thorax and abdomen, giving the animal an overall "greasy" appearance (Fig. 17-70). The lesions rapidly coalesce and become generalized, resulting in greasy, malodorous exudates covering an erythematous skin. If piglets survive, the exudate hardens, cracks, and forms fissures. Subacute disease develops gradually in older piglets, and lesions are generally localized to the skin of the face, pinnae, and periocular regions. Grossly, the epidermis is thickened with scaling. The early histopathologic lesion is subcorneal pustular dermatitis, which extends to the hair follicle, resulting in superficial suppurative folliculitis. In the fully developed lesion the epidermis is hyperplastic and has thick crusts of keratin, microabscesses, and cocci. The term *exudative epidermitis* is descriptive of this condition because the inflammatory changes largely involve the epidermis, and there is an accumulation of exudates on the surface. The dermis is congested and edematous. In the early stages the dermatitis is superficial and perivascular with neutrophils and eosinophils, and in the later stages it is perivascular and mononuclear.

Bacterial Granulomatous Dermatitis (Bacterial Granulomas)

Mycobacterial Granuloma

See the section on Disorders of Domestic Animals, Microbial and Parasitic Disorders, Bacterial Infections, Bacterial Granulomatous Dermatitis (Bacterial Granulomas), Mycobacterial Granulomas.

Bacterial Infections with Toxin-Producing Bacteria

For more mechanistic detail, see Disorders of Domestic Animals, Microbial and Parasitic Disorders, Bacterial Infections, Skin Lesions Secondary to Systemic Bacterial Infections or Infection with Toxin-Producing Bacteria.

Erysipelas

Cutaneous lesions caused by *E. rhusiopathiae* (erysipelas) in pigs are a result of bacterial embolization to the skin during sepsis. Lesions consist of square to rhomboidal, firm, raised, pink to dark purple areas (Fig. 17-71) and are caused by vasculitis, thrombosis, and ischemia (infarction). The rhomboidal shape likely represents the area of skin no longer receiving blood supply from the now thrombosed vessel.

Septicemic Infection with Salmonella *sp.,* Pasteurella multocida, *or* Escherichia coli

Septicemic salmonellosis causes cyanosis of the external ears and abdomen because of capillary dilation, congestion, and thrombosis. The thrombosis leads to necrosis of distal extremities. The mechanism of vascular damage involves endotoxin-induced venous thrombosis. Systemic infection with *P. multocida* can cause similar lesions in pigs. *E. coli* production of Shiga toxin 2e (verotoxin 2e) causes edema disease that primarily affects healthy, rapidly growing nursery pigs. The Shiga toxin is produced in the intestine, is absorbed into the circulation, and targets vascular endothelium with high concentrations of the toxin receptor globotetraosyl ceramide. This results in vascular degeneration, necrosis, edema, and hemorrhage. Gross lesions of the skin in edema disease consist of accumulation of clear fluid (edema) in the subcutis of the snout, eyelids, submandibular area, ventral abdomen, and inguinal areas. Histologically, the subcutis is edematous, and there may be edema, hemorrhage, microthrombi, and smooth muscle necrosis and hyaline degeneration of the tunica media of small arteries and arterioles in the skin and other areas of the body.

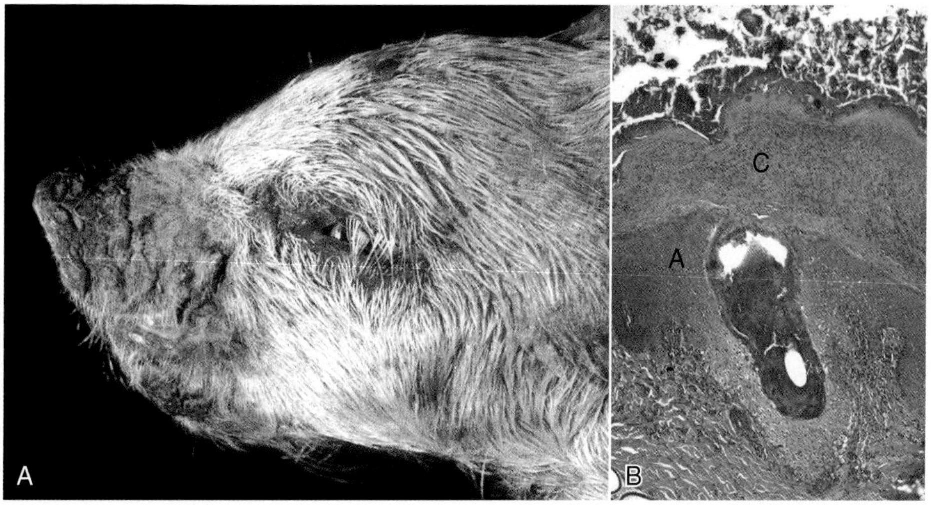

Figure 17-70 Exudative Epidermitis, *Staphylococcus hyicus (hyos)*, Skin, Piglet. A, Head. Exudative epidermitis is also called greasy pig disease. The skin in this pig is heavily crusted, lichenified, and fissured. Greasy exudate focally has adhered to the hair and the skin surface. **B,** Note the epidermal hyperplasia (acanthosis *[A]*) and suppurative exudate within the lumen of a hair follicle and on the epidermal surface. The exudate has dried to form a thick pustular crust *(C)* that is fragmenting superficially. H&E stain. (**A** courtesy Dr. M.D. McGavin, College of Veterinary Medicine, University of Tennessee. **B** courtesy Dr. P.E. Ginn, College of Veterinary Medicine, University of Florida.)

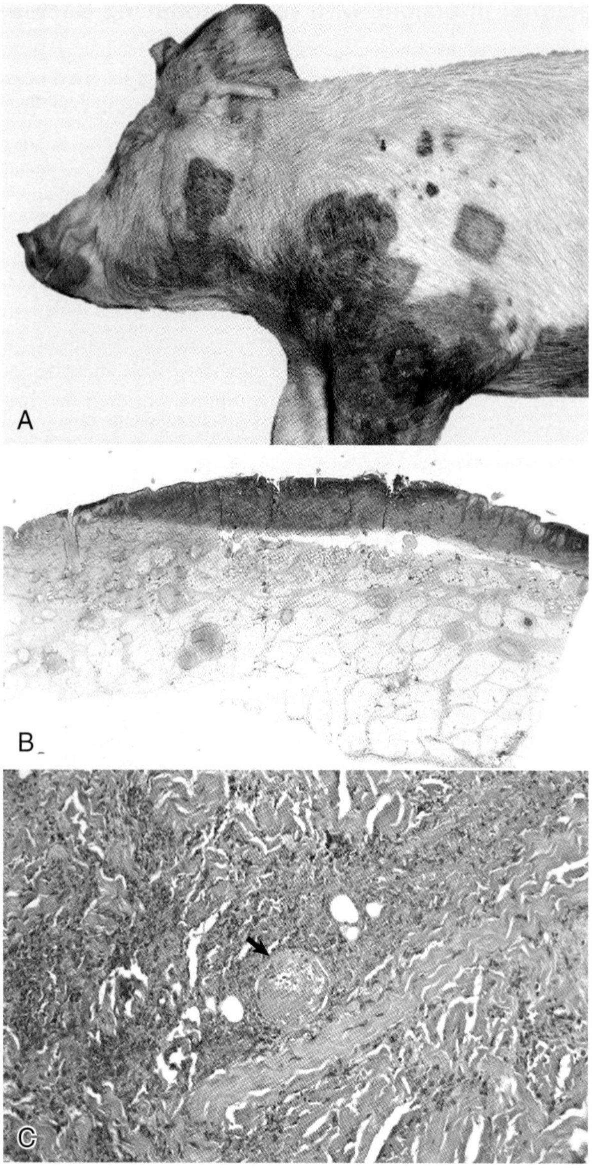

Figure 17-71 ***Erysipelothrix rhusiopathiae*** **Infection, Skin, Haired, Pig. A,** The reddish rhomboidal lesions in the skin are infarcts secondary to thrombosis, from the embolization of septic emboli. **B,** The epidermis and dermis are markedly necrotic from infarction with only a small amount of normal dermis and epidermis at the extreme left. H&E stain. **C,** Note the vascular thrombosis (*arrow*). H&E stain. (**A** and **B** courtesy Dr. M.D. McGavin, College of Veterinary Medicine, University of Tennessee. **C** courtesy Dr. P.E. Ginn, College of Veterinary Medicine, University of Florida.)

Immunologic Skin Disease Resulting from Autoimmune Reactions

Vasculitis

Vasculitis is uncommon to rare in pigs and usually is seen in association with bacterial infection such as *E. rhusiopathiae*, and Gram-negative septicemias caused by *Salmonella*, *Pasteurella*, or *E. coli*. In addition, a condition called *porcine dermatitis and nephropathy syndrome*, predominantly affecting the vessels in the skin and kidneys, has been described. The incidence is usually low (less than 1%); however, epizootics in which the incidence reaches 10% to 20% or higher have been described. Mortality is high (80% to 90%). The cause and pathogenesis are unknown, but the condition may be associated with infection with porcine circovirus 2, porcine reproductive and respiratory syndrome virus, or *P. multocida*. However, the role of these etiologic agents in porcine dermatitis and nephropathy syndrome has not been proven. Immune complex deposition is thought to play a role. Immunoglobulin and complement have been detected in cutaneous vessel walls and glomeruli. Clinical lesions consist of acute-onset cutaneous erythematous to hemorrhagic papules, macules, and plaques that progress to multifocal raised red crusts with black centers that are most severe on the hind limbs, ventral abdomen, flanks, and perineum. Necrosis and ulceration may develop. Histologic lesions are necrotizing neutrophilic vasculitis with hemorrhage, edema, and fibrin deposition affecting small- and medium-sized arteries of the skin, kidney, and other tissues, accompanied by thrombosis and infarction. Systemic signs include fever and lethargy, and the condition is commonly fatal.

Zinc Deficiency

Dietary Zinc Deficiency

Information on this topic is available at www.expertconsult.com.

Predominant Epidermal Hyperplasia (Lichenification or Crusts) Resulting from Disorders of Epidermal Growth or Differentiation

Porcine Juvenile Pustular Psoriasiform Dermatitis (Pityriasis Rosea)

Porcine juvenile pustular psoriasiform dermatitis (pityriasis rosea) develops in suckling and young pigs (3 to 14 weeks of age), usually resolves spontaneously by 4 weeks of onset, and is thought to be inherited. A few piglets in the litter or entire litters can be affected. Lesions are symmetric and develop on the abdomen, groin, and medial thigh and begin as small papules covered by brown crusts. The lesions coalesce and spread and develop into umbilicated plaques with white centers and erythematous, scaly borders that can progress into mosaic patterns (Fig. 17-72). These clinical lesions resemble those of dermatophytosis, swinepox, and dermatosis vegetans, from which they need to be differentiated, but otherwise the clinical lesions are of no significance. Microscopically, the early histologic lesions are superficial and deep perivascular neutrophilic, eosinophilic, and mixed mononuclear dermatitis. Epidermal spongiosis and leukocytic exocytosis result in spongiform pustules. Later, lesions consist of marked psoriasiform epidermal hyperplasia (regular epidermal hyperplasia with epidermal projections of uniform length and width) and parakeratotic cellular crust.

Disorders of Dogs

For disorders occurring in two or more species of animals, see the section on Disorders of Domestic Animals.

Congenital and Hereditary Disorders

Also see the section on Disorders of Domestic Animals, Congenital and Hereditary Disorders.

Mucinosis (Hereditary Cutaneous Hyaluronosis) of the Chinese Shar-Pei Dog

Dermal mucinosis occurs as an inherited dermal connective tissue disorder in the Chinese Shar-Pei dog in which the presence of the dermal mucin causes the thick, wrinkly skin that typifies this breed. The range in degree of dermal mucin deposition varies greatly with some Shar-Pei dogs having small quantities of dermal mucin and minimally wrinkly skin, whereas other Shar-Pei dogs have excessive quantities of dermal mucin, thick wrinkly skin, and "lakes" or pools of dermal mucin that can create clinically evident vesicles. The

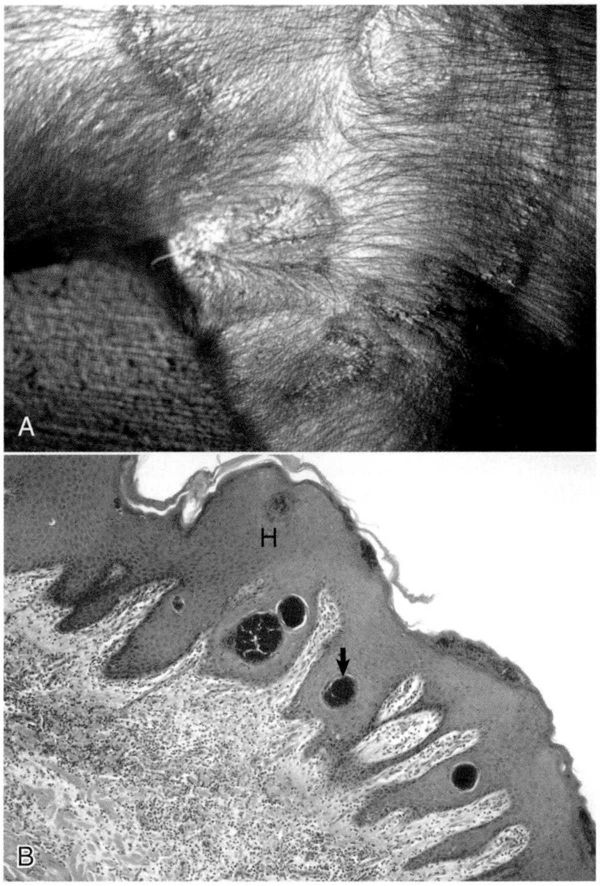

Figure 17-72 **Porcine Juvenile Pustular Psoriasiform Dermatitis (Pityriasis Rosea), Skin, Pig. A,** Abdomen. Note the circular, annular, to serpiginous (wavy) lesions with a distinct raised and erythematous border and adjacent scale. These lesions need to be differentiated from those of dermatophytosis, swinepox, and dermatosis vegetans. **B,** Note the epidermal hyperplasia (acanthosis with elongated rete pegs) *(H)* and intraepidermal pustules *(arrow)*. The dermis contains diffuse accumulations of neutrophils and mixed mononuclear inflammatory cells. The disease receives its name from the juvenile age of onset, the formation of epidermal pustules, and the exaggerated regular epidermal hyperplasia (psoriasiform hyperplasia). H&E stain. (**A** courtesy Dr. M.D. McGavin, College of Veterinary Medicine, University of Tennessee. **B** courtesy Dr. P.E. Ginn, College of Veterinary Medicine, University of Florida.)

main component of dermal mucin is hyaluronic acid (hyaluronan), a glycosaminoglycan produced by many cutaneous cells, including fibroblasts and keratinocytes, and that has a marked ability to retain water, contributing to the dermal thickness noted clinically. The cause of excess hyaluronan in Shar-Pei dogs is thought to be the result of overactivation of the hyaluronan synthase 2 (HAS2) gene. Shar-Pei dogs have increased serum hyaluronic acid concentrations, which may occur as a result of drainage of hyaluronic acid into dermal lymphatic vessels, and subsequently into the blood. Histologically, dermal mucin is an amphophilic amorphous material that separates dermal collagen fibers, sometimes forming lakes of material. In these areas of mucin accumulation, there is a concomitant reduction in dermal collagen fibers, and lymphatic channels may be dilated. These areas of the skin are fragile, and if traumatized, thick, stringy clear or transparent mucin exudes from the dermis.

Mucin deposition, also consisting of glycosaminoglycans, notably hyaluronic acid, may also develop in association with myxedema of hypothyroidism. Myxedema is also present in approximately a third of dogs with hypersomatotropism.

Disorders of Physical, Radiation, or Chemical Injury

Acral Lick Dermatitis (Physical Injury)

Acral lick dermatitis (lick granuloma, acral pruritic nodule, neurodermatitis) usually develops on an extremity (acral = extremity or apex) in dogs and is caused by persistent licking or chewing. The disorder is not uncommon and may be psychogenic in origin or associated with a disease process in the skin (e.g., localized infection or neoplasia) or underlying joint or bone. Boredom may play a role in some cases. The constant licking and chewing of the skin is a form of repeated trauma that leads to the gross and histologic changes. Usually a single lesion develops on the anterior surface of carpal, metacarpal, tarsal, metatarsal, tibial, or radial skin. Grossly, early lesions may be erythematous, haired or hairless, scaly to crusted ovoid to round, occasionally eroded macules or plaques (Fig. 17-73). With time lesions become firm, hairless plaques or nodules that are often extensively or multifocally ulcerated. Ulcers are typically bordered by a raised edge. Microscopically, there is compact hyperkeratosis and acanthosis of the epidermis and follicular infundibulum. Erosions and ulcers may be present, the dermis is thickened by fibrosis, and capillaries and collagen fibers are oriented parallel to hair follicles, called vertical streaking, all the result of chronic irritation from licking. Sebaceous glands and hair follicles are hypertrophic, and there is perivascular and periadnexal plasmacytic dermatitis. Some lesions are complicated by secondary bacterial folliculitis and furunculosis, and severe scarring that may destroy the adnexa.

Pyotraumatic Dermatitis (Acute Moist Dermatitis, "Hot Spots") (Physical Injury)

Pyotraumatic dermatitis, especially common in dogs, is secondary to irritation and principally the result of self-inflicted trauma from biting or scratching because of pain or itching caused by allergies, parasites, matted hair, or irritant chemicals. Dogs with long hair and dense undercoats are predisposed, and lesions develop more commonly in hot humid weather. Flea bite hypersensitivity is a common predisposing cause, and lesions can coalesce to involve large portions of dorsal lumbar and thigh skin (see Fig. 17-53). Type I hypersensitivity reaction to flea bites leads to severe pruritus and self-trauma. Excoriated, moist skin is conducive to bacterial colonization. Grossly the lesions are hairless and red, exude fluid, and have circumscribed edges. Microscopically, affected dogs may have either superficial erosive to ulcerative exudative dermatitis or a deeper suppurative folliculitis (pyotraumatic folliculitis, deep pyoderma). The pyotraumatic folliculitis lesions are considered to represent a deep pyoderma and develop more commonly on the cheek and neck of young golden retriever, Saint Bernard, Labrador retriever, and Newfoundland dogs. Biopsy is required to differentiate the more superficial pyotraumatic dermatitis from the deeper suppurative folliculitis.

Bacterial Infections

Superficial Bacterial Infections (Superficial Pyodermas)

For more mechanistic detail, see the section on Disorders of Domestic Animals, Microbial and Parasitic Disorders, Bacterial Infections, Superficial Bacterial Infections (Superficial Pyodermas).

Superficial Pustular Dermatitis

For more mechanistic detail, see the section on Disorders of Domestic Animals, Microbial and Parasitic Disorders, Bacterial Infections, Superficial Bacterial Infections (Superficial Pyodermas), Superficial Pustular Dermatitis.

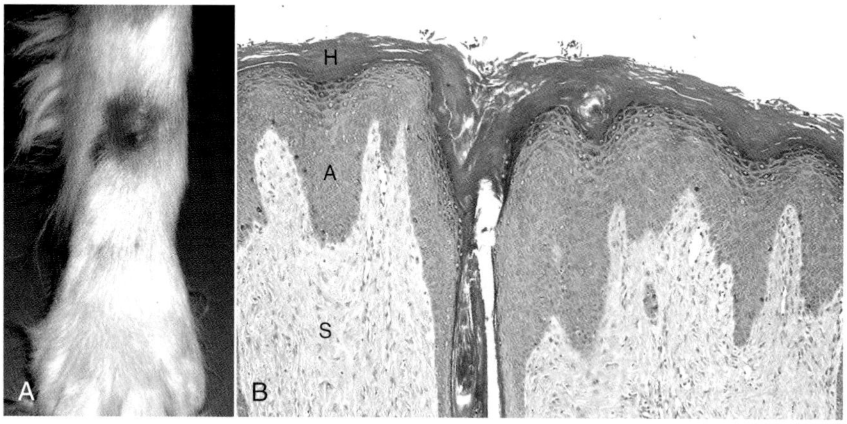

Figure 17-73 **Acral Lick Dermatitis, Skin, Leg, Dog. A,** Chronic licking has resulted in a well-demarcated area of alopecia with a small dark ulcer in the alopecic area. Mechanical removal of the hair or breakage of hair from licking may cause alopecia, and in cases with secondary folliculitis, alopecia can also be caused by follicular inflammation (folliculitis) and sometimes follicular rupture (furunculosis). Mechanical trauma to the skin surface may also cause ulceration. **B,** The epidermis is thickened by compact hyperkeratosis *(H)* and acanthosis *(A)*, and the dermis is thickened by granulation tissue and fibrosis (scarring *[S]*). H&E stain. (Courtesy Dr. A.M. Hargis, DermatoDiagnostics.)

Canine Superficial Pyoderma (Superficial Spreading Pyoderma)

Superficial spreading pyoderma is a common, often pruritic, superficial bacterial infection in dogs caused by *S. pseudintermedius*. Clinical lesions are most frequently recognized in the glabrous ventral thoracic and abdominal skin but can affect the haired skin of the dorsal and lateral trunk as well. Early clinical lesions include erythematous macules, papules, and transient pustules. Older clinical lesions include epidermal collarettes, crusts, alopecia, and hyperpigmentation. Early microscopic lesions are superficial, spongiotic epidermal pustules that rapidly crust and form basophilic debris, often with cocci, on the surface of the epidermis. This basophilic debris can dissect peripherally (laterally) between the epidermis and stratum corneum and is thought to form the rim of scale that clinically represents the epidermal collarette. In this way the lesions "spread" outwardly from the initial lesion. Occasionally, superficial spreading pyoderma can originate from superficial folliculitis in which follicular pustular formation is minor and epidermal collarette formation more prominent. Dermal lesions include superficial perivascular to interstitial accumulations of neutrophils, eosinophils, and mixed mononuclear cells. Some dogs have neutrophilic vasculitis involving superficial venules, possibly caused by immune-complex deposition, a feature suggesting a hypersensitivity response to bacterial antigens. Dermal congestion and edema are usually present.

Mucocutaneous Pyoderma

Mucocutaneous pyoderma is a putative bacterial infection of mucocutaneous junctional skin in dogs. Antibiotic responsiveness suggests that bacteria contribute; however, the etiology is likely more complex and may involve immunologic factors as well. A variety of breeds are affected, but the German shepherd breed is thought to be predisposed. The pathogenesis is unknown. Clinical lesions may be painful and consist of erythema, swelling, and crusting, and in severe cases, fissures and ulcers. Depigmentation may develop in chronic cases. Lesions are most common on mucocutaneous skin and commissures of the lips, but mucocutaneous skin in other sites, including the prepuce, vulva, anus, nares, and eyelids, can be affected. Histologic lesions include a dense band of lymphoplasmacytic inflammation with variable numbers of neutrophils at the dermal-epidermal junction (lichenoid inflammation), typically without basal cell degeneration. Other features include spongiosis and cellular exocytosis into the epidermis, neutrophilic pustular crusts, and folliculitis of adjacent follicles. Over time pigmentary incontinence develops. Although classic cases are said not to have basal cell degeneration, apoptotic keratinocytes above the basal layer can be present. In addition, there can be interface inflammation obscuring the dermal-epidermal interface. These features prevent definitive histologic differentiation from discoid lupus erythematosus. Mucocutaneous pyoderma may coexist with skin fold (intertriginous) pyoderma, and the lesions may appear similar histologically; however, lesions of mucocutaneous pyoderma do not originate in the skin folds.

Bacterial Granulomatous Dermatitis (Bacterial Granulomas)

Mycobacterial Granuloma. See the section on Disorders of Domestic Animals, Microbial and Parasitic Disorders, Bacterial Infections, Bacterial Granulomatous Dermatitis (Bacterial Granulomas), Mycobacterial Granulomas.

Toxic Shock–like Syndrome

See the section on Disorders of Domestic Animals, Microbial and Parasitic Disorders, Bacterial Infections, Skin Lesions Secondary to Systemic Bacterial Infections or Infection with Toxin-Producing Bacteria.

Fungal (Mycotic) Infections

See the section on Disorders of Domestic Animals, Microbial and Parasitic Disorders, Fungal (Mycotic) Infections, Superficial Mycoses. Also see the section on Disorders of Domestic Animals, Microbial and Parasitic Disorders, Fungal (Mycotic) Infections, Cutaneous Mycoses.

Parasitic Infections

Hookworm Dermatitis (Helminth Larva Migrans)

Hookworm dermatitis is caused by cutaneous migration of the larvae of *Ancylostoma* spp. or *Uncinaria* sp. Lesions develop in areas of the skin in contact with an unsanitary environment contaminated by the hookworm larvae, including distal limbs and feet, ventral thorax and abdomen, tail, and caudal thighs. Lesions begin as red papules that coalesce into erythematous areas that later become lichenified and alopecic. Pawpads can become soft, the cornified portion can separate, and secondary bacterial dermatitis and paronychia can develop. Pawpad hyperkeratosis can also be a feature of chronic infection. Hyperplastic spongiotic perivascular dermatitis with eosinophils or neutrophils, serocellular crusts, and migration tracks (tunnels) are the microscopic lesions. Parasitologic evaluation of fresh tissue may allow larval identification.

Other helminth parasites associated with cutaneous larval migration include *Pelodera*, *Necator*, *Strongyloides*, *Gnathostoma*, and *Bunostomum*. Schistosome cercariae, especially of birds, can cause similar lesions.

Immunologic Skin Diseases

Hypersensitivity Reactions

Flea Bite Hypersensitivity. See the section on Disorders of Domestic Animals, Immunologic Skin Diseases, Selected Hypersensitivity Reactions, Insect Bite Hypersensitivity, Flea Bite Hypersensitivity.

Autoimmune Reactions (Vesicles or Bullae as the Primary Lesion)

Pemphigus. See the section on Disorders of Domestic Animals, Immunologic Skin Diseases, Selected Autoimmune Reactions, Reactions Characterized Grossly by Vesicles or Bullae as the Primary Lesion and Histologically by Acantholysis.

Autoimmune Reactions (Depigmentation, Pleomorphic Erythematous Eruptions, Scale/Crusts, or Ulceration)

Proliferative, Lymphocytic, Infundibular Mural Folliculitis and Dermatitis with Prominent Follicular Apoptosis and Parakeratotic Casts. A rare, recently described skin disorder in Labrador retrievers consists of variably extensive, multifocal, verrucous, crusted papules and plaques, and comedones or follicular casts. The lesions develop in haired skin. Histopathologic lesions consist of orthokeratotic and more prominent parakeratotic hyperkeratosis largely of the follicular infundibulum that result in follicular cast formation and a papillary epidermal surface. Histologically, apoptotic keratinocytes and $CD3^+$ lymphocytes (cytotoxic dermatitis) are present in superficial strata of the follicular infundibulum and epidermis. The cause of the condition is unknown, but an immune response directed toward unidentified antigens expressed on the surface of keratinocytes is suspected. The lesions are indistinguishable from those of proliferative and necrotizing otitis externa in cats, which may also affect haired skin in other sites (see Chapter 20), and because of the intraepidermal lymphocytes and apoptotic keratinocytes, this condition histologically resembles erythema multiforme, especially when scales or crusts are prominent.

Autoimmune Reactions (Hemorrhage, Edema, Necrosis, Ulceration, and Infarction)

Vasculitis

Dermatomyositis and Similar Disorders with Cutaneous and Vascular Lesions (Ischemic Dermatopathy). Dermatomyositis is an inherited disease with variable expressivity that occurs in juvenile and adult-onset forms in collies and Shetland sheepdogs (Fig. 17-74). Other breeds are occasionally affected. The pathogenesis involves vasculitis of skin, muscle, and sometimes other tissues. The vascular lesions are subtle and include mild thickening of the vessel wall, occasionally pyknotic cells in the vessel wall, and occasionally lymphocytes within the wall; these changes are termed *cell-poor vasculitis*. Circulating immune complexes have been identified and likely play a role. Dermatomyositis develops in puppies as early as 8 weeks of age. Early lesions include vesicular dermatitis of face, lips, and external ears, which progresses to involve the distal extremities, especially over bony prominences and the tip of the tail. Inflammation of the claw bed may lead to abnormal claw formation or sloughing of the claw. Myositis and atrophy of muscles of mastication, distal extremities, and sometimes of the esophagus develop after the dermatitis (see Fig. 17-74). The myositis is variably severe and multifocal, but more prevalent in peripheral anatomic locations.

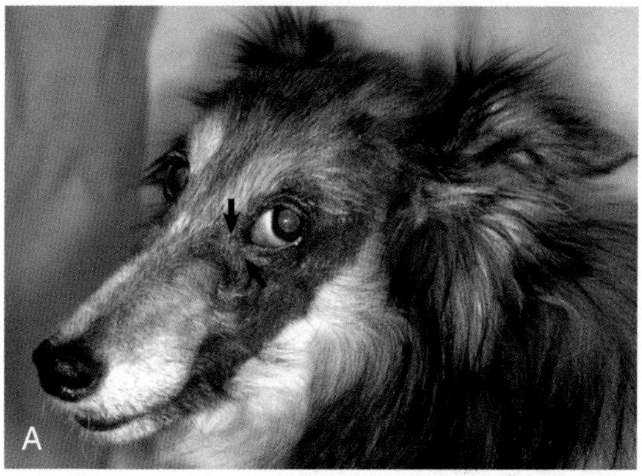

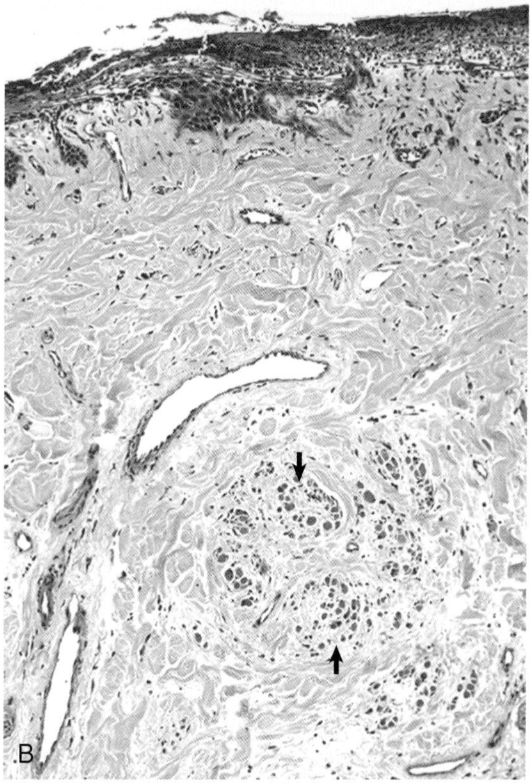

Figure 17-74 **Dermatomyositis, Skin, Dog. A,** Face. Chronic lesions of hair loss, hyperpigmentation, and scarring are present in the skin around the eye and on the lateral side of the face. Interface dermatitis, myositis, and vasculitis have resulted in ischemic follicular atrophy, muscle atrophy, and scarring. The scarring and possibly also some muscle atrophy have contributed to the contraction of the skin of the eyelid and the inability to close the eyelids fully at the medial canthus *(arrows)*. **B,** Lip. Erosion is present on the surface of the lip skin at the far right. Atrophy of the adnexa, not present here, and dermis can predispose to injury of the epidermis and superficial dermis by minor trauma. Muscle atrophy *(arrows)* and scarring around the muscle fibers are present. The diagnosis of dermatomyositis is strengthened if muscle atrophy or myositis is present in the skin biopsy sample. H&E stain. (Courtesy Dr. A.M. Hargis, DermatoDiagnostics.)

The muscle inflammation consists of lymphocytes, plasma cells, histiocytes, and fewer neutrophils or eosinophils. Perifascicular myofiber atrophy (atrophy at the periphery of muscle fascicles) occurs occasionally. The rostral and most superficial portion of the temporalis muscle is the biopsy site of choice to confirm the myositis. Dermatomyositis varies in severity. Mild skin lesions heal without scarring, but moderate skin lesions heal with permanent foci of alopecia, hyperpigmentation or hypopigmentation, and scarring. The hypopigmentation develops from damage to melanin-containing cells in the basal layer of the epidermis. Skin and muscle lesions in dogs with severe disease are progressive and disfiguring, the result of severe scarring of the skin and atrophy of muscle. Microscopic skin lesions include cell-poor interface dermatitis with basal cell degeneration of the epidermis and follicular wall, variable epidermal vesicles and pustules, follicular atrophy, and dermal scarring. Cell-poor vasculitis, a major feature contributing to the lesions in dermatomyositis, is not always identified in small biopsy samples. The combination of interface dermatitis and mural folliculitis with follicular atrophy and cell-poor vasculitis has been considered to represent ischemic lesions and is referred to as *ischemic dermatopathy*.

Skin and vessel lesions indistinguishable from those in dermatomyositis (e.g., ischemic dermatopathy) have developed in other ages and breeds of dogs, sometimes in association with vaccination, and have been organized into the following groups: (1) juvenile dogs other than collies and Shetland sheepdogs without known breed predilection to dermatomyositis, and sometimes with temporal association with vaccination; (2) dogs with localized reactions to subcutaneous injection of killed rabies and sometimes other killed vaccines; (3) dogs with more generalized disease related to rabies vaccination; and (4) dogs with generalized ischemic dermatopathy in which correlation with previous vaccination cannot be documented.

Rabies vaccine–induced ischemic dermatitis develops as a localized form limited to the site of vaccination and as a more widespread form, both developing in the months after rabies vaccination. Poodles, Yorkshire and silky terriers, and other soft-coated breeds of dogs are predisposed to the localized form, but it can occur in any breed. In the localized form an alopecic, hyperpigmented patch of atrophic skin appears at the site of vaccination (see Fig. 17-42).

Microscopically, in addition to lesions of *ischemic dermatopathy*, mild chronic lymphocytic cell-poor vasculitis, a mild diffuse increase in mononuclear cells throughout the dermis, and nodular lymphocytic panniculitis are present. Rabies antigen has been detected in hair follicles and in vessels in affected skin. In the widespread form, lesions are present at the site of vaccination, ear margins, periocular skin, and skin over bony prominences, tip of tail, and pawpads. Lingual erosions and ulcers also occur. In addition, some dogs develop perifascicular muscle atrophy and perimysial fibrosis, with complement components 5b-9 (C5b-9) in the microvasculature. The microscopic lesions are similar to the localized form with the addition of possible muscle lesions, but nodular lymphocytic panniculitis is absent in sites distant from the site of vaccination. The development of lesions after vaccination and the identification of rabies-virus antigen in the vessels and hair follicles in dogs with the localized form of rabies vaccine–induced dermatitis have resulted in the speculation that lesions might be a result of an idiosyncratic immunologic reaction to viral antigen in these sites in genetically predisposed dogs.

Familial Vasculopathy of German Shepherd Dogs. Familial vasculopathy of German shepherd dogs appears to have a genetic basis, but the underlying cause and pathogenesis are unknown. Cutaneous and vascular lesions have similarities to ischemic dermatopathy. Puppies, approximately 1 to 2 months of age, are affected, and some puppies develop lesions after vaccination. The major clinical lesion is swelling of pawpads, and some puppies develop ulcers on the pawpads, ear margins, tail tip, and nasal planum with depigmentation of the nasal planum or nasal commissures. Histologically, early vessel lesions include neutrophil infiltration of small venules and arterioles, but more commonly, vascular lesions are subtle and consist of cell-poor vasculitis (mild thickening of the vessel wall with occasional pyknotic cells and lymphocytes within the wall). In addition, cutaneous lesions consist of mild interface dermatitis with pigmentary incontinence. The nodular lesions in pawpads are in the dermis and subcutis, and early lesions consist of focal collagen degeneration bordered by neutrophils and mononuclear cells. Chronic lesions have dermal and subcutaneous fibrosis sometimes accompanied by degeneration and fibrosis of skeletal muscle bundles.

Cutaneous and Renal Glomerular Vasculopathy of the Greyhound. Greyhounds with cutaneous and renal glomerular vasculopathy are typically from race track environments. The cause and pathogenesis are unknown; however, there is speculation that the disorder is similar to hemolytic-uremic syndrome in human beings in which a verotoxin (Shiga-like toxin) damages vascular endothelium. Most racing greyhounds eat raw meats, which could contain the *E. coli*–producing toxin. Clinical lesions include hemorrhagic macules that progress to deep ulcers of the tarsus, stifle, or inner thigh. Occasionally lesions develop on the front legs, groin, or trunk. Lesions heal slowly (usually over 1 to 2 months) by fibrosis. Histologically, capillaries, venules, and arterioles in the dermis and occasionally the subcutis have degenerate walls with pyknotic or karyorrhectic nuclei, as well as occasional fibrinoid necrosis. Fibrin thrombi can result in cutaneous infarction. Approximately 25% of the affected greyhounds also have systemic signs of renal failure because of glomerular arteriolar inflammation, necrosis, and thrombosis.

Hair Cycle Disorders of Endocrine Origin (Cutaneous Endocrine Disorders)

Hypothyroidism

Deficiency of thyroid hormone develops most commonly in dogs and usually is caused by idiopathic thyroid atrophy and lymphocytic thyroiditis. Thyroid hormones play an essential role in normal growth and development of many organs, including the skin, and can result in a variety of systemic and cutaneous signs and lesions. In dogs the hair follicle is considered to be an important target for thyroid hormones, where the hormones are thought to be necessary for the initiation of the anagen stage of the hair cycle. Clinical lesions of thyroid deficiency consist of a dull, dry, easily epilated hair coat that fails to regrow after clipping. Alopecia develops in areas of wear, including the tail, elbows, hips, around the neck (wear from the collar), and on the dorsal surface of the nose. Symmetric truncal alopecia is not as common as once thought. Microscopically, in areas of advanced alopecia, hair follicles are in the telogen stage of the hair cycle or more commonly, have lost their hair shafts (kenogen). Follicular infundibular hyperkeratosis with plugging of the follicular opening is also present. Other histologic changes include acanthosis of epidermis and follicular infundibulum and a thicker dermis, features that help differentiate lesions of hypothyroidism from other endocrinopathies. Myxedema, an increase in dermal mucin resulting in dermal thickening, is a rare manifestation of canine hypothyroidism. Secondary staphylococcal infection can develop.

Hypothyroidism can also be the result of congenital iodine deficiency. Iodine deficiency develops in fetuses because of maternal ingestion of diets deficient in iodine or containing substances that interfere with production of thyroid hormones (goitrogens). These factors result in insufficient synthesis of thyroxine and reduced blood concentrations of thyroxine and triiodothyronine. The reduced concentrations of these hormones are detected by the hypothalamus and pituitary gland, stimulating secretion of thyrotropin and resulting in hyperplasia of the thyroid follicular cells. Regions of North America that are deficient in iodine include the Great Lakes basin, the Rocky Mountains, the northern Great Plains, the upper Mississippi River valley, and the Pacific Coast region. Paradoxically, maternal diets high in iodine can also result in congenital hypothyroidism. High blood iodine level also interferes with one or more steps of thyroid hormone production, leading to low blood thyroxine concentrations, hypothalamic and pituitary stimulation, and secretion of thyrotropin. Congenital iodine deficiency can occur in any domestic animal but usually is seen in large animals; it is associated with the birth of dead fetuses or weak neonates. These neonates can have alopecia, and thyroid glands are usually enlarged because of the follicular cell hyperplasia.

Hyperadrenocorticism

Hyperadrenocorticism results in cutaneous lesions principally in dogs, less often in cats, and rarely in other domestic animals. It is usually caused by bilateral adrenal cortical hyperplasia secondary to a functional pituitary neoplasm, and less often by a functional adrenal cortical neoplasm or a functional nodule of cortical hyperplasia. Particularly in dogs, the administration of exogenous glucocorticoids is also a cause. Rarely, accidental topical contact with glucocorticoids used on the skin of human beings may cause lesions, particularly in small dogs. In dogs, cutaneous lesions include endocrine alopecia that generally spares the head and extremities, thinning of the skin, comedones, increased bruising, poor wound healing, and increased susceptibility to infection (Fig. 17-75). Dystrophic calcification of the dermis of the dorsal neck region, inguinal areas, and axillary areas can occur in dogs, particularly in iatrogenic hyperadrenocorticism (calcinosis cutis) (Fig. 17-76). Grossly, lesions of calcinosis cutis are firm, thickened, sometimes gritty, often ulcerated and alopecic, crusted plaques or nodules (see Fig. 17-76). In cats affected with hyperadrenocorticism, calcinosis cutis typically does not develop; however, the dermal collagen fibers can be markedly thin and atrophic, resulting in extremely fragile skin that can tear with normal handling. Microscopically, the lesions of hyperadrenocorticism include epidermal, dermal, and follicular atrophy (see Fig. 17-75) and follicular hyperkeratosis with the formation of comedones. Hair follicles are either in the telogen stage of the hair cycle or more commonly, have lost their hair shafts (kenogen). Calcinosis cutis may develop in affected dogs (see Fig. 17-76), and foreign body reaction (granulomatous inflammation) and draining sinuses can develop in association with the calcium deposits. In cats the atrophic hair follicles often have brightly eosinophilic trichilemmal cornification, a feature associated with prolonged telogen and in the cat, considered highly suggestive of hyperadrenocorticism.

Hyperestrogenism

Hyperestrogenism can develop in male and female dogs. In females the estrogen originates from ovarian cysts, rarely an ovarian neoplasm, or from estrogen administration. In males, elevated serum concentrations of estrogen are usually derived from a functional testicular Sertoli cell tumor or less commonly a testicular interstitial cell tumor. Iatrogenic estrogen administration has also caused hyperestrogenism in male dogs (Fig. 17-77). Rarely, accidental topical contact with estrogens used on the skin of human beings may cause lesions, particularly in small dogs. In addition to endocrine alopecia, female dogs have an enlarged vulva and abnormalities of the estrus cycle. Male dogs can develop gynecomastia, pendulous prepuce, or an enlarged prostate because of squamous metaplasia of prostatic ducts. Cutaneous microscopic lesions include orthokeratotic hyperkeratosis, follicular hyperkeratosis, and telogen follicles that have lost their hair shafts (kenogen) (see Fig. 17-77).

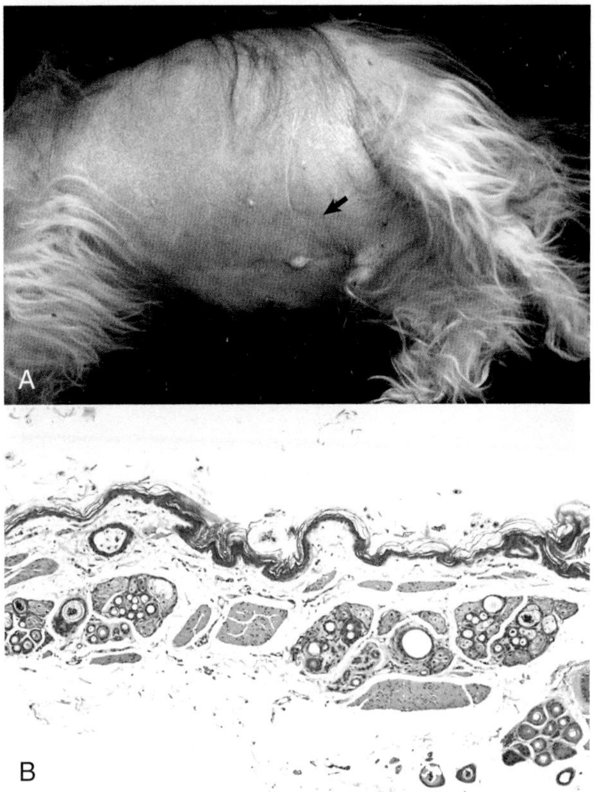

Figure 17-75 **Truncal Alopecia, Hyperadrenocorticism, Skin, Dog. A,** Note the alopecia, distended abdomen, and thin skin in which blood vessels are faintly visible (*arrow*). The distended abdomen and visibility of blood vessels are a result of protein catabolism and loss of muscle and dermal collagen, respectively. The distended abdomen and thin skin with greater visibility of blood vessels in conjunction with symmetric alopecia suggest that a catabolic endocrine disease, such as hyperadrenocorticism, is likely. **B,** Atrophy of dermal collagen fibers is so severe that the collagen has almost disappeared, and the adnexal glands and arrector pili muscles are readily visible. Hair follicles are in the telogen and kenogen stages of the hair cycle. H&E stain. (**A** courtesy Dr. A. Mundell, Animal Dermatology Service. **B** courtesy Dr. A.M. Hargis, DermatoDiagnostics.)

Hypersomatotropism

Hypersomatotropism rarely occurs in adult dogs and is a result of excess concentrations of growth hormone (somatotropin). The excess growth hormone can arise from acidophil tumors of the anterior pituitary gland, injection of pituitary gland extracts, administration of progestins, or with the metestrus (luteal) phase of the estrous cycle in intact female dogs. Elevated concentrations of growth hormone result in increased production of connective tissue, bone, and viscera. Clinical lesions consist of acromegaly (enlargement of parts of the skeleton, especially distal extremities) and thick, folded myxedematous skin over the head, neck, and extremities. The hair coat can be long and thick, and the claws can be thick and hard. Histologic lesions include thickened dermis caused by increased production of glycosaminoglycans and collagen by dermal fibroblasts. Myxedema is present in approximately a third of cases.

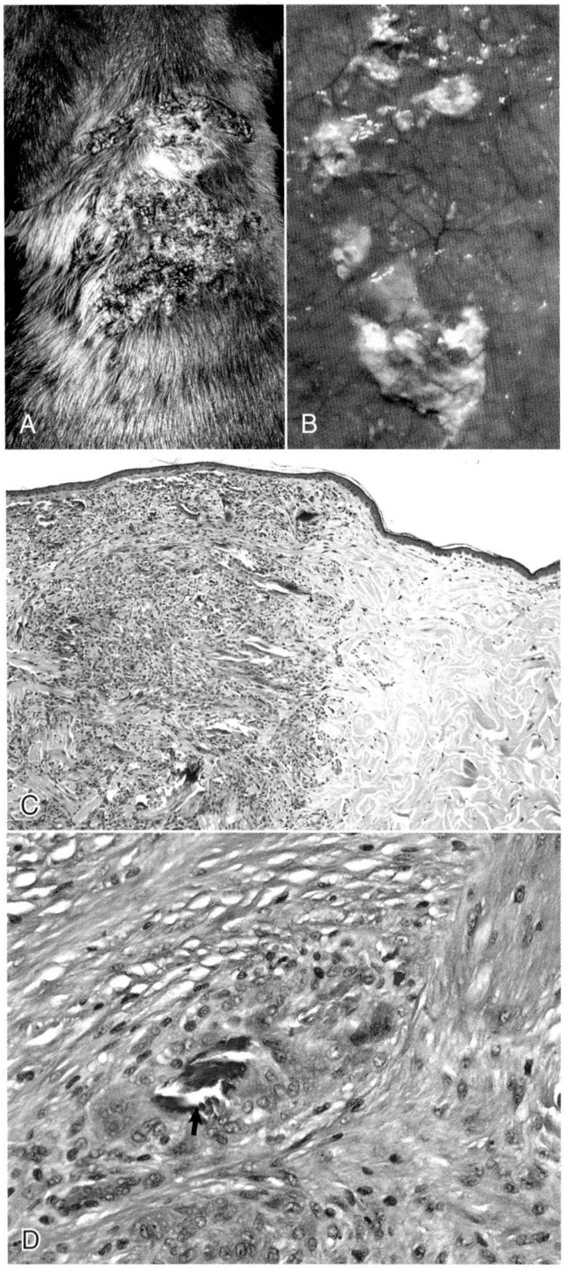

Figure 17-76 **Calcinosis Cutis, Hyperadrenocorticism, Skin, Dog.** **A,** Dorsal neck. The skin is partially alopecic, ulcerated, crusted, and palpably thick and hard. **B,** Subcutis, the skin has been removed from the body and the subcutaneous surface exposed. Mineral deposits are visible as white papules and irregular plaques to nodules. **C,** Skin at the margin of a plaque is thickened by dermal mineralization and granulomatous inflammation *(left half)*. H&E stain. **D,** Higher magnification of dermal mineralization *(arrow)* and granulomatous inflammation. H&E stain. (**A** courtesy Dr. A. Mundell, Animal Dermatology Service. **B** courtesy Dr. M.D. McGavin, College of Veterinary Medicine, University of Tennessee. **C** and **D** courtesy Dr. A.M. Hargis, DermatoDiagnostics.)

Hyposomatotropism

Deficiency of growth hormone in dogs younger than 3 months of age is usually the result of failure of the normal development of the pituitary gland, leading to cyst formation. Deficiencies of thyroid, adrenal, and gonadal hormones are frequent accompanying problems. Pituitary deficiency results in failure to grow, retention of the puppy hair coat, and development of endocrine alopecia. Microscopically, the features are consistent with endocrine alopecia (e.g., hyperkeratosis of superficial epidermis and of hair follicles; normal or atrophic epidermis; follicular dilation from hyperkeratosis; increased numbers of telogen [haired] and kenogen [hairless] follicles; and increased epidermal pigmentation). The numbers of dermal elastic fibers are reduced in the skin of some dogs.

Hair Cycle Disorders of Nonendocrine or Unknown Origin

Prolonged Alopecia Postclipping

Prolonged alopecia postclipping is a failure of the hair to regrow in apparently normal dogs after close clipping. The condition usually occurs in long-haired or heavily coated (plush-coated) breeds of dogs such as the Chow Chow. The pathogenesis of this condition is undetermined, but because hair regrowth may take a year or more, an arrest in the hair cycle is suspected. Alternatively, it is possible that heavily coated breeds of dogs have a prolonged telogen stage of the hair cycle, possibly to conserve energy by avoiding frequent cycles of shedding. Thus clipping when the hair coat is in a prolonged inactive stage of the hair cycle would result in lack of quick regrowth of the hair coat. The hair coat may not regrow until there is another significant growth phase, which may take 6 to 12 months. Most affected dogs regrow the hair coat after they go through a cycle of heavy shedding. Histologic lesions consist of normal epidermis, dermis, and sebaceous glands, and hair follicles in the telogen stage of the hair cycle with retained hair shafts. The follicles may have prominent trichilemmal cornification and resemble flame follicles.

Alopecia X

Alopecia X (adrenal sex hormone alopecia, castration-responsive dermatosis, growth hormone–responsive dermatosis) is seen most often in breeds of dogs with plush hair coats (e.g., Pomeranian, Chow Chow, Samoyed, keeshond, and Alaskan malamute). Toy and miniature poodles and sporadically other breeds of dogs are also affected. Dogs with this condition (or conditions) are grouped together by having in common (1) plush hair coats in the normal state (e.g., when not affected with this condition), (2) alopecia—sparing head and distal extremities, (3) hypothyroidism and hyperglucocorticoidism ruled out, and (4) skin biopsy samples with telogen follicles that retain their hair shafts (haired telogen), and often prominent flame follicles (follicles that have prominent trichilemmal cornification that forms spikes into the follicular stratum spinosum). The alopecia often develops at 1 or 2 years of age in otherwise healthy dogs of either sex. The alopecia is symmetric and involves the perineum, caudal thighs, ventral abdomen and thorax, neck, and trunk. The head and distal extremities are spared. Hyperpigmentation is usually present (Fig. 17-78). Thyroid function testing, adrenocorticotropic hormone response test, low-dose dexamethasone suppression test, and serum chemistry results are normal. Although abnormalities in a number of hormones have been detected, the cause of this condition remains unknown. Microscopic lesions include haired telogen follicles and prominent and diffuse formation of flame follicles (see Fig. 17-78, *B*). Prominent diffuse flame follicle formation is suggestive of alopecia X, but flame follicles can be seen in other endocrine dermatoses (hyperestrogenism and hyperadrenocorticism, particularly in plush-coated breeds), and in follicular dysplasia of the Siberian husky. Follicles similar to flame follicles but with less exaggerated spikes of trichilemmal cornification and with hair shafts retained are seen in normal plush-coated breeds of dogs and in prolonged alopecia postclipping. Epidermal hyperpigmentation and epidermal and dermal atrophy are variable.

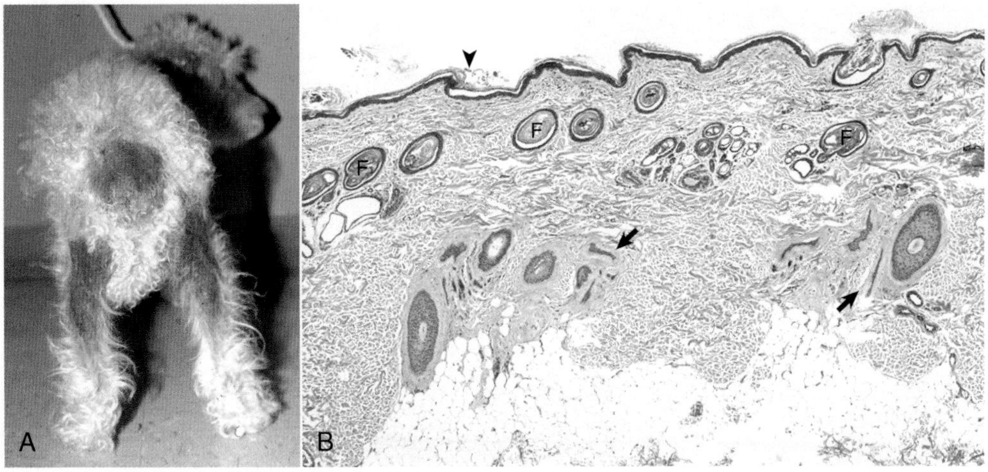

Figure 17-77 **Symmetric Alopecia and Hyperpigmentation, Hyperestrogenism (Iatrogenic From Diethylstilbestrol Therapy), Skin, Male Dog. A,** Note the symmetric alopecia and hyperpigmentation over the caudal dorsal trunk and caudolateral hind legs. In male dogs the symmetric alopecia in conjunction with enlargement of nipples, pendulous prepuce, and attraction of other male dogs suggest the possibility of hyperestrogenism. **B,** Note epidermal orthokeratotic hyperkeratosis *(arrowhead)*, follicles dilated with keratin *(F)*, and small inactive follicles *(arrows)* in the telogen and kenogen stages of the hair cycle. H&E stain. (Courtesy Dr. A.M. Hargis, DermatoDiagnostics.)

Alopecia Related to Chemotherapy

Alopecia related to chemotherapy is best documented in human beings and occurs when there is a severe injury to the anagen (or growing) hair bulbs and is thus called *anagen effluvium*. It is usually diagnosed clinically by examination of pulled hairs, so scalp biopsy sampling is rarely performed. It is the result of an injury that interrupts the mitotic activity of the hair matrix cells in the hair bulb that have the greatest proliferative activity compared to other hair follicle cells. The abrupt cessation of mitotic activity is thought to lead to weakening of the developing anagen hair shaft nearest the hair bulb, which subsequently breaks at its narrowest or weakest point within the hair canal. The consequence of anagen effluvium is hair shedding that usually begins within a week or two after initiation of chemotherapy and is complete by 1 to 2 months after therapy. Because approximately 90% of human scalp hair is in the anagen phase, the hair loss is usually significant and alopecia obvious. Diagnosis can be made early in the course of hair loss by gently pulling out the damaged anagen hairs, which have irregularly narrowed or pointed ends that may contain melanin pigment when examined microscopically. Diagnosis can also be made late in the course of hair loss after anagen hairs have been lost. Because telogen hair follicles are immune to this injury, they remain intact. Thus microscopic examination of hairs pulled during the late stage of hair loss reveals a vast majority of telogen hairs, essentially confirming the presence of anagen effluvium (the anagen hairs have been lost). Alopecia related to chemotherapy also occurs in dogs and cats but has not been well studied. In dogs it has been reported most commonly with doxorubicin therapy and occurs in longer-coated breeds such as poodles and old English sheepdogs and also in some terrier breeds. The prolonged anagen hair phase in some of the longer-haired breeds may explain why they are predisposed. The degree of hair loss varies substantially and depends on drug, dose, method of administration, and treatment schedule, as well as individual animal variables (dogs with long versus short anagen hair cycle phases). Hair loss may begin within 7 to 10 days and is usually apparent within 1 to 2 months. The hair loss may be complete or partial (generalized thinning of the hair coat or loss of primary versus secondary hairs) and can affect different regions of the body (head and site of intravenous injection of the drug; skin of ventral trunk and medial legs; somewhat symmetric involvement of facial skin). Hair loss can include vibrissae in both dogs and cats. With doxorubicin therapy, cutaneous hyperpigmentation is also present. Hair growth resumes after therapy is terminated, but the color or texture of the hair coat may be altered. Diagnosis is based on clinical history, physical examination, and microscopic examination of pulled hairs. Histopathologic examination has rarely been done and is not considered to be diagnostic. It has revealed a prominence of telogen follicles, which is more consistent with an early stage of telogen effluvium. The reason for this discrepancy is unknown but may reflect stage of hair loss at time of biopsy sampling (late in the course of hair loss) or differences in hair follicle cycling, response to chemical injury, or regenerative capabilities between dogs and human beings.

Other Conditions Associated with Alopecia

Acquired Pattern Alopecia (Pattern Baldness)

Acquired pattern alopecia develops in selected toy breeds of dogs with a short smooth hair coat (dachshund, Boston terrier, Chihuahua, Italian greyhound, and whippet). Breed predilections suggest a genetic basis. Generally, before 1 year of age, these dogs gradually develop a bilaterally symmetric thin hair coat in specific areas of the body such as the pinnae, skin caudal to the pinna, caudal thighs, perineal skin, or ventral neck, chest, and abdomen. The dogs are otherwise healthy. Histologic findings reveal miniaturized hair follicles and small (vellus) hair shafts.

Disorders Related to Nutrient Imbalances, Deficiencies, or Altered Metabolism

Zinc Deficiency

Canine Zinc-Responsive Dermatosis. Canine zinc-responsive dermatosis occurs in two forms. One form occurs principally in Siberian huskies and Alaskan malamutes, but other large-breed dogs can be affected. Alaskan malamutes have an inherited reduced ability to absorb zinc from the intestine. Scaling and crusting develop in the skin around the mouth, chin, eyes (Fig. 17-79), external ears, pressure points, and pawpads. The second form of zinc deficiency occurs in rapidly growing pups of large-breed dogs fed diets low in zinc or high in calcium or phytates, which can interfere with zinc absorption. Clinically dogs with this form have scaly plaques located on those areas of the skin subjected to repeated

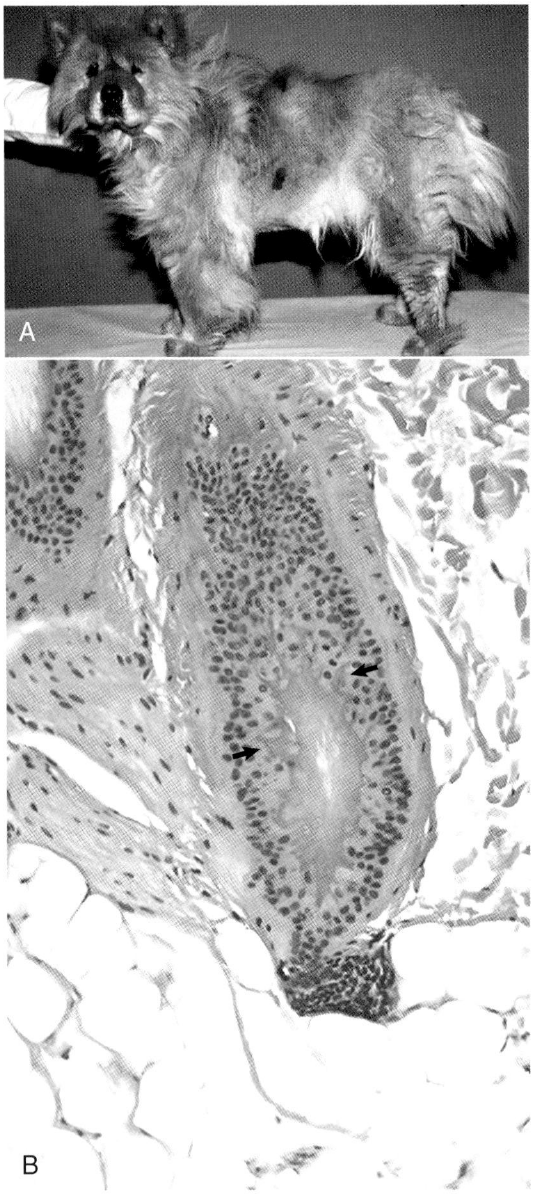

Figure 17-78 **Alopecia X, Skin, Dog. A,** Alopecia X in Chow Chow. Note the partial alopecia and hyperpigmentation of trunk. The alopecia is not diagnostic for a specific condition. The plush-coated breed of dog suggests that alopecia X should be considered as one of the differential diagnoses. **B,** Flame follicle, haired skin. The hair follicle is in the telogen stage of the hair cycle and has excessive trichilemmal cornification resembling the spikes of a flame *(arrows)* and is consistent with a "flame follicle." H&E stain. (**A** courtesy Dr. A. Mundell, Animal Dermatology Service. **B** courtesy Dr. A.M. Hargis, DermatoDiagnostics.)

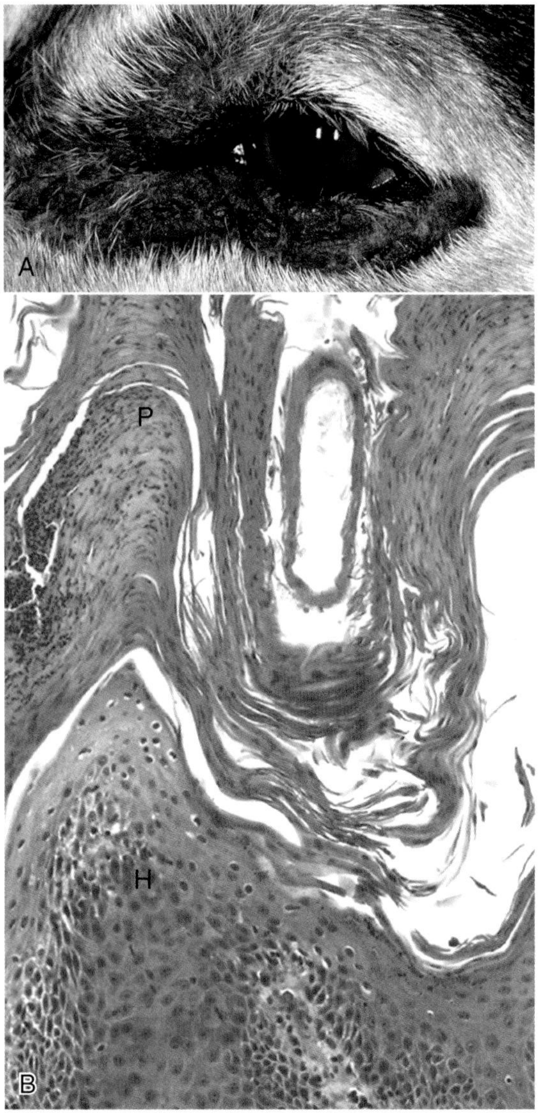

Figure 17-79 **Zinc-Responsive Dermatosis, Skin, Dog. A,** Siberian husky. Periocular skin is thickened, alopecic, pigmented, and covered by tightly adherent scale. In Siberian huskies and Alaskan malamutes in particular, scaling and crusting develop in the skin around the mouth, chin, eyes, external ears, pressure points, and pawpads. **B,** Note the papillary epidermal hyperplasia *(H)* with marked parakeratosis *(P)*. The parakeratotic hyperkeratosis and acanthosis form the thickened adherent scale. Although epidermal hyperplasia and parakeratosis are features of zinc-responsive dermatosis, they also occur in other conditions (such as superficial necrolytic dermatitis, chronic surface trauma, and nasal parakeratosis). Therefore breed, lesion distribution, and other features in the clinical history are important in differential diagnosis. H&E stain. (Courtesy Dr. A.M. Hargis, DermatoDiagnostics.)

trauma (e.g., elbows and hocks), the pawpads, and planum nasale. Microscopically, there is marked diffuse parakeratosis (see Fig. 17-79) that extends into the hair follicles and an accompanying superficial perivascular lymphocytic and sometimes eosinophilic dermatitis. Another disorder, generic dog food dermatosis, a largely historical disease that occurred in the 1980s in dogs fed generic dog foods, has clinical and histologic lesions similar to those of canine zinc-responsive dermatosis. However, dogs with generic dog food dermatosis had a more rapid onset of lesions and also had systemic signs such as fever, depression, lymphadenopathy, and pitting edema of the dependent areas. The acute onset and systemic signs suggested that more than zinc deficiency played a role in generic dog food dermatosis.

Lethal Acrodermatitis of Bull Terriers. Lethal acrodermatitis is an autosomal recessive inherited disease of defective zinc metabolism in white bull terriers. The exact cause or pathogenesis of the disorder is not known. Although defective zinc metabolism and/or absorption are thought to play a role, affected dogs do not respond to oral or parenteral zinc supplementation. The concentrations of serum zinc and copper are low in affected bull terriers compared with those of control dogs, suggesting that copper deficiency might contribute. Lesions generally begin between 6 and 10 weeks of age. Most affected dogs are dead by 15 months of age, usually because of bronchopneumonia. The thymus is small or absent, and T lymphocytes are deficient in lymphoid tissues, likely contributing to immunodeficiency and increasing the potential of infection. Cutaneous lesions begin between the digits and on pawpads and progress to involve mucocutaneous areas, especially of the face. Severe interdigital pyoderma, paronychia (inflammation of the skin around the claws), and villous thickening and fissuring of pawpad keratin ensue. Exfoliative dermatitis can also develop on pinnae, external nose, elbows, and hocks and in some dogs, can become more generalized, with crusting, ulceration, and secondary pyoderma. Microscopically, the principal lesions are extensive diffuse parakeratotic hyperkeratosis, responsible for the exfoliative dermatitis, and accompanying acanthosis. Lesions of secondary infection consist of epidermal pustular dermatitis and folliculitis.

Vitamin A–Responsive Dermatosis

Vitamin A–responsive dermatosis is a rare disorder primarily occurring in cocker spaniels, although a few other breeds of dogs have been affected. Because lesions respond to vitamin A therapy and relapse when treatment is withdrawn, vitamin A plays a role in the pathogenesis. However, vitamin A deficiency is not the cause of the lesions, because plasma concentrations of vitamin A are within the normal range. Vitamin A might contribute to lesion resolution by influencing epithelial differentiation. Gross lesions consist of generalized scaling, dry hair coat, and hyperkeratotic plaques with large "fronds" of stratum corneum extending from distended follicular openings (large open comedones). The plaques are most prominent in the ventral and lateral thorax and abdominal skin but can also occur on the face and neck. Microscopic lesions consist of mild orthokeratotic hyperkeratosis, mild irregular epidermal hyperplasia, and follicles markedly distended by hyperkeratosis.

Predominant Epidermal Hyperkeratosis (Scale) Resulting from Disorders of Epidermal Growth or Differentiation

Hyperkeratosis of Nasal Planum or Pawpads in Dogs

Nasal and/or digital hyperkeratoses have a variety of underlying causes, including infectious disease (e.g., canine distemper [see Chapter 14], leishmaniasis), immune-mediated disorders (e.g., pemphigus foliaceus and lupus erythematosus), familial or inherited disorders (e.g., idiopathic seborrhea, familial pawpad hyperkeratosis of Irish terriers and Dogue de Bordeaux, ichthyosis, nasal parakeratosis of the Labrador retriever, and acrodermatitis of bull terriers), metabolic or nutritional disease (e.g., superficial necrolytic dermatitis, zinc-responsive dermatosis), adverse reaction to drug therapy, and neoplasia (e.g., cutaneous lymphoma) (Box 17-16). In some cases an underlying cause is not determined; thus the condition is considered to be idiopathic (occurs most commonly in old dogs). Some of the disorders in which nasal or digital hyperkeratosis is a feature also have skin lesions in other sites, and systemic disease can be present. Gross lesions on the pawpads or nasal planum include a dry, thick, irregular, and rough surface in which crusts, fissures, or erosions can develop (see Figs. 17-10 and 17-15). The edges of the pawpads and non–weight-bearing pads are more severely affected because friction on weight-bearing surfaces wears through some of the excessively thick stratum corneum. Histologic lesions of nasal and/or digital hyperkeratoses may reflect the underlying cause (e.g., infectious, immune mediated, metabolic, or neoplastic). In the idiopathic nasodigital hyperkeratosis of old dogs, irregular epidermal hyperplasia with marked orthokeratotic to parakeratotic hyperkeratosis is present. In familial nasal parakeratosis of Labrador retrievers, there is variable parakeratotic hyperkeratosis with intraepidermal serum and leukocytic exocytosis. The dermis has perivascular to interface or interstitial mixed inflammation. In familial pawpad hyperkeratosis, there is moderate to extensive epidermal acanthosis and marked diffuse orthokeratotic hyperkeratosis in which the surface stratum corneum forms many papillary projections.

Box 17-16 Hyperkeratosis of the Nasal Planum or Pawpads in Dogs

IMMUNE MEDIATED
Pemphigus foliaceus
Lupus erythematosus
Drug reaction

INFECTIOUS
Canine distemper
Leishmaniasis

METABOLIC
Superficial necrolytic dermatitis
Zinc-responsive dermatosis

INHERITED
Familial pawpad hyperkeratosis (may be a form of ichthyosis)
Ichthyosis
Nasal parakeratosis of the Labrador retriever
Acrodermatitis of bull terriers

IDIOPATHIC
Idiopathic seborrhea
Idiopathic nasodigital hyperkeratosis

NEOPLASTIC
Cutaneous lymphoma

Predominant Follicular Hyperkeratosis (Comedones) Resulting from Disorders of Epidermal Growth or Differentiation

Schnauzer Comedo Syndrome

Schnauzer comedo syndrome affects some miniature schnauzers and probably has an inherited basis. Gross lesions develop on the dorsum of the back and consist of comedones, papules, and crusts. Histologic lesions consist of follicles distended with a plug of follicular stratum corneum and sebum (comedones). Because the follicular opening is connected to the epidermis, the dilated follicles can contain coccoid bacteria. The dilated follicles can rupture (furunculosis) and release contents into the dermis, resulting in a foreign body response and bacterial infection.

Canine Interdigital Palmar and Plantar Comedones and Follicular Cysts

Interdigital comedones and follicular cysts develop on the palmar and plantar skin of dogs and cause recurrent lameness, pain, nodules, or draining sinuses that erupt on the dorsal interdigital surface of the paw (see Table 17-6). The lesions develop most commonly on the palmar and lateral interdigital webs of the front paws, where most weight bearing occurs. The pathogenesis is thought to result from external surface trauma to the palmar/plantar aspect of the haired interdigital skin, which causes follicular plugging and retention of follicular contents. Because canine hair follicles are mostly compound (see Fig. 17-6), 15 or more secondary follicles can exit one common follicular opening, so narrowing or plugging of one follicular opening can result in the formation of multiple comedones or follicular cysts. The cystically dilated follicles can rupture and cause an inflammatory response to the material released from the follicles, and a secondary bacterial infection. Exudate from the ruptured follicles can coalesce and form a draining sinus that ruptures on the dorsal surface of the paw, sometimes providing an erroneous opinion that lesions originate dorsally rather than ventrally. The palmar or planter interdigital skin is usually alopecic, may have callus-like thickening, and has prominent comedones from which follicular contents may be expressed. Histologic lesions consist of comedones and follicular cysts, some of which are ruptured, and pyogranulomatous inflammation containing hair shafts and follicular stratum corneum that form draining sinuses.

Acne

See Disorders of Domestic Animals, Disorders of Epidermal Growth or Differentiation, Predominant Follicular Hyperkeratosis (Comedones), Acne.

Disorders of Pigmentation

Acanthosis Nigricans

Primary idiopathic acanthosis nigricans is considered a genodermatosis (genetically determined skin disorder) of young dachshunds. The disease is manifested by bilateral axillary hyperpigmentation, lichenification, and alopecia, which can involve large areas of skin and also include secondary seborrhea and pyoderma. Histologic lesions are not highly specific, but include hyperplastic dermatitis with orthokeratotic and parakeratotic hyperkeratosis, acanthosis, and rete peg formation. All layers of the epidermis are heavily melanized. Spongiosis, neutrophilic exocytosis, and serous crusts can also be present. The dermal inflammatory reaction is mild, pleomorphic in cell type, and superficial perivascular in location. The term acanthosis nigricans has also been erroneously applied to a variety of inflammatory and pruritic disorders that in their chronic form are clinically manifested by axillary or more diffuse lichenification, alopecia, and hyperpigmentation, and thus overlap with the lesions of primary genodermatosis in young dachshunds. Consequently, the diagnosis of primary idiopathic acanthosis nigricans requires the expected clinical lesions, appropriate breed and age of dog, and histologic evaluation that can rule out other causes of acanthosis and hyperpigmentation.

Disorders Characterized by Infiltrates of Eosinophils or Plasma Cells

Also see the section on Disorders of Domestic Animals, Miscellaneous Skin Disorders, Disorders Characterized by Infiltrates of Eosinophils or Plasma Cells.

Eosinophilic Granulomas (Collagenolytic Granulomas)

See the section on Disorders of Domestic Animals, Miscellaneous Skin Disorders, Disorders Characterized by Infiltrates of Eosinophils or Plasma Cells, Eosinophilic Granulomas (Collagenolytic Granulomas).

Eosinophilic Furunculosis of the Face in Dogs

Eosinophilic furunculosis develops primarily on the dorsal and lateral surfaces of the muzzle of young dogs and is thought to be a result of arthropod bites (bees, wasps, spiders). Lesions develop acutely and are often painful swollen areas that rapidly ulcerate and can drain bloody fluid. Lesions can progress to involve the periocular, pinnal, and sometimes the glabrous ventral abdominal skin. Because lesions develop rapidly and appear clinically severe, biopsy samples are typically collected early in the course of the disease, when microscopic lesions consist of ulceration, superficial and deep interstitial eosinophilic to mixed inflammation with extensive eosinophilic folliculitis and furunculosis.

Hypereosinophilic Syndromes with Systemic Signs or Lesions

Eosinophilic Dermatitis with Edema in the Dog. Eosinophilic dermatitis with edema affects adult dogs of a variety of breeds, although Labrador retrievers may be overrepresented. The cause is not known, but a hypersensitivity reaction to medications, arthropod bites, or other antigens is suspected. Gross lesions consist of extremely erythematous macules that progress and coalesce into arciform and serpiginous plaques. Facial or generalized pitting edema is often seen. Lesions involve the pinnae, ventral abdomen and thorax, and less often the extremities. Histologic lesions consist of diffuse, predominantly eosinophilic dermatitis, vascular dilation, and edema. Eosinophil aggregation and degranulation are seen in some lesions. Depression, hypoproteinemia, gastrointestinal diseases, and pyrexia are present in some dogs.

Nodular Granulomatous Inflammatory Disorders without Microorganisms

Juvenile Sterile Granulomatous Dermatitis and Lymphadenitis (Juvenile Cellulitis, Juvenile Pyoderma, Puppy Strangles)

Juvenile sterile granulomatous dermatitis and lymphadenitis, also known as juvenile cellulitis, juvenile pyoderma, or puppy strangles, is a disorder of unknown cause that occurs in pups younger than 4 months (Fig. 17-80), with one or more of the pups of a litter developing pustular and nodular dermatitis and edema of the face, ears, and mucocutaneous junctions. The pustular and nodular lesions tend to rupture, drain, and crust. Microscopically, early lesions consist of multifocal granulomatous or pyogranulomatous perifolliculitis and dermatitis (see Fig. 17-80). Early lesions are adjacent to but do not primarily involve follicles; however, folliculitis, furunculosis, panniculitis, cellulitis, and granulomatous to pyogranulomatous lymphadenitis develop with disease progression. The lesions initially are considered to be sterile, but secondary bacterial infections develop and can lead to sepsis if not treated. Approximately half of the puppies are lethargic, and anorexia, fever, and joint pain can also occur. This condition occasionally has been reported in adult dogs.

Canine Reactive Histiocytosis

Canine reactive histiocytosis is a poorly understood disorder that occurs in cutaneous and systemic forms in dogs of a variety of ages and breeds, but Bernese mountain dogs, Rottweilers, Labrador retrievers, Irish wolfhounds, and a few other breeds of dogs appear predisposed to the systemic form. The cutaneous form is much more common than the systemic form, which is rare. Reactive histiocytosis is thought to be the result of immune dysregulation, and to be antigen driven, but cultures and special stains have failed to reveal etiologic agents, and no other antigen has been detected. The disorder typically has a slowly progressive, waxing and waning course but can spontaneously resolve and can respond favorably, at least for a time, to immunomodulatory therapy. The lesions require long-term management and often lead to death, particularly if there is systemic involvement. The cutaneous form consists of single or multifocal, nonpainful plaques or nodules composed predominantly of histiocytic cells that are immunophenotypically identified as activated dermal (interstitial) dendritic antigen-presenting cells that express CD1a, CD4, CD11c/CD18, CD90, MHC class II markers. Also intermixed with the histiocytic cells are T lymphocytes, mostly of the $CD8^+$ type, and neutrophils. The role of the $CD8^+$ lymphocytes is unknown. They may be involved in activation of the dendritic cells via release of cytokines such as GM-CSF and TNF-α known to be involved in the proliferation and differentiation of

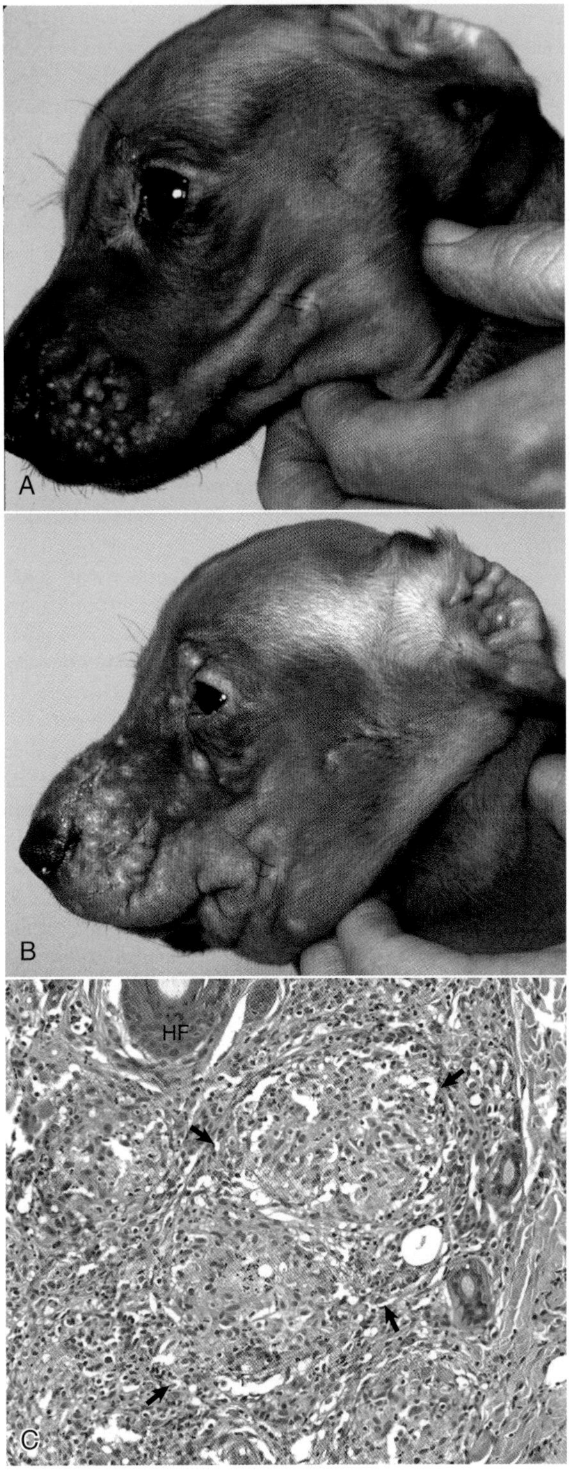

Figure 17-80 **Juvenile Sterile Granulomatous Dermatitis and Lymphadenitis (Juvenile Pyoderma), Granulomatous Dermatitis, Skin, Dog. A,** The pustules on the muzzle are of 1-day duration. The mandibular lymph node (held between thumb and index finger) is markedly enlarged. **B,** The lesions, of 12-days' duration in the same dog as **A,** have progressed to include alopecia, thickening of the skin from edema, crusting, and ulceration. The mandibular lymph node (held between thumb and index finger) has at least doubled in size. **C,** Note the discrete nodular granulomatous dermatitis *(arrows)* that consists of a mixture of macrophages and fewer lymphocytes, plasma cells, and neutrophils is located below and adjacent to a hair follicle *(HF)*. No microorganisms are present. H&E stain. (**A** and **B** courtesy Dr. D. Prieur, College of Veterinary Medicine, Washington State University. **C** courtesy Dr. A.M. Hargis, DermatoDiagnostics.)

dendritic cells. The systemic form is identical immunophenotypically but can also involve the nasal mucosa, eyelids, sclera, lung, spleen, liver, bone marrow, and multiple lymph nodes in addition to the skin. Gross lesions in the cutaneous form are restricted to the skin and subcutis, can be alopecic or haired, and are most often on the nose, face, neck, trunk, perineum, scrotum, and extremities, sometimes including pawpads. Histologically, there are single or multifocal nodular infiltrates of large, round to oval histiocytes mixed with lymphocytes and neutrophils that, in early lesions, are in the mid-dermal perivascular and periadnexal dermis and may be elongate and oriented vertically. Later, the infiltrates coalesce into larger deep dermal and subcutaneous masses. Vessels are often surrounded and invaded by the infiltrates (lymphohistiocytic vasculitis), which can result in thrombosis, necrosis, infarction, and ulcers.

Canine Langerhans Cell Histiocytosis

Canine Langerhans cell histiocytosis is a rare condition in dogs resulting from progression of single or multiple persistent or recurrent canine cutaneous histiocytomas that spread to regional lymph nodes and subsequently to internal organs. The cell of origin is the Langerhans cell, a cell immunophenotypically identified as the intraepithelial dendritic Langerhans antigen-presenting cell that express CD1a, CD11c/CD18, CD45, MHC II, and usually E-cadherin markers. Expression of E-cadherin may diminish as the Langerhans cells lose their connections with the epidermal and follicular cells. The lesions begin with the development of one or more nodular, dome-shaped, often hairless masses (histiocytomas). In contrast to the majority of histiocytomas, the lesions fail to regress and become persistent, or they may recur after excision. The masses extend more deeply into the subcutis. There is enlargement of regional lymph nodes, the result of spread of Langerhans cells to the nodes. With time, infiltrative nodular masses of Langerhans cells develop in internal organs.

Histologically, the initial lesion consists of one or more circumscribed but nonencapsulated dermal to superficial pannicular masses that are broader at the surface than at the base. The masses consist of cords and sheets of round to polyhedral cells with a rounded, sometimes indented or folded nucleus (Langerhans cells). The epidermis may be acanthotic with exaggerated dermal-epidermal interdigitations. Langerhans cells are often present in the epidermis. Ulceration and secondary bacterial infection can develop. In the persistent lesions the cellular infiltrates extend more deeply into subcutis, become less well-differentiated, have increased mitotic index, and lack T lymphocyte infiltrates peripherally and foci of necrosis (features of regression of the typical and more common cutaneous histiocytomas). In addition, clusters of Langerhans cells are located within dermal lymphatic channels. These cells spread to efface architecture of regional nodes and form infiltrative nodular masses in internal organs. The condition has a poor prognosis. Immunomodulatory therapy is not effective and not recommended in cases of Langerhans cell histiocytosis.

Cutaneous Paraneoplastic Syndromes (Manifestations of Systemic Disorders)

Superficial Necrolytic Dermatitis (Diabetic Dermatopathy, Hepatocutaneous Syndrome, Necrolytic Migratory Erythema, Metabolic Epidermal Necrosis)

Superficial necrolytic dermatitis (also known as diabetic dermatopathy, hepatocutaneous syndrome, necrolytic migratory erythema, metabolic epidermal necrosis) is an uncommon disorder reported primarily in older dogs with deranged nutrient metabolism associated with hepatic dysfunction, diabetes mellitus, hyperglucagonemia, malabsorption, or in a small percentage of dogs, glucagon-secreting tumor usually within the pancreatic islets. Long-term anticonvulsant therapy and the rare ingestion of mycotoxins also have preceded the development of superficial necrolytic dermatitis. The disorder is rare in cats and has been associated in some instances with pancreatic carcinoma and/or hepatopathy, and in one cat a glucagon-producing primary hepatic neuroendocrine carcinoma. The pathogenesis of superficial necrolytic dermatitis is not completely understood and may vary with the underlying defect. When glucagon level is elevated, persistent gluconeogenesis is thought to result in a negative nitrogen balance with protein degradation, including proteins in the epidermis. However, when glucagon level is not elevated, as occurs in human beings with some types of hepatic or malabsorptive disease and in dogs with diabetes and multinodular vacuolar hepatopathy, it is thought that deficiencies of certain essential fatty acids, zinc, and amino acids play a role. Ultimately, low blood amino acid concentrations are thought to lead to the development of the cutaneous lesions. In dogs these lesions consist of scales, thick adherent crusts, erythema, alopecia, erosions, and ulcers on the mucocutaneous junctions, genitalia, pinnae, skin subjected to trauma (elbows, hocks), and ventral thorax. Pawpad lesions consist of crusting and fissuring or ulceration (see Fig. 17-10) and result in lameness. In cats, alopecia and scaling of trunk and limbs have been seen; another cat had alopecia of the ventral trunk and medial thighs and ulceration and crusting of the oral mucocutaneous and interdigital regions. Microscopic lesions, when fully developed, are considered diagnostic and consist of trilaminar thickening of the epidermis in which the stratum corneum has marked parakeratosis, the upper stratum spinosum is pale with reticular degeneration, and the lower spinous and basal cell layers are hyperplastic (see Fig. 17-10). Secondary infections with bacteria or yeast frequently complicate lesions, and secondary infection with dermatophytes also has been seen.

Pancreatic Panniculitis (Necrotizing Panniculitis)

Pancreatic panniculitis (necrotizing panniculitis) is an acute rare disorder that has developed in dogs with pancreatic neoplasia or pancreatitis. It is seen less frequently in cats. The lesions are thought to be a result of the release of pancreatic enzymes (e.g., lipases) either from damaged pancreatic exocrine cells or from neoplastic exocrine cells. The lipases enter the systemic circulation and subsequently locate in the panniculus. Gross lesions are mostly truncal and consist of multiple, frequently ulcerated and hemorrhagic nodules or poorly defined swellings within the subcutis. Lesions may drain purulent, oily material. Histologically, there is necrosis of adipose tissue (caused by the lipases) with fine basophilic granularity (caused by mineralization of the necrotic fatty tissue). Suppurative to pyogranulomatous inflammation occurs at the periphery of the necrotic foci. Hemorrhage and fibrin exudation may be evident, and lesions may extend into the dermis and rupture through the epidermis.

Nodular Dermatofibrosis and Renal Disease in the Dog

In nodular dermatofibrosis, multiple cutaneous nodules composed of excessive collagen coexist with renal cystadenomas, cystadenocarcinomas, hyperplastic epithelial cysts, or uterine smooth muscle tumors. Renal lesions are often bilateral and may not be detectable clinically for months or years after the appearance of the cutaneous nodules. The syndrome has been described most commonly in the German shepherd but has been seen in a few other purebred dog breeds and mixed-breed dogs and is thought to have an autosomal dominant mode of inheritance in the German shepherd. Whether the condition is a true paraneoplastic syndrome with the renal neoplasm inducing dermal fibrosis or the simultaneous occurrence of two independent conditions with a common hereditary linkage is undetermined. Gross lesions consist of firm dermal and subcutaneous nodules on legs, head, or ears. Histologic lesions consist of nodular dermal and subcutaneous aggregates of poorly cellular, mature dermal collagen bundles that are slightly thickened. In the dermis the collagen bundles blend often imperceptibly with bordering collagen, but in the subcutis the nodules are usually circumscribed. Adnexa are normal or hyperplastic. The cutaneous nodules are benign but serve as a marker for the more serious renal lesions.

Disorders of Cats

For disorders occurring in two or more species of animals, see Disorders of Domestic Animals.

Disorders of Physical Injury

Feline Ulcerative Dermatitis Syndrome

Feline ulcerative dermatitis syndrome is an uncommon disorder that may have more than one underlying cause. Previous injections and hypersensitivity are thought to initiate the syndrome in some but not all cats. The pathogenesis is not known, but self-trauma appears to significantly contribute to and perpetuate lesions. Lesions develop most commonly in the skin of the dorsal neck or interscapular regions and grossly consist of a nonhealing ulcer with serocellular exudate that can mat the adjacent hair. Microscopic lesions consist of an ulcer covered by fibrinonecrotic crust. The dermis subjacent to the ulcer contains components of necrotic epidermis and adnexa intermixed with degenerate neutrophils. Adnexal effacement by fibrosis is seen in severe cases. Inflammation in adjacent and deeper dermis is variable but often scant and consists of a few neutrophils, eosinophils, and mixed mononuclear cells. Chronic lesions consist of acanthosis of bordering epidermis with a linear band of fibrosis beneath and parallel to the adjacent intact epidermis. In those cases attributed to previous vaccination, nodular lymphoplasmacytic to histiocytic panniculitis is present.

Viral Infections

Cowpox Infection in Cats

Cowpox virus infection in cats is uncommon and usually occurs in outdoor cats living in rural areas, presumably because these cats hunt and have contact with rodents harboring the poxvirus. Primary cutaneous lesions typically develop on the face, neck, or forelegs and consist of an ulcerated or crusted macule or plaque. Lesions can develop into deep ulcers that heal with granulation tissue or less commonly develop into abscesses or cellulitis. Rarely, oral or mucocutaneous junctional areas are affected. Additional secondary cutaneous lesions can develop within approximately 2 weeks after viremic distribution to other cutaneous sites and less commonly to the upper or lower respiratory tract. The microscopic lesions are sharply demarcated, often deep ulcers covered by fibrinonecrotic exudate. Intracytoplasmic inclusion bodies in keratinocytes or follicular or sebaceous glandular cells help establish the diagnosis. Viral infectivity may remain for months in crusts. A variety of species may be infected, including human beings.

Herpesviruses

For more mechanistic detail, see the section on Disorders of Domestic Animals, Microbial and Parasitic Disorders, Viral Infections, Herpesviruses.

Feline Herpesvirus Dermatitis. FHV-1is an uncommon cause of ulcerative, often persistent, facial dermatitis or stomatitis in cats of various ages and sexes. Less commonly, similar lesions have developed in the skin of other sites. Glucocorticoid therapy or stresses, such as overcrowding, are thought to play a role in lesion development. Most lesions, particularly those affecting the face or oral cavity, develop under circumstances suggesting reactivation of latent herpesvirus infection. The pathogenesis is typical of that described for herpesviruses in the previous section. Gross lesions are ulcerative and crusted (see Table 17-6). Histologically, there is extensive necrosis of the epidermis, follicles, and sometimes sebaceous glands accompanied by prominent mixed dermal inflammation that frequently includes numerous eosinophils. Hair follicles can be destroyed, and free keratin in the dermis is associated with eosinophils and foci of eosinophil degranulation bordering collagen fibers and collagen degeneration. Large amphophilic or hyaline intranuclear inclusions are present in the surface and adnexal epithelium. Inclusion bodies are often easily overlooked, variable in number, and sometimes present in small rafts of epithelial cells surrounded by necrotic debris or in crust. The lesions are different from those previously reported in domestic cats in that they persist and many are limited to the skin of the face or oral mucosa and often have significant eosinophilic inflammation. The inflammation in feline herpesvirus dermatitis overlaps with that of the hypersensitivity reactions, including mosquito bite hypersensitivity, and also with that of eosinophilic ulcers, thus warranting close scrutiny of eosinophilic necrotizing cutaneous lesions for intranuclear inclusion bodies or using more sensitive tests such as immunohistochemical staining for feline herpesvirus.

Bacterial Infections

Bacterial Granulomatous Dermatitis (Bacterial Granulomas)

Mycobacterial Granuloma. See the section on Disorders of Domestic Animals, Microbial and Parasitic Disorders, Bacterial Infections, Bacterial Granulomatous Dermatitis (Bacterial Granulomas), Mycobacterial Granulomas.

Feline Leprosy. Feline leprosy is usually caused by M. *lepraemurium* or *Mycobacterium visibile*, which are considered saprophytic organisms that typically do not grow in culture. Definitive diagnosis can be made by use of PCR and DNA sequencing, but not all laboratories perform these tests. Differential diagnoses include potentially zoonotic tuberculosis infections. Feline leprosy typically develops in cats living in cold, wet areas of the world, including the northwestern United States and Canada. Mode of transmission is not known, but bites of cats or rodents, soil contamination of cutaneous wounds, or possible transmission via biting insect vectors may be involved. Lesions develop most commonly on the head, neck, and limbs but can occur anywhere (Fig. 17-81). Histologically, two distinct morphologic patterns of inflammation are present. In one there is diffuse granulomatous inflammation without necrosis and with large numbers of intracellular acid-fast bacilli; some of these infections have been caused by M. *visibile*. In the other pattern there are granulomas with central necrosis surrounded by a zone of lymphocytes. Few to moderate numbers of acid-fast bacilli are generally limited to the areas of necrosis. Some of these infections have been caused by M. *lepraemurium*. However, it has been suggested that the number of mycobacterial organisms may have more to do with the immune competence of the host than the mycobacterial agent itself, with infections in immunocompetent hosts having fewer mycobacteria than infections in hosts with immune compromise.

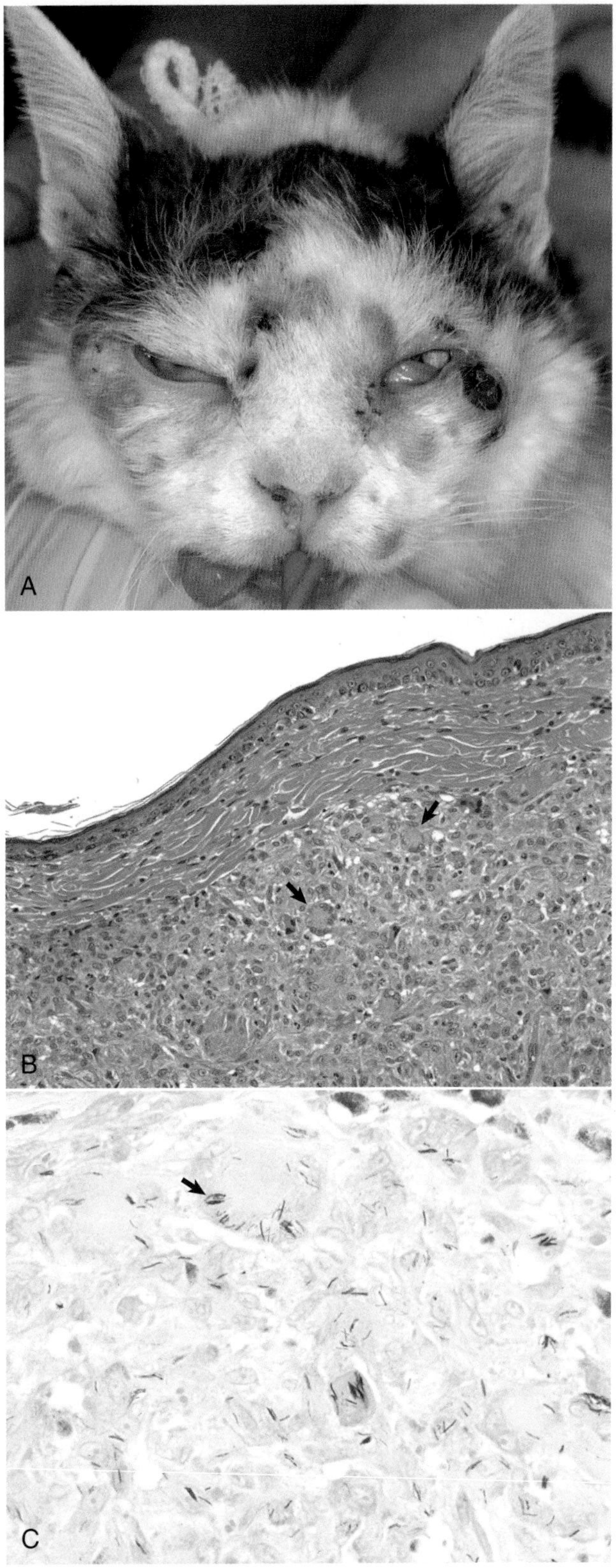

Figure 17-81 **Feline Leprosy Syndrome, *Mycobacterium lepraemurium* (and Sometimes Other *Mycobacterium* sp. Such as *Mycobacterium visibile*), Nodular Granulomatous Dermatitis, Cat. A,** Face and ears. Note multiple partially alopecic and focally ulcerated nodules histologically consisting of granulomatous inflammation. In feline leprosy, slowly growing nodules are present in the skin especially of the face, forelegs, or trunk. **B,** The dermal nodule consists of macrophages and multinucleated giant cells *(arrows)*. H&E stain. **C,** Macrophages contain numerous mycobacteria that are stained red *(arrow)*. Fite Faraco stain. (**A** courtesy Dr. D. Duclos, Animal Skin and Allergy Clinic. **B** and **C** courtesy Dr. A.M. Hargis, DermatoDiagnostics, Edmonds, Washington.)

Fungal (Mycotic) Infections

See the section on Disorders of Domestic Animals, Microbial and Parasitic Disorders, Fungal (Mycotic) Infections, Superficial

Mycoses. Also see the section on Disorders of Domestic Animals, Microbial and Parasitic Disorders, Fungal (Mycotic) Infections, Cutaneous Mycoses.

Dermatophytic Pseudomycetoma

Dermatophytic pseudomycetoma is a rare, deep dermal and subcutaneous infection, usually caused by *Microsporum canis*, that develops predominantly in Persian cats, suggesting the possibility of a specific genetic deficit in innate or adaptive immunity in this breed. It is presumed that follicles rupture, releasing dermatophytes into the subfollicular dermis. Gross lesions are similar to other subcutaneous mycoses. Microscopic lesions are in the subfollicular dermis or subcutis and consist of a granulomatous inflammatory response and intermixed aggregates of fungal hyphae with irregular dilations. Hair shafts within adjacent follicles contain *Microsporum canis* hyphae and spores.

Immunologic Skin Diseases

Hypersensitivity Reactions

Flea Bite Hypersensitivity. See the section on Disorders of Domestic Animals, Immunologic Skin Diseases, Selected Hypersensitivity Reactions, Insect Bite Hypersensitivity, Flea Bite Hypersensitivity.

Mosquito Bite Hypersensitivity in Cats. Mosquito bite hypersensitivity develops in cats hypersensitive to mosquito antigens, presumably present within the injected mosquito saliva. Experimental studies using intradermal skin tests and Prausnitz-Küstner tests in cats indicate that these lesions are initiated by a type I hypersensitivity reaction. A delayed hypersensitivity reaction also may occur but has not been fully characterized. Mosquito bite hypersensitivity develops primarily on the haired skin of the nose, but lesions can involve nasal planum, periocular skin, pinnae, and less commonly the flexor surface of the carpi and margins of pawpads. Lesions begin as erythematous papules and progress to crusts, erosions, ulcers, and alopecia (Fig. 17-82). Inactive lesions can be hypopigmented or hyperpigmented, presumably from damage to or regenerative hyperplasia of melanin-containing cells in the epidermis. Histologic lesions include extensive superficial and deep, perivascular and interstitial eosinophilic to mixed dermatitis, occasionally with foci of degranulated eosinophils (flame figures) and eosinophilic folliculitis and furunculosis. The epidermis is acanthotic with foci of erosion, ulceration, and cellular crusting (see Fig. 17-82).

Autoimmune Reactions with Vesicles or Bullae

Pemphigus. See the section on Disorders of Domestic Animals, Immunologic Skin Diseases, Selected Autoimmune Reactions, Reactions Characterized Grossly by Vesicles or Bullae as the Primary Lesion and Histologically by Acantholysis.

Autoimmune Reactions with Hemorrhage, Edema, Necrosis, Ulceration, and Infarction

Vasculitis

Vasculitis in Cats

Information on this topic is available at www.expertconsult.com.

Hair Cycle Disorders of Endocrine Origin (Cutaneous Endocrine Disorders)

Hyperadrenocorticism

See Disorders of Dogs.

Alopecic Disorders Associated with Normal Follicles

Feline Psychogenic Alopecia

Psychogenic alopecia occurs in cats of the more sensitive or attention-demanding breeds, including Siamese and Abyssinian, and possibly others. A partial alopecia is the result of the breaking of hairs from gentle but persistent licking. Linear or symmetric areas of alopecia are found along the caudal dorsal midline or in the perineal, genital, caudomedial or caudolateral thigh, or abdominal areas. Microscopically, the skin is generally normal, but there may be trichomalacia (twisted or broken hair shafts within hair follicles). The

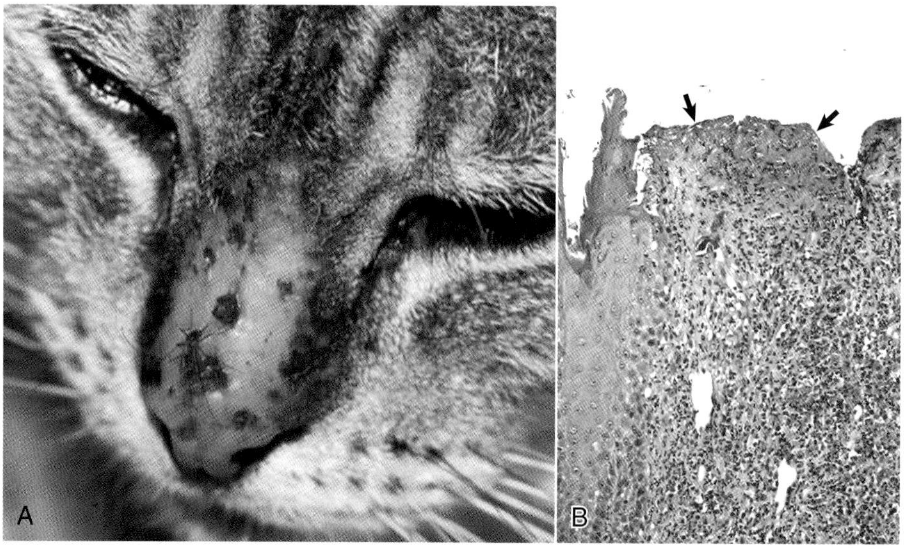

Figure 17-82 **Resolving Mosquito Bite Hypersensitivity Dermatitis, Skin, Face, Cat. A,** Alopecia, erythema, and erosions are present. Note the mosquito that is biting the skin. The two red depressions nearest the mosquito are healing biopsy sites collected previously during a more active stage of the disease. Mosquitoes have been kept away from this cat for 1 week, allowing some of the active lesions of hemorrhagic crusting to resolve. A few small red depressions (erosions and ulcers) remain. **B,** Under the ulcer *(arrows)*, the dermis is heavily infiltrated with eosinophils, lymphocytes, and plasma cells. H&E stain. (**A** courtesy Dr. K.V. Mason, Animal Allergy and Dermatology Service, Springwood, Queensland, Australia. **B** courtesy Dr. A.M. Hargis, DermatoDiagnostics.)

principal differential diagnosis is alopecia resulting from hypersensitivity (see next discussion). Alopecia related to endocrine disease is rare in the cat but has been seen in association with persistent licking in cats with hyperthyroidism.

Alopecia Caused by Hypersensitivity Reactions in the Cat

Clinical signs of alopecia caused by hypersensitivity reactions are often identical to those of feline psychogenic alopecia. Pruritus typically is the result of hypersensitivity reactions to a variety of causes (food allergy, parasitism, or atopic dermatitis). Histologically, there is perivascular dermatitis, usually with eosinophils, mast cells, and lymphocytes. The inflammation helps to distinguish alopecia associated with hypersensitivity from that of feline psychogenic alopecia.

Nutrient Imbalances, Deficiencies, or Altered Metabolism

Vitamin E Deficiency

Cats fed diets containing an excess of dietary polyunsaturated fatty acids, such as canned red tuna, can develop inflammation of the subcutaneous and abdominal fat (pansteatitis). This condition develops when the diet is high in fat and when food processing or oxidation inactivates vitamin E. Vitamin E has a number of functions that contribute to its role as an antioxidant that stabilizes lysosomes. Affected cats may be anorexic, lethargic, and painful on palpation or movement. Grossly, the subcutaneous fat contains firm, nodular, yellow to orange masses. Microscopic lesions consist of fat necrosis that stimulates a lobular to diffuse neutrophilia followed by granulomatous inflammatory response. Macrophages and multinucleated giant cells contain ceroid pigment, which is responsible for the yellow to orange color of the affected fat.

Predominant Follicular Hyperkeratosis (Comedones) Resulting from Disorders of Epidermal Growth or Differentiation

Acne

See the section on Disorders of Domestic Animals, Disorders of Epidermal Growth or Differentiation, Predominant Follicular Hyperkeratosis (Comedones), Acne.

Disorders Characterized by Infiltrates of Eosinophils or Plasma Cells

See the section on Disorders of Domestic Animals, Miscellaneous Skin Disorders, Disorders Characterized by Infiltrates of Eosinophils or Plasma Cells.

Eosinophilic Plaques

Eosinophilic plaques are common lesions of the skin of cats that occur on the abdomen and medial thigh and are thought to be associated with hypersensitivity reactions. Lesions consist of raised, variably sized erythematous, pruritic, and eroded to ulcerated plaques. Microscopically, epidermal lesions include acanthosis, variable spongiosis, erosion, and ulceration, accompanied by superficial and deep, perivascular to diffuse, predominantly eosinophilic dermatitis.

Eosinophilic Granulomas (Collagenolytic Granulomas)

See the section on Disorders of Domestic Animals, Miscellaneous Skin Disorders, Disorders Characterized by Infiltrates of Eosinophils or Plasma Cells, Eosinophilic Granulomas (Collagenolytic Granulomas).

Hypereosinophilic Syndromes with Systemic Signs or Lesions

Feline Hypereosinophilic Syndrome. Feline hypereosinophilic syndrome is a rare multisystemic and progressive disorder of unknown cause that is associated with moderate to marked peripheral eosinophilia and infiltrates of mature eosinophils in multiple organ systems, sometimes including the skin. Middle-aged female cats are more often affected. Gross lesions of the skin include erythema and excoriations associated with severe pruritus. Histologically, there is superficial and deep, perivascular dermatitis with prominent eosinophils. Clinical signs include anorexia, diarrhea, weight loss, and vomiting.

Plasma Cell Pododermatitis

Feline plasma cell pododermatitis is an uncommon condition of undetermined cause or pathogenesis. Immunohistochemical staining with a polyclonal anti–*Mycobacterium bovis* antibody cross-reactive to a broad spectrum of bacteria and fungi, and PCR for a variety of potential feline pathogens, including *Bartonella* spp., *Ehrlichia* spp., *Anaplasma phagocytophilum*, *Chlamydia* (formerly *Chlamydophila*) *felis*, *Mycoplasma* spp., *Toxoplasma gondii*, and FHV-1 have been negative. However, some cats have tested positive for FIV. Affected cats have hypergammaglobulinemia and a response to immunomodulating therapy, leading to the hypothesis that feline plasma cell pododermatitis is an idiopathic immune-mediated disease. It is characterized clinically by soft, painless swelling of multiple pawpads that can lead to collapse of the pawpad and ulceration, hemorrhage, and lameness. Histologically, the skin of the pawpad is heavily infiltrated by plasma cells with variable quantities of intracytoplasmic immunoglobulin (Russell bodies), neutrophils, and lymphocytes. This condition is sometimes accompanied by plasmacytic stomatitis, immune-mediated glomerulonephritis, or renal amyloidosis.

Nodular Granulomatous Inflammatory Disorders without Microorganisms

Feline Progressive Histiocytosis. Feline progressive histiocytosis is a rare condition in middle-aged to older cats resulting in development of cutaneous histiocytic masses most often on the head, distal extremities, or trunk. Immunophenotyping of the histiocytic cells has revealed expression of CD1a, CD11/18, MHC II, and usually a lack of E-cadherin expression. These features are most consistent with interstitial dendritic cells. Also present are reactive lymphocytes that express CD3 and CD8. Feline progressive histiocytosis behaves as a low-grade histiocytic sarcoma. Gross lesions begin with the development of one or more dermal masses that may subsequently enlarge and coalesce into larger plaquelike areas that may remain limited to the skin. In some cases there may be spread to regional lymph nodes. In addition, some masses may become poorly differentiated and develop invasive features of histiocytic sarcoma with spread to one or more internal organs.

Histologic lesions consist of circumscribed, but nonencapsulated masses in the dermis and panniculus that are broader at the surface than the base. The masses consist of large rounded to polyhedral-shaped histiocytic cells with a large central vesicular nucleus. Less than half of the cases have epitheliotropism (extension of the histiocytic cells into the epidermis). In addition to lymphocytes, neutrophils and vacuolated macrophages may be present.

Cutaneous Manifestations of Systemic Disorders

Paraneoplastic Syndromes

Feline Pancreatic Paraneoplastic Alopecia. Feline pancreatic paraneoplastic alopecia associated with internal malignancies in the cat (pancreatic paraneoplastic syndrome) is a rapidly progressive, largely ventrally distributed, symmetric alopecia that develops in older cats with metastatic pancreatic or biliary carcinomas. The pathogenesis of this condition is not known. The alopecia typically affects the ventral abdomen, thorax, and legs. The ears and periocular skin are less frequently involved. Alopecic skin is smooth, soft, and often has a shiny or glistening appearance. The pawpads are dry with circular rings of scale and may be painful. Histologically, affected skin has small inactive hair follicles with a reduction or absence of the stratum corneum. Some cats groom excessively, and it has been suggested that the smooth shiny appearance of the skin is caused by the absence of the stratum corneum. In other areas of the skin, there is variable orthokeratotic and parakeratotic hyperkeratosis in which *M. pachydermatis* is sometimes identified. In addition to the alopecia, the cats have systemic signs of anorexia, weight loss, and lethargy.

Feline Exfoliative Dermatitis with or without Thymoma. A generalized exfoliative dermatitis has been documented as a paraneoplastic syndrome of older cats with thymomas. More recently the condition has been recognized in dogs and rabbits. T lymphocyte immune dysregulation probably plays a role in lesion development. Rarely, identical cutaneous lesions are recognized in cats without evidence of underlying neoplasia or internal disease, suggesting that the histologic lesions in this disease syndrome may represent a cutaneous reaction pattern associated with T lymphocyte immune dysfunction. Gross lesions begin as scaling and erythema of the head, neck, and ears and progress to generalized alopecia with scales, crusts, and ulcers. Histologically, the lesions include basal cell hydropic degeneration, lymphocyte exocytosis, and lymphocyte clustering around apoptotic keratinocytes of the epidermis and outer follicular root sheath. Sebaceous glands may be absent. The histologic lesions are similar, but generally milder, than those in the spectrum of erythema multiforme or a graft-versus-host disease reaction. Pruritus is variable but may be severe in some cats. *M. pachydermatis* is sometimes identified. Cats with this syndrome may have clinical signs referable to an intrathoracic mass resulting in dyspnea.

Suggested Readings

Suggested Readings are available at www.expertconsult.com.

CHAPTER 18

Female Reproductive System and Mammae[1]

Robert A. Foster

Key Readings Index

The reproductive system is arguably the most important organ system for the survival of a species. In production animals, reproduction is essential for the continued supply of product, whether it is meat, fiber, milk, or many other by-products. Our understanding of many of the reproductive processes has progressed dramatically, and many of the accepted "dogmas" have been challenged and/or modified. In addition, the traditional approach of studying diseases of the reproductive system has focused on specific diseases for which information is known rather than taking into consideration the overall significance of the clinical environment. In this chapter, the relative importance of specific diseases or processes in each anatomic component or region of the reproductive system is emphasized. Historically, studies of reproductive diseases often focused on cattle, but no more. During approximately the past decade, diseases of companion animals have been studied in greater detail and are also discussed in this chapter.

Structure[2]

Female Reproductive System

The female reproductive system of domesticated animals consists of paired ovaries each with an accompanying uterine tube, and a bicornuate uterus, cervix, and vagina. Although diverse in anatomy, these structures share many similarities in structure and function. Traditionally, embryologic development of the female reproductive tract has been considered the default outcome when the male reproductive tract does not form, but now we know some of the many unique genes and subsequent processes that determine which gender arises during sexual differentiation.

Genes initiate the pathways of ovarian differentiation and development. *NROB1* (*DAX1*) and *FOXL2* are female-specific genes that promote ovarian development and inhibit testicular development, but neither is an ovary-determining gene like the sex-determining region (i.e., testis-determining gene) of the Y chromosome (*SRY*) in males. In the development of the ovary, the germ cells undergo meiosis and the supporting cells surrounding the oocytes become the granulosa and theca cells of the follicles. The differentiation of a female phenotype requires development of (1) the paramesonephric (Müllerian) ducts to form the uterine tube, uterus, and cranial vagina and (2) the urogenital sinus to form the caudal vagina and vulva.

Ovary

The structural arrangement of the ovary is similar in all species except the mare, which has an ovulation fossa around which are located the cortical structures (i.e., Graafian follicles and cortical stroma). The ovary is supported by the mesovarium, which contains the vascular pampiniform plexus of the ovary. The ovary itself has an outer layer of epithelium, which is of mesothelial origin. Beneath this layer is the capsule of the ovary. The cortex of the ovary contains follicles, stromal connective tissue, blood vessels, and, in some species, interstitial endocrine cells. The medulla has large blood vessels, lymphatic vessels, nerves, and loosely arranged connective tissue. Remnants of the mesonephric tubules, called the *rete ovarii*, are present in this region.

Ova develop within follicles, and follicles are named according to their stage of development: primordial, primary, secondary, and tertiary types. Each developing follicle has multiple layers of granulosa cells and peripheral theca cells. Ovulation occurs when the follicle ruptures, releasing the ovum and allowing the space to fill with blood and then with luteal cells to form the corpus hemorrhagicum and corpus luteum, respectively. Follicles that do not ovulate become atretic. In addition to these various ovarian structures, cats have prominent interstitial endocrine cells. The canine ovary has small ingrowths of the ovarian surface that are called

[1]For a glossary of abbreviations and terms used in this chapter, see E-Glossary 18-1.

[2]See E-Appendix 18-1 for postmortem methods used in the female reproductive system and mammae.

subsurface epithelial structures and structures called *granulosa cell rests* that are aggregates of granulosa cells in a tubular arrangement.

Oogenesis (i.e., the production and/or development of an ovum) is usually complete at birth. At puberty in most species, ovulation occurs through the outer surface of the ovary, and the ovum is collected by the infundibulum of the uterine tube.

The ovary of the mare differs from those of other species in several ways. Equine fetal gonads undergo hypertrophy wherein interstitial endocrine cells, stimulated by equine chorionic gonadotropin (formerly called pregnant mare serum gonadotropin) from the endometrial cups, expand in number and produce an extremely large gonad. The hyperplastic interstitial endocrine cells produce dehydroepiandrosterone (DHA), which is converted to different estrogens including estrone, equilin, and equilenin. The interstitial endocrine cells atrophy and disappear before birth and result in gonadal atrophy that returns the ovary back to a "normal" size. The ovary of the mare has a kidney shape with a depression called the *ovulation fossa*. The ovum is released from this depression. The follicles in the mare can attain a large size—up to 7 cm or more in diameter. Mares can therefore form a large corpus hemorrhagicum. Occasionally, a corpus hemorrhagicum and a corpus luteum can be visible externally as structures that extend outward through the ovulation fossa.

Uterine Tube

The uterine tube has four regions—the infundibulum, ampulla, isthmus, and uterotubal junction (listed in the order in which the ovum passes through each region). It is supported by a mesosalpinx. The mesosalpinx of the dog completely surrounds the ovary to form a bursa and has a large amount of fat; a small hole connects the interior aspect of the bursa to the abdominal cavity. The infundibulum surrounds the ovary of each species, except in the horse, in which it only covers the ovulation fossa. The uterine tube is where fertilization occurs, and the conceptus then moves into the uterus.

Uterus

All species have a bicornuate uterus with uterine horns and a uterine body. The uterus of the mare has longitudinal folds. Endometrial cups are present in the endometrium between 37 and 150 days of gestation and are the site of production of equine chorionic gonadotropin (Fig. 18-1). These typically form around the pregnant horn at the bifurcation. Their disappearance is an immune-mediated event. The placenta of the horse is diffuse and microcotyledonary. In ruminants, each uterine horn contains four rows of protuberances that become the caruncles. These may be pigmented in sheep. The placenta of ruminants is cotyledonary. The placenta of the pig is diffuse with small ridges. Dogs and cats have a zonary placenta with marginal hematomas.

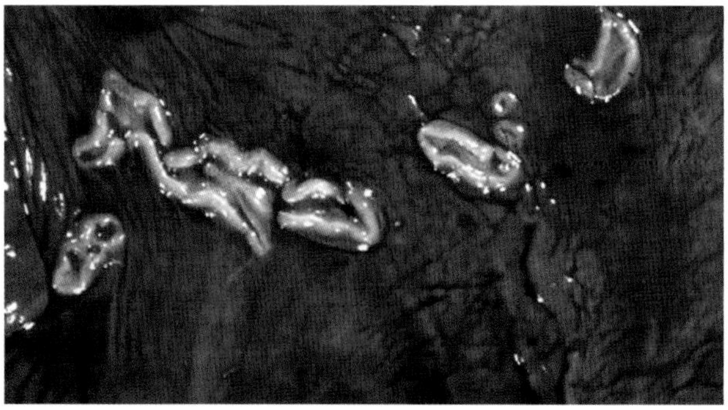

Figure 18-1 **Endometrial Cups, Uterus, Mare.** Endometrial cups are plaque-like structures in the endometrium that form when trophoblasts invade the endometrium early in pregnancy. They are present between 37 and 150 days of pregnancy and secrete equine chorionic gonadotropin. The chorionic surface opposite each cup is called the chorioallantoic pouch and is avillous. (Courtesy Dr. K. Read, College of Veterinary Medicine, Texas A&M University; and Noah's Arkive, College of Veterinary Medicine, The University of Georgia.)

Cervix

The cervix separates the external genitalia from the uterus and is an effective barrier from the external environment. Cervical mucus is viscous except during estrus, when it becomes more plentiful and thinner. The cervix in the mare, dog, and cat does not have transverse folds as it does in ruminants and sows. The cervix of the dog and cat opens on the dorsal aspect of the cranial vagina.

Cell Types of the Female Reproductive System

The epithelia of the tubular parts of the reproductive tract form the main barrier (i.e., barrier system) to the external environment. Modifications of the epithelium and of the responses of innate and adaptive immunity during the estrous cycle and with pregnancy alter the structure and function of these barriers.

Ovary

The cell types of the ovary include the epithelium (surface epithelium, subsurface epithelial structures of the bitch, and the rete ovarii), the stroma, germ cells, and follicular cells. Lymphoid cells are usually absent. Control of ovarian function is through the hypothalamic-hypophyseal- (pituitary gland)-gonadal (ovary) axis through release of gonadotropin-releasing hormone (GnRH) (see Chapter 12), as well as follicle-stimulating hormone (FSH) and luteinizing hormone (LH) (see Fig. 12-3).

Uterus

The endometrium is a unique environment separated from the caudal reproductive tract by the cervix. The endometrium has an epithelial lining of columnar and sometimes ciliated cells. There is also a stroma of the endometrium, where inflammatory and immune cells are present, particularly during estrus, when the cervix is open and the uterus is exposed to contaminants and spermatozoa or semen (horses and pigs have intrauterine insemination). Inflammation is a "normal" part of the estrous cycle, such as that which occurs in postmating endometritis.

Vulva, Vagina, and Cervix

The vulva, vagina, and part of the cervix are lined by stratified squamous epithelium that varies in thickness and cellular morphology with the stage of cycle. This variation is best illustrated in the bitch and queen, in which vaginal cytology is a practical guide to determine the stage of cycle. During anestrus, the epithelium is predominantly of a basal type, as each epithelial cell has a large nucleus and a small amount of cytoplasm. With the progressive approach of estrus (i.e., during proestrus), the epithelium becomes more mature so that at estrus the majority of cells are superficial epithelial cells with either pyknotic nuclei or no nuclei. Lymphoid follicles beneath the epithelium are a normal part of the distal vagina.

Pregnancy causes considerable change to the reproductive system. The maintenance of pregnancy and the exchange of O_2/CO_2, nutrients, and waste by-products between mother and fetus depend on the interactions of the trophoblasts with the endometrium. During pregnancy, the trophoblasts are in direct contact with the endometrial epithelium, and in some species including carnivores, some trophoblasts are in direct contact with the endometrial stroma. Maintenance of pregnancy is dependent on multiple factors that tend to vary with species. For example, cattle rely on the inhibition of prostaglandin $F_{2\alpha}$ production in the endometrium so luteolysis does not occur. Endometrial cups are essential in the mare to stimulate progesterone production by the ovary in the early phases of pregnancy. Trophoblasts must avoid immunologic rejection by the mother (also known as dam) and maintain an operational barrier system, yet provide a mechanism for the effective exchange of nutrients and waste products.

Some cells normally considered "inflammatory" cells have specific functions separate from their usual roles. Thus, uterine macrophages, natural killer cells (NKs), and, in some cases, neutrophils have separate and distinct functions. For example, macrophages are important in maintaining the size and shape of bovine caruncles, $CD2^+$ T lymphocytes and NK–like cells are important in establishing and maintaining early pregnancy in pigs, and neutrophils are involved in cervical relaxation at parturition in sheep. Thus, the usual function of inflammatory cells can be modified or used by the reproductive tract for specific but otherwise unexpected purposes that result in the maintenance of pregnancy. This outcome is likely initiated and regulated by an array of endocrine hormones and other bioactive molecules from trophoblasts as well as from cell types from fetal and reproductive tract tissues and endocrine glands.

The Mammae (Also Known as Mammary Glands)

Mammary Development, Lactation, and Involution

The ventrolateral ectoderm of the embryo becomes the mammary ridge and then the mammary complex. In development, mammary buds push into mesenchyme with their number equaling the number of mammae: mares 2, cows 4, ewes and does 2, sows 14, bitches 10, and queens 8. Sprouts form from each mammary bud, and the number equals the number of papillary ducts (and therefore mammary glands) per mamma: mares 2; cows, ewes, and does 1; sows 2; bitches 8 to 14; and queens 3 to 7. Each mamma has a single papilla (teat). Mammae develop in male embryos, but in domesticated species, they only regress fully in the stallion.

As puberty approaches, there is branching of ducts mediated by estrogen, progesterone, prolactin, growth hormone, insulin-like growth factors, and many other factors. This process is facilitated by an intimate interaction between the mesenchyme and epithelium in the formation of ducts and alveoli. Mammary development is maximal at the onset of lactation. Milk flows from alveoli through the lactiferous ducts to a lactiferous sinus (in large animals) and with suckling, through a papillary duct and the papillary ostium.

There is variation between the species in the amount of regression that occurs when milking ceases. All species reduce the volume of secretary epithelium and increase the relative amount of stroma of the gland. When secretion ceases completely, mammary fluid is resorbed. Bovine mammary glands do not regress as much as in other species, and they complete involution in approximately 2 weeks. Ewes take approximately 4 weeks to involute. Leukocytes, especially macrophages, increase in number in the involuting gland.

Cell Types

Each mammary gland is sequestered from the environment by gatekeeper functions (i.e., barrier systems) of the sphincter of the mammary papillary (teat) ostium and the papillary duct and, at least in the ruminant, its lining of keratinized squamous epithelium. The lactiferous sinus and ducts are lined by columnar epithelial cells, whereas alveoli are lined by secretory epithelium. Secretion of milk occurs in the alveoli. Mammary epithelial cells are of two types: (1) the luminal secretory epithelial cells of the ducts and secretory alveoli and (2) the basal cells. The secretory epithelial cells have receptors for immunoglobulin (Ig) G that allow for transfer of antibody from the circulatory system across (through) the secretory cells and into the milk to form colostrum. The receptors, present for approximately 1 week before parturition, disappear during lactation. These epithelial cells also facilitate the transfer of IgA produced locally by subepithelial plasma cells into alveolar lumens and the milk. The stroma of mammary glands contains capillaries, lymphocytes, and plasma cells.

Lymphoid cells in normal glands are derived from blood, and there is homing of lymphocytes from the intestine (the enteromammary pathway [see Chapter 5]) to the mammae as part of the common mucosal immune system. Lymphocytes of the cellular immune system are also present but in low numbers.

Function

Female Reproductive System

The overall function of the female reproductive tract is to provide a location for the conception, development, and eventual release of viable offspring. One offspring is sufficient for dairy cows, but the largest number possible is required for other production animals. Each anatomic unit (i.e., ovary, uterine tube, uterus, cervix, vagina, and vulva) of the female reproductive system has its own unique function.

The function of the ovary is to develop and release an ovum or ova and to produce hormones, such as estrogen and progesterone, to influence behavior and affect other organs and tissue to maintain pregnancy. It is controlled as part of an endocrine feedback system of the hypothalamic-hypophyseal-gonad loop (see Chapter 12).

The uterine tube acts as a transport system and storage site for spermatozoa. It collects and transports the ovum or ova and provides the optimal environment for fertilization. The conceptus is nourished and eventually transported to the uterus for subsequent development.

The uterus provides a suitable environment for the development of the conceptus. The endometrium and the placenta provide protection, nutrition, respiration, and endocrine activities. Exchange of nutrients, trophic factors, waste products, and immunologic components such as immunoglobulin molecules also occur. This exchange is achieved via placental sites that increase the surface area of the interface between maternal and fetal tissue. At a time appropriate for parturition, the muscles of the uterus contribute to the release and birth of the developed fetus.

The cervix functions as a gatekeeper by holding the products of conception within the uterus until parturition. It also provides a seal that prevents microbes and substances from entering the cranial vagina. Its dilation is an important step in the process of parturition.

The vagina and vulva provide a passageway that allows spermatozoa to be deposited in the reproductive tract and prevents excessive contamination with microbes and materials that would inflame or infect the uterus and uterine tube. The vagina also reduces contamination of the cervix, especially during pregnancy. It is also a portal for the fetus at parturition.

Mammae

The mammae provide nutrients, macromolecules for humoral immunity, and cells for cell-mediated immunity to the neonate. Nutrients include proteins, carbohydrates, and lipids. Milk is also the source of many humoral substances, including antimicrobial, antiinflammatory, and immune-modulating molecules, such as antibodies, complement proteins, and antimicrobial peptides. Components of the cellular immune system, such as lymphocytes and cytokines, are also transferred in milk. During the first 24 hours after parturition, transfer of immunoglobulins via colostrum is an important means of providing immunity to offspring of all domestic animal species. Most domestic animals rely on colostrum as the sole source of serum immunoglobulin in early life because their humoral immune systems are immature and they receive no or limited passive transfer of immunity via the placenta before birth. Dogs and cats have some transplacental transfer, so they are exceptions. After the immediate postnatal period (first 24 hours), substances in ingested milk (including immunoglobulin) provide some local protection against intestinal and respiratory pathogens.

Dysfunction/Responses to Injury

Female Reproductive System

Little is known about the response of the ovary to infection or insults. Observations of neutrophilic and, in viral infections, lymphocytic inflammation indicate that the ovary is capable of inflammatory and immune responses similar to those observed in other parts of the body. Hyperplasia of the surface epithelium is a common response to irritation, injury, and inflammation, just as it is with mesothelium elsewhere.

The uterine tube is such a narrow structure that its function is altered readily with edema, inflammation, and scarring. Exocytosis of neutrophils from blood vessels via the interstitium can be rapid. In sufficient numbers, pus is formed. Local immune responses can develop and result in the presence of lymphocytes, plasma cells, and, in some instances, lymphoid follicles in the supporting stroma. Granulation tissue formation in severe inflammatory conditions leads to scarring, and subsequent obstruction of the uterine tube is followed by an accumulation of fluid (hydrosalpinx) or pus (pyosalpinx).

There are many studies of the response of the uterus to infection. Inflammation varies from mild, in disorders such as postmating endometritis, to severe, in disorders such as bacterial metritis and pyometra. In mild acute inflammation of the endometrium (endometritis) of domestic animal species—apart from the dog and cat (see the following paragraph)—neutrophils and macrophages migrate through the epithelium into the lumen, and the stratum compactum is edematous. This result becomes more florid with an increased severity. Neutrophils and necrotic debris accumulate in the uterus until pyometra forms. Lymphocytes and plasma cells accumulate in the stroma of the endometrium. With chronicity and in severe situations, the epithelium becomes squamous; thus, squamous metaplasia develops (see Chapter 1). Necrosis and erosion of the epithelium results in the formation of granulation tissue, and varying degrees of fibrosis with scarring are commonplace in severe infectious or inflammatory endometritis.

The canine endometrium in particular, as well as the feline endometrium, responds with cystic endometrial hyperplasia (see Fig. 18-19). Any injury or insult, whether inert foreign material or pathogenic infectious microbes, stimulates this hyperplastic response particularly in diestrus. The luminal epithelium becomes papillated and can resemble a placental site.

In the vulva and vagina, inflammation and infection of the external part of the reproductive tract results in hyperplasia and keratinization of the stratified squamous epithelium. Exocytosis of inflammatory cells does occur, predominantly with neutrophils. These inflammatory cells migrate through the epithelium with some difficulty because of the "tight" intercellular junctions (see Chapter 1) between epithelial cells. The inflammatory response is typically lymphocytic and plasmacytic, and these cells can form a thick band of cells beneath the epithelium. Lymphoid follicles often form and give the affected region of the vagina a granular macroscopic appearance.

Placenta

Reactions of the placenta to injury rely heavily on the maternal and, to a lesser extent, the fetal immune systems. Species variability to injury is, in general, related to the type of placentation of the species affected and the route of infection. Trophoblasts are phagocytic, and they take up debris, blood, and infectious microbes. Fluid exudation and connective tissue responses, such as granulation tissue formation and fibrosis, are similar to those that occur in other organ systems. The reactions of fetal macrophages and neutrophils are less obvious than those responses seen where maternal leukocytes are readily accessible. Placentitis occurs when there is sufficient time for a response; fetal death and expulsion can be rapid with fetal distress, and there can be insufficient time to mount an effective immune response. Chronic lesions are much more obvious and occur especially in ruminants. In the cotyledonary placenta of ruminants, the intercotyledonary placenta appears to have a larger area than the cotyledons; however, the extensive papillation of the cotyledon of the placentome produces an extremely large surface area. The intercotyledonary region is a potential space that can accumulate a large volume of exudate. Chronic inflammation in ruminants is common and identified by fibrosis of the placenta. The neutrophils are probably of maternal origin. Lymphoid follicles and plasma cells are a lesser component of the reaction, but lymphocytes do accumulate beneath the layer of trophoblasts and around blood vessels. In the equine placenta, placentitis involves a small area, usually around the cervical star (see Fig. 18-37). There is no potential space within the diffuse microcotyledonary type of placenta, and thus exudates and suppuration are much less prominent; chronic placentitis is rare. The inflammatory reaction in placentas of the pig, dog, and cat are often very mild, and chronic placentitis is rare.

Mammae

The glandular and ductal components of the mammae are usually sterile but can respond rapidly to infection or other irritants. The columnar epithelial cells can become hyperplastic, but the cells are not able to withstand injury to the same extent as stratified squamous epithelium; thus squamous metaplasia is a frequent occurrence when irritants, such as infection or intramammary preparations, are introduced. Necrosis of the epithelium is common in infectious disease, and granulation and scarring of the lining of the ducts and sinus are frequent.

Although the adaptive immune system of normal mammary glands is quiescent, injury quickly results in recruitment of various innate and adaptive elements. Neutrophils and macrophages are rapidly recruited. Humoral and cellular immune responses are typically seen in disorders caused by infectious microbes. The presence of large numbers of plasma cells occurs with the development and response of the local immune system and is an invariable component of the immune response in infection. Edema and subsequent fibrosis are also part of the reaction to injury. The flow of milk is often halted and/or blocked by injury and exudates; thus the normal involutionary processes that result in resorption of secretion (macrophage and epithelial uptake) occur.

Portals of Entry/Pathways of Spread

Female Reproductive System

It is critical that infectious microbes be excluded from the uterus; otherwise fertility or pregnancy can be jeopardized. Portals of entry are listed in Box 18-1. Microbes that cause injury and inflammation

Box 18-1 Portals of Entry into the Female Reproductive System, Especially the Uterus

Ascending infection through cervix
- At insemination
- Excessive vaginal contamination
- Postpartum and with retained fetal membranes

Hematogenous
- Localization in maternoplacental interface

Descending from ovary via uterine tube
Direct penetration with foreign body (setae)
Transneural with recrudescence of herpesvirus infection

of the uterus can enter through the vulva (ascending infection), arrive via the blood (hematogenous infection), or in rare circumstances arrive from penetrating injury through the uterine wall. Reinfection of the external genitalia from nerve endings (axonal transport [see Chapter 14] is a unique feature of infection with some herpesviruses that have latency stages in their life cycles (see Chapter 4).

Ascending Infections

Ascending infections occur at estrus, breeding, and parturition. At estrus, the cervix is open to admit spermatozoa. Contamination of the cranial vagina is very important in determining whether infection of the uterus occurs or not. Conformational and structural changes in the vulva and vagina are also important determinants of infection. These changes are discussed in more detail later. A subcategory of ascending infection is caused by the contamination by infectious microbes of semen used for artificial insemination. There are many microbes, including bacteria, viruses, protozoa, and *Ureaplasma* and *Mycoplasma* spp., that cause uterine disorders via ascending infection. These disorders are discussed further in the sections on disorders of the uterus. Ascending infection is the major portal by which the equine placenta becomes infected with bacteria or fungi. The cervix in the mare is "loose" and can be readily opened with digital pressure. It is virtually impossible to penetrate the cervix of other species with a probe without creating severe trauma. Infection of the uterus and/or placenta by the ascending route with *Streptococcus zooepidemicus* is common in the mare, but most ascending infections in other species include a mixture of bacteria. This outcome is particularly the case with postpartum infections.

Hematogenous Infections

Hematogenous infections are less common and are usually involved in specific microbial disorders, such as in brucellosis, salmonellosis, pestivirus, and herpesvirus infections, and they usually occur during pregnancy. Many of the fungal infections of the placenta occur via the hematogenous route.

Direct Penetration

Direct penetration of the uterus occurs rarely. It is reported in mares that ingest the setae of processionary caterpillars.

Descending Infections

Descending infections may occur and appear to involve bacteria that descend from the ovary through the lumen of the uterine tube to the uterus. Some viral, chlamydial, and *Ureaplasma* infections can also be descending.

Box 18-2 Portals of Entry into a Mammary Gland

Ascending ductular route
- Bacteria, fungi, parasites
- Teat lesions
- Therapeutic agents

Systemic infection and localization
- Systemic fungi, viruses, mycoplasmas, mycobacteria

Direct penetration
- Penetrating injury

Box 18-3 Defenses of the Female Reproductive System

Innate defenses
- Vaginal epithelium
- Cervical barrier
- Conformation
- Myometrial tone and contraction
- Drainage of secretions
- Neutrophils
- Macrophages
- Complement
- Cytokines
- Microbial recognition molecules

Adaptive defenses
- Humoral immunity including common mucosal immune system
- Cellular immunity

Transaxonal Infections

Transaxonal infection of the distal reproductive tract occurs with some herpesviruses, where stressful events such as parturition cause a recrudescence of latent infections. Neonates can be exposed and infected via this route, but clinical disease in the mother is unusual.

Mammae

Portals of entry for the mammae are listed in Box 18-2. Most infectious microbes and foreign material (intramammary preparations) enter the gland in an ascending manner via the papillary duct. Small (bacteria) and large (leaches) pathogens can enter the gland via this route. There are some rare instances in which microbes "target" the mammary glands from systemic infection. Viruses, such as the retroviruses of caprine arthritis and encephalitis, ovine maedi-visna, and *Mycoplasma* spp., are good examples. Penetrating injury is rare.

Defense Mechanisms/Barrier Systems

Female Reproductive System

Innate, nonimmune, and physical (structural) factors are very important in the defense of the reproductive system. An adaptive immune response occurs after these factors have failed. In many instances, failure of these factors results in infection of the reproductive tract, infertility, and failure of pregnancy. Defense mechanisms are listed in Box 18-3.

Innate Immunity (Acute Inflammation)

The reproductive tract requires a defense system that provides a sterile environment for the fetus but also allows entry of antigenic and potentially infectious materials such as semen. It does this by providing a specialized epithelium (see later) in the "contaminated" environment of the vulva and vagina, and it has a specialized structure, the cervix, that excludes most microbes from the cranial "sterile" regions composed of the uterus and uterine tubes. All parts of the tubular reproductive tract are lined by epithelium in which the cells are unified by tight junctions (see Chapter 1) and are anchored to the extracellular matrix (ECM) and stroma by a basement membrane. Mucus bathes the epithelium, especially during estrus. Vaginal epithelium is stratified squamous in type and has many layers of intercellular tight junctions that inhibit the transepithelial migration of microbes and molecules. There is also a normal vaginal microbiota that may inhibit pathogenic bacteria. All parts of the tubular genitalia, including uterus and vagina, have pattern recognition receptor molecules (PRRMs) that detect pathogen-associated molecular patterns (PAMPs) including Toll-like receptors and defensins. These molecules initiate a cascade of inflammatory mechanisms that exclude or kill many pathogens before they can damage or cross the epithelium. Natural killer cells, macrophages, neutrophils, and dendritic cells are all present as cellular components of the innate system and acute inflammation.

The anatomy and "normal" integrity of the cervix are very important in maintaining its functional role (ability to close fully) in excluding infectious microbes from the uterus. In mares, the "normal" conformation of the external genitalia is a physical factor that is very important in minimizing contamination of the cranial vagina. For example, in older multiparous mares, the vulva is frequently higher than the floor of the pelvic canal and tends to become horizontal. Air and contaminants, including feces, are sucked in or allowed entry into the vagina or even into the uterus. Urine can pool in the vagina of mares with defective function of the vestibular and vulval muscles. When contamination and pooling of urine occur, the vestibule and vagina become inflamed. Subsequently, the cervix and uterus become affected either from direct contact with environmental microbes or from local spread of inflammation.

Muscular contractions of the uterus and gravitational drainage of secretions (mucus, lochia) from the uterus and vagina are also physical (functional) factors that can flush out infectious microbes. Congenital malformations and anomalies, such as persistent hymen, can reduce outflow and increase pooling in the vagina and uterus. The altered environment of the vagina in spayed, obese bitches can predispose the vagina and vulva to infection.

After microbial infection or irritation from a substance such as semen, the recognition of PAMPs and damage-associated molecular patterns (DAMPs) by molecular innate pattern recognition receptors such as Toll-like receptors and β-defensins in the endometrium initiates acute inflammation. This process occurs by the release of inflammatory mediators, including cytokines, chemokines, and prostaglandins, that results in both fluidic and cellular events (see Chapter 3). The changes include hyperemia and edema of the endometrium and fluid accumulation in the lumen of the uterus. These processes have the effect of diluting irritant substances and isolating/trapping infectious microbes, so they may be flushed out of the uterus and vagina or acted upon during the cellular phase of acute inflammation. Recruitment of neutrophils from the blood occurs in response to chemotactic substances released by bacteria, complement, and inflammatory mediators from endometrium and leukocytes. Attracted neutrophils infiltrate the endometrium, enter the uterine lumen, and contribute additional amounts of inflammatory mediators, providing additional chemotactic stimuli. Pattern recognition molecules and complement activation, directly by bacteria via the alternate pathway or by specific antibody via the classical pathway, can kill bacteria, either by lysis after attack on their membranes or by phagocytosis and phagolysosomal fusion enhanced by opsonization (see Chapters 3 and 4).

Adaptive Immunity

The reproductive tract is a unique environment because it must respond adequately to challenge from pathogens yet tolerate the allogeneic spermatozoa and fetus. Adaptive immune responses, whether humoral or cellular, have to be carefully controlled. Differing cytokine expression of epithelial cells and their effects on regulatory T lymphocytes make "decisions" as to the types and extent of responses. As a result, the responses in the "sterile" compartments of the uterus and uterine tube are different from those of the "nonsterile" vagina and ectocervix (i.e., vaginal part of the cervix).

Although the upper (cranial) reproductive tract (i.e., ovaries, uterine tubes, and uterus) is part of the common mucosal immune system, it differs from intestinal and bronchial mucosae because it does not have mucosal-associated lymphoid tissue (MALT) analogous to Peyer's patches. This difference occurs because of the lack of continuous antigenic stimulation. Lymphoid follicles, however, are present in the vulva and caudal vagina. The uterus also has the added potential influence of reproductive hormones (i.e., estrogens, progesterones, and androgens) that can modify mucosal immunologic responses.

Little is known about T lymphocyte responses and the cell-mediated immune system of the reproductive tract; much more is known about its humoral immune system. T lymphocytes are critical in determining whether the appropriate adaptive immune response is predominantly humoral or cell mediated. $CD8^+$ T lymphocytes are the most common lymphocytes of the luminal endometrial epithelium and stroma (stratum compactum especially), although there is variation, depending on the location in the uterus. For example, $CD4^+$ lymphocytes are more common in the horns of the uterus of mares, whereas $CD8^+$ lymphocytes are more numerous in the body.

It is generally believed that locally produced antibodies are more important in those diseases that are acquired by ascending infection, such as *Tritrichomonas foetus* in cattle, whereas systemic immunity is more important in systemically or hematogenously acquired infections, such as *Brucella* sp. infection. The generalization that IgA is the main mucosal antibody is not always the case because some species and individuals within a species respond with IgG_1 or IgG_2. The response to specific infectious microbes is not uniform, and there are differing immunoglobulin profile responses between species. Protection against *Tritrichomonas foetus* in cattle, for example, is mostly by IgG_1. Local transfer of immunoglobulin occurs at all levels of the tract.

Leakage of serum into the uterine lumen from an inflamed endometrium also contributes to the antibody content of the uterine fluid. Opsonization of bacteria by antibodies, especially IgG, promotes more efficient phagocytosis by neutrophils and macrophages; thus, they enhance the innate cellular response by phagocytes.

The influence of the estrous cycle on antibody responses and profiles in the uterus is controversial, but data suggest that concentrations of luminal immunoglobulins and immunoglobulin-containing cells in the endometrium are not influenced by the stage of the estrous cycle.

Locally produced IgA (see Chapters 3, 4, and 5) interferes with the attachment of bacteria to mucosal surfaces and can activate complement via the alternate pathway. It is not directly bactericidal and acts neither as an opsonin nor as a macrophage activator. Variations occur among species in the region of the reproductive tract where the concentration of IgA is greatest, but the sites correspond to the sites of semen deposition (uterus in mares, vagina in cows).

Hormonal Influences on Innate and Adaptive Immunity

Infections of the uterus are more easily overcome at estrus than at other stages of the cycle. This resistance to infection at estrus is probably attributable, at least in part, to better drainage of the uterus through an open cervix. Both estrogen and progesterone affect neutrophil and lymphocyte functions, but there is variation in results obtained when the effects of hormones are studied. In some species, such as the mouse, estrogen induces an influx of neutrophils and macrophages (at estrus). Estrogen can also be involved in the upregulation of subsets of T lymphocytes. There is variation in the number of lymphocytes in the reproductive tract during the estrous cycle. Even so, there is evidence that $CD4^+$ lymphocytes increase in number with increases in estrogen concentration. Progesterone, which dominates during the luteal phase and pregnancy, antagonizes the "proinflammatory" activity of estrogen. There is upregulation of both T and B lymphocyte responses in sheep and cattle during the follicular phase of the estrous cycle when estrogen dominates. Major histocompatibility complex II (MHC II) expression is enhanced at estrus in direct correlation with increasing estrogen concentration. The influence of the estrous cycle on antibodies in the uterus is controversial, but data suggest that concentrations of luminal immunoglobulins and immunoglobulin-containing cells in the endometrium are not influenced by the stage of the estrous cycle. Generally, the uterus is more susceptible to infection during the progestational or luteal phase of the estrous cycle and during pregnancy. The nonpregnant uterus is highly resistant to infection. The mechanisms involved in the effect of sex hormones on neutrophils are unknown, and no receptors for sex hormones have been identified.

Prostaglandins are normally produced by the epithelium of the endometrium. In most species (excluding the dog, cat, and primates), prostaglandins are responsible for lysis of the corpus luteum. In acute inflammation, prostaglandin production by the endometrium is increased, and lysis of the corpus luteum occurs. When there is epithelial and mucosal surface loss, production of prostaglandin is decreased, the corpus luteum persists, and the more susceptible (to infection) progestational uterine environment is maintained.

Mammae

As with the body in general, the mammae have a full range of mechanisms to prevent and control infectious disease. Resistance to infection relies heavily on structural isolation of anatomic structures. The structure and function of the papillary duct of the teat and the keratin that accumulates within form a plug that prevents many potential pathogens from entering the gland, ascending into alveoli, and interacting with epithelial cells. Secretions of the gland contain antimicrobial, antiinflammatory, and immune-modulating substances. Innate defense mechanisms are listed in Box 18-4. Within the gland, there also are humoral and cellular defenses.

Box 18-4 Innate or Nonspecific Defenses of the Mammae

Physical factors
- Sphincter and keratin of papillary orifice
- Flushing action of milk

Soluble factors
- Lactoferrin
- Lysozyme
- Complement
- Cytokines

Cellular factors
- Microbial recognition molecules
- Macrophages
- Neutrophils
- Natural killer cells

Innate Immunity (Acute Inflammation)

Physical factors are very important in the resistance to infection. The papillary ostium, with its sphincter, and the papillary duct offer mechanical resistance to the entry of microbes. The keratin and wax-like components of the inner aspect of the papillary duct can be protective. These constituents have bactericidal fatty acids and may also aid in killing and eliminating bacteria that attempt to gain entry to the gland by adsorbing bacteria into the wax-like components and then desquamating the debris when coated with bacteria. Delays in the formation of the keratin plug at drying off following lactation or cracks in the end of the papilla increase the risk of ascending intramammary infection. Regular milking of the lactating mammary glands probably is a natural defense mechanism because of the flushing of microbes and products of inflammation from the gland.

Once bacteria or other microbes enter the gland, sentinel and effector innate immune systems (acute inflammation) operate. Pattern recognition receptors, such as Toll-like receptors and NOD-like receptors, on alveolar and ductal epithelial cells and on leukocytes in the milk (somatic cells) recognize PAMPs on the surface of bacteria. These ligand-receptor interactions (see Chapter 4) begin inflammation and include the release of antimicrobial peptides, proinflammatory cytokines, and acute phase proteins that result in vascular effects (fluidic phase [see Chapter 3]) and the attraction of neutrophils and macrophages (cellular phase [see Chapter 3]). The release of cytokines such as tumor necrosis factor (TNF) is an important component in the eventual outcome of infection.

Soluble factors are numerous and contribute to resistance to infection. Lactoferrin, the major iron-binding protein of saliva and milk, is a nonspecific natural protective factor in milk. Mammary epithelial cells produce the bulk of lactoferrin. Lactoferrin concentration is increased in acute mastitis and in the involuting gland. The binding with lactoferrin withholds iron from pathogenic bacteria and thus has a bacteriostatic effect. The lactoperoxidase-thiocyanate-H_2O_2 system temporarily inhibits some staphylococcal, streptococcal, and coliform bacteria. Lactoperoxidase is synthesized by mammary epithelium, thiocyanate is derived from certain green feeds, and H_2O_2 is produced by exogenous sources or by enzymatic activity of *Streptococcus* spp. on constituents of milk. Hypothiocyanite produced by the lactoperoxidase system damages the inner bacterial membrane, killing the bacteria. Lysozyme, synthesized locally or from blood, destroys bacteria by lysis of cell wall peptidoglycan. Complement activated in mastitis by the alternate pathway in response to the presence of bacterial endotoxin can be important in bactericidal activity, opsonization, and promoting inflammation. Normal milk is antiinflammatory.

Cells that are not part of the adaptive or acquired immune system include macrophages, neutrophils, and natural killer cells (i.e., cells of acute inflammation). Macrophages are usually the most numerous leukocyte in mammary secretions. They phagocytose bacteria and act as antigen-presenting cells. Macrophages can be found free in alveoli and the interstitium, as well as in the lamina propria of the lactiferous sinus and interlobular and intralobular lactiferous ducts. In a lactating cow, at least 500,000 phagocytes per milliliter of milk are necessary for defense of the mammary glands against invading bacteria. In uninfected bovine mammary glands, 50,000 to 200,000 neutrophils and macrophages per milliliter of milk are present, with macrophages predominating. Lymphocytes represent approximately

10% of the leukocytes in lactation. Neutrophils are present only in low numbers unless there is bacterial infection or injury, when their influx can dramatically increase. Neutrophils play an extremely important role in antibacterial action by phagocytosis and the release of antibacterial substances. Their function is inhibited in the periparturient period. Recruitment can be so rapid that neutrophils are the dominant cells as soon as 2 hours after infection. Cell counts in milk can average 700,000 per milliliter in subclinically infected quarters, and millions of neutrophils per milliliter are common in clinical infections.

Although neutrophils recruited from the blood are important in fighting infection in the mammary glands, they do not kill bacteria as well as in milk as they do in blood. Milk seems to be a poor medium for the function of neutrophils. Some possible reasons include the absence of glucose in milk for the glycolytic metabolism of neutrophils, decreased amounts of "stored" glycogen in milk neutrophils, deficiency of opsonins and complement in milk, coating of the surface of neutrophils with casein, loss of neutrophil pseudopodia caused by phagocytosis of fat, and a decrease of hydrolytic enzymes within neutrophils after phagocytosis of casein and fat.

In experimental staphylococcal mastitis, the numbers of inflammatory cells (mostly neutrophils) in milk cycle up and down every several days, with a corresponding inverse cycling of the number of viable bacteria. When phagocytic cell counts are at a peak, phagocytosis is optimal and bactericidal activity per cell is most efficient, by as much as 10,000-fold higher. The frequency and periodicity of the cycle, as well as the amplitude of phagocytic cell and bacterial numbers, are independent for each infected quarter. The likely source of reinfection of the mammary glands is neutrophils that are inefficient at killing phagocytosed bacteria at the time of low cell count. As these cells undergo necrosis and lysis, their previously protected intracellular viable bacteria are released to multiply, and the inverse cycling of neutrophils and bacterial numbers continues.

In the first week after parturition, when neutrophils are most needed to deal with mammary infections, bovine blood neutrophils already are defective before they pass into the mammary glands. They have significantly impaired (1) chemokinesis and decreased superoxide anion production, (2) antibody-dependent cell-mediated cytotoxicity, and (3) phagocytosis of bacteria. The causes are probably some combination of the effects of stress, energy deficiency, and protein demands of early lactation and the hormonal fluxes of this stage of the reproductive cycle. In the parturient period, the concentration of glucocorticoids is increased. This relationship means that leukocyte function is less effective because expression of L-selectin and CD18 on neutrophils is downregulated by glucocorticoids. This outcome downregulates adhesion between neutrophils and vascular endothelium and transendothelial migration of neutrophils into tissues and areas containing bacteria. Neutrophils are also important in creating bystander injury of mammary tissues when the products of neutrophil granules, such as superoxide anions and enzymes, are released during phagocytosis and with neutrophil destruction.

Natural killer cells use perforin to kill bacteria in a major histocompatibility complex–independent way, and this is part of the nonspecific defenses of the mammary gland.

Adaptive Immunity

The humoral immune system operates in the mammae in several ways apart from the transfer of immunoglobulin in colostrum and during lactation. Antibody concentration in normal bovine milk is small, approximately 1 mg/mL, and includes IgA, IgM, IgG_1, and IgG_2. IgA and IgM are synthesized locally in the stromal tissue of the acini of the mammary glands and may be part of the enteromammary link (see Chapter 5) of the mucosal immune system, whereby lymphocytes from gut-associated lymphoid tissue (GALT) home to the gland. Most IgG is serum derived; IgG_1 is selectively transferred into mammary secretions and is the major immunoglobulin class in milk obtained from healthy mammary glands. IgG_2 is both serum derived and locally produced by resident plasma cells, especially in inflammation.

Particulate antigens, such as bacteria, stimulate an antibody response in the mammae of the cow, whereas soluble antigens do not. In colostrum and in milk from inflamed mammae, antibody concentration approaches 50 mg/mL. Early in inflammation, IgG_1 and IgG_2 opsonize bacteria to enhance phagocytosis by macrophages, but later the importance of IgG_2 as an opsonin increases as neutrophils enter the gland. Neutrophils can transport IgG_2 to the mammary glands as they move to the site of inflammation. IgM also functions as an opsonin. IgA does not opsonize, but it can prevent bacterial adherence to epithelium, inhibit bacterial multiplication, neutralize leukocyte-inhibiting bacterial toxins, and agglutinate bacteria. Concentrations of immunoglobulin are reduced in the periparturient period and may contribute to the increased susceptibility of the gland to infection.

Cell-mediated immunity in the gland is stimulated in infectious disease. Interleukins from mammary macrophages stimulate the immune system by activating T and B lymphocytes. Only a few B lymphocytes are present in the normal mammary glands and milk. T lymphocytes in normal mammary tissue and milk of cows and pigs are mostly $CD4^+/CD8^+$ T lymphocytes. The $CD4^+/CD8^+$ ratio is <1, which is reversed from the ratio in blood. The mammae thus have selective lymphocyte trafficking, favoring $CD8^+$ lymphocytes, which have either cytotoxic or suppressor functions. T lymphocytes and macrophages are underrepresented in normal mammary tissue and milk. $CD8^+$ T lymphocytes are found in the lactiferous duct and alveolar epithelium, whereas the lesser numbers of $CD4^+$ (T helper [T_H]) lymphocytes and B lymphocytes are in clusters in the connective tissues. In early lactation, $CD8^+$ lymphocytes in milk function more as suppressor lymphocytes than cytotoxic lymphocytes, but the situation is reversed in mid and late lactation. $CD4^+$ lymphocytes predominate in goat mammary glands and in mastitis. In response to bacterial infection, an influx of $CD4^+$ T lymphocytes occurs in milk, and these lymphocytes eventually outnumber $CD8^+$ T lymphocytes. During the periparturient period, T_H2 lymphocytes (cell-mediated response) secreting IL-4 and IL-10 predominate over T_H1 lymphocytes (humoral-mediated response) secreting IL-2 and interferon-γ. T lymphocytes may be cytotoxic, and they preferentially migrate to epithelial surfaces and can destroy altered epithelial cells. $CD4^+/CD8^+$ T lymphocytes are present in greater numbers in mammary secretions and parenchyma compared with blood. The percentage of $CD4^+/CD8^+$ T lymphocytes of mammary parenchymal lymphocytes decreases in the postpartum period, a time of increased susceptibility of the mammary glands to disease, which suggests that $CD4^+/CD8^+$ T lymphocytes can be important in defense against infection.

Disorders of Domestic Animals

Female Reproductive System

Normal Sexual Development

An understanding of the development of the reproductive tract of domesticated animals is the result of studies in multiple species, including humans, laboratory rodents, and pigs. Sequencing of genomes of animals now makes identification of genes and processes responsible for sexual development applicable to recognizing and understanding reproductive anomalies in veterinary medicine. There is also a pragmatic reason for examining embryology: It is easier to learn the mechanisms of how anomalies occur and to determine their significance rather than memorize every possible disorder.

The nomenclature for describing disorders of sexual development and their clinical manifestations and syndromes has undergone considerable change during the past decade. Reproductive disorders and syndromes were classified based on chromosomal sex, gonadal sex, and phenotypic sex using terminology such as hermaphrodite or pseudohermaphrodite, feminization and masculinization, and sex reversal. During the past decade, a more logical and simplified system of nomenclature has evolved. It is based on determining the karyotype (sex chromosomes), genotype, gonadal type and make up, and arrangement (or phenotype) of the tubular genitalia.

Sexual development occurs in three sequential processes: (1) sex chromosome type is established at conception, (2) gonadal type is established early in development, and (3) the type and arrangement of tubular genitalia and particularly the external genitalia are established after the gonadal type is set. Germ cells migrate from the yolk sac to the genital ridge, and without germ cells the ovaries do not develop and gonadal dysgenesis is the result. During embryologic development, the undifferentiated and bipotential gonad acquires germ cells, mesenchymal cells, coelomic epithelial cells, and mesonephric epithelial cells. These stem cells form the major "adult" cell types in the developed gonad: germ cells; supporting, steroid-producing cells and unspecialized mesenchyme; and epithelium. Before differentiation into a normal male or female phenotype, the embryo has a double set of ducts: the mesonephric (Wolffian) ducts (and tubules) and the paramesonephric (Müllerian) ducts (Fig. 18-2). In individuals with a karyotype of XX (female), without the sex-determining region of the Y chromosome (*SRY*–), there is activation of genes and gene products so that a normal ovary develops.

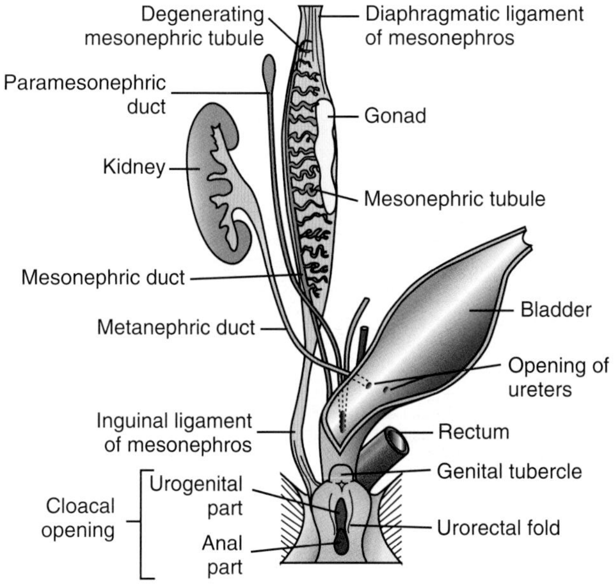

Figure 18-2 **Schematic Diagram of the Normal Components of the Female Reproductive System and the Embryonic Structures, Especially the Paramesonephric (Müllerian) Duct and Urogenital Sinus and Tubercle From Which They Were Derived.** The paired paramesonephric ducts fuse to form the body of the uterus, cervix, and cranial vagina. The mesonephric tubules remain as the microscopic rete ovarii and the mesonephric ducts usually regress completely.

Development of a testis is inhibited. The tubular genitalia of the female develop from the paramesonephric ducts, and the mesonephric ducts and tubules disappear. The paramesonephric ducts are paired and join the urogenital sinus. They fuse to form the cranial vagina and the uterine body. The urogenital sinus forms the vulva and caudal vagina. The external genital tubercle forms the clitoris. All stages of the development of the genitalia are under the control of genes and gene products.

Disorders of the Reproductive Tract[3]

Congenital Disorders of the Reproductive Tract. There are a large number of individual steps involved in sexual development and differentiation, and missing or changing one step in these processes can have major effects on subsequent differentiation. Congenital diseases of the reproductive tract are traditionally separated into those disorders that result in (1) alterations of the anticipated genital appearance or phenotype (intersex, sex reversal, and ambiguous or altered external genitalia), (2) failed or altered development of gonads and/or internal tubular genitalia, and (3) the myriad cystic remnants. From a pathogenesis standpoint, all anomalies of the reproductive system are disorders of sexual development (DSD) and are classified and discussed as such later in this section. It is almost impossible to successfully classify each and every anomaly, be it coincidental (no effect on reproductive potential) or if it results in infertility, based on its macroscopic or histological appearance alone. An abnormal location and/or size of external genitalia can create phenotypic ambiguity of the gender and therefore is often an indication of a major underlying anomaly. The categorization of DSD is based on whether the karyotype is abnormal or normal and requires an assessment of the (1) sex chromosomes, (2) the presence or absence of genes such as the sex determining region of the Y chromosome (*SRY*), (3) gonadal type, and (4) genital phenotype.

There are three major categories of DSD: (1) an abnormal or missing sex chromosome, (2) a normal female karyotype, and (3) a normal male karyotype. *Sex chromosome DSD* are those with an abnormal number and/or mixture of sex chromosomes, including XXY (Klinefelter syndrome), X_ (Turner syndrome), and XX/XY (chimerism). XY disorders of sexual development are those with disorders of testicular development, disorders of androgen synthesis or action, and miscellaneous conditions (see Chapter 19). XX DSD includes disorders of ovarian development, androgen excess, or miscellaneous disorders. The greater availability of tests for the *SRY* gene and other genes means a greater ability to more precisely define the underlying anomaly. Disorders with a normal XX or XY karyotype are subdivided into XY *SRY* positive (+) and XY *SRY* negative (–) genotypes. Once the karyotype and genotype are identified, gonadal type becomes important in understanding the development of a specific type of DSD.

Gonadal anomalies are identified at surgery or postmortem examination. Histologic assessment is necessary to differentiate between rudimentary gonads (gonadal dysgenesis), testis, ovary, and ovotestis (a combination of both male and female gonadal structures in a single gonad). The nature of the gonad often determines the eventual genital phenotype of an animal. Phenotypic females with a mismatch of gonadal type are often identified clinically by the lack of an estrous cycle, have an enlarged clitoris, and/or have an increased distance from the anus to vulva. Descriptions of the phenotypic and gonadal anomalies are often done without the benefit of karyotype, but it is preferable to describe the disorder completely as discussed next.

[3]See E-Table 1-1 for potential, suspected, or known genetic disorders.

Disorders of Sexual Development. The term "disorders of sexual development (DSD)" is now preferred and replaces previously used words such as intersex, hermaphroditism, sex reversal, and the many other pseudonyms. Common DSD are listed in Table 18-1. The disorders are divided into three major categories: the sex chromosome DSD, the XY DSD, and the XX DSD. XX DSD is a major focus of this chapter. When the sex chromosome is unknown, the DSD is classified according to the gonadal type; thus there is gonadal dysgenesis DSD, testicular DSD, ovarian DSD, and ovotesticular DSD. It is always preferable to determine the sex chromosomal complement.

Sex Chromosome Disorders of Sexual Development. True sex chromosome DSD is very rare. Cases of X_ (Turner syndrome) and XXY (Klinefelter syndrome) are reported. They usually have gonadal dysgenesis and a female phenotype. *Chimerism* is more common. Chimeras and mosaics have two or more somatic cell types, each with a different chromosome constitution. Chimeras have two genetically distinct cell types that come from different individuals, whereas *mosaicism* is a different chromosomal constitution from altered mitosis. The most common chimera in domestic animals is the *freemartin* calf (Fig. 18-3, *B*). Blood vessels of the placentas from two different fetuses fuse and exchange blood between fetuses. Each fetus becomes a hematopoietic chimera. Anastomosis of placental vessels occurs most often in bovine species and less frequently in other ruminants and pigs. The freemartin is the female of a set of male and female twins. Gene products from the cells of the male fetus induce fetal Sertoli cells and seminiferous cordlike structures in the ovaries of the female twin. The ovaries are small and can have reduced number of or no germ cells. Some freemartins have ovotestes. The paramesonephric (Müllerian) duct derivatives vary from almost normal to cordlike structures, but their lumens do not communicate with the vagina. The vagina, vestibule, and vulva are hypoplastic. Vesicular glands are always present; other mesonephric (Wolffian) structures are present to varying degrees. Externally, the

Table 18-1 Common Syndromes of Disorders of Sexual Development (DSD)

Category of DSD	Syndrome	Species	Comments
Sex Chromosome DSD	Freemartinism	Bovine, ovine	Chimerism in twinning
XX *SRY* − testicular DSD	XX sex reversal	American cocker spaniels	Autosomal recessive inheritance
XX *SRY* − testicular DSD	XX sex reversal	Polled goats	Linked to the poll gene
XY *SRY* + testicular DSD	Male feminization syndrome	All species	Lack of testosterone receptors
XY *SRY* + testicular DSD	Persistent Müllerian duct syndrome	Miniature schnauzer	Complete internal female tubular genitalia
XY *SRY* + testicular DSD	Failure of testicular descent	All species	Discussed under male genital system
XX *SRY* − ovarian DSD or XY *SRY* + testicular DSD	Segmental aplasia	All species	Rare anomaly often missed at clinical examination
	Gonadal hypoplasia	All species	Males especially

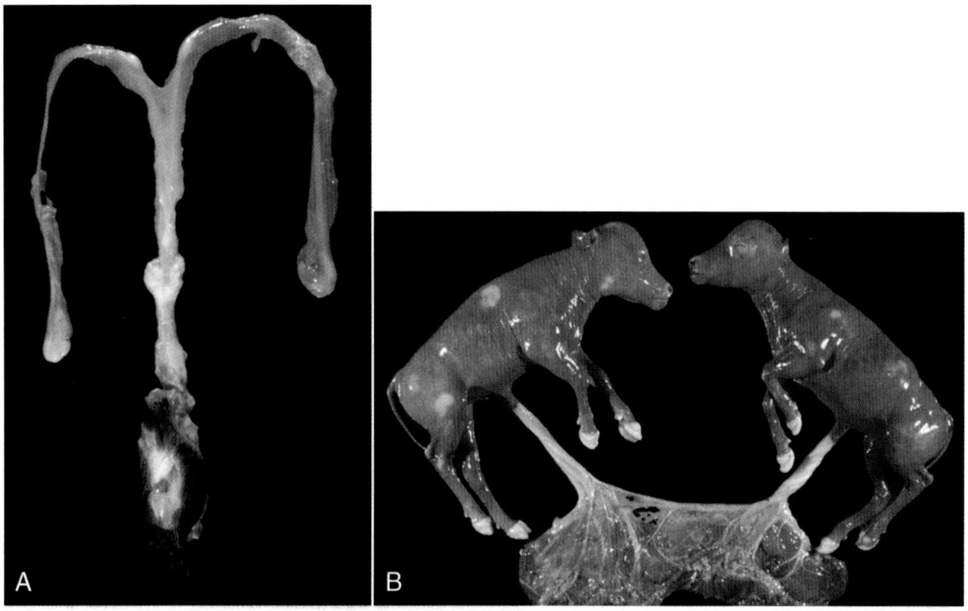

Figure 18-3 **Sex Chromosome Disorder of Sexual Development, Bovine Freemartinism, Cow. A,** Phenotypically female, reproductive tract, cow. The freemartin is the female of a set of male and female twins. Freemartins are chimeras. There is a vulva and vagina with a prominent clitoris. The internal genitalia consist of bulbourethral and vesicular glands, deferent duct, and short incomplete segments of uterus. The gonads are testis with epididymides attached. This major anomaly renders the cow infertile. **B,** Placenta, twin fetuses. Placental vascular anastomosis, which allows exchange of blood between fetuses, is a requirement for freemartinism. These anastomoses occur most often in the bovine species. (Courtesy Dr. R.A. Foster, Ontario Veterinary College, University of Guelph.)

animal has a female phenotype, but the vestibule and vagina are short, the vulva is hypoplastic, and the clitoris is enlarged. The male twin is minimally affected.

XX Disorders of Sexual Development. The more traditional XX DSD has an ambiguous phenotype. The majority of these are XX, SRY– ovotesticular DSD and a female but ambiguous phenotype. They are usually true hermaphrodites with both male and female gonads (Fig. 18-4). They are phenotypically female with masculinization, such as an enlarged clitoris. American cocker spaniels and some other breeds of dog have this autosomal recessive trait. In goats, it is associated with the polled gene. Confirmation of this syndrome requires karyotyping because in the case of goats, the presence of mammary development in bucks is not always an indication of an XX DSD. All DSD with a normal female karyotype (XX) reported in animals are *SRY*– (XX *SRY*– DSD). They are subcategorized based on whether the gonad is an ovary, testis, ovotestis, or has gonadal dysgenesis. Based on prevalence, the majority of XX disorders are of minor or incidental nature, and they are found in otherwise normal females with normal ovaries. These cases are *XX* SRY– *ovarian DSD and female phenotype*. The anomalies, discussed later, vary from insignificant or incidental findings to those that interfere with fertility or parturition.

XY Disorders of Sexual Development. The XY DSD is discussed in more detail in Chapter 19. The XY DSD are divided into subcategories based on their gonadal type, including the presence of testis, ovary, ovotestis, or gonadal dysgenesis. The majority of disorders are XY *SRY*+ testicular DSD and are of an incidental or minor nature, including cystic remnants of embryonic ducts. The more dramatic types have a normal male chromosome (XY) and a female phenotype. They have abnormal gonadal development that drives phenotypic abnormalities, abnormal androgen synthesis, or lack androgen receptors. The common example is XY *SRY*+ testicular DSD and female phenotype. These disorders were called *male pseudohermaphrodites*, *testicular feminization*, or *XY sex reversal* (Fig. 18-5). They usually lack androgen receptors. Serum testosterone is present, but the genitalia are female. A mild form occurs in miniature schnauzers with persistent Müllerian duct syndrome. They are XY males with normal male sex organs and a complete paramesonephric system, including uterine tube, uterus, and cranial portion of the vagina. They lack the anti-Müllerian hormone (AMH; previously called Müllerian inhibitory substance) or its receptor. XY *SRY*– gonadal dysgenesis DSD and female phenotype is another category and is found in horses and other species. They have hypoplastic or undifferentiated gonads and a female phenotype.

Cysts. Minor or incidental disorders are myriad in the reproductive tract. Foremost of these are the numerous cysts and tubular remnants. Periovarian (also called paraovarian) cysts are extremely common and can be confused with cystic neoplasms. They are derived from paramesonephric ducts or mesonephric ducts or tubules. Table 18-1 lists the locations and names of common incidental cystic lesions. They are discussed in more detail later.

Inclusion cysts of the reproductive tract are isolated cysts not derived from embryonic elements. The serosal inclusion cyst of the uterus in bitches is a common type (Fig. 18-6). It arises from a small group of mesothelial cells trapped beneath the serosal surface during involution of the uterus. These grapelike clusters of semitransparent thin-walled cysts are located on the serosal surface of the uterus. Subsequent distention and enlargement result in numerous cysts developing.

Disorders of Growth. More significant disorders include failure of the normal maturation, hypoplasia, or aplasia of parts of the internal or external genitalia. Because normal development requires such intricate timing of events, including regression of some parts, the joining of ducts and tubules, migration of components from one site to another, the interaction of genes, and hormones and local factors, it is no wonder there are myriad anomalies.

Segmental aplasia of the paramesonephric duct can affect any part of the duct, and little is known of its pathogenesis. A genetic basis is implicated in shorthorn cattle, in which it is linked to the recessive gene for white coat color. The simplest form is failure of the paramesonephric duct to make a proper connection with the urogenital sinus, leaving a persistent hymen, a membrane at the site where the two precursor tissues join (Fig. 18-7). A perforated hymen sometimes persists and is not clinically significant. If the hymen is complete and there is no drainage of fluid from the uterus, the cranial portion of the vagina, cervix, and uterus distend with normal

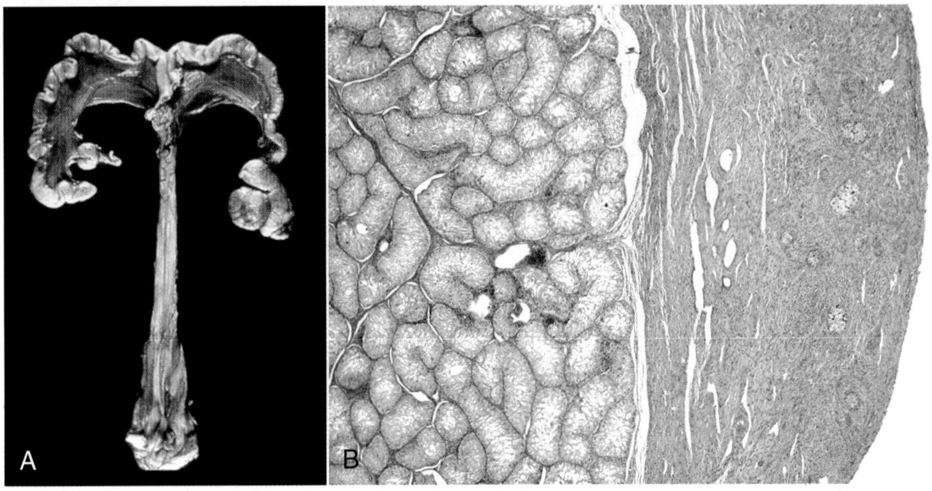

Figure 18-4 **Ovotesticular Disorder of Sexual Development with Female Genitalia, Reproductive Tract. A**, Gilt, an ovotestis is on the left and a testis on the right. Note the well-developed uterus, cervix, and vagina. **B**, Dog, ovotestis, at the periphery *(right half of image)* is the ovarian component with capsule and stroma. No active follicles are visible. The testicular component contains seminiferous tubules lined by Sertoli cells *(left half of image)*. There is no spermatogenesis in these tubules. H&E stain. (**A** courtesy Dr. K. McEntee, Reproductive Pathology Collection, University of Illinois. **B** courtesy Dr. J.F. Zachary, College of Veterinary Medicine, University of Illinois.)

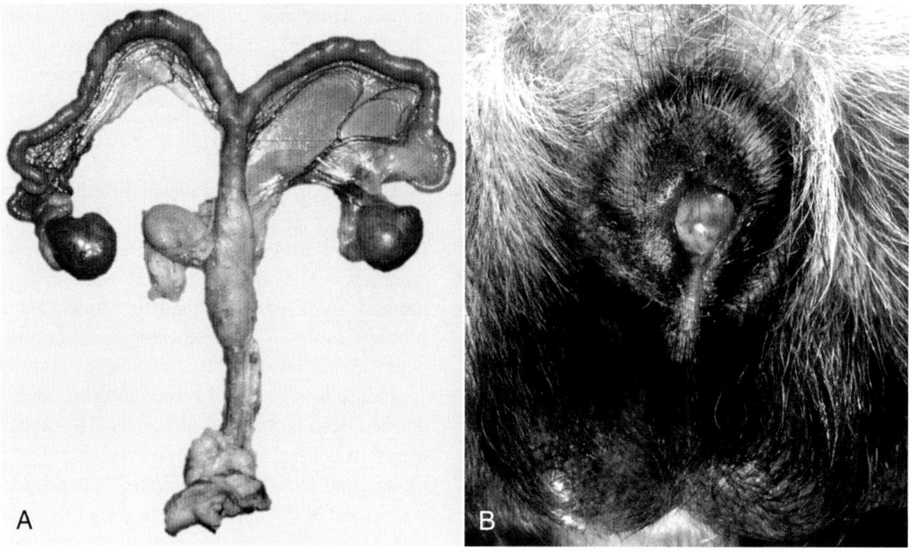

Figure 18-5 **Testicular Disorder of Sexual Development with Female Genitalia, Reproductive Tract. A,** Pig. A testis and epididymis are present on each side. Note the well-developed uterus, cervix, and vagina. No ovarian tissue is present. **B,** Clitoral enlargement, dog. The clitoris protrudes between the labia of the vulva and is visible on the ventral floor of the vulva. Note the formation of a bifid scrotum ventral to the vulva. (Courtesy Dr. K. McEntee, Reproductive Pathology Collection, University of Illinois.)

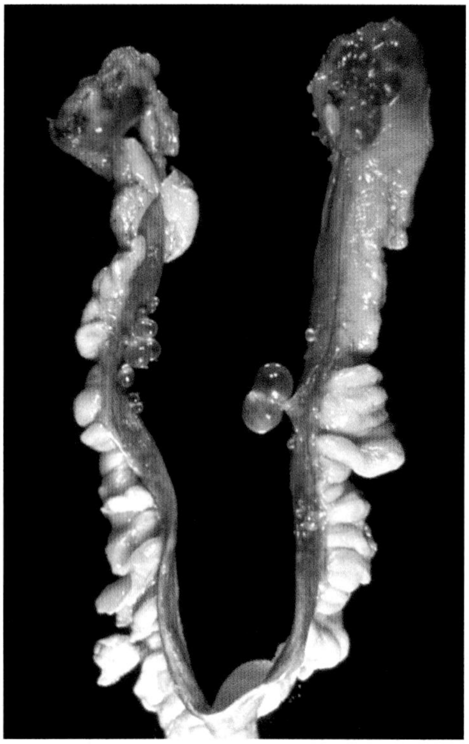

Figure 18-6 **Uterine Serosal Inclusion Cysts, Reproductive Tract, Bitch.** The cysts projecting from the serosal surface of the uterus are believed to arise from mesothelial cells trapped within serosal connective tissue. These cysts are an incidental finding at ovariohysterectomy. Note that there are also multiple thin-walled cysts around the right ovary. These cysts are remnants of embryonal ducts and are called periovarian cysts. (Courtesy Dr. K. McEntee, Reproductive Pathology Collection, University of Illinois.)

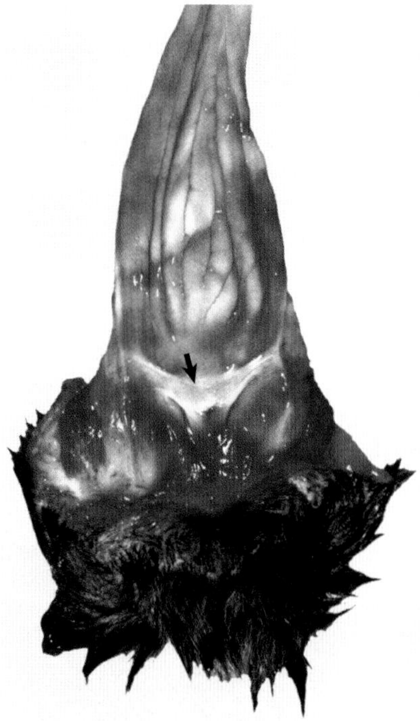

Figure 18-7 **XX Disorder of Sexual Development, Persistent Hymen, Vagina, and Vulva, Bitch.** The membrane *(arrow)* partially separates the vestibule from the vagina and is just cranial to the urethral opening. This minor anomaly is of little consequence and does not interfere with coitus or parturition. (Courtesy Dr. R.A. Foster, Ontario Veterinary College, University of Guelph.)

secretions. In the more severe forms of segmental aplasia, one or more segments of the vagina, cervix, uterine body, and uterine horns are absent or rudimentary. Aplasia of a segment of the uterus (Fig. 18-8) occurs in cattle. Prostaglandin can be synthesized and released from the blind ending uterine horn, just as is produced by a normally connected uterine horn. In those animals with a local utero-ovarian pathway for luteolysis, such as the cow, the absence of a segment of the uterus can result in insufficient $PGF_{2\alpha}$ to cause regression of the corpus luteum. In the pig, in which systemic circulation of $PGF_{2\alpha}$ from the endometrium to the corpus luteum is important,

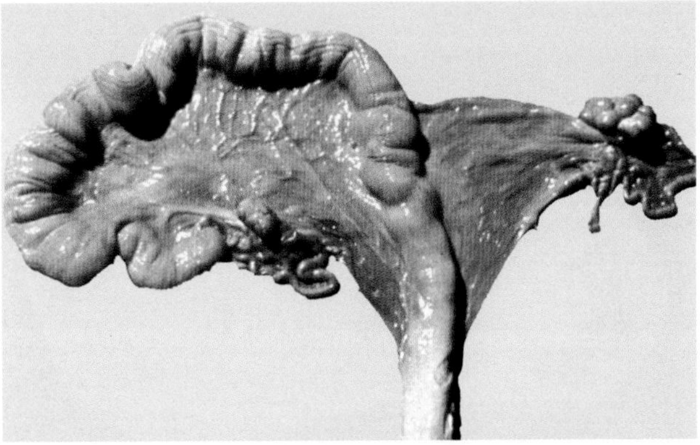

Figure 18-8 XX Disorder of Sexual Development, Segmental Aplasia of a Uterine Horn, Uterus, Pig. The right uterine horn is completely missing. (Courtesy Dr. K. McEntee, Reproductive Pathology Collection, University of Illinois.)

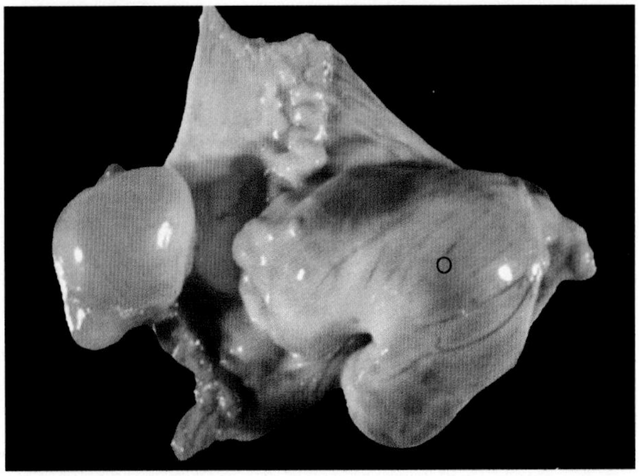

Figure 18-9 Cystic Remnant of Paramesonephric Duct (Hydatid of Morgagni), Ovary, Mare. This cystic structure is located in the fimbria, adjacent to the ovary *(O)*. They are very common in mares and are cystic remnants of paramesonephric ducts. (Courtesy Ontario Veterinary College, University of Guelph.)

prostaglandins from the blind uterine horn can have a lytic effect on the corpora lutea of pregnancy in the contralateral ovary. In the dog and cat, the uterus does not play a role in the regression of the corpus luteum.

Imperfect lateral fusion of the paired paramesonephric ducts results in anomalies. Normally the two ducts unite first at the cloacal end to form the cranial vagina. The fusion moves cranially to form the cervix and the uterine body. Malformations caused by imperfect fusion are most common in and adjacent to the cervix. They range from a dorsoventral fibrous band in the cranial vagina, failure of fusion of the caudal cervix with bifurcation of the cervical canal, to complete duplication of the cervix and body of the uterus (uterus didelphys).

Hypoplasia (and its extreme, aplasia) of a portion of the reproductive tract apart from the tubular genitalia occurs in many different degrees. Gonadal hypoplasia is common, especially in males, and these are discussed in the later sections and in Chapter 19.

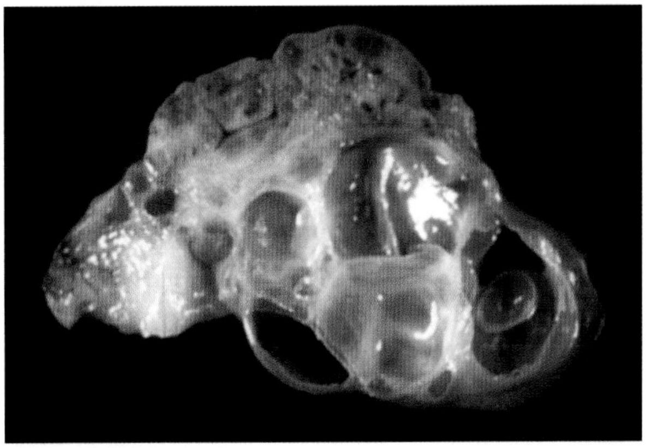

Figure 18-10 Multiple Cystic Rete Ovarii, Ovary, Bitch. Note the multiple cysts *(lower right half of image)* within the ovary at the hilus. They are incidental findings in bitches and are of little consequence. They develop from the rete (mesonephric tubules) of the ovary and become cystically distended. In cats, they can be unilocular and very large and cause pressure atrophy of the ovary. They must be differentiated from cystadenomas and cystadenocarcinomas, histologically. (Courtesy Dr. R.A. Foster, Ontario Veterinary College, University of Guelph.)

Disorders of the Ovary

Developmental Anomalies

Cysts in and around the Ovary. Periovarian (paraovarian) cysts are cysts that are external to the ovary. They are common findings in dogs and cats during ovariohysterectomy (E-Table 18-1). Intraovarian cysts are the cysts within the ovary. They should be differentiated from cystic neoplasms (see later).

Periovarian Cysts. Periovarian cysts are usually cystic remnants of embryonic structures, either paramesonephric ducts or mesonephric tubules or ducts. Location of the cyst helps differentiate them. Cystic remnants of the paramesonephric ducts include the fimbrial cyst and the cystic accessory uterine tube. This morphology is common in the mare and called the *hydatid of Morgagni* (Fig. 18-9). Hydatid of Morgagni measure up to several centimeters in diameter and are cranial to the ovary in the mesovarium. Cystic accessory uterine tubes are located in the mesosalphynx.

Histologically, they resemble the normal uterus and have a thin coat of muscle. There are cysts that arise from mesonephric remnants, either ducts or tubules. Cysts of the mesonephric duct are in the cranial or caudal mesovarium and histologically have a thick smooth muscle coat.

Intraovarian Cysts. Intraovarian cysts are numerous and common. Many are derived from Graafian follicles, but others are epithelial cysts arising from surface epithelium or from intraovarian rete ovarii—that is, embryonic structures of mesonephric tubular origin. The most common cyst in the mare is an epithelial inclusion cyst; the most common cyst in dogs and cats is cystic rete ovarii (Fig. 18-10).

Epithelial inclusion cysts in mares can cause infertility (see E-Table 18-1). They are located in the ovary around the ovulation fossa. Epithelium from the surface of the ovary becomes pinched off and embedded in the stroma during ovulation. This epithelium produces fluid that causes the cyst to enlarge and eventually reach several centimeters in diameter. They are identical in appearance to large follicles, but they do not appear and disappear as follicles should; histologic assessment is necessary to confirm the diagnosis. Their size and number may block ovulation. Epithelial inclusion cysts in other species, or cysts of subsurface epithelial structures in bitches, form in a similar manner, but they are in the capsule of the ovary and are usually small and incidental.

Cystic ovarian (Graafian) follicles, or follicular cysts, are defined as follicles that are larger than normal. They are especially important in cows and sows. The disease in cows is called *cystic ovarian*

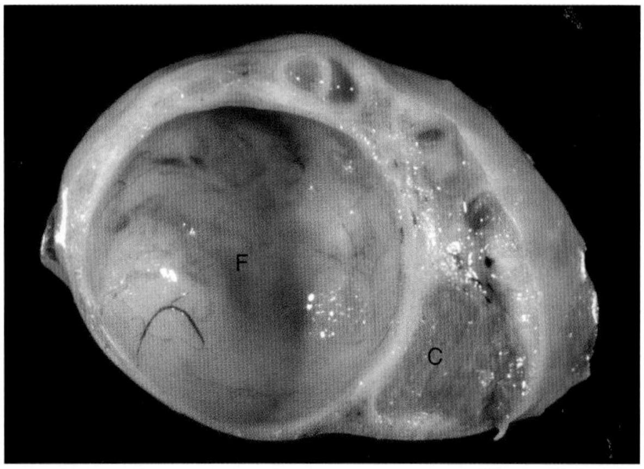

Figure 18-11 Cystic Graafian Follicle, Ovary, Cow (Also Called Follicular Cysts). Follicular cysts *(F)* are larger than normal follicles and usually greater than 2.5 cm in diameter. They are the macroscopic lesions of cystic ovarian disease in the cow. They arise when ovulation of a normal follicle does not occur. C, Corpus luteum. (Courtesy Dr. R.B. Miller, Ontario Veterinary College, University of Guelph.)

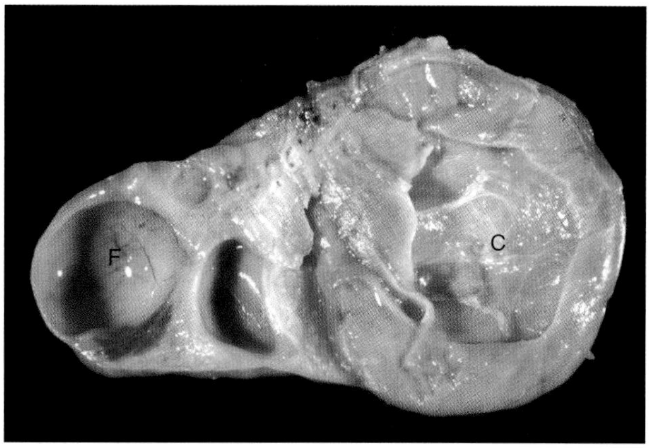

Figure 18-12 Cystic Corpus Luteum, Ovary, Cow. A cystic corpus luteum *(C)* is a normal corpus luteum complete with an ovulation papilla and a prominent cystic center. There is also a normal Graafian follicle *(F)* present. (Courtesy Dr. R.B. Miller, Ontario Veterinary College, University of Guelph.)

degeneration (COD). Bovine cystic follicles are 2.5 cm or more in diameter (Fig. 18-11) and persist for 10 or more days without the formation of a corpus luteum. The prolongation of the postpartum interval to first estrus (so-called *days-open*) is the main consequence of cystic follicles. Ovulation does not occur. These cysts probably develop because of an abnormality of the hypothalamo-hypophyseal-ovarian axis that causes a deficiency of luteinizing hormone (LH) or of the LH receptor in the ovary. Evidence suggests that stress is involved wherein adrenocorticotropic hormone (ACTH) or cortisol inhibits GnRH release from the hypothalamus and prevents upregulation of LH receptors in the ovary. Higher concentrations of progesterone can have a similar effect. The end result is an inadequate LH surge and failure of ovulation. Cystic ovarian degeneration is treated with GnRH, which causes release of LH in the pituitary, and is also treated with chorionic gonadotropin (high in LH). Postpartum uterine infection (endometritis) can cause cystic follicles. Infection of the uterus with *Escherichia coli* increases concentrations of serum $PGF_{2\alpha}$ metabolites and cortisol. Bacterial endotoxins or the prostaglandins produced because of damage caused by endotoxins stimulate the adrenal cortical secretion of cortisol; cortisol excess suppresses the preovulatory release of LH, resulting in the development of follicular cysts.

Luteinized cysts are anovulatory luteinized follicular cysts. They develop from follicular cysts by delayed or insufficient release of LH and are therefore part of COD (see E-Table 18-1). They therefore occur in cows and sows more often than in other species. Luteinized cells line the cystic cavity. Cystic follicles and luteinized cysts can occur in the same ovary.

Cystic corpus luteum is a corpus luteum with a cystic center. It is unknown why the affected follicle fails to luteinize fully. The cystic center is larger than the small central cavity that occurs normally in some corpora lutea. Ovulation occurs in a normal follicle, but a large irregular cystic center develops (Fig. 18-12). The length of the estrous cycle is not affected, and most cystic corpora lutea are incidental.

Miscellaneous Developmental Ovarian Anomalies

Agenesis. Agenesis, a total lack of ovarian tissue, can involve one or both ovaries. The entire reproductive tract also can be absent. In cases of bilateral agenesis, the tubular genitalia remain infantile.

Duplication. Duplication of an ovary is a rare anomaly that arises by two different mechanisms: (1) originating separately or (2) splitting in two of an already developing ovary. The former is a theoretical possibility and is often used to explain cases in which incompletely spayed cats and dogs come into heat (estrus) again (ovarian remnant syndrome). The latter type is close to the normally located ovary and may be connected to it.

Hypoplasia. Hypoplasia of the ovaries is reported most often in cows. It occurs in Swedish Highland cattle as an autosomal recessive trait with incomplete penetrance. It is either unilateral or bilateral. The number of primordial follicles and the proportion of Graafian follicles are fewer than normal. Ovarian hypoplasia occurs with sex chromosome DSD such as XXX and X_ chromosomes in mares and XXX karyotype in cows. It is usually bilateral but not symmetric, and it affects young cows. The affected ovaries are small and lack follicles or surface scars from ovulation. Microscopically, cortical stroma and follicles or ova are absent or poorly developed. The tubular genitalia remain infantile after the expected time of puberty. Other causes of an infantile reproductive tract are malnutrition and debility. Ovaries in these animals, however, have numerous primordial follicles and can respond to gonadotropic hormones after removal of the debilitating factor.

Vascular Hamartomas. Vascular hamartomas of the ovary are incidental findings in the mare, cow, and sow and extremely rare in other species. They appear as a dark red mass on the surface of the ovary and consist of connective tissue and vascular channels lined by mature endothelial cells.

Inflammation of the Ovary

Oophoritis. Oophoritis, or inflammation of the ovary, is rare in domestic animals. Infectious bovine rhinotracheitis virus (bovine herpesvirus 1 [BoHV-1]) viremia in experimental studies can induce necrotizing oophoritis in the postestrus cow. A cloudy fibrinous fluid fills some follicles. Microscopically, the lesions in the corpus luteum range from diffuse hemorrhage and necrosis to focal necrosis and the presence of mononuclear cells. Most affected ovaries also have necrotic follicles and lymphocytes and plasma cells in the stroma. Bovine viral diarrhea (BVD) virus, a vertically and horizontally transmitted virus responsible for mild to fatal enteric disease and reproductive failure, can localize in bovine oocytes and cumulus cells[4] and cause chronic oophoritis. Infection of ovarian oocytes with BVD virus is one of several possible routes of transmission of the virus from cow to fetus. Bacterial perioophoritis occasionally is found in cats and dogs. In cats, it must be differentiated from feline infectious peritonitis (FIP). The inflammation is located around the ovary and within the uterine tube, suggesting that the causative bacteria may ascend from the uterus.

Noninflammatory Disorders

Senescence. As animals age, germ cells are diminished in number until a minimum critical number is reached, whereupon the animal ceases to cycle and ovulate. The hypothalamic-pituitary-gonadal axis stops functioning and estrus no longer occurs. The ovary becomes atrophic and there is no further cyclic change in the tubular genitalia. It too becomes atrophic.

Supernumerary Follicles. Supernumerary follicles occur in bovine ovaries when follicle-stimulating hormone (FSH) is used in doses to cause superovulation in preparation for embryo transfer. There may be more than a dozen well-developed ovarian follicles or corpora lutea.

Adhesions. Adhesions between the infundibulum and the ovary vary from thin bands to large sheets of fibrous connective tissue binding the walls together. The lesion is often bilateral in cows and results from ascending infection after postpartum metritis. Physical trauma from rectal palpation and manipulation of the ovary is another possible cause; infundibular adhesions are common in beef heifers. Adhesions can obstruct or cause retention of fluids and result in a cystic infundibulum.

Hemorrhage. A small amount of hemorrhage is normal at the time of ovulation in all species. The mare is an exception because the follicles are large and the cavity of the ovulated follicle fills with blood to form a large corpus hemorrhagicum. In rare cases, the hemorrhage can be extensive enough to form an ovarian hematoma or even hemoperitoneum, which can be fatal. If the hematoma extends through the ovulation fossa, the corpus luteum develops external to the ovarian capsule. In the mare and cow, a focal area of serositis is detectable at the point of ovulation. Progression through a fibrinous to a fibrous stage is rapid, and an "ovulation tag" is formed. The manual expression of a persistent corpus luteum in the cow sometimes results in severe periovarian hemorrhage. Organization of the hematoma results in adhesions between the ovary and adjacent structures, such as infundibulum of the uterine tube, and causes infertility. Excessive hemorrhage into follicles is sometimes present in calves, and hemorrhage into cystic follicles occurs occasionally in the bitch.

Atretic Follicles. Atretic follicles are those that become arrested at any stage of development and then regress. In any estrous cycle, only one or a small number of follicles is destined to mature, whereas the others undergo atresia at various stages of maturation. A similar process occurs in seasonal anestrus and in all domestic species during pregnancy, except for the mare. Follicular atresia is considered abnormal when it is a part of any disease process that interferes with the release of or the pituitary response to GnRH. Development of the follicle can be arrested at any stage, and after an undetermined amount of time, it degenerates. The ovum undergoes apoptosis (see Chapter 1) first; then the granulosa cells become pyknotic, vacuolated, and desquamate. The follicle either persists as a cyst with a partial thin lining of granulosa cells or is replaced by macrophages, theca cells, and fibrous connective tissue, eventually becoming a small scar.

[4]Cells that surround the oocyte in the follicle and after ovulation.

Neoplasms of the Ovary. There are three main groups of primary ovarian neoplasms in domesticated animals: germ cell, sex cord stromal, and epithelial. Little is known of ovarian carcinogenesis. Neoplasms rarely metastasize to the ovary of domestic mammals.

Germ Cell Neoplasms. Neoplasms arising from germ cells can differentiate along either embryonic or extraembryonic lines and are benign or malignant. The majority of neoplasms of germ cells are benign and undifferentiated (dysgerminoma) or benign with somatic cell (i.e., non–germ cell) differentiation (teratoma).

Dysgerminoma. Dysgerminoma is a rare ovarian neoplasm of all species. It is usually a white solid friable lobulated mass with areas of hemorrhage and necrosis. It is composed of large round cells with a high nuclear to cytoplasmic ratio and many mitoses. This neoplasm is identical to seminoma in the testis. Metastases are rare.

Ovarian Teratomas. Ovarian teratomas are rare and usually well differentiated and benign. They have disorganized elements of at least two of the three embryonic germ layers: ectoderm, including neuroepithelium; mesoderm; and endoderm. Skin with hair is often present (Fig. 18-13). Bone, cartilage, nervous tissue, fat, and respiratory epithelium are frequently seen. Malignant teratomas occur less often, and they are usually poorly differentiated with primitive tissue types.

Sex Cord Stromal Neoplasms. Sex cord stromal neoplasms have a phenotype that resembles tissues derived from sex cords and/or follicles. Most tumors have regions with combinations of granulosa cell, theca cell, luteal cell, Sertoli cell, or interstitial endocrine cell phenotypes. Granulosa cell phenotype usually predominates; thus most are called *granulosa cell tumors*. Most of these tumors produce anti-Müllerian hormone (AMH), estrogens, androgens, and/or inhibin. Inhibin is a protein that inhibits FSH synthesis and FSH secretion. In females, it arises from the gonads, pituitary gland, placenta, or corpus luteum; in males, it arises from Sertoli cells of the testis. The mare can have signs of anestrus (inhibin-producing), nymphomania (estrogen-producing), or stallion-like behavior (androgen-producing); the bitch is likely to have prolonged estrus and may develop pyometra.

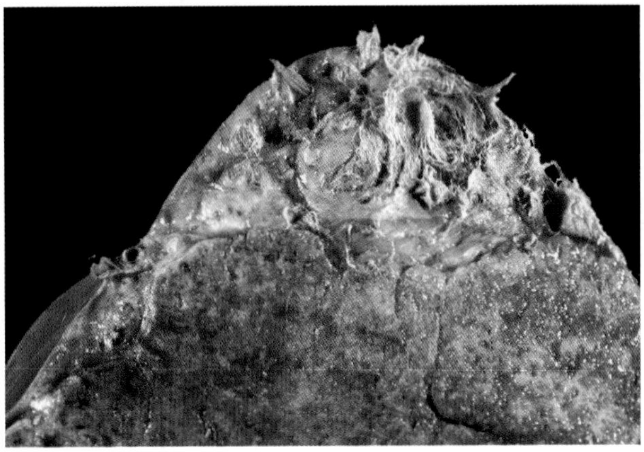

Figure 18-13 **Ovarian Teratoma, Ovary, Bitch.** These tumors have cells from all three germ cell lines: ectodermal (epithelium, including neuroepithelium), mesodermal (mesenchymal tissue), and endodermal (intestine and respiratory tissues). The most common tissues seen macroscopically are hair, cartilage, and bone. This teratoma was 30 cm in diameter and surrounded by a bursa, but residual ovarian tissue was not found. Hair *(top half of image)* and bone are the main structures visible. (Courtesy Dr. R.A. Foster, Ontario Veterinary College, University of Guelph.)

Granulosa Cell Tumors. Granulosa cell tumors are the most common ovarian neoplasms reported in large animals. They are unilateral, smooth surfaced, and round and can be 20 to 30 cm in diameter. They can be solid, cystic, or polycystic (Fig. 18-14, *A* and *B*). The cysts can vary from microscopic size to several centimeters in diameter. Often, the fluid within the cysts is red-brown. Microscopically, the neoplastic cells resemble normal granulosa cells and often are arranged as they would be in normal Graafian follicles: in single or multiple rows of round to columnar cells lining fluid-filled spaces (Fig. 18-14, *C*). In less differentiated areas, the neoplastic cells are arranged in sheets. Call-Exner bodies (i.e., rosettes of granulosa cells around a central space) may be present. The stroma can be sparse or plentiful. Granulosa cell tumors in the mare and cow are usually benign, are sometimes malignant in the bitch, and are often malignant in the queen; prognostic criteria are not established.

Pure thecomas are sex cord stromal tumors with predominantly thecal differentiation. The cytoplasm of cells in a thecoma contains lipid droplets, as do the cells of the internal theca. Areas of luteinization in sex cord stromal neoplasms occur, but pure luteomas, neoplasms with a uniform population of luteinized cells, are rare. Interstitial endocrine cell tumors have also been reported. Sertoli cell tumors are discussed in Chapter 19.

Epithelial Neoplasms. The single layer of cells overlying the ovaries, while contiguous with the mesothelium, is called ovarian epithelium. This coelomic covering is the same tissue that invaginates in early fetal life to form the epithelial cell lining of the internal tubular genitalia. Neoplasms of the ovarian surface epithelium and of the uterine tube and endometrium can have a similar appearance. In some species, ovarian epithelial neoplasia is believed to come from the tubular genitalia. Neoplasms of the ovarian epithelium, adenoma and carcinoma, occur commonly in the bitch (Fig. 18-15, *A*). In dogs, they originate from the subsurface epithelial structures that are invaginations of the epithelium into the capsule of the ovary. They are often multifocal and bilateral, not from metastasis but from multiple de novo development. Macroscopically, the affected ovary is large and multinodular and has a cystic or shaggy appearance. Histologically, they have a combination of papillary and cystic regions (Fig. 18-15, *B*). When predominantly papillary, they are called *papillary adenoma* or *adenocarcinoma*; if they are mostly cystic, they are called *cystadenoma* or *cystadenocarcinoma*. It is very difficult to differentiate some epithelial tumors from sex cord stromal tumors based on histology and immunohistochemistry because of similarities in phenotype and in immunohistochemical staining between the two groups. Most epithelial tumors stain for cytokeratin (CK) 7, and most sex cord stromal tumors stain for inhibin. Malignant forms usually spread over the peritoneal surface by both direct lateral extension and seeding (Fig. 18-15, *C*), or they metastasize to lymph nodes and other organs. Ascites results from obstruction of the diaphragmatic lymphatic vessels, which fail to reabsorb peritoneal fluid, and/or from excess fluid secretion by the neoplasm. Neoplasms that arise in the rete ovarii of the ovarian hilus are extremely rare.

Disorders of the Uterine Tubes

Lesions of the uterine tubes are either from current or previous infection or are incidental cystic remnants of embryonic ducts.

Salpingitis (Including Pyosalpinx). Salpingitis is inflammation of the uterine tube, and pyosalpynx is a pus-filled uterine tube. Both result from infection with bacteria usually. Salpingitis accompanies endometritis, metritis, or pyometra in most species; thus it is the result of ascending infection and is often bilateral. Salpingitis is

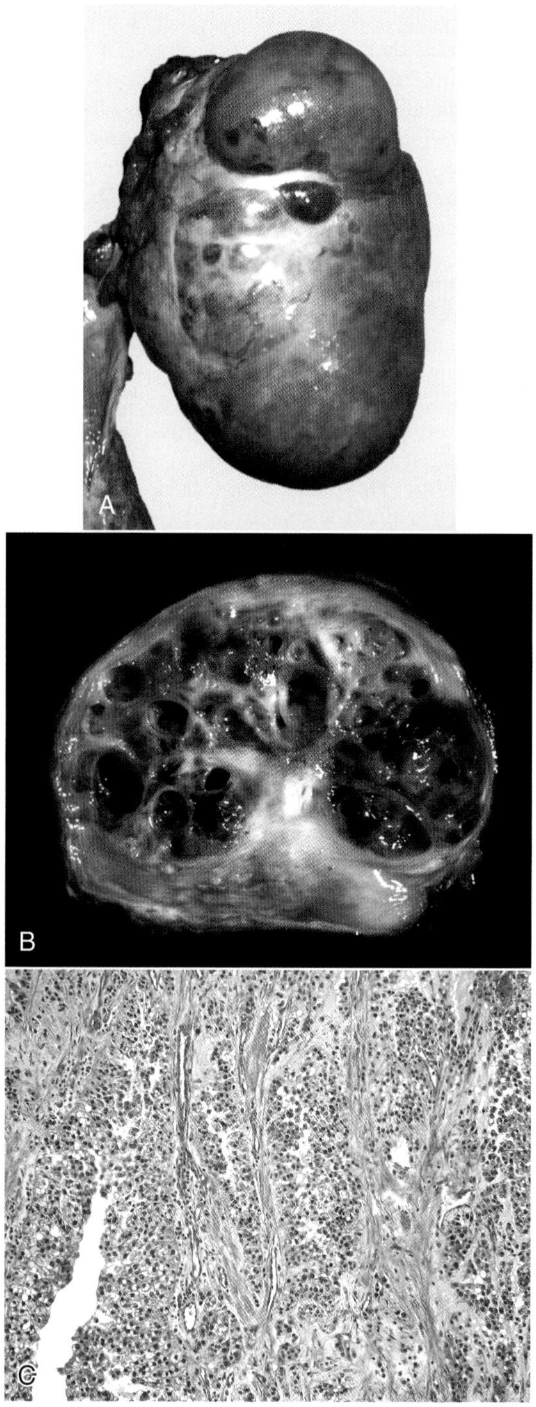

Figure 18-14 **Sex Cord Stromal Neoplasm, Granulosa Cell Tumor, Ovary, Cow. A,** This large, lobulated neoplasm has obliterated the normal structure of the ovary. They can be solid (as in this case) or multicystic. **B,** Multiple fluid-filled cysts and solid areas have caused the dramatic ovarian enlargement. Granulosa cell tumors are part of the group of neoplasms known as sex cord stromal tumors. **C,** This granulosa cell tumor has solid and cystic regions. The cysts are lined by cells that resemble granulosa cells of the follicle. H&E stain. (**A** courtesy College of Veterinary Medicine, University of Illinois. **B** and **C** courtesy Dr. R.A. Foster, Ontario Veterinary College, University of Guelph.)

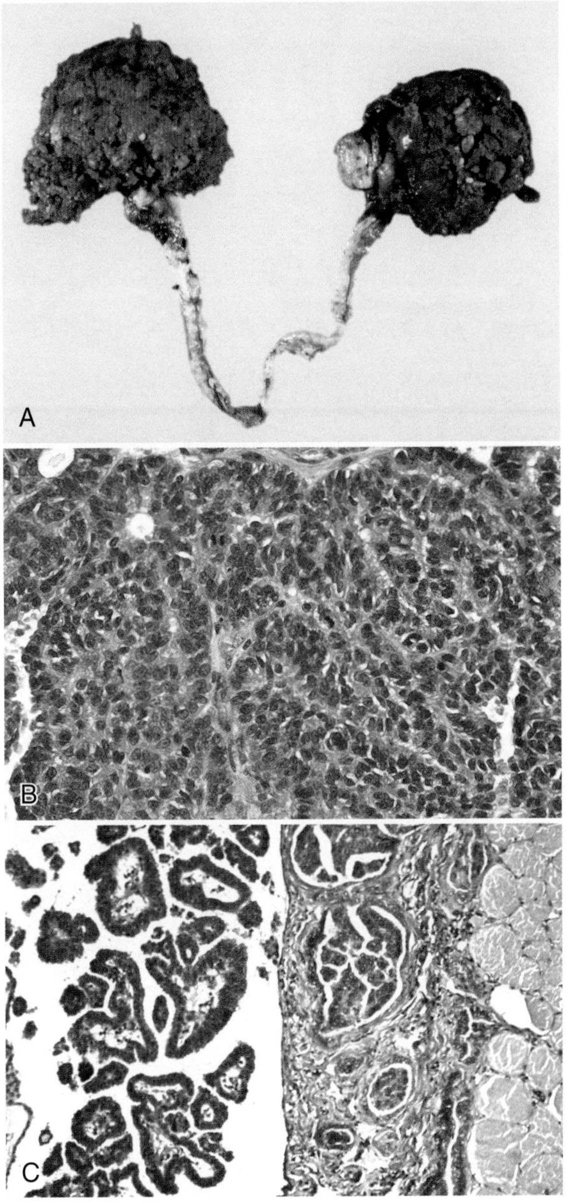

Figure 18-15 Papillary Ovarian Carcinoma, Ovary, Bitch. A, Both ovaries are enlarged by neoplastic epithelium that has formed papillary structures that give the masses a shaggy outer surface. These neoplasms are considered malignant, and they seed the abdomen, producing carcinomatosis. **B,** Neoplastic epithelial cells are arranged in cords and papillae, are pleomorphic, and have many mitoses. H&E stain. **C,** This papillary carcinoma has seeded the abdominal cavity, implanted on the peritoneum, invaded into the muscle of the diaphragm, and is in subserosal lymphatic vessels adjacent to the diaphragmatic skeletal muscle *(right)*. H&E stain. (**A** courtesy Dr. R.B. Miller, Ontario Veterinary College, University of Guelph. **B** courtesy Dr. M.D. McGavin, College of Veterinary Medicine, University of Tennessee. **C** courtesy Dr. K. McEntee, Reproductive Pathology Collection, University of Illinois.)

a rare lesion in the dog. Descending infection from the ovary may occur with viral infection. Direct hematogenous infection is possible. Macroscopic lesions are minimal. There may be hyperemia, thickening of the mucosa, and small amounts of luminal exudate. Inflammation of the infundibulum of the uterine tube accompanies perioophoritis. Microscopically, the inflammation ranges from mild to severe and from acute to chronic. Early mild lesions are loss of cilia and desquamation of epithelial cells at the tips of the mucosal folds. When severe, salpingitis involves other parts of the mucosa and sometimes the muscle layer. Exudate is present in the lumen. When adhesions form between the erosions and adjacent mucosa, the tube becomes cystic, reepithelialized, or replaced by granulation tissue. Obstruction of the uterine tube combined with suppurative inflammation results in pyosalpinx, which is a dilated and pus-filled uterine tube. Neutrophils predominate and form large lakes in the lumen or in mucosal cysts derived from the glands of the tube. As with pyometra, the epithelium is missing or hyperplastic or develops squamous metaplasia.

Hydrosalpinx. Hydrosalpinx is a dilated and fluid-filled uterine tube. Obstruction of the uterine tube prevents normal fluid from exiting to the uterus. Obstruction results from previous salpingitis and scaring, from trauma in cattle after aggressive rectal palpation or manual expression of a corpus luteum, ovarian hematoma, or from cystic dilation of duct remnants of embryonic tissues or segmental aplasia. Macroscopically, there is dilation of the uterine tube with clear fluid so that it becomes thin-walled, tortuous, and appears to be longer than normal.

Lesions commonly encountered in dogs and cats are duct remnants in the mesosalpinx, more often of mesonephric duct (simple tubular structures lined by low columnar to cuboidal cells) than of paramesonephric duct (lined by a folded mucosa similar to the uterine tube mucosa) origin. Mesonephric and paramesonephric duct remnants are described in the discussion on periovarian cysts in the section on the Ovary.

Ectopic Pregnancy. Ectopic pregnancy of human beings occurs when the conceptus develops in the Fallopian (uterine) tube or on the endocervix. An equivalent condition has not been reported in domesticated mammals. Ectopic pregnancy in dogs and cats occurs with traumatic rupture of the pregnant uterus and release of the fetus into the peritoneal cavity.

Disorders of the Uterus

Uterine disease is a significant cause of infertility and mortality. Foremost of these disorders are inflammatory diseases, usually the result of contamination of the uterus with bacteria.

Inflammatory Disorders. Most uterine infections are the result of ascending infection when the cervix is open—at estrus, parturition, or the postpartum period. Infection can also result from a hematogenous route of spread, particularly in pregnancy when the uteroplacental interface is the site for preferential localization of microbes such as *Brucella*, *Coxiella*, *Chlamydia*, and *Ureaplasma* spp. The placenta and/or the endometrium are the targets because their interface is a unique environment that is suitable for many infectious microbes to multiply. Infection can also descend from the ovary and uterine tube or enter the uterus by direct extension from adjacent viscera. Resistance of the uterus to infection is influenced by innate and acquired immune defense mechanisms and further altered by the hormonal environment, as discussed previously.

Endometritis. Endometritis is inflammation of the endometrium. It most commonly occurs from mating (insemination) in nonpregnant animals (postmating endometritis). In pregnancy, microbes that cause placentitis, fetal infection, and failure of pregnancy also cause inflammation of the endometrium. Postpartum endometritis occurs after a normal pregnancy and parturition. It is especially common and more severe after an abnormal parturition (i.e., dystocia) or failure of the uterus to involute. Lochia, the fluid and debris discharged from the uterus for a short time after parturition, is an excellent nutrient medium for bacterial growth.

Mild cases of endometritis are not detectible grossly. In more severe cases, the mucosa is swollen and has a corrugated surface, often with adherent fibrin and necrotic debris. With microscopic examination, lesions of the mucosa range from desquamation of a few surface epithelial cells to severe necrosis of the entire endometrium. Neutrophils are observed in the endometrial stroma and glands. Mild lesions resolve completely or incompletely with residual changes of cystic glands and periglandular fibrosis. Severe endometritis often becomes chronic, and necrotic endometrium is replaced by granulation tissue and subsequently fibrous connective tissue. In large animals (i.e., livestock and horses) with endometritis, the release of $PGF_{2\alpha}$ from the endometrium following 4 or 5 days of progesterone priming causes premature regression of the corpus luteum and shortening of the estrus cycle. The absence of endometrium resulting from endometrial necrosis in severe endometritis decreases the amount of $PGF_{2\alpha}$ released, especially in the mare and the cow, and results in a persistent corpus luteum.

Persistent mating-induced endometritis occurs most commonly in mares, but it also occurs in other domestic animal species. It is normal for inflammation, presumably because of the local effects of seminal fluid, to be resolved in the mare in 24 to 36 hours. However, some affected animals are unable to resolve the inflammation. The position of the uterus appears to play an important role, and normal mares have a more horizontal uterus that allows better drainage of fluid than the more drooped or vertical orientation of "susceptible" mares. Greater susceptibility occurs with repeated pregnancies, loss of body condition, and genetics. Susceptible mares have reduced uterine contractility from intrinsic neuromuscular dysfunction or the release of nitric oxide in the endometrium. Because they fail to clear seminal fluid and resolve the inflammation, persistent edema and endometrial fibrosis result. This situation is the basis for endometrial biopsy in the mare.

Endometrial biopsy is a breeding management tool used most commonly in the mare but also in the cow and bitch. The severity of endometritis and fibrosis is correlated directly with the inability of the fertilized ovum to attach or remain attached to the endometrium and to carry a fetus to term. In mares, prognosis for carrying a foal to term is based on (1) a combination of clinical features such as failure to produce a foal in the previous season and (2) morphologic features of the endometrium. These latter changes include the histologic stage of estrus cycle compared to the clinical stage, luminal contents, morphology of the endometrial luminal epithelium, presence and number of inflammatory/immune cells, and frequency and severity of periglandular fibrosis (Fig. 18-16). In pathology reports, the lesions of the endometrium of mares are categorized into grades 1, 2, or 3, which equate to a high, reduced, or low likelihood of the mare delivering a live foal, respectively.

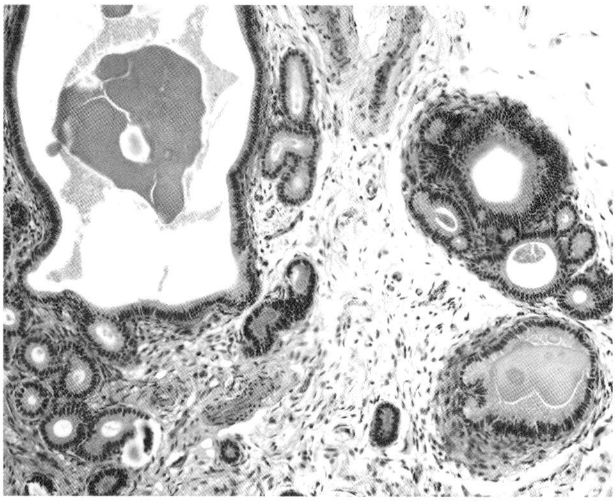

Figure 18-16 **Endometrial Fibrosis, Endometrial Biopsy, Mare.** Fibrosis from endometrial inflammation and edema results in endometrial glands forming nests *(right)* and cysts *(left)*. This fibrosis results in reduced fertility due to a lack of attachment of the conceptus, or a failure of formation of normal microcotyledons and a reduced placental area. H&E stain. (Courtesy Dr. R.A. Foster, Ontario Veterinary College, University of Guelph.)

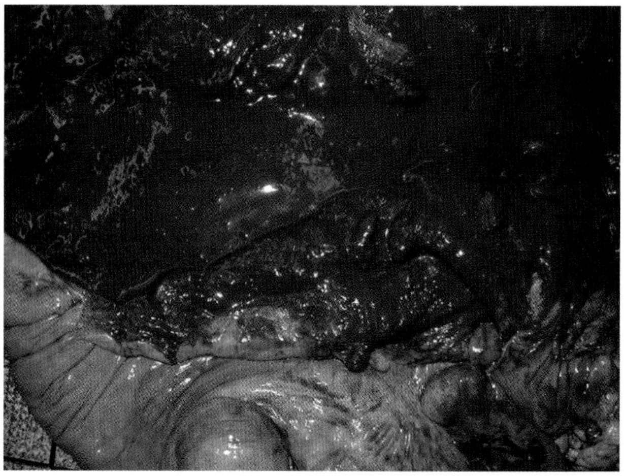

Figure 18-17 **Postpartum Metritis, Uterus, Cow.** The uterus is distended and filled with foul-smelling dark brown fluid. The endometrium was red-black and dull, indicating an endometritis secondary to bacterial infection. This cow developed a severe metritis immediately after calving. (Courtesy Dr. R.A. Foster, Ontario Veterinary College, University of Guelph.)

Metritis (Including Postpartum Metritis). Metritis is literally inflammation of all layers of the uterine wall (Fig. 18-17). In theriogenology, it is usually synonymous with a more severe and advanced form of endometritis. In its initial stage, the serosa is dull, finely granular, and has petechial hemorrhages and fine strands of fibrin adherent to the mesothelium. The endometrium is swollen, red, dull, often ulcerated, and has bloody flocculent and foul-smelling fluid. Microscopically, edema and neutrophils are observed in the endometrium, and this process and the resulting exudate extend through the muscle layers to injure and inflame the serosa.

Pyometra. Pyometra (accumulation of pus in the uterine lumen) occurs as a sequela to endometritis or metritis. It is infection of the uterus with dilation and accumulation of pus in the lumen (Fig. 18-18). The closure of the cervix is not always complete, and if not, exudate is discharged into the vagina. In cows, endometritis and pyometra prevent prostaglandin release and the corpus luteum is retained, thus mimicking pregnancy. In the bitch and queen, pyometra follows endometritis, which requires a corpus luteum for its development (see the discussion on cystic endometrial hyperplasia later in this chapter) (see Fig. 18-18, *A* and *B*). The color and consistency of the exudates vary with the infecting bacteria. Exudate is typically viscid and brown with *Escherichia coli* infection and creamy yellow with *Streptococcus* spp. The uterus can be greatly distended but not necessarily uniformly. Macroscopically, necrotic, ulcerated, and hemorrhagic areas are present in the endometrium, with dry, white, thickened, finely cystic areas. Microscopically, the dry white areas have hyperplasia and squamous metaplasia, a common occurrence in chronic inflammation of any mucous membrane. The cystic areas are cystic endometrial hyperplasia (Fig. 18-19). Lesions outside the genital tract secondary to pyometra include widespread extramedullary hematopoiesis and immune

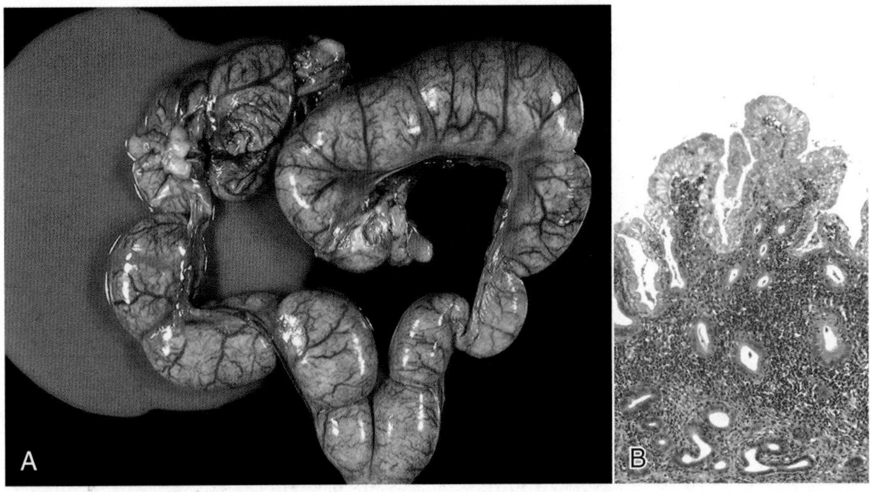

Figure 18-18 Metritis-Pyometra-Endometrial Hyperplasia, Uterus, Bitch. A, Pyometra occurs several weeks after estrus. Bacteria grow in the uterus and induce a suppurative response. The uterus fills with pus and is distended. **B,** Endometritis and pyometra. There are large numbers of lymphocytes and plasma cells in the endometrial stroma. The surface epithelium is hyperplastic and papillary. The luminal epithelial cells are highly vacuolated. Pus in the lumen of the uterus was removed during processing of the histologic section. H&E stain. (**A** courtesy Dr. J. Wright, College of Veterinary Medicine, North Carolina State University; and Noah's Arkive, College of Veterinary Medicine, The University of Georgia. **B** courtesy Dr. R.A. Foster, Ontario Veterinary College, University of Guelph.)

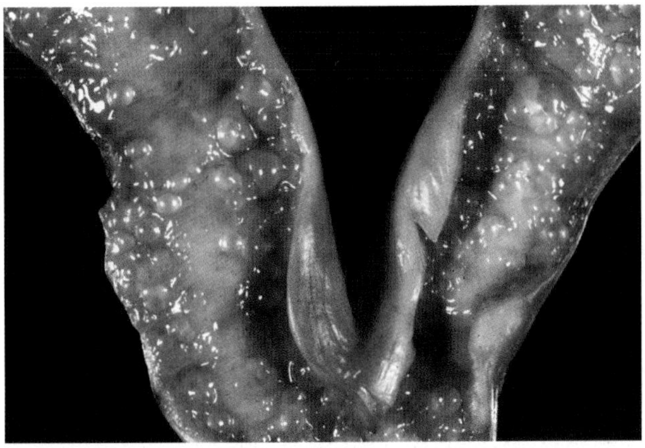

Figure 18-19 Cystic Endometrial Hyperplasia, Uterus, Bitch. Note the cysts in the mucosa of the endometrium. This change occurs under the influence of progesterone after estrus. Cystic hyperplasia may provide a suitable environment for bacteria to grow and cause pyometra, or alternatively, cystic hyperplasia may be secondary to uterine infection and endometritis. (Courtesy Dr. W. Crowell, College of Veterinary Medicine, The University of Georgia; and Noah's Arkive, College of Veterinary Medicine, The University of Georgia.)

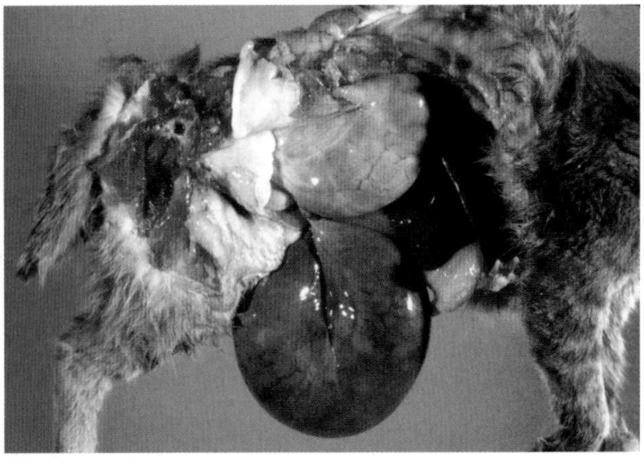

Figure 18-20 Uterine Torsion, Cat. The dark red black structure *(bottom center)* is a twisted uterine horn that contains a fetus. Its color is the result of venous infarction. (Courtesy Dr. R.A. Foster, Ontario Veterinary College, University of Guelph.)

complex glomerulopathy (see Chapter 11) and are common in the bitch.

Noninflammatory Disorders

Aging Changes. The uterus is under hormonal control of the ovary, and with senescence and a lack of estrus cycles, the endometrium becomes atrophic. In addition, with greater parity,[5] the walls of the uterine arteries become thicker and prominent. Histologically, the intima and muscularis layers are thicker and homogenous in staining (hyaline).

Torsion. Torsion of the uterus occurs in pregnant animals and most frequently in the cow. It occurs rarely in the pregnant bitch and queen (Fig. 18-20) but can occur when the uterus is enlarged by pyometra or mucometra (accumulation of mucus in the uterine lumen). The rotation is around the mesometrium and occurs at the level of the cervix in the cow and mare and at the junction of the uterine horn and body in the bitch and queen. Torsion results in circulatory compromise and venous infarction. The veins, which have a lower pressure and are thinner walled, are compressed and occluded before the arteries. The uterine wall and placenta become congested and edematous. The fetus dies and mummifies, or if the cervix is open enough to allow the entrance of bacteria or fungi, the fetus putrefies. The uterine wall is friable and prone to rupture.

Rupture. Rupture of the uterus occurs as a sequel to torsion, in severe dystocia and during treatment of uterine diseases by infusion of drugs and fluids. The torsion and dystocia-related ruptures are likely to be in the caudal part of the uterus and are often fatal because of hemorrhage or bacterial infection. The rupture that

[5]The number of times the dam (female) has given birth to a fetus.

follows over vigorous infusion of medications into the uterus occurs at the lesser curvature of an infused uterine horn, dissects beneath the serosa and into the mesometrium, and results in inflammation around the uterus (perimetritis) or peritonitis.

Prolapse. Prolapse of the uterus after parturition is important in the cow, ewe, and sow. A flaccid uterus and excessive straining are predisposing conditions. Factors that cause uterine inertia, such as prolonged dystocia, hypocalcemia, and ingestion of estrogenic plants, usually contribute to prolapse of the uterus. The anatomic structures that are prolapsed can be restricted to the previously pregnant horn, cervix, or vagina or can include all of the uterus, the bladder, and sometimes some of the small intestine. As the structures prolapse, there is vascular compression and thus compromise, and congestion and edema result (Fig. 18-21). Constriction by the vaginal and vulval tissues exacerbates this process by further compressing blood vessels, and as edema develops, the tissues exposed to the outside environment continue to swell, hang down further (as a result of gravity), dehydrate, and become traumatized. This result further exacerbates the swelling. Constant straining and the effects of gravity on the prolapsed tissues contribute to stretching of internal structures, including ligaments and blood vessels. Hemorrhage and shock can cause death even if the uterus is manually returned to its normal anatomic position in the abdominal cavity. If the animal survives the intervening drying and trauma, the venous infarction and infection that occur may prevent future fertility.

Retention of Fetal Membranes. Retention of fetal membranes for longer than normal after parturition is common, especially in the cow. In cows, membranes are considered retained if not expelled by 12 to 24 hours postpartum. In the mare, it is 3 hours. In cattle, in which this process is studied the most, there are many mechanisms thought to cause separation of the fetomaternal interface (cotyledon and caruncle). These mechanisms include the following:

1. The effects of increasing relaxin and decreasing progesterone concentrations in increasing collagenase activity to favor enzymatic breakdown of collagen linkages
2. Increased expression of MHC-1 by trophoblasts and a maternal immune response to allow leukocytes (especially neutrophils) and cytokines to promote separation

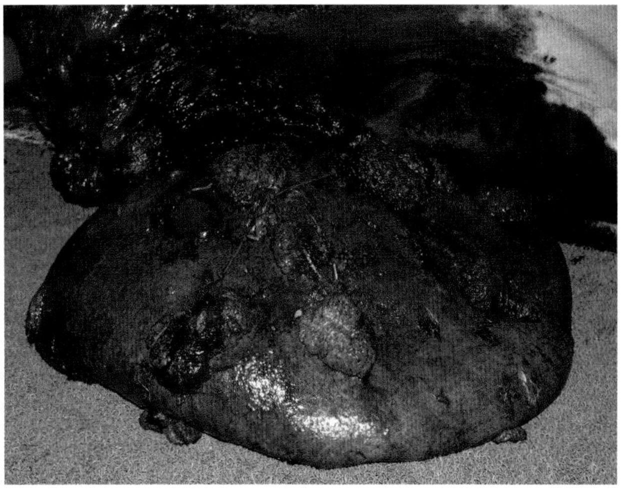

Figure 18-21 **Uterine Prolapse, Vulva, Cow.** The uterus, cervix, and part of the vagina have prolapsed. The uterus has become swollen from dependent edema and from reduced venous outflow. The mucosa, including the caruncles, of the uterus are exteriorized and exposed to the environment, and thus they have become dehydrated and traumatized. (Courtesy Dr. R.A. Foster, Ontario Veterinary College, University of Guelph.)

3. Mechanical effects of uterine contraction induced by prostaglandin and estrogen upregulation of oxytocin receptors
4. A turnover of maternal epithelial cells of the caruncle in normal pregnancy, where as when parturition approaches, there is a gradual loss and flattening of the cells

The normal separation of the fetomaternal unit involves so-called *fetomaternal maturation* with reduced proliferation of mucosal cells, increased apoptosis, increased proteolytic activity, changes in collagen composition, increased activity of enzymes from neutrophils, and local ischemia. Parturition before there is complete "maturation" of the fetomaternal unit results in retention of placental tissues. It is common in cases in which cesarean section is medically necessary before the time of normal parturition because there is insufficient time for complete maturation to occur. In addition, infectious, nutritional, hormonal, circulatory, hereditary, and weather factors may inhibit the "maturation" process. Retained membranes can act as a nutrient medium for growth of contaminant bacteria and for the development of severe endometritis from a transient mild postparturient endometritis. Bacterial endometritis can even cause systemic disease, such as toxemia, septicemia, or disseminated intravascular coagulation (DIC).

Subinvolution of Placental Sites. Subinvolution of placental sites is a disorder unique to dogs and is discussed in the section on Disorders of Dogs, Uterus.

Pseudopregnancy. Pseudopregnancy is a common disorder in dogs and is discussed in the section on Disorders of Dogs, Uterus.

Endometrial Atrophy. Endometrial atrophy usually results from loss of ovarian function. It occurs (1) at anestrus, (2) with malnutrition or cachexia, and (3) in disorders of sexual development. Focal endometrial atrophy of unknown cause sometimes occurs in the mare. Atrophic endometrium is macroscopically thin. In the mare, the longitudinal folds are indistinct, and in the cow, the caruncles are flat. Microscopically, the uterus of the mare is the most studied because data from uterine biopsies are frequently used for the management of breeding. The endometrium of the uterus of the anestrous mare has cuboidal luminal and glandular epithelium, with short, straight glands.

Endometrial Polyps. Endometrial polyps are common lesions in older bitches and queens. The cause is unknown, but they usually occur with cystic endometrial hyperplasia. They are localized and often pedunculated hyperplastic nodules of endometrial stroma and glands that vary from microscopic up to several centimeters long (Fig. 18-22). They can cause obstruction of the uterine lumen and mucometra.

Endometrial Hyperplasia. Endometrial hyperplasia can be localized or generalized; is an important lesion in the ewe, bitch, and queen; and is rare in the mare. Cystic Graafian follicles, ovarian neoplasms (granulosa cell tumors especially), and estrogens from plants are causes of endometrial hyperplasia in the cow. In ewes, it is caused by prolonged hyperestrogenism. Ingested estrogenic clover, such as subterranean (*Trifolium subterraneum*) and red (*Trifolium pratense*) clover, is the most likely source of estrogen. In ewes, endometrial hyperplasia results in reduced fertility, dystocia, and uterine prolapse because of uterine hypotonicity. Glands of the endometrial type can develop in the cervical mucosa. Even when nonpregnant, ewes have mammary gland enlargement. Endometrial cysts develop beside and beneath the caruncles, are approximately 1 cm in diameter, and are filled with clear fluid. The estrogenic mycotoxin zearalenone obtained from moldy feed causes endometrial cysts in the sow. In the bitch and presumably the queen, cystic endometrial hyperplasia (CEH) is a common response of the uterus (see Fig. 18-19) in diestrus. The disease is reproduced experimentally by estrogen priming of dogs followed by progesterone administration, but this result may not be the physiologic mechanism for the lesion. Bacteria are almost always present in the uterus of dogs with CEH and are probably the cause. Increased concentration of progesterone in late estrus or early diestrus and aberrant hormonal function may alter hormonal receptor expression. This outcome may prime the uterus so that inflammation or irritation by bacteria (or other substances, such as suture material and oil) stimulates the uterus to undergo hyperplasia and the type of change seen in early pregnancy.

Simple endometrial hyperplasia can be overlooked macroscopically when the endometrium has patchy or diffuse thickening. When it is cystic, the lesion is readily recognized at surgery or postmortem examination. Microscopically, the main component of endometrial hyperplasia is an increase in the size and area of glands with no change in the stroma except for edema. The glandular epithelium is progestational in appearance (i.e., the cells are columnar, hypertrophic, and hyperplastic and have a clear vacuolated cytoplasm) (see Fig. 18-18, *B*). As the glands become cystic with increased pressure of retained secretion (see the following section on Mucometra and Hydrometra), the epithelium of the glands becomes flattened and simple squamous in type (compression atrophy).

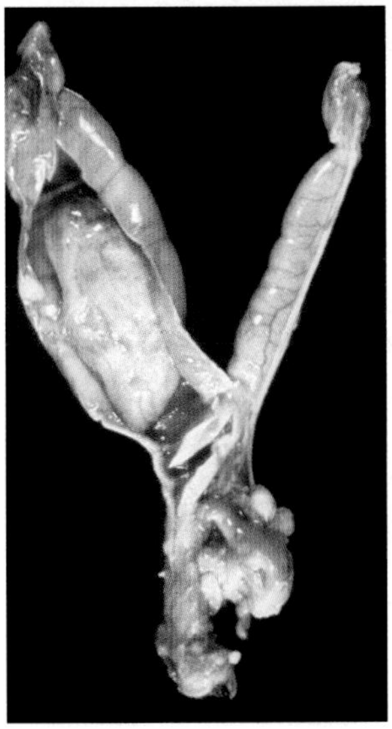

Figure 18-22 **Endometrial Polyp, Cat.** The uterine horn on the left is distended by a solid cylindrical polyp that is connected to the endometrium by a narrow stalk. (Courtesy Dr. G. Foley, Pfizer, Inc.)

Mucometra and Hydrometra. Mucometra and hydrometra are the accumulation of mucus and clear fluid, respectively, in the uterine lumen (Fig. 18-23, *A* and *B*). The cause is congenital or acquired obstruction of the outflow of the fluid and/or mucus produced by the endometrium and released when the cervix opens. However, hydrometra and mucometra can develop with excessive production in hyperestrogenism. Hydrometra and mucometra occur in pseudopregnancy, in which it resolves spontaneously.

Adenomyosis. Adenomyosis is the presence of endometrium within the myometrium, and the effect generally is negligible in domestic animals, which do not menstruate. Adenomyosis is found in the cow, bitch, and queen. It is thought that endometrium is either forced into the myometrium by pressure of pregnancy or pyometra or that the epithelium "migrates." In primates, adenomyosis is considered part of *endometriosis*, which is a general term in which endometrium is found in ectopic locations. Endometriosis, in which endometrium is found on serosal surfaces, around the ovary, or in the chest, is not reported in domestic species. Macroscopic changes in adenomyosis are primarily localized thickening of the myometrium, especially near the cervix. In dramatic cases, cysts form in the myometrium. Sometimes in bitches, the uterus undergoes diffuse symmetric or focal asymmetric enlargement near the cervix (Fig. 18-24). Microscopically, endometrial glands, stroma, or both are within the myometrium.

Neoplasms. Uterine neoplasms are uncommon in domestic animals. Lymphoma, which affects multiples sites of the body, is a common neoplasm in the cow. Of the other types of neoplasms, smooth muscle tumors in the bitch and carcinoma in the cow are more frequently seen.

Lymphoma. Lymphoma of the uterus is a basic disease in cattle so it is discussed in the section on Disorders of Ruminants (Cattle, Sheep, and Goats), Uterus.

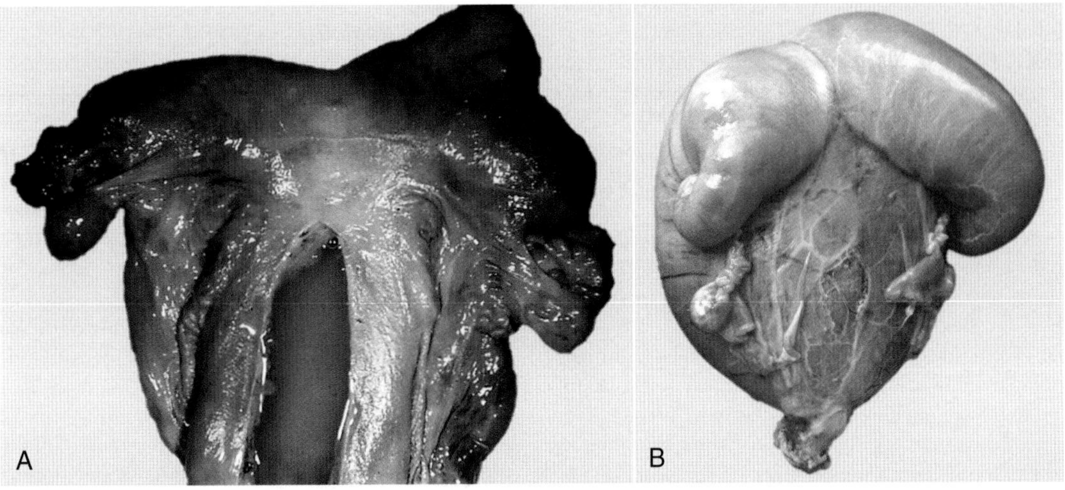

Figure 18-23 **Mucometra and Hydrometra, Uterus. A,** Mucometra, mare. Note the accumulation of mucus within the opened body of the distended uterus. **B,** Hydrometra, goat. The uterine horns and body are filled with clear watery fluid. (**A** courtesy Dr. K. McEntee, Reproductive Pathology Collection, University of Illinois; and Dr. J. King, College of Veterinary Medicine, Cornell University. **B** courtesy Dr. P.W. Ladds, James Cook University of North Queensland.)

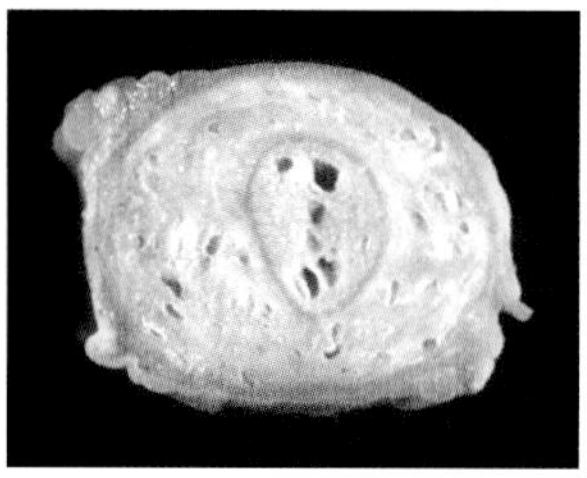

Figure 18-24 **Adenomyosis, Uterine Body, Bitch. Formalin Fixed Specimen.** The myometrium *(outer portion)* contains and is expanded by multiple cysts of endometrial glands. Many of these cysts are filled with pus, and the endometrium is expanded as a result of inflammation secondary to bacterial infection. (Courtesy Dr. R.B. Miller, Ontario Veterinary College, University of Guelph.)

Smooth Muscle Tumors. Uterine smooth muscle tumors are mostly found in dogs and are discussed in the section on Disorders of Dogs, Uterus.

Endometrial Carcinoma. Endometrial carcinoma is a well-known disease of cattle and is less frequently seen in dogs and cats. It is discussed in the section on Disorders of Ruminants (Cattle, Sheep, and Goats), Uterus.

Disorders of the Cervix

Diseases involving only the cervix are rare in domestic animals because most are extensions of uterine disease. There is considerable variation between species in the anatomy of the cervix, and this variation has an impact on uterine and placental health. The equine cervix is thin and easily opened (called "loose"), whereas the cervices of cattle and dogs are not. The responses to injury and inflammation are identical to those of the uterus because the cervix is a part of the uterus. Anatomic features and responses to injury were detailed previously in this chapter. Humans and some primates develop papillomavirus infection and subsequently cervical carcinoma; domesticated species do not.

Noninflammatory Disorders

Anomalies. Anomalies of the cervix are disorders of sexual development and are rare. They occur most commonly in the cow, in which there can be hypoplasia of the whole structure, aplasia of one or more of the rugae, tortuosity, and dilation or diverticulum formation of the cervical canal. Two entire cervices or a single bifurcated cervix have been described. One of these outcomes can occur as the only lesion in the entire reproductive system or as part of a more extensive failure of proper fusion of the paired paramesonephric ducts and can be found with a divided vagina and two compete uteri (uterus didelphis).

Estrogenic Substances. Ewes exposed to estrogenic substances following consumption of subterranean and red clover develop permanent infertility because of alteration of the cervix. Affected animals have a cervix that has fused cervical folds and uterine-like glands that produce less viscous mucus. Alteration of the viscosity of cervical mucus affects spermatozoal migration and results in reduced fertility.

Neoplasms. Neoplastic disease of the cervix of domestic animals is very rare, unlike in human beings, in which cervical dysplasia and neoplasia linked to human papillomavirus types are well recognized. The types of neoplasms that occur in the cervix are the same as those discussed previously for the uterus.

Inflammatory Disorders

Cervicitis. Inflammation of the cervix (cervicitis) usually occurs as a minor lesion concurrently with endometritis or vaginitis. It is observed in specific infectious diseases, such as *contagious equine metritis* caused by *Taylorella equigenitalis*, and in nonspecific postparturient endometritis, metritis, and vaginitis. Inflammation restricted to the cervix can arise from mucosal trauma resulting from poorly performed artificial insemination. In cows with acute cervicitis, the caudal rugae are edematous and may prolapse into the vagina. Inflammatory exudate covers the simple cuboidal epithelium and collects in the vagina. Whereas the cervical mucosa is thin, the underlying fibromuscular tissue is thick and relatively impervious to infection; thus most cases of cervicitis resolve readily. Infections that result from traumatic dystocia with lacerations are likely to involve the muscle layer from the onset and can produce severe lesions, including paracervical abscesses, local peritonitis with granulating tracts into the connective tissue of the pelvic canal, stenosis with adhesions across the lumen of the cervix in areas denuded of epithelium, and/or cervical glandular cysts filled with mucus or neutrophils.

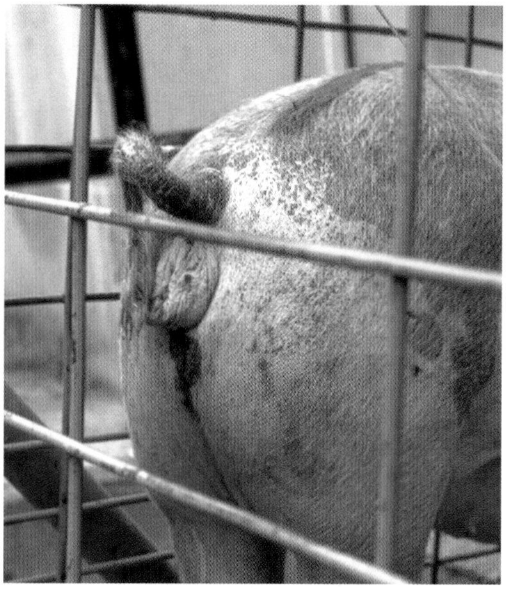

Figure 18-25 **Vulva Hypertrophy and Edema, Estrogenic Effect, Sow.** The vulva of this sow is swollen with edema. This swelling is typical of hyperestrogenism secondary to mycotoxicosis. (Courtesy Dr. J. Simon, College of Veterinary Medicine, University of Illinois.)

Vulva and Vagina

The two main categories of disease of the vagina and vulva are (1) infectious (and inflammatory) disease and (2) noninflammatory conditions. For the majority of diseases, lesions occur sporadically and disease in one species is similar in appearance to that of another species. However, there are a few diseases of the vulva and vagina that are unique to or commonly affect one specific domesticated animal species, and these disorders are discussed later in the sections covering disorders of individual species.

Noninflammatory Disorders. Swelling of the vulva is normal during estrus. Excessive or persistent swelling is abnormal and occurs commonly in dogs (see later) and occasionally in cattle. It also occurs in hyperestrogenism, such as with estrogen-producing ovarian neoplasms or exposure to estrogenic substances (Fig. 18-25) including creams and gels used in estrogen replacement therapy of owners. When the vaginal mucosa swells with edema, it protrudes through the vulva, exposing the mucosa.

Vaginal Polyps. Vaginal polyps occur in most species, but they are particularly common in dogs (Fig. 18-26; also see the section on

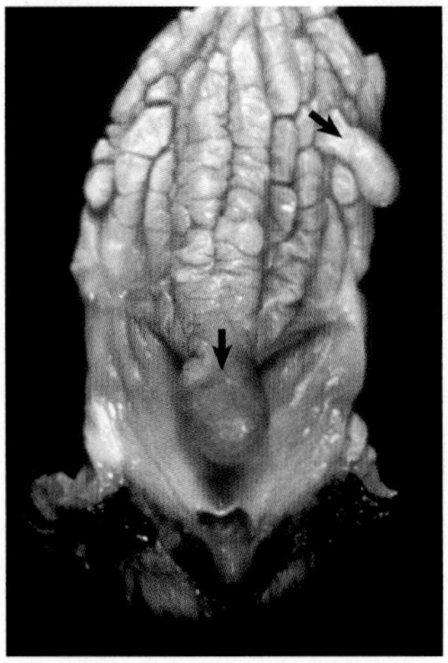

Figure 18-26 **Polyps, Vagina, Bitch.** There are several vaginal polyps *(arrows)* arising from the wall of the vagina. The larger caudal polyp adjacent to the urethra protrudes caudally through the labia of the vulva and is ulcerated. (Courtesy Dr. K. McEntee, Reproductive Pathology Collection, University of Illinois.)

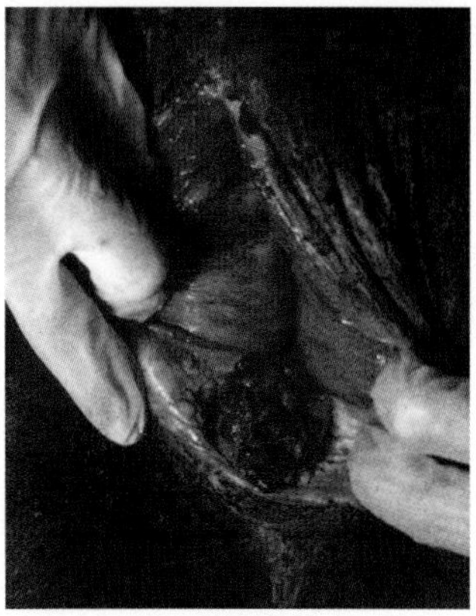

Figure 18-27 **Squamous Cell Carcinoma, Vulva, Mare.** The clitoris has been replaced by a multinodular and ulcerated tumor. (Courtesy Dr. J. King, College of Veterinary Medicine, Cornell University.)

Disorders of Dogs). They begin as focal mucosal edema, and either their stroma (submucosa) is normal but swollen with edema fluid or there is diffuse fibrosis from long-standing edema. As the process progresses over time, the structure elongates to assume the characteristic "polyp" appearance. They may, if large enough, protrude from the vulva and frequently ulcerate.

Cysts. Cysts in the vaginal wall arise from remnants of the mesonephric ducts (Gartner's ducts) or from vestibular (Bartholin's) glands. Causes of cyst formation include inflammation of the lining of the duct or gland and hyperestrogenism, in which edema caused by estrogen stimulation is prolonged. In addition, several minor and major disorders of sexual development occur in the vagina. The cranial vagina is of paramesonephric derivation, and the caudal vagina is of urogenital sinus derivation. Mesonephric ducts are not part of the sexual development of the vagina, but remnants occur in the wall of the vagina. When these remnants become cystic, they form single or multiple cysts or a tortuous tube in the lateral floor of the vagina between the cervix and near the urethral opening.

Major vestibular glands are found on the ventral and lateral walls of the vestibule and become cystic when edema, inflammation, or scar tissue obstructs their openings. Other disorders of sexual development of the vagina and vestibule include persistent hymen and vaginal septum (double vagina). Stricture or stenosis of the vagina or vestibule occurs as a disorder of sexual development or follows traumatic injury at parturition.

Neoplasms. The most common neoplasm of the vagina and vulva is the sunlight-induced squamous cell carcinoma of the vulva. Smooth muscle tumors and carcinoma of the vagina occur sporadically in all species, but they are most common in dogs. They are discussed later in the section on Disorders of Dogs.

Squamous cell carcinoma of the vulva occurs in all species, but especially in the cow, ewe, and mare (Fig. 18-27). Exposure to sunlight (ultraviolet light [UVB radiation]) is a known cause. The vulva of ewes subjected to the Mules operation (surgery of the perineum and inguinal areas intended to prevent urine wetting the wool) and to short tail docking and of cattle with tail docking have greater exposure of the vulva to the sun and a greater incidence of squamous cell carcinoma of the vulva. Lack of pigmentation of the vulva is an additional risk factor. Squamous cell carcinoma originates on the hairless and less pigmented skin of the vulva and has the appearance and biologic behavior of squamous cell carcinomas of the eye and conjunctiva, skin, and other sites (see Fig. 21-33). The neoplasm metastasizes late in the course of the disease to the medial iliac lymph nodes.

Inflammatory Disorders

Postparturient Vulvitis and Vaginitis. Postparturient vulvitis and vaginitis develop from trauma and laceration of mucosae during dystocia, and subsequently, secondary bacterial infection can exacerbate the original injury. Trauma unrelated to parturition, such as during coitus, artificial insemination, embryo transfer, or other human activity, may also progress similarly. Inflammation of the cervix and cranial vagina after dystocia can have a more serious outcome because of local spread of infection into and through the wall of the cervix and/or vagina into the peritoneal cavity.

Granular Vulvitis. Granular vulvitis describes the clinical appearance of the vulva and vagina in inflammatory diseases. Inflammation causes red coloration (hyperemia) and exudates, and the granular appearance is usually the result of development and hyperplasia of lymphoid follicles (Fig. 18-28). Thus, any infectious microbe can be a cause if there is sufficient time for adaptive immunity to develop.

Genital Herpesvirus Infection. Genital herpesvirus infection occurs in most species. The virus is venereally spread and causes death of mucosal epithelial cells in multiple locations leading to the formation of microscopic vesicles and to erosions following rupture. As with the general pathogenesis of herpesvirus infection (see Chapter 4), the virus enters the nerves and remains in neuronal cell bodies and ganglia in a latent state until there is recrudescence and shedding. Macroscopic lesions begin as 1- to 2-mm white, raised foci that soon erode (Fig. 18-29). Clinically visible vesicle formation is unusual. In some species, lesions will expand and coalesce to form large ulcers, up to several centimeters in diameter (Fig. 18-30). Affected pigmented skin loses pigmentation and after healing remains as white regions of depigmentation (Fig. 18-31).

Fetus and Placenta

Normal Pregnancy. Pregnancy begins at conception, and the product of conception is the conceptus. It begins as a fertilized ovum, develops into a blastocyst, and then develops further so the conceptus is composed of fetal membranes and the embryo. The embryo is the part of the conceptus that gives rise to the adult. The time when embryos become fetuses is debated; some believe it is the time when the embryo develops features that allow its species and sex to be determined phenotypically, and others consider it to be when the embryo begins spontaneous movement. This movement occurs at approximately 35 to 45 days of age in large animals.

Maintenance of Pregnancy. Maintenance of pregnancy is one of those miraculous events that defies logic, and there is much to be learned about pregnancy and embryonic/fetal development. The conceptus is allogeneic[6] and therefore foreign to the mother. Yet it survives, even though both fetus and mother could mount an immune response to each other. Tolerance or suppression of the maternal immune system is required, but the mechanisms are incompletely understood. Mechanisms in rodents and primates are studied in detail and involve several potential processes, including the following:

- An active role of systems such as the Fas/Fas ligand system in which active immune cells undergo apoptosis when they contact trophoblasts expressing the Fas ligand.
- The suppression of maternal immunity in the endometrium by production of indolamine 2,3-dioxygenase (IDO), which inhibits tryptophan, an amino acid necessary in the growth and development of T lymphocytes.
- The lack of MHC expression on trophoblasts.
- Alteration of the balance of T_H and T_S lymphocytes.

Immunologic considerations are only part of the maintenance of pregnancy narrative. There are also hormonal influences, especially the maintenance of serum and uterine progesterone concentrations by the corpus luteum and placenta. Stressors and systemic cytokines, such as prostaglandin, can cause luteolysis of the corpus luteum and terminate pregnancy during the time in gestation when pregnancy is dependent on the corpus luteum (all of gestation in cattle, goats, pigs, and dogs, and up to 50 days of gestation in horses, sheep, and cats).

Fetuses of most species are believed to initiate their own parturition, and the process is complex. Disease conditions can mimic the events leading to normal parturition so that with fetal stress, such as occurs with maternal or fetal illness, hyperthermia, and hypoxia, the fetal pituitary gland secretes ACTH, resulting in subsequent glucocorticoid (i.e., corticosteroids) production by the fetal adrenal gland. Corticosteroids increase the synthesis of estrogens in the placenta, which causes upregulation of oxytocin receptors in the smooth muscle of the uterus (myometrium) and the synthesis and release of $PGF_{2\alpha}$ from the endometrium. $PGF_{2\alpha}$ initiates myometrial contraction and causes luteolysis and decreased progesterone production. Lysis of the corpus luteum also results in relaxin secretion and a further decline in progesterone concentration. Relaxin secretion and reduced progesterone promote placental separation from the endometrium by promoting collagenase activity. Initiation of parturition by this process results in a fresh (nonautolyzed) fetus. If there is rapid fetal death, loss of pregnancy occurs by other mechanisms, and the fetus, having spent additional time at body temperature, will be autolyzed.

[6]Animals of the same species that are different enough genetically to interact antigenically via immunologic responses.

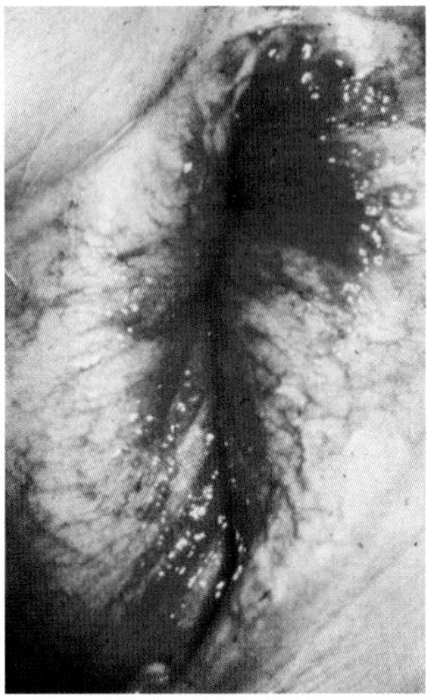

Figure 18-28 **Granular Vulvitis, Vulva, Cow.** Granular vulvitis is a nonspecific condition resulting from development and hyperplasia of subepithelial lymphoid follicles of the vulva and vestibule. Inflammation of the vulva, in the initial stages, causes hyperemia. There is subsequent hyperplasia of lymphoid tissue, visible as 1- to 2-mm raised white nodules on the vulval mucosa. It is commonly seen in cows with infection of the vulva or vagina with *Ureaplasma diversum* and results in a granular appearance of the mucosa. (Courtesy Dr. R.B. Miller, Ontario Veterinary College, University of Guelph.)

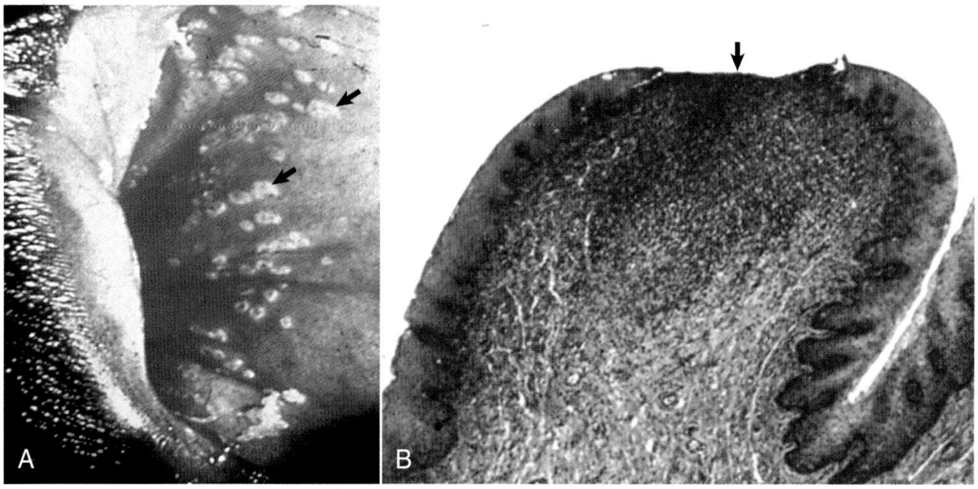

Figure 18-29 **Infectious Pustular Vulvovaginitis (IPV), Bovine Herpesvirus 1 Infection, Cow. A,** Focal ulceration of mucosa of the vestibule. The multiple white regions *(arrows)* are areas of necrotic epithelium and ulceration. **B,** Ulceration of mucosa of the vestibule. Note the ulcer *(arrow)* with loss of the epithelium over an aggregate of lymphocytes. H&E stain. (Courtesy Dr. K. McEntee, Reproductive Pathology Collection, University of Illinois.)

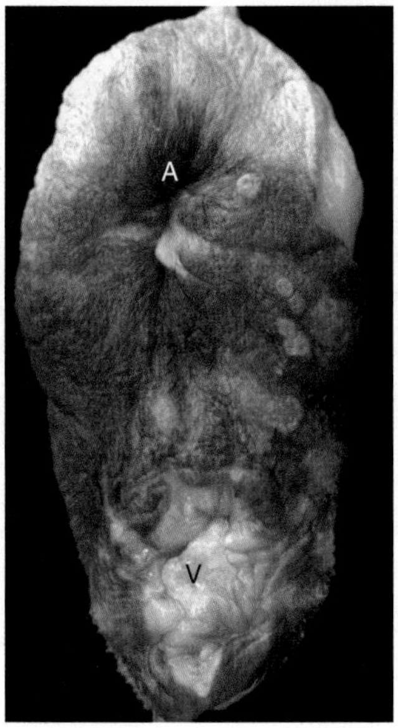

Figure 18-30 **Ulcerative Vulvitis, Caprine Herpesvirus 1 Infection, Goat.** The vulva *(V)* has numerous vesicles on the mucosa. The skin of the perineal region around the anus *(A)* and vulva has multiple circular regions of epithelial necrosis and erosion. Herpesviral infection of the genital tract has the classic lesions of microvesicles that rupture to form ulcers, which are irregularly distributed on the affected areas. (Courtesy Dr. P.W. Ladds, James Cook University of North Queensland.)

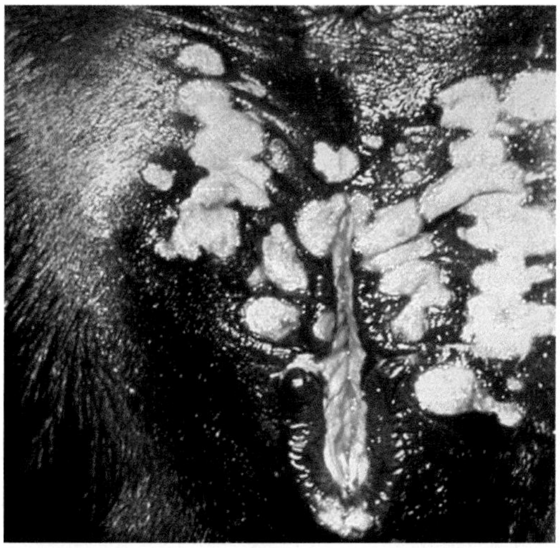

Figure 18-31 **Coital Exanthema, Ulcerative Vulvitis, Equid Herpesvirus 3, Mare.** Large full-thickness ulcers around the perineum and on the vulvar skin heal with depigmented regions. (Courtesy Dr. K. McEntee, Reproductive Pathology Collection, University of Illinois.)

Failure of Pregnancy

Fetal Characteristics. Failure of pregnancy is divided into three subgroups based on fetal development and the potential viability of the fetus as follows:

Early embryonic mortality occurs at the embryonic stage, usually less than 35 to 45 days postconception in large animals and approximately 20 days postconception in dogs and cats.

Fetal loss (abortion) occurs at the stage of fetal development, when the fetus is not independently viable (i.e., cannot live without the placental and uterine environment).

Stillbirth occurs when the fetus is potentially viable.

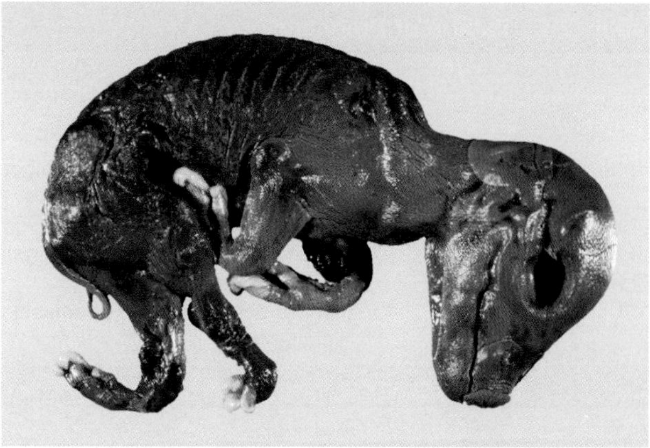

Figure 18-32 **Failure of Pregnancy, Mummified Fetus, Pig.** This fetus died in utero, and the fluids were resorbed. Dehydration of a fetus in utero following death of the fetus usually takes longer than 1 week to occur. (Courtesy Ontario Veterinary College, University of Guelph.)

Maternal Characteristics. The exact outcome of early embryonic mortality and fetal death on the dam is unpredictable and is influenced by the cause of the failure of pregnancy, species affected, stage of gestation, and number of fetuses. The main outcomes are as follows:

1. Embryonic death and return to estrus at the normal interval
2. Embryonic death and delayed return to normal estrus
3. Fetal loss (abortion) with no autolysis
4. Fetal loss (abortion) with autolysis
5. Mummification of the fetus/fetuses
6. Maceration of the fetus/fetuses
7. Stillbirth

Characteristics of Embryonic Mortality and Fetal Loss. *Embryonic mortality* occurs in all species, and the causes are discussed in the section on Causes of Failure of Pregnancy. *Fetal loss* with no autolysis is the norm in horses, sheep, and goats. In the bitch and queen, fetal loss with autolysis is the norm because when embryonic or fetal death occurs, the corpus luteum and products of conception may be retained in the uterus until the time of normal parturition.

Mummification. Mummification is one of the possible outcomes of fetal death. Rather than being expelled soon after death, the fetus is retained and progressively dehydrates to become a firm, dry mass, which is discolored by degraded hemoglobin to brown or black, and consists of leathery skin enclosing the other dehydrated organs (Fig. 18-32). The cause of death can be infectious or noninfectious, and the bacteria that promote lysis of dead tissue must be absent and the cervix must be closed to prevent the entry of putrefactive bacteria. The situations in which mummification mostly occurs are listed in Table 18-2. In twin pregnancy of the mare, the mummified fetus and the longer surviving fetus abort together. In parvovirus infection in the sow, mummified fetuses are retained and can be born at term along with live fetuses. In any species with a "single fetus" pregnancy, the mummified fetus can be expelled at any time or retained indefinitely.

Maceration. Maceration occurs when the fetus becomes liquefied (Fig. 18-33). This outcome requires bacterial infection of the fetus. The bacteria could be the cause of fetal death or they could be contaminants that entered the uterus via an open cervix. In addition to disintegration of the fetus (see Fig. 18-33), the uterus also has lesions. Endometritis or pyometra is present; the type of lesion depends on whether the cervix remains open or closed. Endometritis and pyometra tend to become severe and chronic. Emphysema occurs when the bacteria are gas forming, such as occurs with

Table 18-2 Failure of Pregnancy

GUIDE TO FETAL AUTOLYSIS*	
Time Since Death	**Change**
12 hr	Cornea cloudy, amnionic fluid blood tinged
24 hr	Fluid in body cavities
36 hr	Gelatinous fluid in subcutis
72 hr	Eyes dehydrated
144 hr	Carcass dehydrated, no abomasal contents
COMMON CAUSES OF FETAL MUMMIFICATION	
Mare	Twinning
Cow	Bovine viral diarrhea virus infection, trichomoniasis
Bitch	Canine herpesvirus
Queen	Torsion of a uterine horn
Sow	Parvoviral infection
INFECTIOUS MICROBES COMMON TO ALL SPECIES	
Brucella sp.	
Campylobacter sp.	
Chlamydia abortus	
Coxiella burnetii	
Herpesviruses	
Leptospira interrogans	
Listeria monocytogenes	
Mycoplasma and *Ureaplasma* spp.	
Neospora caninum	
Salmonella sp.	
Toxoplasma gondii	
SOME NONINFECTIOUS CAUSES COMMON TO ALL SPECIES	
Anomalies	
Chromosomal, genetic, and epigenetic	
Macroscopically or microscopically visible	
Proteomic or metabolomic	
Hydramnios, hydroallantois	
Hyperthermia	
Nutritional diseases	
Excessive	
Inadequate	
Deficiency of individual nutrients	
Toxicosis	
Plant	
Elements	
Other	
Hypoluteism and other hormonal dysregulation	
Excessive numbers of fetuses including twinning	
Environmental stress including trauma	

*Data from Dillman RC, Dennis SM: *Am J Vet Res* 37:403-407, 1976.

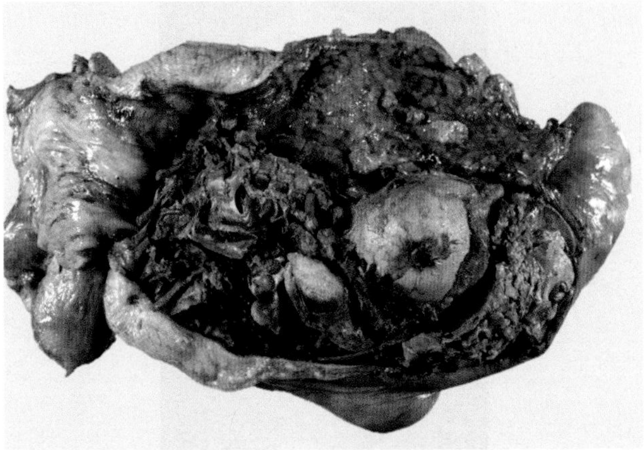

Figure 18-33 **Failure of Pregnancy, Macerated Fetus, Lamb.** Fetal bones, hair, and brown pasty material fill the uterus. The ewe was infertile. (Courtesy Dr. R.A. Foster, Ontario Veterinary College, University of Guelph.)

Clostridia spp. Maternal toxemia and death are likely if the bacteria produce potent exotoxins or endotoxins. Fetal bones resist maceration, and if the uterus eventually regains some muscular tone, the bones can cause perforation.

Veterinary diagnostic laboratories that publish prevalence data of the various causes of *sporadic* failure of pregnancy (specifically abortion) identify a cause in less than 50% (and often approximately 20%) of individual cases. However, the causes of herd outbreaks of abortion are identified in most cases. Many of the recognized causes are infectious (Table 18-3) because infections are usually easy to diagnose. This correlation has led to the general approach of determining if the loss of pregnancy is because of a recognized lesion and if the cause is infectious or not.

Identifying the cause of embryonic death is very difficult because there are seldom embryonic or placental tissues to examine, and most laboratories are only able to identify infectious causes. The embryo is thought to dissolve, but the conceptus is so small that it may not be found. There are recognized infectious causes of early embryonic mortality, and the infection often occurs at or near the time of coitus or conception. Microbes such as *Campylobacter*, *Tritrichomonas*, *Ureaplasma*, and nonspecific endometrial infections are among the common examples. Noninfectious causes of early embryonic mortality appear to be from chromosomal abnormalities and other lethal genetic traits.

Examination of Fetus and Placenta in a Failure of Pregnancy. Investigating failure of pregnancy requires a keen sense of what can be achieved. The investigation may have an economic impact, identify a zoonotic disease, or appeal to scientific curiosity. Maternal, fetal, and placental factors should be considered while simultaneously identifying any lesions and any significant infectious microbes. There are infectious causes common to all species (see Table 18-2), causes that are species specific (Table 18-4), and causes that are geographically important. Those cases without a recognized infectious cause are assumed to be noninfectious.

Examination of the fetus and placenta and sampling of tissues are performed to primarily answer the following question: Are there any fetal or placental abnormalities or lesions to explain the failure of pregnancy? Some of the lack of success in determining the cause of a failure of pregnancy is the failure to examine all organs and to submit the appropriate specimens. Where feasible, send the whole fetus and placenta to the laboratory. When this is not feasible, success in ruling out fetal or placental factors depends on a careful examination of all structures and submission of the correct specimens. Each diagnostic laboratory has a submission guide that recommends samples to submit to maximize diagnostic success.

Each species and breed of animal has an expected rate of fetal development and an average size at birth. Variation from this normal fetal development indicates an abnormality that needs to be explained. Fetal and placenta weight, fetal size including crown-rump length, and degree of development for gestation length (in days) are basic parameters, and changes from "normal" may indicate increased or inadequate maternal nutrition, concurrent disease, or placental sufficiency.

Table 18-3 Occurrence of Causes of Sporadic Failure of Pregnancy in Various Domesticated Species

Cause	Equine (%)	Bovine (%)	Ovine (%)	Caprine (%)	Porcine (%)
No diagnosis	40	60	60	52	53
Noninfectious	26*	3	5	10	1
Infectious	34	37	35	38	46
Placentitis	12	5	9	3	7
Viral	9	3	0	0	20
Bacterial	10	16	25	31	32
Protozoal	0	16	10	7	0

*See Box 18-5.

Table 18-4 Specific or Regionally Important Diseases that Cause Failure of Pregnancy

Species	Cause
Equine	Insufficient serum progesterone
	Equid herpesvirus 1
	Fescue toxicosis (*Neotyphodium coenophialum*)
	Thyroid hyperplasia/musculoskeletal syndrome
Bovine	*Brucella abortus*
	Foothills abortion
	Ponderosa pine abortion
	Campylobacter fetus
	Tritrichomonas foetus
Ovine	*Listeria monocytogenes*
	Brucella ovis
	Wesselsbron disease
	Rift Valley fever
	Cache Valley virus
	Salmonella sp.
	Iodine deficiency
Caprine	*Brucella melitensis*
	Iodine deficiency
Porcine	Leptospirosis

These are not the most common in all areas. Common causes are listed in Table 18-2.

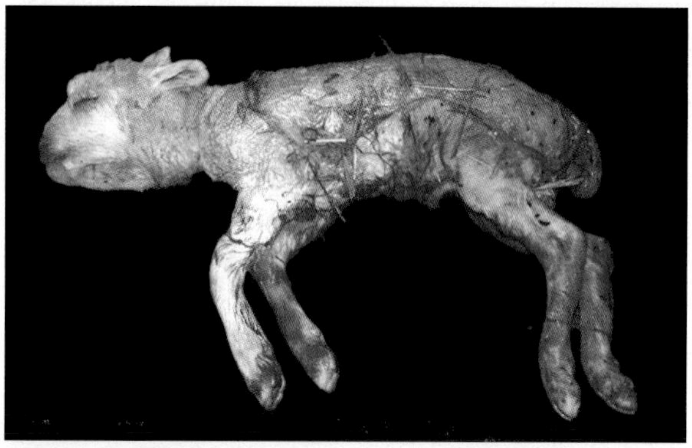

Figure 18-34 Dystocia, Lamb. This large lamb died during parturition. It was trapped in the birth canal by the shoulders and right foreleg, which was flexed (folded back). The lamb became hypoxic and defecated meconium, visible as a yellow deposit on the skin of the body caudal to the shoulder. The head and left foreleg became swollen and the wool is dry. The rest of the body is moist from amniotic fluid (and meconium), indicating that this portion of the body was in the vagina and uterus. (Courtesy Dr. R.A. Foster, Ontario Veterinary College, University of Guelph.)

The degree of fetal autolysis and evidence of fetal distress provide useful information. Fetal autolysis was studied in sheep and gives an approximation of the time of fetal death before expulsion. It is generally believed that an autolyzed fetus dies too quickly to initiate its own parturition, as would occur with septicemia or viremia, whereas a fetus without autolysis is able to initiate its own parturition. When distressed and hypoxic, a fetus gasps and aspirates amniotic contents, and meconium[7] is released into the amniotic fluid. Meconium staining of the skin can be seen at postmortem examination (Fig. 18-34). Keratin squames and meconium from the amniotic fluid are found in the lungs with histologic examination.

A fetus caught in the birth canal for a sufficient period of time (i.e., dystocia) develops localized swellings of the tongue and face (see Fig. 18-34), hemorrhage and bruising, and a swollen limb or limbs. Pressure from the birth canal restricts venous and lymphatic flow, and any fetal part trapped exterior to the birth canal is edematous.

[7]Feces composed of materials ingested during gestation, including intestinal epithelial cells, mucus, amniotic fluid, bile, and water.

The fetus is similar to an adult in general responses to disease, particularly near parturition, but many of the innate (inflammatory) and adaptive immune responses are rudimentary, depending on the stage of gestation. The fetus is in a sterile environment and has no flora or fauna. Exposure to environmental or pathogenic microbes occurs from contact with the external environment or with maternal infection.

Causes of Failure of Pregnancy. Each species has common and known causes and profiles of lesions and conditions that result in the failure of pregnancy. These causes are discussed in detail later in the sections that cover species-specific disorders. Table 18-3 lists the likely laboratory diagnostic success and the types of diseases and conditions to expect.

In most species, the common known causes of failure of pregnancy are infectious diseases, and therefore one of the initial diagnostic processes is to separate the causes into infectious and noninfectious. A similar approach is to divide the causes into those with lesions or not. Determining if there are lesions requires knowing the normal anatomy of both fetus and placenta; these features are listed later.

Many of the known causes of failure of pregnancy are infectious, and some of these infectious microbes affect all species (see Table 18-2). Microbes of the same genus produce similar lesions in different species. It is always important to correlate an infectious microbe with an appropriate lesion and clinical history. In some cases, infectious microbes may be identified by culture or molecular techniques, but they may not be responsible for the presenting signs. Especially challenging are those failures of pregnancy in which the initial lesion is inapparent, difficult to detect, or inaccessible such as occurs with some viral-induced failures of pregnancy. More commonly, however, bacterial infections stimulate a fetal inflammatory response and inflammatory cascade involving cytokines and oxidative stress that results in failure of pregnancy with observable postmortem lesions.

Infectious Causes of Failure of Pregnancy. Important viruses that cause failures of pregnancy include the herpesviruses, pestiviruses, and bunyaviruses. Herpesviruses cause failure of pregnancy in cows, mares, sows, and, less frequently, in other domestic animal species. Generally, the macroscopic lesions in affected fetuses are multiple randomly distributed pale gray to white foci of acute cellular necrosis, most commonly seen in the liver (Fig. 18-35, *A*). Often, the fetal liver is enlarged, and the necrotic foci are large enough to be visible as 1- to 2-mm white areas (Fig. 18-35, *B*). Foci can be red from hyperemia and hemorrhage. Similar lesions occur less frequently in other organs, including the lungs, kidneys, brain, or virtually any other organ. The placenta can be edematous, but in the majority of domestic mammals, there are no other lesions. Pestiviruses in cattle (bovine viral diarrhea virus), sheep (border disease virus), and pigs (classical swine fever virus) also cause failures of pregnancy and produce a similar spectrum of lesions. They cause fetal death or malformation, depending on virus strain, fetal age, and stage of development of the fetal immune system. Placental and fetal lesions either are absent or are restricted to microscopic lymphocyte aggregates in the heart and brain. Fetal malformations caused by these viruses are discussed in the next section and in Chapter 14, which covers the nervous system, and other chapters.

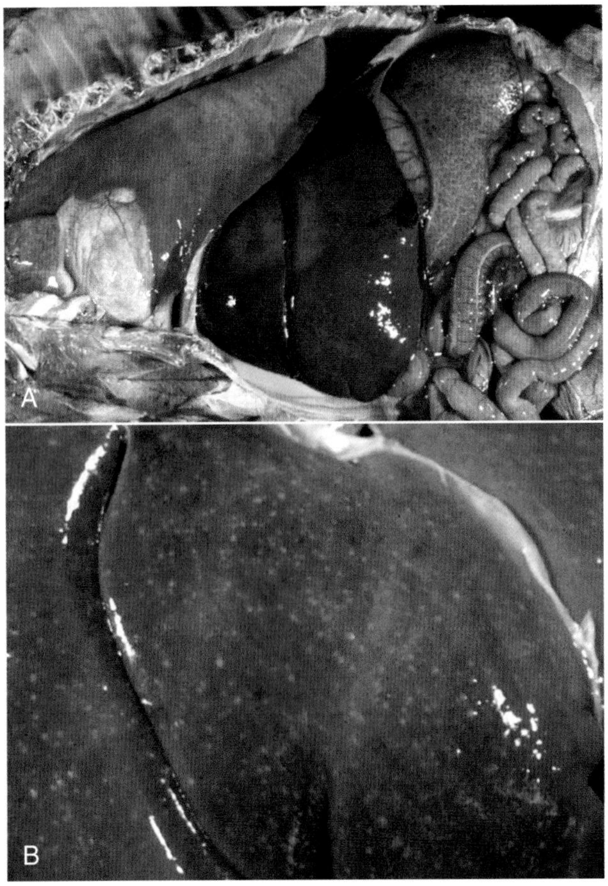

Figure 18-35 Equine Herpesvirus 1 Infection, Aborted Equine Fetus. **A,** The changes typical of herpesvirus abortion include solid rubbery lungs and multiple foci of necrosis in the liver. **B,** Randomly distributed multiple 1-mm white foci in the liver are characteristic of necrosis caused by herpesvirus infection. This case is more florid than most. (**A** courtesy Dr. R.B. Miller, Ontario Veterinary College, University of Guelph. **B** courtesy Dr. J. King, College of Veterinary Medicine, Cornell University.)

Bacterial species causing inflammation of the placenta and fetal sepsis are numerous. Almost any organism that causes bacteremia and septicemia can infect the pregnant uterus; common examples are *Brucella*, *Salmonella*, *Listeria*, and *Campylobacter* spp. Entry into the body is often after fecal-oral transmission and then hematogenous spread. Some microbes gain entry by venereal transmission. The important genera are listed in Tables 18-2 and 18-4. In all species of domestic animals, *Salmonella*, *Campylobacter*, and *Listeria* spp. cause maternal intestinal disease and, if bacteremic, can cause placental and fetal infections. Some bacteria, such as *Brucella*, *Leptospira*, *Chlamydia*, and *Coxiella* spp., have a particular affinity for the reproductive tract, and these are genera that infect virtually every domestic animal species. Important bacterial causes of failure of pregnancy are discussed in later sections covering disorders of individual species.

The protozoa of importance are *Toxoplasma gondii* and *Neospora caninum*. *Toxoplasma gondii* can cause failure of pregnancy in virtually every species except cattle. Likewise, the list of domestic animals affected by *Neospora caninum* is growing. There are also sporadic cases of *Sarcocystis* sp. abortion. The lesions seen with these protozoa include multifocal placental necrosis and microscopic foci of necrosis and inflammation in many fetal organs, especially the brain.

Noninfectious Causes of Failure of Pregnancy. Any failure of pregnancy without an infectious cause is placed into the noninfectious failure of pregnancy category. The potential list is very long, and specific conditions vary with the domestic species. Diagnostic laboratories are able to identify a myriad of infectious microbes, but except in herd outbreaks, the noninfectious causes are responsible for the majority of cases of failure of pregnancy. Noninfectious causes are listed in Table 18-2. Some of the noninfectious causes are obvious because there are lesions present, especially anomalies such as hydrocephalus, arthrogryposis, schistosomus reflexus, fetal hydrops, cyclopia, and myriad others. These disorders are the result of infectious, dietary, toxic, genetic, or unknown causes. Less obvious anomalies such as cleft palate, cardiac anomalies, and congenital hematological disease require careful examination of the appropriate organs. Nutrient deficiencies (and in some cases excesses) such as iodine deficiency and vitamin E and selenium deficiencies can result in lesions affecting the thyroid gland, heart and skeletal muscle, or other tissues. Genetic testing of chromosomes and genes from animals with failure of pregnancy is not routinely done unless there is a special circumstance, and even then, paternal or maternal samples are usually collected. Other known causes include hyperthermia and seasonal infertility of pigs. Careful examination of herd records and knowledge of the local environment and management practices are essential to identify the noninfectious causes of failure of pregnancy.

The Mammae

Mastitis and mammary neoplasia are the major diseases of the mammary glands in all species. Their individual prevalence rates vary considerably from species to species. Important and unique disorders of the mammary gland, including neoplasia, are species specific and are discussed in the sections of the disorders of individual animal species.

Mastitis is inflammation of the mammary gland. Most cases of mastitis begin with *galactophoritis*, which is inflammation of the lactiferous ducts. Mastitis is an economically important disease of animals used for milk production, so considerable time is spent discussing it.

Galactostasis is milk retention and is called failure of milk letdown. The glands become engorged, hot, and painful, mimicking mastitis but there is no systemic illness. It occurs after weaning or in pseudopregnancy and is thought to result from inadequate oxytocin release because of fear, stress, or lack of mammary stimulation.

Agalactia is failure of milk production by the gland and is rare. It is a manifestation of caprine arthritis and encephalitis virus (CAEV) infection in goats and maedi-visna virus infection of ewes. The udders are hard—thus it is called *hard udder*—and no milk is produced. Usually microscopic interstitial inflammation is present.

Galactorrhea (also called inappropriate lactation and precocious lactation) is also unusual. It is seen in male goats of high milk production lines. In bitches, it is part of pseudopregnancy and occurs at the termination of diestrus when there is a prolactin surge in response to a reduction in progesterone concentration. It also occasionally occurs after ovariohysterectomy during diestrus.

Disorders of Horses

Female Reproductive System

Disorders of the female reproductive system that affect the mare, but that are not unique to the mare, are discussed in the section on Disorders of Domestic Animals.

Ovary

Cystic follicles and cystic ovarian disease occur much less often in the ovary of mares compared to those of cows and sows. Mares develop seasonal or anovulatory follicles that grow to a large size before the onset of regular estrus and the maturation of "regular" follicles. They can also develop hemorrhagic anovulatory follicles that resemble a normal corpus luteum except they occur in anovulatory follicles. With ovulation, some mares develop considerable hemorrhage that can result in an ovarian hematoma or, if severe, hemoperitoneum. Of the ovarian neoplasms, sex cord stromal tumors, particularly of the granulosa cell type, occur most commonly.

Uterine Tubes

Disorders of the uterine tube of the mare are rare and are discussed in the section on Disorders of Domestic Animals, Uterine Tubes.

Uterus

The mare is particularly prone to develop postmating endometritis, and both subclinical and clinical endometritis are very common. Endometrial biopsy is used during breeding soundness evaluation to establish the category or "grade" of endometritis and to assess its effect on subsequent pregnancy. These techniques are discussed in the section on Disorders of Domestic Animals, Uterus.

Cervix

The cervix of the mare is extremely important in the pathogenesis of endometritis and placentitis because its structure is different from that of other species. The cervix of the mare does not form as tight and impenetrable barrier as it does in the other species, so it is a "loose" cervix. More details are discussed in the section on Disorders of Domestic Animals, Uterus and Cervix.

Vulva and Vagina

Mares develop a range of diseases of the vulva and vagina as discussed in the section on Disorders of Domestic Animals, Vulva and Vagina.

Equine Coital Exanthema. Equid herpesvirus 3 is the cause of equine coital exanthema. It is a herpesvirus disease of the vulva that is spread venereally and results in transient vesicles and erosions of the external genitalia of both mares and stallions (see Fig. 18-31). Depigmentation of pigmented skin of the vulva occurs with healing of the lesions.

Fetus and Placenta

Failure of Pregnancy

Noninfectious Failure of Pregnancy. The potential list of causes of noninfectious failure of pregnancy is very long, and specific conditions vary with the domestic mammal species. All domestic species have sporadic fetal anomalies, thyroidal hyperplasia and goiter (Fig. 18-36), and dystocia. Horses are unique because they have a large number of noninfectious causes of failure of pregnancy (Box 18-5), related in some instances to the apparent lack of placental reserve and their microcotyledonary placentation.

Fetal anomalies are usually rare and sporadic in horses. In some regions, especially where feed quality during winter is inadequate, foals die in utero because of thyroid hyperplasia and musculoskeletal disease (TH-MSD). The thyroid lesion is microscopic hyperplasia, but there is no macroscopic enlargement of the glands. Routine histologic examination of the thyroid glands is therefore necessary to confirm this diagnosis. Musculoskeletal diseases seen in this syndrome include prognathia, flexural deformity, joint laxity, and tendon ruptures, presumably from hypothyroidism.

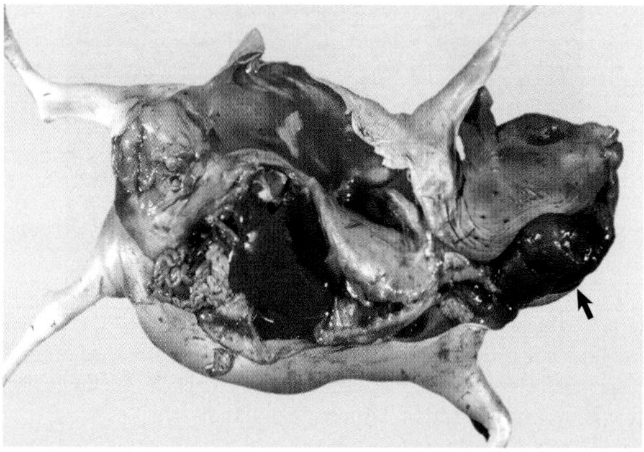

Figure 18-36 **Iodine Deficiency, Goiter, Goat Fetus.** This fetus has bilaterally extremely enlarged thyroid glands *(arrow)*, alopecia, and myxedema evident subcutaneously over the thorax and abdomen, which are the classic lesions of severe hypothyroidism. (Courtesy Dr. R.A. Foster, Ontario Veterinary College, University of Guelph.)

Box 18-5 Noninfectious Causes of Pregnancy Failure Unique to Horses

Twinning
Umbilical cord anomalies
- Excessive length
- Torsion
- Too short

Inadequate villus development
- Endometrial fibrosis

Thyroid hyperplasia and musculoskeletal disease
Premature placental separation
Body pregnancy

Examination of the placenta for lesions requires knowledge of normal anatomy, and there are many features and structures that are normal but have the appearance of being a lesion (Box 18-6). It is important to assess the equine placenta for the following:

- Anything that reduces placental area, such as avillous regions (avillous placenta) and twinning
- Lesions of the cervical star (Fig. 18-37)
- Excessive length (normal is 36 to 83 cm) and torsion (Fig. 18-38) of the umbilical cord

Box 18-6 Normal Structures of the Equine Placenta Confused with Lesions

Amniotic plaques
Avillous regions of:
- Chorioallantoic pouches
- Large vessels
- Insertion of cord
- Location of uterine tube
- Cervical star

Hippomane
Allantoic pouches
Yolk sac remnant

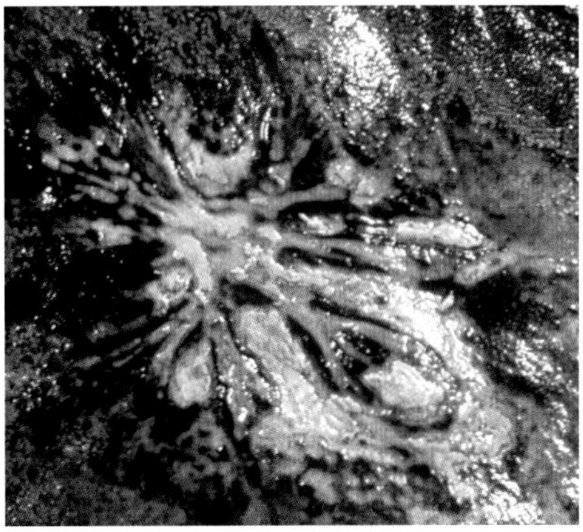

Figure 18-37 Bacterial Placentitis, Cervical Star, Mare. The chorion at the cervical star is thickened by edema, and there is fibrin, necrotic debris, and suppurative exudate on the surface. (Courtesy Dr. K. McEntee, Reproductive Pathology Collection, University of Illinois.)

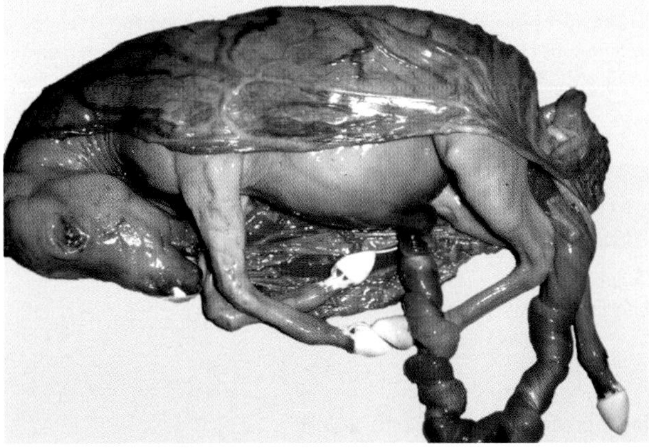

Figure 18-38 Umbilical Cord Torsion, Equine Fetus. This aborted fetus, wrapped in its amnion, has a very long and twisted umbilical cord. Twisted cords are often longer than 83 cm, a risk factor for torsion of the cord. (Courtesy College of Veterinary Medicine, University of Illinois.)

- Lesions of the amnion (allantoic hyperplasia and amnion nodosum)

Normally, chorionic villi develop where contact is made between the endometrium and the chorion. Small and insignificant regions of avillous placenta occur in the following areas:

- At the contact area between chorion and endocervix (cervical star)
- At sites of the endometrial cups (chorioallantoic pouches)
- Where there are folds of the chorion
- Over large vessels in the chorioallantois
- At the site of insertion of the umbilical cord

Structures that often cause confusion are amniotic plaques, hippomanes, and yolk sac remnants. The placentas of all species have amniotic plaques, and they are most prevalent on the umbilical cord near the fetus and on the amniotic membrane (Fig. 18-39, *A*). Almost all equine placentas have a hippomane in the allantoic cavity. These structures are rubbery concrements of allantoic precipitates that vary in color from white to tan to red (Fig. 18-39, *B*). The yolk sac remnant is the remaining tissue of the yolk sac and is a circular cystic structure found in the allantoic portion of the umbilical cord near the chorioallantois. It may be within or extend from the umbilical cord with a stalk (Fig. 18-39, *C*). This remnant is often mineralized and has a fluid-filled center and an ossified wall. The outer surface is smooth, but the inner surface has a pattern that resembles the inner surface of the calvarium. It is sometimes mistaken for the skull of a twin or an amorphous globosus (see the section on Failure of Pregnancy in Ruminants; also see Fig. 18-43). The final common normal finding is allantoic pouches. These are outpouches of the allantois into the allantoic cavity that form a small polyp. Sometimes they have a long stalk.

Twinning is a common noninfectious cause of abortion in mares. Chorionic villi do not develop over the contact area between the two placentas. Thus, the combined functional area of the chorions of both twins is only slightly larger than that for a normal nontwin foal. Twin fetuses often have growth retardation. Aborted twin equine fetuses often appear to have died at different times. Death is thought to be from placental insufficiency. When the available space in the uterus is divided evenly, which is approximately 80% of cases, both twins usually die and are aborted in midgestation. In cases in which great disparity exists in the apportioning of space, the favored twin has a chance of survival, whereas the other dies and mummifies.

There are several common abnormalities of the equine umbilical cord: inadequate length, excessive length, and torsion. In torsion of the umbilical cord, the cord is usually longer than normal and excessively twisted (more than three complete turns). For a twisted cord to qualify as being functionally significant, there must be compromise (occlusion) of the umbilical vessels and urachus. The wall of the urachus is thinner and more pliable than the umbilical arteries or vein and thus is more easily constricted. Local distention of the urachus occurs between the twists and anywhere along its course in the cord from the umbilicus to the allantoic cavity. The cord is edematous and hemorrhagic, and red distended segments alternate with pale constricted twisted segments (see Fig. 18-38). Fibrin is sometimes present on the outer surface of affected areas of the cord. Funisitis, inflammation of the umbilical cord, is a reported lesion in horses affected by mare reproductive loss syndrome caused by the setae of processionary caterpillars.

In the mare, endometrial fibrosis, often the result of a previous endometritis, reduces the area of the endometrium available for the formation of the maternofetal interface (see Fig. 18-16). Chorionic villi–microcotyledons do not fully develop in affected areas. Thus with large areas of endometrial fibrosis, the chorion does not develop

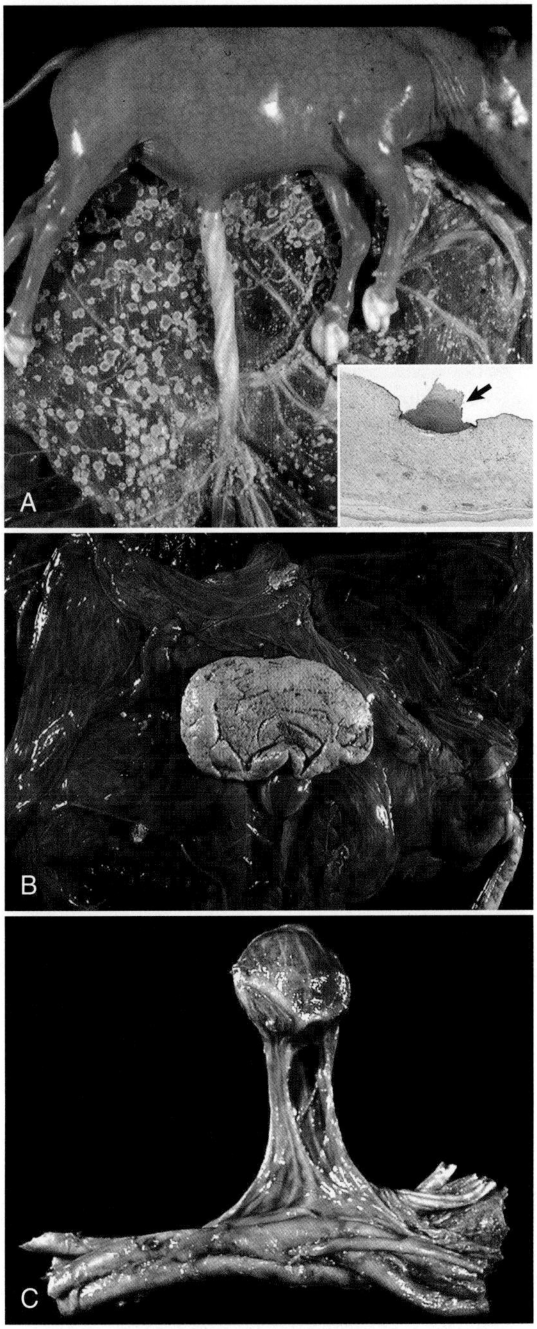

Figure 18-39 Incidental Structures, Placentas. A, Amniotic plaques, bovine fetus and placenta. Multiple white, raised circular plaques up to 1.5 cm in diameter are present on the fetal side of the amnion. They are normal incidental structures composed of stratified squamous keratinizing epithelium. *Inset,* An amniotic plaque *(arrow)*. H&E stain. **B,** Hippomane, allantois, equine placenta. These rubbery flattened discs up to 10 cm in diameter are the end result of aggregation of sediments of allantoic fluid in the horse and other species. They are incidental findings. **C,** Mineralized yolk sac remnant, umbilical cord, equine fetus. Yolk sac remnants seen on the allantoic portion of the umbilical cord are incidental structures. Note that in this case the yolk sac is connected by a stalk containing blood vessels and is located at the junction of the umbilical cord and the chorioallantois. (**A** courtesy Department of Veterinary Biosciences, The Ohio State University; and Noah's Arkive, College of Veterinary Medicine, The University of Georgia. Inset courtesy Dr. M.D. McGavin, College of Veterinary Medicine, University of Tennessee. **B** courtesy Dr. M. McCracken, College of Veterinary Medicine, University of Tennessee; and Noah's Arkive, College of Veterinary Medicine, The University of Georgia. **C** courtesy Dr. J. King, College of Veterinary Medicine, Cornell University.)

sufficient surface area so that severely affected mares may become pregnant but do not carry the fetus to term because the functional area of the placenta is too small.

Premature separation of the placenta in the mare has two forms. One form occurs around the time of parturition, causing the chorioallantois to appear at the vulva with the cervical star intact. This outcome is known as a "red bag" delivery because the exposed chorion is a bright red color. The second form causes tearing of the chorioallantois across the body of the placenta rather than at the cervical star. Tearing occurs when the caudal part of the chorioallantois is detached from the uterus and the cranial part remains in place. This form occurs any time before parturition. Prematurely detached areas become brown and dehydrated.

Another equine placental disease is called *body pregnancy*. Fetal death and abortion occur as a result of placental insufficiency and fetal malnutrition or with infection of the placenta. The initial site of fetal embryonic attachment is in the body of the uterus rather than at the bifurcation of the uterine horns. The fetus occupies the uterine body only rather than the body and horns, and the placenta is underdeveloped in the horns. Some fetuses expand in size so that the placenta extends through the cervix, where it is avillous and becomes infected with vaginal microbes.

Infectious Failure of Pregnancy

Viral Infections

Equine Herpesvirus. Equid herpesvirus 1 (EHV-1) (family Alphaherpesvirinae, genus *Varisellovirus*) is an important cause of failure of pregnancy in mares. EHV-1 infects respiratory epithelium, and after lymph node involvement, the virus is transported to the uterus (and other tissues) in leukocytes where infection of uterine arteriolar endothelial cells occurs. The resultant microvascular damage leads to thrombosis, edema, hemorrhage, and infarction. The endometrium has perivascular lymphocytes, neutrophils, and histiocytes. Fluid that escapes through the damaged endometrium separates the maternal and fetal layers, thus allowing virus from the endometrium to enter the placenta and then fetus. Fetal endothelial cells and the cells of most organs are then infected with the virus. The classic lesion, as with most herpesviruses, is focal hepatic necrosis. Focal necrosis also occurs microscopically in many other organs. Death of bronchiolar epithelial cells and fibrin exudation produce a diffuse pneumonia. Fibrin casts in the trachea are formed in some cases, and this is a characteristic diagnostic lesion. EHV-3 (equine coital exanthema) and EHV-4 produce a similar lesion but much less frequently.

Equine Viral Arteritis. Equine arteritis virus (family Arteriviridae, genus *Arterivirus*) in the mare causes failure of pregnancy, but in the majority of cases, there are no lesions in the fetus. The mechanism is probably fetal hypoxia caused by compression (obstruction) of uterine blood vessels caused by edema and inflammation secondary to virus-induced myometritis, although a few cases of arteritis in the chorion and myocardium of aborted fetuses are described.

Bacterial Infections. In the mare, most bacterial pathogens enter the pregnant uterus from the vagina through the cervix (see Fig. 18-37), and several bacteria are involved. The equine cervix is relatively "loose," and bacteria appear to readily transfer from the vagina to the placenta at the cervical star. The bacteria that are the most common causes of placentitis in mares include hemolytic streptococci, especially *Streptococcus equi subsp. zooepidemicus* (frequently cultured from fetal organs, placentas, and uterine discharges), *Escherichia coli*, and other Gram-negative bacteria. Inflammation of the chorioallantois is most severe at the cervical star, opposite the cervix. Fetal expulsion and death occur because of a reduction in placental area caused by placentitis, fetal sepsis, or an inflammatory cascade resulting in cytokines that enter the fetal fluids and affect the fetus. Because many cases have only a small area of placenta affected, the cervical star must be examined carefully for placentitis. Affected parts of the placenta are edematous and brown and covered by small amounts of fibrinonecrotic exudate. Macroscopic fetal lesions attributable to the infection are rare. Microscopically, the lesions include neutrophils in debris on the surface of affected microcotyledons, and severe inflammation of the stroma of microcotyledons and desquamation of trophoblasts. Microscopic fetal lesions are rare, despite the ease with which bacteria are recovered from many fetal organs.

Mammae

Disorders of the mammae that affect the mare, but that are not unique to the mare, are discussed in the section on Disorders of Domestic Animals.

Mammary disease is sporadic in mares, although the full gamut of disorders of other species does occur. Mastitis is the most prevalent disease of those reported. It is assumed that the pathogenesis of mastitis in mares is similar to that of other species, especially because the microbes are similar, at least in type. *Streptococcus zooepidemicus* is the most prevalent, with Gram-negative species second. Early weaning of foals and spread by seasonal insect feeding are implicated in predisposing a mare to mastitis. Mastitis occurs at any stage of lactation, is usually unilateral, and may just affect one mammary gland in one mamma (mares have two or three mammary glands per mamma); it results in local pain, swelling, and pyrexia in approximately 50% of cases.

Mammary carcinoma is also sporadic and very rare. No cause is known. Case reports indicate they are often metastatic.

Disorders of Ruminants (Cattle, Sheep, and Goats)

Female Reproductive System

Disorders of the female reproductive system that affect ruminants, but that are not unique to ruminants, are discussed in the section on Disorders of Domestic Animals.

Ovary

Cystic ovarian degeneration is a major disease in high producing dairy cows. It and other diseases are discussed in the section on Disorders of Domestic Animals, Ovary.

Uterine Tubes

Diseases of the uterine tubes occur sporadically and are discussed in the section on Disorders of Domestic Animals, Uterine Tubes.

Uterus

Inflammation. The most common and important uterine disease of cattle is postpartum endometritis, also known as postpartum uterine disease. *Escherichia coli*, *Trueperella pyogenes* (formerly called *Arcanobacterium pyogenes*), and *Fusobacterium necrophorum* are commonly found in a large number of disorders affecting dairy cattle and are discussed in the section on Disorders of Domestic Animals, Uterus. Postpartum uterine disease in dairy cows has a major negative effect on the production of calves (and milk) by increasing the critical parturition to conception interval. Although it is normal for the uterus to be contaminated with bacteria after parturition, clearance of the bacterial infection is rapid in "normal healthy" cows.

Neoplasms

Endometrial Carcinoma. Endometrial carcinoma is well known in cattle and is found at the time of meat inspection. Despite this observation, it is rarely identified clinically or at postmortem evaluation in diagnostic laboratories. The cause is unknown. The earliest microscopic lesion is most often in the depths of the endometrial glands of the horns and less often in the body of the uterus. As it increases in size, the neoplasm thickens the uterine wall without altering the luminal epithelium. A scirrhous response, the deposition of large amounts of fibrous tissue, is a characteristic lesion, and this response makes the neoplasm firm and tough and causes localized constriction bands on the serosal surface. The neoplasm can be small and annular or involve a large area of the uterine wall. Microscopically, the neoplasm is readily distinguished from normal endometrium by the increased size, pleomorphism, and disarray of the glandular epithelial cells and the accompanying scirrhous reaction. Metastases occur to the regional (medial iliac) lymph nodes and lungs, and they can seed the serosal surfaces of the abdomen.

Lymphoma. Lymphoma in enzootic bovine lymphoma, caused by bovine leukemia virus (BLV), commonly affects the heart, abomasum, and uterus, as well as the lymph nodes. In the uterus, as in other locations, the neoplastic cells can be focal, multifocal, multifocally coalescing, or confluent. Lesions are up to 3 cm thick (Fig. 18-40). Affected areas are white to light yellow, slightly friable, and sometimes centrally necrotic and involve any or all layers of the uterine wall. An extensively involved uterus can support pregnancy, even to an advanced stage.

Cervix

See the section on Disorders of Domestic Animals because disorders of the cervix of ruminants (cattle, sheep, and goats) are those seen in all species.

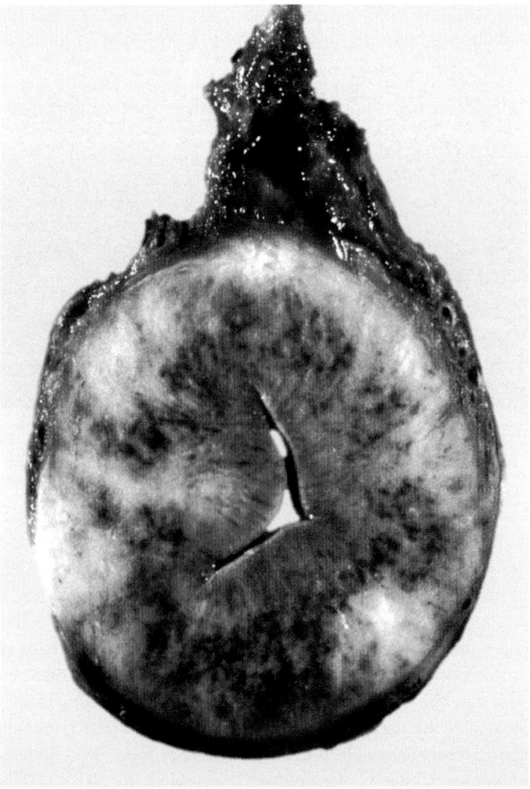

Figure 18-40 **Lymphoma (Lymphosarcoma), Uterus, Cross Section, Cow.** The mucosa, lamina propria, and myometrium are expanded by neoplastic lymphocytes. The dark-red to brown regions are areas of necrosis and hemorrhage. (Courtesy Dr. R.A. Foster, Ontario Veterinary College, University of Guelph.)

Vulva and Vagina

Granular Vulvitis. Many different microbes cause granular vulvitis in cattle. It begins as an acute vulvitis or as a subclinical disease. *Ureaplasma diversum* is the classic cause of granular vulvitis. In the acute stage, there is a purulent vulvar discharge and a hyperemic vulvar mucosa. Two-millimeter raised granules subsequently develop (see Fig. 18-28). Lesions resolve within 3 months. In approximately 10% of infected cows, discrete, raised, white nodules of follicular lymphoid hyperplasia, 2 to 5 mm in diameter, occur in rows or clusters on the dorsolateral wall of the vulva. Infection is usually self-limiting, but herds can have a persistent infection. The prepuce of bulls and their semen can remain infected and spread the infection during mating or artificial insemination. Reduced fertility with return to service or abortion occurs as a sequel to infection of the embryo or placenta with pathogenic strains of the microbe.

Infectious Pustular Vulvovaginitis. Infectious pustular vulvovaginitis (IPV) of cattle is caused by BoHV-1, which is similar to the BoHV-1 that is the cause of infectious bovine rhinotracheitis (IBR). The two diseases behave as separate entities, but their occurrence can overlap in a herd or in an individual animal. Vulvovaginitis is transmitted by coitus, artificial insemination, and possibly nose-to-vulva contact. The first lesions of the disease include hyperemia and edema of the vagina and vulva followed by petechial hemorrhages and slight nodularity (swelling) of mucosal surfaces because of edema within epithelial cells. A rapidly coalescing multifocal erosion of the mucosa follows (see Fig. 18-29). Microscopically, lesions are detected in the epithelium, the lamina propria, and the lymphoid nodules. The epithelium develops eosinophilic intranuclear inclusions and undergoes ballooning degeneration or apoptosis, followed by desquamation, but usually without discrete stages of vesicle or pustule formation. The lamina propria is hyperemic and edematous. The subepithelial lymphoid nodules become prominent and hyperplastic. Resolution of the disease is rapid, and by 7 and 10 days after onset, the lesions are a slightly thickened epithelium and hyperplastic lymphoid nodules. Lesions are similar on the penis of affected bulls. An identical disease occurs in goats (caprine herpesvirus 1) (see Fig. 18-30) and rarely in sheep.

Fetus and Placenta

Failure of Pregnancy. The diagnostic process utilized to determine the failure of pregnancy in ruminants is similar to that of other species. There are many similarities in the pathogenesis and morphology of the lesions of failure of pregnancy among ruminants because they all have cotyledonary placentas. There are several anatomically normal structures that are often mistaken for lesions and include adventitial placentation, mineralization of the fetal membranes and placenta, and amniotic plaques.

Adventitial placentation in cattle is the formation of additional placentomes (Fig. 18-41) and occurs most commonly in cows with higher parity. It is considered to be a hyperplastic response to inadequacy of existing placentome surface area. A reduction in the area of placentomes from the loss of caruncles can occur because of endometritis, removal of cotyledons during aggressive manipulations, removal of retained placental membranes, and chronic placentitis. Compensation for a reduced area is also achieved by enlargement of the existing functional placentomes. Adventitial placentation is also seen in hydroallantois and when fetuses are the result of cloning. These adventitious areas initially form near the normal placentomes but can expand to involve much of the intercotyledonary surface. Mineralization of fetal membranes and the placenta appears as white lacy change, especially of the chorion. All species have amniotic plaques (see Fig. 18-39, *A*). They are small

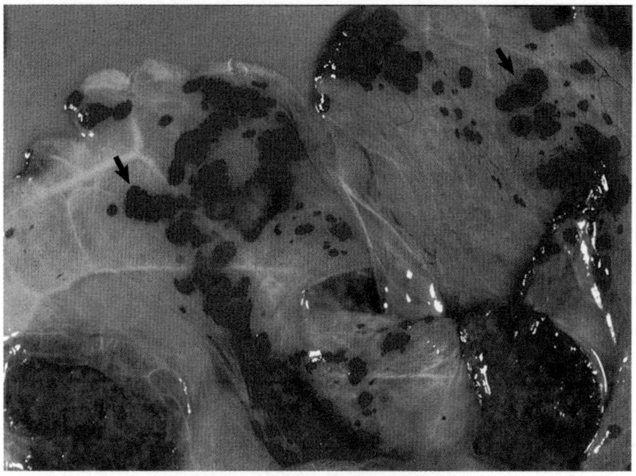

Figure 18-41 Adventitial Placentation, Placenta, Chorion, Cow. Additional sites of placentation are visible in the intercotyledonary chorion. They appear as red plaques *(arrows)*, sometimes with villi, that extend from cotyledons. There is a corresponding change on the endometrium. (Courtesy Dr. W. Crowell and Dr. D.E. Tyler, College of Veterinary Medicine, University of Georgia; and Noah's Arkive, College of Veterinary Medicine, University of Georgia.)

raised areas of epidermal tissue, and some may have hair growing from them. In ruminants, they are up to 2 cm in diameter and are only on the amnion, thus on the same side as the fetus.

Because the placentation of ruminants is cotyledonary, there is a large potential space between the placentomes in which exudate and microbes can accumulate. Chronic placentitis involving the pericotyledonary areas and the intercotyledonary portions of the chorion is common. The lesions are stereotyped and include the following:

1. Placental edema and fibrosis
2. Cupping of the cotyledon
3. Exudate on the chorionic surface
4. Cotyledonary necrosis

Most microbes cause similar lesions, and the etiologic diagnosis depends on microbiologic cultures. The list of possible infectious microbes is long, although there are species of bacteria and fungi that are more prevalent in some geographic locations and in some ruminant species.

Noninfectious Failure of Pregnancy. Noninfectious failure of pregnancy in ruminants, in general, is identical to that which occurs in all domestic animal species. A classic example is prolonged gestation in ewes that ingest the plant *Veratrum californicum* on day 14 of gestation. Along with cyclopia (Fig. 18-42) and holoprosencephaly, the pituitary gland may be absent, and without a normal pituitary-adrenal axis to initiate parturition, prolonged gestation is seen.

In addition, amorphous globosus is a rare and incidental finding, especially in bovine placentas. It is a type of acardiac monster and is a severely anomalous second fetus. Macroscopically, it is usually spheric, covered in hair, and attached to the placenta by a cord (Fig. 18-43). Various organs can be identified within the structure, histologically.

Hydramnios and Hydroallantois. Hydramnios and hydroallantois refer to the excessive accumulation of fluid in the amniotic and allantoic sacs, respectively. These lesions occur mostly in the cow but can occur in any species. The volume and composition of placental fluids are mostly regulated by the membranes of the amnion and allantois, and the nature of the dysregulation in hydramnios and

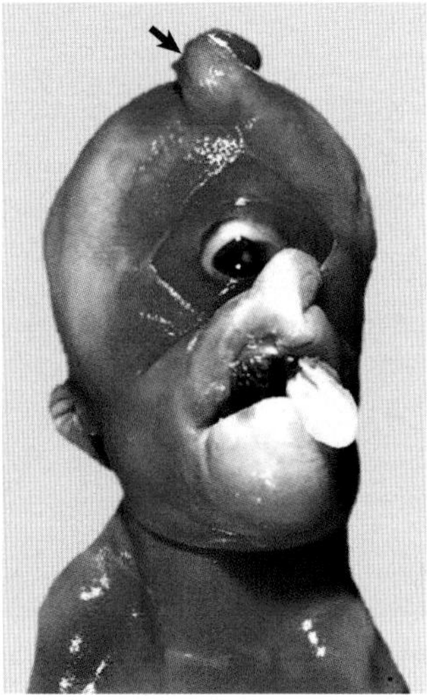

Figure 18-42 **Cyclopia, Porcine Fetus.** A defect of ocular and cranial development has resulted in fusion of the eyes (cyclops) and a proboscis (*arrow*) above the eye. Cyclopia can occur in the lambs of ewes that ingest the plant *Veratrum californicum* on day 14 of gestation. (Courtesy Dr. J. King, College of Veterinary Medicine, Cornell University.)

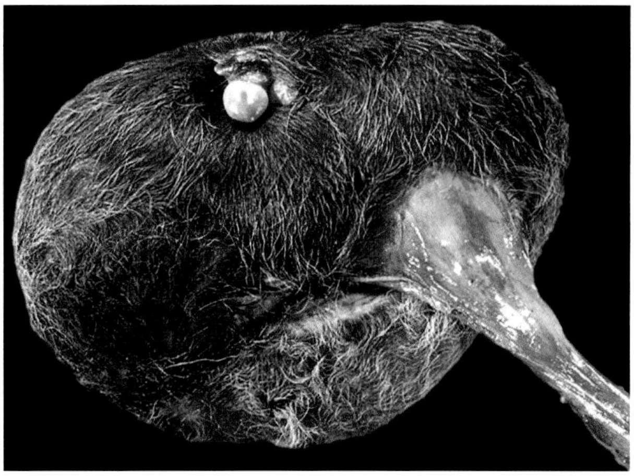

Figure 18-43 **Acardiac Monster (Bovine Amorphous Globosus).** This structure, covered with hair, is the remnant of a twin fetus and is attached to the placenta of the normal twin by a stalk. It is a rare finding in cattle and is usually of little consequence. (Courtesy Dr. J. Edwards, College of Veterinary Medicine, Texas A&M University; and Dr. J. King, College of Veterinary Medicine, Cornell University.)

hydroallantois is unknown. Hydramnios also occurs with some fetal facial muscle and skeletal abnormalities in which impairment of the fetal swallowing reflex reduces amniotic fluid removal by the fetus. Allantoic fluid is formed in part from fetal urine received through the urachus; thus excessive urination is implicated. In the cow, hydroallantois occurs in conjunction with adventitial placentation and in some twin pregnancies. The allantoic fluid composition changes from normal to that closely resembling maternal or fetal extracellular fluid. When these membranes are retained after delivery of a fetus, they sometimes continue to produce fluid.

Infectious Failure of Pregnancy

Diseases of Cattle. In cattle, *Neospora caninum* and specific bacteria (discussed in detail next) are among the most common causes of failure of pregnancy, according to the results from diagnostic laboratories worldwide.

Protozoal Infections

Neospora Caninum. *Neospora caninum* is a major cause of abortion in cows. Fetuses are 3 to 9 months' gestational age and have no gross lesions, except in rare cases in which there is fetal heart failure from myocarditis. There are no macroscopic placental lesions. In the fetal brain, multiple foci of necrosis or clusters of microglial cells are often adjacent to capillaries. *Neospora caninum* zoites in or around these foci are either extracellular or occur in glial or endothelial cells. In the heart, the lesions include multifocal epicarditis, myocarditis, endocarditis, and protozoal organisms in either myofibers or endothelial cells. Lymphocytic portal hepatitis, multifocal hepatocellular necrosis, and fibrin thrombi in hepatic sinusoids are also seen. Foci of lymphocytes are present in additional organs, including the placenta.

Tritrichomonas Foetus. *Tritrichomonas foetus* causes transient vaginitis, cervicitis, and endometritis and therefore infertility. It can cause early embryonic mortality but only occasionally causes abortion. Macroscopic lesions are usually absent. Microscopically, there is placental edema and a mild lymphocytic and histiocytic chorionitis and focal necrosis of trophoblasts. Large numbers of trichomonads are present. Fetal pneumonia with intrabronchiolar neutrophils, macrophages, and some multinucleated giant cells may occur in one-half of cases. The diagnosis is confirmed when trichomonads are seen in the contents of the fetal abomasum or in fetal and placental tissues. Endometritis can be severe and result in pyometra.

Bacterial Infections

Brucella Abortus. Brucellosis caused by *Brucella abortus* has been eradicated from several countries, but it is a disease that is still important economically because of import/export regulations. Cattle are infected by exposure to infected placental fluids at several portals of entry, but most often through ingestion and the alimentary tract. Infection is possible via both conjunctiva and inhalation. After exposure, the bacterium is found in macrophages in the draining mucosal, local, and regional lymph nodes. Bacteremia ensues, and systemic infection and localization in the pregnant uterus, testes (in bulls), and mammae occur. The trophism of *Brucella abortus* for the pregnant uterus appears to be related to some unknown effects of erythritol and steroid hormones on the organ and its tissues and cells. Bacteria enter the erythrophagocytic trophoblasts of the hemophagic organ of the placentome, at the base of the chorionic villi. They replicate in the rough endoplasmic reticulum of the periplacentomal and interplacentomal trophoblasts, a unique mechanism of intracellular parasitism. Macroscopic lesions of the placenta are those typical of placentitis and include thickening and edema of the intercotyledonary chorioallantois, a fibrinonecrotic coating of the intercotyledonary chorion, and cupping of the cotyledon. There are no unique lesions, but histologically, large numbers of bacteria are observed in trophoblasts and there is vasculitis in both maternal and fetal tissues, a lesion that could be a response to endotoxin released from the *Brucella* microbes. Most fetuses develop pneumonia that ranges from minimal to severe. Microscopically, the pneumonia is either bronchopneumonia with numerous macrophages and lymphocytes and some neutrophils or a fibrinous pneumonia. Microscopic granulomas that include multinucleate giant cells occur in organs such as the lung, liver, spleen, and lymph nodes.

Leptospirosis. Leptospirosis is another disease in which failure of pregnancy is a common outcome. Results of serologic studies indicate that a large percentage of cattle are infected, but most do not have clinical signs. Several different serovars are responsible for abortion, especially *Leptospira interrogans* serovar *hardjo*. In adult animals, the bacteria seldom cause clinical disease but localize in the kidneys after the bacteremic phase. Abortion is considered sporadic. Pregnant cows abort weeks or months after the bacteremic phase, usually in the last trimester. Placental lesions are usually limited to edema; fetal lesions often are mild and obscured by autolysis. Some dead fetuses expelled near term have the gross lesions of ascites and fibrinous peritonitis. Microscopic fetal lesions include interstitial nephritis and necrotizing hepatitis. Leptospires can be demonstrated in peritoneal or pleural cavity fluid by dark-field microscopic examination and in renal tubular lumens by silver stains or by immunohistochemistry. Measurement of the leptospiral antibody in fetal fluids (serum, cavity fluids) is also used for diagnosis.

Epizootic Bovine Abortion. Epizootic bovine abortion (EBA), also known as *foothill abortion*, occurs in California and adjacent states. The causative microbe, known as the "agent of EBA," is a novel Deltaproteobacterium and is carried and transmitted by the tick *Ornithodoros coriaceus*. The fetal disease is chronic with notable microscopic lesions 50 days after exposure of the dam to ticks. The lesions are sufficiently specific for a diagnosis in fetuses whose gestational age is greater than 100 days. Gross lesions include petechial hemorrhages of the conjunctiva and oral cavity, an enlarged nodular liver and ascites (both presumably from heart failure secondary to myocarditis), and enlarged lymph nodes and spleen. Microscopically, lymphoid follicles are hyperplastic and have large numbers of histiocytes. The thymus is atrophic because of the loss of cortical lymphocytes. The thymic parenchyma and interstitium contain many histiocytes. Foci of acute necrosis are present in several organs, especially the lymph nodes and spleen. These foci frequently develop into pyogranulomas. Vasculitis occurs in several organs. Deposits of IgG and IgM are present in the vascular lesions.

Ureaplasma Diversum. *Ureaplasma diversum* causes failure of pregnancy at different times of gestation in cattle. The characteristic gross lesion observed in abortions is amnionitis, a change only occasionally seen in other bacterial or fungal infections of fetal membranes. Early in the process, there is focal or diffuse reddening of the amnion and also of the chorioallantois. Later with chronicity, there is thickening and yellow discoloration of the amnion (Fig. 18-44). The lesions are chronic and ongoing with fibrosis, edema, inflammation, and necrosis of the amnion occurring together with focal inflammation and necrosis of the cotyledons and the intercotyledonary chorioallantois. Many fetuses have bronchopneumonia with large lymphoid follicles near bronchi.

Other Bacteria. Other bacterial causes of placentitis produce similar and often identical lesions. *Bacillus licheniformis* is a common cause. The pathogenesis of *Bacillus licheniformis*, based on experimental studies, suggests there is localization in the placentomes after bacteremia. Cotyledonary necrosis and suppurative inflammation occur with fetal infection resulting from fetal bacteremia or ingestion of contaminated amniotic fluid.

Campylobacteriosis is a sporadic disease unless it is newly introduced into a herd. *Campylobacter fetus* var. *venerealis* can be a long-term inhabitant of the preputial cavity of bulls. It is transmitted venereally and can survive on vaginal mucosa, but the cow must become pregnant for it to establish itself in the uterus. Early embryonic death is the most likely manifestation of campylobacteriosis and often the only clinical abnormalities are an irregular estrous cycle or the return to estrus of an animal thought to be pregnant. Much less frequently, abortion occurs. Cows become resistant to subsequent infections by the bacterium. Gross and microscopic lesions in placentas are similar to those described in brucellosis (edema of the intercotyledonary chorioallantois and necrosis of cotyledons with microscopic inflammation of both) but are less severe and with fewer bacteria in the desquamated trophoblasts.

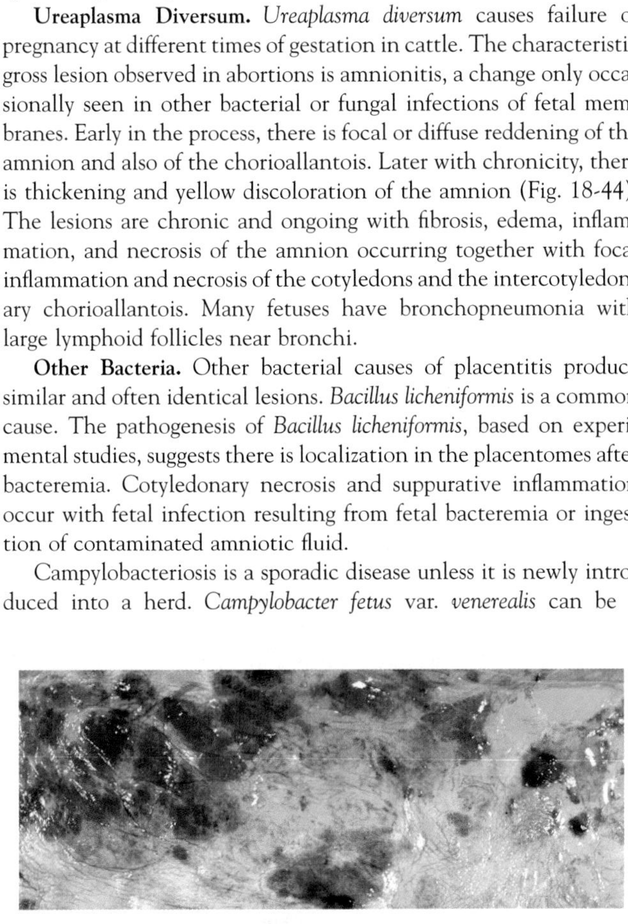

Figure 18-44 Amnionitis, *Ureaplasma Diversum* Infection, Cow. The amnion has large, opaque, red and white areas of granulation and fibrous tissue, respectively *(left half of image)*. Amnionitis without placentitis in cattle is a good indicator of *Ureaplasma* sp. infection. (Courtesy Dr. R.B. Miller, Ontario Veterinary College, University of Guelph.)

In addition, any bacterium with a bacteremic phase in cows could cause lesions in the placenta and fetus. *Salmonella* spp., *Mannheimia* spp., and *Pasteurella* spp. and *Histophilus somni* are therefore potential causes of placentitis, fetal pneumonia, hepatitis or other lesions, and failure of pregnancy.

Viral Infections. The frequency of viral causes of failure of pregnancy in cattle is probably underreported, especially those caused by bovine viral diarrhea virus (BVDV). There are seldom macroscopic or microscopic lesions of BVDV infection in the fetus and placenta, and the virus may not be found. The pathogenesis of BVD is discussed in Chapters 4 and 7.

Bovine Herpesvirus. Bovine herpesvirus 1 (BoHV-1) is a sporadic cause of bovine abortion. Fetal autolysis is usually present because of rapid death of the fetus. Fetal lesions are typical of herpesvirus infection in other species and include multifocal necrosis and hemorrhage (see previous discussion). There are usually no macroscopic or microscopic placental lesions, although necrosis of vascular endothelium and cotyledonary villi with neutrophils in the necrotic tissue occurs in experimental infection. In addition, BoHV-1 and -4 produce an acute necrotizing endometritis in the uterine body or caudal parts of the uterine horns of the cow, particularly in the postpartum period. Microscopically, the lesions range from mild focal lymphocytic endometritis to severe diffuse necrotizing metritis.

Other Viral Infections. Bunyaviruses, such as Schmallenburg virus, Akabane virus, and bluetongue virus, cause fetal infection and abortion and produce a range of lesions in the developing fetal central nervous system, including hydranencephaly, microencephaly, cerebellar hypoplasia, and a lack of spinal cord ventral horn neurons. Spinal lesions cause neuropathic muscle atrophy that leads to arthrogryposis (fixation of limb joints) and skeletal deformities such as torticollis and scoliosis.

Fungal Infections. Fungal abortion caused by *Aspergillus* spp. and the Zygomycetes (*Absidia*, *Mortierella*, *Rhizopus*, and *Mucor*) in cattle is a major cause in some geographic locales but is sporadic in most places. The fungi spread to the placenta hematogenously because the placentomes are involved first and there is multifocal involvement. In some cases, lesions occur in the placenta in the tip of the horn with the degree of fibrosis suggesting movement caudally; this suggests descending intrauterine spread. The placental changes are those of chronic necrotic placentitis as the cotyledons become enlarged, brown, and friable and the intercotyledonary chorioallantois becomes leathery and covered with a brown exudate (Figs. 18-45 and 18-46). In a small number of cases, the amnion may be thick, white, or yellow with leathery areas resembling the lesions caused by *Ureaplasma diversum*. Fetal dermatitis may be present wherein small, white, raised plaques are present on the skin of the fetus, often over the neck and shoulder. Microscopically, the lesions include large numbers of neutrophils, macrophages, and lymphocytes in the amnion (if affected) and chorioallantois, and necrosis and desquamation of trophoblasts. The vessels at the base of the cotyledons have vasculitis and fungal vascular invasion. Lesions in the fetus may include a superficial perivascular and hyperkeratotic dermatitis and bronchopneumonia. Fungal hyphae, septate in *Aspergillus* and nonseptate in the Zygomycetes, are abundant in lesions of the placenta. Fungi can also be recovered from the fetal stomach, presumably from swallowed amniotic fluid.

Diseases of Sheep

Bacterial Infections. In sheep, many cases of failure of pregnancy are caused by bacteria, including *Chlamydia* (*Chlamydophila*) *abortus*, *Campylobacter fetus*, and *Brucella ovis*.

Enzootic Abortion. Enzootic abortion of ewes (EAE) is caused by *Chlamydia* (*Chlamydophila*) *abortus* and is one of the most common abortifacient microbes in sheep. It occurs in all sheep-producing countries and produces late-term abortion. It occurs in two forms: outbreaks when first introduced into susceptible flocks or as an enzootic condition of ewe lambs. The microbe is present in fluids from infected placentas, and the oral cavity is the portal of entry. Ewes abort only once, but they may remain carriers. Ewes infected before 5 or 6 weeks of gestation abort in late gestation, but ewes infected after 5 or 6 weeks of gestation abort in the subsequent pregnancy. Pathogenesis involves infection of susceptible animals and persistence of *Chlamydia abortus* in an unknown site within the body. After approximately day 90 of pregnancy, there is proliferation of *Chlamydia abortus* in the placentome and then in trophoblasts in the intercotyledonary placenta. This process leads to a cytokine and chemokine cascade, with inflammation and thrombosis of placental vessels and subsequent abortion. The placentitis is similar to that described in placentitis of cattle (see the discussion on bacterial disease in the section on Diseases of Cattle). The microbes distend the trophoblasts and are obvious with such special stains as modified Ziehl-Neelsen or Gimenez stains. In the fetus, foci of lymphocytes and macrophages may be present in the liver, lungs, and muscle. *Coxiella burnetii* (see the section on Disease of Goats) and *Brucella ovis* induce a similar placentitis.

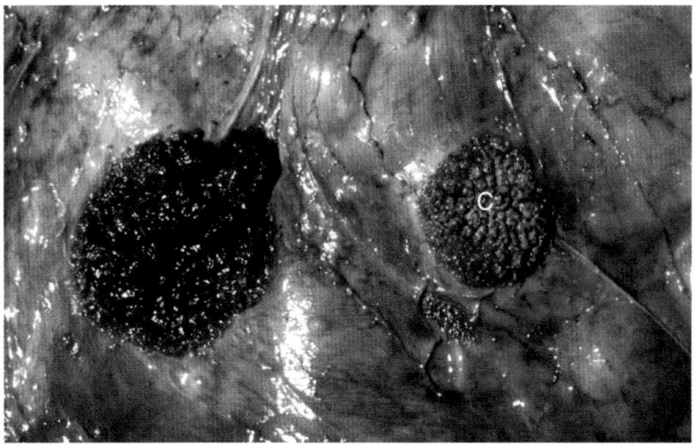

Figure 18-45 **Mycotic Intercotyledonary Placentitis, Cow.** Marked edema, fibrosis, and thickening of the intercotyledonary placenta has caused it to be opaque. The cotyledon (*C*) on the right is necrotic. (Courtesy Dr. R.A. Foster, Ontario Veterinary College, University of Guelph.)

Coxiellosis. Sheep develop coxiellosis (Q fever) caused by *Coxiella burnetii*, but the disease is more common in goats and is described in the section on Diseases of Goats.

Brucellosis. *Brucella ovis* in sheep is transmitted venereally from infected rams with epididymitis and is shed in semen. Gross placental lesions are similar to those that occur with *Brucella abortus* in cattle. There are no specific fetal lesions. Calcified plaques on the hooves are reported, but this is not a specific lesion. Microscopically, as with *Brucella* sp. infections in other species, large numbers of coccobacilli are found in trophoblasts and are free in the chorionic mesenchyme. There is vasculitis that involves the larger chorionic vessels. Lesions in the fetus when present are pneumonia, lymphadenitis, interstitial nephritis, and pericholangitis. In younger fetuses, the cells are histiocytes, whereas older fetuses have well-formed nodules of lymphocytes and plasma cells.

Campylobacteriosis. *Campylobacter fetus* ssp. *fetus* and *Campylobacter jejuni* are primarily intestinal inhabitants. These bacteria are transmitted fecal-orally or from infected placentas or fluid via the oral cavity. Failure of pregnancy occurs in outbreaks and continually cycles through the flock as microbes spread from an aborting ewe to an uninfected ewe. Infection of the pregnant uterus results in late-term abortion or the birth of live but sick lambs. Ewes become immune after the first infection. Placentitis results in an edematous intercotyledonary chorioallantois and friable, yellow cotyledons, as is seen in other cases of acute placentitis. At necropsy, approximately 25% of the fetuses have multiple, well-circumscribed, up to 20 mm in diameter yellow hepatic foci with red depressed centers, which are areas of necrosis. Microscopically, the lesions are those of an acute neutrophilic (suppurative) and necrotic placentitis, as occurs with other bacteria, including *Brucella ovis*. The

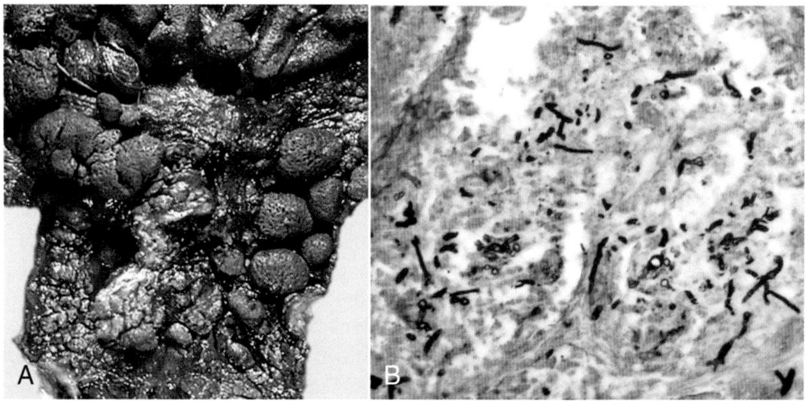

Figure 18-46 **Mycotic Endometritis, Postpartum Uterus, Cow. A,** The endometrial surface of the middle and lower portion of this uterus is irregularly thickened and corrugated. Caruncles are small or missing. **B,** The placenta is necrotic, and the numerous fungal hyphae (*black*) are irregular in diameter, do not have regular septation, and branch at odd angles—all features typical of the Zygomycetes. Gomori's methenamine silver stain. (**A** courtesy Dr. J. King, College of Veterinary Medicine, Cornell University. **B** courtesy Dr. K. McEntee, Reproductive Pathology Collection, University of Illinois.)

chorioallantois and especially the cotyledon have necrotic neutrophils and trophoblasts along the surface. *Campylobacter* microbes are abundant among the inflammatory cells, within trophoblasts, and there may be dense emboli of bacteria in the capillaries of the chorionic villi. The hepatic lesion is a multifocal necrotizing hepatitis with abundant intralesional bacteria. *Flexispira rappini* causes an identical lesion in the ovine placenta and fetal liver, but infections are less common and sporadic.

Listeriosis. Listeriosis of the fetus and placenta, caused by *Listeria monocytogenes*, is a cause of sporadic abortions in many species, including cattle, sheep, and goats, and of outbreaks of abortion in sheep. Although both nervous disease and reproductive disease occur in the same flock or herd, it is rare for both forms to occur concurrently in the same animal. Listerial abortions occur in the last trimester of pregnancy. Some aborting dams are septicemic and also have endometritis. The placental lesion, as with other bacterial placentitis, is severe diffuse necrotizing and suppurative placentitis of both the cotyledons and the intercotyledonary areas. In the aborted fetus, there are multiple 1-mm yellow or white foci in many organs, but they are readily seen in large numbers in the liver. These foci are areas of acute multifocal necrotizing hepatitis in which the Gram-positive *Listeria* microbes are numerous. The microscopic lesions in the placenta are identical to those of campylobacteriosis and brucellosis, except that the trophoblasts, especially in the intercotyledonary areas, are filled with Gram-positive listerial bacilli.

Protozoal Infection

Toxoplasmosis. *Toxoplasma gondii* is an important cause of abortion in ewes. Susceptible ewes eat food contaminated by cat (usually kitten) feces that contain oocysts. Macroscopic lesions in the placenta are white 1- to 2-mm foci of necrosis in the cotyledons (Fig. 18-47). There may be edema of the intercotyledonary chorioallantois. Microscopically, the cotyledonary lesions are distinctive and consist of multiple foci of necrosis with rare groups of *Toxoplasma* microbes within trophoblasts. Immunohistochemical labeling techniques are often needed to detect the microbe. A small percentage of affected fetuses have cerebral leukoencephalomalacia, a nonspecific effect of fetal anoxia secondary to placentitis. Focal necrosis and gliosis and the presence of the protozoa are more likely to be found in parts of the brain rostral to the pons and in the optic tracts, locations that may not be routinely sampled during necropsy.

Diseases of Goats

Bacterial Infections

Coxiellosis. *Coxiella burnetii* infection is extremely important in goats and sheep and potentially in all species. *Coxiella burnetii*, the cause of Q fever in humans, causes abortion or the birth of dead or weak lambs or kids. Abortion occurs in newly exposed does (also known as nannies), and repeat infections resulting in abortion are possible. *Coxiella* is acquired by ingestion or by inhalation. It is shed in vaginal discharges at parturition and in the milk. In affected placentas, the intercotyledonary chorioallantois is thick, leathery, yellow, and covered with tenacious exudate (Fig. 18-48). There are no macroscopic fetal lesions. Microscopically, the placental lesions are most severe in the intercotyledonary areas where there is necrotic inflammatory debris on the chorionic surface and neutrophils, macrophages, and lymphocytes in the chorionic stroma. Hypertrophic trophoblasts contain myriad *Coxiella* microbes. Fetal lesions, if present, consist of peribronchiolar, renal medullary, and hepatic portal lymphocytes.

Other Bacteria. Goats also develop chlamydiosis and campylobacteriosis as described for sheep. *Brucella melitensis* infection in goats (and sheep) occurs mainly in Mediterranean countries. There is an initial bacteremic phase, and subsequently, inflammation is localized to the mammae and pregnant uterus. Goats develop a more severe febrile disease and more severe mastitis than do sheep. The lesions are similar to those caused by *Brucella abortus* in cattle and *Brucella ovis* in sheep. Toxoplasmosis of goats is common but less so than in sheep.

The Mammae

Disorders of the mammae that affect ruminants, but that are not unique to ruminants, are discussed in the section on Disorders of Domestic Animals.

Mastitis of Cows

Mastitis in dairy cattle is an extremely important disease. Most of the microbes responsible for mastitis are bacteria, and the number and range of lesions they cause is large. The majority of cases are caused by *Staphylococcus aureus* and are of subclinical or moderate clinical forms.

Predisposing conditions that may potentially contribute to the development of mastitis include (1) a high producing dairy cow, (2) excessive high vacuum in milking machines, (3) the presence of lesions on the "ends" of papillae, (4) contamination of the mammae

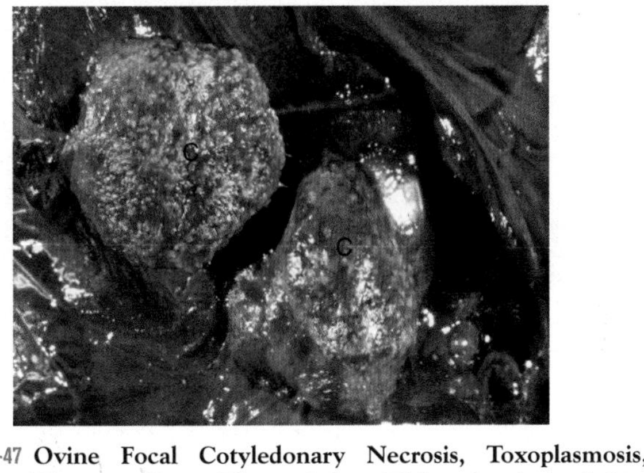

Figure 18-47 Ovine Focal Cotyledonary Necrosis, Toxoplasmosis, Abortion, Placenta, Sheep. The cotyledons (C) have hundreds of white foci of necrosis, a lesion that is characteristic of *Toxoplasma gondii*–induced abortion in sheep and goats. (Courtesy Ontario Veterinary College, University of Guelph.)

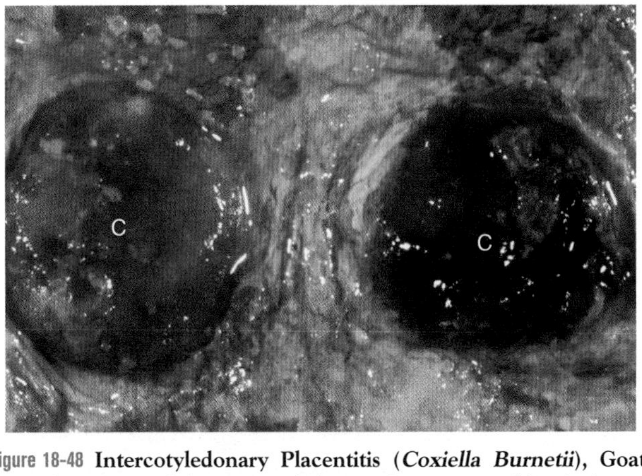

Figure 18-48 Intercotyledonary Placentitis (*Coxiella Burnetii*), Goat. Note the opacity of the intercotyledonary placenta caused by thickening from inflammation and fibrosis. The cotyledons (C) have variable areas of gray discoloration, indicating necrosis and inflammatory exudates. The gross appearance of the lesions of placentitis tends to be similar, regardless of the etiologic microbe identified by microbiological examination. (Courtesy Dr. R.A. Foster, Ontario Veterinary College, University of Guelph.)

with fecal material, (5) poor mammary hygiene while milking, and (6) contact of mammae with certain types of flies.

Mastitis is divided into multiple overlapping groups based on the source of the infection, clinical manifestations, and etiological microbe.

Source of Infection. Determining the source of infection of the mammae is very important in understanding the pathogenesis of mastitis and therefore its treatment and prevention. The infecting bacteria are either obligate mammary pathogens or environmental microbial contaminants. *Streptococcus agalactiae*, *Staphylococcus aureus*, and *Mycoplasma* sp. persist or reside in the mammae and do not survive long in the "farm" environment outside the gland. These microbes are transmitted from cow to cow. The environmental contaminants include coliform microbes such as *Escherichia coli*. They contaminate the end of the papilla and are acquired from the external environment, such as fecal matter, soil, water, or bedding. The occurrence of new mammary infections in dairy cows caused by environmental pathogens is greatest during the first and the last 2 weeks of a 60-day nonlactating period. Environmental bacteria acquired during the nonlactating period are present at the time of parturition and cause clinical mastitis soon afterward. An overlap group capable of persisting in either the mamma or the environment includes *Streptococcus uberis* and *Streptococcus dysgalactiae*.

Clinical Manifestations of Mastitis. Mastitis is divided clinically into severe (with or without necrosis), suppurative, and subclinical mastitis. Granulomatous mastitis is also included in this grouping.

Severe Necrotizing (Gangrenous) Mastitis. Severe necrotizing (gangrenous) mastitis often has concurrent systemic effects and is most commonly caused by Gram-negative pathogens that gain access to the glands and release endotoxins. Massive cytokine release results in necrosis and severe vascular leakage (Fig. 18-49) in the gland. A systemic acute-phase reaction causes fever, anorexia, leukopenia, hyperfibrinogenemia, and hypocalcemia. This latter feature can be mistaken for primary hypocalcemia (milk fever). Edema of the mamma and surrounding areas is often prominent. Local lesions include death and sequestration of glandular tissue, wherein regions of the gland become dry, friable, and surrounded by a red border of hyperemia and hemorrhage (Fig. 18-50). The edema fluid causes a dramatically swollen and hard mamma, and the "milk" is watery and/or contains fibrin. Fibrin can obstruct the lactiferous and papillary ducts. Not only is this type of mastitis potentially life-threatening because of endotoxemia but also the severe effects on the gland often lead to reduced defenses to other pathogens so that secondary, pyogenic pathogens proliferate.

Severe necrotizing mastitis is also caused when necrotizing Gram-positive bacteria, including virulent *Staphylococcus aureus* and streptococci, enter the mamma. With severe staphylococcal mastitis, neutrophils enter the tissue within minutes to hours, and the products of neutrophil granules contribute to the death of the glandular tissue. Cell surface–associated (adhesions, protein A, and capsular polysaccharides) and extracellular secretory (leukotoxins, extracellular enzymes, and coagulase) products of these microbes also contribute to the damage. The combined result is hemorrhage and death of the gland, with the result that all or part of the mamma becomes hard, dry, and red-black (and thus gangrenous). When severe, systemic effects of the acute-phase response caused by cytokines induce fever, anorexia, weight loss, leukopenia, and hyperfibrinogenemia.

Severe Mastitis. Severe mastitis without clinically apparent necrosis of tissue is caused by both Gram-positive and Gram-negative bacteria, but with less damage to the tissue. Exotoxins (Gram-positive bacteria) and endotoxins (Gram-negative bacteria) are released but produce a less dramatic disease, often with only local effects of edema, fibrin exudation, and a predominantly neutrophilic response. Although there is death of ductular and glandular tissue, there is not the formation of necrotic sequestra and the systemic affect is either mild or absent.

Suppurative Mastitis. Suppurative mastitis occurs when pus-forming Gram-positive bacteria do not induce the degree of necrosis, vascular lesions, and systemic effects that occurs with severe necrotizing (gangrenous) mastitis and severe mastitis. *Trueperella pyogenes*, *Mycoplasma bovis*, *Streptococcus dysgalactiae*, and various other aerobes and anaerobes individually may cause suppurative mastitis. Infection with these microbes, especially *Trueperella pyogenes*, can occur with long-acting intramammary preparations used in the nonlactating or dry cow period. The occurrence in dry cows, initially recognized in the summer months, led to the name "summer

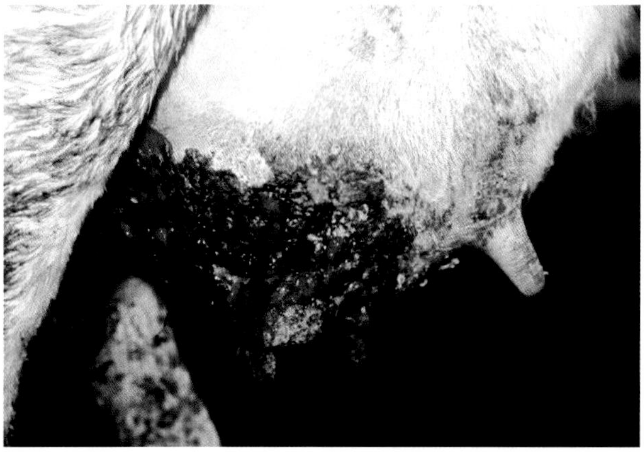

Figure 18-49 **Severe Necrotic Mastitis, Coliform Mastitis, Mamma, Cow.** Serum oozes through the dead skin of the affected right rear quarter. (Courtesy Dr. M.D. McGavin, College of Veterinary Medicine, University of Tennessee.)

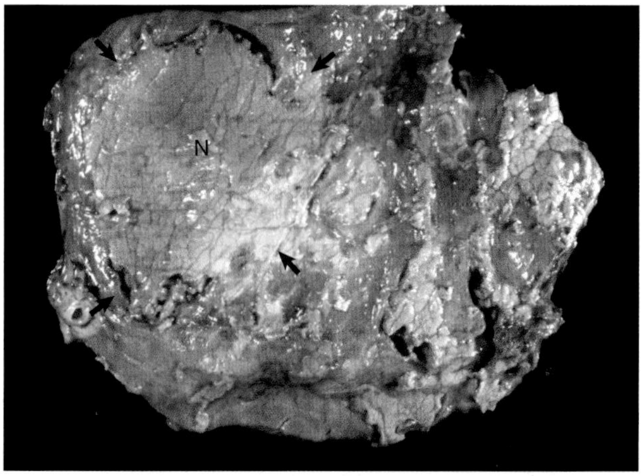

Figure 18-50 **Necrotizing Mastitis, Coliform Mastitis, Mamma, Transverse Section, Cow.** Note the dry and pale gray-white area, typical of coagulative necrosis, to the left of center (delineated by *arrows*). The necrotic tissue (*N*) is partially surrounded by a zone of edema and by a thin light-gray band of fibrous tissue. Encapsulated necrotic tissue is designated a "sequestrum." (Courtesy College of Veterinary Medicine, University of Illinois.)

mastitis." Up to five or six different species of bacteria (*Trueperella*, *Streptococcus*, *Bacteroides*, *Peptostreptococcus*, and *Fusobacterium* genera) may be present concurrently in the disease. These bacteria invoke a neutrophilic response that dominates the lesion and results in a buildup of necrotic leukocytic debris that typifies the suppurative response. The lesions they induce are centered on lactiferous ducts and sinus, which are filled with suppurative exudate (Fig. 18-51). Dry cows are not usually closely monitored, so the mastitis is typically chronic, with thick intramammary exudates and fibrosis.

Granulomatous Mastitis. Granulomatous mastitis in the cow occurs when drugs for the treatment or prevention of mastitis are introduced through the teat and are contaminated with *Nocardia asteroides*, *Cryptococcus neoformans*, atypical *Mycobacterium* sp. (other than *Mycobacterium bovis*), or *Candida* spp. These microbes can also cause spontaneous mammary disease. Nocardial mastitis is the best known because it occurs in outbreaks. Severely affected cows develop pyrexia that may last for several weeks. Cows become lethargic and lose weight, as would be expected with systemic cytokine release. The glands are hot and swollen and may have multiple abscesses or granulomas. Small white particles may be found in the exudate. Lesions are centered on the lactiferous ducts and sinuses because galactophoritis is the prominent lesion. Because the infection is chronic and ascending, lobules are affected to varying degrees. Granulomas and pyogranulomas predominate microscopically. These granulomas are usually surrounded by fibrous tissue, and extensive involvement results in the gland being replaced by a framework of fibrous tissue surrounding pockets of inflammatory cells and central necrotic debris (Fig. 18-52). An udder affected with cryptococcal mastitis has the same yellow gelatinous material that is typical of cryptococcal lesions in other organ systems.

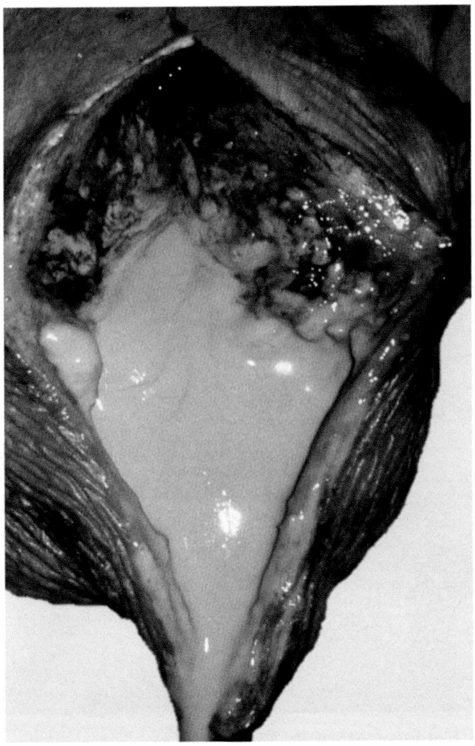

Figure 18-51 Suppurative Mastitis, Mamma, Cow. The lactiferous sinus and ducts are filled with viscous yellow pus. (Courtesy College of Veterinary Medicine, University of Illinois.)

Subclinical Mastitis. Infection and inflammation of the mammary gland at a level too low to result in clinical disease is called subclinical mastitis and is identified by the presence of a higher than normal somatic cell count. Infection rates often exceed 50%. A small percentage of these cows with intramammary infections subsequently develop clinical mastitis.

Mastitis Caused by Specific Bacteria

Streptococcal Mastitis. *Streptococcus agalactiae* was the most important pathogen of the bovine mamma in the era before adequate mammary hygiene and efficient antibacterial drugs. Resistance of cows to mastitis caused by this organism is subject to great individual variation; in general, resistance decreases with age. The mamma is the only organ affected by this organism. *Streptococcus agalactiae* does not persist long in the "farm" environment. Once a cow is infected, however, the organism persists in the lactiferous sinus, with periodic waves of multiplication, increase in virulence, and tissue invasion. The macroscopic appearance depends on the stage of the disease; different stages can occur concurrently in different areas of the gland. Usually more than one mamma is involved. In the initial stage, there is hyperemia of the lactiferous sinus. Milk quality is altered, and strands or clumps of debris or pus are present in the milk. Areas with parenchymal edema are gray and turgid. Groups of alveoli with retained secretion because of duct obstruction resemble small abscesses. Involuting parenchyma and fibrotic parenchyma are similar in appearance and are difficult to differentiate grossly. The lactiferous sinus becomes granular and thickened because of underlying projecting areas of granulation tissue and surrounding fibrosis.

The initial microscopic response to invasion of *Streptococcus agalactiae* is interstitial edema and an influx of neutrophils into the interstitium and alveoli. The alveolar epithelium undergoes either brief hyperplasia or vacuolation and then desquamates. Macrophages appear quickly in infected alveoli, and fibrosis rapidly obliterates the lumen of these alveoli. Edema, inflammatory cells, and fibrosis are lesions found in infected and adjacent alveoli so that pressure is increased within the lobule and within adjacent lobules. The increased pressure causes cessation of milk flow, thereby initiating premature involution of a portion of the gland. After the initial phase, periductal fibrosis occurs and granulation tissue replaces part

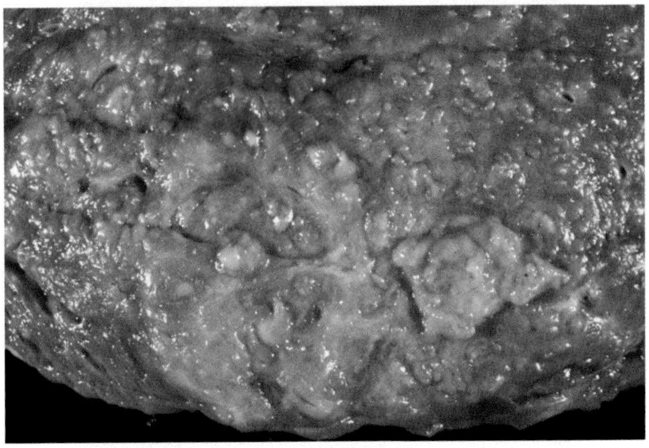

Figure 18-52 Chronic Mastitis and Galactophoritis (*Nocardia* Spp.), Mamma, Transverse Section, Cow. Chronic inflammation of the lactiferous ducts and adjacent mammary gland has resulted in the replacement of most of this gland by pyogranulomas and abscesses containing yellow pus. The adjacent normal glandular tissue has involuted. This cow was infected when the dry cow medication was contaminated by *Nocardia* spp. (Courtesy Dr. R.A. Foster, Ontario Veterinary College, University of Guelph.)

of the normal cuboidal to columnar epithelium of smaller ducts. If severe, fibrous polyps can occur and completely obstruct milk flow. Regeneration of ductal epithelium can occur. The lactiferous ducts and sinus, with their normally two-layered columnar epithelium, are similarly but less severely affected, often going through a phase of squamous metaplasia of the epithelium.

Staphylococcal Mastitis. *Staphylococcus aureus* causes mastitis similar to streptococcal mastitis but has a greater propensity to invade the interstitial tissue between alveoli and induce a more severe disease. Isolates of *Staphylococcus aureus* obtained from bovine mammary glands range from nonpathogenic to highly pathogenic. The most severe form of staphylococcal mastitis is the gangrenous form (Fig. 18-53), usually seen soon after parturition and involving a variable proportion of the udder. Severe inflammation, with classic heat, redness, swelling, and pain, progresses to coldness of the affected area, a blue-black color, and fluid exudation, indicating tissue death. Microscopically, during the first 48 hours after infection with toxigenic *Staphylococcus aureus*, the tissue has severe interstitial edema that increases the interalveolar stromal area. Progressive swelling, vacuolation, and focal erosion of epithelial cells occur throughout the ducts and are prominent near the junction of stratified squamous epithelium and columnar epithelium of the papillary duct. The bacteria attach to epithelial cells, cause focal damage, and later can be seen on, within, and below ductal and alveolar epithelia. The neutrophil response is rapid; they are initially seen in the subepithelial tissues of the duct system, then within the epithelium, and later in the lumen of alveoli.

The less severe form of staphylococcal mastitis follows a course similar to that of streptococcal mastitis. Initially, damage occurs to the epithelium of the lactiferous sinus and larger lactiferous ducts. Bacterial numbers expand rapidly along the ducts and produce inflammation in groups of adjacent terminal alveoli. In chronically infected quarters, macrophages are the principal cell type in the epithelial lining, in lumens, and especially in the glandular interstitium. Lymphocytes increase in number, but some investigators have reported a lack of increase in plasma cells; thus mammary lymphocytes could become hyporesponsive to antigenic stimulation in chronically infected mammary glands. The extent of regeneration of glandular tissue is unknown; it is unclear whether damaged alveoli redevelop secretory tissue or remaining healthy tissue undergoes compensatory hypertrophy, or whether both processes occur.

In suppurative staphylococcal mastitis, abscess formation follows the initial disease. Abscesses vary in size from those that are microscopic to those grossly visible. Sometimes staphylococcal bacteria are surrounded by club-shaped material of the Splendore Hoeppli reaction (the term *botryomycosis* was applied to such lesions [see Fig. 7-51]). Obstruction of milk flow by granulation tissue and pressure from surrounding fibrosis result in involution. Disease caused by less pathogenic strains of staphylococci, such as nonhemolytic coagulase-negative strains, progresses less dramatically and not necessarily with obvious abscess formation. However, the same components of granulation tissue and fibrosis are present, causing obstruction and pressure, which in turn cause atrophy of adjacent lobules.

Coliform Mastitis. Coliform mastitis occurs when Gram-negative bacteria from the environment contaminate the opening of the papillary duct and ascend. Currently, the most common coliform bacteria in veterinary medicine are *Escherichia coli*, *Enterobacter aerogenes*, and *Klebsiella pneumoniae*. Coliform bacteria probably exert their damaging effect via endotoxin and subsequent cytokine release acting on the vasculature. In the severe form of the disease, the lesions are hyperemia, hemorrhage, and edema of the affected areas centered on the lactiferous ducts. The fluid in the lactiferous sinus is cloudy and blood stained and has clumps of fibrin (Fig. 18-54). Microscopically, interlobular septa are edematous and fibrin thrombi form in lymph vessels. Epithelium of ducts and alveoli is necrotic, and only low numbers of inflammatory cells are observed. Coliform bacteria are numerous within both the alveoli and the epithelium. The severity of the disease in postparturient cows is attributed to a delay in the influx of neutrophils. The cow's response to endotoxin is influenced by the stage of the reproductive cycle. Nonlactating mammary glands are much less sensitive to the effects of endotoxin than are lactating glands.

If the cow survives endotoxemia, the necrotic mammary tissue, which can be a large portion of a mamma, separates from the viable tissue and is sequestered or eventually sloughs (Fig. 18-55). Cows in early lactation with less severe coliform mastitis often develop

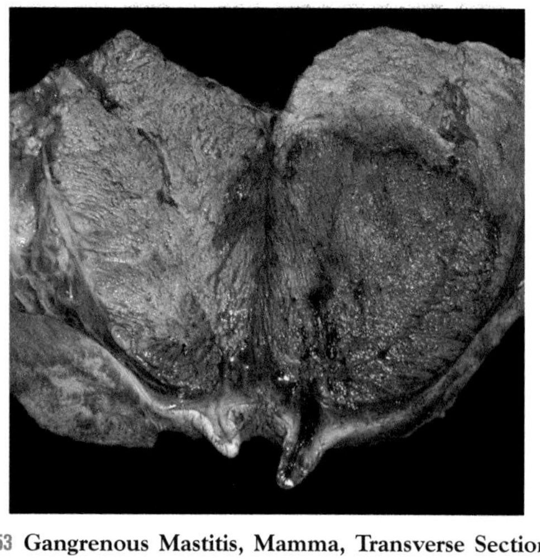

Figure 18-53 Gangrenous Mastitis, Mamma, Transverse Section, Cow. Most of the right quarter and some of the adjacent left quarter are dark red with hemorrhage. A well-demarcated hyperemic (darker red) border has formed at its junction with the adjacent normal gland *(right udder)*. There is also marked subcutaneous edema between the gland and the skin. (Courtesy Dr. R.A. Foster, Ontario Veterinary College, University of Guelph.)

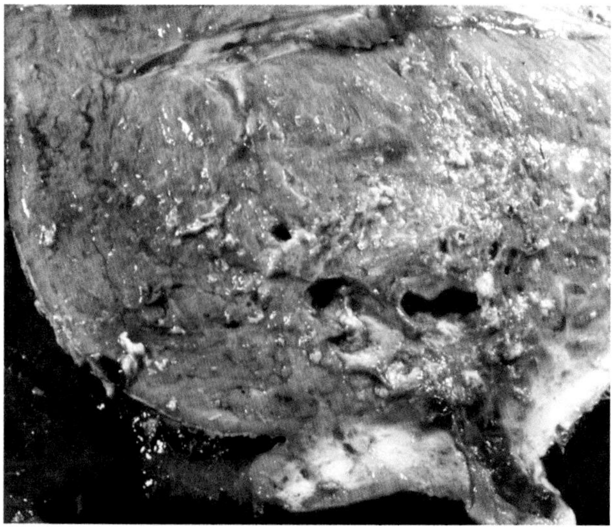

Figure 18-54 Coliform Mastitis, Mamma, Cow. There is marked thickening of the walls of the lactiferous ducts. White to yellow fibrin and pus have collected in the lactiferous ducts and the upper portion of the lactiferous sinus. (Courtesy College of Veterinary Medicine, University of Illinois.)

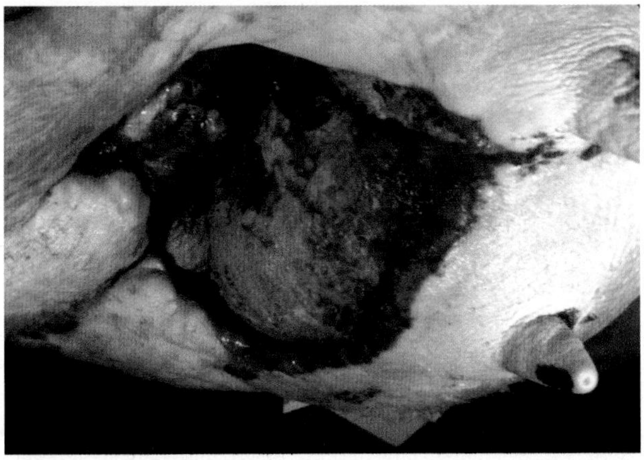

Figure 18-55 **Sloughed Quarter, Necrotizing Mastitis, Mamma, Cow.** The necrotic right rear mamma has recently sloughed, leaving a large ulcerated area covered by a thin gray layer of exudate. The surface of the ulcer is finely granular, indicating the formation of granulation tissue. (Courtesy College of Veterinary Medicine, University of Illinois.)

suppurative or subclinical mastitis that microscopically has hyperplasia, disorganization, and filiform processes of the epithelial lining of the papillary duct and lactiferous sinus.

***Mycoplasma* Mastitis.** *Mycoplasma* mastitis in cows occurs as individual sporadic cases or in outbreaks. Several mycoplasmas are capable of causing bovine mastitis, but *Mycoplasma bovis* is the most prevalent. The disease caused by *Mycoplasma bovis* can affect one, some, or all mammae; mycoplasmas inoculated into one mamma often spread to some or all mammae. Hematogenous spread and contamination of the papilla are therefore routes by which the mammae become infected. Affected quarters initially are enlarged, firm, and light brown and have a nodular parenchyma. The nodules are abscesses that can be up to 10 cm in diameter. Large numbers of neutrophils are found in the lobular interstitium and alveoli in the early stages. This pattern changes with time to include lymphocytes and macrophages. Early vacuolation and degeneration of alveolar epithelium is followed by hyperplasia and then by squamous metaplasia. Eroded ductal epithelium is replaced by granulation tissue. Aggregates of lymphocytes occur in the lobular interstitium and around ducts. Interstitial fibrosis and lobular atrophy occur in the late stages. Spread of the organism to calves and resultant otitis, arthritis, and pneumonia can occur.

***Trueperella* Mastitis.** *Trueperella* (formally called *Arcanobacterium*) *pyogenes* causes mastitis in lactating, nonlactating, and even immature bovine mammary glands. It is a common environmental pathogen affecting cattle, and in mammae it induces abscesses in the small and large lactiferous ducts. Abscesses range from microscopic in size to those grossly visible. Fistulas from the abscesses can form at the base of the papilla. Fibrosis of the walls of the abscesses can result in loss of small unaffected ducts and involution and fibrosis of the parenchyma they drain.

Mastitis in Sheep and Goats

The two main microbes recovered from the mammae of sheep are *Mannheimia haemolytica* and *Staphylococcus aureus*. In many sheep flocks, the main manifestation of infection with these microbes is unexpected death because these bacteria are responsible for a severe necrotizing or gangrenous mastitis. The morbidity can be approximately 5% and mortality 20%. Mastitis in goats is similar, and as with the disease in sheep, it is assumed to have a similar pathogenesis to the disease in cattle. For mycoplasmal mastitis, *Mycoplasma agalactiae* or *Mycoplasma mycoides* ssp. *mycoides* are usually the causative microbes.

Goats infected with caprine arthritis encephalitis virus (CAEV) can develop "hard udder." The udder is hard, and little milk can be expressed from the papilla. Recovery occurs, but milk production is reduced. Histologically, there are large numbers of lymphocytes and lymphoid follicles in the interstitium between the glandular alveolae. The virus grows in mammary epithelium and is present in milk. The newborn is infected through infected milk. A similar disease in sheep is seen with infection with maedi-visna virus (MVV). The pathogenesis is provided in more detail in Chapters 4 and 9. Briefly, the virus is spread through respiratory secretions rather than milk, and the virus replicates in macrophages and results in slowly progressive lesions with large numbers of lymphocytes and plasma cells in many organs, with the mamma being one.

Disorders of Pigs

Disorders of the female reproductive system that affect sows, but that are not unique to sows, are discussed in the section on Disorders of Domestic Animals.

Female Reproductive System

Ovary

The most common lesion of the ovary of pigs is cystic ovarian disease. See the section on Disorders of Domestic Animals, Ovary.

Uterine Tubes

See the section on Disorders of Domestic Animals, Uterine Tubes.

Uterus

Metritis, as part of mastitis, metritis, and agalactia (MMA) syndrome, is an important disease of the sow uterus. See the section on Disorders of Domestic Animals, Uterus.

Cervix

See the section on Disorders of Domestic Animals, Cervix.

Vulva and Vagina

Vaginal and Vulval Hypertrophy. Toxicosis of pigs caused by the mycotoxin zearalenone found in *Fusarium* sp.–infected grain and corn is a cause of vaginal and vulval hypertrophy, particularly in prepubertal gilts (see Fig. 18-25). The toxin is a nonsteroidal estrogen that binds to the estrogen receptor. The vaginal and vulval lesions are stromal edema. Other effects of the mycotoxin are altered time of first estrus, both early and late; reduced numbers of live embryos; prominent ovarian follicles; endometrial hyperplasia; and precocious mammary development.

Fetus and Placenta

Failure of Pregnancy. The principles of diagnosis used in other species apply to pigs (the presence or absence of lesions, the presence or absence of infectious disease, and disease of mother, fetus, or placenta); however, the approach in intensive pig production is different and more epidemiologic in nature. Strict biosecurity has eliminated many potential diseases.

For the majority of causes, there are no fetal or placental lesions and the testing for infectious microbes is more microbiologic and molecular (i.e., polymerase chain reaction [PCR]) in nature.

Noninfectious Failure of Pregnancy. There are many potential noninfectious causes of failure of pregnancy, and approximately 70% of cases have no recognized infectious cause. Many fetal anomalies and goiter are readily identified, but most others are not. There are often no lesions in the mother, placenta, or fetus. Seasonal infertility wherein there is failure of pregnancy at a regular time each year is very common in large production units. It may be in the summer, when heat is implicated, or in the fall or with the onset of cold weather. This diagnosis is based on the appropriate history and a failure to identify other causes.

Infectious Failure of Pregnancy

Viral Infections. Viral diseases are the most important infectious causes of pregnancy failure in pigs. Porcine reproductive and respiratory syndrome virus (PRRSV), porcine parvovirus (PPV), porcine circovirus 2 (PCV-2), and pseudorabies virus (PRV; Suid herpesvirus 1) are the most important viruses.

Porcine Reproductive and Respiratory Syndrome. PRRSV, an Arterivirus, is transmitted horizontally through body fluids and vertically to the fetuses of those sows without immunity. Transplacental infection of pig fetuses causes abortion, usually in the later stages of pregnancy, but there are seldom macroscopic and microscopic lesions in the fetuses or placentas. The diagnosis is based on evidence of herd exposure, maternal serology, and virus isolation. Lesions, when present, are segmental or diffuse hemorrhage in the umbilical cord as a result of necrotizing umbilical arteritis. Ascites, hydrothorax, and edema of perirenal tissue, splenic ligament, and mesentery are seen in some fetuses. Microscopically, a segmental arteritis occurs in the umbilicus and fetal lungs, heart, and kidneys. Alveolar septal walls in the lungs are thickened by lymphocytes and histiocytes and also by proliferation of type 2 pneumocytes. Aggregates of lymphocytes, plasma cells, and macrophages are present in blood vessels in the heart, portal tracts, and cerebellar white matter. Endometritis and myometritis also occur with edema and lymphocytes and histiocytes in the interstitium and around uterine vessels.

Porcine Parvovirus. PPV is an important cause of embryonic and fetal loss and causes death and mummification of affected fetal pigs (Fig. 18-56). Sows usually are not ill, but fetuses are infected and die at varying stages—all in the one pregnancy. This outcome suggests fetus-to-fetus transmission within the uterus. The characteristic findings in fetuses therefore are some fresh fetuses and then varying stages of autolysis and mummification, with the most mummified fetuses being the smallest. This pattern indicates that fetal death occurs at different stages of gestation. Microscopically, fetuses that are infected after immunocompetence has developed have widespread lymphocytes and plasma cells in the liver, lungs, kidneys, and cerebellum.

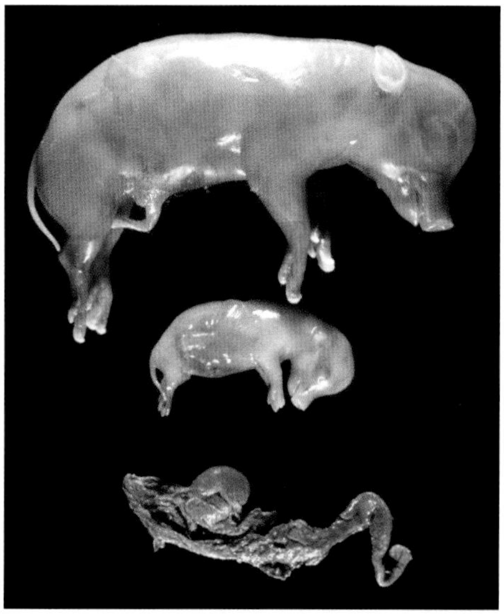

Figure 18-56 **Stillbirth, Mummification, Embryonic Death and Infertility (SMEDI), Abortion, Pig Fetus.** Viruses, such as porcine parvovirus and porcine enteroviruses, induce SMEDI. These viruses affect the fetuses to differing degrees and at different stages of gestation. Those fetuses that die early in gestation are usually mummified *(bottom fetus)* or resorbed. (Courtesy College of Veterinary Medicine, University of Illinois.)

Porcine Circovirus 2. PCV-2 is capable of causing reproductive failure at any stage of gestation. The virus crosses the placenta and replicates in lymphoid tissues. Death of the fetus and expulsion occurs without macroscopic or microscopic lesions. Some affected litters have fresh, autolyzed, and mummified fetuses. Interstitial edema of the heart, a lymphocytic interstitial myocarditis, and ascites and hepatic congestion of heart failure may occur.

Pseudorabies Herpes Virus. PHV (Suid herpesvirus 1; SHV-1) is eradicated from many jurisdictions. It can cause typical herpesviral lesions (see Chapters 4, 8, and 9) in porcine fetuses, and it is one of the few examples in which typical herpes inclusion bodies (see Figs. 8-45 and 9-32) are seen in the chorion.

Bacterial Infections. Numerous bacteria are implicated in pregnancy failure. Any bacteria that become bacteremic could localize in the placenta and cause failure of pregnancy; they are listed in Tables 18-2 and 18-4. The bacteria that are especially important are *Brucella suis* and *Leptospira* sp.

Brucella Suis. Brucella suis causes failure of pregnancy, but the disease in pigs differs in several respects from brucellosis in ruminants. Suppurative endometritis, focal granulomas, and multiple hyperplastic lymphoid nodules may occur in the endometrium of nonpregnant sows. Endometrial glands become distended with neutrophils, and the luminal epithelium is lost and focally has squamous metaplasia. In pregnancy, the lumen of the uterus between placentas has mucopurulent exudate in which trophoblasts contain intracellular bacteria. The chorioallantois has edema and some focal hemorrhage. Microscopically, there are many neutrophils in the tissue, necrotic debris on the chorionic surface, and loss of trophoblasts.

Leptospirosis. Leptospirosis is an important cause of failure of pregnancy. The pathogenesis is similar to that of cattle and is discussed in Chapters 4 and 11. *Leptospira interrogans* serovar *pomona* is commonly isolated. Sows abort after a bacteremic phase, and there are no placental lesions. Fetuses become septicemic, die, and are autolytic. Some develop nephritis and/or neutrophils may be found in the peritoneal serosa.

Mammae

Disorders of the mammae that affect sows, but that are not unique to sows, are discussed in the section on Disorders of Domestic Animals.

Agalactia

Agalactia in sows is often part of a postpartum syndrome known as mastitis, metritis, and agalactia (MMA) or the postpartum dysgalactia syndrome. Affected sows have insufficient production of colostrum and milk during the first days postpartum, and they have mastitis and pyrexia. The piglets get insufficient colostrum and milk with subsequent development of a negative energy balance, secondary infection, diarrhea, and death. Agalactia is thought to be a failure of responsiveness of the mammary gland to oxytocin. There is a genetic predisposition for this disease.

Mastitis

Coliform, staphylococcal and streptococcal mastitis in pigs are presumed to have the same pathogenesis as in cattle and are discussed in the section on Disorders of Ruminants (Cattle, Sheep, and Goats), Mammae.

Disorders of Dogs

Female Reproductive System

Disorders of the female reproductive system that affect bitches, but that are not unique to bitches, are discussed in the section on Disorders of Domestic Animals.

Ovary

The common lesions of the ovary of the dog are mostly cysts within (cystic rete ovarii) and around the ovary (cystic remnants of the paramesonephric duct or mesonephric tubules or duct) and also neoplasms including both sex cord stromal tumors and carcinomas. The carcinomas usually develop in the subsurface epithelial structures of the dog and can be multifocal. These disorders and other diseases are discussed in the section on Disorders of Domestic Animals, Ovary.

Uterine Tubes

Diseases of the uterine tubes of dogs are rare and are discussed in the section on Disorders of Domestic Animals, Uterine Tubes.

Uterus

Noninflammatory Disorders

Subinvolution of Placental Sites. Subinvolution of placental sites is a disease unique to the bitch. It is the persistence of placental sites in the uterus after parturition beyond the normal 12 weeks. In the normal canine placenta, trophoblasts are found in the endometrium and around the blood vessels of the myometrium, but they rapidly degenerate in the postpartum period. Subinvolution of placental sites is identified clinically by an excessive bloody vaginal discharge that lasts for weeks or months after delivery instead of the normal 1 to 6 weeks. Grossly, subinvoluted placental sites are approximately twice as wide as normal sites for the same time after parturition, but their appearance is identical to normal except that fibrin adherent to the site is more prominent (Fig. 18-57). As such, multiple segmental thickenings of the walls of the uterine horns are visible from the serosal surface. The luminal surface of each site is a raised, rough, ragged, gray to brown plaque of hemorrhage and fibrin. Microscopically, the luminal part of the plaque consists of cell debris, hematoma, fibrin, and regenerating endometrium. In the deeper part of the site, the changes are an abundance of an eosinophilic matrix, hemorrhage, distention, and decreased density of endometrial glands. Trophoblasts appear to be more numerous in subinvolution sites than in normally involuting placental sites and are abundant at the deepest portion of the eosinophilic matrix; these cells can invade the myometrium and penetrate the full thickness of and perforate the wall of the uterus. Affected animals have a prolonged bloody discharge and can become anemic, and those dogs with coagulation disorders, such as von Willebrand's disease, can exsanguinate. The uterus is prone to develop ascending infection, endometritis, and open pyometra.

Pseudopregnancy. Pseudopregnancy is an exaggerated form of a normal physiologic process. Every nonovariectomized female dog has a prolonged luteal phase of estrus, and this phase is called *covert pseudopregnancy* or *physiologic pseudopregnancy*. Some dogs, especially of the toy breeds, develop an exaggerated reaction. The mechanism is poorly understood, but prolactin or its receptors play a role. The presence of progesterone is necessary for the tissue changes to occur. Overtly pseudopregnant dogs either have an increased concentration of prolactin or have increased sensitivity to prolactin. This prolactin milieu can occur with a more rapid than usual decline in progesterone when dogs are spayed during diestrus. Hyperprolactinemia that occurs in response to visual stimuli of the presence of surrogate neonates results in the mammary development, lactation, maternal behavior, and other clinically apparent changes of pseudopregnancy. Uterine changes in pseudopregnancy can include the formation of structures that resemble placental sites (now called *localized endometrial hyperplasia of pseudopregnancy* or *pseudoplacentation endometrial hyperplasia*) and mucometra; obviously there are no fetuses.

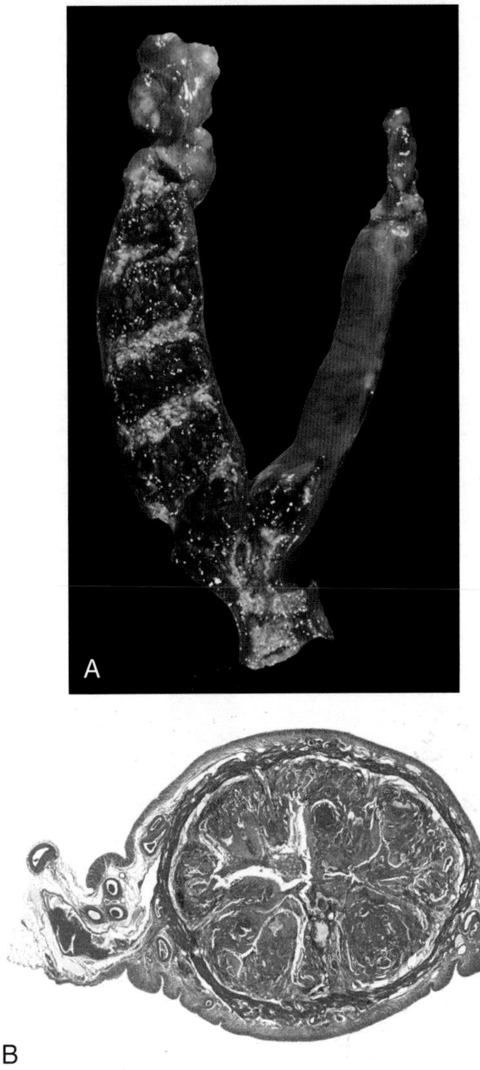

Figure 18-57 Subinvolution of Placental Sites, Uterus, Bitch. A, Incompletely involuted placental sites. The red transverse stripes are placental sites with hemorrhage, fibrin, and necrotic debris. They are larger than normal sites for the same stage after parturition and remain long after normal sites would have disappeared (12 to 15 weeks postpartum). **B,** Transverse section of the uterus at a subinvoluted placental site. The two pink outer layers are normal myometrium and underlying endometrial stroma. Most of the distended lumen is filled with large irregularly sized clots of blood, fibrin, and necrotic debris around which are endometrial epithelium and trophoblasts. H&E stain. (Courtesy Dr. M.D. McGavin, College of Veterinary Medicine, University of Tennessee.)

Adenomyosis. Adenomyosis is the presence of endometrial epithelial tissue within the myometrium. Its appearance is identical to that of the endometrial glands, and it usually is surrounded by endometrial stroma. It becomes cystically distended and contains cell debris, keratin if there is squamous metaplasia, and inflammatory exudate. Some bitches develop such severe adenomyosis that it causes dramatic thickening of the uterine wall particularly in the uterine body.

Neoplasms

Uterine Smooth Muscle Tumors. Smooth muscle tumors in the bitch often occur in the cervix and vagina, and they occasionally occur in the uterus (Fig. 18-58, *A* and *B*). Estrogens likely have a role in maintaining these neoplasms because ovariectomy can result in the disappearance of surgically inaccessible tumors. In other domestic species, however, these neoplasms are rare and tend to be solitary. They are well demarcated, unencapsulated, spheric, and vary in size. If they are small, they are confined within the wall of the vagina, cervix, or uterus or can protrude into the lumen or project to the serosal surface of the uterus or into the pelvic canal. Some luminal neoplasms, especially those in the vagina, are susceptible to trauma or necrosis. They are usually firm, pink or white, and occasionally calcified or edematous. The color is related to the amount of fibrous tissue present along with the whorled smooth muscle cells; in the macroscopically white neoplasms, fibrous tissue is the dominant component. The vast majority of smooth muscle tumors are benign and metastasis is rare. There are no recognizable histological features of malignancy/potential metastasis. Although they are classified as leiomyomas or leiomyosarcomas, the prognosis is the same.

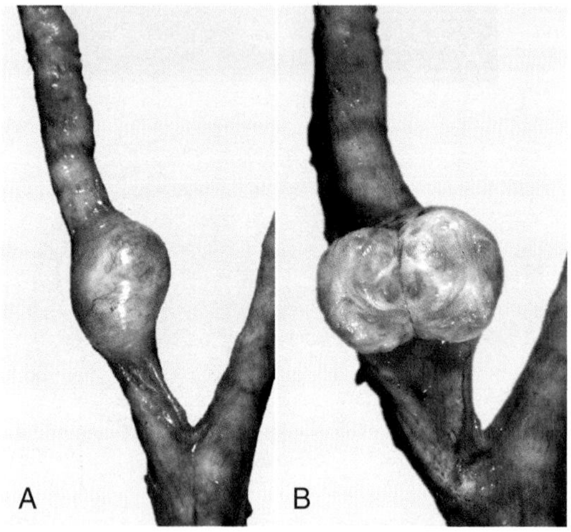

Figure 18-58 Smooth Muscle Tumor, Uterus, Bitch. A, Note the well-circumscribed, firm mass in the left uterine horn. **B,** The cut section of the leiomyoma reveals gelatinous content and bands of smooth muscle and connective tissue. This mass is within and arising from the myometrium. (Courtesy Dr. D.D. Harrington, College of Veterinary Medicine, Purdue University; and Noah's Arkive, College of Veterinary Medicine, The University of Georgia.)

Cervix

Diseases of the cervix, apart from uterine diseases, are very rare. Diseases of the cervix are discussed in the section on Disorders of Domestic Animals, Cervix.

Vulva and Vagina

Vaginitis or Vulvitis. In bitches, so-called nonspecific vaginitis or vulvitis is common. The lesions range from acute vaginitis to chronic granular vulvitis (see previous section).

Vaginal Hyperplasia. Vaginal hyperplasia, hypertrophy, and/or prolapse of bitches are common diseases seen during the follicular stage (proestrus) of the first to third estrus periods in young animals, particularly of the brachiocephalic breeds. An increased sensitivity to estrogen is assumed, and there is excessive edema of the submucosal tissues of the vagina. The vaginal mucosa swells and interferes with coitus. Dramatic swelling can, if severe, result in vaginal tissue protruding from the vulva that becomes excoriated and ulcerated. Spontaneous regression during diestrus is the norm.

Vaginal Polyps. Vaginal polyps are relatively common in older, usually intact bitches (see Fig. 18-26). They are often solitary, up to several centimeters in diameter, and have a thin stalk of attachment to the vaginal wall. Most are located on the ventral floor of the vagina. They are indistinguishable from leiomyomas macroscopically. Excision is usually curative.

Canine Transmissible Venereal Tumor. Canine transmissible venereal tumor (CTVT) of dogs is transmitted at coitus by the transfer of intact neoplastic cells. CTVT cells have 59 chromosomes compared with the normal canine karyotype of 78 chromosomes. Immunohistochemical evaluation suggests a histiocytic phenotype. Both sexes are affected. The neoplasm begins as a nodule beneath the vaginal or vestibular mucosa and when enlarged, breaks through the overlying mucosa. The lesion often begins in the dorsal wall of the vagina at the junction with the vestibule. It bulges into the lumen of the vagina and can protrude through the vulva as an ulcerated, friable mass (Fig. 18-59, *A*). Microscopically, the neoplastic cells are large, round or oval, and uniform in size (Fig. 18-59, *B*) but with occasional large, bizarre nuclei. The cytoplasm is pale staining and may have peripheral vacuoles. Lymphocyte-mediated

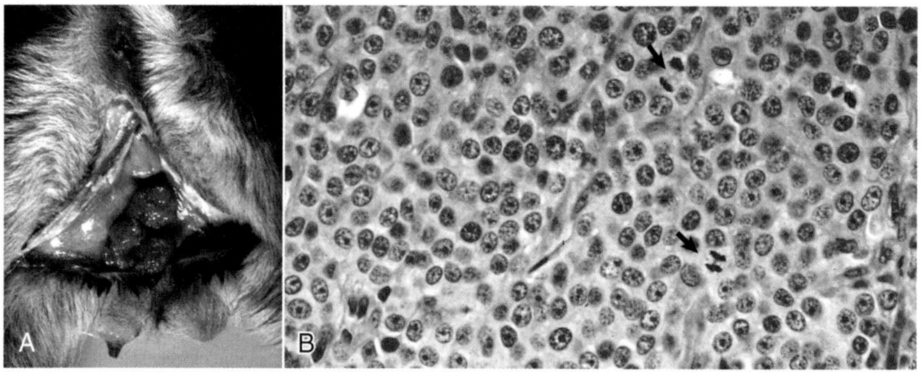

Figure 18-59 Canine Transmissible Venereal Tumor (CTVT), Vulva and Vagina, Bitch. A, The multinodular tumors markedly distend the lumens of the vagina and vestibule and are grossly characteristic of CTVT. **B,** Neoplastic cells are round and often divided into packets by a fine fibrous stroma. Mitoses are frequent *(arrows)*. H&E stain. (**A** courtesy Dr. J. King, College of Veterinary Medicine, Cornell University. **B** courtesy Dr. M.J. Abdy, College of Veterinary Medicine, The University of Georgia; and Noah's Arkive, College of Veterinary Medicine, The University of Georgia.)

cytotoxicity occurs in some cases and results in regression of tumors. This neoplasm is particularly sensitive to vincristine. In countries with stray dogs and dogs in poor health, metastases to other sites, especially the skin, are relatively common.

Smooth Muscle Tumors. Bitches develop single or multiple smooth muscle tumors (leiomyomas) of the vagina. These tumors usually only occur in intact (nonneutered) bitches, so a hormonal link is proposed. Ovariohysterectomy may be curative, further supporting a hormonal dependence. The common differential diagnosis of leiomyoma is vaginal polyps (see previous discussion). Histologic examination is usually required to differentiate them because each is a well-circumscribed nodule up to several centimeters in diameter arising from the vaginal wall (see Fig. 18-58). The likelihood of metastasis is very low.

Carcinomas. Carcinoma of the vagina in bitches is a recognized entity. Some clearly arise from the urethra, especially when they extend from the urethral orifice. Others arise from vaginal epithelium, but little is known of their cause. They are phenotypically similar to transitional cell carcinomas (see Chapter 11). The long-term prognosis is poor, but the prevalence of metastatic disease varies and urethral obstruction often is the complication that is difficult to control.

Fetus and Placenta

Failure of Pregnancy. Very little is published in the peer-reviewed literature about failure of pregnancy in dogs. There is much published about production animals, in which the economic importance of pregnancy failure provides an incentive to identify the cause and prevent further disease.

Noninfectious Failure of Pregnancy. The general approach to and causes of noninfectious failure of pregnancy in dogs are assumed to be similar to those of noninfectious failure of pregnancy as discussed in the section on Disorders of Domestic Animals, Fetus and Placenta, Failure of Pregnancy.

Infectious Failure of Pregnancy

Viral Infections

Canine Herpesvirus. Canid herpesvirus-1 (CaHV-1) is capable of causing failure of pregnancy, although it is far more likely to cause death of puppies up to 8 weeks of age. The lesions of herpesvirus infection of pups are similar to those of herpesviruses discussed in other species. In puppies, infection is acquired in the perinatal period from recrudescence of the virus in the bitch. Chilling of the puppies and the subsequent lower body temperature facilitates viral replication and viremic spread (see Chapter 11). Multifocal hemorrhage of the kidney is a characteristic change, and microscopically, there is widespread focal necrosis and hemorrhage with typical intranuclear herpesviral inclusion bodies (see Fig. 11-74).

Bacterial Infections

Brucella Canis. Brucella canis, as with other brucella, is acquired by the dog through oral (ingestion), nasal, conjunctival, or venereal transmission. Adult dogs acquiring the bacterium by ingestion initially develop lymphadenitis of the head and neck and bacteremia. Epididymitis and testicular degeneration are the lesions in male dogs, and pregnant females develop microscopic placentitis and fetal endocarditis, pneumonia, and hepatitis. Microscopically, there may be multifocal coagulative necrosis of the placenta and adjacent neutrophils and macrophages. Trophoblasts of the marginal hematoma and zonary placenta are packed with *Brucella* microbes, and there may be neutrophils within the chorion. Other possible fetal lesions include portal hepatitis, multifocal renal hemorrhage, and lymphadenitis.

Other Bacteria. There are reports of *Salmonella* sp., *Campylobacter jejuni*, *Streptococcus canis*, and *Leptospira* serovars causing abortion in dogs. Maternal illness and bacteremia result in infection of the placenta, but the lesions are mild and often are limited to a neutrophilic placentitis.

Protozoal Infections. *Toxoplasma gondii* and *Neospora caninum* both are uncommon causes of failure of pregnancy. Macroscopic lesions in fetuses are absent, and microscopically there may be focal necrosis of all tissues, but often protozoa can only be identified immunohistochemically.

Leishmania infantum is a reported cause of failure of pregnancy. Placental lesions are large numbers of amastigotes within trophoblasts of the zonary portion of the placenta. No lesions are reported in other tissues.

Mammae

Disorders of the mammae that affect bitches, but that are not unique to bitches, are discussed in the section on Disorders of Domestic Animals.

Infectious Diseases

Mastitis. In dogs, mastitis occurs early in lactation or pseudopregnancy. *Staphylococci* spp., *Streptococci* spp., and *Escherichia coli* are major isolates. Mycoplasma species are also occasionally identified. It is assumed that the pathogenetic pathways of mastitis in dogs are the same as those for dairy cows. Infection of fissures in papillae and adjacent skin spreads via the lactiferous ducts into the glands and results in suppurative inflammation and/or abscesses. The mamma becomes swollen, large, firm, and edematous because of the toxins and tissue destruction caused by the microbes, neutrophils granule contents, and cytokines. It may be superimposed on mammary hyperplasia or mammary neoplasia, especially with tumors of ducts. Systemic illness is often seen.

Neoplasms

Neoplasia of the mammary glands is common in the dog. The dog has the highest incidence of all domesticated species (Fig. 18-60). Most canine mammary tumors are clinically benign regardless of their phenotype. Even some classified as mammary carcinomas have

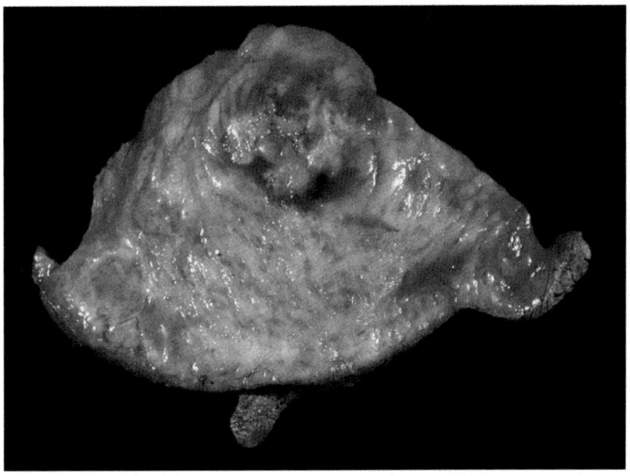

Figure 18-60 **Mammary Carcinoma, Mamma, Bitch.** This mammary carcinoma has infiltrated and replaced normal mammary gland and contiguous soft tissue. The upper nodule is the neoplasm, and the lower and surrounding white tissues are composed of infiltrating neoplastic cells and fibrous tissue, the result of a desmoplastic response. (Courtesy Dr. R.A. Foster, Ontario Veterinary College, University of Guelph.)

a low metastatic rate. However, it is most important to identify those tumors that have a high potential to be metastatic.

There has been much interest in canine mammary neoplasia from the viewpoint of prognosis and treatment, from a logical pathogenetic viewpoint, and as a tool in comparative oncogenesis. Although the phenomenon of mammary neoplasia is well recognized, the cause is not. Ovariohysterectomy after the second estrus dramatically increases the prevalence of this disease. The "window of susceptibility" is up to 2 years of age. A high-protein diet decreases susceptibility, whereas treatment with medroxyprogesterone acetate and being a purebred increase susceptibility.

Mammary neoplasms are a diverse group that are dominated by epithelial and combined epithelial and myoepithelial tumors. Sarcomas, such as fibrosarcoma and osteosarcoma, are much less common, but they are particularly aggressive and metastatic. The embryology of the mammary glands involves a close association between the epithelium and mesenchyme, so it is not surprising that tumors are often combinations of stroma and epithelium; these are the complex adenomas and carcinomas. The mixed mammary tumor is well known in the dog and has, in addition to myoepithelium and epithelium, cartilage and bone.

The development of mammary epithelial neoplasia can proceed from ductal or lobular hyperplasia to dysplasia and on to neoplasia and subsequent progression from benign adenoma to noninvasive carcinoma and to metastatic forms (Fig. 18-61). A bitch that develops a mammary tumor will often subsequently develop multiple mammary masses. The prognosis for each subsequent mass is not dependent on the previous one, and many different types of neoplasia can be found in the mammae of the same animal.

The presence of metastasis is the ultimate indication of a poor prognosis. Predicting the probability of metastasis in carcinomas is an inexact science. There are six main features that are prognostically significant for mammary tumors, and they are listed from worst prognosis to a better prognosis as follows:

- Metastasis to draining lymph node
- Intravascular tumor emboli
- Invasion at the periphery of the mass (peripheral invasion)
- Unique histological phenotypes
- Histologic grade including degree of dysplasia and mitotic rate
- Tumor size

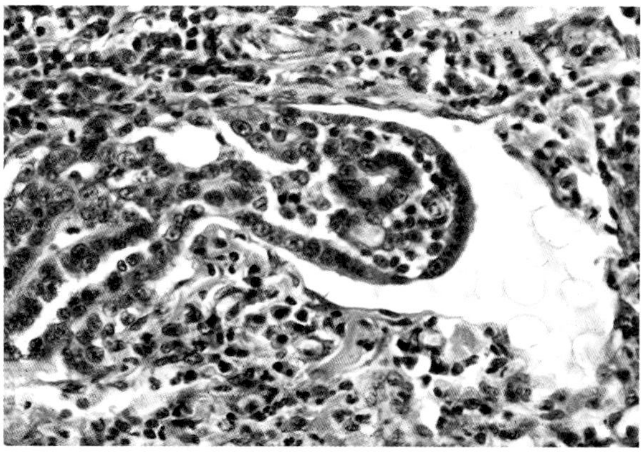

Figure 18-61 **Adenocarcinoma, Invasion Into Lymphatic Vessels, Bitch.** Note the neoplastic cells infiltrating through the wall of the lymphatic *(above left)*. Microscopic invasion by mammary carcinoma into a lymphatic, as depicted here, indicates a poor prognosis. In this case, there are lymphocytes and plasma cells in the perilymphatic tissues. H&E stain. (Courtesy Dr. M. Domingo, Autonomous University of Barcelona; and Noah's Arkive, College of Veterinary Medicine, The University of Georgia.)

Excisional biopsy and evaluation of the draining lymph nodes is the best procedure for diagnosis and prognosis in dogs; cytology can be useful in identifying inflammation and sarcomas but can give a false impression of malignancy in epithelial tumors. The neoplasms that arise are variable in their phenotypes; as such, the widely used World Health Organization classification scheme describes more than 30 types of mammary masses. The following information characterizes the prognostic significance of the behaviors of mammary tumors:

Lymph node metastasis: The presence of the metastasis has a very high correlation with a short survival interval after diagnosis. The 2-year survival is very low.

Intravascular invasion: Intravascular invasion is a prelude to the development of lymph node metastasis and to the survival of circulating neoplastic cells. Survival after diagnosis is much shorter with evidence of lymphatic invasion.

Peripheral invasion: The ability of neoplastic cells to invade the surrounding normal tissue is an early step in the development of metastasis. Those neoplasms that show invasion at the periphery of the neoplasm and, thus, are not well circumscribed are more likely to develop metastasis than well-defined/circumscribed tumors. Invasive carcinomas have a 2-year survival approximately half that of the well-demarcated tumors of the same phenotype.

Histological phenotype of neoplasm: Although there are many different types of mammary neoplasia in dogs, the less differentiated types are more likely to eventually result in death from metastasis. There is a progressive reduction in the survival for 1 or 2 years with papillary, tubular, solid, and anaplastic carcinoma subtypes. There are also some unique mammary carcinomas that have a very poor prognosis. These include the lipid-rich carcinoma, comedocarcinoma, micropapillary invasive carcinoma, and anaplastic carcinomas.

Histological grade: There is a mammary carcinoma grading scheme adapted for use in dogs. Carcinomas are divided into three grades: I, II, and III. The three histological characteristics that form this grade are percentage of tubule formation, nuclear pleomorphism, and mitotic count. Grade III tumors have a very poor prognosis.

Tumor size: Because there is a potential for progression from benign to malignant neoplasms (either because of rapid growth or having additional time to develop), those tumors larger than 3 cm and especially 5 cm in diameter have a poorer prognosis.

Male dogs can develop mammary tumors, but they are rare and usually benign.

Disorders of Cats

Female Reproductive System

Disorders of the female reproductive system that affect queens, but that are not unique to queens, are discussed in the section on Disorders of Domestic Animals.

Ovary

The most common ovarian lesion in the cat is ovarian remnants from inadequate surgical removal in ovariohysterectomy. Ovarian disorders are discussed in the section on Disorders of Domestic Animals, Ovary.

Uterine Tubes

Disease of the feline uterus tube is rare, and the lesions are discussed in the section on Disorders of Domestic Animals, Uterine Tubes.

Uterus

Cystic endometrial hyperplasia, endometrial polyps, and pyometra are the most common diseases of the feline uterus. The lesions are discussed in the section on Disorders of Domestic Animals, Uterus.

Cervix

Primary disease of the cervix is exceptionally rare and is discussed in the section on Disorders of Domestic Animals, Cervix.

Vulva and Vagina

Disorders of the vulva and vagina are rare and are discussed in the section on Disorders of Domestic Animals, Vulva and Vagina.

Fetus and Placenta

Failure of Pregnancy. Failure of pregnancy in cats is approached in an identical manner to that of the dog and other domestic species. Noninfectious failures of pregnancy are similar to those discussed previously for other species. Infectious causes of failure of pregnancy based on direct or epidemiologic data include feline herpesvirus 1, feline leukemia virus, feline panleukopenia virus, and feline infectious peritonitis virus. Failure of pregnancy appears to result from maternal illness rather than from placental or fetal lesions. Bacterial causes of failure of pregnancy include *Coxiella burnetii* and *Salmonella* spp.

Mammae

Disorders of the mammae that affect queens, but that are not unique to queens, are discussed in the section on Disorders of Domestic Animals.

Noninfectious Disorders

Fibroadenomatous Hyperplasia. Fibroadenomatous hyperplasia (mammary hypertrophy) is highly prevalent and is the most common disease of the gland; it occurs in young intact queens. Queens younger than 2 years of age are most likely to develop mammary enlargement, which usually occurs in the spring and with the first several estrous cycles. Much of what is known about this disease is based on its coinciding with the luteal phase of estrus, early in pregnancy, or after progestin therapy. High concentrations of progesterone or progesterone-like substances are the common link. As expected, progestogen treatment of an old neutered male or female can also induce this lesion. What is difficult to explain is the distribution of the lesion because all mammae, only one mamma, or one mammary gland may be affected. The lesion is proliferation of mammary ducts and adjacent stroma (Fig. 18-62). This overstimulation of an otherwise normal process is the result of a dysregulation of tissue growth with the stimulation of receptors by progesterone. Some have theorized an exaggerated response to prolactin as well. Hemorrhages, coagulative necrosis, and/or ulceration of affected areas can occur. In young queens, resolution is spontaneous or ovariohysterectomy is effective. Older neutered queens on a progestogen require drug withdrawal and sometimes mastectomy.

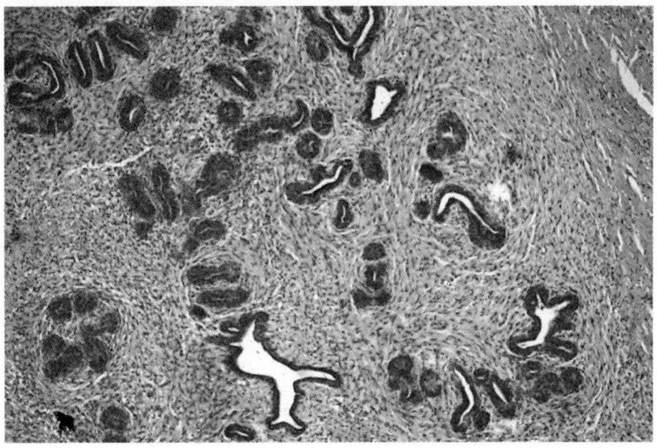

Figure 18-62 **Mammary Hypertrophy (Fibroadenomatous Hyperplasia), Mamma, Cat.** Mammary ducts have proliferated and are surrounded by abundant loosely arranged stromal tissues. Typically, cats with mammary hypertrophy are young and develop enlargement of one or several mammae in the spring. H&E stain. (Courtesy Dr. W. Crowell, College of Veterinary Medicine, The University of Georgia; and Noah's Arkive, College of Veterinary Medicine, The University of Georgia.)

Neoplasms

Mammary neoplasia in cats is relatively uncommon, so studies of causal factors are limited. There is not the same relationship with early neutering as there is with dogs. Progression from focal hyperplasia to adenoma to carcinoma is recognized, but this progression is presumably rapid because many of the carcinomas are small. The majority of neoplasms in cats are carcinomas, and they metastasize. They are usually single and occur in the tissue adjacent to the nipple; 75% to 96% are adenocarcinomas and show rapid growth (Fig. 18-63). They metastasize to regional lymph nodes (axillary or the superficial inguinal nodes), lungs, or other mammary glands. The average age of affected animals is 11 years, and there is a 7- to 9-year-old risk plateau. Intact animals are at a slightly greater risk, but the effect of spaying is controversial. Prognosis is based on the presence of lymph node metastasis, lymphovascular invasion, the histological grade, and the size of the mass. The poorest prognosis is when affected cats are older and have carcinomas with metastasis to regional lymph nodes, lymphovascular invasion, a histological grade III, and neoplasms that are greater than 3 cm in diameter. The interval between diagnosis and death is often short, less than 1 year, but the range is wide. Well-differentiated tumors (histological grade I) have a good prognosis.

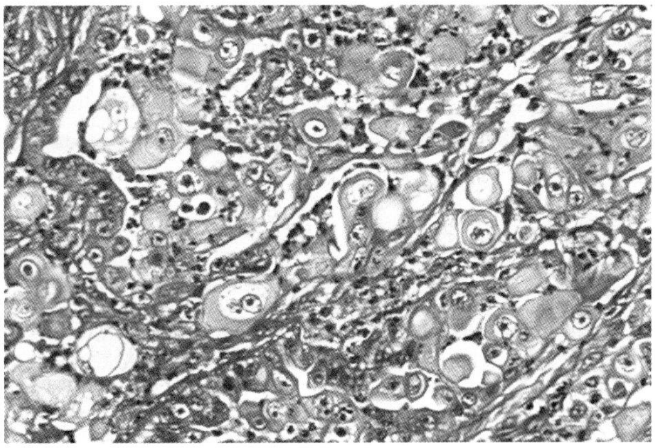

Figure 18-63 **Mammary Carcinoma, Mamma, Cat.** The cells of this anaplastic neoplasm do not resemble those of normal epithelium but are large and round. They are arranged either in clusters or as individual cells within a fibrous stroma. Inflammatory cells, including neutrophils and lymphocytes, are also present. H&E stain. (Courtesy College of Veterinary Medicine, University of Illinois.)

Suggested Readings

Suggested Readings are available at www.expertconsult.com.

CHAPTER 19

Male Reproductive System[1]

Robert A. Foster

Key Readings Index

The male reproductive system is critical for the survival of a species. In production animal industries, successful reproduction is essential for the continued supply of labor, meat, fiber, milk, or other products. Most production animal units rely on a small number of males as breeding stock, so in addition to being 50% of the reproductive team, an infertile male or one carrying an undesirable genetic trait can have a major impact on the unit's productivity.

Infertility in the male is difficult to reverse unless the cause can be readily found and corrected. Determining the cause is where knowledge of disease processes, responses to injury, and prognoses are so important.

Research in understanding disorders of reproduction in production animals is well established and is also increasing in companion animals. Therefore, the aim herein is to emphasize male reproductive disorders of both production and companion animal species and highlight the mechanisms and reactions of the male reproductive tract by examining the disorders of each major anatomic location.

Structure[2]

The male reproductive tract is divided into three major areas based on anatomic location, function, and important disease processes. These areas are the scrotum and its contents, the accessory genital glands, and the penis and prepuce.

The Scrotum and Contents

The purpose of the scrotum and its contents is to produce spermatozoa and hormones, especially testosterone. Although the general focus in this chapter is on the testis and the germinal cells contained in the seminiferous tubules, other parts of the contents, such as vaginal tunics and the spermatic cord (deferent duct, pampiniform plexus, and cremaster muscle), have important functions that allow spermatogenesis and the transportation of sperm to the female to occur successfully. Testicular development is quiescent from birth until puberty when spermatogenesis begins. The testes therefore are small until puberty, when they increase to their adult size. They are covered by a capsule (once called the *tunica albuginea*), which is relatively nonexpansile and usually maintains the testicular contents under slight pressure. Within the testis are interstitial and intratubular regions. The interstitium (i.e., intertubular or interstitial region) contains interstitial endocrine cells (previously called Leydig cells), blood and lymphatic vessels, and immune cells such as macrophages, dendritic cells, mast cells, and T lymphocytes (Fig. 19-1). Each seminiferous tubule has a lining of myoid cells (smooth muscle cell–like functions) and a limiting membrane (see Fig. 19-1). There is a basement membrane between these structures. The arrangement of the seminiferous tubule within the testis varies from species to species, but the end result is the formation of spermatozoa. After spermatogenesis, spermatozoa are transported through rete tubules into the efferent ductules and then into the epididymis, a single and extremely long duct. In doing so, the spermatozoa mature and are concentrated. The pathway out of the scrotal area is through the deferent duct (commonly called the vas).

The purpose of the scrotum, vaginal tunics, and spermatic cord (deferent duct, pampiniform plexus, and cremaster muscle) is to protect and maintain spermatogenesis at a temperature slightly lower than body temperature. The testes are raised or lowered according to ambient temperature by the cremaster and scrotal dartos muscles. Furthermore, there is a countercurrent vascular system that allows the testes to be at a lower temperature than body temperature; the pampiniform plexus assists this process. The pulsatile nature of arterial blood flow is altered to form a continuous and lower pressure system. In addition, the scrotal skin, which is thin, often hairless, and in most species has abundant apocrine sweat glands, helps to dissipate heat and maintain a lower testicular and epididymal temperature. The vaginal tunic, which is an outpouching of the peritoneum, allows for free movement of the testes within the scrotal sac. The scrotum is composed of skin, dartos muscle, and scrotal fascia. It is fused with the parietal layer of the vaginal tunic.

Cell Types

Cell types of the scrotal contents include germ cells and spermatozoa; Sertoli cells; interstitial endocrine (Leydig) cells; epithelial cells lining the various ducts, such as the rete tubules, efferent ductules, and epididymides; and cells forming accessory genital glands.

---

[1]For a glossary of abbreviations and terms used in this chapter, see E-Glossary 19-1.

[2]Methods for examining the male reproductive tract are discussed in E-Appendix 19-1.

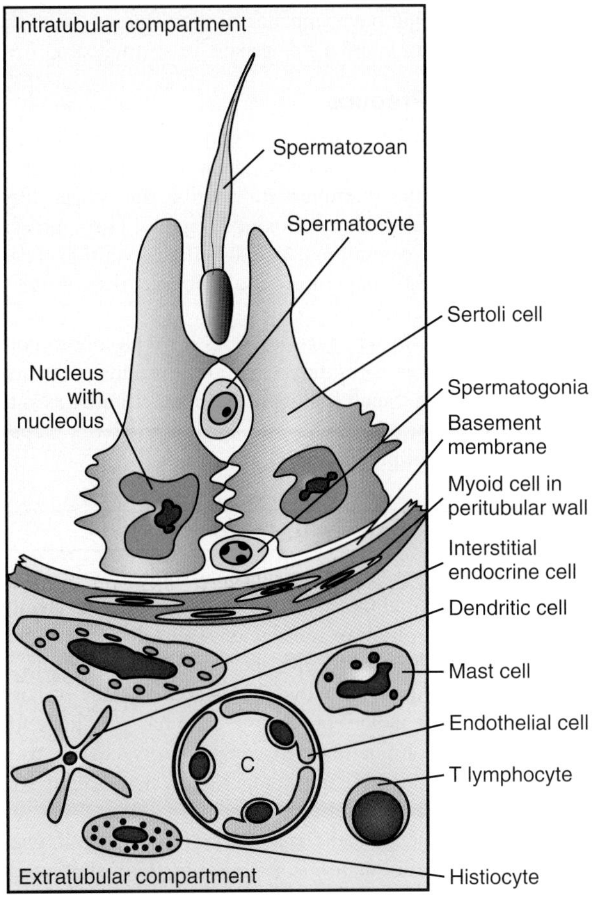

Figure 19-1 Schematic Diagram of the Normal Components of the Testis. The Sertoli cells, germ cells, and interstitial endocrine cells are closely integrated, and considerable messaging occurs between them. The blood-testis barrier is at the level of the Sertoli cells, with contributions from the myoid cells and basement membrane. Spermatogonia are on the interstitial side of the blood-testis barrier. C, Capillary lumen.

Spermatozoa. Spermatozoa are formed from germ (stem) cells by a process called spermatogenesis. Spermatogenesis occurs in three stages: the proliferative, meiotic, and spermatogenic stages. The proliferative phase involves the mitotically active spermatogonia, the stem cells. They are present at the periphery of the seminiferous tubules on the basement membrane. The second phase is the meiotic phase, in which spermatocytes are formed. In the spermatogenic phase, spermatids and finally spermatozoa are formed. Spermatozoa have a head, body, and tail. The head contains the nucleus and an acrosome, which contains enzymes required for the penetration of the zona pellucida of the ovum. The body or midpiece contains mitochondria, and the tail is a flagellum.

Sertoli Cells. Sertoli cells provide support, nutrients, hormones, and cytokines to facilitate spermatogenesis. During spermatogenesis, the spermatogenic cells pass into a region that is separated from and external to the immune system of the body. The barrier is called the *blood-testis barrier*, and it is maintained by the Sertoli cells especially and also the basement membrane and peritubular cells (see Fig. 19-1). Control of spermatogenesis is achieved through a combination of both central (luteinizing hormone [LH] on the interstitial endocrine cells and follicle-stimulating hormone [FSH] on Sertoli cells) and local (paracrine and autocrine molecules, including testosterone) factors, and there is considerable "crosstalk" between germ cells, Sertoli cells, and interstitial endocrine cells. Local modification of spermatogenesis is achieved through increased or decreased apoptosis at any stage of development. Many of the disorders and conditions that affect spermatogenesis increase or decrease the apoptotic rate.

Interstitial Endocrine (Leydig) Cells. Interstitial endocrine cells are essential for normal testicular function. They produce testosterone to maintain secondary sexual characteristics, the accessory genital glands, and spermatogenesis. They also produce cytokines that, with testosterone, maintain the antiinflammatory environment of the testis. Normal crosstalk between interstitial endocrine cells and myoid cells of the seminiferous tubules, Sertoli cells, endothelial cells, and other cells of the intertubular compartment (see Fig. 19-1) is essential for the normal function of all components of the testis.

Epithelial Lining Cells. The cells lining the various ducts, including the rete tubules, efferent ductules, and epididymides, are epithelial cells with a variety of functions, in addition to being a barrier. Absorption, phagocytosis, and secretion are part of their physiologic role. Movement of spermatozoa along these ducts and tubules is achieved through peritubular smooth muscle contraction and cilia.

Cells Forming Accessory Genital Glands. In the accessory genital glands (see the next section), storage of spermatozoa (particularly in the ampulla, where present) and secretion of various substances are the major roles for the epithelium of these glands. From the pelvic urethra and through the penile urethra, the lining cells are urothelial (i.e., transitional epithelium) in type.

The Accessory Genital Glands

The structure of the accessory glands provides the microenvironment for the storage, transport, and release of spermatozoa. Furthermore, the accessory glands provide nutrition and a transport medium for spermatozoa. There are four main accessory glands: the ampullae of the deferent duct, vesicular glands, prostate, and bulbourethral glands. There is considerable species variation in the size, type, and arrangement of these accessory glands. Horses and ruminants have all four glands, although the prostate of ruminants is either very small (bull) or disbursed within the pelvic urethra (ram and buck). Pigs lack ampullae, dogs have only a prostate, and cats have a prostate and bulbourethral glands. The secretion of the vesicular gland and prostate is serous, but the bulbourethral gland typically has a viscous mucoid product.

The Penis and Prepuce

There is considerable structural difference between the penis and prepuce of the various species. In prepubertal animals, the prepuce is completely attached to the penis, but they become separated at sexual maturity. The penis of the horse is erectile and is located within a prepuce that produces a thick, waxy material called *smegma*. Ruminants and pigs have a long fibrous penis that has some erectile tissue, a series of bends called the sigmoid flexure, and a retractor muscle to hold the penis in the prepuce. There is also an extension of the urethra in small ruminants that is called the *urethral process* (was also called the *vermiform appendage*). During ejaculation, this appendage spins and sprays semen onto the cervix. The head of the penis (was called the glans penis) of the boar has a corkscrew shape that allows it to insert into the cervix. The penis of dogs and to a lesser extent cats is erectile and has an os penis (a bone in the penis). When erect, the dog penis has lateral swellings called bulbs. All of the intrapreputial components and the bulbs of the dog penis are part of the head of the penis. The cat has projections of epithelium called *spines* or *barbs* on its penis, and they are testosterone dependent.

Function

The overall function of the male reproductive system is to provide genetic material (haploid number of chromosomes in each spermatozoon) to the female for combination (fertilization) with female genetic material (haploid number of chromosomes in each ovum) to produce offspring (zygotes) with a combined (diploid) and, it is hoped, better genetic makeup. In addition, the functions of the male reproductive system are the production of hormones, especially testosterone, and the production and transportation of spermatozoa. These goals are achieved by several separate areas—the scrotum and contents, accessory genital glands, and the penis and prepuce.

The Scrotum and Contents

The testes function to provide genetic material for transfer to the female. One-half of the chromosomes (haploid number) are produced by the process of meiosis in the seminiferous tubules in the process of spermatogenesis (see the section on cells of the male reproductive system). The interstitial endocrine (Leydig) cells of the testes produce the hormone testosterone to ensure development of male phenotypic, behavioral characteristics, and, where appropriate, the signals that stimulate females to come into heat and become receptive. The testis also produces other molecules for the regulation of spermatogenesis. Spermatozoa leave the testis in a high volume of fluid—the rete testis fluid—and enter the epididymis. The epididymis has the function of supporting and directing spermatozoal maturation and capacitation (the process by which sperm become capable of fertilizing an oocyte), so they can move and fertilize the oocyte, and concentrating spermatozoa for ejaculation. The function of the testis and epididymis depends on unique requirements, including maintenance of a temperature below body temperature and a continuous nonpulsatile blood flow. The scrotum provides protection, support, and, with the cremaster muscle in concert with the dartos muscle of the scrotal wall, thermoregulation by raising the testis and epididymis closer to the body wall. The pampiniform plexus is a countercurrent system that assists in maintaining a lower temperature, and the long and tortuous testicular artery removes the pulses of the arterial supply. The deferent duct is the conduit for taking the concentrated spermatozoa to the urethra, where they are mixed with the secretions of the accessory genital glands.

The Accessory Genital Glands

The function of the accessory glands is to produce ejaculatory fluid to support, nourish, and protect spermatozoa as they are transferred to the female. The energy source of spermatozoa includes fructose produced by the accessory glands, usually the vesicular glands. Accessory genital glands also provide some fluid for territorial scent marking. The domestic species have a differing size and arrangement of accessory glands. The amount and type of fluid vary according to the unique arrangements and mating behavior of the species. Coitus in ruminants is a rapid event, and they produce a small and highly concentrated ejaculate that is deposited around the external os of the cervix. On the other end of the scale are pigs, for which coitus takes approximately 20 minutes, insemination is intrauterine, and the ejaculate is high volume (up to 500 mL). Pigs have large vesicular glands that produce a watery fluid and large bulbourethral glands that produce a viscous mucoid product. The prostate of the dog is the only gland, and it provides all the seminal fluid. All species except the dog and pig have ampullae of the deferent ducts; these glands provide secretion and a storage site for spermatozoa.

The Penis and Prepuce

The penis is designed to enter the vagina of the female and to deposit the ejaculate in a location unique to each species. Pigs and horses are intrauterine inseminators, whereas the others deposit semen around the cervix and proximal vagina. These processes ensure protection of spermatozoa, including the prevention of desiccation. There are also adaptations and functions that ensure the spermatozoa of the dominant male are the ones that fertilize the ova. This need may explain why pigs and dogs have prolonged coitus. The penis of the cat has barbs that stimulate the vagina of the queen and induce ovulation. Small ruminants have a urethral process that sprays spermatozoa around the cervix, and the pig has a preputial diverticulum for scent production.

Dysfunction/Responses to Injury

Injury to the male reproductive system comes in different forms, and there are many potential targets, including the control mechanisms of the hypothalamic-pituitary-gonadal axis (see Chapter 12), interstitial endocrine cells, Sertoli cells, spermatogenic germ cells, and the various ducts. Apart from the obvious redundancy of having bilateral systems, the male reproductive tract has very little functional reserve and cannot undergo compensatory change to any significant degree. Some testicular compensatory hypertrophy is possible and is discussed later in this chapter.

The formation of *spermatic granulomas* (Fig. 19-2) is one of the most dramatic and important responses of the male reproductive system to injury. Spermatic granulomas occur with disruption of a seminiferous tubule or rupture of a duct; spermiostasis (i.e., abnormal stasis and accumulation of spermatozoa within the tubules or ducts of the epididymis and deferent duct) and spermatocele (i.e., a cavity filled with spermatozoa) are the usual preliminary stages. Spermatozoa are "foreign" to the body. Immunity to spermatozoa with the formation of antisperm antibody is a well-recognized phenomenon. The cell wall constituents and the high chromatin (i.e., complex of DNA and protein) content make them resistant to degradation. Any injury that exposes spermatozoa to the interstitial tissue of the body results in severe inflammation, mostly of the granulomatous type. This response can be a foreign body–type response, an immunologic response, or both. The inflammation produced results in severe fibrosis, which further obstructs tubules and ducts, leading to even more inflammation so that it becomes self-perpetuating. It is therefore critical to prevent such injury.

The Scrotum and Contents

Injury to the testis can be the result of a primary attack on a target cell or may be secondary to interruption of hormonal regulation, whether systemic or local. The endpoint of an injury can therefore be far-reaching. Regardless of the primary target, most injurious events result in germ cell degeneration, death, and depletion. Germ cells are sensitive to injury, but Sertoli cells are relatively resistant to injury. As a result, severe injury often results in seminiferous tubules containing only spermatogonia and Sertoli cells. As Sertoli cells degenerate, they become vacuolated and swollen. The spermatogenic epithelium responds to injury by increasing or decreasing apoptosis, resulting in spermatogenic arrest or a complete failure of spermatogenesis. The formation of multinucleated spermatid giant cells and phagocytosis of spermatozoa by Sertoli cells occur. As long as spermatogonia remain, spermatogenesis can restart.

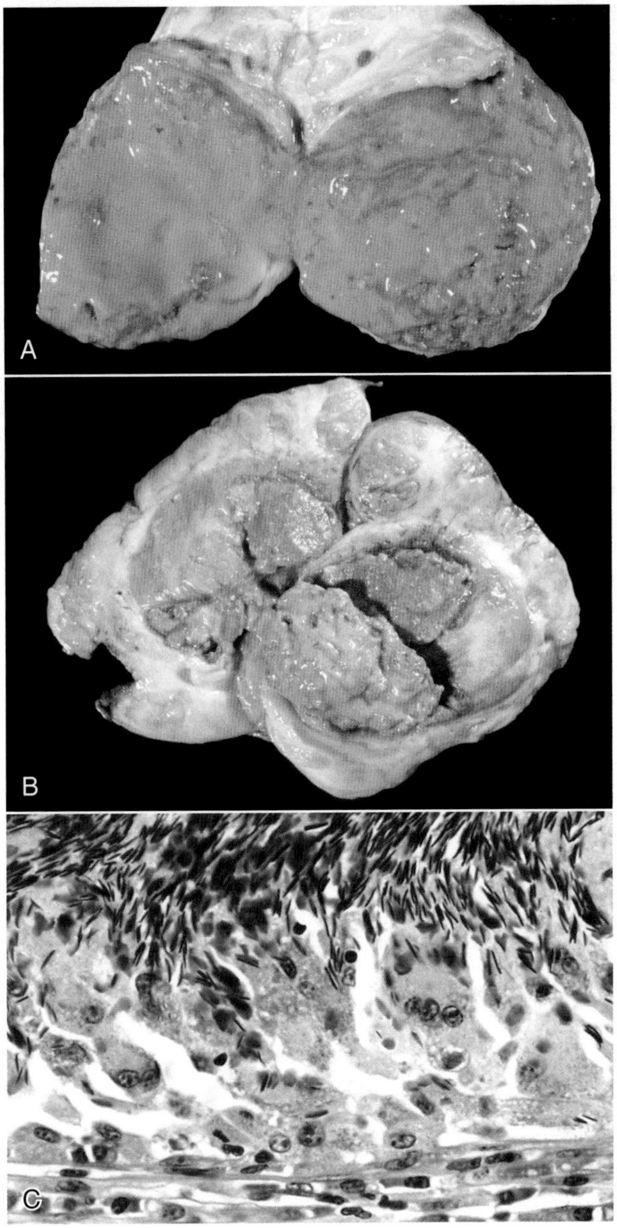

Figure 19-2 **Spermatic Granulomas, Tail of the Epididymis, Ram.** **A,** Most of the tail of the epididymis (bisected and reflected) is replaced by a yellow-tan, semiliquid spermatic granuloma. These granulomas are any color from white to red. They are frequently and incorrectly called abscesses. **B,** Multiple encapsulated (chronic) spermatic granulomas with white caseous centers. **C,** A mass of spermatozoa free in the interstitium *(upper half of image)* is surrounded by epithelioid macrophages and multinucleated giant cells, some of which have phagocytosed spermatozoa. Lymphocytes, plasma cells, and fibrous connective tissue surround these granulomas *(lower half of image)*. H&E stain. (**A** and **B** courtesy Dr. P.W. Ladds and Dr. R.A. Foster, James Cook University of North Queensland. **C** courtesy Dr. R.A. Foster, Ontario Veterinary College, University of Guelph.)

Spermatogenesis and cells of the testis in general are very susceptible to free radical injury, and the balance between oxidant and antioxidant activity is important. A slight imbalance results in free radical damage to membranes and increased apoptosis. Injury, including a slight increase in body temperature, results in greater numbers of free radicals, which explains why injury to one testis affects the contralateral testis and why systemic conditions affect spermatogenesis in general.

A major effect of injury to interstitial endocrine cells (also known as Leydig cells) is the failure of release of testosterone. This result can effectively stop spermatogenesis by increasing apoptosis and by inhibiting maturation of spermatids. Direct damage to spermatozoa can affect motility and fertilizing capability. Recovery from injury, although taking time, is achieved by restarting spermatogenesis from the relatively resistant spermatogonia.

The testis is a specialized immunologic environment and has a reduced immune responsiveness, no doubt because of the importance of not developing an immunologic response to germ cells. Unfortunately, if an inflammatory response does occur within the testis, it is likely to be sustained. It will also generate more free radicals and cause further injury.

Injury to the epididymis can have permanent and devastating effects. Not only does injury affect the functions of the epididymides—including maturation and storage of spermatozoa, resorption of fluid, and secretion of materials—but also severe injury results in inflammation. Any constriction of the epididymal duct results in spermiostasis, potential rupture, and the formation of spermatic granulomas. Because the epididymis is very limited in its responses, alteration to the structure and function of the epididymis is often permanent and affects fertility in a dramatic manner.

The peritesticular tissues, particularly the vaginal tunics, are also prone to injury from intraabdominal peritoneal diseases and local reactions secondary to epididymal disease or from a direct penetrating injury. The reaction of these tissues is identical to that of the peritoneum, and as such, fibrosis and adhesions are common responses to injury. Adhesion can limit the movement of the testes and alter its ability to thermoregulate.

The Accessory Genital Glands

Injury to the accessory genital glands is not common, and they can heal, but often with reduced function. Functional reserve is often sufficient to maintain fertility. If the injury is severe enough for them to not fully heal, they become fibrotic or may be unable to secrete sufficient fluid. Fertility is still possible, but the viability of frozen semen can be altered.

The Penis and Prepuce

The penis is sheltered from most injuries by the prepuce. There is a normal preputial flora that can become excessive and induce inflammation when preputial defenses are reduced. The prepuce has a full array of innate and local immune functions, and the responses to injury include epithelial hyperplasia and metaplasia with keratinization, hyperplasia of lymphoid elements to form lymphoid follicles, and the formation of granulation tissue if the injury is particularly severe or sustained. Adhesion of the penis to the prepuce is an unusual event. Direct trauma to the penis and prepuce can occur during urination or coitus, and the healing response can be particularly exaggerated in the prepuce with edema, eversion, and granulation tissue formation. Subsequent fibrosis and stenosis of the preputial orifice can prevent extrusion of the penis and, if severe, prevent urination. Excessive swelling and eversion/prolapse can produce the same effect. The prepuce is also susceptible to the irritant effects of urine, particularly if there is urine stasis from stenosis or preputial eversion.

Portals of Entry/Pathways of Spread

There are four main portals of entry of infectious microbes and injurious agents to the male reproductive tract (Box 19-1): direct penetration and injury, ascending infection, hematogenous localization, and peritoneal spread.

Box 19-1 Portals of Entry

Direct penetration
Ascending infection
Hematogenous localization
Peritoneal spread

The Scrotum and Contents

Of the four main portals of entry, ascending infection and hematogenous spread of infectious microbes or other agents are the main ways the testis, epididymis, and spermatic cord are affected.

Ascending infection occurs sporadically in adults but curiously is particularly a problem in pubertal animals when hormonal changes make the system more prone to infection from bacteria. This pubertal change has been shown for *Actinobacillus seminis* and *Histophilus somni*, which are resident flora of the prepuce of sheep. Infectious microbes may also ascend to the epididymis. It is exceedingly rare, because of the long length of the epididymis, for the testis to be involved in ascending infection.

Hematogenous localization is a recognized portal of entry for specific pathogens, such as the various *Brucella* spp. The epididymis is the main target, but the testis can be infected by this route.

The vaginal tunics are potentially affected by direct penetrating injury, but apart from bite wounds, this is a rare occurrence. As an outpouching of the peritoneal cavity, any process affecting the peritoneum, whether infectious or neoplastic, affects the peritesticular tissues.

The scrotal skin is exposed to the external environment and is affected by disease conditions just as the skin in general (see Chapter 17). Occasionally fistulae from disease of the vaginal tunics or epididymis affect the scrotal skin.

The Accessory Genital Glands

Ascending infection with pathogens moving from the prepuce retrograde to the flow of spermatozoa is common in the accessory genital glands. They can also be affected secondary to infection of the epididymis with pathogens being transferred with spermatozoa or exudates from the testis or epididymis. Hematogenous localization of pathogens occurs with classic examples including *Brucella* spp., and *Mycoplasma* spp.

The Penis and Prepuce

The external location of the penis and prepuce makes them prone to direct penetrating injury and to blunt force trauma. Although rare, this usually occurs at extrusion during intromission or masturbation. The male reproductive tract is also a target of pathogens that are spread by sexual activity. Venereal spread from females or in some circumstances from other males is well recognized.

Defense Mechanisms/Barrier Systems

The male reproductive tract, and particularly the internal genitalia, is so exquisitely sensitive to injury that it is extremely important to prevent injury rather than respond to injury. The combined effect of the high antigenicity of spermatozoa and the exceedingly long and very narrow duct system means that there is little tolerance for inflammation, necrosis, fibrosis, or other injurious situations. Much of the male reproductive system relies on isolation for protection and the prevention of infection or injury. Therefore, the innate immune system is generally more important than the adaptive or acquired immune system.

Innate Immunity

Each of the general locations of the male reproductive system relies largely on isolation and the barrier functions of the epithelium. Pattern recognition molecules, soluble factors in secretions, and the presence of continuous flushing all contribute to prevent infection. The ability to rapidly acquire nonspecific cellular responses, especially neutrophils and macrophages, provides further protection in infections.

Adaptive Immunity

Much of the reproductive tract can produce an adaptive immune response if antigenically stimulated. This response is particularly important in the accessory genital glands and the prepuce. Unfortunately, development of an adaptive response in the testis and the epididymis is often "too little, too late." Also, development of adaptive responses in the testis is inhibited by local immunosuppressive factors. This arrangement does not, however, prevent adaptive immunity from developing in the testis. The epididymis and deferent duct do not have a developed mucosal immune system, but one does exist in the accessory genital glands, particularly the ampulla and bulbourethral glands. When there is infection, local immunity and transfer of serum immunoglobulins occur. Preputial immunity is also mediated by local humoral and cellular mechanisms. Immunoglobulin G (IgG)- and IgA-based systems are present. Much less is known of cell-mediated immune mechanisms in the male reproductive tract.

Using local immunity to protect against infectious disease, particularly sexually transmitted diseases, has had little success. Response to vaccination has been variable, with some individuals having protective immunity, particularly with *Campylobacter fetus* infection in bulls. Systemic immunity to reproductive disease is of variable effectiveness. Although protecting against systemic infection, challenge to the reproductive tract has in some instances increased the response to the infection and caused more damage than would normally occur.

Inflammation

In general terms, inflammation (see Chapter 3) of the male reproductive tract is similar to that of other systems. What is unique about the male genital tract is the inflammatory response to spermatozoa. Spermatozoa and germ cells outside the blood-testis barrier act as foreign material and are antigenic. There are also antigenic components within seminal fluid. Spermatozoa have antigens that attract immune cells and also nonspecifically bind immunoglobulin. These reactions can have minimal effect on tissues directly and act by agglutinating spermatozoa or by opsonization. In some instances, the effect is much more dramatic, and immunization against spermatozoa can result in a severe inflammatory response. This inflammation is more likely to occur where the tissue-spermatozoal barrier is the weakest. The blood-testis barrier is the strongest, and in many species, the efferent ductules and the epididymis have a relatively weak barrier. This so-called autoimmune reaction to spermatozoa can be experimentally created, but a clinical correlate is infrequent. Local effects, however, are much more recognized. Direct damage to testicular parenchyma can result in granulomatous inflammation centered on the seminiferous tubules, the so-called intratubular orchitis. Where spermatozoa are exposed to the interstitial tissues of the body, the reaction is that of granulomatous inflammation. Macrophages and multinucleate giant cells are found adjacent to spermatozoa (see Fig. 19-2, C). Initially at least, $CD4^+$ T lymphocytes are abundant. Immunoglobulin-producing cells, particularly IgG-containing cells, are found. Granulomas are formed with the characteristic appearance of layers of epithelioid macrophages with multinucleate giant cells and then lymphocytes and plasma cells with a surrounding of fibrous tissue (see Fig. 3-24). In advanced cases, inspissated spermatozoa are found within a fibrous capsule. The production of a fibrous capsule and resultant contraction leads to further obstruction of adjacent ducts and tubules, with spermiostasis and spermatocele and spermatic granuloma formation. This inflammation therefore has devastating effects on fertility. Further complications occur if spermatozoa are released into the cavity of the vaginal tunics because a severe periorchitis develops and results in fibrosis and the lack of ability to adequately thermoregulate the testes.

The Scrotum and Contents

The testes and epididymides are hidden from the external environment by their intrascrotal location and by the extremely long and narrow tube (the deferent duct) that connects them to the outside world. The thin luminal diameter and extreme length of the deferent duct make ascending infection unlikely. Furthermore, there is almost continuous flow of fluid along the epididymis and deferent duct; thus the flushing action is protective.

Testicular and epididymal fluid has antibacterial properties. The high chlorine content may be partially responsible. Antimicrobial proteins in seminal plasma are numerous and include bovine seminal plasmin, lactoferrin, β-defensins, and the antibacterial CXC chemokine granulocyte chemotactic protein-2/CXCL6. Some of these proteins are acquired in the epididymis, where they are bound to spermatozoa. There are also numerous cytokines, such as interleukin (IL)-1β, IL-8, transforming growth factor (TGF)-α, and tumor necrosis factor (TNF)-α, normally produced in the tract. Epithelial cells of the reproductive tract have physical barrier proteins, including mucin, that prevent infection, and Toll-like receptors to stimulate inflammation.

Blood-Testis Barrier

The blood testis barrier was identified as a major barrier between the germinal epithelium and the interstitium of the testis. The physical barrier is predominantly at the level of the intercellular junctions between Sertoli cells (see Fig. 19-1). The basement membrane and peritubular cells contribute. The interstitium of the testis has long been recognized as an antiinflammatory location where immune responses and inflammation are muted. Testosterone and the interstitial endocrine cells are instrumental in maintaining this barrier, and there is considerable "crosstalk" between endothelial cells of capillaries, dendritic cells, mast cells, peritubular cells, and interstitial endocrine cells. Immune functions are suppressed, and the environment is generally antiinflammatory. Neutrophils are not normally present in seminal plasma but can infiltrate rapidly if required. Macrophages are present within male reproductive tissues and particularly within the testes, where they are recruited and maintained by the interstitial endocrine cells. Their presence inhibits the immune response. Cell-mediated responses, such as natural killer cells, lymphocyte-activated killer cells, and cytotoxic T lymphocytes, are inhibited as part of immune privilege and tolerance.

The Accessory Genital Glands

The accessory genital glands are located within the pelvis and are in a protective environment in which direct penetration rarely occurs. The epithelial cells form a barrier to the external environment—the lumen of the glands. In addition, the accessory genital glands are protected by the flushing action of urine and by the length of the urethra, especially in ruminants and pigs.

The Penis and Prepuce

The penis spends most of its time within the prepuce and is in direct contact with the inner lining epithelium of the prepuce. It is covered by epithelium that is stratified squamous in type. It is extruded for urination and intromission. The preputial orifice prevents most external contaminants from entering the preputial space. Little is known of pattern recognition receptors in the prepuce, but urine and genital fluids and their inherent antibacterial activities provide protection. There is humeral adaptive local immunity, and, particularly near the orifice of the prepuce, lymphoid follicles are often present or can form with antigenic stimulation. The preputial cavity has its own flora. The external component of the prepuce is the same as the skin in general.

Disorders of Domestic Animals

Disorders of Sexual Development[3]

All disorders of sexual development (DSD) are now grouped together and categorized according to sex chromosomes, genotype, gonad type, phenotype, and cause. The adoption of uniform nomenclature has eliminated the emphasis on categorizing animals with DSD as male or female. It greatly simplifies classification.

Abnormal sex chromosomes, gonads, or phenotype are usually manifested by abnormalities in sexual dimorphism. Many of the abnormalities result in a female phenotype and are mentioned in more detail in Chapter 18. The focus here is on those disorders that involve animals that have male gonads or are predominantly phenotypic males. The complete definition of a DSD requires knowledge of sex chromosomes, gonads, and phenotype. When the sex chromosomes are not known, the classification begins with the gonadal type.

Pragmatically, the majority of animals with dramatic disorders of sexual development have a female phenotype. In addition, the categorization scheme now in use includes all anomalies of the reproductive tract because each has a basis in sexual development. A much more detailed scheme is provided in Chapter 18.

There are a large number of anomalies of the male reproductive system (Box 19-2). Some have clinical relevance and others do not. Differentiating between these is very important. Some of the anomalies represent the most common disease of a particular species.

[3]See E-Box 1-1 for potential, suspected, or known genetic disorders affecting the male reproductive system of domestic animals.

Box 19-2 Selected Disorders of Sexual Development

IMPORTANT DISORDERS

Ciliary dyskinesia (immotile cilia syndrome)
Cryptorchidism
Hypospadias
PIS (polled intersex syndrome), goat
Retained preputial band
Segmental aplasia of mesonephric duct
Sex chromosome disorders–chimerism, freemartinism
XX Sex reversal syndromes
Spermatic granuloma of the epididymal head
Testicular hypoplasia

INCIDENTAL DISORDERS

Inclusion cysts
Remnants of mesonephric ducts
- Internal and external paradidymis

Persistent Müllerian duct syndrome
Remnants of paramesonephric (Müllerian) ducts
- Appendix testis
- Cystic uterus masculinus

Penile or preputial tags from retained preputial band

Where this is the case, the disease is discussed under disorders of a particular anatomic location because this is the most clinically relevant place. Anomalies are discussed based on effects on fertility and on the future breeding potential of the animal. Some anomalies have a genetic basis and such individuals should not be used as breeding stock, even though the animal may still be fertile.

Normal Male Sexual Development

Chromosome mapping and sequencing the genomes of animals now makes identification of genes and processes responsible for sexual development easier. In normal animals, the sex chromosome type and its genetic arrangement determine sexual development. Normal males have a single X and a single Y chromosome. The differentiation of the bipotential fetal gonad to a testis depends on the presence of a gene called the sex-determining region of the Y chromosome (*SRY*). *SRY* codes for a product (once called the testis-determining factor) that ultimately results in formation of a testis, and acts on genes that cause the germ cells to go into mitotic arrest. Supporting cells become Sertoli cells, steroid-producing cells become interstitial endocrine (Leydig) cells, and the mesenchyme develops the appearance of a testis. Further development requires the activation of many other genes that are not on the Y chromosome. The expression of *SRY* occurs briefly in the somatic cells of the indifferent gonads (or genital ridges). Because expression ceases shortly before Sertoli cells are recognized, it is proposed that the functional gene product of *SRY* influences other genes, such as *SOX9*, that ensure the differentiation and maintenance of Sertoli cells. *SOX9* is upregulated in XY individuals just before gonadal differentiation. Sertoli cells signal the other supporting cell precursor lines to differentiate along the male pathway. Early in differentiation, the embryo has a double set of ducts that arise by invagination of the lining of the celomic cavity. The mesonephric (Wolffian) ducts are male precursors of the epididymides, deferent ducts, vesicular glands, and ampullae. The rete testis and efferent ductules are derived from mesonephric tubules. There are approximately 20 efferent ductules, with the number varying by species (Fig. 19-3).

The testes develop in the tissue of the genital ridge, and the germ cells migrate there from the yolk sac. Sertoli cells secrete the polypeptide hormone anti-Müllerian hormone (AMH; previously called Müllerian inhibitory substance) during development and at lower concentrations postnatally. AMH causes regression of the ipsilateral paramesonephric duct, indirectly through action on mesenchymal tissue. Sertoli cells stimulate differentiation of interstitial endocrine cells from other cells of the testicular interstitium. Interstitial endocrine cells secrete the steroid hormone testosterone, which causes persistence and differentiation of the mesonephric ducts. Testosterone is likely transported down the mesonephric ducts rather than moving by simple diffusion. Dihydrotestosterone, a metabolite of testosterone, is required for formation of the prostate, the closing of the urethral folds, and the formation of the penis and scrotum. The enzyme steroid 5α-reductase is produced by cells in the urogenital sinus, genital tubercle, and genital swellings and reduces testosterone to dihydrotestosterone. Functional androgen receptors on target tissues are necessary for androgen-dependent differentiation and growth. Species differences exist in whether the production of testosterone by interstitial endocrine cells is under the control of gonadotropin produced by the fetal pituitary gland or the placenta. Fetal interstitial endocrine cells are replaced by postnatal interstitial endocrine cells, which are relatively quiescent until puberty. The production of testosterone is regulated by luteinizing hormone (LH), which is under the control of gonadotropin-releasing hormone (GnRH) from the hypothalamus. GnRH also controls follicle-stimulating hormone (FSH), which is produced by the anterior pituitary gland. FSH regulates the activity of Sertoli cells and can thus influence AMH production. Sertoli cells stimulated by FSH produce a glycoprotein, androgen-binding protein, which promotes high testosterone concentration around the germ cells for the progression of spermatogenesis.

The external genitalia form when the genital tubercle is masculinized by the presence of androgens. Elongation of the tubercle forms the phallus, opposing urethral folds form the penile urethra, and the genital swellings fuse to form the scrotum.

Testicular Descent. The testes and epididymides undergo descent from their original location to the scrotum. There are three main phases in testicular descent: abdominal translocation, transinguinal migration, and inguinoscrotal migration. The developing gonads are held in place by cranial and caudal suspensory ligaments. The caudal ligament, the primitive gubernaculum testis, attaches the developing testis to the site of the inguinal canal. It develops

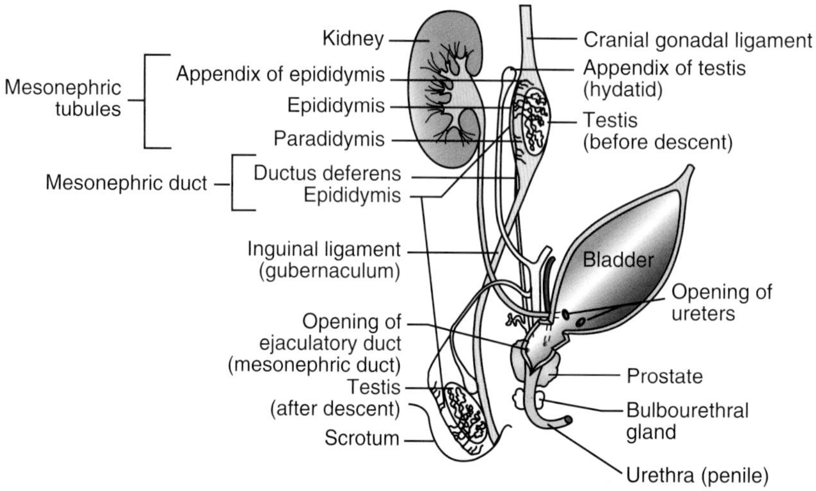

Figure 19-3 **Schematic Diagram of the Normal Components of the Male Reproductive System and the Embryonic Structures, Especially the Mesonephric (Wolffian) Duct and Urogenital Sinus and Tubercle, From Which They Were Derived.** The rete tubules and efferent ductules are formed from the mesonephric tubules; the epididymis, deferent duct, ampullae, and vesicular glands form from the mesonephric duct; the prostate and bulbourethral glands form from the urogenital sinus; and the penis, prepuce, and scrotum form from the genital tubercle and swellings.

into an intraabdominal and extraabdominal part that protrudes into the scrotum. Evagination of the peritoneum forms the inguinal canal and the vaginal tunic.

In the abdominal translocation phase, stimulation of gubernaculum mesenchymal cells is controlled in rodents by the insulin-like peptide (INSL) hormone, INSL3. The receptor for INSL appears to be GREAT/LGR8. Other molecules are likely involved. The subsequent enlargement of the gubernaculum and progressive weakening of the cranial suspensory ligament anchors the testis so that with fetal growth, the testis retains its position near the inguinal canal.

Little is known about the transinguinal phase, apart from the lack of involvement of testosterone or INSL3. Dilation of the inguinal canal by the gubernaculum and then intraabdominal pressure is involved with movement of the testis through the inguinal canal to bring the testis and epididymis into a subcutaneous location. The third and inguinoscrotal phase of testicular descent is mediated by the hypothalamopituitary-induced production of gonadal androgens. However, domestic animals with failure of testicular descent into the scrotum seldom have a deficiency of testosterone or a lack of the androgen receptor. The genitofemoral nerve and calcitonin gene–related proteins or binding sites are involved in rodents.

Sex Chromosome Disorders of Sexual Development

Sex chromosomes can be abnormal in structure or number. Two examples of abnormal structure of the Y chromosome are deletion of the short arm and isochromosome formation (duplication of one arm and loss of the other). Affected individuals have a female phenotype and extremely hypoplastic gonads. A few cattle have been identified with an isochromosome Y. With duplication of one of the sex chromosomes in an individual with a Y chromosome (XYY or XXY), or a mosaic (as occurs with the calico or tricolor male cats), the external genitalia are male in character. Klinefelter syndrome (XXY) is discussed in the section on Testicular Hypoplasia. Chimeras, such as XX/XY, are phenotypically sexually ambiguous, and the degree depends on the relative amounts of each chromosome. Freemartins are chimeras and are discussed in Chapter 18.

XX Disorders of Sexual Development

These are animals with XX sex chromosomes but have testes or ovotestes and a male phenotype. These animals are labeled XX sex reversal. They may be *SRY*-positive or *SRY*-negative. XX *SRY*-negative testicular DSD is reported in many breeds of dogs, in goats, and in horses. It is assumed they have a testis-determining region on another chromosome. XX *SRY*-positive DSD is not reported in domestic mammals.

XX ovotesticular DSD may have ambiguous genitalia and can be phenotypic male, female, or various combinations of the two, depending on the amount of hormones, including testosterone and AMH, during development. Most ovotestes have central testicular tissue with a periphery of ovarian structures. Rarely, ovotestes have an end-to-end arrangement of ovarian and testicular tissue, with clear demarcation between the two.

XY Disorders of Sexual Development

The XY disorders of sexual development are classified as those with abnormal gonads such as gonadal dysgenesis or ovotestes, those with ovaries, and those with testes. XY testicular DSD are the most common. They can be either *SRY*-positive or *SRY*-negative. XY *SRY*-negative DSD usually have primitive and undifferentiated gonads, called *gonadal dysgenesis*, and a female phenotype.

XY SRY-Positive Testicular DSD and a Female Phenotype. Individuals with XY *SRY*-positive testicular DSD and a female phenotype are called *male pseudohermaphrodites* (Figs. 19-4 and 19-5). The differentiation of the genital tract can be slightly or greatly abnormal. In many cases, the mechanism for the abnormal differentiation is unknown, but there are well-recognized syndromes in which the underlying pathogenesis is known. Three such syndromes are persistent Müllerian duct syndrome (PMDS), androgen insensitivity, and steroid 5α-reductase deficiency.

PMDS is a rare disorder of anti-Müllerian hormone (AMH) production or function. AMH can be absent or present in affected human beings; the syndrome can be a result of a mutation in either

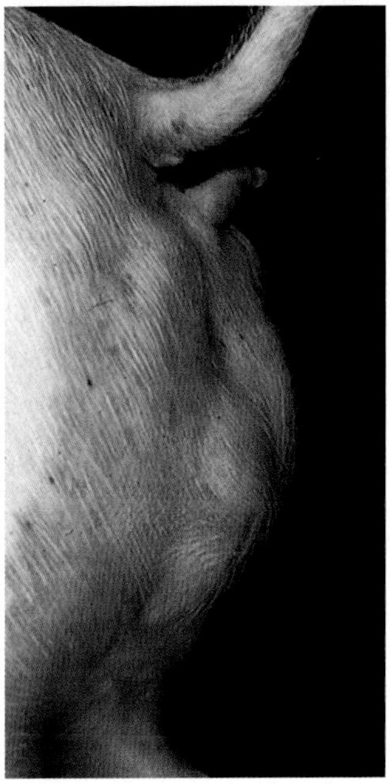

Figure 19-4 XY Testicular Disorder of Sexual Development, Feminized External Genitalia, Boar. This pig has a scrotum and intrascrotal testes, but the penis is small and clitoris-like and has a terminal urethral opening (ventral to the tail). (Courtesy Dr. D. Dodd; and Noah's Arkive, College of Veterinary Medicine, The University of Georgia.)

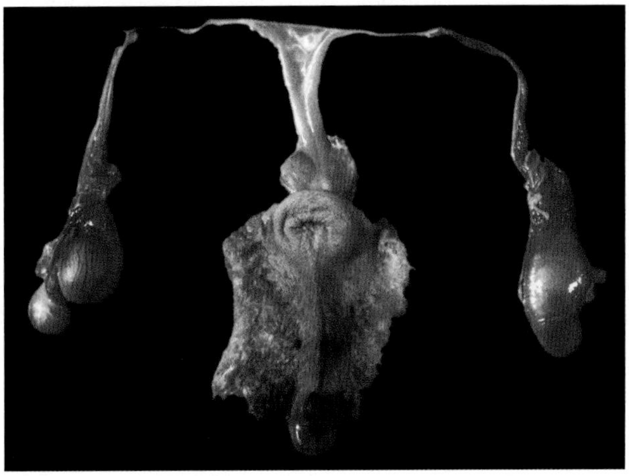

Figure 19-5 XY Testicular Disorder of Sexual Development, Feminized External Genitalia Reproductive Tract, Ram. This sheep has testes, deferent ducts, and accessory genital glands but also a vulva and a prominent clitoris. An androgen receptor defect would explain these anomalies. (Courtesy Dr. R.A. Foster, Ontario Veterinary College, University of Guelph.)

the *AMH* gene or the AMH receptor. In animals, the syndrome is described in miniature schnauzer dogs and basset hounds with an autosomal recessive mode of inheritance and in a goat with an unknown mode of inheritance. Affected dogs have XY chromosomes and testes, and externally they are normal males, with the common exception of unilateral or bilateral cryptorchidism. The testes, however, are attached to the cranial ends of uterine horns. When a testis has descended into the scrotum, the uterine horn passes through the inguinal ring. The deferent duct can be found microscopically within the myometrium. The cranial vagina and the prostate are often present. AMH is present in the testes of normal male dogs up to 143 days of age. AMH is also present in the testes of young affected dogs and is bioactive. A mutation in the structural gene for the AMH receptor results in AMH resistance in PMDS-affected dogs. Dogs with unilateral or bilateral scrotal testes can be fertile. Affected dogs may develop Sertoli cell tumors, hydrometra, and pyometra. Testicular abnormalities in PMDS, such as reduced spermatogenesis and tubular sclerosis, can be attributable to cryptorchidism. Cryptorchidism could be the result of interference with the AMH-controlled function of the gubernaculums in the transabdominal phase of descent.

Androgen receptor disorders are becoming increasingly recognized. Most cases are caused by a mutation in the androgen receptor gene, which is located on the X chromosome and thus in a single copy. Hundreds of mutations have been identified in other species. The normal androgen receptor has a hormone-binding and a DNA-binding domain; once activated by androgen, the domain changes shape and is able to bind to specific DNA sequences and regulate the transcription of other specific genes, leading to normal male differentiation. In human beings with androgen insensitivity, the gene is rarely deleted, but numerous point mutations in the receptor gene have been identified, mostly in the hormone-binding and DNA-binding domains. Whether the result is partial or complete androgen insensitivity depends on the location of the mutation and the change in function of the receptor. Dihydrotestosterone binds to the androgen receptor with greater affinity than that of testosterone, and the receptor, when it acts as a transcriptional factor, might interact with different genes other than the testosterone-bound receptor. In domestic animals, complete androgen insensitivity is described in equine, bovine, and feline species. The testes are often cryptorchid and located in the inguinal area. The first and second phases of testicular migration are normal. The inguinoscrotal third phase, which is under the control of androgens, does not occur. AMH produced by the testes causes regression of the paramesonephric ducts. External genitalia are female in complete androgen insensitivity, with a cranial blind end to the vagina, and neither the paramesonephric nor mesonephric ductal system is present.

Deficiency of 5α-reductase type 2, inherited as an autosomal recessive trait in human beings, has not yet been documented in animals, but in all likelihood, it does exist. The enzyme converts testosterone to dihydrotestosterone, which is required for the masculinization of the urogenital sinus, tubercle, and genital swellings. Without dihydrotestosterone, these structures become caudal vagina, vestibule, clitoris, and vulva. Internally, mesonephric structures (deferent duct, epididymis) develop. The testes are likely to be retained.

XY SRY-Positive Testicular DSD and Male Phenotype. The vast majority of congenital anomalies of the male reproductive tract are in otherwise normal males with testes and a male appearance. There are many well-known syndromes included in this group. They are discussed in the later sections on disorders of the scrotum and contents, accessory genital glands, or penis and prepuce.

Cryptorchidism. Cryptorchidism is a common anomaly and is discussed in detail as a separate entity in the section on the testis in Disorders of the Scrotum and Contents.

Segmental Aplasia of the Mesonephric Duct. Segmental aplasia of the structures of mesonephric ductal origin (epididymis, deferent duct, ampulla, or vesicular gland) can involve any of the structures, but most commonly it involves the epididymis alone (Fig. 19-6) and less commonly other structures. Segmental aplasia is reported mainly in the bull but is seen periodically in dogs. It most commonly involves the body and tail of the epididymis and is unilateral. Its inheritance is thought to be autosomal recessive. Spermatozoa become impacted (spermiostasis) because the epididymal duct has a blind ending; local dilation or rupture occurs secondarily, allowing escape of spermatozoa and formation of spermatic granulomas.

Ciliary Dyskinesia (Immotile Cilia Syndrome). Ciliary dyskinesia is caused by structural defects in the flagellum of spermatozoa and the axoneme of ciliated epithelial cells of numerous organ systems. It is a rare disease identified in human beings, dogs, pigs, mice, and rats. An autosomal recessive mode of inheritance is proposed. In dogs, heterogeneity of ultrastructural abnormalities of microtubule doublets and their dynein arms or central microtubules is reported. The effect on the male reproductive system is (1) immotile or hypomotile spermatozoa caused by flagellar lesions or (2) oligospermia (a subnormal concentration of spermatozoa) or azoospermia (no spermatozoa), presumably because of defective cilia in the epididymis and deferent duct. Female infertility is related to defective function of cilia of the uterine tube (see Chapter 18).

In other organ systems, ciliary dyskinesia effects ciliated epithelium. As examples, defective cilia in the nasal mucosa, bronchial and bronchiolar mucosa, and ependyma commonly cause rhinitis, bronchopneumonia, and bronchiectasis. Defective cilia in the ependyma can lead to hydrocephalus. Ciliary dyskinesia may also be linked to situs inversus, but the pathogenesis of the reversal of the normal left and right orientation of organs is unclear.

Spermatic Granuloma of the Epididymal Head. The development of a spermatic granuloma in the region of the epididymal head is an anomaly that is either missed or confused with infectious epididymitis.

Within the developing gonad are sex cords, which join with remnants of the rete testis and efferent ductules derived from mesonephric tubules. Efferent ductules enter the single duct of the epididymis; there are approximately 20 efferent ductules, but the number varies with the species. Blind efferent ductules result when there is no connection to the epididymis and can be resorbed or persist and enlarge to form cysts or rupture. Blind-ending efferent ductules can be present in sufficient numbers to cause spermiostasis,

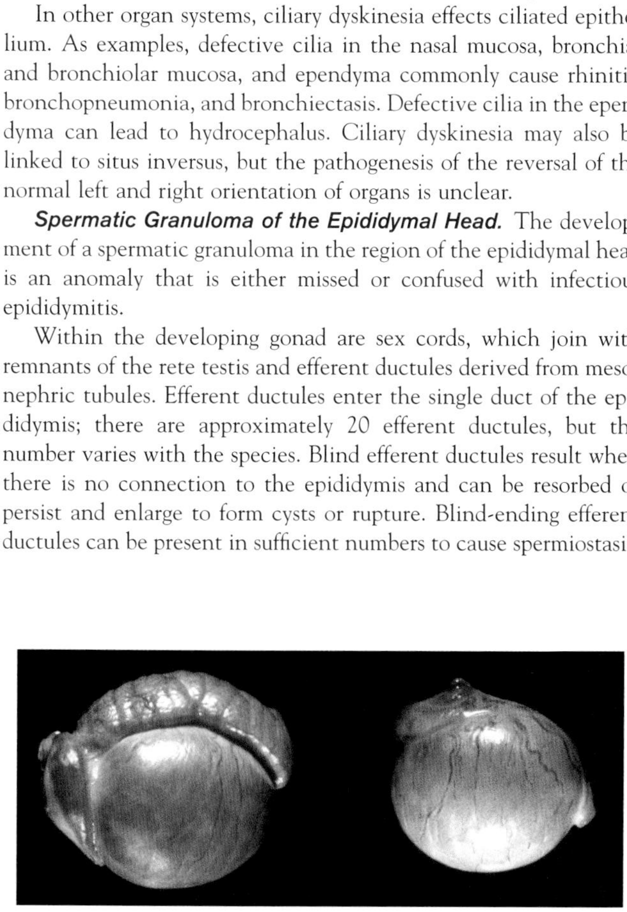

Figure 19-6 Segmental Aplasia of Mesonephric Duct, Epididymis, Dog. There is no tail of the epididymis of the right testis. This portion of the mesonephric duct did not develop. The left testis is normal. (Courtesy College of Veterinary Medicine, University of Illinois.)

spermatocele, and spermatic granulomas. The condition known as *spermatic granuloma of the epididymal head* (SGEH) is thus formed (see the section on Spermatic Granulomas and Epididymitis).

Cysts of the Reproductive Tract. There are myriad minor anomalies that are of little consequence except when they are confused with conditions that do affect fertility. Foremost of the minor anomalies are the various cysts that occur as a result of duplication or failure of regression of embryonic ducts and tubules. It is often difficult to identify the origin of an individual cyst or group of cysts. In many instances, anatomic location is the determining factor. Some of the cysts are simply called *inclusion cysts* (Fig. 19-7). These cysts have a wall of compressed collagen, a thin inner lining of flattened mesothelial-like cells, and a clear fluid content. They are found where mesothelial cells are trapped adjacent to a serosal surface. Inclusion cysts attached to the head of the epididymis are good examples.

Unconnected with the lumen of the epididymal duct and efferent ductules, remnants of mesonephric tubules can form cysts adjacent to the head of the epididymis (external paradidymis) or within the head of the epididymis (internal paradidymis). Cysts, both connected and unconnected with the ductular system, are lined by ciliated columnar epithelium. They are clinically significant if they become large enough to cause spermiostasis in adjacent structures. The remnant of the paramesonephric duct, called the appendix testis, is not clinically significant and is located on the cranial or cranioventral surface (depending on the species orientation of the testes) of the testis near the head of the epididymis. Sometimes, this small nodule of tissue can appear cystic. A similar cystic structure is found in the band of tissue between the ampullae. It is called the *cystic uterus masculinus* (Fig. 19-8). Some prostatic cysts of dogs have a similar origin.

Disorders of the Scrotum and Contents

The clinical examination of the scrotum and its contents begins with observation and palpation of the scrotal skin, vaginal tunics, testis, epididymis, and spermatic cord. The most common and economically important disorders are those that affect the testis and epididymis, but the skin and tunics are critical for thermoregulation and normal function of the testis and epididymis. These structures are exquisitely sensitive to an increase in temperature and oxidative stress, and slight changes can result in infertility. The scrotum and its contents are also prone to trauma. Trauma frequently results from kicks by mares at mating in horses; fighting in bulls, rams, and bucks; and biting in dogs and cats.

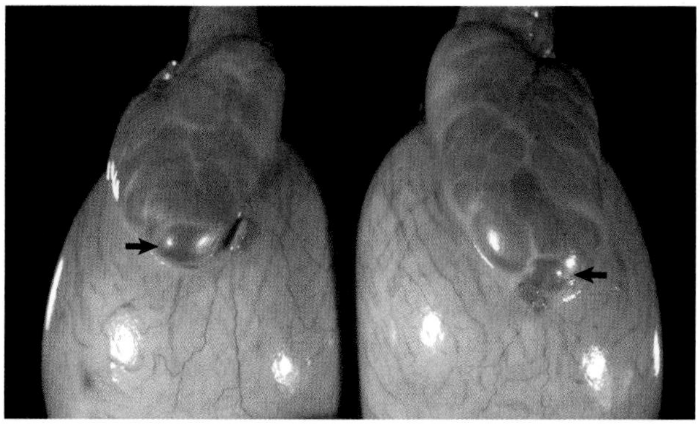

Figure 19-7 Congenital Inclusion Cysts, Testis and Epididymis, Ram. These 7-mm cysts *(arrows)* in the tissue between the head of the epididymis and testis are incidental findings and are not significant. (Courtesy Dr. P.W. Ladds and Dr. R.A. Foster, James Cook University of North Queensland.)

The Scrotum

The fusion of the paired primordia of scrotal skin depends on androgens produced by the interstitial endocrine cells (Leydig cells) of the gonad after it has differentiated into a testis. Altered androgen concentration or a lack of androgen receptors can lead to defects in the scrotum such as failure of fusion, cleft formation, or bifurcation. Defects can be local, confined to the scrotum and penis, or part of a wider range of disorders of sexual development. *Hypospadia*, in which the urethra opens on the ventral side of the penis, can be part of these anomalies.

Dermatitis of the scrotal skin is common (see Chapter 17). Often it is part of generalized dermatopathy. Dermatitis restricted to the scrotum can result from trauma, frostbite (Fig. 19-9), or exposure to environmental irritants such as cement dust. The scrotum is a

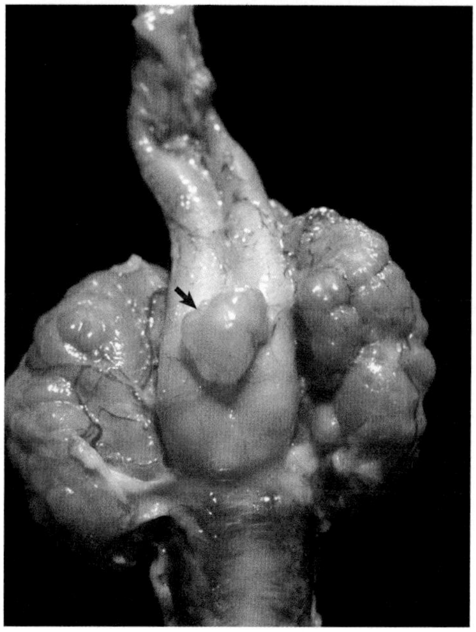

Figure 19-8 Cystic Uterus Masculinus, Accessory Genital Glands, Ram. This sheep has a 1-cm thin-walled cyst in the tissue between the ampullae of the deferent ducts *(arrow)*. (Courtesy Dr. P.W. Ladds and Dr. R.A. Foster, James Cook University of North Queensland.)

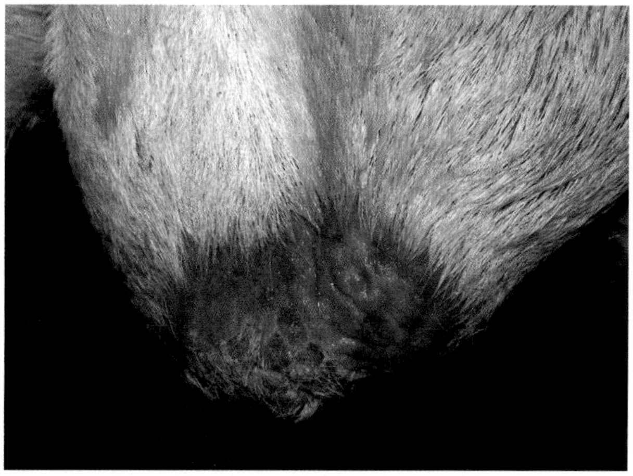

Figure 19-9 Frostbite, Scrotum, Ram. The skin of the lower portion of the scrotal sac has sloughed. The ventral scrotal skin is alopecic or covered by crusts from previous frostbite. (Courtesy Dr. R.A. Foster, Ontario Veterinary College, University of Guelph.)

predilection site for some pathogens. These include *Dermatophilus congolensis* and *Besnoitia besnoiti* in the bull and *Chorioptes bovis* in the ram (Fig. 19-10). Scrotal dermatitis can interfere with the thermoregulatory function of the scrotum by either generating more heat or preventing cooling, leading to testicular degeneration.

Neoplasms of skin can occur but are much less common in the scrotal skin. They include papillomas in the boar and mast cell tumors and hemangiosarcomas in the dog. Testicular tumors, especially Sertoli cell tumors and interstitial (Leydig) cell tumors, occur in the scrotum of previously castrated male dogs and cats, respectively, presumably from cells inadvertently transplanted at surgery. Vascular abnormalities, often called *hemangiomas* and which are probably hamartomas, occur on the scrotum of the boar and dog. The scrotal veins of bulls sometimes become varicose.

Vaginal Tunic

The vaginal tunics are the extension of the peritoneum. They line the scrotal sac as the parietal layer and cover the testis, epididymis, and spermatic cord as the visceral layer. The cavity between the two layers is continuous with the peritoneal cavity. The tunics and the cavity thus are subject to all the disorders of the peritoneum and peritoneal cavity. Ascites therefore results in hydrocele, fluid within the tunics around the scrotal contents. Polyserositis in pigs and feline infectious peritonitis (FIP) are examples of diseases that cause inflammation of the tunics and periorchitis. Neoplasia is uncommon; mesothelioma and peritoneal carcinomatosis are the most frequently encountered. Parasites, especially the metacestode larvae *Cysticercus tenuicollis* in rams, occurs periodically and can be confused with cysts or spermatic granulomas.

Inflammation of the vaginal tunics without initial inflammation of the abdominal peritoneum is from trauma or local infection. The latter case is usually an extension from orchitis or epididymitis. Especially well-known causes are trypanosomiasis in bulls, rams, and bucks; *Brucella abortus* in bulls; *Brucella ovis* and *Actinobacillus seminis* in rams; and *Brucella melitensis* in bucks. Adhesions between the parietal and visceral vaginal tunic are fibrinous at first and later fibrous.

Testis and Epididymis

The testis and epididymis are inseparable, and disease of one usually results in disease of the other. Scrotal palpation is the main clinical method to identify abnormalities, and changes in size are the most obvious. Diseases that cause small scrotal contents are discussed next, followed by those that result in enlargement of one or more of the intrascrotal structures (Box 19-3).

Reduced Testicular and Epididymal Size. Many disorders of sexual development result in a reduction in size or the absence of scrotal contents. Missing or aplastic components are rare. Segmental aplasia of the mesonephric duct, manifested as aplasia of the epididymal tail (see Fig. 19-6), is one example. It was described previously in the section on Disorders of Sexual Development, XY *SRY*-Positive Testicular DSD and Male Phenotype. If one complete side of the scrotal contents is missing, either unilateral castration was performed or the affected animal is a unilateral cryptorchid. Sometimes, the undescended testis and epididymis subsequently descend, or the castration operator may have missed a testis and epididymis. Affected sheep, for example, often have the scrotum removed, and the testis is located beneath the underlying skin. A lack of both sides of the scrotal contents can represent castration or bilateral cryptorchidism and requires additional investigation, including measurements of hormone (testosterone, AMH) concentrations, especially after treatment with GnRH, or surgical exploration. A search for secondary characteristics that are testosterone dependent, such as the barbs on the penis of the cat and the presence of a prostate in dogs, can assist in separating behavioral characteristics from similar behaviors in incompletely castrated males.

A small testicular size is of great importance, especially to production animals, because daily sperm output is correlated to testicular volume and weight. A small size indicates hypoplasia or atrophy. These lesions can be difficult to differentiate unless there is a history of size change. Hypoplasia is a congenital condition in which the testis does not increase to its full size at puberty. It is often seen as part of other disorders of sexual development, most commonly cryptorchidism.

Cryptorchidism. Cryptorchidism occurs when there is incomplete descent of the testis (normal testicular descent is discussed earlier). In most mammalian species, the testis descends into the scrotum by the time of birth. Cryptorchidism is more often unilateral than bilateral, with the side affected being species dependent. Many undescended testes are on the right side. In the horse, the distribution is equal left to right, and in the bull, the left side is

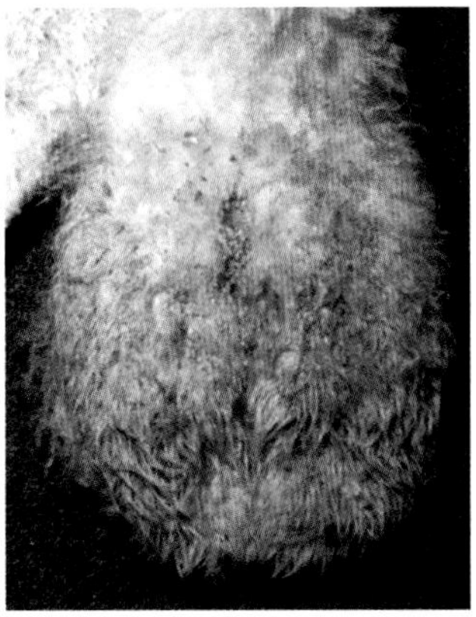

Figure 19-10 **Scrotal Dermatitis (*Chorioptes Bovis*), Scrotum, Ram.** There is extensive crusting and exudation of the skin in response to the irritation and inflammation caused by the mites. (Courtesy Dr. R.A. Foster, Ontario Veterinary College, University of Guelph.)

Box 19-3 Intrascrotal Disease Based on Differences in Size of the Testis and/or Epididymis

DECREASED SIZE

Cryptorchidism
Hypoplasia
Segmental aplasia
Testicular atrophy/degeneration

INCREASED SIZE (INCLUDING MASSES)

Cystic retained embryonic structures
Epididymitis
Inguinal hernia
Orchitis
Periorchitis
Scrotal lymphadenopathy
Spermatic granuloma of epididymal head
Testicular neoplasia
- Seminoma, teratoma
- Sertoli cell tumor
- Interstitial cell tumor

Torsion
Varicocele

usually affected. The undescended testis can be anywhere along its path from caudal to the kidney (Figs. 19-11 and 19-12, *A*) to the scrotum but is commonly within the abdomen near the internal inguinal ring, within the inguinal canal or in a subcutaneous location just outside the external inguinal ring. Epididymal development is coordinated with testicular development and consequently is slowed in cryptorchidism.

Cryptorchidism is the most common disorder of sexual development (DSD). Most disorders are XY *SRY*-positive testicular DSD. It has a polygenetic basis and an autosomal recessive mode of inheritance. It can be the result of failure of normal production of testosterone or failure of regulation by one or more genes for the production of testosterone, androgen receptor, INSL3, INSL3 receptor, and/or calcitonin gene–related protein. Descriptions of cryptorchidism should include whether it is unilateral or bilateral and which stage of descent is abnormal (abdominal translocation, transinguinal migration, and inguinoscrotal migration).

In the horse, left and right testicular retention are almost equal in occurrence, and the left retained testis is more likely to be abdominal than inguinal in location. Three breeds (Percheron, American saddle horse, and American quarter horse), ponies, and crossbred horses are significantly overrepresented in a large hospital-based study of cryptorchidism.

Abnormalities in the gubernaculum can cause cryptorchidism by its failure to develop, improper positioning, excessive growth, or failure to regress. In human beings, some other predisposing or contributing factors for cryptorchidism include testicular hypoplasia; estrogen exposure in pregnancy; breech labor compromising blood supply to the testes; and late closing of the umbilicus, delaying the ability to increase abdominal pressure.

A cryptorchid testis remains small at puberty, probably because of its higher than optimal temperature. Superimposed atrophy occurs in the cryptorchid testis after puberty. The testis is small and fibrotic and has interstitial collagen deposition, hyaline thickening of the tubular basement membranes, and degeneration of germinal epithelium so that only a few spermatogonia remain with the normal complement of Sertoli cells (Fig. 19-12, *B*).

Cryptorchid testes are much more prone to develop neoplasia than are scrotally placed ones. In the dog, Sertoli cell tumors are more likely to occur in the testes present in the abdomen (Fig. 19-13), whereas seminomas tend to develop more commonly in inguinally placed testes. The contralateral testis is also at increased risk for developing a neoplasm, even if that testis is located in the scrotum. A retained testis, especially if enlarged by a neoplasm, is prone to torsion.

Cryptorchidism is a phenotypic DSD. Many animals with other DSD have cryptorchidism, and cytogenetic and genetic testing can identify these disorders. Some of these individuals have ovotestes. The greater the ratio of testicular to ovarian tissue, the more likely

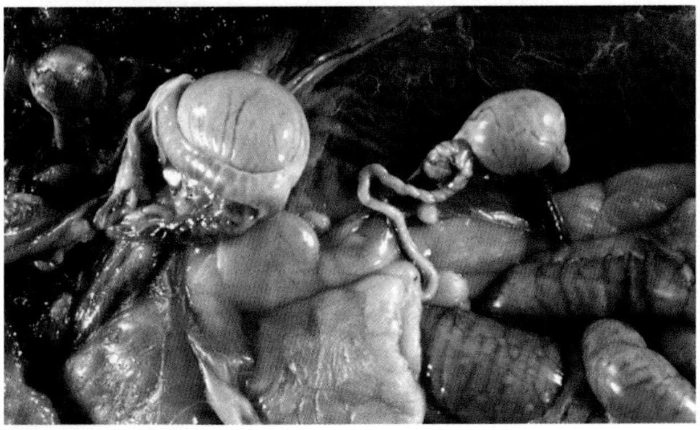

Figure 19-11 Cryptorchid Testis, Intraabdominal, Dog. The retained testis and epididymis *(right)* are hypoplastic. The other descended testis *(left)* is normal. Intestines are below the right testis. (Courtesy Dr. Y. Niyo, College of Veterinary Medicine, Iowa State University; and Noah's Arkive, College of Veterinary Medicine, The University of Georgia.)

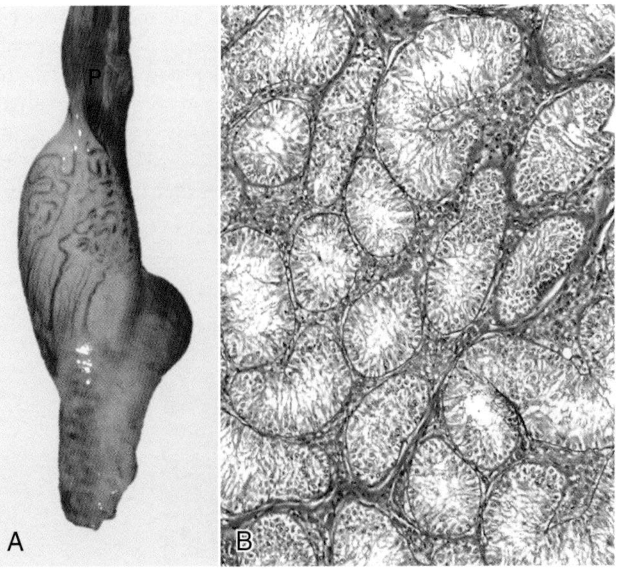

Figure 19-12 Cryptorchid Testis. A, Cryptorchid testis and epididymis, bull calf. The testis and epididymis are hypoplastic and are barely larger than the pampiniform plexus above *(P)*. There are no attachments to the vaginal tunic. **B,** Cryptorchid testis, dog. There is complete absence of spermatogenesis; however, the Sertoli cells are normal. H&E stain. (**A** courtesy Dr. R.A. Foster, Ontario Veterinary College, University of Guelph. **B** courtesy Dr. J.A. Ramos-Vara, College of Veterinary Medicine, Michigan State University; and Noah's Arkive, College of Veterinary Medicine, The University of Georgia.)

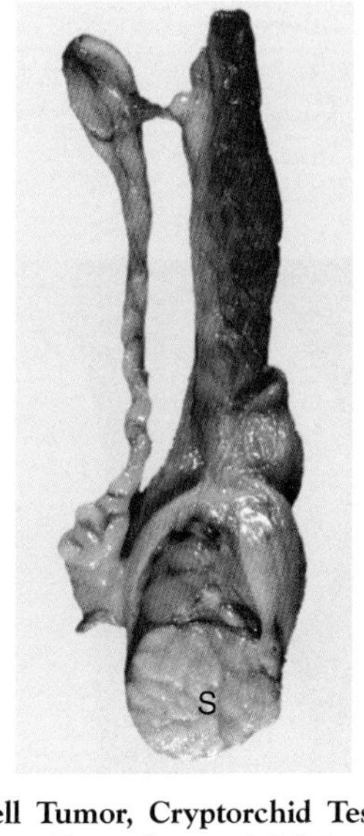

Figure 19-13 Sertoli Cell Tumor, Cryptorchid Testis, Dog. The testicular parenchyma is replaced by a white multilobular Sertoli cell tumor *(S)*. The texture is firm, indicating fibrosis. This dog had bilaterally retained testes and epididymides and bilateral Sertoli cell tumors. (Courtesy Dr. R.A. Foster, Ontario Veterinary College, University of Guelph.)

an ovotestis has descended into the scrotum. The ovary or ovarian portion of an ovotestis is histologically normal, but the seminiferous tubules of a testis or ovotestis are abnormal because of a combination of increased temperature and the effects of estrogen produced by the ovarian tissue.

Testicular Hypoplasia. Hypoplasia of the testes is a common condition and disorder of sexual development. The testis is smaller than normal for the age of the animal, and it is often present in disorders such as cryptorchidism and other DSD. Hypoplasia of the testis and epididymis in an otherwise normal male is the focus here.

It is difficult to distinguish hypoplasia from testicular atrophy by using morphologic features. Both testicular hypoplasia and atrophy can occur alone, with no apparent contributing or influencing factors; either can also be associated with, secondary to, or part of some other lesion. Testicular and epididymal hypoplasia (Fig. 19-14, A and B) is causally linked to poor general nutrition, zinc deficiency, specific genes in the Swedish red and white breed of cattle, and endocrine and cytogenetic abnormalities. Endocrine disturbances causing testicular hypoplasia are those that reduce production of either luteinizing hormone by the pituitary gland, which in turn influences testosterone production by the interstitial endocrine (Leydig) cells, or FSH by the pituitary gland, which stimulates the nurturing function of the Sertoli cells.

A wide range of cytogenetic abnormalities, from translocations and mosaics to nondisjunctions causing polysomes of sex chromosomes, result in testicular hypoplasia. The best known example of polysomy is the XXY karyotype of Klinefelter syndrome seen in stallions, bulls, boars, dogs, and tricolor cats. In cats, the syndrome is recognized in males with the tricolor, tortoise shell, or calico coat types. These cats can be XXY, XX/XXY, or more complex chimeras or mosaics with two or more X chromosomes and one or more Y chromosomes. The gene for black and the gene for orange are carried one per X chromosome, so a normal male cat should not have hair of both colors.

Hypoplasia of the testis can theoretically occur when the number or length of seminiferous tubules is reduced or when there are no or insufficient germ cells. Usually before puberty, the seminiferous tubules have only Sertoli cells and spermatogonia (see Fig. 19-14, B). At puberty, the tubules of hypoplastic testes undergo an irregular progressive sclerosis and become collagenous, presumably from concurrent degeneration. Interstitial endocrine cells appear to be more numerous and clustered.

Hypoplasia of the testes is not apparent until after puberty. Unilateral hypoplasia is more common than bilateral hypoplasia, but this difference in prevalence could be a reflection of the relative ease of recognizing a size difference when the normal contralateral testis is available for ready comparison. Unilateral hypoplasia is difficult to explain because most of the causes seem to act systemically and therefore should produce a bilateral effect.

The size range of a hypoplastic testis generally is from a prepubertal size (see Fig. 19-14, A) to almost normal. The palpation consistency of a hypoplastic testis is near normal. The severity of hypoplasia can be graded histologically by the proportion of hypoplastic tubules scattered throughout the organ. Hypoplastic tubules have a small diameter and are lined only by Sertoli cells and sometimes a few spermatogonia. Interstitial endocrine cells appear proportionally more numerous, but this is only because the tubular area is reduced and the relative amount of interstitium is increased. In severe testicular hypoplasia, most or all of the tubules are abnormal; the tubules have a small diameter and a uniform microscopic appearance with only infrequent vacuolation of Sertoli cells and without a thickened basement membrane. In moderate hypoplasia, fewer tubules are small, those of normal size have some differentiation of the seminiferous epithelium, and a few tubules have complete spermatogenesis. In most tubules, however, when the stage of spermatocyte formation is reached, the spermatocytes undergo apoptosis or degeneration, leaving tubules lined by Sertoli cells with a vacuolated cytoplasm. The lumen of such tubules can contain cellular debris and multinucleate cells that are formed when dividing cells fail to separate. When hypoplasia is mild, only a few small tubules are lined only by Sertoli cells; most tubules have normal spermatogenesis. Mild hypoplasia is difficult to distinguish from testicular degeneration. The number of hypoplastic tubules would not be expected to increase with age because tubules do not arise after puberty. Mild hypoplasia is detected when scrotal circumference is just less than the accepted minimum clinical diameter.

Testicular Degeneration and Atrophy. Testes that reduce in size after puberty are called atrophic, and the microscopic change is called degeneration of the seminiferous tubules. Testicular atrophy is a common lesion. Mild testicular degeneration can be detected only microscopically, but when it is severe and chronic, the testis is small and firm (Fig. 19-15). The causes are many, and in a particular individual, the specific cause is often unknown. Degeneration can be unilateral or bilateral, depending on whether the cause is local

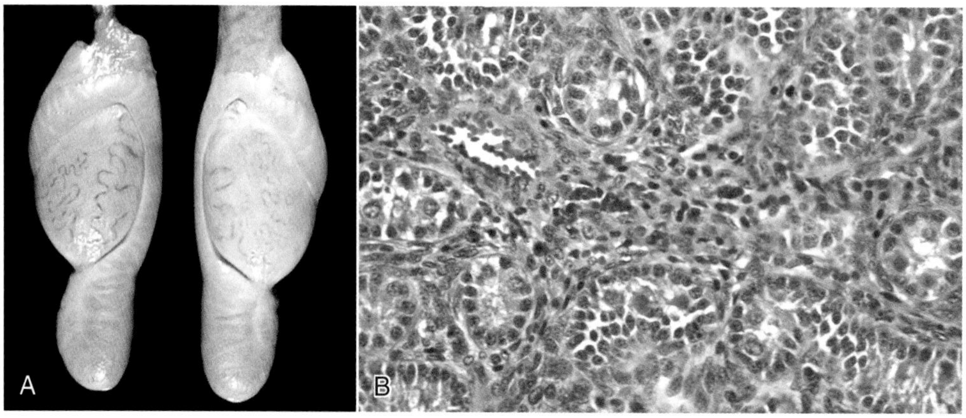

Figure 19-14 **Bilateral Hypoplasia, Testes, Yearling Ram. A,** Both testes and epididymides from this yearling ram are very small compared with normal age-matched controls. **B,** The seminiferous tubules are lined only by Sertoli cells, and there is no spermatogenesis. H&E stain. (Courtesy Dr. R.A. Foster, Ontario Veterinary College, University of Guelph.)

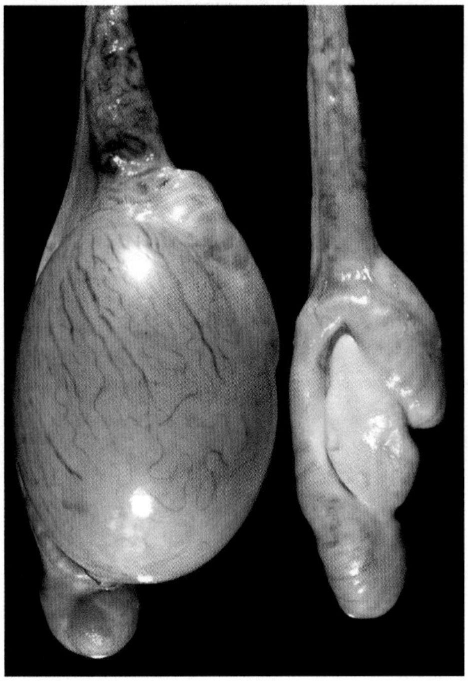

Figure 19-15 **Unilateral Testicular Atrophy and Epididymitis, Testis and Epididymis, Ram.** The affected testis *(right)* is small, and testicular veins are not visible on the capsule of the testis because of fibrosis and contraction of the connective tissue. The other testis *(left)* is bulbous, indicating hypertrophy. (Courtesy Dr. P.W. Ladds and Dr. R.A. Foster, James Cook University of North Queensland.)

or systemic. In young growing males, the distinction between testicular degeneration and hypoplasia is often difficult to make using morphologic features. Both lesions are often present together because hypoplastic testes are prone to degeneration. Inflammation also can be superimposed on degeneration when there is spermiostasis leading to mineralization and spermatic granuloma formation. Healing of a testis with degeneration and return to normal structure and function are possible if the injurious agent is eliminated and damage is not too severe.

Specific causes of testicular degeneration are numerous (Box 19-4). Increased apoptosis of germ cells is a common endpoint of many causes, regardless of whether the initial effect is on the hypothalamo-pituitary-gonadal endocrine axis or on the Sertoli cell–interstitial cell–germ cell axis. Fever or local heat from inflammation of the scrotal skin is a classic cause of degeneration. Obstruction of flow of spermatozoa causes testicular degeneration. Obstruction can be the result of developmental disorders such as segmental aplasia of mesonephric duct derivatives, local injury, or inflammation of the epididymis. Vascular events, such as impairment from aging, torsion, or severe crushing of the spermatic cord, cause degeneration. Systemic injurious factors include nutritional deficiency, hormonal aberrations, toxins, and irradiation. Hypovitaminosis A and zinc deficiency are specific nutritional deficiencies; general malnutrition also causes testicular degeneration. Many of these causes are thought to increase oxidative stress in the testis.

Interference with GnRH, LH and its control of androgen production by interstitial endocrine cells, or FSH and its effect on the production of androgen-binding protein by Sertoli cells can have a deleterious effect on the seminiferous epithelium. Such interference could happen, for example, when a neoplasm of the pituitary gland causes local compression of the pituitary gland, the hypothalamus, or both. Estrogen produced by Sertoli cell tumors induces testicular degeneration. Environmentally acquired endocrine disruptors are also implicated. Some therapeutic drugs, such as amphotericin B, gentamicin, and chemotherapy compounds, cause testicular degeneration.

Many toxins are capable of causing testicular degeneration, and most damage the spermatogonia and dividing primary spermatocytes, but some damage later stages (e.g., spermatocytes and spermatids) or injure Sertoli cells.

A testis undergoing atrophy initially is softer than normal, and as the degeneration progresses, the testis becomes smaller. The cut surface of the normal testis bulges slightly and so will the degenerated testis initially. With time, the degenerated testis becomes firmer and has small flecks or large areas of mineralization, especially in ruminants. Degeneration can be either generalized or regional, occurring in the ventral portion of the testis of bulls or in the dorsal part of the testis (near the head of the epididymis) in rams. If the degeneration is caused by ischemia after a vascular accident in the

Box 19-4 Some of the Known Causes of Testicular Atrophy/Degeneration in Mammals (Including Rodents)

Advancing age
Chlorinated naphthalenes
Epididymitis
Chemicals
- Chemotherapy
- Halogenated compounds, including hexachlorophene
- Nitrogen-containing compounds, including benzimidazoles and nitrofurans

Heat
Hormones
- Dexamethasone
- Estrogen
- Testosterone
- Zeranolone
- Other endocrine disruptors

Metal compound toxicosis
Neoplasia
- Pituitary tumors
- Sertoli cell tumors

Nutritional disorders
- Negative energy balance
- Fatty acid deficiency
- Hypovitaminosis A
- Hypervitaminosis A
- Hypovitaminosis B
- Hypovitaminosis E
- Hypovitaminosis C
- Oxidative stress
- Protein and amino acid deficiency
- Zinc deficiency

Plants
- Locoweed (*Astragalus*)
- Lysine seeds
- Gossypol

Radiation
Scrotal disease
Stress/corticosteroid therapy
Trauma
Ultrasound
Viral infection
- Bovine viral diarrhea virus
- Distemper virus
- Porcine reproductive and respiratory syndrome virus

spermatic cord, small islands of parenchyma beneath the testicular capsule can survive the infarction because of diffusion of oxygen and nutrients from vessels of the epididymis and capsule of the testis. Degeneration can occur locally around a lesion, such as a neoplasm, that expands and causes compression.

Microscopically, the initial change is spermatogenic arrest at one or more stages of the spermatogenic cycle. The seminiferous tubules have a smaller diameter. With further degeneration, there is a thickened and undulating basement membrane, decreased numbers of germinal cells, vacuolated Sertoli cells, intratubular multinucleated spermatids, and interstitial fibrosis (Fig. 19-16, *A* and *B*). A key lesion in the differentiation of testicular degeneration from testicular hypoplasia is the wavy basement membrane found in testicular degeneration because affected tubules had at some stage reached full size and then subsequently collapsed. At the end stage of testicular degeneration, Sertoli cells are the only lining cells remaining, but with time, these also disappear, leaving only the basement membranes. Mineralization can involve intratubular cellular debris, tubular basement membranes, or the interstitium.

Degeneration of the epididymis is less well studied but does occur. In degenerative conditions, the epididymis is much less likely to be reduced in size. This lack of reduction in size can be helpful in differentiating testicular atrophy from hypoplasia macroscopically. In the former, the epididymis approximates adult size, whereas in hypoplasia the epididymis is small in size.

Testicular and Epididymal Enlargement. There are several disorders that result in testicular and epididymal enlargement. Foremost is inflammation, especially epididymitis and orchitis. Testicular neoplasia is a common cause of testicular enlargement in dogs.

Spermatic Granulomas and Epididymitis. Spermatic granuloma of the epididymal head is a unique congenital disorder of most species. It is not an infectious condition, but inflammation dominates as a response to extravasated spermatozoa. It affects the efferent ductule region first and then spreads to involve the head of the epididymis (Fig. 19-17, *A*). All efferent ductules should connect

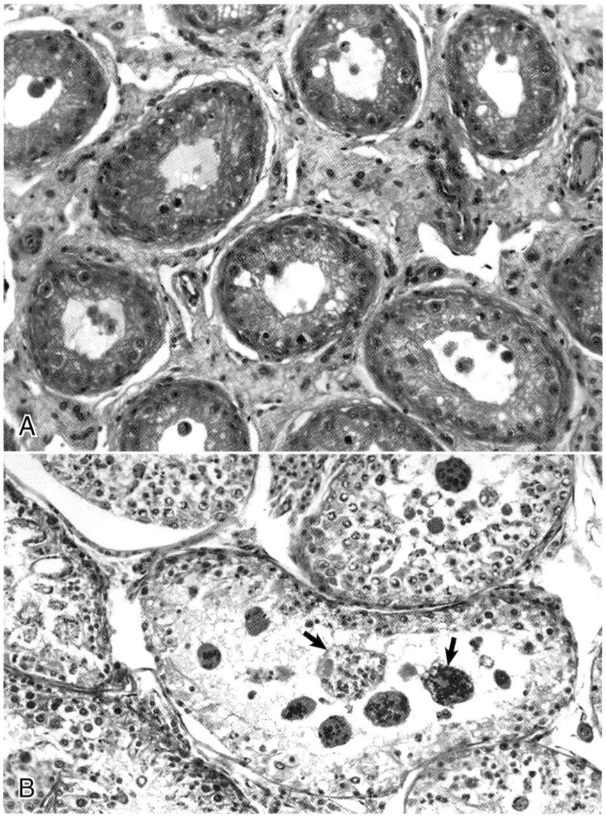

Figure 19-16 **Testicular Degeneration, Testis. A,** Ram. There is interstitial fibrosis that separates the seminiferous tubules. Spermatogenic arrest at the spermatocyte stage, vacuolation of Sertoli cells, and a wavy basement membrane caused by a reduction in tubular diameter are present. H&E stain. **B,** Dog. In addition to reduced spermatogenesis, there is formation of multinucleated spermatids *(arrows)* as a result of failure of spermatids to separate. This is a common change in testicular degeneration. (Courtesy Dr. R.A. Foster, Ontario Veterinary College, University of Guelph.)

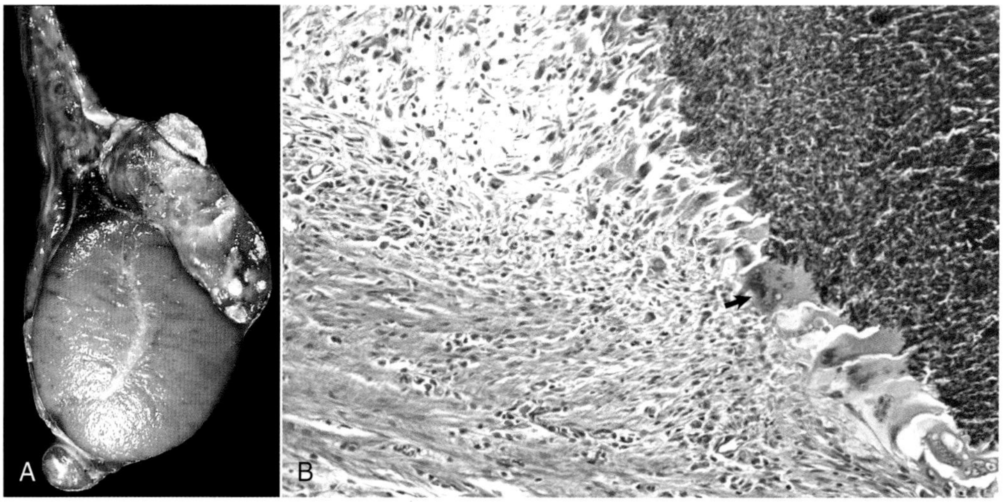

Figure 19-17 **Spermatic Granuloma of Epididymal Head, Head of the Epididymis, Ram. A,** The head of the epididymis is enlarged because of spermatic granulomas *(white-yellow masses)*. The body and tail of the epididymis (ventral) are small, as the spermatic granulomas have obstructed the flow of spermatozoa from the testis to the epididymis. **B,** The mass of spermatozoa *(right)* in the interstitial connective tissue of the epididymis is surrounded by macrophages and multinucleated giant cells *(arrow)*. H&E stain. (**A** courtesy College of Veterinary Medicine, University of Illinois. **B** courtesy Dr. K. McEntee, Reproductive Pathology Collection, University of Illinois; and Dr. J. King, College of Veterinary Medicine, Cornell University.)

to the single epididymal duct in the head of the epididymis, but some are blind-ended. At puberty, the blind-ending ductules fill with spermatozoa and the resultant spermiostasis proceeds to spermatocele and then spermatic granulomas (Fig. 19-17, *B*). These lesions progress over time and result in infertility because of obstruction of the epididymal duct. The back pressure produced by the spermatic granulomas causes dilation of the mediastinum of the testis and testicular atrophy.

Epididymitis is very important in rams (Fig. 19-18; also see the section on Disorders of Ruminants (Cattle, Sheep, and Goats), The Scrotum and Contents, Epididymitis) and dogs (Fig. 19-19; also see the section on Disorders of Dogs and Cats, the Scrotum and Contents, Infectious Epididymitis with Orchitis) and is rare in other species. The tail of the epididymis is almost always affected, allowing the majority of cases to be differentiated from spermatic granuloma of the epididymal head. Because the epididymis is only a single coiled duct, any lesion along its length has the potential to cause obstruction of spermatozoal flow and the formation of spermatic granulomas. Thus epididymitis is frequently accompanied by spermatic granulomas and also periorchitis. Epididymitis is frequently encountered as a unilateral, chronic lesion of the tail of the epididymis and thus can be recognized by comparing the size and shape of the abnormal organ with the contralateral normal one. In acute inflammation, the epididymis is swollen and soft. In chronic inflammation, it is enlarged and firm because of abundant fibrous tissue and the presence of spermatic granulomas. Epididymitis is one of the causes of testicular degeneration, and macroscopically, the testis is atrophic. Focal fibrinous or fibrous adhesions occur between the visceral and parietal vaginal tunics over the epididymis (see Fig. 19-18). If a spermatic granuloma ruptures into the cavity of the vaginal tunic, diffuse inflammation can result (Fig. 19-20), followed by adhesions across the cavity. In some cases, fistulas discharge through the scrotum.

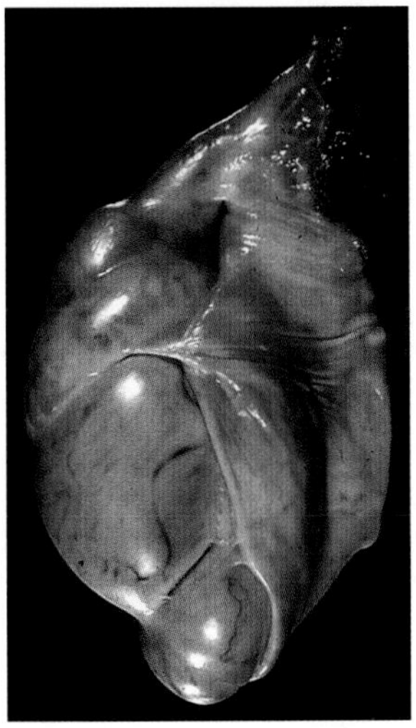

Figure 19-18 **Epididymitis (*Brucella Ovis*), Tunic Adhesions, Epididymis, Ram.** Note the dramatic enlargement of the epididymis *(left upper and lower portions of the image)* and the adhesion of the parietal vaginal tunic to the visceral vaginal tunic around the affected epididymis. (Courtesy Dr. K. McEntee, Reproductive Pathology Collection, University of Illinois; and Dr. J. King, College of Veterinary Medicine, Cornell University.)

Microscopically, the early lesions of epididymitis begin when bacteria are within the lumen of the duct. Neutrophils infiltrate, and their enzymatic and antimicrobial products combined with bacterial products, such as exotoxin and endotoxin, cause ductal and stromal necrosis, fibrin exudation, and edema. Spermatozoa extravasate, and spermatic granulomas form. With time, there will be neutrophils and macrophages within the tubules, epithelial hyperplasia, metaplasia, intraepithelial cavities, or lumina, and many lymphocytes and plasma cells within the interstitium (Fig. 19-21).

Noninfectious causes of epididymitis are exceedingly rare, and frequently cases that have no recoverable agent have spermatic granulomas that remain after a previous infection is otherwise controlled.

Orchitis. True orchitis (inflammation of the testis) is much less common than epididymitis, probably because the testis is much further "upstream" than the epididymis and possibly because of its altered immunologic environment, which is antiinflammatory. Orchitis is, unfortunately, the clinical term for inflammation of the scrotal contents, even though most cases are epididymitis. Orchitis is usually accompanied by epididymitis; it may be an extension of epididymitis. Primary orchitis is usually hematogenous, with examples including *Brucella abortus* infection in bulls, *Corynebacterium pseudotuberculosis* in rams, and *Brucella suis* in boars. Orchitis occurs in several forms. Intratubular orchitis is centered on the seminiferous tubules, so it is assumed that the agent and the inflammatory reaction began there. Intratubular orchitis appears grossly as poorly defined, up to 1-cm yellow foci that become firm and white as the lesions become older. Initially, the affected tubules have acute

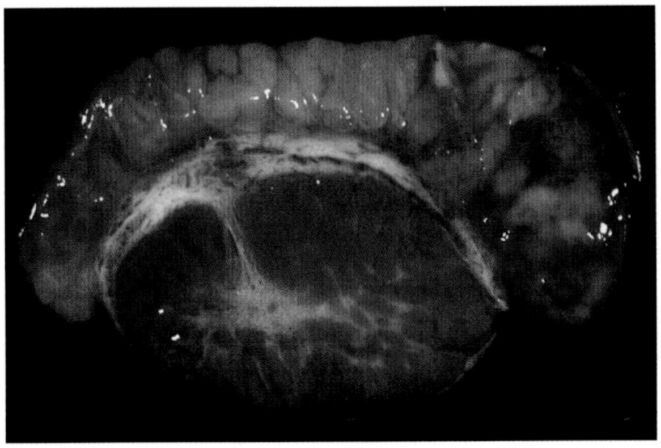

Figure 19-19 **Acute Epididymitis, Epididymis, Dog.** The head *(left)* and tail *(right)* of the epididymis are grossly hyperemic and contain pale foci of suppurative exudate and spermatozoa. (Courtesy Dr. K. McEntee, Reproductive Pathology Collection, University of Illinois; and Dr. J. King, College of Veterinary Medicine, Cornell University.)

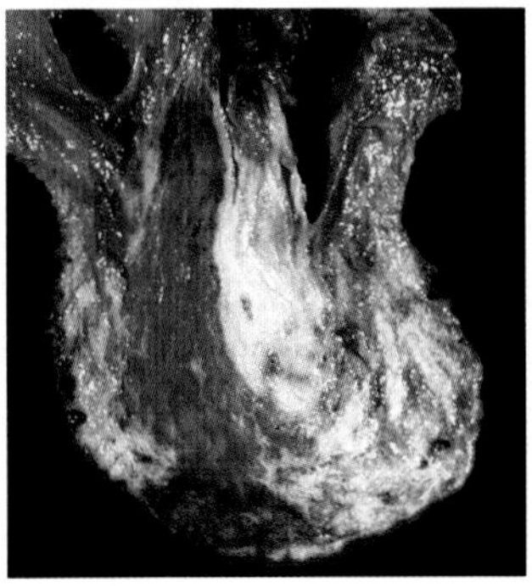

Figure 19-20 **Scrotal Cellulitis and Periorchitis, Scrotum (Testis Has Been Removed), Dog.** The vaginal tunic is thickened by inflammatory exudate, granulation tissue, and fibrous tissue. The inflammation extends into the skin. There is an ulcer in the ventral skin from self-mutilation. (Courtesy Dr. R.A. Foster, Ontario Veterinary College, University of Guelph.)

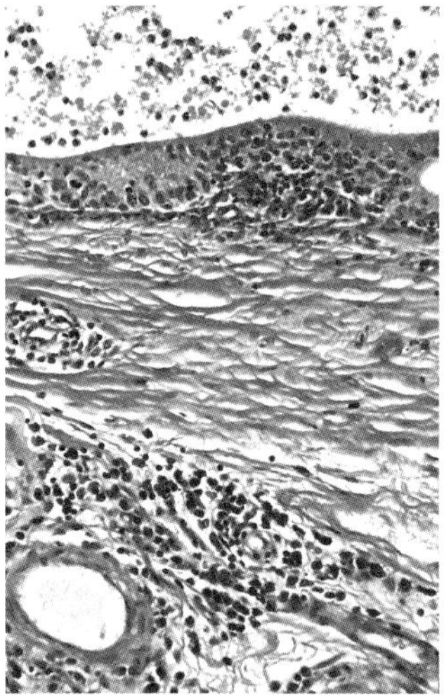

Figure 19-21 Chronic Epididymitis, Epididymis, Ram. Note the intertubular fibrosis and large numbers of lymphocytes and plasma cells in the interstitium *(lower half of image)*. The epithelium of the epididymal duct *(top)* is hyperplastic, and the lumen contains neutrophils and spermatozoa. H&E stain. (Courtesy Dr. R.A. Foster, Ontario Veterinary College, University of Guelph.)

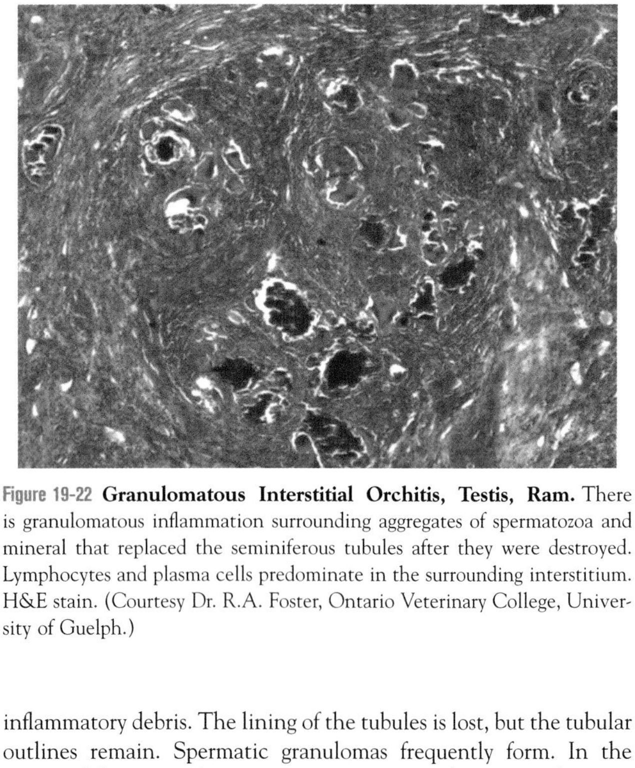

Figure 19-22 Granulomatous Interstitial Orchitis, Testis, Ram. There is granulomatous inflammation surrounding aggregates of spermatozoa and mineral that replaced the seminiferous tubules after they were destroyed. Lymphocytes and plasma cells predominate in the surrounding interstitium. H&E stain. (Courtesy Dr. R.A. Foster, Ontario Veterinary College, University of Guelph.)

inflammatory debris. The lining of the tubules is lost, but the tubular outlines remain. Spermatic granulomas frequently form. In the center of these granulomas, spermatozoa are within macrophages or free within the tissue. Macrophages and lymphocytes surround the spermatozoa and with time, collagen is formed at the edge of the lesion. When the lesion is predominantly in the interstitium, it is called *interstitial orchitis* (Fig. 19-22).

Necrotizing orchitis, such as is caused by *Brucella abortus* and *Brucella suis*, is the most severe form of orchitis. It is a more severe form of intratubular or interstitial orchitis, but in some cases the affected areas are so severely inflamed and the necrosis is so extensive that the original structures form a caseous mass. Gray-brown, initially soft and later firm, necrotic debris replaces an irregular but large portion of the testis. In a few extremely severe cases, a fistula

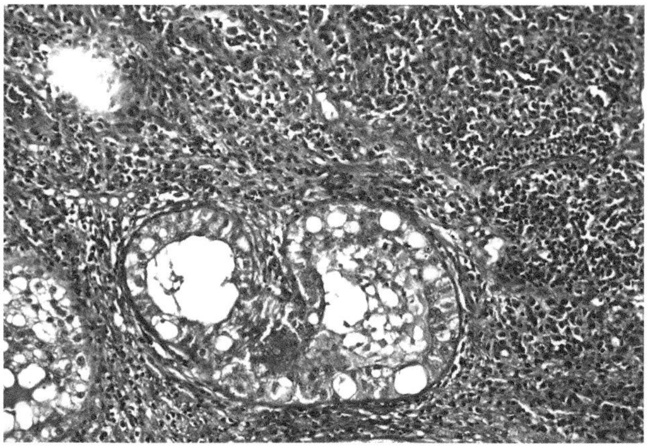

Figure 19-23 Severe Fibrinous Interstitial Orchitis, Feline Infectious Peritonitis (FIP), Testis, Cat. Note the severe orchitis with a mixture of fibrin and plasma cells in the interstitium. The tubules are degenerate and not directly involved. The testicular lesion was the first manifestation of FIP in this cat. H&E stain. (Courtesy Dr. R.A. Foster, Ontario Veterinary College, University of Guelph.)

develops through the scrotum. One manifestation of feline infectious peritonitis (FIP) in cats is a fibrinous and necrotic orchitis (Fig. 19-23).

Granulomatous orchitis, especially tuberculous orchitis, is now very rare as countries eradicate *Mycobacterium bovis*. Mycotic orchitis caused by *Blastomyces dermatitidis* occurs sporadically in dogs in endemic areas.

Neoplasia. Testicular neoplasms are common in older dogs, much less frequent in horses, and rare in other species. They usually arise from germ cells, interstitial endocrine (Leydig) cells, or Sertoli cells. Occasionally, neoplasms of testicular mesenchymal tissues or metastatic neoplasms are found. The three common primary testicular neoplasms are seminoma (germ cell origin), interstitial cell tumor, and Sertoli cell tumor; they occur singly or in combination. These primary neoplasms are almost always benign, and there are no features that indicate the likelihood of metastasis. Metastasis, when it does occur, is identified by nodules in the spermatic cord, scrotal lymph node, or beyond.

Germ Cell Neoplasms. Germ cell neoplasms are seminoma, teratoma, and other less common types such as embryonal carcinoma. *Seminomas* are the most common testicular neoplasm in the aged stallion and the second most common canine testicular neoplasm (Fig. 19-24, *A*). They are more prevalent in cryptorchid testes than in descended testes. Multicentric origin within the testis and local invasiveness are characteristic, but metastasis is rare. The neoplasm is homogenous, white or pink-gray, and firm; bulges when cut; and has fine fibrous trabeculae. Microscopically, seminomas are either intratubular or diffuse, and the neoplastic cells are large round cells with scant cytoplasm and a large nucleus with a prominent nucleolus. Anisokaryosis is up to sixfold, but most cells are large and uniform in size. The mitotic rate is usually high. Giant cells, with either a single nucleus or multiple nuclei, are sometimes present (Fig. 19-24, *B*). Aggregates of $CD8^+$ T lymphocytes are often present around blood vessels in seminomas and are a useful diagnostic feature because they are not seen in other testicular neoplasms. *Teratomas* arise from totipotential primordial germ cells. They are uncommon but occur in the young horse, especially in a cryptorchid testis. The neoplasms can be large, cystic, or polycystic and can contain recognizable hair, mucus, bone, or even teeth. Microscopically, derivatives of two of the three embryonic germ layers

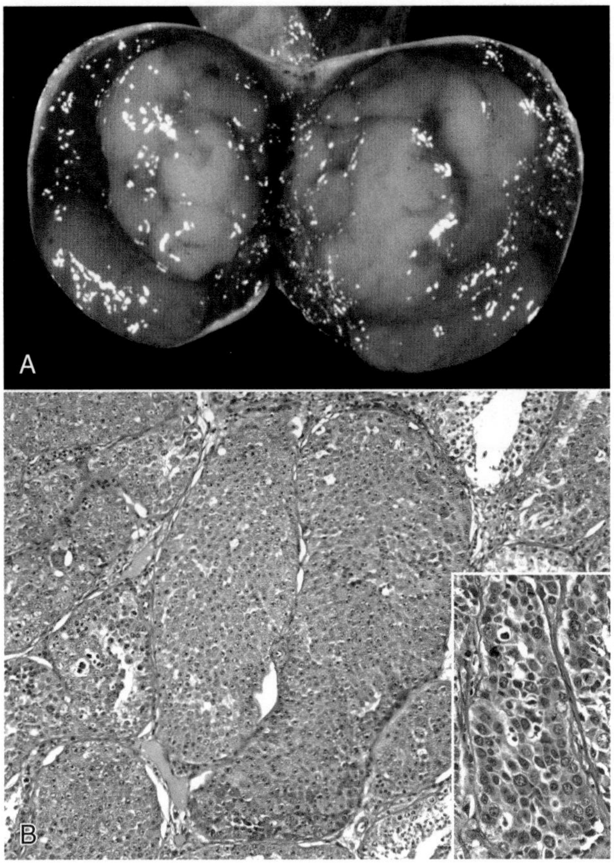

Figure 19-24 Seminoma, Testis, Bisected and Reflected Section, Dog. A, Note the pale pink to beige circumscribed homogeneous mass. The cut surface has a gelatinous texture and has bulged slightly on incision. The contralateral testis was atrophic. **B,** Seminomas consist of round germinal cells with a high nuclear-to-cytoplasmic ratio and frequent mitoses (*not shown here*). Note how the cells have filled and expanded the seminiferous tubules. *Inset,* Higher magnification of the neoplastic cells. Note the mitoses. Despite this "malignant" appearance, most are behaviorally benign. H&E stain. (**A** courtesy Dr. K. Read, College of Veterinary Medicine, Texas A&M University; and Noah's Arkive, College of Veterinary Medicine, The University of Georgia. **B** courtesy College of Veterinary Medicine, University of Illinois. Inset courtesy Dr. R.A. Foster, Ontario Veterinary College, University of Guelph.)

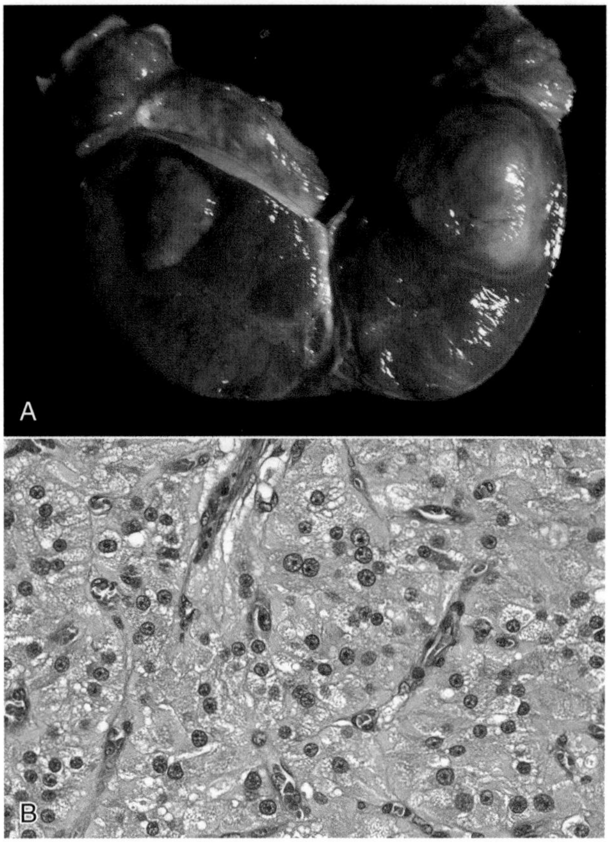

Figure 19-25 Interstitial Cell Tumor, Testis, Bisected and Reflected Section, Dog. A, Note the well-demarcated, yellow-tan mass, which has bulged on incision. Such masses become hemorrhagic when they become large. Atrophy of an affected testis as the result of pressure is common when the tumor is large. **B,** Cells are arranged in packets surrounded by a fine fibrous stroma typical of endocrine cells. Their cytoplasm is pale, eosinophilic, and abundant and often has fine vacuoles. Mitoses are rare. H&E stain. (**A** courtesy Dr. M.D. McGavin, College of Veterinary Medicine, University of Tennessee. **B** courtesy Dr. W. Crowell, College of Veterinary Medicine, The University of Georgia; and Noah's Arkive, College of Veterinary Medicine, The University of Georgia.)

(ectoderm, mesoderm, and endoderm) are present. Most teratomas have well-differentiated tissue and are benign.

Interstitial Endocrine (Leydig) Cell Neoplasms. Interstitial cell tumor is the most common testicular neoplasm of the bull, dog, and cat. These neoplasms are almost always benign. They likely begin as regions of nodular hyperplasia. Some tumors produce hormones, including estrogenic substances. They are readily identifiable grossly because they are spherical and well demarcated (Fig. 19-25, *A*), a tan to orange color, often with regions of hemorrhage. Microscopically, they are noninvasive and finely encapsulated. The neoplastic cells are arranged in solid sheets or packed into small groups by a fine fibrous stroma (Fig. 19-25, *B*). The cells of the bovine neoplasms vary little, but in the dog, the cells can be large, round, and polyhedral or spindle shaped. The cells have abundant cytoplasm that is often finely vacuolated and often has brown lipofuscin pigment. Nuclei are round, and anisokaryosis is usually minimal. Hemorrhage and necrosis are common.

Sertoli Cell Neoplasms. Sertoli cell tumor is the third most common testicular neoplasm of the dog. It is rare in other species. In the dog, more than 50% of Sertoli cell tumors are located in retained testes. The neoplasm is well circumscribed, expansile, firm, white, and lobulated by fibrous bands and can cause dramatic enlargement of the affected testis (Fig. 19-26, *A*). Metastasis is rare, but when present, it is in the spermatic cord and occasionally spreads to the superficial inguinal (scrotal) lymph node. Metastases beyond the regional lymph node are reported but are very rare. Microscopically, the abundant fibrous tissue in Sertoli cell tumors distinguishes them from the other two common types of testicular neoplasm. Neoplastic Sertoli cells have an intratubular or a diffuse arrangement and tend to palisade along the fibrous stroma or form tubular structures (Fig. 19-26, *B*). They either resemble normal Sertoli cells or are pleomorphic. In addition to the effects of pressure and local invasion, approximately one-third of Sertoli cell tumors produce a feminizing effect, causing gynecomastia (enlargement of the mammary glands), alopecia, hyperplasia, or squamous metaplasia of the acini of the prostate (Fig. 19-26, C). The amount of hormone produced is generally proportional to the size of the neoplasm. Although some produce estrogen, many produce inhibin, which inhibits GnRH secretion and subsequently LH and FSH release. This arrangement alters the balance between estrogen and

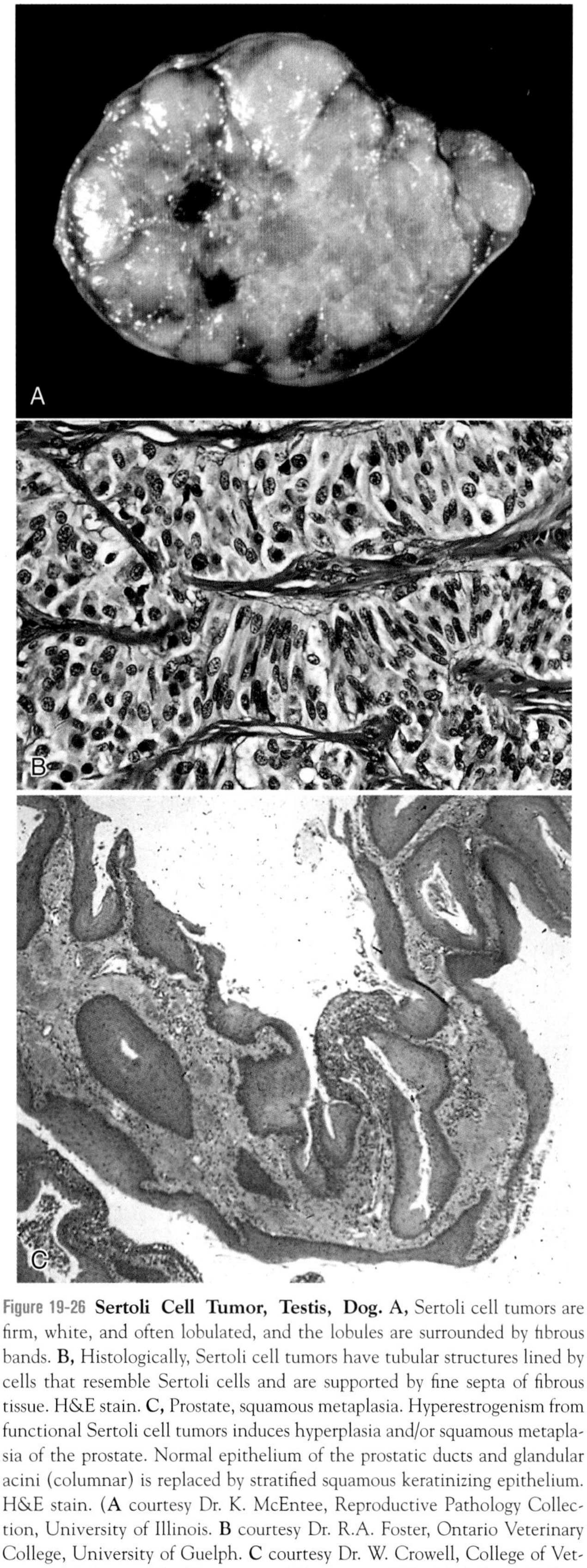

Figure 19-26 Sertoli Cell Tumor, Testis, Dog. A, Sertoli cell tumors are firm, white, and often lobulated, and the lobules are surrounded by fibrous bands. **B,** Histologically, Sertoli cell tumors have tubular structures lined by cells that resemble Sertoli cells and are supported by fine septa of fibrous tissue. H&E stain. **C,** Prostate, squamous metaplasia. Hyperestrogenism from functional Sertoli cell tumors induces hyperplasia and/or squamous metaplasia of the prostate. Normal epithelium of the prostatic ducts and glandular acini (columnar) is replaced by stratified squamous keratinizing epithelium. H&E stain. (**A** courtesy Dr. K. McEntee, Reproductive Pathology Collection, University of Illinois. **B** courtesy Dr. R.A. Foster, Ontario Veterinary College, University of Guelph. **C** courtesy Dr. W. Crowell, College of Veterinary Medicine, The University of Georgia; and Noah's Arkive, College of Veterinary Medicine, The University of Georgia.)

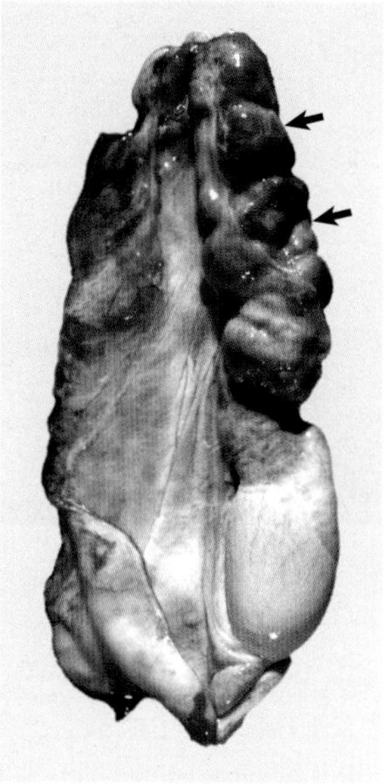

Figure 19-27 Varicocele, Pampiniform Plexus, Ram. This extremely large varicocele *(arrows)* is larger than the testis. It is multinodular from large thromboses filling the dilated veins. (Courtesy Dr. P.W. Ladds, James Cook University of North Queensland.)

testosterone production. A possibly life-threatening effect of hyperestrogenism is myelotoxicity, resulting in a poorly regenerative anemia, granulocytopenia, and thrombocytopenia.

Mixed germ cell–stromal neoplasms are also described. The testis containing the neoplasm is large and often cryptorchid. The testis is partially or completely replaced by a firm, gray-white to tan, single multilobed mass that is almost identical in appearance to a Sertoli cell tumor. Microscopically, germ cells intermingle with Sertoli cells in tubular structures of various sizes, thus it is a mixture of seminoma and Sertoli cell tumor.

Spermatic Cord

The spermatic cord is composed of the deferent duct, pampiniform plexus, and cremaster muscle. The scrotal lymph node and the inguinal canal are adjacent structures. The most common disease is *varicocele* or varicose dilation of veins of the pampiniform plexus (Fig. 19-27) in older rams and is described in the section on Disorders of Ruminants. It can be found in any species.

Torsion of the spermatic cord is usually seen in retained testes, especially when there is a testicular neoplasm present. Torsion also occurs periodically in the stallion and is a cause of colic. Torsion causes venous occlusion with a resultant venous infarction of the testis and less frequently the epididymis.

Inflammation of the spermatic cord (funisitis, scirrhous cord) occurs after contamination of a castration wound. Sometimes the lesion is neutrophilic and necrotizing (acute inflammation), but more often it is chronic and a scirrhous cord is encountered. Great enlargement of the distal part of the cord is caused by exuberant granulation tissue (see Chapter 3) in which numerous small pockets of pus are scattered. Staphylococci are the bacteria frequently recovered from the pus in the horse. The term *botryomycosis* is often used to name these staphylococcal pyogranulomas. Radiating club-shaped eosinophilic deposits (Splendore-Hoeppli reaction [see Chapters 3, 5, and 7]) are present around the central clusters of bacteria. This area is surrounded in turn by neutrophils and multinucleated giant cells and then by granulation and fibrous tissue.

Inguinal hernia is a differential diagnosis for masses or swellings in the region of the spermatic cord and scrotum. Stallions, older rams, and some Pietrain strains of pigs are particularly prone to inguinal hernia. It is an important cause of scrotal enlargement and colic in stallions. Little is known about the cause of inguinal hernia in domesticated animals. The herniated structures are usually a part of the intestine, and they can be free within the vaginal tunics or encased in a second fold of peritoneum. In stallions, the entrapped intestine undergoes venous infarction, causing life-threatening colic. In other species, intestinal infarcts are unusual.

Scrotal lymphadenopathy is another cause of swelling in the region of the spermatic cord. Caseous lymphadenitis in rams and lymphoma in dogs are causes of enlargement of the scrotal lymph nodes.

Disorders of the Accessory Genital Glands

The accessory genital glands include the ampullae, vesicular glands, prostate, and bulbourethral glands. The ampullae and vesicular glands are derived from the mesonephric duct, and the prostate and bulbourethral glands are derived from the urogenital sinus. Because of their location within the pelvis, they are not routinely examined. However, they should be routinely examined.

Ampullae of the Deferent Duct

Diseases of the ampullae are unusual, and the majority are microscopic. Bulls have variation in the patterns of insertion of ampullae at the seminal colliculus. The ampullae can be above or below the vesicular glands. This structural arrangement may contribute to the greater occurrence of ampullitis in bulls. The membrane between the ampullae is also the location for remnants of the paramesonephric duct—the cystic uterus masculinus—in bulls and rams. Hyperestrogenism can cause these duct remnants to become greatly enlarged.

Ampullitis is a feature of infection with microbes that cause epididymitis and vesicular adenitis, including *Brucella abortus*, *Brucella ovis*, *Actinobacillus seminis*, and *Histophilus somni*. It may precede epididymitis as part of an ascending infection or occur when organisms and inflammatory products pass through the deferent duct from an infected epididymis.

Vesicular Glands

The major disease of the vesicular glands (seminal vesicles) is inflammation of the gland, and often it is clinically silent, except in the bull, in which it is an important disease (see the section on Disorders of Ruminants (Cattle, Sheep, and Goats), The Accessory Genital Glands, Vesicular Adenitis).

Vesicular adenitis is occasionally seen in stallions and can be a part of lesions caused by *Burkholderia pseudomallei* in boars and the many *Brucella* spp., especially *Brucella ovis* in sheep (Fig. 19-28).

Prostate

The prostate is derived from the urogenital sinus. Both estrogens and androgens are trophic to the prostate.

The only species with any frequency of prostatic disease is the dog. There are three main disorders and their prevalence is, in descending order, hyperplasia (Fig. 19-29), prostatitis (Fig. 19-30), and neoplasia (Fig. 19-31). These disorders are discussed in the section on Disorders of Dogs and Cats, The Accessory Genital Glands, Prostate (Prostatic) Hyperplasia, Prostatic and Paraprostatic Cysts, Prostatitis, Carcinoma of the Prostate).

Bulbourethral Glands

The bulbourethral glands, as with the prostate, are derived from the urogenital sinus. There are few lesions of the bulbourethral glands, no doubt because of their dense structure and lack of lumina to allow bacterial growth and persistence. The major disease of this gland is seen in castrated male sheep grazing subterranean and red clover pasture with a high estrogen content (phytoestrogens). The glands of these wethers become so large that they cause perineal swellings. The glands have massive hypertrophy, squamous metaplasia, and cyst formation.

Disorders of the Penis and Prepuce

Disorders of the penis and prepuce are relatively rare, but infection is common and extremely important in production animals as a means of disease transmission. Many of the venereally transmitted organisms, such as *Tritrichomonas foetus*, *Campylobacter fetus*, herpesviruses, and papillomaviruses, are present in the prepuce and do not cause severe disease or have a mild and self-limiting course. The penis is protected from trauma and drying by the prepuce, and this environment is permissive of many infections. Only some induce an immune reaction and/or inflammation.

Phimosis is the inability to extrude the penis, *paraphimosis* is the inability to retract the penis into the prepuce, and *priapism* is a persistent erection; all are seen occasionally.

Disorders of Sexual Development

Persistent frenulum is a band of tissue between the ventral raphe of the penis and the prepuce. The raphe of the penis and prepuce are

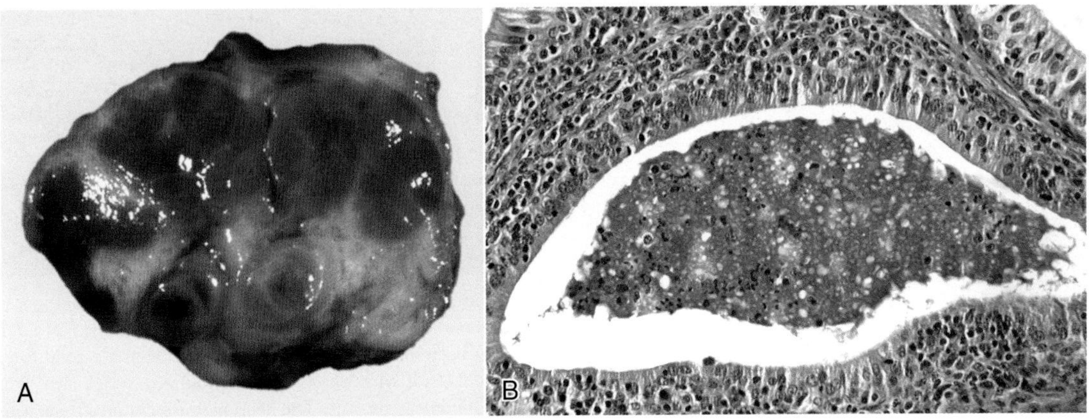

Figure 19-28 Chronic Vesicular Adenitis, Vesicular Gland, Cut Surface, Ram. A, The normal lobulation of the vesicular gland is distorted by white-gray fibrous tissue that surrounds the glandular tissue. **B,** Chronic vesicular adenitis (*Brucella ovis*). Glandular acini are filled with degenerating neutrophils and debris, and neutrophils are migrating through the acinar epithelium. The interstitium contains many plasma cells and lymphocytes. H&E stain. (Courtesy Dr. R.A. Foster, Ontario Veterinary College, University of Guelph.)

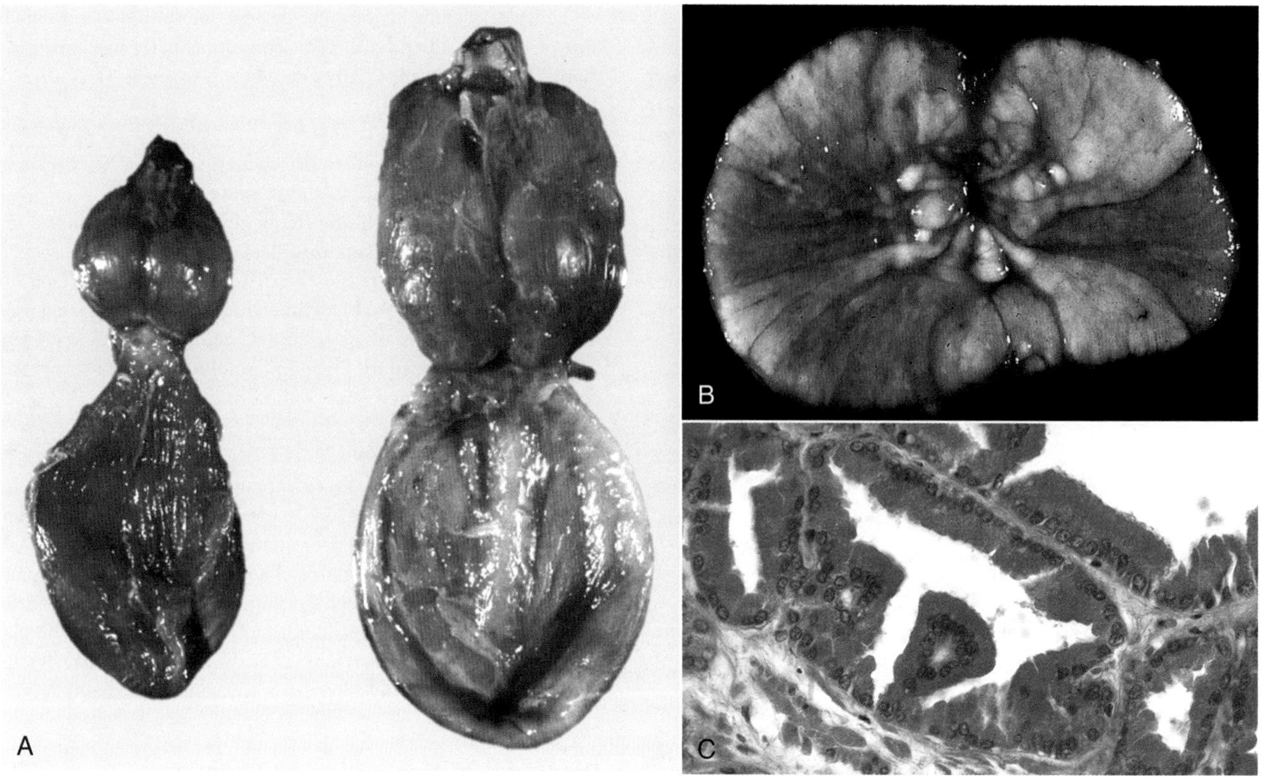

Figure 19-29 Prostatic Hyperplasia, Prostate, Dog. A, Prostates of two dogs of different ages (oldest on the right [age-related growth]). Both prostates are bilaterally and symmetrically larger than normal postpubertal prostates. **B,** The lighter white tissues that in some areas bulge from the cut surface are areas of hyperplasia. A hyperplastic prostate is symmetrically enlarged and detectable on rectal palpation, ultrasonography, or by gross examination at postmortem. **C,** The prostatic acini are larger than normal, as the epithelium is hyperplastic and the cells enlarged (hypertrophy). Note the abundant granular apical cytoplasm and the uniform size and shape of the cells. Mitotic activity is very low. H&E stain. (**A** courtesy Dr. R.A. Foster, Ontario Veterinary College, University of Guelph. **B** courtesy Department of Veterinary Biosciences, The Ohio State University; and Noah's Arkive, College of Veterinary Medicine, The University of Georgia. **C** courtesy Dr. R.K. Myers, College of Veterinary Medicine, Iowa State University.)

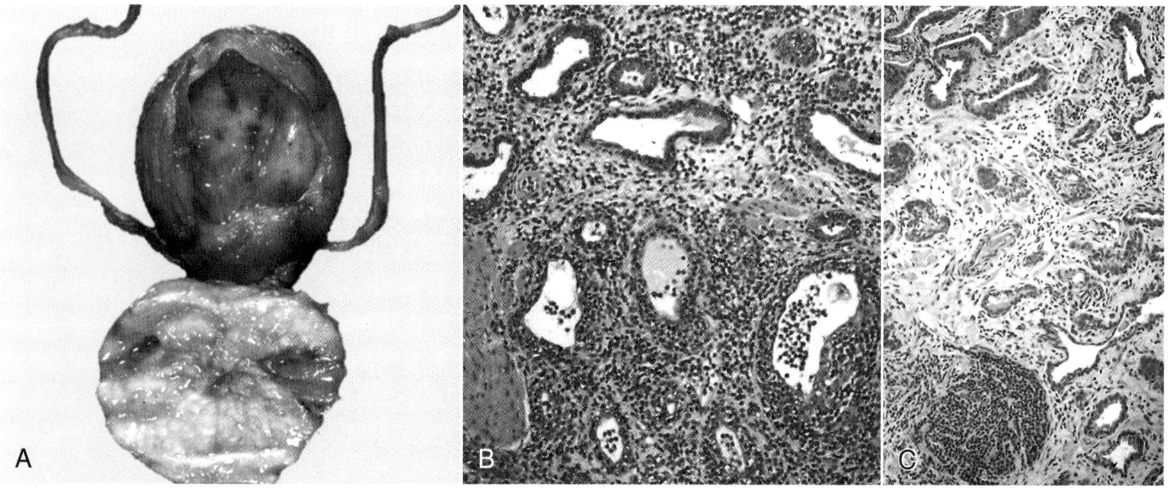

Figure 19-30 Prostatitis, Prostate, Dog. A, Severe acute prostatitis, cut surface. The prostate is enlarged with edema, and there are many white foci of inflammatory cells instead of the usually smooth whitish-pink surface. Clinically, this condition is usually painful. **B,** Acute prostatitis. Note that the glands and interstitium contain large numbers of neutrophils. Most of these infections are of bacterial origin and develop after bacteria ascend the urethra. H&E stain. **C,** Chronic prostatitis. Note that the glands and interstitium contain large numbers of lymphocytes and macrophages and a large lymphoid nodule *(bottom half of image)*. Follicular lymphoid hyperplasia is a common finding in chronically infected tissue. The abundant interstitial stroma is from fibroplasia and chronic inflammation. Most cases of chronic prostatitis have a bacterial origin. H&E stain. (Courtesy Dr. W. Crowell, College of Veterinary Medicine, The University of Georgia; and Noah's Arkive, College of Veterinary Medicine, The University of Georgia.)

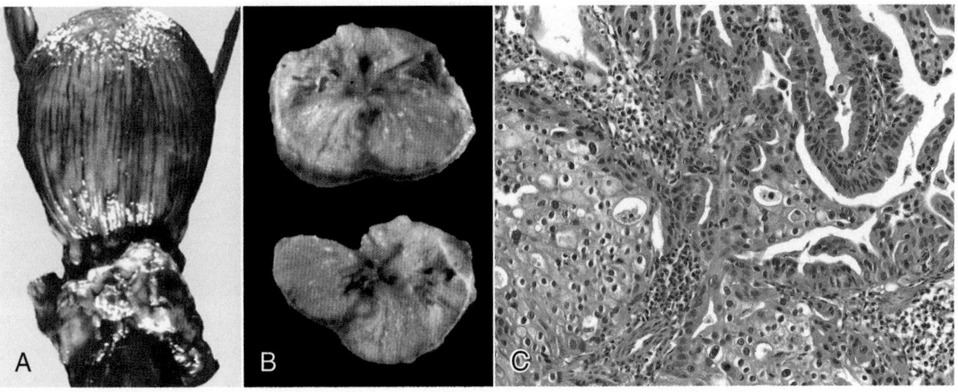

Figure 19-31 **Carcinoma, Prostate, Dog. A,** The adjacent pelvic tissues of this dog contain many coalescing nodules of metastatic carcinoma that have spread from the prostate, which is barely recognizable beneath the bladder *(opened, upper half of image)*. Prostatic carcinomas are usually asymmetric and lobulated white to gray masses that expand the size of the gland and may compress the urethra (dysuria) and the colon (difficulty defecating, ribbon stools). **B,** Cross section. Note the asymmetric enlargement. The focal white areas are regions of necrosis within a gland that is enlarged by neoplastic epithelial cells that induce the abundant fibrous tissue that is also present. **C,** Note the anaplastic prostatic epithelial cells arranged in papillae *(upper right)* and solid nodules *(lower left)*. Mitoses can be frequent in some cases. There also may be stromal or lymphatic invasion and desmoplasia (scirrhous response). H&E stain. (**A** courtesy Dr. M. Howard, College of Veterinary Medicine, Iowa State University; and Noah's Arkive, College of Veterinary Medicine, The University of Georgia. **B** courtesy Dr. J.A. Ramos-Vara, College of Veterinary Medicine, Michigan State University; and Noah's Arkive, College of Veterinary Medicine, The University of Georgia. **C** courtesy Dr. R.A. Foster, Ontario Veterinary College, University of Guelph.)

remnants of the frenulum, a thin membrane ventral to the penis. The penile and preputial epithelium is completely fused before puberty and separate, probably as the result of simple mechanical forces. Balanopreputial bands that do not separate are located elsewhere on the penis. They are relatively common and minor anatomic abnormalities rather than serious defects, but they can have an important deleterious effect in limiting the extent to which the penis can be protruded from the sheath and in causing the erect penis to be curved instead of straight (Fig. 19-32). Persistent frenulum is important in bulls and boars. Judging by the frequent occurrence of large flaps and tags of tissue on the ventral raphe of the penis, transitory persistence of the frenulum is quite common.

The penis is subject to many abnormalities of size and form, such as congenital absence, hypoplasia, duplication, directional deviations, and, in ruminants, absence of the sigmoid flexure and abnormal locations of the insertions of the retractor penis muscles. None of these lesions are common.

Hypospadias and epispadias are malformations of the urethral canal that create abnormal openings of the urethra on the ventral surface (hypospadias) or on the dorsal surface (epispadias) of the penis. In hypospadias, the urinary opening is anywhere from the head to the shaft of the penis, penoscrotal junction, or the perineum. Their importance is in the potential for causing urinary obstruction and in interference with normal insemination.

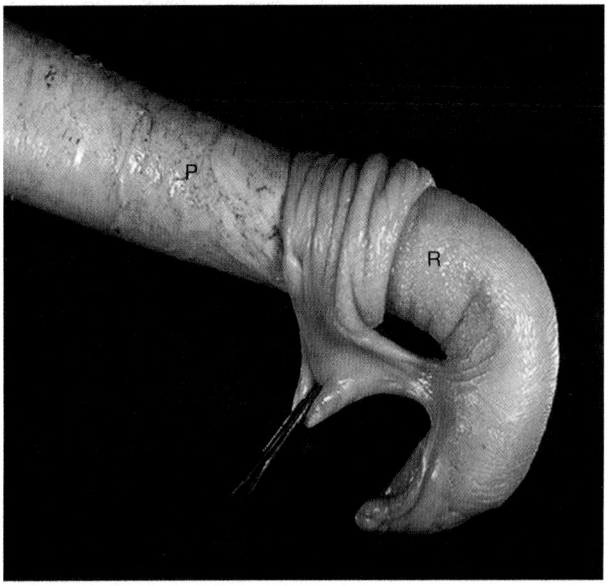

Figure 19-32 **Persistent Frenulum, Penis, Bull.** A band of tissue *(forceps)*, a frenulum remnant, connects the ventral surface of the penis to the prepuce *(R)* at its reflection from the penis and has caused the penis *(P)* to be curved ventrally as the animal has matured, thus making intromission impossible. (Courtesy Dr. W. Crowell, College of Veterinary Medicine, The University of Georgia; and Noah's Arkive, College of Veterinary Medicine, The University of Georgia.)

Hemorrhage and Penile Hematoma

The penis is a highly vascular structure, and the presence of erectile tissue and high pressures during erection and coitus make the potential for severe or even fatal hemorrhage high (Fig. 19-33). Trauma to the penis is usually responsible; cuts, lacerations, and surgical incisions bleed profusely. Forced deviation of the penis in ruminants causes rupture and hemorrhage (see the section on Disorders of Ruminants (Cattle, Sheep, and Goats), The Penis and Prepuce, Penile Forced Deviation and Hematoma) that can be fatal.

Inflammation

Inflammation of the penis is *phallitis*, that of the head (glans) of the penis is *balanitis*, and that of the prepuce is *posthitis*. Inflammation of both the penis and prepuce (*phaloposthitis* or *balanoposthitis*) occurs mostly in castrated animals. This consequence could be the result of alterations to structure because of a lack of testosterone and/or normal development and the tendency of these animals to urinate within their prepuce. Retention of urine in the preputial cavity irritates and damages the mucous membrane and creates an environment for the overgrowth of bacteria. Bacteria that produce urease split urea to ammonia, a toxic molecule that further damages the preputial epithelium, causing erosion and ulceration. Ovine posthitis (discussed later) is a classic disease.

Nonspecific posthitis occurs in all species but is most common in the gelding. In geldings, it is believed to occur because of a lack of extrusion of the penis with a resultant buildup of waxy smegma and bacterial overgrowth. A foul-smelling prepuce and posthitis is the result. Dogs commonly develop a nonspecific and purulent discharge of the prepuce.

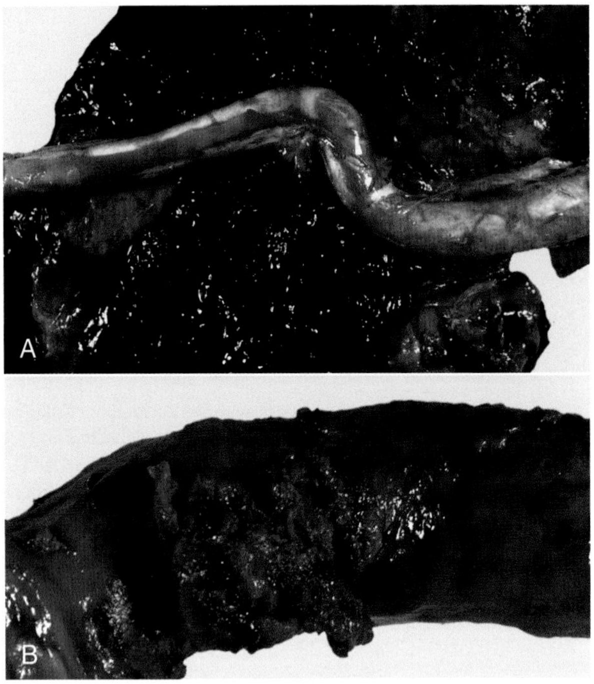

Figure 19-33 **Penile Hematoma, Penis, Bull. A,** The large hemorrhage around the penis at the sigmoid flexure is a hematoma from rupture of the penis during forced deviation. **B,** Illustrated is the site of rupture of the penis with a blood clot filling the rupture site. (Courtesy Dr. M.D. McGavin, College of Veterinary Medicine, University of Tennessee.)

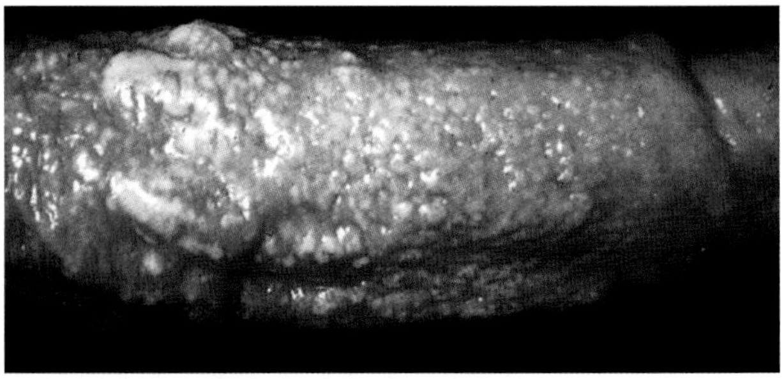

Figure 19-34 **Phaloposthitis, Bovine Herpesvirus 1, Penis (Free Part), Bull.** Note the vesicles and pustules of the mucosa. Bovine herpesvirus 1 causes hyperemia, swelling, vesicles, pustules, and 1- to 2-mm ulcers, especially of the prepuce. Intranuclear inclusion bodies are present microscopically, briefly in epithelial cells of the penis and prepuce during the vesiculopustular stage. (Courtesy Dr. K. McEntee, Reproductive Pathology Collection, University of Illinois; and Dr. J. King, College of Veterinary Medicine, Cornell University.)

Herpesviruses cause multifocal phaloposthitis in several species. Equid herpesvirus 3 is the cause of *equine coital exanthema*, a disease of stallions and mares with a similarly short clinical course but with larger (15-mm) ulcers with a predilection for the body rather than the head of the penis. Bovine herpesvirus 1 (BoHV-1) causes a phaloposthitis in the bull, progressing over the course of a few days from hyperemia and swelling to vesicles and pustules and then to 1- to 2-mm ulcers, especially of the head of the penis (Fig. 19-34). In the vesiculopustular stage, intranuclear inclusion bodies are present briefly in epithelial cells of the penis and prepuce. Ulcerative balanoposthitis with acidophilic intranuclear inclusions has been observed in goats and is considered a result of caprine herpesvirus 1 infection. Canid herpesvirus 1 reportedly causes inflammation at the base of the penis and the reflection of the prepuce but does not cause pustules or ulcers. Resolution of these lesions in the affected species is rapid, leaving only hyperplastic mucosal lymphoid nodules and small areas of depigmented mucosa (see Chapter 18). BoHV-1, suid herpesvirus 1 (pseudorabies virus) in pigs, caprine herpesvirus 1, and canid herpesvirus 1 can persist in a latent state, capable of becoming reactivated by stress or treatment with corticosteroids.

Other organisms are capable of causing phaloposthitis. These organisms include the larvae of *Habronema* spp. in the horse and *Strongyloides papillosus* in the bull. The well-known bovine venereally transmitted diseases of campylobacteriosis and trichomoniasis cause no lesions or minimal nonspecific lesions of the penis and prepuce, even though they reside there.

Foreign material sometimes is found in the prepuce; bulls, rams, bucks, and tomcats can have matted hair around their penis to form a constricting ring (colloquially called *hair ring*). This "ring" can cause a posthitis or even avascular penile necrosis. It is assumed that the deposition of hair in this location is, at least in ruminants, the result of homosexual activity and the rubbing of the penis on the posterior of other animals. Dogs, especially those of the chondrodystrophic breeds with short legs, impact their prepuce with sand.

All species can have traumatic wounds of a variety of types and severity, resulting from mating injuries. Mating or attempting to mate through fences can cause lacerations of varying severities. Owners attempting to "untie" mating dogs can cause degloving injuries (skin is sheared or torn off) to the penis. Horses with penile laceration can develop exuberant granulation tissue ("proud flesh") of the penis.

Many species develop preputial prolapse, but it is well known in the bull and is discussed in the section on Disorders of Ruminants (Cattle, Sheep, and Goats).

Papillomaviruses affect the penis of many species. Typical "warts" are produced in the dog, sarcoids are seen in horses, and the bull develops fibropapilloma (Fig. 19-35, *A* and *B*). The bovine disease is discussed in the section on Disorders of Ruminants (Cattle, Sheep, and Goats), The Penis and Prepuce, Penile Fibropapilloma.

Obstruction of the penile urethra, especially at the sigmoid flexure of all ruminants and the urethral process of small ruminants, is common with urolithiasis (see Chapter 11). The narrowest part of the urethra is the urethral process, and small uroliths that pass through the rest of the urethra become lodged near the tip. Depending on the degree of obstruction, necrosis, and rupture, penile and preputial necrosis can occur. Many animals die of bladder rupture before necrosis of the urethral process or penis occurs.

Neoplasms

Primary neoplasms of the penis and prepuce are mostly restricted to a limited number of types of neoplasms and species affected. Metastatic or multicentric neoplasms affect these tissues rarely. Dogs develop the allotransplanted (i.e., the transplantation of living cells between animals) *canine transmissible venereal tumor* (CTVT; see the section on Disorders of Dogs and Cats, The Penis and Prepuce, Canine Transmissible Venereal Tumor). Cells forming the tumor have 57-64 chromosomes, whereas normal somatic cells in dogs have 78 chromosomes. *Papilloma* and *squamous cell carcinoma* occur in the horse (see Disorders of Horses, Penile Squamous Cell Carcinoma), bull, boar, and dog and are discussed in the sections covering individual species. Horses develop *sarcoids* of the penis, which are described in more detail in the section on Disorders of Horses.

Disorders of Horses

The most common disorders of the male reproductive system of horses are listed in Table 19-1.

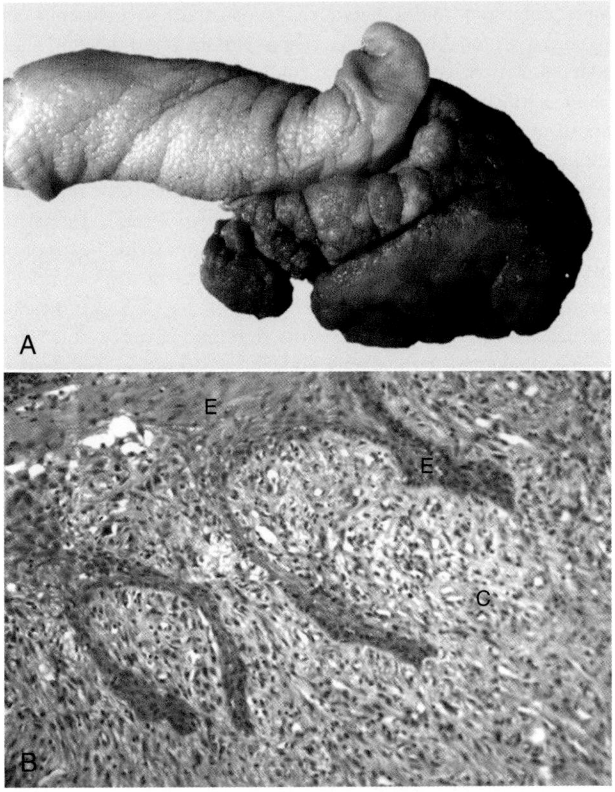

Figure 19-35 **Penile Fibropapilloma, Head of Penis, Bull. A,** There is a large exophytic papillary mass protruding from the penile epithelium. This large proliferative lesion on the penis is typical of a fibropapilloma. **B,** Note the abundant connective tissue *(C)* covered by hyperplastic stratified squamous epithelium *(E)* that is thickened and has elongated epidermal-dermal interdigitations that penetrate deeply into the connective tissue. H&E stain. (**A** courtesy Dr. R.A. Foster, Ontario Veterinary College, University of Guelph. **B** courtesy Dr. J. Simon, College of Veterinary Medicine, University of Illinois.)

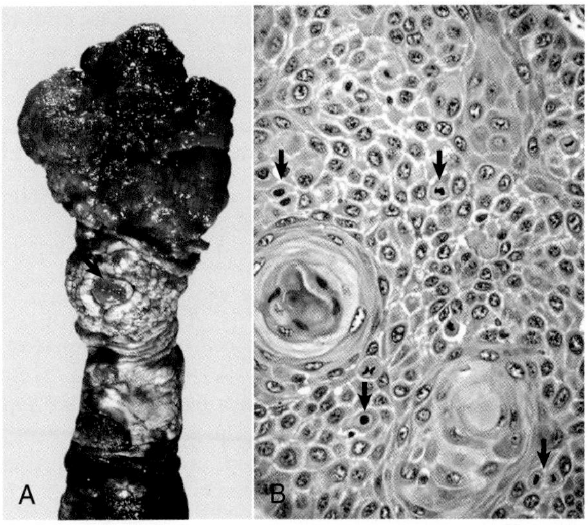

Figure 19-36 **Squamous Cell Carcinoma, Penis, Ventral Surface, Horse (Gelding). A,** A large ulcerated mass protrudes from the glans penis. The urethral opening is visible *(arrow)*. **B,** Neoplastic squamous epithelial cells are often arranged around "keratin pearls." Mitoses are frequent *(arrows)*. H&E stain. (**A** courtesy Dr. R.A. Foster, Ontario Veterinary College, University of Guelph. **B** courtesy Dr. M.J. Abdy, College of Veterinary Medicine, The University of Georgia; and Noah's Arkive, College of Veterinary Medicine, The University of Georgia.)

Table 19-1 Horses: Common and Important Disorders of the Male Reproductive System

Species	Disorders
Stallion	Scrotum and contents
	Cryptorchidism
	Seminoma and teratoma
	Torsion
	Inguinal hernia
	Penis and prepuce
	Squamous cell carcinoma

The Scrotum and Contents

The common and important disorders of the scrotum and contents are trauma, cryptorchidism, testicular and epididymal torsion, scirrhous cord, and inguinal hernia. Young horses can develop testicular teratomas and aged horses can develop seminomas. These disorders are described in greater detail in the section on Disorders of Domestic Animals, Disorders of the Scrotum and Contents.

The Accessory Genital Glands

Disorders of the accessory genital glands are rare in stallions.

The Penis and Prepuce

The range of lesions possible are those described in the section on Disorders of Domestic Animals, Disorders of the Penis and Prepuce. In the penis and prepuce, squamous cell carcinoma, habronemiasis, equine sarcoid, exuberant granulation tissue, and nonspecific posthitis in geldings are common.

Penile Squamous Cell Carcinoma

Both stallions and geldings develop squamous cell carcinoma of the head of the penis (Fig. 19-36, *A*). This neoplasm is causally linked with the equine papillomavirus *Equus caballus* papillomavirus-2 (EcPV-2). Although exophytic masses do occur, the usual pattern of growth is infiltrative. These carcinomas induce abundant fibrous tissue, which results in an enlarged firm penis with focal ulcers. Microscopically, the neoplasm is well differentiated with the classic appearance of invasive nests, cords, and nodules of neoplastic epithelium with differentiation toward the stratum spinosum, often with well-developed keratin pearls (Fig. 19-36, *B*) or keratin squames mixed with neutrophils. The neoplastic cells are surrounded by fibrous tissue, as well as lymphocytes and plasma cells. Metastasis is to the superficial inguinal (scrotal), deep inguinal, and/or medial iliac lymph nodes. The prepuce often becomes edematous because of lymphatic obstruction by the neoplasm, and the preputial cavity becomes distended by retained smegma, inflammatory debris, and urine.

Penile Habronemiasis, Sarcoids, and Exuberant Granulation Tissue

Habronemiasis is the lesion caused by aberrant migration of the larvae of *Habronema muscae* and *Draschia megastoma*, which are deposited by infected flies on wounds (or elsewhere) on the penis or prepuce of horses. The gross lesion is an ulcerated, often exophytic mass on the penis or prepuce. It has the same appearance as exuberant granulation tissue or equine sarcoid. Microscopically, however, the lesions are multiple distinct nodules and tracts containing larvae and/or are filled with debris and eosinophils. Granulation and fibrous tissue surround the nodules and tracts.

Equine sarcoids and exuberant granulation tissue of the penis or prepuce are identical to their dermal counterparts (see Chapters 3 and 17). As with habronemiasis, these disorders form ulcerated proliferative lesions on the penis and prepuce. Histologic evaluation is necessary to differentiate these disorders from each other.

Disorders of Ruminants (Cattle, Sheep, and Goats)

The most common disorders of the male reproductive system of bulls, rams, and bucks are listed in Table 19-2.

The Scrotum and Contents

Bulls, rams, and bucks all develop the range of lesions of the scrotum, vaginal tunics, testis, and epididymis seen in all species (see the section on Disorders of Domestic Animals, Disorders of the Scrotum and Contents). Cryptorchidism, testicular hypoplasia, and atrophy/degeneration are important. In rams, epididymitis and varicocele are important. Those disorders that are both unique and well studied are described here.

Epididymitis

Infectious epididymitis is most common and important in rams. It occurs in two main ways in rams: hematogenously by *Brucella ovis* and by ascending infection with bacteria such as *Actinobacillus seminis*, *Histophilus somni*, and *Escherichia coli*. Regardless of the causative microbe, the lesion is similar and is dominated grossly and microscopically by swelling and then formation of spermatic granulomas. Macroscopically, the lesions are usually restricted to the tail of the epididymis, regardless of the causative bacterium. The tail of the epididymis is enlarged up to 10-fold and is largest when spermatic granulomas form. Microscopically, the duct lumina contain a mixture of spermatozoa, neutrophils, and macrophages and multinucleate foreign body–type giant cells. The epithelium changes from simple columnar and ciliated to pseudostratified columnar and cuboidal with focal hyperplasia. These regions often develop a secondary lumen or intraepithelial lumina. Some of the epithelium becomes stratified squamous in type (squamous metaplasia). The smooth muscle wall of the duct and the interstitium contain many lymphocytes and plasma cells, plus edema and fibrin initially. Fibrous tissue rapidly develops beginning with granulation tissue and eventually forming mature fibrous tissue (see Fig. 19-21). Interstitial abscesses and spermatic granulomas develop after either death of the tissue or rupture of the duct and development of a spermatocele. Spermatocele can rupture into the cavity of the vaginal tunics and produce a severe periorchitis. With time and severity, the tunics become thickened with edema and fibrin deposition, followed by granulation tissue and finally fibrosis.

Varicocele

Varicocele is the local dilation of the spermatic vein in the pampiniform plexus. Older rams are most commonly affected, but the underlying defect is unknown. Approximately half the cases are bilateral, and the unilateral cases are evenly divided between the left and the right side. Thrombosis of affected vessels is common. The dilated veins are located near the inguinal ring; the complex distal part of the pampiniform plexus is not affected (see Fig. 19-27). The thrombosed and dilated vessels are up to 10 cm in diameter and are so large that they interfere with thermoregulation, either by their sheer size or by interfering with the countercurrent system. Venous flow from the testis could theoretically be restricted, and this could subsequently alter testicular oxygen tension and create oxidative stress, thus causing testicular degeneration, poor spermatozoal motility, and immature spermatozoa in the semen.

Table 19-2 Ruminants (Cattle, Sheep, and Goats): Common and Important Disorders of the Male Reproductive System

Species	Disorders
Bull	Scrotum and contents
	Cryptorchidism
	Testicular hypoplasia
	Testicular atrophy/degeneration
	Accessory genital glands
	Vesicular adenitis
	Penis and prepuce
	Fibropapilloma
	Penile hematoma
	Preputial prolapse
Ram	Scrotum and contents
	Epididymitis
	Testicular atrophy/degeneration
	Testicular hypoplasia
	Varicocele
	Accessory genital glands
	Vesicular adenitis
	Penis and prepuce
	Ovine posthitis
	Urolithiasis
Buck	Scrotum and contents
	Testicular atrophy/degeneration
	Penis and prepuce
	Hair ring
	Caprine herpesvirus-1

The Accessory Genital Glands

Bulls, rams, and bucks can develop the range of lesions of the accessory genital glands seen in all species (see the section on Disorders of Domestic Animals, Disorders of the Accessory Genital Glands). Vesicular adenitis is unique and important.

Vesicular Adenitis

Vesicular adenitis (seminal vesiculitis) is a significant disease because it reduces fertility, particularly in young bulls. Inflammation in the vesicular glands contributes inflammatory cells and mediators to the semen. It also reduces the ability of spermatozoa to survive freezing. Young bulls in their first breeding season are especially affected. The cause is most likely infectious; various organisms, including viruses, protozoa, *Chlamydia* sp., *Ureaplasma diversum*, *Mycoplasma* sp., *Brucella abortus*, and other bacteria, have been investigated throughout the years. The pathogenesis is uncertain, but hypotheses include ascending infection, descending infection, hematogenous spread, congenital malformation preventing excretion of fluid and spermatozoa, and reflux of spermatozoa or urine into the glands.

The common form of vesicular adenitis in bulls is a chronic interstitial inflammation (see Fig. 19-28, *A* and *B*). It begins with an acute inflammatory form where the glands are swollen with edema, and they are painful on palpation. Microscopically, neutrophils enter the lumen of glands and there is edema and fibrin in the interstitium. In the more long-standing and interstitial form, both vesicular glands are enlarged and firm and have loss of lobulation. Glandular lumina contain neutrophils and debris, but there are many lymphocytes and plasma cells in the interstitium, and collagen is deposited between the acini (see Fig. 19-28, *B*). Metaplasia of glandular epithelium develops, and a stratified squamous type is common. Vesicular adenitis in rams and bucks cannot be detected with gross observation and thus is diagnosed by microscopy.

The Penis and Prepuce

Bulls, rams, and bucks can develop the range of lesions of the penis and prepuce seen in all species (see the section on Disorders of Domestic Animals, Disorders of the Penis and Prepuce). Those disorders that are both unique and important are described here.

Penile Forced Deviation and Hematoma

Penile hematoma (penile deviation; broken penis) after forced deviation is an important disease in bulls. A similar disease is reported in the ram. During mating, the penis probes for the vulva, and when appropriate, the copulatory thrust and ejaculation is done with great force. If the penis deviates from its intended target, lateral pressure is applied to the region of the sigmoid flexure and insertion of the retractor penis muscles, resulting in rupture and hemorrhage (see Fig. 19-33). The swelling of the hematoma is just cranial to the scrotum and can be up to 50 cm in diameter. In severe cases, hemorrhagic shock occurs. Small hematomas heal without complications, but depending on the extent of the injury and size of the hematoma, granulation and scar tissue is formed and prevents extension of the penis (phimosis). Some hematomas become infected and result in a penile abscess.

Penile Fibropapilloma

Fibropapilloma occurs on the head of the penis of young bulls (see Fig. 19-35, A and B). It is caused by bovine papillomavirus 1 infection, but the pathogenesis is incompletely understood. Affected animals are young, usually in their first breeding season, and the lesions are self-limiting. Larger neoplasms can interfere with breeding by causing pain or by their physical size. Affected bulls can develop an aversion to mating. Macroscopically, the single or multiple warty masses have a papillary epithelial covering and a fibrous core. Surface ulceration is often extensive. They are histologically typical of fibropapillomas elsewhere, with epithelial and stromal hyperplasia and long projections of epithelium into the fibrous tissue. Intranuclear inclusion bodies are seen in the epithelium of some cases. The proportions of epithelial and fibrous tissue vary greatly from case to case.

Preputial Prolapse

Bulls of the *Bos indicus* type have a pendulous prepuce, and many have a small or absent preputial retractor muscle. Temporary eversion of the prepuce for urination is common in bulls, but affected bulls have inadequate muscular control. The everted preputial mucosa is injured and becomes swollen with edema and inflammation. The prepuce remains everted (prolapsed), swells further, dries, and is further lacerated, leading to a cycle of injury and inflammation that is permanent. Affected bulls are unable to mate.

Ovine Posthitis

Ovine posthitis (pizzle rot) is a disease of wethers mostly and is caused by urease-producing *Corynebacterium renale*. When the diet is high in protein and the urine has a high concentration of urea, *Corynebacterium renale* breaks the urea down to ammonia, which is cytotoxic. This condition produces ulceration of the prepuce near the orifice. Lack of testosterone (from castration) is also involved because the disease can be prevented by administration of androgens to wethers. If the preputial orifice becomes blocked by swelling, the disease becomes much more severe, spreading beyond the initial small ulcer on the hairless skin of the prepuce to diffusely involve the mucosa, with ulceration of the head of the penis and loss of the urethral process. Scarring and phimosis can result. In severe cases, the preputial orifice becomes blocked and animals die from the retention of urine.

Table 19-3 Pigs: Common and Important Disorders of the Male Reproductive System

Species	Disorders
Boar	Scrotum and contents Cryptorchidism Scrotal hemangiomas Testicular atrophy/degeneration Penis and prepuce Preputial diverticulitis

Disorders of Pigs

The most common disorders of the male reproductive system of boars are listed in Table 19-3.

The Scrotum and Contents

Boars develop a full range of lesions of the scrotum and its contents, as do other species. These disorders are described in the section on Disorders of Domestic Animals, Disorders of the Scrotum and Contents.

The scrotal skin of boars commonly develops what is called scrotal hamartomas or scrotal hemangiomas. These lesions are multiple focal dark red to black proliferations of the scrotal skin that histologically are clusters of capillaries. They have no known effect on fertility, but they can ulcerate and bleed. Papillomas can also form on the scrotum.

Cryptorchidism is very common in boars, and torsion of a cryptorchid testis is frequently encountered in abattoirs. Testicular hypoplasia and testicular atrophy/degeneration also occur. *Brucella suis* is the common *Brucella* spp. of pigs but is largely eradicated from intensive piggeries (confinement pig production). It causes orchitis and epididymitis.

The Accessory Genital Glands

Although the accessory genital glands of boars, particularly the vesicular glands and bulbourethral glands, are very large, little has been published about their diseases. The range of potential diseases are as outlined in the section on Disorders of Domestic Animals, Disorders of the Accessory Genital Glands.

The Penis and Prepuce

Many different conditions of the penis and prepuce are possible in boars, just as they are in other species (see the section on Disorders of Domestic Animals, Disorders of the Penis and Prepuce).

Of particular note because it is unique to the boar is preputial papilloma virus infection and preputial diverticulitis.

Preputial Diverticulitis

Boars are the only domesticated animal with a preputial diverticulum; it is located dorsal to the preputial orifice. Inflammation of the preputial diverticulum is called preputial diverticulitis and has an unknown pathogenesis. Deflection of the penis into the diverticulum because of malformation or masturbation is suspected, and local infection occurs. Macroscopically, there is swelling above the preputial orifice, and a foul-smelling fluid and exudate can be expressed instead of the normal clear fluid. Histologically, the epithelium is eroded and covered with fibrin, debris, and neutrophils. Lymphocytes and plasma cells and granulation tissue are located in the wall. The diverticulum is also a location for transmissible genital papillomas to develop.

Disorders of Dogs and Cats

The most common disorders of the male reproductive system of the dog and cat are listed in Table 19-4.

The Scrotum and Contents

Dogs and cats develop a full range of lesions of the scrotum and its contents, as do other species. These are described in the section on Disorders of Domestic Animals, Disorders of the Scrotum and Contents.

Cryptorchidism is a common and important disease in both dogs and cats and is the most common testicular disease of cats. In dogs, testicular atrophy/degeneration is very common, particularly in older dogs. Hypoplasia of the testis also occurs frequently. Dogs commonly develop primary testicular neoplasms, and these are described in the section on Disorders of Domestic Animals. Infectious epididymitis with concurrent orchitis is an important disease with some unique features, so it is described next.

Infectious Epididymitis with Orchitis

Infectious epididymitis occurs most commonly in mature dogs, and not just at puberty. The reason for this is unknown. Most cases are caused by Gram-negative bacteria such as *Escherichia coli* and presumably by ascending infection. Infectious orchitis is surprisingly common too, and hematogenous or local spread from infectious epididymitis are both possible. In severe disease, dogs have a large painful and doughy scrotum plus endotoxemia and a systemic response to infection with anorexia, lethargy, and fever. The tail of the epididymis and vaginal tunics are usually affected, but in some cases, a severe necrotizing orchitis also develops. Dogs will lick and chew at an affected scrotum and may create a fistula to the scrotal contents (see Fig. 19-20). *Brucella canis* infection also causes epididymitis by a hematogenous route. The lesions in the testis and epididymis (see Fig. 19-18) are identical to those described previously in the discussion of epididymitis in the section on Disorders of Ruminants (Cattle, Sheep, and Goats). Testicular atrophy and degeneration is an invariable consequence of epididymitis, and many dogs also have prostatitis.

Table 19-4 Dogs and Cats: Common and Important Disorders of the Male Reproductive System

Species	Disorders
Dog	Scrotum and contents
	Cryptorchidism
	Epididymitis
	Testicular neoplasia
	Interstitial cell tumor
	Seminoma
	Sertoli cell tumor
	Accessory genital glands
	Carcinoma of prostate
	Paraprostatic cysts
	Prostatic hyperplasia
	Prostatitis
	Penis and prepuce
	Nonspecific posthitis
	Papilloma
	Transmissible venereal tumor
Cat	Scrotum and contents
	Cryptorchidism
	Penis and prepuce
	Urolithiasis

Testicular Neoplasms

The three most common primary testicular neoplasms in the dog are seminoma, Sertoli cell tumor, and interstitial (Leydig) cell tumor; they occur alone or in combination. For more detail on these important tumors, see the section on Disorders of Domestic Animals, Disorders of the Scrotum and Contents, Testis and Epididymis, Testicular and Epididymal Enlargement, Neoplasia.

The Accessory Genital Glands

The only accessory genital gland of the dog is the prostate, and it develops all the major prostatic diseases that occur in human beings. Cats have a prostate and bulbourethral gland, but disease of those organs is extremely rare. When present, they are similar to the disease in dogs.

Prostate (Prostatic) Hyperplasia

The dog is the only domestic animal species to spontaneously develop prostatic hyperplasia with age (see Fig. 19-29, *A* and *B*). The clinical consequence of prostatic enlargement includes constipation from the "ball valve" effect of a large prostate forced into the pelvis during attempted defecation. Although obstruction of the urethra is a feature of prostatic hyperplasia in human beings, stenosis of the urethra only occasionally occurs in the canine disease. Enlargement of the prostate is hormone related, but the precise mechanisms are unknown. Enlargement of the gland at puberty does not occur in castrated dogs, and removal of androgens by castration of dogs after puberty causes atrophy. Administration of estrogens may initially reduce the size of an enlarged prostate, but it eventually causes enlargement of the gland because estrogen and testosterone operate in concert (see Fig. 19-29, *C*). Enlargement of the gland is usually uniform. Occasionally, the hyperplasia is cystic, and in extreme cases, a large single cyst or multiple small cysts are found. Microscopically, there is hyperplasia of the acinar epithelium, and individual epithelial cells are larger than normal and their apical cytoplasm is expanded and filled with eosinophilic globules. Stromal hyperplasia causes a larger amount of the interlobular and to a lesser extent the intralobular fibromuscular stroma. Some acini are distended with fluid and have a flattened epithelium.

Estrogen-induced hypertrophy of the canine prostate is most often seen with a testicular Sertoli cell tumor. Hyperestrogenism also causes squamous metaplasia of acinar epithelium, ducts, prostatic urethra, and the uterus masculinus (see Fig. 19-26, *C*). Flattened keratinized epithelial cells are desquamated into the acini, and neutrophils and other inflammatory cells are present. Squamous metaplasia of the prostate in dogs is not preneoplastic.

Prostatic and Paraprostatic Cysts

Prostatic and paraprostatic cysts occur periodically in dogs, and their origin is debated. Intraprostatic cysts occur in prostatic hyperplasia, squamous metaplasia, and prostatitis. Paraprostatic cysts are outside the capsule of the prostate. Some are an enlarged cystic uterus masculinus (see the section on Disorders of Sexual Development, Cysts of the Reproductive Tract), and some are scrosal inclusion cysts or pseudocysts that do not have an epithelial lining. Many are probably hyperplastic cysts formed when cystic acini extrude through the incomplete muscular layer of the prostatic capsule, in a manner similar to adenomyosis of the uterus. Paraprostatic cysts can attain giant proportions, as large as 30 cm in diameter. Some cysts become infected and abscessed. They have a thin wall, and some have mineralization and ossification of the collagen in the capsule. Microscopically, they have an inner lining of either flattened cuboidal epithelium, cells resembling mesothelium, or granulation and fibrous tissue. They also have a thin fibrous capsule. Those cysts with mineralization and ossification have normal woven or lamellar bone within the capsule. Most have no inflammation.

Prostatitis

Prostatitis is seen periodically and can be clinically significant if toxemia accompanies the infection or if there is urinary obstruction. Prostatitis is found in older animals, often together with hyperplasia, or in young animals without hyperplasia. Although increased concentrations of zinc in prostatic fluid have antimicrobial properties in human beings and dogs, resistance to infection and resolution of infection are not correlated with zinc concentrations in prostatic tissue in the dog. Prostatitis can be divided into an acute inflammatory form, a chronic inflammatory form, an abscess form, and a form caused by *Brucella canis*. In the acute inflammatory form, bacteria such as *Escherichia coli* and *Proteus vulgaris* ascend from the urethra. The affected prostate can be diffusely or focally involved, swollen, red, and edematous (see Fig. 19-30, *A*). The initial microscopic lesion following bacterial infection is neutrophilic inflammation, and acini contain neutrophils and debris. The degree of necrosis varies and is extensive in some cases. Without resolution of the cause, the acute form transitions to the chronic inflammatory form of prostatitis. Abscesses can also form (see Fig. 19-30, *B*). The abscesses can persist or be replaced by fibrous tissue. With continued infection, lymphocytes and plasma cells are present in the interstitium in large numbers. Usually, fibrosis is an accompanying change (see Fig. 19-30, *C*). Prostatitis is part of the spectrum of lesions caused by *Brucella canis* in the dog, and the prostate can be the site of persistence of the bacterium.

Carcinoma of the Prostate

Canine prostatic carcinoma is the only prostatic neoplasm of importance in domestic animals (see Fig. 19-31, *A*). A similar disease is exceedingly rare in the cat. The cause is not known, and castration is not protective. Prostatic hyperplasia and metaplasia appear not to precede neoplasia, although hyperplasia and carcinoma are found together in intact dogs. Prostatic intraepithelial neoplasia (PIN) is only found in a high-grade form in prostates that already have carcinoma. Low- and intermediate-grade PIN are too rare to suggest progression from one to the next grade. Some of the clinical signs of carcinoma of the prostate are similar to those of prostatic hyperplasia because of the enlargement of the organ. Carcinoma and its metastases cause cachexia and locomotor abnormalities through pressure and invasion of nearby structures, including the bones of the spine and pelvis. Macroscopically, there are two general appearances. The most obvious is the type that causes asymmetric extreme enlargement (see Fig. 19-31, *B*). The prostate becomes very large and attached to other pelvic structures. The second type is mostly periurethral, with a necrotic and cystic cavity within the prostatic capsule. It causes minimal enlargement of the gland, but urinary obstruction and metastatic disease are present. Castrated dogs are usually affected with this latter form.

Much has been written and said about the prevalence of different types of neoplasia of the prostate. Carcinomas probably arise from prostatic ducts and thus have squamous (squamous cell carcinoma), glandular (adenocarcinoma), transitional (transitional cell carcinoma), and mixed carcinoma phenotypes. Attempts to accurately phenotype carcinomas by histologic, immunohistochemical, and molecular methods are unsuccessful or inaccurate because there are no specific markers to separate acinar ductal and urothelial epithelial cell types. This consequence is probably because of the common embryologic origin of prostatic ducts and glands and for urothelium in general. Because of this dilemma and the tendency for carcinomas to have multiple phenotypes within one neoplasm, the term *carcinoma of the prostate* is the preferred general term. Adenocarcinoma, mixed carcinoma, squamous cell carcinoma, and transitional cell carcinoma are subcategories used when the histologic type is purely glandular, mixed, squamous, or urothelial, respectively. The appearance of a carcinoma reflects attempted differentiation toward glandular, urothelial, or epidermal tissues, or mixtures of two or more (see Fig. 19-31, *C*). There are varying degrees of stroma between the neoplastic epithelial cells. Some also contain sarcomatous tissue.

The prognosis for carcinoma of the prostate is generally poor. Approximately 80% of affected dogs have metastases to a lymph node and/or lung at the time of diagnosis, and 20% of these neoplasms have metastasized to bone.

The Penis and Prepuce

Dogs and cats develop a full range of lesions of the penis and prepuce, as do other species. These disorders are described in the section on Disorders of Domestic Animals, Disorders of the Scrotum and Contents. There are unique features of the penis of dogs and cats. Dogs have erectile bulbs, and the intrapreputial part of the penis is entirely the head of the penis. Cats have testosterone-dependent penile barbs on the surface. Dogs develop a nonspecific posthitis. They also develop a unique disease of great importance—canine transmissible venereal tumor.

Canine Transmissible Venereal Tumor

Canine transmissible venereal tumor (CTVT) is a type of allotransplantation. Based on immunologic, cytogenetic, and nucleotide sequence studies, the neoplasm is thought to arise from a specific genetic alteration of canine histiocytes, followed by the transmission of abnormal cells from dog to dog via direct contact with the tumor (see Fig. 18-59). The primary neoplasm is usually on the external genitalia, but extragenital primaries and metastases also occur, particularly in stray dogs and those in poor health. The neoplasm is found on the penis, more often on the proximal parts, and not often on the prepuce (Fig. 19-37, *A*). The neoplasm can be single or

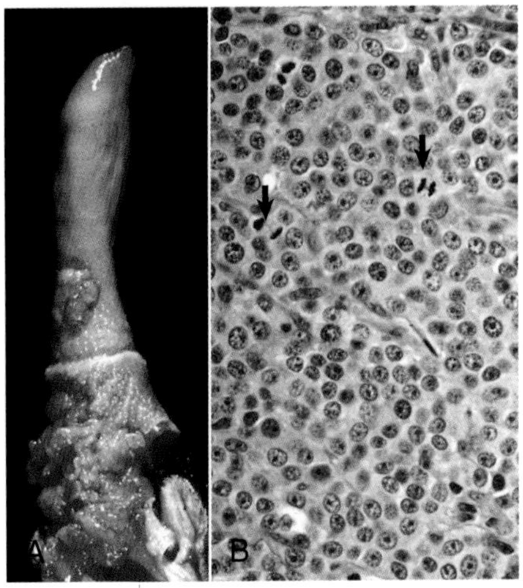

Figure 19-37 **Transmissible Venereal Tumor, Penis, Dog. A,** There is a large multinodular mass involving the penis and the prepuce at its reflection from the penis. **B,** Neoplastic cells are round, uniform in size, and often divided into packets by a fine fibrous stroma. Mitoses are frequent *(arrows)*. H&E stain. (**A** courtesy Dr. M.D. McGavin, College of Veterinary Medicine, University of Tennessee. **B** courtesy Dr. M.J. Abdy, College of Veterinary Medicine, The University of Georgia; and Noah's Arkive, College of Veterinary Medicine, The University of Georgia.)

multiple and up to 10 cm in diameter, with a red, ulcerated, multinodular surface. Microscopically, the neoplastic cells form a diffuse sheet with minimal stroma. The cells are large, round or oval, and uniform in size, thus resembling lymphocytes (Fig. 19-37, *B*). The cytoplasm is pale staining and may have peripheral vacuoles that are readily identified on cytologic preparations. This neoplasm can develop multifocal necrosis and spontaneously regress because of lymphocyte-mediated cytotoxicity.

Suggested Readings

Suggested Readings are available at www.expertconsult.com.

CHAPTER 20

The Ear[1]

Bradley L. Njaa

Key Readings Index

The ear is a specialized sense organ formed by a highly organized mixture of cutaneous, nasopharyngeal, osseous, and neurologic tissues. Within the ear are several air- and fluid-filled interfaces involved in the transduction of sound waves to action potentials that are conducted by the nervous system to the brain for interpretation and appropriate motor and cognitive responses.

In the context of interacting with animals, hearing is often considered of secondary or tertiary importance when compared to vision or olfaction. For many years, specific breeds predisposed to auditory dysfunction were maintained in colonies to facilitate investigation as animal models of human disease. More recently, throughout the world, deaf and hearing-impaired human beings are greatly benefiting from professionally trained hearing dogs. In addition, animal trainers, pet owners, and producers rely on a fully functioning auditory system to train, address, keep safe, or herd their animals. Therefore a much better understanding of conditions affecting this special sense is needed.

Many current textbooks focus on one species or one aspect of the ear. The focus of this chapter is to (1) clarify the anatomy of the ear by comparing and contrasting anatomic features of the domestic animal species, (2) address the responses to injury and the defense mechanisms protecting against injury, and (3) delineate various otic diseases that either affect many different species or are more unique to certain species.

Structure and Function

External Ear

The external ear comprises the auricle (also known as the pinna) and external acoustic meatus terminating medially at the tympanic membrane. Developmentally, the external ear arises from tissue elevations called *auricular hillocks*, three from the first branchial or pharyngeal arch and three from the second branchial or pharyngeal arch. The first pharyngeal groove or cleft between the two arches forms the external acoustic meatus. As they come into apposition early in development, the auricle and external acoustic meatus form. The auricle is a highly mobile and flexible, cartilaginous structure that is covered by haired skin with adnexa more dense on the convex than concave surface. The structural characteristics of auricles are closely tied to breed specifications. Among the species and breeds covered in this chapter, auricles can be erect, semierect, lop-eared, pendulous, microtic, or folded.

The auricle functions to collect, focus, and direct sound down the funnel-shaped external acoustic meatus to the tympanic membrane (Fig. 20-1). Movement of the auricle around its central axis requires coordinated movement of the complex dorsal, rostral, caudal, and ventral groups of auricular muscles. All muscles are innervated by the motor branches of the facial nerve. The position of the auricle can signal an animal's behavior or emotion. Fearful cats often flatten their ears in a defensive posture, whereas angry horses often completely flatten their ears caudally as an initial warning before they strike. Alternatively, a dog may flatten its ears when content or when it is being verbally scolded.

The *external acoustic meatus* (ear canal) is a conical opening made up of elastic cartilage and bone (Fig. 20-2). The more lateral portions are composed of auricular cartilage that narrows and overlaps with annular cartilage. Dense fibrous connective tissue forms a bridge between the annular cartilage ring and the osseus portion of the external acoustic meatus. In cats and dogs the osseous portion (1) is a very narrow rim of bone and (2) is a broad opening exposing the tympanic membrane that is readily visible during otic examination. In horses, ruminants, and pigs the osseous portion of the external acoustic meatus is an elongate cylinder of bone with a narrow lumen (Fig. 20-3). In horses the junction between the cartilaginous and osseous portions of the external acoustic meatus is grossly identified by an abrupt change from pigmented to nonpigmented epithelium. Visualization of the deeper portions of the external acoustic meatus in livestock species requires specialized equipment and heavy sedation.

Although there are wide species variations, the cartilaginous and osseous portions of the external acoustic meatus are lined by a thin epidermis formed by stratified squamous epithelium and a thin dermis that contains a relatively uniform allotment of sebaceous glands, fewer hair follicles, and greater ceruminous glands when comparing medial to lateral portions (Fig. 20-4). Sebaceous glands are composed of 6 to 10 club-shaped acini surrounded by thin fibrous tissue with ducts opening into associated hair follicles. Relative to ceruminous glands, sebaceous glands tend to be located in the more

[1]For a glossary of abbreviations and terms used in this chapter see E-Glossary 20-1.

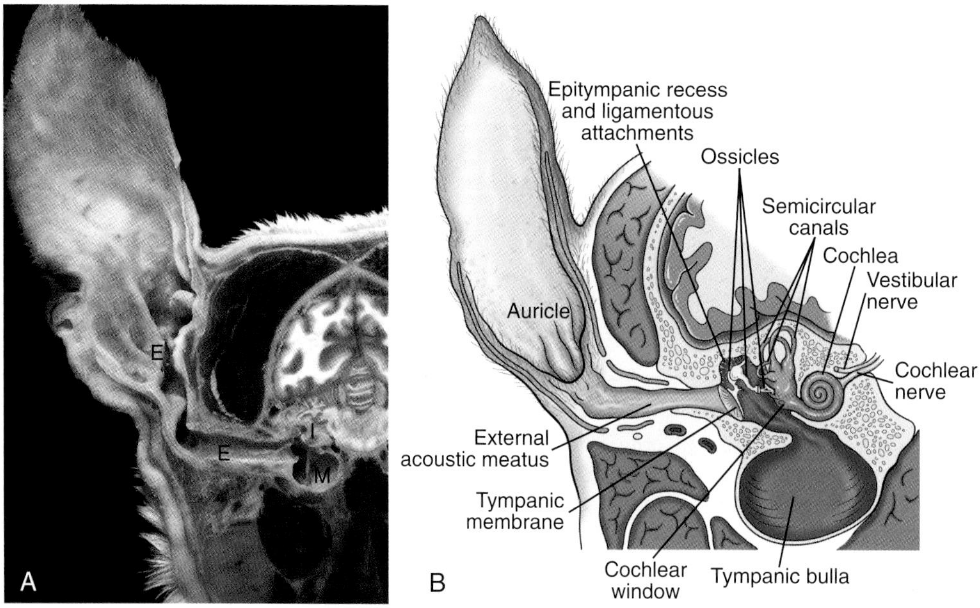

Figure 20-1 **Major Regions of the Ear. A,** Cross section, head through the right ear, rostral surface, dog. External *(E)*, middle *(M)*, and internal *(I)* ear are illustrated. The tympanic membrane has been removed in this section. The external ear consists of the auricle and external acoustic meatus; the middle ear consists of the ossicles, tympanic cavity, and bulla; and the internal ear consists of the cochlea and semicircular canals. **B,** Schematic diagram depicting a cross section through the external, middle, and internal ear of a dog. (**A** courtesy Dr. B.L. Njaa, Center for Veterinary Health Sciences, Oklahoma State University.)

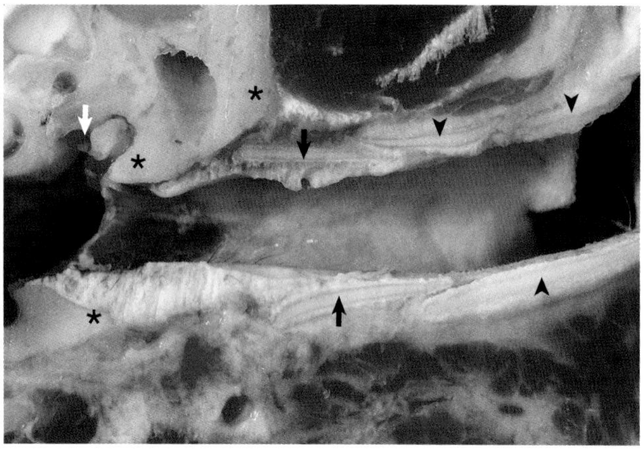

Figure 20-2 **External Acoustic Meatus, Osseous and Cartilaginous Portions, Cross Section Through the Left Ear, Dog.** Annular *(black arrows)* and auricular cartilage *(black arrowheads)* form the structure of the cartilaginous portion of the external acoustic meatus. Dense, white, fibrous connective tissue attaches the annular cartilage to the osseous rim of the external acoustic meatus *(asterisks)*. The incudostapedius joint is visible in this image *(white arrow)*. The tympanic membrane is removed in this section. (Courtesy Dr. B.L. Njaa, Center for Veterinary Health Sciences, Oklahoma State University.)

superficial dermis. Ceruminous glands are simple, coiled, tubular glands that resemble apocrine sweat glands. Their ducts open either into hair follicles or directly to the epidermal surface.

Although motor innervation of muscles of the external acoustic meatus is provided by the facial cranial nerve, sensory innervation is more complex. Branches of the trigeminal, facial, and vagal cranial nerves and branches of the second cervical spinal nerve innervate the skin. Sensory innervation to the dermis and epidermis of the external acoustic meatus is provided by the mandibular branch of trigeminal and auriculotemporal cranial nerves. The primary blood supply to the ear is through the caudal auricular artery, which branches into the lateral, intermediate, deep, and medial auricular arteries. The caudal auricular artery is a main branch of the external carotid artery.

Middle Ear

Tympanic Membrane (Tympanum)

The tympanic membrane, also known as the tympanum, is an extremely thin, three-layered, semitransparent membrane peripherally suspended from the tympanic ring by a fibrocartilaginous to osseous ring. The tympanic membrane is formed when the endoderm of the first pharyngeal pouch comes into close contact with the ectoderm of the first pharyngeal cleft or groove. Most of the tympanic membrane is held under tension so it can be responsive to sound waves (Fig. 20-5). It covers the medial extremity of the external acoustic meatus, demarcating the junction between the external ear and middle ear. Both surfaces of the tympanic membrane have an air interface.

In most species the tympanum is an oval to round structure, whereas in ruminants it is shaped more like a broad triangle (Fig. 20-6). Embedded in the tympanum is the manubrium of the malleus. The placement of the manubrium in the tympanic membrane is highly variable between species. It is more centrally located in horses versus a more rostromedial location in ruminants and pigs.

The tympanum is divided into two portions, the *pars tensa* and the *pars flaccida*. The majority of the tympanic membrane is made up of the pars tensa, which is a very thin, translucent, and taut membrane that bulges convexly into the tympanic cavity (see Fig. 20-6, *E*). The pars tensa is made up of three layers: (1) outer layer of keratinizing squamous epithelium derived from ectoderm of the first pharyngeal groove; (2) middle layer of thin, variably vascularized fibrous connective tissue originating from the pharyngeal wall; and (3) inner layer of very low cuboidal to nonkeratinizing squamous epithelium, which is of pharyngeal pouch origin.

The most dorsal portion of the tympanic membrane is the pars flaccida, which is roughly triangular, thicker, more vascular, and flaccid when compared to the pars tensa (see Fig. 20-6, *E*). Overlain

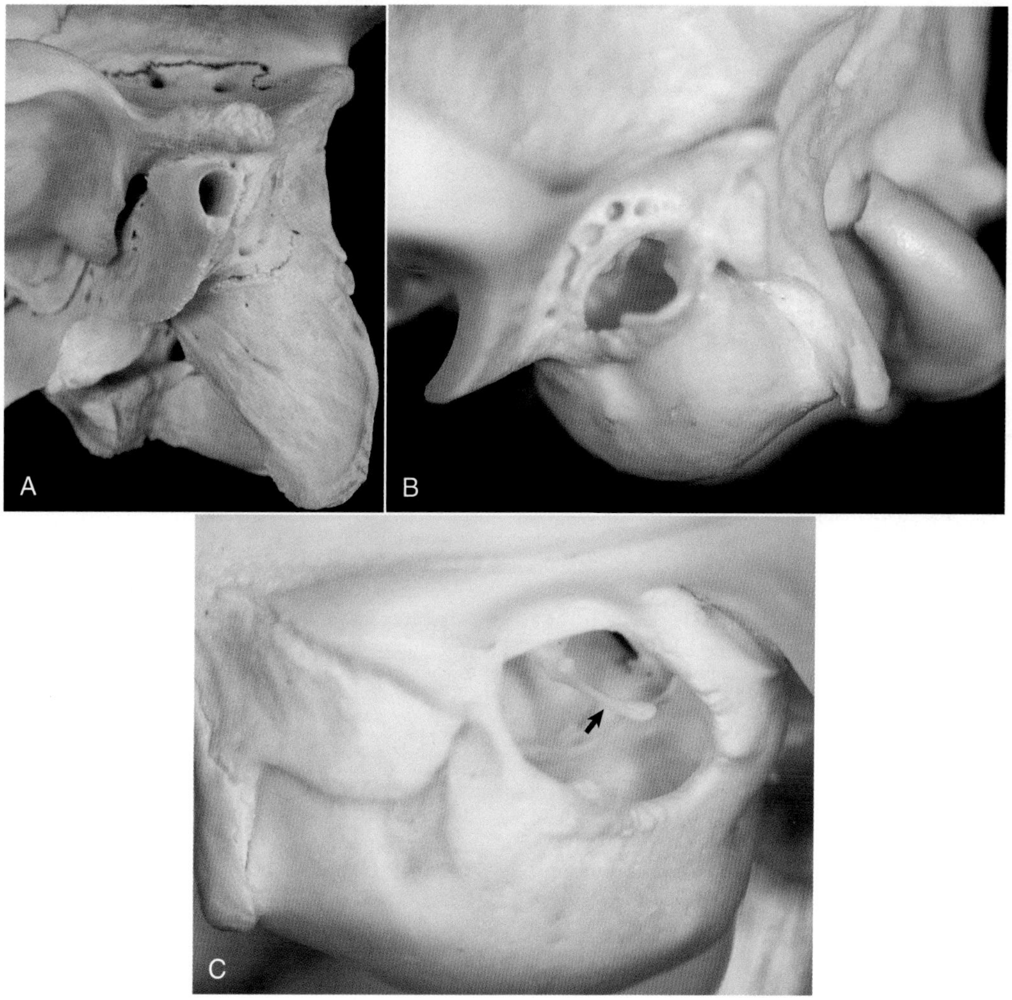

Figure 20-3 **Osseous External Acoustic Meatus, Macerated Specimens. A,** Ox. The bony external acoustic meatus in most livestock is much longer and narrower when compared to dogs and cats. Visualization of the middle ear is obscured by the elongate osseous external acoustic meatus. **B,** Dog. The osseous portion of the external acoustic meatus is a thin rim of bone allowing easy visualization of the middle ear. **C,** Cat. The osseous portion of the external acoustic meatus is very thin and the opening is very large, allowing easy visualization of the middle ear and malleus *(arrow)*. (Courtesy Dr. B.L. Njaa, Center for Veterinary Health Sciences, Oklahoma State University.)

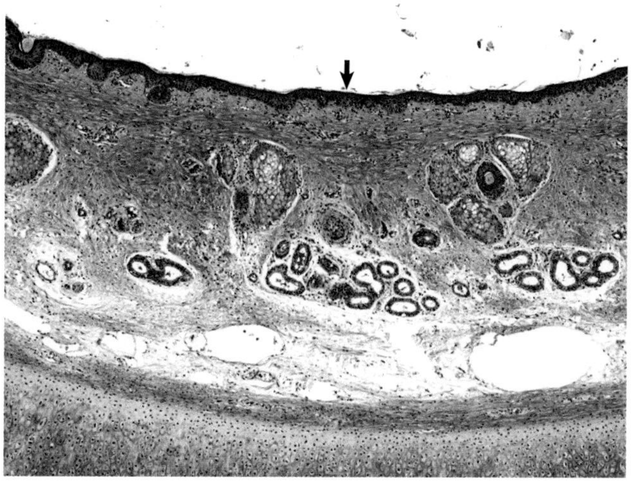

Figure 20-4 **External Acoustic Meatus Epithelium and Adnexa, Pig.** Stratified squamous epithelium *(arrow)* lines the external acoustic meatus. Adnexa present are mixtures of sebaceous glands, most often flanking hair follicles, and deeper eccrine glands referred to as *ceruminous glands*. Auricular cartilage is present along the lower edge of the image. H&E stain. (Courtesy Dr. B.L. Njaa, Center for Veterinary Health Sciences, Oklahoma State University.)

by keratinized epithelium, the underlying stroma of the pars flaccida in dogs is made of loosely arranged collagen, rare mast cells, and few elastin fibers. This latter feature is in direct contrast to human beings, in which there are abundant elastin fibers. Visualized from the external acoustic meatus, this portion of the tympanic membrane may bulge into or away from the middle ear.

The tympanic membrane is placed roughly at a 45-degree angle relative to the central axis of horizontal portion of the external acoustic meatus (Fig. 20-7, A). However, commonly the actual placement of the tympanic membrane is more variable with the external, concave surface of the tympanic membrane angled more rostrally (see Fig. 20-7, B and C). Cats have a similar orientation to their tympanum (Fig. 20-8). Interestingly, the surface area of the tympanic membrane from an approximately 550-kg horse is larger than the tympanic membrane of a Maltese dog but is approximately 15% smaller than the surface area of the tympanic membrane of a German shepherd dog. Additionally, the tympanum of the fetal goat is approximately 20% larger than that of large dog breeds.

Tympanic Cavity

The tympanic cavity is an air-filled compartment surrounded by bone that is separated from the external ear by a thin tympanic membrane (tympanum) and is in direct communication with the

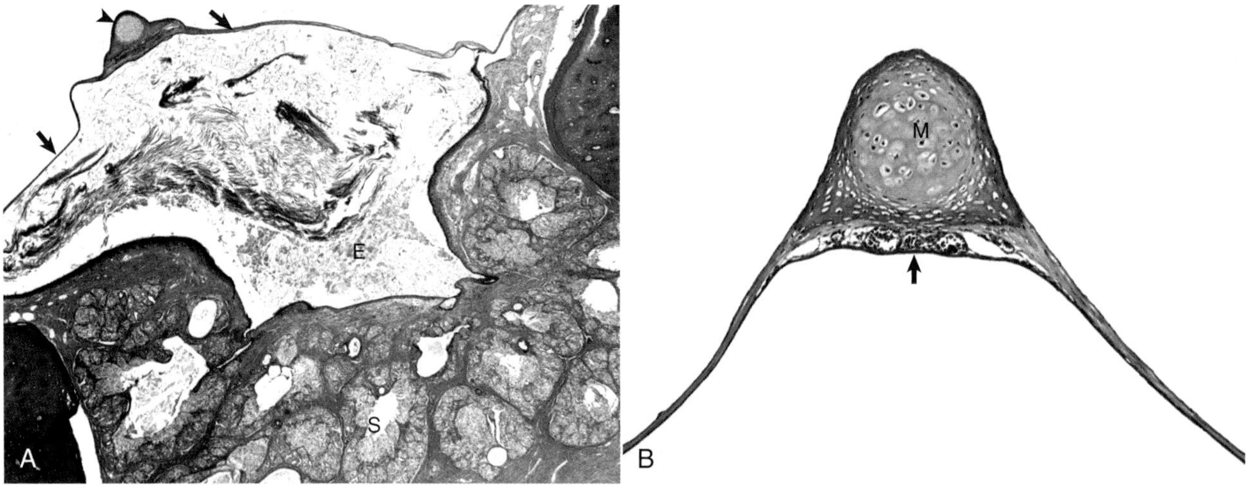

Figure 20-5 Tympanic Membrane. A, Cat. Cross section through the tympanic membrane *(arrows)*, manubrium of the malleus *(arrowhead)*, and external acoustic meatus *(E)*. An intact tympanic membrane at the level of the pars tensa is very thin. It is lined by a single layer of cornified squamous epithelial cells externally, and low cuboidal to noncornified squamous epithelium line the inner surface. The abundant keratin within the external acoustic meatus is not uncommon. The prominent, multiple, branching sebaceous glands *(S)* are common in the deepest portions of the external acoustic meatus. H&E stain. **B,** Higher magnification of the tympanic membrane and malleus, pig. The manubrium *(M)* of the malleus is embedded in the tympanic membrane. Numerous blood vessels are present beneath the manubrium *(arrow)* and are located in the middle layer of the tympanic membrane beneath the external concave surface, which corresponds with the region of germinative epithelium. H&E stain. (Courtesy Dr. B.L. Njaa, Center for Veterinary Health Sciences, Oklahoma State University.)

pharynx via the auditory tube (also known as the eustachian or pharyngotympanic tube). Both the tympanic cavity and the auditory tube are derived from the endoderm of the first pharyngeal pouch. The epitympanic recess is the dorsal extremity of the tympanic cavity, within which lie the head of the malleus and short crus of the incus. Ligaments stabilize and anchor the incudomallearis joint and the short crus of the incus within this recess (Fig. 20-9).

In many species there is a bulbous, ventral portion of the tympanic cavity called the *tympanic bulla* (see Fig. 20-3, *B* and *C*). Within the bulla of the dog and cat is a bony septum referred to as the *septum bulla*. In the cat the septum bulla abuts the petrous portion of the temporal bone and separates the tympanic cavity into two compartments: the dorsolateral epitympanic cavity and the ventromedial tympanic cavity (see Fig. 20-8). This separation is incomplete, which allows communication between the two compartments through a narrow opening between the septum bulla and petrous portion of the temporal bone and a larger opening at its caudal edge. In the dog this septum is a much smaller, incomplete bony ridge that only makes contact with the petrous portion of the temporal bone rostrally. The mucoperiosteum represents a fused mucosa and periosteum lining the surface of bony structures of the middle ear. In cats and dogs the lining epithelium varies, depending on the location. Dorsally, close to the auditory tube opening, the mucoperiosteum comprises mostly ciliated columnar cells mixed with goblet cells and basal cells contiguous with the nasopharyngeal mucosae (Fig. 20-10; see Fig. 20-20). Ventrally, the number of ciliated cells and goblet cells decreases, and the number of cuboidal, less differentiated cells increases. The surfaces of the petrous portion of the temporal bone, auditory ossicles, and tympanic membrane are typically lined by cuboidal to noncornifying squamous epithelium. In cattle, goats, camelids, and pigs, the ventral portion of the tympanic cavity or bulla is made of more numerous bony compartments lined by noncornifying (nonkeratinizing) squamous epithelium (Fig. 20-11). In cattle and pigs these compartments are air filled with direct communication with the tympanic cavity. In camelids and goats the ventral bullae maintain limited communication with the tympanic cavity. Horses have shallow tympanic bullae with several incomplete bony shelves forming small compartments. Sheep have bulbous open bullae similar to dogs and cats.

Auditory Ossicles

A chain of three bones, or auditory ossicles, forms the mechanical transduction system of hearing: the malleus, incus, and stapes (Figs. 20-12 and 20-13). The malleus and the incus, as well as the tensor tympani, are derived from the mesenchyme of the first branchial or pharyngeal arch. The stapes and the stapedius muscle originate from the mesenchyme of the second branchial or pharyngeal arch.

Malleus. The largest of the ossicles is the malleus. The manubrium of the malleus is embedded in the tympanic membrane (see Fig. 20-5). The most ventromedial convexity of the malleus is the "umbo" (see Figs. 20-6, *F*, and 20-12). The muscular process of the manubrium near the neck of the malleus is the attachment site of a thin tendinous portion of the tensor tympani muscle. Various ligaments stabilize the malleus in the epitympanic cavity by anchoring the long, thin rostral process, the neck, and the head of the malleus. The head of the malleus articulates with the articular surface of the body of the incus, forming the incudomallearis joint (see Figs. 20-9, 20-12, and 20-13). In the horse and cow and in aged dogs and cats, the incudomallearis joint capsule is a narrow but thick ligament that makes disarticulation difficult and gives the external appearance of a falsely fused joint. In younger dogs and cats the incudomallearis ligament is not nearly as tenacious, and disarticulation is much less difficult.

Incus. The incus is a bicuspid-shaped bone that lies caudal and dorsal to the malleus. It has two crura, one designated as the short crus, which is anchored in the epitympanic recess along with the body of the incus by a band of narrow connective tissue, and the other designated as the long crus, which transmits vibrations to the stapes. The lenticular process is a bony appendage at the end of the long crus (see Fig. 20-13), and in young animals is a separate bone. In older animals, the lenticular process fuses with the distal end of the long crus of the incus and articulates with the head of

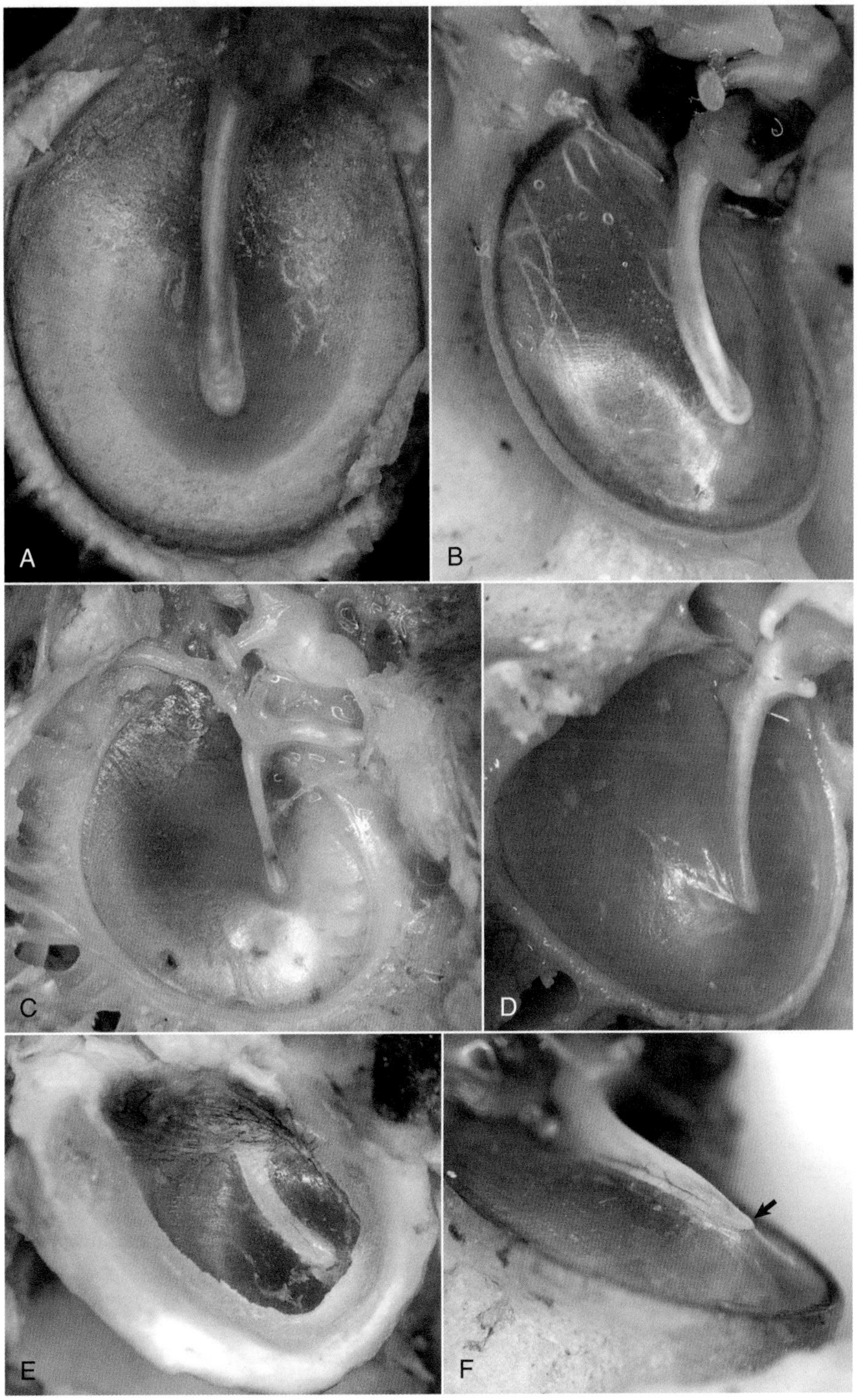

Figure 20-6 Tympanic Membrane. A, Horse. In the horse, the tympanic membrane (tympanum) is more round than other species. The manubrium of the malleus forms a very shallow arc and is centrally located in the tympanum. **B,** Dog. The tympanum is oval to comma-shaped in dogs, and the manubrium of the malleus is C-shaped. **C,** Pig. The shape of the tympanic membrane is similar to that of the dog, but the manubrium of the malleus is shorter and straighter. **D,** Goat. Ruminants tend to have a more triangular-shaped tympanic membrane. In both pigs and ruminants the manubrium of the malleus is more rostral and medial than in other species. **E,** Dog. Lateral view of tympanic membrane. The transparent portion of the tympanic membrane held under tension and associated with the manubrium of the malleus is the pars tensa. The highlights depict the radial striations of the normal pars tensa. Dorsally the tympanic membrane is thicker, highly vascular and is under much less tension, and is designated as the pars flaccida. **F,** Dog. The tympanic membrane is convex on its medial surface in the tympanic cavity. The ventromedial extremity of the manubrium is called the umbo *(arrow)*. (Courtesy Dr. B.L. Njaa, Center for Veterinary Health Sciences, Oklahoma State University.)

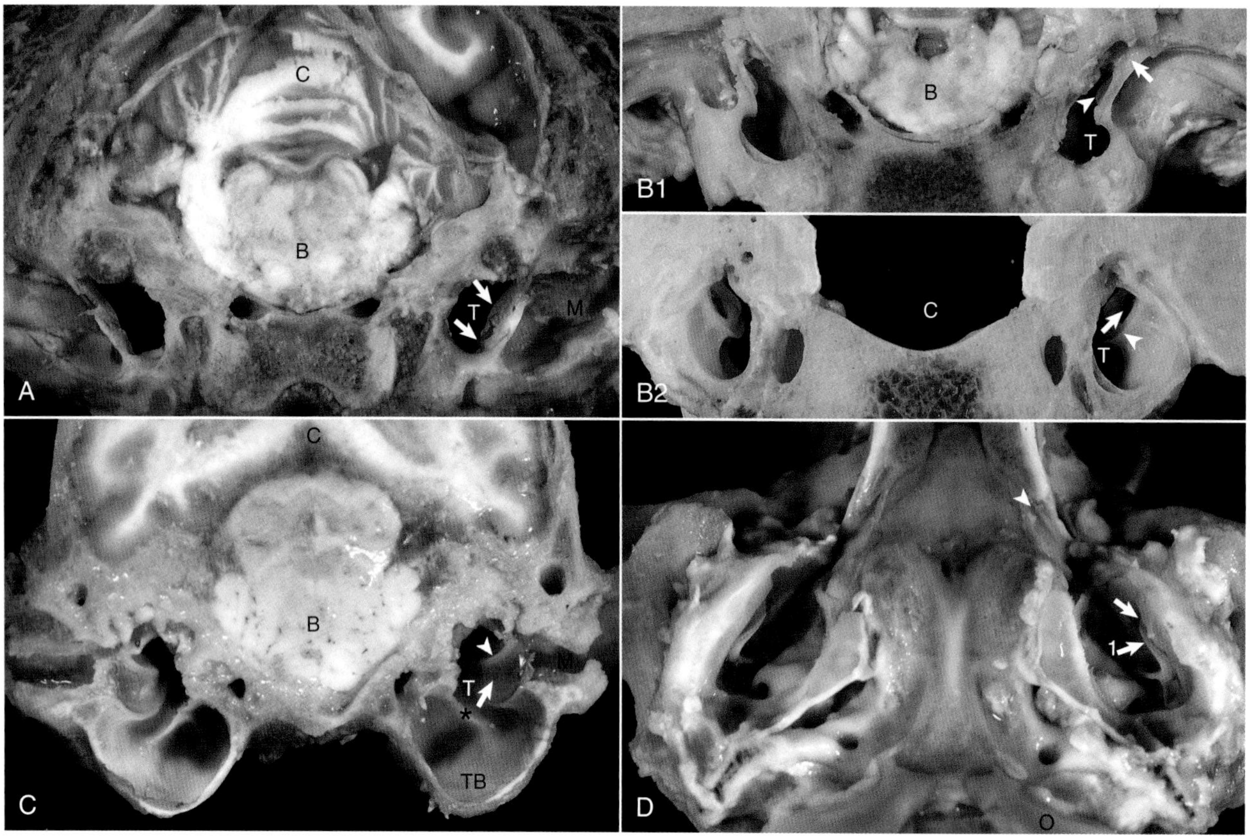

Figure 20-7 **External Acoustic Meatus, Tympanic Membrane, Tympanic Cavity. Compare Unlabeled Contralateral Side with Labeled Side for More Structural Detail. A,** Transverse section, rostral surface, dog. The tympanic membrane *(arrows)* extends medially toward the tympanic cavity *(T)* at an approximate 45-degree angle from dorsal to ventral, in relation to the central axis of the horizontal part of the external acoustic meatus *(M)*. Portions of the rostral edge of the tympanic ring have been inadvertently removed during sample preparation. *B*, Brainstem; *C*, cerebellum. **B,** Transverse section, rostral **(B1)** and caudal **(B2)** surfaces, goat. The tympanic cavity *(T)* has been opened bilaterally. In the cranial view **(B1)**, the tympanic membrane is not visualized because it is hidden by the tympanic ring *(arrow)*, which surrounds the membrane. The manubrium of the malleus *(arrowhead)* is minimally visible. However, from the caudal view **(B2)**, the tympanic membrane *(arrow)* is clearly visible and is positioned so that the concave or external surface is tilted rostrally. *Arrowhead*, Tympanic ring; *B*, brainstem; *C*, calvaria where brainstem would be positioned. **C,** Transverse section, caudal surface, dog. The external or concave surface of the tympanic membrane *(arrow)* is angled almost fully rostral rather than lateral. Note that the septum bullae *(asterisk)* are short and incomplete in the dog when compared with a cat (see Fig. 20-10). *Arrowhead*, Manubrium of the malleus; *B*, brainstem; *C*, cerebellum; *M*, external acoustic meatus; *T*, tympanic cavity; *TB*, tympanic bullae. **D,** Ventral-dorsal view, opened bullae. Bilaterally the concave surface of the tympanic membranes *(arrow)* is tilted rostrally. Occipital condyles *(O)* appear at the bottom of the image. Extending rostrally and medially from the tympanic cavity are the auditory tubes *(arrowhead)*, which provide direct communication between the tympanic cavity and nasopharynx. *Arrow 1*, Manubrium of the malleus. (Courtesy Dr. B.L. Njaa, Center for Veterinary Health Sciences, Oklahoma State University.)

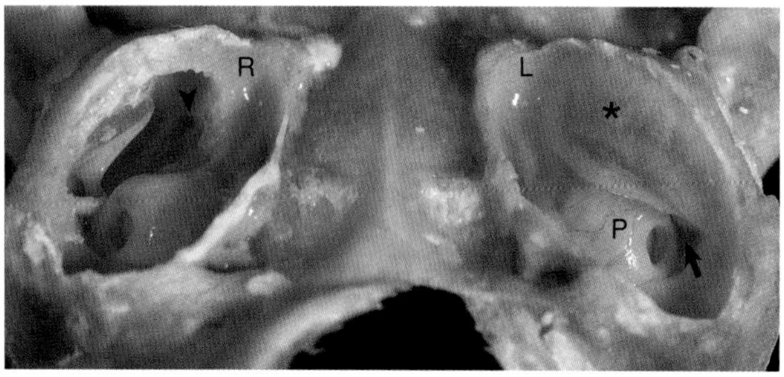

Figure 20-8 **Tympanic Bullae, Cat.** Caudoventral section, with both tympanic bullae opened ventrally. The septum bulla *(asterisk)* is intact in the left bulla *(L)* and opened ventrally in the right bulla *(R)*. From rostral to caudal, the septum bulla dorsally abuts the petrous portion of the temporal bone. At its caudal extreme is an opening that allows communication between the two cavities *(arrow)*. The auditory tube opening into the tympanic cavity is observed in the dorsal, rostral extremity of the right epitympanic cavity *(arrowhead)*. The large bulge rostral to the round window corresponds to the start of the cochlea and is called the promontory *(P)*. In both specimens the tympanic membrane is tilted rostrally. (Courtesy Dr. B.L. Njaa, Center for Veterinary Health Sciences, Oklahoma State University.)

the stapes. Regardless of age, the incudostapedial joint capsular ligament is more translucent than the incudomallearis joint capsule, and there is inherently more joint laxity.

Stapes. The stapes is often considered the smallest bone in the body.[2] However, its size and shape is somewhat variable, depending on species (Fig. 20-14). Its base, or footplate, is convex and firmly seated in the vestibular (oval) window of the petrous portion of the temporal bone and anchored by the annular ligament of the stapes. This arrangement forms a syndesmosis between the stapes base and cartilage of the vestibular window (Fig. 20-15). The stapedius muscle, fittingly referred to as the smallest muscle in the body, is attached to the muscular process of the shorter caudal crus close to the head of the stapes. Vibrations of the tympanic membrane are

[2]This categorization depends on the age of the animal. In young animals, the unfused lenticular process of the long crus of the incus is the smallest bone in the body.

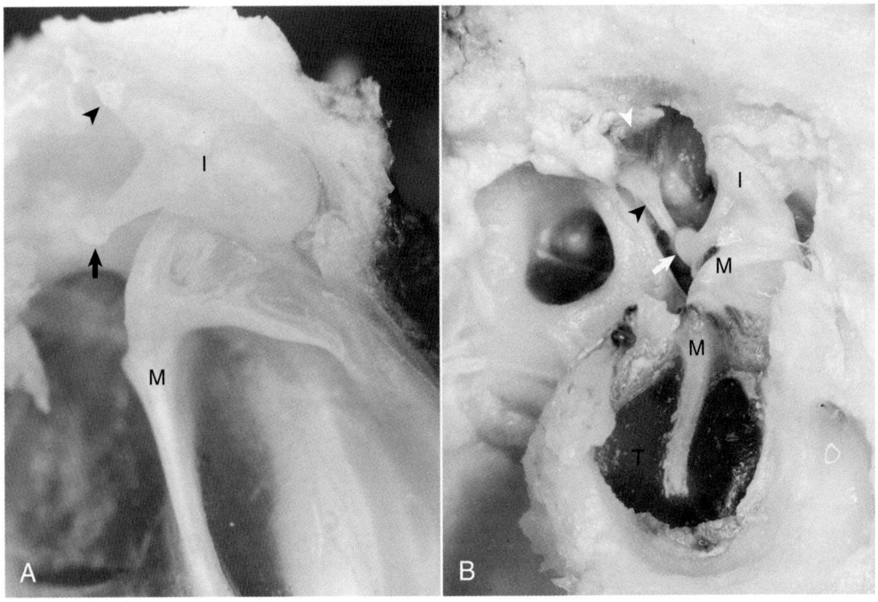

Figure 20-9 **Malleus, Incus, Incudomallearis Joint, Epitympanic Recess. A,** Cat. Medial view. Seated in the epitympanic recess is the rounded head of the malleus *(M)* and the incus *(I)*; together they are articulated to form the incudomallearis joint. The smaller crus of the incus *(arrowhead)* and the head of the malleus are anchored to the epitympanic recess by ligaments (see Fig. 20-1). At the end of the longer crus of the incus is the lenticular process *(arrow)*. **B,** Giraffe. Lateral view, right ear. The tympanic membrane is intact *(T)*. The small crus of the incus *(I)* along with the head of the malleus *(M)* are firmly anchored in the epitympanic recess by ligamentous attachments. The lenticular process of the long crus articulates with the head of the stapes seated in the oval window to form the incudostapedius joint *(white arrow)*. The facial nerve has been removed to expose the stapedius muscle *(white arrowhead)*, which is firmly attached to the stapes via its tendon *(black arrowhead)*. (Courtesy Dr. B.L. Njaa, The Center for Veterinary Health Sciences, Oklahoma State University.)

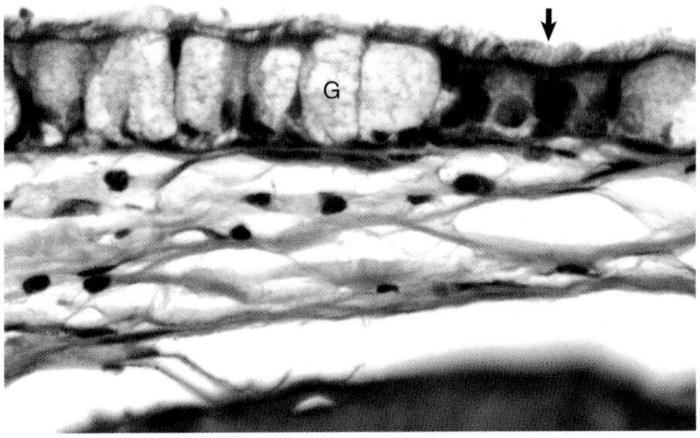

Figure 20-10 **Tympanic Cavity, Mucoperiosteum, Cat.** The mucoperiosteum of the tympanic cavity is not uniform. In cats and dogs the mucosal epithelium in the more dorsal portions of the bullae morphologically mirrors mucosae of the nasopharynx. Included are ciliated columnar epithelial cells *(arrow)* and goblet cells *(G)* mixed with fewer nonciliated columnar epithelial cells. A lattice of connective tissue forms the fused submucosa and periosteum overlying the bone. H&E stain. (Courtesy Dr. B.L. Njaa, Center for Veterinary Health Sciences, Oklahoma State University.)

transduced to stapes vibrations that lead to fluid waves of the perilymph of the internal ear.

Middle Ear Muscles and Nerves

The middle ear has two muscles associated with the auditory ossicles that help modulate auditory transduction and a third muscle group that controls patency of the auditory tube. The tensor tympani muscle originates rostrally and medially from the bony recess in the petrous portion of the temporal bone and makes its tendinous insertion onto the muscular process of the neck of the malleus (Fig. 20-16; see Fig. 20-13, *A*). It receives its innervation via a motor branch of the trigeminal nerve. Contraction of the tensor tympani muscle pulls the tympanic membrane medially and rostrally, placing greater tension on the auditory ossicle chain, which results in an increased resonant frequency of the auditory sound conduction system.

The stapedius muscle originates in the stapedius muscule fossa located dorsomedial to and obscured by the facial nerve as it courses through the facial (Fallopian) canal of the temporal bone (Fig. 20-17). The stapedial branch of the facial nerve innervates this muscle as it converges into a thin tendon that inserts onto the muscular process of the short crus close to the head of the stapes. In the cat the displacement variance of the stapes in its vestibular window is approximately 0.2 μm, whereas the maximal contraction of the stapedius muscle leads to dorsal and caudal stapedial bone displacement of 40 to 60 μm. This displacement, which is perpendicular to the normal movement of the stapes, maximally attenuates sound transmission up to 30 decibels. Contraction of the stapedius and tensor tympani muscles are integral parts of the *acoustic reflex*, defined as consensual, reflexive contraction of the muscles in response to stimuli (typically high-energy sound pressure) that leads to attenuated acoustic transmission.

The tensor veli palatini muscle arises from a groove in the petrous portion of the temporal bone medial and ventral to the tensor tympani muscle. Along with its nerve, the tensor veli palatini nerve, a branch of the trigeminal nerve, this long, slender muscle extends rostrally from the tympanic cavity parallel to the auditory tube. In concert with the levator veli palatini muscle, which is innervated by the facial nerve, coordinated contraction of these muscles opens the pharyngeal orifice of the auditory tube.

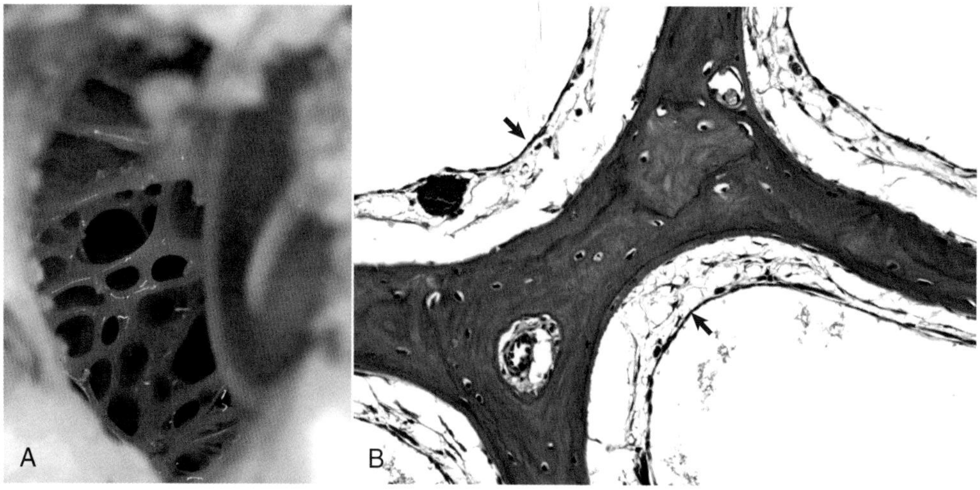

Figure 20-11 **Tympanic Cavity and Bulla. A,** Dorsal view into the middle ear, ox. Cattle, goats, and pigs have small tympanic cavities but much larger tympanic bullae. The bullae are made of multiple, arborizing air-filled channels with numerous bony septa as shown here. **B,** Histologic section of tympanic bulla, pig. Bony septa are lined by low cuboidal to nonkeratinizing squamous epithelial cells *(arrows)*. H&E stain. (Courtesy Dr. B.L. Njaa, Center for Veterinary Health Sciences, Oklahoma State University.)

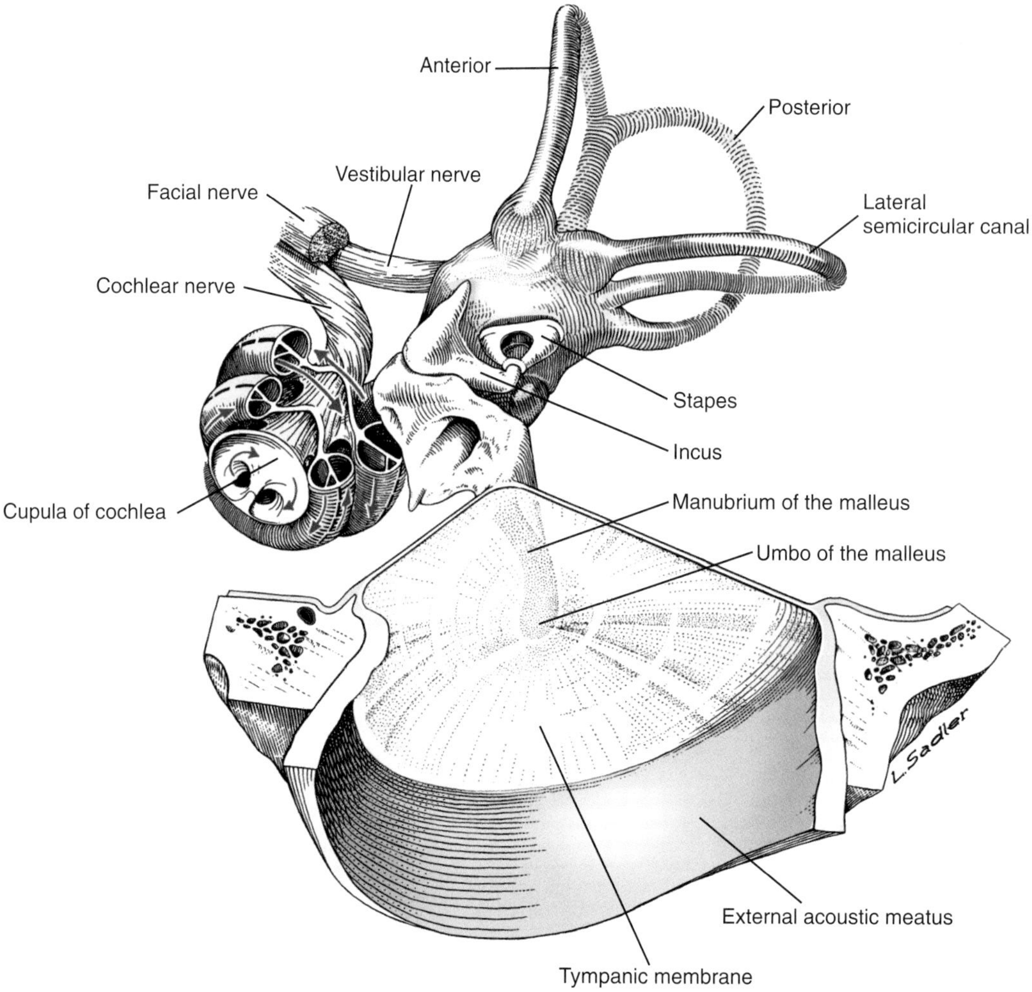

Figure 20-12 **Middle and Internal Ear, Dog.** Tympanic membrane, auditory ossicles, and membranous labyrinth. The bony labyrinth has been removed to demonstrate the orientation of the cochlea and semicircular canals relative to the auditory ossicles and tympanic membrane. The facial nerve and vestibulocochlear nerve enter the ear together through the internal acoustic meatus.

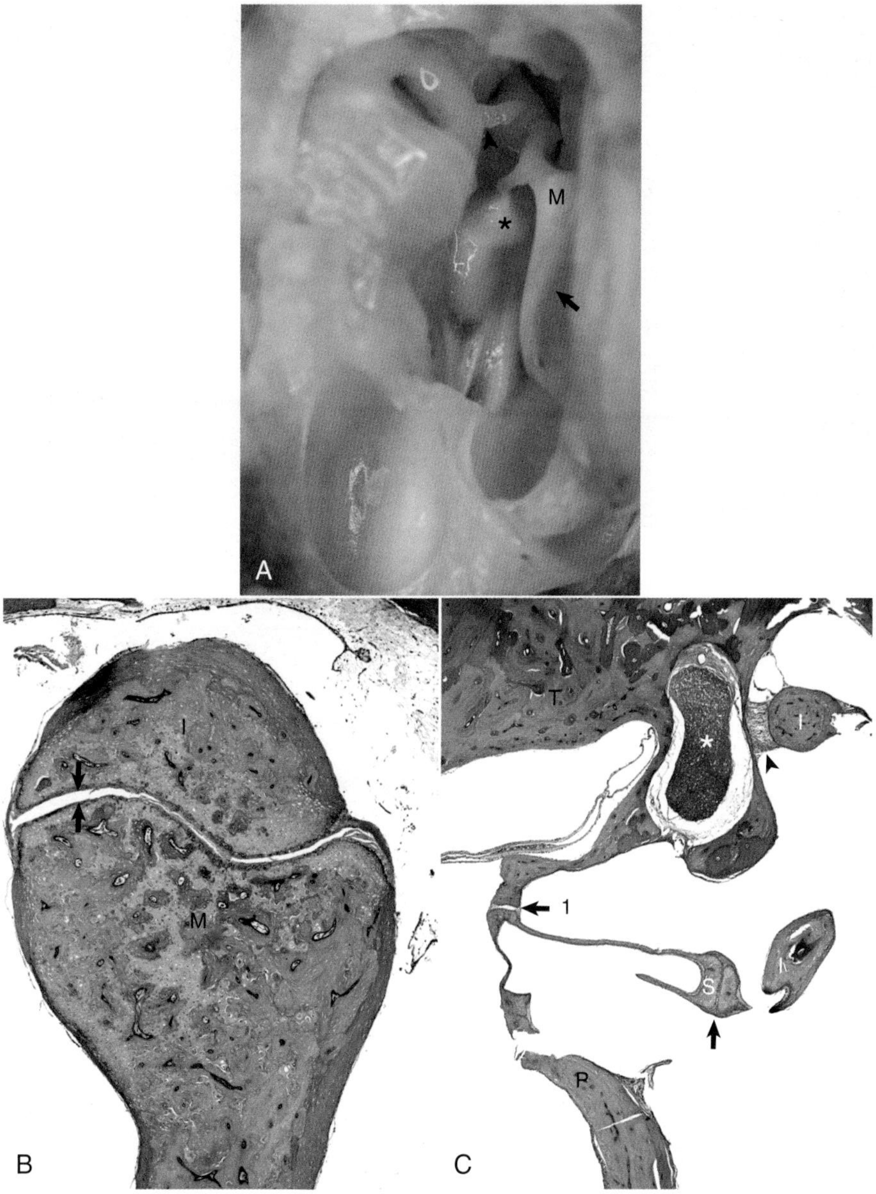

Figure 20-13 Auditory Ossicles and Ossicular Joints, Cat. A, Tympanic cavity, tympanic membrane, auditory ossicles, petrous portion of the temporal bone, auditory muscles, ventral view. The manubrium of the malleus is embedded in the tympanic membrane. The head of the malleus and incus are anchored in the epitympanic recess and form the incudomallearis joint. The long crus of the incus is shown articulating with the stapes to form the incudostapedial joint *(arrowhead)*. Attached to the muscular process of the malleus *(M)* is the tensor tympani muscle *(asterisk)*. *Arrow,* Tympanic membrane. **B,** Histologic section of the incudomallearis joint *(between the arrows)*, normal. The articulation of the malleus *(M)* and incus *(I)* is shown in the epitympanic recess. Similar to the petrous portion of the temporal bone, these ossicular bones lack a medulla. **C,** Histologic section of the incudostapedial joint. Positioned in the vestibular window is the stapes *(S)*, held in place by a syndesmosis *(arrow 1)*. The more ventral edge of the stapes has artifactually fractured. Articulating with the head of the stapes is the lenticular process of the long crus of the incus *(I)* to form the incudostapedial joint *(arrow)*. The lenticular process of the incus is to the right of the incudostapedial joint. A portion of the short crus is positioned in the epitympanic recess and anchored by a ligamentous attachment *(arrowhead)*. The facial nerve is present coursing through the facial canal *(asterisk)*. Note that the opening of the bony canal is called the facial canal foramen, allowing communication with the tympanic cavity. *P,* Promontory; *T,* petrous portion of the temporal bone. H&E stain. (**A** and **B** courtesy Dr. B.L. Njaa, Center for Veterinary Health Sciences, Oklahoma State University.)

Two cranial nerves provide motor branches to the muscles of the middle ear. Branches of the trigeminal nerve named for their respective muscles innervate the tensor tympani and tensor veli palatini muscles within the tympanic cavity. The facial nerve initially leaves the cranial cavity through the internal acoustic meatus (see Fig. 20-17), along with the vestibulocochlear cranial nerve, and then courses through the facial canal of the petrous portion of the temporal bone in close proximity to the vestibular window (Fig. 20-18). Several millimeters medial and lateral to the tendon of the stapedius muscle, the bony casing of the facial canal is incomplete, forming a facial canal foramen. This opening allows an unimpeded connection between the stapedius tendon and the stapes. It also allows direct communication between the epineurial connective tissue of the facial nerve and the tympanic cavity (see Fig. 20-18). This proximity and exposure of the facial nerve to the tympanic cavity potentially explains why middle ear disease can manifest as facial nerve

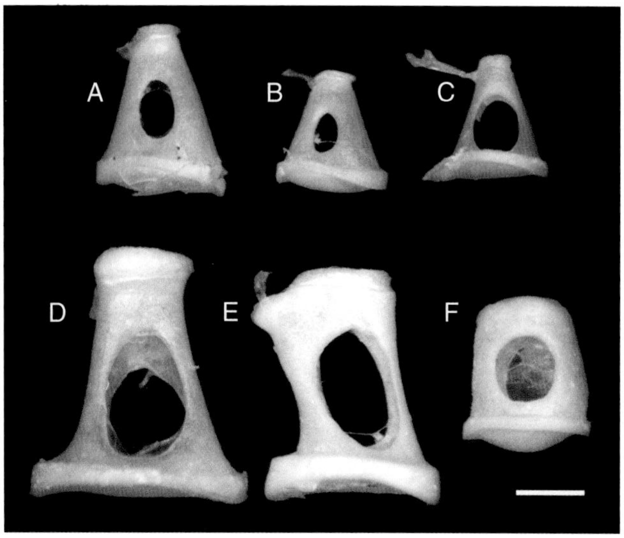

Figure 20-14 **Stapes, Species Variations.** Stapes are highly variable in size and shape, depending on the species. The first two stapes, beginning from the top row left are from different-sized dogs. The larger stapes is from a 20-kg mixed-breed dog **(A)**. The smaller stapes is from a Maltese dog **(B)**. The third stapes of the upper row is from a cat **(C)**. The lower row depicts stapes from a horse **(D)**, cow **(E)**, and slaughter-age pig **(F)**. In all cases the lower plate of the stapes is convex. Also, in each case the tendinous attachment of the stapedius muscle is affixed to the shorter crus or limb of the stapes. Scale bar = 1 mm. (Courtesy Dr. B.L. Njaa, Center for Veterinary Health Sciences, Oklahoma State University.)

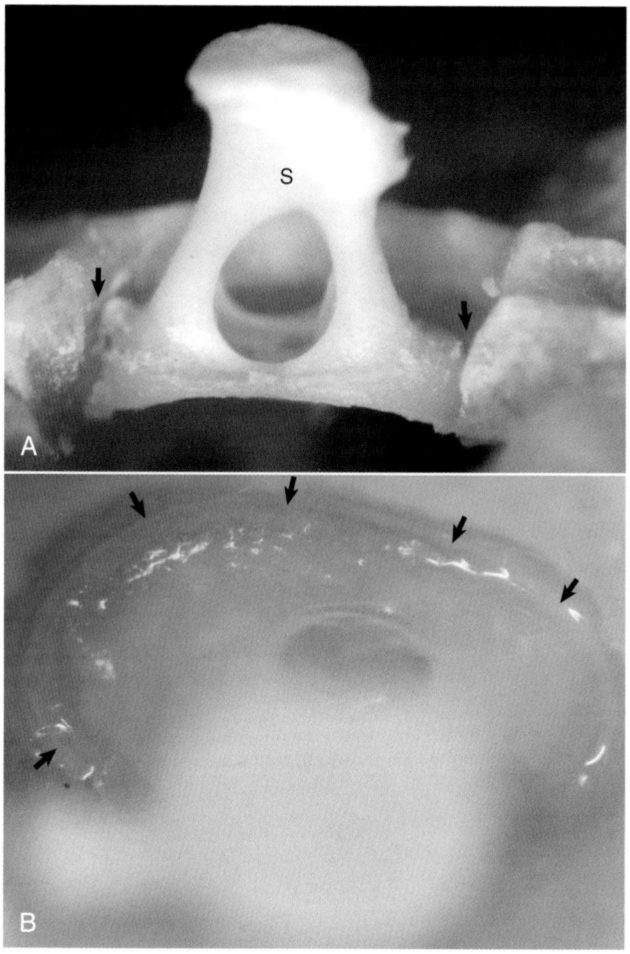

Figure 20-15 **Stapes in Situ, Horse. A,** Partially opened oval window. The stapes *(S)* is seated in the oval window connected to the petrous portion of the temporal bone by the annular ligament *(arrows)*. **B,** Ventrolateral view of the stapes, in situ. A thin rim of annular cartilage is visible, denoting the syndesmosis formed between the stapes and cartilage of the oval window of the petrous portion of the temporal bone *(arrows)*. (Courtesy Dr. B.L. Njaa, Center for Veterinary Health Sciences, Oklahoma State University.)

dysfunction. The facial nerve emerges from the middle ear through the stylomastoid foramen immediately caudal to the external acoustic meatus.

Auditory Tube (Eustachian or Pharyngotympanic Tube)

In most mammalian species the middle ear communicates with the pharynx through the auditory tube, which originates from the first pharyngeal pouch (Fig. 20-19). In the middle ear the auditory tube opens into the most rostral and dorsal portion of the tympanic cavity called the *epitympanic cavity*. In the pharynx the auditory tube originates from a narrow slitlike opening in the nasopharyngeal cavity and is lined by epithelium that is contiguous with the nasopharynx, namely, ciliated columnar pseudostratified epithelium mixed with goblet cells (Fig. 20-20). In a few species, flanking the auditory tube are clusters of lymphocytes referred to as the *tubal tonsil*.

Infectious organisms can migrate via the auditory tube between the nasopharynx and the middle ear, thus serving as a portal of entry for each area. Additionally, the auditory tube is an important route for clearance of an infectious organism from the middle ear via the nasopharynx to the respiratory and alimentary systems.

Unique to the horse and other Equidae, guttural pouches (see Chapters 9 and 17) are enlarged diverticula of the auditory tubes that extend further rostrally, medially, and ventrally when compared to auditory tubes of other mammalian species. Although the precise function of guttural pouches remains controversial, their proximity to internal carotid arteries and their ability to inflate during vigorous exercise makes the idea of an extracalvarial brain cooling apparatus a provocative hypothesis.

Internal Ear

The internal ear is confined to a single bone, the petrous portion of the temporal bone. In most mammalian species it is a triangular, wedge-shaped bone that forms the dorsomedial margin of the tympanic cavity. Often referred to as the hardest bone of the body, it is frequently slightly more yellow than surrounding bone and lacks the cancellous bony arrangement or medullary cavities present in other portions of the temporal bones. The internal ear is derived from a focal area of ectoderm referred to as the *otic placode*. This eventually forms an otic vesicle and through interaction with surrounding embryonic tissues, differentiates into this highly specialized tissue.

The internal ear is essentially made up of several membranous compartments, collectively known as the *membranous labyrinth*, derived from ectoderm, that contain *endolymph*. The membranous labyrinthine compartments include the cochlear duct, sacculus, utriculus, and three semicircular canals arranged in three geometric planes (Fig. 20-21). Surrounding the membranous labyrinth and derived from mesoderm, the *osseous labyrinth* (i.e., petrous portion of the temporal bone) represents a compartment that lacks an epithelial lining and is filled with perilymph. The osseous labyrinth is classically a rostrally coiled tube or duct with an intermediate compartment or vestibule and a caudal semicircular canal region. However, the shape of the petrous portion of the temporal bone is very different. The basal turn of the cochlea is denoted by the prominent bulge in the petrous portion of the temporal bone known as the *promontory*. Caudally, portions of this bone give the

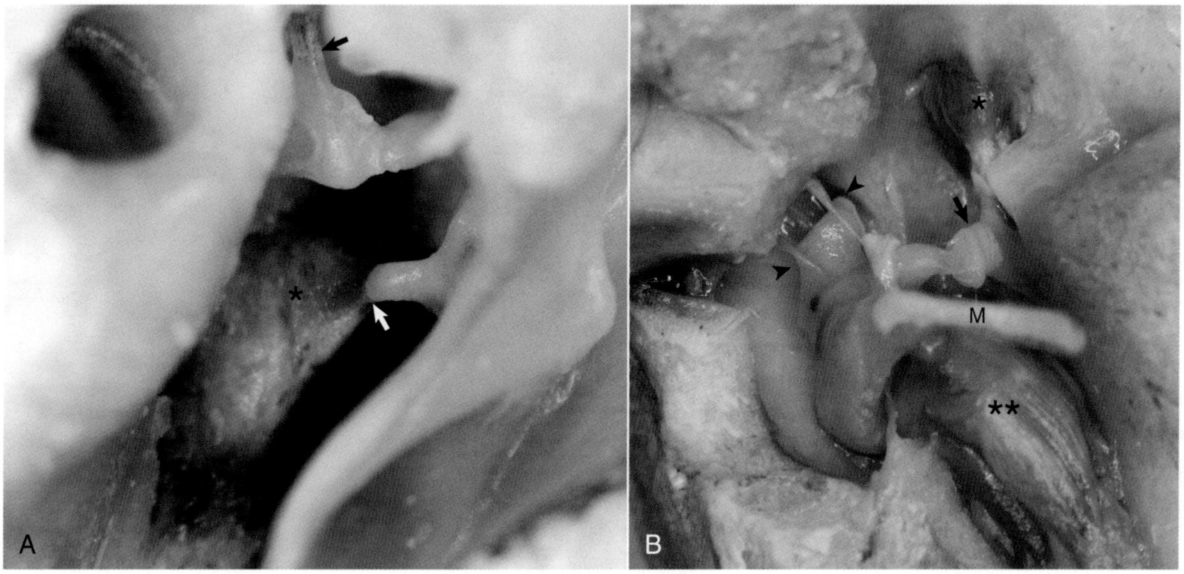

Figure 20-16 **Auditory Ossicular Muscles. A,** Middle ear, caudal view, ox. The external acoustic meatus is to the right on this image with the caudal edge of the tympanic membrane removed. The tensor tympani muscle *(asterisk)* is attached via its tendon to the muscular process of the malleus *(white arrow)*. The tendon of the stapedius muscle *(black arrow)* is attached to the stapes bone near the head of the stapes. **B,** Middle ear, ventral view, horse. The bony external acoustic meatus, tympanic membrane, and associated connective tissue have been removed. The articulated incus and malleus form the incudomallearis joint and are anchored in the epitympanic recess *(arrowheads)*. The incudostapedial joint is opened *(arrow)*. The facial nerve and some of the surrounding bone have been removed to expose the stapedius muscle *(asterisk)* anchored in the facial canal fossa and attached to the stapes. The muscular process of the malleus is obscured by the position of the manubrium (M) of the malleus, which is attached to the tensor tympani muscle *(double asterisk)*. (Courtesy Dr. B.L. Njaa, Center for Veterinary Health Sciences, Oklahoma State University.)

appearance of the tubular membranous labyrinth that likely represent the semicircular canals. Within the membranous labyrinth are biologic mechanosensory hair cells (see later) responsible for hearing (the auditory compartment) and for assessing head position, acceleration, and balance (the vestibular compartment).

Cochlea

The cochlea is the most complex portion of the membranous and bony labyrinths, comprising two closed-end tubular structures that are highly coiled (see Fig. 20-21). The central core of bone around which the cochlea turns is the modiolus. Sound waves vibrate the tympanic membrane and are converted by coordinated movements of the malleus, incus, and stapes to fluid waves within the perilymph by vibrations of the vestibular window. Fluid waves travel through the perilymph of the scala vestibuli toward the cupula, reaching the helicotrema, and then returning within the scala tympani toward the cochlear (round) window. Positioned between the scala vestibuli and the scala tympani is the second closed compartment known as the *cochlear duct*. It is filled with endolymph. The cochlear duct is separated from the scala vestibuli by the vestibular membrane (also known as Reissner's membrane) and the scala tympani by the basilar membrane. The spiral organ (organ of Corti) is the sound transducer within the cochlear duct that transforms mechanical deflection of fluid waves into neurologic impulses (action potentials) that travel via neurons to the brainstem and auditory cortex and are recognized as sound.

Sensory hair cells, inner and outer, basally contact interphalangeal cells that in turn are basally anchored to the basilar membrane. Inner hair cells are closer to the inner modiolus and separated from the outer hair cells by inner and outer pillar cells that form the inner spiral tunnel. Overlying the hair cells is a ribbon-like strip of extracellular matrix called the *tectorial membrane*. It is composed of several genetically distinct types of collagen (collagen types II, IX, and XI) and three distinct noncollagenous glycoproteins (α-tectorin, β-tectorin, and otogelin). The tectorial membrane rests on and is affixed to tips of the outer hair cells that make up the mechanosensory portion of the spiral organ that lies on the basilar membrane (Fig. 20-22). There are a series of three or more rows of outer hair cells and a single row of inner hair cells (see Fig. 20-22). Fluid waves in the scala vestibuli result in distortion of the basilar membrane, leading to distortion of the apical appendages of the hair cells (i.e., stereocilia), resulting in their depolarization and afferent transmission of action potentials via the cochlear branch of the vestibulocochlear cranial nerve to the brainstem and auditory cortex.

The basilar membrane of the spiral organ varies in its thickness and width along its length. Briefly, the cochlea is defined by its turns, with the basal portion in close proximity to the vestibule and vestibular window, whereas the cochlear apex is the most rostral portion, where the scala vestibuli and scala tympani are connected. In the basal portion of the cochlea, the basilar membrane is widest and thinnest, whereas in the cochlear apex the basilar membrane is narrowest and thickest. The basilar membrane in the basal cochlear turn detects high-frequency sounds, whereas the apical portion of the basilar membrane detects low-frequency sounds. Along its entire length, hair cells are "tuned" to the resonant frequency inherent to the section of basilar membrane and correspond to the "tuned" portion of the auditory cortex. Thus sounds of a particular frequency result in distortion of a portion of the spiral organ most in tune to that frequency. Damage to portions of the spiral organ result in impaired sound detection and perception.

Vestibular System

The vestibular system is made of several endolymph-filled compartments located in the caudal third to half of the petrous portion of the temporal bone. It represents a major sensory system that (1) maintains balance in concert with general proprioception and visual systems, (2) coordinates body posture, and (3) helps maintain ocular position in relation to the position or motion of the head. Included

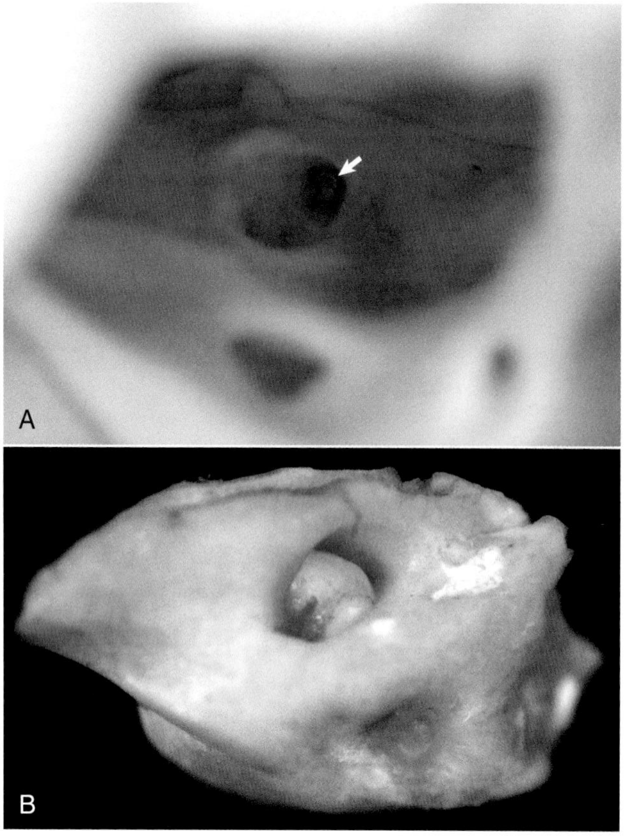

Figure 20-17 Internal Acoustic Meatus, Cat. A, Right internal acoustic meatus. Viewed through the open left external acoustic meatus, the right internal acoustic meatus *(arrow)* represents the bony opening into the petrous portion of the temporal bone, through which the vestibulocochlear nerve and facial nerve exit the cranial cavity. **B,** Petrous portion of the temporal bone, cat. The yellow hue is very typical of this bone in all species. The large central opening is the internal acoustic meatus within which lie the vestibular and cochlear nerves. (Courtesy Dr. B.L. Njaa, Center for Veterinary Health Sciences, Oklahoma State University.)

in the vestibular system are the semicircular canals, utriculus, sacculus, vestibular ganglia, vestibular portion of cranial nerve VIII (vestibulocochlear nerve), vestibular nuclei, and vestibular lobules of the cerebellum.

There are three semicircular canals oriented at right angles relative to each other occupying three planes. Each canal has a terminal dilation, or ampulla, that contains a specialized surface sensory organ called the *crista*. In aggregate, the sensory portion is referred to as *crista ampullaris*. Each crista is lined by specialized sensory hair cells that send continuous tonic neural signals to the vestibular nucleus. Deflection of these sensory hair cells during acceleration, deceleration, or rotation results in variation of the tonic signals sent to the vestibular nucleus. However, the hair cells are not activated during constant velocity.

Maculae are receptors located within the membranous utriculus and sacculus of the vestibule. The saccular macula is oriented in the vertical plane, whereas the macula of the utriculus is oriented in the horizontal plane. Surface-lining neuroepithelial hair cells of the macula project into an otolithic membrane, a mucopolysaccharide filamentous meshwork embedded with calcium carbonate–rich crystalline *otoliths (otoconia)*. Movement of the otolithic membrane causes deflection of the hair cells and triggers action potential. As in the case of the crista ampullaris, macular receptors provide a continuous tonic nervous input, with a net effect of maintaining static head positioning relative to gravity.

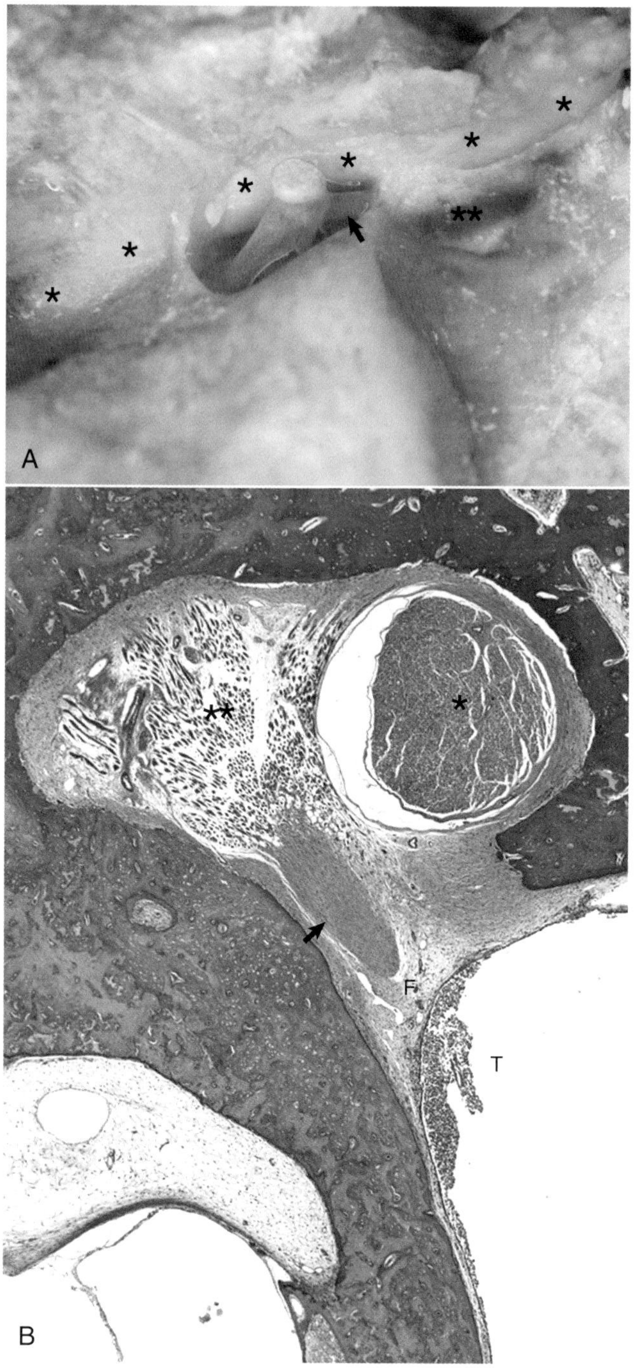

Figure 20-18 Stapedius Muscle, Facial Canal, Facial Canal Foramen and the Facial Nerve. A, Horse. The facial nerve *(asterisk)* courses through the facial canal in close proximity to the stapes and partially obscures the stapedius muscle *(double asterisks)*. The tendon of the stapedius muscle *(arrow)* is shown attached to the short crus of the stapes, near the head of the stapes. **B,** Dog. Histologic section of facial canal, facial canal foramen, facial nerve, stapedius muscle and its fossa and stapedius tendon. The facial nerve *(asterisk)* is present within the facial canal partially obscuring the stapedius muscle *(double asterisks)* anchored in its stapedius muscle fossa. The tendon of the stapedius muscle *(arrow)* is observed in oblique, transverse section, extending toward the stapes through the facial canal foramen *(F)*, but the stapes is not in this plane of section. Within the tympanic cavity *(T)* are moderate numbers of neutrophils, indicative of suppurative otitis media. H&E stain. (Courtesy Dr. B.L. Njaa, Center for Veterinary Health Sciences, Oklahoma State University.)

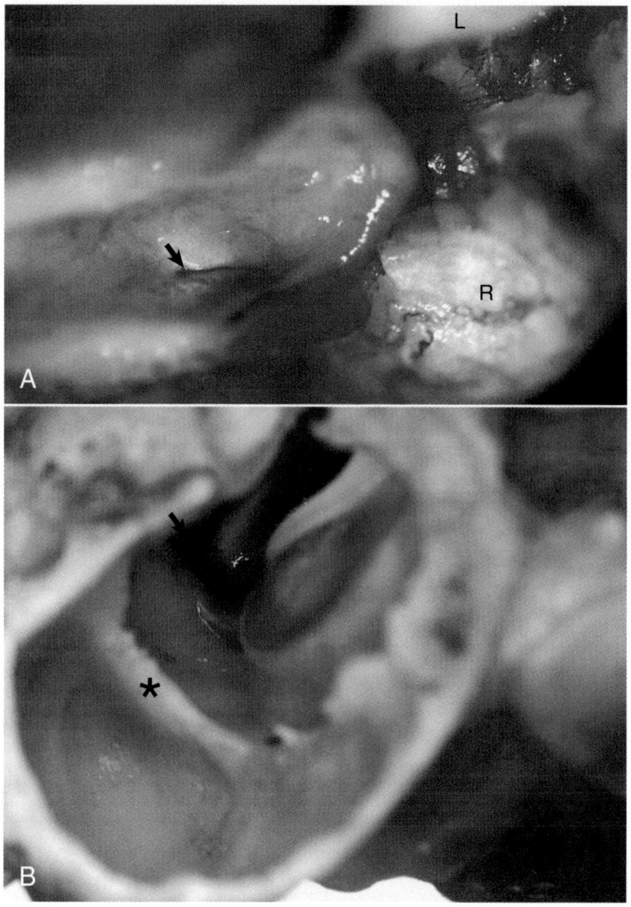

Figure 20-19 **Auditory Tube. A,** Nasopharynx, cat. A thin slitlike opening, normally maintained in a closed position, represents the opening of the right auditory tube into the nasopharynx *(arrow)*. *L,* Left occipital condyle; *R,* right occipital condyle. **B,** Middle ear, tympanic bulla, right ear, caudoventral, oblique view, dog. The auditory tube *(arrow)* is located dorsal, medial, and rostral to the tympanic ring of the tympanic membrane just to the left of the tympanic membrane and manubrium of the malleus. The septum bulla *(asterisk)* is a short and incomplete bony ridge when compared to the cat. (Courtesy Dr. B.L. Njaa, Center for Veterinary Health Sciences, Oklahoma State University.)

On stimulation of sensory nerve endings, action potentials are transmitted through bipolar cells whose cell bodies are located in the vestibular ganglia of the vestibular branch of the vestibulocochlear nerve. Signals travel to the vestibular nuclei in the medulla. From the vestibular nuclei, connections are made with the oculomotor, trochlear, and abducent nuclei of the rostral brainstem via the medial longitudinal fasciculus, the vestibulocerebellum by the caudal cerebellar peduncle, and the spinal cord via the vestibulospinal tract located in the ventral funiculus.

Histologic Evaluation of the Internal Ear

See E-Appendix 20-1.

Dysfunction/Responses to Injury

The ear's responses to injury are listed in Box 20-1.

External Ear

The external ear is an extension of the integument, and it responds to inflammatory stimuli similarly. All of the hallmarks of inflammation occur in otitis externa. Initially there is reddening and warmth of the affected auricle associated with otitis externa caused by vascular dilation and hyperemia. Transudation of fluid out of leaky vessels leads to edema affecting both the auricle (see Fig. 17-15) and external acoustic meatus. Edema within the tissues results in swelling of the tissues and discomfort when the tissues are touched. As the inflammatory response progresses, the transudate becomes an exudate, infiltrating the dermis of the external ear. Epithelial and adnexal changes, described later, result in further expansion of the external ear dermis. Eventually the lumen of the external acoustic meatus may become so stenotic that hearing function becomes impaired.

As has already been described, the external acoustic meatus and auricle are lined by haired skin. Large, abundant, multiple, branching, and actively secreting sebaceous glands are most prominent in the superficial dermis of deeper portions of the external acoustic meatus associated with hair follicles (see Fig. 20-5, A). Smaller, tubular, eccrine sweat glands, referred to as *ceruminous glands*, are located in the deeper layers of dermis. The epidermis, which is best studied in dogs, in response to inflammation, becomes hyperplastic and hyperkeratotic, although in some conditions it becomes ulcerated. Glandular changes include smaller, less abundant, less active sebaceous glands and more numerous, typically large, dilated ceruminous glands. Neutrophils, lymphocytes, and macrophages typically infiltrate the dermis, as well as the ectatic ceruminous glands (Fig. 20-23). Aggregates of lymphocytes form when the process is chronic. With increased chronicity, there is greater infiltration by fibroblasts and collagen, which can lead to more permanent stenotic changes. Late-stage otitis externa is associated soft tissue ossification, arising from the auricular perichondral scaffold depicted as abrupt ossification similar to intramembranous ossification but likely a metaplastic change to severe, chronic inflammation (E-Fig. 20-1).

Auricles of lightly pigmented cats chronically exposed to ultraviolet (UV) light are prone to developing squamous cell carcinoma (described later in the chapter; also see Chapter 17). UVB light leads to cellular transformation of the epithelial cells, leading to a clonal population of neoplastic squamous epithelial cells.

Box 20-1 Responses to Injury of the Ear

EXTERNAL EAR

- Inflammation, acute and chronic
- Epithelial and adnexal hyperplasia
- Fibrosis
- Osseous metaplasia
- Neoplasia (occasionally)

MIDDLE EAR

- Inflammation (myringitis)
- Healing of the tympanic membrane
- Goblet cell metaplasia
- Impaired mucociliary clearance (likely atrophy of ciliated epithelial cells)
- Osteosclerosis of the tympanic bulla
- Formation of inflammatory polyps
- Horner's syndrome/Pourfour du Petit syndrome

INTERNAL EAR

- Sensory cell degeneration/death
- Inflammation: Auditory ossicular chain damage (osteolysis/osteonecrosis)

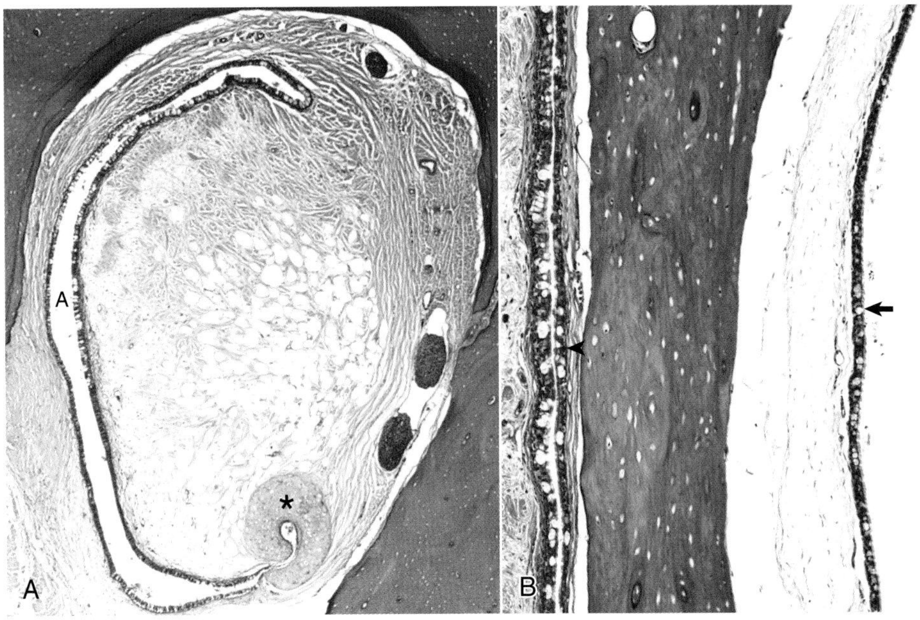

Figure 20-20 **Histologic Section of the Auditory Tube Mucosa, Cat. A,** Rostral opening of the auditory tube. The auditory tube *(A)* in cross section is typically C-shaped. Comma-shaped cartilage *(asterisk)* provides structural support to portions of the auditory tube. The mucosal epithelium is composed of ciliated, pseudostratified, columnar epithelium mixed with goblet cells and nonciliated epithelial cells. H&E stain. **B,** Cross section through tympanic bulla and auditory tube. The mucoperiosteum *(arrow)* and the auditory tube mucosa *(arrowhead)* are composed of pseudostratified, ciliated columnar epithelial cells mixed with goblet cells and basal cells. This epithelium is contiguous with the nasopharyngeal mucosa. H&E stain. (Courtesy Dr. B.L. Njaa, Center for Veterinary Health Sciences, Oklahoma State University.)

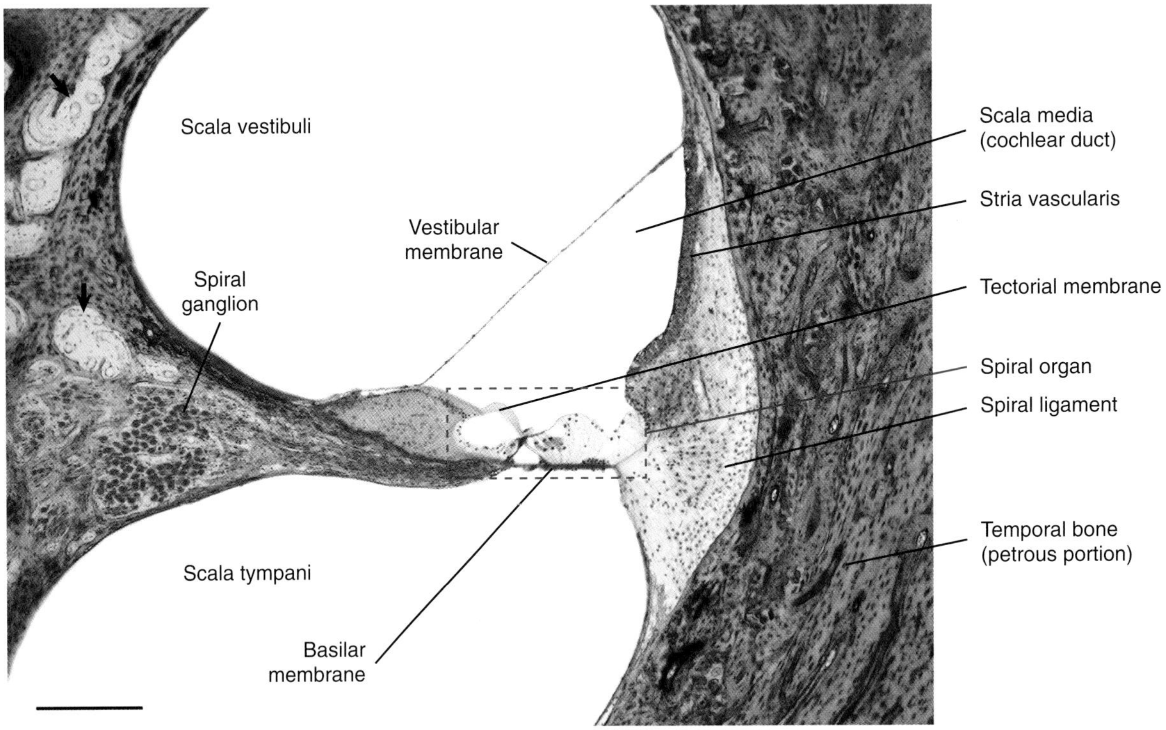

Figure 20-21 **Structure of the Cochlea, Basal Turn of the Cochlea, Cat.** The scala vestibuli and scala tympani are filled with perilymph and represent the bony labyrinth of the cochlea. The cochlear duct is the membranous labyrinth of the cochlea, derived from the otic vesicle and filled with endolymph. The spiral organ is highlighted *(red dashed rectangle)*. H&E stain; celloidin embedded; slow EDTA decalcification. *Arrows*, Bony core remnants of the petrous temporal bone arising from cartilage cores during the formation of the bone. (Courtesy G. Pagonis, Massachusetts Eye and Ear Infirmary.)

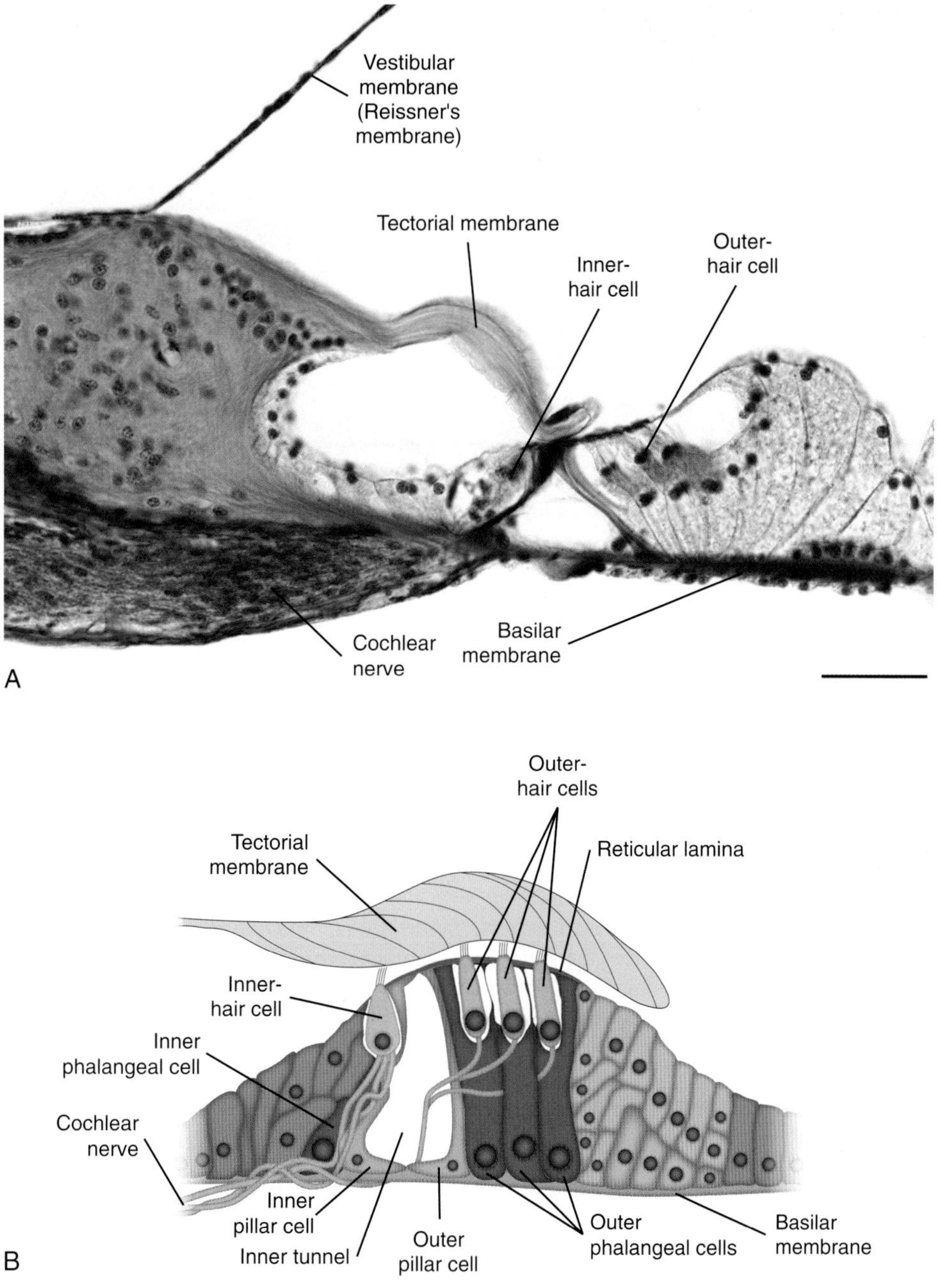

Figure 20-22 **Spiral Organ (Organ of Corti), Cat. A,** Higher magnification of the spiral organ from Figure 20-21. H&E stain; celloidin embedded; slow EDTA decalcification. **B,** Schematic diagram of the spiral organ depicting three rows of outer hair cells and a single row of inner hair cells. Inner and outer hair cells are supported by inner and outer phalangeal cells, respectively, that are anchored to the basal membrane. Pillar cells form a triangular inner tunnel and serve as a fulcrum. Fluid waves traveling in the scala vestibuli result in deviation of the basilar membrane. This structure leads to deflection of the apical hair cell stereocilia. Associated nerve ends at the basolateral edge of hair cells and transduces mechanical deflection into sound detection. (**A** courtesy G. Pagonis, Massachusetts Eye and Ear Infirmary. **B** courtesy Dr. B.L. Njaa, Center for Veterinary Health Sciences, Oklahoma State University; and Dr. J.F. Zachary, College of Veterinary Medicine, University of Illinois.)

Middle Ear

Myringitis

Inflammation of the tympanic membrane is called *myringitis* and is most commonly caused by bacterial infection of the external or middle ear (see Fig. 20-39, *B*). Macroscopically, the tympanic membrane may be congested, hemorrhagic, or thickened, resulting in opacity. Microscopically, the tympanic membrane has all of the characteristics of acute inflammation and if the inciting cause is unresolved, results in chronic inflammation (see Chapter 3). Prolonged and severe myringitis may lead to perforation of the tympanic membrane and prevent its healing.

Healing of the Tympanic Membrane

The tympanic membrane is a regionally well vascularized membrane that has an air interface along each surface. It can be perforated by traumatic injury, sudden exposures to high pressures, degradative enzymes and pressures from acute and chronic inflammation, chronic mite infestations, and neoplasms. Unique to the tympanic

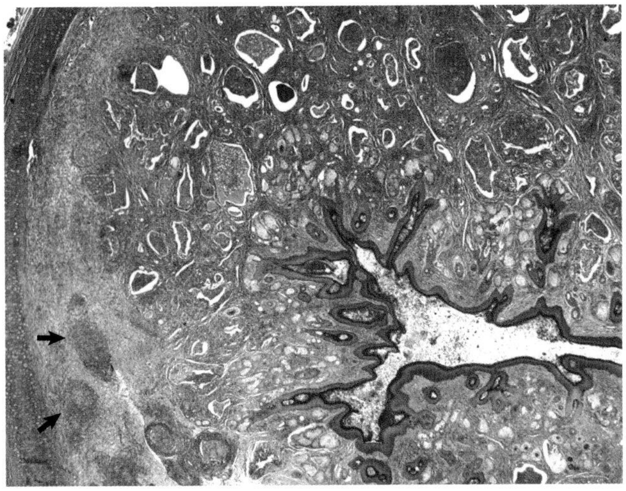

Figure 20-23 **Otitis Externa, External Acoustic Meatus, Dog.** In this histologic section the dermis contains increased numbers of ceruminous glands that are dilated and filled with inflammatory cells, typically neutrophils, macrophages, lymphocytes, and plasma cells. These inflammatory cells are also present in the periadnexal dermis. Lymphoid aggregates form nodules *(arrows)* in the deep dermis near the cartilaginous rings of the external acoustic meatus. The overlying epidermis is mildly to moderately thickened (acanthosis). The luminal diameter has been markedly reduced, which can further exacerbate the problem of otitis externa. H&E stain. (Courtesy Dr. B.L. Njaa, Center for Veterinary Health Sciences, Oklahoma State University.)

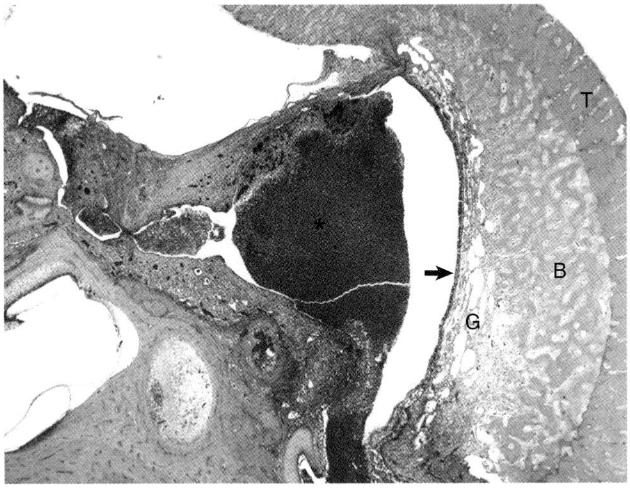

Figure 20-24 **Chronic Otitis Media with Bony Proliferation, Guinea Pig.** The tympanic cavity is partially filled with suppurative exudate *(asterisk, center of image)*. The tympanic bulla has thickened, hyperplastic mucosal epithelium *(arrow)*. The mucoperiosteum is thickened by granulation tissue (G) that overlies the formation of newly proliferative bone *(B)* in response to chronic inflammation. Tinctorially, the tympanic bulla *(T)* is the darker blue area along the right margin of the image. H&E stain. (Courtesy Dr. B.L. Njaa, Center for Veterinary Health Sciences, Oklahoma State University.)

membrane, and likely related to its function, is its inherent ability to heal rapidly while maintaining its thin structure during healing through a process called *epithelial migration*. Unlike most other tissues, in which granulation tissue forms and bridges the defect, followed by reepithelialization, the tympanic membrane closes the defect first with migrating epithelial cells, followed by a granulation tissue response that closes the mesenchymal portion of the tympanic membrane.

Within minutes to hours of the initial perforation, injured tissue at the edge of the perforation initiates an acute inflammatory response. Within hours, epithelial cells proliferate initially along the annulus and along the margin of the manubrium, corresponding to areas in which the blood supply is most prominent and epithelial stem cells of the tympanum are thought to reside. Proliferating epithelium advances toward the perforation using keratin as a scaffolding to initially bridge and reepithelialize the defect. As this epithelium is migrating across the defect, granulation tissue forms on the inner edge of the perforated membrane. Anchored to the epithelium that initially closes the perforation, the middle, mesenchymal layer of the tympanic membrane is repaired by this advancing granulation tissue. As granulation tissue remodels to its normal thin layer, the inner epithelial layer finally bridges the defect to complete the healing process. In an experimental animal model, 2.5-mm perforations were completely healed by 9 days after injury.

Goblet Cell Metaplasia and Impaired Mucociliary Clearance

An important defense mechanism of the middle ear is the mucociliary apparatus of the auditory tube and contiguous tympanic cavity. Chronic otitis media causes a decrease in the number of ciliated cells (ciliary atrophy) in the mucosa of the auditory tube. Studies in cats determined that neutrophil lysate (likely consisting of degradative enzymes) or lipopolysaccharide did not significantly reduce the number of ciliated cells in the auditory tube, but auditory tube obstruction and likely increased pressure in the middle ear resulted in a dramatic decrease in the number of ciliated epithelial cells. In the same study there was a marked increase in the total number of goblet cells in the mucoperiosteum of the middle ear. It was hypothesized that obstruction of the auditory tube elevated partial pressure of carbon dioxide (pCO_2) in the mucus layer of the mucosa, triggering mucosal stem cells to differentiate toward goblet cells rather than ciliated cells. The viscoelasticity of the mucus produced by these goblet cells was greater than normal and resulted in a marked decrease of mucociliary clearance of the middle ear, probably further contributing to auditory tube obstruction, increased pressure in the middle era, and metaplasia of ciliated cells to goblet cells.

Osseous Metaplasia of the Tympanic Bulla

In infections of the middle ear caused by microorganisms, mediators of acute and chronic inflammation, such as cytokines and degradative enzymes, may lead to excessive periosteal proliferation of new bone and thickening of the wall of the tympanic bulla (Fig. 20-24; see Chapter 16). The bulla may become grossly distorted, and the lumen volume typically decreases. Inflammation also can contribute to bone lysis. In the most severe cases, proliferative bone depicts medullary compartments containing bone marrow.

Formation of Aural Inflammatory Polyps

Aural inflammatory polyps are discussed later but are thought to represent both inflammatory and hyperplastic responses to injury induced by otitis media. Acute inflammation of the middle ear results in rapid expansion of the mucoperiosteum by edema, congestion, and acute inflammatory cells (see Chapter 3); chronic inflammation results in mucoperiosteal expansion characterized by aggregates of chronic inflammatory cells and granulation tissue (see Chapter 3). This expansion may also result in the formation of polypoid masses by an undetermined mechanism. These masses then result in clinical disease referable to where they exert their greatest effect. Polyps that involve the auditory tube and the nasopharynx can result in dysphagia and dyspnea, whereas those involving the tympanic membrane and external acoustic meatus lead to signs of otitis externa.

Horner's Syndrome/Pourfour du Petit Syndrome

Postganglionic sympathetic nerve fibers follow the internal carotid as it passes through the tympano-occipital fissure and enters the carotid canal medial to the tympanic bulla. These axons innervate smooth muscle of the periorbital sheath known as the orbital muscle, which extends groups of muscle fibers to the base of the third eyelid, as well as into both the superior and inferior eyelids. Debate currently exists on whether branches of these postganglionic sympathetic nerves course through the middle ear. Otitis media in dogs and cats is believed to induce injury to these axons, resulting in signs of denervation to the eye that include miosis, enophthalmos, a narrowed palpebral aperture, protrusion of the third eyelid, and peripheral vasodilation of the skin of the face on the affected side. This constellation of signs collectively is termed Horner's syndrome. Interestingly and related to a different anatomic trajectory, otitis media in farm animals and horses does not similarly affect these sympathetic fibers.

Irritation of the postganglionic sympathetic fibers can much less commonly result in hyperexcitability or hyperirritability. This is most commonly reported in cats that have had their ears examined, sampled, and flushed while under anesthesia. Clinical signs include mydriasis, exophthalmos, widening of the palpebral aperture, and cool skin over the face. In all cases reported, clinical signs resolved spontaneously. This hyperirritability syndrome is the opposite of Horner's syndrome and is referred to by some as *Pourfour du Petit syndrome*.

Internal Ear

Sensory Cell Degeneration/Death

Within the spiral organ (organ of Corti) are the outer and inner sensory hair cells, as well as spiral ganglion neurons. The sensory hair cells are the most vulnerable to injury. Damage to the sensory cells or ganglion cells results in impaired function that is often permanent. Whether the cause is labyrinthitis, noise-induced hearing loss (85-dB sound pressure level or higher), chemical ototoxins, or the poorly understood disorder called *presbycusis* (i.e., age-related hearing loss), sensory hair cells are targeted and undergo degeneration or death, leading to hearing impairment. Bursts of intense noise are thought to result in disarrangement or breakage of the apical stereocilia, whereas continuous exposure to damaging noise leads to death of the hair cell.

Auditory Ossicular Chain Damage

Chronic otitis media can potentially lead to conductive hearing loss by damaging the auditory ossicles. Chronic exposure to infection, bacterial or fungal toxins, and degradative enzymes from inflammation can result in bony lysis. Excessively lytic bones may develop pathologic fractures. Additionally, chronic inflammation can result in fibrosis, which may restrict the movement of the ossicles. Finally, chronic inflammation can damage the articulations of the ossicles, thus impairing transmission of vibrations.

Aging

Senescence has many manifestations, and sensorineural hearing loss is a common feature of aging. *Presbycusis* is the term used for age-related hearing loss (ARHL). Age-related hearing loss is the aggregate result of sensory and neural changes involving the spiral organ and associated cochlear neurons as well as dysfunction at the level of the auditory cortex. Morphologic features of presbycusis confirmed with audiometry include loss of inner and outer hair cells, loss of supporting cells, accumulation of lipofuscin in remaining hair cells and supporting cells, loss of cochlear neurons, atrophy of the stria vascularis, and atrophy of the spiral ligament. These histologic features have been observed in cats and rodents studied as animal models of age-related hearing loss in human beings and in human temporal bone collections.

Mechanisms that underlie morphologic features of age-related hearing loss are numerous, but a few will be discussed. *KL* is an aging-suppressor gene that encodes for Klotho, a protein involved with calcium homeostasis and located in close proximity to the Na-K-Cl cotransporter in the cells of the stria vascularis. It is postulated to participate in the regulation of the ionic components of the endolymph. The stria vascularis has myriad mitochondria and marginal cells. The mitochondria are important for necessary energy, and marginal cells have a high apical density of potassium channels and pumps, collectively functioning to maintain the endocochlear potential. Both are decreased in age-related hearing loss. Finally, senescent fibrocytes may lead to loss of structural integrity of the spiral organ and reduced mechanical elasticity of the basilar membrane of the cochlea, further leading to age-related hearing loss.

Portals of Entry/Pathways of Spread

Portals of entry into the ear are listed in Box 20-2.

External Ear

Extension from the External Environment

Extension from the external environment is a common portal of entry into the external ear. As the external acoustic meatus gradually narrows, its funnel shape is conducive to directing foreign materials, fomites, parasites, and/or infectious microorganisms into the external ear and toward the tympanic membrane of the middle ear. Additionally, its potentially moist environment may favor colonization of the skin by pathogenic microorganisms (Table 20-1). Although dermatitides can affect any part of the dermis, including the external ear, occasionally involvement of the ear is an important feature used to arrive at a definitive diagnosis.

Hematogenous Spread

Hematogenous spread is a portal of entry into the external ear. Septicemias and/or specific types of viremias are thought to contribute to the development of external ear disease. Otitis externa and possibly deafness have been attributed to canine distemper virus, but it is unclear if the virus is a primary cause or one of several factors

Box 20-2 Portals of Entry into the Ear

EXTERNAL EAR
- Extension from the external environment (acoustic meatus)
- Hematogenous spread
- Extension from the middle ear

MIDDLE EAR
- Extension through perforation of the tympanic membrane
- Ascension of the auditory tube
- Extension via degeneration of the temporohyoid joint
- Extension via erosion through the tympanic bulla
- Migration along vascular or neural pathways

INTERNAL EAR
- Extension from the middle ear
- Hematogenous spread
- Migration along vascular or neural pathways

Table 20-1 Predisposing Factors and Primary Causes of Otitis Externa

Predisposing Factors	Outcomes
Conformation	Stenotic external acoustic meatus Excess hair within the external meatus Pendulous pinnae
Excessive moisture	Swimmer's ear High-humidity climate
Excessive cerumen production	Overactive glands
Treatment effects	Trauma from treatment swabs Irritation from topic products Altering normal microflora
Obstructive ear disease	Neoplasms Polyps Granulomas
Systemic disease	Immune suppression Viral disease Debilitation Catabolic states
Primary Causes	**Outcomes**
Parasites	Ticks, mites, nematodes (see E-Table 20-1)
Hypersensitivity reactions	Atopic dermatitis Food hypersensitivity Contact hypersensitivity Drug reactions
Keratinization disorders	Primary idiopathic seborrhea Endocrine disorders Sex hormone imbalances Lipid-related conditions
Foreign bodies	Plants (especially foxtails) Hair Sand, dirt Hardened secretions, medications
Glandular disorders	Ceruminal gland hyperplasia Sebaceous gland hyperplasia or hypoplasia Altered secretion rate Altered type of secretions
Autoimmune diseases	Lupus erythematosus Pemphigus foliaceus Pemphigus vulgaris Pemphigus erythematosus
Vascular diseases	Cold agglutinin disease Solar dermatitis Frostbite Vasculitis Juvenile cellulitis Aural chondritis
Secondary Causes	**Outcomes**
Bacteria	*Staphylococcus* spp. *Proteus* spp. *Pseudomonas* spp. *Escherichia coli* *Klebsiella* spp.
Yeast	*Malassezia* spp. *Candida albicans*

Modified from Griffin CE, Kwochka KW, MacDonald JM: Otitis externa and media. In *Current veterinary dermatology: the art and science of therapy*, St. Louis, 1993, Mosby; and Scott DW, Miller WH, Griffin CE: *Muller & Kirk's small animal dermatology*, ed 6, Philadelphia, 2001, WB Saunders.

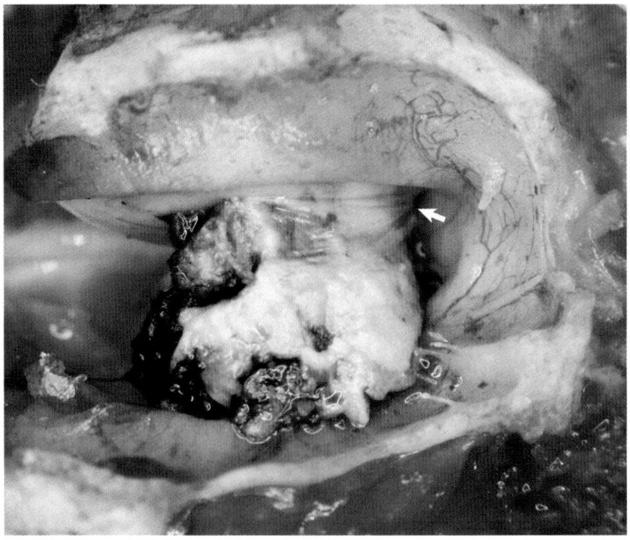

Figure 20-25 **Ruptured Tympanic Membrane, Dog.** A large aggregate of cerumen bulges through a tear in the caudal portion of the pars tensa between the manubrium of the malleus and the caudal bony tympanic ring into the tympanic cavity. The wrinkled flap of the torn pars tensa can be seen *(arrow)*. There was no evidence of otitis media, and likely the tear was acute. A ceruminous gland adenoma was identified in the horizontal portion of the external acoustic meatus unassociated with the tympanic membrane, causing complete obstruction. (Courtesy Dr. B.L. Njaa, Center for Veterinary Health Sciences, Oklahoma State University.)

leading to otic disease. In an animal with septicemia, circulating bacteria have the potential to adhere to the endothelium of the capillary beds of the dermis, colonize the endothelium, and spread into adjacent tissues (see Chapter 4).

Extension from the Middle Ear

Extension from the middle ear is another portal of entry into the external ear, especially in Cavalier King Charles spaniels with primary secretory otitis media. In primary secretory otitis media, the external ear is typically unaffected unless the tympanic membrane is ruptured and mucoid debris is spread into the external acoustic meatus. However, it has been suggested that this breed may have underlying failure of mucosae of the middle ear, predisposing these spaniels to auditory tube dysfunction and thus otitis media, leading to rupture of the tympanic membrane.

Middle Ear

Extension through Perforation of the Tympanic Membrane

Extension from the external ear through a perforated tympanic membrane is a portal of entry into the middle ear (Fig. 20-25). In dogs with chronic otitis externa, secondary otitis media may occur in as many as 80% of affected dogs. At the time of clinical diagnosis, the tympanic membrane is most often intact, although some studies report perforations in over 40% of cases with otitis externa and concurrent otitis media. Based on the results of bacteriologic studies, it has been shown that a majority of dogs with concurrent otitis externa and otitis media have different bacteria isolated from each compartment. Thus it is unclear if the portal of entry in otitis media involves perforation of the tympanic membrane and spread of otitis externa into the middle ear with subsequent healing of the tympanic membrane or if otitis media results from bacteria ascending a poorly functioning auditory tube. Multiple studies implicate the latter mechanism (see later). In cats, a recent study determined that otitis media was rarely associated with concurrent otitis externa, and the tympanic membrane remained intact.

Ascension of the Auditory Tube

Ascension up the auditory tube is a portal of entry into the middle ear. It appears that dysfunction of the auditory tube is a necessary precursor for development of otitis media and likely leads to impaired clearance of middle ear effusions and prolonged periods of negative pressure within the tympanic cavity. Dysfunction may be related to impairment of the opening of the auditory tube into the pharynx during swallowing, when pressure equalization takes place, or it could be related to alterations of mucociliary clearance facilitated by epithelial cells lining the tube. Via either mechanism, it appears that microorganisms can use this portal to reach the middle ear. Auditory tube dysfunction is the presumed mechanism for many cases of otitis media in cats and piglets.

Extension via Degeneration of the Temporohyoid Joint

Direct extension into the middle ear can occur from degeneration of the temporohyoid joint and release of microorganisms. See the discussion on temporohyoid osteoarthropathy in the section on Disorders of Horses.

Extension via Erosion through the Tympanic Bulla

Erosion through the tympanic bullae is a rare portal of entry into the middle ear. Neoplastic processes, such as oral squamous cell carcinomas, regional lymphosarcoma, or local compression by an abscess, can lead to bone remodeling, as well as bone lysis, with subsequent spread into the middle ear.

Migration along Vascular or Neural Pathways

Branches of the caudal auricular artery and the facial nerve traverse within the middle ear and have the potential to serve as pathways for spread of microorganisms and neoplasms from the middle ear to the cranial cavity or vice versa. (Recall that the facial nerve directly communicates with the middle ear through the facial canal foramen. Refer to the earlier section on Middle Ear Muscles and Nerves.) This migratory process likely occurs via the extracellular matrix of arteries and nerves (see Chapters 3, 10, and 14) and via anterograde axonal transport in nerves (see Chapter 14). As an example, cranial nerve sheath tumors (see Chapter 14) in the brain have been reported to migrate along branches of the facial nerve and vestibulocochlear nerves and enter the middle ear via the internal acoustic meatus.

Internal Ear

Extension from the Middle Ear

Extension from the middle ear is a portal of entry into the internal ear; thus otitis interna or labyrinthitis is most commonly thought of as occurring by direct extension from an infection of the middle ear. The most likely portal is the cochlear window. Based on studies in cats, the permeability of the membranous cochlear window is increased for elements (sodium) and macromolecules (tritiated albumin) during mild cases of experimentally induced otitis media. Penetration through the vestibular window is less likely because of the annular syndesmosis that is formed between the petrous portion of the temporal bone and the stapes (Fig. 20-26). Although otitis media may be diagnosed in isolation, otitis interna is rarely diagnosed without concurrent otitis media.

Hematogenous Spread

Entry through hematogenous spread occurs in the internal ear (see the previous discussion on the middle ear in the section on Portals of Entry/ Pathways of Spread for details).

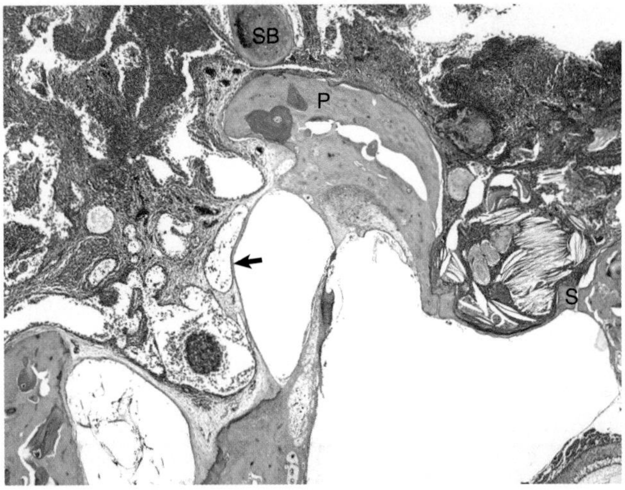

Figure 20-26 **Chronic Otitis Media, Cat.** Histologic section of middle ear, petrous portion of the temporal bone through the cochlear round and vestibular oval windows with the stapes in situ. The syndesmosis formed between the bone of the vestibular window of the petrous portion of the temporal bone and stapes seems to prevent otitis media from spreading into the internal ear. Conversely, the membranous covering of the cochlear window is infiltrated by inflammatory cells. During episodes of otitis media, the permeability of this membrane is increased. Otitis interna was diagnosed in this cat (not depicted in this image). At the top of the image is the edge of the septum bulla (*SB*) abutting the petrous portion of the temporal bone, anatomic indication that this is from a cat. *Arrow,* Cochlear window membrane; *P,* promontory; *S,* edge of stapes. H&E stain. (Courtesy Dr. B. L. Njaa, Center for Veterinary Health Sciences, Oklahoma State University.)

Migration along Vascular or Neural Pathways

Migration along vascular or neural pathways as a portal of entry occurs in the internal ear (see the previous discussion on the middle ear in the section on Portals of Entry/Pathways of Spread for details).

Defense Mechanisms/Barrier Systems

Defense mechanisms of the ear are listed in Box 20-3.

External Ear

Integumentary Defenses

Defense mechanisms of the skin are discussed in Chapters 3, 4, and 17.

Epithelial Migration

Migration of cornified epithelial cells to the periphery of the tympanic membrane and onto the epidermis of the external acoustic meatus continuously replaces the effete epidermal layer of the tympanic membrane. Epithelial migration is thus an important means of maintaining tympanic membrane thickness, clearance of debris and likely microorganisms and parasites from the tympanic membrane and external acoustic meatus, and retaining vibratory sensitivity. Alterations in this epithelial migratory pattern can lead to or may be the cause of disease of the external or middle ear. As discussed previously, epithelial migration is also the method by which perforations of the tympanic membrane are repaired.

Adnexa and Cerumen

Cerumen is an oily emulsion that coats and protects the integument of the external acoustic meatus. Its naturally hydrophobic properties make it an important barrier to the entry of excessive moisture into the epidermal cells or underlying dermis. In normal ears of dogs,

Box 20-3 Defense Mechanisms of the Ear

EXTERNAL EAR
Integumentary defenses
Epithelial migration
Cerumen barrier and acidity
Cerumen immunoglobulins
Commensal organisms
Structural defense from the osseous external acoustic meatus

MIDDLE EAR
Mucociliary apparatus
Surfactant
Auditory tube–associated lymphoid tissue
Commensal microorganisms

INTERNAL EAR
Structural defense from the petrous portion of the temporal bone
Acoustic reflex

cerumen is made of sloughed superficial squamous cells mixed with ceruminous and sebaceous gland secretions. There is a high lipid content in cerumen made up of neutral lipids. In otitic ears the cerumen changes because ceruminous glands are typically more numerous and active during periods of inflammation and thus contribute more to the content of cerumen (see Fig. 20-25). One consequence is a decrease in the lipid content, a decrease in hydrophobicity, and impairment of a natural barrier.

Cerumen in otitic ears becomes more acidic than normal, which is believed to impair bacterial growth. This outcome is due to greater contribution by ceruminous glands during periods of external ear inflammation. The pH of the external acoustic meatus is variable in dogs, ranging from 4.6 to 7.2. During periods of inflammation the mean pH in acute otitis externa may decrease, whereas the mean pH in chronic otitis externa tends to increase. The mechanistic consequences of these changes are poorly understood.

Immunoglobulins A, G, and M (IgA, IgG, and IgM) have been identified in canine cerumen; however, the predominant immunoglobulin is IgG. This high level of IgG is believed to be related to transudation of serum in the inflamed external ear. Lysozyme and interleukins have also been identified in cerumen and provide an antimicrobial function.

Commensal Organisms

A mixture of bacteria and yeast normally populates the external acoustic meatus. Various species of "potentially pathogenic" microorganisms have been cultured from external ears of dogs with no evidence of disease. They include *Bacillus* spp., *Corynebacterium* spp., *Escherichia coli*, *Micrococcus* spp., *Staphylococcus* spp., *Streptococcus* spp., and yeast organisms, most commonly *Malassezia* spp. Rarely, *Pseudomonas* spp. and *Proteus* spp. have been isolated. Based on a single study of horses, *Corynebacterium* spp. and *Staphylococcus intermedius* were isolated from normal ears. Presumably these organisms live symbiotically, and defense mechanisms limit or prevent proliferation of a monoculture. However, the spectrum of microorganisms cultured from diseased external ears closely mirrors this list.

Osseous External Acoustic Meatus

The length and diameter of the osseous portion of the external acoustic meatus are highly variable among species and provide a unique structural defense mechanism. Animals with longer and narrower osseous portions have tympanic cavities and tympanic membranes that are better protected than those with shorter osseous portions.

Middle Ear

Mucociliary Apparatus

Various portions of the middle ear are lined by epithelium similar to that found in the nasopharynx. A combination of goblet cells and ciliated columnar epithelial cells extends through the auditory tube into the tympanic cavity. See Chapters 4 and 9 for discussion of the mucociliary apparatus.

Surfactant

Surfactant in the lung has long been recognized for its central role in reducing surface tension in alveoli, allowing them to expand and collapse normally during inspiration and expiration, respectively (see Chapter 9). However, recently it has been shown that surfactant has other roles, especially in the function of the auditory tube. Surfactant is a complex mixture made up of 90% lipid and phospholipid and 10% surfactant proteins, designated surfactant protein A (SP-A), SP-B, SP-C, and SP-D. Cuboidal epithelial cells lining the auditory tube are the source of surfactant and contain apical secretory granules analogous to what are seen in type II pneumocytes of the lung. One major difference between pulmonary surfactant and auditory tube surfactant is the ratio of phosphatidylcholine to sphingomyelin. Pulmonary surfactant has a ratio of 67 to 1, whereas auditory tube surfactant has a ratio of 2 to 1. This dramatic difference in auditory tube surfactant phospholipid content is reflected in a reduced ability to modify surface tension.

The most abundant surfactant protein in lung surfactant is SP-B, a strongly hydrophobic protein with high surface activity. However, auditory tube surfactant has a paucity of SP-B and relative abundance of SP-A and SP-D, two highly hydrophilic surfactant proteins. This difference may indicate a different function for auditory tube surfactant, namely, acting as a release agent and antiadhesive rather than a surface tension–modifying substance. Antiadhesive properties would facilitate opening of the auditory tube.

Surfactant proteins are collectins that have two domains: (1) a lectin moiety that binds to the surface of foreign substances and organisms and (2) a collagenous domain that functions as a ligand for phagocytosis and complement activation (see Chapters 3, 4, and 5). Finally, surfactant is believed to play a protective role against free radicals by early termination of free radical propagation and protecting against oxidative injury. A lipid-binding pocket in surfactant proteins may prevent free radicals from propagating.

Auditory Tube–Associated Lymphoid Tissue (ATALT)

Dorsal to the opening of the auditory tube is an aggregate of lymphoid tissue. In human beings, horses, and rodents, this aggregate is referred to as the *tubal tonsil*. Previous reports determined that dogs and cats do not have distinct tubal tonsils. Lymphoid tissue in the nasopharynx may proliferate and become locally prominent in response to inflammation or infection.

Commensal Microorganisms

Resident microflora in the middle ear are similar to microbes found in the nasopharynx and the external ear. They include aerobic and anaerobic bacteria and yeast in small numbers. *Staphylococcus* spp., *Streptococcus* spp., *E. coli*, *Branhamella* spp., *Bordetella bronchiseptica*, *Enterococcus* spp., and *Bacillus* spp. have been isolated from the middle ear of normal dogs. *Clostridium perfringens* has also been isolated from tympanic cavities of normal dogs.

Internal Ear

Petrous Portion of the Temporal Bone

Referred to as the hardest bone in the body, the petrous portion of the temporal bone is the bony labyrinth that encases and protects the membranous labyrinth held within. The thick and extremely dense bone ensures maximal protection to the sensory portions of the internal ear. In addition, its dorsomedial location in the body deep to the external acoustic meatus provides one of the most protected sites in the body.

Acoustic Reflex

Reflexive contraction of the tensor tympani and stapedius muscles in response to loud and injurious noise functions to protect the delicate sensory portions of the internal ear by dampening sound conductance. Contraction of the tensor tympani pulls the malleus rostrally and applies tension to the tympanic membrane. The stapedius muscle applies tension to the stapes in a dorsocaudal direction relative to the tensor tympani muscle, parallel to the long axis of the vestibular window and perpendicular to the direction the stapes oscillates in the vestibular window.

Disorders of Domestic Animals

Developmental Anomalies of the External Ear

Auricular Agenesis/Aplasia

Auricular agenesis/aplasia (also known as anotia) has been reported in sheep, cattle, and a dog. Auricular hillocks or ridges of the first and second branchial (pharyngeal) arches, which normally interact to form the auricle and the first groove or cleft that normally forms between the two arches, which becomes the external acoustic meatus, fail to interact properly during embryologic development. This failure to develop normally results in anotia and a lack of an external acoustic meatus. It can manifest as a unilateral or bilateral lesion. In sheep, auricular agenesis has been associated with deafness, as well as other congenital anomalies.

Auricular Hypoplasia

Auricular hypoplasia (also known as microtia) is a normal feature of certain animal breeds. Auricles are what distinguish the La Mancha from other goat breeds. Ear length in goats is inherited as an incompletely dominant trait. Two auricular phenotypes exist in the La Mancha breed: "gopher ears" and "elf ears." Goats with gopher ears have microtic ears that possess little or no auricular cartilage and either fold dorsally or ventrally. La Mancha goats with elf ears have microtic auricles that are larger than gopher ears, up to 5 cm in length with folded, distorted auricular cartilage (Fig. 20-27, A) that either folds upward or downward.

Scottish fold cats have slightly microtic ears with a characteristic forward or rostrally folded auricular cartilage. Cats with this simple autosomal dominant inherited trait have unaffected auricles at birth, but the fold of the auricle begins to develop at 3 to 4 weeks of age. Defective cartilage is believed to be the primary problem in these cats, whereby the auricular cartilage either develops abnormally or lacks resiliency, succumbing to gravitational forces. Presumably, present-day Scottish fold cats are descendants of a single Scottish female cat that had a spontaneous mutation of the folded ear allele (Fd). It is believed that all Scottish fold cats with the folded-ear phenotype have mild (heterozygous) or severe (homozygous) forms of osteochondrodysplasia of their distal limbs and tails. The mode of inheritance for this skeletal abnormality is also believed to be incomplete dominant.

Unilateral microtia was first reported in a 1950s report involving six slaughter-age pigs in Denmark. Affected auricles were one-third

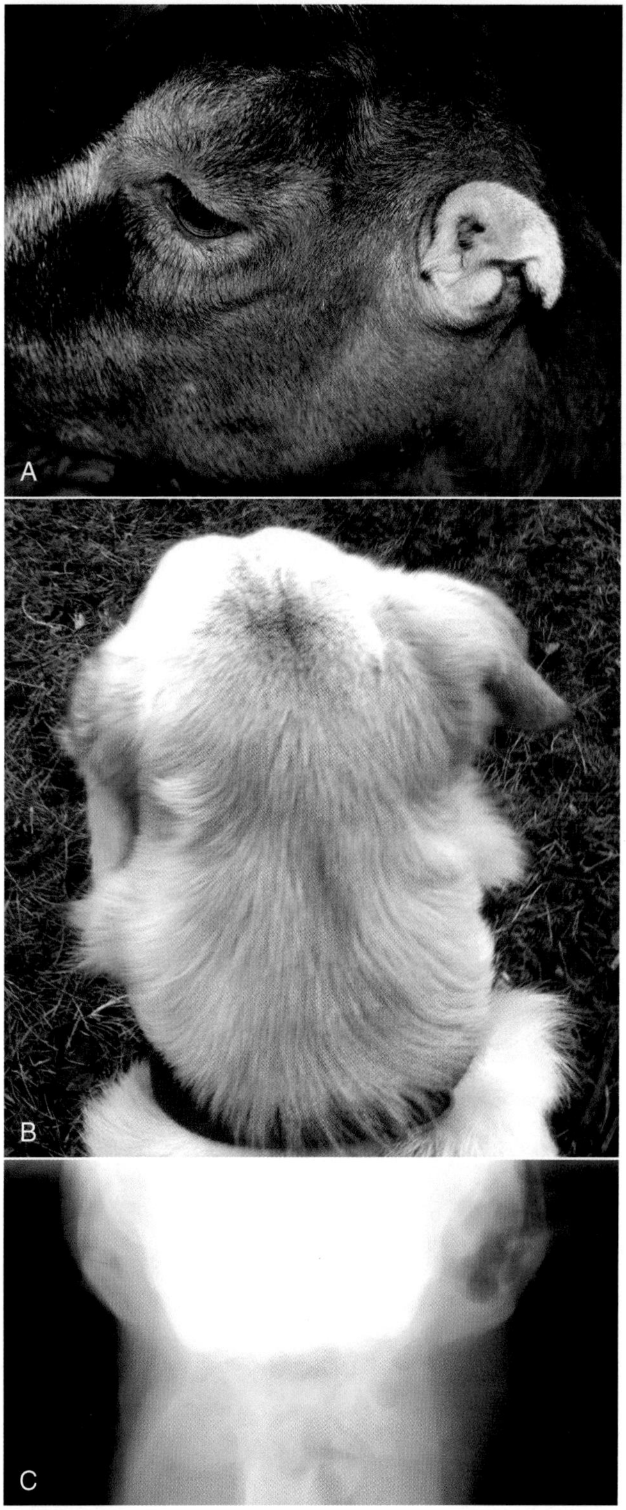

Figure 20-27 **Microtic and Distorted Ears, Goat and Dog. A,** La Mancha doe. Elf ears are one of two breed-standard auricle phenotypes accepted for La Mancha goat registry. **B,** Labrador retriever dog. The left auricle is smaller than the right and has always been. The dog is deaf as a result of impaired development of the ear. **C,** Radiograph of the same dog as in **B**. The left external acoustic meatus, middle ear, and bulla are very small and underdeveloped when compared to the right side. (**A** courtesy Dr. M. Smith, College of Veterinary Medicine, Cornell University. **B** and **C** courtesy Dr. T. Lykins, Pet Pro, and Ms. T. Maxey, owner.)

their normal size, and there was atresia of both the bony and cartilaginous portions of the external meatus. In addition, the tympanic cavity was poorly developed with complete absence of tympanic membranes and auditory ossicles. Specimens were never examined histologically. Other species, such as dogs, may be affected sporadically (see Fig. 20-27, *B*).

Auricular Agenesis/Aplasia

Preauricular malformations (tags, cysts, pits, fissures, and sinuses) are a group of developmentally related disorders of soft tissues that occur rostral to the auricle (E-Fig. 20-2). Preauricular tags are pedunculated outgrowths of skin that contain no bony, cartilaginous, or cystic components and do not communicate with the external or middle ear. The remaining malformations often have an opening rostral to the auricle that is contiguous with a sinus tract that travels under the skin following alongside the cartilage of the external acoustic meatus. These latter malformations are lined by squamous epithelial cells, which may lead to the formation of cysts filled with squamous cell debris or, if infected with microorganisms, can result in abscesses and, with rupture, fasciitis (cellulitis).

Preauricular malformations should be differentiated from branchial cysts that arise developmentally from the first branchial cleft. Cleft malformations are closely linked with other structures that may develop normally from the clefts and arches such as the external acoustic meatus, tympanic membrane, and facial nerve. Animals with preauricular or cleft malformations should be examined for congenital anomalies affecting other organ systems.

Cropped or Notched Ears

Cropped or notched ears was a deformity identified in a group of Highland cattle, affecting 45 of 46 progeny from one breeding sire. The inheritance was determined to be incomplete dominance of a single autosomal gene. Other auricular anomalies that have been reported, primarily in sheep, include polyotia (presence of more than one auricle), macrotia (enlarged auricles), synotia (fusion of auricles), and misplaced auricles (heterotopic otia). A single case report of a Friesian cross calf with epitheliogenesis imperfecta had one ear deformed from rolling of its lateral margins followed by fusion of the surfaces after being brought into close proximity.

Atresia of the External Acoustic Meatus

The external acoustic meatus is normally patent with a very narrow opening for the first few days of life in altricial animals but is more broadly patent at birth in precocial animals.[3] For example, beyond this initial neonatal period, atresia of the external acoustic meatus is reported as congenital or secondary to trauma (Fig. 20-28). When congenital, it occurs in animals as a lone defect or with other congenital abnormalities such as anotia, microtia, middle ear hypoplasia, auditory ossicular malformation or agenesis, agenesis of ossicular musculature, abnormal positioning of the facial nerve, hydrocephalus, and soft palate hypoplasia. The external acoustic meatus arises from the first branchial cleft or groove and disturbances of its embryonic development result in congenital atresia. Atresia has been described in all species typically covered in this text.

[3]Altricial refers to animals that are helpless at birth and require greater parental care (i.e., puppies, kittens). Precocial refers to animals that are active very shortly after birth (i.e., calves, lambs, kids, foals, and piglets).

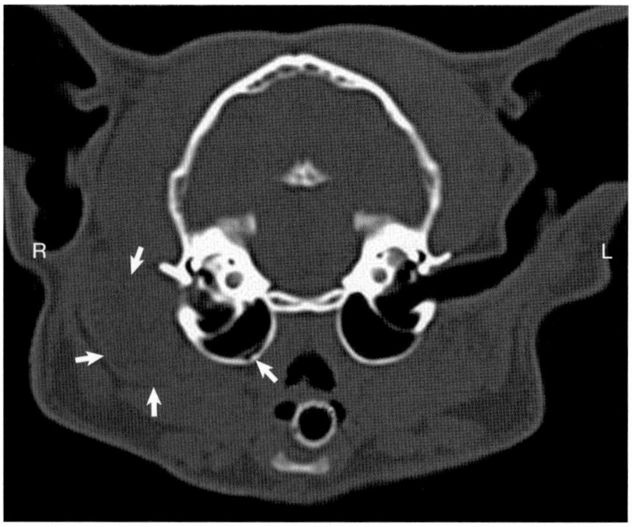

Figure 20-28 **Congenital, Unilateral External Acoustic Meatus Atresia, Right Ear, Cat.** Axial computed tomography scan of the head of the cat demonstrating replacement of the right horizontal canal by a hypodense round, well-marginated fluid-attenuating material located immediately lateral to the right tympanic bulla, outlined by the solid white arrows. The white arrows illustrate the soft-tissue material accumulating in the dependent portion of the bulla. *L*, Left side; *R*, right side. (With permission of *J Feline Med Surg* 11:864-868, 2009.)

Stenosis of the External Acoustic Meatus (Congenital Hypothyroidism)

Stenotic external acoustic meatuses can occur in toy fox terriers that develop goiter caused by a fully penetrant, autosomal recessive nonsense mutation of the thyroid peroxidase gene resulting in dyshormonogenesis and congenital hypothyroidism. Clinically, puppies are lethargic, do not walk, and are able to hear normally.

A congenital hypothyroidism and dysmaturity syndrome with multiple congenital musculoskeletal abnormalities has been described in foals in western Canada. In addition to tendon laxity and bony changes, some foals have floppy ears that likely are caused by congenital defects in the formation of auricular cartilage. External acoustic meatus, middle ear, or internal ear abnormalities have never been investigated in foals affected by this syndrome.

Otognathia

Otognathia, a rudimentary accessory mouth found at the base of the pinna, is an unusual condition reported in sheep and cattle. This accessory orifice is either blind or contiguous with the pharynx, lined by a mucous membrane, and may contain rudimentary teeth, mandible-like bones, and lateral extensions of the tongue. Both unilateral and bilateral otognathia have been reported. Embryologically, the first branchial pouch (endodermal origin) makes contact with the first branchial cleft (ectodermal origin), eventually thinning to form a membrane, which normally becomes the tympanic membrane. In otognathia, during development, this membrane between the developing first pharyngeal cleft and first pharyngeal pouch ruptures and forms persistent fistulae. Dentigerous cysts, most commonly reported in horses and described later, may have a similar embryologic origin.

Inflammation of the External Ear

Otitis Externa

Otitis externa is rarely a primary condition but arises from the interaction of predisposing factors, primary causes, and secondary causes (see Table 20-1). Predisposing factors, such as conformation, auricular phenotype, breed, and external ear moisture, act as inherent risk factors for the development of otitis externa but are not directly causative. Primary causes, such as ectoparasites, keratinization defects, foreign bodies, hypersensitivity reactions, and systemic immune-mediated disorders that affect the integument, may initiate inflammation of the external acoustic meatus. Secondary factors, such as bacterial and fungal infections, tend to intensify the inflammatory reaction and subsequent severity of otitis externa.

Dogs are most severely affected and therefore examined the most. The most common primary causes include atopic dermatitis, adverse food reactions, ectoparasites, and foreign bodies. It is estimated that the prevalence range of otitis externa in dogs is 15% to 20.4%, which is much higher than the estimated prevalence of 4% in cats. Long-standing chronic external ear infections that have excessive healing responses with extensive fibrosis, cartilage remodeling, and para-auricular osseous metaplasia can make an eventual return to normal structure and function difficult or nearly impossible.

Macroscopically, otitis externa may include discharge from the ear (also known as otorrhea), hemorrhage from the ear (also known as otorrhagia), and pain elicited when palpating the ear (also known as otodynia or otalgia). The auricles tend to be red, warm, and edematous (see Fig. 17-15) due to increased congestion of dermal blood vessels (Fig. 20-29). With chronicity the epidermis may become thickened and bosselated, as well as hyperpigmented. The normally pliable auricular cartilage may be modified by fibrosis or osseous metaplasia and become stiffer. The most severely affected ears may develop acquired stenosis of the external acoustic meatus. This feature is an important perpetuating factor that promotes recurrent episodes of otitis externa and prevents satisfactory resolution.

Microscopically, many of the changes have already been discussed. The dermis thickens initially because of edema followed by exudation and infiltration by inflammatory cells. Initially, neutrophils predominate, but later, with more chronic inflammation, macrophages are prominent, mixed with lymphocytes and plasma cells. The formation of multiple lymphoid aggregates is not uncommon (see Fig. 20-25). The adnexa transforms from an initially dominant sebaceous gland population to an overabundance of ceruminous glands that tend to be large, ectatic, and infiltrated by inflammatory cells. The overlying epidermis is typically both hyperplastic and hyperkeratotic, although it may be multifocally eroded or ulcerated in acute episodes. All of this thickening leads to a reduction in the luminal diameter of the external acoustic meatus.

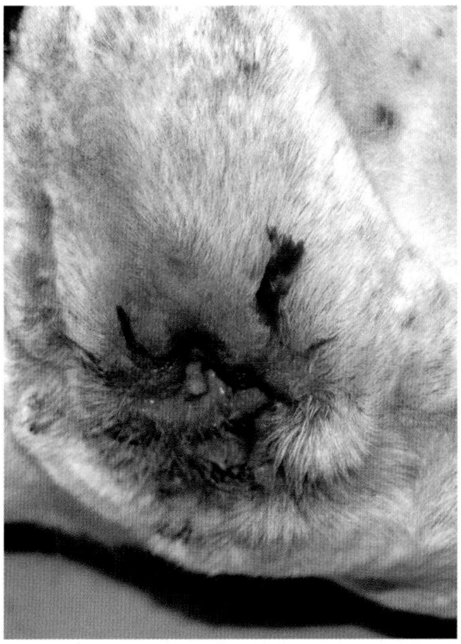

Figure 20-29 Otitis Externa, Dog. The auricle is thickened, reddened, and painful (otalgia) with obvious otorrhea and presumed otomiasma. (Courtesy Dr. W.H. Miller, College of Veterinary Medicine, Cornell University.)

In chronically affected ears, thick bands of dense fibrous connective tissue replace dermal adnexa. The lack of ceruminous and sebaceous glands results in a lack of cerumen production. Without this natural, typically hydrophobic barrier, the epidermal surface is perpetually hyperplastic and hyperkeratotic. The reduced hydrophobicity results in an increased amount of moisture, superficially resulting in more intercellular edema (see Fig. 17-15) of the epidermis. Cartilage may undergo metaplastic change, resulting in the formation of cartilaginous nodules, or more commonly undergo osseous metaplasia. The net effect is a permanent, severe reduction in the luminal diameter of the external acoustic meatus.

Clinically, affected animals have an increased tendency to scratch their ears or shake their heads incessantly. Otitis externa is frequently associated with a malodorous aural discharge or otomiasma (alternatively, miasmic otorrhea).[4] In general, animals have a reluctance to allow examination of affected ears. For those animals that are chronically affected, signs of middle and internal ear disease may develop.

Vascular Injury of the External Ear

Infarction

Vascular injury to the auricle occurs in all domestic animal species and results in responses ranging from ear tip necrosis to sloughing of the entire auricle. Various causes, such as bacterial septicemia, immune-mediated vasculitis, frostbite, and toxins, injure and activate endothelium, platelets, and clotting cascades, often resulting in vascular thrombosis. In pigs, septicemic salmonellosis and its endotoxins can injure vascular endothelium, leading to thrombosis of small vessels and tissue infarction of the ear tip and tail (see Chapter 2 for mechanistic details). Ears initially are dark red to purple-black and painful and then become dry (dry gangrene) and scabbed and eventually slough. In cats with feline infectious peritonitis (FIP), hypothesized in German shepherd dogs with familial vasculopathy (autosomal recessive inheritance pattern), and in drug reactions, especially vaccine reactions, immune complex–mediated vasculitis (type III hypersensitivity) has the potential to cause systemic or cutaneous vasculitides of extremities such as the ears, tails, and potentially feet. Severe drops in ambient temperature in newborn animals or animals that are poorly sheltered can result in frostbite. In these cases, blood is shunted away from the extremities to preserve the core body temperature, and the poorly perfused extremities, such as ears, tails, feet, and nose, are compromised. Affected tissues demonstrate a clear line of demarcation between tissue that has died or has become infarcted as the result of inadequate circulation and the tissue that retained adequate circulation. The dead tissue darkens, is cool to the touch, and becomes dry from dry gangrene (Fig. 20-30). Ingested preformed toxins, such as ergot alkaloids, cause vasoconstriction leading to vascular compromise, infarction, and sloughing of extremities.

[4]*Otomiasma* is a proposed term for foul-smelling otorrhea, derived from two root words: *oto* for ear and *miasma* for noxious odors from putrid organic matter.

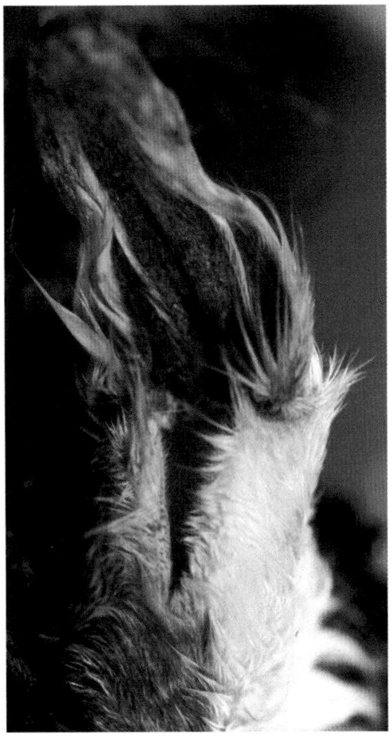

Figure 20-30 Auricular Infarction, Frostbite, Goat. Note that the distal (upper) half of the ear has dry gangrene from frostbite. (Courtesy Dr. B.L. Njaa, Center for Veterinary Health Sciences, Oklahoma State University.)

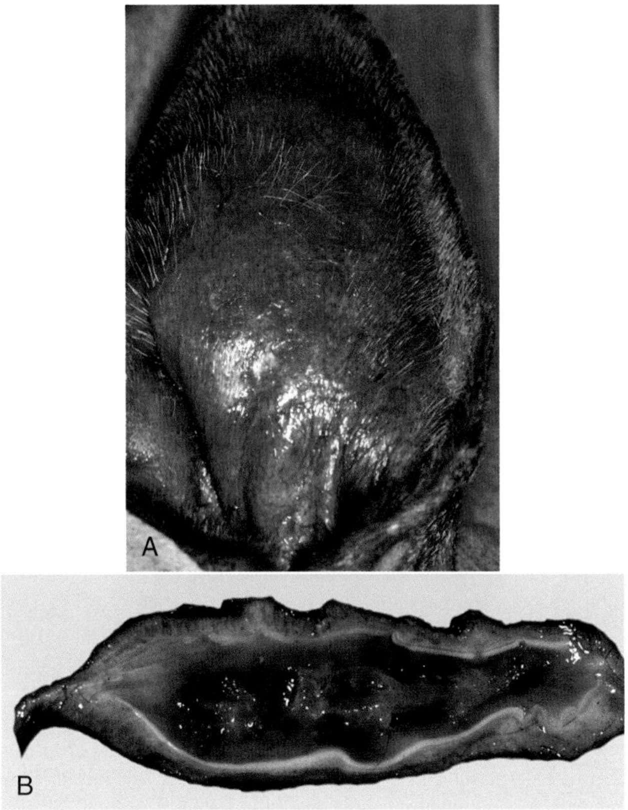

Figure 20-31 Aural Hematoma, Dog. A, Left auricle. The concave aural surface has become convex due to expansion of the underlying connective tissue by mixtures of blood and fibrin. **B,** Auricle, cross section. Portions of the auricular cartilage are present on both sides of the cavity. Within the cavity are abundant strands of lighter, eosinophilic fibrin strands mixed with thicker, larger dark red blood clots. (**A** courtesy Dr. M.C. Rochat, Center for Veterinary Health Sciences, Oklahoma State University. **B** courtesy Dr. D.D. Harrington, School of Veterinary Medicine, Purdue University; and Noah's Arkive, College of Veterinary Medicine, The University of Georgia.)

Hematomas

Animals with chronic external or middle ear disease often respond clinically to discomfort by continuously and vigorously shaking their heads. This action applies severe centrifugal shearing forces (trauma) to blood vessels and auricular cartilage at the sides and tips of the auricles. Auricular cartilage is a single plate of elastic cartilage normally containing perforations through which blood vessels pass between the convex and concave surfaces of the pinnae. Repeated trauma results in fractures of auricular cartilage, most likely at these areas of perforation. Presumably, the sharp edges of the fracture cartilage and the shearing forces lead to laceration of associated blood vessels. Hemorrhage from these ruptured auricular blood vessels is the genesis of aural hematomas with blood collecting either intrachondrially or subparachondrially.

Aural hematomas are most common in dogs, pigs, and cats but have been reported in sheep, goats, a cow, and a foal. Affected auricles are markedly swollen, most obvious on the concave surface, and are warm, hyperemic, painful, heavy, and tend to droop (Fig. 20-31, *A*). Large-breed dogs, in particular golden retrievers and Labrador retrievers, and middle-aged to older dogs with ear disease are prone to develop aural hematomas. If untreated, hematomas eventually heal by fibrosis, resulting in a very firm to hard, thickened, and permanently malformed auricle. When opened, the cavity that forms is filled with clotted blood and a meshwork of fibrin (see Fig. 20-31, *B*). Microscopic changes typically include cartilage fractures and splitting, cartilage erosion, granulation tissue, and hemorrhage.

Parasitic Diseases of the External Ear

Numerous ectoparasites parasitize or infest domestic and wild animals, including mites, ticks, and nematodes (E-Table 20-1). Most affect their hosts by infesting various parts of the integumentary system (see Chapter 17). A small proportion of these organisms preferentially infest the ear. Reactions vary from minimal irritation to gross deformity. External ear infections may be isolated or extend to the middle and internal ears. The clinical signs are prototypic, including head shaking, repeated ear twitching, excessive ear itching, and traumatization of the auricle and base of the ear.

Ear Mite Infestations (Otoacariasis)

Mites are categorized as burrowing or nonburrowing. Many species, such as *Sarcoptes* spp. (see Fig. 17-54) and *Demodex* spp., can cause more generalized lesions with possible involvement of the ear. However, there are few mites that spend much or all of their life cycle within the concave portion of the auricle or in the external acoustic meatus.

Otodectes Cynotis. *Otodectes cynotis* infests the external acoustic meatus of domestic and wild cats, dogs, and occasionally ruminants. The main route of infestation is from dam to offspring. Other routes of spread include contaminated combs, brushes, bedding, or other grooming accessories. They are nonburrowing and feed on the cerumen, keratin, and lipids. These mites are a prominent primary cause of otitis externa with up to 50% of cats and 10% of dogs developing otitis externa. They cause intense irritation by mechanisms not well understood. Copious cerumen production ensues until a thick, waxy, dark brown otorrhea (exudate) obstructs the external acoustic meatus. Auricles are often alopecic and have "scratching" wounds from trauma that form in response to intense pruritus. These areas may also become infected secondarily with bacteria. The epidermis becomes acanthotic with parakeratotic hyperkeratosis and crusts that contain mites and mite detritus mixed with cerumen. Small to moderate numbers of lymphocytes and macrophages infiltrate the dermis and subcutis. Ceruminous glands are typically hypertrophied and hyperplastic and may contain cellular debris and neutrophils.

Although a majority of cats are infested, a minority manifest clinical disease, possibly owing to early exposure as kittens and the development of Arthus- and immediate-type hypersensitivity reactions.

Notoedres Cati. *Notoedres cati* is primarily a cat pathogen but can infest dogs, foxes, rabbits, and rarely human beings. Usually infestations are restricted to the auricles, head, face, neck, and shoulders. Infestation produces alopecia, pruritus, thick crusting, and excoriation of the rostral pinnae as the female mite burrows in the stratum corneum and occasionally penetrates hair follicles and sebaceous glands. Microscopic lesions include epidermal hyperplasia and spongiosis with perivascular eosinophilic dermatitis and crusting.

***Raillietia* Species.** *Raillietia* spp. of mites occur most commonly in cattle, buffalo, and goats of nearly every continent. Cattle are most commonly parasitized by *Raillietia auris*, whereas the mite infesting goat ears is *Raillietia caprae*. *Raillietia flechtmanni* is found in buffalo and cattle ears. These mites often go undetected because of their small size and their tendency to reside deep in the external acoustic meatus adjacent to the tympanic membrane, and they do not commonly cause clinical disease. When clinically apparent, there is often a thick plug of cerumen and debris, with variable suppuration, behind which the mites reside. Additionally, the external acoustic meatus may be ulcerated. Affected animals rarely may develop central nervous system signs related to heavy infestations that penetrate the middle and internal ear. Otitis externa is more severe with concurrent bacterial infections or if the host is additionally infected with *Rhabditis* spp. of nematodes. In goats there are often concurrent infections with *R. caprae* and pathogenic *Mycoplasma* spp.

***Psoroptes cuniculi*.** Psoroptic otoacariasis is most commonly caused by *Psoroptes cuniculi*, infesting sheep, goats, deer, horses, donkeys, mules, and antelope. Although capable of feeding on any part of the animal, it prefers the ear in goats, sheep, and horses. They live on the surface, feeding on lipids, keratin, crusts, and cerumen. Pruritus can be intense and is related to surface irritation by infesting mites and hypersensitivity reactions, leading to self-trauma to the auricle and periauricular skin. As described (see Chapter 17), histologic lesions include eosinophilic perivascular dermatitis that can be spongiotic, hyperplastic, hyperkeratotic, or exudative. In affected goats, care must be taken to check that the infestation is not complicated by *Raillietia* spp.

Ticks

Ticks and tick-borne diseases rank as some of the most important health constraints of livestock in many parts of the world. Ticks serve as vectors for the spread of disease, affect production parameters such as weight gain or milk production, can lead to significant anemia, may impair individual or herd immunity, and can be a source of aggravation or irritation. Sites of attachment and feeding may occur in multiple locations, but many species of ticks have preferred sites. What follows is a discussion of a few species of ticks that preferentially feed in the ears.

***Rhipicephalus* Species.** The brown ear tick, *Rhipicephalus appendiculatus*, is found most commonly in southern and southeastern African countries. Adults primarily attach to the ears of domestic and wild ruminants, whereas larvae and nymphs attach to ears, head, and neck of most ruminant species, as well as equids, carnivores, and hares. *Bos indicus* cattle become fairly resistant to tick infestations, but exotic *Bos taurus* cattle can have severe production losses and very significant ear damage. *R. appendiculatus* secretes proteins in its saliva, some of which react with the host animal enzymes to form a hard feeding cone and others have inherent enzymatic activity. The protein that forms the cone is called *cement*, and it provides an anchor for feeding ticks and may interfere with a robust inflammatory reaction by the host animal. Affected ears can range from minimally injured to very deformed and sometimes can appear shredded. Microscopically, at the feeding sites, neutrophils predominate in the dermis immediately surrounding the brightly eosinophilic cement layer and are also mixed with macrophages and variable numbers of eosinophils. Brown ear tick toxicosis is a poorly understood condition that occurs in susceptible cattle, presumably the result of tick saliva toxins. Some saliva-derived toxins have an immunosuppressive effect, although the exact mechanism is not understood. These animals may have suppression of adaptive immune responses and lose protection against other environmental pathogens that they have encountered and resisted. In some instances, tick toxicosis can be fatal.

Gulf Coast Ear Tick. Another tick that preferentially infests the ear is variably named the Gulf coast tick or Gulf coast ear tick. *Amblyomma maculatum* is native to North, Central, and South America. In North America, this tick can be found all along the Gulf coast, extending as far inland as Oklahoma, Kansas, and Arkansas, and along the southern Atlantic coast. Adult ticks preferentially feed on cattle, sheep, horses, and mules by attaching to the external ears but can also infest deer, cats, foxes, dogs, and pigs. Heavy infestations cause intense auricular inflammation and swelling and may even cause the destruction of the auricular cartilage, resulting in a droopy ear sometimes referred to as "gotch ear"[5] (Fig. 20-32). *A. maculatum* is an experimental vector for transmitting *Ehrlichia ruminantium*, the causative agent for heartwater disease, but it has not been implicated in field outbreaks in North America. It has also been shown that the Gulf coast ear tick in Florida, Georgia, Kentucky, Mississippi, Oklahoma, and South Carolina may serve as a reservoir for *Rickettsia parkeri*.

Spinose Ear Tick. *Otobius megnini*, the "spinose ear tick," has a broad host range, including ungulates, sheep, goats, cattle, horses, dogs, and human beings. Adults are free living and nonparasitic, but nymph and larval stages are parasitic. Newly hatched larvae remain in the environment until they climb onto a suitable host. Owing to their small size and propensity for living very deep in the external acoustic meatus, larvae are rarely identified in host ears. As these ticks molt and mature, some can be found attached to and blood feeding in the more shallow portions of the external acoustic meatus or attached to the auricular skin (Fig. 20-33). After several months of feeding in or on host ears, nymphs drop off the host, seeking dry, sheltered places where they molt into adults. Lesions are attributable to blood feeding, which results in local irritation and secondary otitis externa. As has already been described, local reactions to the

[5]"Gotch ear" is a colloquial term with Spanish roots coined by cowboys and defined as a type of earmark used to identify cattle that resulted in severe rostral, medial, and ventral flexion of the auricle.

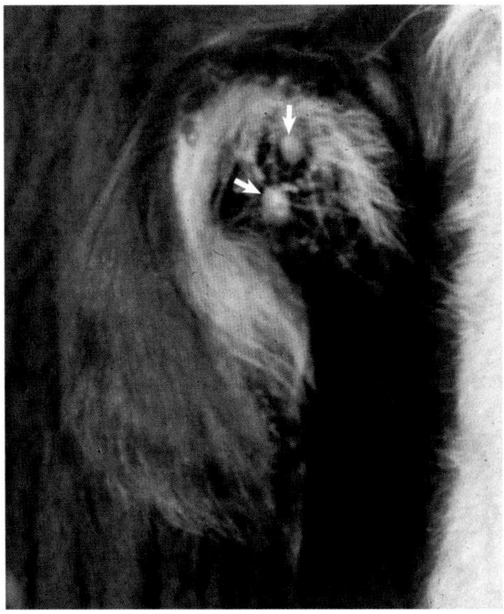

Figure 20-32 **Gotch Ear, Bovine.** The right ear of a Hereford cow is severely deformed because of infestation by numerous Gulf coast ear ticks, *Amblyomma maculatum*. The bodies of several ticks *(arrows)* are attached to the concave surface of the medially, ventrally, and rostrally deviated auricle. (Courtesy Dr. J.A. Hair, Oklahoma State University.)

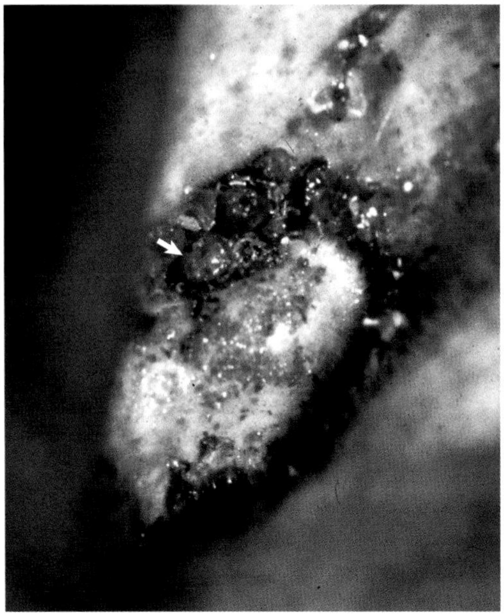

Figure 20-33 **Spinose Ear Tick, Bovine.** Deep within the concave surface of the auricle are numerous *Otobius megnini*, or spinose ear ticks *(arrow)*. Associated with these ticks is an increased amount of brown ceruminous exudate. (Courtesy Dr. J.A. Hair, Oklahoma State University.)

feeding sites include perivascular to interstitial dermatitis laden with neutrophils and eosinophils. Infested animals may develop clinical symptoms such as head shaking and pruritus related to nymph feeding on blood and lymph of the skin of the external acoustic meatus.

Bacterial Diseases of the External Ear

Dermatophilosis (Streptothrichosis)

Dermatophilosis (also known as streptothrichosis) is caused by *Dermatophilus congolensis* and is a zoonotic bacterium of the skin and

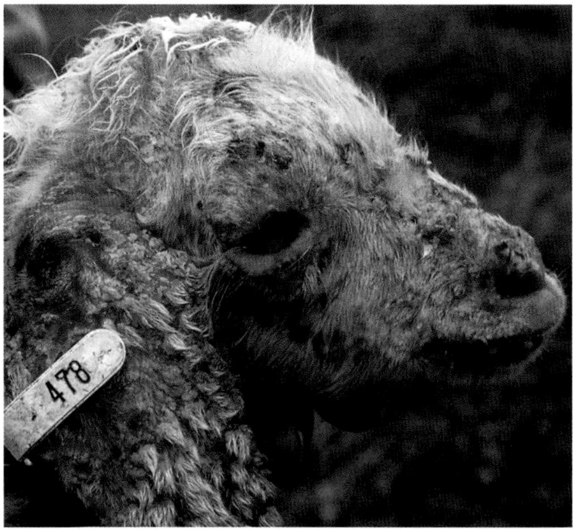

Figure 20-34 **Cutaneous Dermatophilosis, Goat.** The auricular skin, as well as skin of the muzzle, face, and periocular region, is matted from a severely exudative dermatitis caused by *Dermatophilus congolensis*. (Courtesy Dr. K.G. Thompson, Institute of Veterinary, Animal, and Biomedical Science, Massey University.)

mucosae of the nose, commissures of the lips, distal or proximal limbs, and ears but may proliferate virtually anywhere on the body. The bacterium prefers moist areas and requires the integrity (i.e., barrier) of the skin to be impaired. Thus damaged skin with scabs and crusts on the face and ears are sites of colonization by *D. congolensis* in younger animals. *D. congolensis* is transferred during nursing from damp and traumatized skin of the inguinal region of lactating dams to the ears of nursing kids (Fig. 20-34). Colonization begins by invasion of flagellated zoospores that penetrate the epidermis and reach the level of the basement membrane, in which they transform to a filamentous structure. They also penetrate into the dermis and follicular adnexa, inciting a prominent neutrophilic response. This acute inflammation halts further invasion. However, residual bacteria colonies are able to invade nascent, regenerated epidermis. This cycle of bacterial growth, inflammation, and epidermal regeneration leads to the multilaminated pustular crusts so typical of dermatophilosis. Damage to the cutaneous barrier system can also be caused by other invasive bacteria, fungi, or ectoparasites such as mites and ticks. Macroscopically, lesions are characterized by a crusting and exudative dermatitis (see Chapter 17) with thick crusts covering an epidermis that is ulcerated and hemorrhagic. Microscopically, crusts are made of alternating layers of markedly parakeratotic hyperkeratosis, degenerate neutrophils, and coagulative necrosis, all laden with *D. congolensis*. It can be identified by its filamentous structure with longitudinal and transverse septa (see Fig. 17-48).

Neoplasms of the External Ear

Most frequently, aural neoplasia is a unilateral disease; bilateral involvement is rare. Sebaceous gland tumors, histiocytomas, plasmacytomas, and mast cell tumors (see Chapter 6) are the most common types of aural neoplasms in dogs. Sebaceous gland tumors are most often benign, but diagnoses of aural masses resembling sebaceous glands include sebaceous gland hyperplasia, sebaceous adenoma, sebaceous epithelioma, and rarely sebaceous adenocarcinoma. Differentiating between histiocytomas, plasmacytomas, and mast cell tumors requires a surgical biopsy (see Chapters 6 and 17) and histologic examination.

In cats, trichoblastomas, vascular tumors, and squamous cell carcinomas are the most common types of aural neoplasms. Vascular neoplasms and squamous cell carcinomas arise on lightly pigmented pinnae of outdoor cats exposed to the sun for prolonged periods of time as a result of UVB light–induced neoplastic transformation (see Chapter 6). With squamous cell carcinomas the margins at the base and tips of the ears are most often affected (Fig. 20-35; also see E-Table 17-6). However, they can also arise within the external acoustic meatus and the tympanic cavity and bulla. Macroscopically, they are raised, ulcerated, and hemorrhagic neoplasms. Growth is often a combination of local stromal invasion and concurrent vascular invasion with metastasis via regional lymphatic vessels. Initially these tumors can be misdiagnosed as exudative dermatitic lesions.

Neoplasms of the external acoustic meatus in the dog or cat are infrequently diagnosed, but the most common types include ceruminous gland tumors, sebaceous tumors, and epithelial neoplasms of undetermined origin. In fact, the majority (85%) of feline aural neoplasms are malignant compared to 60% of canine aural neoplasms being malignant. Of these, ceruminous gland adenocarcinomas are the most common neoplasm diagnosed in the external acoustic meatus of both dogs and cats. Typically, middle-aged to older animals are affected.

Canine ceruminous gland hyperplasia and ceruminous gland adenomas can be difficult to differentiate. Adenomas are single to multiple, small, pedunculate, irregular, and firm masses. These masses may develop secondarily to recurrent bouts of chronic otitis externa, or their growth may obstruct the external acoustic meatus and result in secondary otitis externa. It was speculated years ago that ceruminous gland hyperplasia and adenomas preceded the development of malignant ceruminous gland tumors, but this conjecture has never been fully substantiated. Ceruminous gland adenocarcinomas tend to be locally invasive and expansile.

By contrast, ceruminous gland adenocarcinomas are more frequently diagnosed in cats than adenomas and account for up to 2% of all feline neoplasms (Fig. 20-36, *A*). Ceruminous gland tumors diagnosed in dogs also tend to be more commonly malignant. They tend to be locally invasive, and up to 50% are reported to metastasize to regional lymph nodes, lungs, or systemic viscera. There is a greater tendency for adenocarcinomas to be diagnosed in aged male cats.

These neoplasms are readily capable of growing between overlapping areas of auricular cartilage extending into the periauricular dermis and subcutis (see Fig. 20-36, *B*). Histologically, the neoplastic cells tend to form acini, small ducts, irregular tubular structures, or small clusters (see Fig. 20-36, *C*). Neoplastic cells are typically basaloid to low columnar with intensely basophilic cytoplasm. The sizes of nuclei and cells are variable, but neoplastic cells may be quite uniform. The occurrence and number of mitotic figures are highly variable. There tends to be a very prominent desmoplastic response to the surrounding tissue. Large areas of necrosis are not uncommon.

Mixed ceruminous gland tumors are rarely observed in dogs. Because ceruminous glands are modified apocrine gland, they are associated with myoepithelial cells. Uncommonly, ceruminous gland tumors may depict cartilaginous or osseus metaplasia in the proliferative myoepithelial tissue. Mixed ceruminous gland tumors can be benign (adenomas) or malignant (adenocarcinomas).

Miscellaneous Disorders of the External Ear

Pinnal Alopecia

Pinnal alopecia occurs as a congenital disease in cattle or an acquired disease in dogs and cats. In polled Hereford calves, this congenital disease begins at birth as an alopecic disease of the muzzle, auricular margins, and base of the ears. Pedigree analysis suggests this disorder is an inherited disease, but the mode of inheritance remains undetermined. A detailed analysis of this condition consistently found evidence of epidermal maturation and keratinization defects. At birth the hair coat was wiry and tightly curled; it epilated easily. Alopecia and hyperkeratosis became generalized by 3 months of age. Marked

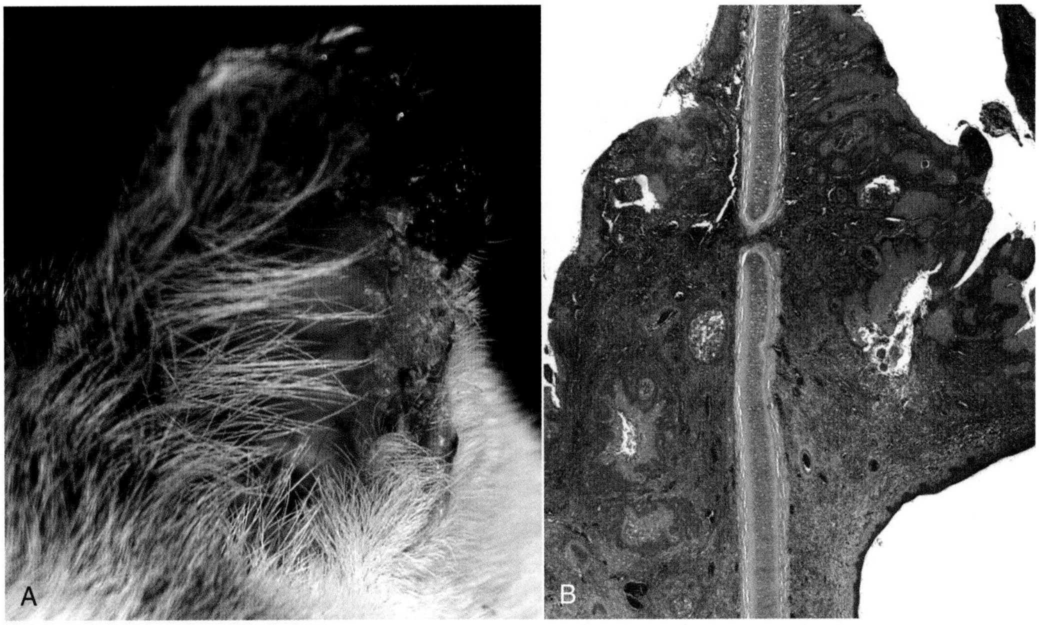

Figure 20-35 **Aural Squamous Cell Carcinoma, Cat. A,** Lateral view. The lateral margin and tip of the left auricle are ulcerated and covered by a serohemorrhagic crust caused by an underlying squamous cell carcinoma. **B,** Histologic section of aural squamous cell carcinoma. Note the cords and islands of anaplastic squamous epithelial cells that have infiltrated the dermis. The tumor may penetrate through the auricular cartilage as it grows. H&E stain. (**A** courtesy Dr. W.H. Miller, College of Veterinary Medicine, Cornell University. **B** courtesy Dr. B.L. Njaa, Center for Veterinary Health Sciences, Oklahoma State University.)

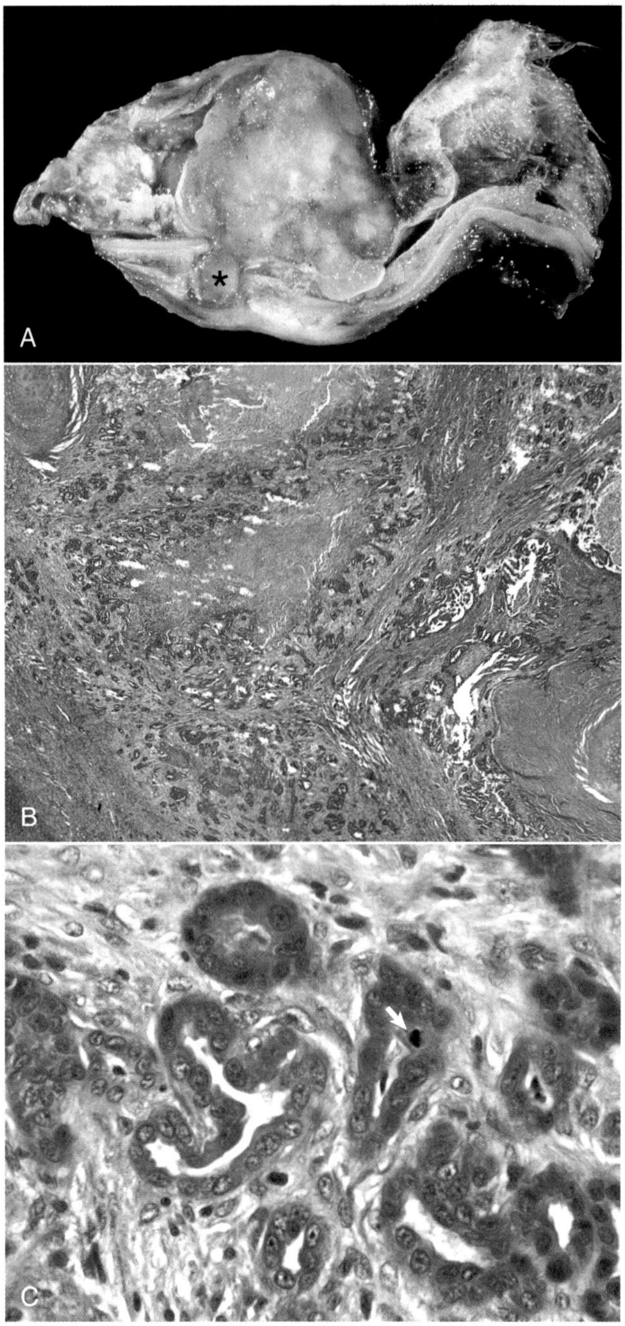

Figure 20-36 Ceruminous Gland Adenocarcinoma. A, Cross section of external acoustic meatus. This ceruminous gland adenocarcinoma fills the external acoustic meatus and expands its luminal diameter. Ventrally there is a small extension of the neoplasm *(asterisk)* either through or between overlapping layers of auricular and annular cartilage. **B,** Histologic section of ceruminous gland carcinoma. Neoplastic ceruminous glands induce a prominent desmoplastic response and are shown invading through the cartilage *(bottom center of image)*. H&E stain. **C,** Higher magnification of **B**. Neoplastic cells are haphazardly arranged and form tubules and acini with evidence of anaplasia and increased mitotic activity *(arrow)*. It is shown growing through the auricular cartilage. H&E stain. (**A** courtesy Dr. W.N. Evering, Pfizer Global Research. **B** and **C** courtesy Dr. B.L. Njaa, Center for Veterinary Health Sciences, Oklahoma State University.)

Box 20-4 Causes of Pinnal Alopecia

Adverse drug reactions
Alopecia areata
Atopy
Canine hypothyroidism
Canine pinnal alopecia
Color dilution alopecia
Congenital anemia, dyskeratosis, and progressive alopecia of polled Herefords
Congenital hypotrichosis
Demodicosis
Dermatophytosis
Epitheliotropic T lymphocyte lymphoma
Estrogen-responsive dermatosis
Feline hypothyroidism
Feline pinnal alopecia
Food allergy
Hyperadrenocorticism
Leishmaniasis
Pattern baldness
Topical steroid–induced alopecia
Vasculitis/ischemic dermatitis

wrinkling of the skin developed over the face and neck as the cattle aged. Microscopically, the density of hair follicles was normal, but a higher proportion of these follicles were in telogen phase. Additionally, there was premature keratinization and degeneration of the internal root sheath of the follicle, sebaceous gland atrophy, and dilated sweat glands that were lined with a thinned epithelium. This process resulted in easy epilation of hair. In older affected calves the hyperkeratotic skin was also inflamed with a mild, superficial, perivascular, lymphocytic perivascular dermatitis. Interestingly, hyperkeratotic lesions also affected the rumen mucosa. Clinically, the anemia was characterized as nonregenerative, normocytic to macrocytic, and normochromic.

Acquired pinnal alopecia occurs primarily in dogs and cats (Box 20-4). The condition in dogs primarily affects dachshunds but has also been reported in Chihuahuas, Boston terriers, whippets, and Italian greyhounds. Siamese cats are more commonly diagnosed with acquired pinnal alopecia that is patchy to complete but unlike the dog spontaneously resolves. In dogs it is often symmetrical, and auricular hair of the convex surface becomes miniaturized. Then gradually over time, auricles become alopecic (Fig. 20-37). Rarely, the auricle becomes completely alopecic; however, the remainder of the body hair coat is typically unaffected. Biopsy results show affected anagen hair follicles that are smaller in diameter or shorter.

Developmental Anomalies of the Middle Ear

Primary Ciliary Dyskinesia (Immotile Cilia Syndrome)

Described most completely in the dog, primary ciliary dyskinesia (also known as immotile cilia syndrome) has also been suspected or confirmed in horses, ruminants, pigs, and cats. Typically, affected animals are under a year of age, have a persistent cough and nasal discharge related to chronic rhinitis, and have chronic recurrent respiratory disease related to impaired or ineffective mucociliary clearance without evidence of immunologic impairment.

In dogs the most common ciliary defects include dynein arm deficiency, abnormal microtubular patterns, random orientation of the microtubules, and electron-dense inclusions in the basal body that anchors the cilium to the cell. In horses the total number of cilia may be decreased, and the vast majority have central microtubule pair defects. The middle ear relies in part on fully functioning

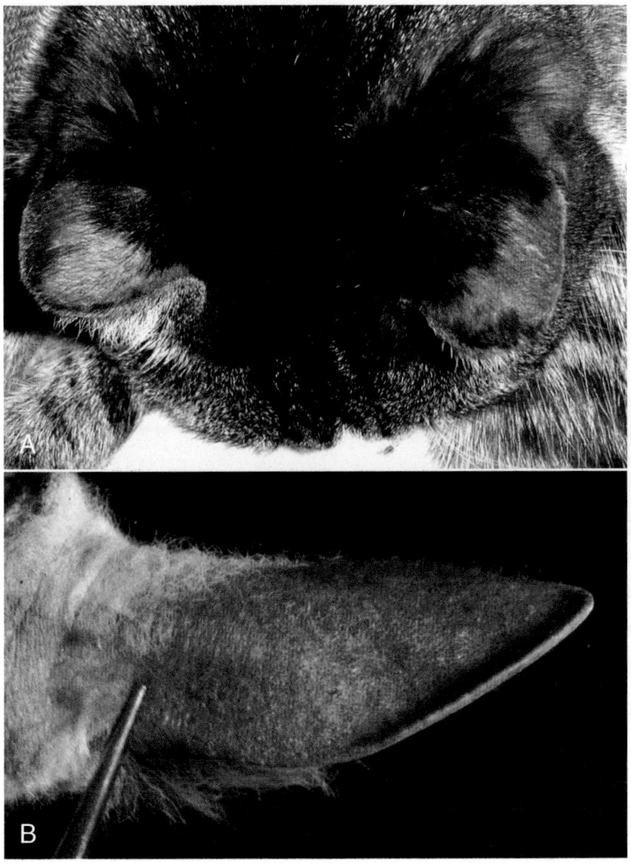

Figure 20-37 **Pinnal Alopecia. A,** Dorsal view, cat. Alopecia is present as bilaterally symmetric lesions most severely affecting the convex surface of the auricles of the distal half of each ear *(light pink areas)*. In the dog this lesion tends to be permanent, whereas in the cat, typically Siamese breeds, this often spontaneously resolves. **B,** Auricle, convex surface, calf. Note the absence of hair on the convex surface of the ear. This case is an example of congenital pinnal alopecia in polled Hereford calves. (**A** courtesy Dr. W.H. Miller, College of Veterinary Medicine, Cornell University. **B** courtesy Drs. W. Crowell and D.E. Tyler, College of Veterinary Medicine, The University of Georgia; and Noah's Arkive, College of Veterinary Medicine, The University of Georgia.)

ciliated epithelial cells and mucus-producing goblet cells for clearance of fluid and debris through the auditory tube. Thus abnormal cilia equates to abnormal auditory tube clearance.

Macroscopic lesions include bilateral mucopurulent rhinitis, sinusitis, and chronic tracheitis. There is frequently unilateral or bilateral otitis media evident with mucopurulent exudate or with sterile, gelatinous material filling the tympanic cavity. Tympanic bullae may be thickened or sclerotic. Microscopically, the tympanic cavity contains proteinaceous material mixed with variable numbers of inflammatory cells, typically neutrophils and macrophages with variable aggregates of lymphocytes and plasma cells.

Clinically, animals present with a chronic cough and persistent nasal discharge, and the symptoms are unresponsive to antibiotics. Typically, middle or internal ear signs are not evident clinically. Frequently animals are neutrophilic, likely caused by persistent secondary bacterial infections of the upper respiratory tract. Affected males are frequently infertile.

Inflammation of the Middle Ear

Otitis Media

Infections of the middle ear affect all domestic animal species but vary in prevalence and which pathogens are isolated. Ruminants and pigs are most severely affected, whereas cats are less commonly affected.

Otitis media in pigs occurs naturally as a result of nasopharyngeal ascent of bacteria through the auditory tubes. *Pasteurella multocida, Trueperella pyogenes*, and *Mycoplasma hyorhinis* are likely pathogens, separately or concurrently, that first colonize the nasopharynx and ascend the auditory tube to gain entry and cause otitis media. Studies of the pathogenesis of otitis media in young piglets suggest that dysfunction of the auditory tube is an initial contributing factor. Dysfunction is linked to acute inflammation, goblet cell hyperplasia of mucoperiosteum, and occasional acute inflammatory exudate of the tympanic cavity. In older pigs, otitis media was more severe and suppurative, and auditory tube lesions were more severe and characterized by interepithelial infiltration by neutrophils, intraluminal exudation of neutrophils and fibrin, marked goblet cell hyperplasia of the mucoperiosteum as well as erosion to ulceration, and infiltration by lymphocytes and macrophages. Bacterial colonies of *P. multocida* and *T. pyogenes* were present in the exudate. Colonization of the tympanic cavity resulted in lysis of bone of the wall and of the osseous septa of tympanic bullae. In severe cases, lesions spread and caused otitis interna and acute fibrinous inflammation of the cochlea and vestibule, as well as extension into the leptomeninges and neuropil of the brain. Pigs older than 4 months more commonly had severe, chronic otitis media with extensive expansion as described earlier.

In ruminants, *Histophilus somni, P. multocida, T. pyogenes, Mycoplasma bovis*, and *Streptococcus* spp. have been isolated from animals with otitis media. Various mites (see earlier discussion) and nematodes may also contribute to the occurrence and severity of disease. As in pigs, otitis media occurs as a result of nasopharyngeal ascent of bacteria through the auditory tubes. In natural infections, potential routes of initial exposure to these bacteria include congenital infection, ingestion of colostrum, ingestion of contaminated milk, exposure to infected vaginal secretions, or ingestion or inhalation of respiratory secretions leading to nasopharyngeal colonization. Other factors include concurrent bacterial or viral infections, nutritional status of the herd, level of contamination in the environment, and host immune status.

Macroscopically, lesions may be unilateral or bilateral. The mucoperiosteum is congested and edematous (see Fig. 17-15). Bullae can be filled with fibrinopurulent to caseous exudate, and the mucoperiosteal epithelium is often ulcerated (Fig. 20-38; E-Fig. 20-3). There may be remodeling of bony septa of the bullae or osteolysis, as well as osteolysis of auditory ossicles. With chronicity the mucoperiosteum becomes markedly thickened by fibrosis and granulation tissue. In severely affected animals, tympanic membranes and auditory ossicles are missing. Microscopic lesions reflect what is seen grossly, namely bony lysis of bullae septa, infiltration by mixtures of neutrophils and macrophages, abundant cellular debris, and variable numbers of bacteria. When examined, auditory ossicles have superficial erosion of bone. The morphologic features of the mucoperiosteal epithelium are highly variable, with areas lined by squamous epithelium, whereas others are lined by ciliated, pseudostratified columnar epithelium mixed with goblet cells. Often embedded in the thickened, inflamed mucoperiosteum are cystic cavities that contain or are surrounded by exudate and lined by goblet cells and pseudostratified epithelium. These structures have been referred to as glandular structures, glands, pseudoglands, or invaginating glands. They likely represent folds that form and are lined by mucoperiosteal epithelium. Additionally, chronically inflamed mucoperiosteum often will contain variable amounts of acicular clefts (cholesterol clefts), the result of cholesterol released from cell membranes of necrotic cells, previous sites of hemorrhage, and from surfactant.

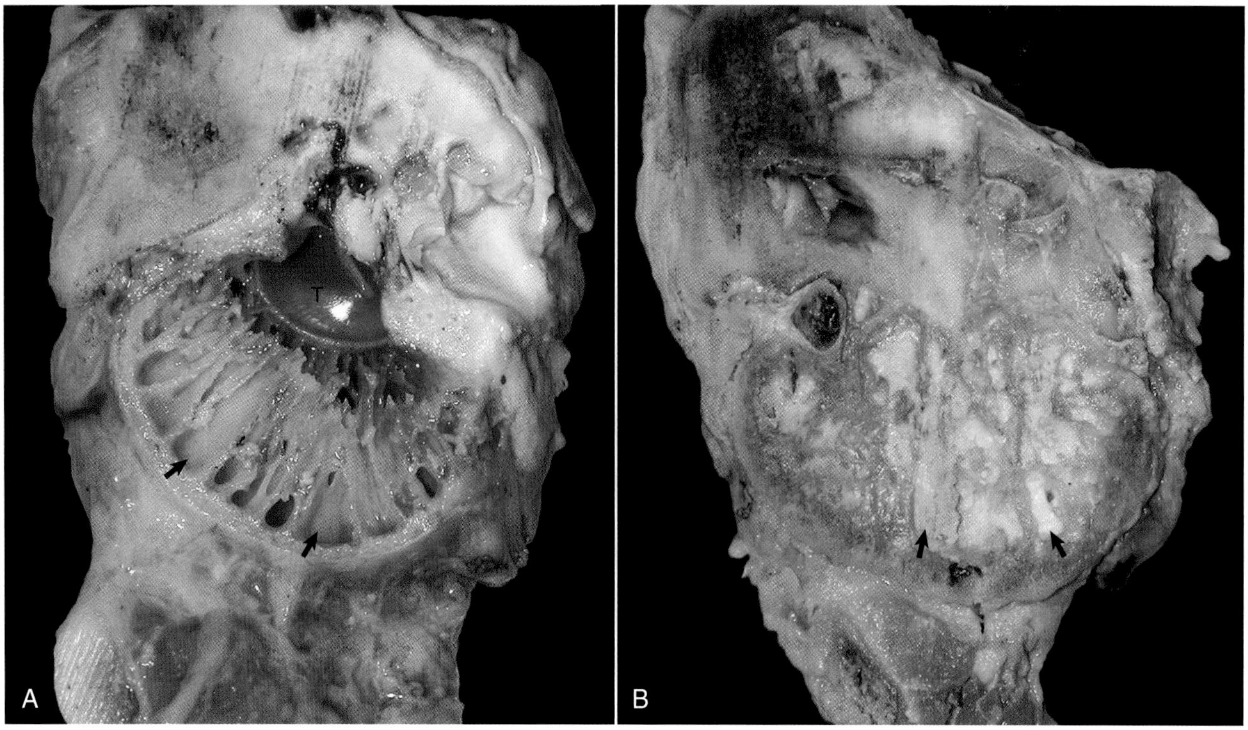

Figure 20-38 **Suppurative Otitis Media, Calf. A,** Medial view. Middle ear from a normal 5-week-old calf. The cavities between the bony septa of the tympanic bulla are empty *(arrows)*. The ventral half of the tympanic membrane, the bony ring, and manubrium of the malleus are partially exposed *(T)*. Dorsally, the yellow-tinged bone is the petrous portion of the temporal bone. **B,** Medial view. Otitis media in a 5-week-old Holstein calf. Necrotic, caseous exudate fills the cavities between the bony septa in the tympanic bulla *(arrows)*. *Mycoplasma bovis* was confirmed by polymerase chain reaction in this ear and a lung sample from this calf. (Courtesy Dr. B.W. Brodersen, University of Nebraska Veterinary Diagnostic Center.)

The propria submucosa of the mucoperiosteum is infiltrated by variable numbers of lymphocytes, plasma cells, macrophages, and neutrophils.

Clinical signs frequently include facial nerve paralysis, head tilt, drooping ears, epiphora, and mucopurulent nasal discharge. Severe otitis media can result in tympanic membrane rupture leading to purulent otorrhea and otomiasma. Rarely, infections spread to cause meningitis.

Otitis media was reportedly a uncommon disease in cats; however, a recent prospective study of cats submitted for autopsy for various reasons determined that otitis media is much more common than originally thought. Otitis media in cats is typically unassociated with otitis externa and is presumed to be the result of impaired auditory tube function. In dogs, otitis media often results secondarily from severe otitis externa that may lead to tympanic membrane rupture; however, at the time of diagnosis, tympanic membranes are commonly intact.

Numerous bacteria have been isolated, including *E. coli*, *Enterobacter* spp., *Enterococcus* spp., *Streptococcus* spp., β-hemolytic *Streptococcus* spp., *Staphylococcus* spp., *Proteus* spp., and *Clostridium* spp. Although more frequently a unilateral disease, bilateral disease is reported. Grossly, any tympanic bulla that contains fluid of any kind should be suspected as being otitis media. Middle ear effusions may be translucent, gray mucoid, yellow-green, red tinged, or hemorrhagic (Fig. 20-39, *A*). Flushing the effusion may allow visualization of ruptured tympanic membranes, bony proliferation of the tympanic bulla, or deformities to the auditory ossicles, when examined with the use of a dissecting microscope. Microscopically, there are abundant neutrophils, typically degenerate, mixed with macrophages, and variable numbers of lymphocytes and plasma cells (see Fig. 20-39, *B*). Often the pseudostratified, ciliated columnar epithelium of the tympanic bulla is undermined by the infiltrate and frequently forms pseudoglands or infolded glands. Areas of cholesterol cleft formation are common, as are areas of hemorrhage. The amount of granulation tissue and fibrosis within the tympanic cavity is variable and relates to the chronicity of the otitis media. Osseous proliferation of the tympanic bulla is seen more often than bony erosions (see Fig. 20-24). As part of a routine autopsy examination, both tympanic bullae should be opened ventrally for any evidence of effusion or other lesions, regardless of clinical signs reported. Unilateral or bilateral otitis media without concurrent evidence of otitis externa or vestibular disease may be clinically silent.

Aural Inflammatory Polyps (Nasopharyngeal Polyps)

Aural inflammatory polyps are the most common nonneoplastic inflammatory masses affecting cats, often under 2 years of age. They also occur much less frequently in dogs and have been reported once in a horse. A confirmed cause has not yet been determined, but proposed causes include chronic upper respiratory tract infections, otitis media, ascending middle ear infections via the auditory tube, or congenital defects such as aberrant growths from remnants of the branchial arches. As their name suggests, inflammatory polyps are pedunculated and polypoid, often with a smooth surface (Fig. 20-40). They may be confined to the middle ear, protrude through the auditory tube into the nasopharynx, or penetrate through a ruptured tympanic membrane into the external acoustic meatus. Histologically, inflammatory polyps have a fibrovascular core that is infiltrated with lymphocytes, plasma cells, and macrophages of varying numbers and are covered by epithelium that may be severely ulcerated. The overlying epithelium reflects the tissue of origin,

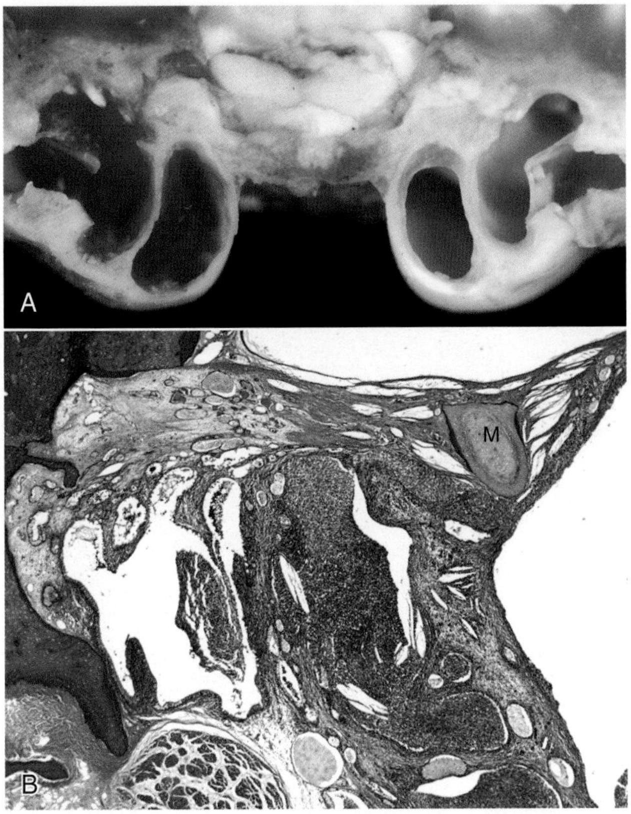

Figure 20-39 **Otitis Media, Cat. A,** Rostral view. Red-tinged, viscous fluid fills the tympanic compartments of the right ear. The left ear is normal with no luminal exudate. The septum bulla is complete and separates the tympanic cavity into the dorsolateral epitympanic cavity and the ventromedial tympanic cavity. **B,** Histologic section of middle ear. The tympanic cavity contains abundant suppurative exudate *(center)* mixed with numerous cholesterol clefts. The mucoperiosteum of the tympanic cavity is thickened by edematous fibrous connective tissue and granulation tissue. Throughout are numerous invaginated, pseudoglands lined by pseudostratified epithelium. The manubrium *(M)* of the malleus is embedded in a tympanic membrane that is thickened as a result of chronic inflammation (myringitis) with fibrosis and cholesterol cleft formation. In aggregate, these are the prototypic morphologic features of chronic otitis media. H&E stain. (Courtesy Dr. B.L. Njaa, Center for Veterinary Health Sciences, Oklahoma State University.)

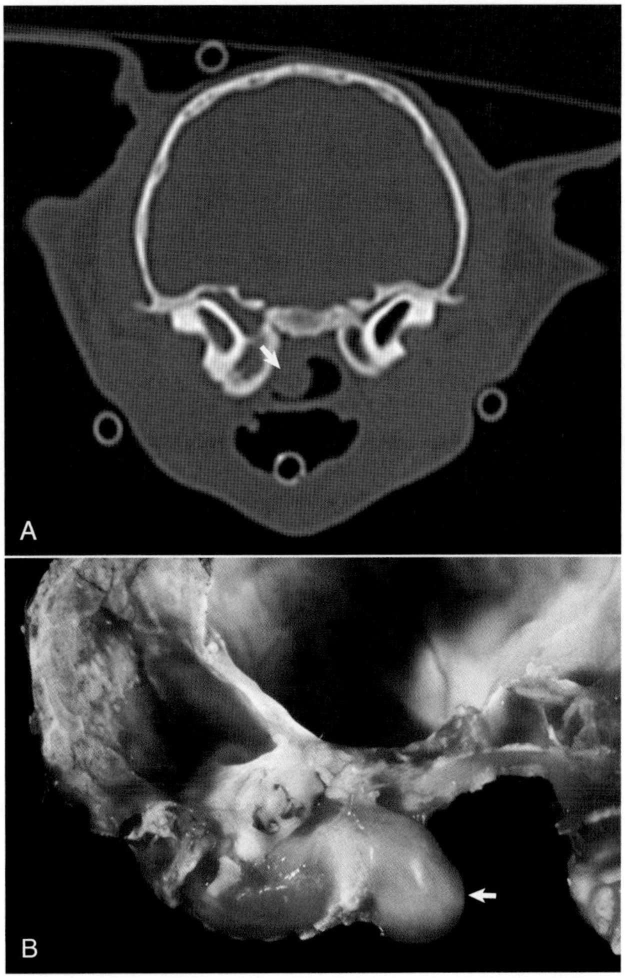

Figure 20-40 **Aural Inflammatory Polyp, Cat. A,** Computed tomography of tympanic bullae and pharynx. A small, central bulge of hypoechoic tissue *(arrow)* extends from the left tympanic cavity into the nasopharynx, presumably through the auditory tube. **B,** Cross section through the left tympanic bulla and nasopharynx. An aural inflammatory polyp *(arrow)* fills the tympanic bulla and extends through the auditory tube into the nasopharynx. The smooth, shiny surface indicates it is covered by epithelium. The internal ear is opened in this view, and the rostral, ventral spiral turns of the cochlea are present. (**A** courtesy Dr. N. Dykes, College of Veterinary Medicine, Cornell University. **B** courtesy Dr. J. Render, North American Science Associates.)

whether arising from the auditory tube, tympanic bulla, or other portions of the tympanic cavity, and varies from stratified squamous epithelium to pseudostratified ciliated columnar epithelium mixed with goblet cells (Fig. 20-41). Inflammatory polyps are most commonly associated with chronic otitis media and therefore have features similar to a chronically inflamed mucoperiosteum, namely, the formation of pseudoglands or invaginating glands connected to the surface of the lining epithelium. Signs of disease vary, depending on the location of the polyps. Signs of otitis externa or otitis media may commonly indicate the presence of polyps. Other symptoms include nasal, otic, or ocular discharge; sneezing; dyspnea; stridor; voice change; dysphagia; head tilt; Horner's syndrome; nystagmus; and ataxia. Much less commonly, obstructing polyps may lead to cyanosis and syncope.

A smaller subset of inflammatory aural polyps originates in the external acoustic meatus. These polyps are typically lined by squamous epithelium with variable inflammation and edema in the fibrovascular core. Invaginating glands or pseudoglands will not develop in polyps that originate from the external ear.

Neoplasms of the Middle Ear

Neoplasms occur rarely in the middle ear. Squamous cell carcinomas have been diagnosed most frequently in cats, whereas carcinomas of undetermined origin more commonly occur in dogs. Neoplasms may originate within the middle ear or arise in the external ear canal and penetrate through the tympanic membrane into the tympanic cavity. Neoplastic growth tends to be expansile and infiltrative with evidence of bony lysis of bullae, lysis of the petrous portion of the temporal bone, or intracranial invasion. Local damage to the facial nerve or vestibulocochlear nerve may lead to vestibular signs, facial nerve paralysis, or Horner's syndrome. In both dogs and cats, pain on opening the mouth is very common.

Jugulotympanic paraganglioma is an uncommon tumor that arises from paraganglia in close proximity to the tympanic bulla or arises within the middle ear. This tumor is only reported in human beings and dogs. In a few instances in dogs, metastatic tumors are found in distant parenchymatous organs.

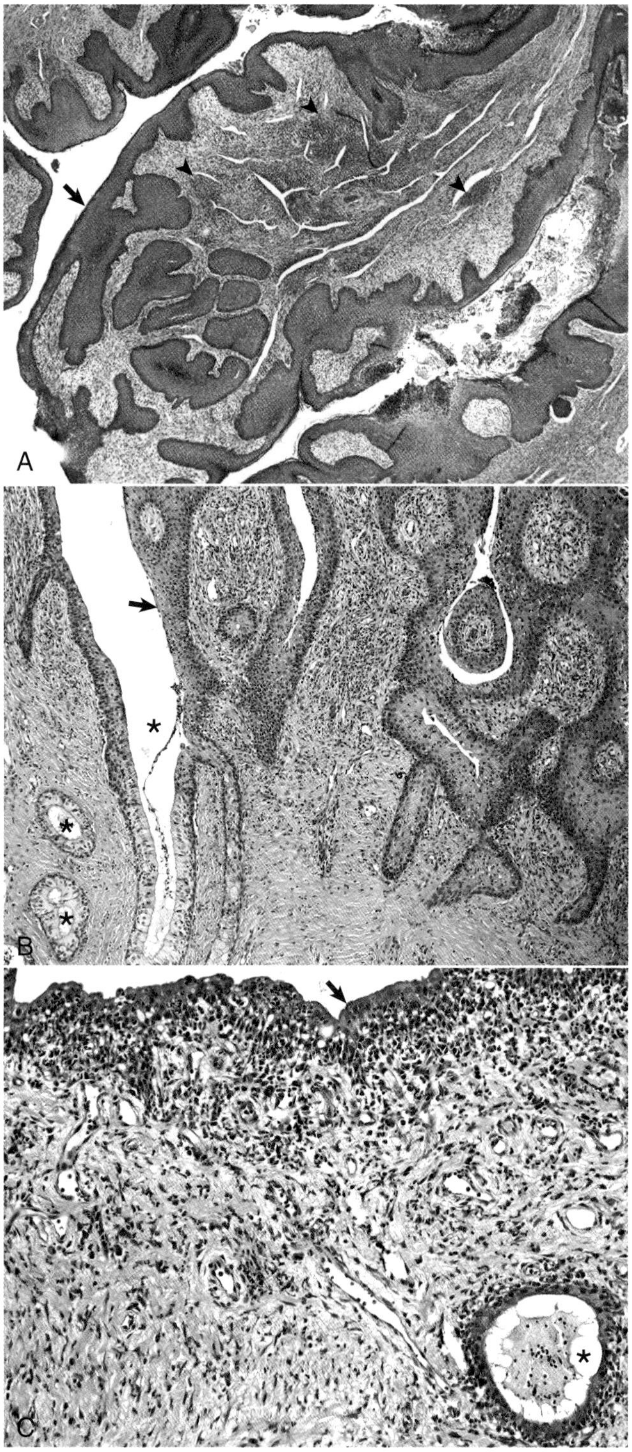

Figure 20-41 Auditory Inflammatory Polyps, Cats. A, The epithelium covering the surface of this polyp is stratified squamous *(arrow)*. The stromal core is infiltrated by mixed population of inflammatory cells that regionally form lymphoid aggregates *(arrowheads)*. The luminal (surface) squamous epithelium forms "folds" that do not form pseudoglands. These features support an aural polyp that likely originated from the epidermis and dermis of the external acoustic meatus. H&E stain. **B,** The surface epithelium is squamous *(arrow)* and infolds to form pseudoglands and transitions from squamous epithelium to pseudostratified, ciliated columnar epithelium mixed with goblet cells *(asterisks)*. The core is richly vascularized and inflamed. These infolded pseudoglands are characteristic of a middle ear mucoperiosteal origin. H&E stain. **C,** The surface epithelium is pseudostratified, ciliated, columnar epithelium *(arrow)*. A single infolded pseudogland is present in the underlying stroma *(asterisk)*. The core is proliferative fibrovascular stoma with prominent inflammation. In aggregate, these morphologic features are characteristic of a middle ear mucoperiosteal origin. (Courtesy Dr. B.L. Njaa, Center for Veterinary Health Sciences, Oklahoma State University.)

Inflammation of the Internal Ear

Otitis Interna (Labyrinthitis)

Otitis interna results from extension of otitis media. It may occur with or without osteomyelitis of the petrous portion of the temporal bone. With time and severity, lesions progress retrograde through the internal acoustic meatus into the cranial cavity, resulting in meningitis, ventriculitis, and encephalitis. Macroscopically, there is typically a middle ear exudate that varies from serosanguineous to suppurative to granulomatous. Microscopically, the inflammatory infiltrate affecting the middle ear is typically composed of neutrophils, macrophages, lymphocytes, and plasma cells. Within the membranous labyrinth, smaller numbers of neutrophils mixed with fibrin can be found in the perilymph (Fig. 20-42). Fewer lymphocytes and plasma cells may infiltrate the lamina propria of the osseous labyrinth. The most plausible portal of entry is through the membranous covering of the cochlear window (see Fig. 20-21).

Vestibular Disease of the Internal Ear

Injury to any portion of the vestibular system (see the earlier section on the Vestibular System) leads to a condition collectively referred to as *vestibular disease*. Although the lesion may be located peripherally (internal ear sensory receptors, vestibular ganglia, or peripheral axons of cranial nerve VIII) or centrally (vestibular nuclei of the medulla, vestibular projections to the rostral brainstem, cerebellum, or spinal cord), affected animals typically exhibit a head tilt, nystagmus, asymmetric ataxia, circling, and variable facial paralysis.

Congenital vestibular disease has been reported to occur in certain breeds of dogs (Doberman Pinschers, German Shepherd dogs, Cocker Spaniels, Beagles, or Akitas) and more commonly in Siamese, Tonkinese, or Burmese cat breeds. The cause of this disease is not well understood largely because most affected animals recover spontaneously or compensate within the first few weeks of life. Gross lesions are typically absent. As a result of the clinical course, histologic lesions are usually not reported. However, in one report a small number of Doberman Pinscher puppies had evidence of intense lymphocytic infiltration of the middle and internal ear propria submucosa. The most common clinical sign is a head tilt with varying degrees of ataxia. Nystagmus is reported but is a less prominent feature. Deafness has been reported in some cases.

Concurrent otitis media and otitis interna is a common cause of peripheral vestibular disease. Otitis media in isolation likely will not result in vestibular disease (potentially, an elevated middle ear temperature related to otitis media could instigate temperature-induced [caloric] vestibular signs), but if deficits are detected that are compatible with peripheral vestibular disease, concurrent internal ear involvement is presumed. Causes include (1) viral infections such as those caused by canine distemper virus and feline infectious peritonitis virus and (2) various bacterial, rickettsial (Rocky Mountain spotted fever, ehrlichiosis, bartonellosis), protozoal (toxoplasmosis, neosporosis), and mycotic (cryptococcosis, blastomycosis, histoplasmosis, coccidiomycosis) infections. A small group of

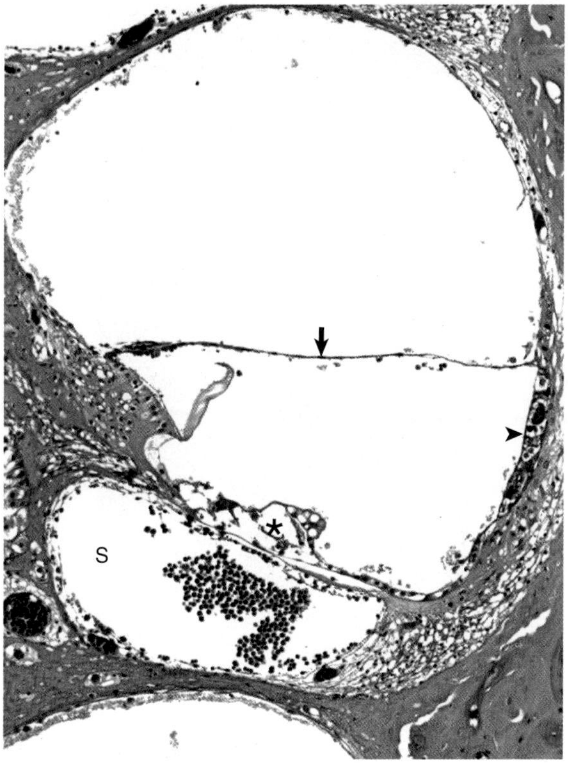

Figure 20-42 **Otitis Interna, Guinea Pig.** The scala tympani (*S*) contains a large luminal aggregate of inflammatory cells, mainly heterophils (neutrophils). Fewer inflammatory cells are present in the cochlear duct and scala vestibuli. The vestibular membrane (*arrow*) is intact. The tectorial membrane is artifactually separated from the spiral organ (*asterisk*) that is also presumably a fixation artifact. See Figure 20-21 for a diagram of the structure. *Arrowhead,* Stria vascularis. H&E stain. (Courtesy Dr. B.L. Njaa, Center for Veterinary Health Sciences, Oklahoma State University.)

affected horses had concurrent facial nerve paralysis as well. Refer to previous discussions of gross and histologic features of otitis media and otitis interna.

Idiopathic peripheral vestibular disease is considered the second most common form of this disease diagnosed in dogs and cats. Dogs are typically geriatric at the time of diagnosis. In cats, age is less important, but most cases are diagnosed in the summer and fall months in the northeastern and mid-Atlantic regions of the United States. A cause has not been determined, and specific lesions have not been identified. One key clinical feature in making this diagnosis is the presence of peripheral vestibular disease signs in the absence of concurrent facial nerve paralysis or Horner's syndrome.

Aural or intracranial neoplasia may arise within, compress on, or infiltrate into the labyrinthine or neural portions of the vestibular system. Vestibular neurofibromas or schwannomas rarely arise within the vestibulocochlear nerve (see Figs. 14-114 and 14-115). Compression or invasion of soft tissues of the head and ear, the skull, brainstem, or cerebellum can result in significant vestibular deficits. Based on diagnostic imaging, lytic lesions of the tympanic bullae or petrous portions of the temporal bone are more often associated with aural neoplasia than with otitis media or otitis interna. Signs associated with intracranial neoplasia depend more on the location of the neoplasm than on the kind of neoplasm. Grossly, the neoplasm may arise within or infiltrate a portion of the central vestibular system. Alternatively, the mass may cause obstructive hydrocephalus or brain herniation, resulting in more widespread neurologic deficits.

Various therapeutic agents can cause vestibular disease. Ototoxic agents, such as aminoglycoside antimicrobials, furosemide, platinum-containing antineoplastic agents, and salicylates, are a few categories of chemicals that cause injury to or degeneration of the hair cells of the membranous labyrinth. In cats, gentamicin leads to damage of hair cells in the vestibular maculae, whereas amikacin damages the hair cells nearly exclusively in the cochlea. Hearing impairment with salicylates and furosemide tends to be transient owing to temporary disruption of membrane conductance and resolves when treatment is stopped. Metronidazole is an antimicrobial agent capable of causing neurotoxicity with resultant vestibular disease. The exact mechanism is not fully known but theorized to be modulated by γ-aminobutyric acid (GABA) receptors in the vestibulocerebellum and may result in axonal degeneration. The signs typically resolve on cessation of therapy. There is very little published documenting lesions associated with metronidazole therapy.

Hearing Loss and Deafness

Hearing loss and deafness can be congenital or acquired, and each type further categorized as conduction or neurosensory deafness. Sound perception can first be detected by audiometrics in 5-day-old kittens and 14-day-old puppies. Animals that are known to hear normally that subsequently undergo hearing loss have acquired deafness. A patent external acoustic meatus, intact tympanic membrane, functioning auditory ossicles, and normal perilymph of the cochlea define the conduction portion of hearing, and thus any damage or loss of these structures leads to conduction deafness. The neurosensory contribution to hearing includes the stria vascularis, normal endolymph, sensory hair cells of the spiral organ, and associated neural connections. Any interference with the neural pathways or injury to the mechanosensory spiral organ and stria vascularis lead to neurosensory deafness.

Causes of conduction hearing loss include (1) external acoustic meatus stenosis that may be congenital or acquired secondary to otitis externa, (2) chronic otitis externa leading to narrowing of the external acoustic meatus or tympanic membrane rupture and impaired sound transmission, (3) auditory ossicle damage or tympanic membrane injury from otitis media, and (4) damage from neoplasms affecting any portion of the conduction system. Repair or removal of the cause of the conduction deafness can result in return to normal function and hearing.

Congenital inherited sensorineural deafness is a common disorder, especially in dogs and cats. Alterations in the function of microphthalmia-associated transcription factor (MITF) occurs in Dalmatian dogs with congenital sensorineural deafness and blue iris color. The merle color pattern is a pigment dilution related to variable expression of the merle allele of the pigment locus, mouse *Silver* pigment locus homolog (*SILV*). Dogs homozygous for the dominant merle allele are significantly more likely to be deaf than heterozygotes. The piebald gene, which results in a coat color that alternates between white and darkly pigmented, also has been linked with deafness. Both the piebald and merle genes cause (1) the blue eye phenotype by suppressing melanocytes in the iris and (2) deafness by suppressing marginal cells in the stria vascularis of the cochlea.

Congenital sensorineural deafness has been classified into two major categories based on mechanism: albinotic and abiotrophic. The albinotic form, or Scheibe deformity, is also known as *cochleosaccular degeneration*. It is associated with hypopigmentation and stria vascularis dysfunction. Deafness due to stria vascularis dysfunction is related to abnormal intermediate cells. Endolymph is produced and maintained by the stria vascularis, but dysfunctional intermediate cells affect endolymph formation. Abnormal endolymph is associated with degeneration of hair cells of the cochlea characterized by atrophy of stria vascularis, collapse of the cochlear

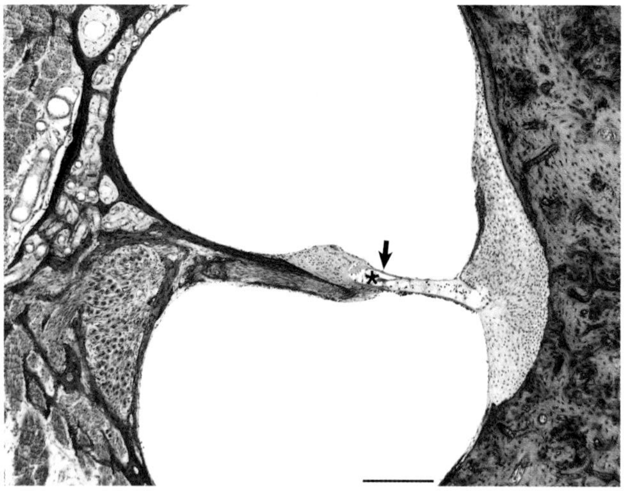

Figure 20-43 **Albinotic Deafness, Cat.** The vestibular membrane *(arrow)* is collapsed onto the spiral organ *(asterisk)*, and the tectorial membrane is difficult to discern in the section. The cochlear duct is obliterated. The spiral organ lacks normal detail due to loss of hair cells and support cells. Compare with Figures 20-21 and 20-22. H&E stain. Scale bar = 200 μm. (Courtesy G. Pagonis, Massachusetts Eye and Ear Infirmary.)

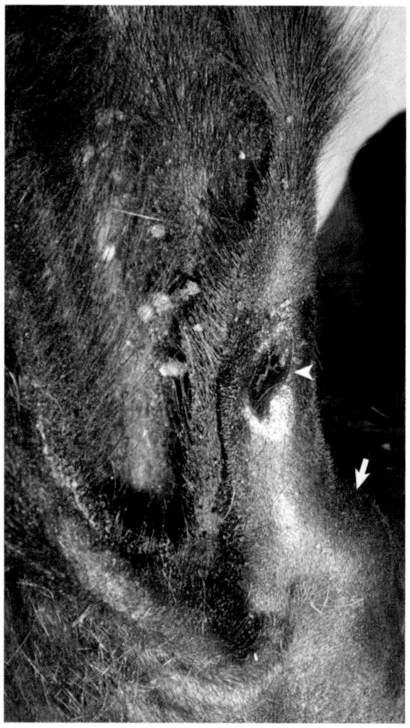

Figure 20-44 **Dentigerous Cyst, Right Auricle, Horse.** Within the craniomedial edge of the right auricle is a firm mass that represents a dentigerous cyst *(arrow)*. Along the craniodorsal edge of this mass is an external opening to a fistulous tract *(arrowhead)*. Scattered over the concave surface of the auricle are several pale, aural plaques (see Fig. 20-46). (Courtesy Dr. P. Fretz, The Western College of Veterinary Medicine, University of Saskatchewan.)

duct, degeneration of the spiral organ, abnormal tectorial membrane, progressive spiral ganglion degeneration, and saccular collapse (Fig. 20-43). Deafness may be unilateral or bilateral with up to 50% of white-coated, blue-eyed cats affected. Dalmatian dogs have a 30% incidence of the albinotic form, which is inherited as an autosomal dominant gene.

The abiotrophic form is caused by abiotrophy of sensory hair cells (neuroepithelial) with subsequent atrophy of the spiral organ, yet the cochlear duct and stria vascularis are morphologically unaffected. Typically a bilateral condition, hair cells of the vestibular system and cochlea are affected. This form of deafness is a progressive condition, most often recognized at a later age. This mechanism may be the cause of deafness in Cavalier King Charles spaniels, which typically is not recognized until 3 to 4 years of age. Although much is known clinically and functionally about this disease, because of the need for rapid fixation and decalcification of affected tissues, little is known about the pathogenesis or histopathologic features of this form.

Acquired sensorineural deafness commonly occurs secondary to otitis media. Inflammation extends through the cochlear window into the compartment of the bony labyrinth. Inflammatory mediators may lead to degeneration of hair cells, resulting in both vestibular signs and deafness.

Presbycusis refers to age-related hearing loss that occurs as an animal ages. Age-related hearing loss represents an acquired form of deafness with a multifactorial pathogenesis. Refer to the section on aging for more details.

Acoustic noise trauma has been studied in cats. Injury is primarily focused on the spiral organ, spiral ligament, limbal fibrocytes, and spiral ganglion cells. Tears form in the supporting structures of the spiral organ, causing release of hair cells into the endolymph and vascular injury resulting in bleeding into the compartments of the cochlea. Several weeks after the initial injury, the spiral organ is completely degenerated, related initially to outer hair cell loss followed by inner hair cell loss. There is also a retrograde degeneration of the associated cochlear nerve tracts.

Ototoxicity is another means of acquired deafness. Many compounds are known to be ototoxic, including aminoglycoside antimicrobials, platinum-containing chemotherapeutic agents, furosemide, salicylates, and otic cleansers. To exert toxicity, ototoxins must reach the internal ear. This process may occur via hematogenous spread, enhanced diffusion through a tympanic membrane under the influence of otitis media, or through a perforated tympanic membrane. Once in the tympanic cavity, ototoxic compounds gain access to the internal ear by diffusing through the cochlear window. The target of most ototoxicants is the hair cells. As has already been discussed, hair cells of the vestibular and cochlear systems succumb and become injured or die from apoptosis. Deafness and vestibular disease may be permanent or transient dependent on the ototoxic agent.

Disorders of Horses

Developmental Anomalies

Dentigerous Cysts (Temporal Odontomatas, Periauricular Cysts)

Dentigerous cysts (also known as temporal odontomatas, temporal teratomas, temporal cysts, ear or aural fistulas, ear teeth, and heterotopic polydontia) are rare, nonheritable, congenital cysts that occur rostral and ventral to the base of the ear pinna (Fig. 20-44). They also occur in the forehead, paranasal sinuses, and petrous portion of the temporal bone. Typically flask-shaped due to a long narrow fistula that drains to the surface, dentigerous cysts are most often unilateral, arising in the temporal region as the result of malpositioned tooth stem cells from the first branchial arch that are displaced within the first branchial cleft. Microscopically, the fistula and cavity are lined by stratified squamous epithelium and teeth of varied stages of differentiation composed of dentin, cementum, and enamel. Teeth are loosely or firmly attached to underlying temporal or parietal bones of the skull. Salivary gland tissue may also be present. When dentigerous cysts do not contain teeth or dental structures, they are called *dermoid cysts*. In sheep, dentigerous cysts occur in the mandibular incisor region and are called *ovine odontogenic cysts*.

Miscellaneous Disorders

Auricular Chondrosis

Auricular chondrosis is a condition in horses with similarities to auricular chondritis (see sections on Disorders of Dogs and Disorders of Cats) but with one main difference and that is a lack of inflammation and chondritis. A cause for this condition has not been determined. The lack of inflammation and lack of response to corticosteroids in the lone case report indicate the pathogenesis is likely distinct from auricular chondritis. Macroscopically, lesions were characterized by nodular thickenings of both pinnae that ranged from 3 to 8 mm in diameter palpable below the surface with no apparent involvement of the overlying epidermis. With the exception of mild parakeratotic hyperkeratosis, microscopic lesions were primarily confined to the auricular cartilage. Cartilage plates were markedly thickened with central areas that lacked chondrocytes and had areas of degeneration and necrosis. Other regions contained adipocytes and were invaded by small blood vessels. Along the margins of the damaged cartilage were areas of nascent cartilage formation with macrocytic chondrocytes and deeply basophilic matrix present at the interface. However, there was no evidence of infiltration of the cartilage or peripheral soft tissue by inflammatory cells. In the lone reported case, nodules were nonpainful and persistent.

Temporohyoid Osteoarthropathy

The temporohyoid joint is a permanent synchondrosis connecting the proximal stylohyoid bone to the petrous portion of the temporal bone via tympanohyoid cartilage. This articulation is in very close proximity to the middle ear. A complete understanding of normal joint movement is lacking, but the temporohyoid joint is believed to function by dampening movement of the hyoid apparatus during tongue movement. Temporohyoid osteoarthropathy is a bony proliferative disease of the temporohyoid articulation that may result from (1) infectious agents inciting the disease by local extension of otitis media/interna, hematogenous spread, ascending infection from the respiratory tract, or extension from guttural pouch disease or (2) degenerative joint disease of the temporohyoid joint.

Infectious Microorganisms. Otitis media causes ventral osteitis of the bone of the tympanic bulla and because of proximity to the temporohyoid joint, osteoarthritis of the joint ensues by extension of inflammation. Osteomyelitis and periosteal proliferation of bone result in ankylosis of the temporohyoid joint and fusion of the stylohyoid bone to the petrous portion of the temporal bone (Fig. 20-45). Additionally, the bony portion of the external acoustic meatus is also in close apposition and may become narrowed as a result of exostosis and osteoarthritis. Infectious agents may also affect this region via other routes leading to similar lesions.

Degenerative Joint Disease. Thickening of the proximal stylohyoid and ankylosis of the temporohyoid joint can result from degenerative joint disease. In a recent study, age-related bony remodeling changes were documented in the temporohyoid joint, including (1) club-shaped development to the proximal stylohyoid bone, (2) rounding of the synostosis with the petrous portion of the temporal bone, and (3) extension of osteophytes from the petrous portion of the temporal bone, typically enveloping the stylohyoid head and in some cases bridging the joint. These proliferative changes were typically observed bilaterally but were never as severe as is seen in temporohyoid osteoarthropathy. Histologic changes were most pronounced in the oldest horses in the study. There was marked disorganization of the joint with marked irregularity in the depth of the joint fibrocartilage, a variation of lipping to fragmentation of the petrous portion of the temporal bone along the joint margin, markedly irregular chondro-osseous junctions, extensive fibrous replacement of periarticular bone, marked periosteal thickening, and marked clustering of chondrocytes with heterogeneity of the surrounding and intervening matrix. There were no areas of active inflammation in any of the examined sections.

Clinical disease is often categorized into two syndromes. In the first scenario, horses demonstrate abnormal behavior, such as shaking their heads, ear rubbing, and problems chewing, and resent having a bit in their mouths. The second syndrome is related to a fracture through the ankylosed joint and possibly fracture of the petrous portion of the temporal bone, leading to signs attributable to acute vestibular or facial nerve injury. Rarely, affected horses may develop meningitis.

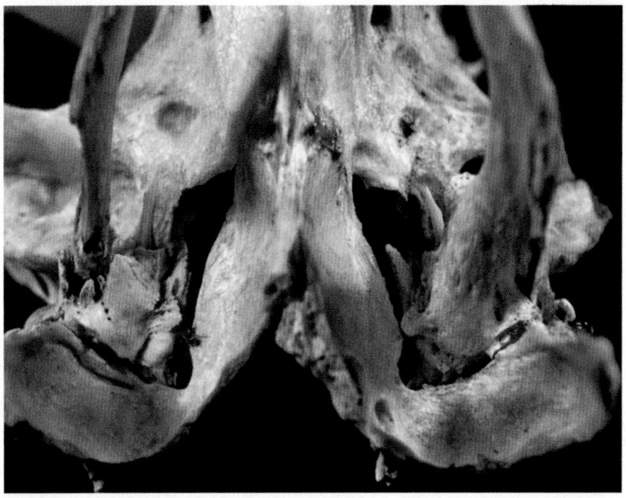

Figure 20-45 **Temporohyoid Arthropathy, Horse.** The left stylohyoid bone from this mature thoroughbred mare is thickened and fused with the temporal bone. (Courtesy Dr. R. Peters, Cummings School of Veterinary Medicine, Tufts University.)

Aural Plaques (Aural Papillomatosis)

Aural plaques (also known as equine ear papillomas, papillary acanthoma, hyperplastic dermatitis of the ear, or "ear fungus") occur in horses over 1 year of age and are caused by papilloma virus spread between horses by fly bites. Macroscopically, lesions are characterized as raised, well-demarcated, hypopigmented, hyperkeratotic plaques arising from the concave surface of the auricle (Fig. 20-46, *A*). Plaques are typically 1 to 3 mm in diameter but can overlap to involve larger areas. Microscopically, the epidermis is moderately hyperplastic with a stratum corneum that is variably hyperkeratotic. The granulosis layer tends to be quite prominent. Scattered through the affected epidermis are singlets or clusters of koilocytes. Basal epithelial cells tend to be more poorly pigmented when compared to peripheral, more normal epidermis (see Fig. 20-46, *B*). Various molecular techniques have been used to demonstrate papillomavirus in the epidermis of the plaques. Clinically, aural plaques rarely resolve spontaneously, but they are usually of little clinical significance unless infected by bacteria secondary to trauma.

Guttural Pouch Disease

See Chapters 9 and 17.

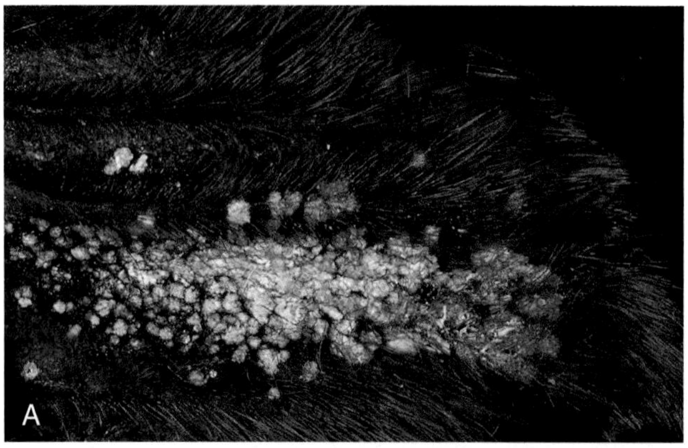

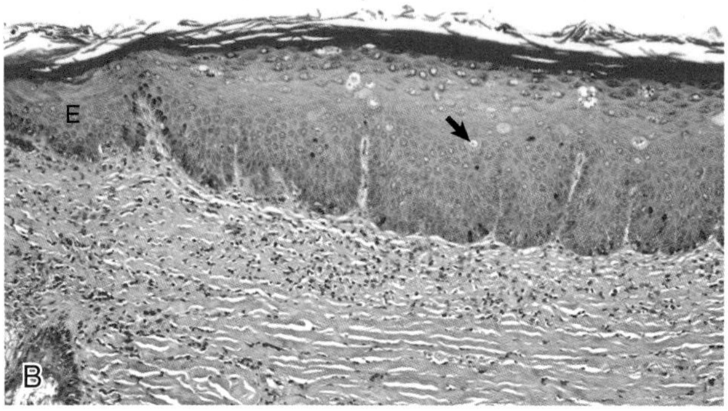

Figure 20-46 **Aural Plaques, Horse. A,** Concave surface of right auricle. Multiple, hypopigmented, exophytic, gray to tan masses cover the central portion of the auricle. Often these plaques coalesce to form a large mass. **B,** Histologic section of an aural plaque. The stratified squamous epithelium is hyperplastic. When compared to the adjacent more normal and basally pigmented epithelium *(E)*, the basal epithelial cells are hypopigmented. Scattered through the sessile mass are koilocytes *(arrow)*. H&E stain. (**A** courtesy Dr. R. Fairley, The Western College of Veterinary Medicine, University of Saskatchewan. **B** courtesy Dr. R. Bildfell, College of Veterinary Medicine, Oregon State University.)

Disorders of Ruminants (Cattle, Sheep, and Goats)

Developmental Anomalies

β-*Mannosidosis of Cattle and Goats*

β-Mannosidosis is an autosomal recessive lysosomal storage disease caused by a deficiency of glucohydrolase β-D-mannosidase leading to the accumulation of oligosaccharide substrates of β-mannosidase in lysosomes of multiple cell types located in nervous, renal, thyroid, and lymphoid tissues. This disease was first described in Nubian kids and has subsequently been reported in Salers calves. Newborn animals were unable to rise and had dome-shaped heads, intention tremors, nystagmus, and bilateral Horner's syndrome. Macroscopically, affected animals have bilaterally kinked and folded auricles that are most severe in Nubian kids but less severe in Salers calves. Additionally, Nubian kids have sensorineural deafness; Salers calves have normal auditory function. In both species there is narrowing of the cartilaginous portions of the external acoustic meatus. Tympanic bullae are normal in the goats but smaller in the calves. Mucosa of the middle ear of the goats forms prominent polypoid projections, thus reducing the volume of the tympanic cavity.

Microscopically in both species, prominent intracytoplasmic vacuoles (lysosomes, see Chapter 14) are present in cells of the cochlear duct, including cochlear hair cells, supportive cells of the spiral organ, cells of the stria vascularis, mesothelial cells covering the scala tympani, neurons of the spiral ganglion, cells of vestibular membrane, endothelial cells, and fibroblasts.

Parasitic Diseases

Stephanofilarial Otitis

Stephanofilarial otitis, commonly referred to as *ear-sore,* occurs in cattle and buffalo and is caused by *Stephanofilaria zaheeri.* Biting flies have been implicated in the transmission of the parasite to the auricle, and infestation is painful. Macroscopic lesions are most evident on the concave surface of the auricle and vary from congestion to inflammation with hemorrhage, to severe crusting (parakeratosis) if chronic, and to alopecia with depigmentation. Microscopically, microfilaria are present in the auricular epidermis and dermis along with lymphocytes, macrophages, hyperplastic or degenerate sebaceous glands, and hemorrhage. Microfilaria in the dermis are usually dead and located in areas that are infiltrated by macrophages, eosinophils, and plasma cells. It has been hypothesized that this lesion may represent a form of immune-mediated response. Chronic cases of "ear-sore" can result in dysplastic or neoplastic transformation of cells of the epidermis, likely linked to excessive cellular mitoses and mutations of genes that arise in rapidly dividing somatic cells (see Chapters 1 and 6).

Rhabditis Species Otitis

A free-living, saprophytic, rhabditiform nematode of the genus *Rhabditis* is a cause of otitis externa in cattle. Concurrent infections with the ear mite *Raillietia auris* and the yeast *Malassezia* spp. are also common. *Rhabditis* spp. occur in tropical and subtropical climate zones of Africa and some regions of Brazil. *Rhabditis* spp. infect and proliferate in the external acoustic meatus. Infested cattle may be asymptomatic or exhibit depression, otorrhea, otitis media and interna, cranial nerve paralysis, meningitis, circling, recumbency, and death. Elevated environmental temperature and high humidity are primary risk factors that contribute to the occurrence of this disease; additional risk factors include the breed, presence of horns, irritation or injury of the auricular skin caused by certain types of insecticide dips, and age. Examples of risk factors are (1) purebred and crossbred *Bos indicus* cattle, such as Gyr, have long, pendulous auricles that provide a more favorable environment for infection; (2) in *Bos indicus* cattle breeds, horns are thought to compress the external acoustic meatus and thus increase their susceptibility to infection; (3) cattle "dip treated" with an acaricide have greater infestations with *Rhabditis* spp. compared to cattle treated by a spray method; and (4) because older cattle accumulate more organic matter in their external acoustic meatuses, it is thought that this outcome provides a better environment for infestation with *Rhabditis* spp.

Neoplasms

Aural Melanomas of Angora Goats

UV radiation (see Chapter 6) plays a significant role in the induction of malignant melanomas on the dorsal surface of the auricle of Angora goats (Fig. 20-47); a less common site is the base of the horns and coronary band of the hooves. Macroscopically, this neoplasm is characterized by single or multiple black nodules either superficially or subcutaneously. Aural melanomas are highly aggressive and spread initially by local invasion to areas such as the frontal sinuses, followed by rapid and widely disseminated metastases to regional lymph nodes and other organ systems, such as the liver. Microscopically, these neoplastic cells are polygonal to spindle shaped, typically heavily pigmented, and moderately pleomorphic. Mitotic figures can be numerous. Typically, neoplastic cells stain strongly for melanin A. One report determined strong expression of p53 in neoplastic cells, but its significance remains undetermined (see Chapter 6).

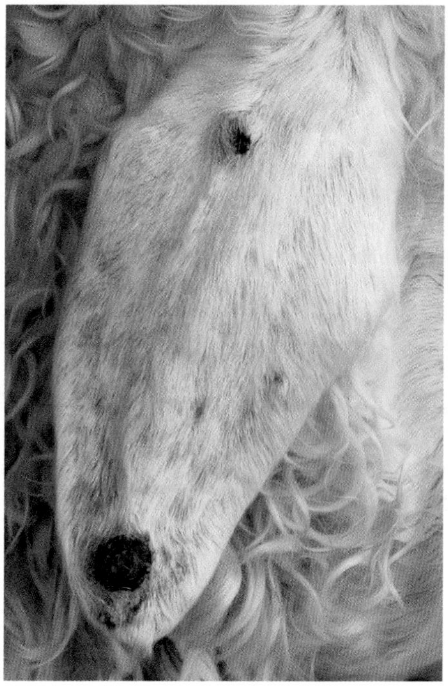

Figure 20-47 **Auricular Melanomas, White Angora Goat.** Two large exophytic, dark black, ulcerated melanomas are growing from the convex surface of the auricle. Closer inspection reveals several smaller melanomas. These neoplasms are highly malignant and are believed to be caused by ultraviolet radiation. (Courtesy Dr. K.G. Thompson, Institute of Veterinary, Animal & Biomedical Sciences, Massey University.)

Disorders of Pigs

Miscellaneous Disorders

Aural Chewing (Ear Chewing or Ear Cannibalism)

Aural chewing (also known as ear chewing or ear cannibalism) appears to be linked to the practice of intensified confinement rearing systems and docking of tails. High population density, heightened competition for food, low protein or inadequate nutrition, boredom, and inadequate microclimatic conditions probably increase the stress on and irritability of piglets, resulting in restlessness and aberrant behaviors. It is likely that tail docking simply redirects the focus of such behavior to the ears, because they represent two protruding and readily assessable objects. Eventually piglets begin to suck or chew the ears of pen mates until they become reddened and ulcerated. The appearance of these lesions and the taste of the serum and blood likely attract additional piglets to suck or chew the ears, thus worsening the lesions. At this stage the affected piglets experience intense pain. Macroscopically, lesions are typically bilateral, most often affecting the ventral portions of the ears, and are characterized by torn and traumatized auricular edges with crusting. The remainder of the auricle is typically red and thickened. Repeated trauma may lead to localized intradermal or intrachondral abscess formation. It may also represent a nidus of infection that disseminates systemically as a septicemia such as *Streptococcus* spp. Microscopically, lesions are consistent with those tissue changes described in acute inflammation (see Chapter 3).

Ear Necrosis (Necrotic Ear Syndrome and Ulcerative Spirochetosis of the Ear)

Ear necrosis, which is also known as necrotic ear syndrome and ulcerative spirochetosis of the ear, occurs in 6- to 9-week-old piglets and is thought to be caused by a spirochetal bacterium of the genus *Treponema* that is transmitted between animals through broken skin caused by biting of ears. Macroscopically, lesions appear as ulcerated, hemorrhagic, and crusted areas along the lower margin of the auricle near the base of the ear. When severe, the entire ear margin may be affected. The dermis and subcutis beneath the crusts are typically thickened due to edema and active hyperemia and vary in color from gray-black to red. Microscopically, thick serocellular crusts, often containing cocci or coccobacilli, cover the ulcerated epidermis that also contains large numbers of neutrophils mixed with cellular debris (acute inflammation). Vasculitis is evident in both arterioles and venules of the deeper dermis with fibrinoid degeneration, medial hyperplasia, and thrombosis. Adjacent, nonulcerated epidermis is hyperplastic with prominent, deeply invaginating epidermal pegs (reparative response). The Warthin-Starry stain (silver impregnation methodology) has been used to identify spirochetes in the junction between necrotic and healing tissues, as well as in the deeper dermis that has vasculitis, edema, and hemorrhage.

Disorders of Dogs

Parasitic Diseases

Auricular Parasitic Dermatitis

Auricular parasitic dermatitis is more commonly referred to as fly-bite dermatitis. Lesions develop in dogs that spend time outdoors during summer months from regions that have *Simulium* spp. (blackflies), *Chrysops* spp. (deerflies), or *Stomoxys calcitrans* (stable flies). Recently fly-bite dermatitis was subdivided into three types: type I lesions were large, 1- to 3-cm, targeted lesions without crusts involving the lateral surfaces of the pinnae; type II were small, 2- to 4-mm, hemorrhagic, crusted lesions that involved the lateral surface of pinnae; and type III were ulcerated, crusted, hemorrhagic lesions on the tips and folds of pinnae. None of the dogs were noted to be pruritic at the time of diagnosis. All lesions spontaneously resolved, but many dogs continued to have seasonal recurrence of lesions. Histologically, there is an intense perivascular to interstitial dermatitis with areas of necrosis and infiltration by numerous eosinophils, plasma cells, and macrophages. The overlying epidermis is irregularly acanthotic with compact orthokeratotic or parakeratotic hyperkeratosis and may be ulcerated dependent on the clinical syndrome.

Inflammation

Otitis Externa, Media, and Interna

See section on Disorders of Domestic Animals.

Canine Leproid Granuloma

Canine leproid granuloma is an uncommon mycobacterial disease affecting the subcutis and dermis of dogs. A causative agent has never been cultured, but through molecular techniques the cause of canine leproid granuloma is a novel, slow-growing mycobacterium of the *Mycobacterium simiae*–related group. The mycobacterium is thought to be an environmental saprophytic organism, and lesions form as a result of dermal inoculation through traumatic wounds or arthropod vectors. Single to multiple, firm, painless nodules most frequently arise on the dorsal surface of the auricle at its base but may affect the auricular tip, the head, or distal forelimbs. The largest lesions, upward of 5 cm in diameter, are alopecic and frequently ulcerated.

Histologically, a multinodular to diffuse, pyogranulomatous infiltrate extends from the dermis into the subcutis (Fig. 20-48). Macrophages may be large with abundant cytoplasm and may form multinucleated giant cells. Neutrophils are intermixed with the macrophages or may aggregate into focal clusters. The occurrence

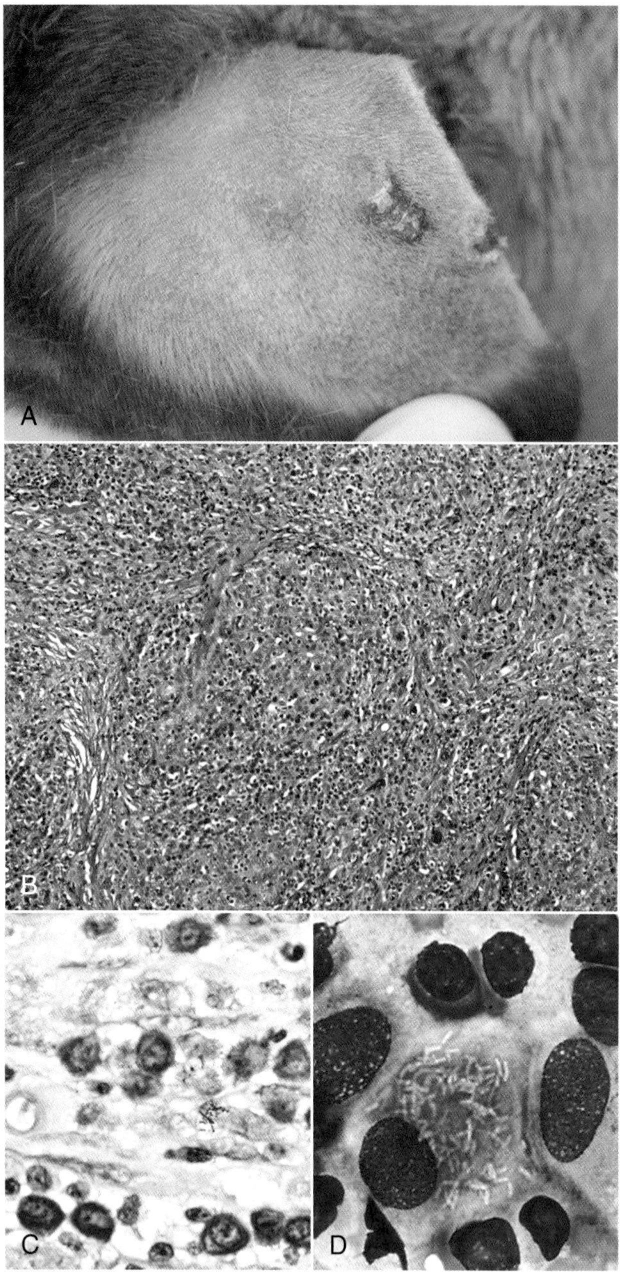

Figure 20-48 **Canine Leproid (Lepromatous) Granulomas, Auricle, Dog. A,** Several pyogranulomas are present in the subcutis of the convex surface of the external ear. Overlying skin is eroded or ulcerated; the leftmost ulcer has healed. **B,** The granulomas contain numerous large macrophages, many lymphocytes, fewer plasma cells and neutrophils. H&E stain. **C,** Higher magnification of **B**. Short to long acid-fast bacilli *(red color)*, some with a beaded structure, are present in the granulomatous exudate. Acid-fast stain. **D,** Fine-needle aspirate of a mass. In this cytologic preparation, there is a large macrophage that contains numerous bacilli consistent with a diagnosis of a canine leproid granuloma. Aqueous Romanowsky stain. (**A** courtesy Dr. D. Crow, Animal Dermatology Clinic, Dallas, TX. **B** courtesy Dr. B.L. Njaa, The Center for Veterinary Health Sciences, Oklahoma State University. **C** and **D** courtesy Dr. R.W. Allison, The Center for Veterinary Health Sciences, Oklahoma State University.)

and number of lymphocytes and plasma cells are highly variable, often scattered throughout, and more prominent along the deep edge of the mass. The morphologic features of the mycobacteria are not uniform and include filamentous to bacilliform forms, with or without beading, to coccoid forms. In contrast to rapidly growing mycobacteria of the Runyon group IV, which typically have discrete pyogranulomas centered on clear spaces that contain acid-fast–positive bacteria, this form is absent in leproid granulomas. In addition, caseous exudation and mineralization are not features typical of leproid granulomas. This condition is a self-limiting disease that typically resolves spontaneously within 6 months of the initial diagnosis. Neither regional lymph node involvement nor systemic disease has been reported. Short-haired dog breeds are predisposed to developing canine leproid granulomas with no sex predilection. Based on Australian studies, more than half of the cases were described in boxers and boxer crossbred dogs. In a much smaller North American study, German shepherds were overrepresented.

Chronic Otitis Media with Cholesterol Clefts (Cholesterol Granulomas)

The mucoperiosteum in chronic otitis media becomes expanded by granulomatous inflammation, granulation tissue formation, fibroplasia, invaginated glands, or pseudoglands and frequently contains cholesterol clefts (Fig. 20-49, *A*). The accumulation of cholesterol in these regions of chronic otitis media has been noted in many species, including dogs, cats, pigs, and cattle. Sources of cholesterol include cell membranes from necrotic cells, previous hemorrhage at the site, and surfactant. Therefore it should be considered inappropriate to designate exuberant granulation tissue with chronic inflammation, pseudoglands, and cholesterol clefts as cholesterol granulomas when this response is the prototypic mucoperiosteal reaction to chronic otitis media. Therefore chronic otitis media with prominent cholesterol clefts is preferred.

Furthermore, cholesterol granuloma and cholesteatoma are consistently confusing terms. Cholesterol granuloma in the middle ear is a designation that should be avoided because chronic otitis media typically is a combination of inflamed granulation tissue embedded with cholesterol clefts. Cholesteatoma should be avoided and replaced with tympanokeratoma, representing an epithelial cyst that originates from the tympanic membrane (refer to the next section). To add to this confusion, chronic otitis media commonly accompanies these lesions and is believed to play a role in the development of tympanokeratomas (see Fig. 20-49, *B*).

Miscellaneous Disorders

Tympanokeratoma (Aural Cholesteatoma)

Tympanokeratomas are epidermal cysts most commonly found in the middle ear of middle-aged to aged dogs, possibly more commonly in cocker spaniels (see Fig. 20-49). Although more commonly referred to as aural cholesteatomas, this term has its origins in very early literature referring to a "pearly" gross appearance. In fact, tympanokeratomas are benign cysts that arise from the epidermis of the tympanic membrane. By virtue of their location, concurrent otitis media, and expansile growth, they can be locally destructive and rarely lead by extension to meningitis.

Two main theories exist that account for the origin of these epithelial cysts. The first and least likely (referable to dogs) is the congenital theory in which embryonic epithelial rests are the genesis for their formation. However, the occurrence of otitis media and otitis externa in nearly all canine cases strongly supports cyst formation as an acquired change. The more likely pathogenesis is a combination of otitis media and otitis externa resulting in prolonged negative pressure within the middle ear, leading to deformity of and likely perforation or invagination of a portion of the tympanic membrane into the middle ear, forming a cyst lined by cornifying, stratified squamous epithelium. Because of the inherent epidermal migration of the external surface of the tympanic membrane, these cysts continue to expand as a result of continuous keratin

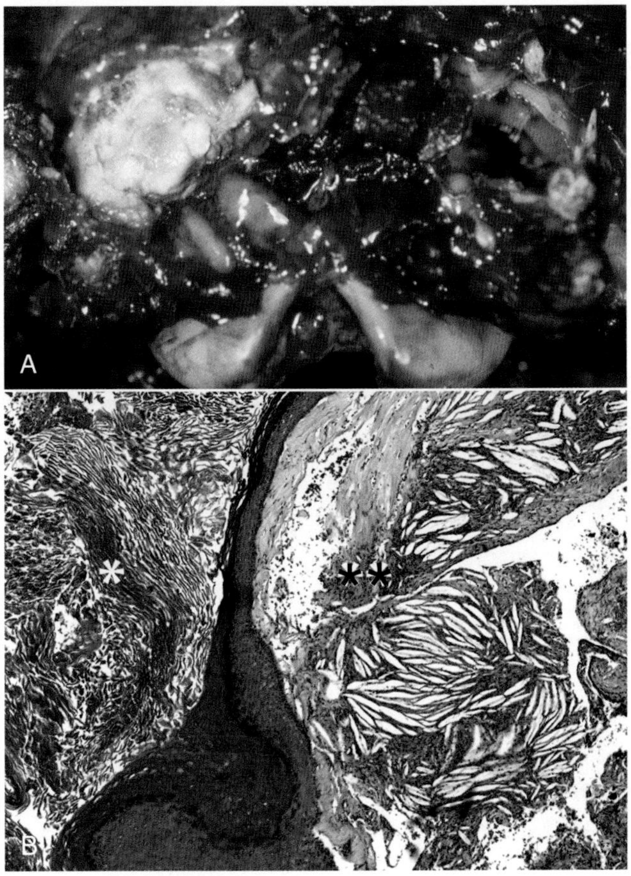

Figure 20-49 **Tympanokeratoma with Chronic Otitis Media, Dog.** **A,** Ventral-dorsal view. The right tympanic cavity is filled with layers of keratin and associated middle ear effusion obliterating the lumen. The left tympanic cavity is considered within normal limits. Numerous slender bony spicules with bulbous ends arising from the incomplete septum bulla represent mucoperiosteal exostoses in dogs. **B,** Histologic section of the right tympanic cavity depicted in **A**. The left half of the figure shows an epithelial-lined cyst filled with keratin flakes. This is a tympanokeratoma *(asterisk)*. The right half of the figure shows granulomatous inflammation and granulation tissue laden with acicular clefts (cholesterol clefts) *(double asterisks)*. Cholesterol clefts are a prototypic feature of chronic otitis media. Tympanokeratomas in dogs are typically associated with chronic otitis media. H&E stain. (**A** courtesy Dr. M. Rozmanec, College of Veterinary Medicine, Cornell University. **B** courtesy Ms. J.M. Cramer and Dr. A. Alcaraz, College of Veterinary Medicine, Cornell University.)

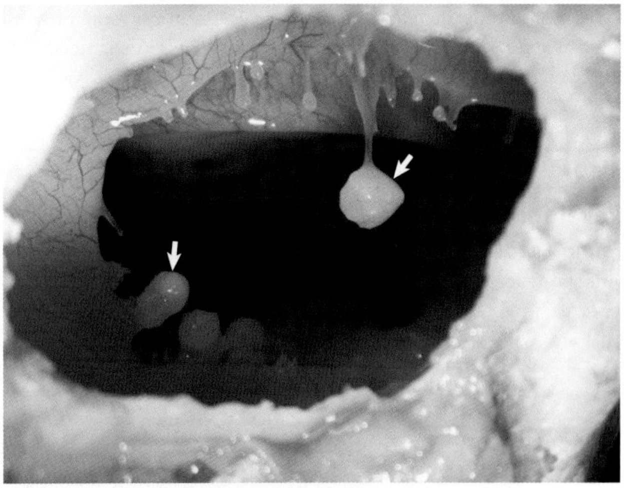

Figure 20-50 **Mucoperiosteal Exostoses, Dog.** Bony spicules extend from the incomplete septum bulla in a dog. These spicules may have sharp ends but often have bulbous ends *(arrows)*. This middle ear has no evidence of otitis media. (Courtesy Dr. B.L. Njaa, Center for Veterinary Health Sciences, Oklahoma State University.)

production. In addition, chronic otitis externa can lead to external acoustic meatal stenosis or obstruction, preventing the normal flow of keratin from the external tympanic membrane out the external acoustic meatus.

Macroscopically, these expansile cysts may have a layered, pearly appearance owing to the abundant laminated keratin. Expansion of the cyst within the middle ear can result in enlargement of the tympanic bulla, as well as bony lysis of bullae. Lysis of the petrous portion of the temporal bone may occur and when severe is associated with neurologic signs. Sclerosis or periosteal reactions of the ipsilateral temporomandibular joint is a common sequela.

Microscopically, tympanokeratomas are simple epidermal cysts commonly diagnosed elsewhere in the skin. The lumen contains abundant layers of keratin flakes. A band of well-vascularized fibrous connective tissue that may contain neutrophils, lymphocytes, and macrophages forms the wall of the cyst. Outside of the wall is mature granulation tissue, most likely a reparative response to chronic, recurrent otitis media. Cholesterol clefts may develop in concert with granulation tissue, which may lead to confusion and misdiagnosis as cholesterol granulomas.

Clinical signs are referable to concurrent otitis externa and otitis media and may include facial nerve palsy, head tilt, ataxia, nystagmus, and circling. Lesions are most typically unilateral. Hearing impairment may be (1) conductive in nature, owing to damage to the tympanic membrane or ossicular chain, or (2) sensorineural in nature, related to lysis of the petrous portion of the temporal bone. Temporomandibular joint involvement often results in pain when opening the mouth.

Craniomandibular Osteopathy

Craniomandibular osteopathy is a proliferative, nonneoplastic lesion affecting bones of the head, in particular of the tympanic bullae (see Chapter 16 for more detail). It is an autosomal recessive disorder of terrier breeds, especially West Highland white terriers. Macroscopically, tympanic bullae are markedly enlarged and filled with new bone. Typically a bilateral lesion, affected bullae fuse with the adjacent mandible, restricting movement of the mandible. Microscopically, normal lamellar bone undergoes osteoclastic resorption and is replaced by a primitive, coarse type of bone that expands beyond the normal confines of the periosteum. Lymphocytes, plasma cells, and neutrophils invade the periphery of the affected bone. Presumably, filling of tympanic bullae with new bone impairs hearing by interfering with auditory ossicular function; however, there is a paucity of confirmatory reports.

Mucoperiosteal Exostoses (Otolithiasis)

Bony spicules arising from incomplete canine septum bullae are poorly defined but referred to as mucoperiosteal exostoses. They appear spiny or may have bulbous ends (Fig. 20-50; see Fig. 20-49, A). The two reports that document this change refer to these bony concretions as otoliths secondary to otitis media, and this erroneous term persists in current editions of radiology texts. Otoliths or otoconia in mammals refer to calcium carbonate–rich crystals that overlay the sensory maculae of the sacculus and utriculus. The earliest report of this bony change is briefly addressed in the largest report on otitis media in dogs and was considered a uncommon change by the authors. However, based on experience, this change is found rather commonly in middle ears opened at autopsy that have no gross evidence of otitis media. Further investigation is needed to better characterize this feature in the middle ears of dogs.

Disorders of Cats

Developmental Anomalies

Feline Lysosomal Storage–Induced Microtia

Mucopolysaccharidosis (MPS) VI is a lysosomal storage disease reported most commonly in cats (see Chapter 14). Affected cats have mutations in their 4-sulfatase gene that leads to the accumulation of dermatan and chondroitin sulphate in lysosomes of cells. This accumulation is thought to lead to inhibition of other lysosomal enzymes and possibly the accumulation of other glycolipids. Aside from other features of facial dysmorphism, one characteristic of mucopolysaccharidosis VI is microtia or small auricles that are typically set lower on their heads (Fig. 20-51). The gross lesions can be extremely subtle unless a direct comparison is made to age-matched, unaffected cats. There are no histologic features specific to the auricles. Clinical disease is referable to neurologic symptoms (see Chapter 14).

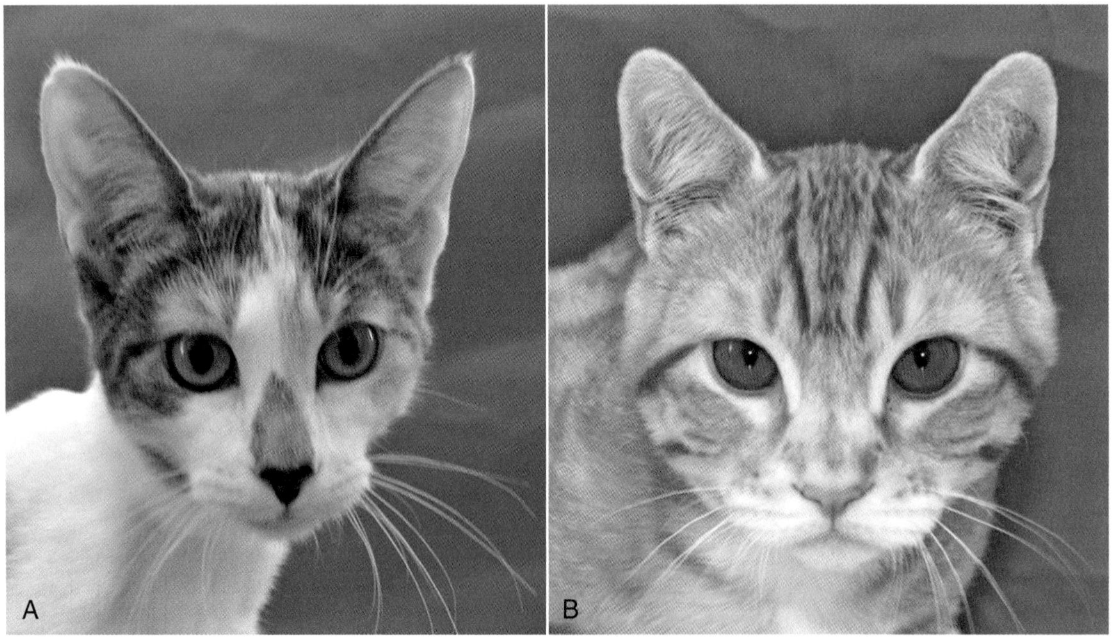

Figure 20-51 **Mucopolysaccharidosis VI, Cat. A,** Normal cat. **B,** Cat with mucopolysaccharidosis VI. The auricles in the cat with mucopolysaccharidosis VI are smaller than the normal cat. The bridge of the nose is also broader in the cat with mucopolysaccharidosis VI when compared with the normal cat. (Courtesy Dr. M.E. Haskins, School of Veterinary Medicine, University of Pennsylvania.)

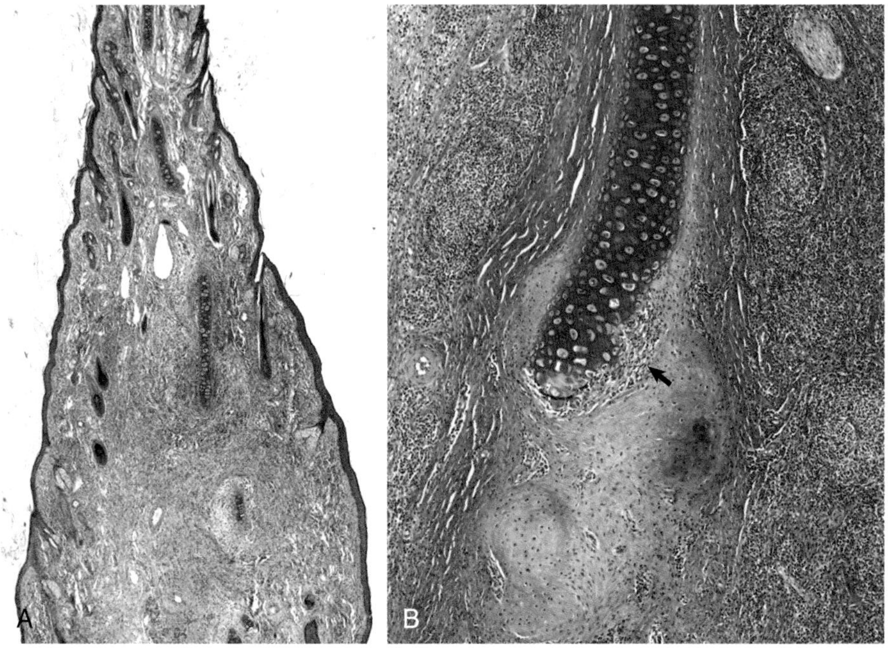

Figure 20-52 **Auricular Chondritis, Cat. A,** Histologic section of an auricle. The auricle is thickened and expanded by chronic inflammation, including lymphocytes, macrophages, and neutrophils. The auricular cartilage is incomplete, surrounded by inflammatory cells, and distinctly hypereosinophilic. Auricular cartilage is normally basophilic, but in auricular chondritis, auricular hyaline cartilage is brightly eosinophilic due to decreased matrical proteoglycans. H&E stain. **B,** Higher magnification of **A.** Auricular cartilage is brightly eosinophilic with multifocal regions of nascent, proliferative cartilage nodules. Abundant lymphocytes infiltrate the dermis and form multiple lymphoid follicles. Neutrophils *(arrow)* are shown invading and destroying the preexisting auricular cartilage. H&E stain. (Courtesy Ms. J.M. Cramer, College of Veterinary Medicine, Cornell University.)

Inflammation

Otitis Externa, Media, and Interna

See section on Disorders of Domestic Animals.

Auricular Chondritis (Relapsing Polychondritis)

Auricular chondritis is the auricular manifestation of a broader, rare inflammatory condition called relapsing polychondritis (RP). In human beings, relapsing polychondritis is thought to be caused by an immune-mediated response to type II collagen and matrilin 1 (MATN1), a cartilage matrix protein. In addition to auricular chondritis, human beings afflicted with relapsing polychondritis may have chondritis of the nose, larynx, trachea and bronchi, as well as conjunctivitis, episcleritis, keratitis, anterior uveitis, cardiovascular disease, and sensorineural hearing loss. Interestingly, ear lobes in human beings remain unaffected.

True relapsing polychondritis has been reported in cats positive for feline leukemia virus and in a single cat dying of lymphoma, raising speculation that other clinical signs may have been paraneoplastic phenomena. However, most affected cats manifest only auricular chondritis. Most cats are 3 years old or younger. Auricles are most often bilaterally swollen, erythematous, painful, pruritic, variably alopecic, and curled. Over time they can become permanently deformed, thickened, and firm. Microscopically, auricular cartilage is distorted and wrinkled rather than being a typical straight band caused by cartilage degeneration (Fig. 20-52). A virtually pathognomonic feature is a transformation of the normally basophilic hyaline cartilage to an eosinophilic matrix. Inflammation characterized by infiltration with lymphocytes, plasma cells, macrophages, multinucleated giant cells, and neutrophils is observed. Distinct lymphoid follicles may form in the periphery. In the severe chronic cases, auricular cartilage is necrotic with areas of regenerative or dysplastic chondroid nodule formation, neovascularization, and extensive fibrosis. A similar condition has been reported in a single dog.

Proliferative, Necrotizing Otitis Externa

A rare, unique condition of unknown etiology is proliferative necrotizing otitis externa that affects cats. Large, well-demarcated erythematous plaques develop over the concave auricular surface and are covered by thick, tan to brown keratinous debris (Fig. 20-53, *A*). These lesions may extend into and partially occlude the external acoustic meatus. Microscopically, these plaques are sharply demarcated from the adjacent normal skin. The key diagnostic features include (1) superficial acanthosis with pronounced hair follicle outer root sheath hyperplasia, (2) marked neutrophilic luminal folliculitis, (3) mild to moderate follicular hyperkeratosis, and (4) scattered individually necrotic keratinocytes of the outer root sheath of hair follicles (see Fig. 20-53, *B*). Cats may range from 2 months to 5 years of age. Lesions may cause no discomfort or mild pruritus and pain. Lesions typically resolve spontaneously.

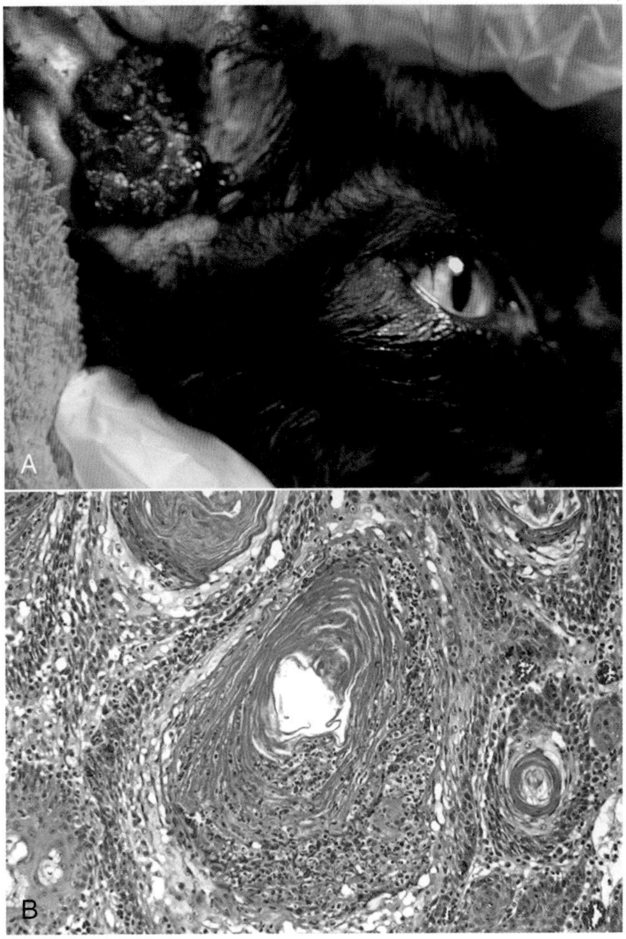

Figure 20-53 **Proliferative, Necrotizing Otitis Externa, Cat. A,** A large, thick proliferative mass grows from the inner, concave surface of the auricle and extends into the external acoustic meatus. **B,** The epithelium of the hair follicle is markedly hyperplastic and hyperkeratotic with luminal folliculitis. Numerous necrotic keratinocytes are present within the follicular lumen mixed with necrotic inflammatory cells and cellular debris. H&E stain. (Courtesy Dr. E.A. Mauldin, School of Veterinary Medicine, University of Pennsylvania.)

Parasitic Diseases

Mammomonogamus auris

Mammomonogamus auris, a strongyloid nematode, is a rare and regionally distinct cause of otitis media in cats of the Asian Pacific region. It is unknown how the adult nematode infects and spreads to and in the middle ears of affected cats. The tympanic membrane is not considered a portal of entry because it is always intact at the time of diagnosis. The need for an intermediate host has been speculated but as of yet has not been identified. However, after infection, some nematodes mature in the trachea, larynx, nasal sinuses, or middle ear and can readily pass in and out of these locations via the auditory tube, nasopharynx, and laryngopharynx. Frequently a unilateral infection with a single worm pair is observed, although bilateral infections occur and up to eight pairs have been recovered from middle ears of affected cats (Fig. 20-54). Samples of the middle ear have never been collected for microscopic or microbiologic examination. Most cats infected with *M. auris* are asymptomatic, although head shaking can be a feature of this disease.

Miscellaneous Disorders

Acquired Folding of the Auricle

Acquired folding of the auricle is a disease of sudden onset in adult cats. In nearly all cases, affected cats have a prolonged history of treatment with otic preparations containing glucocorticoids. Affected cats typically have biochemical evidence of iatrogenic adrenocortical insufficiency. The lesion consists of bilateral rostral and lateral folding of the distal or apical third of the auricles. They are cool and thin and appear to lack palpably normal cartilage. Histologic features have not been reported.

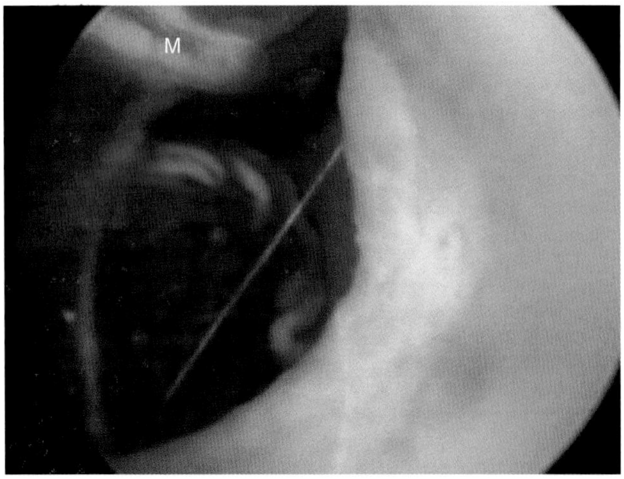

Figure 20-54 ***Mammomonogamus Auris,* Middle Ear, Cat.** *Mammomonogamus auris* is shown through the intact tympanic membrane using video-otoscopy. Manubrium of the malleus (M). (With permission from Tudor EG, Lee ACY, Armato DG, et al: *J Feline Med Surg* 10:501-504, 2008.)

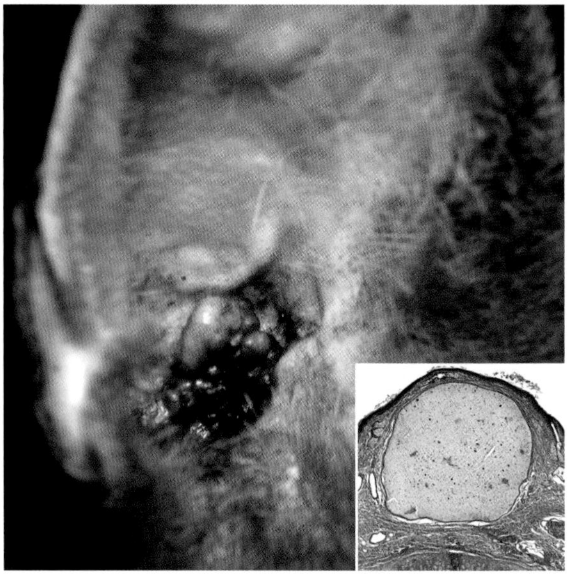

Figure 20-55 **Feline Ceruminous Cystomatosis, Auricle, Abyssinian Cat.** Multiple, dark gray to blue to black nodules aggregate along the concave surface of the auricle and are characteristic of feline ceruminous cystomatosis, a cystic dilation and hyperplasia of ceruminous glands. *Inset,* Cuboidal to flattened epithelial cells line the surface of the cyst. Ectatic lumens are filled with gray to basophilic secretion. H&E stain. (Figure courtesy B. Moyes and Dr. B. Milleson, Briarglen Veterinary Clinic, Tulsa, OK. Inset courtesy Dr. B.L. Njaa, Center for Veterinary Health Sciences, Oklahoma State University.)

Feline Ceruminous Cystomatosis

The cause of feline ceruminous cystomatosis is unknown. It is characterized by benign, cystic, nonneoplastic proliferation of ceruminous glands on the medial surface of the auricle, the base of the auricle, and extending to variable depths into the external acoustic meatus. These glands can be markedly dilated, clustered, and filled with brown to basophilic, inspissated ceruminous secretion. Their dark blue to black appearance can result in a misdiagnosis as melanocytic or vascular neoplasms (Fig. 20-55). Microscopically, ectatic glands and cysts can be massively dilated, surrounded by minimal to moderate plasmacytic and lymphocytic inflammation. Clinical signs vary from inapparent to progressive irritation of the ceruminous glands.

Neoplasms

Squamous Cell Carcinoma

See section on Disorders of Domestic Animals, Neoplasms of the External Ear and Fig. 20-35.

Suggested Readings

Information on this topic is available at www.expertconsult.com.

CHAPTER 21

The Eye[1]

Philippe Labelle

Key Readings Index

The eye is unique among organs in that its superficial anatomic location and the transparency of cornea allows for direct and detailed evaluation in the clinical setting. In fact, complete clinical examination of the eye in the living patient will generally provide as much or more information than evaluation at necropsy or gross assessment of an enucleated globe. Even in eyes in which corneal transparency is lost, the superficial location lends itself well to imaging modalities such as ultrasound. The complex terminology of ophthalmic pathology has roots in the terminology of clinical ophthalmology. Historical terms that are anatomically incorrect are widely used in both clinical and pathological settings. For example, "retinal detachment" is an acceptable diagnosis denoting the separation of the sensory neuroretina from the retinal pigment epithelium despite the fact that the two structures are part of the retina and are truly apposed rather than attached. The term "uveitis" in particular causes confusion between clinicians and pathologists. The histologic diagnosis of uveitis heavily relies on the infiltration of leukocytes in the uveal tract, whereas many of the clinical entities and processes diagnosed as uveitis represent vascular-mediated inflammation. Such clinical lesions can be difficult to evaluate histologically and may go unrecognized. For example, mild fibrin in the aqueous humor of the anterior chamber, easily diagnosed as aqueous flare clinically, may be difficult to appreciate grossly and may not be recognized histologically because the aqueous humor is not typically preserved during sectioning and processing. Furthermore, fibrovascular proliferation secondary to release of vascular mediators within the globe is often considered histologically as a separate event from inflammation with leukocytic infiltration. As such, both clinicians and pathologists must remember that the absence of leukocytes in the globe histologically is not incompatible with a clinical diagnosis of uveitis.

The embryologic development, general reactions to injury, and specific diseases vary significantly between the different components of the globe. There are some diseases affecting the eye as a whole, but most tend to affect one structure of/within the globe predominantly or exclusively. As such, the anatomic, physiologic, and pathologic features of the globe are usually presented separately for each portion: cornea and sclera, uvea, lens, vitreous, retina and optic nerve, and orbit. The features of eyelid, conjunctival, and orbital diseases are similar to those of skin, mucosa, and connective tissue elsewhere in the body, but there are particularities of periocular structures that warrant inclusion as part of a discussion on the eye.

All adult mammalian globes have similar general anatomy, depicted in Fig. 21-1. The globe is a spherical biologic camera with a transparent surface, an elaborate autofocus lens derived from surface ectoderm, and a light-absorbing retina created by an outgrowth of specialized neurons from the brain. The other structures within the globe and those adjacent to it mainly provide support to ensure the optimal function of the cornea, lens, and retina in order to maintain vision.

The eye develops as a outpouching of brain tissue that extends to the skin surface of the developing embryo. The eye's purpose is to gather sensory information in the form of photons of light, which is absorbed by neurons specifically adapted to convert light into electrical energy. To facilitate access by those photons to the light-sensitive neurons of the retina, the surface ectoderm, which elsewhere would normally form ordinary opaque skin, undergoes specialized differentiation into the cornea and lens as the tentacle of the brain comes into proximity with it. Details of embryogenesis are discussed in later sections of this chapter.

Ocular anatomy includes specific features that are particularly relevant to ocular pathology. The globe is a sealed, media-containing organ, which is protected from injury by a bony orbit and mobile eyelids. It has a thick fibrous outer shell of cornea and sclera, and a series of barriers and mechanisms intended to reduce bystander injury.

Proper visual function requires that very precise anatomic relationships be maintained among the constituent parts of the globe. Minor alterations that would be insignificant in most other tissues can have devastating results within the globe. For example, even mild accumulation of fluid behind the retina (serous retinal detachment) can result in blindness; repair with granulation tissue that can restore some function elsewhere can lead to opacity and loss of light perception.

Vision requires that the cornea, lens, and fluid media within the globe remain optically clear. This means that accumulation of

[1]For a glossary of abbreviations and terms used in this chapter, see E-Glossary 21-1.

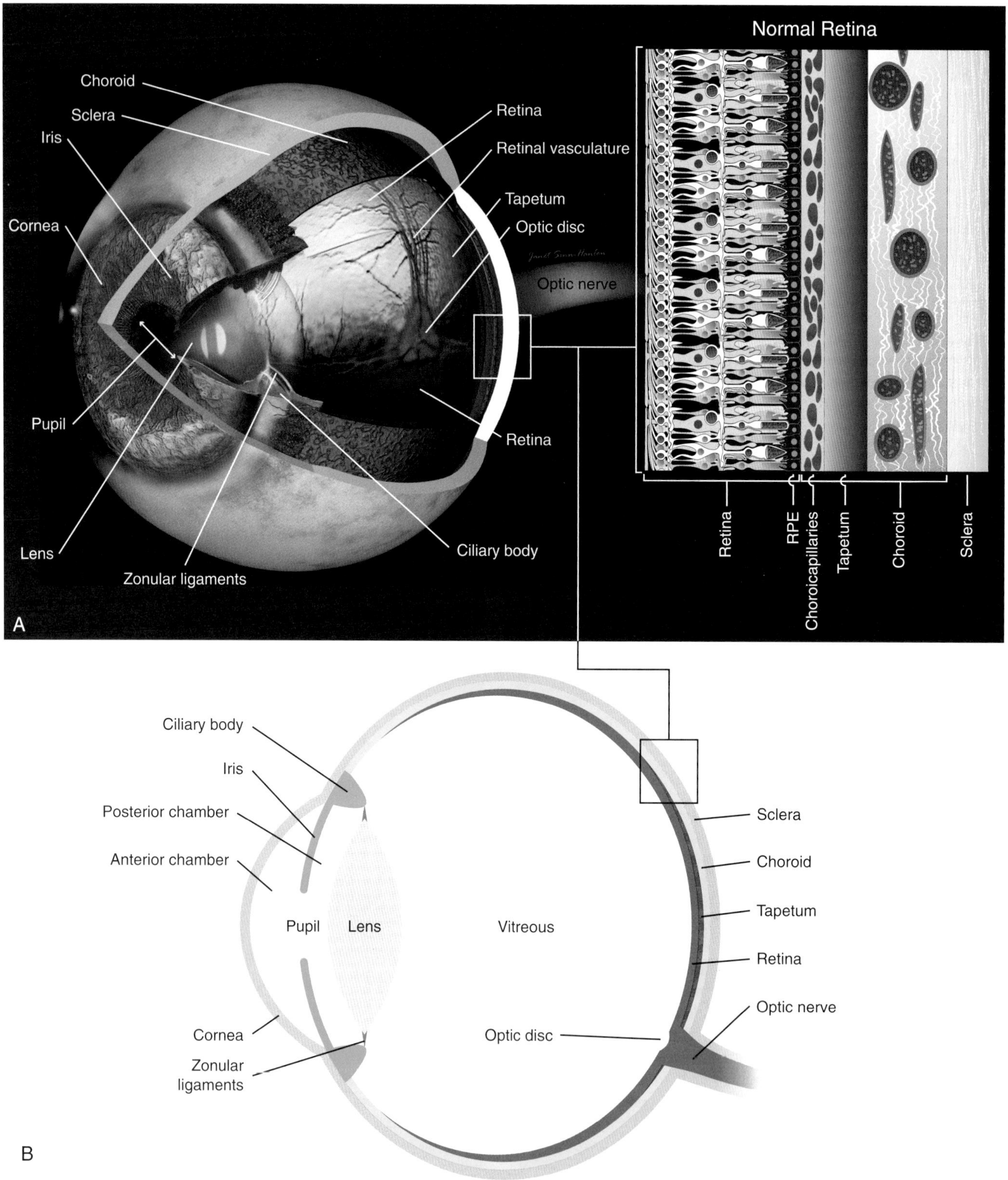

Figure 21-1 **Anatomy of the Eye with Details of the Posterior Segment. A,** The cornea and sclera form the fibrous tunic of the globe. The uvea is the vascular tunic of the globe. It is composed anteriorly of the iris and ciliary body, and posteriorly of the choroid. In some species the choroid dorsal to the optic nerve head includes a specialized layer called tapetum lucidum. The lens is positioned by the circumferential zonular ligaments and the pressure of the vitreous. The retina lines the posterior aspect of the globe, located internally to the choroid. The portion of the optic nerve internal to the sclera is the optic disc. *Inset,* The retina includes the neuroretina on the internal aspect and the retinal pigment epithelium *(RPE)*, which is derived from the outer layer of the optic cup. The retina is apposed to the choroid. **B,** Simplified diagram of ocular structures. Vision requires light to pass through the cornea and aqueous humor of the anterior chamber, within the pupil, and through the lens and vitreous to reach the retina. Light that reaches the retina will pass through multiple retinal layers to be absorbed by the photoreceptors. Light not absorbed by the photoreceptors may be reflected by the tapetum lucidum to further stimulate the photoreceptors. Light is then transduced to neuronal electric signals sent though the optic nerve to the brain. (**A** courtesy Ophthalmology Service and The Design Group, College of Veterinary Medicine, University of Illinois. **B** courtesy Dr. J.F. Zachary, College of Veterinary Medicine, University of Illinois.)

exudates or changes in refractive properties related to conditions such as edema and fibrosis are extremely detrimental to visual acuity. Responses intended to save the globe itself can cause loss of function, essentially defeating the purpose of protecting the globe.

Most of the visually critical tissues within the globe have limited to no regenerative capacity. Some, like the adult retina, are essentially postmitotic and cannot regenerate at all. Others, such as the lens and cornea, are capable of limited regeneration, but the regeneration almost never re-creates a perfect structural or functional replica of the original tissue. Many of the most significant intraocular lesions are related to events of healing, at times from very minor injuries. There are essentially no functionally insignificant lesions within the globe because every injurious event has a visual consequence even if the degree of impairment is not easily measured or depends on a cumulative effect.

The same unique features of ocular anatomy and physiology that serve to protect the globe from injuries affecting other parts of the body also render the globe vulnerable to the propagation of injury once those defenses have been overcome. The same defenses that prevent entry of various types of chemical or biologic agents also prevent or limit drainage of dangerous by-products of tissue injury and inflammation. The fluid media within the globe allows diffusion of infectious toxic agents and chemical mediators of inflammation throughout the globe.

Ocular bystander injury occurs when injury to one component of the globe "spills over" and affects other parts of the globe. Many diseases that predominantly affect one portion of the globe can also cause significant functional impairment by extension in adjacent components. Examples include the following:

- Inflammatory effusion from choroiditis, which can cause retinal detachment
- Alteration in aqueous humor composition and flow, which can lead to cataracts
- Chemical mediators of wound healing in chronic uveitis that stimulate corneal stromal vascularization and fibrovascular proliferation
- Fibrovascular proliferation in turn can cause tractional retinal detachment or glaucoma secondary to pupillary block or peripheral anterior synechia

Structure and Function

Embryology

The globe has a complex embryogenesis involving carefully orchestrated interactions of neuroectoderm, surface ectoderm, and periocular mesenchyme throughout embryogenesis and in early life (Fig. 21-2). In carnivores the ocular development continues into the fifth or sixth week after birth. As such, not all developmental errors are congenital, especially in carnivores. Because the globe is not essential for in utero survival, both mild and severe ocular congenital anomalies are encountered in otherwise normal patients. Selective breeding practices have increased the frequency of ocular anomalies. Those that are important or prevalent are discussed in sections dealing with diseases of the specific ocular segment affected.

The eye begins very early in gestation as an outgrowth from the primitive neural tube ectoderm, essentially the primitive forebrain. This primary optic vesicle grows outwardly from the brain toward the overlying surface ectoderm, remaining connected to the brain by the optic stalk. As the primary optic vesicle approaches, the overlying ectoderm will focally thicken to form the lens placode. The lens placode thickens, invaginates, and separates from the surface ectoderm migrating inwardly as the lens vesicle to indent the spherical optic vesicle. As the lens vesicle pushes into that optic vesicle, the optic vesicle collapses and invaginates to form a bilayered optic cup. When the lens vesicle separates from the surface ectoderm, that ectoderm re-forms to eventually become corneal

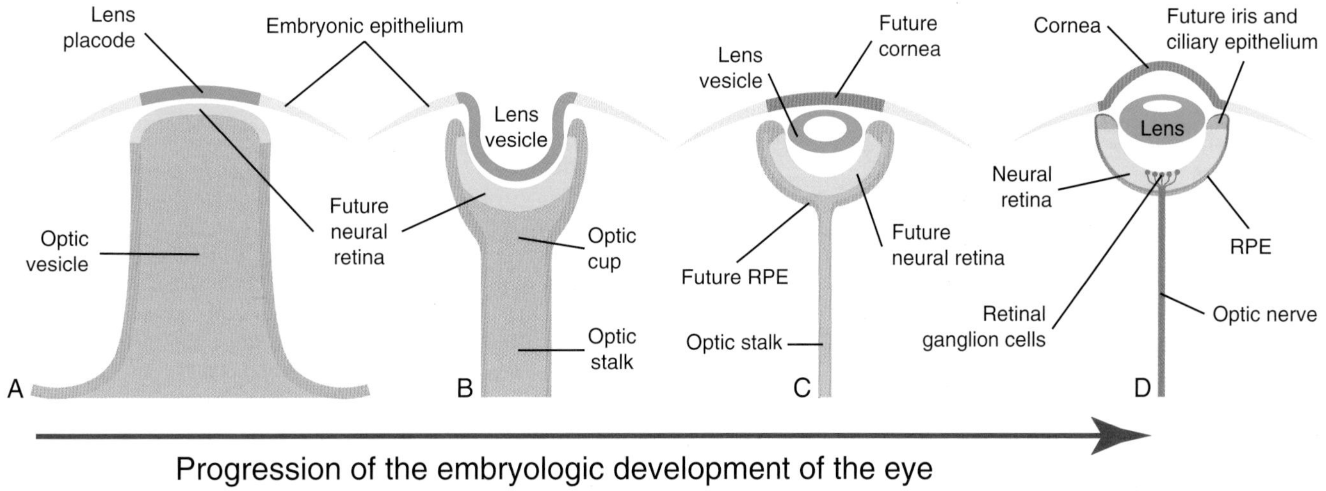

Figure 21-2 **Embryologic Development of the Eye. A,** The primitive neural tube ectoderm forms the primary optic vesicle as an outgrowth. The primary optic vesicle migrates from the brain toward the overlying surface ectoderm while remaining connected to the brain by the optic stalk. The overlying ectoderm will thicken to form the lens placode. **B,** The lens placode thickens and invaginates to form the lens vesicle, eventually pushing into the optic vesicle. The optic vesicle also invaginates to form the bilayered optic cup. **C,** The lens vesicle separates from the surface ectoderm, which re-forms to become the corneal epithelium. The inner layer of the optic cup will progress to form the inner and outer neuroblastic layers and eventually differentiate into the neuroretina. The retinal pigment epithelium *(RPE)* originates from the pigmented outer layer of the optic cup. **D,** Retinal ganglion cells first develop within the inner neuroblastic layer formed by the inner layer of the optic cup. The iris and ciliary body epithelium develop from the anterior rim of the optic cup: The nonpigmented epithelium arises from the inner layer and the pigmented epithelium from the outer layer of the optic cup. The optic nerve is formed by the axons of the ganglion cells and elements of the optic stalk. (Courtesy Dr. P. Labelle, Antech Diagnostics, and Dr. J.F. Zachary, College of Veterinary Medicine, University of Illinois.)

epithelium. The presence of the corneal epithelium seems to stimulate one or more waves of periocular mesenchyme that forms the primitive corneal stroma and endothelium. This periocular mesenchyme is derived from the neural crest and eventually also forms the sclera, the uveal stroma, and a well-developed but transient intraocular network of blood vessels (hyaloid artery and tunica vasculosa lentis) that nourish the developing retina and lens (Fig. 21-3). Following lens placode induction, the inner layer of the optic cup will progress to form the inner and outer neuroblastic layers. These neuroblastic layers will eventually differentiate to form the neuroretina. The retinal pigment epithelium (RPE) originates from the pigmented outer layer of the optic cup. Differentiation of the neuroretina beyond the neuroblastic layers requires a functional RPE. The eyelids, extraocular muscles, lacrimal gland, and orbit mostly develop independent of the globe and are generally not affected by those diseases that impair development of the eye itself.

In the adult globe of domestic animals, only the corneal epithelium and lens epithelium are derived from the surface ectoderm. The neuroretina, retinal pigment epithelium, posterior iris epithelium, iris dilator and sphincter muscles, and ciliary epithelium are derived from the neural ectoderm. The neural crest is the origin of the corneal stroma, corneal endothelium, uveal stroma, ciliary muscle, and trabecular cells. The mesoderm provides the vascular endothelium.

Eyelids and Conjunctiva

The first line of defense for the globe includes the eyelids, conjunctiva, and the soft tissues and bones of the orbit. These create a protective physical barrier against outside forces as well as extension of diseases from surrounding structures (e.g., nasal cavity, oral cavity). This protective wall allows light penetration, but it excludes the many elements of the external environment that might injure the structures responsible for vision (cornea, lens, and retina).

The diseases of the eyelids, conjunctiva, and orbit tend to mimic those of similar tissues at other sites and have fewer unique pathologic features than those of the globe itself. However, the diseases of these structures, the eyelid and conjunctiva in particular, represent a significant proportion of ocular conditions in clinical ophthalmology.

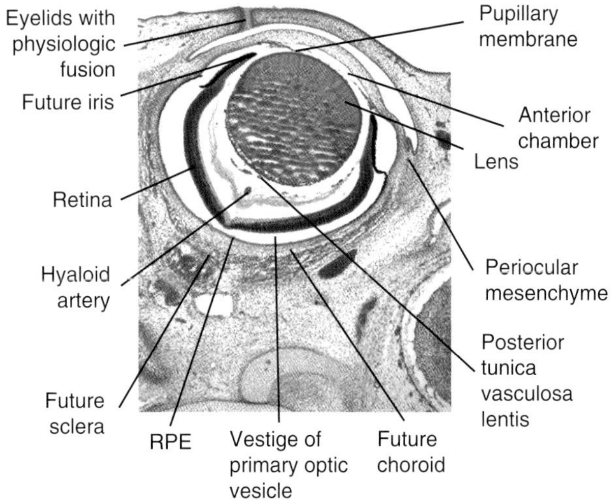

Figure 21-3 Fetal Globe, Gestational Age Day 34, Dog. The periocular mesenchyme is organizing to form the choroid and sclera. The anterior chamber has been formed, but the anterior lip of the optic cup has not yet folded inwardly to induce the formation of the iris and ciliary body. The relatively large lens is surrounded by a rich vascular tunic derived from the hyaloid artery and pupillary membrane. *RPE*, Retinal pigment epithelium. H&E stain. (Courtesy Dr. B. Wilcock, Ontario Veterinary College.)

Eyelids

The epithelium of the eyelids develops from the surface ectoderm adjacent to the cornea. After separation of the lens vesicle, the surface ectoderm regains continuity to form the cornea. Ectoderm at the periphery of the cornea then migrates over the surface of the embryonic cornea, accompanied by underlying periocular mesenchyme to form the eyelids. The ectoderm forms the surface epithelium and glands; the accompanying periocular mesenchyme forms the dermis and the eyelid muscles. These ingrowing eyelids fuse over the central cornea. This fusion provides a physical protection to the globe and provides the immature cornea with a sterile environment in which to complete its embryologic development. Physiologic ankyloblepharon or fusion of the eyelids in the postnatal period is normal in dogs and cats, and it persists 10 to 15 days allowing tear production to reach adequate levels.

The mature eyelids are movable folds of skin that slide across the surface of the cornea on a film of mucus and fluid known as the tear film. This blinking movement serves to help distribute the protective tear film across the corneal surface and to remove unwanted particulate debris from the corneal surface. Each eyelid has an anterior surface of haired skin, with all of the adnexal glands as seen in skin at other sites. The dermis is modified by the addition of striated muscle (orbicularis oculi and levator muscles). The inner surface of the eyelid, which apposes the cornea and bulbar conjunctiva, is covered by a mucous membrane known as the palpebral conjunctiva (see Conjunctiva below). The transition between the eyelid skin and palpebral conjunctiva is termed the eyelid margin. The eyelid margin is characterized by several rows of large modified hairs (eyelid cilia/eyelashes), which serve a direct protective purpose. The cilia are largest and most numerous along the margin of the upper eyelid; they may be infrequent or absent along the lower eyelid. The eyelid margin also includes a row of large modified sebaceous glands known as meibomian glands (or tarsal glands). The meibomian glands produce meibum, which forms the superficial lipid layer of the tear film that prevents evaporation and aids in the dispersal of the aqueous component of the tear film.

Conjunctiva

The conjunctiva is a mucous membrane extending from the palpebral margin of the eyelid to the periphery of the cornea. The conjunctiva is continuous from the inner surface of the eyelid to the surface of the globe. The portion of conjunctiva that covers the posterior surface of the eyelid is the palpebral conjunctiva, and the portion attached to the surface of the globe and continuous with the peripheral cornea at the limbus is the bulbar conjunctiva.

The conjunctival epithelium includes goblet cells, melanocytes, dendritic cells, and other leukocytes. The palpebral conjunctiva is composed of stratified squamous nonkeratinizing epithelium near its origin at the eyelid margin. Most of the palpebral conjunctival consists of stratified columnar epithelium with variable numbers of goblet cells. The bulbar conjunctiva extends over the globe and merges with the corneal epithelium at the limbus. The epithelium of the bulbar conjunctiva lacks goblet cells. At the junction between bulbar conjunctiva and corneal epithelium, there is a population of germinal cells that are the permanent replicative cells of the corneal epithelium (stem cells). They are the source of replacement corneal epithelial cells in both physiologic processes and pathologic responses.

The space between the palpebral and bulbar conjunctiva is the conjunctival sac. The space between the upper and lower eyelid is known as the palpebral fissure. The medial (nasal) limit of the palpebral fissure (where the upper and lower eyelids are continuous) is the medial canthus. The lateral (temporal) margin of the palpebral fissure is the lateral canthus.

The substantia propria of both the palpebral and bulbar conjunctiva resembles the lamina propria of any other mucous membranes. It consists of well-vascularized loose connective tissue. There are both diffuse lymphoid tissue and lymph nodules (mucosa-associated lymphoid tissue [MALT] and conjunctiva-associated lymphoid tissue [CALT]) in the substantia propria. The CALT responds immunologically to the microbial flora within the conjunctival sac.

The ventral conjunctiva, as it transforms from palpebral to bulbar conjunctiva, undergoes an additional specialization to form the third eyelid (nictitating membrane). This large fold of conjunctiva protrudes from the ventral-medial canthus over the anterior surface of the cornea and contains a central supporting plate of cartilage and a stroma of dense fibrous tissue, containing an accessory lacrimal gland (gland of the third eyelid). Both its anterior and posterior surfaces are covered by stratified squamous nonkeratinizing epithelium. In most domestic species, its movement is passive, serving to cover the globe and provide an extra level of protection when the globe is retracted into the orbit by the retractor bulbi muscle.

Cornea and Sclera

The cornea and sclera form the fibrous tunic of the globe. The cornea is the anterior third of the fibrous tunic. At the limbus the cornea merges with the conjunctiva and sclera. The cornea and sclera provide structural support for the globe. In addition, the cornea allows light penetration and therefore vision by its transparency. The cornea has four histologic layers (Fig. 21-4; E-Fig. 21-1):

- Corneal epithelium and basement membrane
- Corneal stroma
- Descemet's membrane, the basement membrane of the corneal endothelium
- Corneal endothelium

The tear film is a clinically important functional layer that covers the corneal epithelium, but it cannot be evaluated histologically. The cornea is 0.5 to 0.8 mm thick, depending on species, regions of the cornea, and age. The corneal epithelium, the anterior most layer, is derived from fetal surface ectoderm and consists of stratified nonkeratinizing epithelium that includes surface (nonkeratinized squamous) cells, intermediate (wing) cells, basal cells, and a basement membrane. The corneal epithelium is 5 to 7 layers thick in dogs and cats and approximately 8 to 15 layers thick in larger animals. The corneal epithelium is completely renewed every 5 to 7 days. The corneal stroma represents roughly 90% of the corneal thickness. The corneal stroma is composed of rare keratocytes, which are modified fibroblasts. The keratocytes are interspersed between the collagen fibrils that form parallel lamellae. The stroma also contains abundant water and the extracellular matrix composed of glycoaminoglycans and other components. The corneal stroma lacks blood vessels. The posterior (inner) surface is covered by a single layer of cuboidal epithelial cells, known as the corneal endothelium, which like the stroma is derived from periocular mesenchyme. The basement membrane of the corneal endothelium, termed Descemet's membrane, lies between the stroma and endothelium and is easily recognizable histologically. The corneal endothelium in adults of most domestic mammals is postmitotic and has no or limited ability to replicate.

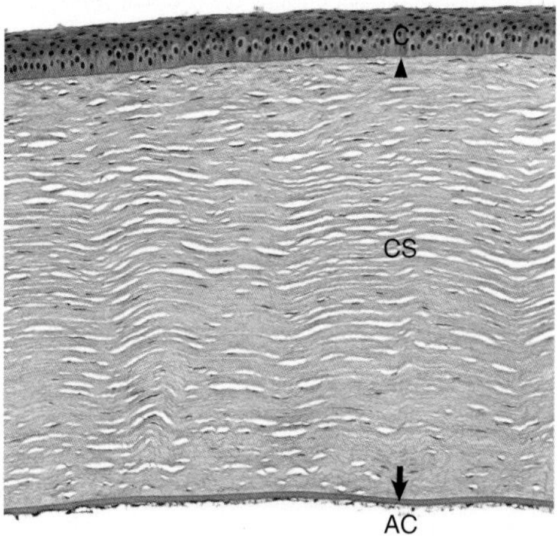

Figure 21-4 **Normal Cornea, Dog.** The cornea has four histologic layers. The corneal epithelium (C) and its basement membrane *(arrowhead)* is the most anterior layer and is composed of basal cells, intermediate cells, and surface cells. The corneal stroma (CS) includes only rare cells called keratocytes but represents approximately 90% of the thickness of the cornea. Descemet's membrane *(arrow)* is the basement membrane of the corneal endothelium. The corneal endothelium is a single layer of cells that separates the aqueous humor of the anterior chamber (AC) from the corneal stroma. The tear film is a functionally important layer that covers the corneal epithelium, but it cannot be evaluated histologically. H&E stain. (Courtesy Dr. P. Labelle, Antech Diagnostics.)

Box 21-1 Factors That Contribute to Corneal Transparency

- Smooth and continuous surface formed by the tear film and corneal epithelium
- Nonkeratinizing, nonpigmented epithelium
- Narrow diameter of the collagen fibrils
- Parallel lamellar arrangement of the collagen fibrils
- Orthogonal arrangement of collagen fibrils in adjacent lamellae
- Low cell density of the stroma
- Relatively dehydrate state of the stroma
- Avascular stroma

Corneal transparency is essential for vision and is the result of a number of anatomic and physiologic features listed in Box 21-1. The corneal epithelium differs from that of the conjunctiva or skin in that there is no keratinization or pigmentation. The corneal stroma resembles conjunctival substantia propria or dermis, but it lacks blood vessels, hair follicles, glands, and leukocytes. The narrow collagen fibrils are arranged in compact lamellae separated by a space that corresponds to the wavelength of visible light. Thus the cornea allows the passage of light without any scattering. To further facilitate the unimpaired passage of light, the corneal stroma is maintained in a dehydrated state compared with that of most other tissue. That dehydrated state is maintained passively by intercellular junctions within the corneal epithelium and endothelium, which exclude water from the tear film and anterior chamber, respectively. It is further maintained by the active removal of solutes (and thus fluid) by energy-dependent sodium potassium membrane pumps within the corneal endothelium. The corneal stroma lacks blood vessels, and the cornea is dependent on the tear films, conjunctival and scleral vessels, and the aqueous humor for nutrition and oxygen.

The sclera represents most of the fibrous tunic of the globe. It consists of three layers. The outermost layer is the episclera, which is a densely vascularized fibrous layer that connects Tenon's capsule to the sclera proper. The sclera proper (scleral stroma) consists of densely packed collagen with elastic fibers, fibroblast, as well as proteoglycans and glycoproteins. The innermost layer is the lamina fusca, which contacts the choroid. Blood vessels and peripheral nerves use channels within the sclera to vascularize and innervate to the uveal tract. The scleral venous plexus that provides some of the outflow for the aqueous humor is located in the anterior aspect of the sclera, within the sclera proper. On the posterior aspect of the sclera, there is a specialized fenestrated area termed lamina cribosa, which allows the axons of the retinal ganglion cells to exit the globe and form the optic nerve.

Uvea

The uvea, or uveal tract, is the vascular tunic of the globe. It is divided into three portions: the iris, ciliary body, and choroid. The iris and ciliary body form the anterior uvea, and the choroid may be termed posterior uvea. The uveal tract contains virtually no resident lymphoid tissue and lacks true lymphatic vessels.

The anterior aspect of the iris consists of a layer of modified stromal cells. Most of the iris consists of connective stroma with blood vessels and nerves. Variable numbers of melanocytes are dispersed in the stroma, mostly in the posterior stroma. Irides of blue eyes have noticeably fewer melanocytes than brown irises. There are two smooth muscle groups within the iris, the constrictor and dilator muscles, which control the size of the pupil and therefore light penetration. The posterior aspect of the iris consists of a layer of neuroepithelium termed posterior iris epithelium, which is continuous with its counterpart in the ciliary body. In horses and ruminants, the posterior iris epithelium forms a nodular and cystic structure termed corpora nigra in horses and granula iridica in ruminants. This protrusion of neuroepithelium further contributes to the control of light penetration.

The ciliary body extends from the base of the iris to the junction with the choroid and retina. The ciliary body consists of connective stroma with blood vessels and nerves and a prominent smooth muscle, the ciliary muscle, which is aligned along a meridional plane. This muscle allows accommodation through changes in the position or shape of the lens, and contraction of the muscle increases the drainage of aqueous humor through the trabecular meshwork. The anterior portion of the ciliary body includes numerous (70 to 100) processes or folds (pars plicata) that are absent in the posterior portion (pars plana). The ciliary body is lined by two layers of neuroepithelium (Fig. 21-5). The inner layer is nonpigmented, whereas the outer layer is pigmented. The ciliary epithelium, specifically the nonpigmented epithelium, contributes to aqueous humor production through both filtration and active transport mediated processes such as the carbonic anhydrase pathway. The ciliary epithelium provides the extracellular matrix that forms the zonular ligaments that suspend the lens and also produces the hyaluronic acid incorporated in the vitreous.

The iridocorneal angle is delimited anteriorly by the pectinate ligament, which extends from the anterior base of the iris to the inner peripheral cornea at the termination of the Descemet's membrane (Figs. 21-6 and 21-7). In the dog and cat, the normal pectinate ligament is difficult to evaluate histologically because the fibers are more slender and more widely dispersed than in other domestic species. Horses and ruminants have robust pectinate ligaments. The pectinate ligaments of pigs are intermediate between those of carnivores and those of herbivores. The iridocorneal angle also includes a network of trabeculae termed ciliary cleft and corneoscleral trabecular meshwork that allow drainage of aqueous humor. The ciliary cleft lies posterior to the pectinate ligament and consists of widely separated collagen beams lined by trabecular cells. The corneoscleral trabecular meshwork is embedded in the inner sclera. It is similar in composition to the ciliary cleft but has smaller trabeculae and smaller intertrabecular spaces.

The choroid is the posterior portion of the uvea and lies between the retina and sclera. The innermost layer is the choriocapillaris, a thin layer of capillaries delimited on the inner aspect by a basement membrane (Bruch's membrane). The choriocapillaris provides nutrition to the outer retina. The choroidal stroma is the middle layer and includes numerous blood vessels supported by connective

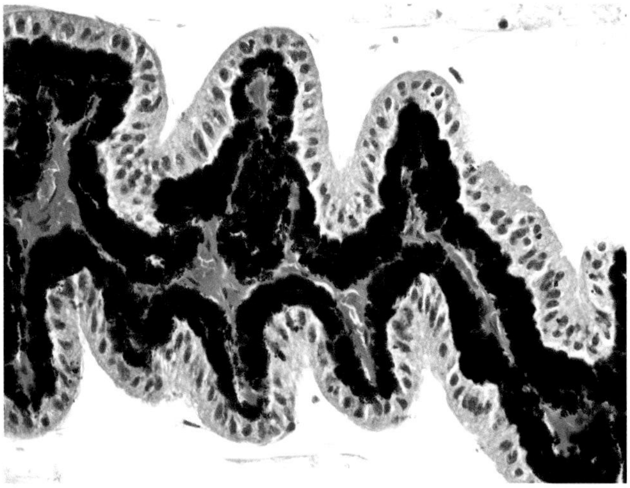

Figure 21-5 **Normal Ciliary Process, Horse.** The ciliary body is lined by a bilayered epithelium (neuroepithelium). The innermost layer, which communicates with the posterior chamber, is nonpigmented. The outer layer is pigmented. H&E stain. (Courtesy Dr. P. Labelle, Antech Diagnostics.)

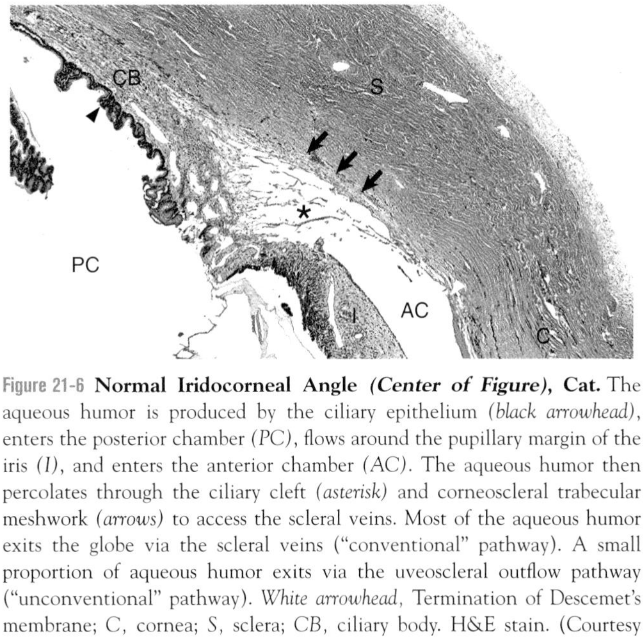

Figure 21-6 **Normal Iridocorneal Angle *(Center of Figure)*, Cat.** The aqueous humor is produced by the ciliary epithelium *(black arrowhead)*, enters the posterior chamber *(PC)*, flows around the pupillary margin of the iris *(I)*, and enters the anterior chamber *(AC)*. The aqueous humor then percolates through the ciliary cleft *(asterisk)* and corneoscleral trabecular meshwork *(arrows)* to access the scleral veins. Most of the aqueous humor exits the globe via the scleral veins ("conventional" pathway). A small proportion of aqueous humor exits via the uveoscleral outflow pathway ("unconventional" pathway). *White arrowhead,* Termination of Descemet's membrane; *C,* cornea; *S,* sclera; *CB,* ciliary body. H&E stain. (Courtesy Dr. P. Labelle, Antech Diagnostics.)

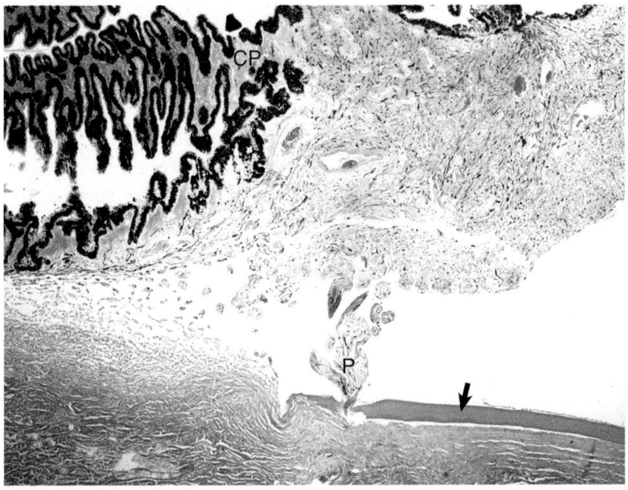

Figure 21-7 **Normal Iridocorneal Angle, Horse.** Horses and ruminants have robust pectinate ligaments *(P)*. *Arrow,* Descemet's membrane; *CP,* ciliary processes. H&E stain. (Courtesy Dr. P. Labelle, Antech Diagnostics.)

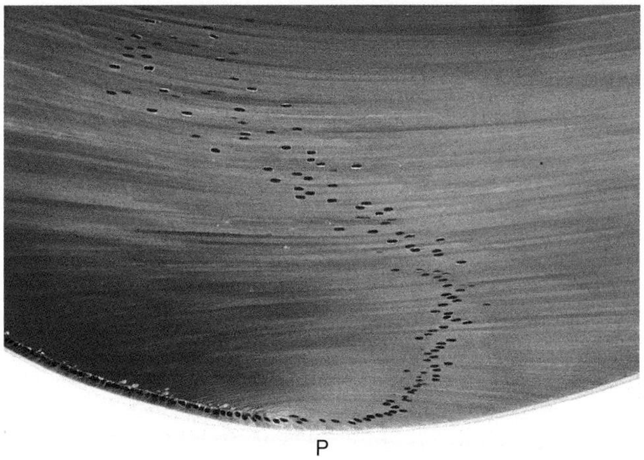

Figure 21-8 **Normal Lens, Rabbit.** The lens epithelium forms a single layer underlying the anterior lens capsule. At the equator, the lens epithelium migrates inwardly to form the lens bow. There is no lens epithelium along the posterior lens capsule *(P)*. (Courtesy Comparative Ocular Pathology Laboratory of Wisconsin.)

stroma that is typically heavily pigmented. In domestic species except the pig, the inner aspect of the choroidal stroma includes the tapetum lucidum. The tapetum lucidum is a specialized layer located only dorsal to the optic nerve in domestic animal species and serves to reflect light that has already passed through the retina further stimulating the photoreceptor cells and improving vision in low light. Domestic carnivores have a cellular tapetum lucidum composed of regularly arranged cells containing reflective rods suggestive of modified melanocytes. Domestic herbivores have a fibrous tapetum lucidum composed of regularly arranged collagen fibers and only rare fibrocytes. The pig does not have a tapetum lucidum. The outer aspect of the choroidal stroma includes larger vessels. The suprachoroid is the outermost layer of the choroid and provides the transition between the choroid and sclera.

Lens

The purpose of the lens is to refract light on the retina and provide focus. The lens is a biconvex, avascular, transparent accumulation of elongated epithelial cells. It is located posterior to the iris and anterior to the vitreous. It is suspended by the zonular ligaments (zonules, zonular fibers) formed by the ciliary epithelium and held in position in part by the presence/pressure of the vitreous. The relative size, shape, and elasticity vary significantly between species and to a lesser extent with age. The lens capsule is the basement membrane of the lens epithelium. It is composed of predominantly type IV collagen and is produced throughout life by the lens epithelium. The lens capsule is impermeable to large proteins but allows diffusion of water and electrolytes that nourish the lens epithelium. The lens contains only one cell type, the lens epithelium, which forms a single layer of cuboidal epithelial cells just internal to the anterior lens capsule. Epithelium is absent from the posterior surface of the lens. At the lens equator, the epithelial cells are mitotically active and more columnar. The cells migrate inwardly, rotate, and elongate to become lens fibers (Fig. 21-8). The lens fibers elongate to reach opposite poles of the lens. As the cells differentiate, they lose most of their cytoplasmic organelles and lose their nuclei. The lens fibers are arranged in layers with interdigitations of their plasma membranes and gap junctions that allow each lens fiber to adhere tightly to adjacent fibers. The lens epithelium arises from the surface ectoderm and expresses cytokeratin early during embryogenesis, but the mature lens epithelium expresses vimentin, a filament typically found in mesenchymal cells.

The lens epithelium produces new lens fibers throughout life. As new fibers are produced, there is a progressive increase in the density at the center of the lens (lens nucleus), which is formed by the oldest lens fibers. The lens is avascular and dependent on the aqueous humor for transport of nutrients and removal of cellular waste products. Lens metabolism is primarily via anaerobic glycolysis and the hexokinase pathway. There is limited aerobic glycolysis via the citric acid pathway. Glucose is delivered by the aqueous humor and is absorbed across the lens capsule.

The purpose of the lens is to further refract light that has passed through the cornea and to focus that light onto the retina. As such, the lens must remain transparent and in its proper location within the pupillary aperture. Lens transparency depends on the precise orientation of the lens fibers, the scarcity of cytoplasmic organelles, unique intracellular crystalline proteins, and on the maintenance of a state of dehydration. This dehydration is maintained primarily by excretion of electrolytes through an active sodium-potassium–dependent adenosine triphosphatase pump, located mostly in the membranes of anterior lens epithelium and in the lens fibers. The location of the lens within the pupillary aperture is maintained by the circumferential zonular ligaments that extend from the ciliary body to the lens equator. Contraction and relaxation of the ciliary muscle alters the tension on the zonular ligaments, resulting in changes in the shape or position of the lens, thus facilitating accommodation/focus.

Vitreous

The vitreous is an optically clear elastic hydrogel. It is a modified extracellular space, not a cavity, and represents approximately 80% of the volume of the globe. It is composed almost entirely of water (99%). The remaining 1% consists mostly of collagen, hyaluronic acid, and widely dispersed cells called hyalocytes. Little is known about the production and turnover of the vitreous humor. The ciliary epithelium produces the hyaluronic acid and other components. Nonneuronal cells of the retina may also contribute. The collagen fibers form a complex network and provide attachment to the adjacent structures including the posterior lens capsule, ciliary epithelium, internal limiting membrane of the retina, and optic nerve head. The hyalocytes are thought to have secretory and phagocytic functions and are the source of fibroblasts in healing responses. Along the anterior surface of the vitreous is a shallow depression known as the hyaloid fossa, in which lies the posterior surface of the lens. The anterior surface of the vitreous undergoes condensation to form the anterior hyaloid membrane, which separates the vitreous from the aqueous humor. The vitreous seems to function mainly to maintain the shape of the globe, help support the lens and retina in normal positions, and provide some cushioning against blunt trauma.

Retina and Optic Nerve

The retina transduces visible light into electrical neuronal impulses, which are transmitted to the visual cortex of the brain. Light passes through the transparent cornea, ocular media, and lens to reach the photoreceptors of the retina. The photoreceptors, the rods and cones, contain photopigment that helps convert light energy in neuronal signals. The electrical signal generated by activation of the photopigment is transmitted in a stepwise manner from the outer nuclear layer to the neurons of the inner nuclear layer, then to the ganglion cells, and finally via the nerve fiber layer to the optic nerve and brain. The number of photoreceptors linked to a single ganglion cell varies greatly among species and is one of the variables determining visual acuity and the efficiency of low-light vision. In all domestic animals except the pig, light not absorbed by the photoreceptors is reflected by the tapetum lucidum to stimulate the photoreceptors a second time. The tapetum lucidum is therefore assumed to be a choroidal adaptation to increase the efficiency of vision in low light. The retina lines the posterior aspect of the globe with the exception of the optic nerve head. It lies between the vitreous and choroid. The neuroretina is not attached to the retinal pigment epithelium (RPE) and/or choroid except at the optic disc and at its very periphery, where it becomes continuous with the epithelium of the pars plana of the ciliary body (the site of transition is known as the ora ciliaris retinae).

The retina includes three layers of neurons (ganglion cell layer, inner nuclear layer, and outer nuclear layer) separated by cell-free layers created by the intermingling of the axons and dendrites of those neurons. The cell types found in the retina include five types of neurons: ganglion cells, bipolar cells, horizontal cells, amacrine cells, and photoreceptors (rods and cones). The retina also includes nonneuronal Müller glial cells. The rods and cones transmit the neuronal signal through the bipolar cells to the ganglion cells. Horizontal and amacrine cells modulate the signal. Müller cells are nonneuronal glial cells that provide support for the retina.

Histologically, the retina is separated in 10 layers (Fig. 21-9). The 9 internal layers comprise the neuroretina (neurosensory retina). The inner limiting membrane is a basement membrane that includes the inner processes of Müller cells. The nerve fiber layer consists of the axons of the ganglion cells. The axons are arranged parallel to the retinal surface and continue to form the optic nerve. The axons exit the globe through a series of perforations, known as the lamina cribrosa, present within the sclera at the posterior pole of the globe. The axons within the nerve fiber layer are unmyelinated in order to maintain transparency. In most species, axons become myelinated at about the level of the lamina cribrosa as they exit the globe. The ganglion cell layer consists of the cell bodies of the ganglion cells and occasionally includes displaced amacrine cells, and it is only one cell layer thick throughout the retina except the central retina (area centralis). The density of ganglion cells varies between species but is lowest in the peripheral retina. The inner plexiform layer is composed of synapses including those between retinal ganglion cells and both bipolar and amacrine cells. There are also synapses between bipolar and amacrine cells. The inner nuclear layer includes the nuclei of the bipolar, horizontal, and amacrine cells. The nuclei of the nonneuronal Müller cells are also within the inner nuclear layer. The outer plexiform layer is composed of synapses between the photoreceptors (rods and cones) and the bipolar and horizontal cells as well as synapses between the adjacent photoreceptors. The outer nuclear layer includes the nuclei

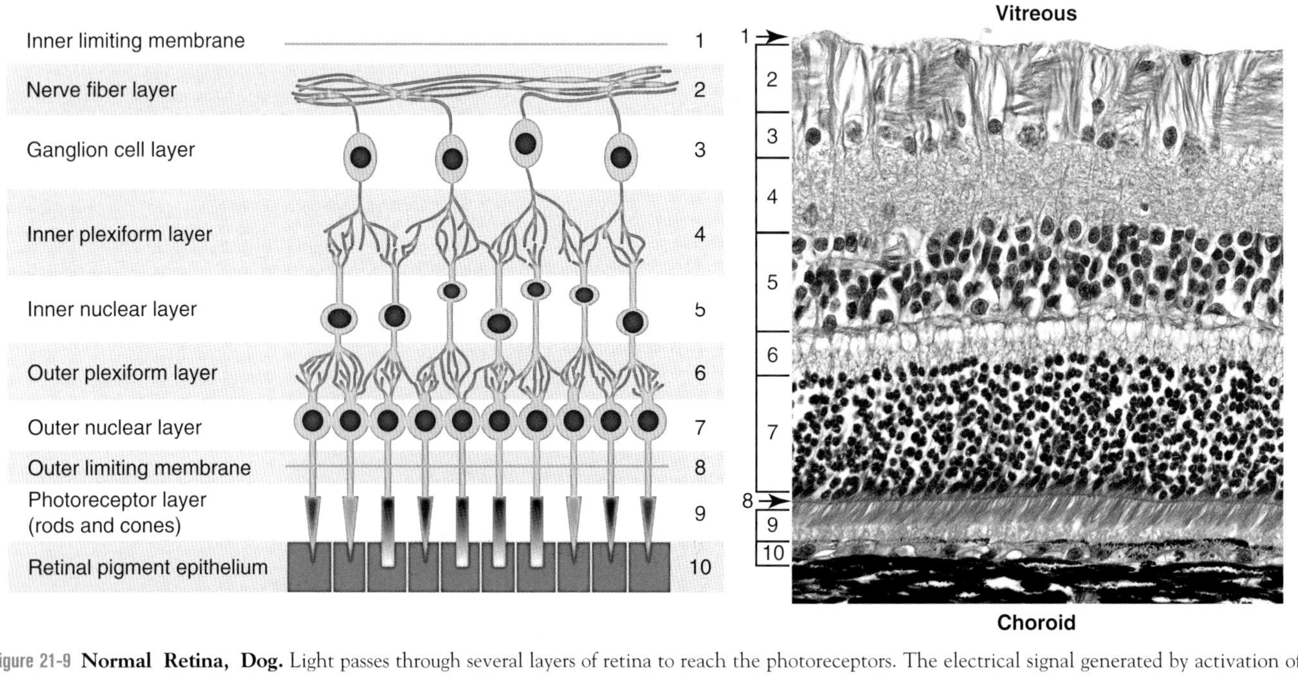

Figure 21-9 **Normal Retina, Dog.** Light passes through several layers of retina to reach the photoreceptors. The electrical signal generated by activation of the photopigment within the photoreceptors is transmitted from the outer nuclear layer to the neurons of the inner nuclear layer, then to the ganglion cells, and finally via the nerve fiber layer to the optic nerve and brain. (Courtesy Dr. E.A. Driskell and Dr. J.F. Zachary, College of Veterinary Medicine, University of Illinois.)

of the photoreceptors. The outer limiting membrane is not an actual structure and is not a basement membrane. It is a band formed by tight junctions between cell membranes of photoreceptors and Müller cells. The outer limiting membrane is a barrier between the potential subretinal space and the outer nuclear layer. The photoreceptor layer is composed of the inner and outer segments of the rods and cones. The inner segments include the cells organelles. The outer segments contain the photopigments where light is converted into a neuronal signal. The retinal pigment epithelium (RPE) is the outermost layer of the retina. It is a single layer of cells continuous with the pigmented ciliary epithelium and located between the neuroretina and choroid. The RPE has a different embryology than the neuroretina and is not directly involved in vision. The photoreceptors are embedded into crevices within the surface of the adjacent RPE, but there are no actual cellular junctions. As such, the potential subretinal space where edema, hemorrhage, and inflammatory cells can accumulate is the remnant of the lumen of the primary optic vesicle and is delimited by the tight junctions between the RPE cells and the outer limiting membrane. The clinically termed "subretinal space" is technically within the retina, not subretinal. The RPE that overlies the tapetum lucidum (dorsally) is nonpigmented, and the RPE may also lack pigment in color-dilute animals. In the pig, which lacks a tapetum lucidum, the RPE is diffusely pigmented. The RPE supports photoreceptor function by reactivating spent photopigments. It also phagocytoses portions of the photoreceptor outer segments that are shed as part of normal renewal. The RPE transports nutrients to the outer retina and removes waste products. It also scavenges free radicals and has antioxidant properties.

In domestic species, the retina has a dual blood supply. Blood vessels within the retina supply the inner aspect, whereas the outer retina, specifically the photoreceptors, is supplied by the choroidal vasculature. The presence of blood vessels makes inner retinal ischemia quite rare, whereas ischemia of the outer retina, which depends on diffusion from choroidal vessels, is more common. In fact, it is expected with retinal detachment. The distribution of blood vessels within the retina varies considerably between species. In domestic ruminants, pigs, and carnivores, the retina contains blood vessels throughout most of the retina (holangiotic pattern). In horses only the area adjacent to the optic disc is vascularized; the remainder of the retina is avascular (paurangiotic pattern), increasing the dependence on choroidal supply. Histologically, blood vessels may be present within the nerve fiber, ganglion cell, and inner plexiform layers.

The optic nerve is the continuation of the nerve fiber layer of ganglion cell axons into the optic chiasm and brain and uses the preexistent tube formed by the embryonic optic stalk (Fig. 21-10). The portion of the optic nerve within the sclera that includes axons, myelin, and supporting glial cells forms the optic nerve head (optic disc [E-Fig. 21-2]). The axons of the retinal ganglion cells exit the globe through a series of perforations, known as the lamina cribrosa, present within the sclera at the posterior pole of the globe. In most species, axons become myelinated just prior to or just after crossing the lamina cribrosa. In dogs, the myelin extends several millimeters within the sclera or internal to the lamina cribrosa, and this extension is responsible for the prominence of the optic disc in that species. The optic nerve is an extension of the brain rather than a true peripheral nerve. The myelin is produced by oligodendrocytes instead of Schwann cells (see Chapter 14).

Orbit

The bony orbit surrounds most of the globe, except the cornea, and separates the globe from the brain. Along its posterior border are numerous foramina through which blood vessels and nerves reach or leave the globe. The orbit is formed by the fusion of five to seven bones, depending on the species. It is a complete bony shell, except in dogs, cats, and pigs, in which the dorsal roof of the orbit is formed only by the supraorbital ligament that extends from the frontal bone to the zygomatic bone, leaving the dorsal orbit incomplete. The orbit contains the globe itself but also the extraocular muscles, abundant fat, lacrimal gland, zygomatic salivary gland, and all the muscles and nerves that support these structures.

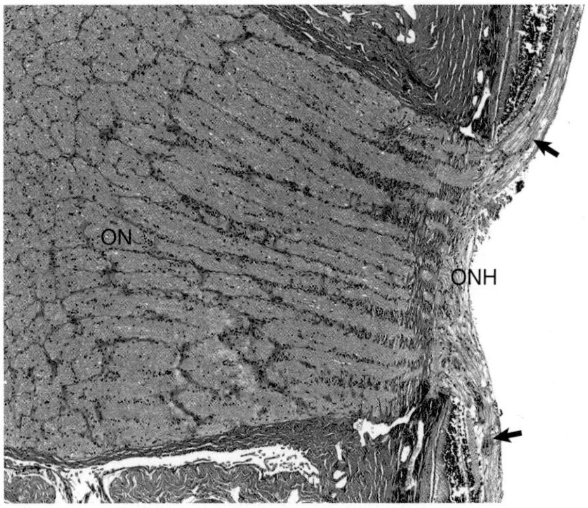

Figure 21-10 Normal Optic Nerve, Dog. The optic nerve *(ON)* is formed by the convergence of the axons *(arrows)* of the ganglion cells, which exit the globe through perforations known as the lamina cribosa. The portion of the optic nerve interior to the lamina cribosa is the optic nerve head (optic disc *[ONH]*). (Courtesy Dr. P. Labelle, Antech Diagnostics.)

The lacrimal gland is a specialized serous salivary gland located in the orbit, dorsolateral to the globe. Along with the histologically similar gland of the third eyelid, it is responsible for the production of the serous component of tears. It empties through 15 to 20 small excretory ducts at the lateral part of the fornix of the superior conjunctival sac.

Dysfunction/Response to Injury

Eyelids and Conjunctiva

Eyelids

The eyelids respond to insult in a manner similar to that of haired skin elsewhere on the body (see Chapter 17). Infections, immune-mediated diseases, and neoplasms with a predilection for the head and neck may affect the eyelids directly or by extension. The eyelids are most often involved as part of multicentric skin diseases or affected by diseases that could affect other areas of skin. The few inflammatory diseases and neoplasms that have a predilection for the eyelids are described later under specific diseases.

Although the responses of the eyelids mimic those of haired skin elsewhere, there may be vision-threatening consequences to altered eyelid structure and function. Changes to the shape of the eyelids as a result of inflammation, fibrosis/scarring, or neoplasia may interfere with proper eyelid closure and function. This may cause inappropriate exposure of the conjunctiva and cornea, changes to tear film distribution and contents, or inability to properly protect the globe from injury. The abnormal eyelid may cause mechanical injury with direct contact to the cornea. There may also be extension of eyelid inflammation or neoplasia to the adjacent conjunctiva or cornea.

Conjunctiva

The reaction of conjunctiva to injury is comparable to that of other mucous membranes. The normal conjunctival surface flora may be altered with conjunctival disease as well as corneal disease. The conjunctival epithelium responds to acute injury with necrosis leading to erosion or ulceration. Chronic injury may cause hyperplasia, squamous metaplasia and keratinization, decrease or increase in the number of goblet cells, and hyperpigmentation. The underlying substantia propria (conjunctival submucosa) typically responds to acute injury with edema and hyperemia. Neutrophils may be present if there is epithelial ulceration. Almost any cause of chronic conjunctival injury will result in the infiltration of lymphocytes and plasma cells in the substantia propria (nonspecific lymphoplasmacytic conjunctivitis). Lymphoid hyperplasia may be present in some chronic conditions, notably in horses, and those lymphoid nodules may become large and easily recognizable clinically. Eosinophils are a feature of hypersensitivity disease/allergic conjunctivitis and foreign body reactions in dogs, cats, and horses, and often numerous with parasitic infections (habronemiasis in horses and onchocerciasis in dogs and cats). Macrophages may infiltrate the conjunctiva with parasitic disease, foreign body injury, and some idiopathic inflammatory disease such as nodular granulomatous episcleritis in dogs. Fibrosis/scarring is the end result of some cases of severe conjunctival injury and healing, and it may interfere with eyelid function as noted previously depending on extent and location. Chronic sun exposure may cause solar elastosis and other forms of solar damage in the superficial substantia propria as it does in the dermis.

Cornea

The cornea responds to injury in a variety of manners, but most diseases provoke a few common processes that may be seen in combination (Box 21-2).

Epithelial and/or Stromal Necrosis

Because most of the corneal injuries are from external insults, the corneal epithelium is most commonly affected. Epithelial necrosis is typically the result of acute injury from trauma, severe dessication, chemical burn, and less frequently infectious diseases. Minor injuries may cause only erosions, but more severe damage will cause full-thickness loss of epithelium (corneal ulcers). There is immediate osmotic absorption of water from the tear film in the anterior stroma after corneal ulceration, resulting in focal superficial stromal edema. Corneal ulcers imply the exposure of the underlying stroma, which can be detected clinically with the use of water-soluble dyes such as fluorescein. Neutrophils from the tear film will rapidly infiltrate the area to protect the cornea against opportunistic infection and provide growth factors for subsequent wound healing. Small uncomplicated lesions with minimal stromal involvement will heal by sliding and proliferation of the epithelium (see Corneal Wound Healing).

Corneal injuries that extend beyond the epithelium will also cause stromal necrosis, recognized clinically as keratomalacia. This is most commonly seen in rapidly progressing ulcers contaminated with bacteria or fungi but may also be observed in sterile wounds. Many organisms produce enzymes that cause stromal necrosis. Furthermore, neutrophils will migrate from the tear film and limbus in large numbers and release lytic enzymes also contributing to the stromal destruction and resulting in neutrophil-induced suppurative keratomalacia. These ulcers, clinically termed melting ulcers, will progress rapidly over just a few days. Corneal healing in those instances will require fibrotic repair. The most severe cases will cause full-thickness stromal necrosis exposing Descemet's membrane. Descemet's membrane may bulge anteriorly into the defect created by the loss of the overlying stroma and epithelium to create a descemetocele. In the absence of immediate medical intervention, this typically leads to rupture of Descemet's membrane (perforating ulcer), leakage of aqueous humor from the anterior chamber, and possibly iris prolapse.

Corneal Edema

Corneal edema (stromal edema) is the presence of excess fluid and alteration of glycoaminoglycans contents within the stroma leading to separation of lamellae and decreased transparency. The causes of stromal edema are numerous, and edema may be present with injury to the epithelium, the stroma itself, or the endothelium (Box 21-3). Any injury that results in interruption of the corneal epithelium may cause stromal edema from osmotic absorption of fluid from the tear film. The excess fluid should be removed by the actions of the endothelium after reepithelialization of the defect. Inflammation/infiltration of leukocytes that reach stroma from the surface, conjunctiva, or anterior chamber may be accompanied by edema. Neovascularization of the stroma from ingrowth of blood vessels at the limbus often results in edema, as new immature vessels tend to be leaky. The corneal endothelium is critical to maintaining the stroma's dehydrated state. The endothelium uses energy-dependent sodium potassium transport pumps to transfer solutes in the anterior chamber (with fluid leaving by osmosis). Cellular tight junctions act as a physical barrier to prevent extension of fluid from the aqueous humor in the stroma. Any injury to the corneal endothelium may cause edema from absorption of fluid from the aqueous humor or decreased ability to respond to edema secondary to epithelial or stroma injury. Common causes of endothelial injury include contact between the lens and corneal endothelium from anterior lens luxation, glaucoma, and intraocular inflammation (leukocytic infiltration).

Corneal Neovascularization

Corneal neovascularization (stromal neovascularization) is the ingrowth of blood vessels from the limbus in the corneal stroma.

Box 21-2 Corneal Responses to Injury

- Epithelial necrosis
- Stromal necrosis
- Corneal edema
- Corneal neovascularization
- Corneal degenerations and depositions
- Corneal inflammation (keratitis)
- Nonspecific chronic keratitis with epidermization
- Corneal wound healing
- Corneal fibrosis/scarring (fibrotic repair)

Box 21-3 Causes of Corneal Edema

- Interruption of the corneal epithelium
- Ulceration
- Penetrating trauma
- Stromal injury
- Inflammation
- Neovascularization
- Disruption or dysfunction of the corneal endothelium
- Anterior lens luxation
- Increased intraocular pressure (glaucoma)
- Primary corneal endothelial dystrophy
- Intraocular inflammation

Because the normal stroma is avascular, stromal neovascularization is always considered a pathologic response. Most instances of corneal neovascularization follow a predictable series of events (Box 21-4).

The potential causes of corneal neovascularization are wide ranging and include trauma (both accidental and surgical), inflammation, infection, degenerative conditions, and others. Corneal neovascularization is primarily mediated by vascular endothelial growth factor (VEGF) in most instances; however, other growth factors may play a role depending on the cause. Following the initiating event, there is a period of latency during which VEGF levels will increase. The latent period lasts approximately 24 hours. This is followed by dilation of limbal blood vessels, which can be recognized clinically and precedes corneal neovascularization. For vascular sprouting to occur there will be multifocal enzymatic digestion of the basement membrane of the limbal vessels accompanied by endothelial cell proliferation. The endothelial cells will then migrate in the direction of the initiating cause, usually dissecting parallel to the corneal stromal lamellae. The growing sprouts become tubes with a lumen followed by adjoining of nearby sprouts to form vascular loops with blood flow. Assuming the initiating cause persists, vessels providing both the afferent and the efferent blood flow will mature into recognizable small arterioles and venules. The process of corneal neovascularization can be interrupted if the initiating cause is removed or controlled. Conversely, the framework of corneal neovascularization may persist for an extended period of time after the initiating cause is removed and blood flow has ceased ("ghost vessels"). These remnant vessel walls may become easily engorged with blood with only mild stimulus and in the absence of new vessel formation. Clinically and histologically, corneal neovascularization is generally characterized as superficial, midstromal, or deep. The distribution of the vessels typically corresponds to the origin of the initiating cause (superficial vs. deep). Midstromal neovascularization can be seen secondary to uveitis, even in the absence of any other overt corneal disease.

Corneal Degenerations and Depositions

A variety of conditions, both inherited and acquired, may cause the accumulation or deposition of excess material within the cornea. Most examples in veterinary medicine represent the deposition of lipids or minerals. Specific examples are discussed under Diseases of the Cornea.

Corneal Inflammation (Keratitis)

Neutrophils are typically the main leukocyte in acute keratitis. Almost any cause of chronic corneal injury will result in the infiltration of lymphocytes and plasma cells in the stroma. Eosinophils are uncommon in the cornea and are usually seen with specific conditions (see Eosinophilic Keratitis).

Box 21-4 Events in Corneal Neovascularization

1. Initiating cause
2. Latent period
3. Dilation of blood vessels at the limbus
4. Dissolution of the basement membrane of capillaries and venules
5. Vascular endothelial cells proliferation
6. Vascular endothelial cell migration toward the initiating cause
7. Formation of a solid sprout, formation of the lumen, and merging of adjacent sprouts
8. Maturation

Nonspecific Chronic Keratitis with Epidermalization. Nonspecific chronic keratitis with epidermalization (cutaneous metaplasia) is an adaptive response to mild but persistent corneal injury. These changes inevitably result in loss of corneal transparency; however, the purpose is to maintain corneal integrity and avoid eventual rupture as a consequence of chronic injury. The most common causes of mild chronic irritation are tear film abnormalities and mechanical irritation. Tear film abnormalities that result in desiccation include diseases such as keratoconjunctivitis sicca, improper distribution of tears because of abnormal eyelid structure or function, and any condition that prevents the eyelids from closing properly (lagopthalmos). Mechanical irritation may be secondary to eyelid diseases such as entropion or eyelid neoplasia, anomalous distribution/direction of eyelashes (distichiasis and trichiasis), or friction from the nasal skin folds. Unlike acute injuries discussed previously, mild persistent irritation does not cause necrosis. The corneal response to mild chronic injury is a stereotypical pattern of epithelial and stromal changes (Fig. 21-11; E-Figs. 21-3 and 21-4). The epithelial changes of nonspecific chronic keratitis consist of hyperplasia with rete peg formation, melanosis, and keratinization. The combination of these changes has been termed corneal epidermalization or cutaneous metaplasia because the corneal epithelium acquires features expected with the skin's epidermis. Corneal melanosis results from centripetal migration of limbal melanocytes and melanin accumulation within the corneal basal cells. The stromal changes of nonspecific chronic keratitis consist of superficial neovascularization and fibrosis. There may be infiltration of inflammatory cells, most often lymphocytes and plasma cells. There may also be significant pigmentary incontinence (leakage of melanin from the epithelial basal cells) resulting in superficial stromal melanosis from pigment accumulation in macrophages and fibroblasts. Not all examples of nonspecific chronic keratitis involve the entire range of adaptive changes; it is possible, for example, to have keratinization without melanosis or epithelial changes without accompanying stromal fibrosis and neovascularization. Some of the lesions of nonspecific chronic keratitis are reversible if the underlying cause can be removed, although there may be permanent loss of transparency. Clinically these changes may be recognized simply as "chronic keratitis" or "pigmentary keratitis" if the changes include melanosis. Nonspecific chronic keratitis that includes melanosis should not be

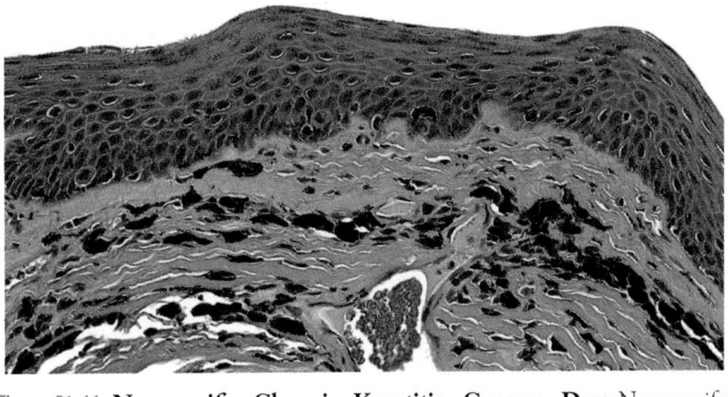

Figure 21-11 **Nonspecific Chronic Keratitis, Cornea, Dog.** Nonspecific chronic keratitis with epidermalization is an adaptive response to long-standing corneal injury. The epithelial changes include hyperplasia and melanosis, and some cases also include keratinization (note the thickened corneal epithelium containing melanin pigment). The stromal changes include pigmentary incontinence (i.e., melanin in the stroma and within macrophages), fibrosis, and neovascularization. Infiltration of lymphocytes and plasma cells is also a frequent finding. H&E stain. (Courtesy Dr. P. Labelle, Antech Diagnostics.)

Chronology of corneal wound healing

	0 hours	12 hours	24 hours	48 hours to > 48 hours	Months to years
Epithelium	• Latent phase • Epithelial cell migration			• Surface closure • Proliferation and return to normal thickness • Attachment to the basement membrane	
Stroma	• Edema • Apoptosis of local keratocytes • Infiltration of neutrophils	• Keratocyte migration • Proliferation of keratocytes and transformation to fibroblasts and myofibroblasts • Collagen and extracellular matrix production	• Infiltration of macrophages	• Myofibroblast and inflammatory cell apoptosis/necrosis • Chronic remodeling and return to normal-near normal state	
Endothelium			• Endothelial cell migration	• Secretion of a new Descemet's membrane	

Figure 21-12 **Chronology of Major Events in Corneal Healing.** (Courtesy Dr. P. Labelle, Antech Diagnostics, and Dr. J.F. Zachary, College of Veterinary Medicine, University of Illinois.)

confused with pigmentary keratopathy of some brachiocephalic breeds such as the pug in which corneal melanosis occurs in the absence of persistent irritation.

Corneal Wound Healing. Skin has provided the model for most basic wound healing studies (see Chapters 3 and 17). Although some of the principles involved in skin wound healing can be applied to the cornea, there are significant differences. Some differences are mechanistic, but, more important, the desired outcome in corneal wound healing includes transparency. The dermis and corneal stroma are analogous, but the corneal stroma has unique and specialized properties, including the parallel lamellar arrangement of the small-diameter collagen fibrils, the low cell density, lack of blood vessels, and relative dehydrate state (see Box 21-1). These specializations are essential for corneal function and transparency. The requirement for such precise structural organization constrains the corneal stroma to undergo a more deliberate homeostatic remodeling than the dermis of the skin and most other collagenous tissues. Corneal stromal collagen is renewed at unusually slow rates compared to dermal collagen, and keratocytes exhibit slow replication. The cornea is much more resistant to stimuli that would initiate fibrotic repair responses in other tissues. In fact, many mechanisms and adaptations of the cornea aim to provide wound healing by regeneration rather than fibrotic repair in order to maintain transparency. The lack of blood vessels in the corneal stroma also significantly affects the healing process. In skin, platelets derived from the vasculature are a major source of fibrotic repair stimulating and modulating factors. The corneal healing response does not involve platelets, and other cells must provide the cytokines, growth factors, and other substances required. The epithelial response also differs between skin and cornea. Epithelial migration and wound surface closure in the cornea are much more rapid than in the skin. Furthermore, the corneal epithelium produces substances that substitute for those contributed by platelets.

The mechanisms that regulate corneal wound healing represent a complex series of events that are determined by the etiology and severity of the injury. The principles of corneal wound healing by regeneration provide the mechanistic framework to understand how the cornea responds to injury (Fig. 21-12). However, few examples in clinical veterinary medicine truly represent wound healing only by regeneration, and most clinical diseases that require intervention include some aspect of fibrotic repair (Fig 21-13). Sterile surgical corneal incisions (cataract surgery or other) are one example in which healing is expected by regeneration despite being a full-thickness corneal interruption. In addition, the response to corneal injury is not limited to the cornea itself. The tear film, for example, is intimately involved in the process contributing various growth factors and proteases, and it provides the means for leukocyte movement and removal of damaged cells. Posteriorly, the aqueous humor of the anterior chamber is the source of the fibrinogen needed to form a fibrin clot that seals a full-thickness interruption allowing the healing process to begin.

Corneal Healing

Favors Regeneration		Favors Scarring
• One-time injury		• Ongoing injury
• Defect is shallow		• Defect is deep
• Stroma is healthy	 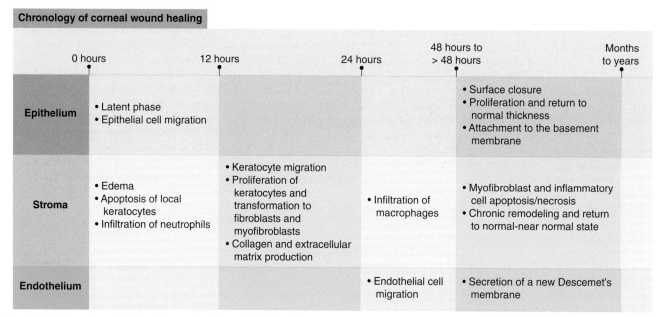 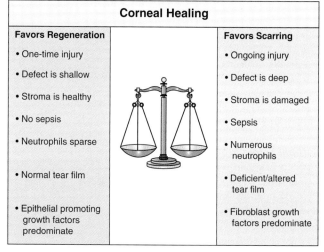	• Stroma is damaged
• No sepsis		• Sepsis
• Neutrophils sparse		• Numerous neutrophils
• Normal tear film		• Deficient/altered tear film
• Epithelial promoting growth factors predominate		• Fibroblast growth factors predominate

Figure 21-13 **Corneal Healing.** The outcome of corneal wound healing depends on a number of factors. Single events that are sterile, mild, and shallow favor regeneration, especially if the cornea was previously healthy in the tear film. Chronic lesions that are deep or infected are more likely to induce fibrotic repair.

Corneal Epithelium. The corneal epithelium is constantly being renewed by centripetal migration of limbal stem cells to replace the basal cells. The basal cells are mitotically active, and surface maturation ends with apoptotic shedding of the superficial cells. When healthy, the corneal epithelium is completely renewed every 5 to 7 days. Corneal epithelial wound healing is divided into four phases. During the first phase, the latent phase, there is no proliferation or cell migration. Damaged cells undergo apoptosis and are shed in the tear film. There is polymerization of fibronectin over the injury site to form a temporary extracellular matrix scaffold that will facilitate cell movement. The injury will initially result in the arrest of mitotic activity, retraction and hypertrophy of the cells at the margins, and disruption of hemidesmosomal attachments to the basement membrane. The latent phase may last for several hours. The second phase is migration, in which basal epithelial cells at the margins of the defect will slide in a centripetal migration to cover the defect, in part under the influence of Slug, a member of the Snail family of transcription factors. The cells remain attached by desmosomes essentially forming a sheet of cohesive cells that can cover the denuded area. The sliding occurs in the absence of cell proliferation (E-Fig. 21-5). The corneal epithelial can slide by as much as 1 mm per day. Once the defect is reepithelialized, the third phase of proliferation begins. Mitoses and maturation will resume restoring normal thickness. The fourth phase is attachment and consists of the formation of hemidesmosomes to provide a strong attachment to the basement membrane. If the basement membrane is damaged, repair may occur simultaneously with hemidesmosome formation. Continued alteration may occur until the integrity of the underlying superficial stroma is restored. Corneal ulcers with interruption of the basement membrane may be reepithelialized quickly, but normal function will be delayed until the basement membrane is repaired (weeks) (Fig. 21-14).

Stroma. Stromal healing requires transformation of keratinocytes, production of matrix, and tissue remodeling (see Fig. 21-12). Stromal injury initially results in edema, apoptosis of local keratinocytes, and infiltration of neutrophils from the tear film within 1 to 2 hours of the injurious event. Apoptosis of keratinocytes is a key event that serves to avoid a fibrotic repair response by removing the mediating cells. Adjacent stromal keratocytes transform to fibroblasts or myofibroblasts, proliferate, migrate to the site of injury, and synthesize collagen and extracellular matrix. Monocytes can also differentiate into fibroblasts to contribute to stromal healing.

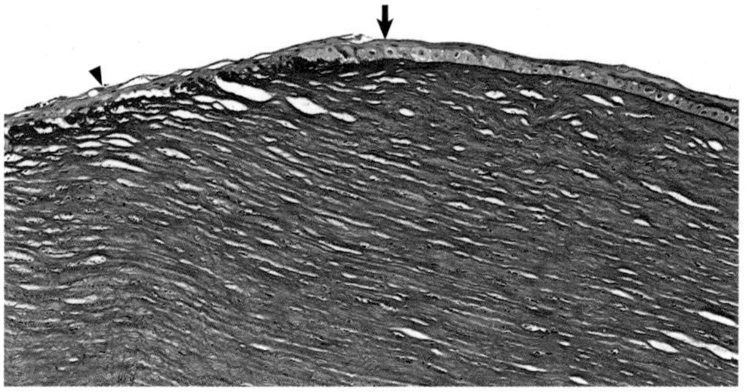

Figure 21-14 Healing Corneal Ulcer, Dog. The *arrow* indicates the site of interruption in the basement membrane of the corneal epithelium corresponding to the edge of the previous ulcer. The corneal epithelium has migrated to cover the stroma *(arrowhead)*. Small numbers of neutrophils remain in the stroma. Periodic acid–Schiff (PAS) reaction. (Courtesy Dr. P. Labelle, Antech Diagnostics.)

Stromal healing initially results in irregular deposition of collagen fibrils and decreased corneal transparency. Remodeling over months to years can often at least partially restore transparency and tensile strength. Regenerative healing can be separated into three phases: keratocyte migration and secretion of growth factors, proteases, and extracellular matrix (ECM); differentiation in myofibroblasts that are contractile and nonmotile and remodel of the ECM; and wound closure and myofibroblasts apoptosis/necrosis. The persistence of myofibroblasts can result in overproduction of ECM and exuberant contraction leading to fibrotic repair and loss of transparency. The final outcome depends on the severity of the lesion, the cause, the contribution of the infectious agent, and the balance of mediators and matrix metalloproteinases.

Endothelium and Descemet's Membrane. The corneal endothelial cells are postmitotic with minimal to no regenerative potential in most species. Defects in the corneal endothelium are healed by sliding and hypertrophy of the adjacent viable endothelial cells. Normal function can be restored by sliding within a few days if sufficient endothelial cell density remains (400 to 700 cells/mm^2). The endothelial cells may secrete a new basement membrane if there is damage to Descemet's membrane. This process is often imperfect and can lead to duplication of Descemet's membrane.

Molecular Regulation and Modulation of Corneal Wound Healing. Cytokines, growth factors, and proteases all play significant roles in modulating corneal wound healing.

Cytokines released following epithelial injury contribute to corneal would healing by (1) stimulating epithelial migration, (2) influencing the production of epithelial growth factors and their release, and (3) initiating stromal responses. Epithelial injury induces the release of cytokines mainly interleukins 1 and 6 (IL-1 and IL-6) and tumor necrosis factor-α (TNF-α). IL-1 and IL-6 are released proportionately to the severity of the epithelial damage. IL-1 promotes wound healing in concert with epithelial growth factor (EGF), upregulates the release of hepatocyte growth factor (HGF) and keratinocyte growth factor (KGF [a member of the fibroblast growth factor {FGF} family]), and potentiates the effects of platelet-derived growth factor (PDGF). IL-1 also stimulates the stromal response including collagenase and matrix metalloproteinase (MMP) production by keratocyte, keratocyte apoptosis, and neutrophil recruitment. IL-6 mediates epithelial cell migration by upregulation of the integrin receptor for fibronectin. TNF-α promotes keratocyte apoptosis, neutrophils recruitment, and influences epithelial healing through transforming growth factor-β (TGF-β). IL-8, upregulated by IL-1 and TNF-α, promotes neutrophil recruitment and angiogenesis. Many other cytokines (RANTES, MCP-1, and others) play a role in corneal wound healing.

Growth factors released following epithelial injury and upregulation by cytokine action induce proliferation and migration of epithelial cells. EGF, HGF, insulin growth factor (IGF), and KGF increase epithelial cell proliferation. HGF and IGF also facilitate epithelial cell migration and inhibit apoptosis. Some members of the EGF family (heparin-binding EGF-like growth factor [HB-EGF] and transforming growth factor-α [TGF-α]) increase proliferation but inhibit corneal epithelial cell terminal differentiation. Nerve growth factor (NGF) and other neurotrophic factors promote both epithelial proliferation and differentiation. PDGF is released from the epithelium and enhances epithelial migration in the presence of fibronectin. PDGF also stimulates keratocytes migration and proliferation, in part by mediating the action of TGF-β. TGF-β is also released from the epithelium and inhibits the epithelial proliferation stimulated by EGF, KGF, and HGF. TGF-β will act on stromal keratocytes when the basement membrane is damaged and induces differentiation into fibroblasts/myofibroblasts, migration and proliferation of keratocytes, as well as alteration in the synthesis of extracellular matrix. Other growth factors play lesser roles in corneal wound healing.

Proteases (proteinases) promote and regulate epithelial cell migration and proliferation during corneal epithelial wound healing and are essential for remodeling of the corneal stroma. Some proteases, including serine proteases urokinase-type plasminogen activator (uPA) and plasmin, contribute to the disruption of epithelial attachments to the basement membrane facilitating migration. Proteases, mainly serine proteases and MMPs, are critical to remodeling the stroma. Injury to the cornea disrupts the physiologic balance of proteases and protease inhibitors that contribute to corneal maintenance and renewal. Corneal injury shifts the balance toward degradation and remodeling and reduces the role of protease inhibitors such as α_2-macroglobulin, α_1-proteinase inhibitor, tissue metalloproteinase inhibitors, maspin, serine protease inhibitors (serpins), secretory leukocyte protease inhibitor, and calpeptin. Proteases secreted by infectious organisms will further promote degradation. MMP-2 and MMP-9 are the most extensively studied of the MMPs. MMP-9 is produced by epithelial cells and leukocytes and is mainly localized at the leading edge of the wound. MMP-9 breaks down collagen and basement membrane proteins, modulates IL-1, and activates TGF-β. MMP-9 also degrades the temporary fibronectin matrix following wound closure. MMP-2 is produced by the corneal epithelium and keratocytes. It is involved in renewal of healthy corneas and increased following corneal injury to influence stromal remodeling. Unlike other MMPs involved in corneal wound healing, epithelial injury is not required for MMP-2 activation. MMP-1 and -7 modulate epithelial migration. MMP-3, -12, -13, and -14 regulate stromal remodeling.

Corneal Fibrosis/Scarring (Fibrotic Repair). Significant stromal injury that overwhelms the cornea's ability to heal by regeneration leads to fibrotic repair, permanently impairing transparency. Many corneal injuries in veterinary patients are beyond the globe's ability to heal in any manner that would allow a return to normal function. In those instances, fibrotic repair that maintains corneal integrity is preferable to corneal rupture. Factors that stimulate fibrotic repair include extensive corneal injury, deep or full-thickness corneal injury, infiltration of large numbers of neutrophils, and the presence of infectious organisms (see Fig. 21-13; E-Figs. 21-6 through 21-10). Histologically, enlargement and hyperchromasia of limbal fibroblasts and angioblasts is visible within 24 to 48 hours of injury, but detectable migration is not evident until approximately 4 days. Fibroblasts and blood vessels migrate as much as 1 mm per day until they reach the site of injury. If the cause of the injury is removed or controlled so that corneal rupture is avoided, the process will evolve to form a bed of granulation tissue covered by epithelium. Remodeling over time may help restore some transparency; however, there will never be a return to completely normal structure and function. Surgical grafting usually serves to facilitate and accelerate fibrotic repair in order to maintain corneal integrity in patients at risk of corneal rupture, or to promote fibrotic repair of a previously ruptured cornea.

Uvea

Uveitis

The nomenclature of uveal leukocytic inflammation is essentially the same as that used in clinical ophthalmology (Box 21-5). Hypopyon is the accumulation of neutrophils and fibrin that typically settles ventrally within the anterior chamber (E-Fig. 21-11). Inflammation within the iris and ciliary body is usually referred to as anterior uveitis (or less commonly iridocyclitis). Inflammation limited to the choroid is choroiditis; inflammation limited to the vitreous is hyalitis; inflammation throughout the uveal tract is panuveitis; and inflammation involving the uveal tract and the adjacent components (anterior chamber, posterior chamber, and vitreous) is endophthalmitis. Uveitis or endophthalmitis that extends in the sclera is known as panophthalmitis. As previously discussed, the histologic diagnosis of ocular inflammation usually implies the infiltration of leukocytes, whereas many of the clinical diagnoses of ocular inflammation often represent predominantly vascular-mediated processes.

Box 21-5 Histologic-Clinical Correlation in Uveitis

The macroscopic manifestations of uveitis detectable by clinical examination are as follows:

- Aqueous flare: An increase in protein content within the aqueous humor increases light scattering
- Iris swelling and color change: Iris stromal hyperemia, edema, leukocyte accumulation, and fibrovascular proliferation
- Conjunctival reddening: Hyperemia of the superficial and deep conjunctival blood vessels in response to vasoactive chemicals generated by the nearby uveitis
- Hypopyon: The accumulation of neutrophils and fibrin that settles ventrally within the anterior chamber
- Keratic precipitates: Small aggregates of inflammatory cells adherent to the corneal endothelium
- Peripheral corneal midstromal neovascularization: Persistent inflammation results in the generation of enough angiogenic growth factors to stimulate "accidental" migration of limbal blood vessels into the peripheral cornea

Uveal inflammation almost always involves all portions of the uvea at least to some degree and readily extends in the ocular media. Furthermore, inflammatory mediators and toxic products are likely to be widely disseminated within the globe. Thus from a purely histologic perspective, almost all cases of uveitis can be technically classified as endophthalmitis. For practical purposes, the terminology chosen typically represents the component(s) most severely affected or the known underlying pathogenesis.

Causes of Uveitis. Uveitis can be initiated by a wide array of infections, immune responses, and trauma. The response obviously varies depending on the cause and severity of the insult. The components of the globe usually act as an integrated unit, and injury to one component almost always extend to other parts of the globe. The iris stroma, in particular, is highly reactive because there is direct communication with the aqueous humor. Any toxins, chemical mediators of inflammation, or growth factors secreted into the aqueous humor are absorbed by the iris, causing that portion of the uveal tract to respond.

Most of the infectious causes of uveitis are ocular responses to systemic viral, bacterial, or fungal diseases in which the uveal tract is only one of many tissues affected. Endophthalmitis as the sole manifestation of infectious disease may be seen as a sequela to penetrating injuries or perforating ulcers that allow the entry of environmental organisms into the globe. There are no viral causes of endophthalmitis, although there are a few systemic viral infections that cause vasculitis or retinitis that result in a uveal inflammatory response (e.g., feline infectious peritonitis). Uveal involvement in systemic mycoses and protothecosis is common in animals in certain geographic regions. Aberrant migration of nematode or trematode larvae occasionally causes endophthalmitis, as does ocular colonization by a variety of protozoal parasites that cause systemic disease (e.g., toxoplasmosis and encephalitozoonosis).

Ocular trauma is a frequent cause of endophthalmitis. The lesion may be transient with mild blunt trauma or noncontaminated penetrating trauma where the perforation is rapidly sealed. Conversely, introduction of bacteria in the globe or rupture of the lens will provoke massive endophthalmitis.

Immune-mediated uveitis is common and presents in various forms. These typically present as chronic conditions with nonspecific lymphoplasmacytic uveitis. In individual cases, it is not known if such a lesion reflects primary immune-mediated disease or simply a response to an infectious agent that is no longer present. Previous inflammation can cause the release of uveal- or retinal-specific antigens that are normally masked intracellularly, thus eliciting an immune response. There are only a few diseases for which the cause is known. Examples include: (1) uveodermatologic syndrome as a reaction to antigen associated with melanocytes and (2) lens-induced uveitis following exposure to normally sequestered lens protein.

The uvea responds to afferent neural signals and chemical mediators released from an injured cornea. Any significant corneal injury can elicit a mild anterior uveitis ("reflex uveitis").

Because the uveal tract is a vascularized tissue, the response to injury is similar to that in other organs. Furthermore, injury that overwhelms the barrier mechanisms will result in loss of immune privilege making the entire globe subject to immune and inflammatory responses similar to that of other sites.

Consequences of Uveitis. The inflammatory reactions in the uveal tract mimic those in other organs for both acute and chronic processes. The consequences of inflammation, both for the uveal tract and for other portions of the globe, are what make uveitis unique. Inflammation of the uveal tract can have injurious consequences for every other component of the globe. Uveitis may result in corneal neovascularization and endotheliitis, synechiae, fibrovascular proliferation, cataract, retinal detachment, and glaucoma.

Midstromal corneal neovascularization is commonly seen with chronic uveitis. The vessels grow inwardly from the limbus as the blood vessels of the limbus respond to angiogenic factors being produced within the globe as part of the ongoing inflammation and healing. Endotheliitis develops when leukocytes extend from the uveal tract in the aqueous humor to reach the corneal endothelium (E-Fig. 21-12). Lymphoplasmacytic uveitis and feline infectious peritonitis are common causes.

Synechiae are adhesions between the inflamed iris and either the cornea or the lens (E-Fig. 21-13). *Anterior synechia* is an iridocorneal adhesion. The adhesions may be focal or diffuse, along the central cornea or peripheral. Central anterior synechia is most commonly seen as a sequela to corneal rupture with or without iris prolapse. Peripheral anterior synechia commonly accompanies preiridal fibrovascular membranes (see later discussion). Adhesion to the anterior capsular surface of the lens (in the normal globe, the iris lies against the lens capsule) is known as *posterior synechia*. Because of the proximity of the iris and lens, posterior synechiae are more common than anterior synechiae. The adhesion is initially fibrinous and often occurs when aqueous humor protein content is high. The adhesions may become a firm fibrovascular membrane if allowed to persist. If that adhesion is sufficiently extensive around the pupillary margin (i.e., approaching the full circumference of the pupil), there will be significant impairment of aqueous humor outflow from the posterior chamber to the anterior chamber (pupillary block) leading to secondary glaucoma. Increased pressure within the posterior chamber in the presence of a circumferential posterior synechia results in anterior bowing of the iris known as *iris bombé*.

Cataracts are frequent sequelae to uveitis, likely from impaired nutrition. The avascular lens entirely depends on the aqueous humor for the delivery of nutrients and the removal of metabolic waste products. Uveitis results in altered composition and decreased production of aqueous humor. Furthermore, cataracts may result from diffusion of inflammatory mediators of inflammation and other toxic products in the aqueous humor of inflamed globes. In some cases, the cause-effect relationship may not be evident and history may be necessary to differentiate between cataracts secondary to uveitis and cataracts that cause lens-induced uveitis.

Retinal detachment is a common sequela to uveitis and endophthalmitis, either from exudation from the choroid or traction from the vitreous. Increased vascular permeability within the choroid results in effusion of fluid and leukocytes in the subretinal space, causing exudative retinal detachment. Because the normal neuroretina is not actually attached to the retinal pigment epithelium (RPE), there is a potential space termed the subretinal space where fluid leaving the choroid during inflammation can accumulate. Choroidal exudation occurs in the subretinal space because the fluid cannot diffuse through the thick sclera. Alternatively, fibrovascular proliferation within the vitreous may contract, causing tractional detachment.

Phthisis bulbi refers to a shrunken, disorganized end-stage globe. It is a sequela not only to uveitis, but severe uveitis is the most common cause.

Fibrovascular Proliferation and Neovascularization. Fibrovascular proliferation (neovascularization) is often considered separately from uveitis involving infiltration of leukocytes. However, fibrovascular proliferation is part of the inflammatory and healing responses, and many of the forms of uveitis commonly diagnosed by clinicians reflect vascular-mediated processes rather than leukocytic infiltration. Fibrovascular membranes may be present with leukocytic uveitis but also with neoplasms, trauma, and tissue damage associated with hypoxia such as retinal detachment and glaucoma. In fact, fibrovascular membranes are present in approximately 75% of all enucleated canine globes and in 20% to 30% of the enucleated globes in other species. Fibrovascular membranes develop when the balance of angiogenic and antiangiogenic factors favors neovascularization. Of the many cytokines that contribute to fibrovascular proliferation, vascular endothelial growth factor (VEGF) is the most significant. Fibrovascular membranes include newly formed vessels, spindle cells compatible with fibroblasts and myofibroblasts, and collagenous extracellular matrix. The contribution of each component to fibrovascular membranes depends in part on cause and chronicity. Fibrovascular membranes are often described by their distribution: retrocorneal, preiridal, posterior iridal, cyclitic, and intravitreal. Retrocorneal membranes line the posterior aspect of the cornea, often effacing the corneal endothelium. Preiridal membranes are the most common form of fibrovascular proliferation in the eye (Fig. 21-15; E-Figs. 21-14 and 21-15). These fibrovascular membranes line the anterior aspect of the iris. The membranes arise from budding and migration of capillaries from the iris stroma (Fig. 21-16) and recruitment of fibroblasts and myofibroblasts, similar to a healing response in other organs. Contraction of preiridal fibrovascular membranes can cause distortion of the iris, most often retraction of the pupillary margin of the iris, either anteriorly (ectropion uveae) or posteriorly (entropion uveae). Preiridal fibrovascular membranes may be continuous with retrocorneal membranes or extend posteriorly. Posterior iridal membranes cover the posterior iris epithelium and may extend to cover the ciliary body. Cyclitic membranes extend from the ciliary epithelium along the anterior vitreous face and may extend to carpet the posterior lens capsule.

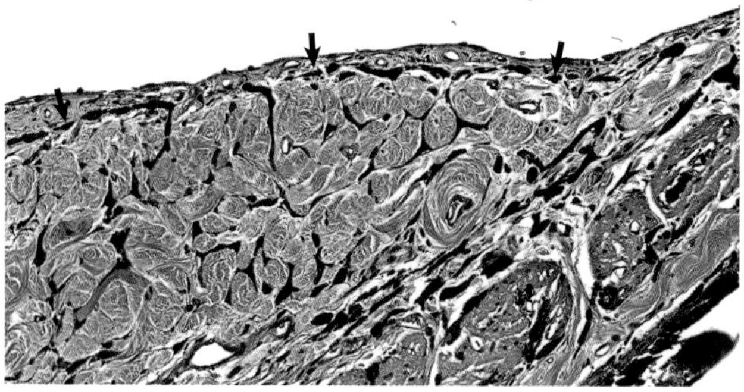

Figure 21-15 **Preiridal Fibrovascular Membrane, Iris, Dog.** The anterior surface of the iris is covered by a membrane including cellular, fibrous, and vascular elements. The anterior surface of the iris can be recognized by the row of melanocytes *(arrows)*. Preiridal fibrovascular membranes (PFIM) can extend over the iridocorneal angle causing obstruction of the aqueous humor outflow. PFIMs can also contract, resulting in retraction of the pupillary margin of the iris (ectropion or entropion uveae). H&E stain. (Courtesy Dr. P. Labelle, Antech Diagnostics.)

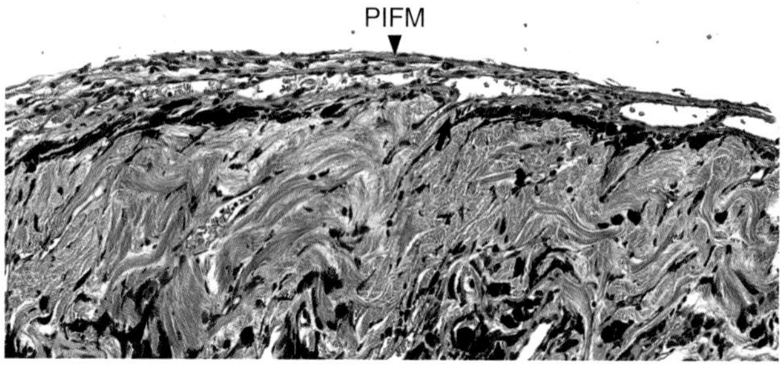

Figure 21-16 **Preiridal Fibrovascular Membrane, Iris, Dog.** The preiridal fibrovascular membrane *(PIFM)* is formed by proliferation of fibroblasts and capillaries that extend from the iris stroma *(arrow)*. Like granulation tissue, these membranes form in response to inflammatory mediators and growth factors within the aqueous humor. PIFMs cover the iris surface and almost never involve the iris stroma. H&E stain. (Courtesy Dr. P. Labelle, Antech Diagnostics.)

Intravitreal membranes typically originate from the pars plana ciliary body. Such membranes may be the cause of vitreal hemorrhage but may also be part of the response to chronic intravitreal hemorrhage. Retinal and epiretinal membranes seen in some human conditions are rare in domestic animals.

The development of fibrovascular proliferation in the globe shares mechanistic features with granulation tissue in other organs. However, unlike granulation tissue elsewhere, intraocular fibrovascular membranes tend to have detrimental rather than beneficial effects on function. The newly formed vessels are fragile and prone to hemorrhage, and fibrovascular proliferation can also contribute to the development of glaucoma. Preiridal fibrovascular membranes may extend to cover and obstruct the iridocorneal angle or extend along the posterior cornea causing a peripheral anterior synechia resulting in secondary glaucoma. Preiridal fibrovascular membranes may also extend on the anterior lens surface contributing to posterior synechiae and pupillary block, which may cause glaucoma. Intravitreal fibrovascular membranes can cause traction within the vitreous resulting in retinal detachment.

Fibrovascular proliferation almost never develops within the uveal stroma itself. Only in instances in which there is massive injury to the globe does fibrovascular proliferation occur in the uveal stroma, where it behaves similar to granulation tissue elsewhere. The mechanisms by which the uveal tract protects itself from fibrovascular proliferation/granulation tissue have not been elucidated but likely include a variety of antiangiogenic factors and likely overlap with the molecular adaptations that keep the cornea avascular.

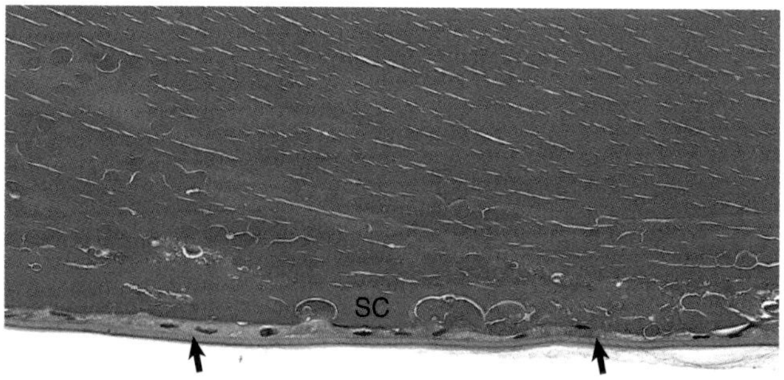

Figure 21-17 **Cataract, Lens, Dog.** Cataracts are the result of any opacification of the lens. Note the liquefaction of the subcapsular cortex *(SC)*. The normal lens lacks epithelium along the thin posterior capsule, and posterior migration of the lens epithelium *(arrows)* is one form of lenticular opacity. H&E stain. (Courtesy Dr. P. Labelle, Antech Diagnostics.)

Box 21-6 Morphologic Features of Cataracts

- Liquefaction of the lens cortex
- Morgagnian globules
- Bladder cells
- Posterior migration of the lens epithelium
- Hyperplasia/fibrometaplasia of the lens epithelium
- Mineralization
- Lens collapse

Lens

The lens can only respond to injury in limited ways. The lens is avascular, lacks any cells other than the lens epithelium, and prevents leukocyte infiltration through the capsule. The response to injury is usually limited to hydropic swelling or degeneration of the lens fibers and attempts at regeneration through proliferation and adaptation of the lens epithelium. The outcome is essentially identical, regardless of pathogenesis. The changes all result in variably severe cataract, broadly defined as an opacification of the lens. Because normal function of the lens requires transparency, any opacification, or cataract, is a pathologic change (Fig. 21-17; E-Figs. 21-16 and 21-17).

The microscopic changes of cataracts are various combinations of the following, listed in order of overall frequency (Box 21-6):

- Fragmentation and liquefaction of cortical lens fibers, creating hypereosinophilic spherical globules of denatured lens protein known as Morgagnian globules. Alternatively, the liquefied cortex may have a "smudgy" appearance.
- Hydropic swelling of cells that retain their nuclei, an ineffective attempt at regeneration. These dysplastic swollen cells are termed *bladder cells*.
- Posterior migration of the lens epithelium. The lens epithelium migrates from the lens equator to line posterior lens capsule. Because the normal adult lens has no epithelium posterior to the equator, the presence of cells along the posterior capsule is a form of opacity.

- Hyperplasia and fibrometaplasia of lens epithelium. The normal lens epithelium is a single layer thick and any epithelial hyperplasia may create plaque-like thickening. In some instances, the lens epithelium may adopt a spindle cell phenotype with or without fibroblastic metaplasia and collagen deposition.
- More variable changes include lens swelling in acute cataracts, lens shrinking with wrinkling of the lens capsule in advanced ("hypermature") cataracts, epithelial cell necrosis/apoptosis, and intralenticular mineralization.

Cataracts are best classified by the clinician who can examine the entire lens. Such classification is most important in the clinical diagnosis of breed-related inherited cataracts in dogs. Cataract may still be classified histologically by extent, location, and cause. Extent can usually be categorized as incipient (<15%), immature (>15%, incomplete), mature (circumferential), and hypermature cataract with evidence of lens collapse or resorption. Cataracts may be cortical with liquefaction, Morgagnian globules and bladder cells, or subcapsular with epithelial hyperplasia, fibrometaplasia, and posterior extension. Cataracts may be inherited or acquired/secondary.

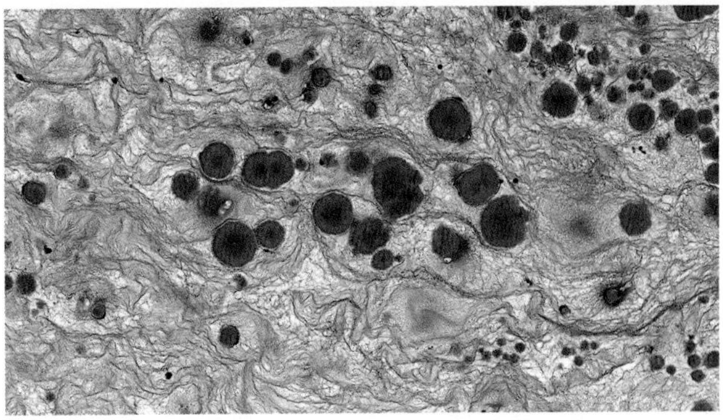

Figure 21-18 **Asteroid Hyalosis, Vitreous, Dog.** Asteroid hyalosis is a form of vitreal degeneration that can be associated with inflammation, neoplasia, and aging. The "bluish purple" asteroid bodies located predominantly in the center of the figure consist of phospholipid and calcium complexes. (Courtesy Dr. P. Labelle, Antech Diagnostics.)

Vitreous

The vitreous has limited ways in which it can respond to injury. The vitreous is avascular and lacks cells other than hyalocytes. Injury, including inflammation and glaucoma, often results in altered composition and loss of viscosity, essentially liquefaction of vitreous. The vitreous is highly susceptible to hemorrhage, and chronic lesions may cause fibrovascular proliferation. The significance of vitreal injury lies on the possible effects on the retina: separation from the retina and increased risk of retinal tearing with liquefaction and traction and retinal attachment with fibrovascular proliferation.

Box 21-7 Features of Vitreal Blood Removal

- Rapid fibrin clot
- Absence of early polymorphonuclear leukocyte infiltration
- Slow fibrinolysis
- Extracellular hemolysis of red blood cells
- Long-term persistence of intact red blood cells
- Low turnover of macrophages

Asteroid Hyalosis

Asteroid hyalosis is one form of vitreal degeneration. The lesion consists of numerous spherical bodies with irregular contours embedded within the collagen framework of the vitreous (Fig. 21-18). Occasionally the asteroid bodies will be bordered by or within macrophages. The asteroid bodies are composed of phospholipid and calcium complexes. The change is nonspecific and can be seen with chronic inflammatory, degenerative, and neoplastic diseases. Asteroid hyalosis can also be an age-related change.

Vitreal Hemorrhage

There are three main pathologic mechanisms for ocular hemorrhages: bleeding from normal vessels (trauma), bleeding from abnormal vessels (systemic hypertension and uveitis), and bleeding from newly formed immature vessels (fibrovascular membranes and neoplasia). Blood disorders (e.g., coagulopathies, anemia, anticoagulants) are a less frequent cause of intraocular hemorrhage. The basic principle of blood catabolism applies to ocular hemorrhage; however, there are features unique to the removal of blood in the eye. Blood in the anterior or posterior chambers is removed through the iridocorneal angle, assuming it is functional and unobstructed. Hemorrhage within the uveal tract is rare and is often associated with significant uveal destruction with breakdown of ocular defense mechanisms and immune privilege. Blood catabolism in those instances is similar to that in other tissues.

Vitreal hemorrhage catabolism is significantly different than hemorrhage removal in any other tissues (Box 21-7). Rapid clot formation is facilitated by the network of vitreal collagen, which enables platelet aggregation and promotes the intrinsic clotting pathway. The absence of polymorphonuclear leukocyte infiltration early in the process decreases fibrinolysis. In turn, the lack of fibrin degradation production limits stimulation of polymorphonuclear leukocyte migration to the site. Low levels of tissue plasminogen activator in the vitreous also contribute to slow fibrinolysis. Some erythrocytes undergo extracellular hemolysis as a result of either lysosomal enzyme release by macrophages or autohemolysis secondary to the lack of required concentrations of oxygen and glucose. Hemolysis may be more important than phagocytosis by macrophages for clearance of vitreal hemorrhage. Some red blood cells will persist for months within the vitreous. These cells must possess a metabolism allowing survival in the altered vitreous and escape phagocytosis by macrophages. These intact cells may be fresh red blood cells that lack the opsonins recognized by macrophages on older red blood cells targeted for phagocytosis. Macrophages will infiltrate the vitreous within days, but the response is measured and will continue for months. The number of macrophages that respond to vitreal hemorrhage is significantly less than that in other organs. Some of the macrophages in the vitreous appear metabolically inert and will undergo cytolysis with phagocytosis by other cells. The measured response is a consequence of reduced chemotactic stimulation, including the lack of fibrin degradation products, and the vitreal properties of hyaluronate that impedes migration and inhibits phagocytosis. The purpose of this measured response may be to maintain ocular immune privilege and ocular function by avoiding a marked response leading to granulation tissue formation. Consequences of vitreal hemorrhage include liquefaction of the vitreous. The presence of ferric and ferrous iron, a decrease in the concentration of hyaluronic acid, and an increase in the concentration of chondroitin sulfate, as well as the effect of plasma proteases, account for the change. Normal viscosity is regained after several months.

Retina and Optic Nerve

The retina responds to injury in a manner similar to that of the central nervous system (see Chapter 14). The neuronal elements of the adult retina do not regenerate; the outer segments of the photoreceptors, however, have a rapid turnover and have among the highest metabolic activity in the body. As long as the cell body within the outer nuclear layer remains viable, photoreceptors can be quickly regenerated. The inflammatory response within the retina is similar to that in the central nervous system: neuronal necrosis, perivascular cuffing, and gliosis. The retinal pigment epithelium (RPE) remains mitotically active throughout life. Like other epithelia, it repairs by sliding viable cells into the area where cells have been lost followed by mitosis. The RPE may undergo fibrometaplasia. The Müller glial cells are less sensitive to injury than retinal neurons and are capable of proliferation. Repair of most cases of retinal necrosis occurs primarily by proliferation of Müller cells, which eventually form a nonfunctional dense glial scar. Occasionally the astrocytes proliferate along the vitreal face of the retina, forming a preretinal fibroglial membrane. Subretinal membranes (between the photoreceptors and the RPE) of a similar microscopic appearance are seen occasionally with chronic detachments and originate from migrating Müller cells or from retinal pigment epithelium that has undergone fibrometaplasia.

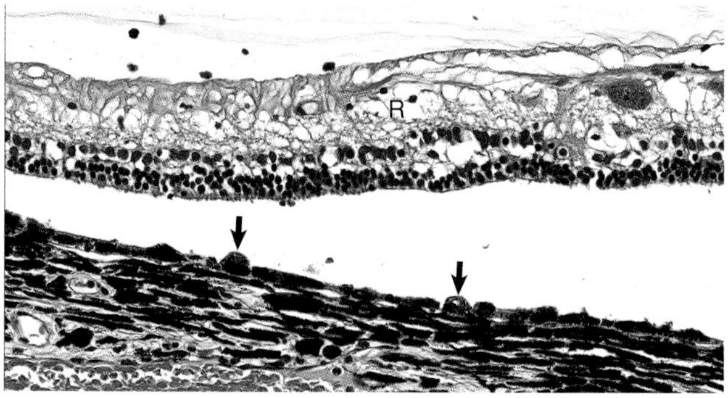

Figure 21-19 Chronic Retinal Detachment, Retinal, Dog Chronic retinal detachment with degeneration of the photoreceptor layer, atrophy of the outer nuclear layer, collapse of the outer plexiform layer, and atrophy of the inner nuclear layer. At this stage, the retinal changes and associated vision loss are permanent. There is also multifocal hypertrophy of the retinal pigment epithelium *(arrows)*. With time, chronic retinal detachment can progress to full-thickness retinal atrophy. *R*, Retina. H&E stain. (Courtesy Dr. P. Labelle, Antech Diagnostics.)

Retinal Detachment

The neurosensory retina (not including the RPE) is physically anchored only at the ora ciliaris retinae and at the optic disc. It is held in apposition to the RPE partly by the physical presence of the vitreous and partially by the membrane forces related to the intricate interdigitations between photoreceptors and surface crevices in the RPE. As such, the term retinal detachment, which is commonly used in both clinical and pathologic settings, may be more accurately described as separation between the neuroretina and RPE. It does not describe a disconnection between the RPE and choroid. The potential space between the photoreceptors and the RPE is the remnant of the lumen of the primary optic vesicle, and it persists throughout life. Retinal detachment is a frequent and serious complication of many different ocular diseases. It may be focal, multifocal, or diffuse. The distance of separation between the photoreceptors and the RPE may only be slight, or the entire retina may be separated and suspended in the vitreous. Retinal tears may develop along with retinal detachment.

The most frequent types of retinal detachment are as follows:

- Exudative retinal detachment: Accumulation of serous, fibrinous, or cellular exudates within the subretinal space as a consequence of choroiditis, retinitis, or neoplasia. Hemorrhagic detachment may be seen with trauma, systemic hypertension, or neoplasia.
- Rhegmatogenous retinal detachment: Leakage of liquefied vitreous into the subretinal space through traumatic or degenerative breaks in the retina.
- Tractional retinal detachment: Vitreal or preretinal membranes that develop as a consequence of uveitis or chronic hemorrhage can pull the neuroretina from the RPE.

Histologically, retinal detachment can be recognized by the presence of material within the subretinal space, atrophy of the outer retina, and hypertrophy of the underlying RPE (E-Figs. 21-18 through 21-21). The presence of serous, fibrinous, hemorrhagic, or cellular exudates within the subretinal space is the most diagnostically reliable feature of retinal detachment. Outer retinal atrophy is an expected consequence of retinal detachment. Within days, there will be atrophy of the photoreceptor layer. Atrophy of the outer nuclear layer suggests chronicity (Fig. 21-19). The progression of outer retinal atrophy is highly variable and depends in part on the nature of the exudate, the presence of inflammatory cells and mediators, the extent of the detachment, and the integrity of the choroidal

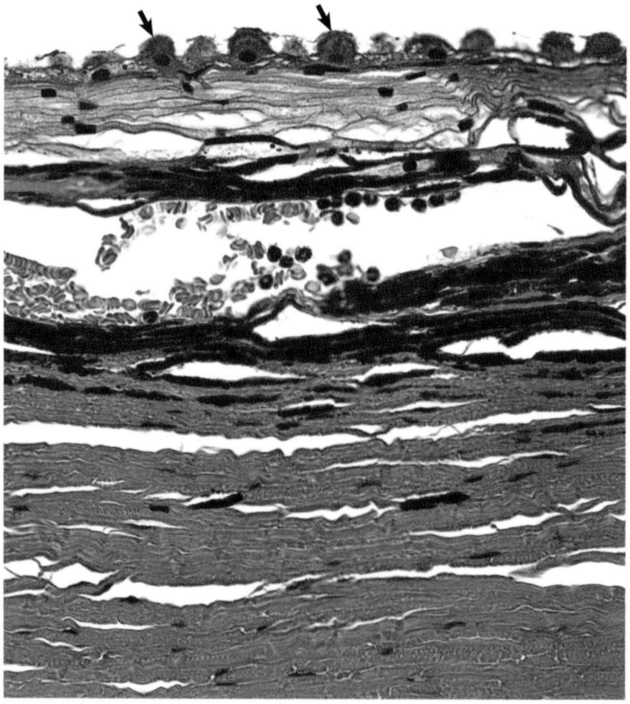

Figure 21-20 Retinal Detachment, Retina, Dog. In some instances of retinal detachment, there will be hypertrophy of the retinal pigment epithelium (RPE). The enlarged cells *(arrows)* bulge toward the subretinal space; the change has been termed "tombstoning." (Courtesy Dr. P. Labelle, Antech Diagnostics.)

vascular supply. As such, it is not possible to accurately age retinal detachments histologically. Hypertrophy of the RPE, so-called "tombstoning," is an indicator of retinal detachment and can be seen as early as 24 hours after retinal detachment (range, 1 to 3 days) (Fig. 21-20: E-Figs. 21-22 and 21-23). However, the change is not always present, and it depends in part on the health of the RPE itself, the health of the choroid, and the nature of the subretinal exudate. Less commonly, the RPE may be multifocally hyperplastic. Retinal detachment that develops prior to glaucoma may have a sparing effect on the inner retina; there may be no inner retinal atrophy despite significant elevation in the intraocular pressure. Histologically, retinal detachment must be differentiated from artifactual separation, which occurs frequently during processing. With artifactual separation, there is no material within the subretinal space; there is no outer retinal atrophy or hypertrophy of the RPE. The presence of photoreceptor segments on the apical surface of the RPE also indicates artifactual separation.

The immediate consequence of retinal detachment is loss of function—that is, loss of vision. The detached hypoxic retina produces angiogenic growth factors, mainly vascular endothelial growth factor (VEGF). This is presumably intended to increase the retinal blood supply; however, there is little evidence of stimulation of retinal angiogenesis in domestic animals. Instead, VEGF diffuses in vitreous and aqueous humor, resulting in vascular/fibrovascular membrane formation. These membranes may cause further damage to the globe because the new vessels may easily hemorrhage. The membranes may also cause secondary glaucoma as a consequence of obstruction of the iridocorneal angle or pupillary block.

The optic nerve responds to injury in a manner similar to that of the central nervous system (see Chapter 14).

Orbit

The response to insult of the bone, adipose tissue, skeletal muscle, and glandular tissue that constitute the orbit is similar to that of the same tissue type elsewhere in the body. Such responses may have significant consequences for the globe and vision. Space-occupying lesions in the orbit, including neoplasia, cysts, inflammation, hematomas, and edema, may cause protrusion of the globe (exophthalmos), which may impair proper eyelid closure resulting in corneal exposure and desiccation. Space-occupying lesions, particularly neoplasia, may also compress the optic nerve causing atrophy and blindness. Extraocular myositis and other conditions that cause damage to the orbital muscle may result in abnormal positioning of the globe with possible eyelid trauma to the cornea or exposure of the cornea with desiccation. Injury to the lacrimal gland, either dacryocystitis or extension of orbital lesions affecting other tissues, can lead to altered tear film production and keratoconjunctivitis sicca. Although rare, severe emaciation with atrophy of orbital adipose tissue can cause the globe to be positioned deeper in the orbit with possible entropion and eyelid trauma to the cornea.

Portals of Entry/Pathways of Spread

Eyelids and Conjunctiva

Eyelids

The outer surface of the eyelid is skin and therefore is susceptible to the same diseases as the skin elsewhere on the body. For palpebral skin, the portals of entry are the same as for skin at other sites:

- Colonization of the skin's surface or adnexal glands by niche-adapted infectious agents
- Penetrating injury
- Hematogenous localization (immune-mediated diseases, infectious)
- Contact injury (physical or chemical)

Conjunctiva

The conjunctiva is a mucous membrane similar in structure to other mucous membranes and is therefore susceptible to injury from the same range of physical and chemical injuries affecting any other mucous membrane. The routes of entry are predictable and as follows:

- Colonization of the epithelial surface by niche-adapted infectious agents
- Penetrating injury
- Hematogenous localization (immune mediated diseases, infectious)
- Contact injury (physical or chemical)

Cornea

Portals of entry into the cornea are listed in Box 21-8. Desiccation is a common form of corneal injury that can be the result of insufficient or altered tear film production. Desiccation can also be caused by any condition that impairs proper eyelid movement and closure, such as exophthalmos, eyelid conformation defect, and eyelid masses. Some eyelid diseases can also cause trauma and chronic irritation if a mass or distorted eyelid directly contacts the corneal surface. Penetrating trauma, essentially foreign body injury, can damage the epithelium, extend in the stroma, or cause a full-thickness breach with intraocular extension. Cat claws, plant material, and, to a lesser extent, bite wounds are common sources of traumatic injuries to the cornea and globe. Chemical injury is rare but includes both accidental exposures to various chemicals and inappropriate administration of preparations not intended for the ocular surface (e.g., skin formulations). Extension of conjunctival disease in the cornea is uncommon but may include spillover of inflammation or neoplasia, or induction of nonspecific reactive changes (corneal hyperplasia, stromal neovascularization). Corneal disease from intraocular extension via damage to the corneal endothelium may be the result of endotheliitis or endophthalmitis, anterior synechia, anterior lens luxation, or glaucoma. The portals of entry for the sclera consist essentially of trauma, hematogenous, extension of intraocular disease, and, less commonly, extension of orbital disease.

Uvea

Portals of entry into the uvea are listed in Box 21-9. Injury to the uvea may occur through the bloodstream (hematogenous), trauma, or by extension of disease elsewhere in the globe (aqueous humor, vitreous, sclera). Hematogenous entry is used by infectious agents,

Box 21-8 Portal of Entry Into the Cornea

External injury
- Desiccation
- Trauma
- Chemical injury

Extension from the conjunctiva
Extension of intraocular disease

Box 21-9 Portal of Entry Into the Uvea

Hematogenous
- Infectious agents
- Neoplastic cells
- Toxins

Trauma
- Penetrating wounds
- Blunt trauma

Extension from other ocular structures

metastatic neoplasia, and, less frequently, toxins. Injury to the blood vessels themselves from thrombosis or occlusion by neoplastic emboli may cause ischemic damage. Traumatic injury may be the result of penetration or blunt force. Penetrating injury may cause direct injury or provide infectious agents entry into the globe and uveal tract. Blunt trauma may result in separation of the uveal tract from the sclera leading to traumatic angle recession or cyclodialysis. Blunt trauma may also damage blood vessels, causing hemorrhage. Corneal and scleral disease may extend to involve the uveal tract. Furthermore, chemical mediators of inflammation released from injured cornea, lens, or retina diffuse through the aqueous humor or vitreous, or directly in the uveal tract eliciting uveal damage as part of the inflammatory response.

Lens

Portals of entry into the lens are listed in Box 21-10. The lens is occasionally injured by a direct perforating injury or blunt trauma. In those instances, other ocular components are expected to be involved. The significance of the lens injury will depend on its severity as well as the severity of damage elsewhere in the globe. Electrocution, albeit a rare event, can cause degeneration of the lens.

Many injuries to the lens reflect the lens' dependence on the aqueous humor. There may be inadequate delivery of nutrients because of defective flow of aqueous humor or chemically abnormal aqueous humor. Metabolic diseases that cause cataracts include excessive glucose levels in animals with diabetes mellitus and cataracts associated with systemic hypocalcemia. The aqueous humor may also contain damaging inflammatory mediators or cataractogenic chemicals including some drugs. Degenerative changes in the lens are also seen in dogs with inherited photoreceptor disorders caused by diffusion of toxic by-products of photoreceptor degeneration. Inherited cataracts in dogs are frequent, although the underlying biochemical pathogenesis has not been elucidated.

Light-induced lens injury is mostly relevant for laboratory animals but nonetheless a potential mechanism of lenticular damage in domestic animals. Similarly, therapeutic radiation is an uncommon cause of cataract in domestic animals.

Because the lens is avascular and surrounded by a dense collagenous capsule, it is relatively resistant to invasion by infectious organisms in the absence of penetrating trauma. One rare exception in domestic mammals is the specific targeting of the lens capsule in some instances of systemic mycosis, typically aspergillosis. These fungi exhibit a tropism for basement membranes throughout the body, including the lens capsule. In rabbits, the lens is frequently affected by the microsporidian *Encephalitozoon cuniculi*, possibly from in utero infection. There are a few reports of *E. cuniculi* causing lenticular disease in cats. In fish, cataracts induced by the intralenticular penetration of fluke larvae are common. Several viral diseases including bovine viral diarrhea are occasionally associated with congenital cataracts as a consequence of systemic infection in utero before the establishment of the blood-eye barrier.

Box 21-10 Portals of Entry Into the Lens

Trauma
- Penetrating trauma
  - Through the cornea
  - Through the sclera
- Blunt trauma
  - Displacement of the lens
  - Lens capsule rupture

Electrocution
Diffusion from the aqueous humor
- Nutritional
- Metabolic
  - Diabetes mellitus
- Toxic
  - Inflammatory mediators
  - Chemicals

Radiation
Light
Therapy (cancer treatment, x-rays)
Infectious

Vitreous

Portals of entry into the vitreous include penetrating trauma, extension of uveal disease, diffusion of inflammatory mediators and other chemicals from the aqueous humor, and extension of retinal disease.

Retina and Optic Nerve

Portals of entry into the retina are listed in Box 21-11. It is important to view this list in perspective. Despite the long list of potentially injurious stimuli and the innumerable routes by which such stimuli can impact the retina, retinal disease is overall infrequent. The vast majority of retinal lesions fall into the following four categories:

1. Destruction of the neural elements of the inner retina (nerve fiber layer, ganglion cells, and inner nuclear layer) as a result of increased intraocular pressure (see Glaucoma). The pathogenesis of the inner retinal destruction and destruction of the optic nerve remain a source of great controversy, and it probably varies among species and with the type of glaucoma (see Glaucoma).
2. Retinal detachment is a common consequence of inflammatory, infectious, and vascular disease. The photoreceptors are therefore likely to become necrotic from ischemia and malnutrition

Box 21-11 Portals of Entry Into the Retina

Increased intraocular pressure (glaucoma)
Hematogenous
- Infectious
- Toxic
- Systemic hypertension
- Thrombosis/thromboembolism
- Metastasis

Radiation
Light
Extension from the vitreous
- Endophthalmitis
- Traction detachment
- Liquefaction

Extension from the choroid
- Exudative retinal detachment
- Choroiditis
- Collie eye anomaly

Extension of the optic nerve
- Retrograde atrophy
- Retrograde infection
- Retrograde malignancy

Genetic
- Retinal dysplasia
- Inherited retinopathies

Storage diseases
Vitreoretinal dysplasia

resulting from their anatomic dislocation from the RPE and decreased access to nutrients supplied by the choroidal vasculature.
3. Inflammation as a result of extension from endophthalmitis. Inflammation targeting the retina specifically is rare and extension of encephalitis is uncommon. Retinal detachment is a frequent complication of inflammation involving the choroid.
4. Noninflammatory photoreceptor degeneration from inherited metabolic disease or, less frequently, toxicity. The inherited photoreceptor diseases vary considerably in pathogenesis but are indistinguishable from one another using routine histologic examination techniques.

Less common causes of retinal injury include: (1) light and other types of radiation arriving through the cornea and lens, (2) hematogenous dissemination of chemical or infectious agents, and (3) objects penetrating through the cornea or through the sclera. Because the retina is an extension of the brain, it is susceptible to most of the infectious, degenerative, and metabolic diseases of the brain, including the storage diseases.

The main portals of entry in the optic nerve are extension of orbital disease and the effects of increased intraocular pressure (glaucoma). Trauma causing traction, with or without proptosis, may result in significant optic nerve damage. Extension of intraocular, retinal, and brain disease are less frequent causes of optic nerve injury.

Orbit

Portals of entry into the orbit are as follows:
- External trauma resulting in orbital fractures
- Penetrating injury through the skin, oral cavity, or nasal cavity
- Direct extension of inflammatory or neoplastic diseases from the oral cavity or the nasal cavity
- Direct extension of intraocular inflammatory or neoplastic disease through the sclera
- Direct extension of inflammatory or neoplastic disease from the conjunctiva or eyelid
- Hematogenous localization (immune-mediated diseases, infectious, neoplasia)

Defense Mechanisms/Barrier Systems

Eyelids and Conjunctiva

Eyelids

Like skin at other sites, the defenses of eyelid against injury include barrier functions, resistance to mechanical force, and immunologic defense mechanisms (see Chapters 3, 5, 13, and 17). Features of note regarding the eyelids include the presence of modified hair (cilia and sinus hairs). Reflexive blinking does not protect the eyelids themselves but does protect adjacent structures.

Conjunctiva

The conjunctiva is protected from most physical and chemical injuries by the eyelids and by the tear film. The epithelial cells are joined by desmosomes and tight junctions to prevent easy access by infectious or chemical agents into the underlying substantia propria. It is capable of rapid replication in the event of injury and readily undergoes squamous metaplasia as an adaptive survival mechanism in response to chronic low-grade irritation of any type. Both innate and adaptive immune responses contribute to the defense of the ocular surface (see Cornea below). The resident mucosal immune system (MALT) of the conjunctiva (CALT) functions similarly to immune systems in other mucosal sites, such as the upper respiratory tract, lungs (bronchus-associated lymphoid tissue [BALT]), and gastrointestinal tract (gut-associated lymphoid tissue [GALT]) (see Chapters 4, 7, 9, and 13).

Cornea

The ocular surface is an intricate integrated functional unit that includes the eyelids, lacrimal gland, tear film, conjunctiva, and cornea. Both innate and adaptive immune responses contribute to the defense of the ocular surface. The innate response is not antigen specific. The cornea is protected from most physical and chemical injuries by the action of the eyelids from several reflexes, the bony orbit, and by the constant flow of the tear film. Multiple reflexes are activated by mechanical stimulation of eyelids or the cornea. The blink reflex causes the eyelids to close when stimulated by contact with any solid material or strong airflow. The menace response causes the eyelids to blink when there is visual perception of a threat to the globe. The corneal reflex causes the eyelids to close when the cornea itself is irritated by external stimuli. Reflex retraction of the globe into the orbit, with subsequent passive sliding of the third eyelid to cover the cornea, occurs in response to corneal trauma.

The tear film is produced by the lacrimal gland and by the gland of the third eyelid, with contributions from conjunctival goblet cells, several accessory glands within the conjunctival substantia propria, and the meibomian glands. The tear film provides nourishment for the avascular cornea, a mucus layer to prevent evaporation of the protective fluid, soluble antibacterial chemicals, and a flushing action to protect the cornea against infectious agents and foreign material.

The production of mucins by goblet cells forms the innermost layer of the tear film and may be increased under the influence of cytokines including interleukin-6 and interferon-γ during inflammation and by several pathways including the nuclear factor-κB pathway during infection. Ocular surface mucins provide an anchor to bond the tear film and corneal epithelium, inhibit bacterial colonization, and help remove foreign material. Transmembrane mucins produced by the corneal and conjunctival cells may help the spread of the tear films and protect against bacterial adhesion. Furthermore, the corneal epithelium has junctional complexes (tight junctions, gap junctions, desmosomes, and hemidesmosomes) to prevent easy access by infectious or chemical agents into the underlying stroma, and it can shed and renew superficial layers that are compromised. Mature and immature dendritic cells are present at the periphery and immature dendritic cells are present in the central corneal epithelium. Toll-like receptors (TLRs) are expressed throughout the ocular surface and can trigger an immediate innate response to the pathogen and activate adaptive immunity. TLR regulation is also critical for ocular surface tolerance of antigen, including sparing of commensal flora.

The innate immune response also includes antimicrobial peptides such as lysozyme, lactoferrin, lipocalin, angiogenin, secretory phospholipase A_2, secreted immunoglobulin A (IgA), complement factors, defensins, and others that inhibit the invasion of infectious organisms (Table 21-1). Lysozyme binds to the outer membrane of the bacteria, creating a pore that leads to cell death. Lactoferrin binds divalent cations such as iron that many microorganisms require for function and growth. Tear lipocalin scavenges bacterial products and binds siderophores that transport iron in microorganisms. Angiogenin has multiple antimicrobial effects. Secretory phospholipase A_2 acts via its lipolytic enzymatic activity. IgA is produced by plasma cells in the lacrimal gland and neutralizes pathogens by preventing their attachment to host cells. IgA also binds to adhesion molecules on pathogens, causing their aggregation and facilitating clearance by the tear film. β-Defensins from epithelium and

Table 21-1 Ocular Surface Antimicrobial Peptides and Their Source

Peptide	Source
Lysozyme	Lacrimal gland
Lactoferrin	Lacrimal gland
Lipocalin	Lacrimal gland
Angiogenin	Epithelial cells
Secretory phospholipase A_2	Lacrimal glands, epithelial cells
Secreted IgA	Plasma cells (lacrimal gland)
Complement factors	Epithelial cells, neutrophils, conjunctival vessels
β-Defensins	Epithelial cells
α-Defensins	Neutrophils

α-defensins from neutrophils help protect against a broad spectrum of organisms through membrane permeabilization.

Antigen-presenting cells, namely the resident dendritic cells of the conjunctival and corneal epithelium, play a pivotal role linking the nonspecific innate response and the development of antigen-specific adaptive immunity. TLRs and other mechanisms also bridge the innate and adaptive immune responses.

The cornea is an immune privileged site. The purpose of this altered immune response as a defense mechanism is to minimize bystander injury. Factors that contribute to the immune privilege in the cornea include the lack of blood and lymphatic vessels and the blood-aqueous barrier (see section below) resulting in separation from circulating immune cells and lack of efferent transport for antigen-presenting cells (APCs). Furthermore, only immature APCs that do not express major histocompatibility complex class II are present in the central cornea. Although mainly relevant to corneal transplantation, the low immunogenicity of the stroma and endothelium and induction of anterior chamber-associated immune deviation (ACAID) by the endothelium (see Uvea) also contribute to the unique immune status of the cornea. The adaptive immune response is also modified by the presence of indolamine dioxygenase in keratocytes and to a lesser extent in the corneal epithelium and endothelium. This intracellular enzyme catabolizes tryptophan, an amino acid essential for the survival of T lymphocytes.

Uvea

The uveal tract is protected from physical injury by the eyelids, fibrous tunic of the globe, and by the bony orbit. The uvea is critical to maintenance of ocular immune privilege. Immune privilege describes anatomic and molecular mechanisms of immune regulation that provide protection against inflammation-induced injury while maintaining protection against pathogens. Within the eye, the anterior and posterior chambers, the vitreous, and the subretinal space are immune privileged sites. Protecting ocular structures against bystander injury from inflammation is critical to maintaining vision. Corneal endothelial cells and some retinal cells, for example, have limited to no capacity for regeneration. Controlling inflammation also helps keep the ocular media clear of cells and molecules that could diminish or scatter light. Ocular immune privilege is dependent on the immunologic phenomenon known as ACAID as well as the blood-ocular barriers. The lack of true lymphatic vessels within the uveal tract also contributes to the unique immunologic status of the globe.

Blood-Aqueous Barrier

The blood-aqueous barrier, one of two main blood-ocular barriers along with the blood-retinal barrier, is created by tight junctions between nonfenestrated endothelial cells of the iris blood vessels and tight junctions between adjacent epithelial cells of the inner nonpigmented ciliary epithelium. In the iris, large molecules such as large proteins are unable to pass the barriers of the blood vessels. In the ciliary body, the blood vessels are fenestrated and allow passage of plasma proteins and molecules into the stroma as part of aqueous humor production. The barrier is thus located at the nonpigmented epithelium where tight junctions are part of junctional complexes that also include adherens and gap junctions. The tight junctions limit the diffusion of large molecules through the paracellular spaces and also prevent the backflow of aqueous humor. Small amounts of plasma-derived protein will reach the aqueous humor by diffusion from the ciliary stroma to the iris stroma and release in the anterior chamber. Ocular inflammation may result from the disruption of the blood-ocular barriers, resulting in increased vascular permeability, but significant inflammation can also be the cause of the disruption of the blood-ocular barriers. In both instances, the disruption allows infectious agents, inflammatory mediators, and leukocytes access to the uveal tract, including the stroma of the iris, followed by extension into the aqueous humor of the anterior chamber and throughout the globe.

Anterior Chamber-Associated Immune Deviation

Anterior chamber-associated immune deviation (ACAID) is a specialized immune response unique to the eye by which infectious agents and other antigens introduced into the anterior chamber induce only a highly controlled immune response that effectively eliminates the provoking antigen while limiting bystander injury. The process involves the absence of certain response mechanisms normally active in other organs as well as augmented tolerance of some antigens. ACAID is not the absence of an immune response but, rather, a vigorous immune response that favors specific effector mechanisms and a form of selective unresponsiveness. ACAID protects the eye from antigen-specific immune-mediated injury from delayed-type hypersensitivity and B lymphocytes that secrete complement-fixing antibodies. ACAID depends on a unique intraocular immune environment and a modified systemic response.

Major histocompatibility complex (MHC) class I molecules are expressed on virtually all nucleated cells, with the exception of the neurons in the central nervous system, and the corneal endothelium and retina. The low expression of classical MHC class I molecules on the corneal endothelium and the retina prevents targeting by cytotoxic T lymphocytes. MHC class I molecules also regulate natural killer (NK) cell-mediated cytolysis. NK cells are programmed to destroy any cell that lacks MHC class I molecules, usually infected cells or neoplastic cells. To avoid NK cell-mediated destruction, corneal endothelial cells and retinal cells express nonclassical MHC class Ib molecules, which can interact with NK cells transmitting an "off" signal and prevent NK activation.

The aqueous humor benefits from multiple soluble and membrane-bound immunosuppressive molecules. These molecules are released or expressed by the corneal endothelium, the trabecular meshwork cells, the iris posterior epithelium, and the ciliary body epithelium. Transforming growth factor-β (TGF-β) is the most important molecular mediator of immune privilege. TGF-β-exposed antigen-presenting cells (APCs) promote the generation of regulatory T lymphocytes (Treg) that suppress immune responses. TGF-β modifies APCs by inhibiting the expression of interleukin 12 (IL-12) and CD40, molecules that support activated T lymphocytes. Soluble TGF-β also induces the expression of TGF-β and IL-10 by APCs. α-Melanocyte-stimulating hormone (α-MSH) also induces Treg generation and synergizes with TGF-β. Transforming growth factor ($TGF\text{-}\beta_2$), α-MSH, and calcitonin gene-related peptide (CGRP) inhibit innate immunity by interfering with nitric oxide production by macrophages. TGF-β, α-MSH, and vasoactive intestinal peptide inhibit interferon-γ expression by activated $CD4^+$ T lymphocytes modulating helper T lymphocyte differentiation. The aqueous humor contains complement regulatory proteins that inactivate the complement cascade. The corneal endothelium, iris, and ciliary epithelium express membrane-bound molecules such as CD86, membrane-bound TGF-β, and thrombospondin-1 to induce the conversion of activated T lymphocytes into Treg by contact. In addition, ocular cell surface expression of programmed death ligand-1/2 (PD-L1/PD-L2) and the Fas ligand (CD95 ligand) can induce apoptosis of activated T lymphocytes. Some complement regulatory proteins are membrane bound.

ACAID can be separated into three phases: ocular, thymic, and splenic. The induction of ACAID begins with the ocular phase and the capture of antigen in the anterior chamber by macrophages serving as APCs. Ocular APCs act under the influence of soluble immune suppressive molecules, chiefly TGF-β. After capturing the antigen, the APCs begin to produce macrophage inflammatory protein-2 (MIP-2). Activated ocular APCs express CD1d. CD1d molecules have a similar structure as MHC class I molecules, but they present lipid antigens rather than peptides. Within 72 hours, the ocular APCs that have captured antigens migrate to and through the iridocorneal angle and enter the scleral venous plexus and the venous circulation. Mobilized ocular APCs leave the globe predominantly via the bloodstream to reach the thymus and the spleen.

The thymic phase of ACAID aims to provide natural killer T (NKT) lymphocytes required for the splenic phase. In the thymus, ocular APCs induce the production of a unique population of NKT lymphocytes (CD4-CD8-NK1.1$^+$ T lymphocytes). Only APCs that express CD1d can initiate the generation of these specialized NKT lymphocytes. Thymic NKT lymphocytes will migrate to the spleen within 4 days of the initiation of ACAID in the globe.

The splenic phase begins when the ocular APCs that have captured antigens reach the spleen. Some of the unique features of the ocular APCs include the expression of CD1d and complement 3b receptor. These cells also show increased production of IL-10, IL-13, and MIP-2 but downregulation of IL-12. Furthermore, the ocular APCs migrate to the marginal zones composed of predominantly B lymphocytes rather than target areas dominated by T lymphocytes. Once established in the spleen, the ocular APCs secrete TGF-β, thrombospondin-1, and interferon-α/β, creating an immunosuppressive environment. They also secrete MIP-2, a chemoattractant for $CD4^+$ NKT lymphocytes. These $CD4^+$ NKT lymphocytes in turn produce RANTES, which interacts with the marginal zone B lymphocytes and recruits $CD4^+$ T lymphocytes, γδ T lymphocytes, and $CD8^+$ T lymphocytes that differentiate to become the end-stage ACAID Tregs. Thymic NKT lymphocytes are necessary to produce Tregs, although their exact role has not yet been determined.

One population of Treg cells is $CD4^+$, considered "afferent" because these cells suppress the initial activation and differentiation of naive T lymphocytes into effector cells. Afferent Treg cells of ACAID act in regional lymphoid tissue. The second population of Treg cells is $CD8^+$, considered "efferent" because this population inhibits the expression of delayed-type hypersensitivity. Efferent Treg cells of ACAID act in the periphery, including the eye.

Lens

The lens is protected from physical injury by the eyelids, fibrous tunic of the globe, and the bony orbit. The lens capsule prevents direct invasion of most infectious agents. In addition, the capsule protects the lens from leukocyte-mediated injury but not from inflammatory chemical mediators. The lens also benefits from defense mechanisms at other sites, including the globe's immune privilege/anterior chamber-associated immune deviation (ACAID) and the blood-ocular barriers.

Vitreous

The vitreous is protected from physical injury by the eyelids, fibrous tunic of the globe, and the bony orbit. The vitreous also benefits from defense mechanisms at other sites, including the globe's immune privilege/ACAID and the blood-ocular barriers. The vitreous has minimal active defense mechanisms. The hyalocytes can dedifferentiate into fibroblasts as part of a healing response.

Retina and Optic Nerve

The retina is protected from physical injury by the eyelids, fibrous tunic of the globe, and the bony orbit. The retina also benefits from defense mechanisms at other sites, including the globe's immune privilege/ACAID. The retina contributes to the blood-ocular barriers. The blood-retina barrier includes two components: the retinal vessels and the retinal pigment epithelium (RPE). In the retinal vessels, there are tight junctions between nonfenestrated endothelial cells. There are also tight junctions between the cells of the RPE, acting as a barrier between the choroidal blood vessels and neuroretina. The retina has essentially no defense against infectious agents, radiation, chemicals, or inflammatory diseases that extend from other ocular sites. Ischemic injury is a major threat to retinal viability. The retina does benefit from an autoregulated vascular system that allows retinal perfusion to remain relatively normal despite wide fluctuations in systemic blood pressure. This system helps reduce the risk of ischemic injury. The injured retina also produces angiogenic growth factors and has a powerful system of scavengers to counteract the damaging effects of excitatory neurotoxins, nitric oxide, and other potentially damaging by-products of ischemia. The retina has no resident phagocytes or other cellular components of the immune system.

The optic nerve is protected from physical injury by the eyelids and bony orbit. The meninges provide both support and protection. The cellular and molecular defense mechanisms in the optic nerve mimic those in the central nervous system (see Chapter 14).

Orbit

The orbit is protected from most physical and chemical injuries by the eyelids and adjacent skin. The connective tissues and muscles of the orbit are also protected by the bones of the orbit. The innate and adaptive immune responses of connective orbital tissues are similar to those of other connective tissues. The lacrimal gland contributes to the production of the tear film and the defense of the ocular surface (see Cornea).

Disorders of Domestic Animals[2]

Developmental Anomalies of the Globe as a Whole

Ocular developmental anomalies are divided into failures of induction, failures in remodeling, and late failures in atrophy. Included in this section are only those anomalies in early induction that affect the eye as a whole. The anomalies that result from defects occurring later in remodeling or from atrophy typically affect one component predominantly and are discussed in the sections covering each component of the eye.

[2]Postmortem examination of the eye is discussed in E-Appendix 21-1.

Anophthalmia is a very rare condition in which there is no detectable development of the globe. It is usually bilateral. The vast majority of the cases clinically diagnosed as anophthalmia are more accurately described as severe microphthalmia, and some remnant of the globe can be found within the orbit. Anophthalmia most often accompanies other developmental anomalies.

Microphthalmia is the presence of a small, disorganized globe in an orbit of relatively normal size (E-Fig. 21-24). In some cases, the anomaly does not reflect a primary maldevelopment but, rather, involution after some type of exogenous injury to a globe that up to that stage was normal in its development. This includes in utero trauma, ischemic injury, and infection. Such globes can be remarkably small, presenting as a pigmented nodule embedded in the orbit tissue. In most instances, there is pigmented tissue that can be recognized as uveal tract and some neural tissue with features suggesting retina.

Cyclopia and synophthalmia present as a single midline ocular structure (Fig. 21-21). They reflect failure of division of the optic primordium into paired symmetric optic stalks and vesicles, which therefore results in a single midline globe. Most resulting globes include duplicates of some intraocular structures and are properly termed *synophthalmia*. Cyclopia and synophthalmia usually accompany other craniofacial deformities and are rare conditions. Cases of induced cyclopia/synophthalmia have occurred in sheep as well as llamas and alpacas that have ingested the plant *Veratrum californicum*. The plant contains three steroid alkaloids: jervine, cyclopamine, and cycloposine. The alkaloids cause anomalies through the inhibition of the sonic hedgehog signal transduction pathway, which plays an important role in cell growth and differentiation including ocular development. Ewes ingesting the plant on day 14 of gestation give birth to lambs with this ocular malformation in addition to others. Ingestion of the plant before day 14 may result in fetal death but no anomalies. Ingestion after day 14 results in various anomalies but not cyclopia/synophthalmia.

Coloboma is the least severe of the developmental abnormalities affecting the globe as a whole (Fig. 21-22). Many result in the failure of the optic fissure to close. The optic fissure normally closes in the last third of gestation, persisting longest near the posterior pole of the globe just ventral to the optic nerve. If it persists for too long, there is the possibility that the developing retina will grow outwardly through this defect. Some colobomas are secondary to defects in the uveal neuroepithelium or retinal pigment epithelium and failure to properly induce the differentiation of the neural crest-derived uveal stroma. In Charolais cattle, bilateral but often asymmetric colobomas at or near the optic nerve are inherited as an autosomal dominant trait with incomplete penetrance. In Australian shepherds, colobomas have been shown to be the result of a primary defect in the retinal pigment epithelium (RPE) causing hypoplasia of the adjacent choroid and sclera. Similar colobomas occur in other merle breeds and have been described in cattle and cats exhibiting subalbinism.

Diseases of the Globe as a Whole

Glaucoma

Glaucoma is not a single disease but a diverse group of diseases sharing specific physiologic and structural characteristics. It is a clinical syndrome characterized by a sustained increase in intraocular pressure that is detrimental to the health of the optic nerve and the retina, resulting in loss of vision and eventual blindness. Glaucoma causes changes in virtually every tissue within the globe, but changes in the retina and optic nerve are the most clinically important because they lead directly to vision loss. The condition is more prevalent in dogs than in cats or horses. Glaucoma is a frequent cause of ocular pain and blindness in dogs. It is the leading reason for surgical removal of the globe (enucleation). It is relatively less common in cats, yet it is still the leading cause for enucleation in

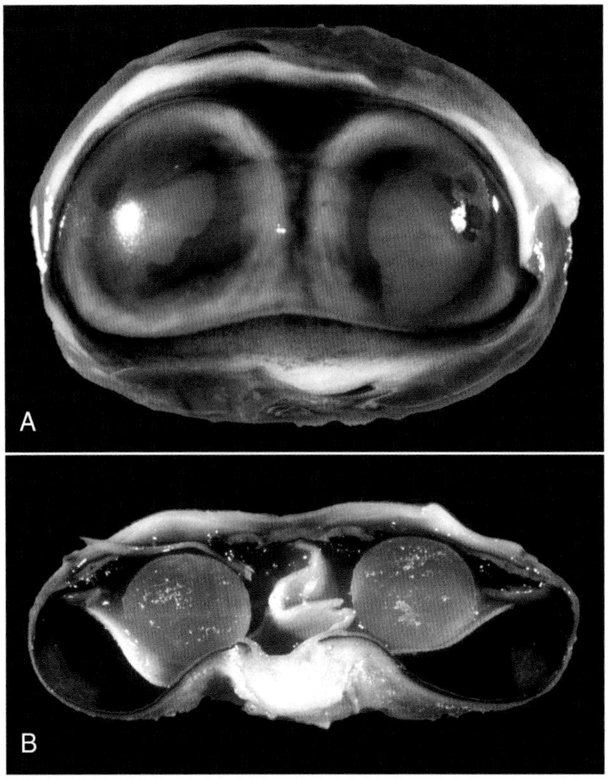

Figure 21-21 **Synophthalmia, Globe, Calf. A,** This fused globe has two lenses, two corneas, and partial duplication of the retina. **B,** Horizontal section of the fused globe revealing two lenses but a shared fused midline retina. (Courtesy Dr. B. Wilcock, Ontario Veterinary College.)

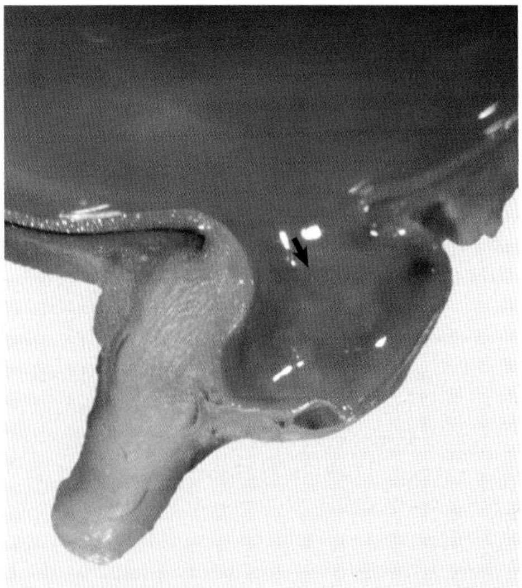

Figure 21-22 **Posterior Coloboma, Collie Eye Anomaly, Globe, Dog.** Failure of closure of the most posterior portion of the optic fissure has allowed outpouching *(arrow)* of the developing retina, adjacent to the optic nerve. The protruding retina is covered by sclera. This result has prevented proper local formation of choroid and sclera, resulting in so-called scleral ectasia. Such globes always have choroidal hypoplasia. (Courtesy Dr. B. Wilcock, Ontario Veterinary College.)

that species. Its frequency in horses may be greatly underestimated because of its variable clinical presentation in that species and because intraocular pressure is not as consistently measured during clinical examination in horses.

Theoretically, glaucoma may result from an increase in the production of aqueous humor or a decrease in its removal. However, there are no known conditions in domestic animals that result from pathologic overproduction of aqueous humor. All examples of glaucoma in domestic animals result from impairment of aqueous outflow. Glaucoma is usually categorized as primary or secondary glaucoma. Primary glaucoma refers to those examples occurring without any known acquired intraocular disease to explain the increase in intraocular pressure. The great majority of these result from developmental errors in the structure and function of the iridocorneal angle and aqueous humor drainage pathways. Secondary glaucoma refers to those examples in which there are acquired lesions responsible for the impairment of aqueous humor outflow such as fibrovascular proliferation, lens luxation, inflammation, or intraocular neoplasia. There are instances in which acquired lesions will occur in globes already predisposed to glaucoma because of developmental structural anomalies. It can be challenging in those instances to determine the relative significance of the developmental and acquired lesions and to characterize the glaucoma as primary or secondary.

The aqueous humor contained in the anterior and posterior chambers is formed continuously by a combination of plasma filtration, diffusion, and active secretion by the ciliary epithelium. The aqueous humor is secreted into the posterior chamber. It circulates near the lens to provide nutrients and remove waste products. The aqueous humor enters the anterior chamber through the pupil, circulates within the anterior chamber to nourish corneal endothelium and stroma, and then exits through the iridocorneal angle at the junction between peripheral cornea and iris. This iridocorneal angle extends circumferentially around the globe and normally has tremendous reserve capacity to accommodate fluctuations in aqueous production and to provide a substantial margin of safety against the development of glaucoma secondary to partial obstruction of aqueous humor outflow by accumulations of blood or inflammatory debris.

The maintenance of intraocular fluid pressure is a balance between aqueous production and outflow and in domestic animals is influenced primarily by resistance to outflow. The outflow pathway is through the iridocorneal angle—a series of perforations in the connective tissue of the peripheral cornea, sclera, and iris stroma that makes up the ciliary cleft and corneoscleral trabecular meshwork (E-Figs. 21-25 and 21-26; see Figs. 21-6 and 21-7). Embryologically, the ciliary cleft and corneoscleral trabecular meshwork are formed by rarefaction of the same mesenchyme that forms iris stroma. In carnivores this remodeling continues for several weeks after birth.

Aqueous humor passing through the iridocorneal angle then enters a network of large veins, known as the scleral venous plexus, which is embedded in the peripheral sclera. The aqueous humor entering these veins is then returned to the systemic circulation. An alternative to this "conventional" drainage pathway is the uveoscleral outflow or "unconventional" pathway. The uveoscleral outflow allows a small percentage of the aqueous humor to percolate through the iris root and ciliary body interstitium to reach the supraciliary space (between the ciliary body and sclera) or suprachoroidal space (between the choroid and sclera) to exit the globe. The proportion of aqueous humor leaving the globe by this more posterior route varies by species: 3% in cats, 15% in dogs, and a larger (but undetermined) percentage in horses. These outflow pathways are not just passive conduits through which the aqueous humor can flow. There is an important physiologic resistance to outflow responsible for the maintenance of normal intraocular pressure. The exact anatomic and physiologic constituents of this outflow resistance remain incompletely defined but include important contributions from the trabecular cells lining the collagen beams within the trabecular meshwork, the glycosaminoglycans embedded in the matrix supporting those trabecular cells, and blood pressure within the scleral venous plexus.

The macroscopic lesions of glaucoma are related to the secondary effects of increased intraocular pressure on the various components of the globe. Although the increase in intraocular pressure is the result of obstruction of aqueous humor outflow, intraocular pressure elevation is distributed throughout the fluid medium of the globe, and the effects are thus felt by all components of the globe. These effects are the same, regardless of the pathogenesis of the glaucoma, and they vary with the rapidity of onset, the severity of the intraocular pressure elevation, and the duration of the elevation. They are also influenced by the age of the patient and by the species. The most obvious of the macroscopic changes include ocular enlargement (buphthalmos), corneal edema, pupillary dilation, and cupping of the optic disc.

Histologic Changes Associated with Glaucoma. The challenge for the pathologist is that many histologic changes that can be secondary to glaucoma can also contribute to the cause of glaucoma. The distinction is not always possible in individual cases. For example, primary lens luxation can lead to pupillary block and glaucoma; conversely, glaucoma causing buphthalmos can damage the zonular ligaments, resulting in lens luxation. As such, ocular changes must always be interpreted in light of history and clinical findings.

The most helpful and frequent histologic changes in the diagnosis of glaucoma are listed in Box 21-12. The changes listed are more frequently observed with chronic glaucoma because globes with acute glaucoma are unlikely to be submitted for histopathologic evaluation.

Buphthalmos is stretching of the globe secondary to increased intraocular pressure (E-Fig. 21-27). It is most obvious in dogs and least obvious in horses. Histologically the sclera becomes thin. Buphthalmos is associated with activation of stretch receptors and pain. Chronic buphthalmos can lead to corneal dessication when the eyelids cannot close over the enlarged globe.

Corneal edema develops when the aqueous pressure exceeds the ability of the sodium pump within the corneal endothelium to dehydrate the cornea (in dogs, at approximately 40 mm Hg). More severe corneal edema then develops as a result of pressure-induced injury to that endothelium, and that injury may become permanent if the endothelial injury is so extensive that it exceeds the capacity of the corneal endothelium to repair itself. Corneal edema secondary to glaucoma is much more frequent in dogs than in cats. Corneal

Box 21-12 Diagnostic Histologic Lesions in Glaucoma

- Inner retinal atrophy
  - Atrophy of the nerve fiber layer and ganglion cell layer
  - Atrophy of the inner nuclear layer (dogs)
- Collapse of the iridocorneal angle
- Optic nerve head cupping
- Atrophy of the ciliary processes
- Scleral thinning

striae (Haab's striae) are breaks in Descemet's membrane occurring secondary to corneal stretching. They are visible on clinical examination as curvilinear to branching tracts of deep corneal stromal opacity. Perilimbal corneal neovascularization is commonly seen secondary to release of angiogenic factors from the injured retina or uveal tract. Chronic keratitis with epidermalization may be present if there is corneal desiccation associated with buphthalmos.

Collapse of the iridocorneal angle is present with almost all forms and almost all cases of glaucoma. The anterior chamber may be shallow. Atrophy of the iris and ciliary processes occurs late in the course of glaucoma, probably as a consequence of chronic pressure-induced ischemia. Atrophy of the ciliary processes eventually leads to normalization of intraocular pressure and even hypotony, seen as part of end-stage glaucoma.

Cataracts are common in glaucoma, presumably as a result of altered aqueous humor dynamics and composition. Lens subluxation or luxation results from stretching and eventual rupture of zonular ligaments secondary to buphthalmos. The luxation may be into the anterior chamber or vitreous. Vitreal liquefaction may be secondary to inflammation preceding the glaucoma, but it also occurs as a consequence of glaucoma.

Retinal atrophy (degeneration) is the most important secondary change in glaucoma. It is important because it causes blindness as a result of damage to the ganglion cells, which cannot regenerate, even if the intraocular pressure returns to normal levels. The degeneration characteristically causes atrophy of the nerve fiber layer and loss of ganglion cells (Fig. 21-23; E-Fig. 21-28). In dogs, there can be later loss of neurons from the inner nuclear layer. The Müller glial cells remain intact, although some functions may be altered. In glaucomatous retinal atrophy, the outer nuclear layer and photoreceptors can remain unaffected for extended periods of time. This pattern of "inner retinal atrophy" with sparing of the outer nuclear layer and photoreceptors is characteristic of glaucoma. Other forms of retinopathy, including inherited, nutritional, and toxic forms, target photoreceptors rather than the inner retina. In some instances, the outer retina may be damaged as part of glaucoma. Acute, severe increases in intraocular pressure can lead to necrosis and apoptosis of photoreceptors, likely as a response to pressure-induced collapse of the superficial choroidal blood vessels and ischemia. In dogs, chronic glaucoma can lead to full-thickness atrophy. In globes with glaucomatous inner retinal atrophy, the retinal degeneration may be more severe ventrally. This is termed "tapetal sparing" but can also be observed in atapetal globes. Tapetal sparing is most common and dramatic in dogs but can be seen in any species.

Optic nerve head cupping is most frequently observed with glaucoma (Fig. 21-24; E-Fig. 21-29). Microscopic changes in the optic nerve include gliosis and degeneration of axons (Wallerian degeneration). Necrosis and malacia can be observed in acute cases. Optic nerve injury occurs more quickly and is more prominent in dogs than in other species.

Pathogenesis of Glaucoma. Glaucoma represents a heterogeneous group of diseases. The exact pathogenesis for the characteristic retinal and optic nerve changes probably varies among species and among different types of glaucoma, and it is the subject of much controversy. Retinal ganglion cell death occurs predominantly by apoptosis. Both the intrinsic, mainly proapoptotic Bcl-2 family members, and extrinsic pathways contribute. Necrosis causes ganglion cell death later in the disease, and likely in specific forms of glaucoma. Multiple mechanisms contribute to the death of retinal ganglion cells. Some of the contributing factors involved in the pathogenesis of glaucoma include the following:

Pressure-induced ischemic damage: This occurs after collapse of blood vessels in the retina, optic nerve, or choroid in response to increased pressure in the vitreous. Pressure-related outward bowing of the lamina cribosa contributes to the altered blood flow. The ischemia and resulting hypoperfusion/hypoxia may contribute to retinal ganglion cell death through multiple mechanisms:

- Direct damage to retinal ganglion cells and the induction of apoptosis
- Excitatory damage from glutamate release (see Excitotoxicity below)
- Oxidative stress and damage
- Mitochondrial dysfunction

Impairment of anterograde and retrograde axoplasmic flow: This interferes with ganglion cell function and is caused by pressure-induced compression of the axons passing through the lamina cribrosa. The altered axoplasmic flow results in disruption of neurotrophic factors from the central nervous system. Neurotrophic factors promote neuron survival by inhibiting apoptosis pathways. Brain-derived neurotrophic factor, ciliary neurotrophic factor, and glial cell line–derived neurotrophic factor all have neuroprotective effects. Endogenous production of neurotrophic factors in the retina can initially protect ganglion cells. However, only neurons exposed to adequate levels of neurotrophic factors can escape apoptosis, and both endogenous neurotrophic factors and those from the central nervous system are

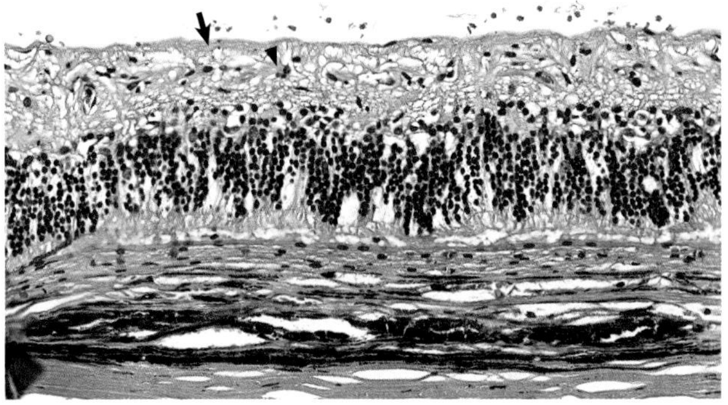

Figure 21-23 **Inner Retinal Atrophy, Glaucoma, Retina, Dog.** Retinal atrophy secondary to glaucoma results in atrophy of the nerve fiber layer *(arrow)* and loss of retinal ganglion cells *(arrowhead)*. In dogs, there may also be atrophy of the inner nuclear layer (as is the case in this image). H&E stain. (Courtesy Dr. P. Labelle, Antech Diagnostics.)

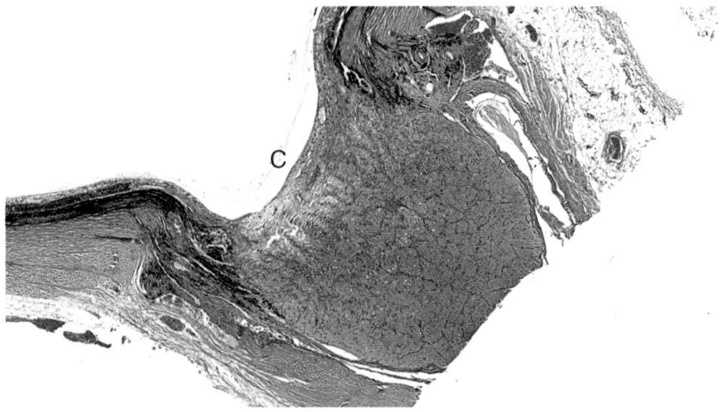

Figure 21-24 **Optic Nerve Cupping, Optic Nerve, Dog.** Atrophy and collapse of the retina results in outward cupping (C) of the optic nerve head in chronic glaucoma. See Fig. 21-10 for the structure of the normal optic nerve. In rabbits, the optic nerve head normally has a deep cup shape. H&E stain. (Courtesy Dr. P. Labelle, Antech Diagnostics.)

required for long-term survival and function of retinal ganglion cells.

Excitotoxicity: Damaged ganglion cells release excitatory compounds, primarily the neurotransmitter glutamate, which then induces apoptosis of previously uninjured ganglion cells. This can lead to a self-perpetuating cycle of neuronal cell death from excitotoxicity. Retinal injury is unlikely to result in massive glutamate release as the case with acute brain injury. Glutamate excess is more likely to only occur in microenvironments representing areas of localized retinal degeneration. Retinal glutamate receptors are located in the outer plexiform layer where glutaminergic synapses connect photoreceptors to bipolar and horizontal cells and in the inner plexiform layer that contains most of the glutaminergic synapses between retinal ganglion cells and bipolar and amacrine cells. Excitotoxic damage occurs when excess glutamate binds to ionotropic glutamate receptors triggering massive calcium influx and activation of proapoptotic pathways. Excitotoxic damage overrides the protective effect of endogenous and exogenous neurotrophic factors. Glial cells that maintain physiologic levels of glutamate are responsible for the uptake of excess glutamate via glutamate/aspartate transporters. As such, deficits in transporter function can contribute to retinal ganglion cell damage. Furthermore, excess glutamate may cause glial cells to exacerbate ganglion cell loss by releasing neurotoxic factors such tumor necrosis factor-α, nitric oxide, and α_2-macromodulin.

The Classification of Glaucoma

Primary Glaucoma. Primary glaucoma occurs without any significant contribution from acquired disease elsewhere within the globe. Primary glaucomas are subdivided into those cases in which there is detectable maldevelopment of the trabecular meshwork (goniodysgenesis) and those cases in which there are no primary histologic lesions (open-angle glaucoma). A very small proportion of these are truly congenital glaucomas in which clinical signs of glaucoma are evident in the first few weeks of life. The vast majority, however, have no clinically detectable increase in pressure or clinical signs related to glaucoma until middle age or even older. The reason for this delay in clinical onset is unclear.

Goniodysgenesis. Goniodysgenesis refers to an abnormal and incomplete development of the iridocorneal angle and aqueous humor draining pathway. It is essentially a canine disease, although reports in other species exist. It mostly occurs as an inherited disease in purebred dogs. It is the result of incomplete remodeling of the solid mass of anterior chamber mesenchyme that gives rise to the stroma of the cornea and anterior uvea. In carnivores, most of this remodeling occurs in the first few weeks of life and involves rarefaction of what was previously a solid mesenchymal mass. The extremely severe cases of goniodysgenesis with essentially no rarefaction of the iridocorneal angle (so-called trabecular hypoplasia) can cause true congenital glaucoma.

The most common histologic anomaly is failure of the most anterior portion of the iridocorneal angle to be adequately remodeled, resulting in thickening of the pectinate ligament with pigmented iris stroma-like tissue that extends from the iris base to the termination of Descemet's membrane (pectinate ligament dysplasia) (Fig. 21-25; E-Figs. 21-30 and 21-31). Arborization of the termination of Descemet's membrane is a common finding, but is not specific for goniodysgenesis. The severity of the lesion may vary significantly along the circumference of the iridocorneal angle. Multiple areas of the iridocorneal angle should be examined histologically before excluding goniodysgenesis, as the lesion may not be recognizable in every section. The risk of developing glaucoma correlates with the extent to which the iridocorneal angle circumference is involved, which must be evaluated clinically. Goniodysgenesis is invariably bilateral but not necessarily symmetric. The robust pectinate ligaments of horses and ruminants, and to a lesser extent pigs, should not be confused with pectinate ligament dysplasia/goniodysgenesis (see Fig. 21-7).

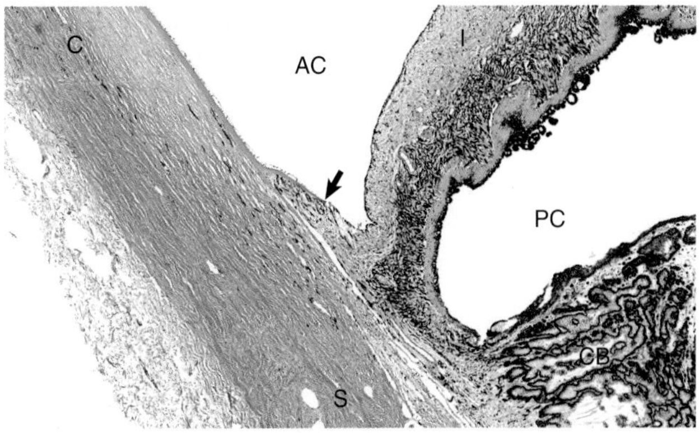

Figure 21-25 **Goniodysgenesis, Primary Glaucoma, Iridocorneal Angle, Dog.** The pectinate ligament is thick with pigmented tissue resembling iris stroma and extends from the base of the iris to the arborizing termination of Descemet's membrane *(arrow)*. The ciliary cleft and corneal scleral trabecular meshwork are collapsed (see Fig. 21-6). AC, Anterior chamber; C, cornea; CB, ciliary body; I, iris; PC, posterior chamber; S, sclera. H&E stain. (Courtesy Dr. P. Labelle, Antech Diagnostics.)

Goniodysgenesis should be considered a risk factor for the development of glaucoma rather than a specific cause. In fact, only a small percentage of affected animals develop glaucoma, including only approximately 15% of the most severely affected dogs. Furthermore, although the lesion is present throughout life, dogs with this condition develop glaucoma as middle-aged to older adults. Dogs that do develop goniodysgenesis-related glaucoma in one eye are at high risk for glaucoma in the contralateral eye. It is likely that there are functional changes associated with goniodysgenesis that do not have a histologic correlate.

The reasons for the delay in the onset of clinical signs of glaucoma are poorly understood. Age-related changes may be contributing factors. Pigment dispersion as a result of contact between the pigmented posterior iris epithelium and the lens capsule has been hypothesized to play a role in the development of goniodysgenesis-related glaucoma in some dogs. Mild uveitis or other minor acquired lesions that might not result in glaucoma in normal globes may be significant in globes with goniodysgenesis. It is possible that any change that decreases the aqueous humor outflow capacity increases the risk of goniodysgenesis-related glaucoma, perhaps in a cumulative manner. The triggering events are unlikely to be the same in each individual.

When goniodysgenesis-related glaucoma does develop, the earliest histologic findings include collapse of the corneoscleral trabecular meshwork, partial and gradual collapse of the ciliary cleft, disruption of the posterior iris epithelium with pigment dispersion, and neutrophilic infiltration within the iridocorneal angle. Early changes in the retina include edema, neutrophilic infiltration, and ganglion cell apoptosis/necrosis. There may be full-thickness injury with severe increases in intraocular pressure. There may be edema and neutrophils within the optic nerve head with eventual infiltration of Gitter cells.

Most globes are examined histologically during the chronic stages of the disease. With chronic goniodysgenesis-related glaucoma, there is complete collapse of the iridocorneal angle including the ciliary cleft and corneoscleral trabecular meshwork. Collapse of the iridocorneal angle can result in a crease at the junction of the pectinate ligament and iris stroma mimicking angle recession (occasionally termed *falsely recessed angle* or *posteriorly displaced angle*). The inner retina is atrophic and there may be full-thickness retinal atrophy in some dogs, with or without tapetal sparing. The optic nerve head is cupped, and the optic nerve is gliotic. Atrophy of the ciliary processes, thinning of the sclera, and other changes associated with chronic glaucoma may be present.

Primary Open-Angle Glaucoma. Primary glaucoma in dogs, cats, and horses can occur in globes in which there is no visible abnormality in the structure of the iridocorneal angle or other portions of the aqueous outflow pathways. These cases represent dysfunction of the iridocorneal angle rather than an anatomic alteration. The best known is heritable open-angle glaucoma described in beagles, and it has been used as a laboratory model of primary glaucoma in human beings. In the early stages of primary open-angle glaucoma, all portions of the aqueous outflow pathways are histologically and ultrastructurally normal. The genetic defect is an autosomal recessive trait that results in accumulation of abnormal extracellular matrix within the trabecular meshwork and resistance aqueous humor outflow. In cats, primary open-angle glaucoma can be unilateral/asymmetric or bilateral. There are no histologic lesions in the iridocorneal angle, but some cases show edema/myxomatous change surrounding the vessels of the scleral venous plexus.

Secondary Glaucoma

Obstruction of the Iridocorneal Angle. The open iridocorneal angle may be blocked by various exudates and cells. Neoplastic cells, hemorrhage/fibrin, and leukocytic infiltrates are the most common forms of open-angle obstruction. Such accumulations of cells and material within the iridocorneal angle are highly unlikely to cause glaucoma unless a significant portion of the iridocorneal angle circumference is affected. Hemorrhage and leukocytic infiltrates in particular will tend to settle ventrally, allowing aqueous humor outflow dorsally. As such, these tend to contribute to the development of glaucoma only in the presence of other lesions.

Neovascular glaucoma is common and occurs when the iridocorneal angle is obstructed by a preiridal fibrovascular membrane. The membrane may also extend on the peripheral posterior cornea (peripheral anterior synechia) and contract to further cause obstruction (E-Fig. 21-32). Neovascular glaucoma is commonly seen with retinal injury, specifically retinal detachment. It is also common with intraocular neoplasia, uveitis, and trauma. Some of the underlying causes of neovascular glaucoma (neoplasia and uveitis) may also contribute directly to aqueous humor outflow obstruction.

Neoplasia often infiltrates the iridocorneal angle directly and can carpet the anterior surface of the iris to cover the iridocorneal angle (E-Fig. 21-33). In addition, tissue damage, uveitis, fibrovascular proliferation, retinal detachment, and lens disease may all contribute to glaucoma secondary to neoplasia. The neoplasms that most frequently cause glaucoma by direct infiltration of the iridocorneal angle are uveal melanocytoma, uveal malignant melanoma, and metastatic lymphoma in dogs and diffuse iris melanoma and metastatic lymphoma in cats.

Pupillary Block. The passage of aqueous humor through the pupil may be blocked or impaired by extension of a preiridal fibrovascular membrane, from adhesions between the iris and lens (posterior synechia) secondary to uveitis, lens luxation, or by massive swelling of the lens part of an intumescent cataract. In pupillary block, aqueous humor accumulates in the posterior chamber, which may result in anterior bowing of the iris (iris bombé), thus displacing the root of the iris and collapsing the iridocorneal angle anteriorly (E-Figs. 21-34 and 21-35).

Aqueous Humor Misdirection. Aqueous humor misdirection (also termed *malignant glaucoma* or *ciliary block*) occurs when aqueous humor accumulates in the vitreous or between the vitreous and retina. This displaces the vitreous, lens, and iris anteriorly, resulting in a shallow anterior chamber and eventually collapse of the iridocorneal angle. Pupillary block develops often as the lens is forced against the iris. It is mostly seen in older cats.

Angle Recession. Angle recession develops following blunt trauma that alters the shape of the globe leading to separation of the ciliary body from the sclera (cyclodialysis). As the ciliary body reconnects with the sclera, there is posterior displacement of the iridocorneal angle. The anterior aspect of the pars plicata of the ciliary body may be thin and lacking ciliary processes. Assuming the aqueous humor outflow pathways remain functional and not obstructed by hemorrhage or fibrovascular proliferation in the immediate period after the trauma, glaucoma can develop later partly because of remodeling of the iridocorneal angle. Fibrosis may be recognized histologically in some cases.

Aging

A number of changes occur as the eye ages. In the cornea, Descemet's membrane becomes thicker while the corneal endothelium is sparser. Senile iris atrophy is common in older animals. Dogs may develop small cysts/cystic degeneration of the posterior iris epithelium. Sclerosis or hyalinization of the collagen at the base of the ciliary processes and pigmentary incontinence in the ciliary body become more prominent in the aging dog (Fig. 21-26). Older cats and horses may have cysts within the pars plana of the ciliary body. The lens capsule thickens and nuclear sclerosis is common in older domestic animals. Senile cataract is common. Older dogs commonly develop hyaluronic acid–containing cysts in the peripheral retina at the ora ciliaris retinae (also termed peripheral cystoid degeneration). Gradual loss of some retinal photoreceptors occurs in older animals. Lipofuscin accumulates in the retinal pigment epithelium as part of normal aging. Foci of mineralization can be found in the sclera of older horses.

Diseases of the Eyelids and Conjunctiva

Developmental Anomalies

Anomalies in the formation of eyelids, including the shape of the palpebral fissure, are common in dogs. In some instances, the "anomaly" is even a feature for the breed (e.g., ectropion in bloodhounds and Saint Bernards). Most of these anomalies are not

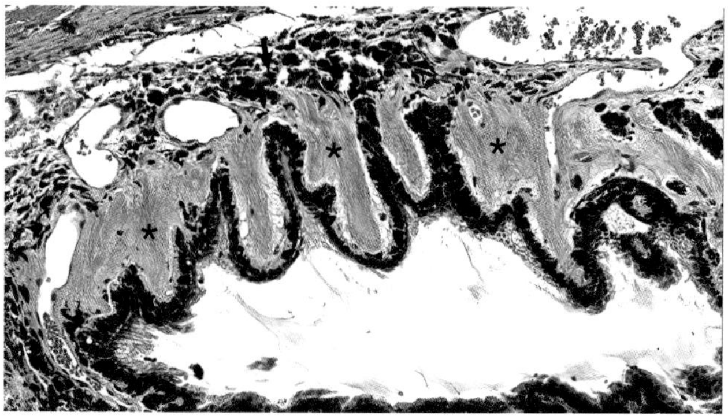

Figure 21-26 **Aging Changes, Ciliary Body, Dog.** As dogs age, the collagen at the base of the ciliary processes becomes hyalinized *(large coalescing pink areas [asterisks])* and there is infiltration of macrophages that phagocytize melanin *(arrow)* that has leaked from the pigmented ciliary epithelium (pigmentary incontinence). H&E stain. (Courtesy Dr. P. Labelle, Antech Diagnostics.)

examined microscopically because they are obvious macroscopically. They are important in clinical ophthalmology, and surgical correction of these anomalies is common, but histologic examination is very rare.

Eyelid Agenesis (Coloboma). There may be partial or complete absence of an eyelid. It occurs in all species but is most common in cats, involving the lateral aspect of the upper eyelid. Dermoids and lacrimal gland aplasia/hypoplasia may be present simultaneously with eyelid agenesis. The eyelid defects may result in inadequate dispersion of the tear film or excessive evaporation leading to chronic keratitis and occasionally corneal ulceration.

Premature Eyelid Separation. In carnivores, the eyelids are normally fused at birth (known as physiologic ankyloblepharon), which is essential to protect the immature cornea from infection and desiccation. Premature eyelid separation predisposes the eye to infectious keratitis, desiccation, and corneal rupture.

Entropion and Ectropion. Conformational entropion is the inward rolling of the eyelid margin because of inadequate overall length. The usual result is irritation of the cornea by the eyelid cilia and/or hair. It is a common bilateral anomaly in purebred dogs that have been selected for breeding based partly on the shape of the palpebral fissure. It is also common in sheep. The extent and magnitude of the defect varies greatly among individual animals but tends to be relatively uniform within an affected breed. Depending on the severity of the irritation, entropion can lead to nonspecific chronic keratitis or progress to corneal ulceration. Entropion may also be acquired as the result of blepharospasm, scarring of the eyelid that is severe enough to cause changes in conformation, or lesions to the globe such as phthisis bulbi or microphthalmia. Surgical correction of entropion is a common procedure.

Ectropion is created by undue laxity of an excessively long eyelid, resulting in an eversion of the eyelid margin. As with entropion, its extent and severity vary greatly among individual animals and among breeds. The lower eyelid is more frequently affected. The anomaly has less significance than entropion because there is no direct corneal irritation, but it can result in chronic keratitis. Like entropion, severe scarring of the eyelid may cause acquired ectropion.

Anomalies of Cilia: Trichiasis, Distichiasis, and Ectopic Cilia. Anomalies of cilia are prevalent in dogs, less so in horses, and uncommon in cats. They may or may not cause clinical signs; their significance lies in the corneal irritation they can cause. These conditions are best diagnosed clinically; there is no need for microscopic evaluation. Distichiasis is the presence of an ectopic cilia originating from the ducts of the meibomian glands. The defect is usually bilateral. Trichiasis is misdirection of the normal cilia so that they contact the cornea. Ectopic cilia are abnormally placed cilia within the lamina propria of the conjunctiva. Their emergence through the palpebral conjunctiva may result in profound corneal irritation and ulceration.

Conjunctival Dermoid. Dermoid is the only conjunctival developmental anomaly that is reasonably prevalent. The bulbar conjunctiva is most commonly affected. It reflects the failure of the fetal ectoderm to undergo complete corneal differentiation with the result that a portion of the conjunctiva remains as skin. Clinically, it is visible as a haired nodule. Histologically, it appears as a segment of conjunctiva that is more or less identical to normal skin. Some dermoids show complete development of skin and hair follicles, whereas others consist only of vestigial hair follicles. Dermoids also occur in the cornea.

Acquired Eyelid Diseases

Acquired diseases that affect the cutaneous aspect of the eyelid are essentially those that affect the skin and those with a predisposition for the head or mucocutaneous junctions (see Chapter 17). Chalazion is sterile lipogranulomatous inflammation in response to the leakage of meibomian secretions into the surrounding dermis of the eyelid margin. It is much more common in dogs than in any other species. In most cases, the inflammation is associated with meibomian gland neoplasia, although it can also occur with other causes of meibomian secretions leakage such as meibomian adenitis. Histologically, the inflammation is an accumulation of macrophages and multinucleated cells bordering the meibomian neoplasm or meibomian gland (Fig. 21-27). In dogs, these cells often contain acicular cytoplasmic clefts that correspond to birefringent material. There may be accumulation of extracellular free lipids (lipid lakes). Similar inflammation with macrophages and multinucleated cells develops in cats (termed lipogranulomatous conjunctivitis). Lipid lakes tend to be prominent. Although feline lipogranulomatous inflammation can be associated with meibomian gland disease, it can also accompany other forms of neoplasia, including malignancies such as squamous cell carcinoma. As such, the lesion is not strictly limited to the eyelid margin and can occur in the bulbar or third eyelid conjunctiva.

Acquired Conjunctival Diseases

Infectious Diseases. Onchocercosis causes conjunctival diseases in dogs, cats, and horses. The life cycle is likely similar for all *Onchocerca* spp., with black flies (*Simulium* spp.) or gnats/midges (*Culicoides* spp.) serving as intermediate hosts. In small animals, the disease is caused by *Onchocerca lupi* and has been reported in dogs and cats from the southwestern United States and dogs from Europe. The condition often presents as conjunctival or episcleral inflammatory nodules centered on adult filarial nematode worms (Fig. 21-28). Orbital nodules may be associated with exophthalmos. The inflammation is predominantly granulomatous. Eosinophils may be present in large numbers, and there may be fibrosis. In some cases, the parasites elicit minimal inflammation and are bordered only by a thin band of fibrous tissue. The paired uteri of the adult female worms typically contain microfilariae, which suggest patent infection. *Onchocerca lupi* must mainly be differentiated from *Dirofilaria immitis*. *Oncocercha* spp. have annular/circumferential cuticular

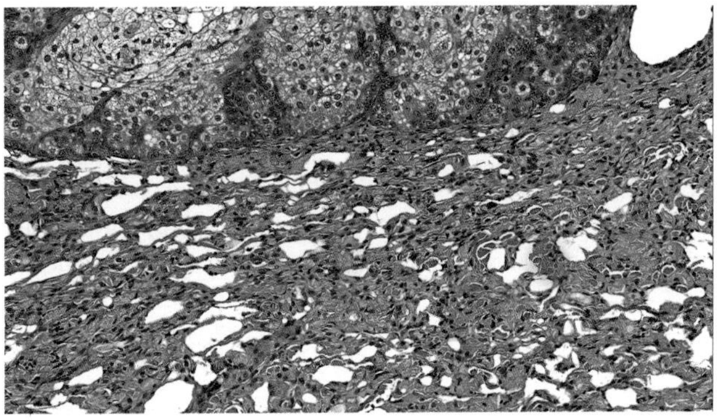

Figure 21-27 Chalazion, Eyelid, Dog. Lipogranulomatous inflammation below a meibomian adenoma located in the top quarter of the figure. The macrophages and multinucleated giant cells often contain cytoplasmic acicular clefts and border lipid lakes (clear spaces in inflammatory response). H&E stain. (Courtesy Dr. P. Labelle, Antech Diagnostics.)

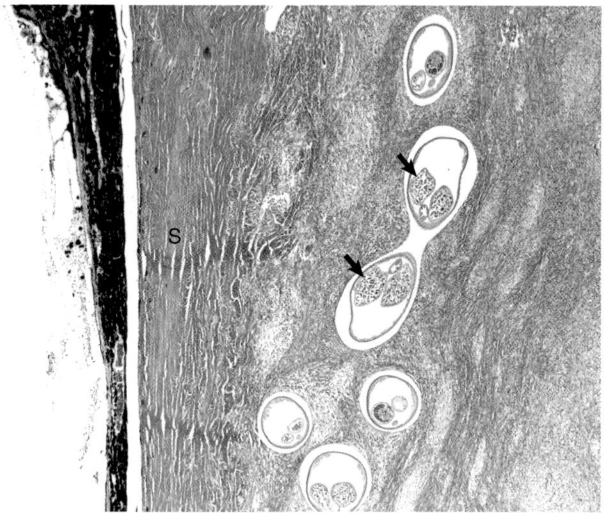

Figure 21-28 Orbital Onchocercosis, Orbit, Dog. Episcleral and orbital granulomatous inflammation centered on nematodes. Microfilariae are present within the paired uteri *(arrows)*. *S*, Sclera. H&E stain. (Courtesy Dr. P. Labelle, Antech Diagnostics.)

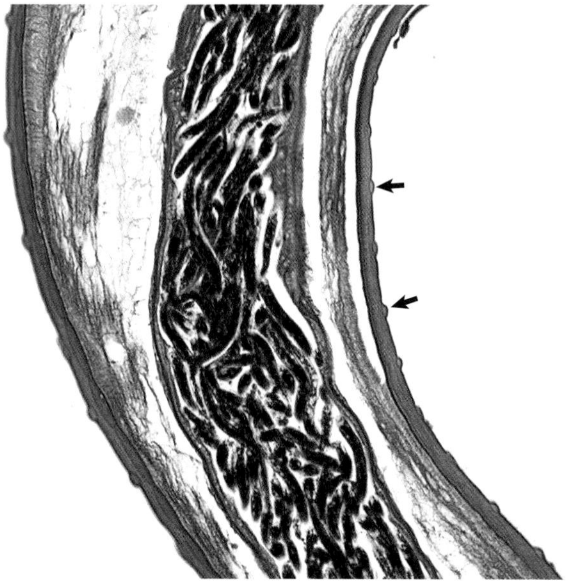

Figure 21-29 Onchocerca Lupi, Dog. Annular/circumferential cuticular ridges *(arrows)* are visible in longitudinal sections of *Onchocerca lupi*. Microfilariae are present within the uterus. H&E stain. (Courtesy Dr. P. Labelle, Antech Diagnostics.)

ridges that are visible in longitudinal section, whereas *Dirofilaria* spp. have longitudinal ridges that are visible in cross sections (Fig. 21-29). In horses, the ocular lesions are caused by *Onchocerca cervicalis* and it is the microfilariae that cause the lesions, not the adult worms. In addition to conjunctivitis, there may be keratitis and uveitis.

Chlamydial conjunctivitis occurs in many species. *Chlamydophyla felis* is often associated with primary conjunctivitis in cats. The lesion is often unilateral initially. It may be seen concurrently with rhinitis and/or respiratory disease. The conjunctivitis is initially neutrophilic but progresses to also include macrophages, lymphocytes, and plasma cells. Early in the disease (between days 7 and 14), intracytoplasmic elementary bodies may be seen on cytology. Because the clinical signs are characteristic, these cases are unlikely to be examined histologically. Histologic examination in chronic cases typically shows nonspecific lymphoplasmacytic conjunctivitis often including lymphoid hyperplasia but no elementary bodies to confirm the diagnosis. In ruminants and pigs, chlamydophilosis causes lesions in multiple organs and may include conjunctivitis. The infection can cause mucopurulent conjunctivitis and polyarthritis in lambs and kids.

Thelazia spp. are thin, rapidly motile nematodes 7 to 20 mm in length that inhabit the conjunctival sac and lacrimal duct of a variety of wild and most domestic animals. Only a small proportion of animals infected with the parasite have clinical disease. They are transmitted from animal to animal by flies, which ingest larvae present in host lacrimal secretions. They are of minor significance as parasites of horses and cattle and cause mild lymphofollicular conjunctivitis. In Asia and Europe, *Thelazia callipaeda* is a cause of conjunctivitis in dogs and cats.

Noninfectious Diseases

Lymphoplasmacytic Conjunctivitis. Lymphoplasmacytic infiltration is the most common inflammatory response of the conjunctiva. This type of inflammation does not suggest a specific etiology and represents the end result of a variety of insults. Chronic or previous infection, physical trauma, immune reactions, chronic irritation, and so on are all possible initiating or contributing causes. Lymphocytes and plasma cells are the predominant cell types. Rare macrophages and mast cells may be present. Mild cases are usually perivascular and superficial in distribution, whereas more severe cases may be diffuse. Some degree of lymphoid follicular hyperplasia will accompany chronic cases. Lymphoid hyperplasia can be quite severe in horses. Lymphoplasmacytic conjunctivitis is typically nonulcerative. The diagnosis of lymphoplasmacytic conjunctivitis is especially common in biopsy submissions, a reflection of the fact that the conjunctiva is sampled late in the disease process and often after treatment using a variety of medications has been attempted.

Eosinophilic Conjunctivitis. Eosinophilic conjunctivitis is the conjunctival counterpart of the eosinophilic keratitis syndrome seen in cats and occasionally in horses (see Disorders of Cats). Rarely, there may be conjunctivitis in the absence of keratitis. Lesions may be unilateral or bilateral. Although eosinophils are required for the diagnosis, the proportion of eosinophils within the inflammatory infiltrate varies greatly between cases. Ulceration is common in severe cases. In chronic cases, especially those in which antiinflammatory medication was used, inflammation is likely to be predominantly lymphoplasmacytic with a scattering of eosinophils. In any species, eosinophils may be present with allergic/hypersensitivity disease and parasitic disease.

Solar-Associated Lesions. As in the skin, chronic ultraviolet exposure results in degenerative lesions in the conjunctiva (see Chapter 17). Factors that contribute to the development of solar-associated lesions include high altitudes, low latitudes, lightly pigmented conjunctiva, and long duration of exposure. The lesions include solar elastosis, solar fibrosis, and solar vasculopathy (Fig. 21-30). The most common and most easily recognizable change consists of solar elastosis. Solar elastosis develops in the superficial substantia propria and is recognized as thick, basophilic, and irregularly aligned fibers. These fibers are visible with standard hematoxylin and eosin staining and do not require special staining for elastin fibers. The fibers of solar elastosis represent mostly newly produced material rather than degeneration of preexisting fibers. The lesions are usually mild in dogs but can form plaques in horses and cattle. Solar fibrosis describes a band of hypocellular, sclerotic altered collagen located immediately underlying the epithelium. Solar fibrosis is not true fibrosis. Solar vasculopathy is uncommonly seen in the

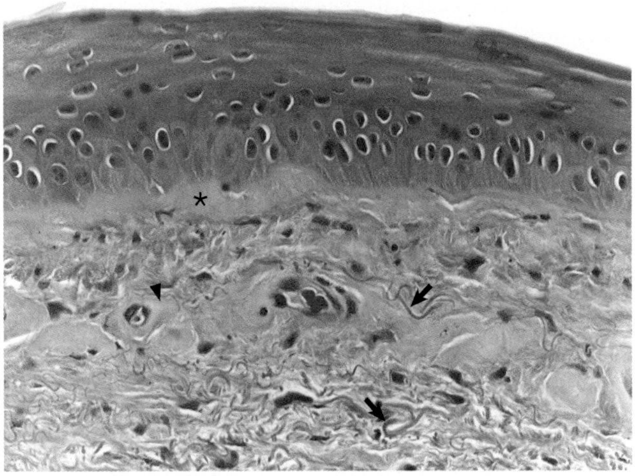

Figure 21-30 **Conjunctival Solar-Associated Lesions, Conjunctiva, Dog.** Solar elastosis consists of thick basophilic irregular fibers *(arrows)*. The band of hypocellular, sclerotic collagen in the superficial substantia propria is solar fibrosis *(asterisk)*. Some of the vessels have thickened, smudgy walls consistent with solar vasculopathy *(arrowhead)*. H&E stain. (Courtesy Dr. P. Labelle, Antech Diagnostics.)

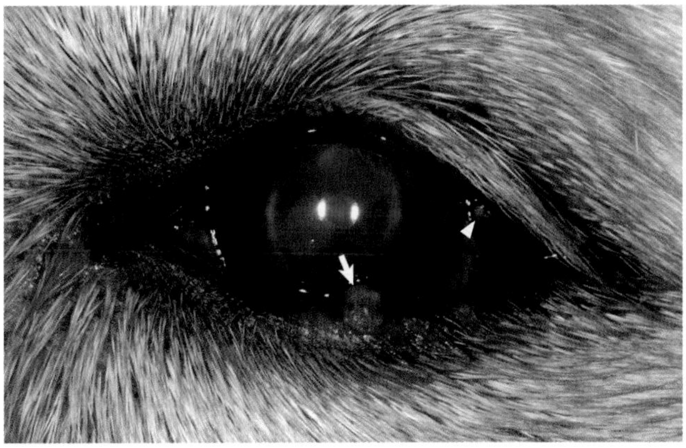

Figure 21-31 **Meibomian Adenomas, Eyelids, Dog.** A poorly pigmented meibomian gland adenoma *(arrow)* is present in the central lower eyelid, and a darkly pigmented meibomian gland adenoma is present in the temporal upper eyelid *(arrowhead)*. (Courtesy Ophthalmology Service, College of Veterinary Medicine, University of Illinois.)

conjunctiva but presents as thickened, hyaline, "smudgy" vessel walls with or without endothelial swelling. Epithelial changes often accompany solar lesions, including hyperplasia, hyperpigmentation, and keratinization. Solar-associated lesions are often seen concurrently with conjunctival squamous cell carcinoma or vascular neoplasia.

Neoplasms of the Eyelids and Conjunctiva

Meibomian Gland Neoplasms. Meibomian adenomas and epitheliomas are very common benign neoplasms and represent up to 70% of all canine eyelid neoplasms. Meibomian gland neoplasms appear clinically as tan, pink, gray, or black masses extending from the meibomian gland orifice or, less frequently, erupting through the palpebral conjunctiva (Fig. 21-31). Histologically, meibomian gland adenomas are similar to sebaceous adenomas of the skin. They are well-circumscribed and often partially exophytic. They are composed of variably sized lobules of meibomian cells that show normal maturation from small basal reserve cells at the periphery to mature large lipid-laden well-differentiated cells centrally (Fig. 21-32; E-Fig. 21-36). Areas of cystic degeneration are common. Meibomian adenomas usually include haphazardly arranged ducts that vary in number and size. Meibomian epitheliomas have histologic features similar to cutaneous sebaceous epitheliomas. They are well-circumscribed masses composed of densely packed sheets of small basal reserve cells with limited differentiation to lobules or single lipid-laden cells or ducts. The mitotic index is typically high, but nuclear atypia and pleomorphism are minimal. Epitheliomas should have a "preponderance" of basal cells. Many meibomian neoplasms are pigmented. Leakage of meibomian secretions can lead to severe granulomatous inflammation (chalazion). Papillary hyperplasia of the overlying epithelium is common.

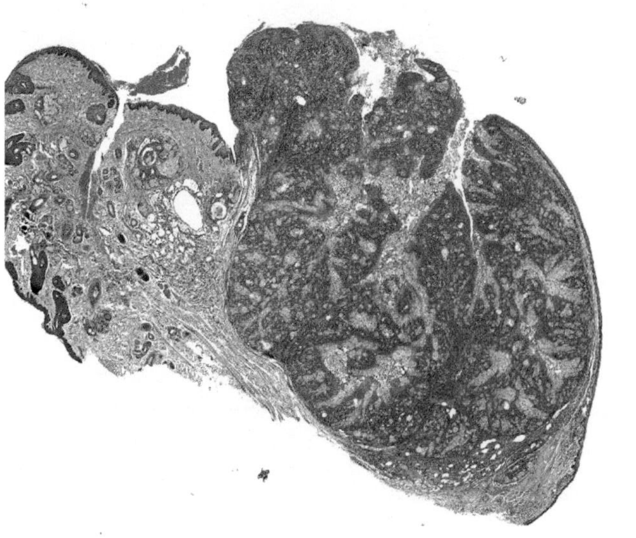

Figure 21-32 **Meibomian Adenoma, Eyelid, Dog.** The well-circumscribed neoplasm is located at the eyelid margin. It is composed of lobules of sebaceous cells with areas of cystic degeneration. H&E stain. (Courtesy Dr. P. Labelle, Antech Diagnostics.)

Conjunctival Squamous Cell Carcinoma. Squamous cell carcinoma of the conjunctiva occurs in all species but is most common in cattle and horses (Fig. 21-33; E-Fig. 21-37). In cattle, it is an economically significant neoplasm. The bulbar conjunctiva, especially at the lateral limbus, is commonly affected. Squamous cell carcinoma is the most common neoplasm affecting ocular structures in horses. The third eyelid and limbus are the most commonly affected conjunctival sites in horses.

In both cattle and horses, the pathogenesis includes a role for ultraviolet light–associated damage. Many/most neoplasms have altered p53 expression. Animals with minimal pigmentation of eyelids and conjunctiva are more susceptible. Actinic keratosis often precedes the development of neoplasia. Viruses, such as bovine papillomavirus and bovine herpesvirus 5, have been detected within bovine ocular squamous cell carcinomas, but their causal role has not been proven. As with sunlight-induced squamous cell carcinoma in the skin, the ocular neoplasms go through a series of precancerous changes in response to actinic injury. The sequence of lesions is as follows: hyperplasia, dysplasia, squamous cell carcinoma in situ, and eventually invasive squamous cell carcinoma. Not all precancerous lesions develop into carcinomas. Solar-associated lesions may be seen concurrently.

In cats, squamous cell carcinoma usually affects the skin of the eyelid itself rather than conjunctiva. Those that do occur in the

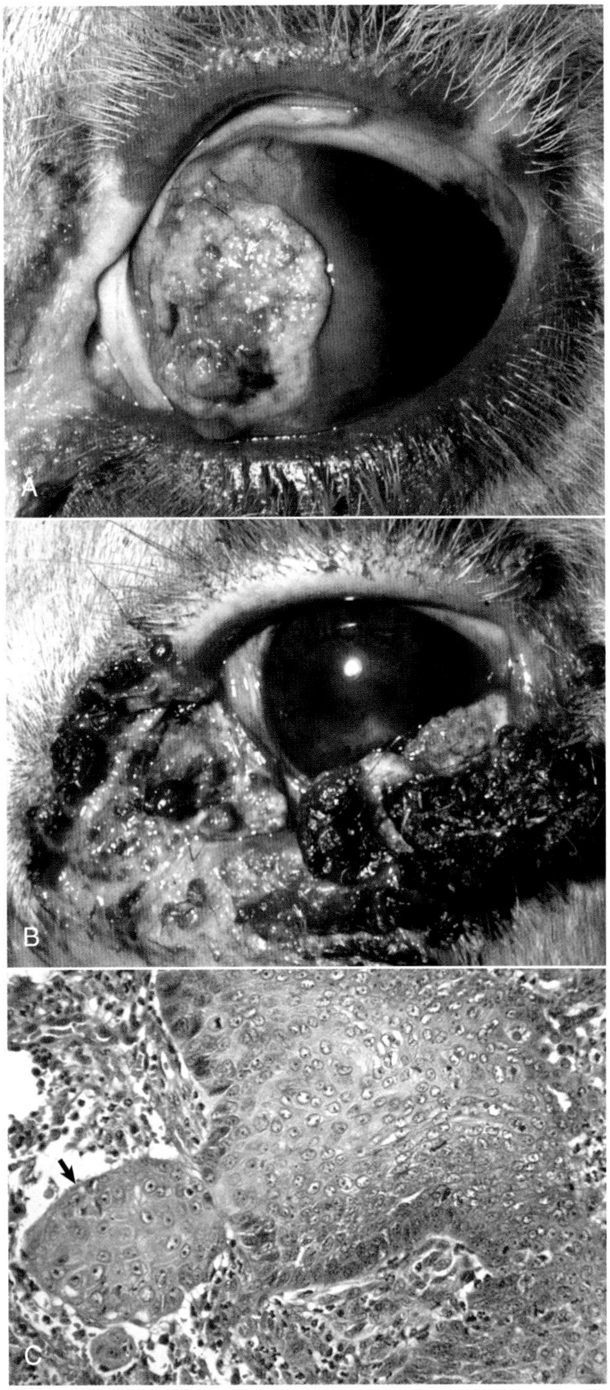

Figure 21-33 **Squamous Cell Carcinoma, Eyelids and Globe, Hereford Cow. A,** Medial limbus. The carcinoma has spread over the cornea as an exophytic growth from its original site on the medial limbus. Note the corneal edema *(gray area)* adjacent to the margin of the carcinoma. **B,** Third and lower eyelids. Note the exophytic squamous cell carcinoma on the third eyelid, acanthosis on the lateral half of the lower palpebral conjunctiva and on the skin of the medial canthus, and keratosis on the lower eyelid. **C,** Early infiltrative squamous cell carcinoma, lower palpebral conjunctiva. A nest of atypical epithelial cells *(arrow)* has infiltrated through the basement membrane of the conjunctival epithelium. H&E stain. (Courtesy Dr. M.D. McGavin, College of Veterinary Medicine, University of Tennessee.)

conjunctiva must be differentiated from conjunctival mucoepidermoid carcinomas, which show some glandular differentiation and are often papillary on the surface. Squamous cell carcinoma is uncommon in the conjunctiva of dogs.

Granular Cell Tumor. Granular cell tumors can affect the eyelid of dogs at the medial canthus. The histologic features are similar to those affecting other sites. The neoplastic cells are characterized by abundant cytoplasm that contains numerous periodic acid–Schiff (PAS)–positive granules. Ultrastructurally, the granules are consistent with lysosomes. The cells show minimal pleomorphism, and mitotic activity is minimal to absent. Excision is usually curative.

Apocrine Cystadenoma. Apocrine cystadenomas (hidrocystomas) are benign lesions that affect the eyelids of cats, most often Persians. Grossly, the lesions present as multinodular to multifocal pigmented masses. Histologically, apocrine cystadenomas consist of multiple variably sized cysts lined by cuboidal to attenuated epithelium. The dark appearance of the nodules is the result of the brown secretions contained within the cysts. Macrophages may infiltrate the cysts. Excision is usually curative, but additional similar lesions may develop.

Adenocarcinoma of the Gland of the Third Eyelid. Adenocarcinomas of the gland of the third eyelid affect dogs and cats. They are expansile and variably infiltrative masses. Some are well-differentiated and composed of tubules that resemble normal gland tissue, and others are mostly solid with only rare tubules. Squamous metaplasia is a common finding. Third eyelid gland adenocarcinomas in dogs tend to recur only with incomplete excision, and they only rarely metastasize. Despite similar histologic features, adenocarcinomas of the gland of the third eyelid are more aggressive in cats and metastasize more readily than in dogs.

Conjunctival Melanocytic Neoplasms. Primary conjunctival melanocytic neoplasia occurs mostly in dogs and cats. In both species, the vast majority of conjunctival melanocytic neoplasms are malignant (E-Fig. 21-38). In dogs, most occur on the third eyelid, whereas the bulbar conjunctiva is the most common site in cats. Conjunctival melanocytic neoplasms appear clinically as pink to lightly pigmented to darkly pigmented masses of the palpebral, bulbar, and third eyelid conjunctiva. Histologically, the cells are polygonal to spindle cells and form various growth patterns. Junctional activity, intraepithelial nests of neoplastic cells, is present in most masses where the overlying epithelium is intact. A mitotic index of at least 4 in 10 400× fields indicates malignancy, although the mitotic index is typically much higher. Foci of necrosis are common, and melanophages may infiltrate the neoplasms. Conjunctival malignant melanomas are invasive with a high rate of recurrence (30% in cats and up to 50% in dogs). Metastasis occurs in 20% to 30% of canine cases and approximately 15% of feline cases.

Conjunctival Vascular Neoplasms. Vascular neoplasms arise within the conjunctival lamina of dogs, cats, and horses. Hemangioma and hemangiosarcoma appear clinically as smooth, raised, pink to red masses on the conjunctival surface. Those tumors that are well circumscribed and consist of attenuated endothelium are classified as hemangiomas, and those with invasion formed by plump endothelium are classified as hemangiosarcomas. However, there is a continuum in the histologic appearance from hemangioma to hemangiosarcoma. Most conjunctival hemangiosarcomas are well differentiated, and distinction from hemangiomas is not always straightforward. Most of vascular neoplasms in dogs and cats are cured by complete excision, although there may be recurrence. The metastatic potential is minimal. In dogs and cats, the pathogenesis includes a role for ultraviolet light–associated damage, and solar-associated lesions may be seen concurrently. In horses, most vascular neoplasms are malignant. Most are poorly differentiated hemangiosarcomas (initially described as angiosarcomas); however, rare lymphangiosarcomas have been reported. These neoplasms are locally infiltrative and may metastasize.

Conjunctival Mast Cell Tumor. Conjunctival mast cell tumors in dogs present clinically as smooth, firm, and subconjunctival and are histologically similar to those in the skin. The conjunctival masses are typically small and well circumscribed, and most are composed of sheets of well-differentiated mast cells. Neither the grading systems nor the prognostic markers established for cutaneous mass cell neoplasia have been investigated in conjunctival masses. Complete surgical excision is reported to be curative for conjunctival mast cell tumors, and metastasis has not been described.

Conjunctival Papillomas. Benign squamous papillomas are frequent lesions of the bulbar conjunctiva of dogs. They are formed by papillary fronds of hyperplastic, often pigmented epithelium supported by fibrovascular stroma continuous with the conjunctival substantial propria. Their significance lies mainly as a differential diagnosis for malignant neoplasms such as squamous cell carcinoma and conjunctival malignant melanoma when pigmented. The vast majority of conjunctival papillomas are not associated with a viral infection; however, papillomavirus-induced lesions can affect the conjunctiva.

Conjunctival Lymphoma. Conjunctival lymphoma occurs sporadically in all species. The conjunctiva may be the primary site or may be part of systemic disease. Conjunctival lymphoma has histologic features and behavior similar to those in the skin.

Diseases of the Cornea and Sclera

Corneal Developmental Anomalies

Dermoid. Dermoid is the only corneal anomaly that is reasonably prevalent. As with conjunctival dermoid, the lesion is composed of ectopic hair follicles and adnexal glands within the cornea (Fig. 21-34; E-Fig. 21-39). The ectopic tissue ranges from just a few scattered sebaceous glands to features of normal skin including mature hair follicle.

Acquired Corneal Diseases

Indolent Corneal Ulcers (Nonhealing/Persistent/Recurrent Ulcers, Spontaneous Chronic Corneal Epithelial Defects). Indolent corneal ulcers mostly develop in dogs, but nonhealing ulcers have also been described in horses and cats. The condition describes superficial ulcers that failed to heal properly despite the absence of an underlying cause. The lesion is likely initiated by trauma. In affected areas, the basement membrane is absent or discontinuous and the stromal surface is covered by fibronectin. Slug expression and other factors involved in epithelial cell migration are absent or decreased at the margins of the ulcer. After ulceration and sliding of the epithelium, permanent adhesion requires the reformation of basement membrane, hemidesmosomes, and hemidesmosomal anchoring filaments, which extend through the basement membrane to anchor into the superficial stroma. If the stroma is abnormal, these filaments cannot anchor the regenerating stroma. Histologically, the lesion is recognized as large flaps of epithelium separated from the stroma (Fig. 21-35; E-Fig. 21-40). The

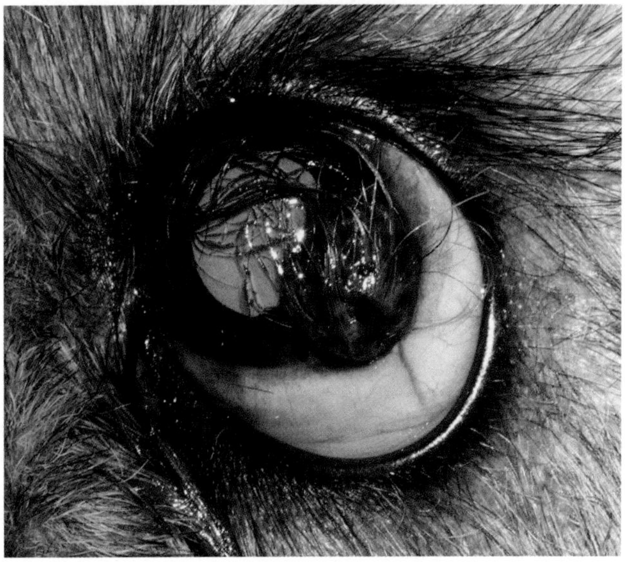

Figure 21-34 **Dermoid, Cornea, Dog.** A pigmented haired nodule is present on the lateral quarter of the cornea and bulbar conjunctiva. (Courtesy Ophthalmology Service, College of Veterinary Medicine, University of Illinois.)

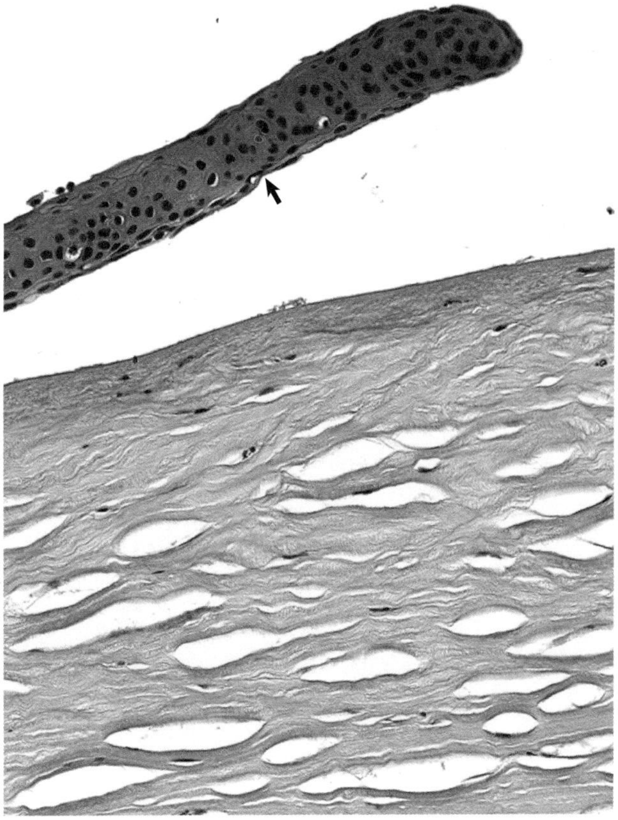

Figure 21-35 **Indolent Corneal Ulcer, Cornea, Dog.** A large flap of corneal epithelium separated from the stroma. The epithelium shows dysmaturation and loss of polarity including a lack of a recognizable basal layer *(arrow)*. The edge of the ulcer is rounded. The underlying superficial stroma is hyalinized and acellular. H&E stain. (Courtesy Dr. P. Labelle, Antech Diagnostics.)

nonadherent epithelium shows dysmaturation and loss of polarity. The epithelial edge tends to be rounded. The underlying superficial stroma is hyalinized and acellular, forming a thin band of pale collagenous tissue. The stromal changes may or may not be present in horses. A variety of corneal stromal diseases, including corneal edema, can, in some cases, cause separation of the corneal epithelium, resulting in a histologic lesion that mimics indolent corneal ulcers. Histologically, indolent corneal ulcers may need to be differentiated from artifactual separation of the corneal epithelium: With artifactual separation, the corneal epithelium maintains polarity and maturation, and the interruption in the epithelium is abrupt.

Corneal Sequestrum. Corneal sequestrum is mainly a condition of cats but it also occurs in horses and dogs (Fig. 21-36; E-Fig. 21-41). The lesion often occurs after chronic ulceration, but the exact pathogenesis is not known. There is imbibition of brown-colored pigment in the superficial stroma. This results in a very characteristic central corneal dark brown pigmentation that is the predominant and essentially pathognomonic feature of this disease. The origin of the pigment remains undetermined; there is evidence to both support and disprove the presence of melanin and iron/porphyrins. Histologically, the lesion is a well-demarcated area where the stroma is devitalized and acellular (Fig. 21-37; E-Fig. 21-42). When present, the brown discoloration is evident histologically. There can be significant, usually neutrophilic inflammation that borders but does not extend in the sequestrum.

Suppurative Keratomalacia ("Melting Ulcer"). Neutrophils from the tear film and limbus can release lytic enzymes, and many organisms produce enzymes that cause stromal necrosis/malacia (Fig. 21-38). Keratomalacia can occur in sterile lesions; however, ulcers that become contaminated with bacteria or fungi are especially prone to destructive suppurative keratomalacia. The most severe cases will progress to descemetocele and corneal perforation. In the absence of immediate medical intervention, this typically leads to rupture of Descemet's membrane (perforating ulcer), leakage of aqueous humor from the anterior chamber, and possibly iris prolapse. Gram-negative bacteria such as *Pseudomonas* spp. are most likely to cause suppurative keratomalacia. Contamination by opportunistic hyphal fungi (especially *Aspergillus* spp. and *Fusarium* spp.) is a particularly frequent cause of keratomalacia in horses (see Equine Fungal Keratitis). Histologically, there is ulceration of the epithelium, often abrupt loss of stromal lamellar organization, and infiltration of mostly degenerate neutrophils.

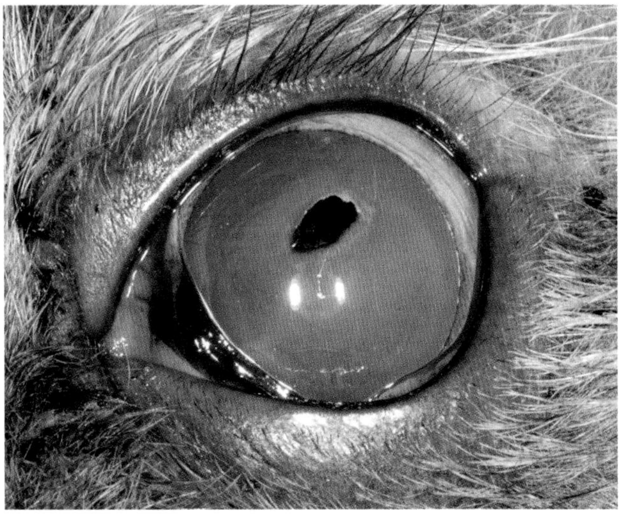

Figure 21-36 **Corneal Sequestrum, Cornea, Cat.** A brown-colored corneal sequestrum is visible in this axial cornea. (Courtesy Ophthalmology Service, College of Veterinary Medicine, University of Illinois.)

Corneal Dystrophies and Depositions. Among the domestic animals, corneal dystrophies and depositions are most often seen in dogs. The lesions may affect the epithelium, stromal, or endothelium. True dystrophies are bilateral and symmetric, often breed related, and occur in the absence of inflammatory or metabolic disease. These deposits often have characteristic clinical features (breed, age, exact anatomic location, and macroscopic appearance)

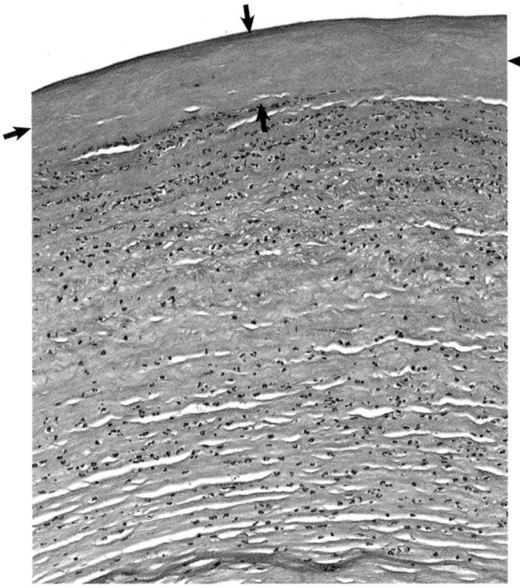

Figure 21-37 **Corneal Sequestrum, Cornea, Dog.** The cornea is ulcerated with a well-demarcated superficial acellular and devitalized sequestrum *(arrows)* bordered by underlying stroma that is infiltrated by neutrophils. This sequestrum is not pigmented. H&E stain. (Courtesy Dr. P. Labelle, Antech Diagnostics.)

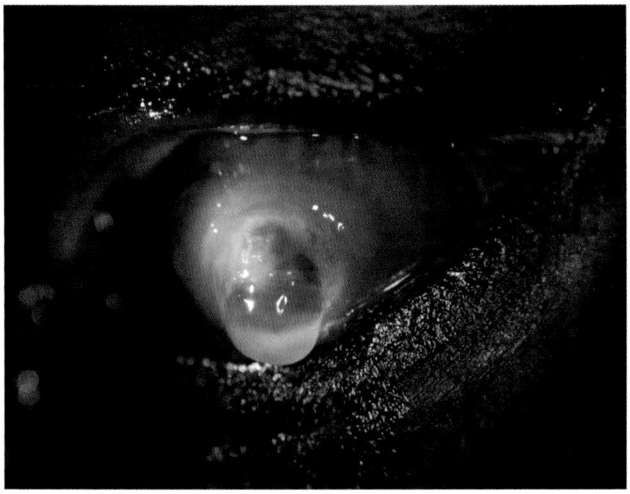

Figure 21-38 **Keratomalacia, Cornea, Horse.** Marked keratomalacia with displacement of the corneal stroma is present in the axial cornea. Corneal edema surrounds the lesion. Fluorescein stain has been applied to the cornea, and the adjacent ulcerated stroma is fluorescein positive *(light green color)*. (Courtesy Ophthalmology Service, College of Veterinary Medicine, University of Illinois.)

that allow a diagnosis to be made without histopathologic examination. Acquired corneal deposits result from previous corneal disease or as incidental manifestations of systemic metabolic disease.

Corneal epithelial dystrophy occurs mainly in dogs. These lesions are unlikely to be examined histologically but consist of abnormalities to the basement membrane of the corneal epithelium with dyskeratosis and necrosis of the epithelial cells. Corneal stromal dystrophies are rare but consist of lipid or mineral deposits within the corneal stroma. Corneal endothelial dystrophy is seen in several breeds of dogs as bilateral, diffuse corneal edema secondary to the progressive destruction of corneal endothelial cells (E-Fig. 21-43). The edema is not accompanied by any evidence of inflammation or stromal fibrosis. The loss of endothelial cells is difficult to evaluate histologically, but subtle attenuation can be recognized. The lesion must be differentiated from acquired endothelial degeneration (e.g., uveitis, glaucoma, surgery, anterior lens luxation). Furthermore, formalin fixation can cause artifactual vacuolation of the endothelium.

Acquired mineral deposition may occur in the basement membrane of the epithelium or in the corneal stroma, usually in the superficial aspect (band keratopathy). Corneal inflammation and hypercalcemia are potential causes of secondary mineral deposition. In horses, it can be seen with uveitis and administration of corticosteroid and phosphate-containing topical solutions.

Acquired corneal lipidosis (lipid keratopathy) results in milky or crystalline stromal deposits of serum lipids within the corneal stroma. It can be seen with primary corneal disease or lesions in adjacent structures that can overflow in the cornea. Hyperlipidemia may be a contributing factor. The lipids are recognized histologically as clear spaces or cholesterol clefts between stromal lamellae. Stromal keratocytes may accumulate small lipid vacuoles. Macrophages may border the foci of lipid deposition. Affected corneas are typically well vascularized.

Neoplasms of the Cornea and Sclera

Corneal Squamous Cell Carcinoma. Corneal squamous cell carcinoma occurs predominantly in dogs and horses. In dogs, lesions are most often limited to the epithelium (squamous cell carcinoma in situ). The neoplasms tend to be exophytic rather than infiltrative. Corneal squamous cell carcinoma is most often seen in brachycephalic breeds and often associated with a history of chronic keratitis. In horses, corneal squamous cell carcinoma tends to diffusely infiltrate the stroma rather than form a distinct mass or an exophytic growth. Some of the corneal stromal invasive squamous cell carcinomas may originate from the limbus. The histologic features of these neoplasms are similar to those at other sites. Most corneal squamous cell carcinomas are well differentiated.

Limbal (Epibulbar) Melanocytic Neoplasia. Limbal (epibulbar) melanocytic neoplasia occurs in dogs and rarely in cats. These neoplasms appear grossly as darkly pigmented masses arising from the limbus and expanding into the adjacent cornea and sclera. Limbal melanocytic neoplasms arise from the melanocytes that demarcate the limbus at the junction of the corneal stroma and sclera. Histologically, almost all are benign melanocytomas. These broad-based, nodular neoplasms are composed of discohesive heavily pigmented plump polyhedral cells often admixed with fewer pigmented spindle cells. There is no atypia, and mitoses are rare to absent. These masses grow by expansion and may extend intraocularly. Rare histologically malignant limbal malignant melanomas have been described, and some otherwise benign neoplasms may include areas with cells that are less pigmented or amelanotic and mitotically active. Limbal melanocytomas have bimodal age distribution, and tumors in older dogs may be particularly slow to progress. Surgical excision or photocoagulation may be considered for larger masses.

Diseases of the Uvea

Uveal Developmental Anomalies

The epithelium on the posterior surface of the iris, the inner surface of the ciliary body, and the retinal pigment epithelium and the inner surface of the choroid are all derived from portions of the original optic vesicle. The uveal stroma is derived from the periocular mesenchyme that originates from the neural crest. After outgrowth and later invagination of the primary optic vesicle to form the optic cup, the intraocular migration of the periocular mesenchyme and its remodeling seem to be guided by soluble factors released from the neuroectoderm.

The anomalies of the uveal tract can be divided into those resulting from a failure of initial induction or migration, a failure of later remodeling, or a failure of eventual atrophy (Table 21-2).

During early embryogenesis, there is a persistent gap between the anterior lip of the optic cup and the overlying corneal epithelium. Several waves of periocular mesenchyme migrate through this gap to form the corneal stroma and endothelium, the stroma of the anterior uvea, and the anterior portion of the perilenticular vascular tunic. The ingrowth of mesenchyme to form the iris stroma is guided by the infolding of the most anterior margin of the optic cup, which will form the two layers of the future iris epithelium (E-Fig. 21-44). Later, papillary proliferation of that iris epithelium gives rise to the epithelium of the ciliary processes. Proper inward migration of the neuroectoderm at the anterior lip of the optic cup seems to be a prerequisite for the subsequent migration of the mesenchyme to form the stroma of the iris and ciliary body. Similarly, proper maturation of the future retinal pigment epithelium from the posterior neuroectoderm of the optic cup is required for the proper maturation of the retina, choroid, and sclera.

Iris Hypoplasia. Failure of ingrowth of the future iris epithelium results in iris hypoplasia, typically affecting only the stroma (E-Fig. 21-45). Cases of extreme iris hypoplasia are clinically referred to as aniridia. This is relatively more frequent in horses than in other species. At least in some cases, it is inherited and may be associated with congenital cataracts.

Other Uveal Developmental Anomalies

Goniodysgenesis. Goniodysgenesis is maldevelopment of the iridocorneal angle and is exceedingly common as a cause of primary glaucoma in dogs, but it is much less frequent in other species. It results from incomplete atrophy of the mesenchyme at the base of the iris. Most of this remodeling occurs in the first few weeks of life. For reasons that are poorly understood, clinical manifestations of glaucoma attributed to this developmental anomaly are not usually detected until middle age or even later. Goniodysgenesis is described in more detail in the section on Glaucoma.

Persistent Pupillary Membranes/Persistent Primary Vitreous. Persistent pupillary membranes and persistent primary vitreous

Table 21-2 Uveal Developmental Anomalies

Failure of Formation	Failure of Remodeling
Iris hypoplasia	Goniodysgenesis
Choroidal hypoplasia	Persistent pupillary membrane
	Persistent hyaloid/primary vitreous
	Anterior segment dysgenesis

refer to abnormal persistence of portions of the perilenticular vascular tunic or the vascular network within the developing vitreous. Such anomalies are common in dogs. The embryonic lens is encased in a network of blood vessels known as the *tunica vasculosa lentis* (E-Fig. 21-46). This network is created by contributions from the same mesenchyme that forms the iris stroma and from vasogenic mesenchyme growing into the developing vitreous through the posterior portion of the slowly closing optic fissure. The latter vessels, growing in from near the optic disc, are the hyaloid artery system. Together with other nonangiogenic mesenchymal elements, these vessels form the primary vitreous. This embryonic hyaloid artery system creates a temporary vascular network along the surface of the developing retina and also joins with the anterior chamber vessels to complete the tunica vasculosa lentis. All portions of this elaborate vascular system undergo atrophy before maturation of the globe. Persistence of one or more portions is common. The most common is persistence of the anterior portion of the tunica vasculosa lentis. This is usually referred to as persistent pupillary membrane. Macroscopically, these are seen as fine threads originating from the minor arterial circle of the iris (Fig. 21-39; E-Fig. 21-47). They are usually bloodless but are often pigmented. They may be inserted into the anterior stroma of the iris, or they may contact the surface of the anterior lens capsule. Occasionally, in what is probably a more significant anomaly, they insert into the cornea. These membranes become clinically significant if they contact the lens or cornea, where they interfere with proper development of corneal or lens epithelium, or their associated basement membranes (Descemet's membrane and lens capsule, respectively). Histologically, persistent pupillary membranes are thin endothelial tubes accompanied by varying amounts of mesenchymal stroma (E-Fig. 21-48). At sites of corneal contact, they may cause fibrous metaplasia of the corneal endothelium. Where they contact the lens, there is usually epithelial proliferation and dysplasia of the lens capsule, resulting in a focal cataract.

Persistence of various portions of the hyaloid artery system, with or without other portions of the primary vitreous, includes much less common anomalies known as persistent hyaloid artery (E-Fig. 21-49) and persistent (hyperplastic) primary vitreous. When persistent blood vessels are accompanied by hyperplastic nonangiogenic mesenchymal spindle cells, the resulting anomaly is known as persistent hyperplastic primary vitreous. It has been described as a prevalent familial lesion in several breeds of dogs. The nonangiogenic mesenchyme undergoes notable fibroblastic proliferation, sometimes with cartilaginous metaplasia. Most affected dogs have concurrent anomalies, such as persistent pupillary membrane, microphthalmia, congenital cataract, and abnormal lenticular shape.

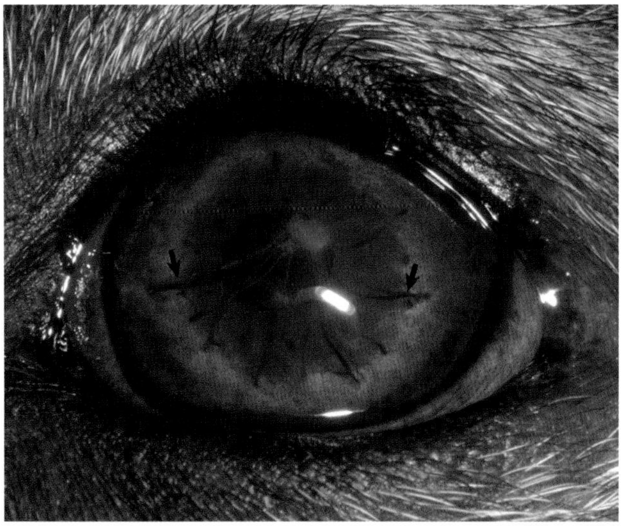

Figure 21-39 **Persistent Pupillary Membranes, Globe, Dog.** Iris-cornea persistent pupillary membranes are visible as normally colored iridal strands *(arrows)* adhering to an axial opacity in the cornea. (Courtesy Ophthalmology Service, College of Veterinary Medicine, University of Illinois.)

Anterior Segment Dysgenesis. Anterior segment dysgenesis is a general term for a variety of rare anomalies in which there is a failure of remodeling of the periocular mesenchyme that normally becomes the corneal stroma, corneal endothelium, iris stroma, and the anterior portion of the tunica vasculosa lentis. The usual clinical observation is absence of anterior chamber and the apparent fusion of the iris stroma to the corneal stroma and no corneal endothelium or Descemet's membrane. True anterior segment dysgenesis must be differentiated from the lesions secondary to perinatal corneal perforation. Perinatal corneal perforation with iris prolapse can result in diffuse anterior synechia and loss of the anterior chamber.

Acquired Uveal Diseases

Idiopathic Lymphoplasmacytic Uveitis. Lymphoplasmacytic uveitis is the most frequent histologic pattern of uveitis. Lymphocytes and plasma cells infiltrate the iris and ciliary body stroma and may also extend in the neuroepithelium. Choroidal involvement is variable but tends to be less severe than in the anterior uvea. Lymphoplasmacytic uveitis is not a specific disease but, rather, a histologic pattern that is shared by many different diseases. It is an indication of the chronicity of the uveitis because microscopic evaluation of globes with uveitis is usually done only in longstanding disease, after attempts at therapy have failed. Some cases may be immune-mediated, associated with trauma or lens disease (termed *lens-induced uveitis* or *phacolytic uveitis*), and a long list of infectious agents may be contributing factors. However, a specific cause is only rarely identified histologically. The diagnosis of lens-induced uveitis (phacolytic uveitis) is often made by exclusion and requires thorough history and clinical details (see below). In dogs, lymphoplasmacytic uveitis typically does not cause glaucoma by itself. In horses and cats, some cases of lymphoplasmacytic uveitis may cause glaucoma and warrant discussion as specific entities (see Disorders of Horses and Disorders of Cats).

Lens-Induced Uveitis. Lens-induced uveitis can be separated between phacolytic uveitis and phacoclastic uveitis. Phacolytic uveitis is a common cause of mild lymphoplasmacytic anterior uveitis that occurs in animals with cataracts in which lens proteins begin to disintegrate and leak through the intact lens capsule. The lesion tends to be mild, and in some cases it may be plasma cell predominant. Posterior synechiae often accompany the inflammation. However, even in globes with cataracts, the final diagnosis of phacolytic uveitis must be made in light of history and clinical findings. Neither the distribution nor the nature of the inflammatory infiltrate is specific to the condition because it mimics idiopathic lymphoplasmacytic uveitis.

Phacoclastic uveitis is an immune-mediated disease in response to the release of large amounts of intact lens protein through a ruptured lens capsule. Because the lens protein is sequestered from the immune system during embryologic development, the release of large amounts of strongly antigenic lens protein into the aqueous humor essentially elicits a foreign body reaction type of response. The histologic lesion is a lens-centric granulomatous endophthalmitis. Phacoclastic uveitis is also seen in dogs that have rapidly progressing diabetic cataracts; however, in those instances, the granulomatous inflammation tends to be more diffuse and may carpet the uveal tract. Phacoclastic uveitis occurs in rabbits as a result of penetration of the lens by *Encephalitozoon cuniculi* (E-Fig. 21-50). Phacoclastic uveitis may be a contributing factor in cases of severe endophthalmitis secondary to the penetrating trauma where there is rupture of the lens capsule (E-Fig. 21-51).

True phacoclastic uveitis must be differentiated from lens septic implantation syndrome. The latter occurs after penetrating trauma where there is lens capsule rupture and seeding of the lens with microorganisms, typically bacteria. The initiating traumatic injury is often a cat scratch. The traumatic event is followed by a period of dormancy of multiple weeks' duration during which there may be a favorable response to treatment. A severe lens-centric suppurative to pyogranulomatous endophthalmitis with suppurative phakitis then develops. The suppurative component distinguish septic implantation syndrome from phacoclastic uveitis, which is predominantly granulomatous.

Systemic Fungal, Algal, and Parasitic Diseases. Systemic mycoses, such as blastomycosis, cryptococcosis, histoplasmosis, and coccidioidomycosis, are frequent causes of severe uveitis in those geographic areas where the organisms are common environmental contaminants. Immunodeficient animals may develop endophthalmitis as part of generalized disease caused by fungi such as *Aspergillus* spp. or *Candida* spp., but these cases are rare; these same agents occasionally cause endophthalmitis when introduced by penetrating plant foreign bodies.

The frequency with which endophthalmitis accompanies systemic mycosis is unknown. The majority of cases are found in dogs, with the exception of cryptococcosis in cats. Ocular involvement is part of systemic disease, but fairly frequently, ocular disease is the initial complaint. Blastomycosis is by far the most prevalent example of an endophthalmitis caused by systemic mycosis.

Blastomycosis is the most frequently reported intraocular mycosis in dogs; it is rare in cats. It is estimated that approximately 25% of dogs with the systemic disease have clinically apparent ocular disease: unilateral or bilateral endophthalmitis with a very high frequency of exudative retinal detachment. The microscopic lesion is severe diffuse pyogranulomatous endophthalmitis, which tends to be more severe in the choroid and subretinal space than in the anterior uvea. The greatest accumulation of both leukocytes and organisms is usually in the subretinal space. The organisms may be numerous or extremely sparse, probably depending on the duration of the disease and on therapy. They are either free or within the cytoplasm of macrophages and have the typical features of *Blastomyces* spp.: thick-walled spherical yeasts, 8 to 25 μm in diameter, with occasional broad-based budding. Some cases may have a predominance of dead organisms where only the thick empty capsule is recognized. The diagnosis can often be made by cytologic evaluation of subretinal exudates, most often performed in eyes that are already blind because of retinal detachment. Other lesions in affected globes are those seen in any severe uveitis: intraocular hemorrhage, posterior synechia, preiridal fibrovascular membrane, and cataract.

Cryptococcosis is similar to blastomycosis in that the lesions are predominantly within the posterior aspect of the globe because the target sites are the retina, choroid, and optic nerve. Ocular cryptococcosis is more prevalent in cats than in any other domestic animal. As is typical of cryptococcosis in other feline tissue, the granulomatous inflammatory response is often minimal. Large collections of poorly stained pleomorphic yeasts, surrounded by wide capsular halos, impart a typical "soap-bubble" appearance in hematoxylin and eosin (H&E)-stained sections. The organisms are usually

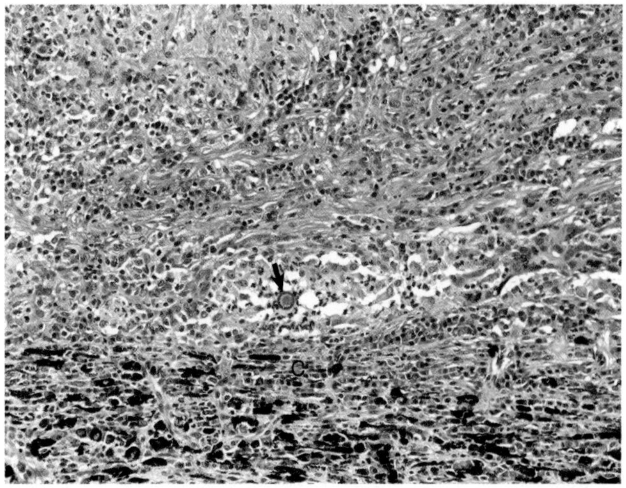

Figure 21-40 Coccidiomycosis, Choroid, Dog. There is severe infiltration of macrophages in the choroid (C) and subretinal space. The granulomatous inflammation is focally centered on a single yeast of *Coccidioides immitis* (*arrow*). H&E stain. (Courtesy Dr. P. Labelle, Antech Diagnostics.)

numerous. The yeasts measure 2 to 10 μm within a capsule up to 30 μm in diameter with rare, narrow-based budding. In a few cases, the granulomatous reaction is much more severe and mimics that seen in blastomycosis. In such lesions, organisms are typically scarce.

The ocular disease caused by *Coccidioides immitis* resembles blastomycosis but can be more suppurative, more destructive, and more likely to progress to panophthalmitis (Fig. 21-40; E-Fig. 21-52). Organisms are often rare and widely dispersed. Involvement of the anterior uvea is more common than in the other systemic mycoses. The disease is seen only in animals that live in (or have visited) the restricted geographic region in which the organism is common. The great majority of cases are seen in dogs from the desert regions of the southwest of the United States and some regions in Central and South America. The organisms measure 20 to 30 μm and may contain endospores. There is no budding.

The lesions caused by ocular infection with *Histoplasma capsulatum* are distinctive and quite different from those of the other systemic mycoses. There is usually a diffuse granulomatous uveitis with little suppuration and without much of the destruction that characterizes blastomycosis and coccidioidomycosis. Organisms measure 3 to 6 μm and are usually very numerous and visible as small spherical bodies within the cytoplasm of macrophages. There is no budding. In cats, histoplasmosis may present as nodular granulomatous conjunctivitis.

Protothecosis is caused by colorless, saprophytic algae capable of causing enteric, cutaneous, or generalized granulomatous disease in a variety of mammalian species. The clinical and histologic features closely resemble those of the systemic mycoses described previously. Ocular lesions have been described only in dogs with the disseminated form of the disease. The lesions are similar to those seen with blastomycosis. In histologic section, the algae are free or within macrophages, and they are typically numerous. The organisms are spherical to oval, from 2 to 10 μm in diameter, and have a refractile cell wall that stains intensely with PAS reaction. Prototheca reproduces by asexual multiple fission, and multiple sporangiospores (endospores) may be present within a single cell wall. Unlike blastomycosis and cryptococcosis, there is no budding.

Leishmaniasis is caused by a protozoan parasite, *Leishmania* spp., and requires transmission by phlebotomine sandflies. Ocular disease usually develops as part of systemic infection, but it can be the predominant or presenting clinical complaint. In dogs, the disease is endemic in the Mediterranean basin as well as areas of Africa, India, and Central and South America. The disease is less commonly seen in cats, mainly in Europe and South America. Although uncommon, there are reports of both canine and feline leishmaniasis in North America. The ocular infection most frequently causes granulomatous nodular conjunctivitis and uveitis; however, the infection may be present in any of the ocular components or periocular tissues. Amastigotes measuring 3 to 5 μm long and 1 to 2 μm wide are found in macrophages.

Iridociliary Cysts. Acquired cysts of the posterior iris or ciliary body epithelium occur sporadically in all species. Most often incidental findings, they can become clinically significant if they are multiple and large and obstructive to flow of aqueous humor. Rarely, individual cysts may become dislodged and displaced in the anterior chamber.

In Golden retrievers, iridociliary cysts represent a specific entity, so-called pigmentary uveitis. The term uveitis derives from the presence of aqueous flare and aqueous debris recognized clinically, but histologically pigmentary uveitis is not associated with infiltration of leukocytes; instead, the condition presents as multiple cysts from the posterior iris or ciliary epithelium, often delimited only by a single cell layer of variably pigmented cells that may be producing a basement membrane (Fig. 21-41). The cysts fill the posterior chamber, contact the lens, and may bulge through the pupil. The cases likely to be examined histologically are those in which secondary glaucoma develops. There is no infiltration of leukocytes, but there may be both preiridal and retrocorneal fibrovascular membrane formation. Posterior synechia is common. Release of pigment from ruptured cyst, obstruction of aqueous humor outflow, fibrovascular proliferation, and forward displacement of the iris are likely contributing factors to the glaucoma. In Rocky Mountain horses, ciliary cyst may be present as part of an inherited condition that includes other ocular anomalies.

Neoplasms of the Uvea

Uveal neoplasms are common only in dogs and cats. In addition to their direct effect on ocular function, neoplasms are commonly associated with secondary changes such as dyscoria, hemorrhage, fibrovascular proliferation, lens luxation, cataract, asteroid hyalosis, and retinal detachment, and they are a frequent cause of secondary glaucoma. Primary neoplasia is more prevalent than metastatic disease in the globe. In all species, melanocytic neoplasms are by far the most common of all ocular neoplasms. However, there are significant intraspecies differences that warrant consideration of melanocytic neoplasia separately for dogs, cats, and horses.

Canine Uveal Melanocytic Neoplasms. In dogs, benign uveal melanocytomas are most common in the iris and ciliary body, typically affecting both. Only 6% of uveal melanocytomas principally affect the choroid. Melanocytomas of the anterior uvea readily efface the iridocorneal angle. Many will expand along the corneoscleral meshwork, which extends anterior to the termination of Descemet's membrane and blends with the deep peripheral corneal stroma. Scleral extension is common for both anterior uveal and choroidal melanocytomas and is not a feature that is indicative of malignancy (Fig. 21-42; E-Fig. 21-53 and 21-54). All melanocytomas have a similar histologic appearance independent of their origin in the iris, ciliary body, or choroid. The neoplasms are composed of variable proportions of heavily pigmented spindle cells and discohesive heavily pigmented plump polyhedral cells. Uveal malignant melanoma is more common in the anterior uvea than in the choroid. Only 3% of uveal malignant melanomas are choroidal in origin. Approximately 25% of anterior uveal melanocytic neoplasms and 15% of choroidal melanocytic neoplasms are malignant. The mitotic index is the most reliable parameter in the diagnosis of malignant melanoma. A threshold of 4 mitoses in 10 high-power fields (HPF) is most widely used to establish malignancy in uveal melanocytic neoplasms (Fig. 21-43). As with uveal melanocytomas, expansion along the corneoscleral meshwork, in the sclera, and in extrascleral tissues is common. Malignant melanomas are less pigmented than their benign counterpart and can be amelanotic. Neoplastic cells containing pigment should not be assumed to be melanocytes because any disruption of the uveal tract can result in pigment dispersion and phagocytosis by neoplastic cells. For any uveal melanocytic neoplasm, necrosis and infiltration of melanophages is common. Choroidal involvement often causes retinal detachment.

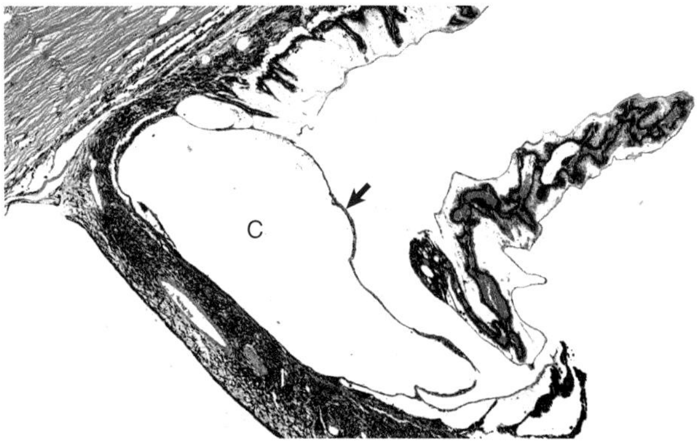

Figure 21-41 **Iridociliary Cysts, Uvea, Dog.** Multiple cysts of different sizes arise from the posterior iris and ciliary epithelium. Most cysts (*C*) are lined by a single layer of variably pigmented epithelium (*arrow*). The condition is also known as pigmentary uveitis and Golden retriever uveitis. There are no leukocytic infiltrates. *I*, Iris. H&E stain. (Courtesy Dr. P. Labelle, Antech Diagnostics.)

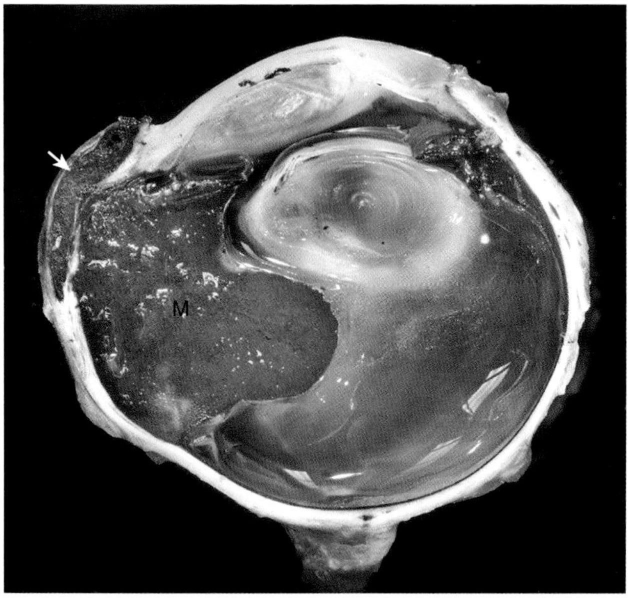

Figure 21-42 **Melanocytoma, Globe, Sagittal Section, Dog.** The iris, iridocorneal angle, ciliary body, and anterior choroid are expanded by a benign melanocytoma (*M*). The neoplasm extends in the sclera (*arrow*), which is not an indication of malignancy. (Courtesy Comparative Ocular Pathology Laboratory of Wisconsin.)

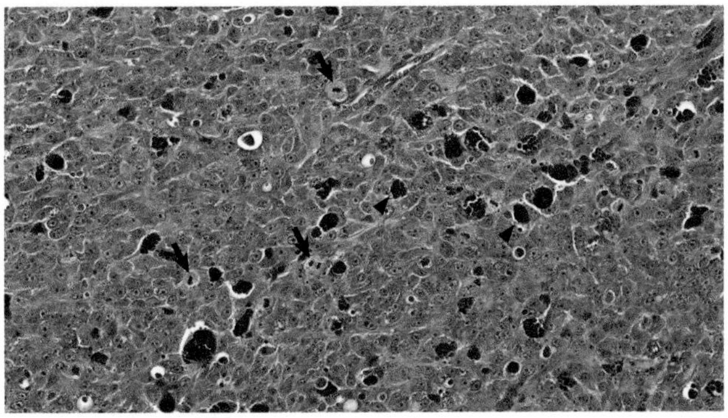

Figure 21-43 **Malignant Melanoma, Uvea, Dog.** Spindle to polygonal neoplastic cells. Most cells are lightly pigmented with melanin. There are numerous mitoses *(arrows)* indicating malignancy. Melanophages are dispersed in the neoplasm *(arrowheads)*. H&E stain. (Courtesy Dr. P. Labelle, Antech Diagnostics.)

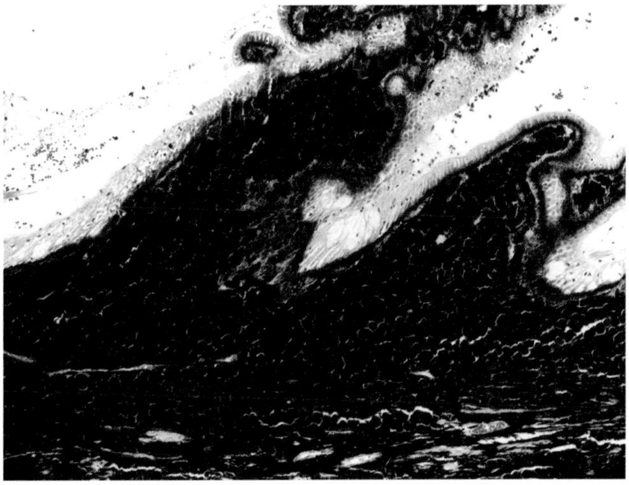

Figure 21-44 **Ocular Melanosis, Ciliary Body, Dog.** There is diffuse expansion of the ciliary body without mass formation. The pigmented cells include both melanocytes and melanophages. It has not been conclusively determined if this proliferative condition is truly neoplastic. H&E stain. (Courtesy Dr. P. Labelle, Antech Diagnostics.)

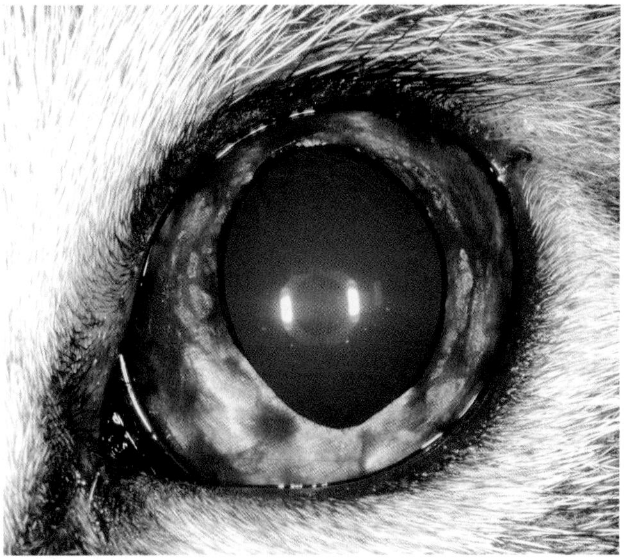

Figure 21-45 **Feline Diffuse Iris Melanoma, Iris, Cat.** Multifocal coalescing irregular pigmentation of the iris stroma is present along with dyscoria of the pupil. (Courtesy Ophthalmology Service, College of Veterinary Medicine, University of Illinois.)

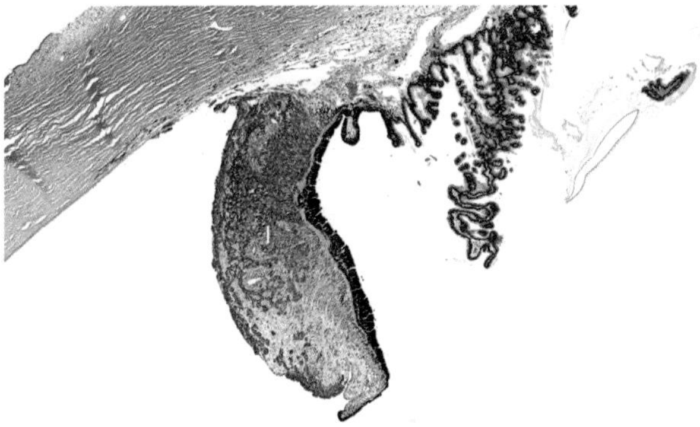

Figure 21-46 **Feline Diffuse Iris Melanoma, Iris, Cat.** The iris *(I)* is expanded by a diffuse iris melanoma. Those limited to the iris are considered "early stage." Neoplasms in the "intermediate stage" infiltrate the iris and ciliary. The "advanced stage" indicates extension in the choroid, sclera, or beyond. H&E stain. (Courtesy Dr. P. Labelle, Antech Diagnostics.)

Ocular Melanosis. Ocular melanosis (pigmentary glaucoma) is a unique condition that must be distinguished from uveal melanocytomas and malignant melanomas in dogs. It is unclear if ocular melanosis is truly neoplastic. It is seen most often, but not exclusively, in Cairn terriers. In that breed, pedigree analysis suggests the trait has an autosomal dominant mode of inheritance. The melanocytes in ocular melanosis have a unique immunophenotype that differs from normal melanocytes with negative staining for Melan-A and S-100. Grossly, ocular melanosis appears as diffuse pigmentation of the uveal tract. Pigment may be visible through the sclera. Histologically, it is characterized by diffuse uveal infiltration of large plump pigment-laden cells without formation of a distinct mass (Fig. 21-44). Both melanocytes and melanophages contribute to the uveal expansion. There may also be extension along the optic meninges. The condition is bilateral in Cairn terriers. In other breeds, it is usually unilateral at presentation, but it may eventually affect the contralateral globe.

Feline Diffuse Iris Melanoma. Feline diffuse iris melanoma (FDIM) is the most common ocular neoplasm in cats. In most instances, diffuse iris melanoma begins as focal or multifocal areas of iris hyperpigmentation. These areas histologically correspond to preneoplastic iris melanosis characterized by one to five layers of well-differentiated heavily pigmented melanocytes that cover the anterior surface of the iris. Iris melanosis may remain stagnant for years or slowly progress by increasing the number and/or size of the foci. Once the melanocytes extend in the underlying iris stroma, it is considered FDIM. The progression of FDIM is highly variable. Some cases can progress slowly over years without clinical signs, whereas others develop rapidly, causing glaucoma and spread to other organs. Almost all instances of FDIM follow a similar progression, albeit at different rates (Fig. 21-45; E-Fig. 21-55). The lesion begins as iris melanosis and then infiltrates and expands the iris stroma, followed by extension in the ciliary body (Fig. 21-46; E-Fig. 21-56). The lesion then extends in the sclera and/or choroid, and some neoplasms infiltrate the scleral venous plexus. Rare cases infiltrate beyond the sclera into the conjunctiva or orbit. Despite this reproducible pattern of growth, the rapidity with which FDIM progresses is unpredictable. As such, there are no definitive criteria to guide veterinarians as to the best time to enucleate. However, there is general agreement that globes with progressing pigmentation compatible with FDIM that develop glaucoma should be enucleated. Histologically, FDIM is composed of neoplastic melanocytes that may be predominantly spindle, polygonal, or round. The amount of pigmentation varies greatly, but very few are amelanotic. Although not prognostically significant, neoplastic cells often exhibit significant pleomorphism with karyomegaly and multinucleated cells. Intranuclear cytoplasmic invaginations may also be a prominent finding. The histologic features that have some prognostic value include extent of the tumor, vascular invasion, mitotic index, and the volume of necrosis within the tumor. FDIM limited to the iris typically does not cause glaucoma, and removal at that time is associated with survival times similar to those of unaffected cats with no risk of metastasis. FDIM with extension in the ciliary body and beyond is more likely to develop glaucoma and more likely to metastasize, especially with extrascleral extension. Vascular invasion typically occurs in the scleral venous plexus and is usually associated with advanced or extensive lesions. A high mitotic index is a poor prognostic indicator, and a threshold of 7 mitoses in 10 400× fields may be used as a guideline. The liver and lungs are the most frequent sites of metastasis. Metastases tend to develop slowly and in some cases may not be recognized for 1 to 3 years after enucleation. FDIM must be differentiated from the much less frequent feline atypical melanoma. Feline atypical melanoma forms multinodular masses in the uveal tract rather than diffuse expansion of the iris. It is composed of well-differentiated, heavily pigmented melanocytes with minimal pleomorphism and a low mitotic index. However, despite these features typically associated with a benign process, feline atypical melanoma may metastasize.

Equine Intraocular Melanocytic Neoplasia. Equine intraocular melanocytic neoplasia (EIMN) is associated with equine cutaneous melanoma. Most EIMNs (67%) are diagnosed in horses known to have cutaneous melanoma. As with cutaneous melanoma, most horses with EIMN are gray horses (85%). Histologically, the iris is often affected, with some cases involving the iris and ciliary body. Fewer cases expand the anterior uvea as well as the choroid and/or sclera. The cellular features of EIMN are similar to those of equine cutaneous melanoma. Almost all EIMNs are moderately to heavily pigmented. The cells are spindle to polygonal with minimal to no mitotic activity. Many masses are necrotic with infiltration of melanophages. Preiridal fibrovascular membranes and pigment within the corneal endothelium are common findings. Glaucoma, however, appears uncommon. The pathogenesis is unknown; however, the strong association with cutaneous melanoma suggests a genetic basis.

Neuroectodermal Neoplasms. Neuroectodermal neoplasia is second only to melanocytic neoplasia in frequency. Most are iridociliary adenomas or well-differentiated iridociliary adenocarcinomas. Medulloepitheliomas are rare. Iridociliary neoplasms arise from the neuroectoderm of the ciliary body or posterior iris. Grossly, they are recognized as nonpigmented to lightly pigmented pink discrete masses that can protrude into the pupillary aperture and displace the iris face anteriorly. The neoplasms are composed of cuboidal to columnar cells that form cords and nests with tubules and occasionally cysts (E-Fig. 21-57). Tubules and cysts may contain hyaluronic acid. Neoplastic cells produce periodic acid–Schiff (PAS)–positive basement membrane material. Most neoplasms include some cells that contain pigment, but heavily pigmented iridociliary neoplasms are uncommon. Approximately 15% invade the sclera and are considered malignant (adenocarcinoma), but the risk of metastasis is low. In cats, many neoplasms are predominantly composed of elongated cells in sheets, and some contain metaplastic bone; these neoplasms are often misdiagnosed as sarcomas. Iridociliary neoplasms typically express vimentin and neuroendocrine markers, but malignant neoplasms in dogs may also express cytokeratin.

Medulloepithelioma is a relatively rare congenital counterpart of iridociliary neoplasms, most commonly seen in horses. They arise most commonly from the ciliary body or optic nerve and less frequently in the retina. The histologic appearance reflects its embryonic origin from primitive neuroectoderm still capable of both iridociliary and retinal differentiation. The neoplasms are composed of small hyperchromatic stellate to round cells that form loose sheets and poorly organized multilayered rosette-like structures with a central cavity. True Flexner-Winterseiner and Homer-Wright rosettes may be present, and some areas may have features resembling ciliary processes or retina. In horses, they often contain heterotopic elements that are not normal derivatives of the ocular embryonic development, such as cartilage and bone. These variants are known as teratoid medulloepitheliomas. Although they are by definition congenital tumors, their growth is slow and they may not be diagnosed until many years later.

Schwannomas. Schwannomas (also termed *spindle cell tumors of blue-eyed dogs* or *peripheral nerve sheath tumors*) occur almost exclusively in dogs, but they have been described in cats. These neoplasms may not form a mass that is recognizable clinically. Histologically, they typically arise in the iris and extend in the ciliary body. The masses are nonpigmented and composed of interlacing bundles, streams, and whorls. Antoni A and B patterns are often recognized. Approximately half of the neoplasms are well-differentiated with a low mitotic index. Metastasis is rare and has only been described in dogs.

Metastatic Neoplasms. Neoplasms metastatic to the globe are much less frequent than primary ocular neoplasia. Lymphoma is the most common secondary neoplasms in all species, but it is particularly prevalent in cats. There are two general patterns of metastasis to the globe. Leukocytic neoplasms such as lymphoma and histiocytic sarcoma will typically cause diffuse expansion and effacement of the uveal tract (Fig. 21-47). Carcinomas and nonleukocytic sarcomas more often will form multifocal masses. Some will carpet the iris and ciliary body and occlude blood vessels. Mammary adenocarcinomas and pulmonary adenocarcinomas are the most common

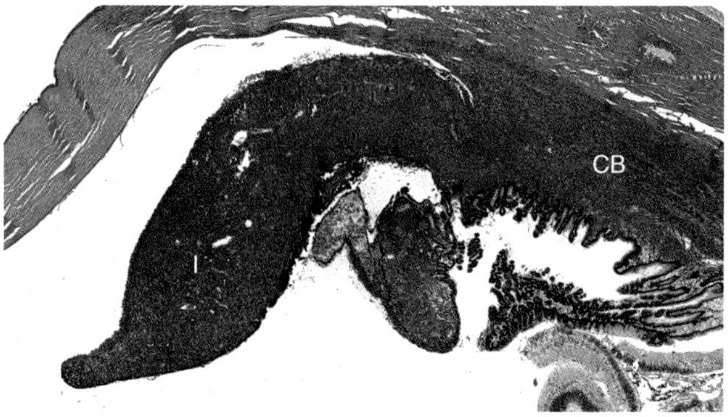

Figure 21-47 **Metastatic Lymphoma, Uvea, Cat.** Diffuse infiltration of neoplastic lymphocytes in the iris *(I)* and ciliary body *(CB)*. This pattern is typical of leukocytic neoplasms. Metastatic carcinomas and nonleukocytic sarcomas more often form masses within the uveal tract, and neoplastic cells may carpet the uvea. H&E stain. (Courtesy Dr. P. Labelle, Antech Diagnostics.)

secondary epithelial neoplasms in dogs and cats, respectively. Hemangiosarcoma, malignant melanoma, fibrosarcoma, and osteosarcoma are common nonleukocytic sarcomas that spread to the eye.

Diseases of the Lens

Developmental Anomalies of the Lens

The lens is derived from the thickening of the ectoderm induced by contact with the primary optic vesicle. This lens placode then migrates inwardly to cause the optic vesicle to invaginate on itself to form the primary optic cup. As it does, the lens placode grows to become a lens vesicle and separates from the overlying ectoderm (see Fig. 21-2). This vesicle initially is just a single layer of cuboidal epithelial cells surrounded by a very thin capsule. The epithelial cells along its posterior surface elongate to obliterate the lumen of this primitive vesicle, creating the primary lens fibers that persist throughout life as the lens nucleus. The subsequent development of the cortical fibers of the postnatal lens depends entirely on mitotic activity from the anterior lens epithelium. No epithelium remains along the posterior half of the lens any time after the stage of the primary lens vesicle.

The lens has a central inductive role in ocular development, so significant anomalies of the lens are almost always accompanied by multiple ocular anomalies such as microphthalmia. It is likely that many of the lens developmental anomalies reflect acquired degenerative changes (even if occurring in utero), resulting in regression of what was a normally developing lens. Such changes include an abnormally small lens (microphakia) or abnormally shaped lens (lenticonus and lentiglobus).

Lens Luxation

Dislocation of the lens may be partial (subluxation) or complete (luxation). The lens may be forced in the anterior chamber, or it may remain trapped in the posterior chamber (Fig. 21-48; E-Fig. 21-58). A completely dislocated lens is likely to develop a diffuse cataract, presumably because of its inadequate access to aqueous humor and nutrition. Anterior lens luxation is much more significant because it causes pain and also predisposes to glaucoma. Lens luxation may be primary or secondary. Care must be taken during the processing of globes not to cause iatrogenic displacement of the lens that could mimic lens luxation.

Primary lens luxation refers to that occurring without any known trauma or other ocular disease. It may be congenital or may be seen later in life. Congenital luxation is usually the result of a developmental error that causes abnormal or insufficient zonules. Much more prevalent are spontaneous luxations that occur in young adult dogs of specific breeds (terriers and others). The luxation is almost always bilateral. In many breeds, primary lens luxation is associated with a mutation in the ADAMTS17 gene. Some cases of primary lens luxation secondary to zonular ligament dysplasia can be recognized histologically. In these cases, there is acellular, hyaline, eosinophilic material that covers portions of the nonpigmented ciliary epithelium (Fig. 21-49). This material stains intensely with the periodic acid–Schiff (PAS) reaction, and the trichrome stain indicates increased collagen compared to normal zonular ligaments.

Secondary lens luxation is most often seen with excessive stretching of the zonular ligaments within a globe that has become greatly enlarged secondary to glaucoma, blunt trauma that causes avulsion of the zonular ligaments, or uveitis that affects the quality of the zonular ligaments. Displacement of the lens can also occur in the presence of space-occupying neoplasms. Severe cataract with intumescence or collapse can also result in excessive stretching of the zonular ligaments.

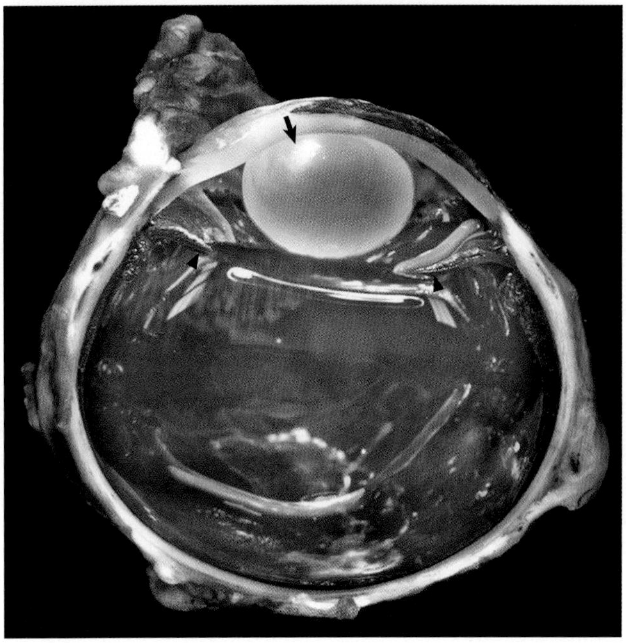

Figure 21-48 Anterior Lens Luxation, Globe, Sagittal Section, Dog. The lens *(arrow)*, which normally lies posterior to the iris *(arrowheads)*, has been displaced anteriorly in the anterior chamber. Most luxated lens show some degree of cataract. Contact with the cornea can damage the corneal endothelium. Fibrovascular membranes along the posterior cornea and iris are common. These lesions can contribute to the development of glaucoma. (Courtesy Comparative Ocular Pathology Laboratory of Wisconsin.)

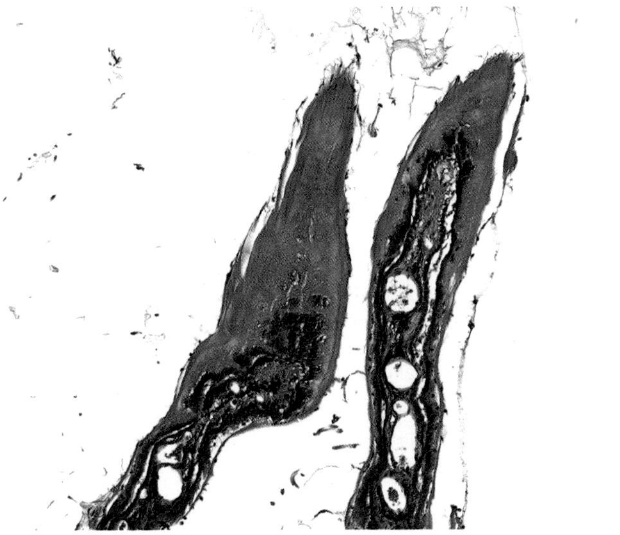

Figure 21-49 Zonular Ligament Dysplasia, Ciliary Processes, Dog. The ciliary processes are covered by thick, hyaline, eosinophilic material. The material is tightly adhered to the nonpigmented ciliary epithelium and much thicker than normal zonular ligaments. H&E stain. (Courtesy Dr. P. Labelle, Antech Diagnostics.)

The distinction between lens luxation as a cause of glaucoma and lens luxation as a consequence of glaucoma is not always obvious in cases in which both lens luxation and glaucoma are diagnosed in the same globe. Lens luxation can cause glaucoma if there is posterior synechia and pupillary block, by obstruction of aqueous humor flow in the anterior chamber or by displacing the vitreous, which can be an obstruction and predispose to retinal detachment. Lens luxation can be a consequence of glaucoma when there is buphthalmos that stretches and tears the zonular ligaments.

Diabetic Cataract

Diabetic cataract is the best-studied form of metabolic lens disease. Rapidly progressing bilateral cataracts develop in most diabetic dogs. After being diagnosed with diabetes mellitus, approximately half of the dogs will develop cataracts within 6 months and 80% within 16 months. Controlling the hyperglycemia and, by extension, the levels of glucose in the aqueous humor can delay the development of cataracts. Once the lesion develops, progression to complete cortical opacity and thus visual impairment usually occurs within days to weeks. The swelling may be so rapid that the lens capsule ruptures. The cataract develops because of high levels of glucose within the aqueous humor. When the hexokinase pathway is overloaded with glucose, the excess glucose absorbed by the lens is shifted to the sorbitol pathway, where it is transformed by the enzyme aldose reductase into sorbitol. This leads to accumulation of sorbitol, which creates a hyperosmotic effect, and the influx of fluid. The result is rapid swelling of the lens and disruption of its architecture. The osmotic stress also induces apoptosis of lens epithelial cells. The histologic features of the cataract itself are similar to those of any other severe cataract, making clinical history critical to the diagnosis. Some cases develop severe granulomatous endophthalmitis (phacoclastic uveitis) that tends to carpet the uveal tract rather than be centered on the lens. This form of inflammation associated with diabetic cataracts must be differentiated from asymmetric uveitis (see Disorders of Dogs). Rarely, diabetic cats can also develop cataracts, but the lesion is less severe than in dogs and appears to have limited clinical significance. Older cats have lower aldose reductase activity than dogs and young cats, which may provide protection by limiting the production of sorbitol.

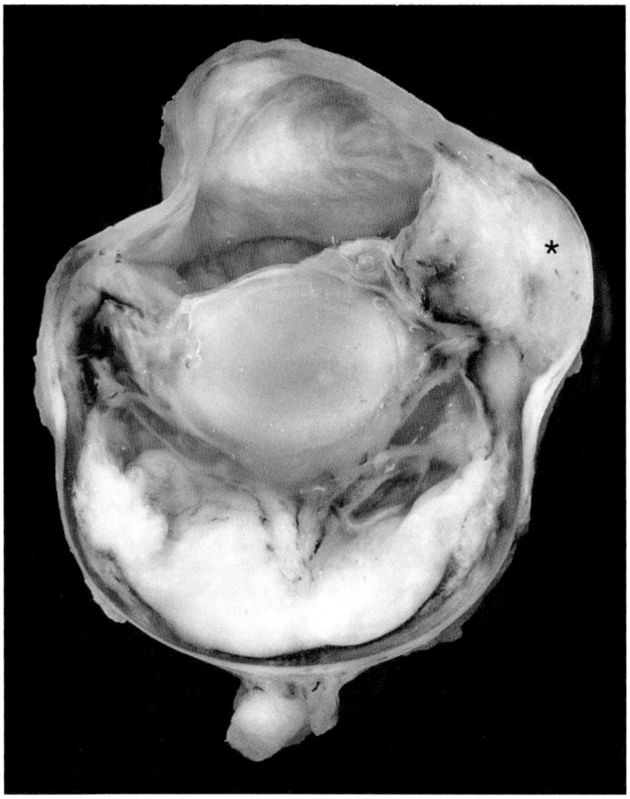

Figure 21-50 **Posttraumatic Ocular Sarcoma, Globe, Sagittal Section, Cat.** A solid multinodular neoplasm partially fills the globe and invades the sclera *(asterisk)*. Early neoplasms will border the lens progressing to line and invade the uvea. In late stages, the lens may be collapsed with only remnants of ruptured capsule entrapped in the mass. (Courtesy Comparative Ocular Pathology Laboratory of Wisconsin.)

Neoplasms of the Lens

Feline Posttraumatic Ocular Sarcoma. Feline posttraumatic ocular sarcoma (primary ocular sarcoma) (FPTOS) is the second most common primary ocular neoplasm in cats. The condition is almost exclusive to the cat, although a few cases have been described in rabbits. The initiating event is presumed to be ocular trauma or severe ocular disease. The neoplasms are recognized following a period of dormancy typically lasting multiple years following the initiating event (average 5 years). Morphologically, the neoplasm is a sarcoma and expresses vimentin. The neoplasm is believed to arise from malignant transformation of the lens epithelial cells. Some neoplasms are immunopositive for the lens structural protein crystallin αA, and lens capsule rupture is recognized in almost all cases. Neoplasms are initially centered on the lens, and neoplastic cells multifocally deposit lens capsule/basement membrane-type material that stains with PAS and is collagen type IV immunopositive. To a lesser extent, immunoreactivity to smooth muscle actin (SMA) is also consistent with lens origin because lens epithelial cells can express SMA especially in diseased states such as cataracts. Similarly, the occasional immunoreactivity to cytokeratin may reflect the origin of the lens epithelium from the surface ectoderm; cytokeratin expression is normally lost during embryogenesis.

Gross findings reflect the fact that most neoplasms are recognized late in the disease process. The globe is often almost filled by the neoplasm, and the lens may be collapsed (Fig. 21-50; E-Fig. 21-59). Scleral and optic nerve extension may be visible grossly. Histologically, early lesions may be recognized as streams of spindle cells bordering the lens in the area of lens capsule rupture. A characteristic feature of FPTOS is that as the neoplasm progresses, the spindle cells will initially line the uveal tract, especially choroid. Eventually, the neoplasm effaces the uvea, and there may be extension in the sclera and optic nerve. In late cases, the globe is essentially filled by the neoplasm. The neoplastic cells are usually spindle with severe pleomorphism and a high mitotic index (E-Fig. 21-60). Multinucleated cells may be present. In some areas of the neoplasm, the neoplastic cells may be separated by basement membrane-type material. A small percentage of neoplasms show osteoid and/or chondroid material deposition. In extensive neoplasms, the lens may only be recognized as fragments of lens capsule. FPTOS are highly infiltrative, and extension beyond the sclera is a poor prognostic indicator. Rare intracranial extension along the optic nerve and metastasis has been described. FPTOS has similarities with vaccine site sarcomas: traumatic initiating event, long period of dormancy between initiation and the development of a neoplasm, and similar histologic characteristics. However, there is no known association between these two entities.

There is a less frequent variant of feline posttraumatic sarcomas composed of pleomorphic round cells. These cases are also associated with previous trauma and lens capsule rupture, and most have a distribution typical of FPTOS. The neoplastic cells have features that most closely resemble pleomorphic lymphoma; however, the exact histogenesis of the round cell variant of FPTOS is unclear. In many cases, the neoplastic cells express both T lymphocyte and B lymphocyte markers.

Diseases of the Retina and Optic Nerve

Retinal diseases categorized by lesion are listed in Table 21-3; retinal diseases categorized by pathogenesis are listed in Table 21-4.

Table 21-3 Retinal Diseases Categorized by Lesion

Ganglion Cell (Inner Retinal) Atrophy	Photoreceptor (Outer Retinal) Atrophy	Full-Thickness Necrosis	Retinitis	Other
Glaucoma Optic nerve injury (retrograde atrophy)	Progressive retinal atrophy Inherited photoreceptor dysplasias/ degenerations Retinal detachment Light-induced retinopathy Toxicity Nutritional deficiency Choroidal ischemia	High-pressure glaucoma (dogs only) Ischemic injury Systemic hypertension Vascular occlusion (thromboemboli, metastasis)	Hematogenous infection Extension of uveitis/ endophthalmitis	Retinal pigment epithelium and neuronal storage diseases Developmental anomalies

Table 21-4 Retinal Diseases Categorized by Pathogenesis

Ischemia	Inflammation	Trauma	Toxic/Metabolic/ Oxidative	Genetic/ Developmental
Glaucoma* Systemic hypertension Vascular occlusion (thromboemboli, metastasis) Retinal detachment Vasculitis	Hematogenous infection Infection via penetrating injury Extension of uveitis/ endophthalmitis	Retinal detachment Hemorrhage/infarction Optic nerve injury (retrograde atrophy)	Nutritional deficiency Toxic retinopathies Light-induced retinopathy	Inherited photoreceptor dysplasias/ degenerations Neuronal storage diseases Retinal dysplasia Retinal detachment (vitreoretinal dysplasia)

*Ischemia is one contributing factor to glaucomatous retinal atrophy.

Retinal Developmental Anomalies

Retinal Dysplasia. Retinal dysplasia is a general term denoting an abnormal retinal differentiation characterized by disorganized retinal layers. Acquired retinal folds, which can develop secondary to retinal detachment and reattachment or following retinal scarring, should be considered as a separate entity.

Retinal dysplasia is a rare anomaly that results from improper induction of retinal maturation by the retinal pigment epithelium (RPE). Most cases of retinal dysplasia are seen in dogs as an inherited disease. Retinal dysplasia may also be one of multiple congenital malformations in severely affected globes. The details of the pathogenesis likely vary depending on the cause, but all involve separation or inadequate apposition between the neuroretina and RPE, or dysfunction of the RPE itself. The result is a retina with multifocal to diffuse disorganization of the retinal layers with variably organized rosettes, variation in thickness, and, in many cases, retinal detachment (Fig. 21-51). Retinal folding is commonly seen with retinal dysplasias (E-Fig. 21-61). In some cases, the retinal folds are present without disorganization of the retinal layers, and those instances may not represent true retinal dysplasia. Those cases may represent a globe where the development of the retina has occurred more rapidly than the development of the supporting choroid and sclera. The implication is that such retinal folds are transient and will disappear as the animal ages and the support structures continue to grow.

In all species, retinal dysplasia may occur following retinal injury during retinal development. Viral infection is most common, but other causes include toxic injury, nutritional deficiencies, radiation exposure, and intrauterine trauma. This typically implies in utero disease. However, in dogs and cats, the period of susceptibility to some of these events extends for at least 6 weeks after birth, during which time the retina continues to develop. In contrast to the adult retina, which retains no mitotic capability, the developing retina can still react with at least some neuronal regeneration. Such regeneration is usually mixed with glial scarring and does not restore normal retinal organization.

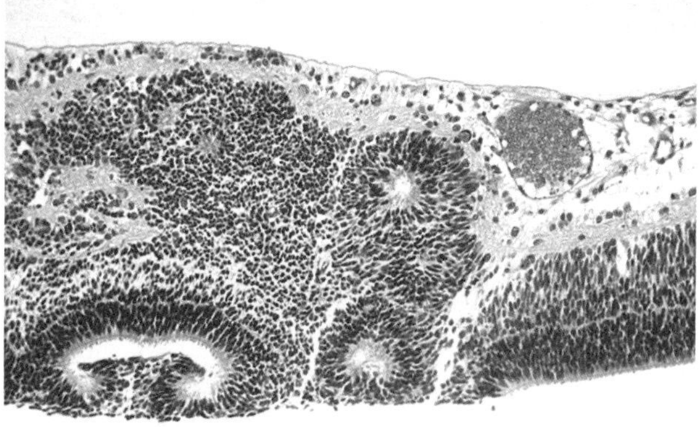

Figure 21-51 **Retinal Dysplasia, Retina, Puppy.** The cells of the retinal layers are poorly organized and arranged haphazardly, sometimes creating acinar-like structures known as retinal rosettes. H&E stain. (Courtesy Dr. B. Wilcock, Ontario Veterinary College.)

The viruses that most often cause retinal dysplasia in domestic animals are bovine viral diarrhea and mucosal disease virus (BVD-MD) in cattle, bluetongue virus in sheep, herpesvirus and adenovirus in dogs, and parvovirus and feline leukemia virus in cats. The viruses typically cause necrosis or inflammation within the retina, and the attempt at regeneration results in retinal dysplasia (E-Fig. 21-62). Retinal dysplasia only occurs if these viral infections damage the retina while its neurons still have proliferative capacity.

Retinal scarring as a result of necrosis and mild inflammation may persist in some cases. The window of susceptibility for the development of retinal dysplasia depends on the species because retinal development varies with the species.

Infection of bovine fetuses with BVD-MD is the most frequent and the most studied of the virally induced retinal dysplasias. Infection between days 79 and 150 of gestation can result in postnecrotic retinal dysplasia. The initial ocular lesion is necrotizing lymphocytic endophthalmitis with random retinal necrosis. The inflammation gradually subsides, and there is often minimal inflammation in fetuses aborted later or in dead neonatal calves. The ocular components that are already well-differentiated at the time of the endophthalmitis, such as cornea, uvea, and optic nerve, may remain normal or exhibit some postnecrotic scarring. Only the retina, which is still developing, will exhibit unsuccessful attempts at regeneration. Because the peripheral retina remains mitotically active for several weeks after the central retina has matured, dysplastic lesions may be found only in the peripheral retina. Calves with BVD-MD–associated retinal dysplasia typically also have cerebellar hypoplasia.

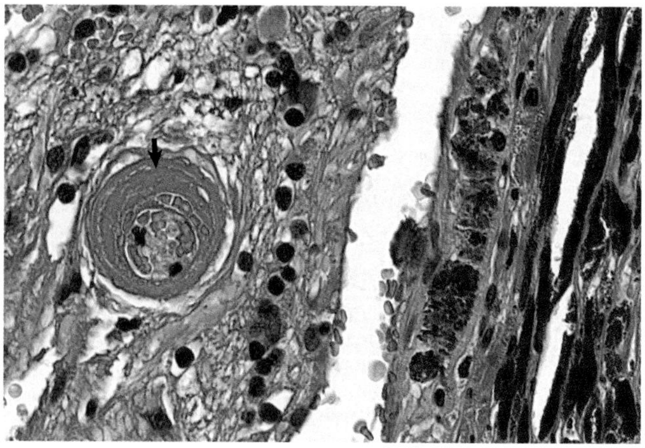

Figure 21-52 **Hypertensive Vasculopathy, Retina, Dog.** There is fibrinoid necrosis of a retinal arteriole *(arrow)*. Normal retinal layering is no longer present following retinal detachment and full-thickness retinal atrophy. (Courtesy Dr. P. Labelle, Antech Diagnostics.)

Optic Nerve Hypoplasia. Optic nerve hypoplasia may be unilateral or bilateral. Primarily documented in dogs, optic nerve hypoplasia also occurs in cats, horses, cattle, and pigs. The lesion is not necessarily associated with visual impairment. It is the consequence of retinal ganglion cell maldevelopment, early loss of retinal ganglion cells, or failure of the axons to exit the globe. It is inherited in some breeds of dogs. Histologically, the optic nerve has a narrow diameter with increased connective tissue in increased numbers of glial cells. The retina has fewer retinal ganglion cells than normal, and the nerve fiber layer is thin. In cattle and pigs, optic nerve hypoplasia must be differentiated from optic nerve atrophy secondary to vitamin A deficiency. Vitamin A deficiency causes abnormal thickening of growing bones, including orbital bones. This results in compression atrophy of the optic nerve. In pigs, the deficiency can also affect the globe with lesions such as microphthalmia. Vitamin A deficiency causes retinal degeneration (see Nutritional Retinopathies).

Acquired Retinal Disease

Ischemic Retinopathies. Ischemic damage to the retina can be the result of occlusion of the retinal vessels or, more often, from interference with blood supply in the choroid. Thromboemboli, metastatic disease, and severe choroiditis may all interfere with proper vascular supply to the retina. Vasculitis in the retina or choroid is uncommon but can be seen with immune disease or infectious diseases such as thrombotic meningoencephalitis of cattle, Rocky Mountain spotted fever, or ehrlichiosis in dogs (E-Figs. 21-63 and 21-64). Ischemia also contributes to retinal injury as part of retinal detachment and is one of the contributing factors to retinal atrophy in glaucoma. Microvascular disease associated with diabetes mellitus may be seen in dogs and cats, but it does not have the same clinical significance as diabetic retinopathy in human beings.

Systemic hypertension is a relatively common cause for retinal ischemic damage in dogs and cats. It is usually secondary to chronic renal disease but can also be associated with endocrine diseases such as hyperthyroidism, diabetes mellitus, hyperadrenocorticism, and pheochromocytoma, as well as cardiovascular disease. The clinical findings often include intraocular and retinal hemorrhage, retinal edema, and retinal detachment. The globes submitted for histopathologic examination are typically glaucomatous. The lesions are usually bilateral but may be asymmetric. The diagnostic histologic lesions are most obvious in the retina and choroid, but they may be found throughout the uvea. The affected arterioles have thickened hyaline walls with narrowed lumen (Fig. 21-52; E-Fig. 21-65). The walls are expanded by periodic acid–Schiff (PAS)–positive material that may be solid or layered concentrically, which represents fibrinoid necrosis of the tunica media. Retinal edema and hemorrhage, segmental retinal necrosis, retinal detachment with outer retinal atrophy, and intraocular hemorrhage commonly accompany the vascular lesions. There can be necrosis of the retinal pigment epithelium (RPE). In cases in which there is severe retinal hemorrhage and necrosis, the diagnostic vascular lesions may be most easily recognizable in the choroid. Fibrovascular proliferation secondary to the release of vascular mediators from the injured retina is present in most cases and often the cause of neovascular glaucoma.

Nutritional Retinopathies. Vitamin A deficiency as a cause for retinopathy has been reported in cattle, horses, and pigs receiving a ration deficient in vitamin A over an extended period of time. The ocular effects of hypovitaminosis A first involve photoreceptor outer segments, specifically rods, in which vitamin A (retinol) is a component of the photopigment rhodopsin. The lesion can slowly progress to diffuse photoreceptor atrophy, loss of the outer nuclear layer, and eventually to complete retinal atrophy. Early lesions can be reversed with vitamin A therapy.

Vitamin E deficiency in dogs and horses manifests as lipofuscin accumulation in various cell types including the RPE, consistent with oxidative damage. Accumulation in the RPE is greater than that expected with normal aging. Histologically, lipofuscin accumulation in the RPE is visible with standard hematoxylin and eosin staining and may be highlighted with PAS stain. The RPE may concurrently be hypertrophic. As a consequence of RPE dysfunction, chronic vitamin E deficiency eventually progresses to degeneration of the photoreceptors. Retinal pigment epithelial dystrophy/central progressive retinal atrophy (RPED), recognized mainly in some populations of dogs in Europe, presents with histologic findings indistinguishable from vitamin E deficiency. With RPED, the lesions occur despite adequate vitamin E intake, suggesting an inability to properly metabolize vitamin E that results functionally in a deficiency at the cellular level.

Toxic Retinopathies. Toxic injury to the retina is a rare event. Locoweed poisoning affects cattle, sheep, and horses. The ocular lesions mimic those in the central nervous system and consist of swelling and vacuolation of retinal neurons as well as axon degeneration (see Chapter 14). The effects of braken fern toxicity are discussed in Disorders of Ruminants, and the effects of enrofloxacin/fluoroquinolone toxicity are discussed in Disorders of Cats.

Retinitis

Retinitis is most often a consequence of direct extension of uveitis or endophthalmitis. Some cases of idiopathic lymphoplasmacytic uveitis also include perivascular cuffing in the retina. The presence of retinal disease in those instances does not provide clues as to the underlying etiology.

Systemic infectious diseases may affect the retina, and the lesions usually mimic those at other sites. The retina may be the target of viral infections such as canine distemper, rabies, pseudorabies, classical swine fever, Borna disease, and malignant catarrhal fever. Bacterial diseases such as canine ehrlichiosis, Rocky Mountain spotted fever, and bovine thromboembolic meningoencephalitis may cause retinal lesions as a consequence of vascular disease. Parasitic diseases of the retina include toxoplasmosis, neosporosis, and ocular larval migrans caused by the migration of the larvae of *Toxocara canis* and *Baylisascaris procyonis*.

Neoplasms of the Retina and Optic Nerve

Ocular Astrocytomas. Ocular astrocytomas have only been described in dogs. Clinically, astrocytomas appear as a discrete mass in the fundus or more frequently as retinal detachment with secondary vitreal hemorrhage, hyphema, and glaucoma. Astrocytomas may arise in the retina or optic nerve and often involve both. The histologic features and classification are similar to those in the central nervous system (see Chapter 14). The prognosis is good with complete excision; however, neoplasms with optic nerve involvement may extend intracranially.

Orbital Meningiomas. Orbital meningioma (optic nerve meningioma, retrobulbar meningioma) is a disease of dogs. Clinically, orbital meningiomas are associated with exophthalmos and vision loss. Orbital meningiomas likely arise from extradural nests of arachnoid cells. The neoplasms efface the orbital connective tissue (Fig. 21-53). The masses may compress but do not invade the optic nerve until late in the disease. Very rarely there may be extension in the sclera or choroid, or through the optic foramen into the calvarium. The histologic features of orbital meningiomas differ from those of intracranial/spinal meningiomas. The neoplastic cells are large with abundant eosinophilic "glassy" cytoplasm. The neoplastic cells form sheets and nests with subtle whorls. In most masses (>90%), there are foci of myxomatous, chondroid, and/or osseous metaplasia. Only rare orbital meningiomas have features typical of intracranial/spinal meningiomas. Optic nerve atrophy and degeneration and retrograde retinal atrophy with loss of ganglion cells are frequent secondary findings. Larger masses may cause bone remodeling.

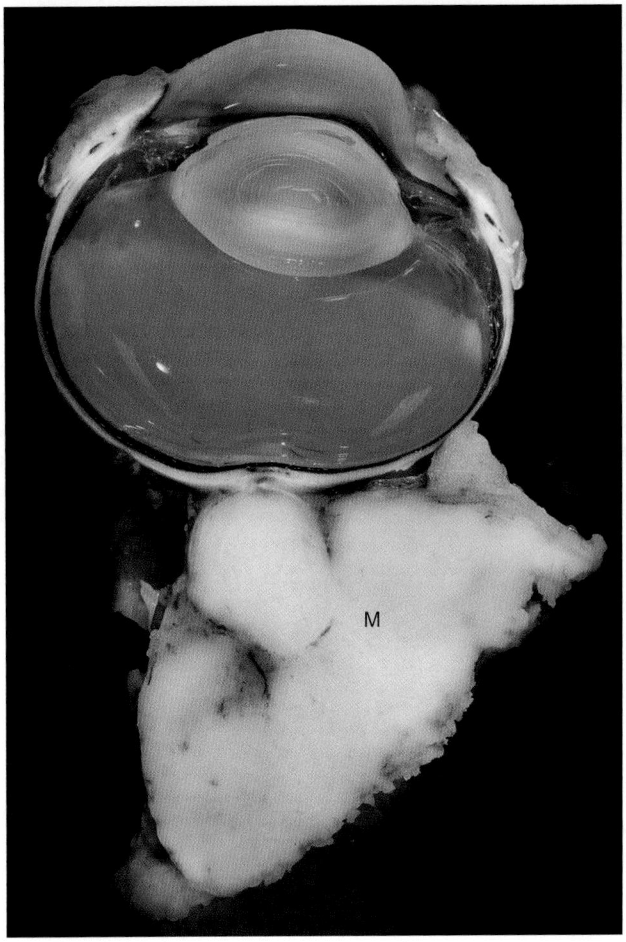

Figure 21-53 Orbital Meningioma, Globe, Sagittal Section, Dog. A multinodular mass (*M*) effaces the orbital soft tissues. Initially the neoplasm will envelop the optic nerve eventually causing atrophy with extensive disease. (Courtesy Comparative Ocular Pathology Laboratory of Wisconsin.)

Diseases of the Orbit

Orbital cellulitis is not a specific disease but inflammation of soft tissue in response to infectious agents introduced via a penetrating wound, a migrating foreign body, or an inflammatory focus from adjacent tissues (e.g., tooth root abscess). Only rarely does panophthalmitis extend into the orbit to cause orbital cellulitis because the sclera is generally an effective barrier to the migration of leukocytes and infectious agents.

Neoplasms of the Orbit

Orbital neoplasms are overall infrequent, perhaps with the exception of orbital lymphoma in cattle. Most orbital neoplasms are not discovered until they are large enough to cause an abnormality of the globe, such as exophthalmos or strabismus. Any of the connective, muscle, and bone components of the orbit may give rise to neoplasms such as multilobular tumor of bone (multilobular osteochondrosarcoma), osteosarcoma, fibrosarcoma, liposarcoma, rhabdomyosarcoma, and salivary-lacrimal adenocarcinoma. There may be direct extension from conjunctival or nasal neoplasia. Metastatic disease to the orbit also occurs on occasion.

Canine Lobular Orbital Adenomas. Canine lobular orbital adenomas arise from the lacrimal gland located dorsally or zygomatic salivary gland located ventrally. Clinically, lobular orbital adenomas present as exophthalmos or subconjunctival mass effect. The masses are soft and friable. Histologically, the neoplasms are multilobular and composed of nests and cords occasionally with acini. The lobules lack ducts, and this feature is essential to making the diagnosis of lobular orbital adenoma. The cuboidal cell population resembles normal tissue, and mitoses are absent. Local recurrence is common because complete excision is unlikely without exenteration.

Hibernomas. Hibernomas are benign neoplasm of brown adipose tissue and occur as subconjunctival or orbital masses. Ocular hibernomas have been described only in dogs.

Histologically, the masses are variably encapsulated and composed of lobules of often vacuolated cells that show mild pleomorphism and minimal mitotic activity. Ultrastructurally, the neoplastic cells have fairly distinct basal laminae, and the cytoplasm contains numerous mitochondria and lipid droplets. The main differential diagnosis is well-differentiated liposarcoma, and distinction may not always be possible without history, especially in incisional samples. Hibernomas are immunopositive for uncoupling protein 1 (UCP1) normally expressed in brown adipose tissue.

Disorders of Horses

Diseases of the Eyelids and Conjunctiva

Habronemiasis

Habronemiasis (summary sores) causes nodular inflammation most often in the medial canthus as the response to infection by larvae of nematodes *Draschia megastoma*, *Habronema muscae*, and *Habronema majus*. The adult nematodes infect the gastric mucosa. The larvae are excreted in feces, ingested by fly maggots, and transferred to the periocular skin and conjunctiva by fly bites. The gross lesion is a firm nodule with yellow caseous debris in the center. Histologically, the lesion is similar to that anywhere in the skin and consists of chronic eosinophilic and granulomatous inflammation targeting live or dead larvae that are often difficult to identify in histologic sections (E-Fig. 21-66). Conjunctival lesions may abrade the cornea and cause keratitis.

Diseases of the Cornea and Sclera

Equine Fungal Keratitis

Fungal keratitis (keratomycosis) occurs frequently in horses and is reported mostly during warmer weather and in warm, humid climates. Similar infections occur much less frequently in dogs, cats, and other species. It is suspected that the use of topical antibiotics is a predisposing factor for fungal keratitis as the result of changes in the normal bacterial microflora with decreasing numbers of Gram-positive organisms and increasing numbers of Gram-negative bacteria. The normally predominant Gram-positive bacteria produce antimicrobial substances including the antifungal natamycin. Topical administration of corticosteroids may also be a predisposing factor, and it can exacerbate the effect of proteases and impair corneal healing. The pathogenesis involves disruption of the corneal epithelium secondary to erosion, ulceration, or penetrating trauma. The epithelial injury allows fungal organisms from the environment or those from the normal microflora to anchor, colonize, and invade. The release of proteases by the organisms and by inflammatory cells contributes to stromal injury and provides access to the deep cornea. Some fungal organisms also produce metabolites that inhibit angiogenesis, altering the cornea's healing response. *Aspergillus* spp. are the most common agents isolated. *Fusarium* spp. and others also cause fungal keratitis. Fungal keratitis typically elicits a suppurative response with keratomalacia (see Fig. 21-38). The inflammation may be superficial but there is most often involvement of the deep stroma, and many fungal organisms show a tropism for the deep stroma and Descemet's membrane (Fig. 21-54; E-Fig. 21-67). These organisms may have an affinity for glycoaminoglycans that are abundant in those areas. Inflammation that is predominantly deep can form a stromal abscess, which may protrude in the anterior chamber. Untreated or unresponsive cases can progress to corneal rupture. Despite extension to and involvement of Descemet's membrane that essentially provides access to the anterior chamber, fungal keratitis does not progress to endophthalmitis in the absence of corneal rupture.

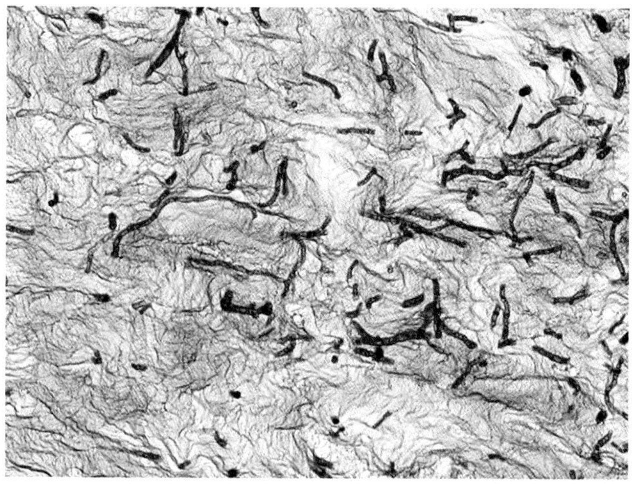

Figure 21-54 **Fungal Keratitis, Cornea, Horse.** Numerous fungal hyphae (*Aspergillus* sp.) infiltrate the corneal stroma. In most cases, fungal hyphae are most numerous in the deep stroma and readily infiltrate Descemet's membrane. H&E stain. (Courtesy Dr. P. Labelle, Antech Diagnostics.)

Eosinophilic Keratitis

Eosinophilic keratitis occurs predominantly in cats and occasionally in horses (see Disorders of Cats).

Immune-Mediated Keratopathies

Immune-mediated keratitis (IMMK) represents a diverse group of nonulcerative, noninfectious corneal diseases. IMMK occurs in the absence of uveal disease. The lesions may be epithelial or stromal (superficial, midstromal, or endothelial). The etiology or initiating cause likely varies between cases, but all are presumed to be at least in part immune-mediated. Histologically, the findings are those of chronic keratitis and include stromal fibrosis and neovascularization with inflammatory infiltrates composed of predominantly lymphocytes and plasma cells. There is a predominance of T lymphocytes, including both $CD4^+$ and $CD8^+$ cells.

Diseases of the Uvea

Equine Recurrent Uveitis

Equine recurrent uveitis (ERU) is a worldwide disease and is the most common cause of glaucoma and blindness in horses. Clinically, it is a complex syndrome defined by repeated episodes of uveitis. The periods of active inflammation alternate with periods of quiescence during which there is little or no recognizable intraocular inflammation. The episodes of uveitis tend to increase in frequency and severity over time, causing cumulative damage. Early lesions of ERU are unlikely to be examined histologically but consist of neutrophilic infiltration of the iris and ciliary body with a rapid transition to lymphocytes and fewer plasma cells and macrophages. Exudation of fibrin and proteinaceous material is a feature of the early disease.

The histologic features of the chronic disease are listed in Box 21-13. The histologic lesions that characterize the chronic disease include variably severe infiltration of lymphocytes and plasma cells in the uveal tract. The infiltrate tends to be most severe in the iris and ciliary body, but there is almost always some degree of choroidal involvement (panuveitis). The inflammation most often includes the formation of lymphoid follicles that become increasingly organized with chronicity (E-Fig. 21-68). During periods of quiescence, the lymphoplasmacytic infiltrate is milder and predominantly perivascular. Many of the diagnostic changes involve the nonpigmented ciliary epithelium. Lymphocytes and/or plasma cells infiltrate the

Box 21-13 Histologic Lesions in Chronic Equine Recurrent Uveitis

Main findings
- Lymphoplasmacytic uveitis often with lymphoid follicles
- Acellular hyaline material (amyloid) expanding/covering the nonpigmented ciliary epithelium
- Eosinophilic linear inclusions within the nonpigmented ciliary epithelium

Secondary findings
- Cataract
- Retinal detachment
- Fibrovascular proliferation
- Anterior and posterior synechiae
- Glaucoma-related changes

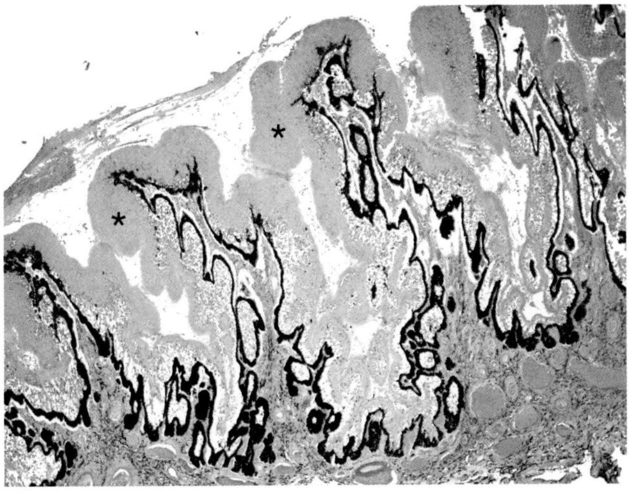

Figure 21-55 **Equine Recurrent Uveitis, Ciliary Body, Horse.** The nonpigmented ciliary epithelium is covered and expanded by hyaline eosinophilic material (amyloid) *(asterisks)*. H&E stain. (Courtesy Dr. P. Labelle, Antech Diagnostics.)

nonpigmented ciliary epithelium. The nonpigmented ciliary epithelium is covered/expanded by acellular hyaline eosinophilic material compatible with amyloid (Fig. 21-55). The eosinophilic material stains positive with Congo red and shows apple green birefringence under polarized light. It demonstrates immunoreactivity to antibodies specific for AA amyloid, and mass spectrometry indicates a predominance of serum amyloid A1 protein. The cytoplasm of some of the nonpigmented ciliary epithelial cells contains eosinophilic linear inclusions (Fig. 21-56). These inclusions are crystalline arrays of protein that appear to develop within mitochondria. Masson's trichrome staining facilitates their identification. Although typical of the disease, the mechanisms involved in the amyloid deposition and formation of the linear eosinophilic inclusions are unknown. There are a number of secondary lesions that can develop as a consequence of ERU and that may or may not be present in every case. ERU is the most common cause of cataract in horses. Retrocorneal and preiridal fibrovascular membranes are frequent and may lead to anterior or posterior synechiae. Many cases show retinal detachment secondary to choroidal disease, which can include thickening of choroidal vessels. The optic nerve may be infiltrated by lymphocytes and plasma cells or exhibit glial scarring. Many of the changes are nonspecific and secondary to the effects of glaucoma. The disease eventually leads to phthisis bulbi.

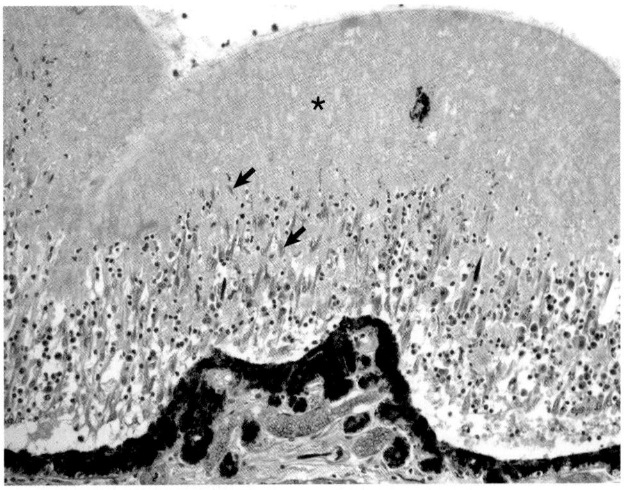

Figure 21-56 **Equine Recurrent Uveitis, Ciliary Body, Horse.** The nonpigmented ciliary epithelium is infiltrated by lymphocytes and plasma cells and covered and expanded by hyaline eosinophilic material (amyloid) *(asterisk)*. There are numerous eosinophilic linear inclusions *(arrows)*. H&E stain. (Courtesy Dr. P. Labelle, Antech Diagnostics.)

Many of the details of the pathogenesis have not yet been elucidated; however, ERU is generally regarded as a multifactorial immune-mediated disease. The majority of the infiltrating cells are $CD4^+$ T lymphocytes and include helper T lymphocytes that secrete IL-2 and interferon-γ. There is also secretion of IL-17 likely by helper T lymphocytes 17, indicating a role for autoimmunity. Many cases of ERU show immune responses to ocular proteins, most often retinal antigens such as interphotoreceptor-binding protein, S-antigen, and cellular retinaldehyde-binding protein. Some horses develop lymphocytic inflammation in the pineal gland, which shares antigens with the retina, including the S-antigen. Furthermore, the disease is associated with specific equine major histocompatibility complex haplotypes.

Infectious agents have been implicated in the development of the disease, and there is some correlation between infection with *Leptospira* spp. and ERU. Antibodies against *Leptospira* spp. are detected in the serum, aqueous humor, and vitreous of some clinically affected horses, and leptospiral organisms have been cultured or identified by polymerase chain reaction in some ERU globes. The disease has also been reproduced experimentally by exposing ponies to *L. interrogans* serovar *pomona*; the ponies recovered from the systemic infection but developed ocular lesions within the following months. Antibodies against *Leptospira* spp. cross-react with the equine cornea, lens, ciliary body, and retina, suggesting that molecular mimicry contributes to the pathogenesis of the ERU. It is therefore possible that beyond the uveitis that occurs as part of systemic leptospirosis, exposure to leptospiral organisms also stimulates autoimmunity.

The mechanisms by which repeated episodes of uveitis develop remain unclear but likely involve epitope spreading. In ERU, there is evidence for both intramolecular and intermolecular epitope spreading. Epitope spreading occurs when immune-mediated damage to the tissue exposes antigens previously unrecognized by the immune system that can now be the target of additional injury.

Disease of the Retina and Optic Nerve

Congenital Stationary Night Blindness

Congenital stationary night blindness in horses predominantly affects Appaloosas, although it has been reported in other breeds. In Appaloosas, it is associated with the leopard complex gene responsible for the white spotted coat patterns. There is abnormal transcription of the gene coding for a cation channel (TRPM1), which is required for normal signaling between rods and bipolar cells. This results in visual deficits, most notably night blindness (nyctalopia). The abnormality does not cause histologically recognizable lesions.

Disorders of Ruminants (Cattle, Sheep, and Goats)

Disease of the Eyelids and Conjunctiva

Infectious Bovine Rhinotracheitis

Infectious bovine rhinotracheitis is caused by bovine herpesvirus type-1 (BoHV-1), a member of the alpha herpesvirus family. The various strains of the disease can cause lesions in multiple organ systems. The ocular signs of the disease include serous to mucopurulent conjunctivitis. The acute lesion consists of serous to mucopurulent conjunctivitis, whereas the chronic disease typically presents as severe follicular lymphoid hyperplasia recognizable both grossly and histologically. Following infection, the main site for BoHV-1 latency is in the neurons of the trigeminal ganglia.

Infectious Bovine Keratoconjunctivitis

Infectious bovine keratoconjunctivitis (also known as pink eye) is a worldwide contagious disease of considerable economic importance. It is caused by the Gram-negative coccobacillus *Moraxella bovis*. The disease is transmitted from animal to animal by mechanical vectors such as flies, by direct contact, and by fomites. Natural outbreaks occur most often during the summer, and the face fly (*Musca autumnalis*) appears to be the most important vector. Ultraviolet light is a contributing factor possibly through damage to the corneal epithelium facilitating colonization by the bacteria. Concurrent infection with bovine herpes virus type-1 (infectious bovine rhinotracheitis) increases the severity of the disease. Other infectious agents that may contribute include *Moraxella ovis*, *Mycoplasma* spp., *Listeria monocytogenes*, and *Thelazia* spp.

The disease initially presents as conjunctival edema and congestion. Within 24 to 48 hours, shallow corneal ulcers develop, likely the result of epithelial cytotoxins produced by the bacteria. Numerous neutrophils infiltrate the affected area, and some may phagocytize the organisms. Keratomalacia is associated with collagenase release from the corneal epithelium, keratocytes, and neutrophils (Fig. 21-57; E-Fig. 21-69). *Moraxella bovis* does not produce collagenases but produces a cytotoxin that damages neutrophils in a dose-dependent manner. The cytotoxin and the release of enzymes by neutrophil contribute to stromal injury. The lesion induces prominent and rapid corneal stromal neovascularization, which reaches and surrounds the affected cornea within 7 to 9 days. Most cases will significantly improve within a few weeks, leaving only mild corneal scarring. In severe cases, the corneal ulcer may progress to corneal rupture with iris prolapse and, in some cases, phthisis bulbi.

Moraxella bovis exhibits several virulence factors, but only the presence of fimbriae (type IV pili) on the bacterial cell surface and the secretion of a β-hemolytic, corneotoxic, and leukotoxic cytotoxin impact clinical disease. Only piliated strains cause clinical signs: The Q pili facilitates the attachment of the organisms to the cornea, and the I pili enables maintenance of an established infection. Hemolytic *Moraxella bovis* strains produce a pore-forming cytotoxin (cytolysin/hemolysin) that induces corneal ulcers by lysis of corneal epithelial cells and neutrophils. Nonhemolytic strains of *Moraxella bovis* are not pathogenic for cattle. Other virulence factors that some strains or isolates may exhibit include phospholipases, hydrolytic and proteolytic enzymes, and iron acquisition systems.

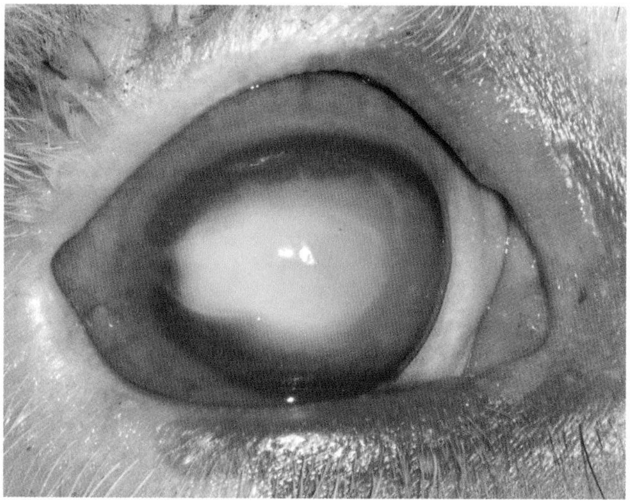

Figure 21-57 **Infectious Bovine Keratoconjunctivitis ("Pink Eye"), Cornea, Cow.** The axial half of the cornea is ulcerated with infiltration of neutrophils (suppurative keratomalacia) and surrounded by a border of red granulation tissue. The initial lesions are shallow corneal ulcers and foci of suppurative superficial stromal keratitis with conjunctival hyperemia, followed by circumferential superficial vascular ingrowth from bulbar conjunctiva toward the central ulcers. (Courtesy Ophthalmology Service, College of Veterinary Medicine, University of Illinois.)

Infectious keratoconjunctivitis in sheep and goats has similar clinical and histologic features to the bovine disease with the same name, but the condition can be caused by a wide range of organisms. *Chlamydophila pecorum* and *Mycoplasma* spp. account for most cases. The lesions initially present with conjunctival edema and congestion, followed by serous to mucopurulent conjunctivitis, and, with chronicity, lymphoid follicular hyperplasia.

Diseases of the Uvea

Malignant Catarrhal Fever

Malignant catarrhal fever is a sporadic, highly fatal systemic infectious disease that affects cattle and, less frequently, other ruminants and pigs. It has a worldwide distribution and is economically significant. The disease is caused by herpesviruses of the gamma herpesvirus family. The sheep-associated form has a worldwide distribution and is caused by ovine herpesvirus 2 (OvHV-2). It is transmitted by sheep and goats to cattle and other susceptible hosts. The wildebeest-associated form is caused by Alcelaphine herpesvirus 1 (AHV-1) and is transmitted by wildebeest. This form occurs mainly in Africa, but it also occurs in wildlife facilities housing wildebeest. The majority of cattle with malignant catarrhal fever have prominent ocular lesions including corneal edema, corneal neovascularization, and anterior uveitis. These lesions can distinguish this disease from bovine viral diarrhea and mucosal disease. In the eye, the lesion consists of necrotizing vasculitis with perivascular cuffing. $CD8^+$ T lymphocytes predominate. The vasculitis is most often identified within the iris, but it can be found anywhere within the uveal tract or retina. Peripheral corneal stromal neovascularization and corneal edema are often marked. Lymphocytic corneal endotheliitis may also contribute to the corneal edema. The pathogenesis of the disease is unclear. A cell-mediated cytotoxic lymphocytic process was initially suspected, but a pathogenesis of direct virus–cell interactions or immune-mediated responses directed against infected cells has also been proposed.

Diseases of the Retina and Optic Nerve

Transmissible Spongiform Encephalopathies

Transmissible spongiform encephalopathies (TSEs) are a group of neurodegenerative disorders caused by infectious protein particles (prions) (see Chapter 14 for general discussion and lesions in the central nervous system). In addition to the lesions in the central nervous system, including some affecting the visual pathway, TSEs also target the neural tissue of the globe. Ovine spongiform encephalopathy (scrapie) causes atrophy of the inner and outer nuclear layers with atrophy of the outer plexiform layer. The outer limiting membrane is less easily defined, and there can be vacuolation of the photoreceptor layer. Müller cells are hypertrophic, and there is increased glial fibrillary acidic protein (GFAP) immunoreactivity. Prions can be detected in the retina of most affected sheep. There can be optic nerve degeneration with vacuolation, Wallerian degeneration, gliosis, and infiltration of Gitter cells. Histologically, the lesion of bovine spongiform encephalopathy includes displacement of nuclei from the outer and inner nuclear layers into the photoreceptor and inner plexiform layers. There can also be loss of retinal ganglion cells. Rare vacuolation/spongiform change can be seen. Prions can be detected in the retina of most affected cattle.

Retinal Toxicity

Braken fern (*Pteridium aquilinum*) toxicity is a potential cause of retinal degeneration in sheep in the United Kingdom. In addition to its effect in other organ systems, the toxin ptaquiloside causes degeneration of the photoreceptor layer that eventually progresses to full-thickness retinal atrophy. Because the severely affected animals are blind and present with dilated pupils and tapetal hyperreflectivity, the condition has been termed bright blindness.

Disorders of Pigs

Diseases of the Eyelids and Conjunctiva

In pigs, conjunctivitis is often a manifestation of systemic diseases. Hog cholera can cause severe conjunctivitis. Pseudorabies, African swine fever, swine influenza, porcine reproductive respiratory syndrome, swine pox, rubulavirus, chlamydophylosis, and mycoplasmosis are also potential causes of conjunctivitis. Some of these conditions may cause keratitis in addition to conjunctivitis. In addition to surface lesions, diseases such as hog cholera and pseudorabies may cause intraocular lesions in some cases. In almost all instances, conjunctivitis is not the most significant clinical sign or lesion.

Diseases of the Cornea and Sclera

Blue Eye Disease

Blue eye disease is caused by porcine rubulavirus, a member of the paramyxovirus family. The disease has been reported only in Mexico; however, closely related paramyxoviruses have been identified in other countries. The virus mainly causes encephalitis, pneumonia, and reproductive failure, as well as ocular disease. The effects of the virus vary by age. Suckling piglets younger than age 21 days are most susceptible. Mortality among affected piglets can be as high as 90%; however, less than half of the piglets within a litter and approximately 20% of litters will be affected during an outbreak. Despite the name of the disease, only a small percentage of piglets develop corneal opacity corresponding to severe corneal edema. Many cases also have mild anterior uveitis, and some present with conjunctivitis. Older pigs tend to develop transient nonfatal disease that can include corneal disease.

Disorders of Dogs

Diseases of the Globe as a Whole

Goniodysgenesis

See Disorders of Domestic Animals, Diseases of the Globe as a Whole, The Classification of Glaucoma, Primary Glaucoma, Goniodysgenesis.

Diseases of the Eyelids and Conjunctiva

Entropion and Ectropion

See Disorders of Domestic Animals, Diseases of the Eyelids and Conjunctiva, Developmental Anomalies, Entropion and Ectropion.

Idiopathic Granulomatous Marginal Blepharitis

Idiopathic granulomatous marginal blepharitis is seen only in dogs as a nodular to multinodular to diffuse thickening of one or both eyelid margins. The histologic lesion consists of coalescing nodules of macrophages and neutrophils with variable numbers of lymphocytes and plasma cells in the subconjunctival tissue of the eyelid margin. Distinct granulomas and pyogranulomas characterize the lesion. The histologic presentation is similar to that of idiopathic sterile granuloma and pyogranulomas (see Chapter 17). The inflammation is not associated with hair follicles or glands. Microorganisms are never identified.

Prolapse of the Gland of the Third Eyelid

Prolapse of the gland of the third eyelid ("cherry eye") is common in dogs and is thought to be the result of laxity in the connective tissue anchoring the third eyelid to the periorbital tissues. The gland is histologically normal, although there may be secondary inflammatory changes.

Nodular Granulomatous Episcleritis

Nodular granulomatous episcleritis (NGE) is a common nodular lesion of the conjunctiva. The lesion is most often solitary and presents as a smooth, tan to red, subconjunctival mass. As the name reflects, the vast majority of cases occur at the limbus, but the lesion may be seen in other conjunctival sites and rarely in the orbit. NGE has distinct histologic features consisting of a well-circumscribed nodule composed of spindle and epithelioid macrophages in variable proportions admixed with lymphocytes and plasma cells (Fig. 21-58). Some spindle cells may be myofibroblasts.

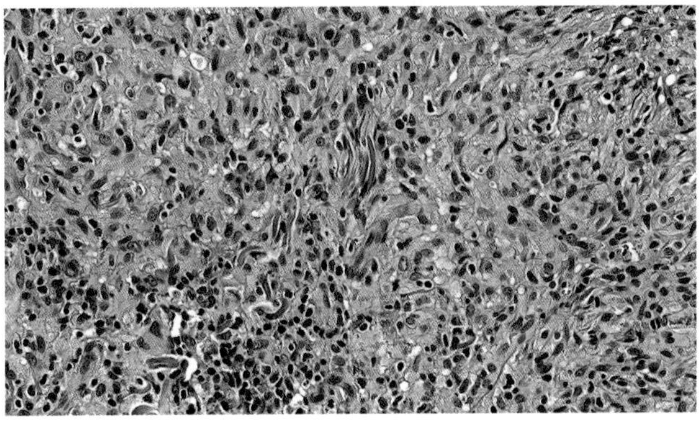

Figure 21-58 **Nodular Granulomatous Episcleritis, Conjunctiva, Dog.** The lesion consists of a distinct nodule of spindle and epithelioid macrophages admixed with lymphocytes and plasma cells. No granulomas are present. No microorganisms are present. H&E stain. (Courtesy Dr. P. Labelle, Antech Diagnostics.)

Multinucleated giant cells and eosinophils are occasionally admixed with infiltrate. Distinct granulomas are not a feature of the condition. It is likely that the histologic lesion represents a reaction to different stimuli rather than a specific disease. NGE is presumed to be an immune-mediated reaction, and most cases respond to immunomodulation.

Ligneous Conjunctivitis

Ligneous conjunctivitis is a rare entity seen predominantly in Doberman pinschers and Golden retrievers and described in other breeds. Grossly, the conjunctiva is bilaterally firm with a pseudomembranous exudate. Histologically, the main finding is the presence of abundant poorly cellular hyaline eosinophilic matrix in the substantia propria. The matrix is positive with phosphotungstic acid–hematoxylin (PTAH) staining and negative for Congo red, indicating fibrin. Similar material may be deposited at other sites. In some dogs, the disease is caused by a plasminogen deficiency.

Diseases of the Cornea and Sclera

Chronic Superficial Keratitis (Pannus)

Chronic superficial keratitis (CSK) is a clinically distinctive superficial keratitis seen primarily but not exclusively in German shepherd dogs and sighthounds. The underlying mechanism appears to be an immune-mediated response targeting cornea-specific antigens that have been altered by environmental factors such as ultraviolet light. There is a genetic component to the disease, and an MHC class II risk haplotype has been identified in German shepherds. Dogs homozygous for the risk haplotype are eight times more likely to develop CSK. The disease usually begins at the lateral limbus as red conjunctival thickening. The lesion spreads toward the axial cornea as a superficial, fleshy, vascularized stromal infiltrate, involving both globes although not always symmetrically (E-Fig. 21-70). Chronic lesions become intensely pigmented, and eventually the entire superficial stroma may be vascularized, fibrotic, and pigmented.

Histologically, the lesion is a dense lichenoid lymphoplasmacytic stromal keratitis with stromal fibrosis and neovascularization. Cases with pigmentation are likely to show pigmentary incontinence. The corneal epithelium is likely to be hyperplastic, pigmented, and keratinizing. There may be single cell necrosis/apoptosis within the corneal epithelium. In commonly affected breeds, the lesion is likely to be recognized clinically, and most cases respond to long-term immunomodulatory therapy. A condition similar in signalment, histopathology, and likely pathogenesis targets the third eyelid (plasmacytic conjunctivitis/plasmoma). The histologic lesion of CSK overlaps with nonspecific chronic keratitis, and the distinction may require clinical information.

Granulomatous Scleritis

Granulomatous scleritis (necrotizing scleritis) is a condition of unclear pathogenesis. It is suspected to be an immune-mediated disease but is not associated with immune-mediated diseases affecting other sites. The inflammation does not form nodules and is always predominantly centered on the sclera. There may be extension in the adjacent uveal tract or anteriorly in the cornea in severe cases. The histologic lesion consists of macrophages with lymphocytes and plasma cells. Rare multinucleated giant cells may be present, and some cases may include neutrophils. Collagenolysis and vasculitis are inconsistent findings. Retinal detachment is common in cases with extension in the choroid. The lesion can be unilateral, but in many cases the contralateral globe will eventually develop a similar lesion.

Diseases of the Uvea

Uveodermatologic Syndrome (Vogt-Koyanagi-Harada–like Syndrome)

Uveodermatologic syndrome is relatively frequent in dogs. Clinically, the disease is most often seen in Akitas, Siberian huskies, Samoyeds, and Australian shepherds, although many other breeds are affected. The globes from less commonly affected breeds are more likely to be examined histologically, perhaps because the disease is less readily recognized clinically. The clinical syndrome of dermal depigmentation and severe bilateral uveitis is distinctive. Ocular lesions typically precede skin lesions. In Akitas, specific dog leukocyte antigen (DLA) class II alleles predispose to the development of the disease. DLA are part of the major histocompatibility complex (MHC). The pathogenesis of the lesion involves immune-mediated inflammation targeting a protein involved in melanin production in melanocytes, likely tyrosinase or tyrosinase-related proteins. Histologically, the lesion consists of severe granulomatous panuveitis with prominent pigment dispersion (Fig. 21-59). The iris, ciliary body, and choroid are typically all affected, but the inflammation may not be as severe diffusely. The inflammation is strikingly uveocentric with very little extension in other parts of the globe. Retinal detachment and glaucoma are common secondary findings.

Asymmetric Uveitis

Asymmetric uveitis describes a condition in which injury to one eye causing a specific pattern of inflammation predisposes the contralateral globe to similar inflammation even in the absence of the initiating cause. The vast majority of cases are thought to be initiated by penetrating trauma to one globe. The lesion consists of granulomatous to pyogranulomatous endophthalmitis where the leukocytes carpet the uveal tract, posterior cornea, and/or inner retina (Fig. 21-60). Retinal detachment and necrosis are common. Usually within weeks, the contralateral globe will develop inflammation with similar distribution and composition without trauma. However, it is not possible to accurately predict if or when the contralateral globe will be affected. Clinicians should be made aware of this risk so that the contralateral globe can be closely monitored and early treatment can be administered. The pathogenesis has not been elucidated in dogs, but asymmetric uveitis may represent a T lymphocyte-mediated delayed-type hypersensitivity reaction targeting a uveal antigen. Clinical information is often required to differentiate asymmetric uveitis from phacoclastic uveitis associated with diabetic cataracts. Unlike uveodermatologic syndrome, in

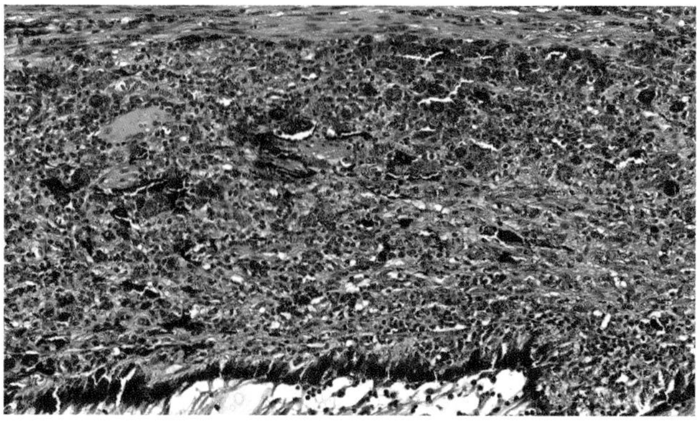

Figure 21-59 **Uveodermatologic Syndrome, Ciliary Body, Dog.** Numerous macrophages with fewer lymphocytes and plasma cells infiltrate the uveal stroma. There is release of melanin granules by uveal melanocytes, which is then phagocytized by macrophages (pigmentary dispersion). H&E stain. (Courtesy Dr. P. Labelle, Antech Diagnostics.)

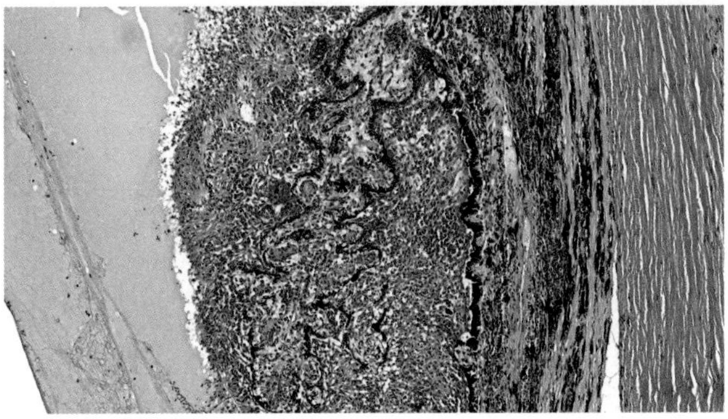

Figure 21-60 **Asymmetric Uveitis, Ciliary Body, Dog.** Numerous macrophages with fewer lymphocytes and plasma cells carpet the ciliary body and ciliary process *(asterisk)*. The inflammation within the uveal stroma is significantly milder. H&E stain. (Courtesy Dr. P. Labelle, Antech Diagnostics.)

which the inflammation is mostly within the uveal tract, asymmetric uveitis predominantly lines or carpets the uveal tract.

Intraocular Xanthoma (Xanthogranuloma)

Intraocular xanthoma is a rare condition mostly seen in Miniature Schnauzers. Grossly, the entire globe is filled with tan material mimicking a mass. Histologically, the material consists of massive numbers of vacuolated "foamy" macrophages and multinucleated giant cells. There are extracellular deposits of lipid presenting as birefringent crystals and clefts. Idiopathic primary hyperlipidemia, diabetes mellitus, and lens-induced uveitis may all be contributing factors.

Diseases of the Retina and Optic Nerve

Collie Eye Anomaly

Collie eye anomaly (CEA) is a bilateral, congenital, recessively inherited syndrome. It is most commonly seen in rough and smooth collies, Shetland sheepdogs, Australian shepherds, border collies, Lancaster heeler, as well as other breeds. The pathogenesis of the defect is thought to be a failure of the outer layer of the optic cup, which eventually becomes the retinal pigment epithelium (RPE), to induce the proper development of the neural crest-derived choroid, tapetum lucidum, and sclera. Molecular signaling between the RPE and periocular mesenchyme is required for melanocyte differentiation and choroidal vasculature development. For example, VEGF from the RPE is required for the development of the choroidal vasculature. The underlying genetic mutation of CEA is an intronic deletion in the NEHJ1 gene.

The histologic findings always include some degree of choroidal hypoplasia (Fig. 21-61). There is choroidal hypopigmentation as a result of a decrease in the number of melanocytes as well as segmental tapetal aplasia/hypoplasia. The choroidal hypoplasia tends to be more pronounced lateral to the optic disc, near the junction of the tapetal and nontapetal choroid. Posterior polar colobomas at or near the optic disc may be unilateral or bilateral and reflect a defect in the lamina cribrosa or sclera adjacent to the optic nerve (E-Figs. 21-71 and 21-72; see Fig. 21-22). The colobomas are lined by retinal/neural tissue. Other findings may include retinal detachment, retinal dysplasia, and intraocular hemorrhage. Of interest, choroidal hypoplasia by itself does not lead to impaired vision.

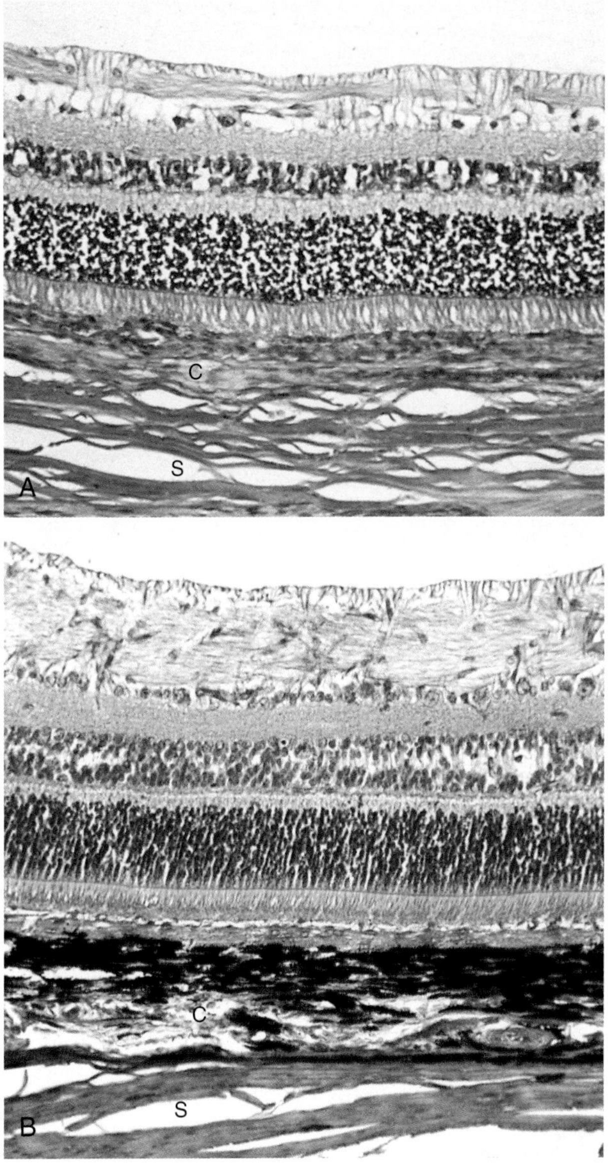

Figure 21-61 **Choroidal Hypoplasia, Collie Eye Anomaly, Choroid, Dog. A,** The choroid is approximately half the normal thickness and has no pigment. H&E stain. **B,** Normal canine retina and choroid, age-matched control. C, Choroid; S, sclera. H&E stain. (Courtesy Dr. B. Wilcock, Ontario Veterinary College.)

Canine Progressive Retinal Atrophy

Canine progressive retinal atrophy describes a group of inherited or suspected inherited photoreceptor disorders of dogs. It is a bilateral progressive degeneration of photoreceptors that leads to blindness, in the absence of an inflammatory or toxic cause. The underlying genetic and biochemical alterations vary greatly, but these disorders share clinical and histologic features. The molecular work in various breeds does not translate to specific histologic findings. This group of diseases includes early onset photoreceptor dysplasias in which photoreceptors fail to develop normally as well as late-onset degenerations that most often become significant in adults. Most of the breed-specific conditions included under the broad term progressive retinal atrophy are autosomal recessive diseases. Many of these conditions initially target rods, and night blindness (nyctalopia) is a common presenting complaint.

Because the initial retinal degeneration does not cause glaucoma, affected globes are only evaluated histologically in the very late stages of the disease or as part of the evaluation for other ocular disorders. At that time, the changes include multifocal loss

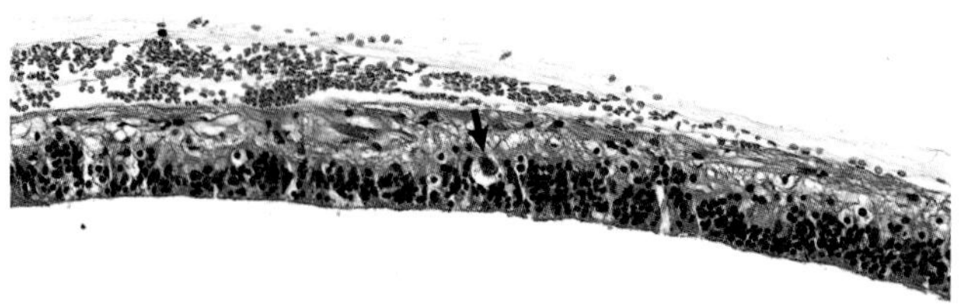

Figure 21-62 **Progressive Retinal Atrophy, Retina, Dog.** With chronic disease, there is diffuse atrophy of the photoreceptor layer and blending of the inner and outer nuclear layer. Note the ganglion cell, which has "dropped" within the nuclear layer *(arrow)*. H&E stain. (Courtesy Dr. P. Labelle, Antech Diagnostics.)

of photoreceptors that progresses to diffuse involvement and eventually includes the outer nuclear layer. As the disease progresses, there is blending of the outer and inner nuclear layers and unaffected ganglion cells may "drop" within that layer (Fig. 21-62). Invariably the disease proceeds to full-thickness retinal atrophy and glial scarring. Complications of chronic progressive retinal atrophy include retinal detachment and cataract, both of which may lead to glaucoma. Only the early multifocal distribution can be helpful to suggest progressive retinal atrophy by histology. Once the lesion diffusely affects the photoreceptors, it is indistinguishable from any other cause of photoreceptor degeneration.

Sudden Acquired Retinal Degeneration

Sudden acquired retinal degeneration (SARD) is a common cause of acute, rapidly progressing, permanent photoreceptor degeneration. Blindness occurs within days to weeks. Affected dogs are adult, and the disease can affect any breed or crossbreed. The lesion is bilaterally symmetric and diffuse across the retina. The cause is unknown. Some dogs are otherwise healthy, whereas others show clinical signs suggestive of metabolic disease, such as weight gain, polyuria, polydipsia, polyphagia, and blood work that at times suggests adrenal dysfunction. Histologically, the lesion begins as thinning of the outer plexiform layer. The lesion progresses to a uniform diffuse loss of photoreceptors and eventually to diffuse full-thickness retinal atrophy. Once the lesion diffusely affects the photoreceptors, it is indistinguishable from any other cause of photoreceptor degeneration. There can be lymphoplasmacytic retinitis; however, the change is histologically minimal. Because the retinal degeneration does not cause glaucoma, affected globes are only evaluated histologically in the very late stages of the disease or as part of the evaluation for other ocular disorders.

Diseases of the Orbit

Orbital Extraocular Polymyositis

Orbital extraocular polymyositis affects all the extraocular muscles except the retractor bulbi muscle. It is a rare disease, typically affecting young dogs. Clinically, the condition presents as bilateral and variably symmetric exophthalmos, retraction of the upper eyelid, and mild chemosis. In the chronic disease, there is enophthalmos (retraction of the globe into the orbit) and strabismus. Histologically, the lesion is a $CD3^{+}$ predominant lymphocytic myositis that results in myonecrosis, followed by attempts at regeneration and eventually muscle atrophy and fibrosis. An immune-mediated attack directed specifically against the extraocular muscles is suspected to be the cause of this disorder. Because the extraocular muscles are a difficult site from which to obtain a biopsy, diagnosis is generally based on the clinical findings.

Disorders of Cats

Diseases of the Cornea and Sclera

Herpesvirus Keratitis

Feline herpesvirus 1 (FHV-1), a member of the alpha herpesvirus family, has a worldwide distribution and causes a combination of upper respiratory disease, conjunctivitis, and keratitis that predominantly affects kittens. The virus causes epithelial cell cytolysis, which can predispose to secondary bacterial infection. The conjunctivitis can also lead to symblepharon, adhesions between the cornea and conjunctiva. Intranuclear inclusion bodies are present only during the early stages of the disease and are therefore almost never seen histologically. After recovery, most kittens develop latent infection primarily in the trigeminal ganglia. FHV-1 is the most commonly clinically diagnosed cause of keratitis in cats, presumed to represent recrudescent disease in most adult cases. However, the causative effect of FHV-1 is difficult to document in clinical cases. Proving FHV-1 as the cause of keratoconjunctivitis is problematic because greater than 95% of cats show serologic evidence of exposure and up to 50% of clinically normal cats contain FHV-1 DNA in the cornea. Clinically, the disease may present as ulcers, either dendritic ulcers considered pathognomonic for the disease or geographic ulcers. FHV-1 can also cause a chronic stromal keratitis with nonspecific infiltration of lymphocytes and plasma cells. Based largely on the presence of viral DNA, some have also proposed a role for FHV-1 in feline corneal sequestrum and feline eosinophilic keratoconjunctivitis. Herpesvirus keratoconjunctivitis is essentially a clinical diagnosis, and affected corneas are unlikely to be examined by a pathologist. Samples that are examined histologically do not show intranuclear inclusions, nor do they demonstrate changes that can be specifically attributed to the cytopathic effect of the virus. It is therefore not possible to confirm FHV-1 infection histologically.

Eosinophilic Keratitis

Eosinophilic keratitis is a unique disease that occurs predominantly in cats but also occasionally in horses. The pathogenesis has not been determined in either species. The clinical presentation varies, but the condition has similar histologic features in both species. In cats, the typical clinical presentation consists of white to pink proliferative plaques, most often involving the lateral cornea initially (Fig. 21-63). Many cases have similar lesions in the adjacent conjunctiva, and in a few cases the lesions are exclusively conjunctival. The disease can be diagnosed by demonstrating the presence of eosinophils on cytology. Histologically, eosinophils are always a component of the inflammation but may not be the predominant cell type (Fig. 21-64; E-Fig. 21-73). Because most cases sampled are chronic, the infiltrate is often predominantly lymphoplasmacytic with variable numbers of eosinophils. Mast cells and macrophages can be present in variable numbers. Some cases present with a band of granular hypereosinophilic material near or at the epithelial basement membrane presumed to represent eosinophilic degranulation. The overlying epithelium is often intact. The histologic diagnosis of eosinophilic keratitis is usually made in keratectomy samples. The disease usually responds favorably to medical treatment, and there is almost never an indication for enucleation, although the disease can be recurrent. The cause and pathogenesis are unknown. There is no known association with cutaneous eosinophilic granuloma complex or systemic diseases. A causative role for feline herpesvirus 1 has not been established.

Acute Bullous Keratopathy

Acute bullous keratopathy occurs almost exclusively in cats, but it has been reported in horses. The condition describes a specific form

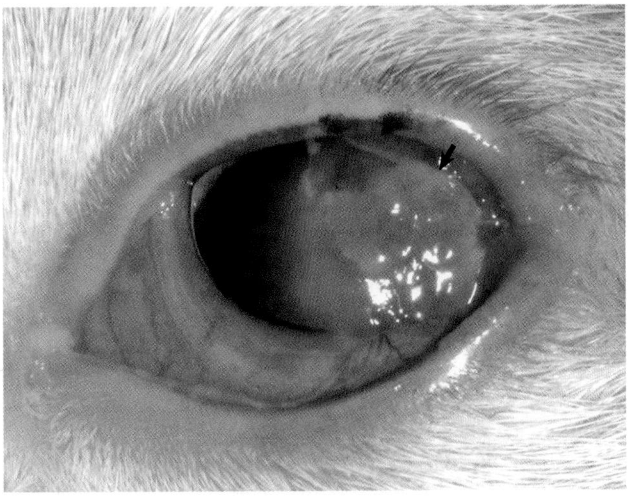

Figure 21-63 **Eosinophilic Keratitis, Cornea, Cat.** The temporal half of the cornea is covered by a raised, pink/white plaque in this cat with eosinophilic keratitis *(arrow)*. Corneal neovascularization surrounds the lesion. Marked conjunctival hyperemia and chemosis is also present. (Courtesy Ophthalmology Service, College of Veterinary Medicine, University of Illinois.)

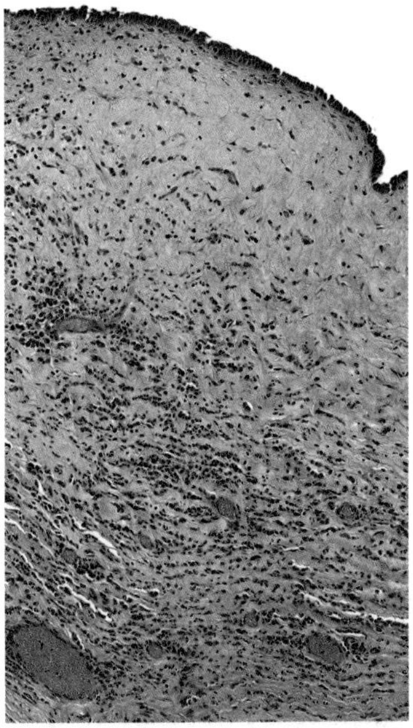

Figure 21-64 **Eosinophilic Keratitis, Cornea, Cat.** Numerous eosinophils admixed with lymphocytes and plasma cells infiltrate the corneal stroma. The stroma is edematous, and there is neovascularization. H&E stain. (Courtesy Dr. P. Labelle, Antech Diagnostics.)

of bullous keratopathy that develops within hours. Acute bullous keratopathy develops in the absence of preexisting corneal disease. Grossly, there is marked corneal edema and formation of stromal bullae. Histologically, there is a relatively well-circumscribed severe expansion of the corneal stroma. There is no associated inflammation. The cause of the lesion appears to be rupture of Descemet's membrane, which may be recognized histologically. Unlike most causes of corneal edema, there is no evidence of injury to the corneal epithelium or corneal endothelium. The underlying pathogenesis is unknown; however, an association with administration of systemic antiinflammatory or immunosuppressive therapy has been proposed.

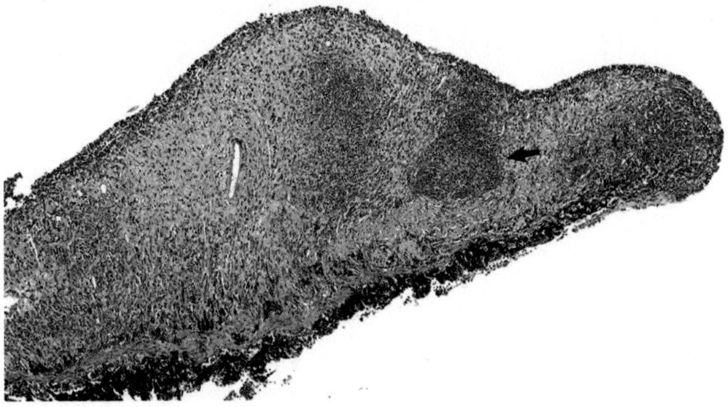

Figure 21-65 **Lymphoplasmacytic Anterior Uveitis, Iris, Cat.** Numerous lymphocytes and plasma cells infiltrate the iris with early follicle formation *(arrow)*. Lymphoid follicles become increasingly organized with chronicity. H&E stain. (Courtesy Dr. P. Labelle, Antech Diagnostics.)

Disease of the Uvea

Feline Lymphoplasmacytic Uveitis

Feline lymphoplasmacytic uveitis is the most frequent histologic pattern of the uveitis in cats. It is not a specific disease but, rather, a common reaction to a variety of insults, including trauma, infectious diseases, and neoplasia. It is presumed to be an immune-mediated disease; however, the cause and pathogenesis likely vary considerably between individual cases. Histologically, there is infiltration of lymphocytes and plasma cells predominantly in the iris, iridocorneal angle, and ciliary body (Fig. 21-65; E-Fig. 21-74). The infiltrate may extend in the posterior iris and ciliary epithelium. Choroidal involvement is variable but tends to be mild. There can also be perivascular infiltration of lymphocytes and plasma cells in the retina, which does not provide any clues as to the initiating cause. Chronic and severe cases often include formation of lymphoid follicles within the iris, iridocorneal angle, or ciliary body. The lesion indicates chronicity, and the initiating cause is almost never recognized histologically. The lesion may be unilateral or bilateral, likely a reflection of the numerous potential causes. The significance of lymphoplasmacytic uveitis is that it is a common cause of glaucoma in cats. The mechanism by which the uveitis causes the glaucoma is unclear. Obstruction and functional distortion of the iridocorneal angle by the inflammation are likely contributing factors. Severe lymphoplasmacytic uveitis may clinically mimic uveal lymphoma.

Feline Infectious Peritonitis

Feline infectious peritonitis (FIP) has a worldwide distribution. The FIP virus is a strain of the feline coronavirus (FCoV) that has acquired virulence, possibly through a mutation that allows replication in macrophages (see Chapters 4, 7, and others). FIP is a common cause of uveitis and endophthalmitis in cats, most often in young cats. Ocular disease may be present with or without obvious systemic signs. Gross lesions include accumulation of highly proteinaceous material within the anterior chamber and/or vitreous. The histologic presentation is highly variable. In most cases, the disease is most severe in the anterior uvea with extension into adjacent anterior and posterior chambers. The inflammation tends to be predominantly neutrophilic with areas of pyogranulomatous or granulomatous inflammation (Fig. 21-66; E-Fig. 21-75). Some cases are plasma cell predominant. Neutrophilic or lymphoplasmacytic endotheliitis is common. Vasculitis may or may not be present.

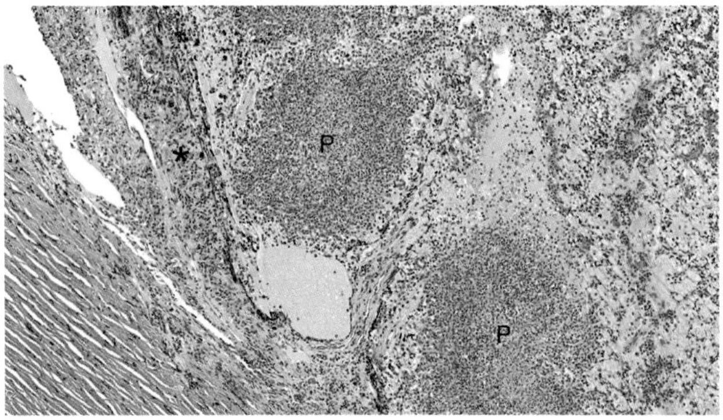

Figure 21-66 **Pyogranulomatous Endophthalmitis, Feline Infectious Peritonitis, Anterior Uvea, Cat.** Multifocal pyogranulomatous inflammation *(P)* within the posterior chamber. Plasma cells and lymphocytes infiltrate the iris *(asterisk)* and ciliary body. (Courtesy Dr. P. Labelle, Antech Diagnostics.)

Inflammation in the choroid tends to be lymphoplasmacytic, and there can be retinal perivascular cuffing. Retinal detachment is common. The inflammation may also extend in the optic nerve and/or optic meninges. In enucleated globes from patients that do not manifest overt systemic signs and present for chronic unresponsive uveitis, the inflammation tends to be plasma cell predominant. Although the changes in the globe are often highly suspicious for FIP, an absolute definitive diagnosis is rarely possible based on ocular histopathology alone.

Diseases of the Retina and Optic Nerve

Inherited Retinal Dysplasias and Degenerations

Inherited retinal dysplasias and degenerations have been reported as sporadic occurrences in a variety of cat breeds. Two separate diseases have been described in the Abyssinian. One is an early onset rod-cone dysplasia with clinical signs of slower pupillary light reflexes, mydriasis, and nystagmus developing as early as 4 to 6 weeks of age. It has an autosomal dominant mode of inheritance and is the result of a single base deletion in the CRX gene. Both cones and rods show abnormal and retarded development. The photoreceptor degeneration begins in the central retina and progresses toward the periphery. Cones are more severely affected than rods. By 1 year of age, the disease is advanced and cats are blind. In contrast, the late-onset retinal degeneration is inherited as an autosomal recessive trait, and affected cats usually show no clinical signs until approximately 2 years of age. There is variable progression to full-thickness retinal atrophy over 2 to 4 years. Rods are more severely affected than cones. The earliest histologic lesions are disorganization of the photoreceptors and loss of neurons from the outer nuclear layer. Late in the disease, there is complete loss of the outer segment of the photoreceptors with loss of some inner segments and thinning of other retinal layers. During all stages of the disease, the central retina is less severely affected.

Taurine Deficiency

Taurine deficiency (also known as feline central retinal degeneration) causes photoreceptor degeneration in cats. Unlike other domestic animals, cats have only limited capacity to synthesize taurine from the precursor amino acid cysteine because of low levels of the enzyme cysteine sulfinic acid decarboxylase. Cats depend on dietary intake to maintain normal tissue concentrations. All ocular components contain taurine, but the concentrations are highest in the retina and even more so in the photoreceptors. Taurine plays a critical role in normal development and function of the retina and also of the visual cortex of the brain. The exact functions of taurine are not clearly defined, but it does provide cytoprotection through its antioxidant properties and also modulates neuronal activity in a neurotransmitter-like manner. In taurine-deficient cats, the earliest lesions consist of cone disorganization. Cones are more sensitive than rods to taurine deficiency, and the rods of the peripheral retina are the last to degenerate. Initially, the histologic lesion is photoreceptor degeneration in the area centralis that progresses to more widely affect the retina dorsal to the optic nerve. In some cases, diffuse retinal atrophy develops, leading to blindness. The cardiac changes associated with taurine deficiency are described in Chapter 10.

Enrofloxacin/Fluoroquinolone Toxicity

Fluoroquinolone toxicity causes photoreceptor degeneration in cats. The lesion develops acutely and can even be seen in cats receiving a single inappropriately high dose. Histologically, there can be swelling and vacuolation of the photoreceptors within the hours of exposure to a toxic dose. Diffuse photoreceptor degeneration is recognizable within days. The susceptibility of cats to fluoroquinolone toxicity has a genetic basis. There are specific amino acid changes to the transport protein ABCG2 at the blood-retinal barrier compared to other species. These changes allow accumulation of fluoroquinolone within the retina. Fluoroquinolones are photoreactive, and exposure to light can generate reactive oxygen species that damage lipid membranes.

Suggested Readings

Suggested Readings are available at www.expertconsult.com.

Photographic Techniques in Veterinary Pathology

M. Donald McGavin

Gross Specimen Photography

Judged by the photographs presented at seminars and conferences, requirements for gross specimen photography are not fully appreciated. Because of space limitations in the sixth edition, the techniques used to obtain these types of images are discussed in detail at www.expertconsult.com, including descriptions of the techniques of gross specimen photography, camera stand and photographic lamps, backgrounds, flash photography, photomicrography, and evaluation of photomicrographs.

Studio Lighting

The optimal arrangement for the photography of isolated organs is a studio setup as depicted in Fig. 1, with a main light to the left to produce shadows and a fill light on the right to illuminate those shadow sufficiently to show detail in them without being so intense as to erase them. To achieve this, the fill light is 1.5 to 3 times the distance of the main light from the subject. A good default is 1.5 times the distance from the average specimen. To cast shadows downward, the axis of the main light should be approximately 30 degrees above the plane of the specimen and at the 10:30 o'clock position (315 degrees) on a clock face around the axis of the camera lens (see Fig. 1). This means that for an anatomically and correctly oriented specimen, the main source of light comes from the left and above. This seems natural to us because for millions of years man has been programmed to interpret images based on the assumption that there is one light source (the sun), and it comes from above. Lighting from below casts shadows upward and appears unnatural or eerie; it is called "spook" lighting and for that reason is used for movies of that name. To emphasize surface "hills and valleys" (i.e., texture) in a flat surface such as intestinal mucosa or skin, the main light is lowered to 15 to 25 degrees above the plane of the specimen to produce a "skimming light." With a digital camera it is simple to try different angles of the main light and immediately review the images in the view finder.

Flash Photography

If studio lighting is not available or if the specimen is too large to fit on the background or cannot be moved, then flash photography is the alternative. Point-and-shoot cameras produce photographs with excellent exposure and color balance, but the built-in flash unit produces axial lighting (i.e., light on the same axis as the axis of the camera lens). Therefore it casts no shadows, and it is shadows on the surface that are responsible for the depiction of three-dimensional shapes (modeling) of organs and the texture of their surface. The only answer is to move the axis of the light beam away from the axis of the camera lens. There are two main ways to do this. For small specimens (a maximum dimension of approximately 9 inches), the flash unit can be mounted on a side bracket (Fig. 2), but for larger specimens the flash will have to be held by hand—either by the photographer or an assistant (Figs. 3 and 4). A black background from a glass-topped black box, painted blackboard, or black construction paper is used. These may become blotchy when wet by fluids, but this is easily corrected by Adobe Photoshop.

The requirements for a photograph of a gross specimen include the following:

- Appropriately dissected specimen
- Correctly anatomically oriented specimen
- Suitable framing so that anatomic landmarks are included and can be recognized and used for orientation by the viewer
- Correctly focused with adequate depth of field
- Lighting from above that renders surface modeling and texture
- Interesting and aesthetically pleasing composition, if possible
- Unobtrusive background—no stainless steel tables, tiled floors, floor drains, or colored backgrounds

Photomicrography

Automatic exposure determination, automatic color balancing, and on-the-monitor focusing have made digital photomicrography easier, but some steps to obtain optimal photomicrographs (Fig. 5) are still the responsibility of the operator. Koehler illumination is particularly important and has two steps that need to be carried out after the microscope has been focused on the specimen: (1) focusing the image of the field diaphragm in the microscope's field of view (easier to do than describe) and (2) setting the position of the aperture diaphragm. The aperture diaphragm controls three important features of the image: (1) resolution, defined as the ability of the lens to separate adjacent points in the image; (2) contrast, the differences between the light and dark tones (gray scale) of colors; and (3) depth of field (i.e., the thickness of the specimen in focus). Maximum resolution occurs when the aperture diaphragm is open so its circle of light in the rear focal plane (RFP) of the objective (visible only when the ocular has been removed) is the same diameter as the circle of light of the objective (Fig. 6). This arrangement is called *100% cone* and is an expression of the relative diameters of the illuminated circles from the objective and condenser as viewed in the RFP. Closing the aperture diaphragm increases contrast (similar to "lowering" the condenser), but if the aperture diaphragm is closed too far, diffraction occurs and resolution is markedly reduced (see Fig. 5, *B*). Thus the choice is a balance between resolution and contrast. There are some rules of thumb for obtaining maximum resolution and good contrast. With thin specimens, such as blood smears and thin tissue sections (3 to 4 μm in thickness),

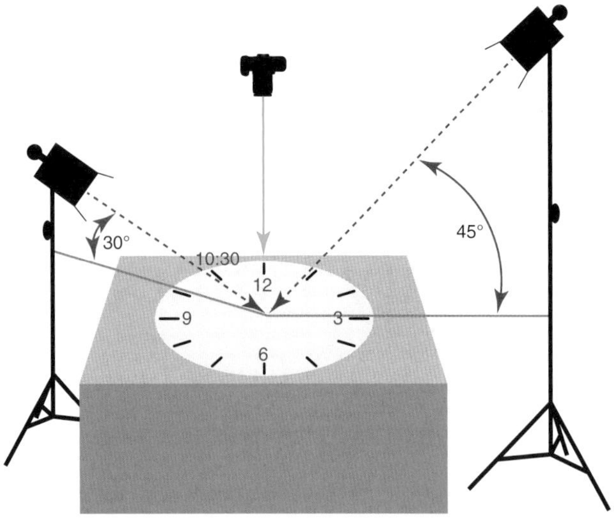

Figure 1 **Studio Lighting Arrangement.** Note that the axis of main light *(left)* is 30 degrees above the plane of the specimen to produce shadows that will show the topography of the surface. Also, the main light is at the 10:30 o'clock position to ensure that the light comes from the top left. The fill light on the right is at the 3 o'clock position, but further away (1.5 to 3 times) from the specimen than the main light, to ensure that the shadows cast by the main light are not obliterated. (Courtesy Dr. M.D. McGavin, College of Veterinary Medicine, University of Tennessee.)

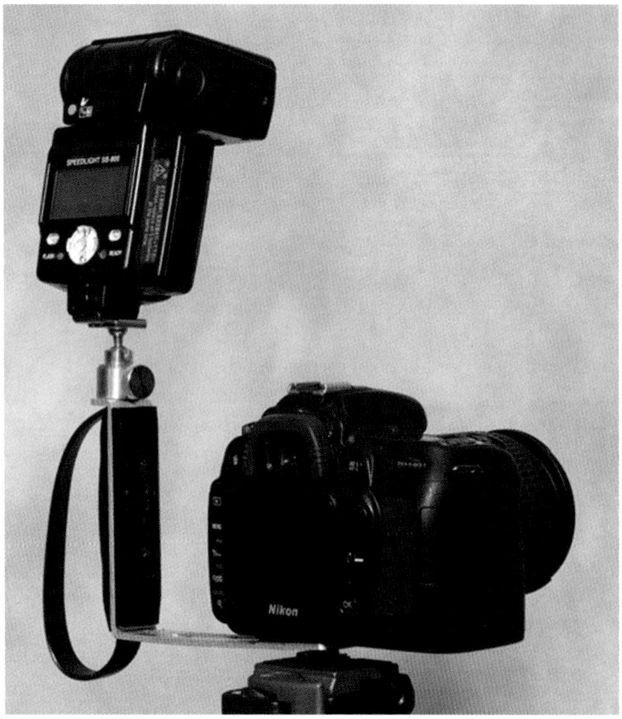

Figure 2 **Camera, Bracket, and Flash Unit.** The bracket holds the flash unit approximately 6 inches to the side of the camera with the result that its light produces shadows and thus modeling for small specimens less than 9 inches in length. At greater distances the flash is so close to the axis of the camera lens that it does not produce shadows large enough to depict modeling. Note also that the axis of the camera lens is directed onto the specimen from approximately the 10:30 o'clock position. The handle is extremely handy when holding the camera in an autopsy laboratory. (Courtesy Mr. P.D. Snow, College of Veterinary Medicine, University of Tennessee.)

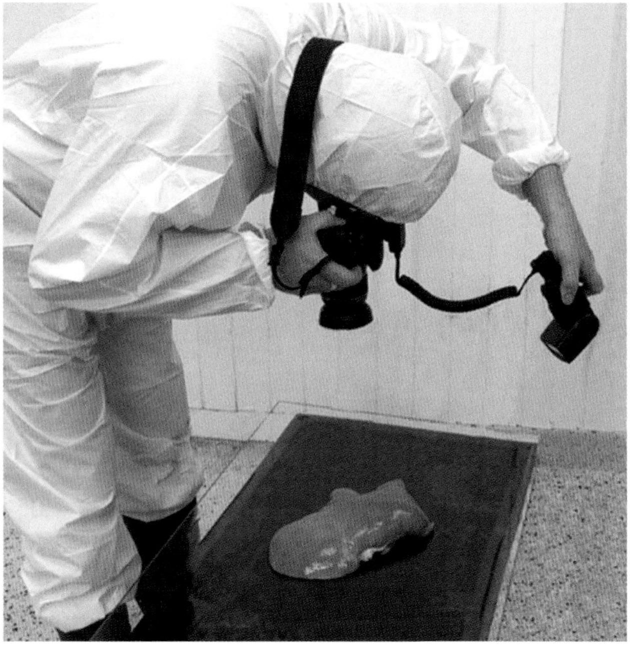

Figure 3 **Flash, Off the Camera.** To obtain modeling for specimens whose dimensions are greater than approximately 9 inches, the main light has to be moved further to the left than is possible using a camera bracket. Thus the flash unit is held by hand at the 10:30 o'clock position and approximately 30 degrees above the specimen plane by the photographer, but for larger specimens an assistant is necessary. The background in this case is a glass-covered black box. (Courtesy Dr. C. O'Muireagain, Regional Veterinary Laboratory, Sligo, Ireland.)

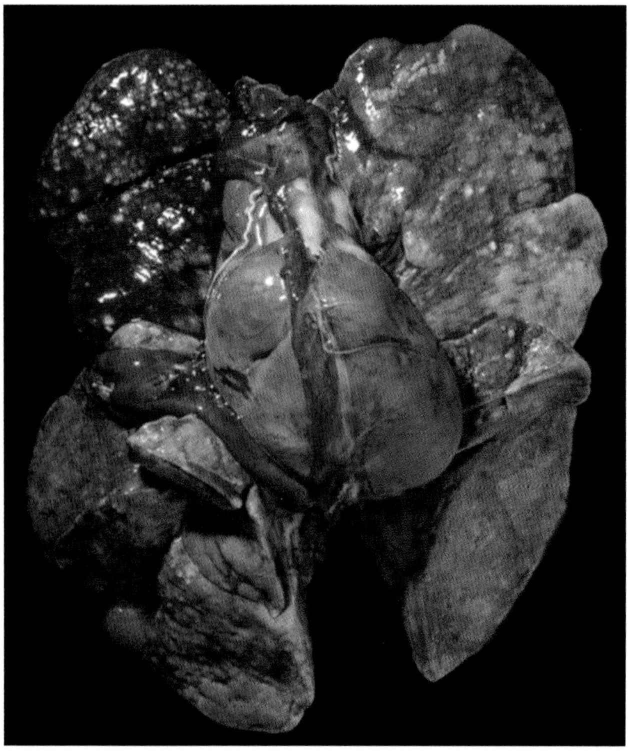

Figure 4 **Thoracic Viscera, Lungs, Badger, Tuberculosis.** The flash unit was held by hand off the camera at the 10:30 o'clock position, as is evident from the shadows cast down by the heart. Note the excellent rendition of modeling of the lung lobes, tuberculosis tubercles in the top left lobe *(right cranial)* and heart. The homogeneous black background was obtained by means of digital editing using Adobe Photoshop. (Courtesy Dr. C. O'Muireagain, Regional Veterinary Laboratory, Sligo, Ireland.)

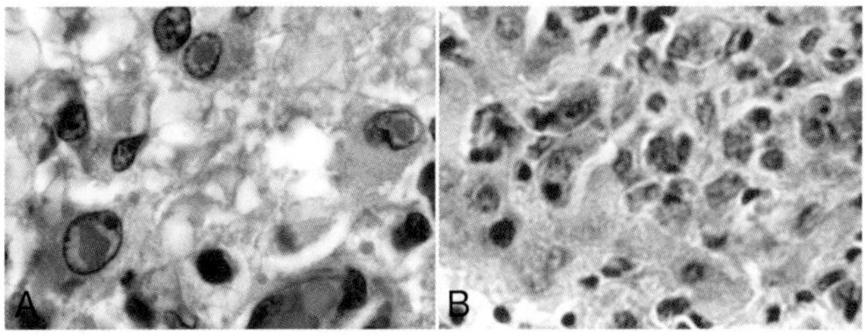

Figure 5 **Outcomes of Koehler Illumination. A,** Koehler illumination with optimal resolution and contrast. Brain, canine distemper, inclusion bodies. H&E stain. 40× planachromatic objective. **B,** Koehler illumination with diffraction and reduced resolution. Caseous exudate. The aperture diaphragm has been closed too far—to 50% cone. 40× planapochromatic objective. (**A** courtesy Dr. M.D. McGavin, College of Veterinary Medicine, University of Tennessee. **B** courtesy Dr. P.W. Ladds, James Cook University, Australia.)

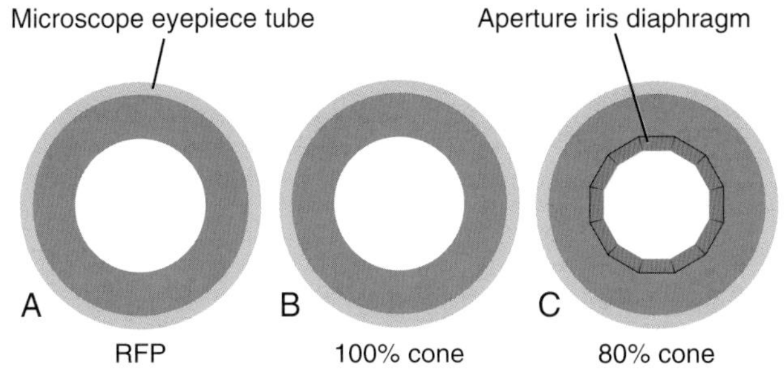

Figure 6 **Koehler Illumination.** The ocular (eyepiece) has been removed from the microscope eyepiece tube to reveal the rear focal plane (RFP) of the objective. **A,** RFP of the objective with the aperture (condenser) diaphragm fully open so that it is not visible and to reveal the full diameter of the objective's aperture. **B,** RFP of the objective with the aperture diaphragm at 100% cone. The internal diameter of the image of the aperture diaphragm matches the internal diameter of the aperture of the objective. **C,** RFP of the objective with the aperture diaphragm at 80% cone. The internal diameter of the image of the aperture diaphragm is 80% of the aperture of the objective *(gray)*. *Yellow,* eyepiece tube; *gray,* inner surface of eyepiece tube; *green,* aperture (condenser) iris diaphragm; *white,* rear focal plane. (Courtesy Dr. M.D. McGavin, College of Veterinary Medicine, University of Tennessee; and Dr. J.F. Zachary, College of Veterinary Medicine, University of Illinois.)

open the aperture diaphragm to 90% cone so the condenser's circle of illumination is just visible inside the RFP. For well-stained histologic sections, use 80% to 90% cone diameter, but if the contrast of the stained section is low, as from inadequate density of the stain, it may be necessary to use 70% to 80% cone diameter. For very low-contrast specimens, it may be necessary to close the aperture diaphragm even more and risk diffraction if the specimen is to be visible. With histologic slides the secret is to have well-stained sections with good color and tonal (gray scale) contrasts. If the specimen is thick (7 to 9 μm in thickness), to have the image in focus it may be necessary to close the aperture diaphragm almost to the point of causing diffraction, particularly with high-magnification objectives, which have the shallowest depth of field (i.e., depth of the tissue in focus).

Evaluation of Photomicrographs

1. **Focus.** The image should be in focus across the entire monitor. If it is out of focus at the edges ("falloff"), this appearance could be caused by poorly corrected flat field (or plan objectives), or the aperture diaphragm has not been closed adequately to increase the depth of field. Before the use of digital cameras and focusing on the screen of the computer monitor, focusing was done on the aerial image of the microscope's image, "floating" in front of the image of the graticule, when viewed through the focusing telescope of the camera. This method had significant problems. Corrections had to be made for the viewer's eyesight and objectives with a large depth of field; the 4× and lower-power objectives were particularly difficult to focus. With these objectives it is necessary to focus on a plane in the section that gives the appearance of the whole field being in focus, and not on a single cell that may or may not be in a plane that would render those cells above and below it also in focus. However, focusing the image on the monitor's screen is relatively reliable and avoids these problems.
2. **Exposure.** Exposure is evaluated by looking at the microscope's clear background in the print or digital image. This background should have a faint density, usually gray unless there is a color cast. In a printed photomicrograph there should be just a faint density, slightly darker than that of the white of the blank page.
3. **Color cast.** The microscope's clear background should be white and have no color casts. The usual color casts are yellow, orange, or blue arising from incorrect color temperature. Occasionally color casts are green from a chromatically uncorrected lens, usually in the lamp house. Color casts can easily be prevented in digital photomicrography by setting the white balance before each exposure, usually by selecting an area of faint density in the microscope's clear background and pressing the "white button."
4. **Uneven illumination.** Uneven illumination can be due to errors in setting up Koehler illumination but is also a common problem with low-power objectives, 4× and lower. To obtain even illumination with low-power objectives of less than 4×, special condensers and highly corrected objectives are frequently required, but an easier method is to use a software program to correct this problem in the image stored in the computer.
5. **Contrast.** The factors involved in controlling contrast are as follows:
   - Quality and staining of the specimen and the specific stain chosen (e.g., trichrome vs. van Gieson).
   - Quality of the objective (e.g., apochromatic objectives have far higher contrast than achromatic objectives).
   - Correct positioning of the aperture diaphragm. With Koehler illumination, positioning of the aperture diaphragm controls resolution, contrast, and depth of field. Its correct positioning is particularly important with high dry and 100× oil immersion objectives.
   - Cover glass and mountant thickness, which together should be 0.17 mm, requiring a No. 1 coverslip.
   - Cleanliness of the surface of the coverslip.
   - Digital camera quality, including image correction software if provided.
   - Magnification of the objective: Lower-magnification objectives and high-power objectives (i.e., high dry and oil immersion) have lower contrast than 10× and 25× objectives of the same optical correction (e.g., all apochromatic objectives or all achromatic objectives).

Troubleshooting of problems with photomicrography is described in the online Appendix. A convenient arrangement is for the operator to make a checklist that applies to the procedure for taking photomicrographs with a specific microscope and digital camera. Checklists may be boring but are essential for ensuring that the correct steps and sequence in Koehler illumination are followed. Unfortunately, Koehler illumination is not an intuitive process. Computer programs are available to correct out-of-focus areas from curvature of field, incorrect density of the microscope's clear background, color casts, and contrast. More information on these topics is available at www.expertconsult.com.

Index

Page numbers followed by *b* indicate boxes; *f*, figures; *t*, tables; and *e*, online only materials.

D

E

H

J

M

P